ORGAN PANELS/LDRGs (Laboratory Diagnosis Related Groups) *Continued**

Chronic Hepatitis Carrier, Immunopathology Panel

HBsAg (hepatitis B surface antigen)
Anti-HBs (anti-hepatitis B surface antigen)
HBeAg (hepatitis Be antigen)
Anti-HBe

Neoplasm (Malignancy) Panel

Alpha fetoprotein (AFP)
Carcinoembryonic antigen (CEA)
Prostatic acid phosphatase (PAP)
B-human chorionic gonadotropin (B-hCG)
Lactate dehydrogenase (LD)
Alkaline phosphatase

Pancreatic Panel

Amylase
Lipase
Calcium
Glucose

Parathyroid Panel

Calcium
Phosphorus
Magnesium
Alkaline phosphatase
Total protein
Albumin
Creatinine
Urinary calcium

Pulmonary Panel

CO_2 content
P_aCo_2
pH
P_aO_2
O_2 saturation
a/A ratio

Renal Panel

BUN/creatinine
Urinary creatinine, 24 hr.
Urinary protein, 24 hr.
Creatinine clearance
Total protein
Albumin
Sodium
Potassium
Chloride
CO_2 content
Glucose

Thyroid Panel

T_4 (thyroxine)
T_3 (triiodothyronine)
FTI (free thyroxine index) or Free T_4
TSH (thyroid stimulating hormone)

Transitional (Metastatic Disease) Panel

Lactate dehydrogenase (LD)
GOT (AST)
Alkalaine phosphate (AP)
Total protein
Albumin
Calcium
Carcinoembryonic antigen (CEA)

TORCH (Toxoplasmosis, Rubella, Cytomegalovirus, Herpes) Panel

Anti-toxoplasmosis
Anti-rubella
Anti-cytomegalovirus
Anti-herpes

---

*Final selection of most cost-effective, sensitive, and specific measurements for each LDRG should be based upon available laboratory equipment and appropriate medical staff consultation with Director of Laboratories.

Henry, J. B.: Focused profiling: selection of laboratory measurements and examinations; videotape or 35-mm slides. Wilmington, E. I. du Pont DeNemours & Co., 1982.

Henry, J. B., and Arras, M. J.: Organ panels: An innovation in health care delivery. Med. Times, 98(2):106, 1970.

Henry, J. B., and Howanitz, P. J.: Organ panels and the relationship of the laboratory to the physician. *In* Young, D. S., Uddin, D., Nipper, H., et al. (eds.), King, J. S. (exec. ed.): Clinician and Chemist: Proceedings of the First Arnold O. Beckman Conference in Clinical Chemistry. Washington, D.C., American Association for Clinical Chemistry, 1979.

Henry, J. B., and Howanitz, P. J.: Organ panels and the relationship of the laboratory to the physician. *In* AMA Council on Scientific Affairs: Laboratory Tests in Medical Practice. Chicago, 1980.

Associate Editors

DOUGLAS A. NELSON, M.D.

Professor of Pathology, College of Medicine, and Deputy Director of Clinical Pathology, University Hospital, State University of New York, Upstate Medical Center, Syracuse, New York

RUSSELL H. TOMAR, M.D.

Professor of Pathology, College of Medicine, Associate Director of Clinical Pathology, University Hospital, State University of New York, Upstate Medical Center, Syracuse, New York

JOHN A. WASHINGTON II, M.D.

Professor of Microbiology and Laboratory Medicine, Mayo Medical School; Head, Section of Clinical Microbiology, Mayo Clinic, Rochester, Minnesota

Assistant Editors

JOSEF V. KADLEC, S.J., M.D., Ph.D.

Assistant Professor of Pediatrics and Microbiology, School of Medicine; Member, International Center for Interdisciplinary Studies in Immunology, School of Medicine, Georgetown University, Washington, D.C.

WILLIAM W. McLENDON, M.D.

Professor of Pathology, School of Medicine; Chairman, Department of Hospital Laboratories, North Carolina Memorial Hospital, University of North Carolina, Chapel Hill, North Carolina

RICHARD A. McPHERSON, M.D.

Assistant Professor of Pathology, School of Medicine; Director of Clinical Chemistry Laboratory, Department of Clinical Laboratories, Georgetown University Hospital, Washington, D.C.

GREGORY A. THREATTE, M.D.

Assistant Professor of Pathology, Schools of Medicine and Dentistry; Associate Director of Clinical Chemistry, Department of Clinical Laboratories, Georgetown University Hospital, Washington, D.C.

Todd • Sanford • Davidsohn

Clinical Diagnosis and Management

by LABORATORY METHODS

SEVENTEENTH EDITION

JOHN BERNARD HENRY, M.D.

Professor of Pathology and Dean, School of Medicine, Georgetown University;
Director of Histocompatibility Laboratory,
Department of Clinical Laboratories,
Georgetown University Hospital, Washington, D.C.

W. B. SAUNDERS COMPANY 1984

Philadelphia London Toronto Mexico City Rio de Janeiro Sydney Tokyo

W. B. Saunders Company: West Washington Square
Philadelphia, PA 19105

1 St. Anne's Road
Eastbourne, East Sussex BN21 3UN, England

1 Goldthorne Avenue
Toronto, Ontario M8Z 5T9, Canada

Apartado 26370—Cedro 512
Mexico 4, D.F., Mexico

Rua Coronel Cabrita, 8
Sao Cristovao Caixa Postal 21176
Rio de Janeiro, Brazil

9 Waltham Street
Artarmon, N.S.W. 2064, Australia

Ichibancho, Central Bldg., 22-1 Ichibancho
Chiyoda-Ku, Tokyo 102, Japan

Library of Congress Cataloging in Publication Data

Henry, John Bernard, 1928-
Clinical diagnosis and management by laboratory methods.

At head of title: Todd, Sanford, Davidsohn.
Includes bibliographies and indexes.
1. Diagnosis, Laboratory. I. Todd, James Campbell, 1874-1928. II. Sanford, Arthur Hawley, 1882- . III. Davidsohn, Israel, 1895- IV. Title. [DNLM: 1. Diagnosis, Laboratory. QY 4 T634c]

RB37.H37 1984 616.07'5 83–20128

ISBN 0–7216–4657–3

Listed here is the latest translated edition of this book together with the language of the translation and the publisher.

Japanese (16/E)—Hirokawa Publishing Co., Tokyo, Japan

Clinical Diagnosis and Management by Laboratory Methods ISBN 0-7216-4657-3

Last digit is the print number: 9 8 7 6 5 4 3 2 1

To Georgette, my wife of 30 years
and mother of our six children
Maureen, Julie, Bill, Paul, John, and David
all of whom accepted patiently
the inconvenience and separation
associated with my long preoccupation
with this work

CONTRIBUTORS

C. A. ALPER, M.D.
The MHC (Major Histocompatibility Complex) and Disease
Scientific Director, Center for Blood Research; Professor of Pediatrics at the Children's Hospital Medical Center, Harvard Medical School; Senior Associate in Hematology and Oncology, Children's Hospital Medical Center; Consultant in Medicine, Brigham and Women's Hospital, Boston, Massachusetts.

Z. AWDEH, Ph.D.
The MHC (Major Histocompatibility Complex) and Disease
Investigator, Center for Blood Research; Assistant Professor of Pathology, Harvard Medical School, Boston, Massachusetts.

PAUL S. BACHORIK, Ph.D.
Lipids and Dyslipoproteinemia
Associate Professor of Pediatrics and Laboratory Medicine, and Head, Lipid and Lipoprotein Analytical Laboratory, Lipid Research–Atherosclerosis Unit, Johns Hopkins University School of Medicine, Baltimore, Maryland.

CHARLIE C. BARNES, Jr., B.A.
Organization and Management of the Clinical Laboratory
Assistant Director, Professional Services Division, North Carolina Memorial Hospital, Department of Hospital Laboratories, University of North Carolina, Chapel Hill, North Carolina.

ROY N. BARNETT, M.D.
Statistical Tests
Clinical Professor of Pathology, Yale University School of Medicine, New Haven; Professional lecturer, Mt. Sinai School of Medicine, New York; Chairman Emeritus, Department of Pathology, Norwalk Hospital, Norwalk, Connecticut.

JOSEPH A. BELLANTI, M.D.
Immunodeficiency Diseases
Professor of Pediatrics and Microbiology and Director, International Center for Interdisciplinary Studies of Immunology, Georgetown University School of Medicine; Director, Immunology and Virology Laboratories, Georgetown University Hospital, Washington, D.C.

MARY BRADLEY, M.D.
Examination of Urine
Associate Professor, Department of Laboratory Medicine and Pathology, University of Minnesota Medical School and University Hospitals. Minneapolis, Minnesota.

DONALD C. CANNON, M.D., Ph.D.
Metabolic Intermediators and Inorganic Ions; Seminal Fluid; Examination of Gastric and Duodenal Contents
Pathologist, Bethania Hospital, Wichita Falls, Texas.

DAVID CHOU, M.D.
Information Management
Assistant Professor, Department of Pathology, School of Medicine, and Director of Computer Services, Department of Hospital Laboratories, The North Carolina Memorial Hospital, University of North Carolina, Chapel Hill, North Carolina.

RONALD P. DANIELE, M.D.
Cells of the Immune System
Professor of Medicine and Pathology, University of Pennsylvania School of Medicine; Attending Physician, Hospital of the University of Pennsylvania, Philadelphia, Pennsylvania.

FREDERICK R. DAVEY, M.D.
Hematopoiesis; Erythrocytic Disorders; Leukocytic Disorders
Professor of Pathology, College of Medicine; Director of Blood Bank and Tissue Typing Laboratory, Clinical Pathology, University Hospital, State University of New York, Upstate Medical Center, Syracuse, New York.

HELEN DOERPINGHAUS, B.A.
Fiscal Management
Business Manager, Division of Laboratory Medicine, School of Medicine, University of North Carolina, Chapel Hill, North Carolina.

MERLE A. EVENSON, Ph.D.
Principles of Instrumentation
Professor, Department of Medicine, Pathology and Laboratory Medicine, University of Wisconsin; Director, Toxicology Laboratory, University of Wisconsin Hospital, Madison, Wisconsin.

HJORDIS M. FOY, M.D., Ph.D.
Mycoplasmal Infection
Professor, Department of Epidemiology SC-36, School of Public Health and Community Medicine, University of Washington, Seattle, Washington.

MICHAEL M. FRANK, M.D.
Complement
Clinical Director and Laboratory Chief, Laboratory of Clinical Investigation, National Institute of Allergy and Infectious Diseases, National Institutes of Health, Bethesda, Maryland.

THELMA A. GAITHER, B.S.
Complement
Research Biologist, Laboratory of Clinical Investigation, National Institute of Allergy and Infectious Diseases, National Institutes of Health, Bethesda, Maryland.

THOMAS L. GAVAN, M.D.
Quality Control on Microbiology
Assistant Clinical Professor of Pathology, Case Western Reserve University; Adjunct Professor, Biology and Health Sciences, Cleveland State University; Chairman, Department of Microbiology, Vice Chairman, Division of Laboratory Medicine, Member, Board of Governors, Chairman, Medical Information Policy Steering Committee, and Vice Chairman, Remodeling and Space Committee, The Cleveland Clinic Foundation, Cleveland, Ohio.

ROBERT GILBERT, M.D.
Spirometry and Blood Gases
Professor of Medicine, College of Medicine; Attending Physician, State University Hospital, State University of New York, Upstate Medical Center, Syracuse, New York.

YEZID GUTIERREZ, M.D., Ph.D.
Medical Parasitology
Assistant Professor of Pathology, Institute of Pathology, Case Western Reserve University School of Medicine; Pathologist, University Hospitals of Cleveland, Ohio.

ROBERT J. HARTZMAN, M.D.
Immunogenetics of HLA Antigens
Staff Scientist, Naval Medical Research Institutes; Associate Professor of Pediatrics and Microbiology, School of Medicine, Georgetown University, Washington, D.C.

JOHN BERNARD HENRY, M.D.
Clinical Pathology/Laboratory Medicine Purposes and Practice; Evaluation of Renal Function and Water, Electrolyte, and Acid-Base Balance; Clinical Enzymology; Immunohematology; Blood Banking and Hemotherapy; SI Units
Professor of Pathology and Dean, School of Medicine, Georgetown University; Director of Histocompatibility Laboratory, Department of Clinical Laboratories, Georgetown University Hospital, Washington, D.C.

MARY JANE HICKS, M.D.
Viruses, Rickettsia, and Chlamydia
Assistant Professor of Pathology, University of Arizona College of Medicine; Chief, Cellular Immunology Section, and Attending in Pathology, Arizona Health Sciences Center, Tucson, Arizona.

JOAN H. HOWANITZ, M.D.
Carbohydrates; Immunoassay and Related Techniques; Tumor Markers; Evaluation of Endocrine Function; Therapeutic Drug Monitoring and Toxicology
Chief, Clinical Pathology, Wadsworth VA Medical Center, Los Angeles, California.

PETER J. HOWANITZ, M.D.
Carbohydrates; Immunoassay and Related Techniques; Tumor Markers; Evaluation of Endocrine Studies; Therapeutic Drug Monitoring and Toxicology
Associate Director of Laboratories, Center for the Health Sciences, University of California at Los Angeles; Attending Pathologist, Wadsworth VA Medical Center, Los Angeles, California.

ARMEAD H. JOHNSON, Ph.D.
Immunogenetics of HLA Antigens
Assistant Professor of Pediatrics and Microbiology, Georgetown University School of Medicine, Washington, D.C.

JOSEF V. KADLEC, S.J., M.D., Ph.D.
Immunodeficiency Diseases
Assistant Professor of Pediatrics and Microbiology, Georgetown University School of Medicine; Member, International Center for Interdisciplinary Studies of Immunology, Georgetown University School of Medicine, Washington, D.C.

YUAN S. KAO, M.D.
Exocrine Pancreatic Function; Malabsorption, Diarrhea, and Examination of Feces
Associate Professor, Department of Pathology, School of Medicine, Louisiana State University Medical Center; Associate Director, Department of Hemotherapy, Charity Hospital of Louisiana, New Orleans, Louisiana.

RICHARD T. KELLY. M.D.
Spirochetes and Spiral Bacteria
Clinical Associate Professor, Department of Pathology, University of Tennessee Center for the Health Sciences; Pathologist in Charge, Microbiology and Serology Sections, Baptist Memorial Hospital, Memphis, Tennessee.

GEORGE E. KENNY, Ph.D.
Mycoplasmal Infection
Professor and Chairman, Department of Pathobiology SC-38, School of Public Health and Community Medicine, University of Washington, Seattle, Washington.

THOMAS F. KEYS, M.D.
Hospital Infection Control
Hospital Epidemiologist and Staff, Department of Infectious Diseases, Cleveland Clinic, Cleveland, Ohio.

CARL R. KJELDSBERG, M.D.
Cerebrospinal Fluid and Other Body Fluids
Professor of Pathology and Head, Anatomic Pathology Division, University of Utah School of Medicine, Salt Lake City, Utah.

ELMER W. KONEMAN, M.D.
Mycotic Disease
Associate Professor of Clinical Pathology, School of Medicine, Northwestern University, Chicago, Illinois.

ARTHUR F. KRIEG, M.D.
Cerebrospinal Fluid and Other Body Fluids; Pregnancy Tests and Evaluation of Placental Function
Professor of Pathology, Chief of Clinical Pathology, College of Medicine; Director of Clinical Laboratories, The Milton S. Hershey Medical Center, The Pennsylvania State University, Hershey, Pennsylvania.

MICHAEL W. LAPINSKI, M.D.
Collection, Processing, and Measurement of Blood Gases
Associate Pathologist at Woman's Christian Association Hospital, Jamestown, New York, and Warren General Hospital, Warren, Pennsylvania.

CHANG LING LEE, M.D.
Immunohematology; Blood Banking and Hemotherapy
Late Professor of Medicine and Pathology, Rush Medical College; Late Director of Charles Hymen Blood Center, Mount Sinai Hospital Medical Center of Chicago; Late Scientific Director, Mid-American Red Cross, Chicago, Illinois.

H. PETER LEHMANN, Ph.D.
SI Units
Professor of Pathology, School of Medicine, Louisiana State University Medical Center, New Orleans, Louisiana.

ROBERT I. LEVY, M.D.
Lipids and Dyslipoproteinemia
Professor of Medicine and Vice President for Health Sciences, Columbia University College of Physicians and Surgeons, New York, New York.

E. GEORGE LINKE, Ph.D.
Clinical Pathology/Laboratory Medicine Purposes and Practice
Scientific Associate, Department of Laboratory Medicine, St. Luke's Hospital, Milwaukee, Wisconsin.

ROBERT P. LISAK, M.D.
Autoantibodies: Autoimmunity and Immune Complexes
Professor, School of Medicine, University of Pennsylvania, Department of Neurology; Attending Neurologist, Hospital of University of Pennsylvania, Philadelphia, Pennsylvania.

EUFRONIO G. MADERAZO, M.D.
Phagocytic Cells: Polymorphonuclear Cells and Monocytes
Assistant Professor of Medicine and Pathology, University of Connecticut School of Medicine, Farmington; Director, Medical Research Laboratory, Department of Medicine, Hartford Hospital, Hartford, Connecticut.

JOHN M. MATSEN, M.D.
Bacterial Susceptibility Testing and Assay
Professor of Pathology and Pediatrics, Chairman, Department of Pathology, University of Utah School of Medicine, Salt Lake City, Utah.

WILLIAM W. McLENDON, M.D.
Organization and Management of the Clinical Laboratory; Fiscal Management; Information Management
Professor of Pathology, School of Medicine, and Chairman, Department of Hospital Laboratories, North Carolina Memorial Hospital, University of North Carolina, Chapel Hill, North Carolina.

RICHARD A. McPHERSON, M.D.
Specific Proteins
Assistant Professor of Pathology, School of Medicine; Director, Clinical Chemistry Laboratory, Department of Clinical Laboratories, Georgetown University Hospital, Washington, D.C.

JONATHAN L. MILLER, M.D., Ph.D.
Blood Platelets; Blood Coagulation and Fibrinolysis
Associate Professor of Pathology, College of Medicine; Assistant Director of Clinical Pathology and Director of Coagulation Laboratory, University Hospital, State University of New York, Upstate Medical Center, Syracuse, New York.

LINDA L. MINNICH, M.S.
Viruses, Rickettsia, and Chlamydia
Supervisor, Virology-Serology Section, Arizona Health Sciences Center, Tucson, Arizona.

MICHAEL W. MORRIS, M.S., SH (ASCP)
Hematology: Basic Methodology
Associate Professor of Medical Technology, College of Health Related Professions; Hematology Supervisor and Assistant Laboratory Manager, Clinical Pathology, University Hospital, State University of New York, Upstate Medical Center, Syracuse, New York.

JOHN E. MURPHY, M.D.
Evaluation of Renal Function and Water, Electrolyte and Acid-Base Balance
Associate Clinical Professor of Pathology, Southern Illinois University School of Medicine; Associate Pathologist, Memorial Medical Center, Springfield, Illinois.

ROBERT M. NAKAMURA, M.D.
Antibody as Reagent
Chairman, Department of Pathology, Scripps Clinic and Research Foundation; Adjunct Professor of Pathology, University of California, San Diego, School of Medicine, La Jolla, California.

DOUGLAS A. NELSON, M.D.
Hematology: Basic Methodology; Hematopoiesis; Erythrocytic Disorders; Leukocytic Disorders
Professor of Pathology, College of Medicine; Deputy Director of Clinical Pathology and Attending Pathologist, University Hospital, State University of New York, Upstate Medical Center, Syracuse, New York.

DANIEL C. NIEJADLIK, M.D.
Sputum
Assistant Professor of Laboratory Medicine, University of Connecticut School of Medicine, Farmington; Associate Pathologist, Middlesex Memorial Hospital, Middletown, Connecticut.

HARRY G. PREUSS, M.D.
Evaluation of Renal Function and Water, Electrolyte, and Acid-Base Balance
Professor of Medicine and Pathology, School of Medicine, Georgetown University Medical Center, Washington, D.C.

DONALD D. RAUM, M.D.
The MHC (Major Histocompatibility Complex) and Disease
Investigator, Center for Blood Research, Assistant Professor, Harvard Medical School; Assistant in Medicine, Beth Israel Hospital, Boston, Massachusetts.

C. GEORGE RAY, M.D.
Viruses, Rickettsia, and Chlamydia
Professor of Pathology and Pediatrics, University of Arizona College of Medicine; Chief, Virology-Serology Section, Arizona Health Sciences Center, and Chief, Pediatrics Infectious Diseases Section, Arizona Health Sciences Center, Tucson, Arizona.

MANUEL J. RICARDO, Jr., Ph.D.
Immunoglobulins and Paraproteins
Associate Professor of Microbiology and Immunology, Bowman Gray School of Medicine of Wake Forest University, Winston-Salem, North Carolina.

BASIL M. RIFKIND, M.D., F.R.C.P.
Lipids and Dyslipoproteinemia
Chief, Lipid Metabolism–Atherogenesis Branch, National Heart, Lung, and Blood Institute, National Institutes of Health, Bethesda, Maryland.

GLENN D. ROBERTS, Ph.D.
Mycotic Disease
Associate Professor of Laboratory Medicine and Microbiology, Mayo Medical School; Director of Clinical Mycology and Mycobacteriology Laboratories, Mayo Clinic and Mayo Foundation, Rochester, Minnesota.

MARY ANN ROBINSON, Ph.D.
Immunogenetics of HLA Antigens
Staff Fellow, Laboratory of Immunogenetics, National Institute of Allergies and Infectious Diseases, National Institutes of Health, Bethesda, Maryland.

JERALD M. ROSENBAUM, M.D.
Assessment of Fetal Condition and Amniotic Fluid Analysis
Instructor in Pathology, University of Massachusetts Medical School, Worcester; Attending Pathologist, Bay State Medical Center, Springfield, Massachusetts.

DAVID T. ROWLANDS, Jr., M.D.
Cells of Immune System
Professor and Chairman, Department of Pathology, University of South Florida College of Medicine, Tampa, Florida.

THOMAS A. RUMA, M.D.
Therapeutic Hemapheresis
Pathologist, Immanuel Medical Center; Director, Midwest Clinical Laboratories, Omaha, Nebraska.

RONALD A. SACHER, B.Sc., M.B.B.Ch., F.R.C.P(C)., D.T.M.&H.
Therapeutic Hemapheresis
Associate Professor of Medicine and Pathology, School of Medicine; Director of Blood Bank and Transfusion Service and Director of Hemapheresis Unit, Department of Clinical Laboratories, Georgetown University Hospital, Washington, D.C.

W. DOUGLAS SCHEER, Ph.D.
Malabsorption, Diarrhea, and Examination of Feces
Assistant Professor, Department of Pathology, Louisiana State University Medical Center; Staff Scientist, Department of Pathology, Charity Hospital of Louisiana, New Orleans, Louisiana.

G. BERRY SCHUMANN, M.D.
Examination of Urine
Associate Professor of Pathology, University of Utah College of Medicine; Director, Cytology Division, Department of Pathology, University of Utah Medical Center, Salt Lake City, Utah.

PESACH SEGAL, M.D.
Lipids and Dyslipoproteinemia
Chief, Diabetes and Lipid Metabolism Unit, Department of Medicine, The Chaim Sheba Medical Center, Tel-Hashomer, Israel.

JAMES W. SMITH, M.D.
Medical Parasitology
Professor of Pathology, Indiana University School of Medicine; Director, Division of Clinical Microbiology, Indiana University Hospitals, Wishard Memorial Hospital, and Veterans Administration Hospital, Indianapolis, Indiana.

HERBERT M. SOMMERS, M.D.
Mycobacterial Diseases
Professor of Pathology, Northwestern University Medical School; Director of Clinical Microbiology, Northwestern Memorial Hospital, Chicago, Illinois.

BERNARD E. STATLAND, M.D., Ph.D.
The Theory of Reference Values; Pre-Instrumental Sources of Variation; Quality Control: Theory and Practice; Assessment of Fetal Condition and Amniotic Fluid Analysis
Professor of Medicine and Pathology, Boston University Medical School; Director of Laboratory Medicine, University Hospital, Boston, Massachusetts.

RUSSELL H. TOMAR, M.D.
Immunoglobulins and Paraproteins; Hypersensitivity Reactions; Immunodeficiency Diseases
Professor of Pathology, College of Medicine; Attending Physician, Director, Diagnostic Immunology Laboratory, Clinical Pathology, University Hospital, State University of New York, Upstate Medical Center, Syracuse, New York.

ERNEST S. TUCKER, III, M.D.
Antibody as Reagent
Associate Clinical Professor of Pathology and Pediatrics, University of California, San Diego; Green Hospital of Scripps Clinic, La Jolla; University Hospital, San Diego, California.

PETER A. WARD, M.D.
Phagocytic Cells: Polymorphonuclear Cells and Monocytes
Professor and Chairman, Department of Pathology, Interim Dean, Medical School, The University of Michigan; Chief, Section of General Pathology, The University of Michigan Hospitals, Ann Arbor, Michigan.

JOHN A. WASHINGTON II, M.D.
Medical Microbiology; Medical Bacteriology
Professor of Microbiology and of Laboratory Medicine, Mayo Medical School; Head, Section of Clinical Microbiology, Mayo Clinic, Rochester, Minnesota.

ROBERT E. WENK, M.D.
Pregnancy Tests and Evaluation of Placental Function; Assessment of Fetal Condition and Amniotic Fluid Analysis
Clinical Associate Professor of Pathology, Pennsylvania State University; Associate Professor of Clinical

Pathology, University of Maryland; Assistant Professor of Laboratory Medicine, Johns Hopkins University School of Medicine; Division Head, Clinical Pathology, Sinai Hospital, Baltimore, Maryland.

JAMES O. WESTGARD, Ph.D.
Quality Control: Theory and Practice
Professor, Department of Pathology and Laboratory Medicine, Department of Medicine, and Medical Technology Program, University of Wisconsin; Associate Director of Laboratories, University of Wisconsin Hospital and Clinics, Madison, Wisconsin.

THERESA L. WHITESIDE, Ph.D.
Cells of the Immune System
Associate Professor of Pathology, Department of Pathology, University of Pittsburgh School of Medicine; Associate Director, Clinical Immunopathology, University Health Center, Pittsburgh, Pennsylvania.

PER WINKEL, M.D., Doc. Med. Sci.
The Theory of Reference Values; Pre-Instrumental Sources of Variation
Director of Clinical Chemistry, Finsen Institute, Copenhagen, Denmark.

JANNIE WOO, Ph.D.
Metabolic Intermediates and Inorganic Ions
Associate Professor of Pathology, College of Medicine; Associate Director of Clinical Pathology, University Hospital, State University of New York, Upstate Medical Center, Syracuse, New York.

WEI T. WU, Ph.D.
Exocrine Pancreatic Function
Associate Professor, Department of Pathology, Louisiana State University Medical Center; Director, Clinical Chemistry Laboratory, Chemical Pathology Section, Department of Pathology, Charity Hospital of Louisiana, New Orleans, Louisiana.

S. Y. YANG, Ph.D
The MHC (Major Histocompatibility Complex) and Disease
Instructor of Pathology, Harvard Medical School; Investigator, Center for Blood Research and Dana Farber Cancer Institute, Boston, Massachusetts.

E. J. YUNIS, M.D.
The MHC (Major Histocompatibility Complex) and Disease
Professor of Pathology, Harvard Medical School; Chief, Division of Immunogenetics, Dana-Farber Cancer Institute, Boston, Massachusetts.

HYMAN J. ZIMMERMAN, M.D.
Function and Integrity of the Liver; Clinical Enzymology
Professor of Medicine, George Washington University School of Medicine and Health Sciences; Clinical Professor of Medicine, Georgetown University School of Medicine and Uniformed Services University of Health Sciences; Director of Gastroenterology, George Washington University Medical Center; Consultant, Veterans Administration Hospital, Walter Reed Medical Center, Washington, D.C., and U.S. Naval Medical Center and N.I.H. Clinical Center, Bethesda, Maryland.

BURTON ZWEIMAN, M.D.
Autoantibodies: Autoimmunity and Immune Complexes
Professor of Medicine and Neurology and Chief, Allergy and Immunology Section, University of Pennsylvania School of Medicine, Philadelphia, Pennsylvania.

PREFACE

For over 75 years, "Todd and Sanford" has served generations of physicians, specialists, and scientists in laboratory medicine/clinical pathology as well as medical laboratory personnel. Its users include medical technologists and medical technicians, medical students, family physicians, internists, surgeons, pediatricians, obstetricians/gynecologists, and, of course, pathologists, both in practice and in training.

The goals of this Seventeenth Edition, in addition to providing an information base in virtually all aspects of clinical pathology or laboratory medicine with sufficient emphasis to promote understanding and critical analysis, include the following:

1. Identification of appropriate measurements and examinations for diagnosis, confirmation of a clinical impression, therapeutic or management guideline data, prognosis, and screening or detection of disease.
2. The order or sequence, and groups when appropriate, in which such measurements and examinations should be requested.
3. Interpretation and translation of laboratory measurements and examinations in light of a patient's particular medical problem(s).
4. Understanding of pathophysiology or natural history of disease as reflected by clinical pathology data.
5. Recognition of pitfalls, problems, and limitations of laboratory data, including quality control (sensitivity, precision, accuracy, specificity) and drug interaction, as well as relative merits in terms of methodology, turnabout time, patient preparation, communication, and cost effectiveness.
6. Appreciation and understanding of the importance of laboratory organization and management for efficient and cost-effective medical care delivery.

Clinicians and pathologists have come to assume or take for granted the quality of laboratory measurements and examinations. The art and science of laboratory medicine have clearly established the validity of laboratory data in terms of accuracy and precision, so that it is now indeed recognized and in a secure position in terms of credibility. Over the past 15 years, the major thrust has been in the achievement of rapid turnabout time, reflected in the prompt reporting of measurements and examinations to the physician at the bedside or in his office. New technology in terms of instrumentation and information processing has accomplished this where there is appropriate laboratory organization and management. At the present time there is a major emphasis on the cost of laboratory measurements and examinations. Regulations, reimbursement, and competition prompt this concentration on costs with the assumption that quality and turnabout time are assured. The advent of reimbursement plans based on Diagnosis Related Groups brings cost effectiveness into sharp focus and undoubtedly will result in LDRGs (Laboratory Diagnosis Related Groups) that will reflect both diagnostic and management applications.

This edition begins with an introduction to the clinical laboratory, the fundamentals of instrumentation, and evaluations of data and quality control; it concludes with management and administration of the clinical laboratory. These two parts are of critical importance to the laboratory physician or scientist, as well as the medical technologist. However, all clinicians and users of laboratory medicine can benefit from an appreciation of these two parts since they are important in effective utilization of the laboratory. Utilization has become a key word in medical practice today and undoubtedly will be a more significant controlling factor in cost containment and reimbursement in the remainder of this decade.

Seven parts with their constituent chapters reflect the organization of the laboratory in a functional manner as well as according to medical problems:

1. The Clinical Laboratory
2. Clinical Chemistry
3. Medical Microscopy
4. Hematology and Coagulation
5. Immunology and Immunopathology
6. Medical Microbiology
7. Administration of the Clinical Laboratory

The chapters emphasize topics that have compelling practical application to the patient. Reorganization of the text should make it more readily accessible to the varied individual users and reflect the thrust of special competence in clinical pathology and subspecialization in medicine. A reduction in the number of pages compared with the previous edition necessitated greater selectivity in emphasis to sustain the comprehensive and intensive development of laboratory medicine/clinical pathology in its application to medical care in recent years. The new technology of medicine reflected in clinical pathology as well as its growth is reviewed, as is the important role of the physician in laboratory medicine.

Virtually all of the material has been either updated or thoroughly revised or newly introduced to reflect current thrusts in laboratory medicine. This is especially prominent in immunopathology. Thus Part Five begins with the major histocompatibility complex and concludes with immunohematology and blood banking. Cellular as well as humoral aspects of the immune response and laboratory applications are emphasized throughout Part Five. Antibody has become an important reagent not only to immunogenetics but also to immunohematology, immunochemistry, serology, hemotherapy, and microbiology as well as medical microscopy and examination of other body fluids.

Clinical chemistry continues to expand in complexity and with an increasing specificity and sensitivity of determinations for diagnosis and management, especially in endocrine disorders and therapeutic drug monitoring. The new biology of medicine—cell biology, molecular biology, and molecular genetics—is evident not only in immunopathology but also in hematology, chemical pathology, and microbiology. Medical microscopy reflects reproductive biology translated into patient care through the clinical laboratory.

In the appendices we continue to present recommendations for the standardized presentation of clinical laboratory data. The appendices also provide information useful to the clinician and laboratorian in terms of reference (normal) values and intervals. An introduction to SI units with conversion to SI units has also been incorporated. Such new terminology has been incorporated not only with the reference intervals but also throughout the text whenever feasible and consistent with optimal patient care.

My own special interest in effective utilization of the laboratory is reflected on the end papers. An alternative strategy for ordering blood in elective surgery including the type and screen is outlined in addition to selected organ panels which may well evolve into LDRGs (Laboratory Diagnosis Related Groups).

In summary, this edition is a complete and thoroughly updated revision consistent with the tradition of this text and the role of the laboratory. I accept full responsibility for any errors of omission or commission and enthusiastically welcome any comments or reactions to the Seventeenth Edition.

JOHN BERNARD HENRY, M.D.

ACKNOWLEDGMENTS

It is with great pleasure and deep satisfaction that I acknowledge the collaboration of my esteemed colleagues and friends as associate editors, Douglas A. Nelson, M.D., John A. Washington II, M.D., and Russell H. Tomar, M.D., and assistant editors, William W. McLendon, M.D., Josef V. Kadlec, S.J., M.D., Ph.D., Richard A. McPherson, M.D., and Gregory A. Threatte, M.D. Each has been most gracious, diligent, and resourceful in his efforts to accomplish our task of both renewal and revision of this text. A work of multiple authors requires a willingness of the contributors to accept the guidance of the editors. Our collaborators have been responsible and responsive in this respect.

Special gratitude is due to Leonard Chiazze, Jr., Sc.D., for his critical assistance in Statistical Tests and Aaron Altschul, Ph.D., for his assistance with Appendix 2. Likewise, I am grateful to Marie L. Foegh, M.D., and Peter W. Ramwell, Ph.D., for their assistance with eicosanoids in Chapter 16.

I also acknowledge with gratitude the stimulus of former medical students, residents, and colleagues who have helped in so many ways over the years to improve this text.

For her sustained loyalty and meticulous attention to detail, I express my deepest gratitude and appreciation to my assistant, Ms. Elisabeth Oles, who has been supportive and has shown commitment and dedication to this edition. Our association for the past four years at Georgetown University School of Medicine and an additional two years at SUNY, Upstate Medical Center in Syracuse, has made it possible for me to undertake this project as well as participate in so many other related activities that have enhanced this effort.

In addition, I am grateful for the excellent clerical support which has been rendered in a superb manner by others, including Mrs. Doris W. Davey, Ms. Judith Kelsey, Mrs. Sara E. Fuoco, Miss Connie Bistrovich, and Mrs. Ivy F. West.

To our entire Georgetown University Medical Center Dahlgren Memorial Library staff, and especially Ms. Naomi Broering, Medical Center Librarian, Nancy Knight, Susan Anderson, and Anne Linton, I am most appreciative and most grateful for assistance in validating references and conducting literature searches. Having access to and support from a superb medical library is an essential prerequisite to writing.

Special thanks and gratitude are due to Dorothea Nelson, Maaja Washington, Karen Tomar, Anne McLendon, Stephanie McPherson, and Stephanie Threatte. Without their understanding and faithful support, the contributions of my associate and assistant editors would not have been possible.

To Dr. James N. Patterson of Tampa, Florida, goes my sincere thanks for introducing me to Dr. Israel Davidsohn. I look back with a great sense of pride and satisfaction on the 15 years shared with Dr. Davidsohn in contributing to this text. Since the last edition, Dr. Davidsohn has died (December 3, 1979) and so has his associate and my colleague Chang Ling Lee, M.D. (August 18, 1983). I especially missed Dr. Lee's help with the galleys and page proofs of our two chapters on immunohematology and hemotherapy. To his widow, Dr. Charlotte Ho, I wish to express my deepest sympathy and gratitude. Many in clinical pathology and, in particular, blood banking and immunohematology will greatly miss her husband.

I am very grateful to Ms. Bettina Martin, whose critical comments and suggestions over the years for management and administration have been most valuable.

To Ms. Karen Lenz I acknowledge my gratitude for assistance in selection of this book's cover, which reflects the Georgetown University colors and tradition.

I sincerely appreciate the cooperation and guidance of Albert Meier, Bill Preston, and Dave Kilmer, as well as the entire staff of W. B. Saunders Company who shared and supported this effort.

There are many others who, in so many ways, have contributed to and assisted in this work. I express my sincere thanks to them though they are not identified. In addition, there are people who have taught me much over the years and from whom I continue to learn. I acknowledge their contributions, and will always be grateful to them.

JOHN BERNARD HENRY, M.D.

CONTENTS

Part I

THE CLINICAL LABORATORY

EDITED BY JOHN BERNARD HENRY, M.D., AND RICHARD A. McPHERSON, M.D.

1

CLINICAL PATHOLOGY/ LABORATORY MEDICINE PURPOSES AND PRACTICE

E. GEORGE LINKE, PH.D.,
and JOHN BERNARD HENRY, M.D.

The clinician uses the laboratory to assist in diagnosis and management of the patient (Table 1–1). In effect, a test requisition is a request for consultative services which sets in motion a vast array of maneuvers to generate a laboratory report. Usefulness of the data in making clinical judgments depends upon prompt, accurate reporting of a result (Chap. 57). Each procedure to generate a result consists of a series of steps, or processes. An adequate understanding of each process enables the laboratorian to achieve more nearly optimal conditions and, consequently, to improve the accuracy and precision of each measurement. Collection, handling, and processing the specimen prior to analysis must receive prime consideration. Validity of data obtained on the specimen itself is highly dependent upon the excellence of laboratory technique, including proper manipulation of equipment, use of reagents of specified purity, and environmental control. The purpose of this chapter is to provide fundamental knowledge prerequisite to skillful technique in each step of an analysis, keeping always in mind resultant improved patient care and reasons or indications for laboratory measurements and examinations (Table 1–1) and activities in clinical laboratories (Table 1–2). Misuse of laboratory tests and diagnostic procedures has been reviewed recently (Griner, 1982). The authors review all the factors responsible for inappropriate or excessive use as well as those that foster overuse.

Table 1–1. INDICATIONS OR REASONS FOR ORDERING LABORATORY MEASUREMENTS AND/OR EXAMINATIONS

1. To confirm a clinical impression or establish a diagnosis.
2. To rule out a diagnosis.
3. To monitor therapy (management guide).
4. To establish prognosis.
5. To screen for or detect disease.

Table 1–2. SCHEMATIC OUTLINE OF ACTIVITIES IN CLINICAL LABORATORIES

	ADMINISTRATION	
	PATIENT CARE SERVICE	
Indications and Selection	Technology and Generation	Interpretation and Translation
	TEACHING	
	RESEARCH	

TEST REQUISITION

The clinician initiates the test requisition by writing an order for laboratory measurements and examinations in the patient's medical record/chart. A hospital unit secretary usually transcribes the test orders from the chart to an appropriate laboratory requisition form supplied by the laboratory to the various nursing stations throughout the hospital. A check for transcription errors and delivery of the requisition forms to the laboratory ensues.

Each laboratory form has a list of tests with reference intervals and a space for the result. Patient demographics, keyed in from a computer or on an addressograph plate, are stamped onto the appropriate requisition forms at either the admitting office or the nursing stations. Patient demographics include patient's name, sex, age, date of admission, date test ordered, hospital number, room number, doctor, and doctor's pharmacy code number. Test requisitions from the nursing stations are received by the laboratory computer center and entered into the computer (Chap. 57, p. 1401). Labels are printed by the computer with patient demographics, accession number, draw time, tube type, and department to which specimen is to be delivered. The requisition slips and computer labels are given to the phlebotomist, who goes to the hospital units to collect the various blood specimens. The phlebotomist records time the specimen is drawn and phlebotomist code on each of three labels. One label is applied to the specimen tube *before the specimen is drawn.* Another label goes back to the computer operator for data entry. A third label is sent with the requisition and specimen to the appropriate department.

It is essential to follow strict quality control procedures through all stages of test requisition to avoid several possible errors (Slockbower, 1982), such as tests entered incorrectly or missing, test priorities entered incorrectly, wrong time or date on the requisitions, and venipuncture charges missing. Test requisition forms that are clear and easy to use reduce errors, as do frequent inservice training and review.

SPECIMEN COLLECTION

Blood

Blood is by far the most frequent body fluid used for analytical purposes. Three general procedures for obtaining blood are (1) skin puncture, (2) venous puncture, and (3) arterial puncture. The technique used to obtain the blood specimen is critical in order to maintain its integrity. Even so, arterial and venous blood differ in important respects.

Blood oxygenated by the lungs is pumped from the heart to all organs and tissues for their metabolic needs. This arterial blood is essentially uniform in composition throughout the body. The composition of venous blood varies, depending on metabolic activity of the organ or tissue being perfused. Site of collection can affect the venous composition (Pryce, 1980). Venous blood is oxygen deficient relative to arterial blood, but also differs in pH, carbon dioxide concentration, and packed cell volume. Glucose, lactic acid, chloride, and ammonia concentrations also may vary. Blood obtained by skin puncture, sometimes incorrectly called capillary blood, is a mixture of blood from arterioles, venules, and capillaries. Skin puncture blood is, therefore, a mixture of arterial and venous blood. Increased pressure in the arterioles yields a specimen enriched in arterial blood. Skin puncture blood also contains interstitial and intracellular fluids.

SKIN PUNCTURE

Skin puncture is the method of choice in pediatric patients, especially infants. The larger amount of blood required for repeated venipuncture may cause anemia, especially in premature infants. Venipuncture of deep veins in pediatric patients may also rarely cause (1) cardiac arrest, (2) hemorrhage, (3) thrombosis, (4) venous constriction followed by gangrene of an extremity, (5) damage to organs or tissues accidentally punctured, and (6) infection. Skin puncture is useful in adults with (1) extreme obesity, (2) severe burns, and (3) thrombotic tendencies. Skin puncture is often preferred in geriatric patients.

Technique for Skin Puncture (NCCLS Pub. H 4-A, 1982; Meites, 1979)

1. Select an appropriate puncture site. For infants this is most usually the lateral or medial plantar heel surface. In older infants the palmar surface of the last digit of the second, third, or fourth fingers may be used. Other sites for skin puncture are the plantar surface of the big toe, the side of a finger adjacent to the nail, and the earlobe. The site of puncture must not be edematous or a previous puncture site.

2. Warm the puncture site with a warm moist towel no hotter than 42°C.; this increases the blood flow through arterioles and capillaries and results in arterial-enriched blood especially useful for pH and blood gas measurements (Chap. 7, p. 100).

3. Cleanse the puncture site with 70 per cent (v/v) aqueous isopropanol solution. Disposable absorbent pads saturated with 70 per cent isopropyl alcohol are especially convenient. Allow the area to dry. Do not touch the swabbed area with any unsterile object.

4. Make the puncture with a sterile lancet. Use a single deliberate motion with the lancet nearly perpendicular to the skin surface. For a heel puncture hold the heel with forefinger at the arch and thumb proximal to the puncture site at the ankle. Use a lancet with blade no longer than 2.4 mm to avoid injury to the calcaneus (heel bone).

5. Discard the first drop of blood by wiping it away with a sterile pad. Regulate further blood flow by thumb pressure. Do not milk the site, as this may hemolyze the specimen and introduce excess tissue fluid.

6. Collect the specimen in a suitable container (NCCLS Pub. H 14-T, 1980). Open-ended, narrow-bore disposable glass micropipettes are most often used in volumes from 1 to 200 μl. The bore may be uniform or tapered at one end (Caraway and Natelson pipettes). Both heparinized and nonheparinized micropipettes are available. Oral aspiration of blood is discouraged for obvious safety reasons; manual aspirators are recommended. Plastic and clay compounds

are available to seal the pipettes. Test tubes are available up to 1000 μl capacity, without anticoagulant. Serum separator tubes with an inert polyester barrier material are also available.

7. Seal the specimen container, e.g., insert clay into each end of the micropipettes.

8. Label the specimen container with date, time of collection, and patient demographics.

9. Indicate in the report that test results are from skin puncture blood, bearing in mind that important differences exist in concentrations of glucose, potassium, total protein, and calcium between skin puncture and venous serum (Blumenfeld, 1977).

VENOUS PUNCTURE

The relative ease of obtaining venous blood makes this a primary source of specimen for clinical laboratory analyses. Also, the analytical chemist recognizes a primary advantage in that most analytes are present in soluble form or a homogeneously dispersed phase. Even so, various sources of bias presenting during preparation of the subject for venipuncture must receive prime consideration (see Chap. 5).

Venipuncture is accomplished with needles attached to glass test tubes under specified vacuum. The system makes possible direct sampling from a vein, economically and efficiently. Tubes come in various sizes (2, 3, 5, 7, 10, and 15 ml). Disposable needles eliminate the hazard of serum hepatitis transmission, provided the phlebotomist uses proper drawing and needle disposal techniques (Walker, 1981). Rubber stoppers are color-coded to distinguish whether the tube contains a specific anticoagulant (heparin, oxalate, citrate, or ethylenediaminetetraacetic acid salts), is a plain

Table 1–3. GUIDE FOR PROPER SPECIMEN TUBE SELECTION*

Blood Bank—7 ml Plain Tube (red top)
- Antibody detection (screen) (2 tubes)
- Antibody identification (2 tubes)
- Antiglobulin (direct and indirect) (DAG and IAG)
- Erythrocyte typing (ABO and Rh)
- Erythrocyte typing (extended)
- Open heart evaluation (ABO, Rh genotype, DAG, IAG) (3 tubes)
- Prenatal evaluation (ABO, Rh genotype, IAG) (2 tubes)
  - (ABO, Rh) and crossmatch (compatibility) (1 tube for 3 units)
  - (ABO, Rh) and screen (antibody detection) (2 tubes)

Blood Bank—Histocompatibility—7 ml Na Heparin (green top)
- HLA (A and B) lymphocyte typing
- HLA (cytotoxic) antibody detection and % reactivity (PRA)
- MLC (HLA-D) mixed lymphocyte culture

Chemistry—7 ml Plain Tube (red top)
- Acetaminophen (Tylenol)
- Acetone
- Albumin
- Aldolase
- Alanine aminotransferase (ALT) or (GPT)
- Alcohol (do not use alcohol swab)
- Amylase (AMS)
- Aspartate aminotransferase (AST) or (GOT)
- Barbiturate screen
- Bilirubin
- Bromide
- BUN (blood urea nitrogen)
- Calcium (total)
- Carotene
- Cholesterol
- Cholinesterase (CHS)
- Copper (acid-washed)
- Cortisol
- Creatine kinase (CK) and CK isoenzymes
- Creatinine
- Digoxin
- Digitoxin
- Electrolytes (Na, K, Cl, CO_2)
- Electrophoresis
- Ethosuximide (Zarontin)
- Folate
- FSH (follicle stimulating hormone)
- Free thyroxine (free T_4)
- Glucose
- Growth hormone
- Iron and iron binding capacity
- Lactate dehydrogenase (LD) and LD isoenzymes
- Leucine aminopeptidase (LAP)
- Lipase (LPS)
- Lipoprotein electrophoresis
- Lithium
- Long acting thyroid stimulator (LATS)
- Luteinizing hormone (LH)
- Magnesium
- Osmolality
- Parathyroid hormone (2 full tubes)
- Phenobarbital
- Phenytoin (Dilantin)
- Phosphatase, acid (ACP)
- Phosphatase, alkaline (ALP)
- Phosphorus
- Primidone (Mysoline)
- Procainamide
- Prolactin
- Propranolol
- Pseudocholinesterase
- Salicylate
- SMA 6-60 (Na, K, Cl, CO_2, BUN, Glu)
- T_3-RIA
- Testosterone
- Theophylline
- Thiocyanate
- Thyroid binding globulin (TBG)
- Thyroid stimulating hormone (TSH)
- Total protein
- Total thyroxine (T_4-RIA)
- Triglyceride
- Uric acid
- Vitamin B_{12}
- Vitamin B_{12} (unsaturated binding capacity)

Chemistry—5 ml Na Heparin (green top)
- Ammonia (on ice)
- Carboxyhemoglobin and oxygen saturation
- Cholinesterase (CHS)
- Erythrocyte potassium (K)
- Methemoglobin
- pH
- Plasma hemoglobin

*Two to three tests can be done per tube, unless otherwise specified.

tube, or is a special tube made chemically clean (e.g., for lead or iron determinations). Tubes also come sterile or non-sterile, and silicone coated or non-silicone coated. Non-glycerine coated tops are available for lipid analysis. Whole blood without anticoagulant yields serum, with anticoagulant, plasma. Plasma contains fibrinogen, which is missing from serum. Heparin in the form of a lithium salt is an effective anticoagulant in small quantities without significant effect on many determinations and is the ideal universal anticoagulant for blood (Table 1–3). For glucose measurements fluoride may be added to heparin. Fluoride inhibits glycolysis of the blood cells that may otherwise destroy glucose at the rate of about 5 per cent per hour. In the presence of bacterial contamination of blood specimens, fluoride inhibition of glycolysis is neither adequate nor effective in preserving glucose concentration. Furthermore, prompt separation of plasma or serum from cells is important to yield a proper specimen for most chemical determinations.

Integrated serum separator tubes are available for

Table 1–3. GUIDE FOR PROPER SPECIMEN TUBE SELECTION* *(Continued)*

Chemistry—5 ml NaF Oxalate (gray top)
- Glucose
- Glucose tolerance
- Lactate (on ice)
- Lactose tolerance

Chemistry—7 ml Versene Tube EDTA (lavender top)
- Carcinoembryonic antigen (CEA) (2 tubes)
- Lead
- Renin (2 tubes, on ice)

Hematology—4.5 ml Na Citrate Tube (blue top)—must be full
- Factor assays (coagulation)
- Fibrinogen level
- G-6-PD assay (also 1 lavender top)
- Partial thromboplastin time (PTT)
- Prothrombin time (PT)
- Thrombin time (TT)

Hematology—7 ml Versene Tube (lavender top)
- CBC (WBC, RBC, Hgb, Hct, MCV, MCH, MCHC)
- Differential count
- Erythrocyte sedimentation rate (ESR)—tube must be full (Westergren)
- Glucose-6-phosphate dehydrogenase screen (G-6-PD)
- Hgb electrophoresis
- Platelet count
- Reticulocyte count
- Sickle cell preparation
- Total eosinophil count
- Zeta sedimentation rate (ZSR)—tube must be full

Hematology—7 ml (red top)
- Haptoglobin
- LE preparation
- Serum viscosity (3 full tubes)

Immunology-Serology—7 ml (red top)
- Alpha-1-antitrypsin
- Alpha-1-fetoprotein
- Anti-DNA
- Anti-DNAse B
- Antihyaluronidase (AH)
- Antinuclear antibody (ANA)
- Antistreptolysin O (ASO)
- Antithyroid antibody
- Aspergillus antibody
- Brucella antibody
- Candida antibody

Immunology-Serology—7 ml (red top) (continued)
- Ceruloplasmin
- C_1 esterase inhibitor
- CH_{50} (total hemolytic complement)
- Cold agglutinins
- Complement
  - C_3
  - C_4
  - C_3A (Factor B)
- Cryoglobulin
- Extractable nuclear antibodies
  - Anti-Sm
  - Anti-DNP
- Farmer's lung antibodies
- Fluorescent treponemal antibody absorption (FTA-ABS)
- Franciscella agglutinins
- Hepatitis associated antigen (HAA, HB_sAg)
- Heterophile antibody
- IgE
- Immunoelectrophoresis
- "Lung" antibodies
- Lysozyme
- Monospot
- Muramidase
- Proteus agglutinins
- Rheumatoid factor
- Rubella antibodies
- Salmonella agglutinins
- Thyroid antibody
- Toxoplasma IFA
- VDRL

Immunology-Serology—7 ml Na Heparin (green top)
- (*Note:* These tests must be scheduled with the Immunology Laboratory)
- Nitroblue tetrazolium (NBT)
- Phagocytosis—2 tubes (1 plain tube must accompany)
- T and B cells—3 tubes (1 versene tube must accompany)

Immunology-Serology—Special tubes from Immunology
- Lymphocyte proliferation
- Phytohemagglutinin (PHA)

*Two to three tests can be done per tube, unless otherwise specified.

isolating serum from whole blood. An evacuated glass tube serves as a closed system for both collection and processing of the blood specimen. During centrifugation blood is forced into a silicone gel material located at the base of the tube, causing a temporary change in viscosity. The specific gravity of the gel is intermediate to that of the red cells and serum, so that the gel rises and lodges between the packed cells and the top serum layer (Spencer, 1976). The gel hardens and forms an inert barrier. Pediatric-sized tubes are also available with the same concept. Advantages of serum separator tubes are (1) ease of use, (2) shorter processing time through clot activation, (3) a higher serum yield, (4) only one centrifugation step, (5) use of the same tube as that into which the patient specimen is drawn, and (6) ease of labeling. A unique advantage for the reference laboratory is that the centrifuged specimen can be transported without disturbing the separation. These tubes must not be spun down in an angle-head centrifuge as the barrier will not be horizontal, allowing red blood cells to escape back into the serum in a relatively short time. Some silica gel serum separation tubes give rise to minute particles which cause flow problems in continuous flow analyzers. Filtering the serum solves the problem.

Technique for Venous Puncture (NCCLS Pub. H 3-A, 1980; Clark, 1981)

1. Verify that computer-printed labels match requisitions at the nursing station or outpatient clinic.
2. Identify the patient by checking identification band against labels and requisition forms. Ask the conscious patient his or her full name and birthdate. Verify identity of an unconscious patient from a nurse, relative, or friend. Positively identify emergency patients when the blood specimen is drawn. If identity is unknown, give the patient a temporary identification. *Do not draw any specimen without properly identifying the patient.*
3. If a fasting specimen is required, confirm that the fasting order has been followed.
4. Address the patient and inform the patient what is to be done. Reassure the patient to avoid as much tension as possible.
5. Position the patient properly, depending on whether the patient is sitting or prone, for easy, comfortable access to the antecubital fossa.
6. Assemble equipment and supplies, including collection tubes, tourniquet, preps for cleansing the area, syringes if necessary, sterile blood collection needle, and holder used to secure the needle and evacuated collection tubes.
7. Ask the patient to make a fist to make the veins more palpable.
8. Select a suitable vein for puncture. Veins of the antecubital fossa, in particular the median cubital and cephalic veins, are preferred. Wrist, ankle, and hand veins may also be used. If one arm has an intravenous line, use the other arm to draw a blood specimen.
9. Cleanse the venipuncture site with 70 per cent isopropyl alcohol solution or 1 per cent iodophor-pvp saturated swabstick. Begin at the puncture site and cleanse outward in a circular motion. Allow the area to dry. Do not touch the swabbed area with any unsterile object.
10. Apply a tourniquet several inches above the puncture site. Never leave the tourniquet in place longer than one minute.
11. Anchor the vein firmly, both above and below the puncture site. Use either the thumb and middle finger or thumb and index finger.
12. Perform the venipuncture. (a) Enter the skin with the needle at approximately a 15° angle to the arm, with the bevel of the needle up. Follow the geography of the vein with the needle. (b) Insert the needle smoothly and fairly fast to minimize patient discomfort. Do not "bury" the needle. (c) If using a syringe, pull back on the barrel with a slow, even tension as blood flows into the syringe. Do not pull back too quickly to avoid hemolyzing the blood or collapsing the vein. (d) If using a vacutainer, as soon as the needle is in the vein, ease the tube forward in the holder as far as it will go. At the same time, hold the needle firmly in place. When the tube has filled, remove it by grasping the end of the tube and pulling gently.
13. Release the tourniquet when blood begins to flow.
14. After all blood has been drawn, have the patient relax his or her fist. Do not allow the patient to pump the hand.
15. Place a clean sterile cotton ball lightly over the site. Withdraw the needle, then apply pressure to the site.
16. Bandage the arm. Usually, a Band-Aid over the ball of cotton is adequate to stop bleeding.
17. Mix tubes with anticoagulant. For syringe-drawn specimens, transfer blood to appropriate tubes, taking precuations to avoid hemolyzing the specimens. Follow any special handling procedures, e.g., chilling certain specimens.
18. Check condition of the patient, e.g., whether patient is faint and that bleeding is under control.
19. Dispose of contaminated material such as needles, syringes, cotton, etc.
20. Initial the labels and record the time specimens were drawn.
21. Deliver tubes of blood for testing to appropriate departments in the laboratory. Time stamp requisition if necessary.

An additional protocol is important in the venipuncture procedure. Follow the recommended "order of draw" when collecting tubes (Calam, 1982). To avoid possible contamination draw specimens into non-additive tubes before tubes with additives. Fill additive-containing tubes in the following order: citrate, heparin, EDTA-K_3, and oxalate-fluoride.

ARTERIAL PUNCTURE

Arterial blood is used to measure oxygen and carbon dioxide tension, and to measure pH. These blood gas measurements (Chap. 7, p. 97) are critical in assessment of oxygenation problems encountered in illnesses such as pneumonia, pneumonitis, and pulmonary embolism. Patients on prolonged oxygen therapy or mechanical ventilation are monitored to avoid extremes in oxygenation which produce either anoxia with respiratory acidosis or oxygen toxicity. Critically ill cardiovascular patients and patients undergoing major surgery, especially cardiac or pulmonary surgery, are closely monitored for hypoxia.

Arterial punctures are technically more difficult to perform than venous punctures. Increased pressure in the arteries makes it more difficult to stop bleeding with development of a hematoma. Arterial spasm is a reflex constriction which restricts blood flow with possible severe effects on circulation. Patients may complain of considerable discomfort associated with radial artery puncture (Clark, 1982). Symptoms of temporary discomfort may be expressed in terms such as aching, throbbing, tenderness, sharp sensation, and cramp.

Technique for Arterial Puncture (NCCLS Pub. H 11-T, 1980; Sumner, 1980; Young, 1981; see Chap. 7, p. 99)

1. Select the puncture site (Chap. 7, p. 99). The radial artery is the most common site. However, establish the presence of collateral circulation to the hand via the ulnar artery using the Allen test. If the ulnar artery is absent, do not puncture the radial artery. The femoral artery and the brachial artery at the antecubital fossa provide alternative sites for puncture. Scalp arteries are used in infants. Catheterization of the umbilical artery is frequently used in neonates up to 48 hours after birth.
2. Anesthetize the puncture site, if necessary. Hyperventilation caused by anxiety may significantly affect the blood gas measurements.
3. Prepare the syringe. Wet the barrel and needle or cannula with sterile anticoagulant (usually heparin) solution. Expel excess solution.
4. Record the patient's temperature and oxygen concentration of inspired air (F_IO_2).
5. Perform the puncture (radial artery). First perform the Allen test. Compress the radial and ulnar arteries at the wrist until the palm of the hand becomes blanched. Release pressure from the ulnar artery. Observe that the hand becomes flushed. If the hand remains blanched, *do not* puncture the radial artery. Palpate the artery. Cleanse the site. Place a finger over the artery. With the bevel of the needle up, puncture the skin 5 to 10 mm distal to the finger which locates the artery. Aim for the artery at a point directly below the finger. Blood rushing into the needle usually forces the plunger back. If not, gently pull back on the plunger. Obtain the required amount of blood. Quickly withdraw the needle and syringe. At the same time place a sterile cotton ball or a dry sterile gauze sponge over the puncture site. Apply firm pressure for at least five minutes, or longer if the patient has a prolonged clotting time. Watch the puncture site an additional two minutes to be certain a hematoma does not develop.
6. Expel any air bubbles from the syringe.
7. Remove the needle and cap the syringe with a tight-fitting Luer cap.
8. Mix the specimen with anticoagulant by gentle inversion of the syringe.
9. Identify the specimen with the patient's name, location, and time of draw.
10. Place the syringe which contains the specimen in an ice water bath.
11. Transport the specimen on ice to the laboratory.

Syringes containing lyophilized (freeze-dried) heparin have distinct advantages: (1) time savings in that prewetting of the barrel with liquid heparin is unnecessary and (2) no dilution problem with underfilling of the syringe. No significant differences were found in blood gas parameters comparing syringes with lyophilized heparin and syringes wetted with solubilized heparin (Madiedo, 1982; Crockett, 1981).

DRAWING OFF INDWELLING LINES

Indwelling catheters provide ready access to the patient's circulation and eliminate the need to puncture the patient repeatedly when ongoing blood studies are required to monitor the patient. They are especially useful in critical care situations and during surgery. Arterial catheters most often are placed in the radial artery, but other arteries are used, e.g., the pulmonary artery. The Broviac or Hickman indwelling catheter is surgically inserted in the cephalic vein and positioned in the lower superior vena cava at the entrance to the right atrium. It is especially useful in selected patients for drawing venous blood, administering drugs or blood products, and total parenteral nutrition (Bjeletich, 1980; Anderson, 1982).

Placement of indwelling catheters is not ordinarily a laboratory function. The primary concern of the laboratorian is that blood specimens drawn from these catheters be uncontaminated with whatever is being fed into the blood stream via the catheter. Solution (usually heparin) being used to maintain patency of the vein must also be cleared. Thus, sufficient blood must be withdrawn to clear the line so that blood testing is accurate.

Laboratory data are reported to be reliable after withdrawal of 2.2 ml from a quadruple-lumen Swan-Ganz catheter in the pulmonary artery (Krueger, 1981). To obtain a blood specimen from the Hickman indwelling catheter, or the double-lumen Hickman catheter, first draw 6 ml of intravenous fluid from the line. In a separate syringe, withdraw the amount of blood required for the laboratory, then put the first 6 ml draw back into the patient. Follow strict aseptic technique to avoid infection. Coagulation tests are extremely sensitive to heparin interference so that even larger volumes of intravenous fluid must be withdrawn before the laboratory specimen is valid. We recommend that the appropriate volume be established by each laboratory. The laboratory is sometimes asked to do blood culture studies on blood drawn from indwelling catheters. This procedure is not recommended because organisms which grow on the walls of the catheter contaminate the blood specimen.

PROBLEM DRAWS

Occasionally, the phlebotomists are unable to obtain blood from a patient by ordinary venipuncture techniques. In some cases a skin puncture may suffice. If not, a physician draws the specimen, using most commonly the femoral vein or, in children, the jugular vein.

Urine

Collection and preservation of urine for analytical testing must follow a carefully prescribed procedure to ensure valid results. Laboratory testing of urine generally falls under three categories, i.e., chemical, bacteriologic, and microscopic examination. In this section, obtaining the specimen for chemical testing is stressed.

There are three kinds of collection for urine specimens: (1) random, (2) timed, and (3) 24-hour total volume. Random specimens are collected any time. Test results for a random collection are expressed per unit volume if the result is a quantitative analysis. Much reporting of testing on a random collection is expressed as "positive" or "negative," indicating the presence or absence of a particular constituent, such as glucose. Random urine specimens should be collected in a chemically clean receptacle, either glass or plastic. The vessel is tightly sealed, labeled with the patient's name and date of collection, and submitted for analysis. Timed specimens are obtained at designated intervals, starting from "time zero." For example, in the glucose tolerance test, collections are made at 0, 30, 60, 120, and 180 minutes. It is important to note the time of collection on each specimen container. Urine specimens for a 24-hour total volume collection are most difficult to obtain and require the utmost cooperation from the patient. Incomplete collection is the major problem. In some instances, overcollection occurs. As in-hospital collection is usually under the supervision of the nursing staff, it is more reliable than outpatient collections. Collection of urine specimens from pediatric patients requires special attention to avoid contamination from the stool. One can avoid problems by giving patients complete instructions with a warning that the test can be invalidated by incorrect sampling. One should give the patient a one-gallon (approximately 4 L), chemically clean bottle with the correct preservative already added. An unbreakable plastic container is preferred. One should remind the patient to *discard* the first morning specimen, record time, and collect every voiding for the next 24 hours, with the last to be 24 hours after timing commenced. Overcollection occurs if the first morning specimen is included in this routine. Measure the total volume collected, record on the request form, thoroughly mix the entire 24-hour collection, and submit for analysis. A 40-ml aliquot is adequate for this purpose. Completeness of collection is difficult to determine. If results appear clinically invalid, this is cause for suspicion. Since creatinine excretion is based on muscle mass, and since a patient's muscle mass is relatively constant, creatinine excretion is also reasonably constant. Therefore, one should measure creatinine on several 24-hour collections and keep this as part of the patient's record. Another approach is to express results relative to the concentration of creatinine when collecting a specimen other than a 24-hour one.

Preservation of a urine specimen is essential in order to maintain its integrity. Unpreserved urine specimens are subject both to microbiologic decomposition and to inherent chemical changes. To prevent growth of microbes, the specimen should be refrigerated during and after collection, and when necessary should contain the indicated chemical preservative. For some determinations, where a chemical additive will affect the assay, use only refrigeration if necessary. The preservative is added to the empty bottle and a warning label is placed on the bottle as well. Warnings are necessary, e.g., acid burns to patient's genitals are not an unknown occurrence with the use of concentrated acids as preservatives. Light-sensitive compounds are protected in either amber glass bottles or plastic bottles wrapped in aluminum foil. Precipitation of calcium and phosphorus occurs unless the urine is acidified adequately before analysis.

It is particularly important to use *freshly* voided urine to test for bilirubin, RBCs, and WBCs, as these undergo decomposition upon standing at room temperature (Chap. 18). One should deliver specimens for these measurements to the laboratory within one hour of collection.

A useful guide for the collection and preservation of urine specimens according to the chemical analyte measured is presented in Table 1–4.

SPECIMEN PROCESSING

Processing of specimens embraces that period between collection of specimens and actual analysis. The sequence involves three distinct phases, pre-centrifugation, centrifugation, and post-centrifugation (NCCLS Pub. H 18-P, 1981). We refer to the last of these as specimen preservation.

Pre-Centrifugation

Ideally all measurements should be performed within one hour after collection. Whenever this is not practical, the specimen should be processed to a point at which it can be properly stored in order to preclude alterations of constituents to be measured. However, some whole blood specimens are initially processed by preparation of a protein-free filtrate with tungstic acid, trichloroacetic acid, or barium sulfate; such filtrates may be stored in a refrigerator at 4 to 6°C. if the interval prior to analysis exceeds 30 minutes. Plasma or serum is preferred to whole blood for most determinations because many constituents are distributed differently in erythrocytes versus serum or plasma; also, the results in the whole blood are different from those obtained in plasma because of a difference in water content between erythrocytes and plasma. Plasma or serum contains about 93 per cent water, whereas whole blood contains about 81 per cent water. The most efficient processing system

Table 1–4. URINE DETERMINATION WITH RECOMMENDED COLLECTION AND PRESERVATION*

Determination	Collection†	No Preservative	Boric Acid (10-15 g)	Glacial Acetic Acid (15 ml)	Hydrochloric Acid (15 ml)	Refrigeration—No Preservative
ALA (delta-aminolevulinic acid)	24				X	
Albumin	24		X			
Aldosterone	24			X		
Alpha-amino nitrogen	24		X			
Amino acids	24		X			
Amylase	2					X
Arsenic	24	X				
Barbiturates	R					X
Bence Jones protein	24		X(mail)			X
Calcium	24				X	
Catecholamines	24			X		
Chloride	24		X			
Chorionic gonadotropin	24					X
Copper	24	X				
Coproporphyrin (see under porphyrins)						
Cortisol	24		X			
Creatine	24		X			
Creatinine	24		X			
Drug abuse screen	R					X
Electrolytes (Cl, K, Na)	24					X
Estriol, pregnancy	24	X	X(Kober)			
Estrogens, total	24		X			
Follicle stimulating hormone	24					X
Glucose	24		X			
Heavy metals	24	X				
17-Hydroxycorticosteroids	24			X		
5-Hydroxyindoleacetic acid (5-HIAA)	24		X			
Hydroxyproline	24		X			
17-Ketogenic steroids (17-KGS)	24			X		
17-Ketosteroids (17-KS)	24			X		
Lead	24	X				
Lithium	24			X		
Mercury	24	X				
Metanephrines	24			X		
Osmolality	24			(mail or store frozen)		X
Phosphorus	24				X	
Porphobilinogen (see under Porphyrins)						
Porphyrins, Total	24					
Coproporphyrin	24	5 g Na_2CO_3				
Porphobilinogen	24	(protect from light;				
Protoporphyrin	24	ship frozen)				
Uroporphyrin	24					
Potassium	24					X
Pregnanediol	24			X		
Pregnanetriol	24			X		
Protein	24		X(mail)			X
Protoporphyrin (see under (Porphyrins)						
Sodium	24					X
Tetrahydro compound "S" (THS)	24			X		
Uric acid	24		X			
Uroporphyrin (see under Porphyrins)						
Vanillylmandelic acid (VMA)	24			X		

*Courtesy of International Clinical Laboratories, Inc., Nashville, Tennessee.
†Time of collection: 24 = 24 hour; 2 = 2 hour; R = Random.

generates a single or as few as possible blood fractions for analyses.

In clinical chemistry, serum and plasma are interchangeable except for very few measurements, e.g., ACTH and renin by radioimmunoassay require plasma. In fact, if serum can be used, it is preferred over plasma because of simplicity of specimen collection and handling. A further advantage is that serum poses no possible interference from anticoagulant. One should not refrigerate blood which is to be used for preparation of serum or plasma, as refrigeration inhibits the sodium-potassium pump, leading to increased potassium in the separated serum or plasma.

The actual steps in processing that must be followed for separation of whole blood into its fractions, components, or derivatives are as follows:

1. Blood should be kept in the stoppered original container until ready for analysis, which should begin within one hour after drawing blood specimen.

2. For plasma preparations, centrifuge blood within one hour after collection, preferably in the original container, for 10 minutes at a relative centrifugal force (RCF) of 850 to 1000 g, keeping the container stoppered to prevent evaporation. Label plasma container and store in refrigerator at 4 to 6°C. until plasma is analyzed, or freeze at −20°C. if analysis is to be delayed more than four hours. The Caraway microcapillary tubes with a maximum volume of 350 μl are occluded with microcaps or vinyl plaster putty at the tapered end prior to centrifugation for one minute at 5000 g; this will yield about 150 μl of plasma.*

3. For serum preparations, allow blood to clot in the original closed container at room temperature (usually 20 to 30 minutes). Allow adequate time for clotting in order to prevent latent fibrin formation which may pose a problem in automated instrumentation. The addition of Li-heparin to the specimen may resolve sampling problems due to fibrin formation (Kapke, 1982). Do not loosen the clot by "rimming" the tube. With technical improvements in tube manufacture this is unnecessary, and may cause hemolysis. Centrifuge blood 10 minutes at an RCF of 850 to 1000 g in the stoppered container. Label and store the serum in a refrigerator at 4 to 6°C. until analyzed or freeze at −20°C. if analysis is to be delayed more than four hours.

Centrifugation

A centrifuge is a machine which uses centrifugal force to separate phases of different densities. The centrifuge has multiple specific uses in the clinical laboratory. One of the most frequent uses of primary importance is in blood processing to derive plasma or serum fractions. Conditions for centrifugation should specify both the time and centrifugal force. In selecting a centrifuge, one should look for the highest possible centrifugal force and not be misled by the high rotational speed. When the radius (r) is known, calculation of the relative centrifugal force (g) may be made from a nomogram (Fig. 1–1) or by the use of the following formula:

$$\text{RCF} = 1.118 \times 10^{-5} \times r \times (\text{rpm})^2$$

in which RCF is the relative centrifugal force in units of g, i.e., multiples of the gravitational force; 1.118×10^{-5} is a constant; r is the radius, expressed in centimeters, between the axis of rotation and the center of the centrifuge tube; and rpm is the speed in revolutions per minute. Several principles must be observed to avoid damage to the centrifuge or the specimen and danger to personnel.

The principle of "balance" must be observed. Tubes and carriers or shields of equal weight, shape, and size should be placed in opposing positions in the centrifuge head, with regard for a geometrically symmetrical arrangement, using water-filled tubes when necessary.

Equipment. A wide variety of centrifuges and accessories are available to meet specific needs in the clinical laboratory. Table-top general laboratory centrifuges develop forces up to about 3000 g, depending on the type of centrifuge head. Angle centrifuge heads are high-speed heads with drilled holes which hold the tubes at a fixed angle. Horizontal centrifuge heads allow the tubes to swing from a vertical to horizontal position during centrifugation. Portable floor-type models, nonrefrigerated, are capable of accepting both angle and horizontal heads, with up to 36 places for the angle heads. Horizontal heads may have 4 to 16 places. By number of places is meant the number of cups or tubes which the head can accept. Generally, the lower the number of places, the larger the volume or capacity of each cup. These portable floor models operate at an RCF (g forces) of 800 to 3500, depending on the type of head. A microhematocrit centrifuge is a special version of a table-top centrifuge which very rapidly generates g forces in the range of 12,000 and also can be stopped in seconds. Tiny capillary tubes fit into a fixed head which may be specially cooled. Refrigerated centrifuges are heavy-duty, non-portable, floor-type centrifuges capable of generating g forces up to 50,000, if angle heads are used. These centrifuges are utilized in the blood bank, and to very good advantage in the radioimmunoassay laboratory, i.e., for spinning down protein precipitates and for handling large numbers of tubes in temperature-sensitive charcoal separations. Ultracentrifuges, generating g forces in the hundreds of thousands, are finding routine clinical use in tissue receptor assays and clarifying lactescent serum for electrolyte and other measurements (Musiala, 1977).

Calibration of Centrifuge. For every procedure requiring a centrifuge operation there should be a written specification in the procedure manual. It is important to define which particular centrifuge to use, at what temperature, the g forces required, and the length of time for spinning. In order to calculate the g forces, the rpm and radius must be known (Fig.

*International Micro-Hematocrit, Centrifuge Model MB with 16-place head. Sample slots are milled down to base. An embroidery hoop may be used as a gasket; tapered ends of Caraway tubes may cut standard rubber gasket (Mabry, 1967).

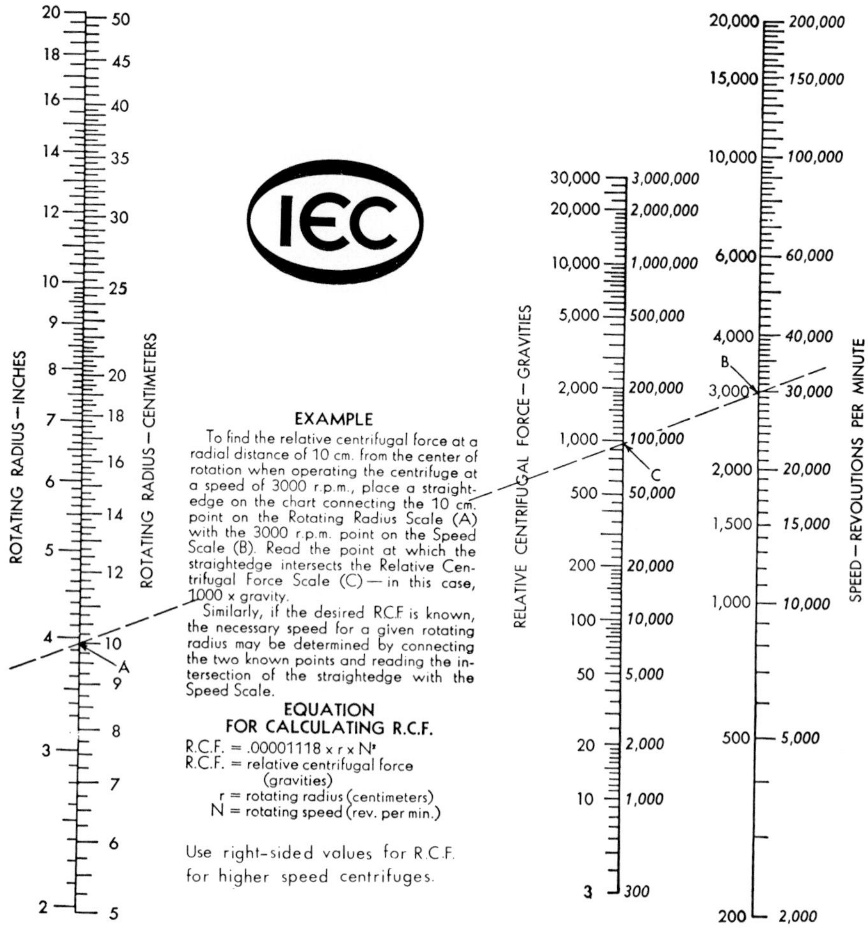

Figure 1–1. Nomogram for calculation of relative centrifugal force (RCF) in g.

1–1). Therefore, a centrifuge has to be calibrated. Koenig (1982) provides an excellent review of function, verification, and adjustment for a centrifuge. To do this, the centrifuge must have a built-in tachometer or a dial on its rheostat. Otherwise, it can be calibrated only at maximum speed. It is very important to calibrate the instrument each time under as nearly identical conditions as possible. Use the same head loaded with the same number of empty cups. Any significant change will indicate deterioration effects, such as wearing of brushes, incipient bearing problems, or a defective tachometer (Koenig, 1982).

Specimen Preservation

A myriad of changes occur in clinical specimens once removed from the patient. Bacterial growth and enzymatic activity can alter drastically the value of blood components. Many biologic compounds are of themselves unstable. Refrigeration or freezing of the biologic specimen is an effective means of retarding many of these degradative reactions (Rossing, 1980). In fact, preservation of specimens is a prime consideration, and increases in importance with increasing time of delay before the analysis is performed.

Effect on Specimen. Generally, the Q_{10} of a reaction, or the increase in reaction rate with an increase in temperature of 10°C., is about two. If we consider that the difference in temperature between room and refrigerated storage is about 20°C., it is immediately apparent that a reaction will occur about four times as fast at room temperature.

The effect of bacterial degradation may be much more dramatic (Simkins, 1978). With long-term storage in the refrigerator, bacterial populations reach significant levels with severe degradative effects on biologic components. These effects are extremely variable, since entirely different bacterial populations may predominate in serum specimens.

Even under frozen storage (−20°C.) a biologic system is unstable. For example, enzymatic reactions occur to alter the concentration of substrate. The enzyme molecule itself may be unstable, so that enzyme activity will change with long standing. Some fairly simple molecules, like folic acid, are unstable at −20°C. The most practical consequence is that control specimens stored at −20°C. can and sometimes do change in concentration with long-term storage. This effect will be seen by a gradually decreasing mean on control charts. The question of the effect of freeze-thaw cycles on stability comes up often. In specimens such as plasma and serum the ice crystals which form cause shear effects which are disruptive to molecular structure, especially large molecules like proteins. Slow freezing allows larger crystals to form, with more serious degradative effects. Therefore, for optimal stability quick freezing is preferred. As for the extent of degradation in freeze/thaw cycles, actual experimentation is necessary to demonstrate the quantitative effect (Plant, 1982).

PERFORMING THE ASSAY

The validity of clinical laboratory data is dependent not only upon proper manipulation of equipment but also upon use of specific reagents and materials and upon environmental control. An understanding of these fundamental issues embracing materials and essential measurements is a prelude to an appreciation of analytical procedures.

Reagents

Grades. Chemicals exist in varying degrees of purity. Even sodium chloride may contain a small amount of potassium sulfate or iodide. Meticulous attention to the label on a bottle as well as to the supplier's catalogue will frequently reveal the maximum limits of impurities in chemicals. Several companies show on the label the actual analysis so that one may identify the exact amount of an impurity present in a particular batch or bottle. For quantitative measurements and preparation of accurate standard solutions, it is important to use pure chemicals and to identify exact amounts of compound or elements desired, as well as amounts of contaminants. The use of "reagent-grade" chemicals, although more expensive than less pure grades of chemicals, is essential for accuracy. Because several grades of chemicals are available, an awareness of the terms used widely is necessary. For the most highly purified chemicals, "reagent grade," "analytical grade," or "ACS" for having met the established standards of purity by the American Chemical Society are terms that should be identified on a label or in the catalogue. Less pure grades are referred to as "purified" and "technical."

U.S.P. and N.F. represent other grades of purity and mean that these chemicals meet the stipulations listed in the United States Pharmacopeia or the National Formulary; while they are adequate for human consumption, they may not be pure enough for specific chemical applications. Radin (1967) has reviewed the use and availability of standards with the limitations of so-called standards.

The National Bureau of Standards (NBS) through the Office of Standard Reference Materials (Alvarez, 1982), the College of American Pathologists (CAP), and the National Committee for Clinical Laboratory Standards (NCCLS) all supply certified clinical laboratory standards. These, plus several suppliers who list the exact composition or maximum limits of impurities in their chemicals, are preferred sources for preparation of many standards used in medical chemistry (Meinke, 1971). Proprietary reagents (such as drugs) of undisclosed composition should be avoided, even though they may give satisfactory results under the usual conditions. With abnormal specimens or under abnormal conditions, confusing results as well as invalid data may be produced by use of such proprietary reagents. It is important to know what compounds are being used in a specific determination to understand what reaction is taking place and to identify as well as anticipate and evaluate abnormal reactions or interferences.

Techniques of Use and Storage. A reagent or chemical will arrive in the laboratory with a certain guarantee of purity. Once the seal is broken, the guaranteed analysis is strictly in the hands of the receiving laboratory. Definite steps must be taken to ensure that the chemical or reagent is handled under optimal conditions: (1) It is extremely important to read the label for proper storage. While most chemical compounds are stable at room temperature without desiccation, some must be refrigerated, frozen, or even stored at $-70°C$. Light-sensitive chemicals and reagents must be stored in brown bottles. (2) Absolutely never sample directly from the reagent bottle. An entire bottle of reagent grade chemical can become contaminated by an unclean spatula or a dirty pipette. Pour slightly more than the required amount of reagent into another vessel, such as a beaker, and sample from that vessel. Discard the excess. It is a common practice to sample directly from standard solutions, largely as a matter of convenience. This can lead to contamination of the standard and a change in its value.

Immunoreagents. Modern clinical immunology and radioimmunoassay require special reagents supplied largely in the form of commercial kits. A typical kit, e.g., for a radioimmunoassay procedure, will contain all essential reagents, including standards, radiolabeled antigen, and antibody, plus ancillary reagents. A critical problem with use of commercial kits is that the laboratory is dependent upon the supplier to produce and maintain components which must meet rigid standards. It is essential that each laboratory first evaluate a kit according to an established protocol (NCCLS Pub. LA1-A, 1982; NCCLS Pub. LA12-P, 1980), then monitor kit performance thereafter by appropriate quality control procedures. Many of the analytes measured by immunochemical methods, such as hormones, are available as reference preparations from the World Health Organization (WHO) or the National Institutes of Health (NIH).

Water

Purification. The two methods in general use for preparation of laboratory reagent grade water are distillation and deionization. To meet standards for reagent water specified by the College of American Pathologists, it will generally be necessary to further purify distilled water. This is most often done by deionization. Many laboratories use deionization without prior distillation for preparation of reagent grade water. Deionizers work on the principle of ion exchange. Insoluble resin polymers are prepared with acid or amine functional groups on the molecule. A cation exchange resin, for example, a phenolformaldehyde polymer with $—SO_3H_3$, $—CH_2COOH$, —COOH, or —OH radicals, will react in the following manner, with R— representing the insoluble backbone of the polymer, and Na^+ as an example:

$$R—\overset{\overset{\displaystyle O}{\|}}{\underset{\underset{\displaystyle O}{\|}}{S}}—OH + Na^+ \rightleftharpoons R—\overset{\overset{\displaystyle O}{\|}}{\underset{\underset{\displaystyle O}{\|}}{S}}—O—Na + H^+ \quad (1)$$

In this reaction, sodium ions are removed from solution and hydrogen ions are ejected into solution. Thus, there is an exchange between sodium and hydrogen ions. In a similar manner, an anion exchange resin such as formed by the condensation of formaldehyde with various amines, for example, *m*-phenylenediamine and urea, will exchange hydroxyl ions for negatively charged ions in solution. One such reaction will be:

$$R_4NOH + Cl^- \rightleftharpoons R_4NCl + OH^- \quad (2)$$

A commercially installed system usually will have a cationic exchange resin followed by an anionic exchange resin, a charcoal filter to remove organic compounds, and a final filter to remove particulate matter. This type can be monitored, for example, at 1 megohm per cm specific resistance with a light to indicate that the system is producing water at least equal to the indicated quality. At peak operation this system will generate water at 10 megohm per cm specific resistance or better.

Specifications. The College of American Pathologists has drawn up specifications and methods of quality control for reagent water (Hamlin, 1978). Three grades of water are defined, Types I, II, and III, with resistance specifications shown in Table 1–5.

Each test established in the laboratory must be judged for the type of water necessary to avoid interference with specificity, accuracy, and precision. It is known, for example, that metal contaminants can have profound effects on enzyme values (Winstead, 1967). The following are recommendations of the Commission on Inspection and Accreditation of the College of American Pathologists (Hamlin, 1978) for reagent water requirements:

Type I Reagent Water
For procedures which require maximum water purity:
- Preparation of standard solutions.
- Ultramicrochemical analyses.
- Measurements at nanogram or subnanogram concentrations.
- Tissue and/or cell culture methods.

Type II Reagent Water
For most laboratory testing in chemistry, hematology, microbiology, immunology, and other clinical test areas.

Type III Reagent Water
For most qualitative testing; most procedures in urinalysis, parasitology, and histology; washing glassware; in general, any laboratory procedures not requiring Type I or II reagent water.

Carbon dioxide (CO_2) free water (reagent water, free of CO_2) is used where such gases as CO_2, ammonia, and oxygen may affect analysis. Boiled Type II water is adequate for such use.

Table 1–5. RESISTANCE SPECIFICATIONS OF REAGENT WATER

Specification	Type I	Type II	Type III
Specific resistance,* megohms @ 25°C., minimum	In-line 10	Effluent 2.0	(As used) 0.1

*Specific resistance is the resistance in ohms of a column of solution 1 cm long and 1 cm^2 in cross-sectional area.

Measurement of Mass

In the modern clinical laboratory, measurements of mass are seldom performed. Reagents, standards, and controls come ready for use, or simply need reconstituting. However, since the measurement of mass is fundamental to every analysis, the technologist will eventually use some sort of balance. It is usual for the toxicologist to prepare drug standards from pure authentic material. Fecal fats may be measured by gravimetric analysis. It is prudent to prepare in-house many laboratory reagents which are much less expensive than if purchased. Of course, volumetric equipment is calibrated by measurement of mass.

Theory and Technique (Natelson, 1971; Fritz, 1974; Hackler, 1970). The basic principle in the measurement of mass is to balance an unknown mass with a known mass. Analytical balances, though extremely sophisticated, use the basic concept of a simple lever which pivots on a knife-edge fulcrum placed at the center of gravity of the lever. From this concept, balances are designed in a variety of ways. *Two pans* of equal mass may be suspended from the ends of the lever, or beam. In this case, *calibrated* weights are placed on one pan to counterbalance an object of unknown mass on the other pan. A rider and/or a chain weight device is generally utilized to avoid fractional weights. Motion of the beam is indicated by a pointer traversing a scale much like a ruler. Macrobalances of this sort generally have a capacity of 200 g and a sensitivity of 0.1 mg.

Single-pan balances offer the speed and accuracy necessary in the clinical laboratory. These balances encompass a range from 1 μg to 1000 g in both analytical and top-loading balances. Although single-pan balances work on the principle of weighing by substitution, they still utilize the basic concept of a lever and fulcrum. The balance is first set at the zero point. In this configuration one end of the beam has a built-in mass just equal to the mass on the other end of the beam, which includes the single pan and a set of built-in calibrated weights. These weights are nonmagnetic chrome-nickel steel rings or cylinders standardized against prototype weights at the National Bureau of Standards. The sample is placed on the pan. As selector knobs are adjusted, weights are removed until the zero point is again reached. Therefore, the mass of the sample is exactly substituted for an equivalent mass of weights originally on the sample side of the beam. Single-pan analytical balances suitable for the clinical laboratory are available as semimicro or macro balances with a scale from 0 to 160 g and a precision (standard deviation) of 0.01 mg or 0.1 mg.

The guiding principle in weighing technique is to regard a balance as a delicate, precision instrument which will function properly only if it is not abused. The knife edge located at the fulcrum of the beam is a synthetic sapphire and can be injured by lowering the beam too hard or through excessive vibration. Make gross weight changes with the balance in the beam arrest position. Release the beam gently. Avoid chemical spills; if these occur, immediately clean up the area. Never weigh a sample directly on the pan. One must not overload the balance.

The sequence in weighing a sample using a single-pan balance is as follows:

1. Check that the balance is level by observing the level indicator. Make appropriate adjustments to the feet.
2. Observe that the balance is not in direct sunlight and is in a draft-free location.
3. Set the balance to its zero point. If taring is used, set the read-out at zero. For the analytical balance, this setting is made with the sliding windows closed and the beam resting on the knife edge.
4. Lock the beam of the analytical balance. Open the window of the balance case and place the object to be weighed on the pan. Close the window.
5. Set the beam arrest knob in the intermediate position.
6. Make gross weight changes until the weight of the object is in the range of the optical scale.
7. Fully release the beam and allow the pan to come to its final point of rest.
8. Record the mass of the object.
9. Fully arrest the beam and remove the object from the pan.

Hygroscropic materials and volatile liquids are difficult to weight accurately. Solids which have been dried *in vacuo* and placed in a desiccator are often hygroscopic and should be weighed in weighing bottles with ground-glass stoppers.

Calibration. The weights in a typical single-pan analytical balance meet individual and group tolerances for Class S weights established by the National Bureau of Standards. These tolerances are defined in the NBS Circular 547 (Lashof, 1954). In order to calibrate a balance, weights conforming to Class S tolerances are available commercially. One such set consists of 12 fractional weights: 1–2–3–5–10–20–30–50–100–200–300–500 mg; and 9 rhodium-plated bronze gram weights: 1–2–3–5–10–20–30–50–100 g. These weights must be handled with forceps supplied with the set. A balance out of calibration will usually require a specialist for adjustment and realignment.

Top-Loading Balances. Single-pan top-loading balances operate on the same principle as single-pan analytical balances, i.e., weighing by substitution. Damping is magnetic rather than air-release. There is an entire line of these balances available covering a dynamic weighing range up to 10,000 g. These balances are especially suitable for rapidly weighing larger masses which do not require as much analytical precision, such as large volume reagent preparation.

Electronic Balances. Modern electronic balances couple the advantage of ease of use with very high resolution. Resolution is an expression of sensitivity in relation to the total dynamic range, defined in points. A scale with 130 kg capacity that reads accurately to ½ kg has a resolution of 260 points. An electronic semi-micro balance has a resolution of 3 million points (30 g accurate to 0.01 mg). An electronic balance operates on the principle of electromagnetic force compensation. A coil, placed between the poles of a cylindrical electromagnet, is mechanically connected to a weighing pan. Mass placed on the pan produces a force which displaces the coil within the magnetic field. A regulator generates a compensation current just sufficient to return the coil to its original position. The more mass placed on the pan, the larger the deflecting force, and the stronger the current required to correct the deflection of the coil. The measuring principle is based on a strict linear relationship between compensation current and force produced by the load placed on the pan.

Balance Maintenance. The two most important factors in balance maintenance are to keep the balance scrupulously clean and to avoid excessive vibrations. The more rugged general utility balances can be taken apart to clean the knife edges, which can become clogged with dust accumulation. Intricate, internal maintenance of analytical and top-loading balances is best left to qualified factory-trained service personnel.

Measurement of Volume

Types of Glassware. By far the most common type of glassware encountered in measurement of volume is borosilicate glass. It is essentially a sodium-aluminum borosilicate with an excess of silica. This glass is characterized by a high degree of thermal resistance. Commercial brands are known as Pyrex (Corning) and Kimax (Kimble). The glass has a low alkali content and is free from the magnesia-lime-zinc group of elements, heavy metals, arsenic, and antimony. It is very poor technique to store concentrated alkaline solutions in borosilicate glass. The caustic conditions will etch, or dissolve, the glass and destroy the calibration. Also, glass stoppers become frozen and are extremely difficult to remove without breaking the neck of the flask. Borosilicate glassware with heavy walls, such as bottles, jars, and even larger beakers, should not be heated with a direct flame or hot plate. Be careful not to heat any glass above its strain point, which for Pyrex is 515°C. If this occurs, and the glass is cooled too quickly, strains will develop and the glass cracks easily when again heated. Also, in the case of volumetric glassware, heating can destroy the calibration.

Corex brand glassware is a special alumina-silicate glass strengthened chemically rather than thermally. Corex is at least six times stronger than borosilicate glass, e.g., Corex pipettes have a typical strength of 30,000 psi, compared to 2000 to 5000 psi for borosilicate pipettes. Corex brand cylinders will outlast conventional cylinders by at least 10 times. Corex is also better able to resist clouding and scratching.

Alkali-resistant glassware should be used to handle strongly alkaline solutions. However, it has only about half the thermal shock resistance of Pyrex glassware and therefore must be heated and cooled more carefully.

Low actinic glassware is a glass of high thermal resistance with a red color added as an integral part of the glass. The density of the red color is adjusted to permit adequate visibility of the contents, yet give maximum protection to light-sensitive materials, such as bilirubin standards.

Specifications. Volumetric glassware is classed A, B, and Student Grade. The tolerances for accuracy of Class A glassware meet or exceed the strict requirements specified by the National Bureau of Standards in Circular C-602. All Class A volumetric ware is the only type acceptable by the College of American Pathologists for use in an approved clinical laboratory.

Pipettes. There are many kinds of pipettes available for use in a clinical laboratory, each intended to serve a specific function. In general, pipettes fall into two classes, volumetric or transfer pipettes and graduated or measuring pipettes. The volumetric pipette is calibrated for one specified volume measurement, either "to deliver" (T.D.) or "to contain" (T.C.). For class A pipettes this distinction is clearly indicated on the pipette. A "to deliver" pipette calibrated for blow-out has an opaque ring near the top. In this case the small amount of liquid remaining in the tip after free delivery has ceased is blown out and added to the initial volume. "To deliver" pipettes are calibrated for the volume delivered, with no attempt to wash out the film which adheres to the inside glass surface. "To contain" pipettes are calibrated for the total volume of liquid held in the pipette, and must be washed out completely for delivery of the correct volume. Most micropipettes, in the range up to 0.5 ml, are calibrated "to contain." Graduated pipettes are long, cylindrical tubes drawn out to a tip and are calibrated in uniform fractional volume measurements. The Mohr type is calibrated between two marks on the stem, while the serologic type is calibrated to the tip. All serologic pipettes are therefore calibrated for blow-out, and accordingly have an opaque ring at the top for identification.

Before using a pipette, be sure it is the correct size, is clean, and is free of chips. Without careful inspection, a broken tip may go unnoticed. Absolutely never pipette by mouth. This is especially critical in the clinical laboratory. There is no guarantee that the stem of the pipette is sterile, so that pathologic organisms can be taken in by this route. Also, in pipetting sera it is very easy to suck serum into the mouth. The same applies for strong acids and alkalis.

The steps in good pipetting procedure include the following:

1. Place a safety pipette filler on the stem of the pipette.
2. Lower the pipette into the solution. Allow sufficient depth to fill the pipette above the calibration mark.
3. Apply suction and load the pipette to a point above the calibration mark. In cases of a critically low volume of solution, fill the pipette slowly and watch carefully to avoid aspiration of air.
4. Remove the pipette from the solution. Wipe the tip with a tissue or gauze.
5. Hold the pipette in a vertical position. Empty the pipette slowly until the lower meniscus just touches the calibration mark. Pay attention to parallax errors.
6. Touch the tip to a clean, dry receptacle to remove any pendant drop.
7. Drain the pipette freely in a *vertical* position. The pipette has been calibrated to deliver its specified volume in a vertical position with a constant rate of delivery. Changing the angle of the pipette changes the rate of delivery and hence the volume of liquid left behind in the pipette. For the same reason, do not attempt to force the liquid from the pipette at a faster rate than free drainage permits.
8. When the liquid enters the stem just below the bulb, touch the tip to the side of the receiving vessel, but not into the liquid. Allow several seconds for the pipette to drain. For blow-out pipettes, manipulate the small bulb of the safety pipette filler to force a gentle blast of air through the pipette. This removes the last bit of liquid from the tip.

Semiautomatic and Automatic Pipettes. Automatic pipetting devices permit rapid, repetitive measurement and delivery of equal volumes. Automatic pipetting and diluting devices have evolved for ensuring the more efficient delivery of equal volumes of specimens followed by diluent at a constant ratio to specimen. Commercial automatic pipettes are either of the sampling type, usually manually operated, or of the sampling-diluting type, usually electrically operated. Manually operated automatic pipettes are generally of the air-displacement variety, with a range in volume capacity from 1 to 6000 μl. Tip-ejector models, variable-setting digital pipettes, and repetitive-dispensing pipettes are available for added convenience. Since proper care and calibration are essential to precise, accurate sampling, it is important to read and follow the manufacturer's instructions. Two common errors include allowing a sample to aspirate into the barrel of the pipette and ignoring lubrication of the piston. The sampling-dispensing automatic pipettes fall into two general classes: (1) the peristaltic type and (2) the piston type. Automatic sampler-diluters are available with sampling volume ranges from 0.1 to 5000 μl and diluting volumes from 0.2 to 25 ml. For maximum accuracy and precision, diluent volumes up to 5000 μl are optimum. Again, it is very important to follow the manufacturer's instructions in the operation and maintenance of these machines.

Automatic pipettes remove much of the tedium associated with repetitive sampling and dilution. Even for a limited number of samples, the speed of an automatic pipette is an advantage. Because operator fatigue is minimized, precision of multiple sampling and dilution is often improved with the automatic pipette. The micro-automatic pipettes, which can sample as little as 2 to 5 μl, offer a unique advantage, especially for radioimmunoassay.

Manufacturers generally claim a pipetting and dilution accuracy in the range of 0.1 to 1.0 per cent. However, it is essential that automatic pipettes be calibrated when new and at regular intervals thereafter. Never assume that factory calibrations are accurate! The random analytical variation of an automatic manual pipette can be established by repetitive pipetting of a radioactive solution and counting the activity of each sample. Calculations are made to determine the mean and standard deviation of the counts. The total variance includes both the variance of the counter and the variance of the pipette. The variances are additive. Therefore, the variance of pipetting is calculated as:

$$\sigma^2 \text{ Total} = \sigma^2 \text{ Counter} + \sigma^2 \text{ Pipetting}$$

In using an automatic pipette, the tip wiping technique is important in obtaining reproducibility. Aspirate the sample into the tip. Then wipe the tip with absorbent cloth or tissue with two downward strokes at 90 degrees with respect to one another. Each stroke should start above the level that the tip was immersed into the fluid sample and proceed downward past the tip. Do not actually touch the fluid in the tip, as this will draw the fluid out of the tip.

With an automatic sampling-diluting pipette, the operator must always beware of possible carry-over. When a sample is introduced into the tip, diffusion of sample occurs. The washout by diluent may be insufficient to remove all the sample, and this becomes mixed with the succeeding sample. The result is that any analyses performed on the first sample dilution are too low, and those done on the the second are too high. In general, the ratio of diluent to sample must be at least 5:1 for quantitative washout. This must be increased if the sample is viscous or oily and the diluent is of an aqueous base. Also, certain components are adsorbed by the tip construction, and the washout must be increased. In general, a Teflon tip absorbs less than a glass tip. Some hormones and drugs, for example, have a high affinity for glass.

Volumetric Flasks. Inspect the flask to be sure that it is clean, dry, and not cracked. For glass-stoppered flasks, be sure the stopper fits properly so as not to leak. It is usually possible to tell by how well the stopper seats in the joint. The steps in using a volumetric flask are as follows:

1. Add to the flask the solution to be diluted or the solid to be dissolved and diluted to volume. A solid is best added to the flask by having first weighed the material in a beaker. Then add enough solvent to the beaker to dissolve the solid. Hold a glass rod across the beaker with one end over the lip. Tip the beaker and allow the solution to pour down the glass rod into the opening of the flask. Keep adding small volumes of solvent to wash the beaker. This will result in a quantitative transfer to the flask.
2. Bring nearly to volume with solvent.
3. Use a Pasteur pipette to wet the neck of the flask. Add solvent drop by drop to bring the meniscus to the final calibration mark.
4. Stopper the flask and mix thoroughly. For adequate mixing turn the flask upside down and shake. Then turn the flask upright. Repeat this four more times. In the case of solutions which foam, mixing must be done more slowly with many more revolutions of the flask. In extreme cases of foaming, the flask can only be rotated, not tipped upside down. Magnetic stirrers may be used.

Calibration. According to the strictest of standards, every piece of volumetric glassware in the clinical laboratory should be coded and a record kept of its calibration. Any piece of glassware which does not meet Class A tolerance should be rejected. To prepare a piece of glassware for calibration, rinse with tap water followed by a thorough rinsing with reagent grade water.

Cleaning of Glassware. Glassware from general laboratory use should be rinsed and immediately placed into a weak detergent solution. Never leave corrosive chemicals in glassware which is later to be picked up by washroom personnel. Serious chemical burns may occur in handling. The glassware will usually be rinsed and placed in a completely automatic glassware washer, which will prewash, wash, rinse, and finally rinse with reagent grade water from a separate plumbing system. The glassware will then be placed in a glassware dryer before distribution to laboratory glassware storage.

The surface of a thoroughly clean glass apparatus will become uniformly wet, with no adhering water droplets. Special treatment is required in cases of stubborn grease and other organic residues. Let the glassware stand overnight in a sulfuric acid–dichromate mixture, prepared by pouring 1000 ml of concentrated sulfuric acid into 35 ml of saturated sodium dichromate. Avoid contact with the skin or clothing. Rinse the glassware *thoroughly* after removal from the mixture.

Bacteriologic glassware should be soaked in 2 to 4 per cent cresol, or a weak Lysol solution. Follow by autoclaving, then pass the glassware through the normal washing procedure.

Glassware used for iron determinations must be soaked in hydrochloric acid solution (concentrated HCl diluted 1:2) or nitric acid solution (concentrated HNO_3 diluted 1:3) and then rinsed with reagent grade water.

Control of Temperature

Precise temperature control in many clinical measurements is an absolute prerequisite. The dependence of enzyme activity on temperature and the requirement for precise temperature control is a classic example. Indeed, any measurement which includes a time/

temperature–dependent reaction must be rigorously controlled with respect to these two variables.

Constant Temperature Baths. For general clinical laboratory use, constant temperature water baths must offer variable temperature control from +5°C. above ambient temperature to 100°C., with accurate control to ±0.2°C. No refrigeration capabilities are required in this type of unit. For precise temperature control at room temperatures or below, refrigeration is necessary. Baths are available with a temperature range from −30° to 100°C., accurate to ±0.02°C. A compressor and heater work in tandem to offer temperature control over this range. An important consideration in the selection of a constant temperature bath is that the model be large enough to accommodate the desired working volume. Models which have independent controlled agitation to maintain a uniform bath temperature are desirable. Heating blocks are more useful for high temperature use.

Maintenance. Maintenance of a constant temperature water bath is improved by filling it with distilled or deionized water. This prevents the accumulation of mineral deposits from regular tap water which can affect the temperature sensing elements and generally lead to poor heat transfer. However, if an accumulation of these minerals does occur, a weak hydrochloric acid solution will dissolve the deposits. Overheating can occur if the bath goes dry, so this should be avoided. At higher temperatures the bath should be covered, both to maintain proper temperature control and to prevent rapid evaporation to dryness.

Quality Control. Accurately calibrated thermometers are issued by the National Bureau of Standards. These have an auxiliary ice-point scale from −0.20 to +0.20°C. to check the calibration (Ween, 1976). A thermometer calibrated against another certified by the National Bureau of Standards must be a component of any constant temperature bath. The temperature should be noted and recorded for each assay. This function by the operator ensures that indeed the temperature of the bath is the same as the reading of the thermometer.

Timing

Timing accuracy is critical in measurement of rate reactions, e.g., in enzyme chemistries and coagulation studies. To assure accuracy of timing devices, such as stopwatches used in coagulation measurements, follow an acceptable quality control protocol. One such procedure is to verify the accuracy of each stopwatch in a department against a stopwatch adjusted for accuracy on an electronic timing machine. This verified "standard" stopwatch, with the balance wheel carefully adjusted, will be accurate to 2 to 3 seconds per day. Modern digital electronic quartz stopwatches are recommended for increased accuracy to 12 to 60 seconds per year.

Evaporation and Specimen Concentration

Evaporation as a batch or unit process is an essential step in many analytical procedures. Solvent extraction is almost always followed by evaporation of solvent to recover the extracted material for further processing. Cerebrospinal fluid, urine, and even serum specimens must be concentrated to bring certain compounds within the range of analytical sensitivity.

Large-volume solvent evaporation is best accomplished with a thin-film rotary vacuum evaporator. Evaporation of test-tube quantities of solvent, in the range of 10 to 15 ml or less, is handled conveniently in an evaporator which concentrates by blowing a stream of an inert gas, usually nitrogen, across the surface of the solvent. Using the same principle, evaporators to handle large numbers of tubes such as required in high volume radioimmunoassay or toxicology laboratories can be designed.

Polymer films, or membranes, constructed with an effective pore size to retain solutes above a selected molecular weight, can be utilized to concentrate proteins, including enzymes, isoenzymes, and hormones. Typical molecular weight cut-off values for these ultrafiltration membranes are 15,000, 25,000, 75,000 and 125,000. Amicon Corporation (21 Hartwell Avenue, Lexington, Mass. 02173) utilizes these films in the construction of clinical sample concentrations. A technique for measurement of ultrafiltrable calcium with demonstrated exclusion of albumin and amylase (Toffaletti, 1981) involves use of a Millipore membrane (Ultra-Free; Worthington Diagnostics, Freehold, N.J. 07728).

Ultrafiltration membranes constructed in the form of a cone can be supported in a tube and placed in a centrifuge. The force of centrifugation will drive liquid and solute past the membrane, below a critical molecular weight cut-off value. Protein-free filtrates can be prepared by this technique. Therefore, it becomes possible to determine the free, or non–protein-bound, fraction of blood components. For instance, using this technique it is possible to measure the concentration of free phenytoin in serum (Booker, 1973).

Filtration

Filtration may be used in place of centrifugation to separate solids from liquids. This is usually performed with filter paper, folded properly, and a funnel. A funnel containing glass wool may be substituted for paper when acids or bases too strong for filter paper require filtering. Many types of filter paper with different degrees of porosity are available for selection according to requirements of separation by filtration.

Dialysis

Dialysis is a technique for the separation of substances in molecular or ionic solution from colloidally dispersed molecules. A dialyzing membrane is a porous diaphragm which acts like a sieve. When an aqueous system to be dialyzed is placed on one side of the membrane and pure water is placed on the other side, the substances in molecular or ionic solution diffuse through the pores of the membrane.

Colloidally dispersed molecules are too large to pass through the pores and therefore are held back. Diffusion of the smaller molecules or ions in solution continues until at equilibrium their respective concentrations on each side of the membrane are equal. Therefore, if the side originally containing the pure water is continuously replaced with pure water, a condition will be reached where the colloidally dispersed molecules are practically free of all diffusible molecules. The material which passes through the membrane during the process of dialysis is referred to as diffusate, or dialysate. The term retentate applies to the substance which does not pass through the membrane.

Membranes used in dialysis are most commonly made of regenerated cellulose, using cotton linters for the source of cellulose. The membrane may be constructed as a tube or sheet. Cellulose membranes are available with a molecular weight cut-off specification ranging from 2000 MWCO (molecular weight cut-off) to 12,000 to 14,000 MWCO. The 12,000 MWCO film will have an average pore diameter of 4.8 nanometers. The 12,000 to 14,000 MWCO membrane has a dialysis rate about three times that of the 6000 to 8000 MWCO membrane. After processing, cellulose membranes have glycerol added as a humectant to keep the film supple. Small amounts (0.1 per cent) of polysulfides are also generally present as a contaminant. Both the glycerol and polysulfide may be removed by proper washing.

Dialysis is a unit process for determinations employing continuous flow analyzers. One such dialyzer component consists of two flat, spirally grooved plates; one is a mirror image of the other. The two plates, separated by a cellulose membrane, are clamped together with the grooves matched. The standard or specimen stream enters the dialyzer and flows parallel to a stream of reagent; the two streams (specimen and reagent) are separated by the cellulose membrane. The constituent for analysis dialyzes through the membrane and enters the reagent stream.

Dialysis is a key step in the analysis for CEA (carcinoembryonic antigen) by radioimmunoassay (Roche Diagnostics, Nutley, N.J. 07110). It is critical that the dialysis be conducted under controlled conditions with uniform adequate agitation during the dialysis. Dialysis is used to remove interfering substances in the radioimmunoassay of FSH and LH in urine. A simplified, reproducible procedure for the determination of serum-free thyroxine by equilibrium dialysis is available (Wilson, 1974).

Technique. Prewet dialysis bags before use. Do this by cutting a desired length of dialysis tubing from the roll and lowering the tubing into a beaker of distilled water. Change the water at intervals to wash away impurities. An hour is adequate time for prewetting. Tie the bag at one end, *using a double knot*. Fill the bag with the solution to be dialyzed. Care must be taken at this point because the solution can be easily spilled. Rub the untied end of the prewetted tube between the thumb and forefinger. The end of the tube will open up. By rubbing the tube farther and farther down from this initial opening a large air space can be made. Bring the beaker, test tube, or pipette to the opening of the bag. The liquid will now easily enter the bag and run to the bottom. It is important to remove all air from the dialysis bag, since the presence of air will retard the rate of dialysis and cause the bag to float. Tie off the bag with a double knot, leaving room for expansion of the liquid volume. Immerse the sac in the dialyzing medium.

Extraction

Theory. Extraction is a separation technique in which a solute is transferred from one solvent to a second immiscible solvent by allowing the solute to form an equilibrium distribution between the two solvent phases. For increased separation efficiency the solute is transferred a fraction at a time by a series of single extractions. The distribution of solute between the two immiscible solvents is quantitatively expressed by the distribution, or partition, coefficient, K, according to equation (3):

$$K = \frac{\text{concentration of A in solvent 1}}{\text{concentration of A in solvent 2}} \qquad (3)$$

Let us consider that X_O g of compound A is being extracted from V ml of solution by repeated extraction with v ml of an immiscible solvent. The number of grams, X_n, of compound A remaining in solution after n extractions can be shown to be

$$X_n = X_O\left(\frac{KV}{KV + v}\right)^n \qquad (4)$$

where K is the partition coefficient. The important principle which this illustrates is that extraction with several smaller volumes of an extracting solvent is more efficient than using the same total volume of solvent in one extraction.

Technique. A separatory funnel is commonly used in the laboratory for extraction, especially for larger volumes. Screw-capped or glass-stoppered centrifuge tubes are convenient for extractions involving large numbers of samples. An entire rack of tubes can be placed in a shaker to rapidly equilibrate the solute being extracted.

The main problem in using screw-capped or glass-stoppered centrifuge tubes for extraction is leakage during the shaking operation. Caps of screw-capped tubes must be lined with Teflon, and the rim of the glass tube must not be chipped. These rims must be examined before each use, as breakage in washing happens frequently. Similarly, the stoppers for glass-stoppered centrifuge tubes must fit properly and must be held firmly in place during shaking. If both layers must be saved, use a Pasteur pipette to draw off the top layer; otherwise, aspirate.

Extremely efficient column extractions are finding use, especially in toxicology. Various types of column materials are (1) diatomaceous earth, (2) silica gel, (3) C-18 bonded silica gel, and (4) ion-exchange resins. Drugs in solution are adsorbed on the surface of the column packing in an extremely thin film of liquid, approaching a monolayer. An extremely large surface area is exposed to the eluting solvent with single-pass extraction efficiencies from 75 to 95 per cent.

1

Chromatography

Chromatography is discussed in detail in Chapter 2. High performance liquid chromatography (HPLC) is growing in popularity and merits special attention. HPLC offers advantages of high resolution with fast, accurate quantitation for polar, non-polar, and heat-labile compounds. With care, columns may last for several thousand injections. A good liquid pumping system and high-resolution column are critical to successful operation. Filtering and degassing the solvent are recommended to remove particulate contamination and to avoid formation of bubbles in the system which affect elution times. A guard column and saturation column usually precede the analytical column. Both columns are packed by hand with the same material used in the analytical column. The shorter guard column traps particulate matter. The saturation column "saturates" the solvent with the column packing to help prevent solubilization of the analytical column. In fact, if this isn't done, a concave depression can occur on top of the analytical column which destroys separation efficiency of the column. In clinical situations isocratic solvent elution, i.e., elution with a solvent of constant concentration, is preferred over gradient elution.

Mixing

Mixing as an operation is intended to form a homogeneous mass, or to create a uniform heterogeneous system. Mixing is used to bring solids into solution; to bring phases into intimate contact, for instance, in extraction procedures; to wash suspended solids; to homogenize liquid phases; and to perform many other operations too numerous to mention. Mixing and centrifuging accomplish opposite objectives. A serious consequence of inadequate mixing can be failure to completely resuspend protein which settles out under long-term frozen storage of serum controls. The result might be a run invalidated because the control is "off." In some instances, mixing must be carefully controlled to avoid protein denaturation. The importance of mixing serum and plasma specimens before sampling for analysis cannot be overly stressed. A phase separation occurs when these specimens stand for a period of time, as can be noted by careful visual observation. The concentration of even small molecules in such a system will be heterogeneous. The reason is that as protein settles and becomes more concentrated at the bottom of the specimen, the effective water concentration decreases in this layer. This produces a water concentration gradient throughout the system and, consequently, a concentration gradient of all components.

Single-tube Mixers. A vortex mixer is capable of a variable speed oscillation which results in a swirling motion to liquid contents of a test tube or other container. The angle of contact and degree of pressure can be regulated for optimal mixing action. A very effective mixing action is created by a multiple touch sequence, i.e., touching and withdrawing the tube from the neoprene oscillating cup of the mixer. The operator must be careful not to fill the container too full or to mix the liquid contents too fast, since spillage can occur.

Multiple-tube Mixers. A whole line of mixers is available to handle a variable number of tubes, with several different types of motion. A Thermolyne Maxi-Mix (Sybron Corporation, Dubuque, Iowa) can conveniently be used for vortex mixing one tube or several tubes at one time. Mixing action is varied by changing the pressure of the container against the foam rubber top, which is replaceable. Circular motion on a tilted disc provides continuous inversion of contents in tubes which are clipmounted at the circumference of the rotating disc. Rotational speed can be varied to provide gentle or more vigorous mixing. Control sera are conveniently reconstituted on this type of mixer. Tube shakers which tilt back and forth at variable speeds provide thorough mixing of, for example, whole blood samples.

Drying

Desiccants or drying agents have a variety of applications in the laboratory (Bermes, 1976). It is apparent from Table 1–6 that several are alkaline and one is

Table 1–6. CHEMISTRY AND ACTIVITY OF DESICCANTS*

Drying Agent	Activity†	Capacity	Deliquescence	Easy Regeneration	Chemical Reaction
Phosphorus pentoxide	0.02	very low	yes	no	acidic
Barium oxide	0.6–0.8	moderate	no	no	alkaline
Alumina	0.8–1.2	low	no	yes	neutral
Magnesium perchlorate (anhydrous)	1.6–2.4	high	yes	no	neutral
Calcium sulfate (Drierite)	4–6	moderate	no	yes	neutral
Silica gel	2–10	low	no	yes	neutral
Potassium hydroxide (stick)	10–17	moderate	yes	no	alkaline
Calcium chloride (anhydrous)	330–380	high	yes	no	neutral

*From Bermes, E. W., Jr., and Forman, D. T.: Basic laboratory principles and procedures. *In* Tietz, N. W. (ed.): Fundamentals of Clinical Chemistry. 2nd ed. Philadelphia, W. B. Saunders Company, 1976.

†Micrograms residual water per liter of air at 30°C.

strongly acidic. Selection of an appropriate desiccant or drying agent for absorption of moisture depends on the composition of materials or gases to be dried, convenience, efficiency, and cost. Some desiccants can be regenerated easily, e.g., silica gel by heating in a drying oven at 120°C.

DETECTION OF ANALYTICAL RESPONSE

For every analytical procedure there is a concentration-response curve, also referred to as a dose-response curve. The response per unit of concentration is the analytical sensitivity. Every measurement system requires a mechanism to detect a response. To achieve maximum sensitivity with accuracy and precision requires optimal response of the detection system. For example, lamps, mirrors, and slits on a spectrophotometer must be properly aligned and cleaned at regular intervals. The pulse height analyzer of a scintillation counter must be adjusted to the correct "window" settings. Much of what is gained by meticulous detail to all other steps of the analytical process will be lost by improper calibration and maintenance of the detection system.

CALCULATION OF RESULTS

Errors in patient or specimen identification as well as transcription errors may well constitute major problems, but errors in arithmetic warrant equal attention. A brief review of the mathematics most frequently utilized by laboratory personnel should clarify and identify principles so essential for accurate work (Rice, 1960; Segel, 1976).

Significant Figures. In addition, subtraction, multiplication, and division, calculation of data should retain as many significant figures as are contained in the quantity having the least number of significant figures.

Example: Sum of 65.12
2.115
1.2222
68.4572
Answer: 68.46

Exponents. The use of exponential forms permits simple calculation involving large or small numbers.

$$5^2 = 5 \times 5 = 25$$

$$5^{-2} = \frac{1}{5^2}$$

$$5^0 = 1$$

$$5^2 \times 5^3 = 5^5$$

$$5^{1/2} = \sqrt{5^1} = \sqrt{5} = 2.23$$
$$5^{2/3} = \sqrt[3]{5^2} = \sqrt[3]{25} = 2.92$$

Logarithms. The common logarithm of a number is the exponent which must be applied to the base 10 in order to produce the number.

Example: $10^3 = 1000$. The exponent 3 is the common logarithm of 1000, since 3 applied as an exponent to 10 = 1000.

In terms of logarithms, this is written as follows: $\log_{10} 1000 = 3$ (logarithm of 1000 to the base 10 equals 3)

Exponents and Logarithms

$\log_{10} 1 = 0$	$1 = 10^0$
$\log_{10} 10 = 1$	$10 = 10^1$
$\log_{10} 100 = 2$	$100 = 10^2$
$\log_{10} 1000 = 3$	$1000 = 10^3$
$\log_{10} 0.1 = -1$	$0.1 = 10^{-1}$
$\log_{10} 0.01 = -2$	$0.01 = 10^{-2}$
$\log_{10} 0.001 = -3$	$0.001 = 10^{-3}$

A logarithm is composed of two parts: (1) the mantissa (found in logarithm tables), which is placed to the right of the decimal point, and (2) the characteristic, which is placed to the left of the decimal point. The mantissa gives the antilogarithm, or the number of which it is the logarithm. The characteristic identifies the decimal point in the antilogarithm. Logs simplify arithmetical calculations. For example:

1. To multiply two or more numbers, add their logs, then look up the antilog (antilog is the number which corresponds to a log).
2. To divide, subtract logs, then look up the antilog.
3. For roots and fractional exponents, multiply the log by the fractional exponent, then look up the antilog.

Examples:

$$\log(5 \times 2) = \log 5 + \log 2$$
$$\log 47/2 = \log 47 - \log 2$$
$$\log 76^{3/8} = \tfrac{3}{8} \log 76$$

To find the characteristics:

Digits to the left of decimal point:	1	2	3	4	5	6
Characteristic is:	0	1	2	3	4	5

Zeros to right of decimal point and preceding first significant figure:	0	1	2	3	4
Characteristic is:	−1	−2	−3	−4	−5

Aqueous Solution. The concentration of a solution may be expressed in a variety of ways, e.g., molarity, normality, and weight/volume (w/v). These are concentrations based on volume. Solutions based on weight and expressed as molality and weight/weight (w/w) are used less frequently in the laboratory.

Molarity (M) is equal to the number of moles of solute per liter of solution. One gram molecular weight of a substance (GMW) is also called 1 mole of the substance. One mole of water (H_2O) = 18.015 g.

$$\text{Moles} = \frac{\text{g}}{\text{GMW}}$$

A 1-molar (M) solution contains 1 mole of solute per liter of finished solution.

$$\text{Molarity} = \text{moles/liter} = \frac{\text{grams/liter}}{\text{GMW}}$$

A millimole (m mole) is 1/1000 of a mole.

$$\text{Millimoles per liter} = \frac{\text{milligrams/liter}}{\text{GMW}}$$

Avogadro's number = number of molecules per g-mole
= number of atoms per g-atom
= number of ions per g-ion
= 6.023×10^{23}

In practice one Avogadro's number of particles (e.g., 1 g-mole, 1 g-atom, or 1 g-ion) is called a "mole" regardless of whether the substance is ionic, monoatomic, or molecular in nature. Thus, 39.0 g of K^+ ion may be called a "mole," instead of a "gram-ion." To make 1 L of a 1M NaCl solution (mol. wt. = 58.5), 58.5 g of NaCl is dissolved in enough water to make 1 L.

When small concentrations are used, they are frequently expressed in millimoles/liter (1000 millimoles = 1 mole). For example, to prepare 10 ml of a 10 mM (0.01M) NaOH solution, 4 mg NaOH are diluted to 10 ml.

Normality (N) is equal to the number of equivalents of solute per liter of solution. One gram equivalent weight of an element or compound equals the gram molecular weight divided by valence.

$$\text{Gram equivalent weight} = \frac{\text{GMW}}{\text{valence}}$$

One gram equivalent weight of a substance is also called one equivalent of the substance.

$$\text{Number of equivalents} = \frac{\text{grams}}{\text{gram equiv. wt.}}$$

Examples: $Ca(OH)_2$ (GMW = 74)
Equivalent wt. = 74/2 = 37
1 mole = 2 equivalents

H_2SO_4 (GMW = 98)
Equivalent wt. = 98/2 = 49
1 mole = 2 equivalents

Therefore, one equivalent (i.e., the equivalent weight) of an acid or base is the weight that contains 1 g-atom (1 mole) of replaceable hydrogen, or 1 g-ion (1 mole) of replaceable hydroxyl.

To prepare 1 L of 1N H_2SO_4 from pure (96.2 per cent) concentrated sulfuric acid having a specific gravity* of 1.84, dilute 27.7 ml H_2SO_4 to 1 L.

Appendix 2 contains useful information about various acids and bases commonly used in the laboratory.

Weight/volume per cent (% w/v) is equal to the number of grams of a solid dissolved in enough solvent to bring the final volume to 100 ml.

A 10 per cent NaOH solution is prepared by dissolving 10 g NaOH in enough water to make a final volume of 100 ml.

Molality (M) is equal to the number of moles of solute per 1000 g of solvent. A molal solution is used in certain physical chemical calculations, e.g., calculations of boiling-point elevation and freezing-point depression.

Weight/weight per cent (% w/w) is equal to the weight in g of a solute per 100 g of solution. The concentrations of many commercial acids are given in terms of % w/w.

Acids, Alkalis, and pH. An acid molecule yields hydrogen ions (protons) in aqueous solutions; an alkali accepts these. At room temperature in pure water:

$$[H^+] = [OH^-] = 1 \times 10^{-7} \text{ molar}$$

In all aqueous solutions, both acid and alkaline:

$$K_w = [H^+] \times [OH^-] = 10^{-14}$$

In an acid solution $[H^+]$ is greater than 10^{-7} M. In an alkaline solution, $[H^+]$ is less than 10^{-7} M.

pH is the exponent which must be applied to 10 in order to give the value of $1/H^+$. That is,

$$\text{pH} = \log_{10} 1/H^+$$

When pH is	H^+ is	and OH^- is
1,	10^{-1}	10^{-13}
2	10^{-2}	10^{-12}
4	10^{-4}	10^{-10}
6	10^{-6}	10^{-8}
10	10^{-10}	10^{-4}
13	10^{-13}	10^{-1}

A change of one pH unit indicates a tenfold change in H^+ concentration.

Buffer Solutions. The theory of buffers and their preparation can be found in Appendix 2. A more extensive description of various buffer solutions is reviewed by Gomori (1955).

REPORTING OF RESULTS

For clinical usefulness a test result must be reported promptly and accurately (Chap. 57). Delay in report-

---

$$\text{*Specific gravity (sp. gr.)} = \frac{\text{weight in g}}{\text{volume in ml}}$$

ing a result can make the data useless, for example, reporting out an acetaminophen concentration in serum 24 hours after the test was requested. Entering data incorrectly into the computer is not an uncommon occurrence. In addition, clarity of the report form is essential. The form should be well organized with all headings and abbreviations easily understood. Interpretive reporting is being emphasized in the modern practice of laboratory medicine (Halsted, 1981). The pathologist is called upon not only to report results but also to assist in interpreting their meaning. This is essential for an effective consultative service.

LABORATORY SAFETY

The Psychology of Safety. Injuries affect the morale and threaten the emotional health of the party involved. Injuries are expensive in terms of lost wages and medical treatment. An injured person cannot work at peak efficiency. Persons in the professions of health care are vital to the needs of others. Injuries impair this ability to serve (see Chap. 55).

Disaster drills are very useful in giving laboratory and hospital personnel practice with simulated real-life possibilities (Greenberg, 1982).

In an excellent study, Stout (1972) investigated the cause of accidents. These findings have important implications for the medical professional. It was discovered that accidents were not caused by inexperience. Rather, accidents occurred when experienced operators consciously accepted *risks* that inexperienced operators would avoid. Contributory causes to accidents were found to be (1) the conscious acceptance of an obvious and familiar risk; (2) hurrying to meet deadlines, some imaginary; (3) carelessness and fatigue; (4) mental preoccupation—planning, worrying, daydreaming.

Accident prevention can therefore be broken down into two components, namely, knowledge factors and emotional factors. It is important to *know* and *practice* the rules of safety (Carlson, 1975). However, Stout (1972) found in his study that the injured parties knew the rules of safety. Therefore, this is not enough. The knowledge factor must be accompanied by emotional or psychological factors. The worker must maintain a constant, cautious, attentive *alertness. Concentration* on the job is imperative. This attitude of safety which encourages an awareness of hazards can help ensure the continued health and productivity of all personnel.

Alvarez, R., Rasberry, S. D., and Uriano, G. A.: N.B.S. Standard Reference Materials: Update 1982. Anal. Chem., *54*:1226A, 1982.

Anderson, M. A., Aker, S. N., and Hickman, R. V.: The double-lumen Hickman catheter. Am. J. Nurs., *82*:272, 1982.

Bermes, E. W., Jr., and Forman, D. J.: Basic laboratory principles and procedures. *In* Tietz, N. W. (ed.): Fundamentals of Clinical Chemistry. 2nd ed. Philadelphia, W. B. Saunders Company, 1976.

Bjeletich, J., and Hickman, R. O.: The Hickman indwelling catheter. Am. J. Nurs., *80*:62, 1980.

Blumenfeld, T. A., Hertelendy, W. G., and Ford, S. H.: Simultaneously obtained skin-puncture serum, skin-puncture plasma, and venous serum compared, and effects of warming the skin before puncture. Clin. Chem., *23*:1705, 1977.

Booker, H. E., and Darcey, B.: Serum concentrations of free diphenylhydantoin and their relationship to clinical intoxication. Epilepsia, *14*:177, 1973.

Calam, R. R., and Cooper, M. H.: Recommended "order of draw" for collecting blood specimens into additive-containing tubes. Clin. Chem., *28*:1399, 1982.

Carlson, D. J.: Gudelines for Laboratory Safety for Medical Technologists. College of American Pathologists, 7400 North Skokie Blvd., Skokie, Ill., 60077, 1975.

Clark, B. A.: Getting those blood samples right. RN, *44*:36, 1981.

Clark, G. S., Latto, I. P., and Davies, J. M.: Symptoms following radial artery puncture. Anaesthesia, *37*:78, 1982.

Crockett, A. J., McIntyre, E., Ruffin, R., and Alpers, J. H.: Evaluation of lyophilized heparin syringes for the collection of arterial blood for acid base analysis. Anaesth. Intens. Care, *9*:40, 1981.

Fritz, J. S., and Schenk, G. H.: Quantitative Analytical Chemistry. 3rd ed. Boston, Allyn and Bacon, Inc., 1974.

Gomori, G.: Preparations of buffers for use in enzyme studies. Meth. Enzymol., *1*:138, 1955.

Greenberg, J. B., and Brennan, R. E.: Diaster drills with a difference. MLO, 14, No. 11, 39, 1982.

Griner, P. F., and Glaser, R. J.: Misuse of laboratory tests and diagnostic procedures. N. Engl. J. Med., *307*:1336, 1982.

Hackler, M.: How to choose a laboratory balance. Am. Lab., March, 1970.

Halsted, J. A., and Halsted, C. H.: The Laboratory in Clinical Medicine, Interpretation and Application. Philadelphia, W. B. Saunders Company, 1981.

Hamlin, W. B.: Reagent Water Specifications. Commission on Laboratory Inspection and Accreditation. College of American Pathologists, 7400 North Skokie Blvd., Skokie, Ill., 60077, 1978.

Kapke, G. F., Philon, M., and Harkness, L.: Do you have sampling problems due to fibrin formation? ASTRA ADVISOR, 18 (May/June), 5, 1982.

Koenig, A. S., Day, J. C., Sodeman, T. M., and Alpert, N. L.: Laboratory Instrument Verification and Maintenance Manual. College of American Pathologists, 7400 North Skokie Blvd., Skokie, Ill., 60077, 1982.

Krueger, K. E., Carrico, C. J., Detter, J. C., Raisys, V. A., and Underhill, S. L.: The reliability of laboratory data from blood samples collected through pulmonary artery catheters. Arch. Path. Lab. Med., *105*:343, 1981.

Lasof, T. W., and Macurdy, L. B.: Precision laboratory standards of mass and laboratory weights. National Bureau of Standards Circular 547. Washington, D. C., United States Department of Commerce, 1954.

Mabry, C. C., Roeckel, I. E., Gevedon, R. E., and Koepke, J. A.: Recent Advances in Pediatric Clinical Pathology. Lexington, Kentucky, The University of Kentucky Medical Center, 1967.

Madiedo, G., Sciacca, R., Hause, L., and Sasse, E.: Use of syringes containing dry (lyophilized) heparin in sampling blood for pH measurement and blood-gas analysis. Clin. Chem., *28*:1727 (1982).

Meinke, W. W.: Standard reference materials for clinical measurements. Anal. Chem., *43*:28A, 1971.

Meites, S., and Levitt, M. J.: Skin-puncture and blood-collecting techniques for infants. Clin. Chem., *25*:183, 1979.

Musiala, T. A., and Dubin, A.: Effects of chylomicrons and their removal on spectrophotometric analyses. Clin. Chem., *23*:1121, 1977.

Natelson, S.: Weighing the sample. *In* Techniques of Clinical Chemistry. 3rd ed. Springfield, Ill., Charles C Thomas, Publisher, 1971.

National Committee for Clinical Laboratory Standards Publication H 4-A: Standard procedures for the collection of diagnostic blood specimens by skin puncture. NCCLS, Villanova, Pa., 1982.

National Committee for Clinical Laboratory Standards Publication H 14-T: Devices for collection of skin puncture blood specimens. NCCLS, Villanova, Pa., 1980.

National Committee for Clinical Laboratory Standards Publication H 3-A: Standard procedures for the collection of diagnostic blood specimens by venipuncture. NCCLS, Villanova, Pa., 1980.

National Committee for Clinical Laboratory Standards Publication H 11-T: Tentative guidelines for the percutaneous collection of arterial blood for laboratory analysis. NCCLS, Villanova, Pa., 1980.
National Committee for Clinical Laboratory Standards Publication H 18-P: Proposed standard procedures for the handling and processing of blood specimens. NCCLS, Villanova, Pa., 1981.
National Committee for Clinical Laboratory Standards Publication LA1-A: Approved guidelines to access the quality of radioimmune systems. NCCLS, Villanova, Pa., 1982.
National Committee for Clinical Laboratory Standards Publication LA-12P: Proposed guidelines for evaluating a B_{12} (cobalamin) assay. NCCLS, Villanova, Pa., 1980.
Plant, S. B., and McCarron, D. A.: Effects of sample freezing on ion-selective electrode determinations of serum calcium. Clin. Chem., *28*:1362, 1982.
Pryce, J. D., and Durnford, J.: Multiple venous samples: A cautionary tale. Clin. Chem., *26*:1369, 1980.
Radin, N.: What is a standard? Clin. Chem., *13*:55, 1967.
Rice, E. W.: Principles and Methods of Clinical Chemistry for Medical Technologists. Springfield, Ill., Charles C Thomas, Publisher, 1960.
Rossing, R. G., and Foster, D. M.: The stability of clinical chemistry specimens during refrigerated storage for 24 hours. Am. J. Clin. Path., *73*:91, 1980.
Segel, I. H.: Biochemical Calculations. 2nd ed. New York, John Wiley & Sons, Inc., 1976.
Simkins, A., and Crawley, M.: Some chemical and bacterial contributions to analytical variation in urinary oestrogen quantitations during pregnancy. Med. Lab. Sci., *35*:325, 1978.
Slockbower, J. M.: Blood collection problems: Factors in specimen collection that contribute to laboratory error. Am. Assoc. Clin. Chem., TDM, October, 1982.
Spencer, W. W., Nelson, G. H., and Konicki, K. A.: Evaluation of a new system ("Corvac") for separating serum from blood for routine laboratory procedures. Clin. Chem., *22*:1012, 1976.
Stout, T. T., and Darby, B. I.: Disabling farm accidents. Ohio Rep. Res. Devel., *57*:35, 1972.
Sumner, S. M.: Refining your technique for drawing arterial blood gases. Nursing, *10*:65, 1980.
Toffaletti, J., Tompkins, D., and Hoff, G.: The Worthington "ultrafree" device evaluated for determination of ultrafiltrable calcium in serum. Clin. Chem., *27*:466, 1981.
Walker, A. M.: How to take blood from patients who have hepatitis B. Br. Med. J., *282*:1316, 1981.
Ween, S.: Correct application of liquid-in-glass thermometers for accurate temperature measurements in the clinical laboratory. Clin. Chem., *22*:1112, 1976.
Wilson, F., Rankel, S., Linke, E. G., and Henry, J. B.: Free-thyroxine—an abbreviated assay. Am. J. Clin. Path., *62*:383, 1974.
Winstead, M.: Reagent grade water: How, when and why? Austin, Tex., The Steck Company, 1967.
Young, P., and Stevens, J.: Step by step through an arterial stick. RN, *44*:46, 1981.

1

2

PRINCIPLES OF INSTRUMENTATION

MERLE A. EVENSON, PH.D.

The purpose of this chapter is to provide a brief non-mathematical explanation of the physical and chemical principles of analytical methods. Textbooks on instrumentation that offer more complete reviews include those by Malmstadt et al. (1981), Willard et al. (1981), and Robinson (1982).

PHOTOMETRY AND SPECTROPHOTOMETRY

The term *photometric measurement* was originally defined as measurement of light intensity of multiple wavelengths, while *spectrophotometric measurement* formerly meant measurement of light intensity in a much narrower wavelength range. It has recently become common usage to refer to instruments that use filters for isolation of part of the spectrum as photometers or colorimeters, whereas instruments that use gratings and/or prisms are called spectrophotometers. The wavelength range of light measured is no longer a valid distinction between colorimeters and spectrophotometers.

Electromagnetic radiation (EMR) includes radiant energy from short wavelength gamma rays to long wavelength radio waves. Frequently, a white light source for the visible region or a deuterium source for ultraviolet (UV) light will provide the wavelengths used. The wavelength of light is defined as the distance between peaks as the light is envisioned to travel in a wavelike manner. The distance between peaks in the ultraviolet and visible ranges is measured in Angstroms (Å), nanometers (nm), or millimicrons (mμ). There are 10^{10} Å, 10^{9} nm, or 10^{9} mμ in 1 meter. The recommended standard international (SI) unit for expressing the wavelength of light is the nanometer (nm). There are 10 Å per nm and a nm numerically equals a mμ. In addition to possessing wavelength characteristics, light also has properties that indicate its composition to be discrete energy packets called photons. The relationship between the energy of photons and their frequency is given by the equation:

$$E = h\nu$$

E refers to the energy in ergs when the frequency ν is given in hertz (cycles per sec.) and h, Planck's constant, is given as 6.62×10^{-27} erg-second. The frequency of light is related to the wavelength by an equation:

$$\nu = \frac{c}{\lambda}$$

where ν is the frequency in cycles per second, c is the speed of light in a vacuum (3×10^{10} cm/sec.), and λ the wavelength in cm. By looking at the above equations we can readily see that as the frequency of light increases, so does the energy. If we substitute the value of ν from the second equation into the first equation we obtain:

$$E = \frac{hc}{(\lambda)}$$

This equation shows that the energy of light is inversely proportional to the wavelength. For example, UV radiation at 200 nm possesses greater energy than infrared radiation at 750 nm.

Table 2–1 shows the relationship of the wavelength

Table 2–1. ELECTROMAGNETIC RADIATION CHARACTERISTICS

	Wavelength Interval Where the Type of EMR Begins						
	Gamma Rays	X-Rays	Ultraviolet	Visible	Infrared	Micro Waves	Radio Waves
Wavelength							
Angstrom (Å)	1	10	1800	3400	7000		
Nanometer (nm) (millimicron) (mμ)			180	340	700		
Micrometer (micron) (μ)					0.7	400	
Centimeter (cm)						0.04	25

to the name assigned to certain areas in the electromagnetic radiation spectrum and also shows relationships between the various units that are used in the measurement of wavelength. Table 2–2 shows similar relationships except that it is limited to the UV and visible range of the spectrum. The areas are classified as to the name of the region, its wavelength, its color, and its complementary color.

If a solution absorbs light between 400 and 480 nm (blue), it will appear yellow to the eye. Therefore, yellow is the complementary color of blue. Likewise, if the green color is absorbed, the solution will appear purple. The human eye responds to radiation only between 350 and 800 nm, but laboratory instrumentation permits measurements at both shorter wavelength—ultraviolet (UV)—and longer wavelength—infrared (IR)—portions of the spectrum.

Spectrophotometric measurements have gained significantly in popularity in recent years. The principal advantages of spectrophotometric measurements are relatively high sensitivity, ease with which rapid measurements can be made, and a relatively high degree of specificity. Specificity is obtained by reacting the substance of interest with the proper reagents, thus producing different colors, or by analytical separations prior to color forming reactions. Spectral isolation of interferences by the monochromators in spectrophotometers is also used but may alone be inadequate for high accuracy measurements. Spectrophotometric methods are widely applicable for both qualitative and quantitative analyses. Nearly all substances of interest will either absorb energy of a specific wavelength themselves or can be chemically converted to compounds which will then absorb energy of a specific wavelength. The specificity of many spectrophotometric procedures used in measurements is not always adequate, and continuous efforts to improve methods are being made. At the same time, other physical measurements are being developed so that dependence of clinical laboratories on spectrophotometric measurements will probably decrease in the future.

Table 2–2. COLORS AND COMPLEMENTARY COLORS OF THE ULTRAVIOLET (UV) AND VISIBLE SPECTRUM

Wavelength (nm)	Region Name	Color Absorbed	Complementary or Solution Color
180–220	Short UV	Not visible	—
220–340	UV	Not visible	—
340–430	Visible	Violet	Yellow green
430–475	Visible	Blue	Yellow
475–495	Visible	Green blue	Orange
495–505	Visible	Blue green	Red
505–555	Visible	Green	Purple
555–575	Visible	Yellow green	Violet
575–600	Visible	Yellow	Blue
600–620	Visible	Orange	Green blue
620–700	Visible	Red	Blue green

Selection of Wavelength for Measurement. When a measurement is made in a spectrophotometer, the color of light that shows maximum or near maximum absorption should be passed through the solution to obtain maximum sensitivity. A blue solution absorbs red strongly; therefore a wavelength in the red portion of the spectrum would be chosen for measurements of blue solutions. Occasionally an absorption measurement will intentionally be made at a wavelength off the absorption maximum to minimize absorption of interfering substances. Although less than ideal, a reduction in sensitivity is often less critical than the interference. This reduction in sensitivity will frequently linearize or extend the linear portion of a working curve. Many chemical methodologies in clinical chemistry use the above approach to reduce nonlinearity in non-specific color reactions.

Most analyses performed in the clinical chemistry laboratory depend upon making measurements of the amount of light absorbed for each of the particular substances being measured. Most of the measurements are made in the visible range of the spectrum, some in the ultraviolet range, and even fewer in the infrared region. However, new instruments and improved methodology are making more and more applications practical in the field of infrared spectrophotometry. In clinical laboratories, infrared instruments are used to determine the composition of renal stones and gallstones and to analyze for purified toxicologic substances.

Beer's Law. Beer's law states that the concentration of a substance is directly proportional to the amount of light absorbed or inversely proportional to the logarithm of the transmitted light.

The mathematical relationship between absorption

of radiant energy and the concentration of a solution is shown by Beer's law:

$$A = abc = \log \frac{100}{\%T} = 2 - \log \%T$$

where A = absorbance
a = absorptivity
b = light path of the solution in cm
c = concentration of the substance of interest
%T = per cent transmittance

Transmittance (T) is defined as the ratio of transmitted light (I) to incident light (I_o).

The above relationship is the basis for all spectrophotometric absorption measurements and results from contributions from several individuals. Lambert, Bouguer, and others independently contributed to the above formula, commonly called "Beer's law."

Beer's law is an ideal mathematical relationship that contains several limitations in practice. There are three areas where deviations from Beer's law can occur—simultaneous absorption at multiple wavelengths, absorption of light by other species, and transmission of light by other mechanisms. Strictly speaking, the absorptivity (a) is different for each wavelength of light. Unless the absorptivity is constant over the range of wavelengths being used, Beer's law will not be followed.

If two or more chemical species are absorbing the wavelength of light being used, each with a different absorptivity, Beer's law will not be followed.

Finally, if the absorption of a fluorescent solution is being measured, Beer's law may not be followed.

Deviations from Beer's law also occur when a very wide range of concentrations is measured. The range of concentrations that are linear with absorbance varies with each substance.

Figure 2–1 shows a plot of per cent transmittance (%T) vs. concentration, illustrating that %T is inversely and logarithmically related to concentration. Also shown is a plot of absorbance vs. concentration, where the absorbance is directly and linearly related to the concentration of interest. From the figure, notice that the absorbance decreases by 50 per cent when the concentration (or light path) decreases by 50 per cent, while %T shows a non-linear relationship to the same condition. Since %T has a reciprocal log relationship to concentration, a decrease in concentration produces a logarithmic increase in %T. Most laboratory instruments produce an electrical signal that is proportional to %T. If one wants to take advantage of the linear relationship between absorbance and concentration, the %T values have to be converted to absorbance either electronically or with the aid of logarithmic scales or tables. Usually the conversion is electronic, and a digital read-out or printer gives the values in absorbance.

In summary, Beer's law will be followed only if the incident radiation on the substance of interest is monochromatic, if the solvent absorption is insignificant compared to the solute absorbance, if the solute concentration is within "linear limits," and if a chemical reaction does not occur between the molecule of interest and another solute or solvent molecule.

Components of Spectrophotometers (Fig. 2–2)

The Light Source. The function of the light source is to provide radiant energy in the form of visible or nonvisible light that may be passed through the monochromator to be separated into discrete wavelengths. The light of the proper wavelength is then made to be incident on the analytical cell holding the solution whose absorption is to be measured.

The tungsten bulb is acceptable for making measurements in moderately dilute solutions where the difference in color intensity varies significantly with small changes in concentration. A common disadvantage with some early photometers was that a considerable amount of electrical energy was necessary to maintain a constant high energy output. As a result, the generated heat may change the geometry of the optical system as well as the sensitivity of the detectors. A thermal change can shift the optics (lenses) so that a different wavelength of light is incident on the cuvette between the standardization and analysis steps. This wavelength change or a sensitivity change of the detectors may produce significant errors.

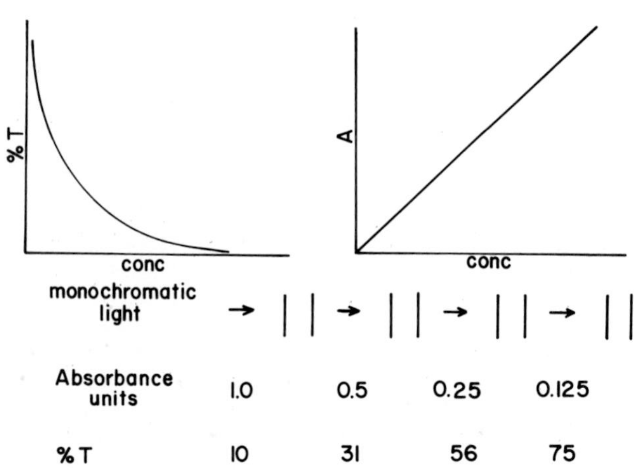

Figure 2–1. The relationship of absorbance (A) and per cent transmittance (%T) to concentration (conc).

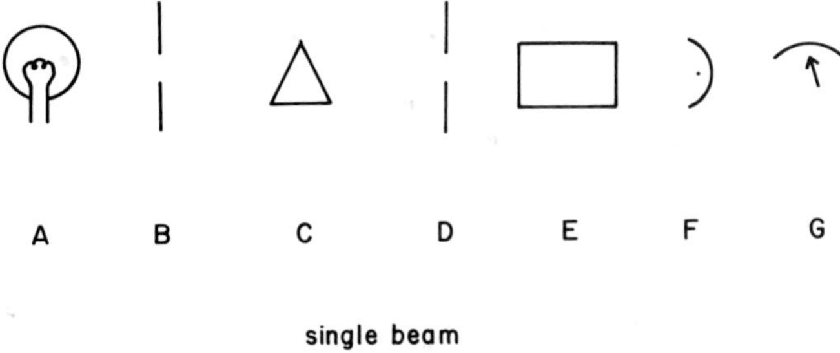

Figure 2–2. Components of a single spectrophotometer. *A,* Light source; *B,* entrance slit; *C,* monochromator; *D,* exit slit; *E,* cuvette; *F,* detector; *G,* meter.

A tungsten light source does not supply sufficient radiant energy for measurements in the ultraviolet region below 320 nm. For this purpose a mercury-arc, hydrogen, or deuterium lamp is suitable. The deuterium light source does not possess as much intensity as the mercury arc, but has approximately three times as much intensity as a hydrogen lamp.

Tungsten iodide sources are frequently used for visible and UV measurements. These sources are high intensity and long lasting. They will frequently operate two to three thousand hours before replacement is necessary.

The Entrance Slit. The function of the entrance slit is to minimize stray light and prevent scattered light from entering the monochromator system. Stray light must be excluded from passing through the cuvette; otherwise Beer's law will not be followed and significant errors may be introduced depending upon how compensations for such design deficiencies are handled.

Monochromators. The monochromator isolates specific wavelengths of light by the use of prisms or gratings or both.

Prisms are wedge-shaped pieces of glass, quartz, sodium chloride, or some other material that allows transmission of light. Because of the variation of the refractive index with wavelength, the light that enters the prism is dispersed to varying degrees, depending upon the wavelength of the light. The red end of the spectrum is refracted least while the blue or violet end is refracted the most.

A grating is a device that has small grooves cut into it at such an angle that each groove behaves like a very small prism. Light is reflected from or transmitted through the grating in such a manner that white light is separated into its various color components. A grating may have 3000 or more small grooves per mm cut into the grating surface. Usually the light is reflected off the grating rather than transmitted through the prism, thereby reducing loss of energy.

The prism or grating may be tilted or rotated in the light beam so as to permit the proper wavelength to be incident upon the cuvette and the detector. Some spectrophotometers obtain the proper wavelength of light by moving the source. In visible spectrophotometry, glass prisms are frequently used, but quartz is required for ultraviolet region measurements. Prisms made of sodium chloride or potassium bromide were frequently used in infrared spectrophotometers before gratings became popular. Some spectrophotometers designed years ago contained only prisms, while certain high-quality, high-performance ultraviolet-visible recording spectrophotometers contained both prisms and gratings. In many of the medium-price-range, medium-quality spectrophotometers, prisms have been replaced with gratings.

Interference Filters. Filter photometers use devices called *interference filters* to obtain spectral purity instead of using prisms or gratings. Interference filters are made by depositing thin semitransparent silver films on each side of a dielectric such as magnesium fluoride. A dielectric is an insulating material that does not allow electric current to flow. When light perpendicular to the silvered surface enters the interference filter, it will pass through the dielectric and be reflected from the second silver surface back through the dielectric to the first silver layer to be reflected again. Finally, the light is transmitted through the semitransparent silver film and into the photometer. Constructive and destructive interference will occur as the light is reflected between the transparent silver films. Constructive interference will occur only when the wavelength of the light is equal to the thickness of the magnesium fluoride layer or a multiple of that thickness. Interference filters will allow transmission of a range of wavelengths between 10 and 20 nm wide and will allow 40 to 60 per cent of incident light to be transmitted. The band of wavelengths allowed to pass is called the "band path." The thickness of the magnesium fluoride can be carefully controlled, and filters of different wavelengths are made by varying this thickness. Multilayer interference filters can be prepared by depositing several layers of dielectrics on each other, each of which is a fraction of a wavelength thick. Multilayer interference filters such as this will have a band path of 5 to 10 nm and will allow 60 to 95 per cent of the incident light to be transmitted. Interference filters are inexpensive individually, but several sets are required to work at different wavelengths. The Technicon AutoAnalyzer colorimeter contains interference filters of this type with individual specifications on the filters. For example, the identification number 530 on a filter means that the peak transmittance occurs at 530 nm. A second number e.g., 18, that appears below the first number refers to the band path transmitted by that filter at one half the height of maximum transmission, i.e., 18 nm.

Analytical Cell or Cuvette. The function of the cuvette is to hold the solution in the instrument where the absorption is to be measured. Cells are made of soft or borosilicate glass, quartz, or plastic. The soft glass cells are used for solutions that are acidic and do not etch glass. Strongly alkaline solutions should be measured in borosilicate cells because of their higher resistance to alkali. As soon as measurements are completed, alkaline solutions must be rinsed from the cells. Glass cells are unsuitable for measurements in the short ultraviolet region of the spectrum. Some glass cells (Corex) can be used to make measurements at 340 nm. Only quartz or plastics that do not absorb ultraviolet radiation can be used for measurements at wavelengths below 320 nm. Recently, some plastic materials have been developed that show little or no absorption of radiant energy from 200 to 700 nm. Generally, these cells are inexpensive and in some cases disposable and will most certainly find increased use in the near future.

Common errors in handling cuvettes are failure to position the cell properly in the photometer and failure to match absorbance readings of the cells. When round cuvettes are used, they should be marked near the top and always positioned in a predetermined manner. If inexpensive unmatched cells are used, blank readings should be taken to measure the tolerance of each cuvette at each wavelength used.

Photomultiplier Tubes as Detectors. A photomultiplier is an electron tube that is capable of significantly amplifying a current. It is constructed by using a light-sensitive material that emits electrons in proportion to the radiant energy which strikes the surface. The electrons produced by this first stage go to a secondary stage (surface) where each electron produces between four and six additional electrons. Each of these electrons from the second stage goes on to another stage, again producing four to six electrons. Each electron produced cascades through the photomultiplier stages; thus, the final current produced by such a tube may be one million or more times as much as the initial current. As many as 10 to 15 stages or dynodes are present in common photomultipliers.

To operate such a tube, voltage is applied between the photocathode and each successive stage. The normal increment of voltage increase of each photomultiplier stage is from 50 to 100 volts larger than that of the previous stage. A common photomultiplier tube will have approximately 1500 volts applied to it.

Photomultiplier tubes have extremely rapid response times, are very sensitive, and do not show as much fatigue as other detectors. Because of their excellent sensitivity and rapid response, all stray light and daylight must be carefully shielded from the photomultiplier. A photomultiplier with the voltage applied should never be exposed to room light because it will burn out. Because of the fast response time of the photomultiplier, this detector is applicable to interrupted light beams such as those produced by choppers and thus provides significant advantages when used as a UV-visible detector in spectrophotometers. The rapid response times are also needed when a spectrophotometer is being used to determine an absorption spectrum of a compound. The photomultiplier also has adequate sensitivity over a wider wavelength range than do photo cell detectors.

When voltage is applied to photomultipliers and all light has been blocked from them, some current will usually be produced. This current is called *dark current*. It is desirable to have the dark current of photomultipliers at their lowest level, as it would also be amplified and would appear as background noise.

Double-Beam Spectrophotometers. Double-beam instruments have been classified as double beam in space (Fig. 2–3) or double beam in time (see Fig. 2–6). Notice in the double beam in space instrument that all components are duplicated except the light source. The two beams pass at the same time through different components separated in space. This arrangement would compensate for changes in intensity of the light source and also compensate for changes in absorbance of the reagent blank as the wavelength is changed in a scanning operation.

A double-beam instrument in time usually uses the same components as a single-beam instrument. The two beams pass through the same components but not at the same time. Duplication of cuvette compartments is sometimes used. A light beam chopper (a rotating wheel with alternate silvered sections and cut-out sections) is inserted after the exit slit. A system of mirrors would pass the reflected portion of the light off the chopper through a reference cuvette

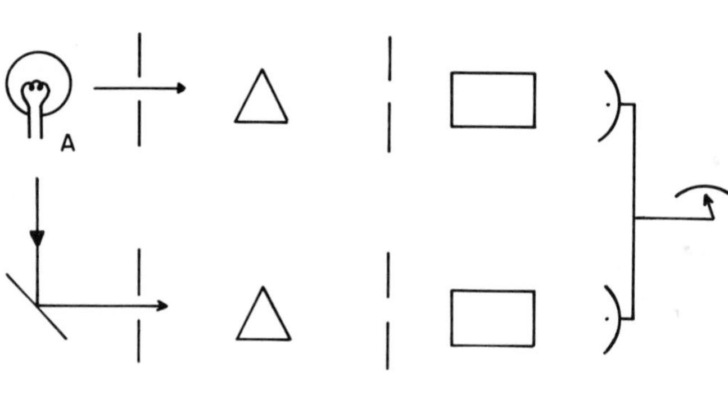

Figure 2–3. Double beam in space spectrophotometer. *A*, Light source; *B*, mirror; *C*, entrance slits; *D*, monochromators; *E*, exit slits; *F*, cuvettes; *G*, photomultipliers; *H*, meter.

and then onto the common detector. Just as a single-beam instrument is adjusted to zero absorbance with the blank before and between sample readings, the double-beam system makes these adjustments automatically. The detector, as in Figure 2–6, is made to look alternately at the sample and then the reference beam of light. The difference or ratio of the timed signals is then amplified and is proportional to the substance of interest in the sample cuvette. The double-beam-in-time approach using one detector compensates for light source variation as well as for sensitivity changes of the detector.

Various other combinations of components and parts of the two approaches presented above have been used in double-beam spectrophotometers. Usually the design is conceived to solve a specific problem.

Although more expensive, double-beam instruments provide increased quality measurements. Some double-beam instruments use a recorder for the output. The recorder traces a plot of the absorbance or per cent transmittance (%T) versus wavelength as the operator desires. The recording double-beam spectrophotometer has its greatest advantage when scanning the spectrum. It automatically compensates when the absorbance of the blank and the intensity of the light source vary with wavelength.

Solid diode array spectrophotometers are now available that use halographic gratings, microprocessor-controlled beam directors, and signal-to-noise averaging techniques that can produce high quality spectra in very short times. Several scans, data acquisition, data manipulation, and output on an electronic screen can be completed in one to ten seconds over the wavelength range of 200 to 800 nm. This type of instrument as a liquid chromatographic detector is expected to give important new information about organic compounds of medical interest.

Selection of an Instrument for Photometry

The most important consideration in the selection of an instrument for spectrophotometric or photometric analysis is the intended use of the instrument. If a high-precision scanning instrument is required, a high quality recording double-beam spectrophotometer is needed. If, on the other hand, it is necessary to measure changes in concentration at a limited number of wavelengths where it is not critical to have spectral purity and wavelength isolation, an inexpensive instrument would work well.

If a UV spectrophotometer is to be used for measuring a barbiturate, it is desirable to have a double-beam recording scanning or a microprocessor-controlled instrument for such a determination. The advantage of a double-beam instrument is that a continuous correction for optical errors or deficiencies can be made automatically as the wavelength changes. In the case of the barbiturate determinations, if a known negative serum sample is inserted in the reference beam and the sample to be analyzed is placed in the sample beam, the instrument automatically makes the correction for unwanted extracted substances and presents to the operator a corrected peak which is directly related to concentration without further calculations. This technique of using a serum sample in the reference beam of double-beam UV-visible recording spectrophotometers also has the advantage of increasing the sensitivity for all measurements. A spectrum scan will usually detect interferences owing to other drugs.

The method of *ultimate precision* may be applied in absorption spectroscopy. This is accomplished by closely bracketing the unknown solution with two solutions of known concentration, then adjusting the darker colored solution to read zero transmittance and the lighter colored solution to read 100 per cent transmittance. The per cent transmittance of the unknown is read and the result obtained by interpolation. The maximum sensitivity and smallest error in measurement are achieved by using this method of *ultimate precision*.

Figure 2–4 is an example of an absorption spectrum showing the plot of absorbance vs. wavelength. If a single well-defined absorption spectrum is obtained, the amount of absorption that occurs at the "peak" wavelength (B) (Fig. 2–4) is to be preferred over an absorption measurement on the "shoulder" (A) of the peak. An increase in sensitivity and specificity results from a measurement at peak absorption. However, if interferences are present, it may be necessary, although less desirable, to make measurements of absorption off the peak wavelength and relate this measurement to concentration. If the absorption peak is sharp or if a shoulder wavelength is selected for absorbance readings, great care must be used in adjusting the proper wavelength each time the instrument is used. Shoulder operation can easily introduce large measurement errors and should be avoided.

Occasionally, by not measuring at the peak absorption, the linear working range of a method can be expanded. This occurs because of the reduction in sensitivity and is frequently used in cholesterol and glucose methods.

A method to correct for background interferences is to measure absorbance at the peak wavelength and at two other wavelengths, usually equidistant from the peak. Values for the latter are averaged to obtain

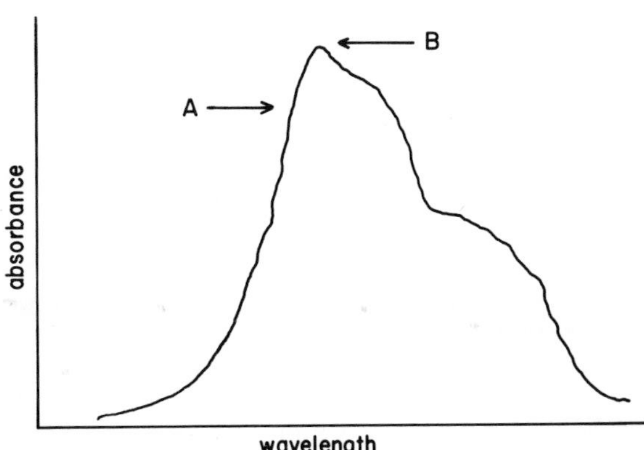

Figure 2–4. Example of an absorption spectrum (see text).

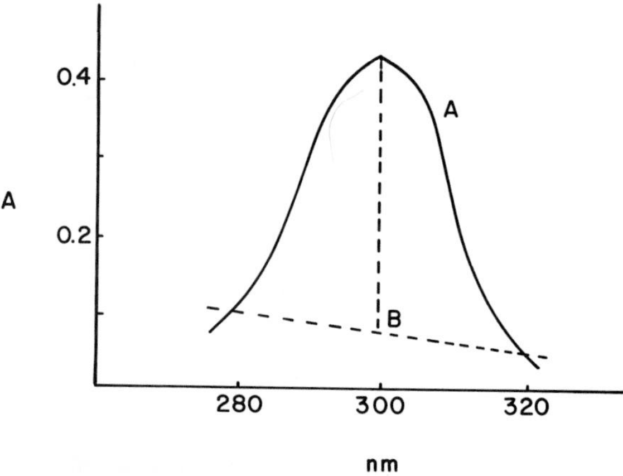

Figure 2–5. Example of an Allen correction for a measurement of salicylate in serum (see text).

a baseline under the peak, which is then subtracted from the peak reading. The value so obtained is known as a "corrected" absorbance and can be related to the concentration, provided that the background absorbance is linear with wavelength over the region in which readings are made. This technique of making corrections for interfering substances is called the *Allen correction* and is illustrated in Figure 2–5.

Salicylate extracted from acidified serum, for example, shows a peak absorbance at 300 nm (see curve A of Fig. 2–5). An extract of salicylate-free serum also exhibits appreciable absorbance at this wavelength, but the absorbance is linear between 280 and 320 nm (line B of Fig. 2–5). The corrected absorbance at 300 nm is obtained from the Allen equation:

$$A_{Corr} = A_{300} - \frac{(A_{280} + A_{320})}{2}$$

Similar corrections are applied in procedures for spectrophotometric determinations of porphyrins, steroids, and other compounds.

Before using the Allen correction, knowledge of the shape of the absorption curve for the substance of interest and of the interferences must be obtained. The linearity of the baseline shift should be verified by measuring the absorption spectrum of commonly encountered interferences. Care should be exercised in use of the Allen correction. If not properly used, it may introduce larger errors than would be observed without correction. For example, such a situation may occur if the background reading is not linear over the region measured.

FLAME PHOTOMETRY

The principle behind flame photometry involves the excitation of electrons in an atom by the heat energy of a flame. The electrons, being unstable in this excited stage, then give up their excess energy to the environment as they change from the higher energy state (excited) to a lower energy state. If the energy is dissipated as light, the light may consist of one or more than one energy level and therefore may possess different wavelengths. These different wavelengths or lines of the spectrum are individually characteristic for each element. The wavelength to be used for the measurement of an element—as in spectrophotometry—depends upon the selection of a spectral line of strong enough intensity to provide adequate sensitivity. It also depends upon freedom from other interfering lines at or near the selected wavelength.

Alkali metals are comparatively easy to excite in the flame of an ordinary laboratory burner. Lithium produces a red, sodium a yellow, potassium a violet, rubidium a red, and magnesium a blue color in a flame. These colors are characteristic of the metal atoms that are present as cations in solution.

Under constant and controlled conditions, the light intensity of the characteristic wavelength produced by each of the atoms is directly proportional to the number of atoms emitting energy, which in turn is directly proportional to the concentration of the substance of interest in the sample. Thus, flame photometry lends itself well to direct concentration measurements of some metals.

Other cations, like calcium, are less easily excited in the ordinary flame. In these cases, the amount of light given off may not always provide adequate sensitivity for analysis by flame emission methods. The sensitivity can be improved slightly by using higher temperature flames. Of the more easily excited alkali metals like sodium, only 1 to 5 per cent of the atoms present in solution become excited in a flame. Even with this small percentage of excited atoms, the method has adequate sensitivity for measurement of alkali metals for most bioanalytical measurements. Most metal ions are not as easily excited in a flame, and flame emission methods are not as applicable for their measurement.

Essential Parts of the Flame Photometer

Gases for Flame Photometry. A mixture of hydrogen and oxygen gas produces a hot temperature commonly used on conventional flame photometers. In addition, natural gas, acetylene, and propane using either air or oxygen are other combinations of gases frequently used. All of these fuel gases and their various oxidants work well, the difference being in the flame temperature and therefore the sensitivity that each combination provides. It is essential that the flame temperature be held constant; otherwise sensitivity changes will result. High quality gas regulation to maintain constant flame temperature is also essential for proper operation. Frequent standardization of flame photometers is essential because thermal changes do occur and affect the response of the flame photometer.

The Atomizer. The function of the atomizer or burner is to break up the solution into fine droplets so that the atoms will absorb heat energy from the flame and become excited. In one type of burner, the gases are passed at high velocity over the end of a capillary suspended in the solution, causing liquid to be drawn up through the capillary into the flame. This type of burner is called the total consumption burner. A second kind of burner involves the gravitational feeding of solution through a restricting capillary into an area of high-velocity gas flow where small droplets are produced and passed into the flame. The large droplets in this type of burner are usually taken to waste and not all the sample is forced to go into the flame as in the capillary type burner.

Monochromator. The monochromator, including the entrance and exit slits, is similar to those previously described for spectrophotometers. Its function is to isolate the wavelength of interest from interfering light before it passes on to the detector. Ideally, monochromators in flame photometers should be of higher quality than those found in absorption spectrophotometers. When non-ionic materials are burned, light of various wavelengths is given off. This is known as *continuous emission* and will be added to the *line emission* of the element being measured. For this reason, the narrowest band path that is achievable should be used to eliminate as much of the extraneous, continuous emission as possible but still permit a maximum amount of the line emission to pass through to the detector.

Detectors. Detectors used in flame photometers operate by the same principle and in the same way as those previously described in the spectrophotometry section. In designing a flame photometer, compensation or design features must be incorporated so that thermal equilibrium is achieved rapidly. Flame photometers that use photomultipliers for detectors have improved sensitivity and, because of improved design, seldom require long times to come to thermal equilibrium. However, even this type of flame photometer usually requires aspirating water and standards to establish flame thermal equilibrium before measurements are taken.

Operation of Flame Photometers

The major problem associated with flame photometers involves inadequate control over the flame and the aspirator. Slight variations in gas pressure will change both the rate of aspiration of the sample and the temperature of the flame. A significant amount of design effort has been exerted to assure constant flame and aspirator conditions. A flame photometer is available that uses an internal standard of lithium. A single flame and multiple detectors are used to monitor the same flame. The ratio of the sample and reference (lithium) detectors is proportional to the sample concentration. Therefore, any change in flame characteristics and aspirator conditions would simultaneously affect the signal to both the lithium reference detector and the sample detector. By using the ratio of the two signals, errors due to flame fluctuations or changes in the aspiration rate are minimized.

The ratio between the lithium and sodium and the lithium and potassium channels is taken, amplified, and fed to a direct digital read-out displayed on the front of the instrument. In addition, the lithium acts as a *radiation buffer*. If potassium is measured, for example, the potassium signal is critically dependent upon the amount of sodium present unless a high concentration of another easily excited cation such as lithium is present. In the absence of a high concentration of lithium, energy will be transferred from an excited sodium atom to a potassium atom. This would produce different percentages of potassium atoms excited, depending upon sodium concentration. The amount of potassium excited would vary and analytical errors would result. A means of compensating for this error is to dilute the samples with an excessively high concentration of lithium, so that the same percentage of potassium becomes excited regardless of the sodium concentration in the sample. The use of an internal standard and radiation buffer, the direct read-out for sodium and potassium concentrations, and the simple dilution of serum make the modern flame photometer highly suitable for use in the clinical laboratory.

1

ATOMIC ABSORPTION SPECTROPHOTOMETRY

Atomic absorption spectrophotometry is basically the inverse of emission methods. In all emission methods—arc, spark, laser, flame, x-ray fluorescence, or neutron activation analysis—the sample is excited in order to measure the radiation energy of interest given off as the sample returns to its lower energy level. Extraneous radiation must be isolated from the energy of interest if interference by these signals is to be avoided.

In atomic absorption spectrophotometry, the element is not excited, but merely dissociated from its chemical bonds and placed in an unexcited, un-ionized, neutral atom ground state. In such a low energy state it is capable of absorbing radiation at the very narrow band path width between 0.001 and 0.01 nm. The source emitting such radiation is the hollow cathode lamp. The energy of the absorbed radiation is equal to that which would be emitted if the element in question were excited. In contrast to emission methods, in which only a small percentage of atoms are excited, nearly all can be converted to the dissociated form in which they are capable of absorbing light emitted by the hollow cathode lamp.

Components of Atomic Absorption Spectrophotometers

Figure 2–6 shows the basic components of an atomic absorption spectrophotometer. The hollow cathode lamp is the light source; the nebulizer (atomizer) sprays the sample into the flame; and the monochromator, the slits, and the detectors have their usual function, as described previously in the spectrophotometer sections.

The Hollow Cathode Lamp. The hollow cathode lamp produces a wavelength of light specific for the kind of metal in the cathode. In some cases, an alloy is used to make a multielement cathode.

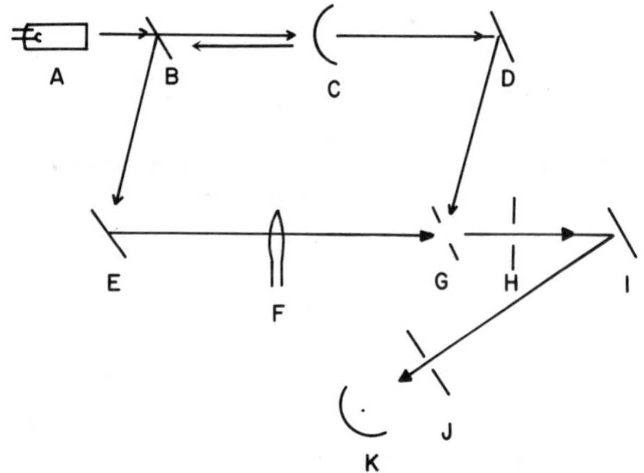

Figure 2–6. Schematic diagram of a double beam in time atomic absorption spectrophotometer. *A*, Hollow cathode lamp; *B*, half silvered mirror that reflects and transmits light; *C*, chopper; *D* and *E*, mirrors; *F*, flame; *G*, half silvered mirror; *H*, slit; *I*, grafting; *J*, slit; *K*, detector.

Neon or argon gas at a few millimeters of mercury pressure is usually used as a filler gas. A neon-filled lamp produces a reddish orange glow during operation, while the argon produces a blue to purple glow inside the hollow cathode lamp. Quartz or special glass that allows transmission of the proper wavelength is used as a window.

A current is applied between the two electrodes inside the hollow cathode lamp, and metal is sputtered from the cathode into the bases inside the glass envelope. When the metal atoms collide with the gases, neon or argon, they lose energy and emit their characteristic radiation. Calcium has a sharp, intense, analytical emission line at 422.7 nm. This line is the most frequently used for calcium analysis. In an interference-free system, only calcium atoms will absorb the calcium light from the hollow cathode as it passes through the flame.

The Burner. Until now, only two types of burners have been used in most clinical applications. With the *total consumption burner,* the gases—hydrogen and air—and the sample are not mixed before entering the flame. One disadvantage of this type of burner is that relatively large droplets are produced in the flame, which cause signal noise by light scattering. Another disadvantage is that the amount of acoustical noise produced is very high and may become uncomfortable after a few hours of operation. An advantage of this type of burner is that the flame is more concentrated and can be made hotter, causing molecular dissociations which may be desirable to minimize some chemical interferences.

A modification of this type of burner is to split the liquid stream aspirated into 10 to 20 smaller streams prior to injection into the flame. This usually results in a flame that may be about 2.0 cm in diameter at the base. This modification produces much less noise than the single-jet total-consumption burner.

In a *pre-mix burner* the sample is aspirated, volatilized, and then burned. An advantage of this system is that the large droplets go to waste and not into the flame, thus producing a less noisy signal. Moreover the path length of the burner is longer than that of the total consumption burner. This produces greater absorption and increases the sensitivity of the measurement. On the other hand, its flame is usually not as hot as that of the total-consumption burner and cannot sufficiently dissociate certain metal complexes in the flame (e.g., calcium phosphate complexes). Another disadvantage is that as much as 90 per cent of the sample may be discarded; hence, the sensitivity may be less than desirable. Nitrous oxide pre-mix burners produce higher temperatures and will dissociate some calcium complexes. This makes unnecessary the addition of competing cations, e.g., lanthanum or strontium, to the solutions. However, an error can be introduced into the calcium determination because calcium becomes excited to a significant extent and thus emits ions in the flame.

The Monochromator and Detector. All atomic absorption systems use monochromators and photomultipliers for isolating a spectrally pure light signal and measuring the intensity of that signal, respectively. The monochromator filters out extraneous light from the flame, while the photomultiplier converts that part of the light from the hollow cathode which was not absorbed in the flame to an electrical current and amplifies this current to drive a read-out device or recorder. The monochromators and the photomultipliers have been discussed previously in the spectrophotometric section of this chapter.

Interferences in Atomic Absorption Spectrophotometry

There are three general types of interferences in atomic absorption spectrophotometry—chemical, ionization, and matrix effects.

When the flame cannot dissociate the sample into neutral atoms, absorption cannot occur. An example is the phosphate interference in the serum determination of calcium caused by the formation of calcium phosphate complexes. These do not dissociate in the flame unless a special high-temperature burner is used or a cation is added which will displace the calcium from phosphate. Usually in atomic absorption determinations of calcium in serum, lanthanum or strontium is added to the serum, releasing the calcium from the phosphate in solution and replacing it. The free neutral calcium atoms are then capable of absorbing the calcium light from the hollow cathode. The freeing of calcium occurs because lanthanum and strontium form more stable complexes with phosphate than does calcium.

Ionization interference results when atoms in the flame become excited instead of only dissociated and then emit energy of the same wavelength as that being measured. Compensation for this condition can be achieved by adding an excess of a more easily ionized substance that will absorb most of the flame energy so that the substance of interest will not become excited. Another way to correct for ionization interference is to operate the flame at a lower temperature.

A third type of interference is the matrix interference. One example of a matrix effect is the enhancement of light absorption by organic solvents. An atom may absorb between two and five times more energy when dissolved in an organic solvent instead of an aqueous solvent. A second kind of matrix effect is the light absorption caused by formation of solids from sample droplets as the solvent is evaporated in the flame. This will usually occur only in concentrated solutions of greater than 0.1 mol/L. Refractory oxides of metals formed in the flame can also be classified as matrix interferences.

Commercial Atomic Absorption Spectrophotometers

Figure 2–6 is a schematic diagram of a type of atomic absorption spectrophotometer manufactured by a number of instrument companies. If one traces the light path in Figure 2–6 from the hollow cathode lamp, we see that the chopper either reflects the light beam or allows the light beam to pass through the flame as the reference beam in the rear (top of Fig. 2–6). The beams then pass alternately through the same monochromator to the one detector. When the beams arrive at the detector, they are out of phase with each other. In other words, the photomultiplier looks first at the reference beam and then uses this value to compare the reference and the sample beams. When more atoms are present in the flame, more light will be absorbed, and the greater the difference will be in light intensity between the sample and reference beams. This difference is then amplified and fed into a read-out device. Note that in the double-beam system, differences between the sample and reference beams are continuously being measured. This double-beam arrangement compensates for changes in the output of the hollow cathode lamp and for changes in the detector system. However, it does not correct for variations in the sample beam that may occur between the sample beam and the reference beam.

Atomic absorption spectrophotometry provides the analyst with a technique that is accurate and precise. To achieve comparable selectivity, sensitivity, and versatility with other instrumentation, the cost would be several times that of atomic absorption spectrophotometers.

Atomic absorption spectrophotometry is sensitive, accurate, precise, and high in specificity. One of the reasons for these advantages is that the method does not require excitation of the sought-for substance, and thus it is less affected by temperature variations in the flame and the transfer of energy from one atom to another. The high specificity results from the fact that the light used has an extremely narrow band path (0.001 to 0.01 nm) which is selectively absorbed by atoms being measured.

The disadvantages of atomic absorption spectrophotometry are few. The most significant difficulty is the elimination of interferences. Although some suggestions have been presented to compensate partially for some of these factors, more work is needed to study and to explain some of the interference problems that remain in atomic absorption spectrophotometry.

OTHER APPROACHES

Fluorometry

Fluorescence is a physical energy process that occurs when certain compounds absorb electromagnetic radiation, become excited, and then return to an energy level slightly higher than or equal to their original energy level. Since the energy given off is less than or equal to that absorbed, the wavelength of the light being given off will be longer or equal to that absorbed for excitation. A delay time of between 10^{-8} and 10^{-4} second occurs between the absorption of the energy and the releasing of part of the energy in the form of light.

If the length of time is longer than 10^{-4} second from the time the chemical species absorbs the energy until the light is emitted, this process is called phosphorescence. The remainder of this discussion will be centered on fluorescence, since it is the more common process used in the laboratory.

Fluorometric Instrumentation. Figure 2–7 shows a schematic diagram of the components of a fluorometer. The energy source of a fluorometer is generally a mercury arc lamp or xenon lamp that will produce enough energy that when absorption occurs, electron

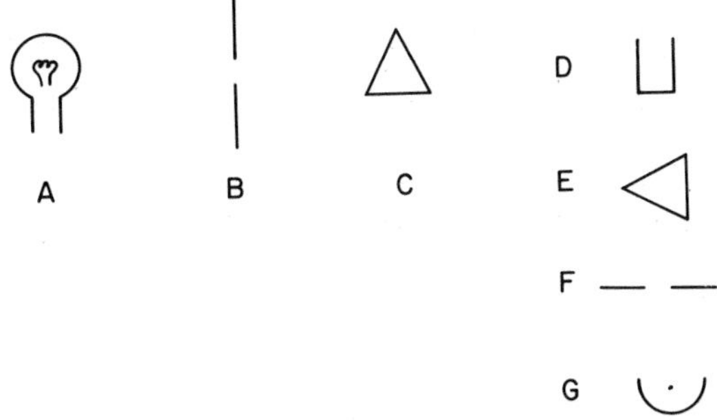

Figure 2–7. Essentials of a fluorometer. *A*, Light source; *B*, slit; *C*, primary monochromator or filter; *D*, cuvette; *E*, secondary monochromator or filter; *F*, slit; *G*, detector.

transitions to higher energy within the molecule will occur. In a fluorometer, the entrance and exit slits are similar to those described in spectrophotometers, except that the exit slit is usually perpendicular to the entrance slit. Fluorometers that use a continuous source like a xenon lamp have a monochromator so that isolation of wavelengths can occur before excitation of the substance in the cell occurs. All fluorometers have another monochromator system that will selectively remove unwanted wavelengths before they fall upon the detector. Fluorometers are designed so that the secondary monochromator and the detector are at right angles to the incident light beam into the cuvette. This arrangement prevents the light from the high-energy source of the mercury or xenon lamp from reaching the detector.

The single most important advantage of fluorometry is its extreme sensitivity. Sometimes the sensitivity may be one thousand times that of colorimetric methods. Some molecules fluoresce directly, but a larger percentage must be complexed or chemically reacted to transform them into fluorescent compounds. The fluorescence of the new compound is then measured. By selection of different complexers, fluorescence of different wavelengths may be produced, making it possible to work at a wavelength significantly removed from interferences.

Fluorescent spectra are not as valuable for qualitative identification as are absorption spectra. Other disadvantages of fluorometry are quenching interferences, extreme sensitivity to pH change, temperature change, and interferences owing to the presence of other foreign undefined fluorescent materials in reagents. Frequently, energy is transferred from one molecule to another in solution and is dissipated in this manner rather than being given off directly as fluorescence energy. Quenching sometimes occurs when foreign materials form unwanted non-fluorescent complexes with the substance of interest.

The use of fluorescent instruments for immunochemistry measurements will probably increase in the near future. A goal of this approach is to use fluorescent labels instead of radioactive tags because it is widely accepted that due to disposal problems the use of radioactive materials in the clinical laboratory should be kept to a minimum (Chap. 38).

Commercial instruments are beginning to become available that bind fluorescent labeled antibodies to glass filters, that use polarized fluorescent light for the output signal, and that use fluorescent labeled substrates for read-out for analysis of drugs, peptides, hormones, and other compounds present at very low concentrations.

Turbidimetry

Turbidimetry measures the amount of light blocked by particulate matter as light passes through the cuvette. Several problems are inherent in making turbidimetric measurements, problems associated mostly with sample and reagent preparation rather than with the operation of the instrument. Turbidimetric measurements can be made with either a colorimeter or a spectrophotometer.

The amount of light that is blocked by a suspension of particles in a cuvette depends not only upon the number of particles present but also upon the cross-sectional area of each particle. If the particle size of the standards is not the same as the particle size in the samples being measured, errors result. Another problem with the turbidimetric measurement is the need to keep the length of time between sample preparation and measurements as constant as possible. Particles may settle out of solution while the measurements are being made, thus producing an error. Control of the rate of settling is usually accomplished by using gum arabic or gelatin. These materials provide a viscous medium which retards particle settling while measurements are being made.

Turbidimetric measurements are acceptable provided that the number of particles and their size are in a reasonably narrow range. A high-intensity light or a very low-intensity light should not fall on the photo detector because errors in instrumentation would then augment other errors in the measurement.

Nephelometry

Nephelometric measurements are similar to turbidimetric measurements. In nephelometry, the light that is scattered by the small particles is measured at right angles to the beam incident to the cuvette. The amount of scatter that occurs is related to the number and to the size of particles in the light beam. The particle size and shape and the wavelength of the incident light are important variables to control. The shorter the wavelength of the incident light, the greater the degree of dispersion. Nephelometry has an advantage over turbidimetric measurements in that nephelometric measurements are usually capable of somewhat greater precision. Specific antigen-antibody complexes and a laser source have been combined to provide high specificity with high precision. As a result turbidimetric and especially nephelometric measurements will be used more in clinical laboratories in future years.

Electrochemistry

Analytical electrochemistry for the clinical laboratory includes potentiometry, amperometry, and coulometry. Generally amperometry and potentiometry are the most commonly used techniques, and these center on blood gas measurements. Potentiometry is the measurement of the potential of a solution, while amperometry refers to the measurement of the amount of current that flows when a constant voltage is applied to the measuring electrode. Ion-selective electrodes for sodium, potassium, calcium, and many other substances of medical importance have increased the amount of interest in electrochemistry for the clinical laboratory (Pelleg, 1975).

Potentiometry. The measurement of the potential

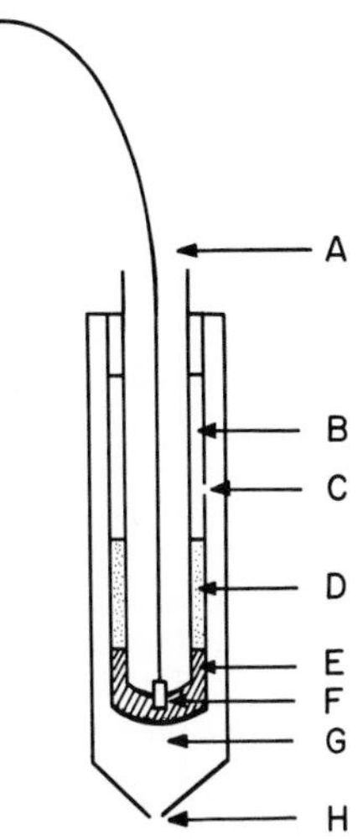

Figure 2–8. Saturated calomel electrode. *A*, Wire; *B*, inner jacket; *C*, port for saturated KCl; *D*, Hg, Hg_2Cl_2, KCl paste; *E*, Hg; *F*, platinum tip; *G*, saturated KCl; *H*, a porous plug.

(voltage) between two electrodes in solution forms the basis for a variety of measurements that can be used to quantitate concentrations of the substance of interest.

Both an indicator and a reference electrode are necessary to measure the potential (E) of a solution. The potential of the indicator electrode can be made to respond proportionally to the concentration of the substance of interest, while the reference electrode must maintain a constant voltage under controlled conditions for a significant length of time. The most frequently used reference electrode in electro-analytical measurements is the saturated calomel electrode (SCE). Figure 2–8 shows the schematic diagram of the components of an SCE reference electrode. A porous plug shown at the bottom of the figure stoppers the outside glass jacket yet allows solution contact with the inner part of the calomel electrode. A small platinum tip is sealed on the end of the inner glass jacket, which is submerged in a saturated solution of potassium chloride. A paste is made of mercury and saturated mercurous chloride. Potassium chloride is next inserted into the inner jacket. Finally, electrical contact is made to the mercury–mercurous chloride interface and the platinum tip electrode by a wire to the measuring device. The standard reduction potential (E_o) of the calomel electrode versus a normal hydrogen electrode is −0.242 volt.

A silver–silver chloride electrode is another common reference electrode and may be easily constructed using a low-voltage (less than 6 volts) battery, a platinum wire, and a silver wire. The silver wire is usually coiled, connected to the positive pole of the battery, and submerged in a dilute chloride solution. The platinum wire is connected to the negative pole of the battery, then submerged in the same solution containing the coil of silver wire. Hydrogen will be liberated at the platinum cathode and silver chloride will be deposited on the silver anode when connected to the battery.

The silver wire will develop a rose to purple color in a few minutes. The silver–silver chloride wire is then placed in a standard chloride solution that has been saturated with silver ions to decrease the solubility of silver chloride and maintain a stable reference potential. A silver–silver chloride electrode has the advantage over the calomel electrode of being less sensitive to temperature changes.

The normal hydrogen electrode (NHE) consists of a platinized platinum electrode in a 1.228 N HCl solution with hydrogen at atmospheric pressure bubbled over the platinum surface. This reference electrode has an assigned E_o of 0.000 volt. Owing to difficult maintenance problems, the NHE is not frequently used in routine measurements.

There are several types of indicator electrodes that can be used with reference electrodes like those described above. Indicator electrodes can be a platinum wire, a planar surface of almost any other metal, a carbon rod, or a thin stream of mercury flowing into the solution where a measurement will be made.

In potentiometry the potential is measured and the relationship between the measured voltage and the sought-for concentration is shown by the Nernst equation:

$$E = E_o + \frac{0.059}{n} \log \frac{[C_{ox}]}{[C_{red}]} \tag{1}$$

where E = the potential measured at 25° C.
E_o = the standard reduction potential
n = the number of electrons involved in the reaction
C_{ox} = the molar concentration of the oxidized reaction form
C_{red} = the molar concentration of the reduced reaction form

Measurement of pH. The pH of a solution is defined by the equation:

$$pH = -\log [H_3O^+] \tag{2}$$

where $[H_3O^+]$ = hydrogen ion concentration in moles/liter.

In buffer solutions, the pH is related to the concentrations of the undissociated acid and its corresponding anion according to the following equation:

$$pH = pK_a + \log \frac{[A^-]}{[HA]} \tag{3}$$

where $[A^-]$ = the molar concentration of anion
$[HA]$ = the molar concentration of acid
K_a = the acid dissociation constant
pK_a = $-\log K_a$

Notice the similarities and relationships between (1) the Nernst equation, (2) the definition of pH, and (3) the buffer equation. A single potential measurement under proper conditions can be directly related to the H_3O^+ concentration in solution.

A pH measurement is usually made with the aid of a glass indicator electrode. One type consists of a bulb of special glass filled with 0.1 mole/liter HCl in contact with a suitable metallic electrode. When immersed in solution, a potential difference develops between the solution inside the glass electrode and the solution being measured for H_3O^+. The magnitude depends upon the hydrogen-ion concentration of the solution. This potential difference is measured by combining the glass electrode with some standard reference electrode, such as the saturated calomel electrode, and measuring the voltage of the system.

Calibration is achieved by using a known buffer solution that has a pH value assigned by the National Bureau of Standards. The pH of an unknown solution is compared to the known buffer solution by potential measurements using a pH meter. A pH meter simply measures the potential produced in a solution using electrodes described above.

The electrode arrangement for a pH measurement may be considered as a special type of concentration cell. A modification of equation (1) that can be used for a concentration cell is:

$$\Delta E = \frac{RT}{nF} \ln \frac{C_1}{C_2} \tag{4}$$

where ΔE = measured change in potential
R = gas constant
T = temperature in degrees Kelvin
n = number of electrons in electrochemical reaction
F = value of the Faraday constant
C_1 = concentration of unknown (outside of glass electrode)
C_2 = concentration of known (inside glass electrode)

At 25°C. for a one-electron reaction and with C_2 equal to one mole/liter, equation (4) becomes $\Delta E = 0.059$ pH. In other words, a 59 millivolt (mv) change will occur when the pH changes 1 unit.

A schematic diagram for a pH meter is shown in Figure 2–9. While making the pH measurement, it is important that the amount of current drawn from the measuring electrodes be very small. Generally 10^{-10} to 10^{-12} ampere or less is drawn. The principle behind the pH measurement involves the adjustment of the high-impedance potentiometer potential to be equal to and in the opposite direction from the potential of the measuring electrodes.

Coulometric Measurements. Coulometry involves the measurement of the quantity of electricity (in coulombs) at a fixed potential where:

$$Q = I \times T \tag{5}$$

Q = coulombs of electricity
I = the current in amperes
T = the time in seconds that the current is flowing

Two approaches can be used in coulometric measurements. When the current is kept constant, the elapsed time is proportional to the total coulombs consumed. Alternatively, the current may be changed in a known manner for a fixed time and the area beneath the current curve integrated with respect to time to obtain the number of coulombs. A coulomb is equal to a current flow of one ampere per second. A Faraday is defined as 96,500 coulombs and corresponds to the electrical charge carried by one gram equivalent of substance. One equivalent is equal to one mole if only one electron is involved in the electrochemical reaction. Thus, the number of coulombs consumed can be related directly to the concentration of the unknown.

In the chloride determination using the Cotlove titrator (Buchler Instruments, Inc., Fort Lee, N.J.), a constant current is applied across silver electrodes, which liberates silver ions into the solution at a constant rate. When all of the chloride ions in solution have been complexed by the liberated silver ions, a pair of indicator electrodes senses the excess silver ions and activates a relay which shuts the timer off and stops the titration. The length of time that the titrator generates silver ions is directly proportional to the chloride ion concentration, since the current has been kept constant.

Ion Selective Electrodes. In the last few years there has been a major shift in methodologies for measuring serum and urine electrolytes from flame photometry to ion-selective electrodes (ISE). There are three different basic ISE classes. *Ion-selective glass* formulated with particular metal additives preferentially allows ions such as H^+, Na^+, or NH_4^+ to cross a hydrated outer layer of glass. This ion diffusion results in an electrical potential change which is related to ion concentration in the sample by the Nernst equation. *Solid state electrodes* such as silver–silver chloride membranes for chloride determination have crystals impregnated in an inactive membrane. The other halides can be measured with electrodes using their specific silver halide crystals in the membrane. This form of membrane has also been adapted for measuring chloride in sweat directly on the surface of the skin.

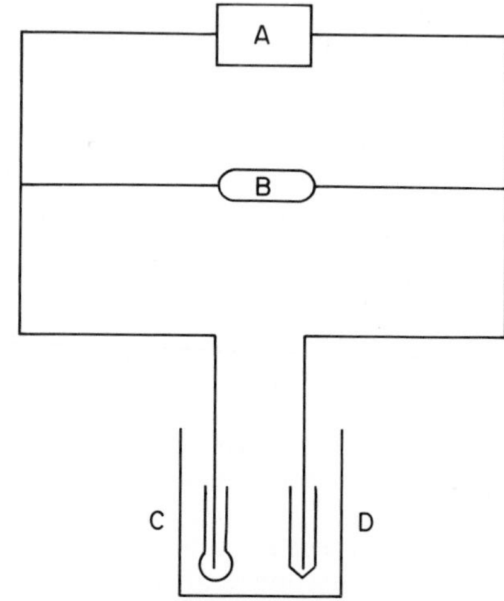

Figure 2–9. Schematic diagram of a pH meter. In making pH measurements one adjusts the potentiometer *(A)* until the voltage across the glass electrode *(C)* and the reference electrode *(D)* is zero, which is indicated by the null meter *(B)*.

Liquid ion-exchange membranes contain a water insoluble and inert solvent which dissolves and isolates an ion-selective carrier. Ions outside the membrane and the same ions bound to the ion-exchange material inside the electrode produce a potential again related to concentration in the sample by the Nernst equation. In the case of an ionized calcium electrode, the solvent is dioctylphenyl-phosphonate and the carrier is dioctyl phosphate. In potassium selective electrodes, the carrier is the cyclic antibiotic valinomycin which has a central cavity in its molecule that approximates the size of an unhydrated potassium ion. Still another variation is the carbon dioxide electrode. It measures the pH in a bicarbonate solution that receives CO_2 gas which passes through a gas-permeable membrane after the CO_2 has been liberated from a sample by acid treatment.

The specificities of electrodes for their stated ions have improved recent automated instruments—on the order of 300 to 1 preference for sodium over potassium in a sodium electrode, and nearly 1000 to 1 for potassium over sodium in a potassium electrode.

Aside from general simplicity of operation, the ISEs which measure monovalent cation activities in whole blood, plasma, or serum have a distinct advantage over flame photometry for specimens that have a lower than normal plasma water content due to marked lipoproteinemia or paraproteinemia (Ladenson, 1981). Instruments which dilute samples several-fold prior to analysis by ISE produce results comparable to flame photometry in that they reflect ion content rather than ion activity in the sample. However, they have the capacity to handle microsamples routinely since the specimen aliquot is normally diluted to a greater volume prior to analysis. Whole blood analyzers are very useful for rapid quantitation of potassium in critical care situations such as cardiac surgery and cardiopulmonary bypass which are followed by intense diuresis and potassium flux. Calcium selective electrodes presently measure only the ionized fraction of calcium and are insensitive to protein-bound and other complexed or chelated calcium. Electrodes for cholesterol, enzymes, amino acids, sulfur compounds, creatinine, urea, uric acid, and other blood constituents have been reported (Covington, 1979).

In 1982 commercial competition in ISE availability widened considerably with instruments available from Beckman Instruments (Brea, Ca.), Nova Biomedical (Newton, Mass.), Worthington Diagnostic Systems (Freehold, N.J.), Corning Medical and Scientific (Medfield, Mass.), Instrumentation Laboratory (Lexington, Mass.), Orion Research (Cambridge, Mass.), and Eastman Kodak (Rochester, N.Y.).

Clinical laboratories should include the development of ISEs for total calcium, total magnesium, and ammonia in serum.

Electrophoresis

Electrophoresis for protein fractionation has been a valuable separation and quantitation technique in the clinical laboratory. It is discussed in Chapter 12, Specific Proteins (p. 205).

Instrumentation Characteristics. The instrumentation for electrophoresis consists basically of a power supply, an electrophoresis cell, electrodes submerged in a buffer compartment isolated physically but not electrically from the gel or cellulose acetate strip, and the densitometer for measuring the amount of each of the fractions after the separation. Staining and destaining are optional. The power supply commonly requires an output of about 200 volts with about 4.5 milliamperes of current being drawn. The buffer must have a carefully controlled ionic strength. A dilute buffer causes heat to be generated within the cell while a high ionic strength does not permit good separation of fractions. The electrodes that are immersed in the buffer are usually placed in separate compartments connected to the cell by salt bridges so that pH changes that occur in the electrode chambers do not alter the pH of the buffer saturating the matrix. Significant care must be taken by the operator to prevent contamination of the cell, the electrodes, or the matrix with fingerprints or any foreign substance that will disturb the even current flow throughout the matrix. Most commercial apparatuses have built-in safety features to protect the operators from the potentially dangerous voltages present in such devices; however, the laboratorian must frequently check to see that these safety features are working properly.

Osmometry

The *osmolality* of a solution is dependent only on the *number* of particles in solution. The size or charge of the ion or molecule does not affect the measurement. One *osmol* of a substance is equal to the gram-molecular weight divided by the number of particles or ions into which the substance dissociates in solution. Thus, since glucose molecules do not dissociate in aqueous solution, 1 osmol of glucose = 1 mole = 180 g. For NaCl, which dissociates into 2 ions in aqueous solution, 1 osmol = 0.5 mole or $\frac{58.5}{2}$ = 29 g = 1 osmol. For Na_2SO_4, 1 osmol = 0.33 mole, etc., assuming 100 per cent dissociation for ions in solution.

A solution containing 1 osmol of solute per kilogram of solvent has a concentration of 1 osmolal. This concentration is independent of temperature, since it is based on weight only. A solution containing 1 osmol of solute per liter of solution has a concentration of 1 osmolar. Osmolar concentrations vary with temperature, since the volume varies with temperature. For aqueous solutions of low concentrations, such as body fluids, the difference between osmolality and osmolarity becomes negligible and it is customary to use milliosmols per liter (1 osmol = 1000 milliosmols).

The freezing point of water is depressed 1.86° C. when solute is added to make a 1 osmolal solution; hence, 1 osmol of any solute is that amount which will depress the freezing point of 1 kg of water by 1.86° C. An osmolality measurement in clinical chemistry provides an estimate of the effective number of particles in solution even though we do not know either the nature or the concentration of the individual substances dissolved in the solution.

Osmolality is determined by measuring the freezing point depression (Chap. 8). The apparatus consists of a cooling bath to freeze the specimen and a thermistor. A thermistor is a device whose electrical resistance decreases as the temperature decreases. With a constant current source and a balancing circuit, the resistance of a potentiometric balance bridge is adjusted to equal the resistance of the thermistor. This resistance of the thermistor is directly related to the temperature being measured. Thus, a thermistor is an electrical thermometer.

The measurement is very accurate and precise and is easily calibrated. The precision of an osmometer is usually of the order of 0.3 per cent or less.

The amount that the freezing point is depressed is related to the concentration by the following equation.

$$\Delta T = \frac{RT_o^2 M_1 W_2}{H_f W_1 M_2} \qquad (7)$$

where ΔT = the change in the freezing point
R = the gas constant, 1.987 cal/mol
T_o = the freezing point of the solvent in °K.
M_1 = the molecular weight of the solvent
W_2 = the grams of the solute
H_f = the heat of fusion of the solvent in cal/mol
W_1 = the grams of the solvent
M_2 = the molecular weight of the solute

The weight of solute (W_2) divided by the molecular weight of the solute (M_2) is equal to the number of moles of solute present; hence, from the equation above, the depression in freezing point is directly proportional to the number of moles of solute and is independent of the molecular weight.

The heat of fusion of water is 1436 calories per mole and the freezing point of water is 273.1 °K. A 1 molal solution of urea, for example, contains 60 g of urea dissolved in 1000 g of water. The change in freezing point, calculated from the above equation, is:

$$\Delta T = \frac{(1.987)\,(273.1)^2(18.02)\,(60)}{(1436)\,(1000)\,(60)} = 1.86°$$

Based on equation (7), the number of moles (m) of solute dissolved in 1000 g of water is:

$$m = \frac{\Delta T}{1.86}$$

Freezing point depression is a colligative property of a solution; that is, its magnitude depends on the number of solute particles per kg of H_2O. Other colligative properties include boiling point elevation and vapor pressure depression. This latter property is exploited by instruments that use dew point (vapor pressure) change to measure osmolality (Chap. 8).

Chromatography

Chromatography began when a Russian botanist named Tswett ground up some green leaves, extracted them, and placed the extract on a sorbent in a column. He observed that the green color was separated into various color bands that were adsorbed onto the solid support in the column. It was because of this experiment and the separation of colors that the word "chromatography" was coined. Today most applications of this technique do not involve separation of substances of different colors, but the term chromatography remains.

The purpose of chromatography in all cases involves separation of a mixture on the basis of specific differences of the physical-chemical characteristics of the components.

In paper chromatography the physical characteristics that determine separations are the rate of diffusion, the solubility of the solute, and the nature of the solvent. In liquid-liquid chromatography, separation is based on differences in solubility between two liquid phases. One of the liquids is often aqueous, while the other is an organic solvent. Solubility can be modified by changes in ionic strength or pH of each of the liquid phases. In gel-permeation chromatography, the molecular weight, the size and charge of the ions, and the hydrophobicity of the molecules are the characteristics that are responsible for separation. In ion-exchange chromatography, the separation of substances depends principally upon the sign and ionic charge density. Ions with greatest charge density will be held most strongly on an ion-exchange material. In an electrophoresis separation, the physical characteristic that differentiates between components is the mobility of the substance of interest in an electric field. In gas-liquid chromatography, the sample volatility, its rate of diffusion into the liquid layer of the column packing, and the solubility of the sample gas in the liquid layer (partition coefficient) determine the separation capabilities of this technique. Thin-layer chromatography, like paper chromatography, depends upon the rate of diffusion and solubility of the substance of interest in solvents as the components migrate through media such as silica gel.

Ion-Exchange Chromatography. Ion-exchange chromatography is a very well-established procedure that has been studied intensively. The natural purification of water as it percolates through soil is an

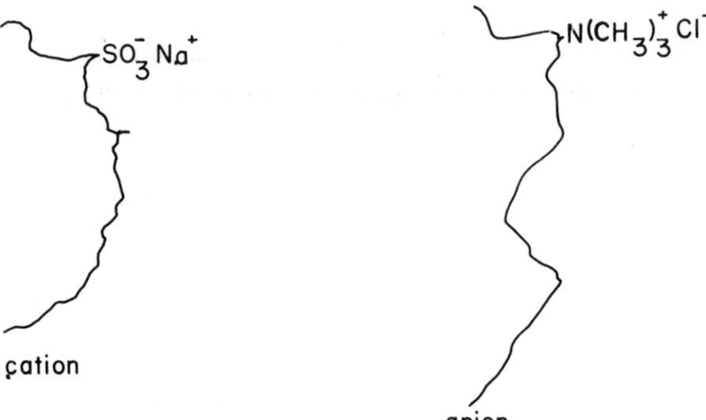

Figure 2–10. Illustration of a strong anion and cation resin with functional groups.

example of this process. Ion-exchange chromatography potentially has many uses in clinical chemistry.

Figure 2–10 shows the functional groups that are attached to the styrene structure cross-linked with divinyl benzene, used in constructing a synthetic strong *anion*-exchange resin. Nitrogen is bonded to the styrene, and three methyl groups are bonded to the nitrogen. The chloride anion is electrostatically attracted to the positive charge that remains on the nitrogen atom. Any anion passing through the solution that has greater affinity for the nitrogen than the chloride ion causes a displacement of the chloride from the resin. The amount and the rate of exchange depend upon the relative affinities of the nitrogen atom for the chloride ion or the other anion in solution. This is a technique to remove an unwanted anion from solution by exchanging it for other more desirable anions.

Figure 2–10 also shows a typical strong *cation*-exchange resin, again with the styrene structure, but with SO_3^- groups bound to the styrene. In this example, any cation that would be more strongly held to the SO_3^- than sodium would be preferentially adsorbed from solution and the sodium ion would be discharged into the solution. As with the anion-exchange material, a cation-exchange process serves to separate unwanted substances from solution. In certain cases, very large volumes of dilute solutions may be passed through ion-exchange materials to effectively concentrate the solute of interest. Ion-exchange chromatography will find increasing uses in the clinical chemistry laboratory, since it materially improves the specificity and accuracy of the method by removal of interfering substances.

Gel-Permeation (Size-Exclusion) Chromatography. Gel-permeation chromatography became widely used in the early 1960's. The trade name of a material that appeared on the market is Sephadex (Pharmacia, Inc., Piscataway, N.J.). Polyacrylamide gels are also often used in size-exclusion chromatography. Sephadex is a dextran material that has been modified so that it contains pores of accurately controlled size. Various pore size materials are currently commercially available. When a mixture of small and large molecules is allowed to pass over small particles in a column, the smaller molecules and ions diffuse into the gel. Larger molecules such as proteins are too large to diffuse into the interstitial cavities of the material and pass rapidly through the column. The smaller molecules and ions are then temporarily retained until they have time to diffuse back out of the gel. Thus, the large molecular weight materials will appear in the effluent first and the smaller molecular weight materials will be delayed in the dextran packing of the column.

The use of gels makes it possible to separate compounds by their molecular weight, provided the pore size of the material is properly selected for the separation.

Gel-permeation chromatography was further improved by introducing ion-exchange groups on the dextran. The ion-exchange characteristics of the dextran, in addition to the size-exclusion chromatography, greatly expanded the separation capability of this material. With the additional ion-exchange characteristics, not only the size of the molecule but the ionic charge of the molecule became important for the separation. Recently, Sephadex has been further modified to allow it to be used with organic solvents. Hydroxypropylation of G-25 produces a dextran material capable of performing separations of compounds dissolved in highly non-polar organic systems.

Agarose gels (Sepharose) are commonly used for the separation of larger molecular proteins, polysaccharides, and nucleic acids. These agarose gels are often the starting material that is modified to produce affinity columns. The use of agarose and six molar guanidine hydrochloride will allow an estimate of the molecular weight of proteins and is a widely used technique.

In addition to Sephadex, other materials have been used in gel-permeation chromatography. Polyacrylamide gels have been manufactured that, like dextran, have a closely controlled pore size. These materials are more suitable for use in a wider pH range. The rate of hydrolysis of Sephadex becomes significant at high pH values, while polyacrylamide gels are more suitable for this type of application. Polyacrylamide has the additional advantage that it will not support bacterial growth, which is frequently a problem when working with biologic fluids.

Gel-permeation chromatography has been used principally for the separation of proteins from lower molecular weight molecules and ions. In addition, gel-permeation chromatography has been used quite extensively in the study of isoenzymes and enzyme chemistry.

High Performance Liquid Chromatography (HPLC). Since the early 1970's the development of pumps, columns, flow monitors, and other instrumentation has allowed aqueous or organic solutions to be pumped through columns with pressures between 500 and 5000 pounds per square inch. Additional technologic advances allowed the preparation of controlled pore size porous glasses for size-exclusion chromatography. The glass beads are spherical and are very small (5 to 8 microns). For size exclusion chromatography glass beads with pore sizes of 60, 100, 500, or 1000 Angstroms (10^{-10} meter) are commercially available.

Very carefully controlled spherical silica gel beads of the same size as mentioned above are also available for adsorption chromatography. Because different molecules adsorb differently, often a separation can be completed in a few minutes using the types of solvents used for silica gel thin-layer chromatography plates. The thin-layer method may take up to an hour to allow separation to occur, while a few minutes is often enough with HPLC. A disadvantage of HPLC adsorption chromatography is that the extent of hydration of the silica gel is critically important. The degree of hydration can easily change as various amounts of solvent are pumped through the column. Hence, exactly reproducing separation conditions is often difficult and equilibration time may be long.

A still more recent development in HPLC is the "reverse phase" column packings that are now commercially available. A very common, widely useful, and universal packing involves the covalent bonding of octadecyl silane (ODS) to small porous spherical glass beads. This ODS material is non-polar, and non-polar molecules will dissolve in the non-polar liquid phase bound to the glass support beads packed in a column. The sample containing a mixture of non-polar molecules (benzene, naphthalene, anthracene, etc.) is dissolved in a solvent like methanol. Using a mobile phase mixture of about 75 per cent methanol and 25 per cent water, the sample is injected on the top of the column. Because of the different solubilities (partition coefficients) between the mobile phase and the liquid phase on the solid support of the different components, the individual components will separate on a pass through the reverse phase column. This same column can be used for many drug analyses as well as for phenylthiohydantoin derivatives of amino acids.

Anion- and cation-exchange coated glass beads are also available in the small bead sizes that are suitable for use in the HPLC instruments. Other types of cyano derivative functional groups and C_8 phases are also becoming commercially available, but their use in clinical laboratories remains to be developed.

Gas-Liquid Chromatography. Gas-liquid chromatography (GLC) is one of the most versatile, powerful analytical tools available. This technique is capable of separating and measuring nanogram and picogram amounts of volatile substances. It is used for the measurement and fractionation of steroids, lipids, barbiturates, drugs, blood alcohol, and measurements of other toxicologic substances. Gas-liquid chromatographic methods are rapid, sensitive, and accurate when compared with other separation techniques.

Although the basic principles are not difficult to understand, the technologic requirements for columns, electronics, and temperature control were difficult to achieve until a few years ago.

The carrier gas is introduced near the top of the column near the point where the sample is to be injected. The carrier gas is an inert gas such as helium, nitrogen, or argon that flows at a constant rate through the column. The column is usually glass or an inert metal and is packed with an inert solid support such as diatomaceous earth that has been coated with a thin layer of a liquid phase. The liquid phase is usually some silicon oil that is non-volatile and does not chemically react with the substance of interest.

The detectors of gas-liquid chromatographs generally are of three basic types: the hydrogen flame, nitrogen-phosphorus, and the electron capture detectors. Since the hydrogen flame detector is most commonly used in the clinical laboratory, it will be discussed in some detail. It consists of a small platinum loop mounted approximately 1 cm above the hydrogen flame. A metal gas jet is mounted directly over the exit port of the column, and a flammable gas such as hydrogen is passed through the gas jet. A small flame is ignited and burns at the tip of the jet where the column effluent and the hydrogen mix. A voltage is applied between the gas jet and the platinum ring mounted above it. The platinum ring is maintained at a voltage of 50 to 125 volts or more. When the hydrogen flame is burning, ions that are formed by burning the effluent in the flame will be collected by the platinum ring and produce a small current between the gas jet and the platinum loop. This current is detected by the electrometer, amplified, and the signal fed to the recorder.

The Electrometer. Basically, the electrometer is an electronic device that is capable of measuring very small currents and amplifying them linearly. The amplified signal is then fed to the read-out device which is a strip chart recorder, an integrator, or a printer.

The Programmer. The programmer is a combination of electronic controls whose basic function is to provide temperature control of the column oven. The oven is usually controlled to within a tenth of a degree and is usually capable of being changed at a linear and constant rate ranging from 1°C. to 50°C. per minute. This change in temperature during a determination is useful in producing separations of materials that have penetrated the liquid phase. The respective components of the sample are then selectively eluted from the column in accordance with their differences in volatility as the temperature changes.

The Recorder. The recorder is simply an electrical mechanical device that measures the voltage output of the electrometer and presents it on a strip chart for interpretation by the operator. The size of the voltage signal introduced to the recorder is usually 1 to 10 millivolts.

Principles of Operation. In a gas-liquid chromatography determination, either the substance of interest must be volatile or a new compound (derivative) must be formed that is volatile. The derivative, in addition to being more volatile, may protect the compound of interest from thermally decomposing by binding with heat-labile groups. A small quantity of the liquid material to be measured is injected onto the column and is immediately volatilized in the entrance port to the column. The carrier gas then transports the volatilized sample to the liquid phase on the solid support within the column. Separation occurs owing to the different solubility and the different diffusion rates of the various components of the sample gas into and out of the liquid phase. Thus, the various fractions of the gaseous sample tend to move through the column at different rates and appear at different times at the detector. This process of going into the liquid phase by solubility, diffusing back out, and going back into the liquid phase is usually repeated 6000 to 8000 times during the one pass through the column. The column is said to have 6000 to 8000 theoretical plates.

As these bands are eluted from the column by the carrier gas, the burning flame produces a large number of ions. The surge of ions causes an increase in detector current, which is amplified by the electrometer and sent to the recorder. Peaks will then appear on the strip chart recording. As each of the bands is eluted from the column, successive peaks will be presented on the strip chart recorder. The length of time for each of the peaks to appear on the strip chart recorder from the injection time is the *retention time* and is usually characteristic for the substance of interest.

Two substances in a mixture generally do not have identical retention times. The retention time, therefore, *qualitates* the substance in the sample while the peak area *quantitates* the amount of each of the fractions present. If good resolution in the gas chromatograph is achieved and if the peaks formed on the strip chart recorder are very sharp, then the peak height may be found to be proportional to the concentration. Temperature changes, type or concentration of the liquid phase, volatility of different derivatives, or some other parameter can be introduced to effect an adequate fractionation of the sample.

In summary, because the gas chromatograph separates, detects, qualitates, and quantitates several fractions of a volatilized sample in a single step, its use has great potential in clinical chemistry, especially in drug analyses.

Liquid-Liquid Chromatography. When two liquid phases are mixed, as is commonly done in a separatory funnel, substances will distribute themselves between the two phases. The solubility principally determines the distribution of the species into the aqueous or the organic layer in a two-phase system. Generally, the solubility will be determined largely by the relative polarity of the substance of interest and the polarity of the two liquid phases. A highly polar substance tends to be more soluble in a highly polar solvent such as water, while the less polar substances tend to be more soluble in the less polar solvents such as organic solvents ("like dissolves like").

The solubility of a species and therefore the control of what phase the species will be found in is most easily managed by changing the pH of the aqueous solution. For example, if an anion is found in the aqueous phase and if that anion is to be extracted into the organic phase, addition of hydrogen ion will usually produce the transfer. When H^+ is added to the aqueous layer and the anion becomes protonated, the polarity of that molecule is much less (less ionic) than it was as an anion. Its solubility will be much greater in the organic phase because of its reduced polarity and the lower polarity of the organic phase compared with the water phase.

An example of how liquid-liquid chromatography is applied to clinical chemistry is the UV barbiturate method. The acid form (non-ionized, non-polar) of the barbiturate is first extracted from the aqueous phase (blood, urine) into an organic phase like chloroform. Next, the chloroform layer is contacted with a NaOH solution and the anion of the barbiturate goes into the alkaline aqueous phase, which then can be analyzed for barbiturates.

The distribution ratio ($D_{o/w}$) defines the amount of material found in each phase at equilibrium.

$$D_{o/w} = \frac{[C_{org}]}{[C_{water}]}$$

where $[C_{org}]$ = concentration in the organic phase
$[C_{water}]$ = concentration in the aqueous phase

A column liquid-liquid chromatography system can be established by impregnating a solid support with one liquid phase, then allowing another liquid to percolate through the column. A solid phase frequently is silica gel, the liquid phase is water, and an organic solvent is allowed to percolate through the column. Separations will occur with such an arrangement in a manner similar to other column chromatographic separations.

Paper Chromatography. In ascending paper chromatography, a strip of filter paper is usually hung vertically into a solvent. The solvent moves up through the paper by capillary action, with the paper serving as a wick. A spot of the substance to be fractionated is placed on the paper just above the solvent level and permitted to dry before the paper is inserted in the jar containing the solvent. As the solvent moves up through the paper, various fractions in the sample move at different rates. The relative solubilities of the components of the sample in the solvent mixture, the polarity of the solvent, and the polarities of the solutes of interest all affect the rate at which different components move. After the separation has taken place, the paper is removed, dried, and sprayed with a chemical for color development. The spots may then be quantitated by measuring their area or intensity or both. In certain cases, the spots may be visible in the ultraviolet region of the spectrum, in which case the paper is examined under such light. In descending chromatography the papers are inserted into a tray and clamped into position to allow the solvent to rise over the edge of the tray by capillary action, then pass down through the paper and drop to the bottom of the tank.

Paper chromatography has been used in clinical laboratories in the past for fractionation of sugars and amino acids and for barbiturates. Today amino acid analyzers involving ion-exchange chromatography are more frequently used for amino acid separations, while barbiturates are usually identified by UV spectrophotometry, HPLC, or thin-layer or gas chromatography. Sugars are usually separated by column chromatography.

Thin-Layer Chromatography. The principles of thin-layer chromatography (TLC) are similar to those described above for ascending paper chromatography. The main difference between the two techniques is that glass or plastic plates to which is attached a thin layer of silica gel, alumina, polyacrylamide gel, or starch gel are used for the matrix instead of filter paper. The edges of the plates are then placed on edge into a solvent solution and the solvent passes up through the thinly layered material on the glass plate in the same manner as it passes up the paper—by capillary action. Again, separation occurs because of differences in solubility, polarity of the solvent, polarity of the substance of interest, and rate of diffusion.

One advantage of thin-layer chromatography is that the spot may be scraped from the plate, easily redissolved in a solvent, and then analyzed on an instrument such as a gas chromatograph or a fluorometer. Another advantage of TLC is that separation can often be completed in 30 to 90 minutes, as compared with 12 to 24 hours for paper chromatography. The main functions of thin-layer chromatography are the identification and separation of unknown substances in one step or preliminary purification of mixtures prior to performing the final analysis by another technique.

Several samples can be spotted on the same plate and a standard can be placed on each plate to test whether the whole system is working properly.

Radiochemical Techniques

Perhaps 50 different compounds important in clinical medicine have been measured using radioimmunoassay (RIA) methods. The largest number of analyses has been in the area of hormones for endocrinology. Peptide hormones and steroids are ideal candidates because of their size and concentration for RIA analysis and account for the focus in endocrinology. Several drug analyses are becoming commercially available that use immunochemical techniques. Several companies are using radioactive labels for these types of methods; hence, radioactivity counting is an important instrumental technique for clinical laboratories.

We will discuss only liquid scintillation counting for beta radiation and sodium iodide activated with thallium for gamma radiation counting. There are higher resolution gamma counters that consist of lithium-drifted germanium solid state detectors. These detectors have lithium metal deposited on one side of a germanium block. The whole detector must be operated at liquid nitrogen temperatures, so clinical laboratories usually do not use these solid state detectors.

When a gamma ray penetrates the NaI (Tl) crystal, a flash of light is generated as the energy is absorbed. These flashes of light can then be measured by a typical photomultiplier (PM) tube. The PM amplification plus additional electronic amplification makes the counting a highly sensitive technique. The NaI (Tl) crystal must be sealed from the air because it is hygroscopic. Another disadvantage is that large amounts of lead shielding are usually necessary, so the counter is heavy and occupies substantial space.

Beta counting, on the other hand, involves mixing the radioactivity directly with a solvent and an organic compound that will absorb the much weaker beta radiation and then give off a flash of light. Two common scintillators are 2,5-diphenyloxazole (PPO) and 2,2-p-phenylene bis-5-phenyl-oxazole (POPOP). Today most service laboratories purchase the scintillation "cocktails" already prepared. When the flash of light is given off by the liquid scintillation fluid again, as with the gamma counter, a photomultiplier detects the signal, amplifies it 10^6 to 10^8 times, and feeds that signal to the electronics.

By adjusting the amplification it is possible to minimize the background count, select a narrow energy range of only the isotope to be counted, or conduct pulse height analysis of the radiation measured by the counter. Quenching is a problem in liquid scintillation counting but usually is not troublesome for gamma counting. Quenching may be the absorption of the light within the sample cocktail prior to PM detection. Most often cleaner glassware, a cleaner sample, or additional separations prior to counting will correct some of the quenching problems.

Several companies now provide excellent counters, have training courses for operators, and offer various types of service contracts. Hence, today radiation counting is not a difficult measurement to make in most service clinical laboratories.

Covington, A. K. (ed.): Ion-selective Electrode Methodology, Vol. 2. Boca Raton, Fla., CRC Press Inc., 1979.

Goldberg, R.: Microcalorimetric determination of glucose in reference samples of serum. Clin. Chem., *22*:1685, 1976.

Horowitz, P., and Hill, W.: The Art of Electronics. Cambridge, Cambridge University Press, 1980.

Kabra, P., and Marton, L. (eds.): Liquid Chromatography in Clinical Analysis. Clifton, N.J., The Humana Press Inc., 1981.

Ladenson, J. H., Apple, F. S., and Koch, D. D.: Misleading hyponatremia due to hyperlipemia: A method-dependent error. Ann. Intern. Med., *95*:707, 1981.

Malmstadt, H., et al.: Electronics and Instrumentation for Scientists. Reading, Mass., The Benjamin/Cummings Publishing Co., Inc., 1981.

McLafferty, F.: Interpreting Mass Spectra. 3rd ed. Mill Valley, Cal., University Science Books, 1980.

Pardue, H., et al.: Applications of a vidicon spectrometer to analytical problems in clinical chemistry. Clin. Chem., *21*:1192, 1975.

Pelleg, A., and Levy, G. B.: Determination of Na^+ and K^+ in urine with ion-selective electrodes in an automated analyzer. Clin. Chem., *21*:1932, 1975.

Robinson, J.: Undergraduate Instrumental Analysis. 3rd ed. New York, Marcel Dekker Inc., 1982.

Skoog, D., and West, D.: Principles of Instrument Analysis. 2nd ed. Philadelphia, Saunders College, 1980.

Snyder, L., and Kirkland, J.: Introduction to Modern Liquid Chromatography. 2nd ed. New York, John Wiley and Sons, Inc., 1979.

Van Loon, J.: Analytical Atomic Absorption Spectroscopy: Selected Methods. New York, Academic Press, 1980.

Willard, H., et al.: Instrumental Methods of Analysis. 6th ed. Belmont, Cal., Wadsworth Publishing Co., 1981.

Friedman, G. D., Siegelaub, A. B., Seltzer, C. C., et al.: Smoking habits and the leukocyte count. Arch. Environ. Health, *26*:137, 1973.

Galteau, M. M., Siest, G., and Poortmans, J.: Continuous *in vivo* measurement of creatine kinase variation in man during an exercise. Clin. Chim. Acta, *66*:89, 1975.

Gambino, S. R., and Schreiber, H.: The measurement of CO_2 content with the Auto-Analyzer. Am. J. Clin. Pathol., *45*:406, 1966.

Giampietro, O., Navalesi, R., Buzzigoli, G., et al.: Decrease in plasma glucose concentration during storage at −20°C. Clin. Chem., *26*:1710, 1980.

Glenn, G. C., and Hathaway, T. K.: Effects of specimen evaporation on quality control. Am. J. Clin. Pathol., *66*:645, 1976.

Hagebusch, O. I.: Automation in the private practice of laboratory medicine. Automat. Anal. Chem., Technicon Symposium, 1965, Technicon, 1966, p. 417.

Keys, A., and Parlin, R. W.: Serum cholesterol response to changes in dietary lipids. Am. J. Clin. Nutr., *19*:175, 1966.

King, S., Statland, B. E., and Savory, J.: The effects of a short burst of exercise on activity values of enzymes in sera of healthy subjects. Clin. Chim. Acta, *72*:211, 1976.

Laessig, R. H., Hassemer, D. J., Paskey, T. A., et al.: The effects of 0.1 and 1.0 per cent erythrocytes and hemolysis on serum chemistry values. Am. J. Clin. Path., *66*:639, 1976a.

Laessig, R. H., Hassemer, D. J., Westgard, J. O., et al.: Assessment of the serum separator tube as an intermediate storage device within the laboratory. Am. J. Clin. Path., *66*:653, 1976b.

Larsson-Cohn, U.: Differences between capillary and venous blood glucose during oral glucose tolerance tests. Scand. J. Clin. Lab. Invest., *36*:805, 1976.

Laurell, C. B., Killander, S., and Thorell, J.: Effect of administration of a combined estrogen-progestin contraceptive on the level of individual plasma proteins. Scand. J. Clin. Lab. Invest, *21* (Suppl.):337, 1967.

Levi, L.: The effect of coffee on the function of the sympathoadrenomedullary system in man. Acta Med. Scand., *181*:431, 1967.

Lubran, M.: The effects of drugs on laboratory values. Med. Clin. North Am., *53*:211, 1969.

Marley, E., and Blackwell, B.: Interactions of monoamine oxidase inhibitors, amines and foodstuffs. Adv. Pharmacol. Chemother., *8*:185, 1970.

Martin, T. J.: The pharmacologic interactions with laboratory test values. August 1970, 596 Burnhamthorpe, Etobiocoke, Ontario, Canada.

McGeachin, R. L., Daugherty, H. K., Haryan, L. A., and Potter, B. A.: The effect of blood anticoagulant on serum and plasma amylase activities. Clin. Chim. Acta, *2*:75, 1957.

Musiala, T. S., and Dubin, A.: Effects of chylomicrons and their removal on spectrophotometric analyses. Clin. Chem., *23*:1121, 1977.

Ong, Y. Y., Boykin, S. F., and Barnett, R. N.: You can draw blood from the "IV arm" below the intravenous needle if you put a tourniquet in between. Am J. Clin. Path., *72*:101, 1978.

Pragay, D. A., et al.: Evaluation of an improved pneumatic-tube system suitable for transportation of blood specimens. Clin. Chem., *20*:57, 1974.

Remes, K., Kuoppasalmi, K., and Adlercreutz, H.: Effect of long-term physical training on plasma testosterone, androstenedione, luteinizing hormone and sex-hormone-binding globulin capacity. Scand. J. Clin. Lab. Invest., *39*:743, 1979.

Rossing, R. G., and Foster, D. M.: The stability of clinical chemistry specimens during refrigerated storage for 24 hours. Am. J. Clin. Path., *73*:91, 1980.

Schiele, F., et al.: The effects of drugs on enzyme reference values. Clin. Chem., *23*:1120, 1977a.

Schiele, F., Guilmin, A. M., Detienne, H., et al.: Gammaglutamyltransferase activity in plasma: Statistical distributions, individual variations, and reference intervals. Clin. Chem., *23*:1023, 1977b.

Schwartz, M. K.: Interferences in diagnostic biochemical procedures. Adv. Clin. Chem., *16*:1, 1973.

Statland, B. E., and Winkel, P.: Problems of precision and accuracy related to specimen collection and handling. Tech. Impr. Serv. *24*:60, 1976.

Statland, B. E., and Winkel, P.: Effects of non-analytical factors on the intra-individual variation of analytes in the blood of healthy subjects: Consideration of preparation of the subject and time of venipuncture. CRC Crit. Rev. Clin. Lab. Sci., *8*:105, 1977.

Statland, B. E., and Winkel, P.: Selected pre-analytical sources of variation. *In* Grasbeck, R., and Alstrom, T. (eds.): Reference Values in Laboratory Medicine. New York, John Wiley and Sons, 1981, pp. 127–137.

Statland, B. E., Winkel, P., and Bokelund, H.: Factors contributing to intra-individual variation of serum constituents: 2. Effects of exercise and diet on variation of serum constituents in healthy subjects. Clin. Chem., *19*:1380, 1973a.

Statland, B. E., Winkel, P., and Bokelund, H.: Serum alkaline phosphatase after fatty meals: The effect of substrate on the assay procedure. Clin. Chim. Acta, *49*:299, 1973b.

Statland, B. E., Winkel, P., and Bokelund, H.: Factors contributing to intra-individual variation of serum constituents: 4. Effects of posture and tourniquet application on variation of serum constituents in healthy subject. Clin. Chem., *20*:1513, 1974.

Steige, H., and Jones, J. D.: Evaluation of pneumatic tube system for delivery of blood specimens. Clin. Chem., *17*:160, 1971.

Stout, R. W., Henry, R. W., and Buchana, K. D.: Triglyceride metabolism in acute starvation: The role of secretin and glucagon. Eur. J. Clin. Invest., *6*:179, 1976.

Sunderman, F. W., Jr.: Drug interference in clinical biochemistry. CRC Crit. Rev. Clin. Lab. Sci., *1*:427, 1970.

Swanson, J. R., and Wilkinson, J. H.: Measurement of creatine kinase activity in serum. Stand. Meth. Clin. Chem., *7*:33, 1972.

Weindling, H., and Henry, J. B.: Drug interaction and clinical laboratory data. Lab. Med., *6*:24, 1975.

Wilkinson, E. J., Cherayil, G. D., and Borkowf, H. I.: L/S ratio and the "g-force" factor. N. Engl. J. Med., *296*:286, 1977.

Wilson, S. S., Guillan, R. A., and Hocker, E. V.: Studies of the stability of 18 chemical constituents of human serum. Clin. Chem., *18*:1498, 1972.

Winkel, P., and Statland, B. E.: Using the subject as his own reference in assessing day-to-day changes of laboratory test results. Contemp. Top. Clin. Anal. Chem., *1*:287, 1977.

Winsten, S.: Collection and preservation of specimens. Stand. Meth. Clin. Chem., *5*:1, 1965.

Young, D. S., Pestaner, L. C., and Gibberman, V.: Effects of drugs on clinical laboratory tests. Clin. Chem., *21*:1D, 1975.

1

6

QUALITY CONTROL: THEORY AND PRACTICE

BERNARD E. STATLAND, M.D., PH.D.,
and JAMES O. WESTGARD, PH.D.

OVERVIEW

Clinical laboratories perform qualitative, semiquantitative, and quantitative tests on a variety of biologic specimens. Qualitative tests, in which a particular characteristic of the specimen is determined to be either present or absent, are called binary descrete variates. Examples of such tests are blood grouping or the identification of microbiologic organisms present in a specimen. The results of such tests are in the nature of "yes" or "no" or "positive" or "negative" answers. That is, the examination shows what particular characteristics are present or absent in the specimen. Semiquantitative tests are those in which the degree of positivity or negativity is roughly estimated, usually by visual observation. An example of such a test is the dipstick test for urinary glucose, in which the degree of reaction is visually estimated and indicated as negative, weakly positive, moderately positive, or strongly positive, or more simply as 0, +, + +, or + + +. In the last example, we are dealing with a discrete variate having four possible values. Quantitative tests are those in which the amount of a particular substance, or property, is measured by some instrument and the result is expressed numerically. Examples of quantitative measurements are the determination of the number of red or white cells in a blood specimen, the number of organisms found in a microbiologic culture, or the concentration of some analyte in a specimen of blood or urine. In the last example, we are dealing with a continuous variate. In this chapter we will be concerned with the techniques for monitoring and assessing the reliability of *quantitative* laboratory measurements (continuous variates) in laboratory medicine.

The basic principles of industrial quality control were set forth by Shewhart in 1931. Measurements were made of items produced by a machine or sequence of machines, and the average value and range of values of the measurements were determined. Tolerance limits that would result in an acceptable product then were established, and product uniformity could be assured by continual surveillance of these critical measurements to detect deterioration of machine performance and by correction of the problems as they become evident. The ways in which these basic principles have been extended to develop systems of quality assurance in clinical chemistry have been reviewed by Grannis (1977).

Most quantitative analytical procedures involve several operations, or steps, and each operation is subject to some degree of inaccuracy or imprecision or to the possibility of a mistake. The immediate aim of quality control is to assure that the end-products—the analytical values regularly produced by a clinical laboratory—are sufficiently reliable for their intended use. A broader objective is to assure that all laboratories produce analytical values that meet acceptable standards of precision and accuracy at all times. The attainment of these intra- and interlaboratory aims requires that all laboratory personnel—technologists, supervisors, and directors—be knowledgeable of the causes of analytical inaccuracies and of the techniques that are available for their detection, correction, and control. In addition, knowledge is required of the degree of the inaccuracy and imprecision allowed if analytical values are to be clinically useful.

Quality control in laboratory medicine has been defined as the study of those errors which are the responsibility of the laboratory, and the procedures used to recognize and minimize them. An alternative term, "quality assurance," has been used to represent the techniques available to ensure with a specified degree of confidence that the result reported by the laboratory is correct. In order to have such confidence, the laboratory director must be assured that there is both "precision control" and "accuracy control" performed in the laboratory.

In this chapter we will consider some of the general principles of quality assurance of clinical laboratory data and some of the specific systems that have been developed for monitoring and improving the quality of clinical laboratory performance. However, before we consider these specific details, it will be helpful to review some basic concepts concerning quantitative measurements.

THE NATURE OF ANALYTICAL BIASES AND RANDOM VARIABILITY

Analytical Bias

It is a basic premise of quality control that the analytical values actually reported by the laboratory ideally should correspond to the correct or expected

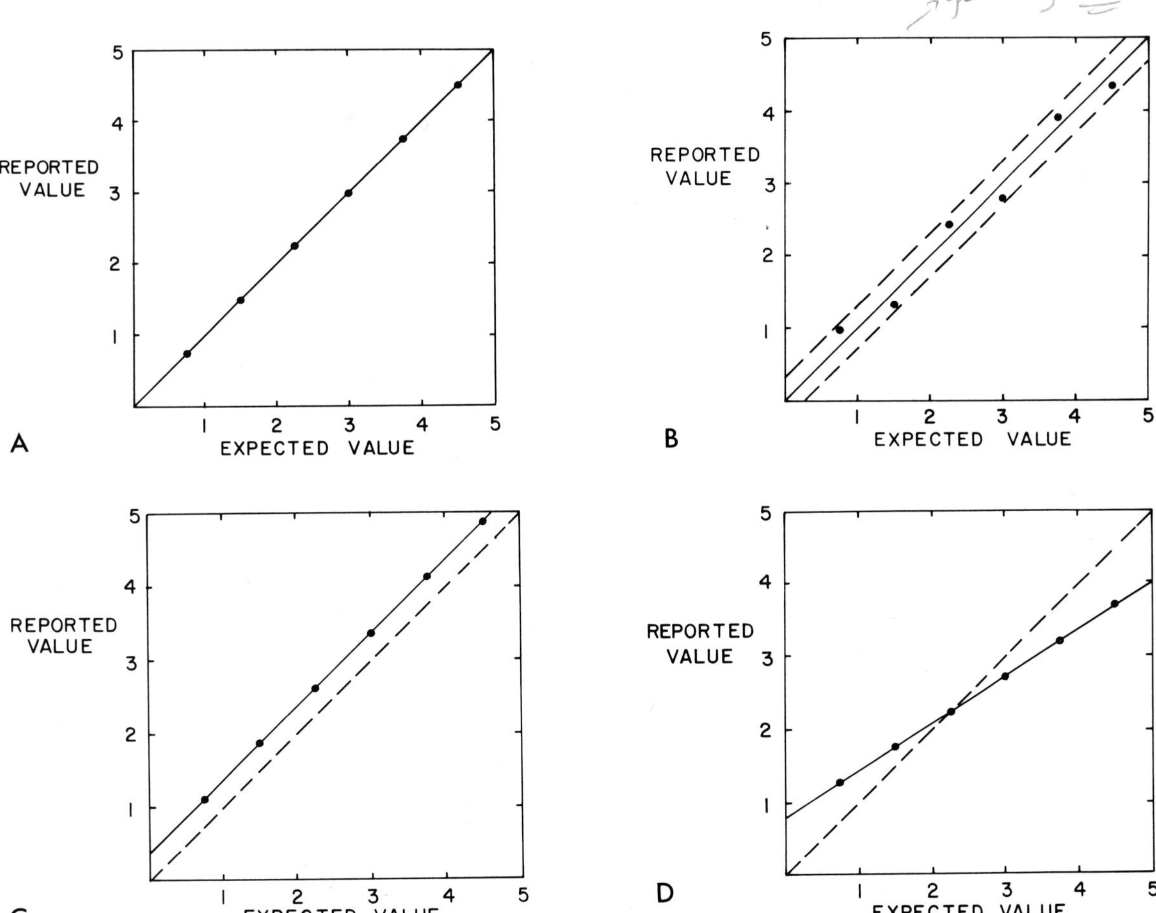

Figure 6–1. Illustration of the concept of the "operational line." When the laboratory's reported values for a series of specimens are plotted against the known, or expected, values, the data should fall along the straight line of slope 1.0, as shown in *A*. *B*, *C*, and *D* respectively illustrate the results observed when proportional, constant, or combined biases are present. The dashed lines in *B*, *C*, and *D* represent the case of no proportional bias and no constant bias. Every laboratory, in every analytical procedure, produces results that fall along some operational line, and one objective of quality control is to determine and optimize the laboratory's operational lines.

values. Let us assume that we do have some specimens for which we know the *true* concentration (expected value) of an analyte. In the optimal case when those specimens are analyzed by the laboratory, the reported values should correspond exactly to the expected values. That is, the reported values should fall along a line of slope 1.00 when graphed as shown in Figure 6–1*A*. However, all analytical procedures are subject to a variety of analytical inaccuracies, or biases. Figure 6–1*B* illustrates the effects of a proportional bias in which the reported values are higher than the expected values. The bias is called proportional because the amount of bias increases in direct proportion to the concentration of analyte in the specimen. Figure 6–1*C* illustrates the effect of a constant bias, in which the reported values are each higher than the expected values by a constant amount, at all concentrations of analyte.

The biases shown in Figures 6–1*B* and *C* are positive biases, because the reported values are greater than the expected values. Of course, negative biases may also occur; furthermore, the reported values may fall along a curve rather than a straight line. Nevertheless, Figures 6–1*B* and *C* illustrate the two major classes of biases that affect the accuracy of clinical analyses. Many analytical procedures are subject to either constant or proportional biases, or to both. Figure 6–1*D* illustrates how combined constant and proportional biases may affect the correlation of reported and expected values. It is worth noting that when combined biases are present, there is frequently one concentration at which the reported value does correspond exactly to the expected value. This phenomenon—that the reported value at some analyte concentration is the same as the expected value while they disagree at all other concentrations—is commonly observed and must be considered when interpreting quality control data. The phenomenon is sometimes used to advantage to minimize analytical bias. For example, when a particular method is found to have a constant positive bias, that bias may be partially compensated by deliberately introducing a negative proportional bias. This principle, of introducing compensatory biases to minimize total bias, although widely employed in some analytical systems, may result in unexpected problems in certain situations.

Charts such as those shown in Figure 6–1 have been called "operational charts," and the lines on which the reported values fall have been called "operational lines," because every laboratory does produce results that tend to fall along some line when graphed as in Figure 6–1 (Grannis, 1972). That is, each laboratory for each analytical procedure customarily operates with a certain degree of bias that causes its results to be distributed along some operational line, as shown in the figures. One primary objective of quality assurance procedures is to determine a laboratory's operational line for each analytical method. Ideally, of course, all laboratories should have an operational line of slope 1.00 (Fig. 6–1*A*), so that their reported values are unbiased and correspond exactly to the known values. But if this ideal cannot be attained, then the laboratory's customary operational line should at least be maintained in a reproducible manner.

Random Analytical Variability

In addition to analytical biases, laboratory analyses are also subject to imprecision, or random variability. The effects of random variation on analyses are illustrated in Figures 6–2*A* and *B*, which show how a laboratory's results may, on the average, fall along some operational line even though the individual results are distributed about the line, within certain limits of variability. Figure 6–2*A* illustrates limits of variability that increase in proportion to the mean analyte concentration, while Figure 6–2*B* illustrates limits of variability that are constant at all concentrations of analyte.

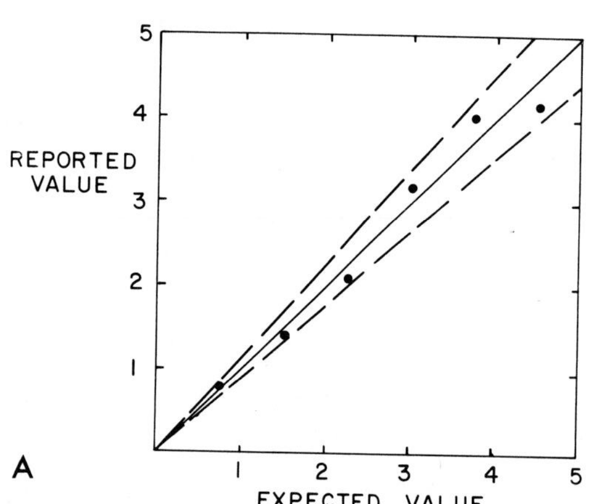

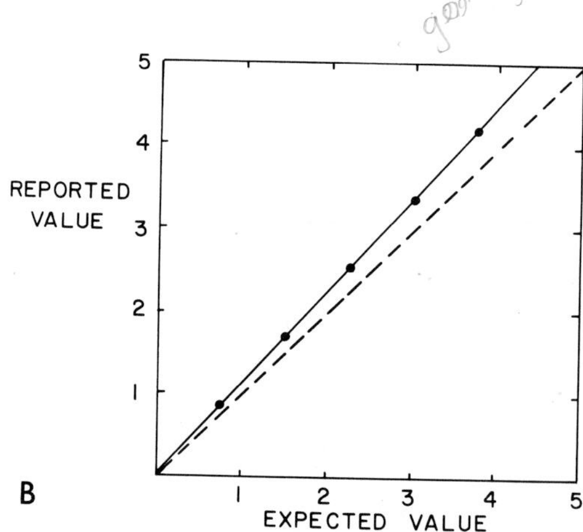

Figure 6–2. Random analytical variability causes results to be dispersed about the operational line, and may increase in proportion to analyte concentration (*A*) or may be constant at all concentrations (*B*).

Knowledge of the kinds of bias and random variability that affect an analytical system is helpful in identifying their causes. For example, proportional limits of variability are commonly caused by imprecision in volumetric dispensing of the sample. An automatic pipettor is a mechanical device and as such there may be a certain amount of "play" in the operation of its parts, which may increase as the parts become worn. Variation in the amount of sample measured by such a pipettor will introduce variation in the analytical results that is proportional to the analyte concentration of the specimen, and will cause proportional variability as shown in Figure 6–2*A*. Similarly, constant limits of variability are commonly observed in analytical procedures that are influenced by the turbidity of the specimen. Sample turbidity is usually independent of analyte concentration, but may vary from specimen to specimen, thus causing results to be distributed between constant limits, as shown in Figure 6–2*B*. Thus, knowledge of how various sources of analytical bias and variability affect the accuracy and precision of the operational line can be most helpful in identifying and in correcting analytical problems as they arise.

Mistakes

In addition to analytical factors that introduce bias and random variability into the analytical procedure, laboratory analyses are also subject to "mistakes." It is sometimes difficult to determine whether an erroneous result was due to an analytical factor or to a mistake, but the differentiation is of some importance if the cause of a problem is to be identified and corrected. Analytical errors are usually systematic in nature. That is, they are caused by some factor in the analytical system which can affect a series of analyses. For example, an erroneously calibrated pipettor might cause a systematic proportional bias, while a pipettor that operates imprecisely will cause random variability of analyses. Mistakes occur rather seldom, however, and usually affect only a few analyses. The pipettor might be used to measure a sample into the wrong tube, or the analytical result might be assigned to the wrong specimen, or the numbers in the analytical value might be transposed. These kinds of incidents are due to human mistakes rather than to deficiencies in the analytical system.

Several studies have indicated that as many as 2 per cen of all clinical chemistry analyses may be erroneous due to mistakes (Grannis, 1972; Whitehurst, 1975; Ladenson, 1975). There are a multitude of steps involved in the processing of a specimen; thus, there are numerous points where a mistake may occur. Even when the probability of a mistake occurring is low at any one point, the probability that at least one error occurs can be quite high.

One important aspect of quality control is to identify those steps in the analytical process where the likelihood of mistakes is high, and to consider ways to minimize that likelihood.

Quality Control Specimens Used in Monitoring Analytical Bias and Variability

The use of samples obtained from the same pool for the comparison of laboratory analyses was introduced nearly three decades ago and is still the most direct and widely applied quality assurance technique (Henry, 1952; Henry, 1959). In a number of studies (Belk, 1947; Shuey, 1949; Wootton, 1953) samples (assumed to be identical) of aqueous solutions of analytes, or of liquid serum or urine, were distributed to several laboratories for analysis. The results revealed clear evidence of substantial systematic differences among the laboratories. Similarly, when samples of the same serum pool were analyzed in a single laboratory over a period of time, variability in the measured values could be documented (Levey, 1950). These early studies established the important principle that a laboratory's analyses could be compared with those of other laboratories, or with its own prior analyses, simply by periodically analyzing samples that had been reserved from a large serum pool. The studies of Belk led directly to the establishment of interlaboratory comparison programs (Dorsey, 1975), and the studies of Levey led to the establishment of intralaboratory quality control programs.

However, the development of these programs was not without difficulty. In order to be effective the samples had to be essentially equivalent one to the other, the analytes in the sample had to be stable in storage over a substantial period of time, and the material had to be available in sufficient quantity to be used by many laboratories or by a single laboratory for a long period of time. It is beyond the scope of this chapter to consider the technical development of samples suitable for use in quality control. Suffice it to say that most samples used today are lyophilized products prepared from large pools of serum. As the interpretation of quality control data requires some appreciation of the limitations of these control specimens, it is worthwhile to consider some of the characteristics of such specimens.

The larger manufacturers of quality control specimens maintain blood plasma collection stations, and the fresh plasma is frozen for transport to a manufacturing plant. When a batch of control serum is to be prepared, as much as 2000 L of plasma is thawed, pooled, defibrinated, supplemented with various analytes to achieve the desired concentrations in the final product, mixed thoroughly, filtered, and dispensed into vials. The vials are then lyophilized and capped under nitrogen. The steps in this manufacturing process which are most critical for assuring that the final specimens will contain essentially the identical quantities of the analyte(s) of interest are the dispensing and lyophilization procedures. In addition, the entire process must be completed expeditiously, to prevent deterioration of the pool. The dispensers used are precision instruments that deliver pre-set volumes with a coefficient of variation (CV) of less than 1 per cent, and can dispense 2000 L in about 10 hours. The serum is processed at cold room temperatures to minimize deterioration. Lyophilization is carried out to a residual moisture content of less than 2 per cent water to assure stability in transport and storage. In general, the final samples are found to have a vial-to-vial variability of about 1 per cent. Except for occasional loss of glucose due to bacterial contamination and occasional changes in enzyme activities, the lyophilized products are generally stable. Some preparations are found to have greater turbidity than is customarily seen with clinical specimens. However, currently available specimens are generally satisfactory for most quality control programs, and we may expect continuing product improvements as manufacturing technology is further developed. In practice, the laboratory should purchase a supply of commercial lyophilized serum pool sufficient to last one year. Unassayed material is less expensive and avoids the pitfalls of erroneous assay values or assay values which show methodology bias. Such unassayed material will be useful for "precision control"; however, it should not be considered adequate for "accuracy control."

INTRODUCTION TO QUALITY CONTROL TECHNIQUES

Quality control can be divided into two major types: internal quality control (intralaboratory quality control) and external quality control (interlaboratory quality control). Intralaboratory quality control can be based either on the results of control specimens or on the results of patient specimens.

INTRALABORATORY QUALITY CONTROL (INTERNAL QUALITY CONTROL) BASED ON USE OF CONTROL SPECIMENS

Quality control within the clinical chemistry laboratory should be thought of as a *system* for assuring the quality of total laboratory performance. The purpose of the control program is to assess realistically the laboratory's usual performance in relation to that of other laboratories, to identify significant problems as they arise, and to document that the problems are solved. This endeavor requires the involvement of all laboratory personnel and is most effectively coordinated by one individual who has the assigned responsibility of maintaining and reviewing the laboratory's quality control records and of making regular reports to the laboratory staff. A coordinated system of quality control provides a mechanism for the open discussion of current laboratory problems and for developing uniform standards of performance throughout the laboratory.

An effective system of quality control was developed by Sax (1967), modified by Allen (1969), and further refined by Grannis (1972). In this system each analyst in the chemistry laboratory routinely includes known quality control specimens in each analytical run. The expected values for these specimens are known to the analyst, and the purpose of these control specimens is to aid the analyst, who is responsible for a particular procedure, in deciding whether the analytical system is producing analytically reliable results for that particular analyte. Other quality control specimens, which may be duplicate patient specimens, commercial control specimens, or specimens with known additives, are prepared by the "Quality Control Laboratory" and interspersed randomly among the clinical specimens. The fact that these specimens are control specimens is unknown to the analysts in the laboratory. The purpose of the latter specimens is to obtain an independent assessment of all the procedures performed in the laboratory. The data from both types of specimens are assessed on a daily basis, and the Quality Control Laboratory prepares a monthly statistical summary and a review of apparent problems. This summary is a permanent agenda item for the regular meeting of the laboratory supervisors and director.

The quality control laboratory also receives and distributes specimens from various interlaboratory surveys and maintains records of the survey reports. Thus, this system provides a mechanism for acquiring a variety of information about laboratory performance, for identifying and resolving problems, and for developing realistic standards of performance.

Although the system just described may appear suitable only for the larger clinical laboratories, the basic concept of having a regular review and discussion of quality control data, whether acquired with known or unknown samples, is applicable to all laboratories. In the following paragraphs we will consider some details in setting up and maintaining the system, but these details should be generally applicable to other systems as well.

Selection of Quality Control Specimens

We suggest that commercial suppliers of control sera target the values of analytes at or near the clinical decision levels (Statland, 1983). Essentially, the clinician should be informed as to the analytical performance at or near those values where clinical decisions will be made (see Chap. 4).

Preparation of Control Specimens

Because an effective quality control program depends on having control specimens that are highly reproducible, it is absolutely essential that the lyophilized samples be reconstituted and handled with good quantitative technique. That is, the reconstitution fluid should be measured with a volumetric pipette or a well-calibrated dilutor; the proteinaceous material must be allowed to dissolve completely; and, as the specimens will be used over the course of several hours, they should be protected from deterioration due to bacterial action (glucose), exposure to light (bilirubin), evaporation (all analytes), or loss of CO_2. The preparation of the daily control specimens is a specialized task, and this task should be included in the laboratory's regular schedule of personnel rotation or assigned to one individual. If precautions such as these are not taken, then each questionable result may be "explained" as an erroneous control sample and real analytical problems may remain undetected. Recently, the advent of stable liquid controls has overcome many of the above-mentioned difficulties.

Selection of Statistical Control Techniques

Many different statistical techniques can be applied to help decide when control data indicate that an analytical run is "in-control" or "out-of-control." One of the difficulties for analysts is to assess the relative advantages and disadvantages of different control techniques, and therefore be able to select the best techniques for their applications. Some knowledge of the characteristics of statistical control techniques is valuable to aid in the selection of control techniques.

Performance Characteristics of Statistical Control Techniques. These techniques are statistical tests that are applied to data having an expected mean and standard deviation, based on the stable performance of the analytical method. The techniques provide some decision criteria to signal the acceptance or rejection of an analytical run. The performance of these statistical techniques must be assessed by determining their statistical properties, in this case their probabilities for rejecting analytical runs containing different sizes of errors.

Probability for rejection refers to the chance that a rejection signal will occur. The numerical value for the probability will be between 0 and 1, a probability of 0 meaning that an event will never occur, and a probability of 1 meaning that an event will always occur. It is also common to express it as a percentage from 0 to 100 per cent.

It is of interest to know the probability for rejection when there are no analytical errors occurring, which is called the "probability for false rejection." Any rejections under these conditions would be false rejections because there are no real problems with the analytical method. Obviously, a high probability for false rejection would cause analysts to waste time searching for problems that don't really exist, repeating laboratory tests on patient specimens, and delaying the reporting of patient results. The probability for false rejection should therefore be low, usually less that 0.05, or 5 per cent.

It is also of interest to know the probability of detecting certain analytical errors, particularly those that would invalidate the medical usefulness of a test result. The "probability for error detection" should ideally be high, approaching 1.00, or 100 per cent. Since both random and systematic errors can occur, it is necessary to assess the probabilities for detecting both kinds of errors.

The probabilities can be determined from calculations based on probability theory, although these calculations become very complex. An alternative approach has been to perform experiments using numbers, adding different amounts of errors to groups of random numbers, then testing hundreds of different sets of these numbers to determine how often the simulated control data give rejection signals. Such "simulation studies" can easily be done with present-day computer facilities, and have been employed to determine the performance characteristics of many of the commonly used statistical control procedures (Groth, 1981; Westgard, 1977a).

"Power function graphs" have been proposed as a way to describe the performance characteristics of statistical control procedures (Westgard, 1979). A power function graph shows the probability for rejection plotted on the y-axis versus the size of the analytical error on the x-axis. Separate graphs are necessary for random and systematic errors. There may be several lines on each power function graph to represent the performance when there are different numbers of control observations (N). Figure 6–3 shows an example of power function graphs.

The probability for false rejection can be read from the point where a power curve intersects the y-axis. This is the probability for rejection for a zero systematic error, or for the background random error (inherent imprecision of the analytical method).

The probability for error detection is determined from a power curve by the y-value that corresponds

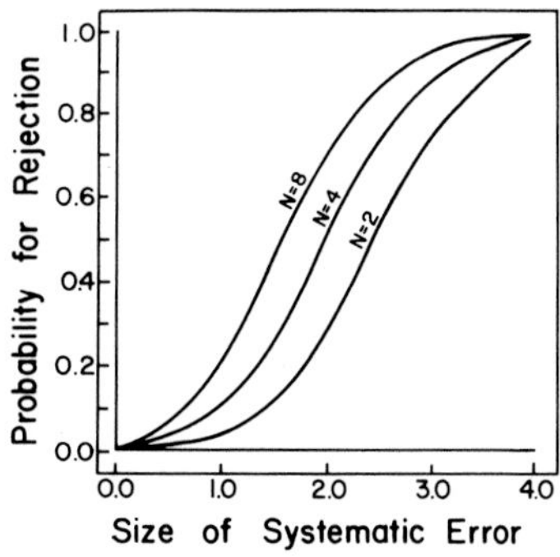

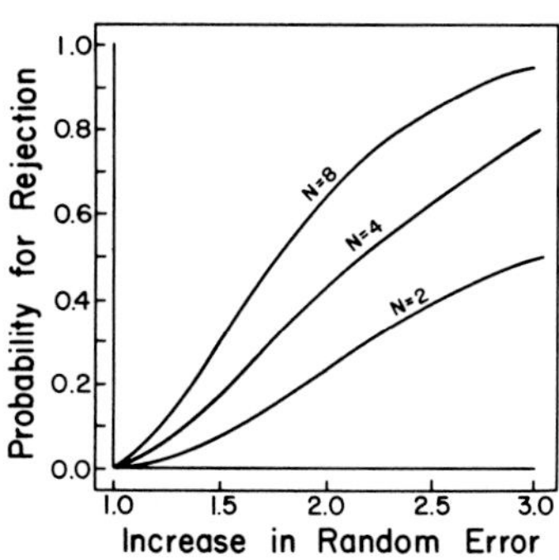

Figure 6–3. Power function graphs for systematic error (top) and random error (bottom). Probability for rejection is plotted on the y-axis vs the size of the errors on the x-axis. For systematic error, a size of 2.0 is equivalent to a shift of 2.0 times the standard deviation of the analytical method. For random error, a size of 2.0 means a doubling of the standard deviation of the method. (Reproduced from Westgard, 1981a, with permission from Clinical Chemistry.)

to the x-value or error of interest. Note that for systematic error the size of the error is given as a multiple of the size of the standard deviation of the method. For example, a "delta SE" of 2.0 corresponds to a systematic shift equivalent to twice the size of the standard deviation. For random error, a "delta RE" of 2.0 corresponds to a doubling of the standard deviation of the analytical method.

In general, control procedures should be selected to have a low probability for false rejection and a high probability for error detection. The relative performance of many of the commonly used control procedures has been presented by Westgard (1977a, 1979). He recommends eliminating those control procedures that have a probability for false rejection greater than 0.05, or 5 per cent, then choosing at least two control techniques (rules, decision criteria), one sensitive to random error and one sensitive to systematic error. Finally, the number of control observations can be chosen to provide the desired probability for error detection. This approach should provide control procedures having a low probability for false rejection and a high probability for error detection.

Predictive Value of Control Signals. How low should the probability for false rejection be, and how high should the probability for error detection be? Ideal values of 0.00 for false rejection and 1.00 for error detection are not attainable and probably aren't really necessary. The performance necessary would seem to depend on the stability of the analytical method that is to be monitored. A very stable analytical method that seldom has a problem should require less control effort than an unstable one that frequently has problems. Different designs or techniques would seem to be appropriate for analytical methods having different frequencies of errors.

The performance of a quality control test can be optimized for frequency of errors in the same manner that performance of a diagnostic test can be optimized for prevalence of disease. A quality control technique is a statistical test from which a yes/no decision is made, in a manner analogous to the yes/no interpretation of a diagnostic test. By employing predictive value theory, the relationship between frequency of errors and the desired probabilities for false rejection and error detection can be understood.

A predictive value model for a "QC test" has been described (Westgard, 1983) and is summarized in Table 6–1. To help understand the model, it is useful to review briefly the predictive value model for diagnostic tests (see Chap. 16, 16th Edition of this text). "Diagnostic sensitivity" describes how often a test gives a positive result when a patient has the problem of interest. Diagnostic sensitivity is determined as the ratio of the number of patients with the problem having positive test results (true positives), divided by the total number of patients with the disease (true positives plus false negatives which were not detected by the test). "Diagnostic specificity" describes how often a patient not having the problem of interest gives a negative test result. Diagnostic specificity is determined as the ratio of the number of non-problem patients having negative test results (true negatives), divided by the total number of non-problem patients in the study (true negatives plus false positives which gave positive results even though they didn't represent the problem of interest).

In the predictive value model for the QC test, the

Table 6–1. PREDICTIVE VALUE MODEL FOR A "QC TEST"

Analytical Run	Reject Signal	Accept Signal	Totals
With error	TR (True Reject) $f(P_{ed})$	FA (False Accept) $f(1\text{-}P_{ed})$	TR + FA f
Without error	FR (False Reject) $(1-f)P_{fr}$	TA (True Accept) $(1-f)\ (1-P_{fr})$	FR + TA $1-f$
Totals	TR + FR $f(P_{ed})+(1-f)P_{fr}$	TA + FA $f(1-P_{ed})+(1-f)(1-P_{fr})$	TR+FR+TA+FA 1

$$P_{ed} = \frac{TR}{TR + FA}$$

$$P_{fr} = \frac{FR}{FR + TA}$$

$$PV(\text{reject}) = \frac{TR}{TR + FR} = \frac{f(P_{ed})}{(P_{ed}) + (1-f)P_{fr}}$$

$$PV(\text{accept}) = \frac{TA}{TA + FA} = \frac{(1-f)(1-P_{fr})}{(1-f)(1-P_{fr}) + f(1-P_{ed})}$$

$$\text{Efficiency} = \frac{TR + TA}{TR + FR + TA + FA} = f(P_{ed}) + (1-f)(1-P_{fr})$$

$$\text{Cost or loss} = Wt_{FA}(FA) + Wt_{FR}(FR) = Wt_{FA}(1-P_{ed})f + Wt_{FR}(1-f)P_{fr}$$

probability for error detection is given by the ratio of the number of analytical runs having problems and having a reject signal, divided by the total number of runs having problems. Probability for error detection is directly analogous to diagnostic sensitivity. Both should be high (probability value approaching 1.00) to provide good detection of the problem situations.

The probability for false rejection is given by the number of non-problem runs misclassified as problems, divided by the total number of non-problem runs. One minus the probability for false rejection is equivalent to diagnostic specificity. A high diagnostic specificity is the same as a low probability for false rejection. For example, a probability for false rejection of 0.05 would be equivalent to a diagnostic specificity of 0.95.

In addition to the concepts of sensitivity and specificity, the concepts of predictive value and efficiency can also be applied. The frequency of errors occurring with an analytical method is analogous to the prevalence of disease in the application of a diagnostic test. The predictive value of accept and reject signals can be calculated to take the frequency of errors into account. The QC test can therefore be optimized for predictive value.

Table 6–1 provides a full description of the predictive value model for a QC test. The typical "two by two" classification table is shown at the top to illustrate the meaning of the classifications true reject, false accept, false reject, and true accept. These terms are also defined based on how they can be determined from the frequency of errors (f), probability for error detection (P_{ed}), and probability for false rejection (P_{fr}). The bottom half of the table gives equations for calculating the predictive value of both "reject" and "accept" results, the efficiency or overall correctness of all control results, and finally the cost or loss function which illustrates how weighting factors (in terms of cost) can be included to evaluate the performance of a QC test.

The predictive value equations are particularly useful in determining appropriate values for the probabilities of false rejection and error detection as related to analytical methods with different frequencies of errors. When the frequency of errors is very low, reject signals are particularly troublesome because they cause much time and effort to be wasted on nonexistent problems. The predictive value of a reject therefore needs to be optimized. Figure 6–4 shows the predictive value of a reject signal varies as a function of the frequency of errors. For low frequencies of error, a high predictive value for a reject signal is obtained only when the probability for false rejection is kept very low, 0.01 or below. The effect of the probability for error detection is secondary, having some influence, but not by itself being able to effect a high predictive value for a reject signal. In short, the optimal control technique for stable analytical methods is one having a very low probability for false rejection, 0.01 or below. The probability for error detection can be in the intermediate range of 0.25 to 0.50.

For unstable analytical methods, those having a high frequency of problems, a high predictive value is desired for an accept signal. Figure 6–5 shows the predictive value of an accept signal as a function of frequency of errors. When the frequency of errors is high, optimal performance depends on having a high

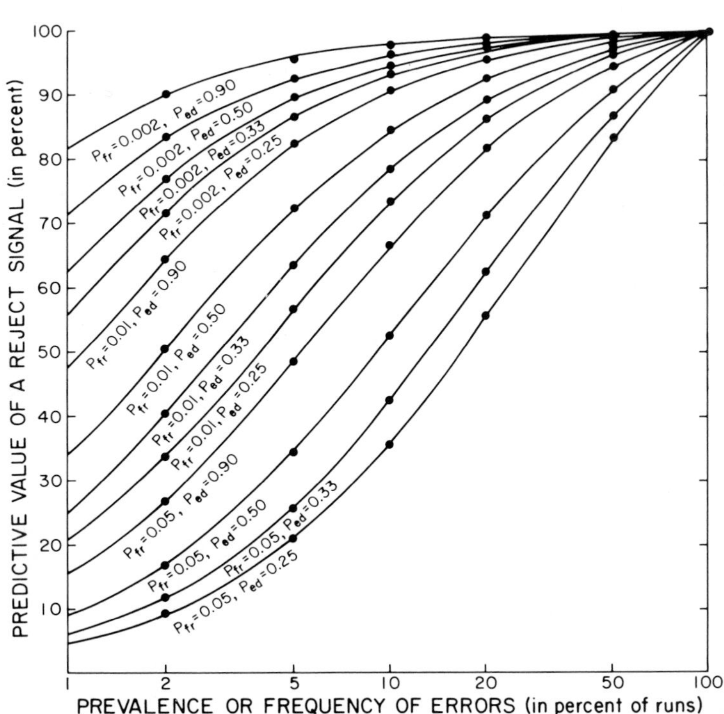

Figure 6–4. Predictive value of a reject signal from a control technique, as a function of the prevalence or frequency of occurrence of analytical errors. Predictive value is plotted on the y-axis in units of percentage. The different lines correspond to control techniques having different probabilities of false rejection (Pfr) and error detection (Ped). Pfr is 0.05 for the bottom four lines, 0.01 for the middle four lines, and 0.002 for the top four lines. Within each of these groups of four lines, Ped is 0.25, 0.33, 0.50, and 0.90 from bottom to top, respectively. (Reproduced from Westgard, 1983, with permission of the American Journal of Clinical Pathology.)

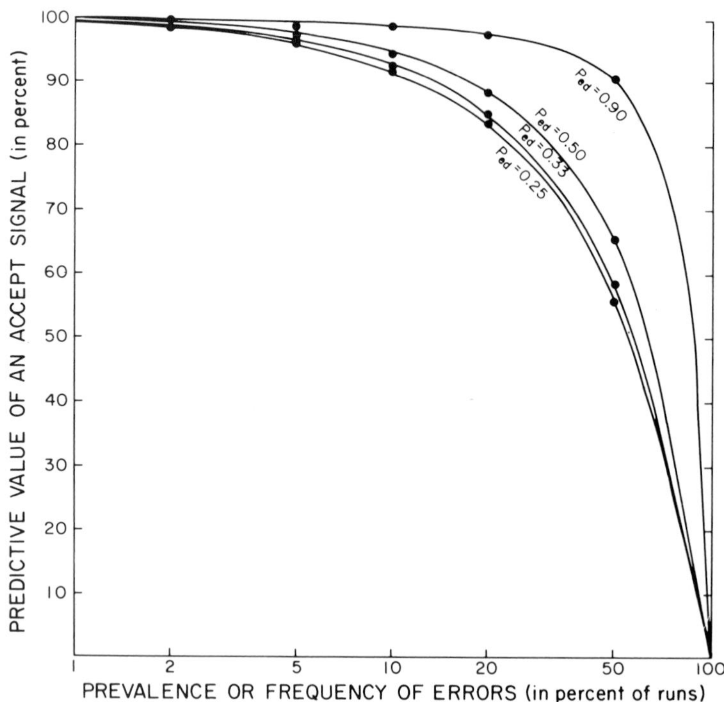

Figure 6–5. Predictive value of an accept signal from a control technique, as a function of the prevalence or frequency of occurrence of analytical errors. Units and scales are the same as in Figure 6–4. The four lines, from bottom to top, correspond to probabilities of error detection (Ped) of 0.25, 0.33, 0.50, and 0.90, respectively. (Reproduced from Westgard, 1983, with permission of the American Journal of Clinical Pathology.)

probability for error detection, 0.50 or greater. The actual probability for false rejection has little effect, and can even be allowed to increase above 0.05, or 5 per cent.

In summary, a low probability for false rejection is the primary consideration when monitoring a stable analytical method having a low frequency of errors. A high probability for error detection is the primary requirement for monitoring unstable analytical methods or new methods whose analytical performance is not well documented. The predictive value model provides a quantitative way of relating the performance of the control technique to the stability of the analytical method itself.

Influence of Quality Goals. Statistical control techniques often compare only present performance (the new run) with previous performance (the runs in the previous month). The acceptability of the new run is judged relative to the performance observed in the previous runs, even if that performance is not really medically acceptable. Initial method evaluation studies help prevent the implementation of analytical methods that do not provide the medically necessary quality. In addition, control techniques can be selected or designed to detect those critical-sized errors which would invalidate the medical usefulness of the test results (Groth, 1981).

Quality goals are very useful for the development of a quality control program and for assessing the suitability of control techniques for their intended applications. Quality goals should be expressed as allowable analytical errors, for example, as an allowable standard deviation for random error and as an allowable bias for systematic error. Alternatively, an allowable total error (95 per cent limit of error) can be defined as the quality goal for both random and systematic errors.

When quality goals have been specified, it is possible to calculate the size of the errors that must be detected if the specified quality is to be achieved. For example, if the allowable SD for a glucose method were specified as 5.0 mg/dl and the analytical method had a stable standard deviation of 2.5 mg/dl, then it would be necessary for the control procedure to detect a doubling of the standard deviation in order to achieve the quality goal. If the allowable bias were 10 mg/dl for this same glucose method (and the stable performance showed no bias), a systematic error equivalent to 4.0 times the standard deviation would need to be detected. Use of a total error specification of 10 mg/dl as a 95 per cent limit of error gives the same sizes of random and systematic errors that must be detected.

Once the critical-sized errors have been determined, power functions can be inspected to determine the performance capabilities of control techniques. The probabilities for false rejection and error detection can be determined, and their suitability judged based on the expected frequency of errors. For more formal assessment, the efficiency and predictive values for accept and reject signals can be calculated. In this way, it is possible to assess the suitability of a control technique for achieving a specified level of quality.

Control Techniques

A variety of statistical control techniques have been used in clinical laboratories, most often on a manual basis. Tabular records with appropriate calculations

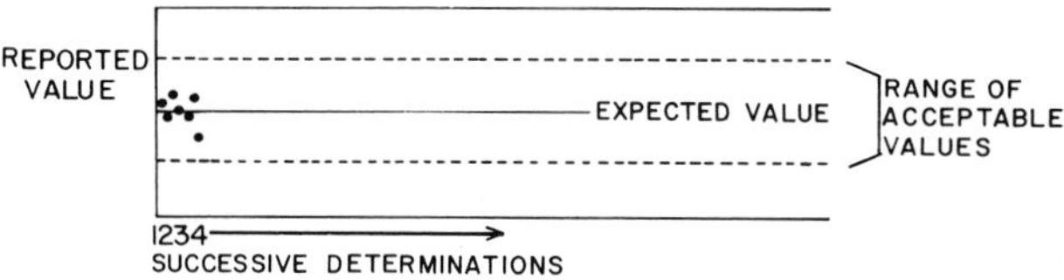

Figure 6–6. A modified Levey-Jennings quality control graph. Control data are graphed as acquired and should fall within the established limits. Values exceeding the limits are indicative of a possible analytical problem or of a mistake.

can be used to implement the techniques, but graphical displays are often easier to interpret. Tabular data do not readily reveal subtle changes that may be occurring with an analytical method. Therefore, control charts have been accepted as a more effective way to implement most control techniques.

Control charts generally display the control observation (or a calculated statistic) as a function or time (date, run number). The Levey-Jennings chart (1950) has been the most widely used technique. Recently, a "multi-rule" technique (Westgard, 1981a) has gained acceptance. Cumulative sum techniques have been used for many years but have never been widely applied in clinical laboratories. In addition, "mean and range" techniques have been used, and more sophisticated techniques employing "trend analysis" (Cembrowski, 1975) are becoming practical when implemented on micro-computers.

These different control techniques provide different criteria for judging control status based on the parameter that is plotted and the control limits that have been chosen. Control limits are usually calculated from the mean and the standard deviation. For convenience in describing these decision criteria or "control rules," we adopt a symbol of the form A:L, where A is an abbreviation for the control parameter or a number of control observations, and L represents the control limits. Control limits will usually be given by xs, where x is a multiplier and s is the standard deviation determined for that control material when analyzed by the analytical method being monitored. For example, 1:2s refers to a control rule where control status is judged based on one control observation exceeding control limits set as the mean plus/minus 2s.

Levey-Jennings Control Chart. The control results are plotted on the y-axis versus time on the x-axis, as illustrated in Figure 6–6. This chart shows the expected mean value by the solid line in the center and indicates the control limits or range of acceptable values by the dashed lines. The usual way of interpreting this control chart is to consider the run to be in control when the control values fall within the control limits, and to be out of control when a result exceeds the control limits.

It is common to use either 1:2s or 1:3s control rules with Levey-Jennings charts, i. e., control limits set as either the mean plus/minus 2s or the mean plus/minus 3s. The 1:2s rule should preferably be limited to applications where N = 1, in order to keep the level of false rejections suitably low. The probability for false rejection increases rapidly with N: 0.05 for N = 1; 0.09 for N = 2; 0.14 for N = 3; 0.18 for N = 4. For the 1:3s rule, false rejections will be less than 0.01 to 0.02, or 1 to 2 per cent, for N up to 8 to 10. Error detection is considerably lower for the 1:3s rule, but will be improved (without causing false rejection problems) by making additional control observations.

In addition to using control rules such as these to interpret the data, experienced analysts can often detect more subtle control problems by visual inspection of the data on control charts. Figure 6–7 illustrates three types of changes that are commonly observed in quality control data. Increased dispersion is observed when random error or imprecision increases. A trend, or systematic drift of the observed values, occurs when the analytical method suffers a progressively developing problem. An abrupt change, or systematic shift, may be observed when there is a sudden development of certain analytical problems.

When changes in control data indicate that the performance of an analytical method has deteriorated, the analyst must determine the cause of the problem. It is generally useful first to try to classify the error as random or systematic because the different kinds of errors suggest different sources. As seen in Figure 6–7, random error shows a wider range of scatter of the points on the control chart. Systematic error can be seen when the points drift or shift to one side of the central line. Further information on the nature of the systematic error can be obtained by remembering the concept of the operational line. Each control material provides one point along the operational line. When data from two or more materials are available, they may be assessed to determine if the error is constant, proportional, or mixed.

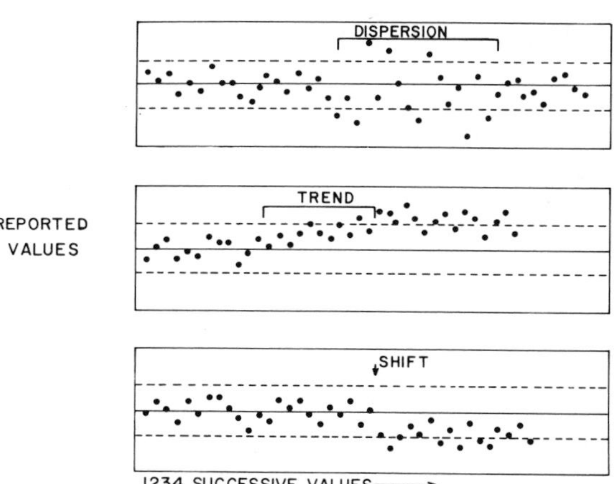

Figure 6–7. Examples of three common changes in quality control data. *Dispersion* is seen when there is an increased frequency of both high and low outliers. A progressive drift of the reported values from the prior mean value is called a *trend.* A *shift* occurs when there is an abrupt change from the established mean value.

Westgard Multi-Rule Technique. Analysts who do not have years of experience interpreting control charts may find it difficult to interpret the more subtle changes occurring in control data. To help uncover these problems, a series of control rules can be applied, some which are sensitive to random error and some which are sensitive to systematic error. The control data are plotted in the same manner as for a Levey-Jennings chart; however, the control chart has several limit lines (drawn at the mean plus/minus 1s, 2s, and 3s) to permit application of additional control rules.

For manual implementation, the 1:2s control rule is recommended as a "warning" rule, which should trigger inspection of the control data, using other rules as rejection criteria. The other rules can be selected to have a very low probability for false rejection; thus the overall false rejection level can be suitably low. The rules can also be chosen for their sensitivity in detecting either random or systematic errors and can therefore provide improved error detection.

The set of rules recommended by Westgard (1981a) includes the following:

1:3s—reject when one observation exceeds the mean plus/minus 3s limit.

2:2s—reject when two consecutive observations exceed the same mean plus 2s limit or the same mean minus 2s limit.

R:4s—reject when one control observation in the run exceeds its mean plus 2s limit, and another exceeds its mean minus 2s limit.

4:1s—reject when four consecutive control observations exceed the same mean plus 1s limit or the same mean minus 1s limit.

10:mean—reject when ten consecutive control observations fall on one side of the mean.

The procedure for employing the multi-rule analysis is outlined by the logic diagram shown in Figure 6–8. When there are no control observations in a run which exceeds a 2s limit, the run can be accepted without further inspection. It is theoretically possible that a 4:1s or 10:mean rule could still be violated, but it is pragmatic with manual implementation to accept the run without further inspection. (With computerized implementation, the 1:2s warning rule can be omitted and all the rules applied automatically.) When any one of the control observations exceeds a 2s limit, it is interpreted as a warning of possible problems. The control data are inspected by applying each of the rules in sequence. If any one rule indicates a rejection, the run should be rejected. If none of the rules indicate a rejection, the run should be accepted.

The multi-rule technique can be applied both "within" a run or material and "across" runs or materials. For example, when collecting two control observations per run, one each on normal and elevated materials, the 2:2s rule can be used to test the two observations obtained within the run (within run and across materials), or to test each of the last two observations on each material by looking back to a previous run (within material and across runs). This can improve error detection by increasing the number of control observations available for inspection, and also makes possible the differentiation of systematic errors, such as a systematic shift occurring throughout the analytical range from a shift occurring in one part of the analytical range. A baseline shift may be detected by observing that the two observations within the run both exceed the same 2s limit (2:2s across materials, within run). A loss of linearity at the high end of the analytical range may be detected by observing that the current observation is low by more than 2s and that the observation from the previous run was also low by more than 2s (2:2s within material, across runs).

The multi-rule technique has been recommended for N from 2 to 4, with 6 being the maximum number of observations to be used. For these N's, the probability for false rejection is much lower than observed for the 1:2s rule alone. When compared to the 1:3s rule, error detection is improved because of the effects of the R:4s, 4:1s, and 10:mean rules.

In addition to the improved performance characteristics, the multi-rule analysis can provide some indication of the type of error occurring. The 1:3s and R:4s rules generally suggest random error, while the 2:2s, 4:1s, and 10:mean rules generally suggest systematic error. With large systematic errors, the 1:3s rule may also be violated, and with very large random

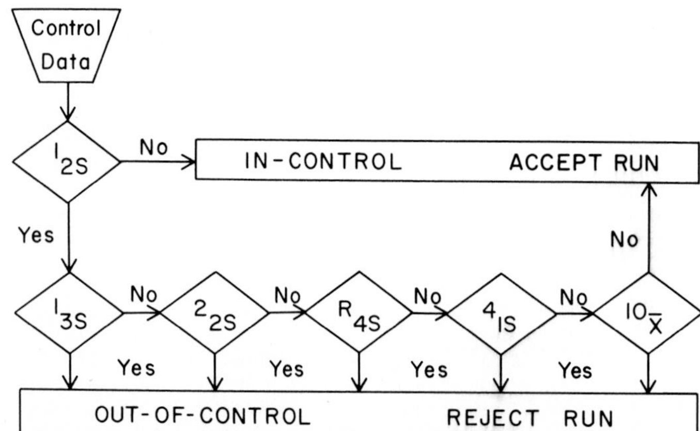

Figure 6–8. Logic diagram for applying the multi-rule control technique. (Reproduced from Westgard, 1981a, with permission from Clinical Chemistry.)

errors, all rules have shown an increased probability for rejection.

Cumulative Sum Techniques. Systematic errors can be observed qualitatively by noticing whether the control points scatter randomly about the expected mean. Counting the number of consecutive observations falling on one side of the mean (or one side of some other limit) provides another way of assessing systematic errors. A more exact and quantitative way is to calculate the actual differences between the individual values and the expected mean value, then sum those differences to determine the cumulative effect for all control observations collected.

Techniques which do this are known as "cumulative sum" or "cusum" techniques. They were introduced in the early 60's by Woodard (1964) and have found widespread application in industrial labs. Their use in clinical laboratories has been limited in part by the need to perform special calculations prior to inspection and in part by the difficulty in judging control status.

The calculation of cusum for a set of control data is illustrated in Table 6–2. The observed serum chloride value is shown in column 2, and its difference from the expected or assigned mean of 100 is given in column 4. The cusum is calculated by adding the values in column 4. For example, the cusum for day 4 is equal to the sum of 0 −2 +2 and −1, which gives a cusum value of −1. The cusum for the next day can be calculated simply by adding the new difference to the previous cusum; for example, for day 5 the cusum is total of +1 (day 5's difference) and −1 (cusum from day 4), giving a new cusum of 0.

Cusum values can be plotted versus time as done with other control charts. However, there is a major difference in the cusum control chart in that control status is generally based on the angle or slope of the cusum line. When control data are randomly scattered about their expected mean value, the cusum value will wander above and below zero, yielding a horizontal line on the cusum chart. When a systematic error is present, the cusum values will steadily increase. The slope of the line will be related to the size of the systematic error that is occurring—the larger the error, the steeper the angle of the cusum line. At a certain size, the error will be too large to be acceptable and the method will be considered out of control. The slope therefore becomes the criterion by which control status is determined.

Table 6–2. CALCULATION OF CUMULATIVE SUMS FOR DAILY OBSERVED VALUES IN CONTROL SPECIMENS OF SERUM CHLORIDE

Day No.	Serum Chloride (mmol/Liter)	Assigned Value	Daily Difference	Cusum
1	100	100	0	0
2	98	100	−2	−2
3	102	100	+2	0
4	99	100	−1	−1
5	101	100	+1	0
6	100	100	0	0
7	98	100	−2	−2
8	101	100	+1	−1
9	97	100	−3	−4
10	99	100	−1	−5
11	98	100	−2	−7
12	101	100	+1	−6
13	100	100	0	−6
14	99	100	−1	−7
15	99	100	−1	−8
16	101	100	+1	−7
17	97	100	−3	−10
18	100	100	0	−10
19	101	100	+1	−9
20	99	100	−1	−10

In the use of cusum techniques in clinical laboratories, the slope of the line has generally been assessed by visual inspection. The criterion therefore has been qualitative and difficult to employ on a uniform basis when many analysts are involved in assessing control status. This difficulty has limited the application of cusum control charts in clinical laboratories.

Even when cusum charts are employed, it is recommended that a Levey-Jennings chart still be used. Cusum responds primarily to systematic errors. Random errors must be monitored by some other technique, such as a Levey-Jennings chart with a 1:3s rule. A combined Levey-Jennings–cusum chart has also been described (Westgard, 1977b), which allows both control procedures to be plotted simultaneously on one control chart. The cusum technique employed is the "decision limit" alternative, which sets control limits for the actual value of the cusum, rather than judging control status by interpreting the slope.

Cusum techniques generally provide better detection of systematic errors than can be obtained from a Levey-Jennings chart. The multi-rule technique provides nearly as good detection of systematic errors, which should not be too surprising in view of how the 2:2s, 4:1s, and 10:mean rules accumulate differences. (In addition, the multi-rule technique has criteria for monitoring random error.)

False rejections can be minimized by proper choice of conditions; thus good performance can be expected from cusum techniques. In spite of these capabilities, the cusum technique is not being widely utilized. This is perhaps due to the difficulty of establishing the technique in busy service laboratories when employed on a manual basis. Implementation via computer should permit its easier utilization.

Mean and Range Techniques. Statistical control procedures were first introduced in industry in the 1930's by Shewhart (1931). He recommended the use of two control charts, one for plotting the mean of a group of control observations and another for plotting the range or standard deviation. A detailed guide to the use of mean and range techniques in a clinical laboratory setting has been provided by Hainline (1982).

Mean and range charts have been limited in use in the clinical laboratory, but they should be given more consideration. They have very good performance characteristics. The probability for false rejection can be set at a chosen level by choice of control limits. For example, control limits for the mean can be chosen to provide 0.05, 0.01, or 0.002 probabilities for false rejection (see Table 1 in Westgard, 1977a), or any other specified value. Error detection is very good; in fact, these charts tend to be more sensitive than the previously discussed techniques. Computer-assisted implementation is probably the key to making these techniques practical for routine applications.

Trend Analysis. An interesting application of mean and standard deviation charts has been developed based on a trend analysis technique (Cambrowski, 1975). By use of an exponential smoothing calculation, new estimates of the mean and standard deviation can be obtained each time a new control observation is added, rather than waiting for a whole group of observations to be obtained and processed as a batch. The most recent observation is weighted most heavily in the calculation, and older observations gradually diminish in importance as their age increases. The estimates for the mean and standard deviation can be plotted on control charts and also tested for significant change (see description of techniques in Westgard, 1981b).

Trend analysis techniques of this kind are impractical unless implemented on computers. Fortunately, the micro-computers widely available now can provide the necessary capabilities. Programs are available to perform trend analysis, making these rather complicated procedures easy to use in clinical laboratories (Westgard, 1982).

Analysis of Variance Techniques. A more thorough analysis of the characteristics of a group of control observations can be made by applying more sophisticated statistical calculations, such as analysis of variance (ANOVA). The basic assumption underlying the use of control specimen results to monitor analytical variation is that the analytical variation obtained from the same control material is an accurate reflection of the analytical variation observed with patient specimens. There are reasons to believe that this assumption is not always correct: there may be additional variation in the control results due to such factors as instability of the control material, variation in reconstitution and aliquoting, or inconsistent handling of the material. Because of these problems, the calculated variance of daily control values might overestimate the day-to-day analytical variance from instrumental sources.

Analytical variance alone, however, can be theoretically computed using multiple control specimens. The ANOVA statistical model permits the partitioning of the variance due to "analytical sources" from the variance due to "control specimens." In practice, with each run of specimens at least two separate control pools should be assayed in replicate. The results are analyzed using a two-way analysis of variance model with the factors being "control material used" and "run number" (Winkel, 1976). This approach has been applied in the clinical setting, and the analysis of the results has been automated using a laboratory-based computer and the ANOVA program (Riddick, 1972).

Forms, Reports, and Records

Quality control programs generate large amounts of data, requiring a variety of forms to organize the data, reports to summarize the data, and records for documentation.

Raw Data Forms. The results from control specimens should be tabulated on a standard form designed for each analyte or each analytical system. Information should be entered for the name of the analyte or system, control material(s), and lot number(s). The form should have columns for each control material, time or date of analysis, the observed results, and space for comments. For the form to be used at the bench to monitor an analytical method, a range of acceptable values should be listed. It is common to use a range calculated as the mean plus/minus 2s (standard deviation) or the mean plus/minus 3s.

The Monthly Report Form. The monthly report form simply lists the mean, standard deviation, and coefficient of variation (CV) for the various controls and the expected mean value and acceptable CV for each procedure. The data are listed in columns, and a new column is added each month, so that prior and current values may be easily compared. It is convenient to arrange the test procedures by supervisory areas of responsibility. The monthly report is accompanied by a summary of apparent problems to be discussed at the supervisors' meeting.

Long-Term Records. The setting of ranges for evaluating the acceptability of the quality control results is a critical aspect of the quality control program. Gooszen (1960) has noted that when the ranges are too narrow there will be frequent out-of-range results, tests will appear to be frequently "out-of-control," and concerned laboratory personnel may spend an inordinate amount of time and effort pursuing insignificant problems. On the other hand, if the ranges are too wide, few out-of-range results will be observed, the test will appear always to be "in-control," and significant problems may go unnoticed. For these reasons, it is customary to define two limits for evaluating results: "warning limits" representing ± 2 standard deviation intervals from the expected value of a control specimen, and "action limits" representing ± 3 standard deviation intervals (Henry, 1959). On a statistical basis, about 19 of every 20 values should be expected to fall within the warning limits, and values exceeding the action limits should rarely be observed unless a real analytical change has occurred (Copeland, 1978b).

The data accumulated on successive monthly reports are an important source of information for setting practical ranges for acceptability of control results.

This policy, when applied to all procedures performed by the laboratory, assures that the established ranges will be realistic, that frequent out-of-range values will be indicative of real problems that merit attention, and that the laboratory's standards for performance must remain constant, or, improve, but may not be relaxed.

Events and Action Records (Mistakes). If it is accepted that quality control specimens can be reproducibly prepared and that practical limits for analytical variability can be established, then it must be accepted that reported values which exceed these limits are exceptional and noteworthy. It is helpful to record the occurrence of these events and, whenever possible, to investigate their causes and to record the corrective action that was taken. Such investigations will reveal that many of these out-of-range values are due to mistakes. When a mistake is found with a control specimen, there is a good likelihood that one or more clinical specimens were also involved, and efforts should be made to identify the specimens involved and correct the mistake. Control specimens make up a small fraction of the laboratory's total workload, and they cannot possibly detect all mistakes. However, the data accumulated in the "Events and Action Book" can be used to estimate the *frequency* of occurrence of mistakes in various work areas of the laboratory and can serve as a reminder to laboratory personnel to be alert to the probability of mistakes. The data of the Events and Action Book should be reviewed periodically and included with the quality control report.

INTRALABORATORY QUALITY CONTROL (INTERNAL QUALITY CONTROL) BASED ON PATIENT SPECIMENS

The reference sample approach to quality control (i.e., the use of identical samples over a long period of time) is widely used because it provides the laboratory with a rather constant frame of reference for the evaluation of its performance. However, commercial control specimens do not exactly simulate genuine clinical specimens, and occasionally changes in the control specimen (e.g., a loss of glucose) may incorrectly lead the laboratory personnel to believe that their analytical method is "out of control." In addition, the analytical biases observed with clinical specimens may not be identical to those observed with control specimens.

In the case of patient specimens, one must take into account the pre-instrumental sources of variation, including specimen collection, specimen transport, and specimen preparation. These same sources of variation are not present in the case of control material. For these reasons, a number of approaches of quality control (quality assurance) using the results observed on patient specimens have been proposed. They include determining the daily mean of certain patient results, using one or more arithmetic checks on multiple results obtained on the same specimen, comparing the "present result" with any previous results from the same patient, noting apparently absurd results and "alert values," evaluating the combination of multiple results for unusual patterns, and assaying randomized duplicate patient specimens. Each of these approaches will be presented.

The Daily Mean

Waid (1955) and Hoffmann (1965) have postulated that if a significant analytical change occurs in a test procedure, that change should be reflected in the clinical data. They proposed several techniques (average of all values, average of values in the reference interval, number of values greater than the mode) for detecting changes in the frequency distribution of the clinical assay values. Although these procedures are basically attractive because they deal with clinical specimens, they have not been widely adopted. Several studies have shown the methods to be relatively insensitive to changes in analytical bias (Henry, 1959; Van Peenen, 1965; Frankel, 1967; Kilgariff, 1968; Amador, 1968). The reason these methods are insensitive may be understood by considering that for many analytes, the clinical assays include values both above and below the reference interval. When either constant or proportional biases are introduced (see Fig. 6–1), some clinical assays will move into the reference interval while others will move out, and the number of values within the central portion of the distribution curve will tend to remain constant (Kilgariff, 1968). In addition, many analytical systems employ the technique known as "single-point calibration." This technique is subject to combined constant and proportional systematic biases, and the "operational line" may pivot about the calibration value (see Fig. 6–1*D*). As the calibration point is often near the mean value of the clinical specimens, most clinical assays will be relatively unchanged even when the method is clearly biased at other concentrations. It is quite possible that in the routine operation of the clinical laboratory, a subtle combination of compensatory biases affects the clinical assays, making the detection of the biases from examination of the clinical data quite difficult. Nevertheless, a number of authors have reported successful application of the techniques, particularly when large biases were present (Dixon, 1970; Begtrup, 1971; Berry, 1973).

Arithmetic Check

Examination of clinical assays does have much value in the detection of mistakes. Whitehurst (1975) has described a computer-assisted program in which the clinical assay results are examined in several ways to detect questionable values. The arithmetic check compares two or more results from the same specimen that are related. For example, the difference between the major anions and cations of serum (i.e., the anion gap) was found most commonly to have a value between 10 and 21 mmol/L.

Let us take the situation where S-sodium = 140 mmol/L, S-potassium = 5 mmol/L, S-bicarbonate = 26 mmol/L, and S-chloride = 100 mmol/L. In such a case the anion gap would be 145 minus 126, or 19 mmol/L.

The analysis as described by Whitehurst (1975) is automated using a computer program. According to the program, differences of less than 10.0 mmol/L or greater than 21 mmol/L are written into the discrepancy file for eventual computer printout. For checking acid-base calculation, actual bicarbonate and total CO_2 are calculated from pH and PCO_2 values by means of the Henderson-Hasselbalch equation, and the calculated values are compared with the observed values. In an analgous manner, when one knows the concentration values of serum sodium, urea, and glucose, one can compute a calculated osmolality and compare this value with the observed serum osmolality. The presence of significant discrepancies may not always be an indicator of analytical error; however, they should be cause for concern and further investigation.

Previous Value Check

The previous value check compares the result obtained for one specimen with the previous result(s) obtained for the same patient. Limits for the usual differences between specimens are entered into the computer program, and specimens having differences greater than these limits are listed for review by laboratory personnel. Here knowledge of the magnitude of the total (physiologic and analytical) intraindividual variation under various conditions is critical (see Chap. 4). The limits can be based solely on a statistical model and the width of the interval is dependent upon the probability value which one is using to decide if a measurement is outside the limits. Of course, finding such a result will not necessarily be associated with an analytical error. In fact, most often it is associated with a change in the disease course or a change in therapy. Some workers have used the term "delta check" to refer to this type of evaluation (Ladenson, 1975).

Alert Check and Absurd Values

The alert check is designed to detect large errors or very unlikely values. For example, serum urea values less than 1.0 mmol/L or greater than 18.0 mmol/L are listed by the computer for review by laboratory personnel. Absurd values must also be recognized; e.g., a serum potassium of 40.0 mmol/L may represent a value in which the decimal point had been misplaced.

Pattern Recognition

Lindberg (1965, 1966) has described the use of pattern recognition techniques to detect unlikely combinations of values. As examples, (1) urea, creatinine, and uric acid values or (2) sodium, potassium, chloride, and bicarbonate values are found to occur in clinical specimens in distinctive combinations, and the frequency of these various combinations can be calculated. The laboratory director should be aware of unusual combinations, e.g., grossly elevated serum alanine aminotransferase in association with a "normal" serum aspartate aminotransferase. An additional example is the situation when the results of the visual inspection of erythrocytes in a blood smear do not correspond to the values of red blood cell indices (see Chap. 29). When such unusual combinations occur, the possibility of laboratory error should be considered.

In all the cases presented, the laboratory-based computer could be programmed to detect unusual combinations of laboratory values. These various data analysis procedures are basically systems for checking and cross-checking the clinical assays for known internal consistencies, and for identifying unusual values. Whitehurst (1975) found that with his system, 8.4 per cent of all clinical assays were listed by the computer for review, 1.9 per cent of the specimens were re-analyzed, and 0.83 per cent were judged to be erroneous.

Randomized Duplicate Specimens

An additional technique, which is useful for *occasional* checks of the reproducibility of a laboratory's analyses, is the use of randomized duplicate specimens (Bokelund, 1974). This technique is applied to serum analytes as follows: (1) Two blood specimens are obtained per venipuncture. (2) Each specimen is uniquely labeled and uniquely processed. (3) All specimens in a batch are placed in a randomized order. (4) The technologist is not informed as to which two samples are members of a duplicate pair. (5) The specimens are assayed for the analyte(s) of interest and the results are recorded. (6) The within-batch random analytical variation is computed on the basis of the "difference of duplicates" approach. (7) Whenever the absolute difference in duplicate values for any particular pair of results is greater than a predefined limit, both specimens are reassayed. The limit is based on the calculated standard deviation. (8) If the difference of the reassayed duplicates is still greater than the limit, the cause for the "apparent discrepancy" is sought. (9) If the difference is within the limit, the average of two replicates is computed and the resultant mean value is sent out to the requesting physician.

The use of randomized duplicates for monitoring within-batch quality assurance has certain advantages. Randomization of the specimens within a batch (as compared to the case where one replicate specimen follows the other) should overcome any possible correlation between "time of assay" and the "order of the specimen"; i.e., any general analytic drift occurring during the assaying of the batch of specimens will be included. In addition, the use of duplicates obtained at venipuncture allows estimation of the *total* (preinstrumental and instrumental) within-batch analytical variation. Thus, this approach provides a realistic assessment of total variability in the entire analytical process and should give a greater degree of confidence in the quality of each particular measurement reported from the laboratory. Of course, the cost-benefit of this approach may be questioned; however, the availability of laboratory-based computers and analyzers with very high throughputs might make this method cost effective.

INTERLABORATORY COMPARISON PROGRAMS (EXTERNAL QUALITY CONTROL)

At present there are two principal types of programs in which laboratories may compare their analytical results. There are *survey programs* (proficiency testing) in which large numbers of laboratories analyze the same specimens several times each year, and there are *regional quality control programs* in which a group of laboratories in a geographical region use the same lots of quality control specimens on a daily basis for their internal quality control programs. The first of the survey programs was initiated in the late 1940's by Sunderman, and the most successful of these (The College of American Pathologists Survey Program) has grown to include more than 9000 of the approximately 13,000 clinical laboratories in the United States as well as several hundred laboratories in other countries (Gilbert, 1975). The first regional quality control program was started by Preston in 1967 (Lawson, 1976). There are now many such regional programs, and by 1981 over 50 per cent of all laboratories in the United States participated in these programs. Thus, both regional quality control programs and survey programs are widely used by clinical laboratories to facilitate interlaboratory comparisons of analyses.

Regional Quality Control Programs

These programs are available from the major manufacturers of quality control specimens, as well as from various professional societies. In a typical program each participant receives a stock of quality control serum that is to be analyzed on a daily basis over a period of about one year. The analytical results are sent weekly or monthly to the supplier of the program for entry into a computer, and the participant receives a monthly report that compares the mean value and standard deviation of his analyses with those of peer laboratories—i.e., laboratories that use a comparable analytical method. Most of these programs also supply computer-generated Levey-Jennings graphs of the data with ample room for the laboratory personnel to manually plot current results. This type of program is very useful to smaller laboratories that lack the personnel or computer facilities to perform the statistical calculations or to prepare the graphs that are necessary to maintain their internal quality control program.

Regional quality control programs are necessarily limited in size because of limitations in the volume of serum that can be processed to prepare the control specimens. However, some of these regional quality control programs have been integrated through the College of American Pathologists (CAP) Computer Center. That is, the data from various regional programs are processed by the CAP computer center. In this way the data from the various programs, even though based on the use of several different serum pools, may be combined for detailed statistical analyses. These data may be used by the individual laboratories in evaluating their acceptable limits for quality control specimens in their internal control program as well as being an indicator of the current level of performance of laboratories throughout the country.

Survey Programs

Although there are many clinical chemistry survey programs available to laboratories through governmental, private, and professional agencies, the program developed by the College of American Pathologists is the largest in scope and is probably the most sophisticated at the present time. Participants in the program receive several specimens several times each year for analysis, and return their results to the CAP Computer Center. Shortly thereafter each participant receives a report that compares this reported value with the mean and standard deviation obtained by peer laboratories, the number of peer laboratories, and the "SDI" of the reported value. (The SDI is the *S*tandard *D*eviation *I*nterval, i.e., the difference between the reported value and mean value, divided by the standard deviation. An SDI of -0.4 means that the reported value is 0.4 standard deviation unit below the group mean value.) Reported values that differ excessively from the mean value are flagged to alert the participant to the possibility of an analytical error. In addition to this statistical summary, each participant receives a concise summary of the performance of all methods for each analyte covered in the survey. The summary lists results according to all method/instrument combinations that were used by 20 or more laboratories. The complete participant report includes data for each of more than 20 analytes. This kind of report provides an overview of the field at the time of each survey and is valuable to participants because it indicates the popularity of various methods and the relative bias and variability of the various methods as they are actually used in the field. As such summaries are provided with each survey, the popularity and performance characteristics of each method over a period of time are continuously documented.

In addition to the regular participant report and method summaries, an annual report (called Survey Data) is also prepared for the participants. The specimens used in the CAP Survey Program are sometimes prepared to have subtle interrelationships. The survey specimens are mailed during the year in various combinations that may include duplicate specimens, interrelated specimens, or unrelated specimens. It is possible to statistically analyze the data from such specimens to obtain estimates of the intra- and interlaboratory variability of analyses, as well as the relative bias between analytical methods as a function of analyte concentration. Such data are most valuable to laboratories and to instrument/reagent manufacturers in comparing the analytical performance of various methods.

There are two other aspects of the CAP Survey Program that have important bearing on quality assurance. First, the specimens used in the survey program are manufactured in excess of survey needs, and after each survey is completed the excess serum is made available as a survey-validated reference material (SVRM). Thus, this reference serum is continuously renewed with each survey, is nationally available, and has consensus mean values assigned for more than 20 analytes and for all methods used by 20 or more laboratories. This reference serum has many practical uses for trouble-shooting analytical problems, comparing methods, or checking analytic values assigned to other reference, calibration, or quality control products. The consensus mean values attached to these reference sera have been evaluated for reliability (Gilbert, 1976; Grannis, 1976) and some specimens have been analyzed by the National Bureau of Standards using definitive (absolute) methods for some constituents (Gilbert, 1978). Second, laboratories that participate in the CAP Inspection and Accreditation Program receive a quarterly report that lists those tests for which the laboratory's reported results differed significantly from the consensus mean value. The report lists all such results for the preceding three years, unless satisfactory results were obtained in four successive surveys. This report serves to alert the laboratory to possible problem areas. As the inspection and accreditation procedure includes a review of such tests, an effective mechanism is established for assuring that these apparent problem areas will receive attention.

Youden Plots

Youden (1960) presented a novel approach in plotting the results obtained from each of two control specimens sent out to various laboratories. The range of possible results of the one specimen, e.g., the "lower level," is marked on the abscissa (x-axis) and the range of the possible results of the second specimen, e.g., the "higher level," is marked on the ordinate (y-axis). The results from many laboratories are plotted on the same graph. The interlaboratory means and standard deviations are computed. The two scales are adjusted so that the actual measured distances of the standard deviations are the same for the two specimens.

Assuming that the mean values of the results represent a reasonable estimate of the "true values," one can determine how his laboratory performed as compared with other laboratories. Furthermore, one can verify the possibility of a consistent positive bias (right upper quadrant of the Youden plot) or of a consistent negative bias (left lower quadrant of the Youden plot). The relationship of the Youden plot to various kinds of operational lines (Fig. 6–1*A* to *D*) has been described (Grannis, 1977).

ACCURACY CONTROL

The maintenance of analytical accuracy (i.e., reproducible method calibration) over extended periods of time is important. Each new analytical method introduced into the laboratory must undergo strict reliability checks before it is used clinically. After being placed into use, a method may become inaccurate (biased) for many reasons, and it is helpful to monitor and occasionally confirm the method's "operational line." This may be done by plotting the difference between the laboratory's monthly mean and the expected value, for each control material (Grannis, 1977). The difference should, of course, be zero. Accuracy problems sometimes arise owing to the widespread use of secondary serum calibrators for some analytical systems. It may be found that the assigned values for some lots of such calibrators are not consistent with those of other lots. When this occurs, the appropriate caliber value may be determined by concomitant analysis with the prior lot of calibrator, as well as with CAP Survey Serum or other well-assayed serum products. Method calibration may also be checked for some analytes by dilution of such well-assayed sera with diluents having weighed-in concentrations of analytes (Grannis, 1978). Using this technique, the method calibration may be checked for correspondence to peer laboratories that established the mean value of the Survey Serum, as well as for ability to recover known amounts of added analyte. In addition, well-defined reference methodologies are becoming available, and these should be useful in providing a reliable reference base from which to determine appropriate calibrator values.

Changes in method calibration may occur when any part of the analytical system is altered, as, for example, by the replacement of instrument parts or the introduction of new reagents or standards. Whenever these kinds of changes are made they should be documented in a log book and the quality control results must be examined critically for the appearance of method bias. In addition, it is good laboratory practice to determine reference values on a defined population of apparently healthy subjects at least annually (Copeland, 1974).

AN INTEGRATED APPROACH TO QUALITY ASSURANCE

We have presented a variety of quality assurance techniques that are available to laboratories. The extent of use of these techniques in any one laboratory will depend on the size and scope of that laboratory's services. However, regardless of the actual techniques used, all quality control programs should include a regular critical review of laboratory performance. The laboratory director, quality control coordinator, chief technologist, and section supervisors should meet regularly to evaluate the quality of measurements produced by the laboratory. On a monthly basis this group should have available various indicators of performance such as the statistical summaries of various control specimens, the control charts for those procedures in which significant change has occurred, and records of results obtained in proficiency survey programs. The possible causes of particular problems are discussed and corrective actions proposed. First, it must be recognized that a problem exists, then the nature of the problem must be clarified, and finally specific remedial action must be developed. When there are inconsistencies in results on performance using control specimens versus patient specimens, these may be explained on the basis of the obvious differences in the preinstrumental sources of variation for the two types of specimens.

The regular review of quality control data by the

senior laboratory staff serves to focus attention on significant laboratory problems and to assure that the problems will be addressed. In the course of such meetings, as the resolution of problems is documented and various laboratory policies are evolved, a confidence in the quality of the laboratory's performance develops. This confidence, which is based on documented, objective data, is necessary for making the many decisions that must be made in the daily operation of the laboratory. The most critical decisions involve whether to release particular batches of results to the requesting physicians. These decisions are aided by full knowledge of the usual analytical performance of the laboratory. Quality control programs provide the objective data base from which these decisions may be made with confidence. And it is through making the correct decisions that the physician-user is assured of the quality of the laboratory result. It should be emphasized that the laboratorian must be sensitive to feedback from the clinics and wards, i.e., is the laboratory result of the patient's specimen consistent with the clinical findings?

ANALYTICAL GOALS IN CLINICAL CHEMISTRY

From an idealistic viewpoint, quantitative clinical laboratory measurements should be highly accurate and precise. But it is a practical reality that the methods and techniques in common use have various degrees of analytical bias and variability. Intra- and interlaboratory quality control programs provide a means for assessing the magnitude of bias and variability of various methods and for documenting changes in quality of performance, but they do not indicate whether laboratory results are in fact sufficiently accurate and precise for maximum clinical usefulness. The basic question we will now consider is "How accurate and precise must clinical laboratory measurements be in order to provide the most clinically useful results?"

Accuracy Goals

Few workers in the clinical laboratory field have attempted to define goals for analytical accuracy. Rather, mechanisms have evolved that assure that analytical biases will, in the course of time, become minimal. For example, the College of American Pathologists' Survey Program provides an excellent assessment of the relative bias among various methods.

As reliable knowledge of the magnitude of analytical bias of various methods becomes known, we may expect the clinical laboratory field to voluntarily adopt such methods that show the least bias and are most cost-effective. Interlaboratory programs provide the data which document these changes in the field and such data provide abundant evidence that inferior methods are readily abandoned as improved methods become available (Gilbert, 1977).

Precision Goals

The question of how precise clinical analyses should be was addressed at a recent conference (Elevitch, 1977). Clinical analyses are used in various medical situations, but the most precise analyses are required when an individual's present value is to be compared with his prior value and a decision must be made as to whether a real change has occurred. Quite clearly, in this situation the laboratory's analytical variability must be less than the intraindividual physiologic variability. The conference recommended the goal that analytical variance ultimately should not exceed one fourth of the physiologic variance. The magnitude of physiologic variability for many analytes has been determined (see Chap. 4), and consequently the maximum desired analytical variability can be calculated. Table 6–3 compares the average coefficient of variation

Table 6–3. COMPARISON OF AVERAGE COEFFICIENTS OF VARIATION (CV) OBSERVED IN THE 1975 CAP SURVEY PROGRAM WITH THE DESIRED ANALYTICAL COEFFICIENT OF VARIATION*

Analyte in Serum	Analyte Concentration	Observed Analytical CV	Desired Analytical CV†
Calcium	2.75 mmol/liter	4.2	0.9
Chloride	110 mmol/liter	2.5	1.1
Cholesterol	6.5 mmol/liter	5.9	2.4
Creatinine	180 μmol/liter	11.7	2.2
Glucose	5.5 mmol/liter	5.4	2.2
Phosphate	1.5 mmol/liter	6.6	2.9
Potassium	3.0 mmol/liter	2.8	2.2
Sodium	130 mmol/liter	1.6	0.4
Protein, total	70 g/liter	3.6	1.5
Urea	10 mmol/liter	9.2	6.2
Urate	350 μmol/liter	6.6	3.7

*Adapted from Elevitch, F. (ed.): Analytical Goals in Clinical Chemistry. Skokie, Ill. College of American Pathologists, 1977.

†Based on the intra-individual day-to-day physiologic variation; that is, the "desired analytical coefficient of variation" is computed as one-half the mean physiologic coefficient of variation (see Chap. 5).

observed in a recent CAP survey with the coefficient of variation desired for maximum clinical usefulness, and it is apparent that for most analytes the average analytical variation at present is somewhat larger than required for maximum clinical utility, at least when following a patient's results sequentially (Elevitch, 1977).

An alternative approach, used to set performance goals for the analytical variation, is to survey clinicians in terms of asking, "At a defined, narrow concentration range, what do you consider to be the minimum change in the concentration of the analyte which would precipitate a change in your treatment/diagnostic plan?" Barnett (1977), Skendzel (1978), and Elion-Gerritzen (1978) have conducted investigations with practicing physicians to determine what levels of precision are utilized. The results of their studies, combined with the results of the regional quality control values throughout the USA compiled by Ross (1976), Gilbert (1975), Kurtz (1977), and Copeland (1978a), yield the major conclusions: that for the most frequently used assays—serum glucose, creatinine, urea, nitrogen, sodium, potassium—the physician's need for precision is easily met by the laboratory; cholesterol and triglyceride measurements meet the requirements, but calcium measurements do not meet the desired precision goals.

SUMMARY

Powerful techniques for monitoring, assessing, and improving the quality of quantitative laboratory measurements have been developed and are widely used by clinical laboratories. Through their participation in interlaboratory comparison programs, the laboratories collectively generate a massive data base that provides information about the analytical bias and variability of the various methods that are in common use. With these data individual laboratories and manufacturers of analytical systems may make informed decisions as to which instrument and method they prefer to use. Through their participation the laboratories also collectively create well-assayed sera that are continually renewed and have well-characterized target values for all of the common analytes. These sera have use in aiding the solution of various problems brought to light in intralaboratory quality control programs, and as reference materials for checking the validity of target values assigned to other reference, calibration, or control materials. As intra- and interlaboratory monitoring programs are ongoing endeavors, they serve continuously to document development of the clinical laboratory field as it evolves toward the goal of fully reliable laboratory measurements. Over the coming years, there will be an increasing greater reliance on the personal small computer to automate many of the data-handling procedures done now in the manual mode.

Allen, J. R., Earp, R., Farrell, C. E., and Gruemer, H. D.: Analytical bias in a quality control scheme. Clin. Chem., *15*:1039, 1969.

Amador, E.: Quality control by the reference sample method. Am. J. Clin. Path., *50*:360, 1968.

Barnett, R. N.: Analytical goals in clinical chemistry. Pathologist, *31*:319, 1977.

Begtrup, H., Leroy, S., Thyregod, P., and Wallow-Hansen, P.: Average of normals used as control of accuracy, and a comparison with other controls. Scand. J. Clin. Lab. Invest., *27*:247, 1971.

Belk, W. P., and Sunderman, F. W.: A survey on the accuracy of chemical analysis in clinical laboratories. Am. J. Clin. Path., *17*:854, 1947.

Berry, A. J., Lott, J. A., and Grannis, G. F.: NADH preparations as they affect reliability of serum lactate dehydrogenase determinations. Clin. Chem., *19*:1255, 1973.

Bokelund, H., Winkel, P., and Statland, B. E.: Factors contributing to intraindividual variation of serum constitutents: 3. Use of randomized duplicates to evaluate sources of analytic error. Clin. Chem., *20*:1507, 1974.

Cembrowski, G. S., Westgard, J. O., Eggert, A. A., and Toren, E. C., Jr.: Trend detection in control data: Optimization and interpretation of Trigg's technique for trend analysis. Clin. Chem., *21*:1396, 1975.

Copeland, B. E., Day, K., Shruhan, C., and Doherty, A.: Long term human reference values in a specific age range: Report of five years' experience. J. Clin. Chem. Clin. Biochem., *5*:252, 1974.

Copeland, B. E.: 1978—An evaluation of the state of the art of the precision of clinical chemistry measurements compared with the state of the art of medical decision making. Panel on Laboratory of the Council on Scientific Affairs. Chicago, American Medical Association, 1978a.

Copeland, B. E., Rosvoll, R. V., and Casella, J. M.: Quality Control in Clinical Chemistry. 3rd ed. Chicago, Commission on Continuing Education. American Society of Clinical Pathologists, 1978b.

Dixon, K., and Northam, B. E.: Quality control using the daily mean. Clin. Chim. Acta, *30*:453, 1970.

Dorsey, D. B.: The evolution of proficiency testing in the U.S.A. *In* Proceedings of the Second National Conference on Proficiency Testing. Bethesda, Md., Information Services, 1975.

Elevitch, F. (ed.): Proceedings of the 1976 Aspen Conference on Analytical Goals in Clinical Chemistry. Skokie, Ill., College of American Pathologists, 1977.

Elion-Gerritzen, W. E.: Medical significance of laboratory results in relation to analytical performance. Thesis. Rotterdam, Erasmus University, 1978.

Frankel, S., and Ahrlen, R. C.: An evaluation of the number plus method of quality control. Am. J. Clin. Path., *37*:248, 1967.

Gilbert, R. K.: The perspective (on proficiency testing) of the College of American Pathologists. *In* Proceedings of the Second National Conference on Proficiency Testing. Bethesda, Md., Information Services, 1975, p. 15.

Gilbert, R. K.: A comparison of participant mean values of duplicate specimens in the CAP chemistry survey program. Am. J. Clin. Path., *66*:184, 1976.

Gilbert, R. K.: CAP interlaboratory survey data and analytic goals. *In* Elevitch, F. (ed.): Analytical Goals in Clinical Chemistry. Skokie, Ill., College of American Pathologists, 1977, p. 63.

Gilbert, R. K.: The accuracy of clinical laboratory study by comparison with definitive methods. Am. J. Clin. Path., *70*:450, 1978.

Gooszen, J. A. H.: The use of control charts in the clinical laboratory. Clin. Chim. Acta, *5*:431, 1960.

Grannis, G. F., Gruemer, H. D., Lott, J. A., Edison, J. A., and McCabe, W. C.: Proficiency evaluation of clinical chemistry laboratories. Clin. Chem., *18*:222, 1972.

Grannis, G. F.: Studies of the reliability of constituent target values established in a large inter-laboratory survey. Clin. Chem., *22*:1035, 1976.

Grannis, G. F., and Caragher, T. E.: Quality control programs in clinical chemistry. CRC Crit. Rev. Clin. Lab. Sci., *7*:327, 1977.

Grannis, G. F.: Use of survey validated reference materials to establish target values of quality control pools. Pathologist, *32*:96, 1978.

Groth, T., Falk, H., and Westgard, J. O.: An interactive computer simulation program for the design of statistical control procedures in clinical chemistry. Comput. Progr. Biomed., *13*:73, 1981.

Hainline, A., Jr.: Quality assurance: Theoretical and practical aspects. *In* Faulkner, W. R., and Meites, S. (eds.): Selected Methods for the Small Clinical Chemistry Laboratory. Washington, D.C., American Association for Clinical Chemistry, 1982.

Henry, R. J., and Segalove, M.: The running of standards in clinical chemistry and the use of the control chart. J. Clin. Path., *5*:305, 1952.

Henry, R. J.: Use of the control chart in clinical chemistry. Clin. Chem., *5*:309, 1959.

Hoffmann, R. G., and Waid, M. E.: The "average of normals" method of quality control. Am. J. Clin. Path., *43*:134, 1965.

Kilgariff, M., and Owen, J. A.: An assessment of the "average of normals" quality control method. Clin. Chim. Acta, *19*:175, 1968.

Kurtz, S., Copeland, B. E., and Straumfjord, J. J.: Guidelines for clinical chemistry quality control based on the long term experience of sixty-one university and tertiary care referral hospitals. Am. J. Clin. Path., *68*:463, 1977.

Ladenson, J. H.: Patients as their own controls: Use of the computer to identify "laboratory error." Clin. Chem., *21*:1648, 1975.

Lawson, N. S., and Haven, G. T.: The role of regional quality control programs in the practice of laboratory medicine in the United States. Am. J. Clin. Path., *66*:286, 1976.

Levey, S., and Jennings, E. R.: The use of control charts in the clinical laboratory. Am. J. Clin. Path., *20*:1059. 1950.

Lindberg, D. A., Van Peenen, H. J., and Couch, R.: Patterns in clinical chemistry. Am. J. Clin. Path., *44*:315, 1965.

Lindberg, D. A., and Van Peenen, H. J.: The meaning of quality control with multiple chemical analysis. *In* Skeggs, L. T., Jr. (ed.): Automation in Analytical Chemistry. New York, Mediad, 1966, p. 433.

Riddick, J. H., Flora, R., and Van Meter, Q. L.: Computerized preparation of two-way analysis of variance control charts for clinical chemistry. Clin. Chem., *18*:250, 1972.

Ross, J. W., and Fraser, M. D.: The effect of analyte and concentration upon precision estimates in clinical chemistry. Am. J. Clin. Path., *66*:193, 1976.

Sax, S. M., Dorman, L., Lebenson, D. D., and Moore, J. J.: Design and operation of an expanded system of quality control. Clin. Chem., *13*:825, 1967.

Shewhart, W. A.: Economic Control of Quality of Manufactured Products. New York, D. Van Nostrand Co., 1931.

Shuey, H. E., and Cebel, J.: Bull. U.S. Army Med. Dept., *9*:799, 1949.

Skendzel, L. P.: How physicians use laboratory tests. J.A.M.A., *239*:1077, 1978.

Statland, B. E.: Decision Levels for Laboratory Testing. Oradell, N.J., Medical Economics Company, 1983.

Sunderman, F. W., and Boerner, F.: Normal Values in Clinical Medicine. Philadelphia, W. B. Saunders Company, 1949.

Survey Data 1975, R. K. Gilbert (ed.). Skokie, Ill., College of American Pathologists, 1976.

Van Peenen, H. J., and Lindberg, D. A. B.: The limitations of laboratory quality control with reference to the "number plus" method. Am. J. Clin. Path., *44*:322, 1965.

Waid, M. E., and Hoffmann, R. G.: The quality control of laboratory precision. Am. J. Clin. Path., *25*:585, 1955.

Westgard, J. O.: Better quality control through microcomputers. Diagnost. Med., *5*:60, 1982.

Westgard, J. O., Barry, P. L., Hunt, M., and Groth, T.: A multi-rule Shewhart chart for quality control in clinical chemistry. Clin. Chem., *27*:493, 1981a.

Westgard, J. O., and Groth, T.: Power functions for statistical control rules. Clin. Chem., *25*:863, 1979.

Westgard, J. O., and Groth, T.: Design and evaluation of statistical control procedures: Applications of a computer 'Quality Control Simulator' program. Clin. Chem., *27*:1536, 1981b.

Westgard, J. O., and Groth, T.: A predictive value model for quality control: Effects of the prevalence of errors on the performance of control procedures. Am. J. Clin. Path., *80*:49, 1983.

Westgard, J. O., Groth, T., Aronsson, T., Falk, H., and de Verdier, C-H.: Performance characteristics for rules for internal quality control.: Probabilities for false rejection and error detection. Clin. Chem., *23*:1857, 1977a.

Westgard, J. O., Groth, T., Aronsson, T., and de Verdier, C.-H.: Combined Shewhart-cusum control chart for improved quality control in clinical chemistry. Clin. Chem., *23*:1881, 1977b.

Whitehurst, P., DiSilvio, T. V., and Boyadjian, G.: Evaluation of discrepancies in patients' results—An aspect of computer-assisted quality control. Clin. Chem., *21*:87, 1975.

Winkel, P., and Statland, R. E.: Two novel approaches combined for quality assurance in the routine clinical chemistry laboratory. Clin. Chem., *22*:1216, 1976.

Woodard, R. H., and Goldsmith, P. L.: Cumulative Sum Techniques. ICI Monograph No. 3. Edinburgh, Oliver and Boyd, 1964.

Wootton, I. D. P., and King, E. J.: Normal values for blood constitutents: Inter-hospital differences. Lancet, *1*:470, 1953.

Youden, W. I.: The sample, the procedure and the laboratory. Anal. Chem., *32*:23A, 1960.

1

3

STATISTICAL TESTS

ROY N. BARNETT, M.D.

1

The manipulation of numerical data which we call statistics is an essential tool in the clinical laboratory. This introductory chapter will serve as a reminder of common concepts particularly applicable to the laboratory; it is not a substitute for an elementary statistics course. Occasional reference is made to other sections of the book where more intensive discussions of specific topics are found.

GENERAL COMMENTS

Only a select few persons think in terms of formulas and mathematical terms. The rest of us think in logical non-arithmetic formulations; this section is written primarily for the latter group.

Arithmetic manipulations have been vastly simplified and expedited by the development of powerful and inexpensive pocket-calculators; these are necessary for statistical calculations. Such calculators determine averages and square roots to many decimal places, a highly desirable step. Before such instruments were available it was necessary to actively encourage carrying out all calculations to at least two places beyond the original figures to avoid the magnification of "rounding-off" errors when numbers are squared. For example we know that plasma glucose is originally calculated to whole numbers, such as 101 mg/dl. However, the average of a series of such values should be carried to at least two decimal places, and if the electronic circuits go to eight places no harm is done.

It is still possible to make arithmetic errors, usually by punching the wrong key, so results should always be double checked. In addition, it is desirable to inspect the numbers to avoid idiotic errors. This permits questioning of results which could be wrong entries as well as applying logic. If the values or conclusions are not in accord with your experience, they should be questioned, no matter how impressive the calculations appear. If, for example, someone claims to achieve a 2 per cent coefficient of variation for an analysis for which you never could do better than 10 per cent, be suspicious. Even looking at the raw data may not solve the mystery; perhaps all the poor results were omitted!

It is also worth noting whether variability of results is due to consistent imprecision or to a few erratic results markedly different from the others. In the first case there is a predictable phenomenon which can be used as the basis for future prediction; in the second case there is erratic performance which cannot be trusted for predictions.

Another excellent way of checking the validity of numbers is by inspection of graphic representations of either individual values or groups of values. Are they distributed as a bell-shaped curve, or are there several peaks, or does the distribution appear quite random? Are there one or more "outliers" which do not appear to be from the same population as the other values?

In inspecting graphs it is useful to check the scale on each axis. It is all too easy to magnify small differences, to minimize large ones, or to make straight lines out of curves by manipulating the scales, particularly through logarithmic transformations. Such conversion may be perfectly legitimate, but you should be aware of them to fully understand the graph.

DEGREES OF FREEDOM

The number of degrees of freedom is the number of ways in which a series of numbers can vary independently. For example, the area of a rectangle is represented by the formula: Area = length × width. If we know that the area is 2 square meters and the length is 2 meters, the width is no longer an independent variable; it must be 1 meter. Or if we calculate the mean of four numbers as 5, the first three numbers being 5, 6, and 4, the fourth must be

5. Because we need to calculate the mean ($\bar{x}$) in calculating standard deviation, we use as a divisor n − 1 to allow for our prior loss of one degree of freedom. The arithmetical importance of this correction diminishes as the series becomes larger.

When we calculate the mean more than once, as in the unpaired t test, we subtract one degree of freedom for each such calculation.

THE NULL HYPOTHESIS AND PROBABILITY STATEMENTS

It is rarely possible to "prove" something by statistical techniques. What we can do is to calculate probabilities that some event could have been a random one and to make statements about this event or predictions about future events based on the greatest likelihood of their occurrence. The formulation of probability statements rests on the "null hypothesis," which states that there is *no* difference between two sets of values which are being compared. The calculated P value after statistical manipulations indicates the probability that there is *no* difference. If the P value is very small, we reject the null hypothesis.

For example, P = 0.01 indicates that such a result would occur only once if the experiment or experience were repeated 100 times. (Probability will be represented in this chapter by the capital P; there are other usages, and P has other meanings in other books.) Or we might write $0.05 > P > 0.01$, indicating that it would occur less often than five but more often than once in 100 tries. The usually chosen critical P values are 0.05 (called significant) and 0.01 (called highly significant). There is nothing sacrosanct about these numbers, but many useful reference tables have been worked out using them. Several facets of probability statements are worthy of further explication.

1. The fact that some event is unlikely (P value of 0.05 or less) does not mean that the event could not occur. It may be unusual for a flipped coin to come up heads ten times in a row, but this certainly can and will occur if you flip coins often enough.

2. It is imperative that there be a definition of what is being compared; e.g., the probability that two reagents give the same results is 0.01. When this is not specifically defined, the assumption is that the two series preceding the probability statement are being compared; unfortunately the author himself may not be certain about his meaning.

3. The level of the P value which should lead to a specific action depends on many factors, including the importance of the decision. For example, if we are seeking the cause of a patient's asthma and we suspect a certain pillow, we would be happy to accept P = 0.5, because all we are going to do is to enclose the pillow in a plastic cover. On the other hand, assume that a 50-year-old man, an inveterate cigarette smoker, develops a cough and bloody sputum and is found to have an abnormal shadow 2 cm in diameter on chest x-ray. We assume from these data that there is a 95 per cent chance that he has a primary lung carcinoma requiring removal of the affected lung. Conversely there is a 5 per cent chance that the lesion is a benign tumor, a metastatic malignant tumor, or an inflammatory lesion, for none of which will lung removal be necessary. Should we proceed with surgery, or should we do more tests to reduce our 5 per cent chance still further, to 4 per cent or 2 per cent? This particular dilemma, how far to go in reducing the chance of being wrong, is a constant occurrence in modern medical practice and greatly increases the costs of medical care.

4. The probability statement itself has an inherent imprecision, based largely on the number of observations or experiments performed to calculate the P value. It may be desirable to define this exactly, i.e., "The probability that these populations are the same is 0.05 (95 per cent confidence limits 0.03 to 0.07)." This facet is described further in Chapter 4 (p. 51).

5. The occurrence of an authentically small and relevant P value, i.e., 0.001, establishes the unlikelihood that the two populations are similar. It does *not* per se indicate that the difference is important. For example, we compare two glucose methods on 200 samples of human plasma. We find that the mean value by method A is 100 mg/dl and by method B is 101, P = 0.001. We can be quite certain that the methods do produce different results, B higher than A, but from the viewpoint of clinical relevance 1 mg is a negligible difference and would not lead to different diagnosis or treatment.

6. We may interpret the null hypothesis incorrectly. If we assume that the null hypothesis is false when it is indeed true, this is called a Type 1 or alpha error. If we assume that the null hypothesis is true when it is false, this is a Type 2 or beta error. To avoid these errors we may make our significant probability levels smaller, i.e., 0.01 rather than 0.05. However, such efforts to decrease one type of error inevitably lead to an increase in the other type. For example, we may find that the central 95 per cent of healthy persons' serum calcium values fall within the range 8.0 mg/dl to 10.2 mg/dl. This means that 2.5 per cent of individuals have a calcium level of over 10.2 mg/dl and are considered hypercalcemic. Therefore they are submitted to further diagnostic investigation. Because not many of these subjects turn out to have significant disease, we might decide this is too expensive so we will only consider the upper 0.6 per cent to be hypercalcemic, and so our upper limit of normal becomes 10.5 mg/dl. In so doing we are now calling "normal" persons whose serum calcium lies between 10.2 and 10.5, thereby missing a population of truly hypercalcemic persons whose values fall at the lower end of the hypercalcemic range. Thus in order to decrease Type 2 errors we increase Type 1 errors. This is also illustrated in Figure 3–1 for enzymes; it is easy to visualize in this figure the effect of moving the critical level from left to right.

TESTS TO COMPARE TWO SERIES OF VALUES

The usual statistical problem is to compare two or more series of numbers to determine whether they are similar or dissimilar. To do this we calculate for each

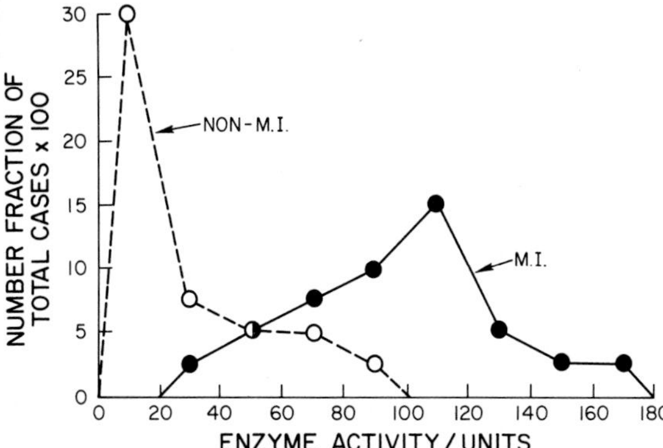

Figure 3–1. Distribution of enzyme activity values for the class of patients independently known to have suffered a myocardial infarction (MI) presented as closed circles and for the class of patients independently known *not* to have suffered a myocardial infarction (non-MI) presented as open circles. It is assumed that the prevalence of myocardial infarction in the total population is 50 per cent. The mean enzyme activity in the class of patients with MI is 97 units. The mean enzyme activity in the class of patients with non-MI is 27 units. However, the overlap of the two groups is very apparent.

series the variability (variance, standard deviation) and the arithmetic mean. These are explained and the calculations illustrated in Chapter 4 (p. 53). These calculations rely on the assumption of a Gaussian distribution. Fortunately, despite the criticisms which have been leveled at this assumption (Elvebach, 1970), the Gaussian distribution is a "rugged" statistic, and small or even moderate deviations from it do not usually alter the inferences drawn to a significant degree.

The F Test

This test is used to answer the question, "Do the two series differ significantly in their variances (or standard deviations)?" After doing the prescribed calculations we compare the F value obtained to those in a table; if the F value exceeds the tabular value, it is correspondingly unlikely that the two series represent the same population. Put another way, the individual values in one series vary more from each other than do the values in the other series. Therefore one cannot reasonably compare the mean values (see t test). Fisher (1974) developed this test during agricultural experiments in which various treatments were given to crops; his question was, "Is the variability of crops given the new treatment significantly *greater* than that of crops given the old treatment?" Therefore the calculation was made as follows:

$$F = \frac{s^2 \text{ (new)}}{s^2 \text{ (old)}}$$

in which s = standard deviation. Only values greater than one were put in the table because he assumed that if the new treatment produced less variability, this was automatically satisfactory. Often in the clinical laboratory the calculation used is:

$$F = \frac{s^2 \text{ (larger)}}{s^2 \text{ (smaller)}}$$

When this is done the standard one-tailed F table (Pearson, 1966) must be converted to a two-tailed table; the 5 per cent becomes a 10 per cent and the 1 per cent becomes a 2 per cent table.

The F test is often used in the analytic laboratory when comparing new methods to old by repeated analyses of stable materials. Inferences may thereby be drawn as to the desirability of new methods based on precision estimates.

Abbreviated F Table

df	5%	1%
20	2.12	2.94

Values exceeding these critical values for 20 df in the numerator and in the denominator are significant at the levels indicated. Complete tables are widely available. Values close to the tabular levels indicate the need for more testing.

The t Test

"Students' " t test (Pearson, 1947) is used to compare the means of two series (or more than two if desired). It determines whether the two means are significantly different and employs the variability (standard deviation) in the calculation. If the two variabilities are significantly different as determined by the F test, it is not proper to calculate t values. If there is no significant difference in variability, we can then proceed with t test calculations, the form of which depends on the exact situation.

1. In the general form of the t test, we wish to know whether the mean value of series A is different from the mean value of series B. The observations going into each series differ and the number in each series may differ. For example, we wish to compare fasting plasma glucose in 50 control women and 40 diabetic women. The formula is:

$$t = \frac{|\bar{x}_A - \bar{x}_B|}{\left[\left[\frac{(n_A - 1)s_A^2 + (n_B - 1)s_B^2}{n_A + n_B - 2}\right]\left[\frac{1}{n_A} + \frac{1}{n_B}\right]\right]^{1/2}}$$

where $\bar{x}_A$ = mean of series A
$\bar{x}_B$ = mean of series B
n_A = number of observations in series A
n_B = number of observations in series B
s_A^2 = variance of series A
s_B^2 = variance of series B
$|\ |$ = the difference between; always a positive number

2. Paired observations are made on identical samples. For example, we analyze four plasma samples for glucose by two methods whose variability we have

demonstrated not to be significantly different by F test. The formula we use is:

$$t = \frac{\bar{d}\sqrt{n}}{s_d}$$

where $\bar{d}$ = mean difference between the two methods
n = number of samples analyzed
s_d = standard deviation of the differences between results by the two methods, calculated as

$$s_d = \left(\frac{\Sigma(d - \bar{d})^2}{n - 1}\right)^{1/2}$$

A sample calculation for s_d and the paired t test is shown in Table 3–1.

$$s_d = \left(\frac{\Sigma(d - \bar{d})^2}{n - 1}\right)^{1/2} = \left(\frac{5}{3}\right)^{1/2} = (1.667)^{1/2} = 1.29$$

$$t = \frac{\bar{d}(\sqrt{n})}{s_d} = \frac{2.5\sqrt{4}}{1.29} = \frac{5}{1.29} = 3.88$$

Looking at a two-tailed t table we find for 4 df the critical value at the 5 per cent probability level is 2.776. Therefore the t value of 3.88 is significant, and we can conclude that method B gives different (and higher) results than method A.

3. We wish to know whether there is a difference in the mean value of a standard material or analysis, known or assumed to be free of bias, and the mean value for some comparative material or analysis. Similar procedures are done on identical materials. The formula is:

$$t = \frac{|\bar{x} - K|\sqrt{n}}{s}$$

where $\bar{x}$ = mean for the test material or method
K = designated true value
n = number of tests performed
s = standard deviation for the test material or method

After the calculation by the appropriate method a t value is found. Values exceeding the tabular value for the appropriate df are used to disprove the null hypothesis that the means are not different.

The t test is primarily useful for small series of observations. If the series are large enough, any difference becomes significant statistically. Whether the difference is important in clinical laboratory practice is another matter and depends on value judgments not made by t tests, such as how physicians use tests, what the physiologic variations are, and so forth. The influence of the number of observations is well shown by a government survey of laboratory tests in which a method which gave results *closer* to the accepted truth was considered *worse* than one which gave results *further* from the truth (Barnett, 1974). This is a mathematical aberration occurring because many more laboratories used the first method, and one which illustrates the importance of knowing something about statistics before publishing articles based on statistics.

Abbreviated t Table

df	5%	1%
20	2.09	2.85

Values exceeding these critical values for 20 df are significant at the indicated levels. Complete tables are widely available. Values close to tabular values indicate the need for more testing.

Table 3–1. SAMPLE CALCULATION FOR s_d AND PAIRED t TEST

	Results				
Patient	*Method A*	*Method B*	d (difference)	$(d - \bar{d})$	$(d - \bar{d})^2$
J	10	11	−1	1.5	2.25
K	18	20	−2	0.5	0.25
L	22	26	−4	−1.5	2.25
M	8	11	−3	−0.5	0.25
	58	68			5.00
$\bar{x}$	14.5	17			

Bias = −2.5($\bar{d}$).

Chisquare Statistics

Chisquare is a useful statistic applied to counts of things. For example, if 20 of 40 men with prostatic carcinoma have elevated serum acid phosphatase (AP) levels, and 5 of 38 normal men have similar elevations, is this really different? The calculation given below assumes a Gaussian distribution and also depends on the null hypothesis. The tabular arrangement of data is made as follows:

a	b	a + b
c	d	c + d
a + c	b + d	n

where a = number of cancer patients with elevated AP
b = number of normal patients with elevated AP
c = number of cancer patients without elevated AP
d = number of normal patients without elevated AP
a + c = total number of cancer patients
b + d = total number of normal patients
n = total number of all patients

Filling in the actual numbers in the example we find:

20	5	25
20	33	53
40	38	78

Calculation is then made using the formula:

$$\chi^2 = \frac{n\left(|ad - bc| - \frac{n}{2}\right)^2}{(a + b)(c + d)(a + c)(b + d)}$$

Substituting:

$$\chi^2 = \frac{78\left(|660 - 100| - \frac{78}{2}\right)^2}{(20 + 5)(20 + 33)(20 + 20)(5 + 33)}$$

$$\chi^2 = \frac{78(560 - 39)^2}{25 \times 53 \times 40 \times 38} = \frac{78 \times 271{,}441}{2{,}014{,}000}$$

$$\chi^2 = \frac{21{,}172{,}398}{2{,}014{,}000} = 10.51$$

Abbreviated Chisquare Table for 1 df

5%	1%
3.84	6.63

Values exceeding the critical values for 1 df are significant at the indicated levels. Complete tables are widely available. Values near the tabular level indicate the need for further testing.

In the example the calculated chisquare of 10.51 exceeds the tabular value at a highly significant level. We have therefore rejected the null hypothesis that patients with prostatic carcinoma do not have acid phosphatase levels exceeding those of normal persons.

Chisquare should ordinarily not be used if any of the boxes for the reference values have numbers smaller than 5, or if either of the series has less than 20 individual numbers. When smaller series are to be used, e.g., 2 of 7 versus 4 of 5, one goes to 2 × 2 tables for testing significance in unequal samples (Natrella, 1976), or one may use other methods of calculation.

Additionally, if one is interested in comparing numbers which form a small proportion of a large population, e.g., 3 of 100, the Poisson distribution is more suitable and is discussed in statistics textbooks (see also Chap. 27, pp. 588, 591, and 593). When the proportion exceeds 10 per cent, the Poisson and the Gaussian distributions become quite similar.

*Correlation Coefficient (r Values)**

This is a widely used statistic which calculates whether two series of numbers are related positively (up to +1), negatively (down to −1), or not at all (0). For example, we might relate the number of cigarettes smoked per day to the risk of developing carcinoma of the lung. Suppose we found an r of 0.6. In the specific context this would be a very strong correlation for the two variables. It does not prove a causal relation; the relation could be coincidental, or related to an associated variable common to both cigarette smoking and to cancer of the lung, or it could fit with a causal relationship.

When we are comparing laboratory data, for example, the same quantitative analysis performed by two different methods, r values should be very near 1, i.e., 0.99 or higher, if the methods truly produce similar results. At one meeting I attended, the purveyor of a novel platelet-counting system proudly proclaimed an r value of 0.7 for his system versus the standard manual counts. On further calculation it became evident that a correct platelet count of 400,000 could actually be determined as anything between 200,000 and 600,000 by the novel method, which was therefore quite useless.

One other feature of r is the attribution of a P value to it. The smaller the P (i.e., 0.01), the more certain you are that there is a difference between the calculated r and 0. The small P value does not prove that the two series are closely or usefully correlated; this depends on the r value itself.

*See formula, Chapter 4, p. 54.

SPECIAL FORMS OF THE STANDARD DEVIATION

Standard Deviation of the Difference, s_d. This is another statistic used in comparing two series of numbers and calculates the spread of individual differences. In the clinical laboratory it is most valuable when one performs analyses of identical samples by two different methods and wishes to compare the results for their agreement. It is an essential part of the calculation of t values. The formula used is:

$$s_d = \left(\frac{\Sigma(d - \bar{d})^2}{n - 1}\right)^{1/2}$$

The bias (mean difference, $\bar{d}$) is subtracted from each individual difference d to ensure that the calculated variance represents only the random differences and not the systematic ones. The smaller this random variance is, the larger the t value will be and the more certain you are that the apparent bias is statistically significant (see t test, Formula 2).

The Standard Error, SE. The standard deviation is a measure of the dispersion of individual values about their mean. Suppose, however, our interest is in the variability of the mean itself, or of a series of means. As an example we find the mean serum uric acid level of 20 men to be 6.3 mg/dl with a standard deviation of 1.0, therefore a central 95 per cent range of 4.3 to 8.3. If we were to analyze the serum of several more groups of 20 men, how close would the means be? The standard deviation of means is called the standard error and is calculated as:

$$SE = \frac{s}{\sqrt{n}} \text{ for n observations}$$

Obviously the variability of means so figured will be smaller than the variability for individual men. In this instance standard error will be:

$$SE = \frac{1.0}{\sqrt{20}} = \frac{1.0}{4.47} = 0.224$$

The range will therefore be 5.85 to 6.75 for the central 95 per cent of the mean values. It would be wrong, however, to expect 95 per cent of individual male values to fall within these narrowed limits, an assumption which has regrettably been made in many published papers extolling the virtues of specific analyses.

ANALYSIS OF VARIANCE

Recall that the variance of a series of numbers is the sum of the squared differences from the mean divided by the degrees of freedom and can be portrayed by the formula:

$$s^2 = \frac{\Sigma(x - \bar{x})^2}{n - 1}$$

(See Chap. 5, p. 61.) If there are multiple (k) components of variability, the contribution of each can be calculated as s^2 (total) $= s^2$ (A) $+ s^2$ (B) $+ \ldots\ldots\ldots s^2$ (k). Further manipulation can be used to find s, but one cannot add and subtract s in the same fashion as s^2. To calculate each component in the formula above, we line up the results so that we can compare them for the single variables under question. To calculate the total variance we use the usual formula given above. After quantitating each known component there usually is a remainder which can be attributed to all of the unknown factors or to one which is assumed to be the only one left.

A good example of the fruitful use of analysis of variance is found in the work of Gilbert (1977) with College of American Pathologists Chemistry Survey Programs. He sent out survey samples so that identical unknown samples were sometimes analyzed in the same run and sometimes at relatively long intervals of three or six months. With stable samples the analysts should theoretically have secured identical results, but of course they did not. By calculating the method variances for the samples done at the same time in the same laboratory, those for samples done at the same time in different laboratories, and the total variance, he came up with the formula:

$$\sigma\, t = \sqrt{\sigma\, st^2 + \sigma\, lt^2 + \sigma\, bl^2 + \sigma\, sp^2}$$

where $\sigma\, t$ = the standard deviation of all the results submitted by all the laboratories
$\sigma\, st^2$ = short term within laboratory variance
$\sigma\, lt^2$ = long term within laboratory variance
$\sigma\, bl^2$ = between laboratory variance
$\sigma\, sp^2$ = variability associated with the specimens used for the analysis

Ordinarily $\sigma\, sp^2$ was assumed to be negligible on the basis of prior studies. The findings indicated that there was approximately an equal contribution by each of these components, varying by method, constituent, and time.

In more formal analysis of variance one makes use of the F ratios of each known variable to the remainder; significant ratios indicate that the specific variable is indeed significant (Barnett, 1979).

MISTAKES CANNOT BE PREDICTED STATISTICALLY

Considering the number of laboratory tests performed (billions), it is inevitable that some substantially incorrect values will be reported. The number of these which reflect the imprecision of the methods can be calculated; unfortunately these are the smallest fraction. The others can be considered as true mistakes. The opportunities for such errors or mistakes are almost limitless, at every point from incorrect patient preparation or wrong identification through analytic mix-ups to decimal point errors or illegible handwriting in the final report. (See Table 5–1, page 61, for a partial listing.) Is there any statistical approach which will pick up such errors?

Unfortunately there is no practical and reliable technique. *Delta checks,* in which patient results are compared with previous results for the same patient, should be useful; in practice they are cumbersome, require much computer time, and give mostly false alarms.

Outlier formulas do exist to help identify discordant values in a set of numbers whose distribution is predictable. Unfortunately we would rarely know when to use them in ordinary practice. Highly unlikely patient results, those which are not compatible with life, are recognized fairly readily and are then usually rechecked, as are other very abnormal values. However, most erroneous results are probably in the normal range because normal values are much more common than abnormals; detection of these may require considerable sleuthing, and most probably go undetected.

Fortunately most mistakes do not cause much trouble for patients. In the first place, laboratory test results are rarely the sole basis for definitive action by the physician but are only part of his whole information about the patient. Secondly, many laboratory results are ignored because of the information overload. Finally, an abnormal result so important that it should lead to action is usually repeated and the mistake thereby uncovered.

APPLICATION OF SOME COMMONLY USED STATISTICAL PROCEDURES AND PRECAUTIONS IN USING THEM

These are presented in Table 3–2.

Table 3–2. APPLICATION OF SOME COMMONLY USED STATISTICAL PROCEDURES AND PRECAUTIONS IN USING THEM

Application	Term	Precaution
I. Find center of a distribution		
Any distribution	Median	Not easy to work with
Distribution reasonably Gaussian	Arithmetic mean (average)	Easily influenced by large outliers or marked skewness
Distribution not Gaussian but skewed	Log mean or geometric mean	Must convert all raw numbers; distribution must thereby be made Gaussian
II. Find variability of a distribution		
Any distribution (indeterminate distribution)	Range	Crude but useful; difficult to use for further manipulations
Any distribution (indeterminate distribution)	Percentiles	Difficult to use for further manipulations
Distribution reasonably Gaussian	Variance	Markedly influenced by large outliers; can manipulate by adding or subtracting; requires conversion to standard deviation for quality control functions
Distribution reasonably Gaussian	Standard deviation	Markedly influenced by large outliers; cannot manipulate by adding or subtracting
Distribution reasonably Gaussian; to find variability of means of a series rather than of individual values	Standard error	Must not be used to indicate distribution of single values
Distribution is of discontinuous events forming a small fraction of the total (less than 10%)	Standard deviation of Poisson distribution	Calculated as the square root of the average number of rare events; above 10% is very close to the Gaussian distribution
III. Compare two sets of values		
Are the variations about the mean different?	F test	The standard F tables (Pearson and Hartley) are one-tailed; when the question is asked as it is here, the 1% table becomes 2% and the 5% table becomes 10%
For independent samples, are the means different?	Unpaired t test	Variances of the two series should not be significantly different by the F test; use two-tailed t table
For paired samples, are the means different?	Paired t test	Same as unpaired t test
Are the two variables correlated?	Coefficient of correlation (r)	Demonstrates positive, negative or no correlation; size of r value gives degree of correlation; very sensitive to narrow range of values and to large outliers
For discontinuous variables, are the two variables independent?	Chi-square	Should not be used when the expected number of individuals in any category is less than five or there are less than 20 in each series; use Fisher's exact test for small frequencies in a 2 × 2 table
Are the two series linearly related?	Linear regression	Unreliable if data points closely grouped in the center of the range
How are the two series related numerically?	t-test statistics	Unreliable if data points widely spread
IV. What is the contribution of each known factor to a variance?	Analysis of variance (ANOVA)	Analysis of variance covers a broad range of techniques; appropriate analysis depends upon number of factors involved, relationship among the factors and the study design

1

Barnett, R. N.: Clinical Laboratory Statistics. 2nd ed. Boston, Little, Brown & Co., 1979.
Barnett, R. N.: NBSIR studies 73–162, 73–163, 73–162 appendix and 73–197. Am. J. Clin. Path., *62*:438, 1974.
Elvebach, L. R., Guillier, C. L., and Keating, F. R.: Health, normality and the ghost of Gauss. J.A.M.A., *211*:69, 1970.
Fisher, R. A., and Yates, F.: Statistical Tables for Biological, Agricultural and Medical Research. 6th ed. New York, Haffner, 1974.
Gilbert, R. K.: CAP interlaboratory survey data and analytic goals. *In* Elevitch, F. R. (ed.): Proceedings of the 1976 Aspen conference on analytical goals in clinical chemistry. Skokie, Ill., College of American Pathologists, 1977.
Natrella, M. G.: Experimental Statistics. National Bureau of Standards Handbook 91. Washington, D.C., U.S. Government Printing Office, 1966, 1976.
Pearson, E. S., and Hartley, H. O. (eds.): Biometrika Tables for Statisticians. 3rd ed. Cambridge, England, Cambridge University Press, 1966.
Pearson, E. S., and Wishart, J.: "Students' " Collected Papers: London, The Biometrika Office, University College, 1947.

4

THE THEORY OF REFERENCE VALUES

PER WINKEL, M.D., DOC. MED. SCI.,
and BERNARD E. STATLAND, M.D., PH.D.

Reference values can be defined as a set of values of a measured quantity obtained from a group of individuals (or a single individual) in a defined state of "health."

We will consider two types of reference values in this chapter: group-based reference values and subject-based reference values.

REFERENCE VALUES CHARACTERIZING A GROUP OF HEALTHY SUBJECTS

The process of obtaining and characterizing reference values includes (1) defining the population of subjects, (2) the selection of subjects, (3) the obtaining, processing, and assaying of the specimens, and (4) the statistical analysis of the data.

The level of health should be specified based on criteria for inclusion or exclusion of subjects from whom reference values are obtained. The population from which reference subjects are selected should be clearly defined, and one of the components of this definition should be the criteria for good health. The latter criteria may have to be established prospectively, as, for example, in a geriatric population based on survival time subsequent to the collection of the specimen (Grasbeck, 1969).

Selection of Subjects

The general problem one faces when collecting reference values is the following: we want to know certain information about a very large number (set) of subjects, but we have to rely on information obtained from a smaller subset of the larger set of subjects. In the statistical sense of the word, a set (also called a population) is a collection of items, in the present case, e.g., the set of all healthy females living in a certain location at a particular time. We are interested in a particular quantity characterizing the subjects, e.g., their weight as measured at a particular point in calendar time. When the total population of values (the set of values) is very large or infinite, we may obtain a smaller sample (or subset) of values upon which to generalize about the values in the original set. To characterize a finite set of values, we may examine a simple, randomly chosen subset of observed values obtained from the set. To obtain a simple, randomly chosen subset of a given size from a finite set, we must be assured that every possible subset of the given size has an equal chance of being selected. If the subset is a simple, randomly chosen one, it may be used for making inferences about (1) certain derived quantities (parameters) characterizing the set and (2) future random subjects obtained from the set. However, if this condition is not fulfilled, such use of the subset is not justified. Harris (1981) pointed out that in the vast majority of cross-sectional surveys for reference values there is no justification for making the assumption that the individuals selected represent a random sample of individuals.

Even if we assume that the sample of individuals selected is random, the comparison between an observed value and the reference values obtained from the selected group of reference individuals is meaningful only if the observed individual sufficiently resembles the reference individuals in all respects other than those under investigation. This condition is usually impossible to fulfill completely in the clinical setting. Even though compatibility can be assured with regard to all easily recognized demographic factors such as sex, age, and race, other factors may be overlooked and/or may be impractical to control.

The reduction of the variability of the group-based

Table 4–1. RATIO OF ANALYTES IN THE BLOOD OF NEONATES TO THOSE IN ADULTS*

Analyte	Ratio of Mean Values
Bilirubin	7.5
Alkaline phosphatase	2.5
Ammonia	2.0
Phosphorus	1.9
Potassium	1.5
Cholesterol	0.5
Immunoglobulin IgM	0.1
Amylase	0.1

*Blood specimens obtained from healthy neonates and healthy adults. Modified from Winsten, S.: CRC Crit. Rev. Clin. Lab. Sci., *6*:319, 1976.

reference values obtained by controlling the abovementioned well defined factors is often surprisingly small, however (Harris, 1975; Williams, 1978). Some of the more striking and important effects are highlighted below.

Age. Winsten (1976) has divided the various age groups into the following categories: *newborns, the prepubertal group, the adult population* (postpubertal and premenopausal), and *the older adult population* (postmenopausal female and the male after the sixth decade). Table 4–1 from Winsten (1976) lists eight analytes in which there is a significant difference between reference values obtained from neonates and from adult subjects. A comparison between a group of subjects in prepuberty and a comparable group of adults showed that the prepubertal subjects exhibited higher values of serum alkaline phosphatase, inorganic phosphate, aspartate aminotransferase, and lactate dehydrogenase, but significantly lower serum urate, cholesterol, creatinine, and total protein values. The mean activity value of alkaline phosphatase in the sera of a group of healthy prepubertal subjects was found to be four times higher than that for a group of healthy young adults (Statland, 1972). The difference was attributed solely to the higher bone isoenzyme activities found in the younger group (Kattwinkel, 1973).

For two other quantities, serum thyroxine and serum IgE, pediatric levels differ considerably from those in adults (Hicks, 1981; Johansson, 1976). For an excellent survey of pediatric reference values, the reader is referred to Meites (1981).

The effects of advanced age upon the mean values of biochemical constituents in serum of adults often depend on the sex of the subjects. After the onset of menopause, the changes observed in females as a function of age are especially pronounced for a number of constituents. Wilding (1972) noted that changes due to or associated with menopause in females include increases in the serum concentrations of cholesterol, urate, and inorganic phosphate and the serum activity of alkaline phosphatase. For both males and females there are common changes noted with advancing age—a decrease in serum albumin and total protein and an increase in serum urea, creatinine, glucose, cholesterol, and alkaline phosphatase. In the case of alkaline phosphatase the increase is mainly due to an increase in the serum concentration of the liver isoenzyme (O'Carroll, 1975).

Sex. The mean values for serum urate, creatinine, and urea are higher in healthy males than in female counterparts. Before the sixth decade males have higher values for serum triglycerides, cholesterol, sodium, and calcium; however, after the fifth decade of life, females generally have higher serum values of cholesterol, calcium, inorganic phosphate, and alkaline phosphatase (Leonard, 1973; Werner, 1975). Obviously, for serum LH, FSH, estradiol, and testosterone, there are differences related to the factor of sex. These differences are most pronounced at and after the onset of puberty (see Chap. 16).

Pregnancy. Pregnant women were found to have significantly lower mean values of serum calcium, glucose, urea, total protein, and albumin as compared with age-matched nonpregnant women; however, the pregnant group's mean values for serum urate, cholesterol, lactate dehydrogenase, aspartate aminotransferase, and alkaline phosphatase were higher (O'Kell, 1970). The difference in alkaline phosphatase values is due to the presence of the placental alkaline phosphatase isoenzyme in the serum of the pregnant woman. In addition, there are dramatic differences in various procoagulant and profibrinolytic values in the healthy pregnant woman as compared to her healthy non-pregnant counterpart (Hellgren, 1981).

Other Factors. The degree of obesity has been correlated positively with urate, glucose, and triglyceride concentration values in serum (Lellouch, 1973) and with the activity value in serum of alanine aminotransferase (Siest, 1975). Smokers as a group tend to have higher values for blood hemoglobin, hematocrit, and mean corpuscular volume than do non-smokers (Statland, 1977a). Recently, it has been reported that serum estradiol values are higher in male smokers than in male non-smokers (Lindholm, 1982). The mean value of intestinal alkaline phosphatase isoenzyme activity in serum is higher in subjects who are blood type O, Lewis positive secretors. It should be noted that, theoretically at least, many of the observed differences between demographically different groups of subjects may be caused by factors other than those under investigation. For instance, observed differences between races may be caused by socioeconomic factors correlated with the racial differences among the subjects.

Obtaining and Assaying Specimens

Having selected an appropriate group of subjects, both the preparation of the subject prior to specimen collection and the analytical process, including the pre-instrumental and instrumental components, should be specified with the reference values. Factors known to influence the quantity should be controlled when the reference values are obtained only if it is at all practical to control them also in the clinical situation. In addition, compatibility with the clinical situation should be assured. For instance, in the case of serum albumin, reference values obtained from blood specimens drawn from subjects in the sitting position should not be used when assessing the serum albumin of a blood specimen drawn from a patient in the supine position, since albumin concentration in serum is markedly influenced by the body position.

Statistical Analysis of the Data

As noted by Harris (1981), very few probability samplings have been undertaken to derive reference values in clinical chemistry. Therefore, one should keep in mind that the relatively trivial issue of analyzing the data statistically is of little practical importance because the basic assumption justifying a statistical analysis is usually not fulfilled. Therefore, a simplistic approach such as using the interval embracing 95 per cent of the observations as a reference and a yardstick to be used on an intuitive basis while gathering the necessary clinical experience is the approach that we would personally recommend. For a detailed exposé of various statistical techniques, the interested reader is referred to Chapter 3.

Table 4–2 presents the classic statistical approach used. One first attempts to fit a parametric probability distribution to the data. If the cumulative number fraction distribution of the data does not fit a cumulative gaussian probability distribution, one of a number of transformations may be successful in changing the data to correspond to a gaussian distribution, and the mean and standard deviations of the subset of values are computed on the transformed data. Alternatively, one may elect to use a non-parametric technique in analyzing the data.

Harris (1972) has discussed various reasons why the data often do not correspond to the classic gaussian

Table 4–2. CLASSIC STATISTICAL APPROACH FOR CALCULATING THE ESTIMATED HYPOTHETICAL POPULATION PARAMETERS BASED ON A RANDOMLY CHOSEN SUBSET OF VALUES*

1. Arrangement and inspection of subset of random observed values.
2. Hypothesis about distribution type of set of possible values.
3. Testing of fit between observed and hypothetical distribution. Assuming the hypothesis (Step 2) is accepted, Steps 4, 5, and 6 are ignored.
4. Rejection of hypothesis.
5. Transformation of observed values (log x; log (x + c); 1/x; $\sqrt{x}$).
6. New hypothesis and testing.
7. Acceptance of hypothesis.
8. Calculation of estimates of hypothetical parameters (e.g., arithmetic mean; standard deviation).

*Modified from Dybkaer, R.: Automatisation and Prospective Biology, 1973.

probabilistic model. On this basis, he has derived a general technique for transforming laboratory data, which was later further modified by Boyd (1982).

The Use of Data Obtained from Unselected Patients

Two major problems present themselves to the investigator interested in producing reliable reference values from a group of healthy subjects: (1) being able to obtain specimens from a sufficiently large number of healthy subjects—Martin (1975) recommends a minimum of 300 subjects—and (2) being certain that the factors involved in the preparation of the subject and in the analytical procedure noted during the production of the reference values are the same (i.e., no bias) as the factors present during the day-to-day routine of obtaining and assaying patient specimens. To overcome these problems, an alternative approach for producing reference values has been recommended, namely obtaining and assaying specimens from each of a number of unselected patients and analyzing the results using indirect methods to characterize a hypothetical subset of the data which is compatible with data obtained from healthy subjects. The unselected patient population may consist of all individuals entering the outpatient department over a stated time interval or all patients admitted to the inpatient ward. The reasoning behind this approach is based on the observation that the number fraction distribution of patient data often has a peak near one end with skewing toward the other end where pathologic values predominate. Based on the assumption that the majority of values stem from subjects whose values are compatible with those of healthy subjects (in the sense that their values have not been altered by disease), various attempts have been made to devise methods to characterize the data set corresponding to these subjects. A number of graphical methods are based on the assumption that the values obtained from the mentioned population, which are compatible with those of healthy subjects, follow a gaussian distribution and are fairly well separated from the pathologic values (Hoffman, 1963; Neumann, 1968; Curnow, 1963).

Cichinelli (1963) assumed that patient data constitute a mixture of two data sets, each of which can be fitted to a gaussian distribution. He fitted a composite probability density function to the data, based on a method programmed for a digital computer. Amador (1969) compared the results obtained by the above-mentioned methods in a hospital setting with the results obtained using healthy volunteers of both sexes covering a wide age span (17 to 82 years). The serum specimens from the latter group were obtained and processed by the same personnel, with the same reagents and equipment, and in the same analytical batches as were the serum specimens from the patients. The estimated means based on patient values were shifted toward pathologic values, and the standard deviations were larger as compared with the estimates based on the results obtained from the healthy subjects. Thus, it is likely that the indirect methods failed for one reason or another. However, theoretically, the discrepancy may be due to differences with regard to preparation of the subjects and/or demographic factors.

Martin (1975) suggested using a computerized least squares technique by which clinical data are fitted to two or more probability density functions. Each function is allowed to have only one peak (i.e., one maximum). But it should be noted that the probability density functions do not have to be gaussian. The proposed technique allows for various degrees of skewness of the probability density functions assumed to generate the data, and is thus made more general than the previously mentioned methods. The data set to be analyzed then is considered to comprise a mixture of data subsets, each of which is generated by a hypothetical probabilistic mechanism characterized by a probability density function. It should be noted that in order for this program to work, the number of data subsets, their relative representation in the total data set, and the parameters of the corresponding probability density functions should first be guessed by the user of the program, and these estimates should then be used as input to the program in addition to the patient data. Furthermore, the guesses, which are usually based on inspection of the number fraction distribution of the data, should not be too much off if the program is to function. This requirement may be difficult or impossible to fulfill as soon as more than two probability density functions are postulated to generate the data. Thus, in practice, the applicability of the method is probably limited to the case of two or, at most, three functions.

The validity of all indirect statistical attempts to characterize a subset of values unaffected by disease may be questioned on the following grounds: first, since many diseases are represented in a sample of patients, it is likely that a large number of different data subsets are represented in the data, and second, the fact that a subgroup of patient results may fit a gaussian or other probability density function does not in itself guarantee that it represents a group of patients whose values are unaffected by their disease.

Multivariate Prediction Regions

If one quantity is measured in a healthy subject, there is a 5 per cent chance that the observed value will be "abnormal" in the sense that it will fall outside the 95 per cent prediction interval. The more assays we perform on a healthy subject, the more likely we are to find an "abnormal" result. Assuming independence of the measured constituents, it can be demonstrated that for "n" constituents, the probability that at least one of "n" constituents will fall outside its 95 per cent prediction interval is: $1 - (0.95)^n$. Table 4–3 indicates the probability of obtaining an "abnormal" result as we increase the number of assays performed. This is a theoretical presentation and assumes independence of laboratory measurements and in this case is based upon the 95 per cent prediction interval. The introduction of multi-assay analyzers into the clinical laboratory has brought this theoretical issue into practical considerations, e.g., how can one justify the apparent occurrence of one or more "abnormal" results in a battery of 20 chemical measurements in 64 per cent of the population of healthy subjects? (Table 4–3). A number of approaches have been offered to resolve this dilemma: first, decrease the number of abnormal results by using a wider interval, e.g., a 99 per cent prediction interval. In the case of a 99 per cent prediction interval for 10 independent quantities, the per cent of "abnormal" results would be: $1 - (0.99)^n$, or approximately 9 per cent as compared to 40 per cent when we use a 95 per cent prediction interval. Second, assume *a priori* that 5 per cent of the population of healthy subjects should be outside the 95 per cent prediction interval irrespective of the number of assays performed. Thus, for "n" assays, we solve the equation: $0.05 = 1 - (x)^n$, with "x" being the probability used for each of "n" prediction intervals. Thus for 40 separate assays ($n = 40$), the computed probability for each quantity would be 99.86 per cent, in that $1 - (0.9986)^{40} = 0.05$.

Table 4–3. RELATIONSHIP OF "EXPECTED ABNORMAL" RESULTS TO NUMBER OF MEASURED CONSTITUENTS*

Number of Measured Constituents	Expected Percentage of One or More "Abnormal" Results
1	5
2	10
4	19
6	26
10	40
15	54
20	64

*Calculated by $1 - (0.95)^n$, where n is equal to the number of tests.

The Multivariate Gaussian Model. Both of the approaches presented above ignore the relationships among the quantities, i.e., the correlations of the various pairs of quantities. We will consider the case of two variates: X and Y, and assume that their joint distribution is gaussian. The two-dimensional gaussian distribution is characterized by five parameters, namely, the mean values of the two quantities and their variances, which together characterize the expected location of the observations, as well as their scatter and the correlation coefficient, which characterizes the expected relationship between the values of the two quantities.

As in the univariate case, where we may compute a tolerance interval, in an analogous manner we can compute a tolerance *region,* which is defined to include, at least, a stated proportion of the population of pairs of values with a specified degree of confidence. This approach can be generalized to include an arbitrary number of quantities. Although such models have been examined from a theoretical perspective (Grams, 1972; Winkel, 1972), their applicability in practice has yet to be demonstrated. Harris (1981) used simulation techniques to study the behavior of these models. He noted that for batteries of highly correlated tests multivariate reference regions are likely to de-emphasize positive findings in one or more of the variables judged against their separate reference ranges.

REFERENCE VALUES CHARACTERIZING A SINGLE SUBJECT

An alternative to the use of reference values characterizing a *group* of subjects is to use the subject's previous values as a reference for any future value. In this latter approach a number of specimens are obtained from a subject over a stated period of time during which the subject is in the same well-defined state of health. All specimens are assayed for the analyte in question, and the results are used to compute an interval which will contain the measured value as assayed in a future specimen with a specified probability, assuming that the individual is still in the same state of health. We shall refer to such an interval as a subject-based prediction interval.

Biologic Time-Series Models

Before we can define and compute a subject-based prediction interval, we must adopt some notion as to the appropriate model of biologic time-series which the concentration of the analyte follows. Must we assume a constant mean value (set point) over a long time interval (homeostatic model)? Should we allow a changing set point over time in a healthy subject (non-stationary model)? If we assume that the former model (fixed set point) is the more correct biologic model, then we should place equal weight on all values observed in a subject over past time. If we assume a nonstationary set point, then we would rely most heavily on the more recent values.

Harris (1975, 1976) reviewed three major statistical time-series models which belong to the class of so-called "auto-regressive models." Two extreme models, the "homeostatic model" and the "random-walk model," as well as an "intermediate (more general) model" were introduced. For many analytes, we may assume that the values obtained from healthy subjects follow the homeostatic model. In the homeostatic model it is assumed that the observed values fluctuate at random around a fixed set point. It is also postulated that these fluctuations are independent of each other. Such models are called *deterministic,* since random components in the models do not create any dependency among the measurements. Random biologic fluctuations relative to a fixed set point take place. However, the organism responds to these fluctuations by changing the concentration back to the set point. The salient point is that this counter-regulation is so fast relative to the time interval between consecutive measurements that the fluctuation reflected in any given measurement is without influence on the value of the subsequent measurement. However, if we shorten the length of the time interval sufficiently (i.e., increase the frequency of timed measurements), we will eventually reach a point at which measurements are no longer independent.

An example of a model where the parameters are based on a more detailed physiological reasoning is that stated by Winkel (1976). He relates the changes in plasma progesterone values during pregnancy to changes in the growth rate of the placenta and suggests that this model be used for the prediction of spontaneous abortion.

Once a model has been chosen, the next step is to predict future measured values on the basis of values already observed in a given subject. The clinician may have introduced a factor, e.g., a new therapeutic maneuver, that may cause a change of the measured value in addition to that induced by random biologic and analytical factors, or alternatively he may suspect that a significant shift has occurred in a patient secondary to a change in the course of the disease. In either of the two situations, the observed value would be compared with that predicted by the model chosen and a decision made whether or not one should act on the assumption that the observed change is due to the influence of random biologic and analytical factors alone. For the model-specific computations involved in this process, the reader is referred to Harris (1975, 1976) for a detailed derivation and application. Before the results of such computations are accepted, at least two conditions should be fulfilled: (1) a well-defined hypothesis alternative to that implied by the model should be formulated by the clinician, and (2) the preparation of the patient and the specimen, as well as the analytical procedure, should be under good control. When assuming either the random-walk model or the intermediate model, it is necessary for the time intervals between consecutive measurements to be constant. Furthermore, in the case of the intermediate model a considerable number of observations must be obtained because one must estimate a parameter specifying the dependency among observations in addition to estimating the usual parameters.

In the clinical situation, usually only a few observations are available and the time intervals between observations may often vary considerably. From a practical point of view therefore, the homeostatic model will probably have to be the model of choice in most situations. Winkel (1982) modified this model for a specific clinical application, namely, the postoperative monitoring of plasma carcinoembryonic antigen (CEA) measured in patients operated on for primary breast cancer. He modified the significance test procedure to make the model more sensitive to persistent deviations believed to be unique for the development of recurrence and less so to unspecific aberrations. He also specified a mathematical model describing the alternative hypothesis, i.e., the growth of a CEA-secreting metastasis (Fig. 4–1). From a theoretical point of view at least, this approach might have applications in monitoring creatinine values in patients who have received renal transplants, in fol-

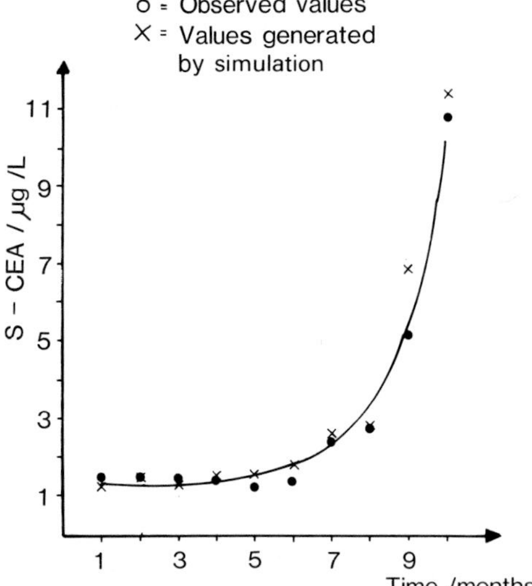

Figure 4–1. Postoperative serum CEA values (•) are presented from a patient who underwent surgery for primary breast cancer. Clinically overt recurrence was noted shortly after the time when the last serum specimen was obtained from the patient. The curve is fitted to the observations according to a mathematical model which states that the serum CEA level is a sum of two components, one which is not related to the tumor and one which reflects the size of the tumor. Values (×) generated by computer simulation and based on this model are also shown.

lowing bilirubin values in the jaundiced neonate, and in monitoring serum complement C3 in a patient with systemic lupus erythematosus, just to mention a few possibilities.

Intra-individual Variation in Healthy Subjects

Over 70 years ago, Rietz pointed out that under apparently identical conditions the quantitative measurement of physiologic functions shows considerable variability within the same subject. An assessment of the magnitude of this intra-individual variation may be obtained from the results determined on multiple specimens obtained from the same individual over time. Using the homeostatic model one would compute the intra-individual variation from the standard deviation of the quantity values as measured in the specimens. The magnitude of the observed intra-individual variation depends, of course, on the particular subject selected but also on the magnitude of the analytical variation and on the control of preparation of the subject prior to specimen collection described in Chapter 5.

For a given quantity, a given individual, a given analytical procedure, and a defined preparation of the subject, the magnitude of the intra-individual variation may also depend on the times at which the specimens are obtained as well as the total time period over which the specimens are obtained. Thus, the term "intra-individual variation" should be further qualified to be meaningful. Accepting the homeostatic model, variation around the subject's set point may still be partially systematic in nature. However, as long as we do not have a meaningful physiologic theory as to what the nature of such a variation may be, the most practical and clinically relevant approach seems to be to relate the variation to time of day and to date of collection of specimen. Therefore, we partition the intra-individual variation into two major components: (1) a within-day variation relative to the daily mean value and (2) a day-to-day variation of the daily mean value relative to the set point.

Within-Day Variation. The within-day variation may be systematic in the sense that the same pattern of variation is repeated from day to day for all the reference subjects (group-specific diurnal variation) and/or for each particular subject (subject-specific diurnal variation). In the latter case each person has a particular pattern of changes that is repeated from day to day. However, the patterns vary from individual to individual. The pattern is a function of the number of specimens obtained from each subject per day as well as the specific times of day at which the specimens are obtained. The remaining nonsystematic within-day biologic variations are referred to as random biologic fluctuations. Thus, the within-day variation is partitioned into three components: (1) group-specific diurnal variation, (2) subject-specific diurnal variation, and (3) random biologic fluctuations.

Winkel (1975) found that for the majority of the more commonly ordered serum constituents (hormones excluded) as measured in healthy subjects, the systematic diurnal components of variation are unimportant from a quantitative point of view as compared with the day-to-day variation or to the random biologic fluctuations. The case of serum potassium is the notable exception. Over 70 per cent of the total biologic variation for potassium is related to the subject's personal diurnal variation, which is consistent from day to day and also independent of any group diurnal variation. A clinically important within-day variation (mainly random biologic variation) has been seen for the serum concentration of iron, triglycerides, fatty acids, bilirubin, and amino acids as well as for a number of hormones in the sera of healthy subjects (Halberg, 1975; Statland, 1977b).

Day-to-Day Variation. Fawcett (1956) assessed the day-to-day variation of the plasma concentrations of electrolytes and total proteins. Williams (1970), using the statistical technique of analysis of variance, examined the day-to-day variation of a number of quantities in healthy subjects. This latter study, as well as the majority of other studies of the intra-individual variation in healthy subjects, is based on assaying multiple specimens obtained from each of a number of subjects with one specimen obtained per subject per day and always at the same time of day (usually in the morning). Using such an experimental design, the observed intra-individual physiologic variation will reflect the variation of the subject's daily means relative to his set point plus any random biologic fluctuations, excluding systematic diurnal variations. Table 4–4 summarizes the results of a

Table 4–4. INTRA-INDIVIDUAL PHYSIOLOGIC DAY-TO-DAY COEFFICIENT OF VARIATION × 100 OF COMMONLY ORDERED CLINICAL CHEMICAL ANALYTES*

Analyte	Coefficient of Variation × 100					Reference†
Electrolytes						
Sodium	0.7,	1.4,	0.5			a, d, f
Potassium	4.3,	5.0,	4.6,	6.2		a, c, d, f
Calcium	1.7,	1.7,	1.6,	1.6		a, c, d, f
Magnesium	1.3,	2.3				c, d
Chloride	2.1,	1.4,	2.1			a, c, d
Phosphate	5.8,	7.5,	9.6,	6.8		a, c, d, f
Metabolites						
Urea	12.3,	13.3,	11.9,	13.6,	11.1	a, b, c, d, f
Creatinine	4.3,	7.5,	4.4			a, b, d
Urate	7.3,	8.3,	10.1,	8.5		a, b, c, d
Bilirubin	22.0,	26.0				a, f
Glucose	5.6,	6.5				c,d
Iron	26.6,	24.5,	29.3			a, g, h
Cholesterol	5.3,	6.4,	8.6,	4.8,	6.6	a, c, d, e, j
Triglycerides	25.0,	18.0,	15.9			e, i, j
Enzymes						
Acid phosphatase	9.9					a
Alkaline phosphatase	4.8,	7.0,	5.7,	3.5,	6.4	a, b, d, e, f
γ-Glutamyl transferase	3.9					e
Lactate dehydrogenase	12.1,	4.7,	9.0,	7.3,	5.5	a, b, c, d, e
Aspartate aminotransferase	24.2,	8.3,	7.8,	10.9		a, b, d, e
Alanine aminotransferase	26.4,	13.2				a, e
Creatine kinase	25.7					e
Proteins						
Total protein	2.9,	2.8,	2.2,	3.0		a, c, d, f
Albumin	2.8,	3.9,	3.0,	3.2		a, c, d, f
Transferrin	2.5					e
α_1-antitrypsin	2.9					e
α_2-macroglobulin	3.1					e
IgG	2.7					e
IgA	3.5					e
IgM	3.1					e
Complement C3	3.8					e
Complement C4	5.9					e
Haptoglobin	8.8					e
Orosomucoid	11.1					e

*Analytes measured in the serum of healthy subjects.

†References:

(a) P. Winkel, H. Bokelund, and B. E. Statland: Clin. Chem., *20*:1520, 1974.
(b) P. Winkel, and B. E. Statland: Clin. Chem., *22*:1855, 1976.
(c) G. Z. Williams, D. S. Young, M. R. Stein, and E. Cotlove: Clin. Chem., *16*:1016, 1970.
(d) D. S. Young, E. K. Harris, and E. Cotlove: Clin. Chem., *17*:403, 1971.
(e) B. E. Statland, and P Winkel: CRC Crit. Rev. Clin. Lab. Sci., *8*:105, 1977.
(f) J. F. Pickup, E. K. Harris, M. Kearns, and S. S. Brown: Clin. Chem., *23*:842, 1977.
(g) K. Hoyer: Acta Med. Scand., *119*:562, 1944.
(h) B. E. Statland, and P. Winkel: Am. J. Clin. Pathol., *67*:84, 1977.
(i) G. R. Warnick, and J. J. Albers: Lipids, *11*:203, 1976.
(j) L. E. Hollister, W. G. Beckman, and M. Baker: Am. J. Med. Sci., *248*:329, 1964.

number of such studies. The results presented in the table are based on studies where the duration varied from two to four weeks and the time interval between the collection of consecutive specimens from the same subject varied from one to seven days. For each serum constituent and for each study the reported average intra-individual variation is expressed in terms of coefficient of variation (i.e., $(s/\bar{x})$) × 100. It is noteworthy that for the majority of constituents, the intra-individual physiologic variation is remarkably consistent from study to study (Table 4–4).

The electrolyte concentrations in serum are controlled within narrow limits by healthy subjects. For electrolytes, the intra-individual physiologic day-to-day variation is relatively small, generally less than 5 per cent. Note how much tighter creatinine is maintained as compared to urea (Table 4–4). The pronounced day-to-day physiologic variations in urea and

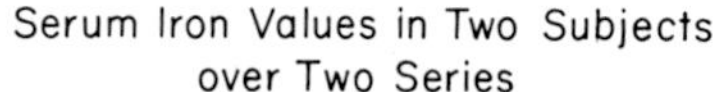

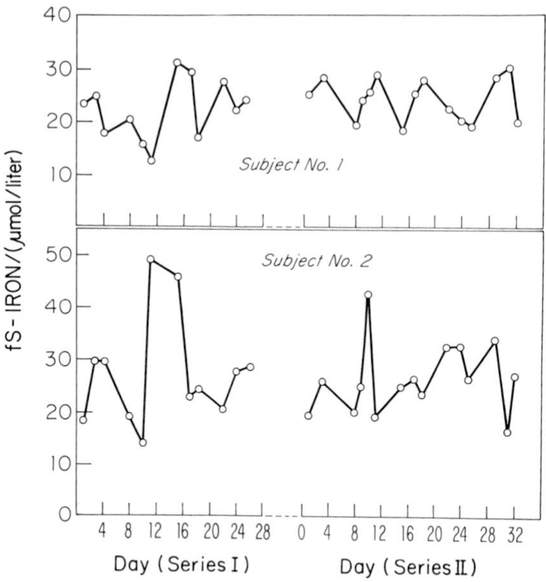

Figure 4–2. Mean concentration values of fasting serum iron in each of two healthy subjects on each of 12 days in Series I and on each of 15 days in Series II. (Modified from Statland, B. E., and Winkel, P.: Am. J. Clin. Pathol., 67:84, 1977.)

triglyceride probably reflect inconsistencies in dietary habits. Figure 4–2 illustrates the dramatic day-to-day variation in serum iron values in two healthy young adults. This variation is almost exclusively of a biologic nature (Statland, 1977b). Apart from alkaline phosphatase and gammaglutamyl transferase, most enzymes in serum which we commonly measure in the laboratory vary greatly from day to day. This may be explained by inconsistent patterns of physical activity from day to day and possibly by variation in food intake and/or ethanol consumption. Furthermore, these enzymes, as well as bilirubin and urea, for example, should probably be regarded as waste products that have no function to carry out in the extracellular space. Therefore, from a teleologic point of view at least, there is no reason for the body to regulate the concentration of these constituents very closely. Note the narrow limits within which the human organism controls specific protein concentrations in serum. This fact, coupled with the relatively large inter-individual variation for specific proteins in serum, demonstrates the insensitivity of group-specific reference intervals for detecting changes in these constituents due to pathologic processes.

LIMITATIONS RELATED TO THE USE OF REFERENCE VALUES

In the clinical setting, group reference intervals based on data from so-called healthy subjects are the predominant type of reference interval used. A common error occurring when such an interval is being used is the practice of using the lower and upper limits of the interval as rigid boundaries within which the patient is considered "normal" and beyond which the patient is termed "abnormal" and thought to be suffering from some pathologic process. This approach may be very misleading for many reasons. For one thing, having a value outside the stated interval might be a sign of *good* health rather than a cause for concern, e.g., a patient having a serum cholesterol value *below* the lower reference limit. For another patient, having a value within the stated interval might *not* be a sign of good health, e.g., a patient on Coumadin with a "normal protein."

Since the alternatives are not usually explicitly defined in the clinical setting, the isolated use of a reference interval may lead to erroneous conclusions. The only question that can be answered when using these intervals is the following: if the subject belongs to the reference group, what is the probability that we would observe the result which we have actually observed? For this reason, we want to discourage the determination and utilization of group-based reference intervals independent of alternative reference intervals for relevant "disease groups."

Another major criticism is that the interval may be too broad. In examining a given patient we are really interested in the interval of values characterizing this particular patient when he or she is in a state of good health.

The error we are making in using a group-based reference interval may be assessed from the so-called ratio value. The ratio value (Harris, 1974) is defined as the ratio of the physiologic intra-individual variation over the biologic inter-individual variation. (For statistical details the reader is referred to Harris, 1974.) The analytical variation should be separated in the computations. The inter-individual variation reflects the variation among the subjects with regard to their mean values or set points, and the intra-individual variation is the average variation over time of the observed values relative to the set point. Figure 4–3 is a good illustration of the problem. This figure, which presents the actual values of serum concentrations of immunoglobulin IgM for nine healthy subjects, illustrates the small magnitude of the intra-individual variation relative to the inter-individual variation for serum IgM.

DECISION LEVELS—AN ALTERNATIVE TO REFERENCE VALUES

In this chapter, we have presented the way in which reference values can be produced, as well as their obvious limitations. An alternative to reference values which is gaining some consideration is that of "decision levels." This concept has been developed and popularized by Statland (1983). Essentially, decision levels represent threshold values above which or below which clinicians will respond to quantitative values. An example of such a decision level would be a

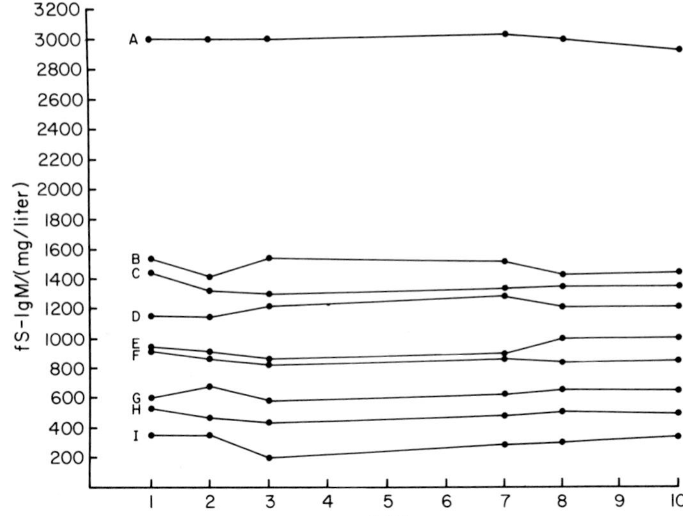

Figure 4–3. Mean concentration values of serum IgM from each of nine fasting healthy subjects (A–I) over a ten-day period. (Modified from Statland, B. E., Winkel, P., and Killingsworth, L.: Clin. Chem., *22*:1635, 1976.)

1

calcium value of 11.0 mg/dl (2.75 mM/L). When the patient's serum calcium value is 11.0 or above, this result should suggest the diagnosis of primary hyperparathyroidism. A *decision* may be taken to repeat the calcium determination as well as to perform additional tests and finally to consider surgery. A second decision level for serum calcium might be 7.0 mg/dl (1.75 mM/L). Values below 7.0 would recommend consideration of tetany or convulsions in a patient. Obviously, one *action* would be to order a serum albumin and a bicarbonate determination.

In the example given above, an expected reference interval for serum calcium may be 9.0 to 10.6 mg/dl. Although one decision level (11.0) is near the upper reference limit, the other decision level (7.0) is somewhat less than the lower reference limit. Thus, in the example given, it should be obvious that the reference limits do not always correspond to limits for action. Statland (1983) has developed a series of decision levels for each of approximately 70 analytes. It is hoped that the use of decision levels rather than reference limits will yield greater clinical usefulness. The reliance on reference limits for clinical decision making has resulted in excessive testing and overutilization of the clinical laboratory (Martin, 1982).

Amador, E., and Hsi, B. P.: Indirect methods for estimating the normal range. Am. J. Clin. Path., *52*:538, 1969.

Boyd, J. C., and Lacker, D. A.: A multi-stage gaussian transformation algorithm for clinical laboratory data. Clin. Chem., *28*:1735, 1982.

Cichinelli, A. L.: The composite of two gaussian distributions as a model for blood pressure distribution in man. Ph.D. Thesis, University of Michigan, 1963.

Curnow, D. H., and Sheard, K.: The use of probability paper in analyzing frequency distribution. Clin. Chem., *9*:462, 1963.

Dybkaer, R.: Production and presentation of reference values. Proc. 2nd Int. Colloquium "Automatisation and Prospective Biology," Pont-à-Mousson, 1972. Basel, Karger, 1973, p. 2.

Fawcett, J. K., and Wynn, V.: Variation of plasma electrolytes and total protein levels in the individual. Br. Med. J., *2*:582, 1956.

Galen, R. S.: The normal range. Arch. Path. Lab. Med., *101*:561, 1977.

Grams, R. R., Johnson, E. A., and Benson, E. S.: Laboratory data analysis system: Section III—Multivariate normality. Am. J. Clin. Path., *58*:133, 1972.

Grasbeck, R., and Alstrom, T.: Reference values in laboratory medicine. The current state of the art. New York, John Wiley and Sons, 1981.

Grasbeck, R., and Saris, N. E.: Establishment and use of normal values. Scand. J. Clin. Lab. Invest., *24*(Suppl. 110):62, 1969.

Halberg, F.: Biological rhythms. Adv. Exp. Med. Biol., *54*:1, 1975.

Harris, E. K.: Effects of intra- and inter-individual variation on the appropriate use of normal ranges. Clin. Chem., *20*:1531, 1974.

Harris, E. K.: Some theory of reference values. I. Stratified normal ranges and a method for following an individual's clinical laboratory values. Clin. Chem., *21*:1457, 1975.

Harris, E. K.: Some theory of reference values. II. Comparison of some statistical models of intra-individual variation in blood constituents. Clin. Chem., *22*:1343, 1976.

Harris, E. K.: Statistical aspects of reference values in clinical pathology. *In* Stefani, M., and Benson, E. S. (eds.): Progress in Clinical Pathology. Volume VIII. New York, Grune and Stratton, 1981, p. 45.

Harris, E. K., and DeMets, D. L.: Effects of intra- and inter-individual variation on distributions of single measurements. Clin. Chem., *18*:244, 1972.

Hellgren, M., and Blomback, N.: Studies in coagulation and fibrinolysis in pregnancy, during delivery, and in the puerperium. Gynecol. Obstet. Invest., *12*:141, 1981.

Hicks, J. M., Hammond, K., and Boeckx, R. L.: Pediatric reference values. *In* Reference Values in Laboratory Medicine. The Current State of the Art. New York, John Wiley and Sons, 1981.

Hoffman, R. G.: Statistics in the practice of medicine. J.A.M.A., *185*:864, 1963.

Johansson, S. G. O., Strawberg, K., and Urnas, B.: Molecular and Biological Aspects of the Acute Allergic Reaction. New York, Plenum Press, 1976, p. 179.

Kattwinkel, J., Taussing, L. M., Statland, B. E., and Verter, J. I.: The effects of age on alkaline phosphatase and other serologic liver function tests in normal subjects and patients with cystic fibrosis. J. Pediatr., *82*:234, 1973.

Lellouch, J., and Claude, J. R.: A study of several biological parameters measured in a large population of a single profession. II. Factors which may affect the 'normal values.' Proc. 2nd Int. Colloquium "Automatisation and Prospective Biology," Pont-à-Mousson, 1972. Basel, Karger, 1973, p. 100.

Leonard, P. J.: The effect of age and sex on biochemical parameters in blood of healthy human subjects. Proc. 2nd Int. Colloquium "Automatisation and Prospective Biology," Pont-à-Mousson, 1972. Basel, Karger, 1973, p. 134.

Lindholm, J., Winkel, P., Brodthagen, U., and Gyntelberg, F.: Coronary risk factors and plasma sex-hormones. Am. J. Med., *73*:648, 1982.

Martin, A. R.: Common and correctable errors in diagnostic test ordering. West. J. Med., *136*:456, 1982.

Martin, H. F., Gudzinowicz, B. J., and Fanger, H.: Normal Values in Clinical Chemistry: A Guide to Statistical Analysis of Laboratory Data. New York, Marcel Dekker, Inc., 1975.

Meites, S.: Pediatric Clinical Chemistry: A survey of Reference (Normal) Values, Methods, and Instrumentation with Commentary. 2nd ed. Washington, D.C., American Association for Clinical Chemistry, 1981.

Neumann, G. J.: Determination of normal ranges from laboratory data. Clin. Chem., *14*:979, 1968.

O'Carroll, D., Statland, B. E., Steele, B. W., and Burke, M. D.: Chemical inhibition method for alkaline phosphatase isoenzymes in human serum. Am. J. Clin. Path., *63*:564, 1975.

O'Kell, R. T., and Ellott, J. R.: Development of normal values for use in multitest biochemical screening of sera. Clin. Chem., *16*:161, 1970.

Rietz, H. L., and Mitchell, H. H.: On the metabolism experiment as a statistical problem. J. Biol. Chem., *8*:297, 1910.

Siest, G., Schiele, F., Galteau, M-M., et al.: Aspartate aminotransferase and alanine aminotransferase activities in plasma: Statistical distributions, individual variations, and reference values. Clin. Chem., *21*:1077, 1975.

Statland, B. E.: Clinical Decision Levels for Lab Tests. Oradell, NJ, Med. Economics, 1983, in press.

Statland, B. E.: Establishing decision levels in clinical chemistry. *In* Grasbeck, R., and Alstrom, T. (eds.): Reference Values in Laboratory Medicine. New York, John Wiley and Sons, 1981, pp. 207–221.

Statland, B. E., and Winkel, P.: Effects of non-analytical factors on the intra-individual variation of analytes in the blood of healthy subjects: Consideration of preparation of the subject and time of venipuncture. CRC Crit. Rev. Clin. Lab. Sci., *8*:105, 1977a.

Statland, B. E., and Winkel, P.: The relationship of the day-to-day variation of serum iron concentration values to the iron binding capacity values in a group of healthy young women. Am. J. Clin. Path., *67*:84, 1977b.

Statland, B. E., Young, D. S., and Nishi, H. N.: Serum alkaline phosphatase: Total activity and isoenzyme determinations made by use of centrifugal fast analyzer. Clin. Chem., *18*:12, 1972.

Werner, M., and Marsh, W. L.: Normal values: Theoretical and practical aspects. CRC Crit. Rev. Clin. Lab. Sci., *6*:81, 1975.

Wilding, P., and Rollason, J. G.: Detection of menopausal changes in biochemical constituents in well population screening. Scand. J. Clin. Lab. Invest., *29*(Suppl. 126):21, 1972.

Williams, G. Z., et al.: Biological and analytical components of variation in long-term studies of serum constituents in normal subjects. I. Objectives, subject selection, laboratory procedures, and estimation of analytical deviation; II. Estimating biological components of variation; III. Physiological and medical implications. Clin. Chem., *16*:1016, 1022, 1028, 1970.

Williams, G. Z., Widdowson, G. M., and Penton, J.: Individual character of variation in time-series studies of healthy people. II. Differences in values for clinical chemical analytes in serum among demographic groups by age and sex. Clin. Chem., *24*:313, 1978.

Winkel, P., Bentzon, M. W., Statland, B. E., Mouridsen, H., and Sheike, O.: Predicting recurrence in patients with breast cancer from cumulative laboratory results: A new technique for the application of time series analysis. Clin. Chem., *28*:2057, 1982.

Winkel, P., Gaede, P., and Lyngbye, J.: Method for monitoring plasma progesterone concentrations in pregnancy. Clin. Chem., *22*:422, 1976.

Winkel, P., Lyngbye, J., and Jørgensen, K.: The normal region—a multivariate problem. Scand. J. Clin. Lab. Invest., *30*:339, 1972.

Winkel, P., Statland, B. E., and Bokelund, H.: The effects of venipuncture on variation of serum constituents: Consideration of within-day and day-to-day changes in a group of healthy young men. Am. J. Clin. Pathol., *64*:433, 1975.

Winsten, S.: The ecology of normal values in clinical chemistry. CRC Crit. Rev. Clin. Lab. Sci., *6*:319, 1976.

Wootton, I. D. P., and King, E. J.: Normal values for blood constituents. Lancet, *1*:470, 1953.

5

PRE-INSTRUMENTAL SOURCES OF VARIATION

BERNARD E. STATLAND, M.D., PH.D.,
and PER WINKEL, M.D., DOC. MED. SCI.

1

THE ANALYTICAL PROCEDURE

The major steps involved in requesting, performing, and evaluating a measured quantity are outlined in Table 5–1. Prior to the analysis, a physician requests a quantitative measurement on a specimen from his (or her) patient. The actual analytical procedure starts with preparing the patient, continues with the collection of the biologic specimen, and ends with the production of a report. Laboratory personnel involved in performing the assay include clerical or health-related personnel who inform the patient what he should do (or refrain from doing) prior to specimen collection; a technologist who collects, processes, stores, and transports the specimen; an analyst who performs the measuring steps; and a laboratorian who decides if the resultant measurement is of adequate quality to be sent to the requesting physician. The final step—that of accepting, evaluating, and acting upon the measurement—is usually done by the physician who originally requested the measurement and/or a laboratory physician as a consultant. This chapter will explore in detail the steps involved in performing the assay (Table 5–1).

Table 5–1. STEPS INVOLVED IN REQUESTING, PERFORMING, AND EVALUATING A MEASURED QUANTITY

I. Physician *requests* a quantitative measurement of a constituent in a biologic specimen
II. Laboratory personnel *perform* the assay
  A. Pre-instrumental phase
    1. Preparation of the patient
    2. Obtaining the specimen
    3. Processing the specimen
    4. Storing the specimen prior to the measuring step
  B. Instrumental phase
    1. Dispensing a sample aliquot into a reaction vessel
    2. Combining the sample with one or more reagents
    3. Recording some physical-chemical consequence of the reaction
    4. Calculating the value of the quantity measured
  C. Post-instrumental phase
    1. Laboratory technical and professional staff accept the value (result of the measurement) as being of good quality
    2. The report of the measurement is sent to the requesting physician
III. Physician *evaluates* the report of the measurement
  A. Physician assesses whether the measurement *could be consistent* with other known patient information
  B. The physician makes a clinical decision at least partially based on the reported measurement

PREPARATION OF THE PATIENT

The total variance of a series of sequential laboratory measurements obtained from the same subject may be considered as the sum of many variances, each having a different source. These may include variability due to analytical imprecision, changes in the health status of the subject, endogenous factors influencing the internal hormonal control, and variability due to stresses originating from the outside environment (exogenous stresses) or activities undertaken by the subject prior to specimen collection. To improve the clinician's ability to classify patients on the basis of laboratory measurements, he may minimize the effect of factors not related to the patient's state of health. Thus, the clinician attempts to decrease the random analytical variation (e.g., by taking specimens at the same time of day when we measure serum cortisol), thus controlling the effect of exogenous factors and activities of the subject (Statland, 1981).

Schwartz (1973) and Statland (1977) have reviewed the many known factors contributing to the variation which are due to the preparation of the subject; however, in this present context we will include only the most pronounced effects and consider the factors of prior exercise, previous diet, drug intake, tobacco smoking, posture of the patient, and tourniquet application time prior to venipuncture.

Exercise

Muscular activity has both transient and longer-lasting effects on various clinical chemical quantities. The transient biochemical changes in plasma constituents induced by exercise include an immediate fall and then subsequent increase in the concentration of free fatty acids, a marked increase (180 per cent) in the concentration of the amino acid alanine, and a profound increase (300 per cent) in that of lactate. The transient changes (within the hour) noted during exercise are related to increased metabolic activity for energy purposes and are corrected to pre-exercise levels soon after the cessation of the exercise (Carlsten, 1962; Statland, 1973a; Galteau, 1975).

The longer-lasting effects of exercise consist of increases in the activities of muscle enzymes measured in serum, e.g., creatine kinase, aldolase, aspartate aminotransferase, and lactate dehydrogenase. King (1976) observed a mean peak increase of 125 per cent as compared to baseline values in serum creatine kinase activity in four subjects 11 hours after a 60-minute exercise challenge of handball training.

Long-term physical training changes the levels of a number of sex hormones. During six months of physical training, the mean plasma testosterone concentration increased by 21 per cent, the androstenedione concentration by 25 per cent, and that of LH by 25 per cent in 39 Army recruits (Remes, 1979). The mean ratio of plasma testosterone to sex hormone binding activity (SHBG) increased by 32 per cent, while the SHBG concentration tended to drop, although not significantly. The increase in the LH concentration fits well with the increase in the testosterone and androstenedione levels and may be secondary to the increase in testosterone concentration.

Prolonged Fasting

Although it has been recommended that the patient be in a fasting state before being subjected to venipuncture to ensure that laboratory measurements are compatible with "reference values," "prolonged" fasting, e.g., more than 24 hours, can lead to unexpected laboratory results. Prolonged fasting has been associated with elevations in serum bilirubin concentration (240 per cent increase after 48 hours of fasting) (Barrett, 1971).

Fasting for 72 hours decreased the concentration of plasma glucose in healthy women to a value of 450 mg/L (2.5 mmol/L) (Statland, 1977). Stout (1976) monitored the concentrations of plasma lipids and hormones in nine healthy volunteers who underwent a 72-hour total fast (only water was allowed). The major conclusions by Stout (1976) were that fasting results in a dramatic increase in the concentrations of plasma triglycerides, glycerol, and free fatty acids, *without* a significant change in the concentration of plasma cholesterol.

Diet

The physiologic (*in vivo*) effects of eating a meal include increase in the plasma concentrations of potassium and triglycerides. The *in vivo* changes are dependent upon the type and quantity of food ingested as well as the timing of the venipuncture in relationship to the meal. Two to four hours after consuming a meal high in fat content, many subjects will demonstrate a significant increase in the serum alkaline phosphatase activity which is primarily an increase in intestinal isoenzyme activity and is most pronounced in patients who are Lewis-positive secretors and have blood type O or B (Statland, 1973b).

In addition to the physiologic changes noted above, the increased turbidity due to hyperchylomicronemia may interfere with a number of assays. This type of *in vitro* error will be discussed below as a source of pre-instrumental variation (see p. 71 on "lactescent serum").

Certain foods or special dietary regimens may affect particular serum and urine constituents. A diet high in protein results in an increase in the serum concentration of urea, ammonia, and urate; however, it does not significantly affect the serum creatinine (Statland, 1977). A diet having a high ratio of unsaturated to saturated fatty acids will result in a decrease in the serum cholesterol concentration (Keys, 1966). Ingestion of a diet rich in purines is followed by an increase in the serum urate concentration (Bishop, 1953). In one study (Marley, 1970), the ingestion of bananas increased the renal 5-hydroxyindoleacetic acid excretion from 5 mg to 54 mg per day. The presence of serotonin in banana, pineapple, tomato, and avocado can lead to an elevated excretion in the urine of 5-hydroxyindoleacetic acid (Schwartz, 1973). Beverages containing caffeine will result in as much as a threefold rise in the concentration of plasma non-esterified free fatty acids (Bellet, 1965), and will cause a release of catecholamines from the adrenal medulla and from brain tissue (Levi, 1967).

Ethanol

The immediate changes induced by ethanol ingestion include increases in the plasma concentration of lactate, urate, and the metabolites of ethanol, namely acetaldehyde and acetate. Belfrage (1977) challenged nine healthy male volunteers with approximately 1.00 g ethanol per kg body weight per day for five weeks. He observed a significant increase of plasma triglyceride concentration (+40 per cent at two weeks) followed by a reduction to baseline values by the fifth week.

It has been noted that chronic alcoholics have higher plasma HDL cholesterol concentrations than do matched control subjects (Belfrage, 1977), which appears to be related to the amount and frequency of ethanol ingestion prior to specimen collection. Abusers of alcohol show increased values of serum γ-glutamyltransferase, serum urate, and mean erythrocyte volume. A number of workers have recommended using various combinations of assays, e.g., serum γ-glutamyltransferase (Freer, 1977), plasma HDL-cholesterol, and mean corpuscular volume (MCV) of erythrocytes, as indicators of alcohol consumption (Schiele, 1977).

Tobacco Smoking

Tobacco smoking results in an increase in the percentage of blood carboxyhemoglobin values. In heavy cigarette smokers who inhale while smoking, it is common to note carboxyhemoglobin values of up to 8 per cent as compared with values of less than 1 per cent in non-smokers.

The acute effects of tobacco smoking include increases in plasma catecholamines as well as increase in serum cortisol. Such changes are probably related to the nicotine in tobacco. The changes in these hormones will also result in important effects on the peripheral leukocyte count (Friedman, 1973): a decrease in eosinophils, an increase in neutrophils, and an increase in monocytes. The changes in hormone values also lead to an increased value for plasma non-esterified fatty acids.

The acute effects of tobacco smoking should be differentiated from the more chronic effects. These chronic effects include increased blood hemoglobin values, increased mean corpuscular volume (MCV), and increased white blood cell count. The physician should be aware of the acute effects when following sequential values for various hormones in the blood stream.

Dalferes (1980) used a procedure for determining thiocyanate concentrations in plasma so as to detect the presence or absence of cigarette smoking in normal volunteers. The mean value of plasma thiocyanate concentrations in adult smokers was 161 μmol/L (SD = 43) as compared with a mean plasma thiocyanate concentration in 24 nonsmokers of 62 μmol/L (SD = 19).

Physiologic Effects of Drugs

Given the large number of drugs available to the physician treating his patient and the variety of assays available in the chemistry laboratory, there exists a very great number of potential drug-assay interferences. Drug interference can be grouped into two general categories: physiologic *in vivo* effects of the drug or its metabolites on the quantity to be measured and *in vitro* effects due to some physical or chemical property of the drug or its metabolites which can cause interferences with the assay (Weindling, 1975).

Young (1975) has compiled a master file of over 2000 references and over 15,000 drug-assay interactions of both types. He has found that the pharmacologic response of a healthy individual to the administration of a drug may very well differ from that of a patient. The *in vivo* response to a drug depends on the individual, the dose of the drug in question, and other medications given concurrently.

A number of drugs are known to affect the liver by inducing hepatic microsomal enzymes, or by producing hepatocellular damage or cholestatic jaundice (Lubran, 1969). Table 5–2 lists the major drugs involved. Cholestasis can be caused by orally active synthetic steroids and sulfonylurea derivatives, including chlorpromazine, thiouracil, propylthiouracil, methimazole, chlorpropamide, and tolbutamide (Young, 1975). Hepatocellular damage resulting in

Table 5–2. SELECTED MEASUREMENTS OF HEPATIC FUNCTION AND A LIST OF DRUGS IMPLICATED IN PHARMACOLOGIC INTERFERENCE*

Effects on Liver Function Tests	
Urine:	Bilirubin: increased
Serum:	Alkaline phosphatase: increased
	Bilirubin: increased
	Bromsulphalein (BSP): increased
	Glucose: decreased
	Alanine aminotransferase (ALT) and aspartate aminotransferase (AST): increased

Drugs That May Affect Liver Function Tests	
Acetohexamide	Methyldopa
Acetophenetidin	Methylthiouracil
Allopurinol	Nicotinic acid
Aminosalicylic acid	Nitrofurantoin
Amodiaquine	Novobiocin
Amphotericin-B	Oleandomycin
Anabolic agents	Oxazepam
Androgens	Oxyphenbutazone
Chlorpropamide	Paraldehyde
Cyclophosphamide	Paramethadione
Desipramine	Phenacemide
Erythromycin	Phenothiazines
Glycopyrrolate	Phenylbutazone
Haloperidol	Progestins
Halothane	Progestins-estrogens (oral contraceptives)
Hydrazine	Propylthiouracil
Imipramine	Quinacrine (mepacrine)
Indomethacin	Sulfonamides
Isoniazid	Tetracyclines
Lincomycin	Thiosemicarbazones
MAO inhibitors	Thiothixene
Mercaptopurine	Tolazamide
Metaxalone	Tolbutamide
Methoxsalen	Trimethadione
Methoxyflurane	Uracil mustard

*Modified from Martin, T. J.: The Pharmacologic Interactions with Laboratory Test Values, 1970. 596 Burnhamthorpe, Etobicoke, Ontario, Canada.

an increase in the activity of aminotransferases in serum can be caused by antineoplastic agents. The list of drugs inducing hepatic microsomal enzymes includes barbiturates, glutethimide, phenytoin, tolbutamide, chlordiazepoxide, and phenylbutazone (Lubran, 1969).

Pharmacologic effects of oral contraceptives include increases in the concentrations in serum of ceruloplasmin, transcortin, thyroxine-binding globulin, α_1-antitrypsin, plasminogen, transferrin, iron, and triglycerides, and decreases in the concentrations of albumin, orosomucoid, and zinc (Laurell, 1967; Sunderman, 1970). These effects are probably related to the estrogen portion of the drug (Sunderman, 1970). Oral contraceptives are reputed to cause an increase of the activities of alanine aminotransferase and γ-glutamyltransferase owing to an induction of the synthesis of the hepatic enzymes (Schiele, 1977a).

Table 5–3 is an abridged compilation of the drugs affecting common clinical chemistry tests, including the direction of the alteration caused by the drugs and the mode of interference, which is either a physiologic effect or a chemical (methodologic) interference. The chemical (methodologic) interferences will be discussed later in this chapter.

Posture

Specimens are usually obtained from a subject in either the supine or upright sitting posture. As a patient goes from the supine to the standing posture there will be an efflux of water and filterable substances from the intravascular space to the interstitial fluid space. The non-filterable substances such as proteins, cellular elements, and compounds associated with either cells or protein will increase in concentration. Thus, for example, the serum albumin value will increase as the individual goes from the supine to the standing posture. Since calcium is bound to a large extent to albumin, it also will increase as the individual goes from the supine to the standing posture. The list of such components in blood having a similar direction of change includes albumin, total protein, various enzymes, calcium, bilirubin, cholesterol, and triglycerides. The changes in cholesterol, triglycerides, and bilirubin are related to the fact that they are all bound to proteins. We also note an increase in the plasma concentrations of those drugs also bound to proteins. The hematocrit, the blood hemoglobin values, and other cellular-related elements will also increase when one goes from the supine to the standing position (Winkel, 1977).

In general, the shift of body water in healthy individuals will result in an 8 to 10 per cent increase in the concentration of total protein in serum. To the extent that substances are more or less filtered as compared to total protein, they also will increase in the same order of magnitude. In those individuals who have an excessive amount of fluid, there will be an even greater difference due to changes in posture. This consideration is very important when comparing outpatient (ambulatory clinic) results with those obtained when the patient is in the hospital bed. For example, on an outpatient basis the serum albumin might be 38 g/L, while in the hospital the value may drop to 34 g/L.

In addition to the changes enumerated above, the action of going from the supine to the standing position also affects a number of hormones. Specifically, when one goes from the supine to the standing position there will be a dramatic increase in plasma norepinephrine—approximately a doubling of baseline. This increase in norepinephrine will also cause an increase in the plasma renin activity. The increase in plasma renin activity may also be partly related to the decreased blood volume presented to the kidney. Another consequence of going from the supine to the erect posture is an increase in plasma aldosterone values. This increase appears to be associated partially with the increased angiotensin II values. However, it is possible to separate these two effects. Finally, going from the supine to the standing position will also result in an increase in the 8-arginine-vasopressin values. The consequences of postural effects are such that conditions of specimen collection should be stated very explicitly when one is interested in evaluating the hormonal status of the patient. In fact, a number of laboratory measurements are based on appropriate stress tests to the patient which include postural challenges as part of the protocol.

Other Factors

The incorrect application of tourniquets, as well as fist exercise, can result in erroneous test results. When obtaining a blood specimen for lactate assay, one should draw the specimen without the use of a tourniquet (Calam, 1977). The lactate values increase as one goes from aerobic to anaerobic metabolism. Prolonged tourniquet application before venipuncture can cause significant changes in the concentration of many serum constituents, especially enzymes, proteins, and protein-bound substances. Examples of analytes which are protein-bound and thus show an increase in the serum concentration after venous stasis include cholesterol, triglyceride, calcium, and iron (Statland, 1974). The mean increases in serum concentrations after a three-minute tourniquet application as compared with a one-minute tourniquet application in healthy subjects include 5 per cent for total proteins, 5 per cent for cholesterol, 6 per cent for iron, 8 per cent for bilirubin, and 10 per cent for aspartate aminotransferase (Statland, 1974).

Stress affects adrenal hormone secretion. Anxiety resulting in hyperventilation prior to venipuncture will lead to disturbances in acid-base balance, an increase in the serum lactate concentration, and a profound increase in the serum concentration of nonesterified fatty acids (Schwartz, 1973).

PREPARATION OF THE SPECIMEN

We have partitioned the analytical procedure into three phases: pre-instrumental, instrumental, and post-instrumental (Table 5–1). The pre-instrumental

Text continues on page 69

Table 5–3. SOME DRUGS WITH PHYSIOLOGIC EFFECT ON AND/OR CHEMICAL INTERFERENCE WITH COMMONLY ORDERED CONSTITUENTS IN BLOOD AND URINE*

Constituent in Blood	Drugs Causing Physiologic Effect	Type of Effect†	Drugs with Chemical Interference	Type of Effect†
Acid phosphatase (ACP)	Androgens (in women)	I	Fluorides	D
			Oxalates	D
Alkaline phosphatase (ALP)	(Refer to Table 5–2)		Albumin from placental sources	I
	Phenytoin	I	Fluorides	D
			Oxalates	D
			Theophylline	D
Ammonia			Isoniazid	I
Amylase (AMS)	Cholinergics	I	Citrate	D
	Ethanol	I	Oxalate	D
	Narcotics	I	Fluorides	D
Bilirubin	(Refer to Table 5–2)		Dextran	I
	Chlordiazepoxide	I	Novobiocin	I
	Gallbladder dyes	I	Ascorbic acid	D
	Phenobarbital	D	Caffeine	D
			Theophylline	D
Bromsulphalein (BSP)	(Refer to Table 5–2)		Heparin	I
	Barbiturate	I	Phenazopyridine	I
	Clofibrate	I	Phenolphthalein	I
	Narcotics (Opiates—meperidine and methadone)	I	Phenolsulfonphthalein	I
	Phenytoin	I		
	Probenecid	I		
Calcium	Androgens	I	Citrate salts	D
	Calciferol-activated calcium salts	I	EDTA (interferes with dye-binding methods)	D
	Dihydrotachysterol	I		
	Progestins-estrogens	I		
	Thiazide diuretics	I		
	Acetazolamide	D		
	Costicosteroids	D		
	Mithramycin	D		
Chloride	Acetazolamides	I	Bromide	I
	Chlorides	I		
	Oxyphenbutazone	I		
	Phenylbutazone	I		
	ACTH, corticosteroids	D		
	Ethacrynic acid	D		
	Furosemide	D		
	Mercurial diuretics	D		
	Triamterene	D		
Cholesterol	ACTH	I	Bromide	I
	Bile salts	I		
	Chlorpromazine	I		
	Heparin	D		
	Thyroxine	D		
Cortisol			Chlordiazepoxide	I
			Dexamethasone	I
			Digoxin	I
			Methenamine	I
			Thorazine	I
Creatine kinase (CK)	Carbenoxolone	I		
	Clofibrate	I		
	Codeine	I		
	Dexamethasone	I		
	Digoxin	I		
	Ethanol	I		
	Furosemide	I		
	Glutethimide	I		

Table continues on following page

Table 5–3. SOME DRUGS WITH PHYSIOLOGIC EFFECT ON AND/OR CHEMICAL INTERFERENCE WITH COMMONLY ORDERED CONSTITUENTS IN BLOOD AND URINE *(Continued)*

Constituent in Blood	Drugs Causing Physiologic Effect	Type of Effect†	Drugs with Chemical Interference	Type of Effect†
Creatine kinase (CK) *(cont.)*	Halothane anesthesia	I		
	Heroin	I		
	Imipramine	I		
	Lithium carbonate	I		
	Meperidine hydrochloride	I		
	Morphine sulfate	I		
	Phenobarbital	I		
	Suxamethonium	I		
Creatinine	Amphotericin B	I	Ascorbic acid	I
	Kanamycin	I	Barbiturates	I
			Cephalosporins	I
			Glucose	I
			Levodopa	I
			Methyldopa	I
			BSP and PSP	I
Glucose	ACTH, corticosteroids	I	Acetaminophen	I
	Epinephrine	I	Aminosalicylic acid (PAS)	I
	Ethacrynic acid	I	Ascorbic acid	I or D
	Furosemide	I	Dextran	I
	Thiazides	I	Hydralazine	I
	Phenytoin	I	Isoproterenol	I
	Propranolol	D	Levodopa	I
			Mercaptopurine	I
			Methimazole	I
			Methyldopa	I
			Nalidixic acid	I
			Oxazepam	I
			Propylthiouracil	I
Lactate dehydrogenase	Clofibrate	D	Oxalate	D
			Theophylline	D
Lipase	Cholinergics	I	Bilirubin	I
	Ethanol	I		
	Narcotics	I		
Phosphate	Calciferol-activated methicillin	I		
	Tetracyclines	I		
	Aluminum hydroxide	D		
	Glucose infusion	D		
	Insulin	D		
	Mithramycin	D		
Potassium	Heparin	I	Calcium	I
	Potassium	I	Penicillin G	I
	Spironolactone	I		
	ACTH, corticosteroids	D		
	Amphotericin	D		
	Glucose infusion	D		
	Insulin	D		
	Oral diuretics	D		
	Salicylates	D		
	Tetracycline	D		
Total protein	ACTH, corticosteroids	I	BSP dye	I
	Anabolic/androgenic steroids	I	Bilirubin	I
			Dextran	I
			Phenazopyridine	I
			Acetylsalicylic acid	D
Transferases AST (GOT) and ALT (GPT)	(Refer to Table 5–2)		*For spectrophotometric assay of AST:*	
	Ampicillin	I		

Table continues on opposite page

Table 5–3. SOME DRUGS WITH PHYSIOLOGIC EFFECT ON AND/OR CHEMICAL INTERFERENCE WITH COMMONLY ORDERED CONSTITUENTS IN BLOOD AND URINE *(Continued)*

Constituent in Blood	Drugs Causing Physiologic Effect	Type of Effect†	Drugs with Chemical Interference	Type of Effect†
Transferases	Colchicine	I		
AST or GOT and ALT	Cephalothin	I	Ascorbic acid	I
(GPT) *(cont.)*	Clofibrate	I	Erythromycin	I
	Gentamicin	I	Isoniazid	I
	Methyltestosterone	I	Levodopa	I
	Nafcillin	I	Paraminosalicylic acid	I
	Opiates	I		
	Oxacillin	I		
Sodium	Androgens	I	Calcium	D
	Rauwolfia alkaloids	I		
	Corticosteroids	I		
	Mannitol	I		
	Methyldopa	I		
	Oxyphenbutazone	I		
	Phenylbutazone	I		
	Ammonium chloride	D		
	Heparin	D		
	Oral diuretics	D		
	Mercurial diuretics	D		
	Spironolactone	D		
Urea	Alkaline antacids	I	Chloral hydrate	I
	Antimony salts	I	Chlorobutanol	I
	Arsenicals	I	Guanethidine	I
	Cephaloridine	I		
	Furosemide	I		
	Gentamicin	I		
	Kanamycin	I		
	Methyldopa	I		
	Neomycin	I		
Urate	Andrenocortical steroids	I	Ascorbic acid	I
	Busulfan	I	Glucose	I
	Ethacrynic acid	I	Methyldopa	I
	Nitrogen mustard	I	Theophylline	I
	Purine analogue antimetabolites	I		
	Pyrazinamide	I		
	Quinethazone	I		
	Thiazides	I		
	Vincristine sulfate	I		
	Acetylsalicylic acid	D		
	Allopurinol	D		
	Chlorpromazine	D		
	Chlorprothixene	D		
	Oxyphenbutazone	D		
	Phenylbutazone	D		
	Probenecid	D		

Constituent in Urine	Drugs Causing Physiologic Effect	Type of Effect†	Drugs with Chemical Interference	Type of Effect†
Catecholamines	Nitroglycerin	I	B-vitamin (high dose)	I
	Phenothiazines	I	Erythromycin	I
	MAO inhibitors	D	Hydralazine	I
			Levodopa	I
			Methenamine hippurate	I
			Methenamine mandelate	I
			Methyldopa	I
			Nicotinic acid	I

Table continues on following page

Table 5–3. SOME DRUGS WITH PHYSIOLOGIC EFFECT ON AND/OR CHEMICAL INTERFERENCE WITH COMMONLY ORDERED CONSTITUENTS IN BLOOD AND URINE *(Continued)*

Constituent in Urine	Drugs Causing Physiologic Effect	Type of Effect†	Drugs with Chemical Interference	Type of Effect†
Catecholamines *(cont.)*			Quinine-quinidine	I
			Salicylate	I
			Tetracyclines	I
Chloride			Bromide	I
Creatinine			Ascorbic acid	I
			Levodopa	I
			Methyldopa	I
			Nitrofuran derivatives	I
Glucose				
1. Enzymatic method (Clinistix, Testape)			Ascorbic acid	D
			Levodopa	D
2. Benedict's solution of Clinitest			Ascorbic acid	I
			Cephalosporins	I
			Chloral hydrate	I
			Nitrofuran derivatives	I
Porphyrins	Progestins-estrogens	I	Acriflavin	I
			Ethoxazene	I
			Phenazopyridine	I
			Procaine	I
			Sulfonamides	I
5-Hydroxyindoleacetic acid (5-HIAA)	Reserpine	I	Mephenesin	I
			Methocarbamol	I
			Phenothiazines	D
17-Hydroxycorticosteroids = (17-OH)				
17-Ketogenic steroids = (17-KGS)				
17-Ketosteroids = (17-KS)				
(17-KS)	Anabolic steroids	I		
(17-KS, 17-OH)	Phenytoin	D		
(17-KS, 17-OH)	Estrogens	D		
(17-KS)	Ethacrynic acid	D		
(17-KS, 17-KGS)	Penicillin	D		
(17-KS)	Probenecid	D		
(17-OH)	Thiazide diuretics	D		
(17-OH, 17-KS, 17-KGS)	Meprobamate	I		
(17-OH, 17-KS, 17-KGS)	Phenothiazines	I		
(17-OH, 17-KS, 17-KGS)	Spironolactone	I		
(17-OH, 17-KS, 17-KGS)	Penicillin G	I		
(17-OH)	Ascorbic acid	I		
(17-OH)	Chloral hydrate	I		
(17-OH)	Chlordiazepoxide	I		
(17-OH)	Hydroxyzine	I		
(17-OH)	Inorganic iodides	I		
(17-OH)	Methenamine	I		
(17-KS)			Phenothiazines	I
(17-OH)			Quinidine, quinine	I
(17-OH)			Reserpine	I
(17-KS)			Ethinamate	D
(17-OH, 17-KS, 17-KGS)			Nalidixic acid	D
Pregnanediol			Mandelamine	I
Phenolsulfonphthalein	Penicillin	D		
	Probenecid	D		
	Salicylates	D		
	Sulfonamides	D		
	Thiazide diuretics	D		

Table continues on opposite page

Table 5–3. SOME DRUGS WITH PHYSIOLOGIC EFFECT ON AND/OR CHEMICAL INTERFERENCE WITH COMMONLY ORDERED CONSTITUENTS IN BLOOD AND URINE *(Continued)*

Constituent in Urine	Drugs Causing Physiologic Effect	Type of Effect†	Drugs with Chemical Interference	Type of Effect†
Vanillylmandelic acid	Epinephrine	I	Anileridine	I
	Lithium carbonate	I	Caffeine	I
	Nitroglycerin	I	Mandelamine	I
	Chlorpromazine	D	Methocarbamol	I
	Guanethidine	D	Salicylates	I
	MAO inhibitors	D		
	Reserpine	D		

*Modified from Martin, 1970, and Young, 1975.
†I indicates an increase and D a decrease.

phase refers to all actions performed on (by) the *patient* during the collection of the specimen and to all actions performed on the *specimen* prior to the measurement step. The preparation of the specimen is not as rigidly controlled as is the measurement of the analytes; thus, it is during the pre-instrumental phase that numerous sources of variation are in operation. Variation may be caused by (1) actions during collection of the specimen, (2) specimen interferences, (3) actions during processing of the specimen, and (4) actions during storage of the specimen.

Collecting the Specimen

Identification Errors. The person collecting the specimen from the patient must feel certain that the correct individual is contributing the appropriate specimen. Questioning the patient for his name and confirming the name with identifying name and number tags on his person are very critical. The correct identification must be recorded on the specimen container and on the request slip. Finally, the correct type of container and the presence (if needed) of the appropriate anticoagulant and/or preservative must be checked before collecting the specimen. The collection of a timed 24-hour urine specimen is often subject to confusion and subsequent errors. For the collection of a timed urine specimen or a timed fecal specimen, proper instructions on the method of collection should be given to the patient and to the nursing staff, and these instructions should then be carried out accordingly.

Site of Blood Drawing. Previously we have discussed the postural considerations as well as the effects of prolonged venous stasis on the concentration in blood of various quantities. The choice of capillary vs. venous blood is not usually of clinical importance except in the case of the glucose tolerance test where the capillary glucose concentration is reported to be 10 to 30 per cent higher than the venous glucose concentration (Larsson-Cohn, 1976). The phlebotomist should be certain to avoid sampling from an extremity in which an indwelling intravenous catheter is delivering parenteral solutions.

Blood samples for analysis of 18 chemical and six hematologic constituents may be drawn from either arm of a patient into whom an intravenous solution is flowing without any clinically important difference in results for any analyte except glucose. The site of venipuncture must be distal to the intravenous needle, and the tourniquet must be placed between the intravenous needle and the site of venipuncture. For glucose, there was an appreciable difference, the value averaging 43 mg/dl higher (range -10 to $+156$) in the "intravenous arm" (Ong, 1978).

Contamination of Specimens. Residual detergent in collecting tubes may contaminate the specimen with inorganic phosphate. Plasticizers in intravenous tubing and in tube stoppers have been implicated in creating spurious peaks in methods based on gas-liquid chromatographic procedures. In addition, cork stoppers and some glass tubes will release calcium when exposed to blood, thereby causing a falsely increased serum calcium concentration. Blood specimens collected for lead analysis must be obtained in lead-free, acid-washed containers. Urine collected for all rare metal analyses demands acid-washed containers free of contaminants. When liver biopsies are obtained for rare metal analysis, the investigator must consider the contamination from the metal in the bore of the needle. When assaying for coagulation factors (e.g., Factor XII, platelets), special precautions regarding specimen collection must be taken (Calam, 1977).

Specimen Interferences

Lysis of or Leakage from Cells. The majority of chemical measurements are performed on specimens obtained from the extracellular fluid, that is, usually on serum or on plasma. Certain analytes are present in the formed elements of the blood in concentrations many times higher or lower than in the surrounding plasma (Table 5–4), and therefore lysis of the cells will "contaminate" the plasma or serum to a measurable amount. "Hemolysis" refers to the abnormal lysis of erythrocytes. Hemolysis can occur before venipuncture (*in vivo* hemolysis) or during the analytical procedure (*in vitro* hemolysis). Factors contribut-

Table 5–4. CHANGES IN THE SERUM CONCENTRATIONS (OR ACTIVITIES) OF SELECTED CONSTITUENTS DUE TO LYSIS OF ERYTHROCYTES (RBC)*

Constituent	Ratio of Concentration (or Activity) in RBC to Concentration (or Activity) in Serum	Change of Concentration (or Activity) in Serum After Lysis of 1% RBC, Assuming a Hematocrit of 0.50
Lactate dehydrogenase	160:1	+272.0%
Aspartate aminotransferase (AST or GOT)	40:1	+220.0%
Potassium	23:1	+24.4%
Alanine aminotransferase (ALT or GPT)	6.7:1	+55.0%
Glucose	0.82:1	−5.0%
Inorganic phosphate	0.78:1	+9.1%
Sodium	0.11:1	−1.0%
Calcium	0.10:1	+2.9%

*Modified from Caraway, 1972, and Laessig, 1976a.

ing to *in vitro* hemolysis when blood is collected in vacuum tubes include vigorous expansion of the blood into the evacuated tube and/or mixing of the blood with an oxalate anticoagulant. Recently it has been suggested that greater hemolysis actually occurs with wider bore needles than with smaller bore needles (Calam, 1977). *In vitro* hemolysis can be minimized by allowing the alcohol applied to the skin to dry before performing the venipuncture. Additional *in vitro* lysis of cells occurs during the centrifugation and separation steps in the processing of the specimen. The effects of hemolysis or leakage from erythrocytes can be divided into two types: (1) the release of erythrocyte constituents, including water, and (2) direct interference of hemoglobin with various assays.

Normal serum appears visibly hemolytic when the concentration of hemoglobin exceeds 200 mg/L, although much higher levels could remain undetected in icteric serum. Assuming that a patient's hematocrit value is 0.50 and that the hemoglobin concentration in the whole blood is 150 g/L, then one can compute the expected concentration of hemoglobin in the contaminated serum for various fractions of erythrocytes lysed. For the following example, we assume that the erythrocytes present in the supernatant are completely lysed and the cellular constituents enter the serum. If we are successful in removing 99 per cent of the erythrocytes, the serum will contain 3 g/L hemoglobin. Laessig (1976a) examined the changes in the serum concentration of various constituents as a result of incomplete removal of erythrocytes and subsequent *in vitro* lysis of the remaining erythrocytes. He studied 99 per cent removal (therefore, 1.0 per cent lysis) of erythrocytes in the blood of 10 healthy subjects. Table 5–4 presents the mean change in the serum concentration for each of a number of constituents in these healthy subjects with 1.0 per cent erythrocytes added (Laessig, 1976a). The table also persents the ratio of the measured value in erythrocytes to the determined value in serum (Caraway, 1972). In addition to the analytes presented in Table 5–4, *in vitro* hemolysis results in an increase in the serum activity of acid phosphatase and in the serum concentration of zinc and magnesium. Lysis of red blood cells also releases a number of the interfering substances into the plasma or serum. The released hemoglobin causes an apparent increase in the serum albumin concentration as determined by the bromocresol green method, an apparent increase in the serum bilirubin concentration as determined spectrophotometrically, an interference with the measurement of sulfobromophthalein and the biuret method of protein determination when primitive one wavelength methods are used, and an apparent decrease of the serum bilirubin concentration as assayed by the diazotization reaction (Schwartz, 1973). Lysis of erythrocytes results in a release of the enzyme adenylate kinase. The presence of adenylate kinase will cause an apparent elevation of the creatine kinase activity in serum when the latter enzyme is assayed with adenosine diphosphate in the reaction mixture (Swanson, 1972). It has been found that a 1 per cent solution of lysed erythrocytes causes a 98 per cent increase in mean creatine kinase activity in sera of healthy subjects (Laessig, 1976a). *In vitro* thrombolysis (platelet lysis) can result in marked increases in the serum concentration of potassium and magnesium and the serum activities of acid phosphatase and aldolase, while *in vitro* granulocytolysis will cause a release of the enzymes muramidase (lysozyme), phosphohexose isomerase, arginase, glucose-6-phosphate dehydrogenase, and glutamate dehydrogenase (Schwartz, 1973).

Anticoagulants and Preservatives. The use of anticoagulants, e.g., potassium oxalate, causes variable dilution of plasma owing to water transport from the cells of the blood into the plasma and should be considered as a source of bias. Anticoagulants that act as chelators of calcium will also cause an inhibition of various plasma enzyme activities if calcium is not added later on. Amylase activity is inhibited by oxalate or citrate (McGeachin, 1957), and lactate dehydrogenase and acid phosphatase by oxalate (Caraway, 1972). Oxalate, citrate, or ethylenediaminotetraacetate (EDTA) will cause a decrease in the calcium concentration in plasma when calcium is determined spectrophotometrically by a dye method but will not affect the result when calcium is assayed by an atomic absorption procedure. The sodium or potassium salt of fluoride, heparin, or EDTA will interfere with the analysis of the electrolyte involved. Fluoride is used as a preservative for plasma being assayed for glucose; however, fluoride will inhibit the action of glucose oxidase in the enzymatic analytical method for glucose, will diminish the activity of acid phosphatase, and will increase the activity of amylase.

Preservatives are often used in preparing urine specimens. As is the case for blood, the purpose for using each of these preservatives must be known so that no error of omission or commission is made.

Icteric Serum. Bilirubin present in serum will result in a noticeable "jaundice" color when the concentration of bilirubin is above 430 μmol/L (25 mg/L). Bilirubin will interfere with albumin assays performed by the HABA (2-(p-hydroxyphenylazo)-benzoic acid) procedure, with cholesterol assays using the ferric chloride reagents, with glucose determinations based on an *o*-toluidine method, and with total protein determinations using the biuret procedure. In each instance the values are artifactually elevated, and in each case the effect can be eliminated or at least minimized with appropriate "blanking procedures" or dual wavelength methods.

Lactescent Serum. The turbidity caused by elevated triglyceride concentration in serum will cause apparently elevated results for those substances whose measurements are based on absorbance at the same wavelengths at which the lipid particles also absorb light and at which the final absorbance reading is used as the index of the concentration value of the analyte. The bromocresol green procedure for albumin, the cresophthalein method for calcium, and the acid-ammonium molybdate procedure for inorganic phosphate are all affected by the increased turbidity. One means of correcting for this interference is the use of a reference (or blanked) assay; i.e., the latter contains the serum, diluent, etc., but is lacking in at least one critical reagent. The net absorbance reading (refer to Chapter 2, Principles of Instrumentation, for details) is the absorbance reading in the total assay mixture minus the reading in the reference mixture. However, even blanking procedures will not eliminate all the interferences.

Plasma appears lactescent when the concentration of triglyceride exceeds 4.6 mmol/L (4 g/L). Amylase activity is inhibited in highly lipemic serum. Whether the lipid fraction or some inhibitor associated with the hyperlipidemic state is the cause of the inhibition is still unresolved. Hyperlipidemia will cause an inhibition of the activities of the enzymes uricase and urease; thus, when these enzymes are used as reagents in the assay of urate and urea, and the measurement is based on the initial rate of the reaction, the results of the assays will be too low. The same phenomenon occurs in the case of creatine kinase, bilirubin, and total protein, i.e., they are decreased in the presence of severe hypertriglyceridemia ($>$ 5.8 mmol/L); moreover, this effect cannot be corrected by "blanking." Ultracentrifugation is particularly useful in pretreating lactescent serum specimens (Musiala, 1977).

Chemical Interferences Due to Drugs and Endogenous Metabolites in Biologic Specimens. In addition to the pharmacologic effects caused by drugs, there are a number of methodology-related drug interferences with the assays which may bias the results. A list of some of these drug-assay interactions is presented in Table 5–3. Endogenous metabolites also may be the cause of bias, e.g., falsely elevated serum aspartate aminotransferase activities have been noted in patients with diabetic ketosis in that acetoacetate interferes with the colorimetric procedure used to measure serum aspartate aminotransferase activity. It will also cause an apparent increase in creatinine results as measured by the Jaffe reaction (Caraway, 1972). Non-specific methods used to quantitate glucose result in apparently elevated values in patients with uremia. The introduction of more specific analytical methods has decreased the frequency of chemical interferences due to drugs or to endogenous metabolites.

1

Processing the Specimen

Transporting whole blood specimens through pneumatic tube systems may result in damage of erythrocytes during the transportation process (Steige, 1971). More recently Pragay (1974) noted that an improved pneumatic tube system which employs carriers that travel at slower speeds and uses only totally filled tubes did not result in any statistically significant changes which were consistent with *in vitro* hemolysis. The centrifugation step and subsequent decanting of the serum or plasma may lead to errors when not properly performed. The leakage of potassium from cells, the transfer of cellular contaminants during the decanting process, and the mislabeling of receiving tubes all can occur during the centrifugation and decanting steps. Recently the introduction of the "serum separator tube" (Laessig, 1976b) has resulted in a reduction of certain of these errors when used. Freezing, subsequent thawing, refreezing, and rethawing can result in denaturation of proteins. The activity of alkaline phosphatase will rise as a previously frozen specimen thaws and is stored at room temperature (Bodansky, 1932).

Storing the Specimen Prior to the Measurement

Evaporation-Induced Errors. Evaporation of water from serum will result in higher concentrations (or activities in the case of enzymes) of all analytes present in the serum sample. Burtis (1975) has investigated various factors influencing evaporative loss of liquid (water) from a specimen after it has been poured into a sample cup. Evaporative loss is increased with higher ambient temperature, the magnitude of air flow within the laboratory, and the time that the specimen is exposed to the environment, and is inversely related to the relative humidity. The size and shape of the sample cup, the fraction of the cup filled with serum, and nature of the cup material all affect the degree of evaporation (Burtis, 1975). Errors caused by evaporative loss of solvent often are not correctly estimated by conventional quality control procedures, as the control material usually is not exposed to the same environmental conditions during the pre-instrumental phase of the analysis as are the patients' specimens (Glenn, 1976).

Stability of Chemical Constituents During Storage. Alteration in the quantity of chemicals during storage may result from a number of causes. Refrigerated centrifugation of amniotic fluid which is being processed for a lecithin:sphingomyelin (L/S) ratio is recommended in order to inhibit the activity of the phospholipases which catalyze the hydrolysis of fatty acids from lecithin. This specimen should also be centrifuged slowly to avoid pulling the phospholipid down with the cellular debris (Wilkinson, 1977). Carbon dioxide in plasma will evaporate from a specimen stored in an open sample cup, causing a drop in concentration of approximately 5 mmol/L in 60 minutes at room temperature (Gambino, 1966). The loss of carbon dioxide from serum results in an increase in the serum pH. The pH of the serum will reach 8.5 two hours after being separated from the blood clot. At this alkaline pH the enzyme acid phosphatase begins to be destroyed. The stability of acid phosphatase can be prolonged by adjusting the pH to 6.2 with citrate buffer. Glycolysis occurring in whole blood will cause a drop in serum glucose concentration when a long time elapses from the collection of the whole blood specimen until the separation of the serum; e.g., serum glucose concentrations determined two hours after collection (serum being in contact with the clot for two hours) were an average of 10 per cent lower than the concentrations obtained when the serum was separated 30 minutes after collection (Hagebusch, 1966). Proteolytic and hydrolytic processes will result in increased concentrations of ammonia in stored blood. Changes in erythrocyte permeability result in increased serum concentrations of potassium, phosphorus, and magnesium when whole blood is stored before separating the serum. Storing blood in a refrigerator (4°C.) will increase the loss of potassium from the erythrocytes as compared to storing the blood at room temperature (25°C.); this difference is due to the greater inhibition of the sodium-potassium pump of the erythrocytes in the cold environment. Phosphorolytic enzymes will cause an increase in inorganic phosphate owing to release of the phosphate from organic phosphates. During the time of storage there may be a loss of enzyme activity in serum. The degree of loss is dependent upon the temperature at which the serum is stored (frozen) and on the total time of storage. An ideal method of storing serum includes rapid freezing in liquid nitrogen and storing at −80°C.; however, for most analytes storage at −20°C. for up to six weeks will not result in clinically important changes (Wilson, 1972).

Giampietro (1980) measured plasma glucose concentrations before and after storage at −20°C. for various intervals. A significant positive relationship was found between the storage interval and the percentage decrease in glucose concentration. Over a period of 20 months, the percentage of glucose decrease was approximately 12 per cent.

Rossing (1980) evaluated the stability of clinical chemistry specimens stored under refrigerated conditions. A total of 18 constituents were analyzed in serum both before and after refrigeration. These analytes included AST, LDH, alkaline phosphatase, direct bilirubin, total bilirubin, creatinine, uric acid, cholesterol, inorganic phosphorus, calcium, albumin, total protein, glucose, BUN, CO_2, chloride, potassium, and sodium. Only one analyte (CO_2) underwent a change that was judged to be clinically significant. The CO_2 mean value dropped by 3.7 mEq/L during overnight refrigeration.

Lyophilized specimens will be stable for most analytes for a period of many years, provided the lyophilization has been complete (Winsten, 1965; Schwartz, 1973). Exposure to light will cause a decrease in the serum bilirubin concentration as well as in the concentration of delta-aminolevulinic acid, porphyrins, and porphobilinogen in urine. Because the stability of many constituents measured in urine is pH-dependent, the urine is often maintained at a certain acidity using one of the following preservatives: concentrated hydrochloric acid (pH 0.2 to 1.6), 6 molar hydrochloric acid (pH 0.7 to 2.6), acetic acid (pH 2.3 to 3.9), or boric acid (pH 5.0 to 6.0).

CONCLUSION

The total variation in results obtained from healthy subjects over time can be partitioned into four components: (1) analytical variation, (2) preparation of the subject, (3) intra-individual physiologic variation, and (4) inter-individual biologic variation of mean values. Appreciating these expected, nonpathologic sources of variations is critical in being able to discriminate a patient's value as signifying pathology vs. merely being evidence of some usual variation in the value of an analyte.

Barrett, P. V. D.: Hyperbilirubinemia of fasting. J.A.M.A., *217*:1349, 1971.

Belfrage, P., Berg, B., Hagerstrand, I., et al.: Alterations of lipid metabolism in healthy volunteers during long-term ethanol intake. Eur. J. Clin. Invest., 7:127, 1977.

Bellet, S., Kershbaum, A., and Aspe, J.: The effect of caffeine on free fatty acids. Arch. Intern. Med., *116*:750, 1965.

Bishop, C., and Talbot, J. H.: Uric acid: Its role in biological process and the influence upon it of physiological, pathological and pharmacological agents. Pharmacol. Rev., *5*:231, 1953.

Bodansky, A., Jaffe, H. L., and Chandler, J. P.: Experimental factors influencing blood phosphatase values. J. Biol. Chem., *97*:66, 1932.

Burtis, C. A., Begovich, J. M., and Watson, J. S.: Factors influencing evaporation from sample cups, and assessment of their effect on analytical error. Clin. Chem., *21*:1907, 1975.

Calam, R. R.: Reviewing the importance of specimen collection. J. Am. Med. Technol., *39*:297, 1977.

Caraway, W. T., and Kammeyer, C. W.: Chemical interference by drugs and other substances with clinical laboratory test procedures. Clin. Chim. Acta, *41*:395, 1972.

Carlsten, A., et al.: Arterial concentration of free fatty acids and free amino acids in healthy individuals at rest and at different work loads. Scand. J. Clin. Lab. Invest., *14*:185, 1962.

Dalferes, E. R., Webber, L. S., Radhakrishnamurthy, B., et al.: Continuous-flow (AutoAnalyzer I) analysis for plasma thiocyanate as an index to tobacco smoking. Clin. Chem., *26*:493, 1980.

Freer, D. E., and Statland, B. E.: The effects of ethanol (0.75 g/kg body weight) on the activities of selected enzymes in sera of healthy young adults: 1. Intermediate-term effects. Clin. Chem., *23*:830, 1977.

Part II

CLINICAL CHEMISTRY

EDITED BY JOHN BERNARD HENRY, M.D., AND RICHARD A. McPHERSON, M.D.

7

SPIROMETRY AND BLOOD GASES

ROBERT GILBERT, M.D.

With a Section on Collection, Processing, and Measurement of Blood Gases by Michael W. Lapinski, M.D.

SPIROMETRY

The primary function of the lung is that of gas exchange; arterial blood gases are the best guide to this function and will be discussed later in this chapter. In order for gas exchange to be a continuous process, alveolar air must constantly be exchanged with environmental air. This is the ventilatory function, the act of breathing. Spirometry is the most widely used guide to impairment of this function.

Equipment

The spirogram is a graph with volume of air on the ordinate and time on the abscissa. In its simplest form a spirometer consists of a hollow cylinder open at the bottom, floating in a water jacket (Fig. 7–1).

The subject breathes in and out of the cylinder, causing it to move up and down. The vertical motion

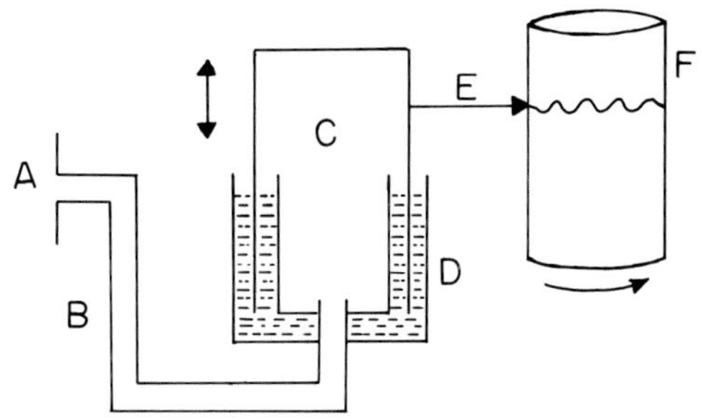

Figure 7–1. Schematic diagram of a simple spirometer. A, mouthpiece; B, conducting tubing; C, Hollow cylinder floating in waterjacket D: E, pen; F, rotating drum containing calibrated paper.

of the cylinder is transcribed onto calibrated paper fixed to a rotating drum, providing a record of volume of air versus time.

The Collins Survey Spirometer (Warren E. Collins Company, Inc., Braintree, Mass.) works exactly as shown in Figure 7–1. It is accurate, relatively inexpensive, and simple to operate. It is an excellent instrument for a physician's office, since an accurate spirogram can be obtained within one or two minutes at each patient visit. In the past two to three years, several computer-controlled spirometry systems have appeared on the market. These range in price between \$10,000 and \$15,000 and provide flow-volume as well as volume-time spirograms. They eliminate operator errors in transcription and calculation of data and, if calibrated carefully, should be sufficiently accurate for clinical purposes. The basic spirometer used in the system should conform to recent American Thoracic Society recommendations (ATS statement, 1979).

Performance

Proper instruction of the patient is vital. Spirometry is a performance test; the patient must understand the test and must be willing to perform at a maximum level. If the patient has not been tested before, both a forced inspiratory and forced expiratory effort should be recorded.

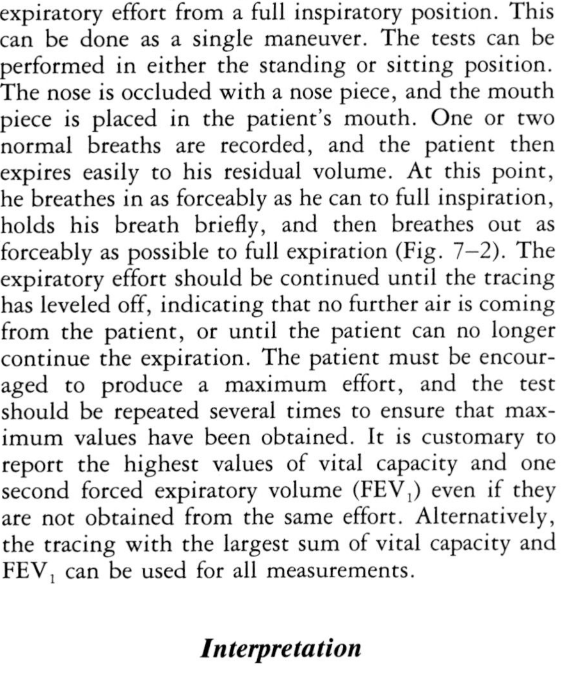

What is required is a maximum inspiratory effort from a full expiratory position, and a maximum expiratory effort from a full inspiratory position. This can be done as a single maneuver. The tests can be performed in either the standing or sitting position. The nose is occluded with a nose piece, and the mouth piece is placed in the patient's mouth. One or two normal breaths are recorded, and the patient then expires easily to his residual volume. At this point, he breathes in as forceably as he can to full inspiration, holds his breath briefly, and then breathes out as forceably as possible to full expiration (Fig. 7–2). The expiratory effort should be continued until the tracing has leveled off, indicating that no further air is coming from the patient, or until the patient can no longer continue the expiration. The patient must be encouraged to produce a maximum effort, and the test should be repeated several times to ensure that maximum values have been obtained. It is customary to report the highest values of vital capacity and one second forced expiratory volume (FEV_1) even if they are not obtained from the same effort. Alternatively, the tracing with the largest sum of vital capacity and FEV_1 can be used for all measurements.

Interpretation

The spirogram contains two basic types of information—the total amount of air which can be moved in or out of the lung (the vital capacity, VC) and the rate of air flow. The most useful measurements of rate of air flow are the volume of air expired during the first second of the forced expiration (FEV_1), the volume of air inspired during the the first second of the forced inspiration (FIV_1), the average flow rate over the middle half of the forced expiratory curve (FEF 25–75), and the instantaneous flow rate after 50 per cent of the vital capacity has been expelled ($\dot{V}$ 50). Figure 7–2 demonstrates the first three of these measurements in a normal spirogram; the volume of air expired is shown equal to the volume inspired. In cases of severe airway obstruction there may be air trapping with forced expiration, so that the total volume expired during this forced expiration, the forced vital capacity (FVC), may be smaller than the vital capacity recorded during inspiration. This is especially likely to be true

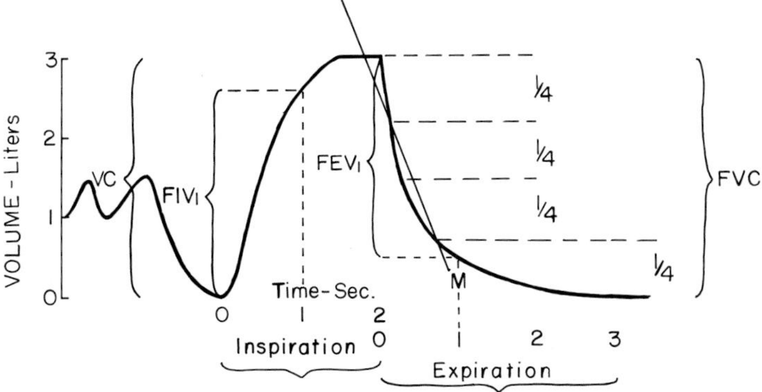

Figure 7–2. Normal shaped spirogram. Slope of line MM is the maximum mid-expiratory flow rate. VC = vital capacity; FVC = forced vital capacity; FEV_1 = one second forced expiratory volume, FIV_1 = one second forced inspiratory volume.

if the inspiratory effort was started from a residual volume reached from a slow, non-forceful expiration. If both the inspiratory and expiratory vital capacities are measured, the larger should be reported as the vital capacity. V 50 is the first derivative of the expiratory volume-time spirogram at 50 per cent of vital capacity. It can be obtained by drawing a tangent to the curve at this point. Since this is a very inaccurate procedure, V 50 is usually obtained directly from the flow-volume curve, and not used if a flow-volume curve is not available (see below).

Reference values for vital capacity, FEV_1, and FEF 25–75 are based on age, height, and sex; the prediction formulas of Morris (1971) and Crapo (1981) are currently in vogue. It has now become customary to consider the lower limit of normal as the predicted value minus 1.64 times the standard error of estimate. The FEV_1 is also expressed as a percentage of FVC, often abbreviated FEV_1%. The lower reference limit for FEV_1% is 70 per cent. It tends to decline slightly with age, but this can be ignored for most purposes. Reference values for FIV_1 are not available, but FIV_1 is normally equal to or nearly equal to the vital capacity.

It is customary to classify abnormal spirograms as "obstructive" or "restrictive." The restrictive pattern or defect refers to a reduced vital capacity with normal or relatively normal flow rates. "Relatively normal" is a vague term, but certainly the FEV_1% should be above 70 per cent. The absolute value of FEV_1, FIV_1, FEF 25–75, or any other measurements may be low with a restrictive defect, especially if the vital capacity is severely reduced. *A spirogram of a restrictive defect looks like a normal spirogram with all volumes reduced proportionally.*

The term "restrictive disease" should not be used, since a wide variety of diseases produce a restrictive pattern. These include heart failure, pneumonia, pulmonary fibrosis and other types of interstitial lung disease, pulmonary embolism, atelectasis, pneumothorax, pleural effusion, crushed chest injuries, and neurological diseases such as poliomyelitis, myasthenia gravis, and Guillain-Barré syndrome. (Rarely, during a severe attack of asthma, clearly a disease involving airway obstruction, a restrictive pattern is seen.) The spirogram, therefore, indicates that a restrictive ventilatory defect is present and provides information as to the severity of the defect, but gives no clue as to the etiology.

The obstructive pattern or defect refers to airway obstruction and its most common cause is the asthma-bronchitis-emphysema group of diseases. FEV_1 and FEF 25–75 will be reduced and FEV_1% will be below 70 per cent. Vital capacity and especially forced vital capacity are usually reduced, but this is primarily the result of an increase in residual volume, rather than loss of lung tissue, increased stiffness of the lung, or chest wall or neuromuscular disease, as in the case of a restrictive defect. A spirogram showing severe airway obstruction with a low vital capacity therefore should not be referred to as a combined restrictive and obstructive defect. In the author's experience, combined defects are relatively rare. Figure 7–3 shows a spirogram of a moderately severe obstructive defect.

The obstructive defects we have been discussing are those of so-called lower airway obstruction, i.e., obstruction of airways within the lung parenchyma. In these cases expiratory flow rates are always more severely reduced than inspiratory flow rates; FIV_1 should always be greater than FEV_1. If both FIV_1 and FEV_1 are reduced, and FIV_1 is smaller than FEV_1, upper airway obstruction must be strongly considered. The most common causes of upper airway obstruction are tracheal stenosis and diseases of the larynx and epiglottis. Tracheal tumor, thyroid compression of the trachea, and obstruction in the posterior pharynx may also cause upper airway obstruction.

A special warning is necessary in the interpretation of the inspiratory spirogram. Although the entire spirogram is effort dependent, this is especially true for inspiration. The inspiratory part of the spirogram must always be interpreted with caution if there is any reason to suspect less than a maximum effort.

There has been a great deal of recent interest in the flow-volume spirogram. It provides an excellent visual display; at a glance one can tell if a defect is present and the nature of the defect. For quantitative measurements for clinical purposes, however, its value in place of or in addition to the volume-time spirogram has yet to be proved. Flow-volume spirograms seem most useful for the detection of upper airway obstruction and for the measurement of instantaneous flow rates such as V 50. A detailed description is beyond the scope of this discussion, but a good review has been published by Kryger (1976).

Limitations of Spirometry

The earliest manifestations of chronic bronchitis and emphysema are probably in the small airways, arbitrarily defined as those with an internal diameter

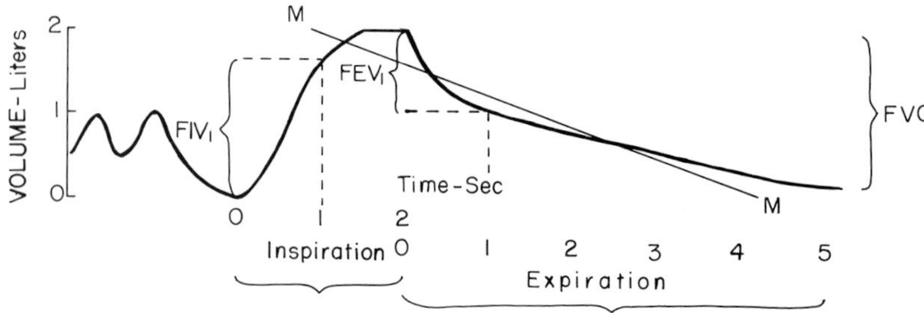

Figure 7–3. Spirogram demonstrating moderately severe airway obstruction. Note that the FVC is less than the vital capacity recorded during inspiration. Note also the difference in slope of line MM compared to that of Figure 7–2.

of less than 2 mm. Furthermore, in the interval between attacks, the asthmatic patient may have obstruction limited to these small airways. Because they are so numerous, their total cross-sectional area is large, and considerable disease can be present in these small airways without contributing significantly to overall airway resistance. In this case, the volume-time spirogram may be normal. There has been considerable effort in recent years to develop more sensitive tests for "early" or small airway obstruction. Many have been reported, but over the course of time they have been found to be too complex, too expensive, too uncomfortable, too unreliable, too time-consuming, or any combination of these for routine use.

The spirogram is used to detect obstructive and restrictive defects when, in fact, it measures neither one. A restrictive defect implies a reduction in total lung capacity, whereas the spirogram, since it does not measure residual volume, uses the vital capacity as an indication of total lung capacity. If there is no evidence of airway obstruction, this is probably a safe approximation. Furthermore, the spirogram does not measure airway obstruction or airway resistance directly. Rather, an "obstructive" defect is reported when there is a reduced rate of maximum air flow. Poor effort, loss of lung elasticity, and loss of lung volume will all produce airflow limitation in the absence of obstruction.

The body plethysmograph will measure the residual volume as well as provide a direct measurement of airway resistance. If the spirogram is entirely normal, residual volume and airway resistance will also probably be normal, and the spirogram, therefore, provides an adequate assessment of ventilatory function. If the spirogram is abnormal, however, the initial pulmonary function evaluation should include a body plethysmograph study as well. Once the physiological defect has been characterized, simple spirometry is an excellent way to follow the course of the illness and to measure responses to bronchodilators and bronchial provocation tests.

2

COLLECTION, PROCESSING, AND MEASUREMENT OF BLOOD GASES

Michael W. Lapinski, M.D.

Specimen Collection Receptacles

Many types of blood specimen collection receptacles have been evaluated and recommended for blood gas determinations. One of the first and still preferred is the glass syringe, which should probably be considered a "reference" receptacle. All others, such as regular plastic syringes, "specialized plastic syringes," vacuum tubes, and capillary tubes, should be compared with glass syringes. The glass syringe and plunger should be matched for best fit. Approximately 1 ml of heparin (1000 or 5000 U/ml) is drawn into the syringe and the barrel lubricated. The plunger is tested to ensure easy mobility, and the heparin should be expelled, leaving the dead space filled with residual heparin (Winkler, 1974). Advantages of the glass syringe include the most accurate results obtainable, a glass plunger that moves upward because of arterial pressure (if 23 gauge or larger needle is used), and reusability. Disadvantages of the glass syringe include relatively high initial cost, need for proper sterilization between patients, and easy breakage. Alternative devices include standard plastic (polypropylene) syringes, special plastic syringes designed especially for blood gases, and vacuum tubes. Plastic syringes eliminate the need for resterilization and are low in cost, readily available in any hospital setting, and relatively unbreakable. Unfortunately, standard plastic syringes have their own disadvantages. A valid question concerns accuracy because of gas leakage through the plastic. A major technical disadvantage is that the plunger will not rise owing to arterial pressure, and a minor problem is that air bubbles are harder to remove.

Leakage of gases through plastic can pose a major problem or a relatively minor problem, depending on the type of plastic and the oxygen and carbon dioxide tensions of the blood specimen collected. The greater the difference between the partial pressures of oxygen and carbon dioxide in the blood and the partial pressures in room air, the larger is the leakage. Scott (1971a, b) does not recommend the use of plastic syringes. Polypropylene plastic syringes are superior to polystyrene plastic syringes (Scott, 1971b). Other authors (Evers, 1972; Winkler, 1974) conclude that plastic syringes are acceptable for patient management and that most clinical problems are not affected by relatively small differences that may exist between glass and plastic syringes.

Recently plastic syringes featuring a plunger which will rise owing to arterial pressure have replaced the standard glass or plastic syringes in many hospitals. Numerous brands are available. The use of these newer syringes has alleviated the major disadvantage of the plastic syringe (the plunger not rising due to arterial pressure) and the major disadvantages of the glass syringe (the easy breakage and need of sterilization).

Another type of blood gas syringe has made an entry into the market. This blood gas syringe has a preheparinized needle-syringe assembly with a vented plunger. An example is OMNISTIK (Marquest Medical Products, Englewood, Col.). Petty (1981) has reported that OMNISTIK has shown no significant errors of analysis introduced by gas exchange at the advancing blood-air interface. Because these syringes use crystalline heparin, the P_{CO_2} dilution artifact is not present, so small samples may be obtained.

Controversy has surrounded the use of vacuum tubes such as the Vacutainer. Fleisher (1971) reported the successful use of a special Vacutainer tube (Becton-Dickinson and Company, Rutherford, N.J.) filled with nitrogen gas at a pressure of 152 mm Hg and containing 143 units of sodium heparin. A special adapter was used to obtain arterial blood gases. Although these specialized vacuum tubes were shown to produce accurate results, the large air space at the top of standard heparin vacuum tubes can produce erroneous results by equilibrating with the blood.

The last type of acceptable container for blood collection and transport (skin puncture blood) is special capillary tubes. However, their accuracy and deficiencies cannot easily be separated from the arterialized capillary blood which they contain.

Blood Specimen Collection and Patient Preparation

The brachial and radial arteries are the preferred vessels for arterial puncture. The femoral artery is relatively large and easy to puncture, but care must be taken in older individuals, in whom the femoral artery tends to bleed more than the radial or brachial. Since the bleeding site is hidden by bedcovers, it may not be noticed until bleeding is massive. The radial artery is more difficult to puncture but exhibits a lower incidence of complications (Mortensen, 1967). When using the radial artery it is essential to test the collateral circulation of the hand using the Allen test (Bedford, 1974; Greenhow, 1972). The Allen test consists of elevating the hand to empty it of blood, occlusion of the radial artery, and observation of the return of blood flow through the ulnar artery as the hand is lowered. This test ensures collateral circulation should the radial artery become occluded as a consequence of manipulation. The major complications of arterial puncture include thrombosis and hemorrhage (Siggaard-Anderson, 1968). Petty (1966) reported no complications except for minimal hematomas with 475 arterial punctures. Using trained registered nurses to perform radial arterial punctures, Sackner (1971) reported 1541 punctures with no morbidity.

The artery to be punctured is identified by its pulsations. The skin is properly cleansed to prepare an aseptic site for puncture. Although a local anesthetic wheal may be made, an anesthetic is not required. Unanesthetized arterial puncture does provide an accurate measurement of resting pH and P_{CO_2} (Morgan, 1979) in spite of the theoretical error possible due to hyperventilation caused by the pain of the arterial puncture. The use of butterfly infusion sets is not recommended (Baegeant, 1975). Using 19 vs. 25 gauge needles does not vary the P_{CO_2} or P_{O_2} more than 1 mm Hg (Baegeant, 1975).

The needle (18 to 20 gauge for brachial artery) should pierce the skin at an angle of approximately 45 to 60 degrees and should approach the artery slowly. Some degree of dorsiflexion of the wrist is necessary with the radial artery for which a 23 to 25 gauge needle is used. The pulsations of blood into the syringe confirm that arterial blood has been obtained. Usually, if a 23 gauge or larger needle has been used, the syringe will fill by arterial pressure alone. If the plunger is pulled back, there is a possibility of aspirating air into the syringe. Any air that is accidently aspirated should be immediately expelled (Ishikawa, 1974). After the blood specimen is obtained, the needle should be removed and an airtight cap placed over the tip of the syringe. Although it is common practice to force the point of the needle into a cork or rubber stopper, this practice should be avoided owing to the danger of the needle's puncturing hospital personnel handling the specimen. After the arterial puncture, compression on the puncture site should be applied for a minimum of two minutes and preferably for five minutes (timed).

The recommended volume of arterial blood obtained varies with different authors, but certainly the greater the specimen volume, the less dilution effect from the heparin. With a 10 ml syringe, the dead space is 1.2 to 2.4 per cent of the maximal volume (Siggaard-Anderson, 1961). The heparin dilution primarily affects the P_{CO_2}. Siggaard-Anderson (1961) reports a 16 per cent fall in P_{CO_2} with a dilution of 12 to 13 per cent, while Bradley (1972) reports an error of 28 per cent on the same dilutional factor.

At times, it is either impractical or impossible to obtain arterial blood from a patient. Under these circumstances, another source of blood can be obtained, but it should always be remembered that the most accurate results are achieved with arterial blood.

While venous blood is more readily obtained, it usually reflects the acid-base status of an extremity, not the body as a whole. Venous blood properly collected will yield adequate pH values, but venous blood yields incorrect values for arterial oxygen saturation and alveolar P_{CO_2} (Gambino, 1959, 1961).

Arterialized skin puncture blood from the finger has been recommended as a suitable substitute for arterial blood for pH and P_{CO_2} but is not acceptable for P_{O_2} (Jung, 1966). In order for it to be a satisfactory substitute for arterial blood, some estimation of the P_{O_2} must be available. The recommended site for obtaining arterialized capillary blood is the earlobe (Langlands, 1965) because of its vascularity, its low metabolic requirements, and the ease with which it can be "arterialized." The earlobe can be arterialized by heat, by flicking with the index finger until definite flushing is observed, or by chemical means of Trafuril paste (Ciba A-G, Basel, Switzerland).

To obtain a blood specimen, the earlobe is cleansed with alcohol and punctured. The puncture area should be adequate to obtain a free flow of blood and the lobe wiped dry. Two heparinized capillary tubes (100 μl) are placed in the center of the drop and filled to capacity without air bubbles. Both ends are sealed in clay after the insertion of a rustproof metal stirrer. Blood in the tubes is stirred by the use of a magnet, thus mixing specimen with heparin (Sadove, 1973). Whenever the cardiac output is severely restricted (Laughlin, 1964) or there is a systolic pressure below 95 mm Hg (Koch, 1968) or vasoconstriction (Sadove, 1973), skin puncture blood yields unreliable data.

The greatest value of skin puncture blood is in the pediatric age group. In the older pediatric population, earlobe blood is available, but in neonates and infants in whom it is impractical to sample the earlobe the heel is often used. A deep heel prick is made at the distal edge of the calcaneal protuberance following a five- to ten-minute period in 45 to 47°C. water (Koch, 1967). The specimen is then handled as described for the earlobe specimen. Skin puncture blood obtained in this manner is unacceptable for PCO_2 and PO_2 determination in the first day of life, probably owing to vasoconstriction and poor perfusion of the extremities (Koch, 1967). In infants with respiratory distress syndrome, heel blood deviates significantly from arterial blood in all parameters except base excess and standard bicarbonate (Gandy, 1964; Bigen, 1975). The best method for blood gas collection in the newborn still remains the indwelling umbilical artery catheter.

The patient's temperature may be taken into account in the determination of blood gas values. For PO_2, there is about a 6 per cent change per degree centigrade (Nunn, 1962). Although correction factors are available for fever (Kelman, 1966), they are rarely used in clinical medicine but should be; with automatic blood gas analyzers, a patient's temperature can be included in the analysis.

Transcutaneous Monitoring

The need for continuous measurement of blood gases has led to the development of transcutaneous monitoring. The skin is arterialized by using electric heat, which causes dilatation of the vasculature causing increasing capillary flow, which leads to the capillary blood being nearly identical to arterial blood. Both oxygen and carbon dioxide are known to diffuse through the skin, so this diffusion would provide a noninvasive medium for the measurement of arterial blood gases.

Transcutaneous monitoring has become common in newborn infants, in delivery with fetal scalp (within Europe), and in adult intensive care patients. Transmucous membrane oxygen monitoring has been advocated (Czech, 1979) intraoperatively. Poor correlation is seen in adult patients undergoing surgery when transcutaneous monitoring is used due to many factors which may include thickness of skin, oxygenation, local perfusion, state of vasodilatation, and skin metabolism.

The use of transcutaneous monitoring has been confined in the past to monitoring oxygen ($P_{TC}O_2$), with the development of monitoring of carbon dioxide ($P_{TC}CO_2$) occurring only recently. The use of transcutaneous carbon dioxide monitoring has been impeded due to technical problems. A rise of 10 mm Hg in PCO_2 is very significant clinically. Unfortunately the usual PCO_2 electrode has a slope of 55 to 60 mV/100 mm Hg, which means a 10 mm Hg change corresponds to a signal change of about 3 to 10 mV, which is difficult to measure reproducibly (Huch, 1979).

The use of transcutaneous oxygen measurement has been standard accepted practice using a Clark electrode and an electric heater. Transcutaneous carbon dioxide measurement usually involves the use of a modified Severinghaus electrode with a heater.

A study by Cubal (1981) reaches the following conclusions concerning transcutaneous blood gas measurements. Patients with intact hemodynamic function have close agreement between $P_{TC}O_2$ and arterial blood tensions. Unheated $P_{TC}CO_2$ sensors measure tissue carbon dioxide. When a high $P_{TC}O_2$ was seen without a clinically apparent cause, the patients later developed manifestations of inadequate tissue perfusion. In patients with hemodynamic compromise, a $P_{TC}O_2$ rise was often the only indication of altered tissue perfusion. In the abnormal tissue, circulation persists and the $P_{TC}O_2$ further increases, with ultimately compromised oxygen delivery with resulting $P_{TC}O_2$ lower than arterial oxygen. Therefore in cardiovascular compromise the $P_{TC}O_2$ reflected tissue perfusion, and the $P_{TC}O_2$ monitored oxygen delivery to the tissues. In patients with ventilatory problems without cardiovascular alterations, $P_{TC}O_2$ and $P_{TC}CO_2$ reliably reflect arterial values.

Conditions such as severe hypovolemia (blood volume $<$ 58 ml/kg), arterial hypotension (systolic blood pressure 10 to 33 mm Hg), anemic hypoxemia (hematocrit 5 to 28 per cent), and/or acidemia (pH 6.72 or less) were associated with poor $P_{TC}O_2$ and arterial oxygen correlation (Versmold, 1979).

The only complication associated with transcutaneous monitoring of blood gases when properly performed is a mild localized erythema at the site of the heated electrode, which usually disappears within a few hours of sensor removal. If a heater temperature rises above normal operating temperatures, burns have occurred. At this time in the United States, no fetal transcutaneous electrodes for fetal scalp attachments have been approved by the Food and Drug Administration. The usefulness of transcutaneous monitoring in obstetrical care has been demonstrated by Huch (1979).

Blood Specimen Handling and Transport

All blood specimens in sealed receptacles should be placed in ice water immediately after they are obtained from the patient. Blood will consume oxygen and liberate carbon dioxide at a rate which is temperature dependent. When the PO_2 of the original blood is above 150 mm Hg, the decay at 37°C. is 2.7 mm Hg/min (Newball, 1973). Although room temperature does not produce as large an error, it is not an acceptable mode of transport. One can appreciate the importance of blood cooling when one considers that in most large hospitals blood gas determinations require between 10 and 15 minutes after blood collection for completion; this means an error of 27 to 40 mm Hg lower for PO_2 at 37°C.

When a specimen is received in the laboratory, it should be placed in ice water, properly identified, and scrutinized for clots and air bubbles. If all these conditions are not met, the specimen should not be analyzed. A clotted specimen aspirated or injected

2

into a modern gas analyzer may necessitate a major cleaning of the instrument. If a specimen arrives only in water, without visible ice, one should be very suspicious of the elapsed time for transport and possible errors from room temperature storage.

Blood Gas Instrumentation

Blood gas instrumentation has advanced tremendously since the development of specific electrodes within the last 20 years. Every modern blood gas instrument contains pH, P_{CO_2}, and P_{O_2} electrodes (see Chap. 2, p. 34).

A glass electrode system is used for pH measurement. This system consists of two halves, the calomel or reference electrode and the glass electrode. The calomel electrode maintains a constant potential, while the glass electrode membrane develops a potential proportional to the hydrogen ion concentration in the solution. This electrode is calibrated by using two phosphate buffers of known pH (Dowd, 1973).

The Severinghaus electrode is used commonly for P_{CO_2}. This is a pH electrode surrounded by an electrolyte solution separated from the blood by a membrane permeable to carbon dioxide. The pH of the solution is dependent on the P_{CO_2} that comes to an equilibrium with the blood. The membrane can be of silicone rubber or Teflon (Severinghaus, 1962, 1968).

For O_2 determination, the polarographic Clark oxygen electrode is used. A constant polarizing voltage is applied to the silver–silver chloride anode and the platinum wire cathode. The anode and cathode are in a KCl electrolyte solution. The blood is separated by an oxygen-permeable membrane of polypropylene or polyethylene. Oxygen is reduced at the electrode, and the potential change is proportional to the rate of oxygen reduction. This rate varies directly with the oxygen tension of the blood.

To calibrate P_{O_2} and P_{CO_2} electrodes, either a gas or a liquid of known oxygen partial pressure must be used. If a gas is used, problems arise because of calibration of the O_2 electrode. Most P_{O_2} electrodes yield a lower P_{O_2} for blood than for the gas with which the electrode was equilibrated. This discrepancy is in the range of 1.8 to 5.6 per cent (Bird, 1974). It is known as the "blood gas factor" and holds the greatest significance at a P_{O_2} over 150 mm Hg (Bird, 1974). Protein contamination of the membranes must periodically be removed; membranes have only limited life before they develop leaks.

The differences among various available blood gas analyzers or instruments center on the degree of automation. A manual instrument properly used will yield results as accurate and reliable as the most automated instrument. In a very busy laboratory where instruments tend to be abused and the number of specimens is great, the more automated analyzers tend to reduce error owing to technical personnel carelessness and abuse; however, they may suffer more from disturbances of electronic circuitry and mechanical parts, which require maintenance and repair. The manual instrument is usually simpler to repair, and repairs can often be accomplished by a well-trained technologist in the laboratory. Usually, most repairs on the automatic instruments necessitate a factory-authorized repair person. All automatic analyzers have automatic calibration. Some of the more advanced instruments have incorporated barometers (strain gauge type) and a photometer to measure hemoglobin. Often the operator can make corrections for a patient's temperature by proper programming. The more manual analyzer generally reports only measured values; thus, the operator uses nomograms for the other parameters such as bicarbonate, base excess, oxygen saturation, total carbon dioxide, standard base excess, and standard bicarbonate. Usually the top-of-the-line instruments will calculate these parameters.

Quality Control

Quality control is difficult to perform adequately. The most accurate instrument is worthless if the specimen is incorrectly obtained or transported. It is imperative that the laboratory receive a proper specimen in every case that is reported. Quality control and preventive maintenance must be performed on a regular schedule. In one large community involving several laboratories, instruments initially showed inaccuracies ranging from −30.8 per cent to +17.3 per cent for P_{O_2} and from −14.0 per cent to +42.9 per cent for P_{CO_2}; by the conclusion of the quality control study, these inaccuracies were greatly reduced (Delaney, 1976).

One method of quality control for a laboratory consists of duplicate determinations of each blood specimen. In our laboratory, all abnormal blood gas results are confirmed on a different instrument and results recorded. If these results agree, we report the results of the first instrument; if they do not agree within 5 per cent, the specimen is reanalyzed with the necessary investigative steps taken to correct the instrument yielding an unacceptable value. All results are maintained as a permanent written record. This method, because of its frequent use, discloses problems which may take hours to identify by other quality control measures. Although duplicate analyses of a single specimen for quality control are useful, they should supplement only another accepted method of quality control.

Other methods of quality control include measuring room air injected into the machine, measuring water equilibrated at 37°C. with room air, and checking the CO_2 channel by another method of analysis.

Two major methods of quality control that should be used employ commercial ampules or equilibrated tonometer blood. All blood gas instruments must be checked with either tonometer blood or commercial ampules each shift at a minimum of three levels. One level should be within the normal range, one level should be alkalotic, and one level should be acidotic. The quality control material must be used when the instrument has been repaired or when suspicion arises concerning accuracy.

The commercial ampules are now available from a multitude of manufacturers with various matrices. Aqueous-based blood gas controls were the first commercially available controls. Examples of the aqueous-based controls include G.A.S. (General Diagnostics—Division of Warner Lambert Company, Morris Plains, N.J.), Confirm (Corning Medical and Scientific, Medfield, Mass.), ContrIL (Instrumentation Laboratory, Lexington, Mass.) and Qualicheck (Radiometer, DK2400, Copenhagen NV, Denmark). Since the development of aqueous controls, other controls have been developed in an attempt to obtain a control more closely resembling the clinical specimen whole blood. Quantra (Dade Division, American Hospital Supply Corporation, Miami, Fla.) is a whole blood tonometer control. Prime (Fisher Scientific, Pittsburgh, Pa.) is a blood-based human hemoglobin control. ABC (Instrumentation Laboratory, Lexington, Mass.) and Gastraka (Curtin Matheson Scientific, Houston, Tex.) are artificial blood controls based on a fluorocarbon. These controls have assigned values for all three levels, usually by the instrument used. Most of the suppliers of control materials, in addition to providing control material, will provide a monthly statistic program, plus periodical proficiency surveys.

The aqueous controls equilibrate easier with room air than do the blood-based controls. For example, once opened for five minutes, the ContrIL, G.A.S., and Quantra changes in pH and Pco_2 were insignificant. After five minutes Po_2 changes of Quantra were up to 3 mm Hg at the low Po_2 tension and up to 3 per cent at higher O_2 tensions. In the 50 to 70 mm Hg range the G.A.S. and ContrIL increased as much as 50 per cent. Therefore, aqueous controls such as G.A.S. and ContrIL must be analyzed immediately after opening. Ampuled controls should not be stored in a syringe because of the possibility of air contamination. By laboratory observation and by hypothesis the lower viscosity of aqueous controls renders them less sensitive to aspiration-related problems than whole blood controls such as Quantra (Leary, 1980).

The only control that behaves similarly to patient blood in all situations is tonometer blood (Leary, 1980). A tonometer equlibrates blood with a known analyzed mixture of gas at a constant temperature of 37°C. (Chalmers, 1974). Major advantages of equilibrated blood from a tonometer are as follows: blood is a biological specimen, which is usually measured in a blood gas instrument; the blood can be equilibrated to specific Po_2 and Pco_2 values which the laboratory desires; and the blood is relatively stable. The disadvantages are that a bulk buffer must be used for pH quality control and technical time must be allocated to prepare a blood sample in a tonometer.

Two major methods of tonometry are in current use. The most widely used method is the thin film approach as used in the IL 237 (Instrumentation Laboratory, Lexington, Mass.). A method which is gaining increased use is a bubble tonometer which bubbles analyzed gas through blood to achieve a more rapid equilibration than is possible in a thin film tonometer. Examples of bubble tonometers include Dynex (Analytical Products, Belmont, Cal.); the Equilibrator (R.S. Weber & Associates, West Lake Village, Cal.); Tri-Channel Bubble Tonometer (Professional Instruments, Glendale, Cal.); and 775 Tonometer (Equilibrated Biosystems, Inc., Syosset, N.Y.).

A new method of tonometry is a syringe tonometer Model 184 (Corning Medical and Scientific, Medfield, Mass.). A syringe tonometer includes a bubble tonometer chamber, a humidifying chamber, and a transport and delivery syringe movable to the analyzing device (Wallace, 1981).

The coefficient of variation with tonometer blood for Pco_2 varies from 2.9 to 6.2 per cent and for Po_2 from 1.2 to 3.6 per cent. Blood obtained from a tonometer is very stable in a plastic syringe for up to 1.5 hours, and for all except the very high Po_2 range most samples remain stable for up to six hours (Leary, 1977).

The use of commercial control ampules or tonometry is a must today for a blood gas laboratory, at three levels each operating shift. This should not be the only method of quality control used. Voluntary proficiency examinations, monthly statistic programs, replicate analysis of patient samples, and instrumentation comparisons should supplement either tonometry or commercial ampules.

ARTERIAL BLOOD GASES

Oxygen

TRANSPORT OF OXYGEN IN THE BLOOD

Partial Pressure. Oxygen and carbon dioxide are generally reported in units of partial pressure. *The partial pressure of a gas in a liquid is the partial pressure of that gas with which the liquid is in equilibrium.* Consider a glass of water in a room. Assuming a barometric pressure of 760 mm Hg, the partial pressure of oxygen (Po_2) in room air is approximately 21 per cent of 760, or 160 mm Hg. Since the water is in equilibrium with the room air, the Po_2 in the water is also 160 mm Hg.

A glass of blood stands next to the glass of water. Since both the water and the blood are in equilibrium with the same gas, in this case room air, the Po_2 of the blood must also be 160 mm Hg. The actual quantity of oxygen in the blood is far greater than that in the water. The *amount* of a gas in a liquid depends on the solubility of the gas in the liquid, as well as on the partial pressure, but the partial pressure of the gas in the liquid depends only on the partial pressure of the gas with which the liquid is in equilibrium.

Oyxgen Saturation. Although the *quantity* of oxygen in the blood can be expressed in absolute terms such as volumes per cent, it is usually reported as oxygen saturation (SO_2). The oxygen saturation is a measure of the amount of oxygen in the blood that is combined with hemoglobin compared with the total amount of oxygen which could combine with hemoglobin in that blood. Oxygen saturation and oxygen content are linearly related through the oxygen capacity, which in turn depends on the amount and type of hemoglobin in the blood.

Oxygen Dissolved in Physical Solution. The oxygen saturation refers to the oxygen carried by the hemoglobin. A very small amount of oxygen will dissolve in the plasma in physical solution, 0.003 ml of oxygen in each 100 ml of plasma for each mm Hg of the PO_2. This amount is ordinarily of no significance; it may assume importance during the breathing of 100 per cent oxygen (approximately 1.95 volumes per cent) and is the key factor in hyperbaric oxygenation.

The Oxyhemoglobin Dissociation Curve. The amount of oxygen combined with hemoglobin is related to the PO_2 by the oxyhemoglobin dissociation curve (Fig. 7–4). Oxygen saturation rather than oxygen content is used for the ordinate so that the curve will apply to any hemoglobin concentration. The reasons for the shape of the curve are complex and will not be discussed here. The implications of the shape are of great importance in the interpretation of blood gas data and will be discussed in the appropriate sections.

The center curve in Figure 7–4 is the so-called standard curve, representing a pH of 7.40 and PCO_2 of 40 mm Hg. Alkalemia shifts the curve to the left, acidemia to the right. A left shift increases the affinity of the hemoglobin for oxygen; for a given PO_2 the content and saturation are greater. A right shift decreases the affinity. Increase in CO_2 will shift the curve slightly to the right; a decrease shifts the curve to the left. This effect is independent of the effect of CO_2 on the pH.

The red cell concentration of 2,3-diphosphoglycerate (DPG) and other organic phosphates will alter the position of the curve; an increase in DPG shifts the curve to the right, for example. These shifts occur in a wide variety of diseases, and therefore there is no standard dissociation curve in clinical medicine. Most of these shifts are minor, however, at least as regards the interpretation of blood gas data; hence it is still useful to think in terms of the standard curve.

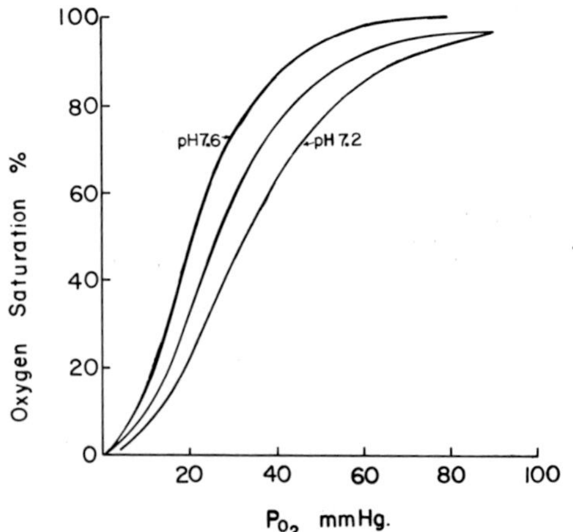

Figure 7–4. Oxyhemoglobin dissociation curve for normal adult hemoglobin. The center curve is a so-called standard curve for a pH of 7.4

THE ALVEOLAR-ARTERIAL OXYGEN DIFFERENCE

The partial pressure of a gas in a liquid is the partial pressure of the gas with which the liquid is in equilibrium. For the arterial blood, what is this gas? The obvious answer is the alveolar air; if this were true, the partial pressures of the arterial blood gases would be the same as those of the alveolar air. This is not the case, however. An understanding of the difference between the partial pressure of oxygen in the alveolar air (P_AO_2) and the arterial blood (P_aO_2), the alveolar-arterial oxygen difference ($P_{A\text{-}aD}O_2$), is vital for the interpretation of arterial blood gas data. This difference is always positive; that is, P_AO_2 is always higher than P_aO_2.

Mixing of Blood. *The* PO_2 *resulting from the mixture of blood samples with different values of* PO_2 *cannot be calculated directly from the* PO_2 *values of the original blood.* Rather, the resulting PO_2 depends upon the oxygen contents of the original samples. The calculation of resulting PO_2 values requires working through the dissociation curve. For example, if equal quantities of two blood samples are mixed, one with a PO_2 of 300 mm Hg and one with a PO_2 of 40 mm Hg, the PO_2 of the resulting mixture is *not* (300 + 40)/2. Instead, the oxygen content or saturation of the two blood samples must be obtained from the dissociation curve and averaged, and the PO_2 then obtained from the resulting content or saturation by referring again to the dissociation curve. When this is done, the PO_2 resulting from equal mixtures of blood at 300 mm Hg and 40 mm Hg is found to be 61 mm Hg.

When *gases* mix, the PO_2 values can be calculated directly, since the concentration or quantity of gas is directly proportional to the partial pressure. Thus, if equal volumes of two gases mix with partial pressures of 300 mm Hg and 40 mm Hg, the resulting PO_2 would be 170 mm Hg.

We can now proceed to a discussion of those factors which produce $P_{A\text{-}aD}O_2$.

Diffusion Gradient. To reach the interior of the red cell from the alveolus, oxygen must pass through the alveolar membrane, an interstitial fluid-filled space, the capillary membrane, the plasma, and the red cell membrane. If these structures are normal, little pressure gradient is required to move the oxygen across this barrier. The normal oxygen pressure gradient between the alveolar air and the *mean* pulmonary capillary blood is about 10 mm Hg, and the gradient between the alveolar air and the *end* pulmonary capillary blood (pulmonary vein) is less than 1 mm Hg. Several factors may increase these gradients: (1) the barrier may be thickened by fibrous or granulation tissue (alveolar capillary block syndrome); (2) the total surface area available for diffusion may become reduced; (3) exercise or other high cardiac output states may reduce the time that the blood spends in the pulmonary capillary bed.

There is a wide margin of safety. A moderate reduction in diffusing capacity will lead to an increase in the alveolar-to-*mean* pulmonary capillary gradient, but will produce only a minor increase in the alveolar-to-*end* pulmonary capillary gradient. At or near sea level, under resting conditions and breathing room air, the diffusion gradient makes only a minor contribution to the total $P_{A\text{-}aD}O_2$. Furthermore, if the concentration of oxygen in the inspired air is raised above that of room air, any hypoxemia owing to a diffusion defect will be abolished.

Ventilation/Perfusion ($\dot{V}/Q$) Inequalities. The normal alveolar ventilation (VA) is approximately 4 L/min and the normal cardiac output (Q) is approximately 5 L/min. The overall V/Q ratio of the lung is therefore approximately 0.8. This ratio, however, does not necessarily apply to every discrete area of the lung. Even in normal lungs, both ventilation and perfusion are unevenly distributed. Part of this is a gravitational effect. In the upright position, there is a gradient of both ventilation and perfusion from the top to the bottom of the lung, so that the lung bases receive more ventilation and more perfusion than the apices. The gradient is much more pronounced for perfusion than for ventilation (West, 1962). At the apex the V/Q ratio is approximately 3.3, in the midportion 0.90, and at the base 0.63. In the supine position a similar condition applies, with the ventilation and perfusion gradients running from ventral to dorsal regions. The magnitude of these gradients would obviously not be as large.

These regional inequalities in V/Q ratios are responsible in part for the normal $P_{A\text{-}aD}O_2$ of about 10 mm Hg. In many diseases, but most prominently in chronic obstructive airway disease, there are marked regional differences in ventilation and perfusion in addition to the gravitational gradients. This nonuniform distribution of ventilation, perfusion, or both leads to a wide spectrum of V/Q ratios throughout the lung. The areas where the ratio is low are underventilated in relation to the blood flow; the P_AO_2 will be low and the blood leaving these areas will have a relatively low PO_2 and oxygen content compared with that of normal arterial blood. The areas with a high V/Q ratio are overventilated in relation to the blood flow; the P_AO_2 will be high, as will the PO_2 of blood leaving these areas. However, the underventilated, overperfused areas contribute a larger proportion of blood to the final mixed arterial blood than do the overventilated, underperfused areas. Furthermore, the blood leaving the overventilated areas is on the high, flat portion of the dissociation curve; although the PO_2 is high, the oxygen content is increased very little above the normal value for arterial blood. Thus, when the blood from areas of low and high V/Q ratios mixes, the resulting blood will *have a lower* PO_2 than if the V/Q ratios were normal. The result will be an increase in $P_{A\text{-}aD}O_2$.

Shunting. Normally, 3 to 5 per cent of the cardiac output is shunted from the right to the left side of the heart without traversing ventilated alveoli. This includes contributions from the thebesian veins which drain directly into the left ventricle, the more distal branchings of the bronchial arteries which drain into the pulmonary rather than the bronchial veins, and blood traveling through alveoli that are not ventilated. This venous blood, when mixed with oxygenated blood, will lower the oxygen content and PO_2 of the resulting arterial blood.

In pneumonia, atelectasis, pulmonary edema, and shock, for example, many lung units may lose their ventilation while retaining their blood supply. In addition, new vascular channels may open which bypass ventilated alveoli. The blood traversing these areas is effectively shunted from the venous to the arterial side of the circulation. This type of right-to-left shunting is an important factor in the extreme widening of $P_{A\text{-}aD}O_2$ in critically ill patients. Since the shunted blood is never exposed to ventilated alveoli, breathing even 100 per cent oxygen does little to improve the hypoxemia resulting from shunting.

Relative Contribution of Diffusion, V/Q Inequalities, and Shunting to $P_{A\text{-}aD}O_2$. Although the diffusion gradient may assume importance during exercise and at high altitudes, even in severe cases of so-called alveolar-capillary block (with the possible exception of the adult respiratory distress syndrome), this gradient makes only a minor contribution to $P_{A\text{-}aD}O_2$ at or near sea level if the patient is at rest breathing at least 21 per cent oxygen. In normal subjects breathing room air, V/Q inequalities and shunting contribute about equally to the normal $P_{A\text{-}aD}O_2$. In chronic obstructive airway disease the abnormally wide $P_{A\text{-}aD}O_2$ is due primarily to the wide spectrum of $\dot{V}/\dot{Q}$ ratios. The widened $P_{A\text{-}aD}O_2$ in critically ill patients is due to varying combinations of V/Q inequalities and shunting.

Effect of Cardiac Output on $P_{A\text{-}aD}O_2$. Cardiac output, oxygen consumption (VO_2), and arterial-venous oxygen content difference ($C_aO_2 - C_vO_2$) are interrelated through the Fick equation: $C_aO_2 - C_vO_2 = VO_2/Q$. If Q decreases without a fall in VO_2, the arterial-venous oxygen content difference widens as the tissues, receiving less blood, extract more oxygen from the blood that is delivered. This results in a fall in the mixed venous oxygen content. Obviously, whatever blood is being shunted, the lower its oxygen content the greater will be its effect on lowering the P_aO_2 and widening the $P_{A\text{-}aD}O_2$.

The Alveolar Air Equation. $P_{A\text{-}aD}O_2$ is the difference between the partial pressure of oxygen in the alveolar air (P_AO_2) and the partial pressure of oxygen in the arterial blood (P_aO_2). P_aO_2 is measured directly. To calculate $P_{A\text{-}aD}O_2$ it is necessary to calculate a value of P_AO_2, since this is cumbersome to measure directly.

There is no single value for P_AO_2, since even in normal lungs the uneven distribution of ventilation and perfusion will cause regional variations in P_AO_2. An average or "ideal" value can be calculated using the ideal alveolar air equation; the derivation for this equation can be found in most textbooks of pulmonary physiology. In clinical medicine the equation is used

2

in a simplified form: $P_AO_2 = P_IO_2 - (1.2 \times P_aCO_2)$, where P_IO_2 is the partial pressure of oxygen in the inspired air. The 1.2 is the reciprocal of an assumed respiratory quotient.

Example: A subject breathing 40 per cent oxygen at a barometric pressure of 750 mm Hg has the following arterial blood gas values: $P_aO_2 = 110$ mm Hg, $P_aCO_2 = 56$ mm Hg; Calculate $P_{A\text{-}aD}O_2$. $P_AO_2 = (750 - 47) \times 0.40 - 1.2 \times 56 = 214$ mm Hg. (47 mm Hg is the vapor pressure of water in the alveolar air. In respiratory medicine it is customary to calculate in terms of dry gas.) $P_{A\text{-}aD}O_2$ therefore will equal 214 − 110, or 104 mm Hg. A final simplification: for practical purposes at or near sea level, barometric pressure − 47 can be assumed to equal 700 mm Hg.

To calculate the P_AO_2, the inspired oxygen concentration must be known. In patients breathing room air, this value is 0.21. The various types of high-flow Venturi masks provide reasonably precise oxygen concentrations. For patients on ventilators, the inspired concentration is set by the operator, and this is usually accurate. If doubt exists, the inspired oxygen concentration can be measured from the inspiration line with one of the inexpensive paramagnetic oxygen analyzers. Unfortunately, with nasal cannulas and catheters, the precise inspired oxygen concentration cannot be determined and $P_{A\text{-}aD}O_2$ cannot be estimated.

The a/A ratio. $P_{A\text{-}aD}O_2$ as an estimate of gas exchange is conceptually appropriate and used widely. A major drawback, however, is that $P_{A\text{-}aD}O_2$ increases with increasing inspired oxygen concentration (F_IO_2), even with all other factors remaining stable. Unfortunately, the precise normal limits for $P_{A\text{-}aD}O_2$ at different values of F_IO_2 have not been reported.

Gilbert and Keighley (1974) described the use of the ratio of P_aO_2 to P_AO_2 (a/A) as a substitute for $P_{A\text{-}aD}O_2$. In normal subjects this ratio remains relatively constant for values of F_IO_2 from 21 to 100 per cent, with the lower limit of normal approximately 0.75. In subjects with pulmonary disease, the ratio is more variable with changing levels of F_IO_2, but more stable than $P_{A\text{-}aD}O_2$ (Gilbert, 1979). a/A therefore can be used (1) to compare gas exchange among patients receiving different inspired oxygen concentrations, (2) to compare gas exchange in the same patient as F_IO_2 is changed, and (3) to estimate the P_aO_2 expected at a given value of F_IO_2 if blood gas data are available at another level of F_IO_2. For example, if P_aO_2 and P_aCO_2 are known for a patient receiving 40 per cent oxygen, the P_aO_2 expected if he were breathing 30 per cent oxygen can be estimated by assuming that P_aCO_2 and a/A will not change as F_IO_2 is lowered. Although this is a rough estimate and these assumptions are not necessarily valid, the calculation is useful for clinical purposes.

The venous admixture (VA) is a calculation used widely in intensive care units where mixed venous blood (pulmonary artery) is usually available. Its formula is $VA = (C_cO_2 - C_aO_2)/(C_cO_2 - C_vO_2)$, where C_cO_2, C_aO_2, and C_vO_2 are the oxygen contents of the pulmonary capillary, arterial, and mixed venous bloods. The oxygen content includes both the oxygen combined with hemoglobin and the oxygen in physical solution. The former is calculated as the saturation multiplied by the hemoglobin multiplied by 1.39. The latter is calculated as the partial pressure multiplied by 0.003. C_cO_2 is calculated by first obtaining P_AO_2 from the alveolar air equation, assuming $P_AO_2 = P_cO_2$, and obtaining the saturation from the dissociation curve.

The venous admixture calculation is influenced by the diffusion gradient, V/Q imbalance, and direct shunting, but expresses the net result of all three as if it were due to direct shunting alone. In other words, the calculation answers the following question: If the $P_{A\text{-}aD}O_2$ were due entirely to shunting, what percentage of the cardiac output would have to be shunted to account for the difference? It is somewhat more precise than a/A or $P_{A\text{-}aD}O_2$ as a measure of gas exchange, since it takes into account the effects of cardiac output; it has the disadvantage of requiring a mixed venous sample. Since V/Q imbalance and the effects of a diffusion defect decline as F_IO_2 increases, whereas the effects of a direct shunt will theoretically remain unchanged, one would expect VA to decline with increasing F_IO_2. The actual results, however, are more complex. VA is highest at an F_IO_2 of 0.21, declines to a minimum at an F_IO_2 of 0.4, then rises again as F_IO_2 approaches 1.0 (Oliven, 1980). The reasons for the rise at high F_IO_2 values are not entirely clear, but may relate in part to atelectasis produced by breathing high oxygen mixtures.

DANGEROUS LEVELS OF HYPOXEMIA

Unlike all other substances that must be obtained from the environment, body stores of oxygen are virtually non-existent and death occurs within a few minutes after complete oxygen deprivation. Any level of hypoxemia, therefore, should be cause for concern. So long as a continuous supply of oxygen is available, however, the defense mechanisms can compensate for surprising degrees of hypoxemia.

The shape of the dissociation curve provides one important line of defense. A fall in P_aO_2 from a normal value of 90 mm Hg to 55 mm Hg produces less than a 10 per cent fall in the oxygen content. Fifty-five mm Hg is the shoulder of the dissociation curve; below this level there is a precipitous fall in oxygen content with further decreases in P_aO_2. For this reason, 50 to 55 mm Hg for P_aO_2 is usually considered the minimum value to aim for in the treatment of respiratory failure; values somewhat higher than this are preferable, since they provide a wider margin of safety.

The arterial oxygen content is only one factor in oxygen delivery to the cells. The cardiac output, regional blood flow, regional oxygen uptake, oxygen extraction, position of the dissociation curve, and hemoglobin concentration all play a role in this vital process. Survival has been reported following values of P_aO_2 as low as 7.5 mm Hg. It is difficult to predict, therefore, in the individual case, at what level hypoxemia becomes life threatening. Additional factors may be decisive. Hypoxemia increases the susceptibility to cardiac glycoside intoxication and may precipitate intractable arrhythmias in patients with severe preexisting cardiac or pulmonary disease. Since oxygen delivery is the product of cardiac output and arterial oxygen content, the combination of hypoxemia and low cardiac output is particularly dangerous.

REFERENCE VALUES

For young healthy subjects breathing 21 per cent oxygen (room air), 80 mm Hg can be considered the lower limit for P_aO_2; for older subjects 70 mm Hg is an appropriate lower limit. For $P_{A\text{-}aD}O_2$, 5 to 20 mm Hg can be considered a reasonable value during room air breathing. On 100 per cent oxygen, values as high as 200 mm Hg have been reported in young healthy subjects, although 35 to 50 mm Hg is generally considered the upper limit. Reference values for $P_{A\text{-}aD}O_2$ while breathing intermediate levels of F_IO_2 are not available. The lower limit for the a/A ratio can be considered to be 0.75 for all values of F_IO_2.

CONCLUSION: GAS EXCHANGE AND VENTILATION

Ventilation is the process by which air moves in and out of the lungs; gas exchange is the process by which oxygen and carbon dioxide are exchanged between alveolar air and pulmonary capillary blood. The defects we have been discussing—V/Q inequalities, shunting, and diffusion defects—produce abnormalities in gas exchange. The result is a wide $P_{A\text{-}aD}O_2$ and a low a/A ratio, which may produce hypoxemia, depending on the F_IO_2 and the severity of the defect. They will also produce an elevated P_aCO_2 (hypercapnia), but only if ventilation is also defective. This will be reviewed next.

Ventilation and Carbon Dioxide

THE ALVEOLAR VENTILATION

The partial pressure of a gas in a liquid is the partial pressure of gas with which the liquid is in equilibrium. For oxygen in arterial blood, the alveolar air is not quite this gas; in fact, there is no single equilibrating gas. Venous to arterial shunting, V/Q inequalities, and, to a lesser extent, the diffusion gradient all lower P_aO_2 and produce a positive $P_{A\text{-}aD}O_2$. This occurs even in normal lungs; in disease the difference is accentuated. The classic approach to blood gas interpretation is that these three factors do not alter P_aCO_2 and that $P_ACO_2 = P_aCO_2$. Since P_ACO_2 (partial pressure of alveolar CO_2) is under control of the alveolar ventilation, P_aCO_2 (partial pressure of arterial CO_2) is considered to give direct information about the state of the ventilation.

The following relationship, the alveolar ventilation equation, exists between carbon dioxide production ($\dot{V}CO_2$), P_ACO_2, and the alveolar ventilation ($\dot{V}_A$): $\dot{V}CO_2 = \dot{V}_A \times P_ACO_2/0.863$. (For simplicity, the constant 0.863 will be omitted subsequently.) Rewriting the equation as $P_ACO_2 = \dot{V}CO_2/\dot{V}_A$, P_ACO_2 emerges as the outcome of the relationship between CO_2 production and alveolar ventilation. A rise in $\dot{V}CO_2$ or a fall in $\dot{V}_A$ without a commensurate change in the other will raise P_ACO_2, and changes in the opposite direction will lower P_ACO_2. Since the classic approach assumes $P_ACO_2 = P_aCO_2$, these statements also apply to P_aCO_2. Thus, P_aCO_2 becomes the indicator of the adequacy of the alveolar ventilation in relationship to the metabolic load; a high P_aCO_2 indicates relative alveolar hypoventilation, and a low P_aCO_2 indicates alveolar hyperventilation.

But what is the alveolar ventilation? It cannot be measured directly; it can be calculated as the total ventilation minus the dead space ventilation, but dead space cannot be measured directly either. Furthermore, there are several different dead spaces, depending on how the calculation is made.

The alveolar ventilation equation can also be written as $\dot{V}_A = \dot{V}CO_2/P_ACO_2$. In this form $\dot{V}_A$ becomes a clearance ratio similar to those used in renal physiology; the alveolar ventilation is the (theoretical) ventilation necessary to excrete the metabolically produced CO_2 at a concentration equal to P_aCO_2/(barometric pressure − 47).

We have been arguing in a circle. P_aCO_2 is high because the alveolar ventilation is low in relationship to the CO_2 production. Since we cannot measure the alveolar ventilation, how do we know that it is low? Answer—because P_aCO_2 is high. Alveolar hypoventilation, therefore, should not be looked on as the cause of hypercapnia. Hypercapnia, rather, should be considered to be synonymous with alveolar hypoventilation.

HYPERCAPNIA AND HYPOCAPNIA

Despite the circuitous reasoning, P_aCO_2 remains the best clinical guide to the effectiveness of ventilation *and the functional integrity of the ventilatory control system.* P_aCO_2 is normally kept within narrow limits (32 to 45 mm Hg) by this rigid control system. The presence of hypo- or hypercapnia indicates a serious defect in ventilatory control.

Any one of three general disturbances may lead to hypercapnia:

1. *The respiratory control centers which set the level of* P_aCO_2 *may be defective.*
2. *The neuromuscular apparatus of breathing may be defective.*
3. *The work of breathing may be markedly increased.* Under this last circumstance, normal respiratory control centers may not be able to force a normal neuromuscular breathing apparatus to maintain the ventilation necessary to excrete the CO_2 produced by tissues at a normal CO_2 concentration; the P_aCO_2 will rise until a new equilibrium is established at the elevated P_aCO_2. Such an increase in the work of breathing is usually the result of severe airway obstruction as seen in the asthma–bronchitis–emphysema group of diseases. It is also common in severe kyphoscoliosis, but is only rarely seen in restrictive defects such as occur in pulmonary fibrosis.

With severe hypercapnia a combination of these factors is often present. Carbon dioxide narcosis in patients with chronic obstructive airway disease is often associated with a high work of breathing owing

2

to the airway obstruction, a defective or inefficient diaphragm, plus respiratory control centers acutely depressed by oxygen and perhaps chronically depressed by a high P_aCO_2.

We have reviewed the relationship of P_aCO_2 to the alveolar ventilation and pointed out the rather elusive nature of the concept of alveolar ventilation. The total minute ventilation, which is the product of the ventilatory frequency and the tidal volume, however, is a clearly definable quantity that can be measured directly. Hypocapnia is always associated with an increase in the total minute ventilation above the normal resting level. With hypercapnia, the total minute ventilation may be low, normal, or high. If the metabolic rate is increased with fever or restlessness, for example, more CO_2 is presented to the lungs for excretion, and a normal ventilation will not keep P_aCO_2 normal. With rapid shallow breathing, the dead space ventilation constitutes a greater proportion of the tidal volume and P_aCO_2 may rise despite a rise in the total minute ventilation. Finally, in many disease states the dead space may be increased. Under all these circumstances only an increased total minute ventilation will keep P_aCO_2 at a normal level. If the ventilatory control system is intact and the work of breathing is not prohibitively high, this increased ventilatory requirement will be met and P_aCO_2 will remain normal. If the work of breathing is excessive or the ventilatory control system defective, only a partial attempt at compensation may occur. In this case, both P_aCO_2 and the total minute ventilation may be high.

The hypocapnic patient always has a total minute ventilation above the normal resting value, whereas the hypercapnic patient may have a ventilation which is low, normal, or high. The importance of hypercapnia is not that it indicates hypoventilation, but that it indicates a serious derangement in the respiratory control centers, a defective breathing apparatus, an overwhelming increase in the work of breathing, or any combination of these.

Hyperventilation with resulting hypocapnia is seen in a wide variety of clinical disorders. Hyperventilation may be secondary to hypoxemia, compensatory to metabolic acidosis, or psychological. In many critical illnesses hyperventilation occurs without acidosis or hypoxemia; if hypoxemia is present, the hyperventilation may persist despite correction of the hypoxemia by oxygen administration. These illnesses include head injuries, liver failure, shock from various causes, and septicemia. The exact stimulus for the hyperventilation is unknown.

EFFECTS OF V/Q INEQUALITIES AND SHUNTING ON P_aCO_2

For several decades, it has been axiomatic that V/Q (ventilation/perfusion) inequalities do not raise P_aCO_2 because the CO_2 dissociation curve is relatively linear in the physiologic range. Furthermore, since the CO_2 dissociation curve is relatively steep (Fig. 7–5) compared with the oxygen dissociation curve, the difference between P_aCO_2 and mixed venous CO_2 ($P_{\bar{v}}CO_2$) is only a few mm Hg, compared with approximately 50 mm Hg for oxygen. Shunting, therefore, has been considered to play an insignificant role in elevating P_aCO_2.

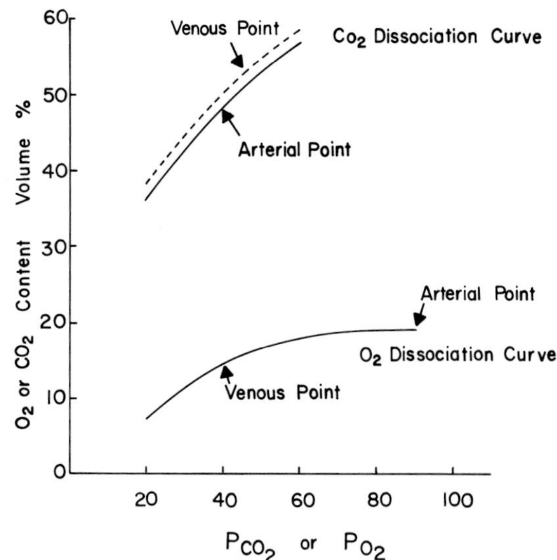

Figure 7–5. Oxygen and carbon dioxide dissociation curves drawn to same scale. The A-V difference for both is approximately the same, but the resulting change in partial pressure is much greater for oxygen than for carbon dioxide.

Although superficially this reasoning seems logical, it does not hold up under close examination. West (1971) has explored these concepts using computer models of the lung. His results show that V/Q inequalities interfere with CO_2 excretion to approximately the same extent as with oxygen uptake and will produce hypercapnia unless compensatory mechanisms intervene. The argument that shunting will not raise P_aCO_2 is also deceptive. If shunting produces a small rise in P_aCO_2, $P_{\bar{v}}CO_2$ will also rise, producing another increment in P_aCO_2, and so on until a new steady state is achieved.

Why then is hypercapnia so much less common than hypoxemia and so intimately bound by tradition to the ventilation? There are several reasons: (1) Because of the steep slope of the CO_2 dissociation curve, an increase in ventilation toward normal of poorly ventilated lung units will lower the CO_2 content of the blood leaving these units to a much greater degree than it will raise the oxygen content. (2) Because the CO_2 dissociation curve does not flatten out at low values of P_aCO_2, overall hyperventilation will lower PCO_2 of blood leaving well-ventilated lung units to compensate for the elevated CO_2 of shunted blood. The hyperbolic nature of the $P_aCO_2 - V_A$ curve (Fig. 7–6 and see below) will make this an inefficient process, but it will occur. The flat shape of the oxygen dissociation curve at high levels of PO_2 will preclude the well-ventilated units from adding appreciable oxygen to the blood (see Fig. 7–5). (3) Hypercapnia is a much more powerful stimulus to ventilation than is hypoxemia. If the respiratory control centers are intact, there will be a strong drive to increase the

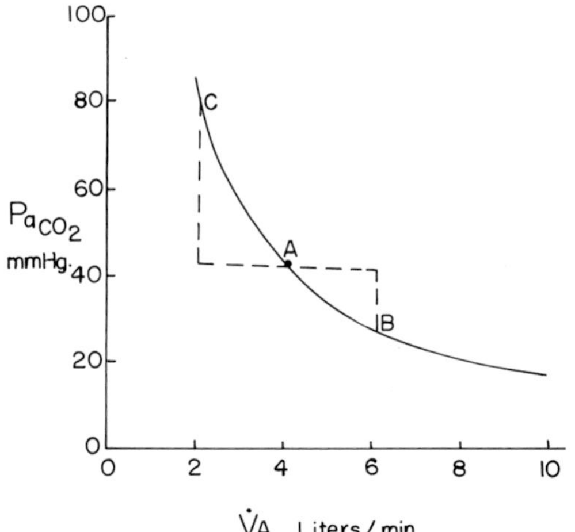

Figure 7–6. Plot of the alveolar ventilation equation. The absolute magnitude of the change in ventilation from A to B and A to C is the same, but the resulting change in P_{CO_2} is much greater on the lower ventilation side.

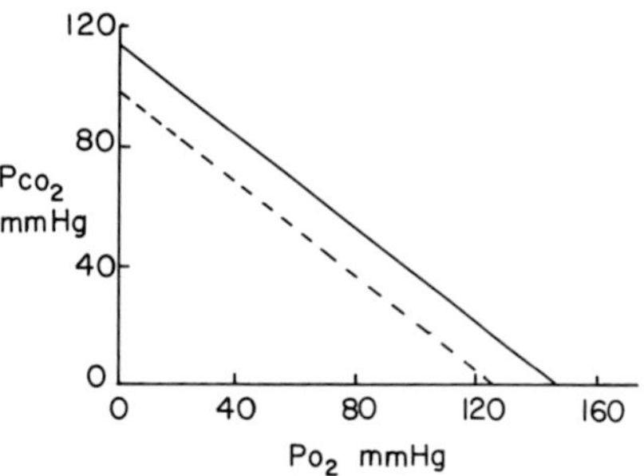

Figure 7–7. The simplified form of the alveolar air equation plotted on an O_2–CO_2 diagram for an F_IO_2 of 21 per cent and an RQ of 0.8. The solid line represents alveolar air; the dotted line represents arterial blood with an A-aDO_2 of 20. Note that for arterial blood, when the P_{CO_2} reaches 80 mm Hg, the Pa_{O_2} has fallen to 20 mm Hg.

2

ventilation so long as hypercapnia persists. Once hypercapnia has been corrected, the remaining hypoxemia will offer less inducement to further increase in ventilation, especially if work of breathing is high.

V/Q inequalities and shunting will lower P_aO_2 and raise P_aCO_2. The important distinction between hypercapnia and hypoxemia in this regard is that an increase in ventilation will correct the hypercapnia but not the hypoxemia.

VENTILATION AND CARBON DIOXIDE

Granting that alveolar ventilation is more a conceptual than an actual quantity, it remains a useful tool for defining the relationship between ventilation and carbon dioxide. Figure 7–6 is a plot of the alveolar ventilation equation substituting P_aCO_2 for P_ACO_2. Hyperventilation is seen as a relatively inefficient process and hypoventilation as a rather critical one. To lower P_aCO_2 from 40 mm Hg to 20 mm Hg requires an increase of 4.1 L/min in alveolar ventilation; to raise P_aCO_2 from 40 mm Hg to 60 mm Hg requires a fall in alveolar ventilation of only 1.4 L/min. From a level of 60 mm Hg, a fall in alveolar ventilation of only 0.7 L/min will raise the P_ACO_2 to 80 mm Hg. Thus, the more hypercapnic the patient becomes, the more sensitive the P_aCO_2 is to further decreases in ventilation.

VENTILATION AND OXYGEN

Hypoxemia, not hypercapnia, is the main threat in respiratory failure. P_AO_2 and P_ACO_2 are related through the alveolar air equation reviewed previously. The simplified form of this equation can be rearranged: $P_ACO_2 = R(P_IO_2 - P_AO_2)$ when R is the respiratory quotient. If constant values are assigned to R and P_IO_2, the equation will be a straight line with the slope equal to $-R$, an X intercept equal to P_IO_2, and a Y intercept equal to $R \times P_IO_2$. In Figure 7–7 the solid line is a plot of this equation for an R of 0.8 and P_IO_2 of 147 mm Hg (room air). If a $P_{A\text{-}aD}O_2$ of 20 mm Hg is assumed, the arterial blood line will be 20 mm Hg to the left, as indicated by the dotted line. With a value of R below 1, the usual case, a rise in P_aCO_2 will produce a fall in P_aO_2 greater than the rise in P_aCO_2. The graph shows why severe hypercapnia rarely occurs in patients breathing room air. With a $P_{A\text{-}aD}O_2$ of even 20 mm Hg, as P_aCO_2 reaches 90 mm Hg, P_aO_2 has fallen to 20 mm Hg, a level often (but not invariably) incompatible with life. The patient may thus die of hypoxia before severe hypercapnia can occur. Furthermore, at very low values of P_aO_2, hypoxemia will become a significant ventilatory stimulus tending to prevent severe hypoventilation. If the patient breathes an enriched oxygen mixture, two things happen. First, the hypoxic stimulus to ventilation will be lessened or abolished and, second, high levels of P_aCO_2 can occur without accompanying severe hypoxemia (the line is shifted to the right).

If $(\dot{V}CO_2 \times 0.863/\dot{V}_A)$ is substituted for P_aCO_2 in the alveolar air equation, this equation becomes: $P_AO_2 = (P_IO_2 - \dot{V}CO_2 \times 0.863)/R \times \dot{V}_A$. With a value of 200 ml/min for $\dot{V}CO_2$, 147 mm Hg for P_IO_2, and a $P_{A\text{-}aD}O_2$ of 20 mm Hg, the curve of P_aO_2 vs $\dot{V}_A$ is shown by the solid line in Figure 7–8. As with hypercapnia, hypoventilation produces an ever-increasing tempo of hypoxemia.

A moderate increase in F_IO_2 provides good protection against the hypoxemia produced by hypoventilation. The broken line in Figure 7–8 shows the same data for an F_IO_2 of 30 per cent and a $P_{A\text{-}aD}O_2$ of 35 mm Hg.

DANGEROUS LEVELS OF HYPOCAPNIA AND HYPERCAPNIA

With the rigid control system for P_aCO_2 which is normally in effect, any abnormal value of P_aCO_2 should cause concern. In contrast to hypoxemia, hypercapnia is important to recognize more for what it indicates about underlying pathophysiology than for its harmful effects per se.

For hypercapnia, there are two aspects to consider. First, what levels indicate a rapidly deteriorating

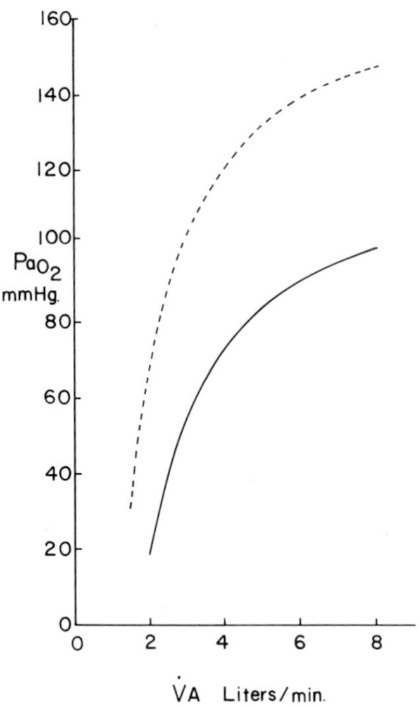

Figure 7–8. A combination of the alveolar air equation and alveolar ventilation equation. The solid line represents an F_IO_2 of 21 per cent with an A-aDO_2 of 20; the dotted line is for an F_IO_2 of 30 per cent with an A-aDO_2 of 35. Note the precipitous drop in PaO_2 as alveolar ventilation falls below 4 L/minute. Note also that although breathing 30 per cent oxygen does not prevent this precipitous fall in PaO_2, the absolute level of PaO_2 is maintained in an acceptable range down to values of $\dot{V}A$ as low as 2 L/minute.

disease process requiring immediate action? This depends on the nature of the disease. When pulmonary function was previously normal, any level of hypercapnia is cause for alarm. In Guillain-Barré syndrome or myasthenia gravis, for example, even mild hypercapnia indicates need for immediate action. During an acute attack of bronchial asthma in a patient known to have a normal P_aCO_2 between attacks, mild hypercapnia (P_aCO_2 of 45 to 55 mm Hg) is cause for concern; moderate to severe hypercapnia often is an indication for intubation and assisted ventilation. In contrast, patients with chronic obstructive airway disease in an acute episode of respiratory failure can usually be managed without intubation or assisted ventilation despite severe elevations of P_aCO_2.

With regard to the harmful effects of hypercapnia per se, it is difficult to be dogmatic for at least two reasons. First, the effects are difficult to separate from hypoxemia and acidosis, which often accompany hypercapnia, and, second, the effects correlate poorly with the level of P_aCO_2. Sieker (1956) found no significant abnormalities in mental state if P_aCO_2 was below 90 mm Hg and pH about 7.25. Coma or a semicomatose state always accompanied P_aCO_2 values above 130 mm Hg and pH below 7.14. Within these limits, however, there was great variability.

A rapid lowering of P_aCO_2 from hypercapnic levels by assisted ventilation has been associated with seizure, coma, and death; the accompanying alkalosis undoubtedly plays an important role. Values of P_aCO_2 above 65 mm Hg have been shown to reduce renal function (Kilburn, 1971) and may account in part for the fluid retention seen in respiratory failure.

Hypocapnia and respiratory alkalosis imposed on the patient by controlled ventilation can cause cardiac arrhythmias refractory to the usual antiarrhythmic measures until the respiratory alkalosis is corrected (Ayres, 1969). In the reported cases, P_aCO_2 varied from 13 to 23 mm Hg and pH from 7.51 to 7.74. Many critically ill patients have spontaneous hyperventilation with resulting hypocapnia. The leftward shift in the oxygen dissociation curve would be expected to interfere with oxygen utilization at the tissue level. Since these patients are critically ill, it is difficult to assign a specific harmful effect to the alkalosis or hypocapnia alone. It is difficult to find convincing evidence that *spontaneously* occurring, as opposed to iatrogenically induced, hypocapnia has significant harmful effects. It is usually unwise to try to treat hyperventilation per se; the attention should be directed to the underlying cause.

CONCLUSION: P_aO_2 AND P_aCO_2

Hypoventilation will lower P_aO_2 and raise P_aCO_2. V/Q inequalities, shunting, and, to a lesser extent, diffusion defects will also lower P_aO_2. V/Q inequalities and shunting have the *potential* to raise P_aCO_2, but will do so only if there is a failure of a compensatory increase in ventilation. P_aO_2 is, therefore, a more sensitive but less specific indicator of abnormal pulmonary function than P_aCO_2; hypoxemia is much more common than hypercapnia. If P_aO_2 is low, there is unquestionably an abnormality in gas exchange, ventilation, or both; the P_aO_2 alone indicates neither the nature of the abnormality nor the underlying disease. A high P_aCO_2 is much more specific; it indicates a defect in the respiratory control centers, a defective breathing apparatus, an overwhelming increase in the work of breathing, or any combination of these.

Acid-Base Balance

This presentation will not follow traditional lines. The Henderson-Hasselbalch equation, base excess, the Singer-Hastings nomogram, and most other familiar concepts will not be considered. Instead, this approach is based on the use of whole body titration curves. The author has found this to be the best method for identification of abnormalities, and it appears to be the way of the future. Only the recognition (or diagnosis) of the abnormalities, based on arterial blood gas data alone, will be reviewed. The various states of acidosis and alkalosis will not be presented in detail, nor will treatment be considered. Acid-base balance is discussed further in Chapter 8, and many other texts are available.

pH AND H^+

There appears to be a gradual replacement of the use of pH by the use of hydrogen ion concentration

Table 7–1. pH vs H^+ (nmol/L)

pH	H^+	pH	H^+
7.00	100	7.40	40
7.05	89	7.45	35
7.10	79	7.50	32
7.15	71	7.55	28
7.20	63	7.60	25
7.25	56	7.65	22
7.30	50	7.70	20
7.35	45	7.75	18

(H^+). Logarithmic notation is convenient when large changes in H^+ occur, but for the narrow range encountered in blood its usefulness is questionable. Furthermore the carbonic acid dissociation equation is manipulated more simply without the logarithmic notation of the Henderson-Hasselbalch equation. The equation is: $H^+ = 24 \times PCO_2/HCO_3^-$, with PCO_2 in mm Hg, HCO_3^- in mmol/L, and H^+ in 10^{-9} mol/L, or nanomoles/L. The reference value for H^+ is 40 mmol/L, corresponding to a pH of 7.40. The scales along the abscissa in Figures 7–9 to 7–12 will give the reader a general idea of the relationship between H^+ and pH in the physiologic range. Table 7–1 presents a more detailed comparison.

NOMOGRAMS

A nomogram is a graphic display of an equation; it contains no information that is not present in the equation itself. Many nomograms have been proposed for the carbonic acid dissociation equation; none are used in this chapter. The acid-base diagram to be presented is not a nomogram, and the whole body titration curves are not expressions of the Henderson-Hasselbalch equation. They are empirical observations that could not have been calculated from any equation; as such they bring additional information to bear on each blood gas determination with which they are compared.

TERMINOLOGY

We will follow the terminology of Winters (1967). The suffix *-emia* will refer to the state of the blood, e.g., acidemia is a condition of excess blood acidity as indicated by the H^+ or pH. The suffix *-osis* will refer to a pathologic process in which acid or base is gained or lost from the body. These processes may or may not be accompanied by acidemia or alkalemia depending upon the degree of compensation. *Compensation* is the physiologic response to the primary disturbance which tends to restore the blood acidity toward normal. This normal or expected physiologic response to a primary disturbance will not be considered a second primary process. Thus the retention of bicarbonate as a compensation for a respiratory acidosis will not be considered a metabolic alkalosis. The acute changes in the blood buffers owing to mass action will not be considered part of the compensation process. Two primary processes occurring together will be considered a *mixed* disturbance.

WHOLE BODY TITRATION CURVES

A whole body titration curve is a graphic representation of the in vivo changes in H^+, PCO_2, and HCO_3^- which occur in the arterial blood in response to a primary acid-base disturbance. The data are obtained by one of two methods. The first involves subjecting normal individuals to an imposed artificial disturbance, for example, breathing a high CO_2 mixture. Blood specimens are drawn at the new steady state. In the second method, arterial blood specimens are obtained from patients with naturally occurring disturbances. These subjects must not have diseases of the organ system responsible for compensation, and they must have only a single primary disturbance. With both methods, data are obtained from a group of subjects and the results expressed as 95 per cent confidence bands. These represent the mean ± 2 standard deviations of the group data at several points, or ± 2 standard errors of estimate of the regression line representing the data. *The 95 per cent confidence band thus represents the primary disturbance plus the expected or normal physiologic response to this disturbance.*

2

The confidence bands will be displayed on a PCO_2-H^+ diagram. These axes have been chosen because they are the two components actually measured by electrodes in blood gas analyzers. Both PCO_2 and H^+ will be displayed as linear scales; pH will also be shown on the same axis as H^+, but will be logarithmic. The normal range will be shown as a square in the center. Bicarbonate isopleths will usually not be shown; the value for bicarbonate can be derived easily from the carbonic acid dissociation equation presented earlier.

ACUTE RESPIRATORY ACIDOSIS

Brackett (1965) studied several normal young subjects exposed to 7 and 10 per cent CO_2 in 21 per cent oxygen in an environmental chamber for periods up to 90 minutes. The 95 per cent confidence band for this disturbance is labeled ARAc in Figure 7–9. Blood gas values falling withing this area are compatible with an acute respiratory acidosis.

Values such as point A in Figure 7–9 which lie to the acid side of area ARAc represent a respiratory acidosis (because the P_aCO_2 is high), but are too acidotic to be explained by the respiratory acidosis alone. Some other primary disturbance must be adding to the acidity, and this can only be a metabolic acidosis. This area, then, represents a mixed disturbance—that is, two primary disturbances, respiratory acidosis and metabolic acidosis.

If a normal value of 24 mmol/L for bicarbonate is entered into the equation $H^+ = 24\ PCO_2/HCO_3^-$, the equation becomes $H^+ = PCO_2$. Thus the $HCO_3^- = 24$ isopleth shown in Figure 7–9 has a slope of one. This line approximates the right margin of the ARAc confidence band, and therefore almost all blood gas determinations in the mixed respiratory and metabolic acidosis area will have a bicarbonate equal to or below 24 mmol/L.

CHRONIC RESPIRATORY ACIDOSIS

Brackett (1969) studied 20 patients with chronic hypercapnia in a relatively stable conditon. The

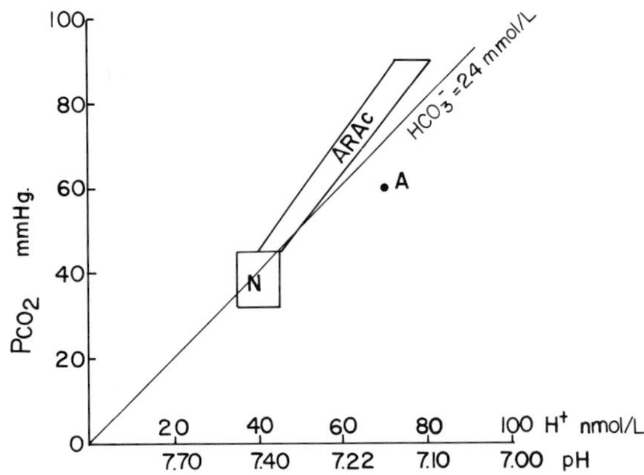

Figure 7–9. A 95 per cent confidence band (ARAc) for the acute respiratory acidosis whole body titration curve. The box labeled N is the normal range. Point A is a mixed disturbance, respiratory and metabolic acidosis. The line is the HCO_3^- isopleth for 24 mmol/L.

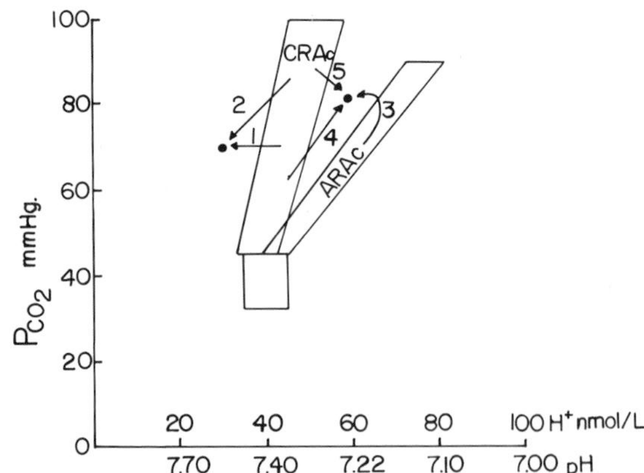

Figure 7–10. CRAc is the chronic respiratory acidosis confidence band. For explanation of points and arrows, see text.

$H^+ - P_aCO_2$ values for these subjects plus seven normal subjects were used to establish the 95 per cent confidence band labeled CRAc in Figure 7–10. Blood gas values within this area are compatible with a *maximally compensated respiratory acidosis*, also referred to as chronic respiratory acidosis. The bicarbonate will always be above 24 mmol/L.

Many patients develop acute CO_2 retention superimposed on a background of chronic hypercapnia. This condition has been duplicated in dogs in an environmental chamber (Goldstein, 1971): the blood gases start from within the CRAc confidence band and change along lines approximately parallel to the ARAc band.

Points to the left (alkalotic side) of the chronic respiratory acidosis confidence band represent a respiratory acidosis but are too alkalotic to be explained even by maximal compensation. A separate primary disturbance must be present, in this case metabolic alkalosis. This will be a true mixed disturbance, metabolic alkalosis and respiratory acidosis. Patients with chronic obstructive airway disease often have blood gas values in this area, the result of CO_2 retention plus a metabolic alkalosis secondary to potassium loss brought on by chronic diuretic therapy. Arrow (1) in Figure 7–10 demonstrates this course.

Rapid correction of hypercapnia may also result in blood gas values to the alkalotic side of the CRAc band. Patients with severe chronic CO_2 retention with a compensatory elevation of bicarbonate may, when placed on a ventilator, change as shown by arrow (2) in Figure 7–10. This occurs because the kidney cannot excrete bicarbonate fast enough to compensate for the rapid fall in P_aCO_2 resulting from assisted ventilation. The chloride depletion which invariably accompanies the bicarbonate expansion accentuates this abnormality, and administration of chloride will help speed the normalization of the acid-base disturbance (Schwartz, 1968).

Values between the acute and chronic respiratory acidosis bands demonstrate the inability to make a specific diagnosis from a single set of blood gas values. Arrow (3) in Figure 7–10 represents a partially compensated respiratory acidosis starting from normal values. Arrow (4) is an acute respiratory acidosis arising from a chronic respiratory acidosis. Arrow (5) shows a metabolic acidosis superimposed on chronic respiratory acidosis. All three clinical disturbances will have the same blood gas analysis at the point shown. It is important to realize that clinical data must usually be added to the blood gas data to make an accurate diagnosis.

CHRONIC METABOLIC ACIDOSIS

Albert (1967) studied 60 patients with metabolic acidosis; most were infants or children with diarrhea, diabetes, or renal disease. The duration of the acidosis exceeded 24 hours, a time sufficient for respiratory compensation by hyperventilation. They had received no medication and had no pulmonary disease. The 95 per cent confidence band for this group is labeled CMAc in Figure 7–11. This is considered to be

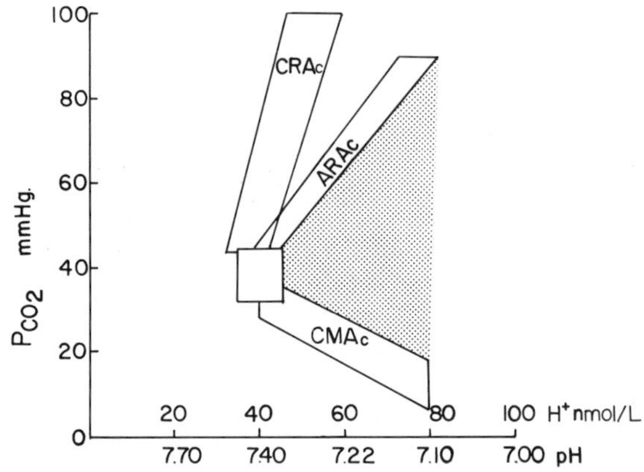

Figure 7–11. CMAc is the 95 per cent confidence band for chronic metabolic acidosis. The shaded area represents a mixed disturbance, respiratory acidosis and metabolic acidosis.

chronic metabolic acidosis, and the slope of the band compared to the slope of the CRAc band indicates that compensation is mush less complete in metabolic acidosis than in respiratory acidosis.

About 24 hours is required for the maximum ventilatory response to metabolic acidosis. Therefore points *above* the metabolic acidosis confidence band may represent an acute metabolic acidosis with insufficient time for the full ventilatory response. Statistical confidence limits for a very acute metabolic acidosis are not available.

If the clinical data suggest that enough time has elapsed for maximum ventilatory compensation, the area above the metabolic acidosis confidence band will then represent an inadequate or defective ventilatory response, and such patients should be suspected of having pulmonary disease. Does this represent a mixed disturbance, metabolic and respiratory acidosis, even when the P_aCO_2 is below 32 mm Hg? If a respiratory acidosis is defined simply as a P_aCO_2 above normal, then the normal P_aCO_2 for a metabolic acidosis is set by the confidence band, and any P_aCO_2 above this band represents a respiratory acidosis. The entire area, then, between the metabolic acidosis band and the acute respiratory acidosis band can be considered an area of mixed respiratory and metabolic acidosis (shaded area in Fig. 7–11). The most critically ill patients will usually be found to have arterial blood gas data within this area.

ACUTE RESPIRATORY ALKALOSIS

Arbus (1969) studied 12 patients who were hyperventilated during general anesthesia; metabolic, endocrine, cardiovascular, pulmonary, and renal diseases were excluded. The 95 per cent confidence band is labeled ARAlk in Figure 7–12; it is essentially a continuation of the band for acute respiratory acidosis. Points to the left (alkalotic side) of this band represent a mixed disturbance, respiratory and metabolic alkalosis. Figure 7–12, incidentally, represents the completed diagram suitable for clinical use.

Metabolic compensation would move the blood gas values to the right (acid side) of the acute respiratory alkalosis band toward normal H^+. Residents at high altitudes and pregnant women have low values of P_aCO_2 with a normal H^+; obviously complete metabolic compensation for respiratory alkalosis is possible. No confidence limits haver been reported for this compensation, however, and complete compensation is unusual in clinical medicine. Patients with blood gas values between the acute respiratory alkalosis confidence band and the $H^+ = 40$ line should be considered to have a mixed disturbance, respiratory alkalosis and metabolic acidosis, rather than a compensated respiratory alkalosis. By taking this approach, one is less likely to miss an important clinical disturbance such as unsuspected uremia or diabetes. If no cause for metabolic acidosis is found and it appears that compensated respiratory alkalosis is the correct diagnosis, no harm has been done.

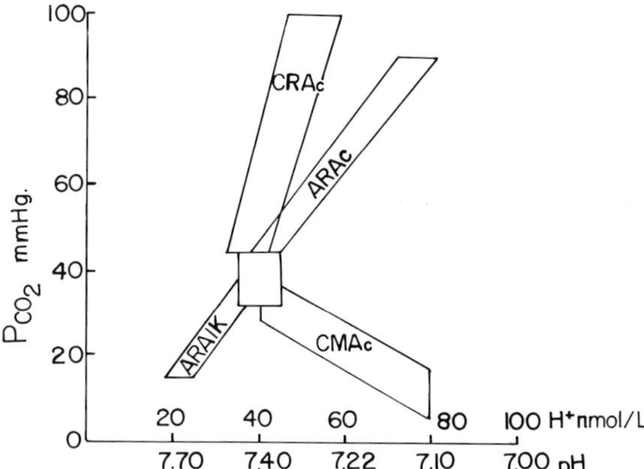

Figure 7–12. ARAlk is the respiratory alkalosis confidence band. This is the completed diagram which can be used for blood gas interpretation. Data for its construction are given in Table 7–2.

METABOLIC ALKALOSIS

An acute, uncompensated metabolic alkalosis would move the blood gas values to the left (alkalotic side) along the $P_aCO_2 = 40$ line. Respiratory compensation would involve a rise in P_aCO_2; does this occur? Kildeberg (1963) has shown that it does occur in infants with persistent vomiting due to pyloric stenosis; comparable data for adults are not available. Data collected up until a few years ago suggested that P_aCO_2 did not rise in adults purely on the basis of metabolic alkalosis. Several recent reports, however, suggest that hypercapnia secondary to severe metabolic alkalosis may be more common than would appear from previous studies. A 95 per cent confidence band for HCO_3^- vs P_aCO_2 based on 14 normal subjects has recently been published (Javaheri, 1982). Regardless of the exact incidence, there seems little doubt that respiratory compensation for metabolic alkalosis (which would require hypoventilation) is much less common than respiratory compensation for metabolic acidosis (requiring hyperventilation). One reason for this may be that most serious illnesses naturally tend to produce hyperventilation.

CONSTRUCTING THE DIAGRAM

The diagram is best constructed on graph paper. The normal area is a box running from PCO_2 32 to 45 and H^+ 35 to 45 (pH 7.45 to 7.35). The confidence bands are bound by straight lines; Figure 7–12 can be used as a guide. Table 7–2 gives the coordinates for these lines.

Several other acid-base diagrams have been published using whole body titration curves. Some have bicarbonate as one of the axes; others have P_aCO_2 on the abscissa and pH on the ordinate. Once the reader has learned the principles behind the use of whole body tiration curves, he will have no trouble adapting to any of the published diagrams.

Precision

The precision of blood gas analysis on a day-to-day basis in a clinical laboratory is difficult to judge; as

Table 7–2. COORDINATES FOR CONSTRUCTING ACID-BASE CONFIDENCE BANDS

	Left Boundary Line			Right Boundary Line		
Disturbance	***Pco_2***	***H^+***	***pH***	***Pco_2***	***H^+***	***pH***
Acute respiratory acidosis	50 90	43.5 73.6	7.36 7.15	50 90	49.5 81.2	7.31 7.09
Chronic respiratory acidosis	50 100	34 45	7.47 7.35	50 100	45 58	7.35 7.24
Metabolic acidosis	30 10	40 72	7.40 7.14	30 20	58 75	7.24 7.13
Respiratory alkalosis	30 15	29.4 18.3	7.53 7.74	30 15	35.7 24.6	7.45 7.61

soon as an assessment begins, techniques tighten up. Reports of reproducibility from research laboratories reflect a minimal workload with special care exerted. Two standard deviations about the mean of replicated samples have been reported as 0.026 for pH, 4.6 mm Hg for PCO_2, and 2.2 mm Hg for PO_2 (Lumley, 1971). Considering that the 95 per cent confidence limits encompass ± 2 standard deviations, these results are disappointing. For example, by these standards, blood with a true PCO_2 of 45 mm Hg could, on a single analysis, have a measured PCO_2 anywhere between 40.5 and 49.5. As noted previously, however, rigorous quality control coupled with preventive maintenance of instruments and meticulous technical attention can yield improved precision and accuracy in blood gas analyses (Leary, 1977).

Uncertainty as to Reference Values

In a survey of 73 laboratories (Leiner, 1969), the accepted lower reference limit for pH varied from 7.35 to 7.39; the upper limit for pH varied from 7.42 to 7.46. The accepted lower reference limit for P_aCO_2 varied from 32 to 38 mm Hg; the accepted upper limit varied from 36 to 46 mm Hg. For P_aO_2 the accepted lower reference limit varied from 68 to 95 mm Hg.

What Arterial Blood Gases Will Not Tell You

Although the blood gases will demonstrate certain abnormalities, they will not indicate how much the patient is suffering from the abnormality. A low P_aO_2 does not necessarily imply tissue hypoxia, nor does a normal P_aO_2 assure adequate tissue oxygenation. The cardiac output, regional blood flow, affinity of hemoglobin for oxygen, capillary perfusion, and tissue oxygen consumption are all important in oxygen utilization. The vital signs and level of mental function are good clinical guides to the adequacy of tissue oxygenation. Mixed venous PO_2 reflects tissue oxygenation much better than does arterial PO_2.

Arterial blood gas values should not be expected to correlate with dyspnea. Dyspnea is a mechanical problem, not a chemical one, usually related to an increase in work of breathing. Unless this work becomes extreme, or the respiratory control system is defective, dyspnea will occur but not hypercapnia. Hypoxemia is more directly related to the distribution of ventilation and blood flow than to abnormalities in the mechanical properties. During an attack of asthma, patients as dyspneic as any which a physician is likely to see may have normal or only mildly abnormal arterial blood gas values.

Arterial blood gas values cannot give a specific etiologic diagnosis. For example, patients with chronic obstructive airway disease and respiratory failure may have the same blood gas values as cardiac patients with acute pulmonary edema; patients with asthma may have values similar to those of patients with pneumonia.

Resting arterial blood gases are poor screening tests for the exclusion of pulmonary disease. The primary function of the lung is to make arterial blood out of venous blood, and the arterial blood gases therefore are an excellent indication of overall pulmonary function. But like all organ systems, considerable disease can be present before the system fails. A careful history and physical examination, spirometry, and the chest x-ray are the proper screening procedures for pulmonary disease.

Patterns of Arterial Blood Gas Abnormalities in Specific Diseases

CHRONIC OBSTRUCTIVE PULMONARY DISEASE

A wide variety of patterns of blood gas values are seen in this group of diseases, ranging from normal to severe hypoxemia and hypercapnia. In the type A (pink puffer or emphysematous) variety, the most common pattern is mild to moderate hypoxemia with a normal P_aCO_2. In the type B (blue bloater or bronchitic) variety, more severe hypoxemia with hypercapnia is the rule. In both groups V/Q (ventilation/perfusion) inequalities are the primary cause for the hypoxemia.

The hypercapnia is usually ascribed to hypoventilation but, as noted previously, this is an oversimplification. It is more likely that the V/Q inequalities produce hypercapnia and the marked increase in the work of breathing precludes the ventilation response required to keep the P_aCO_2 normal.

BRONCHIAL ASTHMA

In the symptom-free intervals the blood gases are normal. During a moderately severe attack, hypoxemia with a normal or low P_aCO_2 is the usual finding. Hypercapnia may be seen during a severe attack and indicates a rapidly deteriorating clinical state, often with exhaustion. Intubation and assisted ventilation may be required at this stage.

DIFFUSE INTERSTITIAL PULMONARY DISEASES

This group of diseases has a wide variety of names (pulmonary fibrosis, fibrosing alveolitis, chronic interstitial pneumonitis, Hamman-Rich disease). Although the diffusion defect (alveolar capillary block) has received a great deal of attention, at rest the P_aO_2 is usually normal or only mildly reduced. A marked fall in P_aO_2 may occur with exercise. The P_aCO_2 is usually normal or low.

SHOCK

Hypoxemia with normal or slightly low P_aCO_2 is the usual finding in septic and hemorrhagic shock (Bredenberg, 1969); the hypoxemia is primarily the result of shunting. Hypercapnia may occur terminally despite high minute ventilation delivered by a ventilator. Metabolic acidosis is a frequent finding.

MYOCARDIAL INFARCTION

There has been a great deal of recent interest in the arterial blood gases in this disease. One of the unexpected findings has been mild hypoxemia even in patients without complications. This mild hypoxemia results from V/Q imbalance, with poor aeration of the lung bases a major factor. When shock, pulmonary edema, or pulmonary embolism occurs in the course of myocardial infarction, these complications will dominate the blood gas picture.

PULMONARY EDEMA

Moderate to severe hypoxemia with normal or low P_aCO_2 is a frequent finding. However, Anthonisen (1965) reported four cases of severe respiratory acidosis in pulmonary edema. This type of disturbance has subsequently been shown to be a mixed respiratory and metabolic acidosis, and to be much more common than previously thought.

PULMONARY EMBOLISM

Szucs (1971) reported the results of 50 patients with pulmonary embolism. P_aCO_2 ranged from 38 to 80 mm Hg. Values of P_aO_2 above 80 mm Hg are seen occasionally, but hypoxemia is the rule. Respiratory alkalosis is the usual acid-base disturbance. Only six of Szucs' patients had a P_aCO_2 above 40 mm Hg; three of these had chronic obstructive airway disease.

EXERCISE

In normal subjects and cardiac patients, the P_aO_2 is normal even at the breaking point of severe exercise, and higher than the resting P_aO_2 (Gilbert, 1970). By contrast, patients with type A emphysema show a fall in P_aO_2 with severe exercise; patients with type B disease usually show a slight rise, presumably the result of more uniform distribution of blood flow and ventilation during exercise. Normal subjects invariably show a metabolic acidosis, often uncompensated, at the breaking point of severe exercise; cardiac and pulmonary patients have less severe degrees of metabolic acidosis than do normal subjects, presumably because they are unwilling or unable to push themselves to extreme limits of endurance. A respiratory alkalosis at the exercise breaking point usually indicates a hyperventilation syndrome or neurocirculatory asthenia.

ADULT RESPIRATORY DISTRESS SYNDROME

Early in the illness the arterial blood gases show mild hypoxemia, hypocapnia, and a mixed respiratory and metabolic alkalosis. Later more severe hypoxemia develops, the result of shunting plus an extreme reduction in diffusing capacity. Metabolic and respiratory acidosis are seen in the terminal stages.

ASPIRIN INTOXICATION

Within the first few hours there is a respiratory alkalosis due presumably to a direct effect of salicylate on the central nervous system. This is followed (especially in infants and young children) by a metabolic acidosis due to a defect in intermediary metabolism, and therefore represents a true mixed disturbance, respiratory alkalosis and metabolic acidosis. A low P_aCO_2 with a normal pH, especially in a young child, should immediately bring to mind the possibility of aspirin intoxication.

RESPIRATORY FAILURE

This commonly used term has no generally accepted meaning. It is often defined in terms of the blood gases; that is, respiratory failure is present when the arterial blood gases are abnormal. Since the major function of the respiratory system is that of gas exchange, there is certainly justification for this usage. But does it require both an abnormal P_aO_2 and P_aCO_2? Many critically ill patients with severe pulmonary disease have a low P_aO_2 and a low or normal P_aCO_2. This implies defective gas exchange but a ventilatory control system sufficiently intact to prevent hypercapnia. Certainly hypercapnia implies ventilatory failure, that is, a ventilation either abnormally low or one that has not responded or is unable to respond sufficiently to the hypercapnia produced by defective gas exchange, increased metabolic activity, or both. The reader should be aware of the various facets of so-called respiratory failure and of the imprecise nature of the term.

Summary

The arterial blood gas interpretation should answer three questions:

1. Is gas exchange defective? This is determined by the P_aO_2 in conjunction with the a/A ratio or $P_{A-aD}O_2$.
2. What is the state of the ventilatory control system? This is determined by the P_aCO_2 with consideration of the acid-base state.
3. What is the state of acid-base balance? This is determined by reference to appropriate whole body

titration curves plus all other available clinical and laboratory findings.

Albert, M. S., Dell, R. B., and Winters, R. W.: Quantitative displacement of acid-base equilibrium in metabolic acidosis. Ann. Intern. Med., *66:*312, 1967.

Anthonisen, N. R., and Smith, H. J.: Respiratory acidosis as a consequence of pulmonary edema. Ann. Intern. Med., *62:*991, 1965.

Arbus, G. S., Hebert, L. A., Levesque, P. R., Etsten, B. E., and Schwartz, W. B.: Characterization and clinical application of the "significance band" for acute respiratory alkalosis. N. Engl. J. Med., *280:*117, 1969.

Ayres, S. M., and Grace, W. J.: Inappropriate ventilation and hypoxemia as causes of cardiac arrhythmias. Am. J. Med., *46:*495, 1969.

Baegeant, R. A.: Variations in arterial blood gas measurements due to sampling techniques. Resp. Care, *20:*565, 1975.

Bedford, R. H., and Wollman, H.: Arterial puncture for blood gas studies: Sites, complications, personnel. J.A.M.A., *228:*763, 1974.

Bigen, R., Racine, T., and Roy, J. C.: Value of capillary blood gas analysis in the management of acute respiratory distress. Am. Res. Respir. Dis., *112:*879, 1975.

Bird, B. D., Williams, J., and Whitwam, J. G.: The blood gas factor: A comparison of three different oxygen electrodes. Br. J. Anaesth., *46:*249, 1974.

Brackett, N. C., Jr., Cohen, J. J., and Schwartz, W. B.: Carbon dioxide titration curve of normal man. N. Engl. J. Med., *272:6,* 1965.

Brackett, N. C., Jr., Wingo, C. F., Muren, O., and Solano, J. T.: Acid-base response to chronic hypercapnia in man. N. Engl. J. Med., *280:*124, 1969.

Bradley, J. G.: Errors in the management of blood Pco_2 due to dilution of the sample with heparin solution. Br. J. Anaesth., *44:*231, 1972.

Bredenberg. C. E., James. P. M., Collins, J., Anderson, R. W., Martin, A. M., Jr., and Hardaway, R. M.: Respiratory failure in shock. Ann. Surg., *169:*392, 1969.

Chalmers, C., Bird, B. D., and Whitwam, J. G.: Evaluation of a new thin film tonometer. Br. J. Anaesth., *46:*253, 1974.

Crapo, R. O., Morris, A. H., and Gardner, R. M.: Spirometric values using techniques and equipment that meet ATS recommendations. Am. Rev. Respir. Dis., *123:*659, 1981.

Cubal, L., Hodgman, J., Siassi, B., and Plajstek, C.: Factors affecting heated transcutaneous Po_2 and unheated transcutaneous Po_2 in preterm infants. Crit. Care Med., *9:*298, 1981.

Czech, K., Lackner, F., and Porges, P.: Intraoperative transmucous Po_2 monitoring ($tmPo_2$). Birth Defects, *15:*551, 1979.

Delaney, C. J., Leary, E. R., Raisys, V. A., and Kenny, M. A.: Proficiency testing for blood gas quality control. Clin. Chem., *22:*1675, 1976.

Dowd, F., and Jenkins, L. C.: Some problems associated with measurement of physiological blood gases. Can. Anaesth. Soc. J., *20:*129, 1973.

Evers, W., Raez, G. B., and Levy, O. A.: A comparative study of plastic (polypropylene) and glass syringes in blood gas analysis. Anesth. Analg. (Cleve.), *51:*92, 1972.

Fleisher, M., and Schwartz, M. K.: Use of evacuated collection tubes for routine determination of arterial blood gases and pH. Clin. Chem., *17:*610, 1971.

Gambino, S. R.: Comparisons of pH in human arterial, venous and capillary blood. Am. J. Clin. Path., *32:*298, 1959.

Gambino, S. R.: Collection of capillary blood for simultaneous determinations of arterial pH, CO_2 content, Pco_2 and oxygen saturation. Am. J. Clin. Path. *35:*175, 1961.

Gandy, G., Grann, L., Cunningham, H., Adamson. K., and James, L. S.: The validity of pH and Pco_2 measurements in sick and healthy newborn infants. Pediatrics, *34:*192, 1964.

Gardner, R. M.: Report of Snowbird workshop for standardization of spirometry. Am. Rev. Respir. Dis., *119:*831, 1979.

Gilbert, R., and Auchincloss, J. H.: Arterial blood gases and acid-base balance at the exercise breaking point. Arch. Intern. Med., *125:*820, 1970.

Gilbert, R., Auchincloss, J. H., Kuppinger, M., and Thomas, M. V.: Stability of the arterial/alveolar oxygen partial pressure ratio: Effects of low ventilation/perfusion regions. Crit. Care Med., 7:267, 1979.

Gilbert, R., Auchincloss, J. H., Jr., Peppi, D., and Ashutosh, K.: The first few hours off a respirator. Chest, *65:*152, 1974.

Gilbert, R., and Keighley, J. F.: The arterial/alveolar oxygen tension ratio. Am. Rev. Resp. Dis., *109:*142, 1974.

Goldstein, M. B., Gennari, F. J., and Schwartz, W. B.: The influence of graded degrees of chronic hypercapnia on the acute carbon dioxide titration curve. J. Clin. Invest., *50:*208, 1971.

Greenhow, D. E.: Incorrect performance of Allen's test ulnar-artery flow, erroneously presumed inadequate. Anesthesiology, *37:*356, 1972.

Huch, A., Huch, R., and Schneidor, H.: Fetal transcutaneous Po_2—current knowledge. Birth Defects, *15:*185, 1979a.

Huch, R., Fallenstein, F., Seiler, D., Lubbers, D., and Huch, A.: $tcPco_2$—state of development. Birth Defects, *15:*413, 1979b.

Ishikawa, S., Fornier, A., Borst, E., and Segal, M.: The effects of air bubbles and time delay on blood gas analysis. Ann. Allergy, *331:*72, 1974.

Javaheri, S., Shore, N. S., Rose, B., and Kazemi, H.: Compensatory hypoventilation in metabolic alkalosis. Chest, *81:*296, 1982.

Jung, R. C., Balchum, O. J., and Massey, F. J.: The accuracy of venous and capillary blood for the prediction of arterial pH, Pco_2 and Po_2 measurements. Am. J. Clin. Path., *45:*129, 1966.

Kelman, G. R., and Nunn, J. F.: Nomograms for correction of blood Po_2, Pco_2, pH, and base excess for time and temperature. J. Appl. Physiol., *21:*1484, 1966.

Kilburn, K. H., and Dowell, A. R.: Renal function in respiratory failure. Arch. Intern. Med., *127:*754, 1971.

Kildeberg, P.: Respiratory compensation in metabolic alkalosis. Acta Med. Scand., *174:*515, 1963.

Koch, G., and Wendel, H.: Comparison of pH, carbon dioxide tension, standard bicarbonate and oxygen tension in capillary blood and in arterial blood during the neonatal period. Acta Paediatr. Scand., *56:*10, 1967.

Koch, G.: The validity of Po_2 measurements in capillary blood as a substitute for arterial blood. Scand. J. Clin. Invest., *21:*10, 1968.

Komjathy, Z. L., Mathies, J. C., Parker, J. A., and Schreiber, H. A.: Stability and precision of a new ampuled quality control system for pH and blood gas measurements. Clin. Chem., *22:*1399, 1976.

Kryger, M., Bode, F., Antic, R., and Anthonisen, N.: Diagnosis of obstruction of the upper and central airways. Am. J. Med., *61:*85, 1976.

Langlands, J. H. M., and Wallace, W. F. M.: Small blood-samples from earlobe puncture. Lancet, *2:*315, 1965.

Laughlin, D. E., McDonald, J. S., and Bedell, G. N.: A microtechnique for measurement of Po_2 in "arterialized" earlobe blood. J. Lab. Clin. Med., *64:*330, 1964.

Leary, E. T., Graham, G., and Kenny, M. A.: Commercially available blood-gas quality controls compared with tonometered blood. Clin. Chem., *26:*1309, 1980.

Leary, T. E., Delaney, C. J., and Kenny, M. A.: Use of equilibrated blood for internal blood-gas quality control. Clin. Chem., *23:*493, 1977.

Leiner, G. C., Abramowitz, S., and Small, M. J.: Pulmonary function testing in laboratories associated with residency training programs in pulmonary diseases. Am. Rev. Resp. Dis., *100:*240, 1969.

Lumley, J., Potter, M., Newman, W., Talbot, J. M., Wakefield, E., and Wood, C.: The unreliability of a single estimation of fetal scalp blood pH. J. Lab. Clin. Med., *77:*535, 1971.

Morgan, E. J., Baidwan, T., Petty, T. L., and Zwillich, C. W.: The effects of unanesthetized arterial puncture on Pco_2 and pH. Am. Rev. Respir. Dis., *120:*795, 1979.

Morris, J. F., Koski, A., and Johnson, L. C.: Spirometric standards for healthy nonsmoking adults. Am. Rev. Respir. Dis., *103:*57, 1971.

Mortensen, J. D.: Clinical sequelae from arterial puncture, cannulation and incision. Circulation, *35:*1118, 1967.

Newball, H.: Arterial blood samples should be stored in ice for gas analysis. J.A.M.A., *223:*696, 1973.

Noonan, D. C., and Komjathy, Z. L.: Long term reproducibility of a new pH/blood-gas quality control system compared to two other procedures. Clin. Chem., *22:*1817, 1976.

Nunn, J. F.: Measurement of blood oxygen tension: Handling of samples. Br. J. Anaesth., *34:*621, 1962.

Oliven, A., Abinader, E., and Bursztein, S.: Influence of varying inspired oxygen tensions on the pulmonary venous admixture (shunt) of mechanically ventilated patients. Crit. Care Med., *8:*99, 1980.

Petty, T. L., and Bailey, D.: A new, versatile blood gas syringe. Heart Lung, *10:*672, 1981.

Petty, T. L., Bigelow, D. B., and Levine, B. E.: The simplicity and safety of arterial puncture. J.A.M.A., *195:*181, 1966.

Sackner, M. A., Avery, W. G., and Sokolowski, J.: Arterial punctures by nurses. Chest, *59:*97, 1971.

Sadove, M. S., Thompson, R. D., and Jobsen, E.: Capillary versus arterial blood gases. Anesth. Analg. (Cleve.), *52:*724, 1973.

Schwartz, W. B., van Ypersele de Strihou, C., and Kassirer, J. P.: Role of anions in metabolic alkalosis and potassium deficiency. N. Engl. J. Med., *279:*630, 1968.

Scott, P. V., Horton, J. N., and Mapleson, W. W.: Mechanism and magnitude of leakage from blood and water samples stored in plastic syringes. Br. J. Anaesth., *43:*717, 1971a.

Scott, P. V., Horton, J. N., and Mapleson, W. W.: Leakage of oxygen from blood and water samples stored in plastic and glass syringes. Br. Med. J., *3:*512, 1971b.

Severinghaus, J. W.: Electrodes for blood and gas Pco_2, Po_2 and blood pH. Acta Anaesth. Scand. (Suppl. XI):207, 1962.

Severinghaus, J. W.: Measurement of blood gases, Po_2 and Pco_2. Ann. N.Y. Acad. Sci., *148:*115, 1968.

Sieker, H. O., and Hickan, J. B.: Carbon dioxide intoxication: The clinical syndrome, its etiology and management with particular reference to the use of mechanical respirators. Medicine, *35:*389, 1956.

Siggaard-Anderson, O.: Acid-base and blood gas parameters—arterial or capillary blood. Scand. J. Clin. Lab. Invest., *21*:289, 1968.

Siggaard-Anderson, O.: Sampling and storing of blood for determination of acid-base status. Scand. J. Clin. Lab. Invest., *13*:196, 1961.

Szucs, M. M., Brooks, H. L., Grossman, W., Banas, J. S., Meister, S. G., Dexter, L., and Dalen, J. E.: Diagnostic sensitivity of laboratory findings in acute pulmonary embolism. Ann. Intern. Med., *74:*161, 1971.

Versmold, H. T., Linderkamp, O., Holzmann, M., Strohhacker, I., and Riegel, K.: Transcutaneous monitoring of Po_2 in newborn infants: Where are the limits? Influence of blood pressure, blood volume, blood flow, viscosity and acid base state. Birth Defects, *15:*285, 1979.

Wallace, W. D., Cutler, C. A., and Clark, J. S.: New gas-liquid equilibration method: Syringe tonometer. Clin. Chem., *27:*681, 1981.

West, J.: Regional differences in gas exchange in the lung of erect man. J. Appl. Physiol., *17:*893, 1962.

West, J. B.: Causes of carbon dioxide retention in lung disease. N. Engl. J. Med., *284:*1232, 1971.

Winkler, J. B., Huntington, C. B., Wells, D. E., and Befeler, B.: Influence of syringe material on blood gas determinations. Chest, *66:*518, 1974.

Winters, R. W., Engel, K., and Dell, R. B.: Acid Base Physiology in Medicine. Cleveland, The London Company, 1967.

2

8

EVALUATION OF RENAL FUNCTION AND WATER, ELECTROLYTE, AND ACID-BASE BALANCE

JOHN E. MURPHY, M.D.,
HARRY G. PREUSS, M.D.,
and JOHN BERNARD HENRY, M.D.

In order that intracellular metabolic processes occur at maximal efficiency, the internal cellular composition has to be controlled within narrow limits. Intracellular composition is influenced greatly by the composition of the surrounding extracellular fluid (ECF), which is precisely regulated by the respiratory and renal systems. The lungs control the partial pressures and concentrations of the blood gases and, therefore, the respiratory component of the acid-base system (see Chap. 7). In addition to eliminating toxic metabolites and drugs, the kidneys control the tonicity, volume, and chemical composition of the ECF.

RENAL FUNCTION

The initial and most cost effective laboratory evaluation of renal function is the urinalysis (see Chap. 18). Depending on the preliminary findings or the clinical situation, further studies may be indicated on accurately timed urine collections, including protein and nitrogen-containing excretory products (creatinine and urea nitrogen). Simultaneous measurements of these analytes in serum may help to quantitate or to detect subtle abnormalities (e.g., creatinine clearance). Individual serum protein studies (electrophoresis) (Chap. 12) and blood lipid studies (Chap. 11) may have diagnostic or prognostic importance. Provocative testing and concentration and dilution studies can also be done on timed urine collections. If there is a significant reduction in the glomerular filtration rate (azotemia or uremia), measurements of electrolytic and acid-base status are in order. Serum K^+ is critically important to evaluate because of the potential adverse consequences of hyperkalemia and hypokalemia.

Excretory urographic and retrograde pyelographic contrast (radiologic) studies can provide evaluation of renal size, shape, presence of filling defects, and the urinary drainage system. Renal radionuclide scanning studies may complement contrast studies. Additional anatomic data can be derived from ultrasound, computed tomographic, and angiographic studies. If the urinary sediment is abnormal, more sensitive evaluation of the sediment, including the use of special stains and specialized microscopy, may be useful (Chap. 18). Finally, renal biopsy to delineate the specific pathologic lesion(s) may be necessary. Besides light microscopy, immunofluorescent and electron microscopy studies are routinely performed on the same biopsy specimen.

Evaluation and management of patients with chronic disorders of renal function are achieved by periodic measurements of urinary volume, urinalyses, serum urea, creatinine, electrolyte determinations, and clearance studies. These parameters, used alone or combined, aid in the determination of appropriate fluid and electrolyte replacement as well as deciding the frequency of dialysis and the constitution of dialysate.

Renal Clearance Studies

Overall renal function and some aspects of kidney physiology can be determined by simultaneously measuring concentrations of substances in both blood and urine. By measuring substances such as creatinine in the urine and the volume of urine formed during a timed collection as well as the concentration of the substance in the plasma (serum) from a midperiod blood collection, the volume of plasma (serum) that contained the measured substance excreted into the urine per unit of time (usually one minute) can be calculated. This volume, expressed in ml/min, is defined as renal clearance. The formula for calculating renal clearance is:

$$\text{Clearance (ml/min)} = \frac{\text{U(mg/dl)}}{\text{P(mg/dl)}} \cdot \text{V(ml/min)}$$

U = concentration of measured substance in urine
P = concentration of same substance in plasma
V = urine volume expressed as ml/min

It is necessary that the concentration units for U and P be identical for calculation. Milligrams per deciliter are used above, as this is the commonly reported value for creatinine. Since clearance is proportional to the total number and size of glomeruli, which correspondingly are proportional to renal parenchymal mass, it is customary to correct the absolute clearance by a factor, 1.73/A for surface area. This is done in order to standardize clearance values. 1.73 is the external surface area (square meters) of the average-sized person; A is the body surface area of the patient. This correction ratio is used because total kidney mass is roughly proportional to body surface area. This correction factor is obviously necessary if the body surface area of the patient (e.g., child, obese adult) differs markedly from the average. The corrected formula for clearance is:

$$\text{Clearance (ml/min/std. surface area)} = \frac{\text{U} \times \text{V}}{\text{P}} \times \frac{1.73}{\text{A}}$$

The surface area, A in the equation, can easily be determined from nomograms or from formulas which relate weight and height to surface area (see Appendix 2).

Small molecules that are not bound to protein and therefore are freely filtered by glomeruli, neither reabsorbed nor secreted by the tubules, can be used to determine the glomerular filtration rate (GFR), i.e., the amount of ultrafiltrate passing from the blood into the tubular lumen over a given period of time.

Inulin, a polysaccharide with a molecular weight of 5100 daltons, is an ideal substance to measure GFR. While the clearance of inulin is used commonly to estimate GFR under experimental conditions, it is not routinely employed in a clinical setting because of the necessity for continuous intravenous infusion. It is, however, the "gold standard" for evaluating other assessments of GFR. Inulin is measured colorimetrically. The average inulin clearance is 125 ml/min/1.73 m^2 for men and 110 ml/min/1.73 m^2 for women (Smith, 1951). The difference between the sexes is due to the larger kidneys in males. GFRs are lower in neonates (even corrected for surface area) until the age of three to five months (West, 1948) because of the physiological and anatomical immaturity of developing glomeruli. Immaturity can be identified histologically by the presence of a cuboidal or columnar visceral epithelial layer lining the glomerular capillaries. The GFRs also progressively decrease as individuals pass middle age (Wesson, 1969). There is a progressive decrease in the number of glomeruli from senile arteriolonephrosclerosis. During pregnancy the GFR increases approximately 50 per cent and returns to normal after delivery (Semple, 1974). This results in increased blood volume and renal plasma flow. In addition, a direct hormonal (placental) influence on the kidneys is possible (Matthews, 1960). Increased GFRs and overall renal mass have been demonstrated in early juvenile diabetics (Mogensen, 1973). The approximately 25 per cent augmentation results from increased glomerular size. Compensatory renal growth in diabetes mellitus has been attributed to high circulating glucose concentrations, as adequate control with insulin results in the return of GFR and renal mass back toward baseline (Seyer-Hansen, 1976). GFRs are increased in patients with major burns, perhaps due to both hypoproteinemia and increased renal blood flow secondary to extensive volume replacement (Loirat, 1978).

The endogenous substance used most commonly in the clinical assessment of GFR is creatinine. Creatinine, a degradation product of creatine, is formed at a relatively constant rate by muscle, the major storage site of creatine phosphate. Thus, creatinine production and excretion relate directly to muscle mass. Accordingly, males and muscular athletes produce greater amounts of creatinine than do nonmuscular women, children, and elderly individuals (Jackson, 1966). Creatinine excretion is not routinely affected by diet. However, large quantities of creatinine are present in sterilized canned meats (Jackson, 1966) and cooked meats (Camara, 1951). If excessive quantities (i.e., >75 g) of these meat sources of exogenous creatinine are consumed, both serum and clearance values of creatinine will be increased for 48 hours (Camara, 1951). However, this will not influence creatinine clearance after a 48-hour interval..

Besides free glomerular filtration, there is also active tubular secretion of creatinine in man that results in an overestimation of the true GFR when compared to inulin clearance. If the GFR is within the normal range, the creatinine clearance estimated by "true" creatinine (see below) exceeds the inulin clearance by 5 to 10 per cent (Renkin, 1974). As the GFR decreases in renal disease, relative tubular secretion compared to glomerular load increases, making the estimate of GFR by creatinine clearance more uncertain. It has also been shown that glomerular filtration of creatinine is increased in patients with nephrotic syndrome (Carrie, 1980). As a result, the "true" creatinine clearance may at times exceed the actual GFR by 50 per cent or more (Renkin, 1974). Another variable to be considered in evaluation of creatinine clearance is drug interference. Salicylates (Burry, 1976), cimetidine (Tagamet) (Larrson, 1980), and trimethoprim (Lee, 1981) interfere with tubular secretion of creatinine. Thus, while the GFR may not change, the creatinine clearance is lowered and gives a false impression of GFR.

In spite of the many variables that influence creatinine clearances, this estimate of GFR has good clinical utility since reliable creatinine methods are available in the clinical laboratory. Serial measurements can demonstrate progression of renal disease and/or response to therapy. However, precisely timed and complete urine collections are required. The usual urine collection is over 24 hours with blood being drawn at the beginning or end of the collection for convenience. Many clinicians perform a hydrated clearance over two hours (three periods of 40 minutes) with blood drawn at the midpoint of the second urine collection. Hydration is performed by giving the patient 20 ml H_2O/kg body weight at the initiation of the test and replacing urine volume throughout. Routinely, the assessment should be performed within a given time of the day because of the diurnal variation in GFR known to occur. Normal values using nonspecific methods to measure creatinine which also include the measurement of other serum chromogens are 85 to 125 ml/min for males and 75 to 115 ml/min for females. If a specific method is used to measure true creatinine concentrations (e.g., use of Lloyd's reagent or the kinetic Jaffe reaction [Chap. 9]), normality is 97 to 137 ml/min for males and 88 to 128 ml/min for females (Fig. 8–1). Falsely low values will be obtained if the collected urine is not refrigerated and/or a bacterial inhibitor (e.g., thymol) is not added to the collection container. Ideally, the urine creatinine concentration should be determined no later than 24 hours after collection. Changes in the acidity or alkalinity of the urine (a result of bacterial metabolism) may promote the conversion of creatinine to creatine. Creatine is not measured directly by the Jaffe reaction. Bacteria may also produce creatininases which degrade creatinine.

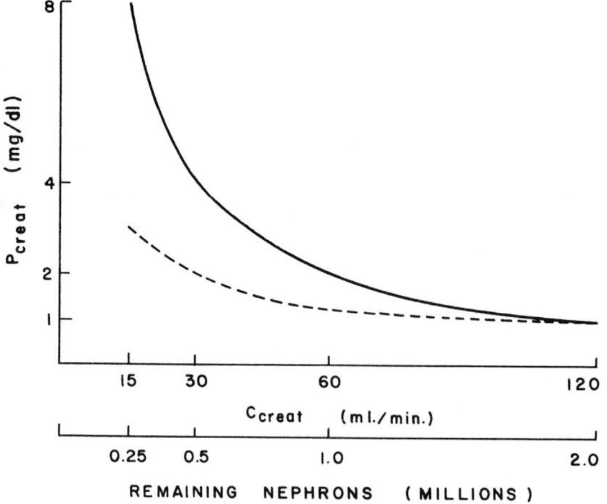

Figure 8–1. Plasma creatinine (P_{creat}) concentration as a function of creatine clearance (C_{creat}) and remaining nephrons.

GFR can also be measured by intravenous or subcutaneous administration of radiolabeled substances, including [^{14}C] inulin. The more commonly used substances are [^{51}Cr] ethylenediaminetetraacetic acid (EDTA), [^{169}Yb] diethylenetriaminepentaacetic acid (DPTA), and [^{125}I] iothalamate. These radioactive substances are similar to inulin—they are not significantly protein bound, are freely filtered by glomeruli, and are neither secreted nor reabsorbed by renal tubules.

Because gamma radiation can be measured easily and since these studies correlate more closely with inulin clearance than creatinine clearance, they are being performed at many large medical centers (Ward, 1981). Additional advantages include the ability to scan the bladder externally to evaluate bladder emptying and the capability to measure GFR by serial measurements of timed blood samples, obviating the necessity for urine collection (Groth, 1977). There are, however, disadvantages to consider (Duarte, 1980). These include the necessity of a priming intravenous dose, constant intravenous infusion, nonconstant absorption of subcutaneous injection, significant radiation exposure to the patient (if multiple studies are required), contraindication of *in vivo* radioisotopic administration in pregnant and lactating women, and analytical interference by recent previous radionuclide administration (e.g., renogram). Although not as practical as creatinine clearance, these radioactive tests to estimate GFR can be useful if more accurate information is desired.

To evaluate secretory function of the renal tubules, exogenous organic anions and/or cations can be injected into the circulation and clearance values determined. At low circulating concentrations, approximately 90 per cent of para-aminohippurate (PAH) is cleared in one passage through the kidney so that the resultant plasma concentration does not exceed threshold. If tubular function is normal, the clearance value for PAH is a rough estimate of renal plasma flow. PAH clearance is often referred to as the effective renal plasma flow (ERPF). Normal PAH clearance is 600 to 700 ml/min. PAH is measured colorimetrically in the laboratory, and it is the reference for ERPF against which all methods are compared. The actual renal plasma flow (RPF) is 8 to 10 per cent greater, the percentage of blood not directly bathing the glomeruli or tubules.

If the circulatory concentration of PAH is raised, the TmPAH can be measured. This specialized test allows an estimation of proximal tubular function. Obviously, by oversaturating the tubular transport mechanism for organic anions, less than 90 per cent of PAH load is excreted in a single passage. Clearance of PAH approaches inulin clearance as the filtered load of PAH rises more in relation to the secreted portion. Under these conditions PAH clearance is not a valid measurement of ERPF.

The GFR/RPF ratio is commonly referred to as the

filtration fraction (FF) and is normally 0.16 to 0.20. Analogous to the GFR, the ERPF is lower in infants until the age of seven to eight months (West, 1948) and progressively decreases after middle age (Wesson, 1969). Since the change in ERPF is greater than the change in GFR, the FF increases progressively with age (Davies, 1950). The ERPF increases 25 per cent in the first and second trimesters of pregnancy and returns to normal in the last trimester (Wesson, 1969). The FF remains unchanged in the first two trimesters as GFR and RPF both increase proportionately but increases 25 per cent in the last trimester as the GFR remains elevated while the RPF returns toward baseline.

Sodium ^{131}I iodohippurate can also be used to measure secretory function and/or ERPF. The clearance values for radiolabeled sodium ^{131}I iodohippurate correlate well but are consistently lower when compared to PAH clearance studies (Duarte, 1980). Simultaneous measurements of GFR using different isotopic labels, e.g., ^{125}I, can be performed on the same collected samples. Hippurate clearance studies are used mainly for very accurate investigational purposes because of the need to maintain constant blood levels using continuous intravenous infusions.

The phenolsulfonphthalein (PSP) test is a simpler measurement of secretory function and renal plasma flow that may be employed clinically. This test detects early impairment in the ERPF but does not allow for accurate and precise serial evaluation (Wesson, 1969). Only in advanced renal failure is renal excretion limited by decreased secretion (van Ypersele, 1979), and therefore this test primarily measures the ERPF rather than tubular secretory capacity. Penicillin, Diodrast, thiazides, and azotemic byproducts interfere with the secretion of PSP and other organic anions (Taggart, 1958; Preuss, 1966), and clearance studies will be falsely decreased if patients are azotemic or receiving these substances. Fifty to 60 per cent of this dye is removed during a single passage through the kidneys, with active tubular secretion accounting for approximately 95 per cent of that cleared. If renal plasma flow is optimal and secretory function is not severely impaired, approximately 35 per cent of the injected dye is excreted in the first 15 minutes and 65 per cent by the end of the first hour (van Ypersele, 1979). The dye concentration is measured colorimetrically (540 mm) after alkalization.

The urea clearance test is an infrequently used and often difficult to interpret measurement of total renal function (i.e., glomerular and tubular function). Urea, having a very small molecular weight of 60 daltons, is freely filtered by the glomerulus but variably reabsorbed by the tubules. Reabsorption depends upon the transit time of filtrate in the tubules. Accordingly, interpretation of urea clearance is evaluated keeping the urine flow rate in mind. If the flow rate is 2 ml/min or greater, the normal urea clearance is 65 to 100 ml/min. This is referred to as the maximal clearance (C_m). If the flow rate is less than 2 ml/min, the normal urea clearance is 40 to 70 ml/min. This is referred to as the standard clearance (C_s). The standard clearance is calculated by substituting $\sqrt{V}$ for V in the formula for clearance. Mathematically, these two clearance values can be compared by dividing each by the average value for each respective clearance (i.e., mean C_m = 75 ml/min; mean C_s = 54 ml/min) and converting to per cent by multiplying by 100. The reference intervals for both clearances expressed as per cent of normal are 75 to 125 per cent. As the number of functioning nephrons decreases in chronic renal disease, less urea is reabsorbed and the urea clearance approaches the inulin clearance. Because of the many factors influencing urea clearance (Chap. 9), this test has been replaced by the creatinine clearance. The urea clearance, however, may have some value when interpreted with the creatinine clearance in severe renal failure (i.e., GFR less than 20 ml/min). The difference between the urea and inulin clearances is approximately the same as the difference between the creatinine and inulin clearances (Lubowitz, 1967). Therefore, an average of urea and creatinine clearances may be a better approximation of the actual GFR in advanced renal disease.

Although clearance studies are technically demanding, requiring accurately timed and complete urine collections, they are very sensitive indices of kidney function. Measurements of plasma metabolic waste substances alone may be insufficient. A steep hyperbolic relationship between clearance values and plasma concentrations exists. In many instances, 65 to 75 per cent of renal function must be lost before the various non-protein nitrogen substances exceed the level of normality of the clinical laboratory. BUN/creatinine serum ratios, however, can be very useful guidelines in differentiating the various etiologies of azotemia. (Chap. 9).

Measurements of Urinary Solute Concentration

The ability of the kidneys to maintain both the tonicity and water balance of the ECF requires that the tubules be functional and responsive to vasopressin (antidiuretic hormone [ADH]). These specific functions can be evaluated by measuring the solute concentrations of the urine either randomly or under well controlled conditions (i.e., concentration and dilution tests). Additional important information concerning renal function, pathology, and etiology behind hydration and electrolyte perturbations can be obtained when urinary and serum measurements are compared. Solute concentrations of fluid are most conveniently and economically quantitated in the clinical laboratory by measuring either specific gravity or osmolality.

Specific Gravity. Specific gravity is the ratio of the mass of a solution compared with the mass of an equal volume of water. Since this is actually a comparison of weights, it is not an exact measurement of the number of solute particles. However, there is a good correlation between specific gravity and osmolality under most circumstances. The specific gravity of plasma is fairly constant and ranges from 1.010 to 1.012. Urine specific gravity varies from 1.003 to 1.035, reflecting either dilution or concentration of the glomerular ultrafiltrate. Urine specific gravity is measured with a calibrated hydrometer, called a urinometer, or more commonly a temperature compensated refractometer calibrated in specific gravity units. Both of these techniques are discussed in detail in Chapter 18.

Osmolality. Osmolality is a measure of the number of dissolved solute particles in solution (Chap. 2). Dissolved solutes change four physical properties of solutions, called colligative properties. They are osmotic pressure, vapor pressure, boiling point, and freezing point. The extent of these changes at a constant temperature is determined only by the number and *not* by the nature or mass of the particles in solution. One gram molecular weight (mole) of a non-electrolyte (e.g., glucose) which contains 6.023×10^{23} particles (Avogadro's number), if dissolved in 1 kg of water, will increase the boiling point of water 0.52°C. and the osmotic pressure 17,000 mm Hg, and lower the vapor pressure 0.3 mm Hg and the freezing point 1.858°C. This solution is defined as having an osmolality of 1 (or 1 osmol/kg H_2O). A related expression is osmolarity, defined as 1 osmol of non-electrolyte dissolved in 1 L of distilled water. Osmolality is the preferred unit of measurement since it is a constant weight/weight relationship. In contrast, osmolarity varies owing to the volume-expanding effect of dissolved solute and the direct proportional effect of temperature on fluid volume.

The osmolality of a one-molal solution of an electrolyte (e.g., NaCl) is greater than 1 owing to the dissociation of electrolyte into component atoms when in solution. The osmolality of an electrolyte solution is determined by the formula:

$$\text{Osmolality} = \phi n C$$

Where n is the number of atoms that dissociate in solution, C is the concentration of the electrolyte in moles/kg H_2O, and ϕ is the osmotic coefficient.

Differing coefficients for each electrolyte arise because the dissociation of electrolyte into individual atoms is not complete and the individual particles may form secondary chemical bonds with solvent molecules. ϕ is derived from dividing the measured osmolality by the theoretical osmolality of the electrolyte solution. ϕ for NaCl is 0.93.

The electrolytes Na^+, Cl^-, and HCO_3^-, because they are present in high concentrations in the ECF and are monoionic, contribute to over 92 per cent of the serum osmolality. The other ECF electrolytes, serum proteins, glucose, and urea are responsible for the remaining 8 per cent. The normal osmolality of the serum is between 285 and 310 mosmol/kg H_2O. Many simple formulas have been devised to convert serum solute concentration to osmolality (Weisberg, 1975). The formula with good clinical utility and most easily remembered is:

$$\text{Osmolality (mosmol/kg } H_2O) = 2\ Na^+ + \frac{(\text{Glucose})}{20} + \frac{(\text{BUN})}{3}$$

which is a simplification of the formula:

$$\text{Osmolality (mosmol/kg } H_2O) = 1.86\ (Na^+) + \frac{(\text{Glucose})}{18} + \frac{(\text{BUN})}{2.8}$$

The number 1.86 is derived from 0.93×2 (ϕn), since each Na^+ in solution is balanced by a corresponding anion (Cl^- or HCO_3^-). The number 18 is used since the molecular mass of glucose is 180 daltons and the expression $\frac{(\text{Glucose})}{18}$ converts the units from mg/dl to mmol/L. Similarly, 2.8 is used because the molecular mass of the two nitrogen atoms in urea is 28 daltons and the expression $\frac{(\text{BUN})}{2.8}$ converts the units from mg/dl to mmol/L.

Urine osmolality varies of course depending on the state of hydration. Maximally diluted and concentrated urine shows osmolalities between 50 and 1400 mosmol/kg H_2O. Urine osmolality corresponds well with urinary specific gravity in non-disease states. However, the correlation is not good in renal disease states owing to the greater contribution of high molecular weight substances such as glucose and protein to specific gravity than to osmolality (Holmes, 1962). Often the physician is perplexed by the high urine specific gravity found after intravenous pyelogram (IVP) studies; this is due to the dye in the urine.

Osmometry. Osmolality can be estimated by measuring the freezing point depression of a solution using an osmometer or cryoscope (Chaps. 2 and 18). Serum or heparinized plasma may be used, but plasma anticoagulated with chelating or precipitating agents is unsuitable. Urine is centrifuged to remove all large particulate matter. The solution is supercooled (i.e., cooled below its freezing point) in an insulated freezing bath and then crystallized, using a vibrator which agitates the solution. As crystallization occurs, heat of fusion is produced and the temperature of the solution increases, reaching a plateau which is slightly below the freezing point. This temperature is compared with plateau temperatures obtained with known standards; therefore, no correction factor is necessary. The temperature changes are measured by a thermistor and converted to mosmol/kg H_2O.

An alternative method for measuring osmolality is to use a vapor pressure or dew point osmometer (Wescor Inc., Logan, Utah 84321). The sample to be tested (see above) is absorbed into a small disk of filter paper which is inserted into a sample holder and then sealed in an enclosed chamber. A temperature-sensitive thermocouple is incorporated into the chamber. Initially, the thermocouple is cooled electrically below the dew point. Water in the chamber air condenses and forms a thin film on the surface of the thermocouple. The dew point is the temperature of the atmosphere at which water begins to condense. As water condenses on the junction, heat of condensation is given off, the thermocouple temperature is increased to the dew point temperature, and water ceases to condense.

When this temperature is stabilized, it is compared to the initial chamber temperature. This measured temperature change is proportional to the vapor pressure of the evaporating fluid in the filter disk and is calibrated in mosmol/kg H_2O by use of known standards.

Vapor pressure osmometers are simpler in design than the freezing point instruments and use smaller volumes of sample (i.e., 8 μl). Although both instruments give identical results with clear sera and urine, there is a positive bias with the dew point instruments if the serum is lipemic (Mercier, 1978). The reason for this difference is not well understood but may be either kinetic or thermodynamic in origin. Comparison studies have indicated that dew point instruments are less precise than the freezing point instruments (Juel, 1977). Another major difference between the two instrument types is that dew point instruments cannot detect the presence of volatiles (e.g., alcohols) in solution, whereas freezing point instruments can (Weisberg, 1975; Rocco, 1976) because *volatile* solute increases the total vapor pressure of solutions, eliminating the direct solute depression of vapor pressure (Barlow, 1976). If significantly different values are obtained by the two methods, the difference in osmolality is an indirect measure of the concentration of volatile present.

Clinical Utility of Osmolality Studies

Comparison of measured and calculated serum osmolality has clinical significance. Calculated osmolalities of serum (and plasma) are usually a little lower than measured osmolalities (Weisberg, 1975). This is referred to as the delta-osmolality. If this calculation is more than 40 mosmol/kg H_2O in critically ill patients, there is a poor prognosis (Weisberg, 1975); the difference arises from the accumulation of osmotically active metabolites, including lactic and keto acids. The delta-osmolality also may be helpful in evaluating acutely ill or comatose patients. An increased gap between the measured (freezing point instrument) and calculated osmolality may indicate the presence of an ingested volatile or poison. Common causes of increased gap are ethanol overdose and azotemia (Loeb, 1974). Other important considerations, if ethanol and azotemia can be ruled out, are methanol, isopropanol, and ethylene glycol poisoning.

In the evaluation of renal function, the ratio of urine to serum/plasma osmolality (U/P osmol ratio) together with urinary electrolyte studies can be especially useful (Levinsky, 1976). Under usual circumstances, the ratio of urine osmolality to serum osmolality is between 1 and 3. In acute tubular dysfunction (including necrosis) and in chronic renal insufficiency, the U/P osmol ratio is equal to or less than 1.2 and the urinary Na^+ is greater than 20 mEq/L (mmol/L). In diseases in which the GFR is primarily impaired (e.g., congestive heart failure, acute glomerulonephritis, acute obstructive uropathy), the U/P ratio is greater than 1.2 and the urinary Na^+ is less than 20 mEq/L (mmol/L).

More recently, physicians confronted with the differentiation of pre-renal and parenchymal acute renal failure have turned to the renal failure index (RFI) and/or the fractional sodium excretion (FeNa) for more complete differentiation.

$$\text{RFI} = \text{Urine Na} \div \text{Urine Cr/Plasma Cr}$$

$$\text{FeNa} = \frac{\text{Urine Na} \times \text{Plasma Cr}}{\text{Urine Cr} \times \text{Plasma Na}} \times 100$$

An RFI or FeNa below 1.0 indicates pre-renal failure and above 1.0 suggests acute tubular necrosis. These simple tests clearly differentiate the type of renal failure, more so than osmolality or sodium excretion alone (Espinel, 1976.)

The U/P osmol ratio can differentiate among etiologies of polyuria. The U/P osmol ratio is greater than 1 in osmotic diuresis and less than 1 in water diuresis. In complete central or nephrogenic diabetes insipidus, the ratio is less than 1 and remains unchanged with water deprivation. In patients with incomplete or partial (i.e., decreased release of ADH) central diabetes insipidus and in psychogenic diabetes insipidus, the ratio will increase and be greater than 1 with fluid restriction (Ruddy, 1981). After Pitressin (vasopressin) administration, the ratio will increase significantly in patients with severe central diabetes insipidus. In addition, the urine osmolality increases at least 50 per cent above that obtained by fluid restriction alone (Ruddy, 1981). Patients with partial defects of ADH release will show an increase but not to the same extent (i.e., between 10 and 50 per cent). In those with nephrogenic diabetes insipidus, there is no increase in either the U/P osmol ratio or urine osmolality after vasopressin administration. If hypertonic saline is administered to patients with psychogenic diabetes insipidus, there is a sharp decline in free water clearance (see below) when the serum osmolality is less than 290 mosm/kg H_2O (Ruddy, 1981). In patients with partial diabetes insipidus, there is a similar response but only when the serum osmolality is greater than 290 mosm/kg H_2O. No change, however, is noted in those individuals with complete central or nephrogenic diabetes insipidus.

Urine osmolality studies are the best method to determine maximal concentration and dilution of urine. Concentration studies can be performed (as above) by restriction of water intake, administration of hypertonic saline, or injection of vasopressin. When both kidneys are functioning maximally and there has been a normal intake of salt and protein, the urine osmolality should exceed 800 mosm/kg H_2O after 16 hours of fluid restriction (Isaacson, 1960). If there is still doubt concerning concentration, vasopressin may be given.

Maximal urinary dilution can be evaluated by observing the change in urine osmolality after water loading. The accepted response after drinking 500 ml of water in an already normally hydrated subject is a reduction in the urine osmolality to 40 to 80 mosm/kg H_2O (Schreiner, 1971). This test is not considered a useful procedure to elucidate the etiology of hyponatremia (van Ypersele, 1979).

A slightly different approach to evaluate concentration and diluting capacities of the kidneys is to calculate osmolar and free water clearances. The U/P osmol ratio can be converted to a clearance value when it is multiplied by the urinary volume (V).

$$C_{osmol} = \frac{U_{osmol} \times V}{P_{osmol}}$$

The osmol clearance is a measure of the amount of water that is cleared from the plasma resulting in urine that has the same osmolality as plasma. The difference between the total urine volume and osmol clearance is called the free water clearance (C_{H_2O}).

$$C_{H_2O} = V - C_{osmol}$$

If the value is positive, this indicates that the urine is dilute compared with serum; conversely, if the value is negative, this indicates that the urine is more concentrated than serum.

Renal handling of H_2O and electrolytes can be studied in greater depth if certain assumptions are accepted. Using osmolality and electrolyte measurements in urine and plasma (i.e., clearances) the following estimations can be made:

a. Delivery of Na and K from the proximal segments to the distal tubular segments

$$= C_{H_2O} + C(Na + K)$$

b. Per cent of Na + K reabsorbed by the diluting segment of the nephron

$$= \frac{C_{H_2O}}{C_{H_2O} + C(Na + K)}$$

c. Per cent of chloride reabsorbed at the diluting sites

$$= \frac{C_{H_2O}}{C_{H_2O} + C_{Cl}}$$

The last two equations give equivalent results and have been used to detect a defect in the chloride pump in Bartter's syndrome (Gill, 1978).

Serum and urinary osmolality studies are also extremely valuable in evaluating the cause(s) of both hyper- and hyponatremia (see Sodium, p. 125).

WATER BALANCE

Water balance is controlled by mechanisms responsive to the tonicity and volume of the ECF. They are (1) the effect of ADH on the collecting tubules, (2) the renin-angiotensin-aldosterone system, and (3) the thirst center. Disorders of these mechanisms and hence water balance are seen frequently in clinical medicine.

If water losses exceed replacement, dehydration or hypovolemia develops. Sodium (Na^+) is usually lost with water, but the relative amount may vary depending on the Na^+ content of the fluid lost. The more common causes of volume depletion are vomiting, diarrhea, surgical drainage, internal pooling (third spacing) of the fluids (e.g., peritonitis, ileus), renal disease, diuretic administration, fever, excessive sweating, and hypoadrenocorticism (i.e., Addison's disease).

There are no laboratory measurements that can quantitate the amount of fluid loss. Laboratory measurements (concentration measurements) are relative measurements (i.e., comparison of amounts of substances in specific volumes of fluid). The hematocrit and serum protein concentrations fluctuate, and these changes may be helpful in estimating a change in plasma volume. The BUN is usually increased to a greater extent than serum creatinine (pre-renal failure). The U/P osmol ratio is greater than 1, and the urine Na^+ concentrations less than 20 mEq/L (mmol/L) except in Addison's disease and renal diseases where there is Na^+ loss. The diagnosis of dehydration and hypovolemia is made clinically (tissue turgor, cardiac and renal dynamics), and treatment consists of administering appropriate fluids to correct both fluid and electrolyte losses.

The opposite situation, an increase in total body H_2O or volume overload is usually associated with an increase in total body Na^+. This occurs frequently in cardiac failure and in conditions associated with hypoalbuminemia such as cirrhosis or the nephrotic syndrome. The common denominator in the latter conditions is "forward failure," i.e., a decrease in renal blood flow. In turn, this causes increased aldosterone and ADH production with Na^+ and H_2O retention. More H_2O than Na^+ is retained. As a result of the impaired hemodynamics, fluid may accumulate in the interstitial spaces, resulting in edema, ascites, and pleural effusions.

For the reason discussed above, there is no practical laboratory measurement to quantitate the amount of overhydration. Assessment is made clinically, and treatment is directed at correcting the underlying pathology and in some cases by the use of diuretics.

ELECTROLYTES AND ELECTROLYTIC BALANCE

Electrolytes are ions that exist in body fluids. In the ECF, the major cation is Na^+ and the major anions are Cl^- and HCO_3^-. Metabolic events are affected, to some degree, by the relative and absolute concentrations of these electrolytes, which are important determinants of osmolality, state of hydration, and pH of both the intracellular fluid (ICF) and the extracellular fluid (ECF). In addition, membrane potentials and normal functioning of nervous tissue and muscle (including cardiac) are regulated by the concentration differences between the ICF and ECF electrolytes. Electrolyte concentrations, formerly expressed as milliequivalents/liter (mEq/L) are now expressed in SI units (Système International d'Unités). In the SI units of measurement, the units are millimoles/liter or mmol/L (Lehmann, 1976). Since 1 mEq is equal to 1 mmol for monovalent ions, the numerical values for the four major electrolytes are the same using either system of units.

Sodium

Na^+ is the major cation of the ECF. Serum Na^+ concentration varies between 135 and 145 mmol/L in healthy individuals. The normal daily intake of Na^+ is 100 to 250 mmol. Ordinarily, the amount of Na^+ loss is balanced by the daily intake. The usual Na^+ level in urine varies from 30 to 280 mmol/day.

Hyponatremia, or low serum Na^+, can be found in a variety of conditions. It can occur with Na^+ (solute) loss or H_2O (solvent) excess. In these situations the serum osmolality is decreased. Excess Na^+ loss relative to water loss can occur via renal or extrarenal routes. Renal etiologies behind hyponatremia include (1) diuretic therapy, (2) salt-wasting nephropathies, (3) adrenal insufficiency, (4) bicarbonaturia, and (5) ketonuria. The urinary Na^+ concentration is usually greater than 20 mmol/L despite hyponatremia. Extrarenal etiologies include (1) vomiting, (2) diarrhea, (3) "third-space" losses, and (4) burns. The urinary Na^+ concentration is less than 10 mmol/L. Therapy to correct this electrolyte imbalance includes Na^+ and fluid replacement.

Excess total body water (edema) is present in (1) the nephrotic syndrome, (2) cirrhosis, (3) cardiac failure, and (4) acute and chronic renal failure. Total body Na^+ is also increased, but the excess of retained water is greater. The urinary Na^+ concentration is less than 10 mmol/L except in renal failure, in which the value may exceed 20 mmol/L. Hyponatremia *without* a visible increase in ECF volume (euvolemia) can be seen in (1) hypothyroidism, (2) glucocorticoid deficiency, (3) chronic disease, and (4) persistent or inappropriate secretion of vasopressin. Patients with hypothyroidism are not able to maximally dilute their urine (Deruberitis, 1971). They may also secrete increased levels of vasopressin (Showsky, 1978). Free water excretion is inhibited in patients with glucocorticoid deficiency (i.e., Addison's disease). The explanation for this is not understood. Hyponatremia is common in patients with chronic diseases and is felt to be a result of the secretion of ADH which is stimulated despite lower than normal plasma osmolalities. Inappropriate secretion of vasopressin has been demonstrated in patients under severe emotional or physical stress or in pain, and in some receiving various medications—central nervous system–acting agents, antineoplastic drugs, and diuretics (Ruddy, 1981). The syndrome of inappropriate ADH secretion (SIADH) refers to the continued secretion of ADH even though the plasma osmolality is subnormal and the plasma volume is normal or increased (Cooke, 1979). This syndrome is associated with a wide variety of neoplasms, inflammatory pulmonary disorders, and inflammatory, traumatic, and metabolic central nervous system disorders. Therapy for situations in which hyponatremia with excess total body water or euvolemia exists includes water restriction. In situations in which acute water intoxication is a possibility, loop diuretics with sodium replacement may be necessary. Lithium and demeclocycline base also have been used by some physicians.

Artifactual hyponatremia is encountered in the laboratory in two situations. Hyperglycemia increases serum osmolality, with a subsequent shift of ICF to the ECF, decreasing ECF electrolyte concentration. Roughly, for each 100 mg/dl increase in blood glucose, there is a 1.6 mmol/L decrease in the serum sodium concentration (Schrier, 1981). Hyponatremia (pseudohyponatremia) may also be present if the serum specimens are lactescent or contain abnormally large amounts of protein (e.g., Waldenström's macroglobulinemia). Na^+ concentrations are restricted to the water space which is proportionately decreased by the lipid or protein volume. Na^+ concentration in the serum/plasma volume is correspondingly less. Importantly, the serum osmolality is normal in pseudohyponatremia. Actual or true Na^+ values can be found by redrawing the serum after fasting, by using nonpolar solvents to extract the lipids, or by using an ultracentrifuge to separate the aqueous from the lipid or protein phases (Steffes, 1976).

Hypernatremia, or increased serum Na^+, is seen when there is an excessive loss of H_2O, relative to Na^+, from the body and when the total amount of Na^+ *per se* in the body is increased. Hypotonic fluid loss may occur via renal or extrarenal routes. Renal losses occur because of osmotic diuresis; the urine osmolality is low or normal and its Na^+ concentration is greater than 20 mmol/L. Extrarenal etiologies are (1) profuse sweating and (2) diarrhea in children without adequate fluid replacement. In these situations, the urine has an increased osmolality and an Na^+ concentration less than 10 mmol/L.

Hypernatremia can also result from loss of H_2O alone. Again, losses may occur by renal or extrarenal routes. Renal losses occur because of (1) central diabetes insipidus or (2) nephrogenic diabetes insipidus. In the latter condition, the kidneys are not able to respond to circulating vasopressin. Etiologies are diverse and include parenchymal diseases affecting the renal medullae, electrolyte disturbances such as hypercalcemia and hypokalemia, and drug therapy, e.g., lithium (Ruddy, 1981). Hereditary nephrogenic diabetes insipidus, a sex-linked disease with variable penetrance, is much rarer (Ruddy, 1981). The osmolality of the urine is either normal or decreased (see Osmolality, above). Pure extrarenal water losses are primarily insensible losses from the lungs and skin (e.g., fever). The osmolality of the urine in these conditions is increased.

Slight hypernatremia may also be observed in (1) Cushing's syndrome or (2) hyperaldosteronism. This is a result of the increased renal Na^+ reabsorption in these conditions. Excessive Na^+ intake may also result in hypernatremia. This is occasionally encountered in clinical medicine (e.g., $NaHCO_3$ administration during a cardiac arrest). The urine osmolality in these situations is normal or increased.

Therapy for hypernatremia consists of appropriate fluid replacement combined with the use of diuretics to rid the body of excess Na^+.

Potassium

K^+ is the major intracellular cation; only 2 per cent of the total body K^+ is extracellular. The diet normally contains 50 to 150 mmol K^+/day. The kidneys usually excrete 80 to 90 per cent of the ingested K^+. The expected range of serum K^+ concentration is 3.8 to 5.5 mmol/L. Unlike Na^+, however, there is no renal threshold for K^+, and some continues to be excreted into the urine even in K^+ depleted states (10 to 20 mmol/day). In normal subjects, daily urinary excretion is 25 to 120 mmol.

Hypokalemia, or decreased serum K^+, can occur even when the total amount of K^+ in the body is normal. Intracellular movement from the ECF into the ICF occurs during alkalemia, insulin therapy, and periodic paralysis. Hypokalemic periodic paralysis is a familial disease with autosomal dominant inheritance characterized by intermittent attacks of weakness or paralysis of limb and trunk muscles when the serum K^+ is markedly decreased.

Depletion of total body K^+ stores and hypokalemia occur as a result of (1) gastrointestinal fluid losses (e.g., vomiting, diarrhea) or (2) renal losses. Diuretics are the most common cause of renal losses. Other important etiologies are losses secondary to metabolic alkalosis, renal tubular acidosis (RTA) (see below), and mineralocorticoid excess.

Hyperkalemia, or increased serum K^+ concentration, can result from transfer of K^+ from the ICF to the ECF and from an actual increase in total body K^+. Cellular efflux occurs in acidemia and from cellular damage (e.g., fever, hemolysis, rhabdomyolysis). Increased total body potassium and hyperkalemia occur typically in acute and chronic renal failure and in mineralocorticoid deficiency (e.g., Addison's disease).

Artifactual hyperkalemia may be encountered when the platelet count is elevated (Weissman, 1974). As clotting occurs in the test tube, intraplatelet K^+ is released and measured in the serum. In these cases heparinized plasma can be used for K^+ determination. False high K^+ values are also seen if a prolonged tourniquet application causes juxtavenular cellular injury with leakage of K^+ into the plasma (Skinner, 1961). The effect is markedly enhanced if the fist is repeatedly clenched prior to and during drawing. A hemolyzed specimen will yield an elevated K^+ value owing to the high concentration of K^+ within erythrocytes (105 mmol/L).

Elevated and depressed serum K^+ concentrations may have profound adverse effects on the neuromuscular system (apathy, weakness, paralysis) and on the myocardium. Serious arrhythmias may eventuate in death. Hypokalemia is treated by parenteral and/or nonparenteral administration of K^+. Acute hyperkalemia is treated by Ca^{++} infusion, which antagonizes the effect of K^+ on cardiac tissue; by $NaHCO_3$ infusion, which causes the movement of K^+ into cells; by glucose infusion, which stimulates insulin production with resultant intracellular sequestration of glucose and K^+; by oral or rectal administration of the cation exchange resin Kayexalate, which binds K^+ (removing it from the ECF); and by dialysis. Chronic hyperkalemia is treated by use of oral Kayexalate, diuretics, and reduction of dietary K^+.

Measurement of Na^+ and K^+

The most frequent means for measuring Na^+ and K^+ in the clinical laboratory are emission photometry and potentiometric (i.e., ion-specific) electrodes (Chap. 2). The alkali metals lithium and cesium are used as internal standards in flame photometry. Cesium is used in instruments that quantitate lithium.

Ion-specific electrodes have been incorporated into many automated systems. The most practical Na^+ electrode is made of specialized glass, selective for Na^+. A liquid ion-exchange membrane electrode, incorporating the antibiotic valinomycin as the K^+ binder, is the most selective for K^+.

It has been demonstrated in intra- (Ladenson, 1979) and interlaboratory surveys (MacDonald, 1981) that the direct measuring (i.e., undiluted specimens) potentiometric instruments give values approximately 1 to 3 per cent higher than those from flame emission instruments. This difference is not great enough to interfere with clinical correlations. The difference may result from the physiochemical properties of the two analytic techniques because ion-specific electrodes may not be affected, to the same extent, by slight variations in plasma water from increases in protein or lipid content (Ladenson, 1979).

Chloride

Cl^- is the major extracellular anion. Most ingested Cl^- is absorbed, and the excess is excreted in the urine. The normal serum concentration is 98 to 106 mmol/L. Slightly lower values are observed in postprandial serum specimens. This occurs from increased synthesis of hydrochloric acid (HCl) by the parietal cells of the stomach. The usual daily urinary output of Cl^- is 110 to 250 mmol.

Hypochloremia, or low serum Cl^-, is seen when there is excessive loss of Cl^- from the body: (1) gastrointestinal (HCl) losses, (2) diabetic ketoacidosis, (3) mineralocorticoid excess, and (4) salt-losing renal diseases. Low serum values may also be encountered in diseases in which there is a high serum HCO_3^- concentration (i.e., compensated respiratory acidosis, metabolic alkalosis). This is a result of the intracellular shift and increased renal excretion of Cl^- in these conditions. Finally, hypochloremia is seen with low serum Na^+ concentrations in chronic diseases (see Sodium, above).

Hyperchloremia may occur during metabolic acidosis resulting from excess loss of HCO_3: (1) gastrointestinal losses, (2) renal tubular acidosis (see below), and (3) mineralocorticoid deficiency. Infrequently, excess administration of NH_4Cl or acidic salts of amino acids (e.g., hyperalimentation) can cause hyperchloremia. Elevated serum Cl^- values have been reported in some cases of hyperparathyroidism (Wells,

1971). This may be a result of PTH decreasing proximal renal tubular reabsorption of HCO_3^- (Karlinsky, 1974).

Measurement of Cl^- concentration in sweat is useful in diagnosing the exocrine glandular disorder cystic fibrosis (Littlewood, 1980). The secretion of sweat Cl^- is increased above the normal range, which is approximately 5 to 45 mmol/L in children (Shwachman, 1981) and slightly higher in adults. Affected infants characteristically have concentrations greater than 60 mmol/L, and affected adults have levels greater than 70 mmol/L. When the disease is mild, it may not be diagnosed until adult life (Boye, 1980). The patient is induced to sweat by iontophoresis or the introduction of pilocarpine into the skin (method of Gibson and Cooke). Sweat Cl^- activity is measured directly using ion-specific electrodes, or the Cl^- concentration is measured after the sweat is weighed. It is recommended that the sweat Na^+ also be quantitated. This serves as an internal quality control check since the Na^+ and Cl^- concentrations should be close to each other (i.e., within 10 mmol/L). Repeat studies and clinical correlations are recommended to rule out false positives.

Measurement of Cl^-

Cl^- is measured in the laboratory by mercurimetric titration, by coulometric titration, by colorimetry using Hg $(SCN)_2$, and by the use of ion-specific electrodes.

In the mercurimetric method, Cl^- combines with added Hg^{++} to form the soluble complex $HgCl_2$. Excess added Hg^{++} combines with the indicator diphenylcarbazone to form a blue color, the endpoint of the titration.

Coulometric titration is described in Chapter 2. This is very accurate; small volumes are required; and it is suitable for pediatric work, including sweat chloride determination.

In the automated thiocyanate method, Hg $(SCN)_2$ is added to the sample and dissociates owing to the complexing of Hg^{++} with Cl^-. The free thiocyanate ion (SCN^-) reacts with added Fe^{+++} to form the colored complex Fe $(SCN)_3$, which is measured photometrically.

Cl^- electrodes are solid-state electrodes using membranes composed of AgCl.

All chloride methods measure bromide to some extent (Driscoll, 1966; Elin, 1981). The electrode methods are influenced to the greatest extent and the mercurimetric and coulometric methods the least. Patients with bromide toxicity will likely have increased "chloride" levels as determined by colorimetric and ion-specific electrode methods. The levels will be less elevated if determined by mercurimetric and coulometric methods.

Surveys have demonstrated that all methods provide comparable clinical data (Geisinger, 1980). However, ion-specific electrodes are the most precise and the manual mercurimetric methods the least precise.

Total CO_2

HCO_3^- is quantitatively the second most important anionic fraction in serum. Its production in the body results from the dissociation of H_2CO_3 produced from the formation of CO_2 during metabolism. HCO_3^- is reconverted to H_2CO_3 and hence to H_2O and CO_2 as the blood perfuses the lungs. HCO_3^- is filtered freely by the kidneys, but little or no HCO_3^- is present in the urine (pH <6.1) when the diet is acidic. Most HCO_3^- is reabsorbed by the proximal tubules (85 per cent) and a small amount (15 per cent) by the distal tubules. HCO_3^- in serum or plasma can be measured directly by titration with acid or indirectly by using the measured P_{CO_2} and pH (H^+) in an equation or a nomogram. However, HCO_3^- is most commonly measured with other combined forms of CO_2 (CO_2, H_2CO_3, carbamino groups) as total CO_2. This value approximates the actual HCO_3^- very closely, since 89 to 90 per cent of all the CO_2 in serum is in the form of HCO_3^-. The reference intervals for total CO_2 are 19 to 25 mmol/L for arterial blood and 23 to 30 mmol/L for venous blood.

Total CO_2 determinations are useful, along with pH and P_{CO_2} measurements, in evaluating acid-base disorders. Discussion of high and low values and their etiologies are included in this chapter under Acid-Base Balance.

Measurement of Total CO_2

Total CO_2 measurements are performed in the clinical laboratory volumetrically, manometrically, or colorimetrically, or by using a P_{CO_2} electrode to measure the rate of formation of released CO_2.

A syringe with a reaction chamber in which serum and acid are mixed and a calibrated barrel (Harleco) has been found to be convenient and also to have suitable clinical accuracy and precision (Lam, 1978). The heights to which the acid-liberated CO_2 pushes the barrel are compared between specimen and standard and the ratio is converted to mmol/L.

Automated methods have been developed (Instrumentation Laboratories) that measure pressure (by means of a pressure-transducer) of the acid-released CO_2, vacuum-extracted into an enclosed space. Another automated method (Technicon) measures the liberated CO_2 after it permeates a silicon rubber membrane into a recipient stream containing the pH indicator phenolphthalein and Tris buffer. The intensity of the color produced from acidification of the buffer is proportional to the total amount of CO_2 present. A third automated method (Beckman Instruments) uses two P_{CO_2} electrodes to monitor the rate of formation of acid-released CO_2 gas. One electrode is the reference electrode. The resulting voltage change is converted to a digital readout in mmol/L. The principle of the CO_2 electrode is discussed in Chapter 2.

The specimen to be analyzed must be handled anaerobically to minimize atmosphere losses of CO_2 and HCO_3^- (converted to CO_2), which would cause a falsely low total CO_2 value. In the laboratory, this can be accomplished by covering the specimen container with plastic or Parafilm. Another method to prevent loss of CO_2 is to add one drop of 1 N NH_4OH to both standards and samples, decreasing the P_{CO_2} in the sample to that of the atmosphere, thereby preventing loss of CO_2 and a reduction of HCO_3^- (Gambino, 1966).

Anion Gap

The anion gap is a mathematical approximation of the difference between the anions and cations routinely measured in serum. Routine electrolyte measurements include Na^+, K^+, Cl^-, and HCO_3^- (as total CO_2). The unmeasured cations (i.e., Ca^{++}, Mg^{++}) average 7 mmol/L, and the unmeasured anions (i.e., $PO_4^=$, $SO_4^=$, protein$^-$, and organic acids) average 24 mmol/L. If the Cl^- and the total CO_2 concentrations are summed and subtracted from the total of the Na^+ and K^+ concentrations, the difference should be less than 17 mEq/L. If the anion gap exceeds 17 mmol/L, this usually indicates significantly increased concentrations of unmeasured anions. Etiologies for this are (1) uremia with retention of fixed acids, (2) ketotic states (e.g., diabetes, alcoholism, starvation), (3) lactic acidosis (e.g., shock), (4) toxin ingestion (e.g., methanol, salicylate, ethylene glycol, paraldehyde), and (5) increased plasma proteins (e.g., dehydration). An increased anion gap occurs occasionally in metabolic alkalosis (Madias, 1979). This is felt to be due to the titration of plasma proteins, resulting in loss of H^+ and the consequent increase in the proteins' net negative charge. In addition, plasma protein concentrations may increase from the ECF deficit that occurs in metabolic alkalosis.

Decreased anion gaps (<10 mmol/L) can result from either an increase in unmeasured cations or a decrease in unmeasured anions. An increase in unmeasured cations can be seen in (1) Li^+ intoxication, (2) hypermagnesemia, (3) multiple myeloma, (4) polyclonal gammopathy, and (5) polymyxin B therapy, since this drug is polycationic (O'Connor, 1978). The reason for the decreased gap due to the presence of increased gamma globulins is the fact that these proteins may have a net positive charge at physiologic pH (Murray, 1975; Keshgegian, 1978). Decreased unmeasured anions occur in (1) hypoalbuminemia and (2) hyponatremia with normal or increased ECF (e.g., SIADH) (Oh, 1978). This is postulated to result from the selective renal excretion of unmeasured anions in this condition. Finally, a spurious increase in measured Cl^- caused by bromide intoxication can cause a spurious decrease in the calculated gap (see Chloride).

The anion gap is useful also for quality control of laboratory results for Na^+, K^+, Cl^-, and total CO_2. If an increased or decreased anion gap is calculated for a set of electrolytes from a healthy individual, this would indicate that one or more of the laboratory results are erroneous. Another possible explanation is that a mixed acid-base disturbance is present.

ACID-BASE BALANCE

A large quantity of acid is ingested daily in the normal diet and produced endogenously as a result of metabolism. Thirteen thousand to 20,000 mmol of CO_2 largely converted to carbonic acid (H_2CO_3) is formed resulting from oxidation of carbohydrates, proteins, and fats (Valtin, 1973). Another 40 to 60 mmol of acid, ketoacids from incomplete oxidation of lipids, and sulfuric and phosphoric acid from oxidation of sulfur-containing amino acids and phosphorus-containing compounds are produced also (Valtin, 1973).

H_2CO_3 is called a volatile acid because it can be converted to CO_2, which can be excreted by the lungs. However, the other acids produced by the body cannot be converted to a gaseous state and are called nonvolatile or fixed acids. The latter must be excreted in the urine.

Many metabolic reactions are catalyzed by enzymes which function at optimal hydrogen ion concentrations. Accordingly, it is necessary that the body possess efficient mechanisms to maintain the pH of both the ECF and ICF within narrow limits (7.35 to 7.45). This is accomplished by the blood buffering, by respiration (Chap. 7), and by renal mechanisms.

A buffer is a weak acid in solution with its conjugate base, which is in the form of a salt. When acid is added to a solution, it combines with the conjugate base to form more weak acid. The result is a small decrease in pH instead of a large one. The ECF buffers, which account for a little less than half of the systemic buffering capacity, are, in descending order of buffering capacity: (1) bicarbonate/carbonic acid, (2) hemoglobin, (3) plasma proteins, and (4) erythrocyte and plasma phosphate. The bicarbonate/carbonic acid equilibrium ($H_2O + CO_2 \leftrightarrows H_2CO_3 \leftrightarrows H^+ + HCO_3^-$) can be conveniently expressed as the derived Henderson-Hasselbalch equation:

$$pH = pK_a + \log \frac{(HCO_3^-)}{(H_2CO_3)}$$

pK_a is the negative logarithm of the dissociation constant, K_a, of H_2CO_3. The pK′ of normal plasma at 37°C. is 6.1.* The pK′ varies inversely with both pH and ionic strength and directly with temperature. This equation can also be expressed as

$$pH = pK'_a + \log \frac{(\text{total } CO_2) - 0.03\ P_{CO_2}}{0.03\ P_{CO_2}}$$

In normal plasma, 0.03 is the solubility coefficient (α) of CO_2 gas at 37°C. This value (0.03) times the P_{CO_2} is equivalent to the small amount of H_2CO_3 found dissolved in plasma. The solubility coefficient varies inversely with temperature and/or concentration

*pK′ refers to the pK_a for given conditions (i.e., pH, ionic strength, temperature, etc.).

of salt or protein and varies directly with lipid concentration. The product, $0.03 \times P_{CO_2}$, subtracted from the total CO_2 value is a close approximation of the HCO_3^-. Although the pK'_a of this buffer system is low (6.1) compared with the pH of plasma (7.4), it is an extremely effective buffer because the ratio of base to acid is finely regulated by respiration.

It is easier to think of acid-base balances in terms of H^+ concentrations (normally 40 nmol/L). Since a pH is actually measured in and reported from the laboratory, a conversion from pH to $[H^+]$ is made (see Chap. 7). There exists a close inverse relationship of pH to $[H^+]$ between pH 7.25 and 7.50. An increase of 0.01 pH unit represents a decrease in $[H^+]$ of approximately 1 nmol/L, and a decrease of 0.01 pH unit represents an increase in $[H^+]$ of 1 nmol/L; i.e., at pH 7.30 $[H^+] = 50$ mmol/L, and at pH 7.50 $[H^+] = 30$ nmol/L. After conversion, the physician commonly uses the Henderson equation to evaluate acid-base perturbations:

$$[H^+] \text{ nmol/L} = 24 \frac{P_{CO_2} \text{ (mm Hg)}}{[HCO_3^-] \text{ mmol/L}}$$

Hemoglobin is the second most important blood buffer owing to the fact that each hemoglobin molecule contains 38 histidine residues that are able to bind with H^+ and owing to the high concentration of hemoglobin (15 g/dl).

Plasma proteins act as buffers because both their free carboxyl and amino groups are able to bind H^+.

Least important is the buffering capacity of the inorganic and organic phosphates present in blood. At a pH of 7.4, the $HPO_4^{=}/H_2PO_4^-$ ratio is 4/1.

The sum of all blood buffers is called the buffer base. The reference values are between 46 and 52 mmol/L, with an average value of 49 mmol/L. If this average value is subtracted from the actual buffer base, base excess is derived. The reference interval for base excess is $\pm$ 3.0 mmol/L. A negative base excess, or decrease in blood buffering capacity, is sometimes referred to as base deficit.

Although the blood buffers act instantaneously to minimize the change in pH, their capacity to do so is limited. Respiratory compensation is prompt, but ultimate regulation of acid-base balance, with regeneration of free buffers, is a function of the renal tubular cells. Renal compensation is gradual and occurs over a three- to four-day period after the acid-base imbalance occurs. HCO_3^- is freely filtered by the glomeruli and at normal plasma levels is completely reabsorbed by the renal tubules with approximately 85 per cent being absorbed by the proximal tubules. There is a renal threshold for HCO_3^-, and this electrolyte will normally be present in the urine if the total plasma CO_2 ($[HCO_3^-]$) is greater than 30 mmol/L (Stenzel, 1981).

During the process of HCO_3^- reabsorption, H^+ is excreted by the proximal tubules into the urine. H^+ is also excreted by the distal tubules. Filtered dibasic phosphate ($HPO_4^{=}$) combines with H^+ to form monobasic phosphate. This is referred to as titratable acidity. H^+ also combines with NH_3 to form NH_4^+. NH_3 is produced in the proximal tubular cells from the deamidation and deamination of glutamine and other amino acids by glutaminase and glutamate dehydrogenase. The total amount of H^+ excreted by these mechanisms is 1 to 2 mmol/kg body weight (Stenzel, 1981). The mechanisms of respiration that control the P_{CO_2} (therefore, the H_2CO_3 concentration) are discussed in Chapter 7.

Laboratory Measurement of Acid-Base Parameters

In order to evaluate the acid-base status of the patient and to identify causes (i.e., metabolic, respiratory, or both) responsible for imbalances, it is necessary to determine, besides pH ($[H^+]$), one or both of the following parameters: (1) total CO_2 and (2) P_{CO_2}. The collection and processing of blood specimens used for these determinations and the methods of their laboratory measurements are discussed in Chapter 7. In addition, the anion gap determination can be useful if metabolic acidosis is present (see Anion Gap, above). Finally, renal function studies that measure the ability of the kidneys either to excrete an acid load or to reabsorb an alkali load are useful for confirming renal tubular diseases resulting in hyperchloremic acidosis. These are discussed under Renal Tubular Acidosis.

2

Acid-Base Imbalances

Acidemia. Acidemia is defined as a blood pH of less than 7.35, $[H^+] > 45$ mmol/L. It can result from the accumulation of CO_2 in the body. This is called respiratory acidosis since it is a result of hypoventilation or ventilation/perfusion inequalities (Chap. 7). The kidneys, by reabsorbing HCO_3^-, are able to compensate somewhat, the degree of compensation depending on the chronicity of the ventilatory insufficiency and the functional capacity of the renal tubules. This is reflected by an increase in total CO_2 and in HCO_3^-.

Acidemia can also occur from an accumulation of fixed acids or a decrease in HCO_3^-. This results in a primary decrease in total CO_2 and is referred to as metabolic acidosis. Clinically, metabolic acidosis can be divided into two types: acidemia with an increased anion gap (>17 mmol/L) and acidemia with a normal anion gap (≤17 mmol/L) or hyperchloremic metabolic acidosis. Causes of metabolic acidosis with an increased anion gap have been listed previously. Likewise, etiologies resulting in hyperchloremic acidosis also have been reviewed previously. Renal tubular acidosis is discussed in greater detail later (see Renal Tubular Acidosis). As a result of metabolic acidosis, the rate and depth of respiration compensate by increasing, with the degree of compensation dependent on the adequacy of respiratory function. Treatment of acidemia is directed at correction of the underlying disease process(es), with the administration of HCO_3^- to acutely ill and symptomatic patients and simultaneous correction of existing electrolyte and fluid imbalances.

Alkalemia. Alkalemia is defined as a blood pH greater than 7.45, $[H^+] < 35$ mmol/L. Alkalemia can occur from decreased $P\text{CO}_2$ concentrations in the blood. This is called respiratory alkalosis because it is secondary to hyperventilation. Etiologies are discussed in Chapter 7. As a result of respiratory alkalosis, the kidneys compensate to varying degrees depending on the chronicity of the alkalemia by decreasing the reabsorption of HCO_3^-. Correspondingly, the total circulating $[HCO_3^-]$ is decreased from baseline by this renal compensatory response. Alkalemia also occurs when there is loss of fixed acids or an increase in blood alkali (e.g., HCO_3^-). There is a primary increase in HCO_3^-, referred to as metabolic alkalosis. Loss of HCO_3^- is most often due to prolonged vomiting or to nasogastric suctioning. Alkali excess can occur in excessive ingestion of basic substances, such as antacids. Metabolic alkalosis can also occur in disease states in which there is excessive intracellular accumulation of $H^+$and/or excess excretion of H^+ into the urine. This occurs with mineralocorticoid excess syndromes (e.g., hyperaldosteronism, Cushing's syndrome, prolonged administration of corticosteroids) and in hypokalemia. Respiratory rate decreases in metabolic alkalosis with a compensatory increase in $P\text{CO}_2$. Treatment, as in all acid-base imbalances, is directed toward the correction of the underlying disease process(es) with the replacement of K^+ defects with KCl and the correction of fluid imbalances.

Renal Tubular Acidosis

Renal tubular acidosis (RTA) is defined as defective secretion of H^+ by the renal tubules in the presence of a normal GFR (Quintanilla, 1980). Either the collecting ducts or the proximal tubules can be responsible. If the collecting ducts are to blame, this is referred to as distal or type 1 RTA. If the proximal tubules are malfunctional, this is referred to as proximal or type 2 RTA. Both types of tubular defects can be a result of primary (both sporadic and familial) tubular defects or secondary resulting from a variety of unrelated diseases.

In type 1 RTA, there is impaired excretion of H^+ resulting in a urinary pH that is inappropriately high (>pH 5.4) even though acidemia is present. The distal tubular defect may result from a gradient or secretory defect (Arruda, 1977). The acidemia that develops in this condition results in extensive buffering by $CaCO_3$ in bone with resultant osteomalacia and hypercalcemia and nephrocalcinosis. Hypokalemia also develops due to increased renal excretion of K^+, enhanced by increased aldosterone secretion resulting from decreased ECF secondary to urinary Na^+ loss. An incomplete form of type 1 RTA has also been identified in which patients have osteomalacia, hypercalciuria, and renal stones, but acidemia is not present. Acidemia, however, will develop when these individuals are challenged with an acid load. Apparently, the tubular defect is mild, and the retained H^+ is completely buffered. Secondary causes of type 1 RTA are many and include (1) cirrhosis, (2) renal diseases resulting from nephrocalcinosis and nephrotoxic drugs (e.g., amphotericin B, Li^+), (3) kidney transplant rejection, and (4) diseases characterized by hypergammaglobinemia (Quintanilla, 1980). In cirrhosis, there is decreased urinary filtration of Na^+ which results in reduced H^+ secretion.

In type 2 RTA, there is reduced reabsorption of HCO_3^- resulting in a significant bicarbonaturia. The tubules are able, however, to reabsorb all of the filtered HCO_3^- if the plasma HCO_3^- falls below 14 mmol/L. Type 2 RTA may be associated with a more generalized dysfunction of the proximal tubules called Fanconi's syndrome. Glycosuria, phosphaturia, aminoaciduria, and uricosuria may, therefore, be associated with loss of HCO_3^-. Mild hypokalemia may be seen in type 2 RTA. This is a result of the increased exchange of K^+ for the increased Na^+ delivered with the nonabsorbed HCO_3^- to the distal tubules and collecting ducts. Nephrocalcinosis is rare, probably due to hypercitruria. Secondary causes of type 2 RTA include (1) diseases characterized by hypergammaglobulinemia, (2) renal diseases (e.g., medullary cystic disease, transplant rejection), (3) proximal tubular defects associated with diseases of inborn errors of metabolism (e.g., cystinosis, Wilson's disease), and (4) drugs and toxins (e.g., outdated tetracycline, heavy metal intoxication) (Quintanilla, 1980).

Combined type 1 and type 2 defects are referred to as type 3 RTA. Another category of RTA is referred to as type 4 RTA (Sebastian, 1977). This condition is characterized by mild to moderate renal insufficiency, hyperchloremic acidosis, and *hyperkalemia*. Many of these patients have reduced mineralocorticoid secretion or decreased renal tubular responsiveness to mineralocorticoids. This condition is probably due to the decreased renal ammoniagenesis produced by the hyperkalemia (Szylman, 1976; Sleeper, 1982).

Treatment of RTA is individualized and involves administration of alkalinizing salts and K^+ (type 1 and 2). Secondary etiologies, if identified, are treated if possible.

Laboratory Diagnosis of RTA

The initial laboratory evaluation in diagnosing RTA includes simultaneous measurement of the serum HCO_3^- ($P\text{CO}_2$ and $[H^+]$) and urinary pH. A urine pH of 5.6 or higher when the blood pH is low and the serum HCO_3^- is less than 22 mmol/L establishes the diagnosis of distal RTA. Heavy urinary HCO_3^- loss associated with hyperchloremic acidosis suggests proximal RTA. It is important to make sure that urea-splitting organisms (e.g., Proteus) are not present resulting in an alkaline pH (normal pH should not exceed 7.8). A urinary tract infection has to be treated before an accurate assessment of urinary pH can be made.

Types 1 and 2 RTA can be differentiated by administration of $NaHCO_3$. If large amounts (i.e., 5 mmol/kg/day) are needed to normalize the serum HCO_3^- concentration, this is typical of type 2 RTA. The hypokalemia occurring in type 2 RTA and not type 1 RTA is also aggravated by HCO_3^- administration.

Specialized studies may occasionally be helpful and confirmatory. An approximation of the tubular HCO_3^- reabsorption threshold can be accomplished by giving increasing doses of oral HCO_3^- and measuring the urinary pH at regular intervals (Greenhill, 1976). When the pH is found to be greater than 6 (no HCO_3^- in urine below pH 6.1), a sample of blood plasma is drawn and its HCO_3^- concentration is measured. This value approximates the HCO_3^- excretion threshold which normally is 25 to 28 mmol/L and is decreased in type 2 RTA.

Type 1 RTA can be confirmed by the NH_4Cl blood test. NH_4Cl is given orally until the serum HCO_3^- level decreases below 15 mmol/L. Urine is collected hourly for six hours, and the urinary pH is measured in each sample. In type 1 RTA, the urinary pH does not decrease below pH 5.4.

An additional confirmatory test for the presence of type 1 RTA is the measurement of the difference between urinary and blood P_{CO_2} (Halperin, 1974). This test is performed by giving orally 0.5 to 2.0 mmol NaHCO/kg and measuring P_{CO_2} in blood and urine samples collected one hour later. The P_{CO_2} in urine is a result of both the diffusion of CO_2 from the blood into the urine forming in the renal tubules and the formation of H_2CO_3 from the excreted H^+ and filtered HCO_3^-. CO_2 is poorly reabsorbed in the lower urinary tract. If the calculated difference which normally is greater than 30 mmol/L (urine > blood) is decreased, this indicates that type 1 RTA exists.

Arruda, J. A. L., and Kurtzman, N. A.: Metabolic acidosis and alkalosis. Clin. Nephrol., 7:201, 1977.

Barlow, L. K., et al.: Volatiles and osmometry (continued). Clin. Chem., *22*:1230, 1976.

Boye, N. P., et al.: Cystic fibrosis in adult patients. Eur. J. Respir. Dis., *6*:227, 1980.

Burry, H. C., and Dieppe, P. A.: Apparent reduction of endogenous creatinine clearance by salicylate treatment. Br. Med. J., *12*:16, 1976.

Camara, A. A., et al.: The twenty-four hourly endogenous creatinine clearance as a clinical measure of the functional state of the kidneys. J. Lab. Clin. Med., *37*:743, 1951.

Carrie B. J., et al.: Creatinine: An inadequate filtration marker in glomerular diseases. Am. J. Med., *69*:177, 1980.

Cooke, R. C., et al.: The syndrome of inappropriate antidiuretic hormone secretion (SIADH): Pathophysiologic mechanisms in solute and volume regulation. Medicine, *58*:240, 1979.

Davies, D. F., and Shock, N. W.: Age changes in GFR, effective RPF and tubular excretory capacity in adult males. J. Clin. Invest., *29*:496, 1950.

Deruberitis, F. R., et al.: Impaired water excretion in myxedema. Am. J. Med., *51*:41, 1971.

Driscoll, J. L., and Martin, H. F.: Detection of bromism by an automated chloride method. Clin. Chem., *12*:314, 1966.

Duarte, C. G.: Glomerular filtration rate and renal plasma flow. *In* Renal Function Tests: Clinical Laboratory Procedures and Diagnosis. Boston, Little, Brown and Co., 1980.

Elin, R. J., et al.: Bromide interferes with determination of chloride by each of four methods. Clin. Chem., *27*:778, 1981.

Espinel, C. H.: The FeNa test. J.A.M.A., *236*:579, 1976.

Gambino, S. R., and Schreiber, H.: The measurement of CO_2 content with the AutoAnalyzer. Am. J. Clin. Path., *45*:406, 1966.

Geisinger, K. R., et al.: Serum chloride: A CAP survey. Am. J. Clin. Path. (Suppl.), *74*:546, 1980.

Gill, J. R., Jr., and Bartter, F. C.: Evidence for a prostaglandin-independent defect in chloride reabsorption in the loop of Henle as a proximal cause of Bartter's syndrome. Am. J. Med., *65*:766, 1978.

Greenhill, A., and Grusk, A. B.: Laboratory evaluation of renal function. Pediatr. Clin. North Am., *23*:661, 1976.

Groth, T., and Tengstrom, B.: A simple method for the estimation of glomerular filtration rate. Scand. J. Clin. Lab. Invest., *37*:39, 1977.

Halperin, M. L., et al.: Studies on the pathogenesis of type 1 (distal) renal tubular acidosis as revealed by the urinary P_{CO_2} tensions. J. Clin. Invest., *53*:669, 1974.

Holmes, J. H.: Measurement of osmolality in serum, urine, and other biological fluids by the freezing point determination. *In* Workshop Manual on Urinanalysis and Renal Function Studies, ASCP—Commission on Continuing Education, 1962.

Isaacson, L. C.: Urinary osmolality in thirsting normal subjects. Lancet, *1*:467, 1960.

Jackson, S.: Creatinine in urine as an index of urinary excretion rate. Health Phys., *12*:843, 1966.

Juel, R.: Serum osmolality: A CAP survey analysis. Am. J. Clin. Path., *68*:165, 1977.

Karlinsky, M. L., et al.: Effect of parathyroid hormone and cyclic adenosine monophosphate on renal bicarbonate reabsorption. Am. J. Physiol., *227*:1226, 1974.

Keshgegian, A. A.: Decreased anion gap in diffuse polyclonal hypergammaglobulinemia. N. Engl. J. Med., *299*:99, 1978.

Ladenson, J. H.: Evaluation of an instrument (Nova-1) for direct potentiometric analysis of sodium and potassium in blood and their indirect potentiometric determination in urine. Clin. Chem., *25*:757, 1979.

Lam, C. W. K., and Tau, I. K.: Evaluation of the Harleco micro CO_2 system for measurement of total CO_2 in serum or plasma. Clin. Chem., *24*:143, 1978.

Larrson, R., et al.: The effects of cimetidine (Tagamet) on renal function in patients with renal failure. Acta Med. Scand., *208*:27, 1980.

Lee, J., Hollyer, R., Rodelas, R., and Preuss, H. G.: Influence of trimethoprim, sulfamethoxazole, and creatinine on renal organic anion and cation transport in rat kidney tissue. Toxicol. Appl. Pharmacol., *58*:184, 1981.

Lehmann, H. P.: Metrication of clinical laboratory data in SI units. Am. J. Clin. Path., *65*:2, 1976.

Levinsky, N. G., and Alexander, E. A.: Acute renal failure. *In* Brenner, B. M., and Rector, F. C. (eds.): The Kidney. Philadelphia, W. B. Saunders Company, 1976, p. 809.

Littlewood, J. M.: The diagnosis of cystic fibrosis. Practitioner, *224*:305, 1980.

Loeb, J. N.: The hyperosmolar state. N. Engl. J. Med., *290*:1184, 1974.

Loirat, P., et al.: Increased glomerular filtration rate in patients with major burns and its effect on the pharmacokinetics of tobramycin. N. Engl. J. Med., *299*:915, 1978.

Lubowitz, H., et al.: Glomerular filtration rate determination in patients with chronic renal disease. J.A.M.A., *199*:252, 1967.

MacDonald, N. F.: Sodium and potassium measurements: Direct potentiometry and flame photometry. Am. J. Clin. Path., *76*(CAP Suppl.):575, 1981.

Madias, N. E., et al.: Increased anion gap in metabolic alkalosis: The role of plasma-protein equivalency. N. Engl. J. Med., *300*:1421, 1979.

Matthews, B. F., et al.: Effects of pregnancy on inulin and para-aminohippurate clearances in the anesthetized rat. J. Physiol., *151*:385, 1960.

Mercier, D. C.: Comparison of dewpoint and freezing point osmometry. Am. J. Med. Tech., *44*:1066, 1978.

Morgensen, C. E.: Elevated glomerular filtration rate in insulin-treated short-term diabetes: Non-dependence on blood sugar value. Acta Med. Scand., *194*:559, 1973.

Murray, T., et al.: Multiple myeloma and the anion gap. N. Engl. J. Med., *292*:574, 1975.

O'Connor, D. T., and Stone, R. A.: Hyperchloremia and negative anion gap associated with polymyxin B administration. Arch. Intern. Med., *138*:478, 1978.

Oh, M. S., and Carroll, H. J.: Decreased anion gap and hyponatremia. N. Engl. J. Med., *298*:111, 1978.

Preuss, H. G., Massry, S. G., Maher, J. F., Gilliece, M. B., and Schremer, G. E.: Effects of uremic sera on renal tubular P-aminohippurate transport. Nephron, *3*:265, 1966.

Quintanilla, A. P.: Renal tubular acidosis: Mechanisms and management. Postgrad. Med., *67(4)*:60, 1980.

Renkin, E. M., and Robinson, R. R.: Glomerular filtration. N. Engl. J. Med., *290*:785, 1974.

Rocco, W. V.: Volatiles and osmometry. Clin. Chem., *22*:399, 1976.

Ruddy, M. C., and Stenzel, K. H.: Disorders of water, sodium and potassium metabolism. *In* Cheigh, J. S., et al. (eds.): Manual of Clinical Nephrology. Martinus Nijhoff, 1981.

Schreiner, G.: Renal biopsy. *In* Strauss, M. B., and Welt, L. G. (eds.): Diseases of the Kidney. Boston, Little, Brown and Co., 1971.

Schrier, R. W.: The patient with hyponatremia or hypernatremia. *In* Manual of Nephrology. Boston, Little, Brown and Co., 1981.

Sebastian, A., and Morris, R. C., Jr.: Renal tubular acidosis. Clin. Nephrol., 7:216, 1977.

Semple, P. F., et al.: Serial studies of the renal clearance of urate and insulin during pregnancy and after the puerperium in normal women. Clin. Sci. Mol. Med., *47*:559, 1974.

Seyer-Hansen, K.: Renal hypertrophy in streptozotocin diabetic rats. Clin. Sci. Mol. Med., *51*:551, 1976.

Shwachman, H., et al.: The sweat test: Sodium and chloride values. J. Pediatr., *98*:576, 1981.

Skowsky, R. W., and Kikuchi, T. A.: The role of vasopressin in the impaired water excretion of myxedema. Am. J. Med., *64*:613, 1978.

Sleeper, R. S., Belanger, P., Lemieux, G., and Preuss, H. G.: Effects of in vitro potassium on ammoniagenesis in rat and canine kidney tissue. Kidney Int., *21*:345, 1982.

Steffes, M. W., and Frier, E. F.: A simple and precise method of determining true sodium, potassium and chloride concentrations in hyperlipemia. J. Lab. Clin. Med., *88*:683, 1976.

Stenzel, K. H.: Acid-base disturbances. *In* Cheigh, J. S., et al.: Manual of Clinical Nephrology. Martinus Nijhoff, 1981.

Szylman, P., Better, O. S., Chaimowitz, C., and Rosler, A.: Role of hyperkalemia in the metabolic acidosis of isolated hypoaldosteronism. N. Engl. J. Med., *294*:361, 1976.

Taggart, J. V.: Mechanisms of renal tubular transport. Am. J. Med., *24*:774, 1958.

Tobias, G. J., et al.: Endogenous creatinine clearance. N. Engl. J. Med., *266*:317, 1962.

Valtin, H.: Renal Function: Mechanisms Preserving Fluid and Solute Balance in Health. Boston, Little, Brown and Co., 1973.

van Ypersele, C., et al.: General techniques in clinical nephrology. *In* Hamburger, J., et al. (eds.): Nephrology. New York, Wiley Flammanon, 1979.

Ward, P. C.: Renal dysfunction 1: Urea and creatinine. Postgrad. Med., *69(5)*:93, 1981.

Weisberg, H. F.: Osmolality-calculated, "delta," and more formulas. Clin. Chem., *21*:1182, 1975.

Weissman, N., and Pileggi, V. J.: Inorganic ions. *In* Henry, R. J., et al. (eds.): Clinical Chemistry, Principles and Technics. 2nd ed. Hagerstown, Md., Harper and Row, Publishers, Inc., 1974, p. 645.

Wells, M. R.: Value of plasma chloride concentration and acid-base status in the differential diagnosis of hyperparathyroidism from other causes of hypercalcemia. J. Clin. Path., *24*:219, 1971.

Wesson, L. G.: Renal hemodynamics in physiological states. *In* Physiology of the Human Kidney. New York, Grune and Stratton, 1969.

West, J. R., et al.: Glomerular filtration rate, effective renal blood flow, and maximal tubular excretory capacity in infancy. J. Pediatr., *32*:10, 1948.

9

METABOLIC INTERMEDIATES AND INORGANIC IONS

JANNIE WOO, PH.D.,
and DONALD C. CANNON, M.D., PH.D.

2

NON-PROTEIN NITROGENOUS COMPOUNDS

There are more than 15 different non-protein nitrogenous (NPN) compounds in plasma with a total nitrogen concentration of 250 to 400 mg/L. The NPN of whole blood is approximately 75 per cent greater than that of plasma, largely because of the high glutathione content of erythrocytes. Urea is the major NPN constituent in plasma and constitutes about 45 per cent of the total. Other major constituents in decreasing order of nitrogen contribution are amino acids, uric acid, creatinine, creatine, and ammonia. Until about 15 years ago, the NPN determination was widely used as an index of renal function. Increased concentrations of several of the major components, i.e., urea, uric acid, and creatinine, do occur as a consequence of diminished renal function. The NPN, however, is a relatively non-specific index of renal disease because other diseases can cause significant alterations in the plasma concentrations of the various constituents. For example, gout or excessive catabolism of purines will increase the uric acid concentration in plasma. Liver disease can cause diminished amino acid metabolism and a corresponding rise in plasma amino acid nitrogen. In contrast, urea synthesis is diminished in severe liver disease. Consequently, most clinical laboratories no longer perform NPN determinations on a routine basis but instead offer determinations of serum urea nitrogen and creatinine, which are more sensitive and specific indices of renal function, uric acid, creatine, ammonia, and alpha amino nitrogen, which reflects the concentration of amino acids.

Urea

Physiologic Chemistry. Urea is the major end product of protein and amino acid catabolism and is generated in the liver through the urea cycle. From the liver, urea enters the blood to be distributed to all intracellular and extracellular fluids, since urea is freely diffusible across most cell membranes. Most of the urea is ultimately excreted by the kidneys, but minimal amounts are also excreted in sweat and degraded by bacteria in the intestines.

Urea is freely filtered by the glomeruli. Depending upon the state of hydration and therefore the rate of urine flow, 40 to 80 per cent of the filtered urea is passively reabsorbed with water, mostly in the proximal tubules. There does not appear to be active tubular reabsorption or secretion of urea by mammalian kidneys. Urea ordinarily constitutes about half (25 g) of the total urinary solids and 80 to 90 per cent of the total urinary nitrogen. Although most cell membranes and capillary walls in the body are freely permeable to urea, the renal nephrons can concentrate urea with a gradient of up to 50-fold greater than plasma.

In the United States, the urea concentration of blood is often expressed in terms of the blood urea nitrogen content (BUN). In Europe, however, it is expressed as units of urea itself. The molecular weight of urea is 60, including two nitrogen atoms with a weight of 28. Consequently, urea nitrogen can be converted to urea by multiplying by 60/28 or 2.14. Thus a BUN of 20 mg/dl is equal to a urea of 20 × 2.14 or 42.80 mg/dl. The concentration of urea nitrogen in whole blood is somewhat less than that in plasma or serum, chiefly because of the lower water content of erythrocytes as compared with plasma. Plasma or serum is the specimen of choice for technical reasons. Nevertheless, the analytical measurement is still termed by convention the BUN. The normal BUN in adults is about 8 to 26 mg/dl (2.9 to 9.3 mmol/L) using either serum or plasma (Reed, 1972).

Clinicopathologic Correlations. The serum concentration of urea varies rather widely in health and is influenced by such diverse factors as dietary intake of protein and the state of hydration. Glucocorticoids have an anti-anabolic effect and the thyroid hormones have a catabolic effect on protein and thus tend to raise the BUN. Androgens and growth hormone have an anabolic effect and thus decrease the formation of urea.

Azotemia is a biochemical designation referring to any significant increase in the plasma concentration of non-protein nitrogenous compounds, principally urea and creatinine. Azotemia is frequently categorized as prerenal, renal, and postrenal. *Prerenal azotemia* is the result of inadequate perfusion of the kidneys and, therefore, diminished glomerular filtration in the presence of otherwise normal renal function. Important etiologies include dehydration, shock, diminished blood volume, and congestive heart failure. Although the increased serum urea or BUN accompanying many cases of massive gastrointestinal hemorrhage is sometimes explained on the basis of greatly increased absorption of amino acids following the digestion of blood proteins, it is probable that hypovolemia resulting from the hemorrhage is the single most important factor. An additional cause of increased serum urea (BUN) is increased protein catabolism, e.g., with fever, stress, and burns.

The pathogenesis of *renal azotemia* is primarily diminished glomerular filtration and, therefore, urea retention as a consequence of acute or chronic renal disease. Other complicating factors frequently present are dehydration or edema, which cause diminished renal perfusion, increased catabolism of proteins, and the general anti-anabolic effect of glucocorticoids. Uremia is a clinical syndrome that can occur with protracted severe azotemia and includes acidosis, water and electrolyte imbalance, nausea, vomiting, anemia, neuropsychiatric changes, and a variety of other clinical manifestations, including coma. The elevated BUN varies in magnitude but usually is in excess of 100 mg/dl, or approaching 200 mg/dl with deep coma or stupor. The progressively rising, but at times fluctuating, BUN is in contrast to the more slowly rising creatinine, which rarely exceeds 20 mg/dl and uric acid, which in the absence of gout does not usually rise above 12 mg/dl in chronic renal failure.

Post-renal azotemia is usually the result of urinary tract obstruction so that urea is reabsorbed into the circulation. An uncommon cause is perforation of the lower urinary tract with extravasation of urine into soft tissues.

From the foregoing discussion, it is evident that the BUN can at best be a rough guide to renal function. Even in the presence of normal dietary intake, hydration, renal perfusion, and integrity of the lower urinary tract, the BUN will ordinarily not be significantly increased until the glomerular filtration is decreased by at least 50 per cent (p. 120). This is a reflection of the fact that the glomerular filtration rate is related to the BUN in a hyperbolic instead of a linear fashion.

A significantly decreased BUN or serum urea occurs in only a few conditions. In addition to poor nutrition, high fluid intake or excessive administration of intravenous fluids in the presence of normal renal function will result in a decreased BUN because relatively little urea will be reabsorbed by the renal tubules. A tendency to a decreased BUN in pregnancy is probably the result of an augmented glomerular filtration rate. Severe liver disease can cause a decrease in urea synthesis because of diminished activity of the urea cycle.

There is some advantage in terms of clinical interpretation to determine both the serum urea and creatinine concentrations and calculate their ratio (Baum, 1975). Creatinine is affected very little by diet and minimally if at all by the state of hydration. Although there is slight tubular secretion of creatinine, tubular reabsorption is minimal if it occurs at all under normal circumstances. Ordinarily the BUN/serum creatinine ratio is about 10:1. Pre-renal azotemia typically results in a ratio greater than 15 because of augmented tubular reabsorption of urea in the presence of diminished glomerular filtration. Similarly, post-renal azotemia also results in a ratio greater than 15 because urea is reabsorbed to a much greater extent than creatinine, whether from the urinary tract in the case of acute obstructive uropathy or from the tissues in the case of extravasation of urine. In patients with reduced muscle mass, creatinine production is subnormal and the BUN/creatinine ratio will be high. A high BUN/creatinine ratio can occur in patients with compromised renal function who have a high protein diet, tissue destruction, thyrotoxicosis, or Cushing's syndrome.

A decreased BUN/creatinine can occur in any of the previously mentioned conditions in which urea production is decreased. Because of their greater creatinine formation, muscular individuals who develop renal failure can also have a low ratio. Renal dialysis causes a decreased ratio because urea is more readily dialyzed than creatinine.

Analytical Techniques. There are two general procedures used to determine urea nitrogen in biologic fluids. A direct method involves the formation of acetyl from diacetyl monoxime and the subsequent condensation of diacetyl with urea to form a colored chromogen, which can be quantitated by photometry. The liberated hydroxylamine accompanying diacetyl formation interferes with quantitation and is usually eliminated with appropriate oxidizing agents such as ferric ammonium sulfate, potassium persulfate, or arsenic acid. The diacetyl reaction, although simple to perform, lacks specificity. Other limitations include instability of the reaction color, deviation from Beer's law, and the irritating odor of the reagents, which can necessitate working in a fume hood.

The alternative indirect procedure utilizes the action of enzyme urease on urea to produce ultimately ammonia and carbonic acid.

Various methodologies have been developed for the measurement of the liberated ammonia, including acidimetric titration, coulometric titration with hypobromide, Nesslerization, and the indophenol reaction of Berthelot. In the Berthelot procedure, catalysts such as nitroprusside are added to facilitate the conversion of ammonia to indophenol.

For ease of adaptation to automation, the ammonia released from the urease reaction is reacted with α-ketoglutaric acid in the presence of glutamic dehydrogenase. The decrease of absorbance at 340 nm, corresponding to the oxidation of NADH to NAD, is proportional to the ammonium concentration. This procedure is currently used on most automated analyzers.

Semi-automated procedures for the determination of urea nitrogen include (1) the conductivity rate measurement of NH_4^+ and HCO_3^- generated from the action of urease on urea, and (2) the measurement of ammonia eluted from immobilized urease with use of an ammonia-sensing electrode.

Since hemoglobin causes colorimetric interference, measurement of urea nitrogen using serum or plasma is preferred over blood. The urease reaction has also been shown to be inhibited by a high concentration of sodium fluoride. Although urea is stable in plasma, serum, or urine for several days under refrigeration, samples, especially urine, should be assayed within a few hours to avoid bacterial contamination, which can result in rapid loss of urea.

Creatine and Creatinine

Physiologic Chemistry. Creatine is important in muscle metabolism in that it provides storage of high-energy phosphate through synthesis of phosphocreatine. Creatine is synthesized in a two-step process involving the initial synthesis of guanidoacetate (glycocyamine), which takes place in the kidneys, small intestinal mucosa, pancreas, and probably the liver. This reaction between glycine and arginine is catalyzed by a transaminidase, which is subject to feedback inhibition by increased creatine. Guanidoacetate is transported to the liver where it is methylated to creatine. Creatine then enters the blood to be widely distributed, chiefly to muscle cells. The body content of creatine is proportional to the muscle mass.

Creatinine is an anhydride of creatine and is formed by a spontaneous and irreversible reaction. Free creatinine is not reutilized in the body's metabolism and thus functions solely as a waste product of creatine. Formation of creatinine is reasonably constant, and about 2 per cent of the creatine is so transformed every 24 hours. Consequently, creatinine formation also has a direct relationship to muscle mass.

Creatine is filtered by the glomeruli but is largely or completely reabsorbed by the proximal tubules. Consequently, there is only a very small net excretion, i.e., from 0 to 40 mg/24 h (0 to 0.30 mmol/24 h) for adult males and 0 to 100 mg/24 h (0 to 0.76 mmol/24 h) for adult females. Creatinine is also freely filtered by the glomeruli but is not reabsorbed to any appreciable extent if at all under normal circumstances. A small but significant amount of creatinine is also excreted by active tubular secretion, which increases with increasing plasma creatinine concentration. Although ranges are frequently quoted for total creatinine excretion, e.g., 1.0 to 2.0 g/24 h (8.8 to 17.6 mmol/24 h) for adult males and 0.6 to 1.5 g/24 h (5.3 to 13.2 mmol/24 h) for adult females, a better index would relate creatinine excretion to muscle mass or lean body weight. A reasonable compromise is to relate creatinine excretion to total body weight, i.e., 21 to 26 mg/kg body weight/24 h (0.18 to 0.23 mmol/kg/24 h) for adult males and 16 to 22 mg/kg body weight/24 h (0.14 to 0.19 mmol/kg/24 h) for adult females. Although creatinine excretion is usually considered to be reasonably constant in a given individual, one study indicated an intraindividual coefficient of variation of 10 per cent (Scott, 1968). Severe exercise and a high meat diet will cause significantly increased creatinine excretion. Total creatinine measurement is commonly used as an index of the completeness of 24-hour urine collections. Some investigators have concluded, however, that this is an unreliable practice (Tocci, 1972).

The serum concentration of creatinine is relatively constant and somewhat greater in males than in females, i.e., 0.6 to 1.2 mg/dl (53 to 106 μmol/L) for males and 0.5 to 1.0 mg/dl (44 to 88 μmol/L) for females when specific analytical methods are used (true creatinine). Less specific, i.e., total chromogen, methods for creatinine result in ranges that are about 0.3 mg/dl higher. The plasma creatine concentration is more variable than creatinine and is higher in females than in males, i.e., 0.2 to 0.6 mg/dl (15 to 45 μmol/L) for males and 0.6 to 1.0 mg/dl (45 to 76 μmol/L) for females. Increased levels occur in children and pregnant women. Ingestion of creatine will cause a rapid rise in plasma concentration.

Clinicopathologic Correlations. Serum or plasma creatine concentration and urinary creatine excretion are increased significantly by skeletal muscle necrosis or atrophy (Pennington, 1971), e.g., trauma, the rapidly progressing muscular dystrophies, poliomyelitis, amyotrophic lateral sclerosis, amyotonia congenita, dermatomyositis, myasthenia gravis, and starvation. Methyltestosterone stimulates increased creatine synthesis by the liver. Increased creatine is also associated with hyperthyroidism, diabetic acidosis, and the puerperium.

The constancy of creatinine formation and excretion makes creatinine a useful index of renal function, primarily of glomerular filtration. By virtue of its relative independence from such factors as diet (protein intake), degree of hydration, and protein metabolism, the plasma creatinine is a significantly more reliable screening test or index of renal function than is the BUN. The plasma creatinine tends to increase somewhat more slowly than the BUN in renal disease but also decreases more slowly with hemodialysis. The usefulness of plasma creatinine and the creatinine clearance test are discussed in detail in Chapter 8.

Analytical Techniques. Most of the commonly used methods for the determination of creatinine and creatine are based on the Jaffe reaction, in which creatinine is treated with an alkaline picrate solution to yield a bright orange-red complex. Unfortunately, this simple procedure is subject to interferences from a variety of substances, e.g., glucose, proteins, and other non-creatinine chromogens. The reaction is also sensitive to temperature and pH changes. To increase specificity, Lloyd's reagent, an aluminum silicate, has been used to separate creatinine from other chromogens prior to the Jaffe reaction. This modification is commonly regarded as the reference method for measuring "true" creatinine. There are numerous modifications of the picrate reaction that are designed to improve assay specificity. One modification, based on the fact that the color resulting from true creatinine is less resistant to acid than the color from non-creatinine chromogens, involves measurement of the impact of acidification on color following total color development. In another approach, the change in color intensity of the picrate reaction is measured before and after bacterial-enzyme destruction of creatinine. In still another version, the proteins are removed by heat prior to treatment with Lloyd's reagent, purportedly to avoid loss of creatinine caused by protein precipitation with tungstic acid. Lloyd's reagent has also been replaced by other adsorbing agents or cation-exchange resin. The eluted creatinine fraction is quantitated directly by ultraviolet absorption, usually at 234 nm.

More specific methods based on principles other than Jaffe's reaction have been developed in the last decade. They include colorimetric determinations of complexes formed with 3,5-dinitrobenzoic acid and with *o*-nitrobenzaldehyde. The use of 3,5-dinitrobenzoic acid as a complexing agent has been shown to optimize complex formation and is superior to the picrate reaction in terms of linearity, precision, and susceptibility to interferences. Creatinine determinations based on enzymatic reactions have also been developed in recent years, and an enzyme-selective electrode coupled to tripolyphosphate-activated creatininase has been described for measuring creatinine in both urine and serum. The high cost and limited availability of creatinase continues to limit the use of enzymatic procedures. The activation mechanism is believed to improve electrode sensitivity.

A recently developed kinetic-rate modification of Jaffe's reaction is applicable to routine automation and is relatively free of interfering chromogens. It has been adapted for use on centrifugal analyzers.

Creatine is usually measured by the difference in creatinine before and after conversion of creatine to creatinine, generally by heat.

Since considerable amounts of non-creatinine chromogens are present in the erythrocytes, plasma and serum are preferred over whole blood for measuring creatinine. While hemolysis does not affect the determination of creatinine, it increases the creatine value by 100 to 200 per cent. Because of the lability of creatine and creatinine, fresh specimens are recommended. Also, specimens should be maintained at pH 7 during storage to minimize interconversion. Substances that can interfere with creatinine determination by Jaffe's reaction include acetoacetate acetone, barbiturates, phenolsulfonphthalein, sulfobromophthalein, and protein.

Uric Acid

Physiologic Chemistry. Uric acid is the major product of purine catabolism in man and the anthropoid apes and is formed from xanthine by the action of xanthine oxidase. In lower mammals uric acid is further oxidized by the action of uricase to allantoin, which is their main excretory product of purine catabolism. Interestingly, birds and reptiles synthesize uric acid as an end product of both purine and protein catabolism, with the distinct advantage that these animals can excrete the sparingly soluble uric acid as crystals and thereby conserve water. The metabolism of uric acid has been reviewed by Balis (1976).

The average adult has a total body content of about 1.2 g of uric acid, which may be considered to be a miscible pool with high turnover. Uric acid in this pool is derived from three sources: (1) catabolism of ingested nucleoproteins, (2) catabolism of endogenous nucleoproteins, and (3) direct transformation of endogenous purine nucleotides (Ryckewaert, 1974). Approximately 60 per cent of this pool is replaced daily by concomitant formation and excretion. Most uric acid formation occurs in the liver, which has a high activity of xanthine oxidase, as does the intestinal mucosa. Only traces of xanthine oxidase are present in other tissues. On a low purine diet, about 275 to 600 mg of uric acid will be excreted by the average adult in a 24-hour period. This is somewhat less than the amount formed by endogenous metabolism. It is probable that most, if not all, of the remaining uric acid excretion occurs through biliary, pancreatic, and gastrointestinal secretions followed by degradation by the intestinal flora. Human tissues have very limited uricolytic capability.

Uric acid is a weak acid with a pKa_1 of 5.75 and a pKa_2 of 10.3. Consequently, at the pH of body fluids uric acid exists almost entirely as the urate anion. Although there is some difference of opinion, it appears that urate binding to plasma proteins is minimal. The stated normal range for serum or plasma urate varies considerably as a consequence of differences in analytical methods and in age, racial, sex, social, and geographic factors. One recent study of 1419 clinically healthy Americans revealed a 95 per cent non-parametric normal range of 4.0 to 8.5 mg/dl (0.24 to 0.50 mmol/L) for males and 2.7 to 7.3 mg/dl (0.16 to 0.43 mmol/L) for females when uric acid was analyzed by a phosphotungstate method (Reed, 1972). This study included adult subjects from age 20 to old age, but there was no statistically significant effect of age except for an increased upper limit of normal of about 0.5 mg/dl for females at the time of menopause. Urate concentration in male children is approximately 1 mg/dl less than that in adult males, but this difference disappears between ages 15 and 20 (Ryckewaert, 1974).

The average adult excretes approximately 0.4 to 0.8 g of uric acid in the urine every 24 hours. On a low purine diet, about 275 to 600 mg of uric acid will still be excreted as a result of catabolism of endogenous purines (Ryckewaert, 1974). Uric acid excretion can exceed 1.0 g/24 h as a consequence of high purine diet or any of the various causes for increased synthesis or catabolism of endogenous purines. Urate is freely filtered by the glomeruli. The renal clearance of urate is, however, less than 10 per cent of inulin clearance, thus indicating considerable tubular reabsorption. The renal handling of urate is, however, extremely complex and involves not only glomerular filtration and active reabsorption by the proximal tubules but also active tubular secretion and a second tubular reabsorption. It has been estimated that 98 to 100 per cent of the filtered urate is actively reabsorbed in the tubules, as is 90 to 94 per cent of that subsequently secreted by the tubules (Rieselbach, 1977).

At least twice as much uric acid will dissolve in urine as in water at the same pH and temperature. Uromucoid is probably one of the most important solubilizers.

Clinicopathologic Correlations. Numerous diseases, physiologic conditions, biochemical changes, and even social and behavioral factors are associated with alterations in the urate concentration of plasma. Increased serum urate concentration is much more frequent and clinically more significant than decreased concentration. Among the most common etiologies of hyperuricemia are renal failure, ketoacidosis, lactate excess, and the use of diuretics. Hyperuricemia also has a poorly understood but positive relationship to hyperlipidemia, obesity, atherosclerosis, diabetes mellitus, hypertension, social class, exercise, and achievement-oriented behavior. Dietary intake of purine-rich foods, e.g., meat, viscera, leguminous vegetables, and yeast, causes mild hyperuricemia as well as significantly increased urinary excretion of urate.

Gout is a disorder of purine metabolism or renal excretion of uric acid characterized by (1) hyperuricemia; (2) precipitation of monosodium urate as deposits (tophi) throughout the body except for the central nervous system, but with a special predilection for joints and the periarticular cartilage, bone, bursae, and subcutaneous tissue; (3) recurrent clinical attacks of arthritis, which typically respond to colchicine; and (4) nephropathy and frequently nephrolithiasis. Although genetic in origin, fewer than one third of all patients have a family history of clinical gout. Hyperuricemia is frequently found in asymptomatic close relatives. Although some investigators have considered gout to be an autosomal dominant trait with incomplete penetrance, the mode of inheritance is not known with certainty. Gout may well be of polygenic origin. Males constitute more than 90 per cent of all cases. Gout is uncommon in females prior to menopause. The peak age of onset is in the fifth decade, and the disease is very rare prior to age 20.

2

Gout is frequently categorized as primary or secondary on the basis of whether the disease is presumed to be an inborn error of metabolism directly involving uric acid synthesis or excretion or whether it is associated with hyperuricemia from any of numerous other etiologies. Considering the frequency of hyperuricemia, secondary gout is a very uncommon complication. The miscible pool of uric acid is greatly increased in gout and can exceed 30 g. The concentration of urate in plasma is roughly correlated with clinical severity, but it is not known why one individual will have clinical gout while another in the same kinship with an equally elevated concentration of urate in the plasma can be asymptomatic. The increased body burden of uric acid is a result of significantly increased synthesis of uric acid from endogenous purines, diminished renal excretion of urate, or a combination of both defects. Most investigators have in the past emphasized the importance of overproduction of uric acid in the pathogenesis of gout, but more recently it has been suggested that cases of gout are about equally distributed in the three categories of overproduction, underexcretion, or a combination of the two defects (Klinenberg, 1977). The pathogenesis of the acute inflammation accompanying uric acid deposits in gout is unclear. It is possible that the monosodium urate crystals enhance bradykinin synthesis through activation of the Hageman factor.

A rare but interesting etiology for primary gout is a deficiency in the enzyme hypoxanthine-guanine-phosphoribosyl-transferase (HGPRT), which results in overproduction of purines and marked accumulation of uric acid. HGPRT is normally present in all tissues and converts hypoxanthine and guanine to their respective nucleotides, inosinic acid and guanylic acid. This disease, commonly termed the Lesch-Nyhan syndrome, is characterized by mental retardation, choreoathetosis, spastic cerebral palsy, aggressive behavior, and compulsive self-mutilation in addition to the pathologic manifestation of hyperuricemia, gouty arthritis, tophi, nephrolithiasis, and nephropathy (Nyhan, 1974).

Urate retention and hyperuricemia are early consequences of azotemic renal disease. Although previously considered to be a reflection of decreased glomerular filtration, the urate retention is more likely the result of decreased tubular secretion of urate or altered postsecretory reabsorption or both factors (Steele, 1975). The plasma urate seldom increases much above 10 mg/dl in renal failure, probably because of increased gastrointestinal secretion and uricolysis. Clinical gout is an uncommon complication of the hyperuricemia of renal disease and occurs in fewer than 5 per cent of all cases. There are two interesting exceptions, however. Chronic lead nephropathy is associated with gout (saturnine gout) in about half of all cases. Polycystic kidney disease predisposes to both hyperuricemia and secondary gout even before renal function deteriorates enough to cause azotemia.

Various drugs and chemical substances interfere with renal excretion of urate. Ethacrynic acid, furosemide, and the benzothiadiazide diuretics have a definite anti-uricosuric effect. *p*-Aminohippurate, lactate, acetoacetate, and β-hydroxybutyrate competitively inhibit tubular secretion of urate. Some drugs such as salicylate, probenecid, sulfinpyrazone, and phenylbutazone are of particular interest in that they inhibit uric acid excretion in low doses but have a marked uricosuric effect in high doses. This is explained by the fact that these drugs inhibit tubular secretion of urate in low doses but are able to inhibit tubular reabsorption only at significantly higher levels.

Increased nucleoprotein production and catabolism are important in the hyperuricemia occurring with leukemia, lymphoma, macroglobulinemia, polycythemia, multiple myeloma, neuroblastoma, and various other widely disseminated neoplasms. Chemotherapeutic agents and ionizing radiation therapy of malignant neoplasms can greatly increase the formation of uric acid. Psoriasis is also associated with hyperuricemia, which is the result of increased proliferation of epidermal cells. Hyperuricemia occurs frequently in sickle cell anemia.

Ethanol intake will frequently increase the plasma concentration of urate and can cause attacks of gout in susceptible patients. The pathogenesis is related to lactate excess, which is produced by the alcohol dehydrogenase catalyzed oxidation of ethanol to acetaldehyde and which competitively inhibits renal excretion of urate. Lactate excess is also associated with hyperuricemia in severe exercise, toxemia of pregnancy, and ethylene glycol intoxication. Increased acetoacetate and β-hydroxybutyrate similarly contribute to hyperuricemia in diabetic ketoacidosis and starvation. Glycogen storage disease type 1 is regularly accompanied by hyperuricemia as a consequence of both lacticacidemia and increased formation of purines.

Hyperuricemia occurs in many other conditions in which the pathogenetic relationship is less well defined. Included are Down's syndrome, barbiturate overdose, chloroform, carbon monoxide, ammonia and beryllium poisoning, hypoparathyroidism, acromegaly, nephrogenic diabetes insipidus, sarcoidosis, and liver disease.

Causes for hypouricemia are relatively few. Renal tubular reabsorption defects, either congenital as in the Fanconi syndrome and Wilson's disease, or acquired, particularly through toxic damage, can cause increased urinary loss of urate and low plasma levels. Hypouricemia has also been described in association with malignant disorders, e.g., Hodgkin's disease, multiple myeloma, and bronchogenic carcinoma. Xanthinuria, a rare condition, is caused by a congenital deficiency of xanthine oxidase so that xanthine and hypoxanthine are excreted instead of uric acid. Vigorous treatment of gout with the xanthine oxidase inhibitor allopurinol can have a similar effect. Another rare congenital condition, phosphoribosylpyrophosphatase deficiency, also causes extremely low plasma urate concentrations. Severe liver disease can seriously impair the conversion of xanthine to uric acid.

Uric acid is an important constituent of renal calculi, but only a small minority of patients with either primary or secondary gout form renal calculi. The risk in primary gout is estimated to be 10 to 30 per cent. In one series of 207 patients with renal calculi, 22 had uric acid calculi, but only four of these patients had primary gout (Melick, 1958). The most important factors in the formation of uric acid calculi are probably increasing concentration of uric acid in urine and increasing acidity of the urine.

Analytical Techniques. Most methods are based on the oxidation of uric acid to allantoin by either chemical or enzymatic means. The older methods are mainly photometric procedures involving the reduction of tungstate to a blue complex. The most commonly used oxidizing agent is alkaline phosphotungstate, the reduction product of which, tungsten blue, can be measured photometrically at 700 nm. However, there are several inherent difficulties with this method, including the coprecipitation of uric acid with plasma proteins, the formation of turbidity during color development, and the presence of endogenous, potentially interfering substances such as ascorbic acid, free thiols, methylated purines, homogentisic acid, and glucose in very high concentrations. The use of a protein-free filtrate for color formation has eliminated most of the interferences. The sodium carbonate reagent initially used to provide the alkaline medium has been replaced by sodium cyanide in order to increase assay sensitivity. Furthermore, the inclusion of urea has been shown to reduce turbidity in the final color solution.

In spite of numerous modifications of the basic colorimetric method aimed at improving specificity, the oxidation of uric acid to allantoin using the enzyme uricase remains the most specific method available. Since uric acid, but not allantoin, absorbs at 293 nm, the difference in absorbance before and after treatment of the sample with uricase is proportional to the uric acid concentration. The advantages of this method are that it avoids protein precipitation and has superior sensitivity and specificity. It is adapted for use on most automated analyzers.

Several modifications making use of the H_2O_2 formed during the enzymatic reaction include the formation of chromogen via coupling with the enzyme catalase and the formation of fluorescent compounds either by self-coupling of *p*-hydroxyphenylacetic acid or by the oxidation of homovanillic acid. Other methods of quantitation include the measurement of oxygen uptake during the formation of H_2O_2, coulometric titration, and chromatographic determinations.

Uric acid is stable in both serum and urine for about three days at room temperature. Stability can be increased with the addition of fluoride or thymol. All anticoagulants can be used except potassium oxalate, which forms insoluble potassium phosphotungstate, resulting in turbidity.

Ammonia

Physiologic Chemistry. Ammonia is a product of amino acid metabolism and therefore of protein catabolism. Considerable ammonia is also absorbed from the intestinal tract, where it is formed by bacterial degradation of dietary proteins and the urea present in gastrointestinal secretions. Ammonia is formed principally in the liver by the oxidative deamination of amino acids, chiefly by the glutamic dehydrogenase catalyzed deamination of L-glutamate to form α-ketoglutarate. Net synthesis of L-glutamate occurs as a result of transamination involving other amino acids, which are transformed in the reaction to their corresponding alpha-keto acids. Smaller amounts of ammonia are formed by non-oxidative deamination of amino acids and aerobic oxidation of various physiologic amines, such as epinephrine and dopamine.

Most ammonia is ultimately disposed of as urea, which is formed in the urea cycle subsequent to the synthesis of carbamyl phosphate. Considerable ammonia is temporarily stored as glutamine, which is formed from glutamic acid principally in the liver but also to some extent in the brain and in skeletal muscle. The kidneys take up glutamine from plasma and form ammonia by the action of glutaminase. The ammonia thus formed is excreted in the urine as one of the two most important urine buffers of hydrogen ions, the other being phosphate. The human kidneys excrete about 30 to 50 mmol (mEq) of ammonia each day, accounting for about 5 to 10 per cent of all nitrogen excreted and buffering most of the 40 to 80 mmol of metabolic acid produced and excreted by the body (Goldstein, 1976).

Ammonia concentration in plasma is ordinarily less than 120 μg/dl (67 μmol/L).

Clinicopathologic Correlations. The most frequent etiology of altered ammonia metabolism is severe liver disease. It is also elevated in Reye's syndrome. When liver function is no longer adequate to metabolize ammonia, the plasma concentration increases, with various toxic manifestations, particularly in the brain. This is discussed in more detail in Chapter 13.

Deficiencies in any of the principal enzymes in the urea cycle, i.e., carbamyl phosphate synthetase, ornithine transcarbamylase, argininosuccinic acid synthetase, argininosuccinase, and arginase, are an important but rare cause for increased plasma ammonia and toxic manifestations (Shih, 1978).

In metabolic acidosis the renal excretion of ammonia rises precipitously, provided that normal renal function is maintained. In chronic renal disease the ability of the kidneys to excrete ammonia and, therefore, to excrete metabolic acid is compromised. This is discussed further in Chapter 8.

Analytical Techniques. The measurement of ammonia in blood involves the conversion of NH_4^+ to gaseous NH_3. This initial reaction can be conducted directly in blood or in a protein-free filtrate. The liberated NH_3 can be separated from the plasma or serum by reabsorption on a cation exchange resin followed by quantitation either with Nessler's reagent or by the indophenol reaction, in which NH_4^+ reacts with sodium phenoxide in the presence of hypochlorite and nitroprusside to yield a stable blue color. An alternative and more widely used procedure in separating ammonia from blood or plasma is isothermal diffusion. The isolated NH_3 can be measured by acidimetric titration, Nesslerization, photometric determination of the color produced with ninhydrin or with the indophenol reaction, coulometric titration with electrolytically produced hydrobromite, or a variety of other means. Another approach for determining blood ammonia is the enzymatic reaction of ammonia with α-ketoglutaric acid in the presence of glutamic dehydrogenase. The decrease of absorbance at 340 nm from the corresponding conversion of NADH to NAD is proportional to the ammonia concentration.

The *in vitro* formation of ammonia in blood, which results from enzymatic action on labile amides such as glutamine, poses a problem in ammonia determinations. The ammonia content in freshly drawn blood increases at the rate of 0.003 μg/ml blood/min at room temperature. The ammonia concentration will remain constant for at least 24 hours if the sample is frozen at −20°C. If analysis is delayed for more than a few minutes, quick freezing of arterial rather than venous blood samples in dry ice and acetone is recommended.

Amino Acids

Physiologic Chemistry. An examination of Figure 9–1 reveals that the α-amino acid molecule contains an amino group ($—NH_2$), a carboxyl group ($—COOH$), and an R group or side chain, which is

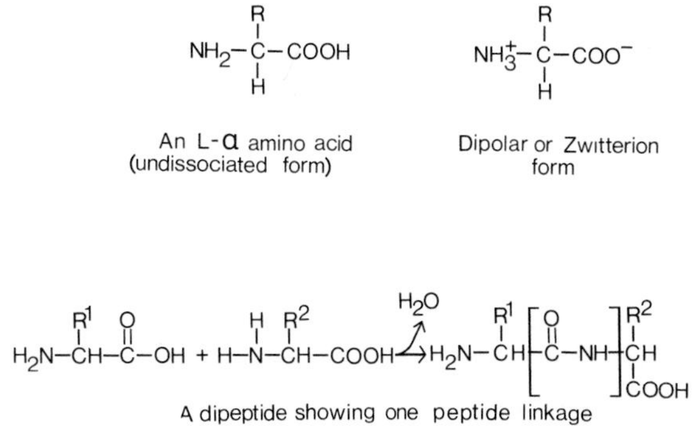

$$NH_2-\underset{H}{\overset{R}{C}}-COOH \qquad NH_3^+-\underset{H}{\overset{R}{C}}-COO^-$$

An L-α amino acid (undissociated form) — Dipolar or Zwitterion form

$$H_2N-\overset{R^1}{CH}-\overset{O}{\overset{\|}{C}}-OH + H-\overset{H}{N}-\overset{R^2}{CH}-COOH \xrightarrow{H_2O} H_2N-\overset{R^1}{CH}\left[-\overset{O}{\overset{\|}{C}}-NH-\right]\underset{COOH}{\overset{R^2}{CH}}$$

A dipeptide showing one peptide linkage

Figure 9–1. Chemical characteristics of amino acids.

responsible for specific characteristics of the particular amino acid. Although more than 150 different amino acids are known biologically, only 21 are present in the body as significant constituents of proteins. Some of these amino acids must be supplied by dietary intake, while others can be synthesized by various metabolic pathways. Those amino acids that have to be supplied by dietary intake because endogenous synthesis is inadequate to meet normal requirements are termed essential amino acids. This distinction implies only a necessity for supply from an external source and does not imply that these amino acids are more important for metabolism and growth than the remaining non-essential amino acids. The essential and non-essential amino acids are shown in Table 9–1.

Amino acids that possess an asymmetric carbon atom, i.e., those with four different substituent groups, have dextrorotatory (D) and levorotatory (L) optical specificity. All amino acids in human proteins are of the L configuration, which is diagrammatically shown in Figure 9–1.

Amino acids in their crystalline state have melting points above 190°C. and are more soluble in water than in other less polar solvents. At a pH that is specific for each amino acid, the molecule is doubly charged, i.e., the carboxyl group is negatively charged and the amino group is positively charged, thus resulting in a net charge of zero. Dipolar ions of this type are referred to as zwitterions (Fig. 9–1). Amino acids thus behave as both weak acids and weak bases, i.e, they are amphoteric.

Proteins are composed of long chains of amino acids joined by peptide linkage. The peptide or amide linkage is formed by the condensation of the α-amino group of one amino acid with the carboxyl group of another. A molecule of water is removed in the formation of the amide bond (Fig. 9–1). After the peptide linkage has been formed, a carboxyl group of one amino acid and the amino group of the other are still available to form additional peptide linkages.

Proteins in ingested foods are not absorbed intact to any significant degree. In the process of digestion, enzymatic cleavage of peptide linkages occurs. In the stomach and proximal small intestine, endopeptidases hydrolyze the inner portions of the polypeptide chains while exopeptidases attack the terminal linkages.

Table 9–1. AMINO ACIDS AS SIGNIFICANT CONSTITUENTS OF BODY PROTEINS

Essential	Non-essential
Valine	Glycine
Leucine	Alanine
Isoleucine	Serine
Methionine	Cysteine
Threonine	Cystine
Arginine	Aspartic acid
Lysine	Glutamic acid
Phenylalanine	Hydroxylysine
Histidine	Tyrosine
Tryptophan	Proline
	Hydroxyproline

The action of the endopeptidases, pepsin, trypsin, chymotrypsin, and elastase, and the exopeptidases, carboxypeptidases A and B, results in a mixture of amino acids and small peptides, which can be absorbed by the intestine. After absorption into the microvilli, further enzymatic hydrolysis converts oligopeptides into the constituent amino acids. The molecules of essentially all the amino acids are much too large to diffuse passively through the membrane pores of the intestinal mucosal cells. The amino acids are absorbed by at least three stereospecific active transport systems: (1) neutral amino acids are absorbed competitively by a single transport system, (2) basic amino acids are absorbed but at a slower rate by a second active transport system, and (3) proline and hydroxyproline are absorbed by a third transport system. After absorption, amino acids enter the portal venous blood to be transported to the liver, where some are utilized for protein synthesis while others enter the systemic amino acid pool. Protein synthesis throughout the body utilizes amino acids from the systemic pool, while protein catabolism contributes additional amino acids. The usual process of catabolism involves initial removal of the amino group. The resultant keto acids enter the Krebs aerobic cycle to be oxidized to CO_2 and water with the production of energy, which can be stored as ATP (adenosine triphosphate). Amino acids exist in the systemic circulatory pool but cannot be stored as such. The adult normal range of plasma amino acids will vary according to the method of analysis. Goodwin (1968), using a method involving the formation of colored complexes, established an adult normal range of 3.6 to 7.0 mg amino acid nitrogen/dl (2.6 to 5.0 mmol/L).

Amino acids are filtered by renal glomeruli and are very efficiently reabsorbed by active transport processes in the proximal tubules. Ordinarily less than 5 per cent of the filtered amino acids are not reabsorbed and are thus excreted in the urine. In the normal adult, urinary excretion of amino acids is fairly constant and averages 200 mg of alpha-amino nitrogen per 24 hours.

Clinicopathologic Correlations. Amino acids are the second largest constituent of the plasma non-protein nitrogen. Significant decreases in either the plasma concentration of amino acids or the urinary excretion rate are rare. Even in severe cachexia the plasma amino acid pool is relatively well maintained as a consequence of the catabolism of intrinsic body proteins.

Increased concentrations of plasma amino acids and especially their urinary excretion rates are of considerable medical importance, particularly in newborns and children. More than 50 hereditary diseases of amino acid metabolism have now been described, most of which have an autosomal recessive mode of inheritance. All of these diseases are uncommon to extremely rare, which is fortunate in view of the fact that many of the diseases are associated with mental retardation, severe metabolic derangements, and failure to thrive. Typically, a hereditary amino acid disorder is directly related to the absence of an enzyme involved in the metabolism of one or more amino acids so that these amino acids increase greatly in both plasma concentrations and urinary excretion rates. Phenylketonuria, for example, is the result of an inherited deficiency or absence of phenylalanine hydroxylase, which is necessary for the metabolic conversion of phenylalanine to tyrosine, with a resulting increase in both phenylalanine and its deaminated metabolite phenylpyruvic acid in plasma and urine. Phenylketonuria is one of the most common hereditary amino acid disorders and affects about one in 10,000 newborns. Early diagnosis is essential so that diets lacking in phenylalanine can be instituted and thereby decrease or avoid the cerebral damage that otherwise invariably occurs.

Increased concentrations of amino acids in plasma can be categorized as primary (hereditary) metabolic defects and secondary metabolic responses. Secondary responses involve most or all amino acids. Significant increases are usually a consequence of severe liver disease that inhibits the oxidative deamination of amino acids. Small increases in the plasma concentration of many amino acids occur after ingestion of a protein-rich meal.

In general, measurement of urinary concentration of amino acids is of a more clinical value than plasma concentrations. Urine amino acids are discussed in Chapter 18. Increased urinary excretion of amino acids is of two major types, viz., overflow and renal. Overflow aminoacidurias are those that accompany increased plasma concentrations of amino acids when normally functioning kidney tubules are unable to reabsorb the increased concentrations of amino acids in the glomerular filtrate, i.e., the renal tubular maximum reabsorption capacity is exceeded.

Renal aminoacidurias are those conditions associated with increased urinary excretion of one or more amino acids while plasma amino acid concentrations are normal. These various conditions have in common a defect in the renal tubular transport mechanism that causes decreased reabsorption of amino acids from the glomerular filtrate. Primary or hereditary renal aminoacidurias are those involving a hereditary defect in renal tubular transport of one or several amino acids. For example, cystinuria results in an inability of the renal tubules to reabsorb not only cysteine but also lysine, arginine, ornithine, and occasionally other amino acids as well. Secondary renal aminoacidurias are those resulting from acquired renal tubular disease, often of a toxic etiology, e.g., heavy metal poisoning. Other etiologies include acute renal tubular necrosis, severe malnutrition, and various metabolic diseases otherwise unrelated to amino acid metabolism, e.g., galactosemia, hereditary fructose intolerance, and Wilson's disease. The renal threshold for amino acid excretion is lowered in pregnancy and in newborns.

Other than plasma and urine, amino acid analysis is of no significant clinical importance except for the quantitation of glutamine in cerebrospinal fluid. Glutamine, the most abundant amino acid in plasma, is of major importance as a source of ammonia in the renal tubules for buffering hydrogen ion in urine. Glutamine is, however, increased in the cerebrospinal fluid in association with hepatic encephalopathy (see Chap. 19).

Analytical Techniques. Analytical techniques are of two basic types in terms of the information generated, viz., those that quantitate total amino acids and those that separate and quantitate individual amino acids or groups of amino acids. Analytic methods for total amino acids rely on the unique reactivity of the amino group attached to the alpha carbon of the basic amino acid structure. The classical reference method for the measurement of alpha amino nitrogen is the gasometric ninhydrin procedure of Van Slyke, but this method is technically demanding and seldom utilized in spite of its exquisite reliability. A reliable and rapid procedure developed by Goodwin (1968) utilized 1-fluoro-2,4-dinitrobenzene, which forms a yellow dinitrophenyl derivative of the amino acids, which can be quantitated spectrophotometrically at 420 nm. The procedure is applicable to both plasma and urine. Other methods use 2,4,6-trinitrobenzene sulfonate or sodium β-naphthoquinone-4-sulfonate.

In many metabolic disturbances, it is not the total concentration of amino acids that is of clinical importance, but rather the altered concentration of one amino acid or a group of related amino acids. In many such instances, the abnormalities can be readily detected by simple screening tests of urine using chromatography (paper or thin layer) or high voltage electrophoresis (HVE). These techniques, along with their interpretation, are fully discussed in Chapter 18. For more accurate quantitative studies, the amino acids in plasma or urine can be separated on an automated high-pressure column chromatography system (amino acid analyzer) using an ion-exchange resin followed by gradient elution. In the original amino acid analyzer, quantitation was achieved by spectrophotometric analysis following ninhydrin derivatization. Refinements in the original procedure, particularly improved column technology and the development of new fluorescent detection systems (fluorescamine and phthaldealdehyde), have resulted in increased sensitivity and reduced analysis time (Hammond, 1976).

Reasonably specific methods that avoid the high cost of column chromatography have been developed for some amino acids including thyroxine, triiodothyronine, hydroxyproline, glutamine, phenylalanine, and tyrosine. Thyroxine and triiodothyronine, though structurally amino acids, are important as thyroid hormones and not as protein constituents. They are discussed in Chapter 16. Hydroxyproline excretion in urine is an important index of collagen catabolism and is discussed later in this chapter. Cerebrospinal fluid glutamine is discussed in Chapter 19.

By virtue of its application to biochemical screening of the newborn, phenylalanine is frequently determined in plasma during the first few days after birth. The Guthrie screening test is a microbiological assay that measures the ability of phenylalanine in the test sample to overcome the metabolic inhibition of β-2-thienylalanine on a strain of *Bacillus subtilis*. A more commonly performed assay today involves a fluorometric reaction between phenylalanine, copper, and ninhydrin with enhancement by any of several dipeptides. Other chemical methods include gas-liquid chromatography and ultraviolet spectrophotometry.

Phenylalanine and phenylketonuria are discussed further in Chapter 18.

Tyrosine can be quantitated fluorometrically following its reaction with 1-nitroso-2 naphthol. The procedure is adaptable to automated continuous flow analysis.

PORPHYRINS

Physiologic Chemistry

The porphyrins are metabolic intermediates in the biosynthetic pathway that has heme as its principal product. The basic structure common to all porphyrins is the porphin nucleus, which consists of one pyrrolenine, one maleimide, and two pyrrole type rings. These rings are joined together by four methene bridges, as shown in Figure 9–2. The porphyrins are differentiated by the substituents found in the eight peripheral positions. There are many kinds of porphyrins known, but very few are found in nature and only three are of clinical significance: uroporphyrins, coproporphyrins, and protoporphyrins. Four isomeric forms can exist for each porphyrin. All naturally occurring porphyrins are of either the I or III isomer type. Only the type III isomers have been shown to play a functional role in the biosynthesis of heme.

The biochemistry of porphyrins and heme synthesis has been the subject of numerous reviews (Elder, 1972; Moore, 1980). A brief sequence of the heme biosynthetic pathway is shown in Figure 9–3. The initial rate-limiting step in hepatic porphyrin synthesis is the formation of δ-aminolevulinic acid (ALA) which requires the presence of pyridoxal phosphate and involves the enzyme ALA synthetase. The condensation of ALA to porphobilinogen (PBG) involves ALA dehydratase, which is present in relatively high levels in both hepatic and bone marrow cells. The formation of uroporphyrinogens I and III from PBG occurs under the influence of enzymes uroporphyrinogen I synthetase and uroporphyrinogen III cosynthetase. Both isomers undergo decarboxylation to yield the respective coproporphyrinogens. The type III isomer undergoes oxidative decarboxylation to form protoporphyrin, which reacts with ferrous ion to produce heme.

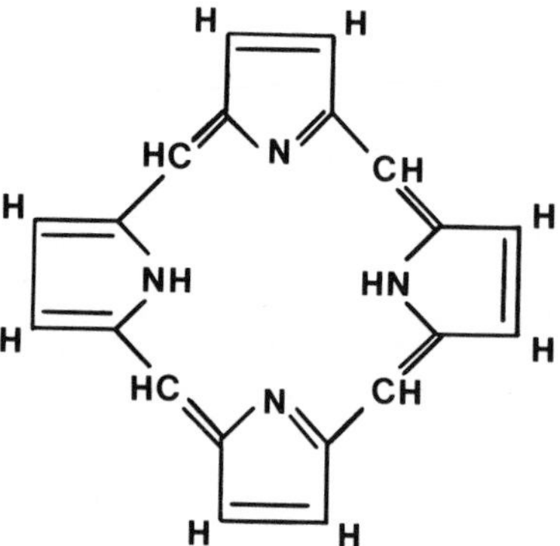

Figure 9–2. Structure of porphin.

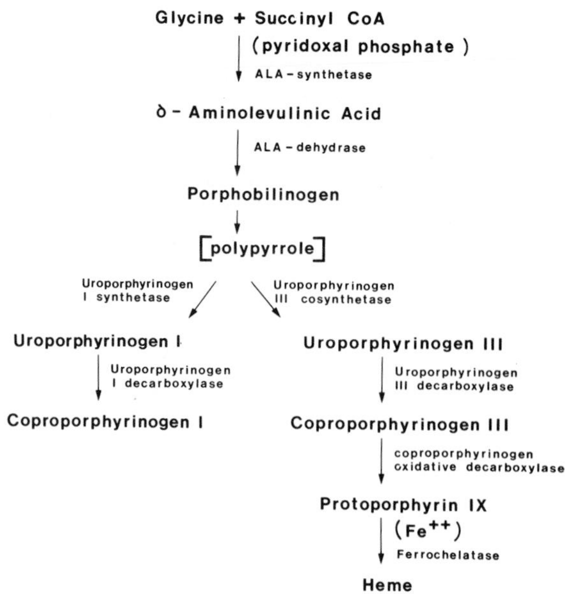

Figure 9–3. Biosynthetic pathway of heme.

It is worth noting that the biosynthetic intermediates between PBG and protoporphyrin are not porphyrins but rather their reduced forms, the porphyrinogens. They are colorless non-fluorescent compounds readily converted to porphyrins by weak oxidizing agents, such as air in the presence of light. Thus uroporphyrin and coproporphyrin are merely the oxidation of their respective porphyrinogens, which are the true substrates in the biosynthetic pathway.

Clinicopathologic Correlations

The porphyrias comprise a group of inherited and acquired disorders characterized by aberrations in the activities of specific enzymes of the heme biosynthetic pathway. Various classifications of porphyrin disorders according to the sites of biochemical and pathologic lesion have been proposed (Elder, 1972). Recent advances in the understanding of the porphyrias have led to the conclusion that the principal control of the heme biosynthetic pathway lies at the level of ALA synthetase, the activity of which is normally low, but is readily inducible by drugs and steroids and is susceptible to negative feedback by heme. It is further recognized that a secondary control point resides with the activity of uroporphyrinogen I synthetase. Decreased levels of this enzyme result in the accumulation of porphyrin precursors (ALA and PBG), while increased levels bring about excessive production of free porphyrins. In light of these findings, Moore (1980) differentiated the acute porphyrias from the non-acute porphyrias on the basis of their clinical manifestation as well as the pattern of production and excretion of porphyrins and their precursors. In Moore's classification, acute intermittent porphyria, hereditary coproporphyria, and variegate porphyria, which display similar abdominal, autonomic, and neuropsychiatric features, are grouped as acute porphyrias, while cutaneous hepatic porphyria, erythropoietic protoporphyria, and congenital porphyria, typically associated with solar photosensitivity of the skin, are classified as non-acute porphyrias.

Acute Intermittent Porphyria. This is the most common of the inherited porphyrias. It is transmitted as an autosomal dominant trait but affects three females to every two males. This disease typically presents with colicky abdominal pain often associated with vomiting, constipation, fever, and leukocytosis. Hypertension, peripheral neuritis, behavioral changes, and frank psychosis can occur. Enzyme defects that have been proposed to account for this disorder include increased levels of ALA synthetase, decreased levels of uroporphyrinogen I synthetase, and a reduced activity of the enzyme Δ^4-5α-reductase. Laboratory findings include elevated urinary ALA and PBG, inappropriate secretion of ADH, and overt liver function abnormalities, e.g., transient elevation of bilirubin and alkaline phosphatase.

Hereditary Coproporphyria. This hepatic porphyria is transmitted as an autosomal dominant. Affected patients either are asymptomatic or present with mild neurologic, abdominal, or psychiatric symptoms. Acute attacks have also been reported. Coproporphyrin III is excreted virtually constantly in the feces, while coproporphyrin, ALA, and PBG appear intermittently in the urine. A block in the conversion of coproporphyrinogen III to protoporphyrin and/or an induction of ALA synthetase has been implicated in the mechanism of this condition.

Variegate Porphyria. This autosomal dominant porphyria affects females and males equally and is particularly prevalent in the white population of South Africa. The disease onset is usually in the third or fourth decade of life and is somewhat variable in its clinical manifestations. The symptoms and signs of acute attacks are similar to those of acute intermittent porphyria, and patients are commonly presented with cutaneous lesions. Elevated urinary ALA, PBG, and porphyrins and highly elevated fecal porphyrins can be found during acute attacks. Increased ALA synthetase has also been demonstrated.

Congenital Erythropoietic Porphyria. This extremely rare autosomal recessive disorder is manifested shortly after birth. It is associated with red pigmented urine, erythrodontia, hemolytic anemia, and severe cutaneous photosensitivity. Splenomegaly and hemolytic anemia typically develop and early death usually occurs. The red urine is the result of excessive excretion of coproporphyrin and uroporphyrin, mainly of type I. The responsible enzyme defects have been attributed to increased activity of ALA synthetase and decreased activity of uroporphyrinogen III cosynthetase.

Erythrohepatic Protoporphyria. This is thus far the only known inherited disorder in which the biochemical lesions are localized in both hepatic and erythropoietic cells. Transmitted as an autosomal dominant trait, it is associated with mild skin photosensitivity. The onset of disease occurs during the first few years of life or adulthood. Laboratory findings are those of abnormally high protoporphyrin in circulating erythrocytes and elevated fecal coproporphyrin and protoporphyrin, which cause the feces to be fluorescent. Overactivity of ALA synthetase appears to be important in the pathogenesis of this disease. It has been proposed that deficient synthesis of heme from protoporphyrin results in deficient production of a specific heme protein that is important in a feedback suppression of ALA synthetase.

Cutaneous Hepatic Porphyria. Except for rare familial cases this group of porphyrias is acquired. Skin lesions are the most obvious clinical feature. The condition has been reported in association with liver disease, particularly with alcohol as the inciting agent, with estrogen therapy, and with ingestion of hexachlorobenzene. Elevated urinary uroporphyrin is the characteristic biochemical finding, while excretion of PBG and ALA is usually normal.

Lead Intoxication. Many of the clinical features of lead poisoning, such as abdominal pain, constipation, and other manifestations of neuropathy, are similar to those of the acute porphyrias. The abnormalities in porphyrin metabolism appear to be the result of the lead inhibiting certain of the enzymes of the heme biosynthetic pathway, including decreased ALA dehydratase, ferrochelatase, and coproporphyrinogen oxidase activity and increased activity of ALA synthetase as a consequence of decreased heme production. Characteristic laboratory findings include elevated urinary ALA and coproporphyrin. The clinical manifestations and laboratory tests of lead intoxication are further discussed in Chapter 17 (p. 372).

Analytical Techniques

A complete laboratory investigation of any disorder of porphyrin generally begins with screening tests for porphyrins or their precursors, ALA and PBG, in urine, feces, and blood. This is usually followed by the appropriate quantitative determinations should the preliminary investigation suggest further study. The typical biochemical findings associated with disorders of porphyrin metabolism are shown in Table 9–2.

All porphyrins have in common a characteristic type of absorption spectrum in the near ultraviolet and visible region, resulting primarily from the conjugated bond system of the tetrapyrrole ring. Hence, all porphyrins have an intense absorption band near 400 nm, known as the Soret band. When irradiated with light of this wavelength, all free porphyrins exhibit an intense red fluorescence. This property enables porphyrins to be detected and quantitated in the laboratory at concentrations of 2×10^{-4} μmol/L. Reference values for porphyrins and their precursors are listed in Table 9–3.

The solubility of both the porphyrins and their precursors decreases with decreasing number of hy-

Table 9–2. TYPICAL BIOCHEMICAL FINDINGS ASSOCIATED WITH DISORDERS OF PORPHYRIN METABOLISM

Disorders	Erythrocyte			Urine				Feces		
	UP	*CP*	*PP*	*ALA*	*PBG*	*UP*	*CP*	*UP*	*CP*	*PP*
Acute intermittent porphyria (AIP)	N	N	N	↑↑	↑↑	↑	↑ or N	N	N	N
Hereditary copro-porphyria	N	N	N	↑	↑	N	↑	N	↑	N
Variegate porphyria (acute attacks)	N	N	N	↑	↑	↑ or N	↑ or N	N	↑	↑↑
Congenital erythropoietic porphyria	↑↑	↑↑	↑	N	N	↑↑	↑	N	↑	N
Erythropoietic proto-porphyria	N	N	↑↑	N	N	N	N	N	↑	↑
Symptomatic porphyria	N	N	N	N	N	↑↑	↑	N	↑ or N	↑ or N
Lead poisoning	N	↑ or N	↑	↑	↑ or N	N	↑	N	N	N

UP = uroporphyrin; CP = coproporphyrin; PP = protoporphyrin; ↑ = increased; ↑↑ = large increase; N = normal.

droxyl and carboxylic groups. Consequently PBG and uroporphyrin are excreted mainly in the urine, while protoporphyrin is excreted exclusively in the bile and thus appears in the feces. Coproporphyrin is excreted mainly in the bile, but also in urine as coproporphyrinogen. The solubility difference plays an important role in the choice of specimen to be analyzed and in the method of measurement.

ALA and PBG. The most widely used screening procedure for excess ALA and PBG was first introduced by Watson (1941). PBG condenses with *p*-dimethylaminobenzaldehyde in hydrochloric acid (HCl) (Ehrlich's reagent) to form a magenta color complex. A description of the analytical techniques and possible interferences is presented in Chapter 18 (p. 443).

Porphyrins. The characteristic red fluorescence exhibited by all porphyrins serves as the basis for the screening tests of porphyrins in urine, feces, and blood. The general procedure involves the extraction of porphyrins into an organic solvent system, e.g., acetic acid/ethyl acetate, followed by re-extraction into HCl. The fluorescence is read with an ultraviolet light source. Comprehensive and rapid porphyrin screening procedures applicable to urine, feces, and blood have been described (Elder, 1980).

Table 9–3. REFERENCE VALUES OF PORPHYRINS AND THEIR PRECURSORS

Analyte	Reference Interval
Erythrocyte	
Coproporphyrin	0.5-2.0 μg/dl (0.75-3.00 nmol/L)
Protoporphyrin	4-52 μg/dl (7.2-93.6 nmol/L)
Urine	
ALA	1.5-7.5 ml/24 h (11.2-57.2 μmol/24 h)
PBG	<1.0 mg/24 h (<4.4 μmol/24 h)
Coproporphyrin	50-160 μg/24 h (0.075-0.24 μmol/24 h)
Uroporphyrin	10-30 μg/24 h (0.012-0.037 μmol/24 h)
Feces	
Coproporphyrin	0-500 μg/24 h (0-0.75 μmol/24 h)
Protoporphyrin	0-600 μg/24 h (0-1.08 μmol/24 h)

Most quantitative measurements of porphyrins are based on preliminary extraction and differentiation by solvent partition followed by spectrophotometric or fluorometric measurement. Although improved resolution of porphyrin fractionation has been achieved in recent years by electrophoresis and by thin layer chromatography after extraction and esterification, these methods are nevertheless technically demanding and time-consuming. With the advent of high-pressure liquid chromatography, rapid identification and quantification of porphyrins have been possible in both urine and feces.

Although the determination of ALA dehydratase has been emphasized as a diagnostic test for lead intoxication, it has met with limited acceptance. Recent interest has focused on the use of erythrocyte protoporphyrin determination as a screening test for lead poisoning. This was motivated in part by the discovery that erythrocyte protoporphyrin exists in "free" form in erythropoietic protoporphyria but is found as zinc protoporphyrin (ZPP) in lead intoxication and in iron deficiency anemias. The prominent fluorescent porphyrin in erythrocytes in chronic lead intoxication has been identified as zinc protoporphyrin, which can be assayed fluorometrically in diluted whole blood. Similar methods employing small sample volumes (10 to 40 μl whole blood) have been proposed by other investigators as screening procedures for lead exposure in children (Orfanos, 1977).

ALA Dehydratase. Clinical tests that have been used for the diagnosis of lead intoxication include blood lead, coproporphyrin, and ALA. Because of inadequate specificity these tests have in recent years been replaced by the determination of ALA dehydratase, particularly since the inhibitory action by lead on this enzyme has been shown to occur long before other biologic effects are measurable. The procedure of choice for measurement of ALA dehydratase appears to be that of Bonsignore or its modifications. This method measures the amount of PBG formed in the crude enzyme assay. However, partial conversion of PBG to porphyrin during the crude enzyme assay has been shown to result in underestimation of its activity and an alternate procedure of measuring the ALA consumed has been proposed (Tomokuni, 1974).

CALCIUM AND PHOSPHORUS

Physiologic Chemistry

Calcium Homeostasis. Calcium is the most abundant mineral element in the human body and the fifth most abundant of all elements. Approximately 98 per cent of the 1000 to 1200 g of calcium in the adult is present in the skeleton, primarily as hydroxyapatite, which is a crystal lattice composed of calcium, phosphorus, and hydroxide. Of the remaining calcium, about half is present in extracellular fluid and the remainder in a variety of tissues, particularly skeletal muscle. Of critical importance to calcium homeostasis is the fact that less than 1 per cent of the total skeletal reservoir of calcium is readily exchangeable with extracellular fluid. In addition to its obvious importance in skeletal mineralization, calcium plays a vital role in such basic physiologic processes as blood coagulation, neuromuscular conduction, maintenance of normal tone and excitability of skeletal and cardiac muscle, stimulus-secretion coupling in various exocrine glands, and preservation of cell membrane integrity and permeability, particularly in terms of sodium and potassium exchange.

The calcium level in serum is maintained within a relatively narrow range of about 9.2 to 11.0 mg/dl (4.6 to 5.5 mEq/L or 2.3 to 2.8 mmol/L) (Reed, 1972). Quoted normal ranges or reference values vary among laboratories, partly as a result of different analytical methods. Three distinct fractions compose the total calcium in serum: (1) free or ionized calcium accounts for about 50 per cent of total calcium; (2) about 5 per cent of total calcium is complexed with a variety of anions, particularly phosphate and citrate; (3) the remaining 45 per cent of calcium is bound to plasma proteins, especially to albumin but also to globulin to a limited extent. Both ionized calcium and the calcium complexes are freely dialyzable. The physiological importance of ionized calcium concentration in extracellular fluid was first established by McLean and Hastings (1935), who observed that the amplitude of contraction of the isolated frog heart is proportional to the ionized calcium concentration. Ionized calcium is also important in such physiologic functions as neuromuscular conduction and blood coagulation. The relative distributions of the three calcium species are altered as a result of change either in pH of the extracellular fluids or in the protein concentration. Acidosis promotes an increase in ionized calcium, while alkalosis causes a corresponding decrease. If ionized calcium is to remain within its normal physiologic range, an increased concentration of plasma proteins will result in a corresponding increase in total calcium, which reflects an increase in bound calcium. Similarly, decreased plasma protein concentration will ordinarily result in decreased total calcium.

The binding of calcium to plasma proteins is a freely reversible process, which is governed by a dissociation constant. The process is thus analogous to the dissociation of a weak acid or base. This was long ago recognized by McLean and Hastings (1935), who represented the relationship as follows:

$$\frac{[Ca^{++}][Pr^{=}]}{[CaPr]} = K$$

where $[Ca^{++}]$ is the concentration of ionized calcium, $[CaPr]$ is the concentration of protein-bound calcium, $[Pr^{=}]$ is the concentration of free protein capable of binding calcium, and K is a constant, which is specific for each protein species and varies with pH and temperature. Simple transposition of this equation serves to emphasize that the concentration of ionized calcium will remain constant and is thus independent of bound calcium as long as the ratio of the concentrations of protein-bound calcium to free protein remains constant:

$$[Ca^{++}] = K\frac{[CaPr]}{[Pr^{=}]}$$

Use has been made of this relationship to construct various equations and nomograms for estimating ionized calcium from measurements of total calcium and protein concentrations. Direct measurement of ionized calcium is now technically reliable and has many clinical applications (Robertson, 1979).

Maintenance of calcium homeostasis involves the participation of three major organs—the small intestine, the kidneys, and the skeleton. The mammary gland is also important during lactation, as are the placenta and fetus during gestation. Although usually ignored in balance studies, the sweat glands are responsible for a small but significant excretion of calcium. In the adult there is no persistent net gain or loss of calcium in health. During growth and pregnancy, a positive calcium balance must be maintained. Calcium homeostasis is regulated by various hormones that act principally upon the major organs involved in calcium metabolism (Lutwak, 1975; Raisz, 1981). The most important hormones are parathyroid hormone and the hormones derived from renal metabolism of vitamin D_3, notably 1,25-dihydroxycholecalciferol. Quite possibly calcitonin plays a role in the regulating process, although its significance in man is still controversial. Other hormones that affect calcium metabolism but whose secretion is determined primarily by factors other than changes in plasma calcium and phosphate include thyroid hormones, growth hormone, adrenal glucocorticoids, and gonadal steroids. Present concepts of the major hormonal regulations of calcium metabolism are summarized in Figure 9–4.

Dietary calcium varies widely for adults from about 200 to 1500 mg/day, most of which in the American diet is derived from milk or other dairy products. The minimum daily dietary requirement for calcium is commonly stated to be 800 mg, but it has been sufficiently demonstrated that calcium balance can be maintained in adults who ingest as little as 200 to 400 mg of calcium daily. It is commonly recom-

2

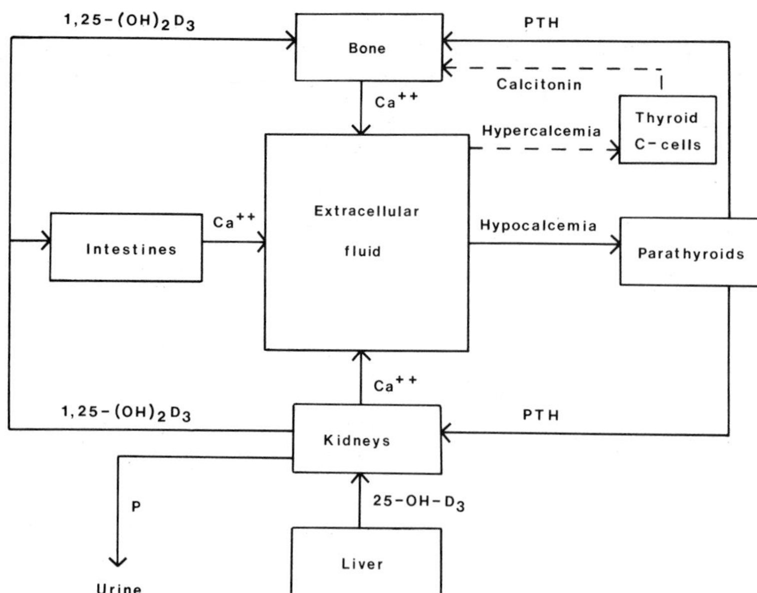

Figure 9–4. Major hormonal regulators of calcium metabolism.

mended that the daily dietary intake of calcium should be about 1200 mg during pregnancy and lactation and 800 to 1200 mg during childhood.

Calcium is absorbed by an active transport process that occurs mostly in the duodenum and upper jejunum. The major stimulus to calcium absorption is vitamin D. Absorption is also enhanced by growth hormone, an acid medium in the intestines, and increased dietary protein. The ratio of calcium to phosphorus in the intestinal contents is also important in that a ratio greater than two tends to inhibit calcium absorption because of the formation of insoluble calcium phosphates. Phytic acid derived from various cereal grains can also form insoluble calcium compounds as can dietary oxalate and fatty acids. Cortisol and excessive alkalinity of the intestinal contents are both inhibitory to calcium absorption. The net absorption of calcium from the intestinal tract is only about 10 to 20 per cent of dietary intake. This approximation is grossly misleading, however, because considerable calcium is actively secreted into the intestines.

Estimates of the daily calcium excretion in sweat vary widely—from 15 to more than 100 mg. The loss can greatly exceed this range during extreme environmental conditions. The major net loss of calcium is urinary excretion, which accounts for 50 to 200 mg or more each day depending on dietary intake. Urinary calcium excretion is enhanced by hypercalcemia, phosphate deprivation, acidosis, and glucocorticoids. Urinary calcium excretion is diminished by parathyroid hormone, certain diuretics, and probably vitamin D.

Phosphorus Homeostasis. Phosphorus is also an abundant element in the body and is omnipresent in its distribution. About 85 per cent of the 500 to 600 g of phosphorus (measured as inorganic phosphorus) in the adult is present in bone as hydroxyapatite. The remaining phosphorus is mostly combined with lipids, proteins, carbohydrates, and other organic substances to fill vital roles as phospholipids, nucleic acids, nucleotides, constituents of cell membranes and cell cytoplasm, and compounds that are important in biochemical energy storage and exchange.

Most of the phosphorus in extracellular fluid is inorganic, predominantly as two species, $HPO_4^{=}$ and $H_2PO_4^-$. Negligible amounts of $PO_4^{\equiv}$ exist in the physiologic pH range. The relative amounts of the two phosphate ions are obviously pH-dependent (Table 9–4). At pH 7.4, the ratio of $HPO_4^{=}$ to $H_2PO_4^-$ is about 4:1. Because of the effect of pH on the relative concentrations of the two phosphate species serum phosphorus should be expressed as milligrams per deciliter. In health, serum phosphorus varies over a rather wide range of 2.4 to 4.7 mg/dl (0.78 to 1.51 mmol/L) (Reed, 1972). Higher phosphorus levels

Table 9–4. pH CONVERSION FACTORS FOR INORGANIC PHOSPHORUS*

pH	Factor
7.10	0.537
7.15	0.546
7.20	0.555
7.25	0.563
7.30	0.570
7.35	0.577
7.40	0.583
7.45	0.589
7.50	0.594
7.55	0.599
7.60	0.603
7.70	0.611

*Milligrams per deciliter × factor = mEq per liter. (With permission of Sunderman, F. W.: Inorganic Phosphorus, Proficiency Test Service, April, 1973, p. 3.)

occur in growing children (4 to 7 mg/dl or 1.30 to 2.25 mmol/L). Ingestion of food can significantly alter serum phosphorus concentration. Ingestion of phosphate-rich food can increase serum phosphorus, while a high carbohydrate meal can cause a significant decrease. Adult values are lower than normal during menstruation.

Three major organs are involved in phosphorus homeostasis: the small intestine, the kidneys, and the skeleton, which functions as a storage reservoir. Phosphorus is present in virtually all foods. Consequently, dietary deficiencies do not occur. The average dietary intake for adults is about 800 to 1000 mg, most of which is derived from milk and dairy products. About two thirds of ingested phosphate is absorbed, mostly in the jejunum. The remaining dietary phosphate is excreted in the feces, mostly as insoluble calcium compounds. Intestinal absorption of phosphate is an active, energy-dependent process. Absorption is increased in association with decreased dietary calcium and increased acidity of the intestinal contents. Absorption is also augmented by the action of vitamin D and growth hormone. The action of parathyroid hormone on the intestinal absorption of phosphate is probably purely indirect through its effect on the metabolism of vitamin D.

Most of the phosphorus absorbed from the intestines of adults who are in phosphorus balance is excreted in the urine. This is equivalent to about 0.35 to 1.0 g of inorganic phosphorus daily. About 90 per cent of plasma phosphorus is filterable by the glomeruli. Ordinarily about 85 to 95 per cent of the filtered phosphate is reabsorbed. Parathyroid hormone inhibits renal tubular reabsorption of phosphate. Whether phosphate is secreted at all by the renal tubules is uncertain.

Parathyroid Hormone. Parathyroid hormone (PTH) is secreted primarily as a single chain polypeptide consisting of 84 amino acids with a molecular mass of 9500 daltons. It is derived from a larger precursor, Pre-ProPTH, of 115 amino acids (Habener, 1981), which undergoes two successive cleavages both at the amino-terminal sequences to yield, first, an intermediate precursor, ProPTH, and then the hormone itself.

Earlier radioimmunoassay studies revealed distinct immunochemical differences between PTH found in the circulation and that present in the glandular extracts. The suggestion of heterogeneous circulating immunoreactive forms of PTH has since been unequivocally confirmed. It is now well known that the circulating immunoreactive PTH exists as a mixture of the intact hormone and lower molecular mass hormonal fragments: the amino-terminal fragments (N-fragment) where the biological activity resides, and the carboxy-terminal fragments (C-fragment) which are inactive. The C-fragment, with a molecular mass of 6000 to 7000 daltons, constitutes the major part of the immunoreactivities of circulating PTH. The intact hormone and the N-fragments are believed to have short half-lives of minutes, while the C-fragment is reported to persist for hours or even days with renal impairment. Although the origin of the C-fragments is not entirely settled, it is generally agreed that while some production may take place in the gland, the major fraction is produced by peripheral conversion. Whereas the liver and the kidneys are the principal organs involved in the metabolism of PTH, the kidneys are the primary site for the removal of C-fragments from circulation.

The primary physiologic function of PTH is to regulate the concentration of ionized calcium in extracellular fluids. PTH secretion ordinarily causes a rise in serum ionized calcium concentration and a fall in phosphorus concentration. By way of an effective negative feedback mechanism, hypercalcemia leads to PTH suppression. The interaction between calcium and phosphorus is complex and involves magnesium in an incompletely understood manner. In severe hypomagnesemia, for example, the action of PTH is impaired. Patients with low serum magnesium concentration often require magnesium to increase the serum PTH levels before the serum calcium concentration can be restored to the desired interval.

The best known effect of PTH is bone resorption to restore extracellular fluid calcium concentration. The site of action of PTH on bone appears to be directed primarily to the stable or established component of bone rather than to the labile component. Bone resorption induced by PTH is mediated by increased activity of osteoclasts. Increased conversion of osteoprogenitor cells to osteoclasts occurs as a consequence of more prolonged PTH stimulation. Additional effects of PTH on bone are increased formation of collagenase, which degrades the matrix of bone, and increased breakdown of the ground substance of bone. The end result of PTH action on bone is thus true bone resorption and not simply demineralization.

The major actions of PTH on the kidneys are the simultaneous reduced reabsorption of sodium, phosphorus, calcium, and bicarbonate ions in the proximal tubule, and the enhanced reabsorption of calcium at the distal tubule. The net effect is a rise in serum calcium concentration and phosphaturia. Although the biochemical mechanisms involved in the renal handling of calcium and phosphorus reabsorption are not completely understood, evidence accumulated thus far is consistent with the hypothesis that the action of PTH in kidney and in bone is mediated through the stimulation of adenyl cyclase activity, which ultimately leads to enhanced cyclic AMP production. These effects precede and presumably mediate changes in phosphorus and calcium transport in kidney and in bone.

The effect of PTH on intestinal absorption of dietary calcium is indirect. PTH stimulates the renal synthesis of the active vitamin D metabolite, 1,25-dihydroxycholecalciferol, which, in turn, acts as a regulator of intestinal calcium absorption.

Vitamin D Compounds. Vitamin D is a generic designation for a group of fat-soluble, structurally similar sterols, several of which are vitally important in calcium and phosphorus metabolism. Some of these sterols appropriately are termed provitamins because they can be transformed into physiologically active compounds by irradiation with ultraviolet light. The two most important vitamins are vitamin D_2 or ergosterol and vitamin D_3 or cholecalciferol. Ergosterol is present in yeast and a variety of plant substances and can be transformed into the antirachitic ergocalciferol by irradiation. Ergocalciferol is the active vitamin D in various commercial vitamin preparations and in irradiated bread. Cholecalciferol, in contrast, is found in certain animal tissues and products, particularly fish livers, the livers of fish-eating mammals, and irradiated milk. Approximately 94 per cent of the vitamins D_2 and D_3 in plasma are bound to a specific inter-alpha globulin with a molecular mass of 60,000 daltons. Excess vitamin D can be stored in tissues, metabolized to inactive products, or excreted in the bile. One reduction product, dihydrotachysterol, is formed from either ergocalciferol or cholecalciferol and has therapeutic uses.

In addition to dietary sources, cholecalciferol is synthesized in the skin by ultraviolet irradiation of 7-dehydrocholesterol. Cholecalciferol is transported to the liver where it undergoes hydroxylation to produce 25-hydroxycholecalciferol (25-$(OH)D_3$). Although 25-$(OH)D_3$ has limited biologic activity, it is the major circulating metabolite of vitamin D_3. In the kidney 25-$(OH)D_3$ undergoes further hydroxylation to form the dihydroxymetabolites 1,25-$(OH)_2D_3$, 24,25-$(OH)_2D_3$, and 25,26-$(OH)_2D_3$. The formation of trihydroxymetabolites, 1,24,25-$(OH)_3D_3$ and 1,25,26-$(OH)_3D_3$, has also been described. Of these, interest has been focused on 25-$(OH)D_3$, 24,25-$(OH)_2D_3$, and 1,25-$(OH)_2D_3$. These metabolites circulate at concentration ratios of approximately 1000:100:1 with reference intervals of 30 ng/ml, 2 ng/ml, and 30 pg/ml, respectively.

It is now known that the formation of 1,25-$(OH)_2D_3$ is regulated by negative feedback mechanism depending on the need for calcium in the circulation. Formation of 1,25-$(OH)_2D_3$ is enhanced by decreased serum phosphate, by PTH, and consequently by any factors that cause augmented secretion of PTH, e.g., hypocalcemia (DeLuca, 1981). Although several specialized functions have been proposed for 24,25-$(OH)_2D_3$, such as normal mineralization of bone, suppression of PTH, and cartilage growth and development, convincing evidence in support of these roles is still pending. On the other hand, 1,25-$(OH)_2D_3$ has been proved to be the most potent metabolite of vitamin D. Under conditions of hypocalcemia, PTH released from the parathyroid glands activates renal 25-hydroxylase to produce 1,25-$(OH)_2D_3$, which independently stimulates intestinal calcium absorption and calcium-dependent phosphate transport. In the bone, 1,25-$(OH)_2D_3$ facilitates the action of PTH to cause mobilization of calcium. The relatively minor effect of 1,25-$(OH)_2D_3$ on the kidneys is to promote reabsorption of calcium and probably also phosphorus. The biochemistry of vitamin D has been extensively reviewed by DeLuca (1981).

Calcitonin. Calcitonin is a peptide hormone produced and secreted by specialized C-cells which are part of the APUD cell system derived embryologically from the neural crest (Chap. 16). In man, the C-cells are represented predominantly as parafollicular cells in the lateral lobes of the thyroid gland. There is evidence of a larger precursor form of calcitonin with a molecular mass of 15,000 daltons, which undergoes several cleavages to yield the major C-cell secretory product, calcitonin monomer of 32 amino acid residues with a molecular mass of 3500 daltons. Available data have also suggested that human calcitonin in the circulation is immunochemically heterogeneous. Structural differences in the hormone among animal species, human, rat, cow, salmon, porcine, and bovine, are reflected in differences in their relative potency. Presently, salmon calcitonin is the only form available in the United States for therapeutic uses.

Although calcitonin was viewed as a major calcium-regulating factor because of its calcium-lowering and phosphorus-lowering properties, evidence accumulated thus far in support of this role has not been conclusive. The major difficulties have been the lack of clearly defined syndromes of calcitonin excess or deficiency under physiological conditions. Secretion of calcitonin is stimulated by an increase in ionic calcium concentration. Many gastrointestinal hormones, such as pentagastrin, glucagon, pancreozymin, and cholecystokinin, are also potent stimuli to calcitonin secretion, thus suggesting a possible physiological role for calcitonin in modulating postprandial hypercalcemia.

The pharmacological action of calcitonin is more definitive. By inhibiting osteoclastic bone resorption, calcitonin causes a decrease in urinary excretion of hydroxyproline. The administration of calcitonin decreases renal tubular resorption of calcium and phosphorus as well as sodium, potassium, and magnesium. Calcitonin decreases gastrin and gastric acid secretion and increases small bowel secretion of sodium, potassium, chloride, and water. Currently, synthetic salmon calcitonin is available as a prescription drug for long-term treatment of Paget's disease of bone and for emergency treatment of hypercalcemia.

Clinicopathologic Correlations

Scientific and technical advancements in clinical laboratory science have been such that precise and accurate determinations of calcium, inorganic phosphate, and alkaline phosphatase in serum are now commonly included in routine health screening or hospital admission profiles. This has resulted in an increasing challenge to the practicing physician, who is more frequently confronted with the interpretation of relatively minor abnormal variations of these analytes. Additional laboratory data are ordinarily required. Determinations of the timed urinary excretions of calcium and inorganic phosphate have long been available but are of limited diagnostic value unless the dietary intake is carefully controlled. Within the past few years, radioimmunoassay of parathyroid hormone has become readily available from reference laboratories. Improved instrumentation is facilitating the routine availability of ionized calcium determinations at least in larger hospitals. Determination of various other analytes can provide valuable information in selected cases, e.g., growth hormone, cortisol, vitamin D metabolites, and hydroxyproline. Nevertheless, the entire constellation of laboratory data related to aberrations in calcium and phosphorus metabolism is seldom both pathognomonic of the disease etiology and indicative of its extent of involvement. Meaningful interpretation of the relevant laboratory data often requires various special studies in addition to a complete history and physical examination. In particular, roentgenographic examinations can provide valuable information regarding both the etiology and extent of disease. Renal function tests and studies of acid-base balance may be indicated. Histopathologic examination of bone biopsies from appropriate sites such as the iliac crest in generalized bone disease or directly from localized lesions can be of unique value in selected cases.

The effects of various diseases on calcium and phosphorus metabolism are summarized in Table 9–5. It is to be emphasized that dietary inadequacies of calcium and phosphorus are seldom the cause of significant metabolic derangements. The high phosphate content of cow's milk can result in deficient calcium absorption and tetany in the newborn. Other factors incriminated in neonatal hypocalcemia include prematurity, vitamin D deficiency, transient physiologic hypoparathyroidism, and decreased ability of the kidneys to excrete inorganic phosphate.

A rare dietary problem affecting calcium and phosphorus metabolism is vitamin D intoxication, which is usually the result of excessive intake of vitamin supplements over a prolonged period of time. Large amounts of vitamin D can be stored in the body, since it is fat-soluble. Clinically the disease is manifested by weakness, irritability, nausea, vomiting, and diarrhea. Plasma calcium is typically elevated, while inorganic phosphorus is variable. The hypercalcemia is the result of both increased intestinal absorption of calcium and increased mobilization from bone. Metastatic calcification of soft tissues and viscera, compromised renal function with frank azotemia, and osteoporosis can occur.

Bone Disease. Most of the body content of calcium and phosphorus is present in bone as a highly structured crystal lattice similar to hydroxyapatite, the general formula of which is $Ca_{10}(PO_4)_6(OH)_2$. Bone minerals also include 70 per cent of the body content of magnesium, 30 per cent of the sodium, and smaller amounts of potassium, carbonate, citrate, and fluoride. The dry weight of compact bone consists of approximately 75 per cent inorganic mineral salts and 25 per cent organic matrix as shown in Table 9–6. Mineralization of bone matrix is not a simple precipitation of salts but rather is a complex, incompletely understood physiochemical process (Parfitt, 1976a). In previous times, the importance to bone mineralization of the solubility product of calcium phosphate, $Ca^{++} \times HPO_4^{=}$, was emphasized. Although the initial salt that is formed may well be $CaHPO_4$, the solubility product explanation is overly simplistic, particularly since extracellular fluid is supersaturated with these ions.

Even in adult life, bone is in a dynamic state, as evidenced by the fact that perhaps 3 to 5 per cent of the bone mass is undergoing active remodeling at any one time. The processes of bone formation and resorption are controlled by various hormonal and metabolic influences (Lutwak, 1975; Deftos, 1975). Bone is formed by the action of osteocytes and osteoblasts, the activity of which is reflected in the alkaline phosphatase level in serum. Bone resorption occurs predominantly as a result of the action of osteoclasts and ordinarily involves dissolution of both minerals and organic matrix. The urinary excretion of hydroxyproline is elevated in association with increased bone resorption, as it is in other etiologies of increased

Table 9–5. TYPICAL CHEMICAL PATHOLOGY FINDINGS IN METABOLIC BONE DISEASES

	Serum				Urine	
Disease	***Ca^{++}***	***$HPO_4^{=}$***	***PTH***	***Alkaline Phosphatase***	***Ca^{++}***	***$H_2PO_4^{-}$***
Primary hyperparathyroidism	↑	↓	↑	N, ↑	↑	↑
Renal osteodystrophy	↓ , N	↑	↑	↑	↓	↓
Vitamin D deficiency (rickets or osteomalacia)	N, ↓	↓	↑	↑	↓	↑
Hypoparathyroidism	↓	↑	↓	N	↓	↓
Pseudohypoparathyroidism	↓	↑	↑	N	↓	↓
Vitamin D resistant rickets	N, ↓	↓	N, ↑	↑	↓	↑
Renal tubular acidosis	N, ↓	↓	N, ↑	↑	↑	↑
Fanconi's syndrome	N, ↓	↓	N, ↑	↑	↑	↑
Idiopathic osteoporosis	N	N	N, ↑	N	N, ↑	N
Paget's disease	N, ↑	N	N	↑	N, ↑	N
Hypophosphatasia	N, ↑	N	—	⇊	N	N
Vitamin D intoxication	↑	N, ↕	↓	N	↑	↑
Fibrous dysplasia	N	N	N	↑	N	N
Osteogenesis imperfecta	N	N	—	N	N	N
Osteopetrosis	N	N	—	N	↓	N

↑ = increase; N = normal; ↕ = increase or decrease; ↓ = decrease; ⇊ = great decrease.

Table 9–6. COMPOSITION OF BONE

Mineral inorganic crystalline salts (75 per cent of dry weight)	Phosphate and carbonate salts of calcium (compressional strength) Small amounts of magnesium, sodium, potassium, hydroxide, fluoride, and sulfate
Organic matrix (25 per cent of dry weight)	94 per cent collagen fibers (tensile strength) (hydroxyproline and proline constitute a third of total amino acid composition of collagen fibrils) 5 per cent ground substance: Extracellular fluid Mucoprotein Chondroitin sulfate Hyaluronic acid 1 per cent citrate

collagen turnover (Table 9–7). This is a result of the fact that collagen is the only mammalian protein that contains significant amounts of hydroxyproline.

Osteoporosis is the most common metabolic disease of bone. It is not a single etiologic entity but rather is associated with a variety of epidemiologic, clinical, and biochemical factors that result in decreased bone mass. The term bone atrophy is sometimes applied to this pathologic process, but this term is imprecise because osteoporosis can occur as a consequence of increased bone resorption, decreased bone formation, or a combination of both factors. Normal mineralization of existing osteoid is a critical feature that distinguishes osteoporosis from osteomalacia. The roentgenographic appearance of diffusely diminished bone density is reflected in the histopathologic appearance of thinned bone cortices and delicate trabeculae. Skeletal deformities, fractures, especially compression fractures of the vertebral bodies, and bone pain are common sequelae.

Table 9–7. ELEVATION OF URINARY HYDROXYPROLINE IN DISEASE*

Marked
- Paget's disease
- Fibrous dysplasia
- Osteomalacia
- Neoplastic bone disease
- Rickets
- Hyperthyroidism
- Hyperparathyroidism (primary and secondary)
- Severe burns
- Acute osteomyelitis
- Congenital hypophosphatasia

Moderate
- Acromegaly
- Marfan's syndrome
- Active rheumatoid arthritis
- Active scleroderma

Normal to slight
- Inflammatory skin diseases
- Osteoporosis
- Pregnancy
- Aseptic bone necrosis
- Diabetes mellitus
- Renal disease

*Niejadlik, D. C.: Postgrad. Med. *51* (No. 5):214, 1972.

The various etiologies of osteoporosis are shown in Table 9–8. The most common type by far is postmenopausal or senile osteoporosis, which is far more common with aging and is three to four times more frequent in females than in males. There are various theories as to the etiologic factors in senile osteoporosis, including diminished physical activity, deficiency of gonadal hormones, and dietary inadequacies. Urinary calcium and hydroxyproline excretions are frequently increased. Other parameters of calcium and phosphorus metabolism are usually normal. In contrast, both calcium and inorganic phosphate in plasma can be elevated in rapidly developing osteoporosis of disuse such as occurs following immobilization or paralysis in a previously active individual.

Osteomalacia refers to deficient mineralization of bone resulting from various disturbances in calcium and phosphorus metabolism. Osteoid formation continues, but the bones become softened. Weakness, skeletal pain and deformities, and fractures can occur as the disease progresses. Roentgenographic examination reveals generalized rarefaction of the skeleton with an accentuated trabecular pattern. Rickets is the designation for osteomalacia that occurs prior to cessation of growth, i.e., closure of the epiphyses of bones. The skeletal deformities in rickets are accentuated as a consequence of compensatory overgrowth of epiphyseal cartilage, wide bands of which remain unmineralized and unresorbed. In severe cases of rickets, decreased growth can be associated with such evident deformities as swellings of the costochondral

Table 9–8. ETIOLOGIC CLASSIFICATION OF OSTEOPOROSIS

Primary (idiopathic, postmenopausal, senile)

Secondary
- Hyperparathyroidism
- Cushing's syndrome
- Hyperthyroidism
- Acromegaly
- Heparin therapy (prolonged high dosage)
- Vitamin D excess
- Immobilization
- Pregnancy (rare cause)
- Miscellaneous (diabetes, liver disease, sickle cell anemia, various lipid or carbohydrate storage diseases)

junctions of the ribs (rachitic rosary), a protuberant sternum, frontal bossing, and delayed closure of the anterior fontanelle.

There are various etiologies of osteomalacia. Vitamin D deficiency is particularly important in childhood and can be caused by inadequate dietary intake, intestinal malabsorption, or diminished synthesis of active metabolites as a consequence of inadequate exposure to sunlight. Dietary deficiency is very uncommon in America because of the widespread use of fortified milk and bread and vitamin supplements. When vitamin D deficiency occurs in adults it is usually a consequence of malabsorption. Because vitamin D is a fat-soluble vitamin, its absorption is impaired in sprue, biliary or pancreatic disease, or steatorrhea from other causes. A systemic resistance to vitamin D can be of major importance in the osteomalacia that accompanies chronic renal disease. Dietary inadequacy of calcium is a rare cause of osteomalacia, while dietary deficiencies of phosphorus do not occur. Increased loss of inorganic phosphorus in the urine occurs in various renal tubular disorders and can result in osteomalacia. These diseases include vitamin D–resistant rickets (phosphate diabetes), renal tubular acidosis, and the Fanconi syndrome.

A rare cause of osteomalacia is hypophosphatasia, an inherited autosomal recessive disease characterized by a significant depression of alkaline phosphatase in both plasma and tissues. Concentrations of calcium and phosphorus in plasma are normal or increased. Urinary excretion of hydroxyproline is decreased. A curious finding is the presence of significant amounts of phosphoethanolamine in urine.

It is not currently possible to designate a common denominator in the pathogenesis of osteomalacia. Formerly, the criticality of the solubility product of calcium phosphate, $Ca^{++} \times HPO_4^{=}$, was emphasized. In chronic renal disease, however, osteomalacia can progress in the presence of a normal or even elevated solubility product. Other etiologies, including vitamin D deficiency, can cause severe osteomalacia in the presence of normal or only slightly decreased serum calcium concentration. Phosphate depletion is probably of greater importance than decreased calcium.

Osteitis deformans or Paget's disease of bone is a disorder of varying severity, which can involve only one bone or be more or less generalized. Osteoclastic resorption of bone, extensive production of abnormal, poorly mineralized osteoid, and fibrous tissue proliferation result in bone that is structurally weak and prone to deformities and fractures. Osteogenic sarcoma is a late complication in a small percentage of cases. Serum calcium and inorganic phosphorus concentrations are usually normal but occasionally are elevated. Of particular significance is the greatly elevated alkaline phosphatase activity in plasma, which reflects the active but pathologic osteoblastic proliferation. Urinary excretion of calcium and phosphorus is normal or increased, while excretion of hydroxyproline is usually significantly increased.

Osteitis deformans frequently responds both clinically and pathologically to therapeutic administration of calcitonin.

Parathyroid Diseases. Primary hyperparathyroidism is characterized by excessive secretion of parathyroid hormone (PTH) in the absence of an appropriate physiologic stimulus, i.e., hypersecretion co-existent with normal or elevated serum ionized calcium. The etiologic frequency of primary hyperparathyroidism has been reported to be single parathyroid adenomas in 92 per cent, multiple adenomas in 4 per cent, hyperplasia in 3 per cent, and carcinoma in fewer than 1 per cent of cases (Goldman, 1971). Uncomplicated primary hyperparathyroidism is characteristically associated with elevated serum calcium and decreased serum inorganic phosphorus (Table 9–5) and frequently accompanied by a mild systemic acidosis. PTH acts directly on bone to cause increased resorption and consequent increase in serum calcium (Parfitt, 1976b). Two other factors also contribute to the elevated serum calcium. PTH stimulates increased renal biosynthesis of 1,25-$(OH)_2D_3$, which increases intestinal absorption of calcium. PTH also augments renal tubular reabsorption of calcium. The decreased concentration of inorganic phosphate is primarily the result of PTH-induced phosphate diuresis caused by decreased renal tubular reabsorption.

The bone lesions of hyperparathyroidism, often termed osteitis fibrosa cystica or von Recklinghausen's disease of bone, are of particular clinical and pathologic importance (Parfitt, 1976c). Increased osteoblastic activity leads to extensive bone resorption with thinning of both cortical and cancellous bone. In addition to severe osteoporosis, extensive fibroblastic proliferation occurs in the marrow spaces and can cause cystic lesions. Bone pain, skeletal deformities, and fractures can result.

In the past, the general assumption was that patients with primary hyperparathyroidism have autonomous PTH secretion. Data from PTH radioimmunoassays, however, clearly reveal that most if not all patients with primary hyperparathyroidism exhibit a suppression of PTH secretion with calcium infusion (Murray, 1972). It can thus be concluded that the set point in the feedback mechanism operates at a higher than normal level. Plasma PTH values obtained by radioimmunoassay cannot always differentiate between hyperparathyroidism and healthy individuals because considerable overlap occurs between the two groups. This discrepancy is resolved in most cases, however, when serum PTH values are compared with plasma ionized calcium concentrations. The discrimination is made on the basis that in a healthy individual, serum calcium concentration bears an inverse relationship to the PTH concentration. Thus, while the plasma PTH concentration can be within the reference range for patients with primary hyperparathyroidism, this level is inappropriately high when coexistent with hypercalcemia (Arnaud, 1971). Hence, the demonstration of detectable amounts of circulating PTH in the presence of elevated calcium is strongly indicative of primary hyperparathyroidism.

Detection of excessive phosphate diuresis is sometimes helpful in distinguishing hyperparathyroidism from other etiologies of hypercalcemia (Gordan, 1968). This can be achieved by determining the tubular reabsorption of phosphate (TRP) or the renal phosphate clearance (C_p) according to the following equations:

$$TRP(\%) = 100\left[1 - \frac{P_u \times Cr_s}{P_s \times Cr_u}\right]$$

$$C_p(ml/min) = \frac{V/t \times P_u}{P_s}$$

where P_u and P_s are the inorganic phosphate concentrations (mg/dl) in urine and serum.
Cr_u and Cr_s are the creatinine concentrations (mg/dl) in urine and serum.
V is the urine volume collected in an established time interval (t).

The TRP is not applicable even in mild azotemia. The TRP is normally 80 to 90 per cent, while the C_p is normally 5 to 15 ml/min. In hyperparathyroidism the TRP is usually less than 78 per cent, while the C_p is greater than 18 ml/min.

Secondary hyperparathyroidism is characterized by an appropriately excessive secretion of PTH in response to chronic hypocalcemia. In the United States and Europe most cases of chronic hypocalcemia are the result of either vitamin D deficiency or renal disease; hypocalcemia is rarely caused by an inadequate dietary intake of calcium. Vitamin D deficiency leads to decreased absorption of both calcium and phosphate so that both the serum calcium and inorganic phosphorus are low. Increased PTH secretion tends to increase calcium toward normal but to suppress inorganic phosphorus even further because of the increased renal loss of phosphate under the influence of PTH (Table 9–5).

Chronic renal failure can result in compensatory hyperparathyroidism, which in turn causes diffuse bone disease, including osteoporosis, osteomalacia, osteosclerosis (areas of increased bone density), osteitis fibrosa cystica, and metastatic calcification. The disease complex is sometimes termed renal osteodystrophy or, when it occurs in children, renal rickets. The bone manifestations of chronic renal disease are seen more often now that life is prolonged with maintenance hemodialysis. The interrelationships in hyperparathyroidism secondary to chronic renal disease are very complex, as shown in Figure 9–5. The pathogenesis varies somewhat, depending upon the nature and severity of the renal disease. Decreased renal excretion of phosphate as a consequence of impaired glomerular filtration is of paramount importance. Diminished responsiveness to vitamin D and probably decreased renal biosynthesis of 1,25-$(OH)_2D_3$ are also important. The effectiveness of PTH is compromised by the functional deficiency of vitamin D and the inability of the renal tubules to respond with a phosphate diuresis. Increased fecal loss of calcium also occurs. There is evidence that normal calcification is impeded by circulating inhibitors.

Hypoparathyroidism is usually the result of parathyroidectomy, frequently as an unintentional consequence of thyroidectomy. Uncommonly it can result from an idiopathic lack of parathyroid function. Lack of parathyroid hormone from whatever cause leads to a fall in plasma calcium and a corresponding rise in plasma inorganic phosphorus concentration. There is increasing evidence that the biosynthesis of 1,25-$(OH)_2D_3$ can be impaired as a result of PTH deficiency and perhaps also hyperphosphatemia. The most important clinical manifestations are directly attributable

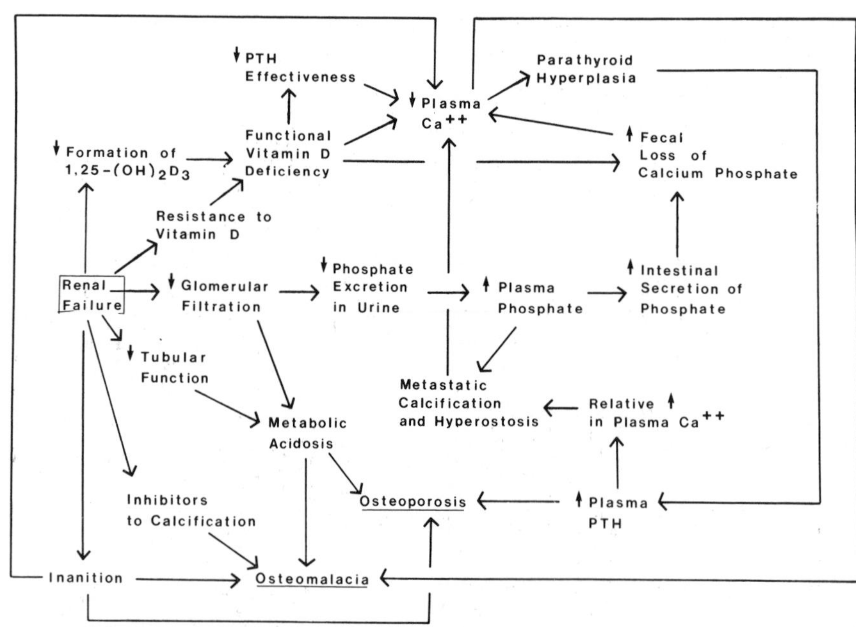

Figure 9–5. Pathophysiologic interrelationships in hyperparathyroidism associated with chronic renal disease.

to decreased ionized calcium concentrations in plasma, which can cause increased neuromuscular excitability and tetany.

Pseudohypoparathyroidism is a rare genetic disorder characterized by signs and symptoms of hypoparathyroidism. It is, however, distinguishable from true hypoparathyroidism in that plasma calcium concentration is low and plasma phosphorus high in spite of an increased concentration of PTH in plasma. Moreover, while infusion of PTH into patients with hypoparathyroidism generally results in a marked increase in both urinary cyclic AMP and inorganic phosphate excretion, PTH infusion into patients with pseudohypoparathyroidism causes a distinctly subnormal response in both urinary phosphate excretion and cyclic AMP production. This has been interpreted as a genetically determined inability of the renal tubules to respond to PTH. The term pseudo-pseudohypoparathyroidism has been used to describe patients with skeletal manifestation of the disease whose plasma calcium and phosphorus metabolism are normal. These are only variations in the same basic genetic defect, as evidenced by the fact that both manifestations can occur in a single kindred.

Hypercalcemia commonly accompanies the metastases of malignant neoplasms to bone, usually as a consequence of rapid bone resorption as the metastases enlarge. Occasional malignant neoplasms, particularly those of the lung, kidney, and ovary, secrete parathyroid hormone to such an extent that true hyperparathyroidism develops. This condition has been termed the ectopic PTH syndrome. Hypercalcemia can also be caused by vitamin D–like compounds produced by neoplasms, especially carcinoma of the breast. One feature that is sometimes useful in distinguishing the two neoplastic etiologies of hypercalcemia is the inorganic phosphorus level in plasma, which tends to be low in association with ectopic PTH production and normal or elevated in association with simple bone resorption secondary to metastases.

Renal Diseases. Chronic renal failure, discussed previously as an important etiology of secondary hyperparathyroidism, is by far the most important renal disease affecting calcium and phosphorus metabolism. In addition, however, several uncommon or rare renal tubular defects can significantly affect calcium and phosphorus metabolism.

Vitamin D–resistant rickets, also termed familial hypophosphatemia and phosphate diabetes, is inherited, usually as a sex-linked dominant character. The exact pathogenesis of the disease is not known with certainty but is believed to be a primary defect in the ability of the renal tubules to reabsorb inorganic phosphorus. Renal phosphate clearance is definitely increased and accounts for the associated hypophosphatemia. Plasma calcium is usually normal, while alkaline phosphatase is moderately elevated. The disease can be asymptomatic or manifested by severe osteomalacia or rickets and growth retardation. The disease can be treated with some success using dietary phosphorus supplementation and high doses of vitamin D.

Renal tubular acidosis consists of both inherited and acquired conditions having in common a metabolic acidosis resulting from decreased ability of the renal tubules to secrete hydrogen ions. The defect can involve primarily either the proximal or distal tubules. The disease inherited as an autosomal dominant and involving the distal tubules is of particular importance to calcium and phosphorus metabolism. Increased calcium excretion occurs, but plasma calcium is usually normal, probably as a consequence of compensatory stimulation of the parathyroids to secrete PTH. Increased phosphate excretion typically leads to low plasma inorganic phosphorus. These factors lead to osteomalacia, which is aggravated by the systemic acidosis. Renal calculi are common sequelae.

The Fanconi syndrome consists of inherited renal diseases characterized by increased urinary excretion of phosphate, glucose, and amino acids, low plasma inorganic phosphorus, and systemic acidosis. Acquired diseases can have identical manifestations. The pathogenesis of the osteomalacia that develops is not well understood.

Calcitonin and Other Hormones. No essential physiologic role has yet been established for calcitonin. The only known cause for excessive secretion of calcitonin is medullary carcinoma of the thyroid, which originates from the parafollicular C-cells. This neoplasm is frequently familial, and kindred of affected patients frequently have elevated levels of calcitonin in their plasma. The elevated levels of calcitonin are associated with decreased skeletal remodeling, but there is no appreciable effect on plasma calcium and phosphorus.

Hyperthyroidism is associated with hypercalciuria, hyperphosphatemia, elevated alkaline phosphatase activity, and occasionally hypercalcemia. There is marked increase in bone turnover and in skeletal remodeling. It is believed that thyroxine acts directly on bone to cause greater bone resorption than formation. This results in a decreased PTH secretion, which accounts for the diminished activity of PTH and vitamin D (Raisz, 1981).

The effect of growth hormone upon skeletal growth has recently been revealed to be mediated indirectly via somatomedin. In adults growth hormone is not necessary for the maintenance of mineral homeostasis. Growth hormone induces an increase in both intestinal absorption and renal reabsorption of calcium and phosphorus. Because of this positive balance with regard to skeletal mass, growth hormone has been proposed as a therapeutic agent for the treatment of osteoporosis.

Administration of glucocorticoids results in a decrease in both intestinal absorption and renal tubular reabsorption of calcium. Consequently PTH secretion is stimulated and increased bone resorption occurs. Osteoporosis is indeed a prominent sign of Cushing's disease. However, the mode of action of cortisol, either in bone or in the intestine, is still unclear.

The effects of estrogens upon bone metabolism are still not clearly defined. While short-term estrogen administration seems to favor bone formation, long-term administration can apparently result in hypocalcemia and secondary hyperparathyroidism. Recent evidence has further suggested that the prostaglandins can also play a role in bone metabolism (Raisz, 1981).

Analytical Techniques

Total Calcium. The oldest procedure for the determination of total serum calcium concentration is that of Clark and Collip. Calcium in serum is precipitated as calcium oxalate, which is subsequently redissolved with acidification. The resulting oxalic acid is titrated against potassium permanganate in a redox reaction, in which the purple $Mn_2O_7^{=}$ is reduced to the colorless Mn^{++}. This method, although highly reliable and regarded for many years as the reference procedure, requires meticulous attention in order to achieve good accuracy and is time consuming. The Clark-Collip procedure has in recent years been replaced by the more convenient and accurate methods involving photometry, fluorometry, and atomic absorption spectrophotometry.

The first direct determination of serum calcium involved titration with the calcium chelating agent ethylenediaminetetraacetic acid (EDTA), using a fluorescent indicator, calcein, to which calcium is complexed. Alternatively, the fluorometric determination of calcium-calcein complex provided a sensitive method for calcium determination which is suitable for pediatric specimens. However, this method is susceptible to interferences by copper, iron, zinc, and certain drugs such sulfadiazine, heparin, and acetylsalicylic acid.

Attempts at determining serum calcium concentration by flame photometry have not met with much success because of positive interference by sodium and potassium, inhibitory interference by phosphates and sulfates, and the fact that excitation of the calcium atom itself is difficult. Isolation of calcium as the oxalate to eliminate interfering substances has not been successful because oxalate itself lowers the emission, probably as a result of the introduction of degradation products with low excitation potential.

With the advent of the automated analyzers, simple chemical methods for the determination of calcium based on color complex formation have found wide application. For example, color complex formation between calcium and *o*-cresolphthalein complex and its subsequent spectrophotometric quantitation is now the most popular automated method. In this procedure, 8-hydroxyquinoline is added to bind magnesium, which otherwise would cause interference. Other automated methods include color complex formation of calcium with alizarin, subsequent quantitation by spectrophotometry, and complex formation of calcium with calcein plasmo-corinth B and glyoxal-dis-(2-hydroxyanil)-GBHA. The precision obtained with automated instruments is in the magnitude of $\pm$ 3 per cent.

In terms of accuracy, precision, and speed, the determination of serum calcium concentration by atomic absorption spectrophotometry is undoubtedly the method of choice both for routine analysis and as a reference procedure. Calcium in serum and urine is diluted sufficiently with lanthanum chloride solution, which binds interfering substances such as protein and phosphates. When introduced into a flame, the dissociated free calcium atom absorbs light from the characteristic wavelengths (e.g., 422.7 nm) produced by a hollow cathode lamp with a calcium filament. A small fraction of calcium atoms (about 1/1000) is raised to high energy level, and on returning to the ground state emits radiation, the intensity of which is proportional to the calcium concentration in the sample. Precision achievable on standard instruments is about $\pm$3.5 per cent. Serum calcium determination has been extensively reviewed by Robertson (1979).

In general, specimens for total calcium determination should be serum or heparinized plasma collected in the fasting state. Oxalate and EDTA interfere with most determinations, since the former causes precipitation and the latter results in chelation of calcium, thus rendering it unavailable for analysis. Total calcium concentrations are known to be affected also by prolonged venous occlusion and by posture. The former leads to hemoconcentration, thereby causing an increase in the calcium values while patients in a recumbent posture have lower calcium concentrations. Both factors, however, appear to affect mainly the protein-bound fraction of the calcium concentration.

Ionized Calcium. A prerequisite for the determination of ionized calcium is that the equilibrium between ionized and protein-bound calcium in serum not be affected at all stages of the procedure. The development of calcium ion selective electrode for the measurement of ionized calcium has largely replaced the earlier colorimetric methods with use of calcium-sensitive dyes murexide and tetramethyl murexide, since the ion selective electrode technique offers speed, simplicity, and improved assay precision. Several types of electrodes are now commercially available. Although each differs in its ion selectivity characteristics, all appear to operate satisfactorily in serum, and in some cases in blood, to give moderately fast and fairly accurate ionized calcium results. An automated system, Orion model SS-20, based on a flow-through electrode with liquid ion-exchange impregnated membrane, permits simple and rapid determinations on relatively small sample volumes (0.5 ml), and is amenable to stat operation. The AMT Electrion system measures ionized calcium using solid-state, specific calcium ion dip electrodes. This system provides temperature regulation and adjustment of pH with CO_2 gas. It enables the use of serum standards on routine runs since all samples are titrated to pH 7.4 prior to measurement. This eliminates protein contamination of the liquid membrane and allows assay of samples which have not been collected anaerobically. The between-run precision is generally within the range of 2 per cent CV. The reference interval is 2.0 to 2.4 mEq/L (1.0 to 1.2 mmol/L).

Because the ionized calcium fraction is pH dependent, the most important condition throughout the analysis is the maintenance of a constant pH. Unless the sample is analyzed on an instrument that permits re-equilibration of pH, blood collection and specimen handling procedure should be conducted anaerobically, and the red cells separated as soon as clotting is complete to obviate pH changes. Variations in serum ionized calcium concentration due to the effect of pH changes can be corrected for, provided that the values both at the time of collection of blood sample and at the time of analysis are known (Wybenga, 1976). The requisite equation is applicable to wide fluctuations in pH and is independent of protein concentration. Hyperventilation sufficient to cause an increase of 0.1 to 0.2 pH unit of blood pH is known to produce up to a 10 per cent reduction in ionized calcium concentration. It is therefore imperative that the state of ventilation be normal during sampling. Prolonged venous occlusion will influence the total serum calcium concentration if pH changes occur as a result. While short-term change in posture does not affect the ionized calcium concentration, long-term bed rest increases both the total and the ionized calcium concentration as a result of increased mobilization from bone.

Ionized calcium in serum is also temperature dependent, and measurement at 37°C. is recommended. Although serum, plasma, and blood are all purported to be acceptable specimens for ionized calcium determination, common anticoagulants, e.g., heparin and citrate, have been shown to decrease ionized calcium concentration. The use of plasma and heparinized blood is therefore not recommended. Because the ion selective electrode responds to the presence of other ions in the sample, serum or aqueous standard should contain ionic compositions of sodium and magnesium similar to those in the serum of healthy individuals. The topic of ionized calcium in serum is extensively reviewed by Robertson (1979).

Although ionized calcium concentration is generally proportional to that of the total calcium over a wide range of serum calcium concentration, its determination may be of use in certain clinical conditions. These include disorders of acid-base balance in which ionized calcium is altered without affecting total calcium concentration, hemodialysis where change in protein concentration may affect total calcium but not ionized calcium, myeloma and renal failure, cirrhosis, and treatment with thiazide diuretics.

Phosphorus. Most methods for phosphorus determination are based on the principle that under suitable conditions molybdates react with phosphate to form various heteropoly compounds, such as ammonium phosphomolybdate, which is believed to have the formula $(NH_4)_3[PO_4(MoO_3)_{12}]$. Different techniques have been employed in the quantitation of this complex. An ultramicro-method has been described in which the phosphomolybdate is determined by acidimetric titration. Direct measurement of this complex at 340 nm is now adapted for use as an automated procedure. To improve assay sensitivity, the phosphomolybdate has also been extracted into xylene-isobutanol prior to spectrophotometric determination at 310 nm. However, most of the techniques for the determination of phosphorus involve photometric measurement of the molybdenum blue formed by reduction of phosphomolybdate under conditions that do not reduce the excess molybdate present. Various reducing agents have been introduced, including stannous chloride, *p*-aminonaphtholsulfonic acid, ascorbic acid, *p*-methylaminophenolsulfate (Elon), N-phenyl-*p*-phenylenediamine, and ferrous sulfate. Most procedures involve proteinization with trichloroacetic acid. The protein-free filtrate is mixed with molybdic acid to form phosphomolybdate that is reduced with the appropriate reducing agent to produce molybdenum blue. Quantitation is usually carried out at 660 nm. A modification using iron (Fe^{++}) and thiourea is the method of choice because of its color stability, improved sensitivity, and conformity to Beer's law over a wide range of concentrations. The precision of this method is reported to be in the range of ±5 per cent.

Complex formation between phosphomolybdate and the triphenylmethane dye malachite green appears to be the most sensitive procedure known for phosphorus determination. Unfortunately, the high acidity at which complex is formed also causes hydrolysis of organic phosphates. An enzymatic method for phosphorus determination is also described whereby phosphorus undergoes successive enzymatic reactions catalyzed by glycogen phosphorylase, phosphoglucomutase, and glucose-6-phosphate dehydrogenase. The NADPH produced can be quantitated fluorometrically or spectrophotometrically. The reaction takes place at neutral pH, thus permitting the measurement of inorganic phosphorus in the presence of unstable organic phosphates. Since organic phosphates exist principally in the erythrocytes, it is important to separate serum from the red cells as soon as clotting is complete.

2

Hydroxyproline. Since more than 90 per cent of the hydroxyproline in urine is present as a component of oligopeptides, almost all laboratory procedures begin with acid hydrolysis of the sample. The liberated hydroxyproline is then oxidized by chloramine T to pyrrole, which reacts with Ehrlich's reagent to form a red chromogen that is determined colorimetrically. However, most hydrolysates of urine also contain ammonium chloride, glucose, and mannitol, which interfere with color formation. Various modifications to this procedure have been developed in an effort to improve assay specificity. For example, the use of a cation-exchange resin is recommended for the separation of hydroxyproline from interfering contaminants prior to hydrolysis, oxidation, and color development. Alternately, the isolation of the oxidized product by distillation or extraction with toluene has successfully eliminated interferences caused by non-volatile color compounds produced by tyrosine and tryptophan. This procedure is found to yield accurate results, provided care is taken to avoid loss of the volatile oxidation products.

Another method using charcoal-butanol extraction of an acid hydrolysate of urine followed by colorimetric determination with *p*-dimethylaminobenzaldehyde has been described (Ritchie, 1977). Results obtained by this procedure compare favorably with those obtained from a more specific method requiring ion-exchange chromatography.

For the determination of free hydroxyproline, the initial acid hydrolysis step is omitted.

Parathyroid Hormone. Although the measurement of PTH by radioimmunoassay was first described by Berson in 1963, only in recent years has this assay found widespread clinical application. The theoretical and technical problems contributing to this delay are many. Important considerations include the heterogeneous nature of PTH in the circulation. insufficient availability of highly purified human PTH for general use, and the limited supply of well characterized antisera. Thus earlier RIA's have been plagued with lack of sensitivity to detect PTH in all healthy individuals, significant overlap between healthy subjects and surgically proven hyperparathyroid patients, and highly discrepant assay results from different laboratories. In recent years, greater understanding of PTH physiology and improved technology have helped in the production of antisera of desired specificity, enabling reliable assays to be developed and meaningful interpretations be made on the assay results (Hawker, 1978).

Currently, two basic types of assays are available in several specialized reference laboratories and medical centers. Bovine PTH is generally used as the assay standard and the antibodies used are directed predominantly against either the N-terminal or the C-terminal sequences of the PTH molecule. These determinations are respectively termed N-terminal or intact PTH and C-terminal assays. Either assay can generally differentiate patients with primary hyperparathyroidism from healthy subjects. However, the assay for intact hormone or the N fragments relies on the use of simultaneous determination of calcium and the formal discriminate analysis of calcium versus PTH. Primary hyperparathyroidism is characterized by an inappropriately high concentration of PTH in the presence of an increased concentration of total calcium. This degree of differentiation can more frequently be achieved with the C-terminal assay alone. Overlap between these two groups is also less with the C-terminal PTH assay, presumably because of the longer half-life of the C-fragments in circulation and of the relatively low ratio of C-fragment/intact hormone in healthy individuals. Ectopic hyperparathyroidism, distinguished from primary hyperparathyroidism by lower PTH values at higher calcium concentrations, can be better differentiated by the C-terminal PTH assay, which is also useful in detecting secondary and tertiary hyperparathyroidism in chronic renal failure because C-fragment values are characteristically extremely elevated and can increase earlier than values for intact hormone after onset of the disease. Because the C-fragments are dependent on renal function, C-terminal assays may not reflect the state of PTH glandular function while the patient is under treatment. To this end, the intact hormone assay is a more meaningful guide to the response of patients to therapy. The intact hormone assay is also useful in the venous catheterization procedure for the preoperative localization of hyperparathyroid tissue. Either the intact or the C-terminal PTH assay can be useful for hypocalcemic disorders. The reference intervals reported for these assays vary according to the nature of the antisera used. Some of the reference values are 210 to 310 pg/ml for intact PTH, 230 to 630 pg/ml for N-terminal assay, and both 180 to 280 pg/ml and 410 to 1760 pg/ml for the C-terminal assays as quoted by separate reference laboratories.

Vitamin D Compounds. The laborious classical bioassay of vitamin D, the rat-line test, which measures the concentrations of all vitamin D precursors and metabolites, has in recent years been replaced by specific assays for the individual metabolites.

Since 25-(OH)D_3 is the most abundant metabolite in the circulation, several competitive protein binding methods using high-affinity binding protein to this metabolite have been developed. This technique provides exquisite sensitivity, requires small sample volume, and is amenable to assaying a large number of samples simultaneously. Unfortunately, interferences from other metabolites that compete with the binding protein compromise method precision, and partial chromatographic separation prior to assay is necessary. High pressure liquid chromatography (HPLC) is rapidly becoming the technique of choice for measuring 25-(OH)D_3 levels in biological fluids because this method offers sensitivity, precision, and specificity without being technically cumbersome. As the major circulating metabolite, 25-(OH)D_3 provides an index of vitamin D status. The reference intervals, however, are subject to seasonal variations because its concentrations are affected by solar exposure. Circulating 25-(OH)D_3 levels are also affected by prior administration of vitamin D. Although both reduced 25-(OH)D_3 and osteomalacia are encountered in anticonvulsant therapy, lowered 25-(OH)D_3 level itself does not appear to cause osteomalacia since these drugs directly inhibit calcium transport in bone and intestine. Measurement of 25-(OH)D_3 is of limited use in patients with renal disorders because of interference to the conversion to 1,25-$(OH)_2D_3$ in the kidney. Although increased levels of 25-(OH)D_3 are associated with vitamin D intoxication, a precise level at which intoxication occurs has not been established.

Much attention has recently been focused on the determination of 1,25-$(OH)_2D_3$ because of its physiological importance as well as its clinical uses. Patients with disturbed calcium metabolism tend to show significantly different mean values compared with those of the healthy individuals. Lowered 1,25-$(OH)_2D_3$ concentrations are associated with renal osteodystrophy, vitamin D–resistant rickets, hypoparathyroidism, rickets, and pseudohypoparathyroidism. Elevated levels of 1,25-$(OH)_2D_3$ are found in hyperparathyroidism and in acromegaly. The low circulating level of this metabolite necessitates extensive purification prior to its measurement. Radioimmunoassay has been attempted, but the lack of antibody specificity precludes its use in distinguishing 1,25-$(OH)_2D_3$ from other metabolites. Recently, quantitative separation of 25-(OH)D_3, 24,25-$(OH)_2D_3$, and 1,25-$(OH)_2D_3$ from the same sample by HPLC followed by individual measurement of these metabolites using appropriate competitive protein binding assays has been reported. One source of specific cytosolic receptor for assaying 1,25-$(OH)_2D_3$ is from the intestinal mucosa of a rachitic chick; the preparation of the receptor protein requires three distinct chromatographic steps. This assay is available in several specialized reference laboratories and medical centers. The reference values are in the range of 30 pg/ml. The clinical implications of measurements of circulating vitamin D metabolites have been extensively reviewed by Mawer (1980).

Calcitonin. Calcitonin was previously measured by a bioassay based on the ability of calcitonin to lower serum calcium concentration in rats. This method was subsequently replaced by the more sensitive radioimmunoassays, which utilize antisera prepared against calcitonin from extracts of medullary thyroid carcinoma. Earlier radioimmunoassays, however, still failed to detect calcitonin in most healthy individuals. The availability of synthetic human calcitonin in recent years has increased assay sensitivity to enable definitive measurement of calcitonin levels in healthy individuals (reference interval $<$ 100 pg/ml). Nevertheless, extremely variable reference intervals of up to 600 pg/ml have also been reported. The issue is further complicated by the finding that heterogeneity of immunoreactive calcitonin occurs in patients with medullary carcinoma, which adds uncertainty to the interpretation of assay results. Other techniques for measuring calcitonin have also been reported. They include a specific receptor assay which utilizes cell membrane preparation from renal tissue, and a calcitonin receptor assay linked to an adenylate cyclase system. Calcitonin measured by either assay is presumably biologically active. However, assay sensitivity does not appear adequate for routine use (Austin, 1981).

The most valuable aspect of the calcitonin assay is in the diagnosis and management of medullary carcinoma of the thyroid. This neoplasm is calcitonin producing and is familial. In a significant number of patients affected with the disease, the baseline levels of calcitonin are normal. However, stimulation with an appropriate secretagogue, such as calcium infusion or pentagastrin injection, or both, usually results in an abnormally large increase in serum calcitonin levels (Hennessy, 1974). These provocative tests have proved useful in the diagnosis of medullary thyroid carcinoma even in the premalignant and hyperplastic phase of the disease, and facilitate identification of individuals with abnormal C-cell mass at a sufficiently early stage. It is recommended that the stimulation test be conducted on kindreds of affected patients. In case of a normal response, the procedure should be repeated periodically.

Other disease states associated with increased concentration of calcitonin include the Zollinger-Ellison syndrome, pyknodysostosis, chronic hypocalcemia, carcinoid neoplasms, and non-thyroidal neoplasms such as breast cancer and oat-cell and squamous cell carcinomas of the lung.

Cyclic AMP. Sensitive assays are available for the determination of urinary cyclic AMP. A competitive protein-binding procedure utilizes a binding protein from either the muscle or the adrenal cortex which is presumably cyclic AMP–activated protein kinase. The assay is based on the competition between cyclic AMP and the radioiodinated nucleotide for binding sites on the binder. Assay sensitivity is 0.05 to 0.1 pmole. The binder, however, cross-reacts with cyclic GMP, which can be removed by separation on a Dowex 1 ion-exchange column. The chromatographic separation step can be eliminated if the measurement is performed using radioimmunoassay because antisera prepared for this purpose have shown adequate specificity for cyclic AMP (Steiner, 1969). Assay sensitivity has been reported to be 0.01 pmole. Both assays are now available commercially in kit packages. However, cyclic AMP measurements have not proved to be as useful as anticipated for hyperparathyroidism.

OTHER INORGANIC IONS

Magnesium

Physiologic Chemistry. Magnesium is one of the most abundant cations in the body and is essential to many physiochemical processes. The body of an adult contains 20 to 30 g of magnesium, about 50 per cent of which is present in bone, 45 per cent in intracellular fluid, and 5 per cent in extracellular fluid. As an intracellular cation, magnesium is second in abundance only to potassium, and its concentration in intracellular fluid is about 10 times that in the extracellular fluid. Magnesium is an activator of various enzymes including phosphatases, transphosphorylases, pyrophosphatases, carboxylases, and hexokinase. Magnesium is also essential for the preservation of the macromolecular structure of DNA, RNA, and ribosomes.

The dynamics of magnesium exchange and homeostasis are rather poorly understood. About one third of the average adult daily dietary intake of 20 to 40 mEq (10 to 20 mmol) is absorbed, predominantly in the small intestine, and excreted in the urine. The absorption process appears to be poorly controlled, and homeostasis is maintained largely by renal excretion, which is regulated by tubular reabsorption. The plasma concentration is not significantly affected by dietary intake over a rather wide range (Agarwal, 1976). The pharmacology of magnesium has been recently reviewed (Massry, 1977).

Reference serum levels vary somewhat depending on the analytical method employed. Using atomic absorption, the reference range is 1.3 to 2.1 mEq/L (0.7 to 1.1 mmol/L). There appears to be no sex difference, but levels are somewhat higher in females during menstruation. The concentration in newborns is essentially the same as in adults. The concentration in erythrocytes is about three times that in serum. About 70 per cent of the magnesium in serum is freely diffusible and the remainder is bound to plasma proteins, largely albumin. The magnesium content of cerebrospinal fluid is 2.0 to 2.7 mEq/L (1.0 to 1.4 mmol/L).

Clinicopathologic Correlations. Magnesium depletion is clinically more significant and frequent than an excess but is nevertheless relatively uncommon. Signs and symptoms of magnesium depletion do not usually appear until extracellular levels have fallen to 1 mEq/L (0.5 mmol/L) or less. Manifestations of significant magnesium depletion include weakness, irritability, tetany, delirium, convulsions, and cardiac arrhythmias. Causes for symptomatic hypomagnesemia include malabsorption, severe diarrhea, nasogastric suction with administration of magnesium-free parenteral fluids, alcoholism, acute pancreatitis, early chronic renal disease, malnutrition, excessive lactation, chronic dialysis, digitalis intoxication, hyper- and hypoparathyroidism, hyperaldosteronism, diabetes mellitus, diuretic therapy (mercurial, thiazides, and ammonium chloride), and porphyria with inappropriate secretion of antidiuretic hormone.

Elevated serum concentrations of magnesium are rarely encountered, largely as a consequence of the ability of the kidneys to excrete systemic excesses. Signs of magnesium toxicity include anesthesia, flaccidity, paralysis of voluntary muscles, and hypotension. Symptomatic hypermagnesemia can be caused by advanced renal failure, acute diabetic acidosis, Addison's disease, severe dehydration, overly aggressive administration of magnesium sulfate enemas, or ingestion of excessive amounts of magnesium-containing antacids.

Analytical Techniques. The oldest method for the determination of magnesium in biological fluids, but one which is occasionally still used, involves precipitation of magnesium as the ammonium phosphate salt after removal of calcium as calcium oxalate. Phosphorus in the precipitate is then quantitated by any of several methods, usually photometry as molybdenum blue or as the molybdivanadate complex.

Precipitation of magnesium with 8-hydroxyquinoline is the basis for many procedures. The precipitate is quantitated by titrimetry, colorimetry, flame photometry, or fluorometry. Calcium, which will interfere, is eliminated by complexing with ethylene bis(oxyethylenenitrilo) tetraacetic acid (EGTA). In the fluorometric determination, the use of 8-hydroxyquinoline sulfonate is preferred because of its greater stability and enhanced sensitivity.

Photometric measurement of the red colored complex formed with titan yellow in an alkaline medium was the first method for the direct determination of magnesium. However, color instability and lack of sensitivity and specificity limit its usefulness.

In terms of accuracy, speed, and convenience, the determination of magnesium by atomic absorption spectrophotometry is the method of choice. After deproteinization and removal of phosphate ions with a lanthanum salt, the diluted filtrate is analyzed using the 285.2 nm line of a magnesium hollow cathode lamp. The determination of magnesium in serum is sometimes performed directly without deproteinization.

Other methods for magnesium determination include complex formation with Magon, 1-azo-2-hydroxy-3-(2,4-dimethyl-carboxanilido)naphthalene-1-(2-hydroxybenzene) and EDTA titration. Flame photometry has not gained widespread application because of interferences from other anions.

Iron

Physiologic Chemistry. Iron is essential to most living organisms and participates in a variety of vital processes varying from cellular oxidative mechanisms to the transport of oxygen to the tissues. It is a constituent of the oxygen-carrying chromoproteins, hemoglobin and myoglobin, as well as various enzymes, e.g., cytochrome oxidase, xanthine oxidase, peroxidase, and catalase. The remaining body iron is present in the flavo-proteins (NADH dehydrogenase and succinic dehydrogenase), the iron-sulfur proteins, as well as the storage (ferritin) and transport (transferrin) forms of iron. The approximate distribution of iron in the normal adult male is presented in Table 9–9.

Table 9–9. APPROXIMATE DISTRIBUTION OF IRON IN THE NORMAL ADULT MALE

Compound	Iron Content (mg)	Per Cent
Hemoglobin	2800	68.3
Myoglobin	135	3.30
Ferritin	520	12.7
Hemosiderin	480	11.7
Transferrin	7	0.17
Enzyme iron	8	0.19
Remaining organic iron (by difference)	150	3.65
Total	4100	100

Unlike other trace elements, iron homeostasis is unique in that it is regulated primarily by absorption and not by excretion. Because the capacity of the body to excrete iron is very limited, its absorption from the intestine must be controlled so that tissue accumulations do not reach toxic levels. For a review of iron metabolism, the reader is referred to Chapter 29. Salient features of iron homeostasis are presented in Figure 9–6.

In adult males, iron is lost by way of the gastrointestinal tract (0.6 mg), sweat and exfoliation of squamous cells (0.2 mg), and the urinary tract (0.1 mg) for a total of 0.9 mg daily. In the female, losses through normal menstruation add an additional average daily increment of 0.4 mg, giving a total daily loss of 1.3 mg. During pregnancy and lactation additional demands of up to 4 mg/day are placed on maternal iron stores.

The recommended allowance of 10 mg/day for adult males is readily obtainable from a well-balanced diet. It is difficult for women to obtain the recommended allowances (18 mg/day) from dietary sources unless fortified foods or supplements are included. The richest dietary source of iron is animal viscera, e.g., liver, kidney, heart, and spleen. Other good sources include egg yolk, fish, oysters, clams, and dried legumes.

Since the body conserves iron extremely well, only 6 to 12 per cent of dietary intake need by absorbed in order to maintain iron equilibrium. However, in iron deficiency states and during growth and pregnancy, the normal gastrointestinal absorption will be increased from 1.3 mg daily to perhaps 4 mg/day (Jacobs, 1977).

Aside from a small amount of iron that is absorbed from the stomach, most iron absorption takes place in the duodenum and jejunum. In order to be absorbed, iron must be in its reduced or ferrous form. The acid pH of the stomach, along with reducing

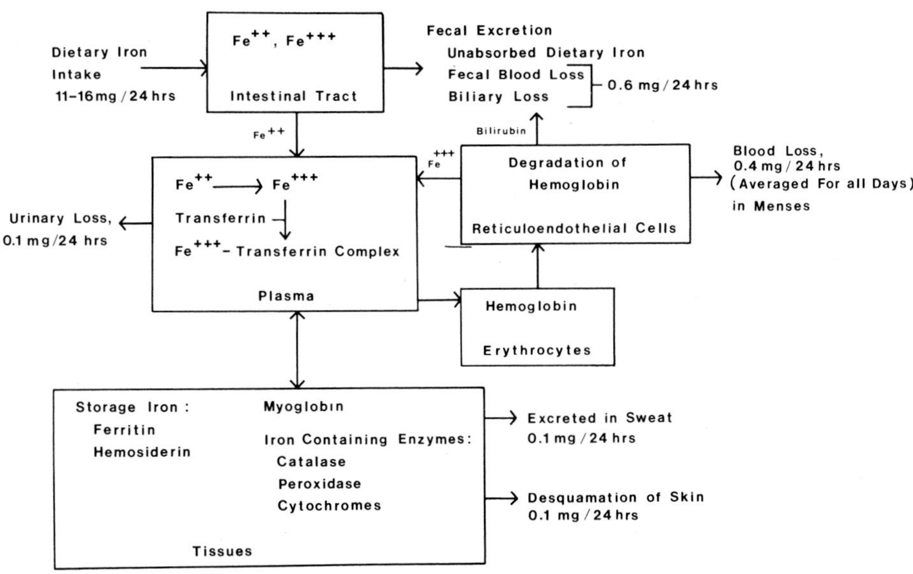

Figure 9–6. Interrelationships in iron homeostasis.

substances and ascorbic acid, enhances iron absorption by maintaining iron in a reduced, more soluble form and by forming a chelate with ferric iron, which remains soluble as the pH rises in the small intestine. The regulation of iron absorption is largely carried out by the intestinal epithelial cells, and a mucosal control mechanism has been proposed in which solubilized ionic iron in the intestinal lumen adsorbs to specific receptors in the brush border of the mucosal cells. The iron then passes from these receptors into the cytosol of the mucosal cell by an energy-dependent process. Controversy still exists concerning the mechanism of transport across the mucosal cell to the serosal surface. Several possible explanations of the process have been proposed. In addition to the classic apoferritin theory, it was recently suggested that iron is solubilized by chelation to low molecular weight endogenous substances, and that transport of iron across the cell is effected by chelation to amino acids. Most absorbed iron becomes attached to the plasma protein, transferrin, for transport in the plasma. Any remaining iron is retained within the cell, where it combines with the protein apoferritin (M.W. 460,000) to form ferritin. Ferritin also occurs in hepatic parenchymal cells and reticuloendothelial cells of the bone marrow, liver, and spleen. If the amount of apoferritin is insufficient to bind the remaining iron, it is deposited in tissues as small iron oxide granules known as hemosiderin. Approximately 25 per cent of the iron in the body is in the storage forms of ferritin and hemosiderin. These storage forms represent a ready reserve of iron that can be mobilized to meet homeostatic needs.

The plasma iron transport protein, transferrin (formerly known as siderophilin), has the electrophoretic mobility of a β_1 globulin and is formed in the liver. It has a molecular weight of approximately 90,000. Each molecule is able to bind two atoms of ferric iron. The half-life of this protein is about 10 days. By contrast, the iron in the plasma pool has a half-life of 60 to 120 minutes.

Iron is carried to storage sites and to the bone marrow. Transferrin is not itself assimilated by the target tissues. Indeed, transferrin may bind briefly to normoblast membranes where the iron is passed directly into the developing erythrocyte for incorporation into heme. Subsequently, transferrin returns to plasma to take up unbound iron. From effete erythrocytes, iron is split from hemoglobin by reticuloendothelial system cells and returns to plasma, where it is again bound to transferrin. A small portion of the emergent iron may enter the plasma in the form of ferritin. Free iron is extremely toxic and little, if any, is present in the body.

Clinicopathologic Correlations. Transferrin is usually measured indirectly by the amount of iron that it can bind; this is referred to as the total iron-binding capacity (TIBC). The total circulating apo-transferrin (protein capable of binding additional iron) is generally about a third saturated with iron; this iron is measured in the serum iron determination. The unsaturated iron-binding capacity (UIBC) is that amount of additional iron that transferrin can bind above that which is already complexed. This relationship can be expressed as TIBC = UIBC + serum Fe.

Another useful expression of this relationship is percentage saturation, which relates the amount of iron present in the serum to the amount of transferrin present (TIBC). The formula for this relationship is:

$$\%\ \text{saturation} = \frac{\text{serum Fe}}{\text{TIBC}} \times 100$$

Percentage saturation is a better index of iron stores than serum iron alone. It is a useful clinical concept but must always be reported along with both the iron and TIBC for optimal clinical interpretation. The

Table 9–10. SERUM IRON, TIBC*, AND PERCENT SATURATION IN VARIOUS CONDITIONS

	Serum Fe (μg/dl)	TIBC (μg/dl)	Saturation (%)
Normal	*60-150*	*300-360*	*20-50*
Iron deficiency	↓	↑	↓
Chronic infections	↓	↓	↓
Malignancy	↓	↓	↓
Menstruation	↓	N	↓
Iron poisoning	↑	↓	↑
Hemolytic anemia	↑	N, ↓	↑
Hemochromatosis	↑	N, ↓	↑
Pyridoxine deficiency	↑	N	↑
Late pregnancy	↓	↑	↓
Oral contraceptives	N, ↑	↑	N
Viral hepatitis	↑	↑	N, ↑
Nephrosis	↓	↓	↑
Kwashiorkor	↓	↓	↑
Thalassemia	↑	↓	↑

↓ = decrease; ↑ = increase; N = normal.
*TIBC = Total iron binding capacity.

relationship between serum iron, transferrin (TIBC), and per cent saturation as it occurs in various conditions and diseases is presented in Table 9–10. Additional clinicopathologic correlations are reviewed in Chapter 29.

Normal values for the TIBC in healthy adults average between 300 and 360 μg/dl (54 to 64 μmol/L). There is no diurnal variation in the level of the TIBC as there is for serum iron. TIBC values tend to decrease with age (250 μg/dl in individuals above 70 years of age). At birth the average newborn levels are about 275 μg/dl and reach a peak by the eighth month.

Common causes for an increase in TIBC include iron deficiency anemia, infancy, ingestion of oral contraceptives, and possibly hepatitis (Table 9–10). Decreased transferrin and, therefore, TIBC can be found in association with a generalized decrease in plasma proteins from various causes, e.g., reduced protein synthesis, nephrosis or other direct loss, and increased catabolism (malignancy or starvation). In common with albumin, but unlike many of the glycoproteins of plasma, transferrin tends to be decreased by inflammatory conditions. Patients with iron overload from repeated blood transfusions also have a depression of transferrin. The average serum iron level is about 125 μg/dl in adult males and 100 μg/dl in adult females. The range varies between 60 and 150 μg/dl (11 to 27 μmol/L). There is no seasonal variation in iron levels, although a diurnal variation has been observed. Serum iron levels can be one third higher in the morning than at night. The average plasma and serum iron levels at birth approach 200 μg/dl. There is a drop to about 45 μg/dl during the first few hours of life and then an increase to 125 μg/dl after the first three weeks of life. In the elderly, the serum iron level decreases to 40 to 80 μg/dl (7 to 14 μmol/L). In pathologic states, elevations of serum iron can be seen in (1) conditions of increased erythrocyte destruction (hemolytic anemia), (2) decreased blood formation (lead poisoning or pyridoxine deficiency), (3) increased release of iron from the body stores (release of ferritin in acute hepatic cell necrosis), (4) defective iron storage (pernicious anemia), and (5) increased rate of absorption (hemochromatosis and transfusion siderosis).

Decreased serum iron occurs in association with (1) generalized iron deficiency (lack of sufficient dietary iron), inadequate absorption, or chronic loss as a result of bleeding or nephrosis, and (2) impaired release of iron from the reticuloendothelial system (infection). Moderate depression of serum iron can occur in association with conditions such as malignancies and rheumatoid arthritis.

The ratio of serum iron level to plasma transferrin level (percentage saturation) is altered in various diseases (Table 9–10). An increase in the saturation can occur in conditions of decreased circulating protein (chronic liver disease, nephrosis, kwashiorkor), in conditions associated with ineffective erythropoiesis or blocks in hemoglobin synthesis (thalassemia, lead poisoning, pyridoxine deficiency anemia), in disease associated with iron overload (idiopathic hemochromatosis and hemosiderosis), and in acute blood loss. A decrease in the percentage of saturation (less than 15 per cent) is present in iron deficiency anemia and in late pregnancy. In conditions such as infection and malignancies, both serum iron and total iron-binding capacity are decreased, but the serum iron depression is proportionately greater, so the percentage of saturation is lower.

In evaluating patients for iron deficiency or iron overload, the work-up should include a complete hematologic profile, including an examination of peripheral blood smear, as well as measurements of serum ferritin, serum iron, and iron-binding capacity (TIBC), with calculation of percentage saturation. A single measurement of serum iron, except in iron poisoning, is inadequate for confirmation of iron overload or iron deficiency.

Analytical Techniques. ***Serum Iron.*** The assessment of iron stores has traditionally been dependent on the colorimetric determination of serum iron. The first step in any analytic procedure for iron is the dissociation of iron from its binding proteins by exposure to strong acids. In manual methods this is accomplished either by removal of proteins by precipitation with hot trichloroacetic acid or by providing conditions that allow the protein to remain in solution without interfering with subsequent analytical manipulations. In automated methods iron is dialyzed from the transferrin. The next step in most procedures is the reaction of the reduced iron with a chromogen to produce an iron-chromogen complex. Reagents with superior sensitivity for complexation with iron include sulfonated bathophenanthroline 2,4,6-tripyridyl-S-triazine (TPTZ), ferrozine, and terosite. Addition of the color reagent results in the formation of a deeply colored Fe-chromogen complex with an absorbance maximum in the visible region.

The determination of serum iron by atomic absorption spectrophotometry has had only limited success primarily because of the relatively low sensitivity and the interference from other iron containing compounds such as hemoglobin-Fe and dextran-Fe. Other attempts at serum iron determination include emission spectrography, flameless atomic absorption spectrophotometry, and x-ray fluorescence spectrometry (Zak, 1980).

TIBC. While serum iron determination reflects iron bound to transferrin, transferrin is usually only 30 per cent saturated with iron. The latent or unsaturated iron-binding capacity (LIBC or UIBC) is estimated also in measurements of total iron-binding capacity. Most commonly the UIBC is determined indirectly by subtracting the serum iron from the TIBC. TIBC is determined by saturating the transferrin with iron, removing the excess, unbound iron with an iron absorbent, and measuring the iron in the filtrate. Absorbents serve to remove any unbound iron excess and ideally should not remove iron that has become bound to the transferrin molecule. Effective absorbents include activated charcoal, magnesium carbonate, and Amberlite resin.

Serum Ferritin. Because the concentration of circulating ferritin in healthy individuals is proportional to the size of iron stores, serum ferritin values, obtained by sensitive immunoradiometric assay, radioimmunoassay, and enzyme-linked immunoassay, are used in the assessment of iron status. Serum ferritin levels of <12 μg/L are usually considered to be diagnostic of iron deficiency anemia. However, in the presence of inflammation, infection, and chronic disease, serum ferritin tends to outproportion the level of iron store; a more prudent value of 50 μg/L is used to identify iron deficiency. Iron overload, i.e., in patients with idiopathic hemochromatosis or thalassemia major, is associated with elevated serum ferritin concentration. However, elevated values can result from liver pathology, e.g., viral hepatitis and malignancy as in Hodgkin's disease (Sayers, 1981).

Copper

Physiologic Chemistry. Copper is an essential trace element that is a constituent of certain metalloenzymes and proteins. It is required for hemoglobin synthesis and is a constituent of cytochrome oxidase, tyrosinase, monoamine oxidase, ascorbic acid oxidase, uricase, galactose oxidase, and amino-levulinate dehydratase.

The major portion of copper in the erythrocyte (at least 80 per cent) occurs as a constituent of the enzyme superoxide dismutase (erythrocuprein). This enzyme, also found in liver (hepatocuprein) and brain (cerebrocuprein), has the unique role of protecting cells by catalytically scavenging the toxic-free radical superoxide ion (O_2^-) generated during aerobic metabolism. The remainder of erythrocyte copper is dialyzable and is believed to consist of complexes with amino acids, which function to maintain dismutase activity. The total copper content of erythrocytes tends to remain constant, on the average 98 μg/dl (15 μmol/L), despite deficiencies of dietary copper or increases in plasma or hepatic copper (Burch, 1975).

The concentration of copper in the plasma is somewhat higher than in the erythrocyte. The normal range for serum copper in adults is 70 to 140 μg/dl (11 to 22 μmol/L) for males and 80 to 155 μg/dl (13 to 24 μmol/L) for females. Copper in plasma occurs in two main forms, one loosely bound and the other firmly bound to plasma proteins. Only trace amounts of copper remain free or dialyzable in plasma. Loosely bound copper is a minor fraction and includes copper bound predominantly to serum albumin.

The albumin-bound copper probably represents copper in transit and increases promptly after copper is ingested, then falls exponentially as a result of hepatic uptake. Firmly bound copper, composing 80 to 95 per cent of the total plasma copper, is incorporated into an α_2-globulin, which is called ceruloplasmin because of its blue color. Serum ceruloplasmin concentration increases as albumin-bound copper decreases. Ceruloplasmin, a multifunctional enzyme, aids in the mobilization of iron from storage sites and functions as a ferroxidase enzyme during the ferrous-ferric conversion of iron. Reference values for ceruloplasmin range from 25 to 43 mg/dl (250 to 430 mg/L).

Clinicopathologic Correlations. The most important abnormality in copper metabolism is Wilson's disease or hepatolenticular degeneration. This disease is of autosomal recessive inheritance with onset usually in the second or third decade but occasionally as early as four or five years of age. As suggested by the name, the disease is characterized by degenerative changes, particularly in the liver and the basal ganglia of the brain as a result of excessive deposition of copper. The most common presenting signs and symptoms are those of central nervous involvement—rigidity, dysarthria, dysphagia, tremor, incoordination, choreoathetotic movements, and ataxia. Some patients, especially those in the younger age ranges, may present with liver insufficiency ranging from weakness and anorexia to jaundice and progressing to ascites and other features of portal hypertension as a consequence of cirrhosis. Other patients present with a combination of central nervous system and hepatic disease. A pathognomonic finding is a brown ring near the limbus of the cornea, termed the Kayser-Fleischer ring, which results from deposition of copper in Descemet's membrane (Clayton, 1980).

The biochemical defect in Wilson's disease has not been elucidated. Plasma ceruloplasmin is ordinarily greatly decreased, usually to less than 20 mg/dl. It is unlikely, however, that the depression of ceruloplasmin is a causative factor in the disease because a few patients with Wilson's disease have normal levels of ceruloplasmin. Furthermore, 10 to 20 per cent of heterozygote carriers and other patients with the nephrotic syndrome or sprue have significantly decreased ceruloplasmin but are free of the manifestations of Wilson's disease. Plasma copper is correspondingly decreased. Patients with Wilson's disease have a persistently positive copper balance in spite of increased renal excretion. The fact that biliary and, therefore, fecal excretion of copper is abnormally low may be of pathogenetic importance. Copper is also increased in the cerebrospinal fluid.

Prompt diagnosis of Wilson's disease is important so that therapy can be instituted. Progression of the disease can be abated and manifestations at least partially reversed by a diet low in copper and therapy with D-penicillamine, which promotes copper excretion.

Hypercupremia is usually observed during pregnancy, with ceruloplasmin concentrations in serum reaching values at parturition that are twice those found in non-pregnant women. Extremely high concentrations of ceruloplasmin, and therefore of copper, have been found in various lymphomas, particularly Hodgkin's disease. Increased ceruloplasmin also occurs in acute and chronic infections, rheumatoid arthritis, biliary cirrhosis, and thyrotoxicosis.

There are several other conditions in which subnormal concentrations of copper are found in the serum. Hypocupremia has been observed in conditions associated with hypoproteinemia, e.g., protein malnutrition (kwashiorkor), protein malabsorption syndrome (sprue), and nephrosis.

Hypocupremia is also a characteristic feature of Menkes' kinky hair syndrome or trichopoliodystrophy, a sex-linked recessive disorder characterized by progressive mental deterioration, retardation of growth, defective keratinization and pigmentation of hair ("kinky hair or pili torti"), hypothermia, degenerative changes in aortic elastic, scorbutic bone changes, and cerebral gliosis with cystic degeneration. In addition to hypocupremia this syndrome is associated with profound hypoceruloplasminemia and diminished concentrations of copper in the hair. The copper deficiency may be responsible for the alterations in the elastic fibers of arterial walls and the scorbutic bone deformities, as well as the changes in hair. Although orally administered copper was ineffective, parenteral administration of copper was therapeutically beneficial as a result of stimulation of ceruloplasmin formation. The role of copper in metabolic disorders has been reviewed by Evans (1981).

Analytical Techniques. While spectrophotometry, neutron activation, and radioisotopic dilution techniques have been used to determine copper in biologic fluids, atomic absorption spectrometry remains the method of choice for the determination of copper in serum, plasma, or urine (Sunderman, 1973). Atomic absorption spectrometry provides the sensitivity, specificity, speed, and ease of analysis required for routine clinical use. Methods of sample preparation for measurements of copper in serum, plasma, and/or whole blood by flame atomic absorption include (1) simple dilution and aspiration in the flame, (2) dissociation of copper from the proteins (albumin and ceruloplasmin) by treatment with acid followed by protein precipitation and aspiration of the supernatant, or (3) liberation of plasma and erythrocyte copper by acid digestion followed by chelation with ammonium pyrrolidine dithiocarbamate (APDC) and extraction into an organic solvent (methyliobutylketone, MIBK) for flame atomic absorption measurement. Copper determination by flameless atomic absorption has also been reported.

Zinc

Until recent years zinc metabolism received relatively little attention in clinical medicine although it is known to be an essential component of many important enzymes, including alcohol dehydrogenase, carbonic anhydrase, alkaline phosphatase, procarboxypeptides, and superoxide dismutase. The importance of zinc in several diseases has now been clearly established.

Low plasma levels of zinc occur as a nonspecific finding in association with a variety of diseases, including alcoholic cirrhosis, sickle-cell anemia, carcinoma of the lung, acute myocardial infarction, chronic renal failure, cutaneous burns, corticosteroid therapy, and oral contraceptive therapy (Prasad, 1981). A pathogenetic association of zinc deficiency with taste and olfactory acuities was suggested earlier, on the basis of beneficial effects observed with supplemental zinc sulfate in some patients with idiopathic hypogeusia. However, evidence cumulated by more recent studies, including those of the same investigators, appears to be less than conclusive (Henkin, 1976; Solomons, 1979). Improvement in healing of extensive burns or wounds has been observed following administration of zinc sulfate to patients with zinc depletion or dietary inadequacy. Zinc deficiency in children is associated with anorexia, impaired taste perception, pica, lethargy, failure to thrive as infants, growth retardation of older children, and delayed sexual maturation.

Acrodermatitis enteropathica is a disease with onset in early childhood characterized by various gastointestinal and cutaneous manifestations including alopecia, diarrhea, and vesiculopustulous dermatitis, particularly of the extremities and around mucous membranes. This disease, which is inherited as an autosomal recessive trait, has been attributed to a defect related to zinc metabolism (Clayton, 1980).

Although deficiencies of zinc have received greater attention than overdoses, acute zinc intoxications from industrial exposure, consumption of acidic foods or beverages from galvanized containers, illicit spirits, or children's toys have been reported. Symptoms from accidental ingestion include gastrointestinal irritation with fever, nausea, vomiting, diarrhea, abdominal pain, and a metallic taste. With industrial exposure via inhalation, metal fume fever is the predominant symptom. Other toxic effects include dry throat, cough and chest discomfort, tachycardia, hypertension, and pulmonary edema. Considerable discrepancies exist in the literature concerning normal zinc levels. Improper specimen collection and/or non-specific colorimetric methods explain part of the disparity. The normal plasma concentration of zinc by atomic absorption is approximately 100 μg/dl, with a range of 55 to 150 μg/dl (8.42 to 22.95 μmol/L). Platelet disintegration is thought to account for the higher level in serum. Plasma level of zinc can be affected by its binding affinity to albumin, exogenous steroid administration, and hemolysis (Solomons, 1979).

Chromium

Although chromium as a component of several enzyme systems may be important in nucleic acid metabolism, its physiological role in man remains unclear. Chromium appears to play a role in potentiating the action of insulin, and a trivalent chromium nicotinic acid complex has been referred to as "glucose tolerance factor." It is not certain whether chromium deficiency is a factor in the etiology of diabetes or merely a consequence of the disease, since chromium supplementation has not been shown to be beneficial in adult diabetes (Clayton, 1980).

Chromium toxicity is seen primarily in occupational exposure to chromium compounds. Toxic exposure to the skin results in dermatitis and persistent ulceration. Accidental ingestion has resulted in vertigo, abdominal pain, vomiting, anuria, convulsions, shock, and coma. Chromium levels in blood are extremely low. A serum level of 1.58 ± 0.08 μg/L in a group of 15 healthy adults was reported. Levels of chromium in hair are substantially higher than in serum and may be used as an index of chromium nutrition.

Agarwal, B. N., and Agarwal, P.: Magnesum deficiency in clinical medicine—a review. J. Med. Wom. Assoc., *31*:72, 1976.

Arnaud, C. D., Goldsmith, R. S., Bordier, P. J., and Sizemore, G. W.: Influence of immunoheterogeneity of circulating parathyroid hormone on results of radioimmunoassays of serum in man. Am. J. Med., *56*:785, 1974.

Arnaud, C. D., Tsao, H. S., and Littledike, T.: Radioimmunoassay of human parathyroid hormone in serum. J. Clin. Invest., *50*:21, 1971.

Austin, L. A., and Heath, H., III: Calcitonin: Physiology and pathophysiology. N. Engl. J. Med., *304*:269, 1981.

Balis, M. E.: Uric acid metabolism in man. Adv. Clin. Chem., *18*:213, 1976.

Baum, N., Dichoso, C. C., and Carlton, C. E., Jr.: Blood urea nitrogen and serum creatinine: Physiology and interpretations. Urology, *5*:583, 1975.

Berson, S. A., Yalow, R. S., Aurbach, G. D., and Potts, J. T., Jr.: Immunoassay of bovine and human parathyroid hormone. Proc. Natl. Acad. Sci. USA, *49*:613, 1963.

Burch, R. E., Hahn, H. K. J., and Sullivan, J. F.: Newer aspects of the roles of zine, manganese, and copper in human nutrition. Clin. Chem., *21*:501, 1975.

Clayton, B. E.: Clinical chemistry of trace elements. Adv. Clin. Chem., *21*:147, 1980.

Deftos, L. J., Roos, B. A., and Parthemore, J. G.: Calcium and skeletal metabolism. West. J. Med., *123*:447, 1975.

DeLuca, H. F.: The vitamin D system: A view from basic science to the clinic. Clin. Biochem., *14*:213, 1981.

Elder, G. H., The porphyrias: clinical chemistry, diagnosis and methodology. Clin. Haematol., *9*:371, 1980.

Elder, G. H., Gray, C. H. and Nicholson, D. C.: The porphyrias: A review. J. Clin. Pathol., *25*:1013, 1972.

Evans, G. W.: The role of copper in metabolic disorders. Adv. Exp. Med. Biol., *135*:121, 1981.

Goldman, L., Gordan, G. S., and Roof, B. S.: The parathyroids: Progress, problems and practice. Curr. Prob. Surg., 1, August, 1971.

Goldstein, L.: Ammonia production and excretion in the mammalian kidney. *In* Thurau, K. (ed.): Kidney and Urinary Tract Physiology II. Baltimore, University Park Press, 1976.

Goodwin, J. F.: The colorimetric estimation of plasma amino nitrogen with DNFB. Clin. Chem., *14*:1080, 1968.

Gordan, G. S., and Roof, B. S.: Laboratory tests for hyperparathyroidism. J.A.M.A., *206*:2729, 1968.

Habener, J. F.: Recent advances in parathyroid hormone research. Clin. Biochem., *14*:223, 1981.

Hammond, J. E., and Savory, J.: Advances in the detection of amino acids in biological fluids. Ann. Clin. Lab. Sci., *6*:158, 1976.

Hawker, C. D., and DiBella, F. P.: Human parathyroid hormones: A review of the radioimmunoassay procedures and clinical interpretation. *In* Natelson, S., Pesce, A. J., and Dietz, A. A. (eds.): Clinical Immunochemistry, Vol. 3 of Current Topics in Clinical Chemistry (Series ed., King, J. S.). AACC, Washington, D.C., Chapter 30, 1978, p. 329.

Henkin, R. I., Schechter, P. J., Friedewald, W. T., Demets, D. L., and Raff, M.: A double blind study of the effects of zinc sulfate on taste and smell dysfunction. Am. J. Med. Sci., *272*:285, 1976.

Hennessy, J. F., Wells, S. A., Jr., Ontjes, D. A., and Copper, C. W.; A comparison of pentagastrin injection and calcium infusion as provocative agents for the detection of medullary carcinoma of the thyroid. J. Clin. Endocrinol. Metab., *39*:487, 1974.

Jacobs, A.: Serum ferritin and iron stores. Fed. Proc., *36*:2024, 1977.

Klinenberg, J. R.: Hyperuricemia and gout. Med. Clin. North Am., *61*:299, 1977.

Lutwak, L.: Metabolic and biochemical considerations of bone. Ann. Clin. Lab. Sci., *5*:185, 1975.

Massry, S. G.: Pharmacology of magnesium. Ann. Rev. Pharmacol. Toxicol., *17*:67, 1977.

Mawer, E. B.: Clinical implications of measurements of circulating vitamin D metabolites. Clin. Endocrinol. Metab., *9*:63, 1980.

McLean, F. C., and Hastings, A. B.: The state of calcium in the fluids of the body. 1. The conditions affecting the ionization of calcium. J. Biol. Chem., *108*:285, 1935.

Melick, R. A., and Henneman, P. H.: Clinical and laboratory studies of 207 consecutive patients in a kidneystone clinic. N. Engl. J. Med., *259*:307, 1958.

Moore, M. R.: The biochemistry of the porphyrias. Clin. Haematol., *9*:227, 1980.

Murray, T. M., Peacock, M., Powell, D., Monchik, J. M., and Potts, J. T., Jr.: Non-autonomy of hormone secretion in primary hyperparathyroidism. Clin. Endocrinol., *1*:235, 1972.

Nyhan, W. L.: The Lesch-Nyhan syndrome. Adv. Nephrol., *3*:59, 1974.

Orfanos, A. P., Murphey, W. H., and Guthrie, R.: A simple fluorometric assay of protoporphyrin in erythrocytes (EPP) as a screening test for lead poisoning. J. Lab. Clin. Med., *89*:659, 1977.

Parfitt, A. M.: The actions of parathyroid hormone on bone: Relation to bone remodeling and turnover, calcium homeostasis, and metabolic bone disease. Part I. Mechanisms of calcium transfer between blood and bone and their cellular basis: Morphological and kinetic approaches to bone turnover. Metabolism, *25*:809, 1976a.

Parfitt, A. M.: The actions of parathyroid hormone on bone: Relation to bone remodeling and turnover, calcium homeostasis, and metabolic bone diseases. Part II. PTH and bone cells: Bone turnover and plasma calcium regulation. Metabolism, *25*:909, 1976b.

Parfitt, A. M.: The actions of parathyroid hormone on bone: Relation to bone remodeling and turnover, calcium homeostasis, and metabolic bone disease. Part III. PTH and osteoblasts: The relationship between bone turnover and bone loss, and the state of the bones in primary hyperparathyroidism. Metabolism, *25*:1033, 1976c.

Pennington, R. J.: Biochemical aspects of muscle disease. Adv. Clin. Chem., *14*:409, 1971.

Prasad, A. S.: Zinc deficiency in human subjects. Prog. Clin. Biol. Res., 77:165, 1981.

Raisz, L. G.: Calcium regulation. Clin. Biochem., *14*:209, 1981.

Reed, A. H., Cannon, D C., Winkelman, J. W., Bhasin, Y. P., Henry, R. J., and Pileggi, V. J.: Estimation of normal ranges from a controlled sample survey. 1. Sex and age-related influence on the SMA 12/60 screening group of tests. Clin. Chem., *18*:57, 1972.

Rieselbach, R. E.: Renal handling of uric acid. Adv. Exp. Med. Biol., *76B*:1, 1977.

Ritchie, J. C., Smith, S. F., and Castor, C. W.: Measurement of urinary and serous-fluid glycosaminoglycans and urinary hydroxyproline. Am. J. Clin. Path., *67*:585, 1977.

Robertson, W. G., and Marshall, R. W.: Calcium measurements in serum and plasma—total and ionized. CRC Crit. Rev. Clin. Lab. Sci., *11*:271, 1979.

Ryckewaert, A., and Kuntz, D.: Etiologic varieties of hyperuricemia and gout. Adv. Nephrol., *3*:29, 1974.

Sayers, M. H.: Iron. Symposium on laboratory assessment of nutritional status. Clin. Lab. Med., *1*:729, 1981.

Scott, P. J., and Hurley, P. J.: Demonstration of individual variation in constancy of 24-hour urinary creatinine excretion. Clin. Chim. Acta, *21*:411, 1968.

Shih, V. E.: Urea cycle disorders and other congenital hyperammonemic syndromes. *In* Stanbury, J. B., Wyngaarden, J. B., and Fredrickson, D. S. (eds.): The Metabolic Basis of Inherited Disease. 4th ed. New York, McGraw-Hill Book Co., 1978.

Solomons, N. W.: On the assessment of zinc and coppe nutriture in man. Am. J. Clin. Nutr., *32*:856, 1979.

Steele, T. H.: Renal excretion of uric acid. Arthritis Rheum., *18*:793, 1975.

Steiner, A. L., Kipnis, D. M., Utiger, R., and Parker, C.: Radioimmunoassay for the measurement of adenosine 3′,5′-cyclic phosphate. Proc. Natl. Acad. Sci. USA, *64*:367, 1969.

Sunderman, F. W.: Atomic absorption spectrometry of trace metals in clinical pathology. Hum. Path., *4*:549, 1973.

Tocci, P. M., Phillips, J., and Sager, R.: The effect of diet upon the excretion of parahydroxyphenylacetic acid and creatinine in man. Clin. Chim. Acta, *40*:449, 1972.

Tomokuni, K.: New method for determination of aminolaevulinate dehydratase activity of human erythrocytes as an index of lead exposure. Clin. Chem., *20*:1287, 1974.

Watson, C. J., and Schwartz, A simple test for urinary porphobilinogen. Proc. Soc. Exp. Biol. Med., *47*:393, 1941.

Wybenga, D. R., Ibbott, F. A., and Cannon, D. C.: Determination of ionized calcium in serum that has been exposed to air. Clin. Chem., *22*:1009, 1976.

Zak, B., Baginski, E. S., and Emanuel, E.: Modern iron ligands useful for the measurement of serum iron. Ann. Clin. Lab. Sci., *10*:276, 1980.

10

CARBOHYDRATES

PETER J. HOWANITZ, M.D., AND JOAN H. HOWANITZ, M.D.

Carbohydrates are compounds of carbon, hydrogen, and oxygen, usually with hydrogen and oxygen present in a proportion of two hydrogen atoms to one oxygen atom, as in water. These "carbohydrates" (carbon hydrates) have the general formula $C_n(H_2O)_n$. The medically important carbohydrates that contain six carbons (hexoses) are glucose, fructose, and galactose, whereas lactose (glucose and galactose) and sucrose (glucose and fructose) are important disaccharides.

Abnormalities in the quantity or structure of enzymes involved in carbohydrate metabolism are numerous; the most important are discussed under disorders of fructose, galactose, and glycogen metabolism.

Measurements of carbohydrates are performed using whole blood, serum, or plasma. Frequently, measurements of carbohydrates in urine, cerebrospinal fluid, and other body fluids are important clinically; these are discussed in Chapters 18 and 19. The concentration of carbohydrates in blood is controlled within narrow limits by many hormones, the most important of which are produced by the pancreas.

PANCREATIC HORMONES

The cells of the endocrine pancreas secrete three hormones involved in glucose homeostasis: insulin, glucagon, and somatostatin. Each hormone is made by an individual cell type physically contiguous with the other types of hormone-producing cells. It is thought that secretion of a hormone by one cell type can influence secretion of the other cells.

Under physiologic circumstances, the availability of energy sources necessitates release of insulin, or glucagon, such that a reciprocal relationship occurs between them. Insulin acts to store carbohydrates as energy and inhibit mobilization of these energy stores from endogenous sources, such as liver, fat, and muscle. In contrast, during fasting periods, glucagon enhances catabolic functions such as hepatic glycogenolysis, and, in conjunction with other catabolic hormones, stimulates the formation of glucose. This bihormonal control of glucose regulation requires appropriate secretion of varying amounts of these two hormones, which act in concert on adipose tissue, liver, and muscle to maintain a steady concentration of plasma glucose. Somatostatin acts locally to regulate release of insulin and glucagon from the pancreas. Additionally, maintenance of plasma glucose concentrations is mediated through adrenergic, cholinergic, and possibly peptidergic mechanisms.

Insulin

Insulin is a small peptide with a mass of about 6000 daltons consisting of an A-chain of 21 amino acids with a B-chain of 30 amino acids connected by two disulfide bonds. A polypeptide precursor of insulin, termed proinsulin, is synthesized in the microsomal fraction of the pancreatic beta cell as a long single chain with a mass of 9000 daltons. During storage in the cell, two disulfide bonds are formed within the chain. It is converted to a double-chain molecule by a proteolytic process that removes the 31 amino acid C-peptide, thus forming insulin (Fig. 10–1). A molecule even larger than proinsulin has been identified and is called pre-proinsulin: this may be a precursor for proinsulin. Equimolar amounts of C-peptide, along with native insulin, are secreted into the blood. In the fasting state, insulin secretion is minimal and proinsulin secretion is only about 15 per cent that of insulin. This ratio stays about the same when there is an acute stimulus to insulin secretion. However, an increased percentage of circulating proin-

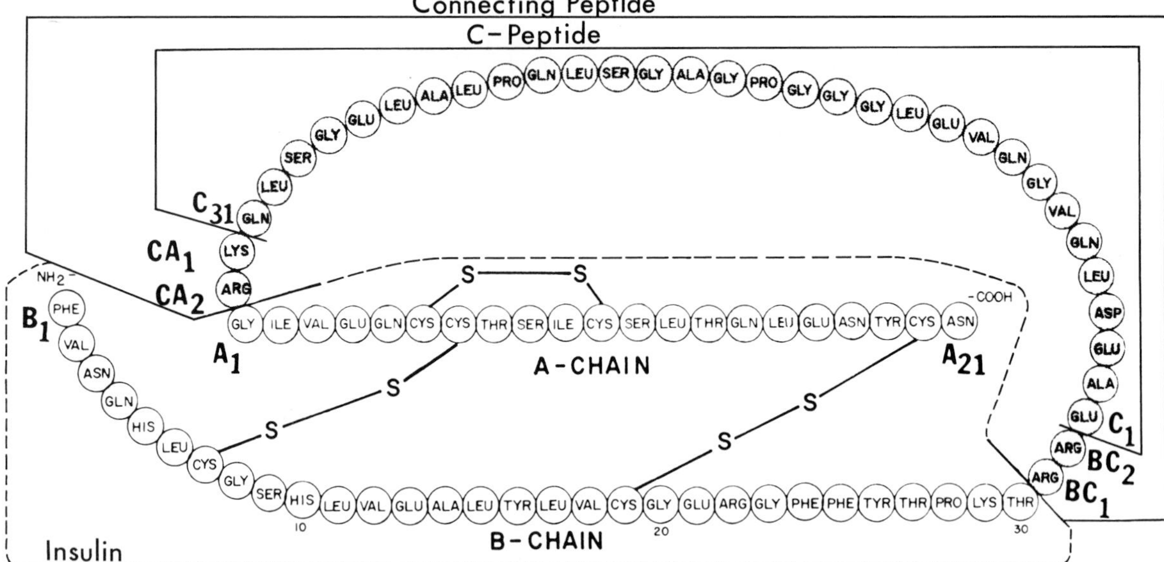

Figure 10–1. Proposed amino acid sequence of human proinsulin (Modified from Kitabchi, Metabolism, *26*:547, 1977). Connecting peptide is the amino acid residue connecting the carboxy end of the B chain to the amino end of the A chain of insulin. "C" peptide is formed when two basic residues BC_1-BC_2 and CA_1-CA_2 have been removed from connecting peptide. Insulin (broken line) consists of the A and B chain.

sulin is found in older patients, pregnant diabetics, obese diabetics, patients with insulinomas, some patients with functional hypoglycemia, and those with a rare syndrome called hyperproinsulinemia. *In vivo* studies of proinsulin have shown that it has about 10 per cent of the biologic activity of insulin; however, it has a half-life three times as long.

The reference interval for fasting serum insulin by radioimmunoassay is usually less than 20 μU/ml, but this is dependent on the antibody used in the assay. It has been shown that antibodies used in the radioimmunoassay of insulin cross-react with proinsulin. The extent of cross-reactivity depends on the individual antibody but usually is in the range of 30 per cent. Measurement of insulin appears to have little clinical value except in diagnosis of spontaneous hypoglycemia (Marks, 1976). The utility of the assay is discussed in sections on hypoglycemia and insulinomas (pp. 170 and 171). In general, the sensitivity of the insulin radioimmunoassay is such that it is impossible to differentiate low insulin levels from those within the reference interval. Assays for proinsulin are not readily available.

Although the secretory ratio of C-peptide to insulin is 1:1, the ratio in serum is about 5 to 15:1. This occurs because insulin is rapidly removed by its initial passage through the liver, but hepatic extraction of C-peptide is negligible. The function of C-peptide in the peripheral circulation is unknown.

Measurement of C-peptide has been used in a few clinical settings (Table 10–1). In certain hypoglycemic states, such as insulinoma, C-peptide is elevated. A diagnostic test for insulinoma has been developed in which insulin is injected and C-peptide quantitated. This is discussed in the section on insulinoma (p. 171). The most important use of C-peptide measurements is in the diagnosis of surreptitious injection of insulin resulting in "factitious" hypoglycemia. Since C-peptide is removed during purification of commercial insulin preparations, those patients who have injected insulin will have demonstrable insulin by radioimmunoassay, but no C-peptide. The absence of C-peptide, high serum insulin, and hypoglycemia point to injection of exogenous insulin. Other uses of C-peptide assays include follow-up evaluation of total pancreatectomy for carcinoma and demonstration of the remission phase of "recovery" from diabetes. Patients with complete loss of beta cell capacity have no C-peptide and are frequently "brittle" diabetics, whereas diabetics with residual beta cell function, and thus C-peptide, tend to have stable diabetes mellitus.

Fasting serum C-peptide concentrations in healthy subjects range from 1.0 to 2.0 ng/ml. After administration of a glucose load, levels rise five- to six-fold. In diabetics, C-peptide may be decreased or nondetectable; in diabetic ketoacidosis, C-peptide is not measurable. In the usual C-peptide assays, cross-

Table 10–1. CLINICAL INDICATIONS FOR C-PEPTIDE MEASUREMENT

Hypoglycemic states
Diagnosis of insulinoma
Diagnosis of surreptitious injection of insulin
Euglycemic states
Demonstration of remission phase or "recovery" from diabetes
Hyperglycemic state
Follow-up evaluation after pancreatectomy
Evaluation of the "brittle" diabetic patient

reactivity of proinsulin may be as high as 20 per cent that of C-peptide. However, since the serum concentration of proinsulin in a reference population is about 10 per cent that of C-peptide, cross-reactivity of proinsulin in C-peptide assays usually is negligible. In insulin-requiring diabetics, endogenous insulin antibodies are produced which bind proinsulin. In the presence of these antibiodies, residual beta cell function results in accumulation of proinsulin in the circulation. It has been found that in some diabetics up to 80 per cent of measured C-peptide is due to proinsulin cross-reactivity. Thus, the presence of C-peptide indicates only that beta cell secretion is taking place, and values which are obtained cannot be compared with those in a reference population to quantitate insulin secretion (Horwitz, 1976).

Glucagon

Glucagon is formed by the alpha-2 (or A cells) that make up about 25 per cent of pancreatic cells. Glucagon-like polypeptides of varying molecular weights also are formed by the gastrointestinal tract. Based on reactivity with glucagon antibodies, polypeptides that react with both C- and N-terminal antibodies are termed "immunoreactive glucagon" (IRG), whereas polypeptides that react only with N-terminal specific antibodies are termed "glucagon-like immunoreactivity" (GLI) (Conlon, 1980). Based on this classification, IRG is associated with the pancreas and GLI with the gut. Thus measurements of pancreatic glucagon in serum require antibody that is specific for the C-terminal region of glucagon.

There appears to be heterogeneity of circulating plasma pancreatic glucagon. The four fractions that are found include a component with a mass of 160,000 daltons ("big plasma glucagon"), others with masses of 9000 and 3500, and one component with a mass less than 2000 daltons. The last of these has been found in plasma and is thought to be a degradation product of glucagon. In healthy individuals, fasting plasma pancreatic glucagon concentrations are about 50 to 150 pg/ml, with 54 per cent comprising the 160,000 dalton component and the remainder the 3500 dalton fraction. The various components show marked differences in response to agents that are known to stimulate or suppress plasma pancreatic glucagon secretion. Hypoglycemia results in a two- to three-fold increase, whereas hyperglycemia results in a decrease by one half in plasma glucagon levels. In patients with renal failure, glucagon levels are increased up to five-fold with the 9000 dalton component predominating, because the kidneys are responsible for removal of this fraction. Although not characterized chemically, the 3500 dalton glucagon is thought to be the physiologically important fraction.

Glucagon concentrations are important in the diagnosis of alpha cell tumors of the pancreas (glucagonomas). This tumor is associated with mild diabetes mellitus and plasma glucagon concentrations ranging from 900 to 7800 pg/ml. The presence of a very high glucagon level in a diabetic suggests this diagnosis. Clinically these patients present with a characteristic necrotizing migratory rash, weight loss, anemia, stomatitis, and glossitis, and about two thirds of the patients have metastases at time of presentation. An autosomal dominant disorder, familial hyperglucagonemia, also has been described in which glucagon is elevated mainly due to the increase of the 9000 dalton component.

In insulin-dependent diabetics, immunoreactive glucagon levels are within the reference interval but inappropriate for plasma glucose concentrations and show an exaggerated response to such stimuli as protein loading. Since recent evidence has indicated that glucagon is stable, precautions such as collection in cold tubes containing a protease inhibitor such as Trasylol, and immediate centrifugation at 4°C. may be superfluous (Hendriks, 1981).

2

Somatostatin

Somatostatin, a tetradecapeptide with a disulfide bond, first was isolated from the hypothalamus. It was originally thought that somatostatin was strictly a hypothalamic hormone that inhibited growth hormone secretion, but the discovery of somatostatin in the islets of Langerhans provided new impetus for investigation of its function in the endocrine pancreas. Subsequently, somatostatin also was found in gastric mucosa and intestine. It inhibits pituitary, gastrointestinal, and pancreatic hormones as well as possessing non-endocrinologic functions (Table 10–2).

The D cells of the pancreas, which make up 10 per cent of the total islet mass, are thought to be the site of somatostatin synthesis. The D cells are distributed asymmetrically such that they are in close proximity to glucagon-producing or A cells, and thus can affect glucagon by diminishing its release. Its short half-life of one minute, diverse actions, and failure to detect it in peripheral circulation argue against the function of somatostatin as a circulating hormone and point to its action as a local modulator. Somatostatin is measured by radioimmunoassay, but the assay is not widely available.

A few tumors of somatostatin-producing D cells of the pancreas have been described; in these cases, patients present with hyperglycemia, hypoglucagonemia, malabsorption, and achlorhydria.

Table 10–2. FUNCTIONS OF SOMATOSTATIN

Endocrine	Non-Endocrine
Inhibition of secretion or diminution of	
Growth hormone	Gastric acid secretion
Thyrotropin	Gastric emptying time
Gastrin	Gallbladder contraction
Secretin	Pancreatic bicarbonate release
Vasointestinal peptide	Pancreatic enzyme release
Glucagon	Acetylcholine release from peripheral nerve endings
Insulin	

GLUCOSE MEASUREMENTS

Specimen Considerations

Diagnosis of disorders of carbohydrate metabolism rests in part on the measurement of plasma glucose either in the fasting state or following stimulation or suppression tests. Venous blood is the specimen of choice for glucose analysis, but in infants and others in whom venipuncture is difficult, capillary blood can be used. After an overnight fast, capillary glucose values are only 2 to 3 mg/dl (0.1 to 0.2 mmol/L) higher than venous concentrations, but after carbohydrate loading, capillary values may be 20 to 30 mg/dl (1.1 to 1.7 mmol/L) higher. Glucose concentrations in arterial and capillary blood are similar.

Although early manual laboratory determinations of glucose were performed using whole blood, these measurements are no longer used. Because some criteria for the laboratory diagnosis of diabetes mellitus were developed using whole blood glucose values, it is important to have a least some knowledge of these determinations. In addition, whole blood measurements have new importance because bedside continuous glucose monitors such as the Biostator[R] (Miles Laboratories) and home glucose monitoring devices use whole blood specimens.

Whole blood glucose levels vary with the hematocrit; as the hematocrit decreases, the aqueous content of blood increases (erythrocytes contain 73 per cent water, whereas plasma contains 93 per cent). For example, if the hematocrit is 45 per cent and whole blood glucose is 100 mg/dl (5.6 mmol/L), then an increase in hematocrit to 60 per cent or a decrease to 20 per cent would result in whole blood glucose in this specimen of 104 or 91 mg/dl (5.8 and 5.1 mmol/L), respectively. Other reasons for laboratories abandoning the measurement of whole blood glucose include lack of an easy automated approach; interference by nonglucose reducing substances from erythrocytes, called saccharides; and the need for inclusion of an inhibitor of glycolysis in the specimen to prevent erythrocytes and leukocytes from metabolizing glucose.

At room temperature, glucose in whole blood specimens without added inhibitors of glycolysis is metabolized at approximately 7 mg/dl/hr (0.4 mmol/L/hr); at 4°C., the loss is approximately 2 mg/dl/hr (0.1 mmol/L/hr) (Weissman, 1958). Although erythrocytes and platelets use glucose, leukocytes and bacterial contamination are the usual sources of glycolysis. A serum specimen is appropriate for glucose analysis if serum is separated from the cells within 30 minutes, but if serum is in contact with cells for longer than 30 minutes a preservative such as fluoride should be added. However, in those serum specimens without bacterial contamination or leukocytosis, a delay up to 90 minutes in separation of serum and cells still produces clinically acceptable results (Sazama, 1979). If whole blood is refrigerated, 2 mg of sodium fluoride per ml of whole blood prevents glycolysis for up to 48 hours. When refrigerated, glucose is stable in serum or plasma for a period of 48 hours. With long-term specimen storage even at −20°C., there is a significant and progressive decrease in glucose values.

Glucose Methods

Glucose methods can be divided into two groups, chemical and enzymatic. Most chemical measurements of glucose depend upon its reducing properties, and because of lack of specificity most are no longer used. Ortho-toluidine is the only chemical method still used widely and is based on the condensation of aldosaccharides, such as glucose, with an aromatic amine and glacial acetic acid. The stable green color that develops then is measured spectrophotometrically. This method can be used for plasma, urine, or cerebrospinal fluid without protein precipitation. Galactose and mannose react as well as glucose, whereas lactose, maltose, sucrose, and fructose react but to a much lesser extent. Hence, values for this method are slightly higher than for more specific enzymatic methods; in patients with uremia, this difference is even more marked. A major disadvantage of ortho-toluidine is the corrosiveness of the reagent to laboratory equipment as well as its toxicity (Indriksons, 1975). (For discussion of other chemical methods see Chapter 7 of the 16th edition of this book.)

Enzymatic methods yield maximum specificity for glucose estimations. Glucose can be measured by its reaction with glucose oxidase, in which gluconic acid and hydrogen peroxide (H_2O_2) are formed. Hydrogen peroxide then reacts with an oxygen acceptor, such as ortho-dianisidine, phenylamine-phenazone (Trinder's reagent), or other chromogenic oxygen acceptors, in a reaction catalyzed by peroxidase to form a color.

$$(1)\ \beta\text{-D-Glucose} + O_2 \xrightarrow[\text{oxidase}]{\text{Glucose}} \text{Gluconolactone} \xrightarrow[O_2]{H_2O} \text{Gluconic acid} + H_2O_2$$

$$(2)\ H_2O_2 + \begin{matrix}\text{Ortho-dianisidine } (or)\\ \text{phenylamine-phenazone}\\ (\text{chromogenic } O_2 \text{ acceptor})\end{matrix} \xrightarrow{\text{Peroxidase}} \text{color (chromogen)} + H_2O$$

Glucose oxidase is highly specific for β-D-glucose, and any glucose present in the α form must be converted to the β form before reacting. Some preparations of glucose oxidase contain the enzyme mutarotase which accelerates this process. The second step involving peroxidase is less specific than the first, and numerous reducing substances inhibit oxidation of the chromogens used in the peroxidase reaction. Although uric acid and creatinine cause little interference in most of these methods, ascorbic acid leads to spuriously decreased values. One of the chief advantages of a glucose oxidase method is its inexpensiveness.

A useful approach to glucose methodology has been the glucose oxidase–oxygen electrode method. In this method, reaction of glucose with oxygen is monitored by an oxygen-sensing electrode, while H_2O_2 generated is removed by reaction with ethanol and iodide. By determining the rate of oxygen consumption (reaction 1 above), glucose can be estimated accurately. This method is precise, linear, and free from important interferences. Results approximate those of the Proposed Product Class Standard hexokinase glucose method (Passey, 1977).

A hexokinase method, which provides a high degree of specificity for estimating glucose, has been proposed as the reference method for glucose. In this method, glucose is measured by quantitating NADPH formation from the following reactions:

$$\text{(1) Glucose} + \text{ATP} \xrightarrow[\text{Mg}^{++}]{\text{Hexokinase}} \text{Glucose 6-phosphate} + \text{ADP}$$

$$\text{(2) Glucose 6-phosphate} + \text{NADP} \xrightarrow{\text{G6PD}} \text{6-phosphogluconolactone} + \text{NADPH} + \text{H}^+$$

The main disadvantage of hexokinase is its cost; in an extended comparison, it produced the best between-run and within-run precision. No major interferences have been demonstrated with a large number of substances that are known to interfere with other methods (Passey, 1977).

Fasting Plasma Glucose

Plasma specimens collected after a 12- to 14-hour fast show less variation among individuals than specimens collected at other times. Plasma glucose results can be classified as either hyperglycemic or hypoglycemic, but both these definitions are rather arbitrary, with no clear-cut distinction between what is normal and abnormal. An overnight fasting glucose between 50 and 110 mg/dl (2.8 to 6.2 mmol/L) is accepted by most workers as within the reference interval. A large number of syndromes and diseases are associated with an inappropriately high fasting plasma glucose level. Some of them are listed in Table 10–3, where they are separated into primary (diabetes mellitus) and secondary causes. Hyperglycemia may result from a total absence of insulin secretion, such as after surgical pancreatectomy; it may occur from infiltration pancreas as in hemochromatosis, or occur intermittently during periods of stress, such as with severe infection, dehydration, or pregnancy. Hyperglycemia may be secondary to other endocrine diseases, or even be due to an antibody to the insulin receptor. Some drugs, such as propranolol, thiazide diuretics, and phenytoin, block insulin release and cause hyperglycemia.

Table 10–3. CLASSIFICATION OF HYPERGLYCEMIA

- Primary
  - Insulin-dependent diabetes mellitus
  - Non-insulin-dependent diabetes mellitus
- Secondary
  - Hyperglycemia resulting from disease of the pancreas
    - Inflammation
      - Acute pancreatitis (rare)
      - Chronic pancreatitis
      - Pancreatitis due to mumps
      - ? Cell damage due to coxsackievirus B_4 infection
      - ? Autoimmune disease
    - Pancreatectomy
    - Pancreatic infiltration
      - Hemochromatosis
      - Tumors
    - Trauma to pancreas (rare)
- Hyperglycemia related to other major endocrine diseases
  - Acromegaly
  - Cushing's syndrome
  - Thyrotoxicosis
  - Pheochromocytoma
  - Hyperaldosteronism
  - Glucagonoma
  - Somatostatinoma
- Hyperglycemia caused by drugs
  - Steroids
  - Thiazide diuretics, propranolol, phenytoin, and diazoxide
  - Oral contraceptives
  - Alloxan and streptozotocin
- Hyperglycemia related to other major disease states
  - Chronic renal failure
  - Chronic liver disease
  - Infection
- Miscellaneous hyperglycemia
  - Pregnancy
  - Related to insulin receptor antibodies (acanthosis nigricans)
  - Abnormal insulin

The diagnosis of diabetes mellitus can be made by measurement of plasma glucose when the patient is fasting. A plasma glucose of 140 mg/dl (7.7 mmol/L) or greater is considered abnormal; if plasma glucose is abnormal on two or more occasions, the diagnosis of diabetes mellitus can be made in accordance with criteria of the National Diabetes Data Group (1979).

Diabetes mellitus is a chronic disease characterized by abnormally high concentrations of plasma glucose, glucosuria, and a thickening of capillary basement membranes. Diabetes mellitus affects about 10 million Americans (5 per cent of the population) and is the third leading cause of death in the United States. Individuals with diabetes have an increased risk of blindness, kidney disease, peripheral vascular disease, and heart disease.

Diabetes mellitus is clinically divided into two groups, non-insulin-dependent and insulin-dependent. Patients with insulin-dependent diabetes mellitus classically present at an early age (usually before 30) and have a rapid onset of the disorder, occasional remissions, and episodes of ketosis. In contrast, patients with non-insulin-dependent diabetes mellitus are commonly obese; they usually first present at an age over 40, the onset is insidious, and ketosis is rare. In insulin-dependent diabetics, there is an increased incidence of histocompatibility antigen HLA-B8 and W15, whereas HLA-B7 is significantly less common. There is some evidence that the D locus, which is involved in cellular immunity, has a close association with insulin-dependent diabetes mellitus. There appears to be no association with the HLA antigens and non-insulin-dependent diabetes mellitus (see Chap. 33).

Hypoglycemia is defined as a syndrome characterized by low plasma glucose and an associated group of symptoms which are relieved by ingestion of food or carbohydrate. Overnight fasting plasma glucose levels below 45 mg/dl (2.5 mmol/L) are clearly abnormal, whereas those above 55 mg/dl (3.0 mmol/L) usually are accepted as "normal." During the first week of life, hypoglycemia is defined as plasma glucose concentrations <25 mg/dl (1.4 mmol/L) in the preterm or low birth weight infant. In the full term infant, plasma glucose values <35 mg/dl (1.9 mmol/L) from birth to 72 hours of age and <45 mg/dl (25 mmol/L) thereafter are considered to represent hypoglycemia. Not all pediatricians agree with these statistical definitions and vigorously treat patients when plasma glucose is <40 mg/dl (2.2 mmol/L) (Aynsley-Green, 1982).

In adults, two different groups of symptoms occur, depending on whether the hypoglycemia is acute or chronic. If low plasma glucose occurs rapidly, homeostatic mechanisms release epinephrine and symptoms of sweating, shakiness, trembling, weakness, and anxiety are produced. If the reduction of plasma glucose occurs slowly, headache, irritability, lethargy, and other central nervous system symptoms predominate. Widespread publicity in the news media has led the public to believe that hypoglycemia is exceedingly common but often goes unrecognized. In a statement on hypoglycemia, the American Diabetes Association and other medical societies conclude that these claims are not substantiated. However, many patients continue to present with the self-diagnosis of hypoglycemia. It is important that, if the diagnosis is not confirmed after a proper workup, these patients be assured that their initial notions of hypoglycemia were wrong. However, if hypoglycemia has been documented, it is essential that a full investigation of its cause be undertaken.

Fasting values also need to be interpreted in relationship to the preparation of the patient. For instance, Felig (1982) has shown that fasting healthy individuals when exercised to exhaustion commonly have plasma glucose values which are considered hypoglycemic; some of these were lower than 35 mg/dl (1.9 mmol/L). Merimee (1974) has attempted to define the criteria for laboratory diagnosis of hypoglycemia during extended fasting. In a group of healthy subjects who had fasted for 24 hours, lower reference limits of plasma glucose were found to be 55 mg/dl (3.1 mmol/L) in men and 35 mg/dl (1.9 mmol/L) in young women. Men who fasted for 72 hours had plasma glucose values as low as 50 mg/dl (2.8 mmol/L). It became virtually impossible to define a reference plasma glucose that was meaningful for discrimination of hypoglycemia in premenopausal women who had fasted more than 36 hours. In these studies, after a 72-hour fast, plasma glucose in this reference population was considered to be as low as 15 mg/dl (0.8 mmol/L). These and other studies have raised a question of the definition of hypoglycemia. Merimee (1977) concludes that what has been called "functional" hypoglycemia (a variety of hypoglycemia provoked by modest withholding of food) is in fact normal, and in this instance false standards have created a false disease.

Table 10–4. CLASSIFICATION OF SOME OF THE MORE COMMON CAUSES OF HYPOGLYCEMIA

No anatomic lesion present
- Fasting plasma glucose normal
  - Reactive hypoglycemia
    - Functional hypoglycemia
    - Alimentary hypoglycemia
    - Diabetic and impaired glucose tolerance
- Fasting plasma glucose low
  - Ethanol-induced hypoglycemia
  - Drug-induced hypoglycemia
    - Sulfonylurea
    - Phenformin
    - Insulin
    - Ethanol
    - Salicylates
    - Combinations of the above
  - Factitious—fasting glucose normal or low

Anatomic lesion present
- Insulinoma
- Extrapancreatic neoplasms
- Adrenocortical insufficiency
- Hypopituitarism
- Massive liver disease

Classification of the causes of syndromes presenting with hypoglycemia is seen in Table 10–4. In the first group, there is no anatomic lesion, hypoglycemia usually occurs in relationship to a meal, and fasting plasma glucose is within the reference interval. The causes of reactive hypoglycemia fall into this category, and may be evaluated by five-hour glucose tolerance testing (see p. 174).

Ethanol and other drugs can cause fasting hypoglycemia. Ethanol-induced hypoglycemia occurs only after prolonged ingestion of alcohol and when the liver supply of glycogen is depleted concurrently. The most common causes of drug-induced hypoglycemia are hypoglycemic agents (sulfonylureas, insulin, etc.), which account for more than half of the drug-induced causes; others are salicylates, sulfonamides, propranolol, or a combination of these (Seltzer, 1972). Factitious hypoglycemia is another phenomenon which may occur without relationship to meals.

Insulinomas or other tumors such as mesotheliomas, hepatic carcinomas, adrenocortical tumors, and gastrointestinal carcinomas may cause hypoglycemia. The hypoglycemia caused by lesions such as tumors generally is profound and unremitting. About 30 to 50 per cent of tumors, such as large mesenchymal tumors, hepatomas, and adrenocortical carcinomas, produce insulin-like substances that cause hypoglycemia. The activity of these substances is not suppressed by insulin antibodies *in vitro;* therefore, this material has been appropriately called non-suppressible insulin-like activity. Other diseases that have commonly been found to present with hypoglycemia include adrenocortical insufficiency, hypopituitarism, and diffuse liver disease.

Random Plasma Glucose

In healthy individuals, plasma glucose concentrations vary only slightly throughout the day and generally are in the range of 45 to 130 mg/dl (2.5 to 7.3 mmol/L). The only rise that occurs is found following a meal, but even then there is rarely a rise of more than 10 to 15 mg/dl (0.6 to 0.8 mmol/L) (Alberti, 1975). This degree of elevation is quite different from that obtained during a glucose tolerance test. When healthy middle-aged and older subjects are given a glucose load, plasma glucose concentrations may range from 20 to 50 mg/dl (1.1 to 2.8 mmol/L) higher than when the same subjects are given a breakfast with 75 g of carbohydrate.

In insulin-treated diabetics, plasma glucose concentrations may be grossly abnormal during the day, with fluctuations in plasma glucose as great as 150 mg/dl (8.3 mmol/L). Although 130 mg/dl (7.3 mmol/L) is considered the upper normal for a random plasma glucose, healthy individuals who are over 65 years old commonly have values of up to 180 mg/dl (10.0 mmol/L).

Random plasma glucose levels below 45 mg/dl (2.5 mmol/L) are unusual and warrant further investigation, especially if the individual is symptomatic. Low values may reflect normal physiologic response in plasma glucose concentrations such as occur following a meal, or they could be the first and only clue to a disorder in glucose homeostasis. It is unlikely that symptoms attributable to hypoglycemia occur when plasma glucose concentrations are greater than 45 mg/dl (2.5 mmol/L).

INSULINOMA

The most important cause of hypoglycemia is excessive and inappropriate secretion of insulin by pancreatic beta (islet cell) tumors. These tumors, called insulinomas, have been reported to occur in every age group, but are most common in the fourth to sixth decades. The many clinical features associated with these tumors are caused by hypoglycemia which they induce. The diagnosis of hypoglycemia should be made using the criteria known as Whipple's triad: (1) hypoglycemic attacks precipitated by fasting, (2) plasma glucose <45 mg/dl (2.5 mmol/L) during the attack, and (3) symptoms relieved promptly by the administration of glucose. Approximately 80 per cent of insulinomas are benign, 10 per cent are multiple, and another 10 per cent are malignant. Malignant insulinomas also have been reported to produce other hormones, including ACTH, glucagon, and gastrin.

Since the cause of hypoglycemia is the excessive and inappropriate production of insulin, the use of the insulin radioimmunoassay is essential in confirming this diagnosis. Normally, fasting is associated with progressive fall in serum insulin concentrations; however, patients with insulinomas usually do not have a fall of insulin levels even with hypoglycemia. Although the absolute insulin concentration in the patient with an insulinoma may actually be within the reference interval, values are inappropriately high for the degree of hypoglycemia. An overnight fast may not be sufficient to demonstrate inappropriate insulin secretion in those patients with tumors; however, three consecutive overnight fasts or a fast for up to 72 hours identifies almost all insulinoma patients. Apart from factitious hypoglycemia, the only other disorder in which inappropriate insulin secretion has been documented during fasting is idiopathic hypoglycemia of childhood.

During a fast, as the glucose concentration falls, serum insulin values decline steadily to reach low levels. The ratio of immunoreactive insulin (μU/ml) to glucose (mg/dl) after an overnight fast, or during a 72-hour fast, usually is less than 0.30 (Fajans, 1976). The use of insulin-to-glucose ratios has become important in the definition of inappropriate insulin secretion and the definition of hypoglycemia.

A ratio of insulin-to-glucose has been developed that corrects for technical problems involved in the insulin assay and has led to an "amended" insulin-to-glucose ratio. Since insulin secretion from the healthy beta cell is reduced to basal levels with hypoglycemia, insulin will be non-detectable by radioimmunoassay at glucose concentrations of about 30 mg/dl (1.7 mmol/L). Therefore, a value of 30 mg/dl is subtracted from the glucose value. This amended ratio is seen below (in μU/ml):

$$\frac{\text{Insulin } (\mu\text{U/ml})}{\text{glucose (mg/dl)} - 30 \text{ (mg/dl)}} \times 100$$

In a reference population the amended ratio extends up to 100 μU/mg, whereas in insulinoma patients a mean ratio of 180 was found (Frerichs, 1976). A similar study by Fajans (1976) has suggested that an amended ratio up to 50 μU/mg is normal. In both these studies a few patients with insulinomas have been found to have normal amended ratios. Some workers have not found these formulas clinically useful and simply use a serum insulin level of greater than 10 μU/ml in the presence of fasting hypoglycemia as diagnostic of an insulinoma.

For patients in whom the diagnosis cannot be confirmed during a 72-hour fast, stimulatory procedures can be used. Manifestations of inappropriate insulin release are exaggerated by responses to insulin secretagogues such as tolbutamide, an oral hypoglycemic agent. When given as a rapid intravenous infusion, tolbutamide causes an immediate release of insulin resulting in hypoglycemia. The depth and length of hypoglycemia have been used to indicate the presence of an insulinoma. The criteria used are (1) a decrease in plasma glucose of more than 65 per cent, or to levels below 30 mg/dl (1.7 mmol/L), (2) plasma glucose of <40 mg/dl (2.2 mmol/L) persisting up to 180 minutes or longer, and (3) significant increase of serum insulin concentrations above the reference interval (Frerichs, 1976). A false positive tolbutamide test may occur in obese subjects and patients with nesidioblastosis, whereas false negative tests occur in up to 50 per cent of patients with insulinomas. A stimulatory test using leucine causes insulin release in about 50 per cent of insulinoma patients. Although other secretagogues such as glucagon and calcium infusions have been used, experience with them is limited and results inconsistent. False positive results for leucine and glucagon procedures may approach 40 per cent (Seyer-Hansen, 1979). The GTT is of little use in diagnosis of an insulinoma, because no diagnostic pattern is found.

Use of the C-peptide assay also has been helpful in diagnosis of insulinomas; the suppressibility of beta cell secretion with insulin-induced hypoglycemia maintained for one hour is monitored by C-peptide measurements. Since commercial insulin preparations have C-peptide removed during purification, presence of C-peptide levels in the circulation is good evidence of autonomous insulin secretion. Healthy individuals suppress their C-peptide secretion to less than 1.2 ng/ml, whereas patients with insulinomas have C-peptide concentrations of greater than 1.9 ng/ml (Service, 1977). Some patients with insulinomas, however, show decreased or absent C-peptide secretion.

GLUCOSE TOLERANCE TESTING

In order to define diabetes chemically, clinicians commonly use the response of a patient to a glucose load or challenge. This challenge has been standardized: after either an oral or an intravenous load of glucose, plasma glucose values are determined. Although the glucose tolerance test (GTT) is very sensitive, it suffers from lack of specificity. It is abnormal in a wide variety of diseases and influenced by diet as well as other variables. In an effort to standardize oral glucose tolerance testing, the Committee on Statistics of the American Diabetes Association (ADA) has recommended a set of conditions under which the test should be performed (Klimt, 1969). When a GTT is carried out without regard to these requirements, proper interpretation is impossible.

Preparatory Phase

If meaningful data are to be obtained, conditions of performing the test must be controlled rigidly. For three days prior to the GTT, a diet containing at least 150 g per day of carbohydrate is required. Two additional days of this diet are essential if the patient previously has not been on a diet sufficient in carbohydrates. The presence of anorexia or any other condition precluding adequate food intake automatically invalidates the test. Inactivity, such as bed rest, has been reported to reduce glucose tolerance; thus a GTT should not be performed in non-ambulatory patients. During the 12 hours prior to a test, the patient must fast and avoid even black coffee. In addition, smoking and even mild exercise are not permitted. The test should not be performed in those patients who have had an illness during the prior two weeks. Endocrine disorders such as acromegaly, hyperthyroidism, or Cushing's syndrome frequently are associated with abnormal glucose tolerance. Thus, dysfunction of the endocrine system should be evaluated and corrected before a GTT is performed. Many drugs such as salicylates, diuretics, and anticonvulsants decrease insulin secretion; they should be avoided for at least three days prior to the performance of the test. Oral contraceptives should be omitted for one complete cycle prior to the test.

Procedures

The size of the glucose load employed is variable, with a 50 g, 75 g, or 100 g load currently used. Some workers recommend a glucose load of 1.75 g/kg body weight; this has been used in pediatric patients. Recently the National Diabetes Data Group (1979) has recommended that the oral glucose tolerance test should be standardized to a 75 carbohydrate dose for non-pregnant adults. Since pure glucose is extremely unpalatable, commercial products such as Glucola, which consist of a hydrolyzable saccharide of corn syrup and carbonated water with cola, grape, or cherry flavoring, commonly are used. Although not recommended because of possible differences in intestinal absorption, these products are tolerated better by patients who experience gastrointestinal upset with pure glucose solutions. Seven ounces of the commercial product is equivalent to 75 g of glucose.

Between 7 and 9 A.M. and after 30 minutes of rest, a blood sample for baseline glucose is obtained and the patient ingests the glucose load. The glucose is ingested over five minutes, and the first blood specimen is drawn at a specified time after baseline, depending on the criteria used for interpretation (see Table 10–5). If nausea, fainting, sweating, or other autonomic nervous system overactivity occurs, a specimen for glucose should be drawn immediately and the procedure discontinued and repeated at a later date if indicated. If a GTT is performed in the morning and repeated 12 hours later, some patients who are judged normal in the morning would be defined as diabetic based on the evening test. Other patients tested on different days may be found to have a GTT consistent with diabetes on one day but not on the second day.

Evaluation of Results

Most of the data used to establish criteria for glucose tolerance testing are based on measurements of whole blood glucose. However, it is current practice to perform glucose determinations only on serum or plasma specimens. Many different glucose methods have been used in determining reference intervals for the GTT; these different methodologies result in dissimilar glucose values and add further confusion to the interpretation of results. The most widely used criteria are those of the Wilkerson point system, Fajans-Conn, Siperstein, and the recent criteria proposed by the National Diabetes Data Group. Many other criteria have been proposed, but for the sake of brevity they have been omitted. The Fajans-Conn criteria were developed using whole blood as the specimen source, but have been modified so that plasma values of >185 mg/dl (10.3 mmol/L) at one hour, 160 mg/dl (8.9 mmol/L) at one and a half hours, and 140 mg/dl (7.8 mmol/L) at two hours are used as the criteria to diagnose diabetes. Six commonly used criteria for diagnosis of diabetes were compared in a study by Valleron (1975); it was found that since only 48 per cent of subjects were classified in the same way by the commonly used criteria, diagnostic interpretation was dependent on the criteria used.

Criticism of the GTT has been made by Siperstein (1975). He points out that the reference population used for the Fajans-Conn criteria were young subjects; that glucose intolerance increases with age; and that if these criteria are accepted, from 35 to 60 per cent of the general population over age 40 would be labeled diabetic. Siperstein recommends that a glucose of greater than 260 mg/dl (14.4 mmol/L) at one hour and 220 mg/dl (12.2 mmol/L) at two hours should be the criteria used for the diagnosis of diabetes mellitus. He recommends that a fasting plasma glucose of 140 mg/dl (7.8 mmol/L) or greater on two and preferably three separate occasions also can be used to establish the diagnosis of diabetes mellitus. At present, some workers even recommend that the GTT be abandoned, and the trend has been away from criteria established by Fajans and Conn toward more liberal criteria (Siperstein, 1975). The most recent criteria proposed by the National Diabetes Data Group (1979) reflect this trend and have been endorsed by the American Diabetes Association as well as the World Health Organization. They recommend that diabetes be diagnosed only when (1) fasting plasma glucose is >140 mg/dl (7.8 mmol/L), (2) the two-hour value = or >200 mg/dl (11.1 mmol/L), and (3) a level between 0 and two hours is >200 mg/dl (11.1 mmol/L). Their reference population of nonpregnant adults have glucose levels during fasting, at two hours, and at intermediate times that are >115, 140, and 200 mg/dl (6.4, 7.8, and 11.1 mmol/L), respectively. Those patients who have glucose values between the reference and diabetic groups are placed in a category called "impaired glucose tolerance."

In many laboratories, urine is collected at frequent intervals during the GTT for measurement of glucose. Although this practice may be of some value in detection of renal glycosuria, it is of no value in diagnosis of diabetes and may actually be an additional stress on the patient, thereby adversely affecting performance of the test. For these reasons, it should not be used (Sherwin, 1977).

It is important to identify mild gestational diabetic women, because perinatal mortality in infants of these patients exceeds that observed in infants of nondiabetics and treatment significantly decreases this loss. In pregnancy, diabetic patients have been identified by the presence of an abnormal glucose tolerance using a 100-g glucose load. Throughout pregnancy, a lower fasting glucose normally is found, but during the second and third trimesters glucose intolerance is increased. O'Sullivan (1964) established reference values during pregnancy as a fasting plasma glucose up to 105 mg/dl (5.8 mmol/L), and one-, two-, and three-hour levels up to 190, 165, and 145 mg/dl (10.6, 9.2, and 8.1 mmol/L), respectively. If two of these values are exceeded, then the diagnosis of diabetes is made (Table 10–5). A one-hour plasma glucose value > 155 mg/dl (8.5 mmol/L) following an oral glucose load has been used as the screening criterion for performing the GTT in pregnant women (O'Sullivan, 1973). It has been recommended that in pregnancy the intravenous GTT not be performed (see below) (Lavine, 1977).

Table 10–5. DIAGNOSTIC CRITERIA FOR DIABETES MELLITUS

	Criteria Based on Plasma Glucose mg/dl (mmol/L)
Fajans and Conn	1 hr—>185 (10.1) 1½ hr—>160 (8.9) 2 hr—>140 (7.8) All three values are abnormal for diagnosis
Wilkerson Point System	Fasting—>125 (6.9) = 1 point 1 hr—>195 (10.8) = ½ point 2 hr—>145 (7.9) = ½ point 3 hr—>125 (6.9) = 1 point Points for abnormal values; 2 points for diagnosis
Siperstein	Fasting—>140 (7.8) 1 hr—>260 (14.4) 2 hr—>220 (12.2) Elevated fasting on two occasions or abnormal 1 and 2 hour values
Pregnancy—O'Sullivan; 100 g to all subjects National Diabetes Data Group	Fasting—>105 (5.8) 1 hr—>190 (10.6) 2 hr—>165 (9.5) 3 hr—>145 (8.1) Two or more values abnormal for diagnosis of gestational diabetes
National Diabetes Data Group; 75 g to all nonpregnant subjects	Diabetes = Fasting ≥140 (7.8) 2 hr and ½, 1, or 1½ >200 (11.1)

Additional Diagnostic Procedures

Although a GTT of three hours' duration has been used for the diagnosis of hyperglycemia, a five-hour GTT traditionally has been used for the diagnosis of reactive hypoglycemia. Because symptoms of hypoglycemia are so transient, specimens are obtained every 30 minutes and when the patient becomes symptomatic. During a five-hour GTT, 2.5 per cent of asymptomatic patients have glucose concentrations of <40 mg/dl (2.2 mmol/L); therefore, chemical hypoglycemia may be considered to occur when the plasma glucose falls below this level (Lev-Ran, 1981). During the five-hour GTT, Park (1972) demonstrated that about one fourth of healthy individuals had plasma glucose values <60 mg/dl (3.3 mmol/L), whereas diabetics had about the same incidence. An occasional individual in these groups had plasma values <40 mg/dl (2.3 mmol/L).

Hypoglycemia that occurs following a meal is classified as "reactive" hypoglycemia and has been divided traditionally into (1) alimentary, (2) functional, and (3) that in diabetics and those with impaired glucose tolerance. Alimentary hypoglycemia usually, but not necessarily, occurs in those patients who have had gastrointestinal surgery. Accelerated absorption of a glucose load leads to marked postprandial hyperglycemia with a corresponding exaggerated insulin release; the ensuing hypoglycemia typically occurs from one and one half to three hours after eating. This pattern of glucose intolerance and a history of gastrointestinal surgery are suggestive of the diagnosis. Patients who are diabetics or who have impaired glucose tolerance also may experience reactive hypoglycemia. In these patients, hypoglycemia occurs later than in the group with the alimentary disorder, and insulin response is delayed and exaggerated.

Functional hypoglycemia is quite common in adults; it may be characterized by abnormally low plasma glucose and symptoms of lightheadedness, shakiness, diaphoresis, weakness, and fatigue occurring with the modest withholding of food. Complaints suggestive of this syndrome commonly are seen in those who have emotional problems. However, when the five-hour GTT is used to diagnose this disorder, these patients are indistinguishable from healthy individuals. Because these patients have unremarkable plasma glucose values during the occurrence of symptoms, the five-hour GTT seems unreliable for the diagnosis of functional hypoglycemia (Johnson, 1980). Patients with functional hypoglycemia do not develop diabetes mellitus at a greater rate than the general population.

It is exceedingly important to obtain plasma for a glucose determination if and when symptoms occur. During the GTT a significant number of patients will experience the symptoms which resulted in their referral, but these symptoms may not occur in relationship to low plasma glucose values. These patients should be evaluated for anxiety states and should receive supportive therapy with de-emphasis of hypoglycemia. Often these patients improve when their food intake is divided so that they eat many small meals rather than several large ones.

Insulin determinations have been suggested in conjunction with glucose measurements in order to improve the diagnostic accuracy of the GTT; however, they have not been widely used. Expense of performing multiple insulin measurements and difficulties in data interpretation probably have been responsible for lack of widespread use. The extreme variability of the insulin response to identical glucose loads also has cast doubt on the appropriateness of insulin measurements during a GTT (Olefsky, 1974).

The intravenous GTT has been used to diagnose diabetes mellitus in patients who are unable to ingest an oral glucose load. In this test 0.5 g glucose/kg body weight is given as a rapid intravenous infusion within a three-minute period. Blood is drawn for glucose before infusion and at 1, 3, 5, 10, 20, 30, 40, 60, and 120 minutes following the end of the infusion. Glucose disappearance constants (k values) are calculated from a plot of the log of the glucose concentration in relationship to time. A k value of less than 1.2 is considered to be diagnostic of diabetes mellitus. In a comparison of the oral GTT and the intravenous test, Olefsky (1973) found these two tests gave different diagnostic information 40 per cent of the time, and it was concluded that the intravenous GTT is a poor method for estimating glucose disposal. For this reason, as well as lack of standardization, the results are even more difficult to interpret than are those of an oral GTT.

Another test of glucose tolerance involves the use of cortisone and glucose (cortisone GTT). Since cortisone promotes gluconeogenesis, it may accentuate carbohydrate intolerance in latent or mild diabetics. After two doses of cortisone, an oral GTT is performed. A two-hour specimen yielding a plasma glucose value >165 mg/dl (9.1 mmol/L) is used to discriminate between diabetics and nondiabetics. Use of this single two-hour value for the upper reference limit has proved to be unreliable, because it results in the diagnosis of diabetes mellitus in a large number of people (Pozefsky, 1965). The prognostic implication of this test is uncertain, not only in the elderly but also in other age groups.

Two-Hour Postprandial Plasma Glucose

Two-hour postprandial glucose levels have been used to screen for diabetes mellitus, to diagnose diabetes, and to monitor glucose control. Usually the maximum increase in plasma glucose following a meal occurs at about 60 to 90 minutes, and by two hours the levels are similar to the fasting values. In older individuals, however, the two-hour level may be slightly higher than the fasting glucose level. Many studies have shown that the two-hour postprandial plasma glucose is the most sensitive of the values of the GTT in establishing a diagnosis of diabetes.

The significance of the two-hour postprandial value is limited by the lack of rigidly controlled conditions such as the amount of carbohydrate, the age of the patient, and intercurrent infection. These factors are responsible for the differences in the interpretation of the results. As with the GTT, the diagnostic value of the two-hour postprandial glucose is debatable. However, if it is to be used, some workers suggest that a formal GTT should be performed when a two-hour postprandial plasma glucose level greater than 140 mg/dl (7.8 mmol/L) is obtained. Good control of diabetes has been defined as a two-hour plasma glucose value of <130 mg/dl (7.2 mmol/L).

HEMOGLOBIN A_{1c}

Current methods of assessing diabetic control include measurement of blood, plasma, and urine glucose. These measurements reflect acute changes and may not be adequate indicators of the long-term aspects of diabetic control. A more useful technique for assessing diabetic control may prove to be the measurement of glycosylated hemoglobins, i.e., hemoglobin A with glucose or glucose phosphate moieties on the amino terminal valine of one or both beta chains. Although many other proteins such as albumin are glycosylated, measurements of glycosylated hemoglobins are performed routinely to monitor glucose control.

When hemolysates of human red cells are chromatographed using cation-exchange resins, three or more small peaks named hemoglobin A_{1a}, A_{1b}, and A_{1c} elute before the main hemoglobin A peak. These hemoglobins are made by post-synthetic modification of hemoglobin A at a slow rate directly dependent on the glucose concentration during the 120-day life span of the red cell. Hemoglobin A_{1c}, which composes 3 to 6 per cent of the total hemoglobin in healthy individuals, may double or even triple in diabetics depending on the level of hyperglycemia. Other hemoglobin variants, Hb A_{1a} and Hb A_{1b}, usually account for about 1.6 and 0.8 per cent of the total hemoglobin, respectively; these hemoglobins also are increased in diabetics. When the total fraction of Hb_{1a}, Hb_{1b}, and Hb_{1c} is measured as a group (fast hemoglobins), this fraction is referred to as hemoglobin A_1 or $A_{1a\text{-}c}$.

Synthesis of increased amounts of hemoglobin A_{1c} has been shown to correlate with glucose control in diabetics; with good diabetic control, the amount of hemoglobin A_{1c} returns to the reference interval. Peterson (1977) has postulated that hemoglobin A_{1c} is proportional to the time-average concentration of glucose; thus A_{1c} assays provide a useful means of evaluating the extent to which satisfactory diabetic control has been achieved.

The validity of hemoglogin A_{1c} measurements depends in part on the method used. Methods of measurement include electrophoresis, isoelectric focusing, radioimmunoassay, chromatography, or colorimetry, with the latter two the most common. With most column chromatography methods, methemoglobin, hemoglobin F, and hemoglobin Wayne co-elute with the glycohemoglobins, whereas methemoglobin falsely elevates electrophoretic measurements. Isoelectric focusing methods avoid interference from abnormal hemoglobins but are tedious to perform. Column methods that measure "fast hemoglobins" also measure pre-A_{1c}, a labile intermediate in the synthesis of hemoglobin A_{1c}. This component may constitute up to 25 per cent of the fast hemoglobins and changes significantly within 12 to 48 hours following alterations in plasma glucose concentrations. These rapidly occurring changes may reduce the degree of correlation between "fast hemoglobin" and diabetic control. At present none of the methods available for quantitating glycosylated hemoglobins is ideal, nor is there consensus on either a reference method or glycosylated hemoglobin standard (Goldstein, 1982).

HOME GLUCOSE MONITORING

Substantial improvements in diabetic control have been achieved with self-monitoring of blood glucose by patients at home. These techniques require patients to take a more active role in managing their disease. Although patients have to obtain a drop of their own capillary blood by needle or lancet, most prefer it to urine testing.

The procedures involve measurement of whole blood glucose (see Chap. 18, p. 397) using reagent strips similar to those for measuring glucose in urine. These strips use glucose oxidase methodology, and either are interpreted visually with the aid of a color chart as with the urine tests or are read with a reflectance colorimeter. Serum or plasma values are an average of 1.18 times whole blood glucose values.

DISORDERS OF FRUCTOSE METABOLISM

Disorders of fructose metabolism are divided into three groups: essential fructosuria, hereditary fructose intolerance, and fructose 1,6-diphosphatase deficiency. All are transmitted as autosomal recessives. Only in essential fructosuria are there no outward signs or symptoms and the patient leads an essentially normal life.

Normally fructose is found in small quantities in serum, usually in the range of 1 to 6 mg/dl (0.1 to 0.3 mmol/L). A major source of fructose is the disaccharide sucrose, which contains one molecule of glucose and one molecule of fructose, and is present in fruits and vegetables. The relationship of the enzymes involved in fructose metabolism is shown in Figure 10–2. After fructose loading, values as high as 100 mg/dl (5.5 mmol/L) are seen in patients with disorders of fructose metabolism.

Essential fructosuria is a benign condition resulting from a relative lack of hepatic fructokinase. This deficiency results in high serum fructose levels after meals containing either sucrose or fructose. The presence in urine of the reducing sugar fructose can be detected by non-specific glucose methods. Neither serum glucose nor serum phosphorus falls in these patients following a fructose load.

Hereditary fructose intolerance is characterized by the development of nausea, abdominal pain, hypoglycemia, aminoaciduria, hyperuricemia, uricosuria, and fructosuria following ingestion of fructose, sucrose (glucose and fructose), or sorbitol (an alcohol which is converted to sucrose). Infants with hereditary fructose intolerance develop normally as long as they are fed only human or cow's milk; however, they become acutely ill exhibiting vomiting and hypoglycemia

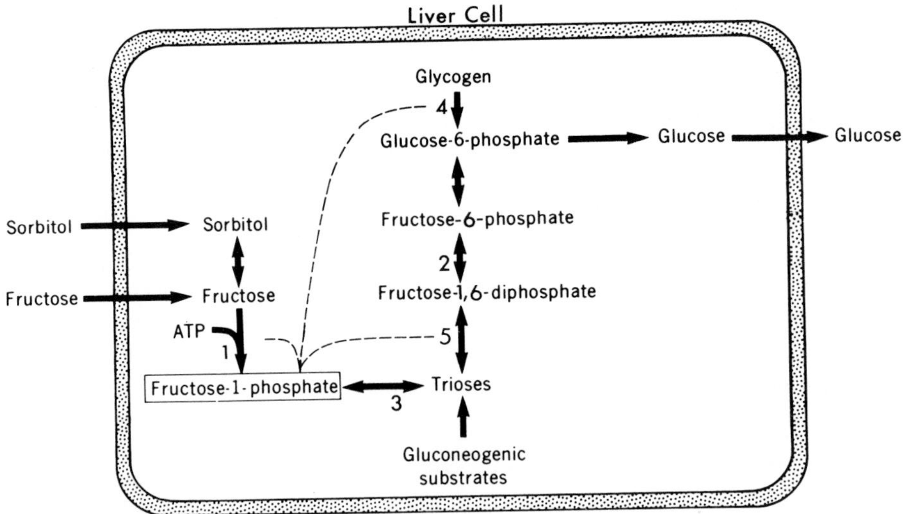

Figure 10–2. Hereditary defects in fructose metabolism (Modified from Steiner, 1977).
1-Primary defect in fructosuria (fructokinase).
2-Primary defect in fructose 1,6-diphosphatase.
3-Primary defect in hereditary fructose intolerance (fructose diphosphate aldolase).
Defects secondary to accumulation of fructose 1-phosphate
1-Fructokinase.
4-Phosphorylase and phosphoglucomutase.
5-Fructose diphosphate aldolase.

when fed formulas high in fructose or fruit juices. Diagnosis of hereditary fructose intolerance is made by the intravenous (IV) fructose tolerance test (Marks, 1976). After the IV infusion of 0.25 g/kg body weight of fructose, blood is obtained at frequent intervals, such as 0, 10, 20, 30, 45, 60, 75, and 90 minutes thereafter, and glucose as well as phosphorus is measured. Healthy individuals respond with only a small, short-lived fall in phosphorus concentrations. Patients with hereditary fructose intolerance show a persistent decrease in the plasma concentrations of glucose and phosphorus and usually become hypoglycemic. A definitive diagnosis can be made by liver biopsy and the measurement of fructose 1-phosphate aldolase, the enzyme that is markedly decreased in this disease. In newborns, the fructose tolerance test may not be as helpful as in adults.

Other enzymatic defects have been associated with hereditary fructose intolerance and account for hypoglycemia (Fig. 10–2). Renal tubular acidosis (Type I or the distal type) has been described in some patients, whereas in others a proximal defect (Type II) occurs during periods of hyperfructosemia.

Patients with fructose 1,6-diphosphatase deficiency tend to present with symptoms indistinguishable from those of type I glycogen storage disease. Lactic acidosis, ketoacidosis, hyperlipidemia, hyperuricemia, and hepatomegaly occur, but skeletal and mental growth are normal. This disease results from a total lack of functioning fructose 1,6-diphosphatase. Since fructose 1,6-diphosphatase is absent, fructose 6-phosphate cannot be formed, and glyconeogenesis cannot occur. The liver can produce glucose as long as glycogen is present, but once glycogen is depleted, the child becomes hypoglycemic. Symptoms usually occur in response to an infection or a prolonged fast. Fructosuria and hypoglycemia without vomiting may occur in response to a large fructose load. Lactic acidosis is found, because fructose enters the glycolytic scheme below the enzyme deficiency. Once the disease is recognized, the patient is treated with frequent meals.

GALACTOSEMIA

Galactosemia is a rare genetic disorder transmitted as an autosomal recessive. The prevalence of the homozygotic state is between 1 in 18,000 and 1 in 180,000. It is characterized by low plasma glucose and inability to metabolize galactose, a monosaccharide that is contained in milk as a constituent of the disaccharide lactose. The classic syndrome develops in infants who appear normal at birth but, after ingestion of milk, develop vomiting, diarrhea, jaundice, failure to thrive, cirrhosis, cataracts, and mental retardation. Many states now require galactosemia screening for newborns; the New York State experience has been described (Kelly, 1980). The metabolism of galactose involves three enzymatic steps as follows:

$$\text{Galactose} \xrightarrow{\text{I}} \begin{matrix}\text{Galactose 1-PO}_4\\+\\\text{UDP Glucose}\end{matrix} \xrightarrow{\text{II}} \begin{matrix}\text{Glucose 1-PO}_4\\+\\\text{UDP Galactose}\end{matrix}$$

$$\text{UDP Galactose} \xrightarrow{\text{III}} \text{UDP Glucose}$$

The three enzymes involved in the metabolism of galactose are galactokinase (I), galactose 1-phosphate uridyl transferase (II), and UDP glucose 4-epimerase (III), with almost all defects involving the transferase.

Symptoms of classic transferase (II) deficiency include mental retardation, failure to thrive, jaundice, and juvenile cataracts, whereas with galactokinase (I) deficiency, juvenile cataracts are the only manifestation. Epimerase (III) deficiency is rare and relatively asymptomatic. There is some evidence that the liver and lens changes which occur in the transferase deficiency are reversible, but that mental retardation resulting from low glucose is not. It is imperative that the diagnosis be documented early in the course of the disease and treatment begun because dietary restriction of galactose intake is effective treatment if started before irreversible damage has occurred. The laboratory diagnosis of the homozygotic state is suggested by the presence of a reducing sugar which is not glucose as detected by specific enzymatic glucose methods in plasma and urine.

Widespread screening programs for galactosemia are based on measuring transferase (II) activity in red blood cells using the method of Beutler (1966). The enzyme is monitored by the generation of fluorescent NADPH with a coupled enzymatic reaction. Glucose 1-phosphate formed by the transferase is converted to glucose 6-phosphate and then to 6-phosphogluconate with formation of NADPH. Absence of transferase results in failure to produce glucose 1-phosphate and subsequently fluorescent NADPH. With this methodology, false positives (absence of fluorescent NADPH) occur with a frequency of 1 in 100 to 1 in 5000. Some of these are due to the presence of other enzyme deficiences such as glucose 6-phosphate dehydrogenase or phosphoglucomutase, two enyzmes that are required in the coupled enzymatic assay for NADPH formation. False positives may be caused by heat inactivation of the transferase occurring during shipping of the specimen to a central laboratory. Specimens from asymptomatic individuals who have enzymatic variants give abnormally low assay results. For confirmation of the diagnosis, a positive by this method requires quantitative measurement of galactose or galactose 1-phosphate.

If a patient has clinical findings compatible with galactosemia and transferase activity is present, an elevated serum galactose can be used to diagnose galactokinase deficiency. The Guthrie or the Paigen test, each of which monitors growth of *Escherichia coli* in the presence of elevated galactose concentrations, is used. Measurement of the enzyme galactokinase is a more specific technique available for making this diagnosis. Management of transferase deficiency involves monitoring the level of erythrocyte galactose-1-phosphate: levels >110 μg/g of hemoglobin indicate noncompliance (reference interval <40 μg/g hemoglobin) (Pesce, 1982). Recently, it has been reported that prenatal diagnosis of galactosemia is possible by measuring transferase activity in cultured amniotic cells.

GLYCOGEN STORAGE DISEASES

Glycogen storage diseases result from specific deficiencies of enzymes involved in metabolism of glycogen. As a consequence of these deficiencies, glycogen accumulates in liver, but with some defects this deposition is generalized. The incidence of all forms of glycogen storage diseases combined is about 1 in 40,000. There are ten distinct types of glycogen storage disease; however, several are extremely rare. Most are inherited as autosomal recessives, with only a few also exhibiting other forms of inheritance. In all glycogen storage diseases, definitive diagnosis can be made by assay of the enzyme from the appropriate tissue and by a characteristic microscopic appearance of the affected tissues. A prenatal diagnosis can be made in those disorders in which the defect is present in all tissues. Generally, in those in which the defect is present in one or two tissues, a prenatal diagnosis is not possible. The classification presented in Table 10–6 employs Roman numerals for each type. In many descriptions of these diseases, eponyms are used; they also are listed.

Those diseases which can be diagnosed by the intramuscular injection of 0.5 mg glucagon include Type I (von Gierke's), Type III (Cori-Forbes), and Type VI (Hers'). A usual response is a glucose rise of 60 to 80 mg/dl (3.3 to 4.4 mmol/L) in 10 to 20 minutes with no change in lactate, but in these three types fasting patients show no increase in glucose during this procedure. With refeeding and retesting two hours later, patients with Type III respond similarly to the reference population. During the glucagon test, plasma lactate increases 3 to 6 mEq/L (3 to 6 mmol/L) in patients with von Gierke's disease. Laboratory diagnosis of McArdle's disease is made by applying a blood pressure cuff on the exercising forearm and sampling blood lactate one minute after the exercise has begun. In this disease no rise in blood lactate occurs. Glycogen storage diseases have been reviewed extensively; for further details see Mahler (1976).

L-LACTATE

Lactic acid, which is a strong acid with a pK of 3.9, is dissociated at physiologic pH. Therefore, practically all of plasma L-lactic acid is in the form of L-lactate and hydrogen ion. Lactate is the end product of anaerobic metabolism and its level is related to oxygen availability. When the supply of oxygen is limited, the cytochrome system is unable to function as an intermediate in transfer of hydrogen to molecular oxygen. In this situation, reduced nicotinamide adenine dinucleotide (NADH) accumulates and is oxidized by lactate dehydrogenase with production of lactate by the following reaction:

$$\text{Pyruvate} + \text{NADH} + \text{H}^+ \leftrightarrow \text{L-lactate} + \text{NAD}$$

Lactate is a dead-end branch of the energy metabolism chain and, following its accumulation, is metabolized back to pyruvate when oxygen again becomes abundant. As lactate increases in skeletal muscle, liver, and erythrocytes, diffusion out of these tissues occurs and blood lactate begins to rise. In non-exercising man, liver and to a certain extent kidneys are the chief organs responsible for lactate metabolism to

Table 10–6. GLYCOGEN STORAGE DISEASES

Type	Major Clinical Features	Enzyme Deficiency (Tissue Affected)	Plasma Glucose Response to I.M. Glucagon (0.5 mg)
I von Gierke's	Hepatomegaly, lactic acidosis, hyperlipidemia, severe fasting hypoglycemia	Glucose 6-phosphatase (Liver, kidney)	No response
II Pompe's	a. Cardiomegaly, muscle weakness, death in infancy b. Adult	Alpha 1,4-glucosidase (All tissues) (Muscle)	Normal Normal
III Cori-Forbes	Variable degrees of hepatomegaly, muscle weakness, fasting hypoglycemia	Debrancher (All tissues)	Normal after food; poor after fasting
IV Anderson's	Portal cirrhosis; usually death in infancy	Brancher (All tissues)	Normal
V McArdle's	Pain and stiffness after exertion; myoglobinuria in 50% of cases	Phosphorylase (Muscle)	Normal
VI Hers'	Hepatomegaly, mild fasting hypoglycemia	Phosphorylase (Liver)	No response fasting or after food
VII Tarui's	Pain and stiffness on exertion	Phosphofructokinase Muscle (? liver)	Normal
VIII	Spasticity, decerebration, high urinary catecholamines, death in infancy	Adenyl kinase (Liver, brain)	Normal
IX	Hepatomegaly, occasional fasting hypoglycemia	Phosphorylase kinase (Liver)	Normal, poor
X	Hepatomegaly only	Cyclic AMP-dependent kinase (Liver, muscle)	Normal

glucose, or oxidation to CO_2 and H_2O. In the presence of elevated concentrations, cardiac and skeletal muscle also may oxidize lactate.

Shock is perhaps the most widely recognized cause of lactic acidosis; however, in some cases, excess lactate production may precede shock. Such conditions as myocardial infarction, severe congestive heart failure, pulmonary edema, and blood loss are the common causes of shock associated with lactic acidosis. The oral hypoglycemic drug phenformin was discontinued because of frequent reports of inducing lactic acidosis. Other causes of lactic acidosis include intravenous infusion of substances such as fructose, sorbitol, or epinephrine and large doses of drugs such as ethanol or acetaminophen (Table 10–7). Hepatic necrosis, neoplasms, lymphomas, and various forms of leukemia have been reported to cause lactic acidosis. In diabetic coma, lactic acidosis is common. In some cases, lactic acidosis is secondary to causes such as shock, phenformin ingestion, or epinephrine release, but in other instances it has been reported secondary to ketoacidosis. A few cases with D-lactic acidosis due to abnormal gut flora have been described (Stolberg, 1982).

An anion gap in a patient with metabolic acidosis suggests the diagnosis of lactic acidosis. It can be suspected when the sum of anions minus the sum of cations $[(Na^+ + K^+) - (Cl^- + HCO_3^-)]$ exceeds 18 mEq/L (18 mmol/L) in the absence of other causes of an increased anion gap, such as renal failure, salicylate ingestion, methanol poisoning, or significant ketonemia.

Lactate values are determined by enzymatic methods employing lactate dehydrogenenase; however, several precautions are necessary in collection of a satisfactory specimen for lactate analysis. Although a venous blood specimen may yield higher results than an arterial specimen, venous specimens often are used for convenience. If prior to obtaining the specimen the patient remains at complete rest, venous and arterial levels are virtually alike. Venostasis formed from applying a tourniquet has little effect, but such minor movements as hand clenching can raise blood lactate significantly (Braybrooke, 1975). Blood may be collected in a syringe and deproteinized immediately by adding the blood to a tube containing percholoric acid. Plasma kept at 25°C. is also a satisfactory specimen if tubes containing sodium fluoride and

Table 10–7. COMMON CAUSES OF L-LACTIC ACIDOSIS

- Shock
- Exercise
- Drugs
  - Phenformin
  - Sorbitol
  - Fructose
  - Ethanol
  - Epinephrine
  - Acetaminophen
- Seizures
- Hepatic disease
- Neoplasms
- Diabetic ketoacidosis
- Idiopathic
- Congenital
  - Glucose 6-phosphatase deficiency (Type I glycogen storage disease)
  - Fructose 1,6-diphosphatase deficiency

potassium oxalate are used for the blood collection and separation of the plasma is completed within 15 minutes (Westgard, 1972), or when specimens are collected and stored in 0.5 g/L iodoacetate for up to two hours (Kaplan, 1980). If blood is not collected by these or comparable methods, lactate will increase rapidly from glycolysis by red cell enzymes. When the specimen is not collected in the correct tube, lactate increases may be as great as 20 per cent in 3 minutes or 70 per cent within 30 minutes at 25°C.

Plasma lactate concentration has a reference interval of 0.6 to 1.7 mEq/L (0.6 to 1.7 mmol/L) for venous blood, but even mild exercise will increase lactate levels substantially. In lactic acidosis, values exceeding 7 to 8 mEq/L (7 to 8 mmol/L) usually are associated with fatal outcome (Oliva, 1970). The absence of a rise in lactate levels after mild exercise is an important criterion in the diagnosis of patients with McArdle's disease (Type V glycogen storage disease), as discussed elsewhere (p. 177). The findings of elevated lactate in CSF can discriminate between meningitis of bacterial and viral etiology. Its measurement also can aid in differentiating septic from other forms of monoarticular arthritis. For further information see Chapter 19.

Alberti, K. G. M. M., Dornhorst, A., and Rowe, A. S.: Metabolic rhythms in normal and diabetic man. Isr. J. Med. Sci., *11*:571, 1975.

Aynsley-Green, A.: Hypoglycaemia in infants and children. Clin. Endocrinol. Metabol., *11*:159, 1982.

Beutler, E., and Baluda, M. C.: A simple spot screening test for galactosemia. J. Lab. Clin. Med., *68*:137, 1966.

Braybrooke, J., Lloyd, B., Nattrass, M., and Alberti, K. G. M. M.: Blood sampling techniques for lactate and pyruvate estimation. A reappraisal. Ann. Clin. Biochem., *12*:252, 1975.

Conlon, J. M.: The glucagon-like polypeptides—order out of chaos? Diabetologia, *18*:85, 1980.

Fajans, S. S., and Floyd, J. C.: Fasting hypoglycemia in adults. N. Engl. J. Med., *294*:766, 1976.

Felig, P., Cherif, A., Minagawa, A., and Wahren, J.: Hypoglycemia during prolonged exercise in normal men. N. Engl. J. Med., *306*:895, 1982.

Frerichs, H., and Creutzfeldt, W.: Hypoglycaemia. 1. Insulin secreting tumours. Clin. Endocrinol. Metabol., *5*:747, 1976.

Goldstein, D. E., Parker, K. M., England, J. D., England, J. E., Wiedmeyer, H-M., Rawlings, S. S., Hess, R., Little, R. R., Simonds, J. F., and Breyfogle, R. P.: Clinical application of glycosylated hemoglobin measurements. Diabetes, *31*:70, 1982.

Hendriks, T., and Benraad, T. J.: On the stability of immunoreactive glucagon in plasma samples. Diabetologia, *20*:553, 1981.

Horwitz, D. L., Kuzuya, H., and Rubenstein, A. H.: Circulating serum C-peptide. A brief review of diagnostic implications. N. Engl. J. Med., *295*:207, 1976.

Indriksons, A.: Hazards of o-toluidine. Clin. Chem., *21*:1345, 1975.

Johnson, D. D., Dorr, K. E., Swenson, W. M., and Service, J.: Reactive hypoglycemia. J.A.M.A., *243*:1151, 1980.

Kaplan, L. A., Gau, N., and Stein, E. A.: Collection and storage of serum lactic acid samples at room temperature without deproteinization. Clin. Chem., *26*:175, 1980.

Kelly, S.: Galactosemia identified in newborn screening program. Clinical and biochemical characteristics. N.Y. State J. Med., *80*:1836, 1980.

Kitabchi, A. E.: Proinsulin and C-peptide: A review. Metabolism, *26*:547, 1977.

Klimt, C. R., Prout, T. E., Bradley, R. F., Dolger, H., Fisher, G., Gastineau, C. F., Marks, H., Meinert, C. L., and Schumacher, O. P.: Standardization of the oral glucose tolerance test. Diabetes, *18*:299, 1969.

Lavine, R. L.: Diabetes and pregnancy. *In* Rose, L. I., and Lavine, R. L. (eds.): New Concepts in Endocrinology and Metabolism: Hahnemann Endocrinology Metabolism Symposium, 1976. New York, Grune and Stratton, 1977.

Lev-Ran, A., and Anderson, R. W.: The diagnosis of postprandial hypoglycemia. Diabetes, *30*:996, 1981.

Mahler, R. F.: Disorders of glycogen metabolism. Clin. Endocrinol. Metabol., *5*:579, 1976.

Marks, V., and Alberti, K. G. M. M.: Selected tests of carbohydrate metabolism. Clin. Endocrinol. Metabol., *5*:805, 1976.

Merimee, T. J.: Spontaneous hypoglycemia in man. Adv. Intern. Med., *22*:301, 1977.

Merimee, T. J., and Tyson, J. E.: Stabilization of plasma glucose during fasting. Normal variations in two separate studies. N. Engl. J. Med., *291*:1275, 1974.

National Diabetes Data Group: Classification and diagnosis of diabetes mellitus and other categories of glucose intolerance. Diabetes, *28*:1039, 1979.

Olefsky, J. M., Farquhar, J. W., and Reaven, G. M.: Do the oral and intravenous glucose tolerance tests provide similar diagnostic information in patients with chemical diabetes mellitus? Diabetes, *22*:202, 1973.

Olefsky, J. M., and Reaven, G. M.: Insulin and glucose responses to identical oral glucose tolerance tests performed forty-eight hours apart. Diabetes, *23*:449, 1974.

Oliva, P. B.: Lactic acidosis. Am. J. Med., *48*:209, 1970.

O'Sullivan, J. B., Charles, D., Mahan, C. M., and Dandrow, R. V.: Gestational diabetes and perinatal mortality rate. Am. J. Obstet. Gynecol., *116*:901, 1973.

O'Sullivan, J. B., and Mahan, C. M.: Criteria for the oral glucose tolerance test in pregnancy. Diabetes, *13*:278, 1964.

Park, B. N., Kahn, C. B., Gleason, R. E., and Soeldner, J. S.: Insulin-glucose dynamics in nondiabetic reactive hypoglycemia and asymptomatic biochemical hypoglycemia in normals, prediabetics and chemical diabetes. Diabetes, *21*:321, 1972.

Passey, R. B., Gillum, R. L., Fuller, J. B., Urry, R. M., and Giles, M. L.: Evaluation and comparison of 10 glucose methods and the reference method recommended in the proposed product class standard (1974). Clin. Chem., *23*:131, 1977.

Pesce, M. A., and Bodourian, S. H.: Clinical significance of plasma galactose and erythrocyte galactose-1-phosphate measurements in transferase-deficient galactosemia and in individuals with below-normal transferase activity. Clin. Chem., *28*:301, 1982.

Peterson, C. M., Koenig, R. J., Jones, R. L., Saudek, C. D., and Cerami, A.: Correlation of serum triglyceride levels and hemoglobin A_{Ic} concentrations in diabetes mellitus. Diabetes, *26*:507, 1977.

Pozefsky, T., Colker, J. L., Langs, H. M., and Andres, R.: The cortisone-glucose tolerance test. The influence of age on performance. Ann. Intern. Med., *63*:988, 1965.

Sazama, K., Robertson, E. A., and Chesler, R. A.: Is antiglycolysis required for routine glucose analysis? Clin. Chem., *25*:2038, 1979.

Seltzer, H. S.: Drug-induced hypoglycemia. A review based on 473 cases. Diabetes, *21*:955, 1972.

Service, F. J., Horwitz, D. L., Rubenstein, A. H., Kuzuya, H., Mako, M. E., Reynolds, C., and Molnar, G. D.: C-peptide suppression test for insulinoma. J. Lab Clin. Med., *90*:180, 1977.

Seyer-Hansen, K., and Lundbaek, K.: The clinical diagnosis of insulinoma. Scand. J. Gastroent., *53*:39, 1979.

Sherwin, R. S.: Limitations of the oral glucose tolerance test in diagnosis of early diabetes. Primary Care, *4*:255, 1977.

Siperstein, M. D.: The glucose tolerance test: A pitfall in the diagnosis of diabetes mellitus. Adv. Intern. Med., *20*:297, 1975.

Steiner, G., Wilson, D., and Vranic, M.: Studies of glucose turnover and renal function in an unusual case of hereditary fructose intolerance. Am. J. Med., *62*:150, 1977.

Stolberg, L., Rolfe, R., Gitlin, N., Merritt, J., Mann, L., Linder, J., and Finegold, S.: D-Lactic acidosis due to abnormal gut flora. N. Engl. J. Med., *306*:1344, 1982.

Valleron, A-J., Eschwège, E., Papoz, L., and Rosselin, G. E.: Agreement and discrepancy in the evaluation of normal and diabetic oral glucose tolerance test. Diabetes, *24*:585, 1975.

Weissman, M., and Klein, B.: Evaluation of glucose determinations in untreated serum samples. Clin. Chem., *4*:420, 1958.

Westgard, J. O., Lahmeyer, B. L., and Birnbaun, M. L.: Use of the Dupont "Automatic Clinical Analyzer" in direct determination of lactic acid in plasma stabilized with sodium fluoride. Clin. Chem., *18*:1334, 1972.

11

LIPIDS AND DYSLIPOPROTEINEMIA

PESACH SEGAL, M.D., PAUL S. BACHORIK, PH.D., BASIL M. RIFKIND, M.D., F.R.C.P., and ROBERT I. LEVY, M.D.

CHEMISTRY

Plasma Lipids

Lipids are organic substances insoluble in water but soluble in organic solvents. The main lipids in human plasma are cholesterol, triglycerides, phospholipids, and non-esterified fatty acids (NEFA). Lipids are transported in plasma and other body compartments in the form of lipoproteins, which are macromolecular complexes composed of a hydrophobic lipid core and a hydrophilic phospholipid and protein surface.

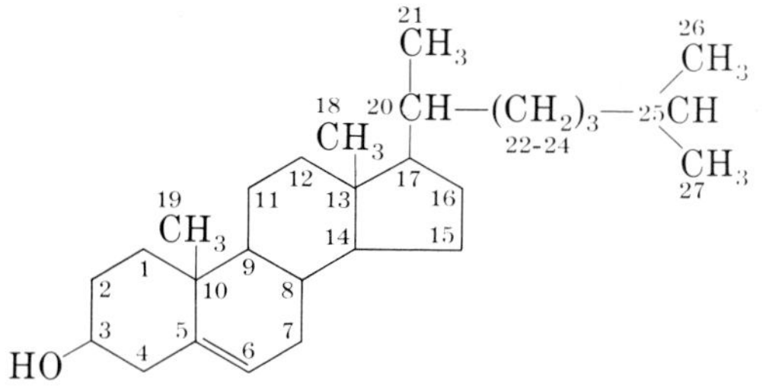

Cholesterol

Figure 11–1. Molecular structure of cholesterol.

Cholesterol. Cholesterol is an unsaturated steroid alcohol (Fig. 11–1). It is an important structural component of cell plasma membranes and a precursor for the biosynthesis of bile acids and steroid hormones. Two thirds of the plasma cholesterol is esterified, and one third is free. Sixty to 70 per cent of it is transported by low density lipoproteins (LDL), 20 to 35 per cent by high density lipoproteins (HDL), and 5 to 12 per cent by very low density lipoproteins (VLDL).

Triglycerides (Triacylglycerol). Triglycerides are esters of glycerol and, usually, three different fatty acids (Fig. 11–2). They constitute about 95 per cent of adipose tissue and are the main form of lipid storage in man. Triglycerides are transported in plasma, mostly in the form of chylomicrons and VLDL.

Phospholipids. Phospholipids are esters of glycerol, two acyl groups, and phosphatidic acid. The main plasma phospholipids are sphingomyelin, lecithin, and the cephalins (Fig. 11–3). Phospholipids constitute about 25 per cent of LDL mass (lecithin:sphingomyelin ratio 2:1), and about 30 per cent of HDL mass (lecithin:sphingomyelin ratio of 5:1).

Non-esterified Fatty Acids (NEFA). NEFA are a very important source of energy. Quantitatively they are a very small fraction of total plasma lipids. However, several grams of the rapidly turning over NEFA are transported in the plasma every day complexed with albumin.

Plasma Lipoproteins

Four major lipoprotein classes can be identified based on particle size, chemical composition, physicochemical and flotation characteristics, and electrophoretic mobility (Table 11–1).

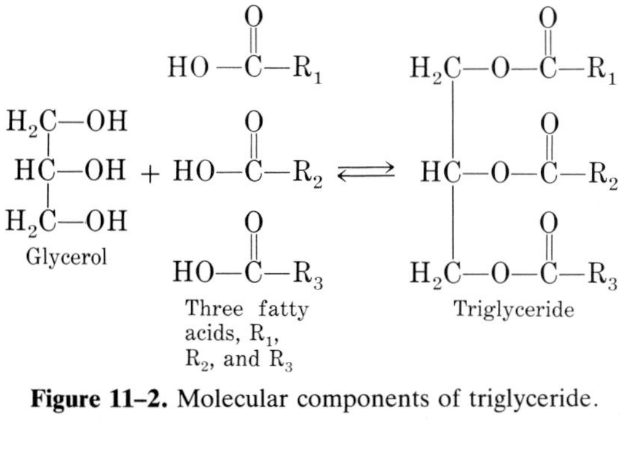

Glycerol + Three fatty acids, R_1, R_2, and R_3 ⇌ Triglyceride

Figure 11–2. Molecular components of triglyceride.

Chylomicrons. Chylomicrons are large particles produced by the intestine, very rich (85 to 95 per cent) in triglycerides of exogenous (dietary) origin, poor in free cholesterol and phospholipids, and containing about 1 to 2 per cent (by weight) of protein. The very high lipid:protein ratio renders the chylomicron very light, and it tends to float even without centrifugation. High chylomicron content results in a "milky" plasma. Chylomicrons contain apoB-48, apoA, apoC, and apoE. Interaction of chylomicrons and lipoprotein lipase results in a smaller particle, depleted in triglycerides and some surface elements, which is sometimes referred to as the chylomicron remnant.

Very Low Density Lipoproteins (VLDL). VLDL particles are somewhat smaller than chylomicrons, and are also rich in triglycerides, though to a lesser extent. They have a lower lipid:protein ratio, and thus float at a somewhat higher density. Excessive amounts of VLDL result in a turbid plasma. VLDL triglycerides are of endogenous, mainly hepatic origin and constitute about 60 to 70 per cent of the particle mass. Cholesterol and phospholipids are minor constituents, and about 10 per cent of the mass is protein—mostly apoB-100 and apoC, but also some apoE. There is a wide range of VLDL particle sizes, with a concomitant variation of the chemical composition; the larger particles are richer in triglycerides and in apoC, and the smaller particles poorer in these two elements. The smaller triglyceride- and surface material–depleted remnant particle resulting from the interaction of VLDL and lipoprotein lipase is often referred to as intermediate density lipoprotein (IDL).

Low Density Lipoproteins (LDL). LDL constitute about 50 per cent of the total lipoprotein mass in human plasma. The particle size is much smaller than that of the triglyceride-rich lipoproteins, and even greatly increased concentrations of LDL do not refract light and thereby alter the clarity of plasma. Cholesterol accounts for about half of LDL mass, most of it esterified. About 25 per cent of LDL mass is protein—mostly apoB-100 with traces of apoC. (For details see Tables 11–1 and 11–3.)

High Density Lipoprotein (HDL). HDL is a small particle consisting of 50 per cent protein (mostly apoA, but also some apoC and apoE), 20 per cent cholesterol (mostly esterified), 30 per cent phospholipids, and only traces of triglycerides. HDL is often subdivided into HDL_2 and HDL_3, varying in density, particle size, composition, and possibly also physiologic role (see Tables 11–1 and 11–2).

LP(a) Lipoprotein. This lipoprotein is found in the density range 1.055 to 1.085 g/ml. It is composed of 27 per cent protein, 65 per cent lipid, and 8 per cent carbohydrate. The apoprotein content of LP(a) consists of 65 per cent apoB, about 20 per cent LP(a) protein, and the rest albumin. The lipid composition is similar to that of LDL. The electrophoretic mobility of LP(a) is usually pre-β but can occur anywhere between LDL and albumin.

Concentrations in normal subjects may vary from

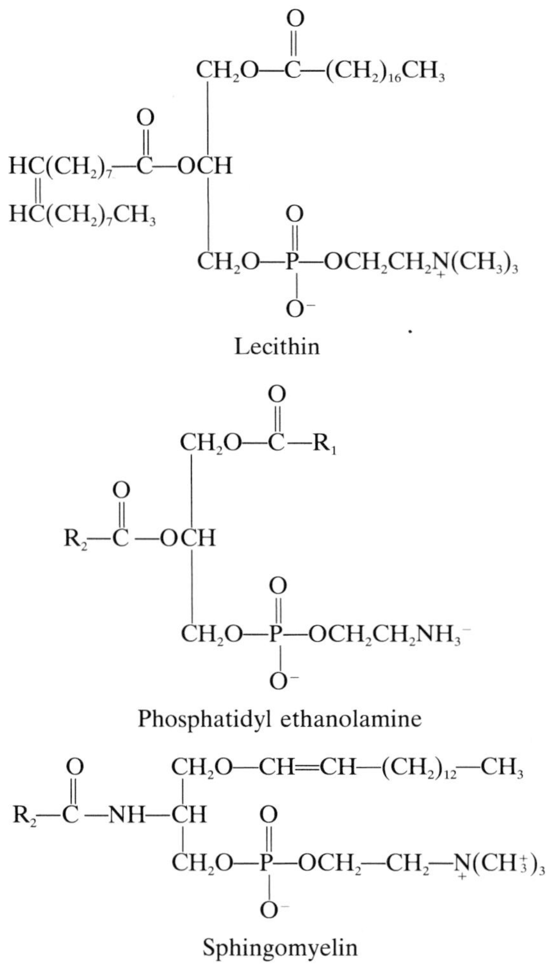

$$\begin{array}{l} \qquad\qquad\qquad\qquad\quad O \\ \qquad\qquad\qquad\qquad\quad \| \\ \qquad\qquad\qquad CH_2O{-}C{-}(CH_2)_{16}CH_3 \\ \qquad\qquad O \qquad\quad | \\ \qquad\qquad \| \qquad\quad\; | \\ HC(CH_2)_7{-}C{-}OCH \\ \;\; \| \qquad\qquad\qquad\;\; | \qquad\quad O \\ HC(CH_2)_7CH_3 \qquad\; | \qquad\quad \| \\ \qquad\qquad\qquad\quad CH_2O{-}P{-}OCH_2CH_2\overset{+}{N}(CH_3)_3 \\ \qquad\qquad\qquad\qquad\qquad\;\; | \\ \qquad\qquad\qquad\qquad\qquad\; O^- \end{array}$$

Lecithin

$$\begin{array}{l} \qquad\qquad\qquad\qquad O \\ \qquad\qquad\qquad\qquad \| \\ \qquad\qquad\quad CH_2O{-}C{-}R_1 \\ \qquad O \qquad\quad | \\ \qquad \| \qquad\quad | \\ R_2{-}C{-}OCH \\ \qquad\qquad\quad\; | \qquad\quad O \\ \qquad\qquad\quad\; | \qquad\quad \| \\ \qquad\qquad\quad CH_2O{-}P{-}OCH_2CH_2NH_3^- \\ \qquad\qquad\qquad\qquad\;\; | \\ \qquad\qquad\qquad\qquad\; O^- \end{array}$$

Phosphatidyl ethanolamine

$$\begin{array}{l} \qquad O \qquad\quad CH_2O{-}CH{=}CH{-}(CH_2)_{12}{-}CH_3 \\ \qquad \| \qquad\qquad\; | \\ R_2{-}C{-}NH{-}CH \qquad O \\ \qquad\qquad\qquad\;\; | \qquad\quad \| \\ \qquad\qquad\qquad CH_2O{-}P{-}OCH_2{-}CH_2{-}\overset{+}{N}(CH_3^+)_3 \\ \qquad\qquad\qquad\qquad\quad\;\; | \\ \qquad\qquad\qquad\qquad\quad\; O^- \end{array}$$

Sphingomyelin

Figure 11–3. Molecular structures of selected phospholipids.

20 to 760 mg/L, and increased levels are familial with autosomal dominant inheritance. When concentrations in the plasma are increased, LP(a) appears as a lipid-staining pre-beta lipoprotein band and may be confused with VLDL.

LpX Lipoprotein. LpX is an abnormal lipoprotein found in patients with obstructive biliary disease. Lipids account for more than 90 per cent of its weight (mostly phospholipids, unesterified cholesterol, and very little esterified cholesterol). Proteins, primarily apoC and some albumin, constitute less than 10 per cent of LpX by weight.

Apolipoproteins

The protein moiety of the lipoproteins is composed of several specific proteins called apolipoproteins. Each lipoprotein has a specific and relatively constant apolipoprotein composition. The apolipoproteins play important roles in lipid transport by activating or inhibiting enzymes involved in lipid metabolism, and/or by binding lipoproteins to cell surfaces. The apolipoprotein composition of the various lipoprotein fractions is summarized in Table 11–3. A useful

Table 11–1. MAJOR CLASSES OF HUMAN PLASMA LIPOPROTEINS—PHYSICOCHEMICAL CHARACTERISTICS

	Diameter (Å)	Density (g/ml)	Sf	Electrophoretic Mobility*
Chylomicrons	750–12,000	< 0.95	400	Origin
VLDL	300–700	0.95–1.006	20–400	Pre-beta
LDL	180–300	1.006–1.063	0–12	Beta
HDL_2		1.063–1.125		
	50–120			Alpha-1
HDL_3		1.125–1.210		

*Agarose-gel or paper electrophoresis.

Table 11–2. MAJOR CLASSES OF HUMAN PLASMA LIPOPROTEINS—CHEMICAL COMPOSITION

	Protein (%)*	Cholesterol		Triglyceride (%)	Phospholipid (%)
		Free (%)	*Esterified (%)*		
Chylomicrons	1–2	1–3	2–4	80–95	3–6
VLDL	6–10	4–8	16–22	45–65	15–20
LDL	18–22	6–8	45–50	4–8	18–24
HDL	45–55	3–5	15–20	2–7	26–32

*Percentage of dry weight.

alphabetical classification was proposed by Alaupovic (1971).

Apolipoprotein A (apoA). ApoA is the major protein component of HDL. It is also present in small amounts in intestinal chylomicrons. The two major components of apoA are apoA-I and apoA-II. They are both synthesized by the liver and intestine, and catabolized in good part by the liver and kidney.

ApoA-I. ApoA-I constitutes about 75 per cent of apoA in HDL. It consists of 243 to 245 amino acids with a molecular weight of 28,300. ApoA-I is thought to be an activator of the enzyme LCAT.

ApoA-II. ApoA-II constitutes about 25 per cent of apoA in HDL. It consists of 154 amino acids and has a molecular weight of 17,000. Each apoA-II molecule consists of two identical peptides linked by a single disulfide bond. The physiologic role of apoA-II is not known.

Apolipoprotein B (apoB). ApoB is the major protein constituent (95 per cent) of LDL and also constitutes about 40 per cent of the protein moiety of VLDL and chylomicrons. It is very difficult to study the physical and chemical characteristics of apoB because it is insoluble in water. However, recent studies have elucidated the fact that apoB is a heterogeneous group of proteins (Kane, 1980). The two major components known today are apoB-100 with a molecular weight of approximately 549,000, probably synthesized by the liver and found in lipoproteins of endogenous origin (VLDL and LDL), and apoB-48 with a molecular weight of approximately 264,000, of intestinal origin and found mostly in chylomicrons, carrying fat of exogenous origin.

Apolipoprotein C (apoC). ApoC is the major protein component of VLDL, and is also a minor constituent of HDL and LDL. Three different groups of C apolipoproteins are known to date:

ApoC-I. ApoC-I consists of 57 amino acid residues with a molecular weight of 6500. It is a minor constituent of chylomicrons and VLDL and HDL proteins.

ApoC-II. ApoC-II has a molecular weight of 8800 and is made of 78 or 79 amino acid residues. It constitutes 5 to 10 per cent of VLDL protein and less than 2 per cent of HDL protein. ApoC-II is a potent activator of the enzyme lipoprotein lipase (LPL) (LaRosa, 1970).

ApoC-III. Several forms of apoC-III exist differing in the molar content of sialic acid residues. ApoC-III is a major component of VLDL protein (25 to 30 per cent), as well as the main apoC of HDL, constituting about 2 per cent of its protein moiety. Its molecular weight is 8750, and it is made of 79 amino acid residues. The physiologic role of apoC-III is not known.

Minor Apolipoproteins. ApoD, sometimes also referred to as apoA-III or "thin line" apoprotein, is a minor constituent of HDL protein (5 per cent or less). It is also present in very small amounts in other lipoproteins. The molecular weight of apoD is about 32,000. ApoD was shown to activate the LCAT reaction, possibly by serving as a specific lysolecithin carrier. ApoA-IV has a molecular weight of 46,000 and is found mostly in the d>1.21 fraction, but also in very small amounts as a constituent of chylomicrons.

Apolipoprotein E (apoE). This arginine-rich apolipoprotein is an important constituent of VLDL and HDL proteins. It is found in chylomicrons, VLDL, and HDL, and to a lesser extent also in LDL. ApoE exists in several forms; they can be identified by isoelectric focusing, and are designated E2-4 isoforms (Utermann, 1975; Pagnan, 1977). Several post-translational modifications of the major E isoproteins,

Table 11–3. MAJOR CLASSES OF HUMAN PLASMA LIPOPROTEINS—APOLIPOPROTEIN COMPOSITION

	Plasma Concentration (mg/dl)	Chylomicrons (%)*	VLDL (%)	LDL (%)	HDL (%)	d > 1.21
ApoA-I	90–130	1	—	—	90	< 10
A-II	30–50		—	—	95	
B-100	80–100	—	< 10	90	Lp(a)	—
B-48	< 5	~100	—	—	—	—
C-I	4–7	Major	Major	Minor	Minor	—
C-II	3–8	Major	Major	Minor	Minor	—
C-III	8–15	Minor	25	Minor	60	—
E	3–6	Minor	Major	Minor	Minor	—

*Percentage of total plasma concentration in fraction.

2

which differ in the number of sialic acid residues in the carbohydrate side chains of the polypeptides, can also be identified using two-dimensional isoelectric focusing (Zannis, 1980). The molecular weight of apoE is 35,000 to 39,000 and it consists of 299 amino acid residues. The charge differences between the various apoE isoforms are caused by cysteine-arginine interchanges at well-characterized locations along the molecule. The synthesis of the various apoE isoforms is under genetic control (see discussion under dysbetalipoproteinemia). ApoE seems to play an important role in the binding of lipoproteins to cell surface receptors.

Enzymes Participating in Lipoprotein Metabolism

The major enzymatic systems that are known to participate in lipoprotein metabolism are the lipolytic enzymes and lecithin:cholesterol acyltransferase (LCAT).

Lipolytic Enzymes. In fasting human plasma, lipolytic activity is barely detectable. A few minutes following the intravenous injection of heparin, several lipolytic activities are discerned. At least two triglyceride hydrolases are detected in this so-called post-heparin plasma. They differ in their pH optimum, inhibition by protamine or concentrated saline solution, activation by specific apoprotein co-factors, and substrate specificity.

Lipoprotein Lipase. This enzyme, derived mainly from adipose tissue, hydrolyzes chylomicron and VLDL triglycerides. It is normally located on the surface of capillary endothelial cells of adipose tissue and of skeletal and heart muscles. Hydrolysis of chylomicron triglyceride occurs following the attachment of these particles to the capillary endothelial cells. Phospholipids and apoC-II are essential co-factors for triglyceride hydrolysis by this enzyme.

Hepatic Lipase. Hepatic lipase is probably secreted by hepatocytes and associates with the surface membrane of non-parenchymal liver cells. The function of the enzyme is not clear. It has only a limited capacity to hydrolyze triglycerides in intact chylomicrons and VLDL, and it does not require apoC-II as a co-factor. It has been postulated that hepatic lipase may participate in the conversion of apoC-poor IDL and LDL (Eisenberg, 1976). However, the enzyme seems to be most active in hydrolysis of phospholipids and triglycerides of HDL_2, and thus may play some role in HDL metabolism (Tikkanen, 1981).

Lecithin:Cholesterol Acyltransferase (LCAT). Normally present in human plasma, this enzyme system catalyzes the esterification of cholesterol by promoting transfer of fatty acids from lecithin to cholesterol, which results in the formation of lysolecithin and cholesterol ester. The enzyme is synthesized in the liver and circulates in plasma associated with HDL, which seems to be the preferred substrate. It is activated by apoA-I. Recently, it was suggested that this enzyme system also plays a role in removing surface material of chylomicrons and VLDL. LCAT may also be involved in removal of excess free cholesterol and lecithin from the circulation.

ApoA-I is an activator of LCAT, but enzyme activity can be detected even in the absence of apoA-I. Thus, the enzyme is not dependent on apoA-I presence for all its activity. LCAT in plasma can be measured either in terms of its enzymatic activity or in terms of its mass, using specific antibodies to the enzyme (Albers, 1981).

LIPOPROTEIN METABOLISM

Lipid Transport in Lipoproteins

The major function of the plasma lipoproteins appear to be the transport of energy-rich and otherwise insoluble triglycerides from sites of origin in the intestine (exogenous origin 70 to 100 g per day) and the liver (endogenous origin 25 to 50 g per day) to sites of energy storage and utilization (Fig. 11–4).

Triglycerides and cholesteryl esters enter the plasma in the form of triglyceride-rich lipoprotein particles (chylomicrons and VLDL) that supply the tissues with fatty acids for energy requirements and storage. Exogenous dietary fat is transported from its intestinal absorption site, in chylomicrons, which are composed of a hydrophobic lipid core surrounded by a surface of polar lipids and apolipoproteins. Endogenously synthesized triglyceride is transported from the liver in VLDL. The general structure of the two triglyceride-rich particles is similar, but they differ in size, lipid composition, and apolipoprotein content. Apolipoprotein B (apoB) is the major protein component in both, but as mentioned previously there are differences between the apoB of intestinal origin (B-48) present in chylomicrons and that of hepatic origin (B-100) present in VLDL. Both particles contain the E apolipoproteins and acquire the C apolipoproteins in the plasma, but only chylomicrons include the A apolipoproteins as a major surface protein component. Chylomicrons and VLDL undergo intravascular change almost immediately after their entry into the circulation through the action of lipoprotein lipase, an enzyme present on the luminal surface of capillary endothelial cells, which hydrolyzes triglycerides and diglycerides into fatty acids and monoglycerides. Lipoprotein lipase is activated by apolipoprotein C-II (apoC-II is present on the surface of triglyceride-rich particles). As a result of lipoprotein lipase action, the triglyceride lipid core is depleted and diminishes in size, and both surface lipid and apolipoproteins are transferred to HDL. The depleted chylomicron particle or remnant, as it is called, subsequently binds to the surface of hepatocytes and is then internalized by means of a highly specific receptor-mediated endocytotic process, and then degraded. Apolipoprotein E (apoE) is thought to play an important role in the binding of the chylomicron remnant to its receptor.

The particle resulting from the interaction of VLDL with lipoprotein lipase is referred to as intermediate density lipoprotein (IDL). Surface materials, namely

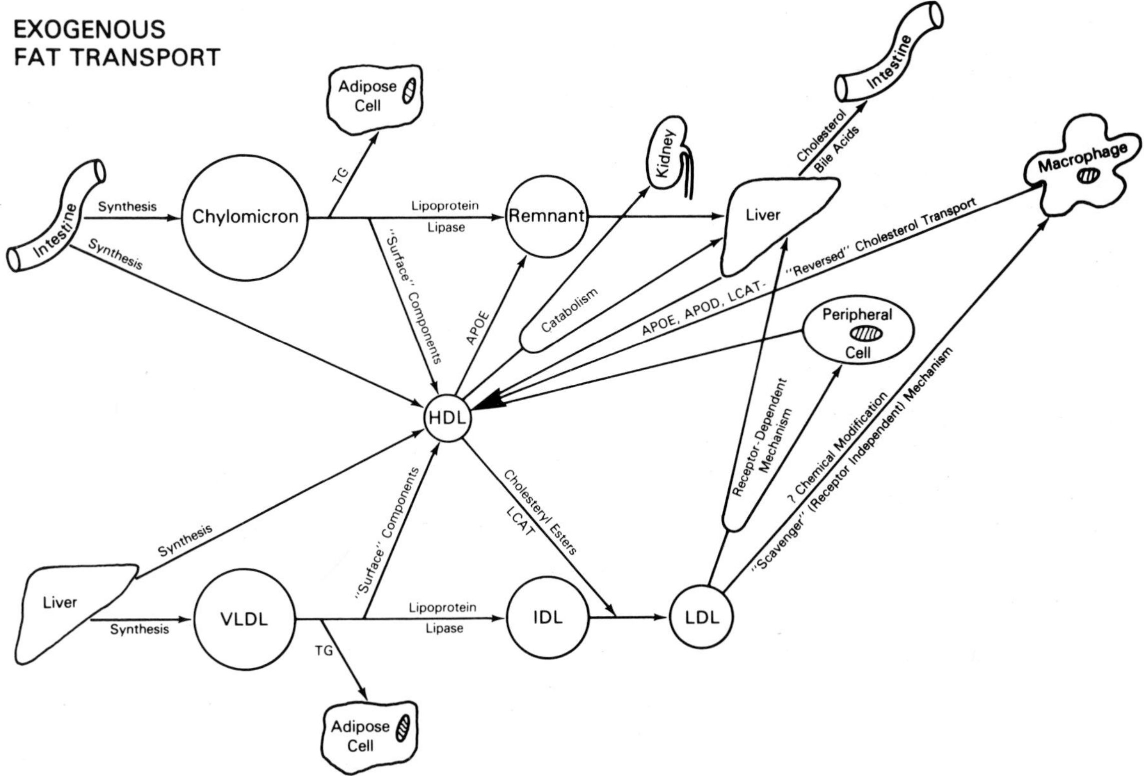

Figure 11–4. Fat transport in man: Roles of lipoproteins in lipid metabolism. Abbreviations: APOE = apolipoprotein; E; APOD = apolipoprotein D; HDL = high density lipoproteins; IDL = intermediate density lipoproteins; LCAT = lecithin:cholesterol acyltransferase; LDL = low density lipoproteins; TG = triglycerides; VLDL = very low density lipoproteins.

free cholesterol, phospholipids, and apolipoproteins, are transferred from VLDL to HDL, which interacts with lecithin:cholesterol acyltransferase (LCAT), an enzyme found in the plasma and responsible for the transfer of an acyl group from lecithin to free cholesterol, to form cholesteryl esters and lysolecithin. The former are subsequently transferred to IDL, which is converted into cholesteryl ester–rich LDL. LDL is thus the end product of intravascular VLDL metabolism. LDL is subsequently removed from the plasma via a specific cell receptor–mediated endocytotic process, which takes place in hepatic as well as extrahepatic tissues (Brown, 1981). HDL is thought to be the vehicle for reversed cholesterol transport and esterification. Not only does it serve as a scavenger picking up cholesterol apoproteins and other surface components during the intravascular catabolism of the triglyceride-rich lipoproteins but it also adsorbs free cholesterol from cells, which is then esterified by plasma LCAT and delivered to VLDL and IDL to form LDL. Receptors on cell surfaces recognize both the B and E apolipoproteins, and thus the apoE content of HDL could play a role in the reversed cholesterol transport process (Fielding, 1982).

LIPID AND LIPOPROTEIN MEASUREMENT

Lipoprotein concentrations have been expressed in several ways. When expressed in terms of particle mass, the values account for the contributions of both the protein and lipid components of the particles. Mass concentrations are generally determined with the analytical ultracentrifuge or from chemical measurements of the protein and each of the major classes of lipids. Neither of these technically demanding approaches is easily applied for screening or routine clinical purposes.

Because the cholesterol composition of each lipoprotein class (VLDL, LDL, and HDL) is generally similar in a variety of individuals, lipoprotein cholesterol is most commonly determined as a measure of lipoprotein concentration. Lipoprotein-cholesterol concentrations correlate fairly well with analytical ultracentrifuge values, and are often determined in most population studies relating lipoprotein concentration to cardiovascular risk. More recently, the growing interest in measuring the apolipoproteins acknowledges their role in lipoprotein metabolism, the link between apolipoprotein abnormalities and clinically identifiable problems, and the possibility that apolipoproteins are better discriminators than other lipoprotein components for coronary heart disease risk.

The analysis of plasma lipoproteins usually requires, first, the separation of the lipoprotein classes, and second, measurement of the lipoprotein or lipoprotein component of interest. Both steps contribute to the error in the measurements, and, as a rule, the more complicated the analytical procedures, the greater the error and variability of the analyses. Lipoprotein analyses must therefore be monitored using some formal system of quality control, and it is useful for individuals who must interpret lipid and lipoprotein data to have some idea of the laboratory quality control limits. Consider the example of how laboratory variability affects the results reported for a plasma sample with a known cholesterol concentration of 250 mg/dl. If a laboratory operating with a coefficient of variation of 3 per cent were to analyze the sample once, in 95 per cent of the cases that laboratory would report a value ranging between 235 and 265 mg/dl. Two additional points should be made. First, as mentioned above, lipoprotein-cholesterol analyses will generally be more variable than total cholesterol analyses because of the additional manipulations required to prepare the lipoprotein-containing fractions. Second, a number of factors contribute to the measured lipid and lipoprotein levels. Some of these factors operate before the sample reaches the laboratory. In the broadest sense, "quality control" begins outside the laboratory and runs as a common theme through all phases of lipoprotein analysis regardless of the methods used or components measured.

Blood Sampling and Storage

Certain kinds of physiological variations and errors can be introduced before or during venipuncture, or when the samples are handled and stored before analysis (Lipid Research Clinics Program, 1982), and it is important to standardize as much as possible the conditions under which blood specimens are drawn and prepared for analysis.

The patient is requested to fast for 12 hours before venipuncture. Chylomicrons are usually present in postprandial plasma and, depending on the type and amount of food ingested, can markedly increase the plasma triglyceride concentration. Chylomicrons are cleared within a few hours, and their presence after a 12-hour fast is considered abnormal. Fasting has little effect on plasma total cholesterol levels.

When a standing patient reclines, extravascular water transfers to the vascular system and dilutes nondiffusible plasma constituents. Decreases of as much as 10 to 15 per cent in total cholesterol concentrations have been observed after a 20-minute period of recumbence. The effect is smaller in a standing subject who sits. The position of the patient should therefore be standardized for venipuncture. Prolonged application of a tourniquet during venipuncture can increase apparent lipid concentrations, and the tourniquet should be released as soon as possible.

Either plasma or serum can be used. Plasma is generally preferred because the samples can be cooled to 4°C. immediately to retard changes that can occur in the lipoproteins at room temperature. The choice of anticoagulant is important, however. Some anticoagulants exert rather large osmotic effects that result in artifactually low plasma lipid and lipoprotein concentrations. Heparin, because of its relatively large molecular weight, has little effect on plasma volume, but can alter the electrophoretic mobilities of the lipoproteins. EDTA is the preferred anticoagulant, even though cholesterol and triglyceride concentrations in EDTA plasma are about 3 per cent lower than in serum (Lipid Research Clinics Laboratory Methods Committee, 1977). This anticoagulant retards certain kinds of oxidative and enzymatic alterations that can occur in the lipoproteins during storage. Blood is cooled in an ice bath as soon as it is drawn, and the cells are removed as soon as possible, generally within three hours. Plasma should not remain in contact with the cells overnight. The plasma is then stored at 4°C. until it is analyzed. Samples can be frozen if only total cholesterol and/or triglyceride will be measured. In general, samples in which lipoproteins are analyzed should not be frozen, and the analyses should be performed promptly.

Other factors can influence lipoprotein measurements, including seasonal variations in plasma lipoprotein levels, recent weight change, intercurrent illness, especially if accompanied by fever, vigorous exercise, and certain kinds of drugs. For example, heparin, when injected intravenously, causes the release of tissue lipases that act on plasma lipoproteins to produce marked transient decreases in triglyceride concentrations, increases in free fatty acids, and alterations in the composition and electrophoretic mobilities of the lipoproteins. Another example is the use of estrogens as contraceptive drugs, or as postmenopausal replacement therapy. Both have a very profound effect on plasma lipid and lipoprotein concentrations.

Changes also occur after a myocardial infarction. There is an immediate decrease of 10 to 60 per cent in LDL concentration and a gradual increase in the concentration of VLDL within 10 to 30 days. It is therefore recommended that lipoprotein measurement be postponed for two to three months after a myocardial infarction.

Estimation of Plasma Lipids

Cholesterol and triglycerides are the plasma lipids of most interest in the diagnosis and management of lipoprotein disorders. Phospholipid analyses are seldom required because they generally provide little additional information, but they may be requested occasionally in cases of obstructive liver disease or disorders associated with abnormally low lipoprotein levels.

Cholesterol. Cholesterol accounts for almost all of the sterol in plasma. It exists as a mixture of unesterfied (30 to 40 per cent) and esterified (60 to 70 per cent) forms, and the proportion of the two forms is fairly constant within and between normal individuals. Total cholesterol and lipoprotein-cholesterol concentrations are usually expressed in terms of the sterol nucleus without distinguishing the esterified and unesterified fractions. In general, it is not necessary to distinguish the two forms except in cases in which total lipoprotein mass is to be calculated, in which case the contribution of the fatty acid moiety to cholesteryl ester mass must be accounted for, or when the cholesterol/cholesteryl ester ratio is decidedly abnormal, which can affect the estimate of total sterol nucleus, depending on the cholesterol method used.

The present discussion considers colorimetric and enzymatic assays because they are used most widely for clinical purposes.

Colorimetric Methods. Cholesterol has long been determined colorimetrically using one of three sets of reagents: acetic anhydride–acetic acid–sulfuric acid (Liebermann-Burchard reagent); iron salt–sulfuric acid; or p-toluenesulfonic acid. With the Liebermann-Burchard and iron salt–sulfuric acid reagents, the absorbance of the chromophores produced from cholesterol and cholesteryl esters differs. Cholesteryl esters produce more color than unesterified cholesterol with the Liebermann-Burchard reagent and lead to a positive bias of 10 to 15 per cent when the analyses are based on unesterified cholesterol standards (Bachorik, 1979). Cholesteryl esters develop slightly less color than cholesterol with the iron salt–sulfuric acid reagent, and the assayed values are slightly lower than reference values (Wood, 1980).

The most accurate chemical methods are those in which cholesteryl esters are hydrolyzed and interfering substances such as hemoglobin, bilirubin, and others are removed. In the Schoenheimer-Sperry method, which is an accepted reference procedure, cholesteryl esters are hydrolyzed. Cholesterol is extracted with organic solvents, precipitated with digitonin, and analyzed using the Liebermann-Burchard reagent. This method is laborious, and has been largely replaced by the technically easier Abell-Kendall method (Abell, 1952). Cholesteryl esters are hydrolyzed, and cholesterol is extracted with petroleum ether and measured with the Liebermann-Burchard reagent. This method is currently accepted as the reference method for total cholesterol. Although simpler than the Schoenheimer-Sperry procedure, it is still rather time consuming, and is not ordinarily applied on a clinical scale.

Most of the chemical procedures that have been used on a large scale omit the hydrolysis of cholesteryl esters, and many of them, the so-called "direct" methods, omit the extraction of cholesterol from the sample as well. These procedures, particularly the direct methods, are rapid and easily automated, and they have been used frequently in the routine clinical laboratory or in other situations in which large numbers of samples must be analyzed. They are, however, subject to error from the sources mentioned above, and when accurate cholesterol values are required it is necessary to correct for the error. It is difficult, however, to appropriately apply correction procedures to methods in which both hydrolysis and extraction are omitted, because without extraction a number of possible interfering substances remain. Much of the error in the analysis of extracts is contributed by the differential development of color by cholesterol and cholesteryl esters, and since the ratio of these two forms is relatively constant in plasma, a correction procedure can be more readily applied. One such procedure was successfully used in the studies of the Lipid Research Clinics Program (1982; Bachorik, 1979). This procedure was based on the use of calibration sera in which the total cholesterol concentrations were determined with the Abell-Kendall reference method. Plasma was extracted with isopropanol, and the extract was treated with a mixture of zeolite, copper sulfate, calcium hydroxide, and Lloyd's reagent. These steps removed proteins, heme pigments, bilirubin, and other interfering substances. The treated extracts were analyzed with the Liebermann-Burchard reagent, using as standards solutions of pure cholesterol. The calibration pools were analyzed with the samples. A calibration factor was calculated from the observed and reference cholesterol concentrations of the pools and used to convert assayed values to reference values in the samples.

2

The success of any calibration procedure depends on the use of calibration pools for which the cholesterol concentrations are determined with a reference method. Such pools are becoming more widely available from commercial sources.

Enzymatic Methods. In completely enzymatic methods for cholesterol analysis (Allain, 1974), total cholesterol is determined directly in plasma or serum in a series of reactions in which cholesteryl esters are hydrolyzed, the 3-OH group of cholesterol is oxidized, and hydrogen peroxide, which is one of the reaction products, is determined enzymatically.

$$(1)\ \text{Cholesteryl ester} \xrightarrow[\text{hydrolase}]{\text{cholesteryl ester}} \text{cholesterol} + \text{fatty acid}$$

$$(2)\ \text{Cholesterol} + O_2 \xrightarrow[\text{oxidase}]{\text{cholesterol}} \text{cholest-4-en-3-one} + H_2O_2$$

$$(3)\ H_2O_2 + \text{Phenol} + \text{4-aminoantipyrine} \xrightarrow{\text{peroxidase}} \text{quinoneimine dye} + 2H_2O$$

The absorbance of the dye is measured at 500 nm.

The enzymatic methods are less subject to interference by non-sterol substances that react in the chemical methods. They are not absolutely specific for cholesterol, however, since cholesterol oxidase can react with other sterols that have been reported as being present in plasma, and with plant sterols present in appreciable concentrations in the circulation of patients with β-sitosterolemia. However, most chemical methods for estimating cholesterol measure these sterols as well.

Reducing substances such as ascorbic acid and bilirubin can interfere with the measurements by consuming H_2O_2 (Witte, 1978). Interference by bilirubin is complex and, depending on the reagent concentrations, can produce artifactually high or low cholesterol values. Bilirubin itself absorbs light at 500 nm, which would tend to increase the assayed cholesterol values. It is, however, oxidized by H_2O_2. Furthermore, when oxidized, bilirubin loses its absorbance at 500 nm, which complicates the application of a serum blank to correct for bilirubin absorbance. Bilirubin may also interfere directly by reacting with an intermediate in the peroxidase reaction. Interference by bilirubin seems to be significant only at concentrations exceeding 5 mg/dl, at which level it has been reported to decrease apparent cholesterol values by 5 to 15 per cent (Deacon and Dawson, 1979; Pesce and Bodourian, 1977). Sample turbidity due to elevated triglyceride concentrations can interfere with the enzymatic methods (Pesce and Bodourian, 1977). Uric acid, hemoglobin, and a large number of other substances in abnormally high concentrations apparently do not affect the cholesterol measurements (Deacon and Dawson, 1979).

The enzymatic methods consume only microliter quantities of sample and do not require a preliminary extraction step. They are quite rapid and, if cholesteryl ester hydrolase is omitted, also provide a measurement of unesterified cholesterol. Finally, the enzymatic methods appear to be quite precise, with coefficients of variation generally in the range of 1 to 2 per cent. For the most part they employ serum calibration standards, and, as mentioned earlier, the cholesterol concentration of the calibration pool must be known accurately. Enzymatic values agree with reference values within about 1 per cent when the enzymatic method is calibrated with serum pools that have been assigned reference cholesterol values (Cooper, 1982).

Triglycerides. A wide variety of methods have been used to measure plasma triglycerides (Bachorik, 1977), but the methods most commonly used for clinical or epidemiological purposes are based on the hydrolysis of triglycerides and the measurement of glycerol that is released in the reaction.

$$\text{(4) Triglyceride} + 3H_2O \longrightarrow \underset{\text{Glycerol}}{\begin{matrix} H_2COH \\ | \\ HCOH \\ | \\ H_2COH \end{matrix}} + \underset{\text{Fatty acids}}{3RC\begin{matrix} \nearrow O \\ \searrow OH \end{matrix}}$$

The reactions are performed chemically or enzymatically.

Chemical Methods. In the chemical methods, triglycerides and other lipids are first extracted into polar organic solvents, such as chloroform or isopropanol, which disrupt the lipoprotein complex and precipitate the proteins. One widely used method is the extraction and washing procedure described by Folch et al. (1957). The triglycerides are then isolated by silicic acid chromatography. In other methods, adsorbents such as alumina or zeolite are added to the lipid extract to remove interfering substances. One commonly used method is the automated procedure described by Kessler and Lederer (1966). An isopropanol extract of plasma or serum is treated with a mixture of zeolite, Lloyd's reagent, copper sulfate, and calcium hydroxide to remove phospholipids and glucose, which would interfere with the triglyceride-glycerol measurements. The adsorbent partially removes free glycerol and reduces potential interference from this source. It also concentrates the extract somewhat by removing some of the water that is introduced with the sample. For this reason the standards should be prepared to contain an equivalent amount of water and should be similarly treated with the zeolite mixture (Lipid Research Clinics Manual of Laboratory Operations, 1982).

Glycerol is released from triglycerides by saponification with alcohol potassium hydroxide or by transesterification with alcoholic solutions of sodium methoxide, and then it is oxidized with sodium periodate.

$$\text{(5) Glycerol} \xrightarrow[4]{NaIO} \underset{\text{Formaldehyde}}{2\,HC\begin{matrix} \nearrow O \\ \searrow H \end{matrix}} + \underset{\text{Formic acid}}{HC\begin{matrix} \nearrow O \\ \searrow OH \end{matrix}}$$

The formaldehyde produced has been most commonly measured either by reaction with a sulfuric acid solution of chromotropic acid to produce a pink chromophore, or by reaction with ammonium ions and acetylacetone to form 3,5-diacetyl-1,4-dihydrolutidine, which is measured colorimetrically or fluorometrically.

Periodate oxidation is not specific for glycerol; formaldehyde is also formed from substances with hydroxyl and amino groups on adjacent carbon atoms, or substances such as glucose that have adjacent hydroxyl groups. Furthermore, glycerol-containing phospholipids such as phosphatidylcholine are susceptible to alkaline hydrolysis to produce α-glycerophosphate, which is also oxidized by periodate to form formaldehyde. These particular substances are removed during the extraction and adsorption steps and do not interfere with triglyceride measurements.

Enzymatic Methods. Completely enzymatic methods are available for triglyceride analysis (Bucolo, 1973). They are relatively specific, rapid, and easy to use, and will probably replace the chemical methods entirely for most purposes.

The analyses are performed directly in plasma or serum, and are not subject to interference by phospholipids or glucose:

$$\text{(6) Triglycerides} \xrightarrow{\text{lipase}} \text{glycerol} + \text{fatty acids}$$

$$\text{(7) Glycerol} + \text{ATP} \xrightarrow{\text{glycerokinase}} \text{glycerophosphate} + \text{ADP}$$

$$\text{(8) Glycerophosphate} + \text{NAD}^+ \xrightarrow[\text{dehydrogenase}]{\text{glycerophosphate}} \text{dihydroxyacetone phosphate} + \text{NADH} + \text{H}^+$$

(9) NADH + tetrazolium dye $\xrightarrow{\text{diaphorase}}$ formazan + NAD^+

The NADH formed in reaction (8) can be measured spectrophotometrically. In most methods, reaction (9) has been added so the absorbance readings can be made in the 500 to 600 nm region of the spectrum, using instruments that are most commonly available in the clinical laboratory.

Enzymatic triglyceride methods have not yet been evaluated as extensively as the enzymatic cholesterol methods, but available information indicates that they generally perform well. The reagents are available commercially as lyophilized preparations that need only be reconstituted before use. For the most part, enzymatic methods correlate highly with the chemical methods. Not all enzymatic methods perform identically, however. For example, the precision of enzymatic methods, when used according to the manufacturers' recommendations, seems to vary about threefold (coefficients of variation of approximately 3 to 10 per cent), depending on the method. It is therefore prudent before selecting an enzymatic method to evaluate its accuracy and precision over the range of triglyceride concentrations likely to be encountered most frequently (50 to 500 mg/dl).

Triglyceride Blanks. The estimation of triglyceride blanks continues to be an area of uncertainty in triglyceride measurements. Increased blank readings can arise from a number of sources, depending on the samples, the methods used, or the physiological state of the patient. Calculations should take into account the non-glyceride substances that would add to the triglyceride measurements. As mentioned earlier, phospholipids and glucose interfere with chemical methods that employ periodate oxidation, but not with the enzymatic methods. Free glycerol, on the other hand, would interfere with both. Glycerol is normally present in plasma in concentrations below 1.5 mg/dl, but can be present in higher concentrations after extremely vigorous exercise, in some patients with uncontrolled diabetes, by chance contamination with the glycerol lubricant used on the stoppers of some blood collection tubes, after recent ingestion of glycerol-containing medications, or in a recently described disorder, hyperglycerolemia.

Partial glycerides are generally present in very low concentrations in fresh plasma or serum, but can form from the slow hydrolysis of triglycerides when samples are stored. They present a more complex problem, since they are detected in the chemical and enzymatic methods and add to the triglyceride measurements. It is common practice to determine triglyceride blanks by omitting the hydrolysis step. This procedure is satisfactory for correcting blanks that arise from many non-glyceride sources, but it can underestimate blanks due to the partial glycerides. In chemical methods that employ periodate oxidation, 1-monoglycerides, which have vicinal hydroxyl groups, are oxidized to form one, rather than two, molecules of formaldehyde (see reaction 5 above), and diglycerides do not react at all. In the enzymatic methods, neither partial glyceride would be detected. Furthermore, it is not clear whether blanks due to partial glycerides should be subtracted at all. As mentioned above, triglycerides are slowly hydrolyzed when samples are stored. Subtraction of the blank in these circumstances would underestimate triglycerides to the extent that the blank was formed from triglycerides that were originally present in the sample.

Fortunately, as complex as the blanking problem is, it is usually of little practical importance, and blanks are not determined routinely in many laboratories. The magnitude of the blanks encountered in most fresh samples is on the order of a few mg/dl and only uncommonly exceeds 8 to 10 mg/dl. Blanks can assume some importance, however, in the standardization and quality control of triglyceride measurements, since they can be of the order of 20 to 30 mg/dl or more in serum pools used for these purposes, probably due in part to the partial hydrolysis of triglycerides during the preparation of the pools. In the reference methods, triglycerides are isolated before analysis; the reference values reflect the actual concentrations of triglycerides at the time of analysis, and do not include the partial glycerides or glycerol that may have been produced during the preparation of the pools. Methods in which monoglycerides or free glycerol are measured along with triglycerides would therefore exhibit higher levels if blanks were not employed.

Phospholipids. Phosphatidyl choline and sphingomyelin constitute over 90 per cent of the phospholipids in human plasma, and of this about 80 per cent is phosphatidyl choline. The remaining phospholipids include phosphatidyl serine and phosphatidyl ethanolamine (3 to 6 per cent) and lysophosphatidyl choline (4 to 9 per cent). Although phospholipid analyses usually provide little additional information, it may be desirable on occasion to determine total phospholipids or individual phospholipid classes in patients with certain kinds of disorders such as obstructive jaundice, abeta- or hypobetalipoproteinemia, Tangier disease, or LCAT deficiency, in which the concentration, composition, and/or lipoprotein distribution of the phospholipids are altered.

Total phospholipids are most conveniently determined by measuring phospholipid phosphorus. Lipids are extracted from the sample and oxidized completely to convert phospholipid phosphorus to inorganic phosphate, which is then determined colorimetrically. Various extraction media have proved satisfactory, such as ethanol-diethylether (Ellefson, 1976) or chloroform-methanol used as described by Folch (1957). Oxidation is generally performed with concentrated H_2SO_4 used in conjunction with H_2O_2 or perchloric acid, at temperatures of 150 to 250°C. (Ellefson, 1976; Bartlett, 1959). The released phosphate is converted to phosphomolybdate by reaction with ammonium molybdate and the mixture is treated with a mild reducing agent (aminonaphthalsulfonic acid, p-methylaminophenol, stannous chloride, or one of several others) to form heteropolymolybdenum blue, which has an intense blue color. The procedures are

2

reproducible and sensitive and can be adapted to measure total phospholipid phosphorus in 100 μl or less of plasma or serum. Phospholipid concentration (mg/dl) is calculated as 25 times phospholipid phosphorus concentration in mg/dl. The analysis of individual phospholipid classes is seldom required for the evaluation of the dyslipoproteinemias and is not discussed here.

Estimation of Lipoproteins

Since the lipoproteins share common lipid and apolipoprotein components, the primary problem in lipoprotein analysis is the separation of the lipoprotein classes from each other. The methods that have been applied to lipoprotein separation include ultracentrifugation, adsorption, gel filtration, affinity chromatography, electrophoresis in various media, polyanion and alcohol precipitation, immunochemical procedures, and various combinations of methods. Some of these methods require special skills and equipment, and are not easily adapted for clinical or epidemiological purposes. The present discussion is limited to several procedures that have been used by the routine or special clinical laboratory that participates in the diagnosis and management of disorders of lipoprotein metabolism. It should be emphasized, as will become evident below, that no single method is capable of providing a patient's complete plasma lipoprotein profile.

Ultracentrifugal Methods. Ultracentrifugal methods take advantage of two properties of the lipoproteins. First, by virtue of their lipid content, they have lower densities than the other plasma macromolecules. Second, each class of lipoproteins has a different density. Thus, VLDL floats at d 1.006 g/ml, the density of plasma; LDL and HDL are sedimented at this density. LDL and VLDL both float at d 1.063 g/ml, and these lipoproteins as well as HDL float at d 1.21 g/ml. The lipoproteins can thus be separated from the other plasma proteins, and from each other, by ultracentrifugation at the appropriate density.

Analytical Ultracentrifugation—the "Reference Method." The lipoproteins have classically been defined in terms of their rates of flotation under specified conditions in the analytical ultracentrifuge (Lindgren, 1972). Although this method is not used in most clinical laboratories or very many research laboratories, analytical ultracentrifugation remains the reference method with which other methods are compared. It has the capability of breaking down the lipoprotein spectrum (especially VLDL, LDL, and HDL) into several different subclasses that can be accurately quantified.

The lipoproteins are first isolated from plasma by preparative ultracentrifugation and then centrifuged in the analytical ultracentrifuge, VLDL and LDL at d 1.063 g/ml, and HDL at d 1.210 g/ml. The lipoprotein classes and subclasses migrate at different rates, and the resulting optical Schlieren patterns can be used to calculate the concentration of lipoproteins. Lipoprotein concentrations are expressed in terms of total lipoprotein mass using calculations that take account of the empirically determined relationships between refractive index and dry weight for each of the major lipoprotein classes. Conditions of sample preparation, temperature, density adjustments, and other factors must be controlled rigorously, and the measurements must be corrected for various effects, such as variations in flotation rate with concentration, Ogston-Johnson effects, the redistribution of salts which changes the background density during ultracentrifugation, and correction of the measurements to standard conditions of temperature and density. The calculations are generally performed by computer.

Preparative Ultracentrifugation. Individual classes of lipoproteins can be quantitatively separated by ultracentrifugation at different densities (Havel, 1955). The separated lipoproteins are then measured in various ways, commonly in terms of their cholesterol content. In one approach, plasma is centrifuged sequentially at d 1.006 g/ml and d 1.063 g/ml. The cholesterol concentrations of the respective floating VLDL and LDL fractions are measured as an index of the concentrations of these lipoproteins. Cholesterol in the d 1.063 g/ml infranatant is associated almost entirely with HDL, and the cholesterol concentration of this fraction can be measured without separating HDL from the other plasma proteins. If it is desirable to isolate HDL, the d 1.063 g/ml infranatant is adjusted to d 1.21 g/ml and HDL is removed in the same way. With appropriate density adjustment, similar procedures can be used to determine subclasses of lipoproteins, for example, HDL_2 (d 1.063–d 1.12 g/ml) and HDL_3 (d 1.12–1.21 g/ml).

Another approach is to centrifuge aliquots of the plasma simultaneously at d 1.006 g/ml, d 1.063 g/ml, and d 1.21 g/ml. The cholesterol contents of the floating layers are determined and the individual lipoprotein concentrations are calculated by difference.

Preparative ultracentrifugation can provide reasonably accurate estimates of the concentrations of VLDL, LDL and HDL in samples that do not contain appreciable concentrations of Lp(a) or other unusual lipoproteins, or in which the densities of the major lipoproteins are not altered. Lp(a) overlaps the LDL and HDL density ranges and would contribute to cholesterol in both fractions. β-VLDL is manifested in Type III hyperlipoproteinemia. It is rich in cholesterol, floats at d 1.006 g/ml, and, when present, greatly enhances the cholesterol in the VLDL fraction.

Electrophoretic Methods. Electrophoresis has been widely used in the routine clinical laboratory to separate and measure lipoproteins. It should, however, be mentioned here that limitations of this methodology (which will be discussed subsequently), and the realization that it is not really needed for diagnosis of most dyslipoproteinemias, have considerably limited the use of electrophoresis for routine clinical practice. The most commonly used supporting media have been paper and agarose gel. In recent years, agarose gel electrophoresis has almost completely replaced paper electrophoresis because of its speed, greater sensitivity, and better resolution of the lipoprotein classes. The relative mobilities of the lipoproteins in both media are the same. Chylomicrons, if present, remain at the origin, and the other major lipoproteins migrate at rates that increase in the order of HDL>VLDL>LDL. The electrophoretically separated lipoproteins have been named according to their mobilities: HDL (α-lipoprotein) moves with the α_1-globulins; LDL (β-lipoprotein) migrates with the β-globulins, and VLDL (prebeta lipoprotein) migrates with the (α_2) globulins. Different properties of the lipoproteins form the basis for electrophoretic and ultracentrifugal separation, and analogous fractions separated by the two techniques may not be identical. For example, β-VLDL is isolated with VLDL by ultracentrifugation but moves electrophoretically with LDL. In the absence of additional information, a sample containing β-VLDL would appear to have an elevated VLDL-cholesterol concentration by ultracentrifugation and an increased LDL concentration by electrophoresis. Another example is Lp(a); ultracentrifugally it is isolated in the LDL-HDL density range, but it has an electrophoretic mobility similar to VLDL. This dichotomy is responsible for naming Lp(a) "sinking" pre-β lipoprotein.

Lipoprotein electrophoretograms are usually visualized with a lipid-staining dye such as Oil Red O, Fat Red 7B, or Sudan Black B, and electrophoresis can be performed in unfractionated plasma, or in plasma fractions that contain other serum proteins. These lipid stains are reacting primarily with the ester bonds in triglycerides and cholesterol esters. Lipoproteins rich in free cholesterol and phospholipids (such as LpX) stain very poorly and thus are grossly underestimated by electrophoretic techniques.

Attempts have been made to quantitate the lipoproteins by densitometry. Lipoprotein levels have been expressed in terms of the percent distribution of lipid-staining material in β, pre-β, and α-lipoproteins, or have been converted to lipoprotein-cholesterol concentrations according to calculations that incorporate assumptions about cholesterol content and dye uptake of the lipoproteins. In general, these approaches have not been successful for reasons that include incomplete resolution of beta and prebeta lipoproteins, the presence of minor or unusual lipoproteins, and differences in the intensity of staining. Electrophoresis has been most successfully used in conjunction with other methods (see below).

Polyanion Precipitation Methods. Lipoproteins are precipitated with polyanions such as heparin sulfate, dextran sulfate, phosphotungstate, and others, in the presence of divalent cations, such as Ca^{+2}, Mg^{+2} and Mn^{+2}. Precipitation is influenced by factors such as reagent concentration, pH, ionic strength, the presence of other serum proteins and anticoagulants, the relative amounts of lipid and protein in the lipoprotein particles, and the duration and conditions of sample storage. Conditions have been established in which the major classes of lipoproteins can be precipitated in stepwise fashion beginning with the lower-density, lipid-rich lipoproteins (Burstein, 1982). The more dissimilar the lipoproteins, the more satisfactorily they can be separated from each other. Thus, while apoB-containing lipoproteins can be precipitated from most samples under conditions in which virtually all the HDL remains soluble, it is more difficult to separate VLDL from LDL. Similarly, HDL can be isolated from the lower density lipoproteins much more satisfactorily than HDL_2 can be separated from HDL_3. In part, the more similar in composition the lipoprotein classes or subclasses to be separated are, the more critically the conditions of precipitation must be controlled to separate them. The likelihood therefore increases that a reagent concentration suitable for some samples may not be suitable for others, and the frequency of inadequate separations becomes unacceptably high. While theoretically attractive, lipoprotein quantitation schemes based entirely on precipitation methods have not gained wide acceptance, and polyanion precipitation has been most commonly used to remove apoB-containing lipoproteins prior to the analysis of HDL-cholesterol.

2

Methods for Determining HDL-Cholesterol Values. In the methods most commonly used, apoB-containing lipoproteins (chylomicrons, VLDL, IDL, LDL, Lp(a)) are removed by polyanion–divalent cation precipitation, and HDL-cholesterol is analyzed directly in the supernatant. Several combinations of polyanion–divalent cation have been used, and not all of them give precisely the same results. HDL-cholesterol values determined with heparin sulfate–Mn^{+2} procedures agree closely with those obtained with the analytical or preparative ultracentrifuge (Bachorik, 1976; Warnick, 1979). Dextran sulfate (Mr-50,000)–Mg^{+2} and sodium phosphotungstate–Mg^{+2} apparently give results about 5 per cent lower than ultracentrifugation, and heparin-Ca^{+2} appears to give results that are about 10 per cent higher. The differences arise, in part, from the extent to which apoB-containing lipoproteins and HDL are separated with the different precipitants. In some cases, traces of apoB-containing lipoproteins remain unprecipitated and can lead to a gross overestimation of HDL-cholesterol. In other cases, some HDL may be precipitated and cause an underestimation of HDL-cholesterol. In addition, the adequacy of seperation may also be influenced by factors such as the concentration of apoB-containing lipoproteins in the sample, the age of the sample, and others. It should be mentioned that the heparin sulfate–Mn^{+2} method has been most extensively studied and has also been most widely used in major population surveys and epidemiological studies in which the relationship between plasma HDL–cholesterol concentration and cardiovascular risk has been examined.

Combined Methods. Evaluation of the hyperlipidemic patient can include measurements of plasma cholesterol, VLDL, LDL, HDL, and triglyceride levels, an assessment of whether the patient has chylomicrons in the fasting state, and an assessment of the presence or absence of β-VLDL ("floating beta" lipoproteins, characteristic of overt Type III hyperlipoproteinemia). In addition, it may be necessary on occasion to assess the activity of lipoprotein lipase or the presence and nature of one or more of the apoproteins. Two approaches are in common use. The more extensive of the two employs a combination of preparative ultracentrifugation, polyanion precipitation, and electrophoresis (Fredrickson, 1968; Lipid Research Clinics Laboratory Manual, 1982).

Plasma total cholesterol, HDL-cholesterol, and triglyceride concentrations are determined as described above. A separate aliquot of plasma is ultracentrifuged without density adjustment. The floating layer containing VDL (and, if present, chylomicrons and β-VLDL) and the infranatant fraction, which contains LDL and HDL, are recovered. The cholesterol content of the infranatant fraction is determined. The lipoprotein cholesterol concentrations are calculated as follows:

1. HDL-cholesterol, measured directly.
2. LDL-cholesterol = (infranatant cholesterol) − (HDL-cholesterol).
3. VLDL-cholesterol = (total cholesterol) − (infranatant cholesterol).
4. A simplified procedure that does not require the ultracentrifuge was described by Friedewald (1972). In this method the plasma total cholesterol, triglyceride, and HDL-cholesterol concentrations are determined as described above. Since most of the plasma triglycerides are carried in VLDL, VLDL-cholesterol concentration is estimated from the ratio of triglyceride to cholesterol in VLDL:

$$\text{VLDL-chol} = \frac{\text{plasma TG}}{5}$$

This assay must be done on a fasting sample. The method assumes that essentially all the plasma triglycerides are carried in VLDL and that the TG/cholesterol ratio of VLDL is invariant. Neither assumption is entirely true, and can lead to fairly large percentage errors in estimates of VLDL-cholesterol. This does not normally produce errors of more than 5 to 10 per cent in LDL-cholesterol measurements, however, because VLDL generally carries only a small proportion of plasma total cholesterol. There are some limitations on the kinds of samples to which the equation can be applied. It is not suitable for use with samples in which triglyceride concentrations exceed 400 mg/dl, or in samples that have chylomicrons or β-VLDL. Compared with VLDL, the ratio of triglycerides/cholesterol in chylomicrons is much higher and that in β-VLDL is much lower, and the presence of either can lead to gross error in LDL-cholesterol estimates. Provided its limitations are appreciated, the method has broad usefulness both as a screening tool and for following patients whose lipoprotein patterns are known from more extensive analyses.

VLDL-cholesterol can be measured directly in the d<1.006 g/ml fraction, but tends to be inaccurate because of the difficulty in recovering VLDL quantitatively.

Standing Plasma Test. Chylomicrons, if present in appreciable quantities, are detected using the "standing plasma" test. An aliquot of plasma (2 ml) is placed into a 10 × 75 mm test tube and allowed to stand in the refrigerator at 4°C. undisturbed overnight. Chylomicrons accumulate as a floating "cream" layer and can be detected visually. The presence of chylomicrons in fasting plasma is considered abnormal. Turbid plasma which does not float after overnight chilling contains excessive amounts of VLDL.

Detection of **β*-VLDL.*** The ultracentrifugal fraction of d <1.006 g/ml is examined electrophoretically for the presence of β-VLDL ("floating beta" lipoproteins). In practice, unfractionated plasma and the two ultracentrifugal fractions are examined at the same time; each sample thus serves as its own control to establish the relative migration of the lipoprotein bands. In normal plasma, the β-, pre-β, and α-lipoprotein bands are visible in unfractionated plasma. Only the pre-β band is present in the d <1.006 g/ml fraction, and the β- and α-lipoprotein bands are seen only in the d >1.006 g/ml fraction. In addition, if Lp(a) is present in sufficient concentration, an additional band with pre-β mobility is also observed in the d >1.006 g/ml fraction (hence the name sinking pre-β). When present, β-VLDL is observed as a band with β-mobility in the d <1.006 g/ml fraction. Its presence is considered abnormal and it is usually associated with dysbetalipoproteinemia, although it is occasionally seen in other disorders as well. Chylomicrons, which are often seen in Type III, remain at the origin on paper and agarose gel.

VLDL-Cholesterol: Plasma Triglyceride Ratio. Finally, the ratio of VLDL-cholesterol to plasma triglycerides is calculated. This ratio is generally in the range of 0.1 to 0.25 in samples without β-VLDL, depending on the relative amounts of VLDL, LDL, and HDL present, and on the errors in the VLDL-cholesterol and plasma triglyceride measurements. Type III subjects generally manifest ratios greater than 0.3, usually in the range 0.3 to 0.4, although higher ratios are observed. Again, because of the error in the measurements, the observation of a ratio of 0.3 on a single occasion may or may not be significant. Overt Type III patients manifest both β-VLDL and a VLDL-chol/plasma TG ratio of 0.3 or greater.

Apolipoprotein Analysis

Quantitation of apolipoproteins is not performed as a routine clinical procedure at present, primarily because it is not clear how useful this information would be to practicing physicians. However, apolipoprotein measurements are being increasingly performed as a research tool and methodologies are being developed to achieve this goal. Some of these studies have already produced results pointing to the possibility that at least a few apolipoproteins are better discriminators of atherosclerotic disease risk than other lipid or lipoprotein determinations (Ishikawa, 1978; Avogaro, 1979; Sniderman, 1980; Kwiterovich, 1981). Most of the quantitation methods are based on immunological identification of the apolipoproteins. Immunoreactivity must then be related to mass, determined by other means. Simple chemical determination is not very useful since even carefully separated lipoprotein fractions contain more than one apolipoprotein, and the chemical determination will not discriminate between the various determinants. Apolipoprotein B can be determined chemically in certain narrow cuts of LDL (d 1.019 to 1.050) which do not contain significant amounts of other apolipoproteins.

Apolipoprotein Immunoassays. These determinations are based on recognition of the apolipoprotein antigen by an antibody or a group of antibodies against one or more of the antigenic sites on the molecule. Several immunoassays are available to date:

Radioimmunoassay (RIA). Sensitive and precise RIA's have been described for measurement of apoA-I (Schonfeld, 1974), apoA-II (Schonfeld, 1977), apoB (Albers, 1975), apoC-II and apoC-III (Schonfeld, 1979), apoE (Falko, 1980), and Lp(a) (Albers, 1977). The advantages of this technique are its sensitivity, its need for only small amounts of antibody, and its being amenable to automation. However, RIA's require special and expensive equipment, and create radioactive waste. Radiolabeling may also damage the antigen, shorten its shelf life, and cause the labeled standard to be different from the unlabeled standard or the unknown sample.

Radial Immunodiffusion (RID). This is a relatively simple method in which an antigen is allowed to diffuse from a well into the surrounding gel (usually agarose) which contains an antibody to it, and thus form a precipitin disc the area of which is proportional to the amount of antigen in the sample. RID does not require complicated and expensive equipment; however, it is not amenable to automation and thus cannot be performed on a very large scale. It also requires large amounts of antibody. Another problem that limits the usefulness of this method is the size-related diffusion differences between the various particles containing the antigen. RID for apoB, for instance, may be quite accurate for measurement of LDL apoB, but it may underestimate VLDL apoB and thus be inaccurate for lipemic samples due to incomplete and slow diffusion of the large VLDL particles. RID assays have been described for apolipoproteins of the A (Cheung, 1977) and B (Sniderman, 1980) groups.

Electroimmunoassay (EIA). This is a rather simple and relatively accurate method based on principles similar to those for the RID, except that the samples are subject to electrophoresis and the precipitin lines are in the form of "rockets" rather than discs. Most of the advantages and disadvantages of RID are valid also for this method. Electrophoresis improves the diffusion of large particles into the gel, but it also has its own inherent problems. EIA's have been described for most of the A (Curry, 1976a), B (Curry, 1978), C (Curry, 1980, 1981), D (Curry, 1977), and E (Curry, 1976b) apolipoproteins.

Immunonephelometry. This method is based on measurement of the turbidity caused by the antigen (apolipoprotein)-antibody complex (Lopes-Virella, 1980). A severe limitation of the method stems from the inherent turbidity of lipemic samples, or even non-lipemic samples subjected to repeated freezing and thawing.

Enzyme-Linked and Fluorescence Immunoassays. Enzyme-linked (ELISA) and fluorescence immunoassays are being developed for apolipoprotein analysis (Fruchart, 1978). ELISA may be particularly useful for clinical application. They are competitive binding assays but do not require radiolabeled reagents. The sample or standard solution is incubated with antibody in a tube that has been precoated with the antigen. The amount of antibody in the solution available for binding to the precoated-tube antigen depends on the sample antigen concentration. The higher the sample antigen concentration, the more antibody is bound, and less of it is left to react and bind to the precoated antigen on the tube. The tube-bound antibody is reacted with a second peroxide-conjugated antibody which enables colorimetric measurement. The assays are sensitive and precise, are amenable to automation, usually using well characterized antibodies, and lack some of the problems inherent in the use of radiolabeled reagents. They hold a very significant hope for future use in clinical practice and/or large-scale population studies.

There are many unsolved methodological problems in apolipoprotein immunoassays. Isolation techniques and molecular properties of the antigens should be standardized. The need for use of proteinase inhibitors immediately after collection of plasma was advocated by some researchers but disputed by others. The effect of long-term storage of samples, antibodies, and standard antigens (labeled and unlabeled) has yet to be established. The question of whether measurement of the standards and the unknown samples should be performed in the same milieu is still open. Related to this problem is the need to delipidate or treat samples with a detergent in order to expose more antigenic sites and improve sensitivity and accuracy. Other unresolved problems relate to the role of monoclonal antibodies in quantitation of apolipoproteins, and the specificity of antibodies. Several antibodies produced against apolipoproteins that are delipidated to various degrees may be reactive with different sites on the same apolipoprotein, or even interactive only with the lipid bound to the apolipoprotein.

Qualitative Apolipoprotein Analysis. Several qualitative analyses of apolipoproteins may supply extremely important information to the researcher or even to the clinician. A simple immunodiffusion technique can determine the existence or absence of a given apolipoprotein. It is especially useful in evaluating a hypolipoproteinemic patient (Tangier disease, abetalipoproteinemia, etc.) or a patient with chylomicronemia possibly due to apoC-II deficiency. Gel electrophoresis techniques (in polyacrylamide, agarose, or other media), which separate apolipoproteins by molecular weight, isoelectric focusing, which separates them by charge, and especially the combination of the two in a bidimensional system have considerably improved our understanding of dysbetalipoproteinemia, and some of the lipoprotein deficiency states (Utermann, 1975; Zannis, 1980, 1981). For detailed description see section on Dysbetalipoproteinemia—Type III hyperlipoproteinemia. The application of these techniques has gone beyond their usefulness as

Table 11–4. PLASMA TOTAL CHOLESTEROL (mg/dl)—WHITE MALES*

	Percentiles				
Age	***Mean***	***5***	***75***	***90***	***95***
0–19	155	115	170	185	200
20–24	165	125	185	205	220
25–29	180	135	200	225	245
30–34	190	140	215	240	255
35–39	200	145	225	250	270
40–44	205	150	230	250	270
45–69	215	160	235	260	275
70+	205	150	230	250	270

*LRC Program Prevalence Study. Values for mean and selected cutpoints were rounded to nearest 5 mg/dl.

a research tool, and by now they already have clinical importance, especially as they readily allow the apoE analysis now employed in the diagnosis of Type III.

FACTORS AFFECTING VARIATION OF PLASMA LIPID AND LIPOPROTEIN CONCENTRATIONS IN INDIVIDUALS AND IN POPULATIONS

Plasma lipid and lipoprotein concentrations vary within and among populations and under different conditions within a given individual.

Limited space precludes a detailed description of all demographic, environmental, genetic, and physiologic determinants of blood lipids and lipoproteins. It should be noted, however, that this variability in the concentrations of lipids and lipoproteins makes the use of universally accepted "upper reference limits" difficult.

Both genetic and environmental factors influence cholesterol concentrations (Segal, 1982). Family and twin studies have shown that genetic components (including polygenic effects as well as the mutant allele responsible for familial hypercholesterolemia) account for a small proportion of the total variability. Environmental factors, although not always clearly understood, markedly influence the variability in the distribution of cholesterol between populations. For example, immigrants who come to the United States from countries in which the mean cholesterol level is low usually acquire the higher levels characteristic of North America. Nutritional factors have important effects upon lipid metabolism in man and probably play the dominant role in the pathogenesis of hyperlipidemia so commonly found in western populations.

In healthy subjects dietary cholesterol raises LDL cholesterol levels. The amount and type of dietary fat (saturated or polyunsaturated) also have well-documented effects upon plasma lipid and lipoprotein concentrations. In general, saturated fat elevates and polyunsaturated fat decreases the plasma and LDL cholesterol levels. The mechanisms by which such fats influence plasma lipid levels are unclear.

The amount and type of carbohydrate consumed appear to have little long-term effect on lipid levels. In short-term (a few days to a few weeks) experimental studies, increased carbohydrate intake (to about 75 per cent of total calories) has usually resulted in a sharp increase in plasma triglyceride and sharp decrease in HDL. Long-term studies, however, have indicated that in spite of continuation of the high carbohydrate diet, triglyceride concentrations and, more slowly, HDL will return to baseline levels.

Excessive caloric consumption of any source of food with an associated weight gain may lead to hypertriglyceridemia through VLDL increase; this is particularly true in individuals with already elevated triglycerides. Even moderate reduction in caloric intake in hypertriglyceridemic overweight patients usually leads to lower VLDL levels. Excessive alcohol intake increases plasma triglycerides. Heavy alcohol consumption is responsible for a considerable proportion of hypertriglyceridemia in many countries. On the other hand, moderate alcohol consumption causes a considerable increase in HDL concentrations.

Various medications are known to influence plasma lipid distribution. Of these, sex hormones (oral con-

Table 11–5. PLASMA TOTAL CHOLESTEROL (mg/dl)—WHITE FEMALES*

	Percentiles				
Age	***Mean***	***5***	***75***	***90***	***95***
0–19	160	120	175	190	200
20–24	170	125	190	215	230
25–34	175	130	195	220	235
35–39	185	140	205	230	245
40–44	195	145	215	235	255
45–49	205	150	225	250	270
50–54	220	165	240	265	285
55+	230	170	250	275	295

*LRC Program Prevalence Study. Values for mean and selected cutpoints were rounded to nearest 5 mg/dl.

Table 11–6. PLASMA TRIGLYCERIDES (mg/dl)—WHITE MALES*

Age	Percentiles			
	Mean	*5*	*90*	*95*
0–9	55	30	85	100
10–14	65	30	100	125
15–19	80	35	120	150
20–24	100	45	165	200
25–29	115	45	200	250
30–34	130	50	215	265
35–39	145	55	250	320
40–54	150	55	250	320
55–64	140	60	235	290
65+	135	55	210	260

*LRC Program Prevalence Study. Values for mean and selected cutpoints were rounded to nearest 5 mg/dl.

Table 11–7. PLASMA TRIGLYCERIDES (mg/dl)—WHITE FEMALES*

Age	Percentiles			
	Mean	*5*	*90*	*95*
9	60	35	95	110
10–19	75	40	115	130
20–34	90	40	145	170
35–39	95	40	160	195
40–44	105	45	170	210
45–49	110	45	185	230
50–54	120	55	190	240
55–64	125	55	200	250
65+	130	60	205	240

*LRC Program Prevalence Study. Values for mean and selected cutpoints were rounded to nearest 5 mg/dl.

traceptives and estrogen replacement therapy) are epidemiologically the most important. For example, the Lipid Research Clinics Program of the National Heart, Lung, and Blood Institute reported that in an aggregate of 11 U.S. populations (Wallace, 1979), 50 per cent of the women in the 20- to 24-year-old age group used combined estrogen-progestogen oral contraceptive medication, and this was associated with increases in plasma cholesterol, triglyceride, and LDL and VLDL levels. HDL was unchanged in this age group. Mean plasma triglyceride concentration was 48 per cent higher in hormone users under age 40 than in non-users in the same age group. Use of sex hormones was the most common cause of hypertriglyceridemia in women 20 to 50 years old. On the other hand, in postmenopausal women the use of estrogen alone as replacement therapy, which was also quite prevalent, was accompanied by a decrease in plasma cholesterol, triglycerides, and LDL and VLDL, and by an increase in HDL.

REFERENCE VALUES FOR PLASMA LIPIDS AND LIPOPROTEINS

The variability in plasma lipids and lipoproteins among populations precludes the establishment of universally acceptable limits of "reference intervals." What may be considered "normal" for one population group may not necessarily be applicable to another. Even within a country, these reference intervals may vary from one region to another and are markedly age-, sex-, and race-dependent.

It should also be mentioned here that a "normal" lipid level, i.e., less than the upper 5 per cent of the distribution, is not synonymous with "healthy" and does not imply absence of risk. Therefore, different cutoff points may be used for different purposes. Traditionally the ninetieth or ninety-fifth percentile is used to define hyperlipoproteinemia. However, it should not be used to define normality, since no clear cutoff point for coronary heart disease exists, and in fact the relationship between plasma cholesterol levels and coronary heart disease risk is continuous.

Total plasma lipid and lipoprotein-cholesterol distributions are presented in Tables 11–4 through 11–11, based on cross-sectional data obtained at 10 Lipid Research Clinics in North America (Lipid Research Clinics Program, 1980.) Means and selected percentiles are given for white males and females, ages 0 to 70+ years, thus demonstrating the effects of age and sex. (No information is given for blacks because of insufficient data.)

LIPIDS, LIPOPROTEINS, AND DISEASE

Abnormal concentrations of plasma lipoproteins are sometimes associated with acute morbidity and with immediately related signs and symptoms. These will be discussed in the section on familial LPL deficiency. However, a great deal of the interest in plasma lipids

Table 11–8. PLASMA LDL CHOLESTEROL (mg/dl)—WHITE MALES*

Age	Percentiles				
	Mean	*5*	*75*	*90*	*95*
5–19	95	65	105	120	130
20–24	105	65	120	140	145
25–29	115	70	140	155	165
30–34	125	80	145	165	185
35–39	135	80	155	175	190
40–44	135	85	155	175	185
45–69	145	90	165	190	205
70+	145	90	165	180	185

*LRC Program Prevalence Study. Values for mean and selected cutpoints were rounded to nearest 5 mg/dl.

Table 11–9. PLASMA LDL CHOLESTEROL (mg/dl)—WHITE FEMALES*

Age	Percentiles				
	Mean	*5*	*75*	*90*	*95*
5–19	100	65	110	125	140
20–24	105	55	120	140	160
25–34	110	70	125	145	160
35–39	120	75	140	160	170
40–44	125	75	145	165	175
45–49	130	80	150	175	185
50–54	140	90	160	185	200
55+	150	95	170	195	215

*LRC Program Prevalence Study. Values for mean and selected cutpoints were rounded to nearest 5 mg/dl.

stems from the alleged association between lipid and lipoprotein levels and atherosclerotic cardiovascular disease (CVD). The "lipid hypothesis" of atherosclerosis is based on the following facts:

1. The human atherosclerotic plaque contains lipids, most of which are derived from plasma lipoproteins.
2. Atherosclerotic lesions can be produced in experimental animals made hypercholesterolemic by dietary means. Some of these lesions can be made to regress by changing the diet to return to normocholesterolemia.
3. Hyperlipidemia is more prevalent among groups of subjects with clinically manifested atherosclerotic disease.
4. Clinical manifestations of atherosclerosis are more prevalent among subjects with certain familial hyperlipidemias.
5. Cross-sectional and, most important, prospective epidemiologic population studies usually reveal a relationship between atherosclerotic disease morbidity and mortality and plasma lipids and lipoprotein levels.

In recent years there have been several attempts at primary prevention of atherosclerotic CVD by modifying the levels of plasma lipids (Committee of Principal Investigators, 1978). At least some of the already completed studies lend support to the "lipid hypothesis" of atherosclerosis. Atherosclerosis is a multifactorial disease. Several habits, traits, and abnormalities associated with a sizable increase in susceptibility to atherosclerotic CVD have been designated as "risk factors." Age, male sex, cigarette smoking, hypertension, and increased serum cholesterol and decreased HDL cholesterol levels were identified as important independent risk factors. Obesity, increased serum triglyceride concentrations, glucose intolerance, and sedentary lifestyle are also associated with atherosclerotic disease, but epidemiologic studies have not established them as independent risk factors beyond reasonable doubt (Hulley, 1980). The risk of coronary heart disease (CHD) in a seemingly healthy population is directly related to plasma cholesterol concentrations. Subjects with the highest cholesterol levels are at greater risk of developing CHD, but low levels do not represent immunity to it. There is a continuous relationship between total plasma cholesterol (and LDL cholesterol) and CHD risk. The arbitrary "cutoff" points that designate "abnormal" levels for the diagnosis of hyperlipoproteinemia are just a tool of convenience to the practitioner faced with the need to make clinical decisions that are based on categorical definitions. The need to consider change in lifestyles and/or take over appropriate prophylactic measures exists throughout the cholesterol distribution of the population.

Increasingly HDL is measured, mainly because it has emerged in recent years as a very strong, independent, inverse correlate of CHD. Increased HDL levels are also solely responsible for hypercholesterolemia in 5 per cent of adults and 20 per cent of children. It is usually quantitated as HDL cholesterol, and it remains to be seen whether some of its protein

Table 11–10. PLASMA HDL CHOLESTEROL (mg/dl)—WHITE MALES*

Age	Percentiles			
	Mean	*5*	*10*	*95*
5–19	50	35	40	70
20–24	45	30	30	65
25–29	45	30	30	65
30–34	45	30	30	65
35–39	45	30	30	60
40–44	45	25	30	65
45–69	50	30	30	70
70+	50	30	35	75

*LRC Program Prevalence Study. Values for mean and selected cutpoints were rounded to nearest 5 mg/dl.

Table 11–11. PLASMA HDL CHOLESTEROL (mg/dl)—WHITE FEMALES*

Age	Percentiles			
	Mean	*5*	*10*	*95*
5–19	55	35	40	70
20–24	55	35	35	80
25–34	55	35	40	80
35–39	55	35	40	80
40–44	60	35	40	90
45–49	60	35	40	85
50–54	60	35	40	90
55+	60	35	40	95

*LRC Program Prevalence Study. Values for mean and selected cutpoints were rounded to nearest 5 mg/dl.

components are better predictors of CHD risk. Total HDL cholesterol measurements may not detect important variability among HDL subfractions. HDL_2, its subfractions, and HDL_2/HDL_3 ratios were employed in various studies, which seem to indicate that HDL_2 is the main "antiatherogenic" lipoprotein (Eder, 1982). The epidemiology of HDL has recently been extensively reviewed in a large population sample in the United States (Heiss, 1980). Genetic as well as environmental and socioeconomic factors affect HDL levels, and should be regarded in the context of any prophylactic measures against CHD. Maleness, progestogens, obesity, high carbohydrate intake, sedentary lifestyle, Type II diabetes, hypertriglyceridemia, and cigarette smoking are associated with lower levels of HDL. Femaleness, estrogens, exercise, and moderate alcohol consumption and nicotinic acid use are associated with higher levels of HDL.

The possible association of very low levels of plasma cholesterol with increased cancer mortality has received some attention in recent years. While some natural history studies suggest this association in men, others do not. The information available to date does not appear to justify any deviation from the prevailing general policy of trying to reduce plasma cholesterol levels in the at-risk population by dietary means (Feinleib, 1981).

DYSLIPOPROTEINEMIA

This is a group of disorders characterized by quantitative and/or qualitative abnormalities of plasma lipoproteins. The term dyslipoproteinemia is preferable to hyper- or hypolipoproteinemia; excessive accumulation of one lipoprotein is not infrequently accompanied by decreased concentrations of another, and absence of low levels of one lipoprotein are sometimes accompanied by elevated levels of another. Accumulation in the plasma of excessive amounts of lipoproteins is usually the result of failure of the catabolic apparatus. This is caused by either an abnormality of the catabolic system (enzymes, cell surface receptors, etc.) or an abnormal structure of the lipoprotein particle, which decreases its ability to interact with the catabolic mechanism. Only seldom is accumulation of lipoproteins due to increased synthesis. Complete absence or extremely decreased concentration of a particular lipoprotein is usually caused by a genetically determined failure of the synthetic mechanism for a certain apolipoprotein or, less commonly, the formation of an altered one. In either case, this leads to complete absence from the plasma of particles that usually contain this apolipoprotein, or to the synthesis of small amounts of abnormal particles, which are quickly removed from the circulation by the body's usual cellular defense mechanisms (see discussion of Tangier disease).

Only a small proportion of the patients with clinically recognized dyslipoproteinemias have well characterized single gene mutations. Most of the dyslipoproteinemias encountered in clinical practice are either polygenic or a product of the interaction of genetically determined susceptibility with environmental factors. Other terms used to characterize the nature of dyslipoproteinemia are "primary" or "secondary." Abnormal plasma lipoprotein concentrations have long been associated with conditions such as diabetes mellitus, hypothyroidism, nephrotic syndrome, obstructive biliary disease, pancreatitis, alcoholism, dysglobulinemia, non-nephrotic renal failure, glycogen storage disease, and others. It should, however, be noted that the finding of the two disorders in the same individual does not automatically mean a causal relationship between them. Not every patient with the above-mentioned disorders is dyslipoproteinemic, and the treatment of the primary disorder may not always lead to the disappearance of dyslipoproteinemia if present. In some cases the metabolic abnormality causes an aggravation of the otherwise dormant genetic tendency to develop primary dyslipoproteinemia. The use of certain drugs is also associated with abnormal plasma lipoprotein concentrations; estrogen- and progestogen-containing drugs, as well as diuretics, antibiotics, β-blockers and others are known to alter lipoprotein metabolism and cause dyslipoproteinemia in some patients. The clinical evaluation of a patient with dyslipoproteinemia should include the identification of clinical conditions or drugs used that are known to cause or aggravate the disorder.

The work of Fredrickson (1967) was the first attempt to classify the dyslipoproteinemias according to genetically determined lipoprotein molecular abnormalities, and precipitated the tremendous research activity in this field. Recent advances in methods of protein chemistry, and of molecular and cell biology, have led to a better understanding of the pathogenesis and the genetics of some of the dyslipoproteinemias. Based on these recent advances, an updated modification of the original system is presented here, but the basic concepts of Fredrickson are still valid today (Fig. 11–5).

Hyperchylomicronemia

This is a heterogeneous group of disorders characterized by accumulation of excessive amounts of chylomicrons in the plasma. At least two familial disorders are known to result in hyperchylomicronemia; one is caused by a deficiency of the lipoprotein lipase enzyme, and the other by a deficiency of its activator. Both result in a very similar clinical syndrome.

Familial Lipoprotein Lipase (LPL) Deficiency (Type I Hyperlipoproteinemia). This is a rare disorder, which usually presents in childhood with abdominal pain and pancreatitis. On examination it often exhibits eruptive xanthoma, lipemia retinalis, and hepatosplenomegaly. Premature atherosclerosis is not a feature of this disease. Recurrent bouts of pancreatitis are the major causes of morbidity and mortality in this disorder. In patients on a regular diet after an overnight fast, chylomicrons are present in huge amounts and cause the cloudy-milky appearance of the plasma. Serum triglycerides are extremely elevated, whereas cholesterol concentrations may be nor-

2

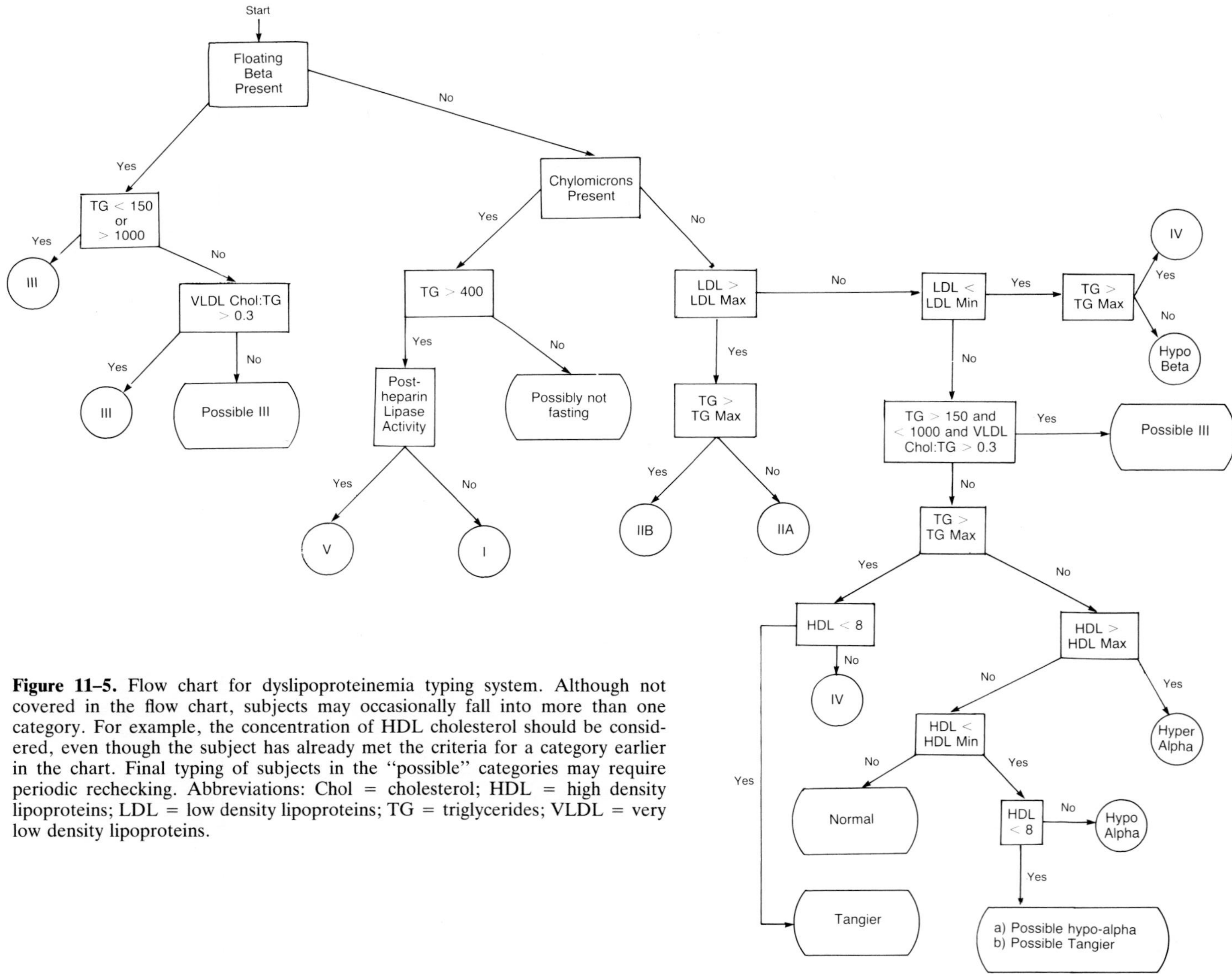

Figure 11–5. Flow chart for dyslipoproteinemia typing system. Although not covered in the flow chart, subjects may occasionally fall into more than one category. For example, the concentration of HDL cholesterol should be considered, even though the subject has already met the criteria for a category earlier in the chart. Final typing of subjects in the "possible" categories may require periodic rechecking. Abbreviations: Chol = cholesterol; HDL = high density lipoproteins; LDL = low density lipoproteins; TG = triglycerides; VLDL = very low density lipoproteins.

mal or only slightly high. Plasma post-heparin lipolytic activity (PHLA), which is a crude estimate of the activities of various lipases (including lipoprotein lipase) released into the plasma following the intravenous injection of heparin, is markedly decreased, because of lipoprotein lipase deficiency. The disease is inherited as an autosomal recessive trait, and the lipoprotein lipase–deficient patients are homozygotes for the mutant allele (Fredrickson, 1978).

Familial Apolipoprotein C-II Deficiency. This syndrome is clinically indistinguishable from the familial LPL deficiency. However, the apparent lipolytic enzyme abnormality is not caused by an enzyme deficiency but rather by a severe deficiency of apo-C-II in the plasma of affected subjects (Breckenridge, 1978). Apo C-II is a potent activator of LPL and, when supplied from the outside in the form of plasma or blood transfusion, restores the lipolytic activity of these patients to the normal range. Inheritance is as an autosomal recessive trait (Cox, 1978).

Familial Hypercholesterolemia (Type II Hyperlipoproteinemia)

Familial hypercholesterolemia, which is a common disorder of lipoprotein metabolism, manifests itself clinically by xanthomata, corneal arcus, and premature atherosclerotic (especially coronary) disease. Plasma cholesterol concentrations are elevated due to increased LDL concentrations. Triglyceride and VLDL concentrations are either normal (Type IIa) or increased (Type IIb). Inheritance is as an autosomal dominant trait with high penetrance of the mutant allele. The gene frequency is estimated to be 0.2 to 0.5 per cent of the white population. It should be noted that most of the subjects with Type II hyperlipoproteinemia seen in clinical practice do not have familial hypercholesterolemia but rather other less well characterized monogenic or polygenic lipid disorders.

Goldstein and Brown (summarized in Goldstein, 1982) showed that subjects with familial hypercholesterolemia have one of several genetic defects in the cell surface LDL receptor that normally controls intracellular cholesterol metabolism as well as the degradation of LDL. Based on these studies three mutant alleles were postulated at the LDL receptor locus: the R^{b^o} allele that specifies the receptor-negative form, the R^{b^-} allele associated with the receptor-defective form, and the R^{b+,i^o} allele responsible for the internalization defect variety. Homozygotes for any given mutant allele have very marked elevations of plasma cholesterol and LDL (>600 mg/dl), which can be detected at a very young age. They also develop xanthomatosis and accelerated CHD as early as the first decade. Heterozygotes to any given mutant allele show *in vitro* LDL binding and/or internalization intermediate between normals and homozygotes. Their clinical manifestations are also not as severe as in homozygotes.

LDL receptor assays are not used as a routine clinical tool. The assays should be performed in specialized laboratories on patients suspected to be homozygotes for the familial hypercholesterolemia gene. However, at our present stage of knowledge, there is no justification to perform the tests routinely in order to characterize heterozygosity because of the wide overlap between these patients and normal subjects.

Treatment of this disorder consists of a diet low in cholesterol and saturated fat and sequestrant resins such as cholestyramine with or without nicotinic acid. Surgical procedures such as partial ileal bypass and portacaval shunt are sometimes used, especially in homozygotes who do not respond to the more conventional forms of therapy.

Familial Dysbetalipoproteinemia (Type III Hyperlipoproteinemia)

Dysbetalipoproteinemia is a disorder of lipid metabolism manifested clinically by accelerated atherosclerosis of the coronary and peripheral arteries and by characteristic tuberoeruptive and planar xanthomas. The palmar areas are very often affected by typical yellowish discoloration along the creases. Affected subjects are commonly overweight and often show abnormal glucose tolerance, including frank diabetes mellitus.

Plasma triglyceride levels are elevated, and usually so are cholesterol concentrations, bringing the ratio of these plasma lipids close to 1. This reflects the presence of an abnormal form of VLDL, which shows beta mobility on electrophoresis (β-VLDL, floating betalipoprotein). The β-VLDL particle is smaller and heavier than normal VLDL, and contains a high proportion of cholesterol relative to its triglyceride content. This results in a high VLDL-cholesterol to plasma triglycerides ratio (≥0.3),which is often used as a diagnostic criterion.

The biochemical abnormality of dysbetalipoproteinemia has recently been characterized as a quantitative and qualitative abnormality of apoE (Havel, 1973; Utermann, 1975; Zannis, 1980; Ghiselli, 1981). The total amount of apoE in VLDL of patients with dysbetalipoproteinemia is increased; however, these patients usually have a typical apoE isoforms phenotype. The synthesis of three major apoE isoforms (apoE^2, apoE^3, and apoE^4) is under the control of three alleles (E^2, E^3, and E^4, respectively) at a single genetic locus. Homozygosity for the E^2 allele gives rise to the E 2/2 phenotype, which predisposes the subject to dysbetalipoproteinemia. VLDL remnant particles (IDL) containing apoE^2 as the major apoE isoprotein bind poorly to cell surface receptors, and thus are not taken up and not catabolized by cells, but rather accumulate in the plasma. The heterogeneity of the three major apoE isoforms is due to structural differences. Cysteine-arginine interchanges at positions 112 and 158 in the amino acid sequence of apoE are responsible for the charge differences between the apoE isoforms (Weisgraber, 1981). ApoE^2 contains cysteine and apoE^4 contains arginine at both positions, while apoE^3 contains a cysteine at position 158 and arginine at position 112. Chemical modification of the apoE[2] charge results in improved binding of this protein to cell surface receptors (Weisgraber, 1982).

The frequency of the E 2/2 phenotype in the population, estimated to be about 1 to 3 per cent, is considerably higher than the prevalence of Type III hyperlipoproteinemia. This has led to the hypothesis that gross hyperlipidemia in dysbetalipoproteinemic patients results from the coincidence, in one individual, of the genetically determined E 2/2 phenotype, and either another monogenic or polygenic dyslipoproteinemia or another environmental factor. The relationship of the E 2/2 phenotype to normolipidemic dysbetalipoproteinemia is not known at present, nor is the significance of the various apoE phenotypes with or without hyperlipidemia known with respect to CHD in the general population.

Dysbetalipoproteinemia, more than other forms of dyslipoproteinemia, is sensitive both to dietary changes and to lipid-lowering medications such as nicotinic acid and clofibrate.

Familial Hypertriglyceridemia (Type IV Hyperlipoproteinemia)

This is a common disorder of lipid metabolism characterized by increased levels of plasma triglycerides and VLDL without any other specific clinical or biochemical features. It is often associated with obesity and/or with various degrees of glucose intolerance. The role it plays as an independent risk factor for the development of atherosclerosis is not clear. Many Type IV patients are non-familial, and some show the characteristics of the other monogenic or polygenic disorders. The inheritance is thought to be autosomal dominant with low penetrance in the early years of life.

Type V Hyperlipoproteinemia. Fredrickson (1968) used the term familial Type V hyperlipoproteinemia to identify a group of patients with familial hypertriglyceridemia who had elevated levels of both VLDL and chylomicrons, lipemia retinalis, eruptive xanthoma, and pancreatitis. These patients are readily distinguishable from those with familial lipoprotein lipase deficiency by the higher age at onset of symptoms, and also by their normal lipoprotein and hepatic lipase activities (Greenberg, 1977). In some, an abnormal apoE isoforms phenotype has been reported (Ghiselli, 1982). The question of whether they represent severe forms of familial hypertriglyceridemia or a separate disorder is still unanswered.

Familial Combined Hyperlipidemia

Genetic analysis of families of hyperlipidemic subjects led to the identification of a new disorder characterized by elevated levels of either VLDL or LDL, or both, in affected members (Goldstein, 1973). The diagnosis of familial combined hyperlipidemia cannot be made until all the family members and their lipid profiles have been examined. Goldstein (1973) postulated monogenic dominant inheritance based on the study of several affected families. Recent studies suggest that increased plasma apoB levels and elevated apoB synthesis characterize individuals with familial combined hyperlipidemia. It should be noted, however, that the increased apoB level is not specific for this disorder.

Familial Hyperalphalipoproteinemia

Increased concentrations of HDL inherited as an autosomal dominant trait were described in a few families. This innocuous hyperlipoproteinemia was associated with longevity and decreased incidence of coronary artery disease. This pattern agrees very well with the role of HLD as an anti-risk factor.

Familial β-Lipoprotein Deficiency

Apolipoprotein B has thus far been difficult to study because of its self-aggregating tendencies when delipidated. Recent studies suggest that it may represent a heterogeneous group of proteins. Sharing a few common features, the various apoB proteins may differ nonetheless in molecular weight, site of synthesis, physiologic role, and possibly other characteristics. Their metabolism could also be under different genetic control mechanisms. Betalipoprotein deficiency syndromes are characterized by deficiency or complete absence of one or more of the apoB proteins.

Recessive Abetalipoproteinemia. This is a rare disorder, characterized clinically by fat malabsorption, neuromuscular abnormalities, retinitis pigmentosa, acanthocytosis, and fat-soluble vitamin deficiencies. Jejunal biopsy is usually pathognomonic, showing fat-laden mucosal cells in well formed villi. Biochemically, the disorder is manifested by hypocholesterolemia and total absence of plasma apoB and hence the lipoproteins (chylomicrons, VLDL, and LDL) that usually contain it. Inheritance is as an autosomal recessive trait. Plasma lipid and lipoprotein levels are not unusually low in obligate heterozygotes. A patient was recently described (Malloy, 1981) who absorbed triglycerides and formed chylomicrons and transported them, and in whom the intestinal form of apoB (B-48 apolipoprotein) was present in the plasma. No hepatic form (B-100 apolipoprotein) could be identified in this one patient with normotriglyceridemic abetalipoproteinemia.

Familial Hypobetalipoproteinemia. This disorder is clinically, biochemically, and genetically different from abetalipoproteinemia. The gastrointestinal, neurologic, ophthalmologic, and hematologic manifestations are mild, if present at all, in affected subjects. The disease is inherited as an autosomal dominant trait. Heterozygotes present with plasma lipid concentrations, definitely overlapping the normal range, and with low but detectable apoB levels. Homozygotes have very low blood lipids and no detectable apoB, and are sometimes indistinguishable from abetalipoproteinemic patients, although the clinical features may be milder.

Familial HDL Deficiency

Low HDL syndromes appear to be a heterogeneous group of disorders, sharing a severe deficiency and sometimes abnormal structure or complete absence of one or more of the HDL apolipoproteins.

Tangier Disease. This rare disorder is characterized by severe deficiency of plasma HDL, and by an accumulation of cholesteryl ester–laden cells in the reticuloendothelial tissue, resulting in enlarged and distinctively colored tonsils, splenomegaly, hepatomegaly, and lymphadenopathy. Corneal infiltration and neuropathy often occur. Patients with Tangier disease frequently develop premature atherosclerotic disease, but this tendency may be attenuated by the concomitant low levels of LDL. The unique plasma lipid pattern of patients with Tangier disease includes a markedly low cholesterol and a moderately raised triglyceride level. HDL levels are extremely low or undetectable, and LDL levels are also reduced, though not to the same extent. HDL from Tangier disease patients differs from normal HDL by having a very low apoAI:apoAII ratio (Assmann, 1977), and an abnormal apoAI isoprotein composition due to a structural defect (Zannis, 1982; Kay, 1982). These abnormal apolipoproteins are probably responsible for the increased and altered catabolism of HDL in Tangier disease patients (Schaefer, 1978).

Inheritance is as an autosomal recessive trait, and affected individuals are homozygous for the mutant allele. With the advancement of methodologies for protein isolation and characterization, other low HDL syndromes are being described (Franceschini, 1980; Weisgraber, 1980; Schaefer, 1982), many of which are associated with increased incidence of CHD. The exact nature of the biochemical abnormality, the genetic transmission, and the pathophysiology of these disorders need further eludication.

Familial Lecithin:Cholesterol Acyltransferase (LCAT) Deficiency

This disorder is characterized by corneal opacities, anemia, proteinemia, and hyperlipidemia. Both cholesterol and triglyceride concentrations are increased, and most of the cholesterol is unesterified. Plasma levels of LCAT are very low. Premature atherosclerosis is also a feature of this disease, which is inherited as an autosomal recessive trait (Glomset, 1982).

Abell, L. L., Levy, B. B., Brodie, B. B., and Kendall, F. E.: A simplified method for the estimation of total cholesterol in serum and demonstration of its specificity. J. Biol. Chem., *195*:357, 1952.

Alaupovic, P.: Apolipoproteins and lipoproteins. Atherosclerosis, *13*:141, 1971.

Albers, J. J., Adolphson, J. L., and Chen, C. H.: Radioimmunoassay of human plasma lecithin:cholesterol acyltransferase. J. Clin. Invest., *67*:141, 1981.

Albers, J. J., Adolphson, J. L., and Hazzard, W. R.: Radioimmunoassay of human plasma Lp(a) lipoprotein. J. Lipid Res., *189*:331, 1977.

Alberts, J. J., Cabana, V. G., and Hazzard, W. R.: Immunoassay of human plasma apolipoprotein B. Metabolism, *24*:1339, 1975.

Allain, C. C., Poon, L. S., Chan, C. S. G., Richmond, W., and Fu, P. C.: Enzymatic determination of total serum cholesterol. Clin. Chem., *20*:470, 1974.

Assmann, G., Simantke, O., Schaefer, H. E., et al.: Characterization of high density lipoproteins in patients heterozygous for Tangier disease. J. Clin. Invest., *60*:1025, 1977.

Avogaro, P., Bittolo Bon, G., Cazzolato, G., and Quinci, G. B.: Are apoproteins better discriminators than lipids for atherosclerosis? Lancet, *1*:901, 1979.

Bachorik, P. S., and Wood, P. D. S.: Laboratory considerations in the diagnosis and management of hyperlipoproteinemia. *In* Rifkind, B. M., and Levy, R. I. (eds.): Hyperlipidemia: Diagnosis and Therapy. New York, Grune & Stratton, 1977.

Bachorik, P. S., Wood, P. D. S., Albers, J. J., Steiner, P., Dempsey, M., Kuba, K., Warnick, G. R., and Karlsson, L.: Plasma high-density lipoprotein cholesterol concentrations determined after removal of other lipoproteins by heparin/manganese precipitation or by ultracentrifugation. Clin. Chem., *22*:1828, 1976.

Bachorik, P. S., Wood, P. D. S., Williams, J., Kuchmak, M., Ahmed, S., Lippel, K., and Albers, J.: Automated determination of total plasma cholesterol: A serum calibration technique. Clin. Chim. Acta, 96:145, 1979.

Bartlett, G. R.: Phosphorus assay in column chromatography. J. Biol. Chem., *234*:466, 1959.

Breckenridge, W. C., Little, J. A., Steiner, G., et al.: Hypertriglyceridemia associated with deficiency of apoprotein C-II. N. Engl. J. Med., *298*:1265, 1978.

Brown, M. S., Kovanen, P. T., and Goldstein, J. L.: Regulation of plasma cholesterol by lipoprotein receptors. Science, *212*:628, 1981.

Bucolo, G., and David, H.: Quantitative determination of serum triglycerides by the use of enzymes. Clin. Chem., *19*:476, 1973.

Burstein, M., and Legmann, P.: Lipoprotein precipitation. *In* Clarkson, T. B., Kritchevsky, D., and Pollak, O. J. (eds.): Monographs on Atherosclerosis, Vol. II. Basel, S. Karger, A. G., 1982.

Cheung, M. C., and Albers, J. J.: The measurement of apolipoprotein A-I and A-II levels in men and women by immunoassay. J. Clin. Invest., *60*:43, 1977.

Committee of Principal Investigators: Report on a cooperative trial in the primary prevention of ischaemic heart disease using clofibrate. Br. Heart J., *40*:1069, 1978.

Cooper, G. R., Duncan, P. H., Hazlehurst, J. S., Miller, D. T., and Bayse, D. D.: Cholesterol, enzymic method. *In* Faulkner, W. R., and Meites, S. (eds.): Selected Methods of Clinical Chemistry, Vol. 9. Washington, D.C., Am. Assn. Clin. Chem., 1982.

Cox, D. W., Breckenridge, W. D., and Little, J. A.: Inheritance of apolipoprotein C-II deficiency with hypertriglyceridemia and pancreatitis. N. Engl. J. Med., *299*:1421, 1978.

Curry, M. D., Alaupovic, P., and Suenram, C. A.: Determination of apolipoprotein A and its constitutive A-I and A-II polypeptides by separate electroimmunoassays. Clin. Chem., *22*:315, 1976a.

Curry, M. D., Gustafson, A., Alaupovic, P., and McConathy, W. J.: Electroimmunoassay, radioimmunoassay, and radial immunodiffusion assay evaluated for quantification of human apolipoprotein B. Clin. Chem., *24*:280, 1978.

Curry, M. D., McConathy, W. J., and Alaupovic, P.: Quantitative determination of human apolipoprotein D by electroimmunoassay and radial immunodiffusion. Biochim. Biophys. Acta, *491*:232, 1977.

Curry, M. D., McConathy, W. J., Alaupovic, P., Ledford, J. H., and Popvic, M.: Determination of human apolipoprotein E by electroimmunoassay. Biochim. Biophys. Acta, *439*:413, 1976b.

Curry, M. D., McConathy, W. J., Fesmire, J. D., and Alaupovic, P.: Quantitative determination of human apolipoprotein C-III by electroimmunoassay. Biochim. Biophys. Acta, *617*:503, 1980.

Curry, M. D., McConathy, W. J., Fesmire, J. D., and Alaupovic, P.: Quantitative determination of apolipoproteins C-I and C-II in human plasma by separate electroimmunoassays. Clin. Chem., *27*:543, 1981.

Deacon, A. C., and Dawson, P. J. G.: Enzymic assay of total cholesterol involving chemical or enzymic hydrolysis—a comparison of methods. Clin. Chem., *25*:976, 1979.

Eder, H. A., and Gidez, L. I.: The clinical significance of the plasma high density lipoproteins. Med. Clin. North Am., *66*:431, 1982.

Eisenberg, S., and Levy, R. I.: Lipoprotein metabolism. Adv. Lipid Res., *13*:1, 1976.

Ellefson, R. D., and Caraway, W. T.: Lipids and lipoproteins. *In* Tietz, N. W. (ed.): Fundamentals of Clinical Chemistry. Philadelphia, W. B. Saunders, 1976.

Falko, J. M., Schonfeld, G., Witztum, J. L., Kolar, J. B., Weidman, S. W., and Steelman, R.: Effects of diet on apoprotein E levels and on the apoprotein E subspecies in human plasma lipoproteins. J. Clin. Endocrinol. Metab., *50*:521, 1980.

Feinleib, M.: On a possible inverse relationship between serum cholesterol and cancer mortality. Am. J. Epidemiol., *114*:5, 1981.

Fielding, C. J., and Fielding, P. E.: Cholesterol transport between cells and body fluids. Role of plasma lipoproteins and the plasma cholesterol esterification system. Med. Clin. North Am., *66*:363, 1982.

Folch, J., Lees, M., and Sloan-Stanley, G. H.: A simple method for the isolation and purification of total lipids from animal tissues. J. Biol. Chem., *226*:497, 1957.

Franceschini, G., Sirtori, C. R., Capurso, A., et al.: A-I Milano apoprotein. Decreased high density lipoprotein cholesterol levels with significant lipoprotein modifications and without clinical atherosclerosis in an Italian family. J. Clin. Invest., *66*:892, 1980.

Fredrickson, D. S., Goldstein, J. L., and Brown, M. S.: The familial hyperlipoproteinemias. *In* Stanbury, J. B., Wyngaarden, J. B., and Fredrickson, D. S. (eds.): The Metabolic Basis of Inherited Diseases. 4th ed. New York, McGraw-Hill Book Company, 1978.

Fredrickson, D. S., Levy, R. I., and Lees, R. S.: Fat transport in lipoproteins—an integrated approach to mechanisms and disorders. N. Engl. J. Med., *276*:32, 94, 148, 215, 273, 1967.

Fredrickson, D. S., Levy, R. I., and Lindgren, F. T.: A comparison of heritable abnormal lipoprotein patterns as defined by two different techniques. J. Clin. Invest., *47*:2446, 1968.

Friedewald, W. T., Levy, R. I., and Fredrickson, D. S.: Estimation of the concentration of low density lipoprotein cholesterol in plasma without use of the preparative ultracentrifuge. Clin. Chem., *18*:499, 1972.

Fruchart, J. C., Desreumaux, C., Dewailly, P., Sezille, G., Jaillard, J., Carlier, Y., Bout, D., and Capron, A.: Enzyme immunoassay of human apolipoprotein B, the major protein moiety of low-density and very-low-density lipoproteins. Clin. Chem., *24*:455, 1978.

Ghiselli, G., Schaefer, E. J., Gascon, P., et al.: Type III hyperlipoproteinemia associated with apolipoprotein E deficiency. Science, *214*:1239, 1981.

Ghiselli, G., Schaefer, E. J., Zech, L. A., Gregg, R. E., and Brewer, H. B., Jr.: Increased prevalence of apolipoprotein E in Type V hyperlipoproteinemia. J. Clin. Invest., *70*:474, 1982.

Glomset, J. A., Norum, K. R., and Gjone, E.: Familial lecithin:cholesterol acyltransferase deficiency. *In* Stanbury, J. B., Wyngaarden, J. B., Fredrickson, D. S., Goldstein, J. L., and Brown, M. S. (eds.): The Metabolic Basis of Inherited Diseases. 5th ed. New York, McGraw-Hill Book Company, 1983.

Goldstein, J. L., and Brown, M. S.: Familial hypercholesterolemia. *In* Stanbury, J. B., Wyngaarden, J. B., Fredrickson, D. S., Goldstein, J. L., and Brown, M. S. (eds.): The Metabolic Basis of Inherited Diseases. 5th ed. New York, McGraw-Hill Book Company, 1982.

Goldstein, J. L., Schrott, H. G., Hazzard, W. R., et al.: Hyperlipidemia in coronary heart disease. II. Genetic analysis of lipid levels in 176 families and delineation of a new inherited disorder, combined hyperlipidemia. J. Clin. Invest., *52*:1544, 1973.

Greenberg, B. H., Blackwelder, W. D., and Levy, R. I.: Primary Type V hyperlipoproteinemia. A descriptive study of 32 families. Ann. Intern. Med., *87*:526, 1977.

Havel, R. J., Eder, H. A., and Bragdon, J. H.: The distribution and chemical composition of ultracentrifugally separated lipoproteins in human serum. J. Clin. Invest., *34*:1345, 1955.

Havel, R. J., and Kane, J. P.: Primary dysbetalipoproteinemia: Predominance of a specific apoprotein species in triglyceride-rich lipoproteins. Proc. Natl. Acad. Sci. USA, *70*:2015, 1973.

Heiss, G., Johnson, N. J., Reiland, S., Davis, C. E., and Tyroler, H. A.: The epidemiology of plasma high density lipoprotein cholesterol levels. Circulation, *62*:IV–116, 1980.

Hulley, S. B., Rosenman, R. H., Bawol, R. D., et al.: Epidemiology as a guide to clinical decisions. The association between triglyceride and coronary heart disease. N. Engl. J. Med., *302*:1383, 1980.

Ishikawa, T., Fidge, N., Thelle, D. S., Førde, O. H., and Miller, N. E.: The Tromsø heart study: Serum apolipoprotein A-I concentration in relation to future coronary heart disease. Eur. J. Clin. Invest., *8*:179, 1978.

Kane, J. P., Hardman, D. A., and Paulus, H. E.: Heterogeneity of apolipoprotein B: Isolation of a new species from human chylomicrons. Proc. Natl. Acad. Sci. USA, *77*:2465, 1980.

Kay, L. L., Ronan, R., Schaefer, E. J., et al.: Tangier disease: A structural defect in apolipoprotein A-I (apoA-I Tangier). Proc. Natl. Acad. Sci. USA, *79*:2485, 1982.

Kessler, G., and Lederer, H.: Fluorometric measurement of triglycerides. *In* Skeggs, L. T. (ed.): Automation in Clinical Chemistry, Technicon Symposia. New York, Mediad, 1966.

Kwiterovich, P. O., Jr., Bachorik, P. S., Smith, H. H., McKusick, V. A., Connor, W. E., Teng, B., and Sniderman, A. D.: Hyperapobetalipoproteinaemia in two families with xanthomas and phytosterolaemia. Lancet, *1*:466, 1981.

LaRosa, J. C., Levy, R. I., Herbert, P., et al.: A specific apoprotein activator for lipoprotein lipase. Biochem. Biophys. Res. Commun., *41*:57, 1970.

Lindgren, F. T., Jensen, L. C., and Hatch, F. T.: The isolation and quantitative analysis of serum lipoproteins. *In* Nelson, G. J. (ed.): Blood Lipids and Lipoproteins—Quantitation, Composition and Metabolism. New York, Wiley-Interscience, 1972.

Lipid Research Clinics Laboratory Methods Committee: Cholesterol and triglyceride concentrations in serum-plasma pairs. Clin. Chem., *23*:60, 1977.

Lipid Research Clinics Program: Manual of laboratory operations. Lipid and lipoprotein analysis. U.S. Department of Health and Human Services, Publication No. (NIH) 75. Revised September 1982.

Lipid Research Clinics Program. Population Studies Data Book. Vol. I. The Prevalence Study. NIH Publication No. 80–1527. Washington, D.C., U.S. Department of Health and Human Services, 1980.

Lopes-Virella, M. F. L., Virella, G., Evangs, G., Malenkos, S. B., and Colwell, J. A.: Immunonephelometric assay of human apolipoprotein A-I. Clin Chem., *26*:1205, 1980.

Malloy, M. J., Kane, J. P., Hardman, D. A., et al.: Normotriglyceridemic abetalipoproteinemia—absence of the B-100 apolipoprotein. J. Clin. Invest., *67*:1441, 1981.

Pagnan, A., Havel, R. J., Kane, J. P., et al.: Characterization of human very low density lipoproteins containing two electrophoretic populations: Double pre-beta lipoproteinemia and primary dysbetalipoproteinemia. J. Lipid Res., *18*:613, 1977.

Pesce, M. A., and Bodourian, S. H.: Interference with the enzymatic measurement of cholesterol in serum by use of five reagent kits. Clin. Chem., *23*:757, 1977.

Schaefer, E. J., Blum, C. B., Levy, R. I., et al.: Metabolism of high density lipoprotein apolipoproteins in Tangier disease. N. Engl. J. Med., *299*:905, 1978.

Schaefer, E. J., Heaton, W. H., Wetzel, M. G., et al.: Plasma apolipoprotein A-I absence associated with a marked reduction of high density lipoproteins and premature coronary artery disease. Arteriosclerosis, *2*:16, 1982.

Schonfeld, G., Chen, J. S., McDonnel, W. F., and Jeng, I.: Apolipoprotein A-II content of human plasma high density lipoproteins measured by radioimmunoassay. J. Lipid Res., *18*:645, 1977.

Schonfeld, G., George, P. K., Miller, J., Reilly, P., and Witztum, J.: Apolipoprotein C-II and C-III levels in hyperlipoproteinemia. Metabolism, *28*:1001, 1979.

Schonfeld, G., and Pfleger, B.: The structure of human high density lipoprotein and the levels of apolipoprotein A-I in plasma as determined by radioimmunoassay. J. Clin. Invest., *54*:236, 1974.

Segal, P., Rifkind, B. M., and Schull, W. J.: Genetic factors in lipoprotein variation. Epidemiol. Rev., *4*:137, 1982.

Sniderman, A. D., Shapiro, S., Marpole, D., Skinner, B., Teng, B., and Kwiterovich, P. O.: Association of coronary atherosclerosis with hyperapobetalipoproteinemia (increased protein but normal cholesterol levels in human plasma low density lipoproteins). Proc. Natl. Acad. Sci. USA, *77*:604, 1980.

Tikkanen, M., Nikkila, E. A., and Sipinen, S.: Reduction of plasma high-density lipoprotein$_2$ (HDL_2) and increase in postheparin plasma hepatic lipase activity during progestin treatment. Clin. Chim. Acta, *115*:63, 1981.

Utermann, G., Jaeschke, M., and Menzel, J.: Familial hyperlipoproteinemia Type III—defiency of a specific apolipoprotein (apoE-III) in the very low density lipoproteins. FEBS Lett, *56*:352, 1975.

Wallace, R. B., Hoover, J., Barrett-Connor, E., Rifkind, B. M., Hunninghake, D. B., Mackenthun, A., and Heiss, G.: Altered plasma lipid and lipoprotein levels associated with oral contraceptive and oestrogen use. Lancet, *2*:111, 1979.

Warnick, G. R., Cheung, M. C., and Albers, J. J.: Comparison of current methods for high-density lipoprotein cholesterol quantitation. Clin. Chem., *25*:596, 1979.

Weisgraber, K. H., Bersot, T. P., Mahley, R. W., et al.: A-I Milano apoprotein. Isolation and characterization of a cysteine-containing variant of the A-I apoprotein from human high density lipoproteins. J. Clin. Invest., *66*:901, 1980.

Weisgraber, K. H., Innerarity, T. L., and Mahley, R. W.: Abnormal lipoprotein receptor-binding activity of the human E apoprotein due to cysteine-arginine interchange at a single site. J. Biol. Chem., *257*:2518, 1982.

Weisgraber, K. H., Rall, S. C., and Mahley, R. W.: Human E apoprotein heterogeneity—cysteine-arginine interchanges in the amino acid sequence of the apo-E isoforms. J. Biol. Chem., *256*:9077, 1981.

Witte, D. L., Brown, L. F., and Feld, R. D.: Effects of bilirubin on the detection of hydrogen peroxide by use of peroxidase. Clin. Chem., *24*:1778, 1978.

Wood, P. D., Bachorik, P. S., Albers, J. J., Stewart, C. C., Winn, C. C., and Lippel, K.: An investigation of the effects of sample aging on total cholesterol values determined by the automated ferric chloride–sulfuric acid and Liebermann-Burchard procedures. Clin. Chem., *26*:592, 1980.

Zannis, V. I., and Breslow, J. L.: Characterization of a unique human apolipoprotein E variant associated with Type III hyperlipoproteinemia. J. Biol. Chem., *255*:1759, 1980.

Zannis, V. I., and Breslow, J. L.: Human very low density lipoprotein apolipoprotein E isoprotein polymorphism is explained by genetic variation and post-translational modification. Biochemistry, *20*:1033, 1981.

Zannis, V. I., Lees, A. M., Lees, R. S., et al.: Abnormal apoprotein A-I isoproteins composition in patients with Tangier disease. J. Biol. Chem., *257*:4978, 1982.

12

SPECIFIC PROTEINS

RICHARD A. MCPHERSON, M.D.

Measurements of plasma protein content provide information reflecting disease states in many organ systems. The primary determination, that for total protein, is usually performed on serum which has no fibrinogen and no anticoagulant that may slightly dilute proteins in plasma. Although total protein determination gives the physician some information as to a patient's general status regarding nutrition or severe organ disease, as in protein-losing states, further fractionations yield far more clinically useful information.

Additional quantitation of albumin, for example, is more informative regarding nutritional status, liver synthetic capacity, or protein-losing nephropathy. It also allows the clinician to interpret high or low calcium and magnesium levels since albumin binds about one half of each of those ions. Finally the difference between total protein and albumin yields the value of all globulins, a mixture of the other fractions which individually can rise several-fold in severe disorders.

Protein electrophoresis separates the globulins from albumin and resolves the major proteins of serum into patterns that may be highly specific for some diseases. High resolution techniques can provide a display of all the components in concentrations down to about 1 g/L; however, at that level quantitation by scanning of stained proteins is not highly reliable and alternative methods should be employed. Such techniques, involving immunologic detection of individual proteins, have the dual advantages of specificity and sensitivity.

Yet there is much to be appreciated from visual inspection of an electropherogram of proteins, since the human eye is still the best scanning device for detecting subtle variations in patterns which should be identified in order to suggest more specific tests on the road to diagnosis. Protein electrophoresis can also be a useful tool for monitoring patients over long periods of time when there are marked alterations in levels of particular proteins such as in myeloma, nephrotic syndrome, cirrhosis, or extensive body burn.

This chapter reviews protein structure, methodologies of measurement and separation, the major plasma proteins (except for immunoglobulins and the complement system, which are covered elsewhere), and some of the patterns encountered in particular disease states.

PROTEIN STRUCTURE

The backbone of all protein molecules is a continuous chain of carbon and nitrogen atoms joined together through peptide bonds between adjacent amino acids. Although the peptide backbone is invariant between different proteins (except for total length, equivalent to total number of amino acids), proteins have structural identity by virtue of the side groups or residues of the amino acids. The linear sequence of its amino acids is called the protein's primary structure. These side chains are conventionally grouped according to chemical nature (hydrogen: glycine; aliphatic: alanine, valine, leucine, and isoleucine; hydroxyamino: serine and threonine; aromatic: tyrosine, phenylalanine, and tryptophan; imino: proline and hydroxyproline; acidic: aspartate and glutamate; basic: arginine and lysine; amides: asparagine and glutamine; sulfur-containing: cysteine and methionine). Attractions between the carbonyl oxygens and the hydrogens bonded to nitrogens along the peptide backbone force a protein molecule to form either an alpha-helical conformation (in which the attractions are internal to the same molecule) or a beta-pleated sheet (in which the hydrogen-oxygen attractions extend between protein molecules). This configuration of a protein is its secondary structure. It results in the side chains pointing to the exterior of an alpha-helix, thereby leading to a specific arrangement of chemical sites in local space.

Molecular regions with clusters of hydrophobic side groups tend to remain inside the whole protein, while those with clusters of charges or other hydrophilic moieties tend to appear on the protein's surface. This bending and turning of the regions of a protein into larger domains is termed its tertiary structure. Individual proteins or monomeric subunits may form more stable complexes as dimers, trimers, tetramers, etc., which is termed quaternary structure.

The average molecular weight of an amino acid is 120 daltons. Serum proteins range from roughly 66 kilodaltons (kd) to over 700 kd.

Cysteine moieties form disulfide bonds with one another to help stabilize the final structure, which probably generates spontaneously as a nascent peptide extends from a ribosome. If a protein folds back on itself, the disulfides hold together peptide loops on stems with anti-parallel orientations of their peptide backbones (e.g., albumin). If it loops around on itself, there can be parallel orientation (e.g., proinsulin) of adjacent peptide segments. The acidic and basic amino acids determine the net charge on a protein and hence its electrophoretic mobility. The charge on carboxyl and amino groups is a function of pH, whether a hydrogen ion is attached or dissociated from the group. Combining all the different side groups and their different degrees of dissociation, the pH at which a particular protein has net charge equal to zero is called its isoelectric point or pI. Proteins with pI less than 7 are acidic, while those with pI greater than 7 are basic.

Additional modifications to protein structures occur post-translationally: enzymatic phosphorylation, proteolysis to remove segments of precursors, and glycosylation by attachment of a string of neutral monosaccharides terminating usually with sialic acid. These changes affect antigenicity, specific activities, bindability to receptors, and electrophoretic mobility.

TECHNIQUES OF PROTEIN SEPARATION

Modern understanding of the protein composition of serum derives from the electrophoretic techniques introduced by Tiselius whereby proteins were separated in an electrolyte solution contained within a quartz U-shaped tube through which an electric current was passed. At pH 7.6, four fractions designated albumin, alpha, beta, and gamma were identified and quantified by change in refractive index at the boundaries between these bands. Because separation was achieved in a homogeneous solution without solid support medium, convective forces prevented resolution into distinct zones. Hence this technique has been termed moving boundary or frontal electrophoresis. Introduction of filter paper as an anti-convection support medium permitted separation of the protein fractions into discrete bands or zones termed zonal electrophoresis. At pH 8.6, the alpha fraction split into two groups of proteins, alpha-1 and alpha-2. Other support media have been used such as cellulose acetate membrane, agarose gel, starch gel, and polyacrylamide gel. Cellulose acetate and agarose have predominated in the clinical laboratory because of ease of use, low cost, and commercial availability (Jeppsson, 1979).

When such an electrophoretic support medium has a negative charge, the electromotive force tends to move it toward the anode. However, since the solid support medium is fixed and stationary, buffer flows toward the cathode instead. This buffer flow is termed electro-osmosis or endosmosis, which also carries the proteins with it to some extent. When the electroosmotic force is greater than the electrophoretic force acting on weakly anionic proteins (e.g., gamma globulins), those proteins move from the application point toward the cathode, although their charge is slightly negative.

Through critical manipulations of buffer salt composition, endosmotic properties of the medium, and application of sample, commercially available electrophoretic agarose plates now achieve consistently high resolution qualities which allow routine separation of all the major serum protein species (Fig. 12–1).

Polyacrylamide is an inert support whose porosity is easily adjusted by changing the composition of acrylamide solution prior to polymerization. Although polyacrylamide gel electrophoresis (PAGE) is applicable to standard separation of native proteins, it can also be used for separating proteins according to molecular weight when they are denatured in the presence of sodium dodecyl sulfate (SDS). SDS-PAGE is presently the most widely used protein electrophoretic technique for research in molecular biology. However, its very power for resolving proteins and separating them into multitudinous subunits has virtually excluded it from use in the clinical laboratory except for highly individualized investigations. Nevertheless there is promise for two-dimensional electrophoresis (2-DE), which uses standard separation in one direction followed by SDS-PAGE in the perpendicular direction. 2-DE results in perhaps hundreds of identifiable protein peaks from which it may be possible to obtain important diagnostic information by sophisticated pattern analysis.

Isoelectric focusing affords superior resolution of closely migrating proteins or various forms of a single protein which differ in charge due to minor modifications. By this technique, proteins migrate through a gel containing a gradient of pH established with a mixture of ampholytes. As each protein reaches the gel location where the pH is equal to its pI, the net charge on it becomes zero, and it comes to rest. Thus the final pattern is strictly according to pI.

Chemical precipitations of serum proteins have been devised to resolve albumin and the globulins into two or more fractions which can then be measured for protein content. With the addition of sodium sulfate, sodium sulfite, ammonium sulfate, or methanol, the globulins tend to precipitate, leaving albumin in solution. By measuring total protein in the original serum and protein in either the precipitate or the supernatant, values for albumin and globulin can be derived. The ratio of these values (A/G ratio) has been extensively used because it accentuates abnormalities in serum protein composition which in disease generally involve depression of albumin and elevation of one or more globulin fractions. Precipitation methods are not as accurate as zonal electrophoresis since some alpha globulins may fail to precipitate and thus lead to an overestimate of the albumin.

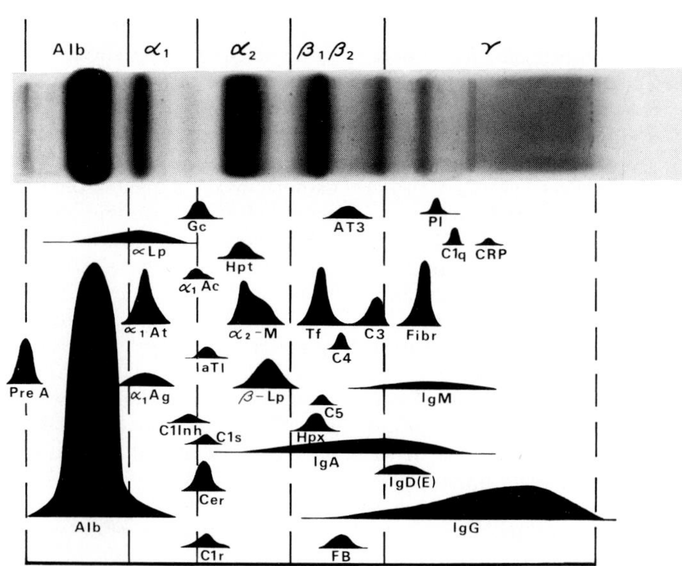

Figure 12–1. Plasma protein electrophoresis pattern in agarose gel is composed of 5 fractions, each composed of many individual species (see Fig. 12–2). Some of the major proteins are shown here in an artist's rendition for clarity. (Adapted from Laurell, C. B.: Clin. Chem., *19*:99, 1973.)

α_1Ac = Alpha$_1$-antichymotrypsin
α_1Ag = Alpha$_1$-acid glycoprotein
α_1At = Alpha$_1$-antitrypsin
α_2 − M = Alpha$_2$-macroglobulin
αLP = Alpha lipoprotein
Alb = Albumin
AT3 = Antithrombin III
β-Lp = Beta lipoprotein
Complement components:
C1q, C1r, C1s, C3, C4, C5 = As designated
C1Inh = C1 Inhibitor
Cer = Ceruloplasmin
CRP = C-reactive protein
FB = Factor B
Fibr = Fibrinogen
Hpt = Haptoglobin
Hpx = Hemopexin
Immunoglobulins:
IgA, IgD, IgE, IgG, IgM = As designated
Pl = Plasminogen
Pre A = Prealbumin

Preparative procedures for the isolation of a single minor protein constituent usually begin with a precipitation step to remove the bulk of other undesired serum proteins. The next step in protein isolation is typically a column which separates on the basis of molecular size (gel filtration) or charge (ion exchange). Gel filtration media such as Sephadex or agarose beads are rated according to pore sizes, which in turn determine what size molecules can pass through the interior of each bead or particle of the column.

After application of a sample composed of various sized proteins in aqueous solvent containing buffer and salt, more of the buffer is applied to drive the sample through the column. Very large molecules tend to flow through interstices without entering the beads and emerge first from the bottom of the column in the "void volume." Slightly smaller molecules enter the largest pores and are slightly retarded in passing through the column so that they elute next. Small protein molecules pass into still smaller pores and are retained still longer. Finally, particles the size of dissolved salt penetrate farthest into the interior of gel filtration beads and come out after all the proteins have emerged in an amount of applied buffer called the "salt volume." Thus in gel filtration, the order of protein elution is by molecular weight or size from largest first to smallest last. Since all protein species continuously move through a gel filtration column all at the same time but with different rates, it is necessary to apply the sample in a small and uniform volume in order to optimize separation between peaks. Gel filtration requires that the medium be inert and not interact chemically or by charge with the proteins.

Ion exchange chromatography, on the other hand, takes advantage of the charge on proteins to bind them to beads of a charged support medium such as DEAE or QAE. In anion exchange chromatography, proteins are usually applied at a basic pH such as 8.6 at which they are either negatively charged (albumin, alpha-1, alpha-2, and beta globulins are anions) or have no net charge (gamma globulins). The neutral proteins pass immediately through an anion exchange column, while the anionic ones stick to the positively charged column matrix. By passing through buffer with a higher salt concentration, anions of the salt displace the anionic proteins and exchange for them in binding to the support medium allowing the proteins to elute from the column. By utilizing a steadily increasing gradient of salt concentration in the eluting buffer, the proteins can be resolved according to charge. The ones with a small amount of charge will elute first, while those with the most charge (e.g., albumin) will elute only when displaced by higher salt levels.

Alternatively, by lowering the pH while holding salt concentration low, anionic proteins will acquire a net neutral or slightly positive charge and will pass through the column. A gradient of falling pH can be used to resolve anionic proteins, with the order of elution being roughly beta, alpha-2, alpha-1 globulins, and albumin. Note that this order of elution is the reverse order of electrophoretic migration at pH 8.6 since in anion exchange chromatography mobility is retarded according to net negative charge, while in electrophoresis the mobility is enhanced.

Cation exchange chromatography begins at an acid pH with the proteins being positively charged (cations) and adhering to a negatively charged column matrix. They can be displaced by the cations of high salt in an eluting buffer or by increasing the pH which will reverse the charge on the proteins to negative. By cation exchange, albumin should elute first, followed by alpha-1, alpha-2, beta, and gamma globulins. Another separation modality by column is hydrophobic chromatography, in which samples are applied at high salt and eluted with low salt. The support medium interacts with proteins according to hydrophobic nature and is a good complementary technique to follow ion exchange chromatography, in which the sample was eluted with high salt.

If the protein of interest has a specific binding property such as an immunoglobulin for an antigen, affinity chromatography is a very powerful tool for selecting from all of the immunoglobulins in a sample only the specific ones that bind to the antigen which is covalently coupled to the support medium. After washing off all the proteins which do not adhere, the high affinity material is usually eluted with very high salt or some chemical denaturant such as urea. Other affinity chromatography gels utilize binding which mimics natural molecular interactions. Thus some dyes coupled to agarose are able to bind albumin for removing it selectively from serum. Immunoglobulins can also be adsorbed using staphylococcal protein A coupled to Sepharose. Many other separation schemes exist which effect a high degree of purification in a single step with affinity chromatography medium coupled to dyes, drugs, nucleotide cofactors, sugars, etc.

PROTEIN DETECTION AND QUANTITATION (Layne, 1957)

The ultimate reference method for determining concentration of protein is the analysis for nitrogen content. The Kjeldahl technique consists of an acid digestion to release ammonium ions from nitrogen-containing compounds. The ammonium can then be quantitated by conversion to ammonia gas and titration as a base or by nesslerization, in which double iodides (potassium and mercuric) form a colored complex with ammonia in alkali. While determination of nitrogen content can be extremely precise, its use for calculation of protein concentration depends on the exact protein composition of a sample, since each protein has a somewhat different nitrogen content according to amino acid composition. However, for a sample of a purified protein, nitrogen content is accurate for estimating protein concentration but must, of course, have been measured previously, although knowledge of a protein's exact amino acid sequence allows an accurate calculation of nitrogen content. Since clinical samples consist of unpredictable mixtures of different proteins and measurement of nitrogen content is not a simple procedure, it is not commonly used in clinical laboratories.

Refractive index is accurate for measuring serum protein concentration as dissolved solute for levels above 2.5 gm/dl. Hemolysis, lipemia, icterus, and azotemia produce erroneously high results. Refractive index cannot be used for urine protein measurement because of excess solutes in relation to the protein.

Formerly, specific gravity (and thus by inference protein content) was estimated by pipetting drops of serum or blood into a graded series of copper sulfate solutions. A protein-copper shell formed about the drop to prevent dissolution for a short interval, during which the drop fell to the bottom, remained stationary, or rose to the top. The protein concentration was estimated by using the specific gravity of the copper sulfate solution in which the drop remained stationary. This technique was simple and was used widely as a screening test for hemoglobin concentration in whole blood, but it has been supplanted by more specific methods.

Proteins in solution absorb ultraviolet light at 280 nm (A_{280}) due mostly to tryptophan but also due to tyrosine and phenylalanine. For accurate conversion of A_{280} readings to concentration, the molar absorptivity must be used, since each protein contains a different amount of these three amino acids. However, the A_{280} of a mixture of proteins is not an accurate measure of protein content, since molar absorptivities vary greatly between different proteins. Because nucleic acids which absorb strongly at 260 nm may be present in protein preparations, total protein can be estimated by the equation:

$$\text{Protein concentration (mg/ml)} = 1.55 \times A_{280} - 0.76 \times A_{260}$$

so that absorbance can be used for quantitating proteins in the range of 0.05 to 1.5 mg/ml.

Turbidimetric methods are often used for a similar concentration range in CSF or urine. Protein precipitates upon the addition of trichloroacetic acid, sulfosalicylic acid, or acetic acid–potassium ferrocyanide for quantitation by increment in optic density in comparison with similarly treated standards. However, these techniques are not specific to proteins since other acid-insoluble substances such as nucleic acids also precipitate.

A colorimetric technique highly specific for proteins and peptides is the biuret method by which copper salts in alkaline solution form a purple complex with substances containing two or more peptide bonds. Interferences are minimal, although ammonium ion may acidify the reaction while hemoglobin and bilirubin absorb in the same regionas the biuret complex (540 to 560 nm). The biuret method is extensively used in clinical laboratories, particularly in automated analyzers in which protein concentration can be measured down to 10 or 15 mg/dl.

Greater sensitivity can be obtained using the Folin-Ciocalteu reagent (or phenol reagent, phosphotungstomolybdic acid) which oxidizes phenolic compounds such as tyrosine and in addition tryptophan and histidine to give a deep blue color.

Lowry (1951) used the biuret method followed by the phenol reagent which greatly enhanced color formation since the phenol reagent can react with biuret complexes involving all the peptide bonds. The Lowry assay has been extensively used for research purposes.

Further sensitivity down to 1 μg of protein can be obtained using Coomassie brilliant blue dye, which is free of interferences from a very wide range of substances.

Comparable sensitivity is also obtained with ninhydrin, which develops a violet color by reacting with primary amines. This reagent is widely used for detection of peptides and amino acids after paper chromatography.

Quantitation of albumin in the presence of other proteins is possible by virtue of the specific binding albumin exerts on some dyes such as bromphenol blue, methyl orange, HABA, bromcresol purple, and bromcresol green (BCG). BCG is extensively used in automatic analyzers for determining serum albumin in parallel with biuret reagent for total protein.

The standard dyes used for staining in electrophoresis are Coomassie brilliant blue, Pontceau S, and amido black. For detection of minor components in high resolution gels, silver staining is very sensitive down to nanogram quantities (Merril, 1981).

In addition, special dyes such as oil red and Sudan black stain lipoproteins and periodic acid–Schiff stains glycoproteins separated in special electrophoretic applications.

Since electrophoresis followed by staining does not afford explicit identification of serum proteins, immunologic measurements have been instituted for quantitation of individual proteins (Laurell, 1966; see Fig. 12–2). The most promising of these newer methodologies are nephelometry, which detects the turbidity produced by an antibody and its target protein, and enzyme-linked immunoassay (ELISA), which detects antigen by alteration of fluorescent or colorimetric changes resulting from activity of a specific enzyme attached to antigen or antibody.

SPECIFIC PLASMA PROTEINS

Major Components

First will be considered the serum proteins readily detected on stained electrophoretic strips.

Prealbumin. Prealbumin migrates in a position faster than albumin toward the anode. Prealbumin has a tetrameric structure with total molecular weight of 62,000. Each monomer can bind a molecule of thyroxine. As such, it is also called thyroxine-binding prealbumin (TBPA), although only a small fraction

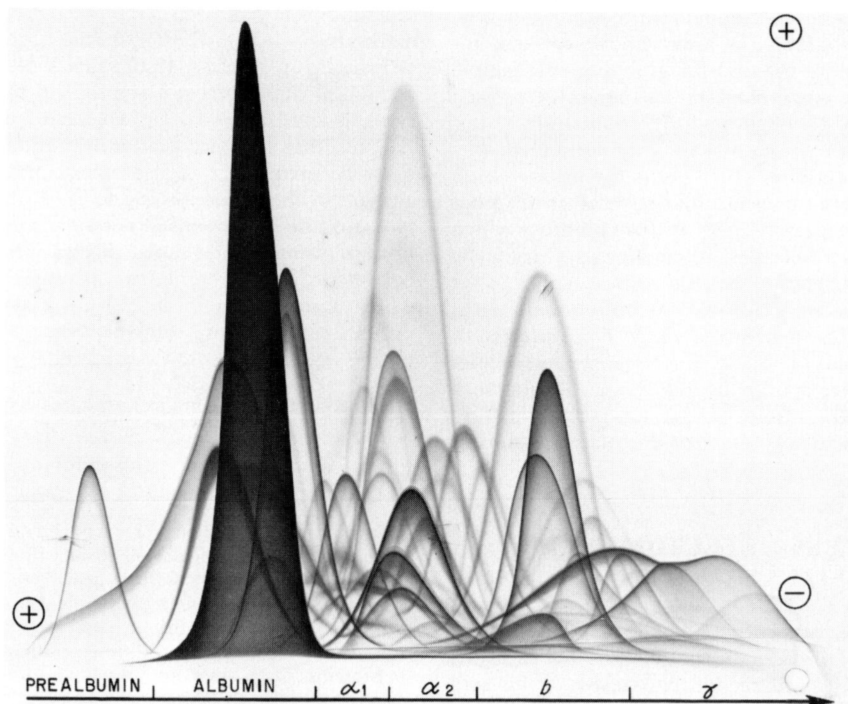

Figure 12–2. Two-dimensional crossed immunoelectrophoresis in a gel containing high quality anti-whole serum shows a complex population of proteins spread from prealbumin to gamma globulin. Each electrophoretic fraction can be seen to contain all or part of many individual species each identified as separate "rocket." The dense peak at left is albumin, and the broadest peak at the right is IgG. Without specific studies it is impossible to unequivocally identify any of the others. (Plate courtesy of DAKOPATTES, A-F, DK-2000, Copenhagen, Denmark.)

Table 12–1. CHARACTERISTICS OF MAJOR PLASMA PROTEINS

Protein	Concentration Range (g/L)	Molecular Weight	Actions
Prealbumin	0.15–0.36	62,000	Binds thyroxine; transports vitamin A
Albumin	39–51	66,000	Oncotic pressure; amino acid reservoir; carries small molecules
Alpha-1-antitrypsin	2.0–4.0	54,000	Protease inhibitor
Alpha-2-macroglobulin	1.5–3.5	725,000	Protease inhibitor
Haptoglobin	0.4–2.9	100,000 (type 1–1)	Binds hemoglobin
Beta-lipoprotein	2.7–7.4	380,000	Lipid transport
Transferrin	2.0–4.0	80,000	Transports iron
C3	0.6–1.4	185,000	Component of complement system
Fibrinogen	1.0–4.0	340,000	Clot formation
Immunoglobulin A	0.4–3.5	160,000	Surface immunity
Immunoglobulin D	0.1–0.4	180,000	
Immunoglobulin E	50–600 (μg/L)	180,000	Binds to mast cells; hypersensitivity reactions
Immunoglobulin G	7–15	150,000	Humoral immunity
Immunoglobulin M	0.25–2.0	850,000	Humoral immunity primary response

of thyroxine is actually bound to TBPA in normal individuals since thyroxine binding globulin has a 100-fold greater affinity for thyroxine (Oppenheimer, 1968). However, there is at least one molecular variant of prealbumin inherited in a familial pattern which has a greatly increased affinity for thyroxine resulting in elevated serum thyroxine content in euthyroid individuals (Moses, 1982). Prealbumin also binds retinol-binding protein (RBP), which in turn complexes with vitamin A so that prealbumin plays a role in the transport and metabolism of vitamin A (Peterson, 1971).

Prealbumin is rich in tryptophan and also has considerable beta-pleated sheet conformation. A portion of prealbumin is the source of the beta-fibrillar amyloid component in Portuguese polyneuropathy type I (Glenner, 1980).

Although low prealbumin levels in serum may be a marker for poor nutritional status, measurement of prealbumin has not been widely used for clinical management. Because of its compactness, prealbumin crosses more easily into the CSF than do the other serum proteins. Therefore concentrating CSF prior to electrophoresis allows visualization of a distinct prealbumin band in CSF while it is below the level of detection in serum electrophoresis (see Chap. 19).

Albumin. The single most abundant protein in normal plasma is albumin, usually constituting up to two thirds of total plasma protein (Peters, 1975). For that reason, depressions in albumin level due to impaired synthesis (Rothschild, 1972) or to losses (e.g., ascites or protein-losing nephropathy or enteropathy) result in serious imbalance of intravascular oncotic pressure and hence peripheral edema (Slater, 1975). However, the congenital absence of albumin (analbuminemia) does not lead to such problems, presumably because of lifelong compensatory mechanisms (Waldmann, 1964). Another major function ascribed to albumin is as a mobile repository of amino acids from the liver, where it is synthesized, to other tissues, where it is broken down intracellularly into free amino acids for incorporation into other proteins. A third function ascribed to albumin is as a general transport or carrier protein which derives from the observation that many organic and inorganic ligands (e.g., thyroxine, bilirubin, penicillin, cortisol, estrogen, free fatty acids, Coumadin, calcium, magnesium, heme) complex with different regions of the albumin molecule in either covalent (e.g., delta bilirubin) (Lauff, 1982) or dissociable binding (Koch-Weser, 1976). These binding interactions with very different ligands are possible because of a wide variety of binding sites on the albumin molecule, which consists of 585 amino acids arranged in nine loops held together by the disulfide bonds between cysteine residues (Meloun, 1975). The primary sequence of albumin suggests that it arose from gene duplication which is preserved in tandem arrangement of three major regions containing three loops each (Peters, 1977). It is also interesting to note that alpha-fetoprotein has regions of homology with serum albumin which may indicate common genetic origin.

In addition to kindreds with analbuminemia, there are many genetic variants which differ from the most common allotype albumin A by single amino acid mutations. These variants can be either rapid or fast migrating compared to albumin A, leading to two distinct albumin peaks in the heterozygous state. None of the variant albumins appears to affect health, but a recently described variant does have greatly enhanced affinity for thyroxine which leads to elevated thyroxine content in serum of such euthyroid persons (Ruiz, 1982). Elevated levels of serum albumin occur in dehydration and artifactually by prolonged application of a tourniquet for venipuncture.

Analysis of newly synthesized albumin from intracellular sites has revealed the existence of a precursor "proalbumin," which has an additional hexapeptide at its amino terminal end. Up to 8 per cent of albumin circulating in normal persons becomes glucosylated non-enzymatically, while up to 25 per cent becomes glucosylated during hyperglycemia in analogy with glucosylated hemoglobin (Guthrow, 1979). The half-life of circulating albumin is about 17 days so that measurement of the glucosylated form may be useful in monitoring diabetic control during a short interval. The primary structure of albumin has 35 cysteine residues, of which 34 form intramolecular disulfide bonds. Upon storage for many days, albumin forms covalently linked dimers through the free cysteines resulting occasionally in an extra band of albumin on electrophoresis.

Alpha-1-Antitrypsin. The major component of the alpha-1 globulins is the protease inhibitor alpha-1-antitrypsin (AAT), which has the capacity to combine with and inactivate trypsin (Eriksson, 1965). The first clue to this function came with the discovery that the serum of some young adults with pulmonary emphysema was deficient in alpha-1 globulin. Further investigations revealed a similar deficiency of AAT in children with cirrhosis (Sveger, 1976). While there are no appreciable circulating levels of trypsin in blood, other related proteases such as collagenase are released from leukocytes responding to irritants or inflammation. AAT is able to neutralize the activity of these proteases too, and hence is an intrinsic factor in the homeostatic mechanism modulating endogenous proteolysis.

The majority of people are homozygous for the normal fully active M allele of AAT, or phenotype MM (Lieberman, 1972). About 10 per cent of Caucasians (and fewer of other races) are heterozygous for M and some other allele of the protease inhibitor or Pi system. More than 2 per cent carry the PiZ allele and have phenotype MZ. Although these individuals are asymptomatic, their ZZ offspring are susceptible to pulmonary or hepatic disease. Since serum protein electrophoresis is not quantitative for AAT, it is necessary to perform ancillary tests such as trypsin inhibitory capacity (TIC) and phenotyping by cross electrophoresis or isoelectric focusing (Jeppsson, 1982) in order to rule out the presence of some other alleles such as PiS or PiF which migrate differently. These alleles result in lower TIC but probably are sufficient to prevent the abnormalities seen with ZZ phenotype which has a very low TIC corresponding to low concentration of antigenic AAT. There is no specific treatment for this disorder by transfusion. However, avoidance of cigarette smoking by homozygous ZZ individuals is essential since cigarette smoke is a major source of irritants which trigger leukocytes in the lung to release proteases (Gelb, 1976). The cirrhosis in young children is reversible by hepatic transplant, as the liver is the site of AAT synthesis. AAT is one of the serum glycoproteins which rise in response to acute inflammation.

An interesting aspect of cirrhosis and ZZ phenotype is the presence of unsialylated Z AAT granules in the hepatocytes, implying a defect of secretion. The alpha-1 fraction never appears completely empty in AAT deficiency, since other proteins migrate there but do not resolve into separate bands.

Alpha-2-Macroglobulin. Alpha-2-macroglobulin (AMG) is one of the largest non-immunoglobulin proteins in plasma with a molecular weight of 725,000. The serum concentration in normals is comparable to the other major protease inhibitor, AAT, although women have higher levels than men in response to estrogen (Horne, 1970). The concentration of AMG rises ten-fold or more in the nephrotic syndrome when other lower molecular weight proteins are lost (Weeke, 1973). The loss of AMG into urine is prevented by its large size. The net result is that AMG reaches serum levels equal to or greater than albumin (about 2 to 3 g/dl) in nephrotic syndrome, which has the effect of maintaining oncotic pressure. There may also be enhanced synthesis of AMG in nephrotic syndrome, which accounts for its absolute increase in concentration. AMG inactivates proteases by complexing with them, changing its own conformation, which enhances clearance by the reticuloendothelial system. There are at least four molecular forms of AMG that differ in sialic acid, mannose, and galactose content and which can be separated by isoelectric focusing. Other molecular variations probably are the result of proteases linked to AMG prior to removal from the circulation. The spectrum of inhibition by AMG is very wide, including virtually all types of serine, carboxyl, thiol, and metal proteases. While it has such widespread action, no single function has been ascribed to AMG. It is noteworthy that no human deficiency states of AMG have been reported, suggesting some crucial role in regulation of proteolysis.

Haptoglobin. The other major protein migrating in the alpha-2 region is haptoglobin, which has the function of combining with hemoglobin released by lysis of red cells in order to preserve body iron and in addition protein stores. Hemoglobin-haptoglobin complexes are taken up by the reticuloendothelial system where the hemoglobin is broken down into globin and heme, which further degrades to iron and bilirubin. Haptoglobin has two heavy chains and two light chains linked by disulfide bonds in analogy to the basic structure of immunoglobulins. Some persons have a light chain gene which is duplicated in a head to tail arrangement (type 2). Normal haptoglobin (type 1–1) gives rise to a single molecular species of molecular weight 100,000. Heterozygous individuals (1–2) have, in addition to type 1–1 haptoglobin, a series of multimers (e.g., dimers, trimers) by virtue of intermolecular disulfide linkages through the duplicated light chain. Type 2–2 haptoglobin consists of a different series of multimers, since type 2 light chain has a different molecular weight from the type 1 light chain (Konigsberg, 1974).

Haptoglobin can be quantitated in terms of its hemoglobin binding capacity or by immunologic means, although discrepancies exist between these two measurements when comparing the different phenotypes.

Serum haptoglobin rises in response to stress, infection, acute inflammation, or tissue necrosis, probably by stimulation of synthesis (see Acute Phase Reactants, below). After a hemolytic episode, haptoglobin concentrations fall as the complexes with hemoglobin are cleared from the circulation. This effect is dramatic following massive hemolysis in situations of hemolytic transfusion reaction, thermal burns, or autoimmune hemolytic anemia. It is also a useful measurement for serially monitoring patients who have a slow but steady rate of red cell breakdown such as by mechanical heart valves, hemoglobinopathies, or exercise-associated trauma. Low haptoglobin concentrations may accompany liver disease when hepatic synthetic capacity is impaired. There are also individuals with congenital deficiency of haptoglobin who must utilize other mechanisms to conserve body iron stores.

Beta-Lipoprotein. Beta-lipoprotein (low density lipoprotein, LDL) migrates with a characteristic sharp leading edge and feathery trailing edge. While it is better quantitated by stains for lipid, there is sufficient apoprotein content to be a distinct band upon staining for protein. The other lipoproteins (VLDL, HDL, and chylomicrons) occur in electrophoretic positions with other serum proteins so that these fractions are not appreciated upon protein stain. Lipoproteins are discussed more thoroughly in Chapter 11.

Transferrin. The major beta-globulin is transferrin (siderophilin), which transports ferric ions from the iron stores of intracellular or mucosal ferritin to bone marrow where erythrocyte precursors have transferrin receptors on their surfaces.

Transferrin consists of 687 amino acids with calculated molecular weight 79,550 (MacGillivray, 1982). Analysis of the amino acid sequence shows that transferrin has two homologous domains that may have arisen by contiguous duplication of an ancestral transferrin gene. Each domain has an iron-binding site.

In normal serum, transferrin ranges in concentration from 200 to 400 mg/dl, which is conveniently measured as iron-binding capacity (IBC) (Tsung, 1975). In response to short-term iron deficiency, transferrin levels rise markedly to twice normal level or more. Since transferrin is a single molecular species with a tight electrophoretic mobility, it can have the appearance of a paraprotein (pseudoparaproteinemia) in cases of severe iron deficiency (Zawadzki, 1970). At least some iron deficiency and elevation of transferrin should be expected with pregnancy (Mendenhall, 1970). Administration of iron to deficient patients increases the saturation followed by return of transferrin to normal. Chronic saturation of transferrin occurs in idiopathic hemochromatosis and transfusional hemosiderosis. Since there is nearly no unsaturated IBC in those situations, iron cannot be mobilized normally for excretion, resulting in the disorders of deposition which also occur in congenital deficiency of transferrin. By chelating iron, transferrin can be a factor in restricting bacterial growth that requires iron (McFarlane, 1970; Weinberg, 1978). Transferrin loss in protein-losing nephropathy may contribute to development of hypochromic anemia.

In addition to prealbumin and albumin, CSF contains a small peak of normal transferrin plus an altered transferrin that differs in carbohydrate content and may be useful as a marker for identifying CSF.

Complement. A separate fraction of beta globulin consists of the C3 component of complement. Although this protein can be resolved easily with a fresh serum sample, in stored specimens and commercial control serum which has been lyophilized, C3 is cleaved to form C3c which migrates anodally to native C3 as a band non-distinct from other beta globulins. Depression of C3 occurs in autoimmune disorders when the complement system is activated and C3 becomes bound to depositions of immune complexes in tissues removing it from serum. The complement system and its inhibitors are discussed further in Chapter 37.

2

Fibrinogen (Doolittle, 1975). Plasma contains 100 to 400 mg/dl of fibrinogen, which is the most abundant of the coagulation factors and which forms the fibrin clot. With an overall molecular weight of 340,000, fibrinogen is a dimer consisting of three pairs of peptide chains (A alpha, B beta, and gamma) linked with multiple disulfide bonds near their amino terminal ends. This region of the molecule is termed the E domain or disulfide knot (DSK). The chains extend outward into two other identical domains (D) at their carboxyl ends, where all three chains are intertwined. Thrombin cleaves fibrinopeptides A and B from the amino ends of the A alpha and B beta chains resulting in fibrin monomer which polymerizes into fibrils that macroscopically form a fibrin clot. Factor XIII then produces covalent bonds between lysine and glutamine residues on adjacent gamma chains of different fibrin molecules, making the fibrin clot essentially a single molecule refractory to dissolution by high molarity urea.

Numerous hereditary variants of fibrinogen (dysfibrinogenemias) have been identified, some with impairment of clotting and hemorrhagic diathesis, others with increased tendency to thrombosis (Menache, 1973).

Fibrinogen levels become elevated with the other acute phase reactants, occasionally to over 1.0 g/dl. In such instances, the erythrocyte sedimentation is also markedly elevated due directly to fibrinogen content. Fibrinogen levels also rise with pregnancy and use of birth control pills. Low levels generally indicate extensive activation of coagulation with consumption of fibrinogen. During this process, plasminogen is also activated into plasmin, which degrades fibrin and fibrinogen into split products which are measured for the assessment of intravascular coagulation. Normally, clots that form are removed by action of plasmin, which in turn is inactivated by antiplasmin and the other protease inhibitors.

Congenital afibrinogenemia results in a hemorrhagic disorder, which paradoxically is not as severe as the hemophilias in terms of joint abnormalities secondary to hemorrhage, perhaps because extremely slow clotting of fibrinogen creates a disarrayed meshwork which is nearly impervious to degradation.

Fibrinogen is absent from normal serum but should

appear in plasma electrophoresis as a distinct band between the beta and gamma globulins. Not infrequently, blood drawn from heparinized patients does not clot fully so that a fibrinogen band is present. It can be distinguished by examining the specimen for a fine clot and by repeat electrophoresis of a thoroughly clotted sample.

Minor Components

The next group of individual proteins are those not usually detected by standard protein electrophoresis due to low levels in serum.

Ceruloplasmin. Migrating in the alpha-2 globulins is a copper-binding protein, ceruloplasmin, whose precise physiologic function is unknown. Synthesized in the liver, it has a molecular weight of 132,000 and consists of a single polypeptide chain. Although lower at birth (Al-Rashid, 1971), serum levels are 20 to 40 mg/dl in normal adults, with two-fold elevations found in oral contraceptive therapy and pregnancy (Burrows, 1971), or as an acute phase reactant. Each molecule of ceruloplasmin can bind six atoms of copper, which imparts a blue tint to the protein and a greenish color to plasma with elevated ceruloplasmin concentration (Schenker, 1971). Iron is oxidized from ferrous to ferric ions by ceruloplasmin, which may be a means of releasing iron from ferritin for binding to transferrin (Roeser, 1970). Wilson's disease (hepatolenticular degeneration) results from disordered copper metabolism and toxic tissue deposition of copper associated with a reduction in the rate at which ceruloplasmin binds copper. Whether abnormal copper transport is the primary defect has not been determined, since there are at least five other copper-containing enzymes in the body. The oxidase activity of ceruloplasmin can be utilized in a colorimetric assay with p-phenylenediamine as substrate for quantitating it. Additionally, immunochemical methods are used since the band is too faint to be used reliably on protein electrophoresis.

Gc-Globulin. Vitamin D binds to the group-specific component (Gc) globulin (Daiger, 1975), which migrates as an alpha-1 globulin and has molecular weight about 51,000. Normal serum concentration is 20 to 55 mg/dl. It may be decreased in severe liver disease. Gc-globulin has two autosomal codominant alleles expressed as three phenotypes: 1–1, 2–2, and 1–2 (Giblett, 1969). Congenital absence of this protein may be a lethal mutation due to impairment of vitamin D transport since vitamin D has low solubility in aqueous medium. Gc-globulin binds vitamin D and metabolites on a mole per mole basis, but in plasma probably is not fully saturated. As a minor component of plasma proteins, Gc-globulin must be quantitated by radioimmunoassay, radioimmunodiffusion, or rocket immunoelectrophoresis (Walsh, 1982).

Hemopexin (Muller-Eberhard, 1970). The beta-migrating globulin hemopexin binds heme released by degradation of hemoglobin to prevent that small porphyrin molecule from being excreted, thereby losing iron from body stores. Normal serum concentration is 50 to 120 mg/dl so that it must be quantitated by immunologic means. It has a molecular weight of 70,000, of which 20 per cent is carbohydrate and consists of a single polypeptide chain. Although low levels of hemopexin can occur with nonspecific urinary loss or due to decreased synthesis in liver failure, the most profound decreases occur following intravascular hemolysis when the amount of free hemoglobin exceeds the binding capacity of haptoglobin. The circulating plasma hemoglobin can then degrade to release heme, which is bound by hemopexin one molecule per molecule. Heme-hemopexin complexes are cleared from the circulation by hepatocytes, which markedly lowers hemopexin concentration. Excess heme then binds to albumin as methemalbumin. As more hemopexin is made available by new synthesis, heme passes from methemalbumin to hemopexin, which continues to depress its level. As such it can be an additional aid for diagnosing earlier hemolysis when haptoglobin levels have returned to normal but before full clearance of the heme (Wochner, 1974).

Alpha-1-Acid Glycoprotein (Schmid, 1975). This protein, also known as orosomucoid, has a very high carbohydrate content, which minimizes its visibility by standard protein stains. With molecular weight roughly 44,000, it passes into the glomerular filtrate to a large extent, resulting in a half-life of only about five days in the circulation. Serum levels are normally 40 to 105 mg/dl with elevations during pregnancy. It is an acute phase reactant, but its biological function is not known. As a binder of progesterone, it may be important in the transport or metabolism of that steroid hormone. There are also some genetic polymorphisms which may be additionally complicated by isomorphic forms of this protein from specific tissue source, although the primary site of its synthesis appears to be the liver.

C-Reactive Protein (Hokama, 1982). This serum constituent was discovered by interacting the serum of patients who had recovered from pneumococcal infections with C-polysaccharide of that bacterium. Visible flocculates formed, which allowed extensive study and purification of this C-reactive protein (CRP) of serum in the 1940s. It was found that CRP is present in serum of patients with disorders other than pneumococcal infections, but that it rises strikingly whenever there is tissue necrosis. Many other substances react with CRP, such as DNA, nucleotides, various lipids, and other polysaccharides. Its molecular weight is between 118,000 and 144,000 with substantial carbohydrate content. The normal serum concentrations are about 100 ng/ml at birth, 170 ng/ml in children, and 470 to 1340 ng/ml in adults. Despite these low concentrations, CRP has major significance as a highly sensitive acute phase reactant. It is generally measured by capacity to precipitate C-substance or by immunologic methods, including precipitations, RIA, and enzyme immunoassay (Saxstad, 1970; Claus, 1976). By electrophoresis, CRP is a gamma-migrating protein that may form a distinct monoclonal appearing band in patients having a severe inflammatory response.

Protease Inhibitors
(Daniels, 1974; Laurell, 1975)

In addition to alpha-1-antitrypsin and alpha-2-macroglobulin already considered, other distinct inhibitors of different proteases are present in serum. They include alpha-1-antichymotrypsin (AAC), inter-alpha-trypsin inhibitor (IATI), anti-thrombin III (AT3), antiplasmin, and C1 inhibitor. None of these five proteins attains serum concentrations appreciable on stained protein electrophoresis. While the other inhibitors show inhibition over a rather wide range of proteases, AAC is highly specific for neutralizing chymotrypsin, which cleaves peptide bonds at the carboxyl side of tyrosine and phenylalanine residues. AAC has a molecular weight of 68,000 with about 25 per cent carbohydrate content. Normal serum concentration is 40 to 60 mg/dl, but AAC can rise rapidly to five times normal as an acute phase reactant that remains elevated throughout a period of inflammation (Kosaka, 1976).

IATI is a glycoprotein of 160,000 molecular weight. Its concentration normally is about 50 mg/dl. IATI does not rise appreciably as an acute phase reactant. Its role in disease states is probably similar to that of the major protease inhibitors in preventing autodigestion of tissues by endogenous cellular enzymes (Steinbuch, 1975).

AT3 is of special clinical interest because of the role it plays in neutralizing thrombin, which normally becomes activated intravascularly from prothrombin during clot formation. This 62,000 molecular weight protein forms a covalently bonded complex with thrombin over a period of several minutes when mixed in solution. Upon addition of heparin, the complex formation occurs almost instantaneously (Rosenburg, 1975). While AT3 is probably essential for successful therapeutic administration of heparin, only those rare individuals with marked deficiencies seem to have thrombotic disorders (Carvalho, 1976). The action of AT3 extends to the other vitamin K dependent factors in addition to thrombin. Serum levels of AT3 may be depressed in severe liver disease or in protein-losing disorders when the similar-sized molecule albumin is lost.

Although AAT, AMG, and AT3 provide the bulk of antiplasmin activity in serum (Harpel, 1976), there is a distinct antiplasmin which migrates as an alpha-2-globulin. This cross-reactivity of serum protease inhibitors for plasmin illustrates the difficulty in sorting out the precise physiologic function of each molecular species, since each one appears capable of substituting for another in different instances.

Acute Phase Reactants

This group of proteins shares the relationship of showing elevations in concentrations in response to stressful or inflammatory states that occur with infection, injury, surgery, trauma, or other tissue necrosis. They include alpha-1-antitrypsin, alpha-1-acid glycoprotein, haptoglobin, ceruloplasmin, fibrinogen, and C-reactive protein (CRP). Other clinical parameters may in fact be as sensitive as these and far easier to measure (e.g., fever, leukocytosis, or erythrocyte sedimentation rate). However, these proteins provide another dimension of quantitation which can be useful for monitoring the course of a patient by serial determinations (van Oss, 1975). Of course, those patients with congenital deficiencies (Gitlin, 1975), other impairment of synthesis due to drugs or organ disease, or newborns who normally have lower levels of many constituents (Gitlin, 1969) may not show the dramatic increases expected. However, a generally useful acute phase reactant (APR) for monitoring at least postsurgical response is CRP, which is the fastest rising APR and one which returns to normal following successful therapies (Fisher, 1976). While new techniques have made measurement of CRP easy and fast, there is still no general consensus among physicians for its widespread use, and there will undoubtedly remain a long-term need for sedimentation rate determinations.

2

PATTERNS OF PROTEIN ABNORMALITIES (Ritzmann, 1975)

Some of the most frequently encountered protein abnormalities in electrophoresis are shown by actual appearance in Figure 12–3 and as densitometric scans in Figure 12–4. While scanning allows quantitation of each fraction, visual inspection of the electrophoretic strip provides more detailed information in high resolution systems.

Patterns of hypoproteinemia due to malnutrition or gross loss of protein show reduction of all fractions, but the most dramatic reduction is often seen in albumin because of its normally high value (Fig. 12–3*A*, inanition in an elderly patient). Specific loss on a molecular weight basis such as in nephrotic syndrome shows a complementary pattern of proteins in the serum (Fig. 12–3*B*, decreased albumin and other fractions except increased alpha-2-macroglobulin and elevated beta-lipoprotein) and in urine (Fig. 12–3*C*, glomerular proteinuria with albumin and other fractions present but without alpha-2-macroglobulin). Tubular proteinuria due to impaired renal tubular reabsorption of small proteins shows a pattern of alpha, beta, and gamma losses with only minimal albumin in the urine (Killingsworth, 1982). Increases in haptoglobin indicate some form of response, whether acute or chronic, to stressful stimulus (Fig. 12–4*B* and *C*). Decreases in haptoglobin secondary to hemolysis may also show an independent band of hemoglobin migrating in the beta or alpha-2 region. Striking elevations of transferrin in the beta region occur in patients suffering from iron deficiency anemia (Fig. 12–3*D*). Broad elevations of gamma with reduction of albumin occur in the cirrhotic pattern (Fig. 12–3*E*). When a few clones of immunoglobulin are active, an oligoclonal pattern results (Fig. 12–3*F*). Deficiency of gamma can occur as a variant in neonates or in adults as an acquired immunodeficiency (Fig. 12–3*G*). One of the most explicit patterns comes

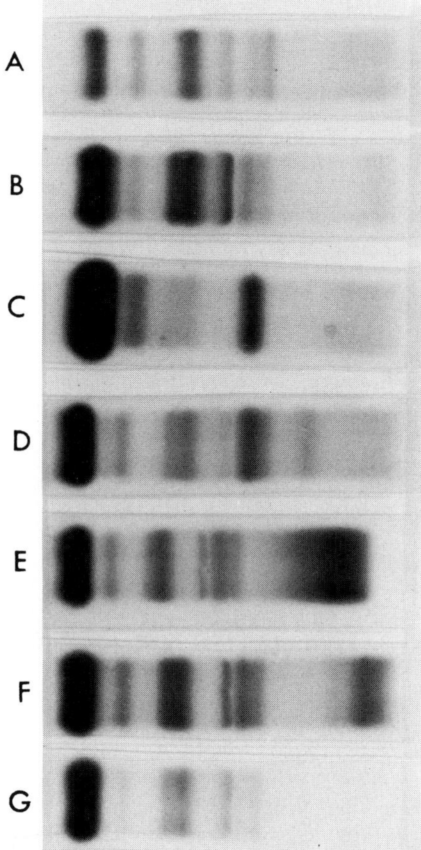

Figure 12–3. Abnormal protein patterns by agarose gel electrophoresis. Anode is to the left; fractions are as labeled in Figure 12–1; all samples are serum except for *C. A,* Inanition in an elderly patient with low total protein and markedly depressed albumin. *B,* Nephrotic syndrome with elevated alpha-2-macroglobulin and beta lipoprotein. *C,* Urine from protein-losing nephropathy. *D,* Iron deficiency with elevated transferrin. *E,* Broadly elevated gamma and low albumin due to liver disease. *F,* Oligoclonal gamma fraction in patient with renal disease. *G,* Hypogammaglobulinemia.

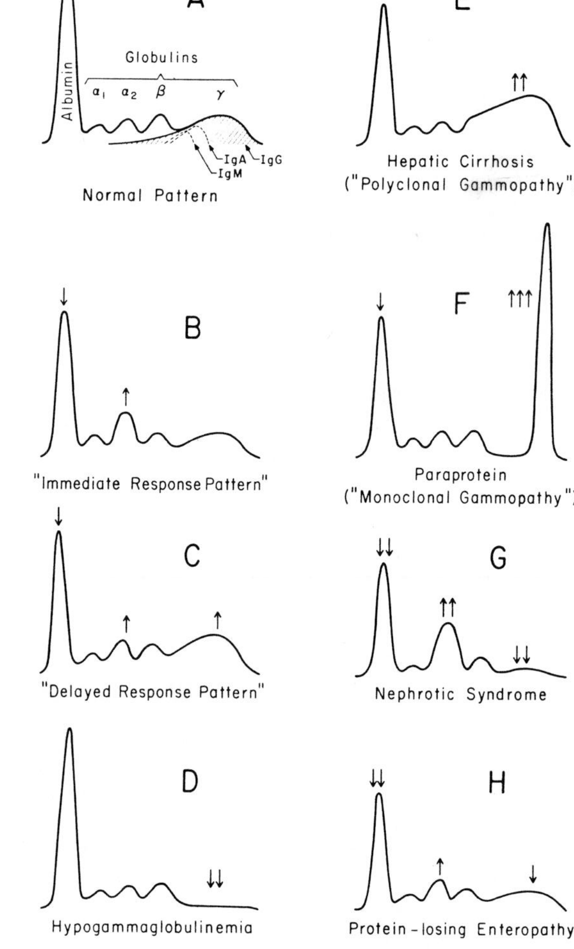

Figure 12–4. Serum protein electrophoresis: clinicopathologic correlations. (Courtesy of Dr. A. F. Krieg.)

from a paraprotein due to a monoclonal proliferation of plasma cells (Fig. 12–4*F*).

Immunoglobulins, disorders of the immune system, and abnormalities of complement are presented in Chapters 36, 37, and 39.

Al-Rashid, R. A., and Spangler, J.: Neonatal copper deficiency. N. Engl. J. Med., *285*:841, 1971.

Burrows, S., and Pekala, B.: Serum copper and ceruloplasmin in pregnancy. Am. J. Obstet. Gynecol., *109*:907, 1971.

Carvalho, A., and Ellman, L.: Hereditary antithrombin III deficiency. Effect of antithrombin deficiency on platelet function. Am. J. Med., *61*:179, 1976.

Claus, D. R., Osmand, A. P., and Gewurz, H.: Radioimmunoassay of human C-reactive protein and levels in normal sera. J. Lab. Clin. Med., *87*:120, 1976.

Daiger, S. P., Schanfield, M. S., and Cavalli-Sforza, L. L.: Group-specific component (Gc) proteins bind vitamin D and 25-hydroxy-vitamin D. Proc. Natl. Acad. Sci. U.S.A., *72*:2076, 1975.

Daniels, J. C., Larson, D. L., Abston, S., and Ritzmann, S. E.: Serum protein profiles in thermal burns. II. Protease inhibitors, complement factors and C-reactive proteins. J. Trauma, *14*:153, 1974.

Doolittle, R. F.: Fibrinogen and fibrin. *In* Putnam, F. W. (ed.): The Plasma Proteins, Vol. II. 2nd ed. New York, Academic Press, 1975, p. 110.

Eriksson, S.: Studies in alpha 1-antitrypsin deficiency. Acta Med. Scand., *177*:Suppl. 432, 1965.

Fisher, C. L., Gill, C., Forrester, M. G., and Nakamura, R.: Quantitation of "acute phase proteins" postoperatively. Value in detection and monitoring of complications. Am. J. Clin. Pathol., 66:840, 1976.

Gelb, A. F., Klein, E., and Lieberman, J.: Pulmonary function in nonsmoking subjects with alpha-1-antitrypsin deficiency (MZ phenotype). Am. J. Med., *62*:93, 1976.

Giblett, E. R. (ed.): Genetic Markers in Human Blood. Oxford, Blackwell Scientific, 1969.

Gitlin, D., and Biasucci, A.: Development of gamma G, gamma A, gamma M, C′1 esterase inhibitor, ceruloplasmin, transferrin, hemopexin, haptoglobin, fibrinogen, plasminogen, alpha 1-antitrypsin, orosomucoid, beta-lipoprotein, alpha 2-macroglobulin, and prealbumin in the human conceptus. J. Clin. Invest., *48*:1433, 1969.

Gitlin, D., and Gitlin, J. D.: Genetic alterations in the plasma proteins of man. *In* Putnam, F. W. (ed.): The Plasma Proteins, Vol. II. 2nd ed. New York, Academic Press, 1975, p. 321.

Glenner, G. G.: Amyloid deposits and amyloidosis. The beta-fibrilloses. N. Engl. J. Med., *302*:1283, 1980.

Guthrow, C. E., Morris, M. A., Day, J. F., Thorpe, S. R., and Baynes, J. W.: Enhanced nonenzymatic glucosylation of human serum albumin in diabetes mellitus. Proc. Natl. Acad. Sci. U.S.A., *76*:4258, 1979.

Harpel, P. C., and Rosenberg, R. D.: Alpha-2-macroglobulin and antithrombin-heparin cofactor: Modulators of hemostatic and inflammatory reactions. *In* Spaet, T. H. (ed.): Progress in Hemostasis and Thrombosis, Vol. 3. New York, Grune and Stratton, 1976, p. 145.

Hokama, Y.: Methods of assay and role of acute phase C-reactive protein in human diseases. *In* Nakamura, R. M., Dito, W. R., and Tucker, E. S. (eds.): Immunologic Analysis. Recent Progress in Diagnostic Laboratory Immunology. New York, Masson Publishing U.S.A., Inc., 1982, p. 239.

Horne, C. H. W., Weir, R. J., Howie, P. W., and Goudie, R. B.: Effect of combined oestrogen-progestogen oral contraceptives on serum levels of alpha-2-macroglobulin, transferrin, albumin and IgG. Lancet, *1*:49, 1970.

Jeppsson, J.-O., and Franzen, B.: Typing of genetic variants of alpha-1-antitrypsin by electrofocusing. Clin. Chem., *28*:219, 1982.

Jeppsson, J.-O., Laurell, C.-B., and Franzen, B.: Agarose gel electrophoresis. Clin. Chem., *25*:629, 1979.

Koch-Weser, J., and Sellers, E. M.: Drug therapy. Binding of drugs to serum albumin. N. Engl. J. Med., *294*:311, 1979.

Killingsworth, L. M.: Clinical applications of protein determinations in biological fluids other than blood. Clin. Chem., *28*:1093, 1982.

Konigsberg, W.: Molecular diseases. *In* Bondy, P. K., and Rosenberg, L. E. (eds.): Duncan's Diseases of Metabolism. 7th ed. Philadelphia, W. B. Saunders Company, 1974, p. 86.

Kosaka, S., and Tazawa, M.: Alpha-1-antichymotrypsin in rheumatoid arthritis. Tohoku J. Exp. Med., *119*:369, 1976.

Lauff, J. J., Kasper, M. E., Wu, T. W., and Ambrose, R. T.: Isolation and preliminary characterization of a fraction of bilirubin in serum that is firmly bound to protein. Clin. Chem., *28*:629, 1982.

Laurell, C.-B.: Electrophoresis, specific protein assays, or both in measurement of plasma proteins? Clin. Chem., *19*:99, 1973.

Laurell, C.-B.: Quantitative estimation of proteins by electrophoresis in agarose gel containing antibodies. Anal. Biochem., *15*:45, 1966.

Laurell, C.-B., and Jeppsson, J.-O.: Protease inhibitors in plasma. *In* Putnam, F. W. (ed.): The Plasma Proteins, Vol. I. 2nd ed. New York, Academic Press, 1975, p. 299.

Layne, E.: Spectrophotometric and turbidimetric methods for measuring proteins. *In* Colowick, S. P., and Kaplan, N. O. (eds.): Methods in Enzymology, Vol. III. New York, Academic Press, 1957, p. 447.

Lieberman, J., Gaidulis, L., Garoutte, B., and Mittman, C.: Identification and characteristics of the common alpha-1-antitrypsin phenotypes. Chest, *62*:557, 1972.

Lowry, O. H., Rosebrough, N. J., Farr, L., and Randall, R. J.: Protein measurement with Folin phenol reagent. J. Biol. Chem., *193*:265, 1951.

MacGillivray, R. T. A., Mendez, E., Sinha, S., Sutton, M. R., Lineback-Zins, J., and Brew, K.: The complete amino acid sequence of human serum transferrin. Proc. Natl. Acad. Sci. U.S.A., *79*:2504, 1982.

McFarlane, H., Reddy, S., Adcock, K. J., Adeshina, H., Cooke, A. R., and Akene, J.: Immunity, transferrin, and survival in kwashiorkor. Br. Med. J., *4*:268, 1970.

Meloun, B., Moravek, L., and Kostka, V.: Complete amino acid sequence of human serum albumin. FEBS Letters, *58*:134, 1975.

Menache, D.: Abnormal fibrinogens: A review. Thromb. Diath. Haemorrh., *29*:525, 1973.

Mendenhall, H. W.: Serum protein concentrations in pregnancy. I. Concentrations in maternal serum. Am. J. Obstet. Gynecol., *106*:388, 1970.

Merril, C. R., Goldman, D., Sedman, S. A., and Ebert, M. H.: Ultrasensitive stain for proteins in polyacrylamide gels shows regional variation in cerebrospinal fluid proteins. Science, *211*:1437, 1981.

Moses, A. C., Lawlor, J., Hallow, J., and Jackson, I. M. D.: Familial euthyroid hyperthyroxinemia resulting from increased thyroxine binding to thyroxine-binding prealbumin. N. Engl. J. Med., *306*:966, 1982.

Muller-Eberhard, U.: Hemopexin. N. Engl. J. Med., *283*:1090, 1970.

Oppenheimer, J. H.: Role of plasma proteins in the binding, distribution and metabolism of the thyroid hormones. N. Engl. J. Med., *278*:1153, 1968.

Peters, T., Jr.: Serum albumin. *In* Putnam, F. W. (ed.): The Plasma Proteins, Vol. I. 2nd ed. New York, Academic Press, 1975, p. 133.

Peters, T.: Serum albumin: Recent progress in the understanding of its structure and biosynthesis. Clin. Chem., *23*:5, 1977.

Peterson, P. A.: Studies on interaction between pre-albumin, retinol-binding protein and vitamin A. J. Biol. Chem., *246*:44, 1971.

Ritzmann, S. E., and Daniels, J. C. (eds.): Serum Protein Abnormalities. Diagnostic and Clinical Aspects. Boston, Little, Brown and Company, 1975.

Roeser, H. P., Lee, G. R., Nacht, S., and Cartwright, G. E.: The role of ceruloplasmin in iron metabolism. J. Clin. Invest., *49*:2408, 1970.

Rosenburg, R. D.: Actions and interactions of antithrombin and heparin. N. Engl. J. Med., *292*:146, 1975.

Rothschild, M. A., Oratz, M., and Schreiber, S. S.: Albumin synthesis. N. Engl. J. Med., *286*:748, 816, 1972.

Ruiz, M., Rajatanavin, R., Young, R. A., Taylor, C., Brown, R., Braverman, L. E., and Ingbar, S. H.: Familial dysalbuminemic hyperthyroxinemia. A syndrome that can be confused with thyrotoxicosis. N. Engl. J. Med., *306*:635, 1982.

Saxstad, J., Nilsson, L.-A., and Hanson, L. A.: C-reactive protein in serum from infants as determined with immunodiffusion techniques. Acta Paediatr. Scand., *59*:676, 1970.

Schenker, J. G., Jungreis, E., and Polishuk, W. Z.: Oral contraceptives and serum copper concentration. Obstet. Gynecol., *37*:233, 1971.

Schmid, K.: Alpha-1-acid glycoprotein. *In* Putnam, F. W. (ed.): The Plasma Proteins, Vol. I. 2nd ed. New York, Academic Press, 1975.

Slater, L., Carter, P. M., and Hobbs, J. R.: Measurement of albumin in the sera of patients. Ann. Clin. Biochem., *12*:33, 1975.

Steinbuch, M., Audran, R., Lambin, P., and Fine, J. M.: New data concerning inter-alpha-trypsin inhibitor. Protides Biol. Fluids, *23*:115, 1975.

Sveger, T.: Liver disease in alpha 1-antitrypsin deficiency detected by screening of 200,000 infants. N. Engl. J. Med., *294*:1316, 1976.

Tsung, S. H., Rosenthal, W. A., and Milewski, K. A.: Immunological measurement of transferrin compared with chemical measurement of total iron-binding capacity. Clin. Chem., *21*:1063, 1975.

van Oss, C. J., Bronson, P. M., and Border, J. R.: Changes in the serum alpha glycoprotein distribution in trauma patients. J. Trauma, *15*:451, 1975.

Waldmann, T. A., Gordon, R. S., and Rosse, W.: Studies on the metabolism of the serum proteins and lipids in patients with analbuminemia. Am. J. Med., *37*:960, 1964.

Walsh, P. G., and Haddad, J. G.: "Rocket" immunoelectrophoresis assay of vitamin D–binding protein (Gc globulin) in human serum. Clin. Chem., *28*:1781, 1982.

Weeke, E. O. B.: Urinary serum proteins. Protides Biol. Fluids, *21*:363, 1973.

Weinberg, E. D.: Iron and infection. Microbiol. Rev., *42*:45, 1978.

Wochner, R. D., Spilberg, I., Atsushi, I., Liem, H. H., and Muller-Eberhard, U.: Hemopexin metabolism in sickle cell disease, porphyrias and control subjects—effect of heme injection. N. Engl. J. Med., *290*:822, 1974.

Zawadzki, Z., and Edwards, G.: Pseudoparaproteinemia due to hypertransferrinemia. Am. J. Clin. Path., *54*:802, 1970.

13

FUNCTION AND INTEGRITY OF THE LIVER

HYMAN J. ZIMMERMAN, M.D.

The liver is a complex organ which performs many metabolic functions. More than 100 measures of hepatic function have been based on the hundreds of reactions that have been shown to occur in the liver. Many of these have been abandoned after early study. A few tests have been found to be clinically useful. Table 13–1 contains a classification of the hepatic tests arranged according to their physiologic basis.

Classic experiments in hepatic physiology have shown that removal of large portions of the liver of normal animals may leave some types of hepatic function unimpaired. This has led many authors to emphasize the great reserve power of the liver and to suggest that mild hepatic disease will not be exposed by examination of hepatic function. The relevance of such experiments to clinical problems, however, is questionable. Diffuse though mild disease, such as viral hepatitis or early cirrhosis of the liver, produces impairment of several measures of hepatic function, with the severity of disease reflected in the degree of hepatic dysfunction. Indeed, disturbed hepatic function does not necessarily mean hepatic disease, since physiologic effects of some non-hepatic diseases also may produce apparent impairment of liver function. Nevertheless, the occurrence of abnormal hepatic function can usually be found to have a rational basis when considered in the light of the clinical problem.

Clinicians tend to refer to all biochemical determinations that reflect hepatic disease as "liver function tests." Only some, however, actually measure hepatic function. For example, the imposition of an exogenous load for clearance by the liver (e.g., foreign dyes, drugs, galactose, or infused bile acid) or the estimation of the ability of the liver to excrete an endogenous load (e.g., bilirubin, bile acids, ammonia) are indeed tests of liver function. Measurement of the ability of the liver to metabolize a drug, to conjugate a foreign compound with glycine, and to synthesize prothrombin, albumin, or urea also measures hepatic function, although factors other than liver function can affect the results. Distortions of intermediary metabolism wrought by hepatic disease are of physiologic interest, and some hepatic function determinations have been based on the distortions.

Another group of biochemical determinations are of great help in the recognition of hepatic disease but do not measure liver function. These include measurement of blood constituents that, when elevated, reflect hepatocyte injury or biliary tree impatency. Serum activity of several enzymes (aminotransferases [transaminases], ornithine carbamoyl transferase, etc.), iron, ferritin, and vitamin B_{12} are elevated in patients with hepatic necrosis, to a degree that may assist in diagnosis. Conversely, the levels of other enzymes (alkaline phosphatase, 5′-nucleotidase, etc.), cholesterol, trihydroxy bile acids, and lipoprotein-X are elevated to a diagnostically helpful degree in patients with biliary tree obstruction.

A third group of biochemical and serologic measurements are useful for the diagnosis of specific hepatic diseases. In this group, for example, are serum alpha-fetoprotein, alpha-1-antitrypsin, ceruloplasmin, iron and transferrin, serologic markers of viral hepatitis, antimitochondrial antibodies, anti–smooth mus-

Table 13–1. PHYSIOLOGIC CLASSIFICATION OF HEPATIC FUNCTION AND RELATED DETERMINATIONS

Physiologic Basis	Measurements	Comments
Excretion and detoxification		
Bilirubin metabolism	Serum bilirubin (direct and indirect)	Very useful
	Urine bilirubin	Very useful
	Urine urobilinogen	Useful
	Fecal urobilinogen	Useful but neglected
Clearance of exogenous load		
Dye excretion	Sulfobromophthalein (BSP)	Very sensitive test of hepatic function; largely abandoned because of reactions; has special uses
	Indocyanine green (ICG)	Used extensively in research to measure hepatic function and blood flow; has seen little clinical use
	Rose bengal	Obsolete test; recently revived as radioactive RB and used for differential diagnosis of infantile jaundice to limited degree
Other	^{14}C-bilirubin	
	^{14}C-cholic acid	Experimental
	Galactose tolerance	See carbohydrate tests
Clearance of endogenous load	Bile acid levels (fasting and postprandial)	Very promising, but limited by technology
	Bilirubin levels	See bilirubin metabolism
	NH_3 levels	See protein metabolism
Xenobiotic metabolism		
Conjugating ability	Hippuric acid excretion	Formerly widely used; now obsolete
Drug metabolism (mixed function oxidase activity)	Drug metabolism measured by $^{14}CO_2$	Promising; thus far use is limited
Metabolic		
Carbohydrate metabolism	Glucose tolerance test Fructose tolerance test	Not useful in measuring hepatic function
	Lactate tolerance test	
	Galactose tolerance test	Used little in U.S.A.; used in other countries
	Epinephrine tolerance tests	Not used
	Glucagon tests	
Lipid metabolism	Plasma or serum cholesterol level	Limited usefulness
	Plasma or serum cholesterol ester level	Little clinical value
Protein metabolism	Serum protein levels	Very useful in analysis of hepatic and non-hepatic diseases
	Albumin, globulin, electrophoretic fractions; gamma globulin levels, immunoglobulins	
	Mucoproteins and haptoglobin	Have seen little use
	Flocculation and turbidimetric tests	Largely obsolete
	Lipoprotein-X	Marker of cholestasis
	Alpha-1-antitrypsin	Specific value for diagnosis of metabolic error
	Alpha-fetoprotein	Specific value for hepatic carcinoma
	Amino acid levels of blood and urine	Of research interest
	Blood ammonia levels and CSF (cerebrospinal fluid) glutamine	Useful in understanding diagnosis and management of hepatic encephalopathy

cle antibodies, and immunoglobulins (IgM, IgG, and IgA).

No one measurement or test of liver function is sufficient for clinical analysis of most problems. From the available measurements and examinations, a group of procedures that are most applicable to a particular clinical problem should be selected. These determinations and the various radiographic, radioisotopic, ultrasonic, and endoscopic procedures, as well as liver biopsy, constitute a panel of measurements and examinations that should permit diagnosis of almost all patients with hepatic disease.

Table 13–1. PHYSIOLOGIC CLASSIFICATION OF HEPATIC FUNCTION AND RELATED DETERMINATIONS *(Continued)*

Physiologic Basis	Measurements	Comments
Biosynthetic activity	Albumin level	See protein metabolism
	Blood urea levels	Of clinical value, but not useful to measure liver function
	Rate of urea synthesis	Research interest thus far
	Prothrombin time and response to vitamin K	Very useful
	Plasma level of other coagulation factors	Reflected in prothrombin time; individual factor measurement of research interest
Serum enzyme levels		
Large number of enzymes normally present in the liver because of multiple metabolic reactions that occur there; enzymes released to blood as a result of hepatocyte injury, biliary tree impatency, or both	Alkaline phosphatase (and related tests)	Very useful
	Aspartate aminotransferase (AST) or GOT	Very useful
	Alanine aminotransferase (ALT) or GPT	See Chapter 14 for other serum enzymes
Other substances released from damaged liver	Iron	Limited use
	Vitamin B_{12}	Limited use
Determinations that reflect special hepatic diseases		
Serum levels of	Alpha-fetoprotein	Hepatocellular carcinoma*
	Alpha-1-antitrypsin	Alpha-1-antitrypsin-liver disease*
	Iron, transferrin, and ferritin	Hemochromatosis*
	Ceruloplasmin	Wilson's disease*
	Serologic tests for	
	Viral hepatitis	See Table 13–13 and Chapter 50
	"Autoimmune" liver disease	See Chapter 40

*Condition for which determination is particularly helpful.

In the following pages, the physiologic basis for examination of hepatic functions is discussed, a number of individual tests are analyzed, and the batteries of tests that are considered useful are presented. The results obtained in various diseases also are described.

HEPATIC TESTS BASED ON EXCRETORY FUNCTION

An important physiologic role of the liver is the removal from the blood of potentially noxious endogenous and exogenous substances, and, thereafter, excretion into the bile or conversion to products suitable for excretion by the kidney or lung. Measurement of the concentrations of some of the endogenous substances in the blood, urine, or feces, or of the rate of uptake and excretion of exogenous substances, has provided useful tests of hepatic function (Table 13–1). Some of these are discussed in this section (related to bilirubin metabolism, dye excretion, bile acid metabolism). Others are discussed in the section devoted to intermediary metabolism (tests based on uptake by the liver of galactose, ammonia, and amino acids).

Bilirubin Metabolism

Knowledge of bilirubin metabolism (Fig. 13–1) is essential for the proper understanding of hepatic disease. Bilirubin is a product of the catabolism of hemoglobin, from which it is formed in the cells of the reticuloendothelial system. Here the protoporphyrin is separated from the iron and globin portions of the molecule, and the ring is opened oxidatively, leading to the quantitative release of the α-carbon bridge as carbon monoxide* and to the formation of biliverdin. The biliverdin is rapidly reduced to bilirubin (Fig. 13–2). Approximately 80 per cent of the bilirubin is derived from senescent erythrocytes. Most of the remainder is produced by intracorpuscular degradation of the hemoglobin of immature erythrocytes in the bone marrow (ineffective erythropoiesis), and from the degradation of heme-containing enzyme proteins derived from the liver and, perhaps, from other organs.

Bilirubin is transported through the blood (bound to albumin) to the liver. Transport of bilirubin from sinusoidal blood into the hepatocyte involves dissociation of bilirubin from albumin and translocation of the bilirubin to the inner surface of the plasma membrane, a process that probably depends on binding proteins located in the membrane. The process is saturable and shows mutually competitive inhibition by other organic ions, such as sulfobromophthalein (BSP), indocyanine green, and iodipamide, suggesting that bilirubin uptake is a carrier-mediated transport process.

*Measurement of CO production can serve as a measure of heme catabolism.

CATEGORY

UNCONJUGATED
PREHEPATIC
(hemolytic)

RE SYSTEM
Hemoglobin → Bilirubin + Iron + Globin

BLOOD
Bilirubin - Albumin

HEPATIC
Gilbert, S.
Crigler-Najjar S.

LIVER
Bilirubin + 2 UDP Glucuronate
Glucuronyl Transferase
Bilirubin Diglucuronide (Conjugated, Direct)

CONJUGATED
HEPATIC
Hepatocellular
Cholestatic

POSTHEPATIC

BILIARY TREE
Bilirubin Diglucuronide

INTESTINES
Bilirubin or Bilirubin Diglucuronide
Bacterial Enzymes
"Urobilinogens" → Urobilins

FECES
Urobilinogens and Urobilins
(50-250 mg. per day)

PORTAL BLOOD
Urobilinogen

KIDNEY

URINE
Urobilinogen
(1-4 mg. per day)
(<1.0 Ehrlich units per 2 hours)

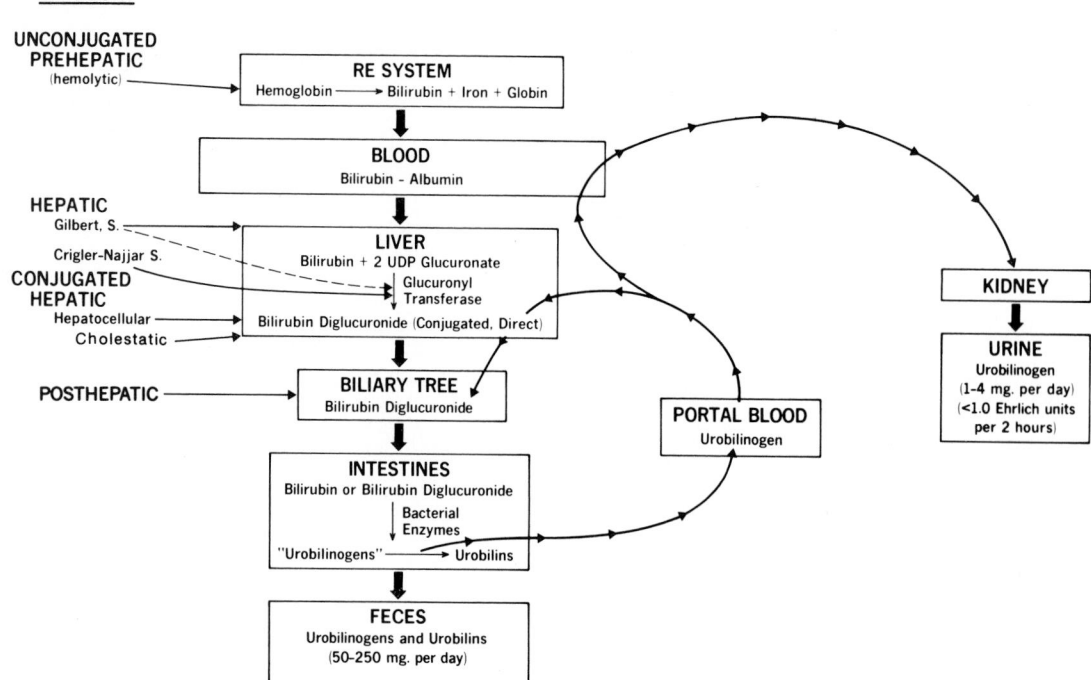

Figure 13–1. Schematic representation of bilirubin metabolism. The classification of jaundice (see Table 13–3) is shown on the left, the arrows pointing to the site of the physiologic defect responsible for the respective category of jaundice.

In the hepatocyte, bilirubin binds mainly to the proteins in the cytosol, ligandin (glutathime-S-transferase B) and Z protein. Formerly considered to play a key role in the uptake of bilirubin, these proteins appear to modulate uptake of bilirubin by binding it within the cell and to be responsible for the intrahepatocytic transport and detoxification of many substances in addition to bilirubin.

In the liver bilirubin is rendered water-soluble by conjugation with glucuronate to form mono- and diglucuronide.* Esterification with one proprionyl group occurs first, under the influences of the microsomal enzyme bilirubin–UDP–glucuronyl transferase. Up to 80 per cent of the monoglucuronate thus formed is then converted to the diglucuronide. The site for

*A fraction of the bilirubin excreted by the liver is conjugated with other groups. The conjugates of bilirubin that are formed differ in different species.

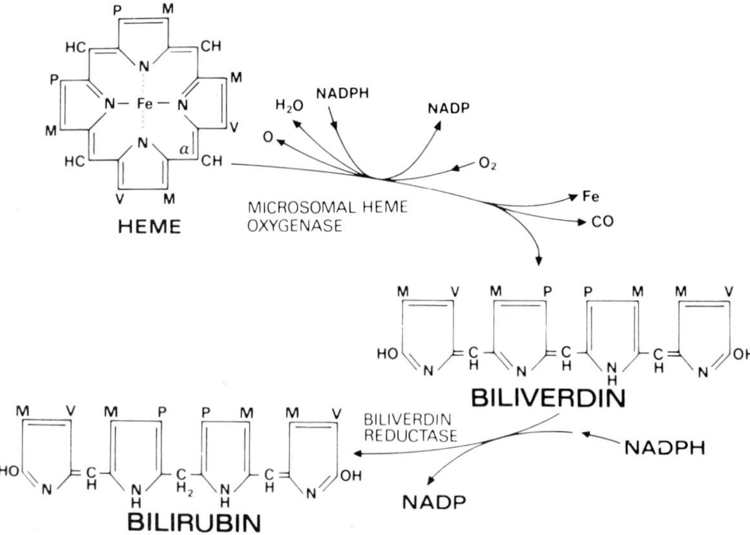

Figure 13–2. Biochemical pathway for conversion of heme to bilirubin via the intermediate biliverdin. (From Tenhunen, 1976, with permission.)

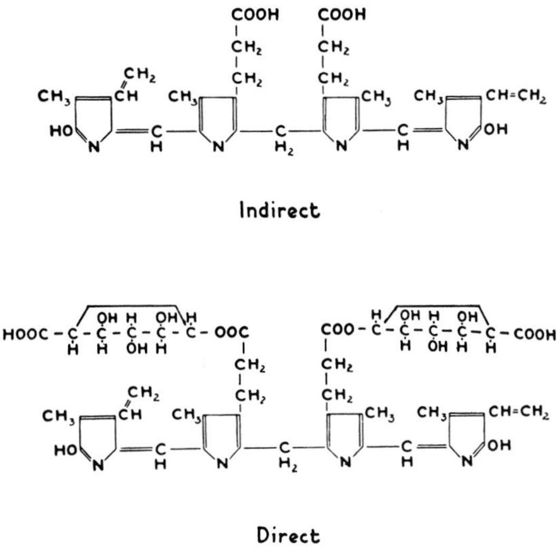

Indirect

Direct

Figure 13–3. The structure of indirect and of the predominant form of direct bilirubin. Approximately 80 per cent of direct bilirubin is the diglucuronide shown, and the remainder is monogluronide. Note that indirect bilirubin is unconjugated. (This schematic representation of bilirubin as a linear tetrapyrrole is the conventional model, although a ring-shaped structure is more accurate.)

the conversion to the diglucuronide is probably also the endoplasmic reticulum, although evidence has been offered in support of an enzyme system in the plasma membrane which can catalyze conversion of two molecules of monoglucuronide to one of diglucuronide and one of unconjugated bilirubin (Billing, 1982).

In the intestines bacterial enzyme action converts bilirubin through a group of intermediate compounds to several related compounds collectively referred to as "urobilinogen" (Fig. 13–1). A portion (estimated to be 10 per cent or more) of the urobilinogen is reabsorbed into the blood and re-excreted by the liver. Normally, small amounts (1 to 4 mg/24 hr) are excreted in the urine. Fecal urobilinogen levels in normals range from 50 to 250 mg/day. Some of the urobilinogen is oxidized to urobilin in the intestines or later in the feces. Measurement of fecal urobilinogen usually includes the sum of urobilinogens and urobilins. The metabolism of bilirubin is summarized in Figure 13–1.

Bilirubin was first demonstrated in serum by van den Bergh and Muller. They found that bilirubin in normal serum reacted with the Ehrlich diazo reagent (diazotized sulfanilic acid) only when alcohol was added. Their observation that bile pigment in human bile reacted with the diazo reagent without the addition of alcohol led to the recognition that some change in bilirubin had been effected by the liver. Van den Bergh called the form of bilirubin that reacted with the diazo reagent without the addition of alcohol "direct" and the variety that reacted only in the presence of alcohol "indirect." Serum from patients with jaundice caused by hemolysis gave the indirect reaction, while in the serum of patients with jaundice due to obstruction of the biliary tree the increased serum bilirubin levels gave the direct reaction. The response of the serum to the van den Bergh test has been the basis for several classifications of jaundice.

The properties of indirect and of direct bilirubin are summarized in Table 13–2. It is clear that the indirect bilirubin is "free" or unconjugated bilirubin bound to albumin en route to the liver from the reticuloendothelial system, where it has been formed. The unconjugated bilirubin is non-polar and therefore not soluble in water. Consequently it will react with the diazo reagent only in the presence of an agent (alcohol) in which it and the diazo reagent are soluble.* The non-polar nature of unconjugated bilirubin bound to albumin is also the basis for the failure of indirect bilirubin to appear in the urine in more than trace amounts. Unconjugated bilirubin is so tightly bound that it cannot be filtered at the glomerulus, and there appears to be no known tubular secretion of bilirubin. Accordingly, unconjugated bilirubin is not excreted in the urine. Direct (conjugated) bilirubin

*The alcohol also enhances the intensity of the color formed by the bilirubin reaction with the van den Bergh reagent.

Table 13–2. COMPARISON OF PROPERTIES OF DIRECT AND INDIRECT BILIRUBIN

	Direct (Conjugated)	Indirect (Unconjugated)
Structure	Bilirubin diglucuronide	Bilirubin
Type of compound	Polar	Nonpolar
Solubility		
Water	+	−
Alcohol	+	+
Van den Bergh reaction	Direct	Indirect
Affinity for brain tissue	Low	High*
Presence in urine of patients with jaundice	+	−
Associated with jaundice		
Hemolytic	−	+
Obstructive and hepatocellular	+	+

*Kernicterus (deposition of bilirubin in brain tissue) occurs only in association with very high levels of unconjugated bilirubin.

is a polar compound. It is therefore soluble in water solution, reacting directly with the diazo reagent and able to appear in the urine when the blood levels are increased. Conjugated bilirubin is, in part, not protein-bound; hence, it can be filtered at the glomerulus and excreted in the urine.

Qualitative analysis of serum bilirubin as indirect or direct according to the type of van den Bergh reaction has long been replaced by quantitative determination of the amount of direct and of total bilirubin, the difference being presumed to represent indirect bilirubin. Commonly used procedures for measuring bilirubin and its fractions are modifications of the method of Malloy (1937). These methods depend on the speed of the reaction with the diazo reagent and on the solvent in which it occurs. The pigment that reacts promptly without the addition of ethanol or methanol is "direct," and that which reacts later and with the addition of the alcohol is the "total" bilirubin (indirect plus direct). Many laboratories supplement their diazotization method with one of the direct spectrophotometric techniques. An excellent review of bilirubin methodology is available (Sunderman, 1978).

The level of bilirubin in the serum is less than 1.0 mg/dl in 99 per cent of normals. This is almost entirely unconjugated. Up to 20 per cent of the unconjugated bilirubin, however, can react with the van den Bergh reagent, simulating the presence of up to 0.2 mg/dl of conjugated bilirubin in normal plasma. Accordingly, values for direct bilirubin above 0.2 mg/dl by the method of Ducci (1947) are suspect. The upper reference limit for direct bilirubin may, however, vary from 0.2 to 0.4 mg in different laboratories, and each laboratory should determine the reference interval for its method and conditions. Levels of total serum bilirubin above 2.5 mg/dl usually produce jaundice.

Jaundice has been classified by various authors according to pathophysiology, etiology, or both. The classification of McNee (1923), which was based on etiology, that of Rich (1930), which was based on mechanisms, and that of Ducci (1947), which was based on both, are now only of historic interest.

The currently employed classification of jaundice (Table 13–3; Fig. 13–1) is rational and simple. It divides hyperbilirubinemia into the two categories of *unconjugated* and *conjugated.* The *unconjugated* category includes the forms of jaundice in which at least 80 per cent of the serum bilirubin is indirect. This may be *prehepatic,* in which excess bilirubin production (hemolysis) is responsible, or *hepatic,* in which either removal of bilirubin from the blood or conjugation of bilirubin by the liver is defective. The *conjugated* category also includes two groups: *hepatic,* which includes a number of genetic and acquired defects of the liver, and *posthepatic,* which refers to anatomic obstruction of the extrahepatic biliary tree.

The *prehepatic* type of unconjugated hyperbilirubinemia commonly referred to as hemolytic jaundice occurs because excessively rapid destruction of erythrocytes results in the production of bilirubin at a rate exceeding the ability of the liver to conjugate and excrete it. It may result from any of the genetic or acquired types of hemolytic disease. Tissue hematomas or collection of blood in body cavities may also be the source of increased amounts of bilirubin produced. The hyperbilirubinemia, accordingly, is largely the indirect (unconjugated) type. The increased production of bilirubin usually results in an increase in the amount of fecal urobilinogen, a characteristic of hemolytic jaundice. Often there is also an increase in the urine content of urobilinogen. Presumably this results from the reabsorption from the intestines of greater amounts of urobilinogen than can be re-excreted by the liver. Bilirubin does not appear in the urine in hemolytic jaundice, since the elevated level of blood bilirubin consists largely of the unconjugated (bound to albumin) type.

The *hepatic* type of unconjugated hyperbilirubinemia includes the Gilbert syndrome (constitutional hepatic dysfunction) and the Crigler-Najjar syndrome (constitutional hyperbilirubinemia with kernicterus). The Gilbert syndrome is a mild condition that appears to result from a genetic defect in the transport of bilirubin from sinusoidal blood into the hepatocyte. (The Gilbert syndrome probably includes several different conditions, all of which present a similar benign syndrome of mild unconjugated hyperbilirubinemia.) The Crigler-Najjar syndrome is a severe disease with marked hyperbilirubinemia that results from a genetic deficiency of the hepatic microsomal enzyme, glucuronyl transferase (bilirubin-UDP glucuronyl-transferase), which is needed for the conjugation of bilirubin. Another form of glucuronyl transferase deficiency, which is a clinically much more benign syndrome, has been described. Hepatic unconjugated hyperbilirubinemia resembles that of hemolytic (prehepatic) hyperbilirubinemia in that it is largely unconjugated. The fecal and urine urobilinogen content in the hepatic type of *unconjugated* hyperbilirubinemia, in contrast to that of the prehepatic type, is normal or reduced, since the rate of bilirubin entry into the duodenum is depressed rather than increased (Fig. 13–4*B* and *C*). Unconjugated hyperbilirubinemia may also be due to immaturity of the glucuronyl transferase system in the neonate, to the interference with uptake of bilirubin by the hepatocyte induced by drugs (e.g., flavaspidic acid), and to transiently impaired bilirubin conjugation seen in newborns as a benign genetic disorder ("breast milk jaundice" and the Lucey-Driscoll syndrome).

Posthepatic jaundice, commonly called obstructive jaundice, usually is the result of obstruction of the common bile or hepatic duct by carcinoma of the head of the pancreas, papilla of Vater, or common duct, by choledocholithiasis, or by pancreatitis. Rarely, diseased lymph nodes surrounding the duct or neoplastic invasion of the *porta hepatis* may produce posthepatic jaundice. Obstruction of the biliary tree produces jaundice by preventing the entry into the duodenum of bilirubin that has been conjugated. The bilirubin is "regurgitated" into the blood, raising the serum level of direct-reacting bilirubin, which then

Table 13–3. CLASSIFICATION OF JAUNDICE

			Tests of Bilirubin Metabolism*			
Classification of Hyperbilirubinemia	**Physiologic Defect**	**Examples of Etiology**	***Serum Bilirubin Direct: Total in %***	***Urine Bilirubin***	***Urobil-inogen†***	***Fecal Urobil-inogen‡***
Unconjugated						
Prehepatic	Excessive production of bilirubin	Hemolytic states Extensive hematoma	<20	–	(↑)	↑
Hepatic	Defective transport of bilirubin from sinusoidal blood into hepatocyte	Gilbert syndrome§ Some toxins (e.g., flavaspidic acid)	<20	–	N	N
	Inability to conjugate	Crigler-Najjar syndrome Neonatal jaundice Some drugs (e.g., Novobiocin)	<20	–	N	N
Conjugated						
Hepatic						
Hepatocellular	Hepatocyte injury	Viral or toxic hepatitis, cirrhosis, alcoholic hepatitis, other causes of hepatocyte injury	>40	+	N, ↑, or ↓	↓
Cholestatic	Intrahepatic cholestasis owing to defective transport of bilirubin into canaliculus	Some drugs (e.g., chlorpromazine, anabolic steroids), viral hepatitis, primary biliary cirrhosis, some forms of familial jaundice	>50	+	N, ↑, or ↓	↓
Posthepatic	Mechanical obstruction of biliary tree	Carcinoma of pancreas or common bile duct Choledocholithiasis Other anatomic obstruction	>50	+	↓	↓

*Arrow indicates direction of change. Parentheses indicate that change may or may not occur. N = normal; ↑ = elevated; ↓ = depressed; + = positive reaction or present.

†Normal urine contains very small amounts of urobilinogen.

‡Normals show a very wide range of fecal urobilinogen content. Levels above 250 mg/day are considered increased and those below 5 mg/day are decreased to a diagnostically useful degree.

§May also include impaired conjugation.

appears in the urine. The exclusion of bilirubin from the duodenum results in clay-colored feces and very low levels of urobilinogen in the feces and urine (Fig. 13–4*F*).

Hepatic (conjugated) jaundice or hyperbilirubinemia can be divided into two subcategories: the hepatocellular and cholestatic types. *Cholestatic jaundice* closely resembles posthepatic jaundice in its clinical and biochemical features. This is also commonly referred to as *intrahepatic cholestasis*.

The hepatocellular types of hepatic jaundice result from injury to the parenchyma (viral hepatitis, toxic hepatitis, cirrhosis). Hepatic damage theoretically might be expected to produce an unconjugated hyperbilirubinemia because of presumed impaired conjugating ability in view of the manifold impairment of other parenchymal functions. The pattern of hyperbilirubinemia in hepatocellular jaundice differs little from that of posthepatic jaundice (Table 13–3; Fig. 13–4). Accordingly, it may be inferred that even in severe hepatocellular disease, the ability to conjugate remains unimpaired; and there is a distinct increase in the direct-reacting bilirubin fraction of the blood and there is bilirubin in the urine. The degree of exclusion of bilirubin from the duodenum, however, is much less marked than in posthepatic jaundice. Stools usually are only somewhat lighter than normal but may be clay colored. The urobilinogen content of the stool is usually decreased, but rarely to the levels characteristic of posthepatic jaundice. Even though amounts of bilirubin entering the duodenum are less than normal, liver damage prevents adequate hepatic clearing from the blood of the urobilinogen reabsorbed from the duodenum. Urine urobilinogen, therefore,

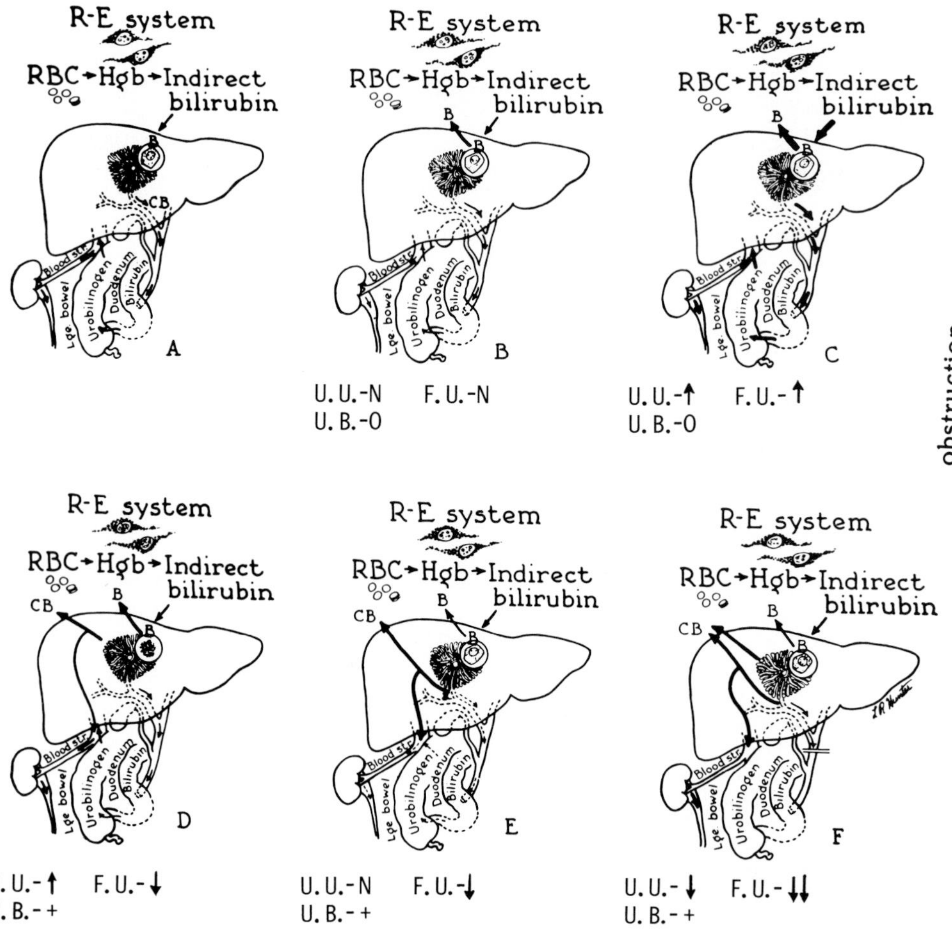

Figure 13–4. Diagrammatic representation of *(A)* normal bilirubin metabolism and the type of defect in *(B)* Gilbert or Crigler-Najjar syndrome, *(C)* hemolytic jaundice, *(D)* hepatocellular jaundice, *(E)* cholestatic jaundice (intrahepatic cholestasis), and *(F)* posthepatic jaundice. In the diagrams, B represents unconjugated and CB conjugated bilirubin; U.U. represents urine urobilinogen, U.B. urine bilirubin, and F.U. fecal urobilinogen. N represents normal; + indicates present; 0 indicates absent; number of upward- or downward-directed arrows indicates increase or decrease, respectively.

is often increased in some stages of hepatocellular jaundice (Figs. 13–4*D* and 13–5). There are, however, changes in the apparent pathophysiology of bilirubin metabolism during the course of acute viral hepatitis (Fig. 13–5). Early in the course, the level of direct bilirubin of the blood is increased, representing 40 to 60 per cent of the total bilirubin, and urine contains bilirubin. Latter in the course, the hyperbilirubinemia may be mainly indirect. Even at the peak of the jaundice, the degree of exclusion of bilirubin from the intestines is much less marked than in posthepatic jaundice. Stools usually are only slightly lighter than normal, although they may be as pale as those of posthepatic jaundice ("clay-colored"). Urobilinogen content of the stool is usually decreased, but rarely to the level characteristic of posthepatic jaundice. Urobilinogen levels of urine are usually increased despite the reduction in bilirubin entry into duodenum, since liver damage prevents adequate clearing from the blood of even the reduced amounts reabsorbed from the intestine.

It has been presumed, therefore, that in hepatitis (as in posthepatic jaundice) much of the bilirubin presented to the liver cell is conjugated, excreted into the canaliculi, and then regurgitated into the blood, perhaps through altered "tight" junctions between hepatocytes. Another possible mechanism is impairment of synthesis of bile acids necessary to permit adequate transport of conjugated bilirubin into the canaliculus.

The cholestatic type of hepatic jaundice simulates posthepatic jaundice very closely (Fig. 13–4*E*). It has also been called *intrahepatic cholestasis,* a term that describes the fact that bile flow into the duodenum is inhibited by intrahepatic disease. This type of jaundice is seen most commonly with certain drug reactions (chlorpromazine, organic arsenicals, methyltestosterone); it is thought to occur occasionally as a result of viral hepatitis or it may be "idiopathic." There are, however, a large number of possible causes of intrahepatic cholestasis (Zimmerman, 1979).

Determinations

Total serum bilirubin level is useful in evaluating the depth and progress of jaundice. Direct and indirect

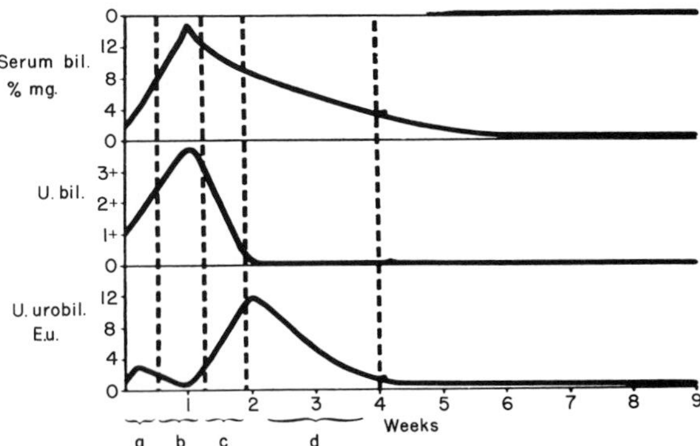

Figure 13–5. Diagrammatic representation of laboratory abnormalities during the course of acute icteric viral hepatitis. Note that early in the course (phase *a*) there is presence of bilirubin and increased amounts of urobilinogen in the urine with elevated serum bilirubin levels. This is followed by the phase *(b)* of deepening jaundice with decreased urine urobilinogen and increased urine bilirubin, after which there is an increase in urine urobilinogen (phase *c*) as the serum and urine bilirubin begin to decrease. In phase *d* bilirubin often disappears from the urine, but serum bilirubin levels are still distinctly elevated. Most patients show or are observed only in phases *c* and *d*, but some show this complete pattern. (Modified from Watson: Ann. Intern. Med., *25*:195, 1947.)

bilirubin measurements have been of some value in the differential diagnosis of jaundice. When the direct fraction is less than 20 per cent of the total bilirubin value, the jaundice is considered to be a manifestation of unconjugated hyperbilirubinemia—due either to hemolysis or to one of the types of constitutional hyperbilirubinemia (Table 13–3). Little specific aid in the distinction of hepatic from posthepatic causes of conjugated hyperbilirubinemic jaundice can be obtained from the relative levels of direct and indirect bilirubin. The direct fraction may constitute 40 to 60 per cent of the total bilirubin in either hepatic or posthepatic jaundice. Levels of the direct fraction that constitute between 20 and 40 per cent of the total bilirubin, however, are more characteristic of hepatic than of posthepatic jaundice. Levels in excess of 50 per cent of the total are somewhat more characteristic of posthepatic than of hepatic jaundice.

Most commonly used methods are the Malloy (1937) or modifications of it such as Ducci and Watson or Michaelsson (1961). In these methods the bilirubin reacts with diazotized sulfanilic acid to form azobilirubin, the intensity of the purple color being proportional to the quantity of bilirubin. In the Ducci and Watson method, the amount of bilirubin that reacts with the diazo reagent (in aqueous solution) at the end of one minute is determined. This "one-minute" bilirubin is equivalent to the "prompt," direct-reacting bilirubin of van den Bergh. The total bilirubin is measured 15 minutes after the addition of methanol. The difference between the total and the direct is the indirect. Other methods employ the same principle.

Urine bilirubin (urine "bile") measurements are useful in the differential diagnosis of jaundice. The presence of bilirubin in the urine of a patient with jaundice shows that the hyperbilirubinemia is of the conjugated type, i.e., hepatic or posthepatic. Bilirubin may also be present in the urine of patients without jaundice, as in early or anicteric hepatitis, in metastatic carcinoma, or in early obstruction of the biliary tree.

A number of methods have been devised for the measurement of bilirubin in the urine. The most sensitive depend on concentration of bilirubin by absorption, followed by oxidation or diazotization to yield a characteristic color reaction. In this country, simplified methods involving tablets or "dip-sticks" impregnated with diazo reagent have superseded other procedures. The impregnated tablets can detect bilirubin concentrations of 0.05 to 0.1 mg/dl. Dip-sticks are somewhat less sensitive. There should be no bilirubin demonstrable by any of these methods in normal urine (see Chap. 18).

Decreased *fecal urobilinogen* is characteristic of obstructive (posthepatic) jaundice but may also be found in patients with hepatocellular jaundice. An extremely low level (below 5 mg per day) of fecal urobilinogen is evidence that the jaundice is posthepatic. An increased level (above 250 mg per day) is evidence of hemolysis. When fecal urobilinogen levels are being determined as measures of hemolysis, they should be correlated with the degree of anemia (see Chap. 29).

Measurement of urobilinogen content of feces and urine can be useful but has lost popularity in recent years. The several compounds which are collectively referred to as urobilinogens give the same cherry-red color with Ehrlich's aldehyde reagent. The intensity of the color permits ready quantitation of total urobilinogen content. Urine urobilinogen can be measured by the simple two-hour test of Watson and even more simply with Ehrlich's aldehyde reagent. By the method of Watson, normal urine should contain less than 1 Ehrlich unit (1 mg urobilinogen) per two-hour specimen. Measurement of fecal urobilinogen involves the same color reaction but is somewhat more arduous.

Urine urobilinogen levels are decreased in posthepatic jaundice and in some phases of hepatic jaundice. Increased levels are observed usually in hemolytic jaundice and with subsiding hepatitis. Increased levels may also be a sensitive measure of hepatic damage even in the absence of jaundice, as in some patients with cirrhosis of the liver, metastatic carcinoma, or congestive heart failure.

Studies of urine and stool pigments are useful to the clinician, but there are several pitfalls in the application of bile pigment study to the analysis of jaundice. Very low levels of urobilinogen in the stool are characteristic of posthepatic jaundice but may also occur in patients who have received "broad-spectrum" antibiotics. These agents suppress the intestinal bacteria which convert bilirubin to urobilinogen. On the other hand, normal levels of urine urobilinogen may be found in patients with incomplete obstructive jaundice. During the course of acute viral hepatitis (Fig. 13–5), urobilinogen and bilirubin content of the urine may be characteristic of hepatocellular jaundice (phases a and c) and of obstructive jaundice (phase b) and may even simulate prehepatic icterus (phase d). Mixed forms of jaundice may yield potentially confusing patterns. For example, hemolytic icterus may be complicated by hepatic necrosis (as in sickle cell anemia) and thus by hepatocellular jaundice or by pigment stones obstructing the common duct and producing posthepatic jaundice.

Other tests based on bilirubin metabolism have been devised but have found little clinical application. The *bilirubin tolerance test* consists of administering a known amount of bilirubin and observing the rate of disappearance from the blood. This test is a sensitive measure of hepatic function but has not been adopted widely because it is laborious and expensive. Use of ^{14}C-bilirubin makes the test far easier to perform, but it is used only in research.

EXCRETION OF FOREIGN DYES

It has been recognized for many years that extraction of foreign dyes from the blood by the liver can be applied to the testing of hepatic function. Three dyes which have been employed for this purpose are rose bengal, sulfobromophthalein (BSP), and indocyanine green (ICG). BSP and ICG also have been used to measure hepatic blood flow. The technique, which is used primarily as a research tool, involves hepatic vein catheterization, measurement of the fraction of dye extracted by the liver per unit volume of blood perfusing it, and application of the Fick principle.

Rose Bengal Excretion. Rose bengal excretion was the first test of liver function, based on the elimination of dyes by the liver, that received significant clinical application. In this test the dye is administered parenterally, and either excretion of the dye into the duodenum or retention in the blood is measured. For technical reasons, this procedure was considered inferior to the BSP test and abandoned. Rose bengal excretion has been revived recently with the introduction of rose bengal "tagged" with ^{131}I. The rate of accumulation of the radioactivity over the liver and its rate of disappearance from the liver have been used to help detect hepatic disease. A test based on the fecal and urinary excretion of injected radioactive rose bengal and its products has been helpful in distinguishing hepatocellular from obstructive jaundice, particularly in infants. It is of little assistance in distinguishing intrahepatic cholestasis from extrahepatic obstruction, particularly in adults. I-131-rose bengal clearance has found little use as a test of liver function.

Sulfobromophthalein (BSP) Excretion. The BSP excretion test has been one of the most widely used and most sensitive tests of liver function. Normal results with this procedure virtually rule out a significant degree of parenchymal hepatic disease.

Recent years have seen decreased use of the procedure, in part because of adverse reactions and in part because the information sought is provided by other tests. Nevertheless, it has been so widely used that an adequate description of its physiologic basis is in order.

The dye is administered intravenously and its disappearance from the blood is determined. The BSP is almost completely cleared from the blood by the normal liver. (In hepatectomized animals, up to 20 per cent of the dye may be removed by extrahepatic tissue.) The two factors involved in BSP excretion by the liver are normal hepatic function and an adequate hepatic circulation.

Excretion of BSP by the liver involves four steps: (1) The dye is transferred from the blood to the hepatic parenchymal cell. (2) It is stored there briefly bound to ligandin and the z protein. (3) It is *conjugated* with glutathione. (4) The conjugate* is excreted by active transport into the bile. Refined techniques are available for the measurement of clearance from the blood and excretion into the bile and for the estimation of storage capacity. Excretion into the bile is the rate-limiting step for which a transport maximum (Tm) has been defined. These measurements and the determination of blood levels of conjugated and unconjugated BSP are research tools useful for unraveling the relative roles of hepatic uptake, conjugation (and storage), and biliary excretion in the clearance of BSP. They are, however, too elaborate for ordinary clinical use. Simplified techniques have been used to demonstrate defective transport of conjugated BSP into the bile in the Dubin-Johnson syndrome and in individuals with impaired hepatic function induced by methyltestosterone and other C-17 alkylated steroids.

Several standardized tests have been based on the ability of the liver to remove BSP from the blood. In the most widely used procedure a dose of 5 mg/kg of body weight is administered intravenously, and a blood specimen is obtained 45 minutes later. The level of dye at 45 minutes is expressed as the per cent of dye "retained," i.e., not excreted. A level of 10 mg/dl is considered to represent 100 per cent retention.

The determination of the rate of disappearance (percentage disappearance rate [PDR]) by obtaining multiple serum samples after administration of the dye provides a greater degree of accuracy than does the single-specimen method. It is too elaborate for routine clinical application, however.

Healthy individuals can remove from the blood over 95 per cent of the injected dose by 45 minutes. "Retention" in the blood of over 5 per cent of the dose, accordingly, is evidence of abnormal hepatic function or impaired blood flow.

Abnormal retention occurs in a number of hepatobiliary and systemic conditions. In hepatic and posthepatic jaundice, values are abnormal. In unconjugated hyperbilirubinemia, however, whether of the prehepatic (hemolytic) or hepatic (Crigler-Najjar and Gilbert's syndromes) type, BSP excretion is usually normal. (One form of Gilbert's syndrome is associated with impaired BSP excretion.)

Excretion of BSP also is abnormal in non-jaundiced patients with hepatic, biliary tract, or extrahepatic disease (Table 13–4). In patients with cirrhosis, excretion is rarely normal. Those with ascites or portal hypertension usually show a high degree of BSP retention. Nevertheless, in rare instances of inactive cirrhosis,† even when accompanied by severe portal hypertension, hepatic function, as measured by BSP excretion, may be normal or only slightly abnormal.

It is apparent that the BSP excretion test is of greatest value in the patient with little or no jaundice. A normal result is helpful in excluding the presence of hepatic parenchymal disease. This test is also useful in measuring the severity of liver disease and in assessing the completeness of recovery (e.g., in hepatitis). It is of aid in detecting early hepatic damage in patients who have been exposed to hepatotoxins. It is of help in recognizing the presence of metastatic hepatic carcinoma.

The BSP excretion test is particularly helpful in diagnosing the Dubin-Johnson syndrome and in distinguishing it from the Rotor syndrome, which it resembles. In the Dubin-Johnson syndrome a genetic defect leads to impaired transport of BSP, after conjugation, into the canaliculus and, consequently, regurgitation of conjugated BSP into the

*A small fraction (<30 per cent) of the dye is excreted in the unconjugated form.

†Absence of necrosis and little or no inflammation.

Table 13–4. DISEASES CHARACTERIZED BY ABNORMAL BSP EXCRETION

I. Parenchymal hepatic disease
   A. Cirrhosis
   B. Fatty metamorphosis
   C. Viral hepatitis
   D. Toxic hepatic injury
   E. Infectious mononucleosis
II. Biliary tract disease
   A. Common bile duct obstruction (with or without jaundice)
   B. Cholelithiasis and cholecystitis
III. Extrahepatic disease
   A. Circulatory
      1. Congestive heart failure
      2. Hepatic vein occlusion (Chiari's syndrome)
      3. ? Shock
      4. Spinal cord injuries
   B. Systemic disease producing infiltrative lesions of liver
      1. Metastatic carcinoma
      2. Lymphomas and leukemias
      3. Granulomatous disease (tuberculosis, histoplasmosis, sarcoidosis)
      4. Amyloidosis
   C. Nonspecific (fever, chronic and debilitating diseases)

blood. Removal from blood and hepatic storage, however, are normal. Accordingly, in the Dubin-Johnson syndrome the BSP values at 45 minutes may be normal or only slightly increased, while the value subsequently (90, 120, or 150 minutes after administration) may be much higher. In the Rotor syndrome, also due to a genetic defect in bilirubin metabolism, storage and excretion of BSP are abnormal and the BSP value in the blood is abnormal at 45 minutes and less abnormal thereafter.

Pitfalls in the application of this test lie in its great sensitivity and, accordingly, in the large number of extrahepatic causes of abnormal values, although clinical correlations are of help in this regard. Conversely, some forms of intrinsic hepatic disease may be associated, though infrequently, with normal BSP excretion. These include occasional instances of hemochromatosis, polycystic disease of the liver, amyloidosis, and inactive macronodular cirrhosis. An additional source of error in interpreting results of the BSP test is the interference with excretion of the dye induced by some gallbladder dyes. Accordingly, an unexpectedly abnormal value within 24 hours of a cholecystogram should not be accepted until confirmed by repetition at another time. Some drugs (e.g., rifampin) also compete with hepatic uptake of BSP.

The irritative effect of BSP on extravascular tissue is great. Extravasation of the dye in the course of intravenous administration can lead to a severe cellulitis and slough. This can be prevented by meticulous technique in administration.

The most important disadvantage is the extremely rare but serious complication of anaphylactic (or anaphylactoid) shock caused by BSP administration. Although this test has almost disappeared from clinical use, it remains useful in the recognition of the Dubin-Johnson syndrome and for special studies of hepatic function and disease.

Indocyanine Green Excretion. Excretion of indocyanine green (ICG) has been utilized as a test of hepatic function during the past two decades. Excretion of this dye by the liver does not involve conjugation. Furthermore, there is virtually no extrahepatic removal from the blood of ICG, which is removed almost exclusively by the liver. Accordingly, this dye has been studied as a possible substitute for BSP. Results of the ICG excretion test in the dose ordinarily used (0.5 mg/kg) are comparable to those of the BSP test in patients with severe hepatic disease, but the BSP test appears to be a more sensitive indicator of mild hepatic abnormality than does the ICG in this small dose. The larger dose of ICG (5 mg/kg) appears to be as sensitive as BSP, but is far more expensive. It is probable that the ICG test will prove to be useful in the settings which have employed the BSP. Nevertheless, a large amount of clinical experience and testing will be required to validate the assumption that results with the ICG test can be considered equivalent to those formerly obtained with the BSP test. Thus far, clinical use of ICG excretion as a test of hepatic function has been confined to a few clinics.

2

SERUM BILE ACIDS

Bile acids are generally referred to as *primary* and *secondary* (Fig. 13–6). The principal *primary* bile acids, cholic and chenodeoxycholic acid, are synthesized in the liver from cholesterol (Chap. 11). Cholic acid is a trihydroxy (3-α, 7-α, 12-α) and chenodeoxycholic acid is a dihydroxy (3-α, 7-α) bile acid. The primary bile acids are conjugated with glycine and taurine prior to their active transport into the bile. The conjugated primary bile acids, after secretion into the bile, are stored in the gallbladder during the fasting state. During digestion the bile acids are excreted into the lumen of the intestinal tract.

The bile acids undergo an efficient enterohepatic circulation involving the following three pathways: (1) passive jejunal reabsorption of the conjugate of chenodeoxycholic acid; (2) active ileal reabsorption of conjugated bile salts; (3) passive colonic reabsorption of "secondary" bile acids formed by bacterial deconjugation and chemical alteration of the conjugated bile salts. Of the many secondary bile acids formed in the colon, deoxycholic and lithocholic (LCA) acids are the most important. The pathophysiologic ramifications of bile acid metabolism are great and beyond the scope of this chapter. The promise that bile acid measurement offers for evaluation of liver function, however, warrants further discussion.

Small amounts of primary bile acids are present in the portal blood at any time. Bile acids are almost completely removed from the portal blood by hepatocyte extraction and are then rapidly re-excreted into the bile. Accordingly, the quantity of bile acids present in the peripheral or portal blood or within the liver normally represents a very small fraction of the total bile acid pool. Almost all of the bile acid pool is within the gallbladder in the fasting state and within the intestinal lumen during digestion (Javitt, 1982).

Removal of bile acids from sinusoidal blood is a concentrative, saturable, and carrier-mediated process (Palmer, 1982). It resembles in some ways the uptake and excretion of bilirubin, BSP, and ICG but differs in that the uptake of bile acids appears not to depend on the y and z carrier proteins. The highly efficient uptake of bile salts by the normal hepatocyte permits

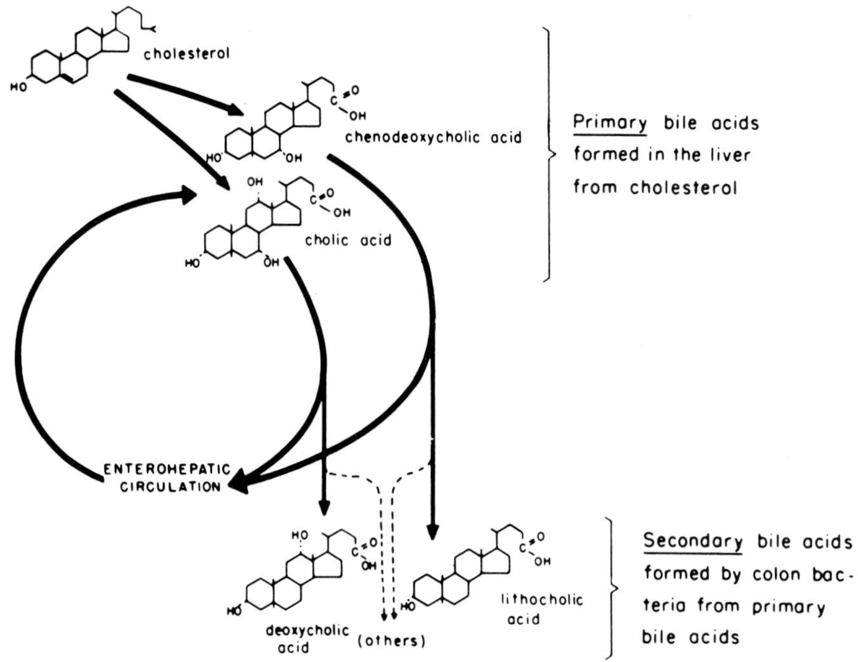

Figure 13–6. Schematic representation of relationship of cholesterol to primary and secondary bile acids and of enterohepatic circulation of bile acids. (From Javitt, 1982, with permission.)

this phenomenon to be utilized as a test of liver function. Indeed, hepatic bile salt uptake and peripheral bile salt concentration have turned out to be highly sensitive indicators of hepatocellular dysfunction. It is clear that decreased or altered hepatic blood flow, such as can occur in cirrhosis, also would lead to abnormalities of this function.

It has long been recognized that levels of bile acids are increased in the blood and urine of patients with obstructive (posthepatic) jaundice, as shown in the past by simple qualitative methods (Hay's and Pettenkofer's tests). The lack of satisfactory quantitation in the past and the demonstration that bile acids may also be found in the urine of patients with hepatocellular jaundice had prevented the clinical application of these procedures. Quantitative methods which have been applied recently, however, have yielded characteristic patterns in patients with hepatobiliary disease. Unfortunately, the methods for the measurement of total serum bile acid and of the individual bile acids thus far available have seemed too difficult and time-consuming or insufficiently reliable for regular clinical application. Nevertheless, rapid advances in the theory and technology of bile acid measurement suggest that assay of bile acid levels will become a routine clinical determination.

There have been four approaches to the utilization of bile acid levels for the diagnosis of hepatobiliary disease. Two of these have involved measurement of total bile acid levels, another has consisted of measuring removal from the blood of an infused bile acid, and the fourth has involved fractionation into the di- and trihydroxy acids.

Total Bile Acid Level. Measurements of total bile acid levels of the serum have been done in the fasting and postprandial states. Fasting levels are elevated in patients with acute and chronic hepatitis, alcoholic hepatitis, cirrhosis, posthepatic jaundice, and intrahepatic cholestasis. Indeed, as a measurement of acute and chronic hepatic disease, the total bile acid level has appeared to be almost as sensitive as the 45-minute BSP excretion test.

Thus far three types of methods have been employed. One has involved the enzymatic measurement employing 3-hydroxysteroid dehydrogenase. Another method has utilized gas liquid chromatography. The third has employed radioimmunoassay (RIA). Of the three, the one which will probably prove to be most suitable for routine application is RIA.

Postprandial Serum Bile Acid Levels. Measurement of serum bile acid concentrations two hours after a meal may be considered an endogenous loading test. The presence during the fasting state of the major portion of the bile acid pool in the gallbladder, the postprandial contraction of the gallbladder, and the efficient enterohepatic recirculation of bile acids provide a setting in which the postprandial bile acid level appears to be an extremely sensitive measure of hepatobiliary disease. Clinical testing suggests that the postprandial value is more sensitive than the fasting concentration. Sufficient clinical application to evaluate the usefulness of the procedure, however, remains to be conducted. Current assessment suggests that the test is most useful for the detection of hepatobiliary disease but not for differential diagnosis, since it yields equivalently abnormal values in a variety of conditions (Combes, 1982).

Bile Acid Tolerance Test. Exogenous bile acid

load tests have utilized infusion of unlabeled cholylglycine or of radiolabeled bile acids. The cholylglycine or other bile acid tolerance tests have involved measuring a fractional disappearance rate or a 10-minute "retention" value utilizing RIA for measurement of the cholylglycine levels. This has been reported to be a sensitive indicator of impaired hepatic function. Indeed, it has been alleged to be more sensitive than serum levels of bilirubin, aspartate aminotransferase (AST or GOT) or alkaline phosphatase, and more sensitive than the levels of cholylglycine. These clearance tests, however, have not been subjected to any significant clinical evaluation, and it remains to be seen whether clinical use will endorse their value.

Ratio of Serum Trihydroxy to Dihydroxy Bile Acids. Theoretically this ratio has much to recommend it. Synthesis of the trihydroxy bile acids requires adequate hepatic function. Patients with posthepatic jaundice or intrahepatic cholestasis are likely to have elevated serum total bile acid concentrations because of excretory blockade, and, because hepatic function is preserved, to have a high ratio of serum trihydroxy to dihydroxy bile acids. The patient with hepatocellular jaundice, however, who may be expected to have impaired hepatocellular function, will have a lesser proportion of bile acids in the trihydroxy form. Accordingly, the ratio may be of help in the differential diagnosis of jaundice. The technical difficulties involved in measuring bile acid levels, however, have precluded extensive efforts to apply this determination.

Accordingly, despite the promise of clinical value of measuring bile acid levels of endogenous and exogenous "tolerance" tests and of fractionating them, clinical application has been delayed. Problems of technology and the lack of a sufficient body of clinical data supporting the applicability preclude their being a part of routine batteries of liver function tests.

DETOXIFICATION AND DRUG METABOLISM

The liver has long been recognized to effect metabolic changes in foreign compounds. Viewed broadly, these changes consist of conversion of non-polar to polar compounds to permit their excretion. While enzymatic machinery for metabolic changes in xenobiotics can be found in extrahepatic tissues, the liver accounts for almost all of the biotransformation of foreign compounds.

The biotransformation consists of two phases. *Phase I* involves oxidation or other reactions that introduce a polar group into the molecule. *Phase II* consists of conjugation of the product of Phase I or the original compound, if it already has a polar group, with glucuronate, glycine, or other moieties. *Phase II* reactions have long been recognized and termed the *conjugating* or *detoxifying* function of the liver. It is the basis of an obsolete measure of hepatic function, the *hippuric acid excretion* test. Conjugation of bilirubin with glucuronide to form "direct" bilirubin and formation of conjugates of steroids and other endogenous substances are other examples of Phase II xenobiotic metabolism. During the past several years, hepatic function tests based on Phase I metabolism also have been introduced.

TESTS BASED ON DRUG METABOLISM

Experimental hepatic disease in animals impairs drug-metabolizing ability, and the degree of impairment reflects the severity of hepatic injury and parallels other measures of hepatic failure. Studies in humans utilizing a variety of indirect measures, including rate of clearance of drugs from the blood and appearance of metabolic products in the blood and urine, also have demonstrated adverse effects of hepatic disease on drug metabolism. These measurements, however, are too cumbersome for regular clinical use and pose problems of interpretation.

The recently introduced "breath analysis" test permits quantitative measurement of drug metabolism and appears to provide a useful type of hepatic function test. It consists of administration by mouth of a drug labeled with a trace dose of ^{14}C. Most extensively studied thus far has been aminopyrine labeled at the 2 N-methyl positions. The labeled methyl groups undergo demethylation, after which they are converted through formaldehyde and formate to CO_2. Accordingly, expired $^{14}CO_2$ becomes a measure of the metabolic conversion of the drug, and of the hepatic microsomal mass (Combes, 1982). Indeed, the studies of Hepner (1976) suggest the breath test of drug-metabolizing activity to be a simple and useful measure of hepatic function (Fig. 13–7). Further experience with this test using this and other drugs and correlating the results with other tests of hepatic function are required to appraise fully the clinical usefulness of this promising approach to hepatic function testing.

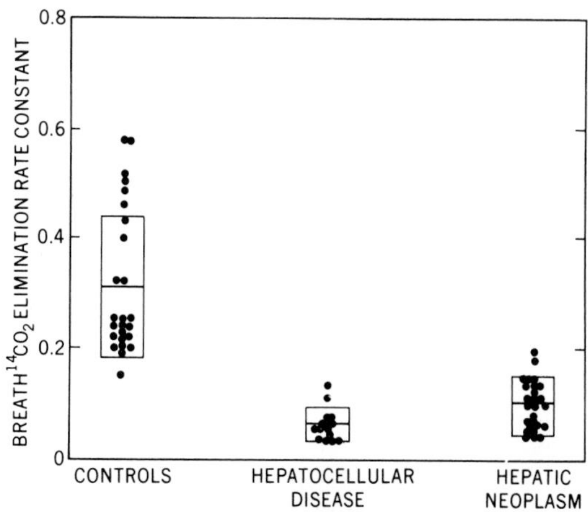

Figure 13–7. Rate of metabolism of ^{14}C-labeled aminopyrine in patients with hepatocellular disease and hepatic neoplasm compared with that of normals as reflected in elimination of $^{14}CO_2$. (From Hepner and Vesell, 1976, with permission.)

2

TESTS OF HEPATIC SYNTHETIC ABILITY

The liver is responsible for a variety of synthetic activities. Some (e.g., conjugations) have been discussed in the preceding section. Others, e.g., synthesis of serum proteins and urea, are discussed in Chapters 9 and 12. A synthetic activity useful for the testing of hepatic function and of clinical importance is the role of the liver in the manufacture of plasma coagulation factors. For testing of hepatic function, the *prothrombin time* and related assays described in Chapter 32 (p. 781) are used.

Prothrombin Time and Vitamin K Response

It has been known for a long time that patients with severe hepatic disease, as well as those with obstructive jaundice, may have coagulation defects. The pathogenesis of the clotting defect is complex and may include deficient or defective platelets, circulating anticoagulants, intravascular coagulation, and deficiency in plasma clotting factors. Demonstration of deficiency of plasma clotting factors, as reflected in the one-stage prothrombin time, has been a valuable tool for the diagnosis of liver disease.

Identification of vitamin K in 1940 and the demonstration that vitamin K deficiency leads to coagulation defects and to hypoprothrombinemia were promptly followed by the recognition that bleeding tendencies in obstructive jaundice could be repaired by the parenteral administration of vitamin K. Vitamin K is fat-soluble and requires bile salts for absorption. The hypoprothrombinemia of obstructive (posthepatic) jaundice, accordingly, was clearly attributable to the deficiency of vitamin K resulting from lack of its absorption. Hypoprothrombinemia, found in patients with parenchymal hepatic disease, however, was not restored to normal by parenteral administration of vitamin K and was recognized to reflect defective hepatic synthesis.

These observations led to the formulation of a test which has been used for the differential diagnosis of jaundice for several decades. The test employs the one-stage prothrombin time (PT). If it is abnormally prolonged, the effect of vitamin K administration can distinguish between deficiency of vitamin K or deficient hepatocyte synthetic ability as the cause of the abnormal PT. Administration of a standard dose of vitamin K to a patient with posthepatic jaundice usually restores a prolonged PT to normal, whereas it fails to do so in patients whose abnormal values are due to intrinsic hepatic diseases. The test is usually performed by measuring the PT, and, if it is prolonged, by administering 10 mg of vitamin K intramuscularly daily for one to three days. In a patient with deep jaundice, the restoration of an abnormal PT to normal by this regimen provides helpful evidence that the abnormality is due to malabsorption of vitamin K and that the jaundice is obstructive. Lack of normalization of a markedly prolonged PT strongly suggests that jaundice is hepatocellular in origin. Normalization characteristically occurs by 24 hours after the first dose but may take up to three days.

There are several pitfalls in the application of this procedure. Patients with obstructive jaundice may have only a mildly prolonged PT; the difference after administration of vitamin K, therefore, may be insufficient to provide a conclusive answer. Furthermore, in intrinsic hepatic disease which mimics posthepatic jaundice (intrahepatic cholestasis), parenchymal dysfunction may be relatively slight, and the response of the "hypoprothrombinemia" may be similar to that of posthepatic jaundice. Also, a patient with a cause for malabsorption other than posthepatic jaundice or one who had been taking an oral antibiotic that inhibits bacterial flora may have an abnormal PT response to vitamin K. Indeed, the PT and its response to vitamin K administration is a relatively anachronistic test for the distinction of posthepatic jaundice from that due to hepatic disease in an era of ultrasonographic and cholangiographic techniques for the precise differential diagnosis of jaundice. Nevertheless, a prolonged PT value, in a patient with presumed posthepatic jaundice, that is not normalized by vitamin K should cast doubt on the diagnosis.

The degree of prolongation of the PT in a patient with parenchymal hepatic disease is a useful measure of the severity of the hepatic injury. In patients with acute hepatitis, marked prolongation of the value is an ominous sign and may herald a fatal outcome. In cirrhosis it is also a reflection of severely impaired parenchymal function.

Originally the one-stage PT was considered to be a specific measurement of prothrombin (factor II). We now know that it depends on factors I (fibrinogen), II (prothrombin), V (proaccelerin), VII (proconvertin), and X (Stuart factor). All of these factors are synthesized in the liver and all but factors I and V require adequate amounts of vitamin K in the liver for their synthesis. Indeed, we now speak of the "prothrombin complex," referring to factors that affect the one-stage PT (Table 13–5).

Coagulation defects in patients with hepatic disease or with obstructive jaundice usually include deficiency of other factors as well as prothrombin (Table 13–5), and the prolonged one-stage PT reflects depression of multiple factors of the prothrombin complex (Chap. 32). Measurable deficiency of factor V, however, is

Table 13–5. CLOTTING ABNORMALITIES IN PATIENTS WITH LIVER DISEASE

Deficiency of plasma factors	
Prothrombin	Measured by one-stage prothrombin time
Factors VII	
X	
V	
Fibrinogen	
(XIIIa)	
Thrombocytopenia (as result of hypersplenism)	
Decreased platelet adhesiveness	
Disseminated intravascular coagulation (DIC)	
Fibrinolysins	

found only in association with severe liver disease. Deficiency of fibrinogen synthesis is a preterminal event and of little clinical significance. Indeed, measurement of individual plasma coagulation factors (Chap. 32), while useful in the management of hemorrhagic phenomena, has been applied to the diagnosis of hepatic disease to only a limited and experimental degree.

Excess fibrinolysis, either as a direct reflection of liver disease or more probably as the result of the disseminated intravascular coagulation syndrome (DIC), may be responsible for a hemorrhagic tendency in patients with terminal cirrhosis (Chap. 32). Thrombocytopenia secondary to hypersplenism and decreased platelet adhesiveness also contributes to hypocoagulability of the blood.

METABOLIC TESTS

A number of hepatic function tests have been based on the role of the liver in intermediary metabolism. Those tests related to carbohydrate metabolism have been least useful and those related to protein metabolism most useful. Only one commonly used test relates to lipid metabolism.

Carbohydrate Metabolism

Patients with hepatic disease may have hypoglycemia. They also may show diminished tolerance for administered glucose, galactose, fructose, or lactate. Their hepatic glycogen stores may be decreased as measured by plasma glucose response to administered epinephrine or glucagon.

Hypoglycemia occurs regularly in hepatectomized animals. It occurs in about 10 per cent of patients with acute hepatic necrosis. The incidence of hypoglycemia in other forms of hepatic disease, however, is low. It has been described in rare instances of biliary cirrhosis, in primary or metastatic carcinoma of the liver, and in the hepatic congestion of heart failure. Hypoglycemia is particularly characteristic of two peculiar forms of fatty livers, one associated with a febrile state in children referred to as *Reye's syndrome,* and the other, the rare *fatty liver of pregnancy.* The hypoglycemia that occurs in alcoholic patients results from acute direct and indirect metabolic effects of alcohol, not from the liver disease of alcoholism.

Glucose tolerance is characteristically abnormal in patients with cirrhosis of the liver. There is a rapid rise of plasma glucose to values above the upper reference limit and then a slow return to normal. This pattern in patients with liver disease can be distinguished from that of diabetes mellitus by the normal or low fasting plasma glucose in liver disease and the occurrence of subnormal values by the fifth hour after the glucose has been given. The oral or intravenous glucose tolerance test is of little value in diagnosis of hepatic disease.

The *galactose tolerance test* has been applied to the study of liver for many years. The normal liver is able to convert galactose to glucose, which is stored as glycogen. In patients with hepatic disease, this ability is defective. Administration of galactose results in persistence of abnormal blood levels for several hours and in urinary excretion of abnormal amounts of galactose. This test yields abnormal results in patients with hepatocellular jaundice but normal results in patients with obstructive jaundice of brief duration (less than three weeks). Although formerly recommended by some authors for the differential diagnosis of jaundice, this test was never widely employed and today is used in few centers in this country. It continues to be employed in some European centers as a measure of functioning liver mass (Ramsoe, 1980).

The *fructose tolerance test,* based on a principle similar to that of galactose tolerance, has found no clinical application. Elevated blood levels of lactic acid have been described in patients with severe liver disease. This observation and a *lactic acid tolerance test* have been described as tests of hepatic function but also have found no regular clinical application.

The *epinephrine tolerance test* was used many years ago to estimate hepatic glycogen stores by observing the plasma glucose response to a standard dose of epinephrine. Normal individuals would show a blood glucose rise of 40 to 60 mg/dl within one hour after the epinephrine has been given. Patients with hepatic disease (cirrhosis, hepatitis) and patients with genetic deficiency in glycogenolytic enzymes (glycogen storage disease) would show a subnormal response. The test has found little use in the diagnosis of liver disease but was employed in clinical research and for the diagnosis of glycogen storage disease. The *glucagon tolerance test,* a modification of this test, has involved the use of glucagon instead of or combined with epinephrine to produce glycogenolysis. Today the diagnosis of glycogen storage disease rests on measuring enzyme activity in liver tissue.

Recent extensive studies on hepatic uptake of circulating asialoglycoproteins in health and disease give promise that useful diagnostic methods may be based on the phenomena, but the available data are not sufficient to evaluate the possibility at this time (Ashwell, 1981).

Lipid Metabolism

The liver is importantly involved in many phases of lipid metabolism, including the synthesis, esterification, and excretion of cholesterol. Only the determination of serum-free and esterified *cholesterol* has been applied intensively to the study of hepatic disease. In normal individuals (in the United States) the serum cholesterol level ranges between 150 and 250 mg/dl,* approximately 70 per cent of which is esterified. Esterification of cholesterol is largely catalyzed by lecithin-cholesterol acyltransferase (LCAT), an enzyme found in the blood and liver.

In general, serum cholesterol is normal or depressed in hepatocellular jaundice and elevated in obstructive jaundice. In patients with hepatitis, the serum cholesterol may be mildly depressed or normal, but the level of esterified cholesterol is usually moderately decreased. In severe hepatitis or cirrhosis the serum cholesterol (total and esterified) levels may be markedly depressed. In patients with posthepatic jaundice or intrahepatic cholestasis, the serum cholesterol value is usually elevated as high as 500 mg/dl.† Even greater elevations occur occasionally, especially in chronic intrahepatic cholestasis, i.e., "primary biliary

*4.9–6.5 mmol/L.

†13 mmol/L.

cirrhosis," in which levels up to 1800 mg/dl* may be observed. It is generally stated that patients with obstructive jaundice usually have a normal (2/3) serum cholesterol-ester/total cholesterol ratio. Strictly speaking, this is not true. Although the degree of depression of the ratio is characteristically less than that seen in hepatic disease, moderate degrees are regularly seen. Determination of total serum cholesterol is widely used in the diagnosis of hepatic disease, but determination of the ester fraction is of little diagnostic value.

Abnormal values of other plasma lipids occur in patients with hepatic and biliary tract disease. Increased plasma levels of triglycerides are observed in patients with obstructive jaundice, in alcoholic patients with hemolytic anemia, hyperlipemia, and fatty liver (the Zieve syndrome), and in those with pancreatitis. Values of plasma non-esterified or free fatty acids are increased in patients with all forms of parenchymatous hepatic disease. Plasma concentrations of phospholipids are increased in obstructive jaundice and in biliary cirrhosis. While measurement of the several lipid fractions has been of investigative interest, it is too time-consuming and complex for routine clinical application.

Protein Metabolism

Amino acid metabolism, urea synthesis, and protein metabolism occur in the liver. Evidence of defects in each of these areas may be observed in patients with hepatic disease. These include abnormal plasma levels of amino acids, proteins, urea, and ammonia as well as abnormal urine (and cerebrospinal fluid) levels of amino acids. Several measurements of hepatic function and disease have been based on these phenomena.

Plasma Protein Values. A number of plasma proteins are formed in the liver. These include albumin, fibrinogen, and some of the alpha and beta globulins.

*47 mmol/L.

Accordingly, changes in the plasma (or serum) proteins form the basis for important laboratory aids to the diagnosis of hepatic disease. Changes in the plasma concentration of an individual protein, however, may be due to altered rate of synthesis or catabolism, to dilution by an expanded plasma volume, or to abnormal losses into the gut. Indeed, the expanded plasma volume associated with cirrhosis exaggerates the hypoalbuminemia owing to impaired synthesis. Nevertheless, the depressed serum albumin level which is characteristic of chronic hepatic disease is a valuable clinical tool. The *serum globulin* level is often elevated in patients with chronic hepatic disease (cirrhosis) and chronic hepatitis, representing mainly the immunoglobulins or gamma globulin fractions and reflecting largely immune responses.

The procedures which have been used to evaluate serum protein changes in patients with liver disease include determination of serum albumin and globulin levels, serum electrophoresis, and several turbidimetric ("flocculation") tests. The turbidimetric tests reflect largely changes of the gamma globulin and albumin levels. Immunochemical methods have been used to measure the various immunoglobulins.

The *serum albumin* level is an index of severity and prognosis in patients with chronic hepatic disease. In patients with cirrhosis there is a positive correlation between the degree of hypoalbuminemia and the severity of the ascites. Patients who show a rise of serum albumin have a more favorable prognosis than those whose levels remain low. In patients with acute hepatic disease (viral or toxic hepatitis), serum albumin levels are usually normal or only mildly depressed. Those who develop subacute hepatic necrosis ("subacute yellow atrophy") frequently have moderate to marked hypoalbuminemia.

The total serum globulin level is often elevated in patients with cirrhosis. The degree of elevation is usually moderate in alcoholic and in biliary cirrhosis, with levels of 3 to 5 g/100 ml. In active macronodular cirrhosis and in chronic active hepatitis (CAH), elevations also may be moderate but at times are marked, with values in the range of 4 to 9 g/dl occasionally

Table 13–6. ABNORMALITIES OF SERUM PROTEINS IN LIVER DISEASE*

	Acute Hepatitis	Cirrhosis (Laennec's)	CAH† with or without Cirrhosis	Cirrhosis (Biliary)	Obstructive Jaundice	Primary or Metastatic Carcinoma
Albumin	N or ↓	↓ ↓	↓ ↓	↓	N or ↓	↓
Globulin	N or ↑	↑	↑	↑	N	N
Alpha-1‡						↑
Alpha-2		N	N	↑	↑	↑ ↑
Beta	↑	↑	↑	↑ ↑ ↑	↑ ↑	N
Gamma§	↑ (IgG or IgM)¶	↑ ↑ (IgA or IgM)	↑ ↑ ↑ (IgG)	↑ (IgM)	N	N

*Direction and magnitude of change indicated by number of arrows.

†Chronic active hepatitis (CAH).

‡Alpha-1-antitrypsin low in one type of familial liver disease (see text). A majority of patients with primary hepatic carcinoma have the abnormal protein, alpha-fetoglobulin, in their serum (see text).

§Main type of immunoglobin (Ig) shown in parentheses.

¶Mainly IgG in virus B hepatitis; mainly IgM in virus A hepatitis.

Table 13–7. SOME FLOCCULATION TESTS INCLUDING SERUM PROTEIN ABNORMALITIES THAT THEY REFLECT*

Test	Precipitating Reagent	Protein Fractions Producing Abnormality	Albumin† Inhibition
Cephalin flocculation	Cephalin-cholesterol emulsion	γ	+
Thymol turbidity	Supersaturated solution thymol	γ (β)	(+)‡
Colloidal gold	Colloidal gold	γ	+
Zinc sulfate turbidity	$ZnSO_4$	γ	(+)
Takata-Ara	$HgCl_2$	γ (β)	+
Cadmium sulfate	$CdSO_4$	γ ($\alpha\beta$)	+

*Modified from Maclagan, N. F.: J. Clin. Path., 5:1, 1952. γ = gamma globulins; β = beta globulins; α = alpha globulins.

†Indicates that addition of albumin *in vitro* can convert a positive to a negative result.

‡(+) Indicates that addition of albumin is less effective in decreasing the degree of abnormal results.

2

observed. Very high levels of serum globulin are particularly likely to be seen in patients with the hepatitis B antigen (HbsAG)-negative, "autoimmune" type of chronic active hepatitis. Levels in patients with acute hepatitis are usually normal or only mildly elevated, uncommonly in excess of 4 g/100 ml. In patients with posthepatic jaundice the globulin level is usually normal, although it may be elevated.

The *total serum protein* level in patients with cirrhosis is occasionally low, often normal, and at times even elevated. Reversal of the albumin·globulin (A/G) ratio has been emphasized in this and in other hyperglobulinemic diseases. Reference to the A/G ratio, however, is needlessly awkward and imprecise. A low A/G ratio may occur because there is hyperglobulinemia or hypoalbuminemia or both. The term should be abandoned and the depression or elevation of the respective protein values described.

Serum protein electrophoresis (Chap. 12) is useful to demonstrate the globulin fraction which is elevated. In active macronodular cirrhosis and in chronic active hepatitis, hyperglobulinemia represents largely increases in the immunoglobulins of the gamma globulin fraction. In biliary cirrhosis the alpha-2 and beta fractions are prominently increased, and often the gamma fraction also shows an increase. In posthepatic jaundice, the gamma globulin level is usually normal but may be increased; the alpha-2 and beta fractions are increased. The patterns of abnormality of serum proteins in patients with hepatic disease are outlined in Table 13–6.

Application of quantitative immunochemical techniques (Chap. 39) has demonstrated characteristic changes in the gamma globulin fractions among the several forms of chronic liver disease. The increased gamma globulin level of chronic active hepatitis (CAH), cryptogenic cirrhosis, and "subacute" viral hepatitis consists mainly of the immunoglobulin gamma (IgG) proteins and includes only minor elevations of other immunoglobulins (Ig). In alcoholic cirrhosis, IgA and to a lesser extent IgM and IgG proteins are increased. In primary biliary cirrhosis (PBC), the elevated gamma globulin value consists mainly of IgM accompanied by minor elevations of IgG and IgA proteins. While the patterns of abnormality are suggestive rather than diagnostic, they can be clinically useful. Thus, an elevated gamma globulin level which consists mainly of IgM protein would favor the diagnosis of primary biliary cirrhosis (PBC) in a difficult-to-distinguish clinical setting.

Special Protein Tests

Flocculation Tests. A large number of tests which reflect abnormality of plasma proteins have been developed. These reactions, which have been called the "flocculation tests," "globulin reactions," or tests of the "serum colloidal stability," have been useful to the clinician. In Table 13–7 are listed a few of these procedures with an indication of the presumed related protein abnormalities.

These tests have in common the tendency to be abnormal in patients with intrinsic hepatic disease (hepatitis, cirrhosis) and to be normal in patients with obstructive jaundice. Indeed, serum from patients with obstructive jaundice has the property of inhibiting the flocculation or turbidity tests when mixed with serum that gives a positive reaction. The responsible factor for this inhibition may be a phospholipid. In patients with various systemic diseases characterized by hyperglobulinemia (Table 13–8), the flocculation tests also may yield abnormal results. The various tests differ in the relative incidence of abnormality in various diseases.

Table 13–8. CLASSIFICATION OF DISEASES ASSOCIATED WITH HYPERGLOBULINEMIA

I. Infections (especially chronic)
  A. Bacterial (subacute bacterial endocarditis, chronic suppurative infections, granulomatous infections)
  B. Spirochetal (syphilis)
  C. Viral (lymphogranuloma venereum, psittacosis)
  D. Fungal (histoplasmosis, coccidioidomycosis)
  E. Protozoal (leishmaniasis, malaria)
  F. Helminthic
II. Liver disease (cirrhosis, chronic hepatitis)
III. Collagen disease (rheumatoid arthritis, lupus erythematosis, polyarteritis nodosa, scleroderma)
IV. Neoplastic (multiple myeloma, macroglobulinemia, lymphomas, and leukemia, but rarely in carcinoma except for bronchogenic carcinoma)
V. Miscellaneous (sarcoidosis)

Today the flocculation tests are generally regarded as too non-specific for clinical application, and they have been abandoned in most centers. Nevertheless, they are interesting reflections of changes in serum protein fractions which are not completely exposed by electrophoretic techniques. Their physiologic interest and their continued use in some clinics warrant this brief description.

Turbidimetric Estimation of Gamma Globulin Levels. There are several turbidimetric procedures in which the turbidity produced correlates quantitatively with the gamma globulin concentration of the serum. Some of these tests depend on the tendency for gamma globulin to be precipitated by low concentrations of metallic or other ions in solutions of low total ionic strength or by high concentrations of salts. One of these, the zinc sulfate turbidity test (Kunkel test), has been applied to the distinction of hepatocellular from obstructive jaundice and in following the levels of gamma globulin in cirrhosis and other hyperglobulinemic diseases. Most laboratories today, however, choose to measure gamma globulin electrophoretically.

Serum Haptoglobin. This protein migrates with the alpha-2 globulins. Serum haptoglobin is elevated in patients with posthepatic jaundice and depressed in those with hepatocellular disease. Measurement of serum haptoglobin level has seen little clinical testing.

Lipoprotein-x (L_p-x). This abnormal lipoprotein is found in the serum of patients with cholestatic jaundice, whether owing to hepatic disease or to obstruction of the biliary tree. It is also found in patients with deficiency of the enzyme lecithin-cholesterol acyltransferase (LCAT). While presence of L_P-x in the serum is a sensitive measure of cholestasis (in the absence of LCAT deficiency), it is of no aid in distinguishing intrahepatic cholestasis from posthepatic jaundice (see Chap. 11).

Alpha-fetoprotein (AFP). This alpha-globulin is present in appreciable amounts in the serum of the fetus, infant, and normal pregnant female. The serum of normal adults and children beyond the age of one year contains less than 30 ng/ml, an amount that is detectable only by radioimmunoassay. High values in amounts detectable by the relatively insensitive technique of Ouchterlony gel diffusion (>1000 ng/ml) are almost diagnostic of hepatocellular carcinoma in adults. In children, such high values may reflect teratoblastomas of the testes and ovary. A small proportion of patients with carcinoma of the pancreas, stomach, colon, and lung have also been reported to show elevated serum AFP, but usually below 500 ng/ml.

Hepatocellular carcinoma is the entity which, among adults, is most characteristically associated with increased levels of AFP. Studies using radioimmunoassay have demonstrated increased levels in over 70 per cent of patients with this tumor, and values in excess of 3000 ng/ml in many of those with elevated levels. Even higher values are found in patients from parts of Asia, Africa, and the Mediterranean littoral who have hepatocellular carcinoma.

Measurement of alpha-fetoprotein (AFP), of course, is not a test of hepatic function or even of hepatic injury *per se*. It is a useful clue in adults to the presence of hepatocellular carcinoma. If the relatively insensitive method of gel diffusion yields a positive result, indicating a probable value above 1000 ng/ml, the likelihood of hepatocellular carcinoma is increased, and a value above 3000 ng/ml as demonstrated by radioimmunoassay is virtually diagnostic. A very low value or absence of AFP from the serum does not exclude the diagnosis of hepatocellular carcinoma, since 30 to 50 per cent of patients may lack the abnormal protein.

Levels of AFP may also serve to monitor the course of hepatic carcinoma in response to treatment. Surgical removal can lead to a dramatic fall from a high value, as may effective chemotherapy.

Non-neoplastic hepatocellular disease can lead to modestly elevated serum AFP levels, almost always below 500 ng/ml (e.g., chronic active hepatitis; alcoholic cirrhosis, especially after a period of abstention; and the early convalescent phase of severe acute hepatitis). Indeed, some of the data from patients with non-neoplastic hepatic disease are consistent with the concept that elevated serum AFP levels reflect regenerative activity of hepatocytes. The impression that presence of elevated levels in patients with fulminant hepatic failure augurs a favorable prognosis, however, has not been confirmed.

Alpha-1-antitrypsin. A recently discovered genetic disease is characterized by a markedly depressed plasma level of alpha-1-antitrypsin, apparently the result of defective assembly of the molecule. The abnormal protein formed, which lacks the sialo groups present in the normal alpha-1-antitrypsin, is not released to the blood from its site of synthesis, the hepatocyte. The accumulated protein can be seen in periportal hepatocytes as diastase-resistant, periodic acid–Schiff positive inclusion bodies. Indeed, their presence provides the histologic hallmark of alpha-1-antitrypsin deficiency.

The manifestations of the condition include liver disease of infancy, childhood, or even maturity, and in some of the involved adults precocious pulmonary emphysema. Deficiency of alpha-1-antitrypsin is reflected in a low or absent alpha-1-globulin peak on a serum protein electrophoretogram (Chap. 12, p. 210).

Measurement of the serum concentration of alpha-1-antitrypsin cannot be considered a test for liver disease, in the ordinary sense. It is a test useful in identifying liver disease in an infant with unexplained cholestasis or in a patient of any age with chronic liver disease of unknown cause. Even more useful for diagnosis is demonstration of the "antitrypsin bodies" in the periportal hepatocytes.

If a low serum concentration of alpha-1-antitrypsin is found, it is desirable to determine the patient's phenotype with respect to the molecular form of the alpha-1-antitrypsin, protease inhibitor (Pi) phenotype (Sharp, 1978). The molecular forms of alpha-1-antitrypsin revealed by special electrophoretic techniques have been designated F (fast), M (medium), S (slow), and Z (ultra-slow) according to their relative electrophoretic mobilities. The patterns specific for particular Pi phenotypes are designated by two of these letters. Most normal people are of the Pi phenotype MM. Patients with hepatic lesions owing to alpha-1-antitrypsin deficiency usually have the rare Pi phenotype ZZ, although subjects with other rare Pi phenotypes (MZ, FZ, and SZ) may have hepatic lesions which are similar to those associated with the Pi ZZ phenotype.

Serum alpha-1-antitrypsin is usually normal or somewhat increased in other forms of liver disease. Indeed, a well-maintained or increased value in fulminant liver failure has been interpreted as a clue to hepatic regenerative activity and, hence, possibly a favorable prognosis.

Ceruloplasmin. Ceruloplasmin is the copper-containing protein in plasma. It also has enzymatic (oxidase) activity. The latter property is utilized in one of the standard methods of measuring the concentration of this protein. Its main function is presumed to be transport of copper (Chap. 12). A low serum concentration of ceruloplasmin (less than 0.2 g/L) occurs in about 95 per cent of patients who are homozygous and in about 10 per cent of subjects who are heterozygous for Wilson's disease (Scheinberg, 1973). Low serum concentrations of ceruloplasmin in these individuals presumably reflect a selective defect in the synthesis of this protein in the liver cell.

Other forms of liver disease (viral hepatitis, cirrhosis) can lead to increased serum levels of ceruloplasmin. As a similar phenomenon, the level may become normal in Wilson's disease once liver damage is advanced. Accordingly, a normal value for this protein in the presence of overt liver disease does not exclude the diagnosis of Wilson's disease. A low value, of course, offers strong support for the diagnosis.

Tests Related to Disordered Nitrogen Metabolism

Aminoaciduria. It has been known for a long time that patients with acute hepatic necrosis ("acute yellow atrophy") have leucine and tyrosine crystals in the urine. These amino acids represent, at least in part, products of autolyzed hepatic tissue. Other amino acids are found in the urine of patients with severe cirrhosis or hepatitis (toxic or viral). This aminoaciduria reflects the elevated levels of blood amino acids that result from impaired amino acid metabolism by the liver as well as from the release from necrotic tissue.

These observations may be applied to the study of hepatic disease. Demonstration of aminoaciduria by paper chromatography is preferable to and more reliable than the laborious search for characteristic tyrosine and leucine crystals. Amino acid content of the blood and urine, however, has found less routine than research application. Tests of hepatic function that have been based on the impaired ability of the damaged liver to metabolize amino acids include the *tyrosine tolerance,* the *methionine tolerance,* the *glycine tolerance,* and the *protein hydrolysate tolerance* tests. Each of these procedures may reveal a defect in the disappearance of administered amino acids from the blood of patients with hepatic disease, but they have not been applied to the study of clinical problems.

Blood Ammonia Determination. A relationship between elevated levels of blood ammonia and liver disease has been recognized for the past 30 years and suspected for over 60 years. It is uncertain whether ammonia, as measured in the blood, represents this substance as such or is ammonia released from some bound state by chemical manipulation.* At any rate, the amount of ammonia released from blood or plasma by treatment with alkali has been shown to be related to the severity of the liver disease.

A variety of methods are available for ammonia determination. A simple and widely used method is that of Seligson (1951), which uses whole blood. By that method, as modified by Bessman (1959), the normal levels are under 100 μg/dl† of whole blood. An adaptation of the glutamate dehydrogenase enzymatic method of van Anken (1974) employing ACA (Dupont Automatic Clinical Analyzer, Dupont Instruments, Wilmington, Del.) has been satisfactory and efficient.

Studies have shown conclusively that the major source of blood ammonia is the gastrointestinal tract, although a minor contribution is made by the kidney. Bacteria, particularly those in the area of the cecum, release ammonia from nitrogen-containing foods. This ammonia, as well as ammonia ingested as ammonium salts or released from urea by bacterial or other urease, is absorbed into the portal vein. The liver normally removes most of the ammonia from the portal vein blood, converting it to urea. Little ammonia normally escapes from the liver into the hepatic vein to be carried to the systemic circulation.

Elevated blood ammonia levels in patients with hepatic disease appear to depend on two mechanisms, "shunting" of portal blood past the liver and impaired parenchymal function (Fig. 13–8). In patients with cirrhosis and extensive collateral portal circulation, elevation of the ammonia levels has been ascribed largely to the shunting of portal blood past the liver. Hepatic vein catheterization studies have shown that patients with severe hepatitis or cirrhosis remove less than normal amounts of ammonia from the portal blood, perhaps as a manifestation of defective urea synthesis.

Elevated ammonia levels are seen in impending or fully developed hepatic coma, owing to cirrhosis or severe hepatitis, and occasionally in severe heart failure, azotemia, cor pulmonale, and erythroblastosis fetalis. They have also been described in animals and humans with Eck fistulas and in animals in shock. Recent focus on biochemical factors in hepatic encephalopathy has drawn attention to elevated blood levels of short chain fatty acids, sulfhydryl compounds, "false neurotransmitters," and gamma-aminobutyric acid. The levels of none of these, however, appear to offer the diagnostic help provided by blood ammonia levels in the recognition of hepatic encephalopathy.

Indeed, the use of the blood ammonia determina-

---

*Almost all the blood "ammonia" is present as NH_4^+ ion rather than NH_3 at the pH of normal blood. Alkalosis increases the levels of free NH_3 by its effect on the equilibrium

$$NH_4^+ \leftrightarrows NH_3 + H^+$$

This has a bearing on the effect of alkalosis on the neurotoxicity of hyperammonemia, since free NH_3 crosses cell membranes more readily than does NH_4^+ ion.

†55μmol/L.

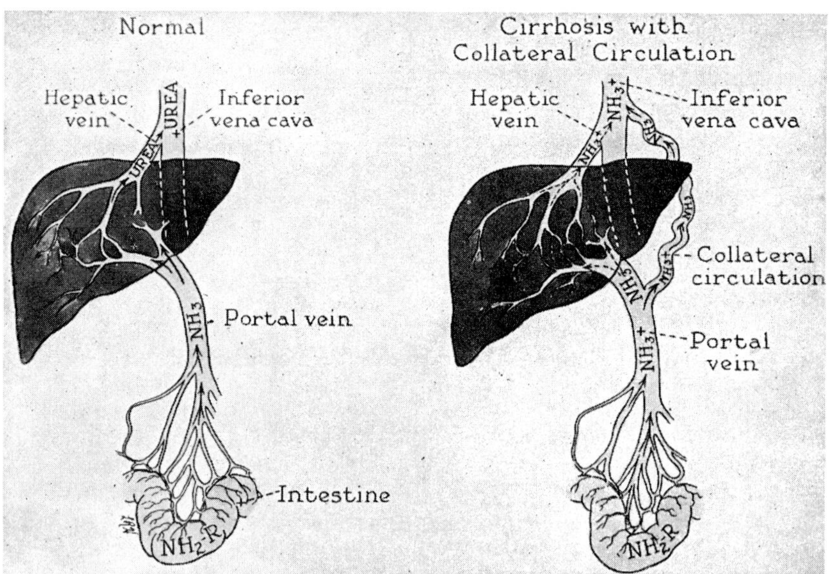

Figure 13–8. Pictorial representation of intestinal formation of ammonia in normal and cirrhotic individuals and of the role of the normal liver in removing ammonia brought to it by the portal blood. Figure also shows the production of elevated plasma ammonia levels by "shunting" of blood through the collateral circulation or by impaired hepatic parenchymal function.

tion has been of assistance in the recognition of impending or established hepatic coma (Chap. 9). Blood ammonia determination may be useful for monitoring the efficacy of treatment of hepatic coma. In Reye's syndrome the level of ammonia appears to relate directly to level of consciousness and survival (Glasgow, 1972). An additional application has been suggested. In patients with cirrhosis and hemorrhage from esophageal varices or from any other source in the esophagus, stomach, or small intestine, blood ammonia levels are elevated, whereas in non-cirrhotic patients with gastrointestinal bleeding the ammonia levels are usually normal. Measuring the plasma ammonia level after a standard dose of an ammonium salt has been recommended as an aid in estimating the patency of a portacaval shunt.

Cerebrospinal Fluid Glutamine. A number of authors have shown that the level of cerebrospinal fluid (CSF) glutamine also correlates well with the degree of hepatic encephalopathy (Chap. 19). Glutamine is synthesized in brain tissue from ammonia and glutamic acid. As more and more glutamic acid is diverted toward the synthesis of glutamine, intermediates of oxidative metabolism such as α-ketoglutaric acid are depleted. Depletion of these intermediary metabolites of cerebral metabolism was at one time thought to be one of the etiologic factors in hepatic encephalopathy. The upper reference limit for CSF glutamine is 20 mg/dl (1.5 mmol/L). Glutamine levels can be measured by a simple method involving hot acid hydrolysis which releases ammonia, in turn measured by a colorimetric reaction (Hourani, 1971). This measurement has seen little clinical use.

*Serum Enzyme Values**

A large number of enzymes are found in normal serum or plasma, to which they gain access from the tissues. The characteristically abnormal serum enzyme levels produced by various diseases and the general aspects of serum enzymology are considered in Chapter 14. The following discussion describes the type of change in serum enzyme levels caused by hepatic disease and deals with the clinical usefulness of a few enzyme assays for the diagnosis of disease of the liver and biliary tree.

Serum enzymes can be arranged into four categories according to the changes in their levels produced by posthepatic jaundice and acute hepatitis (Table 13–9). *Group I* includes enzymes whose levels are higher in obstructive jaundice than they are in acute hepatitis. The prototype of this group is alkaline phosphatase (ALP). This category also includes leucine aminopeptidase (LAP), 5′-nucleotidase (5′-N), and gamma glutamyl transpeptidase (GGT). *Group II* includes enzymes whose levels are much higher in acute hepatitis than in obstructive jaundice. The best known members of this group are the aspartate aminotransferase (AST)† and the alanine aminotransferase (ALT).‡ Ornithine carbamoyl transferase (OCT), isocitric dehydrogenase (ICD), aldolase (Ald), iditol (sorbitol) dehydrogenase (IdD), and a number of other

*References relevant to this section will be found at the end of Chapter 14.

†Also refered to as glutamate oxaloacetic transaminase (GOT).

‡Also referred to as glutamate pyruvic transaminase (GPT).

Table 13–9. CATEGORIES OF SERUM ENZYMES* ACCORDING TO THEIR BEHAVIOR IN HEPATITIS AND OBSTRUCTIVE JAUNDICE

Characteristics	Prototype	Other Enzymes in Group
I Higher in obstructive jaundice than in hepatitis	ALP	LAP, 5′-N,GGT
II Higher in hepatitis than in obstructive jaundice	AST (GOT), ALT (GPT)	OCT, ICD, IdD, Ald
III Normal or only slightly elevated in hepatitis and obstructive jaundice	LD, CPK	Lipase Lecithinase Amylase
IV Depressed in hepatitis and normal in obstructive jaundice	Cholinesterase	LCAT

*See Table 14–1, pp. 252–253, for meaning of abbreviations.

enzymes are also in this category. In *Group III* are enzymes whose levels are elevated only slightly or not at all in hepatitis and in posthepatic jaundice. This group includes lactate dehydrogenase (LD), creatine phosphokinase (CPK), lipase, lecithinase, and a number of other enzymes. A fourth main type of serum enzyme response to hepatic disease *(Group IV)* is seen with cholinesterase, the levels of which are *decreased* in acute hepatitis and normal or only slightly decreased in obstructive jaundice.

The selection of serum enzyme assays for the diagnosis of hepatic and biliary disease has been based on sufficient experience in correlating the serum values with other measures of hepatic function and disease to assure adequate sensitivity and specificity, and on the technical ease of performing the procedure. These considerations have led to the widespread adoption of alkaline phosphatase, aspartate aminotransferase (AST or GOT), and alanine aminotransferase (ALT or GPT) for the diagnosis of hepatic and related disease. These virtually routine hepatic tests and a few related enzyme tests are discussed in the following pages. The levels of other serum enzymes in hepatic and other types of diseases are considered in Chapter 14.

ALKALINE PHOSPHATASE (ALP)

Alkaline phosphatase (ALP) (EC 3.1.3.1), formally designated orthophosphoric monoester phosphohydrolase, was the first serum enzyme to be studied in hepatic disease. It has been extensively applied to the differential diagnosis of jaundice. Early interest in this enzyme focused on the elevated levels seen in patients with osteoblastic bone disease, presumably as a reflection of increased activity of the osteoblasts, which are rich in phosphatase. This was soon followed, however, by the observation that values were also increased in patients with obstructive (posthepatic) jaundice. When the obstruction is complete, the serum enzyme activity is almost always increased to levels that are three to eight times the upper reference limit. Lower values, however, may be observed in obstructive jaundice, especially when the obstruction is incomplete. Biliary obstruction resulting from carcinoma produces higher values than those observed in patients with gallstones producing obstruction. One variety of posthepatic jaundice with normal ALP levels in the serum is that seen in infants with congenital atresia of the extrahepatic biliary tree. In these patients the serum ALP activity may not be elevated unless bony lesions of hepatic rickets develop. In contrast, infants with intrahepatic biliary atresia show striking elevations of serum ALP activity (Table 13–10).

Elevated levels of serum ALP also occur in hepatocellular jaundice. Approximately 90 per cent of patients with viral hepatitis or with toxic hepatocellular jaundice have elevated values. Almost all these have values that are elevated less than three-fold and often less than two-fold. Approximately 5 per cent of

Table 13–10. ALKALINE PHOSPHATASE VALUES (ALP) IN HEPATOBILIARY DISEASE

Disease	Incidence ALP Elevation	Usual Range of Values*
Jaundiced states		
Hepatic jaundice		
Hepatocellular	80–100%	1–3 ×
Hepatocanalicular	100%	3–8 ×
Posthepatic		
Obstruction due to neoplasm	95–100%	3–8 ×
Obstruction due to gallstone	95–100%	1–8 ×
Congenital atresia of bile ducts		
Intrahepatic	100%	10–15 ×
Extrahepatic	20– 30%	1–4 ×
Jaundice absent or present		
Infectious mononucleosis	60– 70%	1–8 ×
Cirrhosis, Laennec's	40%	1–3 ×
Cirrhosis, postnecrotic	50%	1–5 ×
Cirrhosis, biliary, primary	100%	3–20 ×
No jaundice		
Space-occupying lesions		
Carcinoma	80%	1–10 ×
Tuberculosis	50%	1–10 ×
Sarcoidosis	40%	1–10 ×
Amyloidosis	Frequent	1–10 ×
Stone in common duct or one hepatic duct	Frequent	1–10 ×

*Degree of increase over normal (upper reference limit).

patients with hepatocellular jaundice, however, have values that are increased more than three-fold. Nevertheless, values in this range should lead to the suspicion that the jaundice may be posthepatic. In jaundiced patients with higher levels, posthepatic jaundice should be considered.

Some forms of hepatic disease may present a laboratory and clinical picture simulating that of posthepatic jaundice. This has been called "intrahepatic cholestasis" or *cholestatic jaundice* (Table 13–3). Although it has been considered to be a form of viral hepatitis ("cholangiolitic hepatitis"), more often it is a manifestation of drug-induced hepatic injury or is cryptogenic. Indeed, a large number of conditions that can lead to cholestatic jaundice have been recognized (Zimmerman, 1979). Patients with intrahepatic cholestasis may have values of ALP at least as high as those observed in patients with posthepatic jaundice.

The serum ALP activity is of value in the differentiation of hepatocellular from posthepatic jaundice, but there are several caveats. As stated previously, ALP activity in the "obstructive" jaundice range may occur in intrinsic hepatic disease, and levels in the "hepatocellular" range may be seen in patients with incomplete biliary obstruction. When taken with other measurements of liver disease and clinical features, however, the ALP level is a useful diagnostic aid.

Serum ALP elevation may also occur in non-jaundiced patients with hepatobiliary disease. In patients with "space-occupying" lesions of the liver, such as granulomatous disease, metastatic or primary carcinoma of the liver, liver abscess, and amyloidosis, the degree of alkaline phosphatase elevation may at times be striking (up to 20-fold), with little or no rise in the serum bilirubin values. This pattern of hepatic dysfunction is useful in the recognition of these lesions, particularly of metastases to the liver in patients with carcinomatosis (Table 13–10).

There is another type of disease associated with normal or only slightly elevated serum bilirubin levels but with distinctly increased alkaline phosphatase levels. This is occlusion of one hepatic duct or incomplete occlusion of the common bile or hepatic duct. This condition should be kept in mind, particularly in dealing with patients with cholelithiasis who develop this "dissociated" pattern of hepatic dysfunction. Osteoblastic bone disease is also an important cause of elevated ALP levels without evidence of liver disease.

Levels of ALP in micronodular cirrhosis are usually normal or only mildly elevated. In macronodular cirrhosis the levels are generally somewhat higher. In primary biliary cirrhosis elevated levels of ALP are regularly seen. They range from three- to 20-fold the normal or upper reference limit. In obstructive biliary cirrhosis, the elevations are modest, usually elevated less than three- or four-fold, except during bouts of ascending cholangitis.

Most patients with hepatic steatosis have only slightly elevated levels. The occasional instances of deep jaundice in alcoholics with fatty liver accompanied by high ALP levels are probably due to common bile duct obstruction due to concomitant alcoholic pancreatitis or to intrahepatic cholestasis caused by severe steatosis. In alcoholic hepatitis, usual values for ALP are also less than three-fold elevated (Zimmerman, 1970).

The basis for elevated serum levels of ALP in patients with hepatobiliary disease is obscure. Impaired hepatic excretion of enzyme formed in bone or liver or both was formerly considered to be the mechanism. *Increased formation* of the enzyme by hepatic parenchymal or ductal cells, perhaps supplemented by impaired disposition, is the apparent mechanism.

ALP is found in many tissues. In a number of these tissues the molecular form of the enzyme is distinctive. Recognition that hepatobiliary rather than osseous disease is responsible for an elevated ALP level is relatively simple in the patient with jaundice or other overt clinical or laboratory evidence of hepatic or biliary tree disease. In patients whose clinical and biochemical data provide inconclusive evidence for liver disease as the cause of the hyperphosphatasemia, or who show evidence of both hepatic and osseous disease, elucidation of the cause of the elevated ALP level may be difficult. Distinction of ALP isoenzymes by electrophoresis or by the effects of chemical or physical factors on the ALP activity has found selected, if not limited, clinical application. Indeed, of the four isoenzymes of ALP that appear in the serum, the hepatic and osseous are the most difficult to distinguish from each other (see Chap. 14, Table 14–7). Several other serum enzymes, however, are helpful in identifying the source of an elevated ALP level to be hepatic or biliary tree disease (see Table 14–8). Serum values of leucine aminopeptidase (LAP), 5′-nucleotidase (5′-N), and gamma glutamyl transferase (GGT)* appear to parallel those of ALP in hepatobiliary disease and have been considered to approximate the degree of elevation of the hepatic isoenzyme of ALP.

AMINOTRANSFERASES (TRANSAMINASES)†

Enzymes that catalyze the reversible transfer of an alpha amino group from an amino acid to an alpha keto acid (Fig. 13–9) were first demonstrated in animal tissue by Braunshtein in 1937. He called the enzymes *aminopherases*. Although a large number of substrate-specific transaminases have been demonstrated in various animal tissues, only two have been described in the serum: *aspartate aminotransferase* (AST; *glutamate oxaloacetic transaminase* [GOT]) and *alanine aminotransferase* (ALT; *glutamate pyruvate transaminase* [GPT]). Abnormal levels of AST (GOT) are seen in patients with hepatic disease, myocardial and skeletal muscle necrosis, and other diseases to be described. ALT (GPT) elevations are absent or slight in disease that does not involve the liver.

---

*Gamma glutamyl transpeptidase.

†See Chapter 14 for further discussion of transaminases and other enzymes.

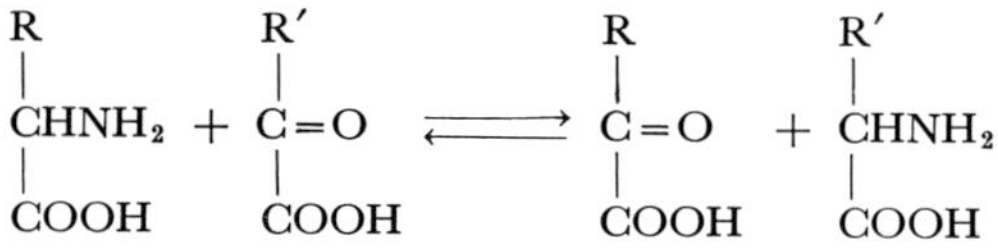

$$\begin{array}{c} R \\ | \\ CHNH_2 \\ | \\ COOH \end{array} + \begin{array}{c} R' \\ | \\ C{=}O \\ | \\ COOH \end{array} \rightleftharpoons \begin{array}{c} R \\ | \\ C{=}O \\ | \\ COOH \end{array} + \begin{array}{c} R' \\ | \\ CHNH_2 \\ | \\ COOH \end{array}$$

Figure 13–9. Prototype of aminotransferase (transamination) reactions.

Aspartate aminotransferase (AST; *glutamate oxaloacetic transaminase* [GOT]) (2.6.1.1) catalyzes the reversible transfer of the amino group from aspartate to α-ketoglutarate (Fig. 13–10). It has been demonstrated in the serum and tissues of all animals studied. In man it is found in cardiac, hepatic, skeletal muscle, renal, and cerebral tissue in decreasing concentrations. The recognition of the high myocardial content of this enzyme led to the observation, in 1953, that patients with acute myocardial infarction had elevated levels in the serum for a few days after the infarction. Shortly thereafter, studies in several laboratories showed high serum levels of this enzyme in patients and animals with acute hepatic necrosis.

The activity of this serum enzyme was first demonstrated by a chromatographic technique, which was too laborious for routine use. The methods that have been used for routine determination have included the spectrophotometric procedure of Karmen (1955) and several simplified colorimetric and fluorometric procedures (Fig. 13–10 and Chap. 14). Many laboratories continue to express the value in "Karmen units." The normal range is 6 to 40 units/ml of serum, but this is temperature-dependent. Conversion of these units to International units may be accomplished by dividing the value by a factor (1.95). Indeed, use of International units (I.U. or U/L) is desirable. For simplicity, the correction factor of 2 can be used with introduction of negligible error, i.e., 5–30 U/L at 30°C.

The range of values of AST (GOT) in patients with various types of hepatic disease and in myocardial infarction is shown in Figure 13–11. Striking elevations (10- to 200-fold increased) are observed in the serum of patients with acute hepatic necrosis (viral hepatitis, carbon tetrachloride poisoning, drug-induced injury). Patients with posthepatic jaundice and intrahepatic cholestasis have more modest elevations (usually less than 10-fold increased). In patients with cirrhosis of the liver there is a 60 to 70 per cent incidence of elevated AST levels (also below 10-fold increased).

Alcoholic liver disease leads to very modestly ele-

ASPARTATE AMINOTRANSFERASE (AST) OR GLUTAMATE OXALOACETATE TRANSAMINASE (GOT)

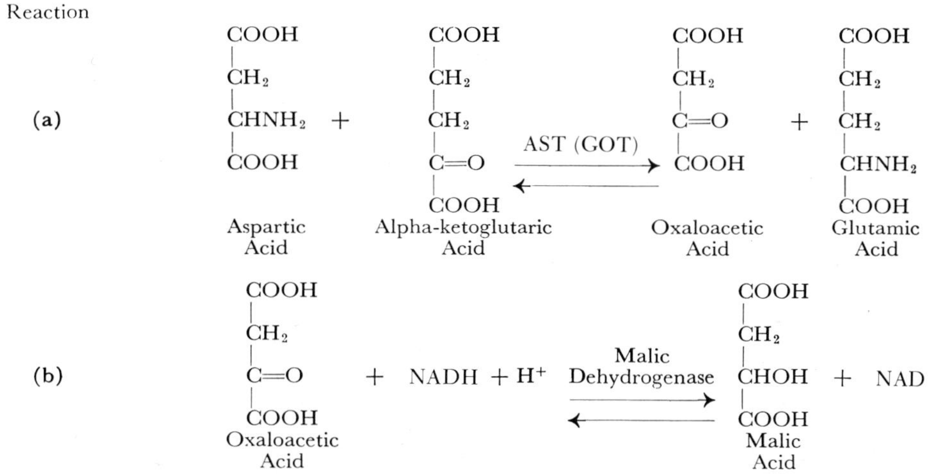

Reaction

(a)

$$\underset{\text{Aspartic Acid}}{\begin{array}{c} COOH \\ | \\ CH_2 \\ | \\ CHNH_2 \\ | \\ COOH \end{array}} + \underset{\text{Alpha-ketoglutaric Acid}}{\begin{array}{c} COOH \\ | \\ CH_2 \\ | \\ CH_2 \\ | \\ C{=}O \\ | \\ COOH \end{array}} \xrightleftharpoons{\text{AST (GOT)}} \underset{\text{Oxaloacetic Acid}}{\begin{array}{c} COOH \\ | \\ CH_2 \\ | \\ C{=}O \\ | \\ COOH \end{array}} + \underset{\text{Glutamic Acid}}{\begin{array}{c} COOH \\ | \\ CH_2 \\ | \\ CH_2 \\ | \\ CHNH_2 \\ | \\ COOH \end{array}}$$

(b)

$$\underset{\text{Oxaloacetic Acid}}{\begin{array}{c} COOH \\ | \\ CH_2 \\ | \\ C{=}O \\ | \\ COOH \end{array}} + NADH + H^+ \xrightleftharpoons{\text{Malic Dehydrogenase}} \underset{\text{Malic Acid}}{\begin{array}{c} COOH \\ | \\ CH_2 \\ | \\ CHOH \\ | \\ COOH \end{array}} + NAD$$

Figure 13–10. Reaction catalyzed by AST (GOT) principles of assay methods, and conditions in which increased serum levels are observed.

Method of assay is based on measurement of rate of formation of product (oxaloacetic acid) of the reaction. This may be done (1) indirectly, by the coupled reaction (b) in which the rate of NADH oxidation, in the presence of added malic dehydrogenase, is a measure of oxaloacetic acid formed (method of Karmen), or (2) directly, by one of several colorimetric methods that depend on the formation of dinitrophenylhydrazone of oxaloacetate or its decarboxylation product (pyruvate) or other colorimetric reactions.

Conditions in which abnormal serum levels of enzyme are observed include the following:

A. *Hepatic Disease*
- Hepatic necrosis
  - Hepatitis (infectious, toxic), infectious mononucleosis
  - Cirrhosis
  - Hematogenous tuberculosis
  - Hepatic congestion
- Metastatic carcinoma
- Obstructive jaundice

B. *Other Disease*
- Myocardial infarction
- Skeletal muscle necrosis
- Hemolysis (slight)
- Pancreatitis (acute)
- Renal necrosis
- Cerebral necrosis

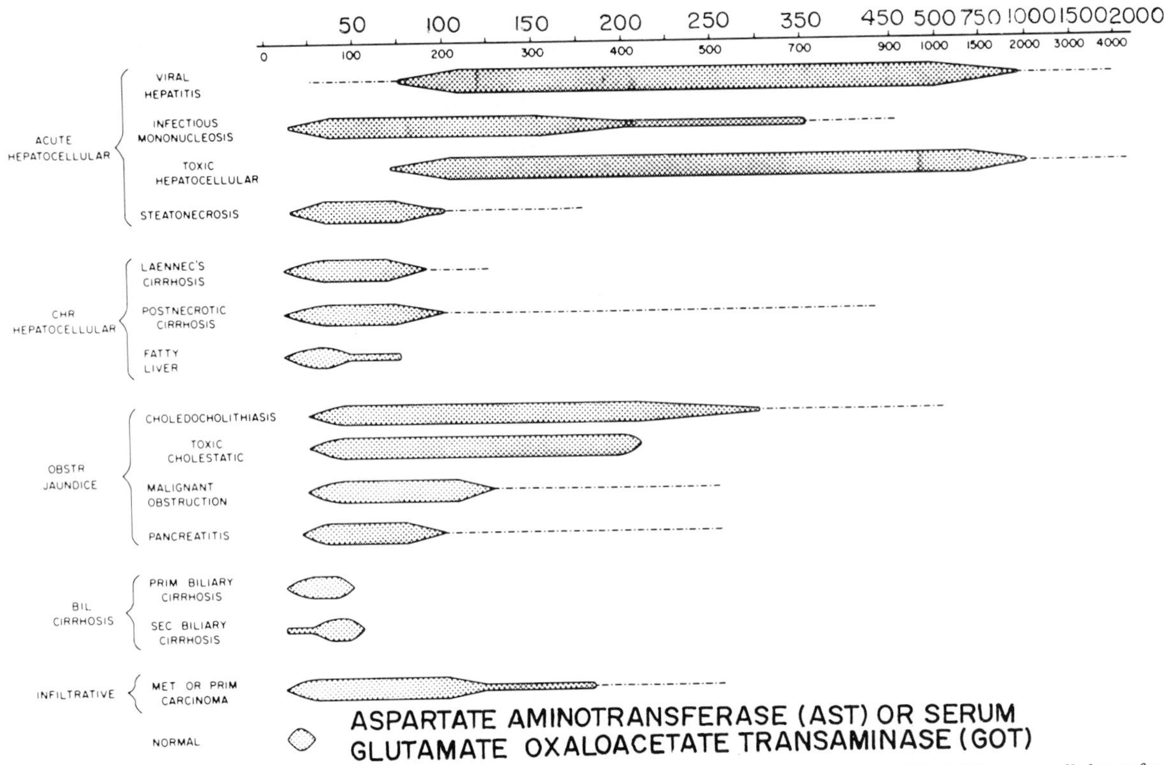

Figure 13–11. Levels of AST in U/L observed in patients with various types of liver disease. "Toxic" hepatocellular refers to some types of drug (e.g., halothane) toxicity or CCl_4 poisoning. Steatonecrosis refers to "alcoholic hepatitis." Values shown for postnecrotic cirrhosis are also characteristic of chronic active hepatitis. Toxic cholestatic jaundice refers to drug-induced or other acute intrahepatic cirrhosis. "Prim" biliary cirrhosis also is called "chronic intrahepatic cholestasis." "Sec" biliary cirrhosis refers to the cirrhosis that follows prolonged obstruction of the common bile or hepatic duct. "Met" refers to metastatic and "prim" refers to primary carcinoma of the liver, respectively. (From Zimmerman, H. J. and Seeff, L. B.: *In* Coodley, E. L. [ed.]: Diagnostic Enzymology. Philadelphia, Lea and Febiger, 1970, with permission.)

vated values. Those with cirrhosis have levels below 10-fold increased and the value may be normal. Patients with hepatic steatosis have even lower values. Even in alcoholic hepatitis, values for serum AST are below 10-fold increased in almost all patients. Higher values in alcoholic patients are usually the result of an accompanying myopathy, delirium tremens, or shock (Zimmerman, 1970).

Patients with chronic active hepatitis with or without cirrhosis may have AST values as low as those of alcoholic cirrhosis or as high as those of patients with acute hepatitis. In general, serum AST values tend to mirror the severity of the chronic hepatitis.

Approximately half the patients with metastatic carcinoma have elevated serum AST levels, usually in the same range as patients with cirrhosis and posthepatic jaundice. Less frequently such moderately elevated serum AST values are observed in patients with lymphoma and leukemia. In 80 per cent of patients with infectious mononucleosis, moderate (one- to 10-fold, but occasionally greater) serum AST elevations are observed. Patients with myocardial infarction usually show AST levels of less than 10-fold. The incidence and significance of AST elevations in patients with this and other non-hepatic conditions are discussed in Chapter 14.

Alanine aminotransferase (ALT) or *glutamate pyruvate transaminase* (GPT) (2.6.1.2) catalyzes the reversible transfer of an amino group from alanine to α-ketoglutarate (Fig. 13–12). It also has been found to be widely distributed in humans. The high hepatic content, compared with the relatively low concentration in myocardial and other tissues, has led to the application of ALT (GPT) determination to the study of hepatic disease.

The methods used for determination of this enzyme in the serum are similar to those used for AST (GOT) assay. Both spectrophotometric and colorimetric methods have been employed. The reference interval for this enzyme is almost the same as that for the serum AST (4 to 24 U/L at 30°C.).

Patients with viral hepatitis and other forms of hepatic necrosis usually show striking elevations of the serum ALT level. Values of ALT are modestly elevated (10- to 200-fold increased) in most patients with posthepatic jaundice and intrahepatic cholestasis. They are even lower (less than 10-fold) in most patients with metastatic carcinoma, cirrhosis, or al-

ALANINE AMINOTRANSFERASE (ALT) OR GLUTAMATE PYRUVATE TRANSAMINASE (GPT)

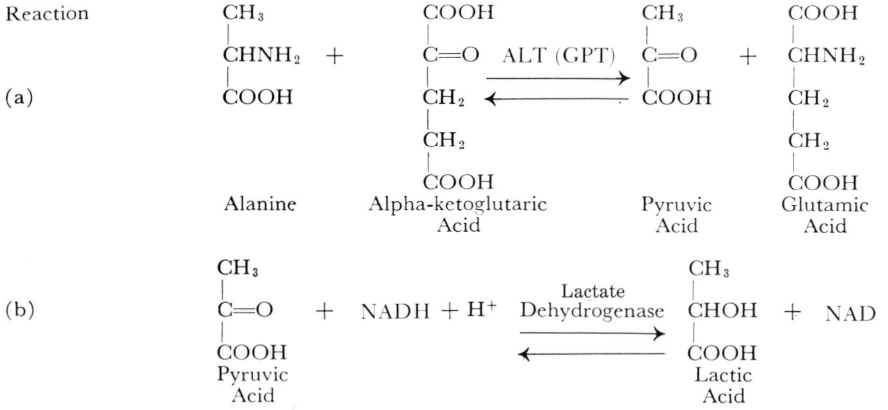

Reaction

(a)

$$\underset{\text{Alanine}}{\begin{matrix} CH_3 \\ | \\ CHNH_2 \\ | \\ COOH \end{matrix}} + \underset{\text{Alpha-ketoglutaric Acid}}{\begin{matrix} COOH \\ | \\ C{=}O \\ | \\ CH_2 \\ | \\ CH_2 \\ | \\ COOH \end{matrix}} \underset{}{\overset{\text{ALT (GPT)}}{\rightleftharpoons}} \underset{\text{Pyruvic Acid}}{\begin{matrix} CH_3 \\ | \\ C{=}O \\ | \\ COOH \end{matrix}} + \underset{\text{Glutamic Acid}}{\begin{matrix} COOH \\ | \\ CHNH_2 \\ | \\ CH_2 \\ | \\ CH_2 \\ | \\ COOH \end{matrix}}$$

(b)

$$\underset{\text{Pyruvic Acid}}{\begin{matrix} CH_3 \\ | \\ C{=}O \\ | \\ COOH \end{matrix}} + NADH + H^+ \overset{\text{Lactate Dehydrogenase}}{\rightleftharpoons} \underset{\text{Lactic Acid}}{\begin{matrix} CH_3 \\ | \\ CHOH \\ | \\ COOH \end{matrix}} + NAD$$

Figure 13–12. Reaction catalyzed by ALT (GPT) principles of assay methods, and conditions in which increased serum levels are observed.

Method of assay is based on measurement of rate of formation of product (pyruvic acid) of reaction. This may be done (1) indirectly by the coupled reaction (b) in which the rate of NADH oxidation, in the presence of added lactate dehydrogenase, is a measure of pyruvic acid formed (method of Karmen), or (2) directly, by one of several colorimetric methods that depend on formation of the dinitrophenylhydrazone of pyruvate.

Conditions in which abnormal serum levels of enzyme are observed, arranged in the order of decreasing levels:

A. *Hepatic Disease Abnormalities*
- Hepatic necrosis; e.g., hepatitis (infectious, toxic), infectious mononucleosis, cirrhosis
- Obstructive jaundice
- Metastatic carcinoma
- Hepatic congestion (centrilobular liver cell necrosis) secondary to heart failure or hepatic vein thrombosis

B. *Other Abnormalities (Slight)*
- Myocardial infarction
- Acute pancreatitis

coholic steatonecrosis (alcoholic hepatitis). Values for ALT are as high as or higher than those of AST in most patients with viral hepatitis, posthepatic jaundice, or intrahepatic cholestasis, while they are much lower than the respective values for AST in patients with cirrhosis, alcoholic hepatitis, or metastatic carcinoma. Levels of ALT are normal or only minimally elevated in patients with myocardial infarction (Fig. 13–13).

Clinical Value of Serum Aminotransferase (Transaminase) Measurements. The determination of serum aminotransferases is of distinct clinical aid. Differentiation of hepatic (hepatocellular) from posthepatic jaundice is facilitated by determining serum AST and ALT values, since values more than 10-fold increased are rare in patients with posthepatic jaundice. In the cholestatic type of hepatic jaundice (intrahepatic cholestasis), the serum AST or ALT values are like those of posthepatic jaundice. Likewise, in cirrhosis of the liver, even with deep jaundice, the moderate AST level and the lower ALT level are in contrast to the high levels of both transaminases* observed in acute viral hepatitis. Determination of AST, ALT, or both is useful in the early recognition of viral or toxic hepatitis and is, therefore, helpful in studying patients exposed to hepatotoxic drugs. Elevations of the ALT activity appear to reflect acute hepatic disease somewhat more specifically than is true of the AST values. The level of either enzyme, particularly the AST, may be elevated in patients with extrahepatic disease (see Chap. 14).

The levels of alkaline phosphatase (ALP), AST, and ALT are individually helpful in the differential diagnosis of hepatic disease. Their diagnostic usefulness is enhanced by observing the patterns of abnormality obtained by measuring all three, especially when combined with lactate dehydrogenase (LD) levels (see Chap. 14). In Figure 13–14 are shown diagrammatically the patterns obtained with a variety of hepatic lesions. The very high values for AST and ALT and relatively slightly elevated ones for alkaline phosphatase (ALP) observed in acute hepatitis and other necroinflammatory diseases of the liver differ sharply from the lower transaminase* and higher alkaline phosphatase values of posthepatic jaundice. The pattern of the "incomplete" posthepatic jaundice of choledocholithiasis overlaps with that of hepatitis, while the pattern of acute cholestatic jaundice or of biliary cirrhosis simulates that of posthepatic jaundice.

The patterns of cirrhosis are characteristically different. In alcoholic cirrhosis, AST elevations are slight, ALT values even lower, and lactate dehydrogenase (LD) and alkaline phosphatase (ALP) values very slightly elevated or normal. In inactive macronodular cirrhosis, the values resemble those of alcoholic cirrhosis; but in active macronodular cirrhosis and chronic active hepatitis, the AST values may be as low as those of alcoholic cirrhosis or as high as

*Aminotransferases.

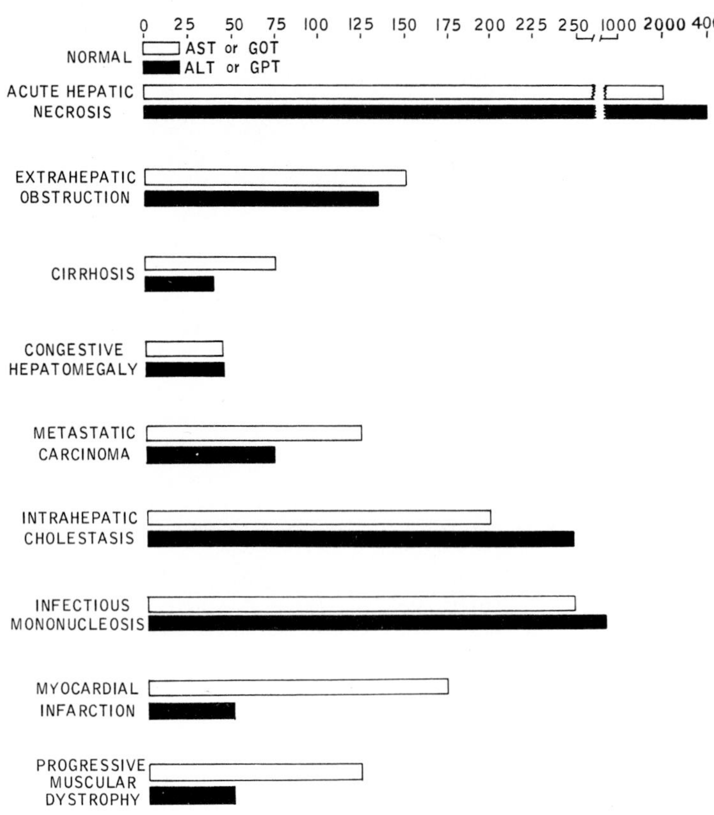

Figure 13–13. Relative levels of aspartate aminotransferase (AST) (glutamate oxaloacetate transaminse [GOT]) and alanine aminotransferase (ALT) (glutamate pyruvate transaminase [GPT]) in patients with hepatic, biliary, and other diseases.

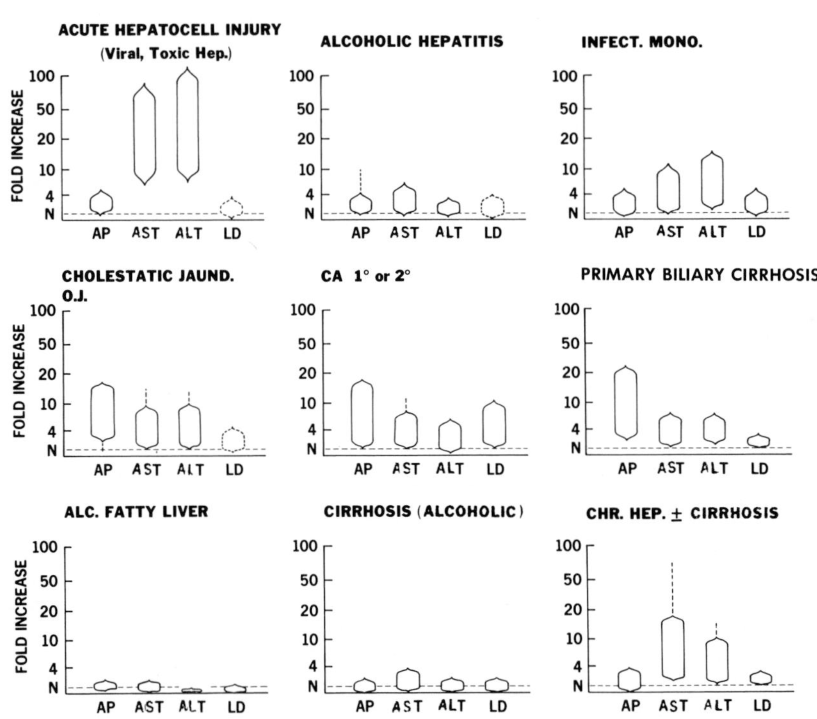

Figure 13–14. Patterns of abnormality in various types of hepatic and biliary disease provided by levels of alkaline phosphatase (AP), aspartate aminotransferase (AST), alanine aminotransferase (ALT), and lactate dehydrogenase (LD). HEPATOCELL = Hepatocellular; INFECT MONO = Infectious mononucleosis; JAUND = Jaundice; CA 1° or 2° = Primary or metastatic carcinoma; ALC = Alcoholic; CHR. HEP ± CIRRHOSIS = Chronic active hepatitis with or without cirrhosis.

those of acute hepatitis, and the values of the two transaminases* may be approximately equally elevated. The pattern of metastatic or primary carcinoma of the liver is distinctive in that the transaminase levels resemble those of alcoholic cirrhosis, while the LD and alkaline phosphatase levels are much higher. (See Chapter 14 for LD values in carcinomatosis.) These patterns, when accompanied by other diagnostic measures and careful clinical assessment, are of great diagnostic assistance.

SERUM "METALS" AND RELATED PROTEINS

Abnormal serum values of certain metallic substances are found in patients with some hepatic diseases. Elevated serum *iron* levels and reduced iron-binding capacity are observed in patients with hemochromatosis and transfusion hemosiderosis and may be of aid in diagnosis. Even more indicative of increased tissue stores of iron are elevated blood levels of ferritin, the tissue iron-binding protein. Indeed, a serum with increased levels of ferritin and iron and decreased iron-binding capacity is strongly predictive that liver biopsy would demonstrate sufficient increase in iron stores to permit the diagnosis of hemochromatosis. Acute elevations of serum iron levels are observed in patients with viral hepatitis and in others with acute hepatic necrosis. It has been observed that patients with posthepatic jaundice usually have normal serum iron levels. This has led to the application by European and South American workers of the serum iron level determination to the differential diagnosis of jaundice. This application, however, has not been adopted widely in the United States.

Elevated blood levels of "free" *copper* and increased amounts of tissue copper have been observed in patients with Wilson's disease (hepatolenticular degeneration). The levels of free copper are increased in most patients with this disease, accompanied by decreased levels of ceruloplasmin, a copper-carrying protein that is also an enzyme (copper oxidase). Diagnosis of Wilson's disease is aided by the demonstration of depressed levels of ceruloplasmin in the plasma. Increased levels of serum and hepatic copper are also observed in primary biliary cirrhosis.

Abnormal levels of other metallic ions of the blood have been described in patients with chronic hepatic disease. Depressed serum levels of *zinc* have been reported in patients with alcoholic cirrhosis. The significance of this observation remains to be determined. Lower than normal serum *magnesium* levels have been reported in alcoholic patients with delirium tremens and with cirrhosis. Among the factors considered responsible is malnutrition. In cirrhotics with ascites the *hyponatremia* commonly observed is considered to be a manifestation of water retention, not sodium loss. *Hypokalemia* is frequent in patients with severe hepatic disease.

*Aminotransferase.

TESTS BASED ON THE ROLE OF LIVER IN VITAMIN ECONOMY

Deficiency in a number of vitamins is prone to occur in the malnourished alcoholic patient. Accordingly, in alcoholic cirrhosis evidence of beriberi, pellagra, and scurvy may be observed. In addition, abnormal levels of vitamins A and B_{12} have been described in patients with hepatic disease.

Depressed plasma levels of vitamin A are characteristic of patients with parenchymal hepatic disease. The observation that patients with early obstructive jaundice usually have normal levels has led to the former application of vitamin A determination to the differential diagnosis of jaundice. The dependence of the absorption of this fat-soluble vitamin on an adequate concentration of bile salts in the duodenum, however, also leads to depressed levels in posthepatic jaundice; accordingly, this determination is of little value in the differential diagnosis of jaundice.

Vitamin B_{12} is stored in the liver. In patients with acute viral hepatitis very high plasma levels of this vitamin are observed, presumably resulting from release by necrotic hepatic cells. Somewhat elevated values are observed in cirrhosis also. A test of hepatic function based on the estimation of the hepatic "uptake" of an oral dose of vitamin B_{12} labeled with radioactive cobalt has been described. None of these tests has been used extensively in the clinical setting.

SPECIAL PROCEDURES

The diagnostic armamentarium of hepatology consists of some of the biochemical tests described in the foregoing pages and a few special procedures (Table 13–11). These include percutaneous biopsy of the liver, scintiscanning employing radionuclides, and serologic tests. Not discussed in this chapter, but of great usefulness in the study of special hepatologic problems, are cholangiography (intravenous, percutaneous, or endoscopic), ultrasonography, peroral endoscopy, laparoscopy, and celiac axis arteriography.

Liver Biopsy

Needle biopsy of the liver, a procedure which has been widely used for more than three decades, is very helpful in the diagnosis of hepatic and non-hepatic disease (Table 13–12). It is useful in defining the cause of hepatocellular jaundice and of hepatomegaly and in demonstrating the presence of cirrhosis, steatosis, alcoholic hepatitis, chronic hepatitis, biliary cirrhosis, and carcinoma. Indeed, it serves to define the hepatic disease, attention to which has been drawn by clinical or biochemical clues. It is an important part of the evaluation of poorly resolving hepatitis. Biopsy may also be of help in distinguishing between intrahepatic cholestasis and posthepatic jaundice, although the distinction is at times difficult and the safety of needle biopsy in the face of posthepatic

Table 13–11. USUAL PANEL OF MEASUREMENTS AND EXAMINATIONS AVAILABLE FOR DIAGNOSIS OF HEPATIC DISEASE*

Bilirubin	Serum levels, direct and total Urine bilirubin (and urobilinogen)
Serum protein levels and electrophoresis	Immunoglobulins (Alpha-1-antitrypsin)† (Alpha-fetoprotein)† (Ceruloplasmin)† (Iron, transferrin, ferritin)†
Serum enzyme activity	ALP (5′-N, LAP, GGT) AST (GOT) ALT (GPT)
Prothrombin time (+ vitamin K)	
Serum cholesterol	
Special procedures	Serology for viral hepatitis (see Table 13–13) Serology for "autoimmune" factors (see Chap. 39) Liver biopsy Scintiscanning Cholangiography Ultrasound Arteriography

*List includes only those available at most hospitals in U.S.A.

†Tests used for special diagnostic purposes.

jaundice somewhat controversial. Liver biopsy is particularly useful in establishing the diagnosis of systemic disease, e.g., tuberculosis, sarcoidosis, amyloidosis. The indications and contraindications for liver biopsy, as we view them, are shown in Table 13–12.

Table 13–12. INDICATIONS AND CONTRAINDICATIONS FOR LIVER BIOPSY

I. Possible applications
   A. Finding the cause of hepatomegaly, jaundice, ascites, gastrointestinal bleeding, or abnormal liver function or serum enzyme values
   B. Establishment of precise diagnosis in patients with probable hepatic disease, e.g., chronic hepatitis, cirrhosis, fatty liver, or carcinoma (metastatic or primary)
   C. Recognition of systemic disease, e.g., hematogenous tuberculosis, sarcoidosis, amyloidosis, and lymphoma (may be helpful in "staging" in known Hodgkin's disease)
   D. Evaluation of response to therapy of acute or chronic liver disease

II. Relative contraindications
   A. Clotting defects (abnormal bleeding time, coagulation time, or partial thromboplastin time), prothrombin time (>5 seconds greater than control), or history of recent hemorrhagic tendency
   B. Firm clinical diagnosis of posthepatic jaundice
   C. Severe anemia
   D. Uncooperative or unduly apprehensive patient
   E. Bacterial infection in area to be traversed by biopsy needle, e.g., right lower lobe pneumonia

Radioisotopes in Diagnosis of Liver Disease

The availability of radioisotopes has contributed much to the study of hepatic physiology and disease. They have been used to measure liver function and blood flow, to define the configuration and size of the liver and spleen, to demonstrate "space-occupying" lesions in the liver (tumor, cysts, and abscesses), and to provide indirect evidence of the presence of portal hypertension.

Four types of radiopharmaceuticals are available. One group consists of tagged molecules that are taken up by normal hepatocytes. A second group consists of substances phagocytized by reticuloendothelial (RE) cells. A third group remains in the blood, and a fourth group is selectively taken up by malignant hepatocytes and by the leukocytes of an abscess.

Tagged molecules taken up by hepatocytes include such substances as ^{14}C-bilirubin, ^{14}C-cholylglycine, ^{58}Co- or ^{60}C-labeled cyanocobalamine, ^{131}I-rose bengal (RB), and ^{131}I-BSP. These have been used to measure hepatic function by the rate of disappearance of the radioactive molecule from the blood or by the rate of its accumulation in the liver. These tests of hepatic function, however, have been largely of research interest. None of these has found regular clinical use. To a limited degree, ^{131}I-RB has been applied to the differential diagnosis of jaundice, especially in infants. The demonstration that the radioactivity is taken up by the liver but fails to enter the duodenum and instead appears in the urine is taken as evidence of biliary obstruction. Even for this limited purpose, the value of ^{131}I-RB is controversial. For visualization of the diseased liver, agents that are selectively accumulated by normal hepatocytes, are, of course, satisfactory. Rose bengal, which was used in the early years of scintiscanning, was discarded after it was found not to be adequately accumulated by diseased hepatocytes. ^{131}I-RB has been replaced by a group of ^{99}m Tc-compounds, of which ^{99}m TC-HIDA is prototypic. These compounds undergo uptake by the hepatocyte and excretion into the biliary tree. Accordingly, they can measure hepatic function and patency of the biliary tree. Their main use, however, has been in the diagnosis of acute cholecystitis.

Radioactive colloids taken up by RE cells are most suitable for nuclear imaging, since parenchymal hepatic disease would not preclude concentration of the agent by the liver. Those which have been used include radioactive gold (^{198}Au or ^{199}Au), indium (^{113m}In), and technetium sulfur colloid (^{99m}Tc). Today ^{99m}Tc is the most widely used in hepatology; and gamma camera imaging is, by far, the most useful application of radiopharmacology to the study of liver disease.

Nuclear imaging with a scintillation camera provides a pattern of the radioactivity concentrated in the liver. Areas within boundaries of the organ that fail to accumulate radioactivity ("cold" areas) represent pathologic processes. They may be produced by primary or metastatic tumors of the liver, cysts, abscesses or the broad scars of macronodular cirrhosis. "Cold" areas also may be caused by a normal gallbladder fossa or some prominent portal veins in the hepatic hilus rather than by an intrahepatic mass. Multiple small cold areas usually represent diffuse disease (cirrhosis), although they may be caused by diffuse carcinomatous involvement. This pattern of diffusely decreased hepatic uptake, accompanied by splenomegaly and increased uptake by the spleen and bone marrow, is common in moderate to advanced cirrhosis.

Gallium (^{67}Ga) citrate is taken up selectively by neoplastic and inflammatory tissues. Areas that appear "cold" with ^{99m}Tc sulfur colloid may concentrate ^{67}Ga if due to primary or metastatic carcinoma or abscess.

Radioactive agents that remain in the blood are useful to measure hepatic perfusion. ^{131}I-labeled albumin, ^{99m}Tc albumin, and ^{133}Xe have been used, largely for research purposes.

Nuclear imaging is an important diagnostic procedure for the study of hepatic disease. Like ultrasonography, it is useful for the detection of masses in the liver, such as metastatic carcinoma, hepatoma, cysts, or abscesses. In a patient suspected of having one of these lesions or with unexplained hepatomegaly, imaging may confirm the diagnosis or indicate the site for biopsy if a carcinoma is suspected. Recognition of a single mass in the liver is possible if it is 2 cm in diameter or greater. Smaller masses cannot be recognized unless they are coalescent. Even larger masses, if multiple, may escape identification, since multiple infiltrative masses and cirrhosis may give a similar pattern. Conversely, the scan of a coarse nodular (postnecrotic) cirrhosis may be mistaken for that of multiple infiltrative masses.

Scanning of the liver is also useful in defining hepatic size, contours, and extent. This is especially important in patients who are extremely obese, in those with marked ascites, and in those with an abnormal contour of the right leaflet of the diaphragm observed on chest roentgenography.

SEROLOGIC TESTS

A number of serologic tests for the diagnosis and prevention of hepatic disease are available. The most important ones are those used to detect current or past infection with hepatitis B virus (HBV).

The antigens of HBV include the surface antigen (HBsAg), the "core" antigen (HBcAg), and the "e" antigen (HBeAg), to each of which demonstrable antibodies are formed. The antigens and antibodies demonstrated in the serum can be correlated with the type of hepatic disease produced by the infection (Table 13–13).

Acute HBV hepatitis is characterized by presence of HBsAg and anti-HBc in the blood and often by HBeAg. Recovery is attended by disappearance of HBsAg and HBeAg, persistence of anti-HBc, and appearance of anti-HBs and often of anti-HBe. Persistence of HBsAg beyond three months of onset of acute illness is a hallmark of chronic hepatitis or of the carrier state. Presence of HBeAg in a presumed carrier of HBsAg enhances the likelihood that the "carrier" is actively infective. The observation that many patients with hepatocellular carcinoma have HBsAg in their blood (and liver) and associated studies have provided convincing evidence of the hepatocarcinogenic role of HBV.

Testing for HBsAg is available in almost all medical centers for the diagnosis of acute and chronic virus B hepatitis and in blood banks for the detection of carriers of HBV. It has also served to demonstrate a probable role of HBV infection in the etiology of hepatocellular carcinoma. Presence of anti-HBs, anti-HBc, and anti-HBe is evidence of former infection with HBV and probably immunity. Of these, anti-HBc is the first to appear during acute infection.

Tests for hepatitis A virus (HAV) infection have also become available. Early in the disease, HAV can be identified in the feces by immunoelectron microscopy or immunofluorescent techniques. This is of no clinical use since the virus usually has disappeared from feces by the time hepatitis appears. Furthermore, the procedure is too technically difficult for routine use. More widely applied to diagnosis, thus far, has been the demonstration of rising titers of anti-HA antibodies.

Circulating antibodies to various tissue components have been found in patients with chronic hepatic disease. These "autoantibodies" in patients with chronic active hepatitis (antinuclear antibodies, LE factor, anti–smooth muscle antibody) and in patients with primary biliary cirrhosis (antimitochondrial antibody) provide indirect evidence of autoimmune pathogenesis of these syndromes, and are clinically useful. The serological features of viral hepatitis and the serological aspects of other hepatic disease are considered in Chapter 39. HLA antigens and their association (susceptibility) to hepatic disease, e.g., hemochromatosis, are reviewed in Chapter 33.

Table 13–13. SEROLOGIC FACTORS RELATED TO HEPATITIS B VIRUS

	HbsAg*	Anti-HBs	Anti-HBc*	HBeAG*	Anti-HBe
Acute hepatitis					
Early acute phase	+	–	+	±	–
Early convalescence	–	–	+	–	–
Recovery	–	+	+	–	±
Chronic HBV hepatitis	+	–	+	±	–
Carrier state	+	–	+	±	±
Hepatocellular carcinoma	+	–	+	±	±

*HBsAG = hepatitis B antigen; HBc = "core" antigen; HBeAg = "E" antigen; HBV = hepatitis B virus.

Table 13–14. APPLICATION OF LIVER FUNCTION TESTING

I. Diagnosis
   A. Recognition of presence or absence of hepatic disease
   B. Differential diagnosis
      1. Hepatomegaly
      2. Jaundice
      3. Ascites
      4. Gastrointestinal hemorrhage
   C. Testing for hepatotoxicity of drugs or industrial hepatotoxins
   D. Recognition of non-hepatic disease, e.g., hematogenous tuberculosis, sarcoidosis, amyloidosis, and infectious mononucleosis
II. Estimating severity in known hepatic disease
   A. Monitoring convalescence (hepatitis, cirrhosis)
   B. Preoperative evaluation

CLINICAL APPLICATION OF LIVER FUNCTION TESTS

Some of the clinical settings in which hepatic tests are applied are listed in Table 13–14. They are useful for the diagnosis of hepatic disease and specifically for the differential diagnosis of jaundice, hepatomegaly, ascites, and gastrointestinal hemorrhage. Systematic monitoring of selected tests of hepatic function is necessary in testing for the hepatotoxicity of new drugs or of industrial exposure to chemicals. Characteristic patterns of abnormality are observed in extrahepatic diseases and assist in their recognition. Estimation of the severity of known hepatic disease and response to treatment is facilitated by testing of liver function.

A large number of tests have been described or mentioned in the preceding material. Only some of these are readily applicable to clinical problems. A "battery" or panel of tests, which we use regularly in the diagnosis of hepatic disease, is shown in Table 13–11. With this group, patterns of hepatic dysfunction are observed that are useful in the differential diagnosis of jaundice (Table 13–15), hepatomegaly (Table 13–16), ascites (Table 13–17), and gastrointestinal hemorrhage (Table 13–18) and that can even be helpful in the recognition of extrahepatic disease (Table 13–19). The patterns shown represent those most frequently observed in each instance. Exceptions occur, and the patterns should be regarded only as guides.

HEPATIC FUNCTION IN NON-HEPATIC DISEASE

Abnormal results with one or more tests of hepatic function may be obtained in patients with a variety

Table 13–15. LABORATORY APPROACH TO DIFFERENTIAL DIAGNOSIS OF JAUNDICE*,†

	Bilirubin Tests					**Serum Enzymes**			**Prothrombin Time**	
Type of Hyperbilirubinemia	***Serum* *(Dir/Tot) × 100***	***Urine* *B***	***Urine* *U***	***Feces* *U***	**Serum Cholest.**	***ALP***	***AST (GOT)***	***ALT (GPT)***	***1°***	***+K***
Unconjugated										
Prehepatic	20	0	↑	↑↑	N	N	N	N	N	NA
Hepatic			N	N						
Conjugated‡										
Hepatic—Hepatocellular										
Viral or toxic hepatitis	40	+	↑	N	N	↑	↑↑↑	↑↑↑↑	(↑)	
Alcoholic hepatitis							↑↑	(↑)		
Cholestatic										
Acute—drug or viral§			(↑)	(↓)	↑↑	↑↑	↑↑	↑↑	↑	+
Chronic (primary biliary cirrhosis¶)	50	+	(↑)	N	↑↑↑↑	↑↑↑	↑	↑	↑	+
Familial cholestatic jaundice			N	N	N	N	N	N	N	NA
Posthepatic—Complete (carcinoma)	50	+	N	↓↓↓	↑↑	↑↑↑	↑↑	↑↑	↑↑	+
—Incomplete (stones)			(↑)	↓	(↑)	↑– ↑↑↑	↑↑↑	↑↑↑	↑↑↑	

*Dir/Tot. = direct/total bilirubin; B = bilirubin; U = urobilinogen; cholest. = cholesterol; ALP = alkaline phosphatase; GOT = glutamate oxaloacetate transaminase; GPT = glutamate pyruvate transaminase; 1° = prior to administration of vitamin K; + K = after administration of vitamin K.

†Arrows indicate direction, degree, and incidence of abnormal results. Arrow in parentheses indicates that abnormality may or may not occur. N indicates normal. NA = not applicable.

‡Distinction between hepatic and posthepatic jaundice may at times require special procedures, e.g., biopsy, ultrasound, cholangiography.

§Serologic studies helpful in diagnosis.

¶The Dubin-Johnson syndrome is a genetic disorder characterized by a black pigment in the hepatocytes and a special form of "dissociated" intrahepatic cholestasis in which there is defective excretion of bilirubin into the canaliculus but other components of bile apparently are normally excreted, thus differing from other forms of hepatic canalicular jaundice. The Rotor syndrome resembles the Dubin-Johnson syndrome in some but not all features. Other familial forms of hepatocanalicular jaundice include "benign intermittent juvenile cholestatic jaundice" and cholestatic jaundice of pregnancy.

Table 13–16. LABORATORY AIDS IN THE DIFFERENTIAL DIAGNOSIS OF HEPATOMEGALY OR OTHER PRESENTATIONS SUGGESTING HEPATIC DISEASE IN THE ANICTERIC PATIENT*

	BSP†	Bilirubin	Alb	Globulin Tot.	Globulin Fract.	Globulin Ig‡	ALP	AST (GOT)	ALT (GPT)	LD	Special§ Procedures
I. Acute hepatitis	↑↑↑	↑	N	(↑)	β,γ	IgG	↑	↑↑–↑↑↑↑	↑↑–↑↑↑↑	↑	Serol (V) B
II. Chronic active hepatitis ± cirrhosis	↑↑↑	(↑)	↓	↑–↑↑↑	γ	IgM	↑–↑↑	↑–↑↑	↑–↑↑	(↑)	Serol (V) Serol (A-I) B
III. Primary biliary cirrhosis	↑↑↑	(↑)	(↓)	(↑)	α_2,β,γ	IgG	↑↑↑	↑	↑	(↑)	AMA, B
IV. Alcoholic cirrhosis	↑↑↑	(↑)	↓	↑,N,↓	γ	IgM IgA	↑	↑↑	(↑)	(↑)	B
V. Steatosis	(↑)	(↑)	N	N		N		↑	N	N	B
VI. Alcoholic hepatitis	↑↑↑	↑	↓	↑,N,↓	γ	IgM IgA	↑–↑↑	↑↑	↑	(↑)	B
VII. Carcinoma, primary	↑↑	(↑)	(↓)	↑,N,↓	α_2	N	↑–↑↑↑	↑↑	↑	↑↑	Scan, US Art, B; AFP
VIII. Carcinoma, metastic or lymphoma	↑↑↑	(↑)	(↓)	(↓)	α_2	N	↑–↑↑↑	↑↑	↑	↑–↑↑↑	Scan, B
IX. Infectious mononucleosis	↑↑	(↑)	N	N	β,γ	IgG	↑–↑↑	↑↑	↑–↑↑	↑–↑↑	Serol
X. Amyloidosis	↑↑	(↑)	↓	↑,N,↓	α_2,γ	IgG	↑–↑↑↑	↑		N,(↑)	B
XI. Congestive heart failure	↑↑↑	(↑)	(↓)	(↓)	–	N	↑	↑↑	↑–↑↑	↑↑	Clinical
XII. Granulomatous disease	(↑)	(↑)	N	↑↑	γ	IgG	↑–↑↑↑	↑	↑	(↑)	B

*Arrows indicate direction, degree, and incidence of abnormal results. N indicates normal. (↑) = may or may not be elevated.
†Normal value would virtually exclude diagnosis in all conditions with two or three arrows. Test, however, has been largely abandoned.
‡IgG in virus B hepatitis. IgM in acute or recent virus A hepatitis.
§Special procedures: serol = serology; V = viral; A-I = autoimmune; B = biopsy; AMA = Antimitochondrial antibody; Scan = scintiscanning; Art = arteriography; AFP = alpha-fetoprotein.
Alb = albumin; Tot. = total.

2

Table 13–17. TYPE OF HEPATOLOGIC BIOCHEMICAL ABNORMALITY IN PATIENTS WITH ASCITES*

Cause of Ascites	Type of Abnormality (See Table 13–16)
Alcoholic cirrhosis	IV
Macronodular cirrhosis	II
Alcoholic hepatitis	VI
Chronic active hepatitis	II
Primary biliary cirrhosis	III
Peritoneal carcinomatosis†	None or VIII
Tuberculous peritonitis†	None or X
Amyloidosis	X
Congestive heart failure	XI

*Decisive diagnostic procedures include laparoscopy and peritoneal and liver biopsy.

†Degree of biochemical abnormality depends on presence and extent of lesions in the liver; if peritoneal without hepatic lesions, may be no helpful biochemical abnormality.

of extrahepatic diseases. These have been considered at times to reflect on the value and specificity of liver function testing. Even in non-hepatic disease, however, fairly consistent patterns of hepatic function may be observed. In Table 13–19 is shown a classification of non-hepatic diseases in terms of the type of hepatic dysfunction observed and the presumed basis for it.

CONCLUSIONS

The foregoing discussion has attempted to review the basis for liver function testing and has listed a large number of laboratory procedures for this purpose. A small number of useful determinations have been selected from this group and their applications in a clinical setting have been considered.

Table 13–19. PATTERNS OF BIOCHEMICAL ABNORMALITY SUGGESTIVE OF LIVER DISEASE IN EXTRAHEPATIC DISEASE

Pattern of Abnormality Suggesting	Example of Condition
Acute hepatic disease Increased level bilirubin, AST, ALT with or without jaundice	Pneumococcal pneumonia[H] Legionella pneumonia[H] Toxic shock syndrome[H] Toxoplasmosis[H] Sickle cell disease[H] Severe heart failure[H] Gram-negative bacterial systemic infection[C]
Chronic hepatic disease Increased level bilirubin; ALP: slight increase AST, ALT, with or without jaundice	Sarcoidosis[C] Hodgkin's disease[H, C] Ulcerative colitis[C] Amyloidosis[C]
Infiltrative lesions of liver High levels of ALP, slight increase AST, ALT, little or no elevation bilirubin	Granulomatous disease Myloidosis Abscess Lymphoma

H = Jaundice, if present, hepatocellular.
C = Jaundice, if present, cholestatic.
H,C = Jaundice, if present, either hepatocellular or cholestatic.

It should be recalled that there are a number of pitfalls in the application of the tests to the diagnosis and management of hepatic disease (Table 13–20). Correlation of laboratory results with clinical features should obviate most of these potential difficulties.

Table 13–18. TYPE OF HEPATOLOGIC BIOCHEMICAL ABNORMALITY IN PATIENTS WITH GASTROINTESTINAL HEMORRHAGE*

Cause of Hemorrhage	Type of Abnormality (See Table 13–16)
Peptic ulcer	None†
Alcoholic or other chemical gastritis	None, or IV, V, or VI
Esophageal varices	
Intrahepatic portal obstruction	
Alcoholic cirrhosis	IV
Macronodular cirrhosis	II
Alcoholic hepatitis‡	VI
Chronic active hepatitis‡	II
Primary biliary cirrhosis	III
Extrahepatic portal obstruction	None†

*Endoscopy, radiography, and at times arteriography are the diagnostically decisive procedures.

†Unless there is coincidental liver disease.

‡Accompanied by cirrhosis.

Table 13–20. SOME COMMON PITFALLS IN APPLICATION OF LIVER TESTS

1. Dependence on results of one test rather than patterns of abnormality.
2. Assumption that normal results signify no parenchymal disease (e.g., values for AST (GOT) normal in 25 per cent and for ALT (GPT) normal in 50 per cent of patients with alcoholic cirrhosis).
3. Assumption that abnormal values for "liver function" tests mean only liver disease.
4. Failure to recognize acute jaundice as:
    a. *Hepatocellular* because AST (GOT) and ALT (GPT) values are unexpectedly low (below 200 U/L in some patients with acute viral hepatitis) or because ALP values are unexpectedly high (more than three times the ULN* in 5 per cent of patients with acute hepatitis).
    b. *Posthepatic* because values for AST (GOT) and ALT (GPT) are unexpectedly high (above 200 U/L in 15 per cent of patients with choledocholithiasis) or because values for ALP are unexpectedly low.
5. Failure to reconcile results of tests with clinical features.

*ULN = upper limit of normal or upper reference limit.

Liver Function (General)

Burke, M. D.: Liver function. Human Path., *6*:273, 1975.

Combes, B., and Schenker, S.: Laboratory tests. *In* Schiff, L., and Schiff, E. R. (eds.): Diseases of the Liver, 5th ed. Philadelphia, J. B. Lippincott Co., 1982, pp. 259–302.

Demers, L. M., and Shaw, L. M. (eds.): Evaluation of Liver Function. A Multifaceted Approach to Clinical Diagnosis. Baltimore-Munich, Urban and Schwarzenberg, 1978.

Goldberg, D. M.: Hepatobiliary Disease. *In* Golden, D. M. (ed.): Clinical Biochemistry Reviews, Vol. II. New York, John Wiley & Sons, 1981, pp. 361–398.

Jones, E. A., and Berk, P. D.: Liver Function. *In* Braun, S. S., Mitchell, F. L., and Young, D. S. (eds.): Chemical Diagnosis of Disease. Amsterdam-New York, Elsevier, 1979, pp. 525–661.

Rosoff, L., Jr., and Rosoff, L., Sr.: Biochemical tests for hepatobiliary disease. Surg. Clin. North Am., *57*:257, 1977.

Sherlock, S.: Diseases of the Liver, 6th ed. Oxford, Blackwell Scientific Publications, 1981.

Bilirubin Metabolism and Jaundice

Berk, P. D., and Berlin, N. I. (eds.): Chemistry and Physiology of Bile Pigments. Fogarty International Proceedings No. 35, DHEW Publication No. (NIH) 77–1100, 1977.

Billing, B. H.: Bilirubin metabolism. *In* Schiff, L., and Schiff, E. R. (eds.): Diseases of the Liver, 5th ed. Philadelphia, J. B. Lippincott Co., 1982, pp. 349–378.

Boucher, I. A. D.: Diagnosis of jaundice. Br. Med. J., *283*:1282, 1981.

Bradley, B. W. D.: A physiological approach to jaundice. Clin. Biochem., *9*:144, 1976.

Ducci, H.: Contribution of the laboratory to the differential diagnosis of jaundice. J.A.M.A., *135*:694, 1947.

Gollan, J. L., and Schmid, R.: Bilirubin Update: Formation, Transport and Metabolism. *In* Popper, H., and Schaffner, F. (eds.): Progress In Liver Disease, Vol. VII. New York, Grune & Stratton, 1982, pp. 261–284.

Jendrassik, L., and Grof, P.: Vereinfachte photometrische Methoden zur Bestimmung des Blutbilirubins. Biochim. Z., *297*:81, 1938.

Malchow-Moller, A., Matzen, P., Bjerregard, B., Hilden, J., Holst-Christensen, J., Staehr-Johansen, T., Altman, L., Thomsen, C., and Juhl, E.: Causes and characteristics of 500 consecutive cases of jaundice. Scand. J. Gastroent., *16*:1, 1981.

Malloy, H. T., and Evelyn, K. A.: The determination of bilirubin with the photoelectric colorimeter. J. Biol. Chem., *119*:481, 1937.

McNee, J. W.: Jaundice: A review of recent works. Q. J. Med., *16*:390, 1923.

Michaelsson, M.: Bilirubin determination in serum and urine. Scand. J. Clin. Lab. Invest., *13* (Suppl. 56):5, 1961.

Moody, F. G.: Diagnosis and treatment of obstructive biliary tract disease. West. J. Med., *136*:530, 1982.

Rich, A. R.: Pathogenesis of forms of jaundice. Bull. Johns Hopkins Hosp., *47*:338, 1930.

Sunderman, F. W.: Proficiency test service. Bilirubin, January, 1978.

Thompson, R. P. H.: Recent advances in jaundice: Physiology. Br. Med. J., *1*:223, 1970.

Watson, C. J.: The importance of the fractional serum bilirubin determination in clinical medicine. Ann. Intern. Med., *45*:351, 1956.

White, T. T.: Obstructive biliary tract disease. West. J. Med., *136*:484, 1982.

Zimmerman, H. J.: Intrahepatic cholestasis. Arch. Intern. Med., *139*:1038, 1979.

Serum Proteins and Related Abnormalities

Alpert, E.: Human alpha-1-feto protein (AFP). *In* Popper, H., and Schaffner, F. (eds.): Progress in Liver Diseases, Vol. V. New York, Grune & Stratton, 1976, pp. 337–349.

Bloomer, J. R.: Serum alpha-fetoprotein in nonneoplastic liver disease. Dig. Dis. Sci., *25*:241, 1980.

Carlson, J., and Eriksson, S.: α_1-Antitrypsin and other acute phase reactants in liver disease. Acta Med. Scand., *207*:79, 1980.

Eliakim, M., Zlotnik, A., and Slavin, S.: Gammopathy in liver disease. *In* Popper, H., and Schaffner, F. (eds.): Progress in Liver Diseases, Vol. IV. New York, Grune & Stratton, 1972, pp. 403–418.

Glynn, L. E.: Immunopathology of liver disease. *In* Popper, H., and Schaffner, F. (eds.): Progress in Liver Diseases, Vol. V. New York, Grune & Stratton, 1976, pp. 311–325.

Owen, J. A., Padangi, R., and Smith, H.: Serum haptoglobins and other tests in the diagnosis of hepatobiliary disease. Clin. Sci., *21*:189, 1961.

Purves, L. R., Bersohn, I., and Geddes, E. W.: Serum alpha-feto-protein and primary cancer of the liver in man. Cancer, *25*:1261, 1970.

Scheinberg, I. H.: Adult Wilson's disease. Arch. Neurol., *29*:449, 1973.

Seidel, D., Gretz, H., and Ruppert, C.: Significance of the LP-X test in differential diagnosis of jaundice. Clin. Chem., *19*:86, 1973.

Sharp, H. L.: Alpha-1-antitrypsin: An ignored protein in understanding of liver disease. Sem. Liver Dis., *2*:314, 1982.

Simon, J. R., and Poor, R. W. M.: Lipoprotein-X levels in extrahepatic versus intrahepatic cholestasis. Gastroenterology, *75*:177, 1978.

Smith, J. B.: Alpha-feto-protein, occurrence in certain malignant diseases and review of clinical applications. Med. Clin. North Am., *54*:797, 1970.

Blood Ammonia Levels and Related Abnormalities

Bessman, S. P.: Blood ammonia. *In* Sabotka, H., and Stewart, C. P. (eds.): Advances in Clinical Chemistry, Vol. 2. New York, Academic Press, Inc., 1959, pp. 135–166.

Fischer, J. E., and Baldesserani, R. J.: Pathogenesis and therapy of hepatic coma. *In* Popper, H., and Schaffner, F. (eds.): Progress in Liver Diseases, Vol. V. New York, Grune & Stratton, 1976, pp. 363–397.

Flannery, D. B., Hsia, Y. E., and Wolf, B.: Current status of hyperammonemic syndromes. Hepatology, *2*:495, 1982.

Galambos, J. T., Warren, W. D., and Rudman, D.: Portal surgery and liver function. A new look at an old problem. Mt. Sinai J. Med., *43*:219, 1976.

Glasgow, A. M., Cotton, R. B., and Dhiensiri, K.: Reye's syndrome. Blood ammonia and consideration of the nonhistologic diagnosis. Am. J. Dis. Child., *124*:827, 1972.

Hourani, B. T., Hamlin, E. M., and Reynolds, T. B.: Cerebrospinal fluid glutamine as a measure of hepatic encephalopathy. Arch. Intern. Med., *127*:1033, 1971.

Seligson, D., and Seligson, H.: A microdiffusion method for the determination of nitrogen liberated as ammonia. J. Lab. Clin. Med., *38*:324, 1951.

Van Anken, H. C., and Schiphorst, M. E.: A kinetic determination of ammonia in plasma. Clin. Chim. Acta, *56*:151, 1974.

Zieve, L.: Hepatic encephalopathy: Summary of present knowledge with an elaboration on recent developments. *In* Popper, H., and Schaffner, F. (eds.): Progress in Liver Diseases, Vol. VI. New York, Grune & Stratton, 1979, pp. 327–341.

Galactose Tolerance and Other Tests Related to Carbohydrate Metabolism

Ashwell, G., and Steer, C. J.: Hepatic recognition and catabolism of serum glycoproteins. J.A.M.A., *246*:2358, 1981.

Blaauwen, D. H., and Thijs, L. G.: The bromosulfalein and galactose tolerance tests in patients with various liver diseases. Acta Gastro-Enterologica Belgica, *36*:345, 1973.

Felig, P., and Sherwin, R.: Carbohydrate homeostasis, liver and diabetes. *In* Popper, H., and Schaffner, F. (eds.): Progress in Liver Diseases, Vol. V. New York, Grune & Stratton, 1976, pp. 149–171.

Menesholme, E. A.: Role of the liver in integration of fat and carbohydrate metabolism and clinical implications in patients with liver disease. *In* Popper, H., and Schaffner, F. (eds.): Progress in Liver Diseases, Vol. V. New York, Grune & Stratton, 1976, pp. 125–135.

Ramsoe, K., Buch-Andreasen, P., and Ranek, L.: Functioning liver mass in uncomplicated and fulminant acute hepatitis. Scand. J. Gastroent., *15*:65, 1980.

Drug Metabolism as a Measure of Hepatic Function

Bircher, J., Küpfer, A., Gikalov, I., and Preisig, R.: Aminopyrine demethylation measured by breath analysis in cirrhosis. Clin. Pharmacol. Ther., *20*:484, 1976.

Hepner, G. W., and Vesell, E. S.: Aminopyrine disposition: Studies on breath, saliva, and urine of normal subjects and patients with liver disease. Clin. Pharmacol. Ther., *20*:654, 1976.

Schenker, S., Hoyumpa, A. M., and Wilkinson, G. R.: The effect of parenchymal liver disease on the disposition and elimination of sedatives and analgesics. Med. Clin. North Am., *59*:887, 1975.

Dye Excretion Tests

Bircher, J., and Häcki, W.: A practical approach to quantitate hepatic excretory function. Yale J. Biol. Med., *3*:196, 1974.

Brody, D. H., and Leichter, L.: Clearance tests of liver function. Med. Clin. North Am., *63*:621, 1979.

Javitt, N.: Clinical and experimental aspects of sulfabromophthalein and related compounds. *In* Popper, H., and Schaffner, F. (eds.): Progress in Liver Diseases, Vol. III. New York, Grune & Stratton, 1970, pp. 110–117.

Paumgartner, G.: The handling of indocyanine green by the liver. Schweiz. Med. Wochenschr., [Suppl.] 105, 1975.

Serum Bile Acid Levels

Barnes, S., Gallo, G. A., Trash, D. B., and Morris, J. S.: Diagnostic value of serum bile acid estimations in liver disease. J. Clin. Path., *28*:506, 1975.

Boucher, I. A., and Pennington, C. R.: Serum bile acids in hepatobiliary disease. Gut, *19*:492, 1978.

Demers, L. M., and Hepner, G.: Radioimmunoassay of bile acids in serum. Clin. Chem., *22*:602, 1976.

Hofman, A. F.: Enterohepatic circulation of bile acids in man. Adv. Intern. Med., *21*:501, 1976.

Javitt, N. B.: Bile acid and hepatobiliary disease. *In* Schiff, L., and Schiff, E. R. (eds.): Diseases of the Liver, 5th ed. Philadelphia, J. B. Lippincott Co., 1982, pp. 119–150.

Korman, M. G., Hofman, A. F., and Summerskill, W. H. J.: Assessment of activity in chronic active liver disease: Serum bile acids compared with conventional tests and histology. N. Engl. J. Med., *290*:1399, 1974.

Palmer, R. H.: Bile salts and the liver. *In* Popper, H., and Schaffner, F. (eds.): Progress in Liver Diseases, Vol. VII. New York, Grune & Stratton, 1982, p. 221.

Blood Clotting in Liver Disease

Aledort, L. M.: Blood clotting abnormalities in liver disease. *In* Popper, H., and Schaffner, F. (eds.): Progress in Liver Diseases, Vol. V. New York, Grune & Stratton, 1976, pp. 350–362.

Dymock, I. W., Tucker, J. S., Woolf, I. L., Poller, L., and Thomson, J. M.: Coagulation studies as a prognostic index in acute liver failure. Br. J. Hematol., *29*:385, 1975.

Green, G., Poller, L., Thomson, J. M., and Dymock, I. W.: Factor VII as a marker of hepatocellular function in liver disease. J. Clin. Path., *29*:971, 1976.

Liebman, H. A., Furie, B. C., and Furie, B.: Hepatic Vitamin K-dependent carboxylation of blood-clotting proteins. Hepatology, *2*:488, 1982.

Ratnoff, O. D.: Disordered homeostasis in liver disease. *In* Schiff, L., and Schiff, E. R. (eds.): Diseases of the Liver, 5th ed. Philadelphia, J. B. Lippincott Co., 1982, pp. 237–258.

Radioisotopic and Other Special Procedures Employed in Diagnosis of Hepatobiliary Disease

Bragg, D. G., and Evans, J. A.: Roentgen aspects of liver and biliary tract diseases. *In* Schiff, L. (ed.): Diseases of the Liver, 4th ed. Philadelphia, J. B. Lippincott Co., 1975, pp. 1246–1277.

Brill, A. B., and Palton, D. D.: Radioisotope methods in diagnosis and assessment of liver metabolism. Int. J. Radiation Oncology Biol. Phys., *1*:981, 1976.

Edmonson, H. A., Schiff, L., and Schiff, E. R.: Needle biopsy of the liver. *In* Schiff, L., and Schiff, E. R. (eds.): Diseases of the Liver, 5th ed. Philadelphia, J. B. Lippincott Co., 1982, pp. 303–332.

Parks, S. N., Blaisdell, F. W., and Lim, R. C.: Special diagnostic tests for the evaluation of liver and biliary tract disorders. Surg. Clin. North Am., *57*:295, 1977.

Pereirus, R.: Special radiologic procedures in liver diseases. *In* Schiff, L., and Schiff, E. R. (eds.): Diseases of the Liver, 5th ed. Philadelphia, J. B. Lippincott Co., 1982, pp. 1451–1506.

Taylor, K. J. W., Neumann, R. D., and Russo, R. D.: Ultrasonography, scintography and computerized tomographic scanning of the hepatobiliary system. *In* Schiff, L., and Schiff, E. R. (eds.): Diseases of the Liver, 5th ed. Philadelphia, J. B. Lippincott Co., 1982, pp. 1349–1394.

Virologic and Other Serologic Tests for Diagnosis of Hepatic Disease

Glynn, L. E.: Immunopathology of liver disease. *In* Popper, H., and Schaffner, F. (eds.): Progress in Liver Diseases, Vol. V. New York, Grune & Stratton, 1976, pp. 311–325.

Hoofnagle, J. H.: Viral hepatitis. *In* Hook, E. W., Mandell, G., Gwaltney, J., and Sande, M. (eds.): Current Concepts of Infectious Disease. New York, John Wiley & Sons, 1977, pp. 243–261.

Husby, G., Skrede, S., Blomboff, J. P., Jacobsen, C. D., Berg, K., and Gjone, E.: Serum immunoglobulins and organ nonspecific antibodies in diseases of the liver. Scand. J. Gastroent., *12*:297, 1977.

Serum Levels of Iron, Ferritin, and Vitamin B_{12} in Liver Disease

Powell, L. W., and Holliday, J. W.: Iron, ferritin and the liver. *In* Popper, H., and Schaffner, F. (eds.): Progress in Liver Diseases, Vol. VII. New York, Grune & Stratton, 1982, pp. 599–614.

Rachmilewitz, M., and Eliakim, M.: Serum B_{12}—a diagnostic test in liver disease. Israel J. Med. Sci., *4*:47, 1968.

Serum Enzymes in Liver Disease

Karmen, A.: A note on the spectrophotometric assay of glutamic-oxaloacetic transaminase activity in human blood serum. J. Clin. Invest., *34*:131, 1955.

Kontinnen, A.: Serum enzymes as indicators of hepatic disease. Scand. J. Gastroent., 6:667, 1971.

Skrede, S., Blomboff, J. P., and Gjone, E.: Biochemical features of acute and chronic hepatitis. Ann. Clin. Res., *8*:182, 1976.

Zimmerman, H. J., and Seeff, L. B.: Enzymes in hepatic disease. *In* Coodley, E. L. (ed.): Diagnostic Enzymology. Philadelphia, Lea & Febiger, 1970, pp. 1–38.

Also see references for Chapter 14.

14
CLINICAL ENZYMOLOGY

HYMAN J. ZIMMERMAN, M.D.,
and JOHN BERNARD HENRY, M.D.

Enzymes, organic catalysts that are responsible for most of the chemical reactions of the body, are found in all tissues. Some have been identified in the plasma (or serum), to which they gain access from injured cells or even perhaps from intact cells. Interest of clinicians in serum enzymes began more than a half century ago with the demonstration of the usefulness of alkaline phosphatase levels in the diagnosis of osseous and hepatobiliary disease, of acid phosphatase levels in the diagnosis of carcinoma of prostate, and of amylase and lipase levels for the diagnosis of pancreatic disease. Despite the clinical usefulness of these parameters of disease and the demonstration, during the next 25 years, of a number of other enzymes in the serum, clinical interest in serum enzymology remained relatively dormant until 1953. The demonstration in that year of glutamate oxalacetate transaminase (GOT; aspartate aminotransferase [AST]) in the serum of normals and the subsequent observations that increased levels of this enzyme were helpful in the diagnosis of cardiac and hepatic disease led to a marked intensification of interest in serum enzymology.

By now, well over 50 enzymes have been identified in the serum (Zimmerman, 1970). The levels of many of these enzymes have been studied extensively in a variety of conditions (Table 14–1). Some serum enzyme tests have been applied so widely to clinical problems as to be considered routine laboratory procedures (Table 14–2, Group A). Others (Table 14–2, Group B), though clearly shown also to reflect various diseases reliably, are performed in relatively few clinical laboratories because the assay is technically difficult or because the information provided appears to add too little to that provided by the enzymes in Group A. Others are of investigative rather than regular clinical interest (Group C) or of importance only in special clinical situations (Group D). A fifth group (Group E) includes enzymes that have not been studied sufficiently to assess their clinical usefulness. In Table 14–1 are shown the main conditions in which abnormal values of the enzymes listed are found.

The usefulness of several serum enzymes (alkaline phosphatase, glutamate oxalacetate transaminase [GOT]—now called aspartate aminotransferase [AST], glutamate pyruvate transaminase [GPT]—now called alanine aminotransferase [ALT]) in the diagnosis of hepatic disease and of several other enzymes (amylase, lipase) in the diagnosis of pancreatic disease is considered in the chapters devoted to liver (Chapter 13) and pancreas (Chapter 24). In this chapter the more general aspects of serum enzymology are considered. The

Table 14–1. CLASSIFICATION OF ENZYMES DEMONSTRATED IN SERUM WITH TYPE AND DEGREE* OF ABNORMALITY IN DISEASE

	Condition†								
Type of Enzyme	***Hepatitis***	***Inf. Mono.***	***Cirrhosis***	***Met. Ca.***	***Obst. Jaundice***	***Heart Failure***	***Myocard. Infarct.***	***Prog. Musc. Dyst.***	***Comments or Other Abnormalities***
I. Carbohydrate metabolism									
A. Glycolytic									
1. Phosphoglucomutase	↑↑		N	↑	↑				
2. Phosphohexoisomerase (PHI)	↑↑↑	↑↑	↑	↑	↑	↑	↑↑	↑	Fig.14–7
3. Fructose 1,6-diphosphate aldolase (ALS)	↑↑↑	↑	↑	↑	N or ↑	↑	↑↑	↑↑↑	Fig. 14–7
4. Fructose-P-aldolase	↑↑↑			N	N		N	N	
5. Lactate dehydrogenase (LD)	↑	↑↑	↑	↑↑	N or ↑	↑	↑↑	↑↑	Table 14–11
6. Pyruvate kinase (PK)	↑↑			↑↑					
7. Enolase	↑						↑		Fig. 14–7
8. Triose-P-isomerase				↑					
9. Glyceraldehyde 3-P-dehydrogenase	↑	↑							
B. Hexose monophosphate shunt (pentose phosphate pathway)									
1. Glucose-6-phosphate dehydrogenase (GPD)	N		N		N		↑↑		Fig. 14–10
2. 6-P-Gluconate dehydrogenase (6-P-GD)	↑	↑							
3. 5-Phosphoriboisomerase	N		↑↑	↑↑	↑				
4. Transketolase	↑								
C. Citric acid cycle									
1. Malate dehydrogenase (MD)	↑↑↑	↑	↑	↑	↑	↑	↑↑		
2. Isocitrate dehydrogenase (ICD)	↑↑↑	↑	N or ↑	↑↑	N or ↑	↑	N	N	Fig. 14–9
3. Fumarase	↑		↑						
D. Other									
1. Amylase (AMS)	N	N	N or ↓	N	N	N	N	N	Chapter 24
2. β-Glucuronidase	↑↑						N or ↑		Ca, Pregnancy
3. Iditol dehydrogenase (ID)	↑↑↑	↑	↑	N or ↑	N or ↑		N	N	Fig. 14–13
II. Esterases									
A. Lipid									
1. Lipase (LPS)	N	N	N	N	N	N	N	N	Chapter 24
2. Aliesterase	N	N	N	N	N	N	N	N	Acute pancreatitis
3. Cholesterol esterase	↓		↓	N or ↓	N				
4. Lipoprotein lipase (LPL)	↑↑		↑↑		↓				
5. Lecithinase	N		N	N	N				Acute pancreatitis
6. Lecithin-cholesterol acyl transferase‡									
B. Nonlipid									
1. Cholinesterase (pseudo)	↓	↓	↓		N or ↑	N or ↑		N	Fig. 14–11
2. Phosphatases									
a. Alkaline phosphatase (ALP)	↑	↑	↑	↑↑	↑↑↑	↑	N	N	Increase in bone disease Table 14–6
b. Acid phosphatase (ACP)	N	N	N	N	N	N	N	N	Ca. of prostate
c. 5′-Nucleotidase (5′-N)	↑		↑	↑↑	↑↑↑				Normal in bone disease
d. Adenosine triphosphatase (ATPase)	↑		↑	↑	↑↑				Elevated in bone disease
3. Deoxyribonuclease I (DNase)	↑	±			N			N	Acute hemorrhagic pancreatitis
4. Ribonuclease (RNase)	N		N	N	N	↑	↑		Uremia, myeloma Leukemia
5. Adenosine deaminase	↑↑	↑↑↑	↑↑	↑↑↑		↑↑	N		
III. Protein and amino acid enzymes									
A. Proteolytic enzymes (trypsin)									Acute pancreatitis
B. Peptidases									
1. Leucine aminopeptidase (LAP)	↑	↑↑↑	↑	↑↑	↑↑↑	↑↑	N	N	Pregnancy Ca. of pancreas Pancreatitis
2. Aminotripeptidase	↑↑	↑↑	↑	↑↑	↑↑				
3. γ-Glutamyl transpeptidase (GGTP) (γ-Glutamyl transferase [GGT])	↑		↑	↑↑↑	↑↑	↑	↑↑		
C. Pepsinogen									Duod. ulcer
D. Amino acid substrate									
1. Aminotransferase (transaminases)									
a. Aspartate aminotransferase (AST) (Glutamate oxalacetate transaminase [GOT])	↑↑↑	↑↑	↑	↑	↑	↑	↑↑	↑↑	Table 14–10 Fig. 14–6
b. Alanine aminotransferase (ALT) (Glutamate pyruvate transaminase [GPT])	↑↑↑	↑↑	↑	↑	↑	↑	N or ↑	↑↑	Chapter 13
c. Glutamate dehydrogenase (GD)	↑↑	N	N or ↑	N	N	N	N	N	
2. Urea cycle									
a. Ornithine carbamoyl transferase (OCT)	↑↑↑		↑	↑↑					Acute cholecystitis
b. Arginase	↑↑		↑						Fig. 14–12

Table 14–1. CLASSIFICATION OF ENZYMES DEMONSTRATED IN SERUM WITH TYPE AND DEGREE* OF ABNORMALITY IN DISEASE *(Continued)*

	Condition†								
Type of Enzyme	***Hepa-titis***	***Inf. Mono.***	***Cirrho-sis***	***Met. Ca.***	***Obst. Jaundice***	***Heart Failure***	***Myocard. Infarct.***	***Prog. Musc. Dyst.***	***Comments or Other Abnormalities***
IV. Other enzymes									
A. Glutathione reductase (GR)	↑↑		↑	↑↑			↑		
B. Ceruloplasmin	↑↑		↑	↑↑	↑↑				Wilson's disease
C. Creatine kinase (CK) (Creatine phosphokinase (CPK))	N		N	N	N	N	↑↑↑	↑↑↑	Derma-tomyositis
D. Benzidine oxidase	↑		↑	↑↑↑	↑↑	↑	↑↑↑		Fig. 14–13
E. Hydroxybutyrate dehydrogenase (HBD)	↑	↑	±	↑	±	↑	↑↑↑	±	Isoenzyme of LD
F. Guanase	↑↑↑	↑	↑	↑	↑				
G. Alcohol dehydrogenase‡									
H. Acylase	↑↑		N	N	N	N	N	N	
I. Angiotensin-converting enzyme (ACE)‡									Elevated in sarcoidosis
J. Catalase‡									
K. Amine oxidase‡									
L. Prolyl hydroxylase‡									

* ↑-slight increase.
↑↑-moderate increase.
↑↑↑-marked increase.
N-no change.
±-variable
†Inf. Mono.—infectious mononucleosis.
Met. Ca.—metastatic carcinoma.
Obst. Jaundice—obstructive jaundice.
Prog. Musc. Dyst.—progressive muscular dystrophy.
Myocard. Infarct.—myocardial infarction.

principles of the methods for measuring enzyme activity are discussed, the possible factors responsible for abnormal values are analyzed, and special attention is devoted to a few of the enzymes found in the serum. Brief reference is made to enzymes of other body fluids and to the clinical significance of enzymes in the formed elements of the blood.

PRINCIPLES OF ENZYME ACTIVITY DETERMINATIONS

Because they are proteins that exist in very small amounts in biologic fluids and are so similar chemically, enzymes are measured for the most part by their activity rather than their concentration. Enzyme ac-

Table 14–2. CATEGORIZATION OF SERUM ENZYMES ACCORDING TO CLINICAL USEFULNESS

Group	Enzymes*
A. Routinely employed in most hospitals	ALP, ACP, lipase, amylase, AST (GOT), ALT (GPT), LD, CPK (CK), GGT
B. Clinically useful, but employed much less widely than enzymes in Group A	Pseudocholinesterase, LAP, 5′N, GGT, ALS, PHI, ICD, OCT, HBD, ID, LPS
C. Primarily of investigative interest; employed for routine clinical purposes in few or no hospitals	α-Lecithinase, LPL, aliesterase, fructose-6-P aldolase, MD, β-glucuronidase, GD, guanase, GR
D. Employed only in special circumstances	Ceruloplasmin (for diagnosis of Wilson's disease): pseudocholinesterase (to study patients with insecticide poisoning and patients with prolonged apnea after muscle relaxants), muramidase in patients with leukemia. ACE for diagnosis of sarcoidosis.
E. Data too scanty to evaluate prospective usefulness or indicative of no clinical utility	ATPases (alk. and acid), heroin esterase, procaine esterase; DNases (I and II), cholesterol esterase, glucokinase, phosphoglucomutase, triose-P-isomerase, glyceraldehyde-3-P dehydrogenase, phosphoglycerate dehydrogenase, enolase, 3-P-glyceric acid kinase, pyruvate kinase, malic enzyme, fumarase, succinic dehydrogenase, G-6-PD, 6-PGD, 5-P-riboisomerase, transketolase, tripeptidase, dipeptidases, oxytocinase, amine oxidases, arginase, adenosine deaminase, benzidine oxidase, et al.

*See Table 14–1 for meaning of abbreviations.

tivity is expressed in units that usually represent one of the following: (1) increase in concentration of one of the products, (2) decrease in concentration of substrate, or (3) change in concentration of coenzyme. The rate of change of any of these is a measure of rate of reaction.

Although a great deal of confusion has resulted from the lack of uniform terminology in the expression of units, attention has been directed to this problem and recommendations have been made by the Commission on Enzymes of the International Union of Biochemistry (Tables 14–3 and 14–4).

Immunochemical methods for the measurement of enzyme levels have found limited clinical application. Assays of levels of isoenzymes of LD, CK, ALP, and pepsinogen employing specific antisera have thus far been of mainly research interest. It is likely, however, that advances in purification of enzymes for the development of antisera and employment of radioimmunoassay will yield clinically useful methods for quantitation of amounts of circulating enzyme protein. Enzyme levels would then be expressed in concentration of enzyme rather than catalytic activity.

The numerical designation for each enzyme consists of four numbers separated by periods, e.g., E.C. 1.1.1.27 for lactate dehydrogenase. EC stands for "Enzyme Commission," the first number defines class (one of six reactions) to which the enzyme belongs while the next two numbers indicate subclass and sub-subclass to which the enzyme is assigned (Table 14–3). A specific serial number is the last number given each enzyme in its sub-subclass.

An enzyme may be considered as follows:

Holoenzyme = apoenzyme + coenzyme

Apoenzyme is the protein portion subject to denaturation, as are all proteins. This denaturation, due

Table 14–3. CLASSIFICATION OF ENZYMES: SIX CLASSES WHICH REFLECT SUBCLASSES AND SUB-SUBCLASSES

- I. Oxidoreductases
  - Oxidases
    - Cytochrome oxidase
  - Dehydrogenases
    - Iditol dehydrogenase (ID)
    - Lactate dehydrogenase (LD)
    - Malate dehydrogenase (MD)
    - Isocitrate dehydrogenase (ICD)
    - Glucose-6-phosphate dehydrogenase (GPD)
    - Hydroxybutyrate dehydrogenase (HBD)
- II. Transferases
  - Aspartate aminotransferase (AST) or glutamate oxalacetate transferase (GOT)
  - Alanine aminotransferase (ALT) or glutamate pyruvate transaminase (GPT)
  - Creatine kinase (CK) or creatine phosphokinase (CPK)
  - Gamma glutamyl transferase (GGT)
  - Ornithine carbamoyl transferase (OCT)
- III. Hydrolases
  - Esterases
    - Phosphatase, acid (ACP)
    - Phosphatase, alkaline (ALP)
    - Cholinesterase (CHS)
    - Lipase (LPS)
  - Peptidases
    - Leucine aminopeptidase (LAP)
    - Trypsin (PTS)
    - Pepsin (PPS)
  - Glycosidases
    - Amylase (AMS)
    - Amylo-1,6-glycosidase
    - Glucoside
    - Galactosidase
- IV. Lyases
  - Aldolase (ALS)
  - Glutamate decarboxylase
  - Pyruvate decarboxylase
  - Tryptophan decarboxylase
- V. Isomerases
  - Glucose phosphate isomerase
  - Ribose phosphate isomerase
- VI. Ligases

Table 14–4. UNITS FOR EXPRESSING ENZYME ACTIVITY

International unit (U)

1 unit (U) = the amount of enzyme that catalyzes the conversion of 1 micromole (microequivalent) of substrate or coenzyme per minute under the defined conditions of the test (temperature with optimal pH and substrate concentration). Activity may be expressed in units, milliunits, microunits, etc., per milliliter of sample. Concentration should be expressed in terms of U/ml or mU/ml = (U/L), whichever gives the more convenient minimal value.

1 unit = 1 micromole per minute (μ mol/min)

1 milliunit (mU) = 1 millimicromole per minute (mμmol/min)

1 microunit (μU) = 1 micromicromole per minute ($\mu\mu$mol/min)

Example:

Lactate dehydrogenase 25°C.

O. D. unit = O. D. of (.001)/min/ml

$$\text{Standard unit} = \frac{\text{O.D.}}{6.25} \times \frac{3.0}{0.2} = \text{O.D./min} \times 2.4$$

Standard unit = difference of 5 min lines on graph
= $\text{O.D.}_5 \times 0.48$
= O.D. × ½

Example:

Test gave O.D. = 0.020/min for 0.2 ml sample

Old method: O.D. = 20 × 5 = 100 O.D. units

Standard method: 0.020 × 2.4 = 0.048 units, or 48 mU

Normal range:

80 to 120 O.D. units

40 to 60 standard milliunits (mU)/ml

Recently, the katal has been recommended. One unit (U) is equal to one micromole catalyzed per minute. One katal is equal to one mole catalyzed per second. Thus, one U is equal to 16.67 nanokatals.

to physical and chemical agents, is associated with a loss of enzyme activity.

Coenzyme is the dialyzable portion and is essential for catalytic activity. It is tightly bound to enzyme and is not a protein. An example of a coenzyme is NAD (nicotinamide adenine dinucleotide). Another coenzyme (organic co-factor) is pyridoxal-5-phosphate, which is derived from pyridoxine; it is essential for aminotransferase (transaminase) activity.

Activators are substances which modify reactions catalyzed—metal ions such as zinc and magnesium, for example.

Enzymes display specificity with regard to substrate (substance which is acted on) and effect (chemical action). Lactate dehydrogenase catalyzes the following reaction:

$$\text{Lactate} + \text{NAD}^+ \rightleftharpoons \text{Pyruvate} + \text{NADH} + \text{H}^+$$

It catalyzes both the forward and reverse reactions as indicated. It acts virtually only on L-lactic acid and pyruvic acid as substrates and catalyzes the reversible transfer of hydrogen between lactate and NAD. Other enzymes are required for the decarboxylation or amination of pyruvic acid.

Many chemical and physical agents exert a marked influence on enzymes. Temperature and hydrogen ion concentration are probably the two best-studied agents. Inactivation of most enzymes will occur in the neighborhood of 65°C. Freezing, however, does not usually destroy enzymes. For each 10°C. rise in temperature (Q_{10}), some enzymes will demonstrate a two-fold increase in activity, but the increase in denaturation may be even greater. Hence, the temperature activity curve for an enzyme will show a maximum, depending on the opposed activating and denaturing effects of rising temperature. Although there is not complete agreement, 37°C. appears to be the best single choice of reaction temperature, followed by 30°C. for the majority of clinical serum enzyme assays. Statland (1977) has reviewed the arguments regarding one temperature versus another. These fall into chemical, technical, and economic categories.

A bell-shaped curve will also often describe the optimal pH for an enzyme (Fig. 14–1). This may also reflect the cumulative effects of hydrogen ion concentration on activation and denaturation of enzyme protein.

Although an enzyme reaction represents very complex mechanisms that are not fully understood, it can be stated that an enzyme reversibly forms a transitory complex with its substrate. Functional groups of coenzymes or prosthetic groups or both may play a role in the formation of the enzyme-substrate complex. The enzyme-substrate complex decomposes to enzyme and product. The enzyme is not altered in the overall reaction. The Michaelis-Menten hypothesis describes

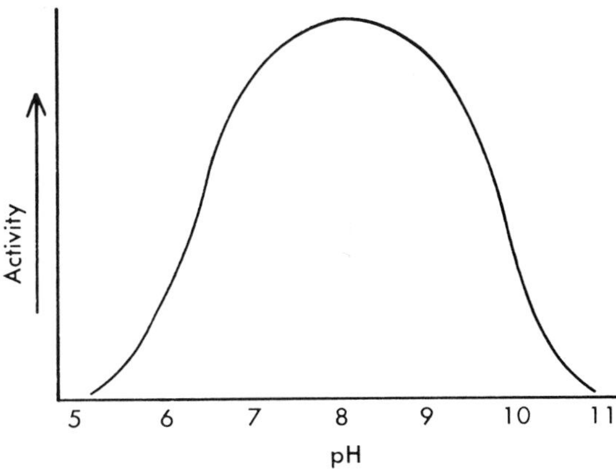

Figure 14–1. Typical curve of activity versus pH for an enzymatic reaction. (From Henry, J. B.: Postgrad. Med., *33*:A-66, 1963.)

this sequence of events, as shown at the bottom of this page.

In addition to a high substrate concentration, with the important assumption of an intermediate enzyme-substrate complex, this theory further states that the rate of conversion of the substrate to the products of the reaction is determined by the rate of conversion of the enzyme-substrate complex to reaction products and the enzyme.

Units of enzyme activity are best expressed in terms of rate of the catalyzed reaction. The rate of reaction can be considered graphically (Figs. 14–2 and 14–3). In Figure 14–2, the relative rate of reaction is expressed as a function of substrate concentration [S]. At low concentration, the rate is first order* with respect to [S]. The rate is zero order,* independent of [S], at a high concentration. In measuring enzyme activity, one should use this part of the curve.

In an enzyme assay, one may measure activity as ΔP (increase in product) or ΔS (decrease in substrate) depending on which is more convenient analytically (Fig. 14–3). Often the product or substrate may be colored and, if so, may be quantitatively determined by colorimetry or spectrophotometry. The concentration of coenzyme (e.g., NAD with virtually no absorption at 340 nm; NADH with maximal absorp-

*A first-order enzyme reaction is one in which the rate of reaction is determined by the concentration of substrate as well as of enzyme. Accordingly, the reaction rate changes continuously with time as the substrate is consumed, and measurement of enzyme activity is difficult. In zero-order enzyme reaction, the rate of reaction is linear with time, independent of the concentration of substrate and directly proportional to the concentration of enzyme (Fig. 14–4). The greater ease of measuring enzyme activity in a zero order, than in a first-order reaction, is shown in Figure 14–5.

$$\text{Enzyme (E)} + \text{substrate (S)} \underset{k_2}{\overset{k_1}{\rightleftharpoons}} \text{enzyme-substrate complex (ES)}$$

$$\downarrow k_3$$

$$(k_1, k_2, k_3 = \text{rate constants}) \qquad \text{products (P)} + \text{enzyme (E)}$$

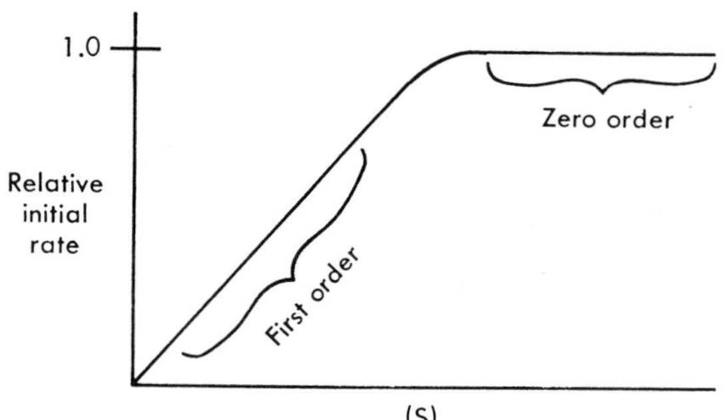

Figure 14–2. Relative rate of reaction expressed as function of substrate concentration *(S)*. (From Henry, J. B.: Postgrad. Med., *33*:A-66, 1963.)

tion at 340 nm) can be measured spectrophotometrically as in the lactate dehydrogenase assay.

An enzyme exerts maximal influence when substrate concentration is highest and product concentration nil. This is most likely to be the case at the beginning of the reaction, when the rate is described as zero order with respect to substrate, followed by a progressive decrease in reaction velocity as equilibrium is reached. Zero-order reaction rate simply means in this case that the rate is constant and independent of substrate and product concentrations. If reaction is zero order, concentration of product will rise linearly with respect to time (Fig. 14–3*a*). Ideally, enzyme assays are performed under conditions which permit reaction to approach zero order with respect to product and substrate during the entire measuring period. Multiple or serial determinations of substrate or product concentration against time are recorded in the assay.

To be valid, an enzyme assay must be so designed that the enzyme concentration is the only limiting factor; i.e., the result reflects the amount of enzyme and is not influenced by other substances present. This is illustrated graphically in Figure 14–4. The rate of product formation increases proportionately with enzyme concentration, e.g., one unit of product formed per minute per each 0.1 ml of serum. Ultimately, the concentration of enzyme exceeds the amount of substrate available; i.e., substrate concentration becomes a limiting factor and proportionality is no longer present. At this point, the assay is no longer a reflection of enzyme activity.

Figure 14–5 illustrates potential hazards of utilizing a single measurement. With a single or one-point (E) measuring system, three different reaction rates would have given the same apparent activity.

An assay system must progress in a zero-order reaction during its entire period of observation if the measurement is to reflect true enzyme activity. Performance of multiple determinations has the advantage of permitting assessment of kinetics and confirmation of zero-order reaction.

Multiple-point or serial measurements of the concentration of products per unit time permit the recognition of rapid attainment of equilibrium and substrate exhaustion with samples of biologic fluids containing very high concentrations of enzyme. In such instances it is preferable to use a smaller volume of sample rather than to make dilutions of sample in repeat assays. In the lactate dehydrogenase assay, the volume ratio, i.e., volume of sample to volume of total assay, should be reduced when very high concentrations of enzyme activity are suspected. Inhibition of enzyme may be suspected when the enzymatic reaction is proceeding at a rate less than expected (Fig. 14–5, curve D). Partial, total, reversible, or irreversible inhibition may occur. Competitive reversible inhibition occurs when the inhibitor resembles the substrate sufficiently to combine with it and form a complex (EI); this complex does not break down to form products. A higher substrate concentration may overcome such inhibition.

Numerous pitfalls are encountered in enzyme assays

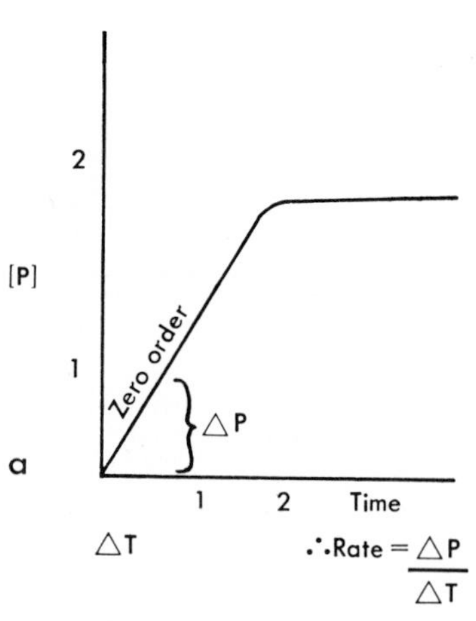

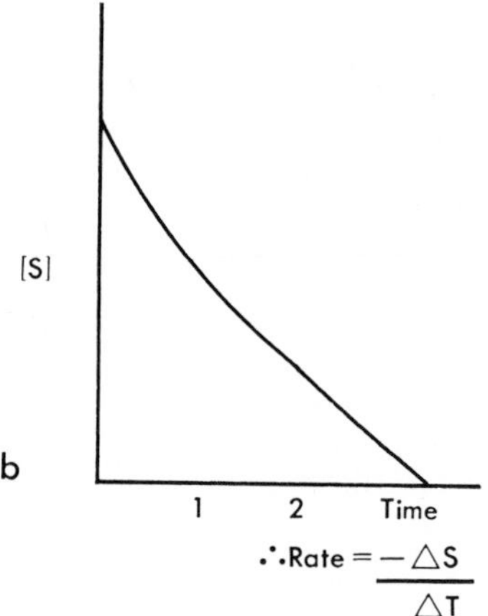

△P = Change in product concentration
△S = Change in substrate concentration
△T = Change in time
[P] = Product concentration
[S] = Substrate concentration

Figure 14–3. Rate of product formation *(a)* and substrate disappearance *(b)*. (From Henry, J. B.: Postgrad. Med., *33*:A-68, 1963.)

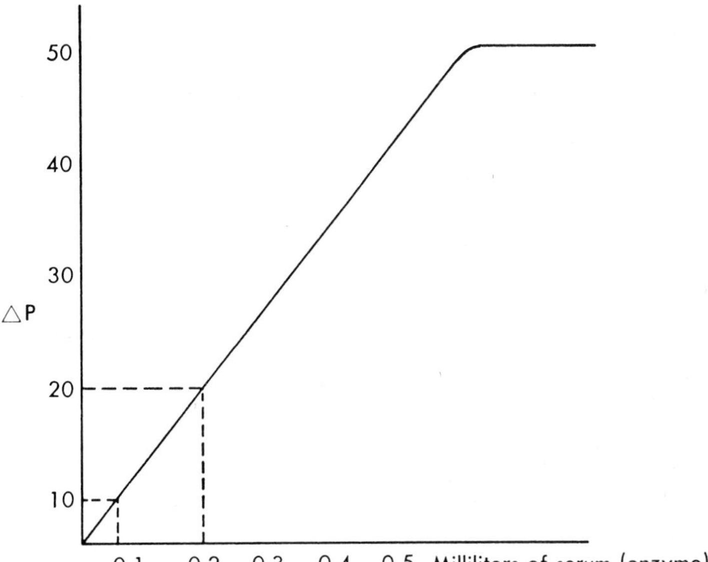

Figure 14–4. Change in product concentration *(ΔP)* as a function of enzyme concentration. The abscissa represents increments of serum added to reaction mixture. (From Henry, J. B.: Postgrad. Med., *33*:A-70, 1963.)

2

in the clinical laboratory. Hemolysis may be associated with the release of enzymes from red blood cells into the serum, causing falsely high serum values. Because of the adverse effects on enzyme activity of various anticoagulants, serum rather than plasma is the preferred specimen for clinical enzyme assays. Lactescence, or milky serum, may result in variable absorbance readings in spectrophotometric assays. Most

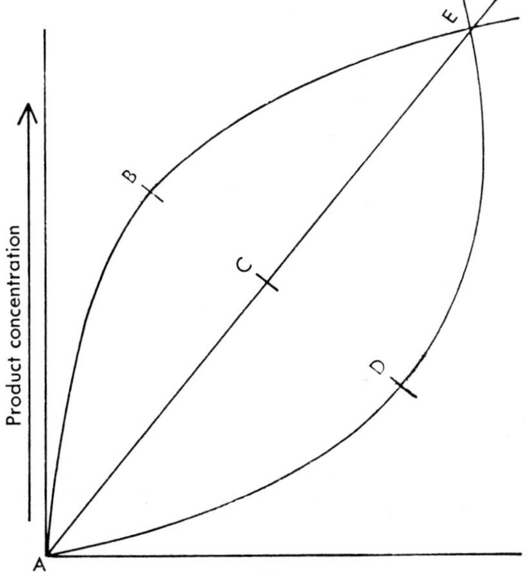

Figure 14–5. Illustration of potential hazards of using a single determination in enzyme assays. Line *ACE* is a zero-order reaction that permits accurate determination of enzyme activity for the entire reaction time. Curve *ABE* shows initial zero-order reaction of high rate followed by falling off of rate of reaction. This is possibly due to exhaustion of substrate prior to termination of assay at point *E*. Curve *ADE* reveals an initial lag phase which masks true activity. (From Henry, J. B.: Postgrad. Med., *33*:A-72, 1963.)

enzymes in biologic fluids are quite stable at 6°C. for at least 24 hours and at room temperature for lesser periods. For prolonged storage, temperatures of −20°C. or lower* must be used in order to assure preservation of enzyme activity. Heat lability must be considered with respect to each enzyme to be assayed as well as other components in the entire enzyme system, especially coenzymes and substrates. Accuracy in timing each assay and use of meticulously clean glassware are essential.

Enzyme assays requiring kinetic measurements in the ultraviolet wavelength region pose new problems for many clinical laboratories. Most of these procedures depend on the changes in absorption at 340 nm of pyridine nucleotides ($NAD^+ \rightarrow NADH$). Owing to the increasing number of nucleotide-dependent enzymes of clinical importance, the ability to work in the 340 nm range is more important. Indeed, a spectrophotometer which measures accurately in the ultraviolet range is virtually essential in clinical enzymology.

A review of the lactate dehydrogenase determination underscores salient features of clinical enzyme assays. In the pH range 7 to 8, the equilibrium favors reduction of pyruvate to lactate, whereas the reverse reaction is favored in the pH range 9 to 10. Wacker (1956) has reported a lactate dehydrogenase assay incorporating a buffer at pH 8.8, lactate as the substrate, and NAD^+ as the coenzyme. The addition of serum provides enzyme, and the assay is conducted at 25°C. Spectrophotometric measurements of absorbance (optical density) are made each minute for 5 minutes at wavelength 340 nm. Lactate is oxidized

*Some enzymes (e.g., CK) do not remain reliably preserved at −20°C. and must be kept at −70°C. to retain activity. A few enzymes are inactivated at refrigerator temperatures, e.g., lactate dehydrogenase (liver isoenzymes, LD4 and LD5) is least stable at lower temperatures. Hence, sera for LD assays should not be refrigerated.

to pyruvate with conversion of coenzyme (NAD^+) to reduced coenzyme (NADH). The multiple measurements at 1-minute intervals provide an assessment of adherence to zero-order reaction. One unit of activity represents a change in absorbance of 0.001 optical density units per ml of serum per minute at 25°C. This in turn can be converted to International Units (U/L) as shown in Table 14–4.

Cabaud (1958) reported a colorimetric assay for lactate dehydrogenase in which the substrate pyruvate is converted to lactate at 37°C. Pyruvic acid reacts with 2,4-dinitrophenylhydrazine to form a colored hydrazone. The amount of pyruvate remaining after the incubation is inversely proportional to the amount of lactate dehydrogenase present in the reaction.

To ensure accuracy and precision in clinical enzyme determinations, one must be aware of the pitfalls and informed regarding the principles of enzyme assays. A quality control program for clinical enzyme assays should include the following: (1) adherence to zero-order kinetics, (2) proportionality studies with increments of sample, (3) use of pooled frozen serum or stable reference materials (lyophilized) as control solutions, and (4) replicate measurements to evaluate precision of assay.

PRINCIPLES OF DIAGNOSTIC SERUM ENZYMOLOGY

All the serum enzymes have their origin in cells. Some enzymes are found in many tissues (e.g., lactate dehydrogenase [LD], aldolase [ALS], phosphohexoisomerase [PHI], malate dehydrogenase [MD]). Other enzymes are uniquely concentrated in one or two tissues. For example, ornithine carbamoyl transferase (OCT) and iditol dehydrogenase (ID) are found almost exclusively in the liver; significant amounts of creatine kinase (CK) are found only in skeletal muscle, myocardium, and brain. Increase in the serum levels of an enzyme which is ubiquitous in its distribution is a less specific biochemical clue to the site of injury than increased levels of an enzyme normally found in only one or two tissues. In order to enhance the diagnostic value of serum enzymology, attention has been directed to the different molecular forms of a given enzyme (isoenzyme) that may be found in different tissues. Isoenzymes of amylase, alkaline phosphatase (ALP), acid phosphatase, glutamate oxalacetate transaminase (GOT)—now called aspartate aminotransferase (AST)—leucine aminopeptidase (LAP), LD, MD, isocitric dehydrogenase (ICD), creatine kinase (CK), cholinesterase, and other enzymes have been demonstrated in different tissues and are of interest to the biochemist, physiologist, geneticist, and clinical investigator. Only the isoenzymes of the LD, CK, and ALP, however, have been of important clinical relevance. These are discussed and the types of methods available for their demonstration are listed in a subsequent portion of this chapter. Some enzymes are found in the cytoplasm of cells and reach the plasma with relatively slight injury (LD, ALS). Enzymes that are found only in mitochondria (e.g., glutamate dehydrogenase) gain entry to the serum as the result of sufficient injury to those organelles. At present, the efforts to define the organelle injury by correlation of the intracellular source of the enzyme with the serum levels are of investigative rather than clinical relevance.

The use of serum enzymes as diagnostic aids has been largely empirical; but the values observed in clinical and experimental circumstances permit speculative analysis of the factors that lead to abnormal levels in diseased subjects (Table 14–5). The serum levels of a particular enzyme may be increased in diseases that lead to increased rates of release from tissue, increased amount available for release, or decreased rate of disposition. The levels of an enzyme may be decreased in disease that interferes with its production.

Increased rate of release is clearly responsible for the high serum levels of hepatic, pancreatic, and myocardial enzymes in diseases that produce necrosis of the respective tissue. The pattern of abnormality of serum enzyme values that results depends on the normal enzyme content of the tissue involved, on the extent and type of necrosis, and on other poorly understood factors. Thus, high serum levels of a number of digestive enzymes are found in acute pancreatitis, and a number of enzymes of intermediary metabolism are found in myocardial infarction or acute hepatitis. Although these enzymes are richly concentrated in both liver and myocardium, higher levels are produced by hepatitis than by myocardial infarction, presumably because the necrosis and degeneration of hepatitis are diffuse and those of infarction, discrete.

High serum levels of enzymes* in which liver is uniquely rich (ALT or GPT, OCT, ID) are produced almost exclusively by acute hepatic disease. The minimal degree of elevation of serum ICD levels in myocardial infarction, despite the rich myocardial content of this enzyme, has been attributed to the rapid removal of this enzyme from the circulation. The relatively slight increase of LD levels in hepatic necrosis, despite the high hepatic content of this enzyme, remains to be explained adequately. Conceivably, it may relate to the simultaneous release of an inhibitor of LD.

Increased rate of release of enzyme into the circulation may occur even without apparent tissue necrosis. Increased permeability of cell membranes seems to account for the elevated serum levels of aldolase, CK, and other enzymes in progressive muscular dystrophy. The high serum levels of CK, GOT, ALS, PHI, LD, and MD in patients with delirium tremens or alcoholic myopathy, but without recognizable liver disease, also may depend upon increased permeability of skeletal muscle membrane.

An increase in the tissue source of enzymes because of increased rate of production per cell or increase in the number of cells may be responsible for increased serum levels. This seems to be the mechanism for the increased levels of pepsinogen, ALP, and acid phos-

*See Table 14–1 for meaning of abbreviations.

Table 14–5. HYPOTHETICAL MECHANISMS FOR ABNORMAL SERUM ENZYME LEVELS

Mechanism	Example	Enzymes	Comments
I. Increased serum levels			
A. Increased release			
1. Necrosis	Myocardial infarction	AST (GOT), LD, ALS, MD, GR, CK, HBD, RNase, and others	
	Acute hepatitis	AST (GOT), ALT (GPT), OCT, ICD, ID, GD, LD, ALS, PHI, MD, GR, ALP, LAP, and others	Increased levels of some enzymes (ALP) may represent increased production as well as release from necrotic cells and decreased excretion
	Acute pancreatitis	Amylase, lipase, lecithinase, trypsin, DNase I	
2. Increased permeability; cell membranes without necrosis	Progressive muscular dystrophy, delirium tremens, dermatomyositis	CK, ALS, LD, PHI, MD, AST (GOT), ALT (GPT)	
B. Increased tissue source of enzymes; increased release from tissue or both	Neoplastic disease (carcinoma, lymphoma), granulocytic leukemia	LD, ALS, PHI, MD, GR, glucuronidase	
	Megaloblastic anemia	LD, ALS, PHI, MD	May be result of increased numbers of megaloblasts, increased intramedullary destruction, or both
	Osteoblastic lesions (Paget's disease, osteogenic sarcoma, healing fractures, rickets, etc.)	ALP, ATPase	
C. Impaired excretion of enzyme	Peptic ulcer	Pepsinogen	
	Uremia	Amylase	Elevated amylase levels secondary to renal failure rare and of uncertain origin
	Obstructive jaundice	ALP, LAP, 5-N, GGT	Increased production main factor in increased levels of ALP in obstructive jaundice
II. Decreased serum levels			
A. Decreased formation			
1. Genetic	Hypophosphatasia	ALP	
	Wilson's disease	Ceruloplasmin	
	Acholinesterasemia	Pseudocholinesterase	
2. Acquired	Hepatitis	Pseudocholinesterase	
	Starvation	Amylase (AMS)	
B. Enzyme inhibition	Insecticide poisoning	Pseudocholinesterase	
C. Lack of cofactors	Pregnancy? Cirrhosis?	AST	? Pyridoxine deficiency or defective pyridoxine metabolism

phatase in patients with peptic ulcer, osteoblastic bone lesions, and prostatic carcinoma, respectively. The serum levels of glycolytic and other enzymes associated with neoplastic diseases seem to reflect the total mass of tumor. Increased serum levels of angiotensin-converting enzymes (ACE) in sarcoidosis and leprosy reflect the rich content of the enzyme in the macrophages and epithelioid cells of the granuloma and in Gaucher's disease. There is evidence that the increased ALP levels of the serum in obstructive jaundice are primarily the result of increased hepatic production of the enzyme, although decreased biliary excretion may play a role.

Impaired disposition of serum enzymes has been considered to contribute to the increased levels of ALP and AST (GOT) in biliary obstruction and for increased amylase levels in renal failure. Evidence for this thesis is lacking. Experimental studies with the "LDH" agent suggest that the mechanism by which this virus causes increased serum levels of LD in mice is by interfering with the uptake of the enzyme by the reticuloendothelial system (Zimmerman, 1970).

Abnormally low levels of some serum enzymes are also observed, presumably as the result of decreased synthesis. Levels of cholinesterase and cholesterol esterase may be low in hepatic disease; levels of amylase are low in chronic hepatic or pancreatic disease or in starvation; levels of pepsinogen are low in gastric mucosal atrophy; levels of ALP are low in hypophosphatasia; and levels of ceruloplasmin are low in Wilson's disease.

The selection of serum enzyme tests for clinical use has depended on historical circumstance, the experience gained in correlating the values with other measures of disease, and the technical ease of performing the respective procedure. A serum enzyme, the diagnostic value of which has been established for a clinical setting, is not likely to be supplanted by a subsequently discovered one, unless the diagnostic usefulness of the more recent candidate is far superior to that of its predecessor. Alkaline phosphatase, a time-honored aid for the diagnosis of hepatobiliary disease, has not been replaced by leucine aminopeptidase* or 5′-nucleotidase,* despite recent reports of the diagnostic advantages of the latter two enzymes. Ornithine carbamoyl transferase* and iditol dehydrogenase,* more recent arrivals than ALT (GPT) to the serum enzyme scene, have not replaced the latter as measures of hepatic disease, despite reports of somewhat greater specificity,

The serum enzymes discussed in detail in this chapter are those which have been of the greatest clinical usefulness or interest in the past or which hold the most promise. Particular attention is given to the phosphatases, transaminases (aminotransferases), lactate dehydrogenase and its isoenzymes, and cholinesterase. Many of the other serum enzymes are described, and their clinical relevance is discussed briefly.

Phosphatases

The phosphatases of the blood, more properly called phosphomonoesterases or orthophosphoric ester monohydrolases, include two main types. The "alkaline phosphatase" has a pH optimum of approximately 9, while the "acid phosphatase" has its optimal activity at a pH of approximately 5. Although there is evidence that alkaline and acid phosphatases each include several different enzymes (isoenzymes), it has been convenient for clinical purposes to consider each a single enzyme.

Alkaline Phosphatase (EC 3.1.3.1). The application of ALP determination to the study of hepatic disease is discussed in Chapter 13. The demonstration that bone is rich in alkaline phosphatase and that normal plasma (or serum) contains the same or a similar enzyme led to the study of serum ALP levels in patients with diseases of bone. Elevated levels of the enzyme occur in patients with bone diseases characterized by increased osteoblastic activity (Table 14–6). These include osteitis deformans, rickets, osteomalacia, hyperparathyroidism, healing fractures, and osteoblastic bone tumors, both primary and secondary. Growing children and pregnant women in the third trimester have "physiologically" elevated serum ALP levels.

Lower than normal levels are observed in patients with hypophosphatasia (an inborn error of metabolism), and in malnourished patients.

The alkaline phosphatase determination is useful in the recognition of diseases of bone, especially osteitis deformans, hyperparathyroidism, and bone neoplasms. Hepatic disease as a cause of serum ALP elevation usually can be distinguished by other laboratory procedures and clinical features. The increased levels of this enzyme in normal, growing children should be kept in mind when attempting to apply the serum alkaline phosphatase levels to diagnosis.

Isoenzymes of Alkaline Phosphatase. Studies of the properties of ALP isolated from various tissues (liver, bone, spleen, kidney, intestine) indicate that each differs from the others. Total serum ALP in normals consists of isoenzymes contributed by liver, bone, and, in some individuals, intestine. During the last trimester of pregnancy 40 to 65 per cent of the serum ALP derives from placenta. Isoenzymes from these four sources have been distinguished from each other by electrophoretic analysis, differential inhibition by chemicals and heat, and immunochemically, although there are also differences in substrate dependence and reaction kinetics.

The degrees of inhibition of isoenzymes of hepatic, osseous, intestinal, and placental origin produced by heating to 56°C. for 15 minutes, exposure to 3 M urea for 18 minutes, incubation with 5×10^{-3} M L-phenylalanine, and the relative electrophoretic migration of these isoenzymes are shown in Table 14–7. (Note that the Regan isoenzyme, found in the serum of about 5 per cent of patients with carcinomas of various types, resembles the placental ALP). These properties are helpful in identifying placental and intestinal ALP (both phenylalanine-inhibited) and in distinguishing them from hepatic and bone isoenzymes. Distinction of hepatic from osseous ALP is aided by heat or urea inhibition, but the overlapping effects lead to imprecision. Nevertheless, the susceptibility of the osseous isoenzyme to heat inactivation has been applied quite widely to distinguish it from the hepatic isoenzyme. Electrophoretic analysis of ALP isoenzymes employing acrylamide gel will also, in most instances, permit identification of the main isoenzyme contributing to an elevated level. Quantitation of the fractions, however, is prevented by the lack of distinct separation of the two rapidly moving isoenzymes (hepatic and osseous). None of the physicochemical methods employed is reliable in distinguishing between hepatocellular and posthepatic jaundice as a cause of elevated ALP levels, although an isoenzyme which migrates more slowly than any of the others has been described in the serum of patients with posthepatic jaundice. Regular clinical application of ALP isoenzymology, however, has awaited better

*See later section of chapter for description of these enzymes.

Table 14–6. CONDITIONS IN WHICH THE SERUM ALKALINE PHOSPHATASE LEVEL IS INCREASED*

Hepatobiliary Disease		Bone Disease		Other Conditions	
Obstructive jaundice	↑↑↑	Osteitis deformans	↑↑↑	Healing fractures	↑
Biliary cirrhosis	↑↑↑	Rickets	↑↑	Normal growth	↑
Intrahepatic cholestasis	↑↑↑	Osteomalacia	↑↑	Pregnancy (last trimester)	↑
Space-occupying lesions (granuloma, abscess, metastatic carcinoma)	↑↑	Hyperparathyroidism	↑↑		
		Metastatic bone disease	↑↑		
		Osteogenic sarcoma	↑↑↑		
Viral hepatitis	↑				
Infectious mononucleosis	↑↑				
Cirrhosis (alcoholic)	↑				

*Degree of increase indicated by number of arrows. Depressed values: hypophosphatasia, malnutrition.

2

means of quantitation of the individual isoenzymes and adequate extensive testing of quantitative values in clinical circumstances (Gorman, 1977).

As discussed in Chapter 13, the probable hepatic origin of an elevated serum ALP level can be recognized by assay of LAP, 5′-N, or GGT activity. Values for these enzymes are high in patients whose hepatobiliary disease leads to high ALP levels but not in those with osseous disease responsible for this increased phosphatase value (Table 14–8).

Study of placental ALP has yielded interesting data. It appears in plasma at the beginning of the second trimester of pregnancy, rises to a maximum during the third trimester, when it contributes 40 to 65 per cent of ALP activity, and then declines to normal during the first postpartum month.

Acid Phosphatase (ACP) (EC 3.1.3.2). This enzyme, first demonstrated in the urine in 1925, was found to be much more prevalent in male than in female urine. It was soon shown that prostatic tissue contains this enzyme in high concentration. Another acid phosphatase, which differs from that found in the prostate (Table 14–9), is present in erythrocytes and platelets. The methods used for determination of acid phosphatase are similar to and include the same substrates as those used for alkaline phosphatase assay.

Elevated serum levels of acid phosphatase (ACP) are seen in patients with prostatic carcinoma that has metastasized. One half to three fourths of patients with carcinoma of the prostate that has extended beyond the capsule have elevated acid phosphatase levels. Patients with prostatic carcinoma still confined within the capsule usually have normal serum levels of this enzyme. However, patients with benign prostatic hypertrophy may have slight elevations of the serum ACP level after vigorous prostatic "massage." Since other tissues, such as erythrocytes, may also release acid phosphatase into the serum, minor elevations of enzyme levels may reflect such an origin rather than the prostate. Accordingly, efforts have been made to distinguish "prostatic" ACP from the isoenzymes that are of erythrocyte and other origin. The efforts to distinguish "prostatic" acid phosphatase from erythrocyte acid phosphatase have been based on the differential effect of various substrates and various inhibitors on enzymes from these two sources (Table 14–9). The inhibition of prostatic acid phosphatase by tartrate and the lack of inhibition by cupric ion, compared with the lack of inhibition of erythrocyte ACP by tartrate and the inhibition by cupric ion, are the properties most commonly utilized (Table 14–9). Acid phosphatase (ACP) released from platelets, however, resembles prostatic enzyme in its response to inhibitors (Wilkinson, 1976).

Elevations of the serum ACP using the method of Bodansky (β-glycerophosphate as substrate) usually reflect carcinoma of the prostate (as discussed previously), especially if the levels exceed 5 Bodansky units. When the method of Gutman (phenylphosphate as substrate) or the King-Armstrong method is used,

Table 14–7. CHARACTERISTICS OF ISOENZYMES OF ALKALINE PHOSPHATASE

	Inhibition* by		
Source of Enzyme	***L-Phenylalanine*† (%)**	***Heat‡ or Urea§* (%)**	**Order Anodal Migration**
Liver	10	60	1
Bone	10	90	2
Intestine	75	60	4
Placenta	80	0	3
Regan (carcinoma)	80	0	3

*Approximate figures.
†L-Phenylalanine (5×10^{-3} M).
‡56°C for 15 minutes.
§3M concentration.

Table 14–8. RELATIVE VALUES* FOR ALKALINE PHOSPHATE AND ENZYMES THAT REFLECT ITS HEPATIC ISOENZYMES IN SEVERAL CLINICAL SETTINGS

	Hepatobiliary Disease				
	Hepatocellular	*Cholestatic or Posthepatic*	*Infiltrative*	**Osseous Disease**	**Alcoholism or Inducing Drugs**
ALP†	1+	3+	3+	1–3+	±
5′N†	1+	3+	3+	—	—
LAP†	1+	3+	3+	—	—
GGT†	1+	3+	3+	—	1–3+

*Number of +'s indicates relative degree of elevation.
†ALP = Alkaline phosphates.
5′N = 5′ Nucleotidase.
LAP = Leucine aminopeptidase.
GGT = 2-Glutamylpeptidase.

other diseases may yield abnormal levels occasionally. Such elevations are frequent in Gaucher's disease and occasional in osteitis deformans.

Acid phosphatase (ACP) determination has been useful in detecting metastases from carcinoma of the prostate. As a diagnostic clue to the presence of resectable carcinoma of the prostate, however, it is of no value.

Schumann (1976) has confirmed that quantitative ACP determination of vaginal specimens may substantiate the allegation of rape.

Leucine Aminopeptidase (LAP) (EC 3.4.1.1)

A number of peptidases have been identified in the serum of patients with various diseases. One of these, leucine aminopeptidase (LAP, naphthylamidase*), has been studied more extensively than the others. Elevated levels of this serum enzyme have been reported in most types of hepatobiliary disease. These include hepatitis, cirrhosis, obstructive jaundice, metastatic carcinoma of the liver, and pancreatitis. Patients with carcinoma of the pancreas have increased levels only if obstructive jaundice or metastases to the liver have developed. The elevated values observed during the last trimester of pregnancy appear to be of placental origin. Although several isoenzymes of LAP have been identified, there has been no clinical application of LAP isoenzymology.

*Recent usage has favored the term "naphthylamidase" rather than LAP, since the enzyme is usually assayed by employing an acyl-β-naphthylamide as substrate.

Table 14–9. EFFECT OF INHIBITORS ON ACID PHOSPHATASE OF PROSTATE AND OTHER TISSUES*

Inhibitor	Inhibition of Prostatic Phosphatase	Inhibition of Erythrocyte Phosphatase
L(+)−Tartaric acid 0.02 M	+	−
Formaldehyde 2%	−	+
Cupric sulfate 0.001 M	−	+

* + represents marked inhibition.
− represents minimal inhibition.

The serum values for this enzyme in patients with hepatobiliary disease appear to parallel those of alkaline phosphatase, with the highest levels in obstructive biliary disease and only moderately elevated levels in hepatocellular injury. Values for LAP, however, are normal in patients with bone disease. This has led to the suggestion that distinction between osseous and hepatobiliary disease as a cause of elevated alkaline phosphatase levels can be provided by assay of LAP activity (Table 14–8), but LAP determination has enjoyed a limited popularity.

5′-Nucleotidase (5′-N) (EC 3.1.3.5)

A serum esterase that has been the subject of a number of recent reports is 5′-nucleotidase. Introduced as a measure for the differentiation of obstructive from hepatocellular jaundice and of hepatobiliary from osseous disease, 5′-N has been the subject of a number of studies. The effects of disease on serum levels of 5′-N are similar to those on LAP. The highest values are observed in patients with posthepatic jaundice, intrahepatic cholestasis, and infiltrative lesions of the liver. Relatively slightly elevated levels are observed in patients with hepatocellular disease. Values in patients with osseous disease, like those of LAP, are normal. Measurement of 5′-N also has been proposed as a diagnostic aid, more specific than alkaline phosphatase, in patients with hepatobiliary disease (Table 14–8).

Gamma-Glutamyl Transferase (Gamma-Glutamyl Transpeptidase, GGT) (EC 2.3.2.1)

This enzyme catalyzes the transfer of a γ-glutamyl group from a γ-glutamyl peptide to another peptide or an amino acid. Kidney and, to a lesser extent, liver and pancreas are rich in GGT. A number of other tissues contain small amounts. Although several isoenzymes of GGT have been demonstrated, the isoenzymology of this enzyme has found no clinical application.

Table 14–10. TISSUES RICH IN AST (GOT) AND CONDITIONS IN WHICH THE SERUM ENZYME IS ABNORMAL*

	Usual Values U/L
A. Tissue content of AST (GOT) (descending order of concentration)	
1. cardiac	
2. hepatic	
3. skeletal muscle	
4. kidney	
5. brain	
6. pancreas	
7. spleen	
8. lung	
9. serum	
B. Conditions in which serum AST (GOT) is elevated	
1. *Cardiac disease*	
myocardial infarction	20–200
pericarditis	<100
cardiac arrhythmias	<200
acute rheumatic fever (?)	<100
postcardiac surgery and catheterization	<100
heart failure	<100
2. *Hepatic disease*	
acute hepatitis (viral, toxic)	500–4000
infectious mononucleosis	50–800
cirrhosis	<100
hepatic congestion	<100
space-occupying lesions (granuloma, metastatic carcinoma)	<200
obstructive jaundice	<200
3. *Other diseases*	
shock	20–1000
pulmonary infarction	<50
acute pancreatitis	20–1000
renal infarction (experimental animals)	<200
cerebral necrosis	<50
dermatomyositis	<200
progressive muscular dystrophy	<200
delirium tremens	<100
hemolysis (slight)	<50
gangrene (slight)	<50
C. Conditions in which serum AST (GOT) is depressed	
1. Pregnancy	0–6

*In acute hepatitis, values above 300 U/L are usual and above 500 are frequent. In all the other conditions shown the levels are usually below this value, although higher values are occasionally observed in infectious mononucleosis and shock. Almost all patients with acute myocardial infarction have elevated values during the first few days. In the other cardiac diseases listed, elevations are less frequent and usually are slight.

The chief clinical value of measuring GGT is in the study of hepatobiliary disease. Values parallel those of ALP, LAP, and 5′-N in obstructive (posthepatic) jaundice and infiltrative disease of the liver. Accordingly, assay of GGT, like that of 5′-N and LAP, serves as an estimate of the level of the hepatic isoenzyme of ALP. Since GGT is a microsomal enzyme, its tissue levels increase in response to microsomal enzyme induction (Table 14–8). This phenomenon may explain the elevated serum levels in chronic alcoholics and in patients taking drugs (e.g., phenytoin) known to induce the microsomal enzyme system (Rosalki, 1975). Serum GGT has thus been advocated in the evaluation of patients with alcoholism. Specifically, the alcoholic who has become abstinent should show a reduction of previously elevated GGT levels.

Aminotransferases (Transaminases)

2

The application of serum aminotransferases (transaminases) to the study of hepatic disease and the principles of assay for these enzymes are discussed in Chapter 13. Aspartate aminotransferase (AST) or glutamate oxalacetate transaminase (GOT) levels of the serum are elevated in patients with hepatobiliary disease, cardiovascular disease, muscle disease, and some miscellaneous conditions. Alanine aminotransferase (ALT), formerly known as glutamate pyruvate transaminase (GPT), levels are elevated in the serum of patients with hepatic disease. In other conditions elevations are negligible unless there is hepatic involvement.

Aspartate Aminotransferase (AST) (Glutamate Oxalacetate Transaminase) (EC 2.6.1.1).* This enzyme is elevated in diseases involving the tissues that are rich in it. In Table 14–10 are also shown the tissues with the highest AST concentration, the categories of disease that may show abnormal levels, and the range of values seen in many of these conditions. The AST levels in patients with liver disease are discussed in Chapter 13.

Extensive studies have shown that patients with acute myocardial infarction have elevated serum AST levels, if measured at the proper interval after infarction (West, 1966). The values are usually 4 to 10 times the upper limit of normal. These usually develop within 12 hours of the time of infarction and reach the peak by the second day; the levels usually return to normal by the fifth day after infarction (Fig. 14–6). Secondary rises may reflect extension or recurrence

*Currently accepted nomenclature for the glutamate oxalacetate transaminase (GOT) is *aspartate transaminase* or *aspartate aminotransferase* (AST).

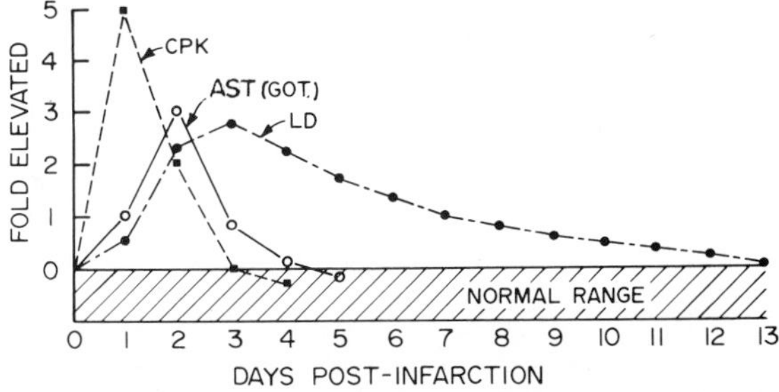

Figure 14–6. CPK, AST (GOT), and LD levels after myocardial infarction (means of values for 200 patients). Note that the CPK rise is earliest, the LD rise is latest, and the LD elevations are present longer than those of CPK and AST (GOT).

of myocardial infarction. Experimental work with animals suggests that the degree of rise of serum AST is related to the extent of myocardial necrosis.

Our experience confirms that of Galen (1975a); in the laboratory diagnosis of myocardial infarction, creatine kinase (CK), CK isoenzymes, lactate dehydrogenase (LD), and LD isoenzyme determinations are sufficient and reliable indicators of myocardial necrosis. Indeed, the combined sensitivity and specificity have resulted in the AST being labeled as a diagnostically redundant cardiac enzyme (Galen, 1975b). Thus, AST assays have been discontinued in some hospitals for the laboratory diagnosis of myocardial infarction.

In patients with electrocardiographic and clinical criteria of "coronary insufficiency" rather than myocardial infarction, elevated serum AST levels may occur. It is not clear whether this phenomenon represents myocardial necrosis which has not been recognized by other means or "leakage" of the enzyme into the serum even without frank myocardial necrosis.

Mild elevations of the serum AST levels have been reported in some patients with pulmonary infarction. The incidence has varied from 0 to 30 per cent, and the elevations are slight to moderate. Animal studies have also yielded inconclusive results on the occurrence of elevated serum AST levels in experimental pulmonary infarction. The incidence of increased values in humans is low, the degree of abnormality slight, and the rise delayed for three to five days after the onset of pain.

In patients with congestive heart failure and in those with marked tachycardia, mild to moderate degrees of AST elevation may occur. These have been attributed to the hepatic necrosis secondary to hepatic congestion. Patients with pericarditis have also been reported to have a 50 per cent incidence of slightly elevated AST levels. The incidence and mechanism of occurrence of elevated enzyme levels in patients with rheumatic fever are not clear. Slight serum AST elevations have been reported after cardiac catheterization and mitral commissurotomy (Galen, 1975a).

Determination of AST or other enzyme levels is not necessary for the diagnosis of myocardial infarction in most patients with classic clinical and electrocardiographic evidence of this condition. Enzyme determinations are of value in patients whose electrocardiographic changes are insufficiently helpful, e.g., those with left bundle branch block or Wolff-Parkinson-White syndrome or in those with electrocardiographic abnormalities remaining from previous infarction, which may obscure acute changes. Measurement of serum enzymes is also of value in recognizing the recurrence or extension of an infarction during convalescence. Normal values obtained at the proper time are of value in excluding a diagnosis of myocardial infarction.

Patients with disease or injury producing inflammation or destruction of skeletal muscle may also have elevated serum AST levels. Patients with progressive muscular dystrophy, dermatomyositis, and trichinosis may have elevated levels, while those with amyotrophic lateral sclerosis, myasthenia gravis, and nerve section do not. Gangrene of the extremities and surgical or other trauma may produce slight AST elevations. In less than 50 per cent of patients with cerebrovascular accidents serum AST elevations may be found.

Elevated serum AST levels in patients with hepatic disease are discussed in Chapter 13. In acute pancreatitis, levels may be elevated. It has been suggested that obstruction of the biliary tree by the edematous pancreas and the presence of associated hepatic disease or of delirium tremens may contribute to the elevated AST levels in these patients.

Alanine Aminotransferase (ALT) (Glutamate Pyruvate Transaminase) (EC 2.6.1.2).* This enzyme is also discussed in Chapter 13. In patients with myocardial infarction, elevations of the serum levels of ALT are slight or absent. Heart failure or shock with the attendant hepatic necrosis, however, may lead to elevated ALT levels. The chief application of determination of this serum enzyme is in the diagnosis of hepatocellular destruction.

Glycolytic Enzymes

The glycolytic pathway, which is found in virtually all tissues, includes a number of enzymes (Fig. 14–7). Almost all of these have been demonstrated in the serum. In patients with extensive carcinoma, elevated levels of several of these enzymes (phosphohexoisomerase, aldolase, and lactate dehydrogenase) have been observed. These elevations have served as a guide to chemotherapy, particularly in carcinoma of the breast and prostate.

Elevated levels of these enzymes also have been observed in patients with megaloblastic and hemolytic anemias and in granulocytic and acute leukemias but not in patients with chronic lymphocytic leukemia, aplastic anemia, or iron deficiency anemia. The most extensively studied of the glycolytic enzymes in the serum are lactate dehydrogenase (LD), aldolase (ALS), and phosphohexoisomerase (PHI). The serum levels of all three are elevated to approximately the same degree in patients with extensive carcinomatosis, megaloblastic anemia, granulocytic leukemia, infectious mononucleosis, hemolytic states, and myocardial infarction (Table 14–11). Levels of PHI seem to reflect carcinomatosis more sensitively, and those of LD seem to be a more sensitive reflection of megaloblastic anemia than are those of the other two. Aldolase is the most sensitive of the three as a reflector of muscle diseases (progressive muscular dystrophy, trichinosis, and dermatomyositis). Levels of ALS and PHI are much more strikingly elevated than those of LD in patients with hepatic necrosis. Indeed, the very insensitivity of the serum LD level to parenchymal hepatic damage coupled with its sensitivity as a measure of carcinomatosis enhances its usefulness for the recognition of metastatic or primary carcinoma of the liver. Other glycolytic enzymes have not been studied suf-

*The currently accepted term for glutamate pyruvate transaminase is *alanine aminotransferase* (ALT).

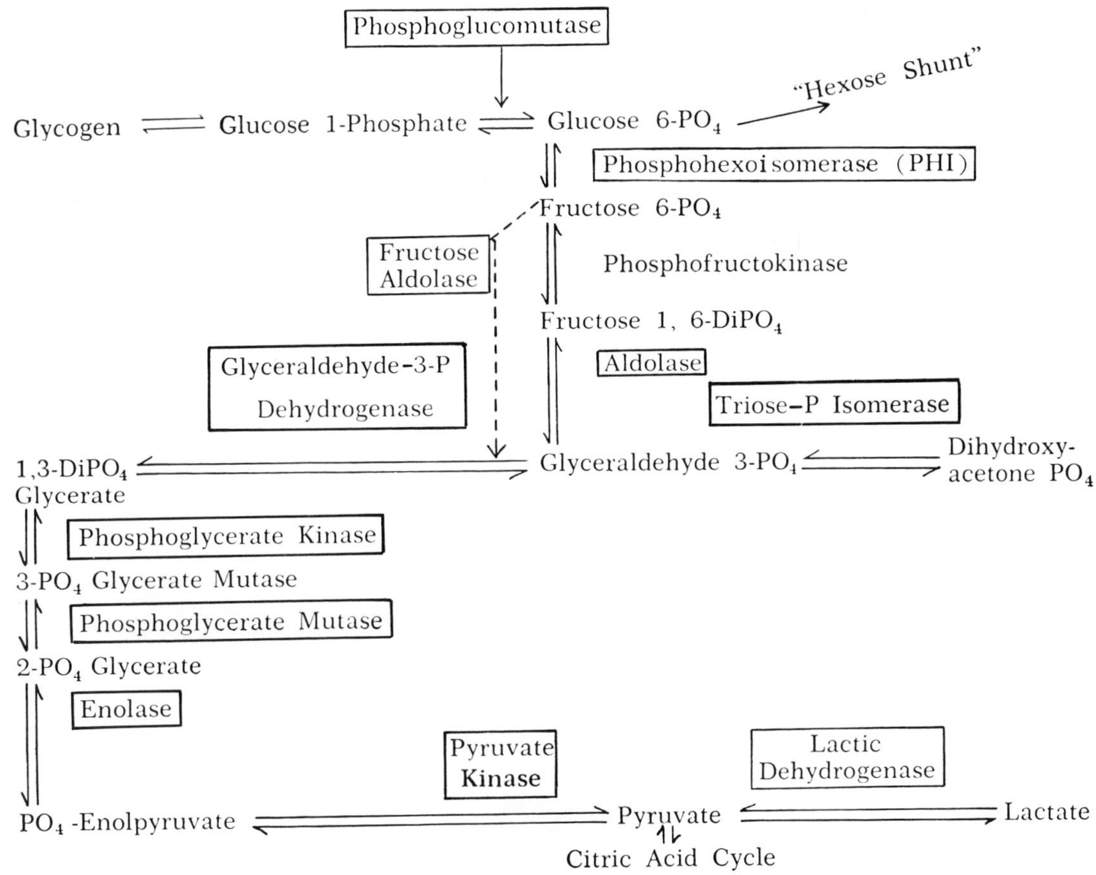

Figure 14–7. Scheme of glycolytic pathway of carbohydrate metabolism. Enzymes demonstrated in human serum are shown in boxes.

ficiently to delineate their value in clinical circumstances.

Phosphohexoisomerase (PHI) (EC 5.3.1.9). This glycolytic enzyme catalyzes the conversion of glucose-6-phosphate to fructose-6-phosphate (Fig. 14–7). First studied in the serum of tumorous rats by Warburg and Christian, PHI levels of the serum have been investigated in patients with carcinoma and other diseases during the past few years.

The activity of PHI is assayed by using glucose-6-phosphate as substrate. The rate of formation of fructose-6-phosphate using the Seliwanoff reaction (resorcinol) is a measure of PHI activity.

Table 14–11. RELATIVE SENSITIVITY OF GLYCOLYTIC ENZYME LEVELS TO VARIOUS TYPES OF DISEASES

	LD	ALS	PHI
Myocardial infarction	↑ ↑	↑ ↑	↑ ↑
Pulmonary infarction	↑	↑	↑
Carcinoma, granulocytic leukemia	↑ ↑	↑ ↑	↑ ↑ ↑
Megaloblastic anemia	↑ ↑ ↑	↑ ↑	↑ ↑
Hepatic necrosis	↑ or N	↑ ↑ ↑	↑ ↑ ↑
Muscle disease	↑ ↑	↑ ↑ ↑ ↑	↑ ↑

Phosphohexoisomerase levels have been used as an index of metastases in patients with carcinoma of the breast and prostate and to monitor the response to therapy. Other diseases in which elevations are observed are listed in Tables 14–1 and 14–11. Determination of this serum enzyme, however, has not been applied extensively to clinical medicine.

Aldolase (EC 4.1.2.13). This glycolytic enzyme catalyzes the cleavage of fructose-1-6-diphosphate into two triose molecules (glyceraldehyde phosphate and dihydroxyacetone phosphate) (Fig. 14–7). Several methods have been devised for this assay, based on the rate at which the trioses are formed. One involves measuring the colored dinitrophenylhydrazone.

Serum aldolase (ALS) levels are elevated in skeletal muscle disease, carcinomatosis, granulocytic leukemia, megaloblastic anemia, hepatitis, other types of hepatic necrosis, and the other conditions that are listed in Figure 14–8 and Tables 14–1 and 14–11. The aldolase levels reflect particularly sensitively progressive muscular dystrophy and inflammatory muscle disease (dermatomyositis, trichinosis), in which strikingly elevated values can be seen. Patients destined to develop progressive muscular dystrophy usually have elevated aldolase levels before any overt clinical manifestation of muscle disease. The chief clinical application of aldolase assay has been in the study of muscle disease.

Lactate Dehydrogenase (LD) (EC 1.1.1.27)

This enzyme catalyzes the reversible oxidation of lactate to pyruvate (Fig. 14–7). It is widely distributed in mammalian tissues, being rich in myocardium, kidney, liver, and muscle.

Methods. Spectrophotometric, fluorometric, and colorimetric methods have been applied to the assay of this enzyme. In the spectrophotometric method, the rate of change in concentration of NADH (DPNH) is determined. The reaction may be measured by following the disappearance of NADH (pyruvate + NADH $\xrightarrow{LD}$ lactate + NAD) at a pH of 7.4 or by following the appearance of NADH (lactate + NAD $\xrightarrow{LD}$ pyruvate + NADH) at a pH of 8.8 or higher. The results should be expressed as U/L, that is, μmoles/minute of NADH reacting per liter of specimen assayed (Table 14–4).

Elevated serum levels of LD are observed in a variety of conditions (Fig. 14–8). The highest values (two- to 40-fold elevations) are seen in patients with megaloblastic anemia, in those with extensive carcinomatosis, and in those with severe shock and hypoxia. Moderate elevations (two- to four-fold) occur in patients with myocardial infarction, pulmonary infarction, granulocytic or acute leukemia, hemolytic anemia, infectious mononucleosis, and progressive muscular dystrophy. Relatively slight elevations occur in patients with hepatitis, obstructive jaundice, or cirrhosis, but higher values occur in those with delirium tremens. Patients with chronic renal disease, especially those with nephrotic syndrome or hemolytic anemia, also have increased values. In patients with

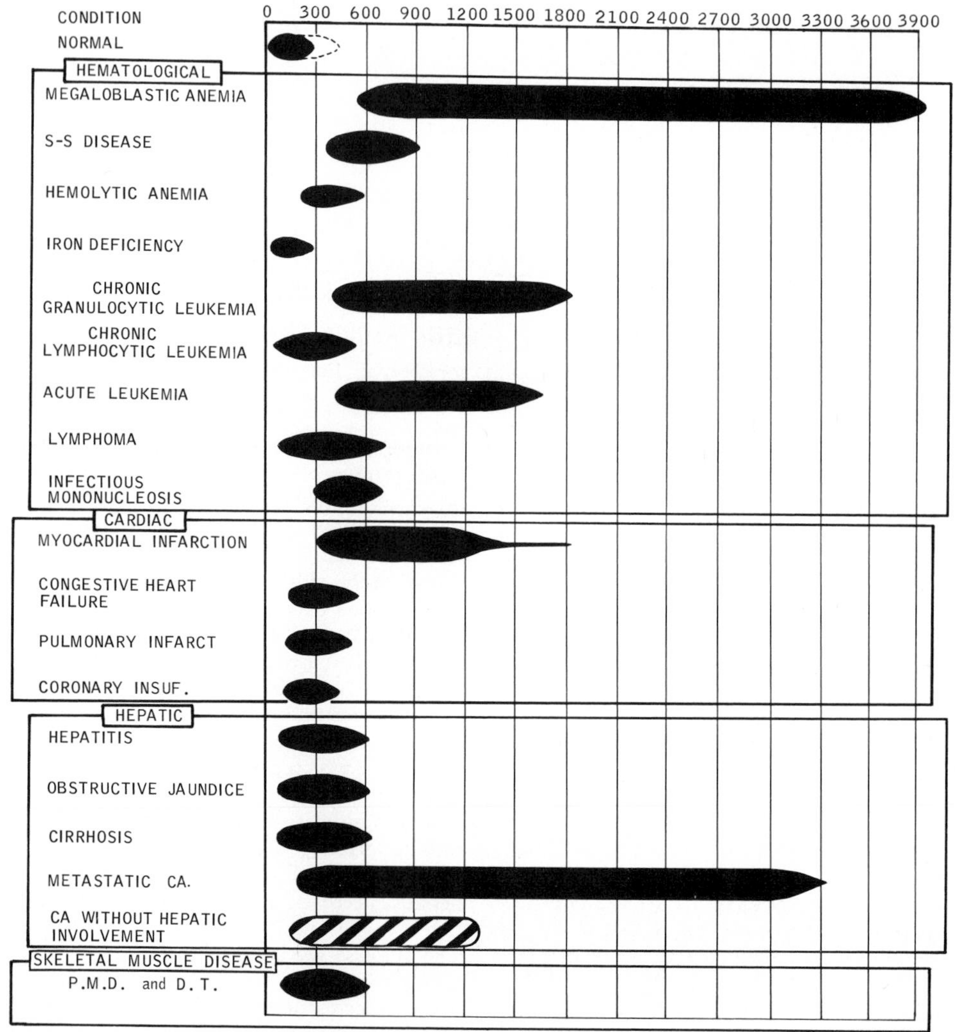

Figure 14–8. Diagrammatic representation of lactate dehydrogenase values (U/L or Units/liter) in normals (dotted line represents higher values in children) and in various diseases. Equivalent degrees of elevation of ALS and PHI occur in all these conditions with the exceptions of megaloblastic anemia, in which levels of LD are relatively higher, and acute hepatitis, in which levels of LD are relatively lower than those of PHI and ALS. Values for ALS are higher than those of PHI and LD in muscle disease.

myxedema, the LD values are also elevated, presumably because of muscle abnormality.

The pattern of elevated serum LD levels in patients with myocardial infarction is quite characteristic. High levels are observed in almost all patients within 24 hours of the apparent onset of infarction. Although the degree of elevation is not so striking as that of AST, the elevated levels persist longer (10 to 14 days). The characteristically prolonged period of elevated LD values with an increase of LD isoenzymes, i.e., LD_1 higher than LD_2 ("flipped" LD), yields a pattern that is useful in the laboratory diagnosis of myocardial infarction (Galen, 1975a). The "flipped" LD pattern usually appears within 12 to 24 hours and is present within 48 hours in sera of 80 per cent of patients with a myocardial infarction (Galen, 1975a) (Fig. 14–6).

Most patients with pulmonary infarction have elevated levels of LD, usually within 24 hours of the onset of pain. The pattern of normal AST and elevated LD levels within one to two days after an episode of chest pain provides suggestive evidence for pulmonary infarction.

Almost all patients with megaloblastic anemia have elevated LD levels. Often the values are strikingly increased. Possible factors in the production of the high values include the large number of megaloblasts, presumably rich in LD, and the intramedullary destruction of these cells. As the anemia responds to treatment, the LD levels return to normal. Hemolytic anemias yield slightly elevated levels. Patients with aplastic and iron deficiency anemias usually have normal values.

Patients with granulocytic and acute leukemia have moderately elevated LD levels. In lymphocytic leukemia, the values are usually normal, unless there is an associated hemolytic state. In patients with lymphosarcoma and Hodgkin's disease, LD levels are normal or moderately elevated, depending on the total mass of tumor and the presence of hemolysis.

Patients and animals with small, localized carcinomas usually have normal serum levels of LD, while those with distant metastases or even local extension have increased levels. The highest values occur in patients with metastases to the liver, although increased levels are also found in some patients with only extrahepatic metastases or extension.

The serum LD level does not provide a sensitive measure of hepatic disease. Patients with viral hepatitis have slightly elevated (one- to two-fold) values. In patients with infectious mononucleosis, LD levels are usually somewhat higher, perhaps released from the aggregates of immature mononuclear cells throughout the body. Only slightly increased values are seen in patients with obstructive jaundice and in those with cirrhosis. Interestingly, almost all patients with delirium tremens have increased values, perhaps of skeletal muscle origin, since, like the elevated LD levels of progressive muscular dystrophy, they are accompanied by increased serum levels of creatine kinase (see later).

The large number of conditions in which LD levels are elevated detracts from the diagnostic usefulness of its measurement. The LD level is clinically useful in the recognition of myocardial infarction and pulmonary infarction. It is often a somewhat superfluous clue to extensive carcinomatosis, but it may be used to monitor the course of cancer chemotherapy, since response to therapy is often mirrored by decreasing serum levels. Other clinical applications entail analysis of the clinical problem in the light of conditions known to cause elevated LD levels.

Isoenzymes of Lactate Dehydrogenase. The LD of normal human serum has been found to be separable into five different components by appropriate electrophoretic techniques. Each of these isoenzymes is distinguishable from the others by serologic, electrophoretic, and various other chemical procedures (Table 14–12). Indeed, the great current interest in isoenzymology derives from the observations on the multiple molecular forms of LD. The isoenzymes of LD are designated according to their electrophoretic mobility. The fraction with the greatest mobility (anodic) is called LD_1, the one with least anodic mobility is called LD_5, and the other three are designated accordingly as LD_2, LD_3, and LD_4, respectively.

The five LD isoenzymes have the same molecular weight (135,000) but differ in the charge that they carry. Each isoenzyme is a tetramer made up of four subunits, each of 34,000 daltons. There are two types of these subunits, designated H and M, respectively, for heart polypeptide chain (H) and skeletal muscle chain (M). The five isoenzymes of LD consist of the five possible combinations of monomers H and M (Table 14–13). Hence there are two homotetramers (LD_1 and LD_5) and three hybrids. The H and M chains differ significantly in their amino acid composition and thus in their structural and kinetic properties; they are probably under the control of two distinct genes.

Tissue LD consists of the five isoenzymes in varying proportions, and the LD activity of each tissue has a characteristic isoenzyme composition (Table 14–13). Thus, the LD of myocardium and erythrocytes consists largely of the fastest moving isoenzymes (LD_1 and LD_2).

In liver and skeletal muscle, the principal isoenzymes are LD_4 and LD_5. In general, tissues exhibiting aerobic metabolism demonstrate predominantly faster moving isoenzymes (LD_1) with more H subunits, while tissues exhibiting anaerobic metabolism demonstrate predominantly slower moving isoenzymes (LD_5) with more M units. A number of tissues (lung, spleen, pancreas, thyroid, adrenals, and lymph nodes) consist mainly of LD_3. The relative concentration of the several isoenzymes in normal serum is LD_2, LD_1, LD_3, LD_4, and LD_5 in descending order. Normal serum LD has been presumed to derive mainly from erythrocytes with LD_2 higher than LD_1.

Studies of the isoenzyme composition of the elevated serum LD levels of various diseases have revealed abnormal patterns that reflect the tissues involved (Table 14–14). In acute myocardial infarction, the elevated serum LD levels consist largely of LD_1 and LD_2 (classically $LD_1 > LD_2$ or "flipped" LD), the isoenzymes in which myocardium is particularly rich.

2

Table 14–12. PRINCIPLES OF SOME OF THE TECHNIQUES EMPLOYED TO MEASURE ISOENZYMES OF LACTATE DEHYDROGENASE

Method	Comment	Clinical Applicability
I. Physical		
A. Electrophoretic	Demonstrates the five isoenzymes	Somewhat cumbersome and not sufficiently quantitative, but clinically useful
B. Selective absorption on DEAE cellulose	Selective absorption of fast ($LD_{1,2}$) isoenzymes, leaving slow ($LD_{3,4,5}$)	Remains to be demonstrated
C. Solvent precipitation techniques in which acetone or chloroform is used	Selective precipitation of slow isoenzymes, leaving fast in supernatant	Remains to be demonstrated
D. Heat denaturation at 65° C. for 30 minutes	Destroys activity of all isoenzymes except most rapid (LD_1)	Useful in the diagnosis of myocardial infarction
II. Chemical		
A. Substrate-product relationship		
1. Measurement of ability to dehydrogenate α-hydroxybutyrate dehydrogenase (HBD) activity	1. HBD activity is largely equivalent to LD_1 activity	1. Suitable for demonstrations of approximate LD_1 activity
2. Relative inhibition by various concentrations of pyruvate or lactate	2. Individual isoenzymes show different degrees of inhibition by high pyruvate concentration	2. Of theoretical interest, but no clinical applicability as yet
B. Coenzyme affinity Measurement of relative activity isoenzymes with DPN and its analogues	Each isoenzyme shows characteristic rates of activity with various analogues of NAD	Extremely useful research tool. Remains to be clinically applicable
C. Differential chemical inhibition of LD activity	Individual isoenzymes are characteristically and differentially inhibited by several chemical agents (urea, sulfate, oxamate, chloroform)	No clinical application as yet
III. Immunologic	Specific antibody to LD_1 and another to LD_5	Evolving

When lactate dehydrogenase is elevated and the ratio of LD_1:LD_2 is greater than 1 (LD_1 greater than LD_2 is called "flipped" LDH), three diagnostic possibilities emerge: it is seen after acute myocardial infarction, acute renal infarction, and in hemolysis such as hemolytic anemia. Following acute myocardial infarction, the LD isoenzymes assume the "flip" profile within 12 to 24 hours with LD_1 greater than LD_2. "Flipped LD" is present in 80 per cent of patients with myocardial infarction within 48 hours after the acute episode. It is not necessarily maintained, since it is present in less than half of such patients (who earlier had a flipped LD) at the end of a week even though the serum LD is elevated (Galen, 1975a). Likewise, an increased LD_5 indicates other hepatic or skeletal muscle injury. LD patterns with intermediate hybrid fractions are found in several pathologic conditions but are less specific than the homotetramer elevations and, thus, are less diagnostic in value. Such patterns are seen in pulmonary embolism as well as in disease states in which levels of all five isoenzymes are increased but their relationship to one another is

Table 14–13. NOMENCLATURE, COMPOSITION, ISOENZYMES, AND TISSUE SOURCE OF LACTATE DEHYDROGENASE FOUND IN HUMAN SERUM BY ELECTROPHORETIC TECHNIQUES

Nomenclature of Isoenzyme Starting with Most Anodic	Composition Proportion of Monomers* in Each Isoenzyme	Relative Content† of Isoenzyme					
		Myocardium	*Liver*	*Skeletal Muscle*	*Brain*	*Kidney*	*RBC*
1	HHHH	+ + + +	±	±	+ +	+	+ + +
2	HHHM	+ + + +	±	±	+ +	+	+ + +
3	HHMM	+	+	+	+ +	+ +	+
4	HMMM	±	+ +	+ +	+ +	+ +	±
5	MMMM	±	+ + + +	+ + + +	±	+ +	±

*Monomer H (myocardial). Monomer M (skeletal muscle).
†Content graded from ±, which represents almost no activity, to + + + +, which represents high activity.

Table 14–14. RELATIVE DEGREE OF INCREASE OF LACTATE DEHYDROGENASE AND PATTERN OF ABNORMALITY OF ISOENZYME IN VARIOUS DISEASES

Disease	Relative Degree Increase Total LD Activity	Isoenzyme Fraction Most Abnormal: Most Anodic (+) LD_1	LD_2	LD_3	LD_4	(−) LD_5
Myocardial infarction	↑↑	X	X			
Pulmonary infarction*	↑				X	X
Congestive heart failure	↑				X	X
Viral hepatitis	↑				X	X
Toxic hepatitis	↑				X	X
Cirrhosis	↑				X	X
Leukemia, granulocytic	↑↑		X	X		
Pancreatitis	↑		X	X		
Carcinomatosis (extensive)	↑↑↑		X	X		
Megaloblastic anemia	↑↑↑↑	X	X			
Hemolytic anemia	↑	X	X			
Muscular dystrophy†	↑	X	X			

*In pulmonary infarction, LD_3 may be elevated.
†In muscular dystrophy, LD_1 and LD_2 are elevated only in a relative sense because LD_4 and LD_5 are depressed.

virtually unchanged (isomorphic elevation). In acute viral hepatitis, the serum LD shows a higher proportion of LD_4 and LD_5 than does the normal. Some of the isoenzyme patterns observed in other diseases are indicated in Table 14–14. Approximations of LD_1, the myocardial isoenzyme, however, may be accomplished by techniques that are as simple as the measurement of total LD activity. Isoenzyme LD_1 resists denaturation at 65°C. for 30 minutes, while the activity of the other four isoenzymes is destroyed under these conditions. Accordingly, the relative amounts of LD_1 can be estimated by comparing the heat-stable LD to the total LD activity. A number of clinical laboratories determine "heat-stable" LD as a relatively routine aid in the diagnosis of acute myocardial infarction. An estimate of the serum level of LD_1 can also be obtained by measuring the level of α-hydroxybutyrate dehydrogenase (HBD). At one time considered to be the activity of a separate enzyme, HBD activity is now recognized to represent that of isoenzymes of LD (largely LD_1 with smaller amounts of other isoenzymes). The measurement of HBD activity is accomplished by a technique similar to that for measuring LD. Measurement of HBD is much less widely employed than that of heat-stable LD for clinical purposes. Electrophoresis employing cellulose acetate or agarose is the best way to determine LD isoenzymes. Fluorescent excitation or tetrazolium reduction by NADH permit visual display and measurement of LD isoenzymes by scanning. Indeed, this has made possible application of LD isoenzymology to clinical problems, especially in evaluation of patients with ischemic heart disease.

"Citric Acid Cycle" Enzymes

Several of the enzymes identified in the serum have been considered to be citric acid cycle enzymes (Fig. 14–9) released into the blood. Although they are shown as such in this discussion, this is an oversimplification for convenience. Enzymes of the citric acid cycle are located in the mitochondria, and are less likely to enter the blood than the cytoplasmic enzymes. Furthermore, the isocitrate dehydrogenase (ICD) found in the serum requires NADP as the coenzyme, while the mitochondrial ICD is a NAD-linked enzyme. Malate dehydrogenase activity has been demonstrated in the cytoplasm and mitochondria. Fumarase appears to be a mitochondrial enzyme.

Isocitrate Dehydrogenase (ICD) (EC 1.1.1.42). ICD catalyzes the conversion of isocitric acid to alpha-ketoglutarate. The serum levels have been reported to be increased up to 40-fold in patients with viral hepatitis. Values are moderately elevated in patients with cirrhosis, obstructive jaundice, and metastatic carcinoma of the liver. Carcinoma, even without metastatic involvement, megaloblastic anemia, and congestive heart failure are also associated with mildly elevated levels of this enzyme. Levels have been reported to be normal in patients with myocardial infarction despite the rich content of ICD in the myocardium. Apparently, the myocardial isoenzyme of ICD disappears shortly after release into the blood. While ICD levels are sensitive reflections of acute hepatic necrosis, this serum enzyme test has not been widely adopted. It is not as sensitive and is no more specific a test of acute hepatic injury than is ALT. It is likely that this procedure will continue to be of investigative interest rather than a clinical tool.

Malate Dehydrogenase (MD) (EC 1.1.1.37). This enzyme catalyzes the reversible oxidation of malate to oxaloacetate. Elevated values have been observed in patients with myocardial infarction, hepatic necrosis, hemolytic syndromes, megaloblastic anemia, and neoplastic disease. In general, the abnormalities of this enzyme appear to parallel those observed with the glycolytic enzymes, but the degree of abnormality is

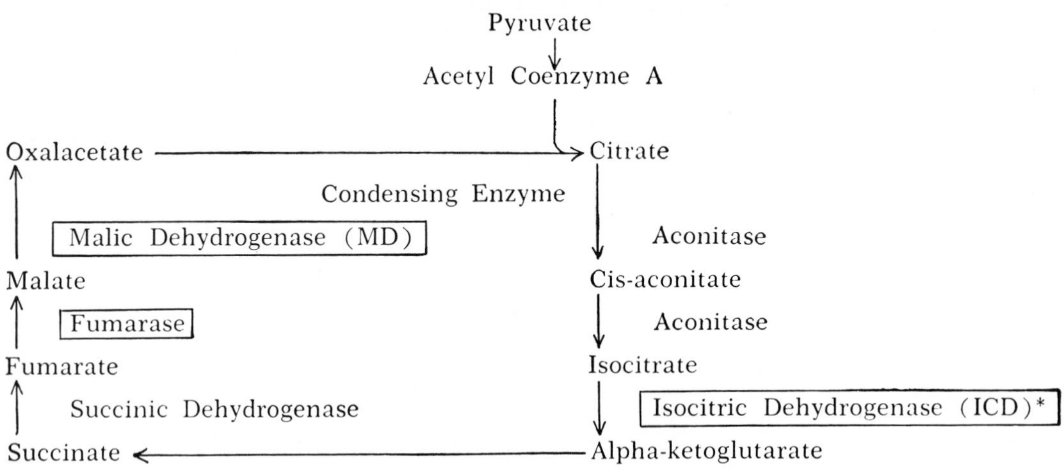

*Strictly speaking, the ICD of the serum differs from that of the citric acid cycle. The ICD demonstrated in the serum is TPN-linked, while that of the citric acid cycle is DPN-linked.

Figure 14–9. The tricarboxylic acid cycle. Scheme of citric acid cycle pathway of carbohydrate metabolism. Enzymes demonstrated in human serum are shown in boxes.

usually less. This enzyme test is also of investigative rather than clinical usefulness.

Hexose "Shunt" Enzymes

Several of the enzymes of the hexose monophosphate shunt have been demonstrated in the serum (Fig. 14–10). Reports have appeared on the occurrence of elevated serum levels of glucose-6-phosphate dehydrogenase and of 6-phosphogluconic dehydrogenase in patients with hepatic disease. 5-P-ribose isomerase and transketolase have also been reported to be found in the serum; but the clinical significance and applicability of assay of these serum enzymes remain to be established. See Tables 14–1 and 14–20.

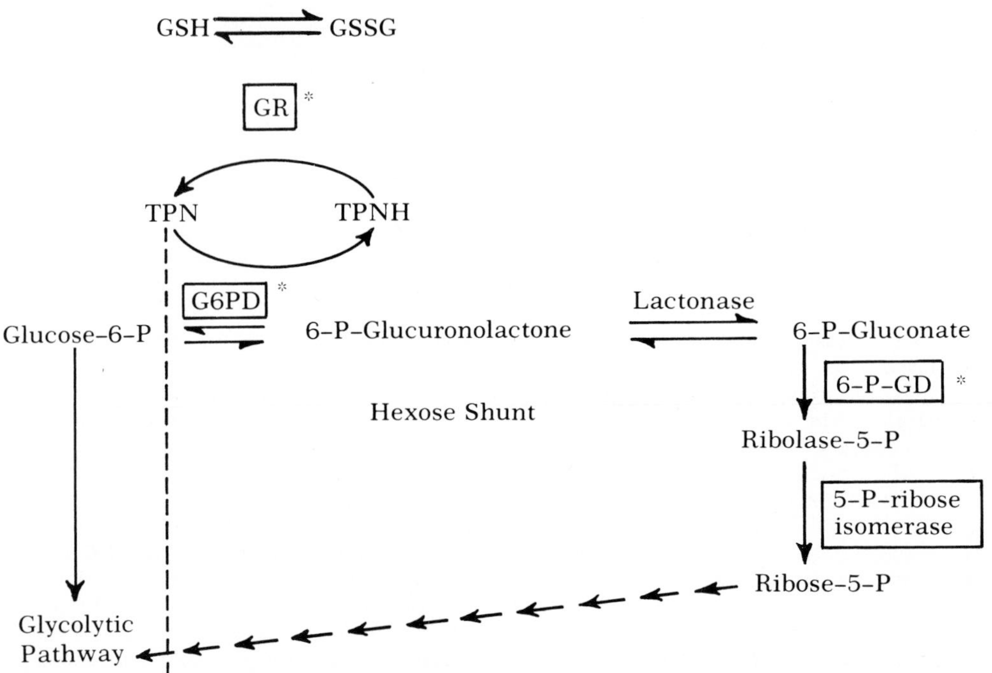

Figure 14–10. Initial reactions of hexose monophosphate shunt showing the rate of generation of TPNH in maintaining reduced glutathione. Enzymes in boxes (GR, G6PD, 6-P-GD, 5-P-ribose isomerase) may be found in serum. Transketolase (not shown) also reported in serum. *Assays performed most frequently on hemolysates of erythrocytes. (After Carson and Frischer, 1966.)

$$RCOOCH_2CH_2N^+(CH_3)_3Cl^- + H_2O \xrightarrow{CHS} RCOOH + HOCH_2CH_2N^+(CH_3)_3Cl^-$$

R = CH_3 optimally for acetylcholinesterase.
R = CH_3 and many other alkyl or aryl groups for cholinesterase.

Method of assay is based on pH change (electrometric titration) that results from acid liberated.

Tissue content: acetylcholinesterase, RBC, nerve cells, synapses, and motor end plates. *Cholinesterase (pseudo):* serum or plasma, pancreas, and liver.

Conditions characterized by abnormal levels:

Depressed		*Elevated*	
Insecticide poisoning	↓	Nephrotic syndrome	↑
Hepatitis	↓		
Cirrhosis	↓		
Abscess	↓		
Metastatic carcinoma	↓ or N		
Obstructive jaundice	↓ or N		
Malnutrition	↓		
Anemias	↓		
Acute infections	↓		
Myocardial infarction	↓		
Dermatomyositis	↓		
Genetic acholinesterasemia	↓		

Figure 14–11. Reaction catalyzed by cholinesterases (CHS), principle of assay, and list of conditions that cause decreased (↓) or increased (↑) serum levels.

Cholinesterase (CHS)

The cholinesterase of the serum (CHS) (EC 3.1.1.8) has been referred to as pseudocholinesterase to distinguish it from the true cholinesterase (AcCHS) (EC 3.1.1.7) of the erythrocytes and nerve tissue. The tissue enzyme acts optimally on acetylcholine and on acetylbetamethyl choline, while the serum enzyme hydrolyzes acetylcholine and other cholinesters even more rapidly (Fig. 14–11; Table 14–15). Alkylphosphates are potent inhibitors of both serum and tissue cholinesterases. Simplified electrometric, manometric, and colorimetric methods have been devised for cholinesterase assay.

Serum CHS values are characteristically depressed in patients with parenchymatous liver disease, including viral hepatitis, cirrhosis, metastatic carcinoma, the hepatic congestion of heart failure, and amebic hepatitis and abscess. In acute hepatitis, levels of the enzyme are lowest at the peak of the disease. Since, with recovery, the CHS level returns to normal, it has been suggested that the enzyme level may serve as an index of recovery and prognosis. In cirrhosis with jaundice, ascites, or other evidence of parenchymal insufficiency, CHS levels are usually depressed. In cirrhotics without these manifestations, the enzyme levels may be normal. Persistent depression of the CHS level in cirrhotics has been considered a poor prognostic sign.

In patients with obstructive jaundice, serum cholinesterase (CHS) levels are often normal. After prolonged obstruction, or when there is cholangitis, the level of CHS may be low.

Low values are also observed in patients with malnutrition, acute infections, anemias, myocardial infarction, and dermatomyositis (Fig. 14–11). In these nonhepatic diseases and in hepatic disease, the CHS level is depressed in those patients who also have a low serum level of albumin. Accordingly, it has been suggested that the low CHS level reflects impaired hepatic protein synthesis. Some support for this concept is derived from the observation that patients with the nephrotic syndrome, in whom the rate of albumin synthesis is increased, may have increased CHS levels, even though serum albumin levels are low.

As a measure of hepatic function and status, the determination of CHS is hardly used today. It is not sufficiently consistent to be useful in the differential diagnosis of jaundice. As an index of parenchymal function during the course of hepatic disease, it appears to add little to more commonly used laboratory measurements.

Assay of serum CHS has found several applications other than in the diagnosis of hepatic disease. The

Table 14–15. SUBSTRATE RELATIONSHIP OF BLOOD CHOLINESTERASES

Enzyme	Source in Blood	Substrates Hydrolyzed				Kinetics with Acetylcholine	
		Acetylcholine	Acetylbetamethylcholine	Butyrylcholine	Benzoylcholine	Optimal concentration	Inhibition by excess
Acetylcholinesterase (true cholinesterase)	RBC	+	+	–	–	3×10^{-3}	+
Cholinesterase (pseudocholinesterase)	Plasma or serum	+	–	+	+	2×10^{-2}	–

organophosphorous insecticides are potent inhibitors of the cholinesterases. Depression of the acetylcholinesterase of the tissue (reflected in levels of erythrocyte AcCHS) and of the pseudocholinesterase of the serum CHS occurs. Serum CHS, which is depressed before erythrocyte AcCHS, is a sensitive measure of overexposure to these agents. Severe exposure is usually reflected in depression of both erythrocyte AcCHS and serum CHS. Serum levels appear to return to normal earlier than do the erythrocyte values.

The genetic control of serum CHS activity has been of great theoretical interest and is of some practical importance. At least two forms of serum CHS have been recognized. One has been called "normal" and the other "atypical." The genes controlling their synthesis are allelic to each other. Individuals homozygous for the "atypical" gene can be distinguished readily from the homozygous normal. The homozygous abnormal has very low CHS levels and the abnormal CHS is not inhibited by dibucaine. The homozygous normal has much higher levels of serum cholinesterase (CHS) activity, inhibitable by dibucaine, while the heterozygote has intermediate levels and response to the inhibitors. Not only is hereditary hypocholinesterasemia an interesting genetic state to study, it is also of clinical importance in regard to the administration of muscle relaxants (succinylcholine). Homozygous abnormals may develop prolonged apnea after they receive succinylcholine. Accordingly, patients who become apneic under these circumstances should have their CHS studied. Indeed, it has been proposed that one of the simple screening methods for CHS be performed prior to administration of an acetylcholine antagonist in order to exclude subjects who should not receive the agent.

Ornithine Carbamoyl Transferase (OCT) (EC 2.1.3.3)

This enzyme, which catalyzes the reversible conversion of ornithine to citrulline (Fig. 14–12), is intimately involved in urea synthesis. It is found almost exclusively in the liver. The intestine has an OCT content of about 1 per cent that of the liver. There is virtually no activity in other tissues. Serum levels are very low in normal individuals, but are markedly elevated (ten- to 200-fold) in those with acute viral hepatitis and other forms of hepatic necrosis. Relatively slight elevations occur in obstructive jaundice, cirrhosis, metastatic carcinoma, heart failure, delirium tremens, cholecystitis, and intestinal infarction. Indeed, serum OCT activity appears to be quite a specific and sensitive measure of hepatocellular injury. The first methods proposed for measurement of OCT activity did not lend themselves to routine assay. The recent introduction of a simplified colorimetric method has made OCT measurement a practical routine procedure. Nevertheless, it is performed in relatively few centers.

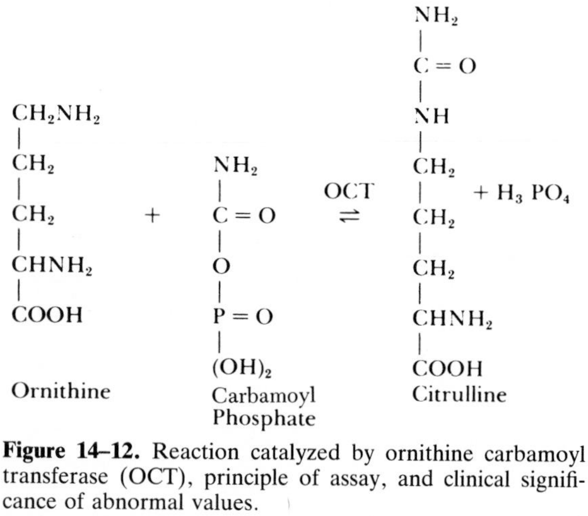

				NH_2	
				|	
				$C=O$	
				|	
CH_2NH_2				NH	
|				|	
CH_2		NH_2		CH_2	
|		|	OCT	|	$+ H_3PO_4$
CH_2	+	$C=O$	$\rightleftharpoons$	CH_2	
|		|		|	
$CHNH_2$		O		CH_2	
|		|		|	
COOH		$P=O$		$CHNH_2$	
		|		|	
		$(OH)_2$		COOH	
Ornithine		Carbamoyl Phosphate		Citrulline	

Figure 14–12. Reaction catalyzed by ornithine carbamoyl transferase (OCT), principle of assay, and clinical significance of abnormal values.

Iditol Dehydrogenase (ID)

Iditol (sorbitol) dehydrogenase (ID) (EC 1.1.1.14) catalyzes the reaction shown in Figure 14–13. It resembles OCT in that it is almost restricted to the liver. It is also found in prostate, and small amounts are present in the kidney. Accordingly, elevated values strongly suggest hepatic injury. Normal serum has negligible activity. The highest values are observed in patients with acute hepatitis or other forms of acute hepatic necrosis. Most of the studies of this serum enzyme have been largely investigative, however, and there is little likelihood that it will replace or routinely supplement the established enzyme tests.

Creatine Kinase (CK) (Creatine Phosphokinase [CPK]) (EC 2.7.3.2)

This enzyme, also referred to as ATP-creatine-N-phosphotransferase, catalyzes the reversible reaction shown in Figure 14–14. Its concentration in skeletal muscle and myocardium is very high. Appreciable amounts are found in the brain. Tiny amounts are found in a few other organs. None is found in the liver. Many studies have shown that CK values are high in patients with myocardial infarction, progressive muscular dystrophy, alcoholic myopathy, and delirium tremens, but normal in patients with hepatitis and other forms of liver disease. The high values in patients with hypothyroidism reflect the muscle changes in this condition. Although CK is found almost exclusively in myocardium, muscle, and brain, and early reports suggested it to be an almost specific index of injury of myocardium and muscle, more recent reports indicate that inexplicably high serum CK values can occur in patients with pulmonary infarction and pulmonary edema. Other causes of CK elevation include exercise, intramuscular injections, and acute psychotic reactions. Further studies are required to define the degree of specificity of high serum CK values. At present, it should be regarded as a useful but not completely specific adjunct in the diagnosis of myocardial and muscle disease. Specificity

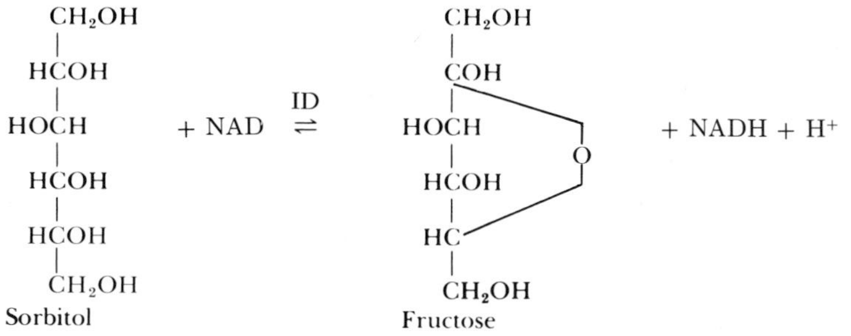

$$\begin{array}{c} CH_2OH \\ | \\ HCOH \\ | \\ HOCH \\ | \\ HCOH \\ | \\ HCOH \\ | \\ CH_2OH \\ \text{Sorbitol} \end{array} + NAD \overset{ID}{\rightleftharpoons} \begin{array}{c} CH_2OH \\ | \\ COH \\ | \\ HOCH \\ | \\ HCOH \\ | \\ HC \\ | \\ CH_2OH \\ \text{Fructose} \end{array} + NADH + H^+$$

Figure 14–13. Reaction catalyzed by iditol dehydrogenase (ID), principle of method of assay, and conditions in which abnormal values are found.

Method of assay depends on measuring the rate of reduction of coenzyme (NAD), which is measured spectrophotometrically.

Abnormal levels

Acute hepatitis	↑↑ ↑
Cirrhosis	↑ or N
Obstructive jaundice	↑

of CK assay is enhanced by measurement of its isoenzymes.

Isoenzymes (Roberts, 1979). The physiochemical properties of CK found in extracts of the human heart, brain, and skeletal muscle differ. Enzyme in the brain (CK_1 or BB) moves most rapidly toward the anode; that in skeletal muscle (CK_3 or MM) moves most slowly. The CK found in myocardium has two components, one moving as slowly as the muscle isoenzyme and the other somewhat faster. The isoenzyme is a dimer; the form found in the brain consists of two similar units, termed accordingly BB or CK_1. The CK found in the muscle consists of two other identical subunits and is called the MM (CK_3) isoenzyme. Myocardial extracts consist mainly of the MM isoenzyme and of another which is the MB (CK_2) isoenzyme. Normal serum CK is virtually 100 per cent CK_3 or MM as is skeletal muscle. Heart yields about 40 per cent CK_2 (MB) and 60 per cent CK_3 (MM). Brain tissue yields about 90 per cent CK_1 or BB and 10 per cent CK_3 or MM. The brain fraction CK_1 (BB) is almost never observed in sera even after cerebrovascular accidents, since the enzyme does not appear to cross the blood-brain barrier (Galen, 1975a). However, CK (BB) has been noted in sera of patients with carcinoma of prostate, colon, lung, and esophagus.

The presence of CK_2 (MB) in sera indicates damage to the myocardium; it is found during the 48-hour period following acute myocardial infarction in all patients (Galen, 1975a). However, it is also found to a lesser degree in patients with severe angina and coronary insufficiency without evidence of infarction. CK_3 (MM) is found in sera of patients with muscle trauma, including intramuscular injections, shock, and postoperatively following major surgical procedures. After acute myocardial infarction, CK_2 (MB) appears within approximately four to eight hours and peaks at 12 to 24 hours; it may persist throughout the initial 72-hour period. CK_2 (MB) activity never exceeds 40 per cent of the total CK serum activity, with the remainder being CK_3 (MM) (Galen, 1975a). However, CK_3 (MM) level of serum remains elevated for four to five days following the onset of chest pain (Galen, 1975a). CK isoenzyme determinations performed subsequent to day four even with an elevated CK level will reveal only CK_3 (MM) activity, and its origin in heart or muscle cannot be established.

The presence of CK_2 (MB) in the serum is not unequivocally specific for myocardium because CK_2 is found in patients with certain muscular dystrophies, polymyositis, and significant myoglobinuria.

We emphasize CK_2 (MB) presence qualitatively following electrophoretic separation; the precision leaves much to be desired. At best, electrophoresis is a semiquantitative procedure in which the presence or absence of CK_2 (MB) should suffice. Among the available methods for CK isoenzymes (Griffiths, 1977) we have found the Corning ACI (agarose film) electrophoresis of CK isoenzyme (catalog No. 470114, Palo Alto, Cal. 94306) acceptable. Interpretation using appropriate fluorometric equipment yields adequate visualization for noting presence or absence of CK_2 (MB).

$$\text{Creatine-P} + \text{ADP} \overset{CK}{\rightleftharpoons} \text{Creatine} + \text{ATP}$$

Method of assay: Several are available. One depends on measuring creatine-P formed by measuring phosphorus after liberating it. Another involves several coupled reactions in which ADP formed is utilized to convert phosphoenolpyruvate to pyruvate in the presence of pyruvate kinase. Pyruvate formed is measured by following disappearance of NADH (at 340 mμ) under influence of added lactate dehydrogenase.

Conditions characterized by increased levels:
Progressive muscular dystrophy
Dermatomyositis
Myocardial infarction
Delirium tremens
Crush syndrome
Hypothyroidism

Figure 14–14. Reaction catalyzed by creatine phosphokinase (CK), principle of assay, and significance of abnormal serum levels.

Angiotensin-Converting Enzyme (ACE) (EC 3.4.15.1)

This enzyme, also called peptidyldipeptide hydrolase, converts angiotensin 1 to angiotensin 2, by splitting off the last two amino acids of angiotensin 1. Assay is usually performed by employing a synthetic substrate, benzoyl-glycyl-histidyl-leucine, and measuring spectrophotometrically the rate of release of the dipeptides benzoylglycine and histidyl-leucine. A radioassay has been developed recently.

Serum levels are elevated in patients with active sarcoidosis and leprosy, reflecting the fact that the main tissue sources of serum ACE are macrophages and epithelioid cells and that there is rich concentration of enzyme in sarcoid granulomas. Values are particularly high in patients with active pulmonary sarcoidosis and usually normal in inactive disease, as well as in other granulomatous disease of the lung, including tuberculosis, mycotic infections, and berylliosis (Rohrbach, 1982).

High values of ACE also are found in patients with Gaucher's disease, a phenomenon attributed to increased synthesis in Gaucher or other macrophage-derived cells in this disease (Silverstein, 1978). Other conditions with increased levels of ACE are primary biliary cirrhosis and amyloidosis (Rohrbach, 1982).

This is an interesting serum enzyme which provides help in the diagnosis of sarcoidosis and in monitoring its activity and in the recognition of Gaucher's disease. Nevertheless, its clinical employment has been limited.

Other Serum Enzymes

Many other enzymes have been demonstrated in the serum (Table 14–1). These are too numerous for individual description in this discussion, but there are a few that warrant special mention. These include guanase, an enzyme that has been reported to reflect, sensitively and specifically, hepatic disease; beta glucuronidase, considered a biochemical clue to neoplastic, hepatic, and other diseases; alcohol dehydrogenase, proposed as a measure of hepatic disease; plasma pepsinogen, an enzyme precursor that reflects function and disease of the stomach (high levels in patients with peptic ulcer, low levels in patients with pernicious anemia); and ceruloplasmin, a copper-carrying protein that is also an enzyme and the serum levels of which are depressed in patients with hepatolenticular degeneration (Wilson's disease). Ceruloplasmin measurement is useful in the diagnosis of Wilson's disease. The practical role that the other enzymes cited and others listed in Tables 14–1 and 14–2 may play in clinical medicine remains to be demonstrated.

CLINICAL APPLICATION OF SERUM ENZYME ASSAYS

Serum enzymology provides aid in making the diagnosis, monitoring the course, and demonstrating subclinical evidence of disease. Diseases that are characterized by distinctly abnormal values of one or more enzymes (Table 14–16) can be readily distinguished from clinically similar states in which abnormal values for the respective enzymes do not occur. The diagnostic circumstances that are most clearly aided by serum enzymology are the distinction of myocardial infarction from other causes of chest pain, the differential diagnosis of hepatobiliary and muscle disease, the diagnosis of pancreatitis, and the recognition of metastases of neoplastic disease to bone or liver (Table 14–17).

The diagnostic application of serum enzyme assays is based on the accumulated clinical experience and experimental data that permit formulation of factors that lead to abnormal enzyme levels (Table 14–5) and correlation of particular serum enzymes with the nature of the pathologic process and the organ involved (Table 14–16). This type of assessment serves to epitomize most of the foregoing material. It permits selection of the enzyme tests most likely to be of diagnostic value and of the clinical circumstances most likely to be benefited by current knowledge of serum enzymology. Some disease processes are characterized by abnormal values of one or more enzymes (Table 14–16). Thus, osteoblastic lesions lead to elevations of ALP values that range from slight to marked. Obstruction of the biliary tree (or intrahepatic cholestasis) leads to markedly elevated values of ALP, LAP, 5′-N, and GGT; relatively slightly elevated values of transaminases, OCT, ID, ICD, LD, HBD, MD, ALS, and PHI; and normal values for CK. Hepatic necrosis leads to lesser values of ALP, LAP, 5′-N, and GGT, but very high values of AST (GOT), ALT (GPT), OCT, ID, ICD, MD, ALS, and PHI; and normal values for CK. In myocardial necrosis, moderately elevated levels of AST, LD, HBD, MD, ALS, PHI, and CK are noted. Skeletal muscle disease of the progressively degenerative or inflammatory type (progressive muscular dystrophy, dermatomyositis, trichinosis) leads to striking elevations of CK and LD levels; moderate elevations of LD, ALS, PHI, and MD, with more modest increase in the AST (GOT) level and even lesser values of ALT (GPT) and normal levels of the other enzymes listed in Table 14–16. Neoplastic disease is characterized by increased values of LD, ALS, PHI, and MD, with the increase seemingly dependent on the tumor having reached sufficient total mass. Reports of GGT suggest that this enzyme is also increased in the serum of patients with carcinomatosis. Metastatic carcinoma of the liver leads to moderate or marked elevations of ALP, LAP, 5′-N, and GGT and to slightly or moderately elevated values of AST (GOT) and ALT (GPT). These abnormalities are also seen with other "space-occupying" lesions of the liver (granuloma, abscess, amyloidosis). The pattern of serum enzyme abnormality of hepatic metastases also includes increased values of enzymes that reflect neoplastic growth. Metastases to various sites from prostatic carcinoma lead to high acid phosphatase levels. Metastases of carcinoma to the bone, if osteoblastic, lead to high alkaline phosphatase levels but to normal values of AST (GOT) and ALT (GPT).

Table 14–16. ABNORMAL VALUES OF SOME SERUM ENZYMES IN VARIOUS PATHOLOGIC PROCESSES*

			Necrosis of				Neoplastic Disease†	
Enzyme	**Osteoblastic Activity**	**Biliary Obstruction**	***Liver***	***Heart***	***Skeletal Muscle***	***Pancreas***	***Neoplastic Growth***	***Hepatic Metastases***
ALP	1–4+	4+	+	–	–	–	–	1–4+
ACP	–	–	–	–	–	–	+(prostate)	
LAP	–	4+	+	–	–	–	–	1–4+
5′-N	–	4+	+	–	–	–	–	1–4+
GGT	–	4+	+	+	–	–	+	1–4+
AST (GOT)	–	+	4+	2+	1+	±	–	2+
ALT (GPT)	–	+	4+	±	±	±	–	1+
ID	–	+	4+	–	–	–	–	1+
ICD	–	+	4+	–	–	–		1+
LD	–	+	+	2+	2+	±	3+	3+
HBD	–	±	±	2+	±	±	+	+
MD	–	+	2+	2+	2+	±	2+	2+
ALS	–	+	3+	2+	4+	±	3+	3+
PHI	–	+	3+	2+	2+	±	3+	3+
CK	–	–	–	4+	4+	–	–	–
Amylase	–	±	–	–	–	4+	–	–
Lipase	–	±	–	–	–	4+	–	–

*1–4+ represents grades of elevated values; – represents values within the expected reference interval.
†Includes granulocytic leukemia.

Table 14–17. PATTERNS OF ABNORMAL SERUM ENZYME VALUES IN SEVERAL CLINICAL SETTINGS*

		AST (GOT)	**ALT (GPT)**	**LD**	**LD_1 (Heat Stable) (HBD)**	**CK (CPK)**	**ALS**	**ALP**
Chest Pain and Related Circumstances	Myocardial infarction	↑↑	±	↑↑	↑↑	↑↑↑	↑↑	N
	Pulmonary infarction	±	±	↑↑	±	±	↑↑	N
	Heart failure	±	±		±	±	↑	↑
	Shock	↑↑	↑	↑↑	±	±	↑↑	N
Muscle Disease	Progressive muscular dystrophy, Trichinosis, Dermatomyositis, Polymyositis, Delirium tremens	↑↑	↑	↑↑	↑	↑↑↑	↑↑↑	N
	Neurogenic muscle disease	N	N	N	N	N	N	N
Jaundice (see Chapter 13)	Acute hepatitis	↑↑↑↑	↑↑↑↑	↑	±	N	↑↑	↑
	Cirrhosis (Laennec's)	↑	±	±	±	±	±	↑
	Obstructive jaundice	↑↑	↑↑	↑	±	±	↑	↑↑↑
Neoplastic Disease	Localized carcinoma of small size	N	N	N	N	N	N	N
	Extensive carcinoma without hepatic or bone metastases	N	N	↑↑	±	±	↑↑	N
	Carcinoma with metastases to liver or hepatoma	↑↑	↑	↑↑	±	±	↑↑	↑↑↑
	Carcinoma with osteoblastic metastases to bone	N	N	↑↑	±	±	↑↑	↑↑↑
	Leukemia (granulocytic or acute)	N	N	↑↑	±	±	↑↑	N
	Leukemia (chronic lymphatic)	N	N	N	N	N	N	N
Anemia	Megaloblastic	N	N	↑↑↑↑	↑	N	↑↑↑	N
	Iron deficiency	N	N	N	N	N	N	N
	Hemolytic	N	N	↑↑	↑	N	↑↑	N

*Number of arrows indicates magnitude of increase; N indicates no change; ± = variable.

Monitoring the course of disease by serial determinations of serum enzyme levels is useful in the management of hepatitis, in the chemotherapy of neoplastic disease, in the treatment of dermatomyositis, and in the recognition of recurrent infarction or other complications during convalescence from acute myocardial infarction. Detection of subclinical disease by serum enzyme assay is exemplified by the use of serum aldolase or CK levels to recognize individuals destined to develop progressive muscular dystrophy, or the employment of AST, ALT, and alkaline phosphatase to monitor patients exposed to known or potentially hepatotoxic agents. In Table 14–17 are shown the patterns of abnormality obtained in various clinical circumstances utilizing a small panel of enzyme tests.

Serum Enzymes in Myocardial Infarction

Serum enzyme analysis has become as routine a measure as electrocardiography in the diagnostic approach to patients suspected of having sustained a myocardial infarction. Distinction is usually readily made from pulmonary infarction, which is characterized by elevated LD levels and usually by normal AST values. In a small proportion of patients with pulmonary embolism, slightly elevated values for AST occur by three or four days after the bout of chest pain.

The complication of myocardial infarction by shock leads to higher values of AST and LD and to abnormal levels of enzymes that reflect hepatic injury (ALT, ICD). Indeed, shock of any origin, or severe hypoxia, leads to high levels of a large number of enzymes presumably released from the liver and perhaps from other tissues.

Of the large number of enzymes released to the blood from infarcted myocardium (Table 14–5 and 14–16), only a few have been regularly applied to the diagnosis of infarction (Table 14–17). Most extensively employed are the total serum activity of CK and LD, each of which yields abnormal values in almost all patients with proven infarction. The degree, onset, and duration of rise of each enzyme are characteristic. CK values increase within four to six hours following myocardial infarction, with a peak value up to 12 times greater than normal CK value occurring at approximately 24 hours. A return of CK to normal activity is found usually by the third day. Within the first 48 hours CK_2 (MB) is present in virtually all patients with myocardial infarction, as well as in some cases of severe coronary insufficiency (Galen, 1975a). The determination of CK isoenzymes with demonstration of a CK_2 (MB) isoenzyme during this period is virtually diagnostic of myocardial infarction. At 72 hours only 66 per cent of patients with myocardial infarction exhibit MB (CK_2 fraction) with significantly lower levels of activity. CK_2 (MB) then disappears rapidly, although the serum CK_3 (MM) fraction may still be elevated.

Serum LD activity increases two- to four-fold following myocardial infarction, with persistence of elevation considerably longer (10 to 14 days). The measurement of LD isoenzymes, as noted previously, provides a further refinement in laboratory assessment of patients with myocardial infarction. However, the "flipped LDH" ($LD_1 > LD_2$) is a more variable phenomenon which may become evident at 12 hours and be present in approximately 80 per cent of patients with myocardial infarction within the first 48 hours (Galen, 1975a). It is not necessarily maintained, since in less than half of the patients with myocardial infarctions there may not be a "flipped LDH" at the end of one week, even though serum LD level may still be elevated.

Combined Criteria Isoenzyme Analysis

The simultaneous use of CK and LD isoenzyme determinations combines the high degree of sensitivity offered by CK with the high degree of specificity offered by LD (Galen, 1975a) (Table 14–18). Combined criteria are met when there is a "flipped LDH" pattern ($LD_1 > LD_2$) present in a patient exhibiting CK_2 (MB) in specimens drawn during the first 48 hours following an acute episode of suspected myocardial infarction (Galen, 1975a). Ideally, three separate specimens are collected; first on admission, a second at 24 hours, and a third at 48 hours. Both CK and LD serum assays are measured. If total enzyme activity is elevated, isoenzyme analyses are performed. The "flipped LD" comes after the appearance of CK_2 (MB). Galen has also emphasized that the criteria do not have to be demonstrated in a single specimen. Indeed, they are frequently met by examining serum patterns in 24- and 48-hour specimens together. Table 14–18 displays the format for interpreting combined isoenzyme data during the initial 48-hour period (Galen, 1975a).

To be used most efficiently the combined criteria must be evaluated during the initial 48 hours of suspected onset of ischemic heart disease. Once diagnostic criteria are met, there is no need for further determinations to document the diagnosis. Indeed, if at 24 hours both criteria are met, the diagnosis is affirmative (Galen, 1975a). A CK_2 (MB) determination may then be done to estimate the infarct size or detect extension or reinfarction (Roberts, 1979). If combined criteria are not met by 48 hours, the diagnosis is then presumptively not myocardial infarction (Table 14–18). It should be emphasized, however, that the combined criteria after a 48-hour interval do not rule out myocardial infarction with the same high degree of certainty present during the acute phase (initial 48-hour period) of potential ischemic injury. Indeed, it is possible that a myocardial infarction may reveal CK_2 (MB) and the usual LD profile on day four.

Galen has also emphasized the application of combined isoenzyme analysis to special conditions in which confirmation of acute myocardial infarction is hampered by non-specific enzyme elevation. In electroshock cardioversion, there is no CK_2 (MB); furthermore, with intramuscular administration of drugs,

Table 14–18. COMBINED ISOENZYME ANALYSIS: RULE OUT MYOCARDIAL INFARCTION (MI)*

CK-MB absent	CK-MB present Usual LDH	CK-MB present Flipped-LDH
↓	↓	↓
100 per cent predictive value that there is no MI	Both MI and non-MI cases†	100 per cent predictive value that there is MI

*During acute 48 hour period following episode.
†Non-MI cases reflect clinical and electrocardiographic evidence of ischemia.
From Galen, R. S.: Hum. Path., *6*:2, 1975. With permission of R. S. Galen, M.D.

serum total CK elevation reflects only CK_3 (MM). Major operative procedures lead to no elevation of CK_2 (MB) but only to that of the MM. Pre- and postoperative total serum LD and CK, however, are not helpful in the postoperative period. In that setting evaluation of myocardial infarction requires the combined isoenzymes "flipped LD" and CK_2 (MB). With cardiopulmonary bypass, patients undoubtedly have a high risk of myocardial infarction; with manipulation of heart, etc., ischemic injury probably takes place during surgery. Hence, discrimination between myocardial infarction and non-myocardial infarction following open-heart surgery is extremely difficult. Indeed, Galen (1975a) has noted, as we have, that an overlap is present between the two groups. Despite these pitfalls, the enzymologic approach to diagnosis in this setting is useful. There are additional caveats to its use in cardiologic diagnosis. There is also myocardial injury with cardiac valve replacement and aneurysmectomy surgery. Hence, LD and CK isoenzymes are less specific and must be interpreted with caution. Furthermore, a "flipped LDH" pattern may appear in 25 per cent of non-myocardial infarction patients secondary to hemolysis from extracorporeal circulation (Galen, 1975a). Indeed, CK levels and measurement of the CK_2 (MB) band appear to be the most sensitive and specific available clinical tests for the diagnosis of acute myocardial infarction (Fisher, 1983).

Serum Enzymes in Liver Disease

The enzymologic approach to liver disease is discussed in Chapter 13. It remains to be proved that employment of the apparently liver-specific OCT, ID, or guanase or of the isoenzymes of LD will add a significant measure of sensitivity or specificity to that provided by the simple panel of AST and ALT. Similarly, the distinction of the elevated ALP levels of hepatobiliary disease from those caused by osteoblastic lesions offers little difficulty if consideration is given to other laboratory measurements and clinical features of hepatic and biliary tract disease. This distinction may be aided by assay of the LAP, GGT, or 5′-N, the levels of which parallel those of ALP in hepatobiliary disease but are normal in diseases of bone. Studies of isoenzymes of ALP by electrophoretic, kinetic, or other techniques for the purpose of distinguishing bone from hepatic phosphatase seem at present to be of greater theoretical interest than clinical benefit. Cholinesterase levels, at one time considered a valuable enzymologic tool for the management of hepatic disease, have been supplanted by the more readily measurable, more sensitive, and more specific transaminases.

Enzyme analysis in hepatobiliary disease is useful in differential diagnosis, as discussed in Chapter 13. Monitoring the course of serum enzyme levels is helpful in following the course of acute or chronic hepatitis or of active macronodular cirrhosis. For this purpose AST and ALT assays may be employed. Alcoholic hepatitis is reflected more sensitively by AST levels than by ALT values. Monitoring of patients exposed to possible hepatotoxins is usefully accomplished by a simple panel consisting of ALP, AST, and ALT. If evidence of mitochondrial injury is sought, glutamate dehydrogenase levels also may be measured.

Serum Enzymes in Muscle Disease

Measurement of serum enzyme levels has become a major component of the diagnostic approach to muscle disease. The enzymes that have been studied most extensively are ALS, AST, LD, and CK. The last named is the most reliable measure of skeletal muscle disease, since, as discussed previously, elevated values are relatively specific for disease of striated muscle (skeletal muscle and myocardium). Aldolase levels appear to be as sensitive to disease of muscle, although somewhat less specific.

Elevated levels of these enzymes occur in patients with dystrophic or myositic processes. In the progressive muscular dystrophies, especially the Duchenne type, the values are particularly high. Moderate or marked elevations are seen in dermatomyositis, in polymyositis, in scleroderma with an associated myositis, and in trichinosis. Slightly or moderately increased levels of these enzymes are also observed in myotonic dystrophy, in myotonia congenita, in the crush syndrome, and in McArdle's disease. High values of these and other enzymes occur in patients with delirium tremens, irrespective of associated hepatic disease, and presumably arise in muscle (LD_5

and CK_3). The muscle involvement of myxedema appears to be responsible for the elevated serum enzyme levels seen in this condition. Strenuous muscle activity in untrained individuals also leads to increased levels of these enzymes. Serum enzyme levels are normal in patients with neurogenic muscle disease. Disease of the upper motor neuron, the anterior horn cell, or the peripheral nerve does not lead to elevated values.

For the clinical application to the diagnosis of muscle disease, both aldolase (ALS) and CK should be measured. If values for both are abnormal, the results can be interpreted with greater confidence. These tests are of help in recognizing early muscular dystrophy before clinical manifestations appear and may be useful clues to the carrier female. They are also of value in the differential diagnosis of the other muscular diseases cited and in following the course of inflammatory disease of the muscle.

Isoenzymes of CK (MM) and LD (LD_5) also reflect skeletal muscle injury. In Duchenne's muscular dystrophy, CK_2 (MB) appears in sera as well as in heart disease with LD_1.

Serum Enzymes in Neoplastic Disease

A large number of studies have demonstrated high serum levels of glycolytic and other enzymes (Table 14–16) in the serum of animals and humans with a variety of carcinomas and other neoplastic lesions. In general, the levels of enzymes studied are normal in patients with small localized tumors; increased values are seen when the local tumor has become large, has extended to surrounding tissue, or has reached distant metastatic sites. Data from several laboratories indicate that the serum levels of these enzymes reflect and are proportional to the total mass of tumor rather than the involvement of tissue at specific metastatic sites. Measurement of levels of any of the glycolytic or other enzymes that are elevated in patients with carcinomatosis fails to provide a means of detecting early neoplasms that are resectable; however, perhaps the search for such an enzymologic clue should continue to be pursued. Patterns of serum enzyme abnormality are of value in supporting the diagnosis of carcinomatosis, and the monitoring of serum enzyme levels is useful in following the response to chemotherapy of patients with inoperable neoplasms.

Increased levels of the same enzymes are observed in patients with Hodgkin's disease, lymphosarcoma, and granulocytic and acute leukemia. Adequate response to chemotherapy is reflected in decreasing values. The values are normal in patients with chronic lymphocytic leukemia and in most patients with multiple myeloma.

The enzymes that have been most extensively studied in neoplastic states and that can be used to monitor the course of widespread neoplastic disease are lactate dehydrogenase, phosphohexoisomerase, and aldolase; however, the others listed in Table 14–17 also reflect the process.

Table 14–19. TYPES OF HEREDITARY NON-SPHEROCYTIC HEMOLYTIC ANEMIA (HNHA) WHICH ARE KNOWN OR SUSPECTED TO BE DUE TO ENZYMATIC DEFECTS OF ERYTHROCYTES*

Condition (Names indicate missing enzymes)
Most important and frequent conditions
1. Glucose-6-phosphate dehydrogenase (G-6-PD) deficiency
2. Pyruvate kinase (PK) deficiency
3. Phosphohexoisomerase (PHI) (Glucose phosphate isomerase) deficiency
Rare conditions
4. Hexokinase (HK) deficiency
5. Phosphofructokinase (PFK) deficiency
6. Triosephosphate isomerase (TPI) deficiency
7. Phosphoglycerate kinase (PGK) deficiency
Very rare conditions
8. Pyrimidine-5′-P-nucleotidase (5-5′-PN) deficiency
9. Aldolase deficiency†
10. GSH synthetase deficiency
11. GSH peroxidase deficiency
Very rare or equivocal conditions
12. Glutathione reductase (GR) deficiency
13. Glyceraldehyde phosphate dehydrogenase deficiency
14. 6-Phosphoglycerate dehydrogenase (6-PGD) deficiency
15. 2,3-Diphosphoglycerate mutase (2,3-DPGM) deficiency
16. ATPase deficiency
17. Adenylate kinase (AK) deficiency
18. Diphosphoglycerate phosphatase (DPGP) deficiency
19. Enolase deficiency

*See Beutler, 1976.

†At one time aldolase deficiency was considered to be responsible for familial spherocytic anemia; now known not to be true.

ENZYMES OF THE FORMED ELEMENTS OF THE BLOOD

During the past few years, considerable attention has been devoted to the metabolic activity and enzyme content of erythrocytes and leukocytes. The extensive studies related to the employment of these elements as *in vitro* metabolic models and to the factors involved in blood preservation are beyond the scope of this discussion. This section attempts to summarize some of the studies of erythrocyte enzymes that have unraveled several genetic hemolytic syndromes (Table 14–19) and the studies of erythrocyte and leukocyte enzymes that have been useful in the diagnosis of several genetic and acquired systemic conditions (Table 14–20).

Hemolytic Anemia Associated with Deficiency of Erythrocyte Enzymes

Genetic defects in erythrocyte metabolism have been found or suspected to be responsible for well over a dozen forms of hemolytic anemia (Table 14–

Table 14–20. SYSTEMIC DISEASES IN WHICH DIAGNOSIS CAN BE ESTABLISHED BY ANALYSIS OF ENZYME ACTIVITY OF FORMED ELEMENT OF BLOOD

Condition	Formed Element	Enzyme Assay
Genetic		
Methemoglobinemia	RBC	NADH-methemoglobin reductase
Acatalasemia	RBC	Catalase
Galactosemia		Gal-1-P-uridyl transferase
Glycogenosis (Type III)	WBC	Amylo-1,6-glucosidase
(Type IV)	WBC	Phosphorylase
(Type VII)	RBC	Phosphofructokinase
Hypophosphatasia	WBC	Alkaline phosphatase
Lipid storage diseases		
Gaucher's	WBC	β-Glucosidase
Niemann-Pick	WBC	Sphingomyelinase
Krabbe's leukodystrophy (globoid)	WBC	β-Galactosidase
Metachromatic leukodystrophy	WBC	Sulfatidase
Fabry's disease	WBC	α-Galactosidase
Tay-Sachs disease	WBC	Hexosaminidase
Acquired		
Thiamine deficiency	RBC	Transketolase
Pyridoxine deficiency	RBC	Alanine aminotransferase
Hyperthyroidism	RBC	Carbonic anhydrase
Leukemia, granulocytic	WBC	Alkaline phosphatase
Lead poisoning	RBC	δ-Aminolevulinic acid dehydrase

19). Some of the demonstrated or assumed enzymatic defects relate to the hexose monophosphate shunt (G-6-PD, 6-PGD, GR, GSH-synthetase, GSH-peroxidase), and some of the enzymatic defects relate to the anaerobic glycolytic pathway (HK, PHI, PFK, ALS, TPI, 2-3DPGM, PGK, PK) and ATP-ase. The hemolytic syndromes associated with enzymatic defects are listed in Table 14–19.

Hemolytic Anemia Secondary to G-6-PD Deficiency. Deficiency of erythrocyte G-6-PD activity has been estimated to involve 2 to 3 per cent of the world population and to be responsible for almost one third of the cases of chronic or recurrent non-spherocytic hemolytic anemia. The defect is sex-linked and appears in a number of genetic variants. The first to be recognized is the relatively mild condition observed almost exclusively in blacks and characterized by deficient concentration of G-6-PD in erythrocytes but normal concentration in leukocytes and platelets. These individuals develop hemolysis on exposure to a number of drugs, including primaquine, sulfonamides, and other agents, and to other stresses, including various infections. A more severe form of G-6-PD deficiency, characterized by deficiency of the enzyme in leukocytes and erythrocytes, by more severe anemia, and by sensitivity to fava beans and to various drugs, is seen in Caucasians, particularly Sephardic Jews, other ethnic groups of the Mediterranean littoral, American Indians, and Orientals. Studies of the various forms of G-6-PD deficiency have shown not only differences in the severity of the clinical illness and the degree of depression of enzyme levels of erythrocytes and leukocytes, but also that there are different molecular variants (isoenzymes) of G-6-PD. The mechanism whereby G-6-PD deficiency permits drug-induced hemolysis remains incompletely understood but is indirectly related to the inability to maintain adequate levels of reduced glutathione in the erythrocyte on exposure to offending agents.

Assay of G-6-PD activity has become a routine procedure in patients with hemolytic anemia, especially if it occurs after administration of a drug or during an acute illness. A precise assay of G-6-PD activity of hemolysate involves measuring the rate at which NADP is reduced in the presence of glucose-6-phosphate. Simplified assays suitable for screening large populations are available.

Deficiency of 6-PGD. Decreased erythrocyte levels of 6-PGD have been reported, but the role of this abnormality in inducing susceptibility to hemolysis remains to be proved. The principle of assay of 6-PGD activity of erythrocytes is similar to that of G-6-PD.

Hemolytic Anemia Secondary to Deficiency of Glutathione Reductase (GR), Glutathione Peroxidase (GSH-Px), or Glutathione Synthetase

A few instances of mild hemolytic anemia have been reported in patients with genetic deficiency in erythrocyte levels of GR. Some have been instances of chronic hemolysis and others of hemolytic anemia after exposure to drugs (primaquine). Thus far, the condition appears to be rare and primarily of genetic interest. Almost complete absence of glutathione from erythrocytes as a genetic abnormality has been found to occur in several genera. The deficiency of glutathione in these individuals appears to be transmitted as an autosomal recessive and presumably results from subnormal glutathione synthetase activity. The erythrocytes of patients with GSH deficiency, like those of patients with G-6-PD and GR deficiency, are susceptible to drug-induced hemolysis. A similar syndrome has been attributed to deficiency of GSH-Px, the enzyme presumed to be mainly responsible for destroying H_2O_2 in human erythrocytes.

Hemolytic Anemias Secondary to Deficiency in Glycolytic Enzymes

Pyruvate kinase (PK) deficiency is the most frequent and important form of hemolytic anemia due to deficiency of glycolytic enzymes in the erythrocyte. It is transmitted as an autosomal recessive and characterized by a non-spherocytic, chronic hemolytic anemia. The hemolysis is attributable to the inability of the PK-deficient erythrocyte to maintain normal ATP levels and the resulting membrane defect. Enzyme activity of the erythrocyte can be assayed by measuring the ability of hemolysate to form pyruvate from ADP and phosphoenol pyruvate.

Similar syndromes appear to result from deficient erythrocyte content of hexokinase, phosphohexoisomerase, phosphofructokinase, triose phosphate isomerase, 2,3-diphosphoglycerate mutase, phosphoglycerate kinase, and ATPase and other enzymes. These are rare and, at present, of little clinical importance (see Chapter 29 for further discussion).

Systemic Diseases Reflected in Abnormal Erythrocyte and Leukocyte Enzymes

Several genetic diseases are reflected by abnormal levels of enzymes in the erythrocytes (Table 14–20). Acatalasia, also called Takahara's disease or oral gangrene, is a condition characterized by marked deficiency in the concentration of catalase in the tissues and in the erythrocytes. Deficiency of catalase, an enzyme which destroys hydrogen peroxide ($2H_2O_2 \xrightarrow{\text{catalase}} 2H_2O + O_2$), leads to the accumulation of hydrogen peroxide when it is produced in excess. This is often asymptomatic and becomes of clinical importance only in some patients with oral sepsis, in whose oral cavities peroxide formed by bacteria can accumulate and lead to gangrene. It is a self-limiting state which disappears after the teeth are lost. Transmitted as an autosomal recessive, the condition is of greater genetic interest than clinical importance. Homozygous abnormals who have almost no catalase in the erythrocytes can be distinguished from the heterozygotes whose values are midway between the homozygote abnormal and normal. Hereditary methemoglobinemia secondary to deficiency of erythrocyte diaphorase is a rare oligosymptomatic condition which is transmitted as an autosomal recessive. The methemoglobinemia, which leads to cyanosis, is the result of deficiency of NADH-methemoglobin reductase (diaphorase).

Glycogenosis of types III, IV, and VII and hypophosphatasia can be identified by measuring the leukocyte content of the relevant enzyme. Confirmation of the diagnosis of type IV glycogenosis, which is due to *hepatophosphorylase* deficiency, can be obtained by measuring the phosphorylase activity of leukocytes. Type III glycogenosis, which is a manifestation of deficiency of the glycogen *debrancher* enzyme (amylo-1-6-glucosidase), can also be diagnosed by measuring the leukocyte content of that enzyme. Type VII glycogenosis, which is associated with a hemolytic anemia, can be identified by demonstrating deficient phosphofructokinase activity in the erythrocytes. *Hypophosphatasia* is characterized by a genetic deficiency of alkaline phosphatase content of tissues and blood. Measurement of alkaline phosphatase levels of the leukocytes can in the proper clinical setting assist in establishing the diagnosis.

Galactosemia is an inborn error of metabolism characterized by a specific defect in the utilization of galactose which results in widespread tissue damage. The defect has been found to be deficiency of the enzyme phosphogalactose-uridyl-transferase. The resulting accumulation of galactose-1-phosphate is considered responsible for the development of cataracts, liver disease, renal disease, and other abnormalities. The hereditary enzyme deficiency can be demonstrated by studying the erythrocyte. The ability of hemolysate to catalyze the conversion of galactose-1-phosphate to UDP-galactose in the presence of UDP-glucose is measured by following the disappearance of UDP-glucose. The test, which can be readily performed, yields very low values in patients with galactosemia, who are homozygous for the abnormal gene. Heterozygote carriers can usually be identified by this test, which yields values intermediate between the normal and the homozygous abnormal.

A number of lipid storage diseases can be identified by demonstrating deficient activity of the related enzyme in circulating leukocytes (Table 14–20). Several acquired diseases can also be identified by studying enzyme activity of the formed elements. Thiamine deficiency can be confirmed by demonstrating depressed transketolase activity of hemolysate. Pyridoxine deficiency can be demonstrated by measuring the ALT activity of erythrocytes before and after incubation with pyridoxal-5-phosphate. Abnormal levels of cholinesterase, carbonic anhydrase, and several other enzymes have been demonstrated in the erythrocytes of patients with a variety of acquired systemic diseases, but these are of pathophysiologic rather than diagnostic importance. The recent description of depressed erythrocyte levels of δ-aminolevulinic acid dehydrase as a measure of blood levels of lead suggests that measurement of this enzyme may be useful in the diagnosis of lead poisoning. Measurement of leukocyte alkaline phosphatase helps in distinguishing granulocytic leukemia from leukemoid states. Alkaline phosphatase levels are very low in the leukocytes of granulocytic leukemia, but they are normal or elevated in patients with non-leukemic leukocytosis.

ENZYME CONCENTRATIONS IN OTHER BODY FLUIDS

Measurement of enzyme activity in serous effusions, gastrointestinal juices, cerebrospinal fluid, and urine has been applied to the diagnosis of various diseases.

Localized release of enzyme from neoplastic cells has been considered responsible for the high levels of LD (and other glycolytic enzymes) in malignant pleural and peritoneal effusions, in the gastric juice of patients with carcinoma of the stomach, and in the urine of patients with renal carcinoma. The glucuronidase in the urine of patients with carcinoma of the bladder and in the vaginal fluid of patients with carcinoma of the cervix may also be considered to be enzyme shed by neoplastic cells.

Determination of levels of LD in serous cavity effusions has been proposed as a method of demonstrating neoplastic involvement of serosal surfaces (Chap. 19). In such circumstances, the serous fluid usually shows higher levels of LD than does the serum. High levels of LD, however, are also found in patients with inflammatory and hemorrhagic effusions. Accordingly, measurements of enzyme content of serous effusions appear to be of limited clinical value. Measurement of LD levels of gastric juice or urine to detect renal or gastric carcinoma, respectively, or of glucuronidase in the urine or vaginal fluid to detect carcinoma of the bladder or cervix, respectively, remains to be proven of clinical value.

The demonstration of a high amylase value in pleural or ascitic fluid is useful in making the diagnosis of pancreatitis. The demonstration of increased levels of amylase in the urine is also a useful supplement to the measurement of serum levels of the enzyme in the diagnosis of pancreatitis (Chap. 24).

Measurement of urinary levels of lactate dehydrogenase, alkaline phosphatase, muramidase (lysozyme), catalase, β-glucuronidase, and pepsinogen has been proposed for the diagnosis or monitoring of a number of conditions. Increased levels of lactate dehydrogenase, alkaline phosphatase, and β-glucuronidase are frequent in patients with carcinoma of the urinary tract but may also be caused by hematuria, urinary tract infection, or glomerulonephritis and are, accordingly, too non-specific to be clinically useful. Catalase may be found in the urine when there is bacteriuria, pyuria, or hematuria. Muramidase activity of the urine may be very high in patients with monocytic or monomyelocytic leukemia. For monitoring the course of the disease, however, serum levels of this enzyme are probably more useful. Urinary (and plasma) pepsinogen values are increased in patients with peptic ulcer and low in those with pernicious anemia. These observations are of pathophysiologic interest rather than clinical value.

Increased levels of β-glucuronidase and 6-phosphogluconate dehydrogenase have been demonstrated in the vaginal fluid of a high proportion of patients with carcinoma of the uterus, especially the cervix. However, the normal values found in some patients with cancer and the elevated values found in some patients with benign conditions prevent useful application of assay of vaginal fluid enzyme activity for the recognition of carcinoma. Measurement of tartrate inhibitable acid phosphatase in vaginal fluid is a useful procedure for the diagnosis of rape, since this isoenzyme is of prostatic origin and therefore high in semen.

Cerebrospinal fluid enzyme levels are relatively independent of the serum levels. Increased spinal fluid levels of glutamate oxaloacetate transaminase, lactate dehydrogenase, ribonuclease, and glutathione reductase have been described in patients with various diseases of the central nervous system. The levels of one or more of these enzymes are increased in patients with cerebrovascular hemorrhage, thrombosis or embolism, meningitis, and neoplasms of the central nervous system. The clinical application and value of spinal fluid enzyme determinations remain to be established. (Also see Chapter 19.)

2

General

Abderhalden, R.: Clinical Enzymology. Princeton, N.J., D. Van Nostrand Co., 1961.

Cabaud, P. G., and Wroblewski, F.: Colorimetric measurement of lactic dehydrogenase activity of body fluids. Am. J. Clin. Pathol., *30*:234, 1958.

Coodley, E. L. (ed.): Diagnostic Enzymology. Philadelphia, Lea & Febiger, 1970.

Goldberg, D. M., and Weiner, M. (eds.): Progress in Clinical Enzymology. New York, Masson Publishing USA, Inc., 1980.

Shugar, D.: Enzymes and Isoenzymes, Structure, Properties and Function, Vol. 18. New York, Academic Press, Inc., 1970.

Statland, B. E.: The case for standardizing enzyme assays. Lab. Manage., *15*:46, 1977.

Wilkinson, J. H.: The Principles and Practice of Diagnostic Enzymology. London, Edward Arnold, 1976.

Wolf, P. L., Williams, D., and Von der Muehle, E.: Practical Clinical Enzymology. New York, John Wiley & Sons, Inc., 1973.

Serum Enzyme Levels in Liver Disease

Ellis, G., Goldberg, D. M., Spooner R. J., and Ward, A. M.: Serum enzyme tests in diseases of the liver and biliary tree. Am. J. Clin. Path., *70*:248, 1978.

Hutterer, F.: Recent progress in clinical enzymology for the diagnosis of liver disease. *In* Schaffner, F., Sherlock, S., and Leevy, C. M. (eds.): The Liver and Its Diseases. New York, International Universities Press, 1974, p. 876.

Patel, S., and O'Gorman, P. O.: Serum enzyme levels in alcoholism and drug dependency. J. Clin. Path., *28*:714, 1975.

Schmidt, E., and Schmidt, F. W.: Fundamentals and evaluation of enzyme patterns in serum. *In* Popper, H., and Schaffner, F. (eds.): Progress in Liver Diseases, Vol. VII. New York, Grune & Stratton, 1982, pp. 411–428.

Skreder, S., Blomkoff, J. P., and Gjone, E.: Biochemical features of acute and chronic hepatitis. Ann. Clin. Res., *8*:182, 1976.

Wacker, W. E. C., Ulmer, D. D., and Vallee, B. L.: Metalloenzymes and myocardial infarction. N. Engl. J. Med., *255*:449, 1956.

Zimmerman, H. J., and Seeff, L. B.: Enzymes in hepatic disease. *In* Coodley, E. L. (ed.): Diagnostic Enzymology. Philadelphia, Lea & Febiger, 1970, p. 1.

Creatine Phosphokinase and Other Enzymes in Myocardial Infarction and Muscle Disease

Auvinen, S.: Evaluation of serum enzyme tests in the diagnosis of acute myocardial infarction. Acta Med. Scand. [Suppl. 539], 1972.

Cohen, L., and Morgan, J.: The enzymatic and immunologic detection of myocardial injury. Med. Clin. North Am., *57*:105, 1973.

Doran, G. R., and Wilkinson, J. H.: The origin of the elevated activity of creatine kinase and other enzymes in the sera of patients with myxoedema. Clin. Chim. Acta, *62*:203, 1975.

Fisher, M. D., Carliner, N. H., Becker, L. C., Peters, R. W., and Plotnick, G. O.: Serum creatine kinase in the diagnosis of acute myocardial infarction. Optimal sampling frequency. J.A.M.A., *249*:393, 1983.

Galen, R. S.: The enzyme diagnosis of myocardial infarction. Hum. Path., *6*:141, 1975a.

Galen, R. S., Reiffel, J. A., and Gambino, S. R.: Diagnosis of acute myocardial infarction: Relative efficiency of serum enzyme and isoenzyme measurement. J.A.M.A., *232*:145, 1975b.

Griffiths, J., and Handschuh, G.: Creatine kinase isoenzyme MB in myocardial infarction: Methods compared. Clin. Chem., *23*:567, 1977.

Konttinen, A., and Somer, H.: Specificity of serum creatine kinase isoenzymes in diagnosis of acute myocardial infarction. Br. Med. J., *1*:386, 1973.

Roberts, R.: Creatine kinase isozymes as diagnostic and prognostic indices of myocardial infarction. *In* Rattazzi, M., Scandallos, J. G., and Whitt, G. S. (eds.): Isozymes: Current Topics in Biological and Medicine Research, Vol. 3. New York, Alan R. Liss Inc., 1979, pp. 115–154.

Roe, C. R., Limbird, L. E., Wagner, G. S., and Nerenberg, S. T.: Combined isoenzyme analysis in the diagnosis of myocardial injury: Application of electrophoretic methods for the detection and quantitation of the creatine phosphokinase MB isoenzyme. J. Lab. Clin. Med., *80*:557, 1972.

West, M., Eshchar, J., and Zimmerman, H. J.: Serum enzymology in the diagnosis of myocardial infarction and related cardiovascular conditions. Med. Clin. North Am., *50*:171, 1966.

Phosphatases

Angellis, D., Ingles, N. R., and Fishman, W. H.: Isoelectric forming of alkaline phosphatase isoenzymes in polyacrylamide gels: Use of Triton x-100 and improved staining technique. Am. J. Clin. Path., *66*:929, 1976.

Bromhult, J., Fridell, E., and Sunblad, L.: Studies in alkaline phosphatase isoenzymes. Relation to γ-glutamyltransferase and lactate dehydrogenase isoenzymes. Clin. Chim. Acta, *76*:205, 1977.

Fishman, W. H.: Perspectives on alkaline phosphatase isoenzymes. Am. J. Med., *56*:617, 1974.

Gorman, L., and Statland, B. E.: Clinical usefulness of alkaline phosphatase isoenzyme determinations. Clin. Biochem., *10*:171, 1977.

Kaplan, M. M.: Alkaline phosphatase. N. Engl. J. Med., *286*:200, 1972.

Marshall, G., and Amador, E.: Diagnostic usefulness of serum and β-glycerophosphatase activities in prostate disease. Am. J. Clin. Path., *32*:83, 1969.

Schumann, G. B., Badawy, S., Peglow, A., and Henry, J. B.: Prostatic acid phosphatase. Current assessment in vaginal fluid of alleged rape victims. Am. J. Clin. Path., *66*:6, 1976.

Warnes, T. W.: Alkaline phosphatase. Gut, *13*:926, 1972.

Woodard, H. Q.: The clinical significance of serum acid phosphatase. Am. J. Med., *27*:902, 1959.

γ-Glutamyltransferase

Davidson, D. C., McIntosh, W. B., and Forg, J. A.: Assessment of plasma glutamyl transpeptidase activity and urinary D-glucaric acid excretion as values of enzyme induction. Clin. Sci. Mol. Med., *47*:279, 1974.

Rosalki, S. B.: Enzyme tests in diseases of the liver and hepatobiliary tract. *In* Wilkinson, J. H. (ed.): The Principles and Practice of Diagnostic Enzymology. London, Edward Arnold Publication, 1975, p. 303.

Cholinesterase

Juul, P., and Leopold, I. H.: Human plasma cholinesterase isoenzymes. Clin. Chim. Acta, *19*:205, 1968.

Vorhaus, L. J., and Kark, R. M.: Serum cholinesterase in health and disease. Am. J. Med., *14*:707, 1953.

Aminotransferases (Transaminases)

Clermont, R. J., and Chalmers, T. C.: The transaminase tests in liver disease. Medicine, *46*:197, 1967.

DeRitis, F., Coltori, M., and Giusti, C.: Diagnostic value and pathogenic significance of transaminase activity changes in viral hepatitis. Minerva Med., *47*:101, 1956.

Wroblewski, F.: Clinical significance of alterations in transaminase activities of serum and other body fluids. Adv. Clin. Chem., *1*:313, 1958.

Angiotensin-Converting Enzyme

Rohrbach, M. S., and DeRemee, R. A.: Pulmonary sarcoidosis and angiotensin converting enzyme. Mayo Clin. Proc., *57*:64, 1982.

Silverstein, E., Friedland, J., and Vuletin, J. C.: Marked elevation of serum angiotensin-converting enzyme and hepatic fibrosis containing long-spacing collagen fibrils in Type 2 acute neuronopathic Gaucher's disease. Am. J. Clin. Path., *69*:457, 1978.

Enzymes of Erythrocytes and Leukocytes

Beutler, E.: Enzyme tests in hematological diseases. *In* Wilkinson, J. H. (ed.): The Principles and Practice of Diagnostic Enzymology. Chicago, Year Book Medical Publishers, 1976, pp. 423–454.

Brady, R. O., Johnson, W. G., and Uhlendorf, B. W.: Identification of heterozygous carriers of lipid storage diseases: Current status and clinical applications. Am. J. Med., *51*:423, 1971.

Mentzer, W. C., Jr.: Pyruvate kinase deficiency and disorders of glycolysis. *In* Nathan, D. G., and Oski, F. A. (eds.): Hematology of Infancy and Childhood. 2nd ed. Philadelphia, W. B. Saunders Co., 1981.

Piomelli, S., and Vora, S.: G6PD deficiency and related disorders of the pentose pathway. *In* Nathan, D. G., and Oski, F. A. (eds.): Hematology of Infancy and Childhood. 2nd ed. Philadelphia, W. B. Saunders Co., 1981.

Stanbury, J. B., Wyngaarden, J. B., and Fredrickson, D. S.: The Metabolic Basis of Inherited Disease. 5th ed. New York, McGraw-Hill Book Co., Inc., 1983.

Weisberg, J. B., Lipschutz, F., and Oski, F. A.: δ-Amino-levulinic acid dehydratase activity in circulating blood cells: A sensitive laboratory test for the detection of childhood lead poisoning. N. Engl. J. Med., *284*:565, 1971.

15

IMMUNOASSAY AND RELATED TECHNIQUES; TUMOR MARKERS

JOAN H. HOWANITZ, M.D., AND PETER J. HOWANITZ, M.D.

2

IMMUNOASSAY

Development of the technique of immunoassay has made an immense impact on many areas of medicine. The sensitivity and specificity of this technique allow accurate quantitation of a wide variety of biologically important compounds, such as peptides, hormones, vitamins, and drugs, which may occur in biologic fluids or tissues in low concentrations. Immunoassay or variations of it based on the same principles have been used to measure hundreds of different substances, some of which occur in blood in ng/ml or pg/ml amounts. Before the development of immunoassay many of these substances could be assayed only with great difficulty, and in some cases no practical assay was available.

The diversity of terminology used to describe this technique may lead to confusion. Some expressions such as saturation analysis or displacement analysis relate to the general principle, whereas other terms such as radioimmunoassay, radioassay, radioligand assay, radioreceptor assay, fluoroimmunoassay, and enzyme immunoassay refer to the specific reagents used in a given assay system. The terms competitive protein binding assay and ligand assay have been used as well, but neither these nor other designations have gained wide acceptance for the group of assays as a whole.

In the 1950's Berson and Yalow, while studying the behavior of ^{131}I-labeled insulin, made several observations that led to development of a radioimmunoassay for plasma insulin. They found that when patients with diabetes mellitus were treated with insulin, insulin-binding antibodies were formed to the injected insulin. Using an *in vitro* system, they subsequently observed that unlabeled insulin displaced radioactive labeled insulin from insulin antibody, and when the antibody concentration was kept fixed, binding of the label was a quantitative function of the amount of unlabeled insulin present (Yalow, 1978b). This work, for which Dr. Yalow shared the 1977 Nobel Prize, formed the basis of radioimmunoassay. The principle of radioimmunoassay is summarized in Figure 15–1.

Reagents necessary to perform a typical radioimmunoassay for a given substance (antigen) include an antibody specific for the antigen, labeled antigen, a standard preparation of antigen, and a system to separate the fraction which is bound to antibody from that which is unbound or free. Thus an assay for plasma insulin would require (1) an antibody to insulin, (2) labeled insulin, (3) a preparation of insulin for use as standard, and (4) a separation system. The assay is performed by using a series of tubes containing a fixed concentration of antibody, a fixed amount of label, and an aliquot of either standard, control, or unknown.

The substance to be measured (unlabeled antigen) in the patient specimen competes with labeled antigen for antibody binding sites. The percentage of antigen bound to antibody is related to the total antigen present and is reflected by the distribution of the radioactive label. With increasing amount of unlabeled antigen, corresponding decreased amount of labeled antigen becomes bound to antibody. The percentage of total radioactive label that is bound to antibody or that is unbound (free) is monitored after the two fractions are separated. By comparing the distribution of label obtained with the unknown to that observed with standards, the concentration of

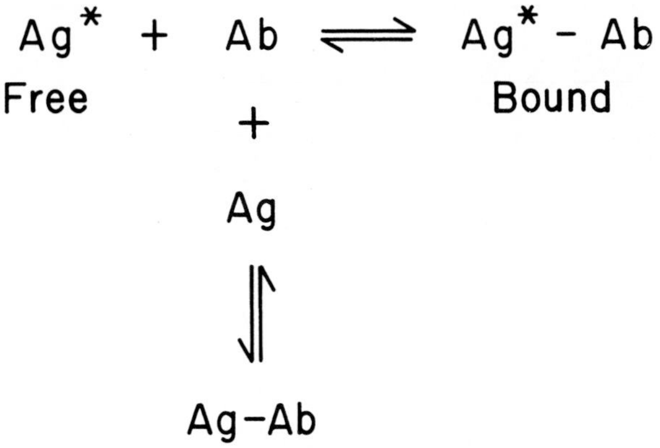

$$\begin{array}{ccccc} Ag^{*} & + & Ab & \rightleftharpoons & Ag^{*}-Ab \\ \text{Free} & & + & & \text{Bound} \\ & & Ag & & \\ & & \Updownarrow & & \\ & & Ag-Ab & & \end{array}$$

Figure 15–1. Principle of radioimmunoassay. Ag* represents the labeled antigen; Ab, the antibody; Ag, the unknown antigen (or standard); Ag*-Ab and Ag-Ab, the complexes formed.

unknown can be determined. The distribution of the radioactive label can be expressed in a number of ways, such as percentage of total counts that are bound (%B) or free (%F), or the ratio of counts in the two fractions (B/F). A standard curve then is prepared by plotting the percentage or ratio obtained with the standard against the concentration of standard; unknown values then are determined using this standard curve.

Immunoassays are dependent on the degree of similarity of behavior of the standard and the unknown, but they fundamentally do not rely on the use of antibodies or a radioactive label. In general terms, the principle involves partitioning of the substance to be measured into two moieties by the reaction with a specific binding reagent of limited capacity (Ekins, 1974). The ratio of the two moieties depends on the amount of unknown, control, or standard in the system. For example, the assay of thyroxine, described by Ekins at about the same time the insulin assay was developed, was based on principles identical to those governing the insulin method (Ekins, 1974). However, this assay relied on a naturally occurring protein, thyroxine binding globulin (TBG), rather than on an antibody as the specific binding reagent. Since this type of assay uses a binding protein instead of an antibody, it is referred to as a radioassay rather than a radioimmunoassay.

Although superficially different, the fundamental principle on which all these assays are based depends on the use of a limited amount of specific binding reagent that is held constant in the system. The technique requires a means of separating, or identifying, the bound or free label.

Specific Binding Reagents

Antibodies, certain naturally occurring binding proteins, enzymes, and receptors have been used as specific binding reagents, each having its advantages and disadvantages. Two important characteristics of the binder are its specificity and affinity (Table 15–1). Specificity denotes the degree of uniqueness with which the substance being assayed is bound. The association constant or K is a measure of the affinity or strength of binding. High affinity binders form a relatively stable complex with limited dissociation.

ANTIBODIES

Antibodies are the most widely used binding reagents, because they can readily be prepared against a large variety of compounds, including proteins, hormones, drugs, and intracellular metabolites. Some disadvantages of their use are difficulty in making antibody to some substances, measurement of immunologic rather than biologic activity, and serious problems with cross-reactivity. In addition, the variability of antibodies made to the same substance makes it necessary to characterize antisera individually.

Antibodies can be used to obtain highly sensitive and specific assays for a wide variety of compounds. The sensitivity of an immunoassay depends predominantly on the affinity of the antibody employed. Specificity of an antiserum may be assessed by reacting it with a number of compounds with which it may be expected to cross-react. Cross-reactivity occurs because of structural similarity of the compounds; for example, antibody to digitoxin may cross-react with digoxin and antibodies to L-thyroxine may cross-react

Table 15–1. PROPERTIES OF SPECIFIC BINDING REAGENTS

Properties	Antibody	Receptors	Binding Proteins
Stability	Stable	Unstable	Stable
Source	Immunized animals or hybridomas	Cells	Naturally occurring proteins
Type of Specificity	Immunologic	Biologic	Biologic
Association constant or K* (L/mole)	10^{10} to 10^{12}	10^{8} to 10^{11}	10^{8} to 10^{10}

*A measure of affinity or strength of binding; large K values reflect strong bonds, and high affinity binders form a relatively stable complex with limited dissociation.

with D-thyroxine. One approach to increasing specificity has been to select the most specific antibodies available and to absorb out the cross-reacting antigens. This can be accomplished if only a small proportion of the antibody population cross-reacts or if the cross-reacting substance differs in affinity for the antibody.

Immunologic activity may have little to do with biologic activity. For example, an inactive precursor or degradation product of an antigen may be relatively inactive biologically but react with the antibody. In addition to assessment of cross-reactivity, the identity of the behavior of the unknown and standard must be evaluated. A necessary but not sufficient condition for proof of identical behavior of standard and unknown in an assay system is that the concentration of the unknown decreases linearly with dilution, and that a dilution curve of unknown is superimposable on a dilution curve of the standard over a wide range of concentrations.

Preparation of antibody for use as an immunoassay reagent usually is done by injecting animals with the antigen of interest. Low molecular weight compounds that are not immunogenic can be attached to a carrier such as a protein before injection. Antibodies also can be produced using hybridomas, which are formed by fusion of antibody-forming spleen cells and myeloma cells. A hybridoma produces antibody against a single antigenic determinant, that is, homogeneous or monoclonal antibody as compared to heterogeneous or polyclonal antibody normally produced when an antigen is injected into animals. Large quantities of monoclonal antibody can be produced by a colony of cells derived from a single hybridoma; cross-reactivity is eliminated during the process of selection of the hybridoma (Sevier, 1981).

BINDING PROTEINS

Naturally occurring binding proteins also have been used as specific binding agents. Binding proteins have the advantage of requiring little or no preparation; in addition, their characteristics are uniform from preparation to preparation. However, binding proteins generally have lower affinity constants than do antibodies and may or may not show good specificity. Serum contains binding proteins for a number of substances, including cortisol, thyroid hormones, testosterone, and vitamin B_{12}. In assays which use binding proteins it is important to eliminate any interference from endogenous binding proteins prior to assay. Heating the sample, for example, commonly is employed to eliminate interference due to endogenous binding proteins in the case of vitamin B_{12} assays.

Advantages in the use of naturally occurring binding proteins include stability, relative inexpensiveness, ease of preparation, and consistency from preparation to preparation. Disadvantages of using naturally occurring binding proteins are that they are available for only a limited number of compounds, and they may not show good specificity. In addition, since their affinity is relatively low, assays with a high degree of sensitivity are difficult to obtain.

Enzymes also have been used in competitive protein-binding assays; an assay was developed for methotrexate based on the binding of the drug to the enzyme dihydrofolate reductase (Myers, 1975).

RECEPTORS

Another source of specific binders is cellular membrane, cytoplasmic, or nuclear receptors. In general, the term receptor refers to a molecule or a molecular complex capable of recognizing and selectively interacting with a substance such as a hormone, neurotransmitter, or drug. A receptor has specificity directed toward the biologically active portion of the molecule.

Receptors tend to be unstable, and they must be obtained by isolation from tissue where they exist in low concentration. Intact cells or cell fractions may be used as a source of receptors; preparations can be made from blood, enzymatically or mechanically disrupted tissues, or tissue cultures. The techniques employed to isolate cells can profoundly affect the concentration and affinity of receptors. Receptor assays have been developed for a number of substances such as hormones, neurotransmitters, and cyclic nucleotides. Receptors from bovine adrenal cortex, bovine skeletal muscle, or calf uterus, for example, have been used to assay cyclic AMP (Parker, 1976).

Advantages of receptor assays include measurement of biologic rather than immunologic activity and uniformity among preparations. However, in practice, uniformity among preparations may not always be achieved.

Disadvantages of using receptors are the instability of receptor preparations and problems which occur due to non-specific binding. Receptors may be more sensitive than other binders in distinguishing changes in a molecule introduced by labeling. Since the equilibrium constant for receptors is in the range of 10^8 to 10^{11} L/mole, receptor assays may show lower sensitivity than a corresponding immunoassay employing an avid antibody (Parker, 1976).

Labels

The indicator molecule employed in the assay system may be labeled in a number of ways including with radioactivity, enzyme activity, or fluorescence (Table 15–2). In order to have a valid assay, it is not necessary for the label to behave identically to the unlabeled unknown; however, the unlabeled unknown and the standard must show identical behavior in the assay system. Provided that both labeled and unlabeled antigens react at the same binding site, some difference in affinity may be acceptable. However, if the affinity of the label is less than that of the unknown, maximal assay sensitivity cannot be achieved. In addition, labeled material that has different properties from the unknown may give rise to unexpected effects such as interaction with assay constituents in an unpredictable manner (Hunter, 1974). Ligand assays can be divided into homogeneous (free label can be distinguished in the presence of bound label) and

Table 15–2. NONRADIOISOTOPIC LABELS*

Labels	Detection System
Bacteriophage	Bacterial culture
Chemiluminescence	Photon counter
Enzymes and enzyme cofactors, inhibitors and substrates	Photometry, fluorimetry
Fluorochromes, fluorogens, and fluorescence quenchers	Fluorimetry, fluorescence polarization
Metal containing compounds and metal chelates	Atomic absorption, fluorimetry
Particles such as latex	Particle (blood cell) counter
Stable free radicals	Electron spin resonance

*Modified from Schall, R. F., and Tenoso, H. J.: Clin. Chem., *27*:1157, 1981.

heterogeneous (free and bound label must be physically separated before detection) assays.

RADIOACTIVE LABELS

Although they have several disadvantages, radioactive labels have been employed widely because of their flexibility and sensitivity. Disadvantages of radioactive labels include potential health hazards, instability, and expense of detection equipment and of waste disposal. Radioactive labels fall into two groups: (1) beta-emitting isotopes such as tritium (^{3}H) and (2) gamma-emitting isotopes such as iodine-125 (^{125}I).

The half-life of a population of radioactive atoms is the time interval in which half of the original number of atoms will have decayed. The term "specific activity" refers to radioactivity expressed in millicuries per mass of element (1 millicurie is equal to 3.7×10^{7} disintegrations per second). In addition, the term specific activity is employed for radioactivity divided by the mass of the compound of which the element forms a part. When a radioactive marker of low specific activity is used, relatively high concentrations are required to obtain a practical level of radioactivity in the immunoassay. If an attempt is made to increase specific activity by maximizing the number of radioactive atoms incorporated per molecule, rapid decomposition sometimes occurs. The radioactivity usually is counted to 10,000 counts to ensure a high degree of precision in counting (Ekins, 1974). Approximately 10,000 atoms of carbon-14 or 100 atoms of ^{3}H produce the same number of disintegrations per minute as one atom of ^{125}I (Landon, 1976).

Beta emitters are detected by using liquid scintillation counting systems. The beta emitting radioisotope is added to a scintillation fluid; when it decays emitting radiation, excitation of the scintillation fluid or fluor occurs. As the fluor returns to ground state, light is emitted. Advantages of using beta-emitting labels such as ^{3}H include the ease with which compounds can be labeled and the long half-life of the isotopes. Disadvantages of beta-emitters include the necessity of expensive scintillation fluids or fluors, and considerable time in sample preparation. In addition, interference with the emission of light (that is, quenching) results in decreased counts detected by the liquid scintillation counter.

There are a number of advantages to employing material labeled with gamma-emitting isotopes, including that the assay tubes can be directly counted without need for quench correction. The counting time may be reduced as compared to beta emitters because of the higher specific activity obtainable. Iodine-125 (^{125}I) is the most commonly employed gamma-emitting isotope.

The shelf life of preparations of ^{125}I depends on a number of factors. When specific activity of the labeled antigen is increased, it is more likely that the preparation will have decreased immunoreactivity and increased susceptibility to radioactive damage. As specific activity is increased, an increased number of molecules will have two radioactive iodine labels. When radioactive disintegration occurs from one atom, it disrupts part of the molecule resulting in the production of labeled molecular fragments or free iodide; therefore, the remaining portion with the other radioactive iodine can expect to have decreased immunoreactivity (Yalow, 1978a). This phenomenon is called decay catastrophe.

A variety of methods have been used to introduce iodine into compounds for use as labels. Hunter and Greenwood (1962) showed that low concentrations of chloramine-T promoted highly effective incorporation of inorganic iodine into protein. The mechanism of this reaction probably involves generation of ionic iodine, which is a potent oxidizing agent. Introduction of radioactive iodine atoms into proteins occurs through a substitution in the tyrosyl residue, but substitution of iodine in other groups such as histidyl also is possible. Other iodination techniques include lactoperoxidase (Marchalonis, 1969), electrolytic iodination (Rosa, 1964), and introduction of iodinated acyl group as described by Bolton and Hunter (1973). The lactoperoxidase method is useful for proteins that are subject to damage during the chloramine-T iodination. The advantages of the Bolton-Hunter method are that it provides a procedure which reduces iodination damage and the method may be used to label peptides that contain no tyrosine.

During iodination, the antigen undergoing labeling can be damaged. Causes of iodination damage include partial degradation of the antigen during labeling, introduction of the isotope into the antigenic determinant, and damage to the antigen caused by radiation during or after iodination. A variety of physiochemical techniques, such as gel chromatography, have been employed for purification of the label, and several methods have been used to assess the suitability of the iodinated compound. Incubation of the label with excess antibody has been used to indicate the suitability of the label; a satisfactorily labeled preparation will be bound to the extent of 90 to 98 per cent when incubated with excess high avidity antibody (Hunter, 1974). In addition, the sensitivity of the assay calibration curve obtained with tracer should be checked.

Other gamma emitting isotopes also can be used.

Cobalt-57 (^{57}Co) is commonly is used in vitamin B_{12} assays, and selenium-75 (^{75}Se) has been used to label steroids (Eckert, 1976).

LABELED BINDER

In order to improve assay systems with respect to sensitivity and precision, the immunoradiometric assay (IRMA) technique was developed. Immunoradiometric assays differ from conventional radioimmunoassay systems in that the compound to be measured combines with radioactive labeled antibody which is present in excess. In one variation of this type of assay, the standards or samples are reacted with excess labeled antibody; separation of free labeled antibody is accomplished by use of an immunosorbent consisting of antigen coupled to a solid phase. The radioactivity present in the bound fraction relates directly to antigen concentration. Use of labeled antibody can overcome problems such as difficulty in antigen iodination and loss of immunologic reactivity or instability when the antigen is labeled (Woodhead, 1974). Disadvantages of the technique are that it requires large amounts of antibody and preparation of reagents is demanding.

A so-called two-site immunoradiometric assay (or "sandwich" technique) also may be used in which sample is reacted with two different antibodies that bind to different parts of the antigen. One antibody usually is adsorbed to a solid phase support and the other labeled. A three site IRMA also can be used in which two antibodies (A and B), one of which is attached to a solid phase, react with the antigen and a third antibody (C) reacts with antibody B (Fig. 15–2).

The high-dose "hook" effect may occur with the two-site assay; that is, as the concentration of antigen increases, there is a paradoxical fall in the bound fraction. The mechanism by which this occurs is controversial; the effect can be avoided by use of sufficient solid-phase unlabeled antibody (Al-Shawi, 1981). If unrecognized, the hook effect can lead to spuriously low values.

Procedures which use enzyme or fluorescent labels also have been developed; they are called immunoenzymometric assays (IEMA) and immunofluorometric assays (IFMA), respectively.

ENZYME LABELS

Enzymes may be used in place of radioactive isotopes to label either antigen or antibody. Enzyme immunoassays generally are of two types: heterogeneous assays known as enyzme-linked immunosorbent assays (ELISA), and homogeneous assays as with the Syva EMIT system.

In a method analogous to radioimmunoassay, enzyme-labeled antigen is employed (Engvall, 1971). The enzyme activity then is determined in the bound or free fraction. The antibody can be labeled with enzyme and employed in assays that are analogous to the immunoradiometric or two-site "sandwich" technique (Engvall, 1972). Homogeneous enzyme assays have been developed in which labels are made by covalently linking antigen to enzyme (Rubenstein, 1978). When the enzyme molecule that is covalently bound to antigen reacts with antibody to that antigen, the enzymatic activity is inhibited. Inhibition of enzyme activity by antibody probably is caused either by conformational changes induced by antibody binding to the active group or by prevention of conformational changes necessary for catalytic activity (Rowley, 1975). Enzyme-labeled antigen and unknown antigen compete for antibody binding sites; the enzyme-labeled antigen that remains free is enzymatically active and can be determined in the presence of the bound label (Fig. 15–3).

A disadvantage of enzyme labels, which can lead to decreased sensitivity, is steric hindrance of the antigen-antibody reaction due to presence of the enzyme. In addition, enzyme labels are technically more difficult to prepare (Yalow, 1978a). A number of enzymes, including glucose-6-phosphate dehydrogenase, alkaline phosphatase, and lysozyme, have been used as labels. It is important that the enzymes employed not be subject to large interferences and that convenient, rapid means of measuring their activity are available. Several methods have been used to link enzymes to antibodies and protein antigens, including glutaraldehyde linkage and dimaleimide linkage (Wisdom, 1976).

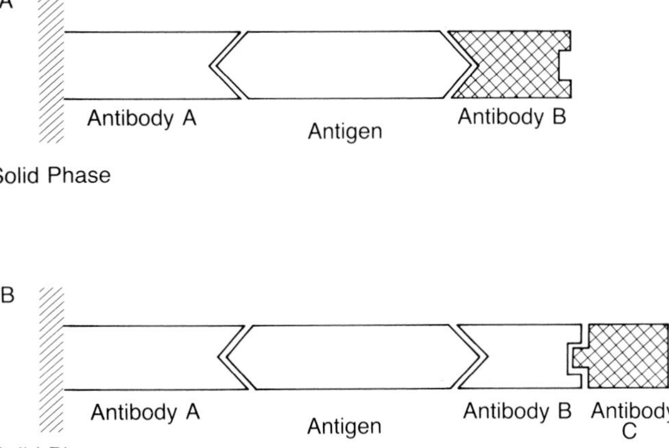

Figure 15–2. Schematic representations showing *(A)* a two-site immunometric assay in which two antibodies react with different sites on the antigen (antibody A is attached to a solid phase, antibody B is labeled); and *(B)* adaptation of the assay with the use of a third antibody (antibody A is attached to solid phase, antibody B attaches to second site on antigen, and antibody C, which is labeled, reacts with antibody B). (Modified from Al-Shawi, A., Mohammed-Ali, S., Houts, T., Hodgkinson, S., Nargessi, R. D., and Landon, J.: Ligand Quart., *4*:43, 1981.)

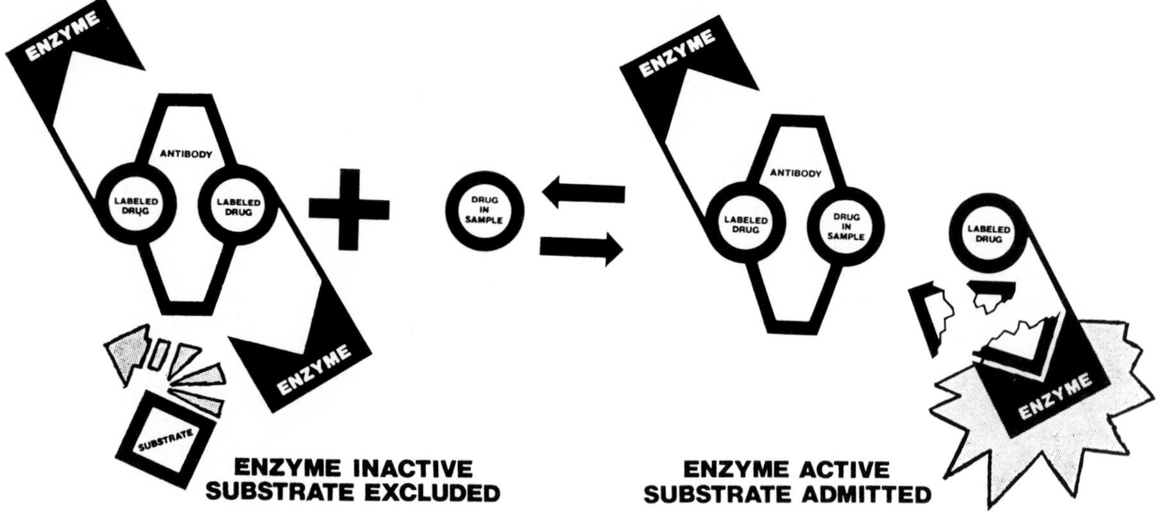

Figure 15–3. Principle of homogeneous enzyme immunoassay. When the enzyme-ligand conjugate is complexed to the antibody (left), the enzyme substrate is excluded from the active site and enzyme activity is reduced. The presence of ligand releases a portion of the enzyme conjugate, which is then active (right). (From Rubenstein, K. E.: Scand. J. Immunol., *8*[Suppl. 7]:57, 1978. With permission.)

FLUORESCENT LABELS

Fluorescent labels have several advantages: they are inexpensive and stable, and fluorescence can be measured quickly with relatively inexpensive instrumentation. Because of background fluorescence and scattering in patient specimens, immunoassays employing fluorescent labels tend to be less sensitive than those using radioisotopes. However, a variety of techniques have been developed to overcome these problems.

By optimizing the instrumentation used for detection of the fluorescent probe, sensitivity can be increased and background decreased. In time-resolved fluorometers, a light pulse excites the label and the fluorescence is measured after a certain time has elasped from the time of excitation. Rare earth metal chelates, such as europium, show promise as probes for use with time-resolved fluorometry (Soini, 1979).

A variety of assays using fluorescence labels have been developed in which separation of the bound and free fraction is unnecessary. In the fluorescence polarization method, a label is excited with polarized light, and the degree of polarization of the emission is measured. As label is bound, its rotation is slowed and the degree of polarization increases. Disadvantages of this method include non-linear response as a function of concentration and the limited range of the response (Soini, 1979). Homogeneous immunoassays have been developed using carefully selected fluorogens which function both as enzyme substrates and nonfluorescent precursor molecules of fluorescent compounds (Schall, 1981).

Separation Systems

The assay endpoint involves determining the relative proportion of antigen which is free (unbound) or bound to specific, saturable binding reagent (bound). In order to determine this distribution, the bound or free fraction is quantitated, often after physical separation of the two components. The separation step is not essential, however, if one of the components is detectable in the presence of the other as in homogeneous enzyme or fluorescent immunoassay system.

When radioactive labels such as ^{125}I are used, the fraction bound to antibody does not spontaneously precipitate; separation of the bound and free is necessary before the fractions are counted. Various systems have been developed to take advantage of differences in properties of bound and free fractions. The choice of method for separating the two moieties depends on a number of factors, such as adsorption properties of the label.

There are a number of characteristics or criteria of an ideal separation system, including the following: (1) the separating agent does not interfere with the equilibrium state of the completed reaction; (2) complete separation of bound and free moieties is obtained; (3) the separation system is reproducible from assay to assay and is uniform within the assay; (4) the separation has a wide margin of error in the condition used; (5) the separation is fast, simple, inexpensive, and performed with readily available equipment and reagents; and (6) the separation is not influenced by nonspecific substances in samples. Other characteristics that may be helpful include wide applicability to a variety of systems and the ability to distinguish between damaged and undamaged label (Ratcliffe, 1974).

A wide variety of separation systems are available (Table 15–3). Some of the first separation methods used, such as electrophoresis, generally are not employed for routine assays because of certain technical disadvantages. Methods that involve adsorption, usu-

Table 15–3. METHODS OF SEPARATING FREE AND BOUND TRACER

Classification	Principle	Example
1. Differential migration of bound and free	a. Mainly due to differences in charge	a. Electrophoresis
	b. Mainly due to differences in molecular weight	b. Gel filtration
2. Adsorption	a. Non-specific adsorption of free moiety	a. 1. Charcoal 2. Silicates—Quso G-32, talc, Florisil, Fuller's earth 3. Resins (Amberlite)
	b. Adsorption of bound	b. Resins (DEAE-cellulose)
3. Precipitation of bound	a. Non-specific precipitation	a. 1. Ammonium sulfate 2. Polyethylene glycol (PEG) 3. Ethanol
	b. Immunologic	b. Double (second) antibody
4. Solid phase	a. Usually antibody attached to solid material	a. Antibody-coated tubes or disks b. Antibody coupled to dextran or cellulose particles
5. Combinations	a. More than one of the above	a. 1. Mixture of PEG and second antibody 2. Second antibody linked to a solid phase
6. Other	a. Internal sample attenuation	a. Addition of bismuth oxide

ally of the free fraction, commonly have been employed in assays for steroids, small peptides, and drugs such as digoxin. Generally the adsorption methods are most satisfactory for antigens with a molecular weight of 30,000 or less (Yalow, 1978a). Separations can be performed rapidly, but several factors, including timing of the separation and amount of adsorbent added to each tube, must be carefully controlled. Adsorption is determined by many factors, including relative surface area of the adsorbent, size and charge of the antigen, protein concentrations in the assay system, temperature, ionic strength, and pH (Ratcliffe, 1974).

Certain types of charcoal such as Norit A have satisfactory characteristics for adsorption of the free fraction. Charcoal, which usually is pretreated with dextran or protein, has a high affinity for a wide variety of substances. However, it may adsorb bound as well as free fractions; the affinity of charcoal for the free fraction may be so high as to disturb the equilibrium of the reaction. The effects of this stripping phenomenon on the assay system can be minimized by keeping the temperature of the incubation mixture low during the period of charcoal addition and by ensuring that time of exposure to charcoal is identical in all tubes (Ekins, 1976).

A number of steps for systematically optimizing conditions of the separation, such as varying the amounts of charcoal and the reaction times, have been suggested by Binoux (1973). Other substances may be used to adsorb the free fraction, including various silicates such as talc, Florisil, and Quso G-32.

The bound fraction may be precipitated, leaving the free fraction in solution. This may be accomplished by a non-specific precipitating system employing ammonium sulfate, ethanol, polyethylene glycol, or a number of other substances. The double antibody or second antibody, which also precipitates the bound fraction, is a commonly used system that depends on the ability of anti-immunoglobulin antibodies to bind the soluble antigen-antibody complex and cause precipitation. For example, if the antibody against the unknown antigen (first antibody) is made in a rabbit, the antibody for the separation (second antibody) is made to rabbit gamma globulin. This technique requires that antigenic determinants of gamma globulin are distinct from the antigen-combining sites and that the relative concentration of reagents in the system favors precipitin formation. This type of separation system often is employed in the assay of polypeptide hormones such as prolactin and growth hormone. The second antibody must be carefully screened for cross-reactivity with human gamma globulin before use.

The double antibody system may be used in several ways. Commonly the so-called post-precipitation method is employed; in this method second antibody and carrier serum or non-immune gamma globulin is added after the first antibody reaction is completed. Major factors affecting the separation include conditions of the second antibody incubation, centrifugation, carrier protein concentration, and characteristics and concentration of the second antibody, as well as non-specific effects due to serum and anticoagulants. In general, interfering factors may be minimized by using a prolonged incubation of 24 to 48 hours in the precipitation step (Ratcliffe, 1974).

In the pre-precipitation method, the first antibody is precipitated by the second before the reaction is carried out. The double antibody system may also be combined with the solid phase system (see below). In addition, separation systems have been devised in which sub-precipitating concentrations of materials such as ammonium sulfate are used in combination with second antibody.

Antibody can be insolubilized through covalent or

non-covalent bonding to solid supports such as test tubes, disks, or other materials. These so-called solid phase systems provide rapid, versatile, and efficient separation of fractions. In general, disadvantages of solid phase separation systems include the requirement for relatively large amounts of antibody and difficulties in ensuring uniformity. Other separation methods have been developed, including use of bismuth oxide, a radiation-absorbing material which can shield the radiation from either antibody-bound or free radioligand fractions (Thorell, 1981).

A new approach, radial partition radioimmunoassay, has been developed in which the entire immunochemical procedure is conducted on a solid phase (Giegel, 1982). A specimen containing the antigen of interest is applied to a small central area of filter paper where it reacts with immobilized antibody. Subsequently enzyme labeled antigen is applied to react with remaining antibody sites. After incubation, substrate for the enzyme is applied to the center of the reaction area and washes out unbound label to the periphery of the paper. Bound antigen remains attached to the immobilized antibody in the center reaction area. The washing step also initiates the enzyme reaction which, in its current application, is quantified by front-surface fluorescence.

For each assay developed, the exact conditions of the separation procedure must be investigated, including the amount of reagent used, the length of reaction, and the speed and length of the centrifugation step. Separation systems, such as ammonium sulfate, are sensitive to assay protein concentration. It may be difficult to obtain serum free of the substance to be assayed for use in keeping the protein concentration in the standard curve tubes constant. Substitutions, for example, animal serum or human serum treated with charcoal to remove the substance measured, have been employed. These maneuvers, however, may not be entirely satisfactory. In addition, anticoagulants may affect the separation system.

Iodination or incubation damage may influence some separation systems. In double antibody methods, generally damage causes a reduction in the bound fraction; however, if the damaged tracer aggregates or adsorbs to the precipitate more than the intact label, the apparent bound fraction will increase (Hunter, 1971). Adsorption systems also tend to be sensitive to alterations in label.

Standards

In order to have a valid assay, standards and specimens must behave in the same manner in the system. Some difficulties that may be encountered in preparation of a suitable standard include variations in the substance in question, for example, precursor forms or degradation products. Synthetic peptides, especially those with more than 20 amino acids, are likely to contain error peptides and racemized residues (Bangham, 1974). There may be artifacts produced in the standard during its preparation or storage; for example, alterations may occur with freezing or thawing. Any differences between binding sites of the standard and the unknown may yield differences in affinity for the binder; differences in affinity thus are likely to affect assay results.

Stability of the standard is important, because ideally it will be used over a long period of time. Loss of activity may be due to a number of causes, including adsorption to surfaces, contamination with bacterial or tissue enzymes, and oxidation (Bangham, 1971). Assay validity also depends on the control of non-specific factors which may influence the reaction, including ionic strength, pH, buffer, and protein concentration of incubation medium. Thus it is desirable to prepare standard solutions in such a way as to control effects of these factors; for example, if the analyte is to be assayed in serum, the standards should be serum based.

Assay Development and Validation

For many clinical laboratories, it is more efficient to purchase reagents in assay kit or component form than to maintain facilities for generation and evaluation of binding reagents and labels. In selecting assay kits many aspects should be considered, including cost, separation technique, type of label, and cross-reacting substances. For example, rapid turn-around time may be particularly important for a determination; thus, a separation step such as a double antibody procedure with a long incubation may not be appropriate.

After proper preparation of the reagents according to the manufacturer's directions, the assay can be performed following the instructions provided. However, the kit performance must be evaluated before it is used routinely. Although the general principles of assay development, validation, and quality control are the same as for other types of determinations, certain aspects warrant special emphasis.

Sensitivity is defined as the minimum amount of antigen that can be measured with acceptable precision (Ekins, 1971). The limits of sensitivity are determined by the affinity of the specific binding reagent employed. The antibody dilution usually is chosen so that 20 to 70 per cent of the label is antibody-bound in the absence of unlabeled antigen. With excess antibody, loss of sensitivity occurs (Hurn, 1971). Other measures designed to increase sensitivity include prolongation of the incubation period, use of small quantities of label, and delayed addition of label (Chard, 1971). Although sensitivity can be increased by delayed addition of label, that is, with "non-equilibrium" assays, failure to reach equilibrium may lead to loss of precision (Rodbard, 1971). If label affinity differs from that of the unlabeled material, the full sensitivity of the assay cannot be achieved. Another approach is to extract and concentrate the specimen. In general, attempts to employ assays at the extreme limits of sensitivity can introduce problems.

Parameters of assay validity include quantitative recovery of added antigen and demonstration that, in

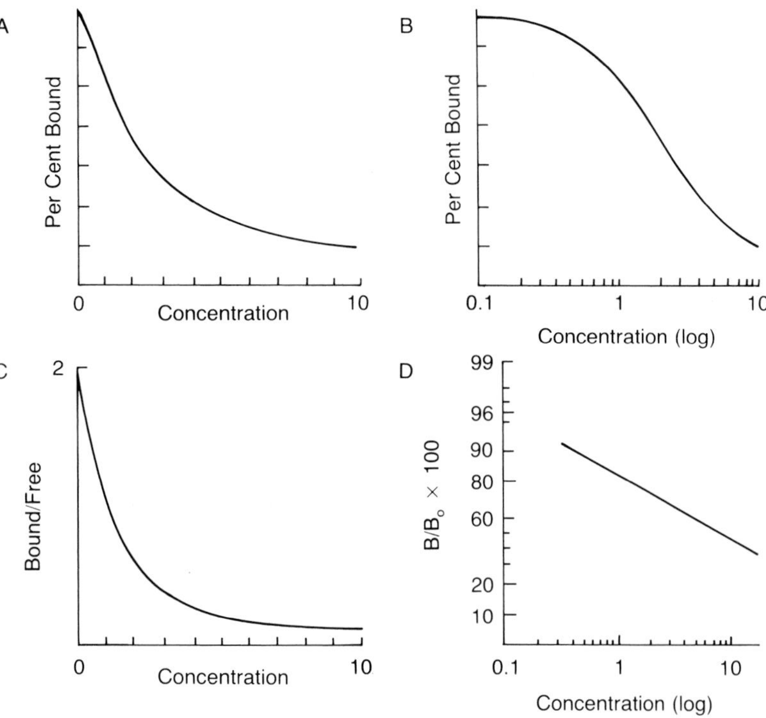

Figure 15–4. Methods of plotting dose-response curves. *A*, Percentage or fraction of label bound versus concentration of standard. *B*, Percentage or fraction of label bound versus log concentration of standard. *C*, Ratio of bound to free label versus concentration of standard. *D*, Logit B/B_0 (where B is the fraction of label bound and B_0 is the fraction bound when there is no unlabeled antigen in the system) versus log concentration of standard.

the absence of antigen, an appropriate response is obtained. It is essential to demonstrate that the apparent antigen content in the unknown is independent of the dilution at which it is assayed. This requires that the concentration of the unknown decreases linearly with dilution and that a dilution curve of unknown sample be superimposed on a dilution curve of standard.

Two types of "blanks" should be included with every assay: one containing labeled antigen, antibody, and antigen-free serum or plasma; the other, labeled antigen and antigen-free serum or plasma but no antibody. The first type of blank provides information on the reaction of label and antibody and the completeness of the separation step (Challand, 1974). The second yields information regarding non-specific binding of the label.

Other considerations when using a radioactive label include counting error, adsorption of the label to glassware, and the possibility of radioactive contamination of the specimen.

To have a valid assay, cross-reactivity studies using appropriate substances should be performed, and nonspecific factors, such as pH and assay protein content, must be controlled. Because of their variability, it is necessary to characterize each polyclonal antibody individually. When the antibody used in a particular assay is changed, it is important that this antibody be recharacterized. Assay values must show appropriate response under various physiologic conditions. This is particularly important to demonstrate with the use of antibody as the specific binding reagent.

Since antibody measures immunologic rather than biologic activity, it should be understood that measurements by immunoassay may not always reflect true *in vivo* activity. For example, proinsulin, which is relatively inactive, may cross-react with antibody to insulin. Also, antibodies in patient sera may affect radioimmunoassays by reacting with the ligand being measured or with reagent antibody (Howanitz, 1982).

Ligand assay precision is less than that achieved with most routine chemical assays; the coefficient of variation of between-batch replicates is usually not less than 6 per cent (Challand, 1974). Precision also is not the same in each portion of the standard curve; the phenomenon of changes in precision is called nonuniformity of variance or heteroscedasticity.

Plots of the dose-response curve, such as percentage bound versus log dose, yield a sigmoidal curve (Fig. 15–4). A wide variety of techniques have been used to automate data reduction; many of these involve linearization of the standard curve. The most commonly employed technique is that of logit transformation in which the logit B/B_0 is plotted versus the log concentration of standard, where B equals the fraction of tracer bound and B_0 equals the fraction bound when there is no unlabeled antigen in the system. The linearization by this method is an empirical finding (Rodbard, 1968). The method has the disadvantage of resulting in marked heteroscedasticity.

RECEPTOR ASSAYS

In addition to their use as specific binding reagents, receptors have a growing importance for the clinical laboratory. For example, there are a number of conditions in which receptor dysfunction appears to have

2

a pathogenic role. Tentative classification of these disorders has been proposed: (1) inherited abnormalities of receptor function, such as occur in some androgen-resistant states, for example, testicular feminization; (2) receptors as targets for autoantibodies, for example, in myasthenia gravis, in Graves' disease, and in a small group of patients with insulin-resistant diabetes; and (3) tolerance and hypersensitivity (Jacobs, 1977). In addition, receptor assays may be useful in evaluating certain treatment modalities.

Estrogen and Progesterone Receptors

The most important practical application of receptor assays at present is the quantitation of receptors in breast cancer tissue. Approximately one third of unselected patients with metastatic breast carcinoma respond with objective remission of disease to either ablative or additive endocrine therapy. Therapeutic modalities include ovariectomy, adrenalectomy, and hypophysectomy (ablative therapy), as well as treatment with antiestrogens, pharmacologic doses of estrogens, androgens, progestin, or glucocorticoids (additive therapy). Regardless of the type of endocrine therapy employed, objective tumor regression occurs in approximately 20 to 40 per cent of patients (McGuire, 1977).

Studies of classic estrogen-dependent tissue, such as uterus, have led to the discovery of a cytoplasmic protein that binds estrogen with high affinity and specificity. The interaction of the estrogen molecule with this cytoplasmic protein is believed to be the initial event leading to the complex series of responses characteristic of estrogen stimulation. An extension of these studies was the search for estrogen receptors in breast tumor tissue. Subsequently the relationship of the presence of estrogen receptor and response of the tumor to endocrine therapy was studied.

Although estrogen receptors cannot be readily detected in non-lactating human breast tissue, the amount of estrogen receptor in primary malignant breast tumors ranges up to 1000 femtomoles/mg of cytosol protein (McGuire, 1977). With estrogen-positive tumors (greater than 3 femtomoles/mg of cytosol protein with the dextran-coated charcoal method), response to endocrine therapy occurs in about 50 to 60 per cent of patients, whereas fewer than 10 per cent of patients with estrogen receptor negative tumors respond to this type of therapy (McGuire, 1980).

Several reasons have been proposed to explain why all patients with estrogen-positive tumors do not respond to endocrine therapy. It is known, for example, that patients with tumors that are positive for both estrogen and progesterone receptors respond to hormonal therapy better than those with tumors that are estrogen-receptor positive but progesterone-receptor negative. Patients with tumors containing both estrogen and progesterone receptors have a response rate to endocrine therapy of greater than 75 per cent (Osborne, 1979).

Receptor measurements for other hormones, including prolactin and androgens, also may be of value in making a prediction of a favorable outcome with hormonal therapy. Tumors may contain a heterogeneous population of hormone-dependent cells and, therefore, display a mixed response to hormonal therapy. Other reasons proposed for the non-responsiveness of patients with estrogen-positive tumors include possibility of defective cytoplasmic receptor proteins; these may prevent the induction of the sequence of biochemical events that ultimately lead to tumor regression with hormonal therapy. Also, there may be absent or defective specific nuclear estrogen receptors. Many tumors have been found to contain nuclear estrogen receptors that are not occupied by estrogen but that may be capable of inducing biological events (Howanitz, 1981).

Methods

One of the most important aspects of receptor assays is the handling of the tumor tissue. Since estrogen and progesterone receptors are labile at room temperature, tissue must be kept cold and frozen in liquid nitrogen immediately after excision. It has been suggested that dextran-coated charcoal assay or some modification of it is the most practical method for routine assay of estrogen and progesterone receptors in breast tissue.

The frozen tissue is pulverized, homogenized, and centrifuged at 4°C. to obtain the supernatant cytosol fraction. Binding data are obtained from incubating aliquots of the cytosol preparation with various concentrations of labeled hormone. After addition of charcoal and centrifugation, the amount of receptor-bound hormone remaining in solution is plotted against the ratio of bound to free label. In this so-called Scatchard plot, the slope of the line gives a measure of the association constant (Fig. 15–5). Scatchard plots of binding generally reveal a single class of receptor sites with high affinity binding. The intercept on the abscissa gives the receptor concentra-

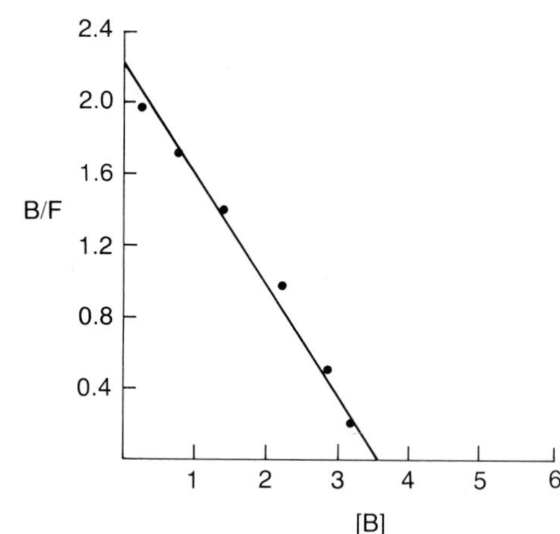

Figure 15–5. Scatchard plot where B = bound and F = free.

tion. Results usually are expressed in terms of mg of cytosol protein.

Other approaches to measurement of estrogen receptors include cytochemical techniques and immunoradiometric assays using monoclonal antibodies. Cytochemical techniques using fluorescent steroid conjugates and tumor tissue slices have been subject to a number of problems such as poor reproducibility and difficulty in fixing the tissue.

Detection and measurement of specific progesterone receptors have been difficult because of instability of the progesterone-receptor complex and interferences by plasma binding proteins. The use of a highly potent synthetic progestin R5020 has helped resolve this problem (Raynaud, 1977).

TUMOR MARKERS

Introduction

Cancer is responsible for almost 500,000 deaths in the United States per year. With early detection and treatment, significant decrease in morbidity and mortality certainly will occur. Early detection of cancer with techniques based on cytological examination, for example, the Papanicolaou technique for cervical cancer, has led to great success in treatment for some tumors. However, cytologic techniques do not lend themselves to detection of many tumors; therefore, the search for markers of cancer has focused on tumor products in blood, urine, and other body fluids, and a wealth of clinical and experimental data is now available. Marker substances are classified as tumor-specific or tumor-associated. Tumor-specific antigens are considered a direct result of the oncogenesis; they may be thought of as neo-antigens specific to tumor cells. Tumor-associated markers include various enzymes and proteins which occur in the blood and are mediated by the tumor itself, or by the influence of the tumor on uninvolved tissue. Examples of tumor-associated markers are production of oncofetal antigens by tumors, and tumor metastasis to liver and bone resulting in increased serum alkaline phosphatase. Table 15–4 lists some clinically useful tumor markers.

Oncofetal antigens are a group of substances which are detected in fetal blood and reach peak levels early in gestation. By time of delivery, these antigens are at low concentration and usually become non-detectable shortly thereafter. However, they may occur during adult life; as a healthy individual grows older, they may appear in serum in low concentrations and can be detected by relatively sensitive techniques. Two of the best known oncofetal antigens are alpha-fetoprotein (AFP) and carcinoembryonic antigen (CEA) (see below).

Among the proteins that have diagnostic utility in the assessment of patients with cancer are those associated with pregnancy such as human chorionic gonadotropin. In patients with breast, lung, and gastrointestinal carcinoma, casein can be found in high concentration in serum, whereas in patients with leukemias and Hodgkin's disease, such protein markers as serum ferritin may be markedly elevated. Enzymes are valuable markers of malignancy. For example, prostatic carcinoma is associated with high concentrations of serum acid phosphatase and the BB isoenzyme of creatine kinase. Certain lung tumors have been found to make a placental-like alkaline phosphatase.

The polyamines, spermine and spermidine, and their diamine precursor, putrescine, are highly basic compounds which may reflect cell turnover. These compounds have been studied as potential tumor markers; however, polyamine assays are not routinely available in clinical laboratories. Many hormones are produced by tumors; when non-endocrine tissue is responsible for the production of hormone, it is called ectopic hormone production (see below). Cellular markers, such as B or T cell antigens, are useful in non-Hodgkin's lymphoma, whereas prognosis and therapy of breast and other carcinomas are based on the detection of specific cellular proteins such as estrogen and progesterone receptors in tumor homogenates (see above).

Hormones as Tumor Markers

Benign and malignant tumors, derived from tissues that usually are not considered to be endocrine in nature, may produce hormonal substances. The so-

Table 15–4. TUMOR-ASSOCIATED MARKERS

Type	Example	Tumors
Oncofetal antigens	CEA	GI
	AFP	Lung, hepatoma, teratoma, GI
	Pancreatic oncofetal antigen	Pancreas
Proteins	Casein	Breast, lung, GI
	Ferritin	Leukemia, Hodgkin's disease
Enzymes	Creatine kinase (BB)	Prostate
	Acid phosphatase	Prostate
	Alkaline phosphatase	Lung
Polyamines	Spermine, spermidine, putresceine	Leukemia, lymphoma, colorectal cancer
Ectopic hormones	Peptide hormones	Many (see Table 15–5)
Cell markers	T, B cell markers	Lymphoma
Receptors	Estrogen, progesterone	Breast

2

called ectopic hormone syndromes were first described over 50 years ago, but until recently were thought to be a clinical rarity. The availability of radioimmunoassay for measurement of small amounts of circulating hormones has made possible documentation of a large number of these syndromes. The ectopic hormone produced may be indistinguishable from the native hormone or may be a fragment or a larger molecular weight form such as a prohormone. Although the ectopic hormone produced may not be chemically identical to the native hormone and may not have full biologic activity, it may be measured as the hormone by a given radioimmunoassay. Rarely syndromes have been described in which a substance is produced that has the biologic activity of a certain hormone but bears no structural relationship to it. Activity of these substances can be demonstrated only by tedious bioassays; this probably accounts in part for the description of only a few of these syndromes.

Ectopic hormone production is important, because it may lead to confusion in making the correct diagnosis or instituting proper treatment in certain endocrine disorders. In other situations, measurement of ectopic hormone production can be used as a biochemical marker for monitoring patients with documented or suspected tumors.

Of the ectopic hormones isolated, most have been peptides and none have been steroid or thyroid hormones (Table 15–5). Many theories have been proposed for the occurrence of these syndromes. One is that depression of the DNA code and subsequent m-RNA production leads to synthesis of polypeptides at an unregulated rate. Hormones such as thyroxine or steroids require a number of enzymatic steps for their formation; for these to be produced by a tumor, a series of ectopically produced enzymes located in a specific compartment presumably would be essential. Obviously, this is a much more complex requirement than the production of a simple polypeptide chain and may possibly account for the type of hormone produced. Another theory widely held is that secretion of hormones by neoplastic cells represents the persistence of a function normally present in a more primitive cell but which has been arrested in its differentiation process. According to this theory, with varying degrees of maturation arrest, tumor cells produce one or many peptide hormones or markers.

Another popular theory, the "endocrine cell" hypothesis, suggests that a change in gene function occurs in a cell that already possesses structural and biochemical characteristics of polypeptide secreting cells. Evidence supporting this theory has been accumulated by Pearse (1974) for a group of potential endocrine cells which have their origin in the neural crest. These cells, which migrate to various locations in the embryo, have been called APUD cells (Amine content, amine Precursor Uptake, amino acid Decarboxylase) based on their cytochemical properties. Ectopic secretion of ACTH by pheochromocytomas, medullary carcinomas of the thyroid, pancreatic islet cell neoplasm, and carcinoid tumors clearly can be interpreted as a change in the role of the APUD cell. Recent evidence indicates that APUD function of these cells is not linked with peptide hormone secretion and that occasionally tumors that secrete these hormones do not possess APUD characteristics.

Cushing's syndrome, associated with an ACTH-producing tumor, was the first description of ectopic polypeptide hormone production. Although features of Cushing's syndrome initially may not be apparent in these patients, signs and symptoms of the disorder become obvious within a short period. The syndrome develops rapidly and as it progresses, extreme muscle wasting, abnormal glucose tolerance, hypertension, and marked hypokalemic alkalosis may occur. Serum cortisol measurements are often >40 μg/dl (104 nm/L) and ACTH >200 pg/ml; usually neither cortisol nor ACTH is suppressed by administration of dexamethasone. In approximately two thirds of patients, ectopic ACTH production is associated with oat cell carcinoma of the lung, whereas tumors such as bronchial carcinoids and pancreatic and thymic tumors account for the other cases. A large number of tumors produce an ACTH with a molecular weight that is

Table 15–5. COMMON ECTOPIC HORMONE SYNDROMES

Hormone	Type of Neoplasm
Adrenocorticotropin (ACTH) and β-lipotropin (β-LPH)	Lung (oat cell, bronchial adenoma), thymus, pancreatic islets
Parathyroid hormone (PTH)	Kidney, lung (squamous cell), pancreas, ovary
Antidiuretic hormone (ADH)	Lung (oat cell)
Human chorionic gonadotropin (hCG)	Testicle (embryonal, choriocarcinoma), GI tract
Growth hormone (GH)	Lung (bronchogenic), stomach
Human placental lactogen (hPL)	Lung
Erythropoietin	Cerebellar (hemangioblastoma), pheochromocytoma, hepatoma
Renin	Lung (oat cell)
Thyrocalcitonin (TCT)	Lung, stomach
Enteroglucagon	Kidney
Non-suppressible insulin-like activity (NSILA)	Hepatoma, sarcoma, fibroma
Insulin-proinsulin	Nerve cell
Thyroid stimulating hormone (TSH)	Lung, breast
Growth hormone releasing hormone	Lung (carcinoid)
Corticotropin releasing hormone	Lung (carcinoid)

greater than that of the native hormone (big ACTH). Since this immunoreactive ACTH has little activity in receptor or bioassays, a clinically recognizable ectopic ACTH occurs only when tumors are able to produce biologically active ACTH. In addition, small ACTH, CLIP (corticotropin-like intermediate lobe peptide) and fragments of ACTH also have been reported to occur. Since both ACTH and β-lipotropin originate from the same precursor molecule, it is not surprising that ACTH-producing tumors have almost consistently been reported to elaborate β-LPH.

Hypercalcemia, one of the most common biochemical abnormalities, is associated with a variety of malignant lesions. It may be clinically manifested in subtle ways, such as anorexia, nausea, vomiting, constipation, and weakness, or may be the cause of life-threatening arrhythmias or coma. Since treatment is effective and relatively benign, all patients with tumors should have serum calcium determinations (see Chap. 9). Hypercalcemia may result from bony metastasis or may be secondary to production of hormonal factors including ectopic parathyroid (PTH) production. When hypercalcemia, hypophosphatemia, and decreased tubular reabsorption of phosphorus occur in the absence of bony lesions, ectopic PTH production should be suspected. Clinically this syndrome is different from primary hyperparathyroidism in that weight loss and constitutional symptoms are profound, hypercalcemia tends to be greater, and hyperchloremic metabolic alkalosis is less frequent. In patients with the syndrome, bony lesions of hyperparathyroidism are uncommon; renal stones and peptic ulceration are absent. Renal cell carcinoma and squamous cell carcinoma of the lung account for about two thirds of ectopic PTH producing tumors, whereas the remainder of tumors originate in a variety of sites. Because of the development of sophisticated radioimmunoassays for PTH, it has become apparent that several different fragments as well as prohormones of PTH occur. Depending on the assay system used, ectopic PTH production has been found to be associated with 30 to 90 per cent of all squamous cell carcinomas of the lung. Other cases have been described in which hypercalcemia and hypophosphatemia occur without an increased arteriovenous PTH gradient across the tumor bed; however, removal of the tumor results in the normalization of the calcium and phosphorus. In some of these patients, the hypercalcemia may be due to prostaglandins (Metz, 1981) or to osteocyte activating factor (OAF) (Mundy, 1974).

Tumors responsible for the production of antidiuretic hormone (ADH) are manifested by the cardinal signs of hyponatremia, depressed serum osmolality, and inappropriately elevated urine osmolality. To fulfill the criteria for diagnosis of inappropriate ADH secretion, renal and adrenal function must be normal. The detailed diagnostic criteria for the inappropriate ADH syndrome may be found in a discussion of the posterior pituitary (p. 304). Lung tumors and pancreatic tumors are most often responsible for this syndrome. Hamilton (1975) has reported that neurophysin, the normal protein carrier for ADH, is found in some tumors that have ectopic ADH synthesizing ability. Depending on the level of serum sodium, patients with the syndrome of water intoxication may present with virtually no symptoms or they may be comatose. Mild symptoms of water intoxication are most often characterized by lethargy, weakness, or confusion.

Of the gonadotropins, only ectopic production of luteinizing hormone (LH) and human chorionic gonadotropin (hCG) is likely to lead to clinically recognizable syndromes. Manifestations include precocious puberty occurring in prepubertal boys or gynecomastia occurring in men. Adenocarcinomas of the stomach, testicle, ovary, and pancreas and hepatomas are tumors most commonly associated with ectopic hCG secretion. Recent observations have indicated that hCG is distributed widely in various normal human tissues (Yoshimoto, 1979). Although this ubiquitous hCG-like substance is reported to lack carbohydrate, it is immunologically indistinguishable from hCG, and if this can be confirmed, these syndromes may no longer be considered ectopic.

The glycoprotein hormones are made up of nearly identical alpha subunits, but differ in beta subunit structure; it has been found that an isolated subunit may be produced by a particular tumor. A few carcinoid or pancreatic tumors have been reported to produce free alpha subunit, free beta subunit, or both; isolated increased alpha chain production is the most common abnormality observed. In another group of patients, alpha subunits have been correlated with the course of the disease and response to chemotherapy. Trophoblastic tumors have been reported to secrete hCG, but these tumors are not ectopic, since the secretion of this hormone is the normal physiologic function of the trophoblast (see below).

Growth hormone (GH) production has been reported rarely and only in association with a few tumors, most commonly bronchogenic and gastric carcinoma. In patients with bronchogenic carcinoma, human placental lactogen (HPL) as a tumor marker has been observed. HPL has an amino acid sequence very similar to that of growth hormone, but in a group of patients clinical features of hormone excess were not found.

Erythropoietin has been found in association with neoplastic renal disease, but since the kidney is normally responsible for its production, these tumors are not ectopic syndromes. However, erythropoietin has been secreted by hepatomas, pheochromocytomas, and 10 to 20 per cent of cerebellar hemangioblastomas; lung tumors are conspicuous by their absence in the production of this hormone. Serum thyrocalcitonin (TCT) is increased in some patients with lung, colon, breast, pancreas, /or gastric carcinoma (Schwartz, 1979). Tumors have been identified to contain high concentrations of prolactin; however, secretion of prolactin resulting in elevated serum prolactin levels does not appear to occur (Molitch, 1981). Other ectopically produced hormones such as thyroid stimulating hormone (TSH), growth hormone releasing hormone, and corticotropin releasing hormone, have been found in only a few cases, and each from a variety of human neoplasms (Table 15–5).

2

Alpha-Fetoprotein (AFP)

Alpha-fetoprotein, an oncofetal antigen, is a glycoprotein present in serum of healthy individuals at concentrations of <10 ng/ml. Values of >10 ng/ml but <400 ng/ml sometimes occur in malignant disease, whereas values >400 ng/ml usually are associated with hepatomas. The occurrence of elevated alpha-fetoprotein values also is found in other diseases of the liver, including cirrhosis and hepatitis, but usually values are relatively lower. Elevations of serum alpha-fetoprotein also are associated with germ cell tumors which contain yolk sac elements. In such tumors as teratoblastoma or embryonal carcinoma of the testes or ovary, alpha-fetoprotein concentrations are elevated in almost 90 per cent of cases and are in the same range as in hepatomas. Small elevations of alpha-fetoprotein may be found in association with tumors of the gastrointestinal tract or lung.

A collaborative study in the United Kingdom (1977) has indicated the value of elevated serum and amniotic fluid alpha-fetoprotein measurements in the antenatal diagnosis of neural tube defects. For further information, see Chapter 21. However, the large number of false positive results found in antenatal screening programs delayed until 1983 the licensing of alpha-fetoprotein assays in the United States (Sell, 1981).

Human Chorionic Gonadotropin (hCG)

Human chorionic gonadotropin (hCG) is a glycoprotein hormone usually found in high concentration in serum and urine during pregnancy. Increases in hCG can be found in serum and other body fluids in patients with gestational trophoblastic disease including hydatidiform mole and choriocarcinoma as well as with other tumors. The hormone is made up of an alpha and beta subunit, the alpha subunit of which is very similar to that of the other glycoprotein hormones, whereas the beta subunit of hCG has large areas of homology with luteinizing hormone (LH). Tumors may produce not only hCG but increased amounts of alpha or beta subunit. Although it was thought that hCG occurred only in pregnant patients or those with carcinoma, it is now known that urine from healthy individuals contains low levels of a substance with hCG immunoreactivity. In addition, non-pregnant individuals with non-neoplastic gastrointestinal disorders may have immunoreactive hCG or its subunits in their serum.

A variety of techniques are available for measurement of hCG and its beta subunit. When hCG is used as a tumor marker, it is necessary to employ immunoassays for the beta unit that have high specificity and a sensitivity of less than 10 IU. Cross-reactivity with LH precludes use of assays for intact hCG, and the usual pregnancy tests are not sufficiently sensitive for use in this capacity. Most antibodies raised against the beta subunit also react with intact hCG (Hussa, 1982).

Assays for β-hCG have been useful in monitoring patients with gestational trophoblastic disease and in monitoring of patients with testicular choriocarcinoma, particularly in conjunction with alpha-fetoprotein assays. Other tumors have also been associated with elevated β-hCG levels, including a variety of testicular tumors in addition to choriocarcinoma of the testes; gastrointestinal carcinoma, including hepatomas and pancreatic carcinoma; ovarian carcinoma; and occasionally leukemia, lymphomas, and a variety of other tumors such as melanoma and bronchogenic carcinoma.

Some patients with testicular choriocarcinoma have had elevated levels of β-hCG without apparent progression of their disease (Light, 1982). This, coupled with reports of false positive immunoassays for serum β-hCG, makes it imperative to interpret elevated β-hCG levels cautiously. In monitoring patients with trophoblastic disease, serum assays for β-hCG often are used, but assays using concentrates of 24-hour urine specimens have been reported to be more sensitive. Assay of β-hCG in cerebrospinal fluid has been used to study patients who may have central nervous system (CNS) metastases from choriocarcinoma. Most patients with CNS metastases show a larger ratio of CSF/serum β-hCG than those without metastases.

The alpha subunit of hCG can be measured by immunoassay, and these assays have been used to monitor patients with various tumors. Although in some patients alpha subunit levels have correlated with the course of disease and response to chemotherapy, this is not the case for all individuals (Kourides, 1981).

Carcinoembryonic Antigen (CEA)

Carcinoembryonic antigen (CEA), which is an example of an oncofetal antigen, is a glycoprotein present in abundance during fetal life in entodermally derived tissue such as intestine and lung. In adult patients with various types of cancer, increased levels can be found in cells and plasma. Although CEA is tumor associated, it is not specific for malignancy or for tumor type. CEA has been isolated from plasma of healthy adults and can be increased in a variety of disorders, including hypothyroidism and inflammation such as occurs with pneumonia and pancreatitis. CEA may be elevated in patients with a wide variety of malignancies, in particular those of the gastrointestinal tract, pancreas, lung, breast, and ovary.

Assay of CEA in plasma can be carried out by radioimmunoassay or enzyme immunoassay. CEA molecules produced by various tumors are not identical; thus results may differ depending on the specificity of antibody used in the assay. There is no agreement as to what the reference interval is for CEA in plasma or serum; some workers have considered the upper limit to be 2.5 ng/ml, but others have used higher values. CEA levels tend to increase with age and to be higher in smokers. CEA levels within the reference interval are not proof of absence of malignancy, and elevated levels are not specific for malignancy. CEA levels also have been measured in body fluids; for example, Satler (1982) reports ascitic fluid CEA levels may be helpful in differentiating malignant and nonmalignant ascites.

Because plasma CEA measurements do not possess the sensitivity or specificity to discriminate between malignant and nonmalignant disease, plasma CEA levels should not be used independently to establish the diagnosis of cancer. In a statement from a Consensus Development Conference of the National Institutes of Health, however, further diagnostic efforts were recommended for patients with symptoms and grossly elevated CEA values (greater that five to ten times the upper limit of the reference range for the particular laboratory) in order to establish the presence or absence of cancer (National Institutes of Health, 1981).

CEA levels may be especially useful in patients with colorectal carcinomas. In about 50 to 90 per cent of patients with colorectal carcinoma CEA levels are above 2.5 ng/ml, and the majority have values above 5.0 ng/ml. Poorly differentiated colorectal carcinomas, however, tend to be associated with lack of elevation in plasma CEA levels. Preoperative CEA levels are recommended in patients with colorectal carcinoma as an adjunct to other staging methods. Following complete surgical removal of a colorectal malignancy, an elevated CEA value usually should return to within the reference interval by six weeks. CEA is helpful in detection of recurrent colorectal cancer and in monitoring treatment of patients with metastatic disease. In patients with colorectal carcinoma, a rapid rise in CEA following treatment is suggestive of hepatic or bony metastasis, whereas slowly rising levels are more indicative of local recurrence. However, elevated CEA levels due to factors such as smoking and intercurrent infection can occur in patients in whom the tumor is stable, and decreasing CEA levels are not invariably a sign of successful therapy. About 10 per cent of patients with rising levels of CEA have stable disease (Reynoso, 1981).

In patients with significant CEA elevations and metastatic lung cancer, particularly small cell carcinoma, or metastatic breast cancer, changes in CEA levels may be of value in assessing response to chemotherapy. CEA may be elevated in a variety of other malignancies; however, the role of CEA in monitoring patients with tumors other than colorectal, bronchial, or breast carcinoma is less well established. In patients with carcinomas of the head and neck, about 50 per cent show elevations of CEA, whereas in patients with malignancies such as sarcomas and lymphomas, CEA is elevated in only about 25 to 35 per cent.

Al-Shawi, A., Mohammed-Ali, S., Houts, T., Hodgkinson, S., Nargessi, R. D., and Landon, J.: Principles of labeled antibody immunoassays. Ligand Quart., *4*:43, 1981.

Bangham, D. R., and Cotes, P. M.: Reference standards for radioimmunoassay. *In* Kirkham, K. E., and Hunter, W. M. (eds.): Radioimmunoassay Methods. Edinburgh, Churchill Livingstone, 1971.

Bangham, D. R., and Cotes, P. M.: Standardization and standards. Br. Med. Bull., *30*:12, 1974.

Binoux, M. A., and Odell, W. D.: Use of dextran-coated charcoal to separate antibody-bound from free hormone: A critique. J. Clin. Endocrinol. Metab., *36*:303, 1973.

Bolton, A. E., and Hunter, W. M.: The labelling of proteins to high specific radioactivities by conjugation to a ^{125}I-containing acylating agent. Biochem. J., *133*:529, 1973.

Challand, G., Goldie, D., and Landon, J.: Immunoassay in the diagnostic laboratory. Br. Med. J., *30*:38, 1974.

Chard, T.: Observations on the uses of a mathematical model in radioimmunoassay. *In* Kirkham, K. E., and Hunter, W. M. (eds.): Radioimmunoassay Methods. Edinburgh, Churchill Livingstone, 1971.

Eckert, H. G.: Radioimmunoassay. Agnew Chem. Int. Ed. Engl., *15*:525, 1976.

Ekins, R. P.: Basic principles and theory. Br. Med. Bull., *30*:3, 1974.

Ekins, R. P.: General principles of hormone assay. *In* Loraine, J. A., and Bell, E. T. (eds.): Hormone Assays and Their Clinical Application. Edinburgh, Churchill Livingstone, 1976.

Ekins, R. P.: Mathematical treatment of data. *In* Kirkham, K. E., and Hunter, W. M. (eds.): Radioimmunoassay Methods. Edinburgh, Churchill Livingstone, 1971.

Engvall, E., Jonsson, K., and Perlmann, P.: Enzyme-linked immunosorbent assay. II. Quantitative assay of protein antigen, immunoglobulin G, by means of enzyme-labelled antigen and antibody-coated tubes. Biochim. Biophys. Acta, *251*:427, 1971.

Engvall, E., and Perlmann, P.: Enzyme-linked immunosorbent assay, ELISA. III. Quantitation of specific antibodies by enzyme-labeled anti-immunoglobulin in antigen-coated tubes. J. Immunol., *109*:129, 1972.

Giegel, J. L., Brotherton, M. M., Cronin, P., D'Aquino, M., Evans, S., Heller, Z. H., Knight, W. S., Krishnan, K., and Sheiman, M.: Radial partition immunoassay. Clin. Chem., *28*:1894, 1982.

Hamilton, B. P.: Presence of neurophysin proteins in tumors associated with the syndrome of inappropriate ADH secretion. Ann. N.Y. Acad. Sci., *248*:153, 1975.

Howanitz, J. H.: Hormone receptors and breast cancer. Hum. Path., *12*:1057, 1981.

Howanitz, P. J., Howanitz, J. H., Lamberson, H. V., and Ennis, K. M.: Incidence and mechanism of spurious increases in serum thyrotropin. Clin. Chem., *28*:427, 1982.

Hunter, W. M.: Preparation and assessment of radioactive tracers. Br. Med. Bull., *30*:18, 1974.

Hunter, W. M., and Ganguli, P. C.: The separation of antibody bound from free antigen. *In* Kirkham, K. E., and Hunter, W. M. (eds.): Radioimmunoassay Methods. Edinburgh, Churchill Livingstone, 1971.

Hunter, W. M., and Greenwood, F. C.: Preparation of iodine-131 labelled human growth hormone of high specific activity. Nature, *194*:495, 1962.

Hurn, B. A. L., and Landon, J.: Antisera for radioimmunoassay. *In* Kirkham, K. E., and Hunter, W. M. (eds.): Radioimmunoassay Methods. Edinburgh, Churchill Livingstone, 1971.

Hussa, R. O.: Clinical utility of human chorionic gonadotropin and α-subunit measurements. Obstet. Gynecol., *60*:1, 1982.

Jacobs, S., and Cuatrecasas, P.: Cell receptors in disease. N. Engl. J. Med., *297*:1383, 1977.

Kourides, I. A., and Schorr-Toshav, N. L.: Alpha subunit of the glycoprotein hormones: Secretion by human malignancies. Clin. Bull., *11*:106, 1981.

Landon, J.: The radioimmunoassay of drugs. Analyst, *101*:225, 1976.

Light, P. A., Felton, T., and Eckert, H.: False-positive markers in testicular tumours. Lancet, *2*:1214, 1982.

Marchalonis, J. J.: An enzymatic method for the trace iodination of immunoglobulins and other proteins. Biochem. J., *113*:229, 1969.

McGuire, W. L.: Steroid hormone receptors in breast cancer treatment strategy. Rec. Prog. Horm. Res., *36*:135, 1980.

McGuire, W. L., Horwitz, K. B., Pearson, O. H., and Segaloff, A.: Current status of estrogen and progesterone receptors in breast cancer. Cancer, *39*:2934, 1977.

Metz, S. A., McRae, J. R., and Robertson, R. P.: Prostaglandins as mediators of paraneoplastic syndromes: Review and update. Metabolism, *30*:299, 1981.

Molitch, M. E., Schwartz, S., and Mukherji, B.: Is prolactin secreted ectopically? Am. J. Med., *70*:803, 1981.

Mundy, G. R., Raisz, L. G., Cooper, R. A., Schechter, G. P., and Salmon, S. E.: Evidence for the secretion of an osteoclast stimulation factor in myeloma. N. Engl. J. Med., *291*:1041, 1974.

Myers, C. E., Lippman, M. E., Eliot, H. M., and Crabner, B. A.: Competitive protein binding assay for methotrexate. Proc. Natl. Acad. Sci. U.S.A., *72*:3683, 1975.

National Institutes of Health Consensus Development Conference Statement—CEA (Carcinoembryonic Antigen): Its role as a marker in the management of cancer. Md. State Med. J., *30*:48, 1981.

Osborne, C. K., and McGuire, W. L.: The use of steroid receptors in the treatment of human breast cancer: A Review. Bull. Cancer, *66*:203, 1979.

Parker, C. W.: Radioimmunoassay of Biologically Active Compounds. Englewood Cliffs, N.J., Prentice-Hall, Inc., 1976.

Pearse, A. G.: The APUD cell concept and its implications in pathology. *In* Summers, S. C. (ed.): Pathology Annual. New York, Appleton-Century-Crofts, 1974.

Ratcliffe, J. G.: Separation techniques in saturation analysis. Br. Med. Bull., *30*:32, 1974.

Raynaud, J. P., Ojasoo, T., Delarue, J. C., Magdelenat, H., Martin, P., and Philibert, D.: Estrogen and progestin receptors in human breast cancer. *In* McGuire, W. L., Raynaud, J. P., and Baulieu, E. E.: Progesterone Receptors in Normal and Neoplastic Tissues. New York, Raven Press, 1977.

Reynoso, G.: CEA basic concepts, clinical applications. Diagnostic Med., *4*:41, 1981.

Rodbard, D., Rayford, P. L., Cooper, J. A., and Ross, G. T.: Statistical quality control of radioimmunoassays. J. Clin. Endocrinol. Metab., *28*:1412, 1968.

Rodbard, D., Ruder, H. J., Vaitukaitis, J., and Jacobs, H. S.: Mathematical analysis of kinetics of radioligand assays: Improved sensitivity obtained by delayed addition of labeled ligand. J. Clin. Endocrinol. Metab., *33*:343, 1971.

Rosa, U., Scassellati, G. A., and Pennisi, F.: Labelling of human fibrinogen with ^{131}I by electrolytic iodination. Biochim. Biophys. Acta, *86*:519, 1964.

Rowley, G. L., Rubenstein, K. E., Huisjen, J., and Ullman, E. F.: Mechanism by which antibodies inhibit hapten-malate dehydrogenase conjugates. J. Biol. Chem., *250*:3759, 1975.

Rubenstein, K. E.: Homogeneous enzyme immunoassay today. Scand. J. Immunol., *8*:57, 1978.

Satler, J. J., and Herzog, B.: CEA serum values controversy. Am. J. Proctol. Gastroenterol. Colon Rectal Surg., *33*:24, 1982.

Schall, R. F., and Tenoso, H. J.: Alternatives to radioimmunoassay: Labels and methods. Clin. Chem., *27*:1157, 1981.

Schwartz, K. E., Wolfsen, A. R., Forster, B., and Odell, W. D.: Calcitonin in nonthyroidal cancer. J. Clin. Endocrinol. Metab., *49*:438, 1979.

Sell, S.: Diagnostic applications of alpha-fetoprotein: Government regulations prevent full application of a clinically useful test. Hum. Path., *12*:959, 1981.

Sevier, E. D., David, G. S., Martinis, J., Desmond, W. J., Bartholomew, R. M., and Wang, R.: Monoclonal antibodies in clinical immunology. Clin. Chem., *27*:1797, 1981.

Soini, E., and Hemmilä, I.: Fluoroimmunoassay: Present status and key problems. Clin. Chem., *25*:353, 1979.

Thorell, J. I.: Internal sample attenuator counting (ISAC). A new technique for separating and measuring bound and free activity in radioimmunoassays. Clin. Chem., *27*:1969, 1981.

United Kingdom collaborive study on alpha-fetoprotein in relation to neural tube defects. Lancet, *2*:1323, 1977.

Wisdom, G. B.: Enzyme immunoassay. Clin. Chem., *22*:1243, 1976.

Woodhead, J. S., Addison, G. M., and Hales, C. N.: The immunoradiometric assay and related techniques. Br. Med. J., *30*:44, 1974.

Yalow, R. S.: Heterogeneity of peptide hormones: Its relevance in clinical radioimmunoassay. Adv. Clin. Chem., *20*:1, 1978a.

Yalow, R. S.: Radioimmunoassay: A probe for the fine structure of biologic systems. Science, *200*:1236, 1978b.

Yoshimoto, Y., Wolfsen, A. R., and Odell, W. D.: Glycosylation, a variable in the production of hCG by cancers. Am. J. Med., 67:414, 1979.

16

EVALUATION OF ENDOCRINE FUNCTION

JOAN H. HOWANITZ, M.D., and PETER J. HOWANITZ, M.D.

2

Most of the hormones of the endocrine system are presented in this chapter; those not presented here are found in other chapters relating to the endocrine system. These include Chapter 9, calcium metabolism (parathyroid hormone, calcitonin, and the D vitamins); Chapter 10, hormones associated with glucose metabolism; Chapter 15, ectopic production of hormones; Chapter 20, placental hormones; and Chapter 25, intestinal hormones.

PITUITARY GLAND

The pituitary gland, which is located at the base of the skull, is divided into an anterior lobe, a rudimentary intermediate lobe, and a posterior or neural lobe. The anterior lobe secretes growth hormone (GH), corticotropin (adrenocorticotropic hormone [ACTH]), thyrotropin (thyroid stimulating hormone [TSH]), follicle stimulating hormone (FSH), luteinizing hormone (LH), and prolactin. The pituitary also synthesizes β-lipotropic hormone. The intermediate lobe of the pituitary is thought to contain most of the β-lipotropic hormone, but it has been found in the anterior lobe as well (Chrètien, 1977). Beta-melanocyte stimulating hormone (β-MSH) appears not to exist as a separate peptide in the human pituitary gland, but as a part of β-lipotropic hormone.

The hypothalamic region of the brain produces releasing and inhibiting hormones that play a role in controlling synthesis and release of anterior pituitary hormones. Feedback mechanisms, in which a hormone influences its own secretion or secretion of another hormone, operate at both pituitary and hypothalamic

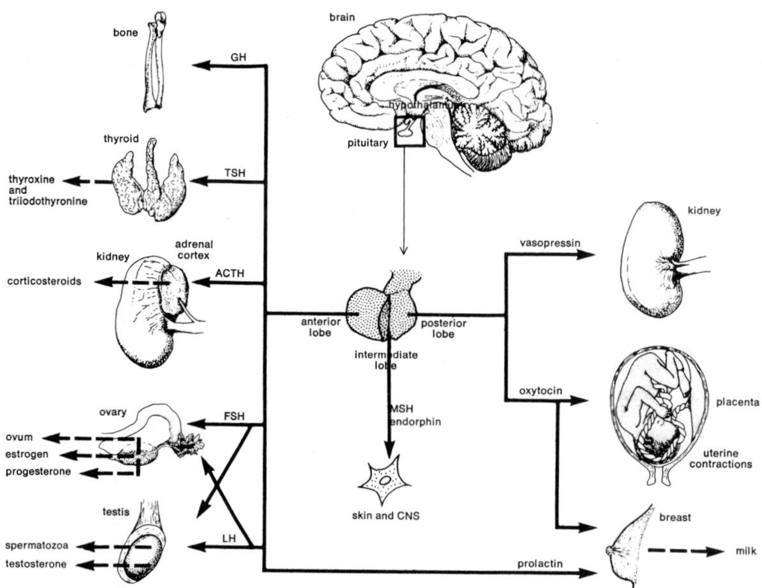

Figure 16–1. Target organs for the pituitary hormones GH, TSH, ACTH, FSH, LH, MSH, vasopressin and oxytocin. (From Schally, A. V., Kastin, A. J., and Arimura, A.: Hypothalamic hormones: The link between brain and body. Am. Sci., *65*:712, 1977. Reprinted by permission of American Scientist, Journal of Sigma Xi, The Scientific Research Society of North America.)

levels. After hormones of the anterior pituitary reach their targets, they regulate various processes, as indicated in Figure 16–1. Vasopressin, also called antidiuretic hormone (ADH), and oxytocin are synthesized in the hypothalamus and then transported to the posterior pituitary gland where they are stored until release.

Hypopituitarism, that is, decreased function of the anterior pituitary, refers to a wide spectrum of entities ranging from isolated lack of one trophic hormone to complete absence of all hormones. Some of these syndromes are not due to lack of hormone-producing cells in the pituitary gland, but are caused by deficiency of hypothalamic releasing hormones. Hypopituitarism may result from pituitary ablation by surgery or radiation, pituitary tumors, metastatic tumors, infarction, and infiltrative granulomatous processes. Hypothalamic disorders and pituitary tumors can lead to excessive secretion of one or more of the hormones of the anterior pituitary. In addition, ectopic production of some of these hormones has been reported.

Anterior Pituitary

GROWTH HORMONE

Although a number of hormones are necessary for growth, the most important hormonal regulator is growth hormone (GH), also called somatotropin. In the absence of GH, growth in children proceeds at one third to one half the usual rate. Importance of human GH has been confirmed by the finding that children of small stature who lack measurable serum levels of the hormone can be stimulated to grow at rates approaching those of healthy children by administration of GH. The function of GH in the adult has not been clarified fully.

The secretion of growth hormone from the anterior pituitary appears to be regulated by hypothalamic releasing and inhibiting factors or hormones; growth hormone release–inhibiting hormone also is called somatostatin (see Chap. 10). Growth hormone–releasing factor (GRF), which recently has been isolated from a human pancreatic tumor that produced clinical evidence of acromegaly, has enormous potential in diagnosis and treatment of GH deficiency (Editorial, 1983). Growth hormone probably exerts its major effects by influencing hepatic production of somatomedins, which in turn act on target tissues; however, GH also appears to have direct action on tissues.

Serum GH levels routinely are measured by radioimmunoassay; in general, antisera with suitable specificity for GH readily can be obtained. For most of a given 24-hour period in non-stressed healthy individuals, serum GH values are undetectable or at very low concentrations, with most values <3 ng/ml (<3 μg/L) (Weitzman, 1976). During the day, short bursts of GH secretion occur in no consistent temporal pattern; however, the day-to-day pattern appears to be fairly constant in a given individual. In premature and newborn infants, basal serum GH levels are elevated.

Increases in serum GH levels occur in association with a number of events, including sleep. During the first two hours of sleep, GH is secreted in substantial amounts, usually with the peak secretion occurring between the first and second hour. Following this major spike in GH secretion, serum concentrations rapidly fall to low levels. There sometimes is a second and even a third secretory peak during the remaining hours of the sleep period. The sleep onset–related GH peak may be delayed or prevented for many hours when sleep is delayed, and in adults over 50 years of age sleep-associated GH release may be absent.

Bursts of GH secretion also may occur with exercise, especially in patients who are fasting. In the healthy adult, a glucose load suppresses GH secretion, but a secondary rise in GH levels occurs several hours later. The sleep-onset serum GH peak cannot be suppressed by glucose infusion. With hypoglycemia, such as occurs with an insulin tolerance testing, GH is released. Protein ingestion and infusion of amino acids, such as arginine, also are associated with increased serum GH. Growth hormone is frequently, but not reproducibly, secreted following stress; major surgery can produce an increase in serum levels despite hyperglycemia.

Somatomedins. The somatomedins are a group of small peptides with similar biologic actions which are transported in plasma bound by carrier proteins. Factors other than GH, such as nutritional state, are important in regulation of somatomedins, and sometimes their influence overrides that of GH. Elevation of serum GH levels in conjunction with low somatomedin levels occurs in Laron dwarfs, newborns, and patients with kwashiorkor or liver disease. In these situations increased GH levels may reflect lack of feedback from somatomedin (Phillips, 1980). Although immunologically distinct from insulin, members of the somatomedin family show many insulin-like metabolic activities *in vitro*. The somatomedin family includes (1) somatomedin A; (2) somatomedin B; (3) insulin-like growth factor 1 (IGF-1), which was formerly known as nonsuppressible insulin-like activity 1 (NSILA-1) and which is probably identical to somatomedin C (somatomedin C and IGF-1 are immunologically identical, and thus immunoassays are referred to as "somatomedin C/IGF-1" [SM-C/IGF-1]); and (4) insulin-like growth factor 2 (IGF-2), which was formerly known as NSILA-2 and is similiar, if not identical, to multiplication stimulating activity (MSA).

Somatomedin C/IGF-1 and IGF-2 are the two major somatomedins in plasma; somatomedin immunoassays have been developed in which the antibody reacts mainly with SM-C/IGF-1, the somatomedin more closely linked to GH action than IGF-2 (Daughaday, 1979). Assays for SM-C/IGF-1 have been used in a variety of clinical situations (see below).

Growth Hormone Hyposecretion. GH hyposecretion in adults is a sensitive indicator of pituitary dysfunction. In children, GH deficiency is a relatively uncommon but important cause of short stature. Patients may have isolated GH deficiency, partial GH deficiency, or GH deficiency associated with deficiency of at least one other pituitary hormone. In most cases of isolated idiopathic GH deficiency, the primary defect is probably hypothalamic. The birth weights of patients with GH deficiency are normal, but decreased growth rates occur within the first few months of life. Most children with GH deficiency have growth velocities below the third percentile, and delay in skeletal maturation almost always occurs. The diagnosis of GH deficiency is made using clinical and radiographic criteria in conjunction with provocative tests of GH function (see below). Because a significant portion of GH deficient children have SM-C/IGF-1 levels within the reference interval, the assay is not sensitive as a diagnostic test for GH deficiency. In addition, SM-C/IGF-1 cannot be used to predict response to GH therapy, because levels do not increase in all individuals who are responsive to GH therapy (Dean, 1982).

Other individuals have some clinical features of GH deficiency, but the defect appears to be in generation of somatomedins. Laron (1966) described a familial form of dwarfism with clinical features of GH deficiency in the presence of high serum GH levels. These patients, called Laron dwarfs, have low somatomedin levels which fail to rise with GH administration. Pygmies have several clinical and biochemical features of isolated GH deficiency, but the major defect appears to be a deficiency of SM-C/IGF-1 (Merimee, 1981).

Provocative Tests of GH Function. Undetectable fasting GH levels occur frequently in healthy subjects, and thus are not diagnostic of hypofunction. Laboratory assessment of GH deficiency is performed by measuring serum growth hormone in the fasting state, following the onset of deep sleep, after exercise, and during stimulation tests.

An insulin tolerance test (ITT) may be used to assess GH as well as ACTH reserve in both children and adults. Performance of an ITT is contraindicated in certain individuals, including those with a history of ischemic heart disease and those with evidence of myocardial infarction, cerebrovascular disease, epilepsy, and low basal serum cortisol levels. The test is performed by injecting a bolus of insulin (0.05 to 0.15 U/kg) intravenously. Blood specimens are drawn before the start of the test and should be collected at least at 15-minute intervals the first hour after insulin is given.

An essential feature of the ITT is that an adequate degree of hypoglycemia must be obtained. This usually is defined as a drop in plasma glucose concentration to <40 mg/dl (2.2 mmol/L) or a depression to less than 50 per cent of the fasting glucose level. The patient must be under constant supervision during the entire procedure, and glucose must be available for immediate intravenous administration. The test should be terminated by giving glucose if the patient has serious signs and symptoms such as chest pain or loss of consciousness. Glucose, GH, and cortisol are determined on each specimen (Fig. 16–2). In healthy subjects, adequate hypoglycemia generally results in a rise in serum GH to levels >20 ng/ml (>20 μg/L).

Arginine infusion also may be used alone or following an ITT (arginine-insulin test). Arginine, 30 g for adults, and 0.5 g/kg body weight (up to 30 g) for children, is infused over a 30-minute period. Baseline serum GH levels are obtained before the start of the infusion and then at 15- to 30-minute intervals for one to two hours. Other stimulation tests have been

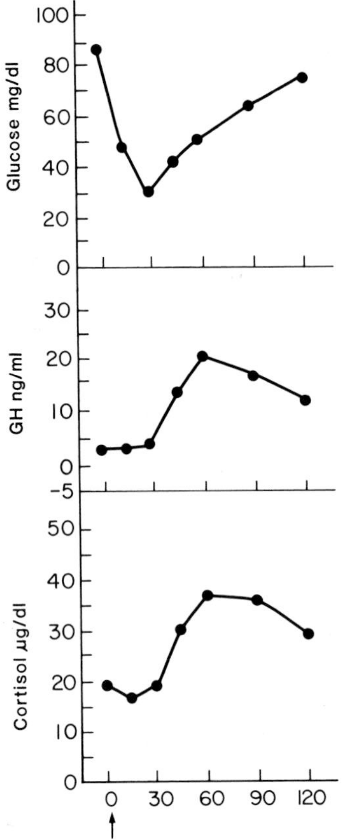

Figure 16–2. Typical response of glucose, cortisol, and growth hormone during an insulin tolerance test with 0.10 unit insulin/kg given intravenously at time zero (↑). To convert to SI units multiply glucose by 0.0555 to yield mmol/L, growth hormone by 1.0 to yield μg/L, and cortisol by 27.59 to yield nmol/L. Abscissa is time in minutes.

employed, using a variety of agents including vasopressin, glucagon, and L-dopa. Collu and colleagues (1978) have reported that use of the combination of L-dopa and propranolol appears to be more effective in releasing GH than other commonly used tests of GH reserve, including the arginine-insulin test. Hypoglycemia can occur with this test, but is much less common than with the arginine-insulin test.

Although the ITT usually is regarded as the definitive test of GH reserve, an ITT may not cause GH release whereas arginine infusion can cause a response, or vice versa; this dissociation may occur in healthy children and less commonly in healthy adults. The absolute value of serum GH which must be exceeded in order to be classified as a normal response is defined differently by various investigators. Failure of GH levels to rise above these limits after at least two stimulation tests is indicative of GH deficiency. Generally, peak post-stimulus GH values of <5 ng/ml (<5 μg/L) are considered subnormal; values from 5 to 10 ng/ml (5 to 10 μg/L), indeterminate; and values of 10 ng/ml (10 μg/L) or greater, normal (van Wyk, 1980).

Patients with normal variant short stature (NVSS) are those with normal birth weight and no apparent organic cause for growth retardation, but whose current height and predicted adult height are below the third percentile. They show normal GH response to stimulation tests such as the ITT and have normal nocturnal GH levels when GH is measured by radioimmunoassay. In some of these patients, when nocturnal GH levels by radioreceptor assay and by radioimmunoassay are compared, a subnormal ratio is found. It has been proposed that these children are secreting GH which is immunologically, but not biologically, active. These children have been reported to have low serum SM-C/IGF-1 levels that are restored to normal after treatment with GH (Rudman, 1981).

Results of pituitary function tests can be altered by numerous factors. Hypothyroidism and hyperthyroidism may cause impaired GH response to stimulatory tests. Hypothyroidism often is associated with short stature; such patients must be maintained in the euthyroid state for a considerable period before their true GH status can be assessed properly. Obesity has an inhibitory effect on GH dynamics; a significant serum GH elevation does not occur in half the patients following an ITT, and similar results are reported using arginine, L-dopa, and glucagon. Abnormal GH dynamics also have been reported in patients with diabetes mellitus, starvation, and cirrhosis and in patients taking certain drugs. For example, GH response to insulin hypoglycemia is blunted in patients taking pharmacologic doses of glucocorticoids.

Growth Hormone Hypersecretion. Acromegaly and gigantism are clinical expressions of GH hypersecretion, which, in nearly all cases, is caused by presence of a GH-secreting pituitary tumor. If excess GH secretion occurs before puberty, gigantism results; in adults, excess GH secretion leads to acromegaly. Gigantism is a rare disorder characterized by generalized overgrowth of the skeleton and soft tissues. Acromegaly is usually first manifested by overgrowth of the head, hands, and feet, resulting in facial changes and changes in hat, glove, or shoe size. Local effects of the tumor may cause headache and visual difficulties. The disease is associated with a number of other disturbances, including impaired glucose tolerance or diabetes mellitus and occasionally hyperthyroidism.

Since GH release occurs in pulsatile bursts or in response to stress, a single GH determination is not useful in making the diagnosis of GH excess, because it may reflect these peaks. In healthy individuals, serum GH levels are suppressed with an oral glucose load such as given with a glucose tolerance test (GTT). In these subjects, serum GH levels at the beginning of the test period are usually <10 ng/ml (<10 μg/L) and suppress to <5 ng/ml (<5 μg/L) at some time during the procedure. This suppression is followed by a secondary rise occurring several hours later and related in magnitude to the amount of glucose ingested (Hunter, 1976).

In most patients with acromegaly or gigantism, GH levels are elevated throughout the day and fail to suppress following a glucose load. In patients with active acromegaly, basal serum GH levels usually are <5 ng/ml (<5 μg/L), and often GH levels do not fall to <10 ng/ml (<10μg/L) during a GTT. With a GTT, some patients with acromegaly may have a paradoxical rise in serum GH, whereas others show normal response or partial suppression of GH. In patients treated for acromegaly, it has been suggested that serum GH should suppress to <2 ng/ml (<2 μg/L) after glucose administration if a patient is considered cured (Schuster, 1981). Failure to suppress serum GH with a glucose load may occur in conditions other than acromegaly or gigantism, including renal failure, cirrhosis, and starvation.

Thyrotropin releasing hormone (TRH) stimulates GH secretion in 50 per cent of patients with acromegaly, but not in healthy subjects. TRH infusion also may cause GH increases in patients with a variety of other disorders, including renal disease, hypothyroidism, anorexia nervosa, depression, and liver disease. L-Dopa and bromocriptine stimulate GH secretion in healthy individuals, but can produce a paradoxical fall of serum GH in acromegalic patients. Those patients who remain responsive to TRH after treatment for acromegaly have a greater chance of relapse than those who do not (Pearson, 1981).

There is evidence that measurement of serum SM-C/IGF-1 may be helpful in the diagnosis and assessment of activity of acromegaly. Measurements of SM-C/IGF-1 appear helpful in patients who are suspected of having active acromegaly, but who do not have increased basal GH or who show normal suppression of GH with glucose administration (Clemmons, 1979). Somatomedin C/IGF-1 measurements, however, probably cannot substitute for study of GH dynamics in assessing cure; some patients treated for acromegaly have basal GH and SM-C/IGF-1 levels within the reference interval, but show abnormal responses to dynamic testing (Pearson, 1981).

PROLACTIN

Prolactin is an anterior pituitary hormone necessary for initiation and maintenance of lactation. There are several forms, including "big" and "little" prolactin; the significance of this heterogeneity remains in question. Prolactin secretion is influenced by prolactin inhibiting and releasing factors from the hypothalamus and, in addition, prolactin attenuates its own secretion. Prolactin is under inhibitory control of the hypothalamus.

Prolactin, which is usually measured by radioimmunoassay, has a reference interval in serum of about 1 to 25 ng/ml (1 to 25 μg/L) for females and 1 to 20 ng/ml (1 to 20 μg/L) for males. Serum prolactin levels are influenced by a wide variety of physiologic, pharmacologic, and pathologic factors (see below). In addition, methodologic factors, such as standardization, assay precision, and reference interval employed, are important in interpreting serum prolactin levels (Jeffcoate, 1978)

There is diurnal variation in serum prolactin levels. With sleep, prolactin levels begin to rise after 60 to 90 minutes, reaching their highest values four to five hours later. Alteration in timing of the sleep period results in changes in the prolactin secretory pattern, indicating it is not an inherent neural rhythm. Prolactin levels also show marked random fluctuations of a brief episodic variety. In pregnancy, maternal serum prolactin levels rise progressively, falling to basal levels within about three weeks after delivery in mothers who do not breast feed. In nursing mothers, basal levels remain somewhat elevated and breast feeding frequently, but not uniformly, causes dramatic increases in serum prolactin levels. The physiologic hyperprolactinemia that occurs with lactation following parturition is associated with delay in restoration of cyclic ovarian function. Serum prolactin levels also rise after stress; for example, increases in prolactin levels are associated with exercise and the hypoglycemia that occurs during insulin tolerance testing.

Hyposecretion and Hypersecretion. In clinical situations, prolactin is rarely deficient; deficiency is seen after pituitary necrosis or infarction and in some patients with pseudohypoparathyroidism. In addition to idiopathic elevations, serum prolactin levels are increased in patients treated with a wide variety of drugs and under certain physiologic and pathologic conditions (Tables 16–1 and 16–2).

Prolactin-secreting pituitary tumors are thought to be the most common of all pituitary tumors, with about 70 per cent of chromophobe adenomas associated with hyperprolactinemia. The height of serum prolactin levels has been correlated with the likelihood of the presence of a pituitary tumor. In the series of Kleinberg (1977), 57 per cent of patients with prolactin levels >100 ng/ml (>100 μg/L) had pituitary tumors; in those with serum levels >300 ng/ml (>300 μg/L), all patients had pituitary tumors. Because patients with prolactin-producing pituitary microadenomas may have serum prolactin values of <100 ng/ml (<100 μg/L), radiographic studies including polytomography are the most important means of identifying patients who might have pituitary tumors (Rogol, 1979). If a pituitary tumor cannot be demonstrated radiographically in a patient who has no other cause for an elevated prolactin level, the hyperprolactinemia is regarded as functional. However, in these patients a very small pituitary microadenoma cannot be excluded.

Prolactin-secreting pituitary adenomas are associated with multiple endocrine neoplasia type I syndromes. An elevated prolactin level in a patient with a pituitary tumor does not necessarily mean the patient

Table 16–1. SOME PHARMACOLOGIC CAUSES OF ELEVATED SERUM PROLACTIN LEVELS

Type of Drug	Example(s)
Antiemetics	Metoclopramide
Antihypertensives	α-Methyldopa, reserpine
Calcium channel blockers	Verapamil
Histamine receptor blockers	Cimetidine (intravenous)
Hormones	TRH, estrogens
Opiates	Morphine
Psychotropic agents	Chlorpromazine, haloperidol, sulpiride, clorgyline

2

Table 16–2. SOME CAUSES OF ELEVATED PROLACTIN LEVELS

Physiologic	Pathologic
Exercise	Acromegaly
Newborn	Cirrhosis (alcoholic)
Nursing	"Empty sella syndromne"
Pregnancy	Hypothalamic disorders
Sleep	Hypothyroidism
Stress	Nelson's syndrome
	Neurogenic (ex. chest wall lesions)
	Pituitary stalk section
	Prolactin-secreting pituitary tumors
	Renal failure

has a prolactinoma; the patient may have a nonsecretory pituitary adenoma with suprasellar extension, thus suppressing prolactin inhibiting factor (PIF). In 20 to 40 per cent of patients with active acromegaly, prolactin secretion is increased; this may occur because of mixed tumors or interference with PIF activity.

Stimulation of prolactin secretion, with agents including thyrotropin releasing hormone (TRH) and chlorpromazine, as well as suppression, with L-dopa and bromocriptine, has been used to try to distinguish patients with prolactinomas from those with functional hyperprolactinemia. Considerable controversy exists regarding the diagnostic value of these dynamic tests in patients with hyperprolactinemia, but in general they are regarded as not clinically useful. Cowden et al. (1979) report that the combination of loss of the normal prolactin circadian rhythm and impaired response to TRH and metoclopramide stimulation is useful in diagnosing occult prolactin-producing microadenomas. However, the number of patients reported was small and contradictory results have been obtained by others (Flückiger, 1982).

Gonadal dysfunction frequently is associated with elevated serum prolactin levels in both men and women. In hyperprolactinemic males, symptoms including impotence, galactorrhea, and gynecomastia are late occurrences, whereas hypogonadism can occur at an earlier phase (Carter, 1978). Most men with gynecomastia do not have elevated prolactin levels, and the gynecomastia associated with prolactin-producing tumors, if present, is slight.

Hyperprolactinemia in women is often accompanied by galactorrhea or oligo/amenorrhea or both. Galactorrhea is more common in women than men with pituitary tumors; however, galactorrhea may fail to occur in some women even when serum levels of prolactin are very high. In a series of 51 patients with galactorrhea and oligo/amenorrhea, 84 per cent had prolactinemia, 68 per cent had radiographic abnormalities of the sella, and 39.2 per cent had surgically proven prolactinomas. Less than 10 per cent of women with diagnosed prolactinomas have neither amenorrhea nor galactorrhea (Molitch, 1980). Patients with prolactinomas also may present with hirsutism or infertility with regular periods. It is important to exclude pituitary tumor as the cause of hyperprolactinemia before induction of ovulation, because during pregnancy pituitary tumors can expand rapidly, causing complications necessitating neurosurgical intervention.

Although the mechanism is uncertain, galactorrhea may occur with use or discontinuation of oral contraceptives. A wide range of prolactin levels, 4.8 to 180 ng/ml (4.8 to 180 μg/L), has been reported in a series of patients in whom galactorrhea appeared to be related to taking oral contraceptives (Kleinberg, 1977). In some patients with primary hypothyroidism, marked hyperprolactinemia may occur. With thyroid hormone replacement, the prolactin levels return to the reference interval in the majority of patients. There is no clear evidence that prolactin is secreted ectopically (Molitch, 1981) (see p. 295).

Posterior Pituitary

ANTIDIURETIC HORMONE (ADH)

The posterior pituitary peptide antidiuretic hormone (ADH), which also is called vasopressin, plays a major physiologic role in control of water reabsorption by the distal convoluted and collecting tubules of the kidney. ADH increases water permeability, allowing hypotonic fluid in the distal tubules to equilibrate with hypertonic fluid in the interstitial space of the renal medulla. Water reabsorption occurs, leading to concentration of the urine.

Antidiuretic hormone together with neurophysin, which appears to serve as a binding protein for ADH during its transport and storage, is synthesized in the hypothalamus. Both then are transferred to the posterior pituitary where they are stored until release. Three major stimuli control release of ADH: (1) changes in osmolality of the blood, (2) alterations in blood volume, and (3) psychogenic stimuli. Under ordinary circumstances, osmotic factors probably predominate in regulating ADH secretion.

Plasma and urinary ADH can be measured by radioimmunoassay, but assays are not readily available because of technical reasons that include low basal levels for plasma ADH (1 to 5 pg/ml). Prompt handling and freezing of the specimen prior to analysis are important because ADH is unstable. Plasma and urine osmolality measurements are the principal laboratory methods used in diagnosis and management of patients with ADH abnormalities. ADH measurements, however, may improve the accuracy in delineating certain polyuric states.

Disorders of ADH can be divided into hypofunction (diabetes insipidus and other polyuric states) and hyperfunction, the so-called syndrome of inappropriate ADH (SIADH).

Diabetes Insipidus. Diabetes insipidus (DI) is characterized by polyuria and polydipsia resulting from inadequate ADH secretion or inability of the renal tubules to respond to the hormone. Causes of decreased ADH secretion (neurogenic or hypothalamic DI) include head trauma, pituitary lesions, and an inherited form of the disorder. Nephrogenic DI (renal resistance to ADH) may be inherited or be associated with such entities as hypercalcemia, hypokalemia, renal disease, and lithium therapy.

In order to diagnose the various polyuric states, water deprivation tests usually are used. Measurement of the antidiuretic response to infusion of hypertonic saline also has been used to establish the diagnosis of DI, but is more cumbersome and less reliable than dehydration tests (Moses, 1976).

Before dehydration tests are undertaken, conditions such as diabetes mellitus, hypercalcemia, and hypokalemia must be ruled out. Patients who excrete large volumes of urine must be closely observed during the test period for signs of vascular collapse. Dehydration tests should be discontinued if patients lose more than 3 to 5 per cent of body weight. An overnight dehydration test has been used; at the end of eight hours of water deprivation, healthy subjects generally have a urine osmolality >800 mOsm/kg (>800 mmol/kg) and a plasma osmolality which is within the usual reference interval (285 to 295 mOsm/kg [285 to 295 mmol/kg]). In patients with DI, the urine osmolality is usually less than that of plasma, and plasma osmolality is >300 mOsm/kg (>300 mmol/kg) (Edwards, 1977).

With water deprivation, osmolality of urine collected hourly usually reaches a plateau (two and preferably three consecutive hourly urine samples with about equal osmolalities). In healthy subjects approximately 16 to 18 hours are necessary to reach a plateau, but in patients with polyuria exceeding 5 L per day usually only four to eight hours are necessary. After a plateau in urine osmolality is reached, ADH is administered, and urine is collected 30 and 60 minutes later. Usually there is less than 5 per cent increase in urinary osmolality after administration of ADH, whereas in patients with severe neurogenic DI the increase is greater than 50 per cent.

The main diagnostic difficulty occurs in differentiating partial neurogenic DI from primary polydipsia. In addition, some patients with nephrogenic DI, with only partial resistance to ADH, may be difficult to differentiate from those with neurogenic DI. In these patients, plasma ADH levels may be helpful in diagnosis of the underlying disorder (Zerbe, 1981). Plasma ADH levels should be obtained under conditions of dehydration or saline infusion and carefully interpreted in the context of concurrent plasma and urinary osmolalities as well as basal urine flow (Stern, 1981).

Inappropriate ADH Secretion. The syndrome of inappropriate ADH (SIADH) is associated with a wide variety of disorders, including cerebral and pulmonary disorders, ectopic production, and as a side effect of treatment with certain drugs (Table 16–3). Characteristic features of SIADH are (1) hyponatremia, (2) continued renal excretion of sodium, (3) absence of clinical evidence of volume depletion, (4) urine less than maximally dilute, (5) normal renal function, and (6) normal adrenal function. Urinary sodium concentrations greater than 20 mEq/L (20 mmol/L) provide support of the diagnosis of SIADH.

Water loading studies often are useful in establishing the diagnosis of SIADH. An oral water load of 20 ml/kg body weight is given over a 15- to 20-minute period while the patient remains recumbent, and urine is collected hourly for five hours. Patients with SIADH usually excrete less than 40 per cent of the water load in five hours and fail to dilute urine maximally. Water loading is dangerous unless the patient has no symptoms of hyponatremia and has received appropriate treatment to raise serum sodium to a safe level, generally above 125 mEq/L (125 mmol/L) (Moses, 1976).

Table 16–3. POSTULATED CAUSES, SYNDROME OF INAPPROPRIATE ANTIDIURETIC HORMONE (SIADH)

Condition	Examples
Ectopic production by tumors	Oat cell carcinoma of bronchus, pancreatic carcinoma
Pulmonary disorders	Tuberculosis, pneumonia
Cerebral disorders	Trauma, neoplasms
Drugs	Chlorpropamide, vincristine
Miscellaneous	Adrenal insufficiency, acute intermittent porphyria

Plasma and urinary ADH levels reveal that the hormone is inadequately suppressed in most patients with SIADH. However, in over 80 per cent of the patients, ADH levels are comparable to those found in normally hydrated healthy adults and thus can be recognized as inappropriate only in relation to low plasma osmolalities (Zerbe, 1980).

OXYTOCIN

Oxytocin is responsible for milk ejection in humans and probably has a role in uterine contractions during parturition. Both oxytocin and ADH are thought to have effects on cognitive functions. Ectopic secretion of oxytocin by tumors such as oat cell carcinoma of the lung and adenocarcinoma of the pancreas has been reported (Edwards, 1977).

THE THYROID GLAND

Physiology

The follicles of the thyroid gland contain colloid, the main constituent of which is thyroglobulin. Thyroglobulin is the storage site of the thyroid hormones. Iodide is actively taken up by thyroid cells; iodination of tyrosine residues in thyroglobulin results in formation of monoiodotyrosine (MIT) and diiodotyrosine (DIT). When two DIT residues couple, thyroxine (T_4) is formed, whereas when one DIT residue couples with one MIT residue, triiodothyronine (T_3) is formed. Thyroxine and triiodothyronine are cleaved from thyroglobulin before secretion from the thyroid gland (Fig. 16–3). Under usual circumstances, T_4 secretion predominates.

The thyroid hormones circulate attached to plasma proteins. About 70 per cent of T_4 is bound to thyroxine binding globulin (TBG), 20 per cent to

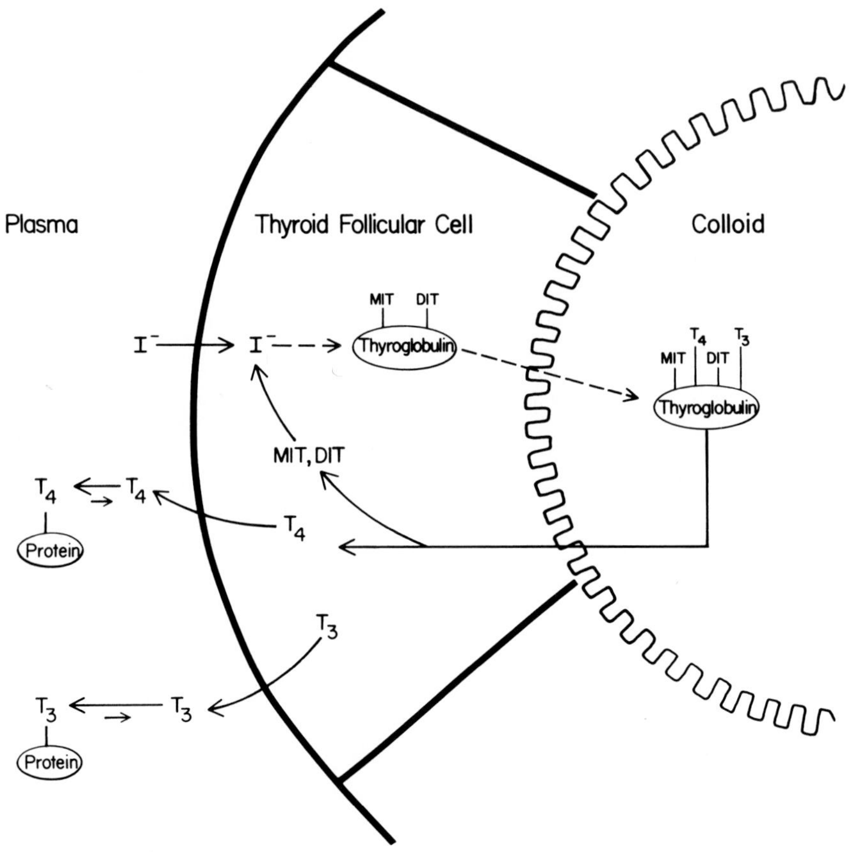

Figure 16–3. Schematic diagram of a thyroid cell outlining formation and release of T_4 and T_3.

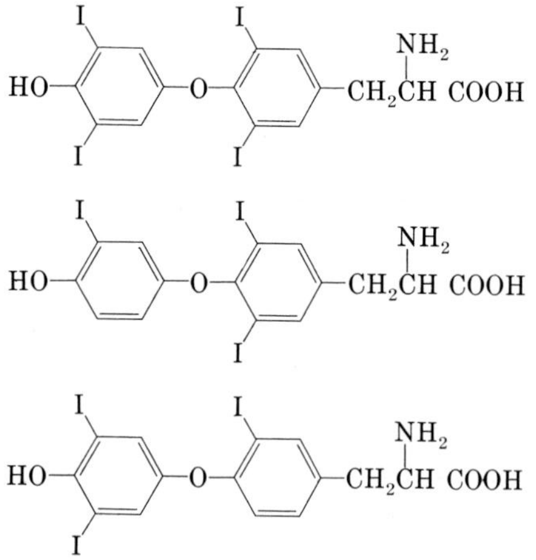

HO–(I, I)–O–(I, I)–$CH_2CH(NH_2)$ COOH — 3,5,3′,5′-Tetraiodothyronine (T_4 or Thyroxine)

HO–(I, I)–O–(I, I)–$CH_2CH(NH_2)$ COOH — 3,5,3′-Triiodothyronine (T_3)

HO–(I, I)–O–(I)–$CH_2CH(NH_2)$ COOH — 3,3′,5′-Triiodothyronine (Reverse T_3)

Figure 16–4. Structure of T_4, T_3, and reverse T_3 (rT_3).

thyroxine binding prealbumin (TBPA), and 10 per cent to albumin, whereas most T_3 is bound to TBG. A small percentage of the thyroid hormones remains unbound to protein, with about 0.03 per cent of T_4 and approximately 0.3 per cent of T_3 remaining free. It is the free fraction that presumably is the active hormonal form. The majority of T_3 arises by peripheral deiodination, with liver and kidney having an important role in this transformation. About 35 per cent of T_4 is monodeiodinated to T_3; 15 to 20 per cent is changed to tetraiodothyroacetic acid ("Tetrac") or conjugated and excreted in urine or bile. The remainder of T_4 is deiodinated to 3,3′,5′-triiodothyronine (reverse T_3 or rT_3) (Fig. 16–4). Further deiodination then occurs: 3,3′-diiodothyronine (T_2) is formed from both T_3 and rT_3.

Biosynthesis and release of thyroid hormones from thyroglobulin are controlled by thyrotropin (thyroid stimulating hormone [TSH]), a glycoprotein hormone synthesized in the anterior pituitary gland. TSH in turn is regulated by hypothalamus through thyrotropin releasing hormone (TRH) and possibly somatostatin.

Thyroid Disease

Thyroid disease may be classified on a functional basis into hyperthyroidism, hypothyroidism, and euthyroidism. When tissues are exposed to excessive quantities of thyroid hormones, hyperthyroidism results. Signs and symptoms include heat intolerance, tachycardia, weight loss, weakness, emotional lability, and tremor. The most common clinical syndrome associated with hyperthyroidism is Graves' disease, which most probably is due to circulating antibodies to the TSH receptor (see Thyroid Stimulating Immunoglobulins). The underlying defect appears to be a defect in suppressor T lymphocytes which allows production of an antibody to this receptor (Strakosch, 1982). Other disorders that lead to hyperthyroidism include toxic multinodular goiter, toxic adenoma, and, rarely, TSH-secreting pituitary tumors and thyroid carcinoma.

Hypothyroidism results from lack of thyroid hormone action on tissues; signs and symptoms include hoarseness, cold sensitivity, dry skin, and muscle weakness. Myxedema coma is an advanced stage of thyroid hormone deficiency characterized by progressive stupor, hypothermia, and hypoventilation. Cretinism is the term employed for functional failure of the thyroid in the newborn period. Failure of the thyroid itself to secrete an adequate amount of thyroid hormone is called primary hypothyroidism and most commonly is due to ablation of the gland. Secondary hypothyroidism results when TSH secretion is decreased due to a pituitary gland disorder. Hypothalamic lesions also may lead to hypothyroidism.

A variety of diseases of the thyroid usually are characterized by euthyroidism. These include goiter, benign tumors such as follicular adenomas, and malignant tumors.

In conjunction with clinical evaluation of the patient, laboratory determinations are valuable in diagnosing and following the course of patients with hyper- or hypothyroidism. The patient's serum thyroid hormone binding capacity, age, drug therapy, and intercurrent illness can all influence results of various laboratory determinations of thyroid function (see below). Wenzel (1981) has published a review on the pharmacologic interferences with the *in vitro* tests of thyroid function.

Clinical judgment together with the patient's history and findings on physical examination is very important in correctly interpreting thyroid function tests. In general, the most useful measurements to confirm or exclude hyperthyroidism are serum T_4, free T_4 (or free thyroxine index), and T_3; for hypothyroidism, they are serum T_4, free T_4 (or free thyroxine index), and TSH. In equivocal cases, a TRH test may be valuable in establishing the patient's thyroid functional status.

2

Laboratory Measurements

THYROXINE

Estimation of circulating levels of thyroid hormones became possible when, in the 1940's, the protein bound iodine (PBI) method was developed. Small amounts of non-hormonal iodine are present in serum of healthy subjects; under most clinical circumstances, 80 to 90 per cent of the PBI is derived from thyroxine. The PBI, which has a reference interval of about 4 to 8 μg/dl, is largely a reflection of the serum T_4 concentration, because serum T_3 expressed in terms of iodine is only about 0.10 μg/dl. The major problem with PBI determinations is spurious elevations due to inorganic or organic iodine contamination. In such circumstances, the PBI becomes invalid as an estimate of circulating thyroxine. Although the PBI has been abandoned for most purposes, it still may be useful in certain clinical situations such as thyroiditis.

Serum T_4 by competitive protein binding or displacement analysis, developed in the 1960's, is based on specific binding properties of TBG, thus allowing determination of T_4 independent of its iodine content. Serum T_4 by competitive protein binding, however, is subject to a number of limitations, including variability in the extraction step used to eliminate interference by endogenous thyroxine-binding proteins. Serum T_4 by radioimmunoassay (T_4 [RIA]), which also is not affected directly by iodine, employs an antibody to thyroxine. Antisera to T_4 can be produced readily and have satisfactory specificity for T_4, but commonly cross-react with D-thyroxine. To quantitate total levels, T_4 must be released from its endogenous binding proteins; this may be accomplished by use of blocking agents, such as 8-anilino-1-naphthalene sulfonic acid (ANS) or heat denaturation. Advantages of serum T_4 (RIA) include its sensitivity and elimination of the extraction step. The reference interval for serum T_4 (RIA) in adults is approximately 5.5 to 12.5 μg/dl (72 to 163 nmol/L) expressed as thyroxine.

Confusion has arisen concerning the reference in-

Table 16–4. SOME CAUSES OF INCREASED SERUM T_4

Cause	Comment
Increased serum binding proteins	See Table 16–5
Isolated hyperthyroxinemia	Some patients with nonthyroidal illness (↑ T_4 but T_3 not increased)
Familial dysalbuminemic hyperthyroxinemia	Increased affinity of albumin for T_4
Familial euthyroid thyroxine excess	Increased affinity of TBPA for T_4
Psychiatric disease	? Mechanism
Target organ resistance: (a) familial (Refetoff's), (b) acquired	Intracellular resistance to thyroid hormone
Other syndromes: (for example, decreased peripheral T_3 production)	(Miscellaneous: ? inhibition of T_4 transport into tissues or reduced T_4 to T_3 conversion)
Spurious	Circulating antibody to T_4
Drugs (excluding those which ↑ TBG): amiodarone,* amphetamine, heparin, heroin, iodine-containing radiocontrast media,* propranolol*	

*Indicates those drugs which block T_4 to T_3 conversion.
For further information see Wenzel (1981) and Cavalieri (1981).

terval for serum T_4. As procedures such as the Murphy-Pattee competitive protein binding assay for serum T_4 were introduced, results were expressed in terms of the T_4 molecule rather than T_4 iodine, as had been done previously. About 65 per cent of the weight of T_4 is contributed by iodine; the reference interval expressed as iodine thus is approximately two thirds as great as when expressed as T_4. Further confusion arose when determinations based on iodine were recalculated to correspond to the T_4 molecule by dividing by 0.65. To avoid any confusion in the interpretation of serum T_4 determinations, it is recommended that those T_4 values reported as iodine be clearly designated as such (i.e., T_4I).

Serum T_4 measurements are used in patients suspected of having hyperthyroidism or hypothyroidism. Most patients with hyperthyroidism have elevated serum T_4 and T_3 values. Hyperthyroidism has been reported in patients with serum T_4 values within the reference interval and elevated serum T_3, so-called "T_3 thyrotoxicosis." Some patients with hyperthyroidism may have an elevated serum T_4 but serum T_3 levels that are within the reference interval or low. This so-called "T_4 thyrotoxicosis" can occur in patients with iodine-induced thyrotoxicosis and in patients with nonthyroidal illness. Other patients with nonthyroidal illness have these findings for thyroid function tests, but are clinically euthyroid (see below). Increased serum T_4 levels can occur from a variety of other causes (Table 16–4). In these clinical situations, the patients generally are euthyroid but further laboratory determinations are necessary to confirm the patient's metabolic status. Serum T_4 levels are affected by changes in serum T_4 binding proteins. In situations in which drugs or other factors cause increased protein binding, there is an increased serum T_4 level; when decreased binding capacity occurs, there is a decreased serum T_4 (Table 16–5). These effects, however, are not reflected at the physiologic level, and in these situations the free or unbound concentration of T_4 correlates better with thyroid functional status than total levels of serum T_4. It is presumably the free fraction which is the active form of T_4 and the moiety which is homeostatically controlled.

In addition to patients with increased TBG, several types of familial euthyroid hyperthyroxinemia have

Table 16–5. SOME CAUSES OF ABNORMALITIES IN PROTEIN BINDING CAPACITY

	Increased Binding Capacity	Decreased Binding Capacity
TBG	Acute intermittent porphyria	Active acromegaly
	Estrogens	Androgens
	Genetic	Genetic
	Hepatic disease	Hepatic disease
	Hypothyroidism	Nephrotic syndrome
	Newborn infants	Phenytoin
	Oral contraceptives	Prednisone
	Perphenazine	Severe illness or surgical stress
	Pregnancy	Thyrotoxicosis
TBPA	Active acromegaly	Nephrotic syndrome
	Androgens	Salicylates
	Prednisone	Severe illness or surgical stress
		Thyrotoxicosis

been described, including peripheral resistance to thyroid hormone, albumin with increased affinity for T_4 (dysalbuminemic hyperthyroxinemia), or TBPA with increased affinity for T_4. Although serum T_4 is usually within the reference interval in patients with nonthyroidal illness, many patients have a decreased serum T_4 level and, less commonly, serum T_4 may be increased. More than 20 per cent of patients with nonthyroidal disease who are critically ill have low serum T_4 levels, but TSH levels are within the reference interval (Slag, 1981). Patients with acute hepatitis may have increased serum T_4 levels secondary to increases in TBG (Gardner, 1982). In hospitalized patients, isolated hyperthyroxinemia in euthyroid patients is about as common as true hyperthyroidism.

Evaluation of serum T_4 values in infants is complicated by TBG elevations in the neonatal period and a TSH surge occurring at the time of birth, both of which lead to increased levels that may remain elevated for a number of weeks (Larsen, 1975). At birth, healthy infants have been reported to have serum T_4 concentrations in the range of 7.8 to 16 μg/dl (101 to 208 nmol/L) (Burman, 1976). Serum T_4 concentrations are remarkably constant throughout the day in hypothyroid patients chronically treated with T_4 (Saberi, 1974). Patients treated with T_3 preparations have very low or undetectable serum T_4 levels.

TRIIODOTHYRONINE

Serum triiodothyronine (T_3) levels usually are measured by immunoassay using highly specific T_3 antisera with little T_4 cross-reactivity and a blocking agent, such as sodium salicylate, to eliminate endogenous T_3 protein binding. The reference interval for serum T_3 varies widely among laboratories, but is typically in the range of 60 to 160 ng/dl (0.92 to 2.46 nmol/L). Triiodothyronine is much less tightly bound to serum proteins than T_4; a relatively greater proportion of T_3 than T_4 exists in the free, diffusible state. It is estimated that approximately 0.3 per cent of T_3 is free (non-protein bound). Serum free T_3 has been measured by methods analogous to those used for serum free T_4.

Serum T_3 measurements may be helpful in confirming the diagnosis of hyperthyroidism, especially in patients with minimal elevations of serum T_4 or ambiguous clinical manifestations. In over 90 per cent of patients with hyperthyroidism, both serum T_3 and T_4 values are increased, with the increase in serum T_3 usually greater than the increase in serum T_4. Serum T_3 levels, however, may be within the reference interval or low in patients with hyperthyroidism and coexistent nonthyroidal illness (T_4 thyrotoxicosis).

Hyperthyroidism with elevated serum T_3 levels in the presence of T_4 and free T_4 values that are within their respective reference intervals is termed T_3 thyrotoxicosis. Patients with this syndrome are a heterogeneous group with no distinctive signs or symptoms of hyperthyroidism. Although most of the patients have Graves' disease, T_3 thyrotoxicosis may occur in patients with other causes of hyperthyroidism such as toxic nodular goiter or toxic adenoma. T_3 hyperthyroidism occurs in about 4 per cent of hyperthyroid patients, except in regions of iodine deficiency, where it is more common. Elevated serum T_3 levels and T_4 levels within the usual reference interval also may occur in patients with hyperthyroidism early in the course of treatment with antithyroid drugs or during relapse after treatment. In clinically euthyroid patients, there are a number of situations in which serum T_3 concentrations are elevated in the presence of increased TSH levels; for example, this is seen in some patients with endemic iodine deficiency in the presence of low serum T_4 concentrations. Elevated T_3 levels occur in patients with elevated TBG levels.

Generally serum T_3 levels are not useful in patients suspected of having hypothyroidism, because serum T_3 levels are within the reference interval in 20 to 30 per cent of hypothyroid patients. Serum T_3 levels are depressed only in patients who are severely hypothyroid, that is, those with serum T_4 levels less than about 2 μg/dl (26 nmol/L) (Bigos, 1978). In addition, low values for serum T_3 along with other changes in thyroid function tests may occur in patients with a wide variety of non-thyroidal illness (Table 16–6). In patients with acute illness such as myocardial infarction, the decrease in serum T_3 occurs rapidly, declining to about 50 per cent of the reference value within three or four days (Utiger, 1980). Serum T_3 concentrations also are low in cord blood, but increase rapidly during the first few hours of life, attaining values higher than those in healthy adults (Abuid, 1974). It has been reported that there is a progressive decrease in T_3 concentrations with advancing age.

Patients receiving thyroid preparations containing T_3, such as desiccated thyroid and synthetic T_3 and T_4 combinations, or those patients treated with T_3 alone will have uninterpretable serum T_3 results unless the time of the hormone administration is known. Administration of T_3 results in a rise in T_3 concentrations with peak serum values occurring between two and four hours. In patients treated with daily doses of T_4 alone, serum T_3 levels do not show a peak after ingestion of the medication. Stable levels of serum T_3 from the peripheral conversion of the T_4 are reached only after weeks of treatment.

REVERSE T_3

Reverse T_3 (rT_3), which is a major metabolite of thyroxine, is produced by 5-deiodination of T_4 and is thought to have little or no metabolic activity. The

Table 16–6. NON-THYROIDAL ILLNESS—TYPICAL FINDINGS FOR THYROID FUNCTION TESTS

Determination	Findings
T_4	Within reference interval*
FTI or free T_4	Method dependent
T_3	Decreased
rT_3	Increased
TSH	Within reference interval

*Some patients with non-thyroidal illness have increased values, and more than 20 per cent of critically ill patients with nonthyroidal illness have decreased serum T_4 levels.

reference interval for serum rT_3, which is measured by radioimmunoassay, is in the range of about 10 to 50 ng/dl (0.15 to 0.77 nmol/L). In general, the specificity of the radioimmunoassay for rT_3 is such that cross-reactivity with T_3 assays is not significant.

In many clinical situations, serum T_3 and serum rT_3 have been found to vary reciprocally. Serum rT_3 often is elevated in patients with nonthyroidal illness in whom serum T_3 concentrations are decreased; this mainly is due to decreased rT_3 degradation to 3,3′-diiodothyronine (Utiger, 1980). Serum rT_3 is decreased in hypothyroidism; thus the finding of an elevated rT_3 in a patient with non-thyroidal illness is indicative that the patient is not hypothyroid (Chopra, 1979). Serum rT_3 is increased in healthy newborns and in patients with hyperthyroidism. Drugs, including amiodarone and propranolol, cause increases in serum rT_3 levels (Cavalieri, 1981).

FREE THYROXINE

With changes in thyroxine binding proteins (Table 16–5), high or low levels of serum thyroxine occur that are not reflected in corresponding alterations in clinical state. In these situations, free (unbound) thyroxine is more closely correlated with the patient's clinical status. Free thyroxine may be quantitated using equilibrium dialysis or radioimmunoassay; the T_4 to TBG ratio (T_4/TBG) also has been employed to correct for changes in binding proteins. In addition, free thyroxine can be estimated using serum T_4 and T_3 uptake values to calculate the free thyroxine index (FTI). The T_3 uptake provides information about free binding sites on TBG; the "T_3" refers to the radioactive label used in the determination and not to the measurement of serum T_3 levels. The reference interval for the T_3 uptake varies not only with the individual laboratory but also with the test procedure employed. Values for T_3 uptake may be expressed in a number of ways, which has led to confusion in calculating the FTI. The Committee on Nomenclature of American Thyroid Association recommends that T_3 uptake be expressed as a ratio and considers this mandatory when calculating the FTI (Solomon, 1976).

Typically, in hyperthyroid patients serum free T_4 (or FTI) is elevated, whereas in hypothyroidism it is decreased. Increases or decreases in serum free T_4 without concomitant changes in metabolic state have been reported in patients treated with certain drugs. For example, prolonged administration of phenytoin results in a 15 to 30 per cent decrease in both serum T_4 and free T_4; carbamazepine has been reported to have similar effects (Cavalieri, 1981). Some drug effects may be related to the assay method employed; for example, heparin may cause an increase or decrease in free T_4, depending on the type of assay used (Boss, 1982).

In certain clinical circumstances, free T_4 results will differ, depending on the method employed. Theoretically any free T_4 method is appropriate for use in the presence of TBG abnormalities; however, at least in certain clinical circumstances, radioimmunoassays for free T_4 have been reported to correct for binding protein abnormalities better than free T_4 index or T_4/TBG ratio (Wellby, 1981). In addition, the FTI may be low in patients with non-thyroidal disease, whereas free T_4 values as determined by equilibrium dialysis are either within the reference interval or high (Chopra, 1979). An unidentified substance in the serum of critically ill individuals inhibits binding of thyroid hormones to ion exchange resins, leading to a normal T_3 resin uptake; when these values are used in conjunction with the patient's low serum T_4, a low result for FTI is obtained. In patients with non-thyroidal illness, values for free T_4 by radioimmunoassay are within the reference interval or low, depending on the particular assay used (Kaptein, 1981). Although a variety of changes in thyroid function tests occur in patients with non-thyroidal illness (Table 16–6), most clinicians agree that the majority of these patients are euthyroid.

Free T_4 measured by equilibrium dialysis and FTI do not yield comparable results in patients with familial dysalbuminemic hyperthyroxinemia. Patients with this disorder are clinically euthyroid, but they have high serum T_4 due to increased binding of thyroxine by a protein which migrates similarly to albumin on electrophoresis. These patients have free T_4 levels within the reference interval as measured by equilibrium dialysis, but they have elevated values for FTI (Ruiz, 1982). In patients with familial dysalbuminemic hyperthyroxinemia, many radioimmunoassay methods for free T_4 give high values as compared with those obtained by equilibrium dialysis (Rajatanavin, 1982).

THYROTROPIN (THYROID STIMULATING HORMONE [TSH])

Thyrotropin (thyroid stimulating hormone [TSH]) usually is measured by radioimmunoassay; the TSH antibody used may cross-react with the glycoprotein hormones, giving falsely elevated values for TSH in such clinical situations as pregnancy (elevated hCG levels) and postmenopausal states (elevated FSH, LH). A variety of techniques, however, have been used to overcome difficulties with cross-reactivity. Sensitivity of TSH assays as well as their reference intervals vary from laboratory to laboratory; with sensitive TSH assays, the mean value in healthy subjects is 1.5 μU/ml (1.5 mU/L) (Pekary, 1975). About 5 to 10 per cent of healthy individuals have undetectable TSH levels (that is, less than 0.5 mU/L) (Lorenz, 1979). TSH shows a circadian rhythm with maximum levels around midnight and minimum levels about noon. In addition, bursts of TSH occur, but levels remain within the reference interval (Lamberg, 1978).

In most patients with primary hypothyroidism, serum TSH levels are markedly elevated. In hypothyroidism secondary to hypothalamic or pituitary disease, basal TSH levels characteristically are not elevated. The major value of serum TSH levels is in diagnosis of primary thyroid failure and as a guide to adequacy of therapy in such patients. Although hyperthyroid patients generally have values below the detection limits of even the most sensitive assays, TSH levels usually are not helpful in these patients because healthy individuals may have undetectable TSH levels. A small number of patients have been reported with hyperthyroidism and an elevated TSH; most of these patients have a TSH-producing pituitary adenoma as the cause of TSH hypersecretion.

TSH values may be elevated in newborn infants during the first few days of life and may be increased in patients who are clinically euthyroid but have conditions such as lymphocytic thyroiditis, severe iodine deficiency, or post-treatment with radioactive iodine for hyperthyroidism.

TRH Tests. TSH values following administration of thyrotropin releasing hormone (TRH) are used as a test of thyroid function. The TRH test may be helpful in individuals who have equivocal signs and symptoms of thyroid dysfunction but whose routine tests of thyroid function do not clarify the diagnosis. A TRH test may be performed in a number of ways which vary as to dose and route of TRH administration, as well as parameter measured, but the intravenous test is most commonly used.

Usually a single bolus of TRH (200 to 500 μg) is administered intravenously after blood has been drawn for a baseline TSH. Another specimen for TSH is obtained 30 minutes (or at 20 and 60 minutes) after TRH administration. Within about five minutes of intravenous administration TRH causes a rise in serum TSH which reaches a peak in 20 to 30 minutes and returns to baseline in two to four hours (Fig. 16–5). A typical response to intravenous injection of 500 μg of TRH is a rise in serum TSH to a concentration of about 16 to 26 μU/ml (16 to 26 mU/L) in women (slightly lower in men) from a mean value of about 6 μU/ml (6 mU/L) (Sterling, 1977). In men, there is a decline in TSH response with age, and in healthy men over 60 years of age a TSH increase of only 2 to 3 μU/ml (2 to 3 mU/L) may be a normal response (Jackson, 1982). In euthyroid subjects, serum T_3 increases to about 70 per cent above baseline levels one to four hours after administration of TRH, and serum T_4 increases but to a lesser extent. TRH usually stimulates prolactin secretion and causes GH release in patients with a variety of conditions, including

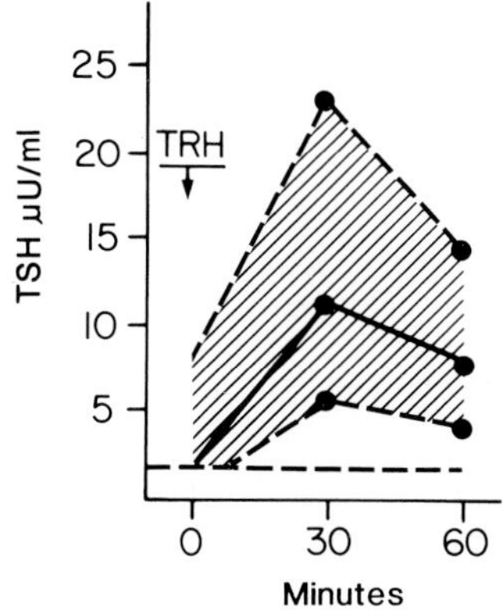

Figure 16–5. The TSH response to 500 μg of intravenous TRH in healthy subjects. (Modified from Jackson, I. M. D.: N. Engl. J. Med., *306*:145, 1982.)

acromegaly (see p. 302). Serum T_3, T_4, prolactin, and GH usually are not measured during a TRH test.

Sometimes, healthy subjects may fail to respond to TRH on one occasion, yet respond normally on subsequent occasions. The response of TSH to TRH usually is suppressed in hyperthyroid patients. Although presence of an impaired response to TRH commonly is due to hyperthyroidism, it may occur in a number of conditions, including patients with multinodular goiter or patients with Graves' disease who are euthyroid after therapy. The TRH test has been used as a reliable index of TSH suppression in patients treated with thyroxine for such disorders as thyroid carcinoma and thyroid nodules (Hoffman, 1977). A number of other disorders may give rise to a suppressed or blunted TSH response, including renal failure, Cushing's syndrome, and depression. The TSH response to TRH also is blunted by a number of drugs, including corticosteroids, L-dopa, and large doses of salicylate (Lamberg, 1978). There is a significant time interval following withdrawal of long-term thyroid hormone therapy before the normal response to TRH is restored (Burger, 1977).

Patients with primary hypothyroidism have a high basal serum TSH level and an exaggerated serum TSH response to TRH. In patients with hypothyroidism secondary to pituitary or hypothalamic disease, basal serum TSH levels usually are within the reference interval; however, some patients with hypothalamic hypothyroidism may have slightly elevated basal serum TSH values. Absent TSH response to TRH in a patient who does not have hyperthyroidism suggests a pituitary rather than hypothalamic lesion, but an intact response of TSH to TRH may be seen in patients with pituitary disease (Burger, 1977). The response to TRH in patients with hypothalamic disease is usually within normal limits or exaggerated, and it may be prolonged (Lamberg, 1978). The frequency with which aberrant responses to TRH occur reduces its usefulness in distinguishing between hypothalamic and pituitary disorders (Jackson, 1982).

THYROXINE BINDING GLOBULIN (TBG)

Thyroxine binding globulin (TBG), which can be measured by radioimmunoassay, is the principal serum carrier protein for T_4 and T_3; levels in healthy individuals are in the range of 12 to 30 μg/ml. The thyroxine binding capacity of TBG also can be determined using electrophoresis or an ion-exchange resin method. Table 16–5 summarizes some of the causes of binding capacity changes in TBG; factors such as estrogen influence the level of binding proteins, whereas certain drugs compete for binding sites leading to displacement of T_4.

Measurement of TBG may be helpful in patients who have serum T_3 and T_4 levels which do not agree with other laboratory parameters of thyroid function, or which are not compatible with clinical findings. TBG:T_4 ratios have been used for diagnosis of hyper- and hypothyroidism in patients with binding protein abnormalities. Some workers have reported that the T_4:TBG ratio better compensates for high TBG levels than measurements of free thyroxine, whereas others

2

disagree (see Free Thyroxine). In patients with dysalbuminemic hyperthyroxinemia, the electrophoretic method has been used to demonstrate the excess binding of thyroxine to the albumin fraction of their sera.

THYROGLOBULIN

Thyroglobulin, which usually is measured by radioimmunoassay, is present in serum of most healthy individuals with levels ranging up to about 30 to 40 ng/ml. It is elevated in a variety of diseases, including Graves' disease, thyroiditis, and nodular goiter.

Measurement of thyroglobulin is not recommended in preoperative identification of thyroid malignancy, but is useful in monitoring the course of disease or response to treatment. It is helpful in patients with well-differentiated carcinoma of the thyroid, but not in patients with undifferentiated or with medullary carcinoma of the thyroid. During treatment with exogenous thyroid hormone, Ashcraft (1981) found that no metastases occurred in thyroidectomized patients with undetectable thyroglobulin levels (<1 ng/ml), whereas detectable thyroglobulin levels (even as low as 4.2 ng/ml) occasionally were associated with metastases. After withdrawal of T_4 treatment in these patients, thyroglobulin levels <10 ng/ml were found to be indicative of successful therapy for thyroid carcinoma, whereas levels >10 ng/ml suggested presence of metastases, even in individuals with negative iodine-131 total body scans. Thyroglobulin levels also have been used to identify individuals with thyrotoxicosis factitia. These patients have undetectable thyroglobulin levels, in contrast to elevated levels found in patients with hyperthyroidism due to a wide variety of other causes (Mariotti, 1982).

THYROID STIMULATING IMMUNOGLOBULINS (TSIs)

Thyroid stimulating immunoglobulins (TSIs), TSH binding-inhibiting immunoglobulins (TBIs), thyroid stimulating antibody (TSAb), and Graves' immunoglobulins are the terms used for circulating immunoglobulins that appear to be antibodies directed against the TSH receptor sites or a closely related membrane antigen in the thyroid. These circulating immunoglobulins act as thyroid stimulators and play an important role in pathogenesis of the hyperthyroidism of Graves' disease. Long-acting thyroid stimulator (LATS) and LATS protector both are thyroid stimulating immunoglobulins which can be demonstrated by stimulation of radioactive turnover in mouse thyroid and competition with LATS for binding to human thyroid membranes, respectively. The terms LATS and LATS protector now usually are applied only for these bioassays. The bioassay procedures employing mouse thyroid tissue have a low detection rate for thyroid stimulating immunoglobulins; for example, only about 50 per cent of patients with Graves' disease can be demonstrated to have LATS in their serum. A variety of assays have been introduced which are better able to demonstrate thyroid stimulating immunoglobulin activity. Many of these assays use human thyroid tissue; however, Davies (1981) has reported that porcine thyroid may be substituted for human tissue.

Assays for TSIs are among the determinations which have been used to predict response of patients with Graves' disease to antithyroid therapy (Editorial, 1980). Most patients with persistently positive TSIs during the course of therapy relapse when therapy is stopped. For further information on TSIs and other thyroid antibodies, see Chapter 39.

Screening Programs for Detection of Neonatal Hypothyroidism

Neonatal hypothyroidism is estimated to occur in about one of 4000 live births. The goal of early detection and treatment of neonatal hypothyroidism is to eliminate severe mental retardation which is associated with thyroid hormone deficiency in early infancy. Various approaches to screening have been employed, including T_4 and TSH measurements using dry blood spots or cord serum. Screening has been performed using T_4 alone, TSH alone, and various combinations of laboratory determinations such as T_4 and TSH, or T_4 with testing of TSH on those specimens with the lowest T_4 levels.

Originally, screening programs relied on estimation of T_4 using either cord blood or dried blood spots collected for phenylketonuria tests. Measurement of only T_4 leads to a high false positive rate, necessitating recall of a large number of infants for retesting. Causes of false positive results include low T_4 levels, which occur in both premature infants and those with congenital deficiency of TBG. Screening with only T_4 may miss infants with compensated or partial thyroid insufficiency. About 15 per cent of infants with primary thyroid disorders have compensated hypothyroidism, that is, they have the serum T_4 within the reference interval and an elevated TSH. A marked increase in T_4 occurs during the first 24 hours of life due to TSH surge at delivery, but in hypothyroid infants T_4 levels do not increase during this period. Thus, testing the newborn infant two to five days after birth has been proposed in order to obtain a clearer separation of serum T_4 levels in euthyroid and hypothyroid infants.

Elevated TSH is the most sensitive test for the diagnosis of congenital hypothyroidism; however, false positive results are occasionally seen, for example, in premature or severely stressed infants. In addition, by screening with TSH alone, those infants with congenital hypothyroidism caused by hypothalamic or pituitary disease will be missed. Some investigators have recommended screening with T_4 levels complemented with TSH measurements on specimens with the lowest 3 to 5 per cent of T_4 results. This combination lowers the recall rate but is expensive and still some infants may be missed. In some screening programs, TBG determinations are performed on samples with low T_4 levels to identify infants with TBG deficiency. For details concerning thyroid hormone levels in term and newborn infants, see Fisher (1981) and Howanitz (1981).

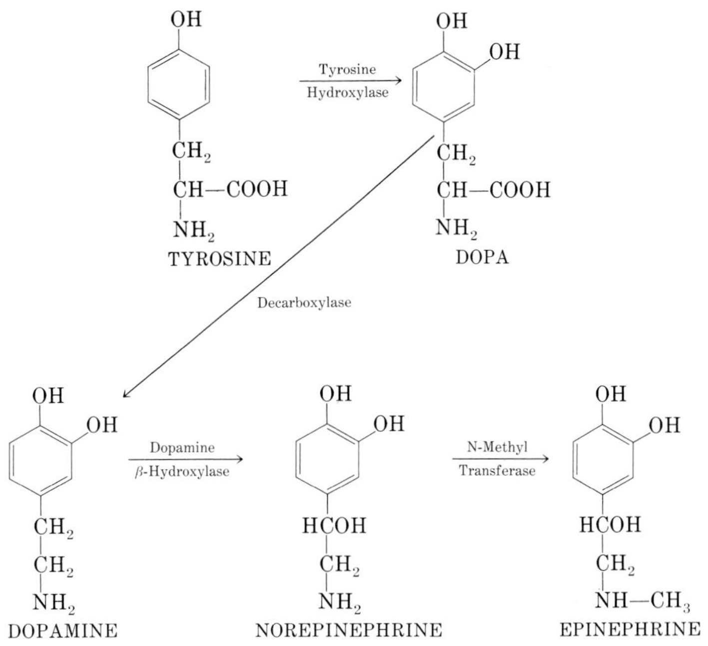

Figure 16–6. Pathway for the biosynthesis of the catecholamines.

ADRENAL MEDULLA

The hormones of the adrenal medulla and sympathetic nervous system are epinephrine (adrenaline), norepinephrine (noradrenaline), and dopamine. In the central nervous system, neurons produce dopamine and norepinephrine which act as neurotransmitters. The adrenal medulla produces both epinephrine and norepinephrine, whereas norepinephrine is the catecholamine liberated by postganglionic sympathetic nerves. The major catecholamine biosynthetic pathways are shown in Figure 16–6; the amino acid precursor of the catecholamines is tyrosine. Conversion of norepinephrine to epinephrine occurs mainly in the adrenal medulla.

When catecholamines are released from sympathetic tissue, other than the adrenal medulla, the primary means of physiologic inactivation is return of unaltered catecholamines into nerve endings by an active transport mechanism. Two enzymes are important for catecholamine metabolism: monoamine oxidase (MAO), which is responsible for oxidation deamination, and catechol-O-methyltransferase (COMT), which is responsible for O-methylation. Methylation may precede deamination or vice versa. COMT is principally responsible for inactivating circulating catecholamines, whereas MAO is thought to play a role in disposing of excess catecholamine stores. The major end product of metabolism of epinephrine and norepinephrine is vanillylmandelic acid (VMA) (Fig. 16–7). The other major urinary metabolites of the catecholamines are metanephrine and normetanephrine. In addition, small amounts of epinephrine and norepinephrine are excreted in the urine in the free form as well as conjugated and excreted as sulfates or glucuronides. Derivatives of dopamine give rise to the metabolites 3,4-dihydroxyphenylacetic acid (DOPAc) and 3-methoxy-4-hydroxyphenylacetic acid (homovanillic acid, HVA). The metabolite 3-methoxy-4-hydroxyphenylethylene glycol (MHPG), which appears in urine as well, is apparently derived mainly from the brain catecholamines (Kopin, 1977).

Catecholamine-Producing Tumors

PHEOCHROMOCYTOMA

Pheochromocytoma is a catecholamine-producing tumor which may arise at the same locations in the body where chromaffin tissue occurs. Although pheochromocytoma is rare, its diagnosis and successful treatment are of great importance, because it causes a potentially curable form of hypertension, which may be fatal if left untreated.

The most characteristic, but not the most common, manifestation of pheochromocytoma is paroxysmal hypertension. Attacks may occur several times a day or at infrequent intervals, and may last for only a minute or as long as a week. Signs and symptoms accompanying the attacks include headache, tachycardia, palpitations, sweating, nervousness, and tremor. Clinical manifestations of pheochromocytoma, however, are variable, and the patient may present simply with sustained hypertension. About two thirds of untreated pheochromocytoma patients show orthostatic hypotension, which appears to be related to a type of autonomic dysfunction simulating ganglionic blockade (Engelman, 1977).

Approximately 60 per cent of pheochromocytomas occur within the adrenal medulla, with greater than 90 per cent of the tumors lying between the dia-

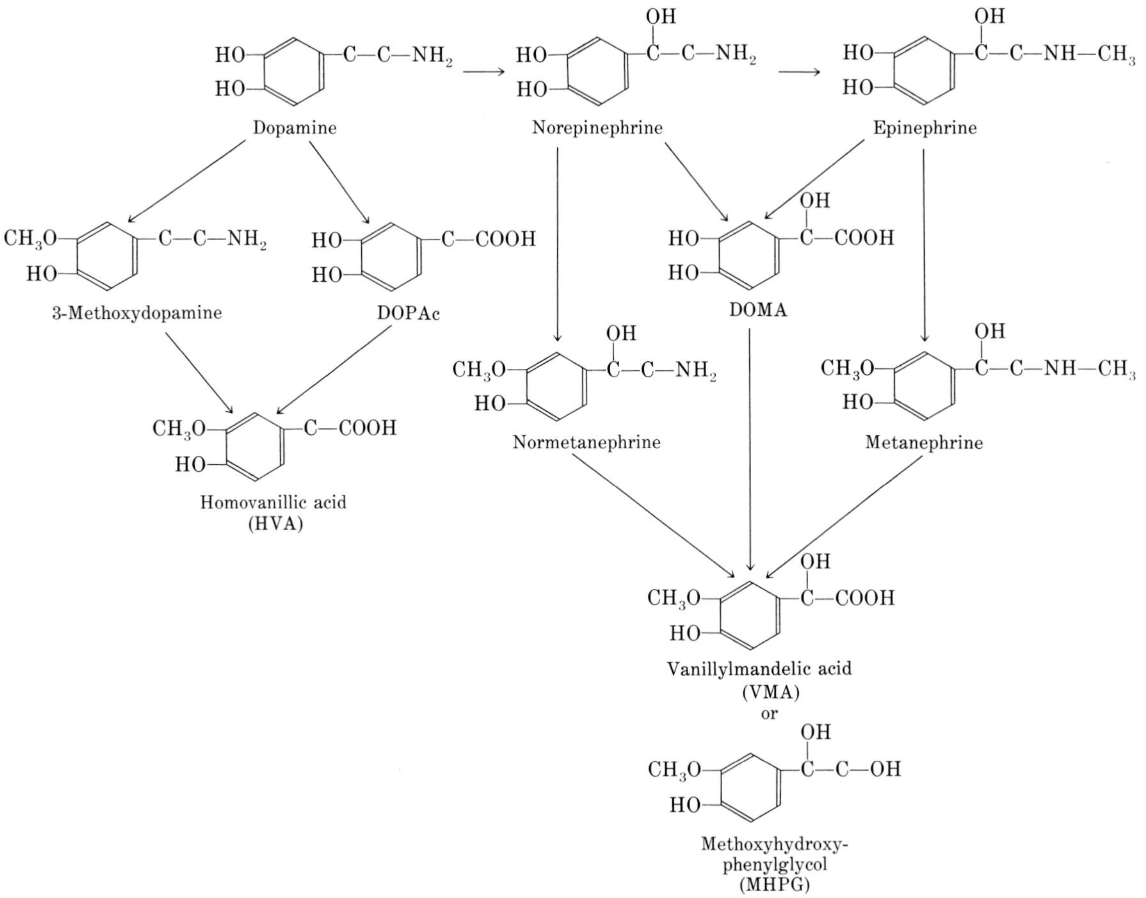

Dopamine → Norepinephrine → Epinephrine

3-Methoxydopamine

DOPAc

DOMA

Normetanephrine

Metanephrine

Homovanillic acid (HVA)

Vanillylmandelic acid (VMA) or Methoxyhydroxyphenylglycol (MHPG)

Figure 16–7. Catecholamine metabolism. DOPAc = 3,4-dihydroxyphenylacetic acid. DOMA = 3,4-dihydroxymandelic acid.

phragm and pelvic floor. In less than 10 per cent of patients, the tumors are malignant as evidenced by metastasis to non-chromaffin tissue. Multiple primary tumors occur in about 20 per cent of patients. Approximately 10 per cent of the patients with pheochromocytoma have associated inherited disorders of neuroectodermal origin, including von Recklinghausen's syndrome (neurofibromatosis), von Hippel–Lindau disease, and Sturge-Weber syndrome. In Sipple's syndrome (multiple endocrine neoplasia [MEN], type 2a), bilateral pheochromocytoma may be associated with medullary carcinoma of the thyroid and hyperparathyroidism; pheochromocytomas also occur in patients with MEN, type 2b. In addition to catecholamines, pheochromocytomas can produce a number of hormones, including vasoactive intestinal peptide (VIP), calcitonin, and ACTH.

NEUROBLASTOMA AND GANGLIONEUROMA

Neuroblastoma is the second most common solid tumor in children, usually occurring before age six. A frequent mode of presentation is that of a mass which may cause symptoms secondary to invasion or compression of surrounding tissues. With neuroblastoma, the course is primarily that of metastatic malignancy, and hypertension is often modest or absent. It has been suggested that neuroblastomas lack the ability to store catecholamines, and thus catecholamines are released from the tumor cells and inactivated soon after their formation. It has been postulated that this inactivation may account for the paucity of sympathetic nervous system symptoms in patients with neuroblastoma. Ganglioneuromas are well-differentiated tumors of the sympathetic nervous system which rarely metastasize. They occur in older children and young adults.

Laboratory Measurements

The diagnosis of pheochromocytoma can be confirmed by demonstrating increases in catecholamines or their metabolites, metanephrines, and VMA. These biochemical determinations usually are performed using an aliquot of a 24-hour urine specimen which has been collected in acid. Urinary metanephrine determinations have been recommended as the most accurate screening method for patients suspected of having pheochromocytoma; however, recently plasma catecholamines have been recommended (see below).

Most patients with pheochromocytoma will have elevated urinary VMA, metanephrines, and free catecholamines. In some patients with pheochromocytoma, however, one or more of these determinations may be within the reference interval. Patients with pheochromocytomas that secrete mainly epinephrine excrete relatively small amounts of VMA. Carefully timed urine collections over the period associated with the symptoms suggestive of pheochromocytoma or plasma catecholamines may be useful in confirming the diagnosis in patients without elevated levels between attacks. Excessive urinary excretion of MHPG commonly has been observed in association with pheochromocytoma; in some patients, excessive urinary excretion of dopamine and HVA may occur as well.

Elevated urinary VMA is the most common abnormal laboratory finding in patients with neuroblastoma. About 20 per cent of patients will not show an elevated urinary VMA, but may have elevated urinary MHPG, HVA, metanephrine, dopa, or dopamine. About 95 per cent of patients with neuroblastoma have an increase either in urinary VMA or HVA Knight, 1975). Other compounds such as cystathionine and beta-amino isobutyric acid can be produced as well (Seeger, 1982).

Since local tumor recurrences and distant metastases may secrete catecholamines, elevated levels of catecholamine metabolites have been used not only to assist in diagnosis of neuroblastoma but also to follow the patient during the course of tumor treatment. In following patients with neuroblastoma, it has been recommended that 24-hour urines be used for determinations of catecholamines and their metabolites. Excessive urinary excretion of catecholamines or their metabolites occasionally is detected in patients with ganglioneuroma or ganglioneuroblastomas. The most consistent abnormal finding in these patients is elevated urinary VMA (Moskowitz, 1977).

In interpreting the results of any determination of catecholamines or catecholamine metabolites, the possibility of false negative and positive results should be considered. Generally, interferences fall into three categories: (1) excess catecholamines not due to production by tumor, i.e., as occur with use of nasal sprays or increased endogenous catecholamine secretion due to stress; (2) drugs which influence catecholamine metabolism (i.e., α-methyldopa); and (3) substances which interfere with assays (i.e., fluorescent compounds). In some cases, discordant results occur, depending on the method used; for example, L-dopa has been reported to both increase and decrease VMA, depending on the assay employed. Degree of assay sensitivity, overlap of values with those of healthy individuals, and accuracy of urine collections add further difficulty in interpreting results.

METANEPHRINES

Metanephrines can be measured by a variety of techniques including the Pisano method, which involves extraction and subsequent oxidation to vanillin. The reference interval for total urinary metanephrines is about 0 to 2 mg/24 hours (0 to 11 μmol/day) for adults, with levels tending to be higher and more variable in children until about age 15. The major disadvantage of the total urinary metanephrine assay is variability of excretion during illness. Patients subjected to severe stress, including hemorrhagic shock, sepsis, and widespread metastatic disease, may have elevated values (Gitlow, 1970). Various drugs can lead to increases in urinary metanephrines; some of these increases apparently are method dependent.

VMA

The most widely used assay for VMA involves its oxidation to vanillin with subsequent determination of this compound by UV spectrophotometry (Pisano method) or by coupling it to indole to form a colored product. It has been reported that diet does not significantly change the determination of VMA excretion by the Pisano method (Rayfield, 1972). However, screening techniques such as those employing diazotized *p*-nitroaniline are interfered with by dietary phenolic acids, including those that occur in coffee, vanilla, and certain vegetables and fruits.

The adult reference interval for VMA is <6.8 mg/24 hours (34 μmol/day), with levels tending to be higher and more variable in children until about age 15. It has been recommended that VMA be expressed per mg urinary creatinine; healthy adult subjects have a mean excretion of 1.4 mg VMA (7.1 μmol) per mg creatinine (Gitlow, 1968). The effect of drugs on VMA results varies considerably with the technique employed for measurement; for example, L-dopa has been reported to both increase and decrease VMA excretion. In studies in which VMA was reported as decreased, the Pisano technique was employed, whereas in those studies in which increased values occurred, VMA was purified and quantitated by gas chromatography or thin layer chromatography (Feldman, 1974).

URINARY CATECHOLAMINES

Catecholamines are excreted into the urine in unconjugated (free) form as well as glucuronide or sulfate. Total catecholamines (unconjugated and conjugated forms) are measured by removing glucuronide and sulfate groups from the conjugated catecholamines prior to assay. There are several disadvantages in measuring total urinary catecholamines; for example, the wide reference interval may obscure the diagnosis of a minimally secreting tumor. In addition, dietary catecholamines, which occur in the conjugated form, may interfere with total catecholamine determinations. For these reasons, urinary free catecholamine measurements are preferred.

Urinary free catecholamines may be assayed by a modification of the trihydroxyindole fluorometric technique; the method also may be used to assay epinephrine and norepinephrine separately. Urinary free catecholamines usually represent approximately 2 to 4 per cent of the total catecholamines produced. The usual reference interval for urinary free catecholamines is up to about 100 μg/24 hours (590 nmol/day); the reference interval for epinephrine and norepinephrine is up to about 20 μg/24 hours (109 nmol/day) and 80 μg/24 hours (473 nmol/day), respectively. Stress may increase urinary free catecholamines, and catecholamine-containing medication can cause high urinary levels. Method dependent interferences occur with drugs; for example, α-methyldopa causes spuriously high values in urinary free norepinephrine when measured by the trihydroxyindole procedure, but low values are obtained with a HPLC technique, presumably because the pharmacologic action of the drug leads to a decrease in urinary norepinephrine (Mell, 1977).

In those patients with rare intermittent attacks, it may be useful to measure catecholamine output fractionated into norepinephrine and epinephrine in carefully timed urine collections from the period associated with the attack (Engelman, 1977). Measurement of urinary epinephrine has been reported as a sensitive and reliable screen for detection of pheochromocytoma in families with multiple endocrine neoplasia, type 2a (Hamilton, 1978).

PLASMA CATECHOLAMINES

The plasma catecholamines, norepinephrine and epinephrine, can be measured using radioenzymatic procedures. Measurements of plasma catecholamines have several advantages. Blood can be sampled immediately following development of symptoms in a patient suspected of having a pheochromocytoma. Plasma catecholamines also are of value in localization of extra-adrenal tumors not found by abdominal exploration and in the diagnosis of pheochromocytomas that secrete episodically (Juan, 1981). The disadvantages of plasma catecholamine determinations are as follows: (1) a specimen at one point in time may fail to reveal evidence of a tumor which is secreting intermittently, (2) there is a large overlap of values between individuals with and without pheochromocytomas, and (3) a wide variety of conditions may elevate plasma catecholamines.

For healthy subjects plasma norepinephrine values range up to about 500 ng/L (2.96 nmol/L) and plasma epinephrine levels up to about 100 ng/L (0.55 nmol/L). Since the catecholamine levels that occur in plasma are dependent on the sampling technique, certain precautions must be taken. Plasma catecholamine values increase with a change in posture from reclining to standing and increase even further with exertion. High plasma catecholamines can be found after emotional or physical stress, after shock, or in patients taking a variety of drugs. In addition, there is some evidence to indicate that there is a diurnal variation of catecholamine levels with highest levels of plasma epinephrine and norepinephrine observed in late morning and early afternoon, whereas lowest levels occur during the evening hours (Prinz, 1979). Plasma norepinephrine levels also increase with age (Kopin, 1977).

Plasma catecholamines are increased in most patients with pheochromocytomas, but diagnostic levels are difficult to establish because of variable levels found in individuals without the disorder (Engelman, 1977). Patients with essential hypertension have elevated plasma catecholamine levels.

Recently, measurement of resting, supine plasma catecholamines, using a radioenzymatic method, has been reported as more useful than VMA or metanephrines in the diagnosis of pheochromocytoma (Bravo, 1979). A plasma catecholamine value (norepinephrine and epinephrine) of 1000 ng/L (5.91 nmol/L) or less generally excluded the diagnosis of pheochromocytoma, whereas values between 1000 and 2000 ng/L (5.91 and 11.82 nmol/L) are considered equivocal (Bravo, 1979). Measurements of plasma catecholamines before and after administration of certain pharmacologic agents may increase specificity of the measurement. In patients with symptoms suggestive of pheochromocytoma and borderline increases in plasma or urinary catecholamine, clonidine suppression tests may prove useful (Bravo, 1981). Pentolinium also has been used in attempts to separate patients with pheochromocytomas from those without the disorder (Brown, 1981).

Measurement of plasma epinephrine appears to be superior to norepinephrine in the detection of small adrenal pheochromocytomas (Brown, 1981). In some patients with large pheochromocytomas, plasma catecholamine concentrations may be within the reference interval because the tumors secrete considerable amounts of pharmacologically inactive metabolites.

PLATELET CATECHOLAMINES

Plasma epinephrine and norepinephrine levels may be elevated in patients who do not have pheochromocytomas; a study by Zweifler (1982) indicates that platelet catecholamine measurements may be helpful in distinguishing these patients from those with pheochromocytomas. In their study patients without tumor had normal platelet catecholamine levels, whereas patients with pheochromocytomas had elevated levels.

ADRENAL CORTEX

The adrenal cortex is divided into three distinct zones; the zona fasciculata, the zona glomerulosa, and the zona reticularis, each of which produces a different group of steroid hormones. The zona fasciculata is responsible for the formation of glucocorticoids; the glomerulosa and reticularis are mainly responsible for mineralocorticoids and sex hormones, respectively. The general effects of the adrenocortical hormones are seen in Table 16–7, while the synthetic pathway for these groups of hormones is seen in Figure 16–8. For the sake of simplicity, many of the minor pathways involving interconversion of the various adrenal hormones are not shown.

The enzymes involved in the formation of steroids are of four general types: (1) hydroxylases, (2) dehydrogenases, (3) desmolases, and (4) isomerases. These enzymes are named depending on the carbon atom transformed. Since most of the inborn errors of metabolism affecting the adrenal cortex involve the

Table 16–7. EFFECTS OF ADRENOCORTICAL HORMONES

Representative Hormone	Biologic Effects
Cortisol (as a representative glucocorticoid)	Protein nitrogen catabolism increased Gluconeogenesis Increased blood glucose concentration Decreased glucose tolerance Increased liver glycogen Increased liver glycogenolysis Decreased peripheral uptake and utilization of glucose Decreased synthesis of acid sulfated mucopolysaccharides Fat synthesis and redistribution Cellular or tissue effects: Anti-inflammatory (retardation of inflammatory reactions) Dissolution of lymphoid tissue Lymphopenia Eosinopenia Increased erythropoiesis Alteration of cellular permeability, especially decreased membrane permeability to water Increased gastric (HCl and pepsin) secretion
Aldosterone (as a representative mineralocorticoid)	Electrolyte regulation Sodium (Na^+) retention Potassium (K^+) excretion Retention of water and expansion of extracellular fluid volume Increases in blood pressure
Androgens (as representative sex hormones)	Protein nitrogen anabolism Growth and maturation—osseous and muscular Body hair (pubic and axillary) Seborrhea

hydroxylases, clinically they constitute the most important group and are discussed under Congenital Adrenal Hyperplasia (p. 327). The end product of the glucocorticoid pathway is cortisol, which has a negative feedback on the pituitary, thereby regulating corticotropin (adrenocorticotropic hormone [ACTH] secretion. Although cortisol is the most important glucocorticoid, corticosterone (mineralocorticoid pathway) also has glucocorticoid activity.

The mineralocorticoid pathway involving most of the same enzymes is located in the zona glomerulosa, and it is responsible for the formation of aldosterone. The mineralocorticoid pathway differs from the glucocorticoids in that the 17-hydroxylase enzyme is absent and there is a final enzymatic step involving hydroxylation at position 18. Although the most important mineralocorticoid is aldosterone, desoxycorticosterone (DOC) and 11-desoxycortisol (glucocorticoid pathway) have mineralocorticoid activity and are responsible for hypertension in some of the congenital adrenal hyperplasia syndromes.

The zona reticularis is responsible for synthesis of sex hormones: steroids containing either 17 or 18 carbons and a hydroxyl at position 17. Those 17-carbon compounds that have an unsaturated A ring are estrogens, whereas the C-18 carbon steroids that do not have an unsaturated A ring are androgens. For discussion of sex hormones see pages 336 to 341.

Regulation of Cortisol Secretion

Secretion of cortisol by the adrenal cortex occurs in response to three identifiable influences: ACTH, a diurnal rhythm, and stress. ACTH and other corticotropin-related peptides compose a family of simple peptides that are synthesized in a single chain as part of a large prohormone with a mass of about 31,000 daltons (Fig. 16–9). This prohormone has been referred to by a variety of names, including pro-opiocortin, ACTH-endorphin precursor, and ACTH/β-LPH precursor. In the anterior pituitary pro-opiocortin is processed predominantly to ACTH and β-lipotropin (β-LPH). Within the ACTH sequence are α-MSH and the CLIP peptide; β-LPH is subject to proteolytic cleavage to yield γ-LPH and endorphin. The endorphin peptide appears to act on neurons in the brain and comprises a distinct peptidergic system related to pain perception. Although β-endorphin is secreted in parallel with ACTH, the significance of this is unknown.

ACTH consists of 39 amino acid residues, with the amino terminal end of 1 to 24 amino acid residues possessing full steroidogenic activity. Occasionally processing of pro-opiocortin is incomplete; other forms of ACTH thus occur, including "big" ACTH, a form with a mass of 20,000 daltons or greater, which has little biologic activity, "little" ACTH, and an "inter-

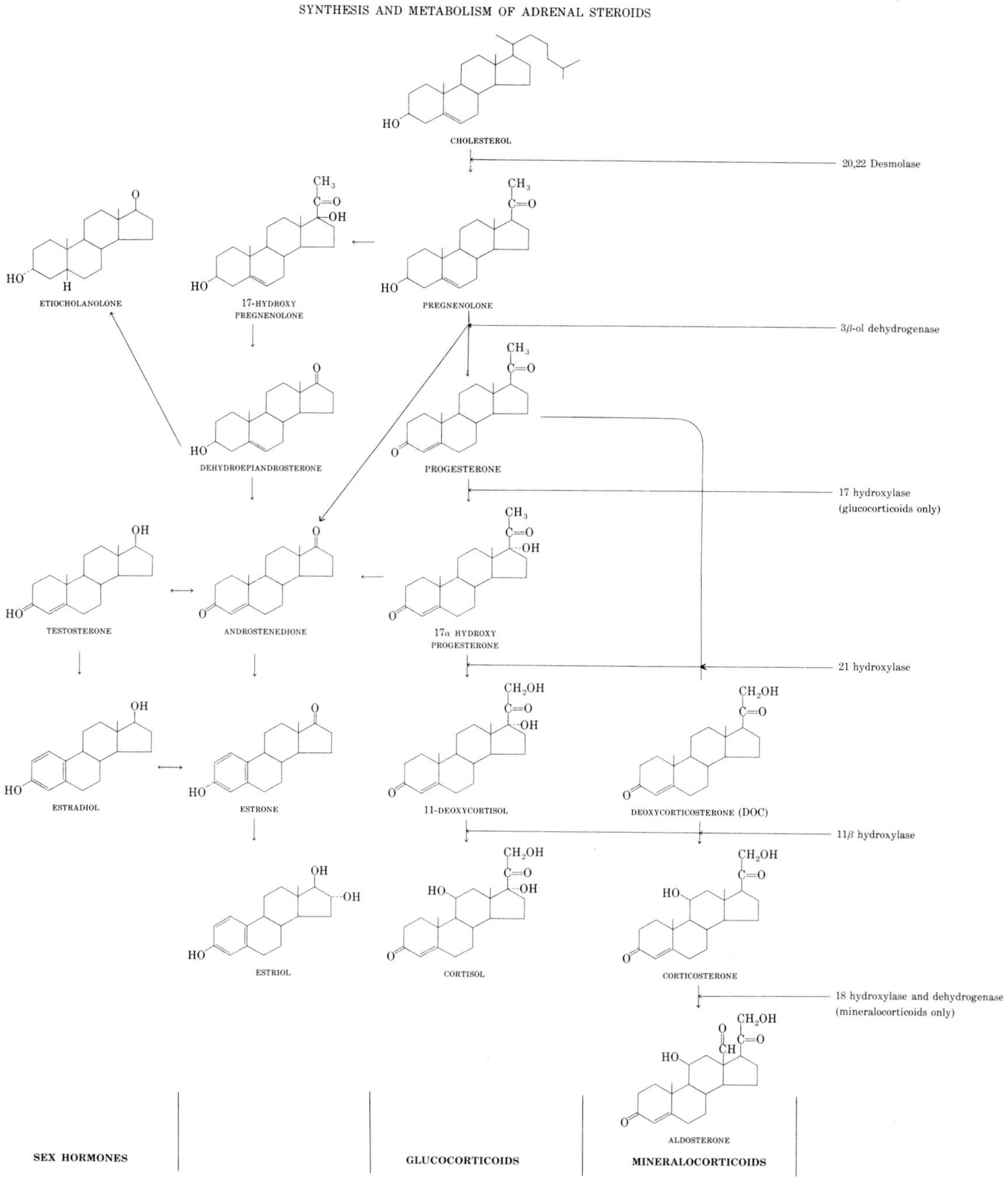

SYNTHESIS AND METABOLISM OF ADRENAL STEROIDS
CHOLESTEROL
20,22 Desmolase
ETIOCHOLANOLONE
17-HYDROXY PREGNENOLONE
PREGNENOLONE
3β-ol dehydrogenase
DEHYDROEPIANDROSTERONE
PROGESTERONE
17 hydroxylase (glucocorticoids only)
TESTOSTERONE
ANDROSTENEDIONE
17α HYDROXY PROGESTERONE
21 hydroxylase
ESTRADIOL
ESTRONE
11-DEOXYCORTISOL
DEOXYCORTICOSTERONE (DOC)
11β hydroxylase
ESTRIOL
CORTISOL
CORTICOSTERONE
18 hydroxylase and dehydrogenase (mineralocorticoids only)
ALDOSTERONE
SEX HORMONES
GLUCOCORTICOIDS
MINERALOCORTICOIDS

Figure 16–8. Simplified pathways of adrenocortical hormone synthesis and metabolism.

Pro-γ-MSH
ACTH
β-LPH
γ-MSH
α-MSH
CLIP
γ-LPH
Endorphin
β-MSH

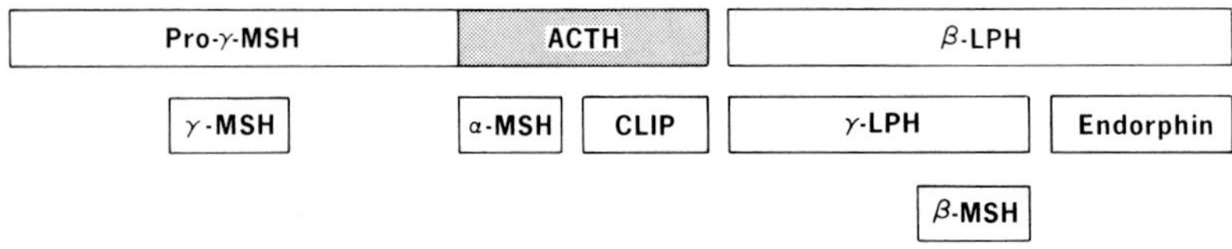

Figure 16–9. Structure of pro-opiocortin and peptides derived from it. MSH indicates melanocyte-stimulating hormone; β-LPH, lipotropin; CLIP, corticotropin-like intermediate lobe peptide.

mediate" variety. These forms may predominate under certain conditions, for example, ectopic production of "big" ACTH by primary or metastatic lung carcinoma and "little" ACTH or the "intermediate" form in some patients with Nelson's syndrome (Orth, 1977). Nelson's syndrome is the occurrence of a pituitary tumor and skin pigmentation following bilateral adrenalectomy for adrenal hyperplasia.

Although several substances which have ACTH releasing capacity are used clinically, corticotropin releasing hormone (CRH) has been identified and may have diagnostic utility in the future. Vasopressin (ADH), which is one of the peptides which releases ACTH, currently is used in studying patients with Cushing's syndrome (Table 16–8).

Cortisol, by direct action on the pituitary, inhibits ACTH directly and probably inhibits the release of CRH as well. When plasma cortisol becomes elevated, it suppresses release of ACTH (and probably CRH), thereby ultimately lowering cortisol. Conversely, when serum cortisol reaches a nadir, the pituitary responds with increased ACTH production, resulting in stimulation of cortisol formation. By this mechanism, ACTH and cortisol control the concentration of each other within a very narrow range, and a small change in one results in a concomitant change in the other. When the adrenal is unable to respond to ACTH because of damage or disease, cortisol levels are low and ACTH levels high. In those conditions in which the pituitary is destroyed, ACTH is not formed and cortisol levels tend to be low. If the pituitary-adrenal axis is interrupted by administration of large amounts of exogenous glucocorticoids, these glucocorticoids feed back on the hypothalamus and pituitary, suppressing ACTH production. If this suppression is continued, the pituitary may become permanently unable to respond or may respond to stress in an inadequate manner.

The second influence on plasma cortisol levels is the diurnal pattern, which in turn is due to a circadian pattern of ACTH release. There is a major increase in secretion occurring between 0400 and 0800 hours and then a decrease during the day. In subjects with a normal sleep-wake schedule, the lowest ACTH concentrations are found from 2100 hours to early morning (Fig. 16–10). Sudden changes in the sleep-wake patterns have little effect on the diurnal pattern, but permanent changes in daily sleeping habits will result in the gradual change in diurnal pattern. Superimposed on the circadian periodicity is an ultradian rhythm of five to ten secretory bursts. The level of serum cortisol gradually falls from its highest concentration (up to 25 μg/dl [690 nmol/L]) in the early morning to a 2100-hour level that is about one half of the 0800-hour level. The level of cortisol from 2100 hours to about 0400 hours is relatively constant. Although cortisol generally follows ACTH, it cannot be assumed that serum cortisol concentration exactly mirrors that of ACTH. Krieger (1977) points out that cortisol levels do not necessarily reflect ACTH levels because of episodic secretion of ACTH and the lag of cortisol secretion, differences in half-lives (the half-life of ACTH is exceedingly short, i.e., about five minutes; for cortisol, about 65 minutes), and an occasional ACTH surge which may not result in a rise of cortisol.

The third important influence on cortisol secretion is stress. Stimuli such as surgical trauma, pyrogens, hypoglycemia, and hemorrhage are capable of bringing about an acute increase in ACTH and cortisol secretion. Response to stress may be absent or decreased in magnitude in patients in whom large doses of steroids have been administered for some time. The initiation of any stressful response also is dependent on an intact nervous system. For example, trauma results in the acute release of ACTH and cortisol; however, in patients with spinal cord transections, the same trauma applied to an extremity will not elicit any ACTH or cortisol response. There is evidence that the stress-response of cortisol is mediated through excitatory and inhibitory inputs which become integrated at the level of the hypothalamus and modulate corticotropin releasing hormone.

Laboratory Measurements

ACTH

The first peptide hormone measured by radioimmunoassay was ACTH; however, widespread popularity and utility of ACTH measurements in clinical medicine have not occurred. Although ACTH by radioimmunoassay has diagnostic usefulness, technical and practical limitations, as well as expensiveness, have restricted its use. Of these, instability of ACTH in plasma probably has been the greatest limitation of its use. ACTH appears to be rapidly deactivated by proteolytic enzymes in plasma, and even addition of the usual proteolytic enzyme inhibitor (Trasylol) has little effect on its preservation. An inhibitor of SH-peptidases, N-ethylmaleimide (NEM), has been used in Great Britain; it has been reported to inhibit degradation of plasma ACTH for up to 72 hours (Jubiz, 1978). Although no current method completely arrests the destruction of ACTH, storing specimens at 4°C. greatly reduces enzymatic degradation of ACTH. Specimens should not be allowed contact with glass during collection, storage, and assay because ACTH can be adsorbed to glass.

Timing of specimen collection is important because of the circadian variation in ACTH. If plasma cannot be analyzed immediately, it should be stored at −20°C or colder. Other problems associated with the measurement of ACTH are incubation damage during assay, poor sensitivity, and poor precision of the assay at low concentrations. Plasma ACTH concentrations in healthy adult subjects are usually <50 pg/ml (11 pmol/L), whereas stressed individuals may have values up to about 500 pg/ml (110 pmol/L).

West (1977) has presented evidence that ACTH levels are useful in differentiating primary from secondary adrenal insufficiency. In primary adrenal insufficiency low cortisol concentrations are found; because of the negative feedback mechanism and an intact functioning pituitary, high ACTH levels are expected. In secondary adrenal insufficiency (pituitary

Table 16–8. SERUM CORTICOSTEROID RESPONSES TO DIAGNOSTIC MANEUVERS DESIGNED TO DEMONSTRATE NON-AUTONOMY OR AUTONOMY OF ADRENAL FUNCTION*

	Serum Cortisol Concentrations					
Condition	***Basal (0800-Hour)***	***Circadian Variation***	***0800 Hour Response to Dexamethasone (1 mg at 2300 hours)***	***Response to Aqueous Pitressin (10 Units IM)***	***Response to Cosyntropin***	**0800-Hour Plasma ACTH**
Normal	10–25 μg/dl (276–690 nmol/L)	A.M. greater than P.M.	<6 μg/dl (166 nmol/L)	≥15 μg/dl (414 nmol/L) increase above baseline	Doubling of baseline value	20–100 pg/ml (4.4–22 pmol/L)
Adrenal hyperplasia	Normal or increased	Absent	>6 μg/dl (166 nmol/L)	Increased	Increased	Normal or increased
Adrenal adenoma	Normal or increased	Absent	>6 μg/dl (166 nmol/L)	Absent	None or normal	Decreased
Adrenal carcinoma	Increased	Absent	>6 μg/dl (166 nmol/L)	Absent	None	Decreased
Pituitary tumor	Increased	Absent	>6 μg/dl (166 nmol/L)	Absent	None to slight	Markedly increased
Ectopic ACTH syndrome	Increased	Absent	>6 μg/dl (166 nmol/L)	Absent	Usually none	Markedly increased

*Modified from Krieger, 1976.

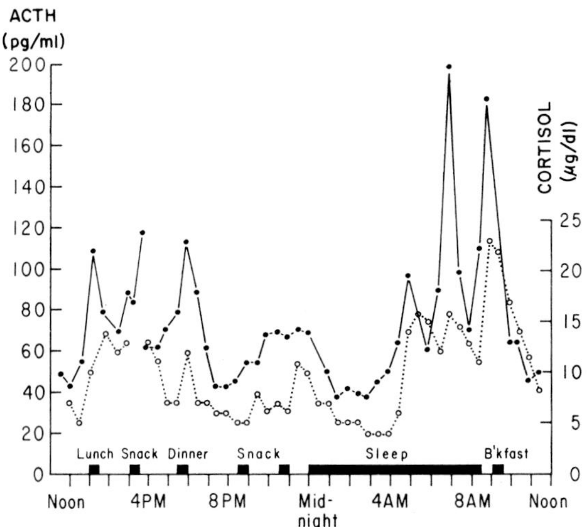

Figure 16–10. Circadian periodicity of plasma cortisol and plasma ACTH levels over a 24-hour period as determined by half-hourly sampling. ACTH and cortisol are lowest at about 4 A.M. and rise to highest level when awakening. Solid line indicates ACTH; dotted line indicates cortisol. (Modified from Krieger, D. T., et al.: J. Clin. Endocrinol. Metabol., *32*:266, 1971.)

insufficiency), normal to non-detectable ACTH levels are the rule. Although in the past stimulatory tests such as cosyntropin and ACTH infusions have been used, a single ACTH level will distinguish between primary and secondary adrenal insufficiency. In the primary disorder, ACTH levels usually are >200 pg/ml (44 pmol/L), whereas in pituitary insufficiency, ACTH concentrations are usually <50 pg/ml (11 pmol/L). ACTH levels best discriminate between healthy individuals and those with adrenal insufficiency when specimens for ACTH are collected between 0800 and 1000 hours.

ACTH measurements may be of great value in establishing the differential diagnosis of patients with Cushing's syndrome (see below). Those patients with ectopic ACTH secreting tumors characteristically have an elevated plasma ACTH (usually >200 pg/ml [44 pmol/L]) and an elevated serum cortisol. Occasionally neoplasms may be occult, and because of diagnostic difficulties ACTH measurements using blood specimens obtained by selective catheterization of the venous system may be useful in localization of the lesion.

In patients with increased levels of circulating glucocorticoids due to adrenal adenomas or carcinomas, ACTH secretion is inhibited; hence circulating ACTH levels are low or undetectable. In patients with pituitary induced adrenal hyperplasia, plasma ACTH may be at or above the upper reference interval at 0900 hours, but fail to show the expected fall near midnight. It should be emphasized that ACTH best discriminates between patients with suspected Cushing's syndrome and healthy individuals when the blood specimens are obtained between 2100 and 2400 hours.

Another use of ACTH assays is determination of adequacy of cortisol replacement in congenital adrenal hyperplasia syndromes. When replacement therapy is optimal, ACTH values are similar to those seen in a reference population.

SERUM CORTISOL MEASUREMENTS

About 90 per cent of the circulating cortisol is bound to serum protein, whereas the remainder is unbound or free. It is estimated that 10 to 20 per cent is loosely attached to albumin, and the remainder is bound to the glycoprotein transcortin (cortisol binding globulin), an alpha-1-globulin. It is believed that only free cortisol is active, and that the protein bound fraction is metabolically inert, probably serving as a reservoir of free cortisol. Protein binding also may protect cortisol from deactivation by the liver or filtration by the kidney.

2

One of the earliest and simplest methods used to determine serum cortisol was a fluorometric assay. Cortisol simply was extracted from serum with dichloromethane, and, after the addition of an ethanol–sulfuric acid mixture, fluorescence was measured. Corticosterone is the most important interfering substance, contributing about 4 µg/dl (110 nmol/L) with this method, but other adrenal steroids, such as dihydroepiandrosterone, testosterone, and 11-desoxycortisol, contribute about 2 µg/dl (55 nmol/L). Spironolactone, tetracycline, and birth control pills containing estrogen lead to spuriously high cortisol levels by this method.

Cortisol can be determined by competitive protein binding (CPB) (Murphy, 1967), but this technique lacks specificity. Competitive protein binding (CPB) assays make use of the naturally occurring cortisol binding protein, transcortin, from various species. Specificity of the method depends on binding characteristics of transcortin; cortisone and 11-desoxycortisol, for example, compete equally well with some binders. Progesterone, which is present in increased amounts in pregnancy, also competes with cortisol for transcortin. The CPB method has a major advantage in that 11-deoxycortisol can be extracted with carbon tetrachloride and subsequently measured in the assay. The competitive protein binding technique gives results which are about 25 per cent lower than those as measured in the Porter-Silber reaction (see below) and 25 to 50 per cent lower than those obtained with the fluorometric procedure.

A more specific method for cortisol estimation is immunoassay. Other advantages of immunoassay include small specimen volume and rapid turnaround time. When radioimmunoassay is used, cortisol is released from its endogenous binding proteins by blocking agents such as 8-anilino-1-naphthalene sulfonic acid (ANS). Some of the antibodies that are used show a large degree of cross-reactivity with steroids such as 11-deoxycortisol, desoxycorticosterone, and synthetic steroids such as dexamethasone. Although cross-reactivity does not pose a problem with baseline testing, in stimulatory and suppressive maneuvers such as metyrapone or dexamethasone suppression, this can lead to spuriously high values. With deterioration of renal function, various steroids and their glucuronides accumulate in blood. Because of their structure, conjugates may cross-react with some cortisol antibodies, producing an interference which can be of the same magnitude as the actual cortisol concentration (Nolan, 1981). In congenital adrenal hyperplasia, high concentrations of cortisol precursors occur in serum because of an enzyme defect. Since these precursors cross-react with assay antibodies, spurious elevations of cortisol concentrations are found; the degree of interference varies with the assay used and cannot be predicted easily. The major disadvantage of cortisol assays continues to be lack of specificity; however, the specificity of the immunoassay is better than that of either the fluorometric or the CPB method.

HPLC assays appear to offer the ultimate in specificity. Simultaneous determinations of other steroids such as occur in congenital adrenal hyperplasia or following metyrapone testing are major advantages of this technique.

Reference values for serum cortisol are in the range of 5 to 25 μg/dl (138 to 690 nmol/L) at 0800 to 1000 hours and by 2000 hours are about 2 to 12 μg/dl (55 to 331 nmol/L). There also is less clinical reliance on absolute cortisol values than on most other laboratory determinations because the diurnal and circadian variation is large. Serum assays are most useful in evaluating responses to adrenal stimulation or suppression tests (see below).

ESTIMATION OF GLUCOCORTICOIDS IN URINE

17-Hydroxycorticosteroids (17-OHCS). One of the first procedures for estimation of glucocorticoids in urine was the method described by Porter (1950). When phenylhydrazine and sulfuric acid are added to urine, those steroids which contain 21 carbons and have a characteristic dihydroxyacetone side chain produce a color with a peak absorption at 410 nm (Porter-Silber chromogens). Methodologic improvements, such as extractions with various organic solvents, purification of urine extracts by chromatography, or the correction for a high blank (Allen corrections), have increased the accuracy of this measurement. Since most glucocorticoids are excreted in urine as conjugates, hydrolysis with a glucuronidase is performed prior to measurement. The glucocorticoids which are measured include 11-deoxycortisol, cortisol, and cortisone (a metabolite of cortisol). Other metabolites of cortisol and cortisone, in which the A ring of the steroid is saturated (tetrahydro derivatives), also are included in this measurement. Although this method has been used to estimate 17-hydroxycorticosteroids (17-OHCS) in urine, in certain pathologic states it does not measure all the 17-OHCS that are excreted. For example, compounds such as pregnanetriol (a metabolite of 17-OH progesterone) and certain 20-OH compounds may be extremely elevated, but are not measured by this technique. Many drugs, including reserpine, chlorpromazine, meprobamate, and spironolactone, interfere with measurement of Porter-Silber chromagens. Elevated 17-OHCS have been reported in patients treated with carbamazepine; this occurs because of formation of a metabolite that reacts with assay reagents (Arisue, 1976). In newborns or neonates with congenital adrenal hyperplasia, this measurement is relatively unreliable; this is due to interference by steroids and their metabolites that usually do not occur in the urine, but that are excreted in large amounts by these patients.

Reference intervals for urine measurements are 5 to 15 mg/24 hours (13.8 to 41.4 μmoles/day) for adult males and 5 to 13 mg/24 hours (13.8 to 36.9 μmoles/day) for adult females. Values for 17-OHCS may be low or within the reference interval in pituitary insufficiency and adrenal insufficiency, whereas in adrenocortical hyperfunction, they may be increased. More definitive diagnostic information is obtained by using these determinations in conjunction with dexamethasone suppression (see below). The Porter-Silber method usually is not used for glucocorticoid estimations in serum because of its lack of specificity, requirements for large serum volumes, and the need for a prior extraction step.

Urinary Free Cortisol. Only 1 per cent of the total adrenal secretion appears in urine as cortisol, but it is this fraction which provides a valuable aid in diagnosis of adrenal disease. In the kidney, glomerular filtration of free cortisol is followed by passive tubular reabsorption without a demonstrable reabsorption maximum.

At serum cortisol levels of about 20 to 25 μg/dl (552 to 690 nmol/L) (the upper 0800-hour reference value), the binding capacity of transcortin is exceeded; this leads to a very rapid and disproportionate increase in the unbound fraction compared to the total serum cortisol. For example, a doubling of the cortisol from 20 to 40 μg/dl (552 to 1104 nmol/L) results in at least a five-fold increase in the unbound cortisol in serum. At these levels, free cortisol clearance by the kidneys is directly proportional to the unbound serum cortisol concentration and leads to a steep rise in cortisol clearance. Thus, when urinary free cortisol excretion rather than serum cortisol is used, it is easier to discriminate between patients with adrenal hyperfunction and a reference population.

Urinary free cortisol levels are unaffected by alterations of hepatic metabolism of cortisol. Although total cortisol production and urinary 17-OHCS may be increased, the serum cortisol and urinary free cortisol remain within the reference interval. In pregnancy and estrogen therapy, as a result of the increased serum concentration of transcortin, serum cortisol is increased. This increase is not reflected by an elevation of cortisol metabolites in urine, but urinary free cortisol may be increased. Since the renal clearance of cortisol is dependent on normal kidney function, it is not surprising that patients with renal disease may have low values. Conditions in which spuriously elevated values occur include starvation, application of topical steroids, and perhaps hydration in the form of water loading.

The techniques used for urinary free cortisol measurement include competitive protein binding (CPB) and radioimmunoassay. The specificity of the competitive protein technique is limited by specificity of transcortin used as the binding protein. Similarly, the measurement of urinary free cortisol using radioimmunoassay is dependent upon the antibody used. Reference intervals for urinary free cortisol by RIA or by CPB are 20 to 90 μg/24 hours (352 to 2530 nmol/day). For increased specificity, radioimmunoassay is performed following chromatography or extraction of urine specimens. Without chromatography to purify the urinary steroids, CPB and radioimmunoassay methods overestimate the amount of cortisol present. For example, when antigentically interfering compounds are removed by HPLC, followed by radioimmunological quantification, a reference interval of 10 to 42 mg/24 hours (28 to 117 nmol/day) is obtained (Schöneshöfer, 1980). Because of nonspecificity of these methods, Murphy (1981) concludes that there is no practical method available for urinary free cortisol; however, the measurement in urine can afford an accurate reflection of adrenocortical function provided that there are no gross metabolic abnormalities present and that the reference interval is established carefully for each method used.

A low urinary free cortisol is suggestive of adrenal hypofunction, such as occurs in Addison's disease, but overlap of values with the reference interval is large. The greatest use of urinary free cortisol determinations is for states of adrenal hyperfunction, such as Cushing's syndrome, in which patients have urinary free cortisol values greater than the reference interval.

Hypercortisolism: Cushing's Syndrome

Cushing's syndrome is a clinical and metabolic entity characterized by adrenocortical hyperfunction; it is associated with excessive production of glucocorticoids, or glucocorticoids and androgens. Patients with severe forms of the syndrome are easily recognizable when the disorder is florid. In less severely afflicted individuals, the vague signs and symptoms which occur may not easily be recognized as caused by hypercortisolism. The lesion responsible for excessive adrenal cortical secretion may reside in the adrenal, pituitary, or hypothalamus, or the increased glucocorticoids may be caused by a tumor (ectopic ACTH production). Since the therapeutic modality and prognosis differ depending on location of the cause, it is important that a specific diagnosis be reached. Adrenal Cushing's (adenoma or carcinoma) accounts for less than 20 per cent of the cases, whereas pituitary Cushing's (with or without pituitary tumor) accounts for about 70 per cent, and ectopic production of ACTH by tumors is the cause in slightly less than 15 per cent of cases. Although many patients with ectopic ACTH–producing tumors have elevated ACTH and glucocorticoids, the patient's demise may occur before clinical signs of the syndrome become evident because of rapid growth of these tumors.

Hallmarks of Cushing's syndrome are (1) excessive and persistent production of cortisol measured as elevated serum cortisol, urinary free cortisol, or 17-OHCS; (2) loss of usual circadian rhythm of ACTH and cortisol; and (3) loss of suppression of cortisol production by administration of the synthetic glucocorticoid dexamethasone. Of the findings that suggest Cushing's syndrome, the most common are obesity, hypertension, and hirsutism.

Serum cortisol concentrations >30 μg/dl (830 nmol/L) at 0800 hours and >15 μg/dl (415 nmol/L) at 1600 hours provide useful guidelines for selecting patients for further diagnostic evaluation (Gold, 1979). Based on review of the literature, Zadik (1980) concludes that use of only a baseline urinary 17-OHCS measurement would result in a 11 per cent false negative and a 24 per cent false positive rate for the diagnosis of Cushing's syndrome. Therefore, before diagnosis of Cushing's syndrome can be substantiated, suppressive or stimulatory procedures are necessary. Suppressive testing usually involves oral administration of dexamethasone, a steroid that has at least 25 times more glucocorticoid potency than cortisol. It is administered in small quantities to suppress ACTH, but provokes little interference with glucocorticoid measurements by any of the commonly used methods. Suppressive testing procedures are divided into two groups: those in which only a serum cortisol is obtained following a single dose of dexamethasone, and those in which serum cortisol and a 24-hour urine are collected prior to and following various doses of dexamethasone (see below). Because of difficulty in collection of a complete 24-hour urine and in administration of dexamethasone on a regularly scheduled basis, those tests which involve urine collection are usually reserved for hospitalized patients. The response of serum and urine determination to dexamethasone suppression is shown in Tables 16–8 and 16–9.

A simple screening test is the overnight dexamethasone suppression test. One mg of dexamethasone is ingested by the patient at 2300 hours, and at 0800 hours a serum cortisol level is obtained. In healthy individuals a serum cortisol < 5 μg/dl (138 nmol/L) is observed, but in patients with Cushing's syndrome there rarely is suppression to <10 μg/dl (276 nmol/L). Psychiatric disease, alcoholism, and stress can cause non-suppressibility in patients without Cushing's syndrome. Since phenytoin causes increased metabolism of dexamethasone, a cortisol level at 0800 hours may be outside the reference interval in a healthy individual taking this drug. Drugs such as estrogens cause increased transcortin (serum transport protein for cortisol); this results in a higher than usual cortisol level at 0800 hours. Although the overnight dexamethasone suppression test is relatively easy to perform, 1 per cent of healthy individuals, 13 per cent of obese, and about 25 per cent of hospitalized or chronically ill patients give false positive results. The incidence of false negative results is less than 2 per cent (Crapo, 1979).

"Low dose" dexamethasone is used to differentiate healthy individuals from those with Cushing's syndrome. At least two baseline 24-hour urine collections are obtained for 17-OHCS (reference interval 3 to 11 mg/24 hours [8.3 to 30.4 μmoles/day]). For two days, 0.5 mg of dexamethasone is given orally every six hours and the response of urinary 17-OHCS (or

Table 16–9. URINARY CORTICOSTEROID RESPONSES TO DIAGNOSTIC MANEUVERS DESIGNED TO DEMONSTRATE NON-AUTONOMY OR AUTONOMY OF ADRENAL FUNCTION*

	Urinary 17-Hydroxycorticosteroids				**Urinary 17-Ketosteroids**
		Suppression with Dexamethasone			
Condition	***Basal***	***2 mg***	***8 mg***	***ACTH Stimulaion***	***Basal***
Normal	3–10 mg/24 hr (8.3–27.6 μmol/day)	<3 mg/24 hr (8.3 μmol/day)	<50% initial value	Two- to three-fold baseline increase	Female: 5–15 mg/24 hr (13.8–41.4 μmol/day) Male: 8–20 mg/24 hr (22.1–55.2 μmol/day)
Adrenal hyperplasia	Increased	Not suppressed	<50% initial value, occasional "paradoxical" response	Hyper-responsive	Normal or increased
Adrenal adenoma	Increased	Not suppressed	Not suppressed	None or normal response	Decreased or normal
Adrenal carcinoma	Markedly increased	Not suppressed	Not suppressed (rare exceptions)	No response (rare exceptions)	Markedly increased
Pituitary tumor	Markedly increased	Not suppressed	Not suppressed	No to slight response	Increased
Ectopic ACTH syndrome	Markedly increased	Not suppressed	Usually not suppressed	Usually no response	Increased

*Modified from Krieger, 1976.

urinary free cortisol) measured. On the second day of dexamethasone, a reference group population suppresses urinary 17-OHCS to <3 mg/24 hours (8.3 μmoles/dl) (urinary free cortisol <20 μg [552 nmol] per 24 hours), whereas patients with Cushing's syndrome fail to suppress to this level. A number of patients with Cushing's syndrome, however, have been described whose response is within the reference interval.

"High dose" dexamethasone suppression test (2 mg given orally every six hours for two days) is used to differentiate patients with adrenal hyperplasia from others with hypercortisolism. A reference population and those with adrenal hyperplasia show urinary 17-OHCS levels which are less than 50 per cent of the initial value (urinary free cortisol is less than 20 per cent of baseline value). However, occasionally a "paradoxical" response of non-suppression occurs in patients with adrenal hyperplasia. Most patients with adrenal adenomas, carcinomas, pituitary tumors, or ectopic ACTH syndromes will not show suppression. Patients with adrenal carcinoma usually have 17-ketosteroids >20 mg/24 hours (69.3 μmol/day) and signs of virilization in contrast to those patients with adrenal adenomas. Pituitary and ectopic tumors can be identified by appropriate radiographic procedures. Although urinary 17-OHCS may be elevated in obesity, urinary free cortisol and serum cortisol are within the reference interval and suppress in response to overnight dexamethasone (see below). This response and usual circadian variation of plasma cortisol make it possible to differentiate obese individuals from patients with Cushing's syndrome.

Ashcraft (1982) has found serum cortisol and urine measurements during dexamethasone suppression tests of equal accuracy in making the diagnosis of Cushing's syndrome. During the second day of the suppression test, non-suppressed cortisol values at 1600 hours are considered >5 μg/dl (138 nmol/L) with the low dose and >10 μg/dl (276 nmol/L) with the high dose dexamethasone. In those patients whose serum cortisol values were non-suppressible, a baseline dehydroepiandrosterone value at 0800 hours of <0.4 μg/ml (1.4 μmol/L) indicated an adrenal adenoma. The laboratory findings in patients with hypercortisolism are summarized in Tables 16–8 and 16–9.

Vasopressin, which releases ACTH probably because its structure is similar to that of CRH, has been of value in the diagnosis of adrenal and pituitary disease. A normal response following the administration of 10 units of vasopressin intramuscularly is a doubling of ACTH levels and an increase in serum cortisol of 15 μg/dl (414 nmol/L) over baseline values. In patients with adrenal carcinoma, adenoma, or pituitary tumor, high circulating levels of cortisol from the autonomously secreting lesion suppress the intact hypothalamic-pituitary-adrenal axis; therefore, a response to vasopressin does not occur. Another aid to localization of the lesion responsible for Cushing's syndrome is the cortisol response to stimulatory testing. Those patients whose Cushing's syndrome is due to adrenal hyperplasia have an increased response of serum cortisol to vasopressin and cosyntropin, a synthetic ACTH analogue. Patients with other forms of the syndrome have little or no response to these stimuli (Table 16–8).

Two modifications of the dexamethasone suppression test result in improved accuracy in the diagnosis of Cushing's syndrome. When the dose of dexamethasone is administered in terms of body weight (i.e., 5 μg/kg/6 hours for the low dose) and urinary excretion of 17-OHCS is expressed in mg/g creatinine, better discrimination between Cushing's syndrome and a reference population is observed (Streeten, 1976).

Plasma ACTH levels are suppressed in patients with adrenal tumors, are elevated (>200 pg/ml [44 pmol/L]) in most patients with ectopic ACTH production, and are within the reference interval despite hypercortisolism in about one half of patients with pituitary Cushing's syndrome (see p. 319).

2

Dexamethasone Suppression Test in Depression

Excessive activity of the hypothalamic-pituitary-adrenal axis similar to that seen in pituitary Cushing's syndrome has been demonstrated in some patients with primary affective disorders. Recently, the suppression of this axis by dexamethasone has been used as a biochemical indicator of melancholia (endogenous depression).

Although many protocols are employed, the one developed by Carroll (1981) is used most widely. The patient ingests 1 mg of dexamethasone at 2300 hours, and serum cortisol measurements are obtained at 1600 and 2300 hours the following day. Approximately 50 per cent of patients with melancholia demonstrate abnormal early escape from suppression (i.e., serum cortisol levels ≥5.0 μd/dl [138 nmol/L] by CPB at 1600 or 2300 hours). If, for practical reasons, sampling is limited to only the 1600-hour specimen, then there is about a 20 per cent loss in procedure sensitivity. Many drugs interfere with interpretation of this test, including alpha-methyldopa, meprobamate, spironolactone, reserpine, and cyproheptadine. Other drugs interfere by accelerating the metabolism of dexamethasone; these include phenobarbital and phenytoin. Illnesses such as cardiac failure, uncontrolled diabetes mellitus, pulmonary disease, fever, and anorexia also interfere with test results. A few patients with psychiatric disease, such as dementia, schizophrenia, character disorders, and manic depression, have been reported to have non-suppression. The use of this test has been reviewed recently (Gwirtsman, 1982).

Hypocortisolism: Addison's Disease and Pituitary Insufficiency

Primary adrenocortical insufficiency (Addison's disease) usually occurs from an autoimmune process (Chap. 39) or from tuberculosis and other granulomatous diseases, or is iatrogenic. When hypocortisolism results from a pituitary lesion, it is termed secondary adrenal insufficiency. Patients with primary adrenal insufficiency have deficiencies of both glucocorticoids and mineralocorticoids in contrast to individuals with secondary adrenal insufficiency, who have only a glucocorticoid deficiency. Since mineralocorticoid deficient patients have a higher plasma renin activity than those with only a glucocorticoid deficiency, renin measurements may be of some value in diagnosis. Although most patients with hypocortisolism have low serum cortisol values, a serum cortisol level within the reference interval obtained when a patient is stressed does not exclude the diagnosis. Rather, it may support this diagnosis because a suboptimal cortisol level may have risen into the reference interval in response to a very high ACTH level induced by stress.

Both primary and secondary adrenal insufficiency can be demonstrated by failure of the adrenal to respond to various stimulatory procedures. The most convenient procedure for studying patients suspected of having hypocortisolism is the injection of a commercially available ACTH analogue, cosyntropin. This peptide is the biologically active amino terminal end of the ACTH molecule and contains amino acids 1–24. Serum specimens for cortisol determinations are drawn as a baseline as well as 30 and 60 minutes following cosyntropin injection. A normal response is a doubling of serum cortisol, but more stringent criteria, such as a baseline of 5 μg/dl (138 nmol/L), with an increase of at least 7 μg/dl (195 nmol/L) at 30 minutes, and 11 μg/dl (304 nmol/L) at 60 minutes, or the 30-minute level exceeding 18 μg/dl (50.7 nmol/L) (Dluhy, 1976), have been applied. Recent evidence indicates that the cosyntropin test accurately reflects integrated hypothalamic, pituitary, and adrenal function.

The diagnosis of pituitary and/or adrenal insufficiency can be made by the insulin tolerance test (ITT); this is described in the section on the pituitary (p. 301). When compared to the cosyntropin procedure, the insulin tolerance test is equally accurate for diagnosis of hypocortisolism (Lindholm, 1978).

Other stimulatory testing involves infusion of ACTH or its analogues for two to five days, with the response of 17-hydroxysteroids (or urinary free cortisol) measured. Patients with either primary or secondary adrenal insufficiency may present with low serum cortisol and not respond to cosyntropin. To substantiate diagnosis of primary or secondary adrenal insufficiency indisputably, prolonged exposure of the adrenal to ACTH is essential. An intravenous infusion of ACTH or its analogues for two days, as proposed by Rose (1970), appears to be the most advantageous in this regard. With this procedure, a normal response is an elevation of urinary 17-hydroxycorticoids three to five times the baseline value, whereas patients with primary adrenal insufficiency have extremely low baseline values that fail to exhibit this degree of stimulation. Patients with secondary adrenocortical insufficiency (hypopituitarism) or patients receiving suppressive doses of steroids for a protracted period of time usually have an inadequate or absent response in urinary 17-hydroxycorticosteroids on the first day of testing and a slight rise on the second day to about 10 mg/24 hours (27.6 μmol/day). It should be noted that the ACTH infusion test can be performed on patients presenting with signs of acute adrenal insufficiency, a medical emergency. If this diagnosis is suspected, a baseline cortisol and ACTH should be obtained and a stimulation test performed over two days, with dexamethasone used to provide the patient with an immediate source of glucocorticoids.

Metyrapone has been used to assess pituitary ACTH reserve. For the performance of this procedure, metyrapone is ingested in divided doses over two days and urinary excretion of glucocorticoids is measured. Since metyrapone is an inhibitor of the 11-hydroxylase enzyme, it blocks the formation of cortisol from 11-deoxycortisol causing cortisol levels to fall and resulting in increased ACTH secretion. If metyrapone is continued for a period of time, the blockade is overcome and glucocorticoids rise. Patients with reduced pituitary reserve, such as those with pituitary tumors, are unable to increase ACTH secretion to maintain cortisol levels. In patients with decreased pituitary reserve, acute adrenal insufficiency may be precipitated if glucocorticoids are not provided during testing. In contrast to the rapid evaluation of pituitary reserve provided by insulin tolerance or cosyntropin testing, this provocative test requires three days to perform. Because of this and the severe side effects which may occur, the metyrapone test has fallen into disfavor. Metyrapone, however, has been used as a single dose in an overnight procedure. A dose of 30 mg/kg body weight is given at bedtime; plasma 11-desoxycortisol and ACTH are measured the following morning. In a reference population, 11-desoxycortisol increases to greater than 7 μg/dl (193 nmol/L) and ACTH to greater than 100 pg/ml (22 pmol/L), whereas in those patients with secondary adrenal insufficiency response is poor. A recent study in a small group of patients indicates that the overnight metyrapone test is superior to the high-dose dexamethasone test in the differential diagnosis of Cushing's syndrome (Sindler, 1983).

The majority of severely ill patients lying in intensive care units have elevated serum cortisol values. Those patients whose 0800-hour serum cortisol values were below 13 μg/dl (350 nmol/L) were found to have an extremely bad prognosis. When these patients were given cosyntropin at 0800 hours, an increase in serum cortisol to less than 7 μ/dl (200 nmol/L) suggested adrenocortical insufficiency (McKee, 1983).

As the use of steroids for the treatment of many malignant and immunologic disorders increases, iatrogenic adrenal insufficiency is becoming more common. The use of glucocorticoids for treatment of systemic diseases results in adrenal suppression of variable duration after withdrawal of steroids. The degree of adrenal suppression is dependent upon the specific glucocorticoid dose, as well as the duration, frequency, and route of administration. A protocol has been developed by Byyny (1976) for tapering steroids and testing for adrenal insufficiency; at four-week intervals the morning exogenous glucocorticoid is omitted and the 0800-hour serum cortisol measured. If it is above

10 μg/dl (276 nmol/L), routine supplementation of steroids can be ended. Since the adrenal cortex lags behind the pituitary in recovery from steroid suppression, recovery can be certain to be complete when an 0800-hour cosyntropin infusion results in an appropriate serum cortisol increase.

Congenital Enzyme Disorders of the Adrenal

At least eight different metabolic defects in the synthesis of cortisol and aldosterone have been described; each is recognized by a deficiency of a specific adrenal enzyme. These enzymatic deficiencies all are inherited as autosomal recessive traits with variable degrees of penetrance. Depending on severity and location of the enzymatic defect in the metabolic pathway, deficiency of glucocorticoids, mineralocorticoids, or sex hormones occurs, resulting in shock, salt wasting, or anomalous sexual development. Other findings such as hypertension, which occurs from accumulation of mineralocorticoids, or virilization, which occurs from shunting of metabolism toward the sex hormone pathway, are clinically useful in differentiating the various enzyme deficiencies. Due to decreased cortisol production, the usual feedback mechanism is interrupted in these syndromes and there is a compensatory increase in ACTH, the magnitude of which may be sufficient to prevent adrenal insufficiency. This compensatory increase in ACTH leads to hypersecretion of steroid precursors and is responsible for development of hyperplastic adrenal glands. Important features of the most common of these syndromes are summarized in Table 16–10.

The 21-hydroxylase (21-OH) is the most common deficiency, accounting for about 95 per cent of all cases of congenital enzyme defects of the adrenal. The 21-OH deficiency involves the enzyme that converts 17-α-hydroxyprogesterone (17-OHP) to 11-deoxycortisol (Fig. 16–8). If the deficiency is mild, as commonly seen, patients will not have markedly increased aldosterone secretion and will not lose sodium. Some affected patients who have mild defects may not develop symptoms until early childhood, adolescence, or late adulthood, whereas in others the defect may even be cryptic. The severe form of the 21-OH deficiency results in almost complete salt wasting and adrenal collapse in the first few weeks of life. Females have ambiguous genitalia, whereas males may have a normal appearance. The diagnosis can be confirmed by demonstrating elevated levels of 17-ketosteroids >5 mg/24 hours (7.2 μmol/day) or pregnanetriol in the urine, or elevated levels of 17-OHP in serum. In healthy individuals, serum 17-OHP levels are <1.0 ng/ml (3.2 mmol/L), but in affected individuals they may be >10 ng/ml (32 mmol/L). Amniotic fluid 17-OHP levels >2.7 ng/ml (8.6 mmol/L) have been used to distinguish an affected from a non-affected fetus. A neonatal screening program has been developed to identify 21-OH deficiencies in newborns by measuring 17-OHP in using blood spots collected on filter paper (Pang, 1982). By measuring plasma 17-OHP following synthetic ACTH (cosyntropin) infusion, heterozygotes can be identified from individuals who are homozygotic for 21-OH deficiency. Close genetic linkage between congenital adrenal hyperplasia attributed to 21-OH deficiency and HLA-B locus makes possible use of HLA typing to identify sibs of patients who are heterozygous carriers of 21-OH deficiency and sibs who are homozygous. By typing families with some affected individuals, this technique can be used to distinguish family members who are carriers from those who are unaffected. Successful HLA typing for 21-OH deficiency using amniotic cells has been reported. In treated patients with 21-OH deficiency, when 17-OHP levels are <2.0 ng/ml (6.4 mmol/L) and ACTH levels are <100 pg/ml (22 pmol/L), normal adrenal secretion of the sex hormones occurs. However, the most sensitive indicator of the adequacy of adrenal suppression is measurement of β-4-androstenedione.

The 11-hydroxylase (11-OH) deficiency is the second most common defect and frequently results in hypertension due to increased deoxycorticosterone (DOC) and 11-deoxycortisol levels. Virilization is the most prominent feature of this syndrome, but the clinical expression is variable; severe and mild forms of the defect have been identified. Two types of defects are recognized, one in which conversion of both 11-deoxycortisol and DOC is impaired and the other in which only the conversion of 11-deoxycortisol is impaired. The findings of elevated serum 11-deoxycortisol concentrations and elevated urinary 17-hydroxycorticosteroids and 17-ketosteroids are diagnostic. A large series of patients with the 11-OH deficiency recently has been reported (Zachmann, 1983).

The 3-beta-hydroxysteroid-dehydrogenase deficiency is an extremely rare defect involving conversion of the delta-5-steroids to delta-4-steroids. In the neonatal period these patients have adrenal insufficiency which invariably results in death if untreated. Males are born without complete masculinization and females with clitoromegaly. The diagnosis is confirmed by the finding of elevated urinary 17-ketosteroids and dehydroepiandrosterone values.

The 17-hydroxylase enzyme (17-OH) is not required for mineralocorticoid synthesis; hence, patients with this defect have increased mineralocorticoid with decreased glucocorticoid and sex steroid secretion. Because these patients cannot convert pregnenolone or progesterone to 17-hydroxy derivatives, affected individuals present with hypertension, exceedingly high DOC levels, and hypokalemic alkalosis. Lack of sex hormone synthesis results in the absence of secondary sexual characteristics in the female and incomplete masculinization in the male neonate. Decreased urinary 17-ketosteroids and 17-hydroxycorticosteroids as well as decreased serum androgens in these subjects confirm the diagnosis.

Cholesterol desmolase (20,22) deficiency also is rare and involves the inability to convert cholesterol to pregnenolone in the adrenal and testes. Consequently, affected males present with complete lack of masculinization, salt wasting, and marked adrenal insufficiency. The absence of adrenal steroids in urine and plasma suggests this diagnosis.

Table 16–10. CONGENITAL ENZYME DISORDERS OF THE ADRENAL: CLINICAL AND BIOCHEMICAL FEATURES

Enzyme Deficiency	Virilization	Adrenocortical Insufficiency (Salt Losing)	Hypertension	Anomalous Sexual Development	Laboratory Findings
21-Hydroxylase	Present	Present in <1/3	Absent	Female virilized	Greatly increased urinary pregnanetriol and 17-KS; increased plasma 17-OHP
11-Hydroxylase	Present	Absent	Present in majority	Female virilized	Increased serum 11-deoxycortisol and urinary 17-OHCS and 17KS
3-Beta-hydroxysteroid dehydrogenase	Slight (in female)	Present	Absent	Female normal or slight virilization	Increased dehydroepiandrosterone; increased 17-KS
17-Hydroxylase	Absent	Absent	Present	Absent secondary sex characteristics	Metabolites of corticosterone and DOC increased; urinary 17-OHCS, 17-KS decreased
20,22-Desmolase	Absent	Present	Absent	Lack of masculinization	All urine and plasma adrenal steroids decreased
18-Hydroxylase and 18-hydroxysteroid dehydrogenase	Absent	Present	Absent	Normal	Metabolites of corticosterone and 11-desoxycorticosterone increased; 17-OHCS increased in 18-dehydrogenase defect

Deficiency of 18-hydroxysteroid dehydrogenase and hydroxylase results in the impaired production of aldosterone, but virilization and adrenal hyperplasia do not occur. These patients, however, are salt losers, and metabolites of corticosterone and 11-deoxycorticosterone that are found in the urine are useful in making diagnosis of this disorder. For further information on these and other, rarer congenital adrenal enzyme defects, see New (1981).

RENIN-ALDOSTERONE AXIS

Hypertension is a major affliction of modern society, striking at least 10 to 15 per cent of the adult population of the industrialized nations of the world. At least 20 million people in the United States have hypertension, with 90 to 98 per cent of the cases classified as essential hypertension. Because of the mortality and morbidity from associated myocardial and cerebrovascular complications, the necessity of treating this disorder has become obvious. Investigation of the etiology of hypertension has indicated the importance of the renin-angiotensin-aldosterone system, not only in the origin and maintenance of hypertension but also as a guide to treatment.

Renin is a proteolytic enzyme formed and stored by juxtaglomerular cells of the kidney and released into the lymph and the renal venous blood. Renin acts with its substrate (renin substrate or angiotensinogen), an α_2 globulin made by the liver, to split off a decapeptide angiotensin I. Angiotensin I is converted within the circulation into an octapeptide, angiotensin II, by an enzyme (converting enzyme) system found mainly in the lung. It is believed that angiotensin II is the peptide responsible for the physiologic effects on target tissues. Evidence indicates that the octapeptide angiotensin II is further split to a heptapeptide, angiotensin III, or that angiotensin I may be changed directly to angiotensin III without being converted to angiotensin II. Although the functions of angiotensin III are speculative, it appears to play a role in the modulation of aldosterone secretion. The active angiotensins are rapidly cleared by various aminopeptidases (angiotensinases) within the circulation and during transit through tissues. These relationships are shown in Figure 16–11. Renin is synthesized in a larger form (prorenin or big renin) and converted to its active form. Circulating prorenin has been associated with some renal tumors, and has been found to increase in parallel with renin in patients undergoing various diagnostic and therapeutic maneuvers.

Renin, through its product, angiotensin II, directly stimulates the synthesis and secretion of aldosterone by the adrenal zona glomerulosa. Renin release is dependent on changes in "effective" plasma volume, which in turn is dependent on tubular reabsorption of serum sodium by the kidney. Low plasma volume and low serum sodium stimulate the secretion of renin, resulting in aldosterone release which causes sodium retention with an increase in plasma volume, and elevated blood pressure and potassium loss. Conversely, increased "effective" blood volume or acute elevation in blood pressure results in low renin, low angiotensin II, low aldosterone, and subsequent sodium loss. Potassium loss stimulates aldosterone secretion and suppresses renin release, whereas elevated potassium has the opposite effect. Although a number of studies have demonstrated that ACTH stimulates aldosterone secretion, it has been found to be less important than potassium and the renin-angiotensin system in the control of aldosterone production.

Renin and Hypertension

The work of Laragh (1972) has indicated that essential hypertension can be classified on the basis of

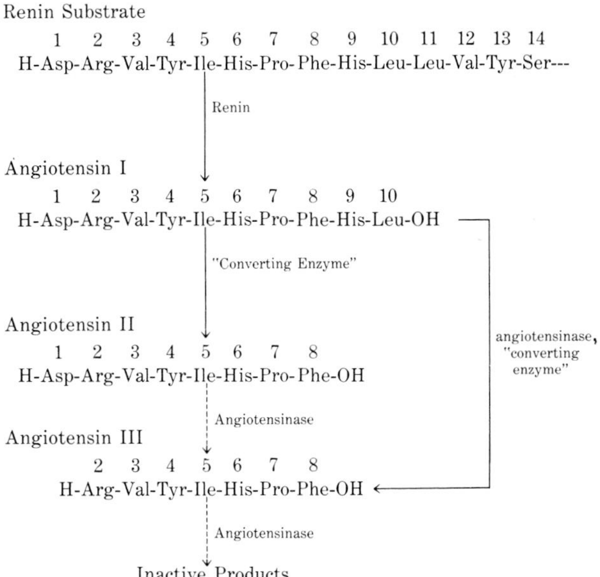

Figure 16–11. The renin-angiotensin system. Angiotensin II is thought to modulate vasoconstriction and is formed from angiotensin I by "converting enzyme." Angiotensin III is formed from angiotensin II; however, it can also be formed from the action of an angiotensinase and converting enzyme without being converted to angiotensin II. (Modified from Oparil, S.: Clin. Chem., *22*:583, 1976.)

2

renin measurements as (1) high renin, (2) low renin, or (3) normal renin, and that drug selection can be based on this classification. About 15 per cent of patients with essential hypertension have high renin hypertension; this excessive renin, which is secondary to lesions found in kidney or its vascular supply, ultimately leads to increased aldosterone production and subsequent changes in sodium and potassium excretion. The increased aldosterone (secondary aldosteronism) may contribute significantly to the symptomatology and course of high renin hypertension. Some of the causes of high renin hypertension are listed in Table 16–11.

Renin secreting tumors are an extremely rare finding; markedly elevated plasma renin and hyperaldosteronism with hypokalemia in the absence of a renovascular lesion are almost pathognomonic of this lesion. Malignant hypertension is associated with an elevated plasma renin and plasma aldosterone; when these patients are given antihypertensive therapy, the increased activity of renin usually can be normalized. In unilateral renal disease, both plasma renin and aldosterone are elevated. The most firmly established clinical application of the renin assay occurs in these patients. Asymmetry in the renin levels obtained during renal vein catheterization offers one of the best measurements to judge likelihood of blood pressure response to corrective surgery. It has been established that when the ratio of plasma renin in the renal vein of the affected to non-affected side is at least 1.5 to 1, surgery may lead to improvement. With suppression of renin release from the non-affected side, renal vein renin levels approximating those found in specimens obtained from the inferior vena cava also indicate likelihood of curative surgery. In patients with renovascular hypertension and a ratio of at least 1.5 to 1, almost 40 per cent have peripheral plasma renin activity that is within the reference interval (Streeten, 1975). Consequently, peripheral plasma renin has not been a useful predictor of response to surgery.

When there is an acceleration of hypertension, renin is usually markedly increased; however, with chronic renal failure, almost any renin level can be expected. A small number of hypertensive patients on dialysis have intractable, accelerated hypertension. In those patients in whom dialysis cannot control the hypertension, markedly elevated plasma renin levels can be lowered by nephrectomy. In those renal transplant patients with rejection, elevated plasma renin may be indicative of renal ischemia. Systemic hypertension has been found to be present in patients with Cushing's syndrome. In some patients, plasma renin and renin substrate are increased (Krakoff, 1975). In other patients with Cushing's syndrome and hypokalemia, it has been found that the secretion of a minor mineralocorticoid such as DOC or corticosterone is responsible for the hypertension. A suppressed plasma renin in a patient with Cushing's syndrome is presumptive evidence that a mineralocorticoid is present in excess. Other causes of a high renin hypertension include treatment with medications such as diuretics, vasodilators, or antihypertensives. Hormonal agents such as glucocorticoids as well as some estrogen-containing oral contraceptives have been found to increase renin substrate activity.

Table 16–11. SOME CAUSES OF HYPERTENSION ASSOCIATED WITH HIGH LEVELS OF PLASMA RENIN

Renin secreting tumor
Malignant accelerated hypertension
Renovascular hypertension
Major arterial lesions
Segmental lesions
Chronic renal failure
End stage
Transplant rejection
Cushing's syndrome
Iatrogenic
Volume depleting agents
Vasodilating agents
Glucocorticoids
Estrogens

Although plasma renin, aldosterone, and urinary sodium excretion may be normal in 60 per cent of hypertensive patients, evidence has accumulated which indicates that the renin-angiotensin plays a significant part in normal renin hypertension. The response of hypertensive patients with normal renin to converting enzyme inhibitors or angiotensin II antagonists (saralasin) has implicated renin and angiotensin II in sustaining hypertension in these patients.

It was found that low renin essential hypertension, which involves chronic expansion of plasma and extracellular fluid volume, is characterized by aldosterone oversecretion and responds to diuretic therapy. At least 25 per cent of patients with essential hypertension are found to have "low renin hypertension." Most investigators have characterized this state as "hyporesponsive," meaning low renin hypertensive patients fail to stimulate as vigorously as healthy subjects with upright posture, sodium restriction, diuretics, vasodilators, or a combination of these. It has been found that renin suppression increases with age, appears to be more common in women, and is more frequently found in older black individuals.

Listed in Table 16–12 is a group of syndromes associated with low levels of plasma renin. These have been divided into a subgroup that is of adrenal origin (primary) and a subgroup that is non-adrenal or "secondary" in origin. Primary aldosteronism is characterized by (1) arterial hypertension caused by oversecretion of aldosterone by an adrenal adenoma, (2) low renin, (3) potassium wastage, and (4) sodium retention. Removal of the adenoma is curative. Pseudoprimary aldosteronism is bilateral adrenal hyperplasia which microscopically has been described as micronodular. Since removal of micronodules has not been found to be curative, it has been postulated that perhaps there may be some unknown extra-adrenal stimulus. Aldosterone is markedly elevated and renin usually suppressed in patients with these lesions. In addition, suppressed renin may occur in situations such as ingestion of licorice, which has a high content of glycyrrhizic acid; excessive sodium intake; and a

Table 16–12. SOME CAUSES OF HYPERTENSION ASSOCIATED WITH LOW LEVELS OF PLASMA RENIN

"Primary" excess of mineralocorticoids
Primary aldosteronism
Pseudoprimary (idiopathic) aldosteronism
Glucocorticoid suppressible aldosteronism
11-Deoxycorticosterone excess
18-Hydroxy-11-deoxycorticosterone excess
Adrenal carcinoma (mineralocorticoid excess)
"Secondary" excess of mineralocorticoids
Licorice ingestion
Excess unsupervised sodium intake
Low renin, low aldosterone syndrome
1. Longstanding essential hypertension
2. Diabetes mellitus

syndrome of low renin and low aldosterone, which is most commonly seen patients with diabetes mellitus and renal disease.

Secondary aldosteronism results from non-adrenal disease in which both adrenal glands are stimulated, producing increased aldosterone secretion. Typically, these patients are not hypertensive. Such conditions as nephrosis, cirrhosis, and heart failure are usual causes. In all these, renin and aldosterone are increased. The response of the renin-aldosterone system in pregnancy is especially complex; there appears to be increased renin, renin substrate, angiotensin II, and aldosterone.

Aldosterone Measurements

Since the concentration of aldosterone in plasma is low (1000-fold lower than cortisol), it has been difficult to measure. Recent developments have made it possible to measure aldosterone directly in unextracted plasma after treatment to remove aldosterone from plasma proteins. An isolated aldosterone measurement with no attention to patient preparation, however, is of little clinical value. Even when time of sampling, posture, and dietary sodium and potassium are controlled, it is difficult to discriminate with certainty between primary aldosteronism and other forms of hypertension by using plasma aldosterone measurements. Direct aldosterone assays without chromatography are now available in the kit form using ^{125}I. In a reference population, plasma aldosterone concentrations are of the order of 10 ng/dl (278 pmol/L) and urinary aldosterone concentrations usually are 6 to 25 μg/24 hours (16.6 to 69.4 nmol/day).

Several potential screening tests to detect primary aldosteronism and to separate unilateral aldosterone-producing adenomas from other causes of primary aldosteronism have been used. Since only patients with adrenal adenomas predictably respond to surgical treatment, accurate diagnosis is imperative.

Low salt diet (<2 g/day), stress, upright posture, and diuretics all increase plasma aldosterone, whereas a high salt diet and lying in a supine position suppress aldosterone secretion in healthy subjects. Combinations of these manuevers are used in diagnosis of excessive aldosterone secretion. When healthy subjects are placed on a high salt diet and lie in the supine position, they suppress their plasma aldosterone levels to less than 10 ng/dl (278 pmol/L). After one hour in the upright position aldosterone levels in patients with Addison's disease are not stimulated to more than 5 ng/dl (139 pmol/L). However, aldosterone measurements for diagnosis of adrenal insufficiency are of little value (see p. 325).

Demonstration of the relative autonomy of the aldosterone secretion may be done in two different ways: administration of sodium or a synthetic mineralocorticoid. With administration of large amounts of sodium chloride (in one procedure, 2 L of isotonic saline infused over a four-hour period) a reference population of those individuals with hypertension not caused by primary aldosteronism suppress their plasma aldosterone to below 5 ng/dl (139 pmol/L). In contrast, those patients with primary aldosteronism have values above 8.5 ng/dl (236 pmol/L). This has been found to be the single best screening technique for outpatients, but it has a false-positive rate of 48 per cent. When four screening tests for primary aldosteronism—(1) serum potassium <3.5 meq/L (3.5 mmol/L), (2) plasma aldosterone concentration after saline infusion, (3) no depressor response to the administration of saralasin (angiotensin II analogue), and (4) stimulated plasma renin activity—are combined (see below), the diagnostic yield is enhanced substantially, but aldosterone-producing adrenal adenomas and idiopathic hyperaldosteronism still cannot be separated accurately (Streeten, 1979).

An alternative diagnostic maneuver is the administration of 200 ng of synthetic mineralocorticoid, fluorocortisone, three times a day for three days, and the demonstration of non-suppressibility of plasma aldosterone (Horton, 1973). A reference population suppresses plasma aldosterone to less than 4 ng/dl (111 pmol/L). In patients with primary aldosteronism, distinguishing patients with aldosterone-producing adenomas from the group with idiopathic hyperaldosteronism who usually are managed medically remains the major diagnostic challenge. Confirmation of an aldosterone-producing adrenal adenoma can best be accomplished by measurement of aldosterone in adrenal venous plasma and by computed tomography.

Renin Measurements

There are important technical differences in determination of renin using current methodology. Renin measurements are of two types: plasma renin activity and plasma renin concentration. In the past, bioassays of the precursor activity of angiotensin were used, but now radioimmunoassay of generated angiotensin I is commonly employed. A plasma specimen containing renin is allowed to react with its substrate; then, after a specified period of time, the reaction is terminated and measurement of generated angiotensin I (or II) made. To ensure stability of the angiotensin I (or II) which is generated, angiotensinases are inactivated by acid, chelation, or specific enzyme inhibitors.

For the estimation of what has become known as plasma renin activity (PRA), the endogenous substrate is not eliminated. Therefore, the rate of generation of angiotensin I is influenced by both the concentration of endogeneous renin and its substrate. This type of assay is the most widely used method for the determination of renin. Comparison of results among laboratories is an impossibility because of procedural differences such as variations of pH, ionic strength, the length of the assay, the angiotensinase inhibitor, lack of a specific reference preparation, and the conditions under which the specimen was obtained. In addition, literature on renin assays reveals confusion regarding units of measurements employed, and even when an attempt is made to express the many arbitrary units in the same terms (ng angiotensin liberated/ml/hour), there are wide ranges reported for human plasma renin activity in reference populations.

When measuring renin concentration rather than plasma renin activity (PRA), the effect of substrate is eliminated. To accomplish this, the specimen may be treated in a number of ways; for example, the plasma may be incubated at a low pH, denaturing the substrate. Then highly active ovine substrate is added, and since substrate is in excess, angiotensin I generation occurs linearly with increasing renin concentrations. Under these conditions, angiotensin generation is independent of substrate concentration and proportional to renin concentration (zero order kinetics). An international reference standard has been developed for this method, and plasma renin activity, which is expressed in Goldblatt units/dl (GU/dl), can be compared among different laboratories.

Assays of plasma renin activity and plasma renin concentration provide similar information except in a few clinical situations. With oral contraceptive administration, plasma renin concentration remains within the reference interval, whereas plasma renin activity increases owing to the increase in substrate. Other procedures such as freezing, thawing, and acidification have been found to convert prorenin to renin and thereby increase values in plasma renin concentration assays.

The direct measurement of renin substrate, angiotensin I, or angiotensin II is not used widely in clinical practice, because of tedious extraction or concentration steps as well as difficulty in eliminating formation or degradation of these compounds by proteases and other enzymes involved in the renin system.

Since renin release is controlled by many physiologic and pharmacologic variables, it is extremely important to know the conditions under which the specimen was obtained. Such conditions as upright posture, the administration of diuretics, or low sodium diets are potent stimuli of renin release and should be adequately controlled prior to the measurement of plasma renin. Renin also appears to be extremely labile so that the variables involved in specimen processing should be vigorously controlled. Blood should be drawn into iced tubes containing chelating agents for inactivation of enzymes (angiotensinases) and centrifuged in the cold, and the plasma frozen to avoid substantial losses from angiotensinase activity; with this technique, the specimen is stable for several months at −20°C.

Plasma renin has been interpreted in individuals relative to a simultaneous 24-hour urine sodium excretion after several days on a stable sodium intake and off diuretics. With normal kidney function, urinary sodium excretion is related to the extracellular or fluid volume and inversely related to the plasma concentration of renin (Fig. 16–12). From this nomogram it should be possible to distinguish low, normal, and high plasma renin groups.

Because the 24-hour renin-sodium profile is cumbersome, various stimuli for renin release have been used. One of the simplest is the procedure described by Kaplan (1976); plasma renin activity is determined in fasting subjects after 30 minutes in an upright position following 40 mg of furosemide (Lasix) given intravenously. This test does not require hospitalization, a special diet, or prolonged standing. In this study, a reference population of whites and blacks had plasma renin activities >1.0 and 0.5 ng/ml/hour, respectively, while low-renin hypertensive patients were unable to respond as well. Although different methods of renin categorization do not always similarly classify the same patients, this test correlates well with other procedures being used to identify low renin hypertensives.

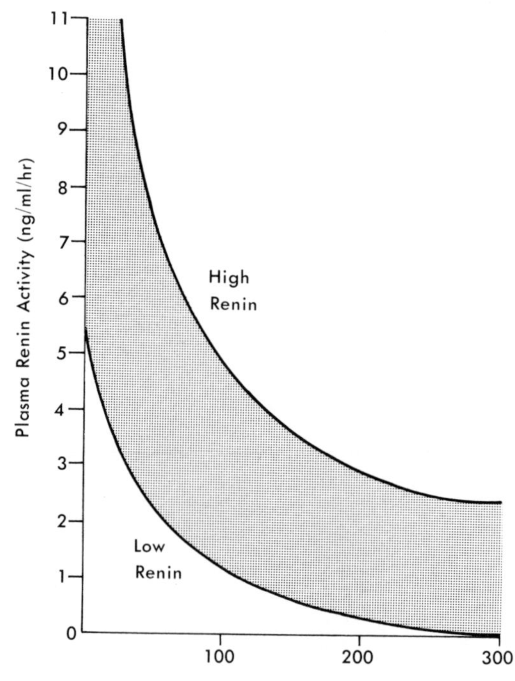

Figure 16–12. Plasma renin activity as a function of the 24-hour urinary sodium excretion. Normal renin hypertension is represented by shaded area. (Modified from Brunner, H. R., et al.: N. Engl. J. Med., *286*:441, 1972.)

Because of conflicting views of the usefulness of routine renin-sodium profiling for the evaluation of hypertension, this procedure is one of the most controversial areas of medicine today. Many feel there is little justification for its use because of the effort and financial resources which it requires without clear-cut diagnostic and prognostic benefit, as well as lack of usefulness in drug selection. For further information on this view, see Gifford (1980).

Angiotensin-Converting Enzyme Activity

The measurement of angiotensin-converting enzyme activity, although of limited usefulness in diagnosis and treatment of hypertension, has been found of value in other circumstances. Recently, increased values have been found in patients with active sarcoid, while in patients with other granulomatous diseases and those whose sarcoid is dormant, it is within the reference interval. Diagnostic usefulness of this determination, however, has been decreased by finding elevated serum activity in a number of other disorders. For example, serum angiotensin-converting activity has been shown to be increased in many liver diseases, including chronic persistent hepatitis, chronic aggressive hepatitis, fatty liver, and obstructive jaundice. Other diseases such as neonatal respiratory distress, silicosis, asbestosis, hyperthyroidism, diabetic retinopathy, Gaucher's disease, and leprosy also may give rise to elevated serum enzyme activity. For further information on methods of measurement, see Rohrbach (1982).

GONADOTROPINS AND SEX HORMONES

Luteinizing Hormone and Follicle Stimulating Hormone

The hypothalamus secretes a single peptide releasing hormone that controls secretion of the gonadotropins luteinizing hormone (LH) and follicle stimulating hormone (FSH) from the anterior pituitary. This hormone, which is a decapeptide, releases both LH and FSH from the same population of pituitary cells. Because it releases LH to a greater extent than FSH, it has been called luteinizing releasing hormone (LRH), but also is known as LH/FSH or gonadotropin releasing hormone (GnRH).

Both LH and FSH consist of a glycopeptide framework to which carbohydrate side chains are attached. Structurally LH and FSH are related to the other glycoprotein hormones, thyrotropin (TSH) and human chorionic gonadotropin (hCG); these hormones are made up of two non-identical, non-covalently bound, biologically inactive subunits designated alpha and beta. It has been found that alpha and beta subunits can be separated and then recombined to give an active hormone. The alpha subunit is nearly identical for all glycoprotein hormones, but the beta unit differs for each, i.e., this subunit is responsible for hormone specificity. Stimulation with LRH causes release of free alpha subunits in addition to LH and FSH. LH and FSH are secreted from the pituitary and are carried in the blood to their site of action, the testes or ovary.

During infancy, serum levels of both gonadotropins are low and relatively constant. In children of both sexes, FSH levels are higher than LH and the FSH response to LRH is greater than LH. During puberty, both gonadotropins increase, with FSH reaching a plateau during mid-puberty and LH reaching a maximum at the end of puberty. In pubertal children, a major increment in serum LH concentrations first occurs in an episodic pattern during sleep. In general, these episodes closely follow onset of non-REM (rapid eye movement) sleep and terminate in relation to REM sleep. As puberty proceeds daytime secretory episodes also begin, and by completion of puberty sleep and wake patterns are equivalent.

In the adult male, secretion of LH and to a lesser degree FSH is episodic, with 9 to 14 such secretory surges of LH per 24 hours corresponding to a 200 to 300 per cent increase over the mean value. FSH also is secreted in a pulsatile manner, but the oscillations are of low magnitude, representing only 25 per cent of the mean.

In adult females, all ovulatory menstrual cycles have a pattern of LH and FSH similar to that seen in Figure 16–13. The female menstrual cycle is divided into a follicular phase and a luteal phase by the midcycle surge of the pituitary gonadotropins. There is a single major sharp peak in LH concentration at about mid-cycle near the time of ovulation. The peak in FSH concentration occurs coincident with the peak of LH, but is of lesser magnitude and briefer duration. Both gonadotropin levels are generally higher during the preovulatory period than during the luteal phase; however, there is a fall in FSH concentration antecedent to the mid-cycle surge. FSH levels generally are higher during the follicular phase than during the luteal phase. Following the mid-cycle surge of LH and FSH, there is a drop in the concentration of both hormones to lower, more irregular levels with occasional "spikes" of LH unaccompanied by "spikes" of FSH. At and after menopause, the gonadotropins continue to be secreted in episodic fashion. FSH levels, however, are higher than those seen during the course of the menstrual cycle; this probably is due to lack of inhibition of an ovarian substance similar to inhibin, which is responsible for the feedback suppression of FSH. Evidence suggests this inhibin-like substance is a protein that is produced by the ovary and selectively inhibits FSH secretion. Serum LH levels after menopause may be similar to or slightly higher than those during the menstrual cycle; this may be a reflection of the persistence of the episodic pattern of LH release as well as a suppressive effect of estradiol, which is secreted from the adrenal.

Estradiol exerts a negative feedback effect on FSH release. In contrast, LH release varies with concentration and duration of exposure to estrogen. At all levels

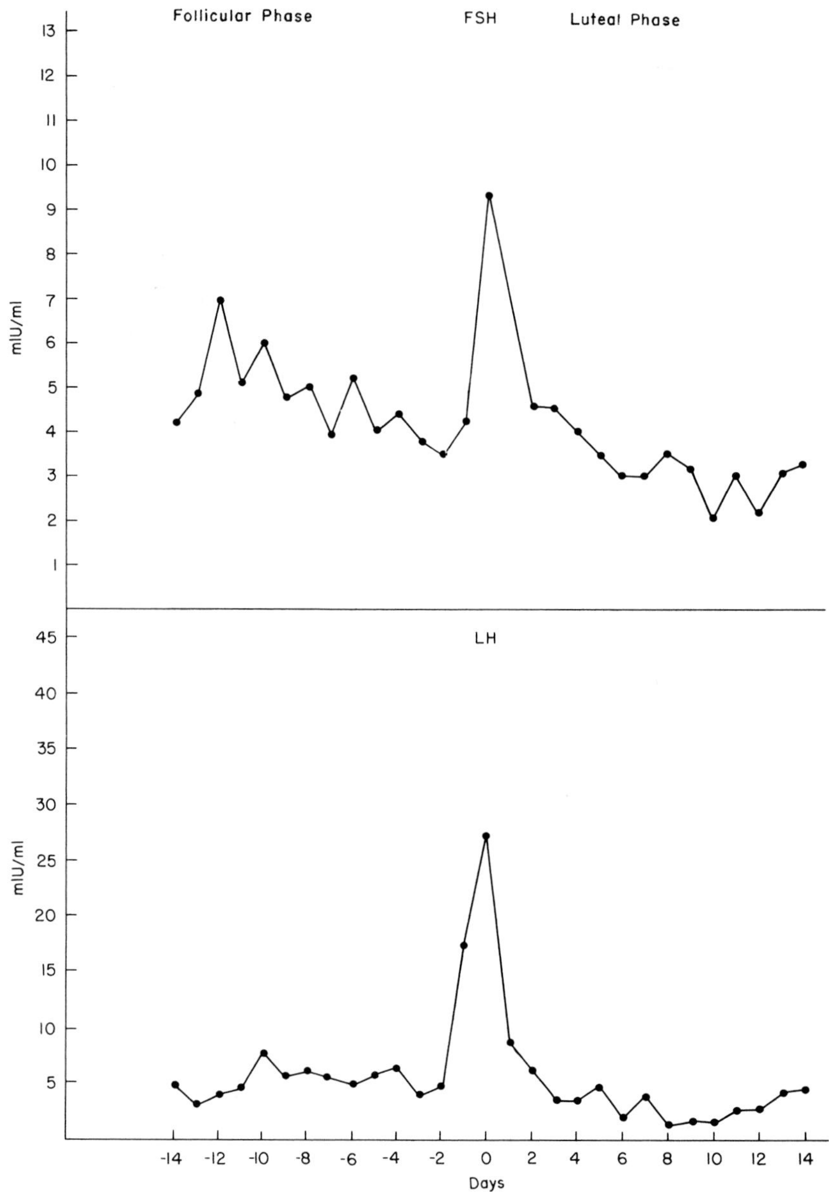

Figure 16–13. Dynamics of serum FSH and LH levels during the course of the menstrual cycle.

estrogen exerts a negative feedback on LH, but at higher levels over a long period of time it stimulates LH release. The transition from suppression to stimulation of LH release occurs during the LH surge of the follicular phase and requires estradiol concentrations in serum of at least 200 pg/ml (734 pmol/L).

In men, at about the sixth decade, there is a gradual increase in LH and FSH; however, there are large individual variations. Testosterone exerts negative feedback effects on the gonadotropins at the hypothalamic and pituitary levels. In addition, testosterone is aromatized into estradiol which also inhibits secretion at the same sites.

The intravenous administration of LRH in healthy individuals results in prompt increases in serum LH, with maximal levels occurring at about 30 minutes. Serum LH then declines gradually over the next few hours. A similar response of FSH also occurs, but it is not as marked and is more variable between individuals. Although LRH potentially has diagnostic and therapeutic value, because of a variety of doses and multiple routes and varying lengths of administration, results have been disappointing. It was hoped that patients with hypothalamic disease would have a brisk response to LRH, while patients with pituitary lesions would have a blunted response. However, many patients with pituitary tumors have a normal response, while hypogonadotropic individuals have a blunted or absent response unless treated with LRH for several days. For further information, see Taymor (1979).

FSH and LH usually are measured by radioimmunoassay. Since the glycoprotein hormones are structurally similar, antibody cross-reactivity may be a problem. In addition, because of the cyclic pattern of gonadotropin release, it is possible to obtain an isolated sample at either the peak or nadir of secretion. For these reasons, some workers have advocated obtaining at least six serum specimens for LH over a six-hour period; the specimens may be assayed individually or pooled. However, in those patients in whom gonadotropins are high, such as those with anorchia or testicular failure or those who are postmenopausal, only one specimen may be necessary. Measurement of the gonadotropins in timed urine specimens has been advocated by some workers as an alternative to pooling serum specimens.

Reference values for serum LH are up to 12 mIU/ml (12 IU/L) for children, up to 15 mIU/ml (15 IU/L) for adult males, and between 30 and 200 mIU/ml (30 to 200 IU/L) in postmenopausal females. In menstruating females, LH values of up to 10 mIU/ml (10 IU/L) occur, except during the mid-cycle peak, when they may reach 80 mIU/ml (80 IU/L). Reference values for FSH are up to 12 mIU/ml (12 IU/L) for children, up to 15 mIU/ml (15 IU/L) for adult males, and up to 200 mIU/ml (200 IU/L) for postmenopausal patients. Menstruating females have FSH values up to 10 mIU/ml (10 IU/L) except during the mid-cycle peak when FSH values as high as 20 mIU/ml (20 IU/L) may occur. In patients with ovarian failure, such as occurs with menopause, high levels of FSH >40 mIU/ml (40 IU/L) and LH occur, with FSH almost always exceeding LH. Absolute levels of LH and FSH can be used to aid in the diagnosis of polycystic ovary syndrome in which elevated levels of LH >35 mIU/ml (35 IU/L) and normal or depressed <15 mIU/ml (15 IU/L) levels of FSH are found. Patients with hypogonadotropin-hypoestrogenic states, such as psychogenic amenorrhea or anorexia nervosa, have gonadotropin levels that are depressed, with FSH being slightly higher than LH. In a series of patients with pituitary tumors, about 20 per cent were found to have high levels of FSH, although serum LH levels were either within the reference interval or low (Snyder, 1979). LH and FSH measurements also have been used for the diagnosis of ectopic tumor production. This is discussed in Chapter 15.

Although patients with lesions in the hypothalamus or pituitary usually have low gonadotropins and low sex hormone levels, those with a primary lesion in the gonads have low sex hormone levels but elevated gonadotropins. The findings in some disorders of the hypothalamic-pituitary-gonadal axis are summarized in Table 16–13.

Clomiphene Testing

Clomiphene, an anti-estrogen which is used as a diagnostic or therapeutic agent, has achieved widespread clinical use. It competes with estrogens or testosterone at the hypothalamus by blocking the uptake of estrogens in the female and testosterone in the male; thus the feedback of estrogens or testosterone on the hypothalamic-pituitary system is interrupted. In the female this results in secretion of larger amounts of LH and FSH, which, in turn, induce follicular maturation and initiate an ovulatory cycle.

A functioning hypothalamic-pituitary-ovarian axis is essential for successful therapy with clomiphene; thus it is indicated in anovulatory females in whom there is evidence of follicular function, estrogen production is adequate (in that they bleed after administration of progesterone), and the gonadotropins are within the reference interval or only slightly diminished.

Table 16–13. BASAL HORMONE LEVELS IN DISORDERS OF THE HYPOTHALAMIC-PITUITARY-GONADAL AXIS IN MALES*

Diagnosis	LH	FSH	Testosterone	Estradiol
Hypothalamus and pituitary (hypogonadotropic syndromes)				
Hypopituitarism	↓ or N†	↓ or N	↓ or N	↓ or N
Kallmann's syndrome	↓ or N	↓ or N	↓ or N	↓ or N
Isolated gonadotropin deficiency	↓ or N	↓ or N	↓ or N	↓ or N
Simple delayed puberty	↓ or N	↓ or N	↓	↓
Gonad (hypergonadotropic syndromes)				
Primary testicular failure	↑	↑	↓	↓ or N
Anorchia	↑	↑	↓	↓ or N
Cryptorchidism	N	N or ↑	N	N
Azoospermia and oligospermia	N or ↑	N or ↑	N	N
Varicocele	N	N	N	N
Klinefelter's syndrome	↑ or N	↑	↓ or N	N or ↑
Complete testicular feminization syndrome	↑	↑ or N	N or ↑	↑
Precocious puberty				
Idiopathic or CNS lesion	↑	↑	↑	↑
Adrenal tumors or congenital adrenal hyperplasia	↓	↓	↑	↑ or N

*Modified from Marshall, J. C.: Clin. Endocrinol. Metab., *4*:545, 1975.
†Normal represented by N, increases and decreases by arrows.

Clomiphene citrate usually is given in a dosage of 50 to 100 mg daily for five to ten days. Therapy is usually begun at the lower dose and, if the patient fails to ovulate after two or three cycles, the dose or the length of therapy is increased. A convenient starting point is the fifth day of menstrual bleeding induced by progesterone administration. Although induction of bleeding prior to administration of clomiphene is not essential, it gives the advantage of simulating a normal menstrual cycle.

A reference population (those with adequate pituitary gonadotropin reserve) shows a 50 per cent increase of LH over baseline and an 85 per cent increase of FSH over baseline on the last day of clomiphene testing. The rise in gonadotropins may continue for one to two days beyond the last dose. In a manner analogous to a normal ovulatory cycle, estrogen levels following a decline rise and trigger the preovulatory LH surge as a result of positive feedback. If ovulation results from the seven-day test, it will occur about 11 days after beginning clomiphene. Although only a single LH determination as a baseline and on the sixth day is considered adequate by some, others recommend two baseline specimens and a specimen for LH and FSH on days four, five, six, and seven (Franchimont, 1974).

Ovulation is induced in up to 70 per cent of anovulatory patients; the pregnancy rate in several large series ranges from 27 to 40 per cent. Clomiphene also can be used in males who have signs and symptoms of androgen deficiency, but in whom the measurement of gonadotropins and testosterone has not led to diagnosis of the underlying disorder. The minimum normal response is an increase over baseline of 30 per cent for LH and 22 per cent for FSH (Walsh, 1977). Clomiphene administration also improves the quantity and motility of spermatozoa.

Estrogens

The estrogens are steroids which have an A ring containing three unsaturated double bonds. Although over 30 estrogens have been identified, measurements of only three estrogens—estradiol, estrone, and estriol—are used in clinical practice. Estriol measurements are important in assessment of the feto-placental unit and are discussed in Chapter 20. The structure of the three common estrogens and their interrelationships are shown at the bottom of this page.

The ovary, as well as the testes and adrenal, has the capacity to synthesize estrogens from the androgens androstenedione and testosterone. During the follicular phase of the menstrual cycle, ovarian secretion represents only one third of total estrogen production. In contrast to estradiol, which is secreted almost entirely by the ovary, most estrone is derived from peripheral conversion of androstenedione and from estradiol metabolism. In healthy postmenopausal women, the ovaries do not secrete significant quantities of estrogens; virtually all estrogen produced is from peripheral conversion of androstenedione made by the adrenal. Although estradiol is the most abundant estrogen in premenopausal women, estrone is the estrogen in highest concentration in postmenopausal females.

In men, the testes secrete significant quantities of estradiol and small amounts of estrone. Testicular secretion, however, probably accounts for only one third of the total production of estradiol in men, with the remainder arising from testosterone and estrone by extraglandular conversion. Thus, the testes are indirectly responsible for most of the estrogen production in men.

A wide range of organs in the body, including skin, fat, red blood cells, uterus, and liver, have enzymes that metabolize estrogens, but liver plays the most important role. Estradiol and estrone are conjugated in the liver and excreted as sulfates and glucuronates. Estrone sulfate and other estrogen conjugates are excreted in the bile and then hydrolyzed in the gut and reabsorbed into the peripheral circulation. The metabolic pattern or rate of estrogen metabolism apparently does not change during various disease states.

Estradiol, estriol, and estrone are bound to sex hormone binding globulin (SHBG), the same carrier protein that binds testosterone. In serum, estradiol is largely in the conjugated form and is bound to sex hormone binding globulin (SHBG). In contrast, most serum estrone is present as estrone sulfate.

Measurements of serum and urinary estrogen concentrations are important in assessing disorders of the menstrual cycle or for monitoring ovulation. Estrogens occur in urine as water-soluble conjugates, glucuronate or sulfate; these groups must be hydrolyzed before the estrogens are extracted with organic solvents. Following extraction, the method of Brown (1968) usually is used to estimate total estrogens in urine (also see Chap. 21). The endpoint reaction depends on the ability of the phenolic group of estrogens to react

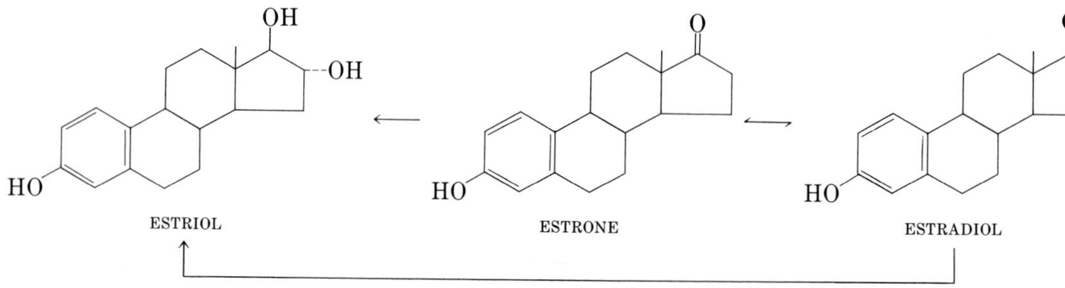

OH
--OH
HO
ESTRIOL
←
O
HO
ESTRONE
⟶
OH
HO
ESTRADIOL

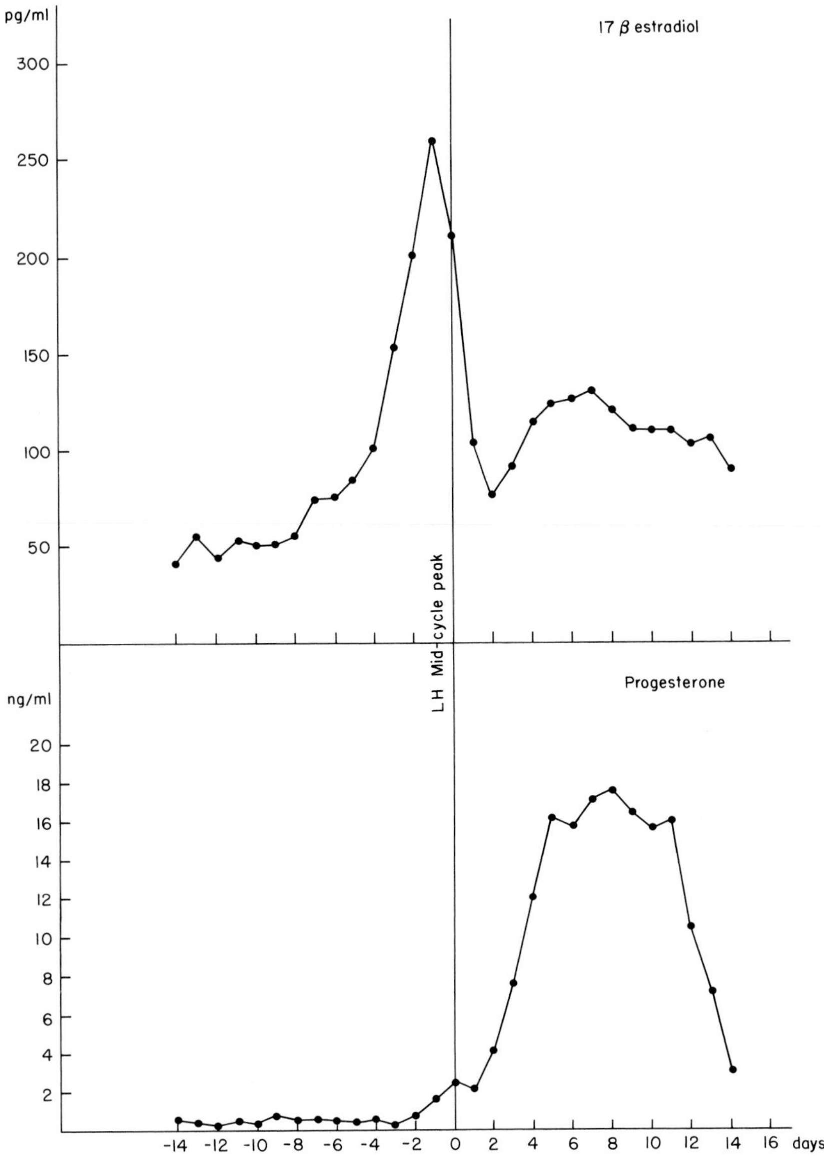

Figure 16–14. Evolution of progesterone and 17-β estradiol during the course of the menstrual cycle.

with Kober reagent (a mixture of phenol and sulfuric acid) to produce a pink color.

For estimation of total estrogens in serum, the method of Brown usually is too insensitive for most purposes, and often radioimmunoassay of estradiol is used. Like other steroid hormones measured by radioimmunoassay, estradiol usually is quantitated after extraction and chromatographic purification. Antibody prepared with estradiol conjugated protein at the C-3 or 17 position may show up to 30 to 50 per cent cross-reactivity with other estrogens, whereas antibody produced using conjugation at the C-6 position is more specific.

When measurement of serum estradiol was compared with total estrogens in urine, serum estradiol determinations were found a more accurate reflection of ovarian function than urinary excretion of total estrogens. At those times when ovarian secretion of estradiol is high, correlation between serum and urinary levels is good; but if the ovarian secretion is low, correlation is poor. When urinary estrogen measurements are compared with serum estradiol to monitor ovulation, the peaks and nadirs of the urinary measurements are delayed one to two days with respect to the corresponding serum profiles (Roger, 1980).

Estradiol is the most potent of the estrogens and is present in concentrations <50 pg/ml (18.4 pmol/L) in the preovulatory period. Concentrations rise during the second half of the follicular phase and reach a peak of 150 to 500 pg/ml (550 to 1836 pmol/L) on the day prior to or the day of the LH surge. The mid-cycle surge of LH may be related to these rising estrogen levels if they are present for the appropriate amount of time. Following the LH surge, serum estradiol drops precipitously almost to preovulatory levels, but then rises slightly to 100 to 200 pg/ml (367 to 734 pmol/L) during the luteal phase (Fig. 16–14). During menopause, estradiol concentrations steadily decrease to approximately 15 per cent of premenopausal levels, and estrone, primarily produced by peripheral aromatization of adrenal androsterone, becomes the predominant estrogen. Estrone concentration in the late follicular phase is in the range of 150 to 200 pg/ml (550 to 730 pmol/L), whereas levels in postmenopausal females are approximately 35 pg/ml (130 pmol/L).

In prepubertal children, reference values for estradiol by RIA are up to 20 pg/ml (73.4 pmol/L); in adult males they are usually 10 to 80 pg/ml (36.7 to 293.7 pmol/L). A few patients with Leydig cell tumors of the testes present with feminization; these patients have elevated serum estrogen levels. For further information on the elevated estrogen levels produced by these tumors, see Perez (1980). The most common tumor-producing signs of estrogen excess in females are the granulosa-theca cell tumors. In order to classify hypogonadism, estrogen determinations usually are interpreted with gonadotropin measurements. This is discussed on page 335.

Progesterone

In menstruating females, progesterone is secreted mainly by the corpus luteum of the ovary; it is partially responsible for cyclic changes in the endometrium which are necessary for attachment and growth of an embryo. Progesterone levels are low prior to the mid-cycle gonadotropin surge. Shortly after the gonadotropin surge, they begin to rise rapidly, reaching peak levels during the middle of the luteal phase. Thereafter a progressive fall occurs with barely detectable progesterone levels reached prior to menses (Fig. 16–14). Although progesterone in large amounts produces a negative feedback on gonadotropin secretion, it is not the major component in the negative feedback system for ovarian steroids.

The small amounts of progesterone in the male and non-menstruating females are derived mainly from extraglandular conversion of adrenal pregnenolone and pregnenolone sulfate to progesterone, and by secretion of progesterone by the adrenals. In serum, about 18 per cent of progesterone is bound to cortisol binding globulin and 79 per cent to albumin, whereas the remainder is free (unbound).

Progesterone production by the corpus luteum can be indirectly assessed by measurement of the basal body temperature. During the luteal phase there is about a 0.5°C. rise in body temperature which lasts about 10 to 12 days (hyperthermic portion of the luteal phase) and parallels the increase in progesterone concentration. For information on progesterone measurements during pregnancy, see Chapter 20.

Function of the corpus luteum can be assessed by measuring serum progesterone concentration. Although conventional radioimmunoassays involving extraction of progesterone with organic solvents have been used, recent approaches include displacement of progesterone from binding sites with danazol or cortisol, freeing progesterone for assay without extraction. With radioimmunoassay methods, serum progesterone concentrations of <1 ng/ml (3.2 nmol/L) are found during the preovulatory phase. At the time of the LH surge, serum progesterone levels begin to rise and about four to six days later reach a peak of about 10 to 20 ng/ml (31.8 to 63.6 nmol/L). After remaining more or less stable for about one week, progesterone concentrations drop rapidly to about 1 ng/ml (3.2 nmol/L) a short time before the onset of menstruation. A mid-luteal phase serum progesterone of 5 ng/ml (15.9 nmol/L) or more is satisfactory index of ovulation. In the adult male, progesterone levels are usually <1 ng/ml (3.2 nmol/L); levels are fairly constant and slightly lower than those in the female during the follicular phase of the menstrual cycle. In children, progesterone concentrations are about 0.3 to 0.4 ng/ml (10.5 to 12.8 nmol/L) until the second half of puberty, at which time they rise by about 50 per cent.

Luteal function has been assessed by measuring progesterone in a serum specimen drawn during the mid-luteal phase; a value of 10 ng/ml (31.8 nmol/L) has been used to delineate adequate and inadequate luteal function. However, because of a large overlap of progesterone levels in individuals with normal and abnormal luteal function, this demarcation has been questioned (Rosenfeld, 1980). Hence, it is recommended that luteal phase defects be identified by progesterone measurements on more than one serum specimen obtained during the luteal phase. The protocol of Abraham (1974) uses the sum of three progesterone levels obtained during an interval from 11 to 4 days preceding menstruation; a sum of 15 ng/ml (47.7 nmol/L) or greater indicates adequate luteal function. Luteal phase defects may be demonstrated in a wide variety of patients, including those who present with habitual miscarriages, those receiving clomiphene, and approximately 4 per cent of infertile females.

Ability of the corpus luteum to secrete steroids can be assessed with administration of human chorionic gonadotropin (hCG). Starting on the third day of the hyperthermic portion of the luteal phase, a dose of 3 mg of dexamethasone is given daily for six consecutive days. On the first, third, and fifth days, 5000 units of hCG is injected intramuscularly. Baseline and post-hCG urinary or serum steroids are measured; serum estradiol or progesterone, urinary estrogens, or pregnanediol may be used. The normal response is a doubling of the baseline value on the last (sixth) day of dexamethasone administration (Franchimont, 1974).

Progesterone can be monitored by measuring its metabolite, pregnanediol, in urine. Urinary pregnanediol, which is essentially all conjugated to glucuronide, is hydrolyzed and measured by colorimetry or gas chromatography, or measured directly by radioimmunoassay using antibody highly specific for the conjugate. Reference values for urinary pregnanediol excretion are <1 mg/24 hours (3.0 μmol/day) during the preovulatory phase, rising to between 2.5 and 6 mg/24 hours (7.4 and 17.8 μmol/day) during the luteal phase. In young adult males, the reference interval is 0.1 to 1.8 mg/24 hours (0.3 to 5.3 mmol/day), decreasing by up to 75 per cent with advancing age. Serum progesterone or urinary pregnanediol has been found to be elevated in those rare patients with feminizing interstitial (Leydig) cell tumor of the testes (see Estrogens, p. 336).

Androgens

TESTOSTERONE

The testes have two main functions: (1) spermatogenesis, the production of germ cells, and (2) steroidogenesis, the synthesis and subsequent secretion of the androgenic hormones. In the male, LH binds to testicular Leydig cell receptors enhancing conversion of cholesterol to testosterone (Fig. 16–8). Once testosterone is formed in the Leydig cell, capillaries and veins carry it to the periphery, or it traverses testicular myoid cells and enters the seminiferous tubules where it is involved in spermatogenesis. FSH is responsible for activation of the seminiferous tubules, resulting in production of sperm (see Chap. 22) as well as the conversion of testosterone to estradiol. The testosterone that diffuses from the Leydig cell into the seminiferous tubules is bound to a binding protein and occurs in concentrations 20 times that of the peripheral circulation. In the seminiferous tubules testosterone stimulates primary spermatocytes to form secondary spermatocytes and finally young spermatocytes. Testicular secretion accounts for 95 per cent of the circulating testosterone present in men. In addition to testosterone, the testes also secrete dihydrotestosterone, progesterone, 17-hydroxyprogesterone, and androstenedione.

In the female, the ovary and adrenal secrete small amounts of testosterone; however, the majority of testosterone in the blood derives from metabolism of androstenedione.

About 60 per cent of circulating testosterone binds strongly to sex hormone binding globulin (SHBG), a β-globulin synthesized in liver, which also binds estradiol and other steroids containing a 17-β hydroxy substitution. It has been postulated that free testosterone feeds back on LH at the level of the pituitary and hypothalamus, and that testosterone metabolites may have similar feedback effects. Almost 40 per cent of testosterone is bound loosely to albumin and about 2 per cent is free (unbound). A recent study has indicated that not only free testosterone but also the albumin bound fraction is able to traverse the blood-brain barrier.

Hormones and drugs which affect testosterone binding are important because they may lead to changes in free testosterone. (When there is a decrease in sex hormone binding globulin, an increased concentration of free hormone occurs, and an increase in the binding protein leads to a decrease in free hormone concentration.) Excess thyroid hormones and growth hormone decrease the concentration of SHBG and concentration of androgens, whereas estrogens and inadequate thyroid hormone levels increase SHBG. Anticonvulsants increase SHBG and decrease free testosterone levels (Dana-Haeri, 1982).

Testosterone is metabolized by the enzyme 5α reductase to another biologically active androgen, dihydrotestosterone. Other testosterone metabolites include androsterone, etiocholanolone, and their sulfates and glucuronides as well as estradiol. Although in the male 70 per cent of serum dihydrotestosterone derives from testosterone, the major prohormone for serum dihydrotestosterone in the female is androstenedione.

The androgens have widespread effects on sexual and non-sexual tissue. Testosterone is the dominant androgen in brain, pituitary, kidney, and testes, whereas dihydrotestosterone is the major androgen in skin, prostate, seminal vesicles, and epididymis. Androgens cause an increase in total body mass, with such tissues as muscle, bones, kidney, and larynx relatively sensitive to their effects. The androgens also have specific effects on hair growth. Under the influence of the androgens, hair at specific sites becomes replaced with longer, coarser, and darker terminal hair. The amount of androgen necessary for the change depends on the race, sex, and age of the individual as well as the site of the hair follicle.

Despite large oscillations in LH concentrations, serum testosterone levels are relatively constant. In young men there is a circadian pattern of testosterone secretion with highest levels occurring at about the time of awakening, but this pattern disappears with advancing age. During periods of stress such as illness, serum testosterone values decrease, but the mechanism for this decrease is not known. Although studies have demonstrated an age-related decrease in serum testosterone in men, healthy individuals probably show no significant age-related decrease.

Excessive growth of body hair is called hirsutism and results from inordinate secretion of testosterone or its precursor androstenedione. Etiologically the two categories of hirsutism, androgen dependent and androgen independent hirsutism, can be separated by hair distribution over the body. Androgen dependent hirsutism is restricted to the chin, upper lip, chest, and other androgen sensitive areas, while these areas as well as the forehead, abdomen, arms, and legs are involved in androgen-independent hirsutism.

Shown in Table 16–14 are the most common causes of androgen-dependent hirsutism. In these patients free testosterone is usually elevated; other measurements of lesser reliability are serum testosterone and dihydrotestosterone, serum androstenedione, dehydroepiandrosterone sulfate, and urinary 17-ketosteroids. Dynamic testing involving dexamethasone suppression has been used in diagnosis and treatment, but results have been conflicting. A recent series has been reported by Abraham (1981).

Reagent antibodies used for measurements of testosterone by radioimmunoassay are subject to major cross-reactivity by dihydrotestosterone. Danazol, a synthetic androgen used for treatment of endometri-

Table 16–14. CAUSES OF ANDROGEN-DEPENDENT HIRSUTISM

Ovarian causes
Neoplastic
Sertoli-Leydig cell tumors (arrhenoblastoma)
Granulosa-stromal cell tumors
Gynandroblastoma
Lipoid cell tumor
Gonadoblastoma
Non-neoplastic
Polycystic ovarian disease
Hyperthecosis
Idiopathic hirsutism
Adrenal abnormalities
Neoplastic
Adrenocortical carcinoma
Virilizing adrenal adenoma
Non-neoplastic
Congenital adrenal hyperplasia
21-Hydroxylase deficiency
11-Hydroxylase deficiency
Cushing's disease
Medications
Androgens (such as danazol, Halotestin)
"19-Nor" progestins

osis, also has been reported to cross-react with some antibodies used for testosterone estimation thereby elevating values (Sharp, 1981). In assays where this cross-reactivity does not occur, low values have been reported because danazol displaces testosterone from SHBG. Other synthetic steroids which displace testosterone from SHBG are methyltestosterone, fluoxymesterone, and norgestrel. Reference intervals for prepubertal children are <1.0 ng/ml (3.5 nmol/L) for males and <0.4 ng/ml (1.4 nmol/L) for females. In adults, reference values are >3.0 ng/ml, (10.4 nmol/L) for males and <0.8 ng/ml (2.8 nmol/L) for females. Low values in a male are suggestive of hypogonadism such as occurs with Klinefelter's syndrome; they warrant further evaluation with gonadotropin measurements to localize the cause of hypogonadism. In the adult female, testosterone values above 1.6 ng/ml (5.5 nmol/L) usually are reflected by virilization. Although virilized female patients with androgen-producing adrenal and ovarian tumors generally have serum testosterone levels higher than 2.5 ng/ml (8.7 nmol/L), some patients have been reported who have serum concentrations less than this value (Muechler, 1978).

Free serum testosterone measurements correlate better with biological activity than does total testosterone. Many indirect methods have been used whereby free testosterone is estimated as the product of total serum concentration and the fraction of testosterone free in serum, but most of these methods have one or more shortcomings. The most commonly reported methods involve equilibrium dialysis or ultrafiltration. A typical range of free testosterone concentrations in healthy individuals as found by Moll (1981) are 1.5 to 11.4 pg/ml (5.2 to 39.5 pmol/L) for menstruating females, and 56 to 240 pg/ml (204 to 832 pmoles/L) for males.

17-KETOSTEROIDS

The 17-ketosteroids (17-KS) are a group of steroid compounds that have a ketone at position C-17 of the steroid nucleus. In women the adrenals secrete almost all of these compounds, whereas in men the adrenals are responsible for two thirds and the testes the remainder. Quantitation of 17-ketosteroids is important because of their androgenic properties. However, not all of the 17-ketosteroids measured are androgens; nor are the most important androgens measured as 17-ketosteroids. For example, androsterone and dehydroepiandrosterone both have androgenic properties and are measured as 17-ketosteroids, whereas etiocholanolone, although measured, does not have androgenic properties. The structures of these compounds are shown at the top of page 341.

Both etiocholanolone and androsterone have saturated B rings and are derived from dehydroepiandrosterone (unsaturated B ring), but differ in that the hydrogen on position 5 is oriented in a different plane. The most potent androgens, testosterone and dihydrotestosterone, are not measured as 17-ketosteroids. Other compounds such as the estrogens, although possessing a ketone group at C-17, are not measured as 17-ketosteroids, because they are removed during the extraction procedure. Most of the 17-ketosteroids are excreted as sulfate or glucuronide conjugates. Measurement of the 17-ketosteroids involve a cleavage of the conjugates with acid prior to extraction, and reaction with m-dinitrobenzene and alcoholic alkali, to produce a reddish purple color with an absorption of 520 nm (Zimmermann reaction). This reaction is pictured at the bottom of page 341.

When a keto group occurs on another carbon such as the 3-keto group in progesterone, a less intense color with a different absorption maximum occurs with the Zimmermann reaction.

Because of the interference by other chromogens, a variety of approaches have been used to improve the specificity of the 17-ketosteroid determination. Extractions which remove interfering chromogens have been used, but a more common approach has been the use of a mathematical formula relating to the different wavelengths near the absorption peak (Allen correction) to eliminate this problem. A variety of drugs have been reported which either spuriously increase or decrease 17-ketosteroid values, including carbamazepine, cephalothin, and tiaprofenic acid (Nahoul, 1979).

The reference values for 17-ketosteroids are 6 to 15 mg/24 hours (20.7 to 51.9 μmol/day) and 8 to 20 mg/24 hours (27.7 to 69.2 μmol/day) in women and men, respectively. In children who have not undergone puberty, reference values are much lower, usually less than 3 mg/24 hours (10.4 μmol/day) and gradually increasing until puberty. Elevated urine 17-ketosteroids are associated with some adrenal, testicular, and ovarian tumors, Cushing's syndrome, some congenital adrenal hyperplasia syndromes (see p. 327), and pregnancy. Decreased 17-ketosteroids occur after adrenalectomy or castration and in Addison's disease, nephrotic syndrome, and hypothyroidism.

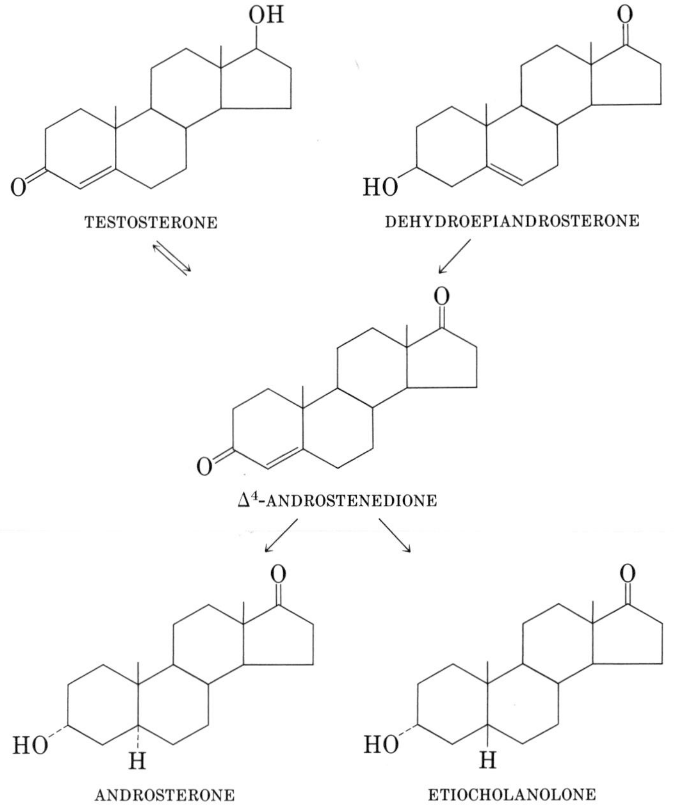

TESTOSTERONE

DEHYDROEPIANDROSTERONE

Δ^4-ANDROSTENEDIONE

ANDROSTERONE

ETIOCHOLANOLONE

2

The principal contribution to 17-ketosteroids is from dehydroepiandrosterone sulfate (DHEA-sulfate) which occurs in healthy individuals in concentrations of between 0.5 and 2.8 μg/ml (1.7 and 9.7 μmol/L). Some believe assay of serum DHEA-sulfate is a more reliable indicator of adrenal androgen secretion than the 24-hour urinary 17-ketosteroids (Lobo, 1981).

THE EICOSANOIDS (PROSTAGLANDINS AND LEUKOTRIENES)

Certain polyunsaturated fatty acids such as arachidonate are oxidized by cyclo- and lipoxygenases to yield a cascade of products (Fig. 16–15). The products include prostaglandins (PG), thromboxane A_2, prostacyclin, and the leukotrienes (LK), all of which are potent intercellular and intracellular chemical transmitters that mediate a variety of physiological and pathological functions. The cyclooxygenase enzyme, which is blocked by aspirin, yields prostaglandins E_2, D_2, and $F_{2\alpha}$ as well as prostacyclin (PGI_2) and thromboxane (TXA_2). The 5′ lipoxygenase enzyme forms a leukotriene (LTA_4), which yields the highly potent chemotactic factor LTB_4 on the one hand and LTC_4, LTD_4, and LTE_4 on the other. These products are powerful bronchoconstrictors. They are derived by LTA_4 combining with glutathione. Collectively the leukotrienes constitute SRS-A (slow reacting substance of anaphylaxis).

Specific and nonspecific stimulation releases arachidonate (Fig. 16–15). The initial step is release of Ca^{++}, which activates acyl hydrolases. The release mechanism is blocked by corticosteroids. The nature of the products formed depends upon the tissue source. For example, platelets mainly synthesize thromboxane, whereas endothelial cells synthesize prostacyclin. In contrast, human peritoneal macrophages synthesize most of the products.

The physiological role of the eicosanoids is to preserve homeostasis. Prostacyclin and PGE_2 appear

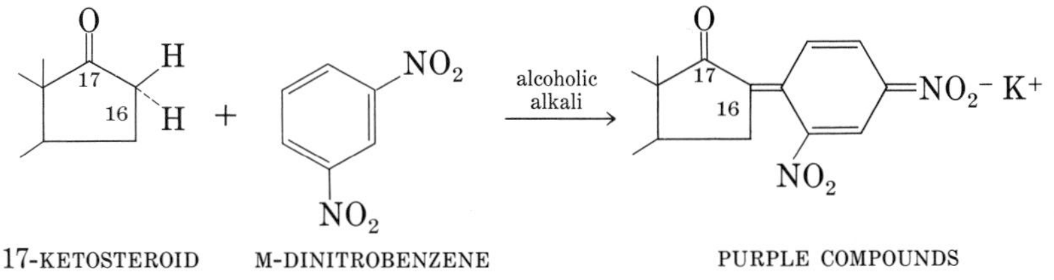

17-KETOSTEROID + M-DINITROBENZENE $\xrightarrow{\text{alcoholic alkali}}$ PURPLE COMPOUNDS

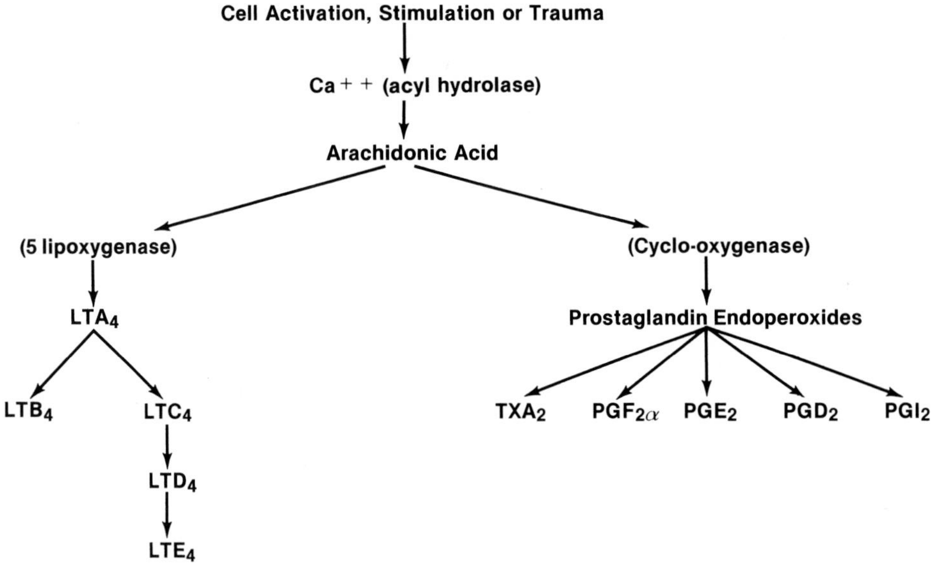

Figure 16–15. Leukotriene and prostaglandin metabolites of arachidonic acid.

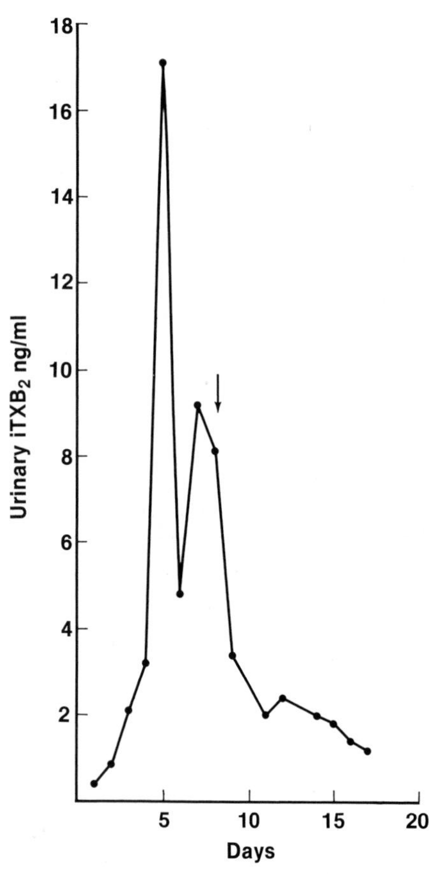

Figure 16–16. Daily levels of urinary i-thromboxane B_2 in a kidney transplant patient in whom a deep venous thrombosis was diagnosed on day 8 (arrow). The patient had subjective symptoms on day 5 (peak level of i-TXB_2). Normal level in kidney transplant patients without rejection is 0.54 ± 0.04 (S.E.M.) ng/ml urine.

to be cytoprotective in the stomach and vessels, as well as most cells. Trauma of any kind provokes the release of large amounts of arachidonate, which is then readily oxygenated. During this process highly destructive free radicals are generated. In addition, some of the arachidonate products generated mediate the four cardinal signs of inflammation. In addition to physiological and pathological roles, some prostaglandins are being developed for therapeutic purposes for treating ulcers, inducing delivery, and treating peripheral vascular disease.

Diagnostic methods are still in their infancy. Urinary analysis may prove a useful starting point. Urinary i-TXB_2 (immunothromboxane B_2) appears to be an immunological indicator of renal allograft rejection and is markedly elevated in deep venous thrombosis. Excessive PGE_2 production mediates hypercalcemia produced by certain solid tumors, and overproduction of PGD_2 occurs in patients with mastocytosis. Elevated excretion of prostaglandins also is observed in Bartter's syndrome and in patients with watery diarrhea associated with medullary thyroid carcinoma. Since most tissues have the ability to synthesize prostaglandins and many drugs modify arachidonate metabolism, caution must be exercised in interpreting assay results.

Abraham, G. E., Maroulis, G. B., Boyers, S. P., Buster, J. E., Magyar, D. M., and Elsner, C. W.: Dexamethasone suppression test in the management of hyperandrogenized patients. Obstet. Gynecol., *57*:158, 1981.

Abraham, G. E., Maroulis, G. B., and Marshall, J. R.: Evaluation of ovulation and corpus luteum function using measurements of plasma progesterone. Obstet. Gynecol., *44*:522, 1974.

Abuid, J., Klein, A. H., Foley, T. P. and Larson, P. R.: Total and free triiodothyronine and thyroxine in early infancy. J. Clin. Endocrinol. Metab., *39*:263, 1974.

Arisue, K., Katayama, Y., Ogawa, Z., Hayashi, C., Miyata, M., Shimada, K., and Nambara, T.: Mechanism for interference of carbamazepine in Porter-Silber reaction for determination of urinary 17-hydroxycorticosteroids. Chem. Pharm. Bull., *12*:3093, 1976.

Ashcraft, M. W. and Van Herle, A. J.: The comparative value of serum thyroglobulin measurements in iodine 131 total body scans in the follow-up study of patients with treated differentiated thyroid cancer. Am. J. Med., *71*:806, 1981.

Ashcraft, M. W., Van Herle, A. J., Vener, S. L., and Geffner, D. L.: Serum cortisol levels in Cushing's syndrome after low- and high-dose dexamethasone suppression. Ann. Intern. Med., 97:21, 1982.

Bigos, S. T., Ridgway, E. C., Kourides, I. A., and Maloof, F.: Spectrum of pituitary alterations with mild and severe thyroid impairment. J. Clin. Endocrinol. Metab., *46*:317, 1978.

Boss, M., Kingstone, D., Chan, M. K., and Varghese, Z.: Contradictory findings in the measurement of free thyroxin after administration of heparin. Clin. Chem., *28*:1238, 1982.

Bravo, E. L., Tarazi, R. C., Fouad, F. M., Vidt, D. G., and Gifford, R. W.: Clonidine-suppression test. A useful aid in the diagnosis of pheochromocytoma. N. Engl. J. Med., *305*:623, 1981.

Bravo, E. L., Tarazi, R. C., Gifford, R. W., and Stewart, B. H.: Circulating and urinary catecholamines in pheochromocytoma. Diagnostic and pathophysiologic implications. N. Engl. J. Med., *301*:682, 1979.

Brown, J. B., MacLeod, S. C., MacNaughtan, C., Smith, M. A., and Symyth, B.: A rapid method for estimating oestrogens in urine using semi-automatic extractor. J. Endocrinol., *42*:5, 1968.

Brown, M. J., Jenner, D. A., Allison, D. J., Lewis, P. J., and Dollery, C. T.: Increased sensitivity and accuracy of phaeochromocytoma diagnosis achieved by use of plasma adrenaline estimations and a pentolinium suppression test. Lancet, *1*:174, 1981.

Brunner, H. R., Laragh, J. H., Baer, L., Newton, M. A., Goodwin, F. T., Krakoff, L. R., Band, R. H., and Buhler, F. R.: Essential hypertension: Renin and aldosterone, heart attack and stroke. N. Engl. J. Med., *286*:441, 1972.

Burger, H. G., and Patel, Y. C.: Thyrotrophin releasing hormone—TSH. Clin. Endocrinol. Metab., *6*:83, 1977.

Burman, K. D., Read, J., Dimond, R. C., Strum, D., Wright, F. D., Patow, W., Earll, J. M., and Wartofsky, L.: Measurement of 3,3′, 5′-triiodothyronine (reverse T_3), 3,3′-1-diiodothyronine, T_3 and T_4 in human amniotic fluid and in cord and maternal serum. J. Clin. Endocrinol. Metab., *43*:1351, 1976.

Byyny, R. L.: Withdrawal from glucocorticoid therapy. N. Engl. J. Med., *295*:30, 1976.

Carroll, B. J., Feinberg, M., Greden, J. F., Tarika, J., Albala, A. A., Haskett, M. B., James, N. M., Kronfol, Z., Lohr, N., Steiner, M., de Vigne, J. P., and Young, E.: A specific laboratory test for the diagnosis of melancholia. Standardization, validation, and clinical utility. Arch. Gen. Psychiatry, *38*:15, 1981.

Carter, J. N., Tyson, J. E., Tolis, G., VanVliet, S., Faiman, C., and Friesen, H. G.: Prolactin-secreting tumors and hypogonadism in 22 men. N. Engl. J. Med., *299*:847, 1978.

Cavalieri, R. R., and Pitt-Rivers, R.: The effects of drugs on the distribution and metabolism of thyroid hormones. Pharmacol. Rev., *33*:55, 1981.

Chopra, I. J., Solomon, D. H., Hepner, G. W., and Morgenstein, A. A.: Misleadingly low free thyroxine index and usefulness of reverse triiodothyronine measurement in nonthyroidal illness. Ann. Intern. Med., *90*:905, 1979.

Chrètien, M., Seidah, N. G., Benjannet, S., Dragon, N., Routhier, R., Motomatsu, T., Crine, P., and Lis, M.: A βLPH precursor model: Recent developments concerning morphine-like substances. Ann. N.Y. Acad. Sci., *297*:84, 1977.

Clemmons, D. R., van Wyk, J. J., Ridgway, E. C., Kliman, B., Kjellberg, R. N., and Underwood, L. E.: Evaluation of acromegaly by radioimmunoassay of somatomedin-C. N. Engl. J. Med., *301*:1138, 1979.

Collu, R., Brun, G., Milsant, F., Leboeuf, G., Letarte, J., and Ducharme, J-R.: Reevaluation of levodopa-propranolol as a test of growth hormone reserve in children. Pediatrics, *61*:242, 1978.

Cowden, E. A., Thomson, J. A., Doyle, D., Ratcliffe, J. G., MacPherson, P., and Teasdale, G. M.: Tests of prolactin secretion in diagnosis of prolactinomas. Lancet, *1*:1155, 1979.

Crapo, L.: Cushing's syndrome: A review of diagnostic tests. Metabolism, *28*:955, 1979.

Dana-Haeri, J., Oxley, J., and Richens, A.: Reduction of free testosterone by antiepileptic drugs. Br. Med. J., *1*:85, 1982.

Daughaday, W. H.: New criteria for evaluation of acromegaly. N. Engl. J. Med., *301*:1175, 1979.

Davies, T. F.: Autoantibodies to the human thyrotropin receptor are not species specific. J. Clin. Endocrinol. Metab., *52*:426, 1981.

Dean, H. J., Kellett, J. G., Bola, R. M., Guyda, H. J., Baumick, B., Posner, B. I., and Friesen, H. G.: The effect of growth hormone treatment on somatomedin levels in growth hormone–deficient children. J. Clin. Endocrinol. Metab., *55*:1167, 1982.

Dluhy, R. G.: Diagnosis and treatment of adrenocortical insufficiency. *In* Rose, L. I., and Lavine, R. L. (eds): The Thirty-ninth Hahnemann Endocrinology-Metabolism Symposium. New York, Grune and Stratton, 1976.

Editorial: Growth-hormone-releasing factor. Lancet, *2*:143, 1983.

Editorial: Prediction of relapse of hyperthyroidism. Lancet, *1*:1393, 1980.

Edwards, C. R. W.: Vasopressin and oxytocin in health and disease. Clin. Endocrinol. Metab., *6*:223, 1977.

Engelman, K.: Pheochromocytoma. Clin. Endocrinol. Metab., *6*:769, 1977.

Feldman, J. M., Butler, S. S., and Chapman, B. A.: Interference with measurement of 3-methoxy-4-hydroxylmandelic acid and 5-hydroxyindoleacetic acid by reducing metabolites. Clin. Chem., *20*:607, 1974.

Fisher, D. A., and Klein, A. H.: Thyroid development and disorders of thyroid function in the newborn. N. Engl. J. Med., *304*:702, 1981.

Flückiger, E., del Pozo, E., and von Werder, K.: Prolactin. Physiology, Pharmacology and Clinical Findings. Berlin, Springer-Verlag, 1982.

Foegh, M. L., Winchester, J. F., Zmudka, M., Helfrich, G. B., Cooley, C., Ramwell, P. W., and Schreiner, G. E.: Urine i-TXB_2 in renal allograft rejection. Lancet, *2*:431, 1981.

Franchimont, P., Valcke, J. C., and Lambotte, R.: Female gonadal dysfunction. Clin. Endocrinol. Metab., *3*:533, 1974.

Gardner, D. F., Carithers, R. L., and Utiger, R. D.: Thyroid function tests in patients with acute and resolved hepatitis B virus infection. Ann. Intern. Med., *96*:450, 1982.

Gifford, R. W.: Is the renin-sodium profile helpful in evaluating hypertension? J.A.M.A. 244:35, 1980.

Gitlow, S. E., Mendlowitz, M., and Bertani, L. M.: The biochemical techniques for detecting and establishing the presence of a pheochromocytoma. Am. J. Cardiol., *26*:270, 1970.

Gitlow, S. E., Mendlowitz, M., Wilk, E. K., Wilk, S., Wolf, R. L., and Bertani, L. M.: Excretion of catecholamine catabolites by normal children. J. Lab. Clin. Med., *72*:612, 1968.

Gold, E. M.: The Cushing syndromes: Changing views of diagnosis and treatment. Ann. Intern. Med., *90*:829, 1979.

Gwirtsman, H., Gerner, R. H., and Sternbach, H.: The overnight dexamethasone suppression test: Clinical and theoretical review. J. Clin. Psychiatry, *43*:321, 1982.

Hamilton, B. P., Landsberg, L., and Levine, R. J.: Measurement of urinary epinephrine in screening for pheochromocytoma in multiple endocrine neoplasia type II. Am. J. Med., *65*:1027, 1978.

Hoffman, D. P., Surks, M. I., Oppenheimer, J. H., and Weitzman, E. D.: Response to thyrotropin releasing hormone: An objective criterion for the adequacy of thyrotropin suppression therapy. J. Clin. Endocrinol. Metab., *44*:892, 1977.

Horton, R.: Aldosterone: Review of its physiology and diagnostic aspects of primary aldosteronism. Metabolism, *22*:1525, 1973.

Howanitz, J. H., and Howanitz, P. J.: Disorders of the endocrine system. Clin. Lab. Med., *1*:399, 1981.

Hunter, W. M.: Growth hormone. *In* Loraine, J. A., and Bell, E. T. (eds.): Hormone Assays and Their Clinical Application. Edinburgh, Churchill Livingstone, 1976.

Jackson, I. M. D.: Thyrotropin-releasing hormone. N. Engl. J. Med., *306*:145, 1982.

Jeffcoate, S. L.: Diagnosis of hyperprolactinaemia. Lancet, *2*:1245, 1978.

Juan, D.: Pheochromocytoma: Clinical manifestations and diagnostic tests. Urology, *27*:1, 1981.

Jubiz, W., and Nolan, G.: N-Ethylmaleimide prevents destruction of corticotropin (ACTH) in plasma. Clin. Chem., *24*:826, 1978.

Kaplan, N. M., Kem, D. C., Holand, O. B., Kramer, N. J., Higgins, J., and Gomez-Sanchez, C.: The intravenous furosemide test: A simple way to evaluate renin responsiveness. Ann. Intern. Med., *84*:639, 1976.

Kaptein, E. M., MacIntyre, S. S., Weiner, J. M., Spencer, C. A., and Nicoloff, J. T.: Free thyroxine estimates in nonthyroidal illness: Comparison of eight methods. J. Clin. Endocrinol Metab., *52*:1073, 1981.

Kleinberg, D. L., Noel, G. L., and Frantz, A. G.: Galactorrhea: A study of 235 cases, including 48 with pituitary tumors. N. Engl. J. Med., *296*:589, 1977.

Knight, J. A., Fronk, S., and Haymond, R. E.: Chemical basis and specificity of chemical screening tests for urinary vanilmandelic acid. Clin. Chem., *21*:130, 1975.

Kopin, I. J.: Catecholamine metabolism. Clin. Endocrinol. Metab., *6*:525, 1977.

Krakoff, L., Nicolis, G., and Amsel, B.: Pathogenesis of hypertension in Cushing's syndrome. Am. J. Med., *58*:216, 1975.

Krieger, D. T.: Diagnosis and management of Cushing's syndrome. 28th Postgraduate Assembly of the Endocrine Society. Syllabus, Bethesda, Maryland, 1976.

Krieger, D. T.: Regulation of circadian periodicity of plasma ACTH levels. Ann. N.Y. Acad. Sci., *297*:561, 1977.

Krieger, D. T., Allen, W., Rizzo, F., and Krieger, H. P.: Characterization of the normal temporal pattern of plasma corticosteroid levels. J. Clin. Endocrinol. Metab., *32*:266, 1971.

Lamberg, B. A., and Gordin, A.: Abnormalities of thyrotropin secretion and clinical implications of the thyrotropin releasing hormone stimulation test. Ann. Clin. Res., *10*:171, 1978.

Laragh, J. H., Baer, L., Brunner, H. R., Buhler, F. R., Sealey, J. E., and Vaughan, E. D.: Renin, angiotensin and aldosterone system in pathogenesis and management of hypertensive vascular disease. Am. J. Med., *52*:633, 1972.

Laron, Z., Pertzelon, A., and Mannheimer, A.: Genetic pituitary dwarfism with high serum concentration of growth hormone: A new inborn error of metabolism? Isr. J. Med. Sci., *2*:152, 1966.

Larsen, P. R.: Tests of thyroid function. Med. Clin. North Am., *59*:1063, 1975.

Lindholm, J., Kehlet, H., Blichert-Toft, M., Dinesen, B., and Riishede, J.: Reliability of the 30-minute ACTH test in assessing hypothalamic-pituitary-adrenal function. J. Clin. Endocrinol. Metab., *47*:272, 1978.

Lobo, R. A., Paul, W. L., and Goebelsmann, U.: Dehydroepiandrosterone sulfate as an indicator of adrenal androgen function. Obstet. Gynecol., *57*:69, 1981.

Lorenz, L., Ridgway, C. E., and Malouf, F.: Hospital lab reports lower TSH normals. Lig. Quart., *2*:12, 1979.

Mariotti, S., Martino, E., Cupini, C., Lari, R., Giani, C., Baschieri, L., and Pinchera, A.: Low serum thyroglobulin as a clue to the diagnosis of thyrotoxicosis factitia. N. Engl. J. Med., *307*:410, 1982.

McKee, J. I., and Finlay, W. E. I.: Cortisol replacement in severely stressed patients. Lancet, *1*:484, 1983.

Mell, L. D., and Gustafson, A. B.: Urinary free norepinephrine and dopamine determined by reverse-phase high pressure liquid chromatography. Clin. Chem., *23*:473, 1977.

Merimee, T. J., Zapf, J., and Froesch, E. R.: Dwarfism in the pygmy. An isolated deficiency of insulin-like growth factor I. N. Engl. J. Med., *305*:965, 1981.

Molitch, M. E., and Reichlin, S.: The amenorrhea, galactorrhea and hyperprolactinemia syndromes. *In* Stollerman, G. H. (ed.): Advances in Internal Medicine. Chicago, Year Book Medical Publishers, 1980.

Molitch, M. E., Schwartz, S., and Mukherji, B.: Is prolactin secreted ectopically? Am. J. Med., *70*:803, 1981.

Moll, G. W., Rosenfield, R. L., and Helke, J. H.: Estradiol-testosterone binding interactions and free plasma estradiol under physiological conditions. J. Clin. Endocrinol. Metab., *52*:868, 1981.

Moses, A. M., Miller, M., and Streeten, D. H. P.: Pathophysiologic and pharmacologic alterations in the release and action of ADH. Metabolism, *25*:697, 1976.

Moskowitz, M. A.: Diseases of the autonomic nervous system. Clin. Endocrinol. Metab., *6*:745, 1977.

Muechler, E. K., Grove, S., and Kohler, D.: Steroid hormones in ovarian vein and cyst fluid of a virilizing stromal tumor. Obstet. Gynecol., *52*:609, 1978.

Murphy, B. E. P.: Some studies on the protein binding of steroids and their applications to the routine micro and ultramicro measurement of various steroids in body fluids by competitive protein-binding radioassay. J. Clin. Endocrinol. Metab., *27*:973, 1967.

Murphy, B. E. P., Okouneff, L. M., Klein, G. P., and Ngo, S. C.: Lack of specificity of cortisol determinations in human urine. J. Clin. Endocrinol. Metab., *53*:91, 1981.

Nahoul, K., Dehennin, L., and Scholler, R.: Interference of tiaprofenic acid in Zimmermann reaction. J. Steroid Biochem., *10*:471, 1979.

New, M. I., and Levine, L. S.: Congenital adrenal hyperplasia. Clin. Biochem., *14*:258, 1981.

Nolan, G. E., Smith, J. B., Chavre, V. J., and Jubiz, W.: Spurious overestimation of plasma cortisol in patients with chronic renal failure. J. Clin. Endocrinol. Metab., *52*:1242, 1981.

Orth, D. N., and Nicholson, W. E.: Different molecular forms of ACTH. Ann. N.Y. Acad. Sci., *297*:27, 1977.

Pang, S., Murphey, W., Levine, L. S., Spence, D. A., Leon, A., LaFranchi, S., Surve, A. S., and New, M. I.: A pilot newborn screening for congenital adrenal hyperplasia in Alaska. J. Clin. Endocrinol. Metab., *55*:413, 1982.

Pearson, O. H., Arafah, B., and Brodkey, J.: Management of acromegaly. Ann. Intern. Med., *95*:225, 1981.

Pekary, A. E., Hershman, J. M., and Parlow, A. F.: A sensitive and precise radioimmunoassay for human thyroid stimulating hormone. J. Clin. Endocrinol. Metab., *41*:676, 1975.

Perez, C., Novoa, J., Alcañiz, J., Salto, L., and Barcelo, B.: Leydig cell tumour of the testis with gynaecomastia and elevated oestrogen, progesterone and prolactin levels: Case report. Clin. Endocrinol., *13*:409, 1980.

Phillips, L. S., and Vassilopoulou-Sellin, R.: Somatomedins (second of two parts). N. Engl. J. Med., *302*:438, 1980.

Porter, C. C., and Silber, R. H.: A quantitative color reaction for cortisone and related 17,21-dihydroxy-20-ketosteroids. J. Biol. Chem., *185*:201, 1950.

Prinz, P. N., Halter, J., Benedetti, C., and Raskind, M.: Circadian variation of plasma catecholamines in young and old men: Relation to rapid eye movement and slow wave sleep. J. Clin. Endocrinol. Metab., *49*:300, 1979.

Rajatanavin, R., Fournier, L., DeCosimo, D., Abreau, C., and Braverman, L. E.: Elevated serum free thyroxine by thyroxine analog radioimmunoassays in euthyroid patients with familial dysalbuminemic hyperthyroxinemia. Ann. Intern. Med., *97*:865, 1982.

Rayfield, E. J., Cain, J. P., Casey, M. P., Williams, G. H., and Sullivan, J. M.: Influence of diet on urinary VMA excretion. J.A.M.A. *221*:704, 1972.

Roger, M., Grenier, J., Houlbert, C., Castanier, M., Feinstein, M.-C., and Scholler, R.: Rapid radioimmunoassays of plasma LH and estradiol-17β for the prediction of ovulation. J. Steroid Biochem., *12*:403, 1980.

Rogol, A. D., and Eastman, R. C.: Prolactin and pituitary tumors. Am. J. Med., *66*:547, 1979.

Rohrbach, M. S., and DeRemee, R. A.: Measurement of angiotensin converting enzyme activity in serum in the diagnosis and management of sarcoidosis. Clin. Lab. Annu., *1*:435, 1982.

Rose, L. I., Williams, G. H., Jagger, P. I., and Lauler, D. P.: The 48-hour adrenocorticotrophin infusion test for adrenocorticol insufficiency. Ann. Intern. Med., *73*:49, 1970.

Rosenfeld, D. L., Chudow, S., and Bronson, R. A.: Diagnosis of luteal phase inadequacy. Obstet. Gynecol., *56*:193, 1980.

Rudman, D., Kutner, M. H., Blackston, R. D., Cushman, R. A., Bain, R. P., and Patterson, J. H.: Children with normal-variant short stature: Treatment with human growth hormone for six months. N. Engl. J. Med., *305*:123, 1981.

Ruiz, M., Rajatanavin, R., Young, R. A., Taylor, C., Brown, R., Braverman, L. E., and Ingbar, S. H.: Familial dyalbuminemic hyperthyroxinemia. A syndrome that can be confused with thyrotoxicosis. N. Engl. J. Med., *306*:635, 1982.

Saberi, M., and Utiger, R. D.: Serum thyroid hormone and thyrotropin concentrations during thyroxine and triiodothyronine therapy. J. Clin. Endocrinol. Metab., *39*:923, 1974.

Samuelsson, B., Paoletti, R., and Ramwell, P. W. (eds.): Advances in Prostaglandin, Thromboxane and Leukotriene Research, Vols. 11 and 12. Fifth International Prostaglandin Conference. New York, Raven Press, 1983.

Schally, A. V., Kastin, A. J., and Arimura, A.: Hypothalamic hormones: A link between brain and body. Am. Sci., *65*:712, 1977.

Schöneshöfer, M., Fenner, A., Altinok, G., and Dulce, H. J.: Specific and practicable assessment of urinary free cortisol by combination of automatic high-pressure liquid chromatography and radioimmunoassay. Clin. Chim. Acta, *106*:63, 1980.

Schuster, L. D., Bantle, J. P., Oppenheimer, J. H., and Seljeskog, E. L.: Acromegaly: Reassessment of the long-term therapeutic effectiveness of transsphenoidal pituitary surgery. Ann. Intern. Med., *95*:172, 1981.

Seeger, R. C., Siegel, S. E., and Sidell, N.: Neuroblastoma: Clinical perspectives, monoclonal antibodies, and retinoic acid. Ann. Intern. Med., *97*:873, 1982.

Sharp, A. M., Fraser, I. S., Robertson, S., and Turtle, J. R.: Positive interference by danazol in a testosterone radioimmunoassay kit procedure. Clin. Chem., *27*:603, 1981.

Sindler, B. H., Griffing, G. T., and Melby, J. C.: The superiority of the metyrapone test versus the high-dose dexamethasone test in the differential diagnosis of Cushing's syndrome. Am. J. Med., *74*:657, 1983.

Slag, M. F., Morley, J. E., Elson, M. K., Crowson, T. W., Nuttall, F. Q., and Shafer, R. B.: Hypothyroxinemia in critically ill patients as a predictor of high mortality. J.A.M.A., *245*:43, 1981.

Snyder, P. J., Bigdeli, H., Gardner, D. F., Mihailovic, V., Rudenstein, R. S., Sterling, F. H., and Utiger, R. D.: Gonadal function in fifty men with untreated pituitary adenomas. J. Clin. Endocrinol. Metab., *48*:309, 1979.

Solomon, D. H., Benotti, J., DeGroot, L. J., Greer, M. A., Oppenheimer, J. A., Pileggi, V. J., Robbins, J., Selenkow, H. A., Sterling, K., and Volpe, R.: Letter to the editor: Revised nomenclature for tests of thyroid hormones in serum. J. Clin. Endocrinol. Metab., *42*:595, 1976.

Sterling, K., and Lazarus, J. H.: The thyroid and its control. Annu. Rev. Physiol., *39*:349, 1977.

Stern, P., and Valtin, H.: Verney was right, but. . . . N. Engl. J. Med., *305*:1581, 1981.

Strakosch, C. R., Wenzel, B. E., Row, V. V., and Volpé, R.: Immunology of autoimmune thyroid diseases. N. Engl. J. Med., *307*:1499, 1982.

Streeten, D. H. P., Anderson, G. H., Freiberg, J. M., and Dalakos, T. G.: Angiotensin II blockade in the hypertensive patient. Hosp. Pract., *10*:83, 1975.

Streeten, D. H. P., Dalakos, T. G., and Anderson, G. H.: Diagnosis and treatment of Cushing's syndrome. *In* Rose, L. I., and Lavine, R. L. (eds.): The Thirty-ninth Hahnemann Endocrinology-Metabolism Symposium. New York, Grune and Stratton, 1976.

Streeten, D. H. P., Tomycz, N., and Anderson, G. H.: Reliability of screening methods for the diagnosis of primary aldosteronism. Am. J. Med., *67*:403, 1979.

Taymor, M. L.: The use of luteinizing-hormone–releasing hormone in gynecology. Obstet. Gynecol. Annu., 7:285, 1979.

Utiger, R. D.: Increased extrathyroidal triiodothyronine production in nonthyroidal illness: Benefit or harm? Am. J. Med., *69*:807, 1980.

van Wyk, J. J., and Underwood, L. E.: Growth hormone, somatomedins, and growth failure. *In* Kreiger, D. T., and Hughes, J. C. (eds.): Neuroendocrinology. Sunderland, Mass., Sinauer Assoc. Inc., 1980.

Walsh, P. C.: Endocrine evaluation of the infertile male. *In* Amelar, R. D., Dubin, L., and Walsh, P. C. (eds.): Male infertility. Philadelphia, W. B. Saunders Company, 1977.

Weitzman, E. D.: Circadian rhythms and episodic hormone secretion in man. Annu. Rev. Med., *27*:225, 1976.

Wellby, M. L., Guthrie, L., and Reilly, C. P.: Evaluation of a new free-thyroxin assay. Clin. Chem., *27*:2022, 1981.

Wenzel, K. W.: Pharmacological interference with in vitro tests of thyroid function. Metabolism, *30*:717, 1981.

West, C. D., and Dolman, L. I.: Plasma ACTH radioimmunoassays in the diagnosis of pituitary-adrenal dysfunction. Ann. N.Y. Acad. Sci., *297*:205, 1977.

Zachmann, M., Tassinari, D., and Prader, A.: Clinical and biochemical variability of congenital adrenal hyperplasia due to 11β-hydroxylase deficiency. A study of 25 patients. J. Clin. Endocrinol. Metab., *56*:222, 1983.

Zadik, Z., de Lacerda, L., de Carmargo, L. A. H., Hamilton, B. P., Migeon, C. J., and Kowarski, A. A.: A comparative study of urinary 17-hydroxycorticosteroids, urinary free cortisol, and the integrated concentration of plasma cortisol. J. Clin. Endocrinol. Metab., *51*:1099, 1980.

Zerbe, R. L., and Robertson, G. L.: A comparison of plasma vasopressin measurements with a standard indirect test in the differential diagnosis of polyuria. N. Engl. J. Med., *305*:1539, 1981.

Zerbe, R., Stropes, L., and Robertson, G.: Vasopressin function in the syndrome of inappropriate antidiuresis. Annu. Rev. Med., *31*:315, 1980.

Zweifler, A. J., and Julius, S.: Increased platelet catecholamine content in pheochromocytoma. A diagnostic test in patients with elevated plasma catecholamines. N. Engl. J. Med., *306*:890, 1982.

17

THERAPEUTIC DRUG MONITORING AND TOXICOLOGY

PETER J. HOWANITZ, M.D., and JOAN H. HOWANITZ, M.D.

PHARMACOKINETIC AND PHARMACODYNAMIC PRINCIPLES

Drug dosage regimens necessary for optimal therapeutic effect differ widely among individual patients. Depending on the individual treated, the usual drug dosage may lead to toxicity or lack of efficacy. With some therapeutic agents, such as antihypertensives, the drug dosage may be adjusted depending on the patient's clinical response. In many situations, however, the best dosage schedule of a drug for an individual patient is difficult to determine, because the pharmacologic response cannot be quantitated readily. For some drugs, the intensity of pharmacologic action and severity of side effects correlate better with steady-state concentrations in serum than with daily dosage. Thus serum drug levels may be useful in determining the optimal drug dosage for a given individual.

For a drug to be therapeutically effective, it must reach the site of its intended pharmacologic activity within the body at a sufficient rate and in a sufficient amount to yield an effective concentration. Factors that are important in determining the serum drug concentrations attained and eventually reflected at receptor sites include (1) compliance, (2) bioavailability, (3) drug pharmacokinetics (absorption, distribution, biotransformation, and elimination), (4) physiologic factors, (5) genetic factors, (6) intercurrent disease, and (7) drug interactions. Factors associated with good compliance (taking medications as prescribed) include explanation of reasons for treatment, simplicity of regimen, and monitoring of drug levels. Bioavailability describes the extent and rate at which an active drug reaches the systemic circulation and ultimately the receptors or sites of action.

Absorption

Absorption of drugs from the gastrointestinal tract is a complex process that is subject to many variables, such as pH, gastric emptying time, intestinal transit time, and mesenteric blood flow. When taken with food, drugs usually are absorbed more slowly, and the total amount absorbed may be decreased. Presence of other drugs in the gastrointestinal tract may enhance or decrease absorption. Drug absorption may be altered in patients with gastrointestinal disease; even in healthy volunteers under well-controlled conditions, wide individual differences occur in rates of absorption.

Even when drugs are administered by intramuscular or subcutaneous injection, the rate of absorption varies not only from individual to individual but also from site to site in the same patient. Orally administered drugs traverse the hepatic portal system before reaching the systemic circulation; thus if a drug is extensively cleared by the liver, only a small fraction of it will reach the systemic circulation. This so-called "first pass elimination" occurs with a number of therapeutic agents and is one explanation why an intravenous dose of a drug may give a greater response than an equipotent oral dose. Propranolol is an example of a drug which is removed extensively on the first passage through the liver.

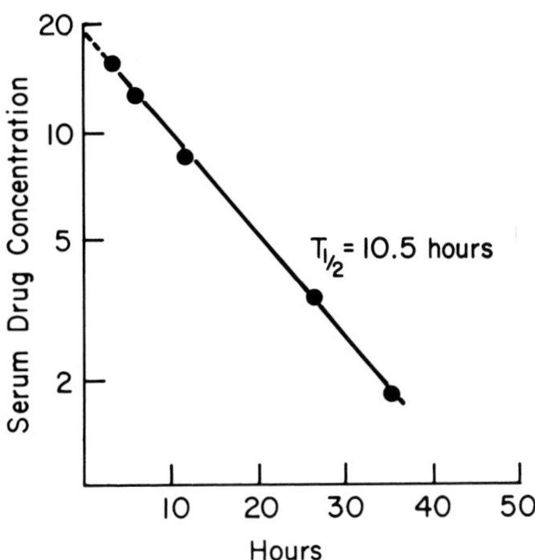

Figure 17–1. Serum concentrations of a drug which is eliminated by a first-order process.

Distribution

After absorption, distribution of a drug will depend largely on its physicochemical properties, including lipid solubility, the extent to which it is ionized, and its molecular size. Often drugs are transported in the blood attached to carrier proteins, albumin being the most important protein for many therapeutic agents. For some drugs other carriers are important; for example, α_1-acid glycoprotein binds cationic drugs such as quinidine and imipramine (Piafsky, 1978). Interaction between serum binding proteins and drugs is reversible, with many drugs existing in the blood in two forms: protein-bound and unbound (free). Presumably only unbound drugs can diffuse into tissues because the drug-protein complex is unable to traverse cell membranes.

Biotransformation and Elimination

Drugs may be divided into water soluble (or polar) compounds and lipid soluble (or nonpolar) compounds. Water soluble drugs are excreted mainly unchanged by the kidney, whereas lipid soluble drugs initially are filtered by the glomerulus and may be fully reabsorbed in the distal nephron. The lipid soluble drugs generally are metabolized to more polar compounds before they are excreted into the urine. Metabolites that are formed are usually, but not always, less active than the parent compound. In some cases, metabolism in the liver is necessary to produce an active metabolite, and sometimes metabolites may account for the toxicity of a drug.

Although the liver is the main site of drug metabolism, other tissues such as lung, kidney, blood, and intestine may metabolize drugs. In general, there are two types of metabolic processes in the liver: one in which more polar groups are introduced into the drug molecule by processes such as oxidation, reduction, or hydrolysis; and the other, a synthetic reaction which involves conjugation of the drug with glucuronic acid, sulfate, glycine, or other groups. Some drugs undergo both types of reactions before being excreted.

Most drugs are eliminated from the body by a process which can be expressed in first-order mathematical terms, that is, elimination is proportional to drug concentration (Van der Kleijn, 1980). When the fraction of drug that is eliminated from the body after a given time is constant, it is meaningful to speak about elimination or serum half-life. If the concentration is plotted on a logarithmic scale versus a linear time scale, a straight line describes the decrease in serum level (Fig. 17–1). The elimination half-life actually depends on both clearance and volume of drug distribution (Greenblatt, 1982). With some drugs, however, zero order kinetics applies; that is, elimination capacity is limited and the drug is eliminated at a constant rate rather than a rate proportional to the amount of remaining drug. When zero order kinetics occurs (for example, with drugs such as phenytoin), the time required for a 50 per cent decrease in initial level increases as the serum drug concentration increases. Clinical use of this type of drug may be difficult because small increments in dose may result in disproportionately large increases in serum levels and result in toxicity (Howanitz, 1981c).

Physiologic Factors

The patient's age has important effects on drug pharmacokinetics; drug elimination is slower in neonates than in adults. During the neonatal period, there is functional immaturity in metabolism and renal excretion of drugs, but the activity of these systems rapidly increases as a function of postnatal age. The time and rate after birth at which adult rates of elimination are achieved vary with the drug and the individual.

Pharmacokinetic changes also have been found in the elderly. Aging is associated with many physiologic alterations, including decreases in cardiac output, renal function, degradative enzyme activity, and density of tissue receptors. In the elderly, serum albumin and lean body mass also tend to decrease. These changes can influence absorption, distribution, metabolism, and excretion of drugs.

Under certain circumstances, such factors as diet, nutrition, environment, and alcohol ingestion can influence drug pharmacokinetics. For example, enhanced metabolism of some drugs occurs with environmental exposure to benzpyrene or with diets containing a high protein-to-carbohydrate ratio.

Genetic Factors

Control of drug metabolism is recognized as an important mechanism by which genetic differences in response to drugs occur. For example, the ability to acetylate drugs in the liver by the N-acetyltransferase system is inherited as an autosomal recessive trait; based on the activity of this enzyme, individuals fall into two groups, fast and slow acetylators. About 45 per cent of the individuals in the United States are fast acetylators. Procainamide, a drug that is acetylated by this enzyme system, is metabolized to an active metabolite N-acetylprocainamide (NAPA). Rapid acetylators have higher serum concentrations of NAPA than do slow acetylators.

Intercurrent Illness or Concomitant Drug Treatment

Important causes of pharmacokinetic alterations are intercurrent illness and the administration of other drugs. For example, in renal insufficiency, there are changes in binding of drugs to plasma proteins, and drugs or drug metabolites may be poorly excreted, thus accumulating in serum. Hepatic disease may influence drug metabolism significantly; for example, decreases in production of serum albumin can lead to decreases in drug binding and rapid increases in free drug levels. Inflammation can cause changes in binding of certain drugs as the result of increases in α_1-acid glycoprotein. Gastrointestinal diseases can alter the rate and amount of drug absorption.

Concomitant administration of more than one drug can lead to a variety of interactions in absorption, distribution, metabolism, and elimination. Antacids have been reported to decrease gastrointestinal tract absorption of digoxin, whereas quinidine causes displacement of digoxin from tissue binding sites and decreases its renal excretion leading to elevated digoxin levels. Drugs that stimulate the microsomal enzyme system in liver will cause increases in metabolism of other drugs that are eliminated from the body by this system.

Table 17–1. PREREQUISITES FOR THERAPEUTIC DRUG MONITORING

The analytical method is specific, sensitive, accurate, and accomplished in an appropriate time frame
The active drug and important metabolites are measured
Development of tolerance at receptor sites does not occur
Concentration of drug in serum is proportional to the concentration of drug at receptor sites
There is reasonably good correlation between serum concentration and therapeutic effects
The therapeutic range is well defined
Proper precautions are taken in interpretation of drug levels

THERAPEUTIC DRUG MONITORING

The therapeutic range of a drug is defined by an upper limit above which adverse effects are likely and a lower limit below which the drug most often is not effective. In general, when serum concentration of a drug exceeds the therapeutic range, the frequency and severity of toxic effects increase. Drug levels below the therapeutic range can exert beneficial effects but are inadequate in most patients, whereas some patients require levels above the therapeutic range for a fully satisfactory response. For drugs, such as digoxin and digitoxin, which have a low therapeutic index (that is, a small difference between median toxic and effective concentrations), therapeutic and toxic ranges can overlap to a significant degree. Also, the effective range of serum concentrations may differ according to the therapeutic goal. Tables 17–1, 17–2, and 17–3 list the prerequisites for therapeutic drug monitoring and situations in which it is useful, as well as precautions necessary in interpretation of values.

If plasma or serum levels are to be indicative of the intensity of the drug's action, it is necessary that equilibrium take place between serum and tissue compartments. With repetitive administration of a drug, serum drug concentrations gradually increase and eventually reach a plateau. When a state of equilibrium between rate of drug administration and rate of elimination is reached, "steady state" is said to exist (Fig. 17–2). When the dosage interval of a

Table 17–2. SITUATIONS IN WHICH THERAPEUTIC DRUG MONITORING MAY BE USEFUL

When:
- there is wide pharmacokinetic variation among individuals
- zero order kinetics apply
- the therapeutic index of a drug is low (small difference between the median toxic and effective concentrations)
- signs of toxicity are difficult to recognize clinically
- physiologic factors are present which may affect drug pharmacokinetics
- intercurrent illness is present which may affect drug pharmacokinetics
- the usual dose does not give expected results
- noncompliance is suspected
- surreptitious use is suspected
- drug interactions are suspected

Table 17–3. PRECAUTIONS IN INTERPRETING SERUM DRUG CONCENTRATIONS

Relationship between times of dosing and sampling must be known and taken into account
Important active metabolites must be measured
Therapeutic goals must be defined clearly
Possible changes in relationship between drug concentration in serum and the site of the action must be considered

drug is equal to the half-life of the drug, four to seven doses are required to reach 95 per cent of the steady state concentration. At steady state, fluctuations in serum drug concentrations that occur reflect the drug's absorption, distribution, and elimination.

Serum drug levels can be used properly only if timing of drug administration and serum sampling is known. The serum half-life of a drug must be sufficiently long that minor differences in timing of specimen collection have only a small effect on interpretation of the results. Even with drugs that have relatively long half-lives, timing of the specimen collection is critical to interpretation of the value. Following administration of a drug, serum concentrations rise, reflecting entry into the circulation. The rise in serum drug concentration is followed by a decrease reflecting an equilibrium phase that occurs as the drug is taken up by tissues (Fig. 17–2). Generally, it is preferable to obtain the specimen at the end of the dosage interval, that is, when equilibrium is complete and serum levels have reached a plateau. By measuring serum levels at the end of the dosage interval, information is obtained about drug elimination; measurement of peak levels gives more information about absorption. The difficulty in attempting to measure peak levels is that sampling at a standard time after dosing often will miss the peak.

Usually total drug concentrations are measured; that is, the methods normally used in measuring serum drug levels do not discriminate between drug molecules that are bound to serum proteins and those that are unbound. Since in most therapeutic situations free drug concentration is a fairly constant percentage of the total, total serum drug levels are indicative of active (free) drug concentrations. However, small changes in binding, especially with drugs that are highly protein bound, cause changes in free drug concentration which result in alteration in pharmacologic effects (Pippenger, 1980).

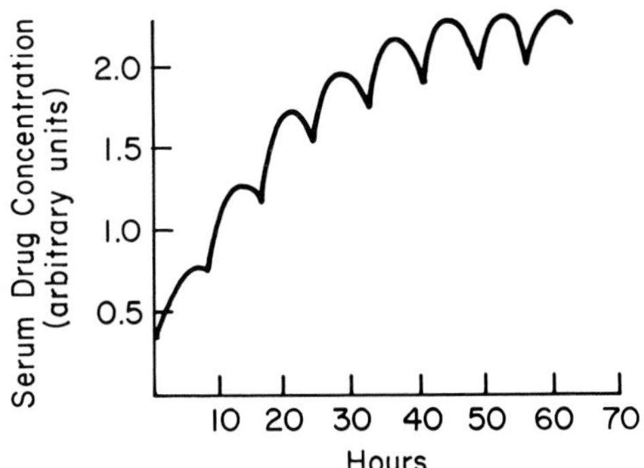

Figure 17–2. The accumulation of drug in the serum after repeated oral dosing.

For a number of therapeutic agents, it has been found that drug transfer between serum and saliva is a passive, pH-dependent process with salivary levels proportional to the concentration of free drug in serum. It has been found that for several drugs, such as phenytoin, salivary levels are a good estimate of the free drug in serum. Although not useful for routine therapeutic drug monitoring, cerebrospinal fluid (CSF) represents an ultrafiltrate of plasma, and thus for many drugs the total CSF drug concentration is essentially the same as free drug concentration in serum.

The serum concentration of a drug in a given patient cannot indicate the intensity of a drug's actions with complete precision under all circumstances; concentration of a drug at the site of action and the degree of tissue responsiveness can affect the relationship between serum concentration and pharmacologic effect. Thus, information about serum levels must always be interpreted in the context of all available clinical information and never applied rigidly or uncritically.

CARDIAC GLYCOSIDES: DIGOXIN AND DIGITOXIN

Cardiac (digitalis) glycosides have the ability to increase the force as well as the velocity of myocardial contraction. They are used in treatment of congestive heart failure and arrhythmias such as atrial fibrillation and atrial flutter. Each cardiac glycoside is a combination of one or more sugars and an aglycone, which is the pharmacologically active residue. Table 17–4 shows a comparison of two commonly prescribed cardiac glycoside preparations, digoxin and digitoxin. Digoxin differs from digitoxin by a hydroxyl group at carbon 12; this results in increased polarity and decreased lipid solubility.

Serum levels of the cardiac glycosides usually are measured by immunoassay; other methods, however, including gas chromatography, are available (Butler, 1972). Most assay procedures employ antiserum with specificity for the aglycone portion of the digitalis molecule. Metabolic breakdown products of the cardiac glycosides that occur in serum and contain intact aglycone thus will react in the immunoassays. In

Table 17–4. COMPARISON OF DIGOXIN AND DIGITOXIN

	Digoxin	Digitoxin
Absorption (%)	60–85	90–100
Serum protein binding (%)	20–30	97
Hepatic metabolism (%)	10	90
Half-life (mean)	35–40 hours	7.6 days
Therapeutic range (serum) ng/ml (nmol/L)	0.5–2.0 (0.6–2.6)	15–25 (19.2–32)

addition, antisera to one digitalis compound may cross-react to some extent with other cardiac glycosides and aglycones. Because of this cross-reactivity, digitalis immunoassays are meaningful only if it is known with certainty which glycoside the patient is receiving. Under certain conditions, for example, in patients with renal insufficiency, metabolites may accumulate in serum. Since it has a higher serum concentration and longer half-life than digoxin, digitoxin may interfere with digoxin assays for up to several weeks after it has been discontinued.

Cardiac glycoside toxicity has a mortality of 5 to 10 per cent, which increases to 20 to 25 per cent with massive overdoses such as occur with suicide attempts. Cardiac manifestations of digitalis toxicity include increasing severity of congestive heart failure and alterations in cardiac rate and rhythm. Acute accidental or suicidal poisoning with digoxin commonly is associated with vomiting, bradycardia, and hyperkalemia.

Factors such as electrolyte abnormalities and types of myocardial disease are associated with increased or decreased sensitivity of myocardium to effects of digitalis glycosides. A variety of drug interactions also have been reported. Absorption of digoxin tends to be enhanced by drugs that decrease gastrointestinal motility and decreased by drugs that increase motility. In addition, compounds such as cholestyramine, Kaopectate, and antacids can interfere with gastrointestinal absorption of digoxin. Concomitant administration of quinidine or verapamil leads to significant increases in serum digoxin concentration. Spironolactone leads to decreased digoxin secretion by the kidney and may interfere with some immunoassays for the drug (Soyka, 1981). Digitoxin is metabolized in the liver to compounds with varying degrees of cardiac activity. Induction of microsomal enzymes by various drugs leads to increased metabolism of digitoxin resulting in increases in dosage requirements. For further information of changes in sensitivity and potential drug interactions with the cardiac glycosides, see Howanitz (1981b).

Digoxin

The major site of digoxin deposition in the body is skeletal muscle, with low concentrations found in fat. The amount of digoxin in heart muscle is approximately 30 times the amount in serum; however, the ratio varies considerably among individuals. Since digoxin is bound to tissue to a high degree, it is not removed effectively by dialysis; in addition, it has been shown that cardiopulmonary bypass and exchange transfusion remove only small amounts from the body.

After oral administration of digoxin, the maximum serum concentration usually occurs within one to two hours (Fig. 17–3). However, in some individuals, absorption takes three to four hours and tissue equilibrium may not be completed until four to six hours. Therefore, it is recommended that blood specimens for serum digoxin levels be collected at least six and preferably eight hours after the last oral dose. Serum plateau levels of digoxin occur 10 to 12 hours after intramuscular administration and two to four hours after intravenous administration.

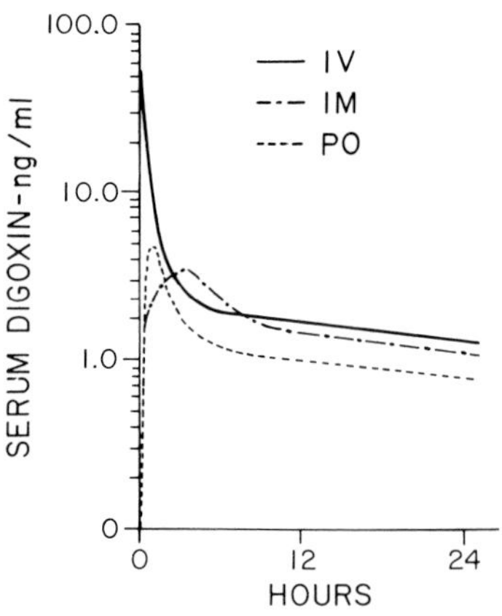

Figure 17–3. Comparative composite serum digoxin levels after oral, intramuscular, and intravenous administration. (Modified from Doherty, J. E., de Soyza, N., Kane, J. J., et al.: Clinical pharmacokinetics of digitalis glycosides. Prog. Cardiovasc. Dis., *21*:141, 1978).

The usual therapeutic range for serum digoxin in adults is 0.5 to 2.0 ng/ml (0.6 to 2.6 nmol/L). In most adult patients with evidence of digoxin toxicity, serum concentrations are $>$ 2 ng/ml (2.6 nmol/L), but some patients have levels in the range 1.4 to 2 ng/ml (1.8 to 2.6 nmol/L). A significant number of non-toxic patients have serum digoxin concentrations $>$2 ng/ml (2.6 nmol/L), usually in the 2 to 4 ng/ml (2.6 to 3.8 nmol/L) range (Butler, 1972). In the presence of supraventricular arrhythmias, some patients require high doses of digitalis to control their cardiac rate; these patients may have serum digoxin concentrations in the range of 2 to 4 ng/ml (2.6 to 5 nmol/L) without evidence of clinical toxicity. It has been reported that erythrocyte digoxin concentrations may be helpful in distinguishing toxic and nontoxic patients (Kawai, 1982).

Although infants have been found to tolerate high digoxin concentrations in serum without developing signs of toxicity, it is unclear if these levels are necessary for adequate inotropic effect. Results of several studies have indicated that, in infants, digoxin concentrations between 2.0 and 3.5 ng/ml (2.6 and 4.5 nmol/L) may or may not be associated with toxicity, but levels $>$3.5 ng/ml (4.5 nmol/L) usually are associated with signs of toxicity (Wettrell, 1977). Some nontoxic infants, however, may have serum digoxin values as high as 5 ng/ml (6.4 nmol/L). In older children, therapeutic values for serum digoxin are similar to those found in adults. Some investigators have suggested that, to avoid toxicity, digoxin dosage schedules in neonates and infants should be adjusted to maintain serum digoxin steady-state concentrations $<$2.0 ng/ml (2.6 nmol/L).

Digitoxin

As with digoxin, there is an overlap between the toxic and therapeutic ranges in patients treated with digitoxin. The therapeutic range for digitoxin generally is considered to be 15 to 25 ng/ml (19.2 to 32 nmol/L). In most adult patients without evidence of toxicity, serum digitoxin concentrations are <30 ng/ml (38.4 nmol/L), whereas most patients with digitoxin intoxication have digitoxin values >25 ng/ml (32 nmol/L). Patients taking digitalis leaf have serum digitoxin concentrations comparable to those taking digitoxin.

Because of the long half-life, differences in serum concentration after various routes of administration are not significant. However, it has been recommended that blood specimens for serum digitoxin levels be collected at least six to eight hours after the last oral or parenteral dose.

ANTIARRHYTHMIC DRUG MONITORING

Antiarrhythmic agents usually are classified based on mechanism of action as seen in Table 17–5. Most antiarrhythmic drugs suppress automaticity in Purkinje fibers as well as increase the effective refractory period in relation to the duration of the action potential. Class I drugs are membrane-stabilizing agents and depress maximal rate of depolarization of the cardiac action potential. These drugs antagonize the fast sodium channels which are responsible for depolarization of the myocardial cell; they exert their effect by slowing the rate of depolarization. Class II agents (β-blockers) are useful because they are antagonists to the action of catecholamines, whereas those in class III increase the depolarization time and the refractory period of the myocardial cell. This increases the duration of the action potential. Class IV agents are antagonists to calcium flux and affect the slow response fibers, sinus node, and atrioventricular node. Antiarrhythmic drugs from the same class are not used together, whereas combinations of drugs from different classes generally have synergistic efficacy.

Disopyramide

Disopyramide phosphate (Norpace), a class I antiarrhythmic agent, reduces the incidence of ventricular and, to a lesser extent, atrial arrhythmias. Disopyramide is N-dealkylated in the liver to form N-desisopropyl disopyramide, which has activity of about 25 per cent of the parent drug. The pharmacokinetic parameters of disopyramide are found in Table 17–6.

The majority of common side effects are related to the drug's anticholinergic properties, the most serious of which is obstructive uropathy occurring in about 5 per cent of patients. Cholestatic jaundice and fasting hypoglycemia have been associated with the drug, and in a pregnant woman disopyramide has been reported to induce uterine contractions. In a series of 100 patients, 16 had manifestations of acute congestive heart failure during disopyramide therapy. If heart failure has occurred at any time in the past, a recurrence may be precipitated by the drug in as many as 50 per cent of patients (Podrid, 1980). In those with no history of congestive heart failure, the likelihood of circulatory failure appears to be less than 5 per cent. Cardiogenic shock and severe arrhythmias also may be precipitated by the drug. The side effects are discussed at length in a review by Morady (1982).

Direct spectrophotometric and spectrofluorometric methods are non-specific because the major metabolite is measured, whereas homogeneous enzyme immunoassay and gas chromatography procedures show little cross-reactivity with this metabolite. High-performance liquid chromatography (HPLC) procedures which measure disopyramide alone or simultaneously with N-desisopropyl disopyramide have been described.

Studies correlating serum levels with clinical effects are few, but present information suggests that serum disopyramide levels of 2 to 5 μg/ml (5.9 to 14.8 μmol/L) represent the therapeutic range. Patients with serum concentrations >7 μg/ml (20.7 μmol/L) have a considerable risk of toxicity. With overdosage, serum levels have been reported as high as 114 μg/ml (336 μmol/L); in these patients, the most common clinical finding is loss of consciousness after an apneic episode. Since levels this elevated are associated with a high fatality rate, charcoal hemoperfusion has been advocated for these patients.

Table 17–5. CLASSIFICATION OF ANTIARRHYTHMIC DRUGS*

Class	Mechanism of Action	Drugs
I	Membrane stabilizing agents Inhibition of fast Na^+ channel Complex action including some inhibition of fast Na^+ channel	Quinidine, disopyramide, procainamide, lidocaine, phenytoin, mexiletene, tocainide
II	β-blocking agents†	Propranolol and other β-blockers
III	Agents widening duration of action potential	Amiodarone, bretylium
IV	Calcium antagonists	Verapamil, nifedipine, diltiazem

*Modified from Singh, 1972.
†Some β-blockers have membrane stabilizing activity.

2

Table 17–6. ANTIARRHYTHMIC DRUGS

	Class	Total Protein Binding (%)	Bound to (Amount)	% Renal Excretion	Elimination Half-Time (Hours)	Active Metabolites	Miscellaneous	Usual Therapeutic Range (SI Units)
Disopyramide	I	Variable (50–90%)	(1) Albumin (10%) (2) α_1-glycoprotein (most)	55	8	N-desisopropyl disopyramide	% free concentration varies in therapeutic range	2–5 μg/ml (5.9–14.8 μmol/L)
Lidocaine	I	70	(1) Albumin (20%) (2) α_1-acid glycoprotein (50%)	10 (maximum)	2 (MEGX: 2) (GX: 10)	(1) Monoethylglycinexylidide (MEGX) (2) Glycinexylidide (GX)	(1) See * (2) MEGX: activity similar to parent (3) GX: 10–26% as potent as parent	1.2–5.5 μg/ml (5.1–23.5 μmol/L)
Procainamide	I	14–23 (NAPA: similar binding)	Albumin	50	3.5 (NAPA: 7–10)	N-acetylprocainamide (NAPA)	NAPA: activity similar to parent compound	Procainamide: 4–8 μg/ml (17–34 μmol/L) Procainamide plus NAPA: 5–20 (or 30) μg/ml
Propranolol	II	85–90	(1) Albumin (2) α_1-acid glycoprotein (75%) (3) Lipoproteins	Negligible	3–6	4-OH propranolol	(1) See * (2) 4-OH propranolol activity similar to parent	50–100 ng/ml (193–386 nmol/L)
Quinidine	I	Variable (80–90)	(1) Albumin (most) (2) α_1-acid glycoprotein (3) Lipoproteins	15–40	2.2–16.2	(1) (3S)-3-Hydroxyquinidine (2) 2-Oxoquinidinone (3) O-Desmethylquinidine	(1) See * (2) Dihydroquinidine occurs in preparations due to manufacturing (activity equivalent to parent) (3) For further information on metabolites see Howanitz (1981a)	2–5 μg/ml (5.9–14.8 μmol/L)

*Contact with rubber stoppers in certain types of blood collection tubes displaces the drug from protein binding sites. For further information, see Howanitz (1981a).

When used with other class I antiarrhythmic drugs, disopyramide toxicity may summate with the toxicity of these agents. Phenytoin and rifampin have been reported to increase the rate of metabolism of disopyramide, resulting in decreased serum disopyramide and increased N-desisopropyl disopyramide levels.

Lidocaine

Lidocaine commonly is used in the prevention of ventricular arrhythmias in patients with acute myocardial infarction. Lidocaine usually is administered parenterally, because about 70 per cent of an oral dose is metabolized during the first passage through the liver.

At usual therapeutic levels, about 70 per cent of lidocaine is bound to serum proteins. Metabolism of lidocaine occurs in the liver mainly to N-dealkylated metabolites such as monoethylglycinexylidide (MEGX) and glycinexylidide (GX), which are pharmacologically active (Table 17–6). MEGX appears to have antiarrhythmic activity similar to that of the parent drug, whereas GX is 10 to 26 per cent as potent (Benowitz, 1978). Usually about 50 per cent of GX is excreted by the kidney; in patients with poor renal function, this metabolite may accumulate.

A variety of methods have been used to determine serum lidocaine levels; HPLC has been used to measure lidocaine and its active metabolites. Rapid generation of serum lidocaine levels can be accomplished by enzyme immunoassay (Lehane, 1979). Generally, serum lidocaine levels correlate well with antiarrhythmic and toxic effects; the usual therapeutic range of lidocaine is considered to be between about 1.2 and 5.5 μg/ml (5.1 and 23.5 μmol/L). Levels of 2.0 to 4.0 μg/ml (8.5 to 17.0 μmol/L) are considered optimal (Salzer, 1981). The minimal effective concentration for suppression of premature ventricular contractions ranges from 0.6 to 2.0 μg/ml (2.6 to 8.5 μmol/L); however, some patients require levels up to 10 μg/ml (42.7 μmol/L) (Benowitz, 1978). Central nervous system toxicity may occur before antiarrhythmic effects have been achieved. Drowsiness and dizziness may occur at lidocaine concentrations >4 μg/ml (17 μmol/L). At levels >9 μg/ml (38.4 μmol/L), convulsions, central nervous system depression, and hypotension may occur, but occasionally similar toxic manifestations may be seen at lower levels.

Increased elimination half-time is seen in elderly patients and in those in whom the drug has been infused longer than 24 hours. Patients in shock show markedly decreased clearances of the drug. Decreased clearance also occurs in patients with liver or heart disease, and in those treated with coadministration of propranolol or cimetidine. Monitoring lidocaine levels is useful in patients in shock, during prolonged (>24 hours) infusion, in patients who are refractory to usual doses, and in patients who have ambiguous signs and symptoms of toxicity (Benowitz, 1978).

Procainamide

Procainamide is an antiarrhythmic agent used to treat both atrial and ventricular cardiac arrhythmias. Side effects include nausea, vomiting, weakness, and mental depression; hypotension and cardiac disturbances, such as ventricular fibrillation, may occur following intravenous administration.

Important features of its pharmcokinetics are seen in Table 17–6. The major metabolite of procainamide is N-acetylprocainamide (NAPA), which has a half-life about two to three times that of procainamide and similar antiarrhythmic activity. It has been shown that there is considerable individual difference in the ratio of NAPA to procainamide in serum. In individuals with the genetic ability to acetylate the drug rapidly, the ratio of NAPA to procainamide in serum has a mean value of 1.8, whereas in those who are slow acetylators the mean is 0.6.

Procainamide and NAPA can be measured by enzyme immunoassay and fluorimetry or determined simultaneously using HPLC. The determination of procainamide and NAPA by HPLC was published in the Proposed Selected Methods section of Clinical Chemistry* (Stearns, 1981). The usual effective serum concentration of procainamide has been reported as 4 to 8 μg/ml (17 to 34 μmol/L) with only an occasional patient showing a better therapeutic response at 8 to 12 μg/ml (34 to 51 μmol/L). At levels >16 μg/ml (68 μmol/L), 40 per cent of patients have minor side effects, whereas 30 per cent have serious cardiovascular toxicity. In most patients, satisfactory clinical response to procainamide therapy is associated with procainamide and NAPA levels that total between about 5 and 20 to 30 μg/ml.

A drug-related systemic lupus erythematosus–like syndrome develops in up to about 30 per cent of patients on long-term procainamide therapy and is associated with the presence of antinuclear antibodies. Studies indicate that the drug-induced lupus syndrome develops in slow acetylators of procainamide after a lower cumulative dose and a shorter period of treatment than in fast acetylators. NAPA appears to cause few or no lupus-like reactions: it has been postulated that acetylation of the aromatic amino group on procainamide prevents induction of the lupus-like syndrome.

Renal insufficiency greatly prolongs the half-life of procainamide, and the accumulation of NAPA is greater than that of procainamide. Impairment of acetylation of procainamide may occur in patients with hepatic disease (Howanitz, 1981a). Co-administration of cimetidine has been reported to prolong the elimination half-life of procainamide by decreasing renal clearance of the drug.

*Although they do not bear the official imprimatur of the American Association for Clinical Chemistry, methods appearing in the Proposed Selected Methods section of Clinical Chemistry are those that seem generally useful and have been checked by several evaluators (see Clin. Chem., *19*:1207, 1973).

Propranolol

Propranolol is a β-adrenegric blocking agent used in treatment of many clinical conditions, including cardiac arrhythmias, angina pectoris, thyrotoxicosis, and hypertension. Propranolol produces most of its important effects, both beneficial and adverse, by blocking the effects of catecholamines at β-adrenergic receptor sites. Adverse effects of propranolol include precipitation of heart failure, bronchospasm, bradycardia, and hypoglycemia. Generalized seizures and intraventricular conduction defects have been reported with overdoses of propranolol, and with severe overdosage death occurs in asystole. When the drug is withdrawn suddenly, adverse effects, including severe angina, ventricular arrhythmias, and myocardial infarction, have been reported. To prevent these effects, Smulyan (1982) has maintained therapeutic serum levels by intravenous infusion in postoperative patients who are unable to take medication orally.

Pharmacologic parameters for propranolol are given in Table 17–6; about 75 per cent of propranolol is bound to α_1-acid glycoprotein at therapeutic levels. Propranolol is metabolized in the liver to a large number of metabolites with the 4-hydroxy (4-OH) propranolol having β-blocking effects similar to that of the parent drug. Liver disease decreases clearance of propranolol.

A variety of techniques are available for measurement of serum propranolol levels, including a fluorometric method (Ambler, 1974). Serum propranolol levels of 50 to 100 ng/ml (193 to 386 nmol/L) at the end of the dosage interval confer a high degree of β-blockade in most patients. These levels have been associated with antiarrhythmic activity. Propranolol levels of 40 to 80 ng/ml (155 to 309 nmol/L) have been shown to be effective in a large percentage of patients with ventricular arrhythmias, but some patients may require levels up to 1000 ng/ml (3860 nmol/L) to abolish ventricular arrhythmias. Although in some patients with ventricular arrhythmias, serum concentrations >100 ng/ml (386 nmol/L) are required to suppress arrhythmias, in other patients levels >100 ng/ml (386 nmol/L) are associated with the recurrence of arrhythmias (Routledge, 1979). Serum propranolol levels of 75 to 100 ng/ml (290 to 386 nmol/L) generally are effective in patients with angina pectoris.

There is increased clearance of propranolol in patients with thyrotoxicosis, and in patients treated with cimetidine there is a reduction in propranolol clearance.

Quinidine

Quinidine, which is the prototype class I antiarrhythmic agent, is used to treat both supraventricular and ventricular cardiac arrhythmias. The most common quinidine side effects are gastrointestinal, whereas the most serious toxicity is manifested by cardiac arrhythmias. Cinchonism, a syndrome characterized by tinnitus, headache, and deafness, and hypersensitivity reactions occur as well.

Pharmacokinetic parameters for quinidine are shown in Table 17–6. Commercial preparations of quinidine contain variable amounts of dihydroquinidine, which has antiarrhythmic activity equivalent to that of quinidine. Both compounds are hydroxylated in liver to form more polar metabolities which are excreted by the kidney. The elimination half-time of quinidine is variable among individuals, ranging from 2.2 to 16.2 hours; this may be due to variability in serum protein binding of the drug.

Therapeutic effectiveness has been reported to be associated with serum quinidine levels of 2 to 5 μg/ml (6.2 to 15.4 μmol/L) as measured by double extraction fluorescence spectrometry technique. Levels measured by homogeneous enzyme immunoassay have been reported to correlate well with the double extraction method. The fluorometric determination of quinidine was published in the Selected Methods section of Clinical Chemistry* (Broussard, 1981); recently the commonly used quinidine methods including fluorescent spectroscopy, liquid chromatography, and homogeneous enzyme immunoassay, have been compared (Drayer, 1981). Since dihydroquinidine is therapeutically active, it is important that methods include measurement of this compound as well as quinidine. Because of variability in the extent to which quinidine metabolites are measured, large method dependent differences in serum quinidine levels occur. Interpreting quinidine levels is complicated by these methodological factors and because the cardiac activity of the metabolites has been incompletely investigated (Howanitz, 1981a). In addition, individuals vary considerably in their levels of unbound quinidine, and thus total quinidine levels must be interpreted cautiously.

Quinidine interacts with a variety of drugs. Coadministration of phenobarbital and phenytoin leads to a shortened quinidine elimination half-time. A two- to three-fold rise occurs with concomitant administration of quinidine and digoxin, whereas co-administration of quinidine and amiodarone apparently leads to increased serum quinidine levels (Tartini, 1982).

ANTICONVULSANTS

Phenytoin

Phenytoin (Dilantin) is the drug of choice for tonic-clonic (grand mal) seizures. It appears to inhibit spread of seizure activity in the motor cortex by stabilizing neurons against hyperexcitability. Phenytoin also exerts stabilizing effects on membranes, which may underlie its effectiveness for relief of pain in neuralgias and its reduction of ventricular ectopic activity in digitalis intoxication.

Absorption of phenytoin from the gastrointestinal tract usually occurs within 3 to 12 hours, but it may be decreased by food or antacids. Since neonates cannot absorb phenytoin for the first few months of life, other anticonvulsants are used in this age group. Slow and

*See footnote on page 353.

erratic absorption following intramuscular injection is probably a consequence of its precipitation in muscle; it has been shown that absorption may occur for up to four or five days after a single intramuscular dose. For those patients who cannot take oral medication, therapeutic phenytoin levels can be maintained by using the intravenous route, but close supervision of the patient is necessary because of potential adverse cardiovascular effects.

Although phenytoin is one of the most thoroughly investigated anticonvulsants, its metabolism still is not elucidated fully. Less than 5 per cent is excreted unchanged in the urine, whereas the remainder is metabolized primarily by the hepatic microsomal enzyme system. About two thirds of the administered dose is hydroxylated, forming para-hydroxyphenylhydantoin (HPPH), which then is conjugated to glucuronide and eliminated in the urinary and biliary tracts. The rate of hydroxylation of phenytoin is dose-dependent at low concentrations. In therapeutic range (15 to 20 μg/ml [59.4 to 79.3 μmol/L]) metabolism becomes independent of the serum concentration, because the hydroxylating system for phenytoin metabolism is saturated. This results in large increases in serum levels with only small increments in dose. About 90 per cent of phenytoin is bound to serum albumin, with the remainder free or unbound (Table 17–7).

Methods of phenytoin analysis include gas chromatography, HPLC, radioimmunoassay, homogeneous enzyme immunoassay, fluoroimmunoassay, fluorescence polarization, and spectrophotometry. Homogeneous enzyme immunoassay values have been reported to overestimate serum phenytoin values by up to 90 per cent in uremia (Burgess, 1981); this is because HPPH glucuronide accumulates and has significant cross-reactivity in the assay. Rapid turnaround time for phenytoin assays are necessitated because both low and high serum levels are associated with lack of seizure control. Over half the laboratories participating in the College of American Pathologists' (CAP) therapeutic drug monitoring in 1982 used homogeneous enzyme immunoassay (CAP, 1982).

The therapeutic range of phenytoin usually is regarded as 10 to 20 μg/ml (39.6 to 79.3 μmol/L). Occasionally, levels of 14 to 20 μg/ml (55.5 to 79.3 μmol/L) are associated with nystagmus on lateral gaze, but this usually is observed with levels >20 μg/ml (79.3 μmol/L). Other signs of intoxication, such as slurred speech and ataxia, develop when serum concentrations approach 30 μg/ml (18.9 μmol/L); mental changes such as somnolence occur at about 40 μg/ml (158.6 μmol/L). At levels >60 μg/ml (237.9 μmol/L), some patients are unable even to sit up. Elderly patients show greater mental changes at a given serum concentration of phenytoin than do younger patients. Paradoxical intoxication has been described in which increased seizure activity occurs as the serum level of phenytoin increases into the toxic range. The therapeutic range for the antiarrhythmic effect of phenytoin appears to be about the same as the therapeutic range for its anticonvulsant effects. About three fourths of responsive arrhythmias are abolished at serum levels of 10 to 18 μg/ml (39.6 to 71.4 μmol/L) (Bigger, 1968).

With decreased serum proteins, differences in quantity of protein-bound and free phenytoin affect the relationship between total serum concentrations and the degree of clinical intoxication. Specimens such as saliva or cerebrospinal fluid are used because these sources represent an estimate of free drug. The therapeutic range for saliva is 1 to 2 μg/ml (4 to 9 μmol/L) (Knott, 1982).

Acetylsalicylic acid (aspirin), sulfisoxazole, phenylbutazone, and chlorothiazide as well as uremia reduce the amount of phenytoin binding to albumin, whereas other drugs known to bind albumin, such as penicillin G or phenobarbital, have little effect on this binding. In about 10 per cent of patients, isoniazid (INH) has been reported to inhibit degradation of phenytoin to HPPH, thereby producing increases in phenytoin concentrations. Patients who genetically are slow in-

Table 17–7. PHARMACOLOGIC PROPERTIES OF SIX ANTIEPILEPTIC DRUGS

	Dosage		Days to Achieve	Serum	Serum Levels		
Drug	*mg/kg*	*mg/day*	**Steady-State Serum Levels**	**Half-Life (Hours)**	***Therapeutic* μg/ml (μmol/L)**	***Toxic* μg/ml (μmol/L)**	**Active Metabolites**
Phenytoin	3–15	—	5–10	24 ± 12	10–20 (39.6–79.3)	20 (79.3)	HPPH†
	—	300–400					
Phenobarbital	2–8	—	14–21	96 ± 12	10–30 (43–129)	40 (172)	Parahydroxy-phenobarbital
	—	180					
Primidone	10–25	—	4–7	12 ± 6	5–12 (23–55)	15 (69)	PEMA‡
	—	750					
Phenobarbital	Derived		14–21	—	—	—	
Ethosuximide	15–40	—	8–10	60 (30 ±)*	40–100 (283–708)	100 (708)	—
	—	1000					
Carbamazepine	15–20	—	2–4	12 ± 3	4–12 (16.9–50.8)	8 (33.8)	10,11 epoxide
	—	1200					
Valproic acid	20–30	1500	2–4	12 ± 3	50–100 (347–693)	100 (693)	

*In children and adolescents.
†Para-hydroxyphenylhydantoin.
‡Phenylethylmalonamide.

Table 17–8. DRUGS THAT ELEVATE SERUM PHENYTOIN LEVELS

Drug	Probability of Significant Elevations of Phenytoin Level
Disulfiram	High
Isoniazid	Moderate
Dicumarol	Low
Chloramphenicol	Low
Chlordiazepoxide hydrochloride or diazepam	Low
Sulfamethizole	–
Phenylbutazone	Low
Sulfaphenazole	?Low
Sulfamethoxazole	Low
Chloropromazine	Low
Chlordiazepoxide	Low
Propoxyphene	Low
Phenobarbital	Low

activators of INH are most susceptible. In addition, elevations in serum phenytoin levels occur with concomitant administration of disulfiram, a drug that inhibits the hydroxylating system from forming HPPH. Drugs that increase serum levels of phenytoin by increasing the half-life include dicumarol and chloramphenicol. Some drugs, including carbamazepine, ethanol, and folate, decrease phenytoin concentrations, presumably by stimulation of its metabolism. Phenobarbital has been reported to stimulate the enzymes that metabolize phenytoin to compete with phenytoin for these enzymes, or to have no effect on phenytoin metabolism. Thus, administration of phenobarbital to a patient receiving phenytoin can decrease, increase, or have no effect on phenytoin concentrations. Phenytoin increases phenobarbital concentrations, but causes decreases in serum digitoxin, dicumarol, metyrapone, dexamethasone, cortisol, 25-OH-calciferol (25-OH-D_3), and folate. Its effects on thyroid hormone assays are reviewed in Chapter 16, and its interaction with other drugs is found in Table 17–8.

Carbamazepine

Carbamazepine (Tegretol) is used for tonic-clonic (grand mal) seizures, complex partial seizures, and trigeminal neuralgia, alone or in combination with other drugs. It depresses convulsive activity, alleviates paroxysms of trigeminal neuralgia, and depresses digitalis-induced cardiac arrhythmias. It has pharmacologic properties similar to those of phenytoin, but its mechanism of action is still unknown. Gastrointestinal absorption is variable, with peak levels usually occurring between four and eight hours after an oral dose, but peaks as late as 24 to 32 hours have been reported. About 25 per cent of carbamazepine is found in the unbound form in serum, whereas the rest is bound to serum proteins, mainly albumin. The half-life (8 to 20 hours) after two to four weeks of treatment is considerably shorter than with an acute dose, and is due to autoinduction of drug metabolizing enzymes.

Carbamazepine is metabolized almost completely, with less than 1 per cent occurring unchanged in the urine. The major pathway is thought to be metabolism to a 10,11 epoxide which then is converted to a 10,11 dihydroxide. The epoxide is important because it has anticonvulsant activity, and production of this metabolite can be enhanced by other antiepileptic drugs.

The side effects of carbamazepine include drowsiness, hyperirritability, granulomatous hepatitis, water intoxication, and seizures. Methods of measurement of carbamazepine include homogeneous enzyme immunoassay, gas chromatography, and HPLC. Some HPLC methods are available which measure carbamazepine simultaneously with the 10,11 epoxide or other commonly used anticonvulsants. Because of requirements for rapid turn-around time, homogeneous enzyme immunoassay is favored by over half the laboratories participating in therapeutic drug monitoring surveys in 1982 (College of American Pathologists, 1982).

Although the therapeutic range is not known with any certainty, 4 to 12 μg/ml (16.9 to 50.8 μmol/L) currently is accepted (Table 17–7). Epoxide concentrations are usually 20 to 40 per cent of those of the parent drug (Cereghino, 1982). Carbamazepine may cause nystagmus at serum levels from 1.5 to 6 μg/ml (6.3 to 25.4 μmol/L), and headache, feelings of inhibition, and disturbances of vision occur at levels of 8.5 to 10 μg/ml (36.0 to 42.3 μmol/L) or greater. Serum concentrations greater than 10 μg/ml (42.3 μmol/L) often are associated with unsteadiness of gait, but data are still incomplete.

The serum concentration is decreased by concurrent administration of phenytoin, phenobarbital, or primidone. A few drugs have been shown to cause episodes of carbamazepine intoxication by inhibiting its metabolism; these include propoxyphene, triacetyloleandomycin, and erythromycin.

Barbiturates

Barbiturates are a group of sedative-hypnotic drugs which are frequently the cause of accidental and intentional poisoning. One of the barbiturates, phenobarbital, is used extensively as an antiepileptic agent.

Based on their duration of action, barbiturates are divided into long-acting (six hours or more), intermediate-acting (three to six hours), short-acting (less than three hours), and ultrashort-acting (10 to 15 minutes) (Table 17–9). Ultrashort-acting agents are used as intravenous anesthetics, short- and intermediate-acting agents as sedative hypnotics, and long-acting barbiturates as antiepileptic agents. Anticonvulsant and hypnotic activities are independent properties and dependent on the individual barbiturate.

Barbiturates reversibly depress activity of excitable tissue in the central nervous system, and all degrees of depression are seen—from mild to sedation to coma—with the degree of depression depending on dose, route of administration, and particular barbit-

Table 17–9. CLASSIFICATION OF SELECTED BARBITURATES ON THE BASIS OF DURATION OF HYPNOTIC ACTION AFTER AVERAGE ORAL DOSE

Generic Name	Trade Name	R_1	R_2	R_3	X
Long-acting (6 or more hours)					
Phenobarbital	Luminal	Ethyl	Phenyl	H	O
Mephobarbital	Mebaral	Ethyl	Phenyl	CH_3	O
Barbital	Veronal	Ethyl	Ethyl	H	O
Short-acting (less than 3 hours) to intermediate-acting (3 to 6 hours)					
Amobarbital	Amytal	Ethyl	Isopentyl	H	O
Butabarbital	Butisol	Ethyl	Isopentyl	H	O
Secobarbital	Seconal	Allyl	1-Methylbutyl	H	O
Pentobarbital	Nembutal	Ethyl	1-Methylbutyl	H	O
Ultrashort-acting (intravenous anesthetic)					
Thiopental	Pentothal	Ethyl	1-Methylbutyl	H	S

H = Hydrogen.
O = Oxygen.
S = Sulfur.

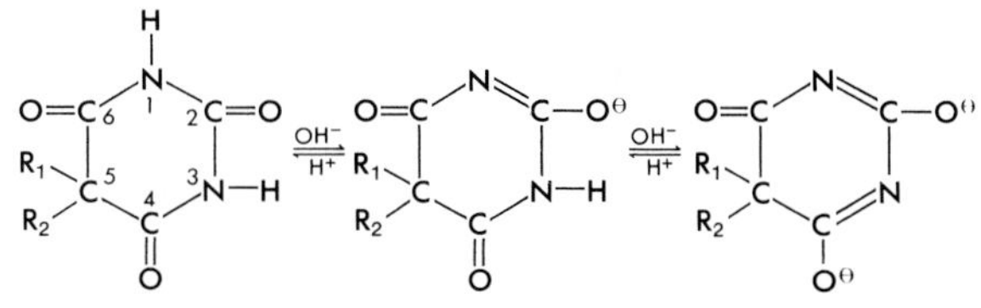

Acid form
Non-ionized acid pH

First ionized form
pH 10

Second ionized form
pH 14

urate. Absorption of short-acting barbiturates is much more rapid than that of long-acting barbiturates, with peak levels obtained within 30 minutes. Long-acting barbiturates such as phenobarbital peak in 12 to 18 hours or longer, with a serum half-life in adults of about two to five days.

Phenobarbital is one of the least toxic and most effective of the anticonvulsants. It is useful for treating tonic-clonic (grand mal) and complex partial seizures. When tonic-clonic seizures are suppressed incompletely by phenytoin alone, phenobarbital may be added. The drug may be used alone for tonic-clonic seizures in infants and preschool children, for whom it is the drug of choice because of adverse effects with phenytoin. The major side effect is drowsiness; but at low serum levels, tolerance occurs within a few weeks and the drowsiness disappears. In the elderly, phenobarbital may cause stimulation of the central nervous system with confusion and delirium, whereas in young children irritability may occur. Nystagmus and ataxia also occur acutely, but diminish as sedation decreases.

About 25 per cent of the phenobarbital dose is excreted unchanged in the urine. The major metabolite is parahydroxyphenobarbital, a compound with weak anticonvulsant activity of its own. Since this metabolite is removed rapidly from the blood by conjugation and renal filtration, it does not contribute significantly to the anticonvulsant activity of phenobarbital.

Analysis of phenobarbital is accomplished readily by gas chromatography, homogeneous enzyme immunoassay, fluoroimmunoassay, fluorescence polarization, and HPLC. Each method is specific and sensitive. Because of the need for a rapid determination and high frequency of phenobarbital overdoses, over 50 per cent of laboratories participating in a therapeutic drug monitoring survey in 1982 have chosen homogeneous enzyme immunoassay as the method of choice (College of American Pathologists, 1982).

Serum concentrations of 10 to 30 μg/ml (43 to 129 μmol/L) are effective for control of seizures (Table 17–7). Higher doses are required in children, because the rate of elimination is greater. Serum levels of phenobarbital <15 μg/ml (65 μmol/L) are frequently ineffective in controlling seizures, whereas values between 40 and 60 μg/ml (172 and 258 μmol/L) may be associated with somnolence. Withdrawal of phenobarbital in patients taking high doses can lead to precipitation of status epilepticus. Adverse effects are not observed with chronic therapy when serum concentrations are <30 μg/ml (129 μmol/L). About 20 per cent of those taking phenobarbital have a depressed serum calcium and elevated alkaline phosphatase; osteomalacia due to increased vitamin D_3 metabolism may occur.

Phenobarbital is the prototype inducer of the hepatic mixed-function oxidase system, which effects biotransformation of numerous drugs, some of which are listed in Table 17–10. Not only does phenobarbital increase metabolism of hydroxycoumarin; it also decreases its absorption. Phenobarbital serum levels usually are increased by coadministration of valproic acid and occasionally of phenytoin.

Barbiturate poisoning is a common problem which remains one of the leading causes of coma secondary to drug ingestion. Phenobarbital, pentobarbital, and secobarbital are the most commonly abused barbiturates. A screening method commonly used for barbit-

Table 17–10. SOME DRUGS WHOSE CLEARANCE IS INCREASED BY PHENOBARBITAL

Dexamethasone	Griseofulvin
Quinine	Doxycycline
Digitoxin	Chloramphenicol
Clonazepam	Chlorpromazine
Aminopyrine	Carbamazepine

urate identification is based on differential absorption of the barbiturate in the ultraviolet range at acid solutions, at pH 10 and pH 14. Other methods of specific barbiturate identification include thin layer chromatography, gas chromatography, radioimmunoassay, homogeneous enzyme immunoassay, and HPLC.

In some respects, the serum barbiturate level in an overdose patient is an unreliable guide to therapy. Patients who have used barbiturates habitually, particularly those who are addicted to such agents, may tolerate far larger doses and higher levels than persons who are not habitual users. For example, a secobarbital addict may be alert with a serum secobarbital level of 20 μg/ml (84 μmol/L), while a person who has not developed tolerance to secobarbital probably would be comatose with a similar serum level.

In spite of these shortcomings, a recent study has indicated that the clinical presentation of non-addicted patients who have short acting barbiturate overdoses can be related to serum levels. Table 17–11 shows the relationship between the state of intoxication and serum concentrations of short-acting barbiturates. The clinical implication for the same concentration of a shorter-acting barbiturate is more serious than for phenobarbital. In general, a serious reaction is likely to occur when the acute dose is more than 10 times the oral hypnotic dose. Potentially lethal serum levels are >80 μg/ml (344 μmol/L) for phenobarbital, >50 μg/ml (215 μmol/L) for amobarbital and butabarbital, and approximately 30 μg/ml (126 μmol/L) for secobarbital. Barbiturate addiction diminishes, whereas

Table 17–11. SHORT-ACTING BARBITURATE OVERDOSE: CLINICAL PRESENTATION*

Level of Consciousness	Short-Acting Barbiturate Level μg/ml	(μmol/L)
Alert	<6	(25.2)
Drowsy	6–10	(25.2–42.0)
Stuporous	11–17	(46.4–71.4)
Stages of coma:		
1 (Responds to pain)	16–20	(67.2–84.0)
2 (Not responsive to pain)	20–24	(84.0–100.8)
3 (Not responsive to pain, shallow respirations	24–28	(100.8–117.6)
4 (Not responsive to pain, inadequate respirations, blood pressure)	28–40	(117.6–168.0)

*From McCarron (1982).

other ingested sedatives potentiate the stage of barbiturate-induced coma.

Because the majority of barbiturate-related deaths are due to respiratory causes, close observation of the unconscious patient for apnea is necessary. If a barbiturate is found in a seriously ill patient, a determination of the barbiturate as long-, medium-, or short-acting should be made, because this may influence treatment. With long-acting barbiturates, alkaline diuresis is helpful in renal elimination, but with intermediate and short-acting barbiturates, diuresis is of little value. Hemodialysis can remove large quantities of long-acting barbiturates from the body with reduction in serum concentration and an associated clinical improvement. In a small study, multiple doses of activated charcoal administered through a nasogastric tube have been shown to reduce the duration of the coma (Goldberg, 1982).

Primidone

Primidone (Mysoline), a desoxy barbiturate, has been used for tonic-clonic seizures (grand mal) and partial seizures with complex symptomatology (psychomotor). It is metabolized to phenobarbital by oxidation and to phenylethylmalonamide (PEMA) by ring cleavage. Both metabolites have anticonvulsant activity. The ratio of phenobarbital to the parent drug during steady-state equilibrium in serum of patients taking primidone alone is usually about 1.5:1, but in patients receiving phenytoin and primidone, this ratio can be over 4:1 possibly because of induction of the enzyme system responsible for conversion of primidone to phenobarbital.

Primidone is absorbed rapidly and has a half-life of about 12 to 14 hours. The half-life of its active metabolites, phenobarbital and PEMA, are 96 hours and 24 to 48 hours, respectively. Primidone and PEMA are minimally bound to protein, whereas phenobarbital is about 60 per cent protein bound.

The major side effect is sedation, which commonly is observed on initiation of treatment and may persist for several days. However, patients usually adapt to this and other acute side effects such as dizziness, nausea, diplopia, and nystagmus. Chronic side effects are very similar to those of phenobarbital.

Methods of choice for measurement are gas chromatography, HPLC, and homogeneous enzyme immunoassay. In the enzyme immunoassay, no cross-reactivity with PEMA occurs, but phenytoin and phenobarbital react to a small extent. These methods recently have been reviewed (Schäfer, 1982).

The therapeutic range for primidone is 5 to 12 μg/ml (23 to 55 μmol/L), but in some patients effective control may require serum concentrations above this range. Toxic effects occur with levels >15 μg/ml (69 μmol/L). In some patients, primidone levels are increased after administration of carbamazepine. Concomitant isoniazid treatment elevates serum primidone levels by inhibiting metabolism of primidone to its active metabolites.

Although relationship of serum levels of primidone, phenobarbital, and PEMA in acute toxicity has not been delineated, Brillman (1974) suggested that acute toxicity correlates best with primidone levels. In some patients with acute primidone intoxication, hexagonal primidone crystals have been identified in the urine (Turner, 1980).

Valproic Acid

Both alone and in combination with other anticonvulsants, valproic acid (Depakene), a branched-chain carboxylic acid, has found increasing use in treatment of tonic-clonic seizures (grand mal epilepsy) and absence seizures (petit mal epilepsy) in children. Its mode of action may be mediated, in part, through its effects on the function of brain gamma-aminobutyric acid (GABA). The main side effect is fatigue, but thrombocytopenia, pancreatitis, hepatic failure, coma, and death also have been reported.

Valproic acid is absorbed rapidly after oral administration, with peak serum levels occurring one to three hours after ingestion. Since it has a biologic half-life which is between 8 and 15 hours, it is given in several doses during the day. About 90 per cent of the drug in serum is bound to proteins, but there is large individual variation in binding. Although metabolic pathways of degradation still have not been elucidated, at least eight active metabolites have been identified. When used in pregnancy valproic acid crosses the placenta, and it has been associated with spina bifida in exposed fetuses.

The most widely used methods of determination are homogeneous enzyme immunoassay and gas chromatography. The accepted therapeutic range is between 50 and 100 μg/ml (347 and 693 μmol/L); however, the relationship between serum levels and clinical efficacy still is debated. Because of large interindividual variation in protein binding (Roman, 1982), free valproic acid levels may prove to be useful in the future. A syndrome of altered behavior, confusion, and deteriorating seizure control may occur when serum concentrations are >100 μg/ml (693 μmol/L).

Because valproic acid inhibits phenobarbital metabolism, phenobarbital (and primidone) dosage must be reduced by approximately one third when administered with valproic acid. Valproic acid increases ethosuximide levels by 50 per cent and also displaces phenytoin from its binding sites on plasma proteins. It may cause a false positive test for urinary ketones by dipsticks.

Ethosuximide

Ethosuximide (Zarontin) is considered the drug of choice for absence seizures (petit mal epilepsy). Despite its frequent use, the site and mechanism of action still are unexplained.

Peak serum levels of ethosuximide are found within four hours after ingesting a dose, whereas the half-life is about 60 hours in adults and 30 hours in children. There appears to be very little protein binding, and cerebrospinal fluid concentrations are quite similar to serum levels. About 30 per cent of ethosuximide appears unchanged in the urine along with at least three hydroxylated derivatives. Most common side effects are gastric distress, loss of appetite, fatigue, lethargy, headaches, and dizziness; these appear to be related to the dose.

Gas chromatography, HPLC, and homogeneous enzyme immunoassay are the methods most widely used to measure ethosuximide levels. Desmethylmethsuximide, the active metabolite of methsuximide (Celantin), has been reported to cross-react in the homogeneous enzyme immunoassay for ethosuximide (Pippenger, 1978).

Clinical control of seizures occurs when serum levels are from 40 to 100 μg/ml (283 to 708 μmol/L), although an occasional patient may need levels of up to 150 μg/ml (1067 μmol/L) for adequate seizure control. In children levels as high as 190 μg/ml (1445 μmol/L) may be tolerated without evidence of toxic effects. The relationship of serum concentration to adverse effects has not been completely established. Two recent reports indicate that co-administration of ethosuximide with carbamazepine or with valproic acid may decrease and increase levels, respectively.

2

ANALGESICS

Acetaminophen

Acetaminophen, or paracetamol (N-acetyl-para-amino-phenol), is an antipyretic and analgesic. Its therapeutic action appears to be related to inhibition of the enzymatic mechanism for synthesis of prostaglandins. In the United States, it is available without prescription and marketed in over 200 formulations, of which the most common are Tylenol, Datril, Tempra, and Liquiprin. A comprehensive list of these formulations has been prepared by Ameer (1977). Phenacetin, an analgesic used with salicylates in a common formulation, is metabolized to acetaminophen. The major adverse reaction related to acetaminophen is hepatotoxicity.

Acetaminophen is absorbed rapidly from the gastrointestinal tract with peak concentrations occurring one to two hours after ingestion. The drug may be up to 50 per cent bound to plasma proteins, but there appear to be no major sites of tissue binding. Approximately 80 per cent of an administered dose is conjugated by hepatic enzymes to glucuronic and sulfuric acids, and these metabolites are excreted into the urine. The remainder is eliminated by other pathways such as the cytochrome P_{450} mixed-function oxidase system; these pathways are increased by microsomal-inducing drugs such as phenobarbital and ethanol.

Although the oxidation pathway accounts for very little of the acetaminophen metabolized, it is postulated that an oxidation product, N-acetyl-imidoquinone, by covalently binding to hepatocellular macromolecules, causes hepatic necrosis. Usually this toxic metabolite is detoxified by conjugation with hepatic glutathione and subsequently excreted into the urine. When large amounts of acetaminophen are ingested, hepatic glutathione becomes depleted, N-acetyl-imidoquinone accumulates, the macromolecular structure of the liver is arylated, and hepatic necrosis results.

Acetaminophen can be measured by ultraviolet spectrophotometry, homogeneous enzyme immunoassay, and HPLC. Some ultraviolet spectrophotometric methods are relatively non-specific and show interferences from salicylates. Phenacetin and acetaminophen have been measured simultaneously by an HPLC procedure which does not require specimen preparation (Gotelli, 1977). A homogeneous enzyme immunoassay method is now available and probably will become the method of choice.

For analgesia in adults, doses of 325 to 650 mg usually are given every three to four hours. Serum concentrations of 5 to 20 μg/ml (31 to 124 μmol/L) are associated with analgesia, but levels are not monitored routinely because there is not a good correlation between serum concentration and intensity of analgesic action.

Hepatotoxicity may occur when large amounts of the drug are acutely ingested accidentally or in suicide attempts. Initially nausea, vomiting, and abdominal pain may result, and within the first two days liver function tests become abnormal. Hepatic abnormalities, however, may not occur until four to six days after ingestion. Hepatotoxicity may occur with a single dose as small as 10 g. When serum acetaminophen concentrations and time after ingestion are plotted on a semilogarithmic scale, toxicity can be predicted if the serum value falls above a line connecting the 200 μg/ml (1240 μmol/L) point at four hours with the 50 μg/ml (310 μmol/L) point at 12 hours (Fig. 17–4). Rumack (1981) recommends that patients whose serum values are 25 per cent below those which may be expected to cause hepatotoxicity should be treated as having taken a potentially toxic dose. This allows for possible errors in assay values or errors in estimating the time elapsed since acetaminophen ingestion.

The serum acetaminophen half-life is probably the best guide to the prediction of extent of hepatic injury and should be determined especially in those patients who have achieved a serum level in the toxic range. It has been shown that hepatic necrosis may occur when the serum half-life exceeds four hours, and hepatic coma is very likely if the half-life exceeds 12 hours. When acetaminophen half-lives are less than four hours, patients are able to metabolize the toxic products and usually do not develop hepatic insufficiency. Patients taking enzyme-inducing drugs such as phenobarbital are at a greater risk of developing hepatotoxicity, probably from increased formation of the toxic metabolite. Observations made from management of over 2000 patients with potentially toxic serum levels have indicated that treatment with sulfhydryl-containing compounds such as N-acetylcysteine may reduce hepatotoxicity; however, to be efficacious these compounds must be given within 24 hours of the time of acetaminophen ingestion (Rumack, 1981). A few patients have been reported who develop hepatic failure after chronic acetaminophen administration for analgesia.

Propoxyphene

Propoxyphene, as the hydrochloride (Darvon) or napsylate (Darvon-N) salt, is an analgesic which is one of the five most commonly prescribed drugs in the United States. Propoxyphene is a congener of the narcotic methadone, but is classified as a non-narcotic.

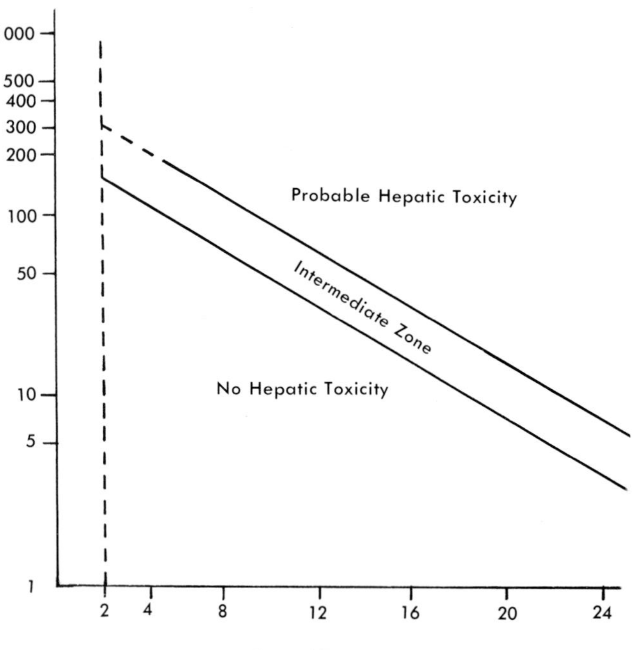

Figure 17–4. Semilogarithmic plot of serum acetaminophen levels vs. time. The serum half-life can be estimated using two specimens obtained several hours apart. To convert to μmol/L, multiply μg/ml by 66.16. (Modified from Krenzelok, E. P., Best, L., and Manoguerra, A. S.: Am. J. Hosp. Pharm. *34*:391, 1977.)

Accidental or intentional ingestion of large amounts of propoxyphene may cause death; dependence and parenteral abuse are additional problems associated with the drug.

Following ingestion of the hydrochloride salt, propoxyphene reaches a peak serum level in one to two hours, but with the napsylate salt the peak occurs in three to four hours. Most propoxyphene is metabolized on the first pass through the liver, with only about 20 per cent reaching the systemic circulation unchanged. The major route of biotransformation is N-demethylation to norpropoxyphene, a pharmacologically active compound which is eliminated by renal excretion. At least seven other metabolites have been identified, but none appears to be important. With chronic dosing, the half-lives of propoxyphene and norpropoxyphene (about 12 and 39 hours, respectively) are considerably longer than with a single dose. Because of its longer half-life, norpropoxyphene serum concentrations are about twice those of propoxyphene. The half-life of propoxyphene is variable in acute overdose patients because both propoxyphene and norpropoxyphene inhibit propoxyphene metabolism (Inturrisi, 1982). Rapid tissue binding of propoxyphene occurs, resulting in immediate and almost complete disappearance of the drug from blood with relatively high concentrations in brain, lung, liver, and kidney.

Following the ingestion of a toxic dose of propoxyphene, symptoms of nausea, vomiting, and drowsiness, which can progress to central nervous system depression, occur within about 30 minutes. Convulsions, cardiovascular collapse, and respiratory depression then usually occur within about one hour. The finding of miotic pupils serves to differentiate intoxication with propoxyphene from that with non-narcotic drugs. The usual modalities of treatment for an overdose, such as dialysis or diuresis, have been of little benefit probably because tissue levels are about 10 to 20 times greater than serum concentrations. However, the toxic respiratory effects can be neutralized by administration of morphine antagonists. Although death in an adult has been reported with a propoxyphene dose as low as 800 mg, 1000 mg of the hydrochloride salt or 1500 mg of the napsylate preparation usually is lethal.

A spectrophotometric method has been used, but it is relatively insensitive and measures both norpropoxyphene and propoxyphene. With gas chromatographic methods, both propoxyphene and norpropoxyphene can be quantitated simultaneously.

In a controlled clinical trial, analgesia and serum concentrations of propoxyphene did not show significant correlation; however, with usual doses a serum level of about 0.3 μg/ml (0.9 μmol/L) is reached. The minimum potentially fatal propoxyphene level is thought to be about 1.0 μg/ml (2.9 μmol/L).

Salicylates

Salicylates are non-addictive analgesics which also have remarkable antipyretic, anti-inflammatory, and antirheumatic effects in man. Despite use of safety containers since 1970, accidental ingestion of salicylates remains the single most common cause of drug toxicity in preschool children, with one of every four cases of childhood poisoning being due to ingestion of salicylates. Toxicity also has been observed in chronic users, both children and adults, but it may not always be obvious. In the study of Anderson (1976), 27 per cent of adult salicylate intoxication occurred in patients on chronic salicylate therapy and went unrecognized for up to 72 hours. Salicylates are one of the drugs most commonly ingested in suicide attempts.

Salts of salicylic acid are rapidly absorbed, mainly from the small intestine, with peak levels achieved in two to four hours. However, absorption is quite variable and dependent on tablet dissolution. Salicylic acid salts, such as acetylsalicylic acid (aspirin), are rapidly hydrolyzed in the circulation to free salicylic acid, which then is bound principally to albumin. Although usually up to 90 per cent of the salicylic acid is bound, protein binding is exceeded at toxic serum levels leading to an increased percentage of the unbound salicylate. Salicylates are metabolized to salicyluric acid and a phenolic glucuronide through two major pathways which become saturated when the concentration of salicylate is in the therapeutic range. When this occurs, the major route of elimination is by renal excretion. Saturation of these metabolic pathways results in a more than proportional increase in serum salicylate levels with increases in dosage. Renal excretion of salicylic acid, a weak acid, is dependent upon hydrogen ion concentration, with a more alkaline environment favoring salicylic acid dissociation and promoting more rapid excretion. This mechanism is sensitive to even small changes in urine pH, and increased excretion can be promoted by infusions of bicarbonate. Use of certain antacids to prevent gastric irritation also results in an increased urinary pH and increased salicylate excretion. Decreases in urine pH can decrease the excretion markedly, resulting in toxicity.

Major toxic effects are gastrointestinal irritation, vomiting, epigastric discomfort, and hemorrhage, but frank bleeding is uncommon. The hemorrhage may be related to decreased levels of clotting factors, impairment of platelet function, and perhaps an increased capillary fragility. Other symptoms of toxicity include tinnitus, irritability, and irrationality similar to that which occurs with alcohol intoxication but without euphoria. Toxicity may progress to coma and death. One of the most important side effects of salicylates is the direct stimulatory effect on the central nervous system. Early in the course of intoxication, hyperpnea may occur, lowering the P_{CO_2} and causing a respiratory alkalosis. A metabolic acidosis soon intervenes from renal compensation for the respiratory alkalosis and from an accumulation of salicylic acid itself. Other metabolic acids accumulate because salicylate interferes with intermediary metabolism and increases lipid metabolism, producing an accumulation of fatty acids and ketones. Salicylates also act to uncouple oxidative phosphorylation, causing an increased metabolic rate and producing mild hyperglycemia which rarely exceeds 200 mg/dl (11.0 mmol/L). Patients on chronic salicylates have been reported to develop hepatotoxicity. Non-cardiogenic pulmonary edema has been recognized as a complication of salicylate intoxication and carries a high fatality rate.

The classic screening test for urinary salicylates involves use of ferric chloride in acid. Even if a small amount of salicylate is present, such as occurs after ingestion of one tablet, a purple color develops. This color reaction is non-specific in that many substances such as amino acids, keto acids, and certain drugs also react to produce a colored product (see Chap. 18). Serum salicylate levels commonly are measured using an automated ferric nitrate technique.

The usual dose of two tablets of salicylates yields serum concentrations <60 μg/ml (0.4 mmol/L). Toxicity is associated with serum salicylate levels of about 300 μg/ml (2.2 mmol/L), but severe toxic effects occur when serum levels approach 500 μg/ml (3.6 mmol/L). Patients with serum concentrations ranging from 550 to 1400 μg/ml (4.0 to 10.1 mmol/L) have a high mortality rate. In older children and adults, there is good correlation between serum salicylate levels and severity of the toxic state, but young children display a variable response to a given salicylate level. Done has published a nomogram which relates severity of salicylate toxicity with serum level when time after ingestion of the potentially toxic dose is known (Fig. 17–5).

Dialysis, plasmapheresis, and exchange transfusion are effective means of achieving a reduction in serum salicylate concentrations and clinical improvement; one of these modalities should be used when levels are >100 μg/ml (0.7 mmol/L) and the patient has failed to respond to supportive therapy. The mean lethal dose of salicylate lies between 20 and 30 g in an adult; however, 1 g of aspirin has been fatal, and

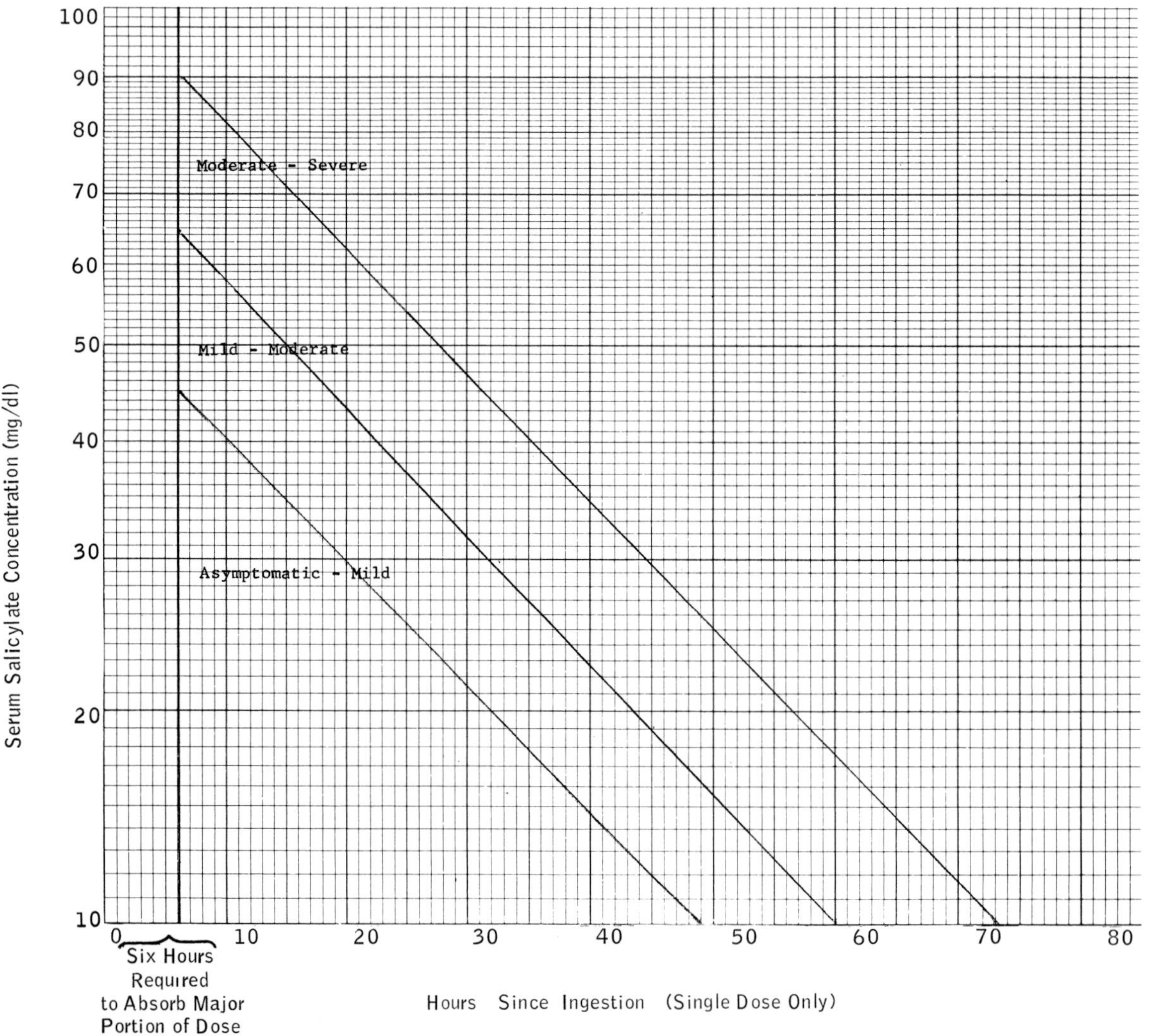

Figure 17–5. Toxicity in children (salicylism) vs. serum concentration as related to time since ingestion. To convert to mmol/L, multiply mg/dl by 1.45. (Modified from Done, A. K.: Pediatrics, *26*:800, 1960).

survival with a dose as high as 130 g has been reported. Methyl salicylate (oil of wintergreen) is the most toxic member of the salicylate family, and the mortality from overdoses is close to 60 per cent.

When salicylates are used in rheumatoid arthritis, the optimal therapeutic effect occurs with serum levels of about 150 to 300 μg/ml (1.1 to 2.2 mmol/L). Tinnitus, the most common salicylate-induced side effect in patients treated with the drug for rheumatoid arthritis, is associated with salicylate levels between about 200 and 450 μg/ml (1.4 and 3.3 mmol/L). In those with pre-existing hearing loss, however, tinnitus is not a reliable guide to toxicity. Hyperventilation usually occurs at levels >350 μg/ml (2.6 mmol/L) (Mongan, 1973), whereas acidosis and other side effects are seen at concentrations >460 μg/ml (3.3 mmol/L).

PSYCHOACTIVE DRUGS

Tricyclic Antidepressants

Amitriptyline, imipramine, and related compounds are used for treatment of a wide variety of disorders, including endogenous depression. The most frequent side effects caused by tricyclic antidepressants are those attributable to anticholinergic effects, for example, dry mouth and urinary retention. Acute toxicity which occurs with overdosage may lead to coma, cardiac arrhythmias, and seizures. Children and the elderly may require conservative dosage schedules of the tricyclic antidepressants. It has been suggested that elderly patients may show severe adverse effects from high doses at least in part because of decreased drug metabolism, decreased protein binding, and increased receptor sensitivity.

There is a high degree of plasma protein binding of the tricyclics. Tricyclic antidepressants are metabolized by the liver; the tertiary amine compounds such as amitriptyline and imipramine are N-demethylated to secondary amines which are pharmacologically active. Amitriptyline is metabolized to nortriptyline, imipramine to desipramine. The metabolites, nortriptyline and desipramine, have been used as tricyclic antidepressants. Amitriptyline, imipramine, and their secondary amine metabolites also are hydroxylated.

A number of problems have been encountered in determining therapeutic ranges for tricyclic antidepressants, including difficulties in performing drug analyses, in determining which metabolites are important to monitor, and in assessing clinical response. Tricyclics can be measured by a variety of methods, including gas chromatography and radioimmunoassay. Care must be exercised in blood collection because the plasticizer tris (2-butoxyethyl) phosphate inhibits protein binding of the tricyclics, thus leading to redistribution and lowering of plasma levels.

The tricyclic antidepressants show a wide variation in steady-state plasma concentration among patients. For several of these drugs, a curvilinear concentration response curve or therapeutic window has been described: a poor response below and above a given plasma level is found. Table 17–12 lists therapeutic ranges for some tricyclic antidepressants. Quantitation of urinary 3-methoxy-4-hydroxyphenylglycol (MHPG) has been proposed as an objective measure of depression as well as an aid to drug selection and monitoring of efficacy of therapy. It has been suggested that endogenously depressed patients with low MHPG respond better to imipramine, but that patients who excrete normal to high levels of MHPG are more likely to respond to amitriptyline (Cutler, 1978).

Table 17–12. POSTULATED THERAPEUTIC RANGES FOR TRICYCLIC ANTIDEPRESSANTS*

	ng/ml	μmol/L
Amitriptyline	120–250	0.43–0.90
Desipramine	150–300	0.56–1.13
Doxepin	75–200	0.27–0.72
Imipramine	150–250	0.54–0.80
Nortriptyline	50–150	0.19–0.57
Protriptyline	70–260	0.27–0.99

*From Orsulak, P. J., and Schildkraut, J. J.: Ther. Drug Monitor, *1*:199, 1979.

The triad of coma, seizures, and cardiac arrhythmias should raise the suspicion of tricyclic overdose. Poisonings with as little as 2.5 g of tricyclics are potentially fatal. Serious tricyclic overdose has been reported when plasma levels are ≥1000 ng/ml. Plasma levels may remain elevated for several days after the acute ingestion, particularly if the patient has ingested a tertiary amine tricyclic antidepressant. Some patients have maintained toxic drug levels for five to six days. Prolonged elevation of tricyclic antidepressant plasma levels following an overdose has several clinical implications. It has been suggested that sustained drug levels may play a role in unexpected cardiac death, which has been reported three to six days after an overdose. In patients with total tricyclic antidepressant levels >1000 ng/ml, the QRS interval of the ECG has been reported to be at or above the upper limit of normal (100 milliseconds). If a serious overdose is suspected, it has been recommended that patients have continuous cardiac monitoring for five to six days (Spiker, 1976).

Lithium

Lithium salts are employed mainly in the control of manic-depressive disorders. Lithium therapy may cause a number of side effects, including goiter, leukocytosis, and polyuria; however, lithium toxicity primarily affects the central nervous system and kidneys. Acute intoxication is characterized by vomiting, diarrhea, ataxia, coma, and convulsions. Chronic toxic manifestations include nausea, vomiting, abdominal pain, diarrhea, and sedation, as well as tremors, seizures, focal neurologic signs, and arrhythmias. Protracted coma, anuria, or circulatory failure may ensue before death occurs.

Lithium is not bound to serum proteins and is not metabolized; its distribution in the body is complicated and achieved slowly. It is eliminated almost entirely by renal excretion, but also is secreted into saliva and breast milk. For practical purposes, lithium can be considered to have a half-life between 24 and 48 hours, but the elimination half-time is dependent on duration of drug therapy. In patients taking the drug for more than one year, the mean elimination half-time is greater than 48 hours (Goodnick, 1981). The elimination half-time is decreased by a diet high in sodium and increased by sodium deprivation or renal damage.

Atomic absorption spectrophotometry and emission flame photometry may be used to determine serum lithium levels. The therapeutic range for lithium is approximately 0.5 to 1.2 mEq/L (0.5 to 1.2 mmol/L). Although toxic side effects can occur at almost any serum level, they are seldom serious <1.5 mEq/L (1.5 mmol/L). Steady-state lithium levels >3.0 mEq/L (3.0 mmol/L) are life threatening, and levels >4.5 mEq/L (4.5 mmol/L) are almost invariably fatal.

Lithium concentration in erythrocytes or the ratio of lithium in erythrocytes to that in serum has been reported to correlate better than serum lithium concentration with clinical response. The ratio of erythrocyte to serum lithium is about 0.35, but it increases at higher serum lithium levels and varies greatly among patients (Guelen, 1980). The erythrocyte to serum lithium ratio, however, is relatively stable in individual patients.

Phenothiazines

Chlorpromazine and related phenothiazine derivatives are employed in treatment of psychoses, but they have other important uses such as control of nausea and vomiting. Side effects include weakness, orthostatic hypotension, palpitations, and neurologic manifestations such as a parkinsonian syndrome. Although phenothiazines have a high therapeutic index, occasionally they may cause serious side effects such as respiratory depression.

Monitoring of phenothiazine levels is not practiced widely. Plasma levels are not correlated consistently with clinical outcome. In addition, analysis is complicated because many phenothiazine derivatives are employed therapeutically, and phenothiazines undergo extensive metabolism in the body. For example, less than 1 per cent of chlorpromazine is excreted unchanged; over 150 metabolites have been postulated, and as many as 12 metabolites of chlorpromazine may occur in plasma in appreciable quantities (Speicher, 1981).

Screening methods are available for detection of phenothiazines in urine; these methods are used to determine compliance and to detect surreptitious use. One commonly used procedure employs FPN reagent (mixture of ferric chloride, perchloric acid, and nitric acids); this reagent is mixed with urine and the color observed immediately. A pink or purple color indicates that phenothiazines may be present. Ascorbic acid has been reported to give false negative results with this method (James, 1980).

SEDATIVES AND HYPNOTICS

Benzodiazepines

Benzodiazepines are the most commonly prescribed drugs in the United States. They are used mainly for treatment of anxiety; however, other uses include treatment of status epilepticus, alcohol withdrawal, and induction of anesthesia for minor surgical procedures. A high incidence of excessive ingestion of these compounds is seen alone and in combination with ethanol in hospital emergency rooms.

Diazepam. When given by the intravenous route, peak serum diazepam (Valium) levels occur in 15 minutes, whereas by the intramuscular or oral route, peak levels occur in 30 and 60 minutes, respectively. Diazepam, which is about 98 per cent bound to albumin, has a biologic half-life of about 40 hours with chronic dosing. It is metabolized to desmethyldiazepam, which is active and has a half-life about twice as long as diazepam. A hydroxylated metabolite of desmethyldiazepam, oxazepam, also is active. Oxazepam, marketed commercially as Serax, has a much shorter half-life than diazepam and shows very little accumulation in serum with chronic dosing.

Specific methods for diazepam analysis include gas chromatography and HPLC. With ultraviolet spectrophotometric methods, values obtained are higher than those by gas chromatography, because the active metabolite, desmethyldiazepam, is measured. A homogeneous enzyme immunoassay is available; it has significant cross-reactivity with 12 other benzodiazepines. Qualitative identification of diazepam in serum from an overdose patient can be performed using thin layer chromatography.

Serum diazepam concentrations associated with clinical efficacy or toxicity have not been clearly established. The concentrations of diazepam and its metabolite are between 0.1 and 1.0 μg/ml (3.5 and 35 μmol/L) with chronic therapy, whereas after a single oral dose of 10 to 15 mg, peak levels range from 0.2 to 0.3 μg/ml (7.0 to 10.5 μmol/L). Whereas acute administration of diazepam may cause profound symptoms when serum levels are >0.4 μg/ml (14.0 μmol/L), with chronic dosage these levels result in few symptoms. When diazepam is given acutely, desmethyldiazepam concentrations are about one third that of the parent drug, but with chronic therapy desmethyldiazepam may be found in equal or higher concentrations.

In a recent series, patients presented with lethargy, stupor, or light coma after ingesting a large diazepam dose in suicide attempts. Since none were found to have absent reflexes or respiratory depression, these findings suggest an etiology for the coma other than a diazepam overdose (Jatlow, 1979). Finkle (1979), in his survey of over 1200 deaths in which diazepam was ingested, could substantiate only two which were related directly to diazepam. Concomitant administration of valproic acid, isoniazid, or cimetidine and liver disease have been reported to prolong the half-life of diazepam.

Chlordiazepoxide. Chlordiazepoxide (Librium) is a

benzodiazepine which is used as an antianxiety agent, as a hypnotic, and for the treatment of acute alcohol withdrawal. It is absorbed slowly from the gastrointestinal tract and may take several hours to reach peak concentrations. About 95 per cent of the drug is bound to serum proteins, and its half-life is from 6 to 30 hours. The major metabolite, N-desmethylchlordiazepoxide, is active, but at least three other inactive metabolites occur in serum in low concentrations. Ethanol has been found to inhibit both chlordiazepoxide and desmethylchlordiazepoxide metabolism, whereas cimetidine inhibits only chlordiazepoxide metabolism.

Qualitative identification of chlordiazepoxide in serum of an overdose patient can be performed using thin layer chromatography. The usual methods of quantitation are ultraviolet spectrophotometry, fluorimetry, gas chromatography, and HPLC.

After chronic oral therapy with total daily doses of 75 to 150 mg, serum levels are in the range of 3.2 to 6.9 μg/ml (10.6 to 22.8 μmol/L), and at this level patients are profoundly sedated. When up to 2 g of chlordiazepoxide was ingested in overdose situations, drowsiness or stupor occurred with serum levels >20 μg/ml, (66 μmol/L), but even at levels of about 60 μg/ml (198 μmol/L), coma did not ensue (Cate, 1973).

Regardless of the level, if a patient is comatose following chlordiazepoxide overdosing, another drug or cause of the coma should be suspected. Since about three fourths of all cases of overdosage with chlordiazepoxide involve a second drug, the additive central nervous system depressant effects are exceedingly important.

MISCELLANEOUS

Theophylline

Theophylline (1,3-dimethyl xanthine) is an effective bronchodilator frequently used in treating asthma and recurrent apnea in premature infants. Although it was once accepted that theophylline-induced bronchodilation was mediated by inhibition of phosphodiesterase and accumulation of cyclic AMP, the exact mechanism remains undetermined. Absorption of some oral preparations may be rapid and complete; however, it may be delayed, slow, or incomplete for other preparations. Following absorption, theophylline is distributed widely in extracellular fluid and tissues. About 60 per cent of theophylline is bound to plasma proteins, whereas the other 40 per cent is free. Theophylline metabolism involves oxidation and methylation by the liver, mainly to inactive metabolites 3-methylxanthine, 1-methyluric acid, and 1,3-dimethyluric acid. In infants, it is metabolized partially to caffeine, which has pharmacologic actions similar to theophylline. About 10 per cent of the administered dose of theophylline is excreted in the urine unchanged.

The half-life of theophylline is about 3.5 hours in children and about 4.5 to 10 hours in healthy adults. Recent evidence has indicated that patients who are ill have prolonged metabolic degradation rates and, when given a theophyline infusion at rates developed for healthy young adults, toxicity occurs frequently. For example, following a loading dose, a maintenance infusion of 0.9 mg/kg/hour resulted in toxic serum levels in about 30 per cent of patients (Hendeles, 1980). A nomogram has been employed to reduce the maintenance dose by one third in patients over the age of 50 and by one half in patients with congestive heart failure or liver dysfunction (Jusko, 1977). In patients chronically taking theophylline, the intravenous infusion is adjusted depending on the baseline theophylline level.

Methods of theophylline measurement include ultraviolet spectrophotometry, homogeneous enzyme immunoassay, homogeneous fluoroimmunoassay, fluorescence polarization, gas chromatography, and HPLC. For many years ultraviolet spectrophotometry was the most commonly used method, but this method is subject to interferences by furosemide, barbiturates, and xanthines. Xanthines such as caffeine, commonly found in tea and coffee and theobromine, a major constituent of chocolate, co-extract and are measured as theophylline. A major advantage of some HPLC theophylline assays is that they simultaneously measure caffeine. However, in a population other than newborns, homogeneous enzyme immunoassay is the method of choice.

Serum therapeutic levels for treatment of asthma are 10 to 20 μg/ml (56 to 112 μmol/L), but at 5 to 10 μg/ml (28 to 56 μmol/L) therapeutic effects do occur. At concentrations >20 μg/ml (112 μmol/L), side effects invariably occur, but patients with serum theophylline values in the range of 15 to 20 μg/ml (83 to 112 μmol/L) occasionally experience anorexia, nausea, vomiting, and abdominal discomfort. In most patients with gastrointestinal symptoms, serum theophylline concentrations usually are >25 μg/ml (139 μmol/L). Severe toxicity, manifested by cardiac arrhythmias, respiratory arrest, cardiac arrest, and seizures, occurs in the range of 30 to 70 μg/ml (168 to 392 μmol/L). In a small series, seizures were fatal in 50 per cent of patients, and were not preceded by gastrointestinal symptoms (Zwillich, 1975). Charcoal hemoperfusion should be considered when serum concentrations are >40 μg/ml (224 μmol/L) and is recommended when serum concentrations are >60 μg/ml (336 μmol/L). For neonatal apnea, theophylline is maintained within a therapeutic range of 6 to 12 μg/ml (33 to 67 μmol/L).

In young cigarette smokers, the half-life is significantly shorter than in non-smokers. Chronic phenytoin therapy has been reported to decrease the theophylline half-life. The half-life tends to be significantly longer in patients with heart failure, acute pulmonary edema, liver dysfunction, or chronic obstructive pulmonary disease and in those patients receiving concomitant treatment with cimetidine, allopurinol, or macrolide antibiotics (troleandomycin and erythromycin).

Methotrexate

Methotrexate, a folic acid antagonist, has been used in low doses for cancer chemotherapy for 35 years.

Since 1973, methotrexate, administered as intravenous infusions lasting from six hours to almost two days, has been used for treatment of osteogenic sarcomas, childhood leukemias, and many other highly malignant tumors. Methotrexate inhibits the enzyme dihydrofolate reductase, thereby reducing the pool of folates available as methyl donors for production of thymidylate, one of four precursors of DNA. The lethal effect occurs when available thymidylate is reduced, resulting in inhibition of DNA synthesis, RNA synthesis, and cell division. The most rapidly proliferating cells, such as those of bone marrow, gastrointestinal tract, and hair roots, are most affected. Methotrexate also can be administered by intrathecal injection with neurotoxicity the most common side effect.

High dose methotrexate is followed within a few hours by administration of leucovorin (5-formyl tetrahydrofolate, also called citrovorum factor). By administering leucovorin, the product of the enzyme inhibited by methotrexate, the block is circumvented and cellular functions are allowed to continue. Use of leucovorin permits administration of about 100 times more methotrexate than when the drug is given alone. Leucovorin cannot "rescue" normal cells if the rescue is delayed, and if serum methotrexate levels are too low, tumor cells are not killed. Thus, the cytotoxic action of methotrexate on target tissue requires the intracellular presence of the drug above a specific threshold for an extended period of time.

Methotrexate is about 95 per cent bound to serum proteins. It exhibits a triphasic serum disappearance with extensive intrahepatic circulation and probably enteric bacterial metabolism; however, most is excreted within the first eight hours, mainly unchanged in the urine. If serum concentrations are in the toxic range and urine pH less than 5.5, methotrexate may precipitate in the kidney, causing renal insufficiency. For this reason, patients treated with high dose therapy not only must have their urine alkalinized but also must have adequate renal function. With high dose therapy, a metabolite, 7-hydroxymethotrexate, is formed, which may precipitate in the kidney because it has a lower solubility than methotrexate at neutral and acid pH.

Methods for measuring methotrexate include HPLC, radioimmunoassay, enzyme immunoassay, radioassay using dihydrofolate reductase as the binding protein, and an enzymatic method using inhibition of the dihydrofolate reductase as the endpoint. The specificity of these assays in the presence of folates and their analogues has not been characterized completely. All methods appear to have sensitivity sufficient to measure methotrexate levels which occur with high dose infusion protocols, but HPLC has the advantage of simultaneously measuring 7-hydroxymethotrexate and methotrexate. Because serum methotrexate concentrations vary over such a large range, serial dilutions of specimens are required to produce values which fall within the assay range. Most laboratories performing methotrexate assays use homogeneous enzyme immunoassay.

Following high level methotrexate infusion, serum levels are obtained that range from 1×10^{-4} M (45.4 μg/ml) to 1×10^{-8} M (0.00454 μg/ml), depending on the time after infusion at which the level is measured. The serum concentration of methotrexate during the infusion correlates with hematologic, gastrointestinal, and hepatic toxicity as well as with the efficacy of treatment (Table 17–13). At levels $<4.5 \times 10^{-6}$ M (2.1 μg/ml) 48 hours following the start of an infusion, severe toxicity is unlikely. Methotrexate determinations also are used to adjust the dose of leucovorin used in the "rescue" (Bertino, 1981).

Nitroprusside

Nitroprusside (Nipride) is an antihypertensive used as a hypotensive agent during surgical procedures or hypertensive crisis, and to facilitate correction of abnormal hemodynamics occurring with acute myocardial infarction and congestive heart failure. It is available in the United States only for intravenous therapy; it is infused initially at an average rate of 3 μg/kg/minute with careful monitoring of the blood pressure.

The structure of nitroprusside is unusual in that it is a hydrated nitrosyl pentacyanoferrate compound (Fig. 17–6). Although nitroprusside is known to cause vasodilation of vascular smooth muscle, the mechanism of action at the cellular level is not fully understood. Nitroprusside initially reacts with sulfhydryl groups in either erythrocytes or other tissues yielding cyanogen (CN^-). This cyanide group rapidly is detoxified to thiocyanate (SCN^-) in the presence of a sulfur donor, thiosulfate, in a reaction catalyzed by the hepatic enzyme rhodanase. If cyanide accumulates, it combines with cytochrome C of the respiratory chain. In individuals with normal renal function, thiocyanate, which is removed almost entirely by the kidney, has a half-life of approximately one week.

Manifestations of acute nitroprusside toxicity are anorexia and nausea followed by vomiting, disorientation, psychotic behavior, trembling, labored respiration, rigidity, convulsions, and finally death. In some fatal cases, high doses of nitroprusside were used (>10 mg/kg/minute); in several of these cases, the

Table 17–13. HIGH DOSE SERUM METHOTREXATE LEVELS*

Time After Dose	Nontoxic	Toxic
24 hours	$<1 \times 10^{-5}$ M (22.8 μg/ml)	$>10^{-5}$ M (22.8 μg/ml)
48 hours	$<5 \times 10^{-7}$ M (1.140 μg/ml)	$>10^{-6}$ M (0.228 μg/ml)
72 hours	$<5 \times 10^{-8}$ M (0.114 μg/ml)	$>10^{-7}$ M (0.023 μg/ml)

*Toxicity dose related and dependent on time after infusion.

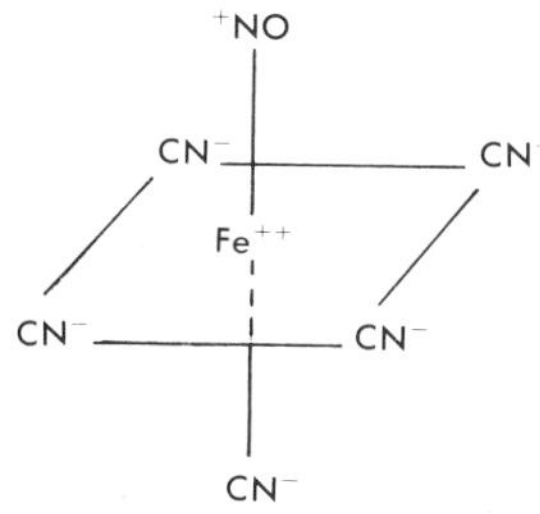

Figure 17–6. Schematic representation of the iron coordination complex of nitroprusside. In sodium nitroprusside, the overall complex has a net negative charge and must be associated with cations such as the two sodiums.

drug was rapidly increased to maintain hypotension, because a resistance was noted five to ten minutes after beginning the infusion. In other fatal cases, tachyphylaxis occurred from 30 to 60 minutes after beginning the infusion. Of the patients treated, young adults and children are most susceptible to tachyphylaxis. In all fatalities, an associated severe metabolic acidosis was found.

Because of rapid detoxification of nitroprusside, serum thiocyanate levels have been used to monitor therapy, with 80 to 120 μg/ml (1.4 to 2.0 μmol/L) considered therapeutic. Recent evidence has shown that thiocyanate levels are unreliable indicators of acute exposure, but may be of value in chronic dosing.

Although cyanide measurements are advocated, there is little agreement on the proper choice of a specimen. In patients receiving nitroprusside, about 98 per cent of the blood cyanide is found in erythrocytes. A recent study found an adequate physiologic response occurred when red cell cyanide levels were 0.6 to 1.0 μg/ml (23.1 to 38.5 μmol/L) and plasma levels were 0.025 to 0.045 μg/ml (1.0 to 1.7 μmol/L) (Cottrell, 1978). Whole blood cyanide concentrations which ranged up to 1.8 μg/ml (69.2 μmol/L) with a mean of 0.333 μg/ml (12.8 μmol/L) were found in a large series of patients who showed therapeutic responses at the end of a constant infusion (Bogusz, 1979). Fatal cyanide poisoning has been reported with blood cyanide levels averaging 24 μg/ml (922 μmol/L): it has been prevented by infusions of thiosulfate or hydroxycobalamin. The potential dangers and safety requirements of cyanide measurements have made this assay impractical for the routine clinical laboratory.

Cyanide

Cyanide poisoning results from inhalation or ingestion of compounds that release cyanide ions. Prolonged contact with cyanide solutions or exposure to hydrogen cyanide gas may result in absorption of toxic amounts through the skin. Cyanides are used in industries and have been employed as rodenticides, and cyanide gas can be released from burning synthetic material. Cyanide poisoning has been reported after the ingestion of the cyanogenic glycoside amygdalin, which is present in kernels of stone fruit, such as apricots, and Laetrile (also called nitriloside or vitamin B_{17}). Nitroprusside is another potential source of cyanide toxicity.

Acute cyanide poisoning causes headache, dizziness, tachycardia, and tachypnea followed by stupor and finally apnea, general convulsions, and death. Diagnosis of cyanide poisoning requires a high index of suspicion; it should be suspected in patients with altered levels of consciousness in the presence of lactic acidosis. Although the scent of bitter almonds is a classic sign of cyanide poisoning, the ability of individuals to recognize the smell is genetically determined and lacking in a large percentage of the population.

Cyanide acts by inhibiting the cytochrome oxidase system, thus blocking cellular respiration. About three fourths of blood cyanide is in cells. Cyanide is metabolized rapidly within the body, and up to about 50 per cent of absorbed cyanide may be inactivated within one hour after exposure. Most is converted by the liver rhodanase system to thiocyanate, which itself is toxic but to a lesser degree than cyanide.

Spectrophotometric methods are available for quantitation of cyanide in blood and plasma. Blood cyanide levels of 0.1 to 0.15 μg/ml (3.85 to 5.77 μmol/L) can occur in healthy individuals from cigarette smoking, food, and industrial pollution (Herbert, 1979). Any blood cyanide level >0.2 μg/ml (7.69 μmol/L) suggests cyanide toxicity. However, because of tight binding to cytochrome oxidase, severe cyanide poisoning can occur with relatively low blood levels, especially if specimens are obtained several hours after exposure. Fatal poisoning has been reported with blood levels >3.0 μg/ml (11.54 μmol/L). Cyanide in plasma rather than red cells may be the critical factor in cyanide intoxication, and a value >0.1 μg/ml (3.85 μmol/L) is suggestive of acute cyanide toxicity, assuming a hematocrit of 50 per cent (Herbert, 1979). Thiocyanate levels are useful when chronic cyanide intoxication is suspected (see Nitroprusside, p. 366).

Bromide

Although use of bromides has declined, sporadic cases of bromide intoxication continue to occur even though they have been removed from over-the-counter drugs. The bromide ion has anticonvulsant activity, but the disadvantage of its use is the low ratio between the therapeutically effective and toxic dose. Acute bromide intoxication is rare because bromide causes gastrointestinal irritation, and thus it is difficult to ingest and retain an amount sufficient to attain toxic levels without vomiting. Chronic ingestion of bromide may lead to toxic levels, because bromides are excreted slowly by the kidney and thus may accumulate. Bromide is not bound to plasma proteins and does not undergo biotransformation.

The features that suggest the presence of bromide intoxication include fever, neurologic disturbances, skin rash, and a history of ingesting proprietary bromide-containing drugs. Toxic manifestations which frequently appear are irritability, agitation, and delirium. Sedation and psychic disturbances as well as tremors and motor incoordination also occur. Chronic bromide intoxication may be associated with elevated cerebrospinal fluid pressure and protein. Spuriously elevated serum chloride levels can be found in patients with bromism; however, the elevation is dependent on the chloride method employed.

A good correlation between the severity of bromide intoxication and serum bromide levels does not always exist; some patients may show signs of severe intoxication when the drug is present in relatively low concentrations. Bromide intoxication should be considered as the possible cause of mental or neurologic symptoms when serum levels exceed 9 mEq/L (9 mmol/L). Most patients show unmistakable signs of poisoning when serum bromide levels are in the range of 19 to 25 mEq/L (19 to 25 mmol/L) (Sharpless, 1965).

Carbon Monoxide

Carbon monoxide (CO) is a colorless, odorless gas which is generated by incomplete combustion of organic matter. It is present in tobacco smoke, fumes from fires, and exhaust of gasoline engines. Carbon monoxide combines with hemoglobin to form carboxyhemoglobin, which impairs the ability of blood to transport oxygen to tissues. Affinity of hemoglobin is over 200 times greater for CO than it is for oxygen; thus, exposure even to low concentrations of CO can reversibly inactivate a significant percentage of oxygen-carrying capacity of blood. In addition, presence of carboxyhemoglobin interferes with release of oxygen carried by the hemoglobin molecule. Tissue oxygen tensions therefore must fall to lower levels before oxyhemoglobin gives up its oxygen. Carbon monoxide also may affect heme-containing enzymes.

The toxic manifestations of CO are primarily the results of hypoxia and include headache, weakness, nausea, confusion, convulsions, and coma. Signs and symptoms of acute CO toxicity depend on the proportion of hemoglobin that is combined with CO; this is a function of the concentration of CO in inhaled air and the volume of inspired air. Toxicity also is governed by a number of other factors, including the patient's cardiac output, hemoglobin level, and tissue oxygen demands. When high concentrations of CO are inhaled, loss of consciousness may occur without classic symptoms of headache, nausea, and vomiting. Late complications which may occur in survivors include demyelinization and neuropsychiatric damage.

A sensitive gas chromatographic method and a rapid differential spectrophotometric technique are available for measurement of carboxyhemoglobin.

Carbon monoxide is produced endogenously from the metabolism of heme pigments, and the concentration is increased in a number of conditions including hemolytic disease. In healthy non-smokers living in cities, 0.25 to 2.1 per cent of hemoglobin is present as carboxyhemoglobin, whereas in smokers, levels of 0.7 to 6.5 per cent carboxyhemoglobin occur. Carboxyhemoglobin levels as high as 16 per cent have been reported in cigarette smokers, and even higher levels can occur in cigar smokers who inhale (Hebbel, 1978).

Symptoms of acute carbon monoxide poisoning generally occur at about 20 per cent carboxyhemoglobin and become severe at 30 per cent. However, individual response to a given level of carboxyhemoglobin is extremely variable. Generally at 40 to 50 per cent carboxyhemoglobin, headache and confusion occur; at 60 to 70 per cent, unconsciousness and convulsions ensue (Winter, 1976). In fatal poisoning, carboxyhemoglobin usually ranges from 60 to 80 per cent, but death has been reported at lower levels.

VOLATILES

Alcohols

Ethanol. Alcoholism is one of the major health problems of this country. It has been estimated that in the United States 95 million people drink ethyl alcohol (ethanol), and 9 million of these can be classified as chronic abusers. One in 25 hospital admissions is associated with ethanol abuse, and 50 per cent of all drivers involved in fatal automobile accidents have been drinking. Combined effects of alcohol are believed to constitute the third or fourth leading cause of death of adults in the United States.

The overall effect of ethyl alcohol on central nervous system function is that of a depressant and an anesthetic. The initial effect is loss of inhibition, followed by loss of judgment and personality change, impairment of memory, and loss of coordination. Additional alcohol ingestion leads to disorientation and then stupor, followed by coma and death. In addition to the need for blood alcohol levels as legal evidence, ethanol measurements commonly are used in cases of coma. In a study in a large city hospital, 42 per cent of specimens sent by the emergency room staff for six common analyses were found to contain ethanol (Senior, 1981).

Ethanol usually is ingested as beer (2 to 6 per cent), wine (10 to 20 per cent), or whiskey (40 to 50 per cent). Proof is twice the percentage of ethanol content; i.e., 100 proof whiskey is 50 per cent ethanol. The amount of ethanol in 1 ounce of whiskey is about the same as in one bottle of beer or in 4 ounces of wine. On an empty stomach, the absorption is so rapid that at least half of the ingested load is absorbed and the peak level is reached in 40 to 70 minutes. Ethanol is one of the few substances that is absorbed in the stomach. Approximately 20 to 25 per cent of that ingested will pass through the stomach with absorption affected by factors such as gastric emptying time as well as concentration and volume of ethanol ingested. Eating immediately prior to ethanol intake is associated with prolonging the peak blood level by one to two hours and reducing the peak level attained. Absorption from the skin, bladder, and inspired air contributes little to blood alcohol levels.

About 10 per cent of the ingested alcohol is excreted in the urine, sweat, and breath, whereas 90 per cent is metabolized in the liver first to acetaldehyde, and then to CO_2 and water. Alcohol dehydrogenase, the first enzyme in this pathway, is the rate-limiting metabolic step and becomes saturated at a blood ethanol concentration of about 16 mg/dl (3.5 mmol/L). At levels higher than this, the rate of metabolism remains constant. A 70 kg person metabolizes about 7 to 10 g of ethanol per hour, which is equivalent to an average of about 20 to 30 ml of 90 proof spirits (2/3 to 1 ounce), 8 to 12 ounces of beer, or 3 to 4 ounces of wine. Very little can be done acutely to increase ethanol metabolism.

Another pathway of ethanol metabolism is the microsomal system, which metabolizes not only ethanol but also such drugs as barbiturates and other sedatives. Drugs that are capable of inducing activity of the microsomal enzyme system increase the capacity for degradation of ethanol. Interaction of various drugs and ethanol with this enzyme system is responsible for the increased mortality which occurs with combined ethanol and benzodiazepine ingestions (see p. 364).

Three different groups of analytical procedures are used for determination of ethanol: (1) chemical oxidation with acid dichromate, (2) enzymatic oxidation with alcohol dehydrogenase, and (3) gas chromatography. These techniques have been reviewed by Dubowski (1980).

Dichromate methodology is dependent on oxidation of ethanol by dichromate in acid solution. The amount of dichromate reduced is proportional to the concentration of ethanol as seen below:

$$2\ Cr_2O_7^{-2} + 16\ H^+ + 3\ C_2H_5OH \rightarrow 4\ Cr^{+3} + 3\ CH_3COOH + 11\ H_2O$$

However, this reaction is not specific in that other alcohols, such as methanol and isopropanol, and aldehydes also reduce dichromate. Methanol is lethal at ethanol levels of 100 mg/dl (21.7 mmol/L), that is, the level required for the legal definition of intoxication. Isopropanol is more intoxicating than ethanol; a patient who appears intoxicated and has an "ethanol level" less than 100 mg/dl (21.7 mmol/L), should be suspected of isopropanol ingestion. Since acetone is the end product of isopropanol metabolism, an acetone determination can be used to help confirm ingestion of isopropanol. Paraldehyde, a drug used in the treatment of agitation, is metabolized to acetaldehyde, which also is capable of reducing dichromate; therefore, it results in a positive test for ethanol. Adaptation of this methodology is used in the Conway diffusion plate, in which dichromate and a patient's specimen are placed in different wells. If ethanol is present, it diffuses from its well and reacts with dichromate to form a green color. This method can be performed fairly quickly and is a semiquantitative estimate of ethanol when read at 30 minutes. When diffusion is allowed to continue for 16 to 18 hours, quantitation is quite precise.

The alcohol dehydrogenase (ADH) method is simple, accurate, and fairly specific; for many clinical laboratories, it is the method of choice for diagnostic purposes, especially when it is available on large, discrete, automated clinical analyzers, e.g., the DuPont aca. Ethanol is converted to acetaldehyde by alcohol dehydrogenase, and NADH is generated. NADH can be quantitated by its increased absorbance at 340 nm in the following reaction:

$$C_2H_5OH + NAD^+ \xrightarrow{ADH} CH_3CHO + NADH + H^+$$

Because equilibrium of this reaction lies far to the left, acetaldehyde is removed by coupling it with a semicarbazide to drive the reaction to the right. This methodology is not specific, since other alcohols such as isopropanol react to a variable degree depending on the source of the alcohol dehydrogenase.

Chromatography of the alcohols has been the method of choice for forensic and toxicologic laboratories. This methodology is qualitative as well as quantitative and, because of its specificity, has become the reference method. Specimens can be directly injected, extracted, or distilled, or a vapor phase (head space) can be prepared and injected.

Breath analysis (Breatholizer) is used in some states as a portable method of alcohol detection. The subject blows through a mouth piece, forcing his breath into an ampule containing potassium dichromate in acid solution. Ethanol is oxidized, and the reduction of dichromate can be quantitated. This method is subject to interferences by other alcohols, as well as recently ingested alcohol remaining in the mouth.

Serum or plasma is the most useful specimen for medical management; when compared to whole blood levels, the values obtained average about 1.18 times higher. However, whole blood is the only specimen required for analysis for medicolegal reasons in the United States, since systemic effects of ethanol have been correlated with blood concentrations. Arterial, venous, or capillary blood properly collected in a closed system is the preferred specimen. The specimen tube should be completely filled and must be kept tightly stoppered for centrifugation and storage to avoid loss of volatile constituents. If serum or plasma measurements are made, the specimen should be removed from blood cells and either analyzed promptly or stored under refrigeration in a stoppered tube. Cleaning of the puncture site should be performed with a non-alcoholic solution. If isopropanol is used as the disinfectant, it may be aspirated into the blood collection tube from the skin or gauze used for cleansing, artifactually raising serum ethanol levels when measured by non-specific techniques.

The relationship between blood and urine ethanol is ordinarily quite constant since kidneys do not have the ability to concentrate ethanol. In a group of volunteers given ethanol, the average urine to blood ratio was 1.35. Thus, if a urine level is obtained, a serum level equal to the urine level $\div$ 1.35 must have occurred. However, assumptions that are necessary to use urine determinations are that peak blood alcohol level has been passed and that the bladder has been emptied in the preceding 30 minutes prior to specimen collection. Determination of ethanol in urine is accepted as legal evidence in some European coun-

Table 17–14. INFLUENCE OF ACUTE ETHANOL INGESTION ON ETHANOL LEVELS AND BEHAVIOR

Whiskey (Ounces)	Blood Concentration	Influence
1–2	10–50 mg/dl (2.2–10.9 mmol/L)	None to mild euphoria
3–4	50–100 mg/dl (10.9–21.7 mmol/L) or greater	Mild influence on stereoscopic vision and dark adaptation
	100 mg/dl (21.7 mmol/L)	Legally intoxicated
4–6	100–150 mg/dl (21.7–32.6 mmol/L)	Euphoria; disappearance of inhibition; prolonged reaction time
6–7	150–200 mg/dl (32.6–43.4 mmol/L)	Moderately severe poisoning; reaction time greatly prolonged; loss of inhibition and slight disturbances in equilibrium and coordination
8–9	200–250 mg/dl (43.4–54.3 mmol/L)	Severe degree of poisoning; disturbances of equilibrium and coordination; retardation of the thought processes and clouding of consciousness
10–15	250–400 mg/dl (54.3–86.8 mmol/L)	Deep, possibly fatal coma

tries. For further information on the collection and handling of alcohol specimens, see Kaye (1980).

Table 17–14 shows blood ethanol concentrations and their effects on behavior. One shot of whiskey (1 ounce) will raise the blood alcohol level to about 25 to 35 mg/dl (5.4 to 7.5 mmol/L). At 100 mg/dl (21.7 mmol/L), a driver is legally under the influence of alcohol, and at 150 mg/dl (32.6 mmol/L), most persons appear intoxicated. When between 250 and 500 g of ethanol is ingested, lethal levels of 350 to 400 mg/dl (76 to 87 mmol/L) have been attained. These values apply only to individuals who are ingesting alcohol acutely.

In a group of chronic alcoholics, Lindblad (1976) demonstrated a remarkable degree of tolerance even to potentially lethal ethanol levels ranging from 500 to 780 mg/dl (108.7 to 169.3 mmol/L). His patients not only survived but tolerated ethanol so well that they were not obtunded. In addition, ethanol is metabolized almost twice as fast in alcoholic as in nonalcoholic subjects.

The hepatic degradation system located in the microsomes is a focal point for the interaction of ethanol and such drugs as chlordiazepoxide, diazepam, meprobamate, phenytoin, guanethidine, and isoniazid. When metabolized by the microsomal system in the presence of alcohol, these drugs have increased half-lives and prolonged effects. Interactions with this enzyme system are responsible for the increased mortality of combined alcohol and barbiturate ingestion.

Disulfiram, when used to treat chronic alcoholism, results in symptoms so unpleasant that the patient is unlikely to imbibe any ethanol-containing beverages while on a maintenance dose. This drug is thought to inhibit metabolism of acetaldehyde.

Although elevations of glucose and urea are well recognized as causing increases in serum osmolality, ethanol is the most common cause of this increase. At ethanol levels of 100 mg/dl (21.7 mmol/L), the serum osmolality is increased by 22 mOsm/kg (22 mmol/kg).

Methanol. Methanol, also called wood alcohol or methyl alcohol, is used in a number of industrial processes and as an adulterant of ethyl alcohol to make it impotable. Although single cases occur, poisoning involving methanol tends to occur in clusters; Swartz (1981) has reported an epidemic of methanol poisoning. The toxicity which develops appears not to be related directly to the amount ingested. Although fatalities usually occur from ingestion of 30 to 100 g, an amount as small as 6 g has been fatal and one as high as 200 g was non-lethal.

Following absorption, methanol is widely distributed in the body with the concentration in cerebrospinal fluid exceeding that of serum. Probably very little ingested methanol is eliminated in expired air or excreted in urine. Most is oxidized by the liver to formaldehyde and formic acid by the enzyme alcohol dehydrogenase at a rate independent of the plasma level. Since methanol is metabolized at about one seventh the rate of ethyl alcohol, complete oxidation of a toxic amount may take several days.

Usually there is a latent period of about 24 hours between ingestion and symptoms of toxicity. Patients complain of nausea, vomiting, headache, and blurring of vision which then progresses to blindness; these are followed by stupor, coma, convulsions, and respiratory arrest. Formic acid and other metabolites that accumulate are probably responsible for blindness and the metabolic acidosis that occurs. In those patients without metabolic acidosis, loss of vision is extremely unlikely.

Potential toxicity of alcohols has been predicted by comparison of measured and calculated serum osmolality. For example, a potentially lethal methanol level of 800 μg/ml (24.2 mmol/L), theoretically would increase serum osmolality by 27 mOsm/kg (27 mmol/kg) but would not be reflected in the calculated osmolality.

In order to retard formation of toxic methanol intermediates, treatment of methanol ingestion should include administration of ethanol to compete with the enzyme alcohol dehydrogenase and bicarbonate to correct the acidosis. Hemodialysis has proved to be of benefit in the treatment of patients who have ingested methanol.

Isopropanol. Isopropanol (isopropyl alcohol) is available as a disinfectant in strengths varying from 30 to 99.9 per cent, but a preparation of 70 per cent isopropyl alcohol, also known as rubbing alcohol, is used widely. When ingested, isopropanol is slightly more toxic than ethanol but results in similar symptoms.

Although some alcohol dehydrogenase methods show minimal reactivity with isopropanol, others show cross-reactivity as high as 40 per cent (Vasiliades, 1977). Gas chromatographic methods are precise and specific.

Isopropanol ingestion is suggested by a large difference between the observed and calculated serum osmolality. About 15 per cent of isopropanol is metabolized to acetone, and presence of acetone further substantiates diagnosis of isopropanol ingestion. When the intake of isopropanol is small, acetone may be found only in urine, but when large amounts are ingested, acetone can be found in both blood and urine. Serum isopropanol levels as low as 15 mg/dl (2.5 mmol/L) have been found in fatal poisoning.

Ethylene Glycol

Ethylene glycol (CH_2OH-CH_2OH) is used as a solvent for dyes, pharmaceuticals, and detergents, as well as a substance to lower the freezing point in engine cooling systems (antifreeze). It is colorless and odorless, and has a nonspecific, slightly sweet taste, all of which may contribute to its popularity as a suicide agent or as a poor man's substitute for ethanol. Ethylene glycol by itself has little toxicity; however, it is metabolized to a variety of toxic compounds, including glycoaldehyde, glycolic acid, glyoxylic acid, and oxalic acid. A dose of about 100 ml of pure ethylene glycol is lethal, but some fatal poisonings have been described with only 60 ml.

The earliest symptom of ethylene glycol poisoning is inebriation. By four to eight hours, metabolic acidosis and calcium oxalate crystals in urine are readily apparent, and over the next few hours congestive heart failure and pulmonary edema become prominent. Subsequently acute oliguric renal failure supervenes. Therapy consists of hemodialysis and administration of ethanol to compete for alcohol dehydrogenase, the enzyme responsible for the critical first step in ethylene glycol metabolism.

Laboratory findings include a large anion gap, metabolic acidosis not accounted for by lactate concentrations, and a calculated osmolality which markedly underestimates the measured value. Dihydrate calcium oxalate crystals and monohydrate calcium oxalate crystals, which can be confused with hippuric acid, are found in urine (Godolphin, 1980). Various complex colorimetric, fluorometric, and chromatographic methods have been described for measurement of ethylene glycol; adaptation of a blood ethanol reagent kit for ethylene glycol measurements provides a rapid method which requires no specialized equipment (Eckfeldt, 1980). Serum levels have not been studied extensively, but levels of 300 to 4300 mg/L (4.8 to 69.2 mmol/L) have been reported in fatal cases.

HEAVY METALS

Arsenic

Inorganic arsenicals are employed as insecticides, herbicides, and rodenticides. These as well as the colorless, non-irritating gas arsine (arsenous hydride) can cause arsenic poisoning. Most cases of arsine poisoning have been associated with concomitant use of acid and crude metals, one or both of which contain arsenic as an impurity. Arsenic also may be found in seafood, especially shellfish, which may contain large amounts.

The toxic action of arsenic occurs through its inhibition of sulfhydryl enzyme systems of the body. Acute toxicity is manifested by gastrointestinal symptoms, such as severe gastric pain, vomiting, and diarrhea. In severe poisoning, convulsions, coma, and death occur. Chronic arsenic poisoning has an insidious onset and is manifested by signs and symptoms including diarrhea, skin pigmentation, hyperkeratosis, hepatomegaly, renal tubular damage, and hair loss. As toxicity advances, central nervous system symptoms may occur. Arsenic accumulates mainly in the liver, kidney, gastrointestinal tract, spleen, and lung. Since it has a high affinity for keratin, the concentration of arsenic in hair and nails is higher than in other tissues. Arsenic is excreted mainly in the urine.

Arsenic may be determined by screening techniques in which it forms a black or brown deposit on copper strips. Other metals such as antimony produce the same effect; thus additional steps are necessary for positive identification. A variety of spectrophotometric procedures and atomic absorption methods are available for arsenic quantitation. In acute poisoning, confirmation of the diagnosis is made by finding increased arsenic in vomitus or gastric lavage; also elevated arsenic levels are found in blood and urine. In chronic exposure, urine, hair, or nail clippings are the preferred specimens. Arsenic may be found in hair as soon as 30 hours after ingestion.

Arsenic levels in individuals without industrial exposure to arsenic are <10 μg/L (0.13 μmol/L) for whole blood, <20 μg/L (0.26 μmol/L) for urine, and <1 μg/g (13 mmol/g) of hair. Blood or urine levels >50 μg/L (0.65 μmol/L) should be regarded as suspicious for toxicity (Berman, 1981). However, a wide range of toxic arsenic levels has been reported, and some workers consider urine levels up to 330 μg/L (4.29 μmol/L) as within the reference interval (Berman, 1981).

Iron

Iron tablets vary considerably in the amount of elemental iron they contain; the most common form of ferrous sulfate tablet is 20 per cent elemental iron by weight. The oral dose of elemental iron considered lethal is accepted to be as low as 200 to 250 mg/kg of body weight, and an iron dose of 150 mg/kg is considered dangerous. In a small child as few as ten ferrous sulfate tablets (130 mg of elemental iron) have been reported to cause death (Robotham, 1980).

Signs and symptoms of iron toxicity may occur within 30 minutes after ingestion or may be delayed as long as several hours. Gastrointestinal irritation and abdominal pain often are accompanied by vomiting and bloody diarrhea. If death does not occur within the first few hours after ingestion, a transient, nearly asymptomatic period may occur before death ensues. After the period of quiescence, shock and hypoglycemia may take place. If recovery occurs, sequelae may include severe scarring of the gastrointestinal tract, hepatic cirrhosis, and manifestations of central nervous system damage. Deferoxamine, a highly specific chelator of ferric iron, is used in the treatment of acute iron poisoning; for further details, see Robotham (1980).

Peak serum iron levels usually occur between two and four hours after ingestion. Toxic effects of iron salts result from the presence of unbound serum iron; under usual circumstances, serum iron binding capacity is 250 to 400 μg/dl (44.8 to 71.6 μmol/L). Shock and coma occur in up to 50 per cent of patients with serum iron levels >700 μg/dl (125 μmol/L), and death usually is associated with peak serum iron levels >1000 μg/dl (179 μmol/L). Although iron levels can be a useful index of significant ingestion, values must be interpreted with caution because large doses of iron can result in only minimal elevations in serum levels. This is due to the rapid clearance of iron from serum and its deposition in the liver. Serum iron levels <500 μg/dl (89.5 μmol/L) have been associated with death, and serious toxicity has been reported with serum iron levels <300 μg/dl (52.8 μmol/L) (Robotham, 1980). Thus Robotham (1980) concludes that whereas serum iron levels >300 μg/dl (52.8 mmol/L) should be of concern, levels less than this do not rule out serious toxicity.

Lead

Lead is a heavy metal without any known physiologic function in the human body. Sources of lead are ubiquitous, and lead poisoning is a serious public health problem. The most important cause of severe childhood lead poisoning is ingestion of lead-containing paints, but air, dust, and dirt also are important sources. A single paint chip may contain 10,000 μg (48.3 μmol) of lead. Vulnerability of children to lead poisoning is enhanced by hand-to-mouth activities, pica, and increased intestinal absorption. Other sources of lead include automobile emissions, fumes from burning storage batteries, and some types of tableware.

Lead is absorbed slowly and incompletely from the gastrointestinal tract and can be absorbed from the respiratory tract after inhalation. The distribution of lead in the body is primarily in two pools; an active pool in blood and soft tissues, and a storage pool in bone. In blood, nearly all circulating inorganic lead is associated with erythrocytes. Following absorption, lead is distributed in the soft tissues, with the highest concentrations reached in the kidney and liver. Over a period of time, the lead is redistributed and accumulates in bone, teeth, and hair, with a small quantity of inorganic lead becoming deposited in the brain. Lead is excreted mainly by the kidneys; the rate of excretion of lead is very slow, and thus it tends to accumulate in the body.

Signs and symptoms of lead poisoning include malaise, anorexia, abdominal pain, vomiting, irritability, and apathy. Manifestations of lead poisoning include effects on the hematopoietic, renal, and central nervous systems. The heme biosynthetic pathway is affected by lead at several different sites (Fig. 17–7). Enzymes in the heme pathway that are sensitive to lead include enzyme δ-aminolevulinic dehydratase, which is responsible for condensation of two molecules of δ-aminolevulinic acid to form porphobilinogen, and ferrochelatase, which catalyzes insertion of iron into protoporphyrin IX to form heme. In lead poisoning, the excess protoporphyrin produced exists as a zinc chelate. Increased coproporphyrin production also occurs probably as a secondary effect of lead-induced inhibition of heme synthesis. Fanconi's syndrome, characterized by aminoaciduria, glucosuria, and phosphaturia, may occur, but is reversible with chelation therapy.

Lead encephalopathy is characterized by sudden onset of cerebral edema, coma, and convulsions. Sequelae include mental retardation, seizure disorders, behavioral abnormalities, and occasionally blindness, aphasia, and hemiparesis. Neurologic damage, especially in children, is often irreversible, and acute neurologic toxicity may develop without previous

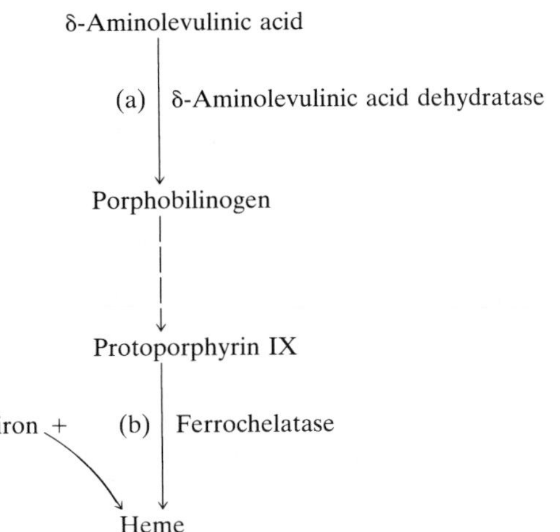

Figure 17–7. Effects of lead on the heme biosynthetic pathway. Lead inhibits most enzymes of the heme synthetic pathway. Inhibition of (a) and (b) leads to accumulation of their substrates, the measurement of which is of diagnostic importance.

symptoms. Therefore, it is important to detect and treat lead poisoning before symptoms become obvious. Lead levels that can be considered as representing excessive exposure are ill-defined. Asymptomatic lead poisoning may cause significant and permanent impairment in nervous system function.

Laboratory Diagnosis of Lead Poisoning. About 90 per cent of circulating lead is associated with erythrocytes, and thus whole blood or erythrocytes are used in lead determinations. Flameless atomic absorption and anodic stripping voltammetry are used to measure lead; they are sensitive and possess a high degree of specifity. The reliability of lead measurement, however, is influenced by the possibility of specimen contamination; thus lead levels are confirmed using a second specimen.

In a statement by the Center for Disease Control (CDC), an elevated blood lead is defined as a confirmed blood lead of 30 μg/dl or more (1.44 μmol/L) (Needleman, 1978). Clinical toxicity, however, does not always relate precisely to blood lead levels; lead encephalopathy may occur at levels as low as about 100 μg/dl (4.83 μmol/L).

For a variety of reasons, including difficulty in obtaining blood specimens which are free of contamination by environmental lead, efforts to identify patients with lead poisoning have been directed toward measurement of effects of lead on heme synthesis. Toxic effects of lead are manifested by (1) increased excretion of δ-aminolevulinic acid, (2) increased coproporphyrin excretion, (3) decreased erythrocyte δ-aminolevulinic dehydratase, and (4) increased erythrocyte protoporphyrin.

The difficulty in using urinary δ-aminolevulinic acid and coproporphyrin as parameters of excess lead burden is in collection of a complete 24-hour urine specimen; random urine specimens are not reliable for screening. In addition, urinary δ-aminolevulinic acid excretion rises slowly until lead levels reach about 40 μg/dl (1.92 μmol/L), and daily excretion is variable in children. Increased excretion of coproporphyrin, which is a byproduct of the heme synthetic pathway, occurs with active lead intoxication. Because it is affected by the lead level at the time of determination, the enzyme δ-aminolevulinic dehydratase, which may be assayed in whole blood, is an indicator of acute exposure to lead. However, usefulness of δ-aminolevulinic acid dehydratase in screening for lead toxicity is limited due to its instability and extreme sensitivity of the enzyme even to minimal lead exposure. Inhibition of the enzyme is so pronounced that differences in enzyme activity in specimens with large differences in lead content cannot be distinguished (Piomelli, 1980). Increased levels of erythrocyte protoporphyrin reflect chronic lead exposure.

The term erythrocyte protoporphyrin is used to refer to zinc protoporphyrin and free erythrocyte protoporphyrin. Both zinc protoporphyrin and free protoporphyrin base have the property of intense red fluorescence; several methods, including direct fluorimetry of whole blood and fluorescence analysis of whole blood extracts, have been developed based on this property. Some extraction methods remove zinc from the protoporphyrin, leaving the free base. Erythrocyte protoporphyrin (EP) levels may be increased in disorders other than lead poisoning, including iron deficiency anemia and erythropoietic protoporphyria. EP levels of 50 to 249 μg/dl (0.90 to 4.48 μmol/L) are generally associated with iron deficiency, whereas markedly elevated values, i.e., ≥300 μg/dl (5.4 μmol/L), usually are due to lead toxicity (Needleman, 1978). In erythropoietic protoporphyria, EP levels also are very high, but this disorder has a number of distinguishing clinical features, including prominent photosensitivity. Since in erythropoietic protoporphyria most of the protoporphyrin is present as the free base, techniques which are highly specific for zinc protoporphyrin such as direct fluorometry may give falsely low results (Piomelli, 1980).

Measurement of EP has been recommended for screening because of its ease of performance and good reproducibility. In addition, there is the benefit of detecting those children who may have iron deficiency. Because EP may be increased by diseases other than lead poisoning and elevated blood lead may be due to specimen contamination, both EP and blood lead are necessary for full evaluation and monitoring of those individuals who have a positive result by either method.

Lead poisoning is defined in a statement by the CDC as existing when a child has one of the following: (1) two successive blood lead levels ≥70 μg/dl (3.36 μmol/L) with or without symptoms; (2) EP level ≥250 μg/dl (4.5 μmol/L) whole blood and a confirmed elevated blood lead level ≥50 μg/dl (2.4 μmol/L) with or without symptoms; (3) EP level >109 μg/dl (1.96 μmol/L) associated with a confirmed elevated blood lead level ≥30 μg/dl (1.44 μmol/L) with compatible symptoms; or (4) confirmed blood lead level >49 μg/dl (2.35 μmol/L) with compatible symptoms and evidence of toxicity (that is, abnormal EP, urinary δ-aminolevulinic acid, urinary coproporphyrin, or calcium disodium EDTA mobilization test) (Needleman, 1978).

Although mobilization tests are good indicators of the body burden of lead, they should be reserved for the asymptomatic patient, and should not be performed in patients with whole blood lead levels >70 μg/dl (3.36 μmol/L). Mobilization (chelation) tests are performed by injecting calcium disodium edathamil (EDTA) and collecting urine for lead measurements. There are several protocols for mobilization tests which vary as to the amount of EDTA used and the timing of the urine specimens. Results are expressed as the ratio of micrograms of lead excreted per milligram EDTA administered; ratios greater than 1.0 are considered indicative of a potentially toxic lead burden (Needleman, 1978).

Mercury

Compounds containing mercury are widely used in agriculture and industry. Most of the biologic properties of mercury are due to its ability to form covalent bonds with sulfur; mercurials even in low concentrations are capable of inactivating sulfhydryl enzymes. Symptoms of mercury poisoning depend on the chemical state of mercury (metallic, inorganic, or bivalent organic) to which the individual is exposed as well as whether exposure is acute or chronic. Bivalent organic mercury compounds containing an alkyl group are the most toxic and the most important of the environmental mercury contaminants. Of these, methyl mercury is the most toxic and is known to be highly resistant to biodegradation. It can be synthesized from other forms of mercury and concentrated in the aquatic food chain.

Inhalation of vapors from metallic mercury leads to pneumonitis, fever, cough, chest pain, and other pulmonary symptoms. Ingestion of inorganic mercury compounds is characterized by gastrointestinal symptoms such as vomiting and bloody diarrhea; shock and death may occur. The signs and symptoms of chronic poisoning from inorganic mercurials include stomatitis, colitis, progressive renal damage, anemia, and peripheral neuritis. Many central nervous system manifestations occur, including behavioral changes, irritability, tremors, and drowsiness. The organic mercurials such as methyl mercury cause mainly neurologic signs and symptoms, including ataxia, tremor, and dysarthria. Severe poisoning may lead to blindness, coma, and death.

The absorption, distribution, and excretion of mercury are determined by the properties and extent of *in vivo* conversion of each compound to inorganic mercury. Although most organic mercurials are excreted quickly, urinary excretion of methyl mercury is slow due to its low decomposition to inorganic mercury, its complete reabsorption when excreted in bile, and its low urinary excretion compared with inorganic mercury. Methyl mercury crosses the blood-brain barrier easily and causes irreversible damage to the nervous system.

Techniques such as the Reinsch test, which depends on the deposition of heavy metals on a copper strip, or one of its modifications can be used to screen for presence of mercury. Mercury can be quantitated by atomic absorption. Although the correlation between urinary mercury excretion and symptoms of mercury poisoning is considered poor, it is the most reliable measurement available to assess exposure to inorganic mercury. Exposure to organic mercury compounds, however, probably is not reliably reflected by urinary levels. In contrast to inorganic mercury, methyl mercury is mainly located in the red blood cells, and thus estimation of levels must be made using red cells or whole blood. Analysis of hair also has been used, and has been reported to help recapitulate the history of exposure.

In healthy subjects, mercury levels are <100 μg/L (0.5 μmol/L) in blood and <30 μg/L (0.15 μmol/L) in urine. Mercury concentrations in whole blood of 500 to 1000 μg/L (2.5 to 5.0 μmol/L) may be associated with symptoms of intoxication. When urinary levels are >300 μg/24 hours (1.5 μmol/24 hours), mercury toxicity should be suspected (Hayes, 1982). Wide fluctuations in excretion of mercury into urine are common in exposed individuals.

DRUG ABUSE

One of the distinguishing features of recent drug use patterns is the variety of drugs abused. In a review of drug trends, Smith in 1974 commented that the only constant in the American drug abuse scene "is that it will change." The drugs abused vary with such factors as geographic location, availability of the substance, and fads. In many cases, two or more drugs are combined to enhance the state of intoxication. In general, abused drugs, excluding alcohol and nicotine, can be placed in the categories of narcotic analgesics, central nervous system stimulants and depressants, cannabinoids, and psychedelics or hallucinogens. The metabolism and physiologic effects of the drugs of abuse, including amphetamines, morphine, cocaine, cannabinoids (marijuana), and lysergic acid diethylamide (LSD), have been reviewed by Lemberger (1976).

Although a number of screening techniques are available, thin layer chromatography is probably the most widely employed method and urine the most commonly used specimen. Many drugs, such as cocaine, barbiturates, glutethimide, morphine, and amphetamines, may be detected using this technique. Confirmatory methods are necessary because of interferences and metabolites. Although some drugs may be excreted in urine unchanged, others may be partially or almost completely metabolized. Use of some drugs may be indicated only by the presence of their metabolites. For example, cocaine is extensively metabolized to benzoylecgonine and ecgonine with little free cocaine available for detection in the urine.

For further discussion of the role of the laboratory in analysis of drugs of abuse, see Frings (1977). Many of the commonly abused drugs, with their street and trade names, are listed in Table 17–15.

DRUG OVERDOSE

Evaluation of a patient in coma with a suspected overdose should include exclusion of entities such as diabetic ketoacidosis, hyperosmolar non-ketotic coma, hypoglycemia, myxedema, hyponatremia, uremia, stroke syndrome, hepatic coma, trauma, and the encephalitides. However, finding a specific cause that could be responsible for the coma does not exclude a drug overdose as a precipitating or associated cause of coma. In addition, presence of an elevated drug level does not obviate another cause or precipitating factor for the coma, such as a second drug, trauma, or metabolic cause. Although coma is the presenting symptom with excessive ingestion of many drugs, potentially fatal toxicity with a few drugs, such as acetaminophen, may not present as coma, and coma may not occur until death is about to ensue. In a non-comatose patient, even though history may be the only means of assessing severity of an overdose at the time of hospital admission, little reliance can be placed on it because overdose patients usually either exaggerate or minimize the situation (Wright, 1980). Hence it is usually left to the laboratory to help

Table 17–15. COMMONLY ABUSED DRUGS

Pharmacological Chemical Class	Generic Name	Rx Trade Name	Street Name
Hypnotics			
Barbiturate			
Rapid acting	Pentobarbital	Nembutal, Carbrital	Nemmies, yellows, yellow jackets
	Secobarbital	Seconal	Reds, pink ladies
	Seco/Amobarbital	Tuinal	Christmas trees, tooies, rainbows
Intermediate acting	Amobarbital	Amytal	Blues, blue angels
	Butabarbital	Fiorinal	
Long acting	Phenobarbital	Primatene tablets	
Nonbarbiturate	Methaqualone	Quaalude	Ludes, 714's, sopers, vitamin Q, love drug, disco biscuits
	Ethchlorvynol	Placidyl	Dyls
	Glutethimide	Doriden	In combination with codeine called "loads"
Benzodiazepine	Flurazepam	Dalmane	Downs
Analgesics			
Narcotic			
Opiate	Diacetylmorphine		H, mexican brown, Harry, dirt, smack, skag, junk
	Morphine		
	Codeine		
Synthetic	Methadone	Dolophine	Dollies
	Propoxyphene	Darvon	
	Pentazocine	Talwin	T's
	Meperidine	Demerol	Demmies
	Salicylate	Aspirin	
	Acetaminophen	Tylenol	
Tranquilizers			
Phenothiazine	Chlorpromazine	Thorazine	
	Thioridazine	Mellaril	
	Trifluoperazine	Stelazine	
	Prochlorperazine	Compazine	
	Promethazine	Phenergan	
Carbamate	Meprobamate	Miltown, Equanil	
	Diazepam	Valium	
Benzodiazepine	Chlordiazepoxide	Librium	
	Oxazepam	Serax	
Antidepressants			
Tricyclic	Amitriptyline	Elavil, Triavil	
	Nortriptyline	Aventyl	
	Imipramine	Tofranil	
	Desipramine	Norpramin	
	Doxepin	Sinequan	
	Amoxapine	Asendin	
Tetracyclic	Maprotiline	Ludiomil	
Stimulants			
Sympathomimetic amines	Amphetamine	Benzedrine	Speed, crystal, whites, crank, crosses, uppers, cart wheels, black mollies, black Cadillacs, Christmas trees, black beauties
	Methamphetamine	Desoxyn	
	Phentermine	Ionamin, Fastin	
	Ephedrine	Bronkaid, Nyquil	
	Pseudophedrine	Primatene tablets, CoTylenol, Novahistine	
	Phenylpropanolamine	Allerest, Comtrex, Contac, Daycare, Formula 44, Sine-Aid, Sinutab, Triaminic, Dexatrim, Dietac, Prolamine, Hungrex	
	Cocaine		Snow, blow, coke, big C, lady, nose candy, toot

Table continued on following page

2

Table 17–15. COMMONLY ABUSED DRUGS *(Continued)*

Pharmacological Chemical Class	Generic Name	Rx Trade Name	Street Name
Stimulants (Continued)	Nicotine		
Xanthine	Caffeine	No-Doz, Vivarin	
	Theophylline	Bronkaid, Primatene	
Hallucinogens	Phencyclidine		PCP, angel dust, crystal, hog, peace pill
	Tetrahydrocannabinol (marijuana)		Grass, dope, THC, pot, weed, smoke, Mary Jane
	Mescaline		Peyote, buttons
	Psilocybin		Magic mushrooms, psychedelic mushrooms, shrooms
	Lysergic acid diethylamide (LSD)		LSD, acid, blotter, microdot, window pane

develop a rational approach to management of these patients by providing drug measurements.

The frequency with which overdoses due to a given drug are found varies not only with the locality but from time to time; for example, acetaminophen was popular in Great Britain in the early 1970's but rarely used in the United States at that time. Glutethimide was a major problem in the 1960s, but by 1980 was not a common cause of an overdose. These factors as well as instrumentation, technical expertise available, and turnaround time are considerations in determining which drug assays are made available. However, since there are over 2500 pharmaceuticals listed in the 1982 edition of the Physicians' Desk Reference (PDR), and because overdose occurs with not only these drugs but with many chemicals as well, it is an impossibility for even the largest laboratory specializing in toxicologic analyses to screen for all available compounds. In several large studies, ethanol, barbiturates, and salicylates account for more than half of the overdoses.

Techniques that are available for screening specimens from overdose patients for drugs include spectrophotometry, paper chromatography, thin layer chromatography, gas chromatography, gas chromatography–mass spectrometry (with computer reference scan), radioimmunoassay, homogeneous enzyme immunoassay, and HPLC. Many of these procedures are time consuming, lack specificity and sensitivity, or are applicable to only a single drug. Some single determinations are available using large automated instruments, e.g., salicylate, phenobarbital, and alcohol assays using the DuPont aca. Because these measurements have a turnaround time of less than 10 minutes and are not labor intensive, they are suitable for rapid detection of these substances. Other specific procedures such as radioimmunoassay are less suitable for use on an emergency basis, because turnaround time is relatively lengthy. However, homogeneous enzyme immunoassay is useful as a screening technique and commonly is employed for barbiturates and narcotics because results can be generated quickly. Techniques in which multiple drug estimations can be made are convenient for screening procedures; these include thin layer chromatography, gas chromatography, and HPLC. A thin layer chromatographic system in kit form is available for detection and identification of a broad spectrum of drugs. This system, Toxi-Lab, (Analytical Systems, Laguna Hills, Cal.) requires very little equipment and has been used successfully by many laboratories.

Table 17–16. TOXIC SUBSTANCES WITH SPECIFIC ANTIDOTES*

Substance	Antidote
Acetaminophen	Acetylcysteine
Iron salts	Deferoxamine
Methanol	Ethanol
Narcotics	Naloxone hydrochloride
Organophosphates	Pralidoxime (PAM)

*Modified from Sohn, D., and Byers, J.: Clin. Toxicol., *18*:459, 1981.

For most drug overdoses, treatment is nonspecific and includes aggressive support of vital functions, evacuation of stomach contents, and administration of activated charcoal when possible. With salicylates and long-acting barbiturates, alkalinization of the urine is an additional therapeutic modality. Specific identification is required for only a few substances when identification and quantitation are necessary to prescribe appropriate doses of specific antidotes (Table 17–16). With some drugs, such as narcotics and propoxyphene, immediate treatment with morphine antagonists may be of benefit. In patients with stage 3 or 4 coma with an unknown intoxicant, hemodialysis may be initiated if improvement is not noted within 24 hours, or if methanol or ethylene glycol intoxication is suspected. When identity of the intoxicant is known, hemodialysis is indicated when criteria outlined by Winchester (1977) are met.

Many factors determine which drug assays should be available for a comatose patient. Because they are present in over 50 per cent of cases and suitable techniques are available, ethanol, salicylate, and barbiturate measurements should be made accessible.

Specific antidotes for those drugs listed in Table 17–16 make availability of measurements of these drugs with an appropriate turnaround time important. Depending on the resources and patient population, screening techniques for hypnotics, opiates, and phenothiazines may be appropriate.

Ambler, P. K., Singh, B. N., and Lever, M.: A simple and rapid fluorometric method for the estimation of 1-(2-hydroxy-3-isopropylamino-propoxy)-naphthalene hydrochloride, propranolol, in blood. Clin. Chim. Acta, *54*:373, 1974.

Ameer, B., and Greenblatt, D. J.: Acetaminophen. Ann. Intern. Med., *87*:202, 1977.

Anderson, R. J., Potts, D. E., Gabow, P. A., Rumack, B. H., and Schrier, R. W.: Unrecognized adult salicylate intoxication. Ann. Intern. Med., *85*:745, 1976.

Benowitz, N. L., and Meister, W.: Clinical pharmacokinetics of lignocaine. Clin. Pharmacokinet., *3*:177, 1978.

Berman, E.: Heavy metals, Lab. Med., *12*:677, 1981.

Bertino, J. R.: Clinical use of methotrexate — with emphasis on use of high doses. Cancer Treat. Rep., *65*:131, 1981.

Bigger, J. T., Schmidt, D. H., and Kutt, H.: Relationships between the plasma level of diphenylhydantoin sodium and its cardiac antiarrhythmic effects. Circulation, *38*:363, 1968.

Bogusz, M., Moroz, J., Karski, J., Gierz, J., Regieli, A., Witkowska, R., and Golabek, A.: Blood cyanide and thiocyanate concentrations after administration of sodium nitroprusside as hypotensive agent in neurosurgery. Clin. Chem., *25*:60, 1979.

Brillman, J., Gallagher, B. B., and Mattson, R. H.: Acute primidone intoxication. Arch. Neurol., *30*:255, 1974.

Broussard, L. A. (submitter); Fendley, T. W., Pellegrino, L., McNair, R. D., and Stearns, F. M. (evaluators); and Frings, C. S. (assigned editor): Fluorometric determination of quinidine. Clin. Chem., *27*:1929, 1981.

Burgess, E. D., Friel, P. N., Blair, A. D., and Raisys, V. A.: Serum phenytoin concentrations in uremia. Ann. Intern. Med., *94*:59, 1981.

Butler, V. P.: Assays of digitalis in blood. Prog. Cardiovasc. Dis., *14*:571, 1972.

Cate, J. C., and Jatlow, P. I.: Chlordiazepoxide overdose: Interpretation of serum drug concentrations. Clin. Toxicol., *6*:553, 1973.

Cereghino, J. J.: Relation of plasma concentration to seizure control. *In* Woodbury, D. M., Penry, J. K., and Pippenger, C. E. (eds.): Antiepileptic Drugs. New York, Raven Press, 1982.

College of American Pathologists: Therapeutic drug monitoring survey. 1982 Set Z-C, Skokie, Ill., 1982.

Cottrell, J. E., Casthely, P., Brodie, J. D., Patel, K., Klein, A., and Turndorf, H.: Prevention of nitroprusside-induced cyanide toxicity with hydroxycobalamin. N. Engl. J. Med., *298*:809, 1978.

Cutler, N. R., and Heiser, J. F.: The tricyclic antidepressants. J.A.M.A., *240*:2264, 1978.

Done, A. K.: Salicylate intoxication; significance of measurements of salicylate in blood in cases of acute ingestion. Pediatrics, *26*:800, 1960.

Drayer, D. E., Lorenzo, B., and Reidenberg, M. M.: Liquid chromatography and fluorescence spectroscopy compared with the homogeneous enzyme immunoassay technique for determining quinidine in serum. Clin. Chem., *27*:308, 1981.

Dubowski, K. M.: Alcohol determination in the clinical laboratory. Am. J. Clin. Path., *74*:747, 1980.

Eckfeldt, J. H., and Light, R. T.: Kinetic ethylene glycol assay with use of yeast alcohol dehydrogenase. Clin. Chem., *26*:1278, 1980.

Finkle, B. S., McCloskey, K. L., and Goodman, L. S.: Diazepam and drug-associated deaths. J.A.M.A. *242*:429, 1979.

Frings, C. S.: Role of the laboratory with regard to drug-abuse treatment facilities. *In* Thomas, J. J., Bondo, P. B., and Sunshine, I. (eds.): Guidelines for Analytical Toxicology Programs, Vol. I. Cleveland, CRC Press, Inc., 1977.

Godolphin, W., Meagher, E. P., Sanders, H. D., and Frohlich, J.: Unusual calcium oxalate crystals in ethylene glycol poisoning. Clin. Toxicol., *16*:479, 1980.

Goldberg, M. J., and Berlinger, W. G.: Treatment of phenobarbital overdose with activated charcoal. J.A.M.A., *247*:2400, 1982.

Goodnick, P. J., Fieve, R. R., Meltzer, H. L., and Dunner, D. L.: Lithium elimination half-life and duration of therapy. Clin. Pharmacol. Ther., *29*:47, 1981.

Gotelli, G. R., Kabra, P. M., and Marton, L. J.: Determination of acetaminophen and phenacetin in plasma by high-pressure liquid chromatography. Clin. Chem., *23*:957, 1977.

Greenblatt, D. J., Sellers, E. M., and Shader, R. I.: Drug disposition in old age. N. Engl. J. Med., *306*:1081, 1982.

Guelen, P. J. M.: Clinical pharmacokinetics of lithium. Excerpta Medica, *501*:106, 1980.

Hayes, W. J.: Pesticides Studied in Man. Baltimore, Williams and Wilkins, 1982.

Hebbel, R. P., Eaton, J. W., Modler, S., and Jacobs, H. S.: Extreme but asymptomatic carboxyhemoglobinemia and chronic lung disease. J.A.M.A., *239*:2584, 1978.

Hendeles, L., and Weinberger, M.: Poisoning patients with intravenous theophylline. Am. J. Hosp. Pharm., *37*:49, 1980.

Herbert, V.: Laetrile: The cult of cyanide. Promoting poison for profit. Am. J. Clin. Nutr., *32*:1121, 1979.

Howanitz, J. H., and Howanitz, P. J.: Antiarrhythmic drug monitoring. Clin. Lab. Med., *1*:501, 1981a.

Howanitz, J. H., and Howanitz, P. J.: Digitalis and vasoactive drugs. Clin. Lab. Med., *1*:523, 1981b.

Howanitz, J. H., and Howanitz, P. J.: Therapeutic drug monitoring: Pharmacokinetic and pharmacodynamic principles. Clin. Lab. Med., *1*:467, 1981c.

Inturrisi, C. E., Colburn, W. A., Verebey, K., Dayton, H. E., Woody, G. E., and O'Brien, C. P.: Propoxyphene and norpropoxyphene kinetics after single and repeated doses of propoxyphene. Clin. Pharmacol. Ther., *31*:157, 1982.

James, G. P., Djang, M. H., and Hamilton, H. H.: False-negative results for urinary phenothiazines and imipramine in Forrest's qualitative assays. Clin. Chem., *26*:345, 1980.

Jatlow, P., Dobular, K., and Bailey, D.: Serum diazepam concentrations in overdose. Their significance. Am. J. Clin. Path., *72*:571, 1979.

Jusko, W. J., Koup, J. R., Vance, J. W., Schentag, J. J., and Kuritzky, P.: Intravenous theophylline therapy: Nomogram guidelines. Ann. Intern. Med., *86*:400, 1977.

Kaye, S.: The collection and handling of the blood alcohol specimen. Am. J. Clin. Path., *74*:743, 1980.

Kawai, S., Ogawa, K., and Satake, T.: Erythrocyte digoxin concentration. Clin. Pharmacol. Ther., *31*:541, 1982.

Knott, C., Hamshaw-Thomas, A., and Reynolds, F.: Phenytoin-valproate interaction: Importance of saliva monitoring in epilepsy. Br. Med. J., *284*:13, 1982.

Krenzelok, E. P., Best, L., and Manoguerra, A. S.: Acetaminophen toxicity. Am. J. Hosp. Pharm., *34*:391, 1977.

Lehane, D. P., Wissert, P. J., Menjharth, P., Levy, A. L., and Kuckucka, M. A.: Enzyme immunoassay for serum lidocaine in antiarrhythmic therapy. Clin. Chem., *25*:614, 1979.

Lemberger, L., and Rubin, A.: Physiologic Deposition of Drugs of Abuse. New York, Spectrum Publications Inc., 1976.

Lindblad, B., and Olsson, R.: Unusually high levels of blood alcohol? J.A.M.A., *236*:1600, 1976.

McCarron, M. M., Schulze, B. W., Walberg, C. B., Thompson, G. A., and Ansari, A.: Short-acting barbiturate overdosage. Correlation intoxication score with serum barbiturate concentration. J.A.M.A., *248*:55, 1982.

Mongan, E., Kelly, P., Nies, K., Porter, W. W., and Paulus, H. E.: Tinnitus as an indication of therapeutic serum salicylate levels. J.A.M.A., *226*:142, 1973.

Morady, F., Scheinman, M. M., and Desai, J.: Disopyramide. Ann. Intern. Med., *96*:337, 1982.

Needleman, H. L., Houk, V. N., Billick, I. H., Buchart, E., Chadzynski, R. S., Challop, R., Curran, A. S., Davidaw, B., Field, P., Graef, J., Greenberg, N. H., Lin-Fu, J. S., Melia, E. P., Piomelli, S., Reigart, J. R., Robinson, B., Sayre, J. W., Soboleskey, W. J., and Welcome, M.: Preventing lead poisoning in young children. A statement by the Center for Disease Control. J. Pediatr., *93*:709, 1978.

Orsulak, P. J., and Schildkraut, J. J.: Guidelines for therapeutic monitoring of tricyclic antidepressant plasma levels. Ther. Drug Monitor, *1*:199, 1979.

Physician's Desk Reference. Oradell, N.J., Medical Economics Company, 1982.

Piafsky, K. M., Borgå, O., Odar-Cederlöf, I., Johansson, C., and

2

Sjöqvist, F.: Increased plasma protein binding of propranolol and chlorpromazine mediated by disease-induced elevations of plasma α_1 acid glycoprotein. N. Engl. J. Med., *299*:1435, 1978.

Piomelli, S., and Graziano, J.: Laboratory diagnosis of lead poisoning. Pediatr. Clin. North Am., *27*:843, 1980.

Pippenger, C. E.: Drug protein binding: An overview. American Association for Clinical Chemistry, June, 1980.

Pippenger, C. E., and Kutt, H.: Common errors in the analysis of antiepileptic drugs. *In* Pippenger, C. E., Penry, J. K., and Kutt, H. (eds.): Antiepileptic Drugs in Quantitative Analysis. New York, Raven Press, 1978.

Podrid, P. J., Schoeneberger, A., and Lown, B.: Congestive heart failure caused by oral disopyramide. N. Engl. J. Med., *302*:614, 1980.

Robert, E.: Letters to the editor. Lancet, *2*:1096, 1982.

Robotham, J. L., and Lietman, P. S.: Acute iron poisoning. A review. Am. J. Dis. Child., *134*:875, 1980.

Roman, E. J., Ponniah, P., Lambert, J. B., and Buchanan, N.: Free sodium valproate monitoring. Br. J. Clin. Pharmac., *13*:452, 1982.

Routledge, P. A., and Shand, D. G.: Clinical pharmacokinetics of propranolol. Clin. Pharmacokinet., *4*:73, 1979.

Rumack, B. H., Peterson, R. C., Koch, G. G., and Amara, I. A.: Acetaminophen overdose. 662 cases with evaluation of oral acetylcysteine treatment. Arch. Intern. Med., *141*:380, 1981.

Salzer, L. B., Weinrib, A. B., Marina, R. J., and Lima, J. J.: A comparison of methods of lidocaine administration in patients. Clin. Pharmacol. Ther., *29*:617, 1981.

Schäfer, H. R.: Primidone. Chemistry and methods of determination. *In* Woodbury, D. M., Penry, J. K., and Pippenger, C. E. (eds.): Antiepileptic Drugs. New York, Raven Press, 1982.

Senior, J. R., and Sloan, B. P.: Emergency measurement of stat, timed, serum ethanol levels for medical management. Alcoholism, *5*:6, 1981.

Sharpless, S. K.: Hypnotics and sedatives. II. Miscellaneous agents. *In* Goodman, L. S., and Gilman, A. (eds.): The Pharmacological Basis of Therapeutics. 3rd ed. New York, The Macmillan Company, 1965.

Singh, B. N., and Vaughan Williams, E. M.: A fourth class of anti-dysrhythmic action? Effect of verapamil on ouabain toxicity, on atrial and ventricular intracellular potentials, and on other features of cardiac function. Cardiovasc. Res., *6*:109, 1972.

Smith, D. E., and Wesson, D. R.: Drugs of abuse 1973: Trends and developments. Ann. Rev. Pharmacol. Toxicol., *14*:513, 1974.

Smulyan, H., Weinberg, S. E., and Howanitz, P. J.: Continuous propranolol infusion following abdominal surgery. J.A.M.A., *247*:2539, 1982.

Sohn, D., and Byers, J.: Cost effective drug screening in the laboratory. Clin. Toxicol., *18*:459, 1981.

Soyka, L. F.: Pediatric clinical pharmacology of digoxin. Pediatr. Clin. North Am., *28*:203, 1981.

Speicher, C. E., and Walters, M. I.: Phenothiazines. Clin. Lab. Med., *1*:547, 1981.

Spiker, D. G., and Biggs, J. T.: Tricyclic antidepressants. Prolonged plasma levels after overdose. J.A.M.A., *236*:1711, 1976.

Stearns, F. M. (submitter); Broussard, L. A., Early, R. J., Shaw, L. N., and Spratt, B. (evaluators); and Frings, C. S. (assigned editor): Determination of procainamide and N-acetylprocainamide by "high performance" liquid chromatography. Clin. Chem., *27*:2064, 1981.

Swartz, R. D., Millman, R. P., Billi, J. E., Bondar, N. P., Migdal, S. D., Simonian, S. K., Monforte, J. R., McDonald, F. D., Harness, J. K., and Cole, K. L.: Epidemic methanol poisoning: Clinical and biochemical analysis of a recent episode. Medicine, *60*:373, 1981.

Tartini, R., Steinbrunn, W., Kappenberger, L., and Meyer, U. A.: Dangerous interaction between amiodarone and quinidine. Lancet, *1*:1327, 1982.

Turner, C. R.: Primidone intoxication and massive crystalluria. Clin. Pediatr., *19*:706, 1980.

Van der Kleijn, E., Baars, A. M., Damsma, J. E., Guelen, P. J. M., Schobben, A. F. A. M., Termand, E., and Vree, T. B.: Pharmacokinetic interpretation of the fate of drugs in body fluids. Excerpta Medica, *501*:18, 1980.

Vasiliades, J.: Emergency toxicology. The evaluation of three analytical methods for the determination of misused alcohols. Clin. Toxicol., *10*:339, 1977.

Wettrell, G., and Andersson, K. E.: Clinical pharmacokinetics of digoxin in infants. Clin. Pharmacokinet., *2*:17, 1977.

Winchester, J. F., Gelfand, M. C., Knepshield, J. H., and Schreiner, G. E.: Dialysis and hemoperfusion of poisons and drugs—update. Trans. Am. Soc. Artif. Intern. Organs, *23*:762, 1977.

Winter, P. M., and Miller, J. N.: Carbon monoxide poisoning. J.A.M.A., *236*:1502, 1976.

Wright, M.: An assessment of the unreliability of the history given by self-poisoned patients. Clin. Toxicol., *16*:381, 1980.

Zwillich, C. W., Sutton, F. D., Neff, T. A., Cohn, W. M., Matthay, R. A., and Weinberger, M. M.: Theophylline-induced seizures in adults. Correlation with serum concentrations. Ann. Intern. Med., *82*:784, 1975.

Part III

MEDICAL MICROSCOPY

EDITED BY JOHN BERNARD HENRY, M.D., AND GREGORY A. THREATTE, M.D.

18

EXAMINATION OF URINE

MARY BRADLEY, M.D., and G. BERRY SCHUMANN, M.D.

The urine specimen has been referred to as a liquid tissue biopsy of the urinary tract—painlessly obtained. It yields a great deal of information quickly and economically. Like any other laboratory procedure, urine tests need to be carefully performed and properly controlled. A physician should be able to perform the necessary screening tests himself and know how to interpret them in relation to the health and management of his patient.

Examination of the urine may be considered from two general standpoints; (1) diagnosis and management of renal or urinary tract disease and (2) the detection of metabolic or systemic diseases not directly related to the kidney.

Among the most important conditions readily detected by chemical means are proteinuria, glucosuria, ketonuria, and the presence of the pigments hemoglobin and bilirubin.

Proteinuria is probably the most common indication of renal disease. It is, for example, an early indication of latent glomerulonephritis, toxemia of pregnancy, and diabetic nephropathy. The finding of proteinuria may strongly suggest the presence of renal disease as opposed to lower urinary tract disease. The finding of large amounts of protein in urine helps define the kind of renal disease present, e.g., with the nephrotic syndrome. When considered with the clinical findings, confirmation of the presence of renal disease can be made by finding casts in the microscopic examination of the urine sediment.

Microscopic examination of the sediment in a properly collected sample of urine may not only provide evidence of renal disease but also indicate the kind of lesion present or the state of activity of a known lesion. The usefulness of the qualitative examination of urine has been discussed in detail by Free (1975), but has also been questioned in terms of cost and significant yield when it is used as a required screening procedure (Fraser, 1977). Laboratories involved in the examination of urine must define responsibilities for both the routine, rapid assessment of urine and the specialized, more time-consuming interpretive tests (Schumann, 1983). It should be considered in every complete medical examination because it provides important morphologic information concerning the kidneys and urinary tract not readily obtainable in any other way. While the value of a required microscopic examination on all routine specimens remains controversial, most laboratorians agree that an accurate urine sediment examination is a front line medical laboratory test for symptomatic patients (Schumann, 1979; Benham, 1982).

FORMATION OF URINE

The kidney has the remarkable ability to select and retain essential substances while excreting end products of metabolism and excess substances from the diet. It maintains water and electrolyte balance and substantially contributes to acid/base homeostasis. To accomplish this balance, the composition of urine will be varied with water and salt intake, protein intake, and metabolic status. This variability creates a practical problem in the timing of collection of urine specimens and in the use of random specimens as representative samples of urinary output. Timed (2-, 12-, 24-hour) urinary collections are therefore preferred to random specimens for quantitative tests.

In the normal adult, 25 per cent of the cardiac output, or more than a liter of blood, perfuses the two kidneys each minute and an ultrafiltrate of the plasma passes through each glomerular capillary tuft into Bowman's capsule. The filtrate has a pH of 7.4 and an osmolality similar to that of plasma (about 285 mOsm/kg water). The specific gravity is about 1.007. Modification of this filtrate to produce excreted urine occurs in the tubules and collecting duct of each nephron. Final concentration will depend upon the state of hydration. Entering the collecting ducts, the pH is usually about 6 with a typical Western diet, and the osmolality may be increased to 800 to 1200 mOsm/kg water. In a very well hydrated person, the osmolality will be much lower as the kidneys excrete a dilute urine. The glomerular filtrate volume of about 180 L in 24 hours (for an 80 kg man) has been reduced to about 1 or 2 L, and water and sodium have been conserved. This is now urine. It will pass from the collecting ducts to the kidney pelvis, ureters, bladder, and urethra to be voided. In disease states, this fluid is altered chemically and cytologically.

COMPOSITION OF URINE

Most of the solute in urine is urea and sodium chloride. Sodium and chloride excretion relate to dietary intake and are, therefore, variable. Protein intake will affect nitrogen excretion as urea. Other substances, such as uric acid, creatinine, amino acids, ammonia, and traces of proteins, glycoproteins, enzymes, and purines, account for the remaining nitrogen excreted. There is a continuous excretion of uric acid even when purine intake is absent. Creatinine excretion is related to muscle mass. It is rather uniformly excreted from day to day; 15 to 25 mg/kg/24 hours or 0.13 to 0.22 mmol/kg/24 hours for adults. Creatinine measurement is therefore (1) a useful gauge of the completeness of timed urinary collections, (2) a basis for a ratio of some other substance being measured, and (3) a basis for the endogenous creatinine clearance measurement most commonly used as an indication of renal (glomerular) function.

Urine contains potassium, which is ubiquitous in the diet, sulfates, and other sulfur-containing substances, such as sulfides, cysteine, and mercaptan. Phosphate excretion is variable and is derived chiefly from nucleic acid in food, casein, and other organic and inorganic phosphates.

Other than the nitrogenous material and salts already mentioned, normal urine contains small amounts of sugars, which, for example, like pentoses, will vary in amount with dietary intake. Intermediary metabolites, such as oxalic acid, citric acid, and pyruvate, are present. Free fatty acids and trace amounts of cholesterol are also found, as are trace amounts of metals.

Hormones such as the ketosteroids, estrogens, aldosterone and pituitary gonadotropins, and the biogenic amines—the catecholamines and serotonin metabolites—are normally found in urine and reflect metabolic and endocrine status. Vitamins such as ascorbic acid are excreted in the urine in amounts that depend on the sufficiency of dietary intake. Trace amounts of bilirubin, hemoglobin from normally excreted red blood cells, porphyrins, and related compounds such as delta amino-levulinic acid are found.

Details on these values are available in Altman (1974).

Microscopic Constituents of Normal Urine. In a concentrated normal urine, uric acid (at an acid pH) and phosphates (alkaline pH) will commonly precipitate at room or refrigerator temperatures and are, therefore, frequently found in routine examination of the urine. Urea and sodium chloride crystals are not seen, although these substances are present in high concentration.

Normal urine also contains "formed" elements; these are red blood cells and leukocytes, renal tubular epithelial cells, transitional epithelial cells, and squamous epithelial cells. The source of the erythrocytes and leukocytes is not known. The proportion of leukocytes to erythrocytes is much greater in urine than in blood; thus, diapedesis of leukocytes through the glomerular membrane or tubules may be postulated. Because of the problems associated with the collection of random specimens and different methods of microscopic examination, there is no good agreement on "normal values." In normal males and females, in most instances, no red cells will be seen on the usual microscopic examination of sediment. In about 10 per cent of the patients, an occasional red cell is seen. The urinary sediment of most normal males will show on microscopic examination an occasional leukocyte or non-squamous epithelial cell. In the normal female, the number may be higher. In the normal person, very few casts are seen; those found are hyaline casts and may show a few fine granules. See Examination of the Urine Sediment for quantitative counts.

Reference values for constituents of urine are shown in Appendix 4.

IDENTIFICATION OF URINE

Occasionally, following abdominal or pelvic surgery, drainage fluid is submitted to the laboratory for identification as urine. After centrifugation, the supernatant may be tested for urea, creatinine, sodium, and chloride. These levels are usually sufficiently concentrated in urine (even when diluted with wound site effusion) to separate probable urine from plasma or serous exudate.

Fistulas. Fistulous connections between the intestine and the bladder will produce fecal contamination in urine. The urine is usually, but not always, brown in color. It may contain food residues, plant material or striated muscle, many bacteria, and an overall yellow-brown color microscopically. When finely divided activated charcoal is given orally to demonstrate a fistula, a few small, dense black granules are found in the urinary sediment. The number found will depend on the size of the fistula, and several 24-hour specimens may have to be centrifuged down to demonstrate the particles. It is useful to have a sample of charcoal in suspension to observe the size of the granules. It is important to use alcohol-cleaned slides and coverslips so that dust particles are not confused with the charcoal.

Amniotic Fluid. Occasionally it is necessary to distinguish between maternal urine and fetal amniotic fluid. Normal amniotic fluid varies in color from clear and colorless to slightly yellow and turbid. Turbidity is due to fetal squamous epithelial cells and fatty material (vernix). The pH of amniotic fluid is usually 7 or more, the specific gravity is usually high, and the protein level is significantly elevated compared with normal urine. Urea and creatinine levels in amniotic fluid are similar to blood levels, whereas the maternal urine will have high levels of these substances.

It should be noted that amniotic fluid constituents vary with the age of the fetus. In late pregnancy, with the addition of fetal urine, the level of urea and creatinine will be approximately two to three times the maternal blood level. Protein levels decrease with fetal age from about 1/10 serum level to 1/20 or less near term (see Chap. 21 and Appendix 4).

COLLECTION OF URINE

There are certain important considerations to be borne in mind relative to the collection of urine specimens for examination. If these are followed, one is less apt to commit serious errors in the interpretation of results obtained.

Deterioration of Specimens. The urine sample must be collected in a clean, dry container and should be examined when freshly voided within one hour of voiding. Red blood cells, leukocytes, and casts decompose in urine that has been allowed to stand for several hours at room temperature. Casts and neutrophils disappear rapidly in hypotonic and alkaline urines (Triger, 1966). Using good collection techniques, Kierkegaard (1980) showed a 35 per cent loss of neutrophils when counted at an average time of 1.4 hours after voiding and again at 4.5 hours after voiding. Bilirubin and urobilinogen will decrease, especially with exposure to light. Glucose is utilized by cells and bacteria; ketones are utilized or volatilized. Bacterial contamination regularly occurs, usually resulting in alkalinization of the urine owing to the conversion of urea to ammonia by Proteus species. pH will also increase as CO_2 is lost. Turbidity develops as bacteria multiply and alkaline precipitates occur. The color will change (usually darken), and the odor will eventually become offensive. However, if much glucose is present, bacteria and yeasts will convert it to acids and alcohol, and the pH will fall.

Collection of Urine for Screening Purposes. For *chemical* and *microscopic* examination, a voided specimen is usually suitable. If the specimen is likely to be contaminated by vaginal discharge or hemorrhage, a clean-voided specimen is collected. It may be necessary to pack the vagina or use a tampon in some cases, especially when examination of the urinary sediment is critical.

For most routine examinations, a fairly concentrated specimen is preferable to a dilute one. The concentration of solutes and formed elements in the urine varies throughout the patient's waking hours, depending upon water intake. Ordinarily the first morning specimen of urine, voided on rising, is the most concentrated specimen. This specimen is the best one to examine for nitrite and protein. An ambulatory person will excrete larger amounts of protein, but for comparison in an individual, the first morning specimens are probably better. Valuable information about the concentrating ability of the kidney may also be gained from the specific gravity of this specimen. However, a randomly collected specimen is often more convenient for the patient and will be suitable for most screening purposes.

Collection of Urine for Quantitative Analysis. A 24-hour specimen is collected for many assays; 2- to 12-hour timed collections are also made, e.g., for urobilinogen, xylose excretion, and quantitative cell counts (Addis, 1948).

Because substances such as hormones, proteins, and electrolytes are variably excreted during a 24-hour period, a better comparison of day-to-day values can be made with 24-hour collections than with random specimens (Schwartz, 1973). *Errors in the results of quantitative urine tests are most often related to collection problems:* loss of a voided specimen, failure to discard the first specimen, poor preservation, or inadequate refrigeration. The adequacy of a 24-hour collection has been related to the creatinine excretion, which is fairly constant in an individual; however, this method for checking on the completion of a collection has been disputed (Edwards, 1969).

When possible, fluids should be moderately restricted during the 24-hour collection period, and alcohol, certain foods, and drugs may have to be withheld. Specifications relating to each assay are available from central or reference laboratories for the more unusual substances to be tested.

Patients should be given *printed instructions* for the collection of timed specimens.

The patient is carefully instructed to empty his bladder at 8:00 A.M. (or a suitable time on rising) and to discard the urine. He collects all subsequent urine up to and including that at 8:00 A.M. the following morning. The total volume of this sample is measured and recorded and the urine thoroughly mixed before a measured sample is withdrawn for analysis.

Collection of Urine for Bacteriologic Examination. A *clean-voided midstream* specimen is desirable; but catheterization or suprapubic aspiration of the bladder is sometimes necessary. Bacteriologic culture should be done immediately. When this is not possible, the urine should be refrigerated at 4°C. until cultured—for a period of not more than 12 hours as a rule, although specimens have been cultured without detriment after four days of adequate refrigeration (Ryan, 1963). Clean voided urine specimens are used for bacterial, mycobacterial, fungal, and viral cultures; 24-hour specimens are used for the detection of Schistosoma and Onchocerca.

In the male the glans should be exposed adequately, thoroughly cleaned with a mild antiseptic solution, and dried. In the uncircumcised male, the foreskin is retracted to avoid contamination from debris under the foreskin. The midstream urine should be collected in a sterile container after the initial flow has been allowed to escape.

The female patient should be instructed to kneel or squat over a bedpan or to stand astride a toilet bowl. While the patient may be able to collect a suitable urine specimen, less contamination occurs when she has trained assistance. Using sterile gloves, the patient or nurse should separate the labia minora widely to expose the urethral orifice and to keep the labia separated throughout the procedure. With sterile, soapy cotton balls, cleanse on each side of urinary meatus; then cleanse the meatus. Rinse the cleansed area with sterile, water-saturated cotton balls. Instruct the patient to void forcibly, and allow the initial stream of urine to drain into the bedpan or toilet, continuing to keep the labia separated. Catch the subsequent midstream specimen in a sterile container, and do not touch any portion of perineum with the container. About 30 to 100 ml of urine should be collected. After obtaining the urine specimen, allow the labia to close. The patient then continues to void into the bedpan or toilet.

Special Collection Techniques

Urethral Catheterization. Catheters introduced into the urethra and bladder may cause infection but are necessary for drainage in some patients, or for urine collection when patients are unable to void.

Suprapubic Aspiration (SPA). Urine is aspirated with a syringe and needle above the symphysis pubis through the abdominal wall into the full bladder. Complications are rare. This method is used for *anaerobic cultures,* for problem cultures (where contamination cannot be ruled out), and in infants. Counts of 5000 to 10,000 ml of a single organism are significant.

Ureteral Catheterization. Ureteral catheters are inserted via a cystoscope into each ureter. Bladder urine is first collected, then a bladder washout specimen; ureteral urine specimens are obtained separately from each kidney pelvis and carefully labeled right or left. This technique may be used to differentiate bladder from kidney infection.

Voided Specimen. A *two or three "glass" technique* is used by urologists to pinpoint roughly the origin of cells and bacteria found in urine in the male:

1. Void the initial 20 to 30 ml into one sterile container; the urine contains urethral washings as well as bladder and kidney elements.

2. Void the remaining urine into a second sterile container. This represents cells, bacteria, etc., from the bladder, ureters, and kidney but few urethral elements.

Note: If a three "glass" collection is made, the patient interrupts completion of voiding and a prostatic massage is done. The specimen then voided will contain prostatic fluid as well as bladder and renal elements. A fourth final urine collection may be made. With prostatitis, higher bacterial counts are found in the last specimens.

Cytology. A two-hour collection of urine, after initial voiding in the morning, will allow the collection of fresh cells from the urinary tract, e.g., the "distorted" red cells and red cell casts from a kidney with glomerulonephritis or casts and cells for special studies.

Urine for evaluation of tumor cells is usually collected into an equal volume of 50 per cent alcohol. Or urine may be mixed in equal volumes with Saccomano's fixative or Mucolexx (Lerner Laboratories). Unfixed urine should be refrigerated immediately upon voiding and should reach the laboratory within one hour to prevent cell loss.

Containers. Disposable plastic containers, 100 to 200 ml with lids, are preferred by many for routine screening urinalysis. Sufficient volume is obtained for repeat or confirmatory tests. Screw caps, if properly applied, are less likely to leak during transit than snap caps. Conical containers are less likely to tip over. Wax-coated cardboard containers should not be used because of the likelihood of contaminating the specimen with fatty material. Paper or plastic cups for urine collection are also available in sets with 12 ml capped, plastic disposable tubes and racks for transportation to the laboratory.* The 12 ml volume may not always be sufficient for special tests.

Rigid brown plastic containers, 3000 ml, with wide mouths and screw caps, are suitable for 24-hour collections for protein, glucose, or creatinine clearance.† Acid may be added to these containers. They are especially preferable for ambulatory patients; the thin-walled collapsible containers are not as sturdy even when supported with an outer cardboard container. One-gallon glass jars with wide mouths and screw caps are also used for 24-hour collections. Bedpans used to collect voided urine for timed specimens should be scrupulously clean.

Pediatric urine collectors of clear pliable polyethylene are available for male and female infants. With these containers, an estimate of the volume excreted may be made. The bag may be folded and self-sealed for transportation. For a 24-hour collection, a tube is attached to the bag and can be connected to a collection bottle. Sterile and non-sterile plastic bags are available.

Sterile containers are used when cultures are to be made. These are usually plastic and disposable with well-fitted lids. Five ml evacuated sterile tubes are available for transportation of urine for culture and may be filled from a collection container or by means of special catheter. A sterile kit for collection of urine for bacteriologic examination is available. It contains a disposable plastic bottle, detergent-impregnated pad, and dry pad. A sterile tray may be prepared for clean-voided specimens for hospital use. Sterile wrapped bedpans should always be available.

TRANSPORTATION, STORAGE, AND PRESERVATIVES

Random specimens for routine urinalysis should be examined fresh, within one hour after voiding, or refrigerated and examined as soon as possible. If delays are anticipated, the laboratory should insist that specimens be refrigerated before delivery. Even at refrigeration temperatures, some cells are lost.

In general, many substances for qualitative or quantitative chemical determinations or cells and casts preserve best when *refrigerated* at an acid pH (about 6) without preservation. Quantitative *creatinine* and *protein* determinations are done on 24-hour urine collections refrigerated between voidings and with no preservative.

Freezing. This is useful for aliquots of urine to be used for quantitative chemistry tests. Freezing will help retard loss of labile substances such as urobilinogen, bilirubin, and porphobilinogen, but not completely. The pigments are stored in dark-colored containers. Frozen aliquots for chemical tests may be mailed in Styrofoam containers in dry ice. Thawing after freezing may reveal some turbidity that does not redissolve (possibly colloidal protein) and may cause assay problems. Freeze-drying is not as suitable for preservation as freezing for the recovery of certain hormones and other constituents in urine (Leach, 1975).

Chemical Preservatives. *Preservatives* used for urine collections will depend on the substance to be tested and the method used. These usually act as antibacterial or anti-yeast agents. Mineral acids or ascorbic acid lowers the pH. Boric acid inhibits bacterial multiplication. Benzoic acid, phenols, thymol, toluol, chloroform, formaldehyde, and mercury compounds have been used to prevent bacterial growth or to preserve cells.

Sodium Fluoride. *Glucose* in 24-hour urine collections is traditionally preserved by using sodium fluoride to inhibit glycolysis by cells and bacteria. Sodium fluoride does not inhibit yeast (*C. albicans*), and glucose will be converted to alcohol (Ball, 1979). About 0.5 g of sodium fluoride* per 3 to 4 L container is used. Sodium fluoride will inhibit the reagent strip test for glucose (if this is used for screening), but at low levels it does not interfere with the hexokinase or other quantitative tests (Onstad, 1975). It does not inhibit the qualitative copper reduction test, and this may be used as a preliminary test to see if dilutions are required. Because of the toxicity of sodium fluoride powder or tablets, satisfactory glucose results have been achieved in 24-hour specimens from pediatric patients using refrigeration alone. For outpatients, the urine may be frozen if there are delays in delivering the 24-hour specimen to the laboratory from the home.† Xylose in urine may be preserved with sodium fluoride.

Chlorhexidine Gluconate. As a 200 g/L solution, it is used to preserve glucose in 24-hour urine collections. About 5 to 10 ml of the solution is added to the container. It is effective against gram-positive organisms, not as effective against Proteus and Pseudomonas species. It does not affect the hexokinase test for glucose but will give a false positive result with the reagent strip for protein. Glucose solutions in urine with chlorhexidine have been stable for weeks at both room temperature and refrigerator temperature (Worth, 1980).

Preservative Tablets. Preservative tablets,‡ used for transportation of urine for routine screening urinalysis, preserve glucose and other constituents by releasing formaldehyde; they also contain benzoate and mercury and have an acid reaction. One 95 mg tablet is used with 20 ml urine. In this concentration, formaldehyde will not react with the copper reduction test (Clinitest), and the preservative, properly used, does not interfere with common reagent strip tests. The specific gravity will be slightly increased (0.002/one tablet/20 ml).

Boric Acid. For many hormones and other substances, boric acid 1 g/dl has been found useful for mailing aliquots of urine to reference laboratories.

*FISHERbrand, Kova, and others.

†Available from Bemis, Sheboygan, Wisconsin.

*Sodium fluoride. Urine preservative tablet. Cambridge Chemical Products/American Scientific Products.

†University of Minnesota Hospitals, Outpatient Clinics.

‡Stabilur Tablets (in three sizes), R. P. Cargille Lab., 55 Commerce Road, Cedar Grove, N.J. 07009.

Estriol and estrogen will be preserved for seven days. Boric acid can also be placed in the collection container. For transport of urine for culture, a solution of 0.5 ml glyceroboric acid with a sodium formate buffer is used to stabilize a bacterial population for 24 hours without refrigeration in evacuated 5 ml sterile tubes (Vacutainer brand).

pH Adjustment. A very low pH (<3) will prevent bacterial growth and stabilize substances such as catecholamines or VMA or 5-HIAA. For a pH of 1 to 2, 30 ml of *6N HCl* (equal parts of concentrated HCl and water) is placed in a 3 to 4 L plastic or glass container and appropriately labeled. Acetic acid is not suitable. For amino acid assay, a pH of 3, using HCl, is desirable. Before transporting or mailing aliquots of acidified urine specimens, a narrow range of pH indicator paper should be used to check the pH.

Urine for 24-hour estimations of porphyrins, porphobilinogen, and delta-aminolevulinic acid is collected and adjusted, if needed, to a pH of 6 to 7, with acetic acid or sodium carbonate (Schwartz, 1951; Bossenmaier, 1968). Dark containers are preferred. The collection is refrigerated between voidings. Aliquots may be refrigerated or frozen.

Formalin. Cells and casts for quantitation (Addis count) may be preserved by "rinsing" the empty container with formalin prior to use or by adding 10 ml of 40 per cent formalin to a 3 to 4 L container. Formalin (40 per cent v/v), 1 drop/10 ml urine, will also preserve sediments. For small quantities of urine, one crystal of *thymol* per 10 to 15 ml is useful; it will help preserve sediments but will interfere with the acid precipitation test for protein. Toluol and chloroform are usually not desirable. Toluol, to be effective, is layered on the surface and clings to pipettes; chloroform at greater saturation levels will sink and may contaminate the sediment.

Sodium azide, 200 mg/L, is used to prevent bacterial growth in urine collected for special protein tests. Usually these are for research-related projects. The urine is refrigerated and usually concentrated within 48 hours.

HAZARDOUS SPECIMENS

Hazardous material from patients with hepatitis and other contagious diseases is always handled with care. Externally contaminated specimen containers should be cleaned with 70 per cent alcohol. Urine is collected in a disposable plastic container with a well-fitted plastic lid. The labeled container is placed in a "zip-lock" plastic bag and sealed. An "isolation" or some other distinctive label should be placed on the bag. Gloves are worn when these specimens are tested, and centrifuge tubes should be capped to avoid the formation of aerosols.

QUALITY CONTROL

Precision and accuracy are essential elements in the conduct of any test. Difficulties arise in the implementation of quality control programs in urinalysis because of the subjective or qualitative nature of many of the tests. This is especially true of the microscopic sediment examination (Winkel, 1974). As seen in other areas of the clinical laboratory, the best results are obtained from better qualified personnel who are performing tests on a regular basis. Surveys have revealed large numbers of false negative results and some false positive results when poorly trained personnel are assigned the task of routine urinalysis (Simpson, 1977). With the implementation of quality control programs and the proper selection of test methods, results should be comparable to those expected in other areas of clinical chemistry (Assa, 1977).

Each laboratory will have to establish its own acceptable range of performance. This is difficult when so much of routine urinalysis involves interpretation of colors, precipitates, or microscopic elements (Becker, 1973). Even in the best hands, there may be as much as ±1 color block difference in the interpretation of positive reagent strip results. However, in most instances one should not expect clearly negative specimens to be called positive or a positive result negative. Laboratory supervisors may wish to introduce positive and negative controls with the daily work load as unknown routine specimens.

Each person should be aware of the principle involved in each test, its sensitivity and specificity, the necessity for quality specimens, the likelihood of interference, and the patterns of expected results for common diseases. This awareness will ensure good quality control in the urinalysis laboratory.

Urinalysis Controls. Urinalysis controls are used as a check on urinalysis reagents and procedures, and as a means of evaluating the laboratory personnel's ability to perform tests correctly and to interpret the results.

New personnel should run reagent strip controls (and confirmatory tests) and check results with a supervisor. It is also useful to have part-time or night staff who do these tests infrequently check controls periodically.

Daily controls are used to monitor reagent strip tests and all qualitative wet chemical tests. When possible, both positive and negative controls should be used. For some procedures, e.g., hemosiderin, known positive urine samples can be saved and refrigerated for use as controls. Samples of urobilinogen and porphobilinogen should be kept frozen and in the dark. In other tests, e.g., for cystine, sugars, and calculi, known chemical solutions are used as positive controls. In addition to chemical tests, it is important to check *daily* the calibration of specific gravity instruments—urinometer or refractometer. Other equipment used in the laboratory should be routinely checked, including refrigerator-freezer temperatures, centrifuge speed, balance, spectrophotometer (daily check), etc.

All reagents should be properly labeled, dated, and stored. When new reagents are made, positive and negative controls are performed; indicate this by a check on the bottle label together with the date. Lot numbers and expiration dates for reagent strips are recorded and periodically checked for outdating.

Daily Procedure. Positive and negative control

solutions are treated as routine urine specimens. See Quality Control Reagents.

1. Measure specific gravity, using distilled water and controls.

2. Test control solutions with a multiple reagent strip (or routine test strips).

3. Do an acid precipitation test for protein, using a suitable control solution.

4. Do a copper reduction test.

5. If the control used has red cells, centrifuge, examine the sediment, and semi-quantitate.

Records

1. Record daily test results of positive and negative "routine" controls.

2. Record daily results of urinometer or refractometer check.

3. Record results of new reagent strips (with lot numbers and expiration dates).

4. Record disposition of outdated reagent strips and tablets.

5. Separate records or charts may be used for other equipment or instruments.

Precautions in Use of Reagent Strips. Protect reagent strips from moisture and excessive heat to prevent loss of sensitivity. Discoloration may indicate significant loss of reactivity; reagent strips with such discoloration should not be used. This also applies to test tablets. Store strips in a cool dry area but not in a refrigerator. Remove only enough strips for immediate use, and recap tightly immediately. Urine should be at *room temperature* when tested with reagent strips.

Avoid contamination of reagent strips. Do not touch test areas with fingers. Do not lay the reagent strip on a bench surface; use a clean sheet of paper or gauze. Do not use strips in the presence of volatile acid or alkali fumes.

Properly moisten the reagent strip in well-mixed urine. Avoid incomplete dipping; all test areas must be completely moistened. Avoid prolonged dipping; excessive dipping may cause leaching of test reagents.

Exercise care in reading reagent strips. Observe the *time elements* indicated in the directions for their use. Hold the reagent strip close to the appropriate color chart when reading. Read only under good lighting conditions.

Quality Control Reagents for Routine Urinalysis. Lyophilized, tablet, liquid, or reagent strip control preparations are available with varying concentrations of the constituents sought in routine urinalysis. Among these are Kova-Trol (ICL Scientific), QC-U (General Diagnostics), Tek-Chek (Ames), and Urintrol (Harleco). The specific gravity test by hydrometer or refractometer, as well as test material for pH, protein, glucose, ketone, and blood, is usually included. Controls containing stabilized red cells for sediment examination (for example, Urintrol) must be properly mixed before use. Chek-Stix (Ames) is in the form of a multiple reagent strip containing seven test substances to be leached off into distilled water. After an appropriate time, the strip is removed and the control solution is then available for checking reagent strips for positive results and interpretation. Lyophilized or liquid controls are used to check the acid precipitation test for protein. Special attention should be given to storage time, temperature, and expiration dates on control preparations.

Formula for Control Solutions. The solutions in Table 18–1 have the advantage of being considerably less expensive than commercially available preparations (see also Bush, 1974).

To facilitate dissolution, pulverize all dry reagents with a mortar and pestle. Dilute to volume with distilled water. Store controls in a stock bottle at room temperature. Remove 50 to 100 ml aliquots periodically to a working control bottle. Solutions are stable for six to nine months.

Chloroform is used as a preservative and allows the reagent to be stored at room temperature. Since chloroform is hepatotoxic, another suitable preservative may be substituted, or vials may be frozen and stored without preservative. Note that chloroform in the control solution will dissolve or etch plastic and should not be used with plastic tubes or instruments containing plastic, such as the refractometer (cover plate) or certain parts of semi-automated urinalysis instruments.

Expected Low Control Result. Multiple Reagent Strip: pH 6, protein 2+, glucose ~1/4 per cent, ketone negative, blood small to moderate. Additional tests: Protein precipitation (SSA) 2+, Benedict's 1+, Clinitest[a] trace, Tes-tape[b] 2+, Acetest[a] negative, specific gravity 1.006 (refractometer), osmolality 305 mOsm/kg water.

Expected High Control Result. Multiple Reagent Strip: pH 6, protein 4+, glucose >1 per cent, ketone small, blood negative. Additional tests: Protein precipitation (SSA) 3 to 4+, Benedict's 3+, Clinitest[a] 3+, Tes-tape[b] 3+, Acetest[a] small, specific gravity 1.020 (refractometer), osmolality 660 mOsm/kg water.

Bilirubin and urobilinogen are negative for each control.

Negative Control. A salt solution containing sodium chloride and urea in distilled water is used as a negative control.

Synthetic Urine. For teaching purposes, a general purpose solution containing NaCl, urea, creatinine, and chloroform can be made in large volumes and stored at room temperature for six months. Reactive substances are then added as required to aliquots. Alternatively, simulated urine solutions may be made in advance (without chloroform) with varying amounts of reactants, frozen in 10 ml amounts, and stored. Solutions should be thoroughly thawed and mixed before use but may remain slightly turbid. The use of simulated specimens in some teaching situations reduces exposure to contaminated patient specimens. Bile or bilirubin solutions may be added just prior to use (see below). A positive Ehrlich reaction is possible with para-aminosalicylic acid as a substitute for urobilinogen. Normal hepatitis-free plasma may be substituted for bovine albumin in an appropriate concen-

[a]Ames Company, Elkhart, Indiana.
[b]Lilly Company, Indianapolis, Indiana.

tration. It is important to include creatinine to obtain good copper reduction test results for sugars. Food coloring may be added to simulate the color of urine.

Note that acetone will not give a positive result with current Ames reagent strips; they are specific for acetoacetic acid. Acetone will give a positive result with Chemstrip[c] reagent strips.

Acetoacetic acid solution may be substituted for acetone. A stock solution of ethyl acetoacetate (5 g/dl) is made by diluting 16 ml ethyl acetoacetate to 250 ml with 2.5 per cent sodium hydroxide solution in distilled water. Let the solution stand for at least 24 hours; it is stable for three months. A working solution (40 mg/dl) is made by acidifying 2 ml of stock solution to pH 5 with approximately one drop of concentrated H_2SO_4 and diluting to 250 ml with distilled water (1:125 dilution). Freeze in small aliquots. Add 8 ml of working solution to 1 L of control solution when ready to use. This control will give a low "moderate" reading when tested with reagent strips for ketones. Stability should be checked.

Bilirubin is available from Matheson, Coleman and Bell, Norwood, Ohio, and other sources. An alkaline stock solution is made to keep the bilirubin crystals dissolved, 20 mg/dl, pH 7 to 7.5. About 70 ml of bilirubin stock solution is added to 500 ml of synthetic urine to produce positive reagent strip and tablet tests. It is necessary to keep the final mixture alkaline in order to have good positive results.

Standardizing Microscopic Urinalysis. Since urine specimens are most often randomly collected, meaningful results for comparison are difficult to obtain. However, each laboratory should adopt a uniform system for both chemical and microscopic analysis. A defined volume (10 to 12 ml) of well mixed urine is centrifuged in a capped tube at a set speed to produce about 450 G for five minutes. The centrifuge should have a horizontal head. Nomograms are available that relate the radius of the centrifuge head, from the center pin to the bottom of a horizontal cup and the speed in revolutions per minute (RPM), to relative centrifugal force (RCF) or use a formula:

[c]Bio-Dynamics/bmc, Indianapolis, Indiana.

Superscripts a, b, and c throughout this chapter refer to these companies.

$$\text{RCF(G)} = 11.18 \times \text{radius in cm} \times \left[\frac{\text{RPM}}{1000}\right]^2$$

Higher RCF and longer centrifugation times, while useful in recovering cells, are apt to break up cellular casts.

It is important that a concentration factor be established and adhered to, e.g., 1:10, 1:12, etc., and reported with the results. Special plastic pipettes or specially contrived tubes hold the sediment in 1 ml or less in the tube while the supernatant is poured off (and saved). Stain may be added to the sediment and the pipette used to mix the sediment well and to place a drop on a molded plastic slide. Cavities in the slide are designed to hold a specific volume of sediment. These systems of plastic tubes, pipettes, and slides have contributed to the standardization of the microscopic method (see Examination of Urine Sediment for manufacturers). When glass slides and coverslips are used, the drop of sediment and the size of the coverslip should be standardized. The sediment is placed on the slide with a disposable pipette so that the drop size is uniform. It should not be poured. For example, with 18 mm square coverslips an appropriate volume of the sediment under the coverslip is about 12 μl. A calculation using the observed microscopic field in millimeters with both high and low power will enable the user to roughly estimate the cell count (allowing for a concentration factor). *Inadequate suspension* of the sediment largely accounts for differences in sediment results between observers when other factors such as volume and coverslip size are kept constant.

It should be noted that although there is a recognized imprecision in the estimation of cells and casts in sediments, there is also a substantial error in the counting of small numbers of cells in leukocyte counting chambers. For example, the error in cell counting is 4.2 to 7.6 per cent (±2 C.V.), depending on skill. Counting chamber calibration error and error due to variation in filling is 4.6 per cent (±1 C.V.). Variability in cell settling becomes smaller as the number of cells counted increases. With 1000 leukocytes per microliter present, and when 80 cells are counted in two chambers on a 1:10 dilution of this in one pipette, the minimal error is ±25.2 per cent

3

Table 18–1. QUALITY CONTROL REAGENTS

Reagent	Low Control		High Control	
	1 L	***Conc.***	***1 L***	***Conc.***
Sodium chloride AR	5.0 g	500 mg/dl	10.0 g	1000 mg/dl
Urea AR	5.0 g	500 mg/dl	10.0 g	1000 mg/dl
Creatinine AR	0.5 g	50 mg/dl	0.5 g	50 mg/dl
Glucose AR	3.0 g	300 mg/dl	15.0 g	1500 mg/dl
30% bovine albumin	5.0 ml	150 mg/dl	35 ml	1050 mg/dl
Whole normal blood (with Hct 40–45) (Hbg 13–15 g/dl)	100 μl	1.3–1.5 mg/dl	—	—
Acetone AR*	—	—	2 ml	160 mg/dl
Chloroform AR†	5 ml	0.5 ml/dl	5 ml	0.5 mg/dl
Distilled water qs	to 1 L		to 1 L	

*For acetoacetic acid, see under Synthetic Urine
†Omit if frozen. Do not use with refractometer or any plastic material.

(2 C.V.) (Cartwright, 1968). (See Quantitative Cell Counts in Urine Sediments for further comments.)

The proper use of the microscope, especially the use of *phase microscopy* to detect casts, is an important aspect of quality performance in examination of the urine sediment. All personnel should be familiar with these procedures. Controls, such as Urintrol (Harleco) contain a known suspension of red blood cells which should be evaluated on a daily basis and used to evaluate new personnel.

Automated Reagent Strip Method. An *automated* system, Clinilab[a] measures specific gravity and seven reagent strip tests—pH, protein, glucose, ketones, bilirubin, blood, and urobilinogen.

The specific gravity is measured by a falling drop method and is related to the time it takes for a drop of urine to pass between two sets of photo cells; the high specific gravity (heavier) drop falls faster than a low specific gravity drop. The reagent strip test methods are similar to those used manually. Urine is automatically aspirated and deposited as drops for specific gravity measurement and then on each reagent strip. The strips issue automatically from a cassette, each reel having the capacity for 400 tests. Colors are read by reflectance, and the results are printed out. The instrument can be interfaced with a computer system.

Calibration is made daily with standard high and low content solutions. A control is supplied with the calibration material.

Bloody or colored specimens are not satisfactory and should be tested by hand; otherwise false positive results will be recorded owing to pigmentation of the reagent areas. Specific gravity measurements of 1.035 or more are duplicated and checked with a refractometer.

The system is useful for high volume laboratories, and with strict attention to cleaning, especially of the specific gravity module, performance is satisfactory. The advantages of the instrument are its speed and objectivity (Wert, 1973).

A *semi-automated* instrument, Clini-Tek[a], is available to read out hand-dipped reagent strips. Color changes are read by reflectance, the amount of light reflected being inversely related to the depth of the color reaction and, in turn, to the concentration of substance being measured. Results are shown on a display panel. A printer is available, and the instrument can be computer interfaced.

The tests performed are the same as those on the multiple reagent strip and include pH, protein, glucose, ketone, bilirubin, blood, nitrite, urobilinogen, and specific gravity. Intensely colored urine specimens may cause false positive results. With these specimens color reactions should be estimated visually.

Controls are similar to those used daily for manual reading. Positive (high and low) and negative controls should be used. Controls containing a chloroform preservative or other organic solvents should not be used with the plastic sample tray.

The advantages of the instrument are those of reproducibility between operators (Peele, 1977) and speed.

Another semi-automated instrument, Uritron[c], reads hand-dipped reagent strips. It has the advantage of testing the urine as a blank and may be updated readily by changing computer cards.

A fast, semi-automated instrument, Vista urine analyzer (American Scientific Products), rotates manually dipped strips into a reader so that seven tests are read in ten seconds. Interference by colored urine is compensated for. The reagent strips used in the instrument are Uriflet 7A. A printer is built in, and the instrument may be interfaced to an on-line computer. It is suitable for high volume work loads.

Proficiency Testing. All laboratories (office, clinic, hospital, etc.) should participate in proficiency testing programs. The small cost involved is more than compensated for by the experience and benefit gained.

Information provided by the College of American Pathologists for each substance tested in their quarterly surveys allows individual laboratory personnel to see results for the many different methods used in hundreds of laboratories. The survey material is provided at basic and more comprehensive levels, allowing the laboratory supervisor to choose the appropriate level of difficulty. The individual can also reflect on the occasional differences among referees and laboratories regarding morphologic material. This emphasizes the difficulty of urine cytology and morphology in general when compared with more uniform morphology occurring in blood.

PROCEDURE FOR ROUTINE SCREENING URINALYSIS

Before any tests are performed, a quality control check should be made as previously described. Precautions in the use of reagent strips should also be noted. An outline of the procedure is shown in Table 18–2.

The Urine Specimen. The volume of urine necessary depends on the number of tests to be performed. As little as 2 ml will suffice; however, 15 ml or more is preferable for routine work (see below).

Specimens must be refrigerated if not examined immediately, but should be brought to room temperature before using enzymatic reagent strips. All specimens should be free from fecal and vaginal contamination. Specimens must be properly identified and two tubes (to be used for centrifuging and supernate) properly numbered.

Screening for Bacteriuria. If only one specimen is available for complete urinalysis, screening for bacteriuria should be done first, provided that the urine has been properly collected into a sterile container. Alternative procedures include a Gram stain of the uncentrifuged, well-mixed specimen, and a quantitative loop culture or miniculture method, all of which require a drop or two of urine.

Color and Appearance. These are recorded, as is odor, if abnormal.

Specific Gravity. At this point, a drop may be used for refractometer estimation of specific gravity.

Chemical Screening (Basic). Using multiple reagent strips, dip and read for all or some of the following on a well-mixed specimen:

pH	bilirubin
protein	urobilinogen
glucose	nitrite
ketones	leukocyte esterase
blood	specific gravity

Refer to Table 18–7 for a list of reagent strips and substances tested (p. 397).

If a multiple reagent strip is not used and bilirubin is suspected, Ictotest[a], a tablet test for bilirubin, is simple, more sensitive, and easier to interpret.

Test for Copper-Reducing Substances (Sugars). It is important that this test be performed on all specimens obtained from *infants* by either Benedict's test or the Clinitest[a] tablet method.

At this point, the specimen should be centrifuged in a numbered disposable centrifuge tube, and the clear supernatant separated from the sediment and saved in an identifiable tube.

The Sediment. Using brightfield and phase microscopy, a drop of the concentrated sediment is examined for red blood cells, leukocytes, renal epithelial cells, casts, and excessive numbers of crystals.

Alternatively, the uncentrifuged, well-mixed specimen may be examined in a counting chamber and reported as cells per microliter.

The Supernatant. The saved supernatant is used for the following tests when they are necessary:

1. A confirmatory protein test, Bence Jones test, and electrophoresis.
2. Separation of sugars carried out by chromatography when a copper reduction test is positive and the glucose oxidase test is negative.
3. To check for ascorbic acid when erythrocytes are present and the reagent strip test for blood is negative.
4. Check a dubious bilirubin result with Ictotest[a]; confirm urobilinogen or porphobilinogen.
5. Confirmation of cystine or sulfonamide crystals by a qualitative test.

The Result. Before any specimen is discarded, the entire report should be examined to determine whether the sediment results match the chemical screen, color, and appearance, and whether all abnormal findings have been followed up through appropriate confirmation. If unusual crystals are found or there are other unexplained findings, a drug list should be obtained.

Volume Needed. At least 10 ml is required for routine urinalysis. However, most tests can be accomplished on a smaller volume when necessary. For volumes between 3 and 10 ml, a multiple reagent strip test, specific gravity (refractometer), copper reducing substances (two to five drops), bilirubin (tablet), and dilution for "large" ketones are possible. Then either 2.5 ml is centrifuged to produce a 0.25 ml sediment or 5 ml is centrifuged to produce 0.5 ml for sediment examination (10:1 concentration). When the volume is less than 2.5 ml, a multiple reagent strip, specific gravity, copper reducing test, and bilirubin test are usually feasible. The urine may

Table 18–2. OUTLINE OF PROCEDURE FOR ROUTINE URINALYSIS*

Appearance		Record turbidity Record abnormal color
Specific gravity		Use refractometer If greater than 1.035, report as "greater than 1.035"
Chemical tests (multiple reagent strip)		
pH		Report as 5, 6, 7, 8, or 9
Protein		Report as Neg, trace, 1+, 2+, 3+ or 4+ Acid precipitation test (SSA) using supernatant urine to confirm positive reagent strip; tests are done in parallel for new patients and outpatients
Glucose	Pediatric patients to six years	Glucose oxidase reagent strip; semiquantitate (g/dl) to 2 g/dl Reducing substances, with Clinitest[a]; semiquantitate (g/dl) to 5 g/dl
	Seven years and up	Glucose Oxidase reagent strip; semiquantitate (g/dl) to 2 g/dl Reducing substance with Clinitest[a] when ketones are moderately positive, and when glucose is 2 g/dl on strip
Ketones		Report as trace, small (1+), moderate (2+); if "large" (3+), dilute until moderate; record as moderate (2+) with dilution factor (1:2, 1:4, etc.)
Bilirubin		If a reagent strip is not a clear cut negative, check with Ictotest,[a] which is more sensitive than the reagent strip; report as 1+, 2+ or 3+
Blood		Report as trace, 1+, 2+ or 3+; use uncentrifuged urine
Ehrlich's reacting substances		If more than 1 EU on the reagent strip (Ames), differentiate with the Watson-Schwartz test (Ehrlich's aldehyde reaction) Watson-Schwartz test: report the result for porphobilinogen and urobilinogen as positive or negative; confirm positive porphobilinogen with Hoesch test
Sediment		Microscopic analysis of a 12:1 concentration of the urine using phase microscopy

*Procedure used at the University of Minnesota Hospitals.

be examined microscopically and the findings reported as uncentrifuged. Occasionally volumes of 0.5 ml or less are tested for specific constituents at the request of the physician.

PHYSICOCHEMICAL TESTS

Possibly because an unwarranted amount of attention was given for many centuries to the appearance of urine, and because the yield in terms of positive results is small, simple gross examination of the urine has been too often ignored by the physician and other health workers. There are certain characteristics of the gross urine specimen, however, which provide useful diagnostic information and should not be overlooked.

Appearance

Appearance of Normal Urine. The amber yellow color of urine is due largely to the pigment urochrome and to small amounts of urobilins and uroerythrin. Urochrome excretion is thought to be proportional to the metabolic rate and is increased during fever, thyrotoxicosis, and starvation. The pink pigment (uroerythrin) may be deposited in uric acid or urate crystals (brick dust deposit), and these should not be confused with blood. *Pale* urine in a normal person follows high fluid intake. Darker urines may be seen when fluids are withheld. Thus, the color roughly indicates the degree of hydration. Note that pale urine of high specific gravity may be found in diabetes mellitus and after the use of radiographic media.

Normal concentrated urine may show a sedimentary deposit if allowed to stand after cooling from body temperature. Precipitation due to phosphates or uric acid may occur. Mucus from the urinary and genital tracts is seen as small cloudy patches (nubeculae) in normal urine.

Certain food and candy dyes will color urine (Levin, 1965), as will drugs used for investigation and therapy. An innocuous red urine associated with ingestion of beets is seen in genetically susceptible persons.

Some of the more important changes in the gross appearance of the urine are described below. For color changes in urine in pediatric patients, see Cone (1968a). A comprehensive listing is given in Table 18–3.

Cloudy Urine. Cloudy urine is most often normal. It may be due to *phosphate* (and occasionally carbonate) precipitation in alkaline urine; the phosphates and carbonates redissolve when acetic acid is added. Uric acid and *urates* cause a white, pink, or orange cloud in acid urine and redissolve on warming to 60°C. Ammonium urates occur in neutral and alkaline urine and dissolve in acetic acid. *Leukocytes* may form a white cloud similar to that caused by phosphates, but in this case the cloud remains after the addition of dilute acetic acid; the presence of leukocytes is confirmed by microscopic examination of the sediment. *Bacterial growth* will cause a uniform opalescence which is not removed by acidification or by filtering through paper. Microscopically, rod-shaped bacteria, sometimes motile, are commonly seen, e.g., *E. coli* and *Proteus*. *Enterococcus* and *Staphylococcus* (a skin contaminant) are coccal forms. Yeasts are prevalent in urine specimens.

Turbidity or smokiness may be due to *red blood cells*—hematuria. This turbidity does not clear on warming, and the presence of erythrocytes may be confirmed microscopically. *Spermatozoa and prostatic fluid* may cause turbidity not cleared by acidification or heating. Prostatic fluid normally contains a few leukocytes and other formed elements. *Mucus* from the urinary passages may cause a fluffy, bulky deposit; this is increased in inflammatory states of the lower urinary tract or genital tract. Turbidity due to blood clots, menstrual discharge, and other particulate material such as pieces of tissue, small calculi, clumps of pus, and fecal material is sometimes seen. Fecal material in urine may result from a fistula between the colon or rectum and bladder. Contamination with powders or with antiseptics which become opaque with water (phenols) will also cause a turbid urine.

Chyluria. This is rare. The urine contains lymph. It is associated with obstruction to lymph flow and rupture of lymphatic vessels into the renal pelvis, ureters, bladder, or urethra. Filariasis (late in the disease), abdominal lymph node enlargement, and tumors have been associated with chyluria. Even with filariasis this is a rare event.

The appearance of the urine varies with the amount of lymph present. It may appear normal, opalescent, or milky. Clots may form. If sufficient lymph is present after a meal, the urine may layer, showing the chylomicrons on top and fibrin and cells beneath. Large numbers of red cells may cause a pink color. Chylomicrons may not be apparent microscopically unless they have coalesced as microglobules. This fat can be extracted from urine using an equal volume of ether or chloroform. If urine is turbid due to phosphates, for example, it will not clear. The protein test is positive; leukocytes and red blood cells are present (Sanjurjo, 1970). Pseudochyluria occurs with the use of paraffin-based vaginal creams for the treatment of Candida infections (Blank, 1982).

Lipiduria. Fat globules appear in urine most often with the nephrotic syndrome; these are neutral fats (triglycerides) and cholesterol. Cholesterol esters polarize. Oily contaminants such as paraffin will float on the urine surface as well as endogenous lipids.

Lipiduria is also present in a significant number of patients who have sustained major skeletal trauma with one or more fractures to major long bones or pelvis. Presumably the source of lipid is exposed fatty marrow. Although in the past the demonstration of fat droplets in the urine has been used as a sign of post-traumatic fat embolism, there is evidence which negates the diagnostic significance of this finding. Quantitative estimations of urinary fat in trauma patients reveal no significant differences between those with fat embolism and those without (Hansen, 1973).

Red Urine. The most common abnormal color is red or red-brown. When seen in the female, contamination with menstrual flow should be considered.

The urine in *hematuria* (presence of red blood cells) may appear cloudy, smoky, pink, red, or brown. The urine in *hemoglobinuria* may be clear red, clear red-brown, or dark brown. *Methemoglobin* has a dark brown color and develops in bladder urine of acid pH or in acid urine on standing. Blood and blood pigments are easily detected by means of a reagent strip. A positive test will indicate the presence of hemoglobin or myoglobin (see Confirmatory Tests).

In the porphyrias, the urine may be normal, red, or purple. It is usually red in congenital erythropoietic porphyria and the cutanea tarda form of porphyria. In acute intermittent hepatic porphyria, it is normal but darkens on standing. In lead porphyrinuria, the urine color is normal. Red urine also may be associated with the use of drugs and dyes in diagnostic tests; for example, phenolsulfonphthalein, which is sometimes used in testing renal function, will cause a red color

Table 18–3. APPEARANCE AND COLOR OF URINE

Appearance	Cause	Remarks
Colorless	Very dilute urine	Polyuria, diabetes insipidus
Cloudy	Phosphates, carbonates	Soluble in dilute acetic acid
	Urates, uric acid	Dissolve at 60°C. and in alkali
	Leukocytes	Insoluble in dilute acetic acid
	Red cells ("smoky")	Lyse in dilute acetic acid
	Bacteria, yeasts	Insoluble in dilute acetic acid
	Spermatozoa	Insoluble in dilute acetic acid
	Prostatic fluid	
	Mucin, mucous threads	May be flocculent
	Calculi, "gravel"	Phosphates, oxalates
	Clumps, pus, tissue	
	Fecal contamination	Rectovesical fistula
	Radiographic dye	In acid urine
Milky	Many neutrophils (pyuria)	Insoluble in dilute acetic acid
	Fat	
	Lipiduria, opalescent	Nephrosis, crush injury—soluble in ether
	Chyluria, milky	Lymphatic obstruction—soluble in ether
	Emulsified paraffin	Vaginal creams
Yellow	Acriflavine	Green fluorescence
Yellow-orange	Concentrated urine	Dehydration, fever
	Urobilin in excess	No yellow foam
	Bilirubin	Yellow foam if sufficient bilirubin
Yellow-green	Bilirubin-biliverdin	Yellow foam
Yellow-brown	Bilirubin-biliverdin	"Beer" brown, yellow foam
Red	Hemoglobin	Positive } reagent strip for blood
	Red blood cells	Positive } reagent strip for blood
	Myoglobin	Positive } reagent strip for blood
	Porphyrin	May be colorless
	Fuscin, aniline dye	Foods, candy
	Beets	Yellow alkaline, genetic
	Menstrual contamination	Clots, mucus
Red-purple	Porphyrins	May be colorless
Red-brown	Red blood cells	
	Hemoglobin on standing	
	Methemoglobin	Acid pH
	Myoglobin	Muscle injury
	Bilifuscin (dipyrrole)	Result of unstable hemoglobin
Brown-black	Methemoglobin	Blood, acid pH
	Homogentisic acid	On standing, alkaline; alkaptonuria
	Melanin	On standing, rare
Blue-green	Indicans	Small intestine infections
	Pseudomonas infections	
	Chlorophyll	Mouth deodorants

3

Table 18–4. URINE COLOR CHANGES WITH COMMONLY USED DRUGS*

Drug	Color
Alcohol, ethyl	Pale, diuresis
Anthraquinone laxatives (senna, cascara)	Reddish, alkaline; yellow-brown, acid
Chlorzoxazone (Paraflex) (muscle relaxant)	Red
Deferoxamine mesylate (Desferal) (chelates iron)	Red
Ethoxazene (Serenium) (urinary analgesic)	Orange, red
Fluorescein sodium (given I.V.)	Yellow
Furazolidone (Furoxone) (Tricofuron) (an antibacterial, antiprotozoal nitrofuran)	Brown
Indigo carmine dye (renal function, cystoscopy)	Blue
Iron sorbitol (Jectofer) (possibly other iron compounds forming iron sulfide in urine)	Brown on standing
Levodopa (L-dopa) (for Parkinsonism)	Red then brown, alkaline
Mepacrine (Atabrine) (antimalarial) (intestinal worms, giardia)	Yellow
Methocarbamol (Robaxin) (muscle relaxant)	Green-brown
Methyldopa (Aldomet) (antihypertensive)	Darken; if oxidizing agents present, red to brown
Methylene blue (used to delineate fistulas)	Blue, blue-green
Metronidazole (Flagyl) (for Trichomonas infection, amebiasis, Giardia)	Darkening, reddish brown
Nitrofurantoin (Furadantin) (antibacterial)	Brown-yellow
Phenazopyridine (Pyridium) (urinary analgesic), also compounded with sulfonamides (Azo-Gantrisin, etc.)	Orange-red, acid pH
Phenindione (Hedulin) (anticoagulant) (important to distinguish from hematuria)	Orange, alkaline; color disappears on acidifying
Phenol poisoning	Brown; oxidized to quinones (green)
Phenolphthalein (purgative)	Red-purple, alkaline pH
Phenolsulfonphthalein (PSP, also BSP)	Pink-red, alkaline pH
Rifampin (Rifadin, Rimactane) (tuberculosis therapy)	Bright orange-red
Riboflavin (multi-vitamins)	Bright yellow
Sulfasalazine (Azulfidine) (for ulcerative colitis)	Orange-yellow, alkaline pH

*Other commonly used drugs have been noted to produce color change once or occasionally; amitriptyline (Elavil)—blue-green; phenothiazines—red; triamterene (Dyrenium)—pale blue (blue fluorescence in acid urine). An extensive list may be found in Young et al.: Clin. Chem., *21*:379, 1975.

in alkaline urine (Table 18–4). In the presence of unstable hemoglobin, such as Hb Köln, the urine has a red-brown color that does not give a positive test for hemoglobin or for bilirubin. The pigment is probably a dipyrrole or bilifuscin.

Yellow-Brown or Green-Brown Urine. Yellow-brown or green-brown urine is most often associated with bile pigments, chiefly bilirubin. On shaking the urine specimen, a yellow foam may be seen which distinguishes bilirubin from a normal, dark, concentrated urine, which will have white foam. In severe obstructive jaundice, the urine may be dark green.

Orange-Red or Orange-Brown Urine. Urine containing large amounts of urobilin may resemble a dark, concentrated normal urine. Excreted urobilinogen is colorless but is converted in the presence of light and acid pH to urobilin which is dark yellow or orange. Urobilin will not color the foam on shaking a urine sample. Urinary analgesics (phenazopyridines) will cause an orange color and will color any foam present.

Dark Brown or Black Urine. An acid urine containing hemoglobin will darken on standing because of the formation of methemoglobin. Other, rarer causes of dark brown urine are homogentisic acid (alcaptonuria) and melanin. Urine containing homogentisic acid will darken more rapidly when alkaline. Dark brown or cola-colored urine is seen in the urine of some patients taking levodopa. See Table 18–3 for causes of colored urines and Table 18–4 for a list of common drugs causing colored urines.

Odor

Normal urine has a faint, aromatic odor of undetermined source. Odor is chiefly important in the recognition of specimens that, due to bacterial contamination on standing, are ammoniacal, fetid, and unsuitable for laboratory examination. Lack of odor in urine from patients with acute renal failure coincides with acute tubular necrosis rather than prerenal failure (Najarian, 1980).

Characteristic urine odors are produced after ingestion of asparagus or thymol.

Urine odors associated with amino acid disorders:

Isovaleric acidemia and glutaric acidemia	Sweaty feet
Maple syrup urine disease	Maple syrup
Methionine malabsorption	Cabbage, hops
Phenylketonuria	Mousy
Trimethylaminuria	Rotting fish
Tyrosinemia	Rancid

Urine Volume

Measurement of the urine volume during timed intervals may be a valuable aid in clinical diagnosis. The average daily volume in the normal adult is 1200 to 1500 ml, the range of normal being from about 600 to 2000 ml. The night urine is generally not in excess of 400 ml. Young children excrete about three to four times as much urine per kilogram of body weight as do adults (Table 18–5). In normal pregnancy, the usual diurnal variation is reversed, causing

Table 18–5. URINARY SPECIFIC GRAVITY AND URINE VOLUME-AGE RELATED REFERENCE VALUES

	Reference Values	Reference
Specific gravity		
Newborn (first few days)	1.012	Rubin, 1964
Infants	1.002–1.006	
Adults	1.001–1.035	
Adults (normal fluid intake)	1.016–1.022	
Volume		
Newborn (1–2 days old)	30–60 ml/24 h	
Infants		
3–10 days	100–300 ml/24 h	
10–60 days	250–450 ml/24 h	
60–365 days	400–500 ml/24 h	
Children		
1–3 years	500–600 ml/24 h	
3–5 years	600–700 ml/24 h	
5–8 years	650–1000 ml/24 h	
8–14 years	800–1400 ml/24 h	
Adults	600–1600 ml/24 h	
Older adults	250–2400 ml/24 h	Howell, 1956

nocturia and the excretion of a dilute urine (Pritchard, 1980).

Increases in Urine Volume. A volume of more than 2000 ml in 24 hours is termed *polyuria*. Any increase in urine volume, even though transitory, is called *diuresis*. Under ordinary physiologic conditions, the chief determinant of urine volume is the intake of water.

Excessive intake of water (polydipsia) will result in polyuria that may be confused with diabetes insipidus. Increased salt intake and high protein diets will also require more water for excretion. Certain drugs exert a diuretic effect. Among these are caffeine, alcohol, thiazides, and other diuretics. Intravenous saline or glucose solutions may increase the urine output.

Classic pathologic states characterized by a continuous polyuria are *diabetes insipidus* and *diabetes mellitus*. They result in excessive thirst and in excessive water intake. In pituitary diabetes insipidus there is a deficiency of antidiuretic hormone, and polyuria with nocturia is marked, up to 15 L per day. In diabetes mellitus there is an excessive amount of glucose excreted, causing a solute diuresis. Compulsive water drinkers will have variable polyuria.

In *chronic progressive renal failure,* functioning renal tissue is lost and the kidney gradually loses its ability to concentrate urine. In order to excrete the daily renal load, an increase in urine volume is inevitable. The urine eventually becomes isosmotic with the plasma ultrafiltrate; the normal day and night volume ratio (2:1) of urine is lost. *Nocturia* is arbitrarily defined as the excretion by an adult of more than 500 ml of urine with a specific gravity of less than 1.018 at night. Polyuria may also result when there is *tubular damage,* and with impairment of the countercurrent mechanism urine will have a low specific gravity.

Decreases in Urine Volume. Oliguria is the excretion of less than 500 ml of urine daily, and anuria is virtually complete suppression of urine formation. Water deprivation will cause a decrease in urine volume even before signs of dehydration appear.

Decreases in urine volume to oliguric levels occur under pathologic circumstances such as the following:

Dehydration. In prolonged vomiting, diarrhea, or excessive sweating, such as may occur in febrile states, loss of body water without adequate replacement results in dehydration and hemoconcentration. Oliguria occurs, and there may even be retention of nitrogenous waste products due to a decrease in the glomerular filtration rate. Urinary specific gravity is elevated to about 1.030. Oliguria will also occur when water is shifted from intravascular to extravascular compartments with edema.

Renal Ischemia. With a poor blood supply to the kidney from heart failure or hypotension, oliguria and anuria occur. These prerenal causes are associated with low sodium excretion and high specific gravity urine. Similar findings are seen when there is decreased filtration in acute glomerulonephritis. Anuria (or oliguria) also follows major hemolytic *transfusion reactions* and also accompanies the "crush" syndrome. Anuria in these conditions is thought to be related to loss of functioning renal mass.

3

Renal Disease. When there is oliguria with *uremia* due to progressive renal disease, urinary specific gravity is low, sodium concentration is elevated, and proteinuria, casts, and cells may be evident. This is in contrast to oliguria due to inadequate renal blood flow. Pyelonephritis or interstitial nephritis will cause predominantly tubular dysfunction with polyuria early in the disease, but later oliguria of chronic renal failure. Toxic agents, such as mercury bichloride, carbon tetrachloride, and diethylene glycol, may result in anuria due to acute tubular necrosis.

Obstruction. Bilateral hydronephrosis, resulting from high-grade or longstanding obstruction of the urinary tract, may be associated with a marked decrease in urine flow and even anuria. This occurs with prostatic hyperplasia and carcinoma. Bilateral ureteral obstruction due to stones, clots, and sloughed tissue and urethral obstruction due to stricture or valves are other forms of obstruction. The anuria associated with sulfonamide therapy and dehydration is due to obstruction caused by the precipitation of crystals in the renal tubules when the urinary pH is acidic.

Specific Gravity and Osmolality

The volume of excreted urine and its concentration of solute are varied by the kidney to maintain homeostasis of body fluid and electrolytes. In order to achieve this, the kidneys produce a urine much more concentrated than the plasma from which it is derived. Inability to concentrate or dilute urine is an indication of renal disease or hormonal deficiency (ADH). See Chapter 8 for a discussion of the concentrating ability of the kidney.

Urines of low specific gravity are called *hyposthenuric,* the specific gravity being less than 1.007. Urines of fixed specific gravity of about 1.010 are known as *isosthenuric.* The specific gravity of the protein-free glomerular filtrate is about 1.007. Its osmolal concentration is about 285 mOsm, or the osmolality of protein-free plasma (the plasma protein makes little contribution to the total osmolality of the plasma, only about 2 mOsm).

The measurement of specific gravity or osmolality should give an indication of the urinary total solute concentration. In critical circumstances, the measurement of osmolality of urine *and* plasma is preferred to the measurement of specific gravity. The reader should refer to Chapter 8 for a discussion of osmolality versus specific gravity of urine.

Osmolality. The normal adult on a normal diet with a normal fluid intake will produce a urine of about 500 to 850 mOsm/kg water. The normal kidney is able to produce urine of osmolality in the range of 800 to 1400 mOsm/kg water in dehydration and a minimal osmolality of 40 to 80 mOsm/kg water during water diuresis. After a period of dehydration, the osmolality of the urine should be three to four times that of the plasma (e.g., with a normal plasma osmolality of 285 mOsm/kg water, the urine osmolality should be at least 855 mOsm/kg water).

Methods for Measuring Osmolality. The freezing point depression method is commonly employed. A solution containing 1 osmol or 1000 mOsm/kg water depresses the freezing point 1.86°C. below the freezing point of water. For method, see Chapters 2 and 8.

Specific Gravity. Useful clinical information can be obtained from the measurement of maximal specific gravity. Urea (20 per cent), sodium chloride (25 per cent), sulfate, and phosphate contribute most to the specific gravity of normal urine. Normal adults with normal diets and normal fluid intake will produce urine of specific gravity 1.016 to 1.022 during a 24-hour period. If a random specimen of urine has a specific gravity of 1.023 or more, concentrating ability can be considered normal.

Urinary specific gravity after taking no fluids for 12 hours overnight should be about 1.022, and after 24 hours without fluid, 1.026. For values in infants, see Table 18–5.

Minimum specific gravity after a standard water load should be less than 1.003. For details of concentration and dilution tests, see Chapter 8.

Specific Gravity Methods. Several methods are available to measure specific gravity—refractometer, hydrometer (urinometer), and reagent strip (see Reagent Strip Methodology).

When only a small amount of urine is available, specific gravity may be measured by using a small volume urinometer, by weighing the urine, by measuring the refractive index, or by using the reagent strip method. The refractometer method is commonly used for routine urinalysis.

Table 18–6 shows the differences in readings for salt solutions used as osmolality standards with three methods for recording specific gravity. Note that the salt solutions have much lower readings on the urine specific gravity scale of the refractometer when compared with the urinometer readings. The refractometer specific gravity scale is *valid only for urine* and cannot be used to indicate the specific gravity of salt or sugar solutions. This should be borne in mind if salt solutions are to be used for calibration. A 5 per cent NaCl solution has a calculated specific gravity of 1.035, but a 7.5 per cent NaCl solution w/v is required to give a reading of 1.035 on the refractometer scale. Special graphs or tables are required to convert refractive index scale numbers to solute concentration in aqueous solutions if this should be required (American Optical Catalog Number 10403).

Refractometer. The refractive index of a solution is related to the content of dissolved solids present. It is the ratio of the velocity of light in air to the velocity of light in a solution. This ratio varies directly with the number of dissolved particles in solution. Measurement of refractive index of urine became feasible and convenient with the development of a clinical refractometer. This device requires only a few drops of urine (unlike the minimum 15 ml of urine necessary with the urinometer). Although the refractometer measures refractive index of a solution, scale readings of the instrument have been calibrated in terms of specific gravity for human urine total solids and for serum protein levels. The specific gravity reading on the refractometer is generally slightly lower than a urinometer reading on the same urine specimen by about 0.002 (Rubini, 1957; Wolfe, 1962).

Procedure. A temperature-compensated hand model is available.* The instrument is temperature compensated between 60 and 100°F. It is damaged by heat above 150°F. and by immersion of the eye-piece and focusing ring in water. It should read zero with distilled water; the zero reading can be reset if necessary by breaking the seal over the setscrew, turning it with a small screwdriver, and resealing. To prevent dropping and lens damage, a stand is recommended to support the refractometer.

Always check calibration daily. If the zero reading is correct for distilled water, it is probably not necessary to check the instrument with high and low specific gravity salt solutions. However, some laboratory personnel may prefer to do this.

To make a specific gravity determination of urine, first clean the surfaces of the cover and prism with a drop of distilled water and a damp cloth and then dry. Close the cover. Hold horizontally and apply a drop of urine at the notched bottom of the cover so that it flows over the prism surface by capillary action.

Point the instrument toward a light source at an angle that gives optimal contrast. Rotate the eye-piece until the scale is in focus. Read directly on the specific gravity scale the *sharp* dividing line between light and dark contrast.

The entire procedure should be repeated with a second drop of urine from the same sample.

Reagent Strip. For specific gravity by reagent strip, see Reagent Strip Methodology.

Urinometer. This is a hydrometer adapted to measure the specific gravity of urine at room temperature. It should be checked each day by measuring the specific gravity of distilled water, which has a specific gravity of 1.000. If the urinometer does not give a reading of 1.000, an appropriate correction must be applied to all readings taken with that urinometer. The accuracy of a urinometer may be further checked in solutions of known specific gravity; e.g., a solution of potassium sulfate with a specific gravity of 1.015 may be prepared by diluting 20.29 g potassium sulfate to 1 L with distilled water.

Procedure. The urinometer vessel is filled three fourths full with urine (minimum volume of urine required is about 15 ml). The urinometer is inserted with a spinning motion to make sure that it is floating freely. (When reading the urinometer, be sure that it is not touching the sides or the bottom of the cylinder. Avoid surface bubbles, which obscure the meniscus.) Read the bottom of the meniscus.

Because temperature influences the specific gravity, urines should be allowed to come to room temperature before a reading is made, or a correction of 0.001 should be made

*TS meter. American Optical Company, Buffalo, New York.

for each 3°C. above or below the calibration temperature indicated on the urinometer, usually 15.6°C. (60°F.).

For accurate determinations of specific gravity in concentration-dilution tests, corrections are made for protein or glucose present. Subtract 0.003 for every 1 g/100 ml of either glucose or protein.

The pH of Urine

The pH of urine is a reflection of the ability of the kidney to maintain normal hydrogen ion concentration in plasma and extracellular fluid. The metabolic activity of the body produces non-volatile acids which cannot be extracted by the lungs—principally sulfuric, phosphoric, and hydrochloric acids, but also small amounts of pyruvic, lactic, and citric acids and some ketone bodies. These acids are excreted by the glomerulus with cations, chiefly sodium. Bicarbonate is reabsorbed. The tubular cells exchange hydrogen ions for sodium of the glomerular filtrate, and the urine becomes acid in reaction. Hydrogen ions are also excreted as ammonium ion (NH_4^+). For a discussion of this exchange process, see Chapter 8.

Normal pH. The average adult on a normal diet excretes about 50 to 100 mEq of hydrogen ions in 24 hours to produce urine of about pH 6. In health, urine pH may vary from 4.6 to 8. When protein intake is high, more phosphates and sulfates are produced; this results in more acid urine. On a predominantly vegetable diet, as in many non-western countries, the urine may have a pH higher than 6. The urine becomes less acid following a meal as a result of secretion of acid into the stomach (the so-called alkaline tide). At night, during the mild respiratory acidosis of sleep, a more acid urine may be formed.

Acid Urine. Acid urine may be produced by a diet high in meat protein and in some fruits such as cranberries. Ammonium chloride, methionine, methenamine mandelate, or acid phosphate is used to produce an acid urine in treatment of some calculi. Acid phosphates with or without antibacterials help keep calcium in solution. Acidifiers are useful for ammonium magnesium stone prevention, since these form in an alkaline urine.

Alkaline Urine. Alkaline urine may be induced by use of a diet high in certain fruits and vegetables, especially citrus fruits. Sodium bicarbonate, potassium citrate, and acetazolamide may be used to induce alkaline urines in the treatment of some calculi. They may also be used in some urinary tract infections (the antibiotics neomycin, kanamycin, and streptomycin are more active in alkaline urine), in sulfonamide therapy, and in the treatment of salicylate poisoning.

Interpretation of Urine pH in Pathologic States. The capacity to exchange hydrogen ion for cation and the formation of ammonia is decreased when tubular function is impaired. In classic *renal tubular acidosis,* glomerular filtration is normal, but distal tubular ability to form ammonia and exchange hydrogen ions for cations is defective. Systemic acidosis results. The urine is relatively alkaline, and the pH cannot be lowered below pH of 6 to 6.5, even with the administration of an acid-loading substance. Titratable acidity and the concentration of ammonium are decreased. In proximal renal tubular acidosis there is bicarbonate wasting. This occurs with proximal tubular diseases such as the Fanconi syndrome.

In metabolic acid-base disturbances, the pH of the urine may reflect attempts at compensation by the kidneys. In *metabolic acidosis* an acid urine is produced and titratable acidity and ammonium ion concentrations are increased. In chronic acidosis, as in diabetic ketoacidosis, very large amounts of hydrogen ions are excreted, much of it as ammonium ion. In *metabolic alkalosis* an alkaline urine with higher levels of bicarbonate is produced and ammonia production is decreased. The kidney may produce urine with a pH as high as 7.8. In *respiratory acidosis* an acid urine is formed and the amount of ammonium excreted is increased; in *respiratory alkalosis* an alkaline urine is produced which is associated with increased excretion of bicarbonate. In *potassium depletion* such as in hypokalemic alkalosis of prolonged vomiting or in hypercorticism, or with prolonged use of diuretics, there may be paradoxical aciduria with slightly acid urine in the presence of a metabolic alkalosis.

For a detailed description of the ammonium chloride loading test in renal diseases, see Wrong (1959). For a description of acidification and bicarbonate loading studies in distal renal tubular acidosis and the

Table 18–6. COMPARISON OF SPECIFIC GRAVITY READINGS OF STANDARD AQUEOUS SOLUTIONS

	Refractometer Urine S.G. Scale 20°C.	Urinometer 20°C.	SG Reagent Strip*	
			Automated	*Manual*
Distilled water	1.000	1.000	1.000	
NaCl solution* 750 mOs/kg H_2O	1.011	1.020	1.015† 1.020†	1.015
NaCl solution* 1000 mOs/kg H_2O	1.015	1.024	1.020 1.025	1.020 1.025
NaCl solution* 1600 mOs/kg H_2O	1.024	1.036	≥1.030	≥1.030

*Standard solutions for osmolality method (pH 5.0).
†Equal numbers of values on repeated tests.

3

use of pCO_2 urine levels for diagnosis, see Halperin (1975).

Measurement of Urine pH. Measurement of urine pH and acidity must always be made on freshly voided specimens. If precise measurements are required, the container should be filled and the urine covered tightly in order to minimize the amount of dead space. The container should be kept cold, preferably on ice, but not frozen. On standing, the pH tends to rise because of loss of carbon dioxide (the pCO_2 of freshly voided urine is approximately 40 mm Hg, that of normal plasma) and because bacterial growth produces ammonia from urea.

A rough estimate of the pH is usually sufficient and may be made with indicator paper. In patients with disturbances of acid-base balance, urinary pH may be accurately measured with a pH meter with a glass electrode.

Procedure. Urinary pH may be measured by means of a closed glass electrode and read directly from the scale of a pH meter. Since the pH meter may tend to drift, it must be standardized with three buffers of known pH immediately prior to use. After standardization, spray the electrodes with distilled water, clean, and dry with tissue. Immerse the electrodes in the urine sample. Report the pH of urine at the temperature of measurement.

Titratable Acidity of Urine. The pH of the urine is largely dependent on the amount of mono- and dibasic phosphate present. Titratable acidity is measured by titrating an aliquot of 24-hour urine (collected on ice) with 0.1 N NaOH with pH 7.4 as an endpoint. The test may be used together with urinary ammonia determination in patients with chronic acidosis of obscure origin.

Procedure. To 25 ml of urine in a flask, add 10 g of powdered potassium oxalate (to precipitate calcium). Mix well. Titrate to pH 7.4 using 0.1 N NaOH with a pH meter and glass electrode. Three reference buffers are used to standardize the pH meter.

Titratable acidity is usually reported as number of milliliters of 0.1 N NaOH required to neutralize a 24-hour specimen.

$$= \frac{\text{ml NaOH} \times \text{24-hour volume in ml}}{\text{25 ml}}$$

For mEq/24 hours, multiply by the normality of NaOH (0.1).

Normal titratable acidity is in the range of 200 to 500 ml 0.1 N NaOH (or 6 ml 0.1 N NaOH per kg body weight) or 20 to 40 mEq/24 hours.

REAGENT STRIP METHODOLOGY

Since reagent strips and multiple reagent strips are so commonly used, their chemical reactants, expected results, and interference problems are summarized below. It should be noted that reagent strip methods are changed periodically, sensitivities and color reactions altered, and new tests added. Manufacturers supply tables of common interfering substances, and these should be consulted. In practice, ascorbic acid and drugs producing colored urines such as phenazopyridine (Pyridium) and other azo compounds and methylene blue are most frequently encountered. As much as 3 g/day of ascorbic acid may be administered in parenteral vitamin preparations with maintenance fluid therapy in an adult. More detailed information on drug interference is listed in Hansten (1979) and Young (1975). For a listing of urine constituents detected by some available reagent strips and tablet tests, see Table 18–7.

pH

Chemistry. Indicators methyl red and bromthymol blue give a range of orange, green, and blue colors as the pH rises. The test permits differentiation of pH values to half a unit within the range of 5 to 9. It should be read immediately, but time is not critical.

pH is not affected by the urinary buffer concentration. Bacterial growth in a specimen may cause a marked alkaline shift and render it unsuitable for testing, usually because of urea conversion to ammonia. Care should be taken not to have excessively wet strips where acid buffer from the protein patch runs into the pH patch, causing it to become orange.

Protein

Tests are based on the principle of protein-error of pH indicators. This is the ability of proteins to alter the color reaction without altering the pH. The test area is buffered to a constant low pH so that color changes reflect the presence and concentration of proteins.

Results may be read in a "plus" system with any plus value indicating significant proteinuria. In concentrated specimens from healthy persons, a "trace" result may be seen with physiological normal excretion of protein.

Chemistry. The reagent strip is impregnated with tetrabromphenol blue[a] buffered to an acid pH of 3, or tetrachlorophenol-tetrabromosulfophthalein.[c] This area is yellow in the absence of protein but changes to a shade of green, depending on the type and concentration of protein present in 30 to 60 seconds. It is important to match the colors closely with the reacted strip.

Five to 20 mg of albumin/dl of urine may be detected. The test area is *more sensitive to albumin* than to globulin, Bence Jones protein, or mucoprotein. For an evaluation, see James (1978a).

High salt levels will lower results (Gyure, 1977). Exceptionally alkaline and/or highly buffered urines may give positive results in the absence of significant proteinuria, e.g., with a patient on alkaline medication or with bacterial contamination. Excessive leaching of the acid buffer by excessive wetting will cause false positive results. False positive results also occur with quaternary ammonium compounds used for cleaning containers and skin (Zephiran) and with amido-amines in fabric softeners and chlorhexidine. The test is unaffected by urine turbidity, radiographic media, most drugs, or their metabolites. Refer to Table 18–11 (p. 407).

Glucose

Tests are based on a specific glucose oxidase and peroxidase method, a double sequential enzyme reaction. Reagent strips differ in the chromogen used. The reagent strips may be used for semiquantitative results. Results should be reported as approximate grams per cent (g/dl) to avoid confusion regarding the relative amounts of glucose represented by the "plus systems" used in the many glucose and sugar tests available. Since these tests are specific for glucose, a copper reduction test such as Benedict's test or Clinitest[a] is included in the chemical screening of young pediatric patients to detect the occasional non-glucose reducing sugars. Diabetics commonly use a combination glucose and ketone reagent strip. This not only detects ketonuria but helps detect the suppression of glucose reaction by ketones.

Chemistry

$$\text{Glucose} + O_2 \xrightarrow{\text{glucose oxidase}} \text{gluconic acid} + H_2O_2$$

$$H_2O_2 + \text{chromogen} \xrightarrow{\text{peroxidase}} \text{oxidized chromogen} + H_2O$$

Clinistix[a]—o-toluidine chromogen. Color changes from pink to purple. This formulation detects 100 mg/dl of glucose and is more sensitive to interfering substances such as ascorbic acid than the following.

Multistix[a]—potassium iodide chromogen. Color changes from blue to brown at 30 seconds. Brown colors are difficult to distinguish.

Chemstrip[c]—an aminopropyl-carbazol chromogen. Color changes from yellow to orange-brown at 60 seconds.

Tes-Tape[b]—o-toluidine chromogen. Color changes from yellow to blue in one to two minutes.

About 50 to 100 mg/dl of glucose in urine is detectable with the above reagent strips. Report as positive or negative, and semiquantitate at 30 to 60 seconds up to 1 or 2 g/dl (as stated by manufacturer) unless moderate or large amounts of ketones are present. If so, confirm with Clinitest.[a]

Chemstrip uG[c]. Reagent pads have different sensitivities to urine glucose, ranging from 60 mg/dl to 5 g/dl. The chromogen is tetramethylbenzidine. Strips are read at two to three minutes and produce results close to a quantitative hexokinase method (Bandi, 1982).

The glucose oxidase test is specific for glucose; it does not react with lactose, galactose, fructose, or reducing metabolites of drugs. False positive readings may be produced by strongly oxidizing cleaning agents in the urine container. Use of sodium fluoride as a preservative will cause false negative readings. See Table 18–8. High specific gravity will decrease color development. All strips should be carefully protected against humidity, which will reduce reactivity. It is important to have the urine at room temperature for these enzyme reactions.

3

Ketones

The test is based on a nitroprusside (sodium nitroferricyanide) reaction. The reagent is very sensitive to moisture and will quickly become non-reactive. With

Table 18–7. URINE CONSTITUENTS DETECTED WITH COMMERCIAL TESTS

	pH	Glucose	Protein	Blood	Ketone	Bilirubin	Urobilinogen	Nitrite	Specific Gravity	Reducing Substances
N-Multistix-SG[a]	×	×	×	×	×	×	×	×	×	
Chemstrip 8[c]	×	×	×	×	×	×	×	×		
N-Multistix[a]	×	×	×	×	×	×	×	×		
Multistix-SG[a]	×	×	×	×	×	×	×		×	
Chemstrip 7[c]	×	×	×	×	×	×	×			
Multistix[a]	×	×	×	×	×	×	×			
Bili-Labstix[a]	×	×	×	×	×	×				
Chemstrip 6[c]	×	×	×	×	×	×				
Chemstrip 5[c]	×	×	×	×	×					
Labstix[a]	×	×	×	×	×					
Chemstrip 4[c]	×	×	×	×						
Hema-Combistix[a]	×	×	×	×						
Combistix[a]	×	×	×							
N-Uristix[a]		×	×					×		
Chemstrip GP[c]		×	×							
Uristix[a]		×	×							
Chemstrip GK[c]		×			×					
Keto-Diastix[a]		×			×					
Diastix[a]		×								
Clinistix[a]		×								
Tes-Tape[b]		×								
Chemstrip G[c]		×								
Albustix[a]			×							
Bumintest (tablets)[a]			×							
Hemastix[a]				×						
Acetest (tablets)[a]					×					
Chemstrip K[c]					×					
Ketostix[a]					×					
Ictotest (tablets)[a]						×				
Clinitest (tablets)[a]										×

This table summarizes reagent strips and tablets used by participants in the College of American Pathologists (CAP) proficiency testing programs during 1982. Other available strips detect leukocyte esterase—Chemstrip L series[c]; Phenistix[a] detects phenylpyruvic acid (and salicylate); Stix[a] and C-Stix[a] are used for ascorbic acid; Urobilistix[a] for urobilinogen.

large (3+) results, urine may be diluted and retested reporting a "moderate" result and the dilution factor.

Chemistry. Chemstrip[c] contains sodium nitroferricyanide and glycine which react with acetoacetic acid and acetone in an alkaline medium to form a violet dye. A positive result is indicated by a color change from beige to violet which is read at 60 seconds. The test detects about 10 mg/dl of acetoacetic acid and 70 mg/dl of acetone. The sensitivity and reaction of the reagent strip are similar to those of the tablet (Acetest[a]), described later.

Multistix[a] contains buffers and sodium nitroferricyanide which react with acetoacetic acid, producing a pink-maroon color in 15 seconds. The reagent area detects 5 to 10 mg acetoacetic acid/dl of urine. It does not react with acetone.

Color reactions (false positives) occur after the use of phthaleins (BSP or PSP dyes) or in the presence of extremely large amounts of phenylketones, and the preservative 8-hydroxyquinoline, or L-dopa metabolites. Acetylcysteine (aerosol) produces a strong red color. The anti-hypertensive drugs methyl-dopa and captopril give positive results. False negative results occur because of loss of reagent reactivity. These tests do not measure the predominant ketone body 3-hydroxybutyrate.

Blood

The test is based on the liberation of oxygen from peroxide in the reagent strip by the peroxidase-like activity of heme from free hemoglobin, lysed red cells, or myoglobin. Intact red cells are lysed on the strip, causing the hemoglobin to react. Therefore *well-mixed* urine must be tested, as intact red cells will be missed if only supernatant urine is used. Because of its reducing properties, ascorbic acid interference is a problem with this test. Hematuria may be missed if only the reagent strip test is used and a microscopic examination is omitted. Refer to Table 18–10 for findings associated with positive reagent strip results.

Chemistry. The reagent area is impregnated with a buffered mixture of an organic peroxide and the chromogen tetramethylbenzidine.

$$H_2O_2 + \text{chromogen} \xrightarrow[\text{peroxidase activity}]{\text{heme}} \underset{\text{(colored)}}{\text{oxidized chromogen}} + H_2O$$

Heme catalyzes the oxidation of tetramethylbenzidine to produce a green color. The test zone is yellow in the absence of blood and green to blue-green in the presence of blood. Timing is important.

Multistix[a] and Chemstrip[c] detect 0.05 to 0.3 mg hemoglobin/dl urine. Read at 40 and 60 seconds, respectively. Sensitivity decreases with age of the reagent strip. Sensitivities shown are those seen in practice. Note that 0.3 mg hemoglobin/dl is equivalent to that from ten lysed red blood cells per μl. These are assumed to be normal erythrocytes containing approximately 30 picograms of hemoglobin per cell. Freni (1977b) found that the most sensitive reagent strip detected about 20 cells/μl.

Sensitivity is reduced in urines with high specific gravity where red cell lysis may not occur and also when protein levels are high. A negative "blood" result for urine containing 5 mg/dl or more of ascorbic acid requires further checking by microscopy. Ascorbic acid in larger concentrations may depress results by approximately one color block. The presence of nitrite in large amounts will delay the test reaction, and formalin used as a urine preservative may cause falsely low or negative reactions. Oxidizing contaminants such as hypochlorites (bleach) may produce false positive results. Microbial peroxidase, associated with urinary tract infection, potentially causes a false positive reading.

Bilirubin

The test is based on a diazo reaction, and tests differ in the diazonium salt used. Urine must be fresh because bilirubin glucuronide in urine quickly hydrolyzes to less reactive bilirubin. Then oxidation of bilirubin in specimens which have stood too long, especially when exposed to light, will result in false-negative findings. With use of this method, normal urine contains no detectable bilirubin. See Confirmatory Tests for diazo *tablet* test.

Chemistry. The reaction is based on the coupling reaction of bilirubin with a diazonium salt in acid medium.

Multistix[a]-diazotized 2,4-dichloroaniline. Color changes from cream-buff to tan at 20 seconds and detects 0.8 mg/dl urine. Colors are hard to read.

Chemstrip[c]-2,6-dichlorobenzene-diazonium tetrafluoroborate. Color changes from pink to violet at 30 to 60 seconds and detects 0.5 mg/dl urine.

Large amounts of ascorbic acid and nitrite lower bilirubin results. Metabolites of drugs such as phenazopyridine (Pyridium) give a reddish color at the low pH of the strip and mask the result. Rifampin and large amounts of chlorpromazine metabolites may give positive tests. Salicylates do not interfere. Urobilinogen does not affect the result.

Urobilinogen

Urobilinogen is normally present in urine. The test is based on the Ehrlich aldehyde reaction or the formation of a red azo dye from a diazonium compound. Urine must be fresh and at room temperature. Urobilinogen is very labile in an acid urine and, with light, forms non-reactive urobilin; a negative result is not significant. Normally 1 Ehrlich unit/dl or 1 mg/dl may be present. Urobilinogen is often designated in units because it represents a mixture of more than one substance. See Tables 18–12 and 18–13 for urobilinogenuria.

Chemistry. Multistix[a]-impregnated with para-dimethyl-amino-benzaldehyde produces a reddish brown color with urobilinogen. The test is read in Ehrlich units/dl. Color blocks representing 0.2 to 12 Ehrlich units/dl are provided. Color varies from light yellow to shades of brown.

Chemstrip[c]-impregnated with 4-methoxybenzene-diazonium-tetrafluoroborate couples with urobilinogen in an acid medium to form a red azo dye. Values are read at 10 to 30 seconds. It detects approximately 0.4 mg/dl. Values up to 1 mg/dl are considered normal. Nitrite or formalin may reduce the color reaction.

The Multistix reagent strip[a] is not specific for urobilinogen and will react with substances known to react with the Ehrlich's reagent. These include porphobilinogen, para-amino-salicylic acid (PAS) metabolites, sulfonamides, procaine, 5-hydroxyindoleacetic acid, indole, and methyldopa (Aldomet). The test is useful as a preliminary test for the detection of porphobilinogen. Porphobilinogen and intermediate Ehrlich reacting substances can be differentiated from urobilinogen by using the Watson-Schwartz test, described later.

Both reagent strips are affected by the metabolites of drugs such as phenazopyridine (Pyridium), which colors the urine orange-red in an acid medium, and other compounds such as Azo-Gantrisin. These may mask the reaction with urobilinogen or give a false positive result. Interfering substances often react faster than urobilinogen.

Bilirubin and blood do not usually affect the test, but bilirubin may occasionally cause a green color.

Nitrite

The test depends upon the conversion of nitrate to nitrite by certain bacterial action in the urine. Because the test requires an overnight (minimum of four hours) bladder bacterial population to convert urinary nitrate to nitrite, a first morning specimen is best. Most Enterobacteriaceae are able to form nitrite from nitrate, but not all bacteria in bladder urine convert nitrate to nitrite, e.g., enterococcus; therefore, false negative results occur. Known nitrate-reducing organisms at significant levels produce false negative results. These organisms reduce nitrate to ammonia, nitric and nitrous oxide, hydroxylamine, and nitrogen, and will therefore give a negative nitrite test. A positive result is a possible indication for culture, unless the specimen has been improperly stored after collection allowing bacterial growth.

Chemistry. Multistix[a]. At an acid pH, nitrite, if present, reacts with para-arsanilic acid to give a diazonium salt, which by coupling with a benzoquinoline forms a pink azo dye. It detects 0.075 mg of nitrite/dl in solution. Read at 40 seconds.

Chemstrip[c] contains a benzoquinoline and sulfanilamide, which produce a pink azo dye with nitrite at 30 seconds. It detects 0.05 mg of nitrite/dl.

False positive readings may be produced by medication that colors the urine red or turns red in an acid medium (e.g., phenazopyridine). Pink spots or edges are interpreted as negative. False negative results occur with nitrite tests due to ascorbic acid, urobilinogen, and low pH (<6) (James, 1978b).

Specific Gravity

With increasing electrolyte concentration in urine, reagents in the strip release hydrogen ions, causing a lowering of the pH of the reagent strip and a subsequent color reaction proportional to the ionic strength. The solute urea, which occurs in large amounts in urine, does not contribute to the reagent strip result as it does for the urinometer and refractometer.

Chemistry. A partially dissociated poly acid (poly methyl vinyl ether/maleic anhydride) reacts with positive ions in the urine (Na^+, etc.) in such a way that neighboring acid groups in the molecule are allowed to dissociate, releasing hydrogen ions and lowering the pH. An indicator, bromthymol blue, changes from blue to yellow with increased acidity which corresponds to a higher specific gravity or salt content. Non-ionic substances such as glucose are not measured.

The color chart provided indicates values of 1.000 (dark blue) to 1.030 (yellow) in increments of 0.005. Read at 45 to 60 seconds.

Interference. Alkaline urines neutralize the released acid, causing a lower specific gravity reading. For urine pH of 6.5 or more, 0.005 should be added to the reading. High levels of protein, contributing to the anions in the urine, may cause an elevation of one color block or less. Glucose and radiographic media do not cause an alteration in the specific gravity recorded on the reagent strip as they do with the urinometer or refractometer. For a comparison of reagent strip and standard salt solutions with other specific gravity methods, see Table 18–6 and the previous section on Specific Gravity and Osmolality.

3

Leukocyte Esterase

Neutrophil granulocytes contain many esterases which catalyse the hydrolysis of an ester to produce its alcohol and acid. The test is similar in principle to the naphthol chloroacetate test used for granulocyte esterases in hematology. The esterase level in urine correlates with the number of neutrophils present. Cells from the urinary tract and red cells do not contribute to this esterase level. The test should be used in conjunction with the microscopic appraisal for leukocytes.

Chemistry. A substrate, indoxyl carbonic acid ester, is catalyzed to indoxyl and by oxidation from atmospheric oxygen forms indigo, a blue color. Reaction time for this formulation is 15 minutes. The reagent has been modified with the addition of a diazonium salt to produce a faster reaction with the indoxyl reacting with diazonium to form a purple color in one to two minutes.

Positive results correlate with "significant" numbers of neutrophils either intact or lysed. Using a chamber count of about 10 neutrophils/μl of fresh urine as a cut-off point, the number of false negatives and false positives was low (Gillenwater, 1981).

Interference. Hematuria and bacteriuria do not affect the reaction. Serum will inhibit the test. Oxidizing agents will give false positive colors. Very large amounts of ascorbic acid may inhibit the reaction. Formalin will inhibit the reaction. Nitrofurantoin and other strong colors affect color interpretation.

CONFIRMATORY TESTS (METHODOLOGY)

Ascorbic Acid

Because of its reducing properties, a large urinary concentration of ascorbic acid from therapeutic doses of vitamin C* or preparations containing ascorbic acid may inhibit some glucose oxidase-peroxidase reactions for glucose and also the tests for occult blood based upon the peroxidase activity of hemoglobin. It is useful to check for the presence of ascorbic acid when the microscopic examination of a urine sediment shows more than two red blood cells per high power field and the screening test for blood on the uncentrifuged urine specimen is negative.

The test has been used as an indication of adequate ascorbic acid therapy. With an adequate diet, 2 to 10 mg/dl is excreted daily. After ingestion of large amounts of ascorbic acid, levels in urine are about 200 mg/dl. Metabolites of ascorbic acid are sulfate and oxalate. With a large intake, 1 g or more per day, oxalate stones may form in susceptible persons.

C-Stix reagent strips[a] have a reagent-impregnated area consisting of phosphomolybdates buffered in an acid medium. Phosphomolybdates are reduced by ascorbic acid to "molybdenum blue." This test detects 5 mg/dl of ascorbic acid in urine after ten seconds. Gentisic acid and L-dopa may cause false positive results.

Stix reagent strips[a] are not as sensitive as C-Stix. They detect about 25 mg/dl of ascorbic acid at 60 seconds. The reagent is methylene green, which is reduced to its colorless form with ascorbic acid. Neutral red provides a background color, and the overall color changes from blue to purple at levels of 150 mg/dl. This test is also part of the Multistix[a] multiple reagent strips. Large amounts of bilirubin and pH greater than 7.5 interfere with the color. False positive results are not seen with urates, salicylates, gentisic acid, or creatinine.

Procedure. Dip the test end of the strip into the specimen. Compare the color of the reagent area of the strip with the color chart supplied by the manufacturer, and report as indicated on the chart.

Bilirubin

The diazo test method, in which bilirubin is coupled to p-nitrobenzene diazonium p-toluene sulfonate to form a blue or purple color (in the form of a tablet or reagent strip) is commonly used. Another test employs a ferric chloride reagent to oxidize bilirubin to a green biliverdin (Watson, 1946; see Henry, 1979).

Bilirubin glucuronide will hydrolyze on standing to less reactive bilirubin, and bilirubin will oxidize to biliverdin, which is not reactive in the diazo test. Hence, urine should be protected from light and examined as quickly as possible. The reagent strip test is much less reactive to the free bilirubin than the tablet test, so that a difference in results becomes more apparent as the urine ages. See section on Clinical Correlations which follows for the interpretation of the bilirubin and urobilinogen tests. The reagent strip method was described earlier.

Diazo Tablet Method (Free, 1953)

Reagents. Tablets containing p-nitrobenzene diazonium p-toluene are used. The tablets also contain sulfosalicylic acid and sodium bicarbonate to provide an acid medium for the reaction and an effervescent mixture that will ensure the solution of a portion of the tablet when water is added. (Ictotest kit, including asbestos-cellulose mats and reagent tablets, is available through Ames Company, Elkhart, Indiana.)

Procedure

1. Place five drops of specimen on an asbestos-cellulose mat provided with the kit. Bilirubin, if present, will be adsorbed onto the mat surface.
2. Place a reagent tablet on the moistened area of the mat.
3. Allow two drops of water to flow over the tablet onto the mat. If bilirubin is present, there will be a coupling of bilirubin with p-nitrobenzene diazonium p-toluene sulfonate from the tablet, as shown by the formation of a blue to purple color within 30 seconds. A pink or red color is negative. The tablet should be moved to reveal the purple color.

The diazo test reacts positively to bilirubin in amounts of 0.05 to 0.1 mg/dl. There is no purple reaction with urobilin or other pigments or with any other known constituent of normal urine. High levels of urobilin or indican will give a red color. Azo compounds cause an atypical color, e.g., Pyridium. Rifampin may interfere. Chlorpromazine metabolites in large amounts produce a purple color. Metabolites of the anti-inflammatory drugs mefenamic and flufenamic acid cause false positive results.

Wash Through Tablet Method (Free, 1978). When false positive reactions are suspected, e.g., with chlorpromazine, the contaminant is diluted out with water in the mat. Prepare duplicate mats with five drops of urine on each. Add ten drops of water to one mat. Place a reagent tablet on each mat and then two drops of water onto each tablet. Bilirubin, if present, is adsorbed into the mat fibers and will appear the same on each mat; an interfering substance produces a light color or no color on the mat with the extra water.

Stability of Reagent. Ictotest[a] reagent tablets are effervescent and somewhat hygroscopic, and, accordingly, they should be protected from moisture or high humidity. The tablets are packed in a brown bottle, since prolonged direct exposure to strong light results in decomposition of the stabilized diazonium compound. Prolonged exposure of several weeks to temperatures of 100°F. or more may also result in deterioration of the tablets. A brown discoloration indicates deterioration, and the tablets should not be used. When each new bottle is opened, tablets should be checked for positive and negative reactions.

---

*L-ascorbic acid, $C_6H_8O_6$, is usually made from dextrose, $C_6H_{12}O_6$ by removing 4 hydrogens. It is a strong reducing agent and is readily converted into dehydroascorbic acid, $C_6H_8O_6$, by oxidizing agents. This is a reversible reaction, allowing oxidation and reduction reactions *in vivo*.

Glucose (and Other Sugars)

Glucose and other reducing substances in urine are detected by a copper reduction test. This non-specific test is useful for semi-quantitation of marked glucosuria when ketone levels are high and for the detection of other sugars early in life. For a discussion of the clinical correlates of glucosuria, see the Clinical Correlations section. Comments on other sugars follow (see Non-Glucose Mellituria).

The glucose oxidase reagent strip test was described earlier.

Copper Reduction Tests. As a screening test, the glucose oxidase test will not detect increased levels of galactose or other sugars in urine. It is therefore important that a copper reduction test be used for young pediatric patients.

Of the copper reduction tests used for screening purposes, the qualitative Benedict test (1909) is more sensitive to reducing substances in urine than the single-tablet copper reduction test (Cook, 1953). Urines containing non-glucose reducing substances may give positive results in healthy persons. Many substances in urine, metabolites, or drug-related metabolites will influence urinary sugar tests (Table 18–8). Strong reducing substances such as ascorbic acid, gentisic acid, or homogentisic acid may inhibit the enzyme test while contributing to the positivity of the copper reduction test. The tablet test is not affected as much as the Benedict test. According to Smith (1977b), very large doses of ascorbic acid do not affect the two-drop copper reduction test. In those instances when the copper test is positive and the glucose oxidase test is negative, glucosuria is ruled out; but before investigating for other sugars the clinical findings and drug history should be evaluated.

Reference Values. Using these tests, the urine of normal children and adults is negative for glucose. Normal neonatal infants during the first 10 to 14 days of life may excrete urine giving a positive reaction due to glucose, galactose, fructose, and lactose (Bickel, 1961). Normal pregnant and postpartum women may give positive reactions to tests for lactose.

Copper Reduction Tablet Test. Clinitest[a] tablets will react with sufficient quantities of any reducing substances in the urine, including reducing sugars such as lactose, fructose, galactose, maltose, and the pentoses.

Both a five-drop and a two-drop Clinitest[a] method have been described (Belmonte, 1967), and corresponding color charts are available for both. The two-drop method was developed in response to a so-called "pass-through" phenomenon, which may occur if more than 2 g/dl of sugar is present in the urine. In the "pass-through" phenomenon, the solution that results after addition of the Clinitest[a] tablet goes through the entire range of colors and back to a dark greenish-brown. This final color does not compare with any section of the color chart; however, it corresponds most closely to a significantly lower result. It is important to observe the entire reaction and for 15 seconds after boiling inside the tube has stopped so that the reversion to a different color is not missed and a falsely low result reported.

Chemistry. Copper sulfate, sodium hydroxide, sodium carbonate, and citric acid are incorporated into a tablet.

3

Table 18–8. REACTIONS OF SUBSTANCES FOUND IN URINE TO TESTS FOR GLUCOSURIA*

Constituent	Glucose Oxidase Reagent Strip	Copper Reduction Tablet Test
Glucose	Positive	Positive
Sugars other than glucose		
Fructose, Galactose, Lactose, Maltose, Pentose	No effect	Positive
Sucrose	No effect	No effect
Ketones (large amounts)	May depress color	No effect
Creatinine, Uric acid	No effect	May cause false positive
Homogentisic acid (alcaptonuria)	No effect	Positive
Drugs†		
Ascorbic acid (large amounts)	May delay color	Trace positive
Cephalosporins (Keflin), etc.	No effect	Positive, brown color
L-Dopa (large)	False negative	No effect
Nalidixic acid glucuronide	No effect	Positive
Probenecid	No effect	Positive
Pyridium	Orange color may affect result	
Salicylate (large)	May lower reading	No effect
X-ray dye (diatrizoates)	No effect	Black color
Contaminants		
Hydrogen peroxide	False positive	May inhibit positive test
Hypochlorite (bleach)	False positive	
Sodium fluoride	False negative	No effect

*Data from Caraway (1962); Wirth (1965); Young (1975).

†Other drugs implicated in copper reduction are amino acids, caronamide, chloral, chloroform, chloramphenicol, formaldehyde, hippuric acid, isoniazid, thiazides, oxytetracycline, p-aminosalicylic acid, penicillin, phenols, streptomycin, phenothiazine, and sulfonamides.

Copper sulfate reacts with reducing substances in the urine, converting cupric sulfate to cuprous oxide. Based on Benedict's copper reduction reaction,

$$Cu^{++} \xrightarrow{\text{hot alkaline solution}} Cu^{+}$$

$$Cu^{+} + OH^{-} \rightarrow CuOH \text{ (yellow)}$$

$$2CuOH \xrightarrow{\text{heat}} Cu_2O \text{ (red)} + H_2O$$

Heat is caused by the reaction of sodium hydroxide with water and citric acid.

Procedure

Five-Drop Method. Place five drops of urine in a dry test tube and add ten drops of water. Add one Clinitest[a] tablet by easing it into the tube without touching it—it contains strong alkali. Watch while boiling takes place, but do not shake or touch the bottom of the tube; it is hot. Wait for 15 seconds after boiling stops, then shake the tube *gently,* and immediately compare the color of the solution with the color scale. Results correspond to the following approximate concentrations: negative; 0.25 g/dl; 0.5 g/dl; 0.75 g/dl; 1.0 g/dl; 2.0 g/dl; pass through. It is important to watch the solution carefully while it is boiling. If at this time the solution passes through orange to a dark shade of greenish brown, it indicates that more than 2 g/dl sugar is present, and this should be recorded as greater than 2 g/dl without reference to the color scale. Urines showing this "pass-through" phenomenon should be retested with the 2-drop method.

Two-Drop Method. Place two drops of urine in a test tube and add ten drops of water. Add one Clinitest[a] tablet. Watch while boiling takes place, but do not shake. Wait 15 seconds after the boiling stops, then shake the tube gently, and compare the color of the solution with the color scale supplied for the two-drop method. The "pass-through" phenomenon may also occur with the two-drop test with large concentrations of sugar, over 5 g/dl. Therefore, it is important to watch the test throughout the entire reaction and waiting period. Report results as negative, trace, 0.5 g/dl, 1 g/dl, 2 g/dl, 3 g/dl, 5 g/dl, and more than 5 g/dl if a "pass-through" reaction occurs.

Clinitest[a] reagent tablets will detect 150 to 250 mg glucose/dl of urine. See Table 18–8 for reactions of sugars and drugs to glucose oxidase and copper reduction.

Precautions. Observe the precautions in the literature supplied with the Clinitest tablets. The bottle must be kept tightly closed at all times to prevent absorption of moisture and kept away from direct heat and sunlight in a cool, dry place. The tablets normally have a spotted bluish white color. If not stored properly they will absorb moisture or deteriorate from heat, turning dark blue or brown. In this condition they will not give reliable results. They are also available individually packaged in aluminum foil to help prevent this absorption of moisture. Although more expensive, such packaging is useful when a limited number of tests are performed.

Sugars

NON-GLUCOSE MELLITURIA

Some hexoses and pentoses cause positive copper reduction tests in urine when the glucose oxidase test is negative. In some rare cases, it is important to identify the sugars so that the patient with persistent mellituria by copper reduction is not mistakenly labeled as diabetic, e.g., in benign essential pentosuria. Fructose, galactose, lactose, maltose, and L-xylulose are found in urine in patients with inherited metabolic disorders (Stanbury, 1983). It should be noted that many drug metabolites, for example in the form of glucuronides, will also give positive copper reduction tests. If an inherited disorder is suspected, the sugar may be identified by thin layer chromatography (Young, 1970). Qualitative confirmatory tests are generally not satisfactory for sugars. The disaccharidase deficiency may be measured on a small intestinal biopsy specimen. Oral tolerance tests and hydrogen breath tests are also used for confirmation. The latter test measures hydrogen gas in expired air 90 minutes after ingestion of the sugar. Bacterial digestion of the excess unabsorbed sugar causes higher than normal hydrogen levels in enzyme deficiencies.

Small amounts of disaccharides are normally excreted in the urine—about 50 mg in 24 hours. With intestinal diseases such as severe sprue or acute enteritis, the level may rise to 250 mg or more. With high levels of sugars in the gut as in lactose intolerance, lactose will be absorbed and excreted unchanged in the urine.

Patients with malabsorption of carbohydrate have symptoms relative to the osmotic activity of the sugars in the gut. Cramping pain and fulness occur shortly after ingestion, and watery diarrhea follows. Bacteria metabolize the carbohydrate to form fatty acids, and the stool pH is lowered to less than 6.

LACTOSE

Lactose may appear in the urine late in normal pregnancy or during lactation.

Intestinal *lactase deficiency* is present in a large number of people, particularly in Africa and Asia. Intolerance increases with age through childhood to adolescence.

In *intestinal disease,* lactase activity may be depressed earlier than the activity of other disaccharidases, e.g., maltase and sucrase. Patients with celiac disease, tropical sprue, and kwashiorkor are most affected.

Lactose intolerance in infancy and failure to gain weight may be associated with lactase deficiency and variable lactosuria. In some cases it can occur as a result of a toxic effect of lactose when lactase is not deficient. In these children there is severe vomiting and diarrhea and high levels of lactose in the urine associated with damage to the intestine. Renal tubular dysfunction and aminoaciduria are present. Milk should be removed from the diet immediately in these infants.

Screening for Lactose. Urine is tested with the glucose oxidase reagent strip and a copper reduction test. A qualitative test may also be used. Thin layer chromatography is used to identify lactose in urine.

Feces from infants and children with sugar intolerances is usually watery; if not, it is suspended in a small amount of water. A Clinitest[a] tablet test for reducing sugar is done using the supernatant of the centrifuged specimen. The watery specimen is smeared onto pH paper and the pH read. With lactose intolerance, reducing sugars may be present and the pH will be low (acid). The same results will be found when there is rapid intestinal transit time associated with infectious or other diarrheas.

Lactase deficiency may be established by means of oral lactose tolerance tests with analysis of blood glucose levels (lactose splits to form glucose and galactose) at half hour intervals. Capillary blood may be used. Normal persons may also give flat blood glucose levels after lactose loading. A lactase enzyme assay of a biopsy of the small intestine will provide a definitive diagnosis.

Lactose Test (Rubner, 1884). To 15 ml urine in a test tube, add 3 g lead acetate. Shake and filter. Boil filtrate, add 2 ml concentrated NH_4OH, and boil. Lactose will cause the formation of a brick red solution and then a red precipitate with clear supernatant. Glucose will cause a yellow solution and yellow precipitate.

FRUCTOSE

Fructose appears in urine during parenteral feedings with fructose and in association with inherited enzyme deficiencies that cause benign essential fructosuria and serious fructose intolerance associated with severe vomiting and liver and kidney disease. (See Table 18–25.) Fructose is identified by thin layer chromatography. A qualitative test, a resorcinol test, is found to be useful by some.

Note. Fructose will form from glucose in alkaline urine, so the specimen should be fresh when testing for fructose.

Quantitative Test. Glucose is removed with glucose oxidase, and a method for inulin (a polyfructose) is used (e.g., Froesch, 1957—a resorcinol method).

Reference Value. Fructose—about 60 mg/24 hours in urine.

Resorcinol Test (Seliwanoff, 1887). Boil 5 ml urine with 5 ml of 25 per cent HCl. Add about 5 mg resorcinol and boil for ten seconds. Fructose will cause the formation of a heavy red precipitate. Separate the precipitate by filtration and dissolve it in ethanol. The precipitate should form a red solution in ethanol for the test to be positive. The fructose is converted to hydroxymethyl furfural; this condenses with resorcinol to form a red color. Use a positive control. Sensitivity is about 100 m/dl urine.

GALACTOSE

Galactose appears in urine due to inherited enzyme deficiencies (see Table 18–25). In these diseases, galactose derived from dietary lactose is not converted to glucose. Galactose in urine causes a positive copper reduction test and may be identified by thin layer chromatography. However, the disease is usually identified by red cell enzyme assay when suspected. (See Urinary Screening for Metabolic Inherited Diseases.)

PENTOSE

Pentosuria may follow the ingestion of large amounts of fruits, causing the excretion of L-xylose and L-arabinose in amounts up to 0.1 g/day. L-Xylulose is excreted in benign essential pentosuria in amounts of 1 to 4 g/day. At concentrations of 250 to 300 mg/dl, L-xylulose will reduce Benedict's qualitative reagent at 50°C. (water bath) within ten minutes or at room temperature in several hours. Fructose will also reduce Benedict's reagent at low temperatures. (See Henry, 1979.) The pentoses are identified by thin layer chromatography.

SUCROSE

Sucrose may appear in the urine after the ingestion of very large amounts of sucrose. Sucrase deficiency is associated with intestinal diseases such as sprue in the same manner as lactase deficiency. Sucrose intolerance is an inherited disorder associated with sucrase and alpha dextrinase (isomaltase) deficiencies. Symptoms are similar to those seen with lactase deficiency and occur in the first few weeks of life when sweetened food is ingested. Tolerance may develop, but sucrose may have to be avoided permanently.

Factitious sucrosuria may create a high specific gravity urine with negative glucose oxidase and negative copper reduction tests. Sucrose will ferment yeast and can be separated by chromatography but needs to be stained with a substance not dependent on reducing properties. See Table 18–9 for sugars and yeast fermentation.

Hemoglobin, Myoglobin, Hemosiderin

The tetramethylbenzidine tests are sensitive to a hemoglobin level of about 0.0003 mg/ml, equivalent to 10,000 red cells/ml or 10/μl. In this test, hemoglobin and other iron porphyrin derivatives, including myoglobin, catalyze the oxidation of tetramethylbenzidine or other colorless dye to a colored product by oxygen release from hydrogen peroxide. (See Reagent Strip Methodology, earlier.) Consult the Clinical Correlations section for causes of hemoglobinuria and myoglobinuria.

HEMATURIA AND HEMOGLOBINURIA

In order to distinguish hematuria from hemoglobinuria, sediment from a fresh urine specimen should be examined microscopically for red blood cells. A markedly hypotonic urine may cause lysis of erythrocytes, and, therefore, the specific gravity of the specimen should also be checked. Microscopic examination is essential to diagnose hematuria; the reagent strip test is likely to be negative in the presence of the ubiquitous ascorbic acid even when hematuria is marked. With low specific gravity and lysis of red cells, ghost forms are easily detected with phase microscopy.

Red blood cell casts and blood pigment casts are seen when there is hematuria associated with glomer-

Table 18–9. QUALITATIVE TESTS FOR SUGARS

Sugar	Copper Reduction	Yeast* Fermentation	Qualitative Tests
Fructose	+	+	Resorcinol, Seliwanoff
Galactose	+	±	
Lactose	+	±	Rubner's lead acetate
Maltose	+	+	
Pentose	+	0	Benedict's at 50°C.†
Sucrose	0	+	

*See Davidsohn (1974) for method.
†See Henry (1979) for method.

3

Table 18–10. DIFFERENTIATION OF HEMOGLOBINURIA, MYOGLOBINURIA, AND HEMATURIA

Condition	Blood Plasma Findings	Urine Findings
Hemoglobinuria	Color—pink (early) Haptoglobin—low	Color—pink, red, brown Red blood cells—occasional Pigment casts—occasional Protein—present or absent Hemosiderin—late
Myoglobinuria	Color—clear Haptoglobin—normal CK*—marked increase Aldolase—increased	Color—red, brown Red blood cells—occasional Dense brown casts—occasional Protein—present or absent
Hematuria	Color—clear	Color—normal, smoky, pink, red, brown Red blood cells—many Renal—red blood cell casts Protein—marked increase Lower urinary tract—no casts Protein—present or absent

*Creatinine phosphokinase.

ular disease. Hemosiderin is found in urine two to three days after an acute hemolytic episode associated with hemoglobinuria, but it is not seen with hematuria. See Table 18–10; refer to Table 18–13.

HEMOGLOBIN AND MYOGLOBIN

The distinction between hemoglobinuria and myoglobinuria is difficult to make on examination of the urine. In both cases, the urine is dark red or brown and some red cells are seen in the sediment. Pigment casts may be found; these may be dark brown with myoglobin. See Table 18–10, comparing hemoglobinuria, myoglobinuria, and hematuria.

The reagent strip test for blood is positive with hemoglobin and myoglobin. If serum can be examined, it will often be pink with hemoglobinemia but a normal color with myoglobinemia because this pigment is cleared so rapidly. None of the qualitative tests have been satisfactory in separating myoglobin and hemoglobin, and both may be present following crush injuries. The salt precipitation method of Blondheim has been used, as have spectroscopic methods. According to Boesken (1979), hemoglobin and some myoglobin are bound to proteins in urine, and this contributes to the difficulty of separating them by salt precipitation or acetate electrophoresis.

Immunochemical tests with antisera to human myoglobin require a human myoglobin standard from muscle or from urine containing myoglobin and an antiserum that does not cross-react with hemoglobin (Kagen, 1967; Markowitz, 1977). The myoglobin antigen is not very stable (Boesken, 1979), but these tests are specific and are preferred. End point and rate nephelometric methods are available.

Qualitative Test for Myoglobin (Blondheim, 1958)

1. Use a fresh urine specimen. Observe the color of urine. Characteristically, urine with myoglobinuria is red when fresh and turns brown on standing, but some myoglobin may be present without color change. Myoglobin is less stable at an acid pH. Neutralize and refrigerate pending testing.

2. Mix 1 ml of urine and 3 ml of 3 per cent sulfosalicylic acid to test for protein. If the pigment is precipitated, it is a protein. Filter. If the filtrate is a normal color, no abnormal non-protein pigment is present. (*Note:* The heat and acetic acid test does not precipitate myoglobin or hemoglobin.)

3. To 5 ml of urine in a test tube, add 2.8 g of ammonium sulfate. Dissolve by mixing. The urine is now 80 per cent saturated with ammonium sulfate. This is optimal for precipitation of hemoglobin. Filter or centrifuge. If the supernatant shows a normal color, the precipitated pigment is hemoglobin. If the supernatant fluid is colored, this is presumptive evidence of myoglobin.

Note that with muscle injury, both pigments may be present. See Table 18–14 for causes of myoglobinuria.

HEMOSIDERIN

Hemosiderin appears in the urine sediment in diseases involving a true siderosis of kidney parenchyma (hemochromatosis). It is also present two to three days after an acute hemolytic episode that caused hemoglobinuria. At this time the reagent strip test for hemoglobin is often negative. Hemosiderin is found as yellow-brown granules that are free or in epithelial cells and occasionally in casts (Fig. 18–1). The Prussian blue reaction is used to demonstrate iron in hemosiderin (Fig. 18–2). A wet preparation (Rous) and a dry smear (Cartwright) are alternative methods.

Wet Procedure (Rous, 1918)

1. Centrifuge a complete morning specimen or random urine samples at 450 G for five minutes and pool the sediment. Examine several drops of sediment microscopically, searching for coarse yellow-brown granules, especially within renal tubular epithelial cells or casts.

2. If such granules are seen, suspend the rest of the sediment in a fresh mixture of 5 ml of 2 per cent potassium ferrocyanide solution and 5 ml of 1 per cent HCl and allow to stand for ten minutes.

3. Centrifuge, and discard the supernatant. Examine the sediment microscopically. Coarse granules of hemosiderin appear blue in this preparation (Fig. 18–2) in cells, casts, and amorphous material. If granules do not stain, re-examine after 30 minutes (occasionally the reaction is delayed).

Dry Procedure (Cartwright, 1968). When stained, hemosiderin appears as blue granules, 1 to 3 μ singly or in groups, in renal tubular epithelial cells, as amorphous sediment, or as blue granules in casts. An iron stain used for siderocytes in blood or bone marrow is also suitable. Urine is collected in an iron-free glass container, overnight. Let stand for two hours. Decant three fourths of it. Centrifuge the remainder. Make a smear(s) of the sediment. Air dry.

Reagents. The Prussian blue reagent is made fresh.

1. Potassium ferrocyanide, 20 per cent in demineralized water. Store in a dark bottle (iron free) at room temperature. Stable for three weeks.
2. Concentrated HCl.
3. *Prussian blue stain:* Add concentrated HCl to an aliquot of the potassium ferrocyanide solution until a white precipitate forms which remains stable on shaking. Filter through Watman No. 5 filter paper.
4. Safranin O, 0.5 g in 100 ml distilled water. Stable stock solution.
5. Phosphate buffer pH 6.4 to 6.7 for counterstain.
6. Working counterstain. Dilute 1 ml safranin O stain to 50 ml with phosphate buffer.

Procedure

1. Fix the smear in methyl alcohol for ten minutes.
2. Rinse with iron-free water (demineralized) and air dry.
3. Stain with Prussian blue reagent for 30 minutes.
4. Wash gently for at least four minutes with iron-free water and air dry.
5. Counterstain with Safranin O for one to five minutes.
6. Rinse with iron-free water. Air dry.
7. Mount a coverslip using a drop of immersion oil.

Note: All glassware, slides, coverslips, etc., should be iron free. Water should be demineralized.

Ketones

Methods for Testing Ketonuria. The Gerhardt *ferric chloride* test has been used for many years as a test for acetoacetic acid (see ferric chloride test for salicylates). However, ferric chloride tests are not very specific and the sensitivity is low—about 25 to 50 mg/dl. The ferric chloride test gives positive results with salicylate and L-dopa.

Acetone and acetoacetic acid react with sodium nitroprusside (nitroferricyanide) in the presence of alkali to produce a purple-colored complex. This reaction was described by Legal (1883) in diabetic urines. In the simplest form of the nitroprusside test, reagent strips impregnated with sodium nitroprusside and alkali are used (see earlier). A tablet form of the test is available with similar sensitivity. A reagent strip without alkali reacts to acetoacetic acid and not to acetone. The *blood* level of ketone bodies may be estimated by the nitroprusside test at the bedside. This is especially helpful in determining the severity of ketosis in the treatment of diabetic acidosis, provided that the reagents are fresh. (See Clinical Correlates for causes of ketonuria.)

Stability of Ketones. In urine, bacterial action will cause loss of acetoacetic acid. This may happen *in vivo* as well as *in vitro.* Acetone is lost at room temperature but not if kept in a closed container in a refrigerator. If a sample cannot be tested immediately, it should be refrigerated.

Reference Values. Depending on the methods used, total ketone bodies (as acetone) range from 17 to 42 mg/dl (Henry, 1964). According to Killander (1962), up to 2 mg acetoacetic acid/dl is normal.

Nitroprusside Tablet Test. A tablet test method may be useful if the urine has an interfering color. The tablets are very sensitive to humidity and will deteriorate if not stored properly. The Acetest[a] tablet contains sodium nitroprusside (nitroferricyanide), glycine, and a strongly alkaline buffer. It can be used to test whole blood, plasma, serum, or urine.

Procedure. Place the tablet on a clean surface, preferably a piece of white paper. Place one drop of urine, serum, plasma, or whole blood on the tablet. For *urine* testing, compare the color of the tablet to a color chart at 30 seconds after application of the specimen. For *serum* or *plasma* testing, compare color of tablet to color chart at two minutes after application of specimen. For *whole blood* testing, ten minutes after application of the specimen remove clotted blood from tablet and compare color of tablet to color chart.

If acetone and acetoacetic acid are present, the tablet will show a color varying from lavender to deep purple. Report the results as negative, small, moderate, or large. If large, a dilution may be made. Report these analyses in a form such as this: undiluted "large," 1:2 dilution "large," 1:4 dilution "moderate," etc.

Acetest[a] will detect 5 to 10 mg of acetoacetic acid/dl of urine and 20 to 25 mg acetone/dl of urine. Like the reagent strips, it does not react with 3 hydroxybutyrate. It will give positive results with L-dopa and large amounts of phenylketones and with BSP and PSP dyes which react with the alkali in the tablets.

Rothera's Test—Urine. See Henry (1979). The test tube nitroprusside test of Rothera (1908) is sensitive to acetoacetic acid, about 1 to 5 mg/dl, and acetone with a sensitivity of 10 to 25 mg/dl.

Protein

Measurement of Proteinuria. Qualitative, semiquantitative, and quantitative methods are available for analysis of protein in urine. Since the positive result of a screening test may have grave significance, it is important to be able to confirm it by a second, different method. See Clinical Correlations for causes of proteinuria.

A comparison of reagent strips and the sulfosalicylic acid method shows that with reagent strips accurate results are obtained only when albumin is measured. Changes in urinary solute concentration affect the reagent strip results but not the sulfosalicylic acid method. High salt levels lower the reagent strip result (Gyure, 1977).

Although not as sensitive as precipitation tests, the reagent strip has the advantage of avoiding false positive reactions with organic iodides, such as those used for x-ray contrast and tolbutamides or other drugs (Table 18–11).

Most other qualitative screening tests rely on a protein precipitation, e.g., with heat and acetic acid, with nitric acid, and with sulfosalicylic (SSA) and trichloroacetic acids. These methods will also precipitate globulins as well as albumin. In practice, negative reagent strips with positive SSA tests in urine specimens are attributable to x-ray dye, to penicillins, and rarely to globulins. Sulfosalicylic and trichloroacetic acids are used to precipitate protein in the cold and are used as convenient screening tests. The sensitivity may be as low as 0.25 mg/dl, depending on the techniques used.

Because of a lack of sensitivity of the reagent strip to globulins, it may be necessary to use an acid precipitation test for screening purposes. This will depend on the patient population and the diseases being screened.

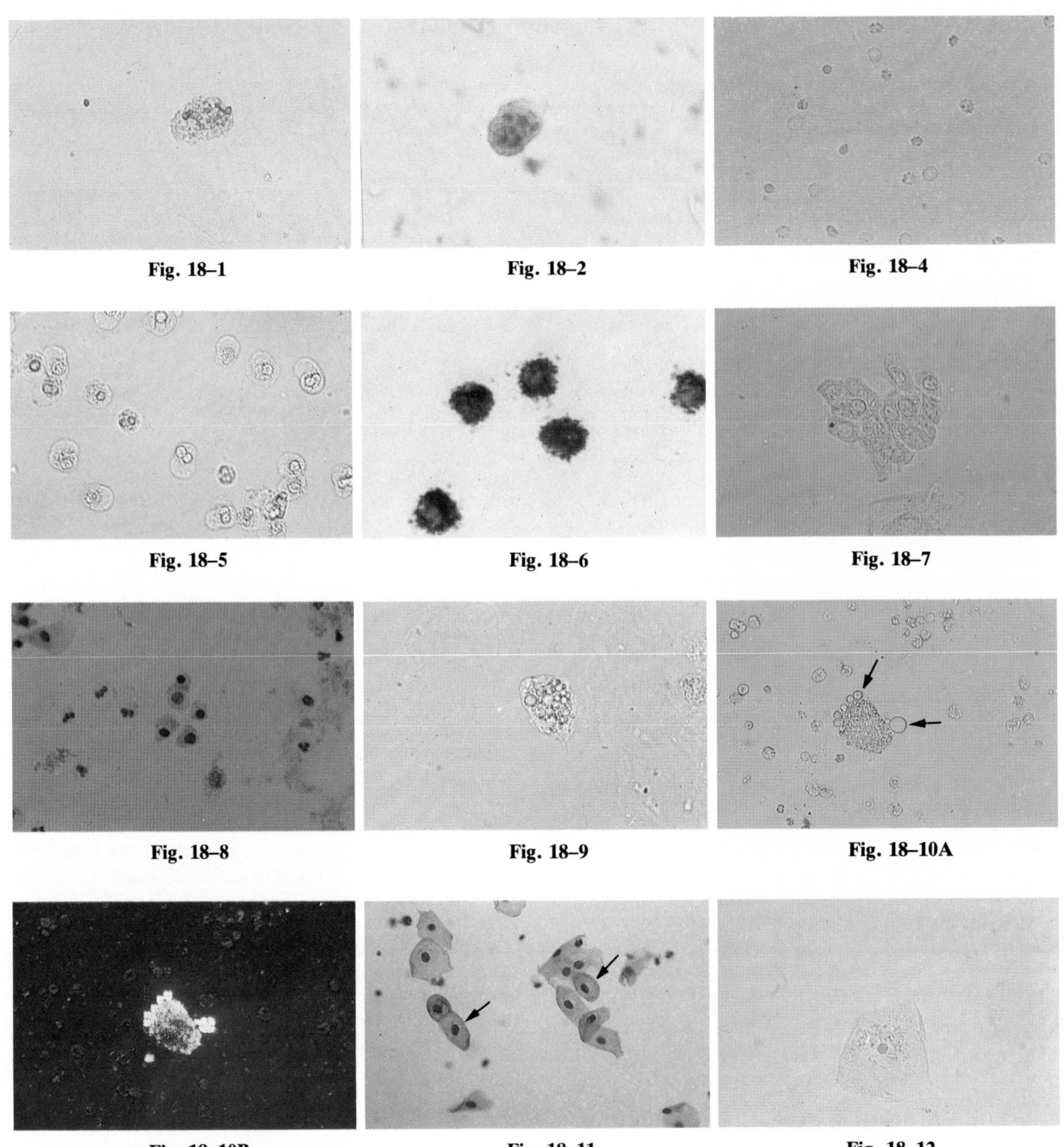

Figure 18–1. Renal tubular epithelial cell containing brown pigment; iron, unstained (×260).

Figure 18–2. Renal tubular epithelial cell positive with Prussian blue stain (hemosiderinuria) (×260).

Figure 18–4. Red cells, some crenated (×160).

Figure 18–5. Neutrophils with dilute acetic acid (×200).

Figure 18–6. Neutrophils, peroxidase positive (×500).

Figure 18–7. Renal tubular epithelial cells (×200).

Figure 18–8. Renal tubular epithelial cells and neutrophils. Papanicolaou stain (×430).

Figure 18–9. Oval fat body (×160).

Figure 18–10. Oval fat body with attached fat droplets (×160): A, brightfield and, B, polarized (×160).

Figure 18–11. Transitional epithelial cells. Papanicolaou stain (×430).

Figure 18–12. Squamous epithelial cell, Pyridium stained (×200).

Table 18–11. FALSE POSITIVE AND FALSE NEGATIVE REACTIONS IN TESTS FOR PROTEINURIA

Urinary Constituents	Reagent Strip	Acid Precipitation*
Radiographic contrast media (diatrizoate)	No effect	May cause false positive
Tolbutamide metabolites	No effect	May cause false positive
Penicillins (massive doses)	No effect	May cause false positive
Sulfisoxazole metabolites (sulfonamide)	No effect	May cause false positive
Tolmetin (Tolectin) (anti-inflammatory)	No effect	May cause false positive
Highly buffered alkaline urine	May cause false positive	May cause false negative
Quaternary ammonium compounds (alters pH)	May cause false positive	No effect
Bilirubin (large amounts) and other strong colors	Interferes with color	No effect

*Drugs in high dosage that are precipitated at an acid pH may cause turbidity.

Sulfosalicylic Acid Method—Qualitative. Different concentrations and proportions of sulfosalicylic acid have been used in the qualitative test and provide different ranges of results.

Specimens should be centrifuged, and a clear supernatant used.

Procedure. To approximately 3 ml of supernatant urine aliquot (about one inch) in a 16 by 125 mm test tube, add an equal amount of 3 per cent sulfosalicylic acid (SSA). Invert to mix. Let stand exactly ten minutes. Invert again twice. Using ordinary room light (not a lamp), observe the degree of precipitation and grade the results according to the following descriptions:

Negative—no turbidity, or no increase in turbidity (approximately 0.005 g/dl or less.*

Trace—perceptible turbidity (approximately 0.020 g/dl).

1^+—Distinct turbidity, but no discrete granulation (approximately 0.050 g/dl).

2^+—Turbidity with granulation, but no flocculation (approximately 0.20 g/dl).

3^+—Turbidity with granulation and flocculation (approximately 0.5 g/dl).

4^+—Clumps of precipitated protein, or solid precipitate (approximately 1.0 g/dl or more).

The method will detect about 5 to 10 mg/dl. Albumin, globulins, glycoproteins, and Bence Jones proteins are detected. High levels of detergents may decrease the result.

When *radiographic dye* is present, the specific gravity of the urine is usually >1.035 and the SSA precipitate will increase on standing. Typical crystals are seen on microscopic examination of the precipitate; a protein precipitate is amorphous. Another urine specimen from the patient should be tested. However, the effects of the radiographic media may persist up to three days. A reagent strip test may be substituted or the heat and acetic acid test used. In the acetic acid test, radiographic contrast media will clear with heat, whereas protein will increase.

Sulfosalicylic Acid Tablet Test Reagent (Bumintest[a]). The tablets contain sulfosalicylic acid and sodium bicarbonate. These are dissolved in deionized water to make a 5 per cent stable solution.

Semiquantitative and Quantitative Methods. More useful information for diagnosis of kidney disease and for following response to treatment is obtained by quantitatively analyzing the amount of protein excreted over a 24-hour period. See Clinical Correlation section for a description of patterns and degrees of proteinuria.

In 1874 Esbach developed a method of urinary protein precipitation in which picric acid was used and by which the amount of precipitated protein could be estimated by volume. The Esbach method, even with modifications, is much less precise and accurate than the turbidimetric methods (Lewis, 1961).

Sulfosalicylic acid (SSA) and trichloroacetic acid (TCA) are commonly used as precipitants; the resultant turbidity is measured by a photometer or nephelometer, or by eye, and compared with known standards. With sulfosalicylic acid, the turbidity produced with albumin is 2.4 times that produced with globulin (Henry, 1956). Polypeptides, glycoproteins, and Bence Jones proteins are also precipitated. Exton's reagent (1925) contains sulfosalicylic acid, sodium sulfate, and an indicator—bromphenol blue. Trichloroacetic acid is a protein precipitant that causes gamma globulin to be precipitated with greater turbidity than albumin. However, the difference is not marked (Henry, 1956). More precise measurements especially suitable for smaller amounts of protein are available. In these tests, a trichloroacetic acid precipitate is dissolved in sodium hydroxide and measured by use of the biuret reaction (Kibrick, 1958). The biuret test as used for serum proteins is not sensitive enough to be used as a test for proteinuria. A modification of the biuret method, the Tsuchyga/biuret method, using a phosphotungstic acid, gives better results. For a comparison of biuret methods with the SSA turbidity test, see Lizana (1977). For comparisons with the dye-binding methods, Coomassie Blue, Ponceau-S, and benzethonium turbidity, see McElderry (1982).

Very small amounts of proteins, such as albumin and β_2 microglobulin, are measured by immunologic means using antibodies to the proteins and nephelometric methods, or radioimmunoassay.

Automated methods for total urine protein include automation of biuret techniques. An automated turbidometric method using benzethonium chloride in an alkaline medium is available (Dupont-ACA).

Methods used to quantitate urinary protein have not been satisfactory. Participants in the College of American Pathologists (CAP) proficiency testing surveys will be aware that test results show that the mean values reported vary two-fold between methods, with the SSA method producing high values. Precision is poor, with the SSA turbidometric method showing the poorest coefficient of variation. The TCA-biuret, Coomassie blue, and trichloroacetic acid turbidity tests show closer agreement and about half the coefficient of variation of the SSA method. Problems arise from non-standardized methods. With turbidity tests, these include different acid concentrations and timing, and variation in the protein standard. There is also variability in the proteins excreted and a primary standard representing this variable mixture of proteins is not possible.

The quantititative TCA/biuret method given below is tedious but gives good precision. A color correction blank

*These values were quantitated by TCA (trichloracetic acid) biuret method with bovine albumin standard solutions.

3

is used. Bovine albumion assayed by Kjeldahl technique is used as the protein standard.

Sulfosalicylic Acid Turbidity Method—Semi-quantitative

Principle. Sulfosalicylic acid precipitates protein in urine with a turbidity that is *approximately* proportional to the concentration of protein in a solution. The turbidity may be measured with a photometer. (See Henry, 1979.)

TCA/Biuret Method—Quantitative

Principle. Protein in urine is precipitated with trichloroacetic acid, redissolved in alkali and measured colorimetrically, using biuret reagent. The color intensity is directly proportional to the number of peptide bonds.

Reagents

1. 100 per cent trichloroacetic acid (w/v). Keep refrigerated. To make 20 per cent trichloroacetic acid, dilute 20 ml of 100 per cent TCA to 100 ml with deionized water. Stable for two days.
2. 0.2 N sodium hydroxide.
3. (a) *Alkaline copper reagent (biuret reagent):*

9.0 g sodium potassium tartrate (Rochelle Salt, $NaKC_4H_4O_6 \cdot 4H_2O$)
3.0 g $CuSO_4 \cdot 5H_2O$
5.0 g KI
0.2 N NaOH (carbonate-free)

Dissolve the Rochelle salt in approximately 400 ml 0.2 N NaOH. Add the copper sulfate and dissolve it. Dilute the solution to 1000 ml with 0.2 N NaOH. Store the solution in a paraffin lined or polyethylene bottle.

(b) *Alternate method for the preparation of the alkaline copper reagent using purchased stock biuret:*

1000 ml biuret reagent (Weichselbaum)
4000 ml blank reagent

Blank reagent: 1600 ml 0.5 N NaOH and 20 g KI. Dilute to 4 L with deionized water. Stable for six months.

4. Albumin solutions: (a) *Stock bovine albumin solution.* Approximately 30 g/dl, available from Metrix, Clinical and Diagnostics Division, Armour Pharmaceutical Company, Chicago, Illinois 60690. The value will differ with each lot number. (b) *Intermediate solution.* 6 g/dl (approximate concentration in 0.9 per cent NaCl. Make 25 ml of a 1:5 dilution of stock bovine albumin solution (a) in 0.9 per cent NaCl. Refrigerate. Stable for six months. The *exact concentration* is measured by the total serum protein biuret method, a procedure standardized by the Kjeldahl N method. The standard is Bovine Albumin Monomer, Standard Protein Solution (Miles Laboratories, Inc., Research Products, Elkhart, Indiana 46514). (c) *Working solution* (make 100 ml of working solution): 1:25 dilution of intermediate solution in 0.9 per cent NaCl. Use at room temperature. The exact concentration of the working solution is calculated using the measured concentration of the intermediate solution. Each new working solution should be checked before it is used. Stable for one month.
5. Control. Use 4 ml of 1:100 dilution of a serum protein control in 0.9 per cent saline. Run in duplicate.

Procedure

1. Measure and record the volume of the 24-hour collection of urine.
2. Perform an acid precipitation test with SSA or TCA for protein on centrifuged urine supernatant. If the qualitative SSA test is:

negative	report as negative.
trace	use 8 ml for precipitation in step 3.
low 1^+	use 8 ml for precipitation in step 3.
1^+	use 4 ml for precipitation in step 3.
2^+	use 2 ml for precipitation in step 3.
low 3^+	use 0.5 ml for precipitation in step 3.

Note: If the 3+ is a high 3+, 0.5 ml of a *1:2* dilution should be done. 0.5 ml of a *1:2* dilution, and 0.5 ml of a *1:5* dilution should also be run on every 4+. Be sure to make immediate note of any of these dilutions or changes.

3. Pipette centrifuged urine, standard bovine albumin working solution, and duplicate controls into *glass* centrifuge tubes. Perform duplicate determinations on selected urine specimens for quality control. Use 1, 2, 3, and 4 ml of standard and 4 ml of control. If a color correction is known to be needed (see step 7), set up a duplicate aliquot at this point.
4. Bring volume in each tube to 4 ml with water unless 8 ml specimen is indicated.
5. Add 1 ml of 20 per cent TCA to each tube (or add 2 ml of 20 per cent TCA to 8 ml of urine). Mix well, using Vortex mixer or by tapping tubes. Do not parafilm. Allow proteins to precipitate for 30 minutes.
6. Centrifuge for ten minutes at 1600 RPM (500 ×G). Use a centrifuge in which the tubes swing into a horizontal position during centrifugation rather than an angle head centrifuge so that the precipitate will be packed in the bottom of the tube. Pour off the supernatant fluid and drain the precipitate by inverting over filter paper for five minutes.
7. Add 5 ml of 0.2 N NaOH to each tube. (If the solution of protein in 0.2 N NaOH is significantly colored, carry a second aliquot of the urine specimen through to this point.) Dissolve the protein precipitate completely by mixing carefully with Vortex mixer or with glass stirring rods before placing in a boiling water bath. Aid solution of protein by placing the tubes in boiling water for one minute. Allow to return to room temperature. Do not use a cold water bath to cool.
8. Add 5 ml of biuret reagent to all the tubes except the color correction tubes. Add 5 ml (more) of 0.2 N NaOH instead of the biuret reagent to the color correction tubes. Mix well with Vortex mixer or stirring rods and transfer the solution to colorimeter tubes if flow-through cuvette is not available.
9. Prepare a blank of 5 ml of 0.2 N NaOH and 5 ml of biuret reagent. Also prepare a color correction blank by pipetting 10 ml of 0.2 N NaOH in a tube.
10. Incubate all tubes in a 30 to 32°C. water bath for 30 minutes. Read per cent T at 550 nm in a Coleman Junior II Spectrophotometer. Use the flow-through cuvette, setting 100 per cent T with water. (If drifting occurs, replace the flow-through cuvette with another acid-cleaned cuvette.) Read all tubes, including reagent blank, against the water. Recheck the center setting after reading the reagent blank. Read any color correction tubes against the NaOH blank. For each specimen requiring color correction, subtract the *absorbance* of the color correction tube from the *absorbance* of the tube to which biuret reagent was added before calculating the protein concentration of the urine.
11. Plot per cent T of standards against their respective concentrations. Use the reagent blank reading for zero concentration on the graph. (The standard line will not go through 100 per cent T.) Relate per cent T of specimens to protein concentration. Apply appropriate dilution factor and report as grams per liter and grams per 24 hours.

Calculations

$$\text{mg per colorimeter tube determined from standard graph} \times \frac{\text{total volume of specimen}}{\text{ml urine used in step 3}} \times \frac{1\text{ g}}{1000\text{ mg}} = \text{g/24 hours}$$

AND

mg per colorimeter tube ×

$$\frac{1000 \text{ ml}}{\text{ml urine used in step 3}} \times \frac{1 \text{ g}}{1000 \text{ mg}} = \text{g/L}$$

Results may be reported as protein per liter or per day. Report results to the nearest 0.1 g.

Normal Value in Urine. 100 to 150 mg/24 hours. Of this, about one third of the protein is plasma albumin, while one fourth represents mucoprotein (Tamm-Horsfall) and the remainder plasma globulins. In a random specimen, this corresponds to 2 to 8 mg/dl at normal flow rate.

Comments

1. Protein excretion rate may be corrected for the patient's deviation from average adult body surface area (1.73 m^2) by:

$$\text{g/24 hours} \times \frac{1.73 \text{ m}^2}{\text{patient's surface area in m}^2}$$

The surface area can be determined from the height and weight of the patient either from the formula of DuBois and DuBois or from a table prepared from this formula.

2. Interfering substances: Drugs may cause precipitates that do not dissolve in NaOH; unusual colors may form with the biuret reagent, depending on therapy. In these instances, the specimen is unsatisfactory for determination.

Bence Jones Proteinuria (Bence Jones, 1848). The presence of Bence Jones globulin is indicated by a single sharp peak in the globulin region on protein electrophoresis. Bence Jones globulin represents either the kappa or lambda immunoglobulin light chain. See Clinical Correlation section for further details.

Measurement of Bence Jones Protein. Globulins are not sensitive to the reagent strip test for protein, which screens predominantly for albumin (Bowie, 1977). Many techniques have been proposed, most of them based on the unusual heat solubility properties of Bence Jones protein. This protein precipitates at temperatures between 40 and 60°C. and redissolves near 100°C. Other tests depend on precipitation in the cold with salts, ammonium sulfate, and acids.

In the presence of *marked* Bence Jones proteinuria, most tests yield positive results. When only a small amount of Bence Jones protein is present, or when other globulins are present, results may be doubtful. With proper pH control and salt concentration, precipitation may be achieved at levels of about 30 mg/dl (Putnam, 1959). False positive reactions are seen when other globulins are precipitated by acetic acid in the heat precipitation method. A false negative reaction may occur if the Bence Jones protein is too concentrated and the precipitate does not redissolve on boiling.

The best method for detection of Bence Jones protein in urine is by protein electrophoresis, when a homogeneous band in the globulin region will be seen. This is followed by immunoelectrophoresis to identify the light chain. For electrophoretic analysis, urine must be concentrated.

Bence Jones Protein—Thermal Method. The qualitative sulfosalicylic acid test for urine protein is performed first; it is negative if no detectable Bence Jones protein is present.

Reagent. Acetate buffer, pH 4.9, 2M. Place 17.5 g sodium acetate trihydrate in a 100 ml volumetric flask, add 4.1 ml glacial acetic acid, and add water to 100 ml.

Procedure

1. Place 4 ml clear urine in a test tube (centrifuge or filter urine if turbid). Add 1 ml acetate buffer and mix. Final pH should be 4.9 ± 0.1.
2. Heat for 15 minutes in a 56°C. water bath. Any precipitation is indicative of Bence Jones protein.
3. If there is a turbidity or precipitate, heat the same tube in a boiling water bath for three minutes and observe for any *decrease* in the amount of precipitate or turbidity. Bence Jones protein will redissolve at 100°C.
4. An increase in turbidity or precipitate on boiling indicates the presence of albumin and globulin. This will mask any dissolving Bence Jones protein. Filter the contents of the tube taken directly from the boiling water and observe the filtrate. If it is clear, becomes cloudy as it cools, and then becomes clear again at room temperature, the test is positive for Bence Jones protein.

Comment. A heavy precipitate of Bence Jones protein at 56°C. may not redissolve on boiling; the test should be repeated with diluted urine. The urine specimen should be fresh or refrigerated, since heat-coagulable protein will denature or decompose if the urine is left at room temperature and give false positive reactions.

Urobilinogen and Porphobilinogen

Urobilinogen. The qualitative test for urobilinogen and porphobilinogen may be performed as a confirmatory test when there is more than one Ehrlich unit shown on the reagent strip test. The Watson-Schwartz test is used to separate causes of a positive Ehrlich reacting strip test and to give an indication of large amounts of urobilinogen or the presence of porphobilinogen. Quantitative tests for urobilinogen in urine are seldom performed. Consult Henry (1979) for two hour quantitative urobilinogen method and Davidsohn (1974) or Schwartz (1944) for 24-hour quantitation.

Normal adult urine contains from about 0.5 to 2.5 mg of urobilinogen in a 24-hour collection; less than one Ehrlich unit in two hours is excreted as measured by a semiquantitative method (Balikov, 1957). See Clinical Correlations for causes of increased urobilinogen in urine, and also see Table 18–12.

Porphobilinogen. The Ames urobilinogen reagent strip is useful for detecting the occasional patient with porphobilinogen in urine. The Chemstrip[c] product for urobilinogen does not detect porphobilinogen. A positive result for porphobilinogen in the Watson-Schwartz test is confirmed by the Hoesch test since the Watson-Schwartz test may show false positive tests for porphobilinogen due to drugs such as methyldopa. Very large amounts are needed to cause false positive results in the Hoesch test. When a qualitative porphobilinogen test is requested or a known porphyric patient is being followed, the simpler Hoesch test is used instead of the Watson-Schwartz test. See Porphyrins in a separate section.

The *urine specimen* for urobilinogen or porphobilinogen must be fresh. If the test cannot be performed at once, the pH should be adjusted to near neutral (pH 7) and stored in a refrigerator where it is stable for about one week (With, 1980). Urine may darken if the patient has porphyria, especially if left at room temperature.

Qualitative Ehrlich's Aldehyde Reaction or Watson-Schwartz Test (Watson, 1941). Methods for measuring urobilinogen and porphobilinogen in urine measure the total chromogens in the urine. Ehrlich's reagent, ρ-dimethyl amino benzaldehyde in concentrated hydrochloric acid, reacts with urobilinogen and porphobilinogen to form a colored aldehyde. The addition of sodium acetate intensifies the red color of the aldehyde and inhibits color formation by skatoles and indoles. Extractions of the colored complex using butanol and chloroform are employed to separate urobilinogen and porphobilinogen from other Ehrlich's-reactive compounds.

Reagents

1. Ehrlich's reagent: Combine 0.7 g ρ-dimethyl amino benzaldehyde, 150 ml concentrated hydrochloric acid, and 100 ml deionized water. Store in brown bottle. Stable for three to six months.
2. Saturated sodium acetate in deionized water.
3. Chloroform.
4. Butanol.

Procedure

1. To one volume (approximately 3 ml) of urine in a test tube, add an equal volume of Ehrlich's reagent. Mix well by inversion.
2. Immediately add two volumes of saturated sodium acetate and mix well by inversion. (When Ehrlich's reagent is added directly to urine, the color produced increases with time owing to slower reacting *non-urobilinogen* substances. The addition of saturated sodium acetate stops these slower reactions.) The color of a positive reaction ranges from a definite light pink to a deep cherry red. Pale peach and light orange colors are often seen, but these are *not* positive reactions. If the test is positive at this stage, split the colored solution into two parts and continue with the next two steps.
3. Add a few milliliters of chloroform to one portion of the colored solution and shake vigorously. Allow layers to separate. Observe whether or not the color is completely extracted into the *lower* chloroform layer. Extract more than once if necessary. Color due to urobilinogen will be extracted into chloroform; that due to porphobilinogen and other Ehrlich's reactive compounds will stay in the aqueous solution on top.
4. If the pink color is not extracted by the chloroform, add a few milliliters of butanol to the other portion of the colored solution. Shake vigorously, then allow layers to separate. Observe whether or not the color is completely extracted into the *upper* butanol layer. If color still remains in the urine-acetate layer, re-extract with more butanol. Color due to urobilinogen will be extracted into the butanol. Color due to other Ehrlich's-reactive compounds will also be extracted into butanol; porphobilinogen will remain in the lower aqueous layer.
5. Report as negative, positive for urobilinogen, positive for porphobilinogen, or positive for both urobilinogen and porphobilinogen (rare). The finding of Ehrlich's-reactive compounds that are neither urobilinogen nor porphobilinogen is due to interfering substances such as sulfonamides, procaine, 5-hydroxyindoleacetic acid, and other compounds that react with Ehrlich's reagent. Methyldopa (Aldomet) will give a positive result similar to porphobilinogen.

Note: Very fresh urine should be cooled to room temperature before the Ehrlich test is carried out. Normal urine contains a chromogen (probably indoxyl) which gives a weak Ehrlich reaction at body temperature—the so-called "warm aldehyde" reaction.

Interpretation of the Watson-Schwartz Test for Urobilinogen and Porphobilinogen. *Urobilinogen* is soluble in both chloroform and butanol. *Porphobilinogen* is not soluble in either chloroform or butanol, always remaining in the aqueous urine-acetate layer. It is the only one of these Ehrlich's-reactive compounds which is not soluble in either one of the solvents. The following sets correspond to the results shown in Figure 18–3:

Set No. 1
+ Urobilinogen
0 Porphobilinogen
0 Other Ehrlich's-reactive compounds

Set No. 2
+ Porphobilinogen
0 Urobilinogen
0 Other Ehrlich's-reactive compounds

Set No. 3
+ Other Ehrlich's-reactive compounds
0 Urobilinogen
0 Porphobilinogen

Set No. 4
+ Urobilinogen
+ Other Ehrlich's-reactive compounds
0 Porphobilinogen

Set No. 5*
+ Porphobilinogen
+ Other Ehrlich's-reactive compounds
0 Urobilinogen

Set No. 6†
+ Urobilinogen
? Porphobilinogen
? Excess urobilinogen

*When the deeper color is in the urine-acetate mixture and the butanol layer is a lighter shade, results can be reported without further examination.

†In this instance, the tube containing butanol is never left with color in both layers. Further extraction of the urine-acetate layer is done with more butanol. If all the color is extracted into the butanol layer, there is no porphobilinogen present (6-a). However, if the color after the re-extraction with the butanol remains in the urine-acetate layer and the butanol layer is colorless, the test is positive for porphobilinogen (6-b). Extract the urine-acetate layer until color remains in only one layer.

Porphobilinogen in Urine—Hoesch Test. The Hoesch test is based on the inverse Ehrlich's reaction (i.e., of maintaining an acid solution by adding a small urine volume to a relatively large reagent volume) eliminating the problem of urobilinogen reaction. The urine specimen must be fresh or stored at neutral pH in a refrigerator. The urine specimen from a patient having an acute porphyric attack may become dark red in color; dilute 1:10 with water, and test.

Reagent. 20 g para-dimethylaminobenzaldehyde diluted to 1000 ml with HCl, 6 mol/L (50 per cent—1:2 dilution of the concentrated HCl in distilled water). It is stable for nine months in a tightly stoppered dark container. Store in a refrigerator.

Procedure. Pour approximately 2 ml of the reagent in a test tube. Add two drops of fresh urine to the reagent. Examine for an instantaneous cherry red color predominantly on the top of the solution, but throughout the tube on brief agitation. Report as positive or negative for porphobilinogen.

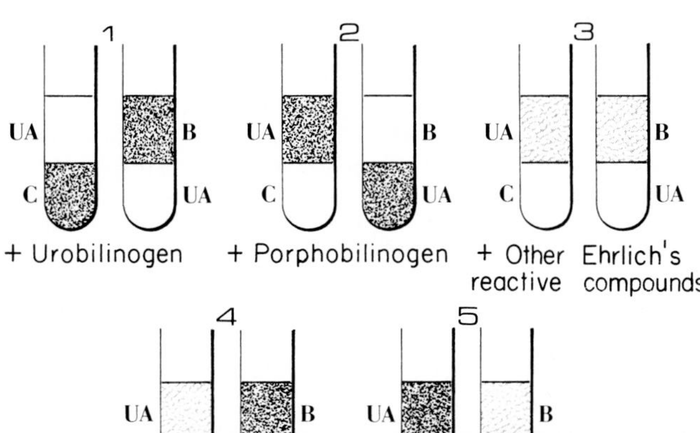

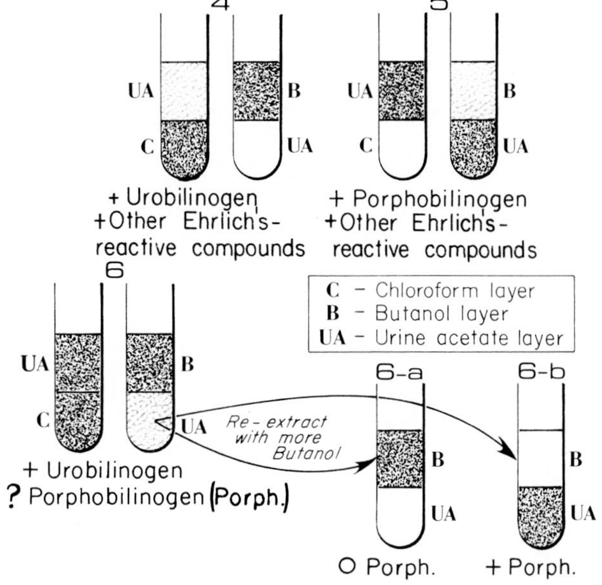

Figure 18–3. Interpretation of the screening method for urine urobilinogen and porphobilinogen (Watson-Schwartz test).

The sensitivity is similar to the Watson-Schwartz test but the reaction is for porphobilinogen (see Lamon, 1974; Hoesch, 1947). The test will detect about 20–100 mg/L of porphobilinogen. A yellow color is caused by urea. Urobilinogen in amounts up to 200 mg/L does not cause a red color.

According to Pierach (1977), the Watson-Schwartz test is more sensitive than the Hoesch test for porphobilinogen, and therefore it may yield a positive result between attacks of acute intermittent porphyria. The Watson-Schwartz test detects greater than 6 mg/L and the Hoesch test greater than 11 mg/L of porphobilinogen. Large doses of methyldopa (Aldomet) gave positive results, as did indoles in some patients with intestinal ileus, and the drug phenazopyridine (Pyridium), which becomes orange with hydrochloric acid. Very large amounts of urobilinogen are needed to give a positive Hoesch test, and this is not a practical problem.

A quantitative porphobilinogen test is necessary if either the Watson-Schwartz test or the Hoesch test result is questionable; this situation may arise because of the instability of porphobilinogen.

The urorosein urinary pigment related to indoleacetic acid will produce a positive Hoesch test (in response to strong HCl), and the rose color may be confused with a positive porphobilinogen result. Some of the false positive problems may be excluded by testing the specimen with concentrated HCl (6 mol/L) separately in conjunction with the Hoesch test.

CLINICAL CORRELATIONS OF CHEMICAL SCREENING TESTS

Some of the common findings are summarized below with some practical comments regarding the tests for *glucose and ketones; protein; bilirubin and urobilinogen; hemoglobin, hematuria, hemosiderin,* and *myoglobin;* and *nitrite and leukocyte esterase.* For specific test information, see Reagent Strip Methodology, Confirmatory Tests, Miscellaneous Tests, and Urinary Screening for Metabolic Inherited Diseases. Clinical correlations for sediment findings and stones are given later. (See Table 18–17).

Clinical correlations and comments regarding color and appearance, volume, specific gravity, and pH are given earlier.

Glucose in Urine

Glucose may appear in the urine at different blood glucose levels, varying in individuals. The blood level, glomerular blood flow, tubular reabsorption rate, and urine flow influence its appearance. Glucosuria usually occurs when the blood level is more than 180 to 200 mg/dl. The glucose oxidase reagent strip test is a

3

specific test for glucose. The glucose oxidase test is more sensitive to glucose than the copper reduction test. Reducing sugars other than glucose may be present when the copper reduction test (Clinitest[a]) is positive and the glucose oxidase test is negative, e.g., with lactosuria and galactosuria. However, the yield for these sugars is extremely low (Potter, 1980). Drugs will give false positive or unusual colors with Clinitest,[a] especially the cephalosporins such as Keflex and radiographic media. While large doses of ascorbic acid do not affect the two-drop Clinitest[a] test for sugars, i.e., do not cause false positive results (Smith, 1977b), delay may occur in color development with the glucose oxidase test. Note that glycolytic enzymes from cells and bacteria will reduce glucose levels in urine; prompt refrigeration or testing is essential.

Diabetes Mellitus. The level and duration of hyperglycemia required to make a diagnosis of diabetes mellitus is variously interpreted by groups in different parts of the world. Although hyperglycemia alone is not necessarily indicative of diabetes mellitus, the appearance of glucose in the urine is regarded as a hallmark of the disease and requires that the patient receive a work-up for diabetes mellitus.

The patient diagnosed as having diabetes mellitus has hyperglycemia which results in glucosuria when the renal threshold for glucose is exceeded. With glucosuria there is polyuria and thirst. With the need to metabolize protein and then fats, ketone levels rise in the blood and urine, and with the excretion of ketones and the accompanying base, metabolic acidosis ensues.

For diabetics, the advantage of a urine test over a blood test for glucose is that it is painless and cheap. However, reagent strips are difficult to interpret at the 1 g/dl (1 per cent) and 2 g/dl (2 per cent) glucose levels, and the Clinitest[a] method is preferred by many to try to offset this problem. Newer reagent strips that discriminate between high urinary glucose levels to 5 g/dl may help. With the Clinitest[a] method, diabetic patients are able to estimate glucose levels in urine to about 10 g/dl, using one drop of specimen rather than two or five drops.

Urine glucose tests are generally useful for the patient who does not have to make frequent dose adjustments. In insulin-dependent diabetes, a negative urine test could correspond to a wide range of blood glucose levels (Malone, 1976); this is attributed to a great variation in renal threshold for glucose in diabetics. In unstable diabetics, therefore, urine tests may be misleading and home blood glucose monitoring is advocated.

In some clinics, the 24-hour urine glucose measurement is found useful for monitoring patients. It represents a defined longer time period, and with blood levels of glycosylated hemoglobin, it contributes to the regular overall long-term management of the disease.

Glucosuria *with hyperglycemia* is also seen in *endocrine disorders* other than diabetes mellitus, e.g., in pituitary and adrenal disorders such as acromegaly and in Cushing's syndrome or hyperadrenocorticism, and with functioning alpha- or beta-cell pancreatic tumors, hyperthyroidism, and pheochromocytoma. Pancreatic disease with loss of functioning islets is also associated with glucosuria, e.g., hemochromatosis, carcinoma, pancreatitis, and cystic fibrosis.

Glucosuria and hyperglycemia may be seen with *central nervous system* disorders; brain tumor or hemorrhage, hypothalamic disease, and asphyxia, and with disturbances of metabolism associated with burns, infection, fractures, myocardial infarction, and uremia. Liver disease, glycogen storage diseases, obesity, and feeding after starvation are also associated with glucosuria, as are certain drugs, e.g., thiazides, corticosteroids and ACTH, and birth control pills.

In pregnancy, there is an increase in glomerular filtration rate and all of the filtered glucose may not be reabsorbed, so that glucosuria may appear at relatively low blood glucose levels. Persistent, or greater than trace, amounts of glucosuria should be investigated. In some patients, diabetes occurs only during pregnancy. There is a decrease in glucose tolerance in the aged, especially when the patients have a poor intake of carbohydrate, but this is not necessarily accompanied by glucosuria.

Glucosuria *without hyperglycemia* is usually associated with renal tubular dysfunction. True inherited renal glucosuria is uncommon; it is associated with reduced glucose reabsorption. In renal tubular transport diseases, glucosuria is not a major finding but one of many. Water, amino acid, bicarbonate, phosphate, and sodium reabsorption are impaired, a pattern seen in the Fanconi syndrome. Galactosemia, cystinosis, lead poisoning, and myeloma are examples of conditions associated with renal tubular dysfunction and possible glucosuria.

Ketones in Urine

In ketonuria the three ketone bodies present in the urine are acetoacetic (diacetic) acid (20 per cent), acetone (2 per cent), and 3-hydroxybutyrate (about 78 per cent) (Henry, 1974). Acetone is formed non-reversibly from acetoacetic acid. Beta-hydroxybutyric acid (3-hydroxybutyrate) forms reversibly from acetoacetic acid.

$$\text{Acetoacetic acid} \xrightarrow{-CO_2} \text{acetone}$$

$$\text{Acetoacetic acid} \underset{-2H}{\overset{+2H}{\rightleftharpoons}} \text{3-hydroxybutyrate}$$

Different tests measure acetoacetic acid or both acetone and acetoacetic acid. Commonly used nitroprusside strip and tablet tests based on Rothera's method detect acetoacetic acid and acetone but not 3-hydroxybutyrate. Ferric chloride (Gerhardt's test) is a wet test that detects acetoacetic acid and one nitroprusside strip test (Ames) detects only acetoacetic acid and does not detect acetone. These reagents are markedly subject to deterioration with humidity and will become non-reactive.

Problems occur with false negative results because

of unstable reagents and labile ketones. Specimens need to be refrigerated if not tested immediately but should be brought to room temperature for testing. Preservatives do not prevent decay of ketones. If results are unexpected, fresh reagents, checked against known positive and negative controls, should be used.

Ketone bodies are the products of incomplete fat metabolism, and their presence is indicative of acidosis. Ketonemia and ketonuria are commonly seen in uncontrolled diabetes mellitus. In *urine*, reagent strips and tablets react to 10 mg of acetoacetic acid/dl and are less sensitive to acetone. In *plasma*, about the same amounts of ketone bodies are detectable. When a patient is being followed with repeated determinations of acetone and acetoacetic acid, the concentrations of these compounds may start at a high level and fall but still give "large" results. Therefore, repeated reports of "large" would not reflect the change taking place. In such an instance, semiquantitative results can be obtained with either the reagent strip or Rothera's tablet test by testing several different dilutions of each specimen. Reagent strips correlate only moderately well with quantitative acetoacetate in plasma and poorly with total blood ketones (Alberti, 1972).

Non-Diabetic Ketonuria. In infants and children, ketonuria commonly occurs in a variety of conditions, such as acute febrile diseases and toxic states accompanied by vomiting or diarrhea (Riekers, 1958). Ketonuria is also present in vomiting of pregnancy, in cachexia, and following anesthesia. In these cases, it is related most probably to increased tissue (especially fat) catabolism in the face of limited food intake. In pregnancy, a normal patient may have a low fasting blood glucose level and mild ketonuria. The use of a low carbohydrate diet for weight reduction will produce ketonuria. Occasionally ketonuria is seen following exposure to cold or severe exercise.

Inherited metabolic disease should be suspected when there is severe neonatal ketoacidosis.

Examination of the urine for ketone bodies is not a necessary part of the routine urine examination except in specimens from young children. However, in the presence of any of the above conditions, or whenever acidosis or ketosis is suspected clinically, urine should be examined for ketones.

Diabetic Ketonuria. The presence of ketonuria indicates the presence of ketoacidosis (ketosis) and may provide a warning of impending coma. Up to 50 mg of acetoacetic acid per deciliter may be present without clinical evidence of ketosis (Killander, 1962). Diabetic children and young adults are prone to episodes of ketosis, often associated with infection as well as other problems in management. It is the usual practice in the management of diabetes to test for ketonuria when the urine, on qualitative examination, displays more than 1 to 2 g/dl of glucose. Combination glucose and ketone reagent strips are useful for patients. Large amounts of ketones will depress the glucose oxidase test and give falsely low results for glucose on some glucose oxidase strips. The urine of diabetic patients controlled with oral hypoglycemic agents should be tested regularly for ketone bodies as well as glucose, especially in the presence of infection, since insulin may then be required for control. Ketonuria should also be checked when changes in diabetic therapy are prescribed.

While there are large amounts of ketones and glucose in urine in diabetic ketoacidosis, ketonuria is not found with the hyperosmolar hyperglycemic coma sometimes occurring in older diabetics.

Lactic Acidosis. Lactic acidosis occurs with shock and with diabetes mellitus, renal failure, liver disease, and infections, and in response to certain drugs, especially phenformin and salicylate poisoning. Acetoacetate and 3-hydroxybutyrate may both be highly elevated in lactic acidosis. Usually the butyrate is high and acetoacetate is low, and it may not be detected by the nitroprusside test (Cohen, 1976; Hansen, 1978).

Protein in Urine

Normally there is a scant amount of protein in urine up to about 150 mg/24 hour or 10 mg/dl, depending on urine volume. The proteins are derived from plasma and the urinary tract. About one third is albumin, and the remaining plasma proteins include many small globulins. Plasma proteins with molecular weight less than 50,000 to 60,000 pass through the glomerular membrane and are normally reabsorbed by proximal tubular cells. Albumin, molecular weight 69,000, is apparently filtered but only in very small amounts. Retinol binding, β_2 microglobulin, immunoglobulin light chains, and lysozyme are excreted in small amounts. Tamm-Horsfall glycoprotein (uromucoid), secreted by distal tubular cells, constitutes about one third or more of the total normal protein loss. Immunoglobulin A in secretions of the urinary tract, enzymes and proteins from tubular epithelial cells, and other desquamated cells and leukocytes are other proteins found in very small amounts in normal urine. Anderson (1979) has demonstrated more than 200 urinary proteins.

Healthy persons may exceed normal levels during exercise or with dehydration. Proteinuria is a consistent finding after strenuous exercise. Proteinuria can occur in the absence of urinary tract disease in patients with hemorrhage or salt depletion and in febrile illnesses. These may cause dehydration and relative renal ischemia.

Screening tests are required to differentiate normal protein excretion from abnormal and therefore should not detect less than about 8 to 10 mg/dl in a normal adult with a normal rate of urine flow. It should be noted that a very dilute random specimen of urine may have a falsely low protein value. Since a positive result for protein is significant, it should be confirmed by a second, different method. The reagent strip method is sensitive to albumin; the acid precipitation tests detect all proteins and will therefore indicate the presence of globulins, as well as albumin.

Detection of an abnormal amount of protein in urine is a reliable indicator of renal disease. When proteinuria is confirmed, a 24-hour collection for

3

protein excretion is made. This will indicate the degree of proteinuria. Repeated measurements may be needed to decide whether the proteinuria is intermittent or persistent. Depending on the history and examination, confirmatory tests for protein are usually accompanied by tests of renal function, examination of the urine sediment, and urine culture. Errors in quantitative protein determinations result from poor collections of 24-hour specimens and variable methods (see Confirmatory Tests). To detect the kinds of protein present in urine requires electrophoretic separation of serum and urine proteins. Based on these and clinical findings, proteinuria may be separated into a *glomerular pattern* and *tubular pattern* indicating which part of the nephron is primarily involved. However, these anatomic entities tend to merge as the diseases progress. A third type has been designated *overflow proteinuria* because the protein material initially results from disease elsewhere, e.g., hemoglobin, following intravascular hemolysis.

Glomerular Disease. This regularly causes proteinuria. A loss or reduction of the fixed negative charge on the glomerular capillary wall allows albumin to permeate into Bowman's space in large quantities, more than can be reabsorbed by the proximal tubular cells (Brenner, 1978). Glomerular disease often causes heavy proteinuria, >3 to 4 g/day. On the other hand, small amounts of albumin are found in urine of insulin-dependent diabetics, and this finding appears to correlate with very early diabetic nephropathy.

Glomerular Pattern. When much serum albumin is lost in urine, other proteins of similar size or charge are also lost, e.g., anti-thrombin, transferrin, prealbumin, α_1-acid glycoprotein, α_1-antitrypsin—i.e., proteins that are usually retained in the plasma. Large proteins are not seen in urine while the glomerulus is still selective, e.g., α_2-macroglobulin and β-lipoprotein. Since tubular function may still be normal, very small plasma proteins are largely reabsorbed. When only albumin or smaller proteins are found, the pattern indicates minimal change disease and generally has a better prognosis. As larger proteins appear, the proteinuria is less selective, indicating greater morphologic changes, for example, with membranous nephropathy and proliferative glomerulonephritis.

Nephrotic syndrome is principally associated with glomerular diseases and diagnosed when the protein excretion is greater than 3.0 to 3.5 g/day or 2 g/m^2/24 hours. Losses of 10 to 20 g/day are found. In addition to heavy proteinuria, the classic syndrome is characterized by low serum albumin level, generalized edema, and increased serum lipids (cholesterol, triglycerides, and phosphatides). Lipoproteins, low density and very low density, are increased in serum while high density lipoprotein, a smaller molecule, has been demonstrated in urine (de Mendoza, 1976). It has been suggested that loss of lipoprotein lipase in urine contributes to the rise of serum lipid levels. Gamma globulin is lost in urine. This contributes to susceptibility to bacterial infections commonly found in the nephrotic syndrome. Lipid is lost in urine; typically many granular casts, fatty casts, and fat-filled renal tubular epithelial cells (oval fat bodies) are found in the sediment. Cholesterol ester droplets are demonstrable by polarization. Common causes of the nephrotic syndrome are mentioned later under Heavy Proteinuria.

Tubular Disease. This is associated with loss of urinary protein that would otherwise be largely reabsorbed. These proteins are usually of low molecular weight, e.g., α_1-microglobulin, beta globulin such as β_2-microglobulin, light chain immunoglobulins, lysozyme. By radioimmunoassay, β_2-microglobulin excretion has been measured in microgram amounts in urine as an indication of tubular damage; its normal excretion is about 100 μg/day. A tubular pattern proteinuria occurs with renal tubular diseases such as the Fanconi syndrome, cystinosis, Wilson's disease, and pyelonephritis and with renal transplantation. The amount of proteinuria is lower than with glomerular diseases and is about 1 to 2 g/day.

Tubular proteinuria may be missed by the reagent strip test because of absence or very low amounts of albumin but will be detected by acid precipitation tests.

Overflow Proteinuria. Excessive production or overflow proteinuria is due to hemoglobin, myoglobin, or immunoglobulin loss into the urine. These proteins are not initially associated with glomerular or tubular disease but may cause renal disease. Myoglobin causes acute tubular necrosis (see under Myoglobin). Hemoglobin is not thought to be toxic unless dehydration is present.

Bence Jones Proteinuria. Bence Jones proteinuria is associated with multiple myeloma, macroglobulinemia, and malignant lymphomas. The incidence of Bence Jones proteinuria in multiple myeloma has been estimated as 50 to 80 per cent; however, its demonstration depends greatly on the technique used. Electrophoresis and immunoelectrophoresis methods are usual. Bence Jones protein may be missed altogether if only a reagent strip test for protein is used. (See Reagent Strip Methodology and Confirmatory Tests—Protein.)

Excretion of Bence Jones protein in large amounts, sometimes several grams/24 hours, causes the tubular cells to become degenerated because of the high levels of protein reabsorbed. Inclusions may form in the cells. Desquamated cells form casts in the tubular lumen. Casts also form from immunoglobulin and Tamm-Horsfall protein mixtures. With renal failure, less protein is reabsorbed and more Bence Jones protein and other proteins appear in the urine. The damaged kidney is sometimes called a myeloma kidney, and the nephrotic syndrome may follow.

Heavy Proteinuria (>3 to 4 g/24 Hours). Heavy protein loss is characteristically seen with the nephrotic syndrome. The syndrome is associated with (1) primary renal diseases, including idiopathic disease, and (2) systemic diseases causing renal involvement. Transient or mechanical causes are severe congestive heart failure, constrictive pericarditis, and renal vein thrombosis. The latter is also a consequence of the nephrotic syndrome because of losses of anticlotting factors in urine and elevation of serum fibrinogen. A common cause of heavy proteinuria is *minimal* *change* (also known as nil lesion, idiopathic) *nephrotic syndrome*. This is a steroid responsive disease usually seen in young children. In adults, diabetes mellitus is a frequent cause of heavy proteinuria. In Africa, malaria is a frequent cause of childhood nephrotic syndrome. Acute, rapidly progressive, and chronic glomerulonephritis are causes of heavy proteinuria. Proteinuria and lipiduria may then be accompanied by red cells. Red cell casts are sometimes seen. The sediment may be "telescoped," that is, display all kinds of cells and casts in lupus nephritis or with a hypersensitivity reaction. Malignant hypertension, toxemia of pregnancy, heavy metals (gold, mercury), drugs (penicillamine), neoplasia in general, amyloidosis (primary, secondary, and with multiple myeloma), sickle cell disease, and renal transplant rejection are all causes of heavy proteinuria.

Moderate Proteinuria (1.0 to 3 or 4 g/Day). Moderate proteinuria may be found in large numbers of renal diseases, primarily glomerular, including those mentioned above, and nephrosclerosis, pyelonephritis, multiple myeloma, and a variety of toxic nephropathies, including radiation nephritis. Leukocytes and leukocyte–tubular cell casts are seen with acute pyelonephritis. Red cells accompany nephrosclerosis and some renal tubular diseases.

Minimal Proteinuria (<1.0 g/Day). Minimal proteinuria may be noted in chronic pyelonephritis, in which case it may be intermittent, and in relatively inactive phases of glomerular diseases. It is also seen with nephrosclerosis, chronic interstitial nephritis, congenital diseases such as polycystic disease and medullary cystic disease, and renal tubular diseases. The urinary sediment is usually not abnormal, but red cells, leukocytes, and tubular cells may be seen with interstitial nephritis. However, as mentioned below, significant sediment findings may sometimes accompany trace protein results. Minimal proteinuria is present in "benign" postural proteinurias and transient proteinuria.

Proteinuria may be absent in phases of acute pyelonephritis, in chronic pyelonephritis, and in the presence of obstructive nephropathy, kidney stones, kidney tumors, and congenital malformations. Cells and casts can be found in the urine in significant numbers when the protein reagent strip screening test is negative. In an analysis of 3152 urine specimens submitted for routine analysis in a tertiary care institution (approximately one third outpatient), 67 per cent had negative protein and 14 per cent had "trace" protein results using a reagent strip. Of the *negative protein* specimens, positive urinary sediment findings are summarized as follows: 2.4 per cent had 3 to 6 RBC/hpf, and 2.2 per cent had 6 to 30 RBC/hpf; 5 per cent had 4 to 15 WBC/hpf, and 1.5 per cent had 15 to 50 WBC/hpf; 4 per cent had positive casts (Bradley, 1978).

Postural Proteinuria. Postural proteinuria (orthostatic) occurs in 3 to 5 per cent of apparently healthy young adults. In these persons, proteinuria is found during the day but not at night when a recumbent position is assumed. Persistent proteinuria may develop in some of these healthy subjects at a later date, and renal biopsies have shown abnormalities of the glomerulus in a few cases (Robinson, 1961). Proteinuria is apparently related to an exaggerated lordotic position and may result from renal congestion or ischemia. The total daily excretion of protein rarely exceeds 1 g. In most instances, no other evidence of renal disease develops.

To evaluate the possibility of postural proteinuria, the patient is instructed to empty his bladder upon going to bed in the evening and to discard the specimen. Immediately upon rising in the morning, the patient voids and saves this specimen. After two hours of standing and walking about, the patient voids again and saves the specimen. The two urine specimens are tested for protein. If the first is negative and the second positive, the patient may have postural proteinuria. Frequent examination of the patient should be made to re-evaluate this condition.

Intermittent, Transient Proteinuria. The history, physical examination, and renal function tests are normal. Except for occasional proteinuria, routine urinalysis is normal. These patients are followed every six months to check for hypertension or other abnormalities. Prognosis is good. A transient proteinuria may occur in normal pregnancy, but any proteinuria in pregnancy is an important finding and requires investigation.

Persistent Proteinuria (1 to 2 g/Day). This finding in an asymptomatic person, or when accompanied by hematuria, has a poorer prognosis than intermittent (transient) or postural proteinuria (Thompson, 1970; Rytand, 1981).

Functional Proteinuria. This is usually less than 0.5 g/day. It is seen with *heavy exercise*, e.g., long distance running, hockey, racketball, and also accompanies congestive heart failure, cold exposure, and fever. Dehydration contributes to the level of protein measured in urine. With strenuous exercise, a mixture of high and low molecular weight proteins appears, and many casts, both hyaline and granular, are seen (Bailey, 1976). Functional proteinuria will resolve with appropriate treatment or rest within two to three days.

Bilirubin and Urobilinogen

Bilirubinuria. A test for bilirubin in urine should be performed when the dark color of the urine indicates its possibility. Experienced personnel become expert in the detection of bilirubin by eye. Because it is so labile, only fresh urine specimens should be tested for bilirubin either by the relatively easy and sensitive diazo tablet test (Ictotest[a]) or the reagent strip test. Biliverdin, an oxidation product of bilirubin, does not give the diazo reaction.

Bilirubin is a breakdown product of hemoglobin formed in the reticuloendothelial cells of the spleen, liver, and bone marrow and carried in the blood by protein. Unconjugated bilirubin in the blood is not able to pass through the glomerular barrier of the kidney. When bilirubin is conjugated in the liver with glucuronic acid to bilirubin glucuronide, it

3

becomes water soluble and is able to pass through the glomerulus of the kidney into the urine. Normal adult urine contains about 0.02 mg of bilirubin/dl (With, 1954), and this is not detected by the usual tests. For a review of bilirubin metabolism, see Billing (1978).

Conjugated bilirubin is normally excreted in the bile into the duodenum. Conjugated bilirubin appearing in urine indicates that there is obstruction to bile outflow from the liver, e.g., gallstones in the common bile duct, carcinoma of the head of the pancreas. The urine is dark and may have a yellow foam. Bilirubinuria is associated with elevated serum bilirubin (conjugated), jaundice, and pale-colored feces. These acholic stools are so called because of the absence of bilirubin-derived pigment. Bilirubin is also found in the urine when intracanalicular pressure rises because of periportal inflammation or fibrosis and from swelling of liver cells. Bilirubin may, for example, appear in the urine in acute viral hepatitis or drug-induced cholestasis before the appearance of jaundice. The test is helpful in diagnosis and in following the course of infectious hepatitis. A positive test for urinary bilirubin with a negative test for urobilinogen in urine is indicative of intra- or extrahepatic biliary obstruction. The test is, therefore, of value in the differential diagnosis of jaundice, since bilirubinuria is not found with hemolytic jaundice. See Table 18–12.

In congenital hyperbilirubinemias, bilirubin will appear in the urine in the Dubin-Johnson type and the Rotor type. It does not appear with Gilbert's disease or Crigler-Najjar disease. In persons exposed to toxins and ingesting certain drugs, a positive test for bilirubinuria may be an early indication of cholestasis or liver damage. Bilirubinuria is found with jaundice of acute alcoholic hepatitis.

Excretion of bilirubin is enhanced by alkalosis.

Urobilinogenuria. After conjugation in the liver cells, bilirubin diglucuronide reaches the duodenum complexed with cholesterol, bile salts, and phospholipids. The conjugated bilirubin is not absorbed from the small intestine. In the colon, glucuronidases from bacteria hydrolyze the conjugate. The free bilirubin is reduced to urobilinogen, mesobilirubinogen, and stercobilinogen. Most of the pigment is excreted in feces as colored urobilins or stercobilin formed after further removal of hydrogen. A small amount of urobilinogen is absorbed into the portal circulation from the colon and travels to the liver where it is re-excreted, unconjugated, in the bile. A small amount normally reaches the kidneys.

Urobilinogen in urine represents more than one closely related tetrapyrrole derived from bilirubin. They are normally present, are colorless and labile, and react to form red-purple compounds with Ehrlich's aldehyde reagent. *Urobilins* are orange-colored oxidation products of urobilinogen that do not react with Ehrlich's reagent but will react with Schlesinger's zinc reagent. Urobilins impart color to normal urine. The Ehrlich reaction with *p*-dimethylamino-benzaldehyde is not specific for urobilinogens; positive reactions occur with indoles and monopyrroles (porphobilinogen) and other substances in urine.

Normal output of urobilinogen is 0.5 to 2.5 mg or units/24 hours. Tubular reabsorption is decreased and output is increased in alkaline urine, such as with the alkaline tide after meals. The level is decreased in acid urine. Since a mixture of substances is measured, the term "units" is frequently used instead of the more precise mg terminology. They are roughly equivalent. For quantitative comparative purposes in the same patient, a two hour test is used. Urine is collected from 2 to 4 P.M. after lunch, making sure the patient is well hydrated. The period after the meal coincides with more excretion of urobilinogen when the pH of the urine is more nearly neutral. Other two-hour periods may be selected, provided that they are the same for each patient, for purposes of comparison.

When there is liver damage or dysfunction, more urobilinogen than normal is excreted through the kidney. With liver cell damage due to viral hepatitis, with drugs or toxic substances, or in some cases of portal cirrhosis, recirculated urobilinogen is not re-excreted in the bile and appears in urine. With congestive cardiac failure and liver congestion, urobilinogen handling and re-excretion in bile are impaired. If there is an infection, such as cholangitis associated with obstruction, large amounts of urobilinogen are excreted in urine together with bilirubin. Urobilinogen is also increased in urine when there is fever; some of this increase is associated with dehydration and concentrated urine.

Persistent excess urobilinogen in urine with negative bilirubin is seen with jaundice due to *hemolytic anemias*. These jaundiced patients have dark-colored stools. For a comparison of urinary and fecal findings in jaundice, see Table 18–12. Increased urobilinogen

Table 18–12. URINE AND FECAL FINDINGS IN JAUNDICE

Finding	**Normal**	**Obstruction to Bile Flow**	**Hemolysis, Hemolytic Anemia**	**Liver Damage, Hepatitis, Cholestasis**
Urinary bilirubin	Absent	Increased, dark urine	Absent	Increased early
Urinary urobilinogen	Present	Neoplasm—low or absent; gallstones—variable	Increased	Decreased early; increased late
Fecal color	Dark	Pale; intermittent with gallstones in common bile duct; persistent with neoplasm in duct or pancreas	Dark	Pale early and dark late in hepatitis; pale with cholestasis

is seen following acute lysis of red cells and with the destruction of red cell precursors in the bone marrow with megaloblastic anemias. There is also an increased urobilinogen accompanying bleeding into tissues and the subsequent formation of excess bilirubin. Persistent *absence of urinary urobilinogen* occurs with complete obstruction of the common bile duct and is associated with pale stools. When also accompanied by blood in feces, carcinoma of the pancreas or the ampulla of Vater is likely. Broad-spectrum antibiotics will cause reduction of urobilinogen formation in the colon and therefore reduce its excretion in feces and urine.

Mesobilifuscin is a dipyrrole that normally contributes to fecal and urine color. It is not derived from bilirubin like urobilinogen but is probably a byproduct of heme synthesis. It causes a dark brown urine color whenever Heinz bodies form in red cells, e.g., with the unstable hemoglobins. This brown pigment in urine also occurs in cases of homozygous beta thalassemia. It does not react to tests for blood or bilirubin.

Hemoglobin, Hemosiderin, and Myoglobin in Urine

Hematuria. The presence of an abnormal number of blood cells in urine is known as hematuria, whereas the term *hemoglobinuria* indicates the presence of hemoglobin in solution in urine. Hematuria is relatively common, hemoglobinuria uncommon, and myoglobinuria rare. Any pink, red, or brown urine is bloody until proved otherwise (refer to Tables 18–3 and 18–4 on color and appearance).

Because of the diagnostic importance of small amounts of hematuria, and because of the tendency of red blood cells to undergo lysis in urine, a screening test for heme is a useful adjunct to the microscopic examination of the sediment. However, a common problem with the test is the inhibition of the heme reagent strip test, often due to ascorbic acid, when red blood cells are present. This problem emphasizes the need for routine microscopic tests in order to make a diagnosis of hematuria.

Because true hemoglobinuria is uncommon, a positive test for hemoglobin with a normal urinary sediment suggests that a fresh urine sample should be examined for red blood cells. Urine specific gravity of 1.010 or less may cause lysis of erythrocytes and an interpretation of hemoglobinuria. The use of phase microscopy permits visualization of "ghost" red cells in questionable cases of hematuria. It is important to search for red cell casts to establish the origin of the cells as renal. When red cell or blood casts are present with significant proteinuria, the red cells are emanating from the kidney and associated with diseases such as acute glomerulonephritis or lupus nephritis. Red cells and small amounts of protein are seen with lower urinary tract bleeding and inflammation.

Hematuria occurs with disease or trauma anywhere in the kidneys or urinary tract, with bleeding diseases and anticoagulants, and with the use of drugs such as cyclophosphamide. Hematuria is also seen in healthy persons undertaking excessive exercise (marathon runners) in whom bleeding emanates from the bladder mucosa. (See Erythrocytes in the section on Examination of the Urine Sediment and Table 18–17.)

Hemoglobinuria. Any cause of hemolysis has the potential of causing hemoglobinuria, but the presence of hemoglobinuria indicates significant *intravascular hemolysis* as opposed to extravascular hemolysis. Free hemoglobin binds to plasma haptoglobin, and once this binding capacity is saturated, dissociated hemoglobin will pass through the glomerulus as $\alpha\beta$ dimers with a molecular weight of 32,000. Some hemoglobin is reabsorbed by proximal tubular cells, and the remaining hemoglobin is excreted. Hemoglobin is metabolized in the tubular cells into ferritin and hemosiderin, which can later be detected in the urinary sediment with Prussian blue stain in desquamated cells and in casts. See Table 18–13.

Thus, the presence of *hemosiderin in urine,* usually two to three days after the acute hemolytic episode, is an indication of significant intravascular hemolysis. Note that hemosiderinuria will also be found with diseases causing siderosis of the kidney, namely, hemochromatosis.

Because of the intermittent presence of hemosiderinuria, urinary iron levels may be quantitated to establish the presence of chronic intravascular hemolysis. Normal urinary iron excretion is about 0.1 mg/day. It is increased with hemochromatosis and in association with red cells traumatized by prosthetic heart valves. Urinary iron levels are normal with pernicious anemia and in hereditary spherocytosis. Refer to tests for hemosiderin in the Confirmatory Tests section.

Hemoglobinuria may follow severe exertion in which there is *direct trauma* to small blood vessels, e.g., marching, jogging, karate, or bongo drum playing. Many other causes of acute red blood cell lysis are summarized under Some Causes of Hemolysis and Hemoglobinuria, below. A comparison of expected urine and plasma findings with moderate and marked hemolysis is shown in Table 18–13. Plasma appears pink at levels of about 50 mg/dl of hemoglobin. With marked hemolysis, plasma levels reach 1 g/dl. The plasma hemoglobin level is more often increased in severe acquired hemolytic anemias than in hereditary hemolytic anemias. However, moderately elevated levels occur with sickle cell disease and homozygous thalassemias. Note that unstable hemoglobins, e.g., hemoglobin Köln, will cause a brown pigmented urine, but this is not due to hemoglobin. It is thought to be a dipyrrole or bilifuscin and does not react with the reagent strip test for heme.

Some Causes of Hemolysis and Hemoglobinuria

Severe hemolytic-uremic syndrome in children. Thrombotic thrombocytopenic purpura.

Trauma to red blood cells. Prosthetic cardiac valves (especially aortic), ostium primum repair with patch causing turbulence, extensive burns, severe exercise, marching, severe trauma to muscle and other vascular tissues.

Organisms. Malaria, bartonella, *Clostridium welchii* toxin, brown recluse spider bite.

Table 18–13. URINE AND PLASMA FINDINGS WITH INTRAVASCULAR RED CELL DESTRUCTION

Test	Moderate Hemolysis	Marked Hemolysis
Urine		
Bilirubin (conjugated)	Absent	Absent
Urobilinogen	Normal or elevated	Elevated
Hemoglobin	Absent	Present
Hemosiderin	Absent	Present (late)
Plasma		
Bilirubin (unconjugated)	Elevated	Elevated
Haptoglobin	Decreased	Absent
Hemoglobin	Elevated	Elevated (marked)

Red cell enzyme deficient (G-6-PD) subjects. With oxidant drugs: acetanilid, sulfamethoxazole, nitrofurantoin, antimalarials (primaquine, etc.); with fava beans *(Vicia fava)* in susceptible groups; with diabetic acidosis; with infections.

Unstable hemoglobin diseases and oxidant drugs.

Normal subjects, oxidative hemolysis due to drugs. Large doses or exposure to naphthalene (mothballs), some sulfonamides, sulfones, nitrofurantoin.

Immune-mediated (see Hemolytic Anemias in Chap. 43). Incompatible blood transfusions. *Warm* antibodies: autoimmune—transient after infection, drug-induced. *Cold* antibodies: IgM—viral anti-i, mycoplasma anti-I; IgG—paroxysmal, Donath-Landsteiner anti-P; may be associated with congenital and acquired syphilis. *Membrane* sensitivity, complement-mediated: paroxysmal nocturnal hemoglobinuria. *Drugs:* as haptens (penicillins), immune complex (quinidine, phenacetin), α-methyldopa.

Myoglobinuria. When there is acute destruction of muscle fibers (rhabdomyolysis), myoglobin is released, rapidly cleared from blood, and excreted in the urine as a red-brown pigment. If large amounts of myoglobin are presented to the kidney, anuria may result from renal damage. (See Table 18–14 for causes of rhabdomyolysis and myoglobinuria.)

Free myoglobin, a monomer with molecular weight of 17,000, is excreted quickly, whereas the hemoglobin-haptoglobin complex is slowly removed and hemoglobin is excreted mostly as dimers of 38,000 molecular weight. Urinary acid pH affects the stability of myoglobin. The specimen should be neutralized and refrigerated as soon as possible.

The distinction between hemoglobinuria and myoglobinuria is difficult to make on examination of the urine. Immunochemical tests may prove to be more useful than qualitative tests. (See Confirmatory Tests.)

The diagnosis of rhabdomyolysis and myoglobinuria is usually made from the history and other laboratory findings as follows. Myoglobinuria has been seen following a number of strenuous exercises, in the military, and with marathon running and karate. Typically, the patient has muscle tenderness or cramps and voids red-brown urine within a day or two after exertion. The reagent strip urine test for heme is markedly positive, and protein and a few red blood cells are present. Serum is clear and has markedly elevated creatinine phosphokinase (CK >100,000 IU/L is typical), and elevated serum aldolase but normal haptoglobin level. Serum creatinine may be slightly increased. The urine usually clears in two to three days and the serum CK level slowly declines. The serum measurements and history help distinguish myoglobinuria from hemoglobinuria. Proteinuria, hematuria, myoglobinuria, and hyaline, granular, and myoglobin casts are all seen following severe exercise, especially in the untrained person (Bailey, 1976).

Strenuous exercise causes a reduction in renal blood flow and glomerular filtration rate. Massive muscle injury associated with alcoholism, drug abuse, especially with seizures, or trauma may result in acute oliguric renal failure with azotemia. Serum phosphorus

Table 18–14. CAUSES OF RHABDOMYOLYSIS (MUSCLE DAMAGE) AND MYOGLOBINURIA

Polymyositis and dermatomyositis (acute, severe)	Toxic substances and drugs
Trauma and ischemia	Acute alcohol overdose, phencyclidine (angel dust), other drugs, especially with seizures
Skeletal muscle injuries	Carbon monoxide, ethylene glycol
Crush injury, surgery	Sea snake bite, hornet's venom
Severe exercise	Diuretics causing hypokalemia
Massive muscle ischemia	Hereditary causes
Cardiac muscle injury	Paroxysmal (Meyer-Betz)
Seizures from any cause	Anesthesia (halothane), malignant hyperthermia
Heat cramps	Phosphorylase deficiency (McArdle's)
Infections	Carnitine palmityl transferase deficiency in children
Influenza, herpes virus	Occasionally in glycogen and lipid storage diseases with myopathies
Epstein-Barr virus	Occasionally in periodic paralysis
Legionnaires' disease and other severe bacterial infections	

levels are increased and serum calcium is low; there are elevations of the serum creatinine phosphokinase and potassium. (See Schulze, 1982.) Myoglobin appears to be more toxic to the kidney than hemoglobin.

Nitrite and Leukocyte Esterase Tests

Nitrite in Urine. A positive nitrite test indicates that bacteria that reduce urinary nitrate to nitrite are present in significant numbers. Many enteric gram-negative organisms will give positive results when their number is greater than 10^6/ml bladder urine. If the test is positive, a culture should be considered provided that the specimen was properly collected and stored prior to testing. A first morning, clean, midstream specimen is best. False positive results occur with poorly collected and stored specimens because of contaminants and bacterial proliferation.

While the first morning specimen will produce higher yields, a positive test on a randomly collected (clean catch) specimen is a very good indication of significant bacteriuria.

According to Kunin (1975), self-administered repeated nitrite tests (three tests) in a small group of patients revealed about 70 per cent overall positive results when compared with cultures. When only *E. coli* was present, bacteriuria detected by a positive nitrite test in any of the three first morning specimens showed 93 per cent agreement with culture results. There were no significant false positive nitrite results in his large test group.

False negative results occur because some nitrate reducing organisms form compounds other than nitrite and will not be detected. (See Reagent Strip Methodology.) Random specimens collected during the day, and urine from patients with draining catheters, do not show good correlation between the nitrite test and significant bacteriuria presumably because of the time required for the chemical reduction to nitrite in the bladder urine.

A negative test for nitrite when combined with a negative leukocyte esterase test might be useful in ruling out significant bacteriuria in a clean-catch concentrated first morning specimen. Refer to the validity of the Gram stain technique at the end of this section.

Leukocyte Esterase in Urine. Esterase activity has been demonstrated in the azurophilic or primary granules of the neutrophil series of leukocytes and is used as a marker for these cells by means of the chloroacetate stain. Extracts of human azurophil neutrophil granules contained up to ten proteins showing esterolytic activity (Dewald, 1975). Since neutrophils and other cells are labile in urine (Triger, 1966), this test is thought to be useful in detecting the enzyme remnants of cells that are not visible microscopically. It is also assumed that granulocytes are the only source of these esterases in urine. (See Reagent Strip Methodology.)

Addis (1926) showed that healthy persons excrete blood cells in urine. A difficulty has arisen in determining suitable cut-off points for normal and abnormal numbers of these cells. Because quantitative counts are so low when compared with blood, precision is poor. (See Quality Control, Microscopic Examination.) Attempts to correlate low urinary chamber cell counts with estimates on sediments and with esterase tests are fraught with difficulties. Values of 10/μl to 30/μl of leukocytes have been used as cut-off points using clinical correlates, usually infection (Stansfeld, 1953; Houston, 1963). Using fresh clean-catch or catheter specimens, Kusumi (1981) found that the esterase test gives a reasonably good indication of the presence of neutrophil esterases when about ten or more cells per microliter are used as an indication of pyuria. Using a concentrated (10:1) urine sediment and a cytocentrifuged stained preparation, Avent (1983) showed that a negative reagent strip test is associated with fewer than 100 neutrophils in ten high power fields (×450).

The esterase test is a useful adjunct to the microscopic examination of the urine sediment. Test results are probably more reliable when clean-catch, midstream specimens are collected. Contamination with vaginal fluid may produce false positive results. The presence of large numbers of squamous epithelial cells and bacteria, indicating vaginal contamination, are easily detected microscopically. Important leukocyte cellular casts indicating renal disease are easily detected in fresh urine using phase microscopy. These would not be differentiated from cells detected by use of the reagent strip alone.

It should be noted that the common finding of leukocytes in urine is not as reliable an indication of urinary tract infection as the detection of bacteriuria by Gram stain or culture of a fresh midstream specimen. In a series of 32,000 tests, Washington (1981) found 94 per cent sensitivity and 90 per cent specificity for the microscopic examination of the Gram stain when compared with significant culture results. A positive microscopic test is defined as even distribution of at least two organisms per oil immersion field throughout at least 20 oil-immersion fields. The microscopic examination was accomplished quickly, but required a carefully collected clean-catch, midstream specimen with experienced personnel assisting the patient. The negative predictive value of this test was 99 per cent and the positive predictive value was 90 per cent.

EXAMINATION OF THE URINE SEDIMENT

The microscopic examination of urine is the most common laboratory procedure utilized for the detection of renal and/or urinary tract disease. Interpretation of urine sediment requires time, skill, training, and experience acquired through constant use of various microscopic methods and continuous pathophysiologic correlation of the sediment findings with the clinical status of the patient. In order to practice with competency, technical staffs must be knowledgeable of numerous morphologic entities, e.g., organisms, hematopoietic and epithelial cells, casts. Also, microscopists must be alert regarding the clinical relevance of urine findings as well as the common chemical abnormalities associated with microscopic interpretations. For a more detailed discussion of urinary findings in urinary system diseases, the reader is referred to Haber (1981), Schumann, (1980, 1981b), Ross (1983), and textbooks of nephrology.

Formed Elements of Urine. Centrifuged urine sediment contains all the insoluble materials (commonly referred to as formed elements) that have accumulated in the urine in the process of glomerular filtration and during passage of fluid through the tubules of the kidney and lower urinary tract. Cells found in urine come from two sources: (1) desquamation or spontaneous exfoliation of epithelial cells lining the upper (kidney) and lower urinary tract and adjacent structures, and (2) cells from the circulating blood (leukocytes and erythrocytes). Casts formed in the renal tubules and collecting ducts are the other formed elements frequently seen.

Organisms (bacteria, fungi, viral inclusion cells, parasites) and neoplastic cells represent elements foreign to the urinary system, and proper identification of these elements may provide important diagnostic clues as to the etiology of certain urinary system disorders.

"Normal" or reference values for formed elements will vary from one laboratory to another because of (1) the variation in concentration of random urine specimens as voided, and (2) the different methods used to concentrate the sediment by centrifugation. Individual laboratories have established their own reference values, often in conjunction with the nephrologists.

Quantitative Counts and Differential Counts. In some laboratories, a hematocytometer is used for quantifying urine sediment findings from random and timed urine specimens. For example, cells and casts from undiluted well-mixed urine are counted in a leukocyte counting chamber and reported as the number of neutrophils per microliter. Gadeholt (1964) describes and reviews factors affecting the quantitative cell count. For example, a very low specific gravity, <1.012, causes a marked reduction in red cells, and a low acid pH reduces red cells slightly. Recovery of cells differed slightly with different centrifuge speeds. Only about half of a known number of red and white cells were recovered in the sediment after centrifugation. When two hour clean-catch specimens from 75 male patients were quantitated, the same specimen counted separately in duplicate showed variations in counts ranging from 10 to 30 per cent. Duplicate chamber counts of the same sediment varied up to 10 per cent. For errors in chamber counts, see Quality Control early in this chapter.

Normal values for neutrophils vary from 5 to 30/μl according to different workers; upper limits for red blood cells vary from 3 to 20/μl (Fassett, 1982; Freni, 1977b), and casts as few as 1 to 2/ml (Wenk, 1981). Freni used centrifugal force of 1230 G for nine minutes and evaluated stained smears of the sediment in a consistent fashion to determine an upper limit for red cells of 20,000/ml in men aged 50 to 65 years. Kesson (1978) provides evidence that chamber counts on centrifuged urine sediments are more reliable in predicting renal functional abnormalities than is a conventional method using cells/high power field. He used values of 2000 WBC/ml, 500 RBC/ml, and 15 casts/ml as upper limits of normal on clean-catch midstream urine specimens. These corresponded to daily urine volumes of 1250 ml and a calculated leukocyte excretion rate of 100,000/24 hours.

As a corollary to quantitation, differential counts from stained cytocentrifuged smears may be performed. While quantitated cell counts differentiate between healthy persons and those with disease, differential counts using phase microscopy or stained sediments help discriminate between diseases (Wahlin, 1977). According to Lindqvist (1975), the percentage of neutrophils seen with bacterial infections of the bladder and kidney was 91 to 97 per cent, and with interstitial nephritis (18 cases) was 85 per cent. With tubular necrosis, renal tubular cells (37 per cent), mononuclear leukocytes (18 per cent), and neutrophils were seen. In ten cases of lupus erythematosus, mononuclear leukocytes 29 per cent, tubular cells 19 per cent, and neutrophils 51 per cent were average differential counts.

Addis Count. The Addis count (Addis, 1948), although a more accurate method of assessing quantitative changes in the sediment, is no longer in general use. Its chief value lies in following the progress of active renal disease, notably acute glomerulonephritis. (For diagnostic purposes, careful examination of the sediment from a random fresh urine sample is usually sufficient.) (For details of methodology, see page 39 of Davidsohn, 1974.)

According to Addis, average rates of excretion for 12 hours (overnight) in 74 medical students were as follows: casts 1040 (range 0 to 4270), red blood cells 65,750 (range 0 to 425,000), and white blood cells with tubular epithelial cells 322,500 (range 32,400 to 1,835,000). The average volume was 352 ml, with an average specific gravity of 1.031 (Addis, 1926).

Methods for Examining Urine Sediment

Specimen. This is most often a randomly collected specimen of urine. For screening purposes this is usually satisfactory. There is less contamination with vaginal elements if the urine is collected as a midstream specimen from women. For better morphology, a two hour voided urine, collected after the first morning voiding has been discarded, is preferable. The urine may be dilute and slightly more alkaline than the overnight specimen (due to the effects of a meal), but the cells and casts are relatively fresh.

The urine specimen must be examined while fresh, since cells and casts begin to lyse within one to three hours. Refrigeration (2 to 8°C.) helps prevent the lysis of pathologic entities. If the urine cannot be examined within one hour of voiding, it should be refrigerated before and after transportation.

Brightfield Microscopy of Unstained Urine. Subdued light is needed to delineate the more translucent formed elements of the urine such as hyaline casts, crystals, and mucous threads. Identification of leukocytes (neutrophils, eosinophils, lymphocytes), histiocytes, renal epithelial cells, viral inclusion cells, neoplastic cells, and cellular casts may be very difficult in unstained preparations. Phase-contrast is strongly recommended for the detection of casts.

Procedure

1. Mix the specimen well (casts tend to settle). Pour exactly 10 ml of urine into a graduated disposable centrifuge tube. Centrifuge at 2000 rpm for five minutes at about 450 × g (see Quality Control section for details). Cellular casts are reasonably well preserved using this method. Remove the supernate by decanting into another tube and resuspend the sediment in exactly 1 ml of urine. A disposable pipette is convenient for this readjustment to 1 ml. Alternatively, one of the commercially available standardized centrifuge tube and pipette systems (mentioned later) can be used.

2. Place a standard drop of resuspended sediment on one area of a slide and cover with an 18-mm square coverslip, avoiding bubbles. Too much fluid will cause the coverslip to float. For this coverslip, approximately 12 μl of sediment supension is used. Alternatively, a plastic disposable slide with suitable wells is used.

3. Examine with both low and high power objectives. Examine with low power (× 100) and subdued light (brightfield) or phase-contrast illumination. The fine focus should be varied continuously while scanning. Systematically progress around all four sides of the coverslip. Either the stained or unstained mount may be used, depending on the kind of specimen and the experience of the examiner. *Casts* are often found along the edge of the coverslip. Count the number of casts per *low* power field in ten fields. Switch to high power (×400) to identify casts present. Casts will not be missed if phase microscopy is used (see Fig. 18–13*A* and *B*).

Erythrocytes, leukocytes, and renal epithelial cells are identified with the high power objective and counted in ten representative fields. Squamous and transitional epithelial cells are noted if a large number are present. Bacteria and yeasts should be noted.

Crystals are reported if the number is unusually large or they are abnormal; these are estimated under low power. The identity of certain abnormal crystals should be confirmed chemically (see cystine and sulfonamide tests).

Report. Average the contents of ten representative fields. A scale for reporting results of examination of urinary sediment is shown below.

RBC and WBC/hpf	*Casts and Abnormal Crystals/lpf*
0–2	neg
2–5	0–2
5–10	2–5
10–25	5–10
25–50	10–25
50–99	25–50
>100	>50

Normal values used for this procedure: 0–2 RBC/hpf, 0–5 WBC/hpf, occasional hyaline casts/lpf.

Brightfield Microscopy with Supravital Staining. Cellular detail is best seen with stained sediments. A crystal-violet safranin stain (Sternheimer, 1951) may be used to aid in the identification of cellular elements.

Reagents

Solution I.	Crystal violet	3.0 g
	Ethyl alcohol (95%)	20.0 ml
	Ammonium oxalate	0.8 g
	Distilled water	80.0 ml
Solution II.	Safranin O	1.0 g
	Ethyl alcohol (95%)	40.0 ml
	Distilled water	400.0 ml

Three parts of Solution I and 97 parts of solution II are mixed and filtered. The mixture should be clarified by filtering every two weeks. Discard after three months. Separately, Solutions I and II keep indefinitely at room temperature. In highly alkaline urines, the stain will precipitate. A similar stain is also available commercially as Sedi-Stain (Clay-Adams), Kova-Stain (ICL Scientific), and others.

Procedure. Add one or two drops of crystal-violet safranin stain to approximately 1 ml of concentrated urine sediment. Mix with a pipette and place a drop of this suspension on a slide and coverslip.

Methylene blue and toluidine blue (Holmquist, 1980) may also be used as simple, quick supravital stains. An improved supravital stain which facilitates identification of cells, casts, and their inclusions is also recommended and available as Cyto-Diachrome (Regis Chemical Company, Morton Grove, Ill. 60053) (Sternheimer, 1975).

3

Phase-Contrast and Interference Microscopy. Many laboratory personnel prefer to use phase-contrast microscopy for the detection of more translucent formed elements of the urinary sediment. Such elements, notably casts (but also mucous threads and bacilli), may escape detection using ordinary brightfield microscopy. Phase-contrast microscopy has the advantage of hardening the outlines of even the most ephemeral formed elements, making detection simple (see Fig. 18–13*A* and *B*) (Brody, 1968). A microscope equipped with 10× and 40× phase objectives plus a 40× brightfield objective and the appropriate rotating phase/brightfield condenser is most useful. Scanning time is decreased and the yield is increased. Even greater morphologic detail of formed elements (notably casts and cells) is afforded by interference-contrast microscopy (Haber, 1972). This technique, however, is not in common use at the present time.

Polarizing filters are used to distinguish crystals and fibers from cellular or protein cast material. Sterols, like cholesterol droplets, will form Maltese crosses with crossed polars. With the addition of a retardation plate, crystals may be further identified as positively or negatively birefringent. (See method for synovial fluid crystals, Chap. 19.)

Combined Cytocentrifugation and Papanicolaou Stain Method. A combined cytocentrifugation (Cytospin, Shandon Southern Instruments, Sewickley, Pa.) and Papanicolaou staining method has been used to evaluate changes in the urine sediment in renal allograft recipients during acute rejection, with acute tubular necrosis, and with other renal parenchymal diseases (Schumann, 1981b). Use of cytocentrifugation permits a simple, rapid, reproducible, and semiquantitative method for preparing urine sediments. Cellular casts, mononuclear cells (plasma cells, lymphocytes, histiocytes, etc.), tissue fragments, and neoplastic cells may be clearly demonstrated with this method.

Procedure. When possible, early morning urine (volumes ranging from 10 to 30 ml) is collected. The container is immediately delivered to the laboratory or refrigerated (2 to 8°C.). An accompanying requisition noting history of transplantation, radiation, and chemotherapy is required with each specimen. A 10 ml sample of urine is immediately spun in a standard centrifuge at 1500 rpm for ten minutes. The supernatant is then discarded by hand-pipetting to 1 ml and the sediment resuspended. Using a cytocentrifuge, four slides are prepared using four drops of resuspended specimen per chamber and spinning at 900 rpm for three minutes. After the filter is discarded, one to two drops of Parlodion* are applied to the cellular area of a horizontally held slide. The slide is then fixed for 15 minutes in acetic acid–alcohol† and stained by the Papanicolaou technique.‡ All four slides are screened, noting background pattern, cellularity, erythrocytes, viral inclusions, and abnormal cells. Ten high power fields are counted on the most cellular slide, differentiating between neutrophils, lymphocytes, renal tubular cells, and casts. Various modifications of the Papanicolaou stain may be used, including a rapid five minute method (Schumann, 1980).

Standardized Slide Methods. The KOVA system (ICL Scientific, Fountain Valley, Calif.), Whale T-System (Whale Scientific, Commerce City, Col.) and Count-10 System (V-Tech, Inc., Palm Desert, Calif.) provide complete standardized procedures that appear more reproducible and reliable than conventional methods. The systems include capped transport centrifuge tubes, transfer pipettes, supravital stain, and plastic slides. The KOVA system uses an optically clear plastic microscopic slide with individual, integrally covered examination chambers. The Whale T-System has a special centrifuge tube allowing the supernate to be decanted without disturbing the sediment; the plastic slide has four separate wells and glass coverslips. The Count-10 System has ten wells per plastic slide.

Microscopic Characteristics of Urine Sediment

CELLS

Erythrocytes. Under high power, unstained erythrocytes or red blood cells appear as pale disks. They vary somewhat in size but are usually about 7 μm in diameter. If the specimen is not fresh when it is examined, the cells will appear as faint, colorless circles or "shadow cells," since the hemoglobin has "dissolved" out. These membranes are more obvious with phase-contrast. Red blood cells may become crenated in hypertonic urine and appear as small, rough cells with "crinkly" edges (Fig. 18–4). Smooth, folded, and crenated cells may be seen in the same specimen. On occasion, red blood cells may be confused with oil droplets or yeast cells. Oil droplets, however, exhibit a great variation in size, are highly refractile, and will not "tumble" when the coverglass is touched with a pencil to set the fluid in motion. Yeast cells usually show budding. If there is doubt about identification, two preparations may be made and a few drops of acetic acid added to one. Red blood cells are lysed in the acidified preparation.

Both erythrocytes and leukocytes are found in small numbers in normal urine. How these cells enter the urine is not known. The proportion of leukocytes to erythrocytes is much greater in urine than in blood; thus, diapedesis of leukocytes through the glomerular membrane or tubular wall may be postulated.

In normal males and females, occasional red cells (0 to 2/hpf or 3 to 12/μl) may be seen on microscopic examination of the sediment. Smoking appears to be related to microhematuria (Freni, 1977a).

When increased numbers of red cells are found in the urine in conjunction with *red blood cell casts,* bleeding may be assumed to be renal in origin. In the absence of casts or proteinuria, increased red blood cells suggest a bleeding site distal to the kidney. Fairley (1982) has observed that aberrant or *dysmorphic erythrocyte* morphology is specific in detecting glomerular bleeding. These distorted cells are also more readily observed using phase-contrast microscopy. When 80 per cent or more of red cells are undistorted and uniform, these are regarded as non-glomerular, i.e., from a tubular source or associated with calculi or lower urinary tract disease. Normal persons also have a mixture of distorted and undistorted red blood cells in urine (Fassett, 1982).

Increased numbers of red blood cells in the urine may be present in (1) renal disease, including glomerulonephritis, lupus nephritis, interstitial nephritis associated with drug reactions, calculus, tumor, acute infection, tuberculosis, infarction, renal vein thrombosis, trauma (including renal biopsy), hydronephrosis, polycystic kidney, and occasionally acute tubular necrosis and malignant nephrosclerosis; (2) lower urinary tract disease, including acute and chronic infection, calculus, tumor, and stricture; and (3) extrarenal disease, including acute appendicitis, salpingitis, diverticulitis, and tumors of the colon, rectum, and pelvis. See Table 18–17.

Hematuria may occur during acute febrile episodes, malaria, subacute bacterial endocarditis, polyarteritis nodosa, malignant hypertension, blood dyscrasias, and scurvy. Hematuria may also reflect toxic reactions to drugs such as sulfonamides, salicylates, methenamine, and anticoagulant therapy. Hemorrhagic cystitis is occasionally noted following cyclophosphamide therapy.

Bloody urine associated with bleeding from the bladder mucosa is seen after strenuous exercise. Addis (1926) found that red cell excretion rate tripled in healthy persons after exposure to a vibrating chair for 30 minutes.

Leukocytes

Neutrophilic Leukocytes. Under high power, neutrophilic leukocytes appear as granular spheres about 12 μm in diameter. In freshly voided urine, nuclear detail is fairly well defined even with brightfield

*200 ml 95 per cent ethanol, 200 ml anhydrous ether, 1 g Parlodion (Mallinckrodt).

†One part glacial acetic acid to nine parts 95 per cent ethanol.

‡Aqueous alum hematoxylin, OG-6, EA-36.

microscopy. Nuclear segments appear as small round discrete nuclei. When cellular degeneration has begun, nuclear detail may be lost. Neutrophils may then become difficult to distinguish from renal tubular epithelial cells. By allowing a small drop of dilute acetic acid to run under the coverslip, one may enhance nuclear detail so that definition may still be possible (Fig. 18–5). Ultimately, however, with continued degeneration, neutrophilic nuclear segments fuse, making distinction from tubular cells difficult or impossible.

Supravital staining may also be helpful in emphasizing nuclear detail. With crystal-violet safranin, neutrophilic nuclei appear reddish purple and cytoplasmic granules violet. Cytochemical definition of neutrophils using the peroxidase reaction has been found especially useful in distinguishing neutrophils (Fig. 18–6) from tubular cells (Bradley, 1968). The stain is described later.

In dilute or hypotonic urine, neutrophils swell and cytoplasmic granules exhibit Brownian movement. Because of the refractility of the moving granules, neutrophils in this setting are known as "glitter" cells. These cells take supravital stains poorly, if at all. Papanicolaou staining also reflects the swelling of neutrophils in hypotonic urine. In addition, the neutrophils show loss of nuclear segmentation (Palmieri, 1977). Clinical studies have shown that the leukocyte esterase reagent strip with a sensitivity of 81 to 94 per cent and a specificity of 69 to 83 per cent is valuable in the confirmation of pyuria in hypotonic urines (Avent, 1983). See Reagent Strip Methodology and Clinical Correlations.

Increased numbers of leukocytes in the urine, principally neutrophils, are seen in almost all renal diseases and diseases of the urinary tract. They may also be transiently increased during fevers and following strenuous exercise (Goldring, 1931). When accompanied by leukocyte casts or mixed leukocyte–epithelial cell casts, increased urinary leukocytes are considered to be renal in origin.

The presence of many leukocytes (more than 50/hpf) and/or clumps of leukocytes in the sediment is strongly suggestive of acute infection. Repeated sterile cultures in this setting may indicate tuberculosis or lupus nephritis. Gross pyuria may reflect rupture of a renal or urinary tract abscess.

Moderate numbers of leukocytes in conjunction with leukocyte casts may reflect either bacterial (chronic pyelonephritis) or non-bacterial (acute glomerulonephritis, lupus nephritis) renal disease. They are frequently absent, however, in chronic pyelonephritis. Calculous disease at any level may give rise to increased numbers of urinary leukocytes because of either stasis-induced ascending infection or localized mucosal inflammatory response. Bladder tumors, as well as a variety of acute or chronic localized inflammatory processes, may also cause leukocytes to be increased in the urine. The latter disorders include cystitis, prostatitis, urethritis, and balanitis. In women, the acute urethral syndrome or dysuria-pyuria syndrome is regularly associated with >8 neutrophils/μl in clean catch urine specimens; however, bacterial colony counts are lower than expected. *Chlamydia trachomatis* as well as staphylococci and coliforms were causative agents (Stamm, 1981). It should be recognized that even in normal circumstances, some leukocytes are found in the secretions of the male and female genital tracts and appear in urine.

Finally, leukocytes are rapidly lysed in hypotonic or alkaline urine. Approximately 50 per cent are lost following two to three hours of standing at room temperature (Triger, 1966). This dramatizes the need for prompt examination of the urinary sediment following collection.

Eosinophils. If clinically indicated, leukocyturia should be further analyzed for the presence of eosinophils (Schumann, 1980). A cytocentrifuge preparation with Wright stain or Diff-Quik stain may be used to demonstrate eosinophils in urine. Appropriately stained, bilobed eosinophils may be noted in patients with tubulointerstitial disease associated with hypersensitivity to drugs such as penicillin and its analogues (Lombardo, 1980). Eosinophils are difficult to find in the cell sediment if the total number of leukocytes is low. Helgason (1972) collected specimens by suprapubic aspiration and prepared cytocentrifuged smears. A total leukocyte count of ten or more cells/μl gave satisfactory smear results. The cell pattern in allergic interstitial nephritis usually includes many red blood cells and some renal tubular epithelial cells.

Lymphocytes and Mononuclear Leukocytes. Small lymphocytes are normally present in urine although not routinely recognized. These cells and histiocytes are more easily differentiated in stained smears. When mononuclear cells (histiocytes, lymphocytes, or plasma cells) constitute 30 per cent or more of a differential count, lupus nephritis or benign endemic nephropathy may be the underlying disease process (Lindqvist, 1975). Many small lymphocytes are found in urine during the first month of renal transplant rejection.

Renal Tubular Epithelial Cells (Figs. 18–7 and 18–8). Small numbers of tubular cells may be seen in normal urine, reflecting the normal sloughing of aging cells (Table 18–15). They are present in somewhat larger numbers in the urine of normal newborns (Cruikshank, 1967).

Table 18–15. NORMAL URINARY EXCRETION RATE OF CELLS*

	Range	Mean
Erythrocytes	0 to 473,000/hr, female	29,000/hr, female
	0 to 915,000/hr, male	38,000/hr, male
Renal tubular cells	5,000 to 243,000/hr, female	68,000/hr, female
	12,000 to 262,000/hr, male	78,000/hr, male
Leukocytes (PMN)	0 to 5,024,000/hr, female	108,000/hr, female
	0 to 956,000/hr, male	28,000/hr, male

*Prescott, 1965. Refer to other quantitative and Addis counts in the text.

3

The Papanicolaou stain has been shown to be especially useful in distinguishing renal tubular cells from other mononuclear cells in urine. Using this method, renal tubular cells from the proximal and distal convoluted tubules have been identified and may be semiquantitated. Renal epithelial cells from the *proximal and distal* convoluted tubules occur singly and are large (14 to 60 μm) oblong or egg-shaped cells with characteristic coarsely granular eosinophilic cytoplasm. Nuclei may be multiple but are small with dense chromatin and rare nucleoli. Increased numbers of proximal and distal convoluted renal epithelial cells are seen in cases of acute tubular necrosis and certain drug or heavy metal toxicity (Schumann, 1981b).

Epithelial cells from the *small and large collecting duct* measure 12 to 20 μm and are identified by their characteristic cuboidal or polygonal shape and large, usually slightly eccentric nucleus. Cytoplasmic properties include a basophilic "endo-ecto" plasmic rim commonly found in transitional epithelial cells. Increased numbers of collecting duct epithelial cells are found in renal transplant rejection, acute tubular necrosis (diuretic phase), and other ischemic injuries to the kidney. They may also be found in increased numbers in malignant nephrosclerosis as well as in some cases of acute glomerulonephritis accompanied by tubular damage. Ingestion of various drugs and chemicals may cause significant tubular desquamation. Collecting duct tubular cells are easily found in the urine following salicylate intoxication.

Renal epithelial fragments of collecting duct origin have been described. Proximal and distal convoluted tubular cells are not found in fragment form. Three or more renal cells of collecting duct origin constitute a renal epithelial fragment and indicate a more severe form of renal tubular injury with basement membrane disruption. Renal epithelial fragments are indicative of ischemic necrosis and are usually found accompanying varying degrees of renal tubular injury and pathologic casts. Five common configurations of renal epithelial fragments have been described (Schumann, 1981a). Proper identification of renal epithelial fragments is essential not only in the diagnosis of a more severe form of renal tubular injury but also in avoiding a false positive diagnosis of low grade transitional cell carcinoma.

Lipids in Renal Tubular Epithelial Cells. Certain tubular cells may be identified with some degree of confidence using brightfield microscopy. These are *oval fat bodies,* i.e., tubular cells which have absorbed lipoproteins with cholesterol and triglycerides leaked from nephrotic glomeruli (Fig. 18–9). Oval fat bodies therefore constitute one form of lipiduria. Lipids may also appear in the urine as free fatty droplets. These, though morphologically similar to red cells, vary considerably in size and do not tumble when pressure is applied to the coverslip. Histiocytes may also ingest lipids and become impossible to distinguish from oval fat bodies. Their clinical significance, however, is similar. Finally, lipids may become incorporated into cast matrices as free fat droplets or as oval fat bodies. Resulting casts are described as fatty (see below). The presence of any or all of these lipid forms is characteristic of the nephrotic syndrome. (See under Protein in Urine, in Clinical Correlations of Chemical Screening Tests.)

Positive identification of lipid is required before reporting lipiduria. When free or incorporated droplets contain large amounts of cholesterol, they exhibit Maltese cross formation under polarized light (Fig. 18–10*A* and *B*). When they contain large amounts of triglycerides, fat stains (Oil red O or Sudan III) are required for positive lipid identification. (See Methods, later.)

Pigment in Renal Tubular Epithelial Cells. With hemoglobinuria, hemoglobin is absorbed into the cells and converted to hemosiderin. The *iron*-laden cells are desquamated and found in the urine sediment. Granules appear yellow-brown and stain for iron with Prussian blue. These cells are also incorporated into cast (Figs. 18–1 and 18–2). (See Causes of Hemoglobinuria and Hemosiderin, in Clinical Correlations of Chemical Screening Tests.)

Melanin granules are absorbed into the tubular cells in rare cases of melanuria. The desquamated pigmented cells may be demonstrated in the sediment. Pigmented tumor cells are also found when there are melanoma metastases to the bladder (Piva, 1964). (See Melanin, in Miscellaneous Tests.)

Bilirubin pigment colors all of the elements of the sediment, including renal tubular epithelial cells. Note that urobilin does not color cells and casts.

Transitional Epithelial Cells. These cells line the urinary tract from the renal pelvis to the trigone of the female bladder and to the distal urethra in the male. In the urine, they are two to four times as large as renal epithelial cells and have round or pear-shaped contours. The nuclei are round and central. Occasionally, these cells may be binucleate. A few are present in normal urine, reflecting normal desquamation. The presence of large clumps or sheets of these cells suggests the need for full cytologic examination with the Papanicolaou stain because of possible transitional cell carcinoma anywhere from renal pelvis to bladder.

Table 18–16. CLASSIFICATION OF CASTS

Matrix
Hyaline—variable size
Waxy—often broad in size
Inclusions
Granules—proteins, cell debris
Fat globules—triglycerides, cholesterol esters
Hemosiderin granules
Crystals—uncommon
Melanin granules—rare
Pigments
Hemoglobin, myoglobin, bilirubin, drugs
Cells
Red blood cells and red cell remnants
Leukocytes—neutrophils, possibly lymphocytes, monocytes, and histiocytes
Renal tubular epithelial cells
Mixed cells—red blood cells, neutrophils, and renal tubular cells
Bacteria

Caudate cells are merely variants of transitional cells in which one or two long cytoplasmic tails are present. These cells derive from either the renal pelvis or the bladder trigone, and have no special diagnostic significance per se.

When stained, transitional cells have dark blue nuclei with variable amounts of pale blue cytoplasm (Fig. 18–11). Another helpful clue to the proper identification of transitional cells is a characteristic "endo-ecto cytoplasmic" rim.

Squamous Epithelial Cells. Much of the female urethra and the terminal 0.5 to 1.0 cm of the male urethra are lined by squamous epithelial cells. In the urine, these cells are large and flat, with abundant cytoplasm and small round central nuclei (Fig. 18–12). Their margins are often folded. Occasionally, the cells are rolled into cylinders. Many of the squamous cells present in female urine may derive from the vagina or vulva. When stained with crystal-violet safranin, nuclei are purple and cytoplasm pink to violet. By and large, squamous cells in female urine have little diagnostic significance.

CASTS

Casts are formed as translucent, colorless gels from protein in the tubules of nephrons. In the normal person, very few are seen in the urinary sediment. In kidney diseases, they may appear in large numbers and in many forms (Table 18–16). Increased numbers of casts usually indicate that kidney disease is widespread and that many nephrons are involved. With chronic renal diseases, some casts become denser in appearance and are known as waxy. Large numbers of casts may also be seen in healthy persons after severe exercise accompanying the proteinuria of exercise.

In normal urine, there is a very small amount of protein—about 150 mg/24 hours. Albumin and small molecular plasma globulins constitute about two thirds of the protein, and about one third is the glycoprotein secreted by the thick part of the ascending loop of Henle and possibly the distal tubule. This is known as Tamm-Horsfall (TH) protein. It is generally held that TH protein forms the matrix of all casts. The protein forms a meshwork of fibrils that may trap cells, cell fragments, or granular material. Cast formation increases with lower pH and when there is stasis or obstruction of the nephron by cells or cell debris. Casts begin to disintegrate in dilute and alkaline urine or in the presence of bacteria which probably contribute to the alkalinity.

Cast formation is increased when larger than normal amounts of plasma proteins enter the tubules. Usually the protein in excess is albumin, but globulins such as the Bence Jones immunoglobulin cause cast formation, as do hemoglobin and myoglobin. The plasma proteins possibly react or combine with TH protein to form less translucent casts and granular casts.

The size and shape of casts depend on the site of formation. Large casts are seen in dilated tubules or with stasis in collecting ducts. Thin casts occur in tubules compressed by swollen interstitial tissue or because of disintegration. Sometimes casts are convoluted and occasionally show a branch. They may be short and stubby or long; long convoluted casts appear when there is diuresis after urinary stasis. Casts have parallel sides and usually have blunt ends. With age they may begin to disintegrate and show thinning and irregularities. Fibrils will separate, causing a frayed appearance. Tails and tapering ends are seen, and these disintegrating forms have been referred to as cylindroids. (See Wenk, 1981, and Haber, 1975).

Casts may be classified according to their matrix, inclusions, pigments, and cells present, as shown in Table 18–16. A detailed discussion, including clinical significance, follows.

Cast Matrix

Hyaline Casts. *Hyaline casts* are translucent with brightfield microscopy but easily seen with phase-contrast microscopy (Fig. 18–13*A* and *B*). With phase-contrast, the typical hyaline cast is seen to contain some fine granules. However, these casts are currently reported as hyaline rather than granular. Increased numbers are seen with renal diseases and transiently with exercise, fever, congestive heart failure, and diuretic therapy (Imhof, 1972).

Waxy Casts. These differ from hyaline casts in that they are easily visualized because of their high refractive index. Early waxy casts are believed by some to reflect the final phase of dissolution of the fine granules of granular casts (Fig. 18–14). Since time is required for granules to undergo lysis, waxy casts imply localized nephron obstruction and oliguria.

With brightfield microscopy, waxy casts are homogeneously smooth in appearance (Fig. 18–15). Their margins are sharp even in subdued light. Their ends are blunt, and cracks or convolutions are frequently seen along the lateral margins, indicating a measure of brittleness. Waxy casts are commonly associated with tubular inflammation and degeneration. They are observed most frequently in patients with chronic renal failure. They are also found during acute and chronic renal allograft rejection. When waxy casts are unusually broad, they are known as renal failure casts. These casts carry the implication of advanced tubular atrophy and/or dilation, in turn reflecting end-stage renal disease.

Inclusion Casts. Granules, small (fine) and large (coarse) represent plasma protein aggregates that pass into the tubules from damaged glomeruli and also cellular remnants from leukocytes, red cell remnants, or damaged renal tubular cells and possibly fine salt precipitates. Protein aggregates include fibrinogen, immune complexes, and globulins. Sometimes lipid droplets are mistaken for large granules. With prolonged stasis, large granules in casts may become smaller.

Granular Casts (Fig. 18–16). These are common. There appears to be no advantage to separating kinds of granular casts. Granular casts appear with glomerular and tubular diseases, but are a feature of tubulointerstitial disease and renal allograft rejection. Granular casts accompany pyelonephritis, viral infections, and chronic lead poisoning. Coarsely granular casts occur, with hematuria, in cases of renal papillary necrosis. It is possible that some fine granules repre-

3

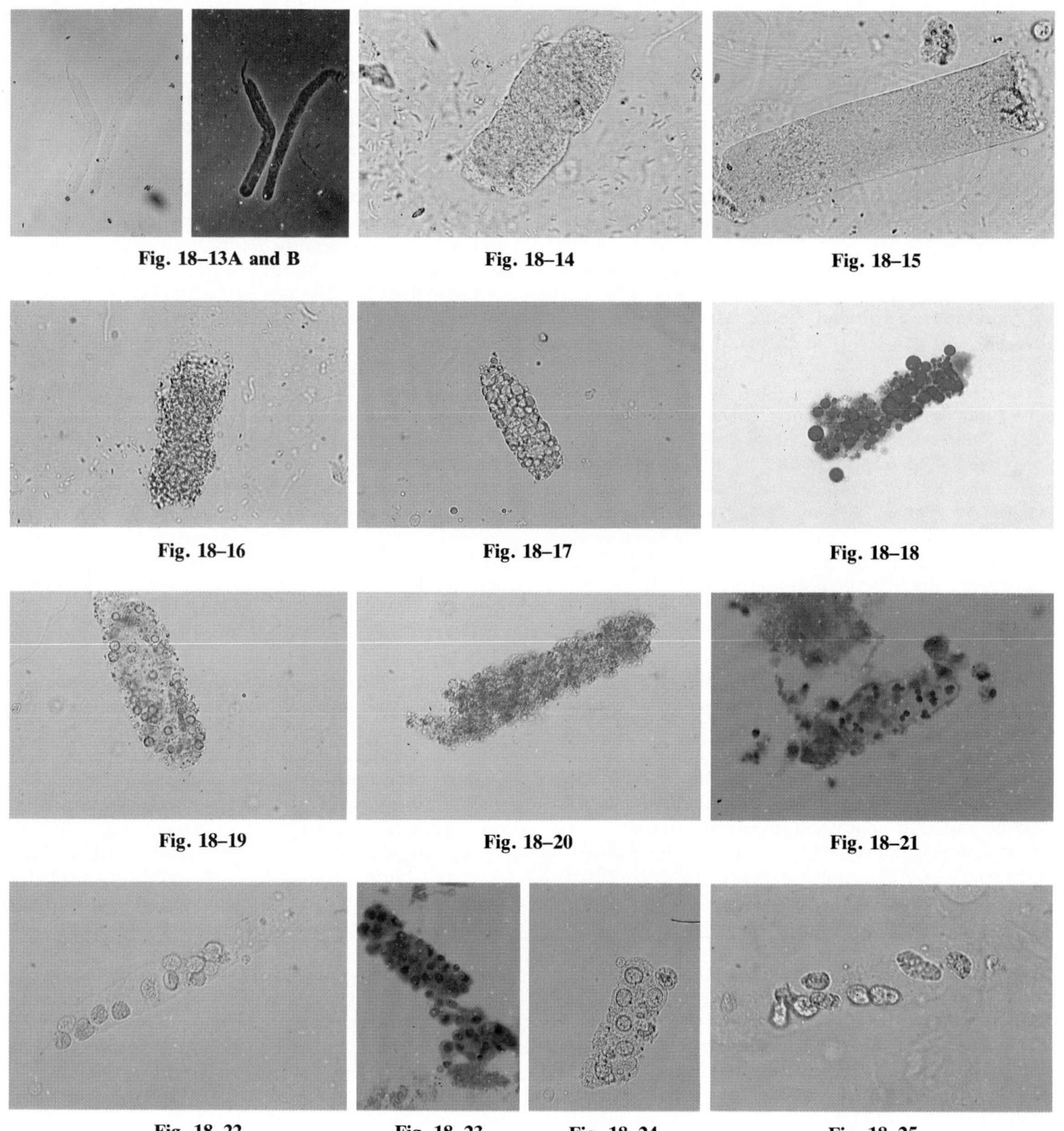

Fig. 18–13A and B

Fig. 18–14

Fig. 18–15

Fig. 18–16

Fig. 18–17

Fig. 18–18

Fig. 18–19

Fig. 18–20

Fig. 18–21

Fig. 18–22

Fig. 18–23

Fig. 18–24

Fig. 18–25

Figure 18–13. Hyaline casts: A, brightfield and, B, phase contrast microscopy (×100).

Figure 18–14. Finely granular cast becoming waxy (×200).

Figure 18–15. Waxy cast (×200).

Figure 18–16. Granular cast (×200).

Figure 18–17. Fatty cast, non-polarizing (×160).

Figure 18–18. Fatty cast, non-polarizing but positive oil red O (×200).

Figure 18–19. Red blood cell cast (×200).

Figure 18–20. Blood or hemoglobin cast (×200).

Figure 18–21. White cell cast. Papanicolaou stain (×430).

Figure 18–22. White blood cell cast (×200).

sent calcium phosphate precipitants in hyperparathyroidism. These fine granules would disappear from the hyaline matrix as the patient's urine was acidified by giving ammonium chloride and would return when the urine was allowed to become more alkaline (Albright, 1935).

Fatty Casts (Figs. 18–17 and 18–18). Fatty material is incorporated into the cast matrix from lipid-laden renal tubular cells. Visible fat droplets are triglycerides or cholesterol esters. These are commonly seen when there is heavy proteinuria and are a feature of the nephrotic syndrome. (See Renal Tubular Epithelial Cells.)

Hemosiderin Casts. Hemosiderin granules in casts derive from pigment-laden renal tubular cells.

Crystal Casts. Casts containing urates, calcium oxalate, and sulfonamides (sulfamethoxazole) are occasionally seen. A matrix is visible in a true crystal cast. The crystals polarize and are readily identifiable in and around the cast. Crystal casts should be carefully distinguished from clumps of crystals forming at room or refrigerator temperatures. These casts indicate deposition of crystals in the tubule or collecting duct. Obstruction occurs, and hematuria, possibly related to tubular damage, is regularly seen with crystal casts. Hyaline casts incorporating calcium deposits have been reported in hyperparathyroidism (see Granular Casts, above).

Pigmented Casts

Hemoglobin (Blood) Casts (see Fig. 18–20). Hemoglobin casts appear yellow to red; sometimes the color is very pale and difficult to interpret. Most often hemoglobin casts, also known as blood casts, accompany red blood cell casts and glomerular disease. Less commonly they are seen with tubular bleeding and rarely with hemoglobinuria (see Hemosiderin).

Myoglobin Casts. These casts are red-brown in color and occur with myoglobinuria following acute muscle damage. These may be associated with acute renal failure.

Bilirubin and Other Drug Casts. *Bilirubin* is seen in urine when there is obstructive jaundice, and will color casts a deep yellow brown. *Drugs,* such as Pyridium, cause a bright yellow to orange color in acid urine and will color casts and cells.

Cellular Casts

Red Blood Cell Casts. Finding these casts in the urine is of singular importance. By and large they are diagnostic of glomerular disease or renal parenchymal bleeding. Glomerular damage (most frequently due to immune injury) allows red blood cells to escape into the tubule. If there is concomitant proteinuria and conditions are optimal for cast formation, red cell casts form in the distal nephron. In urine, these casts appear yellow under the low power objectives. A prerequisite for the identification of a red blood cell cast is that red blood cell outlines be sharply defined in at least part of the cast (Fig. 18–19). If many red cells are present, the matrix may not be visible. However, there may also be delicate hyaline casts with one or two red cells visible in the matrix. These are best seen with phase microscopy. With supravital staining, the red blood cells are colorless or lavender in a pink matrix. When stasis has occurred in the nephron, a red cell cast may degenerate and appear in the urine as a reddish-brown, coarsely granular cast. Such a cast is known as a *blood* (Fig. 18–20) or *hemoglobin cast.* In the absence of concomitant bilirubinuria or Pyridium therapy (both of which spontaneously color formed elements in the urine), a pigmented, coarsely granular cast should raise the suspicion of a blood cast. Rarely there will be myoglobin casts with red-brown pigment resembling blood casts. These occur with rhabdomyolysis.

Disorders reflected in the presence of red blood cell casts in the sediment include many acute glomerulonephritides, IgA nephropathy, lupus nephritis, subacute bacterial endocarditis, and renal infarction. Rarely, tubulointerstitial disease may allow transtubular entry of red blood cells with subsequent incorporation into a cast. This may occur in severe pyelonephritis (Haber, 1975).

White Blood Cell (Leukocyte) Casts. White blood cells usually enter tubular lumina from the interstitium. They enter through and between tubular epithelial cells (Haber, 1975). Hence, diseases which might be expected to be associated with white blood cell casts (Fig. 18–21) in the urine are those in which neutrophilic exudates and interstitial inflammation are present in the kidney. The most common disease satisfying these criteria is pyelonephritis. Although it is also true that white blood cell casts may be present in glomerular disease, this is by no means a common finding. By and large white blood cells casts reflect tubulointerstitial disease.

With brightfield microscopy, leukocyte casts (Fig. 18–22) may be difficult to identify as such, particularly if stasis and nuclear fragmentation or fusion have occurred. Phase microscopy may be helpful in delineating nuclear segments.

In addition to acute pyelonephritis, white blood cell casts may be found in the urine of patients with lupus nephritis. In this disease, urine cultures are sterile. Finally, these casts have been reported in acute glomerulonephritis, interstitial nephritis, and even in the nephrotic syndrome (Schreiner, 1957).

Renal Tubular Epithelial Cell Casts. The difficulties encountered in distinguishing free polymorphonuclear cells from tubular cells are amplified when trying to identify casts in which either or both of these cell types occur. When well preserved, tubular casts contain two parallel rows of cells. This appear-

Figure 18–23. Renal tubular epithelial cast. Papanicolaou stain (×430).

Figure 18–24. Mixed white cell and renal tubular epithelial cast (×200).

Figure 18–25. Cellular cast (×200).

3

ance implies origin in one segment of a damaged tubule. When the tubular cells are randomly distributed throughout a cast, origin of the cells in different parts of the tubule may be postulated. Supravital staining, phase contrast microscopy, and Papanicolaou staining (Fig. 18–23) may be helpful in separating tubular epithelial casts from white blood cell casts.

Renal tubular epithelial cell casts are seen in urine with pure renal tubular necrosis, viral disease (e.g., cytomegalovirus disease), or exposure to a variety of drugs. Heavy metal poisoning and ethylene glycol and salicylate intoxication may cause tubular cells and casts to appear in the urine. In transplant units, these cells and casts constitute one of the more reliable criteria for detecting acute allograft rejection after the third postoperative day (Schumann, 1980).

Mixed Cellular Casts. When tubular cells and white blood cells are identified with certainty in a cast, the resulting hybrid is called a *mixed cast* (Fig. 18–24). This hybrid form implies tubulointerstitial disease. When the cell type cannot be established with certainty, the resulting cast is known as a *cellular cast* (Fig. 18–25). Some inferences as to cell type may be drawn from the dominant population of free cells in the surrounding sediment. If not, the differential diagnosis is additive, i.e., that of white blood cell casts and tubular epithelial cell casts.

Other Miscellaneous Casts or Cast-Like Structures. Bacteria on occasion may be embedded in cast matrices. On supravital staining, they appear dark purple in a pale pink matrix. Mucous threads are commonly confused with casts. However, they are larger, long, and ribbon-like, with poorly defined edges and pointed or split ends. They are readily apparent in the background of the sediment when phase contrast is used.

TELESCOPED SEDIMENT

This term is used to describe the simultaneous occurrence of elements of acute and chronic glomerulonephritis as well as those of the nephrotic syndrome in the same urine. A telescoped sediment might therefore include red cells, red cell casts, cellular casts, broad waxy casts, lipid droplets, oval fat bodies, and fatty casts. Such sediment may be found in collagen vascular disease (notably lupus nephritis) and subacute bacterial endocarditis.

ABNORMAL CELLS AND OTHER FORMED ELEMENTS

Tumor Cells. Malignant tumor cells exfoliated from the renal pelvis, ureter, bladder, wall, and urethra are best identified using cytologic techniques. Occasionally, kidney and metastatic tumor cells may be diagnosed. Myeloma cells have been described with and without apparent renal involvement (Riggs, 1975). For a comprehensive discussion of collection methods, cellular features and types of disease, one should review a standard urinary cytology textbook (Tweedale, 1977; Schumann, 1981b).

Viral Inclusion Cells. Epithelial cells with inclusion bodies may be found in the urine sediment in certain viral diseases (Dewall, 1966). Syncytial giant cells containing eosinophilic, intranuclear inclusion are seen in patients during herpetic infections. In children or immunosuppressed patients with cytomegalic inclusion disease, epithelioid cells with basophilic intranuclear inclusion and/or cytoplasmic bodies may be found in the urine sediment. Cytologic techniques are more sensitive than conventional urine microscopy in detecting virally infected cells (Schumann, 1980).

Platelets. These have been demonstrated in urine. Up to 30,000/μl were found in urine of patients with hemolytic-uremic syndrome before and after therapy. These were found by phase microscopy and confirmed by electron microscopy (Sutor, 1976).

Bacteria, Fungi, and Parasites. *Bacteria* may or may not be significant, depending on the method of urine collection and how soon after collection of the specimen the examination takes place. Well-mixed uncentrifuged urine may be examined with Gram's stain. If bacteria are identified in the uncentrifuged specimen under an oil-immersion lens, it suggests that more than 100,000 organisms per ml are present, i.e., significant bacteriuria. (See Leukocyte Esterase Test under Clinical Correlations.) Most commonly, rod-shaped bacteria are seen, since the enteric organisms are most often found in urinary tract infection. If urinary tract infection is present, many leukocytes will usually be seen in the sediment.

Using direct immunofluorescence as a means of visualizing antibody complexed with the bacteria in the urine, Thomas (1974) found a significant correlation between the presence or absence of antibody-coated bacteria and the localization of the infection in the kidney or the bladder, respectively.

Acid-fast staining of the urine sediment may reveal *tubercle bacilli,* but since the urethra may contain non-pathogenic acid-fast organisms, the presence of tubercle bacilli in urine must be substantiated by culture.

Yeast cells (Candida) are found in urinary tract infection (e.g., in diabetes mellitus), but yeasts are also common contaminants from skin and air. They may be confused with red blood cells; budding is usually seen and helps to identify them as yeast cells (Fig. 18–26). Pseudomycelial forms of *Candida* are occasionally found (Fig. 18–27).

Parasites and parasitic ova may be seen in urine sediments as a result of fecal or vaginal contamination. When these are noted, the examination should be repeated on a fresh, clean-voided urine specimen. In patients with schistosomiasis due to *Schistosoma haematobium,* typical ova may be found in the urine accompanied by red blood cells from the urinary bladder. *Trichomonads* may be present in urine as a result of vaginal contamination. When urethral or bladder infection is suspected, the protozoa should be searched for immediately in a wet preparation of the sediment; the motility of the organism is helpful in making the appropriate identification. *Amebae* are rarely seen in the urine; these may reach the bladder from lymphatics or more likely from fecal contamination of the urethra. The pathogenic *Entamoeba histolytica* is usually accompanied by erythrocytes and leukocytes.

CONTAMINANTS AND ARTIFACTS

Partly digested *muscle fibers* or *vegetable cells* may be found when there is fecal contamination (Fig. 18–28). *Spermatozoa* are occasionally present in the urine of men and are occasionally seen in urine from female patients. They are easily recognized. *Pollen grains* contaminate specimens seasonally.

Cotton, hair, and *other fibers* may be seen and are easily identified. *Wood fibers* from applicator sticks may be found if sticks are used to mix the sediment. Short *fibers from diapers* are easily confused with casts. These are found in disposable diapers. Unlike casts, these fibers polarize brightly.

Granules of starch appear bright and faintly striated and should not be confused with cells. They are irregular in outline with a central depression. With crossed polarizing filters, starch granules exhibit a typical Maltese cross. However, since they are large, several times larger than a red blood cell, they are not likely to be confused with cholesterol droplets. Starch from surgical gloves is the most common contaminant of urine and other body fluids.

Oil droplets from catheter lubricants may be confused with cells, especially red cells, but are structureless. Lipid material from vaginal creams also forms droplets in urine and may aggregate into large amorphous shapes.

CRYSTALS

By and large, crystals in the urine are of limited clinical significance. Phosphates, urates, and oxalates are especially common and occur in normal urine sediment. Their presence often deflects attention from more important formed elements. A few crystals, however, are important. For the purposes of separating these from more commonly occurring "nuisance" crystals, a summary of crystal morphology is presented (Table 18–18).

A prerequisite for the positive identification of crystals is a knowledge of the urinary pH. This helps with the preliminary separation.

Crystals Found in Normal Acid Urine

Amorphous Urates (Calcium, Magnesium, Sodium, and Potassium Urate). The amorphous material precipitates in concentrated urine of a slightly acid pH as yellow-brown small granules. The gross urine specimen precipitate may appear pink-orange to reddish-brown, and is sometimes called "brick dust." Granules form clumps and adhere to fibers and mucous threads. They convert to uric acid crystals with acidification with acetic acid and dissolve with warmth (60°C.) and with dilute alkali.

Crystalline Urates (Sodium, Potassium and Ammonium). Biurates and acid urates. Small brown spheres or colorless needles in slightly acid urine. Spheres cluster in pairs and triplets. Slowly revert to uric acid plates on acidification with acetic acid on the microscope slide (Fig. 18–29).

Crystalline Uric Acid. Low pH, 5 to 5.5. Variety of shapes, usually colored. Typically four sided, flat, yellow or reddish brown. Other shapes: rhombic plates or prisms, oval forms with pointed ends (lemon shaped), wedges, rosettes, irregular plates (Fig. 18–30 and 18–31). Rarely colorless and hexagonal like cystine (Fig. 18–32*A*). Uric acid crystals polarize and show interference colors (Fig. 18–32*B*).

Calcium Oxalates. Dihydrates appear at pH 6 or in neutral urine. Typically small, colorless, octahedrons which resemble envelopes (Fig. 18–33). Also large crystals, sometimes in clusters. Insoluble in acetic acid. Rarely dumbbell, ovoid forms (Fig. 18–34) or longer forms of calcium oxalate monohydrate are seen.

Crystals Found in Normal Alkaline Urine. Phosphates form soluble sodium and potassium salts and less soluble calcium and magnesium salts. Calcium and magnesium phosphate are the least soluble in alkaline urine; calcium and magnesium monohydrogen phosphate are not very soluble, but the dihydrogen phosphates are soluble at alkaline pH. Phosphates, in general, dissolve in acids such as dilute hydrochloric and nitric acid and vary in solubility in acetic acid. They do not dissolve in dilute sodium hydroxide solutions or alcohol.

Amorphous Phosphates (Calcium and Magnesium). Colorless amorphous granules in urine of an alkaline or slightly acidic pH. Clumps or masses seen. Typically form a fine or lacy precipitate macroscopically (Fig. 18–35).

Crystalline Phosphates. *Triple phosphate* (ammonium magnesium phosphate): Alkaline pH, often with infection present. Commonly show a variation in size. Colorless, three- to six-sided prisms with oblique ends referred to as coffin lids, less often flat fern forms. Less common. Forms colorless sheets (Fig. 18–35) or flakes. *Dicalcium hydrogen phosphate:* Long three-sided prisms with pointed end. Seen in neutral or slightly acidic urine. Form clusters or rosettes (Fig. 18–36). *Magnesium phosphate:* Forms colorless rhomboids, some with notched ends or corners. Seldom recognized.

Calcium Carbonate. Uncommon. Small granules or colorless spheres. Forms pairs or fours in alkaline urine. Produces carbon dioxide with acids.

Ammonium Biurate. Crystalline urate forming in alkaline urine. Also seen in neutral and occasionally in slightly acid urine. Usually seen with phosphate crystals and amorphous phosphates. Yellow-brown spheres referred to as thorn apples, showing radial or concentric striations and irregular projections or thorns or horns (Fig. 18–37). Dissolve with heat at 60°C. and with acetic acid, reappearing as typical uric acid crystals after about 20 minutes.

Crystals Found in Abnormal Urine. Always check the patient's drug therapy when unusual crystals are found.

Cystine. Acid pH. Colorless, refractile, hexagonal plates (Fig. 18–38), sometimes twinned. Soluble in water, $<$pH 2, $>$pH 8. Resembles some uric acid crystals. Confirm with cyanide-nitroprusside reaction described under Cystinuria. Both cystine and uric acid are soluble in ammonia water, but cystine will also dissolve in dilute hydrochloric acid and uric acid will not.

Tyrosine. Uncommon. Fine silky needles which may be arranged in sheaves or clumps, especially after

3

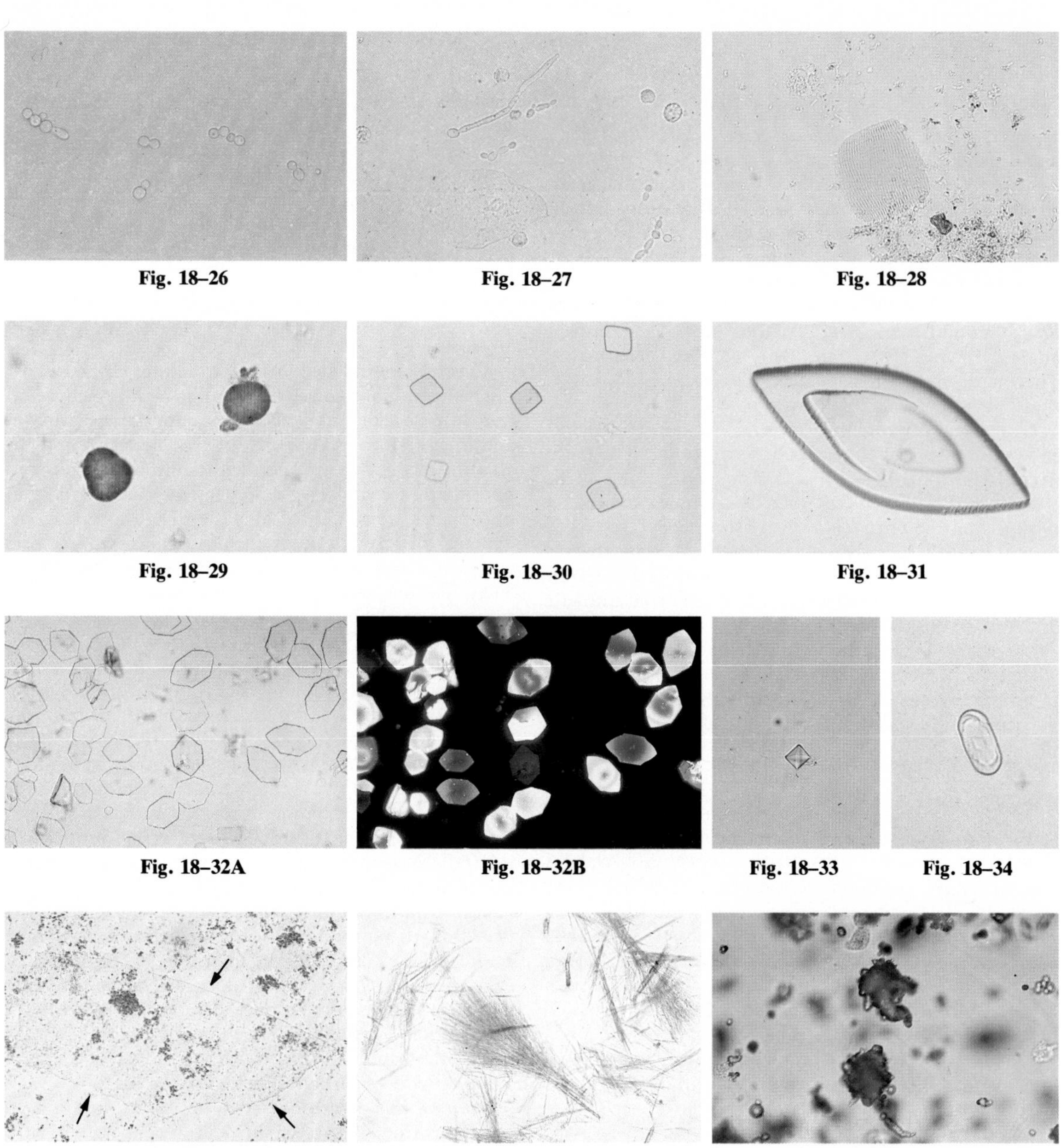

Figure 18–26. Candida: budding spores (×200).

Figure 18–27. Candida: pseudohyphae (×160, unstained).

Figure 18–28. Muscle fiber: patient with rectovesical fistula (×200).

Figure 18–29. Acid urates (×160).

Figure 18–30. Uric acid (×160).

Figure 18–31. Large uric acid plate, laminated (×160).

Figure 18–32. A, Hexagonal uric acid, unpolarized (×50); B, Hexagonal uric acid, polarized (×50).

Figure 18–33. Calcium oxalate (×200).

Figure 18–34. Unusual oval form of calcium oxalate (×200).

Figure 18–35. Large clear plate of calcium phosphate; also amorphous phosphates (×64).

Figure 18–36. Rare fine sheaves of calcium phosphate (×160).

Figure 18–37. Ammonium biurate (×160).

Table 18–17. URINALYSIS ABNORMALITIES FOUND IN VARIOUS URINARY SYSTEM DISEASES

Diseases	Macroscopic Urinalysis	Microscopic Urinalysis
Acute glomerulonephritis	Gross hematuria	Erythrocyte and blood casts
	"Smoky" tubidity	Epithelial casts
	Proteinuria	Hyaline and granular casts
		Waxy casts
		Neutrophils
		Erythrocytes
Chronic glomerulonephritis	Hematuria	Granular and waxy casts
	Proteinuria	Occasional blood casts
		Erythrocytes
		Leukocytes
		Epithelial casts
		Lipid droplets
Acute pyelonephritis	Turbid	Numerous neutrophils (many in clumps)
	Occasional "odor"	Few lymphocytes and histiocytes
	Occasional proteinuria	Leukocyte casts
		Epithelial casts
		Renal epithelial cells
		Erythrocytes
		Granular and waxy casts
		Bacteria
Chronic pyelonephritis	Occasional proteinuria	Leukocytes
		Broad waxy casts
		Granular and epithelial casts
		Occasional leukocyte cast
		Bacteria
		Erythrocytes
Nephrotic syndrome	Proteinuria	Fatty and waxy casts
	Fat droplets	Cellular and granular casts
		Oval fat bodies and/or vacuolated renal epithelial cells occurring singly or as cellular clusters
Acute tubular necrosis	Hematuria	Necrotic or degenerated renal epithelial cells
	Occasional proteinuria	Neutrophils and erythrocytes
		Granular and epithelial casts
		Waxy casts
		Broad casts
		Epithelial tissue fragments
Cystitis	Hematuria	Numerous leukocytes
		Erythrocytes
		Transitional epithelial cells occurring singly or as fragments
		Histiocytes and giant cells
		Bacteria
		Absence of casts
Dysuria-pyuria syndrome	Slightly turbid	Numerous leukocytes, bacteria
		Erythrocytes
		No casts
Acute renal allograft rejection (lower nephrosis)	Hematuria	Renal epithelial cells
	Occasional proteinuria	Lymphocytes and plasma cells
		Neutrophils
		Renal epithelial casts
		Renal epithelial fragments
		Granular, bloody, and waxy casts
Urinary tract neoplasia	Hematuria	Atypical mononuclear cells with enlarged, irregular hyperchromatic nuclei and sometimes containing prominent nucleoli that occur singly or as tissue fragments
		Neutrophils
		Erythrocytes
		Transitional epithelial cells
Viral infection	Hematuria	Enlarged mononuclear cells and/or multinucleated cells with prominent intranuclear and/or cytoplasmic inclusions
	Occasional proteinuria	Neutrophils
		Lymphocytes and plasma cells
		Erythrocytes

Table 18–18. CHARACTERISTICS OF AMORPHOUS AND CRYSTALLINE URINARY SEDIMENTS

Substance	Description	Urine pH Where Found *Acid*	*Neutral*	*Alkaline*	Solubility Characteristics and Comments
Ampicillin	Uncommon—from high dose; colorless; long prisms which form clusters, sheaves	+	–	–	
Bilirubin	Reddish brown; amorphous needles, rhombic plates, or cubes; may color uric acid crystals	+	–	–	Soluble in alkali, acid, acetone, and chloroform
Cholesterol	Rare; colorless; flat plate with corner notch; accompanies fatty casts and oval fat bodies	+	+	–	Very soluble in chloroform, ether, and hot alcohol
Calcium carbonate	Colorless; small granules in pairs, fours; spheres; rarely needles	–	+	+	Soluble in acetic acid with effervescence
Calcium oxalate	Dihydrate—common; colorless; small refractile octahedron Monohydrate—uncommon; dumbbell and ovoid rectangle	+	+	–	Soluble in dilute HCl
Cystine	Colorless; hexagonal plates, often laminated; rapidly destroyed by bacteria; may be confused with uric acid, but cystine is soluble in dilute hydrochloric acid	+	–	–	Soluble in alkali (especially ammonia) and dilute hydrochloric acid; insoluble in boiling water, acetic acid, alcohol, ether; apply cyanide-nitroprusside reaction
Hematin	Small, biconvex whetstone seen with hemoglobinuria	+	–	–	
Hemosiderin	Golden brown; granules in clumps, in cells, casts	+	+	–	Blue with Prussian blue
Hippuric acid	Rare; colorless; needles, rhombic plates and four-sided prisms; distinguish from phosphates	+	+	+	Soluble with hot water and alkali; insoluble in acetic acid
Indigotin	Rare; blue; amorphous or small crystals; colors other crystals	+	+	+	Very soluble in chloroform; soluble in ether; insoluble in acetone
Phosphates					
Amorphous phosphate (magnesium, calcium)	Colorless; fine, granular precipitate	–	+	+	Insoluble with heat; soluble with acetic acid, dilute hydrochloric acid
Calcium hydrogen phosphate	Less common; colorless; star-shaped or long, thin prisms or needles; form rosettes	sl	+	sl	Slightly soluble in dilute acetic acid; soluble in dilute hydrochloric acid
Triple phosphate (ammonium magnesium)	Common form: colorless; three- to six-sided prisms, "coffin lids" Less often: flat, fern leaf form, sheets, flakes	–	+	+	Soluble in dilute acetic acid
Radiographic media (meglumine diatrizoate)	Intravenous: colorless; thin, rhombic plates, some with notch, resemble cholesterol plates; elongated crystals Retrograde: colorless; long, pointed crystals	+	–	–	Soluble in 10% NaOH; insoluble in ether and chloroform; high specific gravity in urine; polarizes with interference colors
Sulfonamides					
Acetyl-sulfadiazine	Wheat sheaves with eccentric binding	+	–	–	
Acetyl-sulfameth-oxazole	Brown; dense spheres or irregular divided spheres	+	–	–	
Sulfadiazine	Brown; dense globules	+	–	–	Soluble in acetone

Table 18–18. CHARACTERISTICS OF AMORPHOUS AND CRYSTALLINE URINARY SEDIMENTS *Continued*

Substance	Description	Urine pH Where Found *Acid*	*Neutral*	*Alkaline*	Solubility Characteristics and Comments
Tyrosine	Rare; colorless or yellow, appear black with focusing; fine silky needles in sheaves or rosettes	+	–	–	Soluble in alkali, dilute mineral acid, relatively heat soluble; insoluble in alcohol, ether
Urates					
Amorphous (calcium, magnesium, sodium, potassium)	Common; colorless to yellow-brown; amorphous, granular precipitate	+	+	–	Soluble in dilute alkali; soluble at 60°C. or lower; change to uric acid crystal with concentrated HCl or acetic acid
Monosodium urate	Colorless; needles or amorphous precipitate	+	–	–	
Urates (sodium, potassium, ammonium)	Brown; small, spherical; clusters resemble biurates	sl	+	–	Soluble at 60°C.; change to uric acid with glacial acetic acid
Ammonium biurate	Common in "old" urine; dark yellow or brown; spheres or "thorn apples" (spheres with horns)	–	+	+	Soluble at 60°C. with acetic acid; soluble strong alkali; change to uric acid with concentrated hydrochloric or acetic acid
Uric acid	Common; yellow, red-brown, brown; large variety of shapes—rhombic, four-sided plates, rosettes, "whetstones," lemon shapes; rarely, colorless hexagonals	+	–	–	Soluble in alkali; insoluble in alcohol and acids; polarizes with interference colors
Xanthine	Rare; colorless; small, rhombic plates	+	+	–	Soluble in alkali, soluble with heat; insoluble in acetic acid

sl = Slight.

refrigeration. Colorless or yellow, appearing black as the microscope is focused (Figure 18–39). Soluble in alkali (ammonia and potassium hydroxide), also soluble in dilute hydrochloric acid. Not soluble in alcohol or ether. Less soluble than leucine; therefore more often precipitated in urine. See nitrosonaphthol test.

Leucine. Rare. Yellow, oily-appearing spheres with radial and concentric striations. Leucine and tyrosine crystals may occur together. Leucine may be precipitated with tyrosine crystals if alcohol is added to the urine. Soluble in acids and alkalis. Unlike fat globules, leucine is not soluble in ether and may be differentiated from fat.

Sulfonamide Crystals. Seen in urine of an acid pH usually less than 6. Various forms are seen depending on the form of drug involved. Occasionally colorless but usually yellow-brown. Seen as sheaves of wheat with central bindings, striated sheaves with eccentric bindings (Fig. 18–40), rosettes, arrowheads, petals, needles, and round forms with radial striations. Apply diazo reaction to confirm. The lignin test is not reliable. See Miscellaneous Tests.

Ampicillin (High Dosage). Acid pH. Long, fine colorless crystals (Fig. 18–41). Form coarse sheaves after refrigeration.

Radiographic Media (Meglumine Diatrizoate). Acid pH. Found briefly after intravenous radiographic studies. Flat, clear, colorless notched rhombic plates or longer slender rectangles. Easily polarized showing interference colors (Fig. 18–42*A* and *B*). Also seen after retrograde cystograms as long colorless needles, forming clusters after refrigeration.

Clinical Significance. Little significance can be attached to crystals detected in urine standing at room temperature. When heated to 37°C., most crystals disappear. Those still present at 37°C. might have some significance when correlated with clinical symptoms.

Phosphate crystals have little if any clinical significance. They are often seen in infected urine of alkaline pH. Large numbers of *uric acid* crystals and urates may reflect increased nucleoprotein turnover, especially during chemotherapy of leukemias or lymphoma. They may provide circumstantial evidence for the nature of small stones lodged in the ureters, especially when radiolucent and found in conjunction with raised serum uric acid levels. They may also herald the urate nephropathy of gout. *Oxalate* crystals in large numbers may reflect severe chronic renal disease or ethylene glycol or methoxyflurane toxicity. Oxaluria has come into prominence as a reflection of the increased absorption of oxalates from food following small bowel diseases and resection, notably for Crohn's disease (Dobbins, 1977). *Cystine* crystals are colorless hexagonal plates which are frequently laminated (see Fig. 18–38). They may, however, be

3

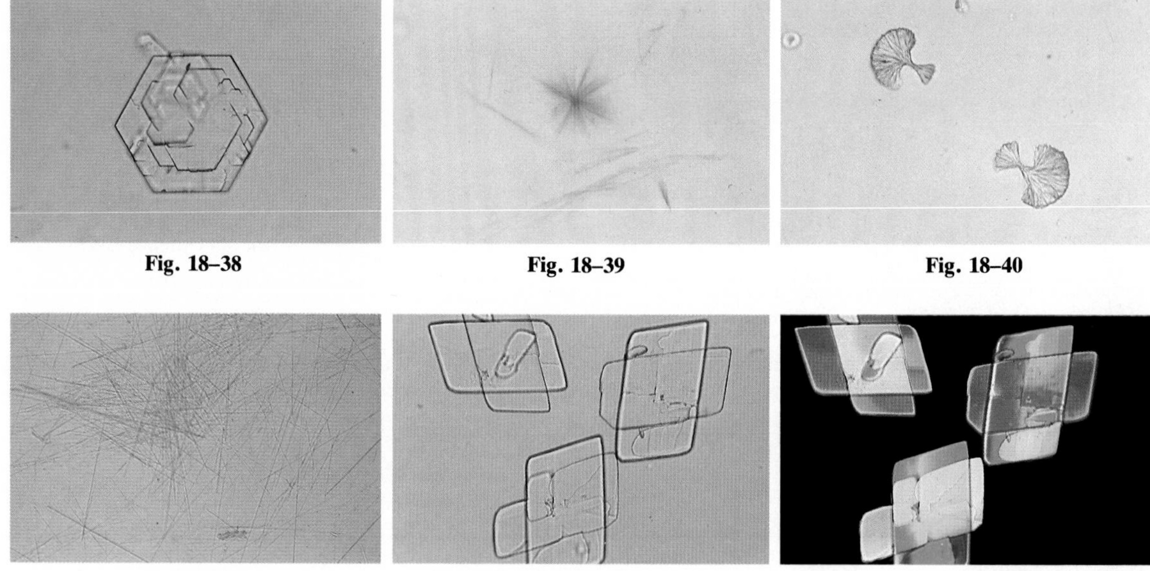

Figure 18–38. Hexagonal cystine, laminated (×200).

Figure 18–39. Tyrosine (×160).

Figure 18–40. Sulfadiazine (×160).

Figure 18–41. Ampicillin (×40).

Figure 18–42. A, Renografin, unpolarized (×160); B, Renografin, polarized (×160).

confused with hexagonal forms of uric acid (Fig. 18–32*A*). Whereas uric acid crystals polarize (Fig. 18–32*B*), thin cystine crystals do not, although thick or laminated forms do polarize. Cystine crystals are among the most important found in the urine. They occur in patients with cystinuria and may be associated with cystine calculi. *Tyrosine* and leucine crystals are occasionally seen in the urine of patients with severe liver disease. With the advent of soluble *sulfonamides,* sulfa crystals (see Fig. 18–40) are not as frequently found in urine, especially when the urine is examined at 37°C. (Alfthan, 1972). However, sulfamethoxazole (Bactrim, Septra) is seen with some regularity. Urinary crystals follow radiographic examinations with diatrizoate dyes (see Fig. 18–42*A* and *B*). *Ampicillin* may crystallize in the urine under conditions of high dosage (see Fig. 18–41). Other drugs are occasionally reported to cause crystalluria when administered in high dosage schedules or following overdosage. Examples include high dosage 6-mercaptopurine therapy (Duttera, 1972), primidone overdosage (Bailey, 1972), and dihydroxyadenine from massive blood transfusion (Falk, 1972). (See Urinary Calculi.)

Special Methods for Examination of Urine Sediment

Method for Examining Refractile Bodies in Urine. Lipid droplets or spherocrystals containing cholesterol esters are anisotropic in polarized light, show up brightly against a dark field, and appear to be divided into four quadrants. This appearance resembles a *Maltese cross.* Visible evidence of anisotropy depends on the orientation of the crystal in the field; not all will be seen. Crystals, hair, and clothing fibers also show up brightly, but do not exhibit Maltese cross forms. Fatty acids and triglyceride do not form liquid spherocrystals and do not show anisotropy, but glycosphingolipids in Fabry's disease are birefringent and may be seen in urinary sediments.

A polarizing microscope with rotating stage may be used in this examination. If one is not available, an ordinary light microscope can be easily made usable by the addition of suitable filters. Polaroid filters, consisting of an analyzer circle and a polarizer circle, are used. Install the analyzer disk in the ocular lens of a microscope by unscrewing the eye lens assembly. Insert the polarizer disk in the slotted opening under the substage condenser. Components are available for the binocular microscopes in common use, e.g., American Optical. A turret can be inserted in the microscope below the binocular head; it carries a polarizing filter (analyzer) and can be rotated in or out. A second detachable polarizing filter with an attached retardation plate is centered over the field lamp below the condenser. The set of filters is useful for the identification of synovial fluid crystals, but can also be used for crystals and lipids in urine.

Sediment from a fresh urine sample is examined. Using a high power magnification and brightfield illumination, turn one polarizing filter until a maximum darkening of the field is produced. Birefringent crystals and fibers will be seen white against a black background. If cholesterol is present, small refractile bodies will have the typical Maltese cross form in cells, casts, or free. If a red retardation plate is inserted, the cholesterol droplet will show typical blue and yellow quadrants against a red background. Starch granules will have a similar appearance when polarized but are much larger.

Method for Examining Fat in Urine

Reagent. Saturated solution of Sudan III in 70 per cent alcohol.

Procedure

1. Urine specimen must be collected in clean, fat-free container (glass, Pyrex, or polyethylene). Waxed cardboard containers are not suitable.
2. Centrifuge about 15 ml of the urine in a clean centrifuge tube for 15 minutes.
3. With a clean pipette, carefully take a drop of urine from the surface of the centrifuged specimen and transfer to a slide, making two deposits. Add a drop of Sudan stain to one and coverslip. Coverslip the unstained deposit.
4. Look at unstained specimen for fat, both brightfield and polarized. Examine the stained deposit microscopically for round droplets of fat which are colored red-orange with Sudan stain. Use the low power objective with subdued light and then the high power objective. The staining reaction may take some minutes. Paraffin oil will stain lightly with fat stains.

3

Leukocyte Peroxidase Stain (Kaplow, 1965). This is a stain for localizing peroxidase activity in which *benzidine dihydrochloride* is used as the indicator compound in a single, stable, reusable staining solution. The method is a rapid and highly sensitive one. The cells are fixed, thereby preserving cell morphology. A method for staining cells in the wet sediment has also been proposed (Prescott, 1964). By this technique, renal epithelial cells and neutrophilic leukocytes are easily differentiated. Since benzidine is carcinogenic, care must be taken in handling the material. (See NIH Guidelines, 1981.)

Reagents. The *incubation* mixture is made as follows:

30 per cent ethyl alcohol	100 ml
Benzidine dihydrochloride	0.3 g
0.132 M (3.8 per cent w/v) $ZnSO_4 \cdot 7\ H_2O$	1.0 ml
Sodium acetate ($NaC_2H_3O_2 \cdot 3\ H_2O$)	1.0 g
3 per cent hydrogen peroxide (must be fresh)	0.7 ml
1.0 sodium hydroxide	1.5 ml
Safranin O	0.2 g

The reagents should be added in the order listed and be mixed well with each addition. The benzidine salt may contain a small amount of inert residue which will not go into solution. A precipitate forms upon addition of the zinc sulfate; this dissolves upon addition of the remaining reagents. The final pH is 6.00 ± 0.05. The solution should be filtered and stored in a capped Coplin jar or bottle at room temperature. The same solution has been used satisfactorily for as long as six months.

Procedure

1. Use fresh smears or cytocentrifuged preparation of the urinary sediment. The urine should be at acid pH. Smears are made by placing a drop of the sediment on a glass slide and making a short smear with another slide edge as for

peripheral blood smears. Dry the preparation by waving it rapidly in the air. Thicker smears are made by placing a drop or two of the sediment on a slide and tilting to spread. Allow these to dry in air. Satisfactory smears have been made from refrigerated sediments up to 24 hours old provided that the pH of the specimen is acid. An albumin adhesive is not usually needed, but may be used with the cytocentrifuge method if protein is low.

2. After proper drying of the smear, fix slides for 60 seconds at room temperature in 10 per cent formol-ethanol (made by adding 10 ml of 37 per cent formaldehyde to 90 ml of absolute ethyl alcohol in a Coplin jar). Wash for 15 to 30 seconds under very gently running tap water. Shake off excess water.

3. Place *wet* slides in incubation mixture in a Coplin jar for 30 seconds at room temperature.

4. Wash briefly (five to ten seconds) in running tap water, dry, and examine.

5. If greater nuclear detail is desired, the stained preparations may be counterstained in 1 per cent aqueous cresyl violet acetate for one minute.

6. After drying, the slides may be rinsed with xylol and mounted with Permount and a coverslip. The stained preparation is stable for at least 12 months. Peroxidase activity is represented by discrete dark blue granules in the cytoplasm of granulocytes and monocytes. The cytoplasm of neutrophils is filled with blue granules (Fig. 18–6). Neutrophils are observed that are weakly stained or unstained, particularly from hypotonic urine specimens. Renal epithelial cells, squamous epithelial cells, and bacteria stain only with the safranin counterstain.

A peripheral blood smear is used as a control.

URINARY CALCULI

Calcium forms insoluble salts with oxalic acid and phosphate, and these salts precipitate as crystals in urine. In some persons crystalluria leads to stone formation. Crystal aggregates form on the surface of the renal papillae, enlarge, sometimes break away, and migrate to the ureter where their passage causes renal colic. It is possible that the mucoprotein (Tamm-Horsfall) secreted by the distal tubule has a role in causing the aggregation of crystals and their attachment to the collecting ducts or papillary tips (Hallson, 1979).

Calcium oxalate is the most commonly found constituent of urinary calculi. It precipitates at an acid or neutral pH. *Calcium phosphate* (hydroxyapatite $Ca_{10}(PO)_6(OH)_2$) forms calculi at the normal urinary pH of 6.0 to 6.5. Less commonly, *uric acid,* which is not very soluble, will crystallize at a low pH (5.3) and form stones. *Magnesium ammonium phosphate* (struvite) forms stones at alkaline pH where the ammonium level is high. They form in the pelvis of the kidney but apparently are not attached to papillae like the calcium stones. They may, however, develop on preexisting nuclei when there is infection from organisms such as Proteus causing alkalinization of the urine. These stones become large, forming casts of the kidney pelvis and showing staghorns. Mixed stones occur because calcium or uric acid crystals or stones may cause obstruction followed by infection and the subsequent deposition of ammonium salts. With the inherited renal tubular transport disease cystinuria, *cystine* stones form. Patients with renal tubular acidosis may form calcium phosphate stones; conversely, patients with renal nephrocalcinosis and stones may have subsequent renal tubular damage resulting in renal tubular acidosis.

In Prien's series (1963), calcium oxalate or a mixture of oxalate and calcium phosphate was most often found in stones (80 to 84 per cent). Mixed calcium phosphate, magnesium ammonium phosphate, and uric acid were the next most common constituents (3 to 10 per cent each), and these were followed by cystine (1 to 2 per cent). Carbonate, which is frequently detected in chemical analysis, probably results from adsorption of carbon dioxide to the calcium phosphate crystal. Rarely, calculi containing *sulfonamides* are found, and *silica* calculi have been reported in patients ingesting silica gel over a long period of time (Levison, 1982). *Triamterene* (Dyazide, Dyrenium), a relatively insoluble diuretic, contributes to stone formation. It will form 1 to 2 mm mustard-colored stones, giving a bright blue fluorescence when dissolved in butanol and with exposure to ultraviolet light (Ettinger, 1979). Although it was anticipated that *adenine* stones would be found after multiple blood transfusions using an ACD-adenine blood preservative, this has not yet been the case. Crystals were found only after enormous amounts of blood were given, 118 units (Falk, 1972). Rare adenine stones have been described in children with an inherited enzyme deficiency disorder and hyperuricemia (Simmonds, 1979). *Xanthine* stones are uncommon and may be associated with a genetic disorder with an absence of liver xanthine oxidase (Stanbury, 1983).

Kidney stones are common, with about 5/1000 person affected; in the United States the average age of onset of common calcium stones is in the 30's (Coe, 1981). Males are more often affected with calcium stones than females. Children are not often affected with calcium stones. Subsequent recurrences are frequent, but with appropriate identification of the stones and the risk factors associated with them, stone formation may be greatly reduced. Upper (renal) stones are common in western industrialized countries, while bladder stones are uncommon. Most of the stones received for analysis are very small calcium oxalate stones; occasionally the larger phosphate stones, cystine stones, and uric acid stones are submitted.

The passage of stones down the ureter produces renal colic, which is characterized by severe pain in the back radiating to the groin. Stones may also be passed through the urethra with great pain. Hematuria is a common urinary finding when symptoms of stone are present. If stones obstruct the pelvis of the kidney or ureter, hydronephrosis will result. Infection is a common consequence.

Laboratory Tests Used to Investigate Stone Formers

1. Urine examinations. (a) Routine urinalysis, qualitative test for cystine, and urine culture. (b) Twenty-four hour urine specimen: Sodium, calcium, phosphorus, uric acid, oxalate, and creatinine clearance. Quantitative urine studies may have to be

repeated. (c) Urine pH determination on a fresh specimen is important in determining the kinds of crystals likely to be precipitated, for example, uric acid with low pH (5 to 5.5), and triple phosphate with alkaline urine.

2. Serum chemistry. Calcium, phosphorus, uric acid, and electrolytes.

3. Stone analysis.

4. Radiologic examination. Asymptomatic stones are sometimes found. All stones are radiopaque except pure uric acid and the rare xanthine; cystine stones are opaque because of their sulfur content.

Urinalysis reveals hematuria. This is a constant finding when stones are present, even when they are asymptomatic. Red cell casts are not found; other casts are unusual. Leukocytes are increased when infection is present. Multiple clusters of non-malignant transitional cells may be found in urine of patients with calculous disease and may be helpful in the diagnosis of unsuspected calculi (Highman, 1982).

Proteinuria is usually not a feature of calculous disease, but with renal tubular damage there may be increased excretion of low molecular weight plasma proteins such as β_2 microglobulin, and some albumin.

Crystals may or may not be found when stones are present. Large calcium oxalate crystals in clusters are said to be associated with stone formation. Both the dihydrate and monohydrate forms are found. Calcium phosphate (apatite) appears as fine granules, whereas calcium hydrogen phosphate (brushite) is seen as colorless, long, thin flat crystals, and triple phosphate in alkaline urine as colorless "coffin lids." Uric acid forms fine granules and a variety of crystal shapes usually yellow to brown in color. Cystine classically presents as hexagonal, colorless flat crystals at an acid pH.

Calcium Stones. Calcium oxalate stones are the most common. Calcium stones form when there is excess oxalate and also with excess uric acid in urine. The uric acid crystals may provide a nidus for stone formation.

Newly formed calcium oxalate aggregates are about 20 to 25 μm in diameter, much smaller than the outlet of the collecting ducts. Adherence to the surface apparently allows them to grow, rather than be excreted. Calcium salts as opposed to uric acid, cystine, and triple phosphate tend to plug the nephrons. Calcium hydrogen phosphate (as brushite) crystallizes more readily in stone formers and may form a nucleus for calcium oxalate stones and for calcium phosphate stones largely composed of the hydroxyapatite form of calcium phosphate. Calcium phosphate stone formation rather than oxalate is favored by a less acid urine as seen in renal tubular acidosis, with infection, and in persons consuming large amounts of alkali. Calcium phosphate stones are also seen in primary hyperparathyroidism, although the urine is in the normal pH range. In a patient exposed to heat and dehydration, these may contribute to a rise in urinary solute levels, followed by crystallization and stone formation.

Causes of Hypercalciuria. Increased calcium in urine results from an increase in intestinal calcium absorption, a lack of appropriate renal tubular reabsorption of calcium, resorption or loss of calcium from bone, or a combination of these. About 10 g of calcium is filtered by the kidneys each day, and all but a small fraction is normally reabsorbed by renal tubular cells.

Calcium homeostasis is maintained by the parathyroid hormone (PTH) and 1,25-dihydroxycholecalciferol [1,25-$(OH)_2D$]. Low serum ionized calcium levels cause increased PTH secretion, and low serum phosphorus stimulates 1,25-$(OH)_2D$ synthesis. Both effect bone resorption by osteoclasts. PTH causes a diminution of phosphorus reabsorption and an increase in calcium reabsorption by renal tubular cells. PTH also causes increased synthesis of 1,25-$(OH)_2D$ which acts on the small intestinal mucosa, causing increased absorption of calcium and phosphorus.

About 40 per cent of patients with calcium stones will have hypercalciuria. Urine calcium levels of more than 300 mg/day in males or 250 mg/day in females are regarded as excessive when the patients are receiving a test diet containing 1 g of calcium per day.

Dietary hypercalciuria is not a common cause of calcium stones; it is associated with large calcium intake, in the order of 3 to 4 g/day, and also with large protein intake. About 800 mg/day is a normal recommended adult intake.

Increased absorption of calcium from the gut and hypercalciuria occur when there is excessive loss of phosphorus from the kidney and low serum phosphorus levels, when there is increased serum 1,25-$(OH)_2D$ with normal serum phosphorus levels, and in an unknown group when serum factors are normal.

3

Table 18–19. QUANTITATIVE TESTS IN INVESTIGATION OF STONE FORMATION*

	mg/24 hours		
	Male	***Female***	**mg/kg/24 Hours**
Urine calcium	300	250	4
Urine oxalate†	50	50	0.73
Urine uric acid	800	750	
Cystine in urine			
Homozygous	>300 mg/g creatinine per 24 hours		
Heterozygous	60–300 mg/g creatinine per 24 hours		

*Usual upper limits of normal range.

†50 mg/24 hours/1.73 m² useful for children.

Patients with *renal loss* of calcium due to a defect in renal tubular calcium reabsorption have increased calcium reabsorption from the gut. Furosemide, a diuretic, also causes renal hypercalciuria.

Increased *resorption of bone* causes hypercalciuria. This occurs with immobilization of the skeleton, rapidly progressive bone disease, thyrotoxicosis, and Cushing's disease. Calcium is lost from bone due to osteolytic tumors and also in the presence of renal disease such as distal renal tubular acidosis and medullary sponge kidney.

Excessive loss of calcium in urine and the possibility of stone formation are therefore secondary to a number of diseases, including sarcoidosis and vitamin D excess, but also to unknown causes.

Primary *hyperparathyroidism* causing increased mineral turnover in bone and hypercalcemia is an important cause of hypercalciuria. It often presents with stone symptoms, and there may be calcium phosphate deposits in the renal tissue, cornea, and other organs. About 5 to 10 per cent of calcium stones are associated with primary hyperparathyroidism. Patients with intermittent hypercalcemia may also have persistent hypercalciuria and stones (Stewart, 1981).

Causes of Hyperoxaluria. The majority of calcium stones (70 to 80 per cent) contain oxalate. Some of the oxalate in urine is *dietary* in origin from beverages (tea, cocoa, coffee, cola), vegetables (beans, rhubarb, spinach), nuts, berries, and citrus fruits. Oxalate is also derived from ascorbic acid. Diseases of the *small bowel* such as Crohn's disease, ileal resection, and intestinal bypass surgery result in excessive oxalate absorption, probably in the colon, and excretion in the urine. Oxalate absorption increases when calcium and magnesium intakes are decreased. Malabsorption with steatorrhea causes loss of calcium as soaps, and malabsorption with increased bile salts remaining in the gut is thought to promote oxalate absorption in the colon. Pyridoxine deficiency is associated with oxalate stones. *Primary hyperoxaluria* is a rare inherited autosomal recessive disease with oxoglutarate carboligase deficiency. There is systemic oxalosis and renal failure in young adulthood. Renal transplantation and large doses of pyridoxine or nicotinamide have been tried for the treatment of these patients. (See Coe, 1978, and Brown, 1982.)

Causes of Hyperuricuria. Uric acid is a weak acid and at pH 5.5 forms free, insoluble, undissociated uric acid and a urate which is more soluble with *some* sodium and potassium present. The amount of free uric acid present in urine will decrease as the pH rises. At pH 7, uric acid is more soluble as urate, but with high salt concentrations the urate becomes less soluble. Solute concentration as well as pH appears to be important in the solubility of uric acid and urate. While large quantities of uric acid crystals are regularly seen in urinary sediment, uric acid stone formation is not common. Uric acid crystals form a sludge that may obstruct the nephron without forming a stone. On the other hand, uric acid and sodium acid urate crystals are found as nuclei for calcium stones. The average uric acid excretion by adults is 500 to 600 mg/24 hours. If the urine volume is low, solubility of uric acid at acid pH will be exceeded. Most normal persons with a pH of 6 will have urine saturated with uric acid but do not form stones. Further acidity or dehydration is apparently required to engender stone formation.

Excessive excretion of uric acid relates to *excessive dietary intake* of purines (liver, dried beans, some fish, meat). Endogenous uric acid production is increased in gout, glycogen storage diseases, Lesch-Nyhan syndrome, myelogenous leukemia, acute leukemia in childhood, and treated tumors with associated cell necrosis. *Chemotherapy* and irradiation cause cell necrosis. Increased breakdown of tumor cells (nucleotide/purine forms uric acid) has caused acute renal failure because of tubular and ureter obstruction by masses of uric acid crystals. In *gout,* about 20 per cent of patients form stones, most of which are pure uric acid and others uric acid and calcium. Heat and dehydration and unusually acid urine contribute to stone formation. There is gouty nephropathy with sodium urate deposits in the medulla even when stones are not present, and masses of crystals may cause obstruction of terminal collecting ducts in the kidney (Cameron, 1979).

Normally about one third of the uric acid formed is degraded by bacteria in the colon. Absence of bacteria or intestinal diversions cause increased absorption of uric acid from the gut. Because ileostomy patients lose large amounts of alkaline fluid from the intestine, they excrete concentrated acidic urine and are likely to produce uric acid stones. Uricosuric drugs cause potential problems with massive uric acid output in the first three to four days of treatment.

Cystinuria. Cystine stones form in patients with an inherited amino acid transport disorder for cystine, ornithine, lysine, and arginine and subsequent excretion of large amounts of these amino acids in the urine. Only cystine forms crystals and stones. Cystine does not become soluble until the urine pH is 7.4, and stones form over a range of normal urinary pH. Heterozygous carriers for the disease will have increased amounts of cystine in urine but do not form stones. Homozygotes are stone formers. A 24-hour quantitative urine cystine measurement is needed to detect the potential stone formers and should always be done when crystals are found in random specimens.

Monitoring Patients. For the common calcium stones, large amounts of fluids and thiazide diuretics are used for treatment. Thiazides plus allopurinol are used for patients with calcium stones who have increased calcium and uric acid in urine. Urine calcium levels are monitored and reduced to below 4 mg/kg/24 hours and urate excretion to below 700 mg/24 hours (male) and 650 mg/24 hours (female) (Coe, 1981). There is some disagreement about the necessity for drug therapy in all of these patients. When applicable for uric acid stones, urinary pH is raised with bicarbonate to 6 to 6.5, or diuretics and allopurinol may be used to reduce hyperuricemia and hyperuricosuria. Alkalinizing urine sufficiently for cystine stone formers is difficult, and large fluid intake is used for treatment.

Stones resulting from infection contain bacteria and are removed surgically and the appropriate fluids and antibiotic therapy instituted.

Analysis of Calculi

Gross Appearance. Calculi may be of various sizes, commonly described as sand, gravel, or stone. Large round stones are characteristic of those found in the bladder; however, large rounded and staghorn shapes derive from the kidney pelvis. The physical characteristics of the various calculi rarely will suffice for their identification, but a few points are worth noting. Uric acid and urate stones are always colored yellow to brownish red and are moderately hard. Phosphate stones are usually pale and friable. Calcium oxalate stones are very hard, often of a dark color, and typically have a rough surface. Cystine stones are the color of old yellow brown soap and feel somewhat greasy.

Several methods are available for the analysis of calculi, such as optical crystallography, x-ray diffraction, and infrared spectroscopy. Electron beam analysis and mass spectroscopy are also used. A review of chemical methods is presented by Beeler (1964).

A quantitative method for five of eight frequently measured substances has been described using available clinical chemistry methods: calcium, phosphorus, magnesium, ammonium, and uric acid. Cystine, oxalate, and carbonate are detected by qualitative means and interpreted with the quantitative results to characterize the stones (Westbury, 1970).

Qualitative Analysis of Urinary Calculi*
Gross Examination of Calculi

1. If not done previously, wash the stone(s) free from blood, mucus, preservation solution, etc. Stones submitted after sonic disintegration have blood and tissue adhering and are difficult to clean. Place stones in a beaker, cover with several thicknesses of gauze held firmly in place with rubber bands, and wash under cold running water. Drain, remove gauze carefully, and dry beaker and stones in an oven. Rinse tiny stones with water from a squeeze bottle (not running water).
2. Record the dimension of the stone.
3. Describe briefly the color and texture of the stone's exterior surface. The stone may be photographed for record purposes.
4. Cut, saw, or break the stone so as to examine the interior. Note whether there is a foreign body which may have acted as a nucleus for its formation. Describe the color and texture of the interior and layers, if present.
5. Reduce small stones to a fine powder by pulverizing with a mortar and pestle.
6. If possible, where there is a very large stone, it may be advisable to make separate analyses of layers which appear to have different constituents.

Reagents. Some of these are for the rarer stones and are not routinely used. Reagent kits are available.†

1. 20 per cent sodium carbonate.
2. 20 per cent sodium hydroxide.
3. 10 per cent ammonium hydroxide.
4. Nessler's reagent: Prepare commercially available Nessler's compound, reagent brand, Koch-McMeekin formula, according to instructions on label. Store at room temperature.
5. Uric acid reagent (phosphotungstic acid) (Harleco). Add 40 g lithium sulfate ($Li_2SO_4 \cdot H_2O$) to each liter.
6. Sulfuric acid–ammonium molybdate reagent (Fiske and Subbarow phosphorus method): Dissolve 2.5 g ammonium molybdate in 50 ml of 10 N sulfuric acid and dilute to 100 ml with distilled water.
7. Amino naphthol sulfonic acid reagent (Fiske and Subbarow phosphorus method): Store this reagent in a dark bottle. Prepare commercially available product according to directions on the label, heating slightly to aid solution.
8. Magnesium reagent: 0.001 per cent nitrobenzene azoresorcinol in 2 N sodium hydroxide. Store in a polyethylene bottle in a dark place.
9. Five per cent sodium cyanide (preserved with 1 ml 28 per cent ammonium hydroxide per 500 ml solution). Prepare under a hood. Refrigerate; stores three months. Dispose of with care.
10. Five per cent sodium nitroferricyanide (nitroprusside). This solution is quite unstable. At the time of testing dissolve a few crystals in a small test tube of distilled water and use fresh. If stored, use a brown glass bottle and store in a refrigerator, but check for reactivity before using in the test.
11. Ten per cent hydrochloric acid.
12. Saturated ammonium oxalate.
13. Manganese dioxide powder (native powder, not reagent grade).

For Rare Stones

1. 0.1 per cent sodium nitrite ($NaNO_2$)—prepared fresh on alternate days for sulfonamide test.
2. 0.5 per cent ammonium sulfamate for sulfonamide test.
3. Sulfa dye reagent: 0.1 per cent (w/v) N-(1-naphthyl) ethylenediamine dihydrochloride. The dye is more soluble in warm water. Store this solution in a dark bottle. Refrigerate.
4. Concentrated nitric acid—xanthine test.
5. Concentrated sulfuric acid—cholesterol test.
6. Acetic anhydride—cholesterol test.
7. Chloroform—cholesterol test.

Controls. Use known stones. It is important to have known positive material to test the reagents.

Sequence of Chemical Determinations in Urinary Calculi. Since most small calculi consist of calcium oxalate, the best way to analyze them is to put all available powder in one test tube. (If the stone is very tiny, it may be placed directly in the test tube and crushed with a spatula.) Add HCl, pour off the supernatant for the calcium, and add MnO_2 to the residue for the oxalate. If the stone is a little larger, then some of the powder could be used to test for phosphates. Perform tests in the sequence shown in Table 18–20 when there is a sufficient amount of stone for all of the analyses.

MISCELLANEOUS TESTS

Indican (Indoxyl Sulfate)

Patients with bacterial overgrowth in the small intestine excrete large amounts of metabolites of amino acids such as tryptophan or tyrosine in urine. These

*Adapted from Winer (1943, 1959).
†Sherwood Medical Industries, Oxford Division, Foster City, California.

3

Table 18–20. SEQUENCE OF CHEMICAL ANALYSIS OF CALCULI

Chemical Group	Reagents and Treatment	Positive Results and Interpretations
1. Carbonates	Relatively large sample of pulverized stone in test tube. 10–15 drops 10% HCl.	Foaming effervescence
	CO_2 is displaced by HCl from the carbonates. $Na_2CO_3 + 2HCl \rightarrow 2NaCl + H_2CO_3 \rightarrow H_2O + CO_2\uparrow$	
	If carbonates are present, allow effervescence to cease. Save most of the supernatant for determinations 5, 6, and 7. Either pour off or take off the acid extract in an aspirating pipette, the tip of which has been lightly plugged with cotton. Remove the cotton by seizing the projecting wisp and divide the "filtrate" into three aliquots for 5, 6, and 7. The original test tube containing the pulverized stone and a few drops of HCl is then used for determination 2.	
2. Oxalates	Test tube from determination 1. Add a pinch of MnO_2; do not mix or shake the tube. It may be necessary to warm the contents of the tube very slightly to obtain reaction of trace quantities.	Effervescence or tiny bubbles of CO_2 popping upward from the sediment of the tube.
	MnO_2 acts as an oxidizing agent in the production of CO_2. $2CaC_2O_4 + 2HCl + MnO_2 \rightarrow 2CaCO_3 + MnCl_2 + CO_2\uparrow$	
3. Phosphates	Pulverized stone in test tube. 1 drop 10% HCl 2 drops $H_2SO_4^-$ molybdate reagent 1 drop amino-naphtholsulfonic acid	Blue color develops. If present in trace quantities, this occurs upon standing in a few minutes.
	The blue color is due to reduced oxides of molybdenum.	
4. Urates and uric acid	Pulverized stone in test tube. 1 drop 20% Na_2CO_3 2 drops uric acid reagent	Prompt *deep* blue color. Pale blue color is negative.
	Uric acid reduces orthophosphoric acid, producing a blue color.	
5. Calcium	Acid extract on microscopic slide. 2–3 drops saturated $(NH_4)_2C_2O_4$	White precipitate or film. The film reaction is most noticeable if slide is held over a dark background.
	Calcium ions in the presence of ammonium oxalate produce a white precipitate of calcium oxalate.	
6. Magnesium	Acid extract in test tube 2–3 drops 20% NaOH 2–3 drops "Mg" reagent	Reddish purple reagent slowly becomes a definite (cornflower) blue and precipitate forms.
	By rendering the acid extract alkaline, $Mg(OH)_3$ is formed. The azo dye is absorbed by the $Mg(OH)_3$ in alkaline solution. The sensitivity is very dependent upon the OH-ion concentration.	
7. Ammonium group	Acid extract in test tube 2–3 drops 20% NaOH 2–3 drops Nessler's reagent	Orange-brown (rusty) precipitate. Positive test differentiates NH_4-urates from uric acid. Positive test indicates triple phosphates vs. Ca or Mg phosphates.
	Ammonia, produced from the ammonium group in alkaline solution, reacts with the double iodide in Nessler's reagent to form dimercuric ammonium iodide (the orange-brown precipitate)	
8. Cystine	Pulverized stone in test tube 1 drop 10% NH_4OH 1 drop 5% NaCN (wait 5 min.) 2–3 drops sodium nitroprusside solution	*Beet-red* color is a positive reaction which may fade to orange-red upon standing.
	Nitroprusside reaction: Proteins with a free SH (cysteine) group yield a reddish color with sodium nitroprusside in an ammoniacal solution. The cystine -S-S- groups in protein may be reduced to -SH groups by reducing agents such as NaCN, after which they give the nitroprusside reaction.	

Table 18–20. SEQUENCE OF CHEMICAL ANALYSIS OF CALCULI *Continued*

Rare Stones	Reagents and Treatment	Positive Results and Interpretations
1. Sulfonamides	Pulverized stone in test tube 2 drops 10% HCl (wait 30 min.) 2 drops 0.1% $NaNO_2$ (wait 30–60 min.) 2 drops 0.5% NH_4-sulfamate 2–3 drops sulfa dye reagent	Magenta color is a positive reaction.
	The presence of any sulfonamide derivative is determined by the diazotization of a free amino group. Excess $NaNO_2$ is destroyed by ammonium sulfamate and the purplish red azo dye is formed by the coupling of the diazotized sulfanilamide with N-(1-naphthyl) ethylenediamine dihydrochloride.	
2. Cholesterol	Pulverized stone in test tube. Add 1 ml chloroform, mix, heat over steam bath. Allow to stand until the insoluble material settles out. Decant into test tube. To this add 3 drops acetic anhydride and 1 drop concentrated H_2SO_4.	Test solution becomes red, then blue, and finally blue-green in color.
	Liebermann-Burchard reaction: Transient colors are probably due to halochromic salts of either the unsaturated sterol or a product of it further dehydrated.	
3. Xanthine	Xanthine is difficult to separate from uric acid, so that the x-ray diffraction method is probably better for identification. Pulverized stone in evaporating dish. Add 2 drops concentrated HNO_3, and evaporate to complete dryness over steam bath. Cool slightly. Add 1 drop 20% NaOH. Warm again.	Residue left after evaporation is yellow. After addition of NaOH, an orange color develops, which becomes red upon warming.
	Xanthoproteic reaction: This is due to the nitration of the phenyl rings present in tryosine, phenylalanine, and tryptophan to give yellow nitro substitution products, which become orange upon the addition of alkali (salt formation).	

In doing the qualitative test for xanthine, colored reactions will also be obtained from uric acid. The dried residue after evaporation is lemon yellow with xanthine, but is orange with uric acid. After addition of NaOH, an orange color develops, becoming red with warming when xanthine is present; if uric acid is present, a cherry red to purple color develops immediately after addition of NaOH.

are used as an indication of the presence of stasis and infection.

Indole is produced by bacterial action on tryptophan in the intestine. Most is eliminated in the feces; the remainder is absorbed and detoxified in the liver to be excreted as *indican* in the urine.

$$\text{Indole} \xrightarrow{\text{oxidized}} \underset{\text{(liver)}}{\text{indoxyl} + H_2SO_4} + K^+ \rightarrow$$

$$\underset{\text{(urine)}}{\text{indican (indoxyl potassium sulfate)}} \rightarrow \text{indigotin (blue)}$$

In normal urine the amount of indican excreted is small; it is increased with high-protein diets. In disease it originates from *bacterial growth,* often in the *small intestine,* and is increased with intestinal obstruction, gastric cancer, hypochlorhydria, biliary obstruction, and malabsorptive syndromes such as sprue and blind loop syndrome. Evidence of bacterial growth in the small intestine is probably most reliably detected by identifying bacterial deconjugation of bile salts with the ^{14}C-glycocholic acid breath test.

In the hereditary *Hartnup disease,* many amino acids are poorly absorbed from the intestine, and this allows bacterial decomposition to take place. Indoxyl sulfate and indole-3-acetic acid are formed from tryptophan and excreted in the urine in large quantities together with large amounts of amino acids that are not reabsorbed. The blue indigo color may appear on diapers.

Tyrosine from dietary protein is degraded to *p*-tyramine by bacterial L-amino acid decarboxylase. Tyramine is deaminated and oxidized to 4-hydroxyphenylacetic acid which is excreted unconjugated in urine. It is determined by gas-liquid chromatography on random urine samples (Chalmers, 1979). Excessive amounts are found in patients with cystic fibrosis, *Giardia lamblia* infestation, ileal resection with a stagnant loop, and hyperoxaluria.

The test for indoxyl potassium sulfate depends upon its decomposition and subsequent oxidation of the indoxyl to indigo blue and its absorption by chloroform.

Procedure. To 5 ml of fresh urine in a test tube, add 5 ml of ferric chloride reagent (0.2 per cent in concentrated HCl). Mix. Add 2 ml chloroform and invert several times. Allow the chloroform to settle and observe. When indican is present, the chloroform layer shows a deep violet to blue color. Normal urine may give a faint blue color. Report as positive or negative. Normally less than 100 mg is excreted in 24 hours.

Comment. Indigo red may form occasionally because of slow oxidation. If iodides are present, iodine will be formed by oxidation and cause a violet color; thymol will also cause a violet color. These are removed by adding a crystal of sodium thiosulfate.

Bile pigments interfere with the reaction and should be removed by shaking the urine with barium chloride and filtering. Formalin will also interfere with the reaction.

Urine from cows and horses will usually give positive reactions and may be used for comparison.

5-Hydroxy Indoleacetic Acid

Serotonin (5-hydroxytryptamine) is produced by the argentaffin cells of the intestines from tryptophan and is carried in the blood by platelets (see bottom of this page).

Carcinoid tumors (argentaffinoma) arising from the argentaffin cells produce excessive amounts of serotonin, especially when metastatic. Serotonin causes intestinal disturbances, vasomotor disturbances, and bronchoconstriction. Edema, right-side valvular heart disease, and neurologic symptoms are seen. The screening test (Sjoerdsma, 1955) is useful for the detection of the serotonin metabolite 5-hydroxy indoleacetic acid in the urine if it appears in fairly large amounts. The quantitative method is more sensitive, since it eliminates the interfering ketoacids and indoleacetic acid (Udenfriend, 1955).

Normal excretion of 5-hydroxy indoleacetic acid in 24 hours is 1 to 5 mg. A random specimen of urine is usually sufficient for screening purposes; if a 24-hour collection is made, it should be acidified with HCl. (See Collection of Urine.) Boric acid may also be used as a preservative. Patients should not take any drugs for 72 hours before the test; phenothiazines, acetanilid drugs, and mephenesin, a muscle relaxant, will interfere with this test.

The principle of the test is based on the development of a purple color specific for 5-hydroxy indoles with nitrous acid and 1-nitroso-2-naphthol. Ethylene dichloride is used to remove interfering chromogens.

Reagents. 1-Nitroso-2-naphthol, 0.1 per cent in 95 per cent ethanol. Nitrous acid prepared fresh by adding 0.2 ml of 2.5 per cent sodium nitrite solution to 5 ml 2 N H_2SO_4. Ethylene dichloride.

Procedure. Pipette into a test tube 0.2 ml urine, 0.8 ml distilled water, 0.5 ml 1-nitroso-2-naphthol solution. Mix well. Add 0.5 ml fresh nitrous acid and mix. Allow to stand at room temperature for ten minutes. Shake with 5.0 ml ethylene dichloride and allow the two layers to separate. A positive test shows a purple color in the upper aqueous layer. Always use known positive and negative controls. Control solutions may be kept frozen. The following control may be used. Dissolve 7 mg 5-hydroxy indoleacetic acid in 5 ml of glacial acetic acid and dilute to 25 ml with deionized water. Use 0.2 ml of control and follow procedure for unknown.

Interpretation. A purple color may appear with as little as 40 mg 5-hydroxy indoleacetic acid in 24 hours. Patients with malignant carcinoid tumors may excrete up to 350 mg 5-hydroxy indoleacetic acid per day, and the test will show a black color. Positive findings should be checked with a quantitative method. Since the quantitative method is more sensitive, it may be necessary to do this when clinically indicated even when the qualitative test is negative. For interfering substances, see Young (1975).

Melanin

Melanin is a pigment derived from tyrosine, which is normally present in hair and skin and in the eye. There are two recognized metabolic pathways for the conversion of tyrosine to melanin, the eumelanin (brown or black) and the pheomelanin (yellow-red) pathways. Normal melanocytes in skin convert tyrosine to dihydroxy phenylalanine (DOPA) and then to dopaquinone and by oxidative steps to eumelanin. The enzyme tyrosinase is required for the first step and is found in the specific organelles of melanocytes called melanosomes. Its formation is stimulated by melanin stimulating hormone. The number of granules present is related to the amount of pigmentation seen. Melanosomes with pigment are normally transferred from melanocytes to skin and mucous membrane cells. Large melanosomes are found in tumor cells, e.g., nevus, melanoma.

An increased urinary excretion of melanin metabolites occurs as malignant melanoma metastasizes. These are called urinary melanogens and include indoles, catechols, and catecholamines. DOPA does not appear in large amounts in urine from melanotic patients, and it is unusual to find a dark color even after standing at room temperature for 24 hours.

Rarely, cells containing melanin pigment are seen in urine sediment when there is melanuria with pigment uptake by renal tubular cells, and when there is metastatic melanoma to the bladder (Piva, 1964). A ferrous ion uptake stain can be used to color the melanin in cells dark blue.

Screening tests for melanin should be made on fresh specimens of urine. Ferric chloride, Ehrlich's aldehyde reagent, and nitroferricyanide will give non-specific color reactions with melanin. There is no simple specific test for melanuria.

A column cation-exchange chromatographic method has been described that allows detection of abnormal metabolites in urine and the early detection of liver metastases (Banda, 1977). Another approach is to measure DOPA-oxidase levels in urine. The enzyme is increased in the urine of patients with melanoma and markedly increased with liver metastases (Roguljic, 1975).

Ferric Chloride Test for Melanin

Procedure. To 5 ml urine in a test tube, add 1 ml 10 per cent $FeCl_3$ in 10 per cent HCl. A gray or black precipitate will form if positive. The HCl prevents phosphate precipitation. Melanogens are oxidized to melanin.

$$\text{Tryptophan} \xrightarrow{\text{hydroxylase}} \text{5-OH tryptophan} \xrightarrow{\text{decarboxylase}}$$

$$\text{5-OH tryptamine} \xrightarrow{\text{monoamine oxidase}} \text{5-OH-indoleacetic acid}$$

Homogentisic acid, which also causes a dark color in urine, gives a transient blue-green color with ferric chloride. This test may be used as a screening test.

Nitroferricyanide Test for Melanin

Procedure. To 2 ml urine in a test tube, add three to four drops fresh solution of sodium nitroferricyanide (nitroprusside) (shake a few crystals in 10 ml water). Add two drops of 10 per cent NaOH to make the solution alkaline. Shake. A red color will develop if acetone, creatinine, or melanin is present. Acidify with two drops of glacial acetic acid. Small amounts of melanogens cause a green color; larger amounts cause a blue, then black color. Acetone causes a purple color and creatinine an amber color (Beeler, 1961). This test is more specific than the ferric chloride test.

Phenothiazine Drugs in Urine

Phenothiazine drugs are used in the treatment of psychiatric disorders. The average daily urinary excretion is about one half of the daily intake; some continues to be excreted over a period of time after therapy has ceased. The screening test has been used to monitor the amount of drug ingested (or not ingested) by the patient. For identification of the drug, spectrophotometric methods are used (see Chap. 17).

Screening Test for Phenothiazine

Reagent. 5 ml 5 per cent ferric chloride in water, 45 ml 20 per cent perchloric acid, and 50 ml 50 per cent nitric acid; mix together.

Procedure (Forrest, 1961). Mix 1 ml urine in a test tube with 1 ml of ferric chloride reagent.

Read immediately. Disregard colors appearing after ten seconds.

Interpretation. Shades of pink to purple indicate dosage levels of 20 to 2000 mg/day. False negative results of up to 25 per cent have been reported (Brownstein, 1966). These may be due to low dose levels, overhydration, and the lack of sensitivity of some related drugs. Prochlorperazine, trifluoperazine, perphenazine, and thioridazine (Mellaril) are not as sensitive to the test as chlorpromazine. Very large amounts of ascorbic acid may cause false negative results when the drug level is low (James, 1980).

False positive results may be seen with high doses of para-aminosalicylic acid, with estrogen therapy, or with phenylketonuria. Indican may cause a purple color. Aspirin does not produce false positive reactions. Phenothiazine drugs may cause positive reactions in other urine tests—for urobilinogen and with ferric chloride test, etc. (Young, 1975).

Porphyrins

The porphyrias are a group of diseases resulting from defects in the synthesis of heme. These are inherited enzyme deficiencies in which the enzyme substrate is usually excreted in excess in urine or feces.

A description of the chemistry and synthesis of porphyrins with clinical pathologic correlation and analytical techniques is given on p. 144.

The patterns of excretion of the various porphyrins vary with the different diseases (Table 18–21). These and the clinical findings help establish the diagnosis. Skin photosensitivity and skin lesions frequently accompany high levels of porphyrins. The one entity without skin lesions is acute intermittent porphyria. In patients presenting with neurologic disease and acute abdominal pain—the hepatic group—there is increased production and excretion of aminolevulinic acid (ALA) and porphobilinogen during the acute porphyric attack. There is probably increased activity of ALA synthase and subsequent increased production of the precursors. Exacerbations of the hepatic diseases are precipitated by drugs known to induce liver enzyme activity, e.g., barbiturates and certain steroids.

Screening Tests. In the patient suspected of having an acute porphyric attack, porphobilinogen is sought in a urine specimen using the *Watson-Schwartz test.* (See Confirmatory Test for Urobilinogen.) Porphobilinogen is insoluble in chloroform or butanol and remains in the aqueous phase of the separation. The Hoesch test is used as a second confirmatory test. During the acute attack, high levels of porphobilinogen are excreted, but the urine is not always colored because about 500 μg/L of porphyrins can be present without causing a red-purple color (Henry, 1974). Between attacks, levels of porphobilinogen may be increased but may also be normal.

Uroporphyrin and coproporphyrin are detected by fluorescence. An orange-red fluorescence is seen if the specimen is placed near an ultraviolet light source. The porphyrins are excreted in most of the porphyrias and in lead poisoning (Table 18–21). Coproporphyrin and uroporphyrin can also be separated by thin-layer chromatography or by extraction and fluorometry and quantitated using ion exchange columns. (See Chapter 9.)

Screening tests together with the clinical findings will indicate whether quantitative tests should be done. These are usually performed by reference or research laboratories.

The urine specimen for quantitative *porphobilinogen* should be kept at a near neutral pH (between 6 and 7) and protected from light (Bossenmaier, 1968). Frozen specimens are fairly stable. *Delta aminolevulinic acid* is more stable if the urine is acidic. However, if both substances are to be tested, the near neutral pH is preferred and the urine aliquot is frozen. These substances are quantitated by eluting from different columns and reacting with Ehrlich's reagent.

The urine specimen for quantitative *porphyrins* is collected in a dark container containing 5 g sodium carbonate for a 24-hour specimen to give a concentration of 0.1 per cent sodium carbonate or to produce urine of *neutral pH.* Urine buffered at pH 7 is preferred to prevent formation of porphyrin from porphobilinogen (Fogstrup, 1979).

Fecal porphyrins can be qualitatively estimated using extraction and UV light, or quantitated. In protoporphyria, the fecal specimen may fluoresce owing to high protoporphyrin levels. In some porphyrias, *red cells* may show fluorescence when an unstained blood smear is examined microscopically. The nucleated bone marrow red cells give greater fluorescence.

Table 18–21. PORPHYRIAS: URINARY FINDINGS AND OTHER SPECIAL DETERMINATIONS*

Porphyrias	Urinary Findings: *Elevated*	Urinary Findings: *Normal*	Special Determinations
Congenital erythropoietic porphyria (rare) Extreme photosensitivity Hemolytic anemia	UP ↑ CP Pink-brown, fluctuates	PBG ALA	Red cell UP ↑ ↑ CP PP (fluoresce) Feces CP ↑
Protoporphyria Skin lesions, liver disease		PGB ALA UP CP	Red cell PP ↑ fluoresce Feces PP ↑ ↑ may fluoresce
Hepatic—inherited			
Acute intermittent porphyria Abdominal pain, drug induced No skin lesions	PBG ↑ ALA PBG→UP on standing → dark color	UP CP variable	
Porphyria variegata (S. African) Photosensitivity, skin lesions Acute abdominal pain, drug induced Neuropsychiatric disorders	PBG ALA with acute attack CP	Variable	Feces UP CP ↑ PP ↑ ↑
Hereditary coproporphyria Photosensitivity occasional Acute abdominal pain, drug induced	CP PBG ALA in acute attack	PBG ALA variable	Feces CP ↑ ↑ UP ↑
Porphyria cutanea tarda Photosensitivity No abdominal pain	UP Pink-brown	PBG ALA	Feces variable Increased body iron
Hepatic—acquired (cutaneous, toxic) Liver disease, etc. Photosensitivity	UP ↑ CP Pink-brown	PBG ALA variable	Feces UP CP ↑
Lead poisoning	CP ALA	PBG UP variable	Red cell PP ↑ ↑ CP ↑

*CP = Coproporphyrin.
UP = Uroporphyrin.
PBG = Porphobilinogen.
ALA = Delta-aminolevulinic acid.
PP = Protoporphyrin.
↑ = Degree increase.

In *lead poisoning,* blood and urinary lead levels, delta-aminolevulinic acid levels in serum and urine, and coproporphyrin levels in urine are all used to help make a diagnosis.

Screening Procedure for Porphyrin. The urine is acidified and the extracted porphyrin exposed to ultraviolet light.

1. Place 5 ml urine in a stoppered glass centrifuge tube. Add 3 ml of a mixture of one part glacial acetic acid with four parts of ethyl acetate.
2. Shake and allow to separate. Centrifuging will accelerate the separation.
3. Using a Wood's lamp, observe the upper layer for fluorescence. Inspect the tube in a dark room with ultraviolet reflected light. A lavender to violet color indicates the presence of porphyrins; pink to red fluorescence indicates higher levels of porphyrin. Pale blue with no pink color is negative. Normal urine may fluoresce blue.

To increase the sensitivity of the test and remove interfering drug metabolites, transfer the upper layer to a glass tube and acidify with 0.5 ml of 3 M HCl (25 ml concentrated HCl diluted to 100 ml with water). Shake. Porphyrins are extracted into the lower aqueous layer and will give a red-orange fluorescence (Haining, 1969).

An alternative screening method utilizes an anion exchange resin column (Dowex column available from Bio Rad Laboratories, Richmond, California). Porphyrins are adsorbed, eluted, and exposed to fluorescent light. This method removes interfering substances and is similar in principle to quantitative method for total porphyrins (Fogstrup, 1979) and coproporphyrin and uroporphyrin (Leahy, 1982). Urinary porphyrin profiles demonstrating more metabolites are detected by high performance liquid chromatography.

Salicylates

Ferric ions react with metabolites of aspirin or other salicylates in weakly acid solutions to form a deep wine-red color (Bordeaux red), which is heat stable. This reaction provides a simple method for the detection of salicylates in cases of suspected overdosage, or in monitoring patients receiving high dosage therapy.

Ferric Chloride Test. To 5 ml urine in test tube, add 10 per cent ferric chloride drop by drop until a stable deep red color forms or any precipitate of ferric phosphate redissolves. (This generally requires only 5 to 10 drops of ferric chloride, and ferric phosphate does not always precipitate.) A red-brown or deep Bordeaux red color develops in the presence of salicylates. This test is also *positive if acetoacetic acid* is present and is known as *Gerhardt's test.*

To confirm a positive reaction for salicylates, divide the test solution in half and boil half for five minutes, or boil 5 ml urine and repeat the test. If the boiled or retested sample still shows the Bordeaux red color, the test is positive for salicylates. If the boiled solution becomes lighter or if the test after boiling is negative, the reaction was due to acetoacetic acid.

Reagent Strip Test. Phenistix[a] reagent strips contain a ferric salt, magnesium sulfate, and cyclohexylsulfamic acid. Although developed for phenylpyruvic acid testing, the strips react with metabolites of aspirin or other salicylates with a color reaction similar to that of the test tube ferric chloride test.

Procedure. Dip the reagent-impregnated portion of the strip into the urine. Immediately compare the color of the dipped end of the strip with a special color chart available from the manufacturer. Metabolites of aspirin or other salicylates will give a pink to Bordeaux red color with Phenistix[a]. In cases of phenylketonuria, phenylpyruvic acid in urine produces a gray to blue-gray color (Johnson, 1963). Phenothiazines also produce a color; this is increased when one drop of strong (50 per cent) H_2SO_4 is added. With salicylates, the strong acid bleaches the color.

Sulfonamides

Sulfonamides are conjugated in the liver by acetylation. Both free and acetylated forms can be found in the blood and urine where they are excreted principally by glomerular filtration. Generally the acetylated forms are less soluble than the free forms. Crystals of sulfonamides are seen in urine at a low acid pH, and usually when the patient is dehydrated. They are yellow-brown and form sheaves and divided spheres.

A problem with older sulfonamides was precipitation of crystals, usually the acetylated form, in the renal tubules and ureters. Crystalline deposits may cause obstruction and anuria, or the drug may cause renal tubular necrosis without obstruction. Adequate fluid should be given with sulfonamides and alkali if the urinary pH is low. Alfthan (1972) showed crystals occurring with acetylsulfisoxazole in concentrated urine at low pH. However, if urine was kept at 37°C. after voiding, crystals were not seen.

Since urine sediments are usually examined at room temperature, other indications of damage by crystals in vivo should be noted: red blood cells, casts, and the occasional crystal cast associated with low volume and high specific gravity urine.

Sulfonamides such as *sulfisoxazole* (Gantrisin) are rapidly absorbed and excreted and are less likely to form crystals in the urine than the older sulfanilamide, sulfapyridine, or sulfathiazole. *Sulfamethoxazole* (Gantanol) is more slowly excreted than sulfisoxazole, and its acetylated form is relatively insoluble and likely to cause crystallluria. These are commonly seen crystals in urine sediments. Sulfamethoxazole is frequently given in combination with trimethoprim as Bactrim or Septra.

With *sulfadiazine,* the acetylated form is unusual in that it is slightly more soluble at 25°C. than the free form, as shown below, and both forms are readily excreted (Jensen, 1943).

Solubility in urine at pH	6.0	7.0	7.5
Sulfadiazine mg/dl	25	110	350
Acetylsulfadiazine mg/dl	40	220	860

Sulfasalazine (Azulfidine) is a poorly absorbed sulfonamide used to treat enteric diseases. It may be absorbed through damaged tissue and appear in urine as the metabolite sulfapyridine or acetyl-sulfapyridine.

For solubility of sulfonamides in solvents, see Table 18–18.

Diazo Test for Sulfonamides. The presence of sulfonamides in urine may be confirmed with a diazo test. Sulfonamides contain a sulfonamide group and a free amino group. The sulfonamide is diazotized with nitrous acid and coupled with N-(1-naphthyl)-ethylenediamine to produce a purple red azo dye. The ammonium sulfamate destroys excess sodium nitrite which would otherwise interfere with the reaction. Since acetylation blocks the amino group, the conjugated form cannot be diazotized. To measure total sulfonamide, the sample is first hydrolyzed with HCl. A protein-free specimen of urine is used. For a quantitative procedure, see Henry (1979) and Bratton (1939).

Procedure. Use a known positive control.

1. To three drops of urine in a small test tube, add two drops of 10 per cent HCl. Mix. Wait 30 seconds.
2. Add two drops 0.1 per cent sodium nitrite. Mix. Wait 30 seconds.
3. Add two drops 0.5 per cent ammonium sulfamate. Mix.
4. Add two drops 0.1 per cent N-(1-naphthyl) diamine dihydrochloride. Mix. A magenta color is a positive test.

Note that the test indicates that sulfonamides are in the specimen; it does not necessarily identify unknown crystals unless they are separated, washed, dissolved, and reacted.

Lignin Test. Sulfonamides react with cellulose or wood fiber in newspaper and paper towels in the presence of strong acid. A drop of urine is placed on a blank piece of paper, and a drop of 25 per cent HCl is added. A yellow to orange color is produced in ten minutes or so. A control drop of urine is also used. Drugs may interfere. Filter paper and bond writing paper are not suitable.

This test is not as satisfactory as the previous diazo test.

URINARY SCREENING FOR INHERITED METABOLIC DISEASES

Urine has been used for many years to screen for metabolic diseases, including those determined by genetic inheritance. In these diseases an abnormal metabolite or a larger than normal amount of a normal metabolite is often excreted in the urine, although the kidney itself is not always involved. Many of these diseases are associated with mental retardation, degeneration of the nervous system, and "failure to thrive."

3

Mass Screening (Bickel, 1980). High levels of some amino acids are detected in *blood* from newborns using the *Guthrie bacterial-inhibition assay* (see Kelly, 1977). An antimetabolite for *Bacillus subtilis* spores inhibits their growth on agar unless an excessive amount of a particular amino acid is present. Phenylalanine (PKU), leucine (maple syrup urine disease), methionine (homocystinuria), tyrosine, histidine, and argininosuccinic acid are all measurable. The Guthrie test is used for PKU testing a few days after birth. Galactosemia and hypothyroidism are also screened at the same time in some programs.

Urine is tested at four and six weeks in programs in Canada (Wong, 1979; 74,521 tested), Australia (Wilcken, 1980; 1,000,000 tested), and U.S. (Levy, 1980; 633,000 tested). The yield from mass screening is about the same for aminoacidurias in Europe, the United States (Massachusetts), Canada (British Columbia), and Australia (New South Wales). In general, phenylketonuria, iminoglycinuria, cystinuria, Hartnup disorder, and histidinemia were found in numbers of about 5 to 10 per 100,000 screened. Cystathioninuria varied from 0.33 to 6.7/100,000. In the Canadian study there were one each of argininosuccinic aciduria, maple syrup urine disease, prenatal diabetes mellitus, and renal glycosuria and three of persistent galactosuria. The yield from mass screening is low, and early detection may benefit only phenylketonuria patients since many disorders are without treatment or do not respond to treatment (Wilcken, 1980). Dietary therapy is used for phenylketonuria, galactosemia, maple syrup urine disease, propionic acidemia, and homocystinuria by withholding the appropriate amino acid or sugar. Large amounts of vitamins are used to supply cofactors. Pyridoxine is used to treat a form of cystathioninuria and cobalamin for some cases of methylmalonic acidemia. Galactosemia was thought to respond to dietary treatment in the neonatal period. However, follow-up on the few diagnosed patients into adolescence shows mental retardation and visual defects in those who were thought to be adequately treated as infants (Editorial, 1982).

Cost-benefit analysis for mass screening has been described in a report from the Massachusetts Department of Public Health (1974). They concluded that there was a substantial net savings resulting from routine screening after estimating the costs of evaluation and treatment and comparing these to projected costs of institutional care for 20 years.

Because of the rarity of these disorders, mass testing is best performed by state or regional public health laboratories. Very careful laboratory and clinical interpretation of screening tests is required because of the number of false positive results, e.g., transient tyrosinuria of the newborn. On the other hand, false negative results will occur if the newborn has not had several days to ingest appropriate protein or carbohydrates. More recently a prospective study by Meryash (1981) in Massachusetts has shown elevated blood phenylalanine levels in infants at risk on day one and day two, and in some cases before feedings. The timing of specimen collections requires further investigation.

Genetic Disease of the Kidney. This is uncommon. Many patients are diagnosed from history and clinical findings; however, in some instances urinary screening may indicate the presence of a specific disease. *Functional abnormalities* are usually associated with a transport defect of proximal renal tubular epithelial cells and include renal glucosuria, cystinuria, and the Fanconi syndrome. The Fanconi syndrome is also caused by a wide variety of inherited diseases, including Wilson's disease, cystinosis, tyrosinemia, hereditary fructose intolerance, glycogen storage disease, and galactosemia where the tubular cells are damaged secondarily. Glucose, phosphate, and amino acids are not reabsorbed by the damaged tubular cells. Other inherited functional renal disorders such as nephrogenic diabetes insipidus are listed in Table 18–22.

With a *structural abnormality* such as polycystic renal disease, microscopic hematuria and mild proteinuria are early signs of a disease which may progress to chronic renal failure in adult life. Urinary concentrating ability is lost early. In various genetic nephritides, proteinuria, hematuria, and increased leukocytes and renal tubular cells may be found. Medullary sponge kidney may be asymptomatic or present because of hematuria, stone formation, and infection. Hereditary nephritis (Alport's syndrome) presents in childhood with hematuria in 80 to 100 per cent of cases; red cell casts are frequent. Other hereditary renal diseases

Table 18–22. METABOLIC RENAL DISORDERS*

Disease	Prevalence	Effects
Renal tubular acidosis Type I	Uncommon	Distal renal tubules not acidifying; metabolic acidosis; hypercalciuria; impaired growth
Familial hypophosphatemic rickets (vitamin D resistant) (not known),† X-linked dominant	≃ 1/25,000	Renal tubular defect in reabsorption of phosphate; loss of calcium from bone; short stature
Nephrogenic diabetes insipidus (not known), X-linked recessive	Uncommon	Renal tubular cells unresponsive to vasopressin; polyuria, thirst
Amyloid nephropathy with familial Mediterranean fever (not known)	1/3000‡	Amyloid in kidney causes nephrotic syndrome

*Adapted from Stanbury (1983).

†Enzyme deficiency is shown in parenthesis when known.

‡Disorder associated with particular geographic or ethnic group and not as prevalent in the general population.

include nephrogenic diabetes insipidus, congenital nephrotic syndrome, and nail-patella syndrome in which there is glomerular disease and an abnormal sediment. Systemic inherited diseases involving the kidney are diabetes mellitus, sickle cell disease with proteinuria and hematuria, and familial Mediterranean fever with hematuria and progressive amyloidosis. In the rare Fabry's disease, renal involvement causes polyuria and then renal failure. Protein, casts, and cells, including an occasional foam cell containing a sphingolipid, appear in the urine.

Kidney stones found in pediatric patients are an indication for investigation of genetic metabolic disease. Crystalluria and stone formation occur with primary hyperoxaluria, and with the purine metabolic diseases gout, xanthinuria, and the rare adenine phosphoribosyl transferase deficiency. Orotic acid crystalluria and stone formation occur with a very rare pyrimidine disorder. Cystine stones occur in children but are more often present in adults.

Acutely Ill Infants; Failure to Thrive. The occurrence of inherited metabolic diseases in these infants is relatively high and will be detected if a suitable protocol for testing is employed in pediatric intensive care units (Krieger, 1982). In the newborn period metabolic acidosis, often associated with severe vomiting and severe ketosis, requires investigation. The infant may be comatose or have seizures. There is a disturbance of acid-base balance with a large anion gap due to organic acids. Screening tests in urine are useful as preliminary tests for sugars and amino acids. The urine will be acidic; *ketones* are present. Organic acids in urine and amino acids in plasma and urine should be measured by chromatography.

Hyperammonemia may occur in premature infants transiently or in association with urea cycle enzyme deficiencies. In some of the organic acidurias there is a neutropenia and thrombocytopenia. Sepsis is seen due to Candida, staphylococcal, and pneumococcal infections. Parenteral feeding and antibiotics used in these patients may cause false results. Ampicillin will cause false positive amino acid chromatography results, and sugars may appear in urine because of dietary or intravenous loading. (See Hill, 1976.)

Other metabolic inherited diseases relating to bilirubin handling by the liver, inherited hemolytic anemias and porphyrias, abnormal metal (iron, copper) and lipid metabolism are discussed in other chapters. These and many other diseases are described in detail in Stanbury (1983).

This segment delineates some of the more commonly screened diseases and describes some of the simpler qualitative, preliminary tests. Tables 18–23 and 18–25 to 18–27 list the diseases, enzyme deficit when known, and disease prevalence for selected amino acid metabolism, carbohydrate, purine, and lysosomal enzyme abnormalities and for some metabolic renal tubular diseases of unknown cause.

Specimen Requirement. Early morning or random fresh urine is used for routine urinalysis and simple screening tests. If urine is to be used for further amino acid analysis or for sugars or organic acids, it should be frozen. Aliquots of measured 24-hour collections should be frozen. If this is not possible, the urine may be acidified for amino acid testing. (See Collection of Urine.)

Bacterial contamination occurs in specimens, especially from young children. Organisms such as *E. coli* will decrease and increase amino acids, and sugars will be utilized. Organic acidurias have been described after bacterial contamination of normal urine (Vidler, 1978).

Urinary Screening Tests and Associated Disorders

1. Odor: See earlier section for odors associated with aminoacidurias, and see Cone (1968b). Ketones produce an aromatic odor.

2. Routine screening:

Color. Refer to Table 18–3. Urates or uric acid in excess may cause a red color to a diaper.

Acid pH and ketones are found with ketoacidosis in a number of disorders.

Glucosuria occurs with diabetes mellitus, renal glycosuria and with renal tubular damage.

Bilirubin is excreted with Dubin-Johnson syndrome and with cholestasis, and is associated with jaundice and liver damage in storage diseases.

Urobilinogen increases with hereditary hemolytic anemias.

Proteinuria occurs with renal diseases.

Blood test is positive with hematuria; myoglobinuria is an occasional feature of McArdle's disease (muscle phosphorylase deficiency).

Red blood cells with stones; also red cell casts with hereditary nephritides (Alport's syndrome).

Leukocytes with infection associated with stones; congenital obstructions in the urinary tract.

Renal tubular cells may show the lipid inclusions of Fabry's disease and congenital nephrotic syndrome.

Crystals: Uric acid in stone formers, Lesch-Nyhan syndrome, gout, and other urate nephropathy. Cystine in cystinuria, rarely in other tubular diseases. Calcium oxalate in primary hyperoxaluria. Tyrosine in tyrosinosis, liver failure. Xanthine in xanthinuria. Extremely rare orotic acid, adenine.

Additional Screening Tests. Consult Thomas (1973) and Kelly (1977) for detailed methods and further information. The qualitative test methods are given later.

1. Reducing substances—see earlier Confirmatory Test section. Copper reduction for sugars. Glucosuria, galactosemia, fructosuria, pentosuria, and homogentisic aciduria are detected.

2. Tests for amino acids: *Ferric chloride* for phenylketonuria, maple syrup urine disease, histidinemia, homogentisic acid. *Dinitrophenylhydrazine* for α-keto acids, for maple syrup urine disease, phenylketonuria. *Nitrosonaphthol* for tyrosinemia. *Methylmalonic acid* for methylmalonic acidemias (ketotic hyperglycinemia).

3. Mucopolysaccharides: *Toluidine blue spot test* for mucopolysaccharidoses.

4. Blood smear for metachromatic granules in leukocyte cytoplasm for leukodystrophy, mucolipidoses, and mucopolysaccharidoses.

Confirmatory Tests. These are also first line tests in infants with unexplained failure to thrive, retardation, and seizures and in severely ill neonates with vomiting, ketoacidosis, and unexplained coma.

Amino acids in plasma, urine: paper chromatogra-

3

phy or high voltage electrophoresis; quantitation with automated ion exchange column chromatography.

Organic acids in urine: gas chromatography.

Sugars in urine: thin layer chromatography.

Specific enzyme assays in red cells, leukocytes, and cultured fibroblasts. Red cells—galactose-1-phosphate uridyl transferase level for galactosuria. Liver biopsy, leukocytes, fibroblasts for branched chain keto acid decarboxylase in maple syrup urine disease. Liver biopsy for phenylalanine hydroxylase if needed.

See Kelly (1977) for confirmatory tests and Stanbury (1983) and Nyhan (1980) for details of individual diseases.

Aminoaciduria

With an enzyme deficiency affecting amino acid metabolism, the substrate and other metabolites in the pathway accumulate causing increased body fluid levels and increased substrate excretion in urine. *Phenylketonuria* is an example of this type of overflow aminoaciduria. In a few instances the substrate or metabolite is found in urine in excessive amounts, but not perceptibly increased in blood. When there is a deficit in cell membrane transport for amino acids, for example in renal tubular cells, certain amino acids are not reabsorbed from the glomerular filtrate and are excreted in excess in the urine. Blood levels are normal. An example of renal transport aminoaciduria is *cystinuria*.

With damage to renal tubular cells by disease or toxic substances, there will be a lack of reabsorption of amino acids as well as glucose and other substances. In this case there is a *generalized aminoaciduria*. This syndrome is seen with the congenital Fanconi syndrome as well as with acquired and inherited diseases causing secondary damage to renal tubules. Generalized aminoaciduria also occurs with severe liver disease because of reduced ability of the liver to metabolize amino acids. Leucine and tyrosine crystals sometimes appear in urine with massive liver failure.

See Table 18–23 for some of the more common amino acid disorders and rarer disorders for which urinary screening is done.

Brief descriptions of cystinuria, homogentisic aci-

Table 18–23. AMINOACIDURIAS*

Disease	*Prevalence*	*Effects*
Amino Acid Disorders with Accumulated Substrates		
Phenylketonuria	1/11,000	Accumulation of phenylalanine and metabolites; retardation (Types II and III milder)
Type I hyperphenylalaninemia (phenylalanine hydroxylase)†		
Type V (dihydrobiopterin synthetase)	1/30,000	Similar to Type I
Tyrosinemia Type I (tyrosinosis)	1/100,000	Accumulation of succinylacetone; liver disease; renal tubular disease; Fanconi syndrome
(fumaryl and maleyl acetoacetate hydrolases)	1/10,000‡	
Alcaptonuria (homogentisic acid oxidase)	≃1/250,000	Homogentisic acid excretion in urine; polymers deposit in cartilage as black pigment
Argininosuccinate lyase deficiency	1/70,000	Accumulation of argininosuccinate in body fluids; CNS dysfunction
Maple syrup urine disease (branched chain 2 ketoacid decarboxylase apoenzyme)	1/200,000	Accumulation of ketoacids; acidosis; growth retarded
Methylmalonic acidemias		
Methylmalonyl CoA mutase	1/20,000	Accumulation of methylmalonate; ketoacidosis; growth retarded
ATP cobalamin-adenosyl-transferase	1/20,000	Similar
Cystathioninuria (α-cystathionase)	≃1/100,000	Accumulation of cystathionine and metabolites
Homocystinuria (cystathionine β-synthase)	1/200,000	Accumulation of homocysteine, homocystine, methionine; affects CNS, lens, bones
Amino Acid Membrane Transport Defects		
Cystinuria (3 variants) (not known)	1/7000	Renal tubular defect in reabsorption of cystine, ornithine, lysine, and arginine; cystine crystals, stones
Iminoglycinuria, benign (not known)	1/15,000	Renal tubular defect in reabsorption of imino acids and glycine
Cystinosis (not known)	1/100,000	Cystine deposits in cell lysosomes in organs; kidney dysfunction, tubular damage; eyes; growth retardation

*Adapted from Stanbury (1983).

†Enzyme deficiency is shown in parenthesis when known.

‡Disorder associated with particular geographic or ethnic group and not as prevalent in the general population.

duria (alcaptonuria), maple syrup urine disease, methylmalonic acidemia, phenylketonuria, and tyrosinemia follow, together with the qualitative tests used to screen for them.

With suspected membrane transport disorders or generalized aminoacidurias, the urine specimen provides the most useful data. Amino acid analyses are expressed as μmol/24 hours or μmol/g creatinine in random urine specimens. The 24-hour specimen is preferred, although it is not always possible to collect this from small children. Although most amino acids found in normal humans have been detected in normal urine, usually not more than about six to eight are detected by paper chromatography or column chromatography in more than trace amounts. In the normal urinary amino acid chromatogram *glycine* is usually most prominent. This is followed by *alanine, serine,* and *glutamine* and then by *taurine, histidine,* and *methylhistidine.* With a high-protein (meat) diet, histidine and methylhistidine are excreted in larger amounts. Other amino acids which may be demonstrated in normal urine, depending on the technique used, are glutamic acid, threonine, tyrosine, lysine, and a trace of arginine; beta-aminoisobutyric acid may also be seen.

In infants the pattern may vary with feeding. The level of amino acid excretion is relatively higher in infants, and increased amounts of cystine, asparagine, glutamine, glutamic acid, and occasionally proline are seen. (See Vaughan, 1979.)

Cystinuria

The defective transport of cystine by the epithelial cells of the renal tubules and gut is transmitted as an autosomal recessive trait. The basic defect is not known. While large amounts of the dibasic acids, ornithine, lysine, and arginine, are also excreted in this disease, cystine is the only one that crystallizes out. Stone formation is a clinical manifestation.

Cystinuria is a common amino acid disorder. It occurs equally in both sexes, with an incidence estimated at about 1 per 10,000 (homozygous) and in larger numbers for heterozygotes. In mass screening programs for infants, the homozygous form is detected at about the same rate as phenylketonuria. Cystinuria is sometimes detected in patients with renal tubular disease. It is excreted with other amino acids in Wilson's disease, in Lowe's disease, and with the aminoaciduria of Hartnup disease. The cyanide nitroprusside test described below is positive in cystinuria.

The classic form of *homocystinuria* is due to deficiency of the liver enzyme cystathionine β-synthase which catalyses the formation of cystathionine from homocystine and serine in the methionine pathway. Homocysteine is rapidly oxidized to homocystine, which accumulates along with methionine and is excreted in the urine. Children with this disease may have seizures and thromboses and become mentally retarded. Urine for testing must be fresh because homocystine is labile. Quantitative urinalysis reveals high levels of homocystine, methionine, and cysteine-homocysteine disulfide. The cyanide nitroprusside test is positive. Urine levels are monitored to follow the effects of the methionine-restricted diet used to treat the disease.

Cystinosis, a recessively inherited disorder of unknown cause, is characterized by cystine crystal deposition in lysosomes in cells. Crystals accumulate in the kidney, eye, bone marrow, and spleen. In the severe form, there is photophobia, renal failure, rickets, and growth failure. With renal tubular involvement, the Fanconi syndrome develops and there is a generalized aminoaciduria and glucosuria. Unlike cystinuria, the cystine loss in cystinosis parallels the loss of other amino acids in the urine.

Cystine Crystals. Examine a first morning urine specimen for colorless, hexagonal crystals of cystine. Urine will be at an acid pH. Note that the solubility of cystine is less in water than in urine and cystine may not always crystallize in a concentrated urine although present in large amounts (Ettinger, 1971).

Cyanide-Nitroprusside Test. This test is Brand's modification of the Legal nitroprusside reaction (Brand, 1930; Legal, 1883). Cystine is reduced to cysteine by sodium cyanide, and the free sulfhydryl groups then react with nitroprusside to produce a red-purple color. Freeing of sulfhydryl groups takes time. Cysteine, cystine, homocystine, and ketones (dark red) will give positive reactions. Smith (1977) evaluated the qualitative test for cystinuria and found that it separated normal, heterozygote, and homozygote ranges of excretion. The lower limit of the test was 35 to 60 μmols of cystine per mol of creatinine, and this corresponded to the heterozygote range. Homozygous stone formers usually excrete more than 300 mg/g creatinine and are detected by this test.

Specimen. A concentrated early morning specimen gives best results. Dilute specimens may be falsely negative. Refrigerate until tested.

Procedure. Place 3 to 5 ml urine in a test tube and add 2.0 ml sodium cyanide solution (5 g/dl water)* and allow to stand for *ten minutes.* Timing is important. Treat a control solution in the same way. Sodium cyanide solution is stable for three months when stored in a refrigerator.

Add fresh, aqueous sodium nitroprusside solution (5 g/dl) dropwise (about five drops), and mix. (In some laboratories, the nitroprusside solution is made weekly and refrigerated.) A stable red-purple color will develop with cystine.

Read immediately as positive or negative. "Trace" results may also be reported. A concentrated normal specimen could give a weak positive "trace" result.

Further identification of cystine is made by chromatography and quantitative amino acid analysis.

Positive Control. Use 5 mg cystine dissolved in 10 ml 0.1 N HCl, diluted to 100 ml with normal urine. Freeze aliquots. To save positive urine specimens, acidify with 0.1 N HCl to pH 1 or 2 and freeze.

Homogentisic Aciduria

Homogentisic acid (dihydroxyphenylacetic acid) is excreted in urine in large quantities in a rare hereditary disease, *alcaptonuria.* Normally, phenylalanine and tyrosine are metabolized to homogentisic acid, which is then oxidized to maleyl acetoacetic acid. With a

**Poisonous.* When disposing of this, discard in the sink, flushing with large amounts of water.

3

deficiency of the liver enzyme homogentisic acid oxidase, there is an accumulation of homogentisic acid.

Patients with alcaptonuria develop dark blue to black pigmentation in cartilage and connective tissue. The disease may not be diagnosed until arthritis develops. A dark color on diapers has been noted in infants (Vaughan, 1979).

Screening. If the urine is allowed to stand, it will very slowly oxidize and *darken* at the surface. Urine at an acid pH is not colored; the addition of alkali will hasten darkening when homogentisic acid is present. If ascorbic acid is present, it will inhibit the oxidation.

Homogentisic acid *reduces the copper reagent* in Benedict's test or with Clinitest[a], and, because of the alkaline reagent, it will also darken to produce a yellow precipitate in an orange to brown solution. This reaction will also take place (more slowly) at room temperature. Glucose oxidase reagent strip is negative, so that the reducing substance should not be confused with glucose.

Ferric Chloride Test. A transient very dark blue color is seen as two drops of 10 per cent ferric chloride solution are added to about 2 ml urine.

Silver Nitrate Test. Add 4 ml of 3 per cent silver nitrate to 0.5 ml urine. Mix, then add several drops of 10 per cent NH_4OH. Homogentisic acid will cause the development of a black color.

Identification of homogentisic acid is made by using paper or thin-layer chromatography. It should be distinguished from gentisic acid, an aspirin metabolite. Normally, there is no homogentisic acid present in urine.

Maple Syrup Urine Disease (MSUD)

MSUD is one of a group of diseases associated with abnormal branched chain amino acid metabolism. These include hypervalinemia, isovaleric acidemia causing "sweaty feet" odor, and other rare diseases. In some of these diseases such as MSUD, the amino acids accumulate and are measured in serum and urine; in others, accumulated organic acids are measured by gas chromatography alone or coupled with mass spectrometry.

There are several forms of MSUD. In the severe form there is severe neonatal vomiting, seizures and stupor, and often episodes of hypoglycemia. Leucine, isoleucine, valine, and their corresponding keto-acids are elevated in the plasma and are excreted in the urine because deficient decarboxylases and other enzymes prevent the conversion of the keto amino acids to fatty acids. The urine has an odor resembling maple syrup, caramelized sugar, or curry, the source of which is not certain. The urinary keto-acids are demonstrable by the first week of life. A screening test with dinitrophenyl hydrazine demonstrates keto-acids and their transformation into keto-acid phenylhydrazones. A microbiologic blood screening test for the elevated leucine is used for mass screening.

Dinitrophenylhydrazine Test. This test indicates the presence of alpha keto amino acids in the urine. Insoluble hydrazones form from the reaction of carbonyl groups with dinitrophenylhydrazine. A positive result is seen with MSUD and possibly in phenylketonuria (phenylpyruvic acid), histidinemia (imidazole pyruvic acid), and methionine malabsorption (oasthouse syndrome). The test is positive with ketonuria due to other inherited diseases and other causes. A preliminary screening test for ketones should be done.

Reagent. 100 mg of 2,4-dinitrophenylhydrazine in 100 ml of 2 N HCl. The reagent should be stored in a brown bottle in the refrigerator.

Procedure

1. Reagent and control should be at room temperature.
2. Add ten drops of reagent to 1 ml of clear urine.
3. After or within ten minutes a yellow or chalky white precipitate indicates a positive reaction. It should be the same as or greater than the control precipitate.

Control. Use ketoglutaric acid, 25 mg in 100 ml normal urine. Freeze in small aliquots.

Methylmalonic Acidemia

A number of enzymes are involved in the conversion of propionyl CoA formed from amino acid metabolism to methylmalonyl CoA. As well as the enzymes, cofactors biotin and cobalamin are needed. Inherited enzyme deficiencies cause (1) ketotic hyperglycinemia and propionic acidemia requiring protein restriction and alkali in the neonatal period and (2) metabolic ketoacidosis due to methylmalonic acidemia.

Normally methylmalonic acid and its precursor propionic acid are found in very small amounts in body fluids.

Methylmalonic acidemia is detected with relative frequency in sick neonates (Krieger, 1982). Table 18–23 lists the enzyme deficiencies involved. It occurs after ingestion of protein has begun. Acidosis and ketosis are prominent features similar to those seen with propionic acidemias.

Methylmalonic Acid Screening Test. Methylmalonic acid excretion is detected by reaction with the diazonium salt of para-nitroaniline in alkaline solution. An emerald green chromogen is formed. See Kelly (1977).

Procedure. Add a single drop of urine to a 10 ml tube. Add 15 drops of 0.1 per cent *p*-nitroaniline and 5 drops of 0.5 per cent sodium nitrite, in that order. Mix and observe partial decoloration. Add 1 ml 1 M sodium acetate buffer (pH 4.3), mix, and place immediately in *boiling water bath* for from one to three minutes. Remove tubes from bath and immediately add 5 drops of 8 N sodium hydroxide. Mix. Use a positive control and a normal negative urine for color comparison.

Large amounts of methylmalonic acid in urine form an immediate emerald green color. Malonic and ethylmalonic acids form green chromogens, but usually are present in trace amounts. Brown colors form with penicillins, creatinine, uric acid, and vitamin K and may mask the green color.

Reagents. Para-nitroaniline, 0.1 per cent: Dissolve 0.1 g *p*-nitroaniline in 100 ml 0.16 N HCl. Stable in dark glass bottle at room temperature for six months or longer.

Sodium nitrite, 5 per cent: Dissolve 0.25 g $NaNO_2$ in demineralized water to final volume of 50 ml. Store in refrigerator.

Sodium acetate buffer, 1 M, pH 4.3: Dissolve 13.6 g sodium acetate in 100 ml demineralized water. Add 158 ml of 1 M acetic acid to give pH 4.3 ± 0.02. Store in a refrigerator.

Sodium hydroxide, 8 N: Dissolve 33.4 g sodium hydroxide in 100 ml demineralized water.

Positive control: Methylmalonic acid standard, 0.025 M: Dissolve 147.5 mg methylmalonic acid in 50 ml demineralized water; add a drop of 6 N HCl. Stable at 4°C. for six months or more.

Phenylketonuria

Phenylketonuria is an autosomal recessive inherited disease associated with an absence of active liver enzyme, phenylalanine hydroxylase. Because dietary L-phenylalanine is not converted to tyrosine, phenylalanine and other metabolites accumulate. Both sexes are affected equally, with an incidence of about 1 in 11,000, with most cases stemming from Northern European stock. Several types of disease occur, varying in severity. Mental retardation is the major clinical finding. Dietary restriction of phenylalanine has shown good results.

In this disease there is an accumulation of normal metabolites in abnormal amounts. Plasma phenylalanine and phenylpyruvic acid levels are elevated; urinary phenylpyruvic acid (highest), phenylacetic acid, and phenylalanine are increased. Urinary indoleacetic acid and other indoles arising from altered tryptophan metabolism and indican (an indole) are also increased. The excretion of 5-hydroxyindoleacetic acid is diminished, paralleling the low level of serum 5-hydroxytryptamine.

Odor is due to phenylacetic acid in urine and sweat and is described as mousy or musty.

Ferric Chloride Test (Table 18–24). The ferric chloride test is non-specific. It will give color reactions with several amino acid disorders, with other metabolites, and with drugs. The ferric ion chelates with the enol grouping and will produce color formation with keto acids from corresponding amino acids. Alcaptonuria (homogentisic acid), histidinemia, tyrosinosis, oasthouse urine disease, and maple syrup urine disease may cause color reaction in urine.

Specimen must be fresh because phenylpyruvic acid is labile. The use of ferric chloride directly on disposable diapers will produce false positive green colors for some brands and is not recommended.

Procedure. Add one drop of 1 N H_2SO_4 to 1 ml of urine in a test tube (also a positive control). Add two drops of $FeCl_3$ solution (10 g/100 ml water) and mix. Observe the color. A green or gray-green color due to phenylpyruvic acid should be observed over a period of two minutes. It will fade slowly. The ferric chloride solution is kept in a brown bottle and refrigerated.

Controls. Positive specimens can be frozen in aliquots. Positive controls are available, e.g., QC-U (General Diagnostics).

The test is positive for phenylpyruvic acid when the plasma level of phenylalanine exceeds 15 mg/100 ml. About 10 mg/100 ml phenylpyruvic acid is detected. Since colored compounds occur with many urinary metabolites, this test should be regarded as a preliminary screening procedure. (See Table 18–24.) Phosphate in urine may interfere with the test, and a modified test using a phosphate precipitating reagent (magnesium) has been advocated (Henry, 1964). Rapidly fading blue-green colors may be seen with homogentisic acid or *p*-hydroxyphenylpyruvic acid (tyrosinosis). Imidazole pyruvic acid will give a green color (histidinemia). Bilirubin, if present, may cause a blue-green color. Ketones, such as acetoacetate, will form a red to red-brown color. It is unlikely that drugs would be present in specimens used for screening for inherited disease, but salicylates (red-purple), phenothiazines, and levo-dopa (brown) are known to interfere with the test (Hansten, 1979; Wirth, 1965).

Table 18–24. FERRIC CHLORIDE TEST IN URINE*

Substance or Disease	Color Change
Acetoacetic acid	Red or red-brown
Bilirubin	Blue-green
Homogentisic acid	Blue or green; fades quickly
o-Hydroxyphenylacetic acid	Mauve
o-Hydroxyphenylpyruvic acid	Red-brown; turns to green or blue then fades to mauve
P-Hydroxyphenylpyruvic acid	Green; fades in seconds
Imidazolepyruvic acid	Green or blue-green
α-Ketobutyric acid	Purple; fades to red-brown
Maple syrup urine disease	Blue
Melanin	Gray precipitate; turns black
Phenylpyruvic acid	Green or blue-green; fades to yellow
Pyruvic acid	Deep gold-yellow or green
Xanthurenic acid	Deep green; later brown
Drugs	
Aminosalicylic acid	Red-brown
Antipyrines and acetophenetidines	Red
Cyanates	Red
Phenol derivatives	Violet
Phenothiazine derivatives	Purple-pink
Salicylates	Stable purple

*Modified from Henry, R. J.: Clinical Chemistry: Principles and Techniques. New York, Harper & Row, Publishers, 1964.

Reagent Strip Test. Phenistix[a] reagent strips contain ferric ammonium sulfate, magnesium sulfate, and cyclohexylsulfamic acid. The cyclohexylsulfamic acid provides optimal acidity for the reaction.

Procedure. Dip the reagent-impregnated portion of the strip into the urine and remove immediately or press it against a wet diaper. At 30 seconds compare the color of the dipped end of the strip with the color chart provided. A positive test is a gray to gray-green color. Report as positive or negative. The test detects 5 to 10 mg/100 ml. (See Kelly, 1977, for a comparison of ferric chloride results and reagent strip results with numerous metabolites.) Salicylates and metabolites of phenothiazine derivatives may cause a pink to purple color.

Tyrosine

Tyrosinemia with tyrosinuria occurs when there is abnormal metabolism of tyrosine derived from the diet or from phenylalanine. This may be part of a

3

generalized amino acid disorder associated with liver disease, or a transitory tyrosinemia seen in premature or low weight infants or, rarely, with the syndrome of hereditary tyrosinemia. The genetic disease tyrosinosis is extremely rare.

Transitory hypertyrosinemia occurs in infants of low birth weight and is found in asymptomatic infants tested in screening programs. There is no liver or renal disease present, and the entity is benign. The elevated tyrosine levels may on occasion be accompanied by transiently elevated phenylalanine levels. Tyrosine and the phenolic acids *p*-hydroxphenyllactic and *p*-hydroxyphenlpyruvic are excreted in larger than normal amounts in the urine.

Hereditary tyrosinemia type I or tyrosinosis is accompanied by a generalized aminoacidemia with a marked loss of *p*-hydroxyphenyllactic acid, glucosuria, ketonuria, proteinuria, and loss of phosphate. (See Table 18–23 for enzyme deficiencies.) Tyrosine is elevated in blood and urine. Cirrhosis of the liver, renal dysfunction, and rickets are the principal findings. Hepatoma occurs in childhood. The clinical entity in some respects resembles those of hereditary fructosemia and galactosemia in which there is liver and kidney involvement and a generalized aminoaciduria because of renal tubular damage. Children do not survive the first decade.

Tyrosine Crystals. Very fine, silky crystals are seen in the urinary sediment in severe liver disease. They are scattered in the field or aggregated to form sheaves. The crystals appear brown to black while focusing. Leucine crystals may accompany the tyrosine. The crystals precipitate at an acid pH and are soluble in alkali.

Nitrosonaphthol Test for Tyrosine. This is a nonspecific screening test and should be confirmed by chromatography or quantitative serum assay of tyrosine. Tyrosine and tyramine form soluble red complexes with nitrosonaphthol. Normal urine contains tyrosine. In tyrosinosis it is about 100 times normal.

Reagents. One volume of concentrated 2.63 N nitric acid in five volumes of water. Nitrosonaphthol—100 mg 1-nitroso-2-naphthol in 100 ml 95 per cent ethanol. Sodium nitrite, 2.5 per cent in water. All reagents are refrigerated.

Procedure. Mix the following reagent in a test tube: To 1 ml of 2.63 N nitric acid add one drop of 2.5 aqueous sodium nitrite solution and ten drops of nitrosonaphthol reagent. Add three drops of urine and mix. Let stand for three to five minutes. An orange-red color will develop. A positive control is tested at the same time.

Control. 50 mg tyrosine in 100 ml water. Refrigerate.

Carbohydrate Disorders

Glucosuria and other melliturias (lactose, fructose, pentose, and sucrose) are described under confirmatory tests for sugars. Table 18–25 lists some of the more

Table 18–25. CARBOHYDRATE DISORDERS*

Disease	Prevalence	Effects
Diabetes mellitus Type I, insulin dependent (not known)†	1/500	Insulin deficiency; glucagon increased; ketosis; blood glucose increased
Fructosuria, essential benign (fructokinase)	≃ 1/130,000	Fructose not converted to phosphate; fructose in urine; no hypoglycemia
Fructose intolerance (fructose-1-phosphate aldolase)	1/20,000‡	Fructose-1-phosphate accumulates in cells; hypoglycemia; reaction to fructose ingestion may be severe
Glycogen storage diseases (8 types)		
Type I (von Gierke's) (glucose-6-phosphatase)	≃ 1/100,000	Accumulation of glycogen in liver, kidney; hypoglycemia
Type V (McArdle's) (phosphorylase)	1/500,000	Accumulation of glycogen in muscle; myoglobinuria
Galactosemia		
(galactose-1-phosphate uridyl transferase)	1/62,000	Accumulation of galactitol and metabolites in organs; cataracts; galactosuria
(galactokinase)	≃ 1/100,000	Accumulation of galactitol; cataracts
Pentosuria, benign (L-xylulose reductase)	1/2,500‡	L-Xylulose in urine continuously
Primary hyperoxaluria, Type I (2-oxoglutarate-glyoxylate carboligase)	Uncommon	Block in glyoxylate metabolism; oxalosis; oxaluria; Ca oxalate stones
Carbohydrate Membrane Transport Disorders		
Transport of lactose (intestinal lactase)	1/10, or more‡	Accumulation of lactose in gut; osmotic diarrhea; occasional lactosuria
Transport of glucose: renal glycosuria, benign (not known)	Uncommon	Renal tubular defect; glucose not reabsorbed; glucosuria
Transport of sucrose (intestinal sucrase–α-dextrinase)	Rare	Accumulation of sucrose and isomaltase in gut; osmotic diarrhea; occasional sucrosuria
Transport of glucose-galactose (intestinal) (not known)	Rare	Accumulation of glucose, galactose in gut; osmotic diarrhea (?); urinary sugars

*Adapted from Stanbury (1983).
†Enzyme deficiency is shown in parenthesis when known.
‡Disorder associated with particular geographic or ethnic group and not as prevalent in the general population.

common disorders and also those associated with intestinal and renal tubular transport defects.

Intestinal lactase deficiency is a very common problem leading to cramping abdominal pain and osmotic diarrhea after ingestion of lactose-containing food. The uncommon lactose, fructose, and sucrose intolerances cause severe illness with vomiting in young infants. Lactose and hereditary fructose intolerances may cause liver dysfunction and renal tubular damage. Removal of the sugar from the diet will alleviate the difficulty. Pentosuria is benign. See confirmatory tests for glucose and other sugars in an earlier section of this chapter.

Galactosuria (Galactosemia). Galactose is found in the urine in genetic disorders of galactose metabolism associated with a deficiency of either galactokinase or, in the classic disease, galactose-1-phosphate uridyl transferase. These diseases are transmitted as autosomal recessives.

Because of the enzyme deficiencies, galactose, which is derived from lactose in the diet, is not converted to glucose in the liver. With galactokinase deficiency, a milder disease ensues: galactose accumulates and is reduced to galactitol in the lens of the eye where cataracts are formed. *Transferase deficiency* causes an accumulation of galactose and galactose-1-phosphate and galactitol. Clinically there is diarrhea with failure to thrive from early infancy. Liver dysfunction and jaundice occur early, and renal toxicity is followed by generalized aminoaciduria, proteinuria, and cataract formation. A lactose (galactose)-free diet may cause regression of symptoms. Early treatment may not prevent retardation (Editorial, 1982). Heterozygotes and Duarte variant carriers have half-normal transferase activity and do not have the disease.

The disease may be diagnosed by means of enzyme studies on cultured cells obtained by amniocentesis (see Chap. 21). Mass screening tests on newborn blood are carried out in some regional or state public health laboratories. A copper reducing test on urine has been recommended for neonates on the day of discharge or at the time of two-week check-up. Galactose oxidase reagent strips have been tried (Dahlquist, 1968). The yield on testing is about one in 40,000 to 70,000 for persistent galactosuria.

Identification. A reducing substance in urine that does not react with glucose oxidase reagent strips may be galactose, lactose, fructose, or pentose (or a number of other substances). In an infant with failure to thrive, the sugar should be identified by chromatography (thin-layer or paper) followed by an assay for red cell enzyme activity.

Reference Value. Normal newborns, premature infants, and some children with high milk consumption may have galactosuria. Reference values for galactose in urine are about 14 mg/24 hours (Dahlquist, 1969).

Lysosomal Disorders

Mucopolysaccharidoses are a group of diseases characterized by excessive amounts of mucopolysaccharide storage in organs. There are seven described groups and some subdivisions according to clinical features and specific enzyme deficiencies. These diseases, except for Type II Hunter (X-linked), are autosomal recessive. Patients have skeletal defects and coarse features which become prominent in the first and second years of life. There is multiple organ disease. Most patients have enlarged liver and spleen and mental retardation. Some have corneal clouding, blindness, and deafness. Hurler syndrome is the classic representative and is due to a deficiency of lysosomal α-L-iduronidase, an enzyme required for metabolism of iduronic acid in the sugars of dermatan and heparan sulfates. (See Table 18–26.)

The mucopolysaccharides and partially degraded mucopolysaccharides excreted in large amounts in urine are dermatan, heparan, and keratan sulfates and, in Type VII, chondroitin sulfate. In Hurler disease, metachromatic staining of large granules of acid mucopolysaccharides in neutrophils, lymphocytes, and histiocytes, especially from the bone marrow, are demonstrated with toluidine blue.

Mucopolysaccharides are also excreted in the rare *mucolipidosis* (pseudo-Hurler disease), a disease with glycoprotein and glycolipid storage in cells as well as mucopolysaccharidosis.

Other lysosomal diseases, including Tay-Sachs, in which glycosphingolipid (ganglioside GM-2) is stored in neuronal cells, and other sugar-lipid storage diseases, e.g., Gaucher's and Krabbe's disease, are not detected by urinary findings. In Krabbe's disease, the tubular cells contain small lipid droplets which stain with toluidine blue, but these are not usually detected

Table 18–26. LYSOSOMAL ENZYME DISORDERS*

Disease	Prevalence	Effects
Mucopolysaccharidoses: Type I (three varieties) (α-L-iduronidase)†	≃ 1/100,000 (Hurler); others less common	Accumulation of dermatan, heparan sulfates in organs; excreted in urine
Leukodystrophies:		
Krabbe's disease (galactosyl ceramidase)	1/50,000‡	Accumulation of glycolipid in CNS; myelin loss; lipid in renal cells
Metachromatic (several) (arylsulfatase A)	≃ 1/100,000	Accumulation of cerebroside in CNS; myelin loss; metachromatic granules in cells and in urine
Fabry's disease (galactosidase A), X-linked recessive	1/40,000	Accumulation of glycolipids in cells; lipid in urine birefringent

*Adapted from Stanbury (1983).
†Enzyme deficiency is shown in parenthesis when known.
‡Disorder associated with particular geographic or ethnic group and not as prevalent in the general population.

Table 18–27. PURINE/PYRIMIDINE DISORDERS*

Disease	Prevalence	Effect
Primary gout (not known)†	1/500 (Western)	Monosodium urate accumulation in body fluids, organs, joints; hyperuricemia; stones
Lesch-Nyhan syndrome: X-linked recessive (hypoxanthine-guanine phospho-ribosyl-transferase) (HPRT)	1/10,000 males	Accumulation of purines; severe CNS disease; uric acid crystalluria; stones
Partial HPRT deficiency	1/1100,000 males	Mild form of disease
Adenine phosphoribosyltransferase deficiency	Very rare	2,8-dihydroxy adenine crystalluria, stones
Xanthinuria (xanthine oxidase or dehydrogenase)	1/45,000	Accumulation of xanthine in muscle; crystalluria; stones
Orotic aciduria (orotidine 5′-phosphate decarboxylase)	Very rare	Orotic acid crystalluria; stones; pyrimidine nucleotide deficiency causing atypical megaloblastic anemia; growth retarded

*Adapted from Stanbury (1983).
†Enzyme deficiency is shown in parenthesis when known.

in the urine. In *Fabry's disease* desquamated lipid-laden cells have occasionally been shown in urine sediment. *Metachromatic leukodystrophy* results from an accumulation of an acid lipid (galactosyl sulfatide) in the central and peripheral nervous system and other organs, including the kidney. Excess galactosyl sulfide is excreted in urine. The sulfatides form granular masses in cells that show metachromatic staining and polarize. A screening test for the deficient enzyme arylsulfatase A can be performed on urine and in leukocytes and serum (Kelly, 1977).

Screening Tests for Mucopolysaccharides. The toluidine blue spot test and turbidity tests have been used. With the spot test, false negative results of 32 per cent were found by Carter (1968) when known patients were tested. The false positive rate in non-Hurler patients was 1.5 per cent.

A turbidity test using cetylpyridium chloride has been found reliable by Pennock (1970). The acid-albumin turbidity test of Dorfman (1958) may be used as a qualitative or semi-quantitative test. In this test, dialyzed, buffered urine is mixed with albumin at an acid pH; a uniform turbidity is seen when acid mucopolysaccharides are present. This test has been more reliable than the spot test in detecting Hurler's disease (Carter, 1968; Pennock, 1970).

Confirmatory tests include column chromatography for the kind and amount of mucopolysaccharide present.

None of the screening tests will detect the keratosulfate excreted in Morquio's disease, group IV, or in generalized gangliosidosis.

Reference Values. In adults, small amounts of chondroitin sulfates and heparan sulfates are excreted in the range of 10 mg/24 hours. Levels increase with rapid growth.

Spot Test Procedure (Berry, 1960). The test is based on the metachromasia produced with the basic groups of the toluidine blue dye in the presence of large amounts of acid mucopolysaccharide.

Equipment

1. Whatman filter paper No. 1. Micropipettes.
2. Control solution of chondroitin sulfate containing 0.1 mg/ml in distilled water.
3. Toluidine blue, 0.04 per cent in 1 M sodium acetate at pH 2. Use a certified buffer tablet.

Method

1. 5, 10, and 25 μl of urine are placed in separate spots on a piece of filter paper. Each spot should be allowed to dry before the next is made. A normal urine may be spotted for comparison.
2. 5 μl of the standard chondroitin sulfate solution is applied separately and dried.
3. The dry paper is dipped into the toluidine blue solution for one minute.
4. Rinse the paper in 95 per cent alcohol two or three times. Dry, then examine.

Result. Urine from children with Hurler syndrome will show a purple spot against a blue background, as will the standard chondroitin sulfate. Normal urine is blue.

Comment. The pH of 2 is important in achieving a good result. Control must be run for comparison. False positive results were obtained in most newborn infants, but after two weeks of age only 0.2 per cent of the normal infants gave positive results (Berry, 1960). Heparan may give false positive results.

Purine/Pyrimidine Disorders

The common disease of primary gout is associated with an overproduction of uric acid, an underexcretion, or both. A specific defect has not been found. Specific enzyme defects have been assigned to some diseases associated with hyperuricemia. See Table 18–27 for examples.

Abnormal purine metabolism in *Lesch-Nyhan disease* is due to a deficiency of hypoxanthine-guanine phosphoribosyl transferase (HGPRT) and affects males. It affects the central nervous system and causes hyperuricemia, gout, stones, and urate nephropathy. The disease is characterized by skin loss due to self-biting. *Urine* contains large amounts of uric acid, which may color the diaper with an orange-red deposit. Hematuria may accompany stone formation. Uric acid blood levels are about 10 mg/dl and urinary uric acid levels are greater than 1 mg/mg creatinine excreted. Enzyme level is measured in red blood cells or fibroblasts.

Addis, T.: The number of formed elements in the urinary sediments of normal individuals. J. Clin. Invest., *2*:409, 1926.

Addis, T.: Glomerular Nephritis. New York, The Macmillan Company, 1948.

Alberti, K. G. M. M., and Hockaday, T. D. R.: Rapid blood ketone body estimation in the diagnosis of diabetic ketoacidosis. Br. Med. J., *2*:565, 1972.

Albright, F., and Bloomberg, E.: Hyperparathyroidism and renal disease with a note as to the formation of calcium casts in this disease. J. Urol., *34*:1, 1935.

Alfthan, O. S., and Liewendahl, K.: Investigation of sulfonamide crystalluria in man. Scand. J. Urol. Nephrol., *6*:44, 1972.

Altman, P., and Dittmer, D. S.: Biology Data Book, Vol. III, 2nd ed. Bethesda, Md., Federation of American Societies of Experimental Biology, 1974.

Anderson, N. G., Anderson, N. L., and Tollaksen, S. L.: Proteins of human urine. I. Concentration and analysis by two-dimensional electrophoresis. Clin. Chem., *25*:119, 1979.

Assa, S.: Evaluation of urinalysis methods in 35 Israeli laboratories. Clin. Chem., *23*:126, 1977.

Avent, J., Schumann, G. B., and Vars, L.: Comparison of the Chemstrip leukocyte test with a standardized Papanicolaou-stained urine sediment evaluation. Lab. Med., *14*:163, 1983.

Bailey, D. N., and Jatlow, P. I.: Chemical analysis of massive crystalluria following primidone overdose. Am. J. Clin. Path., *58*:583, 1972.

Bailey, R. R., Dann, E., Gillies, A. H. B., et al.: What the urine contains following athletic competition. New Z. Med. J., *83*:309, 1976.

Balikov, B.: Urobilinogen excretion in normal adults; results of assays with notes on methodology. Clin. Chem., *3*:145, 1957.

Ball, W., and Lichtenwainer, M.: Ethanol production in infected urine. N. Engl. J. Med., *301*:614, 1979.

Banda, P. W., Sherry, A. E., and Blois, M. S.: Column cation-exchange separation of melanin-related metabolites in urine from cases of melanoma. Clin. Chem., *23*:1397, 1977.

Bandi, Z. L., Meyers, J. L., Bee, D. E., and James, G. P.: Evaluation of determination of glucose in urine with some commercially available dipsticks and tablets. Clin. Chem., *28*:2110, 1982.

Becker, S. M., Ramirez, G., Pribor, H. C., and Gillen, A. L.: A quality control product for urinalysis. Am. J. Clin. Path., *59*:185, 1973.

Beeler, M., and Henry, J.: Melanogenuria—evaluation of several commonly used laboratory procedures. J.A.M.A., *176*:136, 1961.

Beeler, M., Veeth, D., Morriss, R., and Biskind, G.: Analysis of urinary calculus; comparison of methods. Am. J. Clin. Path., *41*:553, 1964.

Belmonte, M. M., Sarkozy, E., and Harpur, E.: Urine sugar determination by the two drop Clinitest method. Diabetes, *16*:557, 1967.

Bence Jones, H.: On a new substance occurring in the urine of a patient with mollities ossium. Phil. Tr. Roy. Soc. (London), *138*:55, 1848.

Benham, L., and O'Kell, R. T.: Urinalysis: Minimizing microscopy. Clin. Chem., *28*:1722, 1982.

Benedict, S. R.: A reagent for the detection of reducing sugars. J. Biol. Chem., *5*:485, 1909.

Berry, H. K., and Spinlanger, J.: A paper spot test useful in the study of Hurler's syndrome. J. Lab. Clin. Med., *55*:136, 1960.

Bickel, H.: Mellituria, a paper chromatographic study. J. Pediatr., *59*:641, 1961.

Bickel, H., Guthrie, R., and Hammersen, G. (eds.): Neonatal Screening for Inborn Errors of Metabolism. Berlin, Springer-Verlag, 1980.

Billing, B. H.: Twenty-five years of progress in bilirubin metabolism (1952–1977). Gut, *19*:481, 1978.

Blank, D. W., and Frohlich, J.: Pseudochyluria caused by vaginal cream. Clin. Chem., *28*:2181, 1982.

Blondheim, S. H., Margoliash, E., and Shafur, E.: A simple test for myohemoglobinuria (myoglobinuria). J.A.M.A., *167*:453, 1958.

Boesken, W. H., Boesken, S., and Marmier, A.: Myoglobinuria: Immunochemical quantitation and electrophoretic separation of free and protein-bound myoglobin (Mb). *In* Dubach, V. C., and Schmidt, V. (eds.): Diagnostic Significance of Enzymes and Proteins in Urine. Current Problems in Clinical Biochemistry, 9. Bern, Huber, 1979.

Bossenmaier, I., and Cardinal, R.: Stability of δ-aminolevulinic acid and porphobilinogen in urine under varying conditions. Clin. Chem., *14*:610, 1968.

Bowie, L., Smith, S., and Gochman, N.: Characteristics of binding between reagent-strip indicators and urinary proteins. Clin. Chem., *23*:128, 1977.

Bradley, G. M.: Differentiating epithelial cells from leukocytes in urine. Postgrad. Med., *43*:245, 1968.

Bradley, P. W.: University of Minnesota Clinical Laboratories: Utilization Study, 1978.

Brand, E., Harris, M. M., and Biloon, S.: Cystinuria: The excretion of cystine complex which decomposes in the urine with the liberation of free cystine. J. Biol. Chem., *86*:315, 1930.

Bratton, A. C., and Marshall, E. K., Jr.: A new coupling component for sulfanilamide determination. J. Biol. Chem., *86*:315, 1939.

Brenner, B. M., Hostetter, T. H., and Humes, H. D.: Molecular basis of proteinuria of glomerular origin. N. Engl. J. Med., *298*:826, 1978.

Brody, L. H., Webster, M. C., and Kark, R. M.: Identification of elements of urinary sediment with phase-contrast microscopy. J.A.M.A., *206*:1977, 1968.

Brown, D. C.: Kidney stones. Current issues in diagnosis and therapy. Postgrad. Med., *72*:124, 1982.

Brownstein, H., and Roberge, A. R.: Detection of phenothiazine derivatives in urine. Clin. Chem., *12*:844, 1966.

Bush, C. L., and Hagen, C. H.: Economical urinology quality control. Lab. Med., *5*:34, 1974.

Cameron, J. S., and Simmonds, H. A.: Gout and crystal related nephropathy. Contrib. Nephrol., *16*:147, 1979.

Caraway, W. T.: Chemical and diagnostic specificity of laboratory tests. Am. J. Clin. Path., *37*:445, 1962.

Carter, C. H., Wan, A. T., and Carpenter, D. G.: Commonly used tests in the detection of Hurler's syndrome. J. Pediatr., *73*:47, 1968.

Cartwright, G. E.: Diagnostic Laboratory Hematology. New York, Grune and Stratton, 1968.

Chalmers, R. A., Valman, H. B., and Liberman, M. M.: Measurement of 4-hydroxyphenylacetic aciduria as a screening test for small bowel disease. Clin. Chem., *25*:1791, 1979.

Coe, F. L.: Nephrolithiasis. Pathogenesis and Treatment. Chicago, Year Book, 1978.

Coe, F. L.: The patient with renal stones. *In* Schrier, R. W. (ed.): Manual of Nephrology. Boston, Little, Brown, 1981.

Cohen, R. D., and Woods, H. F.: Clinical and Biochemical Aspects of Lactic Acidosis. London, Blackwell Scientific Publications, 1976.

Cone, T. E., Jr.: Diagnosis and treatment: Some syndromes, diseases and conditions associated with abnormal coloration of the urine or diaper. Pediatrics, *41*:654, 1968a.

Cone, T. E., Jr.: Diagnosis and treatment: Some diseases, syndromes, and conditions associated with an unusual odor. Pediatrics, *41*:993, 1968b.

Cook, M. H., Free, A. H., and Giordano, A. S.: The accuracy of urine sugar tests. Am. J. Med. Technol., *19*:283, 1953.

Cruikshank, G., and Edmond, E.: "Clean catch" urine in the newborn—bacteriology and cell excretion patterns in the first week of life. Br. Med. J., *4*:704, 1967.

Dahlquist, A.: A test paper for galactose in urine. Scand. J. Clin. Lab. Invest., *22*:87, 1968.

Dahlquist, A., and Svenningsen, N. W.: Galactose in the urine of newborn infants. J. Pediatr., *75*:454, 1969.

Davidsohn, I., and Henry, J. B. (eds.): Todd-Sanford Clinical Diagnosis by Laboratory Methods. 15th ed. Philadelphia, W. B. Saunders Company, 1974.

de Mendoza, S. G., Kashyap, M. L., Chen, C. Y., and Lutmer, R. F.: High density lipoproteinuria in nephrotic syndrome. Metabolism, *25*:1143, 1976.

Dewald, B., Rindler-Ludwig, R., Bretz, V., and Baggiolini, M.: Subcellular localization and heterogeneity of neutral proteases in neutrophilic polymorphonuclear leukocytes. J. Exp. Med., *141*:709, 1975.

Dewall, C. P., Casazza, A. R., Grimley, P. M., Carbone, P. P., and Rowe, W. P.: Recovery of cytomegalovirus from adults with neoplastic disease. Ann. Intern. Med., *64*:531, 1966.

Dobbins, J. W., and Binder, H. J.: Importance of the colon in enteric hyperoxaluria. N. Engl. J. Med., *296*:298, 1977.

Dorfman, A.: Studies in the biochemistry of connective tissue. Pediatrics, *22*:576, 1958.

Duttera, M. J., et al.: Hematuria and crystalluria after high-dose 6-mercaptopurine administration. N. Engl. J. Med., *287*:292, 1972.

Editorial: Clouds over galactosaemia. Lancet, *2*:1379, 1982.

Edwards, O. M., Bayliss, R. I. S., and Millan, S.: Urinary creatinine excretion as an index of the completeness of 24 hour collections. Lancet, *2*:1165, 1969.

Esbach, G.: Dosage practique de l'albumine: Tris méthodes C. R. Soc. Biol. (Paris), *1*:33, 1874.

Ettinger, B., and Kolb, F. O.: Factors involved in crystal formation in cystinuria; *in vivo* and *in vitro* crystallization dynamics and a simple, quantitative colorimetric assay for cystine. J. Urol., *106*:106, 1971.

Ettinger, B., Weil, E., Mandel, N. S., and Darling, S.: Triamterene-induced nephrolithiasis. Ann. Intern. Med., *91*:745, 1979.

Exton, W. G.: A simple and rapid quantitative test for albumin in urine. J. Lab. Clin. Med., *10*:722, 1925.

Fairley, K. F., and Birch, D. F.: Hematuria: A simple method for identifying glomerular bleeding. Kidney Int., *21*:105, 1982.

Falk, J. S., Lindblad, G. T. O., and Westman, J. M.: Histopathologic studies on kidneys from patients treated with large amounts of blood preserved with ACD-adenine. Transfusion, *12*:376, 1972.

Fassett, R. G., Horgan, B. A., and Mathew, T. H.: Detection of glomerular bleeding by phase-contrast microscopy. Lancet, *1*:1432, 1982.

Fogstrup, J., and With, T. K.: Urinary total porphyrins by ion exchange analysis: Reference values for the normal range and remarks on preformed porphyrins in acute porphyria tarda. J. Clin. Path., *32*:109, 1979.

Forrest, F. M., Forrest, I. S., and Mason, A. S.: Review of rapid urine tests for phenothiazine and related drugs. Am. J. Psychiatr., *118*:300, 1961.

Fraser, C. G., Smith, B. C., and Peake, M. J.: Effectiveness of an outpatient urine screening program. Clin. Chem., *23*:2216, 1977.

Free, A. H., and Free, H. M.: A simple test for urine bilirubin. Gastroenterology, *24*:414, 1953.

Free, A. H., and Free, H. M.: Urinalysis in Clinical Laboratory Practice. Cleveland, CRC Press, 1975.

Free, A. H., and Free, H. M.: Rapid convenience urine tests: Their use and misuse. Lab. Med., *9*:9, 1978.

Freni, S. C., Dalderup, L. M., Oudegeest, J. J., and Wensveen, N.: Erythrocyturia, smoking and occupation. J. Clin. Path., *30*:341, 1977a.

Freni, S. C., Heederik, G. J., and Hol, C.: Centrifugation techniques and reagent strips in the assessment of microhaematuria. J. Clin. Path., *30*:336, 1977b.

Froesch, E. R., Reardon, J. B., and Renold, A. E.: The determination of inulin in blood and urine using glucose oxidase for the removal of interfering glucose. J. Lab. Clin. Med., *50*:918, 1957.

Gadeholt, H.: Quantitative estimation of urinary sediment with special regard to sources of error. Br. Med. J., *1*:1547, 1964.

Gillenwater, J. W.: Detection of urinary leukocytes by Chemstrip-L. J. Urol., *125*:383, 1981.

Goldring, W.: Studies of the kidney in acute infection. J. Clin. Invest., *10*:355, 1931.

Gyure, W. L.: Comparison of several methods for semiquantitative determination of urinary protein. Clin. Chem., *23*:876, 1977.

Haber, M. H.: Interference contrast microscopy for identification of urinary sediments. Am. J. Clin. Path., *57*:316, 1972.

Haber, M. H.: Urinary Sediment: A Textbook Atlas. Chicago, American Society of Clinical Pathologists, 1981.

Haber, M. H.: Urine Casts, Their Microscopy and Clinical Significance. Chicago, American Society of Clinical Pathologists, 1975.

Haining, R., Hulse, T., and Labbe, R.: Rapid porphyrin screening of urine, stool and blood. Clin. Chem., *15*:400, 1969.

Hallson, P. C., and Rose, G. A.: Uromucoids and urinary stone formation. Lancet, *1*:1000, 1979.

Halperin, M. L.: Pathogenesis of type I (distal) renal tubular acidosis: Reevaluation of the diagnostic criteria. Ann. Royal Coll. Phys. Surg. Can., *7*:103, 1975.

Hansen, J. L., and Freier, E. F.: Direct assays of lactate, pyruvate, β-hydroxybutyrate and acetoacetate with a centrifugal analyzer. Clin. Chem., *24*:475, 1978.

Hansen, O. H., et al.: The relationship of lipuria to the fat embolism syndrome. Acta Chir. Scand., *139*:421, 1973.

Hansten, P. D.: Drug Interactions. 4th ed. Philadelphia, Lea and Febiger, 1979.

Helgason, S., and Lindquist, B.: Eosinophiluria. Scand. J. Urol. Nephrol., *6*:257, 1972.

Henry, J. B. (eds.): Clinical Diagnosis and Management by Laboratory Methods. 16th ed. Philadelphia, W. B. Saunders Company, 1979.

Henry, R. J.: Clinical Chemistry: Principles and Techniques. New York, Harper & Row Publishers, 1964.

Henry, R. J., et al.: Clinical Chemistry: Principles and Techniques. 2nd ed. New York, Harper & Row Publishers, 1974.

Henry, R. J., Sobel, C., and Segalove, M.: Turbidometric determination of proteins with sulfosalicylic and trichloroacetic acids. Proc. Soc. Exp. Biol. Med., *92*:748, 1956.

Highman, W., and Wilson, E.: Urine cytology in patients with calculi. J. Clin. Path., *35*:350, 1982.

Hill, A., Casey, R., and Zaleski, W. A.: Difficulties and pitfalls in the interpretation of screening tests for the detection of inborn errors of metabolism. Clin. Chim. Acta, *72*:1, 1976.

Hoesch, K.: Über die Auswertung der Urobilinogenurie und die umgekehrte Urobilinogenreaktion. Dtsch. Med. Wochenschr., *72*:704, 1947.

Holmquist, N.: Detection of cancer with urinary sediment. J. Urol., *123*:188, 1980.

Houston, I. B.: Pus cell and bacterial counts in diagnosis of urinary tract infections in childhood. Arch. Dis. Child., *38*:600, 1963.

Howell, T. H.: Urinary excretion after the age of ninety. J. Gerontol., *11*:61, 1956.

Imhof, P. R., et al.: Excretion of urinary casts after the administration of diuretics. Br. Med. J., *2*:199, 1972.

James, G. P., Bee, D. E., and Fuller, J. B.: Proteinuria: Accuracy and precision of laboratory diagnosis by dip-stick analysis. Clin. Chem., *24*:1934, 1978a.

James, G. P., D'Jang, M. H., and Hamilton, H. H.: False negative results for urinary phenothiazines and imipramine in Forrest's qualitative assays. Clin. Chem., *26*:345, 1980.

James, G. P., Paul, K. L., and Fuller, J. B.: Urinary nitrite and urinary-tract infection. Am. J. Clin. Path., *70*:671, 1978b.

Jensen, O. J., and Fox, C. L.: Hydrogen ion concentration and the solubility of sulfonamides in urine; the relation to renal precipitation. J. Urol., *49*:334, 1943.

Johnson, P. K., Free, H. M., and Free, A. H.: A simplified urine and serum screening test for salicylate intoxication. J. Pediatr., *63*:949, 1963.

Kagen, L. J.: Immunologic detection of myoglobinuria after cardiac surgery. Ann. Int. Med., *67*:1183, 1967.

Kaplow, L. S.: Simplified myeloperoxidase stain using benzidine dihydrochloride. Blood, *26*:215, 1965.

Kelly, S.: Biochemical Methods in Medical Genetics. Springfield, Ill., Charles C Thomas, 1977.

Kesson, A. M., Talbolt, J. M., and Gyory, A. Z.: Microscopic examination of urine. Lancet, *2*:809, 1978.

Kibrick, A. C.: Extended use of the Kingsley biuret reagent. Clin. Chem., *4*:232, 1958.

Kierkegaard, H., Feldt-Rasmussen, U., Horder, M., Anderson, H. J., and Jorgensen, P. J.: Falsely negative urinary leukocyte counts due to delayed examination. Scand. J. Clin. Lab. Invest., *40*:259, 1980.

Killander, J., Sjolin, S., and Zaar, B.: Rapid tests for ketonuria. Scand. J. Clin. Lab. Invest., *14*:311, 1962.

Krieger, I., Nigro, M., and Taqi, O.: Screening for metabolic disease in a metropolitan hospital. Am. J. Dis. Child., *136*:125, 1982.

Kunin, C. M., and Degroot, J. E.: Self-screening for significant bacteriuria. J.A.M.A., *231*:1349, 1975.

Kusumi, R. K. Grover, P. J., and Kunin, C. M.: Rapid detection of pyuria by leukocyte esterase activity. J.A.M.A., *245*:1653, 1981.

Lamon, J., Torben, K., and Realker, A.: The Hoesch test: Bedside screening for urinary porphobilinogen in patients with suspected porphyria. Clin. Chem., *20*:1438, 1974.

Leach, C., Rambault, P. C., and Fischer, C. L.: A comparative study of two methods of urine preservation. Clin. Biochem., *8*:108, 1975.

Leahy, D. T., and Brien, T. G.: A simple method for the separation and quantification of urinary porphyrins. J. Clin. Path., *35*:1232, 1982.

Legal, E.: Regarding a new acetone reaction and its use in urinalysis. Chemisch. Zentralbl., *13*:652, 1883.

Levin, S.: Red urine: The Monday morning disorder of children. Pediatrics, *36*:134, 1965.

Levison, D. A., Crocker, P. R., Banim, S., and Wallace, D. M. A.: Silica stones in the urinary bladder. Lancet, *1*:704, 1982.

Levy, H. L., Coulombe, J. T., and Shih, V. E.: Newborn urine screening. *In* Bickel, H., Guthrie, R., and Hammerson, G. (eds.): Neonatal Screening for Inborn Errors of Metabolism. Berlin, Springer-Verlag, 1980.

Lewis, B., and Richards, P.: Measurement of urinary protein. Lancet, *1*:1141, 1961.

Lindqvist, B., and Wahlin, A.: Differential count of urinary leukocytes and renal epithelial cells by phase contrast microscopy. Acta Med. Scand., *198*:505, 1975.

Lizana, J., Brito, M., and Davis, M. R.: Assessment of five quantitative methods for determination of total proteins in urine. Clin. Biochem., *10*:89, 1977.

Lombardo, J. V., Terlinsky, A., Chester, A. C., and Preuss, H. G.: Tubulointerstitial diseases. Am. Fam. Physician, *21*:128, 1980.

Malone, J. I., Rosenbloom, A. L., Grgic, A., and Weber, F. T.: The role of urine sugar in diabetic management. Am. J. Dis. Child., *130*:1324, 1976.

Markowitz, H., and Wobig, G.: Quantitative method for estimating myoglobin in urine. Clin. Chem., *9*:1689, 1977.

Massachusetts Department of Public Health: Cost-Benefit Analysis of Newborn Screening for Metabolic Disorders. N. Engl. J. Med., *291*:1414, 1974.

McElderry, L. A., Tarbit, I. F., and Cassells-Smith, A. J.: Six methods for urinary protein compared. Clin. Chem., *28*:356, 1982.

Meryash, D. L., Levy, H. L., Guthrie, R., et al.: Prospective study of early neonatal screening for phenylketonuria. N. Engl. J. Med., *304*:294, 1981.

Najarian, J. S.: The diagnostic importance of the odor of urine. N. Engl. J. Med., *303*:1128, 1980.

NIH Guidelines for the Laboratory Use of Chemical Carcinogens. NIH Publication #81-2385. Washington, D.C., National Institutes of Health, May 1981.

Nyhan, W. L.: Understanding inherited metabolic disease. Clinical Symposia, Vol. 32, No. 5. Ciba, 1980.

Onstad, J., Hancock, D., and Wolf, P.: Inhibitory effect of fluoride on glucose tests with glucose oxidase strips. Clin. Chem., *21*:898, 1975.

Palmieri, L. J., and Schumann, G. B.: Osmotic effects on neutrophil segmentation. An *in vitro* phenomenon. Acta Cytol., *21*:2, 1977.

Peele, J. D., Gadsden, R. H., and Crews, R.: Evaluation of Ames' "Clini-Tek." Clin. Chem., *23*:2238, 1977.

Pennock, C. A., Most, M. G., and Batstone, G. F.: Screening for mucopolysaccharidoses. Clin. Chim. Acta, *27*:93, 1970.

Pierach, C. A., Cardinal, R., Bossenmaier, I., and Watson, C. J.: Comparison of the Hoesch and Watson-Schwartz tests for urinary porphobilinogen. Clin. Chem., *23*:1666, 1977.

Piva, A. E., and Koss, L. G.: Cytologic diagnosis of metastatic malignant melanoma in urinary sediment. Acta Cytol., *8*:398, 1964.

Potter, J. L.: Simultaneous testing for glucose and total reducing substances in routine urinalysis. Clin. Chem., *26*:172, 1980.

Prien, E. L.: Crystallographic analysis of urinary calculi: A 23 year survey study. J. Urol., *89*:917, 1963.

Prescott, L. F.: Urinary white cell excretion patterns. Lancet, *2*:238, 1965.

Prescott, L. F., and Brodie, D. G.: A simple differential stain for urinary sediment. Lancet, *2*:940, 1964.

Pritchard, J. A., and MacDonald, P. C. (eds.): Williams' Obstetrics. 16th ed. New York, Appleton-Century-Crofts, 1980.

Putnam, F. W., Easley, C. W., Lynn, L. T., Ritchie, A. E., and Phelps, R. A.: The heat precipitation of Bence Jones proteins. I. Optimum conditions. Arch. Biochem. Biophys., *83*:115, 1959.

Riekers, H., and Miale, J. B.: Ketonuria. An evaluation of tests and some clinical implications. Am. J. Clin. Path., *30*:530, 1958.

Riggs, S. A., Minuth, A. N., Nottebohm, G. A., et al.: Plasma cells in urine. Occurrence in multiple myeloma. Arch. Intern. Med. *135*:1245, 1975.

Robinson, R. R., Glover, S. N., Phillippi, P. J., Lecocq, F. R., and Langelier, P. R.: Fixed and reproducible orthostatic proteinuria. Am. J. Path., *39*:291, 1961.

Roguljic, A., and Ruzdic, I.: The DOPA-oxidase activity in urine and its diagnostic importance for malignant melanoma. Clin. Chem., *21*:1025, 1975.

Ross, D. L., and Neely, A. E.: Textbook of Urinalysis and Body Fluids. Norwalk, Conn., Appleton-Century-Crofts, 1983.

Rothera, A. C. H.: Note on the sodium nitro-prusside reaction for acetone. J. Physiol., *37*:491, 1908.

Rous, P.: Urinary siderosis. J. Exp. Med., *28*:645, 1918.

Rubin, M. I.: Urine and urination. *In* Nelson, W. E. (ed.): Textbook of Pediatrics., Philadelphia, W. B. Saunders Company, 1964.

Rubini, H. E., and Wolfe, A. V.: Refractometric determination of total solids and water of serum and urine. J. Biol. Chem., *225*:869, 1957.

Rubner, M.: Über die Einwirkung von Bleiacetat auf Trauben- und Milchzucker. Z. Biol., *20*:397, 1884.

Ryan, W. L., and Mills, R. D.: Bacterial multiplication in urine during refrigeration. Am. J. Med. Tech., *29*:175, 1963.

Rytand, D. A.: Prognosis in postural (orthostatic) proteinuria. N. Engl. J. Med., *305*:618, 1981.

Sanjurjo, L. A.: Parasitic diseases of the genitourinary system. *In* Campbell, M. F., and Harrison, J. H. (eds.): Urology. 3rd ed. Philadelphia, W. B. Saunders Company, 1970.

Schreiner, G. E.: Identification and significance of casts. Arch. Intern. Med. *99*:956, 1957.

Schulze, V. E.: Rhabdomyolysis as a cause of acute renal failure. Postgrad. Med., *72*:145, 1982.

Schumann, G. B.: Urine Sediment Examination. Baltimore, Williams & Wilkins, 1980.

Schumann, G. B., and Greenberg, N. F.: Usefulness of macroscopic urinalysis as a screening procedure. A preliminary report. Am. J. Clin. Path., *71*:452, 1979.

Schumann, G. B., Johnston, J. L., and Weiss, M. A.: Renal epithelial fragments in urine sediment. Acta Cytol., *25*:147, 1981a.

Schumann, G. B., Schumann, J. L., and Schweitzer, S.: The urine sediment examination: A coordinated approach. Lab. Management, *21*:45, 1983.

Schumann, G. B., and Weiss, M. A.: Atlas of Renal and Urinary Tract Cytology and Its Histopathologic Bases. Philadelphia, J. B. Lippincott, 1981b.

Schwartz, M. K.: Interferences in diagnostic biochemical procedures. Adv. Clin. Chem., *16*:1, 1973.

Schwartz, S., Shorov, V., and Watson, C. J.: Studies of urobilinogen. IV. Quantitative determination of urobilinogen by means of Evelyn photoelectric colorimeter. Am. J. Clin. Path., *14*:598, 1944.

Schwartz, S., Zieve, L., and Watson, C. J.: An improved method for the determination of urinary coproporphyrin and an evaluation of factors affecting analysis. J. Lab. Clin. Med., *27*:843, 1951.

Seliwanoff, S.: Ber. Deutch. Chem. Gesellsch., *20*:181, 1887. *In* Essential Fructosuria. Report of three cases with metabolic studies (S. Silberg and M. Reiner, eds.). Arch. Intern. Med., *54*:412, 1934.

Simmonds, H. A.: 2,8-Dihydroxyadeninuria—or when is a uric acid stone not a uric acid stone? Clin. Nephrol., *12*:196, 1979.

Simpson, E., and Thompson, D.: Routine urinalysis. Lancet, *2*:361, 1977.

Sjoerdsma, A., Weissbach, H., and Udenfriend, S.: Simple tests for diagnosis of metastatic carcinoid. J.A.M.A., *159*:397, 1955.

Smith, A.: Evaluation of the nitroprusside test for the diagnosis of cystinuria. Med. J. Aust., *2*:153, 1977a.

Smith, D., and Young, W. W.: Effect of large dose ascorbic acid on the two-drop Clinitest determination. Am. J. Hosp. Pharm., *34*:1347, 1977b.

Stamm, W. E., Running, K., McKeirtt, M., et al.: Treatment of the acute urethral syndrome. N. Engl. J. Med., *304*:956, 1981.

Stanbury, J. B., Wyngaarden, J. B., Fredrickson, D. S., et al. (eds.): The Metabolic Basis of Inherited Diseases. 5th ed. New York, McGraw-Hill, 1983.

Stansfeld, J. M., and Webb, J. K. G.: Observations on pyuria in children. Arch. Dis. Child., *28*:386, 1953.

Sternheimer, R.: A supravital cytodiagnostic stain for urinary sediments. J.A.M.A., *231*:8, 1975.

Sternheimer, R., and Malbin, B.: Clinical recognition of pyelonephritis with a new stain for urinary sediments. Am. J. Med., *11*:312, 1951.

Stewart, A. F., and Broadus, A. E.: The regulation of renal calcium excretion. An approach to hypercalciuria. Ann. Rev. Med., *32*:457, 1981.

Sutor, A. H., Ketelson, V. P., and Schindera, F.: Platelets in the urine: Further evidence. Thromb. Haemostas., *36*:647, 1976.

Thomas, G. H., and Howell, R. R.: Selected Screening Tests for Genetic Metabolic Diseases. Chicago, Year Book Medical Publishers, 1973.

Thomas, V., Shelokov, A., and Forland, M.: Antibody-coated bacteria in the urine and the site of urinary-tract infection. N. Engl. J. Med., *290*:11, 1974.

Thompson, A. L., Durrett, R. R., and Robinson, R. R.: Fixed and reproducible orthostatic proteinuria. Ann. Intern. Med., *73*:235, 1970.

Triger, D. R., and Smith, J. W. C.: Survival of urinary leucocytes. J. Clin. Path., *19*:443, 1966.

Tweeddale, D. N.: Urinary Cytology. Boston, Little, Brown & Company, 1977.

Udenfriend, S., Titus, E., and Weissbach, H.: The identification of 5-hydroxy-3-indoleacetic acid in normal urine and a method for its assay. J. Biol. Chem., *216*:299, 1955.

Vaughan, V. C., III, McKay, R. J., and Behrman, R. E. (eds.): Nelson Textbook of Pediatrics. 11th ed. Philadelphia, W. B. Saunders Company, 1979.

Vidler, J., and Wilcken, B.: Prevalence of unsuspected bacterial contamination: Effects on screening tests for detection of inborn errors of metabolism. Clin. Chim. Acta, *82*:173, 1978.

Wahlin, A.: Differential count of urinary leukocytes and renal epithelial cells. Upsala J. Med. Sci., *82*:43, 1977.

Washington, J. A., White, C. M., Laganiere, M., and Smith, L. H.: Detection of significant bacteriuria by microscopic examination of the urine. Lab. Med., *12*:294, 1981.

Watson, C. J., and Hawkinson, V.: Semiquantitative estimation of bilirubin in the urine by means of barium strip modification of Harrison's test. J. Lab. Clin. Med., *31*:914, 1946.

Watson, C. J., and Schwartz, S.: A simple test for urinary porphobilinogen. Proc. Soc. Exp. Biol. Med., *47*:393, 1941.

Wenk, R. E., Bhagavan, B. S., and Rudert, J.: Tamm-Horsfall uromucoprotein and the pathogenesis of casts, reflux nephropathy and nephritides. *In* Ioachin, H. L. (ed.): Pathology Annual. New York, Raven Press, 1981, p. 229.

Wert, E. B.: The Clinilab automated urinalysis system; six months' experience in a community hospital. Ann. Clin. Lab. Sci., *3*:319, 1973.

Westbury, E. J., and Omenogor, P.: A quantitative approach to the analysis of renal calculi. J. Med. Lab. Technol., *27*:462, 1970.

Wilcken, B., Smith, A., and Brown, D. A.: Urine screening for aminoacidopathies: Is it beneficial? J Pediatr., *97*:492, 1980.

Winer, J.: Practical value of analysis of urinary calculi. J.A.M.A., *169*:1715, 1959.

Winer, J., and Mattic, M. R.: Routine analysis of urinary calculi: Rapid, simple method using spot tests. J. Lab. Clin. Med., *28*:989, 1943.

Winkel, P., Statland, B., and Jorgenson, J.: Urine microscopy, an ill-defined method examined by multifactorial technique. Clin. Chem., *20*:436, 1974.

Wirth, W. A., and Thompson, R. L.: The effect of various conditions and substances on the results of laboratory procedures. Am. J. Clin. Path., *43*:579, 1965.

With, T. K.: Biology of Bile Pigments, Including a Review of Their Chemistry and a Discussion of Analytical Methods. Copenhagen, Arne Frost-Hansen, 1954.

With, T. K.: Diagnostic tests for porphyria. Lab. Med., *11*:446, 1980.

Wolfe, A. V.: Urinary concentrative powers. Am. J. Med., *32*:329, 1962.

Wong, L. T. K., Hardwick, D. F., Applegarth, D. A., and Davidson, A. G. F.: Review of metabolic screening program of Children's Hospital, Vancouver, B.C., 1971–1977. Clin. Biochem., *12*:167, 1979.

Worth, R. D., Harrison, J., and Skillen, A. W.: Stability of glucose in urine (abstract). Clin. Chem., *26*:789, 1980.

Wrong, O., and Davies, H. E. F.: The excretion of acid in renal disease. Q. J. Med. *28*:259, 1959.

Young, D., and Jackson, A.: Thin layer chromatography of urinary carbohydrates: A comparative evaluation of procedures. Clin. Chem., *16*:954, 1970.

Young, D. S., Pestaner, L. C., and Gibberman, V.: Effects of drugs on clinical laboratory tests. Clin. Chem., *21*:386D, 1975.

19

CEREBROSPINAL FLUID AND OTHER BODY FLUIDS

CARL R. KJELDSBERG, M.D., and ARTHUR F. KRIEG, M.D.

CEREBROSPINAL FLUID

Formation, Circulation, and Composition

About 70 per cent of cerebrospinal fluid (CSF) is formed in the ventricular choroid plexuses by a combined process of active transport and ultrafiltration (Hammock, 1976). About 30 per cent of CSF is formed at other sites, which apparently include the ependymal lining of the ventricles and the cerebral subarachnoid space.

Modern studies support the classic view that CSF (1) is formed within the ventricles, (2) exits from the foramina of Lushka and Magendie in the fourth ventricle, (3) circulates upward over the cerebral hemispheres as well as downward over the spinal cord and nerve roots, and (4) is resorbed through arachnoid villi in dural sinuses as well as at dural reflections over cranial and spinal nerves. The arachnoid villi may also function as unidirectional valves capable of clearing particles 4 to 12 μ in diameter from CSF (e.g., cellular debris from leukocytes and erythrocytes) (Plum, 1975).

The concept of a *blood-CSF barrier* accounts for different concentrations of solutes in plasma and CSF. Anatomically, the blood-CSF barrier is represented by the choroid plexus epithelium and the endothelium of all capillaries in contact with the CSF.

CSF also is in equilibrium with interstitial fluid of the central nervous system (CNS) across a *CSF-brain barrier*. Anatomically, the CSF-brain barrier is represented by the pia mater of the CNS (Dunn, 1972).

A third barrier, the *blood-brain barrier,* anatomically is represented by capillary endothelium in contact with astrocyte foot processes.

Total volume of CSF in adults is approximately 150 ml: about 20 ml in the ventricles, about 60 ml in the subarachnoid cisterns, and about 70 ml in the spinal canal. Total volume of CSF in neonates is approximately 10 to 60 ml. Rate of formation is about 500 ml/day, or 21 ml/hour. Rate of formation is independent of pressure, while rate of resorption depends on the pressure gradient between CSF and venous blood in the dural sinuses (about 60 to 80 mm water). In most cases, hydrocephalus appears related to defects in absorption rather than to increased formation of CSF; usually the difficulty is in blockage of the flow of CSF rather than any clearly demonstrated abnormality in the absorption apparatus itself (Collins, 1978).

The CSF concentrations of some substances are regulated within narrow limits, notably the ions K^+, H^+, Mg^{++}, and Ca^{++} (Table 19–1). Regulation of these ions probably depends on (1) active transport across the blood-CSF barrier and (2) exchanges between CSF and CNS interstitial fluid. Water and chloride diffuse rapidly across the blood-CSF barrier. Lipid-soluble drugs, including anesthetics and ethyl

Table 19–1. REFERENCE VALUES FOR LUMBAR CEREBROSPINAL FLUID IN ADULTS*

	Cerebrospinal Fluid	Serum
Protein†	15–45 mg/dl	6.0–7.8 g/dl
Prealbumin	2– 7%	—
Albumin	56–76%	52–67%
α_1 Globulin	2– 7%	2– 5%
α_2 Globulin	4–12%	6–14%
β Globulin	8–18%	8–16%
γ Globulin	3–12%	10–22%
Electrolytes and acid-base measurements		
Osmolality	280–295 mOsm/L	280–295 mOsm/L
Sodium	136–150 mEq/L	136–150 mEq/L
Potassium		
Lumbar fluid	2.6–3.0 mEq/L	3.0–4.5 mEq/L
Cisternal fluid	2.3–2.7 mEq/L	
Chloride	118–130 mEq/L	96–104 mEq/L
Bicarbonate	20–25 mEq/L	21–26 mEq/L
Calcium	2.1–2.7 mEq/L	4.6–5.4 mEq/L
Magnesium	2.4–3.0 mEq/L	1.5–2.4 mEq/L
Lactate	10–22 mg/dl (0.2–0.4 mmol/L)	3–7 mg/dl (arterial)
pH		
Lumbar fluid	7.28–7.32	7.38–7.42
Cisternal fluid	7.32–7.34	(arterial)
P_{CO_2}		
Lumbar fluid	44–50 mm Hg	36–40 mm Hg
Cisternal fluid	40–46 mm Hg	(arterial)
P_{O_2}	40–44 mm Hg	95–100 mm Hg (arterial)
Other constituents		
Ammonia	0.5–1.0 μg/ml	1.0–2.0 μg/ml (arterial)
Creatinine	0.5–1.2 mg/dl	0.5–1.2 mg/dl
Glucose	50–80 mg/dl	70–100 mg/dl (fasting)
Iron	1–2 μg/dl	50–150 μg/dl
Phosphorus	1.2–2.0 mg/dl	3.0–4.5 mg/dl
Urea	6–16 mg/dl	8–20 mg/dl
Uric acid	0.5–3.0 mg/dl	2.0–8.0 mg/dl
Zinc	2–6 μg/dl	50–150 μg/dl

*Data from various sources.
†See also Table 19–7.

alcohol, diffuse from plasma to CSF in proportion to their lipid solubility. Glucose, urea, and creatinine diffuse freely but require several hours for equilibration. Other substances, e.g., drugs such as penicillin and streptomycin, do not normally enter CSF from plasma. Proteins apparently diffuse slowly across a concentration gradient from plasma to CSF, at rates which decrease with increasing hydrodynamic radii (Felgenhauer, 1974).

Studies indicate that the blood-CSF barrier can be reversibly opened by several mechanisms, including acute hypertension, seizures, hypercapnea, and injections of radiographic dyes (Plum, 1975). Functionally as well as anatomically, the blood-CSF barrier is a complex structure not yet fully understood.

LUMBAR PUNCTURE

Indications for lumbar puncture may include:

1. Suspected meningitis, encephalitis (including neurosyphilis), brain abscess, subarachnoid hemorrhage, leukemia involving the central nervous system, multiple sclerosis, Guillain-Barré syndrome, and spinal cord tumor.
2. Differential diagnosis of cerebral infarct vs. intracerebral hemorrhage (xanthochromic CSF found in about 80 per cent of patients with the latter condition).
3. Introduction of anesthetics, radiographic contrast media, or certain drugs (methotrexate in meningeal leukemia and amphotericin in fungal meningitis).
4. Treatment of selected patients with benign intracranial hypertension (the effectiveness of this therapy is not established).

Emergency lumbar puncture may be indicated in patients with suspected meningitis, subarachnoid hemorrhage, or leukemia involving the central nervous system. In most other situations, lumbar puncture is an elective procedure. Elective lumbar puncture should be performed in the morning, with the patient fasting overnight because (1) prompt evaluation by trained laboratory staff may be unavailable during the second and third shifts; (2) glucose levels in CSF can be best evaluated by comparison with blood glucose under fasting conditions; and (3) consultants are more likely to be available in event of unexpected problems.

Potential problems and complications of lumbar puncture include:

1. Herniation of the uncus through the tentorium, or the cerebellar tonsils through the foramen magnum, in patients with increased intracranial pressure. In the presence of papilledema, mortality rate from lumbar puncture may be about 0.3 per cent (Marshall, 1970). Papilledema probably is not a contraindication, provided that (1) the information sought is not available by other methods (e.g., brain scan); (2) there is a high probability that CSF findings will significantly influence both treatment and outcome; and (3) neurosurgical consultation is available.

2. With spinal cord tumor, progression of paresis to paralysis may follow lumbar puncture with removal of CSF. If spinal cord tumor is suspected, it is best to combine lumbar puncture with myelography, and to follow these with surgical exploration, if needed.

3. Extradural or subdural hematoma with resultant paraplegia may follow lumbar puncture in patients who have clotting defects (e.g., thrombocytopenia) or who are receiving anticoagulant drugs (Messer, 1976). Although these conditions are not absolute contraindications, potential benefits should be carefully weighed against risk.

4. In the presence of sepsis, perforation of the meninges enhances development of meningitis (Fischer, 1975). If sepsis is suspected, blood cultures should be obtained prior to lumbar puncture, and repeat examination of CSF performed if the clinical condition warrants.

5. In infants, death may occur from asphyxiation caused by (a) excessive restraint (Campbell, 1968) or (b) tracheal obstruction caused by pushing the head forward (Hinterbuchner, 1968).

6. If no stylet is used, epidermoid tumors may develop after a period of two to ten years (Shaywitz, 1972).

7. Introduction of infection by passing the needle through superficial or deep sepsis in the lumbar regions (e.g., superficial skin infection, cellulitis, or epidural abscess). Indeed, lumbar puncture is contraindicated if there is any infection in the region of the puncture site. If epidural abscess is suspected, aspiration should be performed as the needle is introduced (Alexander, 1967).

8. Postpuncture headache resulting from leakage of CSF has been reported in 13 to 32 per cent of patients (Fishman, 1971). The use of a small needle with stylet (22 gauge) may decrease incidence of postpuncture headache.

Lumbar puncture is performed at L3-L4 or lower to avoid damage to the spinal cord. In small children and infants, the cord may extend as low as L3-L4, so puncture should be performed at L4-L5 or lower.

PRESSURE AND DYNAMICS

Before any fluid is withdrawn, the pressure should be measured by allowing CSF to rise in a sterile, graduated manometer tube. Normal pressure varies between 50 and 180 mm of CSF, measured with the patient in the lateral recumbent position. Should opening pressure exceed 180, reassure the patient, straighten the legs, back, and neck, and ensure that there is no breath holding, jugular compression, or abdominal compression. If pressure then falls to normal, it is probable that the initial elevation was artifactual. When the needle is correctly placed, minor variations in pressure (5 to 10 mm) occur with respiration. Absence of these minor variations may be due to incorrect placement of the needle or to a block between the needle and the dural sinuses.

CSF pressure is directly related to pressure in the jugular and vertebral veins, which communicate with the intracranial venous sinuses. Measured CSF pressure may be decreased with (1) circulatory collapse; (2) severe dehydration; (3) acute hyperosmolality (causes decrease in brain volume owing to passage of water from CNS to systemic circulation); (4) leakage of CSF (e.g., tear in dura following injury to low back, CSF rhinorrhea, previous lumbar puncture); (5) complete spinal subarachnoid block (lumbar fluid does not communicate with fluid at levels above the block). Measured CSF pressure may be increased with (1) congestive heart failure; (2) inflammation of the meninges (interferes with return of fluid through arachnoid granulations); (3) acute obstruction of superior vena cava (before collateral drainage has developed); (4) obstruction of intracranial venous sinuses owing to thrombosis; (5) acute hyposmolality owing to hemodialysis (causes increase in brain volume owing to passage of water from systemic circulation to CNS; (6) impaired resorption of CSF owing to elevated CSF protein, or subarachnoid hemorrhage; (7) mass lesions (e.g., tumor, abscess, or intracerebral hemorrhage); or (8) cerebral edema. If initial pressure is over 200 mm, only 1 to 2 ml of fluid should be removed. A 25 to 50 per cent fall in pressure after removing 1 to 2 ml suggests cerebellar herniation or spinal cord compression above the puncture site. In such cases, *no* additional fluid should be removed, and the patient should be observed closely for several hours. Provided initial pressure is not elevated, and there is no marked fall in pressure when fluid is removed, from 10 to 20 ml of CSF may be obtained without danger to the patient. Ordinarily, three 2 to 4 ml samples are taken in sterile tubes, labeled sequentially as No. 1 (chemistry and serology studies), No. 2 (bacteriologic studies), and No. 3 (cell count).

If the initial pressure is normal and there is clinical suspicion of subarachnoid block or spinal cord tumor, jugular compression (Queckenstedt test) may be performed. This test is contraindicated in suspected intracranial disease, particularly in the presence of increased intracranial pressure! It should *not* be performed as a "routine procedure!"

Normally, if both jugular veins are compressed, CSF pressure increases rapidly to over 300 mm, then rapidly returns to normal when compression ceases. This effect depends on rapid transmission of pressure from the jugular veins, through dural sinuses and arachnoid villi, to intracranial CSF. With sinus thrombosis, obstruction at the foramen magnum, or a mass lesion in the spinal canal, the rise in CSF pressure may be decreased or delayed (a "positive test"). In such cases, normal variations in pressure owing to respiration will be decreased or absent, but straining or abdominal compression results in increased CSF pressure owing to vertebral vein congestion.

About 80 per cent of patients with cord compression have a positive Queckenstedt test. Lesions may include herniated intervertebral disk, vertebral fracture, extradural abscess, adhesions owing to pachymeningitis, and neoplasms.

GROSS EVALUATION AND EXAMINATION FOR XANTHOCHROMIA

Normal CSF is crystal clear, with viscosity comparable to water. However, abnormal CSF may appear "cloudy," "smoky," "hazy," opalescent, turbid, or grossly bloody. Turbidity may be graded from 0 to 4 +:

0 = crystal clear fluid.
1+ = faintly "cloudy," "smoky," or "hazy," with slight (barely visible) turbidity.
2+ = turbidity clearly present, but newsprint easily read through tube.
3+ = newsprint not easily read through tube.
4+ = newsprint cannot be seen through tube.

Turbidity may be caused by leukocytes—at least 200 cells/μl required to cause slight turbidity (Fishman, 1971); erythrocytes—at least 400 cells/μl required to cause slight turbidity (Gooch, 1976; Patten, 1968); microorganisms (bacteria, fungi, amebas); contrast media; or aspiration of epidural fat during lumbar puncture (Mealey, 1962).

Clotting due to elevated CSF protein may occur with Froin's syndrome, which includes (1) subarachnoid block; (2) very high levels of protein in lumbar CSF; (3) xanthochromia due to elevated protein in lumbar CSF; (4) gel formation in CSF after standing. Clot formation is fairly common with protein levels over 1000 mg/dl but also may occur at lower levels. Very fine clots or "pellicles" may be detected by observing the surface of CSF after 12 to 24 hours at refrigerator temperature.

Clot formation is abnormal, and indicates increased amounts of fibrinogen in CSF. This may be due to traumatic tap or to increased protein owing to subarachnoid block, suppurative meningitis, tuberculous meningitis, neurosyphilis, etc.

Increased viscosity of CSF has been reported with metastatic mucinous adenocarcinoma to the meninges (Fishman, 1971).

Gross blood (or red cells on microscopic examination) presents the problem of differentiating traumatic tap from pathologic bleeding owing to spontaneous subarachnoid hemorrhage, intracerebral hemorrhage, or trauma. Crenation of erythrocytes is *not* useful in differential diagnosis of traumatic tap vs. subarachnoid hemorrhage. Differential diagnosis of traumatic tap vs. subarachnoid hemorrhage is based on the following: (1) Findings at the bedside. A traumatic tap usually shows non-homogenous mixing in the manometer, and gradual clearing as several samples are taken (2) Gross appearance of CSF. Visible clearing of blood between the first and third tubes (or a significant drop in erythrocyte count) is evidence of traumatic tap. (3) Clotting. A very bloody specimen (over 200,000 erythrocytes per μl) due to traumatic tap will clot on standing (Calabrese, 1976), while blood from subarachnoid bleeding will not clot *in vitro*. (4) Xanthochromia.

Xanthochromia refers to a pale pink to orange or yellow color in the supernatant of centrifuged CSF. In traumatic samples, the supernatant typically is crystal clear, while in subarachnoid hemorrhage, the supernatant usually is xanthochromic, provided erythrocytes have been present in CSF sufficiently long to cause lysis. Initial lysis of erythrocytes in CSF begins after about one to four hours (Calabrese, 1976). This rapid lysis of erythrocytes in CSF is not caused by an osmotic difference between plasma and CSF, since osmolality of both fluids is essentially the same (Table 19–1). Probably, lysis of erythrocytes in CSF is due to lack of plasma proteins and lipids needed to stabilize the erythrocyte membrane. Thus, examination for xanthochromia requires that CSF be centrifuged *within one hour or less* after collection, to avoid false positives.

A variety of pigments may contribute to xanthochromia as observed visually:

1. Oxyhemoglobin
   a. from lysed erythrocytes present in CSF before lumbar puncture
   b. traumatic tap with lysis of erythrocytes after lumbar puncture:
      (1) detergent in lumbar puncture needle and/or sample tube
      (2) greater than one hour delay prior to centrifuging CSF
2. Methemoglobin
3. Bilirubin
   a. from lysed erythrocytes in CSF
   b. from plasma, due to:
      (1) increased levels of direct bilirubin (e.g., 5 to 10 mg/dl) with normal blood-CSF barrier
      (2) increased levels of indirect bilirubin associated with increased permeability of the blood-CSF barrier
4. Increased concentration of CSF protein
   a. levels of CSF protein over 150 mg/dl
   b. traumatic tap with sufficient plasma in "CSF" sample to produce protein concentration over 150 mg/dl
5. Contamination of CSF by merthiolate used to disinfect the skin
6. Carotenoids in CSF due to systemic hypercarotenemia
7. Melanin in CSF due to meningeal melanosarcoma

Xanthochromia occurs in CSF of normal premature infants owing to combined effects of (a) immaturity of the blood-CSF barrier; (b) elevated bilirubin in blood; (c) elevated protein in CSF (see Total Protein, p. 467).

About two to four hours after subarachnoid hemorrhage, pale pink to pale orange xanthochromia due to oxyhemoglobin appears in CSF, reaching a peak at about 24 to 36 hours, and gradually disappearing at about four to eight days. About 12 hours after subarachnoid hemorrhage, yellow xanthochromia due to bilirubin appears in CSF, reaching a peak at about two to four days, and gradually disappearing at about two to four weeks (Walton, 1956).

Since the early 1960's, there has been increasing interest in spectrophotometric evaluation of xanthochromia. At least two methods have been described:

1. Qualitative estimates of oxyhemoglobin, methemoglobin, and bilirubin based on spectrophotometric scans (Kjellin, 1974).

2. Calculations based on absorbance at specific wavelengths (Kronholm, 1960; Van Der Meulen, 1966).

Spectrophotometric estimates of xanthochromia may be more sensitive and more specific than visual estimates: (1) methemoglobin may be detected in patients with subdural hematomas (one to two weeks duration or longer) despite clear CSF on visual examination; (2) xanthochromia due to bilirubin can be distinguished from xanthochromia due to increased protein. There is evidence that a higher percentage of patients with clinical central nervous system (CNS) hemorrhage have spectrophotometric xanthochromia as compared with visually detected xanthochromia. Although further studies are needed, spectrophotometric evaluation of xanthochromia may well provide a useful supplement to visual evaluation.

Cell Counts and Microscopic Examination

TOTAL LEUKOCYTE COUNT

The generally accepted reference interval or normal range for CSF leukocyte counts in adults is 0 to 5 mononuclear cells (lymphocytes and monocytes) per μl. The reference interval for neonates is somewhat higher: about 0 to 30 mononuclear cells per μl (Dryken, 1975; Sarff, 1976). According to Kolmel (1977), if more than a few milliliters of CSF is taken, the count may rise to 20 or even 30/μl.

Leukocyte counts usually are performed in a Fuchs-Rosenthal counting chamber (depth 0.2 mm), either with undiluted CSF and phase microscopy or with a small amount of acidified crystal violet added to CSF (Skeel, 1968). Using nine large squares on each side of the chamber, a total of $18 \times \frac{1}{5}$ μl (3.6 μl) is examined. If there are 5 cells per μl, then 18 cells will be counted in 3.6 μl.

Assuming a Poisson distribution, the coefficient of variation is given by:

$$CV = \frac{100}{\sqrt{\text{no. of cells counted}}}$$

$$= \frac{100}{\sqrt{18}} = \frac{100}{4.2} = 24\%$$

Thus, at the upper limit of the reference interval (5 leukocytes per μl), we may expect ±2 CV of about ±48 per cent.

CSF cell counts should be performed promptly, since leukocytes, like erythrocytes, begin to lyse within about one hour. For this reason, physicians should be prepared to personally perform CSF cell counts when these cannot be done within one hour by available technical staff.

Increased precision of CSF leukocyte counts is possible by counting larger numbers of cells. Electronic cell counters are not yet practical, since variable background counts cause poor precision in the normal range. However, leukocytes can be collected from 1.0 ml of CSF on a membrane filter, using a Swinney cartridge (Burechailo, 1974). By this method, the upper limit of normal is reported as 2 leukocytes per μl.

Erythrocyte counts on CSF are sometimes used to "correct" CSF leukocyte counts or CSF protein measurements for contamination by peripheral blood associated with traumatic tap. Use of such corrections requires (1) that all measurements (RBC, WBC, and/or total protein) be performed on the same tube; (2) an assumption that *all* RBC present are due to traumatic tap, with *no* contribution from subarachnoid or intracerebral hemorrhage; (3) an appreciation that accuracy of the "corrected" CSF WBC and protein is limited by precision of the CSF erythrocyte count. This last limitation may be appreciated in reference to the following examples. If serum protein is 7.0 gm/dl, hematocrit is 45 per cent, CSF RBC is 10,000 per μl, and peripheral RBC is 4.6 million per μl, added protein due to traumatic tap is:

$$= \frac{(7000 \times 0.55)\ \text{mg/dl} \times 10{,}000\ \text{RBC/μl}}{4{,}600{,}000\ \text{RBC/μl}}$$

$$= 8.4\ \text{mg/dl}$$

Therefore, 8 mg/dl should be subtracted from measured CSF protein to obtain a "corrected" value. Some authorities suggest "correction factors" of 15 mg/dl/10,000 RBC/μl (or 1 mg/dl for every 700 RBC/μl). However, as seen from the foregoing example, these formulas do not take into account the fact that whole blood total protein is about 55 per cent that of plasma protein. A more accurate "correction factor" might be 8 mg/dl/10,000 RBC/μl (or 1 mg/dl for every 1200 RBC/μl), assuming normal hematocrit and normal serum protein.

With a high CSF erythrocyte count, inherent errors of chamber RBC counting become important. If 400 erythrocytes are counted in the hemocytometer,

$$CV = \frac{100}{\sqrt{400}} = \frac{100}{20} = 5\%$$

Thus, 2 CV represents a 10 per cent error owing to inherent limitations of the counting procedure. If serum protein is 7.0 gm/dl, hematocrit is 40 per cent, CSF RBC is 1.0 million/μl, and peripheral RBC is 4.6 million/μl, added protein due to traumatic tap is:

$$= \frac{(7000 \times 0.6)\ \text{mg/dl} \times 1 \times 10^6\ \text{RBC/μl}}{4.6 \times 10^6\ \text{RBC/μl}}$$

$$= 913\ \text{mg/dl}$$

3

However, if there is a 10 per cent error in CSF erythrocyte count, the "true" added protein due to traumatic tap is:

$$= \frac{(7000 \times 0.6)\ \text{mg/dl} \times 0.9 \times 10^6\ \text{RBC}/\mu\text{l}}{4.6 \times 10^6\ \text{RBC}/\mu\text{l}}$$

$$= 822\ \text{mg/dl}$$

Thus in this case, the "correction" is accurate only within a range of ± 10 per cent or ±90 mg/dl.

Similar calculations can be used to correct CSF WBC for traumatic tap:

$$WBC_{added} = \frac{WBC_B \times RBC_{CSF}}{RBC_B}$$

where

WBC_{added} = leukocytes added to CSF for traumatic tap
WBC_B = leukocyte count in peripheral blood
RBC_{CSF} = erythrocyte count in CSF
RBC_B = erythrocyte count in peripheral blood

With normal peripheral blood, this amounts to 1 to 2 leukocytes per 1000 RBC.

DIFFERENTIAL COUNT

Methods. A "chamber differential" may be performed using either a small amount of acidified crystal violet added to CSF (Skeel, 1968) or phase microscopy with unstained fluid (Sornas, 1967, 1971). However, since only a few cells are observed, the "chamber differential" has relatively poor precision. Concentration of leukocytes prior to the differential count can provide larger numbers of cells for improved precision and better staining for more accurate cell identification. Methods for concentrating CSF leukocytes prior to differential counting include:

1. Centrifugation, with Wright's stain of resuspended sediment (Skeel, 1968).
2. Millipore or Nucleopore filter techniques (Gondos, 1976).
3. Sedimentation methods (Kolmel, 1977; Chu, 1977).
4. Cytocentrifuge and related methods (Woodruff, 1973; Ito, 1972).

Centrifugation is relatively rapid (under 1/2 hour) and requires no special equipment. Also, the supernatant fluid is available for further analysis (e.g., total protein, glucose, electrophoresis). Disadvantages include (1) variable and incomplete recovery of sedimented cells; (2) distortion and damage to cells during high-speed centrifugation; (3) the need for careful attention to technique to prepare a high quality film from the sediment. Because of these disadvantages, other methods are now replacing ordinary centrifugation in the United States as well as in Europe.

Millipore (Millipore Corporation, Bedford, Mass.) or Nucleopore (General Electric, Pleasanten, Cal.) filtration, like centrifugation, allows use of supernatant fluid for further analysis. With proper technique, recovery of cells exceeds 90 per cent, so that CSF leukocyte count can be determined from the total number of cells collected (Burechailo, 1974). Although tumor cells are well preserved (Gondos, 1976), other cellular elements are better studied by sedimentation or cytocentrifuge (Sornas, 1967; Krentz, 1972; Hansen, 1974; Castleberry, 1975; Kolmel, 1977). The principal disadvantages of filter techniques include more technical time required than for simple centrifugation, sedimentation, or cytocentrifuge and more technical skill required to cope with problems (e.g., clogging of membranes, staining and clearing techniques).

Sedimentation methods provide better preservation of cellular morphology than filter techniques or cytocentrifuge (Kolmel, 1977; Chu, 1977). The procedure is rapid (1/2 to 1 hour) and technically simple. Disadvantages include loss of cells in the range of 70 per cent owing to absorption on filter paper (Kolmel, 1977); more time required than for cytocentrifuge; and unavailability of the supernatant fluid for chemical analysis.

The cytocentrifuge and related methods provide the following advantages: (1) speed and simplicity superior to other concentration methods, (2) excellent cell preservation, comparable to sedimentation methods, and (3) recovery of cells comparable to sedimentation (though inferior to filtration techniques). Disadvantages include (1) cell recovery inferior to filtration techniques, (2) supernatant fluid unavailable for chemical analysis, and (3) need for special equipment.

For many laboratories, the cytocentrifuge provides an excellent "compromise." The method is rapid, easy to learn, and provides good cytologic detail. Cost of equipment is modest; alternatively, special adapters can be used with an ordinary centrifuge (Ito, 1972). And numerous cells are available for microscopic examination from 0.5 ml CSF.

NOTE: If we assume a "normal" CSF leukocyte count of 1 per μl, a 10 per cent recovery from 0.5 ml would produce 50 cells for study. In actual practice, about 30 to 50 cells are obtained by sedimentation or cytocentrifuge from 0.5 ml of "normal" CSF (Dryken, 1975; Sheth, 1977).

Clinical Correlation. At this time, there is no general agreement on nomenclature for cytologic elements in normal CSF. Sheth (1977) identifies lymphocytes, pia arachnoid mesothelial (PAM) cells, monocytes, and neutrophils (rare) as normally present (Table 19–2). Kolmel (1977) identifies lymphocytes, monocytes, "monocytoid" cells (morphologically similar to the PAM cells described by Sheth), neutrophils (rare), and ependymal cells (rare) as normally present. Dryken (1975) identifies lymphocytes and monocytes in adults, plus a few neutrophils and macrophages also present in normal neonates. The PAM cells described by Sheth appear similar to young monocytes: relatively large nuclei which are round rather than indented; cytoplasm which is more basophilic and less abundant than mature monocytes. These pia arachnoid mesothelial cells have functional similarities to monocytes of peripheral blood (Oehmichen, 1976; Guseo, 1977).

Suggested reference intervals for differential count in CSF (sedimentation or cytocentrifuge technique) are outlined in Table 19–2. These are based on reports by Dryken (1975) and Sheth (1977), as well as on unpublished data from our own laboratory. However, reported normal ranges from the older literature usu-

Table 19–2. REFERENCE INTERVALS FOR CSF DIFFERENTIAL COUNTS BY SEDIMENTATION OR CYTOCENTRIFUGE

Cell Type	Adults	Neonates
Lymphocytes	62% ± 34	20% ± 18
PAM cells* and monocytes	36% ± 20	72% ± 22
Neutrophils	2% ± 5	3% ± 5†
Histiocytes	Rare	5% ± 4
Ependymal cells	Rare	Rare
Eosinophils	Rare	Rare

NOTE: Ordinarily the absolute numbers of cells counted are reported as well as percentages. Since recovery is *not* 100%, the absolute number for each cell type does *not* represent total number for the volume of fluid examined. The CV for a given count can be estimated using the formula

$$CV = \frac{100}{\sqrt{n}} \text{ where n = number of cells counted.}$$

*PAM = Pia-arachnoid mesothelial cells.
†Some authors report high upper limit of normal (McCracken, 1976).

ally specify a lower percentage of monocytes and a higher percentage of lymphocytes (about 14 per cent and 86 per cent, respectively). One possible explanation has been suggested by Kolmel (1977): after the first few milliliters of CSF, the percentage of monocytes increases while the percentage of lymphocytes decreases. A second explanation is that with sedimentation or cytocentrifuge, monocytes are easily recognized, while with other methods, monocytes which are not "spread out" may be classified as lymphocytes. A third explanation is loss of small lymphocytes by sedimentation or cytocentrifuge.

There has been considerable discussion on whether neutrophils are present in "normal" CSF. Some authors consider even one neutrophil as abnormal (Cole, 1969) while others suggest that up to 10 per cent neutrophils (e.g., 5 out of 50 cells counted) are within normal limits (Sheth, 1977). According to Kolmel (1977), neutrophils in CSF probably come from contamination by peripheral blood owing to traumatic tap. At this time, there is no general agreement on the "upper limit of normal." Significance of small numbers of neutrophils should be evaluated in reference to (a) clinical and laboratory evidence of traumatic tap; (b) findings on neurologic examination; or (c) other laboratory findings (e.g., Gram's stain).

Increased numbers of neutrophils may be found in infections, including bacterial meningitis, early viral meningoencephalitis (first one to two days; rarely may persist), early tuberculous or mycotic meningitis, amebic encephalomyelitis, early stages of meningovascular syphilis, and aseptic meningitis owing to septic focus adjacent to the meninges (e.g., septic emboli due to bacterial endocarditis; osteomyelitis of skull or spine; subdural empyema; cerebral abscess; phlebitis of dural sinuses or cortical veins). Noninfectious causes include reaction to CNS hemorrhage (e.g., three to four days after hemorrhagic infarct, subarachnoid hemorrhage, or intracerebral hematoma) (Sornas, 1972), reaction to repeated lumbar puncture (possibly related to hemorrhage caused by traumatic tap), the injection of foreign materials into subarachnoid space (e.g., RISA, xylocaine, methotrexate, or contrast media) (Dramov, 1971; Swartz, 1965), pneumoencephalogram, chronic granulocytic leukemia involving the CNS, lumbar puncture with needles contaminated by detergent, metastatic tumor (necrotic and in contact with CSF), and infarct (hemorrhagic or pale and in contact with CSF).

A neutrophilic reaction classically suggests meningitis owing to pyogenic organisms. During the early acute stage, CSF leukocyte counts frequently exceed 1000/μl and may reach 20,000/μl, with 90 per cent neutrophils. Other neutrophilic reactions (see above) usually are less marked. In viral meningoencephalitis, the cell count seldom exceeds 1000/μl, and usually changes to a lymphocytic response within two to three days. In bacterial meningitis, successful treatment is associated with rapid disappearance of granulocytes. Unsuccessful treatment, with progression to chronic meningitis or cerebral abscess, is characterized by a mixed reaction, i.e., monocytes, lymphocytes, and granulocytes (Kolmel, 1977).

Increased numbers of lymphocytes have been reported in infections, including (1) viral meningoencephalitis (plasma cells and some macrophages also may be present); (2) tuberculous meningitis (the combination of lymphocytes, granulocytes, and plasma cells is characteristic; multinucleate giant cells may be present); (3) fungal meningitis, e.g., cryptococcosis, coccidioides (a mixed reaction with lymphocytes, granulocytes, and plasma cells is characteristic); (4) syphilitic meningoencephalitis (lymphocytes, plasma cells, and monocytes usually predominate); (5) leptospiral meningitis (this may present a mixed reaction with up to 50 per cent granulocytes); (6) partially treated bacterial meningitis (according to Converse [1973], perhaps 10 per cent of patients revert to a lymphocytic reaction following partial treatment with antibiotics); (7) bacterial meningitis due to uncommon organisms (e.g., *Listeria monocytogenes* in infants) (Hyslop, 1975); (8) parasitic disease (e.g., cysticercosis, trichinosis, toxoplasmosis); (9) aseptic meningitis due to septic focus adjacent to the meninges (see above); and (10) subacute sclerosing panencephalitis (SSPE) due to measles virus (cytologic findings similar to multiple sclerosis). Non-infectious causes include (1) multiple sclerosis (about 50 per cent of cases show increased total cell count with lymphocytes and plasma cells); (2) encephalopathy owing to drug abuse (Sheth, 1977); (3) Guillain-Barré syndrome (about 15 per cent of cases may show lymphocytic pleocytosis) (Fishman, 1971); (4) acute disseminated encephalomyelitis; (5) sarcoidosis of meninges; (6) polyneuritis (lymphocytes, plasma cells, and macrophages present during the recovery stage); and (7) periarteritis involving the central nervous system.

Increased numbers of plasma cells may occur in association with lymphocytic reactions. In some cases, e.g., multiple sclerosis, CSF plasma cells may be the only abnormality. Normally, plasma cells are absent from CSF. Morphologic evidence suggests that lymphocytes undergo transformation to plasma cells within the central nervous system (Glasser, 1977). Transitional forms between lymphocytes, "reactive lymphocytes," "plasmacytoid lymphocytes," and classic plasma cells have been described by various observers (Kolmel, 1977; Glasser, 1977).

Increased numbers of eosinophils (over 5 per cent of total leukocytes) have been reported in the following infections: (1) bacterial meningitis (e.g., some cases of pneumococcal meningitis), (2) tuberculous meningitis (a few cases), (3) fungal meningitis (e.g., coccidioidomycosis), (4) syphilitic meningoencephalitis (a few cases), (5) some cases of viral meningoencephalitis (Sheth, 1977), and (6) parasitic infestation (e.g., cysticercosis, hydatid disease). Non-infectious causes include (1) intrathecal injections of foreign protein (e.g., RISA [radioiodinated serum albumin], radiographic contrast media), (2) rabies vaccination, (3) intracranial shunts (reaction to rubber catheter) (4) periarteritis nodosa, (5) acute polyneuritis, (6) drug reactions, (7) food allergies, (8) urticaria, (9) allergic bronchial asthma, and (10) lymphocytic leukemia with spread to CNS. Persistent eosinophilia in CNS suggests the possibility of parasitic infestation, including ascariasis, paragonimiasis, or animal parasites which do not ordinarily affect humans.

Increased numbers of basophils may be seen in chronic granulocytic leukemia involving the meninges.

Increased numbers of ependymal cells may be seen following pneumoencephalography, in hydrocephalus, in specimens obtained by cisternal or ventricular puncture, or following intrathecal administration of chemotherapeutic agents.

Increased numbers of pia arachnoid mesothelial (PAM) cells and/or monocytes usually are seen as part of a "mixed reaction," along with (1) neutrophils, lymphocytes, and plasma cells, or (2) lymphocytes and plasma cells. A "mixed reaction" with neutrophils, lymphocytes, plasma cells, and monocytes is characteristic of tuberculous meningitis, fungal meningitis, chronic bacterial meningitis, rupture of brain abscess, leptospiral meningitis, and amebic encephalomyelitis. A "mixed reaction" with lymphocytes, plasma cells, and monocytes is characteristic of viral meningoencephalitis, syphilitic meningoencephalitis, some cases of partially treated bacterial meningitis, some cases of bacterial meningitis due to uncommon organisms (e.g., *Listeria monocytogenes*), leptospiral meningitis, some cases of parasitic infestation (e.g., cysticercosis), some cases of aseptic meningitis due to septic focus adjacent to the meninges (e.g., encapsulation of brain abscess), subacute sclerosing panencephalitis (SSPE), and non-infectious conditions including multiple sclerosis and polyneuritis. None of these patterns is "diagnostic." The foregoing "lists" of conditions should serve as "reminders" rather than as absolute criteria.

Increased numbers of macrophages, including giant cells, may be associated with tuberculous or mycotic meningitis, reaction to erythrocytes in CSF (following brain surgery, trauma, or subarachnoid hemorrhage) (hemosiderin granules may appear after about four days), reaction to foreign substances in CSF, e.g., contrast media or ventricular drains, and reaction to lipid in CSF derived from CNS injury (e.g., contusion, infarction, brain abscess).

Lupus erythematosus (LE) cells have been described in CSF (Nosanchuk, 1976); however, this finding is rare.

Leukemic cells in CSF are of special importance and have received increasing attention in recent years. Leukemic infiltration of the meninges is related to special characteristics of the blood-CSF barrier, which is almost impermeable to present chemotherapeutic agents. Thus, leukemic cells which enter CSF from blood or from meningeal infiltrates can undergo uninhibited proliferation.

An initial finding of leukemic cells in CSF is uncommon. More often, leukemic cells appear in CSF after the illness has become established, e.g., after several remissions have been achieved by chemotherapy. Indeed, leukemic cells may appear in CSF during apparent remission, and after chemotherapy has been discontinued.

Leukemic cell counts in CSF vary between only a few leukemic cells, and more than 1000/μl. Morphologic appearance is similar to peripheral blood or bone marrow. Meningeal spread is common in lymphoblastic leukemia, acute myeloblastic leukemia, and promyelocytic leukemia (perhaps 30 to 40 per cent of all cases). Meningeal spread is unusual in chronic myeloid and chronic lymphocytic leukemia. Malignant lymphomas may infiltrate the meninges, with appearance of lymphoma cells in CSF. Morphologically these may be difficult or impossible to distinguish from leukemic infiltrates.

Leukemoid reactions in CSF may be associated with coma, which can mimic chronic granulocytic leukemia with promyelocytes present in CSF (Sheth, 1977).

Tumor cells in CSF may be derived from primary or metastatic neoplasms. Primary intracranial tumors include medulloblastoma, retinoblastoma, astrocytoma, ependymoma, pinealoma, oligodendroglioma, meningioma, schwannoma, and pituitary adenoma. Metastatic tumors to CNS include lung, breast, gastrointestinal tract, and melanoma. Examination for "malignant tumor cells" usually is performed in a special tumor cytology laboratory using Papanicolaou stains. The appearance of tumor cells on Wright's stain is well illustrated in Kolmel's atlas (1977).

IDENTIFICATION OF MICROORGANISMS ON MICROSCOPIC EXAMINATION

In bacterial meningitis, the most valuable single examination is a carefully examined Gram's stain of CSF. Reported sensitivity of this procedure ranges from 70 per cent (Hyslop, 1975) to 80 per cent (McCracken, 1976a) to 90 per cent (Carpenter, 1962). Sensitivity depends on the method used for preparing the smears, and is markedly increased when Gram's stain is done on cytocentrifuge slide preparations. Specificity is less well documented, although false positives may occur from (1) gram-positive artifacts in staining solutions or (2) dead bacteria in tubes used for collection or processing CSF specimens (Musher, 1973; Weinstein, 1975).

In fungal meningitis, the classic examination is India ink preparation using centrifuged sediment for detection of *Cryptococcus neoformans* (Fig. 19–1). However, the India ink preparation is positive in only

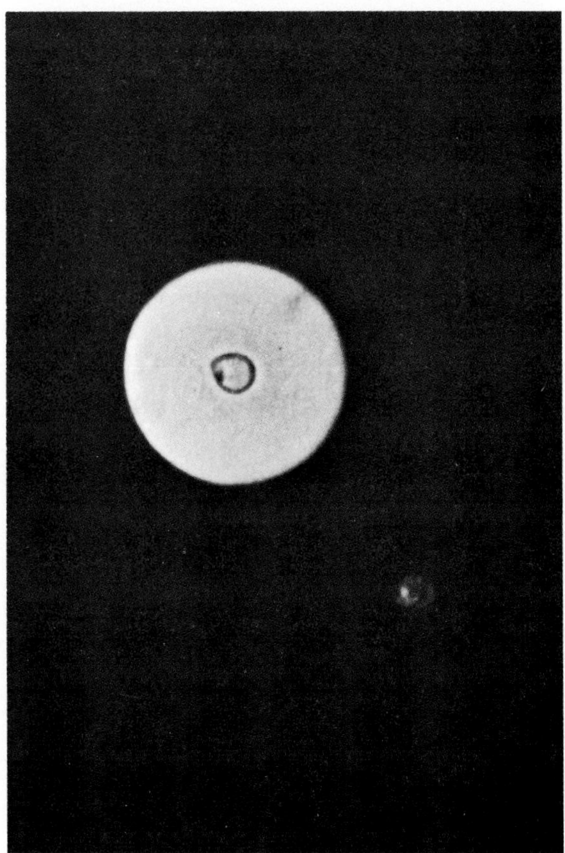

Figure 19–1. *Cryptococcus neoformans* in cerebrospinal fluid. India ink preparation; ×200. (From Anderson, K. F.: The Clinical Practice of Bacteriology. Philadelphia, F. A. Davis, 1966.)

about 50 per cent of cases (Butler, 1964). About 80 per cent of cases can be detected by special stains (PAS, mucicarmine, methenamine silver) on specimens prepared by Millipore filter or cytocentrifuge (Jequier, 1972; Jameson, 1972; Saigo, 1977). The latex agglutination test for cryptococcal antigen in CSF is the recommended method, and is positive in 90 per cent of patients with cryptococcal meningitis. Without special stains, cryptococci may be mistaken for small lymphocytes in "routine" preparations (Sheth, 1977). If initial preparations are negative, fungi sometimes may be detected on cisternal puncture (Gonyea, 1973), or on culture of 10 to 30 ml CSF.

Primary amebic meningoencephalitis, as distinguished from infections by *Entamoeba histolytica,* is a rapidly fatal disease which is uncommon but not rare (Hecht, 1972). The organisms (e.g., *Acanthamoeba* and *Nagleria*) are difficult to detect and identify on Gram's stain or Wright's stain of CSF (Aspock, 1977): frequently the condition is first recognized at autopsy. Motile trophozoites may be recognized by their active movement using a CSF wet mount examined by phase microscopy with a warmed stage or prewarmed counting chamber. However, experience is needed to distinguish amebas from the motility of macrophages and monocytes (Sornas, 1967, 1971).

Acid-fast stains for tuberculous meningitis are frequently performed on CSF. We have found the fluorescent rhodamine stain more sensitive than the Ziehl-Neelsen method. Concentration of 10 ml CSF may further improve sensitivity. In some cases of tuberculous meningitis, a fine clot or pellicle will form over the surface of CSF after standing for 12 to 24 hours in the refrigerator: this pellicle should be carefully examined for organisms with appropriate stain and culture. We have occasionally found false positive stains for tuberculosis due to saprophytic acid-fast organisms in deionized water; these can be eliminated by preparing reagents using sterile water for intravenous infusion.

Total Protein

Protein normally diffuses from plasma to CSF across the blood-CSF barrier. Most of the serum proteins are present in CSF, including fibrinogen and beta lipoprotein in low concentrations (Table 19–3). The concentration ratios between plasma and CSF correlate moderately well with hydrodynamic radii, and somewhat less well with molecular weights. It is apparent from Table 19–3 that the IgM level in CSF is about five times higher than expected: this may be due to IgM monomers in addition to the pentamer. The prealbumin level in CSF is about twelve times higher than expected, and the transferrin level is about two times higher than expected. Reasons for these apparent discrepancies are unknown; selective transport may be involved. The tau protein of CSF, which migrates in the beta-gamma region, represents an altered form of transferrin, which apparently lacks neuraminic acid due to the action of neuraminidase (Bock, 1975).

3

Methods. Methods used to measure total protein in CSF can be classified in six categories:

1. Turbidimetric procedures: (a) sulfosalicylic acid plus sodium sulfate; (b) trichloracetic acid (TCA).
2. Ultraviolet spectrophotometry at 210 nm following: (a) column chromatography; (b) ultrafiltration.
3. Lowry method using Folin-Ciocalteau reagent: (a) blanked; (b) unblanked.
4. Modified biuret procedures with measurement at 330 nm.
5. Dye binding: (a) Ponceau S; (b) other dyes.
6. Immunologic methods.

Turbidimetric methods are widely used in the United States. There is a linear relationship between turbidity and temperature, and accurate temperature control is essential for reproducible results (Schriever, 1965; Pennock, 1968). Sulfosalicylic acid gives greater turbidity with albumin than with globulin; however, variations in the albumin/globulin ratio have no significant effect on the SSA/SS (3 per cent sulfosalicylic acid in 7 per cent sodium sulfate) method of Meulmans or the TCA method of Meulmans (3 per cent trichloracetic acid). Because of variations in reactivity with albumin and globulin, albumin should *not* be used as a standard for turbidimetric methods (Schriever, 1965). Advantages of turbidimetric methods include its simplicity and the fact that some drugs which interfere with the unblanked Lowry and biuret procedures do not cause turbidity with SSA or trichloroacetic acid (TCA). Disadvantages include the fact that about 500 μl CSF is required, compared

Table 19–3. CONCENTRATIONS OF PROTEINS IN PLASMA AND CEREBROSPINAL FLUID*

Protein	Molecular Weight	Hydrodynamic Radius (Å)	Plasma Concentration (mg/L)	CSF Concentration (mg/L)	Plasma/CSF Ratio
Prealbumin	61,000	32.5	238	17.3	14
Albumin	69,000	35.8	36,600	155.0	236
Transferrin	81,000	36.7	2040	14.4	142
Ceruloplasmin	152,000	46.8	366	1.0	366
IgG	150,000	53.4	9870	12.3	802
IgA	150,000	56.8	1750	1.3	1346
α_2 macroglobulin	798,000	93.5	2220	2.0	1111
Fibrinogen	340,000	108.0	2964	0.6	4940
IgM	800,000	121.0	700	0.6	1167
β lipoprotein	2,239,000	124.0	3728	0.6	6213

*Adapted from Felgenhauer, K.: Klin. Wochenschr., *52*:1158, 1974.

with 25 to 200 μl for other methods, and that interference may occur from xanthochromia as well as from intrathecal methotrexate.

Ultraviolet (UV) spectrophotometry at 210 nm is based on the principle that protein solutions exhibit strong absorbance at 210 to 220 nm, reflecting presence of the peptide bond. Interference due to short-chain polypeptides and drugs may be removed by column chromatography (Igou, 1967) or a "blank" prepared by ultrafiltration (Werner, 1969). Disturbances of the albumin/globulin ratio have no effect, since albumin and globulin have comparable absorbance at 210 nm. UV spectrophotometry requires only 100 to 200 μl of CSF, and precision appears somewhat superior to turbidimetric methods. On the other hand, it is more time consuming and difficult than turbidimetric methods; the upper limit of the reference interval by this method is somewhat higher (60 mg/dl) than for other techniques, and instrumentation is not available in all laboratories.

The Lowry method using Folin-Ciocalteau reagent is widely used in Europe. Two reactions are involved: (1) an initial reaction of protein and copper related to the biuret reaction; (2) a second reduction of phosphotungstic and phosphomolybdic acids with the copper-protein complex as well as with tyrosine and tryptophan. The Lowry method requires only 100 to 200 μl of CSF. However, it is more time consuming and difficult than turbidimetric methods, and it experiences variable interference from endogenously produced phenols and drugs (salicylates, chlorpromazine, tetracyclines, and sulfa drugs).

Modified biuret methods have been reported by several authors, including Burgi (1967). However, these seem less widely used than turbidimetric procedures, ultraviolet spectrophotometry, or the Lowry method. Only 100 to 200 μl of CSF is required. Biuret methods are more time consuming and difficult than turbidimetric methods and experience interference from short chain polypeptides (can be compensated by blank using protein-free filtrate).

Dye binding methods have been reported, but experience to date appears limited. Potential advantages include technical simplicity and the fact that only 50 to 100 μl of CSF is required. However, limited experience in comparison with other CSF protein methods is a disadvantage.

Immunologic methods for CSF total protein have also been reported (Heintges, 1973). A major advantage is that only small amounts of CSF (25 to 50 μl) are required. After reaction conditions are established and reagents standardized, the technique is relatively simple and comparable to turbidimetric methods. Disadvantages are that different proteins may give different precipitin curves as well as different light scattering responses when bound to their specific antibodies. Also, variation between different lots of antisera may occur. Although immunologic methods offer significant advantages for CSF total protein, widespread use will require further experience, as well as reliable antisera which react in a uniform manner with all CSF proteins (Bock, 1975).

REFERENCE INTERVALS AND CLINICAL CORRELATION

As noted above, there may be some variation in reference intervals for different methods: UV spectrophotometry apparently gives a somewhat higher upper limit of normal than other procedures (Igou, 1967).

Reference intervals for CSF total protein vary slightly with age. During the neonatal period, reported reference intervals for CSF total protein vary from 30 to 140 mg/dl (Kluge, 1968) to 20 to 170 mg/dl (Sarff, 1976). This relatively high "upper limit" of normal has been attributed to immaturity of the blood-CSF barrier. By age six months, reference intervals fall below normal adult levels, to about 10 to 30 mg/dl (Fishman, 1971), then gradually increase to normal young adult levels of 15 to 45 mg/dl. After age 40, there appears to be a gradual increase with age (Tibbling, 1977). A summary of reference intervals for CSF protein, based on reports in the literature plus our own experience, is outlined in Table 19–4.

Reference intervals for CSF total protein are affected by source of CSF; cisternal and ventricular fluids have

Table 19–4. REFERENCE INTERVALS FOR TOTAL PROTEIN IN CSF*

Age	Reference Interval (mg/dl)
1–30 days	20–150
30–90 days	20–100
3–6 months	15–50
½–10 years	10–30
10–40 years	15–45
10–40 years	15–25 (cisternal fluid)
10–40 years	5–15 (ventricular fluid)
40–50 years	20–50
50–60 years	25–55
60 years and over	30–60

NOTE: These ranges represent a summary of personal experience plus reports in the literature; individual laboratories should establish their own reference intervals before using results for patient care.

*Lumbar fluid unless otherwise specified.

lower levels of total protein than lumbar fluid (Table 19–4). Thus, if several tubes of CSF are collected, the final tubes will have a lower protein concentration than the initial tubes (Bock, 1975). In young children, concentrations of protein are reported as comparable in lumbar and cisternal fluid, possibly owing to (1) increased activity which causes more rapid circulation of CSF; (2) comparable permeability of lumbar and cisternal blood-CSF barriers; or (3) smaller volumes of CSF, so that some cisternal fluid is obtained on lumbar puncture.

Decreased concentration of protein in lumbar CSF (15 mg/dl or less) may be due to (1) leakage of CSF from a dural tear caused by trauma or previous lumbar puncture, or to CSF rhinorrhea or otorrhea; (2) removal of large volumes of CSF (e.g., pneumoencephalography); (3) increased intracranial pressure (may cause increased filtration of CSF through arachnoid granulations of dural sinuses); or (4) hyperthyroidism (mechanism not known). Of the foregoing conditions, leakage of CSF is especially important. A history of repeated meningitis in a patient with normal immunologic function and low CSF protein should suggest the possibility of nasal or aural CSF leakage.

Increased concentration of protein in lumbar CSF may be caused by (1) traumatic tap, with admixture of peripheral blood in CSF, (2) increased permeability of the blood-CSF barrier, (3) obstruction to circulation of CSF, (4) increased synthesis of protein within the central nervous system, or (5) tissue degeneration. Traumatic tap may cause increased CSF protein owing to the marked difference between plasma and CSF protein (ratio about 250:1). If 1 ml of CSF contains 0.1 ml of blood due to traumatic tap, we may expect a CSF RBC of about 0.5 million and a CSF protein of about 400 mg/dl. Although "corrections" for traumatic tap can be performed based on RBC, these may be inaccurate in some cases (pp. 463 and 464).

Increased permeability of the blood-CSF barrier is a common cause for pathologic increases in CSF total protein (Table 19–5). In meningitis there is damage to the blood-CSF barrier, plus decreased removal of protein molecules at the arachnoid villi (Fishman, 1971). Various endocrine, metabolic, and toxic conditions may cause reversible changes in permeability of the brain-CSF barrier; however, the exact mechanisms are not known.

Obstruction to circulation of CSF classically is related to mechanical blockage between the site of lumbar puncture and the foramen magnum, e.g., cord compression due to tumor, herniated disk adhesions, or extradural abscess. Owing to the obstruction, resorption of water (and/or leakage of plasma proteins) produces xanthochromic CSF of high protein content, which may clot spontaneously (Froin's syndrome). A similar syndrome may be caused by leakage of CSF after lumbar puncture to form loculated epidural and/or subdural effusions; subsequent punctures reveal "CSF" protein of progressively higher concentration (Derakhshan, 1973).

Synthesis of immunoglobulins apparently occurs under normal conditions within lymphocytes and plasma cells of the central nervous system (Tourtellotte, 1975). However, no albumin is produced within the CNS. Daily synthesis of IgG in normal humans in minimal: about 3 mg/day (Tourtellotte, 1975). Increased synthesis of IgG within the CNS can occur with lymphocytic and plasmacytic infiltrates involving the central nervous system (Table 19–5).

In some degenerative conditions such as Parkinson's disease, Friedreich's ataxia, or amyotrophic lateral sclerosis (ALS), there is an increase in CSF protein; it is possible that tissue degeneration contributes to such protein elevation (Collins, 1978).

PROTEIN FRACTIONATION

Immunologic Measurements. CSF protein may be derived from two sources: diffusion across the blood-CSF barrier, and synthesis within the central nervous system (CNS). Diffusion across the blood-CSF barrier occurs along concentration gradients between plasma and CSF. Rate of diffusion across these gradients (and plasma-CSF ratios) appears related to hydrodynamic radii for most proteins (Felgenhauer, 1974). The normal plasma:CSF ratio for albumin is generally accepted as about 230. Reported "normal" plasma: CSF ratios for IgG vary from about 370 (Tourtellotte, 1975) to about 500 (Tibbling, 1977) to about 800 (Felgenhauer, 1974). This variation probably is related to different antisera and different standards, which can cause errors in the range of 200 per cent (Bock, 1975; Thompson, 1977). Despite these problems related to standardization, immunologic measurement of CSF albumin and IgG have become widely accepted as methods for evaluating integrity of the blood-CSF barrier and synthesis of IgG within the CNS.

Because albumin is not produced within the CNS, the CSF/plasma albumin ratio is considered to reflect functional integrity of the blood-CSF barrier (Tibbling, 1977; Tourtellotte, 1975). An increased ratio may be due to traumatic tap, increased permeability of the blood-CSF barrier, or impaired resorption of CSF protein caused by subarachnoid block or meningitis (impaired resorption of CSF protein at arachnoid villi). Although variations in plasma albumin may affect the CSF albumin concentration, such variations do not affect the CSF/plasma albumin ratio, which accurately reflects permeability of the blood-CSF barrier. Immediately after birth, the CSF/plasma albumin ratio is relatively high, reflecting immaturity of the blood-CSF barrier (Table 19–6). By age six months, the value falls to adult levels, then gradually increases after age 30 to 40 years (Table 19–6).

The CSF/plasma IgG ratio reflects (1) permeability of the blood-CSF barrier; (2) synthesis of IgG within the CNS. Absolute levels of CSF IgG are relatively high during the first month of life, reflecting an increased permeability of the blood-CSF barrier as well as high levels of plasma IgG (Table 19–6). After age 30 days, CSF IgG falls rapidly, owing to decreasing levels of plasma IgG and increasing maturity of the blood-CSF barrier. The CSF/plasma IgG ratio shows changes with age comparable to the CSF/plasma albumin ratio (Table 19–6).

Table 19–5. DISORDERS ASSOCIATED WITH INCREASED CSF TOTAL PROTEIN

Condition	Comments
Increased plasma protein	Slightly increased CSF protein due to diffusion across blood-CSF barrier
Traumatic tap	Normal pressure; CSF initially streaked with blood, clearing in subsequent tubes
Increased permeability of blood-CSF barrier	
Infectious	
Bacterial meningitis	CSF protein 100–500 mg/dl; Gram's strain usually positive; culture may be negative if antibiotics administered
Tuberculous meningitis	CSF protein 50–300 mg/dl; mixed cellular reaction typical
Fungal meningitis	CSF protein 50–300 mg/dl; special stains helpful
Viral meningoencephalitis	CSF protein usually under 100 mg/dl
Non-infectious	
Subarachnoid hemorrhage	Xanthochromia 2–4 hours after onset
Intracerebral hemorrhage	CSF protein 20–200 mg/dl; marked fall in pressure after removing small amounts of CSF; xanthochromic fluid in 80%
Cerebral thrombosis	Slightly increased CSF protein in 40% of cases (usually under 100 mg/dl)
Endocrine, metabolic, and toxic	
Endocrine conditions: diabetic neuropathy, myxedema, hyperadrenalism, hypoparathyroidism	CSF protein 50–150 mg/dl in about 50% of cases
Metabolic conditions: uremia, hypercalcemia, hypercapnia, dehydration	CSF protein slightly elevated (usually under 100 mg/dl)
Toxic conditions: ethanol, isopropanol, heavy metals, phenytoin	CSF protein slightly elevated in about 40% of cases (usually under 200 mg/dl)
Obstruction to circulation of CSF	
Mechanical obstruction (tumor, abscess, etc.)	Rapid fall in pressure on removal of CSF; Froin's syndrome may be present
Loculated effusion of CSF	Repeated taps may show progressive increase in "CSF" protein; diagnosis by myelography
Increased CNS synthesis of IgG plus increased permeability of blood-CSF barrier	
Meningitis (see above)	About 20% of patients with viral meningoencephalitis have increased CSF IgG as well as increased CSF protein
Guillain-Barré syndrome (infectious polyneuritis)	CSF protein usually 100–400 mg/dl
Collagen diseases (e.g., periarteritis, lupus)	CSF protein usually under 400 mg/dl
Increased CNS synthesis of IgG	
Multiple sclerosis	CSF protein slightly increased in about 40% (usually under 100 mg/dl); CSF IgG elevated in about 80%
Subacute sclerosing panencephalitis (SSPE)	CSF IgG almost invariably increased
Neurosyphilis	CSF protein normal or slightly increased (usually under 100 mg/dl); about 20% have elevated IgG

Table 19–6. CEREBROSPINAL FLUID (CSF): PLASMA PROTEIN RATIOS WITH RESPECT TO AGE*

Age	CSF/Plasma Albumin Ratio × 1000	CSF Albumin (mg/L)	CSF/Plasma IgG Ratio × 1000	CSF IgG (mg/L)	CSF IgG × 1000 / CSF Albumin	CSF IgG Index
1–30 days	14†	450†	5 ± 3	10–100		
30–90 days	8†	300†	3 ± 1	3–15		
3–6 months	6†	220†	1 ± 0.5	3–6		
½–4 years	4†	160†	1.5 ± 1	3–12		
4–30 years	3.7 ± 1.0	120–220	1.7 ± 0.5	10–20	80–130	0.34–0.58
30–40 years	4.0 ± 1.1	130–230	1.9 ± 0.5	15–30	90–140	0.34–0.58
40–50 years	4.6 ± 1.3	140–260	2.1 ± 0.7	15–35	90–140	0.34–0.58
50–60 years	5.5 ± 1.7	160–320	2.5 ± 0.7	20–40	90–140	0.34–0.58
60 years and over	5.6 ± 1.7	160–320	2.6 ± 0.9	20–40	90–140	0.34–0.58

*Adapted from Tibbling, G., Link, H., and Ohman, S.: Scand. J. Clin. Lab. Invest., *37*:385, 1977; Olsson, J. E., and Pettersson, B.: Acta Neurol. Scand., *53*:308, 1976; and Harms, D.: Eur. Neurol., *13*:54, 1975.

†Estimated from total protein measurements (Harms, 1975).

From a clinical point of view, CSF IgG measurements can provide an estimate of IgG synthesis within the CNS. Three methods have been used to "correct" CSF IgG measurements for variation in plasma IgG and permeability of the blood-CSF barrier. (1) CSF IgG expressed as a percentage of CSF total protein or CSF albumin; (2) the CSF IgG/albumin index, with CSF IgG expressed as a ratio to plasma IgG, compared with CSF albumin expressed as a ratio to plasma albumin:

$$\frac{\text{CSF/plasma IgG}}{\text{CSF/plasma albumin}}$$

(Olsson, 1976; Tibbling, 1977); (3) calculation of IgG synthesis within central nervous system (Tourtellotte, 1975). For CSF IgG expressed as a percentage of CSF albumin, the upper limit of normal is about 12 per cent (Thompson, 1977). For CSF IgG expressed as a percentage of CSF total protein, the upper limit of normal is about 8 per cent (Tibbling, 1977). If we assume that increased permeability of the blood-CSF barrier causes increased CSF IgG proportional to increased CSF albumin, then expressing CSF IgG as a percentage of CSF albumin will compensate for increased CSF IgG due to increased permeability of the blood-CSF barrier. Of course, in some cases, damage to the blood-CSF barrier may change the CSF/plasma IgG ratio more than the CSF/plasma albumin ratio. However, in actual practice, this "correction" appears useful.

If the "normal" ratios of plasma: CSF albumin and IgG are known, we can calculate daily synthesis of IgG within the CNS (Tourtellotte, 1975). Although this approach appears promising, it is not yet widely used. Accuracy of such calculations is highly dependent upon accurate "normal values" for CSF/plasma ratios of albumin and IgG. And at this time, different authorities report different reference values or "normal values" for the ratio of CSF/plasma IgG.

In addition to albumin and IgG, other immunologic studies performed on CSF include IgA and IgM measurements, immunoelectrophoresis, evaluation of kappa-lambda ratio, subtyping of IgG (Vandvik, 1976; Palmer, 1976), and immunofixation (Cawley, 1976). At present these techniques are primarily of research interest rather than established clinical value.

Electrophoresis. Three support media are used for CSF protein electrophoresis: cellulose acetate, agarose (agar gel), and polyacrylamide gel. In the United States, cellulose acetate is the most popular technique. This separates CSF into six fractions: prealbumin, albumin, α_1 globulin, α_2 globulin, β globulin, and γ globulin. Concentration of CSF may be performed by vacuum ultrafiltration (Schleicher and Schell, Keene, N.H.) or by Amicon membrane (Amicon Corp., Lexington, Mass.). Reference intervals reported in two different studies are outlined in Table 19–7. Compared with serum, CSF has proportionally less gamma globulin and more albumin. The upper limit of normal for gamma globulin in adults is about 12 per cent of total CSF protein. For children, the upper limit is somewhat less.

In Europe, and in specialized laboratories within the United States, agar gel electrophoresis is preferred over cellulose acetate for CSF (Link, 1971). On agar gel electrophoresis, over 90 per cent of patients with multiple sclerosis have two or more discrete bands in the gamma globulin region, with no corresponding bands on serum electrophoresis (oligoclonal IgG). Recent studies suggest that these bands represent IgG1 (Vandvik, 1976; Palmer, 1976). At present, agar gel electrophoresis is probably the most sensitive single method available to the "routine" clinical laboratory for detection of multiple sclerosis. The technique has been described by several authors, including Johnson (1977a).

Table 19–7. REFERENCE INTERVALS FOR CEREBROSPINAL FLUID (CSF) PROTEIN ELECTROPHORESIS

	CSF (Kaplan, 1967)*	CSF (Windisch, 1970)†	Serum
Prealbumin	3.7– 6.1%	2.2– 7.1%	—
Albumin	56.2–66.8%	56.8–76.4%	52.2–67.0%
α_1 Globulin	3.1– 5.9%	1.1– 6.6%	2.4– 4.6%
α_2 Globulin	4.9– 8.5%	3.0–12.6%	6.6–13.6%
β Globulin	10.1–17.3%	7.3–17.9%	9.1–14.7%
γ Globulin:‡	6.2–11.4%	3.0–13.0%	9.0–20.6%

*Concentration by vacuum ultrafiltration.
†Concentration by Amicon membrane.
‡Children have lower values for CSF and serum γ globulin.

Polyacrylamide gel electrophoresis (PAGE) provides even greater resolution than agar gel (Epstein, 1976). Although PAGE can demonstrate oligoclonal bands in multiple sclerosis (MS) (Thompson, 1977), PAGE is not now widely used for study of CSF.

Isoelectric focusing of CSF proteins also permits demonstration of oligoclonal bands (Thompson, 1977), but further experience is needed before this technique becomes generally accepted.

Qualitative Tests. *Lange's colloidal gold test* is an empirical method for evaluating CSF protein. In this procedure, progressive dilutions of CSF are added to 10 test tubes containing colloidal gold solutions. Precipitation causes the brilliant red colloidal gold color (0) to change to reddish blue (1+), purple (2+), deep blue (3+), pale blue (4+), or colorless (5+). The highest CSF concentration is reported on the left, with progressively decreasing concentrations to the right.

Normal CSF causes either no reaction or only slight precipitation in the middle dilutions, e.g., 0001210000.

A "first zone curve" is found in about 50 per cent of patients with multiple sclerosis, as well as in neurosyphilis, SSPE, CNS hemorrhage, meningitis, polyneuritis, and other conditions. A typical series would be 5554210000. In general, a first zone curve is associated with increased gamma globulin as detected by electrophoresis (Thompson, 1977).

The "mid zone" and "end zone" curves are non-specific and may be found in any CSF with high protein concentration.

The Pandy test requires that one drop of CSF be added to saturated aqueous solution of phenol: turbidity is read as 0 to 3+. Increased concentrations of CSF globulin are associated with increased turbidity.

Since the 1960's, there has been a trend to replacement of these methods by cellulose acetate electrophoresis, agar gel electrophoresis, and immunologic measurements. However, the colloidal gold and Pandy tests are still used for evaluation of CSF in some laboratories.

Clinical Correlation. The most important clinical application of CSF protein fractionation is detection and diagnosis of multiple sclerosis (MS). About 90 to 95 per cent of patients with MS have multiple discrete gamma bands on agar gel electrophoresis (Olsson, 1973; Tibbling, 1977; Johnson, 1977b). However, this finding may also occur in about 90 per cent of patients with subacute sclerosing panencephalitis (SSPE) (Johnson, 1977b), about 60 per cent of patients with neurosyphilis (Link, 1971), about 40 per cent of patients with bacterial or viral meningoencephalitis

(Olsson, 1976), and some patients with acute necrotizing encephalitis (Van Welsum, 1970), Guillain-Barré syndrome (Link, 1975), meningeal carcinomatosis, toxoplasmosis involving the CNS, herpes zoster encephalitis, herpes simplex encephalitis, progressive multifocal leukoencephalopathy, and other neurologic conditions (Johnson, 1977b).

Distinct immunoglobulin bands may occur on agar gel electrophoresis of serum and CSF of patients with infections outside the CNS. For this reason, it is advisable simultaneously to perform agar gel electrophoresis on CSF and serum. An oligoclonal pattern in CSF does not necessarily suggest MS if similar bands are present in serum.

About 75 per cent of patients with multiple sclerosis (MS) have increased CSF gamma globulin on cellulose acetate electrophoresis, when gamma globulin is expressed as a per cent of CSF total protein or CSF albumin. Measurement of CSF gamma globulin on electrophoresis is more sensitive and more specific than older semiquantitative methods such as the Pandy test and colloidal gold curve.

About 75 per cent of patients with MS have increased CSF IgG, when IgG is expressed as a per cent of CSF total protein or CSF albumin.

About 85 per cent of patients with MS apparently have an increased IgG/albumin index (Tibbling, 1977):

$$\frac{\text{CSF IgG/plasma IgG}}{\text{CSF albumin/plasma albumin}}$$

There is suggestive evidence that the IgG/albumin index also may provide improved specificity (Tibbling, 1977).

Increased CSF, gamma globulin (IgG), and/or IgG/albumin index also may occur in about 95 per cent of patients with subacute sclerosing panencephalitis, about 50 per cent of patients with neurosyphilis, about 40 to 50 per cent of patients with meningitis, and some patients with Guillain-Barré syndrome, systemic lupus erythematosus involving the CNS, viral meningoencephalitis, and other neurologic conditions. Among Japanese patients with MS only about 40 per cent have elevated IgG in CSF (Iwashita, 1976). The reason for this relatively low percentage is not known.

Although CSF protein studies currently are of considerable value in the diagnosis of MS, in the future, other approaches may supplement or even supplant evaluation of CSF proteins (Levy, 1976; Cohen, 1976).

At this time, the following procedures are of established value in detection and diagnosis of MS: agar gel electrophoresis of CSF (and serum), immunologic measurements of CSF (and serum) IgG and albumin, and cellulose acetate electrophoresis of CSF (as a method for calculating per cent gamma globulin if the foregoing methods are unavailable).

Glucose

Normal CSF glucose in adults is about 60 to 70 per cent of blood levels, or about 50 to 80 mg/dl in fasting patients with plasma glucose of 80 to 110 mg/dl. Glucose enters CSF from plasma by at least two mechanisms: active transport and passive diffusion. Active transport increases up to plasma levels of about 300 mg/dl, after which the transport system reaches a maximum with CSF glucose in the range of 200 mg/dl (Calabrese, 1976). Thus with plasma glucose in the range of 1000 mg/dl, CSF glucose may be under 300 mg/dl, or less than 30 per cent of plasma levels.

Passive diffusion of glucose from plasma to CSF is influenced by level and duration of elevated plasma glucose. Following a change in plasma glucose, CSF glucose rises or falls slowly over about two hours. Thus accurate evaluations of CSF glucose require a relatively constant level of plasma glucose.

According to Fishman (1971), the CSF/plasma glucose ratio approaches 1.0 during the neonatal period. Although this observation needs further confirmation, immaturity of the blood-CSF barrier might account for such findings.

Elevated CSF glucose (absolute or relative to plasma glucose) is evidence of hyperglycemia two to four hours prior to lumbar puncture.

Decreased CSF glucose is considered present when CSF glucose is under 40 mg/dl in a fasting patient with normal plasma glucose. Decreased CSF glucose may be due to impairment of active transport; to increased utilization of glucose (by CNS, tissue, leukocytes, erythrocytes, and/or microorganisms); or to hypoglycemia. CSF glucose is decreased in about 50 per cent of patients with bacterial meningitis (Swartz, 1965). At least two mechanisms are believed involved: (1) impaired transport of glucose from plasma to CSF; (2) increased utilization of glucose by central nervous system, leukocytes, and microorganisms.

Although CSF glucose is usually considered normal in viral meningoencephalitis, low CSF glucose may occur in about 25 per cent of patients with mumps meningoencephalitis (Azimi, 1975). Impaired transport of glucose has been suggested as a possible mechanism.

Other reported causes of decreased CSF glucose include tuberculous meningitis, fungal meningitis, amebic meningoencephalitis, subarachnoid hemorrhage (decreased CSF glucose typically appears four to eight days after onset), intrathecal administration of radioiodinated serum albumin, viral meningitis including lymphocytic choriomeningitis, herpes simplex meningoencephalitis, herpes zoster meningitis (Wolf, 1974), neurosyphilis (most cases have normal CSF glucose), sarcoidosis involving the meninges, and neoplasms involving the meninges (e.g., leukemia, lymphoma, melanoma, metastatic carcinoma, glioma). In some of these conditions, several different mechanisms probably operate simultaneously to cause decreased CSF glucose. For example, in bacterial meningitis there is evidence of (1) impaired glucose transport, (2) increased CNS utilization of glucose; and (3) increased utilization of glucose by leukocytes in CSF.

CEREBROSPINAL FLUID RHINORRHEA AND OTORRHEA

Occasionally the question arises whether small amounts of clear fluid draining from nose or ear represent cerebrospinal fluid. This question is of especial importance in patients with recurrent meningitis and no evidence of immunologic impairment. Trauma is the most common cause of CSF rhinorrhea, which usually begins within 48 hours, but may not develop for several months.

Glucose oxidase test strips are of *no* clinical value for distinguishing CSF from nasal secretions (Hull, 1975). Diagnosis of CSF rhinorrhea and otorrhea must be made by other means: e.g., intrathecal ^{131}I serum albumin, with cotton pledgets in nose (or ear) counted for radioactivity.

Enzymes

Many different enzymes have been measured in CSF; however, only lactate dehydrogenase (LDH) appears clinically useful at this time.

One source of LDH in normal CSF may be diffusion across the blood-CSF barrier. Normal CSF LDH activity is about 5 to 10 per cent of plasma activity (Mullan, 1969; Morrison, 1971). The "normal range" for the ratio of CSF/serum LDH is not yet well established. And it is not yet customary simultaneously to measure activities in serum as well as in CSF. Indeed, some reports of CSF enzyme activity fail to specify one or more of the following: (1) normal range for enzyme activity in CSF; (2) normal range for enzyme activity in serum; (3) reaction conditions, including assay temperature and source of reagents; or (4) results of simultaneous measurements on serum and CSF.

A second source of CSF LDH is from CNS by diffusion across the brain-CSF barrier. Brain tissue is rich in LDH, and damaged CNS tissue can cause increased levels of CSF LDH.

A third source of CSF LDH activity is cellular elements in CSF: leukocytes, bacteria, and tumor cells.

Based on these considerations, it might seem reasonable to report CSF LDH as a percentage of CSF albumin or total protein, analogous to gamma globulin. However, few reports include CSF LDH activity expressed as a ratio to other proteins.

Increased CSF LDH activity has been reported in many different conditions: about 90 per cent of patients with bacterial meningitis (Beaty, 1968; Nelson, 1975; Feldman, 1975); about 10 per cent of patients with viral meningitis (Beaty, 1968; Feldman, 1975); subarachnoid hemorrhage; leukemia, lymphoma, or metastatic carcinoma involving the CNS.

Measurements of CSF LDH have been used for differential diagnosis of bacterial vs. viral meningitis. High levels of CSF LDH in the latter condition appear associated with encephalitis and a poor prognosis (Beaty, 1968).

LDH isozymes (p. 267) have been used to improve the specificity of LDH measurements in CSF: granulocytes—LDH 5 and 4 predominate; lymphocytes—LDH 3 and 2 predominate; brain tissue—LDH 2 and 1 predominate. With viral meningitis, the LDH isozyme pattern reflects a combined CNS-lymphocytic reaction, with LDH 1–2–3 present. With bacterial meningitis, the LDH isozyme pattern reflects a granulocytic reaction with LDH 4–5 present. In either viral or bacterial meningitis, high levels of LDH 1 and 2 suggest extensive CNS damage and appear associated with a poor prognosis.

Although reports to date appear promising, the value of CSF LDH and LDH isozymes is not yet well established.

Increased CSF creatine kinase (CK) activity has been reported in a wide variety of neurologic disorders, including subarachnoid hemorrhage, cerebral thrombosis, multiple sclerosis and other demyelinating disorders, Guillain-Barré syndrome, following epileptic seizures, primary CNS tumors, metastatic tumors involving CNS, viral meningoencephalitis, and bacterial meningitis. Elevated CSF CK appears to be a sensitive but non-specific index of CNS disease. Owing to poor specificity, the clinical value of CSF CK measurements is not established.

Increased CSF aspartate aminotransferase (AST or GOT) has been reported in a variety of neurologic disorders: bacterial meningitis (elevated levels appear associated with a poor prognosis), intracerebral hemorrhage, subarachnoid hemorrhage, and primary or metastatic malignancy involving the CNS. The clinical value of CSF AST measurements is not established.

3

Lactic Acid

Lactic acid in CSF may vary independently of blood levels: apparently diffusion across the blood-CSF barrier is very slow (Bland, 1974). The source of lactic acid in CSF probably is CNS anaerobic metabolism: CSF lactate appears to be a reliable indicator of brain lactate content (Bland, 1974; Siesjo, 1972).

Reported reference intervals for CSF lactate vary from 10 to 22 mg/dl (0.11 to 0.24 mmol/L) (Pryce, 1970) to 12 to 16 mg/dl (0.13 to 0.18 mmol/L) (Bland, 1974). About 25 mg/dl (0.28 mmol/L) has been suggested as an "upper limit" for clinical purposes (Contronì, 1977). These levels are slightly higher than reference intervals for arterial and venous lactate in adults (3 to 7 mg/dl and 5 to 20 mg/dl), but slightly lower than reference intervals for venous lactate in children (Meites, 1977).

Any condition associated with reduced cerebral blood flow, reduced oxygenation of the brain, or increased intracranial pressure can cause elevated lactate in CSF (Controni, 1977). Conditions associated with increased CSF lactate include traumatic brain injury (Cold, 1975), idiopathic seizures (Brooks, 1975), respiratory alkalosis (hypocapnia), intracranial hemorrhage, hydrocephalus, brain abscess, cerebral ischemia due to arteriosclerosis, low blood pressure, low arterial Po_2, cerebral infarct, multiple sclerosis (less than 50 per cent of patients), and primary or metastatic carcinoma involving CNS. Several reports suggest that CSF lactate may aid in differential diagnosis of bacterial meningitis vs. viral meningitis if other conditions can be excluded (Bland, 1974; Controni, 1977). Over 90 per cent of patients with bacterial meningitis apparently have CSF lactate elevated above 25 mg/dl, while less than 15 per cent of patients with aseptic meningitis have a CSF lactate above this level (Bland, 1974; Contronі, 1977). Measurements of CSF lactate may be useful as a "screening test" to detect CNS disease and as an aid in differential diagnosis of meningitis if other causes for elevated levels can be excluded. With additional experience, it seems likely that CSF lactate may become accepted as a "routine" laboratory procedure.

Serologic Tests

TESTS FOR SYPHILIS

In patients with neurosyphilis, the CSF cell count, CSF total protein, and CSF gamma globulin all may be within normal limits (Hooshmand, 1972; John, 1977). The recommended serologic test for CSF, the VDRL procedure, also may be negative in 40 to 50 per cent of patients with neurosyphilis (Escobar, 1970; Hooshmand, 1972) (see Fluorescent Treponemal Antibody in Chapter 47).

The CSF FTA (fluorescent treponemal antibody) and FTA-ABS (fluorescent treponemal antibody absorption test) have much greater sensitivity, and apparently are positive in 80 to 90 per cent of patients with neurosyphilis (Hooshmand, 1972; McCracken, 1974). However, this increased sensitivity is accompanied by increased false positives: according to Jaffe (1975), the false positive rate may be as high as 4 to 5 per cent.

Some authorities (Jaffe, 1975) regard the CSF FTA and FTA-ABS as still experimental, owing to the high incidnece of false positives. However in patients with clinical findings consistent with early neurosyphilis but a negative CSF VDRL, the CSF FTA may aid in deciding whether to initiate treatment (John, 1977).

OTHER SEROLOGIC TESTS FOR INFECTIOUS DISEASE INVOLVING CNS

Serologic tests on CSF are of established value in diagnosis of cryptococcal meningitis (Kaufman, 1976). The India ink preparation is positive in only about 50 per cent of patients. However, the latex agglutination test for cryptococcal antigen in CSF is positive in about 90 per cent of patients with cryptococcal meningitis. False positives are infrequent.

During the past few years, there has developed increasing interest in diagnosis of bacterial meningitis by countercurrent immunoelectrophoresis (CIE). Sensitivity depends on potency of the antiserum and varies from about 50 per cent to over 90 per cent (McCracken, 1976a; Denis, 1977; Feldman, 1977). Specific antisera are needed for each organism suspected: thus "false negatives" occur with meningitis owing to unusual organisms such as *Listeria monocytogenes, Salmonella,* or diphtheroids (Schlesinger, 1977).

Limulus Lysate Test for Endotoxin

In 1965, Levin and Bang described gel formation of lysate from *Limulus polyphemus* (horseshoe crab) due to endotoxin produced by gram-negative bacteria. The CSF limulus lysate assay is helpful for rapid diagnosis of gram-negative bacterial meningitis, particularly in newborns, in whom rapid diagnosis and treatment are so important (Kjeldsberg, 1982). Positive limulus assays have been reported in CSF of almost all patients with gram-negative meningitis, e.g., *Hemophilus influenzae, Escherichia coli, Neisseria meningitidis, Acinetobacter calcoaceticus, Proteus morganii, Citrobacter freundii, Pseudomonas aeruginosa, Eikenella corrodens,* etc. Negative limulus assays have been reported in CSF of patients with gram-positive meningitis. "False negative" results may occur in some patients with gram-negative bacterial meningitis; false negatives also may be caused by misinterpretation of the gel endpoint (McCracken, 1976a). Because this test detects endotoxin which is ubiquitous and contamination is widespread, adequate precautions must be taken to preclude an apparent "false positive."

Other Measurements and Examinations

Acid-Base Balance. Acid-base balance in CSF has been reviewed by Plum (1975) and by Wichser (1975). Since CSF has little capacity to buffer changes in P_{CO_2}, accurate measurements of CSF pH are difficult: anaerobic conditions must be strictly maintained during and after sampling. And since CO_2 diffuses rapidly across the blood-CSF barrier, reproducible measurements require that the patient be in a respiratory steady state.

Although CSF pH has been suggested as helpful in differential diagnosis of meningitis (Bland, 1974), additional studies are needed before this can be accepted as a "routine" laboratory service.

Hormone Measurements. Many different hormones have been measured in CSF:

Cortisol—normal plasma/CSF ratio approx. 25:1 (Rodriguez, 1976).

Triiodothyronine—normal plasma/CSF ratio approx. 10:1 (Hagen, 1973).

Thyroxine—normal plasma/CSF ratio approx. 40:1 (Hagen, 1973).

TSH—normal plasma/CSF ratio approx. 2:1 (Schaub, 1977).

Growth hormone—normal plasma/CSF ratio approx. 6:1 (Schaub, 1977).

Prolactin—normal plasma/CSF ratio approx. 20:1 (Jordan, 1976).

Insulin—normal plasma/CSF ratio approx. 4:1 (Rodriguez, 1976).

Antidiuretic hormone—normal plasma/CSF ratio approx. 2:1 (Rodriguez, 1976).

ACTH—normal plasma/CSF ratio approx. 1:1 (Jordan, 1976).

LH—normal plasma/CSF ratio approx. 10:1 (Jordan, 1976).

FSH—normal plasma/CSF ratio approx. 8:1 (Jordan, 1976).

Measurements of adenohypophyseal hormones in CSF may provide sensitive indicators for suprasellar extension of pituitary tumors and response of tumors to treatment (Jordan, 1976). However, additional studies are needed to establish normal ranges for plasma/CSF ratios of these hormones.

Measurements of human chorionic gonadotropin (hCG) in CSF have been used for detection and diagnosis of choriocarcinoma metastatic to the CNS. In the absence of CNS metastases, the plasma/CSF ratio for hCG exceeds 60:1 (Chen, 1977). When CNS metastases are present, concentration of CSF hCG rises, and the plasma/CSF ratio falls below 60:1 (Chen, 1977). Additional studies are needed to establish reference values for plasma/CSF ratio of hCG.

SYNOVIAL FLUID

Formation

The synovial membrane lines joints, bursae, and synovial tendon sheaths, but not the articular cartilages or menisci. The synovial lining cells are loosely arranged in a layer one to three cells thick, over a mucopolysaccharide matrix. Unlike other body cavities, there is no basement membrane and no desmosomes joining adjacent synovial cells (Haselwood, 1977). Indeed, the lining presents a discontinuous surface, often with wide gaps between adjacent synovial cells.

The synovial lining cells are classified into three types: (1) A cells, which appear suited for phagocytosis, and morphologically resemble macrophages (numerous mitrochondria, vacuoles, and lysosomes); (2) B cells, which appear suited for protein synthesis (abundant endoplasmic reticulum); (3) C cells, intermediate cells with characteristics of both A and B cells.

Synovial fluid (SF) is believed to be produced by dialysis of plasma across the synovial membrane and by secretion of a hyaluronate-protein complex by the synovial membrane. Only small amounts of higher molecular weight proteins, such as fibrinogen, beta/C globulin, and other globulins have been added to this ultrafiltrate. Thus, SF represents a plasma ultrafiltrate to which a hyaluronate-protein complex has been added (Table 19–8). An excellent review of synovial fluid physiology has been done by Harris (1981).

Hyaluronate is a polymer composed of repeating disaccharide units (glucuronic acid–glucosamine). Molecular weight varies from about 5 to 10 million, depending on the degree of polymerization (Jessar, 1972; Haselwood, 1977). This polymer is linked with about 2 per cent protein. Both hyaluronate and protein probably are produced by the synovial lining cells.

Functions of SF are to provide lubrication and nourishment for articular cartilage.

The most extensive treatise to date on the analyses of normal synovial fluid is that of Ropes and Bauer (1953), which is still a valuable reference.

Arthrocentesis and Sample Collection

Joint aspiration should be performed *only* by an experienced operator under strictly sterile conditions. The technique has been described by various authors (Cohen, 1975; Currey, 1976). Almost any joint can be aspirated, provided an effusion is present. Since even large joints (e.g., knee) normally contain only 0.1 to 2.0 ml SF (Currey, 1976), a "dry tap" is common unless an effusion is present. Synovial fluid aspiration may provide useful information for diagnosis of the following conditions: suspected infection, e.g., acute suppurative arthritis; arthritis due to uric acid (gout) or calcium pyrophosphate (pseudogout); differential diagnosis of arthritis (Tables 19–9 and 19–10). In most cases, synovial fluid examination is not highly specific for any particular type of arthritis. Only in septic arthritis or crystal-induced arthritis is SF examination highly sensitive and specific for a single disease entity.

Table 19–8. REFERENCE INTERVALS FOR CONSTITUENTS OF SYNOVIAL FLUID

	Synovial Fluid	Plasma
Protein	1–3 g/dl	6–8 g/dl
Albumin	55–70%	50–65%
α_1 Globulin	6–8%	3–5%
α_2 Globulin	5–7%	7–13%
β Globulin	8–10%	8–14%
γ Globulin	10–14%	12–22%
Hyaluronate	0.3–0.4 g/dl	
Glucose	70–110 mg/dl	70–110 mg/dl
Uric acid		
Males	2–8 mg/dl	2–8 mg/dl
Females	2–6 mg/dl	2–6 mg/dl
Lactate	10–20 mg/dl (1–2 mmol/L)	3–7 mg/dl (arterial) 5–20 mg/dl (venous)
pH	7.30–7.40	7.38–7.44 (arterial) 7.36–7.42 (venous)
pCO_2	40–60 mm Hg	35–40 mm Hg (arterial) 40–45 mm Hg (venous)
pO_2	40–80 mm Hg	75–100 mm Hg (arterial) 40–50 mm Hg (venous)

Information compiled from Binette, 1965; Lund-Olesen, 1970; Falchuk, 1970; McCarty, 1974; Cohen, 1975; Haselwood, 1977; Kushner, 1977.

Synovial fluid should be collected using sterile disposable needles with a sterile disposable plastic syringe, to avoid contamination from exogenous birefringent material (Phelps, 1968). Ideally, the patient should be fasting for at least 6 and preferably 12 hours to allow equilibration of glucose between plasma and SF. If the patient is not fasting, SF glucose measurements are of little value, except when markedly decreased (under 40 mg/dl).

For routine examination, the syringe can be moistened with about 25 units of heparin per milliliter of synovial fluid as anticoagulant (Naib, 1973); powdered anticoagulants such as oxalate and EDTA should be avoided, since these can present confusing artifacts on microscopic examination (Phelps, 1968).

Detection of Trace Amounts of Synovial Fluid. Occasionally it is important to determine after aspiration whether the synovial space has been entered. In such cases, the material within the needle may be expelled directly into a test tube or flushed into the tube with a small amount of saline. As little as 0.5 μl of this synovial fluid can be identified by (1) turbidity or clot formation with 2 per cent acetic acid or (2) metachromasia with toluidine blue (Goldenberg, 1973). Although the latter method is more sensitive, false positives may result from contact with heparin.

Table 19–9. CLASSIFICATION OF SYNOVIAL FLUID FINDINGS*

	Normal	Non-inflam-matory (Group I)	Inflammatory Mild (Group IIa)	Inflammatory Severe (Group IIb)	Infectious-Septic (Group III)
Appearance	Clear yellow	Clear yellow	Clear yellow to slightly turbid	Turbid	Turbid to purulent
Viscosity	High	High	Decreased	Decreased	Decreased
Mucin clot	Good	Good	Good to fair	Fair to poor	Poor
Leukocyte count (per μl)	0–200	0–5,000	0–10,000	500–50,000	500–200,000
Neutrophils (%)	0–25	0–25	0–50	0–90	40–100
Glucose (blood–synovial fluid difference in mg/dl)	0–10	0–10	0–20	0–40	20–100
Comments				MSU† crystals in gout; CPPD‡ crystals in pseudogout	Gram's stain and/or culture positive in about 50%

*Adapted from Cohen, 1975, and Ropes, 1953.
†MSU = Monosodium urate (p. 478).
‡CPPD = Calcium pyrophosphate dihydrate (p. 479).

Even if no SF is apparent within the syringe, a drop of SF may be present within the needle, and can be used for culture or microscopic examination. In such cases, the needle may be left on the syringe, and inserted into a sterile cork before transport to the laboratory.

Gross Examination, Viscosity, and Mucin Clot Test

Appearance of normal SF is crystal clear and pale yellow. Print should easily be read through normal fluid; cloudiness suggests an inflammatory process. However, not all cloudy fluids are inflammatory, and further microscopic examination is important, in that crystals, fibrin, amyloid and cartilage fragments, or rice bodies can cause cloudy fluid. Turbid yellow fluid may occur with increased numbers of leukocytes due to septic or non-septic inflammation. Turbidity is usually reported as 1+ to 4+ (see section on cerebrospinal fluid) (p. 462).

Milky or "pseudochylous" fluid may occur with tuberculous arthritis (Wallace, 1976), chronic rheumatoid arthritis, acute gouty arthritis (Cracchiolo, 1971), systemic lupus erythematosus (Ryan, 1973), or calcium hydroxyapatite arthropathy.

Grossly purulent fluid may occur with acute septic arthritis, but is often absent, especially during the early stages of infection.

Greenish tinged fluid may occur with *H. influenzae* septic arthritis (Krauss, 1974), chronic rheumatoid arthritis (Jessar, 1972), and acute episodes of crystal synovitis due to gout or pseudogout (Currey, 1976). The SF color is not always an accurate guide to differential diagnosis.

Grossly bloody fluid may occur with fracture through the joint surface, tumor involving the joint,

Table 19–10. SYNOVIAL FLUID ANALYSIS IN DISEASE*

	Osteoarthritis (Degenerative Joint Disease)	Traumatic Arthritis	Rheumatic Fever	Systemic Lupus Erythematosus
Appearance	Clear yellow	Clear yellow (occasionally bloody)	Slightly turbid	Clear yellow to slightly turbid
Viscosity	Variable	Variable	Variable	Variable
Mucin clot	Good-fair	Good-fair	Good-fair	Good-fair
Leukocyte count (per μl)	700 (50–5,000)	1000 (50–10,000)	14,000 (50–50,000)	2000 (50–10,000)
Neutrophils (%)	15 (0–30)	25 (0–30)	50 (0–60)	30 (0–40)
Glucose (blood–synovial fluid difference in mg/dl)	0 (0–10)	5 (0–20)	5 (0–20)	20 (0–30)
Other findings	Collagen fibrils and/or cartilage fragments usually present	Fat globules may be present		LE cells may be present in SF

*Adapted from Cohen, 1975; Jessar, 1972; Owen, 1970; Hollander, 1966; Ropes, 1953.

traumatic arthritis, neurogenic arthropathy, hemophilic arthritis, pigmented villonodular synovitis, or ruptured aneurysm. Occasionally, bloody fluid may be noted with septic arthritis, rheumatoid arthritis, or osteoarthritis (Jessar, 1972). Traumatic tap can be distinguished by (1) decreasing amounts of blood as aspiration is continued (rarely blood may appear as tissues are traumatized later during aspiration); (2) uneven distribution with streaking in the syringe; (3) clotting about blood streaks in the syringe; or (4) lack of xanthochromic supernatant after centrifugation. Although xanthochromia is difficult to interpret, owing to the yellow appearance of normal synovial fluid, a dark red or dark brown supernatant in the presence of gross blood is suggestive evidence of hemarthrosis rather than traumatic tap. In fluid from ochronotic joints, black specks can occur, the "ground pepper" sign.

Viscosity usually is estimated either by allowing synovial fluid to form a string by dropping from a syringe into a beaker or by placing a drop of SF on the thumb, touching this with a finger, and separating the finger to form a string (we prefer to use gloves, since some specimens may be contaminated). Normal SF forms a string 4 to 6 cm in length. If the string breaks before reaching a length of 3 cm, viscosity is lower than normal (Hollander, 1966).

Quantitative measurements of viscosity can be performed using an ordinary white blood cell diluting pipette (Hasselbacher, 1976). However, the additional information gained probably has little clinical significance.

Viscosity is related primarily to the concentration and polymerization of SF hyaluronate. Decreased viscosity may occur in a wide variety of inflammatory conditions including septic arthritis, gouty arthritis, and rheumatoid arthritis. Decreased viscosity also may occur if hyaluronate is diluted by rapid effusion after trauma (Jessar, 1972). Increased viscosity can be seen in effusions from hypothyroid patients. In general clinical practice, however, viscosity is not as reliable as previously thought in the differential diagnosis of joint effusions (Hasselbacher, 1976).

As noted with viscosity, the mucin clot test is only a rough guideline and not as useful as total leukocyte count in differential diagnosis.

Microscopic Examination

Cell Count. *The "upper limit of normal"* or reference value for SF leukocyte count varies in different reports: under 200/μl (Ropes, 1953); under 200/μl (Owen, 1970); under 300/μl (Jessar, 1972); under 600/μl (Hollander, 1966); and under 750/μl (Currey, 1976). However, most authorities accept 200/μl as the upper limit of normal (Cohen, 1975). In this discussion, we will consider 200/μl the "upper limit of normal." The leukocyte count is perhaps the most important clue to differential diagnosis by synovial fluid analyses.

Total leukocyte counts can be performed by examining undiluted fluid in a Fuchs-Rosenthal chamber or a hemocytometer (Currey, 1976). Alternatively, physiologic saline plus a small amount of 0.1 per cent methylene blue can be used as diluent (Cohen, 1975). It is essential that the fluid be thoroughly mixed before adding to the counting chamber. A standard bench vibratory mixer is satisfactory for this purpose. Highly viscous fluids may need to stand for over 30 minutes before the cells can be counted.

A phase contrast microscope provides accurate distinction between leukocytes and erythrocytes without the need for methylene blue as a diluent. If ordinary light microscopy is used, a diluent with 0.1 per cent methylene blue will aid in recognition of leukocytes. For high cell counts (over 50,000/μl), saline dilution may be needed even with phase microscopy.

If the fluid is grossly bloody, one of the following methods may be used to lyse erythrocytes prior to performing a leukocyte count: (1) dilution with 1 per cent saponin in saline (Donaldson, 1972); (2) dilution with 0.3 per cent saline (Jessar, 1972); (3) dilution with 0.1 N HCl (Blau, 1971). If erythrocytes are present, an effort should be made to judge whether these are derived from traumatic tap (see Gross Examination). The erythrocytes should be counted unless it is clear that they are due to traumatic tap.

Table 19–10. SYNOVIAL FLUID ANALYSIS IN DISEASE* *(Continued)*

Rheumatoid Arthritis	Gout	Pseudogout	Acute Bacterial Arthritis	Tuberculous Arthritis
Turbid yellow, milky, or greenish	Turbid yellow to milky	Clear yellow to slightly turbid	Turbid to purulent (occasionally bloody)	Turbid
Decreased	Decreased	Decreased	Decreased	Decreased
Fair-poor	Fair-poor	Fair-poor	Poor	Poor
20,000 (200–80,000)	20,000 (100–100,000)	15,000 (50–75,000)	90,000 (200–200,000)	20,000 (2000–100,000)
70 (0–90)	70 (0–90)	70 (0–90)	90 (50–100)	60 (20–95)
30 (0–60)	10 (0–80)	10 (0–20)	80 (40–100)	70 (0–100)
Leukocyte count occasionally exceeds 100,000; RA§ cells usually present	MSU† crystals in over 90% of patients with acute gouty arthritis	CPPD‡ crystals required for diagnosis	Gram's stain and culture positive in about 50%	Acid-fast stain and culture frequently negative; biopsy may be needed for diagnosis

†MSU = Monosodium urate (p. 478).
‡CPPD = Calcium pyrophosphate dihydrate (p. 479).
§RA = Rheumatoid arthritis (p. 478).

A very high leukocyte count (over 100,000 leukocytes/μl) strongly suggests bacterial infection. However, in the early stages of a bacterial infection, the leukocyte count may be normal. Occasionally, active gout or rheumatoid arthritis may present with SF leukocyte counts over 100,000/μl; in such cases the differential diagnosis from septic arthritis may be difficult.

Differential Count. The percentage of neutrophils can be estimated by: (1) Phase contrast microscopy at the time of leukocyte count. (2) Wright's stain of unconcentrated SF. (3) Wright's stain of centrifuged SF sediment. Hollander (1966) recommends that the sediment be washed by redilution with isotonic saline and recentrifuged to remove most of the mucin. (4) Wright's stain of SF concentrated by cytocentrifuge. We use 0.5 ml SF diluted with 2.5 ml 0.1 per cent methylene blue in saline. (5) SF concentrates prepared by centrifugation or filtration plus Papanicolaou stain (Naib, 1973; Broderick, 1976). Phase contrast is the most convenient method and is adequate for most purposes. However, it is not optimal for detailed morphologic study and does not provide a permanent record. Papanicolaou stain probably is optimal for careful morphologic study but requires considerably more time than the other methods.

The "routine" differential count usually is reported only as the percentage of neutrophils. The generally accepted upper limit is 25 per cent neutrophils (Ropes, 1953; Hollander, 1966; Owen, 1970; Jessar, 1972; Naib, 1973; Scott, 1975; Cohen, 1975), although others report a higher "upper limit of normal" (Currey, 1976). A very high percentage of neutrophils (over 90 per cent) is suggestive evidence of bacterial arthritis, even if the total cell count and other measurements are within normal limits.

Cellular Morphology. ***Rheumatoid Arthritis.*** In about 95 per cent of patients, both phase and ordinary light microscopy reveal small, dark cytoplasmic granules, from 0.5 to 2.0 μ diameter, within 5 to 100 per cent of neutrophils. Such neutrophils are called "RA cells." A given RA cell may contain from 1 to 20 of these granules in its cytoplasm (Hollander, 1965; Cohen, 1975). These granules can be clearly identified using phase contrast with oil immersion, and by immunofluorescent techniques can be shown to consist of immune complexes: IgG, IgM, complement, and rheumatoid factor. RA cells are *not* specific for rheumatoid arthritis, but also occur in other conditions such as gout and septic arthritis (Scott, 1975).

Lymphoblasts and Sézary cells have been reported in SF of rheumatoid arthritis (Traycoff, 1976; Van Leeuwen, 1976); additional studies are needed to confirm these findings and to establish their clinical significance.

Lupus Erythematosus. LE cell formation is a relatively common in vivo phenomenon in synovial fluid (Hunder, 1970). In some cases, LE cells are present in SF with a negative LE test on peripheral blood. A few patients with rheumatoid arthritis also may have "LE cells" in synovial fluid.

Reiter's Syndrome. Large histiocytic cells with intracytoplasmic inclusions have been described on Giemsa and Papanicolaou stains (Naib, 1973; Broderick, 1976). Other workers describe large phagocytic cells with ingested neutrophils visualized on Wright's stain (Pekin, 1967; Cracchiolo, 1971). Additional studies are needed to confirm these reports and to establish their clinical significance.

Osteoarthritis. Multinucleated cartilaginous cells in SF are reported as characteristic (Naib, 1973; Broderick, 1976). Papanicolaou stain may be needed for definitive identification.

Pigmented Villonodular Synovitis. Foreign body giant cells with hemosiderin pigment, and papillary aggregates of synovial cells, are reported as characteristic (Naib, 1973; Broderick, 1976). Papanicolaou stain may be needed for definitive identification.

Septic Arthritis. Gram's stain is positive in about 50 per cent of patients with joint sepsis (Cooke, 1971; McCord, 1977). Depending upon the type of infection, culture may be positive in about 30 to 80 per cent of patients with septic arthritis. If sepsis is suspected but Gram's stain and culture are inconclusive, synovial biopsy may be needed to establish a diagnosis (Bayer, 1977). It is important to remember that septic arthritis can co-exist with other types of arthritis such as lupus, gout, and pseudogout.

Crystals. Five types of crystal-induced arthritis have been reported: (1) arthritis associated with apatite crystals (Schumacher, 1977); (2) gout caused by monosodium urate (MSU); (3) pseudogout caused by calcium pyrophosphate dihydrate (CPPD); (4) chronic arthritis caused by talcum crystals introduced during joint surgery (Naib, 1973); (5) acute synovitis caused by intra-articular injection of crystalline corticosteroid preparations (Schumacher, 1977). Arthritis associated with apatite crystals is now more commonly recognized as a cause of synovitis. The apatite crystals appear as shiny inclusions on wet preparations, or dark cytoplasmic inclusions on Wright's stain (Schumacher, 1977); definitive diagnosis requires electron microscopy or x-ray diffraction of the crystals.

The remaining four types of crystals can be detected and identified by compensated polarized light microscopy (p. 479). Synovial fluid for examination by polarized light should be collected either with no anticoagulant or with a small amount of heparin. EDTA and calcium oxalate crystals are birefringent and can be confused with MSU or CPPD.

Initial examination for crystals should be conducted on a wet preparation, using both plain and polarized light. The slide and coverslip should be cleaned with alcohol or acetone immediately prior to examination, then carefully dried with gauze or lens paper. A few drops of SF are placed on the slide, so that when the coverslip is gently added, the fluid margins barely reach the coverslip periphery. The preparation is promptly rimmed with clear nail polish to prevent drying. Allow the nail polish to dry for about 15 minutes before examination to prevent damage to the microscope objective.

Crystals of MSU appear as birefringent rods or needles under polarized light, varying from 1 to 20 μ in length (McCarty, 1965) (Fig. 19–2*A*). Certain crystalline corticosteroid preparations appear morphologically identical to MSU: e.g., betamethasone

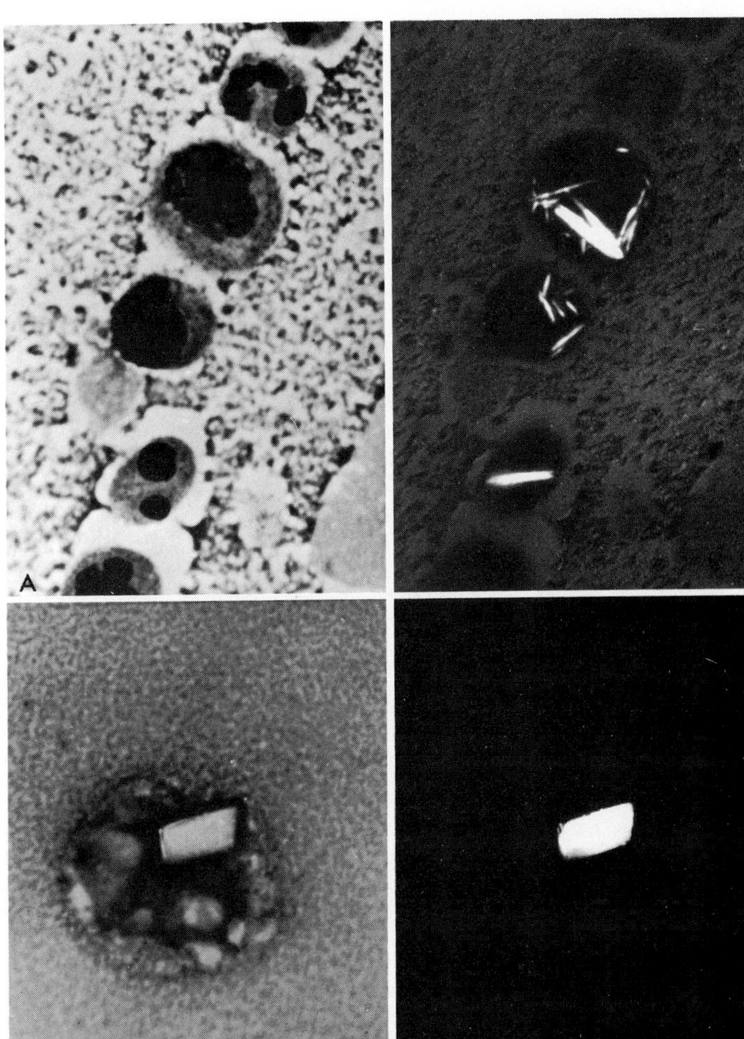

Figure 19–2. *A,* Leukocytes with uric acid crystals under normal and polarized light. *B,* Leukocyte with calcium pyrophosphate crystal under normal and polarized light. (From Good, A. E., and Frishette, W. A.: J.A.M.A., *198*:80, 1966.)

3

acetate (Celestone R), and triamcinolone hexacetonide (Kahn, 1970). Also, cholesterol crystals can appear as birefringent needles in chronic synovial effusions (Nye, 1968). However, cholesterol crystals are usually plate-like in form with a notch in one corner, and are often larger than a leukocyte. Definitive identification of needle-like crystals may be aided by incubation with uricase (McCarty, 1961).

Crystals of CPPD appear as birefringent rods, rectangles, or rhomboids varying from 1 to 20 μ in length and up to about 4 μ in width (McCarty, 1965) (Fig. 19–2*B*). Some corticosteroids used for intra-articular injection can be confused with CPPD (Wild, 1975). Also, cholesterol crystals may appear as rhomboid forms in some chronic effusions (Nye, 1968).

Talcum crystals present a Maltese cross appearance and may be as small as 5 to 10 μ (Naib, 1973). Lipid droplets in SF, associated with chronic inflammation or traumatic arthritis, also may have a Maltese cross appearance under polarized light (Wild, 1975).

Crystalline corticosteroids may appear under polarized light as long needles or rhomboids identical in appearance to MSU or CPPD; they may also appear as short rods, plates, fragments, or clumps, (Kahn, 1970). Calcium hydroxyapatite crystals appear as non-birefringent crystals. Such crystals may persist in SF for a month or longer following intra-articular injection.

Collagen fibrils and fibrin strands vary from 2 to over 100 μ in length. Although these may resemble MSU crystals under ordinary light, they show little or no birefringence with polarized light (Kitridou, 1969). Electron microscopy is required to distinguish definitely collagen fibrils from fibrin (Kitridou, 1969).

Fragments of cartilage may appear birefringent under polarized light (Kitridou, 1969), but unlike MSU or CPPD) do not have parallel margins. These fragments, as well as collagen fibrils, may be present in SF of osteoarthritis or traumatic arthritis.

Cholesterol crystals typically appear as irregular birefringent plates, often with notched margins. However, in chronic effusions, cholesterol crystals may appear either as long birefringent needles or as rhomboids, similar to MSU or CPPD (Nye, 1968). Cholesterol crystals may be present in any chronic effusion, e.g., tuberculous or rheumatoid arthritis.

Gout. MSU crystals can be demonstrated in SF of about 90 to 95 per cent of patients, during attacks of acute gouty arthritis (McCarty, 1965; Schumacher, 1975). Between attacks of acute gouty arthritis, MSU crystals can be demonstrated in about 75 per cent of patients. During attacks of acute gouty arthritis, the majority of crystals are intracellular, within neutrophils or macrophages; between attacks the majority of crystals are extracellular. However, in a few patients with acute gout, even careful examination with compensated polarized light fails to reveal MSU crystals (Abeles, 1977; Schumacher, 1975). Possible reasons for this failure to demonstrate MSU crystals may include crystals loculated within a joint and dissolution of crystals which initiated the acute attack. Occasionally, a 30 to 45 minute search may be required to find one or two MSU crystals in a patient with acute gouty arthritis (Schumacher, 1975). In such cases, there is an obvious need for the attending physician to communicate his clinical impression to the clinical microscopist, and to request a prolonged study of the specimen.

The report should note whether MSU crystals are lying free in SF or have been ingested by leukocytes. Phagocytosis of crystals suggests that these are responsible for acute arthritis. If only extracellular crystals are found, it is unlikely that these are responsible for acute symptoms (Wild, 1975).

Pseudogout. In this condition, clinical symptoms may mimic gout, rheumatoid arthritis, or osteoarthritis (Skinner, 1969). Diagnosis requires the demonstration of CPPD crystals. As in gout, the crystals may be either intracellular or extracellular (Fig. 19–2*B*).

Chemical Examination

Total protein in normal SF averages about 2 g/dl with a range of about 1 to 3 g/dl. Concentration of a specific protein in SF depends upon several factors, including plasma levels, molecular size, permeability of the synovial membrane, local synthesis, and local consumption. As plasma levels of a specific protein increase, levels in SF fluid also tend to increase. Thus, the concentration of a specific protein in SF frequently is expressed as SF: plasma ratio, to compensate for variations in plasma concentration, (Harris, 1981; Ropes, 1953).

Glucose in SF normally is identical to or slightly less than plasma glucose. Since equilibration between blood and SF glucose is slow, samples of blood and SF should be obtained after the patient has been fasting for 6 to 12 hours.

In non-inflammatory arthritis, the blood-SF glucose difference is about 10 mg/dl. With inflammatory arthritis (e.g., rheumatoid, septic, or tuberculous) the blood-SF glucose difference frequently exceeds 25 mg/dl or even 50 mg/dl. If fasting specimens are unavailable, a SF glucose under 40 mg/dl suggests decreased SF glucose; and a SF glucose under 20 mg/dl is considered definitely decreased.

Enzyme measurements in SF appear to have little clinical value, despite extensive investigations during the past 10 to 15 years. Enzymes which have been studied include the lysosomal enzymes (e.g., acid phosphatase and muramidase), alkaline phosphatase, LDH, and the transaminases (Cohen, 1975).

Uric acid measurements in SF (as opposed to microscopic examination for MSU crystals) appear to have little or no diagnostic value. Although some authors have suggested that measurement of SF uric acid might be useful in diagnosing acute gouty arthritis, most investigators feel that gouty effusions have a urate content essentially identical to that of serum (Cohen, 1975).

Lactate and pH measurements in SF may provide a useful but non-specific index of inflammation (McCarty, 1974). A lactate over 20 mg/dl (2/mmol/L) and/or a pH under 7.3 is suggestive evidence of septic or non-septic inflammation. Increased lactate and decreased pH appear to be associated with a rapid change from aerobic to anaerobic metabolism in synovial tissue as the Po_2 falls below 30 mm Hg (Falchuk, 1970). The clinical value of these measurements is not yet well established.

Immunologic Studies

Rheumatoid factor refers to a group of immunoglobulins reacting with the Fc regions of IgG molecules. About 80 per cent of patients with rheumatoid arthritis have rheumatoid factor in serum; about 60 per cent have rheumatoid factor in SF (Cracchiolo, 1972). In early rheumatoid arthritis, rheumatoid factor may appear in SF before becoming measurable in serum (Waxman, 1975). With suspected rheumatoid arthritis and a negative test for rheumatoid factor in serum, measurement of rheumatoid factor in SF may have some clinical value. However, a high incidence of false positive results has been reported (Huskisson, 1971).

Antinuclear antibodies have been demonstrated in SF of patients with systemic lupus erythematosus (about 70 per cent), as well as in SF of patients with rheumatoid arthritis (about 20 per cent) (Cracchiolo, 1972; Cohen, 1975). At present this finding is primarily of research interest rather than practical clinical value.

Complement measurements on SF have excited great interest, particularly over the past few years. The reference interval for SF complement varies with the concentration of SF protein so that SF complement should be expressed in relation to total protein (Bunch, 1974). In general, SF complement is of value when compared to serum complement levels.

In rheumatoid arthritis, decreased SF complement is noted in about 60 to 80 per cent of seropositive patients (rheumatoid factor present in serum), and in about 30 to 40 per cent of seronegative patients (Bunch, 1974). Although measurements of total hemolytic complement (CH 50) are most widely used, measurement of C4 may provide a more sensitive index (Ruddy, 1975). Decreased SF complement is not specific for rheumatoid arthritis: about 80 per cent of patients with systemic lupus have low SF complement. Low levels of SF complement also are occasionally observed in rheumatic fever, bacterial arthritis, gout, pseudogout, and other types of inflammatory arthritis.

Simultaneous measurement of serum and SF complement may be helpful in patients with seronegative rheumatoid arthritis. In about 40 per cent of such patients, serum complement is normal or increased, while SF complement is decreased (Ruddy, 1975). However, SF complement levels can be high in gout, infectious arthritis, and Reiter's syndrome, and in these cases is largely due to elevated serum levels of complement.

Although potentially useful, complement measurements on SF probably should not be considered a "routine" examination at this time.

Clinical Correlation

The "routine" synovial fluid examination includes appearance, viscosity, mucin clot test, microscopic study with compensated polarized light, Gram's stain, culture, and glucose. Except for Gram's stain and crystal identification, the synovial fluid examination is *not* highly specific for any single type of arthritis. Indeed, even Gram's stain and crystal identification do not exclude the possibility of two different diseases, since the following conditions may exist simultaneously in the same joint: septic arthritis and lupus erythematosus (Edelen, 1971); septic arthritis and pseudogout (McConville, 1975); septic arthritis and gout (Smith, 1972); gout and rheumatoid arthritis (Owen, 1966); gout and pseudogout (Jackson, 1965).

According to some authorities (Currey, 1976), small numbers of MSU or CPPD crystals may occur in conditions other than gout or pseudogout; however, this has not been confirmed, and as noted above, steroid or cholesterol crystals may have an appearance very similar to MSU or CPPD.

Even Gram's stain and crystal identification have less than 100 per cent sensitivity; about 50 per cent of patients with septic arthritis have negative Gram's stain, and about 5 to 10 per cent of patients with acute gouty arthritis (about 25 per cent of patients with inactive gouty arthritis) have a negative examination for crystals. The sensitivity of Gram's stain is increased using cytocentrifuge preparations.

The finding of LE cells in synovial fluid is not specific, since these may also occur in rheumatoid arthritis. However, if rheumatoid arthritis can be excluded, the specificity of this finding probably exceeds 95 per cent.

To provide improvèd sensitivity and specificity, two approaches are commonly used for interpretation: classification of synovial fluids into "reaction types" based on multiple findings (Table 19–9), and evaluation of results with regard to "typical" patterns found in different diseases (Table 19–10).

Non-inflammatory effusions (Table 19–9, Group I) usually have leukocyte counts of about 1000/μl and seldom exceed 5000/μl (Cohen, 1975). The percentage of neutrophils is usually under 25 per cent, although some authors report higher levels (Currey, 1976). Non-inflammatory conditions associated with articular effusion include osteoarthritis; traumatic arthritis (may occasionally be hemorrhagic); and neurogenic joint disease. Occasionally, the inflammatory fluids of mild rheumatic fever, systemic lupus erythematosus, or bacterial infection may present similar findings. Under phase microscopy, collagen fibrils and/or cartilage fragments may be seen in osteoarthritis, traumatic arthritis, or neurogenic joint disease.

Mild inflammatory effusions (Group IIa) may be associated with minimal inflammation and synovial fluid findings similar to Group I, e.g., early rheumatic fever; early systemic lupus erythematosus; early bacterial infection; and arthritis accompanying systemic disease such as ulcerative colitis, regional enteritis, or psoriasis. In such cases, the SF leukocyte count seldom exceeds 10,000/μl and the percentage of neutrophils usually is under 50 per cent.

However, with severe *inflammatory effusions* (Group IIb), the synovial reaction may be moderate or severe, e.g., rheumatoid arthritis, gout, and pseudogout. The leukocyte count may exceed 50,000 or even 100,000/μl, with over 90 per cent neutrophils (Frischknecht, 1975; Cohen, 1975).

Infectious effusions (Group III) owing to bacterial sepsis usually are associated with SF leukocyte counts over 50,000/μl and over 90 per cent neutrophils (Cohen, 1975). Counts of over 100,000 to 200,000/μl almost always indicate bacterial infection. However, SF leukocyte counts of under 1000 may be observed in some patients with early infectious arthritis (Brandt, 1974).

Many of the common viral diseases are associated with arthritis and joint effusions. Indeed, arthritis may sometimes precede other manifestations of viral infection. In viral arthritis, the SF leukocyte count commonly is under 10,000/μl with a mononuclear cell response, although exceptions have been reported (Cohen, 1975).

In Reiter's syndrome, the SF leukocyte count tends to be higher than with viral arthritis and associated with increased neutrophils. However, the leukocyte count and neutrophil reaction usually are less marked than with typical bacterial sepsis.

Hemorrhagic effusions may be associated with trauma, fracture, neurogenic joint, tumor (especially hemangioma), pigmented villonodular synovitis, hemorrhagic diathesis (e.g., hemophilia, anticoagulant therapy), or septic arthritis (Hollander, 1966; Jessar, 1972; Cohen, 1975).

Typical SF findings in various diseases are outlined in Table 19–10. With monoarticular effusions, the possibility of bacterial infection (e.g., tuberculosis or gonococcal arthritis) should be considered even if clinical and laboratory findings are atypical. Repeated aspirations, repeated radiologic studies, or even synovial biopsy may be indicated if the diagnosis is in doubt, and there is clinical evidence of progression.

Microscopic Examination of SF: Compensated Polarized Light Microscopy

An ordinary microscope with mechanical stage can be modified for compensated polarized light microscopy (Fig. 19–3):

1. A 32 mm polarizing disk (called "the polarizer") is placed over the light source.
2. A glass microscope slide (called "the compensator") is prepared with two thicknesses of clear cellophane or cellophane tape applied to one side (Fagan, 1974). Streaks in the two layers of cellophane tape must be parallel rather than crossed. Translucent tape is *not* satisfactory. The prepared slide is placed over the polarizer.
3. A second polarizing disk (called "the analyser") is placed either in the barrel of the microscope or in the eyepiece.

The same components are available from most microscope manufacturers (Fig. 19–4):

1. A polarizer which fits over the light source (AO part No. K2108)
2. A compensator which fits over the polarizer (included with AO part No. K2108)
3. An analyzer which fits into the microscope barrel (AO part No. 1114)

A gliding circular stage with mechanical controls for positioning the specimen (AO part No. K2270) greatly facilitates crystal identification, especially for inexperienced observers (Fig. 19–4). An attached camera (AO part No. 668) is useful for preparing permanent records of interesting samples.

With the compensator removed, and the polarizers crossed, the field will appear dark, except for birefringent material such as MSU crystals, CPPD crystals, talc crystals, cholesterol crystals, certain corticosteroid crystals, and oval fat bodies.

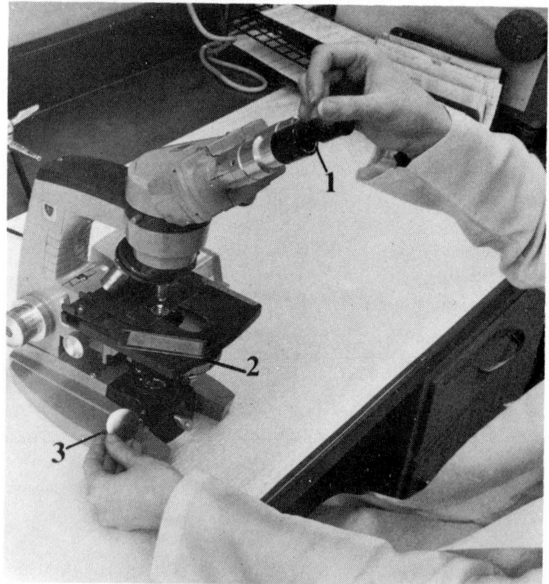

Figure 19–3. Adaptation of ordinary laboratory microscope for compensated polarized light microscopy: *1,* Polarizing disk for eyepiece; *2,* glass slide with two thicknesses of clear cellophane tape to be placed over No. 3; *3,* polarizing disk to be placed over light source.

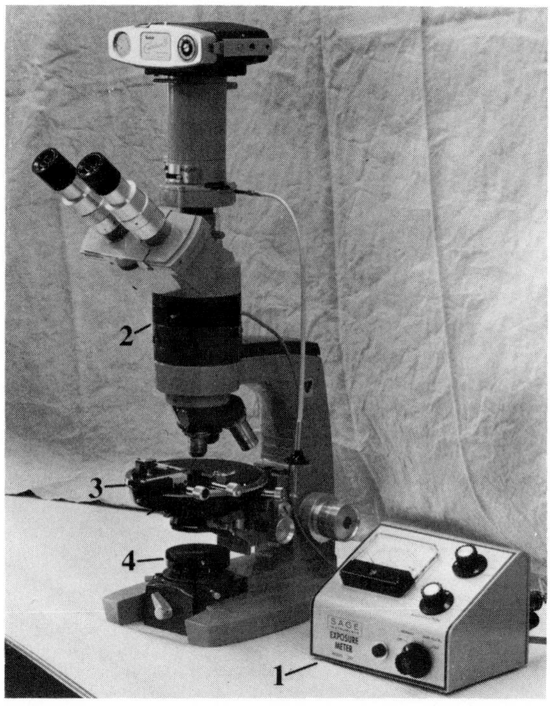

Figure 19–4. Commercial components for compensated polarized light microscopy: *1,* Exposure meter for camera; *2,* analyzer; *3,* circular stage with mechanical controls; *4,* polarizer with compensator.

With the compensator added, the field will appear red, and a given crystal (e.g., MSU) will appear either blue or yellow, depending upon its orientation (Fig. 19–5). A useful mnemonic is "parallel (yellow) gout"; when the long axis of the crystal is parallel to the compensator and the crystal is yellow, it is MSU.

With the compensator in a constant position, a birefringent crystal of MSU will change color (from blue to yellow or vice versa) as the crystal is rotated 90 degrees (Fig. 19–5).

If the crystal is kept in a constant position but the compensator rotated 90 degrees, a similar color change will be observed.

Control slides may be prepared from scrapings of a gouty tophus, a known specimen from acute gouty arthritis, a suspension of betamethasone acetate (appearance under compensated polarized light identical to uric acid crystals), or according to the procedure described by Bartlett (1978). In this last procedure, the control is prepared by adding 5 mg of uric acid to 15 ml of boiling distilled water. After the crystals are dissolved, the solution is cooled and 0.1 g/ml of sodium bicarbonate added until a pH of 7 is reached. This solution is then stored for several days at room temperature, allowing evaporation to dryness. The sediment contains crystals of uric acid which may be resuspended in distilled water for use as a control. The control slides should be rimmed with nail polish and saved for comparison with unknown specimens.

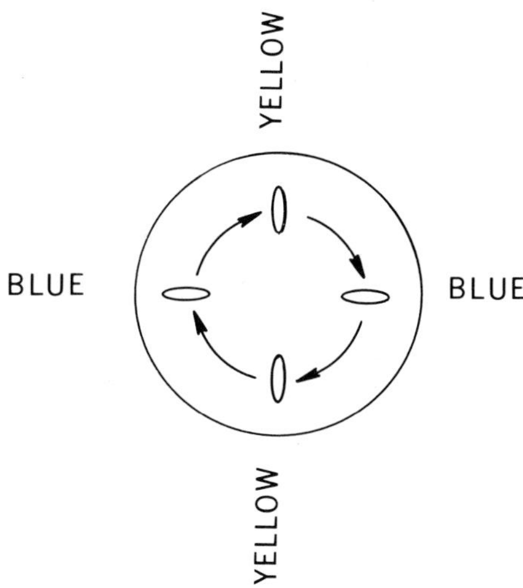

Figure 19–5. Color changes in birefringent crystal observed with compensated polarized light during rotation of microscope stage. (Colors in a given position vary according to setting of compensator and must be checked against a control.)

Immediately before examination of an unknown, use the control slide to sketch the colors of a uric acid crystal in different orientations, with the compensator in a fixed position. Prepare a sketch similar to Figure 19–5 by rotating the stage or by observing crystals lying in different positions. Then observe the unknown: rotate the stage as needed to bring the unknown crystals into the same positions as noted in your sketch. Crystals of MSU will appear identical to those in the control slide, while CPPD crystals will have opposite colors from MSU. Certain corticosteroids may have an appearance identical to MSU under compensated polarized light. Although Nye (1968) describes cholesterol crystals appearing identical to MSU, findings with compensated polarized light were not reported. Digestion with uricase as described by McCarty (1961) may be used to confirm crystal identification in selected cases: (1) Add one part of a saline uricase suspension (minimal activity 0.75 unit per ml) to five parts of SF (as little as 50 μl SF may be used). (2) Add one part of saline control to five parts of SF in a separate tube. (3) Incubate both tubes at 45° C. for four hours. (4) Place a drop of SF from each tube on a glass slide and examine by compensated polarized light microscopy.

PLEURAL, PERICARDIAL, AND PERITONEAL FLUIDS

Transudates and Exudates

Effusions of fluid in the pleural, pericardial, or peritoneal cavity may form on the basis of plasma ultrafiltration. Such ultrafiltrates commonly are classified as transudates and exudates. A transudate is an effusion caused by mechanical factors influencing formation or resorption of fluid, e.g., decreased plasma albumin and/or increased venous pressure. An exudate is an effusion caused by damage to mesothelial linings, e.g., tuberculosis, bacterial or fungal infection, neoplasm, rheumatoid disease, or systemic lupus erythematosus. Effusions also may form owing to escape of chyle from the thoracic duct (chylous effusions, Table 19–11). Some causes for pleural, pericardial, and peritoneal effusions are outlined in Table 19–12.

In pleural fluid, a protein level of 3.0 g/dl classically is used to separate transudates from exudates: about 90 per cent of pleural exudates have a total protein over 3.0 g/dl, and about 80 per cent of pleural transudates have a total protein under 3.0 g/dl. An alternative classification has been suggested by Light (1972) based on three ratios: (1) pleural fluid protein to serum protein (ratio over 0.5 suggests exudate); (2) pleural fluid LDH to serum LDH (ratio over 0.6 suggests exudate); (3) pleural fluid LDH to serum LDH upper limit of normal (ratio over 0.67 suggests exudate). According to Light (1972), over 95 per cent of pleural exudates have at least one of these characteristics, while over 95 per cent of pleural transudates have none of these findings. Additional studies are needed to confirm the value of LDH measurements in laboratory classification of pleural effusions.

In pericardial fluid, the laboratory criteria for transudates are less clearly defined. Indeed, most pericardial effusions are caused by damage to mesothelial linings rather than mechanical factors (Table 19–12). At this time, the clinical validity of total protein measurements to separate pericardial "transudates" from "exudates" is not well established.

In peritoneal fluid, the recommended laboratory criteria for differentiating transudates from exudates vary. Some authorities (Ball, 1976) use a protein level of 2.0 g/dl to separate transudates from exudates, while others use 2.5 g/dl (McClement, 1975; Sabiston, 1974). Both of these recommended "cut-off points" are lower than the generally accepted cut-off of 3.0 g/dl for pleural fluid.

"Routine study" for pleural, pericardial, and/or peritoneal effusion of unknown etiology usually includes gross appearance, total protein, erythrocyte count, leukocyte count, differential count and microscopic study of Wright's stained film, Gram's stain, culture, and cytologic study. Additional studies which may be useful in specific circumstances include glucose (suspected rheumatoid disease or infection), amylase (pleural fluid with suspected esophageal perforation; pleural or peritoneal fluid with suspected pancreatitis), LDH (differential diagnosis of pleural transudate vs. exudate), pH (pleural fluid with suspected esophageal perforation; parapneumonic effusion), ammonia (peritoneal fluid with suspected intestinal necrosis or perforation; differential diagnosis of effusion vs. urinary extravasation), creatinine (differential diagnosis of peritoneal effusion vs. urinary extravasation), alkaline phosphatase (peritoneal fluid with suspected infarction or perforation of small intestine), spot test for bile (peritoneal fluid of greenish appearance), hyaluronate (suspected mesothelioma), and biopsy (suspected tuberculosis with negative acid-fast stain and culture).

Table 19–11. CHYLOUS AND PSEUDOCHYLOUS EFFUSIONS

	Chylous Effusion	Pseudochylous Effusion
Appearance	Milky: may form creamy top layer on standing	Milky to greenish—or "gold paint" appearance
Odor	Odorless	Variable from odorless to foul
pH	Alkaline	Variable
Extraction with ether after acidification with dilute HCl	Clearing and decrease in volume	Does not clear or decrease in volume
Microscopic examination	Lymphocytes plus fine fat droplets	Mixed cellular reaction with cholesterol crystals
Triglycerides	2–8 × serum triglycerides	Lower than serum triglycerides
Cholesterol	Lower than serum cholesterol	May be higher than serum cholesterol
Lipoprotein electrophoresis	Increased chylomicron band in relation to plasma	Chylomicrons scanty or absent
Effect of diet with no long-chain fatty acids	Decreased accumulation of lipid in effusion	No significant change in effusion
Ingestion of lipophilic dye	Dye appears in effusion	Dye does not appear in effusion
Culture	Always sterile	Usually sterile (check for tuberculosis or fungus)
Etiology	Damage or obstruction to thoracic duct	Chronic effusion of any cause (e.g., cyst fluid, rheumatoid disease, tuberculosis, myxedema)

Table 19–12. CAUSES OF PLEURAL, PERICARDIAL, AND PERITONEAL EFFUSIONS

Pleural

Transudate
- Congestive heart failure
- Hepatic cirrhosis
- Hypoproteinemia (e.g., nephrotic syndrome)

Exudates
- Neoplasms
  - Bronchogenic carcinoma
  - Metastatic carcinoma
  - Lymphoma
  - Mesothelioma (increased hyaluronate content of effusion fluid)
- Infections
  - Tuberculosis (high percentage of lymphocytes with under 1% mesothelial cells)
  - Bacterial pneumonia
  - Viral or mycoplasmal pneumonia
- Trauma (may be associated with hemorrhagic effusion)
- Pulmonary infarct (may be associated with hemorrhagic effusion)
- Rheumatoid disease (low pleural fluid glucose in most cases)
- Systemic lupus erythematosus (LE cells occasionally present)
- Pancreatis (elevated amylase activity in effusion fluid)
- Ruptured esophagus (elevated amylase activity and low pH in effusion fluid)

Chylous effusion
- Damage or obstruction to thoracic duct, e.g., trauma, lymphoma, carcinoma, tuberculosis

Pericardial

Exudates
- Infections
  - Bacterial pericarditis
  - Tuberculosis
  - Fungal pericarditis
  - Viral or mycoplasmal pericarditis

Pericardial (continued)

Exudates (continued)
- Neoplasms
  - Metastatic carcinoma or lymphoma
- Trauma (may be associated with hemorrhagic effusion)
- Myocardial infarct
- Hemorrhagic effusion
  - Secondary to anticoagulant therapy
  - Leakage of aortic aneurysm
- Metabolic (uremia, myxedema)
- Rheumatoid disease
- Systemic lupus erythematosus

Peritoneal

Transudates
- Congestive heart failure
- Hepatic cirrhosis
- Hypoproteinemia (e.g., nephrotic syndrome)

Exudates
- Neoplasms
  - Hepatoma
  - Metastatic carcinoma
  - Lymphoma
  - Mesothelioma
- Infections
  - Tuberculosis
  - Primary bacterial peritonitis (may be superimposed on transudate)
  - Secondary bacterial peritonitis (e.g., appendicitis, intestinal infarct)
- Trauma
- Pancreatitis
- Bile peritonitis (secondary to ruptured gallbladder or needle perforation of bile duct)

Chylous effusion
- Damage or obstruction to thoracic duct, e.g., trauma, lymphoma, carcinoma, tuberculosis, parasitic infestation

ASPIRATION OF PLEURAL FLUID

The usual indications for thoracentesis include effusion of unknown etiology, clinical symptoms (e.g., dyspnea) caused by fluid accumulation, intrapleural instillation of drugs for treating infection or malignancy, hemothorax, and empyema. Complications of thoracentesis may include hemothorax due to laceration of the lung and mediastinal shift after removing large amounts of fluid. These complications may be minimized by gradual drainage of fluid via a plastic cannula introduced at the time of thoracentesis (van Heerden, 1968; Wilson, 1975).

ASPIRATION OF PERICARDIAL FLUID

The usual indications for pericardial aspiration include pericardial effusion of unknown etiology and acute or chronic cardiac tamponade. Complications of aspiration include (1) cardiac arrhythmias, (2) infection of pleural spaces by purulent pericardial fluid, (3) laceration of atrium or a coronary artery, and (4) inadvertent injection of air into a cardiac chamber. These complications may be minimized either by open biopsy (Kilpatrick, 1965) or by use of a soft catheter for drainage with EKG monitoring during pericardial tap.

ASPIRATION OF PERITONEAL FLUID

The usual indications for abdominal paracentesis include ascites of unknown etiology; clinical symptoms (e.g., dyspnea) caused by fluid accumulation; suspected intestinal infarct, intestinal perforation, or intra-abdominal hemorrhage; and instillation of cytotoxic drugs for treating malignancy. Combined aspiration and lavage have been described by a number of authors (McCoy, 1971; Olsen, 1972; Perry, 1972; Parvin, 1975; Engrav, 1975; Jergens, 1977). A catheter is introduced through a trocar, and if aspiration is negative (no free blood, bile, feces, or urine), 1 L of normal saline or Ringer's lactate (10 to 20 ml/kg body weight) is infused over 15 to 20 minutes. After manipulation of the abdomen, lavage fluid is siphoned back from the peritoneal cavity into the original container and examined.

Gross Examination

PLEURAL FLUID

Normal pleural fluid is clear, pale yellow, and scanty in amount (under 20 ml). Increased amounts of normal appearing fluid commonly are found with congestive heart failure or chronic liver disease. Cloudy or turbid fluid usually is due to large numbers of leukocytes, associated with septic or non-septic inflammation (e.g., bacterial infection, tuberculosis, rheumatoid disease, rheumatic fever).

"Milky" fluid is characteristic of chylous or pseudochylous effusions. True chylous effusions are due to leakage of thoracic duct contents, while pseudochylous effusions are due to breakdown of cellular lipids in chronic effusions from any cause. Approaches to differential diagnosis are outlined in Table 19–11. With regard to ingestion of lipophilic dye: following oral or gastric tube administration of 1 g lipophilic dye (D and C Green No. 6 Lipophilic Dye, H. Kohnstamn, 161 Avenue of the Americas, New York, NY 10013) in one-fourth pound of margarine, the dye will appear in true chylous fluid after 12 to 24 hours, but will not appear in pseudochylous effusions (Klepser, 1954). With regard to lipoprotein electrophoresis, chylous fluid shows markedly elevated chylomicrons in comparison with plasma, while chylomicrons are scanty or absent in pseudochylous effusions (Seriff, 1977).

It is important to distinguish hemorrhagic fluid from blood-tinged fluid due to traumatic tap. In traumatic tap, the blood typically is non-uniform in distribution and frequently clears with aspiration. Hemorrhagic fluids most often are caused by intrapleural malignancy, but may also occur in some effusions due to pneumonia, closed chest trauma, pulmonary infarct, pancreatitis, and postmyocardial infarction syndrome (Dressler's syndrome). Occasionally, pleural transudates due to congestive heart failure or hepatic cirrhosis may appear hemorrhagic for no apparent cause.

PERICARDIAL FLUID

Normal pericardial fluid is clear, pale yellow, and varies from about 10 to 50 ml in volume.

Interpretation of gross appearance is similar to that for pleural fluid. Hemorrhagic effusions may occur in a wide variety of conditions, including idiopathic hemorrhagic pericarditis, postmyocardial infarction syndrome, postpericardiectomy syndrome, tuberculosis, rheumatoid arthritis, systemic lupus erythematosus, metastatic carcinoma, bacterial pericarditis, or leaking aneurysm. Hemorrhagic pericardial effusion can be distinguished from inadvertent aspiration of blood from the cardiac cavity by observing clot formation; an effusion will not clot, since it has been defibrinated *in vivo.*

Milky fluid presents the problem of differential diagnosis between true chylous and pseudochylous effusion (Hudspeth, 1966). The latter condition may be associated with any chronic effusion of long duration (Table 19–11).

PERITONEAL FLUID

Normal peritoneal fluid is clear, pale yellow, and scanty in amount (under 50 ml).

Cloudy or turbid fluid suggests peritonitis due to appendicitis, pancreatitis, strangulated or infarcted intestine, ruptured bowel following trauma, or primary bacterial infection.

Greenish (bile-stained) fluid has been described with perforated duodenal ulcer, perforated intestine, cholecystitis, perforated gallbladder, and acute pancreatitis (McCoy, 1971). A spot test for bilirubin should be performed in such cases to confirm the presence of bile. Although ruptured gallbladder with bile in the peritoneal cavity can be rapidly fatal, sterile bile may be fairly well tolerated (Diamonon, 1964).

Milky fluid is rare, and may be due to chylous or pseudochylous effusion. These may be differentiated as outlined in Table 19–11. Causes for true chylous ascites include damage to or blockage of the thoracic duct due to lymphoma, carcinoma, tuberculosis, parasitic infestation, adhesions, or hepatic cirrhosis (Lesser, 1970).

Grossly bloody aspirate, or blood-tinged lavage, must be distinguished from traumatic tap. As with other body fluids, traumatic tap is characterized by clearing on continued aspiration.

For lavage fluid, visual quantitation of blood is outlined in Table 19–13. Greater than 25 ml of blood in 1 L of lavage fluid produces bright red fluid sufficiently opaque that newsprint cannot be read through the lavage tubing (Olsen, 1972). This amount of blood (25 ml) corresponds to an erythrocyte count of over 100,000/μl in the lavage fluid. In the series reportedly by Olsen, 98 per cent of patients with 3+ to 4+ lavage fluid had significant intra-abdominal injuries which required exploration, while only 32 per cent of patients with 1+ to 2+ lavage fluid had significant injuries requiring exploration. In the series reported by Engrav (1975), with 100,000 erythrocytes/μl used as the criteria for a "positive" lavage and 50,000 to 100,000 considered "borderline," 85 per cent of patients with erythrocyte counts over 100,000/μl had significant intraperitoneal injury, while only 4 per cent of patients with erythrocyte counts under 50,000/μl had significant injuries requiring exploration.

Microscopic Examination

A leukocyte count, erythrocyte count, and differential count often are considered as part of the "routine" examination for pleural, pericardial, and peritoneal fluids. Undiluted fluid is ordinarily used; however, with grossly bloody pleural fluids it may be necessary to hemolyze the erythrocytes by dilution with 3 per cent acetic acid before performing a leukocyte count. An electronic cell counter should *not* be used, since debris may produce falsely elevated counts.

Cells for differential count may be concentrated by centrifugation and resuspension, by cytocentrifuge, or by Millipore filtration.

The percentage of mesothelial cells has clinical significance in pleural fluid and should be reported (Winckler, 1976). This percentage may be specified either as part of the differential count or as a percentage of total leukocytes (neutrophils, eosinophils, basophils, lymphocytes, monocytes, and macrophages).

In ascitic fluid, the percentage of mesothelial cells ordinarily is specified as a percentage of total leukocytes, rather than as part of the differential count (Kline, 1976).

PLEURAL FLUID

The value of pleural fluid erythrocyte counts, leukocyte counts, and differential counts has been questioned by some authorities (Storey, 1976).

Other workers suggest that careful leukocyte and differential counts are useful in detection and diagnosis of tuberculous effusions. About 90 per cent of such cases are characterized by (1) hypercellularity (leukocyte count over 1000/μl) and/or (2) lymphocytosis (over 50 per cent lymphocytes) and/or (3) scarcity of mesothelial cells (under 1 per cent) (Yam, 1967; Spriggs, 1968; Light, 1973; Winckler, 1976). However, these findings are not specific for tuberculosis, and may also occur with uremic effusions, carcinoma, or lymphoma involving the pleural cavity, chronic lymphatic leukemia, chylothorax, and postpneumonic effusions (Spriggs, 1968; Berger, 1975; Winckler, 1976). Some transudates (perhaps 10 per cent) may present findings similar to tuberculosis, with leukocyte counts over 1000/μl, over 50 per cent lymphocytes, and/or under 1 per cent mesothelial cells (Light, 1973). Tuberculous empyema is *not* associated with lymphocytosis, but is characterized by a change from lymphocytic to neutrophil predominance (Spriggs, 1968).

Pleural fluid leukocyte count and differential may be useful in diagnosis of parapneumonic effusions (effusions associated with pneumonia): about 50 per cent of these have a leukocyte count over 10,000/μl, and about 80 per cent have a predominance of neutrophils (Light, 1973). Less than 10 per cent of transudates have a leukocyte count over 10,000/μl and/or a predominance of neutrophils (Light, 1973).

Eosinophilic pleural effusions are considered by some authors to include cases with 10 per cent eosinophils, while others use this term only for effusions with over 50 per cent eosinophils (Spriggs, 1968). Recently, Askin (1977) described reactive eosinophilic pleuritis as frequently associated with pneumothorax and suggested that pleural eosinophilia is a non-specific reaction to pleural injury. Pleural

Table 19–13. VISUAL QUANTITATION OF BLOOD IN PERITONEAL LAVAGE FLUID*

Appearance of Lavage Fluid in Tubing	Appearance of Lavage Fluid in Bottle	Amount of Blood Necessary to Produce Gross Appearance
Gross blood, opaque	gross blood (4+)	> 100 ml/L
Bright red, opaque	bright red (3+)	> 25 ml/L
Pink, clear	bright red (2+)	5–15 ml/L
Clear	pink (1+)	2 ml/L
Clear	pale pink (trace)	8 drops/L
Clear	clear	0

*Adapted from Olsen, W. R., Redman, H. C., and Hildreth, D. H.: Arch. Surg., *104*:536, 1972. Copyright 1972, American Medical Association.

fluid eosinophilia may be associated with many different conditions, including pneumothorax, postoperative effusions, postpneumonic effusions, closed chest trauma (Kumar, 1975), pulmonary infarct, congestive heart failure, ventriculopleural shunt (Venes, 1974), fungal infections, parasitic disease (e.g., hydatid disease), hypersensitivity syndromes, systemic lupus erythematosus, polyarthritis, Hodgkin's disease, and mesothelioma. Although some authors state that pleural eosinophilia is seldom present with tuberculous effusion, this has limited value for diagnosis, since pleural fluid eosinophilia is unusual and pneumothorax can cause a marked eosinophilic reaction in the presence of co-existing tuberculosis. Thus eosinophilia is quite non-specific and of little diagnostic value.

Rheumatoid arthritis (RA) cells may be seen in rheumatoid pleural effusions, but are non-specific (Boddington, 1971).

LE cells are uncommon, but considered specific when present (Osamura, 1977).

Echinococcosis involving the pleural space may be diagnosed by toluidine blue–stained wet films; the scolices also may be identified on Papanicolaou or Wright's stain (Jacobson, 1973).

PERICARDIAL FLUID

Microscopic findings in tuberculous pericarditis are similar to those in pleural fluid, with a predominance of lymphocytes (Spriggs, 1968).

Increased leukocytes (over 1000/μl) with a predominance of neutrophils are characteristic of bacterial pericarditis but may also be seen in viral pericarditis or postmyocardial infarction syndrome (Soloff, 1971).

Eosinophilia of pericardial fluid is rare: in 1968 Spriggs found no cases either in the literature or in his own experience.

LE cells have been described in pericardial fluid (Seaman, 1952), but this finding is unusual.

Amebic pericarditis has been described; however, the diagnosis is more likely to be made by serologic studies than by microscopic examination of pericardial fluid.

PERITONEAL FLUID

For lavage fluid, an erythrocyte count of over 100,000/μl in lavage fluid is considered "positive," consistent with over 20 to 25 μl whole blood in the peritoneal cavity. Counts in the 50,000 to 100,000 range are considered "borderline." Combined with a history of abdominal trauma, an elevated erythrocyte count may be an indication for celiotomy (Olsen, 1972; Engrav, 1975).

A leukocyte count of over 500/μl in lavage fluid is considered abnormal, but is not in itself diagnostic for peritonitis (Perry, 1972; Engrav, 1975; Parvin, 1975; Jergens, 1977).

For undiluted ascitic fluid, a leukocyte count of over 300/μl in undiluted sterile ascitic fluid is considered "abnormal" (Kline, 1976). Higher counts are seen in over 90 per cent of patients with spontaneous bacterial peritonitis, which may develop either from passage of bacteria from blood into ascitic fluid or from passage of bacteria through the bowel wall. However, about 50 per cent of cirrhotic patients with sterile ascitic fluid may have ascitic fluid leukocyte counts of over 300/μl (Kline, 1976). Although an ascitic fluid leukocyte count of over 300/μl has about 90 per cent sensitivity for spontaneous bacterial peritonitis, if we consider peritoneal transudates due to cirrhosis, specificity is only about 50 per cent. If 500/μl is used as a cut-off level, specificity is increased with a slight loss in sensitivity (Kline, 1976).

A differential count with over 25 per cent neutrophils is considered increased for ascitic fluid. Higher percentages are seen in over 90 per cent of patients with spontaneous bacterial peritonitis (SBP); however, about 50 per cent of cirrhotic patients with sterile ascites due to cirrhosis also have over 25 per cent neutrophils. If 50 per cent is used as a cut-off level, specificity is increased with a slight loss in sensitivity (Kline 1976).

The *absolute* granulocyte count with a cutoff level of 250/μl may provide both sensitivity (about 90 per cent of patients with SBP) and specificity (about 90 per cent in patients with sterile ascites due to cirrhosis have an ascitic fluid absolute granulocyte count under 250/μl) (Jones, 1977).

Conn (1976) concludes that: "When the clinical picture is compatible [with SBP] and the ascitic fluid contains more than 500 WBC's per cu mm,* more than half of which are PMN's, it is in the patient's best interest to begin antibiotic therapy."

A high percentage of lymphocytes should suggest the possibility of tuberculous peritonitis, but also may be seen in chylous ascites. In contrast to pleural fluid, numerous mesothelial cells can occur with tuberculous effusions in the peritoneal cavity.

Eosinophilic ascites is uncommon, but has been reported in association with congestive heart failure, hypereosinophilic syndrome, eosinophilic gastroenteritis, chronic peritoneal dialysis, abdominal lymphoma, ruptured hydatid cyst, atopy, and vasculitis (Adams, 1977).

LE cells have been reported in peritoneal fluid (Metzger, 1974), but this finding is rare.

Rarely, a syndrome of fever and ascites, without infection, may occur several weeks after surgery, caused by talc (from surgical gloves) introduced into the peritoneum. Diagnosis may be made by paracentesis and identification of doubly refractile talc granules on examination with polarized light (Warshaw, 1972).

Rarely, microfilariae may occur in ascitic fluid in the absence of local or systemic symptoms (Figueroa, 1973).

Microbiologic Examination

Acid-fast stain and culture are positive in only about 25 to 50 per cent of tuberculous effusions. This incidence may be increased by special techniques which utilize the sediment from 100 to 500 ml of centrifuged fluid. With the addition of culture and

*1 mm^3 = 1μl.

3

histologic study on biopsy specimens, positive results may be obtained on 90 to 95 per cent of all cases (Levine, 1970).

Chemical Examination

Normal glucose concentration in pleural, pericardial, and peritoneal fluid is approximately equal to whole blood glucose. Changes in blood glucose are reflected in these fluids after lag periods of two to four hours. Thus, systemic hypoglycemia or hyperglycemia may be associated with "false low" or "false high" results, respectively.

PLEURAL FLUID

Glucose under 60 mg/dl, or 40 mg/dl less than plasma glucose, is considered decreased (Light, 1973). Less than 1 per cent of transudates have decreased glucose, while about half of tuberculous effusions, about 10 per cent of neoplastic and septic effusions, and about 80 per cent of rheumatoid effusions are associated with decreased pleural fluid glucose (Light, 1973). Glucose measurements may be helpful in differential diagnosis of rheumatoid effusion vs. systemic lupus erythematosus, since in the latter condition, pleural fluid glucose usually is above 60 mg/dl (Carr, 1970).

Amylase activity is considered elevated in pleural effusions when this exceeds the upper limit of normal for serum or the amylase activity in a simultaneously obtained serum sample. Amylase activity is almost always elevated in pleural effusion associated with pancreatitis. Since pleural effusions are present in about 10 per cent of patients with pancreatitis (Light, 1973), amylase measurements can be helpful in differential diagnosis.

Elevated amylase also is characteristic of effusions associated with esophageal perforation: in these cases the amylase is of salivary origin (Light, 1973).

About 10 per cent of neoplastic effusions, and a smaller percentage of parapneumonic effusions, also may be associated with elevated pleural fluid amylase (Light, 1973).

Measurements of pH have been suggested as an aid in diagnosis of esophageal rupture (Dye, 1974). A pleural fluid pH under 6 is highly suggestive of esophageal rupture.

pH measurements also have been used to guide diagnosis and treatment of pleural effusions (Light, 1973; Potts, 1976). Perhaps 50 per cent of empyemas, loculated effusions, and tuberculous effusions have a pH under 7.30. In parapneumonic effusions with pH under 7.20, intercostal tube drainage usually is needed in addition to antibiotic therapy (Light, 1973).

Hyaluronate measurements in pleural fluid occasionally are helpful in diagnosis of pleural mesothelioma (Hellstrom, 1977).

PERICARDIAL FLUID

Glucose in pericardial fluid may be decreased in bacterial pericarditis, as well as in non-septic inflammation due to rheumatoid disease or malignancy.

PERITONEAL FLUID

Glucose levels in ascitic fluid may be reduced below 60 mg/dl in about 30 to 50 per cent of patients with tuberculous peritonitis (Brown, 1976), as well as in peritoneal carcinomatosis.

Amylase activity in peritoneal fluid is elevated above normal blood levels in about 90 per cent of patients with acute pancreatitis, pancreatic trauma, or pancreatic pseudocyst. Elevated peritoneal fluid amylase also may occur with intestinal strangulation or necrosis (Mansberger, 1964).

Ammonia levels in peritoneal fluid are markedly increased (two times the upper limit of normal for plasma) with perforated peptic ulcer, perforated appendix, or strangulation (with or without perforation) of small or large bowel (Mansberger, 1964). However, peritoneal fluid ammonia is normal in association with pancreatitis. Elevation in both ammonia and creatinine is characteristic of ruptured bladder with urinary extravasation (Mansberger, 1964).

Alkaline phosphatase activity in peritoneal fluid is markedly increased (over two times normal serum levels) in about 90 per cent of patients with strangulation or perforation of the small intestine (Lee, 1969; Delany, 1976). This elevation appears after about two to three hours and progressively increases during the next three to four hours (Rush, 1972). Although other enzymes in peritoneal fluid also increase following injury to the small intestine, these are less specific than alkaline phosphatase measurements.

Measurement of pH in peritoneal fluid has little value in diagnosis of perforated peptic ulcer (Howard, 1963) and is not widely used at this time.

Other Measurements and Examinations

Counterimmunoelectrophoresis for bacterial antigens has been used for detection and identification of bacteria in effusion fluids. However, this technique is not yet generally accepted as a "routine" procedure.

Limulus lysate assays have been used for diagnosis of effusions due to gram-negative organisms. Additional studies are needed to confirm the clinical value of this method.

Lysozyme measurements have been suggested as an aid in diagnosis of tuberculous effusions (Klockars, 1976). The transformation of monocytes into macrophages and epithelioid cells is accompanied by a corresponding increase in lysosomal enzymes, including lysozyme. However, the clinical value of this procedure is not yet established.

Cytologic examination for carcinoma is a highly accurate method for detection and diagnosis of malignant effusions. Sensitivity and specificity are in the range of 90 per cent.

Cerebrospinal Fluid

Alexander, E.: Lumbar puncture, J.A.M.A., *201*:100, 1967.

Aspock, H.: Die Laboratoriumsdiagnostile der Amobeninfektioness des Menschen. Wien. Klin. Wochenschr., *89*:37, 1977.

Azimi, P. H., Shaban, S., Hilty, M. D., and Haynes, R. E.: Mumps meningoencephalitis. J.A.M.A., *234*:1161, 1975.

Beaty, H. N., and Oppenheimer, S.: Cerebrospinal fluid lactic dehydrogenase and its isoenzymes in infections of the central nervous system. N. Engl. J. Med., *279*:1197, 1968.

Bland, R. D., Lister, R. C., and Ries, J. P.: Cerebrospinal fluid lactic acid level and pH in meningitis. Am. J. Dis. Child., *128*:151, 1974.

Bock, E.: Quantitation of plasma proteins in cerebrospinal fluid. *In* Axelsen, N. H., Kroll, J., and Wecke, B. (eds.): A Manual of Quantitative Immunoelectrophoresis. Oslo, Universitetsforlager, 1975, Chap. 14.

Brooks, B. R.: Cerebrospinal fluid acid-base and lactate changes after seizures in unanesthetized man. Neurology, *25*:935, 1975.

Burechailo, F., and Cunningham, T. A.: Counting cells in cerebrospinal fluid collected directly on membrane filters. J. Clin. Path., *27*:101, 1974.

Burgi, W., Richterich, R., and Briner, M.: UV-photometric determination of total cerebrospinal fluid proteins with modified biuret reagent. Clin. Chim. Acta, *15*:181, 1967.

Butler, W. T., Alling, D. W., and Spickard, A.: Diagnostic and prognostic value of clinical and laboratory findings in cryptococcal meningitis. N. Engl. J. Med., *270*:59, 1964.

Calabrese, V. P.: The interpretation of routine CSF tests. Vir. Med. Month., *103*:207, 1976.

Campbell, R. A.: Lumbar puncture in the frail infant. J.A.M.A., *204*:180, 1968.

Carpenter, R. R., and Petersdorf, R. G.: The clinical spectrum of bacterial meningitis. Am. J. Med., *33*:262, 1962.

Castleberry, R. P., Moreno, H., and Wallace, L. S.: Cytologic analysis of cerebrospinal fluid. J. Pediatr., *86*:990, 1975.

Cawley, L. P., Minard, B. J., Tourtellotte, W. W., Ma, B. I., and Chelle, C.: Immunofixation electrophoretic techniques applied to identification of proteins in serum and cerebrospinal fluid. Clin. Chem., *22*:1262, 1976.

Chen, J. H.: Measurement of gonadotropin in cerebrospinal fluid. N. Engl. J. Med., *297*:114, 1977.

Chu, J. Y., Freiling, P., and Wassilak, S.: Simple method for the cytological examination of cerebrospinal fluid. J. Clin. Path., *30*:486, 1977.

Cohen, S. R., Herndon, R. M., and McKann, G. M.: Radioimmunoassay of myelin basic protein in spinal fluid. N. Engl. J. Med., *295*:1455, 1976.

Cold, G., Enevoldsen, E., and Malmros, R.: Ventricular fluid lactate, pyruvate, bicarbonate and pH in unconscious brain-injured patients subjected to controlled ventilation. Acta Neurol. Scand., *52*:187, 1975.

Cole, M.: Pitfalls in cerebrospinal fluid examination. Hosp. Pract., *4*:47, 1969.

Collins, G.: Personal communication, 1978.

Controni, G., Rodriguez, W. J., Hicks, J. M., Ficke, M., Ross, S., Friedman, G., and Kahn, W.: Cerebrospinal fluid lactic acid levels in meningitis. J. Pediatr., *91*:379, 1977.

Converse, G. M., Gwaltney, J. M., Strassburg, D. A., and Hendley, J. O.: Alteration of cerebrospinal fluid findings by partial treatment of bacterial meningitis. J. Pediatr., *83*:220, 1973.

Denis, F., Samb, A., and Chiron, J. P.: Bacterial meningitis diagnosis by counterimmunoelectrophoresis. J.A.M.A., *238*:1248, 1977.

Derakhshan, I., and Kaufman, B.: Subdural effusion of cerebrospinal fluid after lumbar puncture. Arch. Neurol., *29*:127, 1973.

Dramov, B., and Dubou, R.: Aseptic meningitis following intrathecal radioiodinated serum albumin. Cal. Med., *115*:64, 1971.

Dryken, P. R.: Cerebrospinal fluid cytology: Practical clinical usefulness. Neurology, *25*:210, 1975.

Dunn, J. S., and Wyburn, E. M.: The anatomy of the blood brain barrier: A review. Scot. Med. J., *17*:21, 1972.

Epstein, E., Zak, B., Baginski, E. J., and Civin, H.: Interpretation of cerebrospinal fluid proteins by gel electrophoresis. Ann. Clin. Lab. Sci., *6*:27, 1976.

Escobar, M. R., Dalton, H. P., and Allison, M. J.: Fluorescent antibody tests using cerebrospinal fluid. Am. J. Clin. Path., *53*:886, 1970.

Feldman, W. E.: Cerebrospinal fluid lactic acid dehydrogenase activity. Am. J. Dis. Child., *129*:77, 1975.

Feldman, W. E.: Relation of concentrations of bacteria and bacterial antigen cerebrospinal fluid to prognosis in patients with bacterial meningitis. N. Engl. J. Med., *296*:433, 1977.

Felgenhauer, K.: Protein size and cerebrospinal fluid composition. Klin. Wochenschr. *52*:1158, 1974.

Fischer, G. W., Brens, R. W., Alden, E. R., and Beckwith, J. B.: Lumbar punctures and meningitis. Am. J. Dis. Child., *199*:590, 1975.

Fishman, R. A.: Cerebrospinal fluid. *In* Boher, A. B., and Baher, L. H. (eds.): Clinical Neurology. New York, Harper and Row, Publishers, Inc., 1971.

Glasser, L., Payne, C., and Corrigan, J. J.: The in vivo development of plasma cells: A morphologic study of human cerebrospinal fluid. Neurology, *27*:448, 1977.

Gondos, B., and King, E. B.: Cerebrospinal fluid cytology: Diagnostic accuracy and comparison of different techniques. Acta Cytol., *20*:542, 1976.

Gonyea, E. F.: Cisternal puncture and cryptococcal meningitis. Arch. Neurol., *28*:200, 1973.

Gooch, W. M., and Sotelo-Avila, C.: Meningitis in children: Laboratory diagnosis. J. Tenn. Med. Assn., *69*:563, 1976.

Greenblatt, S. H.: Cerebrospinal fluid creatine phosphokinase in acute subarachnoid hemorrhage. J. Neurosurg., *44*:50, 1976.

Guseo, A.: Classification of cells in the cerebrospinal fluid. Eur. Neurol., *15*:169, 1977.

Hagen, G. A., and Elliott, W. J.: Transport of thyroid hormones in serum and cerebrospinal fluid. J. Clin. Endocrinol. Metab., *37*:415, 1973.

Hammock, M. K., and Milhorat, T. H.: The cerebrospinal fluid: Current concepts of its formation. Ann. Clin. Lab. Sci., *6*:22, 1976.

Hansen, H. H., Bender, R. A., and Shelton, B. J.: The cytocentrifuge and cerebrospinal fluid cytology. Acta Cytol., *18*:259, 1974.

Harms, D.: Comparative quantitation of immunoglobulin G (IgG) in cerebrospinal fluid and serum of children. Eur. Neurol., *13*:54, 1975.

Hecht, R. H., Cohen, A. H., Stoner, J., and Irwin, C.: Primary amebic meningoencephalitis in California. Cal. Med., *117*:69, 1972.

Heintges, M. G., Savory, J., and Killingsworth, L. M.: A micro-immunochemical procedure for the measurement of total protein in cerebrospinal fluid. Ann. Clin. Lab. Sci., *3*:265, 1973.

Hinterbuchner, L. P.: Hazards of lumbar puncture in infants. J.A.M.A., *204*:196, 1968.

Hooshmand, H., Escobar, M. R., and Kopf, W. C.: Neurosyphilis. J.A.M.A., *219*:726, 1972.

Hourain, B. T., Hamlin, E. M., and Reynolds, T. B.: Cerebrospinal fluid glutamine as a measure of hepatic encephalopathy. Arch. Intern. Med., *127*:1033, 1971.

Hull, H. F., and Morrow, G.: Glucorrhea revisited. J.A.M.A., *234*:1052, 1975.

Hyslop, N. E., and Swartz, M. N.: Bacterial meningitis. Postgrad. Med., *58*:120, 1975.

Igou, P. C.: An evaluation of a gel filtration–spectrophotometric method for spinal fluid protein. Am. J. Med. Tech., *33*:354, 1967.

Ito, U., and Inaba, Y.: A simple sedimentation chamber adaptable to the laboratory centrifuge. Am. J. Clin. Path., *58*:590, 1972.

Iwashita, H., Bauer, H., and Kuroiwa, Y.: Comparative studies of cerebrospinal fluid proteins of multiple sclerosis patients in Japan and Germany. Neurology, *26*:37, 1976.

Jaffe, H. W.: The laboratory diagnosis of syphilis. Ann. Intern. Med., *83*:846, 1975.

Jameson, B., and Wells, D. G.: Cytologic diagnosis of cryptococcal meningitis. N. Engl. J. Med., *286*:1267, 1972.

Jequier, M., and Dufrensue, J. J.: Diagnosis of cryptococcal meningitis. N. Engl. J. Med., *286*:785, 1972.

John, J. F., and Cuetter, A. C.: Spinal syphilis: The problem of fluorescent treponemal antibody in the cerebrospinal fluid. South. Med. J., *70*:309, 1977.

Johnson, K. P., Arrigo, S. C., and Nelson, B. J.: Agarose electrophoresis of cerebrospinal fluid in multiple sclerosis. Neurology, *27*:273, 1977a.

Johnson, K. P., and Nelson, B. J.: Multiple sclerosis: Diagnostic usefulness of the cerebrospinal fluid. Ann. Neurol. *2*:425, 1977b.

Jordan, R. M., Kendall, J. W., Seaich, L. J., Allen, J. P., Paulsen, C. A., Kerber, C. W., and Vanderlaan, W. P.: Cerebrospinal fluid hormone concentration in the evaluation of pituitary tumors. Ann. Intern. Med., *85*:49, 1976.

Kalin, E. M., Tweed, W. A., Lee, J., and MacKeen, W. L.: Cerebrospinal-fluid acid-base and electrolyte changes resulting from cerebral anoxia in man. N. Engl. J. Med., *293*:1013, 1975.

Kaplan, A.: Electrophoresis of cerebrospinal fluid proteins. Am. J. Med. Sci., *253*:549, 1967.

Kaufman, L.: Serodiagnosis of fungal diseases. *In* Rose, N. R., and Friedman, H. (eds.): Manual of Clinical Immunology. Washington, D.C., American Society for Microbiology, 1976.

Kjellin, K. G., and Soderstrom, C. E.: Diagnostic significance of CSF spectrophotometry in cerebrovascular diseases. J. Neurol. Sci., *23*:359, 1974.

Kluge, H., Winkler, G., and Wieczorek, V.: Results of the comparison of different methods of total protein in CSF. Dtsch. Gesundh., *23*:2039, 1968.

Kolmel, H. W.: Atlas of Cerebrospinal Fluid Cells. New York, Springer-Verlag, 1977.

Krentz, M. J., and Dyken, P. R.: Cerebrospinal fluid cytomorphology: Sedimentation vs filtration. Arch. Neurol., *26*:253, 1972.

Kronholm, V., and Lintrup, J.: Spectrophotometric investigations of the cerebrospinal fluid in the near ultraviolet region. Acta Psychiatr. Neurol. Scand., *35*:314, 1960.

Levy, N. L., Auerbach, P. S., and Hayes, E. C.: A blood test for multiple sclerosis based on the adherence of lymphocytes to measles-infected cells. N. Engl. J. Med., *294*:1423, 1976.

Link, H.: Demonstration of oligoclonal immunoglobulin G in Guillain-Barré syndrome. Acta Neurol. Scand., *52*:111, 1975.

Link, H., and Miller, R.: Immunoglobulins in multiple sclerosis and infections of the nervous system. Arch. Neurol., *25*:326, 1971.

Marshall, J.: Lumbar puncture. Br. J. Hosp. Med., *3*:216, 1970.

McCracken, G. H.: Rapid identification of specific etiology in meningitis. J. Pediatr., *88*:706, 1976a.

McCracken, G. H.: Neonatal septicemia and meningitis. Hosp. Pract., *11*:89, 1976b.

McCracken, G. H., and Kaplan, J. M.: Penicillin treatment for congenital syphilis. J.A.M.A., *228*:855, 1974.

Mealey, J.: Fat emulsion as a cause of cloudy cerebrospinal fluid. J.A.M.A., *180*:246, 1962.

Meites, S. (ed.): Pediatric Clinical Chemistry. Washington, D.C., American Association for Clinical Chemistry, 1977.

Messer, H. D., Forshan, V. R., Brust, J. C. M., and Hughes, J. E. O.: Transient paraplegia from hematoma after lumbar puncture. J.A.M.A., *235*:529, 1976.

Morrison, J. C., Whybrew, D. W., Wiser, W. L., Bucovaz, E. T., and Fish, S. A.: Enzyme levels in the serum and cerebrospinal fluid in eclampsia. Am. J. Obstet. Gynecol., *110*:619, 1971.

Mullan, D. P.: Studies in Clinical Enzymology. St. Louis, C. V. Mosby Co., 1969.

Musher, D. M., and Schell, R. F.: False-positive Gram stains of cerebrospinal fluid. Ann. Intern. Med., *79*:603, 1973.

Nelson, P. U., Carey, W. F., and Pollard, A. C.: Diagnostic significance and source of lactate dehydrogenase and its isozymes in cerebrospinal fluid of children with a variety of neurological disorders. J. Clin. Path., *28*:828, 1975.

Nosanchuk, J. S., and Kim, C. W.: Lupus erythematosus cells in CSF. J.A.M.A., *25*:2883, 1976.

Oehmichen, M.: Characterization of mononuclear phagocytes in human CSF using membrane markers. Acta Cytol., *20*:548, 1976.

Olsson, J. E., and Link, H.: Immunoglobulin abnormalities in multiple sclerosis. Arch. Neurol., *28*:392, 1973.

Olsson, J. E., and Pettersson, B.: A comparison between agar gel electrophoresis and CSF serum quotients of IgG and albumin in neurological diseases. Acta Neurol. Scand., *53*:308, 1976.

Palmer, D. L., Minard, B. J., and Cawley, L. P.: IgG sub-groups in cerebrospinal fluid in multiple sclerosis. N. Engl. J. Med., *294*:447, 1976.

Patten, B. M.: How much blood makes the cerebrospinal fluid bloody? J.A.M.A., *206*:378, 1968.

Pennock, C. A., Passant, L. P., and Balton, F. G.: Estimation of cerebrospinal fluid protein. J. Clin. Path., *21*:518, 1968.

Plum, F., and Siesjo, B. K.: Recent advances in CSF physiology. Anesthesiology, *42*:708, 1975.

Pryce, J. D., Gant, P. W., and Saul, K. J.: Normal concentrations of lactate, glucose, and protein in cerebrospinal fluid, and the diagnostic implications of abnormal concentrations. Clin. Chem., *16*:562, 1970.

Rodriguez, E. M.: The cerebrospinal fluid as a pathway in neuroendocrine integration. J. Endocrinol., *71*:407, 1976.

Saigo, P., Rosen, P. P., Kaplan, N. H., Solan, G., and Melamed, M. R.: Identification of *Cryptococcus neoformans* in cytologic preparations of cerebrospinal fluid. Am. J. Clin. Path., *67*:141, 1977.

Sarff, L. D., Platt, L. H., and McCracken, G. H.: Cerebrospinal fluid evaluation in neonates: Comparison of high-risk infants with and without meningitis. J. Pediatr., *88*:473, 1976.

Schaub, C., Bluet-Pajut, M. T., Szikla, G., Lornet, C., and Talairach, J.: Distribution of growth hormone and thyroid-stimulating hormone in cerebrospinal fluid and pathological compartments of the central nervous system. J. Neurol. Sci., *31*:123, 1977.

Schlesinger, J. J., and Ross, A. L.: *Propionibacterium acnes* meningitis in a previously normal adult. Arch. Intern. Med., *137*:921, 1977.

Schriever, H., and Gambino, S. R.: Protein turbidity produced by trichloracetic acid and sulfosalicylic acid at varying temperatures and varying ratios of albumin and globulin. Am. J. Clin. Path., *44*:667, 1965.

Shaywitz, B. A.: Epidermoid spinal cord tumors and previous lumbar punctures. J. Pediatr., *80*:638, 1972.

Sheth, K. V.: Cerebrospinal and body fluids cell morphology. ASCP Workshop Manual. Chicago, American Society of Clinical Pathologists, 1977.

Siesjo, B. K.: The regulation of cerebrospinal fluid pH. Kidney Internat., *1*:360, 1972.

Skeel, R. T., Yankee, R. A., and Henderson, E. S.: Meningeal leukemia. J.A.M.A., *205*:155, 1968.

Sornas, R.: The cytology of the normal cerebrospinal fluid. Acta Neurol. Scand., *48*:313, 1972.

Sornas, R.: A new method for the cytological examination of cerebrospinal fluid. J. Neurol. Neurosurg. Psychiatr., *30*:568, 1967.

Sornas, R.: Transformation of mononuclear cells in cerebrospinal fluid. Acta Cytol., *15*:545, 1971.

Swartz, M. N., and Dodge, P. R.: Bacterial meningitis—a review of selected aspects. N. Engl. J. Med., *272*:725, 1965.

Thompson, E. J.: Laboratory diagnosis of multiple sclerosis: Immunological and biochemical aspects. Br. Med. Bull., *33*:28, 1977.

Tibbling, G., Link, H., and Ohman, S.: Principles of albumin and IgG analyses in neurological disorders. Scand. J. Clin. Lab. Invest., *37*:385, 1977.

Tourtellotte, W. W., Haerer, A. F., Fleming, J. O., Murthy, K. N., Levy, J., and Brandes, D. W.: Cerebrospinal fluid (CSF) immunoglobulins-G (IgG) of extravascular origin in normals and patients with multiple sclerosis (MS): Clinical correlation. Trans. Am. Neurol. Assoc., *100*:250, 1975.

Van Der Meulen, J. P.: Cerebrospinal fluid xanthochromia: An objective index. Neurology, *16*:170, 1966.

Van Welsum, R. A., and Van der Helm, H. J.: The protein composition of the cerebrospinal fluid in acute necrotizing encephalitis. Neurology, *20*:996, 1970.

Vandvik, B., Natvig, J. B., and Wiger, D.: IgG 1 subclass restriction of oligoclonal IgG from cerebrospinal fluids and brain extracts in patients with multiple sclerosis and subacute encephalitis. Scand. J. Immunol., *5*:427, 1976.

Walton, J. N.: Subarachnoid Haemorrhage. Edinburgh, Livingstone, 1956.

Weinstein, R. A., Bauer, F. W., Hoffman, R. D., Tyler, P. G., Anderson, R. L., and Stamm, W. E.: Factitious meningitis. J.A.M.A., *233*:878, 1975.

Werner, M.: A combined procedure for protein estimation and electrophoresis of cerebrospinal fluid. J. Lab. Clin. Med., *74*:166, 1969.

Wichser, J., and Kazemi, H.: CSF bicarbonate regulation in respiratory acidosis and alkalosis. J. Appl. Physiol. *38*:504, 1975.

Windisch, R. M., and Bracken, M. M.: Cerebrospinal fluid proteins: Concentration by membrane ultrafiltration and fractionation by electrophoresis on cellulose acetate. Clin. Chem., *16*:416, 1970.

Wolf, S. M.: Decreased cerebrospinal fluid glucose in herpes zoster meningitis. Arch. Neurol., *30*:109, 1974.

Woodruff, K. H.: Cerebrospinal fluid cytomorphology using cytocentrifugation. Am. J. Clin. Path., *60*:621, 1973.

Synovial Fluid

Abeles, M., and Urman, J. D.: Acute gouty arthritis: The importance of aspirating more than one involved joint. J.A.M.A., *238*:2526, 1977.

Bartlett, R. C., et al.: *In* Inhorn, S. L. (ed.): Quality Assurance Practices for Health Laboratories. Washington, D.C., American Public Health Association, 1978.

Bayer, A. S., Chow, A. W., Louie, J. S., and Guze, L. B.: Sternoarticular pyoarthrosis due to gram-negative bacilli. Arch. Intern. Med., *137*:1036, 1977.

Blau, S. P.: Leukocyte counts in synovial fluid. Ann. Intern. Med., *74*:638, 1971.

Brandt, K. D., Cathcart, E. S., and Cohen, A. S.: Gonococcal arthritis. Arth. Rheum., *17*:503, 1974.

Broderick, P. A., Corvese, N., Pierik, M. G., Pike, R. F., and Mariorenzi, A. L.: Exfoliative cytology interpretation of synovial fluid in joint disease. J. Bone Joint Surg., *58A*:396, 1976.

Bunch, T. W., Hunder, G. G., McDuffie, F. C., O'Brien, P. C., and Markowitz, H.: Synovial fluid complement determinations as a diagnostic aid in inflammatory joint disease. Mayo Clin. Proc., *49*:715, 1974.

Bunch, T. W., Hunder, G. G., Offord, K., and McDuffie, F. C.: Synovial fluid complement: Usefulness in diagnosis and classification of rheumatoid arthritis. Ann. Intern. Med., *81*:32, 1974.

Cohen, A. S., Brandt, K. D., and Krey, P. R.: Synovial fluid. In Cohen, A. S. (ed.): Laboratory Diagnostic Procedures in the Rheumatic Diseases. Boston, Little, Brown & Co., 1975.

Cooke, C. L., Owen, D. S., Irby, R., and Toone, E.: Gonococcal arthritis. J.A.M.A., *217*:204, 1971.

Cracchiolo, A.: Joint fluid analysis. Am. Fam. Physician, *4*:87, 1971.

Cracchiolo, A., and Barnett, E. V.: The role of immunological tests in routine synovial fluid analysis. J. Bone Joint Surg., *54*:828, 1972.

Currey, H. L. F., and Vernon-Roberts, B.: Examination of synovial fluid. Clin. Rheum. Dis., *2*:149, 1976.

Donaldson, L. E. E.: Technique for performing white cell counts in joint fluids. Med. Lab. Technol., *29*:1, 1972.

Edelen, J. S., Lockshin, M. D., and LeRoy, E. L.: Gonococcal arthritis in two patients with active lupus erythematosus. Arth. Rheum., *14*:557, 1971.

Fagan, T. J., and Lidsky, M. D.: Compensated polarized light microscopy using cellophane adhesive tape. Arth. Rheum., *17*:256, 1974.

Falchuk, K. H., Goetzl, E. J., and Kulka, J. P.: Respiratory gases of synovial fluids. Am. J. Med., *49*:223, 1970.

Frischknecht, J., and Steigerwald, J. C.: High synovial fluid white blood cell counts in pseudogout. Arch. Intern. Med., *135*:298, 1975.

Goldenberg, D. L., Brandt, K. D., and Cohen, A. S.: Rapid, simple detection of trace amounts of synovial fluid. Arth. Rheum., *16*:487, 1973.

Harris, E. D.: Biology of the joint. *In* Kelley, W. N., Harris, E. D., Ruddy, S., and Sledge, C. B. (eds.): Textbook of Rheumatology. Philadelphia, W. B. Saunders Co., 1981, p. 255.

Haselwood, D. M., and Castles, J. J.: The biology of the rheumatoid synovial cell. Western J. Med., *127*:204, 1977.

Hasselbacher, P.: Measuring synovial fluid viscosity with a white blood cell diluting pipette. Arth. Rheum., *19*:1358, 1976.

Hollander, J. L., McCarty, D. J., Astorga, G., and Castro-Murillo, E.: Studies on the pathogenesis of rheumatoid joint inflammation. Ann. Intern. Med., *62*:271, 1965.

Hollander, J. L., Reginato, A., and Torralba, T. P.: Examination of synovial fluid as a diagnostic aid in arthritis. Med. Clin. North Am., *50*:1281, 1966.

Hunder, G. G., and Pierre, R. U.: In vivo LE cell formation in synovial fluid. Arth. Rheum., *13*:448, 1970.

Huskisson, E. C., Hart, F. D., and Lacy, B. W.: Synovial fluid Waaler-Rose and latex tests. Ann. Rheum. Dis., *30*:67, 1971.

Jackson, W. P. U., and Harris, F.: Gout with hyperparathyroidism. Br. Med. J., *2*:211, 1965.

Jessar, R. A.: The study of synovial fluid. *In* Hollander, J. L., and McCarty, D. J. (eds.): Arthritis and Allied Conditions. Philadelphia, Lea and Febiger, 1972.

Kahn, C. B., Hollander, J. L., and Schumacher, H. R.: Corticosteroid crystals in synovial fluid. J.A.M.A., *211*:807, 1970.

Kitridou, R., McCarty, D. J., Prockop, D. J., and Hummeler, K.: Identification of collagen in synovial fluid. Arth. Rheum., *12*:580, 1969.

Kjeldsberg, C. R., and Knight, J. A.: Body Fluids: Laboratory Examination of Cerebrospinal, Synovial, and Serous Fluids. A Textbook Atlas. Chicago, American Society of Clinical Pathologists, 1982.

Krauss, D. S., Aronson, M. D., Gump, D. W., and Newcombe, D. S.: *Hemophilus influenzae* septic arthritis. Arth. Rheum., *17*:261, 1974.

McCarty, D. J.: Selected aspects of synovial membrane physiology. Arth. Rheum., *17*:289, 1974.

McCarty, D. J., Gatter, R. A., Brill, J. M., and Hogan, J. M.: Crystal deposition diseases. J.A.M.A., *193*:123, 1965.

McCarty, D. J., and Hollander, J. L.: Identification of urate crystals in gouty synovial fluid. Ann. Intern. Med., *54*:452, 1961.

McConville, J. H., Pototsky, R. S., Calia, F. M., and Pachas, W. N.: Septic and crystalline joint disease. J.A.M.A., *231*:841, 1975.

McCord, W. C., Nies, K. M., and Louie, J. S.: Acute venereal arthritis. Arch. Intern. Med., *137*:858, 1977.

Meyers, O. L., and Watermeyer, G. S.: Cholesterol-rich synovial effusions. South Afr. Med. J., *50*:973, 1976.

Naib, Z. M.: Cytology of synovial fluids. Acta Cytol., *17*:299, 1973.

Nye, W. H. R., Terry, R., and Rosenbaum, D. L.: Two forms of crystalline lipid in "cholesterol" effusions. Am. J. Clin. Path., *49*:718, 1968.

Owen, D. S., Cooke, C. L., and Toone, E.: Practical synovial fluid examination. Va. Med. Mon., *97*:88, 1970.

Pekin, T. J., Malinin, T. I., and Zvaifler, N. J.: Unusual synovial fluid findings in Reiter's syndrome. Ann. Intern. Med., *66*:677, 1967.

Phelps, P., Steele, A. D., and McCarty, D. J.: Compensated polarized light microscopy. J.A.M.A., *203*:166, 1968.

Ropes, M. W., and Bauer, W.: Synovial Fluid Changes in Joint Disease. Cambridge, Harvard University Press, 1953.

Ruddy, S., and Austen, K. F.: Complement and its components. *In* Cohen, A. S. (ed.): Laboratory Diagnostic Procedures in the Rheumatic Diseases. Boston, Little, Brown & Co., 1975.

Ryan, W. E., Ellefson, R. D., and Ward, L. E.: Lipid synovial effusion. Arth. Rheum., *16*:759, 1973.

Schumacher, H. R., Jimenez, S. A., Gibson, T., Pascual, E., Tragcoff, R., Dorwart, B. B., and Reginato, A. J.: Acute gouty arthritis without urate crystals identified on initial examination of synovial fluid. Arth. Rheum., *18*:608, 1975.

Schumacher, H. R., Smolyo, A. P., Tse, R. L., and Maurer, K.: Arthritis associated with apatite crystals. Ann. Intern. Med., *87*:411, 1977.

Scott, J. T.: The analysis of joint fluids. Br. J. Hosp. Med., *14*:653, 1975.

Skinner, M., and Cohen, A. S.: Calcium pyrophosphate dihydrate crystal deposition disease. Arch. Intern. Med., *123*:636, 1969.

Smith, J. R., and Phelps, P.: Septic arthritis, gout, pseudo-gout and osteoarthritis in the knee of a patient with multiple myeloma. Arth. Rheum., *15*:89, 1972.

Traycoff, R. B., Pascual, E., and Schumacher, H. R.: Mononuclear cells in human synovial fluid: Identification of lymphoblasts in rheumatoid arthritis. Arth. Rheum., *19*:743, 1976.

Van Leeuwen, A. W. F. M., Meyer, C. J. L. M., Van de Putte, L. B. A., de Vries, E., and de Man, J. C. H.: Sézary type cells in rheumatoid synovial fluid. Lancet, *1*:248, 1976.

Wallace, R., and Cohen, A. S.: Tuberculous arthritis. Am. J. Med., *61*:277, 1976.

Waxman, J.: Immunology in rheumatology—1975. J. Louisiana State Med. Soc., *127*:203, 1975.

Wild, J. H., and Zvaifler, N. J.: An office technique for identifying crystals in synovial fluid. Am. Fam. Physician, *12*:72, 1975.

3

Pleural, Pericardial, and Peritoneal Fluid

Adams, H. W., and Mainz, D. L.: Eosinophilic ascites. Am. J. Digest. Dis., *22*:40, 1977.

Askin, F. B., McCann, B. G., and Kuhn, C.: Reactive eosinophilic pleuritis. Arch. Path. Lab. Med., *101*:187, 1977.

Ball, W. C., Jr.: Pleural effusion. *In* Harvey, A. M., Johns, R. J., Owens, A. H., and Ross, R. S. (eds.): The Principles and Practice of Medicine. 18th ed. New York, Appleton-Century-Crofts, 1976, p. 455.

Berger, H. W., Rammohan, G., Neff, M. S., and Buhain, W. J.: Uremic pleural effusion Ann. Intern. Med., *82*:362, 1975.

Boddington, M. M., Spriggs, A. I., Morton, J. A., and Mowat, A. G.: Cytodiagnosis of rheumatoid pleural effusions. J. Clin. Path., *24*:95, 1971.

Brown, J. D., and An, N. D.: Tuberculous peritonitis. Am. J. Gastroenterol., *66*:277, 1976.

Carr, D. T., Lillington, G. A., and Mayne, J. G.: Pleural fluid glucose in systemic lupus erythematosus. Mayo Clin. Proc., *45*:409, 1970.

Conn, H. O.: Spontaneous bacterial peritonitis. Gastroenterology, *70*:455, 1976.

Delany, H. M., Moss, C. M., and Carnevale, N.: The use of enzyme analysis of peritoneal blood in the clinical assessment of abdominal organ injury. Surg. Gynecol. Obstet., *142*:161, 1976.

Diamonon, J. S., and Barnes, J. P.: Choleperitoneum. Am. Surg., *30*:331, 1964.

Dye, R. A., and Laforet, E. G.: Esophageal rupture: Diagnosis by pleural fluid pH. Chest, *66*:454, 1974.

Engrav, L. H., Benjamin, C. I., Strate, R. G., and Perry, J. F.: Diagnostic peritoneal larvage in blunt abdominal trauma. J. Trauma, *15*:854, 1975.

Figueroa, J. M.: Presence of microfilariae of *Mansonella ozzardi* in ascitic fluid. Acta Cytol., *17*:73, 1973.

Hellstrom, P. E., Friman, C., and Teppo, L.: Malignant mesothelioma of 17 years' duration with high pleural fluid concentration of hyaluronate. Scand. J. Resp. Dis., *58*:97, 1977.

Howard, J. M., and Singh, L. M.: Peritoneal fluid pH after perforation of peptic ulcers. Arch. Surg., *87*:483, 1963.

Hudspeth, A. S., and Miller, H. S.: Isolated (primary) chylopericardium. J. Thorac. Cardiovasc. Surg., *51*:528, 1966.

Jacobson, E. S.: A case of secondary echinococcosis diagnosed by cytologic examination of pleural fluid and needle biopsy of pleura. Acta Cytol., *17*:76, 1973.

Jergens, M. E.: Peritoneal lavage. Am. J. Surg., *133*:365, 1977.

Jones, S. R.: The absolute granulocyte count in ascitic fluid. West. J. Med., *126*:344, 1977.

Kilpatrick, Z. M., and Chapman, C. B.: On pericardiocentesis. Am. J. Cardiol., *16*:722, 1965.

Klepser, R. G., and Berry, J. F.: The diagnosis and surgical management of chylothorax with the aid of lipophilic dyes. Dis. Chest, *25*:409, 1954.

Kline, M. M., McCallum, R. W., and Guth, P. H.: The clinical value of ascitic fluid culture and leukocyte count studies in alcoholic cirrhosis. Gastroenterology, *70*:408, 1976.

Klockars, M., Pettersson, T., Riska, H., and Hellstrom, P. E.: Pleural fluid lysozyme in tuberculous and non-tuberculous pleurisy. Br. Med. J. *1*:1381, 1976.

Kumar, U. N., Varkey, B., and Mathai, G.: Post traumatic pleural fluid and blood eosinophilia. J.A.M.A., *234*:625, 1975.

Lee, Y. N.: Alkaline phosphatase in intestinal perforation. J.A.M.A., *208*:361, 1969.

Lesser, G. T., Bruno, M. S., and Enselberg, K.: Chylous ascites. Arch. Intern. Med., *125*:1073, 1970.

Levine, H., Metzger, W., Lacer, D., and Ludmillo, K.: Diagnosis of tuberculous pleurisy by culture of pleural biopsy specimen. Arch. Intern. Med., *126*:269, 1970.

Light, R. W., MacGregor, M. I., Luchsinger, P. C., and Ball, W. C.: Pleural effusions: The diagnostic separation of transudates and exudates. Ann. Intern. Med., *77*:507, 1972.

Light, R. W., and Ball, W. C.: Glucose and amylase in pleural effusions. J.A.M.A., *225*:257, 1973.

Light, R. W., Erozan, Y. S., and Ball, W. C.: Cells in pleural fluid: Their value in differential diagnosis. Arch. Intern. Med., *132*:854, 1973.

Light, R. W., MacGregor, M. I., Ball, W. C., and Luchsinger, P. C.: Diagnostic significance of pleural fluid pH and PCO_2. Chest, *64*:591, 1973.

Mansberger, A. R.: The diagnostic value of abdominal paracentesis with special reference to peritoneal fluid ammonia levels. Am. J. Gastorenterol., *42*:150, 1964.

McClement, J. H.: Diseases of the pleura. *In* Beeson, P. B., and McDermott, W. (eds.): Textbook of Medicine. 14th ed., Philadelphia, W. B. Saunders Company, 1975.

McCoy, J., and Wolma, F. J.: Abdominal tap. Am. J. Surg., *122*:693, 1971.

Metzger, A. L., Coyne, M., and Lee, S.: In vivo LE cell formation in peritonitis due to SLE. J. Rheumatol., *1*:130, 1974.

Olsen, W. R., Redman, H. C., and Hildreth, D. H.: Quantitative peritoneal lavage in blunt abdominal trauma. Arch. Surg., *104*:536, 1972.

Osamura, R. Y., Shioya, S., Handa, K., and Shimiza, K.: Lupus erythematosus cells in pleural fluid: Cytologic diagnosis in two patients. Acta Cytol., *21*:215, 1977.

Parvin, S., Smith, D. E., Asher, W. M., and Virgilo, R. W.: Effectiveness of peritoneal lavage in blunt abdominal trauma. Ann. Surg., *181*:255, 1975.

Perry, J. F., and Strate, R. G.: Diagnostic peritoneal lavage. Surgery, *71*:898, 1972.

Potts, D. E.: Pleural fluid pH in parapneumonic effusions. Chest, *70*:328, 1976.

Rush, B. F., Host, W. R., Fewel, J., and Hsieh, J.: Intestinal ischemia and some organic substances in serum and abdominal fluid. Arch. Surg., *105*:151, 1972.

Sabiston, D. C., Jr.: Diseases of the pleura, mediastinum, and diaphragm. *In* Wintrobe, M. M., Thorn, G. W., Adams, R. D., Braunwald, E., Isselbacher, K. J., and Petersdorf, R. J.: Harrison's Principles of Internal Medicine. 7th ed. New York, McGraw-Hill Book Company, 1974, p. 1327.

Seaman, A. J., and Christerson, J. W.: Demonstration of LE cells in pericardial fluid. J.A.M.A., *149*:145, 1952.

Seriff, N. S., Cohen, M. L., Samuel, P., and Schulster, P. L.: Chylothorax: Diagnosis by lipoprotein electrophoresis of serum and pleural fluid. Thorax, *32*:98, 1977.

Soloff, L. A.: Pericardial cellular response during the post-myocardial infarction syndrome. Am. Heart J., *82*:812, 1971.

Spriggs, A. I., and Boddington, M. M.: The Cytology of Effusions. London, Heinemann, 1968.

Storey, D. D., Dines, D. E., and Coles, D. T.: Pleural effusion: A diagnostic dilemma. J.A.M.A., *236*:2183, 1976.

van Heerden, J. A., and Laufenberg, H. J.: Simplified thoracentesis. Mayo Clin. Proc., *43*:311, 1968.

Venes, J. L.: Pleural fluid effusion and eosinophilia following ventriculopleural shunting. Den. Med. Child. Neurol., *16*:72, 1974.

Warshaw, A. L.: Diagnosis of starch peritonitis by paracentesis. Lancet, *2*:1054, 1972.

Wilson, T., and Lumb, P.: Improved method for aspiration of the pleural cavity. Br. Med. J., *2*:70, 1975.

Winckler, C. F., and Yam, L. T.: Cytologic changes of pleural fluid in pulmonary embolism. Arch. Intern. Med., *136*:1195, 1976.

Yam, L. T.: Diagnostic significance of lymphocytes in pleural effusions. Ann. Intern. Med., *66*:972, 1967.

20

PREGNANCY TESTS AND EVALUATION OF PLACENTAL FUNCTION

ARTHUR F. KRIEG, M.D., and ROBERT E. WENK, M.D.

3

The term "pregnancy test" is actually a misnomer. First, most "pregnancy tests" do not actually determine pregnancy, but human chorionic gonadotropin (hCG) produced by trophoblastic tissue. Second, measurement of hCG is used to diagnose conditions other than pregnancy. Clinical applications of "pregnancy tests" include confirmation of a clinical diagnosis of pregnancy early in the first trimester; identification of pregnant patients before ordering medications or radiographic examinations; diagnosis of ectopic pregnancy in patients with lower abdominal pain; evaluation of threatened abortion during the first trimester; guidance of diagnosis and treatment of trophoblastic tumors; and evaluation of selected non-trophoblastic tumors.

HUMAN CHORIONIC GONADOTROPIN

Human chorionic gonadotropin (hCG) is a glycoprotein consisting of an alpha polypeptide subunit (molecular weight 18,000) and a beta polypeptide subunit (molecular weight 32,000). Alpha subunits for the four human glycoprotein hormones (LH, FSH, TSH, hCG) are nearly identical (Ross, 1977). Beta subunits for these four hormones differ significantly. However, there are similarities between the beta subunits for LH and hCG: about 80 per cent of the first 115 amino terminal residues are identical (Ross, 1977). It is the beta chains that provide the distinctive characteristics of hCG, LH, FSH, and TSH. Under appropriate conditions, beta subunits from hCG can be reassociated with alpha chains from other glycoprotein hormones to reconstitute physiologically active hCG (Ross, 1977). However, the isolated alpha or beta subunits are by themselves physiologically inactive.

As "glycoproteins," the alpha and beta subunits are linked to carbohydrate side chains. These carbohydrate side chains include sialic acid, fucose, galactose, mannose, glucosamine, and galactosamine in varying combinations (Ross, 1977). Progressive removal of sialic acid causes decreased *in vivo* hCG activity, while *in vitro* hCG activity is not affected (Ross, 1977). This discrepancy between *in vivo* and *in vitro* activity is related to the decreased plasma half-life of hCG that accompanies progressive desialylation. The decrease in plasma half-life parallels decreased *in vivo* activity (Ross, 1977).

Since hCG is produced by trophoblastic tissue, it is first detected shortly after implantation (Catt, 1975). Four general methods are available to measure hCG activity: bioassay, agglutination immunoassay (hemagglutination inhibition, latex particle agglutination inhibition, direct agglutination of latex particles), radioimmunoassay, and radioreceptor assay.

Bioassay

The first clinically useful bioassay was introduced by *Aschheim and Zondek* (1928) based on corpus luteum formation induced by hCG in prepubertal female mice. The *Friedman test* (1931) was based on ovulation in mature female rabbits. The *Xenopus laevis* test (Bellerby, 1934) was based on ova release from the South African clawed toad. The *rat ovarian hyperemia* test (Frank, 1941) was based on ovarian hyperemia in prepubertal female rats. The *Rana pipiens frog test* (Wiltberger, 1948) and the *Galli-Mainini toad test* (1948) were based on sperm release using male frogs and toads, respectively. The International Unit is based on bioassays (Storring, 1980).

Limitations of bioassays include interference from LH, high cost (Aschheim-Zondek test), technical difficulty (Friedman and ovarian hyperemia tests), and need for frequent restandardization (frog and toad tests). Although bioassays continue to be performed by some research laboratories, most "pregnancy tests" are now performed by immunoassay, radioimmunoassay, or radioreceptor assay.

Immunoassay

Immunoassays for hCG became available during the early 1960's (Wide, 1960, 1962) and have now largely replaced bioassays. Concentration of hCG may be expressed as:

IU/ml urine or serum
ng/ml urine or serum

The relationship between IU/ml and ng/ml is expressed as:

1 IU/ml = 83.3 ng/ml
1 mIU/ml = 0.08 ng/ml
1 ng/ml = 12 mIU/ml

The International Unit (IU) is related to gonadotropic activity of a powdered urinary gonadotropin standard maintained at the World Health Organization in London, England. Secondary standards are maintained by the National Institutes of Health in the United States.

Three basic types of immunoassay are available: hemagglutination inhibition, latex particle agglutination inhibition, and direct latex particle agglutination.

Hemagglutination inhibition (HAI) is based on the observation that non-agglutinated erythrocytes in low concentration settle in a test tube with a hemispheric bottom to form a sharply demarcated ring or "doughnut," while agglutinated erythrocytes form a uniform film. Progressively increasing agglutination causes the ring gradually to increase in size and decrease in clarity, until it "fades away" into a uniform film (Salk, 1944).

In the HAI procedure, anti-hCG serum and erythrocytes (RBC) coated with hCG are incubated with patient urine. If hCG is present, it will neutralize the antiserum, while if hCG is absent, the antiserum is unaffected. Unaffected antiserum will agglutinate the RBC, so that a diffuse mat of cells forms. However, if the antiserum is neutralized by urine containing hCG, the RBC will form a "doughnut" pattern or ring (Fig. 20–1).

By definition, HAI procedures are "tube tests." Between one and two hours is required for agglutination and settling to occur.

Latex particle agglutination inhibition (LAI) is similar in principle to HAI: anti-hCG serum is briefly mixed with patient urine and latex particles coated with hCG are added. If hCG is present, it will neutralize

1. Anti HCG + urine ➛ incubate
2. Add erythrocytes coated with HCG
3. If urine contains HCG → Positive Test (pregnant) → No hemagglutination; If urine contains no HCG → Negative Test (not pregnant) → Hemagglutination

Figure 20–1. Immunoassay for hCG by hemagglutination inhibition.

the antiserum, while if hCG is absent, the antiserum is unaffected. Unaffected antiserum will cause visible agglutination of the latex particles. However, if the antiserum is neutralized, no visible agglutination occurs (Fig. 20–2).

Most LAI procedures are slide tests that require only a few minutes to perform. One tube test (Placentex) is commercially available; this is more sensitive than the slide tests but requires between one and two hours.

Direct latex particle agglutination utilizes anti-hCG, which is directly adsorbed on the latex particles. If hCG is present, agglutination occurs. In contrast to the LAI procedures, agglutination indicates presence of hCG, while lack of agglutination represents a "negative" result. One direct latex particle agglutination slide test is commercially available.

Radioimmunoassay

Radioimmunoassays (RIA) for hCG are classified by the type of antiserum. The "beta subunit assays" utilize antisera against the beta subunit of hCG and are quite specific. At sensitivities of 5 mIU/ml hCG (0.4 ng/ml), the beta subunit assay described by Vaitukaitis (1972) is unaffected by elevated LH levels during midcycle or menopause. Present antisera for the beta subunit assay have only 1 to 2 per cent cross-reactivity against LH (Ross, 1977).

The "whole molecule" RIA for hCG (antibodies against both alpha and beta subunits) is less specific, showing considerable cross-reaction with both LH and FSH.

Although early methods for the beta subunit RIA required 24 hours' incubation, newer procedures require only one to five hours (Rasor, 1977) (Table 20–1). A serum specimen is usually required.

1. Anti HCG + urine ➛ incubate
2. Add latex particles coated with HCG
3. If urine contains HCG → Positive Test (pregnant) → No latex agglutination; If urine contains no HCG → Negative Test (not pregnant) → Latex agglutination

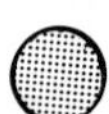

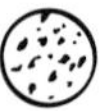

Figure 20–2. Immunoassay for hCG by latex particle agglutination inhibition.

Table 20–1. "PREGNANCY TESTS" BASED ON hCG ASSAY

Product	Incubation Time	Sensitivity IU/ml*	Comments
Hemagglutination inhibition (HAI) (tube tests)			
Pregnosticon (Organon)	1–2 hrs	0.6	Also available in lyophilized form as Pregnosticon Accuspheres
UCG (Wampole)	2 hrs	0.5	Also available in lyophilized form as UCG lyphotest
Latex particle agglutination inhibitor (LAI) (tube test)			
Gravindex (Ortho)	2 hrs	0.5	
Placentex (Roche)	1–2 hrs	1.0	Requires incubation at 37°C.
Latex particle agglutination inhibition (LAI) (slide tests)			
Pregnosticon (Organon)	2 min	1.0–2.0	Also available in lyophilized form as Pregnosticon Dri Dot
UCG (Wampole)	2 min	2.0	
Gravindex (Ortho)	2 min	3.5	
Pregnosis (Roche)	2 min	1.5–2.5	
Direct latex agglutination (slide test)			
DAP test (Wampole)	1 min	2.0	May be used with serum as well as urine
Radioreceptor assay (RRA)			
Biocept-G (Wampole)	1 hr	0.2	
Radioimmunoassay (RIA)			
Beta-hCG (quantitative) (Monitor Science)	5 hrs	0.0005	Continued improvements may provide shorter incubation times for RIA procedures
Beta-hCG (qualitative) (Monitor Science)	1 hr	0.040	
Beta-hCG (Radioassay Systems)	24 hrs	0.006	
Beta-hCG (Serono)	18 hrs	0.005	
Beta-hCG (Serono)	3 hrs	0.009	

*Estimates based on specifications published by manufacturers. Reports in literature suggest that under "routine" conditions tube tests may have sensitivity in the range of 1.0 to 2.0 IU/ml, while the most sensitive slide tests may have sensitivity in the range of 2.0 to 4.0 IU/ml.

Radioreceptor Assay

Radioreceptor assays (RRA) for hCG utilize receptors from the ovaries of pregnant cows (Saxena, 1974). Compared with the beta subunit radioimmunoassay, RRA is more rapid (requires only one hour's incubation) but less specific (shows cross-reaction with LH). Although sensitivity of RRA is about 5 to 10 mIU/ml (Landesman, 1976), "false positives" may occur owing to cross-reactions with LH. Elevated LH may be associated with midcycle peaks or premenopausal status. Ordinarily, a serum specimen is used. Two approaches are available to detect or eliminate such "false positives": repeated RRA on consecutive days to confirm "positive" results (early pregnancy is associated with rapidly increasing hCG, in contrast to midcycle LH peaks or premenopausal status), and use of a "cut off value" sufficiently high to avoid LH interference. The second approach is applied to commercial RRA kits, which are set at "cut off values" of 200 mIU/ml (Wampole Laboratories, Cranbury, N.J.). Although such kits can be used for quantitative hCG measurements with a sensitivity of 30 mIU/ml (Boyko, 1977), this increased sensitivity causes decreased specificity owing to cross-reactions with LH.

Enzyme Immunoassay

A most promising assay is a double-monoclonal antibody (Ab), solid-state ELISA procedure using urine. First Ab is coated onto a tube and affixes hCG by combining with alpha subunit. Washing removes everything but hCG, TSH, LH, and FSH. Second Ab is linked to alkaline phosphatase and affixes to beta subunit of hCG. Blue color is developed with the enzyme's substrate. The test is sensitive to 50 mIU/ml, and the endpoint requires 60 minutes or less. No instrumentation or isotope is required, and it is as specific as RIA and non-invasive. (RIA uses serum.)

Comparison of Methods

Approximate sensitivities for various reagent systems are outlined in Table 20–1. In some cases, sensitivities specified by the manufacturer may vary from those reported in the literature.

It is difficult to assign "absolute" sensitivities with certainty. For HAI, LAI, and direct agglutination procedures, relative sensitivities for different reagents may vary for different urine specimens (Porres, 1975). This may be due to excretion of altered hCG molecules, which are detected with different sensitivities by different reagent systems.

A common approach to classification is "tube tests" and "slide tests." The classic "tube tests" are HAI procedures, with sensitivities in the range of 1.0 to 2.0 IU/ml, which require one to two hours for settling of RBC. Another "tube test," based on latex particle agglutination inhibition, has comparable sensitivity and time requirement (Table 20–1). The classic "slide tests" are LAI procedures, with sensitivities in the range of 2.0 to 5.0 IU/ml, which require only one to two minutes' incubation at room temperature. Another "slide test," based on direct latex particle agglutination, has comparable sensitivity and time requirement (Table 20–1).

Although some slide tests may have slightly better specificity than some tube tests, the decreased sensitivity of slide tests is *not* necessarily associated with improved specificity (Cabrera, 1969; Kerber, 1970; Headden, 1972; Lamb, 1972; Arkin, 1972; Porres, 1975; Lewis, 1977; Roy, 1977).

False negative results in the HAI, LAI, and direct agglutination tests may occur with low hCG levels associated with early pregnancy, ectopic pregnancy, or threatened abortion. False negatives may also occur during the second and third trimesters, when hCG concentrations fall to about 5000 IU/L, close to the limit of sensitivity for LAI procedures (Kerber, 1970). With the direct agglutination slide test, prozoning may account for false negatives in some cases (Horwitz, 1971).

During the week after the first "missed period," or with ectopic pregnancy, the false negative rate is about 50 per cent for conventional immunoassays, but should be less than 10 per cent for the more sensitive beta subunit RIA, RRA procedures, or ELISA.

False positive results in the HAI, LAI, and direct agglutination tests may be due to increased LH at midcycle peak; increased LH in menopausal patients; exogenous administration of hCG; phenothiazine drugs, which may cause increased excretion of LH (Ravel, 1969); promethazine (Phenergan), which may inhibit agglutination, causing false positive HAI or LAI but false negative direct agglutination (Tait, 1971); methadone (Porres, 1975); proteinuria in excess of 1.0 g/24 hours (may cause non-specific inhibition of agglutination or cross-reactions with hCG antisera); ectopic production of hCG and/or hCG-like substances by trophoblastic tumors; ectopic production of hCG and/or hCG-like substances by non-trophoblastic neoplasms (e.g., carcinoma of the lung, ovarian cysts, testicular tumors); tubo-ovarian abscess (Arkin, 1972); deterioration of reagents (deterioration of hCG antiserum will cause "false positive" results in the HAI and LAI procedures, but "false negative" results in the direct agglutination procedure); or slow decline in concentration of hCG following abortion, with residual positive test.

False positive results due to LH, drug interference, or proteinuria have not been reported with the beta subunit RIA method, which has less than 2 per cent cross-reactivity with LH. However, occasional false positives may occur with the RRA owing to cross-reactions with LH.

Reported accuracy of hCG assays is related to prevalence of causes for false negatives (early pregnancy, ectopic pregnancy, threatened abortion, etc.); prevalence of causes for false positives (increased LH, etc.); technical factors (improper shipment and storage of reagents, improper sample collection, quality control); and sensitivity and specificity of the assay procedure.

The incidence of "technical errors" under "normal working conditions" has been estimated to be between 1 and 4 per cent (Hardwick, 1974).

Quality Control

Several authorities recommend that each assay be done in duplicate, using kits from two different manufacturers (Cabrera, 1969). According to Cabrera (1969): ". . . occasional bad lots of reagents are produced which can give very high proportions of false positives as well as false negatives . . . the degree of deficiency (may vary) within the same lot . . . some boxes of a particular lot (are) unusable, while others from the same lot (are) satisfactory . . . this unreliability . . . may result from damage . . . by extreme temperatures . . . (while) immunologic tests are fast and easy to perform . . . many of these tests will go through periods of unreliability . . . we strongly recommend that two . . . immunologic tests be used together . . . one test checking on the other . . . anything less is fraught with danger."

In our opinion, it is desirable periodically to check sensitivities of kits against materials related to the International Standard. "Working Standards" may be provided through quantitative assay of aliquots from a *thoroughly mixed* pool of pregnancy urine by two or more reference laboratories. The remaining pool is frozen in tightly stoppered small aliquots at −70°C. (stable for at least one year).

Using this "working standard," quality control samples can be prepared by dilution to provide a "low positive" (2 to 4 times test sensitivity) and a "high negative" (one-fourth to one-half times test sensitivity) control. These two controls are checked each time a "pregnancy test" is run in order to detect altered sensitivity. If the "high negative" becomes positive, deterioration of HAI or LAI antisera is probable. If the "low positive" becomes negative, consultation with the manufacturer may be indicated.

Dilutions of "working standards" to prepare quality control pools may be performed by direct dilution or serial dilution. The diluent may be urine from males, urine from nonpregnant females, or phosphate buffered saline (pH 6.4) with 0.1 per cent bovine serum albumin. During dilution, reagents may be kept at either refrigerator temperature or room temperature.

Serial dilution tends to give lower values than direct dilutions, possibly owing to hCG adsorption on glass. Either normal urine or buffer with 0.1 per cent albumin tends to protect hCG from denaturation, which may occur in aqueous buffer or saline. The "protective effect" of normal urine seems to vary between different individuals (Tamada, 1969). Reagents should be kept at refrigerator temperature when dilutions are prepared: hCG may undergo slow denaturation at room temperature in dilute solutions (concentrated solutions deteriorate more slowly, possibly due to a "self-protective effect" hCG). The requirements for careful test controls and problems in visualization of endpoints suggest that over-the-counter immunoassay kits for self-testing are problematical.

Diagnosis of Normal Pregnancy

Levels of hCG during pregnancy usually are expressed in relation to days (or weeks) after the last normal menstrual period (LNMP), as shown in Figure 20–3. Concentration of hCG per ml serum is approximately equal to concentration per ml in either a first-voided or a 24-hour urine collection. Concentrations of hCG are somewhat lower in dilute random urine samples. About 6 per cent of serum hCG is cleared in urine and about 94 per cent is cleared outside the kidney. This may be desialated hCG, which is removed quickly by the liver. hCG has a half-life of 1.5 days. It is a small molecule that should readily be passed by the glomerulus into the urine.

Serum hCG first reaches detectable levels (5 mIU/ml) within 24 hours after implantation (Catt, 1975), rapidly increasing to peak levels about 70 days after the LMP (Fig. 20–3). There is considerable variation in rate of rise and peak levels attained. Following the peak at 70 days, hCG levels fall rapidly, reaching a plateau at 5 to 10 IU/ml (Fig. 20–3) about 120 days after the LMP.

During the second and third trimesters, hCG varies over a relatively wide range (Fig. 20–3). Despite this variability, some reports suggest that a small, secondary peak may occur during the third trimester (Braunstein, 1976). Slightly different curves may be obtained for different hCG assays; in actual practice, Figure 20–3 should be modified based on empirical data for a given method.

Since the rate of increase following implantation varies among different individuals, the time at which a given "pregnancy test" becomes positive also varies. The beta subunit RIA procedures with sensitivity of 5 mIU/ml reliably detect pregnancy (approximately 90 per cent sensitivity) at the time of the first missed menses (Kosasa, 1975). Commercial RRA kits, with a sensitivity in the range of 100 to 200 mIU/ml, reliably detect pregnancy (80 to 90 per cent sensitivity) about seven days after the first missed menses (Roy, 1977). The HAI tube tests reliably detect pregnancy (80 to 90 per cent sensitivity) about 14 days after the first missed menses, while the LAI slide tests become reliable (80 to 90 per cent sensitivity) at about 21 days (Roy, 1977). Some "positive results" (at a lower level of reliability) can be expected earlier.

The terms "menstrual regulation" (Brenner, 1975) and "menstrual aspiration" (Kosasa, 1975) have been used to describe vacuum aspiration of uterine contents prior to 14 days after a missed menstrual period. During this time, "standard" pregnancy tests based on LAI and HAI have sensitivities in the range of 70 and 80 per cent, respectively. Greater sensitivity is attainable by RRA or beta subunit RIA, with sensitivities in the range of 90 and 100 per cent, respectively (Roy, 1977). The beta subunit RIA has been used to screen women prior to menstrual aspiration (Kosasa, 1975).

Diagnosis of Ectopic Pregnancy

According to recent reports, even the most sensitive HAI procedures (700 mIU/ml) detect only about 50 per cent of ectopic pregnancies (Saxena, 1975; Milwidsky, 1977a). Although older reports suggest a somewhat lower incidence of false negatives with HAI (Kerber, 1970), there is general agreement that more sensitive procedures are needed to reliably detect ectopic pregnancy.

The hCG levels in ectopic pregnancy usually are in the range of 150 to 800 mIU/ml (Milwidsky, 1977a and b; Saxena, 1975), but levels as low as 10 mIU/ml occur in some cases (Kosasa, 1973, 1974). Several approaches are available to provide increased sensitivity for hCG assays in suspected ectopic pregnancy: beta subunit hCG by RIA, hCG by ELISA, hCG by RRA, and use of HIA procedures with undiluted urine (sensitivity of 300 mIU/ml using UCG test kit). The RIA approach would appear optimal, but it is not always available. ELISA is not widely used as yet. The RRA approach, with commercial reagents, provides somewhat lower sensitivity and specificity than RIA. The approach using HAI procedures with undiluted urine provides even lower sensitivity and specificity, with potential false positives due to cross-reactions with LH.

Evaluation of Threatened Abortion

As previously noted, peak levels of hCG normally occur about 70 days after the LMP (Fig. 20–3). During the first trimester (20 to 90 days after LMP), persistently low or falling plasma hCG (below the

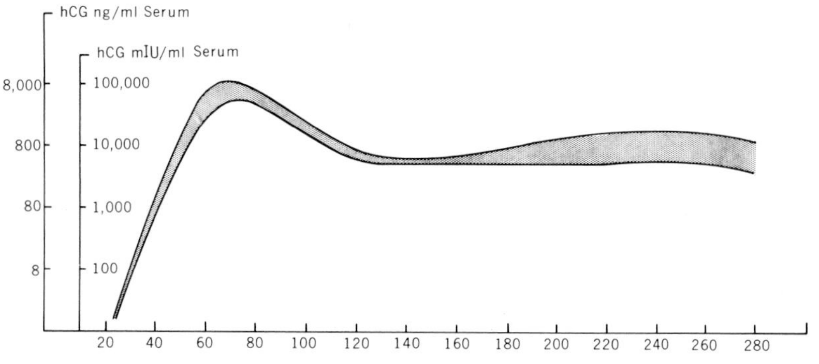

Figure 20–3. Serum hCG levels during normal pregnancy. (Adapted from Lau, H. L.: *In* Practice of Medicine, Vol. II. Hagerstown, Md., Harper & Row, 1975, Chap. 29; and Braustein, G. D., Rasor, J., Adler, D., Danzer, H., and Wade, M. E.: Am. J. Obstet. Gynecol., *126*:678, 1976.)

3

shaded area in Figure 20–3) is associated with inevitable abortion (Rosal, 1975). With regard to urinary measurements, during the period 50 to 90 days after the LMP, hCG levels under 3000 IU/24 hour urine (under 5000 IU/L first-voided morning urine) are associated with inevitable abortion (Salzberger, 1963; Yahia, 1964). In threatened abortion, if hCG levels remain persistently low or are decreasing, probability of inevitable abortion is high.

Evaluation of Trophoblastic Tumors

Trophoblastic tumors such as hydatidiform mole and choriocarcinoma usually present markedly elevated hCG levels, sometimes over 6 million mIU/ml (480,000 ng/ml). However, some patients have relatively low levels, in the range of 5000 mIU/ml.

Evaluation of elevations in the 10,000 to 100,000 mIU/ml range may be aided by sequential assays: normal pregnancy tends to follow the curve depicted in Figure 20–3, while in trophoblastic disease, repeated assays over several weeks usually show irregular fluctuations over a limited range (e.g., 100,000 to 500,000 mIU/ml, or 10,000 to 100,000 mIU/ml).

Several pitfalls should be considered with regard to increased hCG levels and trophoblastic disease:

1. Elevated levels may be associated with multiple pregnancies, polyhydramnios, eclampsia, and erythroblastosis fetalis.

2. hCG levels may be quite variable during the third trimester of normal pregnancy (from 1000 to 20,000 mIU/ml).

3. With titration procedures, a one-tube variation is not significant: thus a level of 2000 mIU/ml should be interpreted as between 1000 to 4000 mIU/ml.

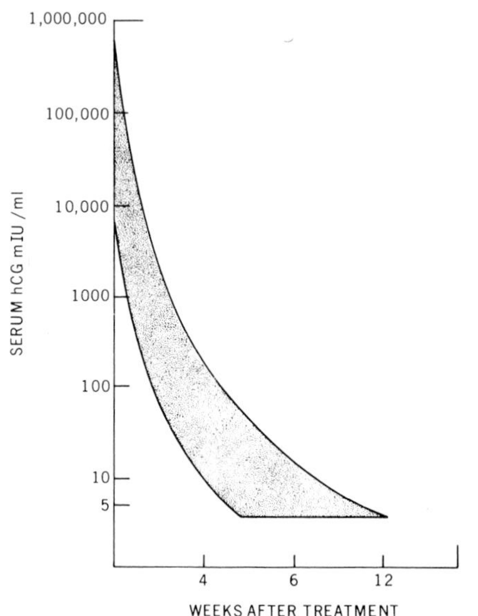

Figure 20–4. Serum hCG levels following complete removal of hydatidiform mole. (Adapted from Morrow, C. P., Kletzky, O. A., Disaia, P. J., Townsend, D. E., Mishell, D. R., and Nakamura, R. M.: Am. J. Obstet. Gynecol., *128*:424, 1977.)

4. On rare occasions, areas of hydatidiform mole may coexist with otherwise normal placental tissue and a normal pregnancy.

Treatment of hydatidiform mole is more effectively monitored by beta subunit RIA than by HAI procedures which may be associated with frequent false negatives (Pastorfide, 1974; Jones, 1975; Yuen, 1977). The higher sensitivity of the RIA procedure provides a more accurate index of remission and more sensitive detection of recurrence. Normal regression of serum hCG, following complete removal of hydatidiform mole, is depicted in Figure 20–4 (modified from Morrow, 1977). Note that qualitative tests for pregnancy can remain positive for long periods following removal of trophoblast.

In a few cases, viable trophoblastic tissue may remain, even after hCG becomes undetectable by beta subunit RIA (Schreiber, 1976). In these patients, alpha subunits, undetectable by beta subunit RIA, may be the only evidence of persisting trophoblastic tissue (Dawood, 1977b).

Treatment of choriocarcinoma should be monitored by beta subunit RIA. As with hydatidiform mole, a few tumors may produce alpha subunits, which are undetectable by beta subunit RIA.

Evaluation of Testicular Tumors

Testicular choriocarcinomas are well known for their association with elevated plasma and urinary hCG. In most cases, hCG can be detected with the HAI or LAI assays. Using the beta subunit RIA, increased plasma hCG can be demonstrated in almost all testicular choriocarcinomas.

Other testicular tumors—notably seminomas, teratomas, and embryonal carcinomas—are well known for their association with elevated plasma and urinary hCG. About 10 to 20 per cent of such cases have elevated hCG by HAI or LAI; about 40 to 60 per cent have elevated hCG by beta subunit RIA. One hypothesis has been that hCG in such cases is produced by small foci of active or "burned-out" choriocarcinoma. However, there is evidence that other cell types also may produce hCG ectopically (Braunstein, 1973).

Sensitive hCG measurements (preferably the beta-subunit RIA) should be performed prior to treatment of testicular tumors; if hCG is found, this can be used as a "tumor marker" to evaluate treatment and/or suspected recurrence.

Ectopic hCG Production in Non-Trophoblastic Tumors

Ectopic hormone production by non-endocrine tumors is well known and has been studied extensively. Indeed, some non-endocrine neoplasms are capable of producing several hormones simultaneously. Also, some endocrine tumors may secrete both the "appropriate" hormone and an ectopic hormone; e.g., medullary carcinoma of the thyroid may produce ACTH as well as calcitonin. Such ectopic hormone production includes adrenocorticotropic hormone (ACTH), melanocyte-stimulating hormone (MSH), parathyroid hormone (PTH), calcitonin, luteinizing hormone (LH), antidiuretic hormone (ADH), insulin-like activity (ILA), vasoactive intestinal polypeptide (VIP), gastrin, erythropoeitin, and thyroid-stimulating hormone (TSH) in a variety of different tumors (Samaan, 1977).

Ectopic hCG production, as determined by beta-subunit RIA, has been described in up to 30 per cent of gastrointestinal neoplasms (especially gastric carcinoma, hepatoma, and pancreatic carcinoma); up to 2 per cent of patients with lymphoma/leukemia/myeloma; and occasional patients with retroperitoneal sarcoma, breast carcinoma, adrenocortical carcinoma, bronchogenic carcinoma, renal cell carcinoma, and melanoma (Braunstein, 1973; Rosen, 1975). In such cases, production of hCG may be as alpha subunits only, beta subunits only, or complete hCG, either alone or with subunits also present. Ectopic hormone lacks sialic acid and is subject to rapid degradation.

Ectopic production of the other placental proteins also may occur in association with various neoplasms, e.g., placental lactogen and placental alkaline phosphatase, either alone or in association with hCG (Braunstein, 1973).

OTHER "PREGNANCY TESTS"

Pregnancy-Associated Plasma Proteins

It is clear that the placenta produces, in addition to hCG, other proteins "specific" to pregnancy. Perhaps the best known is heat-stable alkaline phosphatase, which shows marked elevations in maternal serum during the third trimester. Although heat-stable alkaline phosphatase has been used as a "placental function test," in this role it has largely been replaced by plasma and urinary estriol (Watson, 1973). Like hCG, heat-stable alkaline phosphatase (Regan isoenzyme) may serve as a useful "tumor marker" for a wide variety of neoplasms; however, its clinical value is not yet well established.

Recently, certain alpha and beta globulins known as "pregnancy-associated plasma proteins" (PAPP) have been identified (Lin, 1974; von Schoultz, 1974; Lin, 1975; Grudzinskas, 1977).

Although some of these proteins can be induced by exogenous estrogens or oral contraceptives (von Schoultz, 1974), others may have specificity comparable to hCG (Grudzinskas, 1977). Possible applications include (1) diagnosis of pregnancy during the first trimester and (2) evaluation of placental function (Masson, 1977).

Additional studies are needed to establish the clinical value of these measurements in comparison with measurements of hCG.

PLACENTAL FUNCTION TESTS

Human Placental Lactogen

Human placental lactogen (hPL) is a single chain polypeptide of about 21,000 molecular weight, similar in structure to pituitary growth hormone. Although hPL displays growth hormone effects which contribute to the metabolic changes of late pregnancy, its primary role is a lactogenic hormone functioning in combination with prolactin. hPL is also the major cause of elevated plasma glucose during pregnancy. An alternative name applied to hPL is human chorionic somatomammotropin (hCS).

Like hCG, hPL is produced by the syncytial trophoblast, starting shortly after implantation. During the first trimester, hPL appears in maternal plasma about eight to ten weeks after the LMP (last menstrual period) but is of no practical value for early pregnancy diagnosis, as compared with hCG.

Some reports suggest that hPL measurements may be used as a "placental function test." However, for this purpose, estriol measurements probably provide more useful clinical information than hPL (Watson, 1973; Josimovich, 1973). Possibly, hPL measurements may provide a useful supplement to estriol. At this time, the clinical value of hPL as a "placental function test" is questionable (Wenk, 1979).

In contrast to hCG, hPL is markedly decreased in association with hydatidiform mole and choriocarcinoma. Thus, the combination of high hCG and low hPL possibly may have some diagnostic value (Levitt, 1976). However, for monitoring treatment, measurement of hCG by beta subunit RIA is clearly superior to hPL measurements.

Some non-trophoblastic tumors are associated with increased hPL. Thus hPL, as well as hCG, may provide a useful "tumor marker" in some cases.

Estrogen Measurements

Although estrogen measurements have little value as "pregnancy tests" during the first trimester, in the third trimester, urinary and plasma estriol provide a valuable index of fetal-placental dysfunction (Watson, 1973; Bashore, 1977; Miller, 1977). For further details see Chapter 21.

An approach to management of high-risk pregnancies has been outlined by Crane (1976). Three basic patterns for plasma unconjugated estriol are described: normal pattern ("within normal limits"), chronically low results, and falling values. Chronically low estriol may be unrelated to fetal distress or placental failure. Possible causes include maternal steroid therapy, fetal adrenal insufficiency, congenital anomalies (e.g., anencephaly), and placental sulfatase deficiency.

A day-to-day decrease of 35 to 50 per cent is considered a significant fall in plasma or urinary estriol. Beyond the thirty-fourth week of gestation, values below 4 mg estriol/24 hour urine (3 ng estriol/ml plasma) indicate that fetal death has occurred or is imminent (Fig. 20–5). A single estriol measurement often has limited value; serial measurements in relation to the "normal pregnancy curve" (Fig. 20–5) provide greater sensitivity and specificity than isolated determinations.

About 60 per cent of molar pregnancies are associated with low serum estriol (Dawood, 1977a). However, in some cases, trophoblastic tissue may produce estriol in the absence of viable fetus.

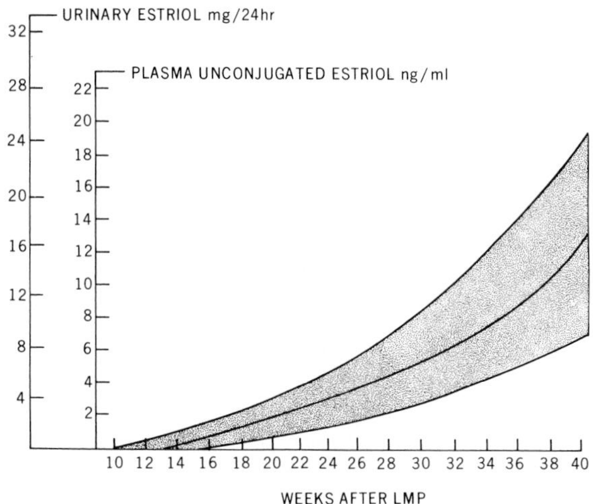

Figure 20–5. Normal ranges for plasma unconjugated estriol and urinary estriol. (Adapted from Bashore, R. A., and Westlake, J. R.: Am. J. Obstet. Gynecol., *128*:371, 1977; and Ansari, A. H., and Fuller, D. G.: South. Med. J., *70*:142, 1977. Reprinted by permission.)

CONCLUSIONS

For most purposes, the term "pregnancy test" is equivalent to "hCG assay." Pregnancy tests may be indicated in a variety of situations, including (1) exclusion of pregnancy in women of childbearing age prior to surgery, drug treatment, rubella vaccination, or radiographic studies; (2) suspected ectopic pregnancy; (3) selection of patients for menstrual regulation; (4) evaluation of threatened abortion; (5) diagnosis and treatment of trophoblastic disease; (6) unexplained cases of gynecomastia or sexual precocity (tumors producing hCG may cause such symptoms in men and children); and (7) regulation of treatment for non-trophoblastic neoplasms which produce hCG. Although other "pregnancy tests" have been described, their clinical value is not yet well established.

Of the various "placental function tests," measurements of urinary and/or plasma estriol appear most useful for evaluating the fetal-placental unit during the third trimester. The clinical value of other procedures, such as hPL and heat-stable alkaline phosphatase, is not yet established.

Arkin, C., and Noto, T. A.: A false positive immunologic pregnancy test with tube-ovarian abscess. Am. J. Clin. Path., *58*:314, 1972.

Aschheim, S., and Zondek, B.: Pregnancy diagnosis with urine by the demonstration of the hormone. Klin. Wochenschr., 7:8, 1928.

Bashore, R. A., and Westlake, J. R.: Plasma unconjugated estriol values in high-risk pregnancy. Am. J. Obstet. Gynecol., *128*:371, 1977.

Bellerby, C. W.: A rapid test for the diagnosis of pregnancy. Nature (London), *133*:494, 1934.

Boyko, W. L., and Russell, H. T.: Application of the radioreceptor assay for human chorionic gonadotropin in pregnancy testing and management of trophoblastic disease. Obstet. Gynecol., *50*:329, 1977.

Braunstein, G. D., Rasor, J., Adler, D., Danzer, H., and Wade, M. E.: Serum human chorionic gonadotropin levels throughout normal pregnancy. Am. J. Obstet. Gynecol., *126*:678, 1976.

Braunstein, G. D., Vaitukaitis, J. L., Carbone, P. P., and Ross, G. T.: Ectopic production of human chorionic gonadotropin by neoplasms. Ann. Intern. Med., *78*:39, 1973.

Brenner, W. E., Edelman, D. A., and Kessel, E.: Menstrual regulation in the United States: A preliminary report. Fertil. Steril., *26*:289, 1975.

Cabrera, H. A.: A comprehensive evaluation of pregnancy tests. Am. J. Obstet. Gynecol., *103*:32, 1969.

Catt, K. J., Dufau, M. L., and Vaitukaitis, J. L.: Appearance of hCG in pregnancy plasma following the initiation of implantation of the blastocyst. J. Clin. Endocrinol. Metab., *40*:537, 1975.

Crane, J. P., Sauvage, J. P., and Arias, F.: A high-risk pregnancy management protocol. Am. J. Obstet. Gynecol., *125*:227, 1976.

Dawood, M. Y., Brown, J. B., and Newman, K. L. H.: Serum free estriol and estriol glucuronide fractions in hydatidiform mole measured by radioimmunoassay. Obstet. Gynecol., *49*:303, 1977a.

Dawood, M. Y., Saxena, B. B., and Landesman, R.: Human chorionic gonadotropin and its subunits in hydatidiform mole and choriocarcinoma. Obstet. Gynecol., *50*:172, 1977b.

Ehrlich, P. H., and Moyle, W. R.: Cooperative immunoassays: Ultrasensitive assays with mixed monoclonal antibodies. Science, *221*:279, 1983.

Frank, R. T., and Berman, R. L.: A twenty-four hour pregnancy test. Am. J. Obstet. Gynecol., *42*:492, 1941.

Friedman, M. H., and Lapham, M. E.: A simple rapid method for the laboratory diagnosis of early pregnancies. Am. J. Obstet. Gynecol., *21*:405, 1931.

Galli-Mainini, C.: Pregnancy test using the male batrachia. J.A.M.A., *138*:121, 1948.

Grudzinskas, J. C., Jeffrey, D., Gordon, Y. B., and Chard, T.: Specific and sensitive determination of pregnancy—specific β1-glycoprotein by radioimmunoassay. Lancet, *1*:333, 1977.

Hardwick, D. F., Brent, R., Burke, M. D., Cohen, H., Falkowski, F., Horwitz, C. A., Lazo-Wasem, E., Perrin, E. U., Poland, B. J., Reiss, A. M., Schenkel, B., Towell, M. E., and Vorherr, H.: Early diagnosis of pregnancy: An invitational symposium. J. Reprod. Med., *12*:1, 1974.

Headden, G. F.: An evaluation of immunological pregnancy tests. Med. Lab. Technol., *29*:332, 1972.

Horwitz, C. A., Polesky, H., Odenbrett, P., Gronli, M., Horowitz, A., Diamond, R., and Ward, P. C. J.: Clinical and immunologic study of a direct agglutination test for pregnancy. Am. J. Obstet. Gynecol., *111*:808, 1971.

Jones, W. B., Lewis, J. L., and Lehr, M.: Monitor of chemotherapy in gestational trophoblastic neoplasm by radioimmunoassay of the β-subunit of human chorionic gonadotropin. Am. J. Obstet. Gynecol., *121*:669, 1975.

Josimovich, J. B.: Placental protein hormones in pregnancy. Clin. Gynecol., *16*:46, 1973.

Kerber, I. J., Inclan, A. P., Fowler, E. A., David, K., and Fish, S. A.: Immunologic tests for pregnancy. Obstet. Gynecol., *36*:37, 1970.

Kosasa, T. S., Levesque, L. A., Goldstein, D. P., and Taymor, M. L.: Clinical use of a solid-phase radioimmunoassay specific for human chorionic gonadotropin. Am. J. Obstet. Gynecol., *119*:784, 1974.

Kosasa, T. S., Pion, R. J., Hale, R. W., Goldstein, D. P., Taymor, M. L., Levesque, L. A., and Kobara, T. Y.: Rapid hCG-specific radioimmunoassay for menstrual aspiration. Obstet. Gynecol., *45*:566, 1975.

Kosasa, T. S., Taymor, M. L., Goldstein, D. P., and Levesque, L. A.: Use of a radioimmunoassay specific for human chorionic gonadotropin in the diagnosis of early ectopic pregnancy. Obstet. Gynecol., *42*:858, 1973.

Lamb, E. J.: Immunological pregnancy tests. Obstet. Gynecol., *39*:665, 1972.

Landesman, R., and Saxena, B. B.: Results of the first 1000 radioreceptor assays for the determination of human chorionic gonadotropin: A new, rapid, reliable, and sensitive pregnancy test. Fertil. Steril., *27*:357, 1976.

Levitt, M. J., and Josimovich, J. B.: Measurement of chorionic gonadotropin and placental lactogen in body fluids. *In* Rose, N. R., and Friedman, H. (eds.): Manual of Clinical Immunology. Washington, D.C., American Society for Microbiology, 1976.

Lewis, C.: Human chorionic gonadotrophin and its detection by immunochemical methods. Can. J. Med. Tech., *39*:58, 1977.

Lin, T. M., and Halbert, S. P.: Immunological comparison of various human pregnancy-associated plasma proteins. Int. Arch. Allergy Appl. Immunol., *48*:101, 1975.

Lin, T. M., Halbert, S. P., Kiefer, D., and Spellacy, W. N.: Three pregnancy-associated plasma proteins. Int. Arch. Allergy Appl. Immunol., *47*:35, 1974.

Masson, G. M., Klopper, A. I., and Wilson, G. R.: Plasma estrogens and pregnancy-associated plasma proteins. Obstet. Gynecol., *50*:435, 1977.

Milwidsky, A., Adoni, A., Palti, Z., Stark, M., and Segal, S.: The significance of human chorionic gonadotropin in blood serum for the early diagnosis of ectopic pregnancy. Acta Obstet. Gynecol. Scand., *56*:19, 1977a.

Milwidsky, A., Adoni, A., Segal, S., and Palti, Z.: Chorionic gonadotropin and progesterone levels in ectopic pregnancy. Obstet. Gynecol., *50*:145, 1977b.

Miller, C. A., Fetter, M. C., Bognslaski, R. C., and Heiser, E. W.: Maternal serum unconjugated estriol and urine estriol concentrations in normal and high-risk pregnancy. Obstet. Gynecol., *49*:287, 1977.

Morrow, C. P., Kletzky, O. A., Disaia, P. J., Townsend, D. E., Mishell, D. R., and Nakamura, R. M.: Clinical and laboratory correlates of molar pregnancy and trophoblastic disease. Am. J. Obstet. Gynecol., *128*:424, 1977.

Pastorfide, G. B., Goldstein, D. P., and Kosasa, T. S.: The use of a radioimmunoassay specific for human chorionic gonadotropin in patients with molar pregnancy and gestational trophoblastic disease. Am. J. Obstet. Gynecol., *120*:1025, 1974.

Porres, J. M., D'Ambra, C., Lord, D., and Garrity, F.: Comparison of eight kits for the diagnosis of pregnancy. Am. J. Clin. Path., *64*:452, 1975.

Rasor, J. L., and Braunstein, G. D.: A rapid modification of the beta-hCG radioimmunoassay. Obstet. Gynecol., *50*:553, 1977.

Ravel, R., Riekers, H. G., and Goldstein, B. J.: Effects of certain psychotropic drugs in immunologic pregnancy tests. Am. J. Obstet. Gynecol., *105*:1227, 1969.

Rosal, T. P., Saxena, B. B., and Landesman, R.: Application of a radioreceptor assay of human chorionic gonadotropin in the diagnosis of early abortion. Fertil. Steril., *26*:1105, 1975.

Rosen, S. W., Weintraub, B. D., Vaitukaitis, J. L., Sussman, H. H., Hershman, J. M., and Muggia, F. M.: Placental proteins and their subunits as tumor markers. Ann. Intern. Med., *82*:71, 1975.

Ross, G. T.: Clinical relevance of research on the structure of human chorionic gonadotropin. Am. J. Obstet. Gynecol., *129*:795, 1977.

Roy, S., Klein, T. A., Scott, J. Z., Kletzky, O. A., and Mishell, D. R.: Diagnosis of pregnancy with a radioreceptor assay for hCG. Obstet. Gynecol.., *50*:401, 1977.

Salk, J. E.: A simplified procedure for titrating hemagglutination capacity of influenza virus and corresponding antibody. J. Immunol., *48*:87, 1944.

Salzberger, M., and Nelken, D.: The immunologic pregnancy test. Am. J. Obstet. Gynecol., *86*:899, 1963.

Samaan, N. A.: Hormone production in non-endocrine tumors. CA, *27*:148, 1977.

Saxena, B. B., Hasan, S. H., Haour, F., and Schmidt-Gullwitzer, M.: Radioreceptor assay of hCG: Detection of early pregnancy. Science, *184*:793, 1974.

Saxena, B. B., and Landesman, R.: The use of a radioreceptor assay of human chorionic gonadotropin for the diagnosis and management of ectopic pregnancy. Fertil. Steril., *26*:397, 1975.

Schreiber, J. R., Rebar, R. W., Chen, H. C., Hodgen, G. D., and Ross, G. T.; Limitation of the specific serum radioimmunoassay for human chorionic gonadotropin in the management of trophoblastic neoplasms. Am. J. Obstet. Gynecol., *125*:705, 1976.

Storring, P. L., Gaines-Das, R. E., and Bangham, D. R.: International reference preparation of human chorionic gonadotropin for immunoassay: Potency estimates in various bioassay and protein binding assay systems; and international reference preparation of the alpha and beta subunits of human chorionic gonadotropin for immunoassay. J. Endocrinol., *84*:295, 1980.

Tait, B.: Interference in immunological methods of pregnancy testing by promethazine. Med. J. Aust., *2*:126, 1971.

Tamada, T., Tsukui, Y., and Matsumoto, S.: On diluent and dilution method in hemagglutination test for human chorionic gonadotropin. Endocrinol. Japan, *16*:399, 1969.

United States Food and Drug Administration: Medroxyprogesterone acetate; norethindrone; norethindrone acetate; progesterone; dydrogesterone; and hydroxyprogesterone caproate. Fed. Reg., *38*:27947, 1973.

Vaitukaitis, J. L., Braunstein, G. D., and Ross, G. T.: A radioimmunoassay which specifically measures human chorionic gonadotropin in the presence of human luteinizing hormone. Am. J. Obstet. Gynecol., *113*:751, 1972.

von Schoultz, B.: A quantitative study of the pregnancy zone protein in the sera of pregnant and puerperal women. Am. J. Obstet. Gynecol., *119*:792, 1974.

Watson, D., Siddiqui, S. A., Stafford, J. E. H., Gibbard, S., and Hewitt, V.: A comparative study of five laboratory tests for faeto-placental dysfunction in late pregnancy. J. Clin. Path., *26*:294, 1973.

Wenk, R. E., London, R., Siegelbaum, M., et al.: A prospective evaluation of placental lactogen as a test for neonatal risk. Am. J. Clin. Path., *71*:1, 72, 1979.

Wide, L.: An immunological method for the assay of human chorionic gonadotropin. Acta Endocrinol., *41* (Suppl. 70:1, 1962.

Wide, L., and Gemzell, C. A.: An immunological pregnancy test. Acta Endocrinol., *35*:261, 1960.

Wiltberger, P. B., and Miller, D. F.: The male frog, rana pipiens, as a new test animal for early pregnancy. Science, *107*:198, 1948.

Yahia, C.: The quantitative toad test in normal and abnormal early gestation. Obstet. Gynecol., *23*:547, 1964.

Yuen, B. H., Cannon, W., Benedet, J. L., and Boyes, D. A.: Plasma β-subunit human chorionic gonadotropin assay in molar pregnancy and choriocarcinoma. Am. J. Obstet. Gynecol., *127*:711, 1977.

21

ASSESSMENT OF FETAL CONDITION AND AMNIOTIC FLUID ANALYSIS

ROBERT E. WENK, M.D., JERALD M. ROSENBAUM, M.D., and BERNARD E. STATLAND, M.D., PH.D.

Amniotic fluid was found to be a source of information in predicting hemolytic disease of the newborn about 30 years ago (Bevis, 1952). Diagnostic amniocentesis is now a fairly safe procedure that can be useful in detecting a great number of teratologic, genetic, endocrine, maturational, and infectious diseases of the unborn (Table 21–1).

A variety of laboratory techniques have been applied to amniotic fluid cells, supernate, fetal tissues, and blood. These include enzyme cytochemistry, cytogenetic, immunologic, and restriction endonuclease analyses. In addition to amniotic sources, samples of parental blood, tissue, and urine can be invaluable in prenatal diagnosis. Technical advances, ethical and legal issues, costs, risks, and social needs have exploded into new major industries that cannot be summarized in this chapter. Brief mention will be made of selected special tests; emphasis will be on common problems and tests of fetal health that can often be resolved at primary and secondary levels of care; prenatal diagnosis of uncommon genetic disorders will be omitted.

AMNIOTIC FLUID: PHYSIOLOGY AND ANATOMY

The amniotic sac arises during the first week of gestation from embryonic tissues. It consists of an outer layer of mesoderm and an inner layer of ectoderm. The amniotic cavity enlarges, reflects over the embryo and its umbilical cord, and may be tapped (amniocentesis) by 14 weeks. At term (40 weeks), the sac contains 0.5 to 2.5 L of fluid, which is apparently produced by the fetal gastrointestinal system, respiratory tract, umbilical cord, amniotic membrane, and kidneys.

Normally, water exchanges between amniotic fluid and mother, between mother and fetus, and between fetus and fluid. As pregnancy advances, the exchange between fetus and mother increases. In hydramnios, however, the fetomaternal exchange decreases, while the fetus increases its water contribution to fluid.

In effect, in the first half of pregnancy, amniotic fluid volume can be regarded as an extension of the fetal extracellular fluid space. Rapidly developing fetal

Table 21–1. CLASSES OF DISORDERS DETECTABLE BY AMNIOTIC ANALYSES

Hemolytic disease of newborn (Rh_o, other isoimmunization)
Fetal immaturity (fetal size, pulmonary)
Anomalies (urinary tract, neural tube, intestinal, other)
Fetal infections (bacterial, viral, other)
Fetal hypoxia and distress
Genetic disorders (of metabolism, coagulation, hemoglobin, lipid, carbohydrate, mucopolysaccharide, steroid, organic acids, thyroid, etc.)
Cytogenetic (Down's, sex chromosomal, autosomal)

edema is, therefore, accompanied by acute hydramnios in disorders such as recipient-twin transfusion syndrome, hydrops fetalis, and fetal heart failure. Chronic hydramnios may develop when the fetus fails to swallow fluid. It is associated with a 20 per cent incidence of fetal malformations such as anencephaly or esophageal atresia. Chronic hydramnios is also associated with maternal disease, commonly toxemia or diabetes mellitus. Oligohydramnios (less than 300 ml) may develop when chronically ill fetuses swallow more frequently than normal. Oligohydramnios often occurs in placental insufficiency, donor-twin transfusion syndrome, and malformation of the fetal urinary tract.

In prolonged pregnancy, amniotic fluid may be obtained to determine if there is oligohydramnios (by hippurate dye dilution measurements). Oligohydramnios is associated with fetal distress and may indicate measurement of fetal blood pH or determination of maternal estriol excretion.

At term, amniotic water is exchanged at the high rate of 400 ml per hour; solutes in the water (1 per cent w/w) exchange at slower rates. A rapid rise in osmolality sometimes occurs in diabetic mothers and predicts a grave fetal outcome (Cassady, 1968).

HEMOLYTIC DISEASE OF NEWBORNS

Sampling of amniotic fluid is a common procedure in the isoimmunization syndrome. Usually amniocentesis is performed beyond 30 weeks, whereas it is a second trimester procedure in genetic and neural tube disorders. Although passive immunization of mothers with anti-Rh_o(D) can effectively prevent isoimmunization in many susceptible women, sporadic cases are expected to occur. Severe hemolytic disease may result when there are untreated mothers, iatrogenic failures, immunizations by transfusion, and abortions that are left untreated. Fetomaternal bleeding at amniocentesis can produce maternal isoimmunization. Rarely, maternofetal bleeding at delivery can cause infant immunization. If these infants become mothers years later, they may transfer antibodies across the placenta, affecting the third generation. Most isoimmunizations will be directed against the Rh system antigens, but others will involve other blood group antigens. The principles of management of these pregnancies are similar to those established for Rh_o(D) isoimmunization.

In the case of non-Rh_o isoimmunization, amniocentesis is performed when (1) an antibody is found which is known to cause severe hemolysis (e.g., Kell) and (2) there is evidence that the father of the child will pass the antigen to his offspring (Weinstein, 1976).

When maternal IgG antibodies cross the placenta to react with fetal erythrocyte antigens, hemolysis is detectable as early as 16 weeks' gestation and may progress at an increasing rate until term. As fetal hemoglobin is catabolized to bilirubin, fetal plasma carries an increased concentration of unconjugated bilirubin to the placenta. The placenta excretes the pigment unless there is severe fetoplacental compromise. When unconjugated bilirubin increases in the fetal circulation, fetal hepatic glucuronyl transferase activity is induced earlier than usual so that conjugated bilirubin can be produced as early as 28 weeks (Brodersen, 1967). The conjugate is not cleared by the placenta and accounts for a variable fraction of the pigment (1 to 50 per cent) found in amniotic fluid. Much of the conjugated bilirubin is excreted via the fetal biliary tract and intestine, where a portion of it is hydrolyzed by intestinal epithelial beta-glucuronidase, reconverted to unconjugated bilirubin, and absorbed by the intestine. In the normal fetus or in one affected by mild hemolytic disease, there is no jaundice *in utero;* but following delivery, in the absence of the placenta, clinical jaundice may become evident. The severity of jaundice is related to increased pigment production found in isoimmunization syndrome. The majority of the pigment is unconjugated bilirubin.

3

Principles of Amniotic Fluid Analysis in Isoimmunization Syndrome

The examination of amniotic fluid in the maternal isoimmunization syndrome is based on the presence of the breakdown products of hemolysis, e.g., bilirubin.

Bilirubin pigment is bound to albumin; its concentration in the amniotic fluid is maintained at a fairly constant level despite the rapid turnover rate of amniotic fluid water, since the turnover of amniotic fluid protein is much slower.

A specimen of amniotic fluid may be aspirated, filtered, and examined with a double beam recording spectrophotometer. If the absorbance of the fluid is recorded continuously between 350 and 700 nm, the resulting curve can be used to (1) detect whether or not the fluid contains bilirubin and/or other pigmented products of hemolysis, and (2) quantitate the bilirubin pigment which is present.

Liley (1963) has shown that the net absorbance at 450 nm from isoimmunized patients who have unaffected babies always decreases as pregnancy progresses. This decreasing net absorbance at the 450 nm wavelength with increasing length of gestation parallels bilirubin pigment concentration, and can be used to measure the severity of hemolytic disease. This is illustrated in Liley's prediction graph (Fig. 21–1). The greater the net absorbance at 450 nm, the more severe is the hemolysis and the lower the umbilical cord hemoglobin of a delivered newborn at any given

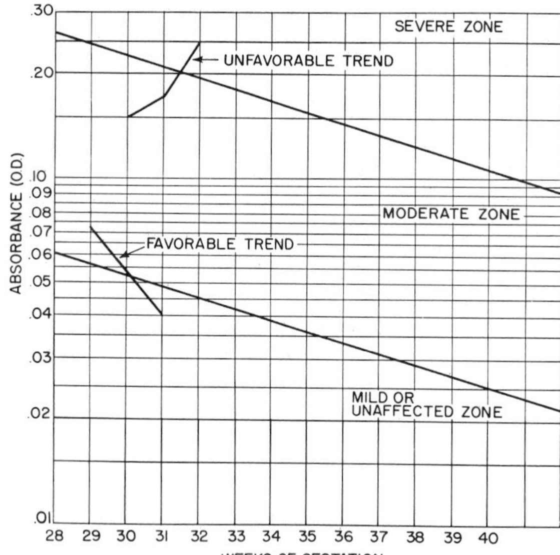

Figure 21–1. Relation of duration of pregnancy and net absorbance of amniotic fluid at 450 nm. Serial spectrophotometric scans at weekly intervals may show increasing, stationary, decreasing, or variable net absorbances.

age of gestation. The slope of the boundaries demarcating the zones of the graph indicates that there is a logarithmic decrease in pigment concentration in the amniotic fluid as pregnancy progresses. These decreases may be the result of a physiologic dilution of bilirubin in the amniotic fluid in the last trimester of pregnancy. Thus, a given net absorbance early in gestation predicts a better outcome than the same net absorbance value at a later date. Accurate dating of gestation is essential for proper interpretation.

Procedure

Approximately 5 ml of amniotic fluid is collected by the obstetrician when he considers the maternal antibody titer critical, or when a possibly severely affected infant is anticipated. "Critical" usually means an antibody titer of 1:16 (± 1 dilution) or higher in the antiglobulin phase of the indirect antiglobulin (Coombs) test when dealing with Rh_0 antibodies. The specimen is sent in an opaque container (bilirubin is light sensitive) to a clinical pathology laboratory, where it is centrifuged in the dark to remove turbidity. If erythrocytes are present, the sediment can be submitted to the blood bank or hematology laboratories, where the cells are identified as maternal or fetal. Specimens may be mailed to reference laboratories for analysis provided they are sterile, centrifuged or filtered before shipment, and sent in opaque containers.

A spectral absorbance curve is made and the net absorbance at 450 nm is determined. This value is related to bilirubin concentration (Gambino, 1966).

An assessment of fetal prognosis (based on net O.D.) is reported (Liley, 1963). A statement regarding current fetal well-being or jeopardy may also be reported (Freda, 1966).

The reader is referred to the previous edition of this text for details of technical procedures (Wenk, 1979b).

Interpretation of Spectrophotometric Tracings

The method of Liley is representative of a predictive type of interpretation. Its reliability and accuracy have been confirmed by considerable experience in many laboratories. Liley subdivided Rh-immunized mothers into five groups.

In this older method, the net O.D. is used to determine the empirically determined, expected initial cord blood hemoglobin concentration of the newborn suffering from hemolytic disease (Fig. 21–1). Predictions are accurate if the child is delivered within a week of the amniocentesis. The rate of hemolysis may be monitored weekly by repeating amniotic analysis, so that trends in disease may be established (Fig. 21–2).

Trends are not always unidirectional. They may graphically change slope or even reverse direction. Trends are used to determine when to reassess the amniotic fluid scan or to decide when to induce labor. A clinical algorithm based on Liley's method has been developed by the American College of Obstetrics and Gynecology (ACOG, 1972).

The method of Freda is a management tool. Rather than predicting severity in terms of cord hemoglobin or number of exchange transfusions, it yields information about severity of anemia and its complications in the fetus (Table 21–2).

Most often, amniotic fluid analysis combines both predictive and management criteria with an assessment of fetal pulmonary surfactant (see below: The Clinical Problem of Assessing Fetal Lung Maturity). The combination of pigment and surfactant analyses permits clinical decision making. If there is no fetal jeopardy secondary to hemolytic disease and the lungs are immature, pregnancy is allowed to continue. If severe hemolytic disease is likely and lungs are mature, delivery is scheduled by the obstetrician. The transfusion service and neonatologist are informed of the probable need for exchange or simple transfusion. Prior to 32 weeks' gestation, *if* fetal lungs are immature, intrauterine transfusion or maternal plasma exchange may be considered as means of improving the chances of fetal survival. Induction of fetal surfactant production may also be attempted pharmacologically by the obstetrician.

It should be stated that pigments other than bilirubin may contribute to the spectrophotometric tracing. Hemoglobin, methemalbumin, meconium, and fetal acidosis produce characteristic absorption peaks and changes (see Fig. 43–7, p. 1054). Tracings are thus subject to interpretation by the clinical pathologist. The amniocentesis may have been a "traumatic tap" resulting in a bloody fluid sample. Erythrocytes may be identified as fetal or maternal by Kleihauer-Betke staining for fetal hemoglobin, and by pheno-

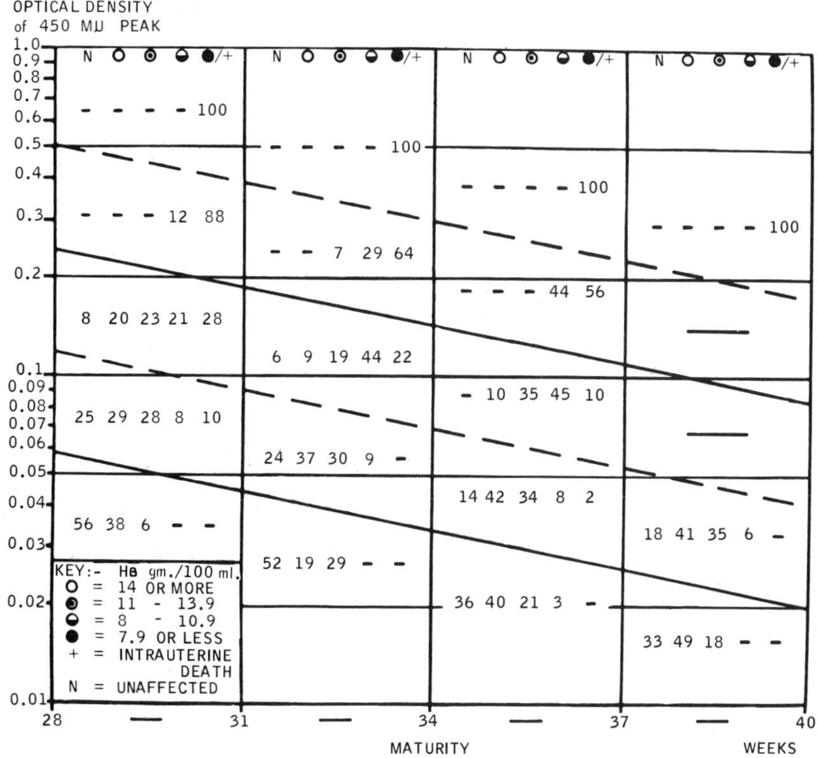

Figure 21–2. Liley prediction table showing the likelihood that a given net absorbance at a given week of gestation will estimate a cord hemoglobin concentration. (From Liley, A. W.: Am. J. Obstet. Gynecol., *86*:485, 1963.)

typing red cells for their surface antigens (Betke, 1958). Presence of fetal cells (1) indicates potential worsening of fetal hemolytic anemia by blood loss, (2) explains subsequent rise in maternal antibody titer and later worsening hemolysis, and (3) explains an immediate and unexpected rise in amniotic yellow pigment caused by admixture of fetal plasma in which bilirubin concentration is increased even in mild disease.

Maternal blood also distorts the normal tracing, but the scan may be interpreted unless the cell/total fluid-volume ratio of the specimen is 0.05 or more. If this ratio is exceeded, hemolysis is usually sufficient to obscure the bilirubin absorbance peak at 450 nm. The amniotic fluid curve is also distorted by maternal plasma contamination with moderate intra-amniotic maternal bleeding. A second clear sample can sometimes be obtained following minor bleeding, immediately after the bloody tap but before diffusion has occurred in the amniotic sac. A major hemorrhage requires about two weeks to clear the amniotic fluid. Major bleeding, with lysis of erythrocytes and release of hemoglobin, shows the three characteristic peaks of oxyhemoglobin at 415 nm, 540 nm, and 575 nm. Minor bleeding may show only the Soret band at 415 nm. Generally the presence of these pigments decreases net absorbance at 450 nm, causing underestimation of fetal disease.

Meconium staining is a sign of fetal distress and is an indication for prompt delivery. Presence of methemalbumin indicates longstanding marked hemolysis and depletion of haptoglobin and is a sign of impending fetal demise.

Table 21–2. FREDA MANAGEMENT TABLE*

Optical Density Difference 450 nm	Grade	Interpretation
0–0.20	1+	Fetus unaffected or mildly affected by hemolysis
0.20–0.35	2+	Fetus definitely affected but not in jeopardy
0.35–0.70	3+	Fetus in distress
0.70 and greater	4+	Impending fetal demise

*Modified from Freda, V. J.: Prog. Hematol., *5*:266, 1966.

Precautions in Interpretation of Pigment Analysis

The clinical pathologist should bear in mind that the obstetrician who performs amniocentesis may have technical problems in obtaining fluid when the placenta and fetus are difficult to localize or when the infant is hydropic. Under these circumstances, the fluid submitted to the laboratory may not be amniotic in origin. Thus, fetal ascitic fluid, fluid from the amnion of an unaffected or affected fraternal twin, amniotic cyst (chorionic bleb) fluid, and urine from the maternal urinary bladder may be aspirated. The most common non-amniotic fluid obtained is maternal urine. (The spectrophotometric tracing is similar to normal amniotic fluid, except that there is a much steeper slope to the curve.) Normal maternal urine may be distinguished from amniotic fluid by urea nitrogen or creatinine measurements. Urine urea nitrogen should approximate a concentration of 300 mg/dl or higher; amniotic fluid urea nitrogen averages about 30 mg/dl. Urine creatinine concentration is over 10.0 mg/dl, whereas amniotic creatinine is about 2.5 mg/dl.

A simple bedside means of distinguishing maternal urine from amniotic fluid is as follows: a protein-glucose dipstick is positive for both solutes when wetted with amniotic fluid, but negative when wetted with urine unless there is maternal diabetes and renal disease. (The dipstick test is also useful as a bedside procedure to determine whether a patient in labor has ruptured membranes or urinary incontinence.) The crystalline arborization test for amniotic fluid may also be used. (Amniotic fluid, when allowed to dry on a glass slide, precipitates a "branching-snowflake" deposit.) Such testing should be confirmed by urea or creatinine analysis. Creatinine or urea analysis should *always* be performed on submitted fluid to establish that the specimen is amniotic in origin. Other pitfalls in analysis involve clinical and laboratory quality control problems.

Specimens may alter with exposure to light or change in pH, or they may contain interfering pigments. There are differences in instruments, calibration, and methods. Varying dilution occurs in fluids of different patients at different gestational ages. Obstetric success is often attributable to the coupling of vigorous clinical management and laboratory monitoring via repeated amniocenteses.

THE CLINICAL PROBLEM OF ASSESSING FETAL LUNG MATURITY

The lungs are among the last of the fetal organs to mature. Accordingly, presence of mature lungs will usually indicate that other organs are also prepared for birth. Fetal lung maturity is evaluated by measurement of a detergent-like substance, surfactant, which lines the alveoli. Intrauterine respiratory movements cause surfactant to diffuse from the unexpanded, nonfunctional lung to the amniotic fluid. Following amniocentesis surfactant may be measured as described below. Once the baby is born, surfactant decreases the work of breathing by lowering the surface tension within the air sacs, reducing resistance to expansion during inspiration, and avoiding alveolar collapse during expiration. A deficiency in the amount and/or function of surfactant in neonates leads to the development of respiratory distress syndrome (RDS). This condition claims 20,000 lives in the United States every year. Babies with RDS struggle to inflate their air sacs during inspiration, and the air sacs tend to collapse completely during expiration. This results in hypoxia, acidemia, and other complications.

Mechanical ventilators assist the newborn with RDS but may overinflate the lungs, causing alveolar rupture, interstitial emphysema, and bronchopulmonary dysplasia. The administration of high concentration of oxygen to the baby can also produce blindness.

Thus, third-trimester amniocentesis and evaluation of fetal pulmonary maturity provide an invaluable method which enables the obstetrician to select among many therapeutic alternatives: await maturation, perform cesarean section, induce labor, allow premature labor to proceed unhindered, administer drugs capable of inducing lung maturity.

Classifying the Small Fetus

The small fetus can be assigned to one of two major groups: the small for gestational age (SGA) fetus and the appropriate for gestational age (AGA) fetus. The SGA fetus is one that is smaller than expected for its gestational age. It often dies *in utero* or at delivery. The SGA fetus produces an adequate surfactant and mature lungs, but usually suffers from placental insufficiency. The appropriate management of the SGA fetus would involve planned delivery as soon as possible. If delivery is delayed, the frequency of stillbirth will increase.

The AGA fetus is small because it is young, i.e., gestation is actually earlier than expected. If the AGA fetus is delivered too soon, it will often suffer from pulmonary immaturity and RDS. The appropriate management of the small AGA fetus is to postpone the delivery. If postponing delivery (i.e., preventing premature labor) is unsuccessful, then it may be possible to give steroids to the mother to induce pulmonary maturation of the fetus.

Establishing the distinction between the SGA and the AGA fetus is critical (Sher, 1983). Amniotic fluid surfactant testing has a particularly important role in distinguishing AGA from SGA fetuses among small babies. Presence of surfactant indicates maturity in the SGA setting but not in the AGA setting. Thus, amniotic fluid surfactant tests are useful in suggesting early delivery in the case of the SGA fetus.

Amniotic Fluid Surfactant

During the last trimester of pregnancy, fetal lung enzyme systems mature, initiating the production and secretion of surfactant by type II alveolar pneumocytes.

Prenatal fetal breathing movements promote the passage of surfactant from the fetal airways into the surrounding amniotic fluid. Approximately 150 ml of tracheal contents reaches the amniotic fluid per day.

Biochemical Properties of Surfactant. Table 21–3 presents the major phospholipid components of surfactant. Approximately 75 per cent of the surfactant consists of lecithin (phosphatidyl choline), about 10 per cent consists of phosphatidyl glycerol (PG), and the remainder consists of various acidic phospholipids and sphingomyelin. The major surface active phospholipid is lecithin. Furthermore, the disaturated form, dipalmitoyl phosphatidyl choline, appears to be the surface active phosphatidyl choline *in vivo*.

Table 21–3. CHEMICAL COMPOSITION OF PULMONARY PHOSPHOLIPIDS AT TERM

Phospholipid	Per cent
Phosphatidyl choline	73–88
Phosphatidyl glycerol	4.9–11
Acidic phospholipids	1.8–4.2
Phosphatidyl ethanolamine	2–7
Sphingomyelin	1.5–1.7

Over the past five years a second phospholipid, PG, has gained importance from a functional and diagnostic point of view.

Sphingomyelin does not appear to have any major surface active properties. Phosphatidyl inositol (PI) tends to have a peak concentration in amniotic fluid approximately five weeks before term and then decreases during the last five weeks of gestation.

Functional Measurement of Surfactant. Table 21–4 lists various laboratory methods used to measure functional surfactant. These methods do not measure the phospholipids specifically, but test the biophysical properties of surfactant present in amniotic fluid.

Tests of Surface Tension-Lowering Ability. In 1975, a simple method was introduced in which surfactant was concentrated by solvent extraction and microliter amounts of the extract were added to a water surface. The surface tension was then measured by means of a DuNuoy tensiometer (Tiwary, 1976). A modification of the method eliminated the need for repetitious measurement, and clinical correlations of surface tension measurements have demonstrated its validity. Measurement of surface tension-lowering ability is subject to the same limitations, with respect to centrifugation and to contamination from blood or meconium, as most other surfactant analyses (see below: Biochemical Assays).

Capillary Flow Rate. Twenty μl of uncentrifuged amniotic fluid may be aspirated into a Pasteur pipette and placed vertically on Whatman filter paper. The retention time of the amniotic fluid in the pipette is directly related to the amount of surfactant in the amniotic fluid (Singh, 1980). This simple method is subject to interference by blood or meconium contamination. Correlation with clinical outcome has not been reported.

Optical Density. The presence of suspended particles of surfactant lamellae in amniotic fluid increases the turbidity of "mature" specimens. In one study, high amniotic fluid optical density correlated well with a mature (over 2.0) L/S ratio. (The L/S ratio is discussed under Biochemical Assays.) Because of potential interferences caused by light absorption of bile pigments, recent studies have compared L/S ratios with the optical density measurement at 650 nm rather than at lower wavelengths. However, correlation of OD_{650} with the L/S ratio has ranged from excellent to poor (Arias, 1978). Polyhydramnios causes dilution and may cause falsely depressed optical density measurements. Class B diabetics show false low optical densities as compared with mature L/S ratios. The assay is simple and rapid, but is subject to problems related to variables in centrifugation. It is likely subject to interference by blood and meconium contamination, although these issues have not been analytically addressed.

Table 21–4. FUNCTIONAL METHODS USED TO MEASURE SURFACTANT

1. Surface-tension lowering ability
2. Capillary flow rate
3. Optical density
4. Microviscosity measurements
5. Foam stability
   a. Simple shake tests
   b. Manual foam stability index (FSI)

Microviscosity Measurements. In 1976, a fluorescent hydrocarbon probe, 1,6-diphenyl-1,3,5-hexatriene (DPH), was used to assess the microviscosity of amniotic fluid (Shinitzky, 1976). DPH polarizes incident light (365 nm) in an aqueous environment, emitting light at a wavelength greater than 418 nm. When mixed with amniotic fluid, DPH becomes embedded in lipid bilayers or liposomes. The extent to which DPH is free to rotate in this hydrophobic environment is dependent upon the microviscosity of the liposomal environment. The greater the viscosity, the more effectively the liposome resists the rotation of the DPH molecule. Restricted rotation of DPH results in depolarization of the incident light which can be measured with a specially designed instrument. This technique is an excellent correlate of the L/S ratio in artificial liposomal dispersions of biologic phospholipids. Physiologically relevant concentrations of PG, phosphatidyl serine (PS), and PI alter microviscosity in a predictable manner, and clinical trials indicate usefulness (Blumenfeld, 1979).

The fluorescence polarization method reportedly is not affected by amniotic fluid dilution (Golde, 1980). The effect of centrifugation on the amniotic fluid prior to analysis has not been evaluated, but lipids in amniotic fluid contributed by the presence of blood or meconium significantly affect the liposomal microviscosity (Blumenfeld, 1979). Instrumentation is specialized and expensive.

Foam Stability Assays. One of the most studied and least understood properties of surfactant is its ability to form stable foams. Proteins, free fatty acids, and other biological materials can form relatively stable foams when air is introduced into an aqueous solution. Adding ethanol to the mixture acts as an antifoaming agent for most biological compounds. Most biochemical compounds are unable to maintain a bubble with lower surface tension than exists at the air-solvent interface when ethanol is present. Surfactant phospholipids, however, produce surface tensions lower than the 29 dynes/cm of ethanol-water mixtures (47.5 per cent vol/vol), and therefore can produce stable bubbles. To the extent that surface tension contributes to the collapse of the bubble structure, the presence of surfactant phospholipids will prolong the life of the bubble.

The Simple Shake Test. The shake test involves adding equal volumes of 95 per cent (vol/vol) ethanol and amniotic fluid, shaking vigorously for 15 seconds, and observing the meniscus of the fluid 15 minutes

3

Table 21–5. ESSENTIAL FEATURES OF THE SIMPLE SHAKE TEST

1. Amniotic fluid is prepared without centrifugation
2. One part amniotic fluid and one part ethanol are combined
3. The mixture is agitated
4. The mixture is allowed to settle for a stated period of time
5. The air-liquid interface is evaluated for the presence or absence of a stated quantity of foam (bubbles)
6. The results are reported as either "positive" (presence of bubbles) or "negative" (absence of bubbles)

later for the presence of a complete ring of bubbles (Clements, 1972). In the absence of interference from other compounds, the presence of stable bubbles is an indication of the presence of saturated phosphatidyl choline: DSPC. The assay is made semi-quantitative by serially diluting the amniotic fluid prior to mixing with the ethanol. Clements' shake test is comparable to the L/S ratio in predicting fetal pulmonary status. Modifications using other concentrations of ethanol change the final alcohol volume fraction of the mixture and the threshold of a positive test. Table 21–5 summarizes the essential features of the simple shake test.

The Manual FSI Test. A more sensitive semi-quantitative assay, the foam stability index (FSI) test followed the shake test (Sher, 1978). Table 21–6 presents the essential features of the manual FSI test.

In practice this assay differs from the Clements test, which is positive for dipalmitoyl phosphatidyl choline values greater than 30 μg/ml (undiluted test at a final ethanol volume fraction of 0.475), while the FSI test also measures surfactant between the ranges of 15 μg/ml and 30 μg/ml in the amniotic fluid. The ability to quantitate in this lower range may provide useful clinical information. An FSI value of 0.48 is analogous to a L/S ratio of 2.0 in correlating with fetal pulmonary maturity. Decreasing FSI values below 0.48 indicate progressively increasing risk of respiratory distress. In general, the FSI and surface tension–lowering ability of amniotic fluid correlate with each other and with DSPC concentration (Statland, 1979).

The FSI test has been used along with measurement of fetal biparietal diameter on ultrasound to discriminate the AGA from the SGA fetus (Sher, 1983). The combination of a fetal biparietal diameter (by ultrasound) less than 8.5 cm and an FSI value of greater than or equal to 47 was detected in SGA in 16 of 19 cases. When the FSI value was less than 47, 19 of 19 were examples of AGA. The 12 cases of RDS in this series occurred only when the fetus was AGA and when the FSI value was less than 47. The discriminating ability of the FSI test separating AGA and SGA is not significant when the biparietal diameter is greater than or equal to 8.5 cm.

Table 21–6. ESSENTIAL FEATURES OF THE MANUAL FSI TEST

1. Amniotic fluid is centrifuged and the supernatant is used for further analysis
2. A series of ethanol–amniotic fluid mixtures are made such that the percentage of ethanol (ethanol volume fraction) will vary between 42 and 55 per cent (0.42 and 0.55)
3. Each mixture is agitated for 30 seconds
4. The individual tubes are evaluated for the presence or absence of a ring of stable bubbles
5. The highest ethanol volume fraction which supports the presence of a stable ring of bubbles is defined as the foam stability index (FSI) value

Biochemical Assays for Fetal Pulmonary Maturity. Gluck and coworkers produced the first practical chemical laboratory test to assess fetal pulmonary status by examination of amniotic fluid surfactant (Gluck, 1971).

Prior to approximately 35 weeks' gestation, the major component of pulmonary surfactant is alpha-palmitic beta-myristic lecithin, but at approximately 35 weeks dipalmitic lecithin (L) predominates (see DSPC, above). Recall that a second major phospholipid is phosphatidyl glycerol (PG), constituting more than 10 per cent of surfactant phospholipids in the adult. While PG is not a necessary component of surfactant, it appears that surfactant with PG maintains alveolar stability (Hallman, 1976). Other minor surfactant components include phosphatidyl inositol (PI) phosphatidylethanolamine (PE), sphingomyelin (S), and phosphatidylserine (PS). *Concentration* of PI in amniotic fluid increases with L/S ratio until about 36 weeks, when PG appears. Before PG appears, PI is an indicator of the concentration of surfactant present in amniotic fluid. However, at this time surfactant is functionally immature. Appearance of PG heralds secretion of mature surfactant. The maturation process is rapid and occurs over several days. The sphingomyelin content in amniotic fluid is relatively constant during the third trimester of pregnancy. Thus, sphingomyelin was proposed as a convenient reference phospholipid against which changes in surfactant lecithin concentration could be measured. The L/S ratio avoids problems associated with expressing surfactant concentration per amniotic fluid volume. Thin-layer chromatography for L/S in amniotic fluid has become the standard against which all subsequent surfactant tests have been compared.

Brief Description of Thin-Layer Chromatography L/S Ratio Test. Surface active phospholipids are extracted from amniotic fluid with organic solvent and purified by precipitation with cold acetone. After redissolving this precipitate in organic solvent, the extract is chromatographed on silica with an appropriate solvent. Phospholipids separate and are visualized by charring on a hot plate, and quantitated by reflectance densitometry.

Problems, Sources of Error, and Limitations of L/S Ratio. Major Pre-analytic Considerations. 1. Amniotic fluid samples collected vaginally, following rupture of membranes, may be dissimilar to samples obtained transabdominally. The L/S ratio in vaginal pool samples is significantly higher (22 per cent) or lower (15 per cent) Bonbroski, 1981). Reasons for this lack of agreement include potential for dilution by vaginal mucus or other secretions, possible contamination by semen, and effects of vaginal epithelium, foreign substances, and urine. (The L/S ratio of urine is 1.0.)

2. Site of amniotic fluid tap: Amniotic fluid specimens sampled near the fetal mouth may be higher in surfactant concentrations than those sampled near the feto-caudal region (Worthington, 1978).

3. Centrifugation time and speed: Phospholipid content of amniotic fluid supernatant will decrease as the centrifugal force, used to prepare the specimen for analysis, is increased. Surfactant is adsorbed to particulates suspended in the fluid.

4. Sample contamination by blood or meconium. Specimens with a hematocrit over 1 per cent yield unreliable results even when there is no visible hemolysis and when the red cells are removed (Badham, 1975). Hemolyzed samples should also be interpreted with great caution, particularly in borderline-mature cases, because the L/S ratio of plasma is approximately 2.0. Obviously mature ratios of 3.0 or more may still be useful in the presence of small amounts of blood or hemolyzed blood contaminants. The effect of meconium on the L/S ratio has been shown by some to be without effect (Gerbie, 1972), while others have found that meconium either increases or decreases the L/S ratio (Brown, 1982). Meconium can also prevent clear separation of lecithin and sphingomyelin on chromatography.

5. Water-soluble dye used in amniography, a radiologic technique used to visualize the fetus, will falsely increase the L/S ratio (Knox, 1976).

Analytic Considerations. Specific conditions of the chromatographic separation, phospholipid visualization, and quantitation may produce significant variations in the L/S result. Methods using cold acetone precipitation may produce results differing from those which do not. Solvent ratios in chromatography affect separations of the lecithin, sphingomyelin, and other phospholipids. Staining agents used to visualize phospholipid spots on the thin layer plate may also produce variability because of differences in the chemical affinity for lecithin and sphingomyelin. Finally, methods of quantitating the lecithin and sphingomyelin vary. Quantitation is usually by visual determination, planimetry, or densitometry.

Clinical Usefulness of L/S. Interpretation of the L/S ratio depends on an understanding of the problems in the test already described and, especially, on which variant of the test is used. One must understand how the laboratory derived its cut-off point which separates a normal fetus from one likely to develop RDS. Many method variants are described in which clinical condition of the neonate was not correlated with the L/S!

While the possible sources of error alluded to above are considerable, it is generally accepted that L/S ratios greater than 2.0 are not associated with life-threatening RDS in more than 95 per cent of cases. Overall, L/S ratios of less than 2.0 may be associated with significant RDS in about 25 per cent of cases.

Although the clinical usefulness of the L/S ratio has been established in uncomplicated gestations in which uncontaminated specimens have been used, three major problems of the L/S ratio have remained and stimulated the search for more reliable tests:

1. There has been a high incidence of false-negativity—i.e., predicted immaturity (L/S less than 2.0) when neonatal respiratory function is normal.

2. In complicated pregnancies such as maternal diabetes, it appears that an L/S ratio of over 2.0 is not a guarantee of functional maturity of neonatal lung (Freer, 1981).

3. L/S has been unreliable in samples contaminated by blood or meconium. This shortcoming of the L/S ratio (and most other tests for surfactant maturity) may be overcome, since *other* surfactant phospholipids may be used to predict pulmonary maturity even in the presence of contamination. PG and PI are virtually absent from blood and meconium. Thus, bloody amniotic fluid may prove to be a particular indication for the "lung profile" over the L/S ratio alone.

Lung Profile. Acetone-precipitated lipid extract is chromatographed in two dimensions on thin layer plates of silica gel H containing 5 per cent ammonium sulfate. Relative amounts of lecithin, sphingomyelin, PG, PI, PS, and PE are measured densitometrically after charring. Density readings for all phospholipids are added together, and relative quantities of PG and PI are expressed as percentages.

Sources of Error and Limitations of Lung Profile. Pre-analytic variables involve the preliminary centrifugation step, site of sampling within the amniotic fluid sac, and type of sample (vaginal vs amniotic sac). Unlike the L/S test, PG detection is affected by dilution of amniotic fluid by water.

Technical variations in test performance, including type of plate, developing solvents, and visualization of spots by charring or color reagents, may significantly affect apparent percentage of PG and whether or not it is detected (Freer, 1981).

Clinical Evaluation. In a study of 215 normal pregnancies there were no cases of RDS following findings of a mature amniotic "lung profile" (Kulovich, 1979b). Only 4 of 43 infants whose amniotic fluid showed immature lung profiles did develop RDS. *Presence of PG indicates no RDS will occur,* but PG in amniotic fluid is a late marker of fetal-lung maturity. Therefore, postponing delivery until PG appears in the amniotic fluid may be unnecessary and even hazardous since delay may lead to fetal deterioration.

In pregnancies complicated by maternal diabetes, the presence of PG in surfactant in amniotic fluid has been offered as the criterion for delivery since it appears to eliminate the risk of RDS regardless of the class of diabetes (Kulovich, 1979a). A concentration of 3 per cent PG or more has been suggested as the point above which RDS will not occur. However, in practice any distinctly visible PG spot on a chromatogram likely indicates fetal pulmonary maturity (Wenk, 1981).

Delayed appearance of PG is of little concern during the 35- to 37-week period when the L/S ratio has just reached the maturity mark of 2.0. This is particularly important in diabetics, especially Class A, B, and C (Kulovich, 1979a). In other common complications of pregnancy such as premature rupture of membranes and severe toxemia there usually is *accelerated* lung maturation. This is reflected by both early increase of

Table 21–7. CONDITIONS IN PREGNANCY AFFECTING FETAL PULMONARY MATURATION*

Conditions Hastening Surfactant Production	Conditions Delaying Surfactant Production
Maternal	
Poor nutrition	Advanced maternal age
Cardiovascular disease	Renal disease
Hypertension (or toxemia)	Collagen disease
	Hepatic disease
Placental abruption	Syphilis
Placenta previa	Toxoplasmosis
Drug addiction	Anemias
Diabetes (some)	Diabetes (some)
Placental	
Premature rupture of membranes	Polyhydramnios
Fetal	
Anomalies (various)	Hypothyroidism
Hemoglobinopathies	Male sex
Intrauterine growth retardation	Twin pregnancy
	Isoimmunization
Female sex	

*From Wenk, R. E.: Check Sample ACC 80–4 (ACC–36) *Amniotic Fluid Phospholipids.* Chicago, The American Society of Clinical Pathologists, 1980. Used by permission.

the L/S ratio to more than 2.0 and early appearance of PG. Table 21–7 summarizes the effects of gestational complications on pulmonary maturation.

Disaturated Phosphatidylcholine (DSPC) Analysis. Biochemically, 70 per cent of surfactant consists of dipalmitoyl lecithin (phosphatidylcholine), the major surface active component of which is DSPC. The selective assay of DSPC is a recent, attractive approach because it measures the primary surfactant phospholipid (Torday, 1979). The test is subject to the same preanalytic considerations as the L/S ratio. Dilution of amniotic fluid *in vivo* or *in vitro* may also affect results. Finally, use of only DSPC ignores possible information from presence of other important surfactant phospholipids, such as PG.

The major advantages claimed for this assay are that blood and meconium contamination of the amniotic fluid samples do not affect the test, and the test is reliable in complicated pregnancies such as diabetes mellitus.

Clinical Usefulness of the Test. With uncontaminated specimens from women with uncomplicated pregnancies, there is no difference in reliability between the L/S and DSPC tests. However, among 322 specimens, 75 per cent of which were either contaminated or obtained from women with complicated pregnancies, the predictive value of an L/S ratio of greater than 2.0 was 95 per cent and the predictive value of a positive DSPC test (greater than 5 mg/L) was 99 per cent. Moreover, the DSPC test may be a significantly better predictor of RDS than the L/S ratio, and may be up to 83 per cent predictive. Acceptance of this procedure must await wider clinical application and confirmation of these initial results.

Table 21–8 summarizes a wide array of tests for amniotic fluid surfactant, only some of which have been discussed. Biochemical, immunologic, ultracentrifugal, and modified coagulation tests have been described.

PERINATAL INFECTION

Congenital Infections. One fifth of perinatal deaths (worldwide) are caused by infections (MacVicar, 1979). Many are congenital, i.e., acquired transplacentally or when the fetus passes through the birth canal (Table 21–9).

Of major concern to the obstetrician is exposure of a pregnant woman to rubella. Presence of antibody (titer 8) indicates immunity. Recent infection is indicated by presence of IgM antibody and rise in titer. (Rubella has also been cultured from amniotic fluid.) Therapeutic intervention in the first trimester may be recommended on the basis of history and laboratory tests.

Syphilis is also of diagnostic concern because treatment of the mother usually prevents congenital infection and its sequelae. Laboratory testing of pregnant women is usually required by law.

The fetus is at risk for herpes throughout gestation when the mother has primary or recurrent disease. Greatest risk occurs during parturition, especially when active genital lesions are present. Diagnosis, by cytologic examination of vesicular fluid or by culture, is possible within hours to several days in many cases. Cesarean section may prevent fetal infection during delivery.

Other congenital infections are difficult to diagnose, prevent, or treat so that screening in pregnancy is controversial (Schoenbaum, 1979).

Premature Rupture of Fetal Membranes. This common event may predispose to amnionitis. Although amniotic fluid is inhibitory to bacterial growth, meconium staining and massive bacterial inoculation predispose to it. The incidence of apparent infection increases with duration of rupture (over eight hours), although many women with intact membranes show bacterial growth and evidence of subclinical infection (Ledger, 1979). Amnionitis places the fetus at risk, but there are currently no certain criteria by which infection is diagnosed.

Currently, positive Gram stains and bacterial culture of amniotic fluid obtained transabdominally are indications for treatment with antibiotics. Amniocentesis is performed in women with premature rupture of membranes whose delivery must be delayed over eight hours (Garite, 1979). Culture of such fluid yields a variety of aerobes and anaerobes, often in mixed culture. Organisms commonly include streptococci, staphylococci, anaerobic cocci (Peptococcus and Streptococcus), coliforms, and anaerobes of the Bacteroides and clostridial groups. Quantitative culture methods, cytologic analysis, and presence of certain organic acids may test for chorioamnionitis in the future (Editorial, 1982).

Determining Amniotic Sac Rupture. Ruptured membranes increase the risk of infection, but it may be difficult to decide clinically if rupture has occurred. To identify released amniotic fluid, appropriate vagi-

Table 21–8. COMPARISON OF REPRESENTATIVE METHODS FOR ANALYSIS OF AMNIOTIC FLUID SURFACTANT*

Method	Principles	Advantages	Disadvantages
1. Thin-layer chromatography	Extraction of amniotic fluid, TLC separation of surfactant phospholipids, detection and quantitation of each component	Long-term tested against clinical outcome; reference procedure	Manual procedure
L/S ratio	Lecithin content compared with sphingomyelin	Simple, rapid, inexpensive; no special instrumentation; dilution no problem	False positives common; imprecise quantitation; amniographic dye interferes
Phospholipid profile	L/S, PG, and PI evaluated	More accurate than L/S; blood interference reduced	Dilution reduces PG content
Disaturated phosphatidyl choline	Extraction of amniotic fluid, OsO_4 treated; TLC separation of phospholipids, stain and quantify	Blood interference reduced; more accurate than L/S	Time consuming or special instrumentation required; dilution may reduce saturated lecithin
2. Other physical methods			
Surface tension foam stability index	Surfactant increases stability of bubbles, interferes with antifoam properties of alcohols, decreases surface tension of air-water interface.	Measures all surfactant phospholipids; simple, rapid bedside test; little blood interference in some methods	Many indeterminate values; false positives; many interferences (blood and vaginal secretions); technique difficult to control
Fluorescence polarization	Fluorescent marker absorbed into phospholipids in a fluid; polarized light induces fluorescence; phospholipid decreases microviscosity of fluids; marker is free of rotate; degree of polarization of fluorescence is increased in proportion to phospholipid surfactant	Rapid; accuracy similar to L/S	Requires special equipment; interference by blood contamination

*From Wenk, R. E.: Check Sample ACC 80–4 (ACC–36) *Amniotic Fluid Phospholipids.* Chicago, The American Society of Clinical Pathologists, 1980. Used by permission.

nal fluid specimens should be subjected to Papanicolaou (Pap) staining and cytologic evaluation. If the Pap stain cannot be performed, a combination of history, alkaline pH (7.0 or greater), and positive crystallization test (see above) are sufficient.

NEURAL TUBE DEFECTS

The development of the spinal cord requires closure of the ectodermal neural tube. Failure of closure results in such defects as anencephaly, spina bifida, encephalocele, and myelocele. Normally, the fetal liver manufactures large quantities of an albumin-like protein, alpha fetoprotein, which circulates in the fetal vasculature and escapes into amniotic fluid from fetal urine. Alpha fetoprotein (AFP) reaches the maternal circulation in very small amounts by diffusion across the amnion and placenta. When there is a severe, open neural tube defect (NTD), the AFP is clearly increased in the maternal circulation about 80 per cent of the time (Brock, 1972). Thus, testing (by

Table 21–9. CONGENITAL INFECTIONS

Viral	Bacterial	Fungal	Parasitic
Cytomegalovirus	Listeria	Candidiasis	*Toxoplasma gondii*
Rubella	Syphilis		Malaria
Hepatitis B	Tuberculosis		Trypanosomiasis
Herpes type 2	Salmonella		
Rubeola	Group B Streptococcus		
Vaccinia	Gonococci		
Western equine encephalitis	Brucella		
Coxsackievirus B	Borrelia		
Chlamydia trachomatis	Tularemia		
	Staphylococci		
	Anthrax		

Table 21–10. CONDITIONS ASSOCIATED WITH INCREASES IN MATERNAL SERUM AFP

Gestational age underestimated	Tetralogy of Fallot
Open neural tube defects	Hydrocephaly
Fetomaternal hemorrhage	Hydrops fetalis
Omphalocele	Twin pregnancy
Congenital proteinuric nephropathies	Turner's syndrome
Sacrococcygeal teratoma	Cystic hygroma
Duodenal atresia	Cyclopia
Intrauterine death	Microcephaly
Esophageal atresia	Gastroschisis
	Maternal malignancy producing AFP

RIA) of the mother's *serum* AFP between 16 and 18 weeks serves as an indicator of possible NTD. Because there is overlap of AFP values in normal cases and NTD cases, because other defects may be associated with increased AFP (Table 21–10), and because AFP concentrations increase markedly during the testing interval, great pains are taken to avoid errors in gestational sampling dates, test procedures, and interpretation. AFP is analyzed in amniotic fluid when it is certain that serum AFP is increased. (Amniotic fluid testing may be carried out without serum testing in families at risk for the disease: families with previously affected children or from certain regions of the world.)

Close patient-physician-laboratory relations are important. When, during general screening, AFP is increased in maternal serum, the test is repeated on a second sample collected a week later. If the second test is positive, sonography is performed to correct gestational age, demonstrate twins, and demonstrate gross anomalies. When normal ultrasound results are observed, AFP concentration is determined in amniotic fluid. (Fetal blood must be absent.) If AFP is increased, acetylcholinesterase activity is determined to confirm the findings (or a second amniocentesis is carried out for AFP retesting). Acetylcholinesterase of fetal origin also escapes into amniotic fluid in neural tube defects. It can be shown to be increased by electrophoretic methods. Nonspecific cholinesterase of fetal plasma does not interfere (Smith, 1979). Since the isoenzyme originating in fetal spinal fluid gives an independent estimate of risk of NTD, it greatly increases the predictive values of amniotic fluid analyses for presence or absence of NTD (Wald, 1982). The isoenzyme analysis has been helpful in samples contaminated with fetal blood, and decreases false positives (Haddow, 1981).

ESTROGEN MEASUREMENTS

Estriol assays have been used to assess fetoplacental function since the early 1960's (Green, 1963). Numerous clinical studies have indicated that maternal plasma (serum) or urinary estriol assays appeared helpful in management of high risk pregnancies, either alone or in combination with antepartum fetal heart rate monitoring and amniotic fluid tests of fetal maturation.

Biosynthesis of Estriol by the Fetoplacental Unit. Estriol is unique among hormones synthesized during pregnancy because its formation depends upon a sequence of biochemical reactions involving both the placenta and fetus. Adequate formation of estriol depends on the integrated function of a fetoplacental unit (Diczfalusy, 1962). In late pregnancy, approximately 90 per cent of the estriol produced and excreted originates in the fetoplacental unit. Estriol is synthesized in the placenta from dehydroepiandrosterone (DHEA) and 16-hydroxydehydroepiandrosterone (16-OHDHEA), which are produced as sulfates by the fetal adrenal cortex.

In the placenta, DHEA sulfate and 16-OHDHEA are hydrolyzed to remove the sulfate and then metabolized to estriol. Estriol then crosses the placenta to reach the maternal plasma, where most of it is conjugated with glucuronic acid in the maternal liver and excreted in maternal bile. Some of the conjugated estriol is excreted in the maternal urine, but that which reaches the intestine is split by bacterial enzymes. This is followed by reabsorption of unconjugated estriol into maternal plasma by the enterohepatic circulation.

In maternal plasma, about 80 to 90 per cent of estriol circulates as the glucuronide conjugate and 10 to 15 per cent as unconjugated or "free estriol." The term "free estriol" is actually a misnomer; in plasma, about 70 per cent of conjugated and unconjugated estriol is bound to sex hormone–binding globulin (SHBG). This protein also binds testosterone, dihydrotestosterone, estrone, and estradiol.

Changes in maternal plasma and urine estriol concentrations reflect fetoplacental unit changes, but biochemical variables in the mother and laboratory procedures influence measured maternal estriol results. Causes of low estriol concentration in maternal plasma or urine are summarized in Table 21–11.

Not all maternal compartment changes result in *low* estriol concentrations. A decrease in maternal hepatic conjugation results in an *increase* in unconjugated plasma estriol but a *decrease* in total plasma and urinary estriol levels. Impaired maternal renal function is associated with an increase in total plasma estriol levels and a decrease in urinary estriol excretion (Goebelsmann, 1979).

Laboratory Aspects of Estriol Measurement. Laboratory methods are available to measure total plasma estriol, unconjugated plasma estriol, or estriol in urine. Commonly used chemical assays for estriol in urine are, in fact, assays for total estrogens, but this lack of specificity is usually not a problem since estriol constitutes about 85 to 90 per cent of all estrogens in the urine of late pregnancy.

A 24-hour urine measurement appears to correlate better with fetoplacental size than either unconjugated or total plasma estriol in diabetic pregnancies and, possibly, in prolonged gestation and intrauterine growth retardation (Distler, 1978).

To avoid the requirement of obtaining accurately timed urine collections, some authors have recommended measurement of estrogen/creatinine ratios in

Table 21–11. CAUSES OF LOW ESTRIOL EXCRETION*

Fetal Compartment	Placental Compartment	Maternal Compartment	Laboratory
Fetal death *in utero* (values rapidly falling)	Placental dysfunction	Incomplete urine collection	Assay error
Anencephaly†	Placental sulfatase deficiency†	Oral antibiotic administration‡	Mandelamine in urine (prevents bacterial splitting or reabsorption of estriol)
Adrenal hypoplasia†	Placental infarcts	Corticosteroid administration§	
Fetal abnormalities	Hydatidiform mole	Renal disease (low urinary estriol)	
Maternal corticosteroid administration§		Liver disease (low total plasma and urinary estriol)	

*Modified from Brown, J. B., Beischer, N. A., and Quinn, M. A.: J. Endocrinol., *89*:95, 1981.
†Values approximately 2 mg per 24 hours and constant.
‡Values may be two thirds normal.
§Values may be half normal.

random urine samples, but both urinary estriol and creatinine excretion appear to vary throughout a 24-hour period. Thus, an estriol/creatinine ratio does not adequately correct for fluctuations in urinary estriol excretion measured in a random urine specimen (Catagiri, 1976).

Plasma estriol measurements have major advantages over urinary estriol. They (1) do not require accurately timed urine collections; (2) are less affected by changes in glomerular filtration rate, which are common in mothers with diabetes, toxemia, and hypertension; and (3) are not affected by drugs, which may cause destruction of urinary estriol during acid hydrolysis (Trolle, 1977).

If plasma measurements are used, measurement of unconjugated estriol may be preferable to total estriol because unconjugated estriol has a plasma half-life of only eight minutes in maternal plasma as compared to a much longer half-life for the conjugates (Klopper, 1978). A sudden decrease of fetoplacental estriol production will result in a rapid fall of unconjugated maternal plasma estriol but a slow decline of conjugates. Thus, there is a more protracted fall of total plasma estriol. Plasma estriol assays are also more convenient for the patient and her physician (who needs fairly rapid turn-around time) and for the laboratory, which now has available commercial immunoassay kits for reliable measurement of unconjugated plasma estriol. Plasma assays of unconjugated estriol will be used more frequently in the future. Urinary excretion of 1 mg/24 hr is approximately equivalent to 0.6 to 0.8 ng/ml of unconjugated plasma estriol. Normal ranges for plasma unconjugated estriol (Bashore, 1977) and urinary estriol (Ansari, 1977) are shown in Figure 20–5 (p. 500).

Clinical Applications. Estriol measurements are used primarily in high risk patients as methods of selecting those pregnancies requiring additional fetal evaluation (fetal heart rate monitoring, ultrasonography, amniotic fluid phospholipid analysis). The clinical indications for estriol testing are (1) poor obstetrical history (fetal abnormalities, stillbirth); (2) intrauterine growth retardation; (3) gestations complicated by pre-eclampsia, hypertension, renal disease, and diabetes mellitus; (4) antepartum hemorrhage; (5) dysmature pregnancy (SGA); and (6) abnormal fetal monitoring studies. The test appears to be of limited or no use in Rh-isoimmunization, trophoblastic disease, and multiple gestation (Goebelsmann, 1979).

Interpretation of Results. Normal plasma or urinary results almost always indicate fetal well-being and avoid unnecessary obstetric intervention that could result in delivery of a premature infant and/or unnecessary cesarean section following failed induction or nonpropagation of labor. An abnormal estriol result, on the other hand, is quite frequently, but not always, associated with increased perinatal morbidity and mortality. With few exceptions, a low unconjugated or total plasma or urinary estriol value (below the 95 per cent confidence limit) suggests intrauterine growth retardation (IUGR) and/or fetal distress. A single estriol determination is of limited use. Serial estriol measurements in relation to the "normal pregnancy curve" (see Fig. 20–5) provide greater sensitivity and specificity than single tests.

In general, a day-to-day decrease of 35 to 50 per cent is considered a significant fall in plasma or urinary estriol measurements. The frequency of estriol testing depends on the underlying complication for which estriol is being measured in a particular pregnancy. In maternal diabetes mellitus, there may be a precipitous decline in fetoplacental estriol production. Serial monitoring is recommended twice weekly during weeks 32 to 34 to establish a baseline, and daily thereafter until delivery (Distler, 1978).

In severe hypertensive disorders of pregnancy and IUGR, estriol levels are decreased but the fall is usually less precipitous than that seen in maternal diabetes. Serial monitoring of estriol levels two or three times per week is sufficient. A reliable sign of IUGR is failure of any one of the three types of estriol measurements to rise during the last four to six weeks of pregnancy (Goebelsmann, 1979).

Prolonged gestation (over 294 days) may produce an increased risk of perinatal morbidity and mortality. Estriol concentrations in plasma and urine normally increase steadily to term and then decline after 40 weeks. This decline proceeds rather slowly, so that estriol assays are performed twice each week. Pattern and absolute estriol levels are useful in identifying pre-term, term, and post-term pregnancies as well as the fetus at risk. Rising serial estriol levels rule out prolonged pregnancy and postmaturity; plateauing estriol results are consistent with 40 to 41 weeks of gestation; and declining estriol levels are consistent with prolonged gestation. Low levels and/or significant falls are observed in postmaturity and fetal distress. Safe levels, above which fetal well-being is virtually assured, have been published for both 24-hour urinary estriol and unconjugated plasma estriol, but laboratory results are dependent on the assay used, particularly for urinary estriol excretion. Measurement of unconjugated plasma estriol levels of over 12 ng/ml rules out postmaturity in prolonged gestations otherwise uncomplicated by diabetes, IUGR, isoimmunization, or other conditions (Goebelsmann, 1979).

OTHER DETECTORS OF FETAL DISEASE

Hormones. Human placental lactogen is of limited value in determining fetal risk, but only when clinical history is unavailable (Wenk, 1979a). Human chorionic gonadotropin, despite its relevance in early pregnancy and in trophoblastic disease, is of almost no value late in gestation.

Antibody-Mediated Disease. Both allo- and autoimmune responses of the mother can affect the fetus. IgG antibodies cross the placenta and combine with fetal antigens. Alloimmune fetal and newborn diseases include hemolytic disease of the newborn (Rh_o, ABO, other), alloimmune thrombocytopenia ($P1^{A1}$), and alloimmune neutropenia (NA1, NA2, NB1, NC1). Autoimmune perinatal diseases include thrombocytopenic purpura, myasthenia gravis, Graves' disease, systemic lupus erythematosus, and autoimmune hemolytic anemia.

Diagnosis of the disease in the mother is important for perinatal management and reduction of fetal risk (Schanfield, 1981).

INTRAPARTUM BLOOD GAS ANALYSIS OF THE PRESENTING FETAL PART

During labor, capillaries of the presenting fetal part (usually scalp) may be sampled to measure pH and Pco_2. These measurements give direct evidence of fetal acidosis (Saling, 1965). Skin surface electrodes are also available to measure tissue Po_2 transcutaneously. Measurements may not be representative of the state of overall fetal oxygenation, since the presenting part may be compressed during labor and the scalp is intermittently ischemic (O'Connor, 1979). Thus, caution is warranted when interpreting laboratory values.

Generally, fetal hypoxia is detected by monitoring of the heart rate. Thirty seconds of bradycardia or tachycardia, late decelerations, or repeated early decelerations of increasing depth and deviation are signs of hypoxia. Scalp pH is measured when indicated by the cardiac monitor. Normal pH is 7.25 to 7.45.

Values below 7.25 should be confirmed by repeat analysis (Lumley, 1971). Spurious results may occur owing to maternal acid-base balance, fetal scalp edema, specimen contamination with amniotic fluid, or improper instrument calibration. On verification, low pH is an indication for obstetrical intervention. Decrease in pH to below 7.20 on *repeat* analysis is a strong indication of fetal deterioration. Clinical decision-making would be faster and technically less problematic when continuous intrapartum pH monitoring becomes available (Simkovich, 1981).

ACOG: Technical Bulletin No. 17: Management of Erythyroblastosis. Chicago, American College of Obstetricians and Gynecologists, 1972.

Ansari, A. H., and Fuller, D. G.: Urinary estriol for assessment of fetoplacental function. South. Med. J., *70*:142, 1977.

Arias, F., Andrinopoulos, G., and Pineda, J.: Correlation between amniotic fluid optical density, L/S ratio, and fetal pulmonary maturity. Obstet. Gynecol., *51*:152, 1978.

Badham, L., and Worth, H. G. J.: Critical assessment of phospholipid measurement in amniotic fluid. Clin. Chem., *21*:1441, 1975.

Bashore, R. A., and Westlake, J. R.: Plasma unconjugated estriol values in high-risk pregnancy. Am. J. Obstet. Gynecol., *128*:371, 1977.

Betke, V. K., and Kleihauer, E.: Foetaler and bleibender Blutfarbstoff in Erythrocyten und Erythroblasten von menschlichen Feten und Neugeborenen. Blut Bank., *4*:241, 1958.

Bevis, D. C. A.: The antenatal prediction of hemolytic disease of the newborn. Lancet, *1*:395, 1952.

Blumenfeld, T. A., Cheskin, H. S., and Shinitzky, M.: Microviscosity of amniotic fluid phospholipids and its importance in determining fetal lung maturity. Clin. Chem., *25*:64, 1979.

Bonbroski, R., MacKenna, J., and Brame, R.: Comparison of amniotic fluid lung maturity profiles in paired vaginal and amniocentesis specimens. Am. J. Obstet. Gynecol., *14*:461, 1981.

Brock, D. J. H., and Sutcliffe, R. G.: Alpha fetoprotein in the antenatal diagnosis of anencephaly and spina bifida. Lancet, *2*:197, 1972.

Brodersen, R., Jacobsen, J., Hartz, H., Rebbe, H., and Sorensen, B.: Bilirubin conjugation in the human fetus. Scand. J. Clin. Lab. Invest., *20*:41, 1967.

Brown, L., and Duck-Chong, C.: Methods of evaluating fetal lung maturity. CRC Crit. Rev. Clin. Lab. Sci., Jan 1982, pp. 85–159.

Cassady, G., and Barnett, R.: Amniotic fluid electrolytes and perinatal outcome. Biol. Neonat., *13*:155, 1968.

Catagiri, H., Distler, W., Friemann, R., and Goebelsmann, U.: Estriol in pregnancy. IV. Normal concentrations, diurnal variations, and day-to-day changes of unconjugated and total estriol in late pregnancy plasma. Am. J. Obstet. Gynecol., *124*:272, 1976.

Clements, J. A., Platzer, A. C. G., and Tierney, D. F.: Assessment of risk of respiratory distress syndrome by a rapid test for surfactant in amniotic fluid. N. Engl. J. Med., *286*:1077, 1972.

Diczfalusy, E.: Endocrinology of the fetus. Acta Obstet. Gynecol. Scand. (Suppl.), *41*:45, 1962.

Distler, W., Gabbe, S., Friemann, R., Mestman, J., and Goebelsmann, U.: Estriol in pregnancy vs unconjugated and total plasma estriol in the management of pregnant diabetic patients. Am. J. Obstet. Gynecol., *130*:424, 1978.

Editorial: The bacteriology of amnionitis. Lancet, *2*:591, 1982.

Freda, V. J.: Recent obstetrical advances in the Rh problem. Bull. N.Y. Acad. Med., *42*:474, 1966.

Freer, D. E., and Statland, B.: Measurement of amniotic fluid surfactant. Clin. Chem., *27*:1629, 1981.

Gambino, S. R., and Freda, V. J.: The measurement of amniotic fluid bilirubin by the method of Jendrassik and Grof. Its correlation with spectrophotometric analysis. Am. J. Clin. Path., *46*:198, 1966.

Garite, T. J., Freeman, R. K., Linzey, E. M., and Bradly, P.: The use of amniocentesis in patients with premature rupture of membranes. Obstet. Gynecol., *54*:226, 1979.

Gerbie, M., Gerbie, A., and Boehm, J.: Diagnosis of fetal maturity by amniotic fluid phospholipids. Am. J. Obstet. Gynecol., *114*:1078, 1972.

Gluck, L., Kulovich, M. V., and Borer, R. C.: The interpretation and significance of the lecithin-sphingomyelin ratio in amniotic fluid. Am. J. Obstet. Gynecol., *120*:142, 1974.

Gluck, L., Kulovich, M. V., Borer, R. C., Brenner, P. H., Anderson, G. G., and Spellacy, W. N.: Diagnosis of the respiratory distress syndrome by amniocentesis. Am. J. Obstet. Gynecol., *109*:440, 1971.

Goebelsmann, U.: The uses of estriol as a monitoring tool. Clin. Obstet. Gynecol., *6*:223, 1979.

Golde, S. H., and Mosley, G. H.: A blind comparison study of the lung phospholipid profile, fluorescence microviscosimetry, and the lecithin/sphingomyelin ratio. Am. J. Obstet. Gynecol., *136*:222, 1980.

Goldkrand, J. W., Varki, A., and McClurg, J. E.: Surface tension of amniotic fluid lipid extracts: Prediction of pulmonary maturity. Am. J. Obstet. Gynecol., *128*:591, 1977.

Green, J. W., and Touchstone, J. C.: Urinary estriol as an index of placental function. Am. J. Obstet. Gynecol., *85*:1, 1963.

Haddow, J. E., Morin, M. E., Holman, M. S., and Miller, W. A.: Acetylcholinesterase and fetal malformations: Modified qualitative technique for diagnosis of neural tube defects. Clin. Chem., *27*:61, 1981.

Hallman, M., and Gluck, L.: Phosphatidylglycerol in lung surfactant. III. Possible modifier of surfactant function. J. Lipid Res., *17*:257, 1976.

Klopper, A. I., Buchan, P. C., and Wilson, G. R.: The plasma half life of placental hormones. Br. J. Obstet. Gynaecol., *85*:738, 1978.

Knox, E., Todd, K., and Cassady, G.: The effect of amniography on amniotic fluid L/S ratio. Obstet. Gynecol., *49*:154, 1976.

Kulovich, M., and Gluck, L.: The lung profile. II. Complicated pregnancy. Am. J. Obstet. Gynecol., *135*:64, 1979a.

Kulovich, M. V., Hallman, M. B., and Gluck, L.: The lung profile. I. Normal pregnancy. Am. J. Obstet. Gynecol., *135*:57, 1979b.

Ledger, W. J.: Premature rupture of membranes and maternal-fetal infection. Clin. Obstet. Gynecol., *22*:329, 1979.

Liley, A. W.: Errors in the assessment of hemolytic disease from amniotic fluid. Am. J. Obstet. Gynecol., *93*:485, 1963.

Lumley, J., Potter, M., Newman, W., Talbot, J. M., Wakefield, E., and Wood, C.: The unreliability of a single estimation of fetal scalp blood pH. J. Lab. Clin. Med., *77*:535, 1971.

MacVicar, J., and Kerr, M. M.: Maternal disease, infection, trauma, rhesus isoimmunization. Lancet, *2*:1284, 1979.

O'Connor, M. C., Hytten, F. E., and Zanelli, G. D.: Is the fetus "scalped" in labour? Lancet, *2*:947, 1979.

Saling, E.: A new method of safeguarding the life of the foetus before and during labour. J. Int. Fed. Gynaecol., *3*:100, 1965.

Sbarra, A. J., Michlewitz, H., and Selvaraj, R. J.: Correlation between amniotic fluid optical density and L/S ratio. Obstet. Gynecol., *48*:613, 1976.

Schanfield, M. S.: Antibody-mediated perinatal diseases. Clin. Lab Med., *1*:239, 1981.

Schoenbaum, S. C.: Specific problems in diagnosis, prevention, and management of congenital infections. Clin. Obstet. Gynecol., *22*:321, 1979.

Sher, G., and Statland, B. E.: Assessment of fetal pulmonary maturity by the Lumadex™–foam stability index test. Obstet. Gynecol., *61*:444, 1983a.

Sher, G., Statland, B. E., Freer, D. E., and Kraybill, E. N.: Assessing fetal lung maturation by the foam stability index test. Obstet. Gynecol., *52*:673, 1978.

Sher, G., Statland, B. E., and Knutzen, V.: Identifying the small for gestational age fetus on the basis of enhanced surfactant production. Obstet. Gynecol., *61*:13, 1983b.

Shinitzky, M., Goldfisher, A., and Bruck, A.: A new method for assessment of fetal lung maturity. Br. J. Obstet. Gynaecol., *83*:838, 1976.

Simkovich, J. W.: Monitoring of fetal scalp pH. Clin. Lab. Med., *1*:215, 1981.

Singh, E. J.: Capillary method for assessment of pulmonary maturity in utero with the use of amniotic fluid. Am. J. Obstet. Gynecol., *136*:228, 1980.

Smith, A. D., Wald, N. J., Cuckle, H. S., Stirrat, G. M., Bobrow, M., and Lagercrantz, H.: Amniotic fluid acetylcholinesterase as a possible diagnostic test for neural tube defects in early pregnancy. Lancet, *1*:685, 1979.

Statland, B. E., and Freer, D. E.: Evaluation of two assays of functional surfactant in amniotic fluid: Surface tension lowering ability and the foam stability index test. Clin. Chem., *25*:1770, 1979.

Tiwary, C. M., and Goldkrand, J. W.: Assessment of fetal pulmonic maturity by measurement of the surface tension of amniotic fluid lipid extract. Obstet. Gynecol., *48*:191, 1976.

Torday, J., Carter, L., and Lawson, E. E.: Saturated phosphatidyl choline in amniotic fluid and prediction of the respiratory distress syndrome. N. Engl. J. Med., *301*:1013, 1979.

Trolle, D., Bock, J. W., and Gaede, P.: The prognostic and diagnostic value of total estriol in urine and in serum and of human placental lactogen hormone in serum in the last part of pregnancy. Am. J. Obstet. Gynecol., *126*:834, 1977.

Wald, N. J., and Cuckle, H. S.: Nomogram for estimating an individual's risk of having a fetus with open spina bifida. Br. J. Obstet. Gynaecol., *89*:598, 1982.

Weinstein, L.: Irregular antibodies causing hemolytic disease of the newborn. Obstet. Gynecol. Surv., *31*:8, 581, 1976.

Wenk, R. E., London, R., Siegelbaum, M., Lustgarten, J. A., and Goldstein, P. G.: A prospective evaluation of placental lactogen as a test of neonatal risk. Am. J. Clin. Path., *71*:72, 1979a.

Wenk, R. E., Lustgarten, J., and Byrd, C.: Simultaneous analysis of lecithin, sphingomyelin, and phosphatidyl glycerol in amniotic fluid using continuous development thin-layer chromatography. Clin. Lab. Med., *1*:210, 1981.

Wenk, R. E., Rosenbaum, J., and Henry, J. B.: Amniotic fluid and antenatal diagnosis. *In* Henry, J. B. (ed.): Clinical Diagnosis and Management by Laboratory Methods. 16th ed. Philadelphia, W. B. Saunders Co., 1979b, pp. 693–711.

Worthington, D., and Smith, T.: The site of amniocentesis and the lecithin spingomyelin ratio. Obstet. Gynecol., *52*:552, 1978.

22

SEMINAL FLUID

DONALD C. CANNON, M.D., PH.D.

Examination of seminal fluid is usually performed as part of a comprehensive infertility investigation involving both partners of a barren marriage. As a result of its relative simplicity, semen examination is often requested before the more complicated and expensive examination of the female. It is now apparent that inadequacies on the part of the male contribute to a significant percentage of infertility problems, estimated to be as high as 40 per cent by some investigators. Some cases of male infertility are now amenable to medical treatment.

In relation to the infertility investigation, it is important to recognize the proper scope of the semen examination. Most importantly, it is but one facet of the medical examination of the male, which must also include a detailed history and general physical examination. Such specialized procedures as studies of thyroid, adrenal, and pituitary functions or testicular biopsy may also be indicated. Not only must the results of the semen examination be interpreted in light of the remainder of the medical examination of the male; the female partner must be considered as well. Indeed, it has been suggested that for purposes of the infertility investigation the male and female involved should be considered not as individuals but as a reproductive unit. An inherent limitation of the semen examination is that the standards of semen quality are the result of population studies of males from fertile and infertile marriages. Consequently the standards of semen quality are relative, not absolute indications of fertility or sterility (with the single exception of complete aspermia). Furthermore, it is usually recommended that semen examination be repeated one or more times if an abnormal result is found.

In addition to infertility studies, the clinical pathology laboratory, particularly one actively engaged in forensic studies, may frequently be requested to examine vaginal secretions or clothing stains for the presence of semen in alleged or suspected rape. The semen examination can also be utilized to evaluate the effectiveness of vasectomy or to support or disprove a denial of paternity on the grounds of sterility.

PHYSIOLOGY OF SEMINAL FLUID

Semen is a composite solution formed by the testes as well as the accessory male reproductive organs and consists basically of spermatozoa suspended in the seminal plasma. The function of the seminal plasma is to provide a nutritive medium of proper osmolality and volume for conveying the spermatozoa to the endocervical mucus, whereupon its contribution to the fertilization process is ended. The seminal plasma also activates the spermatozoa to greater motility.

The components of semen are derived from the following organs:

Testis. Spermatozoa, which constitute less than 5 per cent of the semen volume, are the only cell type present in normal semen in any appreciable number. Spermatozoa are largely stored in the ampullary portions of the vasa deferentia until released in the process of ejaculation. Spermatozoa stored in the ampullae are rather inactive metabolically because of the acid environment and diminished oxygen supply. In this location it has been estimated that spermatozoa can survive for periods of up to one month.

Seminal Vesicles. Approximately 60 per cent of the semen volume is derived from the seminal vesicles. This viscid, neutral, or slightly alkaline fluid is often yellow or even deeply pigmented as a result of its high flavin content, which is responsible for the fluorescence of semen in ultraviolet light. The seminal vesicles are the major source of the high fructose content of semen, which is the major nutrient for the spermatozoa. The importance of other components, such as the relatively high potassium and citric acid content and smaller amounts of ascorbic acid, ergothioneine, and phosphorylcholine, has not yet been established. The seminal vesicle secretion is also important in providing the substrate responsible for the coagulation of semen following ejaculation.

Prostate. The prostate contributes about 20 per cent of the volume of semen. This milky fluid is slightly acid, with a pH of about 6.5, largely as a result of its high content of citric acid, which constitutes the major anion in this component of semen.

The prostatic secretion is also rich in proteolytic enzymes and acid phosphatase. These proteolytic enzymes are responsible for the coagulation and liquefaction of semen. Acid phosphatase can cleave phosphorylcholine present in the semen but the significance of this is not clear.

Epididymides, Vasa Deferentia, Bulbourethral Glands (Cowper's Glands), and Urethral Glands (Glands of Littré). Less than 10 to 15 per cent of the semen volume is contributed by these structures, and little is known of their biochemical significance in man. However, it is becoming increasingly clear that the epididymis secretes a number of proteins into the tubule lumen that are essential for sperm fertilizing capacity.

Fractions of Semen. The process of ejaculation results in the mixing of three distinct fractions of semen, which enter the urethra individually in rapid succession. These fractions differ as to anatomic origin and therefore also in chemical composition. The first fraction, which is of relatively slight amount, consists of a clear viscid fluid believed to originate largely or perhaps exclusively from the urethral and bulbourethral glands. The function of this component is not known with certainty, but it may be to cleanse and lubricate the urethra in preparation for the bulk of the ejaculate that is to follow. The second fraction consists largely of prostatic secretion along with most of the spermatozoa and relatively small amounts of secretions from the epididymides and vasa deferentia, which have been temporarily stored in the ampullae of the vasa deferentia. The final fraction consists almost entirely of a mucoid secretion resulting from emptying of the seminal vesicles.

An understanding of the temporal sequence of mixing of the various fractions in ejaculation is important to the proper conduct of the semen examination. For example, the use of semen samples obtained from the male urethra following coitus, as recommended by some investigators, will result in a specimen which is not only non-representative of the semen as a whole but is also apt to be relatively sperm poor. Furthermore, samples obtained by coitus interruptus can result in loss of part of the sperm-rich middle fraction, although it represents only a minor part of the total volume of ejaculate.

COLLECTION

It is usually recommended that the semen sample be collected following a three-day period of continence. Others have suggested that a more meaningful specimen is one collected after a period of continence equal to the usual frequency of coitus for the couple involved. Prolonged continence prior to the semen collection is to be discouraged because the quality of the semen, especially in regard to sperm motility, will actually diminish. Regardless of what method is employed for collection, the physician will be faced with occasional patients who will not comply because of religious or esthetic standards or who are unable to cooperate because of more complex psychologic considerations. The most satisfactory specimen is that collected in the physician's office or the clinical pathology laboratory by masturbation. This allows a complete examination of the semen, particularly of the process of coagulation and liquefaction, and also eliminates the possibility of cold shock. Acceptable but somewhat less satisfactory are specimens obtained in the patient's home by coitus interruptus or masturbation and delivered soon thereafter to the laboratory. With either method, the specimen can be collected in a wide-mouth clean glass jar supplied by the laboratory (to avoid the possibility of trace amounts of detergents or other harmful contaminants) or in suitable plastic or polyethylene containers such as those used for the collection of urine or sputum specimens. Specimens may be collected in condoms, which are then tied and placed in a clean glass jar. Valid objections to condom collection have been expressed because of the fact that powder or lubricants applied to the condoms or other material used in their manufacture may be actively spermicidal. If the condom is used, it must first be washed with soap and water, rinsed thoroughly, and then dried completely. Plastic sheaths* have been recommended as a means of avoiding the difficulties of condom collection.

In transporting specimens collected elsewhere to the laboratory, several precautions are necessary. First of all, the specimen must be received as soon as possible and in no case after more than two to three hours have elapsed following collection. It is essential that the semen specimen not be subjected to temperature extremes during delivery to the laboratory. The container should be warmed to body temperature prior to collection. It is desirable to keep the specimen at body temperature until liquefaction of the coagulum is complete (about 20 minutes).

GROSS EXAMINATION

Physical Characteristics. Freshly ejaculated semen is a highly viscid, opaque, white or gray-white coagulum, which has a distinct musty or acrid odor. Within 10 to 20 minutes the coagulum will spontaneously liquefy to form a translucent, turbid, viscous fluid, which is mildly alkaline, with a pH of about 7.7. The pH usually does not vary greatly. pH values of less than 7.0 are frequently associated with semen consisting largely of prostatic secretion due to congenital aplasia of the vasa deferentia and seminal vesicles. Increased or decreased turbidity is of little significance except when increased turbidity is the result of leukocytes associated with an inflammatory process in some part of the reproductive tract. With passage of time, colorless, needle-shaped crystals of spermine phosphate may form as a result of the reaction of spermine in the prostatic secretion with phosphoric acid formed from enzymatic cleavage of various organic phosphates.

Viscosity can be assessed while pouring the liquefied specimen from the collection container into the glass

*Milex Seminal Pouch, Milex Products, Chicago, Illinois.

3

graduate for volume measurement. The specimen of normal viscosity can be poured drop by drop. Increased viscosity is of significance if sperm motility is thereby compromised. Occasionally, increased viscosity is associated with poor invasion of the cervical mucus in postcoital studies and is the only demonstrable defect in an infertile couple.

Coagulation and Liquefaction. Coagulation and subsequent liquefaction is believed to be a three-stage process: (1) Coagulation results from the action of a prostatic clotting enzyme on a fibrinogen-like precursor formed by the seminal vesicles. (2) Liquefaction is initiated by enzymes of prostatic origin. (3) The protein fragments are degraded further to free amino acids and ammonia by the action of several poorly characterized proteolytic enzymes, including an aminopeptidase and pepsin. The coagulation process has diagnostic significance in that the semen from males with bilateral congenital absence of the vasa deferentia and seminal vesicles fails to coagulate because of the absence of the coagulation substrate. Liquefaction should be complete within 30 minutes. It is important to distinguish persistently increased viscosity from delayed liquefaction.

Volume. The normal semen volume averages 3 to 4 ml (MacLeod, 1951). Non-parametric analysis of the data of Nelson (1974) indicates a normal range of 0.7 to 6.5 ml. Paradoxically males associated with infertile marriages tend to have an increased rather than a decreased semen volume, which is frequently associated with a significantly diminished sperm count. Postcoital studies suggest, however, that greatly decreased semen volumes can result in poor penetration of the cervical mucus by the sperm. Semen volume does not vary significantly with the period of continence (MacLeod, 1951).

MICROSCOPIC EXAMINATION

Sperm Counts. Following liquefaction of the semen, the spermatozoa can be counted in a hemocytometer chamber following initial dilution in a white blood cell pipette. Mix the semen sample thoroughly and draw an aliquot to the 0.5 mark on the pipette. Dilute to the 11 mark with the following solution:

Sodium bicarbonate	5g
Formalin (neutral)	1 ml
Distilled water	100 ml

After charging the hemocytometer chamber, two minutes are allowed for the immobilized sperm to settle. The spermatozoa in 2 sq mm (two large squares) are counted. This number multiplied by 100,000 gives the number of spermatozoa per milliliter. The entire counting procedure including the initial dilution should be repeated at least once and the results averaged.

Considerable difficulty can be encountered in diluting semen of greatly increased viscosity. Under these circumstances the counting will be facilitated if the semen is diluted 1:1 with the mucolytic agent Alevaire (Breon Laboratories, Inc.) prior to pipette dilution and the final count is multiplied by two (Amelar, 1977).

The hemocytometer method of counting sperm is relatively imprecise. Freund (1964) found that duplicate sperm counts by the same technologist varied by a mean difference of 20 per cent. For counts performed by three technicians, each of whom used duplicate pipettings on the same sample, the 95 per cent confidence limit was ±52 per cent. In the author's experience, however, these variations seem unduly high.

Although it was formerly thought that sperm counts of less than 20 million per ml are abnormal, several recent studies of presumably fertile males clearly refute this assumption. The largest such study (Smith, 1978), involving 2543 males, indicates an overall range of 100,000 to 375 million per ml with a mean of 70 million and 19 per cent of individuals with counts less than 20 million. Sperm concentration increases with abstinence for at least the first 10 days with a daily incremental increase of 13 million per ml (Schwartz, 1979).

Motility. In order for the spermatozoa to penetrate the cervical mucus and subsequently migrate to fertilize the ovum in the fallopian tubes, active motility is necessary. To evaluate motility, a small drop of liquefied semen is placed on a microscope slide prewarmed approximately to body temperature and then covered with a coverslip which has been ringed with petrolatum. Motility can be evaluated by scanning several fields with the high dry objective until a total of at least 200 spermatozoa have been observed. It is essential to focus through the entire depth of a given field so as to include non-motile sperm that have settled to the bottom of the medium. The percentage of sperm showing actual progressive motion should be recorded. Some prefer to render a qualitative estimate of sperm motility. One approach assigns sperm to one of three categories: progressive motility, non-progressive motility, and non-motility. Those showing progressive motility are graded according to the following code: grade I, minimal forward progression; grade II, poor to fair activity; grade III, good activity with tail movements visualized; grade IV, full activity with tail movements difficult to visualize.

In their study of 732 fertile males, MacLeod and Gold (1951) found a mean sperm motility of 61 per cent contrasted with 54 per cent for 869 males associated with infertile marriages. These results are similar to those of a more recent study of 1300 fertile males (Rehan, 1975), which indicated an overall range of 5 to 95 per cent motile sperm with a mean of 65 per cent and a non-parametrically derived 95 per cent normal range of 20 to 90 per cent motility.

Some investigators have previously recommended motility estimates at intervals during the 24 hours following collection, e.g., 3, 6, 12, and 24 hours. The motile forms will decrease by about 5 per cent per hour after the fourth hour following collection. Since sperm must penetrate the cervical mucus within a few minutes following ejaculation (or be inactivated by the relatively low pH of the vaginal secretions), the seminal plasma is not a physiologic medium for prolonged evaluation of sperm activity. Furthermore, the metabolic activity of the sperm as well as bacterial growth will significantly alter the pH of semen after a few hours.

Sperm Morphology. Sperm morphology is evaluated by performing differential counts of morphologically normal and abnormal spermatozoa types on stained smears. Smears are prepared on clean microscope slides in a manner identical to blood films. The best stain for morphologic detail is the Papanicolaou stain (Fig. 22–1). Although somewhat complicated and time consuming, the Papanicolaou technique is to be recommended, particularly in the laboratory that uses this stain routinely for exfoliative cytology. It is essential that the smear be placed immediately into fixative, either 95 per cent (v/v) ethanol or 50 per cent (v/v) ethanol ether, before drying has occurred.

A method which is also satisfactory but gives somewhat poorer differentiation of sperm detail is the hematoxylin method described by Amelar (1977). In this method the film is air dried and then treated as follows: (1) 10 per cent (v/v) formalin, one minute; (2) water rinse; (3) Meyer's (or Harris) hematoxylin, two minutes; (4) water rinse; (5) air dry. Other staining techniques which have been recommended include Giemsa, basic fuchsin, and crystal violet. The last two named require preliminary heat fixing, which has been demonstrated to cause some degree of artifactual distortion of the spermatozoa.

At least 200 spermatozoa should be examined under oil immersion and the percentage of abnormal forms recorded (Fig. 22–2). In addition to sperm morphology, the presence of red blood cells, leukocytes, and epithelial cells should be noted. Immature cells of the germinal line can appear in the semen and must be differentiated from macrophages or leukocytes. Numerous granules and globules are normally present in semen. These presumably originate from the secretion of glandular cells or perhaps from autolysis of epithelial lining cells in the accessory reproductive structures.

As with motility and sperm concentration, previously stated criteria of normality for morphology have been overly rigorous. One study of 100 males of proven fertility indicated a mean of 73 per cent morphologically mature and normal sperm, an overall range of 21 to 90 per cent, and a non-parametrically derived normal range of 40 to 90 per cent (Sobrero, 1975).

OTHER TESTS OF SEMEN

Postcoital (Sims-Huhner) Test. This test consists of the examination of cervical mucus following coitus. It is intended as a measure both of the quality of cervical mucus and the ability of the spermatozoa to penetrate the mucus and maintain activity. The cervical mucus undergoes both quantitative and qualitative changes, which are correlated with the menstrual cycle. In the ovulatory phase at midcycle, the amount of mucus is maximum while the viscosity is significantly diminished, thus facilitating penetration of the mucus by the spermatozoa. Progesterone in the secretory phase causes increased viscosity of the mucus.

During the ovulatory phase, as determined by basal temperature records, the female is instructed to report to the physician within several hours of coitus. The

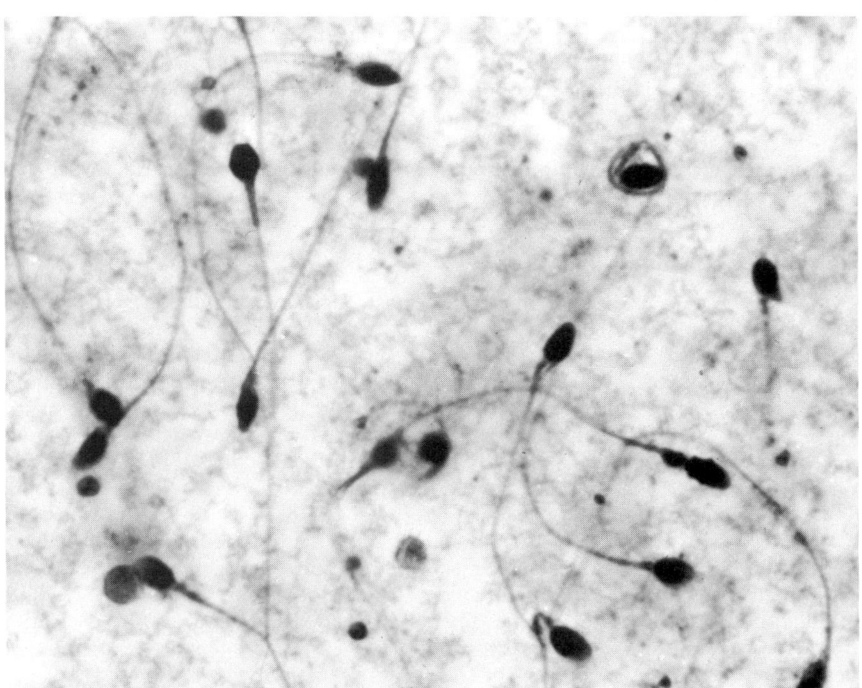

Figure 22–1. Normal spermatozoa. Papanicolaou stain; ×1580.

3

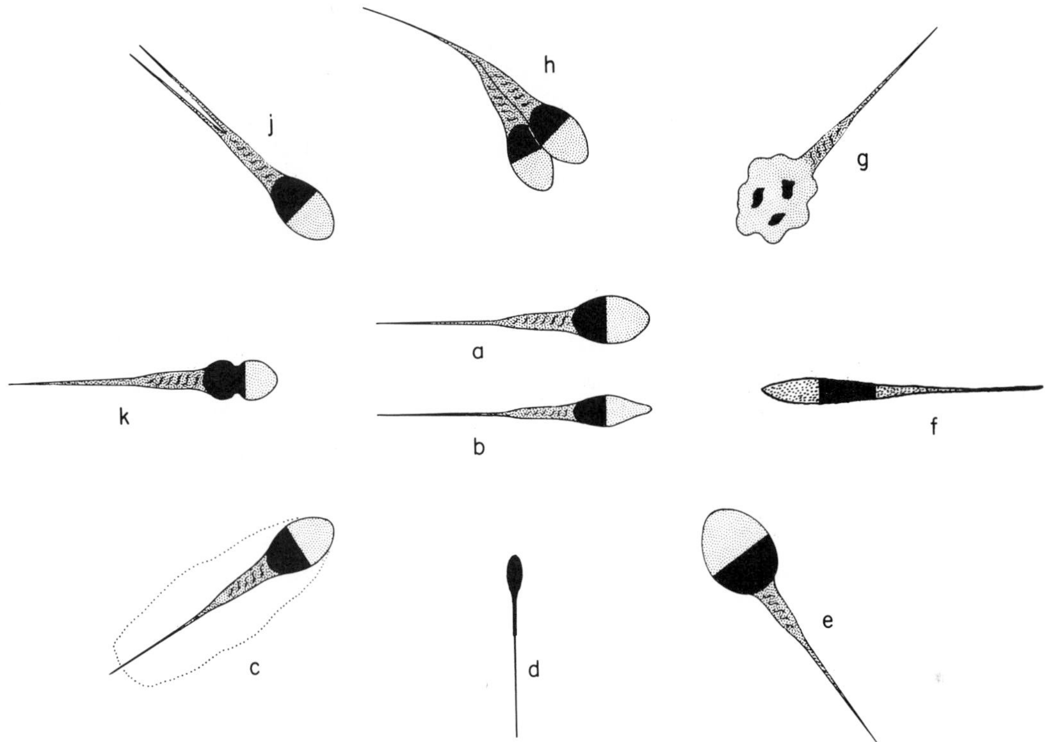

Figure 22–2. Diagrammatic representation of normal and abnormal spermatozoa. *a,* Normal, face view. *b,* Normal, lateral view. *c,* Immature spermatozoon (spermatid). *d-k,* Morphologically abnormal types: *d,* pin-head; *e,* giant head; *f,* acute tapering form; *g,* amorphous form; *h,* double head; *j,* double tail; *k,* constricted head. (Tails on all forms are disproportionately short.)

external cervical os is wiped clear of mucus. The endocervical mucus sample can be obtained by aspiration with a glass cannula attached by a rubber tube to a Luer syringe. The specimen can be delivered to the laboratory in the syringe. The volume of mucus is measured. Following discharge into a Petri dish, its color and viscosity are noted. At midcycle the mucus should be clear and watery. One further property that is commonly evaluated is the spinnbarkeit, which refers to the tenacity of the mucus. This is tested by grasping a portion of the mucus with forceps and noting the distance which it can be drawn before breaking. A good spinnbarkeit, which should prevail at midcycle, is at least 10 cm. A drop of mucus is then placed on a microscope slide, covered with a coverslip, and examined for the presence of sperm. An estimate of the number of sperm per high-power field with percentage of motile forms should be reported. Within six to eight hours after coitus at least 10 motile sperm should be present per high-power field (Moghissi, 1976). The material should also be examined for leukocytes, erythrocytes, and trichomonads.

The postcoital test typically shows better quality of mucus and better sperm penetration at the ovulatory phase than at other times in the ovulatory cycle. The degree of sperm penetration is correlated with the quality of semen as well as with the fertility of the mating, although the differences are usually not striking.

Antibodies to Spermatozoa. During the past two decades considerable interest has focused on the occurrence of antibodies to spermatozoa, both in males with semen abnormalities and in females of infertile marriages. The extensive experimental and clinical work in this complex and as yet rather poorly understood field has recently been reviewed by Jones (1980). Investigations thus far have established a firm immunologic basis for spermatozoal antibodies. There appear to be several antigens that are specific for the sperm cell line. Using immunofluorescence, antibodies have been found to react with four distinct regions of the spermatozoa: the front part of the acrosome, the post-nuclear cap, the equatorial segment of the acrosome, and the tail piece (Husted, 1975). Other techniques for detecting antibodies to spermatozoa include agglutination, immobilization, precipitation, complement fixation, passive hemagglutination, and cytotoxicity. Some of these techniques have not yet proved to be technically reliable, however, and widely variant results often occur among laboratories performing the same test.

A causal relationship between spermatozoal antibodies and disease has not been clearly established. The antibodies are found in some human males with testicular disease and also in association with autoimmune aspermatogenesis experimentally induced by immunization with spermatozoa, semen, or testicular homogenates and appropriate adjuvants. Sperm agglutinins appear in the sera of many men following vasectomy. In one study, sperm agglutinins occurred in 60 per cent of 52 men during the first year following vasectomy (van Lis, 1974). The significance of these antibodies remains an enigma.

There is by no means unanimity of opinion regarding the importance of spermatozoal antibodies in the serum of females, but available evidence strongly suggests a cause and effect relationship to otherwise unexplained infertility. One of the earliest and still controversial reports is that of Franklin (1964), who employed a straightforward agglutination reaction between serum and semen. Results were read microscopically after a four-hour incubation at 37°C. Using this method, antibodies were detected in the serum of 31 out of a group of 43 female partners of infertile marriages in which there was no other demonstrable cause for infertility in either husband or wife. In contrast, such antibodies were present in the female in only two of 35 fertile marriages. Antibodies were variously individual specific, in that they agglutinated only the husband's spermatozoa, or species specific, in that they agglutinated the spermatozoa of all males tested. The clinical importance of this test was further demonstrated by the fact that the antibody levels diminished markedly in each of 13 infertile females who were persuaded to practice continence or to restrict coitus to the use of condoms over a period of two to six months. Nine of these patients eventually became pregnant upon resumption of unrestricted coitus.

EXAMINATION FOR THE PRESENCE OF SEMEN

The clinical pathology laboratory may be requested to investigate material from the vagina or stains from clothing, skin, or hair for the presence of semen. Such cases will usually involve alleged rape or suspected sexual assault in association with homicide. In all medicolegal cases special precautions are indicated to identify specimens properly and to maintain the chain of evidence.

Obtaining the Sample. Secretions from the vagina can be obtained by direct aspiration or saline lavage. A preliminary scan with ultraviolet light is often helpful in selecting specific areas of clothing or other fabrics for further investigation. Semen stains frequently result in a green-white fluorescence, although this can occur with stains from other body fluids as well. A 1 sq cm portion of the stained fabric should be cut out and soaked in 1 or 2 ml of physiologic saline for one hour. The fluid from this washing can be subjected to further tests for semen. It is desirable to include as a control, particularly for acid phosphatase determination and the detection of blood group substances, a piece of fabric remote from the stain.

Examination for Sperm. Prior to aspiration or lavage it is desirable to prepare direct smears from the vagina for Papanicolaou staining. Alternatively, such smears can be prepared from the aspirate or lavage. Contrary to some expressed opinions, well-preserved sperm can be recovered from the vagina many hours after coitus and even from exhumed bodies if they have been properly embalmed. Smears should also be prepared from the washings of fabric stains. The wash fluid can initially be concentrated by centrifugation and a smear prepared from the sediment. Such smears can be stained with hematoxylin and eosin. The fragile tails of the sperm are frequently broken off, thus making identification somewhat more difficult.

Acid Phosphatase Determination. Acid phosphatase should be determined on the vaginal aspirate or lavage or on the wash fluid from stains. High values of acid phosphatase will render positive identification of semen even if the male involved is aspermic. Determination of acid phosphatase is significantly more sensitive than a microscopic search for spermatozoa in detecting intravaginal semen (Schumann, 1976). Seminal fluid averages about 2500 King-Armstrong units per ml of acid phosphatase, while other body fluids and extraneous foreign materials will have well under 5 units per ml. Acid phosphatase can be reliably determined on the wash fluid from stains that are many months old. The acid phosphatase method selected should have a high degree of specificity for prostatic acid phosphatase. (See Chapter 14.)

Detection of Blood Group Substances. In the case of positive identification of fluid or a stain as semen, the presence of A, B, or H blood group substances may be investigated. Approximately 80 per cent of individuals, those having the dominant secretor gene in homozygous or heterozygous state, will secrete the water-soluble form of blood group substances in body fluids, including semen. The identification of the specific substance is based on the ability of the semen partially or completely to neutralize the agglutinating activity of the specific antiserum. With this determination, it is possible on occasion to demonstrate that the seminal fluid of a suspect differs from that recovered from the victim.

Florence Test. This test is a preliminary screening method and has been largely replaced by the far more dependable acid phosphatase determination. It is usually performed on stains from clothing, other fabric, or hair and depends on the presence of choline, which is found in high concentration in seminal fluid. A portion of the stained sample is extracted with distilled water by using gentle heat. Several drops of the extract are placed on a microscope slide and treated with an equal volume of a reagent composed of the following: iodine, 2.54 g; potassium iodide, 1.65 g; distilled water, 30 ml. In a positive test, rhombic or needle-like crystals of periodide of choline will be noted. The test may yield false positive results because of the high choline content occasionally found in other tissue fluids of human or animal origin.

Other Tests. A precipitin test can be used to detect semen of human origin and is therefore helpful in rendering positive identification of semen stains on clothing. The test requires specific antiserum obtained by immunizing suitable animals with human semen and absorbing the non-specific antibodies with human serum. It is performed as a capillary tube precipitin reaction by overlaying the antiserum with washings from the stain.

Determination of the sperm-specific lactate dehydrogenase isoenzyme has been reported to provide a specific differentiation of human semen from other body fluids and from the semen of other animals (Mokashi, 1976).

Amelar, R. D.: Male Infertility. Philadelphia, W. B. Saunders Company, 1977.

Franklin, R. R., and Dukes, C. D.: Further studies on sperm-agglutinating antibody and unexplained infertility. J.A.M.A., *190*:682, 1964.

Freund, M., and Carol, B.: Factors affecting haemocytometer counts of sperm concentration in human semen. J. Reprod. Fertil., *8*:149, 1964.

Husted, S.: Sperm antibodies in men from infertile couples. Analysis of sperm agglutinins and immunofluorescent antibodies in 657 men. Int. J. Fertil., *20*:113, 1975.

Jones, W. R.: Immunologic infertility—fact or fiction. Fertil. Steril., *33*:577, 1980.

MacLeod, J.: Semen quality in one thousand men of known fertility and in eight hundred cases of infertile marriage. Fertil. Steril., *2*:115, 1951.

MacLeod, J., and Gold, R. Z.: The male factor in fertility and sterility. III. An analysis of motile activity in the spermatozoa of 1,000 fertile men and 1,000 men in infertile marriage. Fertil. Steril., *2*:187, 1951.

Moghissi, K. S.: Postcoital test: Physiologic basis, technique, and interpretation. Fertil. Steril., *27*:117, 1976.

Mokashi, R. H., and Madiwale, M. S.: The use of sperm-specific lactate dehydrogenase isoenzyme for the identification of semen in dried stains. Forensic Sci., *8*:269, 1976.

Nelson, C. M. K., and Bunge, R. G.: Semen analysis: evidence for changing parameters of male fertility potential. Fertil. Steril., *25*:503, 1974.

Rehan, N. E., Sobrero, A. J., and Fertig, J. W.: The semen of fertile men: Statistical analysis of 1300 men. Fertil. Steril., *26*:492, 1975.

Schumann, G. B., Badawy, S., Peglow, A., and Henry, J. B.: Prostatic acid phosphatase. Current assessment in vaginal fluid of alleged rape victims. Am. J. Clin. Path., *66*:944, 1976.

Schwartz, D., Laplanche, A., Jouannet, P., and David, G.: Within-subject variability of human semen in regard to sperm count, volume, total number of spermatozoa and length of abstinence. J. Reprod. Fertil., *57*:391, 1979.

Smith, K. D., Stultz, D. R., Jackson, J. R., and Steinberger, E.: Evaluation of sperm counts and total sperm counts in 2543 men requesting vasectomy. Andrologia, *10*:362, 1978.

Sobrero, A. J., and Rehan, N. E.: The semen of fertile men. II. Semen characteristics of 100 fertile men. Fertil. Steril., *26*:1048, 1975.

van Lis, J. M. J., Wagenaar, J., and Soer, J. R.: Sperm-agglutinating activity in serum of vasectomized men. Andrologia, *6*:129, 1974.

23

SPUTUM

DANIEL C. NIEJADLIK, M.D.

PHYSIOLOGY OF SPUTUM

Tracheobronchial secretions are an inconstant mixture of plasma, water, electrolytes, and mucin. As these secretions pass through the lower and upper respiratory tract, they become contaminated with cellular exfoliations, nasal and salivary gland secretions, and normal bacterial flora of the oral cavity. This mixture of secretions and particulate is collectively referred to as sputum.

The principal sources of tracheobronchial secretions are the surface epithelium and the submucous glands. Three secretory cell types can be distinguished within the surface epithelium: the serous cell, the Clara cell, and the goblet cell. The goblet cells are more numerous proximally in the upper respiratory tract. Between the surface epithelial cells and the cartilaginous plates are the submucous gland cells. The goblet cells produce a thick mucin type secretion which is diluted by a more serous mixture of acid glycoproteins, sialoproteins, and sulfoproteins secreted by the submucous glands. Both types of secretions are increased by vagal nerve stimulation and cholinergic drugs, although nerve impulses are not necessary for goblet cells to discharge their content.

Under appropriate immunologic or inflammatory stimulus, mast cells, eosinophils, and plasma cells may contribute to the secretions. An undetermined volume of the sputum occurs as a transudate from the plasma in mucosal capillaries and under normal conditions appears to be quite small. With severe inflammation, though, the tracheal fluid may virtually all be a plasma transudate.

The physical properties of sputum reveal the secretions to be viscoelastic, that is, some of the properties of a liquid and some of a solid. The consistency is dependent mainly on the molecular structure of the glycoproteins and on the degree of hydration. Sialic acid is the most important single component of sputum viscosity. Clinicians have long recognized that patients with chronic obstructive airway disease have greater difficulty in evacuation of secretions and that rehydration by water mist aerosol is followed by easier clearing of the respiratory tract.

Throughout the normal respiratory tract there is a two-layered mucous blanket with a fairly constant depth of 7 μm. The inner 5 μm layer lies beneath a 2 μm higher shear gel of greater viscoelasticity. This gel layer is impermeable to water and contains immunoglobulins to protect the underlying cilia and epithelium from toxic damage (Newhouse, 1976).

Chemical composition of the sputum reveals it to be composed of approximately 95 per cent water and 5 per cent total solids. The solids are primarily carbohydrates, proteins, lipids, and deoxyribonucleic acid (DNA). These solids increase in amount with increasing inflammation. The DNA originates from disrupted leukocytes, macrophages, and bronchial epithelial cells, and in some diseases such as cystic fibrosis may increase to thirty times normal levels. The DNA in sputum has little effect on either viscosity or elasticity. Numerous enzymes have been identified and studied in pathologic and normal sputum; among them are alpha$_1$-antitrypsin, arylsulfatase, complement lysozymes, and lactate dehydrogenase.

Although large numbers of viable microorganisms are inhaled, the lower respiratory tract is maintained virtually sterile. Two mechanisms are responsible: the alveolar macrophage system, and the mucociliary system. The alveolar macrophage system will be discussed later in this chapter.

The mucociliary system provides both a mechanical removal of inhaled organisms and an antimicrobial activity in the secretions within the mucus.

The mechanical removal of inhaled organisms depends on three mechanisms to maintain a continuous outward flow of sputum. The first mechanism is the tapering of the bronchial lumen to produce a vector force directed toward the larger diameter. When sputum impinges upon the wall, this force moves the sputum forward. The second mechanism is the continuous alteration in the diameter of the bronchial lumen produced by respiration. Again, a vector force is formed which leads to the expulsion of sputum. The final and most important mechanism is the effect of the ciliary border of the respiratory epithelium. The cilia move sequentially in metachronal waves and carry the sputum lining the bronchi outward to the oropharynx where it is imperceptibly swallowed. Expectoration of sputum then depends on cough. Excessive mucus can inhibit the action of the cilia. Increased "thickness" is noted in response to irritation or infection, as both gland cells and goblet cells increase in activity and number. Absent mucociliary function is not incompatible with a relatively normal existence, as shown from data in patients with Kartagener's syndrome, in which the cilia have defective radial spokes.

The antimicrobial activity of sputum is composed of many factors (Yeager, 1971). Lysozymes and secretory immunoglobulins are the principal secretions, with the latter the more important. Specific antibodies in the respiratory tract are predominantly dimeric IgA to which is attached an additional structure known as the secretory piece. This immunoglobulin is mostly produced locally by plasma cells in the mucosa, and the secretory piece is added by the epithelial cells in transport of the IgA across the mucosa and into the secretions. Small amounts of IgG are present. IgM is usually undetectable except in pneumonia, when it may be found in high concentrations. IgE reagin is predominantly synthesized locally in the mucous membranes. Currently, the only known function is to sensitize mast cells and basophils involved in the inflammatory response. Deficiency in either IgA production or attachment of the secretory piece significantly reduces the amount of immunoglobulin present and may render the individual more susceptible to increased infections of the respiratory tract. Also, the high or low pH of the secretions contributes to antimicrobial properties. Finally, systemically administered antibiotics diffuse into tracheobronchial secretions fairly effectively and are of importance in the laboratory when interpreting the results of a sputum culture.

SPECIMEN COLLECTION

Specimens labeled "sputum" seldom contain only lower respiratory tract secretions. Saliva, nasopharyngeal secretions, and bacteria or food particles often contaminate these specimens. Prerinsing the mouth prior to collection will remove most of these contaminants and will not affect the result of the bacteriologic examination. Sputum collection should be supervised by professional personnel familiar with the methods discussed later if proper clinical correlations are to be obtained.

For most examinations, a first morning specimen is best, since it represents the pulmonary secretions accumulated overnight. However, most tracheobronchial secretions are not ejected from the mouth, but are swallowed during sleep.

Contamination of the first coughed specimen may occur in catarrhal inflammation of the nasopharynx, as mucus may accumulate in the bronchi at night. Also gastric contents may enter the bronchi in patients with hiatal hernias who have slept in the recumbent position.

To obtain a proper specimen, the most important step is gaining the patient's cooperation and understanding. Usually no problems are encountered in adults, but in children lack of comprehension or cooperation presents a problem. To circumvent this, three different methods are widely used and advocated: In the first method a nasopharyngeal swab is obtained in children with bronchial disease and is said to be representative of the bronchial pathogens. Advocates of this method believe that the viral or bacterial pathogens affect the ciliated columnar epithelium of the nasal passages as well as the respiratory tract. In the second method a cough plate is held before the child's mouth and the child is urged to cough. The third and recommended method, the cough swab technique, is an easy procedure to do and gives the most representative, non-contaminated sputum sample. In this technique the child's mouth is held open with the aid of a tongue blade. The tongue is depressed and the visualized epiglottis is touched with a swab to induce a cough. Material from the trachea expelled from the cough deposits on the swab, and the swab is plated onto the appropriate culture medium. Contamination is avoided if the swab does not touch the nasopharyngeal walls.

In patients who are either non-cooperative or unable to produce sputum spontaneously, sputum induction is becoming a popular means of obtaining specimens. Induction both promotes an increased flow of bronchial secretion and stimulates a cough. Among the popular inductants are 10 per cent sodium chloride and sterile or distilled water aerosols. Propylene glycol in a 10 per cent concentration is usually added to the saline solvent to increase penetration and minimize evaporation of these particles. Acetylcysteine in combination with a bronchodilator is one of the more widely used inductants today. Acetylcysteine and other related drugs act by breaking disulfide bonds which aid in maintaining the gel structure of mucus.

The specimen should be collected in a sterile, disposable, impermeable container with a screw cap or tightly fitting cap or cork. After the patient expectorates the sputum into the container, care should be taken to see that no sputum has been smeared by the patient on the outsides of the container. The sputum specimen should be delivered to the laboratory immediately and not be allowed to stand. However, overnight storage of 4°C. does not affect the recovery of *Mycobacterium tuberculosis*. If 24-hour specimens are being collected for identification of tubercle bacilli or for volume measurements, a large mouth container can be used. Culturing for bacterial organisms is not recommended or suitable from these 24-hour collections.

Finally, to obtain a specimen in problem cases such as the patient with pneumonia who cannot raise a specimen or the patient with equivocal sputum culture findings, transtracheal aspiration is recommended. Contraindications for the procedure include uncooperative patients, hemorrhagic diathesis, severe uncontrolled cough, and cardiac arrhythmias. The major complications include bleeding, paratracheal infections, and subcutaneous emphysema. The clinical usefulness of the procedure must be weighed against the risk.

SPUTUM EXAMINATION

The importance of sputum examination was first documented by Hippocrates in the fifth century B.C. His observations of the sputum sample included color, taste, and smell for diagnostic and prognostic criteria in the treatment of patients. Today, good agreement has been noted between macroscopic type and cell counts, providing a scientific basis for the earlier subjective assessment.

The sputum specimen should be transferred to a sterile empty Petri dish placed against a dark background. Sterile disposable wooden applicator sticks are used to spread it thinly, and the specimen can be examined carefully with the naked eye or a hand lens.

Macroscopic Examination

With gross examination of the sputum the following macroscopic findings are of importance and should be noted.

Consistency and Appearance. Sputum may be described as liquid (serous), mucoid, purulent, bloody, or combinations of these, i.e., seropurulent, mucopurulent. Usually specific diseases have characteristic consistencies and appearances; e.g., in pulmonary edema, the sputum is often described as serous, frothy, and blood-tinged. In most normal sputum specimens, the appearance is clear and watery, and any opaqueness results from cellular material suspended in it. Most opaque particles are masses of pus and epithelium. Other infrequent material seen in sputum can be Curshmann's spirals, lung stones, Dittrich's plugs, caseous material, bronchial casts, or food substances. Particular attention should be paid to the examination of these opaque materials, as their presence may be the initial laboratory clue in the diagnosis of the disease.

Color. The color of sputum is determined by the material contained, and often the color can indicate the pathologic process. Sputum color, though, is an unreliable indicator of the cellular composition. A yellow color indicates pus and epithelial cells are present and is commonly seen in pneumonic processes. When coupled with a green tint, Pseudomonas may be implicated as the etiologic agent. Variation of the color red in sputum can be used as an aid in the differential diagnosis, too. Rust-colored sputum is due to decomposed hemoglobin and is seen in such diseases as pneumococcal pneumonia or pulmonary gangrene, while a bright red is found in recent hemorrhage secondary to a variety of diseases such as acute cardiac failure, pulmonary infarction, or extension of a tuberculous caseous lesion or neoplasm invading and rupturing a blood vessel.

Odor. Usually no odor is present in normal and pathologic sputums, but if bacterial decomposition has taken place within the body or after expectoration, a variety of odors will be present. Suppurative conditions such as lung abscesses, cavitary tuberculosis, or gangrene produce the most putrid odors.

Miscellaneous Findings. Other macroscopic findings which may be observed in sputum in certain diseases are listed below:

Cheesy Masses. These are fragments of necrotic pulmonary tissue primarily seen in such diseases as pulmonary gangrene or tuberculosis.

Bronchial Casts. These are branching treelike casts of bronchi whose size varies with that of the bronchi in which they are formed. They are frequently composed of fibrin and are white or gray in color. At one time bronchial casts were commonly seen during the consolidation stage of lobar pneumonia, but with the advent of drug therapy, they are rarely seen today. Their expulsion is similar to that of a foreign body.

Broncholiths (Lung Stones). These are usually formed by calcification of necrotic or infected tissue within a larger bronchus or cavity. Histoplasmosis is the most common cause for the formation of broncholiths. Other etiologies are tuberculosis, papillary carcinomas, sarcoidosis, and idiopathic microlithiasis. Characterization by analytical scanning electron microscopy may elucidate the underlying disease as the stones have different crystalline compositions (Pritzker, 1981). In addition, histological examination with special stains should be performed to identify possible organisms within the stone. Nevertheless, broncholiths are rarely present in sputum specimens.

Dittrich's Plugs. These are most frequently observed in putrid bronchitis and bronchiectasis. They occasionally are coughed up alone and appear as yellowish or gray caseous bodies which vary in size from the head of a pin to a navy bean. When crushed they are found to be composed of cellular debris, fatty acid crystals, fat globules, and bacteria.

Foreign Bodies. Infrequently, foreign bodies may be expelled during a violent coughing spell. In children, foreign bodies can be any small object a child may place into his mouth and inhale. Among the more common objects are peanuts and buttons. In adults, foreign bodies are either food particles or gastric contents aspirated during convulsions, drug intoxication, or operative anesthesia. Since seeds are frequently part of the average diet, the diagnosis of aspiration is simplified by demonstrating these vegetable particles in the sputum either by gross examination or with a periodic acid–Schiff (PAS) stain on microscopic examination.

Parasites. These are extremely rare in the United States and thus are infrequently seen in sputum. As worldwide travel increases, the laboratory is bound to see more in the future. Among the "common" ones in this country are *Ascaris lumbricoides, Echinococcus granulosus,* and *Toxocara canis.* In Japan *Paragonimus westermani,* the lung flukeworm, may be encountered, with ova found in sputum.

Microscopic Examination

After macroscopic examination is performed, all suspicious particles are transferred by a sterile instrument to a clear slide where they are examined unstained if necessary. The remaining portion of the specimen is cultured.

Examination of the stained specimen reveals best any bacteria and cells (Fig. 23–1). When making smears, it is best to air dry the smear first, then flame it to kill all infectious organisms before applying the Gram stain. Specialized stains for specific cells or organisms can also be made at this time, e.g., Wright's stain for blood cells, buffered crystal violet for bronchial epithelial cells, Ziehl-Neelsen stain for *M. tuberculosis,* Papanicolau stain for malignant cells, and so forth.

The presence of the alveolar macrophage is the best assurance that the material being examined arises from the lower respiratory tract, as macrophages have not been reported in the secretions of the upper respiratory tract. The nuclei of the alveolar macrophage are pyknotic, variable in size, and usually peripherally located. The cytoplasm often contains granules of carbonaceous material or has a foamy vacuolated appearance. Its presence is especially important as to specimen adequacy for cytology and/or culture for mycobacterial, fungal, or mycoplasmal illness.

Three types of cells from the bronchial epithelial layer may be noted. The basal bronchial epithelial cell is usually about the size of a lymphocyte and has the greatest nuclear to cytoplasmic ratio of the three forms. Columnar bronchial epithelial cells are seen in two forms. Both forms are rectangular, with one end tapered and containing a bulging nucleus. One form contains the ciliated border and is more common, while the other is the nonciliated goblet type and is infrequently seen.

Blood cells are best identified with a Wright or Giemsa strain. Neutrophils may be present as partially disintegrated cells in almost every sputum specimen, and their presence intact most frequently indicates a pyogenic infection. Eosinophils are found in large numbers in the sputum of patients with bronchial asthma, but their presence is not pathognomonic of asthma. Erythrocytes are usually present as contaminants in all sputums, but in large numbers indicate an exudate or hemorrhage.

The identification of bacteria in Gram-stained sputum and their significance will be discussed later in the chapter.

SPUTUM CULTURE

Microscopic examination should be performed to determine if sputum is acceptable for culture. Because physicians do not collect sputum from their patients, they are unaware of the adequacy of a specimen for culture. Numerous studies have shown that approximately 50 per cent of submitted specimens are contaminated with or are oropharyngeal secretions.

Bartlett (1974) has reported a procedure for evaluation of specimens collected for culture. Gram stains are examined for the presence of squamous epithelial cells and leukocytes to assess oropharyngeal contamination. Generally, those specimens containing mucus, fewer than 25 squamous epithelial cells, and at least 10 leukocytes per field (× 100 magnification) are acceptable for culture.

If microscopic examination is to be used as a guide for sputum culture, the clinician should be notified before a culture is discarded. Some patients may be immunocompromised and unable to mount an immune response, or the sample may be difficult to obtain, e.g., in children.

When culturing sputum for a possible pathogen, two methods can be used: The first and most popular is the classic technique of streaking on an agar plate. In our laboratory, each specimen is routinely plated in sheep blood agar, chocolate agar, MacConkey's agar, and thioglycolate broth. The plates are incubated

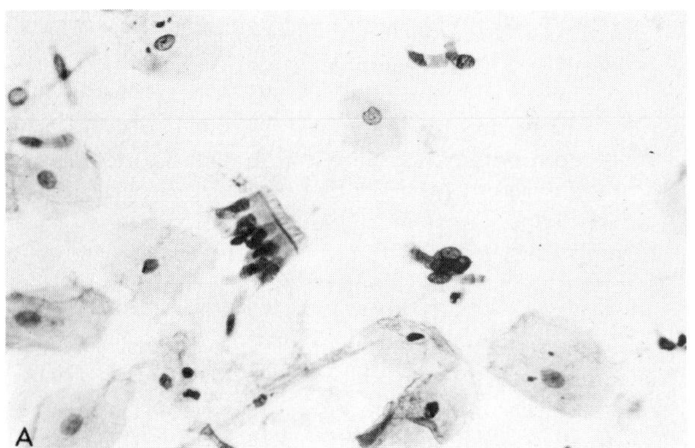

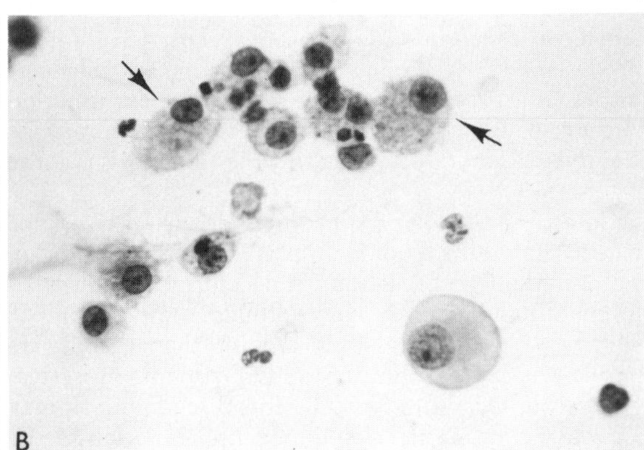

Figure 23–1. Cells commonly seen in sputum. Squamous and respiratory epithelial cells *(A)*. Alveolar macrophages (arrows) and an alveolar cell *(B)*. Appearance of macrophages indicates sample from lower respiratory tract. (Papanicolaou ×650.)

at 37°C. for 24 hours with the chocolate and blood agar plates in a 5 per cent carbon dioxide atmosphere. All known pathogens are identified and semiquantitated as to many, moderate, or few organisms present. The hypothesis underlying the streak method is that the pathogenic organism will be present in greater numbers than any other superficial contaminating organism. Specific identification of all pathogens is performed by standard methods described elsewhere in this book. If no pathogens are present, the predominating organism or normal flora is reported.

The culture should be correlated with the previous Gram stain. If many organisms were seen on Gram stain, but only scant numbers or no growth on culture, then either the culture method was inadequate or the flora was suppressed by antibiotics. Anaerobes require special attention (see Chap. 45).

The second method is quantitative analysis of the organisms present. The sputum is homogenized and various dilutions of the sample are made (Monroe, 1969). The method's hypothesis is that the organisms causing inflammation will be present in greater numbers than any other superficial contaminating organisms. Also, other problems such as overgrowth with *Proteus*, mixed infections, and even superinfections by a single organism are easier to identify.

The reluctance to adopt the method of quantitative analysis centers on the prolonged processing of the specimen required and the numerous agar plates needed.

MYCOBACTERIA

According to the National Tuberculosis Association, any mycobacterial disease of the lungs other than that caused by *M. leprae* can be designated as tuberculosis. In this country the etiologic agent is *M. tuberculosis* in 97 to 99 per cent of the cases, with the remaining ones caused by the atypical mycobacteria. In sputum examination no differentiation by various staining techniques can be made between *M. tuberculosis* and the atypical mycobacteria. For this reason, a culture should always be performed in a previously undiagnosed case of tuberculosis. Treatment and public health procedures are different for these organisms.

In the classic or fulminant forms of the disease, large amounts of mucopurulent sputum are raised. Evidence of pulmonary hemorrhage and particles of caseous and necrotic material are present. Within the caseous material, large numbers of bacilli are usually present. Staining procedures are best performed on this material for bacillus demonstration.

The problem confronting the laboratory centers on the recognition of the disease in its early stages. To aid in the early diagnosis, efforts have involved three parameters: (1) sputum induction and collection, (2) specimen concentration and decontamination procedures, and (3) organism demonstration by smear.

There are six types of respiratory specimens in use today: 24-hour sputum pool, early morning specimen, induced sputum, bronchial washings, transtracheal aspiration, and gastric aspiration.

In recent years, either early morning specimens or induced sputums have come into widespread use since they yield positive culture results earlier and are less contaminated. Gastric aspiration studies are obtained from uncooperative patients. Patients imperceptibly swallow sputum during the night. The aspirated material is obtained early in the morning and should be neutralized immediately since mycobacteria will not survive long periods in gastric acid. Transtracheal aspiration and bronchial washings should be reserved for special cases as in patients with lower lung field tuberculosis.

With the exception of the occasional stat requests for examination of acid-fast organisms, pretreatment of sputum by digestion procedures facilitates organism demonstration by (1) liquefying the sputum for a more even distribution of organisms, (2) lowering the specific gravity for centrifugation of the organism, and (3) decontaminating the specimen of other organisms to allow the maximal survival of the acid-fast organism.

The methods currently in use employ sodium hydroxide, N-acetyl-L-cysteine, Zephiran–trisodium phosphate (Z-TSP), or combinations thereof. Each method has its attributes, whether in preparation time, tubercle bacilli survival, or isolation rate. The various procedures may be found in a 1975 U.S. Department of Health, Education and Welfare publication, Procedures for the Isolation and Identification of Mycobacteria.

Preferably, slides should be stained by a modification of the Ziehl-Neelsen method (Z-N) and/or the auramine-rhodamine (A-R) stain.

Acid-fast staining offers rapid confirmation of infection and enables the clinician to begin chemotherapy immediately. Acid-fast staining should be considered only a screening procedure, the false positive rate varying from 3 to 55 per cent and the false negative rate from 19 to 78 per cent. The variation in detection may be explained by the decreased incidence of tuberculosis in the United States with a secondary deterioration of detection skills in interpreting smears.

The acid-fastness of mycobacteria is attributable primarily to mycolic acid in the outer capsule. At increased temperatures, basic fuchsin in phenol penetrates the capsule. The wax hardens and retains the dye during treatment with acid alcohol.

A second type of acid-fastness is attributable to the free hydroxyl and carboxyl groups of mycolic acid. This type accounts for the staining of pine pollen, keratohyalin, lead inclusion bodies, histoplasma, and lipofuchsin granules. Nocardia and certain proprionibacteria stain acid-fast by an unknown method.

At present the use of fluorescent microscopy is regarded as the most reliable method for the examination of acid-fast bacilli in smears. In 1962 Traunt described the auramine-rhodamine dye combination. Its superiority in comparison with the Z-N staining procedure is due to more intensive binding of mycolic acid of the tubercle bacillus to carbol auramine than to carbol fuschin.

The auramine-rhodamine dye combination stains non-viable bacilli. Since bacilli viability is important

3

in the evaluation of the drug effect, an acid-fast stain should be performed on all positive A-R stains. The acid-fast method stains only viable organisms. In addition, the Centers for Disease Control recommend that A-R stain positive slides be confirmed with a Z-N stain.

Blair (1976) noted that in a series of five A-R stained slides, 94 per cent of all culture positive patients were detected. However, one smear positive and culture negative specimen was obtained in 23 per cent of the patients evaluated. Strumpf (1979) noted the false positive A-R smear rate to be less than 0.17, the true positive rate greater than 0.83, and the specificity (true negative) rate to be 0.99.

With atypical mycobacteria, all strains of Runyon's Groups I, II, and III are auramine-rhodamine fast, while the majority of group IV do not stain by this dye technique.

In summary, the superiority of the A-R staining technique to the acid-fast smear is attributed to the following factors: (1) the tubercle bacilli have a higher affinity for A-R dye; (2) the entire smear can be examined, since the low-power objective is used; and (3) the black background in fluorescent microscopy makes the bacilli stand out more sharply to allow more rapid and accurate slide screening.

MYCOTIC DISEASE

The identification of fungal organisms in sputum plays a vital role in diagnosis of pulmonary lesions of mycotic disease. Mycotic disease of the lungs often mimics either inflammatory or neoplastic disease in clinical symptoms or roentgenographic findings. If the presence of fungi in sputum is noted, valuable time is saved in the diagnosis for both the clinician and the mycologist.

Poor communication between the clinician and mycologist often limits the effectiveness of rapid diagnosis. For example, the identification of *Actinomyces israelii* in sputum requires communication among the following: (1) clinician for the symptoms, (2) roentgenologist for evidence of pulmonary lesion, and (3) mycologist for significance of isolation. Otherwise, a possible pathogenic organism might be considered a "usual" contaminant of sputum.

A first morning specimen is preferred, as it represents the overnight secretions of the tracheobronchial tree. A sterile container should be used to collect the specimen. In the laboratory the specimen should be placed in another sterile container and examined against a dark background. Fungi are usually present in tiny flecks or particles which appear yellow-gray in color and more dense than the surrounding sputum. Structures similar to fungi are illustrated in Figure 23–2.

A direct mount with 10 per cent sodium hydroxide should be made and examined under the low- and high-powered lens. If no fungi are found, the specimen can be concentrated by various techniques. It is recommended that microscopic findings be confirmed by cultural methods. Sputum concentrate should never be cultured, as this procedure kills the fungi.

Pathologic Fungi. *Actinomyces israelii:* Although this is not a true fungus, most clinicians erroneously consider *Actinomyces israelii* and *Nocardia asteroides* to be fungi. *Actinomyces israelii* is a gram-positive organism that tends to grow slowly, with branching filaments. It can be cultured from most of the human tonsils removed at routine tonsillectomy and from scrapings of gum and teeth. Why the organism becomes invasive is not known, as it is a commensal organism. It is the only species of Actinomyces known to cause pulmonary actinomycosis. In sputum *A. israelii* appears macroscopically as yellow sulfur granules, usually less than 1 mm in diameter. Microscopically these granules appear as a mass of gram-positive mycelial filaments surrounded by a sheath of eosinophilic material, which gives a club-shaped appearance to the ends of these filaments.

Nocardia asteroides: In pulmonary nocardiosis caused by *N. asteroides* the pulmonary lesions may resemble tuberculosis or histoplasmosis. Since treatment is radically different in all three diseases, sputum examination can play a vital role in early diagnosis. Nocardia morphology is similar to Actinomyces, but its granules, if present, lack the clubbing of peripheral filaments and are not so compact. The filaments are gram-positive, bacilliform in shape, and in some stains partially acid fast.

Isolation from a solitary specimen is not presumptive of the diagnosis, since it may occasionally be a saprophyte in the upper respiratory tract. Its repeated presence is diagnostic of pulmonary nocardiosis.

Cryptococcus neoformans: The India ink technique is recommended for direct examination of sputum. India ink is mixed undiluted with the specimen; experience indicates the correct amount of ink to use. A negative India ink does not contraindicate performing a culture. The organism appears as a single budding blastospore, 5 to 20μ in diameter, and is surrounded by a capsule from 3 to 5μ in thickness.

Histoplasma capsulatum: The disease frequently starts as a flu-like syndrome; with healing, the pulmonary lesions become fibrotic and calcified, resembling healed primary tuberculosis.

Direct microscopic examination of fresh preparations rarely results in identification of the organism. Staining of sputum with either Wright's or Giemsa's stain often reveals macrophages with characteristic intracellular small yeast cells in the cytoplasm. The specimen should be cultured upon receipt, as sputum contains enzymes fungicidal for the organism.

Coccidioides immitis: The primary pulmonary disease usually has minimal manifestations. Approximately 5 per cent of patients are left with residual lesions of the lung such as nodules, abscesses, and cavities.

Sputum should be examined by wet direct mounts. The organism appears as a spherule, measuring 20 to 60μ in diameter and being filled with endospores (2 to 5μ in diameter). In the chronic cavitary form of the disease, hyphae may be seen.

Blastomyces dermatitidis: The initial infection begins in the lungs, with subsequent hematogenous spread to other organs of the body. In direct wet mounts, the organisms appear as spherical cells 8 to 15 μ in diameter with a thick, double, contoured refractile

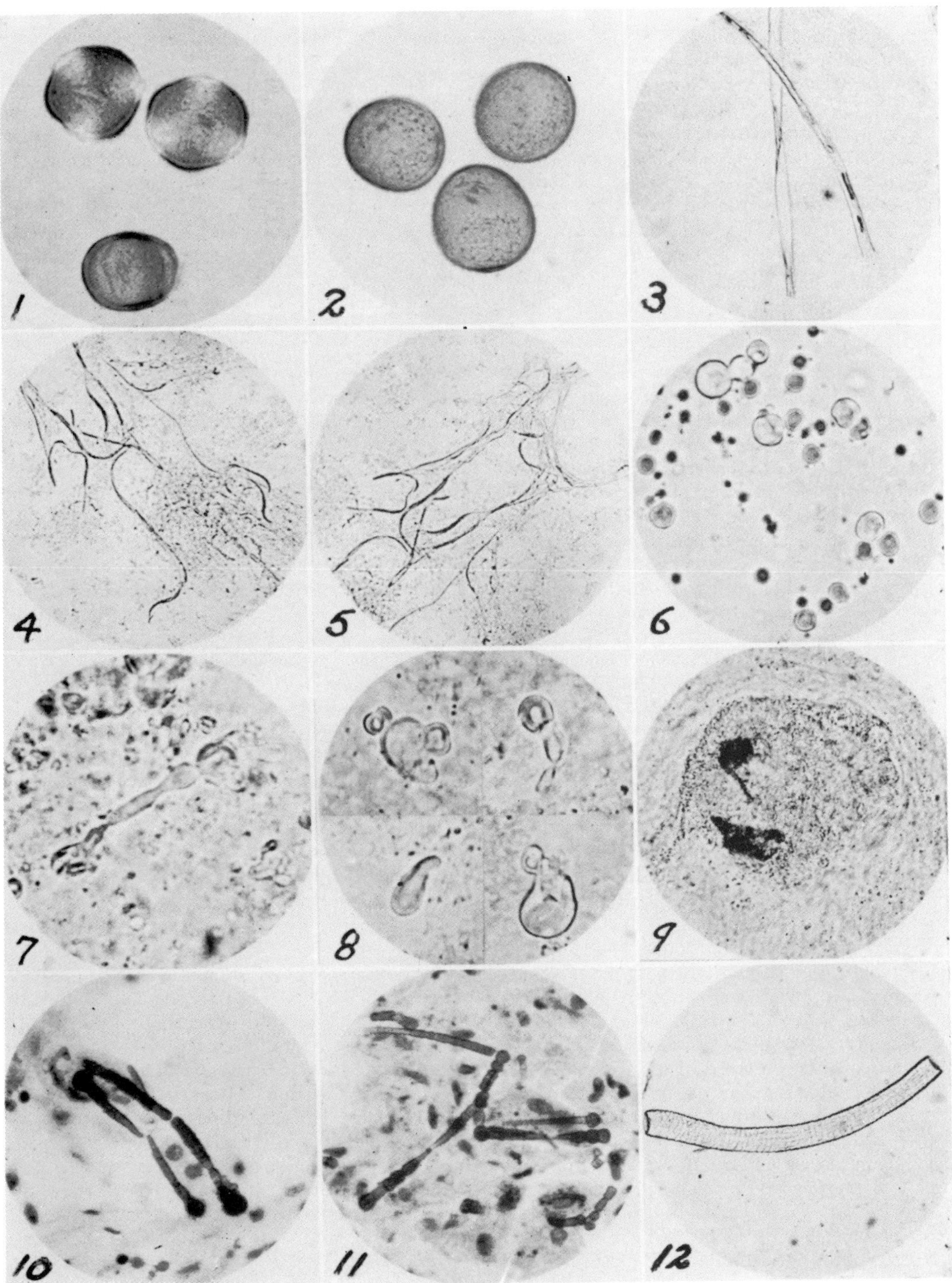

Figure 23–2. Illustrations of structures that resemble fungi found in sputum. *1,* Pollen, timothy grass (×800). *2,* Pollen, maple (×800). *3,* Cotton fibers (×100). *4* and *5,* Elastic tissue (×200). These are slender, highly refractile, wavy fibrils of uniform diameter and double contour. They may appear as single strands or in bundles and frequently show an alveolar arrangement. Their ends are often frayed or split. *6,* Fat cells (×800). *7* and *8,* Myelin globules (×800). Colorless globules occurring in a variety of sizes and bizarre forms. *9,* Bacterial colony (×400). Frequently found in sputum as small, gray or yellowish granules. They consist of a mass of either cocci or bacilli. *10* and *11,* Asbestos bodies (×800). They may occur as single structures or in small bundles and have a yellowish color. *12,* Wool fiber (×100). (From Kurung, J. M.: Am. Rev. Tuberc., *55*:387, 1947.)

wall. Buds are attached to the mother cell by a broad base with a characteristic septum between them. Trumbull (1981) reviewed 30 episodes of pulmonary blastomycosis among 29 patients and noted that the Pap stain ultimately yielded a positive diagnosis in 93 per cent of the patients and a wet smear in 61 per cent, thus markedly reducing the time of diagnostic workup.

Candida albicans: C. albicans is part of the normal throat flora. With widespread antibiotic and immunosuppressive therapy there is often an overgrowth of *C. albicans*. Its appearance on repeated examination indicates it as a possible pathogen. Close communication with the attending physician is needed for proper interpretation of the results.

Candida multiply readily at room temperature, and if the sputum sits at room temperature, the overgrowth may lead to erroneous interpretation. The report should include an evaluation of the number of organisms seen per field. On direct mount the organisms measure about 4 μ in diameter, are thin walled, and may appear singly, in pairs, or in small clusters. Budding forms and pseudomycelia may be formed. The organisms stain intensely positive with Gram stain.

Aspergillus fumigatus: Like *C. albicans,* the organism appears often as a sputum contaminant, and if demonstrated repeatedly in a specimen, it can be implicated as the principal pathogen. Again, communication is essential between the mycologist and the clinician. Pulmonary disease caused by *Aspergillus* may present as either an allergic bronchitis or a localized "aspergilloma."

BRONCHIAL ASTHMA

Laboratory examination of sputum for evidence of bronchial asthma is often neglected, although characteristic patterns can be seen in sputum (Fig. 23–3). The sputum is usually white and mucoid and contains no blood or pus unless an underlying bacterial infection is present. Approximately one third of all asthmatics will have sputum showing evidence of intercurrent respiratory infection. Some of the following findings are frequently observed in sputum.

Eosinophilia. The sputum has distinctive eosinophilic staining properties which have been attributed to an increased number of eosinophils and to the increased accumulation of serum proteins from the inflammation of the allergic reaction. Eosinophil counts above 80 per cent are strongly suggestive of asthma or chronic bronchitis with wheezing (Vieira, 1979). Also, sputum eosinophilia appears to be associated with a better response to corticosteroids; unless there is an underlying infection, neutrophils are not present.

Charcot-Leyden Crystals. These are rarely found in sputum except in cases of bronchial asthma. They may be absent in fresh sputum but make their appearance if the specimen is allowed to sit. The crystals are colorless, pointed hexagons and vary greatly in size. The average length is about three to four times the diameter of a red blood cell. Often they appear needle-like. They are derived from the disintegration of eosinophils; hence, they stain strongly with eosin.

Bronchial Epithelial Cells. The epithelial cells often occur singly and show hydropic degeneration, with poor definition of the original morphology. During acute exacerbations, these cells gather in larger clusters, display a vacuolated cytoplasm with ciliated borders, and are known as Creola bodies. They are seen in approximately one half of the cases. Also present are well-preserved, hypersecretory goblet cells occurring singly or in clusters.

Curschmann's Spirals. These are found most frequently in bronchial asthma and are fairly characteristic of the disease. They may be observed in chronic bronchitis and in heavy cigarette smokers, but in these cases there is nearly always an underlying asthmatic tendency. Macroscopically they can sometimes be recognized by the naked eye and appear as yellow-white, mucoid, wavy threads frequently coiled into little balls. Unraveled, their length rarely exceeds 1.5 cm. Microscopically a central thread is seen around which mucus is wrapped, supported by a fibril network. The central thread is formed by the shedding of the lining epithelium. Often embedded within the mucus are eosinophils and Charcot-Leyden crystals.

BRONCHIECTASIS

Bronchial dilatation of the saccular or cylindrical form *per se* will not cause symptoms unless a superimposed infection is present. The production of a mucopurulent sputum is one of the cardinal symptoms of this disease, and the amount expectorated varies with the posture. In the morning, production of sputum is usually the greatest, as the contents of the dilated lung sacs empty into the larger bronchi.

Characteristically, sputum is putrid, is gray-green in color, and varies in volume from 50 to 250 ml daily. Occasional blood streaking may be present. The source of this blood is usually the chronic granulation tissue of the chronically infected bronchial wall. Microscopic examination reveals the presence of bronchial epithelial cells, fatty crystals, various bacteria, and, occasionally, Dittrich's plugs (see p. 525). Occasionally elongated fatty acid crystals appear to be elastic tissue but lack the characteristic wavy appearance. The presence of elastic fibers may be used to differentiate the sputum of bronchiectasis from that of gangrene or lung abscesses.

CHRONIC BRONCHITIS

In chronic bronchitis the bronchioles as well as the bronchi may be inflamed, and the inflammatory reaction may be either cellular or catarrhal. The mildest and most frequent form of the disease in the United States is smoker's cough. Of all the criteria required to establish the diagnosis of chronic bronchitis, sputum production is accepted as the necessary minimum.

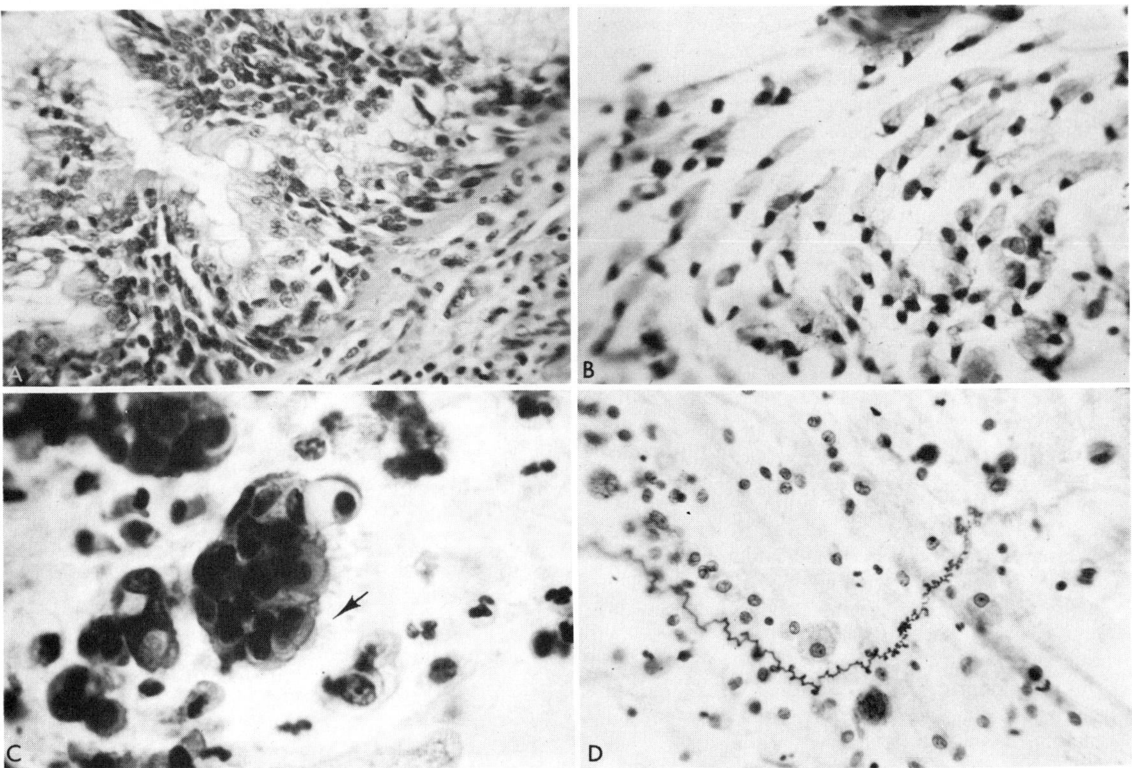

Figure 23–3. Patterns in asthma. *A,* Terminal bronchiole showing goblet cell hyperplasia (H & E stain ×650). *B,* Exfoliated goblet cells (Papanicolaou ×650). *C,* Creola body. Note presence of cilia (arrow) (Papanicolaou ×650). *D,* Curschmann's spiral. Note elongated wavy central thread (Gram stain ×250).

3

Macroscopically the sputum is tenacious, white, and mucoid in appearance. During superimposed infections, the secretions increase in volume and become purulent yellow-green in color. The average volume expectorated is about 60 ml per day, but volumes as high as 600 ml per day have been produced.

Microscopically the presence of histiocytes and monocytes can help in assessing the activity of the disease. In early chronic bronchitis, large numbers of histiocytes and monocytes indicate a stable phase, but during exacerbation these cells disappear. When entering clinical remission again, these cells reappear. A similar pattern holds true for leukocytes and epithelial cells. In remission, a few cells are noted. The presence of necrotic tissue or elastic fibers is an ominous sign, as this indicates a superimposed severe process such as abscess formation or bronchiectasis.

Examination of the Gram stain and subsequent culture usually reveals the presence of mixed organisms without a predominant pathogenic organism. Indeed, there is little difference in the bacterial flora in the sputum of patients in remission or exacerbation.

Chemical analysis of sputum has yet to have practical application in the clinical laboratory.

The activity of the enzyme lactic dehydrogenase (LDH) can be measured in sputum. It originates from serum, the inflammatory cells, and the mucosal surface. Thus, with destructive inflammatory changes in the bronchial mucosa, increased LDH activity may be expected. During exacerbation of chronic bronchitis, total LDH activity increases, with the greatest increase occurring in the electrophoretically faster isoenzyme fractions. With improvement, the reverse is seen.

DNA in sputum can be demonstrated either by fluorescent microscopy or by chemical determination. It originates from disintegrated inflammatory cells and the destruction of bronchial epithelial cells. Thus, in infected secretions, DNA levels are high as a result of extensive cellular damage. Levels fall as improvement is noted.

Immunoglobulin levels reveal low IgA and IgG compared to other disease states. IgM levels are nondetectable.

LUNG ABSCESS

Unless the abscess ruptures into a bronchus, there is little or no sputum production. Most abscesses are initiated by bronchial occlusion, by virtue of either aspirations, tumor, or foreign body occlusion. When rupture occurs, a large amount of bloody, creamy, foul-smelling pus is suddenly and violently expectorated. Close examination reveals the presence of elastic fibers, cellular debris, and leukocytes. Usually more than one organism will be seen with Gram staining. A search for tubercle bacilli or malignant cells must also be made.

PNEUMONIA

Pneumonia has been estimated to occur in 0.5 to 5 per cent of hospitalized patients and is the leading cause of death among all nosocomial infections. In the early diagnosis of pneumonia, Gram stain of the sputum is the most essential examination available in the laboratory. Proper interpretation leads to institution of appropriate therapy at least 24 hours before the results of the culture are available. However, certain hazards in the interpretation of the Gram stain are present. These include the following. Gram-negative organisms are often overlooked, as nonbacterial elements stain gram-negative. Conversely, gram-positive debris is often mistaken for organisms, especially by the novice. Smears are often stained improperly. The occurrence of more than a faint trace of positive stain in the cytoplasm of white blood cells indicates undercolorization. Finally, the description of the Gram stain is often inadequate. For example, "gram-positive cocci" does not distinguish between pneumococcus and staphylococcus, two pathogenic organisms whose antibiotic treatment is different.

Gram-Positive Cocci

Of the gram-positive pneumonias, the principal pathogen is *Streptococcus pneumoniae;* rarely are staphylococci and other streptococci involved.

The diagnosis of pneumococcal pneumonia is based on the presence of gram-positive diplococci on smear and/or the culture of the organism from sputum. Thorsteinsson (1975) has shown that a sputum specimen is as accurate as either a transtracheal or bronchial aspirate in the diagnosis of acute pneumococcal pneumonia.

The sensitivity and specificity of the Gram stain have ranged widely with an overall accuracy of approximately 62 per cent in identifying pneumococci in sputum (Rein, 1978). To increase sensitivity and specificity, the immunodetection of pneumococcal antigens in the sputum has demonstrated strong correlation with the presence of pneumococcal disease. Coagglutination is preferable to counterimmunoelectrophoresis in the detection of pneumococcal antigens, as technique is simpler, cost is less, and sensitivity is higher (Edwards, 1980).

Pneumococci can survive for long periods of time in sputum. At 4°C. refrigerated organisms survive for weeks (Williams, 1978). Unfortunately, cultures of sputum are only presumptive in the diagnosis of clinical disease, as pneumococcal organisms are often carried in the nasopharynx and contaminate the culture.

Even with the above limitations, the Gram stain and culture are widely used to diagnose pneumococcal disease. On Gram stain, the *S. pneumoniae* organisms are gram-positive, lancet-shaped diplococci with the long axis in a straight line. Alpha-hemolytic streptococci are often mistakenly identified as pneumococci.

Daily Gram stains should be performed on patients with pneumococcal pneumonia to follow the effect of treatment on the disease and to rule out secondary infections.

In pneumococcal pneumonia the character of the sputum varies with the stage of the disease. In the early stages of typical lobar pneumonia, the sputum is scanty and transparent, with occasional blood flecks. As the disease progresses to the red-hepatization stage, the sputum becomes rust red, very tenacious, and mucopurulent. Microscopic examination reveals the presence of many intra- and extracellular organisms, epithelial cells, leukocytes, and erythrocytes. During the stages of resolution, the sputum becomes more abundant and less tenacious and assumes the appearance of that seen in chronic bronchitis. The rusty character of the sputum is absent during this stage, and the reappearance of this characteristic should alert the clinician that the disease is progressing or has involved the opposite lung.

In staphylococcal pneumonia, a yellow, purulent, voluminous sputum is present. On Gram stain, large numbers of staphylococci in grapelike clusters and neutrophils are present.

Gram-Negative Bacilli

The initiating event in the development of a gram-negative pneumonia is colonization of the oropharynx by gram-negative organisms. Approximately 2 per cent of normal persons transiently harbor gram-negative bacilli in their throats. Serious illness and antimicrobial therapy through suppression of normal bacterial flora and alteration of bacterial adherence lead to colonization of the oropharynx by gram-negative bacilli. Aspiration of oropharyngeal contents during sleep introduces the organisms into the lower respiratory tract, where they act as pathogens (Penn, 1981).

The gram-negative pneumonias are hard to diagnose initially on sputum examination. Gram stains of sputum may be confusing, since morphologically similar organisms are present in normal throat flora. Almost any of the gram-negative aerobic organisms have the potential to cause disease of the lower respiratory tract, but the more common ones are *Klebsiella, Hemophilus, Enterobacter, Pseudomonas,* and *Escherichia coli.* With the exception of the foul green sputum seen in *Pseudomonas* infections, no "classic" macroscopic findings are present in these sputums.

Hemophilus influenzae is often missed on Gram stain. The organism binds the safranine stain poorly and it is misinterpreted as background debris. *Hemophilus* is particularly important as a pathogen in adults with a diagnosis of chronic bronchitis or bronchiectasis. The methylene blue stain permits easier recognition of *H. influenzae* than does the Gram stain. If the organism suspected is *H. influenzae* and no methylene blue stain is available, 0.2 per cent fuchsin solution can be used as the counterstain instead of safranine.

Klebsiella, Enterobacter, Escherichia coli, and *Pseudomonas* are common gastrointestinal inhabitants which may cause pneumonia. However, these gram-negative organisms may be stable flora in the upper respiratory tract. Therefore, a culture or Gram stain should never be the sole reason for patient treatment without clinical indications.

Various anaerobes such as Bacteroidaceae and anaerobic streptococci have been implicated in essentially all types of pulmonary infections (Bartlett, 1976). The sputum is characteristically putrid. Gram stain usually reveals primarily gram-negative organisms of mixed morphology. In pneumonia caused by the anaerobic streptococci, the sputum is not foul smelling and on Gram stain, tiny gram-positive cocci in chains are noted.

Percutaneous transtracheal aspiration is recommended for specimen collection for culture. Expectorated sputum is often heavily contaminated by the indigenous anaerobic flora of the mouth and oropharynx.

PNEUMOCONIOSIS

The term pneumoconiosis refers to a fibrosis of the lung secondary to inhalation of an organic or inorganic dust. The disease is primarily occupational and its severity differs according to the type of inhaled dust.

To reach the alveoli and initiate a reaction, the particles usually have to be less than 5 μ in diameter. In the alveoli the reaction to the dust particle depends upon its composition. In general, particles are engulfed by macrophages and deposited in peribronchial lymph channels or are carried onto the regional lymph nodes. By far the most common and severe form of pneumoconiosis in the United States is silicosis. Other types of pneumoconiosis are asbestosis, anthracosilicosis, berylliosis, bagassosis, and byssinosis. The latter two are caused by cane sugar and cotton dust, respectively.

The character and production of sputum varies with the severity and stage of the disease. Macroscopically the sputum is tenacious and can sometimes display the color of the dust inhaled. Microscopically various diagnostic features can differentiate the pneumoconiosis, but their presence is difficult to demonstrate.

In anthracosilicosis angular black granules will be both intracellular and extracellular. Unfortunately the presence of these cells is not pathognomonic for anthracosilicosis, as similar cells with smaller carbon particles are abundant in heavy tobacco smokers and people living in highly polluted areas.

In asbestosis the presence of dumbbell-shaped asbestos needles in clusters is diagnostic. They stain yellow to dark brown and measure 10 to 80 μ in size (Fig. 23–4). Numerous multinucleated giant cells and histiocytes may also be observed.

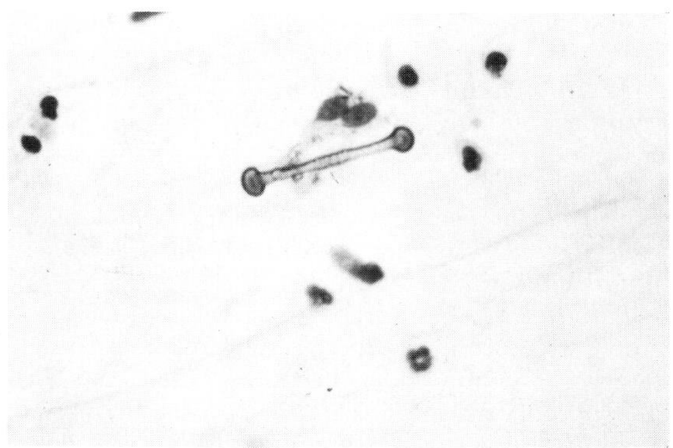

Figure 23–4. Asbestosis body from patient with pneumoconiosis; characteristics may occasionally be overlooked and considered artifact. (Papanicolaou ×650).

In silicosis the particles are detected with polarized light. The crystals appear sharp, elongated, and fragmented. Numerous neutrophils, macrophages, and multinucleated giant cells are present.

In byssinosis polarized light should also be used to demonstrate the crystals. They appear as rectangular, prism-shaped crystals that shine brightly with polarized light.

PULMONARY EMBOLISM

If pulmonary infarction is secondary to thromboembolus, sputum examination shortly afterward reveals the presence of bright red blood in a very tenacious, mucoid background. As the infarction resolves, the sputum becomes progressively darker in color. Microscopic examination reveals erythrocytes, altered hemoglobin, and macrophages with denatured hemoglobin products in the cytoplasm.

Sputum examination in fat embolism is non-definitive. Lipid-laden macrophages and fat droplets may be found in normal persons and especially in persons who are cigarette smokers. Endogenous fat and tobacco tar are positive by oil red O but can be differentiated in that the tar has fluorescent properties.

HEART DISEASE

Sputum examination has characteristic findings in some types of heart disease.

In acute edema, a condition in which large amounts of serous exudate pass from the capillaries into the alveoli, the sputum is abundant, frothy, and pink. As much as 1 liter a day may be expectorated in severe conditions. Microscopically the sputum may be shown to contain numerous erythrocytes and large hyaline masses. These hyaline masses are the protein component of the serous exudate.

In chronic congestive heart failure, the sputum is frothy and rust colored. Microscopic examination reveals the presence of erythrocytes and "heart failure cells." In fresh unstained sputum these cells appear as round colorless bodies filled with various-sized granules of yellow to brown pigment. This pigment may be demonstrated to be hemosiderin by staining with 10 per cent potassium ferrocyanide for a few minutes and then with 0.1 NHCl. Hemosiderin pigment stains a blue color.

PULMONARY ALVEOLAR PROTEINOSIS

In this disease, eosinophilic material which is positive for periodic acid–Schiff (PAS) stain is deposited in the alveoli without serious alteration of lung structure. The disease usually pursues a chronic course ending in death but may resolve spontaneously. Diagnosis is confirmed by lung biopsy but can be made by sputum examination. Microscopic examination reveals numerous macrophages which show abundant quantities of PAS-positive material against a granular protein deposit in the background.

PNEUMOCYSTIS CARINII

Pneumocystis carinii is a protozoan parasite which can cause an interstitial pneumonia in the immunologically impaired host. Expectorated sputum is a poor source to demonstrate the presence of the organism. In a study of patients with known *Pneumocystis carinii* pneumonia, Lau (1976) found the organism present in sputum in approximately 1 per cent of the cases. The best yield for diagnosis is obtained in lung biopsy. Grocott's methenamine silver stain best delineates the cysts of the organism. The cysts measure 4.5 μ in diameter and are round or cup-shaped, with a thin black wall enclosing a cylindrical or comma-shaped structure within the cyst. If one desires a more prompt interpretation, smears made from aspirated specimens and imprint preparations from lung biopsies may be stained by the Gram-Weigert procedure (Rosen, 1977) or by a Giemsa stain. Immunospecific staining will probably be used in the future.

LEGIONNAIRES' DISEASE

Legionnaires' disease is a bacterial illness which primarily affects the lungs. Approximately 5 per cent of the adult population over age 50 have elevated titers indicating previous infection. The organism, *Legionella pneumophila,* is a pleomorphic coccobacillus that stains variably or negative by the Gram stain and positive by the Gimenez stain or Dieterle stain. The organism is difficult to culture and the diagnosis of legionnaire's disease is established by immunofluorescent staining of tissue or sputum or by serological antibody titers.

Broome (1979) reported the rapid diagnosis of

legionnaires' disease by direct immunofluorescent staining of sputum sample. Approximately 10 per cent of sputums were positive in identifying 5 of 21 patients, while there were no false positives in 47 negative controls. Earlier diagnosis is obtained by direct immunofluorescence because the diagnosis can be made within two to seven days of the onset of the symptoms, compared to the three weeks needed for a rise in serological titer. The direct immunofluorescent technique demonstrates both intact bacteria and soluble antigen which affixes to various structures and fibrin.

VIRAL INFECTIONS

Viruses have been estimated to cause between 70 and 90 per cent of all respiratory infections. Six large groups of viruses are capable of causing infections, and almost all the groups include a great number of serotypes. Since the prognosis of respiratory tract infections is usually excellent, little attention has been paid to identifying the specific etiologic viral agents.

Preparation of specimens for viral examination is similar to sputum cytology for malignancy. Instead of examining for malignant changes in cells, the presence of inclusion bodies is looked for.

The inclusion bodies of herpes simplex and adenovirus are intranuclear. Herpes simplex is the easier of the two to identify, and in the bronchial epithelium, the changes involve only the young columnar or squamous exfoliated cells (Fig. 23–5). These mononuclear cells, along with giant cells, develop intranuclear eosinophilic inclusion bodies surrounded by a halo. Decreased nuclear basophilia is also evident in these cells except in areas where the chromatin clump has adhered to the inner surface of the nuclear membrane. In contrast to herpes simplex and other viruses, the adenovirus infection is compatible with cellular life.

Eosinophilic intracytoplasmic inclusions are seen in parainfluenza and measles viral infections, while basophilic intracytoplasmic inclusions are present in respiratory syncytial and cytomegalic viral infections.

CYTOLOGIC EXAMINATION IN MALIGNANCY

The cytologic examination of sputum is the single most reliable method for diagnosis of early pulmonary carcinoma, having a positive yield of approximately 50 per cent as compared to 25 per cent when bronchoscopy and bronchial biopsy are performed. In combination with bronchoscopy and radiography, the number of early cases detected has significantly increased, although unfortunately the survival rate has not improved.

Since methods of specimen collection and preparation vary considerably, it is advisable to consult with the pathologist prior to specimen collection and to follow his instructions.

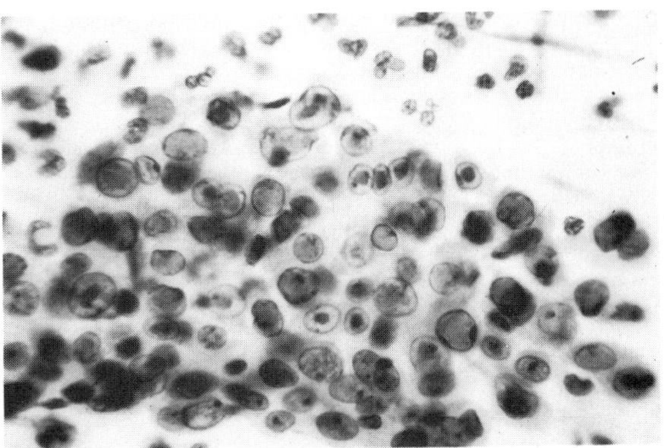

Figure 23–5. Sputum from herpes simplex pneumonia. Note presence of amphophilic intranuclear inclusion, margination of chromatin, and opaqueness of nuclei. (Papanicolaou ×650.)

The most common inpatient specimen is the single, early morning, "deep cough" sputum. These specimens should be collected on a minimum of three and preferably five consecutive mornings and submitted to the laboratory fresh without prior fixation. The fresh specimen is examined, and bloody areas and tissue flecks are selected and smeared onto a slide.

In outpatients, specimen collection should be in widemouth jars containing 50 per cent ethanol and 2 per cent Carbowax fixative. The accepted criterion for a satisfactory sputum sample is the presence of alveolar macrophages. Four slides are prepared for examination and stained with the Papanicolaou stain.

Bartlett, R. C.: Medical Microbiology: Quality Cost and Clinical Relevance. New York, John Wiley & Sons, 1974, pp. 24–31.

Blair, E. B., Brown, G. L., and Tull, A. H.: Computer files and analysis of laboratory data from tuberculosis patient. II. Analysis of six years' data on sputum specimens. Am. Rev. Resp. Dis., *113*:427, 1976.

Broome, C. V., Cherry, W. B., Winn, W. C., Jr., and MacPherson, B. R.: Rapid diagnosis of legionnaire's disease by direct immunofluorescent staining. Ann. Int. Med., *90*:1, 1979.

Charukian, C. J., and Schenk, E. A.: Rapid Grocotts methenamine–silver nitrate method for fungi and *Pneumocystis carinii*. Am. J. Clin. Pathol., *68*:427, 1977.

Edwards, E. A., and Coonrad, J. D.: Coagglutinations and counterimmunoelectrophoresis for detection of pneumococcal antigens in the sputum of pneumonia patients. J. Clin. Microbiol., *11*:488, 1980.

Kurung, J. M.: The isolation and identification of pathogenic fungi from sputum. Am. Rev. Tuberc., *55*:387, 1947.

Lau, W. K., Young, L. S., and Remington, J. S.: *Pneumocystis carinii* pneumonia. Diagnosis by examination of pulmonary secretions. J.A.M.A., *236*:2399, 1976.

Monroe, P. W., Muchmore, H. G., Felton, F. G., and Pirtle, J. K.: Quantitation of microorganisms in sputum. Appl. Microbiol., *18*:214, 1969.

Newhouse, M., Sanchis, J., and Bienenstock, J.: Lung defense mechanisms. N. Engl. J. Med., *295*:990, 1976.

Penn, R. G., Saunders, W. E., and Saunders, C.C.: Colonization of the oropharynx with gram-negative bacilli: A major antecedent to nosocomial pneumonia. Am. J. Inf. Cont., *9*:25, 1981.

Pritzker, K. P., Desai, S. D., Patterson, M. C., and Cheny, P.: Calcite sputum lith. Am. J. Clin. Path., *75*:253, 1981.

Rein, M. F., Gualtney, J. M., Jr., O'Brien, W. M., Jennings, R. H., and Mandell, G. L.: Accuracy of Gram's stain in identifying pneumococci in sputum. J.A.M.A., *239*:2671, 1978.

Rosen, P. R.: Frozen section management of a lung biopsy for suspected Pneumocystis pneumonia. Am. J. Surg. Path., *1*:79, 1977.

Strumpf, I. J., Tsang, A. Y., and Sayre, J. W.: Re-evaluation of sputum staining for the diagnosis of pulmonary tuberculosis. Am. Rev. Resp. Dis., *119*:599, 1979.

Thorsteinsson, S. B., Mosher, D. M., and Fagan, T.: The diagnostic value of sputum culture in acute pneumonia. J.A.M.A., *233*:894, 1975.

Traunt, J. P., Brett, W. A., and Thomas, W.: Fluorescence microscopy of tubercle bacilli stained with auramine and rhodamine. Henry Ford Hosp. Med. Bull., *10*:287, 1962.

Trumbull, M. L., and McChesney, T.: The cytological diagnosis of pulmonary blastomycosis. J.A.M.A., *245*:836, 1981.

Vestal, A. L.: 1975 Procedures for the isolation and identification of mycobacteria. Public Health Service Publications, Center for Disease Control, Atlanta, Ga.

Vieira, V. G., and Prolla, J. C.: Clinical evaluation of eosinophils in the sputum. J. Clin. Path., *32*:1054, 1979.

Williams, S. G., and Kauffman, C. A.: Survival of *Streptococcus pneumoniae* in sputum from patients with pneumonia. J. Clin. Microbiol., *7*:73, 1978.

Yeager, H., Jr.: Tracheobronchial secretions. Am. J. Med., *50*:493, 1971.

24

EXOCRINE PANCREATIC FUNCTION

WEI T. WU, PH.D., and YUAN S. KAO, M.D.

3

PHYSIOLOGY OF PANCREATIC SECRETION

The pancreas produces from 1000 to 2500 ml of juice in 24 hours. This fluid is slightly alkaline and, besides water, contains mainly enzymes, sodium, potassium, sodium bicarbonate, chloride, and phosphate. Secretin, an intestinal hormone produced under stimulation by hydrochloric acid, causes production of fluid high in bicarbonate level and low in enzyme activity, whereas cholecystokinin-pancreozymin, an intestinal hormone produced under stimulation by gastrin, causes production of fluid high in enzyme activity and low in bicarbonate level. Enzymes include amylase, lipase, trypsinogen, chymotrypsinogens A and B, procarboxypeptidases A and B, proelastase, and prophospholipase. Duodenal enterokinase catalyzes formation of trypsin from trypsinogen. Trypsin catalyzes conversion of the proteolytic proenzymes and prophospholipase to their active forms.

SCREENING FOR PANCREATIC DISORDERS

Determination of altered activity of amylase and lipase in body fluids has, for years, been the keystone of the laboratory approach to the diagnosis of acute and relapsing (chronic) pancreatitis, in which there is increased release of these substances into blood and urine; whereas for the diagnosis of pancreatic carcinoma and chronic pancreatitis, examination of stimulated pancreatic fluid through duodenal aspiration has been, until recently, the only reliable means of assessing pancreatic secretory function. These tests are not suitable for detecting the pancreatic disease–prone individual or for screening for the predisease state. However, there are predisposing conditions which can be screened for. For example, alcoholism or gallstone disease is present in over 80 per cent of patients with pancreatitis, so biochemical tests sensitive to liver damage—such as serum aspartate aminotransferase or gamma glutamyl transpeptidase—may be useful. In alcoholics, hypertriglyceridemia may trigger the pancreatitis; therefore, serum triglyceride determinations may also be useful. Serum calcium level measurements may be indicated, since patients with hyperparathyroidism are at increased risk of developing pancreatitis. Hyperparathyroidism merits a screening procedure on its own. Steroids, thiazides, sulfonamides, azathioprine, and birth control pills have also been implicated as causes of pancreatitis, although not commonly. A family history can serve as a good screening test for cystic fibrosis of the pancreas. Pancreatic carcinoma is one of the leading causes of cancer deaths in the United States, and unfortunately there is no established effective screening test for its early diagnosis. Although pancreatic function tests, abdominal ultrasound, computed tomography (CT), endoscopic retrograde cholangiopancreatography, carcinoembryonic antigen, alpha-fetoprotein and pancreatic oncofetal antigen tests have been used, no single test has proved to have both high sensitivity and specificity. Recently, galactosyltransferase isoenzyme II has been found to be elevated in pancreatic carcinoma, and its determination may be useful in the future.

AMYLASE (α-1,4-GLUCAN-4-GLUCANOHYDROLASE, E.C. 3.2.1.1)

Biochemistry and Physiology

Amylases are enzymes that catalyze the hydrolysis of amylopectin, amylose, glycogen, and their partially hydrolyzed products. Alpha-amylase occurs in animal tissue and fluids. It splits α-1,4-glucosidic linkages in polysaccharides containing three or more α-1,4-linked D-glucose units in random fashion. Upon hydrolysis by α-amylase, amylose gives rise to a mixture of maltose and glucose, whereas amylopectin yields a mixture of branched and unbranched oligosaccharides. Since α-amylase is unable to attack α-1,6-glucosidic linkages, the polysaccharides which remain after hydrolysis are dextrins. Alpha-amylase is an endo-enzyme and was so named because all the hydrolysis products have a configuration at C_1 of the reducing glucose unit. Alpha-amylase rapidly decreases the ability of amylose to stain blue with iodine and decreases the viscosity of starch solutions.

Other amylases include β-amylase, found in both animals and plants, an exo-enzyme (α-1,4-glucanomaltohydrolase, E.C. 3.2.1.2), and γ-amylase (α-1,4-glucanglucohydrolase, E.C. 3.2.1.3) found in numerous fungi.

Of these three amylases, only α-amylase is of clinical interest. Alpha-amylase is stable at room temperature for at least one week and at refrigeration temperature for at least six months. It may be kept in the frozen state much longer without appreciable loss of activity.

In humans, α-amylase is normally present in pancreas (approximately 200 mg/kg), salivary glands, liver, muscle, adipose tissue, saliva, blood, urine, feces, milk, semen, kidney, brain, lung, fallopian tube, intestine, spleen, and heart. The α-amylase present in blood and urine of normal individuals is predominantly of pancreatic and salivary origin. Alpha-amylase of pancreatic and salivary origin we abbreviate to P-type and S-type amylase (isoenzyme, isoamylase), respectively, whenever such distinction is needed. These two types of amylase are closely related enzymes but also exhibit organ-specific variations. They yield the same amino acid composition and similar but not identical peptide maps. Each appears to consist of a single polypeptide chain without subunits. Pancreatic amylase has a molecular weight of 54,000 daltons. Higher molecular weights have been reported for salivary amylase. Both amylases contain sulfhydryl groups. Pancreatic amylase is believed to have five binding sites for substrate (Wermus, 1979). Amylases are metalloenzymes containing at least one atom of calcium per molecule and require this metal for their catalytic activities. The pH for optimal activity ranges from 6.9 to 7.0. The pH optimum for salivary amylase varies with the anion used as activator, of which chloride is most important. Optimal chloride concentration is 10 mmol/L and the activation is allosteric. Bromide and iodide ions also activate amylase.

The optimal temperature for α-amylase assay is 50°C., but most determinations are carried out at 37°C. Several automated amylase methods employ 40°C., 45°C., and 50°C. The Q_{10} factors have been reported to be 1.2 between 40°C. and 50°C. (Wu, 1972), and 1.4 between 30°C. and 50°C. (Proelss, 1975).

The isoelectric points (pI) have been reported to be 7.6 and 7.2 for P-type and 6.4 and 5.8 for S-type isoamylases, respectively. Other pI values have also been documented (Scully, 1981; Bossuyt, 1981).

Little is known about the normal mechanism of entrance of pancreatic enzymes, such as amylase, into blood, where normally the pancreatic enzyme appears to account for less than 50 per cent of serum amylase activity. Increased serum activity in acute pancreatitis presumably results from escape of enzyme into the interstitial tissue and peritoneal cavity, with increased absorption through the lymphatics and veins. The renal clearance of amylase has been estimated to be 1 to 3 ml/minute, appearing to be constant over a wide range of urine flow; therefore, increased release into the blood is followed by increased excretion in the urine.

Amylase is first detectable in serum of infants between the ages of two and three months, and by one year of age low normal adult levels are reached.

Interpretation

Determination of serum and urine amylase activities, although not specific indices, has been most extensively used in the laboratory diagnosis of acute pancreatitis. Serum amylase activity rises within 6 to 48 hours of onset in about 80 per cent of patients with acute pancreatitis, but not proportionally to severity of the disease. Values over 600 Somogyi units/dl, or over four times the upper limit of normal, are highly suggestive of the diagnosis. Activity usually returns to normal in three to five days in patients with the milder edematous forms of the disease. Elevated values persisting longer than this suggest continuing necrosis or possible pseudocyst formation. The urine amylase activity rises promptly, often within several hours of the rise in serum activity, and may remain elevated after the serum activity has returned to the normal range. Values over 1000 Somogyi units/hour are seen almost exclusively in patients with acute pancreatitis. False-negative results are often seen when specimen is taken too soon or too late, or in case of fulminating necrosis in which the production of amylase is decreased or ceased. In a majority of the patients with acute pancreatitis, there is always an elevation in serum amylase activity with a concomitant increase in urine amylase activity. There may be instances, however, in which the elevated urine amylase is not accompanied by a concomitant increase in serum amylase.

As may be surmised from this, increased renal clearance of amylase accounts for the greater diagnostic value of the urine amylase activity in the diagnosis of acute and relapsing pancreatitis, and the ratio of amylase clearance to the creatinine clearance expressed as a percentage has been used diagnostically. This ratio (C_{am}/C_{cr}) can be calculated by the following formula:

$$\text{Clearance ratio (\%)} = \frac{\text{Urine amylase activity}}{\text{Serum amylase activity}} \times \frac{\text{Serum creatinine concentration}}{\text{Urine creatinine concentration}} \times 100$$

The normal ratio averages from 1 to 4 per cent, while that for patients with pancreatitis usually exceeds 4 per cent and is often in the range of 7 to 15 per cent. Unfortunately, about one third of pancreatitis patients have normal ratios, and elevated ratios may be found in patients with burns, ketoacidosis, renal insufficiency, heart disease, and duodenal perforation, and after thoracic surgery. Thus, the ratio adds little to the diagnostic armamentarium.

Serum amylase may be elevated in patients with pancreatic carcinoma, but too late to be useful. It is also elevated frequently (over 60 per cent of patients) in diabetic ketoacidosis. Polyacrylamide gel electrophoresis has demonstrated that in this condition it is usually salivary rather than pancreatic amylase that is elevated. Serum amylase activity may also be elevated in patients with cholecystitis or peptic ulcer, or following gastric resection, renal transplant, viral hepatitis, or ruptured ectopic pregnancy; very high activity has been reported in patients with carcinoma of the lung. Fewer hyperamylasemic patients may be found to have intestinal obstruction, mesenteric thrombosis, and peritonitis. In some of these patients, pancreatic secretions find their way into the peritoneal cavity and are absorbed into the bloodstream; in others, there may be inflammation involving the pancreas.

Approximately 20 per cent of patients with pancreatitis have normal or near-normal amylase activity. In hyperlipemic patients with pancreatitis, normal serum and urine amylase levels are frequently encountered. The spuriously normal levels are believed to be the result of suppression of amylase activity by triglyceride or by a circulating inhibitor in serum (Warshaw, 1975).

Less-than-normal serum amylase activity may be found in patients with chronic pancreatitis, and has also been reported in such diverse and unexpected conditions as congestive heart failure, pregnancy (during the second and third trimesters), gastrointestinal cancer, bone fractures, and pleurisy.

The diagnostic sensitivity and diagnostic specificity of serum amylase in acute pancreatitis have been reported to be 70 to 98 per cent and 70 to 76 per cent, respectively, and those of urine amylase, 80 to 98 per cent and 80 to 90 per cent, respectively (Webster, 1974; Lente, 1982).

Macroamylasemia

Macroamylasemia was first discovered by Wilding (1964) and later so named by Berk and coworkers to describe a condition of persistently elevated serum amylase activity with no apparent clinical symptoms of pancreatic disorder. It was attributed to the presence of an amylase-globulin complex whose large size precluded its excretion into urine even though renal function was unimpaired. Macroamylase is a circulating complex of normal amylase linked to an immunoglobulin in most cases, and to a polysaccharide in others. The immunoglobulins involved are IgA and IgG. The composition of macroamylases is heterogeneous. Analysis of the complex after acid dissociation revealed that P-type and S-type isoamylases were present in variable proportions. The molecular weight has been estimated from 150,000 to greater than 1 million daltons. Macroamylasemia may also occur in hyperamylasemic patients with undiminished urine amylase and in patients with normal serum and urine amylase activities. Table 24–1 shows the features of different types of macroamylasemia.

More than 200 cases of macroamylasemia have been reported, with a frequency of 1.05 per cent in randomly selected patients, 2.56 per cent among persons with hyperamylasemia, and 0.98 per cent in persons with normal serum amylase (Klonoff, 1980). Macroamylasemia per se is not a disease entity because no

Table 24–1. TYPES OF MACROAMYLASEMIA*

	Type 1	**Type 2**	**Type 3**
Serum amylase activity	Persistently high	High	Normal
Urine amylase activity	Always diminished	Not always diminished	Normal
Detection of activity after incubation†	Within 10 minutes	Longer than 10 minutes	Longer than 10 minutes
Ratio of macroamylase to normal size amylase in serum	Highest	Much lower than type 1	Low
Relative concentration macroamylase complex in serum	High		
Amylase activity in macroamylase-containing fraction	High	Intermediate	

*Adopted from Fridhandler and Berk (1978).
†Based on Rapid Method (Fridhandler, 1971).

3

clinical symptoms consistently accompany it. It is an acquired and benign condition which may occur in an apparently healthy individual, and is found more frequently in males than in females. The age at time of discovery in most patients is in the fifth to seventh decades. The occurrence of macroamylasemia may be an early sign of disease, either as a marker or as a non-specific disease-induced dysproteinemia with amylase-binding capability, and may be regarded as one of the immunoglobulin-complexed enzyme disorders.

Clinically, it is important to differentiate macroamylasemia from other conditions that are associated with hyperamylasemia. Any patient with hyperamylasemia, a very low (less than 1 per cent) amylase/creatinine clearance ratio, and normal renal function should be suspected of having macroamylasemia. The definitive identification of macroamylasemia, however, requires direct demonstration of the existence of macroamylase molecule by ultracentrifugation, chromatography, or other physical techniques. A detection method by chromatography has been in use for many years (Fridhandler, 1971). Most recently, a rapid and simple assay based on selective precipitation of macroamylase in polyethylene glycol solution has been reported (Levitt, 1982).

Isoenzymes

The fractionation of amylase in serum, urine, or other body fluids may be achieved by physical means, such as electrophoresis, chromatography, and isoelectric focusing, and each isoenzyme is then quantitated either by direct densitometry or by amyloclastic or saccharogenic techniques. A chemical assay employing a salivary amylase-specific protein inhibitor is also being used for isoenzyme determinations (Huang, 1982).

Human pancreatic amylase and salivary amylase, controlled by independent genes, have been found to have the same amino acid composition but also exhibit organ-specific variation. At neutral pH, both amylases exhibit the same action pattern, although there are differences in molecular weight, carbohydrate content, and amide groups. At both high and low temperature extremes, pancreatic amylase is more labile than salivary amylase.

Pancreatic amylase, P-type, is synthesized by the acinar cells of the pancreas, and is tissue specific. Salivary amylase, S-type, is present in and believed to be synthesized by parotid, sweat and lactating mammary glands, lung, fallopian tube, and, possibly, liver.

After electrophoresis of human serum on agar gel, Kamaryt (1965) observed two bands with amylolytic activity. They both appeared in the gamma globulin region. The mobility of the less anodic isoenzyme corresponded to that of the amylase band obtained from pancreas, and the more anodic one corresponded to the band of amylase from salivary gland. A minimum of three and a maximum of five serum amylases were found by De la Lande (1969) using polyacrylamide gel electrophoresis. These isoenzymes were designated as AmySE-1, -2, -3, -4, and -5, respectively, according to their mobilities. It was concluded that AmySE-1 and SE-2 were likely of pancreatic origin and SE-2 and SE-3 were the most active isoenzymes in normal human serum. In his study of 1000 blood donors, Vacikova (1969) reported the presence of four amylase monomers and five possible combinations of isoenzymes designated as SP, sSP, SPp, sSpP, and P.

With refinement of separation techniques, it was found (Spiekerman, 1974) that human amylase of pancreatic origin contained one or two major and one or more minor isoenzymes, whereas salivary amylase generally yielded one or two major and three to six minor amylolytic bands. Otsuki (1976) determined isoamylases in serum and urine of normal individuals and in patients with mumps, pancreatitis, pancreatectomy, and chronic relapsing pancreatitis, as well as in saliva, pancreatic juice, and the homogenates of human pancreas, and found that as many as seven amylase isoenzymes were separated from these specimens. He concluded that essentially all the isoenzymes in human serum and urine were derived from the pancreas and salivary gland, and that the isoenzymes of 98 per cent of normal individuals consisted of two major and two to three minor isoamylases.

Assigning "amylase-1" to the isoenzyme with the slowest mobility, Otsuki found that it also was the major isoenzyme among four pancreatic isoamylases and that "amylase-3" was the major isoenzyme among three salivary isoamylases. This is in agreement with the findings of Spiekerman (1974) that, as a group, human pancreatic isoenzymes migrate more slowly in the electric field toward the anode than do salivary isoamylases.

The assignment of number 1 to the slowest migrating isoamylase and number 7 to the fastest migrating isoamylase is contrary to the commonly accepted isoenzyme numbering practice, in which the fastest migrating isoenzyme is given a subscript 1, such as LD_1. Isoamylase nomenclature is further complicated by other reports (Aw, 1966; Legaz, 1976), in which isoamylases were named either S or P to indicate their origin, and followed by a subscript number to indicate their electrophoretic mobility—for example, S_1 being the slowest migrating salivary isoamylase.

Using DEAE-Sephadex column for the separation, Fridhandler (1972) reported that in normal serum the P-type isoamylase constituted 28 to 49 per cent of the total amylase activity, but in the corresponding urine the percentage of pancreatic amylase was significantly higher. When QAE-Sephadex A-50, a better ion exchanger for the separation of P-type and S-type isoamylases, was used, it was found that in serum the percentage of total amylase activity contributed by P-type ranged from 12.7 to 76.3 per cent, with most of the values falling below 50 per cent; for S-type isoamylase, it averaged 57.6 per cent (Heffernon, 1977). As for the corresponding urines, there was 62.3 per cent (range 30.5 to 94 per cent) of P-type isoamylase and 37.6 per cent of S-type isoamylase. However, according to Gillard (1979), based on polyacrylamide disc-gel electrophoresis, only 43 per cent of total serum amylase was of pancreatic origin. When a selective inhibitor for S-type isoamylase was employed, an average of 48 per cent (range 27 to 70 per cent) of pancreatic isoenzyme in normal individuals was found (Huang, 1982). Conversely, Otsuki (1976) found that for normal adult serum the activity of the P-type amylase averaged 52.3 per cent of the total, and that the P-type activity was higher than that of the S-type in almost all normal adults. Bossuyt (1981) reported that the serum isoamylase pattern was clearly related to age. Using thin-layer gel isoelectric focusing techniques, it was found that the contribution of P-type isoenzyme increases from an average of 25 per cent and peaks to 42 per cent of the total amylase activity at age 40, after which the contribution of P-type decreases rather rapidly, and down to less than 20 per cent after age 70. All these reports agreed that there was no significant difference in results for normal males and females.

The question of whether the isoenzyme determination of amylase is of diagnostic value has been controversial. It certainly adds little additional information to the differential diagnosis of pancreatitis and parotitis, since the clinical symptoms are quite different and easily differentiated. However, in clinically unexplained hyperamylasemia, information obtained from isoamylase determination may be of value in distinguishing acute pancreatitis from other intra-abdominal catastrophes associated with elevated amylase activities.

There have been a great number of reports supporting the finding that, in acute pancreatitis, the P-type amylase is invariably elevated in both serum and urine (Otsuki, 1976; Bossuyt, 1981; Huang, 1982), whereas the S-type isoenzyme is decreased to 0 to 15 per cent of the total activity of hyperamylasemic serum of patients with acute pancreatitis, 12 to 25 per cent in the case of chronic relapsing pancreatitis, and 0 per cent in the case of carcinoma of the head of pancreas. The P-type isoenzyme, however, is elevated in chronic relapsing pancreatitis, hypoparathyroidism, and glomerulonephritis. S-type amylase was found to be increased in serum of patients with chronic pancreatitis, mumps, pancreatic insufficiency, Sjögren's syndrome, cholelithiasis, common duct narrowing, alcohol ingestion, acute gastroenteritis, acute respiratory insufficiency, chronic renal failure, lung cancer, and other cancer-associated hyperamylasemias. Isoenzyme studies on serum, urine, and duodenal fluid from patients with cystic fibrosis revealed that two thirds of the patients had no or little pancreatic amylase (Taussig, 1974).

The relative activity of P-type isoamylase may be highly useful as a diagnostic index of pancreatic pseudocyst (Warshaw, 1980). The P_1 isoamylase (the slowest migrating or least anodic) normally accounts for 80 to 90 per cent of total amylase activity; P_2 and P_3 account for 0 to 4 per cent in both serum and pancreatic juice. The mean ratios of P_2/P_1 and P_3/P_1 in fresh pancreatic juice, normal serum, acute pancreatitis serum, chronic pancreatitis serum, and pancreatic cancer serum were always less than 0.25 and less than 0.04, respectively. The ratio was elevated after incubation of the specimens at 37°C. in about 90 per cent of sera from patients with proven pseudocysts, but not from others. In several cases, this isoamylase analysis ruled out pseudocyst correctly, whereas ultrasound or computed tomography (CT) scan erroneously indicated the presence of pseudocyst.

At present, the clinical usefulness of isoamylase determination is still somewhat limited, especially in pancreatic disorders with concomitant renal insufficiency, which alone may increase P-type isoenzyme to as much as three times the upper limit of normal (Berk, 1979). However, with the availability of a simpler and more reliable isoamylase method, a better defined normal isoamylase pattern, and more clinical information on isoamylase changes in relation to different disease states, the analysis of isoenzyme may provide a new dimension in differential diagnosis of pancreatic diseases in the future.

LIPASE (TRIACYLGLYCEROL ACYL-HYDROLASE, E.C. 3.1.1.3)

Biochemistry and Physiology

Lipase hydrolyzes preferentially glycerol esters of long chain fatty acid at the carbons 1 and 3 ester bonds, producing two moles of fatty acid and one mole of β-monoglyceride per mole of triglyceride. After isomerization, the third fatty acid can be split off.

Lipolysis increases in proportion with the surface area of the lipid droplets, and absence of bile salts in duodenal fluid with resultant lack of emulsification renders lipase ineffective.

Calcium is found to be necessary for maximal lipase activity, but at a concentration higher than 5×10^{-3} M, it has inhibitory effect. It is speculated that the inhibitory effect is due to its interference with the action of bile salts at the water-substrate interface. Bile salts prevent the denaturation of lipase, as does serum albumin, at the interface. Heavy metals and quinine inhibit lipase activity.

Serum lipase is stable up to one week at room temperature and may be kept stable longer if refrigerated or frozen. The optimal reaction temperature is about 40°C. The optimal pH is 8.8, but other values ranging from 7.0 to 9.0 have been reported. This difference probably is due to the effect of the difference in types of substrate, buffer, incubation temperature, and concentrations of reagents used.

Pancreatic lipase is to be differentiated from lipoprotein lipase, aliesterase, and aryl-ester hydrolase, which are related but different enzymes. Lipase is also present in stomach, intestine, white blood cells, fat cells, and milk.

Interpretation

Serum lipase activity tends to become elevated at about the same time as, if not earlier than, the elevation of serum amylase in acute pancreatitis, contrary to the traditional belief that it elevates later than amylase. Serum lipase activity compares very favorably with amylase activity in the frequency of elevated values through the course of acute pancreatitis. There have been a few cases in which (1) the lipase levels remained persistently elevated after serum amylase and urine amylase activities subsided, (2) lipase activity elevated before amylase elevation, and (3) only lipase was elevated (Zinterhoffer, 1973; Lifton, 1974).

The diagnostic sensitivity and specificity of lipase in acute pancreatitis have been reported to be 75 to 100 per cent and 70 to 86 per cent, respectively—both higher than those for serum amylase. Serum lipase activity elevation in patients with mumps strongly suggests significant pancreatic as well as salivary gland involvement by the disease.

In spite of its higher diagnostic values, lipase activity determination is less frequently used in the diagnosis of acute pancreatitis, mainly because of the long incubation period, non-specificity of substrates (some of the substrates are more specific for esterase than lipase), and other technical difficulties.

When both serum amylase and lipase are used in a suspected case of acute pancreatitis, the sensitivity has been reported to be as high as 90 to 97 per cent (Patt, 1966; Lifton, 1974).

OTHER PANCREATIC ENZYMES

Proteolytic enzymes, such as trypsin, chymotrypsin, and carboxypeptidases in pancreatic juices, may, in acute pancreatitis, leak into the interstitial fluid and eventually reach the plasma. Attempts to assay trypsin in the blood of patients with acute pancreatitis by means of conventional enzyme methods have not generally been very successful, because trypsin activity is inhibited by trypsin inhibitors such as α_1-antitrypsin, inter-α-antitrypsin, and α_2-macroglobulin in the serum. Recently, however, radioimmunoassay techniques have been developed to measure circulating trypsins in plasma. It has been found that the measurement of immunoreactive trypsin is a specific and reliable diagnostic test of exocrine pancreatic function. The concentration of immunoreactive trypsin grossly elevates in acute pancreatitis and chronic relapsing pancreatitis without any overlap with normal controls (Masoero, 1980). Serial determinations of immunoreactive trypsin activity showed that the degree and the duration of elevation followed the same pattern as that of serum amylase. However, patients with a two- to five-fold increase in serum amylase without evidence of pancreatic damage have been found to have normal immunoreactive trypsin activity, so this test can supplement in discriminating between pancreatic and non-pancreatic lesions. Serum immunoreactive trypsin levels were found to be very low in chronic pancreatitis and normal in mild or moderate pancreatic insufficiency and in mumps (Gullo, 1980). It has been suggested that the normal ranges of immunoreactive trypsin levels be established according to age groups (Koehn, 1981).

Trypsin and chymotrypsin are nearly always present in grossly measurable quantities in the stools of normal young children. There is frequently much less activity detectable, however, in the adult stool, except when there is rapid transit through the gastrointestinal tract. The enzymes are apparently partially destroyed by bacteria within the gastrointestinal tract, and activity is seldom detectable at all by the cruder tests when there is constipation. The simpler tests are therefore not very useful for adults. On the other hand, many bacteria produce proteolytic enzymes which may give positive tests in the absence of pancreatogenous enzymes. For this reason, results must be interpreted with caution in children also (Ammann, 1968).

A number of methods have been devised for detecting and measuring proteolytic enzyme activity in stools (Wiggins, 1967) and duodenal fluid. These include tests based on ability of stool solutions to digest such substrate as serum proteins, hemoglobin, casein, and gelatin. The methods lack specificity and precision. One has been widely used as a screening test for cystic fibrosis of the pancreas. It depends on the ability of stool suspension to digest the gelatin emulsion of x-ray film.

Serial dilutions are made of stool with barbital buffer, pH 8. Strips of x-ray film are partially immersed in them and are incubated for one hour at 37°C. Proteolytic activity is indicated by digestion and removal of the opaque emulsion from the film.

SECRETIN TEST

The exocrine secretory capacity of the pancreas can be assessed by intubating the duodenum and subjecting the pancreas to stimulation with a test meal, secretin and pancreozymin. However, such testing is now slipping from favor because intubation is so unpopular with patients; in addition, pancreatic disease is usually advanced before exocrine function is appreciably reduced. Therefore, the test is of little help in distinguishing between chronic pancreatitis and carcinoma (Lancet, 1982). In the secretin test, bicarbonate secretory capacity is best expressed in terms of output (secretory rate). It appears that the distribution of bicarbonate output of normal subjects is very skewed, with a sharp cut-off at the lower end of the normal range. Subjects with normal pancreatic function generally secrete more than 15 mmol in 30 minutes. Wormsley (1970) has shown that the diagnostic discrimination between normal and chronic pancreatitis may be improved by considering bicarbonate concentration and volume together or by calculating bicarbonate output. He recommended that the bicarbonate concentration always be assessed in conjunction with the secretory rate.

Dreiling (1950) has published the most extensive study of the secretin test. Using his criteria for the lower limit of normality for volume, bicarbonate concentration, and enzyme output, there were false positives in 5.1 per cent of 2723 patients without pancreatic disease and false negatives in 5.2 per cent of 1725 patients with proven pancreatic disease.

Table 24–2. PATTERNS OF SECRETION OBSERVED FOLLOWING THE AUGMENTED SECRETIN TEST*

	Volume	HCO_3^-		Amylase
		Concentration	*Output*	
Normal	↑ ↑	↑	↑ ↑	↑ ↑
Chronic pancreatitis	↑	= or ↓	↑	↑
Pancreatic cancer	= or ↓	↑	↑	↑

*Modified from Bordalo, O., Noronha, M., Lamy, J., and Dreiling, D. A.: Am. J. Gastroenterol., *64*:125, 1975.

AUGMENTED SECRETIN TEST

(Bordalo, 1975)

The standard test is adequate for the diagnosis of well-established pancreatic lesions causing gross destruction of the parenchyma. The augmented test (4.0 to 5.0 secretin U/kg) is of particular value if the response to 1.0 U/kg is equivocal, inasmuch as augmented stimulation enhances secretory deficiencies in inflammation and cancer. See Table 24–2 for abnormal patterns and Table 24–3 for normal values.

Until recently, attention has been directed largely toward the secretory deficiency pattern. Discordant secretion is a pattern of increased flow after secretin stimulation with lesser increases in bicarbonate secretion. This condition is demonstrated in cases of the Zollinger-Ellison syndrome, hemochromatosis, and alcoholic and non-alcoholic cirrhosis. A preliminary report of the secretory patterns in these patients is as follows: (1) biliary cirrhotics and non-alcoholic cirrhotics had elevated volumes and high normal bicarbonate secretion; (2) patients with the Zollinger-Ellison syndrome, hemochromatosis, and alcoholic cirrhosis had marked increase in volume and a lesser increase in bicarbonate secretion, above the upper limit of normal.

MISCELLANEOUS TESTS

There is usually leukocytosis in patients with acute pancreatitis, white blood cell counts sometimes reaching 30,000/mm³. There may also be signs of hemoconcentration. A falling serum calcium points to the more serious form of pancreatitis, as does turbidity of the serum. The falling calcium presumably results from formation of calcium soaps of the fatty acids liberated by the action of pancreatic lipase. Hyperbilirubinemia occurs in many patients, not only those with gallstones but also those in whom the pancreatitis appears to be related to alcoholism. The reason is not well understood. Results of other liver function tests may also be abnormal. Transient hyperglycemia may also occur.

Table 24–3. NORMAL RANGES FOR STANDARD AND AUGMENTED SECRETIN TEST*

	Standard	Augmented
Volume (ml/kg)	2.0–4.4	4.5–8.1
HCO_3 (mEq/1)	90–130	93–141
HCO_3 (mEq)	12.2–31.0	22.5–58.9
Amylase (U/kg)	6.6–35.2	8.3–65.1

*From Dreiling, D. A.: Scand. J. Gastroenterol., *5*(Suppl. 6):115–122, 1970.

Malabsorption is discussed in Chapter 26. Since it may be caused by inadequacy of pancreatic secretion, and may result from chronic pancreatitis or pancreatic carcinoma, various tests for malabsorption, such as the serum carotenoid level, the glucose tolerance test, the ^{14}C-labeled triglyceride breath test, the starch tolerance test, and the three-day fecal fat determination, may be useful diagnostically, as may gross and microscopic examinations of stool. Only about one third of patients with pancreatic carcinoma are reported to have abnormal starch tolerance test results. A larger percentage may have a "flat" glucose tolerance curve, but this is very non-specific diagnostically. The D-xylose test, discussed in Chapter 26, is a very useful test for distinguishing malabsorption caused by pancreatic disease from that caused by intestinal disorders.

Recently, a few tests have been developed to provide a better indicator of pancreatic function as well as diagnosis of pancreatic carcinoma: (1) Lactoferrin, a protein secreted by the pancreas, is higher in the pancreatic juice of patients with chronic pancreatitis than in that of normal controls or of patients with pancreatic carcinoma (Fedail, 1979; Multigner, 1981). (2) A tubeless technique employs oral administration of a synthetic peptide, N-benzol-L-tyrosyl-p-aminobenzoic acid (BT-PABA). This substrate is broken down in the intestine by pancreatic chymotrypsin and the released PABA is absorbed and excreted in urine. The variation in gastric emptying, absorption, and hepatic metabolism of PABA is then corrected by simultaneous administration of ^{14}C-PABA (Tetlow, 1981). (3) Galactosyltransferase isoenzyme II was found to be raised in pancreatic carcinoma, so it can be used to attempt to distinguish between pancreatic carcinoma and chronic pancreatitis. However, this enzyme is not specific; it may be elevated in the presence of other gastrointestinal carcinomas (Podolsky, 1981).

SWEAT TEST

Principle

Pilocarpine is iontophoresed into the skin to stimulate locally increased sweat gland secretion (Gibson, 1959). The resulting sweat is absorbed by filter paper or gauze, weighed, diluted with water, and analyzed for sodium and chloride concentrations. The method is painless and reliable if performed properly. Total body sweating in patients with cystic fibrosis is hazardous, and a number of deaths from the procedure have been recorded.

When performed properly in duplicate, the Gibson-Cooke test gives a sensitivity of 90 to 99 per cent. However, a study at a cystic fibrosis center (Rosenstein, 1978) and by others (Shwachman, 1979) revealed that up to 43 per cent of the original tests performed on patients referred to the center were incorrect.

Other than iontophoresis, sweat collection may be accomplished without pilocarpine stimulation by placing a weighed gauze pad on the patient's back overnight. The pad is sealed tightly to prevent evaporation and removed in the morning. The pad is then weighed, diluted with water, and analyzed for sodium and chloride.

Interpretation

Cystic fibrosis (mucoviscidosis) of the pancreas is an autosomal recessive disease with an incidence of 1:1600 white births and 1:17,000 black births in the United States. Approximately one in every 20 Caucasians is a carrier. Cystic fibrosis is characterized by abnormal secretion by the various exocrine glands of the body, including pancreas; salivary glands; peritracheal, peribronchial, and peribronchiolar glands; lacrimal gland; sweat gland; mucosal gland of the small bowel; and even the bile ducts.

Involvement of the intestinal glands may result in the presence of meconium ileus at birth. Chronic lung disease and malabsorption resulting from pancreatic involvement are the major clinical problems of those who survive beyond infancy.

Laboratory diagnosis depends largely on demonstration of increased sodium and chloride in the sweat. Unfortunately, unless the sweat test is correctly done, it probably is the least reliable test with a high proportion of false positive and false negative results. Several modifications have been made to render the test more reproducible and results more definitive (Hammond, 1981, 1982). In children, chloride concentrations over 60 mmol/L of sweat on at least two occasions are diagnostic. Levels between 50 and 60 mmol/L are suggestive in the absence of adrenal insufficiency. The sweat sodium concentrations tend to be slightly lower than those of chloride in patients with cystic fibrosis, but the reverse is true in normal subjects (Shwachman, 1981). Sweat chloride concentrations greater than 60 mmol/L may be found in some patients with malnutrition, hyperhidrotic ectodermal dysplasia, nephrogenic diabetes insipidus, renal insufficiency, glucose-6-phosphatase deficiency, hypothyroidism, mucopolysaccharidosis, and fucosidosis. These are usually easily differentiated from cystic fibrosis by their clinical symptoms. Falsely negative sweat tests (elevated electrolyte concentrations) have been reported in patients with cystic fibrosis in the presence of hypoproteinemic edema (MacLean, 1973).

Sweat electrolytes in about half of a group of premenopausal adult women have been shown to undergo cyclic fluctuation, reaching a peak chloride concentration most commonly five to ten days prior to the onset of menses. Peak values were slightly under 65 mmol/L.

METHODOLOGIES

Amylase

Overview. Since the first method for amylase was described in 1831, more than 200 different methods, based on different principles and substrates, have been developed. In clinical laboratory today, the number of amylase methods commercially available probably is greater than that for any other test. In an interlaboratory study of amylase methodologies (Center for Disease Control [CDC], 1979) in which a total of 396 hospital laboratories participated, more than 23 different methods were reported in use. Of these, 31 per cent of the laboratories used three different chromogenic (chromolytic, dyed-starch) substrate methods, 29 per cent used five different couple-enzyme (kinetic) methods, 24 per cent used ten different amyloclastic (iodometric, starch-iodine) methods, 15 per cent used three different nephelometric methods, and 1 per cent used two or more different saccharogenic methods.

One of the most disturbing problems in the determination of amylase activity by different methods is the interconvertibility of the results. Although the use of International Units has been recommended, it is seldom used by the manufacturers of the amylase reagent. Different methods use different expressions of unit based on manufacturer's definition, and most of them are "one of a kind." The interconversion among different units is extremely difficult if possible at all, because many of the substrates used either are ill defined or are not the natural substrate for amylase and, in some cases are the partial breakdown products of starch, the natural substrate for amylase. Some methods use a pH which is not optimal for amylase. As a result, different methods have different "expected normal ranges." For example, the expected normal range for the classic saccharogenic method is 60 to 180 Somogyi units/dl, or 95 to 285 IU/L; the same for the Beckman coupled-enzyme method is 5 to 21 IU/L, and for the Worthington coupled-enzyme method, 51 to 198 U/L for males and 60 to 222 U/L for females. Many efforts have been made to correlate different units but to no avail. Further efforts are necessary to develop improved methods for amylase activity determination that will allow results to be expressed in International Units with a range of normal serum levels corresponding to the results of the saccharogenic assay (Marshall, 1980).

Interestingly, although the determination of serum amylase usually yields results with acceptable precision, it may not be the same for urine amylase. The coefficient of variation of a nearly normal (near upper limit) serum amylase ranged from 6 to 28 per cent by a variety of methods; the same for a normal urine pool ranged from 7 to 44 per cent. The inclusion of 3.0 g/L of human serum albumin to the same urine pool increased the coefficient of variation to 18 to 54 per cent for reasons unknown (CDC, 1979).

A College of American Pathologists Basic Urine Chemistry Survey (CAP, Set U-A, 1982) revealed highly unsatisfactory precisions. The coefficient of variation for one urine pool was 62 to 129 per cent, and the other, 41 to 66 per cent. Improvement of the urine amylase method, therefore, is urgently needed.

With a great number of different methodologies for amylase available today, each with its merits and drawbacks, one must choose a method based on accuracy, precision, ease of operation, and other requirements such as equipment availability and caliber of laboratory personnel. Regardless of the method chosen, cautions must be exercised to avoid contamination of specimens with saliva, since its amylase content is approximately 700 times that of serum. Red cells contain no amylase, so hemolysis generally presents no problem with most of the methods, except those coupled-enzyme methods in which the released peroxide is determined by a coupled peroxidase reaction. Heparinized plasma and serum yield identical results. Oxalated or citrated plasma may give falsely low results by up to 20 per cent. Fasting and postprandial venous blood samples give similar results. For routine determinations, a timed, two-hour urine collection, with activity expressed on a per hour basis, is of greatest clinical value.

It is strongly recommended that the method chosen for the determination of amylase be calibrated against Somogyi's saccharogenic method as modified by Henry (1960) so that results will be more meaningful clinically.

Saccharogenic Method. The saccharogenic method remains the only satisfactory primary method for determination of amylase activity (Marshall, 1980). In this method, the reducing power resulting from the amylase reaction on substrate, starch, (made up of amyloses and/or amylopectins), is measured. The products in the early stage of amylase action on amylose, a linear unbranched polysaccharide, are maltose, maltotriose, maltotetraose, and higher oligosaccharides. In the later stage of amylolysis, the main products are maltose and maltotriose in the ratio of 2.39:1. Maltotriose is further hydrolyzed to glucose and maltose. Maltose itself cannot be hydrolyzed by α-amylase. In amylopectin, a branched polysaccharide with α-1,6-glucosidic linkages at the branching points (which is not attacked by α-amylase), the breakdown products are maltose (42 per cent), maltotriose (28 per cent), and α-limit dextrins (30 per cent). Alpha-limit dextrins contain both α-1,4,- and α-1,6-glucosidic linkages. The amylolysis products of glycogen are the same as those of amylopectin.

In the saccharogenic method, the reducing substances of the reaction products are measured. In the original form (Somogyi, 1960), it employs no buffer for pH control and the color reagent does not always react stoichiometrically with liberated reducing compounds of different chain length. Also, it is a difficult method for inexperienced persons to perform reproducibly. It is not, therefore, an accurate method. However, modification of it (Henry, 1960) serves as the reference method for the iodometric procedure and others. Most clinicians are familiar with the normal range when expressed in Somogyi units, defined as the amount of enzyme in 100 ml of serum which produces reducing substances equivalent to 1 mg of glucose from starch in 30 minutes at 40°C. under the conditions specified in the procedure.

The reducing substances produced by the reaction may be quantitatively determined by copper reduction as described by Somogyi, or, for example, by ferricyanide reduction, picric acid reduction, dinitrosalicylic acid reduction, or any other methods for reducing substances.

Several automated saccharogenic methods have been developed and are routinely used by a number of large hospital and research laboratories (Fridhandler, 1970; Wu, 1972; Matthews, 1973). Except for a few published procedures, in which quantitation of the reducing power is based on the amount of maltose produced by coupled-enzyme reactions, all saccharogenic methods require a blank for each specimen in order to compensate for endogenous glucose and other reducing substances in the specimen. We recommend the saccharogenic method for serum and urine amylases, modified by Henry and Chiamori (1960).

Amyloclastic and Iodometric Methods. The coloration of starch by iodine has been widely used since 1908 for the measurement of amylase activity. Amylose, the linear polysaccharide which is more water soluble and less viscous in solution, is primarily responsible for the blue iodine reaction of starch. The iodine color produced by a given amount of amylose is approximately six times as intense as that produced by an equal amount of amylopectin, which is less water soluble and more viscous in solution. Two factors which influence the iodine color given by a particular starch are the length of glucose chain involved and the degree of branching of the chain. Amylose takes up approximately one iodine molecule per six glucose units, which make up each turn of starch helix. Starches containing 45 glucose residues or more turn blue with iodine. Polysaccharides containing 36 to 48 glucose residues yield a red color; with 12 to 18, a brown color; and with less than 12 residues, no color.

Amyloclastic methods involve measuring the time required to reach the achromic point (the point at which the blue color produced by iodine and starch is no longer visible), and iodometric methods involve measuring photometrically the amount of blue color lost in a given interval of time. The Somogyi amyloclastic method, as modified by Dade Reagents (Miami, Florida), and an iodometric method, also modified by Dade, have been used, and their results can be made to correlate roughly with those of the Somogyi saccharogenic method. Many modifications of the Somogyi starch-iodine method have been developed and made available (Harleco, Biomedix, Cordis, Sigma, American Monitor, Medi-Chem, and others). Unfor-

3

tunately, each employs different types of substrate and uses different expressions for units, making interlaboratory comparison difficult.

With the amyloclastic method it has been shown that (1) the enzyme reaction does not proceed under optimal conditions (Searcy, 1967), (2) it yields elevated amylase values (CDC, 1975) and significantly large variance (CDC, 1979) for specimens with normal amylase activities, and (3) the amyloclastic substrate has a greater activity with pancreatic amylase than with the corresponding salivary amylase (Sampson, 1981). However, in our experience, this method has worked well as a quick screening test and the results have compared closely with those obtained by Somogyi's saccharogenic procedure.

Chromogenic (Chromolytic, Dyed-Starch) Methods. In the past several years, many methods based on dyed-starch substrate, in which a dye is covalently coupled to an insoluble polysaccharide, have been introduced and well received. These include Remazol Brilliant Blue R-Amylopectin (Alpha-Amylase Fast Pack), Reactone Red 2B-Amylopectin (DyAmyl), Procion Brilliant Red M-2BS-Amylopectin, Cibachron Blau F36GA-Amylose (Amylochrome), Cibachron Blau F3GA-d-crosslinked potato starch polymer, and others. The advantages of the dyed-starch methods are their simplicity and sensitivity. However, because different methods use different reaction conditions, enzyme units, and normal ranges, it is virtually impossible to compare results from one method with those from another, although reasonably good correlations with a modified saccharogenic method and an amyloclastic method have been reported.

In a survey of amylase methodology by the CDC (1975), it was shown that dyed-starch methods generally yielded more "accurate" results, both in normal human specimens and in those with elevated activity, than did starch-iodine procedures. A similar report (CDC, 1979) indicated that two of the three dyed-starch kits may yield non-linear results. Sampson (1981) reported that chromogenic substrate demonstrated higher activity with the pancreatic amylase than with the corresponding salivary amylase.

Coupled-Enzymatic (Kinetic) Methods. In coupled-enzyme assay, the substrate, a starch or a better-defined oligosaccharide, yields maltose, maltotriose, and/or dextrins upon the action by amylase. The di- and trisaccharides give rise to glucose by the α-glucosidase externally added. Glucose is then quantitated by glucose oxidase or by any other coupled enzyme systems. The reactions involved in the method originally proposed by Tietz (1972) are as follows:

$$\text{starch} \xrightarrow{\text{amylase}} \text{maltose} + \text{glucose}$$

$$\text{maltose} \xrightarrow{\text{maltase}} \text{glucose}$$

$$\text{glucose} + O_2 \xrightarrow{\text{glucose oxidase}} \text{gluconic acid} + H_2O_2$$

In the last reaction, one molecule of oxygen is consumed, resulting in a decrease of PO_2, which is measured with an oxygen electrode. In another method (Beckman Amylase–DS), maltotetraose is used as substrate:

$$\text{maltotetraose} + H_2O \xrightarrow{\text{amylase}} 2\ \text{maltose}$$

$$2\ \text{maltose} + 2\ PO_4 \xrightarrow[\text{phosphorylase}]{\text{maltose}} 2\ \text{glucose} + 2\ \text{glucose-1-phosphate}$$

$$2\ \text{glucose-1-phosphate} \xrightarrow[\text{glucomutase}]{\beta\text{-phospho-}} 2\ \text{glucose-6-phosphate}$$

$$2\ \text{glucose-6-phosphate} + 2NAD^+ \xrightarrow{\text{G-6-PDH}} 2\ \text{6-phosphogluconate} + 2NADH + 2H^+$$

Other coupled-enzyme methods may use substrates such as maltopentose (DuPont ACA) and short-chain oligosaccharides (about 5 to 15 glucose residues); their results are all based on the quantitation of the glucose or NAD/NADH by the action of the coupled enzyme systems.

In a comparative study of coupled-enzyme methods, Kaufman (1980) concluded that among the four procedures evaluated (Eskalab-amylase, α-Amyl-Harleco, Beckman Amylase–DS, DuPont ACA Amylase), each has its distinct advantages and disadvantages. The day-to-day coefficient of variation ranged from 0.7 to 2.3 per cent for abnormal control serum and 4.4 to 8.9 per cent for normal control serum, much narrower than that for other methods. These narrow coefficients of variation agreed with another survey (CDC, 1979) in which coefficients of variation of 1.4 and 2.0 per cent were reported by 66 laboratories using ACA and 14 laboratories using Beckman–DS procedure. It seems that coupled-enzyme methods have gained much ground in clinical laboratories as DuPont's ACA and Beckman's Astra become widely adopted despite their ill-defined expressions of unit.

A newer coupled-enzyme method using chromogenic substrate consisting of a mixture of glucosidic p-nitrophenyl oligosaccharides of different chain lengths (NPG_X) has been developed (Foldi, 1979; Kaufman, 1980). Amylase hydrolyzes the long chain (4 to 10 glucose residues) p-nitrophenyl glycosides to homologues of shorter chain lengths, which give rise to free p-nitrophenol in the presence of glucosidase. The freed p-nitrophenol may be monitored spectrophotometrically. David (1982) showed that the relative rate of hydrolysis by amylase on p-nitrophenyl oligosaccharides containing four to seven glucose units decreases with the increase in chain length. He defined one unit as "the amount of amylase which causes the ultimate formation of one micromole of free p-nitrophenol per minute from a substrate mixture of NPG_5 and NPG_6 at 37°C.," and recommended that either NPG_5 or NPG_6 or a mixture of both be used as substrate for amylase determinations.

A reagent kit based on nitrophenyl glycosides has recently been introduced (Calbiochem-Behring, La Jolla, Calif. 92037). In this method, interference from endogenous glucose and α-keto acid is circumvented since only the released p-nitrophenol is measured.

Foldi (1979) also reported that when NPG_3 and NPG_4 are the predominating homologues in the substrate mixture, the reactions are highly selective for pancreatic rather than salivary amylase (100:1). Therefore, this method could potentially be used for the determination of pancreatic amylase.

Turbidimetric and Nephelometric Methods. When a starch solution, which is colloidal in nature, is hydrolyzed by amylase, the molecular size of polysaccharides decreases rapidly owing to the fragmentation by amylase action. This results in diminishing turbidity (absorbance) and light scatter of the original solution. The decrease in turbidity can be measured absorptiometrically and the decrease in light scatter can be measured nephelometrically and related to the amylase activity. Turbidimetric and nephelometric methods have the advantages of simplicity and rapidity. The major disadvantages of these procedures have been the lack of proper standards, poor substrate stability, and relatively poor precision at near normal levels of amylase activity, but an amylase-lipase analyzer (Model 91, Perkin-Elmer, Norwalk, Connecticut) is found to yield satisfactory results. Using this method, the decrease in turbidity or light scatter as a function of time is generally recorded continually, and amylase activity is calculated from a calibration curve. Most turbidimetric and nephelometric methods use an amylopectin preparation as substrate, but corn starch, dextrin, and a special liquid laundry starch have been successfully used. Any spectrophotometer (turbidimetry) or nephelometer or fluorometer (nephelometry) of good quality with temperature-controlled cuvettes and a chart recorder may be used. Turbidimetric and nephelometric determinations of amylase have been found to correlate closely with Somogyi units when a conversion factor is applied, although non-linearity has been indicated in a survey (CDC, 1979). Nephelometric methods have an outstanding advantage over turbidimetric methods in that measurement of decreased light scatter is much more sensitive than measurement of decreased activity.

Viscosimetric Method. When the size of the swollen starch granules decreases as a result of amylase action, the viscosity of the starch solution decreases accordingly, because viscosity is a function of interference between granules. This can be made the basis of any amylase assay. However, this method has not been well accepted by clinical laboratories for routine use.

Macroamylase Detection Method

Several methods are available. The direct identification of macroamylase requires ultracentrifugation or chromatography. The indirect methods such as temperature sensitive amylase assay have also been used. A chromatographic screening procedure developed by Fridhandler (1971) is described here.

Reagents

1. Buffer: Contains 50 mmol of Tris, 8.5 g of NaCl, and 0.2 g of sodium azide/L; pH 7.2.
2. Stock substrate solution, 50 g of amylose/L; 100 mg amylose (United States Biochemical Corp., Cleveland, Ohio, 44122) is mixed with 2 ml of dimethylsulfoxide and dissolved with stirring at 80°C.
3. Working substrate solution, 1 g amylose/L; 0.5 ml of stock substrate solution is mixed with 24.5 ml of buffer.
4. Stock iodine solution: A solution of 4 g of KI in 50 ml of water. To this is added 100 mg of iodine crystals. Stir until dissolved, then dilute to 100 ml with water.
5. Working iodine solution: 20 ml of stock iodine solution is mixed with 10 ml of glacial acetic acid and 170 ml of water.
6. Amylase-marker solution: 40 mg of "Blue Dextran" (Pharmacia Fine Chemicals, Inc., Piscataway, N.J. 08854) is dissolved in 2 ml of the buffer solution, and 20 mg of cytochrome C (type VI, Sigma Chemical Co., St. Louis, Mo. 63118) is then added. Gently stir until dissolved.

Equipment

1. Aluminum block incubator (for 37°C.).
2. Microcolumn: 1.2 cm inside diameter, and approximately 12 cm in length. Made of plastic.

Preparation of Microcolumn. Soak Sephadex G-100 (Pharmacia) in buffer solution overnight. Place a porous plastic disk (or other similar restrainer) at the outlet to retain Sephadex in the barrel. Pour the Sephadex suspension into the column and let the buffer flow until the gel beads have settled (8.5 to 9.5 cm high). Plug the outlet with a stopper. Place another porous plastic disk on the top of the gel bed, and press the disk with stainless forceps to compress the gel bed. Keep excess buffer solution on top of the gel bed until use. This column may be reused immediately after the first specimen has totally emerged, as indicated by the red color of cytochrome C in the effluent.

Procedure

1. Mix 200 μl of serum with 20 μl of amylase marker.
2. Remove excess buffer in the column by means of a pipette.
3. Remove stopper to drain residual buffer.
4. Immediately after the residual buffer has migrated into the top porous disk, add sample mixture with a pipette.
5. After sample has entered the disk, add three to four drops of buffer and allow to enter the disk.
6. Fill the top space with buffer.
7. When the blue color (Blue Dextran) reaches the bottom of the column (in about six to ten minutes), examine the appearance of effluent for blue drops.
8. Discard the first two or three faintly blue drops.
9. Use four small cups (such as those used in Technicon AutoAnalyzer) and collect four fractions of nine drops each (approximately 60 μl per drop) of the subsequent blue effluent.
10. Add 200 μl of working substrate solution to each cup. Mix, and incubate fractions at 37°C. in the aluminum block incubator for ten minutes.
11. Add 1.7 ml of working iodine solution to detect residual amylose.

Interpretation of Results. The macroamylase complex emerges along with Blue Dextran. Normal size amylase tends to be retarded through Sephadex, and emerges in approximately the same position as that of cytochrome C.

The absence of macroamylase is shown by the development of blue color after the addition of iodine solution. Discoloration (from blue through purple, brown, and yellow) indicates the presence of macroamylase activity. Should there be any uncertainty, the fractions may be incubated for a longer time. Discoloration is unequivocal in fractions 1 and 2, but less in fractions 3 and 4.

Type 1 macroamylasemia: Discoloration after 10 minutes of incubation.

Types 2 and 3 macroamylasemia: Discoloration requires more than 10 minutes (up to 60 minutes).

3

Isoamylase Fractionation Method

Isoamylase in serum, urine, and other body fluids may be analyzed by electrophoresis, isoelectric focusing, chromatography, heat lability, selective inhibition, and immunologic distinction methods. Most recently, a radioimmunoassay procedure has been published (Ogawa, 1981).

Specimens for isoamylase fractionation may be stored frozen up to 18 months or longer without affecting isoenzyme patterns.

A simplified, readily adaptable chromatographic method (Fridhandler, 1980) is described below.

Reagents

1. Initial buffer: Contains 50 mmol/L of Tris hydrochloride, 1.17 g of NaCl, and 10 mg/L of phenylmercuric acetate; pH 8.1.

2. Second buffer: Contains 50 mmol/L of Tris hydrochloride, 11.7 g of NaCl, and 10 mg/L of phenylmercuric acetate; pH 8.1.

Equipment and Preparation

1. QAE-Sephadex A-50 column: Soak QAE-Sephadex A-50 (Phamacia) in initial buffer (IB) overnight. Pour the Sephadex suspension into a 1.5 × 12 cm column. The Sephadex bed should be approximately 10 cm in height. Store at refrigerator temperature.

2. Sephadex G-100 column: Soak Sephadex G-100 in IB overnight. Pour the suspension into a 2.5 × 10 cm column. This column is to be used for serum specimen only.

3. Sephadex G-25 column: 1.5 × 5 cm. Preparation same as above. This column is to be used for urine specimen only.

Procedure (for Serum Specimens)

1. Add 3.3 ml of serum to Sephadex G-100 column prepared previously.

2. When the sample has entirely seeped into the column bed, IB is added to the reservoir and the effluent collected in a 50 ml graduated cylinder.

3. Discard the first 33 ml of the effluent.

4. Collect the next 10 ml and mix well.

5. Apply 1 ml of this collection to the QAE-Sephadex A-50 column previously prepared.

6. When the applied sample has seeped into the bed, 19 ml of IB is added to the reservoir and 19 ml of the resulting effluent is discarded.

7. Add 19.5 ml of IB to the reservoir and collect the resulting effluent in a test tube containing 10 µl of bovine albumin (50 mg/ml). Mix well and label the tube "P fraction."

8. Add 11.5 ml of second buffer (SB); an equal amount of the effluent is discarded.

9. Add 23 ml of SB and collect 23 ml of effluent in a test tube containing 10 µl of BSA. Mix and label "S fraction."

10. Assay both fractions for amylase activity (see below).

Procedure (for Urine Specimens)

1. Add 50 µl of marker solution (2 per cent Blue Dextran and 1 per cent of cytochrome C in initial buffer) to 0.5 ml of urine.

2. Remove a previously prepared Sephadex G-25 column from cold storage. Remove buffer from the reservoir and allow residual buffer to seep into the bed.

3. Apply the specimen immediately; the effluent colored by the Blue Dextran and cytochrome C (totaling approximately 1 ml) containing all the urine amylase is allowed to drop into the prepared QAE-Sephadex A-50 column directly.

4. Steps thereafter are exactly the same as described in the previous section for serum isoamylase.

The activity of P-type and S-type isoamylases can then be assayed by using Phadebas tablet (Pharmacia) or any other amylase method.

This method requires only a small volume of specimen. One technologist can conveniently perform three or four samples simultaneously. It takes less than 2.5 hours for urine and about 4.5 hours for a serum specimen.

Lipase and Other Examinations

The classic method is that of Cherry (1932), in which olive oil is used as a substrate, avoiding inclusion of non-specific esterase activity in the assay result. Oleic acid released after a 16- to 18-hour incubation at 37°C. is titrated with standard alkali, and results are expressed as ml 0.05 N NaOH (corrected for blank). Normal serum activity is up to 1.5 units/ml. The procedure is too slow to be useful. Many modifications of this procedure have been developed, largely aimed at speeding up the test and improving substrate sensitivity and reproducibility. One of the more successful is the Tietz-Fiereck (1972) modification.

Methods for determination of fecal trypsin, secretin test, augmented secretin test, and sweat electrolytes may be reviewed in the previous edition of this text (pp. 753–756).

Ammann, R. W., Tagwercher, E., Kashiwagi, H., and Rosenmund, H.: Diagnostic value of fecal chymotrypsin and trypsin assessment for detection of pancreatic disease. Am. J. Dig. Dis., *13*:123, 1968.

Aw, S. E., and Hobbs, J. R.: Human isoamylases. Biochem. J., *99*:16P, 1966.

Berk, J. E., Fridhandler, L., and Neww, R. L.: Amylase and isoamylase activities in renal insufficiency. Ann. Intern. Med., *90*:351, 1979.

Bordalo, O., Noronha, M., Lamy, J., and Dreiling, D. A.: Standard and augmented secretin testing in chronic pancreatic disease. Am. J. Gastroenterol., *64*:125, 1975.

Bossuyt, P. J., Bogaert, R. V., Scharpe, S. L., and Maercke, Y. V.: Relation of age to isoenzyme pattern and total activity of amylase in serum. Clin. Chem., *27*:451, 1981.

Center for Disease Control, U.S. Department of Health, Education and Welfare: Alpha-amylase methodology survey I, 1975.

Center for Disease Control, U.S. Department of Health, Education and Welfare: Publication # (CDC) 79–0002. An interlaboratory study of amylase methodologies using purified enzyme materials, 1979.

Cherry, I. S., and Crandall, L. A., Jr.: The specificity of pancreatic lipase: Its appearance in the blood after pancreatic injury. Am. J. Physiol., *100*:266, 1932.

David, H.: Hydrolysis by human alpha-amylase of p-nitrophenyloligosaccharides containing four to seven glucose units. Clin. Chem., *28*:1485, 1982.

De la Lande, F. A., and Boettcher, B.: Electrophoretic examination of human serum amylase isoenzymes. Enzymologia, *37*:335, 1969.

Dreiling, D. A., and Hollander, F.: Studies in pancreatic function. II. A statistical study of pancreatic secretion following secretin in patients without pancreatic disease. Gastroenterology, *15*:620, 1950.

Fedail, S., Harvey, R., Salmon, P., Brown, P., and Read, A.: Trypsin and lactoferrin levels in pure pancreatic juice in patients with pancreatic disease. Gut, *20*:983, 1979.

Foldi, P.: Cleavage of nitrophenyl glucosides by alpha-amylase. *In* Lorentz, K.: Alpha-amylase assay: Current state and future development. J. Clin. Chem. Clin. Biochem., *17*:499, 1979.

Fridhandler, L., and Berk, J. E.: Automated saccharogenic assay of alpha-amylase activity in serum. Clin. Chem., *16*:911, 1970.

Fridhandler, L., and Berk, J. E.: Macroamylasemia. Adv. Clin. Chem., *20*:267, 1978.

Fridhandler, L., and Berk, J. E.: Simplified chromatographic method for isoamylase analysis. Clin. Chim. Acta, *101*:135, 1980.

Fridhandler, L., Berk, J. E., and Ueda, M.: Isolation and measurement of pancreatic amylase in human serum and urine. Clin. Chem., *18*:1493, 1972.

Fridhandler, L., Berk, J. E., and Ueda, M.: Macroamylasemia: Rapid detection method. Clin. Chem., *17*:423, 1971.

Gibson, L. E., and Cooke, R. E.: A test for concentration of electrolytes in sweat in cystic fibrosis of the pancreas utilizing pilocarpine by iontophoresis. Pediatrics, *23*:545, 1959.

Gillard, B. K.: Quantitative gel-electrophoretic determination of serum amylase isoenzyme distributions. Clin. Chem., *25*:1919, 1979.

Gullo, L., Ventrucci, M., Bonora, G., Vezzadini, G., and Vezzadini, P.: Comparative study of serum trypsin levels and pancreatic exocrine function in chronic pancreatitis. Scand. J. Gastroenterol., *15*:Suppl. 62:27, 1980.

Hammond, K. B., and Johnston, B. J.: Sweat test for cystic fibrosis. *In* Faulkner, W. R., and Meites, S. (eds.): Selected methods for the small clinical chemistry laboratory, Vol. 9, Am. Assoc. Clin. Chem., 1982.

Hammond, K. B., and Johnston, B. J.: The sweat test for cystic fibrosis: Improving its reliability. Lab. Med., *12*:56, 1981.

Heffernon, J. J., Fridhandler, L., Berk, J. E., and Shimamura, J.: Assay of amylase and isoamylase activities in serum and urine. Am. J. Gastroenterol., *67*:473, 1977.

Henry, R. J., and Chiamori, N.: Study of the saccharogenic method for the determination of serum and urine amylase. Clin. Chem., *6*:434, 1960.

Huang, W. Y., and Tietz, N. W.: Determination of amylase isoenzymes in serum by use of a selective inhibitor. Clin. Chem., *28*:1525, 1982.

Kamaryt, J., and Laxova, R.: Amylase heterogeneity, some genetic and clinical aspects. Humangenetik, *1*:579, 1965.

Kaufman, R. A., and Tietz, N. W.: Recent advances in measurement of amylase activity—a comparative study. Clin. Chem., *26*:846, 1980.

Klonoff, D. C.: Macroamylasemia and other immunoglobulin-complexed enzyme disorders. West J. Med., *133*:392, 1980.

Koehn, H. D., and Mostbeck, A.: Age-dependence of immunoreactive trypsin concentration in serum. Clin. Chem., *27*:502, 1981.

Lancet: Diagnosis of chronic pancreatitis. Lancet, *1*:719, 1982.

Legaz, M. E., and Kenny, M. A.: Electrophoretic amylase fractionation as an aid in diagnosis of pancreatic disease. Clin. Chem., *22*:57, 1976.

Lente, F. V.: Diagnosing acute pancreatitis the enzyme way. Diagnost. Med., *5*:50, 1982.

Levitt, M. D., and Ellis, C.: A rapid and simple assay to determine if macroamylase is the cause of hyperamylasemia. Gastroenterology, *83*:378, 1982.

Lifton, I., Slichers, K. A., Pragay, D. A., and Katz, L. A.: Pancreatitis and lipase: A re-evaluation with a five minute turbidimetric lipase determination. J.A.M.A., *229*:47, 1974.

MacLean, W. C., Jr., and Tripp, R. W.: Cystic fibrosis with edema and falsely negative sweat test. J. Pediatr., *83*:86, 1973.

Marshall, J. J.: Concerning the measurement of alpha-amylase activity in international units. Clin. Biochem., *13*:4, 1980.

Masoero, G., Andriulli, A., Recchia, S., Marchetto, M., Benitti, V., and Verme, G.: Trypsin-like immunoreactivity in the diagnosis of acute pancreatitis. Scand. J. Gastroenterol., *15*:Suppl. 62:21, 1980.

Matthews, W. S., Sterling, R. E., Boyd, T., and Flores, O. R.: Modified automated saccharogenic determination of serum and urinary amylase activity. Clin. Chem., *19*:1384, 1973.

Multigner, L., Figarella, C., and Sarles, H.: Diagnosis of chronic pancreatitis by measurement of lactoferrin in duodenal juice. Gut, *22*:350, 1981.

Ogawa, M., Takatsuka, Y., Kitahara, T., Matsuura, K., and Kosaki, G.: Radioimmunoassay of human pancreatic amylase. Meth. Enzymol., *74*:290, 1981.

Otsuki, M., Saeki, S., Yuu, H., Maede, M., and Baba, S.: Electrophoretic pattern of amylase isoenzymes in serum and urine of normal persons. Clin. Chem., *22*:439, 1976.

Patt, H. H., Dramer, S. P., Woel, G., Zietung, D., and Seligman, A. M.: Serum lipase determination in acute pancreatitis. Arch. Surg., *92*:718, 1966.

Podolsky, D., McPhee, M., Alpert, E., Warshaw, A., and Isselbacher, K.: Galactosyl transferase isoenzyme II in the detection of pancreatic cancer: Comparison with radiologic, endoscopic and serologic tests. N. Engl. J. Med., *304*:1313, 1981.

Proelss, H. F., and Wright, B. W.: New, simple maltogenic assay for mechanized determination of alpha-amylase activity in serum and urine. Clin. Chem., *21*:694, 1975.

Rosenstein, B. J., Langbaum, T. S., Gordes, E., and Brusilow, S. W.: Cystic fibrosis. Problems encountered with sweat testing. J.A.M.A., *240*:1987, 1978.

Sampson, E. J., Duncan, P. H., Fast, D. M., Whitner, V. S., McKneally, S. S., Baird, M. A., MacNeil, M. L., and Bayse, D. D.: Characterization and intermethod relationships of materials containing purified human pancreatic and salivary amylase. Clin. Chem., *27*:714, 1981.

Sax, S. M.: Interconversion of Enzyme Units. Santa Monica, Clinton Laboratories, 1972.

Scully, C., Eckersal, P. D., Emond, R. T. D., Boyle, P., and Beeley, J. A.: Serum alpha-amylase isozymes in mumps: Estimation of salivary and pancreatic isozymes by isoelectric focusing. Clin. Chim. Acta, *113*:281, 1981.

Searcy, R. L., Wilding, P., and Berk, J. E.: An appraisal of methods for serum amylase determination. Clin. Chim. Acta, *15*:189, 1967.

Shwachman, H., and Mahmoodian, A.: Quality of sweat test performance in the diagnosis of cystic fibrosis. Clin. Chem., *25*:158, 1979.

Shwachman, H., Mahmoodian, A., and Neff, R. K.: The sweat test: Sodium and chloride values. J. Pediatr., *98*:576, 1981.

Somogyi, M.: Modification of two methods for the assay of amylase. Clin. Chem., *6*:23, 1960.

Spiekerman, A. M., Perry, P., Hightower, N. C., and Hall, F. F.: Chromogenic substrate method for demonstrating multiple forms of alpha-amylase after electrophoresis. Clin. Chem., *20*:324, 1974.

Taussig, L. M., Wolf, R. O., Woods, R. E., and Deckelbaum, R. J.: Use of serum amylase isoenzyme in evaluation of pancreatic function. Pediatrics, *54*:229, 1974.

Tetlow, V. A., Herman, H., Kay, G. H., and Braganza, J.: Diagnostic accuracy of the PABA excretion index (using ^{14}C-PABA). Gut, *22*:A4441, 1981.

Tietz, N. W., and Fiereck, E. A.: Measurement of lipase in serum. *In* Cooper, G. R. (eds.): Standard Methods of Clinical Chemistry, Vol. 7. New York, Academic Press, 1972, pp. 19–31.

Tietz, N. W., Mirands, E., and Weinstock, A.: A kinetic method for measuring serum amylase activity. Proceedings of the International Seminar and Workshop on Enzymology, Chicago, May, 1972.

Vacikova, A., and Blochova, L.: Isoamylase in blood donors. Humangenetik, *8*:162, 1969.

Warshaw, A. L., Bellini, C. A., and Lesser, P. B.: Inhibition of serum and urine amylase activity in pancreatitis with hyperlipemia. Ann. Surg., *182*:72, 1975.

Warshaw, A. L., and Lee, K. H.: Aging changes of pancreatic isoamylases and the appearance of "old amylase" in the serum of patients with pancreatic pseudocysts. Gastroenterology, *79*:1246, 1980.

Webster, P. D., and Spainhour, J. B.: Pathophysiology and management of acute pancreatitis. Hosp. Pract., *9*:59, 1974.

Wermus, G., Adams, T., and Menson, R.: A stoichiometric method for the determination of serum amylase. *In* Lorentz, K.: Alpha-amylase assay: Current state and future development. J. Clin. Chem. Clin. Biochem., *17*:499, 1979.

Wilding, P., Cooke, W. T., and Nicholson, G. I.: Globulin-bound amylase. A cause of persistently elevated levels in serum. Ann. Intern. Med., *60*:1053, 1964.

Wormsley, K. G.: Test of pancreatic function. Proc. R. Soc. Med., *63*:431, 1970.

Wu, W. T., and Beeler, M. F.: A simplified semi-automatic saccharogenic method for amylase assay. Am. J. Clin. Path., *57*:497, 1972.

Zinterhoffer, L., Wardlaw, S., Jatlow, P., and Seligson, D.: Nephelometric determination of pancreatic enzymes. II. Lipase. Clin. Chim. Acta, *44*:173, 1973.

25

EXAMINATION OF GASTRIC AND DUODENAL CONTENTS

DONALD C. CANNON, M.D., PH.D.

EXAMINATION OF GASTRIC CONTENTS

Although it is true that analysis of gastric secretion has not fulfilled some of the previous claims and expectations, this procedure maintains a useful role in clinical diagnosis and in the evaluation of therapy. As with most other laboratory examinations, information derived from gastric analysis is by itself seldom of pathognomonic significance but rather must be interpreted in light of the patient's history and with the results of other pertinent clinical, roentgenologic, and laboratory examinations. For example, anacidity does not invariably indicate pernicious anemia, although it is true that adult patients with pernicious anemia invariably have anacidity. Studies of peripheral blood and bone marrow, an investigation of intrinsic factor activity, or measurement of plasma gastrin may be necessary to substantiate or eliminate the diagnosis of pernicious anemia. Furthermore, in interpreting the results of gastric analysis, it must be kept in mind that there exists no sharply delineated normal range such as one is accustomed to use as a reference point for many laboratory measurements in chemistry, hematology, or serology. It is indeed only at the extremes of gastric secretion—anacidity or the marked hypersecretion such as is seen in the Zollinger-Ellison syndrome or in some cases of duodenal ulcer—that one can say with certainty that an underlying disease exists.

Considering both its limitations and its value, it is probable that a properly performed gastric analysis is done too infrequently at the present time. Among the factors that have contributed to this situation is the fact that many of the previously held beliefs regarding gastric secretion have been disproved by newer tests and better controlled surveys, thus adding a note of bewilderment and pessimism in the mind of the physician confronted with a patient having gastrointestinal complaints. For example, studies using the augmented histamine test have disproved the notion engendered by the older and now obsolete tests—standard histamine, alcohol stimulation, or various test meals—that anacidity is frequently a variant of normal. Anacidity, furthermore, is no longer considered to be a reliable screening test for gastric carcinoma, because most afflicted individuals do not have gastric anacidity; when anacidity occurs it is usually only in the more advanced cases. Gastroscopy, roentgenography, and gastric cytology are far more useful in establishing the diagnosis of probable gastric carcinoma than is gastric analysis. Even in the diagnosis of duodenal ulcer, the hypersecretory state that was once considered typical for the disease does not occur in most affected patients. An element of confusion has perhaps been added by the fact that the physicochemical basis for the older concept of "free," "combined," and "total" acid has now been found untenable.

The properly performed gastric analysis requires a relatively large investment of time by the physician who must perform the intubation and supervise the collection of samples. Although in itself a benign procedure, intubation is apt to be an unpleasant experience for the patient, not a few of whom submit to the procedure with reluctance. In view of these facts and the inherent limitations of the information to be gained, it is essential that there be a definite indication for performing routine gastric analysis. In general there are four clear-cut indications:

1. To determine whether or not the patient can secrete any gastric acid. The finding of anacidity is of major importance in three situations: the patient with macrocytic anemia, neurologic disorders, or other signs and symptoms of pernicious anemia; the patient suspected of having pernicious anemia who has been treated with vitamin B_{12} before the diagnosis was unequivocally established; and the exclusion of simple peptic ulceration in a patient with a suspicious ulcerating lesion of the stomach.

2. To measure the amount of acid produced by a patient with symptoms of peptic ulcer, particularly a patient with suspected duodenal or postoperative stomal ulcer who has no roentgenographically demonstrable lesion.

3. To reveal the hypersecretory state characteristic of the Zollinger-Ellison syndrome.

4. To determine the completeness of vagotomy by the insulin test.

In addition, gastric analysis is considered by some to be helpful for judging the efficacy of surgical, medical, or roentgen therapy for peptic ulcer and for determining the proper type of surgical procedure to be performed in the patient with peptic ulcer.

Physiology of Gastric Secretion

Gastric secretion has three major physiologic functions—the initiation of protein digestion, the physical and chemical preparation of ingested food resulting in an optimal mixture for subsequent digestion in the small intestine, and the secretion of intrinsic factor which promotes vitamin B_{12} absorption in the ileum. The first of these functions is not absolutely essential to the welfare of the human body, as shown by the fact that individuals with anacidity of long duration and therefore with failure of gastric protein digestion can exist free of gastrointestinal complaints and in good nutritional status.

Stimuli to gastric secretion are classically considered to occur in three phases, although present information demonstrates a relationship among these various phases. The cephalic or neurogenic phase consists of stimuli that are transmitted by the vagus nerves. This phase consists of anticipatory stimuli that arise from visual or olfactory perceptions associated with the ingestion of food and psychogenic stimuli that are derived from mental processes not related to the ingestion of food. Vagal impulses directly stimulate the parietal cells to secrete acid but also stimulate the antral mucosa to secrete gastrin into the blood. The polypeptide hormone, gastrin, is the most powerful known stimulus to gastric secretion, being many times as potent on a weight basis as histamine. Its elaboration and secretion are the paramount features of the second or gastric phase of secretion. In addition to vagal stimulation, gastrin is released by distention of the antrum with food or fluid and by contact of protein and protein breakdown products, the so-called secretagogues, with the antral mucosa. Secretagogues probably also act to stimulate the parietal and chief cells directly. The gastric phase is thus diminished but not abolished by vagotomy. The intestinal phase is quantitatively the least important phase of gastric secretion and is presumably mediated by humoral substances secreted into the blood by the duodenum in response to the entry of digestive products. It is probable that gastrin, formed by the duodenum, is the major humoral agent in this phase. Gastrin or a very similar substance has also been isolated from non-beta-cell adenomas of the pancreas associated with the hypersecretory state of the Zollinger-Ellison syndrome.

Various mechanisms serve to inhibit gastric secretion. Particularly important is the inhibition of gastrin secretion that occurs when the acidity of antral contents falls below a pH of about 1.5. Various hormonal substances, collectively termed enterogastrone, inhibit gastric secretion and are secreted into the blood by the duodenal mucosa in response to contact with fat and fatty acid breakdown products. The major contributor to enterogastrone activity is gastric inhibitory polypeptide, which is produced by K cells in the intestinal glands of the mid- and distal duodenum and proximal jejunum. Gastric inhibitory polypeptide inhibits gastric motility and gastric secretion as well as directly inhibiting hydrochloric acid and pepsin secretion. Similar action is displayed by vasoactive intestinal polypeptide, which is secreted by H cells in the intestinal mucosa and by certain nerve cells. Psychic mechanisms can inhibit gastric secretion as shown by the diminished secretion reported in patients suffering from chronic depression, and under other circumstances can stimulate gastric secretion.

Composition of Gastric Secretion

Gastric secretion is a complex solution the synthesis of which is not completely understood. Although the cells that secrete hydrochloric acid, pepsin, and mucus have been clearly identified, the varying concentrations of inorganic ions in particular remain the object of speculation.

Hydrochloric Acid. It is a remarkable biochemical feat that the stomach can secrete hydrogen ions at a concentration of more than one million times the plasma concentration—a concentration of about 160 mEq/L prior to dilution with the other secretory components. Hydrochloric acid is secreted by the parietal cells which are located in the isthmus and neck of the gastric glands of the fundus and body of the stomach but not those at either anatomic extreme—the narrow rim of cardia or the pylorus and antrum. The major importance of hydrochloric acid to digestion is to provide the high acidity necessary for the activation of pepsin from pepsinogen but also to a limited extent to hydrolyze polypeptides and disaccharides directly. As a result of the ease of measurement and relatively good correlation with disease states, the determination of gastric acidity is the most commonly used clinical index of gastric secretory activity.

Digestive Enzymes. The major digestive enzyme of gastric secretion is pepsin, which is elaborated by the chief or peptic cells located at the base of the gastric glands of the body and fundus. Pepsin is secreted as the zymogen, pepsinogen, which is activated by gastric acid at an optimal pH of 1.6 to 2.4. Pepsin catalyzes the degradation of proteins to proteoses and peptones but does not liberate free amino acids, this being the function of the more potent proteases in the secretions of the pancreas and small intestine. A small amount of pepsinogen enters the blood, presumably by direct absorption from the peptic cells, and is secreted in the urine as uropepsinogen. It has recently been shown that gastric proteolytic activity is shared by several enzymes. At least one of these, gastricsin, has a higher pH optimum (approximately 3.2) than pepsin. Gastricsin apparently arises from the same zymogen precursor as pepsin, and its concentration in gastric secretion is about one third that of pepsin. The significance of multiple gastric proteolytic enzymes is not yet known.

Other digestive enzymes include rennin and gastric lipase. Rennin has weak proteolytic activity and is best known for its ability to coagulate caseinogen in milk. Its high pH optimum (approximately 5 to 6) would seem to obviate any important contribution to gastric digestion. Gastric lipase, similarly, has a high pH optimum and appears to be of no importance to digestion.

Mucus. Gastric mucus is a chemically complex mixture of mucoproteins and mucopolysaccharides, the physiologic significance of which is poorly understood. Attempts have been made to correlate alterations or deficiencies in gastric mucus with the occurrence of peptic ulcer, but such studies are inconclusive. Mucus is secreted by specialized cells of the gland necks in the fundus and body of the stomach, by cells of the surface epithelium, and by the acinar cells of the cardia, antrum, and pylorus. Mucus secretion is probably stimulated largely by mechanical and chemical stimuli.

Electrolytes. Gastric secretion contains all the electrolytes found in other body fluids in a combined osmolar concentration equal to or slightly greater than plasma. The individual electrolytes vary widely in concentration, and with the exception of hydrogen ion, such variations have no known clinical significance.

Nondigestive Enzymes. Using the technique of intragastric neutralization, various enzymes have been described in gastric secretion, including lactic dehydrogenase, aspartate aminotransferase, isocitric dehydrogenase, leucine amino peptidase, alanine aminotransferase, beta-glucuronidase, alkaline phosphatase, and ribonuclease. These enzymes are doubtless the result of active gastric metabolism and have no function in digestion, particularly since all are inactivated by gastric acid except perhaps ribonuclease.

Serum Proteins. Small amounts of serum albumin and gamma globulin are normally present in gastric secretion. Their presence can usually be detected only in the anacid stomach or by use of intragastric neutralization. Albumin is frequently increased in the gastric secretion in cases of giant hypertrophic gastritis or Menetrier's disease, in carcinoma, and in benign peptic ulcer.

Miscellaneous Substances. The most important component in this group and probably in the gastric secretion as a whole is intrinsic factor, which is elaborated and secreted by the gastric mucosa. It is a mucoprotein with molecular weight of about 17,000. The manner in which intrinsic factor promotes vitamin B_{12} absorption in the ileum is uncertain, but it has been convincingly shown to involve a complex between the two substances.

In approximately 80 per cent of individuals, those possessing the dominant secretor gene in homozygous or heterozygous state, the water-soluble blood group specific substances are present in the gastric secretion. This is of no particular significance to gastric secretion because in these individuals the group specific substances are present in all body fluids.

Nomenclature of Gastric Secretion

It was previously believed that the hydrochloric acid in gastric secretion exists in two distinct phases, the relative amounts of which depend on the pH of the secretion. At high pH values, generally taken to be greater than 3.0 or 3.5, the acid supposedly exists almost exclusively as a mixture of organic salts formed from combination of the acid with proteins and peptones in the gastric secretion. This phase, the "combined acid," was a direct reflection of the buffering capacity of the gastric secretion. Only when the buffering capacity was exceeded could the hydrochloric acid supposedly exist as ions in solution or as "free acid." Acidity was measured in "clinical units" or "degrees of acidity," which were equal to the number of milliliters of 0.1 N NaOH required to titrate 100 ml of gastric secretion to the endpoint of Topfer's reagent (pH 2.8 to 3.5) for "free acid" or to the endpoint of phenolphthalein (pH 8.2 to 10) for "total acid."

The older concept of gastric acidity was supported by titration curves obtained from the neutralization of gastric acid with sodium hydroxide. Such curves were similar to the titration curve of an aqueous solution of hydrochloric acid at pH values below about 2.8, but above this pH the curves resembled more closely those of a buffer mixture composed of a weak acid and its salt. Such studies failed to take into account the buffering effect of the various test meals then in use as gastric stimulants, an effect which could prove considerable. It has, in fact, now been shown that the titration curve of gastric secretion collected after histamine or Histalog stimulation rather closely resembles that of a solution of pure hydrochloric acid, although a slight buffering effect is evident at high pH values, generally above pH 4.0 (Moore, 1965). It is clearly apparent from such studies that a significant amount of "free" hydrochloric acid is present in gastric secretion at pH values greater than 3.5.

It is therefore recommended that the older terms of "free," "combined," and "total" acid be avoided entirely. Gastric secretion can best be described in terms of three measurements to be performed on each sample of gastric secretion:

1. *Volume* in milliliters.
2. *Titratable acidity* expressed in milliequivalents per liter. This is determined by titration of a suitable aliquot of gastric secretion with 0.1 N NaOH to neutrality (pH of 7.0 or 7.4 as preferred by some). The endpoint should be measured electrometrically with a suitable pH meter. If a pH meter is not available, the endpoint can be determined colorimetrically with phenol red (color change of yellow to red in the pH range of 6.8 to 8.4).
3. The *pH* measured electrometrically.

The *acid output* in milliequivalents for each sample can be calculated by multiplying its volume in milliliters by the titratable acidity and dividing by 1000. In addition to reporting the measured *volume, titratable acidity,* and *pH* and the calculated *acid output* for each individual sample, the *total volume* and *total acid output* will usually be reported for a given test by adding the individual sample values. Thus, for the study of basal secretion, a one-hour collection is generally employed consisting of four individually segregated 15-minute samples. The *basal acid output* in milliequivalents per hour is reported as the sum of the acid outputs for the four samples.

Nomenclature related to stimulated gastric secretion has developed in recent years largely in reference to histamine stimulation. The various terms can logically be applied to stimulation using pentagastrin, which is now the preferred gastric stimulant, because the pattern of acid output following stimulation with pentagastrin is similar to that with histamine (Khodadoost, 1972).

The *maximal acid output* was originally defined as the milliequivalents of acid secreted in the hour following injection of histamine in the augmented or maximal histamine test. This is not to be confused with the *maximal histamine response,* which was defined by Kay (1953) as the output of acid in milliequivalents in the period from 15 to 45 minutes after histamine injection. Since these terms are easily confused, the term *maximal histamine response* is best avoided.

The *peak acid output* was originally defined as the greatest acid output in any two successive 15-minute periods in the augmented histamine test (Baron, 1963).

Various terms have been employed to describe qualitatively the results of gastric secretion tests. Most of these terms originated in relation to the older concepts of gastric acid and therefore must be redefined or discarded. Some useful terms have been given different definitions by different investigators. Only with the anticipation of vociferous objection can any definition of these terms be attempted.

Anacidity was previously defined as the absence of "free" acid, usually taken to mean a failure of the gastric secretory pH to fall below 3.5. Most investigators now define *anacidity* as a failure of the pH to fall below either 6.0 or 7.0 in the augmented histamine, pentagastrin, or Histalog tests. It is the most reasonable compromise between clinical usefulness and strict physicochemical definition to define *anacidity* as a failure of the pH to fall below 6.0 following augmented or maximal histamine, pentagastrin, or Histalog stimulation. The reason for choosing 6.0 is that *anacidity* so defined will apply to virtually all adult patients with pernicious anemia. Some of these patients, however, will secrete gastric juice with pH values a fraction of pH unit below strict neutrality, pH 7.0, at some time during the maximal histamine test (Callender, 1960).

Achlorhydria is used synonymously with anacidity by some investigators but is defined differently by others. Some define *achlorhydria* as a gastric secretion with pH persistently above 3.5 and with failure of the pH to fall more than one unit with maximal histamine stimulation (Callender, 1960). *Hypochlorhydria,* on the other hand, has been used to refer to gastric juice with a pH persistently above 3.5 but falling more than one pH unit with maximal stimulation. This fine distinction does not appear justified on clinical grounds. Furthermore, since pH 3.5 has been shown to have neither a unique physicochemical significance nor any particular clinical usefulness, the terms *achlorhydria* and *hypochlorhydria* should probably be avoided entirely.

Hyposecretion and hypersecretion are relative terms referring to the secretion of acid in amounts less than or greater than normal. Since the normal range for gastric secretion is not sharply delineated from that of pathologic states, these two terms, though admittedly useful clinically upon occasion, do not admit to strict definitions.

Gastric Intubation

The general procedure of intubation should be carefully explained to the patient in order to obtain the fullest possible cooperation and to avoid undue apprehension. The best recovery of gastric secretion will be obtained with the patient in a sitting position. Towels or a large apron should be provided to protect clothing. The bedfast patient should lie on his left side with his head elevated approximately 45 degrees. For intubation, a Levin tube, usually number 14F or 16F, can be passed through the nose, or a Rehfuss or similar tube can be passed through the mouth. Whether to use oral or nasal intubation depends largely on the preference of the individual examiner. It is likely that less difficulty will be encountered with nasal intubation if the patient has a hyperactive gag reflex. It is essential for the tube to have a radiopaque tip so that it can be adjusted fluoroscopically.

Many recommend preliminary chilling of the tube with ice in the belief that nausea during intubation is diminished. For oral intubation the patient is instructed to open his mouth and project his chin slightly forward and upward. The tip of the tube is placed on the superior aspect of the posterior portion of the tongue and pushed gently to the posterior pharynx, avoiding the uvula as much as possible. After the patient has closed his mouth gently on the tube he should be encouraged to alternate swallowing and deep oral breathing, the tube being pushed intermittently to its destination as he swallows. It is common for gastric tubes to be calibrated with several measurements, one of which is likely to be 55 cm, which corresponds to the approximate distance from the mouth to the antrum. It is imperative, however, for the position of the tube to be adjusted fluoroscopically so that the tip lies in the most dependent portion of the stomach, which will usually be the antrum if the patient is sitting and in the middle of the greater curvature if he is lying on his left side. Placement of the gastric tube on the basis of measurement, clinical judgment, or trial aspiration will be unsuitable for maximal aspiration in at least half of the intubation attempts. Following correct positioning, the tube should be directed lateral to the third molar tooth and can be maintained in position by taping to the patient's face. Value has been attributed to the water recovery test in positioning a nasogastric tube during gastric secretory studies (Findlay, 1972).

The principles of nasal intubation are similar to those of oral intubation. With the patient's chin elevated, the tube is directed slightly upward and then pushed gently posteriorly into the nasopharynx and esophagus. Some recommend preliminary spraying of the nasopharynx with a local anesthetic, although this should rarely be necessary.

If gastric secretion is to be collected over a period of time, as in the basal one-hour secretion test, continuous aspiration should be employed because intermittent withdrawal of secretion has been shown to result in significantly lower recovery volumes (Kay, 1953). Continuous aspiration can be performed either with a syringe or by mechanical means. In one study in which isotopically (^{131}I) labeled human serum albumin was instilled into the esophagus during gastric intubation in order to simulate gastric secretion, significantly greater recovery was achieved with continuous aspiration with a glass syringe than with suction apparatus (Johnston, 1958). After brief instruction, the patient can usually be depended upon to operate the syringe successfully. It is important to caution the patient to expectorate all saliva and nasorespiratory secretions while aspiration is in progress.

Gastric intubation for secretory studies is contraindicated for patients with esophageal varices, diverticula, stenosis, or malignant neoplasms, aortic aneurysm, recent severe gastric hemorrhage, congestive heart failure, or pregnancy.

Physical Examination of Gastric Contents

Secretion from the normal fasting stomach is a pale gray, translucent, slightly viscous fluid with a faintly pungent odor. The fasting volume varies up to about 50 ml. Following a 12-hour fast the presence of food particles is distinctly abnormal and indicates delayed gastric emptying, often the result of pyloric obstruction.

Bile. Yellow to green coloration is the result of bile, which is occasionally regurgitated in the normal stomach and frequently accompanies excessive gagging during intubation. Large amounts of bile can be present with obstructing lesions of the small intestine distal to the ampulla of Vater.

Mucus. The mucus normally present is largely responsible for the viscosity of gastric secretion. In addition to mucus of gastric origin, important contributions of mucus result from swallowed saliva and nasorespiratory secretions and to a minor degree from the reflux of duodenal contents. The latter is identified by its bile staining. Saliva is identified by its frothy flocculent nature, which causes it to float on the surface of the gastric secretion. Nasorespiratory mucus is highly tenacious and may contain dust particles.

Blood. Flecks or streaks of blood are commonly seen as a result of minor trauma during intubation. Blood of greater amount and longer duration in the acid-secreting stomach will be brown and granular, the so-called "coffee-ground" appearance. Such quantities of blood can be from a gastric lesion such as gastritis, ulcer, or carcinoma or can be swallowed from the mouth, nasopharynx, or lungs. The presence of significant quantities of blood should be confirmed by the orthotolidine (Hematest) or guaiac tests.

pH. pH should be measured electrometrically with a reliable pH meter. There may be occasions when a rapid bedside estimate is indicated, in which case the use of pH indicator paper is permissible if due regard is given to the inherent inaccuracies.

Microscopic Examination of Gastric Contents

A variety of structures can be recognized on microscopic examination. Components that can be present in the normal stomach include erythrocytes, leukocytes, epithelial cells, yeast, bacteria, and particles of mucus. Cellular elements are usually in various stages of autolysis, and their specific identity may be difficult.

As noted previously, small numbers of erythrocytes are of no consequence.

Leukocytes can be of gastric origin or from swallowed secretions. Small numbers of leukocytes are present in normal gastric secretion. Increased numbers can result from inflammation of the gastric mucosa, mouth, paranasal sinuses, or nasorespiratory tract, or, less commonly, from the pancreas, biliary tract, or duodenum.

Epithelial cells will be found in small numbers as a result of desquamation from various mucosal surfaces. Squamous cells can be dislodged from the mouth, nose, pharynx, or esophagus during intubation and can appear in small clumps. Gastritis often results in a significant increase in columnar epithelial cells, but this is usually not a helpful criterion.

As a result of the high acid secretion and perhaps other secretory factors inimical to the survival of bacteria, the normal stomach does not have an established microbiologic flora. Although bacteria and yeasts can be regularly cultured from gastric secretion, these usually reflect the flora of the mouth and nasorespiratory tract from the swallowing of secretions. These same bacteria probably do exist as an established flora in the anacid stomach. Yeasts are often present in large numbers in retention of gastric contents, such as occurs with pyloric obstruction.

In the past, considerable interest has focused on the Boas-Oppler bacillus, a species of lactobacillus. These large, nonmotile, gram-positive bacilli commonly occur in chains or clumps. Although once attributed special significance in the diagnosis of gastric carcinoma, their proliferation is probably the result of a favorable fermentative environment created by retention of gastric contents and decreased or absent hydrochloric acid.

Protozoan and metazoan parasites occur rarely and then usually with reflux of duodenal content. *Giardia lamblia* trophozoites or cysts, strongyloides larvae, or ascaris or hookworm ova can also be found.

Tests of Gastric Function

Basal Gastric Secretion. Basal gastric secretion represents the response of the stomach to endogenous stimuli, which are continually present in the interdigestive or fasting state. These endogenous stimuli include psychoneurogenic influences mediated by the vagus nerves and hormonal stimuli, such as gastrin and perhaps adrenocorticosteroids. For clinical validity it is essential that basal physiologic and environmental conditions be maintained as much as possible during collection of the secretion. Minimum requirements include the following: (1) the patient must be in the fasting state and free from the sight or odor of food. (2) All medications influencing gastric secretion must be withheld for 24 hours. The most obvious medications in this regard include antacids and antisecretory (anticholinergic) drugs and also such secretory stimulants as reserpine, alcohol, adrenergic blocking agents, and adrenocorticosteroids. (3) The patient should be removed from environmental situations evoking untoward psychological reactions such as fear, anger, or depression.

The one-hour morning aspiration is now the standard method of measuring basal secretion, having replaced the cumbersome and inherently less precise 12-hour nocturnal aspiration.

Technique

1. Following a 12-hour overnight fast, the patient is intubated. Water may be taken until 8 hours prior to intubation.
2. The residual volume of gastric secretion is measured and qualitatively examined.
3. Continuous aspiration is begun, preferably manually with a syringe. The aspirate should be segregated into 15-minute samples. Usually the first one or two samples are discarded to allow for adjustment of the patient to the intubation procedure. Subsequent to this adjustment period, four 15-minute samples are taken.
4. For each 15-minute sample, the volume, pH, and titratable acidity are measured and the acid output calculated. The sum of the acid outputs in the four samples, expressed in milliequivalents, represents the one-hour basal acid output.

Clinical Evaluation. The mean basal acid output reported for normal males ranges from 1.3 to 4.0 mEq per hour in various series. This variation among series is a reflection, in part at least, of different collection techniques and methods of measuring titratable acid. Lower values occur in females and with aging. Somewhat lower than normal values are reported in most large series for gastric carcinoma and benign gastric ulcer and distinctly higher values for duodenal ulcer or jejunal ulcer following partial gastrectomy with gastrojejunostomy (Table 25–1). Extremely high acid output is present in patients with the Zollinger-Ellison syndrome. In 25 such patients reviewed by Ellison and Wilson (1964), the one-hour basal acid output varied from 11 to greater than 80 mEq. A high ratio of basal acid output to maximal acid output is of even greater significance, however, in the diagnosis of the Zollinger-Ellison syndrome.

Table 25–1. BASAL AND MAXIMAL ACID OUTPUT IN VARIOUS CONDITIONS*

Condition	Sex	Number of Patients	Acid Output (mEq/hour)	
			Basal	***Maximal***
Controls	Male	35	4.2	22.6
	Female	26	1.8	15.2
Medical students	Male	145	5.3	26.7
	Female	16	3.3	21.4
Duodenal ulcer	Male	256	7.1	35.2
	Female	64	4.2	25.7
Gastric ulcer	Male	117	2.9	19.6
	Female	43	1.6	13.1
Gastric carcinoma	Male	74	1.5	6.7
	Female	32	0.7	3.0
Jejunal ulcer	Male†	10	7.9	25.1
	Female	4	5.5	16.4
	Male‡	4	9.1	36.1

*From Marks, I. N., et al.: S. Afr. J. Surg., *1*:53, 1963.
†Following partial gastrectomy with gastrojejunostomy.
‡Following gastroenterostomy alone.

3

It is important to emphasize that no pathognomonic range exists for any of the disease states listed, with the possible exception of the very high acid output found in patients with the Zollinger-Ellison syndrome. For example, in the series of 20 normal individuals reported by Marks (1962), the acid output in normal individuals ranged from 0 to 13.8 mEq per hour. Nevertheless, a basal acid output greater than 10 mEq per hour is found in only about 4 per cent of normal individuals but in 13 to 19 per cent of duodenal ulcer patients (Marks, 1961).

The volume of gastric secretion in the basal hour, which ranges from about 50 to 100 ml, has by itself little diagnostic significance.

Maximal Stimulation Tests. Maximal stimulation tests are those that result in an output of hydrochloric acid that cannot be increased substantially with additional stimulation. The first such test was the augmented, or maximal, histamine stimulation test introduced by Kay (1953), who demonstrated that a dose of histamine acid phosphate of 0.04 mg/kg of body weight resulted in an acid output that did not increase further with larger doses. In this test the untoward systemic effects of histamine are prevented or ameliorated by prior administration of a suitable antihistamine, which will block the H-1 receptor sites of histamine but will not affect the H-2 receptor sites of the stomach, which stimulate acid secretion. Nevertheless, unpleasant and occasionally serious side effects—erythema, bradycardia, headache, nasal obstruction, lacrimation, hypertension, or hypotension—are unduly frequent.

Histalog (3-β-aminoethyl pyrozole dihydrochloride, betazole), an analogue of histamine, was sometimes used because its side effects are minimal and premedication with an antihistamine is not necessary. It has a longer latency period than histamine, and its effect is more prolonged. The dose of Histalog that results in a maximal acid response is 1.7 mg/kg of body weight (Zaterka, 1964).

Both histamine and Histalog have now largely been replaced by pentagastrin as a stimulus for maximal secretory studies. Pentagastrin is a synthetic pentapeptide derivative that contains the four C-terminal amino acids of gastrin linked to substituted alanine. Pentagastrin retains a significant fraction of the biologic activity of gastrin and therefore is a potent stimulus to the secretion of acid, pepsin, and intrinsic factor by the stomach. It also stimulates secretion of both bicarbonate and enzymes by the pancreas, relaxation of the sphincter of Oddi, and contraction of the gallbladder.

Pentagastrin has been commonly used in Europe for gastric stimulation tests since 1966 but was not approved for routine clinical use in the United States until 1975. It is commercially available as Peptavlon (Ayerst).

A dose of 6 μg/kg of body weight is injected subcutaneously for maximal acid secretion. Side effects following pentagastrin administration are absent or mild and include transitory dizziness, faintness, flushing, and numbness of the extremities.

Technique

1. Following a 12-hour fast from both food and water, basal secretion is collected for one hour as previously described.
2. After the conclusion of the basal secretion study, pentagastrin is administered subcutaneously in a dose of 6 μg/kg body weight.
3. Gastric contents are then collected in 15-minute specimens for one hour.
4. The volume, pH, and titratable acidity are measured for each specimen, and the acid output is calculated. The maximal acid output is calculated as the sum of the four 15-minute specimens.

Clinical Evaluation. Acid output following pentagastrin stimulation is very similar to that following histamine in the maximal secretory tests (Khodadoost, 1972). The duration of histamine stimulation is somewhat longer as evidenced by its greater residual effect on acid output in the second post-stimulation hour. The interpretation of the two tests is the same for all practical purposes and has recently been reviewed by Baron (1979).

The maximum rate of acid secretion is characteristically attained within 15 minutes after histamine or pentagastrin injection and is maintained for approximately 30 minutes. By 60 minutes acid secretion usually will have fallen to basal levels. The maximum acid output, representing the sum of the acid outputs for the four consecutive 15-minute specimens (one hour), is the most generally accepted expression of gastric acid secretion. Values for various conditions are listed in Table 25–1.

As in the case of basal acid secretion, the extended range of the maximal acid output for normal individuals obviates strict diagnostic categorization. Thus, in the series of Marks (1962), the range for maximal acid output in normal males was 4.9 to 38.9 mEq per hour. Some generalizations are useful, however. A maximal acid output of greater than 40 mEq per hour is found in about 40 per cent of males with duodenal ulcer but only rarely in normal individuals (Marks, 1961). In addition to the marked hypersecretion, patients with the Zollinger-Ellison syndrome have a high ratio of basal to maximal acid output. Ratios greater than 60 per cent are strongly indicative of this disorder, while ratios between 40 and 60 per cent are suggestive. The maximal acid output is not of great help in distinguishing benign gastric ulcer from gastric carcinoma unless anacidity is found, in which case benign peptic ulceration can be excluded.

Anacidity in the maximal secretory test is most commonly found in adults with pernicious anemia or gastric carcinoma. Nevertheless, it has been reported in a variety of other conditions, including hypochromic anemia, rheumatoid arthritis, steatorrhea, aplastic anemia, myxedema, nutritional megaloblastic anemia, and the asymptomatic relatives of patients with pernicious anemia. Such cases are uncommon, as indicated by the series of Card (1955) in which, of 500 consecutive patients subjected to the maximal histamine test, all patients with anacidity proved to have pernicious anemia. Pernicious anemia in adults is virtually always accompanied by anacidity, but this does not hold true for the rare cases of juvenile pernicious anemia, in which normal acid secretion may be present. In a series of 30 patients with classic pernicious anemia reported by Callender (1960), the pH of the gastric contents remained above 6.0 in all samples during both the basal and augmented histamine studies. Furthermore, following histamine stimulation, the pH actually increased from basal levels in 25 of the 30 patients, failed to show any change in three, and fell slightly to acid levels in two. In neither of the two cases did the pH fall more than a fraction of one unit.

Anacidity with gastric carcinoma is the exception rather than the rule. In one series, 10 of 38 males and six of 14 females with gastric carcinoma had anacidity in the augmented histamine test (Marks, 1962).

Data from the basal and maximal secretory tests have been used by some physicians as an aid in determining which surgical procedure should be employed in the treatment of peptic ulcer. It has been suggested that an increased functioning parietal cell mass evidenced by an elevated maximal acid output indicates the need for gastric resection. On the other hand, elevated basal secretion with normal or only slightly elevated maximal secretion has been interpreted as an indication for vagotomy with drainage procedure. These are by no means universally accepted dictums.

Insulin Hypoglycemia Test. Hypoglycemia resulting from the administration of insulin is a potent stimulus to gastric acid secretion. The major component of this stimulus is transmitted by the vagus nerves and can be abolished by vagotomy. The hypoglycemia response is complex, however, and probably consists of three phases. For about 30 minutes after insulin injection there is a slight depression of gastric secretion, the mechanism of which has not been explained. The predominant effect during the remainder of the first two hours consists of marked enhancement of gastric secretion. It is believed that this results from stimulation of the anterior hypothalamus by the hypoglycemia and subsequent transmission of this stimulus to the vagal centers of the brain. The final effect, which is manifested after two hours, also stimulates gastric secretion but presumably by a humoral mechanism. This late effect may result from initial stimulation of the posterior hypothalamus, with secondary neurohumoral stimulation of the anterior pituitary to release adrenocorticotropic hormone. The adrenocortical hormones, which are thereby released, probably act directly on the parietal cells because this late effect of insulin hypoglycemia occurs after complete vagotomy.

Technique (Modified from Hollander, 1948)

1. After a 12-hour overnight fast, the patient is intubated. A two-hour basal secretion is obtained in 15-minute samples.
2. Blood samples for glucose determinations are obtained upon completion of the basal secretion study and at 30, 60, and 90 minutes after insulin injection.
3. Insulin is administered intravenously either at a fixed dosage of 15 or 20 units or at a calculated dosage of 0.20 unit/kg body weight. It is essential that a 50-ml syringe filled with 50 per cent (w/v) glucose solution be readily available to counteract any serious hypoglycemic effects.
4. Gastric secretion is collected in 15-minute samples for two hours after insulin.
5. For each basal and postinsulin gastric sample, the volume and titratable acidity are determined, and the acid output is calculated.

Clinical Evaluation. The insulin test is valid only if the blood glucose falls below 50 mg/100 ml at some point in the test, which will usually be 30 minutes after insulin administration. The test is furthermore valid only for the stomach that has been shown to be capable of secreting hydrochloric acid. Therefore, if no acid is present in either the basal or postinsulin periods, it is necessary to perform a maximal stimulation test in an attempt to evoke acid secretion. If the stomach is truly anacid, no conclusion can be drawn regarding the completeness of vagotomy, but the question of simple peptic ulceration is then effectively excluded.

The assessment of gastric function following vagotomy has been reviewed (Read, 1974). There is no clear delineation of normal from abnormal results in the insulin test. Nevertheless, several generalizations can be made. The patient can be considered to be completely vagotomized if the acid output in the greater of the two postinsulin hours is less than the greater of the two basal hours. Incomplete vagotomy is likely if the acid output in the two-hour postinsulin period exceeds that of the two-hour basal period by more than 0.5 mEq (Stempien, 1962). Incomplete vagotomy is also suggested by an acid output of greater than 2 mEq in either basal hour.

The time of increased acid output in the insulin test appears to be of some prognostic significance in incompletely vagotomized patients. Bell (1965) reported the clinical course of 42 patients shown to be incompletely vagotomized by the insulin test. Of 28 patients giving an elevated acid output in the first postinsulin hour, 10 eventually developed recurrent peptic ulceration. In contrast, ulceration recurred in only one of the remaining 14 patients who showed an elevated acid output in the second postinsulin hour.

Tubeless Gastric Analysis. The tubeless gastric analysis is an indirect method for detecting gastric acid secretion and has as its only significant advantage the elimination of gastric intubation. The method utilizes a carboxylic cation exchange resin, the hydrogen ions of which have been replaced by those of an indicator cation. After ingestion the indicator cations are in turn released from the resin by hydrogen ions if acid is present in the gastric secretion. The indicator cations that are released are subsequently absorbed in the small intestine and eventually excreted in the urine. The measurement of the quantity of indicator cations in the urine is thus an indication of gastric acidity.

Initially quininium was used as the indicator but was later replaced by the dye azure A. Azure A has the advantage that its excretion can be estimated by direct visual inspection. For many years this preparation was available as a diagnostic kit (Diagnex Blue Test, Squibb), which has now been discontinued. Tubeless gastric analysis is no longer performed as a clinical test because of the inherent inaccuracies of this method.

Miscellaneous Studies

Mycobacterial Culture. Aspiration of gastric contents for mycobacterial culture is indicated in patients who are suspected of having pulmonary tuberculosis but who are unable to produce adequate sputum samples. The procedure is particularly indicated for young children, since it is not until the age of about seven years that children can effectively expectorate pulmonary secretions. It is essential that the gastric content be collected in the early morning prior to eating or drinking and preferably immediately upon awakening before increased motor activity of the stomach has largely emptied its contents. Because gastric acidity is inimical to the survival of *Mycobacterium tuberculosis,* as well as to most other bacteria, it is important that specimens be submitted immediately for decontamination and culture. Acid-fast stains on gastric contents are unreliable because of the frequent presence of saprophytic acid-fast organisms originating in the mouth.

Exfoliative Cytology of the Stomach. Gastric cytology, gastroscopy, and roentgenography are at present the most useful procedures for investigating lesions of the stomach for possible malignancy. To a large extent the three procedures complement one another, but in the final analysis the most discriminating information is provided by exfoliative cytology. Multiple techniques for obtaining specimens have been reported, including simple aspiration of gastric content, the use of abrasive balloons or brushes, and gastric lavage with saline, buffered salt solutions, or solutions of papain or chymotrypsin. Chymotrypsin is believed to facilitate the exfoliation of cells by liquefying the mucous coating. Accuracies of greater than 90 per cent have been reported for exfoliative cytology in the diagnosis of gastric carcinoma.

Other Procedures in Gastric Analysis

Determination of Hydrogen Ion Concentration from Electrode pH Measurements. Moore (1965) has recommended, on the basis of both practicality and accuracy, the determination of hydrogen ion concentration from electrode pH measurements. This method utilizes the interrelationships between pH, hydrogen ion activity (a_{H+}), the hydrogen ion activity coefficient (γ_{H+}), and hydrogen ion concentration (c_{H+}) represented by the two equations:

$$\mathrm{pH} = -\log_{10} a_{H+}$$

$$\gamma_{H+}\ c_{H+} = a_{H+}$$

The activity coefficient is a function of both total ionic strength and pH. Because the ionic strength of gastric juice is largely determined by the concentration of major cations, sodium, potassium, and hydrogen, it has been possible to tabulate the activity coefficients and therefore the concentration of hydrogen ions for various concentrations of sodium and potassium at a given pH. This method thus requires precise measurement of pH with a glass electrode and determination of the sum of potassium and sodium. This approach has not been widely accepted and does not appear to provide any additional information which is of unique clinical value.

Determinations of Intrinsic Factor. Until recently intrinsic factor activity could be determined only by *in vivo* methods, such as the Schilling test, which measure the absorption of cobalt-60–labeled vitamin B_{12}. Several *in vitro* methods for assaying intrinsic factor have now been reported which utilize various immunologic methods and such techniques as starch-gel or paper electrophoresis, column chromatography, or charcoal absorption. None of these methods has as yet received general acceptance, but it is anticipated that in the near future *in vitro* assays for intrinsic factor will become established as an important supplement to gastric analysis in selected cases.

Determination of Plasma Gastrin. Although not an integral part of gastric analysis *per se,* radioimmunoassay of plasma or serum gastrin is now available as a sensitive (5 pg/ml) and specific clinical laboratory determination. The assay is a valuable adjunct in diagnosis of the Zollinger-Ellison syndrome and pernicious anemia, both of which are associated with marked elevations of gastrin. The two diseases are readily distinguished on the basis of concomitant gastric acid secretion studies and by the fact that intragastric instillation of dilute hydrochloric acid results in a precipitous decrease in plasma gastrin in pernicious anemia, whereas no appreciable change occurs in the Zollinger-Ellison syndrome. In general in normal individuals, fasting plasma gastrin levels, which range up to approximately 300 pg/ml, are inversely related to the rate of gastric acid secretion. Fasting plasma gastrin concentrations in duodenal ulcer patients do not differ from those of normal individuals. Small increases in plasma gastrin are associated with gastric ulcers and with aging (Trudeau, 1971).

EXAMINATION OF DUODENAL CONTENTS

The duodenal contents are composed of exocrine pancreatic secretion, bile, and the succus entericus or secretion of the intestine itself mixed with gastric secretion, which may contain partially liquefied and digested food particles. Clinical examinations are usually performed in the fasting state, and samples are collected in such a manner that gastric secretion is effectively excluded.

Pancreatic Exocrine Secretion

Pancreatic exocrine secretion probably exceeds 1500 ml per day in the normal adult and is thus the major contributor to duodenal contents from the standpoint of volume. It is a colorless, clear, non-viscid, highly alkaline solution with a pH of approximately 8.0. The secretion consists of 1 to 2 per cent organic material, mostly enzymes or their precursors including trypsinogen, chymotrypsinogen, amylase, lipase, lecithinase, elastase, collagenase, leucine aminopeptidase, and various esterases. The secretion contains about 1 per cent inorganic material, with sodium the major cation and bicarbonate the major anion. Compared with serum, sodium and potassium are present in about the same concentrations, while calcium and magnesium are present in lower concentrations. The bicarbonate concentration varies directly with the rate of pancreatic secretion from about 25 to 150 mEq/L, while chloride varies inversely with the rate of secretion, so that the sum of these two ions remains approximately constant (Table 24–2, p. 543).

Pancreatic exocrine secretion occurs in response to both vagal and hormonal stimuli. The vagal component is relatively slight and results in a small volume of secretion that is rich in enzymes. Two hormones, secretin and pancreozymin, which are elaborated in the duodenal mucosa, are potent stimuli to pancreatic secretion. They are released into the blood following the entry of peptones, amino acids, or fluid into the duodenum. Acid by itself can apparently stimulate the release of secretin. Secretin results in a copious flow of pancreatic secretion that is low in enzyme content and high in bicarbonate. Pancreozymin, on the other hand, stimulates the pancreas to secrete enzymes and consequently results in degranulation of the acinar cells. Investigations over the past several decades have established useful clinical tests using these two hormones (see Chap. 24, p. 542).

Bile

Approximately 500 to 1000 ml of bile enters the duodenum daily. Bile is yellow to brown or green and usually alkaline, with a pH of 7.0 to 8.5. In addition to the bile salts, chiefly sodium glycocholate and taurocholate, bile contains the bilirubin pigments, cholesterol, phospholipids, and various inorganic salts. The only enzyme present in a significant amount is alkaline phosphatase, which has no function in digestion. Bile flow is enhanced by two substances which have been termed choleretics and cholagogues. Choleretics are substances, such as bile salts and secretin, which increase the secretion of bile by the hepatic cells. Cholagogues, on the other hand, increase bile flow by causing contraction of the gallbladder and relaxation of the sphincter of the common bile duct. Magnesium sulfate and the hormone cholecystokinin are included in this category. Cholecystokinin is secreted by the duodenum in response to the entry of acid, fats, or partially digested protein, and perhaps also in response to nervous reflex mechanisms. This hormone is of some importance in clinical laboratory tests for the collection of stimulated bile and also for the reason that it is commonly present as an impurity in preparations of pancreozymin.

Succus Entericus

The duodenal secretion, like the pancreatic secretion, contains a variety of digestive enzymes that are capable of breaking down fats, proteins, and carbohydrates. Unlike the pancreatic secretion, however, the enzymatic activity of the succus entericus is considered to be relatively weak. The daily volume of duodenal secretion is not known, but it is mildly alkaline with a pH of about 7.6. Various disease states of the small intestine are not consistently reflected in abnormalities of the succus entericus.

Duodenal Intubation

Duodenal intubation is usually performed in the fasting state by a double-lumen tube, such as the Diamond, Lagerlöf, or Dreiling tube. A simple new device described by Linscheer (1976) eliminates effectively the need for the uncomfortable and prolonged technique associated with use of a Dreiling or Diamond tube. Instruments that have been developed for the purpose of obtaining small bowel biopsies can also achieve rapid duodenal intubation. This allows simultaneous collection of gastric and duodenal contents and largely eliminates entrance of gastric secretion into the duodenum. This same result has been achieved with a variety of other techniques, each of which has its advocates, such as the use of two separate tubes or a three-lumen tube, one lumen of which is used to inflate one or more balloons for sealing the duodenum from the stomach. It is essential for the tube to be equipped with a radiopaque tip so that its position can be verified fluoroscopically.

A rapid method of intubation has been described by Raskin (1958): Following an overnight fast, a sedative dose of pentobarbital is administered parenterally. A double-lumen Diamond tube is inserted into the mouth and passed a distance of 45 cm, which brings the tip approximately to the cardia. The patient is then placed in a left lateral decubitus position on a table, the cephalic end of which is elevated 16 inches. The tube is then slowly swallowed for another 15 cm, which results in its being positioned along the greater curvature. The patient then sits on the edge of the examining table with his body bent forward at the waist as far as possible. Several deep inspirations will assist entrance of the tube into the antrum. Peristalsis will move the tube into the duodenum if the patient lies in the right lateral decubitus position with his feet elevated for about five minutes. Finally the patient lies on his back for another five minutes while the tube is slowly advanced another 10 to 15 cm. The tube is adjusted with fluoroscopic visualization so that its tip is located in the middle of the third portion of the duodenum. Proper location of the tube can be maintained by taping it to the patient's face. This entire procedure can usually be completed in about 15 minutes in contrast to the one or two hours required for many other methods of intubation.

Secretions are collected with continuous suction by a vacuum pump or other suitable apparatus to obtain a pressure of at least 25 mm Hg. During aspiration the patient may lie on either his back or right side. The duodenal aspirate can be collected in suitable containers, such as centrifuge tubes, which can be placed as a trap in the suction line. This will facilitate the frequent changing of containers that is required. The character of the aspirate can be continuously monitored by placing a section of glass tubing in the duodenal tube just before the collection container. The gastric aspirate is discarded.

In addition to the conditions that are contraindications to gastric intubation, duodenal intubation should not be performed as a general rule in patients with acute cholecystitis or acute pancreatitis.

Physical Examination of Duodenal Contents

In the fasting state the residual content of the duodenum varies up to 20 ml. The fluid can be slightly turbid as a result of mixture with gastric secretion; normal duodenal fluid from which gastric juice is excluded is transparent or slightly translucent, pearly gray, and moderately viscid. Bile staining is usually absent, but its presence is of no significance. Slight blood streaking can result from the intubation procedure. Larger amounts of blood suggest neoplasm involving usually the ampulla of Vater. The presence of food particles is distinctly abnormal and usually indicates either intestinal obstruction or a duodenal diverticulum. Sediment or flocculent debris can be seen in inflammation of the duodenal mucosa, pancreas, or biliary tract.

Microscopic Examination of Duodenal Contents

For maximum preservation of cellular elements, the duodenal secretion should be collected in containers chilled in an ice bath and should be examined as soon as possible. Following centrifugation, a drop of sediment may be examined unstained. A few leukocytes or epithelial cells are normal. Increased numbers of polymorphonuclear leukocytes and exfoliated epithelial cells, with or without masses of bacteria, enmeshed in mucus can be found in inflammation of the duodenum, bile ducts, or pancreas. The presence of bile staining may prove of some help in differentiating inflammatory conditions of the biliary tract. Rarely, parasites such as the larvae of *Strongyloides stercoralis*, cysts or trophozoites of *Giardia lamblia* or *Entamoeba histolytica*, or the ova of *Necator*, *Ancylostoma*, or *Ascaris* can be found.

Bacteriologic Examination of Duodenal Contents

Normally the duodenal content is nearly sterile, largely as a result of the bactericidal effect of gastric acid. Elaborate mechanisms have been devised for the collection of culture specimens from the duodenum, but these are not indicated for routine clinical use. One of these utilizes a gelatin cap to cover the sterilized duodenal tube, the cap being forced off after the tube is in place. Although seldom indicated, bacterial cultures can be removed from the aspirate of residual duodenal content or following stimulation of pancreatic or biliary secretion.

Chemical Examination of Duodenal Contents

The most important electrolyte in the duodenal contents is bicarbonate, but its measurement is indicated only in tests of pancreatic function such as the secretin test. Chloride is infrequently determined and provides no useful information.

The determination of amylase, lipase, or trypsin activity in the pancreatic secretion following secretin or pancreozymin stimulation is an important index of pancreatic exocrine function. Variations in the three enzyme levels usually parallel one another so that only one of the determinations is indicated. Amylase is the most commonly measured and has the advantage of greatest stability. Determination of lipase and trypsin, in addition to amylase, is occasionally helpful in infants with suspected cystic fibrosis or with diarrhea or steatorrhea of unknown etiology. Methods for determining either serum amylase or lipase can be easily adapted to duodenal content following an appropriate initial dilution. The Somogyi method for serum amylase, for example, can be adapted to duodenal content by eliminating the initial protein precipitation and substituting a 1:50 or 1:250 dilution of duodenal fluid for the sample (Dreiling, 1955). Trypsin activity can be determined by testing for digestion of the gelatin coating on x-ray film as is done for fecal trypsin. As in the case of fecal trypsin determination, false positive tests can occur as a result of bacterial gelatinase.

Determination of bilirubin and urobilinogen in duodenal contents yields no information that cannot be deduced from measurements of serum bilirubin, urine bilirubin or urobilinogen, or fecal urobilinogen.

Provocative Tests of Pancreatic Secretion

The most important of these are the secretin and pancreozymin tests, which are discussed in Chapter 24.

EXAMINATION OF STIMULATED BILE

Since bile flow into the duodenum is intermittent in the fasting state, it is usually necessary to induce bile flow with a suitable stimulant if examination of bile is indicated. Although secretin is a potent choleretic agent, the increased volume of bile produced by the liver is stored in the gallbladder if the cystic duct is patent. In the presence of normal gallbladder function, secretin can result in a decrease or even disappearance of bile flow into the duodenum. Pancreozymin, on the other hand, will usually result in abundant bile flow as a result of its content of cholecystokinin. Magnesium sulfate, olive oil, and purified cholecystokinin have all been used to stimulate bile flow. Magnesium sulfate functions as an active cholagogue when applied topically to the duodenal mucosa but not when administered orally. Olive oil is probably an even more potent cholagogue but has the disadvantage that the oil interferes with subsequent microscopic examination of the bile. Commercial preparations of cholecystokinin have been used clinically but have no significant advantage over the other more readily available substances.

Technique (Lyon, 1919)

1. Duodenal intubation is performed and the position of the tube confirmed fluoroscopically. The test can be performed following the secretin test for pancreatic function.
2. Following aspiration of the residual duodenal content, slowly introduce 50 to 100 ml of a sterile 25 per cent saturated solution of magnesium sulfate through the duodenal tube.
3. After a minute or so, aspirate the magnesium sulfate and duodenal content. The collections are pooled and

discarded until yellow bile first appears in quantity; this usually requires about two to ten minutes.

4. Three fractions of bile are subsequently collected in separate containers. The first of these to appear, the "A" bile, is light yellow and watery. After one to three minutes, it will normally give way abruptly to a viscid deep yellow-brown bile, the "B" bile. Eventually the bile again becomes pale yellow and watery, heralding the appearance of the "C" bile.

5. If no "B" bile appears after 15 to 20 minutes, stimulation with magnesium sulfate and the entire collection may be repeated one or two times.

Clinical Evaluation. "A" bile will usually amount to 5 to 20 ml and originates in the common duct. "B" bile is the result of concentration and probably comes solely from the gallbladder under normal circumstances. Approximately 30 to 75 ml of "B" bile will normally be recovered. It may be absent in advanced cholecystitis, cholelithiasis with obstruction of the cystic duct, or recent cholecystectomy. Absence of "B" bile is not proof of gallbladder disease, and this finding should be confirmed with cholecystography and other examinations. On the other hand, it has been demonstrated that "B" bile can be obtained following cholecystectomy or in cases of congenital absence of the gallbladder. This is probably the result of other portions of the extrahepatic ducts assuming the function of bile concentration. This explanation is supported by the observation that usually a year or more is required for "B" bile to reappear following cholecystectomy. The hepatic ducts and intrahepatic radicles are presumed to be the source of "C" bile.

Inflammation of the biliary tract is often accompanied by flocculent debris, which will be found to consist of bile-stained epithelial cells and leukocytes in a mucous network, often with clumps of bacteria. The finding of bile sand, often in deep red-brown bile, is highly suggestive of cholelithiasis or calculus elsewhere in the biliary tract.

The importance of microscopic examination of bile for crystals, particularly the transparent rectangular or rhomboidal crystals of cholesterol or the amorphous yellow to orange masses of calcium bilirubinate, is to be emphasized. Bockus (1931) found that the presence of either or both of these crystals was associated with calculi in approximately 90 per cent of patients.

Culture of stimulated bile is occasionally informative. As a consequence of the circumstances of the collection, interpretation is frequently difficult and depends on quantitative as well as qualitative evaluation of cultures. The coliform organisms (*Escherichia coli* and the *Klebsiella-Aerobacter* group), staphylococci, beta-hemolytic or anaerobic streptococci, enterococci, and various species of *Salmonella* are often found in cases of acute or chronic cholecystitis and cholangitis.

Baron, J. H.: Studies of basal and peak acid output with an augmented histamine test. Gut *4*:136, 1963.

Baron, J. H.: Clinical Tests of Gastric Secretion. History, Methodology, and Interpretation. New York, Oxford University Press, 1979.

Bell, P. R. F., Checketts, R. G., Johnston, D., and Duthie, H. L.: Augmented histamine response after incomplete vagotomy. Lancet, *2*:978, 1965.

Bockus, H. L., Shay, H., Willard, J. H., and Pessel, J. F.: Comparison of biliary drainage and cholecystography in gallstone diagnosis with especial reference to bile microscopy. J.A.M.A., *96*:311, 1931.

Callender, S. T., Retief, F. P., and Witts, L. J.: The augmented histamine test with special reference to achlorhydria. Gut, *1*:326, 1960.

Card, W. I., Marks, I. N., and Sircus, W.: Observations on achlorhydria. J. Physiol. (London), *130*:18, 1955.

Dreiling, D. A.: The technique of the secretin test: Normal ranges. J. Mount Sinai Hosp., *21*:363, 1955.

Ellison, E. H., and Wilson, S. D.: The Zollinger-Ellison syndrome: Re-appraisal and evaluation of 260 registered cases. Ann. Surg., *160*:512, 1964.

Findlay, J. M., Prescott, R. J., and Circus, W.: Comparative evaluation of water recovery test and fluoroscopic screening in positioning a nasogastric tube during gastric secretory studies. Br. Med. J., *4*:458, 1972.

Hollander, F.: Laboratory procedures in the study of vagotomy (with particular reference to the insulin test). Gastroenterology, *11*:419, 1948.

Johnston, D. H., and McCraw, B. H.: Gastric analysis—evaluation of collection techniques. Gastroenterology, *35*:512, 1958.

Kay, A. W.: Effect of large doses of histamine on gastric secretion of HCl, an augmented histamine test. Br. Med. J., *2*:77, 1953.

Khodadoost, J., Leitao, O., and Glass, G. B. J.: Comparison of pentagastrin and augmented histamine stimulation as tests of gastric acid secretion. Am. J. Gastroenterol., *57*:311, 1972.

Linscheer, W. G., and Abele, J. E.: A new directable small bowel biopsy device. Gastroenterology, *71*:575, 1976.

Lyon, B. B. V.: Diagnosis and treatment of diseases of the gallbladder and biliary ducts, preliminary report on a new method. J. A. M. A., *73*:980, 1919.

Marks, I. NL: The augmented histamine test. Gastroenterology, *41*:599, 1961.

Marks, I. N., Bank, S., Louw, J. H., and van Embden, B. H.: The augmented histamine test, an analysis of 672 consecutive tests. S. Afr. Med. J., *36*:807, 1962.

Marks, I. N., Bank, S., Moshal, M. G., and Louw, J. H.: The augmented histamine test, a review of 615 cases of gastroduodenal disease. S. Afr. J. Surg., *1*:53, 1963.

Moore, E. W., and Scarlata, R. W.: The determination of gastric acidity by the glass electrode. Gastroenterology, *49*:178, 1965.

Raskin, H. F., Wenger, J., Sklar, M., Pleticka, S., and Yarema, W.: The diagnosis of cancer of the pancreas, biliary tract, and duodenum by combined cytologic and secretory methods. 1. Exfoliative cytology and a description of a rapid method of duodenal intubation. Gastroenterology, *34*:996, 1958.

Read, R. C., and Hall, W. H.: Objective assessment of gastric function after vagotomy. Curr. Probl. Surg. 1, July, 1974.

Stempien, S. J.: Insulin gastric analysis: Technic and interpretations. Am. J. Dig. Dis., *7*:138, 1962.

Trudeau, W. L., and McGuigan, J. E.: Relations between serum gastrin levels and rates of gastric hydrochloric acid secretion. N. Engl. M. Med., *284*:408, 1971.

Zaterka, S., and Neves, D. P.: Maximal gastric secretion in human subjects after Histalog stimulation. Comparison with augmented histamine test. Gastroenterology, *47*:251, 1964.

26

MALABSORPTION, DIARRHEA, AND EXAMINATION OF FECES

YUAN S. KAO, M.D., and W. DOUGLAS SCHEER, PH.D.

THE PHYSIOLOGY OF DIGESTION AND ABSORPTION

Mechanisms of transport of nutrients across the intestinal mucosa include (1) active transport, (2) passive diffusion, (3) facilitated diffusion, and (4) pinocytosis. A brief review of digestion and absorption of major categories of foodstuffs follows.

Amino Acids. Dietary proteins are initially degraded in the stomach by pepsin. The resulting peptides are further degraded by the action of pancreatic enzymes—trypsin, chymotrypsin, aminopeptidase, and carboxypeptidase—to dipeptides and tripeptides plus a small amount of amino acids. Dipeptides and tripeptides are further hydrolyzed by dipeptidase at the brush border of the intestinal epithelium. Only L-amino acids are actively transported.

Carbohydrates. Starch and glycogen are hydrolyzed by salivary and pancreatic amylase to disaccharides. These are split by disaccharidases located on the brush border or within microvilli of the intestinal epithelial cells. Thus, lactose is split into glucose and galactose, sucrose into glucose and fructose, and maltose into two molecules of glucose. The monosaccharides, such as glucose and galactose, are absorbed by active transport.

Fat. Ingested fat is digested mainly in the small intestine. The time interval for gastric emptying is longer following a fatty meal than following a meal containing less fat.

Dietary fat is digested and absorbed in the following sequence: (1) hydrolysis of triglycerides by pancreatic lipase to free fatty acids and two monoglycerides with bile salts, (3) passage of the micelles into jejunal mucosal cells where esterification and chylomicron formation occur, and, finally, (4) transport of chylomicrons from the mucosal cells into the intestinal lymphatics.

Water and Electrolytes. The small intestine absorbs water at an average minimal rate of 200 to 400 ml/hour. Water is absorbed throughout the small intestine, but the main site of absorption following a meal is in the upper part of the small intestine. Water and electrolytes can freely penetrate the membrane through aqueous channels, especially in the jejunum, where the effective pore radius is relatively large. In the ileum and colon the pore size is believed to be smaller; therefore sodium cannot pass freely but rather is absorbed actively. Potassium appears to be passively absorbed in the upper part of the small intestine, but it is secreted in the terminal ileum and colon.

Intestinal Hormones. Secretin, cholecystokinin, VIP (vasoactive intestinal peptide), endorphins, motilin, and enteroglucagon are produced in the intestine. Secretin, synthesized and secreted by duodenal S-cells, is released when the pH of duodenal content is acidic. Secretin then stimulates pancreatic acinar cells to release bicarbonate and water, thus neutralizing the acid content of the duodenum and facilitating the action of the digestive enzymes. Cholecystokinin-pancreozymin (both are an identical enzyme), produced in duodenum and jejunum, stimulates the pancreas to secrete enzymes, water, and electrolytes and increase intestinal motility. VIP is present in all areas of the gastrointestinal tract; it relaxes smooth muscle, inhibits acid secretion, and stimulates pancreatic secretion. Endorphins and related substances are involved in neurotransmission and neuroregulation and have been shown to inhibit secretin- and cholecystokinin-stimulated pancreatic acinar secretion. Motilin, located mainly in the duodenum, is secreted after a mixed meal and fat ingestion. This hormone stimulates gastric and intestinal motility. Enteroglucagon, which differs from pancreatic glucagon chemically and biologically, is mainly produced in ileum and colon. It is released after administration of cholecystokinin, in starvation, in insulin hypoglycemia, or after a mixed meal.

Colonic Physiology. Water and electrolytes, as mentioned, are absorbed from the colon, the other function of which is to serve as a reservoir, allowing storage and evacuation of feces as orderly processes. Up to 1500 ml of water is delivered to the colon daily, depending on the tone of the ileocecal sphincter. Gastrin releases the sphincter as it stimulates propulsive motility of the ileum. The colon itself undergoes slow segmented contractions which impede the flow of contents, followed eventually by mass movements which propel the feces forward into the sigmoid colon. Resulting distention of the rectal walls initiates the defecation reflex, during which contraction of the abdominal muscles and relaxation of the anal sphincter occur.

The average healthy adult defecates at frequencies varying from three times a day to three times a week. The common pattern is once a day. The stool tends to be small and dry on a diet high in meat, soft and bulky on a diet high in vegetables and fiber. Two thirds of the weight of the average stool is attributable to bacteria, indigestible material such as cellulose, undigested or unabsorbed food, gastrointestinal secretions, and desquamated cells. The normal brown color is of still undetermined origin. The odor results largely from indole and skatole, produced by bacteria from tryptophan.

THE MALABSORPTION SYNDROMES

Classification

The malabsorption syndromes result from impaired digestion or assimilation of foodstuffs by the small bowel.

Maldigestion usually results from pancreatic disease (see Chap. 24), such as chronic pancreatitis, carcinoma of the pancreas, or cystic fibrosis of the pancreas, and subsequent lack of pancreatic digestive enzymes. Generally there is associated creatorrhea, evidenced by presence of undigested meat fibers in the feces, and steatorrhea, an increase in fat—largely triglycerides.

Hepatogenous maldigestion results from interference with bile flow. Loss of bile salts interferes with fat emulsification, diminishing the surface area available for lipolytic action. In addition, there is loss of bile salt activation of lipase activity. The diseases with which this syndrome is associated are discussed in Chapter 13. Patients are usually jaundiced, pass dark urine, and have other signs of liver disease. Hepatogenous steatorrhea may coexist with pancreatic steatorrhea, as when there is a neoplasm obstructing the ampulla of Vater.

Enterogenous malabsorption comprises a variety of conditions which have in common normal digestion but inadequate net assimilation of foodstuffs. This may result from competition by bacteria or altered bacterial flora, as in the blind loop syndrome or diverticulosis of the small bowel; from obstruction to the flow of lymph, as in Whipple's disease and lymphoma; from diseases affecting the small bowel mucosa, as in amyloidosis, inflammation following radiation, and other types of small bowel inflammation; from diminished mucosal surface area, as in gastroileostomy or small bowel resection; or from alterations in small bowel mucosal function, as in atrophy secondary to gliadin (a fraction of gluten) sensitivity in celiac disease or secondary to relative vitamin B_6 or B_{12} deficiency. Malassimilation may also occur in patients with vasculitis, diabetes mellitus, the carcinoid syndrome, and hypogammaglobulinemia. In some of these situations it may result from rapid transit of small bowel contents—as diarrheal syndromes may be associated with malabsorption.

The conditions listed above all cause general malabsorption, of which steatorrhea is a major sign. Steatorrhea may be defined as the presence of more than 5 g of lipid (measured as fatty acids) in feces per 24 hours. Normal individuals on a normal fat intake excrete up to 5 g of lipid daily. While the source of fecal lipid is largely dietary, gastrointestinal excretions, cellular desquamation, and bacterial metabolism also contribute. Lipids are normally present as soaps and triglycerides. In addition, lipoids are present, including higher alcohols, paraffins, and vegetable carotenoids. Although diet has some effect on it, the pattern of lipids excreted may be very different from that of the diet, and the quantity of fat ingested by the normal individual has a relatively small effect on the total output of fat. According to one study, the fecal lipid is equal to a constant (2.93 g) plus 2.1 per cent of the dietary fat intake. On the fat-free diet, the output of fat normally varies from 1 to 4 g/day. In severe cases of steatorrhea, stools are generally fluid, semifluid, or soft and pasty, bulky, pale, and foul smelling. They may be foamy and may tend to float on water. Floating stools contain gas, which may also appear in stools from healthy people, so the sign is not specific.

Patients with malabsorption are liable to development of deficiencies of fat-soluble vitamins (A, D, E, and K). Primary and secondary alterations of bowel mucosa may also result in deficiency of water-soluble vitamins. In addition, these patients are liable to weight loss because of large caloric loss, and are likely to have other evidence of nutritional deficiencies, such as hypoprothrombinemia, glossitis, anemia, edema, ascites, and osteomalacia.

Malabsorption may also involve a single foodstuff or vitamin or only a small group of substances. For example, pernicious anemia results from failure to absorb vitamin B_{12} because of deficiency of intrinsic factor. Then, too, different foodstuffs are absorbed primarily in different locations, so that a lesion of regional enteritis localized to the distal ileum may affect only vitamin B_{12} and bile salt absorption. Lactose intolerance caused by lactase deficiency is an example of a specific malabsorption syndrome.

Differentiating Causes

When the diagnosis of malabsorption has been established, differential diagnosis becomes important for determining treatment. The usual problem is differentiation of pancreatogenous from enterogenous malabsorption. In children the definitive test for cystic fibrosis, their main cause of pancreatic malabsorption, is the sweat electrolyte determination described in Chapter 24. This test should be used whenever clinical evidence warrants it, although screening tests based on absent stool trypsin and on semiquantitative demonstrations of increased sweat chloride have been applied. One of the most valuable of the differential diagnostic tests, for adults especially, has been the D-xylose absorption test (Santiago-Borrero, 1971). In this procedure, a 25 g dose of the pentose sugar in water is administered orally, and the amount excreted in the urine over a five-hour period is determined. If the amount excreted is less than 3 g, the diagnosis is most likely enterogenous malabsorption, as pancreatic enzymes are not required for absorption of D-xylose. Poor kidney function may also result in low excretion, and for this reason the test is difficult to interpret in patients with renal disease. If the test is performed under these circumstances, blood levels should also be assayed. High blood values coupled with low urine values are expected in renal disease. Because reference values in this situation are not available, the test is better avoided in patients with renal disease.

There is no fully satisfactory alternative to the D-xylose test, although isotopic techniques and starch tolerance tests have been used by some workers for this purpose. In the latter, absorption of starch is followed by serial blood glucose determinations. The rise in blood glucose is compared with that following a glucose tolerance test. Theoretically, if a patient lacks pancreatic amylase, the glucose tolerance test will yield higher values than the starch tolerance test. Quantitative, specific stool trypsin and chymotrypsin assays may be helpful, as may the Schilling test for vitamin B_{12} absorption, which tends to be abnormal in patients with enterogenous steatorrhea and is not correctable with intrinsic factor. Probably the best alternative laboratory diagnostic aid, although unpleasant for the patient, is duodenal intubation as described in Chapter 25.

Screening Tests

Screening tests are available for detection of steatorrhea, such as determination of serum carotene, which tends, along with fat-soluble vitamin A, to be lower than normal; or microscopic examination of the stool for fat globules. Definitive diagnosis depends upon quantitative demonstration of increased fecal lipid.

Definitive Test for Steatorrhea

The definitive test for steatorrhea is the fecal fat determination. The amount of fat in feces may be determined and expressed as per cent by weight of wet stool, per cent by weight of dry stool, or per cent of ingested fat retained (absorbed), or as a chemically determined amount of fat per 24-hour stool collection. Because of wide variation in water content of the stool, wet weight concentration is the least informative. Dry weight concentration is only slightly less variable because of the effect of diet on bulk. Total output of fat per 24 hours, based on chemical analysis of at least a three-day stool collection, is the most reliable measurement. For this purpose, the patient is placed on a standard diet containing 100 g of fat per day. In infants and children, for whom the standard 100 g diet cannot be used, "per cent coefficient of fat retention" is the more useful expression. This is the difference between fecal fat and ingested fat expressed as a percentage of the ingested fat

$$\left(\frac{\text{dietary fat} - \text{fecal fat}}{\text{dietary fat}}\right) \times 100.$$

The coefficient of fat retention of normal children and adults is 95 per cent or higher, although in premature infants it may be much lower than this. A low value, otherwise, is indicative of steatorrhea.

Protein-Losing Enteropathy

Many gastrointestinal disorders such as Ménétrier's disease, gastric cancer, Crohn's disease of the small intestine and the colon, infectious enteritis, celiac disease, tropical sprue, ulcerative colitis, intestinal lymphangiectasia, and lymphoma may result in some degree of protein malabsorption and excessive transmucosal loss of serum protein. The laboratory test commonly employed in the diagnosis of protein-losing enteropathy has been based on the measurement of fecal radioactive chromium after intravenous injection of radioactive chromium. However, this technique is cumbersome and has numerous disadvantages for routine clinical application. Recently, a relatively simple method, using alpha-1-antitrypsin as an endogenous marker and the determination of the fecal concentration of alpha-1-antitrypsin, has become available for the diagnosis of such disorders. In this method either fecal or blood alpha-1-antitrypsin, or both, is measured by radial immunodiffusion and the results expressed either as mg/g of stool or as clearance (Thomas, 1981, Florent, 1981).

DIARRHEA

General Considerations

The large intestine receives about 500 to 1500 ml of fluid from the ileum daily, but only about 150 ml is normally lost in the stool each day. The large intestine normally absorbs water, chloride, and sodium, but excretes bicarbonate and potassium. Under normal conditions the large intestine of an adult can absorb about double the amount of fluid coming from the ileum daily. If the amount of fluid either entering or secreted into the large intestine exceeds the capacity for absorption, diarrhea will result.

Table 26–1 is an outline of the stool patterns and types of pathophysiology associated with common clinical conditions causing diarrhea.

Stool Examination

When working up a patient for the differential diagnosis of diarrhea, a history is most important. Additionally, establishing presence or absence of fecal polymorphonuclear or mononuclear leukocytes is very useful. Fecal leukocytes are usually present in bacterial

TABLE 26–1. CLASSIFICATION AND CAUSES OF DIARRHEA*

Stool Pattern	Pathophysiology	Common Clinical Conditions
Watery diarrhea	Secretory diarrhea	1. Specific enteric infection *(Salmonella, Shigella, Staphylococcus,* pathogenic *Escherichia coli,* cholera, clostridia, and *Protozoa)* 2. Non-specific enteric mucosal injury (idiopathic ulcerative colitis, regional enteritis, irradiation enteritis, drug injury (methotrexate, lincomycin, clindamycin, digitalis, alcohol, and reserpine) 3. Neoplasms (villous adenoma, abdominal lymphoma, carcinoid, pancreatic islet cell tumors, medullary carcinoma of the thyroid) 4. Hyperthyroidism 5. Post-vagotomy state
	Osmotic diarrhea	1. Post-surgical (pyloroplasty, gastroenterostomy, resection of jejunum and proximal ileum) 2. Primary disease of the intestine (celiac disease, tropical sprue, dermatitis herpetiformis, Whipple's disease, lymphoma, ulcerative colitis) 3. Infestation by parasites (giardiasis, strongyloidiasis) 4. Drug-induced osmotic cathartics (sorbitol, lactulose, antacids, phenformin, tetracycline, lincomycin) 5. Mucosal digestive defects (specific disaccharidase deficiencies) 6. Mucosal transport defect (glucose-galactose malabsorption) 7. Immunoglobulin deficiencies (congenital or acquired) 8. Chloridorrhea
	Altered intestinal transit, hypermotility	1. Secretory and osmotic diarrhea 2. Carcinoid syndrome 3. Post-vagotomy state 4. Functional gastrointestinal disorders 5. Hypocalcemia 6. Hyperthyroidism 7. Hypoadrenalism 8. Hypopituitarism 9. Pancreatic cholera syndrome 10. Gastrin-secreting tumors
Steatorrhea	Maldigestion	1. Pancreatic exocrine insufficiency (chronic pancreatitis, cystic fibrosis) 2. Altered bile salt circulation (steatorrhea of newborn, disorders of liver, blind-loop syndrome, resection of ileum)
	Malabsorption	1. Primary intestinal malabsorption (celiac disease, tropical sprue, Whipple's disease, abetalipoproteinemia, blind-loop syndrome)
Small stool diarrhea	Rectocolic irritability	1. Functional bowel disorder, inflammatory disease of the colon and rectum (ulcerative proctocolitis, Crohn's disease, diverticulitis, irradiation proctocolitis, anorectal tumor)

*Modified from Haubrich, W. S.: *In* Bockus, H. L. (ed.): Gastroenterology, Vol. 2. Philadelphia, W. B. Saunders Company, 1976, pp. 921–922.

infection of the intestines by such organisms as *Salmonella, Shigella, Yersinia,* and invasive *Escherichia coli,* as well as in non-bacterial inflammatory processes, such as ulcerative colitis, and occasionally in antibiotic-associated colitis. Fecal leukocytes are usually not present in the stools of diarrhea secondary to viruses, toxigenic bacteria *(Staphylococcus, E. coli, Clostridium perfringens, Vibrio cholerae)* and parasites *(Giardia, Entamoeba).* A modified version of an algorithm for the differential laboratory diagnosis of diarrhea is shown in Figure 26–1.

INTESTINAL DISACCHARIDASE DEFICIENCY

Many of the previously listed conditions causing malabsorption may also be associated with intolerance to disaccharides. Disaccharide absorption is diminished either from primary disaccharidase deficiencies such as sucrase-isomaltase deficiency, lactase deficiency, primary alactasia, primary trehalase deficiency, or secondary disaccharidase deficiency due to celiac disease, tropical sprue, acute viral gastroenteritis, or drugs such as orally administered neomycin, kanamycin, and methotrexate. These secondary disaccharidase deficiencies are usually transient and usually involve more than one enzyme. Although the incidence of lactose intolerance due to congenital lactase deficiency is low, the prevalence of lactose intolerance in adults is quite high; about 10 per cent of Caucasians and 70 to 80 per cent of American Blacks and even greater percentage of Orientals manifest some degree of lactose intolerance even though they were able to digest lactose well as infants. In these disorders unhydrolyzed and unabsorbed carbohydrates are fer-

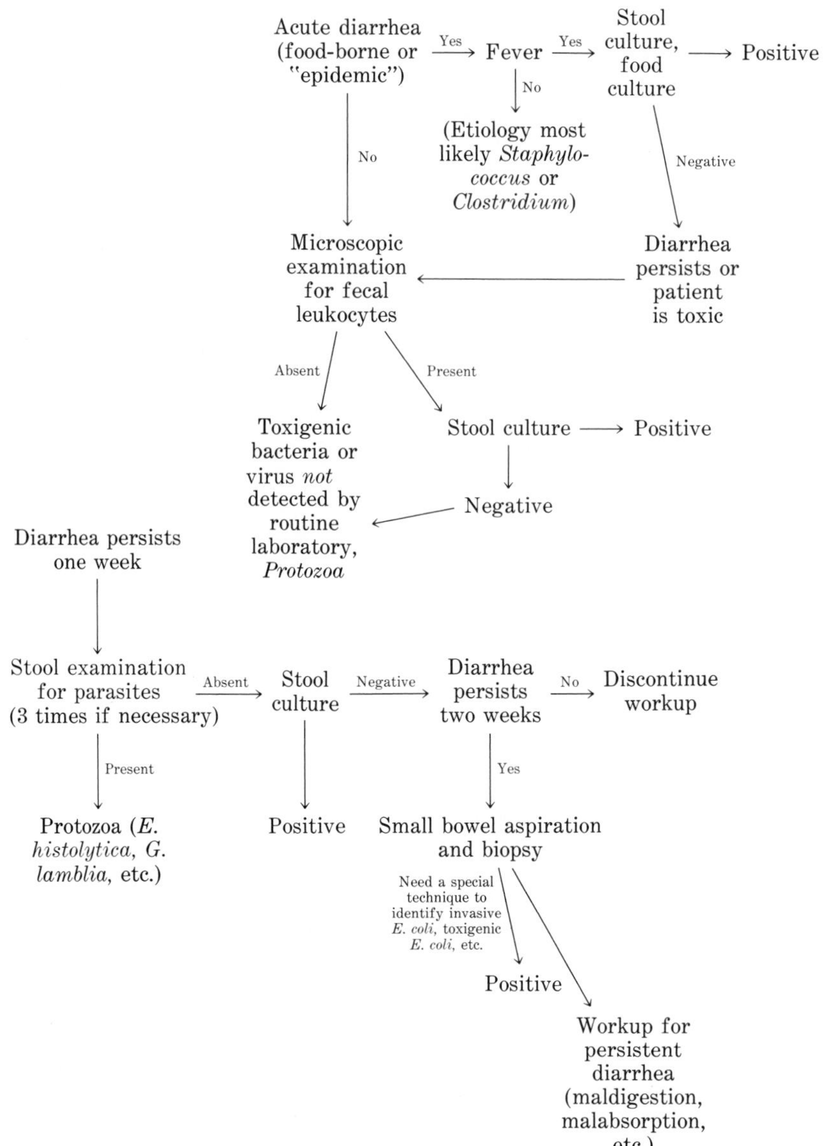

Figure 26–1. Laboratory workup for acute diarrhea. (Modified from Satterwhite, T. K., and Dupont, H. L.: The patient with acute diarrhea: An algorithm for diagnosis. J.A.M.A., *236*:2663, 1976. Copyright 1976, American Medical Association.)

mented by intestinal bacteria, producing gas, lactic acid, or other organic acids. Normally, absorption of digested carbohydrates is rapid and fairly complete in the proximal small intestine. Unhydrolyzed disaccharides or unabsorbed monosaccharides due to deficiency in transport are osmotically active and hence cause secretion of water and electrolyte into the small intestine and large intestine. This often results in protracted diarrhea as well as complaints of bloating and flatulence.

Screening tests for disaccharidase deficiencies include oral challenging of suspected disaccharides to reproduce abdominal symptomatology followed by stool analysis. The stools are usually watery, acid, explosive, and fermentative. Stool pH of less than 5.5 is suggestive but the measurement of pH is not valid if the patient is on oral antibiotics. High pH does not exclude the diagnosis. Abnormally high stool pH is common in normal infants between three and seven days of age. Stools can be analyzed for sugars by chromatography or by one of the semiquantitative non-specific tests for urinary sugar adapted for stool analysis. The Clinitest tablet (Ames Company, Elkhart, Indiana) is suitable for the purpose. Presence of 0.5 g/dl or greater of reducing substance is considered abnormal. In patients with intolerance to sugar, the amount of total reducing substances in the stool usually exceeds 250 mg/dl feces. Children proven to

Table 26–2. RISE IN BLOOD GLUCOSE OVER FASTING LEVEL

Carbohydrate Ingestion	Blood Glucose Increased (mg/dl)		
	Normal	*Lactose Intolerance*	*Idiopathic Sprue*
Lactose, 50 g	14–60 (35)*	2–11 (6)	0–19 (9)
Glucose, 25 g Galactose, 25 g	25–66 (49)	20–71 (40)	24–34 (28)
Maltose, 50 g	(28–80) (52)	57–92 (74.5)	19 (one case)

*Figures in parentheses are average values. (From Basford, R. L., and Henry, J. B.: Postgrad. Med., *41*:A70, 1967.)

be intolerant to sugar can excrete more than 1 g/dl of total reducing substances when fed an offending sugar (Kerry, 1964).

An oral tolerance test using a specific sugar such as lactose or sucrose can be used to establish a specific carbohydrate intolerance (Table 26–2). Although the oral tolerance test is fairly specific and sensitive, in some instances 23 to 30 per cent false positives were noted following administration of lactose—i.e., flat tolerance curve, less than 20 mg/dl (1.1 mmol/L) increase in blood sugar (Krasilnikoff, 1975). Delayed gastric emptying appears to be the cause of the false positive result, since duodenal instillation of lactose eliminates the flat tolerance curve.

Definitive diagnosis of disaccharidase deficiencies depends on demonstrating low specific enzyme activity in the mucosae of small intestinal biopsy material. Assay of disaccharidase has been published (Dahlquist, 1968), and the disaccharidase activity of the small intestinal mucosa is shown in Table 26–3.

GLUCOSE-GALACTOSE MALABSORPTION

Primary glucose-galactose malabsorption is a rare hereditary disorder of active absorption of glucose and galactose from the small intestine. It is inherited as an autosomal recessive trait. Symptoms and signs are similar to those seen in patients with disaccharide malabsorption, diarrhea being the main problem. Stools are watery and always contain several grams per 100 ml of glucose and galactose.

Laboratory Tests. Diagnostic laboratory tests for this disorder include identification of glucose and galactose in the stools, using glucose oxidase, galactose oxidase, or chromatography, and oral glucose tolerance tests and oral galactose tolerance tests, in which a flat curve is expected. Fructose tolerance tests should also be performed, results of which should be normal. A flat glucose tolerance curve alone does not, of course, indicate the presence of this disorder. Many variables affect blood glucose levels (Chap. 10). Flat glucose tolerance curves are normal in newborn babies. Furthermore, blood glucose levels are affected by oral fructose loading (Meeuwisse, 1970). If oral sugar tolerance tests yield equivocal results, intubation and perfusion of a segment of the small intestine may be indicated to establish the diagnosis.

FECAL BLOOD

Bleeding into the gastrointestinal tract may be acute or chronic, massive or slight, obvious or occult, and may originate anywhere from the gingiva or nasal cavity to the rectum. It should never be ignored, although often it results from minor pathology, such as hemorrhoids and anal fissures. Of one group of patients with significant gastrointestinal bleeding, 18 per cent were found to have malignant tumors and 30 per cent benign peptic ulcer. Slightly over 50 per cent had their bleeding source in the esophagus, stomach, or duodenum; 45 per cent in the colon and rectum (Thompson, 1949). Bleeding from the jejunum and ileum was seen in very few of the patients.

Drugs, particularly salicylates, steroids, rauwolfia derivatives, phenylbutazone, and indomethacin, have been shown to be associated with increased gastrointestinal blood loss in normal subjects and even more pronounced increase in blood loss in patients with gastrointestinal tract pathology. This effect may follow even parenteral administration of the drugs. Apparent fecal peroxidase activity has also been shown to increase with use of carmine as a stool marker and occasionally with massive iron therapy. The latter,

Table 26–3. DISACCHARIDASE ACTIVITIES AT THE LIGAMENT OF TREITZ IN 100 HEALTHY SUBJECTS*

Disaccharidase	No. of Subjects	Activity (Wet Wt.)					Activity (Protein)				
		Mean	*SD (units/g)*	*SEM (units/g)*	*Range*	*CV (%)*	*Mean*	*SD (units/g)*	*SEM (units/g)*	*Range*	*CV (%)*
Lactase	100	3.3	2.0	0.2	0–11.1	60.6	29.0	18.6	1.9	0–82.8	64.1
Normal	94	3.5	1.9	0.2	0.7–11.1	54.2	30.9	17.6	1.8	3.0–82.8	56.9
Deficient	6	0.2	0.2	0.07	0–0.5	100.0	1.3	1.4	0.6	0–4.1	108.0
Sucrase	100	5.9	2.3	0.2	1.2–14.0	39.0	51.3	22.9	2.3	4.6–121.0	44.6
Maltase	100	22.3	7.2	2.3	6.5–39.1	32.2	195.2	78.1	7.8	27.7–446.5	40.0
Isomaltase	14	7.2	2.6	0.7	3.0–12.1	36.1	67.3	19.4	5.2	28.5–103.0	28.8

*From Newcomer, A. D., and McGill, D. B.: Gastroenterology, *53*:884, 1967.

3

however, may result from actual bleeding secondary to gastrointestinal irritation produced by some iron compounds.

Loss of more than 50 to 75 ml of blood from the upper gastrointestinal tract generally imparts a dark red to black color and a tarry consistency to the stool. Persistence of a tarry appearance for two or three days suggests loss of at least 1000 ml of blood. Following this amount of bleeding, occult blood may persist for 5 to 12 days. Somewhat smaller quantities entering the lower gastrointestinal tract may produce similar appearing stools, or may appear as bright red blood. Such stools should be considered grossly bloody only after verification with chemical tests to avoid confusion with coloring from dietary substances or medications. Smaller increases in blood content may not alter appearance of the stool. Such stools are said to contain "occult blood," detection of which can be most useful in uncovering or localizing disease. This is especially important because over half of all cancers (excluding skin) are those of the gastrointestinal tract, and early diagnosis and treatment of patients with colonic cancer results in a relatively good prognosis for survival (Greegor, 1971).

According to Winawer (1977), 139 cancers were detected with the Hemoccult test (Smith-Kline Diagnostics, Sunnyvale, Cal.), of which only 20 were within reach of the standard sigmoidoscope. Only one patient had a false negative result. Of 47 "silent" cases, 85 per cent were localized to the bowel wall. The authors noted that only one or two specimens examined out of six are usually positive.

COLLECTION OF FECES

Uninstructed patients sometimes exhibit considerable ingenuity in collecting stool specimens, but a few simple instructions are likely to produce more satisfactory specimens. A scoured, well-rinsed bedpan is a convenient collection container. If the patient does not own one, a carefully cleaned, rinsed, and boiled glass jar of suitable size is a satisfactory alternative. Patients should be warned against passing urine at the same time into the bedpan or container because, among other things, urine has a harmful effect on protozoa. Tongue depressors or pieces of cardboard are reasonably convenient instruments for transferring the stool from bedpan to transport vessel, for which plastic, cardboard, and glass containers are available. We prefer two-ounce ointment jars with screw caps for small stool samples because they are odor free, leak proof, and easy to transport. Patients should be instructed not to contaminate the outside of the container and not to overfill the container. Gas, which frequently accumulates, should be released gradually by careful loosening of the cap. Failure to observe this simple precaution, especially in the case of an overfilled container, can result in an explosive release of contents.

Fecal matter left on the physician's gloved finger at the time of a rectal examination may be transferred to a piece of filter paper for inspection and testing for occult blood.

Because of wide variation in bowel habits, intestinal transit time, and bulk of stool, special consideration must be given to methods of timed stool collection. For collection of timed urine specimens, the urinary bladder can be emptied before and at the end of the collection period; the gastrointestinal tract, however, cannot be emptied completely at will. Therefore, the amount of stool collected in a 24-hour period usually correlates very poorly with the amount of food ingested over a similar period of time. For determining the 24-hour fecal excretion of any substance, stools should be collected over a period of at least three days, and calculations should be based on the entire specimen divided by the number of days of collection. The accuracy of this method can be enhanced somewhat by having the patient ingest carmine dye (0.3 g) at the beginning and charcoal (1 g) at the end of a collecting period, collecting the stools from the beginning of the appearance of the dye to the beginning of the appearance of the charcoal. However, *Salmonella cubana* outbreaks in Massachusetts and California were traced to carmine dye. Another method of signaling the collection period involves use of inert, nonabsorbable stool markers. These are taken in divided, uniform doses for several days prior to the beginning of the collection, continuing through the collection period. The concentration of the material found in the stool specimen is then used to determine the quantity of stool containing one day's ingestion of the material as an indication of the 24-hour output. For this purpose, chromium sesquioxide (Cr_2O_3) has been used and its concentration in the feces determined chemically. The substitution of radioactive chromium or zirconium isotope has made it possible to determine concentration by measurement of radioactivity of the stool, but these methods as currently used are too time-consuming for routine determinations.

Hoffman (1973) has described a sample collection method which has the advantages of ease of transportation and storage, not requiring special equipment, and being acceptable to patients and laboratory staff. A plastic bag is cut halfway down each side seam, with double-sided adhesive tape attached on both sides to the upper outer lip. The bag is opened and placed in a toilet, its top sides attached by adhesive tape, laterally, to an ordinary toilet seat. After collection it can be closed with a twist tie and placed in a paint can. There are problems with this method of collection at home. For example, cultural conditions in rural and ghetto circumstances may make it very difficult for people to collect such samples; and one can not always be sure that the sample brought in actually corresponds to a particular member of the family.

A pediatric method described by Jelliffe (1973) includes using a thick-walled glass tube (¼ inch I.D.), lubricated by dipping into water and then inserted into the young child's rectum. In about two thirds of the cases, a core of feces can be obtained, which can be poked out with an applicator stick into the container. During the procedure, the child can be held on the mother's lap, with the buttocks separated by the operator's left hand, while the tube is inserted with the right hand.

METHODS AND METHODOLOGY

Inspection of Feces

Inspection of the feces is important, for it may lead to a diagnosis of parasitic infestation, obstructive jaundice, diarrhea, malabsorption, rectosigmoidal obstruction, dysentery, ulcerative colitis, or gastrointestinal tract bleeding.

The quantity, form, consistency, and color of the stool should be noted. Normally, 100 to 200 g of stool is passed per day. When there is diarrhea, the stool is watery. Passage of large amounts of mushy, foul-smelling, gray stool which floats on the water is characteristic of steatorrhea. Constipation may be associated with passage of small, firm, spherical masses of stool (scybala). Constipation most often results from the irritable colon syndrome of patients with anxiety or from overuse of laxatives. In such patients, repeated tests for occult (hidden) blood are called for to detect more serious organic problems such as carcinoma, which may also, of course, afflict those patients.

A narrow, ribbon-like stool suggests the possibility of spastic bowel or rectal narrowing or stricture. Clay color suggests diminution or absence of bile or presence of barium sulfate. Blood, especially when originating from the lower gut, may cause the stool to be red; beets in the diet may mimic this. Bleeding from the upper gastrointestinal tract is more likely to cause the stool to be black and of a tarry consistency. Bismuth, iron, and charcoal may also color the stool black. Standing in the air for a time may cause the stool to darken on the surface. Green stools may result from ingestion of spinach and other green vegetables or calomel, or may result from the presence of biliverdin, seen in patients taking antibiotics orally. It is not unusual to see seeds and vegetable skins. Parasites are considered in Chapter 49.

Mucus. Presence of recognizable mucus in a stool specimen is abnormal and should be reported. Translucent gelatinous mucus clinging to the surface of the formed stool suggests spastic constipation or mucous colitis. It is seen in stools of emotionally disturbed patients and may result from excessive straining. Bloody mucus clinging to the fecal mass suggests neoplasm or inflammatory processes of the rectal canal. Mucus associated with pus and blood is found in stools of patients with ulcerative colitis, bacillary dysentery, ulcerating diverticulitis, and intestinal tuberculosis. Patients with villous adenoma of the colon may pass copious quantities of mucus, aggregating up to 3 or 4 L in 24 hours. They frequently develop severe dehydration and electrolyte disturbances, especially hypokalemia.

Pus. Patients with chronic ulcerative colitis and chronic bacillary dysentery frequently pass large quantities of pus with the stool, for the recognition of which microscopic examination is required. This also occurs in patients with localized abscesses or fistulas communicating with the sigmoid colon, rectum, or anus. Large amounts of pus seldom accompany the stools of patients with amebic colitis. Therefore, its presence is evidence against this diagnosis. No inflammatory exudate is seen in the watery stools of patients with viral gastroenteritis.

Microscopic Examination of Feces

Fat (Drummey, 1961). The crudest technique is microscopic examination using Sudan III, Sudan IV, or oil red 0 stains. The procedure has been widely employed for screening because of its simplicity. In our experience, results have correlated well with quantitative measurements when aliquots of the same homogenized stool have been analyzed. For this purpose, a small aliquot of stool suspension is placed on a slide and mixed with 2 drops of 95 per cent ethanol, followed by addition of 2 drops of saturated ethanolic solution of Sudan III, with mixing. It is then coverslipped. Under these conditions fatty acids are present as lightly staining flakes or as needle-like crystals which do not stain and which, therefore, may be missed. Soaps also do not stain, but appear as well-defined amorphous flakes or as rounded masses or coarse crystals. Neutral fats, however, appear as large orange or red droplets. When 60 or more stained droplets of neutral fats per high-power field are seen, one may be reasonably certain that the patient has steatorrhea. (Caution is advisable in interpretation, as mineral oil or castor oil may mimic neutral fat.) The procedure is then repeated, adding several drops of 36 per cent (v/v) acetic acid to the stool mixture and warming the slide several times over a flame until slight boiling occurs. This converts neutral fats and soaps to fatty acids and melts the fatty acids, causing them to form droplets which stain strongly with Sudan III. The slide is then examined while warm. After this procedure, presence of up to 100 stained droplets per high-power field is considered normal. Patients with pancreatogenous steatorrhea are likely to show greater increases in fatty acids and soaps. Use of oil red 0 has been advocated by some because it permits substitution of isopropanol for ethanol.

3

Meat Fibers (Moore, 1971). The technique for sampling is identical to that for Sudan preparations for fecal fat. The stool is mixed thoroughly on a slide with a 10 per cent alcohol solution of eosin, allowed to stain for three minutes, and examined for muscle fibers. The entire area under the coverslip is examined, and only rectangular fibers with clearly evident cross-striation are counted.

It appears that examination for meat fibers yields results that correlate well with chemical determination of fat excretion.

Leukocytes (Harris, 1972)

1. Place a small fleck of mucus or a drop of liquid stool on a glass microscopic slide with a wooden applicator stick.
2. Add 2 drops of Loeffler's methylene blue.
3. Mix thoroughly and carefully.
4. Place a coverslip on the mixture.
5. Let stand for two to three minutes for good nuclear staining.
6. With low-power scanning, make rough quantitative counts by approximating the average number of leukocytes and erythrocytes. All differential counts should be made under high power, counting 200 cells when possible. Only those cells clearly identified as either mononuclear or polymorphonuclear are included in the differential count. Macrophages and epithelial cells that cannot be clearly identified are ignored. The initial cell counts should be performed at the time of presentation of the specimen.

Serum Carotenoids

Carotenoids are a group of compounds which are the major precursors of vitamin A in man. They are synthesized by plants and some animals, excluding man. The absorption of carotenoids in the intestine is dependent on the presence of dietary fat and its normal absorption. Since carotenoids are not stored in the body to any appreciable degree, lack of carotenoids in the diet or disturbances in absorption of lipids from the intestine can result in decreasing levels of serum carotenoids. This is a simple and useful screening test for steatorrhea. In addition to steatorrhea and poor diet, low levels of serum carotenoid may also be caused by liver disease and high fever. Elevated serum carotenoid levels can be caused by hypothyroidism, diabetes, hyperlipidemia, and excessive intake of carotene (such as carrots).

Principle (Levinson, 1969). Carotenoids are normally transported as complexes with lipoproteins in serum. These carotenoid bonds are broken with ethanol and the pigments extracted with petroleum ether. After the absorbance is determined at 440 nm the concentration is calculated by reference to a standard curve.

Reagents

1. Ethanol, 95 per cent.
2. Petroleum ether, boiling point 20° to 40°C.
3. Carotene stock standard. Dissolve 10 mg of carotene in petroleum ether and dilute to 100 ml with petroleum ether.
4. Carotene working standard (100 μg/dl). Dilute 1 ml of carotene stock standard to 100 ml with petroleum ether.

Procedure

1. Add the following amounts (in ml) of serum, water, working standard, ethanol, and petroleum ether to a set of tubes as indicated:

	Reagent Blank	*Patient Sample*	*Standard*
Water	2	—	2
Serum	—	2	—
Working standard	—	—	4
Ethanol*	2	2	2
Petroleum ether	4	4	—

*Add dropwise with continuous shaking of the tube.

2. Stopper all tubes and shake vigorously for five minutes.
3. Remove stoppers, seal tubes with parafilm, and centrifuge for five minutes at 2000 to 2500 rpm.
4. Carefully transfer the petroleum ether extracts to cuvettes and read the absorbance of the standard and unknown solution at 440 nm against the reagent blank.

Calculation

$$\frac{Au}{As} \times 200 = \mu g \text{ carotenoids/dl}$$

where:

Au = absorbance reading of patient's sample, unknown.

As = absorbance of reading of standard.

200 = value of standard solution (100 μg/dl × 2).

Normal values are 40 to 300 μg carotenoids/dl serum (0.74 to 5.58 mmol/L as β-carotene).

Comments

1. The serum for the determination of carotenoids should be free from hemolysis, protected from light, and collected when the patient is in the fasting state.
2. Carotene-loading tests in which serum carotenoids are measured before and after oral administration of carotene have been reported to provide greater diagnostic specificity and sensitivity than a single fasting serum carotenoid value. However, the loading tests are not practical for screening purposes, because they require that blood be collected anywhere from three to seven days after administration of the carotene in order to determine the peak serum value.

Starch Tolerance Test

The starch tolerance test has been used to differentiate pancreatogenous from enterogenous malabsorption. In the presence of pancreatic amylase, starch is hydrolyzed into dextrins, maltose, and glucose. Other enzymes are then able to hydrolyze the dextrins and maltose into their monosaccharide components, which can be absorbed in the intestine. After ingestion of 100 g of soluble starch, in the morning after an overnight (8 hours) fast, hydrolysis and absorption of starch are followed by serial blood glucose determinations. The rise in blood glucose is compared with that following a glucose tolerance test. If the pancreas is unable to synthesize amylase or the ductal system is unable to deliver it to the intestine, the glucose tolerance test will result in significantly higher blood glucose values than those of the starch tolerance test.

Method (Althausen, 1961). One hundred grams of soluble starch (prepared according to the method of Lintner and marketed by Merck and Company, Inc.) is suspended in 150 ml of water by mixing with a spoon. Just before the test this suspension is poured into 300 ml of water which has just ceased boiling and is thoroughly stirred. The fasting patient should ingest the starch as soon as the temperature has cooled sufficiently. Blood specimens are drawn at 30 minutes, one hour, two hours, and three hours after administration of the starch, for glucose determinations. To arrive at the correct answer it is necessary to obtain, in addition, a standard three-hour glucose tolerance test following ingestion of 100 g of glucose. The two tolerance tests should be performed on two consecutive days.

Calculation. The extent to which the maximal rise in blood glucose exceeds that after starch is expressed as a percentage and is calculated as follows:

$$\text{percentage} = \frac{(P' - F') - (P - F)}{P - F} \times 100$$

where:

percentage = the extent to which the maximal rise in blood glucose exceeds that after starch.

P′ = the peak blood glucose value after glucose ingestion.

F′ = the fasting blood glucose before glucose ingestion.

P = the peak blood glucose value after starch ingestion.

F = the fasting blood glucose value before starch ingestion.

Normal Values. Althausen recommended that values below 70 per cent be considered normal. Results falling between 70 and 100 per cent should be considered borderline, whereas values above 100 per cent should be interpreted as definitely abnormal. A positive starch tolerance test (values above 100 per cent) is a reliable indicator of chronic pancreatic disease, but a negative result does not rule out pancreatic disease.

Comments

1. It is absolutely necessary to prepare the starch test meal properly. If the suspension of starch is allowed to boil, the starch may be partially hydrolyzed by heat into a less complex carbohydrate, thereby facilitating absorption in the gastrointestinal tract. Patients with severe pancreatic insufficiency may then exhibit normal responses to the starch tolerance test. If the starch is mixed with cold water and administered at this temperature, normal subjects may have a flat blood glucose curve.

2. The starch test meal must be ingested as soon as prepared and at a temperature of 50° to 55°C. The ingestion of the gel form of the starch meal may result in a flat blood glucose curve even in normal patients.

3. False negative results may be obtained in patients with achlorhydria. It is possible that the lack of hydrochloric acid allows the digestion of starch by salivary enzymes to continue in the stomach and small intestine.

4. It is important to regulate the time of insulin administration on the days prior to the test for diabetic patients. If a single dose of insulin is being used, it should be given at 1 P.M. on the day preceding each tolerance test.

D-Xylose Test

The D-xylose absorption test is a valuable test for the differential diagnosis of malabsorption. In this procedure a 25 g dose of the pentose sugar in water is administered orally, and the amount excreted over a five-hour period in the urine determined. If the amount excreted is less than 3 g, the diagnosis is most likely enterogenous malabsorption, as pancreatic enzymes are not required for absorption of D-xylose. D-Xylose is passively absorbed in the small intestine and is not metabolized by the liver, though a portion of an orally or intravenously administered dose is destroyed. The accuracy of the method depends not only on the rate of absorption of D-xylose but also on the rate of excretion by the kidneys. It is therefore advisable in patients with renal disease to collect a blood sample for xylose quantitation two hours after the administration of xylose.

Method (Reiner, 1965)

Principle. D-Xylose 25 g is administered orally. Blood level is determined two hours later; urine excretion over a five-hour post-administration period is also determined. Chemical determination depends on dehydration of pentose to furfural in the presence of acid, followed by condensation of furfural with p-bromoaniline to form a colored compound.

At 70°C. about 9 per cent of the available pentose is converted to furfural, but at this temperature very little furfural is formed from other percursors. p-Bromoaniline is used because it does not form any appreciable color with other substances; and thiourea, which is an antioxidant, also helps to prevent the formation of interfering colored compounds.

Sample Collection

1. Allow patient nothing by mouth after midnight on the day of the test.

2. Between 8:00 and 9:00 A.M., have patient void. Discard urine.

3. Immediately after patient has voided, give orally 25 g of D-xylose dissolved in 250 ml (8 oz) of tap water, following immediately with an additional 250 ml of tap water. Note time. In the case of children, administer 0.5 g of xylose per pound of body weight up to 25 g, with the amount of water adjusted accordingly.

4. Exactly two hours (one hour for children) after administration of D-xylose, draw 4 ml of venous blood. This should be sent to the laboratory immediately.

5. Allow patient no further fluid or food and keep on bed rest or in a chair until completion of the test. Patient may experience a mild diarrhea later in the day from the D-xylose.

6. Save all urine voided during the test. Five hours after the test was started have the patient void. Add this urine to the rest. Send pooled urine to the laboratory immediately.

Reagents

1. Somogyi deproteinizing reagents: (a) Zinc sulfate; dissolve 5 g of $ZnSO_4 \cdot 7\ H_2O$ in deionized water and dilute to 100 ml with deionized water. (b) Barium hydroxide, 0.3 N. Dissolve 25 g of $Ba(OH)_2 \cdot 8H_2O$ in deionized water and dilute to 500 ml with deionized water.

2. Saturated thiourea: Add about 4 g of thiourea to 100 ml of glacial acetic acid. Shake and decant the supernatant.

3. D-Xylose color reagent: Make fresh before each use. Add 4 g p-bromoaniline to 200 ml of the saturated solution of thiourea in glacial acetic acid.

4. Stock D-xylose standard (2.0 mg/ml). Dissolve 0.20 g D-xylose in 0.3 per cent (w/v) benzoic acid in a 100 ml volumetric flask and dilute to volume with 0.3 per cent benzoic acid.

5. Working D-xylose standard (0.040 mg/ml). Dilute 2.0 ml of the stock D-xylose standard to volume in a 100 ml volumetric flask with 0.3 per cent (w/v) benzoic acid.

6. Working D-xylose standard (0.10 mg/ml). Dilute 5.0 ml of the stock D-xylose standard to volume in a 100 ml volumetric flask with 0.3 per cent (w/v) benzoic acid.

7. Working D-xylose standard (0.20 mg/ml). Dilute 10 ml of the D-xylose stock standard to volume in a 100 ml volumetric flask with 0.3 per cent (w/v) benzoic acid.

Procedure

1. Prepare an appropriate quantity of D-xylose color reagent.

2. Prepare a protein-free supernate 1:10 as follows: Mix 1 volume of serum, 7 volumes of deionized water, 1 volume of zinc sulfate, and 1 volume of 0.3 N barium hydroxide. Mix after the addition of each solution. Centrifuge the solution and collect the supernatant for D-xylose determination.

3. Measure the volume of urine and prepare 1:50, 1:100, and 1:250 dilutions with deionized water.

4. Pipette 0.5 ml of water, standards, serum filtrate, and urine dilutions in a series of duplicate tubes.

5. Add 2.5 ml of p-bromoaniline reagent to all tubes.

6. Incubate one of the duplicate tubes in a water bath at 70° C. ± 2°C. for 10 minutes. Cool tubes in running water to room temperature. Use the unheated set of tubes as blanks.

7. Place the heated and unheated tubes in a dark place for 70 minutes.

8. Read each set of tubes in a spectrophotometer at 520 nm. The unheated tube serves as a blank for each corresponding heated tube. Read within 30 minutes.

9. Construct a standard curve by plotting corrected absorbance vs. D-xylose concentration in mg/ml for the three xylose standards. The corrected absorbance for both standards and samples is absorbance (test) minus absorbance (blank). The standard curve should be linear and pass through the origin.

Calculations

Concentration:

mg D-xylose/dl = mg/ml × 10 × 100

where:

mg/ml is obtained from standard curve using the corrected absorbance.

10 is correction for dilution in preparing protein-free filtrate.

100 converts mg/ml to mg/dl.

Urine Concentration. Read the concentration of D-xylose in mg/ml corresponding to the corrected absorbance for the diluted urine from the standard curve.

For 1:50 dilution:

D-Xylose excreted in g/5 hr = (mg/ml D-xylose) × (50/1) × (urine volume in liters).

For 1:100 dilution:

D-Xylose excreted in g/5 hr = (mg/ml D-xylose) × (100/1) × (urine volume in liters).

3

For 1:250 dilution:
D-Xylose excreted in g/5 hr = (mg/ml D-xylose) × (250/1) × (urine volume in liters).

Normal Values. With a 25 g dose of D-xylose, adults should excrete at least 4 g xylose in the five-hour urine specimen. The blood concentration should be 36 ± 16 mg/dl (2.4 ± 1.07 mmol/L). Children should normally excrete 16 to 33 per cent of the dose in the five-hour urine, and the blood concentration should be greater than 30 mg/dl (2.01 mmol/L).

Laboratory Tests for Fat Malabsorption

The normal fat content of feces consists primarily of fatty acids, fatty acid salts (soaps), and neutral fats, with higher alcohols, paraffins, sterols, and vegetable carotenoids present in significantly smaller amounts. Fractionation of the total lipids into free fatty acids and neutral fats was formerly thought to aid in the assessment of the exocrine functions of the pancreas. However, because of the presence of bacterial lipase and the spontaneous hydrolysis of neutral fats, fractionation of the total lipid provides no additional information about the cause of steatorrhea.

Several laboratory procedures are available for the evaluation of fat malabsorption. Titrimetric methods quantitate various chemical forms of fatty acids, while gravimetric and microscopic procedures evaluate total fecal fat. Breath tests represent a more recent approach to the diagnosis of fat malabsorption. In these tests the specific radioactivity of $^{14}CO_2$ is measured after the ingestion of a test meal containing ^{14}C-labeled triglycerides.

Titrimetric Method. The titrimetric method of Van de Kamer (1949) has been the most widely used chemical procedure for the quantitation of fecal fats and serves as the laboratory procedure for the definitive diagnosis of steatorrhea. In this method fats and fatty acids are converted to soap (saponified) by boiling with alcoholic potassium hydroxide, giving a solution which contains the soaps derived from neutral fats and the fatty acids and the soaps originally present in the stool. After cooling, excess hydrochloric acid is added to convert soaps to fatty acids. These are extracted with petroleum ether. An aliquot is evaporated, taken up in neutral alcohol, and titrated with sodium hydroxide. Fats are calculated as fatty acids.

In some cases of malabsorption, the coefficient of fat retention can be improved by substituting medium chain fatty acids for long chain fatty acids in the diet. The Van de Kamer method does not quantitatively recover medium chain fatty acids. Braddock (1968) has improved the recovery of medium chain fatty acids from feces by slightly modifying the Van de Kamer procedure. He reduced the amount of water during saponification and distilled off the excess of alcohol prior to extraction, resulting in complete recovery of medium chain and long chain fatty acids.

Breath Test. The measurement of $^{14}CO_2$ following the ingestion of ^{14}C labeled tyriglycerides was introduced as a technique for diagnosing fat malabsorption by Schwabe in 1962. Since that time other investigators (Newcomer, 1979; Meeker, 1980) have modified the procedure, employing various labeled triglycerides (triolein, tripalmitin, and trioctanoin) in an attempt to improve its clinical sensitivity and specificity. Steatorrhea from either pancreatic insufficiency or other causes results in a decreased absorption of triglycerides by the digestive system. This in turn results in a decrease in expired CO_2 derived from the metabolism of the triglyceride fatty acids.

Principle. After an overnight fast the patient consumes a ^{14}C labeled triglyceride. Periodically breath CO_2 is collected in a trapping solution containing an indicator which changes color when a predetermined amount of CO_2 is in solution. The radioactivity of the $^{14}CO_2$ is then measured in a liquid scintillation counter and the results reported as per cent dose of $^{14}CO_2$ excreted per hour.

Comment. To distinguish pancreatic insufficiency from other causes of steatorrhea some investigators have developed a two-stage breath test (Goff, 1982). In the first stage of the test the patient consumes a ^{14}C labeled triglyceride, and the $^{14}CO_2$ is measured as described above. The second stage of the test is performed five to seven days later and is the same as the first stage except this time the patient is given an oral dose of pancreatic enzymes along with the dose of ^{14}C labeled triglyceride. In the case of steatorrhea due to pancreatic insufficiency the amount of $^{14}CO_2$ expired should increase relative to the amount of $^{14}CO_2$ expired in the first stage of the test. Patients with steatorhea of other causes should have no significant change in the amount of $^{14}CO_2$ expired due to the oral administration of pancreatic enzymes.

Clinitest for Reducing Substances in Stool

(Kerry, 1964)

Procedure. Add 1 volume of stool to 2 volumes of distilled water and mix thoroughly. Transfer 15 drops of this suspension to a clean test tube and add a Clinitest tablet. The reaction and interpretation of results are described in Chapter 18.

Interpretation. Presence of 0.25 g/dl reducing substances or less is considered normal; from 0.25 g/dl to 0.5 g/dl is regarded as suspicious; greater than 0.5 g/dl is interpreted as indicating abnormal amounts of sugar. Sucrose, of course, is not a reducing sugar and will not react in this test. However, in the case of sucrose intolerance, little sucrose but large amounts of glucose and fructose are found in the stool, presumably due to hydrolysis of sucrose by intestinal bacteria, so that the test is positive nonetheless.

Oral Lactose Tolerance Test

(Gudmand-Hoyer, 1977)

Following an overnight fast, administer, orally, 50 g lactose dissolved in 400 ml of water. Draw fasting blood and blood samples at 30, 60, and 120 minutes after ingestion, as for a glucose tolerance test. Also collect a five-hour stool specimen, examining and recording appearance, consistency, and pH.

Patients with lactase deficiency exhibit a peak rise of less than 20 mg/dl in reducing substances expressed as glucose. In all persons with flat tolerance curves, the test should be repeated within two days and the less abnormal of the two curves used for interpretation. A control test may be performed, using 25 g glucose and 25 g galactose if the lactose test indicates malabsorption. Some investigators use a 100 g dose, which has been reported by some to yield more definitive results. It may cause symptoms in cases of mild lactase deficiency. In children, the dose of lactose or other sugars is 2 g/kg of body weight.

Fecal Blood

Quantitative methods have been developed for study of gastrointestinal bleeding by use of radioactive chromium-51 (Fall, 1971). These methods have greater specificity than peroxidase tests. Furthermore, they can be combined with other techniques to determine the location of bleeding, when present. As they involve considerable time, effort, and expense, their use should be reserved for patients presenting special diagnostic problems.

The procedures are based on ability of radioactive chromium to be bound to red blood cells and on the fact that radioactive chromium is not reabsorbed from the gastrointestinal tract but is excreted in the feces, where it can be measured by gamma-ray spectrometry. For this purpose a sample of blood is withdrawn from the patient, mixed with citrate solution containing ^{51}Cr as sodium chromate, and then reinjected into the patient. Most of the sodium chromate is bound to the red blood cells and remains so bound until they are destroyed or lost through hemorrhage. Subsequently, stools contain quantities of ^{51}Cr quantitatively related to the blood content. Gamma ray activity of the stool specimen is determined and the blood loss is calculated from comparison with activity of patient's blood. Bleeding source may be localized by similarly examining for blood fluid removed from various levels of the gastrointestinal tract through a Miller-Abbott tube or by use of an umbilical tape attached to a small bag of mercury in a lead sinker, swallowed by the patient, located by fluoroscope, and then withdrawn and examined for blood staining. Likewise, injection of autologous erythrocytes labeled *in vitro* with ^{99m}Tc, followed by abdominal nuclear imaging, can very sensitively and accurately depict the source of bleeding (Markisz, 1982).

The commonly applied screening tests depend on the determination of the peroxidase activity of hemoglobin for the semiquantitation of blood in feces. Reagents used include guaiac, benzidine,* ortho-tolidine, and ortho-dianisidine. Peroxidases (including hemoglobin, which can act as either a catalase or peroxidase) catalyze oxidation of the test substance by hydrogen peroxide, causing development of various shades and intensities of blue, depending on reagent, concentration of hemoglobin or other peroxidases, presence of other coloring matter, and presence (or absence) of inhibitors. The reagents differ chiefly in sensitivity. Benzidine gives a positive result with blood in a 1:100,000 dilution with saline; ortho-tolidine is positive in a 1:20,000 dilution, and guaiac is positive in 1:100 to 1:5,000 dilution, depending on the age and hemoglobin concentration of the blood (Hoerr, 1949). The more sensitive reagents can be adapted to provide a less sensitive test by manipulation of techniques. Hematest (Ames Company, Inc.) incorporates ortho-toluidine, while Hemoccult (Smith-Kline Corporation) employs guaiac-impregnated filter paper. These commercial tests have sensitivities intended to be consistent with the uses for which they are designed. The normal individual loses 2.0 to 2.5 ml of blood into the gastrointestinal tract daily (Ebaugh, 1958). Therefore, it is reasonable to use a test which begins to turn positive with a blood loss greater than 5 to 10 ml per day. This corresponds to 5 to 10 mg of hemoglobin/g stool, assuming a blood hemoglobin of 15 g/dl and an average 150 g stool. Morris (1976) found, in comparing three screening procedures (1:60 alcoholic solution of guaiac, Hematest, and Hemoccult) with the quantitative radioassay technique, that guaiac and Hematest detected 95 per cent of stools with more than 5 mg hemoglobin/g stool. Hemoccult detected 37 per cent of stools in 2.0 to 5.0 mg hemoglobin/g stool range, 60 per cent of stools containing 5.0 to 20.0 mg hemoglobin/g stool, and 95 per cent of stools with greater than 20.0 g hemoglobin/g stool. Earlier authors comparing either the volume of ingested blood or fecal quantitation of ingested ^{51}Cr-labeled red cells with different screening methods have, in some cases, confirmed the relative sensitivities of these reagents, while others have come to different conclusions. Ostrow (1973) found that guaiac and Hematest consistently detected as little as 2.0 mg hemoglobin/g stool, while Hemoccult detected only 50 per cent of the stools with 5 to 10 mg hemoglobin/g stool and most of the stools with greater than 10 mg hemoglobin/g stool. However, Peranio (1951) found ortho-toluidine to be more sensitive than guaiac, requiring only 1 ml of ingested blood to yield a positive test, whereas guaiac required 20.0 ml. These differences in relative sensitivity illustrate how the same basic reagents used under different conditions can yield markedly different results.

Stroehlein (1976) found that the ratio of volume of blood loss to stool volume, as well as the amount of blood loss, was an important factor in obtaining a positive fecal occult blood result. Two thirds of the stools were positive for occult blood with Hemoccult when the calculated volume of fecal blood loss was 10 per cent of stool volume, and nearly all specimens were positive when the volume of blood loss was 30 per cent of the stool volume.

Numerous modifications have been developed based on the same fundamental processes in efforts to improve test precision and specificity and diagnostic accuracy. There are at least eight products that are now commercially available to the world (Winawer, 1982). Hemoccult seems to have the lowest percentage of false positive results, approximately 1 to 12 per cent (Stroehlein, 1976; Morris, 1976). The range of false positives reported for other guaiac-based procedures is 6 to 76 per cent (Morris, 1976). Hematest has been reported to have a 27 to 76 per cent false positive rate (Ostrow, 1973; Morris, 1976). The high rate of false positives is influenced by the lack of specificity of the reagents and the presence of peroxidase activity in other fecal constituents, as well as the sensitivity of the different chromogens to peroxidase activity. The myoglobin and hemoglobin of ingested meat and fish have peroxidase activity that may falsely indicate the presence of occult blood. The necessity of eliminating meat from the diet before and during the test period is dependent on the sensitivity of the occult blood test used. In general, the less sensitive test such as Hemoccult test is the least affected by meat in the diet (Ostrow, 1973).

Bacteria in the bowel as well as ingested vegetables, such as horseradish and turnips, and bananas also have

*The use and marketing of benzidine is restricted by federal regulations due to its carcinogenicity, and its use should be eliminated whenever possible. Some or all of the alternative chemicals may also be carcinogenic.

peroxidase and can falsely elevate fecal peroxidase activity. Modifications of tests intended to destroy plant and bacterial peroxidases by boiling or heating the fecal suspension may also denature some of the peroxidase activity of hemoglobin and are therefore not recommended. Recently, a specific test using fluorescein-labeled rabbit anti-human hemoglobin serum to detect fecal occult blood has been developed (Vellacott, 1981). However, its clinical application as a screening test remains to be evaluated.

The possibility of false positives owing to the presence of iron in the diet is widely recognized, but the studies have failed to confirm these findings (Morris, 1976). In fact, in the presence of iron, the percentage of false positives is decreased with Hemoccult and the false negatives tended to be lower with guaiac, Hematest, and Hemoccult. Laxatives and barium do not interfere with the performance of the occult blood test (Morris, 1976). There has been some evidence that false negatives occur with guaiac, benzidine, ortho-toluidine, and ortho-dianisidine in the presence of large amounts of vitamin C (Jaffe, 1975).

As blood traverses the gut, it is broken down into its constituents, which may have decreased or no peroxidase activity. The actual form of hemoglobin most commonly found in the colon is hematin, which has much less peroxidase activity than heme. A source of hemorrhage in the upper gastrointestinal system or an increased transit time through the bowel will, therefore, decrease the peroxidase activity of hemoglobin.

One group found an 80- to 120-fold decrease in the peroxidase activity of blood passing through the gastrointestinal tract as compared to blood added directly to the feces (Ebaugh, 1958). Furthermore, because of inhibiting substances in the stool, similar loss of activity may be found by adding blood to feces, as compared with adding similar quantities of blood to water. Ebaugh and associates suggest that this inhibition results from masking of indicator color by added color from the feces. Another factor may be competition for nascent oxygen by reducing substances in the feces.

Finally, techniques for measuring peroxidase activity are subject to considerable experimental error, particularly when large numbers of stool specimens must be screened by mass production methods. Specimens show marked variability in consistency and in their tendency to disperse in suspensions. This leads to inconsistencies in amount of aliquot used and in the portion of the aliquot actually available to react in suspension. Filter paper techniques are also limited in reproducibility by the tendency for liquid stools to be absorbed into the substance of the paper.

Further errors result from inaccurate measurement of reagents, inaccurate timing of the reaction, and variable interpretation of the color developed. Inconsistencies may also arise from sampling by the patients or incomplete mixing of blood with the stool. Blood arising in the upper gastrointestinal tract is relatively uniformly mixed throughout the specimen, but blood from the lower gastrointestinal tract is likely to be segmental in distribution within the stool, or it may only coat the surface. Anorectal blood frequently produces red streaking of the surface. The presence of such focally distributed blood should be reported after chemical verification. In routine testing for occult blood, an attempt is made to use an aliquot from the center of the formed stool.

In the patient with severe gastrointestinal hemorrhage, the diagnostic problems are not such as to need a very sensitive test to detect blood in feces. The real benefit of these tests is as a screening procedure for hemorrhage which may bleed intermittently. To be valid, the test employed must be repeated at least three and preferably six times with the patient on a diet free of the exogenous sources of peroxidase acitivity. In addition, the patient should be requested to include liberal amounts of high residue foods such as prunes, bran, raw vegetables, corn, and peanuts. This regimen is usually unacceptable to the patient, so that positive tests on a normal diet must be repeated following a three- or four-day period of abstinence from meats, fish, and vegetable sources of peroxidase activity. Only after this regimen can a positive series of tests be considered an indication for further evaluation of the patient.

Methodology. The guaiac method to be described represents a compromise suitable for routine screening. It will detect 0.5 to 1.0 mg of hemoglobin/ml of aqueous solution. If one substitutes 0.2 per cent ortho-tolidine for guaiac and 0.3 per cent hydrogen peroxide for 3 per cent hydrogen peroxide in the same procedure, one obtains approximately the same sensitivity. We have found the Hematest techniques to be capable of detecting as little as 0.1 mg blood in an aqueous solution. It has an unacceptable number of false positive reactions when patients are on a regular diet (Ostrow, 1973; Morris, 1976). Paradoxically, however, Hematest sometimes gives only a trace or 1+ reaction with tarry stools. We believe this results from improper mixing of hematin with reagent, probably because of the tarry consistency of the stool. Mixing (not recommended by the manufacturer) obviates the problem.

We advise use of a saturated solution of guaiac because of the tendency of weaker solutions to fade. Addition of extra powdered guaiac will restore the coloring in these cases. The problem may also be overcome by observing for maximal color development.

Hemoccult, employing guaiac-impregnated filter paper, is of lower sensitivity and begins to turn positive in the presence of about 5.0 mg of hemoglobin/g of stool. This is the upper limit of normal peroxidase activity of stool, and as this represents a significant improvement in methodology false positives can be kept in the range of 1 to 12 per cent (Stroehlein, 1976; Morris, 1976). The Hemoccult test also has the advantage of being so simple and esthetically acceptable that specimens can be collected at home and mailed for evaluation. However, Morris (1976) and Winawer (1977) have found that some specimens may convert from positive to negative after storage for two days.

Guaiac Test for Occult Blood

Reagents

1. 1:60 (w/v) solution of gum guaiac in 95 per cent (v/v) ethyl alcohol or, preferably, a saturated solution.
2. Glacial acetic acid.
3. 3 per cent (v/v) hydrogen peroxide.

Procedure

1. Place about 0.5 g of feces in a 10 × 100 mm test tube.

2. Add about 2 ml of tap water and mix applicator sticks.

3. Add 0.5 ml of glacial acetic acid and mix well.

4. Add about 2 ml of the gum guaiac solution and mix well.

5. Add about 2 ml of hydrogen peroxide and mix; start timer.

6. Observe for two minutes and record the maximal color development during that time as trace, 1+, 2+, 3+, or 4+, depending on the intensity of the blue color. Strongly positive reactions will fade rapidly and should be read according to maximal color development rather than the appearance at the end of the time period.

7. Reagents should be checked daily by testing a sample known to contain blood.

Hemoccult Slide Test for Occult Blood (SmithKline Corp., Sunnyvale, Cal. 94806)

Procedure

1. Collect a very small stool specimen on tip of wooden applicator.
2. Apply thin smear of specimen inside the circle.
3. Close cover; dispose of applicator.
4. Allow specimen to dry (important that specimen dry completely).
5. Open perforated window in back of slide.
6. Apply two or three drops of developing solution to slide opposite specimen.
7. Read results after 30 seconds.

Positive: Reactions that produce a blue color regardless of whether the reaction is weak or strong.

Negative: No detectable blue anywhere on slide indicates test is negative for occult blood. The reactions that do not produce a blue color should not be considered trace but should be considered negative.

Note: The sensitivity of slides can be increased by rehydration prior to adding developing solution. But this results in a high false positivity. Macrae (1982) suggested that the high rate of false positivity resulting from rehydration of the slides can be reduced if the patient is required to maintain a low-peroxidase diet.

Althausen, T. L., and Uyeyama, K.: Further experience with the starch tolerance test for pancreatic insufficiency. Gastroenterology, *40*:470, 1961.

Braddock, L. I., Fleisher, D. R., and Barbero, G. J.: A physical chemical study of the Van de Kamer method for fecal fat analysis. Gastroenterology, *55*:165, 1968.

Dahlquist, A.: Assay of intestinal disaccharidases. Anal. Biochem., *22*:99, 1968.

Drummey, G. D., Benson, J. A., and Jones, G. M.: Microscopical examination of the stool for steatorrhea. N. Engl. J. Med., *264*:85, 1961.

Ebaugh, F. G., Jr., Clements, T., Jr., Rodan G., et al.: Quantitative measurement of gastrointestinal blood loss. Am. J. Med., *25*:169, 1958.

Fall, D. J., Kupier, D. H., and Pollard, H. M.: Use of isotopes for various tests for occult blood in feces. Cancer, *28*:135, 1971.

Florent, C., L'Hirondell, C., Dasmazures, C., et al.: Intestinal clearance of alpha-1-antitrypsin—a sensitive method for the detection of protein-losing enteropathy. Gastroenterology, *81*:777, 1981.

Goff, J. S.: Two-stage triolein breath test differentiates pancreatic insufficiency from other causes of malabsorption. Gastroenterology, *83*:44, 1982.

Goldman, P., Paver, W. K., and Corbett, W. H.: The detection of occult blood in the feces. Med. J. Aust., *1*:755, 1964.

Gregor, D. H.: Occult blood testing for detection of asymptomatic colon cancer. Cancer, *28*:131, 1971.

Gudmand-Hoyer, E., and Simony, K. O.: Individual sensitivity of lactose in lactose malabsorption. Am. J. Dig. Dis., *22*:177, 1977.

Harris, J. C., Dupont, H. L., and Hornick, R. B.: Fecal leukocytes in diarrhea illness. Ann. Intern. Med., *76*:697, 1972.

Hoerr, S. O., Bliss, W. R., and Kaufman, J.: Clinical evaluation of various tests for occult blood in the feces. J.A.M.A., *141*:1213, 1949.

Hoffman, N. E., LaRusso, N. F., and Hoffman, A. F.: An improved method for fecal collection: The fecal field-kit. Lancet, *1*:1422, 1973.

Jaffe, R. M.: False negative stool occult blood tests caused by ingestion of ascorbic acid (vitamin C). Ann. Intern. Med., *83*:842, 1975.

Jelliffe, D. B., and Jelliffe, E. F. D.: Collection of stool sample. Lancet, *2*:618, 1973.

Kerry, K. R., and Anderson, C. M.: A ward test for sugar in feces. Lancet, *1*:981, 964.

Krasilnikoff, P. A., Gudmand-Hoyer, E., and Moltke, H. H.: Diagnostic value of disaccharide tolerance tests on children. Acta Paediatr. Scand., *64*:693, 1975.

Levinson, S. A., and McFate, R. R.: Clinical Laboratory Diagnosis. Philadelphia, Lea and Febiger, 1969, p. 402.

Macrae, F., St. John, D. J. B., Caligiore, P., et al.: Optimal dietary conditions for Hemoccult testing. Gastroenterology, *82*:899, 1982.

Markisz, J. A., Front, D., Royal, H. D., et al.: An evaluation of ^{99m}Tc-labelled red blood cell scintigraphy for the detection of localization of gastrointestinal bleeding site. Gastroenterology, *83*:394, 1982.

Meeker, H. E., Chen, I. W., Connell, A. M., et al.: Clinical experiences in ^{14}C-palmitin breath test for malabsorption. Am. J. Gastroenterol., *73*:277, 1980.

Meeuwisse, G. W., and Linquist, B.: Glucose-galactose malabsorption—study on the intermediate carbohydrate metabolism. Acta Paediatr. Scand., *59*:74, 1970.

Moore, J. G., Engler, E., Jr., Bigler, A. H., et al.: Simple fecal test of absorption—a prospective study and critique. Am. J. Dig. Dis., *16*:97, 1971.

Morris, D. W., Hansell, J. R., Ostrow, J. D., et al.: Reliability of chemical test for fecal occult blood in hospitalized patients. Am. J. Dig. Dis., *21*:845, 1976.

Newcomer, A. D., Hofmann, A. F., DiMagno, E. P., et al.: Tridenin breath test. Gastroenterology, *76*:6, 1979.

Ostrow, J. D., Mulvaney, C. A., Hansell, J. R., et al.: Sensitivity and reproducibility of chemical test for fecal occult blood with an emphasis on false-positive reaction. Am. J. Dig. Dis., *18*:930, 1973.

Peranio, A., and Bruger, M.: The detection of occult blood in the feces including observation on the ingestion of iron and whole blood. J. Lab. Clin. Med., *38*:433, 1951.

Reiner, M., and Cheung, H. L.: Xylose. *In* Meites, S. (ed.): Standard Methods of Clinical Chemistry, Vol. 5. New York, Academic Press, 1965, p. 257.

Santiago-Borrero, P. J., Santini, R., Jr., and Moldonado, N.: The xylose excretion test in normal children and in pediatric patients with tropical sprue. Pediatrics, *48*:59, 1971.

Stroehlein, J. R., Farrbanks, U. F., McGill, D. B., et al.: Hemoccult detection of fecal occult blood quantitated by radioassay. Am. J. Dig. Dis., *21*:841, 1976.

Thomas, D. W., Sinatra, F. R., and Merritt, R. J.: Random fecal alpha-1-antitrypsin concentration in children with gastrointestinal disease. Gastroenterology, *80*:776, 1981.

Thompson, H. L., and McGuffin, D. W.: Melena, a study of underlying causes. J.A.M.A., *141*:1208, 1949.

Van de Kamer, J. H., Ten Bokel Huinink, H., and Weyers, H. W.: Rapid method for the determination of fat in feces. J. Biol. Chem., *177*:347, 1949.

Vellacott, K. D., Baldwin, R. W., and Hardcastle, J. D.: An immunofluorescent test for fecal occult blood. Lancet *1*:18, 1981.

Winawer, S. J.: Screening for colorectal cancer. An overview. Cancer, *45*:1093, 1980.

Winawer, S. J., and Fleisher, J.: Sensitivity and specificity of the fecal occult blood test for colorectal neoplasia. Gastroenterology, *82*:986, 1982.

Winawer, S. J., and Sherlock, P.: Detecting early colon cancer. Hosp. Pract., *12*:49, 1977.

Part IV

HEMATOLOGY AND COAGULATION

EDITED BY DOUGLAS A. NELSON, M.D., AND JOHN BERNARD HENRY, M.D.

27
BASIC METHODOLOGY

Douglas A. Nelson, M.D.,
and Michael W. Morris, M.S., SH(ASCP)

Hematology encompasses the study of blood cells and coagulation. Included in its concerns are analyses of the concentration, structure, and function of cells in blood; their precursors in the bone marrow; chemical constituents of plasma or serum intimately linked with blood cell structure and function; and function of platelets and proteins involved in blood coagulation. Changes in one or more of these characteristics may produce hematologic disease, or may be hematologic manifestations of other disease processes.

BLOOD COLLECTION

Blood sources for hematologic tests are capillary or peripheral blood and venous blood.

Capillary or Peripheral Blood

Free flowing "capillary" or peripheral blood is more nearly arteriolar than capillary.

Venous samples are preferred, but many determinations may be performed on blood obtained from the lobe of an ear, the palmar surfaces of the tip of a finger, or, in the case of infants, the plantar surfaces of the great toe or the heel. The free margin of the ear lobe, not the side, should be punctured. Usually, a finger puncture is more convenient. An edematous or congested site should not be used. Free flow of blood is essential to obtain reproducible results comparable to those from venous blood. Punctures from cold, cyanotic skin result in falsely high figures for hemoglobin and cell counts, but these can be avoided by massage before the puncture until the skin is pink and warm. Vigorous squeezing is another source of errors.

Equipment. Equipment consists of gauze pads, 70 per

cent isopropyl alcohol, and a lancet or scalpel blade, preferably disposable.

Technique. The site is first rubbed vigorously with a gauze pad moistened with 70 per cent alcohol to remove dirt and epithelial debris and to increase blood circulation. After the skin has dried, a puncture 2 to 3 mm deep is made with the blade or lancet. A rapid, firm puncture should be made, but with control of the depth and site. With a sharp blade the puncture gives little pain. A deep puncture is no more painful than a superficial one and makes repeated punctures unnecessary.

The skin at the site of the puncture should be dry. The first drop of blood, which contains tissue juices, is wiped away. The blood must not be pressed out, since this dilutes it with fluid from the tissues. Moderate pressure some distance above the puncture is allowable. To stop blood flow, slight pressure is applied with a gauze.

If the heel is used, it should be warmed by immersion in warm water or with a hot water compress. Otherwise, values significantly higher than in venous blood may be obtained, especially in the newborn.

Precision is poorer in capillary than in venous blood because of variation in flow and dilution with interstitial fluid. Initial capillary samples tend to give lower cell counts. Measurements from freely flowing blood approach those from venous samples, but the cell counts and hemoglobin are still probably slightly lower. Blood from a skin puncture is a mixture of capillary and arteriolar blood, and the venous hematocrit is greater than the whole body hematocrit by a factor of 1/0.9 (ICSH, 1973).

In platelet counting, free flow is critical to prevent platelet clumping, which will result in a decreased count. Blood films made from capillary blood without anticoagulation are preferable; but without free blood flow, leukocyte distribution may be altered.

Venous Blood

The venipuncture is in most instances a relatively simple procedure. The patient's life may depend on vein patency, and care must be taken to preserve these vessels. Hematomas or ecchymoses are usually evidence of the operator's poor technique or judgment.

A few well chosen words will often reassure the patient. The operator's self-assurance and poise will do much to establish the proper rapport. The patient should be made comfortable, with the arm accessible to the operator. Ambulatory patients should be seated comfortably, preferably in a chair provided with a locking armrest for firm support.

Veins should be carefully inspected, particularly with those patients who have already had numerous punctures. A tourniquet makes veins more prominent and should help eliminate blind probing, which is unacceptable.

Equipment. Syringe size is determined by the volume of blood required. Disposable plastic syringes are most widely used.

The gauge and length of the needle used depend on the size and depth of the vein. The gauge number varies inversely with the diameter of the needle. The needle tip should be inspected carefully. A blunt or bent tip will damage the patient's vein and often leads to failure.

Technique. Although few patients faint as a result of venipuncture, this danger must be kept in mind.

To prevent hemoconcentration the tourniquet pressure should not be maintained longer than necessary. The outer end of the tourniquet should be tucked under so that a slight pull will release it. An advantage of the sphygmomanometer (blood pressure cuff) is that it permits adjustment of the compression to a level midway between systolic and diastolic pressures, which reduces the flow of venous blood without stopping arterial circulation. Also, reduction or release of pressure after the needle has entered the vein is facilitated. To distend the veins, the patient is asked to open and close the fist several times. Giving the patient an active role in the procedure helps take his mind off the puncture. Even if not seen, veins can usually be felt beneath the skin. In fat persons, veins that show as blue streaks are usually too superficial and too small.

After the preliminary steps, apply the tourniquet and clean the skin with 70 per cent alcohol and allow it to dry. Fix the vein in position by supporting the patient's forearm with your hand and compressing and pulling the soft tissues just below the intended puncture site with your thumb. Hold the syringe between the thumb and the last three fingers of the other hand, resting the back of these fingers on the patient's arm. Rest the free index finger against the hub of the needle; it serves as a guide. Push the needle into the vein with a single direct puncture of skin and vein.

Entrance into the vein is followed immediately by appearance of blood in the hub of the needle or in the syringe. If that does not occur, withdraw the plunger slightly and in many instances blood appears. Loosen the tourniquet if blood flows freely; otherwise, leave it in place until the desired amount of blood is obtained. At this time, have the patient open his fist, release the tourniquet, withdraw the syringe and needle, and apply gentle pressure to the puncture site with dry gauze or cotton. Instruct the patient to hold the pad and to raise the outstretched arm for a few minutes. This usually stops the bleeding and prevents formation of a hematoma. A small adhesive dressing may be applied, mainly to prevent a stain on the rolled-down sleeve. The operator must see that the patient's condition is satisfactory before he is dismissed. If there is any sign of continued discomfort, anxiety, bleeding, or shock, the patient should be kept lying down and seen by a physician.

There is usually no difficulty in inserting a needle into a vein except in children and in patients in whom the arm is fat or the veins are small.

Instead of syringes, evacuated blood collection tubes may be employed (see Chap. 1, p. 3). Evacuated tubes, sealed with a stopper, are supplied with a measured amount of anticoagulant (or none) and sufficient vacuum to draw a predetermined volume of blood. A disposable needle is screwed into a holder, and the evacuated tube is placed in the holder so that the tube stopped just reaches the guide line. The short shaft is thereby embedded in the tube stopper but does not penetrate through it to break the vacuum. After the needle is inserted into the vein, the tube is pushed all the way into the holder, the vacuum is broken, and blood flows into the tube. After the flow ceases, the tube may be removed and another tube inserted into the holder; or if only one tube is needed, the whole unit is withdrawn as described above for the syringe. This convenient and economical system eliminates the need for syringes and uses disposable needles and tubes.

Hemolysis interferes with many examinations. It can be minimized by using clean glassware and needles that are not too small; by drawing the blood slowly, no faster than the vein is filling; by avoiding admixture of air with frothing; and, after the blood is drawn, by removing the needle and then emptying the blood again slowly and without force into the test tube.

Complications of Venipunctures

Immediate Local Complications. Prolonged application of the tourniquet (i.e., over 60 seconds) will produce measurable increases in the concentration of the blood cells.

Failure of blood to enter the syringe may be the result of several factors. Excessive pull on the plunger may collapse a small vein. Piercing the outer coat of the vein without entering the lumen may also account for failure. This may be remedied by withdrawing slightly and re-entering the vein. This complication may occasionally be followed by hematoma formation. If signs of beginning hematoma are noticed, the tourniquet should be released, the needle withdrawn, and local pressure applied. Venipuncture should then be performed on the other arm. Transfixation of the vein may be remedied by slight withdrawal followed by gentle aspiration to see whether blood appears. If this fails, the puncture may have to be repeated. This complication is frequently followed by formation of a hematoma, and the same remedy is followed as above. Circulatory failure is another cause and is beyond the control of the operator.

Failure to draw blood after two attempts should be an indication to request another operator.

An occasional immediate complication is syncope. This is best treated by having the patient lie down, if he is not already in this position. A physician should check the patient immediately.

Continued bleeding may occur in patients with a hemorrhagic tendency. Local pressure, as a rule, controls the bleeding.

Late Local Complications. Thrombosis of the vein is sometimes due to trauma, especially following many venipunctures at the same site. Rarely, infection results in thrombophlebitis. These complications are rare if the precautions and recommendations discussed in this chapter are observed.

Late General Complications. Use of disposable needles has virtually eliminated transmission of serum hepatitis by contaminated equipment.

Venipuncture in Infants

In infants and children venipuncture presents special problems because of the small size of the veins and the difficulty controlling the patient. Much can be achieved by the same approach that was outlined for adults.

Restraining the infant to reduce mobility, use of sharp needles of appropriate size, careful inspection of the veins, and making certain that the pressure applied with the tourniquet is not excessive (best checked by feeling pulsation of the radial artery) will contribute to a successful venipuncture when others may have failed. After proper training, one may try external jugular puncture in difficult cases.

For hematologic examination, blood obtained by venipuncture is delivered without delay to tubes containing a suitable anticoagulant. Mixing with the anticoagulant is accomplished by thorough but gentle rotation of the container. A drop of blood from the needle or syringe tip is placed on two or more slides, and films are made directly. At the patient's bedside, it is essential that one label the tubes and slides with the patient's name and identification number.

To obtain serum, blood is kept at room temperature or in a 37°C. incubator until a clot has formed and begins to retract; then it is centrifuged and the serum pipetted off. To accelerate retraction the clot may be separated from the wall of the container with a platinum needle, thin glass rod, or wooden applicator. Some commercial evacuated tubes contain a gel which, when spun, forms a barrier between the clot and serum and allows easy decanting of the serum. To obtain serum more rapidly, the blood may be defibrinated with glass beads or a glass rod. Also available are tubes which contain thrombin to enhance clotting.

Anticoagulants

The three anticoagulants commonly used in hematology are trisodium citrate, the tripotassium or disodium salts of ethylenediamine tetraacetic acid (EDTA), and heparin. The first two prevent coagulation by removing calcium from the blood by precipitation or binding in non-ionized form. Heparin acts by forming a complex with plasma antithrombin III, which inhibits thrombin and other stages of clotting factor activation.

Trisodium citrate is used for blood coagulation and platelet function studies. The ratio is one part of a 3.8 per cent or 3.2 per cent aqueous solution to nine parts of whole blood. Buffered citrate (sodium citrate and citric acid) is now commonly used because it helps stabilize plasma pH.

EDTA is used in a concentration of 1 to 2 mg per 1 ml of blood and is the preferred anticoagulant for blood cell counts and for morphological studies if blood films made directly from fresh blood are not practicable. Artifacts form only on prolonged standing. Acceptable blood films can be prepared after two to three hours and cell counts are valid for 24 hours, if the blood is refrigerated. EDTA prevents platelet clumping and is the anticoagulant of choice for platelet counting.

Heparin, 0.1 to 0.2 mg per 1 ml of blood, does not affect cell size or hematocrit. It is the best anticoagulant for prevention of hemolysis and for osmotic fragility tests. It is not satisfactory for leukocyte or platelet counts because of cell clumping. It also produces a troublesome blue background in Wright's-stained blood films.

Sources of Error

Precautions must be taken to prevent errors in analysis of blood cells as a result of *in vitro* change in EDTA-blood.

Blood films should be prepared immediately. If other determinations cannot be performed within two or three hours, the blood should be refrigerated at 4°C. In blood kept at room temperature, swelling of erythrocytes between 6 and 24 hours raises the hematocrit and mean corpuscular volume (MCV) and lowers the mean corpuscular hemoglobin concentration (MCHC) and the erythrocyte sedimentation rate. At 24 hours, however, the white cell count (WBC), red cell count (RBC), hemoglobin, hematocrit, and red cell indices are all unchanged in EDTA-blood stored at 4°C. (Brittin, 1969b). Under these conditions this is true also for the reticulocyte count and the platelet count (Lampasso, 1968). The sedimentation rate should be performed within two hours (Morris, 1975).

Before taking a sample from a tube of venous blood for a hematologic determination, it is important to mix the blood thoroughly. If the tube has been standing, this requires at least 60 inversions of the tube, or two minutes on a mechanical rotator; less than this leads to unacceptable deterioration in precision (Fairbanks, 1971).

HEMOGLOBIN (Hb)

Hemoglobin (Hb), the main component of the red blood cell, is a conjugated protein that serves as the vehicle for the transportation of oxygen and CO_2. When fully saturated, each gram of hemoglobin holds 1.34 ml of oxygen. The red cell mass of the adult contains approximately 600 g of hemoglobin, capable of carrying 800 ml of oxygen. The terminology and

Table 27–1. NOMENCLATURE OF HEMOGLOBIN DERIVATIVES

Term Used	Symbol	Other Terms
Hemoglobin	Hb	
Oxyhemoglobin	HbO_2	
Carboxyhemoglobin	HbCO	
Sulfhemoglobin	SHb	
Carboxysulfhemoglobin	SHbCO	
Hemiglobin	Hi	Methemoglobin
Hemiglobincyanide	HiCN	Cyanmethemoglobin

Modified from van Assendelft, O. W.: Spectrophotometry of Haemoglobin Derivatives. Assen, The Netherlands, Royal Van Gorcum Ltd., 1970.

symbols employed in this discussion are given in Table 27–1.

A molecule of hemoglobin consists of two pairs of polypeptide chains ("globin") and four prosthetic heme groups, each containing one atom of ferrous iron. Each heme group is precisely located in a pocket or fold of one of the polypeptide chains. Located near the surface of the molecule, the heme reversibly combines with one molecule of oxygen or carbon dioxide.

The main function of hemoglobin is to transport oxygen from the lungs, where oxygen tension is high, to the tissues, where it is low. At an oxygen tension of 100 mm Hg in the pulmonary capillaries, 95 to 98 per cent of the hemoglobin is combined with oxygen. In the tissues, where the oxygen tension may be as low as 20 mm Hg, the oxygen readily dissociates from hemoglobin; in this instance, less than 30 per cent of the oxygen would remain combined with hemoglobin.

Reduced hemoglobin (Hb) is hemoglobin with iron unassociated with oxygen. When each heme group is associated with one molecule of oxygen, the hemoglobin is referred to as oxyhemoglobin (HbO_2). In both Hb and HbO_2, iron remains in the ferrous state. With iron oxidized to the ferric state, methemoglobin (hemiglobin; Hi) is formed, and the molecule loses its capacity to carry oxygen or carbon dioxide.

Hemoglobinometry is the measurement of the concentration of hemoglobin in the blood. Anemia, a decrease below normal of the hemoglobin concentration, erythrocyte count, or hematocrit, is a very common condition and is frequently a complication of other diseases. Clinical diagnosis of anemia based on estimation of the color of the skin and of visible mucous membranes is highly unreliable. Anemia is frequently masked in many diseases by other manifestations. To a limited extent similar considerations apply to conditions with abnormally high hemoglobin. For all these reasons the correct estimation of hemoglobin is important and is one of the routine tests done on practically every patient.

Determining the Concentration of Hemoglobin. The cyanmethemoglobin (hemiglobincyanide; HiCN) method, the oxyhemoglobin (HbO_2) method, and the method measuring iron content will be considered. The HiCN method was recommended by the International Committee for Standardization in Hematology in 1966, and was modified in 1977 (ICSH, 1978). It has the advantage of convenience and a readily available, stable standard solution.

Hemiglobincyanide (HiCN) Method

Principle. Blood is diluted in a solution of potassium ferricyanide and potassium cyanide. The potassium ferricyanide oxidizes hemoglobins to hemiglobin (Hi; methemoglobin), and potassium cyanide provides cyanide ions (CN^-) to form hemiglobincyanide (HiCN), which has a broad absorption maximum at a wavelength of 540 nm (Fig. 27–1). The absorbance

4

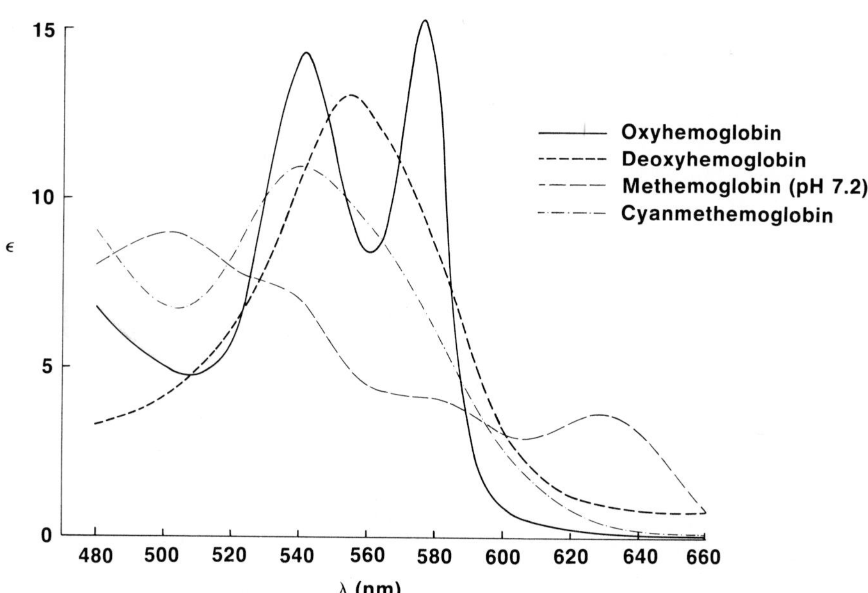

Figure 27–1. Absorption spectra of oxyhemoglobin (HbO_2), deoxyhemoglobin (Hb), methemoglobin (hemiglobin, Hi), and cyanmethemoglobin (hemiglobincyanide, HiCN). (From Bunn, H. F., Forget, B. G., and Ranney, H. M.: Human Hemoglobins. Philadelphia, W. B. Saunders Company, 1977.)

of the solution is measured in a photometer or spectrophotometer at 540 nm and compared with that of a standard HiCN solution.

Reagent. The diluent is detergent-modified Drabkin's reagent:

Potassium ferricyanide, $K_3Fe(CN)_6$	0.200 g
Potassium cyanide, KCN	0.050 g
Dihydrogen potassium phosphate (anhydrous) KH_2PO_4	0.140 g
Non-ionic detergent, e.g.,	
Sterox S.E. (Harleco)	0.5 ml
or Triton X-100 (Rohm and Haas)	1.0 ml
Distilled water to	1000 ml

The solution should be clear and pale yellow, have a pH of 7.0 to 7.4, and give a reading of zero when measured in the photometer at 540 nm against a water blank.

Substituting dihydrogen potassium phosphate, KH_2PO_4, in this reagent for sodium bicarbonate, $NaHCO_3$, in the original Drabkin's reagent shortens the time needed for complete conversion of Hb to HiCN from 10 minutes to 3 minutes. The detergent enhances lysis of erythrocytes and decreases turbidity from protein precipitation.

Care must be taken with KCN in the preparation of the Drabkin's solution, as salts or solutions of cyanide are poisonous. The diluent itself contains only 50 mg KCN per liter, less than the lethal dose for a 70 kg person. However, since HCN is released by acidification, exposure of the diluent to acid must be avoided. Disposal of reagents and samples in running water in the sink is advised. The diluent keeps well in a dark bottle at room temperature, but should be prepared fresh once a month.

Method (Dacie, 1975). Twenty μl of blood is added to 5.0 ml of diluent (1:251), well mixed, and allowed to stand at room temperature for at least 3 minutes. The absorbance is measured, against the reagent blank, in the photoelectric colorimeter at 540 nm or with an appropriate filter. A vial of HiCN standard* is then opened and the absorbance measured, at room temperature, in the same instrument in a similar fashion. The test sample must be analyzed within a few hours of dilution. The standard must be kept in the dark when not in use and discarded at the end of the day.

$$\text{Hb (g/dl)} = \frac{A^{540}\ \text{test sample}}{A^{540}\ \text{standard}} \times \frac{\text{concentration of standard (mg/dl)}}{100\ \text{mg/g}} \times 251$$

It is usually convenient to calibrate the photometer to be used for hemoglobinometry by preparing a standard curve or table which will relate absorbance to Hb concentration in g/dl.

The absorbance of fresh HiCN standard is measured against a reagent blank.

Absorbance readings are made of fresh HiCN standard and of dilutions of this standard in the reagent (1 in 2, 1 in 3, 1 in 4) against a reagent blank. Hb values in g/dl are calculated for each solution as above. When the absorbance readings are plotted on linear graph paper as the ordinates against Hb concentration as the abscissae, the points should describe a straight line which passes through the origin. From this standard curve a table may be prepared giving Hb concentrations for absorbance readings.

*Certified by the College of American Pathologists.

Advantages of the HiCN method are that most forms of hemoglobin (Hb, HbO_2, Hi, and HbCO, but not SHb) are measured. The test sample can be directly compared with the HiCN standard, and the readings can be made at the convenience of the operator because of the stability of the diluted samples.

Increased absorbance not due to hemoglobin may be caused by turbidity due to abnormal plasma proteins, hyperlipemia, large numbers of leukocytes (counts greater than 30 × 10^9/L), or fatty droplets, any of which may lead to increased light scattering and apparent absorbance.

Oxyhemoglobin (HbO_2) Method. No longer widely used but still a satisfactory method is the determination of hemoglobin as oxyhemoglobin. The main disadvantage is the lack of a stable standard for HbO_2. Because of the method's simplicity, it is often used to compare levels of hemoglobin when the absolute quantity is not needed, as in the osmotic fragility or the HbA_2 determinations. The HbO_2 method does not measure carboxyhemoglobin (HbCO), methemoglobin (Hi), or sulfhemoglobin (SHb), all of which are inactive in transporting oxygen.

A 1:251 dilution of blood is made in 0.007 N NH_4OH. The water used in the preparation of the ammonia solution must be glass distilled, because minute amounts of copper in distilled water or other diluents employed in HbO_2 determinations may cause HbO_2 to be converted to Hi and lower the values. Shaking ensures mixing and oxygenation of hemoglobin. The solution is read in a photometer with a green filter (540 nm), and a 0.007 N ammonium hydroxide solution is used as blank. The test can be read within a few seconds or with a stoppered cuvette any time up to three days. The standard curve can be set up with one of the procedures to be listed later.

Chemical Method (Iron Content). Hemoglobin may be measured by determining the iron content of whole blood. The non-hemoglobin iron in blood is negligible compared to hemoglobin iron. Iron must first be separated from hemoglobin, usually by acid or by ashing. It is then either titrated with $TiCl_3$ or complexed with a reagent to develop color that can be measured photometrically. Satisfactory methods are described by van Assendelft (1970) and by Henry (1964).

Based on the molecular structure, the iron content of hemoglobin is 0.347 per cent (ICSH, 1978). The concentration of hemoglobin in blood (g/dl) is calculated by dividing the iron concentration (mg/dl) by 3.47. Determination of the concentration of hemoglobin by measurement of iron content is too complex for routine work, but it can be used for checking other methods, and from it one can construct calibration curves for both the HbO_2 method and the HiCN method. It is used for standardization in hemoglobinometry if desired or if certified cyanmethemoglobin standards are not available. The iron method, of course, measures total hemoglobin; the HbO_2 method measures only Hb and HbO_2; and the HiCN method measures Hb, HbO_2, Hi, and HbCO.

Errors in Hemoglobinometry. The sources of error may be those of the sample, the method, the equipment, or the operator. Some of these have been discussed under the descriptions of the different methods.

Errors Inherent in the Sample. Improper venipuncture technique may introduce hemoconcentration, which will make hemoglobin concentration and cell counts too high. Improper technique in fingerstick or capillary sampling can produce errors in either direction.

Errors Inherent in the Method. The oxyhemoglobin method measures Hb and HbO_2, but not Hi, HbCO, or SHb. It is therefore the method that most closely determines physiologically active hemoglobin. This may be important to recognize in some patients.

The HiCN method is the method of choice. The use of HiCN standard for calibration of the instrument and for the test itself eliminates one major source of error and provides comparability among all laboratories employing it. The broad absorption band of HiCN in the region of 540 nm makes it convenient to use it both in filter-type photometers and in narrow-band spectrophotometers. With the exception of SHb, all other varieties of hemoglobin are converted to HiCN.

Errors Inherent in the Equipment. The accuracy of equipment is not uniform. A good grade of pipette with a guaranteed accuracy of less than 1 per cent is desirable. Calibration of pipettes will lessen errors inherent in the use of reusable glass pipettes. Significant error will be introduced by the use of unmatched cuvettes. Flow-through cuvettes are preferred because they eliminate the error present even in the use of matched cuvettes.

The photometer must be calibrated in the laboratory before its initial use and must be rechecked frequently. The wavelength settings, the filters, and the meter readings require checking.

When used with a properly standardized and regularly checked photometer, the HiCN method's error can be reduced to ± 2 per cent (expressed as $\pm$C.V.).

Operator's Errors. Human errors can be reduced by good training, understanding the clinical significance of the test and the necessity for a dependable method, adherence to oral and written instructions, and familiarity with the equipment and with the sources of error. The technologist should be familiar with the performance of the instrument, and able to identify its misbehavior. Errors increase with fatigue and tend to be greater near the end of the day than at the beginning. The technologist who is patient and critical by nature and by training and who is interested in the work will be less prone to make errors than others.

The above discussion applies to manual techniques of hemoglobinometry. Semiautomated and automated equipment is widely used and eliminates components of the error in individual pipettes and cuvettes and much of the human error.

HEMOGLOBIN DERIVATIVES

The two physiologic hemoglobins, the oxyhemoglobin and the reduced hemoglobin, are readily converted into a series of compounds through the action of acids, alkalies, oxidizing and reducing substances, heat, and other agents. Their gross presence can be distinguished with the spectroscope. For small concentrations (less than 10 per cent) and for quantitative measurements, spectrophotometric, colorimetric, and gasometric methods have to be used.

Hemiglobin (Methemoglobin; Hi). Hi is a derivative of hemoglobin in which the ferrous iron is *oxidized* to the ferric state. The polypeptide chains are not altered.

Hi is unable to combine reversibly with oxygen. Although oxygen affinity increases within the Hb tetramer if only partial oxidation of the heme occurs, the oxygen-hemoglobin dissociation curve does not usually shift to the left; this is probably because of the interaction of remaining ferrous hemes with 2,3-diphosphoglycerate tending to shift the curve to the right (Schwartz, 1978).

Up to 1.5 per cent of the hemoglobin is Hi in the normal individual. Increases of Hi will cause cyanosis and functional "anemia" if high enough, and cyanosis at lower concentrations. Cyanosis becomes obvious at a concentration of about 1.5 g Hi/dl, i.e., 10 per cent of hemoglobin. Comparable degrees of cyanosis will be caused by 5 g Hb/dl blood, 1.5 g Hi/dl blood, and 0.5 g SHb/dl blood. The degree of cyanosis, however, is not necessarily correlated with the concentration of Hi.

A small amount of Hi is always being formed but is reduced by enzyme systems within the erythrocyte. At least four pathways exist by which methemoglobin may be reduced to hemoglobin (Schwartz, 1978). The most important is the NAD-methemoglobin reductase system. Others, which may function mainly as reserve systems, are ascorbic acid, reduced glutathione, and NADP-methemoglobin reductase. The latter requires a natural cofactor or an auto-oxidizable dye such as methylene blue for activity (Fig. 29–15).

Methemoglobinemia, an increased amount of Hi in the erythrocytes, results from either an increased production of Hi or a decreased NAD-reductase activity, and may be hereditary or acquired. The hereditary form is divided into two major categories. In the first, methemoglobinemia is due to a decrease in the capacity of the erythrocyte to reduce the Hi that is constantly being formed back to Hb. This is most often due to *NAD-methemoglobin reductase deficiency,* which is inherited as an autosomal recessive characteristic. The homozygote has methemoglobin levels of 10 to 50 per cent and is cyanotic. Only occasionally is polycythemia present as a compensating mechanism. Hemiglobin concentrations of 10 to 25 per cent may give no apparent symptoms; levels of 35 to 50 per cent result in mild symptoms, such as exertional dyspnea and headaches; and levels exceeding 70 per cent are probably lethal. Therapy with ascorbic acid or methylene blue in this form of hereditary methemoglobinemia will reduce the level of Hi, the latter apparently by activation of the NAP-methemoglobin reductase system. Heterozygotes have intermediate levels of NAD-methemoglobin reductase activity and normal blood levels of Hi. They may become cyanotic because of methemoglobinemia after exposure to oxidizing chemicals or drugs in amounts that will not affect normal individuals.

In the second major category of hereditary methemoglobinemia, the reducing systems within the erythrocyte are intact, but the structure of the hemoglobin molecule itself is abnormal. A genetically determined alteration in the amino acid composition of either alpha or beta globin chains may form a hemoglobin

4

molecule that has an enhanced tendency toward oxidation and a decreased suspceptibility of the methemoglobin formed to reduction back to hemoglobin. Five abnormal hemoglobins have been identified whose principal consequence is asymptomatic cyanosis due to methemoglobinemia; they are designed as various forms of *hemoglobin M (HbM).* They are inherited as autosomal dominants (Bunn, 1977). Methylene blue therapy in these individuals is without effect.

Most cases of methemoglobinemia are classified as secondary or acquired methemoglobinemia. They are due mainly to poisoning with drugs and chemicals that cause increased formation of hemiglobin (Wintrobe, 1974). Chemicals or drugs that directly oxidase HbO_2 to Hi include nitrites, nitrates, chlorates, and quinones. Other substances, which are aromatic amino and nitro compounds, probably act indirectly through a metabolite, since they do not cause Hi formation *in vitro.* These include acetanilid, phenacetin, sulfonamides, and aniline dyes. Ferrous sulfate may produce methemoglobinemia after ingestion of very large doses. Levels of drugs or chemicals that would not cause significant methemoglobinemia in a normal individual may do so in someone with a mild reduction in NAD-reductase activity who, under ordinary circumstances, is not cyanotic. Such individuals are newborn infants and persons heterozygous for NAD-reductase deficiency (Cohen, 1968).

Hemiglobin is reduced back to Hb by the erythrocyte enzyme systems. It can also be reduced (slowly) by the administration of reducing agents, such as ascorbic acid or sulfhydryl compounds (glutathione, cysteine, BAL); these, as well as methylene blue, are of value in cases of hereditary NAD-methemoglobin reductase deficiency. In cases of acquired or toxic methemoglobinemia, methylene blue is of great value; its rapid action is not based on its own reduction capacity but on its acceleration of the normally slow NADP-methemoglobin reductase pathway.

Hemiglobin can combine reversibly with various chemicals (e.g., cyanides, sulfides, peroxides, fluorides, and azides). Because of the strong affinity of Hi for cyanide, the therapy of cyanide poisoning is to administer nitrites to form Hi, which then combines with the cyanide. Thus, the free cyanide (which is extremely poisonous to the cellular respiratory enzymes) becomes less toxic when changed to HiCN.

Hemiglobin and sulfhemoglobin are quantitated by spectrophotometry (Tietz, 1976). If Hi is elevated, drugs or toxic substances must first be eliminated as a cause. Congenital methemoglobinemia due to NADH-methemoglobin reductase deficiency is determined by assay of the enzyme (Hegesh, 1968). An abnormal hemoglobin (HbM; p. 681) may also be responsible for methemoglobinemia noted at birth or in the first few months of life.

Sulfhemoglobin. *In vitro* and in the presence of oxygen, hemoglobin reacts with hydrogen sulfide to form a greenish derivative of hemoglobin called sulfhemoglobin. Since oxygen is necessary for the formation, it is assumed that oxyhemoglobin reacts directly with the H_2S. The role of sulfur or compounds containing sulfur in the *in vivo* production of sulfhemoglobin is unclear. Sulfhemoglobin implies an irreversible change in the polypeptide chains of the molecule. It may form in response to an oxidant stress; further change can result in denaturation and precipitation of hemoglobin as Heinz bodies (Fig. 27–2).

Sulfhemoglobin cannot transport oxygen, but it can combine with CO to form carboxysulfhemoglobin. Unlike methemoglobin, sulfhemoglobin cannot be reduced back to hemoglobin, and it remains in the cells until they break down (see pages 510 and 511 of 16th edition).

Sulfhemoglobin has been reported in patients receiving treatment with sulfonamides, aromatic amine drugs (phenacetin, acetanilid), as well as in patients with severe constipation, and in cases of bacteremia due to *Clostridium welchii,* and in a condition known as enterogenous cyanosis. The concentration of sulfhemoglobin *in vivo* normally is less than 1 per cent, and in these conditions seldom exceeds 10 per cent of the total hemoglobin. It results in cyanosis and is usually asymptomatic. The reason some patients develop methemoglobinemia, some sulfhemoglobinemia, and others Heinz bodies and hemolysis is not well understood.

Carboxyhemoglobin, HbCO. Endogenous carbon monoxide (CO) produced in the degradation of heme to bilirubin normally accounts for about 0.5 per cent carboxyhemoglobin in the blood, and is increased in hemolytic anemia. Hemoglobin has the capacity to combine with carbon monoxide in the same proportion as with oxygen, but the affinity of the hemoglobin molecule for carbon monoxide is 210 times greater. This means that carbon monoxide will bind with hemoglobin even if its concentration in the air is extremely low (e.g., 0.02 to 0.04 per cent). In those cases, HbCO will build up until typical symptoms of poisoning appear (Goldsmith, 1968).

HbCO cannot bind oxygen and therefore is not an oxygen carrier. Furthermore, increasing concentrations of HbCO shift the Hb–oxygen dissociation curve increasingly to the left, thus adding to the anoxia. If a patient poisoned with carbon monoxide receives pure oxygen, the conversion of HbCO to HbO_2 is greatly enhanced. HbCO is light sensitive and has a typical, brilliant, cherry red color.

Acute carbon monoxide poisoning is well known. Chronic poisoning, due to prolonged exposure to small amounts of carbon monoxide, is less well recognized but is of increasing importance. The chief sources of

$$\text{Hb} \underset{\text{tissues}}{\overset{\text{lungs}}{\rightleftharpoons}} \text{HbO}_2 \underset{\text{NAD-reductase}}{\overset{\text{Oxidation}}{\rightleftharpoons}} \text{Hi} \longrightarrow \text{SHb} \longrightarrow \begin{array}{c}\text{Denatured}\\ \text{hemoglobin}\\ \text{(Heinz bodies)}\end{array}$$

Figure 27–2. Simplified concept of oxidation of hemoglobin (Hb) as proposed by Jandl (1960). Reversible binding and release of oxygen occurs in lungs and tissues; oxidation of ferrous ions and formation of hemiglobin is reversible in the red cell to a limited extent; continued oxidation leads to irreversible conformational changes and sulfhemoglobin; still further oxidation results in denaturation of the hemoglobin and precipitation within the erythrocyte as Heinz bodies.

the gas are gasoline motors, illuminating gas, gas heaters, defective stoves, and the smoking of tobacco. Exposure to carbon monoxide is thus one of the hazards of modern civilization. The gas has even been found in the air of busy streets of large cities in sufficient concentration to cause mild symptoms in persons such as traffic policemen who are exposed to it over long periods of time. The chronic exposure to CO through tobacco smoking may lead to chronic elevation of HbCO and an associated left shift in the oxygen dissociation curve; smokers tend to have higher hematocrits than non-smokers and may have polycythemia (Smith, 1978).

Healthy persons exposed to various concentrations of the gas for an hour do not experience definite symptoms (headache, dizziness, muscular weakness, and nausea) unless the concentration of the gas in the blood reaches 20 to 30 per cent of saturation; however, it appears that in chronic poisoning, especially in children, serious symptoms may occur with lower concentrations.

HbCO may be quantitated by differential spectrophotometry or by gas chromatography (Dubowski, 1973).

Tests for Hemoglobin Derivatives. Some information can be obtained by naked eye examination of the blood specimen. Normal appearance of the serum or plasma identifies the red cells as the site of the pigment. Shaking of normal whole blood in the air for 15 minutes imparts to it a bright red color as the Hb is converted to HbO_2. The blood is cherry red when the pigment is HbCO in carbon monoxide poisoning. The color is chocolate brown in methemoglobinemia and mauve-lavender in sulfhemoglobinemia.

Spectrophotometric Identification of Hemoglobins. The various hemoglobins have characteristic absorption spectra, which can be determined easily with a spectrophotometer. The useful absorbance maxima are given in Table 27–2. The maxima for Hi vary considerably with pH. The maxima given in the two right hand columns are useful for distinguishing among these forms of hemoglobin. The absorbance between 405 and 435 nm (the Soret band) is considerably greater and may be used when small concentrations of hemoglobin are to be measured.

The identification of different forms of hemoglobins by determining absorption spectra can be carried out in a very simple way. Approximately one half of a drop of blood is put into a test tube and diluted with approximately 20 ml of de-ionized or double-distilled water. The actual dilution of the hemoglobin depends on the concentration of the hemoglobin. For maximal accuracy, the peak of absorption should be somewhere between 60 and 40 per cent transmittance. After the blood has been diluted with water, samples are read in a spectrophotometer with water as the blank. A recording spectrophotometer is especially convenient for this determination. Otherwise, the absorption is read at intervals of 5 nm (see Fig. 27–1).

Table 27–2. ABSORPTION MAXIMA OF HEMOGLOBINS

	λ	ε	λ	ε	λ	ε
Hb	431	(140)	555	(13.04)		
HbO_2	415	(131)	542	(14.37)	577	(15.37)
HbCO	420	(192)	539	(14.36)	568.5	(14.31)
Hi (pH 7 to 7.4)	406	(162)	500	(9.04)	630	(3.70)
HiCN	421	(122.5)	540	(10.99)		

The wavelength (λ) in nanometers for each maximum is followed by the extinction coefficient (ε) placed in parentheses.

Data are from van Assendelft (1970).

HEMATOCRIT (PACKED CELL VOLUME)

Definition. The hematocrit of a sample of blood is the ratio of the volume of erythrocytes to that of the whole blood. It is expressed as a percentage or, preferably, as a decimal fraction. The units (L/L) are implied. The venous hematocrit agrees closely with the hematocrit obtained from a skin puncture; both are greater than the total body hematocrit. Dried heparin, balanced oxalate, or EDTA is satisfactory as an anticoagulant. The hematocrit may be measured directly by centrifugation with macromethods or micromethods, or indirectly as the product of the MCV × red cell count in automated instruments (q.v.).

Macromethod of Wintrobe

Equipment. The Wintrobe hematocrit tube is a thick-walled glass tube with a uniform internal bore and a flattened bottom. It is graduated in millimeters from 0 to 105 and has a rubber cap to prevent evaporation during the long period of centrifugation. A disposable capillary (Pasteur) pipette with a rubber bulb is used to fill the tube.

The essential requirement of a centrifuge is that it generate a centrifugal field of not less than 2500 g at the bottom of the cup.

Procedure. After adequate mixing of the sample to ensure even distribution and oxygenation of red cells, the hematocrit tube is filled. The tip of the pipette is introduced to the bottom of the tube. As filling proceeds, the tip of the pipette is raised, but it remains under the rising blood meniscus in order to avoid foaming. The level of the blood should be noted and the tubes capped to avoid evaporation during the required centrifugation for 30 minutes at 2500 g.

Reading is done without distributing the specimen. The result is calculated from the formula:

$$\text{Hematocrit} = \frac{L_1}{L_2}$$

where L_1 is the height of the red cell column in mm and L_2 is the height of the whole blood specimen (red cells and plasma). The gray-white layer of leukocytes and platelets above the erythrocytes is not included in L_1.

Micromethod

Equipment. A capillary hematocrit tube about 7 cm long with a uniform bore of about 1 mm is recommended. For blood collection directly from a skin puncture, capillaries are filled with a 1 to 1000 dilution of heparin, dried at 56 or 37°C., and stored. Special centrifuges are available, producing centrifugal fields ranging from 10,000 to 13,000 g. This permits shortening of centrifugation to 5 minutes.

Procedure. The microhematocrit (capillary) tube is filled by capillary attraction, either from a free-flowing puncture wound or a well-mixed venous sample. The capillary tube should be filled to at least 5 cm. The empty end is sealed with modeling clay. The filled tube is placed in the radial grooves of the microhematocrit centrifuge head with the sealed end away from the center.

Place the bottom of the tube against the rubber gasket

4

to prevent breakage. Centrifugation for five minutes at 10,000 to 12,000 g is satisfactory unless the hematocrit exceeds 50 per cent; in this case an additional five minutes' centrifugation should be employed in order to ensure that plasma trapping has been minimized.

The capillary tubes are not graduated. The length of the whole column, including the plasma, and of the red cell column alone must be measured in each case with a millimeter rule and a magnifying lens or with one of several commercially available measuring devices. The instructions of the manufacturer must be followed.

Interpretation of Results. The normal hematocrit for adult males is 0.40 to 0.54, for females 0.37 to 0.47. A value below an individual's normal or below the reference interval for age and sex indicates anemia, and a higher value, polycythemia. The hematocrit reflects the concentration of red cells, not the total red cell mass. The hematocrit is low in hydremia of pregnancy, but the total number of circulating red cells is not reduced. The hematocrit may be normal or even high in shock accompanied by hemoconcentration, though the total red cell mass may be considerably decreased owing to blood loss. The hematocrit is unreliable as an estimate of anemia immediately after a loss of blood, even if moderate, and immediately following transfusions.

Sources of Error

Centrifugation. Adequate duration and speed of centrifugation are essential for a correct hematocrit. The red cells must be packed so that additional centrifugation does not further reduce the packed cell volume. In general, the higher the hematocrit, the greater the centrifugal force required.

In the course of centrifugation, a small proportion of the leukocytes, platelets, and plasma are trapped between the red cells. The error resulting from the former is, as a rule, quite insignificant. The increment of the hematocrit due to trapped plasma is somewhat greater than that due to leukocytes and platelets. The lower the relative centrifugal force, the larger the amount of trapped plasma; therefore, the amount of trapped plasma is larger in high hematocrits than in low hematocrits, and is larger with the macromethod than the micromethod. With the micromethod, trapped plasma accounts for about 1 to 3 per cent of the red cell column in normal blood (about 0.014 in a hematocrit of 0.47), slightly more in macrocytic anemias, spherocytosis, and hypochromic anemias (England, 1972). Even greater amounts of trapped plasma occur in the hematocrits of patients with sickle cell anemia and vary depending upon the degree of sickling and consequent rigidity of the cells. Because less time is necessary for centrifugation, and because there is less error due to trapping of plasma, the micromethod is preferred over the macromethod. In using the microhematocrit as a reference method for calibrating automated instruments, correction for trapped plasma is recommended (ICSH, 1980).

Sample. Posture, muscular activity, and prolonged tourniquet-stasis can cause the same order of changes in hematocrit and cell concentrations as it does for non-filterable soluble constituents (Chapter 1, p. 7; Chapter 28, p. 621). Unique to the hematocrit is the error due to excess EDTA (inadequate blood for a fixed amount of EDTA): the hematocrit will be falsely low due to cell shrinkage, but the hemoglobin and cell counts will not be affected (Lampasso, 1965). The hematocrit of deoxygenated blood is about 2 per cent lower than fully oxygenated blood (Dacie, 1975).

Other Errors. Technical errors include failure to mix the blood adequately before sampling, improper reading of the level of cells and plasma, and inclusion of the buffy coat as part of the erythrocyte volume. Irregularity of the inside diameter of the tubes will also lead to inaccurate hematocrits.

With good technique the precision of the hematocrit, expressed as ± 2 C.V. (coefficient of variation), is ± 1 per cent. With low hematocrit values, the C.V. is greater, especially with the microhematocrit method, owing to reading error.

Macroscopic Examination. When the hematocrit is performed by centrifugation, inspection of the specimen after spinning may furnish valuable information. The relative heights of the red cell column, buffy coat, and plasma column should be noted.

The buffy coat is the red-gray layer between the red cells and plasma; it includes platelets and leukocytes. A buffy coat of 1 per cent of the total volume in the tube indicates a leukocyte count in the range of 10×10^9/L. If the leukocyte count is over 12×10^9/L, a buffy coat of 1 per cent of the total volume represents a leukocyte count closer to 20×10^9/L because of greater packing (Wintrobe, 1974). The size of the cells will alter the estimate if they are much different from normal. These estimates apply best to the macrohematocrit; in the microhematocrit they underestimate the leukocyte count because of the greater packing. The estimates give only a crude idea of the count, but they are sometimes useful.

An orange or green color of the plasma suggests increased bilirubin, and pink or red suggests hemoglobinemia. It should be kept in mind that poor technique in collecting the blood specimen is the most frequent cause of hemolysis. If the specimens are not obtained within an hour or two after a fat-rich meal, cloudy plasma may point to nephrosis or certain abnormal hyperglobulinemias, especially cryoglobulinemia.

BLOOD CELL COUNTING

Counts of erythrocytes, leukocytes, and platelets are each expressed as concentrations—cells per unit volume of blood. The unit of volume for cell counts originally was expressed as cubic millimeters (mm^3) because of the linear dimensions of the hemacytometer (cell counting) chamber. The International Committee for Standardization in Hematology recommends that the unit of volume be the liter. Since $1\ mm^3 = 1.00003\ \mu l$, the preferred mode of expressing blood cell counts for the examples below is on the right:

Erythrocytes

$$5.00 \times 10^6/mm^3 = 5.00 \times 10^6/\mu l = 5.00 \times 10^{12}/L$$

Leukocytes

$$7.0 \times 10^3/mm^3 = 7.0 \times 10^3/\mu l = 7.0 \times 10^9/L$$

Platelets

$$300 \times 10^3/mm^3 = 300 \times 10^3/\mu l = 300 \times 10^9/L$$

Except for platelet counts and low leukocyte counts, the hemacytometer is no longer used for routine blood cell counting in any but the smallest of laboratories. Yet it is still necessary for the technologist to be able to use this method effectively and to know its limitations.

Any cell counting procedure includes three steps: dilution of the blood, sampling the diluted suspension into a measured volume, and counting the cells in that volume.

Erythrocyte Counts

DILUTORS

The method for diluting the blood for hemoglobin or for cell counts can be performed more rapidly and accurately semiautomatically than manually.

Semiautomated Methods. Several instruments are available for precise and convenient diluting, which both aspirate the sample and wash it out with the diluent. In some instruments the volumes are adjustable; in others, one or both volumes are fixed. In either case the dilutor should perform a 1:250 or 1:500 dilution with a coefficient of variation of less than 1 per cent.

A semiautomatic dilutor, the Hem-Aliquanter (Bull, 1968), dispenses the diluent and the sample separately. The sample is dispensed simultaneously for several tests with errors of less than 1 per cent. This dilutor should be considered for the laboratory without a multichannel instrument.

Manual. For capillary sampling, manual methods are still necessary. Accurate disposable pipettes are available, some similar to the classic Sahli pipette. More convenient and reliable are microcapillary pipettes that fill by capillarity and cannot overfill;* when added to the diluent in an appropriate-sized test tube they empty satisfactorily, with sufficient washout of sample by diluent. These pipettes are available with an accuracy of ±0.25 per cent, which is suitable for calibration. Less expensive pipettes with an accuracy of ± 1 per cent are usually used for routine work.

Combining a microcapillary tube with a plastic vial containing a premeasured volume of diluent, the Unopette† is a valuable system for manual dilutions. After the capillary is filled, it is pushed into the container and the sample is washed out by squeezing the soft plastic vial. This system is especially convenient for micro-sampling. Unopettes are available with diluents for counts of red cells, white cells, platelets, eosinophils, and reticulocytes, and for hemoglobin concentrations and osmotic fragility determinations.

ELECTRONIC COUNTING METHODS
(Brittin and Brecher, 1971; Ackerman, 1972)

Electrical Impedance. Cells passing through an aperture through which a current is flowing cause changes in electrical resistance which are counted as voltage pulses. This principle, used in the Coulter Counter,‡ the Celloscope,§ and Sysmex,|| is illustrated in Figure 27–3. An accurately diluted suspension of blood (CS) is made in an isotonic conductive solution (such as Isoton‡) which preserves the cell shape. The instrument has a glass cylinder (GC) that can be filled with the conducting fluid and has within it an electrode (E_2) and an aperture (A) of 100 μm diameter in its wall. Just outside the glass cylinder is another electrode (E_1). The cylinder is connected to a U-shaped glass tube which is partly filled with mercury (M) and which has two electrical contacts (EC_1 and EC_2). The glass cylinder is immersed in the suspension of cells to be counted (CS) and is filled with conductive solution and closed by a valve (V). A current now flows through the aperture between E_1 and E_2. As mercury moves up the tube, the cell suspension is drawn through the aperture into the cylinder. Each cell that passes through the aperture displaces an equal volume of conductive fluid, increasing the electrical resistance and creating a voltage pulse, because its resistance is much greater than that of the conductive solution. The pulses, which are proportional in height to the volume of the cells, are counted.

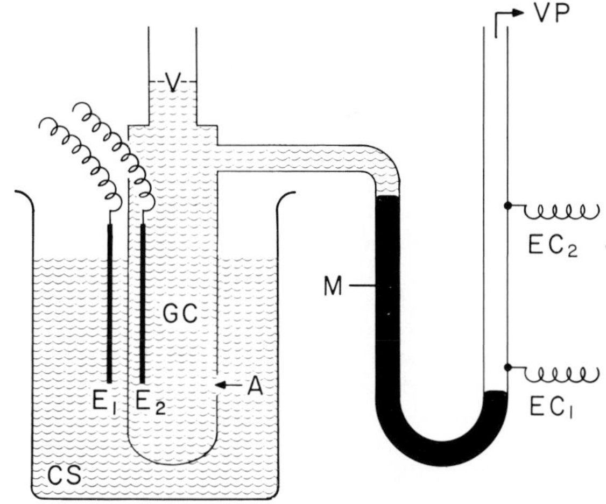

Figure 27–3. Schematic diagram of particle counter in which changes in electrical resistance are counted as voltage pulses. CS = cell suspension, GC = glass cylinder, A = aperture, E_1 and E_2 = platinum electrodes, V = valve, M = mercury column, EC_1 and EC_2 = electrical contacts, VP = vacuum pump. (Diagram adapted from Ackermann, 1972.)

In the simplest system, the counting mechanism is started when the mercury contacts EC_1 and stopped when it contacts EC_2; during this time the cells are counted in a volume of suspension exactly equal to the volume of the glass tubing between contact wires EC_1 and EC_2.

If two or more cells enter the aperture simultaneously, they will be counted as one pulse; this produces a coincidence error for which a correction must be made. The size of the coincidence error can be diminished by decreasing the concentration of cells and decreasing the size of the aperture. However, decreasing the cell concentration increases the effect of errors in dilution, increases the inherent counting error, and makes more critical the error due to the background "noise" of contaminating particles. With decreased aperture size, partial or complete plugging of the aperture with debris becomes a problem. Therefore, a balance is struck, and for a given count above a critical number, a coincidence correction is made by referring to a chart supplied by the manufacturer.

A threshold setting or pulse discriminator allows the exclusion of pulses below fixed heights for red cell

4

*Drummond Hemocaps, Drummond Scientific Company, Broomall, Pa.

†Becton-Dickinson, Rutherford, N.J.

‡Coulter Diagnostics, Hialeah, Fla.

§Lars Ljungberg & Co., Stockholm, Sweden.

||TOA Medical Electronics Co. (USA), Carson, Cal.

and white cell counts on the Coulter Counter Model D, and below an adjustable height on the Models ZF, Fn, and ZBI. On the Model ZBI, a second threshold also excludes the counting of pulses *above* a certain height. One therefore counts only the cells in the "window" between the two settings. Systematically changing each threshold by given increments, one can determine a frequency distribution of relative cell volumes. Such cell size distributions can be automatically plotted by attachments available for the Coulter Counter Model ZBI (Channelyzer) and Model S-Plus series and may be valuable in the study of red cells, white cells, or platelets when two or more changing populations of cells are present.

Instruments that handle the data from the changes in electrical resistance digitally (e.g., the Coulter Counter) are stable and infrequently require calibration. Therefore, properly maintained, they can be relied upon as primary reference machines to give a correct red cell count if the specimens are properly mixed and diluted (Brittin, 1971; Bull, 1971).

Before counting, the adjustment of the threshold is checked by counting the diluted suspension of red cells at successively increasing increments. To ensure that smaller particles (background "noise") are excluded from the count, the adjustment should be in the middle of the plateau. Larger foreign particles in the diluent are quantitated in a background or blank count which may be subtracted from the cell count. However, if the blank count is too high, the accuracy of the cell count will be impaired. The final cell dilution should allow a particle count of at least 5000, which should be at least 20 times the blank count. Specific directions for operation of the instruments are given by the manufacturer.

In the Coulter Counter, the dilution for the red cell count is 1:50,000, usually made in two steps: first, 20 μl of blood in 10 ml (1:500), followed by 100 μl of the first dilution in 10 ml of diluent (1:100). Since 0.5 ml of the cell suspension is counted, 50,000 cells (after correction for coincidence) will be counted for a normal red cell count of 5×10^{12}/L.

For a normal red cell count, therefore, the Poisson error will be about 0.5 per cent $\left(C.V. = \frac{\sqrt{n}}{n}\right)$ and for a very low count, closer to 1 per cent. The actual precision of red cell counting is about twice this, or 1 to 2 per cent (C.V.), and errors of dilution bring the precision achieved in practice to 2 to 4 per cent (Brittin, 1971).

The Celloscope 401 operates on the same principle as the Coulter Counter, but deals with the problem of coincidence in a different way. Instead of counting all the pulses and correcting for coincidence, the Celloscope 401 counts every 64th pulse and no coincidence correction is necessary. The precision of red cell counting is comparable to that of the Coulter Counter; Lappin (1972) found the mean coefficient of variation to be 1.2 per cent.

Light-Scattering. In electro-optical counters (Fig. 27–4) a photomultiplier tube detects light scattering either from external reflections from the surface of cells, from transmitted and refracted light passing through the cells, or from diffracted light which has passed tangential to cell surfaces (Mansberg, 1970). In the Technicon cell counter, the intensity of the diffraction events provides the highest signal-to-noise ratio (about 100:1) in the small scattering angle that is necessary for adequate depth of focus. Because of a uniform pulse amplitude, the high signal-to-noise ratio, and the forward-angle scattering character of the system, there is a broad threshold curve that is the same for leukocytes and erythrocytes. A small sensing volume (44×10^3 fl) is defined by illumination in the flow cell and allows a lesser dilution (1:10,000) than the voltage pulse counter, resulting in minimal coincidence. The characteristics described yield an accuracy and precision in cell counting that is limited only by the qualities of the pumping system.

The Technicon cell counter consists basically of the following modules: sampler, proportioning pump with manifolds having plastic tubing, glass helical mixing and phasing coils, a cell counter, and a single pen recorder. Anticoagulated blood in a tube or sample cup is mixed by two paddles (one minute each) before being sampled during a third minute. (The capacity is 90 samples/hour.) The continuous flow system incorporates dilution with diluent and mixing before the diluted cell suspension reaches the flow cell for counting. The output of the photomultiplier tube is recorded by the pen on moving preprinted paper. The instrument must be calibrated with a known blood or particle suspension at the beginning of each series of counts; since this takes a relatively large volume of known or reference standard blood, it is not practical to run small numbers of samples.

The Technicon red cell counter is now almost always

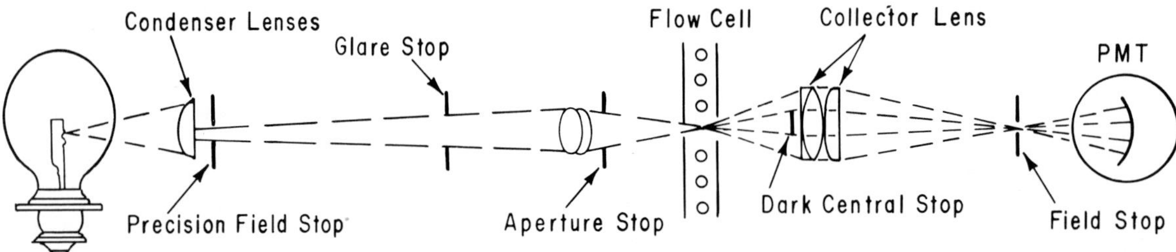

Figure 27–4. Schematic diagram of the electron-optical cell counter. Light is focused on the flow cell. Only light scattered by a cell reaches the photomultiplier tube (PMT), which converts it to an electrical pulse. (From Mansberg, H. P.: Advanc. Automated Anal. *1*:213, 1970.)

used as part of a multichannel instrument, the Hemalog 8/90 or, more recently, the H-6000. The coefficient of variation of the red cell count on these instruments is between 1 and 1.5 per cent (Thom, 1977).

Erythrocyte Indices

Wintrobe introduced calculations for determining the size, content, and Hb concentration of red cells; these erythrocyte indices have been useful in the morphologic characterization of anemias. They may be calculated from the red cell count, hemoglobin concentration, and hematocrit.

Mean Cell Volume (MCV). The MCV is the average volume of red cells and is calculated from the hematocrit (Hct; packed cell volume) and the red cell count (RBC). MCV = Hct × 1000/RBC (in millions per μl), expressed in femtoliters or cubic micrometers. If the hematocrit = 0.45 and the red cell count = 5×10^{12}/L, 1 L will contain 5×10^{12} red cells, which occupy a volume of 0.45 L. The MCV = $\frac{0.45 \text{ L}}{5 \times 10^{12}} = 90 \times 10^{-15}$ L (fl). One femtoliter (fl) = 10^{-15} L = 1 cubic micrometer (μm^3).

Mean Cell Hemoglobin (MCH). The MCH is the content (weight) of Hb of the average red cell; it is calculated from the Hb concentration and the red cell count.

$$\text{MCH} = \frac{\text{Hb (in g per liter)}}{\text{RBC (in millions per } \mu\text{l)}}$$

expressed in picograms. If the Hb = 15 g/dl and the red cell count is 5×10^{12}/L, 1 L contains 150 g of Hb distributed in 5×10^{12} cells.

$$\text{MCH} = \frac{150 \text{ g}}{5 \times 10^{12}} = 30 \times 10^{-12} \text{ g (pg)}$$

$$\text{One picogram (pg)} = 10^{-12} \text{ g} = 1 \text{ micromicrogram } (\mu\mu\text{g})$$

Mean Cell Hemoglobin Concentration (MCHC). The MCHC is the average concentration of Hb in a given volume of packed red cells. It is calculated from the Hb concentration and the hematocrit.

$$\text{MCHC} = \frac{\text{Hb (in g/dl)}}{\text{Hct}}, \text{ expressed in g/dl}$$

If the Hb = 15 g/dl and the Hct = 0.45, the

$$\text{MCHC} = \frac{15 \text{ g/dl}}{0.45} = 33.3 \text{ g/dl.}$$

Discussion. Indices are determined in the Coulter Counter Model S (p. 594) somewhat differently. The MCV is derived from the mean height of the voltage pulses formed during the red cell count, and the Hb is measured by optical density of HiCN. The other three values are calculated: Hct = MCV × RBC; $\text{MCH} = \frac{\text{Hb}}{\text{RBC}}$; $\text{MCHC} = \frac{\text{Hb}}{\text{Hct}}$.

The reference values for the indices will depend on whether they are determined from the centrifuged hematocrit or the Coulter Model S. The values in normal individuals will be similar if both are corrected for trapped plasma. Because of increased trapped plasma in hypochromic anemias and sickle cell anemia, however, the MCHC calculated from the microhematocrit will be significantly lower than the MCHC derived from the Coulter Model S.

With the Coulter Model S, calibrated with correction for trapped plasma, our 95 per cent reference intervals for normal adults are: MCV = 80 to 96 fl; MCH = 27 to 33 pg; and MCHC = 32 to 36 g/dl. In a healthy person there is very little variation, no more than ±1 unit in any of the indices. Deviations from the reference value for an individual or outside the reference intervals for normal persons are useful particularly in characterizing morphologic types of anemia.

In *microcytic anemias,* the indices may be as low as an MCV of 50 fl, an MCH of 15 pg, and an MCHC of 22 g/L; rarely do any become lower.

In *macrocytic anemias,* the values may be as high as an MCV of 150 fl, an MCH of 50 pg, but the MCHC is normal or decreased (Dacie, 1975). The MCHC increases only in spherocytosis, and rarely is over 38 g/dl.

Leukocyte Counts

In the total leukocyte count, no distinction is made among the six normal cell types (neutrophils and bands, lymphocytes, monocytes, eosinophils, and basophils). Although each cell type has its particular function in defending the body against foreign threats, here we are concerned with the total leukocyte concentration in the blood. The reference interval for adults is 4.5 to 11.0 × 10^9/L.

Sample. Heparin is unsatisfactory as an anticoagulant; EDTA should be used.

4

Hemacytometer Method. Although this method is rarely used now in routine leukocyte counting, the technologist should be able to perform it (1) as a check on the validity of electronic methods for calibration purposes; (2) as a check on the validity of electronic counts in patients with profound leukopenia or with leukemia; and (3) as a back-up method.

Equipment. The Thoma glass white cell pipette has a stem and a mixing chamber (Fig. 27–5). The stem has 10 gradations, marked at 0.5 and 1.0. The mixing chamber extends from the mark 1.0 to 11.0. It contains a white bead, which aids in the mixing. When blood is drawn to the 0.5 mark and the diluting fluid to the 11.0 mark, the dilution of the blood sample is 1 to 20 and the dilution factor is 20. When blood is drawn to the 1.0 mark and the diluting fluid to 11.0, the dilution factor is 10. The capillary portion of the pipette contains no blood but only diluting fluid; therefore, it is not included in the total volume, and its contents must be expelled before the cell suspension is introduced into the chamber.

Pipettes with a guaranteed accuracy of ±1 per cent should be used. The rubber tubing that is attached to the pipette should be sufficiently heavy walled to resist collapse during suction and should be long enough (at least 10 inches) to permit easy reading of the graduation marks. A safety mouthpiece with an internal filter should be used to prevent aspiration of specimen into the mouth.*

*Gelman Instrument Company, Ann Arbor, Mich.

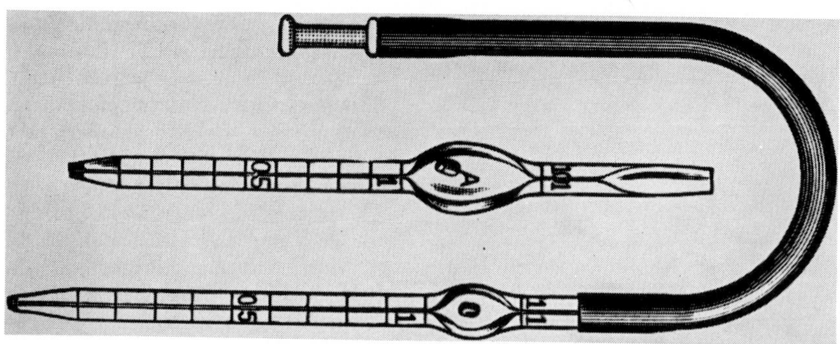

Figure 27–5. Thoma red and white cell diluting pipettes.

After use, pipettes should be rinsed with tap water and then three times with distilled water, filling the bulb through the capillary end, shaking, and emptying through the large-bore end. This is followed by similar treatment with acetone or 95 per cent alcohol and finally with ether, using a water suction pump. The interior of the pipettes should then be dried in an oven or with a current of dry air. The bulb is dry if the bead rolls freely. If the lumen of the capillary pipette contains coagulated blood or other debris, it can be cleaned with a special, delicate, commercially available wire. Washing devices are available that permit cleansing and drying many pipettes simultaneously. Care must be exerted to prevent damage to the bore of the pipette, which leads to inaccuracy in the dilution.

Counting Chamber. The hemacytometer is a thick glass slide, on the middle third of which are fixed three parallel platforms extending across the slide. The central platform is subdivided by a transverse groove into two halves, each wider than the two lateral platforms and separated from them and from each other by moats. The central platforms or "floor pieces" are exactly 0.1 mm lower than the lateral platforms. The central platforms have an improved Neubauer ruling (Fig. 27–6), which is 3 by 3 mm (9 sq mm) subdivided into nine secondary squares, each 1 by 1 mm (1 sq mm). The four corner squares, labeled A, B, C, and D in this figure, are used for the white cell count and are subdivided into 16 tertiary squares.

The central square millimeter is divided into 25 tertiary squares, each of which measures 0.2 by 0.2 mm. Each of these is further subdivided into 16 smaller squares.

A thick coverglass, ground to a perfect plane, accompanies the counting chamber. Ordinary coverglasses have uneven surfaces and should not be used. When the coverglass is in place on the platform of the counting chamber (Fig. 27–6), there is a space exactly 0.1 mm thick between it and the ruled platform; therefore, each square millimeter of the ruling forms the base of a space holding exactly 0.1 cu mm.

Counting chambers and coverglasses should be rinsed immediately after use in lukewarm water, wiped with a clean lint-free cloth, and allowed to dry in the air. The surfaces must not be touched with gauze or linen because they may scratch the ruled areas. A scratch across the chamber or coverglass ruins it. The chamber and coverglass should not be touched because fingerprints are difficult to remove and may be responsible for errors. Before use, the surfaces must be absolutely clean, dry, and free from lint and water marks. After they have been cleaned they must not be touched except at the edges.

Diluting Fluid. The diluting fluid lyses the erythrocytes so that they will not obscure the leukocytes. The simplest diluting fluid is a 2 per cent solution of acetic acid. More satisfactory is the following:

Glacial acetic acid	2 ml
1 per cent aqueous solution of gentian violet	1 ml
Distilled water	100 ml

The fluid must be refrigerated and filtered frequently to remove yeasts and molds.

Procedure

1. The tip of the pipette is placed beneath the surface of the well mixed blood, which is then quickly aspirated just to the 0.5 mark on the red cell pipette. No air bubbles can be in the column of blood. If the blood rises slightly above the mark, it can be drawn back to the mark by touching the tip of the pipette to a tissue or gauze. If a large excess of blood has been drawn up, a clean pipette should be used, because, even if withdrawn, enough blood will adhere to cause significant error. Painstakingly accurate technique is important, because any error is magnified by the subsequent dilution.

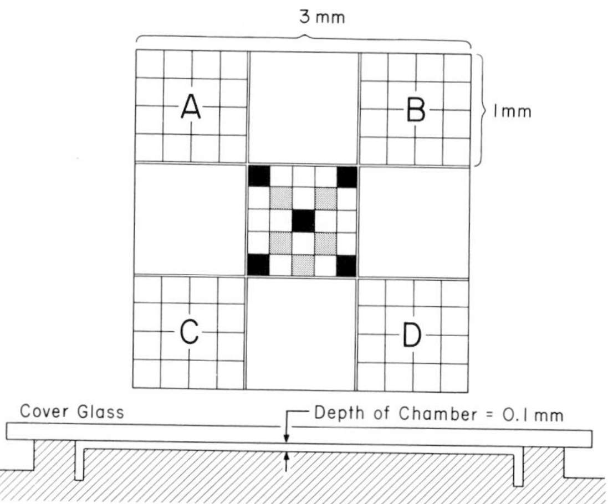

Figure 27–6. The upper figure is a diagram of the improved Neubauer ruling; this is etched on the surface of each side of the hemacytometer. The large corner squares, A, B, C, and D, are used for leukocyte counts. The five black squares in the center are used for red cell counts or for platelet counts, and the 10 black plus shaded squares for platelet counts. Actually, each of the 25 squares within the central sq mm has within it 16 smaller squares for convenience in counting.

The lower figure is a side view of the chamber with the coverglass in place.

2. Blood adhering to the tip is wiped off quickly, the tip is placed into the diluting fluid, and the fluid is drawn up to the mark 11, while rotating the pipette. The pipette is held nearly horizontally to avoid aspiration of air bubbles in the bulb. When the bulb is almost full the pipette is raised to the vertical position. This is a 1 to 20 dilution.

3. The pipette is placed on a rotator for about five minutes to mix. The coverglass is placed on the counting chamber.

4. The first 3 to 4 drops of cell-free diluent are discarded from the pipette. With the pipette at a 35 degree angle, the tip should touch the groove at the edge of the coverglass. The fluid will run under the coverglass by capillary attraction. The fluid is allowed to enter in a controlled manner by pressure from the index finger on the open end of the pipette or from the pressure from the index finger on the open end of the pipette or from the pressure of the tongue on the mouthpiece. Care must be exercised to permit just enough fluid to fill the space beneath the coverglass, without overflowing or creating bubbles.

5. The cells in the chamber are permitted to settle for several minutes, and the ruled area is surveyed with the low-power objective to see whether they are evenly distributed. If not, the procedure must be repeated. If the chamber is filled and the cells not counted promptly, the fluid should be protected against evaporation by placing the chamber under a Petri dish containing a moistened piece of filter paper, which is applied to the top inner surface.

6. Counting. The condenser diaphragm of the microscope is partially closed to make the leukocytes stand out clearly under a low-power (10 ×) objective lens. The leukocytes are counted in each of the four large (1 sq mm) corner squares (A, B, C and D in Fig. 27–6). A total of eight large corner squares from two sides of a chamber are counted.

7. Each large square encloses a volume of 1/10 mm³, and the dilution is 1 to 20. Therefore, in the volume in the chamber over one large square, one is counting the number of leukocytes in 1/10 × 1/20 = 1/200 mm³ of blood. This means that the leukocyte count is the average number of cells in each large square (N) multiplied by 200. A general formula is:

$$\text{Leukocyte count (cells/mm}^3) = \frac{cc}{lsc} \times d \times 10$$

where cc is the total number of cells counted, d is the dilution factor, 10 is the factor transforming value over one large square (1/10 mm³) to the volume in mm³, and lsc is the number of large squares counted.

In leukopenia, with a total count below 2500, the blood is drawn to the 1.0 mark and the dilution factor is 10.

Example: 120 cells counted in eight squares; dilution factor = 10.

$$\text{Leukocyte count} = \frac{120}{8} \times 10 \times 10$$

$$1500/\text{mm}^3 \ (= 1.5 \times 10^9/\text{L}).$$

In leukocytosis, red cell pipettes are used, and the dilution may be 1 to 100 or even 1 to 200.

8. The following rule is suggested to avoid confusion in counting cells that lie on borderlines: Cells that touch any one of the three lines or the single line on the left and the top borders of the small square should be counted as though they were within the squares, but those that touch any of the lines on the right and the bottom borders of the small squares should not be counted. In this way no cell is counted twice. The cells are counted in each small square, first from left to right, beginning with the top of four small squares, and then from right to left for the next row, and so on.

Sources of Error. Numerous possibilities for error exist in all cell counts using the hemacytometer. Errors may be due to the nature of the sample, to the operator's technique, and to inaccurate equipment. Errors that are inherent in the distribution of cells in the counting volume are called "field" errors and can be minimized only by counting more cells.

Errors Due to the Nature of the Sample. Partial coagulation of the venous blood introduces errors by changes in the distribution of the cells or decrease of their number.

The influences of prolonged application of the tourniquet, the patient's posture, and the time relationship to exercise and meals have been discussed (p. 586) and affect all cell counts as well as hematocrit. Failure to mix the blood thoroughly and immediately before drawing the sample into the pipette introduces an error, which depends upon the degree of sedimentation during the interval since the blood was mixed.

Operator's Errors. Errors caused by faulty technique may occur when blood and the diluting fluid are drawn into the pipette, when the chamber is loaded, and when the cells are counted. A frequent source of trouble is faulty application of the coverglass, especially when it is raised by introduction of an excess of diluted blood, or movement of the coverglass after the counting chamber has been filled. Overflowing of the suspension into the moat is another example.

Errors Due to Equipment. Inaccuracies in the graduations of the pipettes and of the ruled areas and depth of the counting chambers are frequent sources of error. They can be diminished by using pipettes and hemacytometers certified by the U.S. Bureau of Standards.

Inherent or Field Error. Even in a perfectly mixed sample, variation occurs in the number of suspended cells that are distributed in a given volume (i.e., come to rest over a given square).

According to Poisson's law of distribution, the variation among the different squares in the chamber is given by the formula S.D. = $\sqrt{m}$, where m is the mean number of cells per unit area and S.D. is the standard deviation of the counts in these areas.

Example: The count per 4 primary squares is 100 (as for a count of 5000 per µl). The S.D. of counts of different sets of 4 squares in the chamber will be $\sqrt{100}$ or 10. Expressed relatively as a per cent, this is $\frac{10}{100} \times 100 = 10$ per cent. This expression of the standard deviation as a percentage of the mean $\left(\frac{\text{S.D.}}{\text{mean}} \times 100\right)$ is known as the coefficient of variation (C.V.), which, for the Poisson distribution $100\,\frac{\sqrt{m}}{m} = \frac{100}{\sqrt{m}}$.

This "error of the field" is the minimal error. Another error is the "error of the chamber," which includes variations in separate fillings of a given chamber, and in sizes of different chambers. Still another is the "error of the pipette," which includes variations in filling a given pipette, and in the sizes of different pipettes.

Berkson (1940) experimentally determined for hemocytometer white cell counts the following coefficients of variation, expressed as a percentage: the field error $= \frac{100}{\sqrt{n_b}}$; the error of the chamber $= \frac{4.6}{\sqrt{n_c}}$; the error of the pi-

4

pette $= \frac{4.7}{\sqrt{n_p}}$, where n_b = number of blood cells counted, n_c = number of chambers examined, and n_p = number of pipettes used. The total

$$\text{C.V.} = \sqrt{\frac{100^2}{n_b} + \frac{4.6^2}{n_c} + \frac{4.7^2}{n_p}}.$$

In performing a WBC count, if 200 cells are counted using two chambers and one pipette, the C.V. = 9.1 per cent, corresponding to 95 per cent confidence limits of ± 18.2 per cent (twice the C.V.). Using four chambers and two pipettes and counting twice as many cells reduces the 95 per cent confidence limits to ± 12.8 per cent. This relatively large percentage error is of little practical consequence because of the physiologic variation of the leukocyte count.

Nucleated Red Cells. Nucleated red cells will be counted and cannot be distinguished from leukocytes with the magnification used. If their number is high as seen on the stained smear, a correction should be made according to the following formula:

$$\text{True leukocyte count} = \frac{\text{total count} \times 100}{100 + \text{No. of NRBC}}$$

where the No. of NRBC = the number of nucleated red cells which are counted during the enumeration of 100 leukocytes in the differential count.

Example: The blood smear shows 25 nucleated red cells per 100 leukocytes. The total nucleated cell count is 10,000.

$$\text{True leukocyte count} = \frac{10{,}000 \times 100}{125}$$
$$= 8000/\mu l\ (8.0 \times 10^9/L)$$

Electronic Counting of Leukocytes (Gagon, 1966; Brittin, 1971). The principle is the same as that of red cells, except that in either electro-optical or impedance counting, the red cells are lysed before counting. Discussion here will be confined to the latter since this is more widely used.

Diluent Solution

1. Physiologic saline, Isoton,* or one of the other commercially available diluting fluids, is used, 10 ml for 20 μl of blood. (a) To this are added two drops of a 3 per cent saponin solution (or one of the commercially available reagents, .e.g., Zaponin*) for lysis of the red cells. Five minutes are required to ensure complete stromatolysis. (b) Alternatively, one can use a commercially available reagent that both lyses red cells and converts Hb to HiCN (e.g., Zapoglobin*); this allows the hemoglobin concentration and the leukocyte count to be determined from the same dilution.

2. Cetrimide-citrate-saline has advantages over saponin in that stromatolysis and dilution occur with one procedure and the leukocytes are stable for several hours (Cartwright, 1968). A 1:500 dilution is made by diluting 20 μl of blood directly in 10 ml of cetrimide-citrate-saline.

Threshold (Pulse Discriminator) Setting. Prior to counting with any new instrument, diluent, or lysing agent, it is necessary to construct a threshold curve. This is done by performing multiple leukocyte counts on a normal blood sample at threshold settings differing by small increments from zero to a point at which the cells are no longer being counted. They may have to be done at different aperture current settings in order to select one that yields a good plateau. The threshold setting is selected so that baseline noise and small particles are not included in the count. The height of the plateau should be checked by several replicate hemacytometer leukocyte counts.

Technique. Details of operation and coincidence correction charts are supplied by the instrument manufacturer. Background counts greater than 100 should be corrected for coincidence and subtracted from the corrected leukocyte count; if less than 100, background counts can be ignored.

Sources of Error. With the Coulter Counter, 0.5 ml of the 1 to 500 dilution of blood is counted, so that 10,000 cells are actually counted for a white cell count of 10,000 per μl. If two counts are made from one dilution and averaged, the error (± 2 C.V.) is approximately ± 10 per cent in the normal range. If two dilutions of blood are made with an automatic dilutor and triplicate counts are done on each and averaged, the error (± 2 C.V.) is ± 4.6 per cent in the normal range. Gagon (1966) showed that the leukocyte concentration in blood anticoagulated with EDTA is stable for 24 hours at 8°C. or 25°C. Counts with heparinized blood may be either higher or lower than those with other anticoagulants and were not reproducible.

The speed of performance, the elimination of visual fatigue of the technician, and the improved precision are decisive advantages of the electronic cell counter over the hemacytometer.

Platelet Counts

Platelets are thin disks, 2 to 4 μm in diameter and 5 to 7 fl in volume (in citrated blood). They function in hemostasis, in maintaining vascular integrity, and in the process of blood coagulation. Reference values for platelet counts are 150 to 400 × 10^9/L.

In EDTA-blood the platelet volume increases with time up to one hour *in vitro,* is relatively stable between one and three hours, and then increases further with time. Change from a discoid to a spherical shape accounts for this increase in apparent volume in EDTA compared to citrate (Rowan, 1982). For reproducible results, platelet volume measurements, obtained with multichannel instruments such as the Coulter Model S Plus series (p. 597), should be made between one and three hours after the blood is drawn. The frequency distribution of platelet volumes in an individual is log normal (see Fig. 27–9). The reference values for mean platelet volumes (MPV) are approximately 6.5 to 12 fl in adults. There is, however, a non-linear, inverse relationship between the MPV and the platelet count within normal individuals (Fig. 27–7). Therefore reference values for the MPV appear to vary with the platelet count (Bessman, 1981).

Platelets are difficult to count, because they are small and must be distinguished from debris. Another source of difficulty is their tendency to adhere to glass, to any foreign body, and particularly to each other. It is often possible to recognize a significant decrease in the number of platelets by a careful inspection of stained films. With capillary blood, films must be made evenly and very quickly after the blood is obtained in order to avoid clumping and to

*Coulter Diagnostics, Hialeah, Fla.

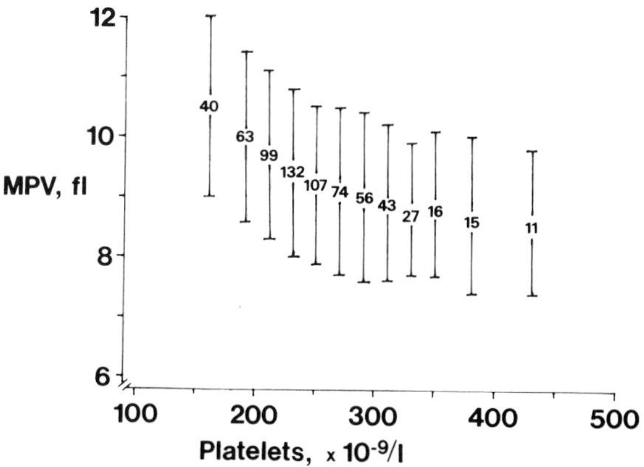

Figure 27–7. Mean platelet volume related to platelet count in 683 normal subjects. Each group is shown as mean (number) 2 S.D. (bar) of subjects grouped by platelet counts of 128–179, 180–199, 200–219, 220–239, 240–259, 260–279, 280–299, 300–319, 320–339, 340–359, 361–403, 406–462 × 10^9/L. The number of the mean position is the number of subjects in the group. (From Bessman, J. D., Williams, L. J., and Gilmer, P. R., Jr.: Am. J. Clin. Path., *76*:289, 1981.)

minimize the decrease due to adhesion of platelets to the margins of the injured vessels. A better estimate is possible by examining stained films made from venous blood with EDTA as an anticoagulant (EDTA-blood), in which platelets are evenly distributed and where clumping normally does not occur. Their morphology on films is described on page 619.

The visual method of choice employs the phase contrast microscope. This is the reference method. Laboratories performing over 20 platelet counts per day can justify electronic platelet counting; both the voltage pulse counting and the electro-optical counting systems are satisfactory.

Hemacytometer Method

Phase Contrast Microscope (Brecher, 1964).

Specimen. Venous blood should be collected in a siliconized glass tube with EDTA as an anticoagulant. Plastic tubes may be satisfactory but should be checked against siliconized glass tubes in a trial before use. Several types of plastic tubes have been found to give significantly lower platelet counts than siliconized glass tubes (Lewis, 1971).

Equipment. Flat bottom counting chamber and a No. 1 or 1½ coverslip. "Long-working distance" phase condenser with 43 × annulus and matching 43 × phase objective and 10 × eyepiece. For American Optical Company equipment, "medium dark contrast" should be specified.

Diluent Solution. One per cent ammonium oxalate in distilled water. Stock bottle is kept in the refrigerator. The amount needed for the day is filtered before use and the unused portion discarded at end of day.

Procedure

1. Though blood collected in plastic or siliconized syringes and test tubes is theoretically preferable, glass tubes in the Vacutainer system have proved satisfactory. Platelet clumping must be avoided by a good venipuncture and prompt anticoagulation. EDTA is the anticoagulant of choice. Although less desirable, blood from a skin puncture wound may be used if only the first few drops are used and the blood is flowing freely.

2. Two red cell pipettes (Fig. 27–5) are used. Each is rapidly filled with blood exactly to the 1 mark, carefully wiped, then filled with ammonium oxalate to the 101 mark, and rotated in a mechanical pipette rotor. The Bryant-Garrey rotors have been found satisfactory. Rotation for as long as eight hours does not affect the counts.

3. The hemacytometer is filled in the usual fashion, using a separate pipette for each side.

4. The chamber is covered by a Petri dish for 15 minutes to allow settling of the platelets in one optical plane. A piece of wet cotton or filter paper is left beneath the dish to prevent evaporation.

5. The platelets appear round or oval and frequently have one or more dendritic processes. Their internal granular structure and a purple sheen allow the platelets to be distinguished from debris, which is often refractile. Ghosts of the red cells which have been lysed by the ammonium oxalate are seen in the background.

6. Platelets are counted in 10 small squares (as for red cell counts, the black squares in Fig. 27–3), 5 on each side of the chamber. If the total number of platelets counted is less than 100, more small squares are counted until at least 100 platelets have been recorded; 10 squares per side (black plus checked squares, Fig. 27–6) or all 25 squares in the large central square on each side of the hemacytometer, if necessary. If the total number of platelets in all 50 of these small squares is less than 50, the count should be repeated with 1:20 or 1:10 dilutions of blood in white cell pipettes.

Calculation. Since each of the 25 small squares defines a volume of 1/250 μl (1/25 mm² area × 1/10 mm depth),

$$\text{the platelet count (per } \mu\text{l)} = \frac{\text{No. cells counted}}{\text{No. squares counted}} \times \text{dilution} \times 250.$$

By adjusting the number of squares so that at least 100 platelets are counted, the field error (the statistical error due to counting a limited number of platelets in the chamber) can be kept in the same range for low platelet counts as for high platelet counts. It has been shown that the coefficient of variation (C.V.) due to combined field, pipette, and chamber errors is about 11 per cent when at least 100 platelets are counted, 15 per cent when 40 platelets are counted. With this method the range of values in 95 per cent of healthy controls is from 150 to 400 × 10^9/L.

Sources of Error. Most of the sources of error are the same as those discussed previously for the red cell and white cell counts. Blood in EDTA is satisfactory for five hours after collection at 20°C. and 24 hours at 4°C., provided no difficulty was encountered in collection. Platelet clumps present in the chamber imply a maldistribution and negate the reliability of the count; a new sample of blood must be collected. The causes of platelet clumping are likely to be initiation of platelet aggregation and clotting before the blood reaches the anticoagulant, imperfect venipuncture, delay in the anticoagulant contacting the blood, or, in skin puncture technique, delay in sampling. Capillary blood gives similar mean values, but errors are about twice those with venous blood, probably because the platelet level varies in successive drops of blood from the skin puncture wound.

Electronic Counting

Electrical Impedance. Relatively inexpensive, stand-alone platelet counters are available. Coulter's Thrombocounter and ZBI, the Baker* MK-4/HC, and the Celloscope 401 require a platelet-rich cell suspension. Red cells must first be removed from the anticoagulated whole blood, either by sedimentation or by controlled centrifugation. To obtain the whole blood platelet count, the count must be corrected for coincidence and erythrocyte plasma trapping, which is proportional to the hematocrit. Favorable coefficients of variation, about 4 per cent, are obtained.

The Baker 810* and Clay Adams† Ultra-Flo 100 perform a whole blood platelet count in less than a minute. An

*Baker Diagnostics, Bethlehem, Pa.

†Clay Adams, Division of Becton-Dickinson & Company, Parsippany, N.J.

initial dilution step is necessary. Both instruments employ hydrodynamic focusing and impedance counting with built-in threshold valley monitoring circuitry to sense excessive noise or small platelets, and large platelets or extremely microcytic red cells. The Baker 810 also provides an MPV and hard copy graph of platelet/RBC size distribution. The Ultra-Flo 100 requires that RBC's be present in the sample and that an accurate RBC count be dialed into the instrument.

Sources of Error. Careful technique is especially important at all steps in platelet counting: collection of blood, having a particle-free diluent, obtaining platelet-rich plasma without losing platelets or having too many red cells remain, microtechnique in diluting, and cleanliness in glassware and in the aperture of the counter.

With instruments using platelet-rich plasma, excessive numbers of red cells in the plasma will give falsely low counts, because platelets entering the aperture at the same time as red cells will not be detected. High leukocyte counts will also produce a falsely low platelet count, because white cells erratically filter out platelets when aspirating into the microcapillary tube. Platelets as large as red cells will be screened out by the upper threshold, also giving a falsely low count. On the other hand, if the sample is hemolyzed, or if red cell fragments are present in the blood, the platelet count is apt to be falsely high.

Always in platelet counting the blood film must be examined before reporting the count, both for concordance of the apparent numbers on the film with that from the machine, and to detect abnormalities such as those just mentioned that are prone to produce erroneous counts.

***Light-Scattering*.** (Brittin, 1971; Simmons, 1971). A semiautomatic instrument for counting platelets, the Autocounter* utilizes the darkfield optical microscope system (Fig. 27–4) described previously for red cell counts. Whole blood is sampled automatically from test tubes or plastic cups, diluted approximately 1:1500 in 2M urea which lyses the red cells. Platelets and leukocytes are counted. For a platelet count of 350 × 10^9/L, about 10,000 light-scattering events are counted in a small optically determined sensing volume (44,000 fl) in the flow cell; this gives a linear response with no significant coincidence. The results are recorded on a moving pen recorder. The instrument is calibrated with fresh normal EDTA-blood, using the average of multiple phase contrast hemacytometer counts. A stable Platelet Reference N (normal)* suspension is available; this should be used as a control or secondary standard rather than to calibrate the instrument. For each sample, the leukocyte count is separately determined and subtracted from the total count.

Compared to the instruments using platelet-rich plasma, the Autocounter has the advantage of using whole blood and automatic mixing, diluting, and counting. Consequently it is easier to use and more reliable, since it is less prone to technical errors in handling samples. In addition, it is readily used for skin-puncture sampling using prediluted whole blood taken with the Unopette system.† A modification in the manifold tubing is necessary, however, to count prediluted specimens.

The Autocounter and the whole blood electrical impedance instruments produce somewhat more precise platelet counts than do those using platelet-rich plasma (C.V. = 1 to 3 per cent versus 4 to 6 per cent).

Sources of Error. Regardless of the method used for platelet counting, the blood film (prepared from EDTA-blood) must be checked to corroborate the height of the count and to detect abnormalities in platelets or other blood elements that may give a false value. If Howell-Jolly bodies or other red cell inclusions are present, they will falsely elevate the count. So too will fragments of leukocyte cytoplasm that are sometimes numerous in leukemias. The phase contrast hemocytometer method must be employed in these cases. Falsely low counts occur if platelets adhere to neutrophils (platelet satellitism) or if there is platelet clumping due to agglutinins, spontaneous aggregation, or incipient clotting. The first two of these phenomena appear to depend upon EDTA (Dacie, 1975).

Platelet counts tend to be the least reproducible of the blood cell counts, and the technologist must use constant vigilance to ensure their accuracy. This also includes the readiness to confirm suspicious or abnormal results with a freshly drawn sample.

*Technicon Corporation, Tarrytown, N.Y.

†Becton-Dickinson, Rutherford, N.J.

Multichannel Instruments

COULTER COUNTER MODEL S

Description. The Coulter Counter Model S produces seven simultaneous measurements (leukocyte count, red cell count, hemoglobin, hematocrit, and the red cell indices) in 40 seconds' time, employing the principles of voltage pulse counting and size analysis together with a photosensitive device for measuring hemoglobin concentration. A power supply provides vacuum and pressure to aspirate the blood and move the diluting fluids and dilutions through the system. The instrument can accept a new sample every 20 seconds, as it counts one sample while diluting the next. The analysis may be performed on whole blood, of which the machine aspirates about 1.3 ml; most is used for flushing, then 44.7 μl is diluted 1:224 with Isoton* (Fig. 27–8). From this (Dilutor I) a second dilution of 1:224 is made, and from the resulting 1:50,000 dilution the red cell count and the MCV are determined by each of three Coulter Counters (C). From Dilutor I, also, the original dilution is brought to a mixing chamber where a lysing agent is added to lyse the red cells and convert the hemoglobin to hemiglobincyanide, and the dilution from 1:224 to 1:250. The hemoglobin concentration is measured, and the suspension of white cells (in dilute HiCN solution) is brought to three counters (C). The red cells and white cells are counted simultaneously, in triplicate, and each group is averaged. This result is printed out unless one result disagrees with the other two by more than 3 standard deviations from the mean, in which case the discordant result is discarded and the mean of the other two is printed out. If all three results disagree by more than 3 standard deviations, none is accepted and the print-out reads zero. The hemoglobinometer is automatically zeroed on an Isoton rinse before each hemoglobin is measured. The MCV is determined directly from voltage pulse heights, and the hematocrit is calculated from the MCV and the red cell count. The other indices are calculated and the seven results appear in digital print-out form on a special card that has been inserted in the printer to receive the data. Simultaneously, the results can pass to a computer.

*Coulter Diagnostics, Hialeah, Fla.

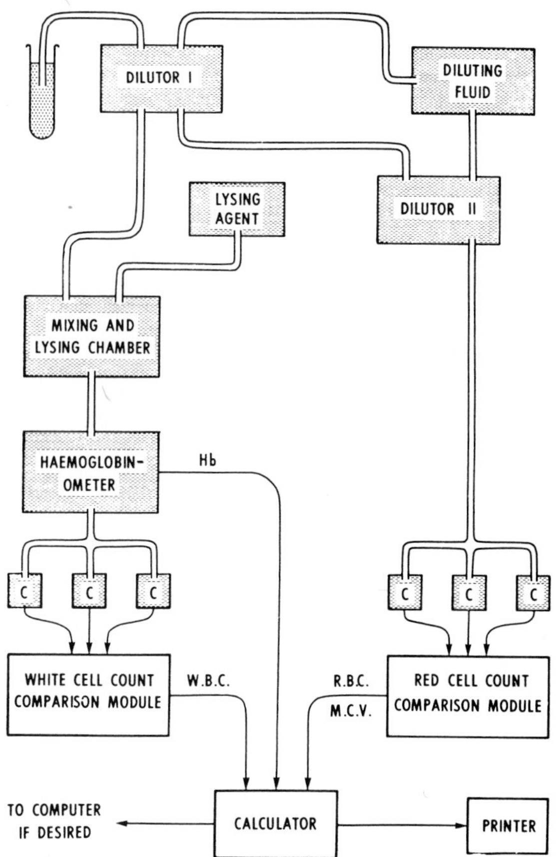

Figure 27–8. Flow diagram of the Coulter Model S. The blood sample is presented manually to the instrument as indicated by the tube, upper left. (From Pinkerton, P. H., et al.: J. Clin. Path., *23*:68, 1970.)

Capillary blood from skin-puncture sampling can be easily handled by diluting 44.7 μ of blood in 10 ml of Isoton. This prediluted sample can then bypass the first dilution step by means of a separate aspirator. The instrument is not fully automatic, in that the technologist must hold the tube of blood up to the aspirator. This allows interruption for the rapid processing of urgent specimens with minimal trouble. Also, the operator is continually watching the oscilloscope screen, the diluting chambers, and other working parts, which helps in early detection of malfunction.

The Coulter Model S has been thoroughly evaluated and found to correlate well with the results from the routine laboratory methods (Brittin, 1969a; Pinkerton, 1970). It is currently the most widely used type of multichannel instrument in hematology. The precision in all the red cell measurements, actual and calculated, has proved to be in the vicinity of 1 per cent (C.V.); the white count slightly higher, 2 to 3 per cent. These values for the coefficient of variation are superior to the routine methods discussed, even when automatic pipettes are used. The reason for this appears to lie in the automatic diluting system which has excellent precision.

Calibration. No certified standard cell suspensions are available, though several stabilized suspensions are commercially available. These stabilized cell suspensions, however, should not be used for calibration. Fresh normal blood should be used for calibration, as emphasized by Brittin (1969a) and Gilmer (1977). Hemoglobin is determined by the HiCN method, using a certified standard and photometer. Hematocrit is measured by the microhematocrit technique. Red cell counts and white cell counts are performed with the Coulter Counter Model F or ZBI. For RBCs, a 1:50,000 dilution is made in a single step to reduce error. A 2 μl ± 0.25 per cent Microcap* pipette is used to deliver the blood into 100 ml (±0.08) of Isoton† in a volumetric flask. (Alternatively, 5 μl, 10 μl, or 20 μl pipettes of similar accuracy may be used to deliver blood into 250, 500, or 1000 ml of diluent, respectively.) The blood for white cell count is diluted 1:500, again with a Microcap, 20 μl ±0.25 per cent of blood in 10 ml of Isoton.

Each of the above is performed in triplicate (each dilution read in duplicate) on fresh blood from 10 to 20 normal individuals. The hematocrit is corrected by subtracting the average proportion of trapped plasma found in hematocrits of normal individuals (ICSH, 1980). This has been estimated to be between 1.5 (Rearson, 1982) and 3 per cent (England, 1972). Our current practice is to subtract 3 per cent, e.g., 0.44 − 0.013 = 0.427. Then the red cell indices are calculated. The white cell count is checked by performing duplicate hemacytometer counts. The normal bloods are run in triplicate on the instrument and the results averaged. The difference between the values from the reference procedure and the Coulter Counter is determined for each specimen so that the per cent difference can be calculated. A normal specimen is then run on the Coulter Counter, and the values are reset in the instrument by multiplying by the proper correction factor. For example, if the Coulter hemoglobin values were on the average 5 per cent lower than the cyanmethemoglobin reference values, the Coulter hemoglobin would be multiplied by 1.05 and this value used to set the instrument. It is important that this calibration not be changed until a "drift" away from these values has been demonstrated on a statistical basis by quality control procedures. At that time, after any necessary maintenance work has been done, the instrument is recalibrated in the same fashion. The calibration settings should not be changed on the basis of a single determination of a control suspension of cells. The Model S and Model S-Plus have been found to be quite stable; recalibration is usually unnecessary more often than every few months.

The method of calibration described gives values for red cell indices from the Model S comparable to

*Drummond Scientific Co., Broomall, Pa.
†Coulter Diagnostics, Hialeah, Fla.

those calculated from the individual methods except that the reference values reflect the slight difference due to correction of the hematocrit for trapped plasma. It is clear that in disorders in which trapped plasma is considerably increased (in the microhematocrit) owing to rigidity or shape of red cells, such as iron deficiency anemia and sickle-cell disease, the hematocrit and MCV are lower and the MCHC slightly higher with the Model S than with conventional methods. It appears quite likely that the Model S gives the more correct values.

Quality Control. Commercially available blood cell control specimens may be used and charted every morning and at intervals during the day, but this is quite expensive and not entirely satisfactory. Brittin (1971) has discussed this problem in his excellent review of instrumentation, and Brittin (1969b) presented a useful method for using patient blood samples in quality control. He demonstrated that all seven values are stable in blood collected in EDTA for at least 24 hours at 4°C. At least five and preferably ten specimens with hematologic values in the normal range are selected on day 1, kept in the refrigerator, and re-analyzed on day 2. A significant change in any channel between the two days can be detected statistically using the Student-t test for paired samples:

$$t_n = \frac{\bar{d}}{S_d}\sqrt{n}, \text{ with } n - 1 \text{ degrees of freedom}$$

n = number of pairs of observations

$\bar{d}$ = mean of the differences (from day to day)

S_d = standard deviation of the differences

$$= \sqrt{\frac{\Sigma(d^2) - \frac{(\Sigma d)^2}{n}}{n - 1}}$$

The t value is calculated for each channel. If the calculated t value exceeds that critical value for the 95 per cent limits found in a statistical table of t-values, the difference is significant at the 5 per cent level. For n = 5, the critical t value is 2.78. For example, if the t score calculated from the five pairs of white cell counts exceeds 2.78, one can be 95 per cent confident that there is a significant difference between the two days. A significant t value should alert one to possible trouble, and persistent significant t scores in the same channel indicate the need for action. Often it is possible to ascertain from simple inspection of the values whether the mean difference from one day to the next differs significantly from zero. The calculations can be easily programmed for a desk top computer, and it is helpful to chart the t values for each channel.

The tendency for drift throughout the day can be monitored by repeating this procedure twice a day, or more simply by running two or three specimens from the first morning batch at intervals throughout the day.

This method will detect a developing loss of calibration, such as may be due to electronic drift. A significant loss of calibration that occurs more abruptly, due to mechanical or electronic breakdown, may not be detected until the following day, however. Bull (1974, 1983) has shown that calculation of a moving average for the MCV, MCH, and MCHC of each successive 20 samples run on the Coulter S throughout the day provides an effective, rapidly available indicator of loss of calibration. It is based on the demonstrated constancy of the mean values for these indices in medium- to large-sized hospitals from day to day and week to week. If the moving average changes by 3 per cent, the calibration must be checked at once. Variations of this method, of increasing complexity, may be performed on a hand calculator or a programmable calculator or be programmed into the laboratory computer system. The moving average is automatically calculated as a part of the quality control program in the Models S-Plus II through V.

Sources of Error. Carry-over is a problem with the Coulter Model S, especially on low white cell counts, since it amounts to about 2 to 3 per cent. If the ratio of successive counts exceeds 3.3:1, the second count will be in error by 5 per cent (Brittin, 1971). It is therefore necessary to repeat any low white count (following a normal or high one) and to use the second value; this should also be done with very low red cell counts.

Increased white cell counts, over $30 \times 10^9/L$, usually produce a slight but significant false elevation of the hemoglobin as a result of turbidity. A very high white count can also elevate the hematocrit and the MCV because the white cells are counted and sized with the red cells.

Errors that influence the MCV determined by voltage pulse analysis have been reviewed by England (1976). From his studies it appears that if the MCV is calibrated in the normal range only, microcytic MCVs will be overestimated when compared with those determined by microhematocrits corrected for plasma trapping. They suggest that the MCV be calibrated with both small cells and normal-sized cells. High glucose concentrations (above 400 mg/dl) and hyperosmolality due to other causes may cause a spuriously high MCV and hematocrit, but low MCHC as measured on the Coulter Counters (Holt, 1982; Beautyman, 1982). Examples are diabetes, hypernatremia, and blood drawn distal to an intravenous glucose line. The probable mechanism is that when diluted in Isoton, the RBCs swell because Isoton is relatively hypotonic to the hypertonic blood sample. Incubating a 1:224 dilution (44.7 μl blood plus 10 ml Isoton) for 10 minutes before analysis will correct the problem.

Cold agglutinins in high titer tend to give spurious macrocytosis and low red cell counts with impossible high MCHCs (Hattersley, 1971). Warming the blood or the diluent eliminates this problem.

In some patients with leukemia the white cells appear to be fragile and escape being counted, giving a falsely low count. Erroneously low white counts may also be found in uremia or in some patients receiving immunosuppressive drugs (Luke, 1971). Hemacytometer counts should be used to check the white counts of such patients. Taft (1973) reported pseudoleukocytosis due to IgG or IgM paraprotein. Whenever the instrument leukocyte count is at odds with an estimate on the blood film, a hemacytometer count should be performed.

Very high lipid levels cause plasma turbidity, which falsely elevates the hemoglobin, MHC, and MCHC (Nosanchuk, 1974). A manual cyanmethemoglobin must be performed, using an appropriate volume of patient plasma in the blank to zero the spectrophotometer. To calculate the appropriate amount of Drabkin's diluent to add to 20 μl of patient plasma to prepare a blank, use the formula:

$$N = \frac{5 \text{ ml}}{(1 - \text{Hct})}$$

where N = ml of Drabkin's to be added to 20 μl of patient plasma. For example, if the patient has a hematocrit of 0.45, then

$$N = \frac{5}{(1 - 0.45)} = \frac{5}{0.55} = 9.1 \text{ ml Drabkin's}$$

As an alternative, a hemoglobin reading can be determined on the patient's plasma, multiplied by the plasmacrit, and subtracted from the whole blood hemoglobin result.

COULTER COUNTER MODEL S-PLUS SERIES

Platelet Counting. The principal new feature of the Model S-Plus is the platelet count. In a 1:6251 dilution (1.6 μl whole blood plus 10 ml Isoton) particles from 36 to 360 fl (μm^3) are counted as RBCs. Particles in the 2 to 20 fl range are counted as platelets. Platelet count and distribution are determined using a 64 channel pulse-height analyzer (Channelyzer). By least squares fitting, an algorithm based on the log normal size distribution of platelets extrapolates to a range of 0 to 70 fl, provided that counting statistics are valid. The platelet size distribution curve can be plotted on the x-y recorder. The mean platelet volume (MPV) is also determined. MPV reference values are 6.5 to 12 fl, but vary with the platelet count (Fig. 27–7).

Red Cell Distribution Width (RDW). A novel calculation, the red cell distribution width (RDW), was introduced as an estimate of erythrocyte anisocytosis. RDW is obtained from the formula; RDW = $\frac{A-B}{A+B} \times K$ where A and B are the red cell volumes at which 20 and 80 per cent, respectively, of the erythrocytes in the sample are larger than that volume. Reference values for the S-Plus I are 10 ± 1.5 (8.5 to 11.5). With the Coulter S-Plus II and subsequent models, the RDW is simply a coefficient of variation for the RBCs. Reference values are 13 ± 1.5 (11.5 to 14.5).

Other S-Plus improvements include a backwash system to reduce carryover to less than 1 per cent; a voting matrix display to monitor "rejects" for each measurement in all three apertures; microprocessor-controlled start up and shut down modes, reagent level sensors, and better checks for electronic stability.

Blood Cell Histograms. The Coulter Models S-Plus II through V provide size distributions (volume in μm^3 [fl] vs. relative number or frequency) for platelets, WBCs, and RBCs. Figure 27–9 shows typical normal distributions for all the cell types. The distributions are displayed on a cathode ray tube and, if desired, printed on the x-y recorder or matrix printer-plotter.

With the quality control (QC) package, per cent lymphocytes (LY%) is determined from the WBC distribution. Using the lyse-treated WBC sample, the pulses between thresholds at 45 and 99 fl are summed and compared to the entire WBC distribution. Per cent lymphocytes and absolute lymphocyte count are determined. These estimations may be useful as a screening test or as a check on WBC differential counts performed. Preliminary work indicates that this lymphocyte analysis should be quite reliable (Oberjat, 1970). Coulter Electronics (1982) claims a correlation coefficient of 0.95 for their "LY%" compared to reference manual differential counts. Note that the volumes do not correspond to those of whole leukocytes, since the lysing solution in the WBC-Hb channel causes partial loss of cytoplasmic contents from the leukocytes.

In Figure 27–10 the WBC of 2.2 × $10^3/\mu l$ is highlighted and the instrument did not calculate LY% or LY# because the specimen "failed the valley check at 45 μm^3." In contrast to normal (Fig. 27–9), in Figure 27–10 the WBCs are considerably above the baseline at 45 μm^3. This sample is from a patient with erythroleukemia who has 44 nucleated red blood cells (NRBC) per 100 WBC. NRBCs usually interfere in the low size range for WBCs, but some may not be counted since they may be smaller than the 45 fl at which the WBC count begins. Any of the cell distributions (WBC, RBC, platelets) can be expanded in size and printed out. Figure 27–11 represents the enlarged WBC curve from Figure 27–10. Figure 27–12 depicts a case of extreme erythrocyte dimorphism, produced by mixing bloods with MCVs of 70 and 107 fl. Similar dimorphism, in varying degree, may be seen following transfusion or specific therapy and in sideroblastic anemias. In this case the RDW is markedly increased. Figure 27–13 shows a microcytic blood with MCV of 70 fl. In the raw platelet curve the extremely microcytic RBCs cause the curve to increase at about 15 μm^3. However, the fitted curve extrapolates out these RBCs, and phase microscopy proved the platelet count to be accurate.

Other Features. The quality control program is comprehensive and allows storage of patient and control values in libraries. Moving averages of red cell indices are calculated every 20 samples, and flagged when acceptable limits are exceeded (p. 596). This permits better instrument monitoring than day-to-day comparisons.

On the Models S-Plus II and III, an optional Coulter Automated Sample Handler allows unattended throughput of up to 32 sealed patient specimens. A cap piercer penetrates the stoppered tubes, decreasing potential contamination.

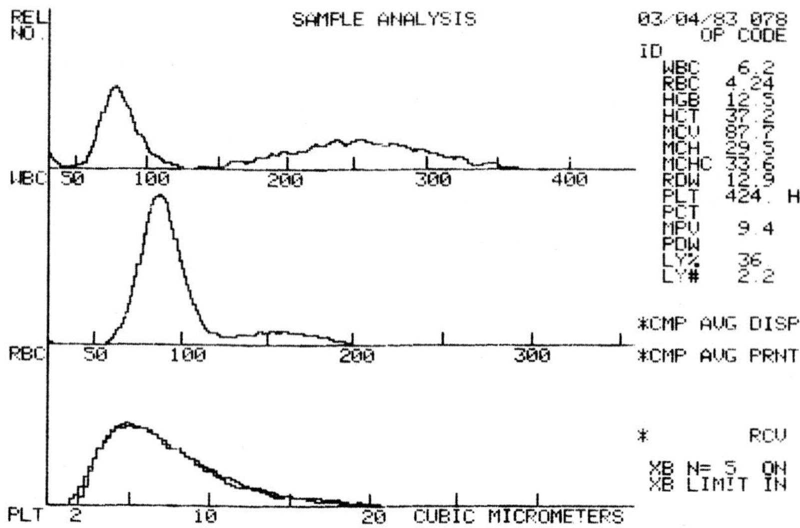

Figures 27–9 through 27–13. Blood cell histograms from the Coulter Counter Model S-Plus IV. More recent models have a three-part "differential": lymphocyte, mononuclear, and granulocyte counts.

Figure 27–9. Normal blood cell histograms. Cells in the WBC channel larger than 45 fl (cubic micrometers) are counted and plotted as WBCs. The small WBC peak (45 to 99 fl) represents lymphocytes. Cells in the RBC channel between 36 and 360 fl are counted and plotted as RBCs; particles in this channel between 2 and 20 fl, extrapolated to 0 to 70 fl, are regarded as platelets. Note the typical skewed (log normal) platelet distribution.

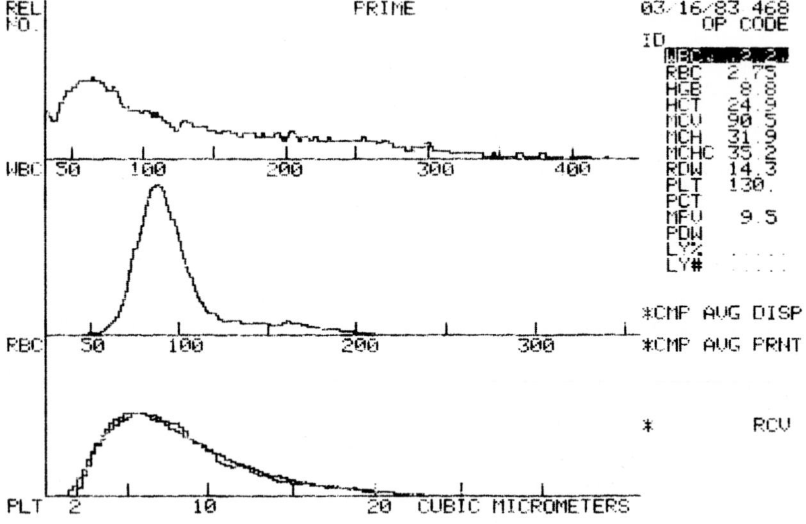

Figure 27–10. Erythroleukemia. Circulating nucleated RBCs are counted with WBCs. When present in large numbers, as here (44 per 100 WBCs) they obliterate the nadir of the curve (normally at 45 fl). This indicates that the smaller cells are not counted. The "WBC = 2.2" is highlighted and serves as a warning.

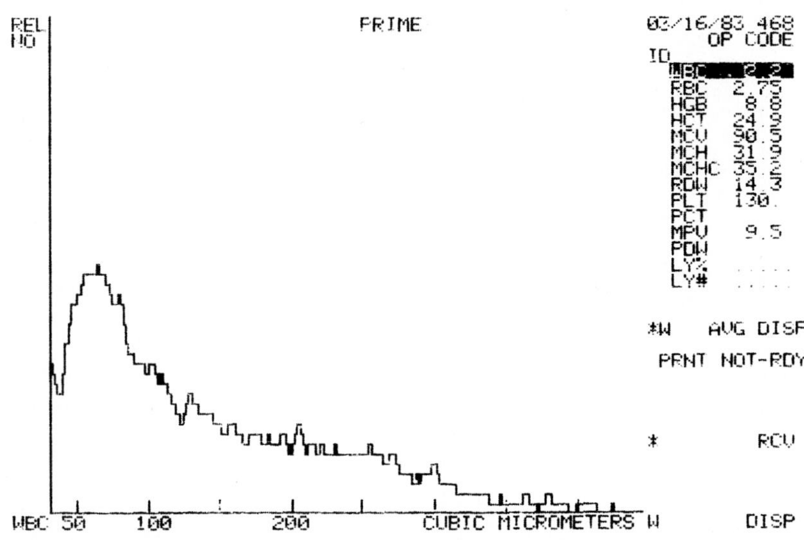

Figure 27–11. Expansion of the WBC histogram from Figure 27–10. Any of the histograms can be amplified in this manner.

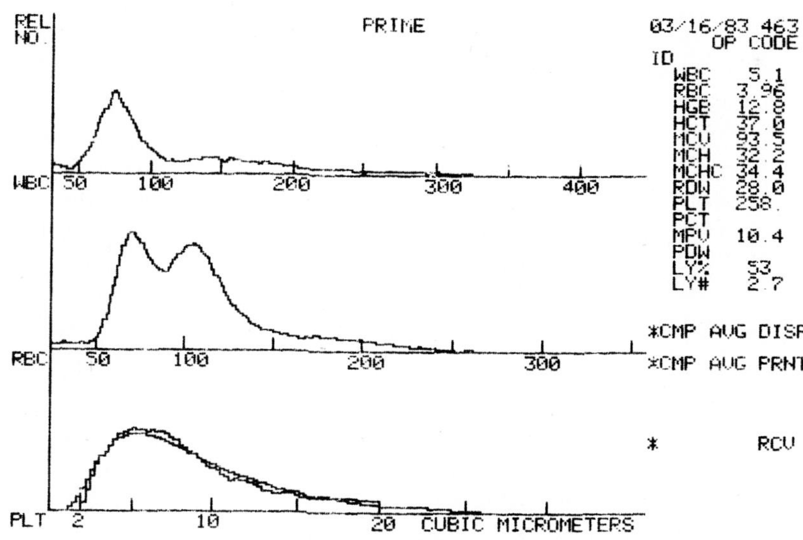

Figure 27–12. Bimodal populations of RBCs produced by mixing blood with MCVs of 70 fl and 107 fl. Because of the great dispersion the RDW is markedly increased.

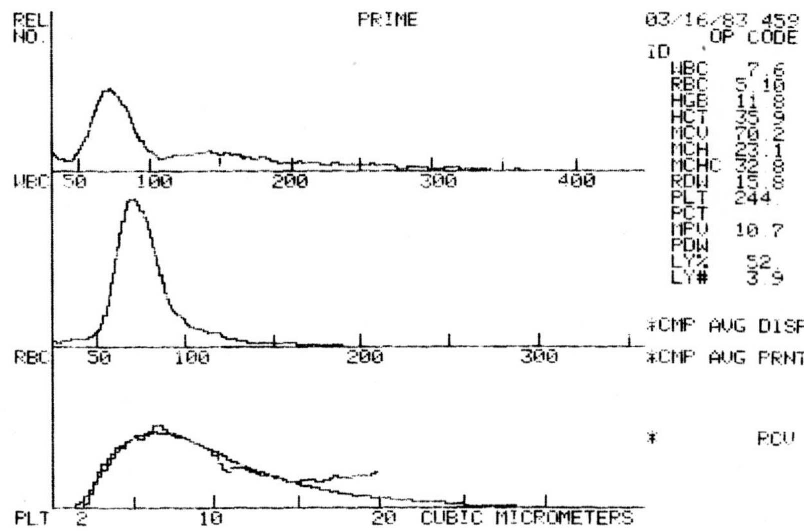

Figure 27–13. Mild microcytic anemia. The rise in the actual platelet curve between 15 and 20 fl (cubic micrometers) is due to microcytic erythrocytes. The extrapolated platelet curve does not include the microcytic RBCs.

The model S-Plus IV has increased throughput (115 to 140/hour) and decreased reagent consumption and requires only 100 μl of whole blood.

SYSMEX CC-800

The Sysmex* CC-800 is an 8 parameter cell counter which employs the impedance principle of detection. Precision is claimed to equal that of the Coulter Model S Plus II. Up to 100 samples on a turntable are analyzed at 80/hour using 0.5 ml whole blood. A quality control program stores control values, calculates moving mean, and plots Levy Jennings charts on a cathode ray tube. A microprocessor monitors and provides alerts for abnormal patient values, manometer performance, reagent supply, aperture clogging, diluent temperature, and electronics. The instrument provides histograms of WBC, RBC and platelets and enumerates subpopulations of each based on size. The CC-720 is a seven parameter instrument, lacking platelet count and histograms, but providing most of the other features at the rate of 110 per hour.

TECHNICON INSTRUMENTS

Hemalog 8. The successor to the Technicon SMA 4A/7A is the Hemalog 8, a continuous-flow system for automation of routine methods in hematology. This instrument uses the electro-optical (light-scattering) principle (Fig. 27–4) to count red cells, white cells, and platelets; it measures hemoglobin by the HiCN method; it incorporates a unique centrifuge method for the microhematocrit, which is read automatically without stopping the centrifuge head. From the three red cell measurements, the MCV, MCH, and MCHC are calculated and the eight results are printed out (Saunders, 1974). This system operates without the need for the constant presence of a technologist, at the rate of 90 samples per hour. It does, however, require calibration for each batch of test samples. Evaluations have shown good correlation with other methods.

H-6000. The Hemalog 8 has been replaced by the Technicon H-6000, which incorporates the 8 parameter CBC and platelet with the cytochemical differential principle of the Hemalog D (p. 618). Stirred whole blood is aspirated and drawn into three manifolds: basophil and alkaline peroxidase for WBC and leukocyte differential count, and RBC/platelet/hemoglobin manifold for CBC and platelets. Hemoglobin is determined using the HiCN reaction. The RBC/PLT optics assembly has two detection channels. A photodiode enumerates RBCs, and the light scatter signals are integrated to determine hematocrit. A more sensitive photomultiplier tube senses scatter from platelets. The differential portion is similar to the Hemalog D except that monocytes are measured in the peroxidase manifold rather than in a separate esterase channel. The H601 printer provides a copy of the CBC and differential, RBC, and platelet histograms, and scatter versus absorption display of the leukocytes in the peroxidase channel (Fig. 27–14).

ORTHO INSTRUMENTS*

ELT-8. In Ortho instruments, cells are counted and sized by laser light scattered by cells focused in a hydrodynamic stream. The Hemac 7 analyzer was replaced in 1979 by the ELT-8, which offered additional features.

At 60 samples per hour, about 100 μl of whole blood is aspirated. Hemoglobin is determined colorimetrically in a separate HiCN channel, different from the other lysed sample for the WBC count. In hydrodynamic focusing, the diluted sample stream of cells is injected in the center of a flowing sheath

*TOA Medical Electronics (USA), Inc., Carson, Cal.; available through American Scientific Products.

*Ortho Instruments, Westwood, Mass.

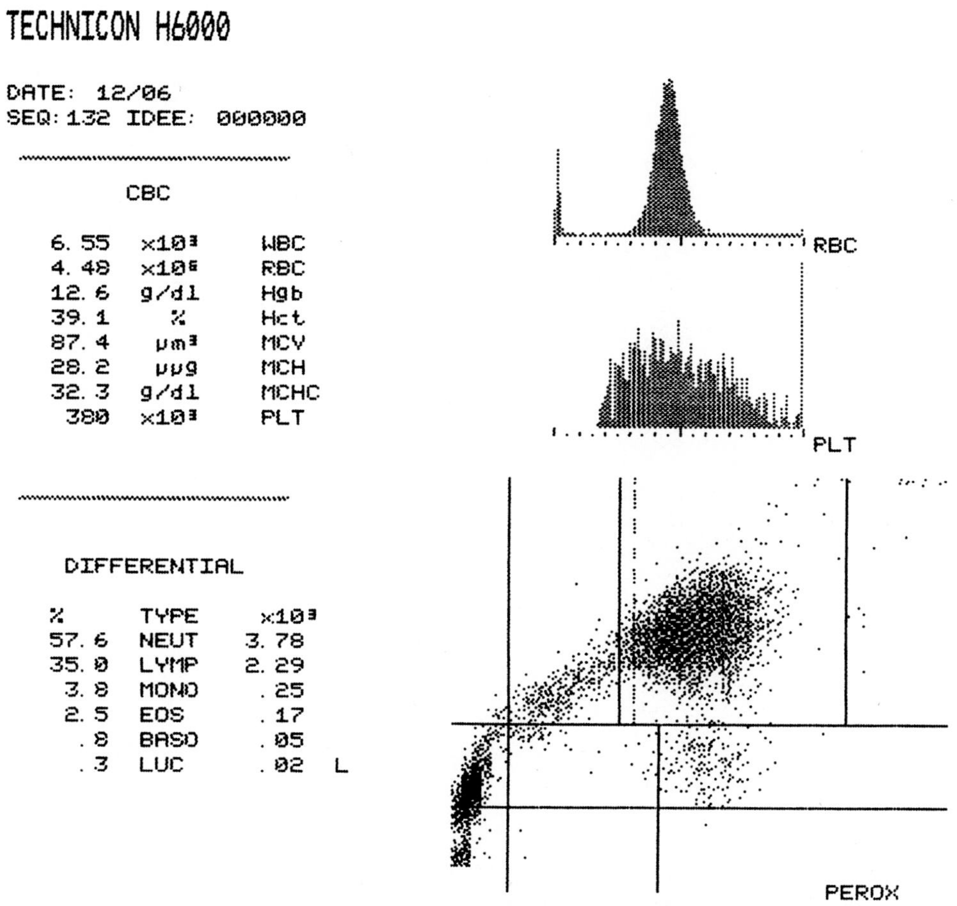

TECHNICON H6000

DATE: 12/06
SEQ: 132 IDEE: 000000

CBC

6.55	x10³	WBC
4.48	x10⁶	RBC
12.6	g/dl	Hgb
39.1	%	Hct
87.4	μm³	MCV
28.2	μμg	MCH
32.3	g/dl	MCHC
380	x10³	PLT

DIFFERENTIAL

%	TYPE	x10³	
57.6	NEUT	3.78	
35.0	LYMP	2.29	
3.8	MONO	.25	
2.5	EOS	.17	
.8	BASO	.05	
.3	LUC	.02	L

RBC

PLT

PEROX

Figure 27–14. Print-out from the Technicon H6000 includes the six RBC measurements and the WBC and platelet counts; the size distributions of the RBCs and platelets; the differential leukocyte count listed as % and as absolute counts (cells × $10^3/\mu l$); and the scatter versus absorption display of leukocytes in the peroxidase channel. In the latter display (which provides most of the information for classifying the leukocytes) the horizontal lines represent low and high thresholds for light scatter, and the vertical lines represent thresholds for light absorbance. See Figure 27–44 for further details.

stream. After entering the 250 μm diameter flow chamber the sample stream narrows to 20 μm. A helium-neon laser beam is focused on the stream of cells to produce a cylindrical sensing zone 7 μm long by 20 μm in diameter. Cells passing through the sensing zone scatter light; the intensity of the forward angle scatter is measured by a photomultiplier tube and processed by the computer.

Discrimination of RBC from platelets depends on cell volume, refractive index, and "time of flight" through the sensing zone. Each cell produces a pulse whose height and width are determined by those three characteristics. The hematocrit represents the sum of the pulses, and indices are calculated.

Inherent advantages of this technology are fewer clogging problems, decreased coincidence permitting enumeration of more cells, and usually a better separation of RBC and platelet pulses. Histogram displays of WBC, RBC, and platelets are available. Ortho was the first manufacturer to take advantage of the instrument's computer to significantly improve quality control and ease of recalibration. Files for storage and analysis of control and patient materials were included. Most importantly, the ELT-8 could automatically accumulate and compute moving average data on patient populations with a selectable batch size of 10 to 99 samples. This feature could quickly notify the operator of potential instrument shifts or drifts. Mayer (1980) found better platelet accuracy in the low (<50,000) range with the ELT-8 than in the Coulter Model S-Plus.

ELT-800. Ortho's latest 8 parameter cell counter is the ELT-800. Increased instrument speed (100 plus samples per hour) and a more powerful and flexible computer for data management are the major areas of improvement.

Reticulocyte Count

Principle. Reticulocytes are immature non-nucleated red cells that contain ribonucleic acid (RNA) and continue to synthesize hemoglobin after loss of the nucleus. When blood is briefly incubated in a solution of new methylene blue or brilliant cresyl blue, the RNA is precipitated as a dye–ribonucleo-

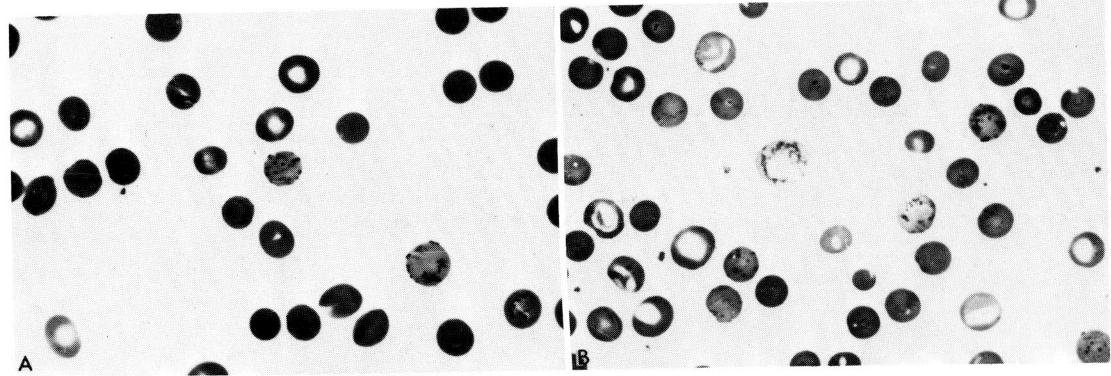

Figure 27–15. Reticulocytes; on air-dried film made after vital staining of blood with new methylene blue dye. RNA precipitates with the dye and appears as blue granules, which are sometimes connected into a network of reticulum.

protein complex. Microscopically, the latter appears as a dark blue network (reticulum) or dark blue granules which allow reticulocytes to be identified and enumerated.

Reagent. One per cent new methylene blue in a diluent of citrate-saline (one part 30 g/L sodium citrate plus four parts 9 g/L sodium chloride).

Procedure. Three drops each of reagent and blood are mixed in a test tube, incubated 15 minutes at room temperature, and remixed.

Two wedge films are made on glass slides and air dried.

Viewed microscopically with an oil-immersion lens, reticulocytes are pale blue and contain dark blue reticular or granular material (Fig. 27–15), and red cells stain pale blue or blue-green.

The percentage of reticulocytes is determined in at least 1000 red cells. A Miller disk inserted in the eyepiece allows rapid estimation of large numbers of red cells by imposing two squares (one 9 times the area of the other) onto the field of view (Brecher, 1950). Reticulocytes are counted in the large square and red cells in the small square in successive microscopic fields until at least 300 red cells are counted. This provides an estimate of reticulocytes among at least 2700 red cells, as follows:

$$\text{Reticulocytes (\%)} = \frac{\text{No. reticulocytes in large squares}}{\text{No. red cells in small squares} \times 9} \times 100$$

The absolute reticulocyte count is determined by multiplying the reticulocyte percentage by the red cell count.

Normal Values. Normal adults have a reticulocyte count of 0.5 to 1.5 per cent or 24 to 84 $\times$ 10^9/L. In newborn infants the percentage is 2.5 to 6.5; this falls to the adult range by the end of the second week of life.

Interpretation. Because reticulocytes are immature red cells that lose their RNA a day or so after reaching the blood from the marrow, a reticulocyte count provides an estimate of the rate of red cell production. An absolute reticulocyte count or reticulocyte production index is more helpful than the percentage (p. 000).

Sources of Variation. Because such a small number of actual reticulocytes are counted, the sampling error in the reticulocyte count is relatively large. The 95 per cent confidence limits may be expressed as $R \pm 2\sqrt{\frac{R\,(100 - R)}{N}}$ where R is the reticulocyte count in per cent and N is the number of erythrocytes examined. This means that if only 1000 erythrocytes are evaluated, the 95 per cent confidence limits for a 1 per cent count are 0.4 to 1.6 per cent; for a 5 per cent count, 3.6 to 6.4 per cent; and for a 10 per cent count, 8.1 to 11.9 per cent.

The automated leukocyte differential counting systems employing digital image processing have programs to perform reticulocyte counts.

BLOOD FILM EXAMINATION

Making and Staining Blood Films

Examination of the blood film is an important part of the hematologic evaluation. The reliability of the information obtained depends heavily on well made and well stained films which are systematically examined.

Three methods of making films are described: the two-slide or wedge method, the coverglass method, and the spinner method.

Wedge Method. Place a drop of blood 2 to 3 mm in diameter about 1 cm from the end of a clean, dust-free slide which is on a flat surface. With the thumb and forefinger of the right hand hold the end of a second (spreader) slide against the surface of the first at an angle of 30 to 45 degrees and draw it back to contact the drop of blood. Allow the blood to spread and film the angle between the two slides. Push the "spreader slide" at a moderate speed forward until all the blood has been spread into a moderately thin film. The spreader slide should be slightly narrower than the first slide so that the edges can be easily examined with the microscope.

The slides should be rapidly air dried by waving the slide or with an electric fan. The thickness of the film can be adjusted by changing the angle of the spreader slide or the speed of spreading, or by using a smaller or larger drop of blood. At a given speed, increasing the angle of the spreader slide will increase the thickness of the film. At a given angle, increasing the speed with which the spreader slide is pushed will increase the thickness of the film. The film should not cover the entire surface of the slide. In a good film there is a thick portion and a thin portion and a gradual transition from one to the other. The film should have a smooth, even appearance and be free from ridges, waves, or holes. The edge of the spreader must be absolutely smooth. If it is rough, the film has ragged tails containing many leukocytes.

In films of optimal thickness there is some overlap of red cells in much of the film but even distribution and separation of red cells toward the thin tail. The faster the film is air dried, the better the spreading of the individual cells on the slide. Slow drying (in humid weather, for example) results in contraction artifacts of the cells.

The slide may be labeled by writing the identification with a lead pencil on the frosted end or directly on the thicker end of the blood film.

Portable instruments that produce consistent wedge films of good quality are commercially available.*

Coverglass Method. No. 1 or 1½ coverglasses 22 mm square are recommended.

Touch a coverglass to the top of a small drop of blood without touching the skin and place it, blood side down, crosswise on another coverglass so that the corners appear as an eight-pointed star. If the drop is not too large and if the coverglasses are perfectly clean, the blood will spread out evenly and quickly in a thin layer between the two surfaces. Just as it stops spreading, pull the coverglasses quickly but firmly apart on a plane parallel to their surfaces. The blood usually is much more evenly spread on one of the coverglasses than it is on the other. Coverglasses should be placed film side up on clean paper and allowed to dry in the air, or they may be inserted back to back in slits made in a cardboard box.

Films from venous blood may be prepared similarly with a drop of blood on a coverslip and proceeding as described.

Spinner Method. Blood films that combine the advantages of easy handling of the wedge slide and uniform distribution of cells of the coverglass preparation may be made with special types of centrifuges known as spinners† (Rogers, 1973). A platen holds the slide in a horizontal plane perpendicular to the rotor. A motor spins the rotor, rapidly accelerates to about 5000 rpm, and quickly stops after a spinning time of a few seconds. About 0.2 ml of EDTA blood is placed on the center of the slide (on the platen). Closing the cover of the centrifuge activates the motor. To produce uniform slides, a knob is used to adjust the duration of spinning depending on the hematocrit.

The spinner slide is covered by a uniform blood film, in which all cells are separated and do not overlap (a monolayer). White cells can be easily identified at any spot in the film, which is ideal for differential counting and is used in several of the automatic white cell differential systems available. The distribution of the different types of white cells in spinner slides equals that of coverglass films and is presumably random. This contrasts with the wedge slide, in which there is a disproportion of monocytes at the tip of the feather edge, of neutrophils just in from the feather edge, and of both at the lateral edges of the film (Rogers, 1973). This is of little practical significance, but it does result in slightly lower monocyte counts in wedge films (see Table 27–5). A minor disadvantage of the spinner slide is the tendency of the red cells to have eccentric central pallor, mimicking the appearance of spheroidocytes.

Blood Stains. The aniline dyes used in blood work are of two general classes: basic dyes, such as methylene blue, and acid dyes, such as eosin. Nuclei and certain other structures in the blood are stained by the basic dyes and, hence, are called basophilic. Structures which take up only acid dyes are called acidophilic, oxyphilic, or eosinophilic. Other structures stained by a combination of the two are called neutrophilic.

Polychrome methylene blue and eosin stains are the outgrowth of the original time-consuming Romanowsky method and are widely used. They stain differentially most normal and abnormal structures in the blood.

The basic components of the Romanowsky-type stains are thiazines, and the acidic components are eosins; this class of stains is known, therefore, as thiazine eosinates (Lillie, 1977). The thiazines present consist of methylene blue (tetramethylthionine) and in varying proportions its analogues produced by oxidative demethylation: azure B (trimethylthionine); azure A (asymmetrical dimethylthionine); symmetrical dimethylthionine; and azure C (monomethylthionine). The acidic component, eosin, is derived from a xanthene skeleton (Baker, 1958).

Most Romanowsky stains are dissolved in methyl alcohol and combine fixation with staining. Among the best known methods are Giemsa's and Wright's.

Wright's Stain. This is a methyl alcoholic solution of eosin and a complex mixture of thiazines, including methylene blue (usually 50 to 75 per cent), azure B (10 to 25 per cent), and other derivatives (Lubrano, 1977). Wright's stain certified by the Biological Stain Commission is commercially available as a solution ready for use or as a powder (Conn, 1960).

The Buffer solution (pH 6.4) contains primary (monobasic) potassium phosphate (KH_2PO_4), anhydrous 6.63 g; secondary (dibasic) sodium phosphate (Na_2HPO_4), anhydrous 2.56 g; and distilled water to make 1 L. A more alkaline buffer (pH 6.7) may be prepared by using 5.13 g of the potassium salt and 4.12 g of the sodium salt.

Procedure

1. To prevent the plasma background of the film from staining blue, blood films should be stained within a few hours of preparation or fixed if they must be kept without staining.
2. Fixation and staining may be accomplished by immersion of the slides in reagent-filled jars or by covering horizontally supported slides or coverslips with the reagents. In the latter method, covering the film with copious stain avoids evaporation, which leads to precipitation.
3. Fixation is for one to two minutes with absolute methanol.
4. The slide is next exposed to undiluted stain solution for two minutes. Then, without removing the stain from the horizontal slide, an equal amount of buffer is carefully added, and mixed by blowing gently.
5. The stain is flushed from the horizontal slide with water. Washing for more than 30 seconds reduces the blue staining. The back of the slide is cleaned with gauze.
6. The slide is allowed to air-dry in a tilted position.
7. Coverglasses are mounted film side down on a slide with Canada balsam or other mounting medium.

Films stained well with Wright's stain have a pink color when viewed with the naked eye. Under low power the cells should be evenly distributed. The red cells are pink, not lemon yellow or red. There should be a minimum of precipitate. The color of the film should be uniform. The blood cells should be free from artifacts, such as vacuoles. The nuclei of leukocytes are blue to purple, the chromatin and parachromatin clearly differentiated, and the cytoplasmic neutrophilic granules tan in color. The eosinophilic granules are red-orange and each distinctly discernible.

The basophil has dark blue to purple granules. Platelets have dark lilac granules. Bacteria (if present) are blue. The cytoplasm of lymphocytes is generally robin's-egg blue; that of the monocytes has a faint blue-gray tinge. Malarial

4

*Miniprep, Geometric Data Corp., Wayne, Pa.

†Hemaspinner, Geometric Data Corp., Wayne, Pa.

parasites have sky-blue cytoplasm and red-purple chromatin. A preparation is usually satisfactory if both the nuclei and the neutrophilic granules are distinct. The colors are prone to fade if the preparation is mounted in a poor quality of balsam or exposed to the light.

Staining Problems

EXCESSIVELY BLUE STAIN. Thick films, prolonged staining time, inadequate washing, or too high an alkalinity of stain or diluent tends to cause excessive basophilia. In such films the erythrocytes appear blue or green, the nuclear chromatin is deep blue to black, and the granules of the neutrophils are deeply overstained and appear large and prominent. The granules of the eosinophils are blue or gray. Staining for a shorter time or using less stain and more diluent may correct the problem. If these steps are ineffective, the buffer may be too alkaline and a new one with a lower pH should be prepared.

EXCESSIVELY PINK STAIN. Insufficient staining, prolonged washing time, mounting the coverslips before they are dry, or too high an acidity of the stain or buffer may cause excessive acidophilia. In such films the erythrocytes are bright red or orange, the nuclear chromatin is pale blue, and the granules of the eosinophils are sparkling brilliant red. One of the causes of the increased acidity is exposure of the stain or buffer to acid fumes. The problem may be in a low pH of the buffer, or it may be in the methyl alcohol, which is prone to develop formic acid as a result of oxidation on standing. A given powder may afford perfect results when dissolved in fresh methanol, but poor results when dissolved in the same lot of methanol after some months of exposure to air. After these steps have been checked, one might suspect that the dye does not have the proper polychrome components and try another lot.

Inadequately stained red cells, nuclei, or eosinophilic granules may be due to understaining or excessive washing. Prolonging the staining or reducing the washing may solve the problem.

Precipitate on the film may be due to unclean slides, drying during the period of staining, inadequate washing of the slide at the end of the staining period, especially failure to hold the slide horizontally during initial washing, inadequate filtration of the stain, or permitting dust to settle on the slide or smear.

Other Stains. Besides Wright's stain, Romanowsky-type stains include a number of others: Giemsa, Leishman, Jenner, May-Grünwald, MacNeal, and various combinations. Some have been particularly recommended for certain purposes, such as Geimsa's stain for excellence in staining malarial parasites and protozoa.

These Romanowsky-type stains (thiazine eosinates) generally vary in the proportions of methylene blue and its demethylated polychrome intermediates (azure B, azure A, etc.). The latter may be developed by "aging" the stain or by adding various oxidizing agents; or they may be more or less purified elsewhere and added. A combination of these thiazine dyes seems to be necessary to produce the subtle varieties of color in well-stained blood cells.

Slight variations in staining quality that are common in most laboratories can be accommodated by the trained observer's eye without difficulty. Automated leukocyte differential counting systems, however, which demanded a much more consistent stain stimulated studies for a better understanding and control of the process.

Marshall (1975a), using thin-layer chromatography, and Lubrano (1977), using high performance liquid chromatography, analyzed the composition of a large number of commercially available Romanowsky dyes. The composition of the dyes in the same stain often varies among different suppliers, and even may vary considerably from batch to batch from the same supplier. In addition, during storage at 25°C. (but not at 4°C.) degradation products that are not polychrome dyes form in methanol; these impair staining intensity but not color (Dean, 1977).

Marshall (1975a) correlated the staining performance of a number of commercial stains with their chemical composition on thin-layer chromatography. Although the results did not show a precise relationship, he was able to determine that methylene blue, azure B, and eosin when used alone produced consistent and satisfactory staining; that poor results were correlated with the presence of methylene violet Bernthsen and methyl thionoline/thionoline; and that the stain must not be contaminated with metal salts. On the basis of these studies a standardized Romanowsky stain has been produced from purified dyes (Marshall, 1975b).

Erythrocytes

In the blood from a healthy person the erythrocytes, when not crowded together, appear as circular, homogeneous disks of nearly uniform size, ranging from 6 to 8 μm in diameter (Fig. 27–16). However, even in normal blood there may be individual cells as small as 5.5 μm and as large as 9.5 μm. The center of each is somewhat paler than the periphery. Erythrocytes are liable to be crenated when the film has dried too slowly. In disease, erythrocytes vary in their hemoglobin content, size, shape, staining properties, and structure.

Color

Hemoglobin Content. The depth of staining furnishes a rough guide to the amount of hemoglobin in red cells, and the terms normochromic, hypochromic, and hyperchromic are used to describe this feature of red cells. *Normochromic* refers to normal intensity of staining (Figs. 27–16 and 27–17). When the amount of hemoglobin is diminished, the central pale area becomes larger and paler. This is known as *hypochromia.* The MCH and MCHC are usually decreased (Fig. 27–18). In megaloblastic anemia, because the red cells are larger and hence thicker, many stain deeply and have less central pallor (Figs. 27–19 and

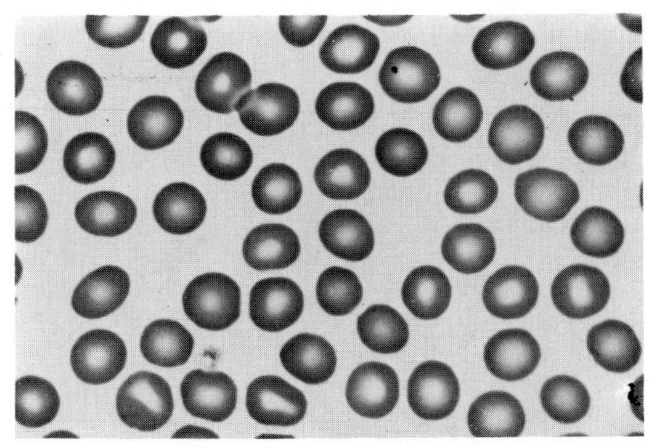

Figure 27–16. Normal blood film (×875).

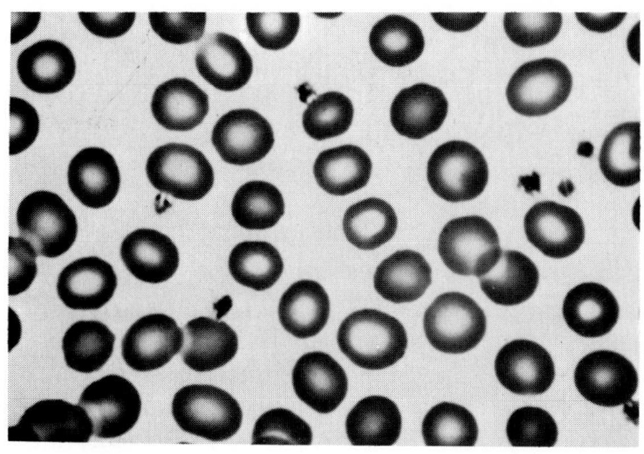

Figure 27–17. This blood film shows a small number of slightly hypochromic red cells; most are normochromic. Cell diameters are normal. MCV and MCHC were normal. The irregular bodies 2 to 3 μm in diameter are normal blood platelets (×875).

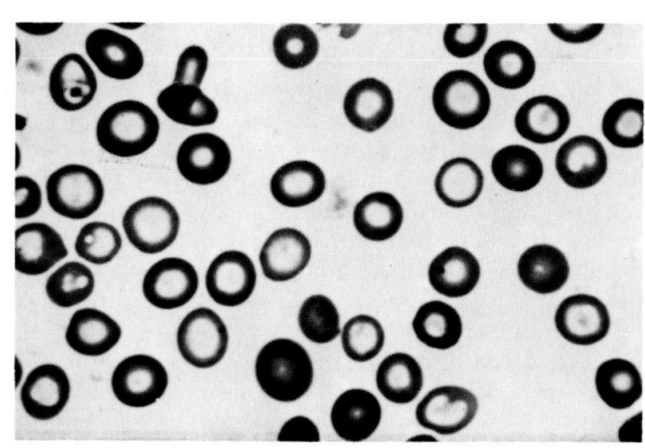

Figure 27–18. Iron deficiency anemia. Most of the cells are hypochromic and microcytic. Note elliptical cells. Anisocytosis is slight in degree (×875).

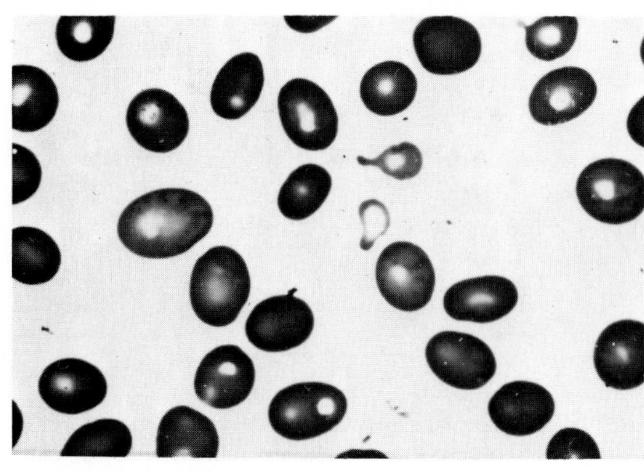

Figure 27–19. Megaloblastic anemia. Macrocytosis. Marked anisocytosis. Note elliptical cells and teardrop-shaped cells (×875).

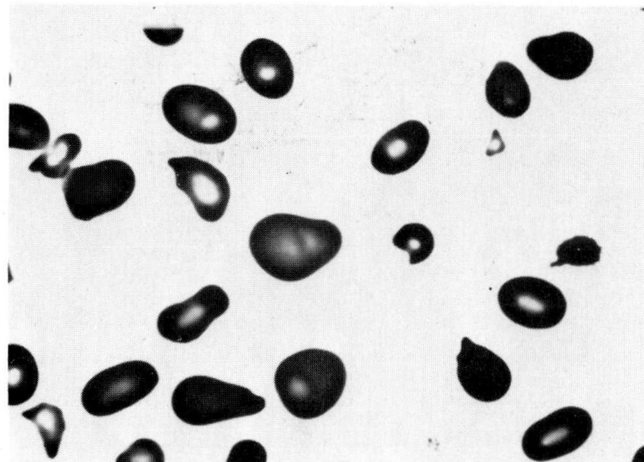

Figure 27–20. Megaloblastic anemia, macrocytosis, marked anisocytosis (×875).

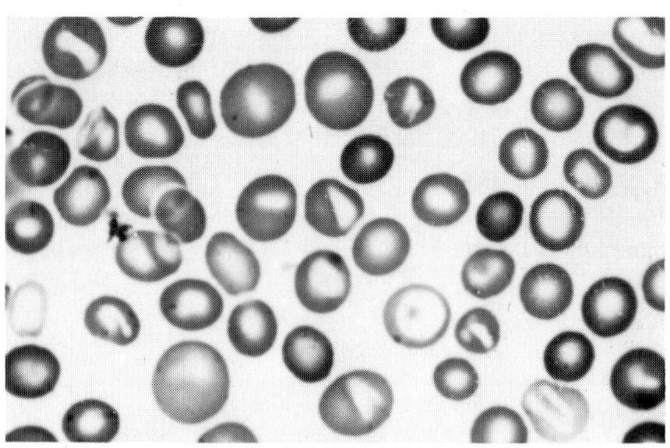

Figure 27–22. Sideroblastic anemia. Dimorphic populations of hypochromic cells and normochromic cells, some of which are macrocytic. Moderate anisocytosis (×875).

27–20). These cells are *hyperchromic* because they have an increased hemoglobin content (MCH), but the hemoglobin concentration (MCHC) is normal. In hereditary spherocytosis the cells are also hyperchromic (Fig. 27–21); though the hemoglobin content (MCH) is normal, the hemoglobin concentration (MCHC) is usually increased because of a reduced surface/volume ratio.

The presence of hypochromic cells and normochromic cells in the same film is called *anisochromia* or, sometimes, a dimorphic anemia (Fig. 27–22). This is characteristic of sideroblastic anemias, but also is found some weeks after iron therapy for iron deficiency anemia or in a hypochromic anemia after transfusion with normal cells.

Polychromatophilia. A blue-gray tint to the red cells (polychromatophilia or polychromasia) is a combination of the affinity of hemoglobin for acid stains and the affinity of RNA for basic stains. The presence of residual RNA in the red cell indicates that it is a young red cell which has been in the blood one to two days. These cells are larger than the mature red cells and may lack the central pallor (Fig. 27–23). Young cells with residual RNA are polychromatophilic red cells on air-dried films stained with Wright's stain but are reticulocytes when stained supravitally with brilliant cresyl blue. Therefore, increased polychromasia implies reticulocytosis; it is most marked in hemolysis and in acute blood loss.

Size. The red cells may be abnormally small or *microcytes* (Figs. 27–18, 27–20, and 27–24), abnormally large or *macrocytes* (Figs. 27–19, 27–20, and 27–22), or show abnormal variation in size (*anisocytosis*) (Figs. 27–18 through 27–24). Anisocytosis is a feature of most anemias; when it is marked in degree, both macrocytes and microcytes are usually present (Figs. 27–19 and 27–20). In analyzing causes of anemia, the terms *microcytic* and *macrocytic* have most meaning when considered as cell volume rather than cell diameter. The mean cell volume, of course, is measured directly on the Coulter Counter Model S, or is calculated from the spun hematocrit and the red cell count. We perceive the diameter directly from the blood film and infer volume (and the hemoglobin content) from it. Thus, the red cells in Figure 27–18 are microcytic; since they are hypochromic they are thinner than normal and the diameter is not decreased proportionately to the volume. Also, the mean cell volume in the blood of the patient with spherocytosis (Fig. 27–21) is in the normal range; though many of

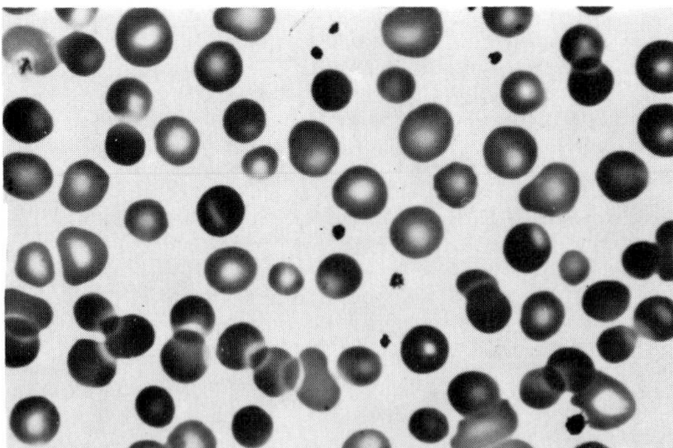

Figure 27–21. Hereditary spherocytosis. The denser cells are more spherocytic. Note that they have minimal and eccentric pallor, moderate anisocytosis. Though the cell diameter is reduced, the MCV is within the normal range (×875).

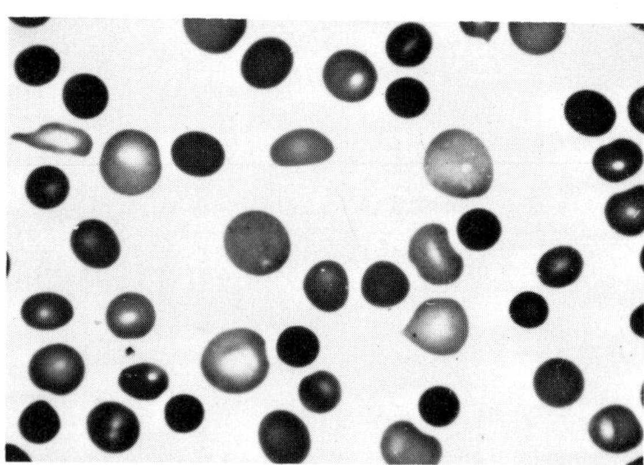

Figure 27–23. Autoimmune hemolytic anemia. The paler, large cells are polychromatic macrocytes (i.e., young reticulocytes.) The small, dense cells are spherocytes. Moderate anisocytosis (×875).

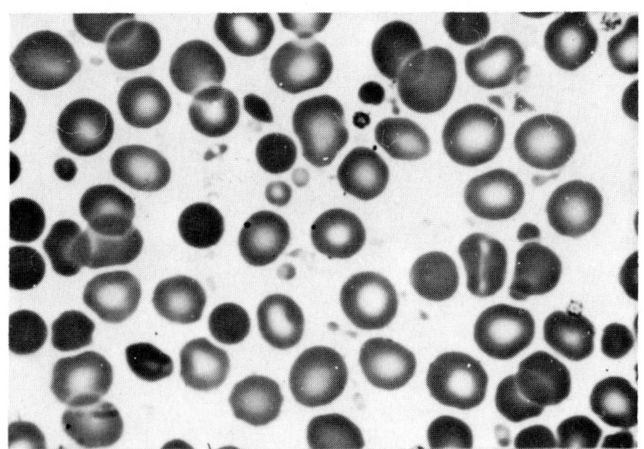

Figure 27–24. Blood film from a patient who has just suffered extensive body burns. Note the many tiny red cell fragments that have budded off the red cells as a result of the heat, leaving spherocytes. Marked anisocytosis (×875).

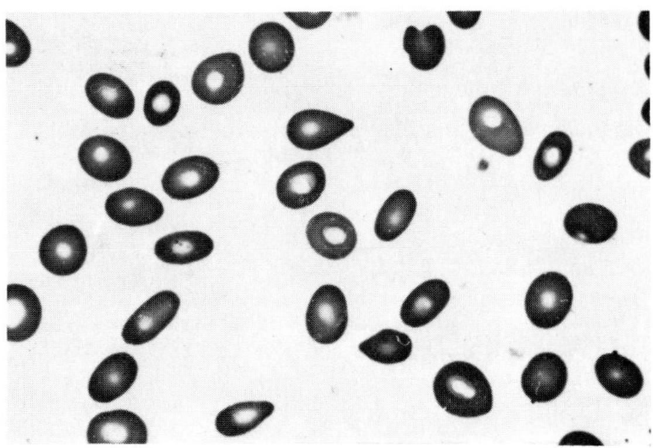

Figure 27–26. Blood film from patients with myelofibrosis with myeloid metaplasia. Numerous elliptocytes. Teardrop-shaped cells (×875).

the cells have a small diameter, their volume is not decreased because they are thicker than normal.

Shape. Variation in shape is called *poikilocytosis.* Any abnormally shaped cell is a poikilocyte. Oval, pear-shaped, tear drop–shaped, saddle-shaped, helmet-shaped, and irregularly shaped cells may be seen in a single case of anemia such as megaloblastic anemia (Figs. 27–19 and 27–20).

Elliptocytes are most abundant in hereditary elliptocytosis (Fig. 27–25), in which the majority of the cells are elliptical; this is a dominant condition that is only occasionally associated with hemolytic anemia. Elliptocytes are seen in normal persons' blood, but number less than 10 per cent of the cells. They are more common, however, in iron deficiency anemia, myelofibrosis with myeloid metaplasia (Figs. 27–26 and 27–27), megaloblastic anemias (Figs. 27–19 and 27–20), and sickle cell anemia.

Spherocytes are nearly spherical erythrocytes in contradistinction to normal biconcave disks. Their diameter is smaller than normal. They lack the central pale area or have a smaller, often eccentric, pale area (because the cell is thicker and can come to rest somewhat tilted instead of perfectly flattened on the slide). They are found in hereditary spherocytosis (HS, Fig. 27–21), in some cases of acquired hemolytic anemia (AHA, Fig. 27–23), and in some conditions in which there has been a direct physical or chemical injury to the cells, such as heat (Fig. 27–24). In each of these three instances tiny bits of membrane (in excess of hemoglobin) are removed from the adult red cells, leaving the cell with a decreased surface/volume ratio. In HS and AHA this occurs in the reticuloendothelial system; in other instances (e.g., the patient with body burns), this may occur intravascularly.

Target cells are erythrocytes that are thinner than normal (leptocytes) and when stained show a peripheral rim of hemoglobin with a dark, central, hemoglobin-containing area. They are found in obstructive jaundice (e.g., Fig. 27–28), in which there appears to be an augmentation of the cell surface membrane; in the postsplenectomy state, in which there is a lack of normal reduction of surface membrane as the cell ages; in any hypochromic anemia, especially thalassemia; and in hemoglobin C disease.

Schistocytes (cell fragments) indicate the presence of hemolysis, whether in megaloblastic anemia (Fig. 27–20), severe burns (Fig. 27–24) or microangiopathic hemolytic anemia (Fig. 27–29). The latter process is associated with either small blood vessel disease or fibrin in small blood vessels and results in intravascular fragmentation; particularly characteristic are helmet cells and triangularly shaped cells. Burr cells are

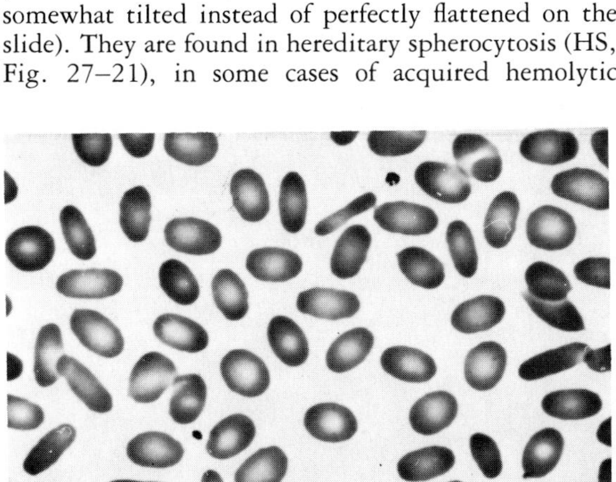

Figure 27–25. Hereditary elliptocytosis. Incidental finding, no anemia (×875).

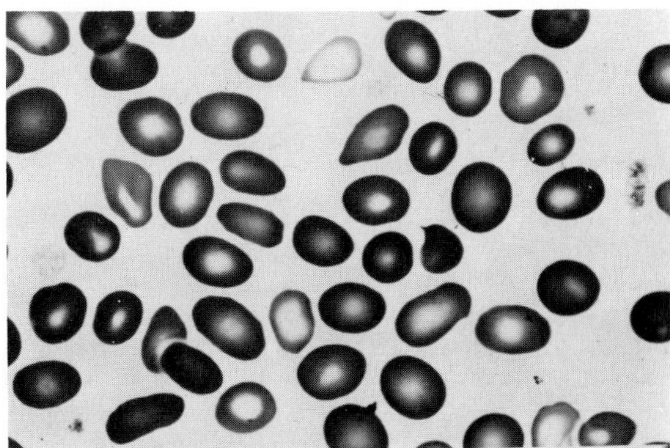

Figure 27–27. Same as Figure 27–26. A few hypochromic microcytic cells are present also (×875).

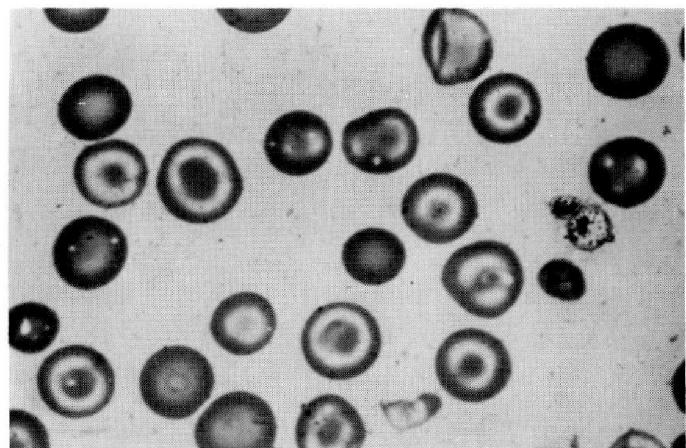

Figure 27–28. Target cells that have an increased cell diameter. Blood film from a patient with obstructive jaundice (×875).

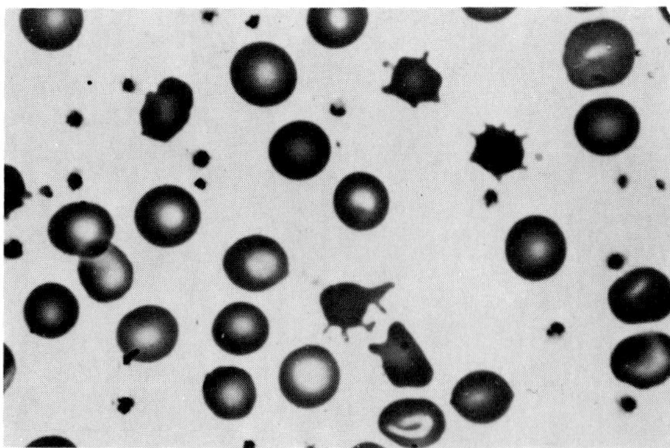

Figure 27–30. Acanthocytes. Note the long spicules, which tend to have bulbous ends (×875).

irregularly contracted red cells with prominent spicules and are seen in the same process; however, this term is used differently by different hematologists, and therefore leads to confusion.

Acanthocytes are irregularly spiculated red cells in which the ends of the spicules are bulbous and rounded (Fig. 27–30); they are seen in abetalipoproteinemia, hereditary or acquired, and certain cases of liver disease. *Crenated cells* or echinocytes (Fig. 27–31) are regularly contracted cells which may commonly occur as an artifact during preparation of films, or may be due to hyperosmolarity, or to the discocyte-echinocyte transformation. *In vivo* the latter may be associated with decreased red cell ATP due to any of several causes (Brecher, 1972).

Artifacts resembling crenated cells consisting of tiny pits or bubbles indenting the red cells (Fig. 27–32) may be caused by a small amount of water contaminating the Wright's stain (or absolute methanol, if this is used first as a fixative).

Structure

Basophilic Stippling (Punctate Basophilia). This is characterized by the presence, within the erythrocyte, of irregular basophilic granules, which vary from fine to coarse (Fig. 27–33). They stain deep blue with Wright's stain. The erythrocyte containing them may stain normally in other respects or it may exhibit polychromatophilia. Fine stippling is commonly seen when there is increased polychromatophilia, and, therefore, with increased production of red cells. Coarse stippling may be seen in lead poisoning or other diseases with impaired hemoglobin synthesis, in megaloblastic anemia, and in other forms of severe anemia; it is attributed to an abnormal instability of the RNA in the young cell.

Red cells with inorganic iron-containing granules (as demonstrated by stains for iron) are called *siderocytes.* Sometimes these granules stain with Wright's stain; if so, they are called *Pappenheimer bodies.* In contrast to basophilic stippling, Pappenheimer bodies are few in number in a given red cell and are rarely seen in the peripheral blood except after splenectomy.

Howell-Jolly Bodies. These particles are smooth, round remnants of nuclear chromatin. Single Howell-Jolly bodies may be seen in megaloblastic anemia, in hemolytic anemia, and after splenectomy. Multiple Howell-Jolly bodies in a single cell (Fig. 27–34) usually indicate megaloblastic anemia or some other form of abnormal erythropoiesis.

Cabot Rings. These are ring-shaped, figure-of-eight, or loop-shaped structures. Occasionally they are formed by double or several concentric lines. They are observed rarely in erythrocytes in pernicious anemia,

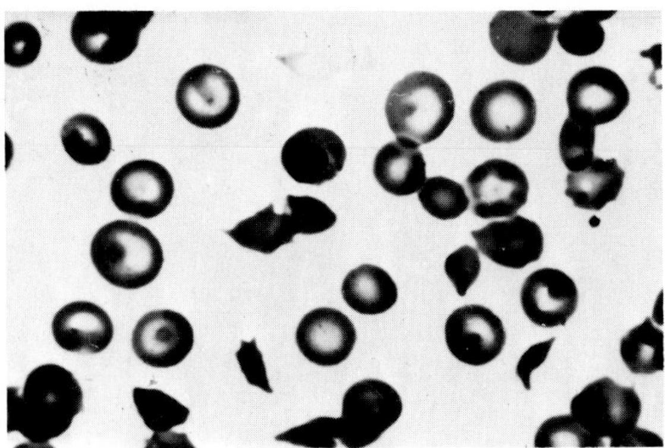

Figure 27–29. Microangiopathic hemolytic anemia; hemolytic-uremic syndrome. Note irregularly contracted cells, schistocytes, a few crenated cells. One nucleated red cell (×875).

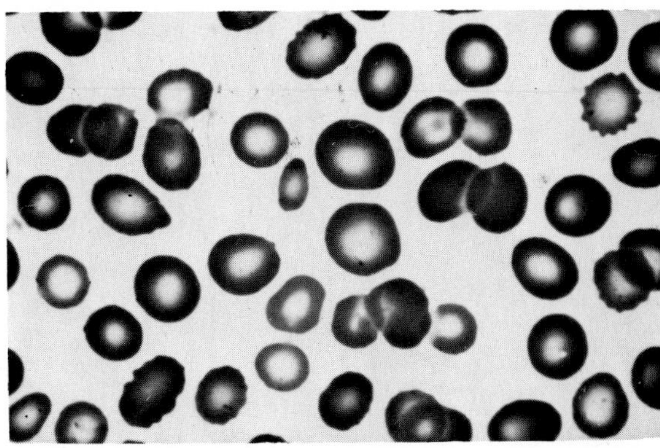

Figure 27–31. Megaloblastic anemia. A few crenated cells are present (×875).

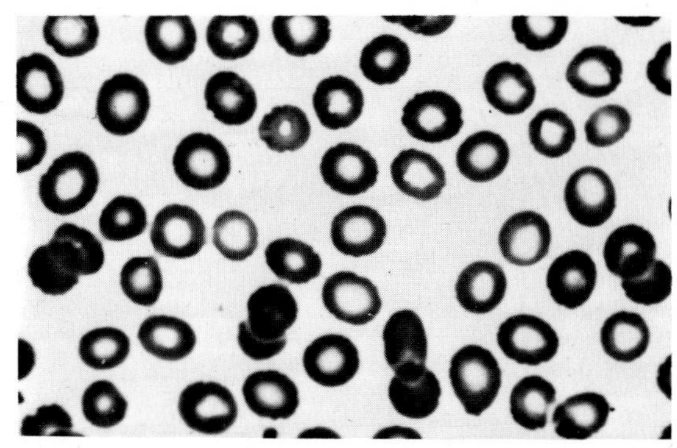

Figure 27–32. Artifact due to water in the methyl alcohol fixative. If bubbles are small in size (as here) they cause an indented appearance which may be confused with crenation (×875).

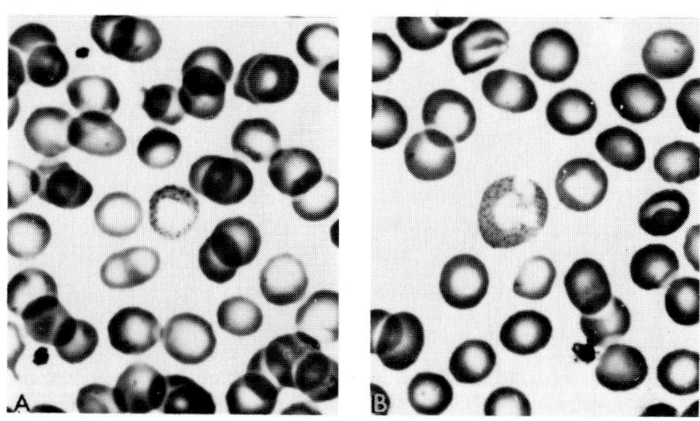

Figure 27–33. Basophilic stippling. One stippled red cell in the center of each field. *A*, thalassemia minor; *B*, lead poisoning (×875).

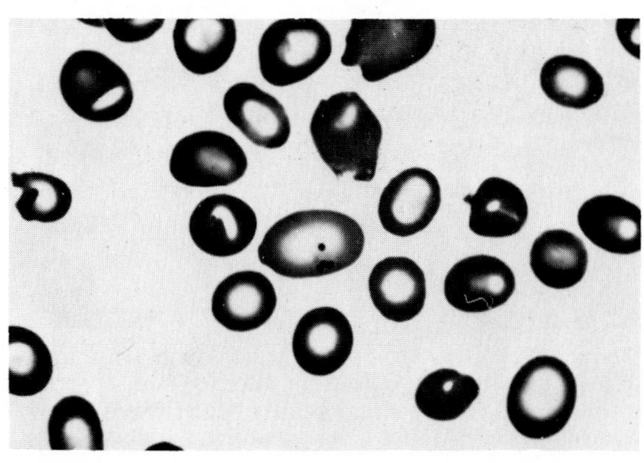

Figure 27–34. Megaloblastic anemia. The central oval macrocyte has four Howell-Jolly bodies; the lower three are touching one another (×875).

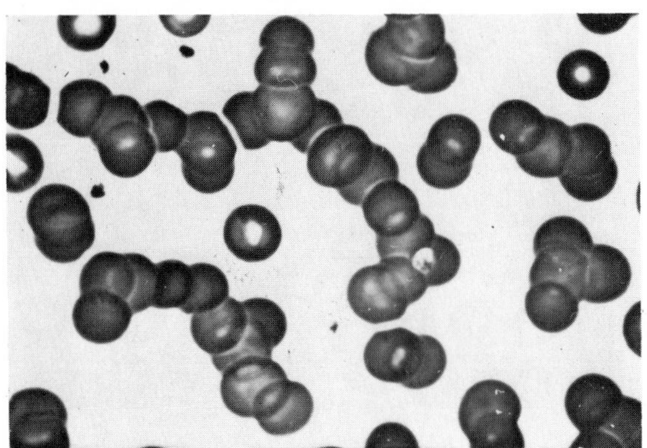

Figure 27–35. Rouleaux in a blood film from a patient with multiple myeloma (×875).

lead poisoning, and certain other disorders of erythropoiesis. They stain red or reddish purple with Wright's stain and have no internal structure. The rings are probably microtubules remaining from a mitotic spindle (Bessis, 1977). They are interpreted as evidence of abnormal erythropoiesis.

Malarial Stippling. Fine granules may appear in erythrocytes that harbor *Plasmodium vivax.* With Wright's stain the minute granules, "Schüffner's granules," stain purplish red. They are sometimes so numerous that they almost hide the parasites. These red cells are, as a rule, larger than normal.

Rouleau Formation. This is the alignment of red cells one upon another so that they resemble stacks of coins in wet preparations. On air-dried films, rouleaux appear as in Figure 27–35. Elevated plasma fibrinogen or globulins cause rouleaux to form and, because of this, also promote an increase in the erythrocyte sedimentation rate. Rouleau formation is especially marked in paraproteinemia (monoclonal gammopathy). *Agglutination* or clumping of red cells is more surely separated from rouleaux in wet preparations, but on air-dried films (Fig. 27–36) tends to show more irregular and round clumps than the linear rouleaux. Cold agglutinins are responsible for this appearance.

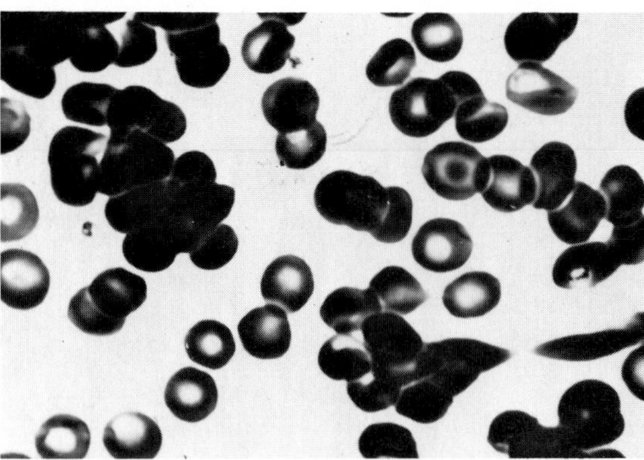

Figure 27–36. Blood film from a patient with a high titer of cold agglutinins. Red cells aggregate in clumps. Separation of cells during making the film may distort the cells (lower right) (×875).

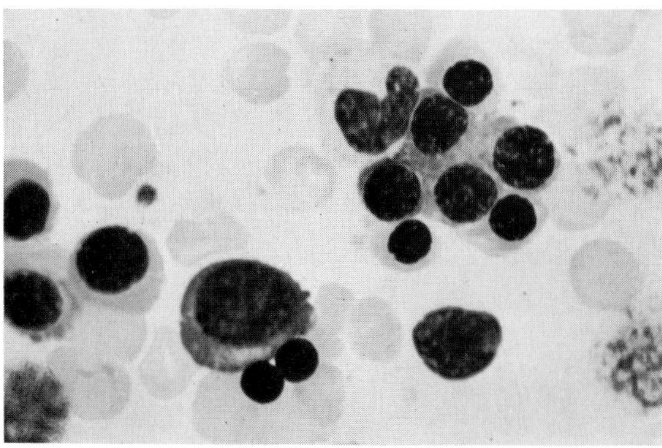

Figure 27–37. Normoblasts in the marrow from a patient with hemolytic anemia. Largest cell is a basophilic normoblast (×875).

Nucleated Red Cells. In contrast to erythrocytes of lower vertebrates and to most mammalian cells, a unique characteristic of the mammalian erythrocyte is the absence of a nucleus.

Nucleated red cells (*normoblasts*) are precursors of the non-nucleated mature red cells in the blood. In the human, normoblasts are normally present only in the bone marrow (Fig. 27–37). The stages in their production (p. 629) from the earliest to the latest are the pronormoblast, basophilic normoblast, polychromatophilic normoblast, and orthochromatic normoblast.

In general, nucleated red cells that might appear in the blood in disease are polychromatic normoblasts. In some, however, the cytoplasm is so basophilic that it is difficult to recognize the cell as erythroid except by the character of the nucleus: intensely staining chromatin, and sharp separation of chromatin from parachromatin. Such erythroid cells are often mistaken for lymphocytes, an error that usually can be prevented by careful observation of the nucleus. The *megaloblast* (Fig. 27–38) is a distinct, nucleated erythroid cell, not merely a larger normoblast. It is characterized by large size and abnormal "open" nuclear chromatin pattern. Cells of this series are not found in normal marrow but are characteristically present in the marrow and sometimes the blood of patients with pernicious anemia or other megaloblastic anemia (p. 657).

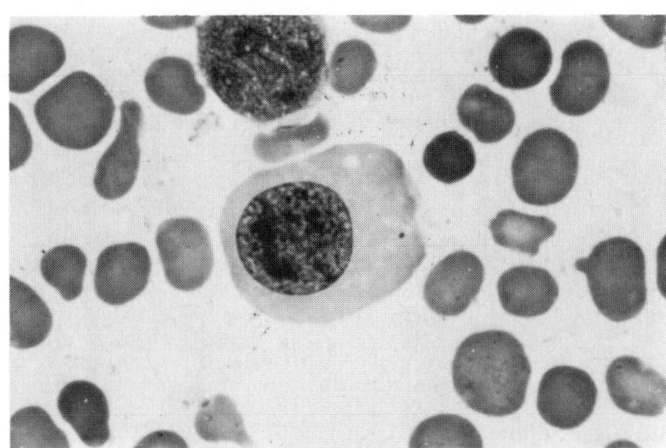

Figure 27–38. Polychromatic megaloblast. Above: "smudge cell" (damaged nucleus; no cytoplasm) (×875).

Significance of Nucleated Erythrocytes. Normoblasts are present normally only in the blood of the fetus and of very young infants. In the healthy adult they are confined to the bone marrow and appear in the circulating blood only in disease, in which their presence usually denotes an extreme demand made on the marrow, extramedullary hematopoiesis, or marrow replacement. Large numbers of circulating nucleated red cells are particularly found in hemolytic disease of the newborn (erythroblastosis fetalis, p. 694) and thalassemia major (p. 683). In the latter, circulating normoblasts may be extremely numerous, which led to an older name for the condition, "erythroblastic anemia."

Leukoerythroblastotic Reaction. The presence of normoblasts and immature cells of the neutrophilic series in the blood is known as a *"leukoerythroblastotic reaction."* This often indicates space-occupying disturbances of the marrow, such as myelofibrosis with myeloid metaplasia, metastatic carcinoma, leukemias, multiple myeloma, Gaucher's disease, and others. Nonetheless, in the study of Weick (1974), over a third of the patients with a leukoerythroblastotic reaction did not have malignant or potentially malignant disease (Table 27–3). In patients with metastatic malignancy, a leukoerythroblastotic reaction is good evidence for marrow involvement by tumor.

The presence of megaloblasts indicates a change in the type of blood formation. This is seen most characteristically in pernicious anemia and other megaloblastic anemias. It indicates the presence of megaloblasts in the marrow and is therefore an important clue.

Leukocytes

DIFFERENTIAL LEUKOCYTE COUNT

Before evaluating leukocytes on the Romanowsky-stained blood film, one should first determine that the film is well made, the distribution of the cells is uniform, and the staining of cells is satisfactory. Learning to identify normal cells with low power (100 × magnification) as well as with the oil immersion lens (1000 ×) will enable one to find abnormal cells readily when they are present.

One first scans the counting area of the slide and in wedge films, the lateral and feather edges where monocytes, neutrophils, and large abnormal cells (if present) tend to be disproportionately represented. Suspicious cells are detected at 100 × magnification, and confirmed at high power. Since nucleated red cells, macrophages, immature granulocytes, immature lymphoid cells, megakaryocytes, and abnormal cells are not normally found in blood, they should be recorded if present.

While scanning under low power, it is advisable to estimate the leukocyte count from the film. Even though it is a crude approximation, it sometimes enables one to detect errors in total count. One then proceeds to determine the percentage distribution of the different types of leukocytes, which is known as the differential leukocyte count. In the crenellation technique of counting, the field of view is moved from side to side across the width of the slide in the "counting area," just behind the feather edge, where the red cells are separated from one another and are free of artifacts. As each leukocyte is encountered, it is classified, until 100, 200, 500, or 1000 leukocytes have been counted. The greater the number of cells counted, the greater the precision (Table 27–4), but for practical reasons 100 or 200 cell counts are usually made. Another technique is to count all the cells as the field of view is moved longitudinally from the thick end of the feather end, encompassing the cells from one part of the original drop of blood. The

Table 27–3. CONDITIONS ASSOCIATED WITH LEUKOERYTHROBLASTOSIS

0.63	0.26	Solid tumors and lymphomas
	0.24	Myeloproliferative disorders including CML
	0.13	Acute leukemias
0.37	0.03	Benign hematologic conditions
	0.08	Hemolysis
	0.26	Miscellaneous, including blood loss

Data are from Weick, J. K., Hagedorn, A. B., and Linman, J. W.: Leukoerythroblastosis: Diagnostic and prognostic significance. Mayo Clin. Proc., *49*:110, 1974.

Proportions are based on a series of 215 cases discovered in a prospective study of 50,277 blood film examinations in a six-month period, a proportion of 0.004.

CML = Chronic myeloid leukemia.

Table 27–4. NINETY-FIVE PER CENT CONFIDENCE LIMITS FOR THE PERCENTAGE OF CELLS WITH A PARTICULAR CHARACTERISTIC, GIVEN THAT *a* PER CENT OF CELLS WITH THIS CHARACTERISTIC ARE FOUND IN A STUDY OF *n* CELLS*

	n							
a	**100**		**200**		**500**		**1000**	
0	0	4	0	2	0	1	0	1
1	0	6	0	4	0	3	0	2
2	0	8	0	6	0	4	1	4
3	0	9	1	7	1	5	2	5
4	1	10	1	8	2	7	2	6
5	1	12	2	10	3	8	3	7
6	2	13	3	11	4	9	4	8
7	2	14	3	12	4	10	5	9
8	3	16	4	13	5	11	6	10
9	4	17	5	14	6	12	7	11
10	4	18	6	16	7	13	8	13
15	8	24	10	21	12	19	12	18
20	12	30	14	27	16	24	17	23
25	16	35	19	32	21	30	22	28
30	21	40	23	37	26	35	27	33
35	25	46	28	43	30	40	32	39
40	30	51	33	48	35	45	36	44
45	35	56	38	53	40	50	41	49
50	39	61	42	58	45	55	46	54

*For n = 100, the confidence limits were calculated exactly; for n over 100, with $a \times n$ over 2000, the normal approximation was applied; and for n over 100 with $a \times n$ under 2000, Poisson's approximation was used.

For x over 50, obtain confidence limits by reading limits for 100 — x in the table and subtracting them from 100. For example, the confidence limits for 75 per cent in a sample of n = 100 are 65 and 84.

From C. L. Rümke: Variability of results in differential counts on blood smears. Triangle, the Sandoz Journal of Medical Science, *4*:156, 1960.

4

Table 27–5. ABSOLUTE LEUKOCYTE COUNTS, 95 PER CENT REFERENCE INTERVALS, ADULTS

	(1)	(2)	(3)
Total leukocytes	4.5 –10.1 Wh 3.6 –10.2 Bl	4.5 –11.0 Wh 3.8 –10.0 Bl	4.5–11.0
Neutrophil bands	0.2 – 2.1 Wh 0.06– 1.6 Bl	0 – 0.96 Wh 0 – 0.6 Bl	0– 0.7
Neutrophils	1.5 – 6.0 Wh 1.1 – 6.7 Bl	1.6 – 6.9 Wh 1.2 – 6.0 Bl	1.8– 7.0
Eosinophils	0 – 0.7	0 –0.6	0–0.45
Basophils	0 – 0.15	0 – 0.19	0–0.2
Lymphocytes	1.5 – 4.0	1.2 – 3.9	1.0– 4.8
Monocytes	0.2 – 0.95	0.12– 1.2 (Sp) 0.1 – 0.8 (We)	0– 0.8

Data from three studies giving absolute leukocyte count (cells × 10^9/L):

(1) Orfanakis, et al., 1970: Based on 200 cell differential counts on coverslip preparations, electronic total leukocyte counts; 226 whites (Wh), 65 blacks (Bl); Salt Lake City, Utah.

(2) Our data: Based on 100 cell differential counts on wedge films (We) and spinner films (Sp) which are similar except for monocytes, electronic total leukocyte counts; 300 white young adults (Wh), 56 black adolescents (Bl); Syracuse, New York.

(3) Altman and Dittmer, 1961: Data compiled from the literature, for 21-year-old individuals.

disadvantage of this latter method is the difficulty in identifying contracted, heavily stained cells in the thicker part of the film.

A record of the count may be kept by placing a mark for each leukocyte on paper, or by using a mechanical or electronic tabulator. Leukocytes that cannot be classified should be placed together in an unidentified group. In some conditions, notably leukemia, there may be many of these unidentified leukocytes. During the differential leukocyte counting procedure the morphology of erythrocytes and platelets is examined and the number of platelets is estimated.

The absolute concentration of each variety of leukocyte is its percentage times the total leukocyte count. An increase in absolute concentration is an *absolute increase;* an increase in percentage only is a *relative increase.* With a low total leukocyte count, for example, the neutrophil count may be relatively normal (normal percentage) but absolutely decreased. Reference intervals are more useful if given as absolute concentrations rather than percentages (Table 27–5).

LEUKOCYTES NORMALLY PRESENT IN BLOOD

Neutrophil (Polymorphonuclear Neutrophilic Leukocyte; Segmented Neutrophilic Granulocyte). Neutrophils average 12 μm in diameter; they are smaller than monocytes and eosinophils and slightly larger than basophils. The nucleus stains deeply; it is irregular and often assumes shapes comparable to such letters as E, Z, and S. What appear to be separate nuclei normally are segments of nuclear material connected by delicate filaments.

A filament has length but no breadth as one focuses up and down. A *segmented neutrophil* has at least two of its lobes separated by a filament. A *band neutrophil* has either a strand of nuclear material thicker than a filament (as described above) connecting the lobes, or a U-shaped nucleus of uniform thickness. The nucleus in both types of neutrophil has coarse blocks of chromatin and rather sharply defined parachromatin spaces. If, because of overlapping of nuclear material, it is not possible to be certain whether or not a filament is present, the cell should be placed in the segmented category (Mathy, 1974). The number of lobes in normal neutrophils ranges from two to five, with a median of three.

The cytoplasm, itself colorless, is packed full of tiny granules (0.2 to 0.3 μm) that stain tan to pink with Wright's stain (Fig. 27–39*A* and Plate 27–1). About two thirds of these are specific granules and one third azurophil granules. The intensity of the red-blue or purple staining of the azurophil granules in the more immature neutrophils (p. 636) has diminished; with light microscopy the two types of granules often cannot be distinguished in the mature cell.

Segmented neutrophils average 56 per cent of

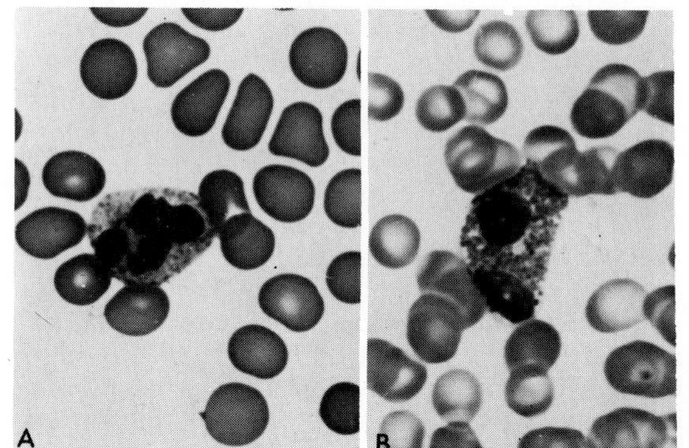

Figure 27–39. *A,* Neutrophil. The cytoplasm is filled with tiny granules, some of which stain more deeply than others (toxic granulation). Note that most of the red cells lack central pallor, an artifact seen near the feather edge of the film. *B,* Eosinophil. Typically this cell has fewer nuclear lobes and larger cytoplasmic granules than the neutrophil (×875).

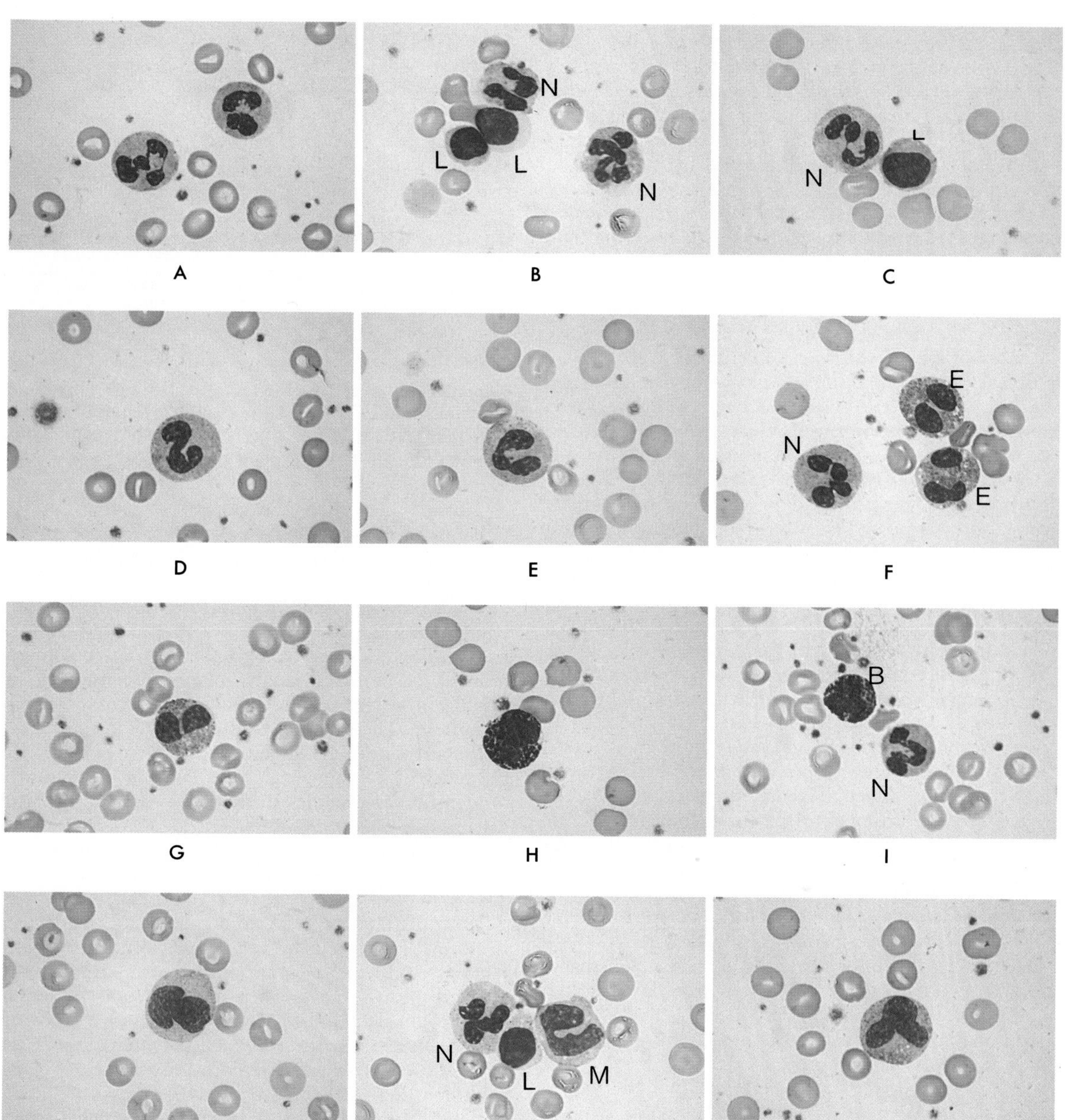

Plate 27–1. These photomicrographs are from buffy coat preparations of blood from a normal individual. The number of leukocytes and platelets per field, therefore, is greater than in blood films made directly. *A,* Neutrophils. The cell on the right has a few nuclear spicules or extensions. These rather pointed spicules are directed toward the centrosomal region of the cell. Such nuclear extensions may be found in normal individuals but are more frequent in those with chronic illnesses (Bessis, 1977). They should be distinguished from the sex chromatin appendages, which have a drumstick appearance. *B,* Lymphocytes (L) of slightly different size and chromatin condensation, and neutrophils (N). *C,* Neutrophil (N) and lymphocyte (L). *D and E,* Band neutrophils. In *E,* note the incomplete segmentation. *F,* Neutrophil (N) and eosinophils (E). Eosinophils have larger granules and, on the average, fewer lobes than do neutrophils. *G,* Eosinophil. *H,* Basophil. *I,* Basophil (B); neutrophil (N). *J,* Monocyte. *K,* Neutrophil (N); lymphocyte (L); monocyte (M). The monocyte has more delicately staining chromatin than the other cells; this usually can be appreciated at low magnification. *L,* Monocyte.

leukocytes; reference intervals are 1.5 to 7.0 × 10^9/L in white adults but have a lower limit of about 1.1 × 10^9/L in blacks. Band neutrophils average 3 per cent of leukocytes; the upper reference value is about 1.0 × 10^9/L in whites and slightly lower in blacks (using the above definition and counting 100 cells in the differential, Table 27–5).

Normally about 10 to 30 per cent of the segmented neutrophils have two lobes, 40 to 50 per cent have three lobes, 10 to 20 per cent four, and no more than 5 per cent have five lobes. A "shift to the left" occurs when there are increased bands and less mature neutrophils in the blood, as well as a lower average number of lobes in segmented cells.

Neutrophil production and physiology are discussed on page 638. Neutrophilia or neutrophilic leukocytosis is an increase in the absolute count, and neutropenia is a decrease; they are discussed in Chapter 30.

Eosinophil (Eosinophilic Granulocyte). Eosinophils average 13 μm in diameter. The structure of these cells is similar to that of the polymorphonuclear neutrophils, with the striking difference that, instead of the neutrophilic granules, their cytoplasm contains larger round or oval granules having a strong affinity for acid stains (Fig. 27–39*B* and Plate 27–1*F* and *G*). They are easily recognized by the size and color of the granules, which stain bright red with eosin. The cytoplasm is colorless. The nucleus stains somewhat less deeply than that of the neutrophils and usually has two connected segments, rarely more than three.

Eosinophils average 3 per cent of the leukocytes in adults and the upper reference value is 0.6 × 10^9/L when calculated from the differential count. If allergic individuals are excluded, and if direct hemacytometer counts of eosinophils are performed, the upper limit is probably 0.35 × 10^9/L or 350/μl (Beeson, 1977). The lower reference value is probably 40/μl; a decrease in eosinophils (eosinopenia) can be detected only by counting large numbers of cells as in direct hemacytometer counts (Dacie, 1975) or with a flow-through automated differential counter (p. 618).

Eosinophilia, an increase in eosinophils, and eosinopenia are discussed on page 710.

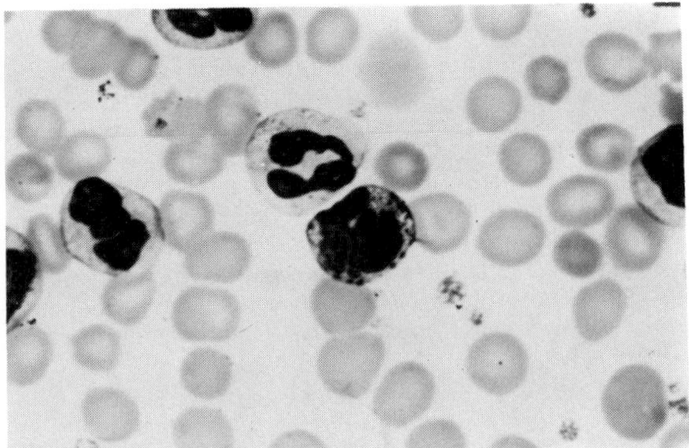

Figure 27–40. Neutrophil (below) and basophil (above). The basophil is smaller, has large deeply basophilic granules which often can be partially washed out, leaving vacuoles (×875).

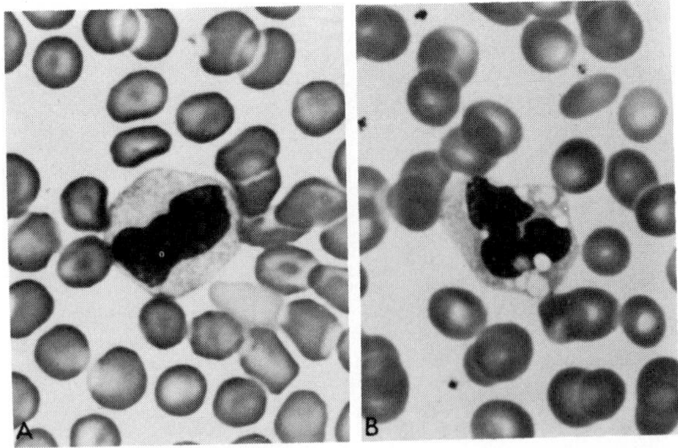

Figure 27–41. *A* and *B*, Monocytes. Of the normal blood cells, the monocyte is the largest and has the most delicate chromatin pattern; it has a propensity to form cytoplasmic vacuoles *(B)* which usually indicate phagocytosis (×875).

Basophil (Basophilic Granulocyte). In general, basophils resemble neutrophils, except that the nucleus is less segmented (usually merely indented or partially lobulated) and granules are larger and have a strong affinity for basic stains (Fig. 27–40 and Plate 27–1*H* and *I*). They are easily recognized. In some basophils, most of the granules may be missing because they are soluble in water, leaving vacuoles or openings in the cytoplasm. The granules then are a mauve color. In a well-stained film the granules are deep purple, and the nucleus is somewhat paler and is often nearly hidden by the granules so that its form is difficult to distinguish.

Unevenly stained granules of basophils may be ring shaped and resemble *Histoplasma capsulatum* or protozoa.

Basophils are the least numerous of the leukocytes in normal blood and average 0.5 per cent of the total leukocytes. The 95 per cent reference values for adults are 0 to 0.2 × 10^9/L when derived from the differential count. Direct hemacytometer counts employing Alcian blue (Gilbert, 1975) or the Hemalog D (p. 618) allow a narrower reference interval of 10 to 80 per microliter (0.01 to 0.08 × 10^9/L).

Basophilia (basophilic leukocytosis) and basopenia (decreased absolute basophil count) are discussed on page 000.

Monocyte. The monocyte is the largest cell of normal blood (Fig. 27–41 and Plate 27–1*J*, *K*, and *L*). It generally is about two to three times the diameter of an erythrocyte (14 to 20 μm), although smaller monocytes sometimes are encountered. It contains a single nucleus, which is partially lobulated, deeply indented, or horseshoe-shaped. Occasionally the nucleus of a monocyte may appear round or oval.

The cytoplasm is abundant. The nuclear chromatin often appears to be in fine, parallel strands separated by sharply defined parachromatin. The nucleus stains less densely than that of other leukocytes. The cytoplasm is blue-gray and has a ground glass appearance and often contains fine red to purple granules that are less distinct and smaller than the granules of neutrophils. Occasionally blue granules may be seen.

When the monocyte transforms into a macrophage, it becomes larger (20 to 40 μm); the nucleus may become oval and the chromatin more reticular or dispersed so that nucleoli may be visible (Plate 27–2*I*). A perinuclear clear zone (Golgi) may be evident. The fine red or azurophil granules are variable in number or may have disappeared. The more abundant cytoplasm tends to be irregular at the cell margins and to contain vacuoles. These are phagocytic vacuoles, which may contain ingested red cells, debris, pigment, or bacteria. Evidence of phagocytosis in monocytes or the presence of macrophages in directly made blood films is pathologic and often indicates the presence of active infection.

Monocytes average 4 per cent of leukocytes and the reference interval for adults is approximately 0.15 to 1.0 × 10^9/L, depending on the method of performing the differential count (Table 27–5).

Monocyte production is discussed on page 640. An increase in monocytes (monocytosis) and a decrease (monocytopenia) are discussed beginning on page 712.

Lymphocyte. Lymphocytes are mononuclear cells without specific cytoplasmic granules. Small lymphocytes are about the size of an erythrocyte or slightly larger (6 to 10 μm) (Plates 27–1 and 27–2). The typical lymphocyte has a single, sharply defined nucleus containing heavy blocks of chromatin. The chromatin stains dark blue with Wright's stain, while the parachromatin stands out as lighter stained streaks; at the periphery of the nucleus, the chromatin is condensed. Characteristically there is a gradual transition or "smudging" between the chromatin and the parachromatin. The nucleus is generally round but is sometimes indented at one side. The cytoplasm stains pale blue except for a clear perinuclear zone.

Larger lymphocytes, 12 to 15 μm in diameter, with less densely staining nuclei and more abundant cytoplasm, are frequently found, especially in the blood of children, and may be difficult to distinguish from monocytes. The misshapen, indented cytoplasmic margins of lymphocytes are due to pressure of neighboring cells. In the cytoplasm of about one third of the large lymphocytes, a few round, red-purple granules are present. They are larger than the granules of neutrophilic leukocytes (Fig. 27–42). It

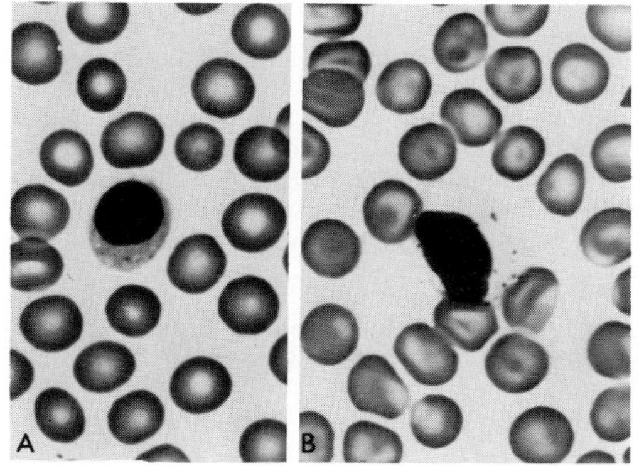

Figure 27–42. *A*, Small lymphocyte. *B*, Larger lymphocyte with granules; note that many of the red cells are target cells (×875).

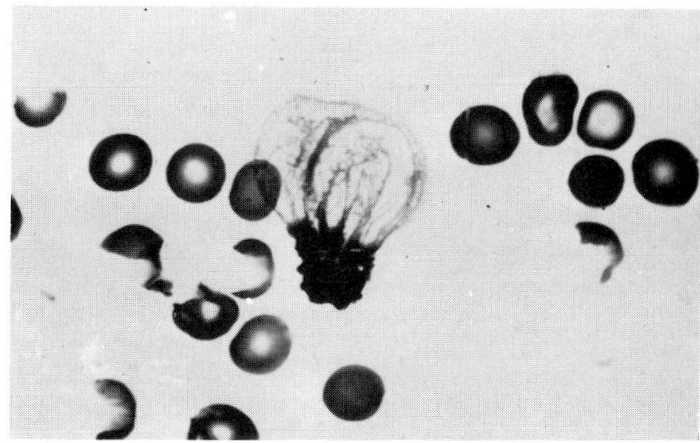

Figure 27–43. Basket cells. This is a nuclear remnant from a damaged or broken cell (×875).

appears that there is a continuous spectrum of sizes between small and large lymphocytes, and, indeed, there can be a transition from small to large to blast forms as well as the reverse (Plate 27–2*J* and K). It does not appear to be meaningful to classify small lymphocytes and large lymphocytes separately in differential counting. The presence of a significant proportion of atypical lymphocytes and the presence of blast forms (non-leukemic lymphoblasts; reticular lymphocytes) must be noted; these findings indicate transformation of lymphoid cells as a response to antigenic stimulation (p. 645).

Plasma cells have abundant blue cytoplasm, often with light streaks or vacuoles, an eccentric round nucleus, and a well-defined clear (Golgi) zone adjacent to the nucleus (Plate 27–2*H*). The nucleus of the plasma cell has heavily clumped chromatin, which is sharply defined from the parachromatin, and often arranged in a radial or "wheel-like" pattern. Plasma cells are not present normally in blood.

Lymphocytes average 34 per cent of all leukocytes, and range from 1.5 to 4 × 10^9/L in adults.

The lymphocytes and their derivatives, the plasma cells, operate in the immune defenses of the body. Lymphocytosis is discussed beginning on page 713, plasmacytosis on page 719.

4

ARTIFACTS

Broken Cells. Damaged or broken leukocytes constitute a small proportion of the nucleated cells in normal blood. Bare nuclei from ruptured cells vary from fairly well preserved nuclei without cytoplasm to smudged nuclear material (Plate 27–2*G*), sometimes with strands arranged in a coarse network, the so-called basket cells (Fig. 27–43). They probably represent fragile cells, usually lymphocytes, that have been broken in preparing the film. They are apt to be numerous when there is an atypical lymphocytosis (p. 718), in chronic lymphocytic leukemia, and in acute leukemias.

Degenerative Changes. As EDTA-blood stands in the test tube, changes in leukocyte morphology begin to take place (Sacker, 1975). The degree of change varies among cells and in different individuals. Within a half hour the nuclei of neutrophils may begin to swell, with some loss of chromatin structure. Cyto-

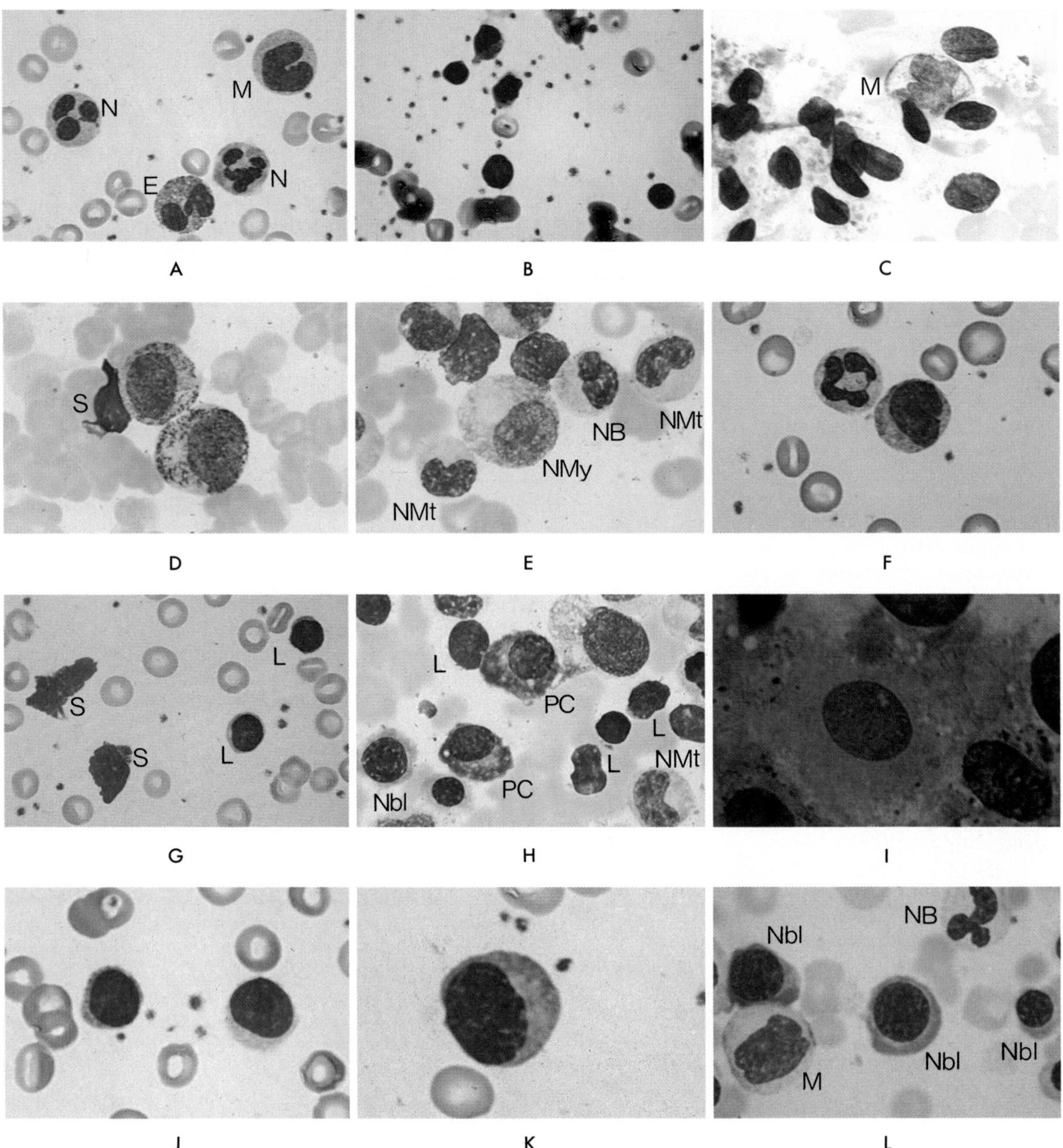

Plate 27–2. Photomicrographs *A, B, F, G, J,* and *K* are from buffy coat preparations from a normal individual. As in Plate 27–1, the number of leukocytes and platelets per field is greater than in blood films made directly. *A,* Neutrophils (N), eosinophil (E), and monocyte (M) are easily identifiable in this thin, well-spread area of film. *B,* Thick area of same film as Plate 27–2*A*, same magnification. Slow drying and shrinkage has made cell identification much less certain. *C,* Endothelial cells and a monocyte (M) at the feather edge of a normal blood film. Endothelial cells have an oval nucleus that is folded or "creased" and abundant, ill-defined cytoplasm. *D,* Two neutrophil myelocytes and the nucleus of a broken or smudged cell (S). Normal marrow. *E,* Neutrophil myelocytes (NMy), neutrophil metamyelocytes (NMt), and neutrophil band forms (NB). Normal marrow. *F,* Monocyte (right) and neutrophil (left). *G,* Lymphocytes (L) and broken, smudged nuclei (S). *H,* Plasma cells (PC), normoblasts (Nbl), lymphocytes (L), neutrophil metamyelocyte (NMt); normal marrow. *I,* Macrophage. These cells have reticular nuclei and abundant cytoplasm containing scattered pigment granules. Bone marrow. *J,* Lymphocytes. *K,* Atypical lymphocyte. Increased cytoplasmic basophilia and more distinct separation of chromatin from parachromatin distinguish this "activated lymphocyte" from resting normal lymphocytes *(J)*. *L,* Normoblasts (Nbl), monocyte (M), and neutrophil band (NB). Normal marrow.

plasmic vacuoles appear especially in monocytes and neutrophils. Nuclear lobulation appears in mononuclear cells; deep clefts may cause the nucleus to resemble a clover leaf (radial segmentation of the nuclei; Rieder cells). Finally, loss of the cytoplasm and a smudged nucleus may be all that remains to be seen of the cell.

Degenerative changes occur more rapidly in oxalated blood than in EDTA-blood. They arise more rapidly with increasing concentrations of EDTA, such as occur when evacuated blood collection tubes (with a given amount of EDTA) are incompletely filled.

Contracted Cells. In the thicker part of wedge films, drying is slow. Obvious changes in the film are rouleaux of the erythrocytes and shrinkage of the leukocytes. Since the leukocytes are contracted and heavily stained, mononuclear cells are difficult to distinguish from one another. Optimal cell identification is usually impossible in these areas (Plate 27–2*B*).

Endothelial Cells. Endothelial cells from the lining of the blood vessel may appear in the first drop of blood from a fingerstick specimen, or, rarely, in venous blood (Plate 27–2*C*). They have an immature reticular chromatin pattern and may be mistaken for histiocytes or for tumor cells.

SOURCES OF ERROR IN THE DIFFERENTIAL LEUKOCYTE COUNT

Even in perfectly made blood films, the differential count is subject to the same errors of random distribution as are other cell counts. For interpretation of day-to-day or slide-to-slide differences in the same patient, it is helpful to see how much of the variation is ascribable to chance alone. Table 27–4 gives 95 per cent confidence limits for different percentages of cells in differential counts performed, classifying a total of 100 to 1000 leukocytes. In comparing the percentages from two separate counts, if one number lies outside the confidence limits of the other, it is probable that the difference is significant (i.e., not due to chance). Thus, on the basis of a 100-cell differential count, if the monocytes were 5 per cent one day and 10 per cent the next, it is quite probable that the difference is due solely to sampling error. Although the difference *could be* real, one cannot be confident that it *is* real, because of the small number of cells counted. If, on the other hand, the differential count totaled 500 cells, the difference between 5 per cent and 10 per cent is significant; one can be reasonably certain (with a 5 per cent chance of being wrong) that the difference is a real one and not due to chance alone. Of course, this is a minimal estimate of the error involved in differential counts, since it does not include mechanical errors (due to variations in collecting the blood samples, inadequate mixing, irregularities in distribution depending on the type and quality of the blood films, and poor staining) or errors in cell identification, which depend upon the judgment and experience of the observer. Meticulous technique and accurate and consistent cell classification are therefore demanded of the technician. The physician who interprets the results must be aware of the possible sources of error, especially the minimal error due to chance in the distribution of cells. The latter is a major source of variation in the absolute leukocyte counts when they are computed from electronically derived total leukocyte counts.

Table 27–5 shows the distribution of the various types of leukocytes in the blood of normal persons. Absolute concentrations are given, as these have considerbly greater significance than percentages alone.

AUTOMATED DIFFERENTIAL LEUKOCYTE COUNTING

Because the differential leukocyte count is nonspecific, non-precise, error-prone, usually labor intensive, expensive to perform, and of limited clinical significance as a screening test, some have suggested that it may be prudent to discontinue use of the differential count as an inpatient screening test for adults (Connelly, 1982; Brecher, 1980). Nevertheless it continues to be among the widely used procedures.

Automation of the differential count may help eliminate some of the detractions. Ideally, requirements for the automated differential leukocyte counting system should include the following: (1) the distribution of cells analyzed should be identical with that in the blood; (2) all leukocytes usually found in blood diseases should be accurately identified, or detected and "marked" in some way; (3) the speed of the process should enable a large number of cells to be counted in order to minimize statistical error; and (4) the instrument should be cost effective (Bentley, 1977).

Two general principles have been employed in the systems available to date: digital image processing systems, which use computer identification of cells on stained blood films; and flow-through systems, which analyze cells suspended in a liquid.

Digital Image Processing. A uniformly made and stained blood film is placed on a microscope stage, which is driven by a motor. A computer controls the movement, scanning the slide and stopping it when leukocyte(s) are in the field. The optical images, e.g., nuclear and cytoplasmic size, density, shape, and color, are recorded by a television camera, analyzed by computer, and converted to digital form; these characteristics are then compared with a memory bank of such characteristics for the different cell types. If the pattern "fits" that of a normal cell type, it is identified as such; otherwise it is classed as "other" or unknown. The coordinates of the unknown cells are kept by the instrument and can be relocated at the end of the count so that the technologist can classify them. Because computerized classifiers can tolerate only limited variation in staining, the manufacturers have made significant improvements in blood stain composition, stability, and reproducibility (Lapen, 1982; Marshall, 1975a, b).

Four pattern recognition instrumental systems have been available commercially and have undergone clinical evaluations: the LARC* (Leukocyte Automatic Recognition Computer), the Hematrak,† the "diff-3 system"‡ and ADC-500.§

*Corning Medical Instruments, Medfield, Mass.
†Geometric Data Corp., Wayne, Pa.
‡Coulter Electronics, Inc., Hialeah, Fla.
§Abbott Laboratories, Dallas, Tex.

4

The *LARC* (Megla, 1973) uses slides made with a spinner (p. 603) and stained in a carefully controlled manner, and classifies 100 cells in about 50 seconds, during which time the operator can evaluate erythrocyte morphology and estimate the number of platelets through the binocular microscope. These observations can be entered on a console. After reviewing and identifying the unclassified cells, which the instrument has relocated on demand, the results are printed out and, if desired, sent to a computer. The results have shown reasonable agreement with "manual" differential counts, including band neutrophil counts and the detection of abnormal cells (unclassified, for review) (Cotter, 1976; Arkin, 1977). A semi-automated reticulocyte program has been added as an optional program. Corning stopped marketing this instrument in 1977.

The *Hematrak* (Dutcher, 1974, 1977; Marchand, 1983) uses Romanowsky-stained wedge films and classifies 100 leukocytes in about 30 seconds. Erythrocyte morphology and platelet estimates are made before or after the count and entered on the console. Programs are available for automated reticulocytes, automated platelet estimate, and automated red cell measurements. The identification of leukocytes, including band neutrophil counts, and the detection of abnormal cells have been reported to be satisfactory (Benzel, 1974; Egan, 1974). Later Hematrak models, such as the 480, 450, 450 QP, and 590, have slide cassettes permitting walk-away performance of leukocyte differentials, including erythrocyte morphology and platelet estimates. With the Hematrak 590, up to 100 label identified blood films are processed per batch in about an hour. Unlike the other pattern recognition instruments, either spun or wedge smears can be accommodated.

The *"diff-3 system"* (Norgren, 1981) requires reproducibly stained blood monolayers, prepared using a specialized diluter/spinner, stainer, and Wright's stain. The instrument can be programmed in one of three modes: review mode with an operator attending; conditional review mode, in which processing continues until an abnormal slide is encountered; or no review–walk away mode, in which abnormal results are flagged for later review. Leukocytes, erythrocytes, and platelets are evaluated. In 1980 the diff 3 was upgraded to the diff 3^{50} system with about 50 per cent faster throughput.

The newer, more compact, diff-4 featured increased throughput, a bar code sample identification system, Winchester hard disk, and floppy disk storage of results. Coulter Electronics withdrew the diff-4 from the field in January 1984.

The *Abbott ADC-500* (Green, 1979) was introduced in 1978 as a third generation automated differential counter. This system also included a spinner for monolayer preparation and a modified Ames Hematek II stainer with a loader mechanism to insert the slides into a plastic holder. An initial problematical encoder which imprinted a digital and bar code on the slide holder was replaced by a typed sticky label. Up to 50 stained, encoded smears could be placed in the analyzer. The instrument, however, did not have the capability of relocating abnormal cells encountered. Therefore, a second analysis in attended review mode was necessary when such cells were present. The approximate fourfold speed advantage allowed statistically more accurate 250 or 500 cell differentials to be performed. This instrument has not been sold since 1981.

Having Romanowsky-stained blood films for verifying cell identification is an advantage in these digital image processing systems. The automated instruments are somewhat more consistent than a group of technologists. Accuracy for mature leukocyte types is acceptable for all the systems. The operating speed, however, is generally too slow to count the large number of leukocytes which would be necessary to improve significantly the random statistical error that has afflicted differential counting. Also, they are only marginally cost effective unless a large volume of samples is analyzed.

Flow-Through Systems. The *Hemalog D** automatically samples blood from cups on a turntable sampler at the rate of 90 per hour. Erythrocytes are lysed, leukocytes are separated into three channels and fixed, and reagents are introduced for cytochemical reactions (Mansberg, 1974). In a photo-optical system, measurements of light scattering and of light absorption are made while the cells are being counted. In the *peroxidase channel* immature neutrophils, neutrophils, and eosinophils (which contain peroxidase) absorb light. A pH of 3.2 is used; eosinophils stain more deeply than neutrophils and are distinguished from them by greater absorption and less scatter. Immature and toxic neutrophils have greater peroxidase activity than mature neutrophils and are designated "high peroxidase cells" (HPX); they are separated by greater absorption and equal or greater scatter. Although it has been generally assumed that an increase in HPX cells is due to increased bands and immature neutrophils, it is likely that an increased HPX count is probably often due to toxic granulation in the neutrophils (Peacock, 1982). Lymphocytes are distinguished by low scatter and low absorption. "Large unstained cells" (LUCs) have high scatter and low absorption and include atypical lymphocytes and blasts. A higher than expected LUC count after initial chemotherapy in acute myelogenous leukemia may be an early means of detecting patients who are unlikely to achieve remission with subsequent therapy (Winkel, 1982). The cells are counted and instantaneously plotted (scatter versus absorption) on a scattergram, which is electronically displayed and may be photographed (Fig. 27–44). Platelets and erythrocyte stroma are excluded by a lower threshold. In the *lipase channel,* monocytes are stained by alpha naphthyl butyrate esterase activity and counted; they are separable from other cells by high scatter and high absorption. In the third channel, basophils are counted as their granular heparin stains with alcian blue. Heparinized blood therefore cannot be used.

Ten thousand leukocytes are counted in each channel; the results are expressed both as percentages and

*Technicon Instruments Corp., Tarrytown, N.Y.

A. DIAGRAM

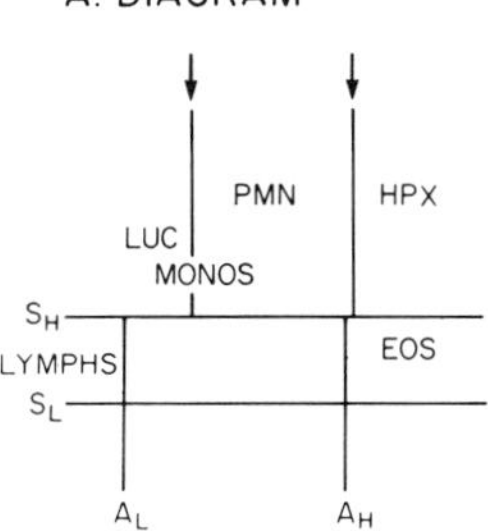

B. NORMAL CONTROL

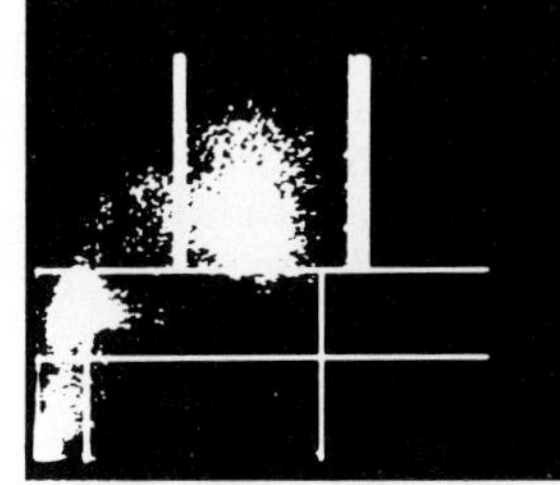

C. INCREASE IN HPX

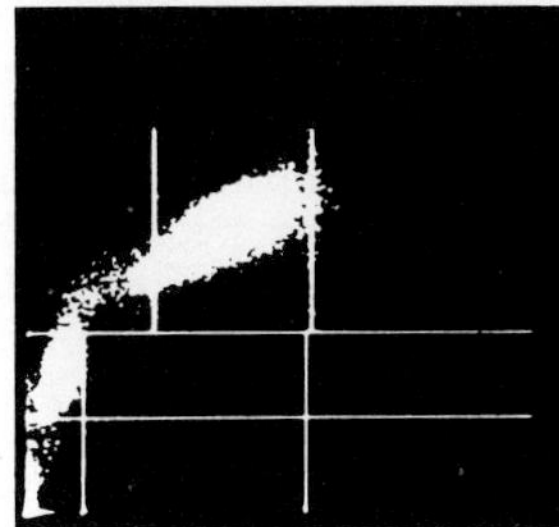

Figure 27–44. The appearance of HPX cells in the peroxidase channel of the Hemalog D. As shown in the line drawing *(A)*, fixed thresholds are set on the horizontal axis for light scatter (S_H = high scatter; S_L = low scatter), and on the vertical axis for light absorbance (A_H = high absorbance; A_L = low absorbance). The neutrophil (PMN) population is identified by size and peroxidase staining; vertical thresholds set to identify PMNs are designated with arrows. Other distinct populations include large unstained cells (LUC), monocytes (MONO), lymphocytes (LYMPH), and eosinophils (EOS). Cells which have the same size (light scatter) as PMNs but fall above the designated absorption threshold are termed high peroxidase cells (HPX). A photograph of the cell distribution from a normal volunteer *(B)* is compared with a donor with an increase (>4%) in HPX cells *(C)*. (From Peacock, J. E., Ross, D. W., and Cohen, M. S.: Am. J. Clin. Path., *78*:445, 1982.)

as absolute concentrations. The total leukocyte count is determined in the peroxidase channel. An optional addition is an automatic slide maker (Autoslide) that makes and stains blood films on a roll of plastic tape, mounts the blood films on glass slides and identifies them by accession number for reference or examination if needed. The reference intervals achieved with the Hemalog D are similar to those with manual technique (Simmons, 1974; Marchand, 1983).

Technicon's later cell counter, the *H6000*, combines the functions of the Hemalog 8/90 and the Hemalog D/90 to provide a CBC, differential WBC, platelet count, and stained blood film from the optional Autoslide from a single sampling at the rate of 90 per hour. Platelets are enumerated using a sensitive photomultiplier tube to detect light scatter in the RBC manifold. The differential is determined primarily from the alkaline peroxidase channel. Monocytes are detected as large cells with weak peroxidase activity instead of in a separate butyrate esterase channel. An optional hard copy printer (H601) allows copies of the CBC and differentials, WBC peroxidase channel, RBC, and platelet size distributions to be produced (Fig. 27–14). A computer system incorporates moving average and control libraries.

Flow cell cytofluorometry (Adams, 1977), using the Cytofluorograf,* can differentiate six classes of cells that appear to represent lymphocytes, monocytes, basophils, eosinophils, neutrophils, and immature neutrophils. The cells are stained supravitally in a hypotonic solution of acridine orange and are identified on a scatter plot of green nuclear fluorescence against red cytoplasmic fluorescence. This system has not been clinically evaluated.

Flow-through systems have the advantage of rapidly analyzing larger numbers of cells, significantly reducing the statistical error of counting. They can be more fully automated than the digital image processors. The disadvantage is that the categories of cells are not completely consonant with those with which we are familiar on Romanowsky-stained films. An "unclassified" category is difficult to interpret. When an abnormal result occurs, a film must be made and examined. Yet this kind of precision in differential leukocyte counting has not previously been available. Analytic variation in the Hemalog D is sufficiently small that physiologic variations previously undetected become apparent, and an individual's own baseline reference values become meaningful (Statland, 1978). For example, the significance of changes in basophil counts in disease appears to become more useful (Gilbert, 1975). As clinical significance of the results of the Hemalog D and H6000 is determined, it is likely that our knowledge of leukocytic changes in disease will increase and the differential leukocyte count will become more useful in diagnostic work.

Platelets

In films made from EDTA-blood and stained with Romanowsky stains, platelets are round or oval, 2 to 4 μm in diameter, and well separated from one another (Plate 27–1). The platelet count may be estimated from such films when the distribution is uniform. On the average, if the platelet count is normal, about one platelet is found per 10 to 30 red cells. At 1000× magnification, this is equivalent to about 5 to 20 platelets per oil immersion field in the areas where red cell morphology is optimal.

4

Platelets contain fine purple granules which usually fill the cytoplasm. Occasionally granules are concentrated in the center (the "granulomere") and surrounded by a pale cytoplasm (the "hyalomere"); these are probably activated platelets, the appearance resulting from contraction of the microtubular band (p. 749). A few platelets may have a decreased concentration of granules (hypogranular platelets).

In EDTA-blood from normal individuals, the fraction of platelets that exceed 3 μm in diameter and the fraction of platelets that are hypogranular are both less than 5 per cent if the films are made at 10 minutes or 60 minutes after the blood is drawn. If films are made immediately or at three hours after blood drawing, the fraction of large platelets and the fraction of hypogranular or activated platelets are

*Bio Physics Systems, Division of Ortho Instruments, Westwood, Mass.

increased (Zeigler, 1978). These artifacts make it necessary to standardize time of film preparation when evaluating platelet size from films.

In patients with immune thrombocytopenia large platelets are increased in number. They are also increased in patients with the rare Bernard-Soulier syndrome (p. 756) and in patients with infiltrated bone marrows or myeloproliferative syndromes; in the latter, the platelets are frequently hypogranular or are "activated", i.e., have a distinct granulomere and hyalomere.

In blood films made from skin puncture wounds, platelets assume irregular shapes with sharp projections and tend to clump together in proportion to the time after the wound is made.

PHYSIOLOGIC VARIATION

Physiologic Variation in Erythrocytes

Changes in red cell values are greatest during the first few weeks of life (Fig. 27–45). At the time of birth, as much as 100 to 125 ml of placental blood may be added to the newborn if tying the cord is postponed until its pulsation ceases. In a study of newborns whose cords had been clamped late, the average capillary red cell counts were 0.4×10^{12}/L higher 1 hour after and 0.8×10^{12}/L higher 24 hours after birth compared with newborns whose cords had been clamped early.

Capillary blood (obtained by skin prick) gives higher RBC and Hb values than venous blood (cord). The differences may amount to about 0.5×10^{12} RBC/L and 3 g Hb/dl. The slowing of capillary circulation and the resulting loss of fluid may be the responsible factor. Examination of venous blood furnishes more consistent results than examination of capillary blood.

In the full-term infant, *nucleated red cells* average about 500/μl. The normoblast count declines to about 200/μl at 24 hr., 25/μl at 48 hours and less than 5/μl at 72 hours. By four days it is rare to find circulating normoblasts (Oski, 1972).

The normal *reticulocyte count* at birth ranges from 3 to 7 per cent during the first 48 hours, during which time it rises slightly. After the second day it falls rather rapidly to 1 to 3 per cent by the seventh day of life.

Hemoglobin concentration in capillary blood during the first day of life averages 19.0 g/dl, with 95 per cent of normal values falling between 14.6 and 23.4 g/dl. In cord blood the average is 16.8 g/dl, with 95 per cent of normals between 13.5 and 20 g/dl (Oski, 1972). There is frequently an initial increase in the hemoglobin level of venous blood at the end of 24 hours compared with that of cord blood. At the end of the first week, the level is about the same as in cord blood and it does not begin to fall until after the second week. During the first two weeks the lower limit of normal is 14.5 g/dl for capillary blood and 13.0 g/dl for venous blood.

The hematocrit in capillary blood on the first day of life averages 0.61, with 95 per cent of normal values between 0.46 and 0.76. In cord blood, the average is 0.53. The changes during the first few weeks parallel the hemoglobin concentration.

The Hb and Hct are highest at birth but fall rather steeply in the first days and weeks of life to a minimum average Hb of 10.7 g/dl and Hct of 0.31 at about two months of age. Though the lower limit of the 95 per cent reference values in some studies is as low as 9 g Hb/dl and 0.26 Hct, these probably include children with nutritional deficiencies. The level to define anemia probably should be no lower than 10.5 g Hb/dl or 0.33 Hct (Williams, 1977).

The normal MCV at birth ranges from 104 to 118 fl, compared with the adult reference interval of 80 to 96 fl. Since the RBC does not fall to the degree the Hb and Hct do, the MCV decreases abruptly, then gradually, during the first few months of life. The lowest value is reached at about one year. In a

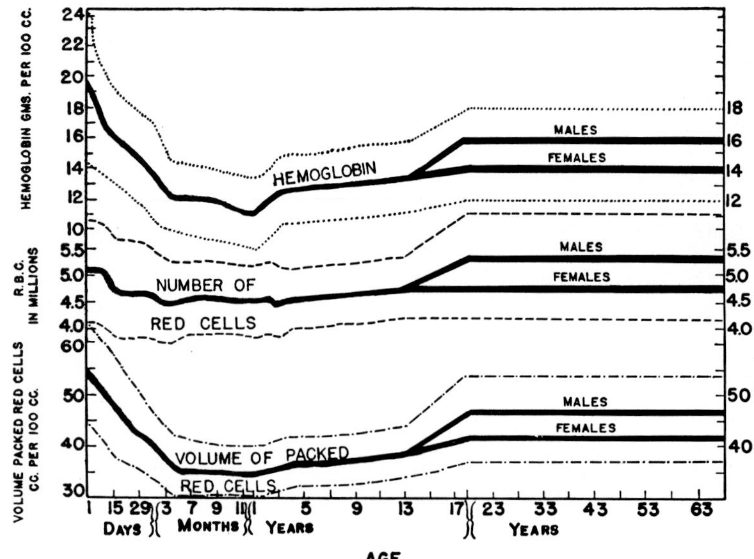

Figure 27–45. Values for hemoglobin, hematocrit (volume of packed red cells), and red cell counts from birth or old age. Mean values are heavy lines. Reference interval for hemoglobin is indicated by dotted lines, for red cell counts by interrupted lines, and for hematocrit by dotted interrupted lines. The scales on the ordinate are similar so that relative changes in hemoglobin, red cell count, and hematocrit are apparent on inspection. The scale for age, however, is progressively altered. (From Wintrobe, M. M.: Clinical Hematology. 6th ed. Philadelphia, Lea & Febiger, 1967.)

Table 27–6. ERYTHROCYTE AND LEUKOCYTE VALUES IN NORMAL ADULTS, 95 PER CENT REFERENCE INTERVALS

	1 Dacie and Lewis (1975)	2 Williams and Schneider (1977)	3 Upstate Medical Center
Leukocyte count ($\times 10^9$/L)	4.0 –11.0	M 3.9 – 10.6 F 3.5 – 11.0	4.5 –11.0
Erythrocyte count ($\times 10^{12}$/L)	M 4.5 – 6.5 F 3.8 – 5.8	4.4 – 5.9 3.8 – 5.2	4.6 – 6.1 4.1 – 5.3
Hemoglobin (g/dl)	M 13.0 –18.0 F 11.5 –16.5	13.3 – 17.7 11.7 – 15.7	13.5 –18.0 11.5 –15.5
Hematocrit (L/L)	M 0.40– 0.54 F 0.37– 0.47	0.40– 0.52 0.35– 0.47	0.41– 0.53 0.36– 0.45
MCV (fl)	77–93	M 80.5 – 99.7 F 80.8 –100.0	80–96
MCH (pg)	27–32	M 26.6 – 33.8 F 26.4 – 34.0	27–32
MCHC (g/dl)	31–35	M 31.5 – 36.3 F 31.4 – 35.8	32–36

Data from Williams, W. J., et al.: Hematology. 2nd ed. New York, McGraw-Hill Book Company, 1977.

study using the Coulter Model S in which iron deficiency and thalassemia were excluded, Koerper (1976) found the following MCVs (average; 95 per cent reference intervals):

Age 10 to 17 months	= 77 fl; 70 to 84 fl
Age 18 months to 4 years	= 80 fl; 74 to 86 fl
Age 4 years to 7 years	= 81 fl; 76 to 86 fl

The MCV very gradually rises until after puberty, when adult levels are reached.

Reference intervals for red cell values in sexually mature adults are given in Table 27–6. The indices are similar in males and females, but the Hb is 1 to 2 g/dl higher in males, with commensurate increments in Hct and RBC. This is believed to be mainly the effects of androgen in stimulating erythropoietic production and its effect on the marrow. Estrogen probably has a slight suppressing effect on red cell production (Erslev, 1977).

In older men the Hb tends to fall and in older women the Hb tends to fall to a lesser degree (in some studies) or even rise slightly (in other studies). In older individuals, therefore, the sex difference is less than 1 g Hb/dl (Dacie, 1975).

Posture and muscular activity change the concentration of the formed elements. The Hb, Hct, and RBC increase by several per cent when the change from recumbency to standing is made (Mollison, 1979; p. 586) and strenuous muscular activity causes a further increase, presumably due primarily to loss of plasma water.

Diurnal variation that is not related to exercise or to analytical variation also occurs (Statland, 1978). The Hb is highest in the morning, falls during the day, and is lowest in the evening, with a mean difference of 8 to 9 per cent (Dacie, 1975).

In persons living at a higher altitude, the Hb, Hct, and RBC are elevated over what they would be at sea level. The difference is about 1 g Hb/dl at 2 kilometers altitude and 2 g Hb/dl at 3 km. Increased erythropoiesis is secondary to anoxic stimulation of erythropoietin production. People who are smokers also tend to have a mild erythrocytosis (p. 698).

Physiologic Variation in Leukocytes

The total white cell count at birth and during the first 24 hours varies within wide limits. Neutrophils are the predominant cell, varying from 6 to 28 $\times$ 10^9/L; about 15 per cent of these are band forms (Altman, 1974), and a few myelocytes are present. Neutrophils drop to about 5 $\times$ 10^9/L and remain at about the same level thereafter. Lymphocytes are about 5.5 $\times$ 10^9/L at birth, and change little during the first week. They become the predominant cell, on the average, after the first week of life and remain so until about age seven, when neutrophils again predominate. The upper limit of the 95 per cent reference interval for lymphocytes at age 6 months is 13.5; at 1 year, 10.5; at 2 years, 9.5; at 6 years, 7.0; and at 12 years, 6.0 $\times$ 10^9/L; for neutrophils at the same ages the values are 8.5, 8.5, 8.5, 8.0, and 8.0 $\times$ 10^9/L, all somewhat higher than those for adults (Table 27–5).

Some studies suggest a slightly higher neutrophil level in adult women, but this has not been found in all studies (England, 1976).

Diurnal variation has been recognized in the neutrophil count, with highest levels in the afternoon and lowest levels in the morning at rest. Statland (1978) has shown, however, using precise methods (Hemalog D), that diurnal variation in neutrophils and in total WBC varies from subject to subject; in some there is very little diurnal variation, but the pattern is quite consistent for the individual.

Exercise produces leukocytosis, which includes an increased neutrophil concentration due to a shift of cells from marginal to circulating granulocyte pool (p. 638); increased lymphocyte drainage into blood also appears to contribute to the total increase.

Both the average and the lower reference value for neutrophil concentration in the black population is lower than in the white (Table 27–5); this difference must be taken into account in assessing neutropenia.

Cigarette smokers have higher average leukocyte counts than non-smokers. The increase is greatest (about 30 per cent) in heavy smokers who inhale, and affects neutrophils, lymphocytes, and monocytes (Corre, 1971).

There appear to be mild changes during the menstrual cycle (England, 1976). Neutrophils and monocytes fall and eosinophils tend to rise during menstruation. Basophils have been reported to fall during ovulation (Mettler, 1974).

The availability of precise automated leukocyte analyzers (p. 619) provides the potential for investigating physiologic sources of variation that have been obscured by the statistical error in traditional microscopic differential counts (Statland, 1978). Reference intervals for each type of leukocyte could be established for an individual. This potential appears promising; its value is beginning to be established in some areas (Gilbert, 1975) and needs to be investigated further.

Physiologic Variation in Platelets

The average platelet count is slightly lower at birth than in older children and adults, and may vary from 84×10^9/L to 478×10^9/L (Oski, 1972). After the first week of life the reference intervals are those of the adult. No sex difference is clearly established. In women, the platelet count may fall at the time of menstruation.

ERYTHROCYTE SEDIMENTATION RATE

Principle. When well-mixed venous blood is placed in a vertical tube, erythrocytes will tend to fall toward the bottom. The length of fall of the top of the column of erythrocytes in a given interval of time is the erythrocyte sedimentation rate (ESR). Several factors are involved.

Plasma Factors. An accelerated ESR is favored by elevated levels of fibrinogen and, to a lesser extent, alpha$_2$-, beta-, and gamma globulins. These asymmetric protein molecules have a greater effect than other proteins in decreasing the negative charge of erythrocytes (zeta potential) that tends to keep them apart. The decreased zeta potential promotes the formation of rouleaux, which sediment more rapidly than single cells. Removal of fibrinogen by defibrination lowers the ESR.

There is no absolute correlation between the ESR and any of the plasma protein fractions. Albumin and lecithin retard sedimentation, and cholesterol accelerates the ESR.

Red Cell Factors. Anemia increases the ESR, because the change in the erythrocyte-plasma ratio favors rouleaux formation, independent of changes in the concentration of the plasma proteins. By any method of measurement, the ESR is most sensitive to altered plasma proteins in the hematocrit range of 0.30 to 0.40 (Bull, 1975; Moseley, 1982).

The sedimentation rate is directly proportional to the weight of the cell aggregate and inversely proportional to the surface area. Microcytes sediment slower than macrocytes which have decreased surface area to volume ratios. Rouleaux also have a decreased surface area to volume ratio and accelerate the ESR. Red cells with an abnormal or irrregular shape, such as sickle cells or spherocytes, hinder rouleaux formation and lower the ESR.

Stages in the ESR. Three stages can be observed: (1) In the initial 10 minutes, there is little sedimentation as rouleaux form. (2) For about 40 minutes settling occurs at a constant rate. (3) Sedimentation slows in the final 10 minutes as cells pack at the bottom of the tube.

METHODS

Westergren Method. Because of its simplicity the Westergren method is widely used. The National Committee for Clinical Laboratory Standards has recommended it as the standard method.

Equipment. The Westergren tube is a straight pipette 30 cm long, 2.5 mm in internal diameter, and calibrated in millimeters from 0 to 200. It holds about 1 ml. The Westergren rack is also used.

Reagent. A 0.105 molar solution of sodium citrate is used as the anticoagulant-diluent solution (31 g of $Na_3C_6H_5O_7 \cdot H_2O$ added to 1 L of distilled water in a sterile glass bottle). This is filtered and kept refrigerated without preservatives.

Technique

1. Four ml of whole blood is added to 1.0 ml of sodium citrate and mixed by inversion.
2. A Westergren pipette is filled to the 0 mark and placed exactly vertical in the rack at room temperature without vibration or exposure to direct sunlight.
3. After exactly 60 minutes, the distance to the top of the column of red cells is recorded in millimeters as the ESR value. If the demarcation between plasma and red cell column is hazy, the level is taken where the full density is first apparent.

Modified Westergren Method. A modification of the Westergren method produces the same results but employs blood anticoagulated with EDTA rather than citrate. This is more convenient, since it allows the ESR to be performed from the same tube of blood as is used for other hematologic studies. Two ml of well mixed EDTA-blood is diluted either with 0.5 ml of 3.8 per cent sodium citrate (Dawson, 1960) or with 0.5 ml of 0.85 per cent sodium chloride (Gambino, 1965). Undiluted blood anticoagulated with EDTA gives poor precision.

The ESR gradually increases with age. Westergren's original upper limits of normal (10 mm per hour for men and 20 mm per hour for women) appear to be too low. Böttiger (1967) recommended that the upper limit of normal should be 15 mm per hour for men and 20 mm per hour for women below the age of 50 and 20 mm per hour for men and 30 mm per hour for women over the age of 50.

Sources of Error. If the concentration of the anticoagulant is higher than recommended, the ESR may be altered. Sodium citrate or EDTA does not affect the rate of sedimentation if used in the proper concentration. Heparin, however, alters the membrane zeta potential and cannot be used as an anticoagulant.

Bubbles left in the tube when it is filled will affect the ESR. Hemolysis may modify the sedimentation. The cleanliness of the tube is important, and all traces of alcohol and ether must be removed.

Tilting the tube accelerates the ESR. The red cells

aggregate along the lower side while the plasma rises along the upper side. Consequently, the retarding influence of the rising plasma is less effective. An angle of even 3 degrees from the vertical may accelerate the ESR by as much as 30 per cent.

Temperature should be within the range of 20 to 25°C. Lower or higher temperatures in some cases alter the ESR. If the blood has been kept refrigerated, it should be permitted to reach room temperature before the test is performed.

The test should be set up within two hours after the blood sample is obtained (or 12 hours if EDTA is used as the anticoagulant and the blood is kept at 4°C.); otherwise, some samples with elevated ESRs will be falsely low. On standing, erythrocytes tend to become spherical and less readily form rouleaux.

There is no effective method for correcting for anemia in the Westergren method.

Zeta Sedimentation Ratio. A centrifugal device (the Zetafuge*) spins capillary tubes in a vertical position in four 45-second cycles (Bull, 1972). This results in controlled compaction and dispersion of erythrocytes, allowing rouleaux to form and sediment in this three-minute period of time. The capillary tube is then read as if it were a standard hematocrit tube, giving a value referred to as a zetacrit. The true hematocrit is divided by the zetacrit, and the result, expressed as a percentage, is the zeta sedimentation ratio (ZSR). It is not affected by anemia, which makes it easier to interpret. Its sensitivity to moderate elevation of the ESR by fibrinogen is the same as the Westergren method. It is perhaps the best ESR method to screen for occult disease and minimal elevation in the sedimentation rate; however, it levels off somewhat in the moderate to markedly elevated range (Moseley, 1982). This ZSR requires only a 100-μl sample and is considerably faster. The adult reference interval is 41 to 54 per cent for both sexes. If the hematocrit is elevated, some of the red cells must be removed and the procedure repeated.

Micro ESR Method. Barrett (1980) described a micro ESR method using 0.2 ml blood to fill a plastic disposable tube 230 mm long with a 1 mm internal bore. Capillary blood values correlated well with venous blood micro ESR and Westergren ESR values. This method may prove especially useful in pediatric patients.

INTERPRETATION

In pregnancy, the ESR increases moderately, beginning in the tenth to twelfth week. Normal rates return about one month post partum.

The ESR tends to be markedly elevated in monoclonal blood protein disorders such as multiple myeloma or macroglobulinemia, in severe polyclonal hyperglobulinemias due to inflammatory disease, and in hyperfibrinogenemias.

Moderate elevations are common in active inflammatory disease such as rheumatoid arthritis, chronic infections, collagen disease, and neoplastic disease. The major use at present is as an indication of the presence of active disease of these sorts. It is a simpler test than protein electrophoresis, which has tended to replace it, and it has few false negative results.

The ZSR has been shown to be a satisfactory alternative to the ESR in a few clinical trials (e.g., Morris, 1977).

The Westergren method is somewhat less useful in the presence of anemia. The sensitivity of the ESR in detecting plasma protein abnormalities is best in the nonanemic state (Bull, 1975). Moseley (1982) described a candidate reference method in which the hematocrit is adjusted to 35 per cent so that the sensitivity of the ESR is linear throughout the range.

*Coulter Diagnostics, Hialeah, Fla.

Ackerman, P. G.: Electronic Instrumentation in the Clinical Laboratory. Boston, Little, Brown and Company, 1972.

Adams, L. R.: Staining for the Cytograf and Cytofluorograf. J. Histochem. *25*:965, 1977.

Altman, P. L., and Dittmer, D. S.: Biology Data Book, Vol. III. 2nd ed. Bethesda, Federation of American Societies for Experimental Biology, 1974, p. 1856.

Arkin, C. F., Sherry, M. A., Gough, A. G., and Copeland, B. E.: An automatic leukocyte analyzer. Validity of its results. Am. J. Clin. Path., *67*:159, 1977.

Baker, J. T.: Principles of Biological Microtechnique. New York, John Wiley & Sons, Inc., 1958.

Barrett, B. A., and Hill, P. I.: A micromethod for the erythrocyte sedimentation rate suitable for use on venous or capillary blood. J. Clin. Path., *33*:1118, 1980.

Beautyman, W., and Bills, T.: Osmotic error in erythrocyte volume determinations. Am. J. Hematol., *12*:383, 1982.

Beeson, P. B., and Bass, D. A.: The Eosinophil. Vol. XIV in the series Major Problems in Internal Medicine, Smith, L. H., Jr. (ed.). Philadelphia, W. B. Saunders Company, 1977.

Bentley, S. A., and Lewis, S. M.: Automated differential leukocyte counting: The present state of the art. Br. J. Haematol., *35*:481, 1977.

Benzel, J. E., Egan, J. J., Hart, D. J., and Christopher, E. A.: Evaluation of an automated differential leukocyte counting system. II. Normal cell identification. Am. J. Clin. Path., *62*:530, 1974.

Berkson, J., Magath, T. B., and Hurn, M.: The error of estimate of the blood cell count as made with the hemocytometer. Am. J. Physiol., *128*:309, 1940.

Bessis, M.: Blood Smears Reinterpreted, trans. G. Brecher. New York, Springer-Verlag, 1977.

Bessman, J. D., Williams, L. J., and Gilmer, P. R., Jr.: Mean platelet volume. The inverse relation of platelet size and count in normal subjects, and an artifact of other particles. Am. J. Clin. Path., *76*:289, 1981.

Böttiger, L. E., and Svedberg, C. A.: Normal erythrocyte sedimentation rate and age. Br. Med. J., *2*:85, 1967.

Brecher, G., Anderson, R. E., and McMullen, P. D.: When to do diffs. How often should differential counts be repeated? Blood Cells, *6*:431, 1980.

Brecher, G., and Bessis, M.: Present status of spiculated red cells and their relationship to the discocyte-echinocyte transformation: A critical review. Blood, *40*:333, 1972.

Brecher, G., and Cronkite, E. P.: Estimation of the number of platelets by phase microscopy. *In* Tocantins, L. M., and Kazal, L. A.: Blood Coagulation, Hemorrhage and Thrombosis. New York, Grune & Stratton, Inc., 1964.

Brecher, G., and Schneiderman, M.: A time-saving device for the counting of reticulocytes. Am. J. Clin. Path., *20*:1079, 1950.

Brittin, G. M., and Brecher, G.: Instrumentation and automation in clinical hematology. Prog. Hematol., *7*:299, 1971.

Brittin, G. M., Brecher, G., and Johnson, C. A.: Evaluation of the Coulter Counter Model S. Am. J. Clin. Path., *52*:679, 1969a.

Brittin, G. M., Brecher, G., Johnson, C. A., and Elashoff, R. M.: Stability of blood in commonly used anticoagulants. Use of refrigerated blood for quality control of the Coulter Counter Model S. Am. J. Clin. Path., *52*:690, 1969b.

Bull, B. S.: Aids to electronic platelet counting. Am. J. Clin. Path., *54*:707, 1970.

Bull, B. S.: Automation in haematology. *In* Goldberg, A., and Brain, M. C. (eds.): Recent Advances in Haematology. Edinburgh, Churchill-Livingstone, 1971, p. 357.

Bull, B. S.: Is a standard ESR possible? Lab. Med., *6*:31, 1975.

Bull, B. S., and Brailsford, J. D.: The zeta sedimentation ratio. Blood, *40*:550, 1972.

4

Bull, B. S., Dutcher, T. F., and Siggard-Andersen, O.: The Hem-Aliquanter: A dispenser-dilutor for hematology. Am. J. Clin. Path., *49*:295, 1968.

Bull, B. S., Elashoff, R. M., Heilbron, D. C., and Couperus, J.: A study of various estimators for the derivative of quality control procedures from patient erythrocyte indices. Am. J. Clin. Path., *61*:473, 1974.

Bull, B. S., and Korpman, R. A.: Autocalibration of hematology analyzers. J. Clin. Lab. Auto., *3*:111, 1983.

Bunn, H. F., Forget, B. G., and Ranney, H. M.: Human Hemoglobins. Philadelphia, W. B. Saunders Company, 1977.

Cartwright, G. E.: Diagnostic Laboratory Hematology. 4th ed. New York, Grune & Stratton, Inc., 1968.

Cohen, R. J., Sachs, J. R., Wicker, D. J., and Conrad, M. E.: Methemoglobinemia provoked by malarial chemoprophylaxis in Vietnam. N. Engl. J. Med., *279*:1127, 1968.

Conn, H. J., and Darrow, M. S.: Staining Procedures Used by the Biological Stain Commission. 2nd ed. Baltimore, The Williams & Wilkins Company, 1960.

Connelly, D. P., McClain, M. P., Crowson, T. W., and Benson, E. S.: The use of the differential leukocyte count for inpatient case finding. Hum. Path., *13*:294, 1982.

Corre, F., Lellouch, J., and Schwarz, D.: Smoking and leukocyte counts. Results of an epidemiological survey. Lancet, *2*:632, 1971.

Cotter, D. A., and Sage, B. H.: Performance of the LARC classifier in clinical laboratories. J. Histochem. Cytochem., *24*:202, 1976.

Coulter Counter Model S-plus IV with Data Terminal. Product Reference Manual No. 4235153D. Hialeah, Fla., November, 1982.

Dacie, J. V., and Lewis, S. L.: Practical Haematology. 5th ed. Edinburgh, Churchill-Livingstone, 1975.

Dawson, J. B.: The E.S.R. in a new dress. Br. Med. J., *1*:1697, 1960.

Dean, W. W., Stastny, M., and Lubrano, G. J.: The degradation of Romanowsky-type blood stains in methanol. Stain Technol., *52*:35, 1977.

Dubowski, K. M., and Luke, J. L.: Measurement of carboxyhemoglobin and carbon monoxide in blood. Ann. Clin. Lab. Sci., *3*:53, 1973.

Dutcher, T. F., Benzel, J. E., Egan, J. J., Hart, D. J., and Christopher, E. A.: Evaluation of an automated differential leukocyte counting system. I. Instrument description and reproducibility studies. Am. J. Clin. Path., *62*:525, 1974.

Dutcher, T. F., Jakubowski, D., and Orser, B.: A comparative evaluation of automated blood cell differential analyzers: Hematrak, LARC and Hemalog D. *In* Koepke, J. A. (ed.): Differential Leukocyte Counting. College of American Pathologists, 1977, p. 161.

Egan, J. J., Benzel, J. F., Hart, D. J., and Christopher, E. A.: Evaluation of an automated differential leukocyte counting system. III. Detection of abnormal cells. Am. J. Clin. Path., *62*:537, 1974.

England, J. M., and Bain, B. J.: Total and differential leucocyte count. Br. J. Haematol., *33*:1, 1976.

England, J. M., and Down, M. C.: Measurement of the mean cell volume using electronic particle counters. Br. J. Haematol., *32*:403, 1976.

England, J. M., Walford, D. M., and Waters, D. A. W.: Reassessment of the reliability of the haematocrit. Br. J. Haematol., *23*:247, 1972.

Erslev, A. J.: Anemia of endocrine disorders. *In* Williams, W. J., Beutler, E., Erslev, A. J., and Rundles, R. W.: Hematology. 2nd ed. New York, McGraw-Hill, 1977.

Fairbanks, V. F., Fahey, J. L., and Beutler, E.: Clinical Disorders of Iron Metabolism. 2nd ed. New York, Grune & Stratton, Inc., 1971.

Gagon, T. E., Athens, J. W., Boggs, D. R., and Cartwright, G. E.: An evaluation of the variance of leukocyte counts as performed with the hemocytometer, Coulter, and Fisher instruments. Am. J. Clin. Path., *46*:684, 1966.

Gambino, S. R., DiRe, J. J., Monteleone, M., and Budd, D. C.: The Westergren sedimentation rate, using K_3EDTA. Am. J. Clin. Path., *43*:173, 1965.

Gilbert, H. S., and Ornstein, L.: Basophil counting with a new staining method using Alcian blue. Blood, *46*:279, 1975.

Gilmer, P. R., Jr., Williams, L. J., Koepke, J. A., and Bull, B. S.: Calibration methods for automated hematology instruments. Am. J. Clin. Path., *68*:185, 1977.

Goldsmith, J. R., and Landow, S. A.: Carbon monoxide and human health. Science *162*:1352, 1968.

Green, J. E.: A practical application of computer pattern recognition research—the Abbott ADC-500 Differential Counter. J. Histochem. Cytochem., *27*:160, 1979.

Hattersley, P. G., Gerard, P. W., Caggiano, V., and Nash, D. R.: Erroneous values on the Model S Coulter due to high titer cold agglutinins. Am. J. Clin. Path., *55*:442, 1971.

Hegesh, E., Calmanovici, N., and Avron, M.: New method for determining ferrihemoglobin reductase (NADH-methemoglobin reductase) in erythrocytes. J. Lab. Clin. Med., *72*:339, 1968.

Henry, R. J.: Clinical Chemistry: Principles and Technics. New York, Harper & Row, 1964.

Holt, J. T., De Wandler, M. J., and Arvan, D. A.: Spurious elevation of the electronically determined mean corpuscular volume and hematocrit caused by hyperglycemia. Am. J. Clin. Path., *77*:561, 1982.

International Committee for Standardization in Hematology: Standard techniques for the measurement of red cell and plasma volume. A report by the International Committee for Standardization in Hematology (ICSH): Panel on diagnostic applications of radioisotopes in haematology. Br. J. Haematol., *25*:801, 1973.

International Committee for Standardization in Haematology: Expert Panel on Blood Cell Sizing: Recommendation for reference method for determination of packed cell volume of blood. J. Clin. Path., *33*:1, 1980.

International Committee for Standardization in Haematology: Recommendations for reference method for hemoglobinometry in human blood. (ICSH Standard EP 6/2:1977) and specifications for international hemiglobin cyanide reference preparation (ICSH Standard EP 6/3:1977). J. Clin. Path., *31*:139, 1978.

Jandl, J. H., Engle, L. K., and Allen, D. W.: Oxidative hemolysis and precipitation of hemoglobin. I. Heinz body anemias as an acceleration of red cell aging. J. Clin. Invest., *39*:1818, 1960.

Koerper, M. A., Mentzer, W. C., Brecher, G., and Dallman, P. R.: Developmental change in red cell volume: Implication in screening infants and children for iron deficiency and thalassemia trait. J. Pediatr., *89*:580, 1976.

Lampasso, J. A.: Changes in hematologic values induced by storage of ethylene diaminetetraacetate human blood for varying periods of time. Am. J. Clin. Path., *49*:443, 1968.

Lampasso, J. A.: Error in hematocrit value produced by excessive ethylenediamine-tetraacetate. Am. J. Clin. Path., *44*:109, 1965.

Lapen, D.: A standardized differential stain for hematology. Cytometry, *2*:309, 1982.

Lappin, T. R. J., Lamont, A., and Nelson, M. G.: An evaluation of the Celloscope 401 electronic blood cell counter. J. Clin. Path., *25*:539, 1972.

Lewis, S. M., and Stoddart, C. T. H.: Effects of anticoagulants and containers (glass and plastic) on the blood count. Lab. Pract., *20*:787, 1971.

Lillie, R. D. (ed.): H. J. Conn's Biological Stains. 9th ed. Baltimore, The Williams & Wilkins Company, 1977.

Lubrano, G. J., Dean, W. W., Heinsohn, H. G., and Stastny, M.: The analysis of some commercial dyes and Romanowsky stains by high-performance liquid chromatography. Stain Technol., *52*:13, 1977.

Luke, R. G., Koepke, J. A., and Siegel, R. R.: The effects of immunosuppressive drugs and uremia on automated leukocyte counts. Am. J. Clin. Path., *56*:503, 1971.

Mansberg, H. P., Saunders, A. M., and Groner, W.: The Hemalog D white cell differential system. J. Histochem. Cytochem., *22*:711, 1974.

Mansberg, H. P.: Optical techniques of particle counting. Technicon International Congress, 1969. Advances in Automated Analysis, *1*:213, 1970.

Marchand, A., Van Lente, F., and Galen, R. S.: Automated differential leukocyte counters: A comparison of three systems. J. Clin. Lab. Automation, *3*:19, 1983.

Marshall, P. N., Bentley, S. A., and Lewis, S. M.: An evaluation of some commercial Romanowsky stains. J. Clin. Path., *28*:680, 1975a.

Marshall, P. N., Bentley, S. A., and Lewis, S. M.: A standardized Romanowsky stain prepared from purified dyes. J. Clin. Path., *28*:920, 1975b.

Mathy, K. A., and Koepke, J. A.: The clinical usefulness of segmented vs. stab neutrophil criteria for differential leukocyte counts. Am. J.Clin. Path., *61*:947, 1974.

Mayer, K., Chin, B., Magnes, J., Thaler, H. J., Lofspeich, C., and Baisley, A.: Automated platelet counters. A comparative evaluation of latest instrumentation. Am. J. Clin. Path., *74*:135, 1980.

Megla, G. K.: The LARC automatic white blood cell analyzer. Acta Cytol., *17*:3, 1973.

Mettler, L., and Shirwani, D.: Direct basophil count for timing ovulation. Fertil. Steril., *25*:718, 1974.

Mollison, P. L.: Blood Transfusion in Clinical Medicine. Oxford, Blackwell Scientific Publications, 1979, p. 128.

Morris, M. W., Pinals, R. S., and Nelson, D. A.: The zeta sedimentation ratio (ZSR) and activity of disease in rheumatoid arthritis. Am. J. Clin. Path., *68*:760, 1977.

Morris, M. W., Skrodzki, Z., and Nelson, D. A.: Zeta sedimentation ratio (ZSR), a replacement for the erythrocyte sedimentation rate (ESR). Am. J. Clin. Path., *64*:254, 1975.

Moseley, D. L., and Bull, B. S.: A comparison of the Wintrobe, the Westergren and the ZSR erythrocyte sedimentation rate (ESR) methods to a candidate reference method. Clin. Lab. Haematol., *4*:169, 1982.

Norgren, P. E.: Leukocyte image analysis in the diff 3 system. Pattern Recog. *13*:299, 1981.

Nosanchuk, J. S., Roark, M. F., and Wanser, C.: Anemia masked by triglyceridemia. Am. J. Clin. Path., *62*:838, 1974.

Oberjat, T. E., Zucker, R. M., and Cassen, B.: Rapid and reliable differential counts on dilute leukocyte suspensions. J. Lab. Clin. Med., *76*:518, 1970.

Oski, F. A., and Naiman, J. L.: Hematologic Problems in the Newborn. 2nd ed. Philadelphia, W. B. Saunders Company, 1972.

Peacock, J. E., Ross, D. W., and Cohen, M. S.: Automated cytochemical staining and inflammation, further assessment of the "left shift." Am. J. Clin. Path., *78*:445, 1982.

Pearson, T. C., and Guthrie, D. L.: Trapped plasma in the microhematocrit. Am. J. Clin. Path., *78*:770, 1982.

Pinkerton, P. H., Spence, I., Ogilvie, J. C., Ronald, W. A., Marchant, P., and Ray, P. K.: An assessment of the Coulter Counter Model S. J. Clin. Path., *23*:68, 1970.

Rogers, C. H.: Blood sample preparation for automated differential systems. Am. J. Med. Technol., *39*:435, 1973.

Rowan, R. M., Fraser, C.: Platelet size distribution analysis. *In* van Assendelft, O. W., and England, J. M. (ed.): Advances in Hematological Methods: The Blood Count. Boca Raton, Fla., CRC Press, Inc., 1982, p. 125.

Sacker, L. S.: Specimen collection. *In* Lewis, S. M., and Coster, J. F. (eds.): Quality Control in Haematology. New York, Academic Press, 1975, p. 211.

Saunders, A. M., and Scott, F.: Hematologic automation by continuous flow systems. J. Histochem. Cytochem., *22*:707, 1974.

Schwartz, J. M., and Jaffé, E. R.: Hereditary methemoglobinemia with deficiency of NADH-dehydrogenase. *In* Stanbury, J. B., Wyngaarden, J. B., and Fredrickson, D. S. (eds.): The Metabolic Basis of Inherited Disease. 4th ed. New York, McGraw-Hill Book Co., 1978, p. 1452.

Simmons, A., Leaverton, P., and Elbert, G.: Normal laboratory values for differential white cell counts established by manual and automated cytochemical methods (Hemalog D). J. Clin. Pathol., *27*:55, 1974.

Simmons, A., Schwabbauer, M. L., and Earhart, C. A.: Automated platelet counting with the Autoanalyzers. J. Lab. Clin. Med., *77*:656, 1971.

Smith, J. R., and Landaw, S. A.: Smoker's polycythemia. N. Engl. J. Med., *298*:6, 1978.

Statland, B. E., Winkel, P., Harris, S. C., Burdsall, M. J., and Saunders, A. M.: Evaluation of biologic sources of variation of leukocyte counts and other hematologic quantities using very precise automated analyzers. Am. J. Clin. Path., *69*:48, 1978.

Taft, E. G.: Pseudoleukocytosis due to cryoprotein crystals. Am. J. Clin. Path., *60*:669, 1973.

Thom, R.: Evaluation of the new model Hemalog 8, which operates at 90 samples per hour, using 400 microliters of blood. *In* Advances in Automated Analysis, Technicon International Congress. Mediad, Inc., Tarrytown, N.Y., 1977.

Tietz, N. W. (ed.): Fundamentals of Clinical Chemistry. Philadelphia, W. B. Saunders Co., 1976.

van Assendelft, O. W.: Spectrophotometry of haemoglobin derivatives. Assen, The Netherlands, Royal Van Gorcum Ltd., 1970.

Weick, J. K., Hagedorn, A. B., and Linman, J. W.: Leukoerythroblastosis: Diagnostic and prognostic significance. Mayo Clin. Proc., *49*:110, 1974.

Williams, W. J., and Schneider, A. S.: Examination of the peripheral blood. *In* Williams, W. J., Beutler, E., Erslev, A. J., and Rundles, R. W. (eds.): Hematology. 2nd ed. New York, McGraw-Hill, 1977, p. 23.

Winkel, P., Olesen, T., and Nissen, N. I.: Automated cytochemistry in the prediction of remission following chemotherapy of patients with de novo acute myeloblastic leukemia. Am. J. Clin. Path., 77:50, 1982.

Wintrobe, M. M.: Clinical Hematology. 7th ed. Philadelphia, Lea & Febiger, 1974, p. 125.

Zeigler, Z., Murphy, S., and Gardner, F. H.: Microscopic platelet size and morphology in various hematologic disorders. Blood, *51*:479, 1978.

28

HEMATOPOIESIS

DOUGLAS A. NELSON, M.D., and FREDERICK R. DAVEY, M.D.

STEM CELLS

In postnatal life in humans, erythrocytes, granulocytes, monocytes, and platelets are normally produced only in the bone marrow. Lymphocytes are produced in the secondary lymphoid organs, as well as in the bone marrow and thymus gland.

Most bone marrow cells are morphologically recognizable precursors of granulocytes, erythrocytes, or platelets. A fraction of cells in adult marrow is identifiable only as lymphocytes. Smaller numbers of monocytes, macrophages, endothelial cells, and plasma cells are noted.

Stem cells can both reproduce themselves and give rise to more differentiated cells. They are not morphologically identifiable as stem cells, but are believed to reside among the small or intermediate-sized lymphocytes.

Hematopoietic Stem Cells

A pluripotential or multipotential stem cell is present in the marrow and gives rise to two major progenitors, the lymphoid stem cell and the myeloid or hematopoietic stem cell (Cline, 1977). The latter is a common precursor cell for granulocytes and monocytes, erythrocytes, and megakaryocytes. Evidence for this in animal models was demonstrated experimentally by Till (1961), who injected isologous bone marrow cells into irradiated mice. Seven to ten days later spleen colonies formed which contained erythroid cells, granulocytes, megakaryocytes, or a mixture of cell types. It could be shown that all the differentiating cells in a single colony were derivatives of a single stem cell (Becker, 1963), and after retransplanting cells from a single colony with only one differentiated cell type present, multipotential stem cells were still present in the individual colonies (Lewis, 1964). These multipotential stem cells have been operationally designated colony-forming units—spleen (CFU-S).

Evidence in the human for a multipotential hematopoietic stem cell derives from myeloproliferative disorders (polycythemia vera, myelofibrosis with myeloid metaplasia, chronic myelogenous leukemia). In these disorders it has been shown that one precursor cell gives rise to the abnormal erythrocytes, granulocytes, and megakaryocytes, but not to marrow fibroblasts, and in most cases not to lymphocytes (Fialkow, 1977).

These multipotential hematopoietic stem cells (HSCs) are present in small numbers in blood and marrow and have a very slow turnover—they comprise a dormant reserve. The mechanism by which HSCs are induced to become committed stem cells for the various cell lines is not known, but there is evidence that it is under the control of environmental factors. Proliferating hematopoietic cells are therefore confined to certain locations in the body (Metcalf, 1977).

Committed Progenitor Cells

Committed progenitor cells (committed stem cells) are characterized by their ability to form colonies *in vitro* in response to a soluble factor. Bradley (1966) and Ichikawa (1966) described *in vitro* culture systems in which granulocytic differentiation occurred from normal mouse hemopoietic cells; the technique was later adapted for human cells by Pike (1970). The cultures consist of two layers of cells in agar: an upper layer of blood or bone marrow contains "target" stem cells (colony-forming cells [CFC] or colony-forming units in culture [CFU-C]); a lower layer of blood cells (feeder layer) contains a diffusible substance (colony-stimulating factor [CSF]) necessary to stimulate the CFC to proliferate and differentiate into colonies. After a period of 7 to 14 days, colonies become visible in the upper layer; these are composed of neutrophils, monocytes (macrophages), a mixture of these two cell types, or eosinophils. The CSF necessary in the feeder layer is produced by monocytes or activated lymphocytes. It was shown that each colony was derived from a single progenitor (stem) cell. Since both neutrophils and monocytes were found in the same colony, it became clear that neutrophils (granulocytes) and monocytes were both derived from a single committed progenitor cell (GM-CFC) in response to a soluble substance (GM-CSF) (Metcalf, 1977).

Modifications in culture systems have permitted *in vitro* colony growth and differentiation of human stem cells: erythroid precursors from erythropoietic progenitor cells, burst forming units—erythroid (BFU-E) and colony forming units—erythroid (CFU-E) in response to erythropoietin (Mladenovic, 1982); eosinophils from eosinophil progenitor cells (Eo-CFC) in response to Eo-CSF produced by activated lymphocytes (Metcalf, 1977); megakaryocytes from colony forming units—megakaryocytic (CFU-Mk), which appear to require a megakaryocytic colony stimulating factor (Mk-CSF) for proliferation and thrombopoietin for maturation (Williams, 1982); and multiple myeloid cell types from pluripotential progenitor cells, CFU-GEMM (Fauser, 1979). Basophil colony forming cells in humans have not been well characterized but have been described recently (Denburg, 1983).

The various CFCs are regarded as committed progenitor cells that have receptors for the appropriate humoral factor (e.g., erythropoietin, CSF) and that respond by proliferation and differentiation (Fig. 28–1). These committed progenitor cells are self-sustaining for long periods of time and are signaled to proliferate by the humoral messenger in response to need.

Neither the multipotential hematopoietic stem cells nor the committed stem cells are morphologically identifiable. Evidence exists that they have the appearance of small to medium-sized lymphocytes, but by immunologic criteria they are neither T cells nor B cells.

HEMATOPOIETIC TISSUES

(Weiss, 1977)

4

Organs or tissues in which blood cell production occurs are known as hematopoietic tissues.

Embryonic and Fetal Hematopoiesis

Beginning in the first month of prenatal life, the first blood cells arise outside the embryo in the mesenchyme of the yolk sac, as *blood islands.* The cells are predominantly *primitive erythroblasts,* which are large and megaloblastic, are formed intravascularly, and retain their nuclei. At the sixth week, hematopoiesis begins in the liver, and this becomes the major hematopoietic organ of early and mid fetal life. *Definitive erythroblasts,* which become non-nucleated red cells, are formed extravascularly in the liver, and granulopoiesis and megakaryocytes are present to a lesser degree. In the middle part of fetal life, the spleen and to a lesser extent lymph nodes have a minor role in hematopoiesis, but the liver continues to dominate. In the later half of fetal life, the bone marrow becomes progressively more important as a site of blood cell production. As this occurs, the liver's role diminishes.

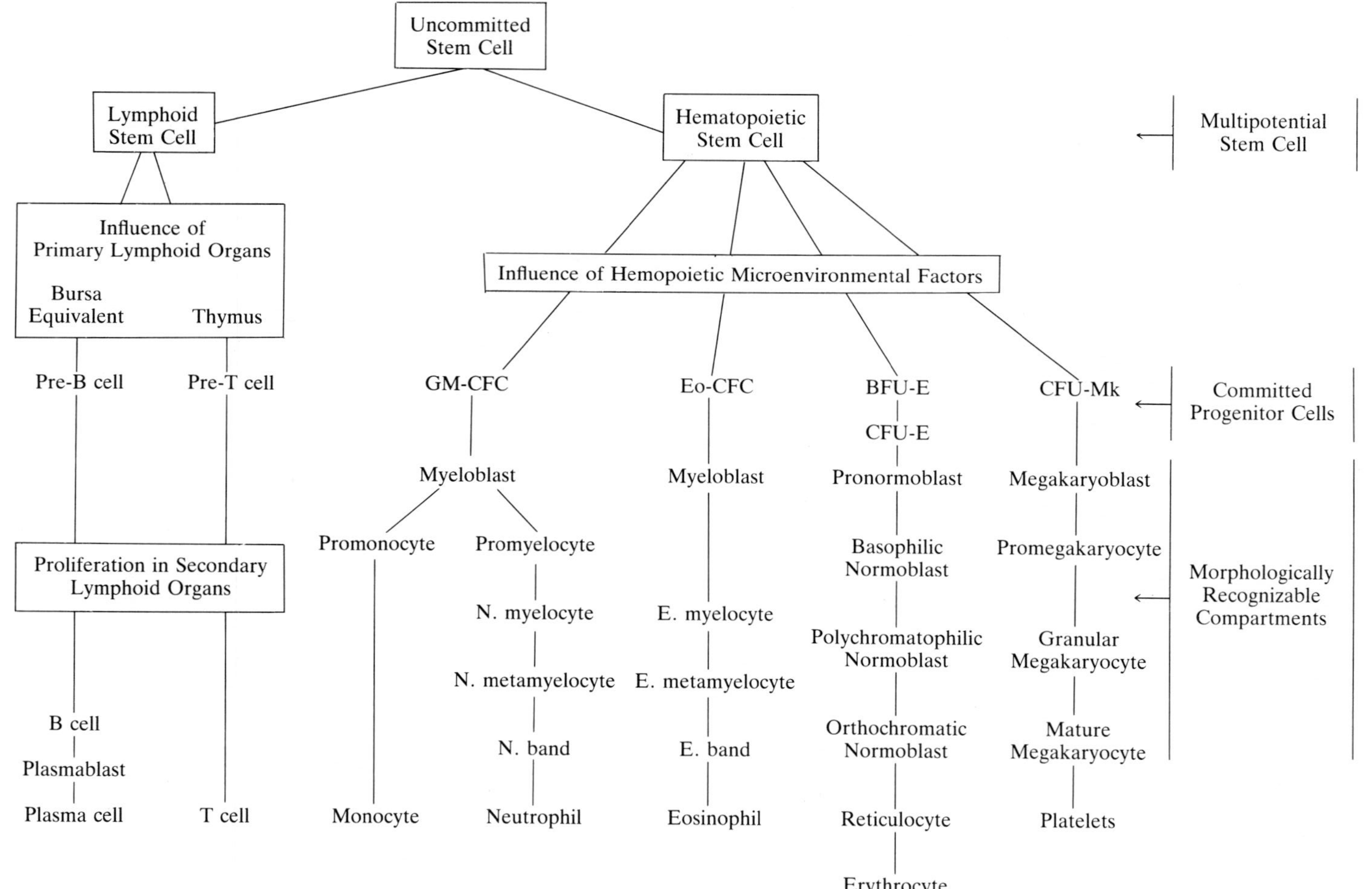

Figure 28–1. Hypothetical scheme of hematopoiesis as discussed in text. Local or short-range factors (or "influences") act on the multipotential stem cells to produce committed progenitor cells.

GM-CFC = granulocyte-monocyte colony forming cell
Eo-CFC = eosinophil colony forming cell
BFU-E = burst forming unit (cell)—erythroid
CFU-E = colony forming unit (cell)—erythroid
CFU-Mk = colony forming unit (cell)—megakaryocytic

The committed progenitor cells of the myeloid lines respond to specific hormones (e.g., erythropoietin for CFU-E, GM-CSF for GM-CFC) by proliferation and differentiation into mature cells of the particular series.

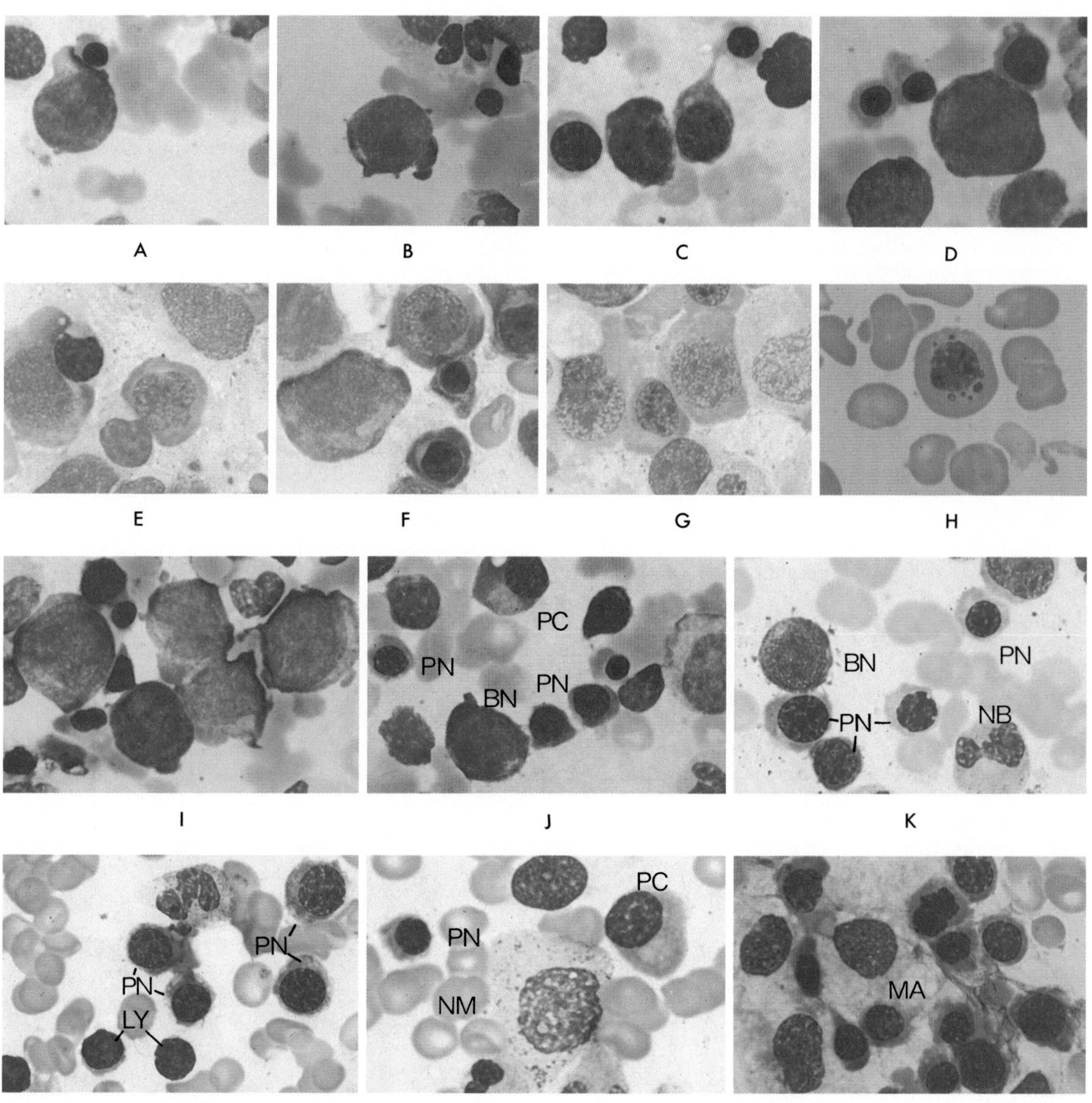

Plate 28–1. Normoblastic series, *A* to *D;* megaloblastic series, *E* to *H;* same magnification. *A,* Pronormoblast, normal marrow. A small orthochromatic normoblast is in contact with the pronormoblast. A broken nucleus of an unidentifiable cell is partly in the field. *B,* Basophilic normoblast, normal marrow. Note the intense cytoplasmic basophilia and irregular cytoplasmic protrusions, which are common. *C,* Basophilic normoblast, center; polychromatophilic normoblasts (PN) on either side. The PN on the right is more mature, having more condensed nuclear chromatin and more cytoplasmic hemoglobin than the PN on the right. *D,* Orthochromatic normoblasts; *left,* normal marrow. Note the pyknotic nuclei. Cytoplasm retains RNA and is polychromatophilic. A basophilic normoblast and a polychromatophilic normoblast are in the field. *E,* Promegaloblast, *left.* Overlying its edge is a small cell with intensely staining nuclear chromatin, probably part of a late polychromatophilic megaloblast. In the center, an earlier polychromatophilic megaloblast is in contact with a lymphocyte. *F,* Basophilic megaloblast, *left;* polychromatophilic megaloblasts, *center. G,* Polychromatophilic megaloblasts. Note, in addition to the large size (compared with *C*), the prominent parachromatin; this is an "open" nuclear chromatin pattern. *H,* Orthochromatic megaloblast with karyorrhexis and multiple Howell-Jolly bodies. *I,* A group of four pronormoblasts, one basophilic normoblast, and a few later forms, from a marrow aspirate showing normoblastic hyperplasia. *J,* Contrast the basophilic normoblast (BN) and the polychromatophilic normoblasts (PN) with the plasma cell (PC); these cells are sometimes confused. *K,* Basophilic normoblast (BN) with several "pseudopods," four polychromatophilic normoblasts (PN), and a neutrophil band form (NB). *L,* Contrast the lymphocytes (LY) with smudged nuclear chromatin, and the polychromatophilic normoblasts (PN) which are sometimes confused. Here, the PN have delayed cytoplasmic maturation (less hemoglobin than expected for the degree of nuclear development). The normoblasts have sharper separation of nuclear chromatin and parachromatin than the lymphocytes. *M,* Small polychromatophilic normoblast (PN), damaged early neutrophil myelocyte (NM), and plasma cell (PC). *N,* Erythroblastic island. The macrophage in the center (MA) has abundant partially vacuolated cytoplasm which is in contact with several normoblasts; one of the latter is in mitosis.

4

Postnatal Hematopoiesis

Shortly after birth, hematopoiesis in the liver ceases and the marrow is the only site for the production of erythrocytes, granulocytes, and platelets. Hematopoietic stem cells and committed progenitor cells are maintained in the marrow. Lymphocytes (of the B cell type) continue to be produced in the marrow, as well as in the secondary lymphoid organs, whereas T-lymphocytes are produced in the thymus and also in the secondary lymphoid organs (p. 643).

At birth, the total marrow space is occupied by active hematopoietic (red) marrow. As body growth progresses and marrow space increases during infancy, only part of that space is needed for hematopoiesis; the remaining space is occupied by fat cells. Later in childhood, only the flat bones (the skull, vertebrae, thoracic cage, shoulder, and pelvis) and the proximal parts of the long bones (femora and humeri) are sites of blood formation. The remaining marrow space is fatty or yellow marrow which can be replaced by hematopoietic cells if continuous, intensive stimulation exists.

The marrow circulation is closed, that is, arterioles deriving from central longitudinal arteries (i.e., in long bones) connect directly with broad venous sinuses which anastomose and eventually empty into central longitudinal veins. The flattened endothelium of the sinuses is partially covered by adventitial reticular cells, a form of fibroblast that elaborates argentophilic reticulin fibers. These reticular cells and fibers form the supporting meshwork of the marrow stroma, where the hematopoietic cells reside. The reticular cells are but minimally phagocytic; they may swell and take up water, may become fat cells, and possibly may induce hematopoietic stem cells to become committed progenitor cells (Weiss, 1977). After proliferation and maturation have occurred in the marrow stroma, blood cells gain entrance to the blood through or between the endothelial cells of the sinus wall. This requires displacement of adventitial cells. Little is known about this process of "release"; in the case of red cells (reticulocytes), erythropoietin appears to play a role.

ERYTHROCYTE PRODUCTION*

The erythrocyte is a vehicle for the transport of hemoglobin, which is produced in precursor cells of the erythrocytes, the normoblasts. The function of hemoglobin is the transport of oxygen and carbon dioxide. The erythrocyte is also metabolically capable of keeping hemoglobin in a functional state.

It is believed that the pluripotential hematopoietic stem cell (HSC) is induced by certain microenvironmental influences to become the committed erythroid progenitor cell. These cell types are not morphologically separable from small lymphocytes.

The committed progenitor cell compartment for erythropoiesis probably consists of two components (Metcalf, 1977; Mladenovic, 1982). These are defined operationally by their behavior in *in vitro* culture systems as burst-forming units (BFU-E) and colony-forming units (CFU-E). The BFU-E is probably the earlier form, responding to uncertain factors (including high concentrations of erythropoietin) by forming CFU-Es. T lymphocytes may be required for optimal BFU-E growth. CFU-Es respond to low concentrations of erythropoietin by forming morphologically recognizable pronormoblasts. BFU-E are present in small numbers in peripheral blood, as well as in marrow.

*See Hillman (1974) and Izak (1977).

Normoblastic Maturation
(Plate 28–1)

The earliest recognizable erythroid precursor is the *pronormoblast* (Fig. 28–1 and Plate 28–1*A* and *I*). At about 20 μm diameter, it is the largest of the erythroid precursors. The nucleus has a fine, uniform chromatin pattern which is somewhat more distinct and more intensely staining than that of the myeloblast. The nuclear membrane is prominent. One or more prominent nucleoli are present. The cytoplasm has a heterogeneous quality and is moderate in amount and moderately basophilic; no granules are present. The pronormoblast undergoes mitosis and forms two basophilic normoblasts.

The *basophilic normoblast* (Plate 28–1*B*, *C*, *J*, and *K*) is somewhat smaller and has slightly coarser chromatin which stains intensely; the chromatin may be partially clumped and the pattern may suggest a wheel with broad spokes. The parachromatin (the non-chromatin part of the nucleus) is distinct and stains pink. Nucleoli are present but not often visible. The nuclear/cytoplasmic (N/C) ratio is moderate; about one fourth of the total cell area appears to be cytoplasm. The cytoplasm is deeply basophilic owing to the abundance of RNA; much of this is evident as polyribosomes in electron micrographs. The cell borders of early normoblasts frequently are made irregular by pseudopodia.

After mitosis of the basophilic normoblast, continuing hemoglobin production becomes visible in the cytoplasm of the two daughter cells as polychromasia, i.e., mixtures of the red-staining of hemoglobin with the blue of RNA in varying shades of gray. This cell is the *polychromatophilic normoblast* (Fig. 27–37 and Plate 28–1*C*, *J*, *K*, *L*, and *M*), which is slightly smaller than the basophilic normoblast. The nucleus occupies about half of the area of the cell, stains intensely, and has moderately condensed chromatin which is sharply distinct from the pink parachromatin. The polychromatophilic normoblast undergoes one or two mitotic divisions.

After the last mitosis, the nucleus becomes small and dense (pyknotic) and the *orthochromatic normoblast* stage is reached (Fig. 27–37 and Plate 28–1*D*). Mitosis is no longer possible. The cell is smaller than the polychromatophilic normoblast and has a lower N/C ratio. The cytoplasm contains more abundant hemoglobin and fewer polyribosomes and remains slightly polychromatophilic.

Finally, accompanied by cytoplasmic contractions and undulations, the nucleus and a small rim of cytoplasm are ejected from the orthochromatic normoblast (Lessin, 1977) forming the *reticulocyte.* On air-dried films with Romanowsky stains, the reticulocyte is polychromatophilic due to the retention of RNA.

In the marrow, developing erythroid cells are usually in contact with macrophages in what are termed "erythroblastic islands" (Plate 28–1*N*). It is likely that ferritin moves from normoblast to macrophage. These erythroblastic islands are usually broken up when aspirated marrow is spread on slides, but fragments of macrophage cytoplasm may sometimes be seen attached to the separated normoblasts, especially on Prussian blue–stained films.

During proliferation and maturation, iron is transferred from plasma transferrin into the cells in the normoblastic series. The pronormoblast and basophilic normoblast have the highest content of RNA, which begins to decline in the polychromatophilic normoblasts as hemoglobin increases in amount. Synthesis of RNA gradually decreases in each stage through the orthochromatic normoblasts. Of course, when the nucleus is no longer present (in the reticulocyte), RNA synthesis ceases, yet the RNA already present remains for a few days, and protein and heme synthesis continue in the reticulocyte until the cell loses its RNA and mitochondria.

During this maturation process, three or four mitotic divisions occur in a period of three days, resulting in the potential production of 16 reticulocytes from each pronormoblast. The reticulocytes are larger than mature red cells and are sticky. They remain in the marrow stroma for one to two days before they are released into the blood.

In the marrow the reticulocytes are about equal in number to the nucleated erythrocytes and slightly greater in number than the reticulocytes in the circulating blood. If sufficiently severe hypoxia is present, this marrow pool of reticulocytes can be released. This approximately doubles the number of circulating reticulocytes.

Normally, reticulocytes remain as such, slowly synthesizing hemoglobin, for one day in the marrow and one day in the blood. Residual ribosomes, mitochondria, and other organelles are then removed, and the mature erythrocytes circulate for about 120 days. During this time they gradually age, certain enzymatic activities diminish, and they are finally destroyed within phagocytic cells of the reticuloendothelial system.

Megaloblastic Maturation
(Plate 28–1)

Abnormal maturation of erythroid precursors that occurs in vitamin B_{12} deficiency or folic acid deficiency (p. 657) is known as megaloblastic maturation, and the abnormal erythroid cells are called *megaloblasts.* Because of impaired ability of the cells to synthesize DNA, the intermitotic and mitotic phases are prolonged. This results in enlarged cells, with nuclear maturation lagging behind cytoplasmic maturation (cytonuclear dissociation). The nuclear chromatin pattern is more delicate and more "open," with prominent parachromatin. Karyorrhexis, or breaking up of the nucleus, and Howell-Jolly bodies are frequently noted. Megaloblastic development parallels normoblastic maturation; the stages of promegaloblast, basophilic megaloblast, polychromatophilic megaloblast, and orthochromatic megaloblast may be recognized (Plate 28–1*E* to *H*).

Regulation of Erythrocyte Production

The number of erythrocytes in the blood may be regulated by changing the rate of production. The rate of erythrocyte destruction does not vary appreciably in normal individuals. Increased production of erythrocytes occurs when oxygen transport to the tissues is impaired, as in anemia, in cardiac or pulmonary disorders, and in the low oxygen tension of high altitudes. On the other hand, production of erythrocytes is decreased when an individual is hypertransfused or exposed to high oxygen tension.

Oxygen affinity of hemoglobin is modulated by the concentration of phosphates, in particular 2,3-diphosphoglycerate (2,3-DPG) in the red cell. These phosphates combine with the beta chains of reduced hemoglobin and diminish its affinity for oxygen (Fig. 28–2). In areas of tissue hypoxia, as oxygen moves from hemoglobin into the tissues, the amount of reduced hemoglobin in the red cells increases, binding more 2,3-DPG, further reducing its oxygen affinity so that more oxygen can be delivered to the tissues. If hypoxia persists, depletion of free 2,3-DPG leads to increased glycolysis, production of more 2,3-DPG, and a persistently lower oxygen affinity of the hemoglobin.

Tissue hypoxia induces formation of *erythropoietin,* a hormone that travels in the plasma to the marrow, where it effects the production of more red cells. Erythropoietin is a glycoprotein that is relatively heat stable but is inactivated by proteolytic enzymes. On electrophoresis, it migrates as an alpha-2-globulin. Erythropoietin is produced mainly in the kidney. It acts by inducing committed progenitor cells in the marrow to proliferate and differentiate into pronormoblasts, by shortening the generation time of normoblasts, and by promoting early release of reticulocytes into the blood. The result is increased numbers of marrow normoblasts, in a normal ratio of cell types, a condition known as normoblastic hyperplasia.

Erythropoietin is measured by bioassay employing mice made polycythemic by hypertransfusion or hypoxia to suppress endogenous erythropoietin production. The test plasma or urine is injected into the mice, and incorporation of radioactive iron into circulating erythrocytes is measured. Normal or increased amounts of erythropoietin can be detected in the plasma of patients with certain types of anemia, but in plasma, decreased levels cannot be detected reliably. Methods for concentrating the urine have been devised, and well-defined levels of erythropoietic activity can be measured in normal urine (Adamson, 1966).

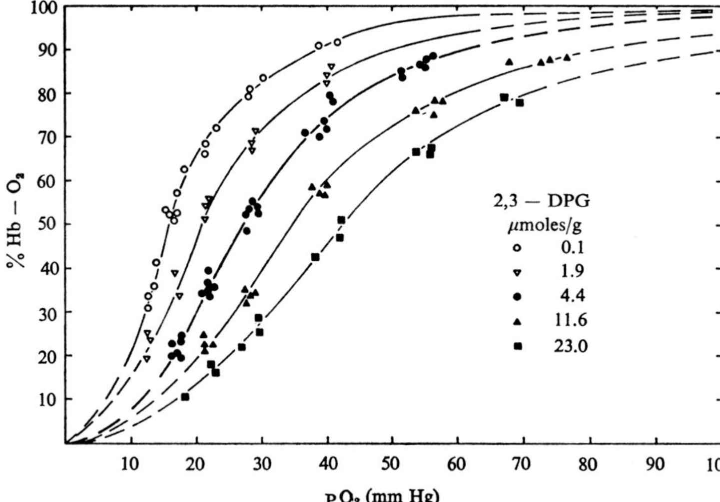

Figure 28–2. Oxygen dissociation curves of hemoglobin at different concentrations of 2,3-diphosphoglycerate (DPG). The curve is sigmoidal and shifts to the right with increasing concentrations of 2,3-DPG: this results in decreased affinity of hemoglobin for oxygen and increased delivery of oxygen to the tissues. (From Duhm, J.: *In* Rørth, M., and Astrup, P. (eds.): Oxygen Affinity of Hemoglobin and Red Cell Acid Base Status. (Alfred Benzon Symposium IV). Copenhagen, Munksgaard International Publishers, 1972, p. 583.)

Elevated levels are detected in patients with erythroid hyperplasia and in aplastic anemia. Decreased levels below the normal range are found in normal individuals after transfusion and in polycythemia vera.

Synthesis of Hemoglobin

Heme Synthesis. Heme synthesis occurs in most cells of the body, except the mature erythrocytes, but most abundantly in the erythroid precursors. Succinyl-coenzyme A condenses with glycine to form the unstable intermediate alpha-amino beta-keto-adipic acid, which is readily decarboxylated to delta-aminolevulinic acid (ALA) (Fig. 28–3). This condensation requires pyridoxal phosphate (vitamin B_6) and occurs in mitochondria.

ALA is excreted normally in small amounts in the urine; but in certain abnormalities of heme synthesis (e.g., lead poisoning) excretion is increased. Two molecules of ALA condense to form the monopyrrole, porphobilinogen, catalyzed by the enzyme ALA-dehydrase. Porphobilinogen is also normally excreted in small amounts in the urine. Markedly elevated

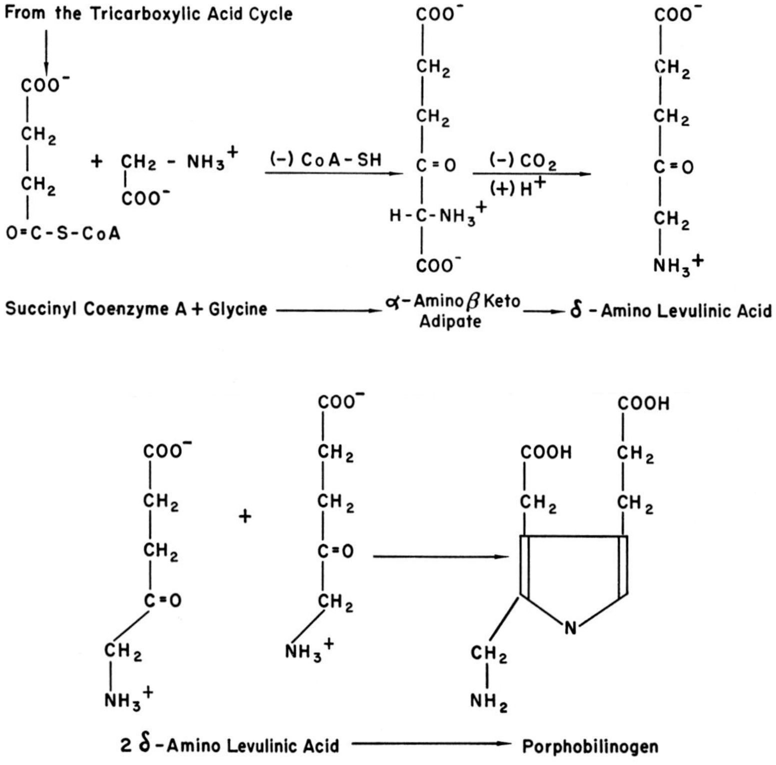

From the Tricarboxylic Acid Cycle

$COO^- - CH_2 - CH_2 - C(=O) - S - CoA$ + $CH_2(NH_3^+) - COO^-$ —(−) CoA-SH→ $COO^- - CH_2 - CH_2 - C(=O) - CH(NH_3^+) - COO^-$ —(−) CO_2, (+) H^+→ $COO^- - CH_2 - CH_2 - C(=O) - CH_2 - NH_3^+$

Succinyl Coenzyme A + Glycine ——→ α-Amino β Keto Adipate ——→ δ-Amino Levulinic Acid

$COO^- - CH_2 - CH_2 - C(=O) - CH_2 - NH_3^+$ + $COO^- - CH_2 - CH_2 - C(=O) - CH_2 - NH_3^+$ ——→ Porphobilinogen (pyrrole ring bearing CH_2COOH, CH_2CH_2COOH and CH_2NH_2)

2 δ-Amino Levulinic Acid ——→ Porphobilinogen

Figure 28–3. Formation of porphobilinogen from succinyl-coenzyme A and glycine. (From Leavell, B. S.: Fundamentals of Clinical Hematology. 4th ed. Philadelphia, W. B. Saunders Company, 1976.)

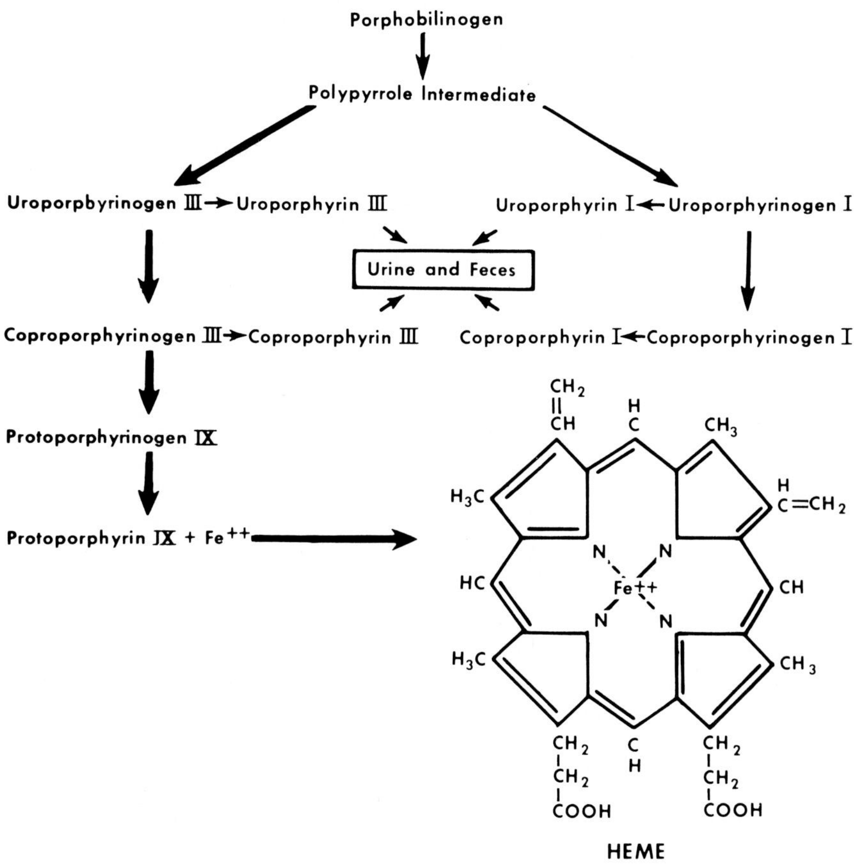

Figure 28–4. Formation of heme from porphobilinogen. (From Leavell, B. S.: Fundamentals of Clinical Hematology. 4th ed. Philadelphia, W. B. Saunders Company, 1976.)

amounts appear in the urine in acute intermittent porphyria, and are easily detected by a color reaction with Ehrlich's aldehyde reagent.

Four molecules of porphobilinogen react to form uroporphyrinogen III or I (Fig. 28–4). The type III isomer is converted, by way of coproporphyrinogen III and protoporphyrinogen, to protoporphyrin. In certain diseases when this pathway is partially blocked, the type I isomers of uroporphyrinogen and coproporphyrinogen are formed and their oxidized excretion products, uroporphyrin I and coproporphyrin I, are increased in amount.

Protoporphyrin is normally found in mature erythrocytes. In lead poisoning and in iron deficiency, levels of free erythrocyte protoporphyrin are increased.

Iron is inserted into protoporphyrin by the mitochondrial enzyme ferrochetalase to form the finished heme moiety.

Globin Synthesis. Globin synthesis occurs in the cytoplasm of the normoblast and reticulocyte. The polypeptide chains are manufactured on the ribosomes. Specific small sRNA (soluble RNA) molecules determine the placement of each amino acid according to the code in the mRNA (messenger RNA). Progressive growth of the polypeptide chain begins at the amino end. This process of protein synthesis occurs on ribosomes clustered into polyribosomes, which are held together by the mRNA. Since the reticulocyte can synthesize hemoglobin for at least two days after loss of its nucleus, it appears that the messenger RNA for hemoglobin is quite stable. The polypeptide chains released from the ribosomes are folded into their three-dimensional configurations spontaneously.

Control of hemoglobin synthesis is exerted primarily through the action of heme. Increased heme inhibits further heme synthesis by inhibiting the activity and synthesis of ALA synthase. Heme also promotes globin synthesis, mainly at the site of chain initiation, the interaction of ribosomes with mRNA (Lodish, 1976).

Structure and Function of Hemoglobin

(Bunn, 1977)

In each hemoglobin molecule, one heme group is inserted into a hydrophobic pocket of one folded polypeptide chain. Normal adult hemoglobin A consists of four heme groups and four polypeptide chains (two alpha chains and two beta chains) which form a roughly globular hemoglobin molecule (Fig. 28–5). The ferrous iron atoms have six coordination bonds, four to the pyrrole nitrogens of heme, one to the imidazole nitrogen of histidine of the globin chain

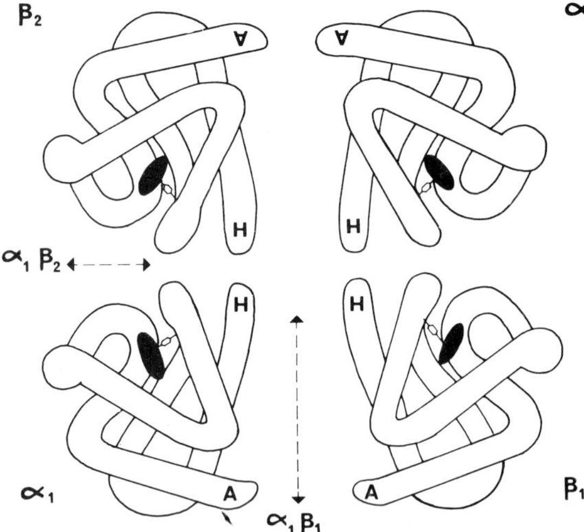

Figure 28–5. Schematic diagram of the hemoglobin molecure (tetramer, molecular weight 64,500 daltons). The heme group for each monomeric polypeptide chain is depicted as a black disk, connected to an imidazole group of histidine, and located near the surface of the molecule in a "pocket" formed by the polypeptide chain. Letters A and H designate alphahelical segments of each polypeptide chain; A is the N-terminal segment and H is the C-terminal segment. The four monomers are separated in this drawing, but actually make contact along a relatively large area (α_1 β_1), which is thought to be the relatively fixed or stabilizing contact area, and a smaller (α_1 β_2) area thought to be the functional contact area, where movement occurs during oxygenation and deoxygenation, changing the molecular configuration. (From White, J. M., and Dacie, J. V.: Prog. Hematol., 7:69, 1971. Grune & Stratton, Inc., New York, by permission.)

(87 alpha or 92 beta), and one that is reversibly bound to oxygen. As the oxygen partial pressure increases, the four heme groups sequentially bind one molecule of oxygen each. In the process, a change in the overall configuration of the hemoglobin molecule occurs, and this altered configuration favors the additional binding of oxygen.

The sigmoid-shaped oxygen dissociation curve of hemoglobin reflects this increasing affinity for oxygen with increasing partial pressure of oxygen in the lungs (Fig. 28–2). In the tissues, the conversion of $HbO_2 \rightarrow Hb$, the decreasing pH and increasing temperature produced by metabolic processes, and the binding of more 2,3-DPG to Hb result in a shift of the Hb-oxygen dissociation curve to the right, favoring the release of oxygen from hemoglobin.

Carbon dioxide (CO_2) is transported in erythrocytes as well as in plasma. A small part of red cell CO_2 is dissolved, a small part is bound to amino groups of hemoglobin as carbamino-CO_2, but most is in the bicarbonate form (Henry, 1964). The enzyme carbonic anhydrase catalyzes the transformation of carbon dioxide to bicarbonate in the red cell while in the tissue capillary bed and catalyzes the reverse reaction (the release of carbon dioxide from bicarbonate) in the erythrocyte when it is in the capillary bed of the lungs.

ERYTHROCYTE DESTRUCTION

The erythrocyte gradually undergoes metabolic changes over the course of its 120-day life span, at which time the less viable senescent cell is removed from the circulation. Certain glycolytic enzymes diminish in activity as the cell ages. Older red cells have a smaller surface area and an increased MCHC compared with younger cells (Ganzoni, 1971). Changes in the cell surface may render the cell more liable to phagocytosis. The exact mechanism by which senescent erythrocytes are recognized and removed by the reticuloendothelial system is unknown. The process may be by phagocytosis of whole erythrocytes or of fragmenting senescent cells. About 3 million cells are normally removed from the blood per second without demonstrable histologic evidence of erythrophagocytosis.

Under normal conditions in man, the major part of erythrophagocytosis appears to occur in the bone marrow (Bessis, 1973). In pathological states when the erythrocyte is damaged and the red cell survival is shortened, the site of destruction depends upon the extent to which the erythrocyte is damaged. If the damage is small, the erythrocytes are removed primarily by the spleen. If the damage is great, the cells are removed mainly by the liver.

Degradation of Hemoglobin

After removal of the red cell from the circulation, hemoglobin is broken down within the macrophages of the reticuloendothelial system into its three constituents—iron, protoporphyrin, and globin. The iron goes into storage and may be completely reutilized. The globin may be degraded and returned to the amino acid pool of the body. In contrast, the protoporphyrin ring is split, converted to bilirubin, and excreted from the body.

In the macrophage, the protoporphyrin ring is cleaved by a heme oxidase enzyme at the alphamethene bridge, yielding one mole of carbon monoxide (CO) and one mole of biliverdin (see Fig. 13–2). The CO appears in the blood as HbCO and is eventually exhaled. Biliverdin is reduced to bilirubin in the macrophage, and bilirubin is transported to the liver by plasma albumin (p. 219). It is removed from the plasma by the liver cell, conjugated mainly with glucuronide and excreted in the bile. In the intestine, reduction by bacteria occurs, and bilirubin is transformed into urobilinogen, mesobilirubinogen, and stercobilinogen, compounds which are collectively designated urobilinogens (see Fig. 13–1).

Estimation of exhaled CO, HbCO, or fecal urobilinogen can be used as measures of hemoglobin breakdown. When production of red cells is diminished and the level of circulating hemoglobin is low, as in aplastic anemia, urobilinogen excretion is reduced. When destruction of erythrocytes is increased, as in hemolytic anemia, all three are increased in amount.

In normal humans about 80 to 90 per cent of the excreted bile pigment measured as fecal urobilinogen is derived from breakdown of senescent erythrocytes which have lived 100 to 120 days. However, about 10 to 20 per cent of the pigment is excreted within the first few days. This early labeled bile pigment comes from non-hemoglobin heme formed in the liver, as well as from the breakdown of newly formed hemoglobin in the bone marrow. Much of this may represent hemoglobin from the nucleus and pieces of cytoplasm of the orthochromatic normoblast that are lost during the process of nuclear extrusion.

In certain hematologic diseases, notably thalassemia, megaloblastic anemia, refractory normoblastic anemia, and erythropoietic porphyria, this early labeled bile pigment fraction may be markedly increased. This excessive intramedullary destruction of hemoglobin, which never appears in circulating erythrocytes, is known as ineffective erythropoiesis.

ERYTHROKINETICS

The balance between delivery of erythrocytes to the blood and removal of erythrocytes from the blood results in a relatively constant hemoglobin mass in the circulation. Anemia occurs when the removal of erythrocytes from the blood is increased and cannot be compensated for by increased production or when the delivery of erythrocytes to the blood is decreased or when both processes exist together.

When anemia develops, the resultant tissue hypoxia leads to elevated levels of erythropoietin in the plasma. Resultant normoblastic hyperplasia produces more erythrocytes for delivery to the circulation. The marrow in a normal individual is capable of six to eight times the normal output of erythrocytes with extreme stimulation. This capacity must be compared with the output actually attained when one is evaluating the marrow response of a given patient.

Measurements that assess effective erythropoiesis (production and delivery of erythrocytes to the circulation), ineffective erythropoiesis, and destruction of erythrocytes may be necessary to determine the mechanism and the cause of anemia (Harris, 1970).

Measurements of Total Production of Erythrocytes or Hemoglobin. The *total mass of erythropoietic cells* in the body cannot be easily measured. An estimate is made by examining a sample of bone marrow from a normally active site and determining the cellularity and the percentage of total nucleated cells that are erythropoietic (see section on bone marrow, p. 647). When marrow activity increases, usually the additional hematopoietic cells replace the fat in the red marrow sites before extension occurs into the yellow marrow of the long bones. One assumes that the sample is representative of the marrow as a whole, an assumption that usually is valid.

The *plasma iron turnover* is calculated from the serum iron level and the rate of removal of injected radioactive iron from the plasma. About 25 to 30 per cent of the iron is not used in erythropoiesis and is probably taken up by the liver. The remaining 70 to 75 per cent is taken up by erythropoietic cells and is therefore a measure of total erythropoiesis, both effective and ineffective.

Measurements of Total Destruction of Erythrocytes or Hemoglobin. Determination of *fecal urobilinogen* is an estimate of the total excretion of bile pigments—the breakdown products of heme. This measurement includes pigment derived from hemoglobin formed and destroyed in the marrow without ever reaching the circulating erythrocytes. Limitations include diminished conversion of bilirubin to urobilinogen because of oral administration of broad-spectrum antibiotics, and failure of pigment to reach the intestine in obstructive jaundice. In severe liver disease less reabsorbed urobilinogen is excreted in the bile and more is excreted in the urine. The urine urobilinogen is not as good a measure of urobilinogen excretion for two reasons: Removal by the kidney is usually a minor component of the total excretion, and with a normally functioning liver, clearance of reabsorbed urobilinogen in the plasma is so effective that considerable increases in the circulating blood may result in little or no elevation of the urine urobilinogen.

Measurements of Effective Production of Erythrocytes. ***Reticulocyte Count.*** Since the RNA of the reticulocyte disappears about a day after its entry into the blood, enumeration of reticulocytes will be a measure of the number of cells being delivered by the marrow to the blood each day, that is, a measure of effective erythropoiesis. If the erythrocyte count is determined, one can calculate the absolute reticulocyte count by multiplying the reticulocyte percentage by the erythrocyte count. To give a meaningful expression of erythropoiesis, the absolute reticulocyte count, or some estimate of it, and not simply the percentage must be used (Hillman, 1967). The normal absolute reticulocyte count is approximately 50×10^9/L or 1 per cent of circulating erythrocytes. Since the normal maturation time for reticulocytes in the blood is one day, production is 50×10^9 reticulocytes per liter per day.

4

A second consideration is an increased maturation time of reticulocytes in the blood due to accelerated release from the marrow, an effect of erythropoietin. The need for this is recognized by the presence of large, polychromatic cells or nucleated red cells in the blood film, indicating a shift of excessively immature reticulocytes from the marrow into the blood. To avoid an overestimate of daily erythrocyte production, a correction factor is used based on estimated maturation time of reticulocytes in the blood. This varies inversely with hematocrit as follows (Hillman, 1974):

Hematocrit (%)	Reticulocyte maturation time (days)
45	1.0
35	1.5
25	2.0
15	2.5

If a patient has a Hct = 0.25, red count = 2.89×10^{12}/L, and a reticulocyte count = 7 per cent, he will have an absolute reticulocyte count = 202×10^9/L. Since the average normal absolute reticulocyte count is 50×10^9/L, he has $\frac{202 \times 10^9/L}{50 \times 10^9/L}$ or four times as many reticulocytes as normal. However, this must be corrected for the increased maturation time (shift): $4 \times 1/2 = 2$. Therefore, two times as many reticulocytes are entering his blood per day as in a normal individual; that is, his red cell production is two times normal.

If only the hematocrit is available, the same correction can be made as follows:

Correction for hematocrit:

$$\text{“Absolute percentage”} = \text{reticulocyte count } (7\%) \times \frac{\text{Patient's Hct } (0.25)}{\text{Normal Hct } (0.45)} = 4\%$$

Correction for shift:

Corrected reticulocyte count

$$= \frac{\text{Absolute reticulocyte percentage } (4\%)}{\text{Maturation time (2 days)}} = 2$$

Corrections are necessary in order to assess the degree of red cell production in response to anemia.

A normal individual with a normal supply of iron can increase red cell production by two times normal within a week if the hematocrit drops to 0.35, or to three times the normal if the hematocrit drops to 0.25. Only if there is a parenteral supply of iron (such as in hemolysis) can the maximal red cell production of six to eight times normal be achieved (Hillman, 1967).

If an appropriate marrow response to anemia has not been reached in one to two weeks, some impairment of red cell production exists.

The *erythrocyte utilization of iron* is a measure of the amount of an injected dose of iron which appears in the hemoglobin of circulating erythrocytes. It is derived from the plasma iron turnover and the percentage of radioactive iron which has been injected and which appears in the circulating erythrocytes after two weeks, assuming that none of the newly formed cells have been destroyed in that time interval. This, too, is a measure of effective erythropoiesis.

Measurements of Effective Survival of Erythrocytes in the Blood. The *erythrocyte survival* can be determined by removing a sample of blood, labeling the erythrocytes with ^{51}Cr, inactivating the excess ^{51}Cr remaining in the plasma, and reinjecting the labeled erythrocytes into the patient. The ^{51}Cr is bound to the beta chain of the hemoglobin molecule and for the most part is not released until the red cell is removed from the circulation and the hemoglobin is degraded. Measurements of radioactivity in the red cells are made at two hours or 24 hours (the zero time, or 100 per cent level) and at one- to three-day intervals until over 50 per cent of the activity has disappeared. The results are usually expressed as the ^{51}Cr half survival time. The normal range is 28 to 38 days. (The reason it is not 60 days is that ^{51}Cr is eluted from the hemoglobin at the rate of about 1 per cent per day.) If the production of erythrocytes equals destruction (i.e., if a steady state exists), the erythrocyte survival is also a measure of effective production of erythrocytes.

Summary. Total erythropoiesis refers to the total production of hemoglobin or red cells; effective erythropoiesis refers to production of hemoglobin or red cells that reach the circulation; and ineffective erythropoiesis refers to production of hemoglobin or red cells that never reach the circulating blood. These concepts of the *erythrokinetic* approach to the study of anemia are useful, especially in situations that defy easy classification.

NEUTROPHILS (Plate 28–2)

The common progenitor cell for neutrophils and monocytes (GM-CFC) divides and gives rise to the myeloblast, the earliest recognizable granulocyte-monocyte precursor, under stimulation by a hormone, colony-stimulating factor for granulocytes and monocytes (GM-CSF).

Morphology of Neutrophil Precursors

The *myeloblast* (Plate 28–2*A*) is a cell about 15 μm in diameter with a moderately high N/C ratio, a large oval to quadrangular nucleus, very fine, uniform chromatin pattern, delicate nuclear membrane, and two to five nucleoli. The cytoplasm is pale, clear blue, and without granules. The appearance of azurophil granules (~0.5 μm diameter) heralds the earliest promyelocyte (Plate 28–2*B*) and indicates that the cell is to be a neutrophil. The *promyelocyte* stage encompasses the entire period of production of azurophil granules. The promyelocyte is slightly larger than the myeloblast. The nuclear chromatin begins to condense a bit, and the nucleoli are less obvious. The cytoplasm is basophilic and is filled by more and more azurophil granules (Plate 28–2*C*). The *neutrophil myelocyte* stage begins with the appearance of specific neurtrophil granules, at first only in the Golgi region; as more specific granules develop they spread throughout the cytoplasm (Plate 28–2*D* to *H*). With successive mitoses the number of azurophil granules (which have ceased production at the end of the promyelocyte stage) are diminished. The early neutrophil myelocyte, therefore, has a rather fine, dispersed nuclear chromatin pattern, many azurophil granules, and few specific granules. The late neutrophil myelocyte has a somewhat more condensed chromatin pattern, a cytoplasm well filled with specific granules, and rather few azurophil granules. The myelocyte is the latest stage capable of cell division. Next is the *neutrophil metamyelocyte,* distinguished by an indented, kidney-shaped nucleus with more condensed chromatin (Plate 28–2*F* and *G*). From this stage on, changes in the cytoplasm are insignificant. In the *band neutrophil* (stab form) the nucleus has more condensed chromatin and a rather uniform elongated shape. Partial constriction of the nucleus occurs in the band stage, until a fine filament (length but no breadth) is formed between two of the lobes, at which point the cell is classified as a *segmented neutrophil.*

The mature human neutrophil has twice as many specific granules as azurophil granules. The azurophil

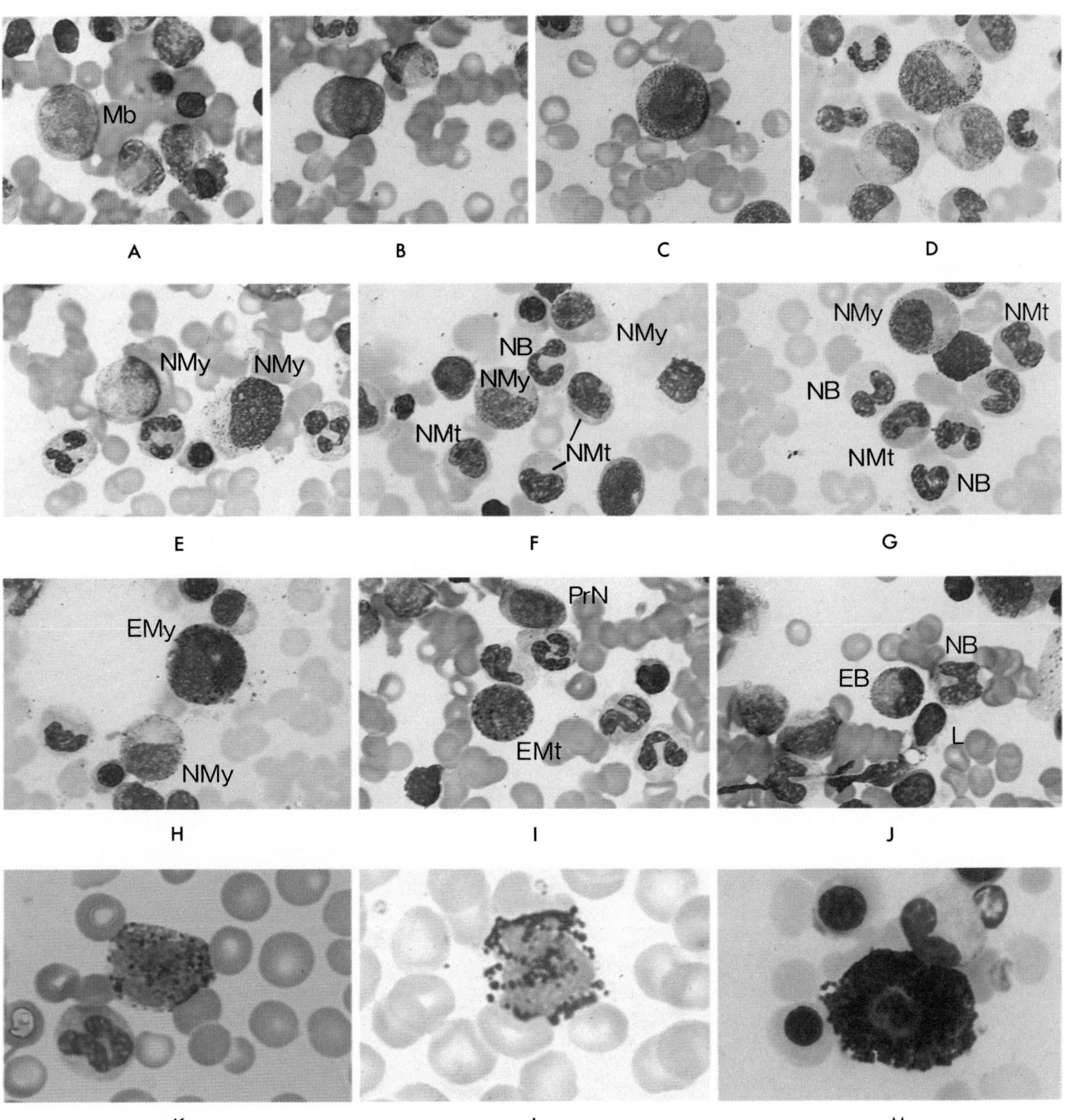

Plate 28–2. *A,* Myeloblast (Mb). *B,* Early promyelocyte has more basophilic cytoplasm than the myeloblast. A few azurophilic granules are in the vicinity of the Golgi zone. *C,* Promyelocyte. Later state has more numerous azurophilic granules. *D,* Neutrophil myelocytes. Newly formed specific granules have appeared in the Golgi zone adjacent to the nucleus. The azurophilic granules, which were formed in the promyelocyte stage, are best seen in the upper cell. As maturation proceeds, the azurophilic staining quality is lost. *E,* Neutrophil myelocytes (NMy), a late polychromatophilic normoblast, and three neutrophils. In the NM on the left, opaque granules overlying the nucleus give it a pale or "moth-eaten" appearance. *F,* N. myelocyte (NMy), N. metamyelocytes (NMt), and N. band form (NB). NMt and monocytes are frequently confused with one another. *G,* N. myelocyte (NMy), N. metamyelocytes (NMt), N. band forms (NB), and a broken or smudged cell. *H,* Eosinophil myelocyte (EMy), contrasted with a neutrophil myelocyte (NMy), is larger and has larger granules. The eosinophil granules that appear early in development have a basophilic staining reaction; as the cell matures they become olive-green, then eosinophilic in their staining characteristics. *I,* Eosinophil metamyelocyte (EMt). Neutrophils and a pronormoblast (PrN) are present. *J,* Eosinophil band form (EB), neutrophil band form (NB), and lymphocyte (L). The granules in the EB have the staining reaction characteristic of the mature cell. *K,* Basophil and neutrophil. *L,* Mature basophil. The nuclei in basophils do not normally segment. Immature basophils have cytoplasmic basophilia (outside the granules) which this cell lacks. *M,* Tissue mast cell; *center*, bone marrow. Mast cell granules are smaller, rounder, less water soluble, and more abundant than basophil granules; they usually obscure the nucleus.

4

granules (formed in the promyelocyte stage) contain lysosomal enzymes (acid hydrolases: acid phosphatase, β-glucuronidase, etc.), acid mucosubstance, peroxidase, one third of the cell's muramidase, and cationic antibacterial proteins. The specific granules (formed in the myelocyte stage) contain lactoferrin, most of the muramidase, and collagenase (Bainton, 1976). Biochemical studies of mature human neutrophils have shown that alkaline phosphatase is not in either of the granule fractions, but is in a lighter membrane fraction (West, 1974).

Distribution and Kinetics

The distribution of this cell series in the body is depicted in Figure 28–6. For each neutrophil in the blood vessels, about 16 precursors are present in the marrow. From the time of differentiation into a myeloblast, through about five mitotic divisions (three of which occur at the myelocyte stage), it takes about 14 days until the progeny of that cell reach the blood. The last eight days are spent in the maturation and storage pool. When a neutrophil enters the blood, it moves readily between a circulating granulocyte pool (CGP), which is sampled in the leukocyte count, and a marginal granulocyte pool (MGP), which is not, but is either marginated along vessel walls or sequestered in capillary beds. In less than a day after it arrives, the neutrophil emigrates from the circulation in a random manner and enters the tissues. From there, if not utilized in an inflammatory exudate, neutrophils leave the body within a few days via secretions in bronchi, saliva, gastrointestinal tract, and urine, or they are destroyed by the reticuloendothelial system.

Function

Neutrophils are able to move in a zigzag manner, but their motion changes to a straight line path if a chemotactic attractant (e.g., a bacterium coated with certain components of complement) is within a certain distance. Neutrophils have receptors for the Fc portion of IgG as well as for complement (C3) and bind and phagocytize the coated particle. Phagocytosis occurs, with the formation of a phagocytic vacuole that contains the ingested particle; accompanying this process is an increase in metabolic activity and energy production. Specific granules, followed shortly by azurophil granules, empty their contents into the phagocytic vacuoles, a process known as degranulation. Bactericidal activity occurs within the vacuole, mediated by H_2O_2, peroxidase, and a halide ion generating the free halogen, or by other enzymatic activity.

Neutrophils are thus important in defense against infectious disease (see Chap. 30). If their enzymes are activated and released outside the cell, neutrophils can cause tissue necrosis, as occurs in the Arthus or Shwartzman reaction. Neutrophils, which are active in inflammation, release an endogenous pyrogen that produces fever by acting on the hypothalamus to set the body's thermostat at a higher level (Murphy, 1976; Cline, 1975).

EOSINOPHILS

Eosinophils are produced in the bone marrow. It seems likely from *in vitro* culture studies that there is a separate eosinophilic committed progenitor cell (colony forming cell, Eo-CFC) in marrow that is distinct from the GM-CFC. The colony-stimulating factor that induces the Eo-CFC to proliferate and differentiate into eosinophil colonies (Eo-CSF) is produced by lymphocytes when stimulated by pokeweed mitogen or mercaptoethanol (Metcalf, 1977).

Morphology of Eosinophil Precursors

The cell that is the precursor for the earliest recognizable eosinophil, the eosinophil myelocyte, is

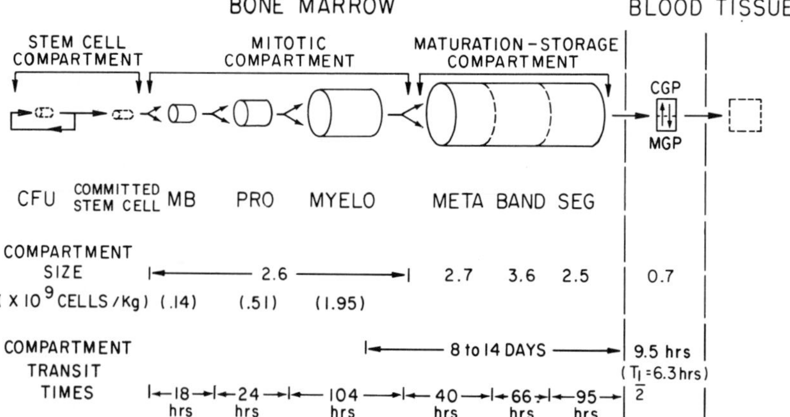

Figure 28–6. Neutrophil production, distribution, and kinetics. CFU = Multipotential stem cell; MB = myeloblast; PRO = promyelocyte; MYELO = myelocyte; META = metamyelocytes; SEG = segmented neutrophil; CGP = circulating granulocyte pool; MGP = marginal granulocyte pool. The cylinders representing the various compartments are drawn proportional to their sizes. The compartment transit times on the next to last line are from $DF^{32}P$ studies; those on the last line are from tritiated thymidine studies. (From Wintrobe, M. M., et al.: Clinical Hematology. 7th ed. Philadelphia, Lea & Febiger, 1974.)

presumably a distinctive myeloblast. However, it is morphologically indistinguishable from that which gives rise to neutrophils and monocytes or to basophils (Fig. 28–1 and Plate 28–2). In the early eosinophil myelocyte the granules are large and take the basophilic stain (Plate 28–2*H*). As the cell matures, the granules appear olive-green (Plate 28–2*I*) and finally the characteristic red-orange color (Plates 28–2*I* and 27–1*F* and *G*). Nuclear maturation is similar to that of the neutrophil. Eosinophils are slightly larger than neutrophils and have fewer nuclear lobes.

Electron micrographs of eosinophils show characteristic granules that have a dense crystalloid core in a less dense matrix. Immature granules, appearing in the myelocyte, at first have no crystalloid but develop them as maturation proceeds. Mature granules are of two types: the larger granule (0.5 to 1.5 μm in largest diameter) with a dense crystalloid; and a smaller granule (0.1 to 0.5 μm diameter) without a crystalloid. The smaller granules appear later during maturation, after the myelocyte stage.

Eosinophil granules contain peroxidase, acid hydrolase, phospholipase, and cathepsin. The small granules contain arylsulfatase; both granule types contain peroxidase and acid phosphatase. In the larger granules, the enzymes are localized in the matrix, not the crystalloid. Eosinophil granules have a different form of peroxidase than do neutrophils; also, eosinophils contain no alkaline phosphatase, muramidase, or phagocytin (Beeson, 1977).

Distribution and Kinetics

The kinetics of eosinophils are less well understood than those of neutrophils, but they are probably similar. They spend about the same half-time in the blood (less than eight hours) as neutrophils, and probably do not re-enter the circulation once they leave it. Eosinophils are considerably less numerous in blood and marrow than are neutrophils. Eosinophils in the tissues, however, are at least 100 times as numerous as the total eosinophils in the blood; they are located primarily in skin, lung, and gastrointestinal tract, i.e., the epithelial barriers to the outside world.

Function (Beeson, 1977)

The function of eosinophils is not completely understood. Eosinophils leave the blood when adrenal cortical hormone increases. Eosinophils proliferate in response to immunologic stimuli; this proliferative response is mediated, at least with some antigens, by T-lymphocytes. Although eosinophils phagocytose foreign particles and antigen-antibody complexes, this may not be their main function. There is evidence that eosinophils modulate reactions that occur when tissue mast cells and basophils degranulate. Among the chemotactic factors that attract eosinophils, ECF-A (eosinophil chemotactic factor of anaphylaxis) is present in basophils and mast cells; also, eosinophils contain substances that inactivate factors released by mast cells and basophils, such as histamine, slow-reacting substances of anaphylaxis, and platelet-activating factor. Except for providing some defense against helminthic parasites, the primary functions of eosinophils seem to be in their reactions with endogenous substances: products from mast cells and from lymphocytes, coagulation factors, complement, hormones, and kinins.

BASOPHILS AND MAST CELLS

Because there is no evidence for basophil development in *in vitro* colonies containing neutrophils and monocytes or eosinophils, it is possible that basophils develop from a separate committed precursor cell; there is, however, no evidence for this.

Morphology

Basophils probably develop from a cell resembling a myeloblast. The first recognizable stage is a *basophil myelocyte,* with the appearance of the specific basophil granules. These granules (about 0.2 to 1 μm in diameter) are larger than the azurophil granules of promyelocyte and often are irregular in shape. As the cell matures, the granules become more metachromatic (red-purple) because of increasing acid mucopolysaccharide (heparin) content. During maturation, cytoplasmic RNA decreases, and the nucleus partially segments. Because of incomplete nuclear segmentation, stages analogous to the neutrophil are not readily identified. In mature basophils the nucleus has condensed but smudged chromatin and the background cytoplasm lacks basophilia (residual RNA) (Plate 28–2*K* and *L*).

In contrast, *tissue mast cells* are connective tissue cells of mesenchymal origin that contain metachromatic cytoplasmic granules. They are widely distributed throughout the organism, including bone marrow, thymus, and spleen, but they do not normally appear in blood. On Romanowsky-stained films (Plate 28–2*M*) they are usually larger than basophils and have a low N/C ratio and a round or oval reticular nucleus which is usually obscured by abundant red-purple granules. The granules are smaller, more round and regular, and less soluble than basophil granules. The cytoplasmic granules are often spindle-shaped rather than round.

Kinetics

Because the basophil is the least numerous of the leukocytes, the kinetics have been difficult to discover and information is sparse. Production is believed to be similar to that of the neutrophil and eosinophil. Its time in the marrow is probably somewhat shorter than that of the neutrophil, and its half-time in the blood is about the same. Its fate in the tissues is not well understood.

4

Function

With regard to circulating numbers, basophils respond to adrenal cortex hormones in similar fashion to eosinophils.

Basophil granules contain histamine, heparin, and peroxidase (Dvorak, 1975). Basophils synthesize and store histamine and eosinophil chemotactic factor of anaphylaxis (ECF-A). They synthesize and release slow-reacting substance of anaphylaxis (SRS-A) and probably platelet activating factor (PAF) at the time of stimulation, but do not store them. Basophils lack hydrolytic enzymes such as alkaline and acid phosphatase, at least in significant amounts. Glycogen is abundant outside the granules. Though ultrastructurally different, mast cells have similar cytochemical characteristics except for the presence of proteolytic enzymes and serotonin, which basophils lack. In tissues the two cell types appear to function in a similar manner.

Basophils (as well as mast cells) appear to be involved in immediate hypersensitivity reactions, such as allergic asthma (Dvorak, 1975). Immunoglobulin E (reagin) binds readily to basophil and mast cell membranes. When specific antigen reacts with the membrane-bound IgE, degranulation occurs with the release of mediators of immediate hypersensitivity, e.g., histamine, SRS-A, PAF, heparin, and ECF-A. The latter leads to the accumulation of eosinophils, which contain substances that tend to counteract these mediators (Beeson, 1977). Basophils are also involved in some delayed hypersensitivity reactions, "cutaneous basophil hypersensitivity," such as contact allergies, in which they appear to undergo a different type of degranulation response (Dvorak, 1975).

MONOCYTES AND MACROPHAGES

Monocytes share the same committed progenitor cell as neutrophils, the GM-CFC (Fig. 28–1).

Morphology

In normal marrow it is not possible to distinguish the "monoblast" from the myeloblast. The earliest recognizable cell in this series is the *promonocyte,* which is 15 to 20 μm in diameter, somewhat larger than the myeloblast. The N/C ratio is moderate, and the nucleus may be oval or indented with a fine uniform or slightly streaked chromatin pattern and two to five nucleoli. The cytoplasm is basophilic with a ground-glass appearance and a variable number of fine azurophilic granules (Plate 28–3*A*). The *monocyte,* which is present in both blood and marrow, is only slightly smaller, has a moderate to low N/C ratio, and an indented or lobed nucleus with a fine streaked, only slightly condensed, delicate chromatin pattern. Nucleoli are indistinct or obscured. The cytoplasm is opaque, more gray than blue, and contains an abundance of fine azurophilic granules (Plate 28–3*B*).

In the promonocyte stage the granules contain acid hydrolase, arylsulfatase, and peroxidase; they represent primary lysosomes. There may be more than one type of granule (Cawley, 1973). As the cell matures, peroxidase activity diminishes and acid phosphatase and arylsulfatase activity increases. The enzyme activity is in the RER, Golgi zone, coated vesicles, and digestive vacuoles, suggesting that in the macrophage the coated vesicles are a second form of primary lysosomes that shuttles hydrolytic enzymes from the Golgi to the digestive vacuoles (Bainton, 1976).

Kinetics

After promonocytes are formed, they undergo two mitotic divisions in a period of about 50 to 60 hours before being released into the blood (Meuret, 1974). Under conditions of increased demand, the cycle time can shorten, with earlier release of more immature cells into the blood. Blood monocytes are distributed in a circulating monocyte pool and a marginal monocyte pool, in a ratio of 1 to 3.5 (Meuret, 1973). Once monocytes enter the blood, they leave randomly with a half-time of 8.4 hours; this time period is shortened in splenomegaly or acute infection, and may be prolonged in monocytosis. After monocytes leave the blood, they spend several months, perhaps longer, in the tissue phase.

Function (Cline, 1975, 1977)

The monocyte is formed in the marrow, transported by the blood, and migrates into the tissues where it transforms into a histiocyte or macrophage (p. 615; Plate 27–2*I*) to spend the majority of its life span. The blood monocytes and tissue macrophages make up a mononuclear phagocyte system (reticuloendothelial system).

The mononuclear phagocyte system has an important role in defense against microorganisms, including mycobacteria, fungi, bacteria, protozoa, and viruses. The cells are motile and respond to chemotactic factors (complement components and factors from activated lymphocytes); they become immobilized by migration-inhibition factor (MIF) from activated lymphocytes. They engage in phagocytosis, a process that is enhanced if the particle is coated by IgG or complement for which the macrophages have membrane receptors. After phagocytosis, they kill ingested microorganisms.

These mononuclear phagocytes are an integral part of both humoral and cell-mediated immunity. They handle or process antigens, providing contact of the antigen (or antigenic information) with lymphocytes. They also respond to various lymphokines and act as effector (e.g., cytotoxic) cells in the cell-mediated immune response.

Macrophages remove and process senescent cells and debris through phagocytosis and digestion: for example, erythrocytes, leukocytes, megakaryocyte nuclei by macrophages in the marrow; inhaled particulate material by alveolar macrophages in the lungs.

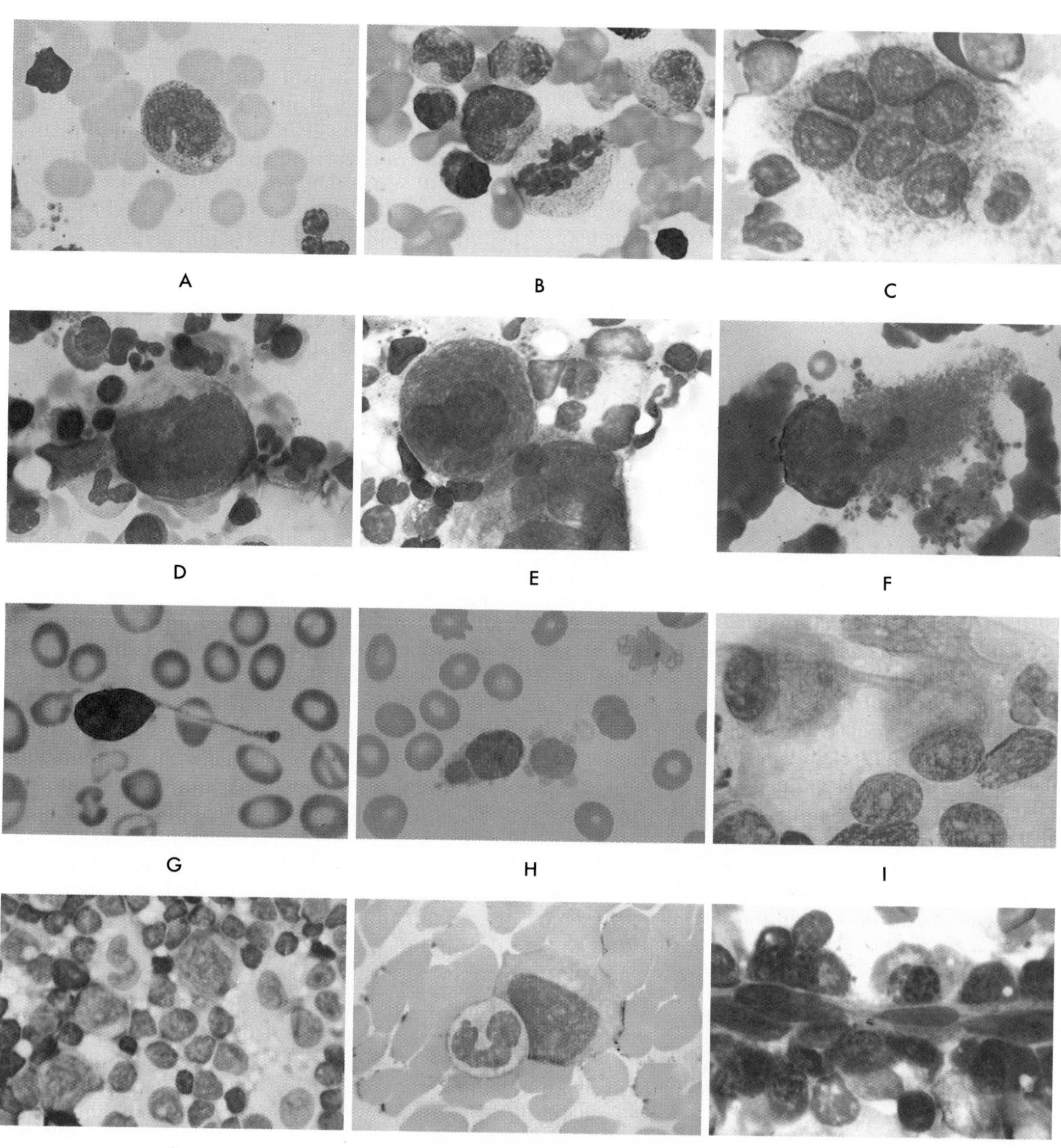

Plate 28–3. *A,* Promonocyte. Multiple fine granules and a deeply indented nucleus help identify this cell as a monocyte. That this is an immature monocyte is evident from the delicate nuclear chromatin, obvious nucleoli, and blue-tinted cytoplasm. *B,* Three neutrophil metamyelocytes at the top, a monocyte in the center of the group of cells, a small plasma cell, and a neutrophil myelocyte in mitosis. *C,* Osteoclast. Separate nuclei with relatively large nucleoli are the major features that distinguish this cell from a megakaryocyte. *D,* Megakaryoblast. *E,* Early megakaryocyte (bottom); the later megakaryocyte at the top has more compact nuclear material and clustering of granules. *F,* Megakaryocyte, releasing platelets. *G,* Megakaryocyte nuclear fragment with long strand of cytoplasmic material. *H,* Dwarf megakaryocyte and two atypical platelets from the blood of a patient with myelofibrosis with myeloid metaplasia. The atypical platelets are large, lack the normal number of granules, and have pseudopods. *I,* Osteoblasts. The eccentric nucleus, reticular chromatin pattern, large nucleolus, basophilic cytoplasm, and large pale Golgi zone separated from the nucleus are characteristic. *J,* Lymph node imprint from a patient with reactive lymph node hyperplasia. Note four or five histiocytes with abundant cytoplasm; numerous small lymphocytes; and stages in blast transformation, including three large reticular lymphocytes (non-leukemic lymphoblasts). *K,* Reticular lymphocyte (non-leukemic lymphoblast) in the blood of a patient with atypical pneumonitis and increased cold agglutinins. Note the large nucleoli, reticular nuclear chromatin, and moderately abundant, opaque, basophilic cytoplasm. *L,* Plasma cells lining sinusoidal endothelium in a marrow film from a patient with rheumatoid arthritis. In reactive plasmacytosis in marrow, plasma cells are frequently oriented in this manner. The chromatin in coarse blocks and the pale Golgi zone immediately adjacent to the nucleus are in contrast to the appearance of osteoblasts (*I*).

Macrophages may be "activated" by either specific factors (e.g., cytophilic antibody) or non-specific factors (e.g., in response to phagocytized material). Activation results in enlargement of the cell and enhanced metabolism, phagocytosis, microbicidal activity, cytotoxicity, etc.

Macrophages also synthesize and secrete several biologically active molecules such as certain complement components, transferrin, muramidase, and interferon. An important role in regulation of hematopoietic activity may be played by GM-CSF, the colony-stimulating factor for neutrophils and macrophages (p. 636; Metcalf, 1977). Although GM-CSF may be found in serum and urine, it is likely that its biologic activity is at shorter range, as it is secreted by macrophages in the marrow. It has been shown *in vitro* that when GM-CSF increases beyond a critical concentration, macrophages then produce prostaglandin E (PGE), which inhibits the response of the GM-CFC, opposing the effect of GM-CSF (Kurland, 1978). Thus, the net myeloproliferative activity of monocyte and neutrophil may be determined by the balance between GM-CSF and PGE, both produced by the mononuclear phagocyte.

This system, therefore, appears to have multiple functions which include host defense, control of hematopoiesis, and policing of the environment within the body (Cline, 1977).

MEGAKARYOCYTES

Platelets originate from polyploid megakaryocytes, the largest of all hematopoietic cells, which number less than 1 per cent of the total nucleated marrow cells. They arise from the multipotential hematopoietic stem cell, probably directly from a committed progenitor cell (Fig. 28–1). Based on *in vitro* and *in vivo* studies, it is likely that megakaryocyte proliferation and maturation are regulated by two humoral factors. *Megakaryocyte colony stimulating factor* (Mk-CSF) induces committed progenitor cells to proliferate, and *thrombopoietin* promotes differentiation and maturation of these as megakaryocytes and influences their ploidy (Williams, 1982).

Morphology

Committed progenitor cells are not morphologically distinguishable from lymphocytes. The different maturation stages of megakaryocytes are illustrated in Table 28–1. Megakaryocyte development is characterized by *endomitosis,* nuclear division without cytoplasmic division, which results in ploidies varying from 2N to 64N. Most are 8N and 16N, with smaller numbers on either side. Nuclear lobes do not correlate precisely with ploidy. Nuclear chromatin is intensely staining, rather dispersed early, more compact and dense later. Nucleoli are small at all stages of megakaryocyte development.

The earliest recognizable *megakaryoblast* has overlapping nuclear lobes and a small amount of basophilic cytoplasm. In the *promegakaryocyte,* nuclear lobes increase and spread out and red-pink granules become visible, first in the center of the cell. The *granular megakaryocyte* is characterized by spreading of the red-pink granules diffusely through most of the cytoplasm and further increase and spreading of nuclear lobes. In the *mature megakaryocyte* the nucleus is more compact, basophilia has disappeared, and the granules are clustered into small aggregates. At an ultrastructural level, this is produced by proliferation in invaginated surface membranes (demarcation membranes) that separate the cytoplasm into individual platelets. Platelets are ultimately shed as cytoplasmic fragments by fusion of demarcation membranes. In the marrow, megakaryocytes are adjacent to sinus walls, and platelets are released into the lumen.

Megakaryocytes in Blood

Whole megakaryocytes or fragments may occasionally be found in normal blood films. If buffy coat films are examined, they are consistently present. Efrati (1960) found megakaryocytes in all of 55 normal individuals studied, an average of 22 per ml of venous blood. Megakaryocytes are frequently found in the capillaries of the lungs. Kaufman (1965a) presented experimental data suggesting that pulmonary megakaryocytes do not originate in the lungs but are carried there in venous blood; it was calculated that 7 to 17 per cent of the body's platelets may be released from pulmonary capillaries (Kaufman, 1965b).

Megakaryocyte fragments in blood films may be as small as lymphocytes and are recognized by the deeply stained chromatin (which has sharper chromatin-parachromatin separation than do lymphocytes) and by fragments of attached megakaryocyte cytoplasm (Plate 28–3*G*). They are found more frequently than normal in myelophthisic processes, myeloproliferative disorders, or after stress or injury to the marrow.

Dwarf or micro megakaryocytes (Plate 28–3*H*), on the other hand, show evidence of abnormal megakaryopoiesis: agranular cytoplasm with hyaloplasmic zones or pseudopods; and association with large atypical platelets having similar cytoplasmic characteristics. These abnormal dwarf megakaryocytes are rarely found in any condition except myeloproliferative disorders.

Kinetics

The maturation time for megakaryocytes in the marrow is about five days in man. Platelets are released into the marrow sinuses over a period of several hours, and the megakaryocyte nuclei are phagocytosed by macrophages. Newly released platelets appear larger, more active metabolically, and more effective hemostatically. Platelets circulate at a stable concentration that averages 275 $\times$ 10^9/L. At any one time, about two thirds of the total platelets are in the circulation, and about one third are present in the spleen. In asplenic individuals, all platelets are circulating; on

Table 28–1. CYTOLOGIC CHARACTERISTICS OF STAGES OF MEGAKARYOCYTIC MATURATION; DIAGRAMS OF NUCLEAR CONFIGURATIONS AND NUCLEAR/CYTOPLASMIC RATIOS AT EACH STAGE ARE IN THE FIRST COLUMN*

	Stage	Nuclear Morphology	Cytoplasmic Staining (Wright-Giemsa)	Approximate Size Range	Demarcation Membranes	Granules	Suggested Name
	I	Compact (lobed)	Basophilic	6–24 μm	Present by electron microscopy	Few present by electron microscopy	Megakaryoblast
	II	Horseshoe	Pink center	14–30 μm	Proliferating to center of cell	Starting to increase	Promegakaryocyte
	III	Multilobed	Increasingly more pink than blue	16–56 μm	Extensive but asymmetric	Great numbers	Granular megakaryocyte
	IV	Compact but highly lobulated	Wholly eosinophilic	20–50 μm	Evenly distributed	Organized into "platelet fields"	Mature megakaryocyte

*From Williams, N., and Levine, R. F.: The origin, development and regulation of megakaryocytes. Br. J. Haematol., *52*:173–180, 1982. Oxford, Blackwell Scientific Publications.

the other hand, in diseases characterized by splenic enlargement 80 to 90 per cent of platelets may be sequestered in the spleen, resulting in a decreased concentration of circulating platelets (thrombocytopenia) on the basis of this altered distribution (Aster, 1977).

Platelets survive 8 to 11 days in the circulation. Some platelets are probably utilized in maintaining vascular integrity and in plugging small vascular injuries (random loss), and others are probably removed by the mononuclear phagocytic system when they become senescent.

Function

Platelets normally function in (1) maintaining the integrity (leak-free state) of blood vessels; and (2) forming hemostatic plugs to stop blood loss from injured vessels, and, in the process, promoting coagulation of plasma factors (Chapter 31).

LYMPHOCYTES

Primary Lymphoid Tissue

According to current concepts (Micklem, 1979), during fetal life lymphocyte precursors originate in the bone marrow and are influenced or programmed to perform a certain function by one of the primary lymphoid organs, either the thymus gland for T-lymphocytes (T cells) or the "bursal equivalent" for B-lymphocytes (B cells).

4

B CELL DEVELOPMENT: BURSAL EQUIVALENT

A distinct organ, the bursa of Fabricius, is present in birds and serves as the primary site of B cell development. In man and other mammals a bursal equivalent probably exists in fetal liver and bone marrow as primary sites of B lymphocyte development. Lymphopoiesis within primary lymphoid organs is vigorous and antigen independent.

B cell differentiation can be divided conveniently into two stages. The initial stage of B cell differentiation involves the antigen-independent generation of diversity. The second stage is regulated by antigen triggering, T cell interactions, and macrophages (Fig. 28–7). This stage occurs predominantly in the secondary lymphoid organs.

A stem cell gives rise to the first recognizable B cell in man and mammals. This cell, known as the large pre-B cell, is characterized by the presence of small amounts of intracytoplasmic immunoglobulin (ICIg) IgM without surface membrane IgM. The large pre-B cell is a rapidly dividing cell and can be found in the fetal liver as early as seven weeks' gestation, two weeks prior to the detection of B cells with surface membrane immunoglobin (SIg). The offspring of the

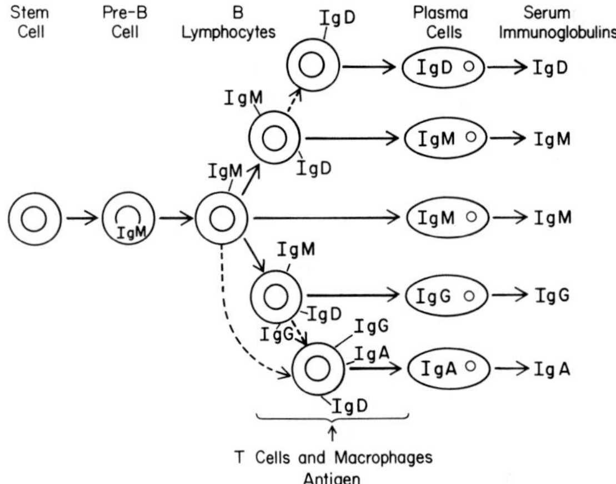

Figure 28–7. Differentiation of B cells. The pre-B cell has intracytoplasmic IgM (ICIgM) without surface immunoglobulin (SIg). B cells have SIg without ICIg. Transformation into plasma cells is characterized by abundant ICIg and reduction of SIg (See text).

large pre-B cell is a small pre-B cell which does not turn over rapidly. Pre-B lymphocytes give rise to B cells with SIgM and receptors for Fc and C3. B cells, producing other classes of Ig, are progeny of cells that formerly expressed only SIgM. SIgD is expressed early in the development of all the B cell subsets, but at a time after IgM has been produced. Cells bearing SIgG and SIgA are first detected at about the twelfth week of gestation. These cells also express SIgM and rarely SIgD. Later on SIgG and SIgA can occur singly on cells or in combination with SIgD and/or SIgM. As maturation proceeds, SIgD is lost. In the second stage of differentiation, B lymphocytes interact with antigen in the presence of T cells and macrophages and transform into plasma cells. These cells are characterized by abundant ICIg reflecting the Ig commitment of the activated B cell. At this stage, Fc and C3 receptors are lost and SIg is reduced. Thus, lymphocytes bearing SIg give rise to cells committed to the synthesis of IgM, IgG, and IgA (Parkhouse, 1977).

T CELL DEVELOPMENT: THYMUS GLAND

The human thymus has two parts. The cortex is populated predominantly by small lymphocytes with a few scattered epithelial cells. In contrast, the medulla is composed mostly of epithelial cells with a small component of lymphocytes. The cortex is subdivided by several fibrous septa extending from the capsule to the medullary region. In the medulla, Hassall's corpuscles are present. Hassall's corpuscles are small islands of partially hyalinized epithelial cells of no known functional significance (Douglas, 1977). The thymus reaches a maximum size (approximately 40 g) during adolescence and then gradually undergoes involutional changes. Some functional activity may be present throughout life.

The microenvironment of the thymus is necessary for the differentiation of T cells in all species. Prothymocytes migrate from the bone marrow to the thymus gland where they are processed into functionally mature T cells for circulation in the blood to the peripheral or secondary lymphoid tissue. As thymic cells mature they acquire and lose certain membrane determinants which are reactive with various monoclonal antibodies (Fig. 28–8). The earliest thymocytes are reactive with anti-T10 and anti-T9 antibodies (Reinherz, 1980). With maturation, however, the T9 antigen is lost; T10 is retained; and antigens T6, T4, and T5 are acquired. With further maturation, thymocytes lose T6 antigen, acquire T1 and T3 antigens, and segregate into T4 positive and T5 positive cells. Following exportation into the circulation, the T10 antigen cannot be detected. T cells with the T4 determinants function as inducer/helper cells, whereas T cells with the T5 antigens include the cytotoxic/suppressor cells.

Secondary Lymphoid Tissue

In late fetal and postnatal life, lymphocytes are produced in the secondary lymphoid tissue: spleen, lymph nodes, and intestine-associated lymphoid tissue. Lymphocytes of the secondary lymphoid organs are progeny from stem cells which have been influenced by primary lymphoid organs. The secondary lymphoid organs are thus composed of a mixture of B cells and T cells. Lymphopoiesis in secondary lymphoid organs depends solely on antigenic stimulation (Miller, 1977). B cells and T cells tend to localize in anatomically distinct parts of the lymphoid tissues, where proliferation can take place.

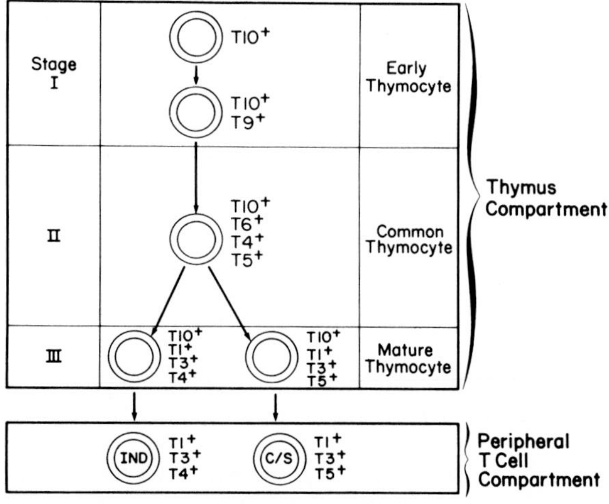

Figure 28–8. Differentiation of T cells. Three stages of intrathymic differentiation are defined on the basis of antigens recognized by monoclonal antibodies. The mature thymocyte (Stage III) gives rise to peripheral T cells, both inducer/helper cells (IND) and cytotoxic/suppressor (C/S) subsets. The cell-surface antigens expressed are shown. (From Reinberg, E. L., and Schlossman, S. F.: N. Engl. J. Med., *303*:370, 1980 Reprinted by permission of the New England Journal of Medicine.)

LYMPH NODES

Lymph nodes are surrounded by a fibrous capsule which is penetrated by afferent lymphatic vessels. These afferent lymphatic vessels carry lymph and lymphoid cells into the subcapsular sinus. The intermediate and radial sinuses bring the lymph from the subcapsular sinus to the efferent lymphatics in the medullary portion of the node. The outer layer of the lymph node (cortex) contains nodules of lymphocytes (primary and secondary follicles). Some of these nodules contain a center (germinal center) composed of macrophages and lymphoid cells of various stages of maturation. When a germinal center is present, the nodule is referred to as a secondary follicle. A strip of loosely packed lymphoid cells is present between follicles (paracortical areas) and as cords extending into the medullary areas (medullary cords). Macrophages capable of phagocytizing antigen line the sinuses. Dendritic reticular cells, located in the germinal center, localize and retain antigen. B cells are located predominantly in the germinal centers and in the medullary cords. Although a few T cells are located in germinal centers, T cells are principally found in the paracortical areas. In addition, the majority of T cells in the paracortical areas are positive for T1, T3, and T4 (inducer/helper) subsets. A small number of helper T cells are located in the germinal centers of follicles. Thus, this subset of T cells is located in appropriate areas to help B cells differentiate and mature (Poppema, 1981).

SPLEEN

The spleen is grossly divisible into white pulp (lymphoid area) and red pulp (vascular sinuses and blood). The *white pulp* is composed of lymphocytes forming a sheath (periarteriolar lymphocyte sheath) around central arteries and its tributaries. T cells are located within the periarteriolar lymphocytic sheath. B cells are present in the primary and secondary follicles, which are in and around the sheath. Surrounding the germinal center is a mantle of small lymphocytes.

The *red pulp* is a network of branching sinuses separated from each other by the splenic cords, which are filled with a variety of cellular blood elements.

The sinuses and cords receive blood from tributaries of the central artery (arteries of the red pulp or penicilliary arteries). Blood cells that have entered the cords must regain the circulation through narrow (3 μm diameter) apertures in the sinusoidal wall. Cells that are inflexible or otherwise abnormal may be trapped and destroyed in the cords. The contents of the venous sinuses, in turn, flow into the pulp veins, trabecular veins, capsular veins, and finally the splenic veins (Weiss, 1977).

The marginal zone represents the junction between the periarterial lymphatic sheath and the red pulp. In the marginal zone small recirculating lymphocytes may leave the venous sinuses and enter the lymphatic sheath.

Lymphocyte Function and Physiology

T cells and their progeny function in cell-mediated immunity, which includes delayed hypersensitivity, graft rejection, graft-versus-host reactions, defense against intracellular organisms (such as tubercle bacillus and brucella), and probably defense against neoplasms. B cells and their progeny perform in humoral immunity, or the production of antibodies, either as a lymphocyte or after transformation into a plasma cell.

The majority of the circulating lymphocytes are T cells, which have a life span of months to years. The B cells are a minor population (10 to 20 per cent of the lymphocytes), probably have a short life span measured in days, and are distinguished by the presence of considerable immunoglobulin on their surface membrane.

Lymphocytes, especially T cells, recirculate from blood to lymph; in the postcapillary venule in lymphoid tissue the lymphocyte travels from the blood through the endothelium and into the lymphoid tissue, where it may stay or percolate through and return to the blood via the thoracic duct lymph. Small lymphocytes (Plate 28–3*J*) have little cytoplasm and, in electron micrographs, few organelles and relatively little RNA. After antigenic stimulation, small lymphocytes (B cells or T cells, depending on the nature of the antigen) become activated, increase their RNA synthesis, and undergo blast transformation. On Wright's stained films, these blasts are large cells (15 to 25 μm) with abundant, rather deep blue cytoplasm, a large reticular nucleus with uniform chromatin, and prominent nucleoli (Plate 28–3*J* and *K*). This is the cell which is called the *reticular lymphocyte* (nonleukemic lymphoblast; "immunoblast"). If the blasts are derived from B cells, the new lymphocytes function in the production of antibodies (B cells, plasma cells); or, if the blasts are derived from T cells, the progeny act in the cellular immune response. The latter is mediated by several soluble factors produced by the activated T cell, including transfer factor, which can transfer the capacity for delayed hypersensitivity to another cell; lymphotoxin, which is directly toxic to cells; and migratory inhibition factor, which promotes adherence of macrophages and keeps them at the site.

Plasma cells have abundant blue cytoplasm, often with light streaks or vacuoles, an eccentric round nucleus, and a well-defined clear (Golgi) zone adjacent to the nucleus. The nucleus of the plasma cell has heavily clumped chromatin, which is sharply defined from the parachromatin and often arranged in a radial or "wheel-like" pattern (Plate 27–2*H* and 28–3*L*).

BONE MARROW EXAMINATION

Marrow aspiration biopsy can be carried out as an office procedure on ambulatory patients with minimal risk. It compares favorably with ordinary venipuncture and is less traumatizing than a lumbar puncture. As for any other special procedure, however, the indications for marrow examination should be clear. In each instance the physician should have in mind some reasonable prediction of its result and consequent benefit to the patient. Without exception, the peripheral blood should be examined carefully first. It is a relatively uncommon circumstance to find hematologic disease in the bone marrow without evidence of it in the peripheral blood.

It is estimated that the weight of the marrow in the adult is 1300 to 1500 g. The marrow can undergo complete transformation in a few days and occasionally even in a few hours. As a rule, this rapid transformation involves the whole organ, as evidenced by the fact that a small sample represented by a biopsy or aspiration is usually fairly representative of the whole marrow. This conclusion is in accord with results of studies of biopsy samples simultaneously removed from several sites. According to these observations, the various sites chosen for removal of marrow for studies are in most instances equally good. Consequently, the difficulty of access, the risks involved, the ease of obtaining a good biopsy, and the discomfort of the patient are the main reasons for selection of a site in the particular patient. Occasionally the failure to obtain quantitatively or qualitatively adequate material in one site may be followed by success in another location. Also, the need for repeated aspirations or biopsies may indicate the use of several different sites. We regard the posterior iliac crest as the preferred site. The large marrow space allows both aspiration and biopsy to be performed with ease at one time. The techniques of marrow aspiration and biopsy have been adequately reviewed (Nelson, 1979; Wintrobe et al., 1981).

Preparation of the Aspirate for Examination

Three commonly used preparations are marrow films, gross quantitative study, and histologic sections.

Marrow Films. Delay, no matter how brief, is undesirable. Films can be made in a similar manner as for ordinary blood counts. Gray particles of marrow are visible with the naked eye. They are the best material for the preparation of good films and serve as landmarks for the microscopic examination of stained smears.

Direct Films. A drop of marrow is placed on a slide a short distance away from one end. A film 3 to 5 cm long is made with a spreader, not wider than 2 cm, dragging the particles behind but not *squashing* them. A trail of cells is left behind each particle.

Imprints. Marrow particles can also be used for preparation of imprints. One or more visible particles are picked up with a capillary pipette, the broken end of a wooden applicator, or a toothpick and transferred immediately to a slide and made to stick to it by a gentle smearing motion. The slide is air dried rapidly by waving and then is stained.

Crush Preparations. Marrow particles in a small drop of aspirate may be placed on a slide near one end. Another slide is carefully placed over the first. Slight pressure is exerted to crush the particles, and the slides are separated by pulling them apart in a direction parallel to their surfaces.

All films should be dried rapidly by whipping them through the air or by exposing them to a fan.

As the aspirated material is being spread, the appearance of fat as irregular holes in the films gives assurance that marrow and not just blood has been obtained.

Gross Quantitative Study. The aspirate is added to EDTA (1.5 mg/ml), mixed, and transferred to a Wintrobe hematocrit tube with a capillary pipette. Some or all of the visible particles are included, depending on their use for preparation of direct smears. The tube is centrifuged at 2500 rpm for 10 minutes. Four layers can be distinguished in the centrifugate: fat, plasma, myeloid-erythroid (M:E) portion, and erythrocytes. Their height is recorded in percentages by reading on the scale of the tube. Normally the fat layer is 1 to 3 per cent of the total volume and the M:E layer, 5 to 8 per cent. The volumes of the plasma and erythrocyte layers vary considerably depending upon the degree of dilution with sinusoidal blood. Smears of the M:E layer may be made by aspirating this complete layer with an equal volume of plasma, mixing in a watch glass, and preparing films.

High myeloid-erythroid and low fat values, in the absence of a significant peripheral leukocytosis, suggest marrow hyperplasia. Low myeloid-erythroid and high fat values suggest hypoplasia, at least of the aspirated sample. If the myeloid-erythroid layer is less than 2 per cent and fat is absent, the sample is mainly sinusoidal blood. Examination of histologic sections is an essential check on the quantitative data. This type of preparation allows an optimal cell density and freedom from erythrocytes and fat cells on the films, and many such slides may be easily prepared.

Histologic Sections. The needle biopsy and the clotted marrow particles (fragments) are fixed in Zenker's acetic acid solution (5 per cent glacial acetic acid; 95 per cent Zenker's) for 6 to 18 hours. The longer time interval promotes adequate decalcification of most biopsies; excessive time in fixative makes the tissue brittle. The tissue is processed routinely for embedding in paraffin. Embedding the tissue in plastic materials allows thinner sections of 1 to 4 μm (Dancey, 1976) and is preferred by many.

Sections provide the best estimate of cellularity and a picture of marrow architecture but are somewhat inferior for the study of cytologic details. Another disadvantage is that particles adequate for histologic sections are not always obtained, especially in conditions in which the diagnosis depends on marrow evidence, e.g., myelofibrosis or metastatic cancer.

Berman (1953) recommended the following technique for marrow particles. The aspirated marrow is deposited in a paraffin-coated vial. A small amount of powdered topical thrombin is placed on a clean glass slide, dissolved in a drop of water, and allowed to dry. The marrow particles in the aspirate tend to stick to the paraffin coating. They are transferred with the broken end of a wooden applicator and placed close to each other on the thrombin-coated area on the slide. A few drops of plasma from the centrifuged aspirate are added. The plasma clots by action of thrombin. The marrow particles are included in the clot, which is transferred to a suitable fixative. The latter is changed repeatedly until it remains water clear and then the tissue is processed.

Staining Marrow Preparations

Romanowsky Stain. Marrow films should be stained with a Romanowsky stain (e.g., Wright-Giemsa) in a similar manner to blood films (p. 603). A longer staining time may be necessary for marrows with greater cellularity.

Perls' Test for Iron. ***Procedure.*** One film containing marrow particles is fixed 10 minutes in formalin vapor, immersed for 10 minutes in a freshly prepared solution which contains 0.5 per cent potassium ferrocyanide and 0.75 per cent hydrochloric acid, rinsed, dried, and counterstained with eosin (Nelson, 1979; Beutler, 1977).

Interpretation. The Prussian blue reaction is produced when hemosiderin or ferritin is present; iron in hemoglobin is not stained. Report as negative or 1+ to 5+. Storage iron, which is contained in macrophages, can be evaluated only in the marrow particles on the smear. In adults, 2+ is normal, 3+ slightly increased, 4+ moderately increased, and 5+ markedly increased.

Storage iron in the marrow is located in macrophages. Normally a small number of blue granules are seen. In iron deficiency, blue-staining granules are absent or extremely rare. Storage iron is increased in most other anemias, infections, hemochromatosis, hemosiderosis, hepatic cirrhosis, uremia, and cancer, and after repeated transfusions (Plate 29–1*D* and *E*).

Sideroblasts are normoblasts which contain one or more particles of stainable iron. Normally, from 20 to 60 per cent of the late normoblasts are sideroblasts; in the remainder, no blue granules can be detected. The percentage of sideroblasts is decreased in iron deficiency anemia (where storage iron is decreased) and also in the common anemias associated with infection, rheumatoid arthritis, and neoplastic disease (where storage iron is normal or increased). The number of sideroblasts is increased when erythropoiesis is impaired for other reasons; it is roughly proportional to the degree of saturation of transferrin (Bainton, 1964). The Prussian blue reaction can also be performed on slides previously stained with a Romanowsky stain (Sundberg, 1955) to identify sideroblasts or to determine whether iron is present in other cells of interest.

Sections. Routine hematoxylin and eosin stains are satisfactory for most purposes. Romanowsky stains can be used to good advantage with Zenker-fixed material. Block (1976) sucessfully relies on the study of routine Romanowsky-stained marrow biopsy preparations almost to the exclusion of marrow films; most people, however, find the combination of marrow films and biopsy specimen to be preferable.

Iron stains may be performed on sections but are less sensitive than films because some iron is lost in the processing of sections (more lost in Zenker's than in formalin-fixed tissue) and much thicker pieces of marrow tissue (whole particles) are visualized on the films.

Examination of Marrow

It is desirable to establish a routine procedure in order to obtain the maximum information from examination of the marrow.

Peripheral Blood. The complete blood cell count, including platelet count and reticulocyte count, should be performed on the day of the marrow study and the results incorporated in the report. The pathologist or hematologist who examines the marrow should also carefully examine the blood film as previously described (p. 602) and incorporate the observations in the marrow report.

Cellularity of the Marrow. The marrow cellularity is expressed as the ratio of the volume of hematopoietic cells to the total volume of the marrow space (cells plus fat and other stromal elements). Cellularity varies with the age of the subject and the site. For example, at age 50 years, the average cellularity in the vertebrae is 75 per cent; sternum, 60 per cent; iliac crest, 50 per cent; and rib, 30 per cent (Custer, 1974). Normal cellularity of the iliac bone at different ages has been well defined by Hartsock (1965), as summarized in Figure 28–9. If the percentage is increased for the

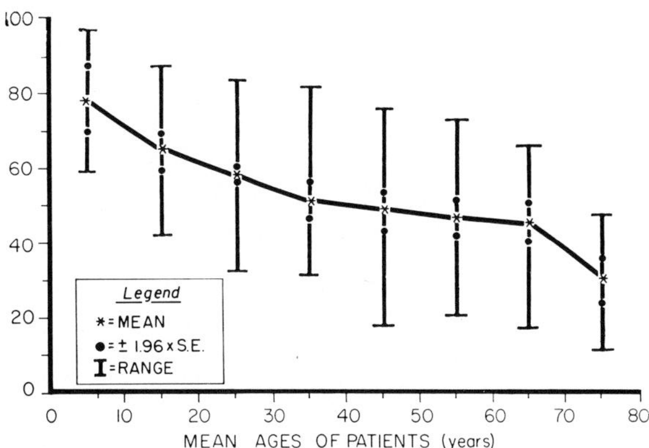

Figure 28–9. Marrow cellularity in hematologically normal individuals. Per cent cellularity on the ordinate, versus age, grouped by decade, on the abscissa. (From Hartsock et al.: Am. J. Clin. Path., *43*:326, 1965.)

patient's age, the marrow is hypercellular, or hyperplastic; if decreased, the marrow is hypocellular, or hypoplastic.

Marrow cellularity is best judged by histologic sections of biopsy or aspirated particles (see Figure 28–10) but should be also estimated from the particles that are present in marrow films. This is done by comparing the areas occupied by fat spaces and by nucleated cells in the particles as well as the density of nucleated cells in the "tail" or fallout of the particles. Comparison of films and sections on each marrow will enable the observer to estimate cellularity reasonably well from films, a skill that is useful in the instances when sectioned material is unavailable.

Distribution of Cells. The distribution of the various cell types can be ascertained in two ways. First, one scans several slides under low, then high magnification; and, on the basis of previous experience, one estimates the number and distribution of cells. Second, one actually makes a differential count of 300 to 1000 cells and calculates the percentage of each type of cell. A combination of both methods is preferred.

The second of these methods, careful differential counting, is an essential part of training in this work without which accuracy in the first method may be difficult to achieve. The differential count also affords an objective record from which future changes may be measured.

One first scans the marrow films under low power (100 × or 200 × magnification), looking for irregularities in cell distribution, the number of megakaryocytes, and the presence of abnormal cells. Then one selects areas on the films where marrow cells are both undiluted with blood cells and separated and spread out sufficiently to allow optimal identification. These areas are usually just behind marrow particles on the direct films, or near the particles on the crushed films. The differential count is performed at 400 × or 1000 × magnification.

Examples of reference intervals for differential counts of the marrow at selected different ages are given in Table 28–2.

Changes in the marrow cell distribution are most

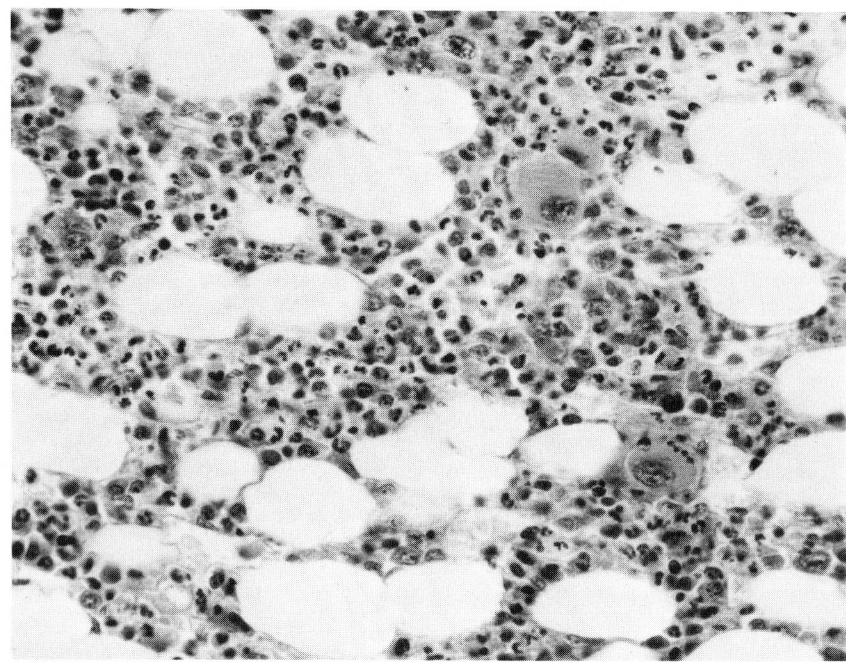

Figure 28–10. Marrow biopsy (×1470). Cellularity here is between 60 and 70 per cent, which is normal for an adult. Three megakaryocytes are present, which is normal for this size field. Granulocytic maturation appears normal with all stages present. Very few normoblasts are noted. (Normoblasts have intensely staining nuclei and tend to occur in clusters.) The M:E ratio is higher than 4:1, indicating erythroid hypoplasia. No other abnormalities are noted.

Table 28–2. DIFFERENTIAL CELL COUNTS OF BONE MARROW IN PER CENT OF TOTAL NUCLEATED CELLS

	Rosse (1977) Birth		**1 Month**		**Mauer (1969) over 4 months**		**Wintrobe (1974) Adult**	
	Mean	***S.D.***	***Mean***	***S.D.***	***Mean***	***Range***	***Mean***	***Range***
Normoblasts, total	14.5	± 7.2	8.0	± 5.0	23.1		25.6	(18.4–33.8)
Pronormoblasts	0.02	± 0.06	0.10	± 0.14	0.5	(0 – 1.5)		(0.2– 1.3)
Basophilic N.	0.24	± 0.24	0.34	± 0.33	1.7	(0.2– 4.8)		(0.5– 2.4)
Polychromatophilic N.	13.1	± 6.8	6.9	± 4.4	18.2	(4.8–34.0)		(17.9–29.2)
Orthochromatic N.	0.69	± 0.73	0.54	± 1.88	2.7	(0 – 7.8)		(0.4– 4.6)
Neutrophils, total	60.4	± 8.7	32.4	± 7.7	57.1		53.6	(49.2–65.0)
Myeloblasts	0.31	± 0.31	0.62	± 0.50	1.2	(0 – 3.2)		(0.2– 1.5)
Promyelocytes	0.79	± 0.91	0.76	± 0.65	1.4	(0 – 4.0)		(2.1– 4.1)
Myelocytes	3.9	± 2.9	2.5	± 1.5	18.3	(8.5–29.7)		(8.2–15.7)
Metamyelocytes	19.4	± 4.8	11.3	± 3.6	23.3	(14.0–34.2)		(9.6–24.6)
Bands	28.4	± 7.6	14.1	± 4.6				(9.5–15.3)
Segmented	7.4	± 4.6	3.6	± 3.0	12.9	(4.5–29.0)		(6.0–12.0)
Eosinophils	2.7	± 1.3	2.6	± 1.4	3.6	(1.0– 9.0)	3.1	(1.2– 5.3)
Basophils	0.12	± 0.20	0.07	± 0.16	0.06	(0 – 0.8)	0.1	(0 – 0.2)
Lymphocytes, total	15.6		49.0		16.0	(4.8–35.8)	16.2	(11.1–23.2)
Transitional	1.2	± 1.1	2.0	± 0.9				
Small (mature)	14.4	± 5.5	47.0	± 9.2				
Plasma cells	0.00	± 0.02	0.02	± 0.06	0.4	(0.2– 0.6)	13	(0.4– 3.9)
Monocytes	0.88	± 0.85	1.01	± 0.89			0.3	(0 – 0.8)
Megakaryocytes	0.06	± 0.15	0.05	± 0.09			0.1	(0 – 0.4)
Reticulum cells							0.3	(0 – 0.9)
M:E Ratio	4.4		4.4		2.9	(1.2– 5.2)	2.3	(1.5– 2.3)

Data from Mauer, A. M.: Pediatric Hematology. New York, McGraw-Hill Book Company, 1969; and Wintrobe, M. M., et al.: Clinical Hematology. 7th ed. Philadelphia, Lea & Febiger, 1974.

dramatic in the first month of life, during which a predominance of granulocytic cells at birth changes to a predominance of lymphocytes. This predominance of lymphocytes characterizes the bone marrow during infancy. A small proportion of "immature" or transitional lymphocytes (fine nuclear chromatin, high N/C ratio, intermediate cell size) is normally present; it may be that included in these are stem cells and progenitor cells, but this has not been demonstrated in human marrow (Rosse, 1977). Normoblasts fall after birth, rise to a maximum at two months, then fall to a stable, relatively low level by four months and remain there during most of infancy.

The myeloid:erythroid (M:E) ratio is the ratio of total granulocytes:total normoblasts. In newborns and infancy it is somewhat higher than in later childhood or adult life (Table 28–2). In adults the range is broad, varying from 2:1 to 4:1.

Both the differential count and the M:E ratio are relative values and must be interpreted with respect to the cellularity or with respect to other evidence that one of the systems is normal.

An *increased* M:E ratio, e.g., 6 to 1, may be found in infection, chronic myelogenous leukemia, or erythroid hypoplasia. A *decreased* M:E ratio, i.e., less than 2 to 1, may mean a depression of leukopoiesis or a normoblastic hyperplasia, depending upon the marrow cellularity.

The number of megakaryocytes is estimated more reliably in sections than in marrow films. In scanning areas of films with good cellularity under low power (100 ×), an average of one to three megakaryocytes should be found in each field in a normal marrow.

Maturation. While examining the cells during the differential count, one should evaluate whether maturation is normal, that is, whether nuclear and cytoplasmic development is in balance. Impaired cytoplasmic maturation in normoblasts, for example, occurs when hemoglobin synthesis is impaired; impaired nuclear maturation occurs in megaloblastic anemias. Bizarre or dysplastic maturation occurs as a result of certain drugs, in some leukemias, and in dysmyelopoietic syndromes.

Presence of Rare Cell Types or Abnormal Cells. In scanning the marrow, one looks for the presence of rare or unexpected cell types.

Tissue mast cells (Plate 28–2*M*) are normally very infrequent. They are increased in number in aplastic or refractory anemias, and in lymphoproliferative disorders.

Osteoblasts (Plate 28–3*I*) are cells which synthesize the collagen matrix of bone. *Osteoclasts* (Plate 28–3*C*) are cells that resorb bone and are thought to result from the fusion of histiocytes. Both cell types are normally present in small numbers in the aspirates of infants and children. They are uncommonly seen in adult marrow, except when bone destruction or repair is occurring, as in hyperparathyroidism, Paget's disease, metastatic tumor, or a recent biopsy at the same site.

Osteoblasts are large cells with a single eccentric nucleus which has reticular chromatin and a prominent nucleolus. The cytoplasm is moderately basophilic; a large pale Golgi zone is separated from the nucleus, rather than abutting it as in plasma cells. Osteoblasts are often present in clusters and may be confused with immature plasma cells or myeloma cells.

Osteoclasts are large, multinucleated cells up to 100 μm diameter that may be mistaken for megakaryocytes. They have multiple nuclei which are separate (not joined as in megakaryocytes). The chromatin is reticular, and a prominent nucleolus is usually present. The cytoplasm may be basophilic but usually has pink-purple granules that resemble megakaryocyte granules. Coarse fragments of purple-staining material are often present.

Clusters of *metastatic neoplastic cells* may be found in one or more marrow films of patients with metastatic tumor in the bone sampled; they may be found in biopsy sections and not films, in both, or less commonly, one or more films and not the biopsy. Some metastatic neoplastic cells resemble myeloblasts or other primitive blasts. The clue to recognizing them is that they almost always appear in clusters or clumps of cells; this is not true of hematopoietic blast cells.

Evaluation of the Biopsy. Histologic sections allow better estimates of the marrow cellularity and the number of megakaryocytes than do marrow films (Fig. 28–10). In good histologic preparations, the cell distribution and maturation abnormalities can be quite reliably determined. In addition to more reliable detection of the presence of lymphomas or metastatic tumor, the histologic pattern can often be diagnostic of the type of neoplasm. Other focal lesions not found in films include granulomas, abscesses, and vascular lesions.

In some conditions, such as myelofibrosis and leukemic reticuloendotheliosis (hairy cell leukemia), the bone marrow cannot be aspirated, and biopsy is necessary to establish a diagnosis.

Trabeculae should always be examined in order to detect bony abnormalities. Osteosclerosis with thickened bone trabeculae may accompany myelofibrosis or be congenital. In osteoporosis the bone trabeculae are thin. Osteomalacia is characterized by a recognizable osteoid seam. Osteitis fibrosa occurs in hyperparathyroidism and is characterized by irregular osteoclastic bony resorption, endosteal fibrosis, and some osteoblastic activity in areas of bone regeneration. Irregularly widened trabeculae with a "mosaic" pattern are typical findings in Paget's disease of bone (Rywlin, 1976).

Interpretation. The *summary* of the marrow report includes an estimate of cellularity, an estimate of the number of megakaryocytes, the M:E ratio, statements about any cytologic or maturation abnormalities, an estimate of the storage iron and proportion of sideroblasts, and statements about any other abnormal findings present. A summary of the abnormalities in the blood cell counts and morphology is also made.

Then an *interpretation* of the observed findings is made, which of course includes a diagnosis if this is possible. In making such an interpretation, one should include an integration of the marrow and blood observations with clinical findings and other laboratory data.

Alterations in blood and marrow cells are discussed with reference to the disease and disorders considered in subsequent chapters.

Indications for Marrow Study

(Wintrobe, 1981)

In the differential diagnosis of macrocytic anemia, there are some cases in which the changes in the blood are minimal, yet the marrow is megaloblastic.

In microcytic anemias, evaluation of the iron stores and sideroblasts allows categorization of the anemia, i.e., iron deficiency, anemia of chronic disease, sideroblastic.

In normocytic anemias, marrow examination is less often useful. Comparing the level of marrow erythroid precursors with the reticulocyte count allows an estimation of the degree of ineffective erythropoiesis, or lack of erythropoiesis, as in pure red cell aplasia.

In neutropenia, thrombocytopenia, or pancytopenia, marrow study is helpful in assessing the presence and normality of the precursor cells in each series. This enables one to assess the probabilities of decreased production, impaired maturation, or increased destruction as the mechanism of the disorder.

In immunoglobulin abnormalities, the diagnosis of plasma cell myeloma or macroglobulinemia may be confirmed if infiltrations of abnormal plasma cells or lymphocytes are present.

If the marrow cannot be aspirated ("dry tap"), biopsy is essential. Marrow biopsy should also be performed if there are blood changes suggesting myelofibrosis with myeloid metaplasia, or if granulomatous disease or metastatic tumor is suspected.

Adamson, J. W., Alexanian, R., Martinez, C., and Finch, C. A.: Erythropoietin excretion in normal man. Blood, *28*:354, 1966.

Aster, R. H.: Thrombocytopenia due to sequestration of platelets. *In* Williams, W. J., Beutler, E., Erslev, A. J., and Rundles, R. W.: Hematology. 2nd ed. New York, McGraw-Hill, 1977, p. 1360.

Bainton, D. F., and Finch, C. A.: The diagnosis of iron deficiency anemia. Am. J. Med., *37*:62, 1964.

Bainton, D. F., Nichols, B. A., and Farquhar, M. G.: Primary lysosomes of blood leukocytes. *In* Dingle, J. T., and Dean, R. T. (eds.): Lysosomes in Biology and Pathology 5. Amsterdam, North Holland Publishing Company, 1976, p. 3.

Becker, A. J., McCulloch, E. A., and Till, J. E.: Cytological demonstration of the clonal nature of spleen colonies derived from transplanted mouse marrow cells. Nature, *197*:452, 1963.

Beeson, P. B., and Bass, D. A.: The Eosinophil. Volume XIV in Major Problems in Internal Medicine. Philadelphia, W. B. Saunders Company, 1977.

Berman, L.: A review of methods for aspiration and biopsy of bone marrow. Am. J. Clin. Path., *23*:385, 1953.

Bessis, M.: Living Blood Cells and Their Ultrastructure. Trans. by R. I. Weed. New York, Springer-Verlag, 1973.

Beutler, E.: Peripheral blood, bone marrow and urine iron stains. *In* Williams, W. J., Beutler, E., Erslev, A. J., and Rundles, R. W. (eds.): Hematology. 2nd ed. New York, McGraw-Hill, 1977.

Block, M. H.: Text—Atlas of Hematology. Philadelphia, Lea & Febiger, 1976.

Bradley, T. R., and Metcalf, D.: The growth of mouse bone marrow cells *in vitro*. Aust. J. Exp. Biol. Med. Sci., *44*:287, 1966.

Bunn, H. F., Forget, B. G., and Ranney, H. M.: Human Hemoglobins. Philadelphia, W. B. Saunders Company, 1977.

Cawley, J. C., and Hayhoe, F. G. J.: Ultrastructure of Haemic Cells. Philadelphia, W. B. Saunders Company, 1973.

Cline, M. J.: The White Cell. Cambridge, Harvard University Press, 1975.

Cline, M. J., and Golde, D. W.: Granulocytes and monocytes: Function and functional disorders. *In* Hoffbrand, A. V., Brain, M. C., and Hirsh, J. (eds.): Recent Advances in Haematology 2. Edinburgh, Churchill Livingstone, 1977.

Custer, R. P.: An Atlas of the Blood and Bone Marrow, 2nd ed. Philadelphia, W. B. Saunders Company, 1974.

Dancey, J. T., Deubelbeiss, K. A., and Harker, L. A.: Section preparation of human marrow for light microscopy. J. Clin. Path., *29*:704, 1976.

Denburg, J. A., Richardson, M., Telizyn, S., and Bienenstock, J.: Basophil/mast cell precursors in human blood. Blood, *61*:775, 1983.

Douglas, S. D., and Ackerman, S. K.: Anatomy of the immune system. Clin. Haematol., *6*:299, 1977.

Dvorak, H. F., and Dvorak, A.: Basophilic leukocytes: structure, function and role in disease. Clin. Haematol., *4*:651, 1975.

Efrati, P., and Rozenszajn, L.: The morphology of buffy coat in normal human adults. Blood, *16*:1012, 1960.

Fauser, A. A., and Messner, H. A.: Identification of megakaryocytes, macrophages, and eosinophils in colonies of human bone marrow containing neutrophilic granulocytes and erythroblasts. Blood, *53*:1023, 1979.

Fialkow, P. J., Jacobson, R. J., and Papayannopoulou, T.: Chronic myelocytic leukemia: Clonal origin in a stem cell common to the granulocyte, erythrocyte, platelet, and monocyte/macrophage. Am. J. Med., *63*:125, 1977.

Ganzoni, A. M., Oakes, R., and Hillman, R. S.: Red cell aging *in vivo*. J. Clin. Invest., *50*:1373, 1971.

Harris, J. W., and Kellermeyer, R. W.: The Red Cell: Production, Metabolism, Destruction: Normal and Abnormal, rev. ed. Cambridge, Harvard University Press, 1970.

Hartsock, R. J., Smith, E. B., and Petty, C. S.: Normal variations with aging of the amount of hematopoietic tissue in bone marrow from the anterior iliac crest. Am. J. Clin. Path., *43*:326, 1965.

Henry, R. J.: Clinical Chemistry: Principles and Technics. New York, Harper & Row, Publishers, Inc., 1964, p. 435.

Hillman, R. S., and Finch, C. A.: Erythropoiesis: Normal and abnormal. Semin. Hematol., *4*:327, 1967.

Hillman, R. S., and Finch, C. A.: Red Cell Manual. 4th ed. Philadelphia, F. A. Davis Co., 1974.

Ichikawa, Y., Pluznik, D. H., and Sachs, L.: *In vitro* control of the development of macrophages and granulocyte colonies. Proc. Natl. Acad. Sci. U.S.A., *56*:488, 1966.

Izak, G.: Erythroid cell differentiation and maturation. Prog. Hematol., *10*:1, 1977.

Kaufman, R. M., Airo, R., Pollack, S., Crosby, W. H., and Doberneck, R.: Origin of pulmonary megakaryocytes. Blood, *25*:767, 1965a.

Kaufman, R. M., Airo, R., Pollack, S., and Crosby, W. H.: Circulating megakaryocytes and platelet release in the lung. Blood, *26*:720, 1965b.

Kurland, J. I., Bockman, R. S., Broxmeyer, H. E., and Moore, M. A. S.: Limitation of excessive myelopoiesis by the intrinsic modulation of macrophage-derived prostaglandin E. Science, *199*:552, 1978.

Lessin, L. S., and Bessis, M.: Morphology of the erythron. *In* Williams, W. J., Beutler, E., Erslev, A. J., and Rundles, R. W. (eds.): Hematology. 2nd ed. New York, McGraw-Hill Book Co., 1977, p. 103.

Lewis, J. P., and Trobaugh, F. E., Jr.: Haematopoietic stem cells. Nature, *204*:589, 1964.

Lodish, H. F.: Translational control of protein synthesis. Annu. Rev. Biochem., *45*:39, 1976.

Metcalf, D.: Hemopoietic Colonies. *In vitro* cloning of normal and leukemic cells. Recent Results in Cancer Research, vol. 61. New York, Springer-Verlag, 1977.

Meuret, G., and Hoffmann, G.: Monocyte kinetic studies in normal and disease states. Br. J. Haematol., *24*:275, 1973.

Meuret, G., Bammert, J., and Hoffmann, G.: Kinetics of human monocytopoiesis. Blood, *44*:801, 1974.

Micklem, H. S.: B lymphocytes, T lymphocytes and lymphopoiesis. Clin. Haematol., *8*:395, 1979.

Miller, J. F. A. P.: The cellular basis of immune responsiveness. Clin. Haematol., *6*:277, 1977.

Mladenovic, J., and Adamson, J. W.: Erythroid colony growth in culture: Analysis of erythroid differentiation and studies in human disease states. *In* Hoffbrand, A. V. (ed.): Recent Advances in Haematology 3. Edinburgh, Churchill Livingstone, 1982, p. 95.

Murphy, P.: The Neutrophil. New York, Plenum Medical Book Co., 1976.

Nelson, D. A.: Hematopoiesis. *In* Henry, J. B. (ed.): Clinical Diagnosis and Management of Laboratory Methods. 16th ed. Philadelphia, W. B. Saunders Company, 1979, Chap. 28.

Parkhouse, R. M. E., and Cooper, M. D.: A model for the differentiation of B lymphocytes with implications for the biological role of IgD. Immunol. Rev., *39*:105, 1977.

Pike, B. L., and Robinson, W. A.: Human bone marrow colony growth in agar-gel. J. Cell. Physiol., *76*:77, 1970.

Poppema, S., Bhan, A. K., Reinherz, E. L., McClusky, R. T., and Schlossman, S. F.: Distribution of T cell subsets in human lymph nodes. J. Exp. Med., *153*:30, 1981.

Reinherz, E. L., and Schlossman, S. F.: Current concepts in immunology: Regulation of the immune response-inducer and suppressor T-lymphocyte subsets in human beings. N. Engl. J. Med., *303*:370, 1980.

Rosse, C., Kraemer, M. J., Dillon, T. L., McFarland, R., and Smith, N. J.: Bone marrow cell populations of normal infants: The predominance of lymphocytes. J. Lab. Clin. Med., *89*:1225, 1977.

Rywlin, A. M.: Histopathology of the bone marrow. Boston, Little, Brown and Co., 1976.

Sundberg, R. D., and Broman, H.: The application of the Prussian blue stain to previously stained films of blood and marrow. Blood, *10*:160, 1955.

Till, J. E., and McCulloch, E. A.: A direct measurement of the radiation sensitivity of normal mouse bone marrow cells. Rad. Res., *14*:213, 1961.

Weiss, L.: The Blood Cells and Hematopoietic Tissues. *In* Weiss, L., and Greep, R. O. (eds.): Histology. 4th ed. New York, McGraw-Hill Book Co., 1977.

West, B. C., Rosenthal, A. S., Gelb, N. A., and Kimball, H. R.: Separation and characterization of human neutrophil granules. Am. J. Path., *77*:41, 1974.

Williams, N., and Levine, R. F.: The origin, development and regulation of megakaryocytes. Br. J. Haematol., *52*:173, 1982.

Wintrobe, M. M., Lee, G. R., Boggs, D., Bithell, T. S., Foerster, J., Athens, J. W., and Lukens, J. N.: Clinical Hematology. 8th ed. Philadelphia, Lea and Febiger, 1981.

Zucker-Franklin, D., Greavey, M. F., Grossi, C. E., and Marmont, A. M.: Atlas of Blood Cells. Function and Pathology. Philadelphia, Lea and Febiger, 1981.

29

ERYTHROCYTIC DISORDERS

DOUGLAS A. NELSON, M.D., and FREDERICK R. DAVEY, M.D.

ANEMIAS

General Manifestations

Anemia is considered to be present if the hemoglobin concentration or the hematocrit is below the lower limit of the 95 per cent reference interval for the individual's age, sex and geographic location (altitude) (see Fig. 27–45, p. 620; Table 29–1). This means that 2.5 per cent of normal individuals will be classified as anemic. Conversely, an individual whose hemoglobin falls within the reference intervals for age and sex yet significantly below his or her own reference values should be considered anemic.

Causes of anemia fall into three major pathophysiologic categories: impaired red cell production, blood loss, or accelerated red cell destruction (hemolysis) in excess of the ability of the marrow to replace these losses. The presence of anemia may be a sign of an underlying disorder whose cause should be identified, since correction may be very important to the individual.

Anemia also may be classified by red cell morphology as macrocytic, normocytic, or microcytic, an approach that is useful in differential diagnosis (p. 696). Both the pathophysiologic and morphologic classifications should be understood. Some anemias have more than one pathogenetic mechanism and go through more than one morphologic stage, e.g., blood loss anemia.

Table 29–1. REFERENCE VALUES BELOW WHICH ANEMIA IS CONSIDERED TO EXIST AT SEA LEVEL

Age (Years)	Hb (g/dl)	Hct (Liter/Liter)
0.6 to 4	11	0.33
5 to 9	11.5	0.345
10 to 14	12	0.36
Adults—men	14	0.42
Adults—women	12	0.36
Pregnant women	11	0.33

From Committee on Iron Deficiency: Iron deficiency in the United States. J.A.M.A., *203*:407, 1968. Copyright 1968, American Medical Association.

CLINICAL SIGNS OF ANEMIA

Clinical signs and symptoms result from the diminished delivery of oxygen to the tissues and, therefore, are related to the lowered hemoglobin concentration and blood volume, and dependent upon the rate of these changes. Modifying factors are compensatory adjustments in the cardiac output, the respiratory rate, and the oxygen affinity of hemoglobin. When anemia develops slowly in a patient who is not otherwise severely ill, hemoglobin concentrations as low as 6 g/dl may develop without producing any discomfort or physical signs as long as the patient is at rest.

In general, the anemic patient complains of easy fatigability and dyspnea on exertion, and often of faintness, vertigo, palpitation, and headache. The more common physical findings are pallor, a rapid bounding pulse, low blood pressure, slight fever, some dependent edema, and systolic murmurs. In addition to these general signs and symptoms certain clinical findings are characteristic of the specific type of anemia.

Blood Loss Anemia

ACUTE POSTHEMORRHAGIC ANEMIA

Blood may be lost from the circulation externally, into the gastrointestinal tract, or into a tissue space or body cavity. If blood is lost over a short period of time in amounts sufficient to cause anemia, *acute posthemorrhagic anemia* occurs.

After a single episode of bleeding, the major manifestations are those due to depletion of blood volume (hypovolemia). After a day or so, blood volume is returned to previous levels by movement of fluid into the circulation, and anemia becomes evident.

The earliest hematologic change is transient fall in the platelet count which may rise to elevated levels within an hour. The next development is a moderate neutrophilic leukocytosis with a shift to the left; a maximum leukocyte count of 10 to 35 $\times$ 10^9/L may occur in two to five hours. The Hb and Hct do not fall immediately, but only slowly as tissue fluids move into the circulation to compensate for the lost blood volume. The fall in Hb and Hct may not reveal the full extent of the red cell loss until two or three days after the hemorrhage.

The anemia that develops at first is normochromic and normocytic, with a normal MCV and MCHC and only minimal anisocytosis and poikilocytosis. Increased erythropoietin secretion stimulates erythroid proliferation in the marrow, and reticulocytes begin to reach the circulation in three to five days, reaching a maximum by 10 days or so. During this period transient macrocytosis (increased MCV), increased polychromasia, and normoblasts may appear in the blood. It takes about two to four days after the blood loss for the leukocyte count to return to normal, and about two weeks for the morphologic changes to disappear. Return of red cell values is slower.

CHRONIC POSTHEMORRHAGIC ANEMIA

If blood is lost in small amounts over an extended period of time, both the clinical and hematologic features that characterize acute posthemorrhagic anemia are lacking. Regeneration of red cells occurs at a slower rate.

The reticulocyte count may be normal or slightly increased. Significant anemia does not usually develop until after storage iron is depleted; the anemia, therefore, is one of iron deficiency (q.v.). The anemia is at first normochromic and normocytic, and gradually the newly formed red cells become microcytic, then hypochromic. The leukocyte count is normal or slightly decreased owing to neutropenia. Platelets are commonly increased, and only later, in severe iron deficiency, are they likely to be decreased.

The cause of blood loss must be identified, for it is toward this that definitive treatment must be directed.

4

Impaired Production—Iron Deficiency

IRON METABOLISM (Hillman, 1974)

The physiologic chemistry of iron and clinicopathological correlations are reviewed in Chapter 9.

Iron is an essential component of hemoglobin, of myoglobin (in muscle cells), and of certain enzymes (in most body cells). The major "pools" of iron in the body are illustrated in Figure 29–1. Two thirds or more of the body's total iron is in the erythron (normoblasts and erythrocytes); each milliliter of red cells contains about 1 mg of iron. Storage iron is present in macrophages of the reticuloendothelial system as ferritin (iron bound to the protein, apoferritin, molecular weight 450,000) and as hemosiderin, a degraded storage form with a lesser proportion of protein than ferritin (Worwood, 1980). Most of the iron utilized in hemoglobin synthesis is that recently released from degraded Hb in macrophages and transported to the normoblasts by plasma transferrin (a beta globulin, molecular weight 80,000).

Very little iron is lost from the body, and this mainly from loss of cells in the gastrointestinal tract and to a lesser extent from the skin and in the urine. The iron excreted in women averages more than that in men because of menstrual blood loss. Iron balance is maintained by control of absorption. In the United

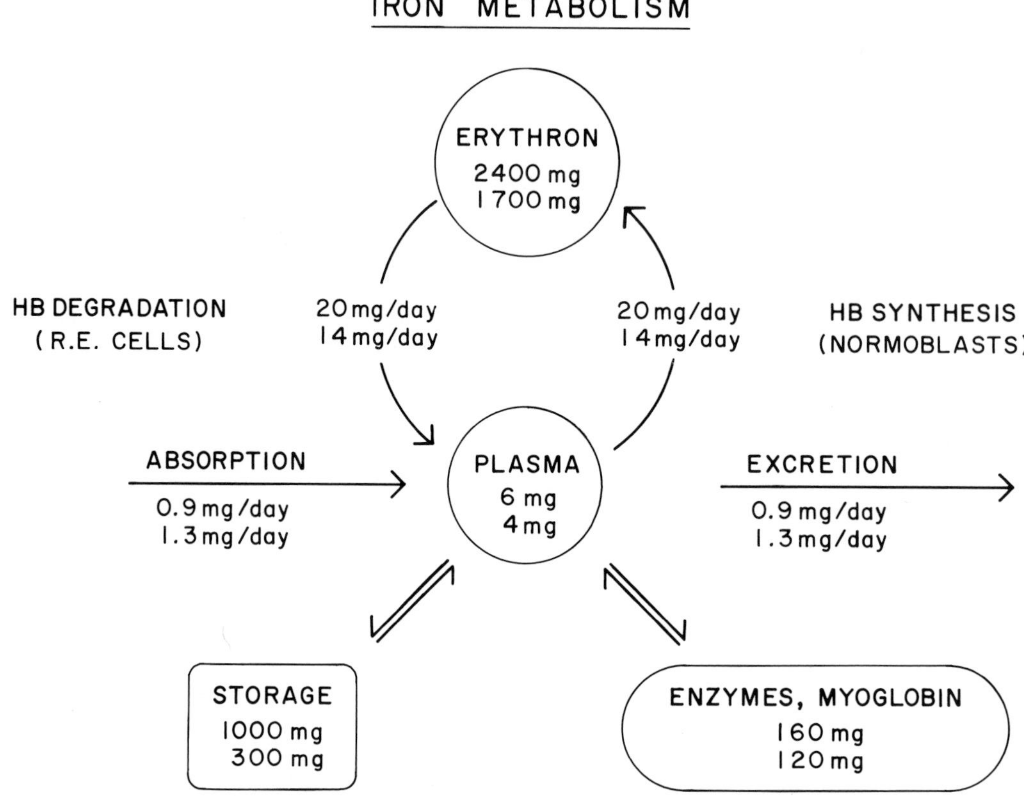

Figure 29–1. Scheme of iron metabolism. The upper figure in each position is average for an 80 kg man; the lower figure is for a 65 kg woman. (Data from Hillman, 1974). The plasma iron, bound largely to transferrin, is central in one scheme. It completely turns over several times a day in supplying iron for heme synthesis.

Each day, about 1/120 of the total circulating red cells are destroyed and the same number of new red cells are delivered to the blood. That proportion of the total erythron iron enters the plasma from the site of Hb degradation, the macrophages of the RE system, and travels (bound to transferrin) to the normoblasts in the marrow. Storage iron largely resides also in the macrophages of the RE system. Absorbed iron enters the plasma pool, bound to transferrin. Excreted iron is largely from loss of cells.

States, dietary iron in men averages 15 mg/day with 6 per cent absorption, and 11 mg/day in women with 12 per cent absorption. Absorption can be increased in iron deficiency, but only to about 20 per cent of ingested iron in meat-containing diets, and less in vegetarian diets. Absorption takes place largely in the small intestine, most efficiently in the duodenum.

In the plasma, the total iron averages 110 μg/dl (1.1 mg/L or 19.7 μmol/L). The great majority of this is bound to the transferrin, which has a capacity to bind 330 μg of iron/dl (or 59.1 μmol/L) and therefore is about one third saturated. A very small amount of iron in plasma is in ferritin. Plasma (or serum) ferritin averages about 100 μg/L in men (less in women, about 50 μg/L). If serum ferritin contained the same proportion of iron as tissue ferritin (20 to 25 per cent), plasma ferritin would normally contain about 20 μg of iron per liter (Siimes, 1974b).

IRON DEFICIENCY ANEMIA

When iron loss exceeds iron intake for a time long enough to deplete the body's iron stores, insufficient iron is available for normal hemoglobin production. When well developed, iron deficiency is characterized by a hypochromic microcytic anemia.

Iron deficiency results only when there is an increased need for iron (e.g., during rapid growth in infancy and childhood or during pregnancy) or when excessive loss of blood has reduced the body's reserves of iron (e.g., following repeated hemorrhages, excessive menstruation, or multiple pregnancies).

Iron deficiency is probably the most common cause of anemia between the ages of six and 24 months. It is caused by insufficient dietary iron to meet the needs of rapid growth. After the first four to six months of life, the iron stores present from birth have been exhausted, and the infant depends on dietary iron. An infant maintained on milk and carbohydrates without supplements of iron-containing foods is likely to develop an iron deficiency anemia, the "milk anemia" of infancy. Defective absorption of iron and eventual iron deficiency anemia occur after total gastrectomy or even subtotal gastrectomy. Except for the sprue syndrome, other causes of malabsorption of iron are extremely rare.

If an adult male had absolutely no iron intake or absorption (which would be extremely unlikely), his body iron stores of 1000 mg would last for three to four years before he would even begin to become iron deficient. Therefore, almost all cases of iron deficiency anemia in adult males are due to chronic blood loss.

The sequence of events in developing iron deficiency anemia is usually as follows (Harris, 1970; Hillman, 1974): When blood loss exceeds absorption, a negative iron balance exists. Iron is mobilized from stores, storage iron decreases, plasma ferritin decreases, iron absorption increases, and plasma iron-binding capacity (transferrin) increases. This stage is known as *iron depletion.* After iron stores are depleted, the plasma iron concentration falls, saturation of transferrin falls below 15 per cent, and the percentage of sideroblasts decreases in the marrow. As a result of lack of iron for heme synthesis, red cell protoporphyrin increases. This second stage is *iron deficient erythropoiesis;* anemia may not yet be present. The third stage is *iron deficiency anemia;* in addition to the above abnormalities, anemia is detectable. The anemia is at first normochromic and normocytic, gradually becomes microcytic, and finally microcytic and hypochromic.

Clinical Features. Clinical findings may be due to the underlying cause of the blood loss itself, to the general manifestations of anemia (p. 653), or to iron deficiency. Those which are probably attributable to lack of tissue iron include paresthesias, such as numbness and tingling; atrophy of epithelium of the tongue with burning or soreness; fissures or ulcers at the corners of the mouth (angular stomatitis); chronic gastritis, which leads to decreased gastric secretions but few symptoms; "pica," which is the craving to eat unusual substances such as dirt or ice; concave or spoon-shaped nails (koilonychia); difficulty swallowing due to "webs" of tissue or partial strictures at the junction of the esophagus and hypopharynx (Wintrobe, 1981). The latter two findings are relatively uncommon. Splenomegaly may occur but is quite uncommon.

Laboratory Features

Blood. In early iron deficiency anemia, the stained blood film often shows normochromic normocytic erythrocytes (Fairbanks, 1971). In later stages the picture is one of microcytosis, anisocytosis, poikilocytosis (including elliptical and elongated cells), and varying degrees of hypochromia (see p. 604). Reticulocytes are usually decreased in absolute numbers except following iron therapy. The MCV is low, and the Hb and Hct are relatively lower than the erythrocyte count. Osmotic fragility may be decreased because the red cells are thinner than normal (Fig. 27–18; Plate 29–1*J*).

The leukocyte count is normal or slightly lowered. Granulocytopenia and a small number of hypersegmented neutrophils may be present. Platelets may be increased, whether the iron lack is due to blood loss or dietary deficiency, but tend to be decreased in severe anemia.

Marrow. Normoblastic hyperplasia occurs early, but in later stages the limiting effect of severe iron deficiency restricts erythropoiesis to the basal level. The normoblasts are smaller than normal, deficient in the amount of hemoglobin in the cytoplasm, and irregular in shape with frayed margins (Plate 29–1*G*). Giant neutrophil bands or metamyelocytes, if present, are rarely due to iron deficiency per se; usually they indicate an associated vitamin B_{12} or folate deficiency (p. 657). Iron stains should be performed routinely (p. 646), Plate 29–1*D* and *E*). *Storage iron* is absent, unless iron has recently been administered in some form. The proportion of normoblasts that are *sideroblasts* is decreased (less than 20 per cent); this proportion is usually about the same as the per cent saturation of transferrin (or TIBC) and is a measure of iron delivery to the normoblasts.

Serum Iron. The reference interval is 50 to 160 μg/dl (9 to 29 μmol/L) in adults. The level is lower in iron deficiency but also in infections and the anemia of chronic disease.

Serum Iron-Binding Capacity. The reference interval for adults is 250 to 400 μg/dl (45 to 72 μmol/L). In iron deficiency anemia, the serum total iron-binding capacity (TIBC) is increased. It is normal or decreased in the anemia of chronic disease. If chronic infection coexists with chronic blood loss, the TIBC may not be increased, even though the patient is iron deficient.

Per Cent Saturation of TIBC. The ratio of serum iron to TIBC is the per cent saturation of the TIBC. Normally this is 20 to 55 per cent; values below 15 per cent indicate iron deficient erythropoiesis.

There is normally a marked diurnal variation in serum iron, with highest values in the morning and lowest values late in the day. Consequently, fasting morning blood specimens are preferred for the diagnosis of iron deficiency.

Somewhat lower reference intervals for serum iron are normal in iron sufficient infants from the second month through the twelfth month. Saarinen (1977) studied infants in whom iron deficiency was excluded by normal hemoglobin, MCV, and serum ferritin values. The TIBC gradually rose during the first year of life. After the first four months of life, through the first year, the lower reference value for per cent saturation in normal infants was 10 per cent rather than 20 per cent as in adults. Thereafter, values slowly rise to adult levels at about the age of two years (Jacobs, 1974).

Serum Ferritin. In adults, the reference values are 12 to 300 μg/L, with higher values in men than women. Serum ferritin appears to be in equilibrium with tissue ferritin and is a good reflection of storage iron in normal subjects and in most disorders (Jacobs, 1975). The equivalence of 1 μg/L of serum ferritin with 8 mg storage iron has been suggested. In patients with some hepatocellular diseases, malignancies, and inflammatory diseases, serum ferritin is a disproportionately high estimate of storage iron. A *low* value, however, below 12 μg/L, indicates low iron stores; falsely low values mimicking iron deficiency have not been found.

In infancy and childhood, between the ages of 6 months and 15 years, the reference interval for serum ferritin is 7 to 142 μg/L (Siimes, 1974a) somewhat

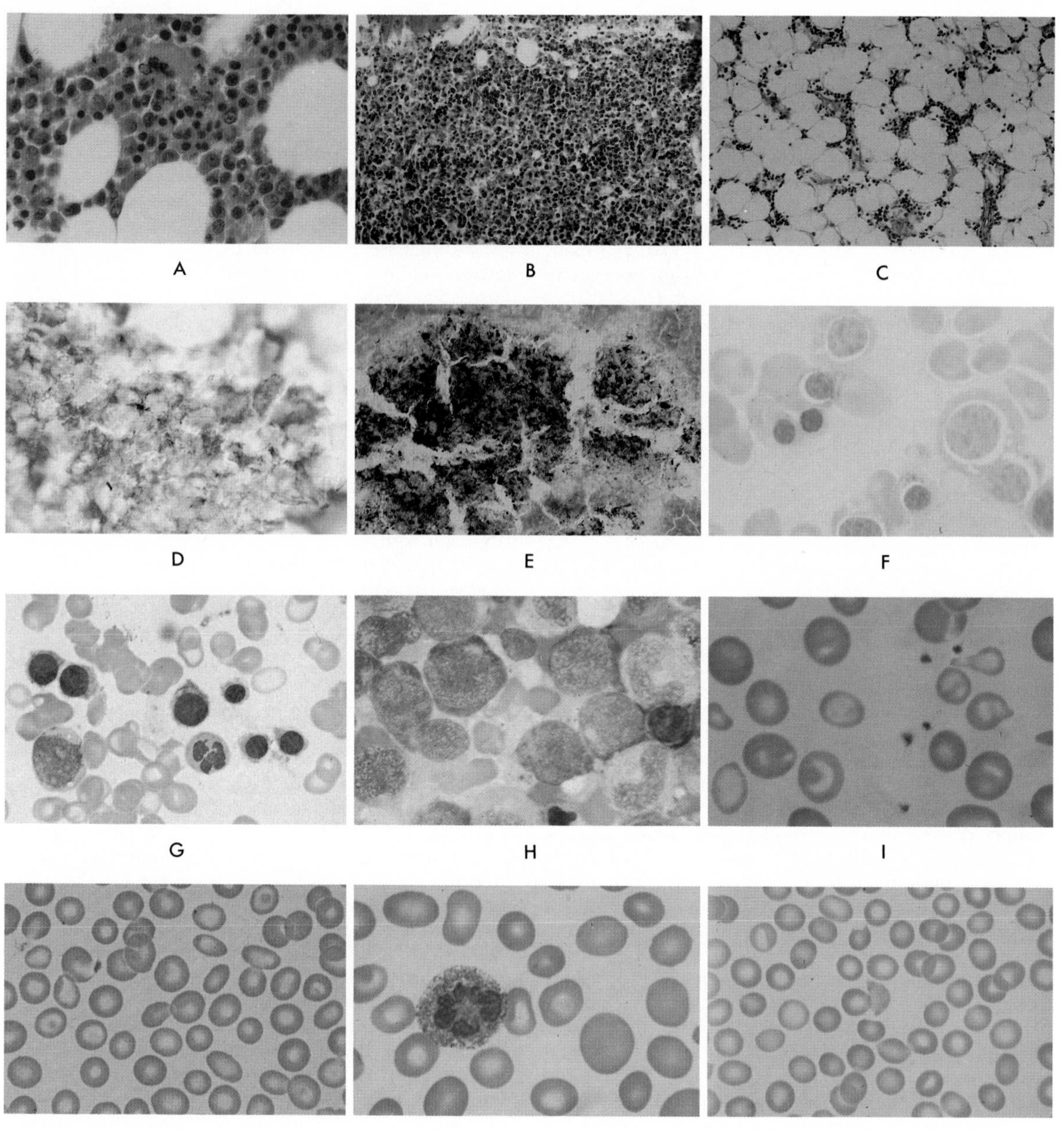

Plate 29–1. *A,* Section of normal marrow. The cellularity (i.e., the ratio of the space occupied by cells to the total) is about 0.5 to 0.6. The E/G ratio is normal, about ⅓. A megakaryocyte is the upper center. *B,* Section of hyperplastic marrow, megaloblastic anemia. The cellularity is over 0.95. *C,* Section of hypocellular marrow, aplastic anemia. The cellularity is about 0.10 or less. Though not discernible at this magnification, most of the cells are lymphocytes and plasma cells. *D,* Marrow film, Prussian blue reaction, no counterstain, normal marrow. Storage iron stains blue-green and is within macrophages. On a scale of 0 to 5+, the amount of storage iron here is judged as 1+, which is in the normal range for a woman, probably somewhat low for a man. In iron deficiency anemia, no blue-green staining iron is visible. *E,* Marrow film, Prussian blue reaction, no counterstain; sideroblastic anemia. On a scale of 0 to 5+, the amount of storage iron is judged at 5+, which is markedly increased. *F,* Marrow film, Prussian blue reaction, counterstained with nuclear fast red, sideroblastic anemia. The normoblasts in the field contain multiple siderotic granules. Two ring sideroblasts are left of the center. The wide perinuclear space in some cells is an artifact. *G,* Marrow film, iron deficiency anemia. The six normoblasts have irregular margins and irregular clear spaces, reflecting lack of hemoglobin synthesis, i.e., defective cytoplasmic maturation. Also in the field are a neutrophil and an immature monocyte. *H,* Marrow film, megaloblastic anemia. Basophilic and polychromatophilic megaloblasts predominate in this field; two giant-band neutrophils are present. The "open," non-condensed chromatin pattern and large cell size are characteristic of defective nuclear maturation. *I,* Blood film, primary acquired sideroblastic anemia. Dimorphic red cell populations: normocytic to macrocytic and normochromic, microcytic, and hypochromic, *J,* Blood film, iron deficiency anemia, same patient as in *G* above. The red cells are microcytic; some are also hypochromic; a few target cells and an increased proportion of elliptocytes are present. *K,* Blood film, megaloblastic anemia. The oval macrocytes and hypersegmented neutrophil are presumptive evidence of megaloblastosis. Note the prominent large neutrophil granules. *L,* Blood film, lead poisoning. The red cells are slightly microcytic with some hypochromic cells. The poikilocyte in the center contains basophilic stippling.

lower than early infancy or adult life. In men, serum ferritin gradually rises between the ages of 18 and 30 years, whereas in women it does not (Finch, 1977); representative geometric mean values of the skewed distribution of reference values were 127 μg/L for men, 46 μg/L for women.

Erythrocyte Porphyrins. Since heme is formed by insertion of iron into protoporphyrin IX, the latter is increased in iron deficient erythropoiesis, whether due to iron deficiency or anemia or chronic disease. It is also increased in lead poisoning and in some cases of sideroblastic anemia but is normal in thalassemia. A relatively simple micromethod measuring "free erythrocyte poryphrins" (FEP) in whole blood (Piomelli, 1973) has been shown to be useful in distinguishing microcytosis due to iron deficiency from that due to beta thalassemia minor (Stockman, 1975). The normal reference interval was 10 to 90 μg/dl of erythrocytes; in iron deficiency, the erythrocyte porphyrins became elevated when the saturation of the TIBC was less than 15 per cent.

Differential Diagnosis. Anemia due to iron deficiency usually must be distinguished from other microcytic or hypochromic anemias (Table 29–10, p. 696). These include the thalassemia traits (p. 683), long-standing anemia of chronic disease (p. 662), and the sideroblastic anemias (p. 667). Bone marrow storage iron and serum ferritin will be decreased in iron deficiency and normal or elevated in all others. In *thalassemia trait,* the FEP is normal, serum iron is normal, and the condition is present in family members. In β thalassemia trait, the Hb A_2 and often the Hb F are increased. Indeed, the Hb A_2 is often decreased in iron deficiency. In *anemia of chronic disorders* (chronic infection, rheumatoid arthritis, or neoplastic disease), although the serum iron is low, as in iron deficiency, the TIBC is low or normal. In the *sideroblastic anemias,* which include chronic lead poisoning, the serum iron and per cent TIBC saturation are increased, and pathologic "ring" sideroblasts are present in the marrow.

Management. The first principle in therapy is that the underlying cause be identified and corrected. Ferrous iron is given orally, about 200 mg per day, in three doses between meals. This will provide 20 to 40 mg of absorbed iron per day, which, with the iron produced by turnover of senescent red cells, will be sufficient to increase production to two or three times normal (Hillman, 1974). The reticulocyte count will reach a maximum at 5 to 10 days, then gradually decrease toward normal. Monitoring the hemoglobin is best; Hb should increase by 0.1 to 0.2 g/dl per day after the fifth day and by at least 2 g/dl each three weeks. After the hemoglobin has returned to normal, iron therapy should be continued for at least two months in order to replenish storage iron.

Impaired Production—Megaloblastic Anemia

MACROCYTOSIS WITH NORMOBLASTIC MARROW

Macrocytic anemias which are not megaloblastic may be due to early release of erythrocytes from the marrow, as in response to acute blood loss or hemolysis; this is a "shift" macrocytosis, since it results from a premature release of reticulocytes from the marrow (Hillman, 1974). Macrocytosis not due to reticulocytosis is found commonly in hypothyroidism and in individuals with an excessive alcohol intake, and in some cases of aplastic or refractory anemias and of non-alcoholic liver disease (Chanarin, 1976).

MEGALOBLASTIC ANEMIA

Blood (Figs. 27–19, 27–20, 27–31, 27–34, 27–38, and 29–2, and Plate 29–1*K*). Macrocytic anemias associated with megaloblastosis differ from non-megaloblastic macrocytic anemia in that macro-ovalocytes and giant hypersegmented neutrophils are present in the blood. Pancytopenia is the rule. The anemia is macrocytic with an elevated MCV and is characterized by macro-ovalocytes and often extreme degrees of anisocytosis and poikilocytosis. Microcytes and dacrocytes are common. Basophilic stippling, multiple Howell-Jolly bodies, nucleated red cells with karyorrhexis, and even megaloblasts may be seen. Leukopenia is present. Granulocytes have increased numbers of lobes, presumably a result of abnormal nuclear maturation. Five or more lobes in more than 5 per cent of the neutrophils constitute hypersegmentation (Herbert, 1975), as do any neutrophils with six or more lobes. Thrombocytopenia is usually encountered and on rare occasions is sufficiently severe to be responsible for bleeding. It is worth noting that significant morphologic changes may occur in the blood in the absence of anemia and also that neurologic symptoms may be present in the absence of anemia.

Marrow (Plate 28–1*E* to *H;* Plate 29–1*B* and *H*). Megaloblastic anemia is characterized by enlargement of all rapidly proliferating cells of the body, including marrow cells. The major abnormality is the diminished capacity for DNA synthesis. The cells have both a prolonged intermitotic resting phase and a block early in mitosis. The number of mitotic figures is increased. RNA synthesis is less impeded than is DNA synthesis; hence, cytoplasmic maturation and growth continue, accounting for enlargement of the

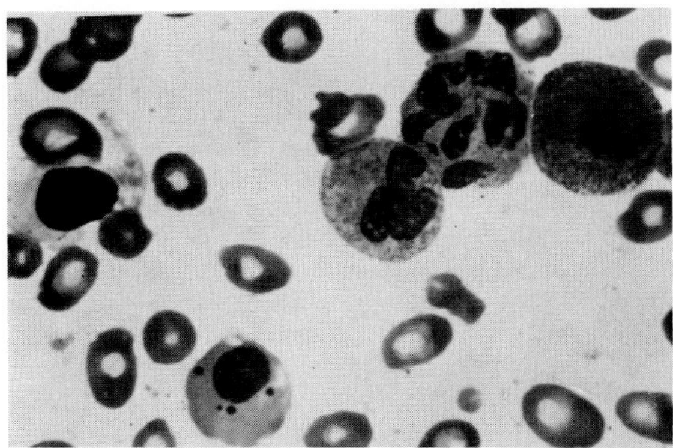

Figure 29–2. Megaloblastic anemia. Below, orthochromatic megaloblast with four Howell-Jolly bodies. Above, right, two giant neutrophils (one of which has nine nuclear lobes and could be called a macropolycyte) and an eosinophil with poor nuclear maturation (×875.)

4

cells. The delicate chromatin and the prominent parachromatin result in a distinctly more "open" chromatin pattern than is seen in the normoblastic series. The nuclei undergo karyorrhexis readily, and multiple Howell-Jolly bodies may be present. There are usually more cells analogous to the pronormoblast and basophilic normoblast (i.e., the promegaloblast and basophilic megaloblast) than are seen in normal erythropoiesis. This has sometimes been termed "maturation arrest," or nuclear-cytoplasmic asynchrony. Giant polychromatic megaloblasts are especially distinctive. The same general features are seen in the other cell lines. In the granulocytic series, the cells are larger, with retarded nuclear maturation and large cytoplasmic mass; often the specific granules themselves are distinctly larger. The chromatin pattern is less condensed (more "open"), and as a result the nucleus appears to stain poorly. Abnormally contorted nuclear configurations are common. The giant metamyelocyte is the most characteristic of the abnormal granulocytes. Megakaryocytes, too, are large and have separated nuclear lobes or nuclear fragments.

The bone marrow is hyperplastic. The fat is replaced, and red marrow extends into the long bones. The number of erythroid precursors (megaloblasts) is increased, and the myeloid-erythroid ratio is decreased. If the megaloblastic process is incompletely developed, or if the patient has been inadequately treated, the findings may be only partial. Since they persist longer, the granulocytic alterations are especially helpful in assessing recently treated megaloblastic anemia. The marrow findings are due to the effects of impaired nucleic acid synthesis giving rise to megaloblastosis, and to hypoxic stress giving rise to increased numbers of erythroid cells. If the patient is transfused with packed red cells, the number of erythroid precursors diminishes but the cytologic abnormalities persist.

Erythrokinetics. In megaloblastic anemias, the mass of erythroid tissue is increased, plasma iron turnover is rapid, and urine and fecal urobilinogen are increased. These measures indicate an *increase of total erythropoiesis* of up to three times normal. Decreased rate of appearance of iron in the Hb of circulating erythrocytes and reticulocytopenia indicate *decreased effective erythropoiesis*. These findings imply a great deal of *ineffective erythropoiesis*. In addition to increased destruction of the defective erythroid precursors in the marrow, survival of circulating erythrocytes is short, indicating hemolysis. Indirect serum bilirubin is increased, serum iron is increased, endogenous carbon monoxide production is increased, and serum lactate dehydrogenase is usually greatly elevated. Serum muramidase may be elevated, and implies ineffective granulocytopoiesis.

Megaloblastic anemia is nearly always due to vitamin B_{12} or folic acid deficiency. The findings described are similar for either.

VITAMIN B_{12} METABOLISM

Vitamin B_{12} (cyanocobalamin) has a molecular weight of 1355. The molecule's two major parts are (1) a "planar group" (the corrin nucleus), a ring structure surrounding a cobalt atom, and (2) a "nucleotide" group, which consists of the base, 5,6-dimethylbenzimidazole, and a phosphorylated ribose esterified with 1-amino, 2-propanol. A cyanide group is in coordinate linkage with the trivalent cobalt. Different forms of vitamin B_{12} result from replacement of the cyanide by hydroxy, aquo, or nitro groups.

Vitamin B_{12} is the only vitamin exclusively synthesized by micororganisms. It is found in practically all animal tissues. It is stored primarily in the liver. The human liver contains approximately 1 μg per gram of liver. Vitamin B_{12}, in its coenzyme form, is released by digestion of proteins of animal origin and then is bound by gastric intrinsic factor (IF), a glycoprotein produced in the parietal cells of the stomach. This vitamin B_{12}–IF complex then adheres to specific receptor sites on the epithelial cells of the ileum, at which site the vitamin B_{12} is absorbed. Several hours are required for absorption.

Once absorbed, vitamin B_{12} is transported in the plasma bound to a group of proteins, called transcobalamin I (TC I), transcobalamin II (TC II), and transcobalamin III (TC III). Ninety per cent of newly absorbed vitamin B_{12} is bound to TC II, which serves as the chief transport protein, rapidly delivering the vitamin to the liver, hematopoietic cells, and other dividing cells. Some vitamin B_{12} attaches to TC I; this appears to be a passive reservoir which is in equilibrium with body stores in the liver. The reference interval for plasma vitamin B_{12}, which varies with different methods of assay, commonly is 200 to 900 mg/L (150 to 670 pmol/L). One third of the vitamin B_{12} binding sites on transcobalamins are normally occupied. TC I is 70 to 90 per cent saturated and binds most of the plasma vitamin B_{12}; this is very slowly cleared from the plasma. TC II is only about 5 per cent saturated; much of newly absorbed vitamin B_{12} bound to TC II is removed from the plasma during the first few hours, but a small fraction remains bound for several weeks (Hall, 1975).

The relative importance of the transcobalamins is illustrated by the effects of congenital deficiency (Hoffbrand, 1981). Lack of TC II results in severe megaloblastic anemia in infancy; yet the serum vitamin B_{12} level is normal. Lack of TC I is not accompanied by anemia or megaloblastosis; yet the serum vitamin B_{12} level is decreased.

TC I and III are R-type proteins, appear to differ only in their carbohydrate proportions, and have been called cobalophilin (Stenman, 1976). Much of the serum TC III is released from granulocytes during blood clotting *in vitro;* TC III does not appear to bind significant amounts of plasma B_{12} under normal conditions. TC I may arise from granulocytes as well as other tissues. Elevation of TC I and III accounts for the elevation of total vitamin B_{12} binding proteins in myeloproliferative diseases. TC II is probably produced in liver, macrophages, and ileum (Hoffbrand, 1981).

The daily requirement of vitamin B_{12} is in the range of 2 to 5 μg per day. The body's stores of 2 to 5 mg will last for several years if intake is cut off, as is the case if total gastrectomy is performed (Beck, 1981).

VITAMIN B_{12} DEFICIENCY

Vitamin B_{12} deficiency is produced by any of several mechanisms.

Inadequate Intake. A dietary deficiency is an *extremely rare* cause of megaloblastic anemia in the United States, and is seen only in persons who completely abstain from animal food, including milk and eggs. For example, strict vegetarians are known to develop this form of vitamin B_{12} deficiency.

Defective Production of Intrinsic Factor. This is the most common cause of vitamin B_{12} deficiency.

Pernicious Anemia (PA). Pernicious anemia is a "conditioned" nutritional deficiency of vitamin B_{12} which is caused by a failure of the gastric mucosa to secrete intrinsic factor. This abnormality is genetically determined but usually is not manifested until late in life; less than 10 per cent of cases occur under age 40.

Clinical Features. The disorder is equally common in males and females. Symptoms of anemia and the combination of skin pallor and jaundice giving a lemon-yellow appearance of the skin are often present. The tongue may be sore, smooth, and pale (atrophic glossitis) or red and raw (acute glossitis). *Gastrointestinal symptoms* may be prominent and include episodic abdominal pain, constipation, and diarrhea. Diffuse and irregular degeneration of the white matter of the *central nervous system* characteristically involves the posterior and lateral columns of the spinal cord (subacute combined degeneration) and sometimes other sites. Symmetrical sensations of "pins and needles" of the distal extremities, numbness and tingling, loss of position sensation (difficulty with balance and gait), and loss of vibratory sensation (perhaps the most constant sign) are indicative of posterior column lesions. Lateral column involvement gives rise to weakness, spasticity, and increased deep tendon reflexes. Sometimes, in advanced cases, the brain may be affected, and the patient shows irritability, emotional instability, or a change in personality, and the term "megaloblastic madness" has been applied.

Gastric Findings. Atrophic gastritis of varying degree is found in most adults with PA, and gastric atrophy involving all coats of the wall in the remainder; they are probably stages of the same process. Intrinsic factor (IF) and HCl are secreted by gastric parietal cells in the human; in adult PA, IF secretion is absent and almost always there is histamine-refractory achylia and achlorhydria—a decreased volume of gastric juice and lack of HCl secretion.

Immune Abnormalities (Hoffbrand, 1981). Two types of autoantibodies have been found in the serum of patients with pernicious anemia. One reacts with gastric parietal cells and is present in 85 to 90 per cent of patients who have been tested. This parietal cell antibody is also present in patients with chronic gastritis, such as that associated with iron deficiency, and in some patients with thyroiditis and myxedema; it may be present in healthy controls, especially in older age groups. This is a non-specific finding that probably indicates the presence of gastritis. The other autoantibodies are directed against intrinsic factor. About 55 per cent of patients with pernicious anemia have in their serum anti-intrinsic factor antibodies of the "blocking" type (which block the binding of intrinsic factor to B_{12}), and 35 per cent have in addition the "binding" type (which inhibit the binding of intrinsic factor to the ileal mucosa). Neither antibody can be found in 45 per cent of patients. Intrinsic factor antibodies in the absence of PA have not been found, except in hyperthyroidism (Graves' disease), where the incidence is 3 to 6 per cent, and in a similar percentage of insulin-dependent diabetics. There appears to be an immunologic relationship of some kind between stomach and thyroid.

Family studies in patients with pernicious anemia have shown an increased incidence of the disease in relatives, and many relatives have achlorhydria and partial defects of vitamin B_{12} absorption. Relatives of patients with pernicious anemia also have a higher incidence of gastric parietal cell antibodies and of thyroid antibodies than normal.

It is possible that adult pernicious anemia is a genetically determined autoimmune gastritis. However, the relationship of the gastric lesion to the antibodies remains unclear.

PA in Children. PA is rare in children, but two forms exist. The more common type occurs usually in the first few years of life. IF secretion is lacking, but acid secretion and the appearance of the gastric mucosa are normal. Antibodies to parietal cells and to IF are absent. The other type of PA occurs usually in older children and is like that of adults, with gastric atrophy, achlorhydria, and serum antibody to IF; antibody to parietal cells, however, is usually absent (Hoffbrand, 1981).

Gastrectomy. Surgical removal of the stomach (total or even subtotal occasionally) will remove the source of intrinsic factor. This will lead to megaloblastic anemia after the body's stores of vitamin B_{12} have been exhausted, in three to six years, if vitamin B_{12} therapy has not been given. Frequently, the anemia is in part due to iron deficiency.

Defective Absorption of Vitamin B_{12}

Malabsorption Syndromes. Celiac disease, tropical sprue, resection of small bowel, or inflammatory disease of the small bowel may be associated with multiple defects of absorption, including other vitamins. Folic acid deficiency (absorbed principally in the upper small bowel) is more commonly seen than vitamin B_{12} deficiency (absorbed principally in the lower small bowel) in diseases leading to malabsorption. The reason for this is probably the lesser time necessary for depletion of body stores of folic acid.

Cases have been reported in which there is specific intestinal failure of absorption of vitamin B_{12} in the presence of normal intrinsic factor, the Immerslund-Gräsbeck syndrome (Cooper, 1976).

Lack of Availability of Vitamin B_{12}. In certain countries infestation with the fish tapeworm *(Diphyllobothrium latum)* is common enough that vitamin B_{12} deficiency may occur occasionally when it is present.

The worm successfully competes with the host for the ingested vitamin B_{12}. Most common in Finland, it is rarely seen in the United States.

Bacteria in a blind-loop of intestine may also preferentially utilize ingested vitamin B_{12} to the detriment of the host.

Diagnosis of Vitamin B_{12} Deficiency. Recognition of megaloblastic anemia indicates the likelihood of vitamin B_{12} deficiency or folic acid deficiency. In addition, evidence of neurologic involvement favors vitamin B_{12} deficiency. This diagnosis can be established by one of four methods.

Therapeutic Trial. With the patient on a diet low in vitamin B_{12} and folate, a parenteral physiologic dose of vitamin B_{12} (1 μ per day) is given. Optimal hematologic response indicates deficiency, and consists of reticulocytosis beginning on the third or fourth day and reaching a peak on the seventh day. Erythropoiesis becomes normoblastic by two days, and leukopoiesis becomes normal by 12 to 14 days (Hoffbrand, 1981). Within a week, leukocyte and platelet counts have returned, and the hemoglobin concentration begins to rise.

Serum Vitamin B_{12} Assay. This is the usual method of detecting a vitamin B_{12} deficient state. Microbiological assay of serum vitamin B_{12} employs an organism (e.g., *Euglena gracilis*) which requires vitamin B_{12} for growth. Radioisotopic dilution assays are more rapid and widely used and give results comparable to the *Euglena* assay, provided that the binding protein is specific for biologically active vitamin B_{12}; a standardized intrinsic factor preparation is most satisfactory. Mollin (1976) discusses the vitamin B_{12} radioassays.

Reference values are 200 to 900 ng/L. In megaloblastic anemia due to vitamin B_{12} deficiency, serum vitamin B_{12} is usually less than 100 ng/L. Individuals with folate deficiency and mild vitamin B_{12} deficiency and who are pregnant have borderline values between 100 and 200 ng/L.

Urinary Methylmalonic Acid. Since a vitamin B_{12} coenzyme is essential for the isomerization of methylmalonate to succinate, excretion of increased amounts of methymalonate is found in vitamin B_{12} deficiency. Provided that the rare inborn error of metabolism methylmalonic aciduria is not present, this is a sensitive test for vitamin B_{12} deficiency, but it is not usually necessary for the diagnosis.

Deoxyuridine Suppression Test. This measures the ability of marrow cells *in vitro* to utilize deoxyuridine in DNA synthesis. Normally, in marrow cells the major source of thymidine for DNA is by *de novo* synthesis from deoxyuridine which requires intact vitamin B_{12} and folate enzymes; therefore, less than 10 per cent of added tritium-labeled thymidine (^{3}H-Tdr) is incorporated into DNA. In megaloblastic marrows due to vitamin B_{12} or folate deficiency, deoxyuridine cannot be efficiently converted to thymidine, and more ^{3}H-Tdr is taken up into DNA. An abnormal deoxyuridine suppression test indicates either vitamin B_{12} or folate deficiency (Chanarin, 1976).

Detecting the Cause of Vitamin B_{12} Deficiency. Clinical history is useful in suggesting whether vitamin B_{12} or folate deficiency is the cause of megaloblastic anemia. Clinical associations of pernicious anemia include a family history of PA in one third of patients, certain endocrine deficiencies (thyroid disease, diabetes mellitus, hypothyroidism, Addison's disease), and certain immune disorders (immune thrombocytopenic purpura, autoimmune hemolytic anemia, and acquired hypogammaglobulinemia). Vitamin B_{12} deficiency is likely in strict vegetarians, and in patients with paresthesias, neuropathy, or a previous gastrectomy (Chanarin, 1976).

Achlorhydria, or absence of gastric acid, is characteristic of adult PA. The volume and pH of gastric juice are measured before and at 15 minute intervals after stimulation by injection of histamine or betazole hydrochloride (Histalog). In PA, the pH is above 3.5 and falls less than 1.0 unit after stimulation. In addition, the basal volume of gastric secretion is low, and fails to increase after stimulation. The presence of HCl virtually excludes the diagnosis of adult PA, but achlorhydria does not establish the diagnosis (Maslow, 1980; Chanarin, 1979).

To demonstrate whether the patient lacks intrinsic factor, absorption of an oral dose of radioactive vitamin B_{12} usually is determined. This can be done in several ways—measuring fecal excretion, hepatic uptake, urinary excretion, plasma uptake, or even whole body counting. Most convenient is the Schilling test, the measurement of radioactivity in a 24-hour sample of urine. Two hours after oral administration of 0.5 to 2.0 μg of radioactive vitamin B_{12}, a large "flushing" dose of non-labeled vitamin B_{12} is given parenterally. Normal individuals will excrete over 7 per cent of a 1 μg dose of ingested vitamin B_{12} in the urine in 24 hours, whereas patients lacking intrinsic factor excrete less. If the excretion is low, the test must be repeated using the same procedure except that hog intrinsic factor is given orally along with the labeled vitamin B_{12}. If the 24-hour excretion is normal, the low value in the first part was due to intrinsic factor deficiency. If the excretion remains abnormal in the second part of the procedure, an explanation for malabsorption of vitamin B_{12} on the basis of intestinal disease must be sought. The validity of the results depends upon good renal function and an accurate urine collection. The Schilling test will be abnormal in PA even after the patient is treated with vitamin B_{12} and is in remission.

Other tests that will establish the diagnosis of PA are direct assay of intrinsic factor demonstrating it to be deficient in gastric juice, and demonstrating the presence of anti-IF blocking antibodies in the serum of a vitamin B_{12} deficient patient (Chanarin, 1979; Hoffbrand, 1981).

FOLIC ACID METABOLISM (Beck, 1981)

Folic acid or pteroyl monoglutamic acid contains three parts: pteridine, para-aminobenzoate, and L-glutamic acid. In nature, folic acid occurs mainly as less soluble polyglutamates, with multiple glutamic acid residues attached to one another. Folic acid is present in a wide variety of foods, such as eggs, milk, leafy vegetables, yeast, liver, and fruits, and also is formed by intestinal bacteria.

Conjugase enzymes in bile and intestine hydrolyze the folylpolyglutamates prior to absorption, which is rapid and occurs in the proximal jejunum. Folate is rapidly removed from plasma to cells and tissues for utilization. The principal form of folate in serum, erythrocytes, and liver is 5-methyl tetrahydrofolate (5-methyl-FH_4); the liver is the chief storage site. The minimal daily requirement is about 50 μg of pteroyl monoglutamate or 400 μg of total folate; the reference interval for serum folate is 5 to 21 μg/L (11 to 48 nmol/L) and for red cell folate 150 to 600 μg/L (340 to 1360 nmol/L) of red blood cells.

FOLIC ACID DEFICIENCY (Hoffbrand, 1981)

Inadequate Intake of Folate

Evolution of Laboratory Abnormalities. Experimental dietary folic acid deficiency in normal man (Herbert, 1962) has elucidated the sequence of events in the onset of folate-deficient megaloblastic anemia. After a folate-deficient diet was initiated, the various abnormalities were established as follows: 3 weeks, low serum folate; 11 weeks, hypersegmentation of neutrophils; 13 weeks, high excretion of formiminoglutamic acid (FIGLU) in urine; 17 weeks, low erythrocyte folate; 18 weeks, macro-ovalocytosis of erythrocytes; 19 weeks, megaloblastic bone marrow; 19 to 20 weeks, anemia.

At this time, changes in the intestinal epithelium had not yet appeared. Therefore, in man, with no dietary intake of folic acid, anemia will appear in three to six months. The peripheral blood and bone marrow features of megaloblastic anemia due to folic acid deficiency are similar to those of vitamin B_{12} deficiency; however, leukopenia and thromboycytopenia are less constant. Folic acid deficiency has usually been found in association with some complicating factor.

Nutritional Folate Deficiency. Megaloblastic anemia due to lack of folate is most commonly associated with insufficient dietary intake. The usual diet does not contain much above the minimal requirements, and body stores in the adult are sufficient for only about three months' needs. Dietary folate deficiency is especially common in the tropics and in India, and even there it is usually associated with increased demand for folate in pregnancy, rapid growth in infancy, infection, or hemolytic anemia.

Folate deficiency in infancy is uncommon in the United States. Human milk or fresh cow's milk contains sufficient folate, but heated milk, powdered milk, and goat's milk do not. If the infant's milk lacks folate, if the diet is low in ascorbic acid, or if infections or diarrhea are a problem, then megaloblastic anemia may occur (Mauer, 1969).

Megaloblastic anemia in pregnancy is not uncommon, because of the fetal requirements for folate. The mother's plasma folate level gradually falls during pregnancy, and at birth the plasma level in the newborn averages five times that of the mother. Megaloblastic anemia is more frequent in multiparae, may be precipitated by infection, and is usually due to folate deficiency rather than B_{12} deficiency. Pregnant women should receive, in addition to iron, folic acid supplements of about 500 μg per day (WHO Report, 1972).

Elderly persons on inadequate diets in this country may develop folate-deficient megaloblastic anemia, a fact increasingly recognized in recent years.

Liver Disease. Liver disease associated with alcoholism may lead to folate-deficient megaloblastic anemia because of the grossly inadequate diet of the alcoholic. With an adequate dietary folic acid intake, however, the anemia that is found with liver disease is macrocytic and normoblastic, not megaloblastic.

Defective Absorption of Folate. Defective absorption of folic acid occurs in association with malabsorption syndromes discussed above and in the blind-loop syndrome, in which bacteria preferentially utilize folate.

Non-tropical sprue, or adult celiac disease, is an important cause of malabsorption in adults or children that is related to dietary gluten (wheat protein). Included among the signs of malabsorption may be megaloblastic anemia due to folic acid deficiency (Beck, 1981). Jejunal biopsy shows villous atrophy. The folate deficiency as well as the malabsorption responds to a gluten-free diet. Folic acid therapy (parenteral) corrects the folate deficiency but not the general malabsorption.

Tropical sprue is common in the Caribbean, India, and Southeast Asia, and is generally similar to non-tropical sprue. It may in part be due to folate deficiency, but bacterial contamination of the small intestine also appears to play a causative role (Sleisenger, 1982). Evidence of malabsorption includes megaloblastic anemia due to folate deficiency. Treatment with folic acid brings considerable improvement in the general malabsorption as well as the anemia, but antimicrobial treatment is recommended in addition.

Megaloblastic anemia or decreased serum and red cell folate without anemia has been associated with the long-term use of anticoagulant drugs, phenytoin, phenobarbital, and primidone. There is considerable evidence that absorption of folate is impaired in the presence of the drug, but the mechanism is not completely understood. Oral contraceptives may adversely affect folate metabolism in a small proportion of women, probably those who have an underlying defect in absorption, utilization, or storage (Stebbins, 1976).

Increased Requirements for Folate. The increased need in pregnancy and in infants (multiple birth) has been mentioned. Increased cell turnover that occurs in neoplasia and in the markedly stimulated hematopoiesis of hemolytic anemias may result in megaloblastic erythropoiesis. The basis for this is increased need for a marginal supply of folate.

Inadequate Utilization of Folate. Inadequate utilization of folic acid is relatively rare.

Folic acid antagonists, such as methotrexate, block folic acid metabolism and because of this are used in therapy of some malignant neoplasms. In addition to inhibiting the growth of the tumor, they will also induce megaloblastic hematopoiesis.

In addition to the previously mentioned nutritional

problem in alcoholics, *alcohol* may exert a direct effect in suppressing hematopoiesis by blocking metabolism of folate.

Diagnosis of Folate Deficiency

Folic acid deficiency or vitamin B_{12} deficiency is suspected when the blood and bone marrow show findings characteristic of megaloblastic anemia; usually serum folate and B_{12} levels are then determined.

Serum and Red Cell Folate. A microbiologic assay for folic acid activity employing *Lactobacillus casei* remains the most reliable method for the definitive diagnosis (Beck, 1981). Radioisotopic methods employing different folate binders are widely used because of rapidity and greater convenience. Although the correlation with the microbiologic assay is generally good, discrepancies seem to be frequent and, on the basis of other data, tend to be resolved in favor of the microbiologic assay (Rudzki, 1976).

The serum folate is decreased (<3 μg/L) in megaloblastic anemia due to folate deficiency but is usually normal in vitamin B_{12} deficiency. A low serum folate level precedes decrease of red cell or tissue folate; it indicates a negative folate balance but does not by itself indicate tissue folate deficiency. In vitamin B_{12} deficiency, serum folate is decreased in 10 per cent of cases, increased in 20 per cent, and normal in the remainder (Tietz, 1983).

The red cell folate is a better test of body folate stores and is decreased in megaloblastic anemia due to folate deficiency. In vitamin B_{12} deficiency, however, red cell folate is low in almost two thirds of cases, so this needs to be excluded before regarding a low red cell folate as proof of severe folate deficiency (Hoffbrand, 1981).

Urinary Formiminoglutamic Acid (FIGLU). Folic acid coenzymes are required for the conversion of FIGLU to glutamic acid in the catabolism of histidine. When oral histidine is given, FIGLU will appear in increased amounts in the urine if folate deficiency is present. However, its value in discriminating between vitamin B_{12} and folate deficiency is lessened by the fact that nearly two thirds of patients with vitamin B_{12} deficiency have increased FIGLU excretion.

Therapeutic Trial. The therapeutic trial remains an excellent way to discriminate between folic acid and vitamin B_{12} deficiency. Physiologic doses of folic acid (parenteral, 50 to 200 μg/day) will allow an adequate reticulocyte response in patients with folic acid deficiency, but not in vitamin B_{12} deficiency.

On the other hand, the usual therapeutic doses of folic acid (5 to 15 mg/day) or larger doses of vitamin B_{12} (500 to 1000 μg) may induce a partial response in a patient with megaloblastic anemia due to the other deficiency.

Deoxyuridine Suppression Test. See p. 660.

THERAPY OF MEGALOBLASTIC ANEMIA

Although it may be necessary to treat severely anemic patients with both vitamins, it is usually possible to determine which is the cause and treat only with it.

The maximal reticulocyte response occurs in five to seven days. Within four to six hours after the initial therapy (if parenteral), the marrow shows decreased early megaloblasts and the appearance of pronormoblasts. Within two to four days the marrow is predominantly normoblastic. Granulocytic abnormalities return to normal more slowly, and hypersegmented neutrophils disappear from the blood only after 12 to 14 days.

PA is treated parenterally on a regular monthly to three-monthly basis with 1000 μg of hydroxycobalamin. Oral vitamin B_{12} therapy can be used only in patients with nutritional deficiency.

In folate deficiency, oral therapy is generally used at a dosage of 5 to 15 mg per day. Vitamin B_{12} deficiency must be excluded, and corrected if present, to avoid the occurrence of vitamin B_{12} neuropathy.

OTHER DEFECTS OF NUCLEOPROTEIN SYNTHESIS

Other defects of nucleoprotein synthesis may lead to megaloblastic anemias which do not respond to vitamin B_{12} or folic acid.

Congenital Defects. Oroticaciduria is a very rare autosomal recessive condition in which certain enzymes required for pyrimidine synthesis are absent. The findings are excessive urinary excretion of orotic acid, failure of normal growth and development, and megaloblastic anemia which is refractory to vitamin B_{12} and folate but which responds to uridine.

Inborn defects in enzymes involved in folate metabolism have also been described.

Synthetic Inhibitors. Synthetic inhibitors of purine synthesis (6-mercaptopurine, thioguanine, azathioprine), of pyrimidine synthesis (5- fluorouracil), or of deoxyribonucleotide synthesis (cytosine arabinoside or hydroxyurea) are used in chemotherapy for neoplasia and may concomitantly produce megaloblastosis.

Refractory Anemias. Anemias that are megaloblastic and that fail to respond to vitamin B_{12} or folic acid are considered with the refractory anemias (p. 668). Usually the megaloblastic changes are not typical and do not include the characteristic granulocytic changes.

Impaired Production—Other

ANEMIA OF CHRONIC DISORDERS

The anemia most commonly seen in chronic infections, rheumatoid arthritis, and neoplastic disease is usually mild and is overshadowed by the basic disease. Usually, the anemia does not progress in severity and has characteristic morphologic, biochemical, and kinetic disturbances (Cartwright, 1966, 1971).

The erythrocytes are usually normocytic and normochromic, but they are often normocytic and hypochromic and occasionally microcytic and hypochromic. Anisocytosis and poikilocytosis are slight. The reticulocyte count is usually not elevated. Leukocytes and platelets are not distinctively altered, except by the causative disease.

The marrow is normocellular or minimally hypocellular or hypercellular, and the cell distribution is not greatly disturbed. The normoblasts may have frayed hypochromic cytoplasm and the appearance of hemoglobin in the cells may be delayed (as in iron deficiency anemia). Sideroblasts are decreased, but storage iron is normal or increased.

The serum iron is characteristically decreased, the total iron-binding capacity (TIBC) is decreased or normal (in contrast to iron deficiency anemia, in which the TIBC is elevated), and the per cent saturation is decreased. Erythrocyte protoporphyrin and serum ferritin are elevated.

Red cell production, though normal or even slightly increased, is insufficient to compensate for a moderately decreased red cell survival. In these patients, the marrow is capable of responding to erythropoietin; but for unknown reasons, erythropoietin production is inappropriately low. Erythropoietin can be produced in response to other types of stimulation, for example, cobalt.

The defect in iron metabolism is principally a block in the movement of iron from the storage sites in the reticuloendothelial cells to the erythroid marrow; this results in the low serum iron and in an iron-deficient type of erythropoiesis, despite the presence of adequate storage iron. The anemia usually fails to respond to therapy with iron or other measures; spontaneous improvement will occur when the underlying disorder is corrected.

ANEMIA OF RENAL INSUFFICIENCY

The correlation between the severity of the anemia and the degree of elevation of the blood urea nitrogen is positive but not strictly linear. When the blood urea nitrogen (BUN) exceeds 100 mg/dl (36 nmol/L), the hematocrit is usually below 0.30 (Erslev, 1977a).

Several factors are often involved in the anemia of chronic renal failure. Decreased production of erythropoietin by the damaged kidney is probably the important factor in most cases in which the blood urea nitrogen exceeds 100 mg/dl. Both ineffective erythropoiesis and impaired ability of the marrow to respond to erythropoietin appear to be present in some degree.

Hemolysis is a significant feature in many cases of chronic renal failure. There appears to be an extracorpuscular factor in uremic plasma which has a detrimental effect on red cell metabolism and results in morphologically deformed cells (echinocytes and spiculated red cells). Numerous irregularly contracted and fragmented cells are seen in the hemolytic-uremic syndrome and in malignant hypertension as a result of traumatic damage incurred by the red cells in traversing the damaged small blood vessels (Brain, 1962).

In addition, bleeding is a common problem in chronic renal disease, probably due either to thrombocytopenia, in some patients, or to platelet functional defects, which are present in most patients. Anemia due to iron deficiency from blood loss should always be suspected. Folic acid deficiency may be a problem in patients in a dialysis program, since folic acid is readily moved into the dialysis bath.

ANEMIA IN LIVER DISEASE

Chronic posthemorrhagic anemia, folate-deficient megaloblastic anemia due to poor nutrition in alcoholic cirrhosis, and acquired hemolytic anemias associated with either Coombs-positive red cells, congestive splenomegaly, or lipid disturbances may occur in liver disease.

In addition to these, there is an anemia associated with liver disease which is characterized by shortened red cell survival and relatively inadequate red cell production. It is exaggerated by an increased blood volume which appears to correlate with the degree of portal hypertension (Wintrobe, 1981). The red cells are normocytic or macrocytic (thin macrocytes). Frequently target cells are present, especially in obstructive jaundice (see Fig. 27–28); these have increased surface membrane with increased cholesterol and lecithin content. Their survival is decreased if there is splenomegaly due to cirrhosis (Cooper, 1977a). Reticulocytes may be slightly increased, and platelets may be normal or decreased. The bone marrow may be slightly hypercellular and erythropoiesis is macronormoblastic rather than megaloblastic. Changes in leukocytes, such as are present in megaloblastic anemias, are not seen, and this type of anemia does not respond to vitamin B_{12} or folic acid. The anemia is of unknown origin.

A small proportion of patients with severe cirrhosis have a hemolytic anemia associated with "spur cells," which are red cells with thorny projections similar to acanthocytes. As with target cells, the spur cells are secondary to lipid abnormalities in the plasma; they have increased surface membrane with increased cholesterol but normal phospholipid content in the membrane. These irregular cells have decreased deformability and tend to be trapped in the spleen and destroyed (Cooper, 1977b).

4

ANEMIA IN ENDOCRINE DISEASE

Uncomplicated anemia in hypothyroidism is mild to moderate; it is normochromic and normocytic without reticulocytosis and with normal red cell survival. It reflects a decreased marrow production due to a smaller tissue oxygen requirement. Since plasma volume is decreased in hypothyroidism, the apparent degree of anemia may not be proportional to the decrease in red cell mass. Hypothyroidism may, of course, be complicated by iron deficiency or folic acid or vitamin B_{12} deficiency. The pathogenesis of a similar anemia in adrenal cortical hormone deficiency is less clear; it is corrected by hormone replacement.

Deficient testosterone secretion in the man results in a decrease in red cell production of 1 to 2 g Hb/dl (to a value comparable to that of the woman); this appears to be due to the effect of androgens on erythropoietin secretion.

Pituitary deficiency tends to result in a greater depression of hemoglobin concentration because of the effect on multiple endocrine glands and possibly the loss of growth hormone effect (Erslev, 1977b).

ANEMIA ASSOCIATED WITH BONE MARROW INFILTRATION (MYELOPHTHISIC ANEMIA)

This anemia is associated with marrow replacement by (or involvement with) metastatic carcinoma, multiple myeloma, leukemia, lymphoma, lipidoses or storage disease, and certain other conditions.

The characteristic finding in the blood is the presence of varying number of normoblasts and immature neutrophils; these are responsible for the descriptive terms *leukoerythroblastotic reaction, leukoerythroblastic anemia,* and *leukoerythroblastosis* (see Table 27–3, p. 611).

Normochromic and normocytic (occasionally macrocytic) anemia of varying severity is present. Reticulocytes are often increased, and the number of normoblasts is usually out of proportion to the severity of the anemia. The leukocyte count is normal or reduced (occassionally elevated), and immature neutrophils and even myeloblasts may be found. Platelets are normal or decreased, and bizarre, atypical platelets can sometimes be seen.

Examination of the marrow will usually reveal the condition responsible for this reaction. Mechanical crowding out of the hematopoietic tissue by the pathologic process has been assumed but not proved and probably is not the usual cause. Often the amount of erythropoietic tissue in the marrow as determined by morphologic and kinetic studies is normal or increased. The mechanism described in the section on anemia of chronic disorders (p. 662) may often play a role, but the reason for the outpouring of immature cells into the blood is not clear.

In addition to myelophthisic anemias, circulating normoblasts and immature neutrophils can also be seen in hemolytic anemias, severe anemias due to other causes, severe infections, and congestive heart failure, but usually the normoblasts are not so numerous.

The *leukoerythroblastotic reaction* associated with myelophthisic anemias cannot always be distinguished from the blood picture of myelosclerosis with myeloid metaplasia (MMM), which is one of the myeloproliferative disorders. In MMM, enlargement of the spleen and liver is almost always found. In the blood film, more severe red cell abnormalities, leukocytosis, myeloblasts and immature granulocytes of all varieties (not just neutrophils), increased basophils, more atypical platelets, more numerous megakaryocyte fragments, and dwarf megakaryocytes are all findings more characteristic of MMM than of a leukoerythroblastotic reaction of some other cause. Examination of the bone marrow by a needle biopsy or surgical biopsy is necessary to differentiate MMM from other myelophthisic anemias.

APLASTIC ANEMIA

The term aplastic anemia usually refers to pancytopenia associated with a severe reduction in the amount of hematopoietic tissue which results in deficient production of blood cells. The marrow, though hypocellular, may have patchy areas of normocellularity or even hypercellularity. The diagnosis of severe aplastic anemia is made in pancytopenic patients when at least two of the following three peripheral blood values—granulocytes less than $0.5 \times 10^9/L$, platelets less than $20 \times 10^9/L$, or reticulocytes less than 1 per cent (corrected for hematocrit)—are present and the bone marrow is either markedly hypocellular or moderately hypocellular with less than 30 per cent of residual hematopoietic cells (Camitta, 1982).

Clinical Features. The clinical course may be acute and fulminating, with profound pancytopenia and a rapid progression to death, or the disorder may have an insidious onset and a chronic course. The symptoms and signs depend upon the degree of the deficiencies: bleeding from thrombocytopenia, infection from neutropenia, and signs and symptoms of anemia. As a rule, splenomegaly and lymphadenopathy are absent.

Etiology. Aplastic anemias are of diverse etiology. In approximately 50 per cent of the cases no specific etiologic agent can be correlated with the disease, and therefore these cases are considered idiopathic. Drug-related aplastic anemias occur in 33 per cent, chemicals and toxins in 4 per cent, and infections including infectious hepatitis in an additional 4 per cent of cases. The remaining 8 to 9 per cent of cases are due to miscellaneous causes (Alter, 1978).

Pathogenesis. Hematopoietic failure may occur at any level in the differentiation of bone marrow precursor cells. There may be insufficient or defective pluripotent stem cells (CFU-S) or committed stem cells (CFU-C). The microenvironment may be unable to provide for the normal development of hematopoietic cells. The appropriate humoral and cellular stimulators for hematopoiesis may be absent. In addition, bone marrow failure could result from excessive suppression of hematopoiesis by T lymphocytes or macrophages. Finally, stem cells could interact among themselves with one clone inhibiting the growth of another (Alter, 1978).

In most cases of aplastic anemia it is likely that damage to the hematopoietic stem cell by a known or unknown agent in some way alters the ability of the cell to proliferate or differentiate. The committed granulocyte-monocyte precursor cells (GM-CFC) are decreased in blood and marrow in most patients with aplastic anemia (Kern, 1977). In a small proportion of cases, it may be that the defect is in the hematopoietic microenvironment which fails to support stem-cell growth; this may be the case when bone marrow transplants repeatedly will not "take." Also, inhibition of stem cell growth may be mediated by blood or bone marrow lymphocytes in some cases of aplastic anemia (Good, 1977). In addition, immunologic mechanisms may suppress hematopoiesis, as is likely in pure red cell aplasias. Excellent reviews of the pathogenesis of aplastic anemias are provided by Young (1981) and Camitta (1982).

Prognosis. Complications are due to infection, bleeding, and problems of iron overload from repeated transfusions. The prognosis appears to depend upon the severity of marrow damage. In a series of 101 patients treated by conventional methods (Williams, 1978), 25 per cent of patients died within four months of the onset of symptoms, 50 per cent died within 12 months, and 71 per cent within five years. Those who died within four months had significantly lower reticulocyte, neutrophil, and platelet counts; a lower percentage of myeloid cells in the marrow; and a shorter interval between onset of symptoms and visit to the physician (Lynch, 1975). Other factors which correlated with a poor prognosis included male gender, but not age of the patient or etiology of the aplasia (Williams, 1978). In some survivors, partial recovery is common. A small proportion of survivors eventually have been found to develop leukemia or paroxysmal nocturnal hemoglobinuria.

Because of the high mortality rate, it may be important to identify early those who have a particularly grim prognosis for marrow transplantation.

Management. Treatment includes blood replacement, stimulation of any residual marrow (androgens, adrenal corticoids), combating infection (antibiotics, isolation), and controlling bleeding problems. Bone marrow transplantation, when a suitable donor is available, is successful in selected patients but as yet requires a vast array of support services and fails in a fair proportion of trials because of marrow graft rejection, graft-versus-host disease, or infections. However, for patients under 25 years of age with an HLA identical sibling donor, bone marrow transplantation may be the treatment of choice (Camitta, 1979).

Idiopathic Aplastic Anemia. In patients with pancytopenia and a hypocellular marrow, search should be made for evidence of significant exposure to radiation, drugs, and chemicals of known or possible propensity to injure the marrow, so that further exposure can be eliminated. Nevertheless, in approximately half the cases of aplastic anemia, no suspected causal relationship to toxic agents can be found, and it is these that are designated as idiopathic.

The symptoms and signs do not differ, but the onset is commonly more insidious than in toxic or hypersensitive aplastic anemias.

Blood. The red cells are usually normal in size and shape, though in some cases there may be varying degrees of anisocytosis and poikilocytosis or macrocytosis. Polychromasia, stippling, and normoblasts are most often conspicuously absent. Leukopenia with marked decrease in granulocytes and a relative lymphocytosis are observed. In severe leukopenia there is often also an absolute lymphocytopenia. Neutrophil granules may be larger than normal and may stain dark red (unlike the "toxic" granules found in infections), and the neutrophil alkaline phosphatase may be elevated. Thrombocytopenia is part of the picture. The serum iron is usually increased. The serum vitamin B_{12} and folate levels are usually normal. Although an occasional patient is hypogammaglobulinemic, most patients have normal levels of serum immunoglobulins.

Bone Marrow. In most cases the aspirate consists of red cells, lymphocytes, some plasma cells, and fatty particles. Marrow sections will show fatty tissue with inconspicuous fibrosis and islands of lymphocytes and plasma cells (Plate 29–1C). Though focal areas of normocellularity or hypercellularity may sometimes be present, the overall cellularity is decreased. Storage iron is increased.

Erythrokinetics. The increased serum iron is a valuable early sign of erythroid hypoplasia and reflects the decreased plasma iron turnover. In addition, the erythrocyte utilization of iron is decreased. Both effective and total erythropoiesis, therefore, are decreased in aplastic anemia.

Aplastic Anemia Associated with Chemical or Physical Agents

Toxic Aplastic Anemias. A number of physical and chemical agents produce marrow damage in all humans and animals exposed to a sufficient dose. Examples are ionizing radiation, mustard compounds, benzene, and antineoplastic agents such as busulfan, urethane, and antimetabolites.

Ionizing Radiation. The effects depend on the radiosensitivity of the cells and the capacity of the cells to regenerate, as well as the survival rate of the cells in the blood. Erythroid cells are most sensitive, granulocytes have intermediate sensitivity, and the megakaryocytes are the least sensitive of the three. Reticulum cells and connective tissue cells are relatively insensitive.

After acute exposure to radiation, the reticulocyte count falls, but the red cells decline slowly because of their long survival. Within the first few hours there is a neutrophilic leukocytosis due to a shift from marginal and probably marrow storage pools. A fall in lymphocytes occurs after the first day and is responsible for the early leukopenia. After five days or so, granulocytes begin to fall. The platelets decrease later. Platelets are often the last to return to normal in the recovery phase.

Hypersensitive Aplastic Anemias. A large number of drugs produce marrow damage in some individuals after single or repeated exposures. Effects are not dose related as they are in toxic aplasia. Agents include antimicrobial drugs (salvarsan, chloramphenicol, sulfonamides, chlortetracycline, streptomycin), anticonvulsants (mephenytoin, trimethadione), analgesics (phenylbutazone), antithyroid drugs (carbimazole), antihistaminics (tripelennamine), insecticides (DDT), and other chemicals—some known (gold compounds, quinacrine, chlorpromazine, hair dyes, bismuth, mercury) and others unknown.

Chloramphenicol is an important drug in this category. Reactions of the marrow to chloramphenicol are of two types which are possibly unrelated (Yunis, 1964).

In about half the patients who receive chloramphenicol, increased serum iron, reticulocytopenia with anemia, neutropenia, and thrombocytopenia are found. The marrow may show decreased erythroid cells and vacuolization of primitive erythroid and granulocyte precursors. These changes are dose related, time dependent, and reversible.

In a very small proportion of persons receiving chloramphenicol, an irreversible aplastic anemia develops which may be fatal. No relationship has been established between the reversible erythropoietic lesion and the development of aplastic anemia; it may be that individual susceptibility is responsible for the latter. For this reason it is essential that restraint be employed in using the drug, because monitoring its administration with blood cell counts is not an effective preventive measure (Wintrobe, 1981).

Aplastic Anemia Associated with Other Disease

Infection. Marrow aplasia has been described as an infrequent sequel to infectious hepatitis, occurring a few months after onset when the hepatitis is resolving. These patients are usually males and under age 20; the prognosis is usually grave (Hagler, 1975). Other viral infections can cause hematopoietic depression and rarely are followed by aplastic anemia.

Paroxysmal Nocturnal Hemoglobinuria (PNH). This rare hemolytic process (p. 672) may be followed by aplastic anemia. Usually in PNH a variable degree of marrow hypofunction coexists. Curiously, in some patients who present with aplastic anemia, the red cell defect of PNH may be present or may appear during the course of the disease. According to Lewis (1967), about 15 per cent of patients with aplastic anemia have a demonstrable PNH red cell defect, with or without clinical hemolysis.

Pregnancy. Pregnancy occurring in a patient with acquired aplastic anemia may make the pancytopenia more severe. Occasionally, however, aplastic anemia occurs during pregnancy and remits following delivery. In some such cases, aplasia recurs during a second pregnancy. The infants may be anemic, thrombocytopenic, or leukopenic (Fleming, 1973).

Thymoma. Although thymomas are usually associated with pure red cell aplasias, other bone marrow elements may also become depressed. Pancytopenia, often with hypoplastic bone marrow, occurs in 10 to 15 per cent of cases with thymoma. Thymectomy results in a good remission in one third of the patients. Most of the patients are women over 50 years of age (Hirst, 1967).

Constitutional Aplastic Anemia. The term constitutional aplastic anemia designates individuals with a congenital or genetic predisposition to bone marrow failure. In a study of 40 patients with constitutional aplastic anemia, 26 had Fanconi's anemia, 10 patients had familial aplastic anemia without classic signs of Fanconi's anemia, and 4 patients presented with a megakaryocytic thrombocytopenia which later developed into complete aplasia (Alter, 1978).

Fanconi's Anemia. In Fanconi's anemia, the pancytopenia becomes obvious after infancy and usually by the eighth year of life. Often more than one member of a family is affected. The anemia is usually normochromic and may be macrocytic; the marrow is generally hypocellular. Developmental anomalies are present and may include hyperpigmentation, short stature, hypogonadism, malformations of the extremities (e.g., aplasia of the radius and abnormalities of the thumbs), microcephaly, and malformation of other organs (e.g., heart and kidneys). Chromosomal defects consisting of random breaks and rearrangements characteristically are present in blood lymphocytes as well as marrow cells.

Familial Aplastic Anemia. In a subset of Fanconi's anemia, patients may have pancytopenia and a hypocellular marrow without major developmental anomalies. In some cases there may be skin hyperpigmentation, a narrow palpebral fissure, or stunted growth. Sometimes the patient with aplastic anemia may have a relative with classic Fanconi's anemia (O'Gorman Hughes, 1974).

However, aplastic anemia may occur in members of a family without the stigmata of Fanconi's syndrome. In this group males are more likely to be affected than females. The age at diagnosis varies from less than 1 year to 77 years.

A few children present with bleeding manifestations secondary to a megakaryocytic thrombocytopenia. As their disease progresses, they develop a pancytopenia and a hypocellular marrow. In some cases, the patients have the developmental abnormalities associated with Fanconi's anemia, whereas in other cases no anomalies are identified.

Pancytopenia and hypoplastic anemia may develop in a subset of patients with other familial disorders. Some patients with dyskeratosis congenita, Shwachman-Diamond syndrome, and amegakaryocytic thrombocytopenia have been reported to develop aplastic anemia (Alter, 1978).

Pure Red Cell Aplasia

Transitory Arrest of Erythropoiesis. This may occur during the course of a hemolytic anemia (often preceded by an infection), and the combination of aplasia and hemolysis becomes a threatening situation (Bauman, 1967). Red cell production may occasionally cease during or following rather minor infections in normal children or adults, at which time the marrow will show absence of all but a few of the most immature erythroid precursors. Since a temporary arrest in production in an individual with normal red cell survival does not cause a drop in hemoglobin sufficient to become symptomatic, it is quite possible that such events are considerably more common than we realize. If the arrest in erythropoiesis persists, anemia will result (Chanarin, 1964).

Congenital Red Cell Aplasia (Diamond-Blackfan Anemia; Congenital Hypoplastic Anemia). This is a rare, constitutional red cell aplasia which usually becomes obvious during the first year of life but may occur as late as six years of age. The severe anemia is normochromic and slightly macrocytic; reticulocyte level is low; leukocytes are normal or slightly decreased; platelets are normal or increased; and the marrow usually shows a reduction in all developing erythroid cells except pronormoblasts, but normal granulocytic and megakaryocytic cell lines. Fetal hemoglobin (Hb F) is elevated (5 to 25 per cent) to a degree not expected for the patient's age, and the antigen "i" (little i) is often present (Diamond, 1976). These findings contrast with those of transient arrest of erythropoiesis (transient erythroblastopenia of childhood). In the latter, the red cells are normocytic, the Hb F is normal, the antigen "i" is absent, and red cell enzymes are at a lower level (characteristic of an older cell population) (Wang, 1976).

The defect appears to be in the erythroid committed

progenitor cells. CFU-Es and BFU-Es are decreased in the marrow, and BFU-Es, which normally circulate, are absent or decreased in the blood (Nathan, 1981).

Most patients respond at least partially to corticosteroids, but only 25 per cent or so achieve long-term remissions without the drug (Diamond, 1976).

Acquired Pure Red Cell Aplasia. In middle-aged adults, selective failure of red cell production occurs rarely. Reticulocytopenia and a cellular marrow devoid of all but the most primitive erythroid precursors are characteristic. Leukocyte and platelet production are normal. About half of the reported cases have been associated with thymoma, usually a noninvasive spindle cell type. However, only 5 to 10 per cent of patients with thymoma have the anemia. Remission of the anemia occurs in about one fourth of the cases following surgical removal of the thymoma. Krantz (1974) has presented evidence for cytotoxic antibody against erythroid precursors and a plasma inhibitor of heme synthesis in the majority of patients he has studied; this kind of humoral activity has not been found in the Diamond-Blackfan anemia.

Sideroblastic Anemia. This is characterized by hypochromic, often microcytic, red cells in the blood usually mixed with normochromic cells so that the appearance is dimorphic (Fig. 27–22). The serum iron is increased, the TIBC is decreased, and the per cent saturation of the iron-binding protein is greatly elevated. The marrow shows markedly increased storage iron, erythroid hyperplasia with evidence of defective hemoglobinization, and increased numbers of sideroblasts. In addition, there are increased numbers of siderotic granules per cell, and granules surround the nucleus (at least two thirds of the circumference) forming "ring sideroblasts" (Fig. 29–3; Plate 29–1*E* and *F*). In the latter, iron loading of mitochondria is seen by electron microscopy. These findings are associated with defective synthesis of heme which may be due to any of several possible enzyme defects (Aoki, 1980). Occasionally, megaloblast-like changes are seen in the erythroid cells, but changes typical of vitamin B_{12} or folate deficiency are not seen in granulocytes unless folate deficiency coexists.

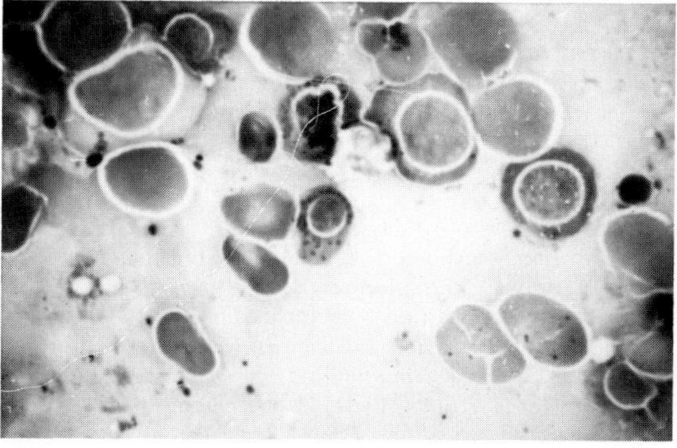

Figure 29–3. Nucleated red cells from the marrow of a patient with sideroblastic anemia. The Prussian blue reaction stains non-hemoglobin iron as blue granules (here shown as dark granules) in the cytoplasm. The perinuclear space is artifactually widened. In the center is a late normoblast with multiple granules of iron, hence, a sideroblast; it is a ring sideroblast, since the granules almost completely surround the nucleus. In the lower right are two siderocytes, i.e., non-nucleated red cells containing stainable iron granules (×875.)

Hereditary Sideroblastic Anemias

Hereditary Sex-Linked. This occurs in males and may not appear until adolescence. It is rare, but a few well documented family studies exist. In contrast to acquired sideroblastic anemia, the ring sideroblast abnormality is usually found in late, non-dividing erythroblasts (Bottomley, 1982).

Inheritance Undetermined. In a few cases, severe sideroblastic anemia has been found in female children, but not in family members. The clinical and hematologic features are similar to those described in males with the sex-linked type. The type of inheritance remains unclear in these patients (Bottomley, 1982).

Acquired Sideroblastic Anemias

Primary (Idiopathic) Sideroblastic Anemia (ISA). When other causes of sideroblastic anemia cannot be identified, the term primary or idiopathic is applied. ISA is more common, has its onset in later adult life, and is seen in either sex. The dimorphic anemia has both hypochromic-microcytic and macrocytic red blood cells, and the MCV is usually high. At least 40 per cent of erythroblasts (early and late forms) in bone marrow are ring sideroblasts. In addition to the marrow findings described previously, megaloblastic alterations are observed in over 50 per cent of the cases, and usually remain after therapy with vitamin B_{12} and folic acid. Many patients have mild leukopenia and/or thrombocytopenia. A small proportion of patients show variable response when treated with folic acid and vitamin B_6.

The etiology of ISA is not yet understood. The activities of both δ-aminolevulinic acid synthetase and mitochondrial serine protease are decreased in erythroblasts and granulocytes of patients with ISA. Deficiencies of these enzymes apparently lead to impaired synthesis of heme (Aoki, 1980). Perhaps 10 per cent of patients with ISA develop acute leukemia.

Sideroblastic Anemia Associated with Other Disorders. In some patients, sideroblastic anemias may precede the development or exist at the time of presentation of a variety of hematologic malignancies. In these cases fewer ring sideroblasts are observed than in the primary form. Sideroblastic anemias have been associated with acute myeloid leukemia, erythroleukemia, myelofibrosis, polycythemia vera, multiple myeloma, and acute lymphoid leukemia. The exact relationship between ISA and hematologic malignancies is not clear. However, in one study using G-6-PD isoenzyme analysis of peripheral blood cells from a patient with ISA, all blood cell lines including B and T lymphocytes were shown to be clonal (Prchal, 1978). This suggests that, at least in some cases, ISA is the result of a clonal abnormality of a pluripotential stem cell.

Sideroblastic anemias have also been described in patients with non-malignant disorders such as pernicious anemia, hemolytic anemia, rheumatoid arthritis, polyarteritis nodosa, and malabsorption.

4

Pyridoxine-Responsive Anemia. Individuals who partially respond to pyridoxine have been included in other categories above. Those in whom the anemia is completely corrected form a smaller group. They are young or middle-aged males with a severe microcytic and hypochromic anemia and are dependent upon extraordinary amounts of dietary pyridoxine to maintain a normal hemoglobin level.

Secondary (Drug- or Toxin-Induced) Sideroblastic Anemia. This form of sideroblastic anemia is secondary to some agent which interferes with heme synthesis; recognition is important because hematologic improvement occurs if the agent is removed.

The *antituberculosis drugs* isoniazid, cycloserine, and pyrazinamide cause sideroblastic abnormalities in some patients on long-term therapy.

Lead poisoning is an important member of this group because environmental exposure to lead is usually unrecognized and needs to be detected. Lead interferes with heme synthesis by blocking the enzymes ALA synthetase, ALA dehydrase, and heme synthetase. These blocks are only partial and of different degree; aminolevulinic acid and coproporphyrin are increased in the urine. *Chloramphenicol* also results in ring sideroblast formation, probably by inhibiting mitochondrial protein synthesis.

Ethanol-induced anemia is perhaps the most common of the reversible sideroblastic anemias. Folate deficiency, hypomagnesemia, and hypokalemia are concomitant findings. After withdrawal of alcohol intake, the abnormal sideroblasts usually disappear within a few days.

Refractory Anemia. There is an ill-defined group of chronic anemias usually occurring in individuals over the age of 50. Normocytic or macrocytic anemia, reticulocytopenia, often pancytopenia, and a hypercellular marrow showing erythroid hyperplasia with a variable degree of dyserythropoiesis are present. The anemia cannot be classified in any of the categories already described. Often the patient has been treated with vitamin B_{12}, folic acid, and iron without response. The process is usually unremitting, and in a small proportion of cases develops additional dysplastic changes in marrow cells and increased blast cells and evolves into an acute leukemia. Refractory anemias, therefore, are considered one of the myelodysplastic syndromes (p. 730).

Congenital Dyserythropoietic Anemia (CDA). Several forms of apparently hereditary anemias characterized by abnormal erythropoiesis with ineffective erythropoiesis and splenomegaly have been identified. They appear to have an autosomal recessive mode of inheritance. In general, they tend to be more benign than β thalassemia major, which forms another group of hereditary anemias with ineffective erythropoiesis.

At least three types have thus far been separated on the basis of marrow and serologic findings (Lewis, 1973). CDA-I has megaloblastic changes with some binuclearity, internuclear chromatin bridges, and a macrocytic anemia. CDA-II shows binuclearity and multinuclearity of erythroid precursors with pluripolar mitoses and karyorrhexis. The anemia is normocytic. CDA-II is distinguished from the others because it has a positive acidified serum test (with some, but not all normal sera) and a negative sucrose hemolysis test. It is known as hereditary erythroblastic multinuclearity with positive acidified serum test (HEM-PAS). The red cells have an antigen not present on normal or PNH cells and about one third of normal sera contain the corresponding antibody. CDA-III, described first by Björkman in 1965, has more pronounced multinuclearity, with giant erythroid precursors and a macrocytic anemia.

Hemolysis—General

Anemias which are due primarily to increased red cell destruction are *hemolytic anemias*. A shortened red cell survival, therefore, proves that hemolysis is present; this measurement is usually unnecessary in practice.

Hemolytic anemias may be due to a defect of the red cell itself, an *intrinsic hemolytic anemia:* these are usually hereditary, and are commonly grouped as *membrane, metabolic,* or *hemoglobin* defects. Or the hemolysis may be due to a factor outside the red cell and acting upon it, an *extrinsic hemolytic anemia:* these are almost always acquired. The terms *intravascular hemolysis* and *extravascular hemolysis* refer to the *site* of the destruction of the red cell: within the circulating blood or outside it, respectively.

Erythrocyte Survival Studies. A shortened red cell survival defines hemolysis. If the hemolytic process is moderate or severe, the studies below will suffice to show that hemolysis is present. If the hemolytic process is mild or obscure, red cell survival studies may be necessary.

Radioactive chromium (^{51}Cr) is convenient and widely used. Labeled chromate is added to a blood sample *in vitro* and binds to β chains of hemoglobin. The chromated red cells are injected intravenously and their disappearance is measured by counting blood which is sampled every 1 to 2 days for 10 to 14 days. Residual activity is an index of the intravascular life span of the labeled red cells. Since ^{51}Cr emits gamma rays, external scanning can detect sites of red cell destruction.

The erythrocyte life span is usually expressed as the period during which one half of the radioactivity remains in the blood (the T 1/2 ^{51}Cr; see Fig. 29–4). Chromium normally elutes from the red cells at a rate of 1 per cent per day. Thus, the half-life of the ^{51}Cr-labeled erythrocytes in normal individuals is 25 to 32 days instead of 60 days. Blood loss, change in hematocrit, and recent blood transfusions significantly complicate the interpretation of survival data; therefore, a steady state is necessary for usable results.

In autoimmune hemolytic anemias the slope of red cell survival produces a straight line when plotted on semilogarithmic paper (Fig. 29–4). In other hemolytic anemias, two cell populations may exist. In these situations the survival curve may be composed of an initial steep slope followed by a flatter component (Fig. 29–5). This type of curve has been seen in hereditary enzyme-deficiency hemolytic anemias, sickle cell anemia, and paroxysmal nocturnal hemoglobinuria (Dacie, 1975).

Hemoglobin Destruction. Laboratory findings differ, depending on the site of blood destruction, the amount of destroyed blood, and the rate of destruction. If the destruction is *intravascular* and the quantity

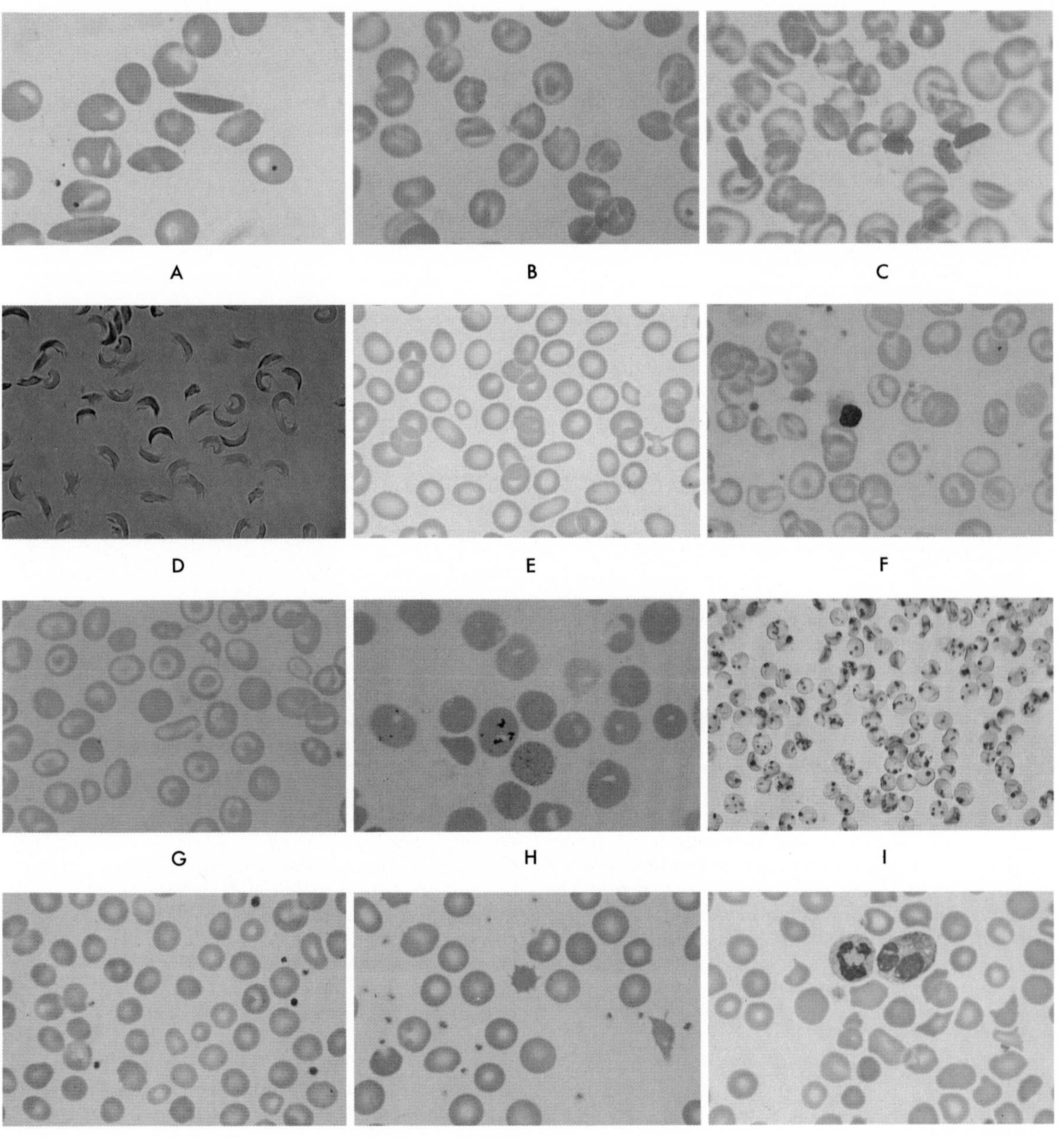

4

Plate 29–2. *A,* Blood film, sickle cell anemia, adult. In contrast to elliptocytes, sickled cells have a densely staining center and pointed ends; three are shown here. Two Howell-Jolly bodies are present, suggesting asplenia. *B,* Blood film, hemoglobin C disease. The numerous target cells and cells with an elongated central density are characteristic. *C,* Blood film, hemoglobin C disease, same patient as in *B* after splenectomy. Four of the red cells here contain densely staining aggregations of Hb C, which tend to become crystals and assume an elongated hexagonal shape. *D,* Sickle cell preparation, in sodium metabisulfite, sickle cell anemia; all the cells are sickled. *E,* Blood film, beta-thalassemia trait. Microcytosis; increased number of elliptocytes. Note that target cells may not be prominent. *F,* Blood film, homozygous beta thalassemia. This patient, a black woman, had a relatively mild hemolytic process, a previous splenectomy, and had not been recently transfused. This is in contrast to the greater severity of the usual homozygous beta thalassemia in Mediterranean peoples. The localized dense hemoglobin in the normoblast suggests precipitation of alpha chains; note the Howell-Jolly body. *G,* Blood film, hemoglobin H disease. A form of alpha-thalassemia, this has the combination of microcytic hypochromic red cells and hemolysis. Target cells are numerous. *H,* Film made after incubation of blood with brilliant cresyl blue, hemoglobin H disease, same patient as in *G.* Two reticulocytes have dark blue precipitates of RNA. Several red cells contain multiple smaller pale blue precipitates of Hb H (*G* and *H:* Courtesy of Dr. McDonald K. Horne). *I,* Heinz bodies. Normal red cells incubated with an oxidant drug, acetyl-phenyldrazine, and stained while in suspension by methyl violet; finally, an air-dried film was made and stained with Wright's stain. Purple-staining Heinz bodies are precipitates of denatured hemoglobin which tend to be attached to the cell membrane. *J,* Blood film, hereditary spherocytosis. In milder cases, the morphologic clues are a decreased red cell diameter and a decreased amount of central pallor which tends often to be eccentric. *K,* Blood film, pyruvate kinase deficiency, post-splenectomy. The contracted, deformed cells were not present prior to splenectomy; they probably represent the most ATP-depleted cells. *L,* Blood film, hemolytic-uremic syndrome. Note the irregularly shaped schistocytes, including helmet cells.

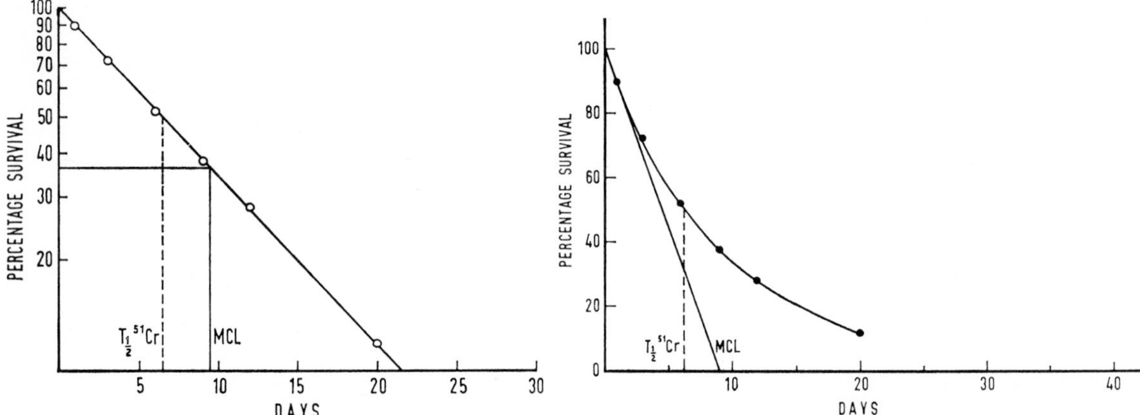

Figure 29–4. Results of ^{51}Cr erythrocyte survival curve in patients with autoimmune hemolytic anemia. The results are plotted on semilogarithmic graph paper. The mean cell life span (MCL) was 9 to 10 days and is recorded at a period when 37 per cent of cells are still circulating. The time of 50 per cent survival ($T_{1/2}$Cr) was 6 to 7 days. (From Dacie, J. V., and Lewis, S. M.: Practical Hematology. 5th ed. Edinburgh, Churchill Livingstone, 1975.)

of destroyed blood is large, free hemoglobin and methemalbumin will be present in the plasma (hemoglobinemia and methemalbuminemia). The urine may contain free hemoglobin and also hemosiderin.

Free hemoglobin readily dissociates into $\alpha\beta$ dimers ($\alpha_2\beta_2 \rightarrow 2\alpha\beta$). These are bound to haptoglobin, an α_2-globulin, and the hemoglobin-haptoglobin complex is rapidly removed from the circulation and catabolized by the liver parenchymal cells. This process prevents hemoglobin from appearing in the urine. However, when the plasma hemoglobin level exceeds 50 to 200 mg/dl (8 to 31 μmol/L), which is the capacity of haptoglobin to bind hemoglobin, the free $\alpha\beta$ dimers of hemoglobin readily pass through the glomerulus of the kidney. Part of the hemoglobin is then absorbed by the proximal tubular cells where the hemoglobin iron is converted to hemosiderin. When these tubular cells are later shed into the urine, *hemosiderinuria* results. If the amount of hemoglobin in the tubular lumen exceeds the capacity of the tubular cell to absorb it, it reaches the urine *(hemoglobinuria).* In the process, it may be oxidized to methemoglobin (hemiglobin). Plasma hemoglobin not bound to haptoglobin nor removed by the kidney is oxidized to hemiglobin. The oxidized heme groups (hemin) are bound to *hemopexin,* a beta globulin, and the complex is rapidly cleared by the hepatic parenchymal cells. If hemopexin is depleted, hemin groups bind to albumin, forming methemalbumin. Once hemopexin again becomes available, it removes the hemin groups from albumin for hepatic clearance (Hillman, 1974).

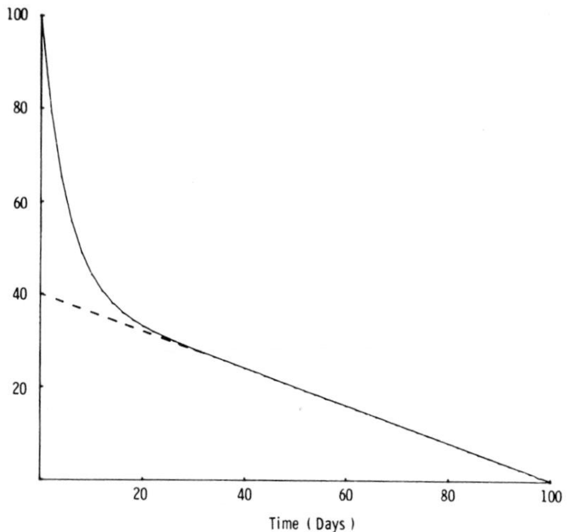

Figure 29–5. Results of ^{51}Cr erythrocyte survival curve in a patient with hemolytic anemia containing two cell populations. The per cent survival is on the ordinate. By extrapolating the flatter curve to time 0, it can be estimated that 40 per cent of the cells have a mean cell life span of 100 days. Sixty per cent of cells have a mean cell life span of five days. (From Bentley, S. A.: Clin. Haematol., *6*:601, 1977.)

Lactate dehydrogenase (LD) is released from red cells and is increased in serum in hemolysis, especially in intravascular hemolysis; it is cleared more slowly than is hemoglobin. If the upper reference value is 207 IU/L, the LD in hemolytic anemia may be increased as much as 800 IU/L. In megaloblastic anemia, for reasons that are unclear, the LD is greatly increased to several thousand units (Chap. 14). Serum LD is also increased in other forms of cellular injury (p. 266).

The normal plasma hemoglobin level is 0.5 to 5 mg/dl (0.08 to 0.78 μmol/L). A rise to 10 mg/dl imparts to the plasma a yellow to orange color. With further increase the color becomes pink. Levels up to 25 to 30 mg/dl are common in hemolytic anemia. Higher levels usually indicate intravascular hemolysis and are seen in hemolytic transfusion reactions and in paroxysmal cold and nocturnal hemoglobinurias.

If hemolysis is primarily *extravascular,* no hemoglobinemia, hemoglobinuria, or hemosiderinuria is present. Hemolysis is detected by measuring an increase in one of the products of heme catabolism (p. 634):

1. An increase in CO expired (a research technique), or in the blood carboxyhemoglobin level.

2. An increase in indirect-reacting serum bilirubin; since this is bound to albumin, it will not appear in the urine.

3. An increase in urine urobilinogen or, more consistently, in fecal urobilinogen.

The normal urobilinogen in a 24-hour specimen is 0.5 to 4 mg (0.8 to 6.75 μmol) in urine and 40 to 280 mg (0.068 to 0.470 mmol) in the stool. Following excessive hemolysis it may increase to 5 to 200 mg in the urine and to 300 to 400 mg in the stool. The examination of feces is more dependable than examination of the urine because it may show an increase when the urine shows none. It may show an increase even when the serum bilirubin is not raised because the normal liver can remove large amounts of (indirectly reacting) bilirubin and of reabsorbed urobilinogen from the blood.

Hemolytic anemia is characterized also by increased red cell production. Because of the availability of maximal amounts of iron for hemoglobin formation, red cell production reaches the maximal degree possible (about eight times normal) in severe chronic hemolytic anemia, if complicating factors such as folate deficiency do not intervene. If red cell destruction exceeds the capacity of the marrow to replace red cells at the same rate, hemolytic anemia occurs. With less severe hemolysis, the marrow may be able to produce enough red cells so that anemia does not occur; this is called compensated hemolysis.

Blood Film. The anemia is normocytic or macrocytic. Macrocytosis is due to the presence of immature red cells, which are larger than normocytes. Polychromasia is usually prominent; it may be excessively basophilic and normoblasts may be present, both of which indicate a "shift" of marrow reticulocytes into the blood.

Other red cell abnormalities may give a clue to the nature of the hemolytic process. Spherocytes suggest hereditary spherocytosis or autoimmune hemolysis (Figs. 27–21 and 27–23); schistocytes suggest traumatic hemolytic anemia (Fig. 27–29); sickle cells, target cells, or crystals suggest a hemoglobinopathy (Figs. 29–13 and 29–14; Plate 29–2). When hemolytic anemia is acute, increased numbers and younger forms of leukocytes and platelets are often released from the marrow together with erythrocytes. The result is leukocytosis with a "shift to the left" and thrombocytosis with both normal and giant platelets.

Bone Marrow. Normoblastic hyperplasia is present and may be striking in degree. Storage iron is usually increased and sideroblasts are normal or increased in number, reflecting the abundance of available iron for hemoglobin synthesis.

Sudden worsening of the degree of anemia may occur in chronic hemolytic anemias and be due to either of two basic mechanisms. Occasionally episodes of bone marrow failure (transient arrest of erythropoiesis, p. 666) characterized by erythroid hypoplasia and reticulocytopenia may upset the equilibrium between production and destruction of red cells. In most instances these *aplastic crises* are thought to be precipitated by infection (Bauman, 1967). On the other hand, a sudden increase in the rate of red cell destruction may occur accompanied by an increased reticulocytosis in an insufficient attempt to compensate. This is called a *hemolytic crisis*.

Hemolysis—Membrane Disorders

Hereditary Spherocytosis (HS). Hereditary spherocytosis is characterized by spherocytic red cells which are intrinsically defective, splenomegaly, and familial occurrence (most often autosomal dominant). The hemolytic process is variable in severity and is corrected by splenectomy, though the spherocytosis remains.

The laboratory findings are those of a chronic extravascular hemolytic process: evidence of increased pigment catabolism, erythroid hyperplasia, and reticulocytosis. The Coombs test is negative. The red cells characteristically have increased osmotic fragility. On the blood film, spherocytes have a smaller diameter and are more intensely stained than normal cells. They have decreased or absent central pallor; if present, the pallor may be eccentric (Fig. 27–21; Plate 29–2*J*). The MCV is normal and the MCHC is often increased, reflecting a decrease in cell surface.

Osmotic Fragility Test. Red cells are suspended in a series of tubes containing hypotonic solutions of NaCl varying from 0.9 per cent to 0.0 per cent, incubated at room temperature for 30 minutes, and centrifuged. The per cent hemolysis in the supernatant solutions is measured and plotted for each NaCl concentration. Cells that are more spherical, with a decreased surface/volume ratio, have a limited capacity to expand in hypotonic solutions and lyse at a higher concentration of NaCl than do normal biconcave red cells. They are said to have increased osmotic fragility. Conversely, cells that are hypochromic and flatter have a greater capacity to expand in hypotonic solutions, lyse at a lower concentration than do normal cells, and are said to have decreased osmotic fragility (Fig. 29–6).

The osmotic fragility of freshly drawn blood is usually increased in HS, but may be normal in mildly affected patients. In blood which is incubated at 37°C. for 24 hours before performing the test, the osmotic fragility is almost always increased (Fig. 29–7).

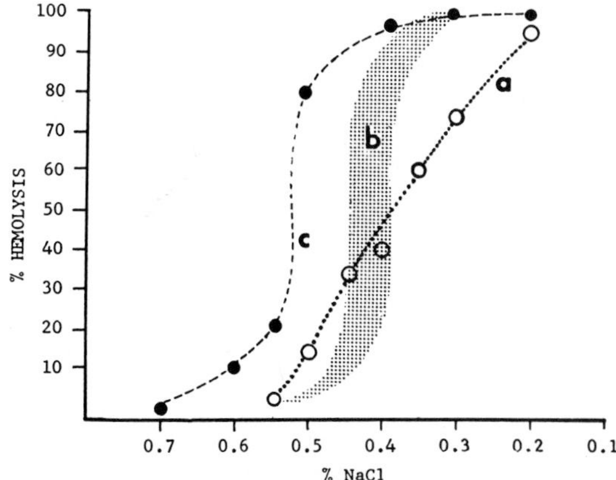

Figure 29–6. Erythrocyte osmotic fragility. *a,* Thalassemia, showing a small fraction of cells with increased fragility (lower left), and a larger fraction of cells with decreased fragility (upper right). *b,* Normal curves fall in shaded area. *c,* Hereditary spherocytosis, showing increased osmotic fragility.

4

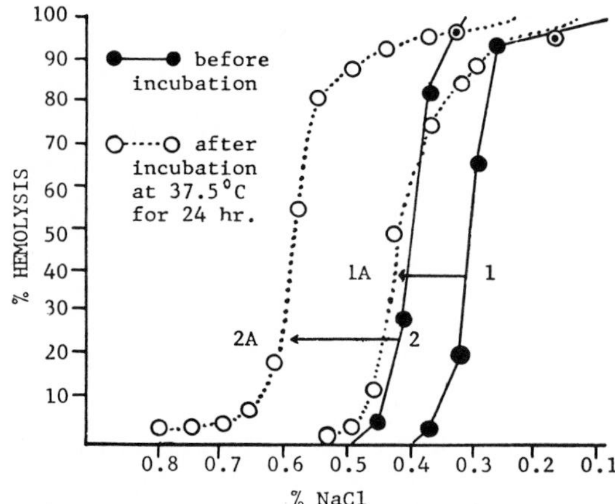

Figure 29–7. The effect of incubation on erythrocyte osmotic fragility. The change in the osmotic fragility curve from "before incubation" to "after incubation" is illustrated for normal blood (1 → 1A), and blood from a patient with hereditary spherocytosis (2 → 2A). Blood in hereditary spherocytosis characteristically shows a greater increase in fragility with incubation than does normal blood or even blood of acquired spherocytosis (e.g., autoimmune hemolytic anemia).

The increased osmotic fragility of freshly drawn blood is characteristic but not specific; it may occur in acquired spherocytic anemias. A greater increase compared to normal after incubation than before incubation is the important finding in the diagnosis of HS.

Autohemolysis Test (Dacie, 1975). Sterile, defibrinated blood is incubated at 37°C. for 48 hours. During this time red cells undergo a complex series of changes, lose membrane, and become more spherocytic. In normal blood, without added glucose, the amount of autohemolysis at 48 hours is 0.2 to 2.0 per cent. In normal blood, incubated with added glucose, the amount of autohemolysis is less, 0 to 0.9 per cent.

In HS, autohemolysis is virtually always increased; with glucose, the lysis is diminished to a variable extent. Rarely, patients with strong clinical and laboratory evidence for HS will have normal incubated osmotic fragility. In these patients the abnormal autohemolysis test is useful in confirming a diagnosis of HS (Fukagawa, 1979).

The erythrocytes are abnormally permeable to sodium, and there is no defect in energy metabolism, which is, in fact, increased. The increased metabolic activity has been explained as an attempt to compensate for a membrane defect which leaks cations, with degenerative changes and the loss of cell membrane accelerated by the metabolic and physical stress of passage through the spleen (Jandl, 1968).

Usually, autosomal dominant inheritance is found, but in about 20 per cent of cases neither parent is affected. The primary defect appears to be heterogeneous and located in the skeletal proteins of the red cell membrane. In very rare patients, the disorder is autosomal recessive and spectrin is deficient; in 10 to 30 per cent of the usual autosomal dominant defects, abnormal spectrin-protein 4:1 interaction has been found; and in most cases, the nature of the membrane defect is yet unknown (Palek, 1983).

Hereditary Elliptocytosis (HE). This autosomal dominant condition probably includes more than one genetic variant. Non-hypochromic elliptocytes are abundant in the blood film, numbering over 25 per cent (see Fig. 27–25), whereas in normal individuals less than 15 per cent of the red cells are elliptical. The deformity is increased in sealed, moist preparations.

Most persons with the common form of HE (about 90 per cent of cases) are non-anemic; a minority of this group (perhaps 10 to 20 per cent) have mild hemolysis. In a subgroup of common HE, especially in black families, affected neonates transiently have moderate poikilocytosis, red cell fragmentation, and budding, with hemolytic anemia; during the first year of life, hemolysis declines and typical HE emerges (Lux, 1981; Zarkowsky, 1979).

Hemolytic HE accounts for 10 per cent of cases. A mild to moderate hemolytic anemia and splenomegaly are present, with both elliptocytes and spherocytes, and abnormal osmotic fragility and autohemolysis tests.

Hereditary Pyropoikilocytosis (HPP). A rare, moderately severe congenital hemolytic anemia is characterized by microcytosis, striking micropoikilocytosis and fragmentation, and autosomal recessive inheritance. It occurs primarily in blacks. In contrast to normal red cells, which show budding and fragmentation when heated to 49°C., HPP red cells fragment at 45 to 46°C. As in some cases of HE, the membrane abnormality involves defective spectrin function (Palek, 1983).

Hereditary Stomatocytosis. Stomatocytes are cells which on air-dried films have a slit-shaped rather than circular pallor; in wet preparations their shape is that of a bowl rather than a biconcave disk. Rh null red cells are stomatocytes and have a shortened survival. A syndrome of hereditary hemolytic anemia with stomatocytes includes cases with considerable variability of hemolysis both within and between families. In some cases, the cells appear as target cells on air-dried films. In common there is increased sodium permeability and flux, but there is variability in ion content and water content (Wiley, 1975).

Paroxysmal Nocturnal Hemoglobinuria (PNH) (Dacie, 1972; Rosse, 1977). PNH is an acquired intrinsic defect of red cells which renders them unusually sensitive to complement. The nature of the defect is unknown, but PNH cells bind more C3 than do normal cells whether complement is activated by the classic or the alternate pathway. Two or three populations of cells of different complement sensitivity are present, and one is almost always normal (Rosse, 1977). Hemolysis *in vivo* probably occurs primarily via activation of the alternate pathway (Götze, 1972). Platelets and neutrophils also appear to be sensitive to complement.

Clinically, PNH usually occurs in young adults and is characterized by chronic intravascular hemolysis with or without obvious hemoglobinuria. Hemosiderinuria is, however, almost constantly present. Typical nocturnal or sleep-related hemoglobinuria is present in less than 25 per cent of patients.

The blood usually shows a normocytic anemia with

a reticulocytosis that is often less than expected for the degree of anemia. Hypochromic microcytic anemia is not uncommon, however, and is due to loss of iron in the urine. Neutropenia occurs in three fifths and thrombocytopenia in two thirds of patients at some time during the course of disease, so that pancytopenia is common. The direct antiglobulin test is usually negative. Red cell acetylcholinesterase and neutrophil alkaline phosphatase are usually decreased. Osmotic fragility is not increased. The autohemolysis test shows increased lysis at 48 hours; with added glucose the degree of lysis is not diminished but may be accentuated.

The marrow is usually hypercellular with normoblastic hyperplasia, but it may be hypocellular. In some patients marrow failure may occur during the course of PNH; in others, aplastic anemia is the initial diagnosis, with signs of PNH later manifesting themselves. An abnormal line of cells probably develops in an aplastic or regenerating marrow (Lewis, 1967).

Thrombotic complications are common. The disease may undergo partial remissions and exacerbations. In over half of patients, both the proportion of abnormal cells and the clinical severity decrease with time.

Sucrose Hemolysis Test (Hartmann, 1970). This test should be performed whenever the diagnosis of PNH is considered, also in hypoplastic anemias, and in any hemolytic anemia of obscure origin. The principle of the test is that sucrose provides a medium of low ionic strength which promotes the binding of complement to the red cells. In PNH, a proportion of the red cells is abnormally sensitive to complement-mediated lysis.

The patient's washed red cells are mixed with ABO compatible normal serum (fresh or properly stored) and isotonic sucrose. The tube is incubated at room temperature for 30 minutes and then centrifuged, and the per cent hemolysis in the supernatant is determined. Two control tubes eliminate the serum, and the cells should be negative. Less than 5 per cent hemolysis in the test specimen is negative, 5 to 10 per cent is suspicious, and over 10 per cent is positive and virtually diagnostic for PNH. Suspicious results can be seen in some other hematologic diseases, especially megaloblastic anemia and autoimmune hemolytic anemia. False negative results occur if the serum lacks complement activity.

Acidified Serum Test (Ham Test) (Ham, 1939; Dacie, 1975). Definitive diagnosis of PNH depends upon a positive acidified serum test. In acidified serum, complement is activated by the alternate pathway, binds to red cells, and lyses the abnormal PNH cells which are unusually susceptible to complement. The patient's washed red cells are mixed with ABO compatible normal serum (fresh or properly stored) and acid; after an hour's incubation at 37°C., the PNH cells are lysed, as indicated in Table 29–2. The patient's own serum may or may not result in lysis, depending on residual complement, and the other tubes provide controls.

In PNH, usually 10 to 50 per cent of the cells are lysed. If lysis also occurs with heat-inactivated serum, the test is not positive, as spherocytic or antibody-sensitized cells may be responsible.

A positive acidified serum test occurs in congenital dyserythropoietic anemia, type II (CDA-II) or HEM-PAS (p. 668). Here, however, lysis does not occur with the patient's own serum, and only with about 30 per cent of normal sera. Also, the sucrose hemolysis test is negative in CDA-II. The hemolysis is probably due to a naturally occurring antibody directed against an as yet undefined antigen.

Hemolysis—Hemoglobin Disorders

In 1949 Pauling and his associates described an electrophoretically abnormal hemoglobin type in patients with sickle cell anemia. Their studies initiated the concept of molecular disease; that is, a molecular variation in a single protein can be responsible for the entire spectrum of clinical, laboratory, and pathologic manifestations that characterize a disease. The subsequent finding that the abnormality was due to the substitution of a single amino acid in a polypeptide chain of hemoglobin inaugurated the field of biochemical genetics.

At present, over 300 different hemoglobins have been described. The great majority of these have been characterized as a single amino acid substitution in one of the polypeptide chains (α, β, γ, or δ), which can be explained by a single base substitution in the corresponding triplet codon of the gene. In a small number of abnormal hemoglobins, the polypeptide chain is abnormally long or short due to termination errors, frame-shift mutations, crossover in phase, deletion of codons, or fused or hybrid chains (Bunn, 1977).

NORMAL HEMOGLOBINS

The heme group is identical in all variants of human hemoglobin. The protein part of the molecule (globin) consists of four polypeptide chains. At least three distinct hemoglobin types are found postnatally in normal individuals, and the structure of each has been determined.

Table 29–2. ACIDIFIED SERUM TEST*

	1	2	3	4	5	6	7
Fresh normal serum	0.5	0.5			0.5	0.5	
Patient's serum			0.5				
Heat-inactivated normal serum				0.5			0.5
0.2 N HCL		0.05	0.05	0.05		0.05	0.05
50% patient's red cells	0.05	0.05	0.05	0.05			
50% normal red cells					0.05	0.05	0.05
Pattern of lysis in positive test	Trace	+ + +	+	–	–	–	–

*Modified from Dacie, J. V., and Lewis, S. M.: Practical Haematology. 4th ed. New York, Grune & Stratton, Inc., 1968.

4

Hb A ($\alpha_2\beta_2$). Hemoglobin A is the major normal adult hemoglobin. The polypeptide chains of the globulin part of the molecules are of two types: two identical alpha chains, each with 141 amino acids, and two identical beta chains, with 146 amino acids each. Each chain is linked with one heme group. The molecule is ellipsoidal, with the four heme groups at the surface of the molecule, where they function by combining reversibly with oxygen (Fig. 28–5).

Hb F ($\alpha_2\gamma_2$). Hemoglobin F is the major hemoglobin of the fetus and the newborn infant. The increased affinity for oxygen of fetal blood over adult blood is not due to the hemoglobin itself, but probably to the environment in the red cell. The two alpha chains are identical to those of Hb A, and two gamma chains, with 146 amino acid residues, differ from beta chains. In normal individuals, Hb F has two types of gamma chains which differ in one amino acid, having either alanine ($^A\gamma$) or glycine ($^G\gamma$) at position 136. The ratio of $^G\gamma$ to $^A\gamma$ chains changes from 3:1 at birth to 2:3 by age 12 months (Weatherall, 1981).

During fetal life, Hb F predominates, as alpha chain production and gamma chain production are high (Fig. 29–8). Beta chain production begins before the twentieth week of prenatal life, so that Hb A is 10 per cent of the total between 20 and 35 weeks and 15 to 40 per cent at the time of birth. After birth, smaller amounts of Hb F are produced; by 6 months Hb F is usually less than 8 per cent and by 12 months less than 2 per cent of the total Hb. In some normal children, however, Hb F may be as high as 5 per cent for 12 to 24 months (Chernoff, 1952). Only traces of Hb F (<1.0 per cent) are found in adults. During fetal life, all red cells produce and contain Hb F, whereas in adults only 0.2 to 7 per cent do so (Weatherall, 1981). The Hb F containing cells (F cells) may increase in number when reactivation of Hb F synthesis occurs in normal pregnancy and in some disorders of erythropoiesis. The total Hb F rarely exceeds 20 per cent in these conditions (Nathan, 1981).

Hb A$_2$ ($\alpha_2\delta_2$). Hemoglobin A$_2$ accounts for 1.5 to 3.5 per cent of normal adult hemoglobin. Its two alpha chains are the same as in Hb A and Hb F; its two delta chains differ from beta chains in only eight of their 146 amino acids.

Delta chain synthesis begins late in fetal life and occurs only in normoblasts (not reticulocytes). The level of Hb A$_2$ gradually increases during the first year of life at which time the adult level is reached. Quantitation has become important, for Hb A$_2$ is increased in some beta-thalassemias. Iron deficiency causes decreased Hb A$_2$ synthesis.

Embryonic Hemoglobins. The zeta (ζ) chain is the embryonic analogue of the α chain and may combine with epsilon (ϵ) chains to form Hb Gower-1 ($\zeta_2\epsilon_2$) or with γ chains to form Hb Portland-1 ($\zeta_2\gamma_2$). The epsilon chain is the embryonic counterpart of the γ, β, and δ chains and combines with α chains to form Hb Gower-2 ($\alpha_2\epsilon_2$). Hb Gower-1, Hb Portland-1, and Hb Gower-2 are the embryonic hemoglobins and are found in normal human embryos and fetuses with a gestational age of less than three months (Figs. 29–8 and 29–9).

Genetics. Analysis of pedigrees has shown that the α and non-α genes are on different chromosomes, and strongly suggested the presence of two α genes on each haploid chromosome (Weatherall, 1981). More recent investigations employing recombinant DNA technology, cloning of specific human DNA fragments, and restriction endonuclease mapping have elucidated more detailed globin gene arrangements (Phillips, 1981; Weatherall, 1982). Two ζ genes and the two α genes are on chromosome 16. Genes for the ϵ chain, the two γ chains, the δ and β chains are located on chromosome 11 (Fig. 29–10). As in other genes, the coding sequences (exons) of the globin genes are interrupted by non-coding DNA sequences (introns). Introns are transcribed into RNA but are removed from the pre-messenger RNA by precise splicing reactions before the resultant mRNA is transcribed into protein.

ABNORMAL HEMOGLOBINS AND NOMENCLATURE

Normal adult hemoglobin is designated Hb A; fetal hemoglobin, Hb F; that found in sickle cell anemia,

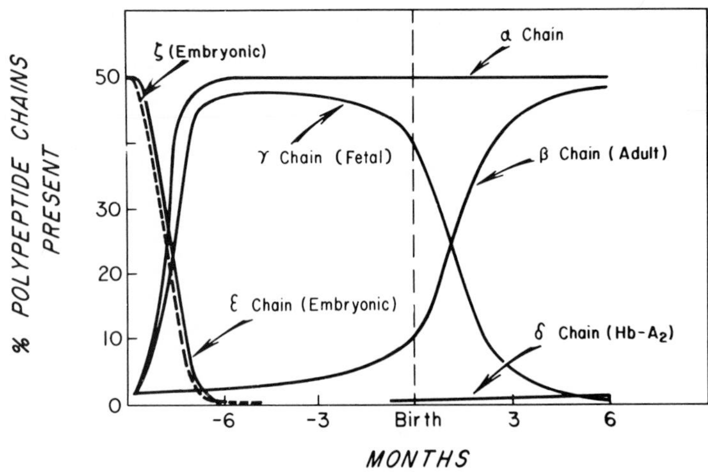

Figure 29–8. Relative proportions of polypeptide chains of hemoglobin present during fetal and neonatal life. (From Bunn, H. F., Forget, B. G., and Ranney, H. M.: Human Hemoglobins. Philadelphia, W. B. Saunders Company, 1977.)

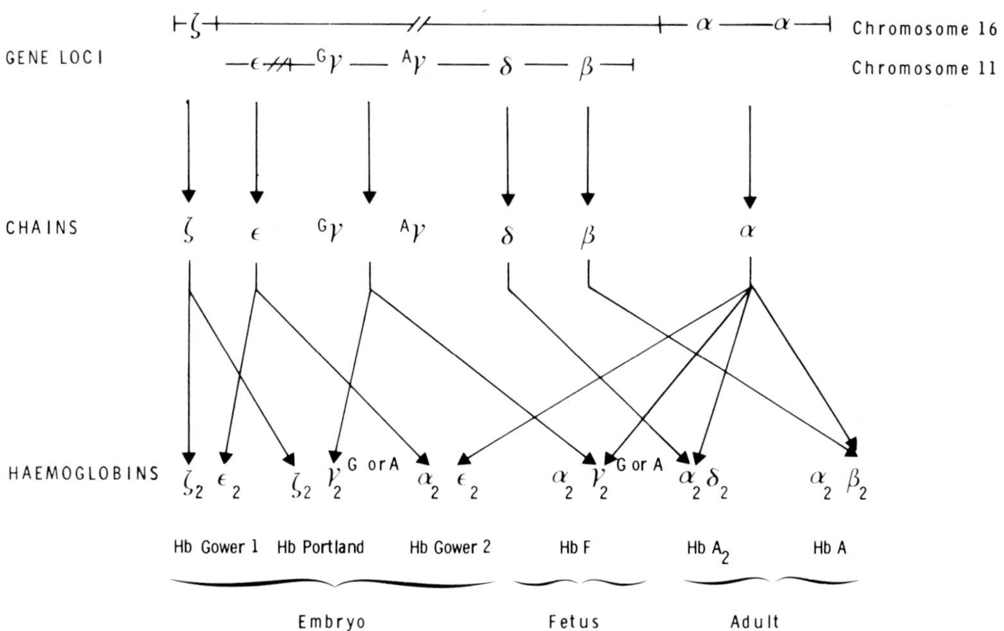

Figure 29–9. The genetic control of human hemoglobin. (From Weatherall, D. J., and Clegg, J. B.: The Thalassemia Syndromes. 3rd ed. Oxford, Blackwell Scientific Publications, 1981.)

Hb S; and those associated with methemoglobinemia, Hb M. Other hemoglobins were assigned letters of the alphabet, then geographical names, or both—usually to distinguish different Hbs with similar characteristics, such as electrophoretic mobilities. There are several variants of Hb D, G, J, and M, for example.

The polypeptide chain on which the abnormality is present can be indicated as a superscript; e.g., Hb S = $\alpha_2{}^A\beta_2{}^S$; Hb I = $\alpha_2{}^I\beta_2{}^A$. The common designation is the number of the amino acid residue in the superscript along with the substituted amino acid; e.g., Hb S = $\alpha_2\beta_2{}^{6Val}$; Hb I = $\alpha_2{}^{16Asp}\beta_2$ (Fig. 29–11). Amino acid substitutions in some of the known hemoglobin variants are listed and classified by functional characteristics in Table 29–3.

Hemoglobin Electrophoresis. Hemoglobin molecules in an alkaline solution have a net negative charge and move toward the anode in an electrophoretic system. Those with an electrophoretic mobility greater than that of Hb A at pH 8.6 are known as the "fast hemoglobins"; these include Hb Bart's and the two fastest, Hb H and Hb I. Hb C is the slowest of the common hemoglobins. A few in order of increasing mobility are Hbs A_2, E = O = C, G = D = S, F, A, Bart's, N, and H (Fig. 29–12).

Different media and different buffers vary in efficiency of separation. None is both practical and adequate for *all* separations and for screening purposes.

A practical method for routine hemoglobin electrophoresis is cellulose acetate at alkaline pH (Briere, 1965). It is rapid and reproducible and separates hemoglobins S, F, C, A, and A_2. Quantification of the major bands is easily accomplished. If an S band is present, a solubility test or sickling test must be performed. Citrate agar electrophoresis at an acid pH (Milner, 1975) provides ready separation of hemoglobins that migrate together on cellulose acetate: S from D and G, and C from E and O (Fig. 29–12) (Schmidt, 1973).

Final characterization of abnormal hemoglobins is beyond the scope of the clinical laboratory. It consists of purification of the abnormal hemoglobin with starch-block electrophoresis, hybridization experiments to determine whether the abnormality lies in the alpha or beta chain, and "fingerprinting." In the latter procedure, the polypeptide chains are split by enzymatic digestion into peptides that are separated by performing horizontal paper electrophoresis and vertical chromatography in sequence. This peptide map, or "finger-

4

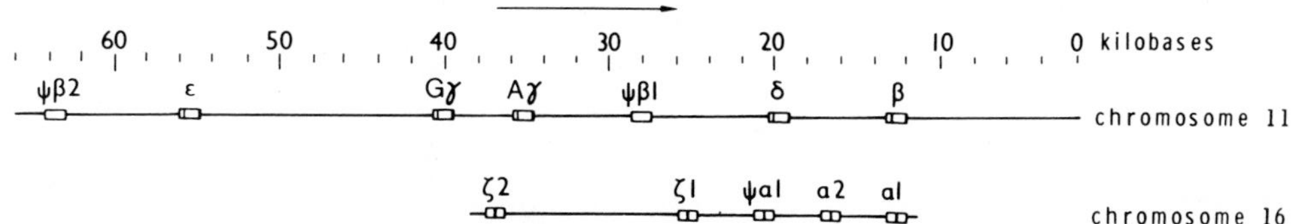

Figure 29–10. The physical arrangement of globin genes on chromosomes 11 and 16. Chromosome 11 has five functional β-like globin genes and two β-like nonfunctional pseudogenes ($\psi\beta_2$ and $\psi\beta_1$). Chromosome 16 has four functional α-like genes and one non-functional α pseudogene ($\psi\alpha_1$). The arrow indicates the direction of transcription of the two clusters of globin genes. (From Weatherall, D. J., and Clegg, J. B.: The Thalassaemia Syndrome. 3rd ed. Oxford, Blackwell Scientific Publications, 1981.)

Hemoglobin	Structure	Nomenclature
A		$\alpha_2 \beta_2$
A_2		$\alpha_2 \delta_2$
F		$\alpha_2 \gamma_2$
S		$\alpha_2 \beta^S{}_2$ $(\alpha_2 \beta_2{}^{6\ Glu \rightarrow Val})$
M (Boston)		$\alpha_2{}^M \beta_2 ; \alpha_2{}^{M(Boston)} \beta_2$ $(\alpha_2{}^{58\ His \rightarrow Tyr} \beta_2)$
Barts		γ_4
H		β_4

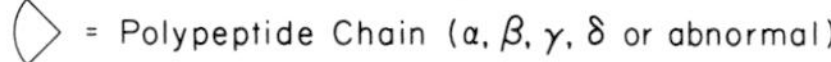

Figure 29–11. Configuration and nomenclature of normal and abnormal hemoglobins. Each triangle represents one folded polypeptide chain; the bar attached to its external surface represents a heme group. The drawing is schematic. Each heme group is near the surface of the molecule, located in a pocket formed by folds of its polypeptide chain and attached to that chain by an imidazole group. In most hemoglobinopathies (e.g., Hb S, Hb $G_{Philadelphia}$), the affected polypeptide chains differs from normal in only one amino acid. In Hb S, the designation could also be written as $\alpha_2\beta_2{}^{6Val}$, and in Hb $G_{Philadelphia}$, $\alpha_2{}^{68Lys}\beta_2$, indicating the site of the substitution and the amino acid which replaces the one usually present. (After Krieg, 1967).

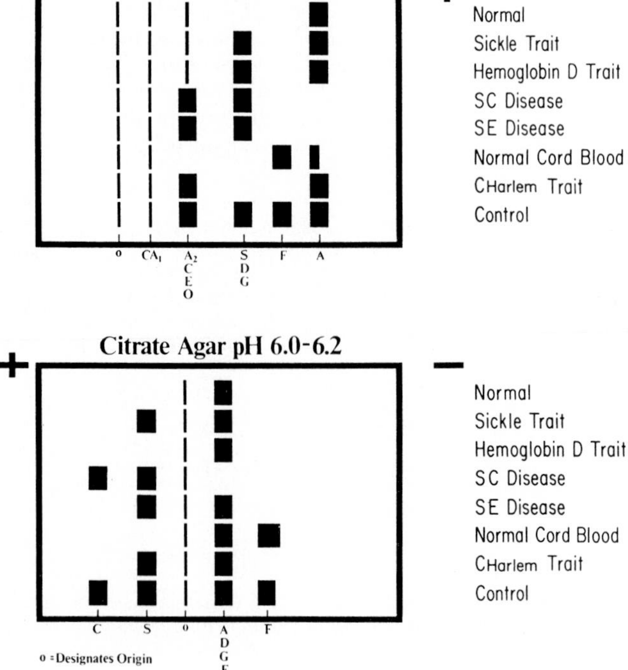

Figure 29–12. Hemoglobin electrophoresis. Comparison of various hemoglobin samples on cellulose acetate and citrate agar, showing relative mobilities. The control is a composite sample. The relative amounts of hemoglobin are not necessarily proportional to the size of the band; for example in sickle trait (Hb AS), Hb A always exceeds Hb S in amount (From Schmidt, 1976.)

Table 29–3. FUNCTIONAL CLASSIFICATION OF HEMOGLOBIN VARIANTS*

I. Homozygous: Hemoglobin polymorphisms; the variants that are most common

Hb S	$\alpha_2\beta_2^{6Val}$	Severe hemolytic anemia; sickling
Hb C	$\alpha_2\beta_2^{6Lys}$	Mild hemolytic anemia
Hb D Punjab	$\alpha_2\beta_2^{121Gln}$	No anemia
Hb E	$\alpha_2\beta_2^{26Lys}$	Mild microcytic anemia

II. Heterozygous: Hemoglobin variants causing functional aberrations or hemolytic anemia in the heterozygous state

A. Hemoglobins associated with methemoglobinemia and cyanosis

1. Hb M Boston $\alpha_2^{58Tyr}\beta_2$
2. Hb M Iwate $\alpha_2^{87Tyr}\beta_2$
3. Hb M Saskatoon $\alpha_2\beta_2^{63Tyr}$
4. Hb M Milwaukee $\alpha_2\beta_2^{67Gu}$
5. Hb M Hyde Park $\alpha_2\beta_2^{92Tyr}$

B. Hemoglobins associated with altered oxygen affinity

1. Increased affinity and polycythemia
   a. Hb Chesapeake $\alpha_2^{92Leu}\beta_2$
   b. Hb J Capetown $\alpha_2^{92Gln}\beta_2$
   c. Hb Malmo $\alpha_2\beta_2^{97Gln}$
   d. Hb Yakima $\alpha_2\beta_2^{99His}$
   e. Hb Kemp $\alpha_2\beta_2^{99Asn}$
   f. Hb Ypsi (Ypsilanti) $\alpha_2\beta_2^{99Tyr}$
   g. Hb Hiroshima $\alpha_2\beta_2^{143Asp}$
   h. Hb Rainer $\alpha_2\beta_2^{145Cys}$
   i. Hb Bethesda $\alpha_2\beta_2^{145His}$
2. Decreased affinity—may have mild anemia or cyanosis
   a. Hb Kansas $\alpha_2^{102Thr}\beta_2$
   b. Hb Titusville $\alpha_2^{94Asn}\beta_2$
   c. Hb Providence $\alpha_2\beta_2^{82Asn,Asp}$
   d. Hb Agenogi $\alpha_2\beta_2^{90Lys}$
   e. Hb Beth Israel $\alpha_2\beta_2^{102Ser}$
   f. Hb Yoshizuka $\alpha_2\beta_2^{108Asp}$

C. Unstable Hemoglobins

1. Hb may precipitate as Heinz bodies after splenectomy; "congenital Heinz body anemia"
   a. Severe hemolysis; no improvement after splenectomy
      Hb Bibba $\alpha_2^{136Pro}\beta_2$
      Hb Hammersmith $\alpha_2\beta_2^{42Ser}$
      Hb Bristol $\alpha_2\beta_2^{67Asp}$
      Hb Olmsted $\alpha_2\beta_2^{141Arg}$
   b. Severe hemolysis; improvement after splenectomy
      Hb Torino $\alpha_2^{42Val}\beta_2$
      Hb Ann Arbor $\alpha_2^{80Arg}\beta_2$
      Hb Genova $\alpha_2\beta_2^{28Pro}$
      Hb Shepherd's Bush $\alpha_2\beta_2^{74Asp}$
      Hb Koln $\alpha_2\beta_2^{98Met}$
      Hb Wien $\alpha_2\beta_2^{130Asp}$
   c. Mild hemolysis; intermittent exacerbations
      Hb L-Ferrara $\alpha_2^{47Gly}\beta_2$
      Hb Hasharon $\alpha_2^{47His}\beta_2$
      Hb Leiden $\alpha_2\beta_2^{6\text{ or }7}$ (Glu deleted)
      Hb Freiburg $\alpha_2\beta_2^{23}$ (Val deleted)
      Hb Seattle $\alpha_2\beta_2^{76Glu}$
      Hb Louisville $\alpha_2\beta_2^{42Leu}$
      Hb Zurich $\alpha_2\beta_2^{63Arg}$
      Hb Gun Hill $\alpha_2\beta_2^{91-97}$ (5 a. a. deleted)
   d. No disease
      Hb Etobicoke $\alpha_2^{84Arg}\beta_2$
      Hb Dakar $\alpha_2^{112Glu}\beta_2$
      Hb Sogn $\alpha_2\beta_2^{14Arg}$
      Hb Tacoma $\alpha_2\beta_2^{30Ser}$
2. Tetramers of normal chains; appear in thalassemias
   Hb Bart's γ_4
   Hb H β_4
   Hb (α_4^A) α_4

*Modified, in part, from Winslow, R. M., and Anderson, W. F.: The hemoglobinopathies. *In* Stanbury, J. B., Wyngaarden, J. B., Fredrickson, D. S., Goldstein, J. L., and Brown, M. S., (eds.): The Metabolic Basis of Inherited Disease. 5th ed. New York, McGraw-Hill Book Company, 1983, Chap. 76.

print," is compared with that prepared from normal hemoglobin, and the peptide in which the abnormality occurs can be located. The abnormal peptide is then eluted and its amino acid content determined. Discussion of techniques for identification of hemoglobins is provided by Huisman (1977).

Hb A_2 Quantitation. The starch block method of Kunkel (1957) is probably most consistently reliable, but it is not practical for routine use.

Estimating Hb A_2 visually or by densitometry from cellulose acetate membranes is unreliable (Schmidt, 1975). Satisfactory methods that can be readily performed in a clinical laboratory are cellulose acetate electrophoresis followed by elution of the Hb A_2 band and measuring this spectrophotometrically as a percentage of the total (Marengo-Rowe, 1965). Somewhat more convenient for large numbers of samples is microchromatography using DEAE-cellulose and inexpensive glassware (Efremov, 1974). This method has been modified to minimize its sensitivity to pH changes of the developer and the ion exchanger (Huisman, 1975; Schleider, 1977).

Reference intervals for Hb A_2 are 1.6 to 3.2 per cent of the total hemoglobin.

Hb A_2 estimation is useful in identifying individuals with β thalassemia trait, in whom it is elevated up to 7 per cent (p. 684). It is also occasionally increased in megaloblastic anemia, and may be decreased in iron deficiency anemia. If an individual with β thalassemia trait has concomitant severe iron deficiency, the usually elevated Hb A_2 may be in the normal range; in this instance, retesting should be performed after the iron deficiency is corrected.

Alkali Denaturation Test for Hb F (Singer, 1951). Fetal hemoglobin resists alkali denaturation; adult hemoglobin does not. A hemolysate is alkalinized and then neutralized, and the denatured adult hemoglobin is precipitated by ammonium sulfate. A filtrate will then contain only alkali-resistant hemoglobin, which is measured and expressed as a percentage of the total.

The modification of Betke (1959) gives reference intervals of 0.2 to 1.0 per cent for adults.

Elevated Hb F is found in some hemoglobinopathies, in β thalassemias, and in hereditary persistence of fetal hemoglobin (HPFH).

In certain acquired hematopoietic disorders, the Hb F level may be elevated. These include megaloblastic anemia, myelofibrosis, aplastic anemia, leukemias, erythroleukemia, refractory anemias, pregnancy, and paroxysmal nocturnal hemoglobinuria.

Acid Elution Slide Test for Hb F. The modification of the original method of Kleihauer and Betke by Shepard (1962) is useful for analyzing the distribution of Hb F among red cells. Hemoglobins other than Hb F are eluted from the red cells on an air-dried blood film by a citric acid–phosphate buffer (pH 3.3). Only Hb F remains in the fixed red cells, and the distribution can be determined after staining.

In normal adults almost all red cells appear as ghosts; 1 per cent or less contain residual hemoglobin (Hb F). If increased Hb F is due to most types of hereditary persistence of fetal hemoglobin (HPFH), the Hb F is distributed evenly among red cells. If the cause is thalassemia or a hemoglobinopathy, the distribution of the Hb F is heterogeneous among red cells.

ABNORMAL HEMOGLOBIN SYNDROMES

In *hemoglobinopathies* the structure of one of the four types of polypeptide chains formed is abnormal; this is usually due to substitution of a single amino acid. A large number of hemoglobin variants which do not cause disease have been discovered in surveys. In clinically significant disease, either the beta chain or the alpha chain is affected. Involvement of the gamma chain and delta chain occurs, but because of the small amount of hemoglobin involved they are less often detected and rarely of any clinical significance. Depending on the type of amino acid and the site involved, the hemoglobin may be functionally abnormal and have altered chemical and physical properties.

In *thalassemias,* globin chains, usually of normal structure, are produced at a decreased rate. Beta thalassemia refers to decreased production of beta chains; therefore HbF ($\alpha_2\gamma_2$) or HbA_2 ($\alpha_2\delta_2$) is often increased with respect to Hb A ($\alpha_2\beta_2$). Alpha thalassemia refers to decreased production of alpha chains: Hb A ($\alpha_2\beta_2$), Hb A_2 ($\alpha_2\delta_2$) and Hb F ($\alpha_2\gamma_2$) are proportionally decreased.

In *homozygous beta hemoglobinopathies,* both allelic genes for the abnormal beta chains are present, so that no normal beta chains (hence, no Hb A) are produced. Examples are sickle cell disease (Hb SS) and hemoglobin C disease (Hb CC). Since alpha, gamma, and delta genes (and chain production) are normal, the Hb F and Hb A_2 formed are structurally normal, though they may be increased in amount.

Homozygous alpha hemoglobinopathies have not been described.

In *heterozygous beta hemoglobinopathies,* the abnormal hemoglobin is present in addition to Hb A; Hb F and Hb A_2 are structurally normal. Examples are sickle cell trait (Hb AS) and hemoglobin C trait (Hb AC). The normal Hb A quantitatively exceeds the abnormal hemoglobin present because of slower production of abnormal beta chains than of normal beta chains, selective early destruction of the red cells with higher concentrations of the abnormal hemoglobin, or selective removal of the abnormal hemoglobin from the cell.

In *heterozygous alpha hemoglobinopathies,* the abnormality in the alpha chain will affect all three hemoglobin types. Therefore, six different hemoglobin types are found—the three normal hemoglobins and the three abnormal forms. Examples are Hb $D_{Baltimore}$, Hb Ann Arbor, and Hb M_{Boston}.

Combinations of abnormalities exist. *Double heterozygotes for two beta chain abnormalities* produce two different abnormal beta chains; therefore, there are two abnormal hemoglobins and no hemoglobin A. An example of this is Hb S-C disease. Double heterozygotes for beta and delta chain abnormalities and for alpha and beta chain abnormalities are rare but have provided important information. The latter will have four major hemoglobin types on electrophoresis: $\alpha_2{}^A\beta_2{}^A$;$\alpha_2{}^X\beta_2{}^A$;$\alpha_2{}^A\beta_2{}^Y$; and $\alpha_2{}^X\beta_2{}^Y$.

Double heterozygotes for beta hemoglobinopathy and beta thalassemia are well known. Here, the quantity of abnormal hemoglobin exceeds the normal hemoglobin, in contrast to the heterozygous beta hemoglobinopathies, in which the reverse is true. Examples are Hb S thalassemias and Hb E thalassemia.

BETA HEMOGLOBINOPATHIES

Hemoglobins S, C, D, and E are believed to be polymorphisms because their frequency is greater than can be explained by mutation alone (Lehmann, 1977). They occur in homozygous as well as heterozygous form and involve the beta chain.

Sickle Cell Disease. Homozygous Hb S disease is a serious chronic hemolytic anemia, first manifest in early childhood and often fatal before the age of 30 years. With modern medical care, however, many patients live longer. Hemoglobin S is found almost exclusively in the black population; 0.1 to 0.2 per cent of the blacks born in the United States have sickle cell anemia (Schneider, 1976).

In hemoglobin S the glutamic acid in the sixth position on the beta chain is replaced by valine. This substitution is on the surface of the molecule and changes its charge and, hence, its electrophoretic mobility. Hemoglobin S is freely soluble when fully oxygenated; when oxygen is removed from Hb S, polymerization of the abnormal hemoglobin occurs, forming tactoids (fluid crystals) which are rigid and deform the cell into the shape which gave the cell its name. In homozygous Hb S disease, sickling occurs at physiologic oxygen tensions and the rigidity of the red cells is responsible for the hemolysis as well as for most of the complications. The rigid cells are more vulnerable to trauma and are readily trapped by the reticuloendothelial system, especially the spleen, accounting for the hemolysis. As a result of the hemolysis, severe continued marrow hyperplasia during childhood produces bone changes: expansion of the marrow space, thinning of the cortex, and radial striations seen in the skull on x-ray. Leg ulcers are common.

Complications. In early childhood, bilateral painful swelling of the dorsa of the hands or feet occurs as a result of sickling and capillary stasis; this is known as the *hand-foot syndrome* or sickle cell dactylitis. It lasts about two weeks, is accompanied by changes of periostitis as observed by x-ray, and does not occur after the age of four.

The spleen is central to three complications: A *sequestration crisis* refers to sudden pooling of blood and rapid enlargement of the spleen, resulting in hypovolemic shock. This may occur in early childhood when splenomegaly is present. *Functional asplenia* (Pearson, 1969) consists of inadequate antibody responses under some conditions and an impaired ability of the reticuloendothelial system to clear bacteria and particulate material from the blood, probably due to reticuloendothelial blockade. This may partly explain the increased risk of infection in children with the disease. Salmonella and pneumococcal infections are unusually prevalent in children with sickle cell anemia. Vaso-occlusive episodes result in progressive infarction, fibrosis, and contraction of the spleen, so-called *autosplenectomy*. Though splenomegaly is present in childhood, a small fibrotic remnant is the rule in the adult.

From early childhood, patients cannot produce a concentrated urine, apparently as a result of anoxic damage in the medullae of the kidneys. Hematuria as a result of papillary necrosis is common.

Vaso-occlusive crises are debilitating episodes of abdominal and bone or joint pain, accompanied by fever, which are probably due to plugging of small blood vessels by masses of sickled cells. Bone necrosis occurs and may be a focus for salmonella osteomyelitis. Aseptic necrosis of the femoral head is occasionally a complication. The various complications as a result of recurring vaso-occlusive crises involve many systems (Diggs, 1965).

Aplastic crises can occasionally afflict any patient with chronic hemolytic anemia. A temporary failure of red cell production which would not be noticed in a person with a normal red cell life span will cause a serious fall in hemoglobin concentration in hemolytic anemia. This may be a result of infection, exposure to toxic drugs, or folic acid deficiency; sometimes no cause can be found. *Hemolytic crises* due to a further increase in hemolysis are rare. Other causes for an increase in jaundice (e.g., gallstones, hepatitis) should be sought.

Blood. The anemia is normochromic and normocytic; polychromasia is increased; normoblasts are present. Target cells are numerous, and Howell-Jolly bodies are regularly seen in older children and adults as a result of asplenia. Sickle cells are often found in the stained smear (Fig. 29–13; Plate 29–2*A*). The microhematocrit as an estimate of degree of anemia is unreliable because of excessive plasma trapping. Osmotic fragility is usually decreased, and mechanical fragility is increased. Neutrophilia and thrombocytosis are usual. The marrow shows normoblastic hyperplasia and increased storage iron.

Sickling Test—Metabisulfite. Adding sodium metabisulfite, a reducing substance, to blood enhances deoxygenation of Hb and sickling of Hb S (Plate 29–2*D*). The test does

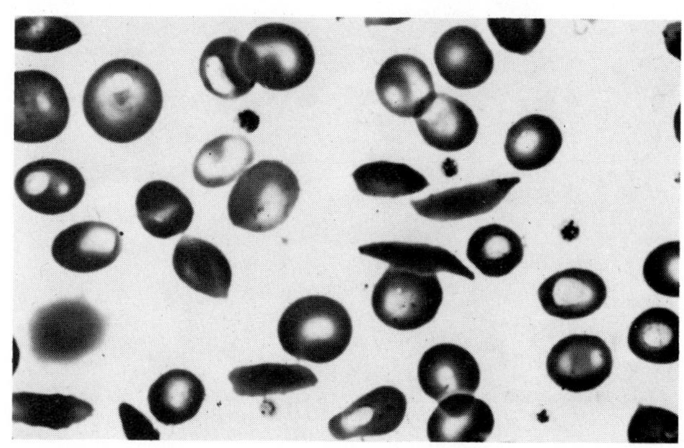

Figure 29–13. Sickle cell anemia. Note that the elongated pointed cells have greater density in the center than near the edges, in contrast to elliptocytes. Linked molecules of reduced Hb S, forming tactoids, distort the cells. (×875.)

4

not distinguish sickle cell anemia from sickle trait or other Hb S syndromes since all red cells sickle; sickling occurs more rapidly, however, with greater amounts of Hb S in the cells. Positive tests may occur with other rare abnormal hemoglobins (e.g., Hb C Harlem and Hb I) and Hb Bart's. False negative tests may occur if Hb S concentration is <10 per cent (as in very young infants) or if deoxygenation is inadequate (e.g., deterioration of reagent).

Solubility Test—Dithionite. Red cells are lysed, Hb S is reduced by dithionite (sodium hydrosulfite), and the reduced Hb S is insoluble in concentrated inorganic buffers. The polymers of deoxy Hb S obstruct light rays and produce opacity. The test is useful in screening large numbers of people for the presence of Hb S or other sickling hemoglobins. Positive reactions (turbid solution) occur also in the presence of many Heinz bodies, as in unstable hemoglobin disorders after splenectomy, and in blood protein disorders due to precipitation of plasma proteins. Negative reactions (clear solution) occur with normal and most abnormal Hbs, and also if the amount of Hb S is too small, as in severe anemia, or if the reagent has deteriorated.

Hb Electrophoresis, pH 8.4. If the patient has not been recently transfused, no Hb A, over 80 per cent Hb S, 1 to 20 per cent Hb F, and 2 to 4.5 per cent Hb A_2 may be found (Wrightstone, 1974). The fetal hemoglobin is distributed unevenly among the red cells. Hb S, Hb D, and Hb G (Philadelphia) have the same electrophoretic mobility but, of these, only Hb S gives a positive sickle cell test. Hb D and Hb G also migrate differently from Hb S in agar gel electrophoresis at an acid pH (Fig. 29–12; p. 676).

Sickle Cell Trait (Hb AS). Sickle cell trait is probably the most common hemoglobinopathy in the United States. This heterozygous condition is present in about 9 per cent of American blacks (Schneider, 1976). Under normal circumstances no clinical signs of disease or hematologic abnormalities are present. However, acidosis or hypoxia due to aircraft flight, respiratory infection, anesthesia, or congestive heart failure may cause sickling and vascular complications with visceral infarcts, including hematuria. Impaired ability to concentrate urine is found in adults with the trait. Sickle cell trait confers protection on children from the lethal effects of falciparum malaria, which may account for the major distribution of Hb S in central Africa.

The stained blood film appears normal, except perhaps for a few target cells. Blood cell counts are normal. The sickle cell preparation is positive, and almost all the red cells eventually sickle. The solubility test is positive.

Electrophoresis. Hb A, 50 to 65 per cent; Hb S, 35 to 45 per cent; Hb F, normal; Hb A_2, normal to slightly increased, up to 4.5 per cent. Less than 35 per cent Hb S often indicates the coexistence of one or more α thalassemia genes (Weatherall, 1981), which is also associated with microcytosis.

Hemoglobin C Disease. Homozygous hemoglobin C disease is a mild hemolytic anemia with splenomegaly which is often asymptomatic but occasionally results in jaundice and abdominal discomfort. In the United States, 0.02 per cent of blacks have Hb C disease (Schneider, 1976).

Blood. Slight normochromic normocytic anemia with an admixture of microcytes and spherocytes, minimal increase in reticulocytes, and numerous target cells (40 to 90 per cent) are seen in the blood. Osmotic fragility is biphasic, with both increased and decreased fragility. Hexagonal or rod-shaped crystals may be seen in erythrocytes in the stained smear, especially after splenectomy or after slow drying of the smear (Fig. 29–14; Plate 29–2*B* and *C*). If red cells are incubated in 3 per cent saline, crystal-like inclusions appear in almost every cell. This tendency of the hemoglobin to form rod-shaped inclusions apparently increases the rigidity of the cells and increases their likelihood of being trapped and destroyed in the spleen (Conley, 1967).

Electrophoresis. No Hb A; over 90 per cent Hb C; less than 7 per cent Hb F. Hb E and Hb O-Arab have the same migration as Hb C on alkaline electrophoresis. They can be separated on agar gel at an acid pH (Fig. 29–12; p. 676).

Hemoglobin C Trait (Hb AC). Hemoglobin C is prevalent in West Africans and in about 2 to 3 per cent of American blacks. The heterozygous state is asymptomatic, without anemia, and mild hypochromia and target cells (up to 40 per cent) may be present.

Electrophoresis. Hb C, 35 to 45 per cent; Hb A, 55 to 65 per cent. Lower proportions of Hb C and microcytosis usually are associated with coexistence of α thalassemia.

Hemoglobin D Disease and Trait. Hemoglobin D is found in India. Hb D-Punjab and Hb D-Los Angeles are the same ($\alpha_2\beta_2{}^{121\ Gln}$) and constitute the most common D-variant in American blacks (<0.02

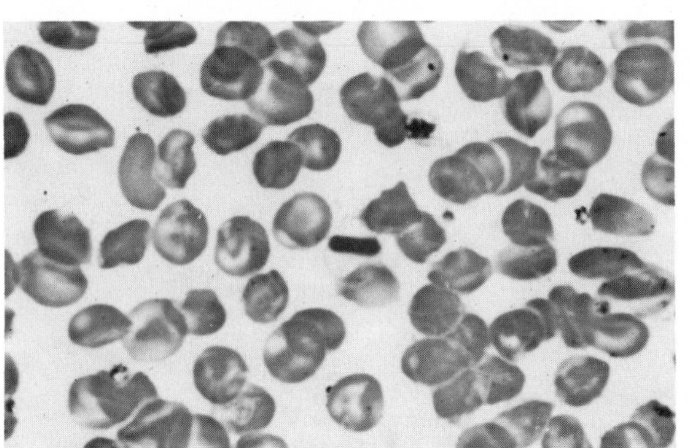

Figure 29–14. Hemoglobin C disease, postsplenectomy. Prior to splenectomy the only morphologic abnormality was the presence of target cells. After splenectomy Howell-Jolly bodies and hemoglobin crystals, such as that in the center, were present. Note that almost all of the hemoglobin in this particular cell is in the dark bar, and the membrane is still visible. Some such crystals are distinctly hexagonal. (×875.)

per cent). The trait is asymptomatic, with no anemia and a normal blood smear. Homozygous Hb D disease is very rare, and has virtually no symptoms and no hemolytic anemia. In some individuals, target cells and decreased osmotic fragility are found.

Electrophoresis. Hb D and Hb G Philadelphia ($\alpha_2{}^{68\ Lys}\beta_2$) have mobilities on alkaline electrophoresis identical to that of Hb S but have negative solubility and sickling tests. Hb D and Hb G migrate differently from Hb S on agar gel at an acid pH. Because alpha chains are affected, Hb G will show a double Hb A_2 band on alkaline electrophoresis. Hb G is probably somewhat more frequent than Hb D in American blacks (Schneider, 1976).

In Hb D disease, Hb D is about 95 per cent, and Hb A_2 is normal. In the trait, Hb D accounts for less than half of the total hemoglobin.

Hemoglobin E Disease and Trait. Hb E is found in Southeast Asia, primarily in Orientals, but does occur in blacks. Hb AE (the trait) is asymptomatic and has no hematologic abnormalities. Individuals homozygous for Hb E have a mild anemia with microcytosis and target cells and a slightly decreased red cell survival. Osmotic fragility is decreased. In Southeast Asia, iron deficiency and thalassemias are prevalent. Hb E-beta thalassemia tends to be a severe disease resembling homozygous β thalassemia; Hb A is reduced or absent. In combination with α thalassemia, the proportion of Hb E is lower than in the trait (Hb AE) (Bunn, 1977).

Electrophoresis. Hb E migrates similarly to Hb A_2, Hb C, and Hb O-Arab on alkaline electrophoresis. On agar gel at acid pH, Hb E migrates with Hb A, Hb O-Arab tends to separate from A, and Hb C is distinct. In the trait, Hb E is 30 to 45 per cent (Lehmann, 1977).

DOUBLY HETEROZYGOUS STATES (BETA HEMOGLOBIN)

A different abnormal beta chain inherited from each parent may result in interaction of Hb C, D, or E with Hb S to produce hemolytic anemia of variable severity.

Hemoglobin SC Disease. The frequency of Hb SC disease is about the same as that of Hb SS disease in American blacks. The severity is intermediate between sickle cell trait and sickle cell disease, with almost all the manifestations of sickle cell anemia appearing but with less frequency. The onset is usually early in childhood, but real difficulties do not occur until the teens or later. Fatigue, dyspnea on effort, frequent upper respiratory infections, attacks of mild jaundice, and arthralgias are seen. Crises are usually rare and mild. Painful crisis occurs more often in joints and muscles than in the abdomen. Constant hip and low back pain may be present with aseptic necrosis of the head of the femur on x-ray. Hematuria and splenic infarcts have been described. Leg ulcers occur only occasionally. In pregnancy there is a tendency toward increased frequency of crises—both clinical and hematologic. Painful crises are related to infarction, and sudden death may occur following childbirth. In contrast to sickle cell anemia, splenomegaly is usually present. The body habitus is normal or stocky in contrast to the asthenic features in sickle cell anemia.

Blood. Anemia varies from moderate to very mild and is normochromic normocytic. Anisocytosis and poikilocytosis are mild to severe, and target cells are numerous—up to 85 per cent of the erythrocytes. Plump and angulated sickled cells are often present on the film. The sickling test is positive.

Electrophoresis. Hb C and Hb S occur in about equal amounts. Hb F ranges from normal to 7 per cent. Because no normal beta chains can be produced, Hb A is absent.

Hemoglobin SD Disease. SD disease simulates but is less severe than sickle cell anemia, and thus may also resemble SC disease. The sickling test is positive.

Electrophoresis. The pattern is indistinguishable from sickle cell anemia because Hb S and Hb D cannot be separated on routine (alkaline) electrophoresis. Agar gel electrophoresis at pH 6.2 will separate Hb S and Hb D; solubility studies (Hb D is more soluble than Hb S) and family studies will help to reveal the true nature of the condition. One parent is likely to have a negative sickling test and an abnormal hemoglobin with the mobility of Hb S.

Other doubly heterozygous beta hemoglobinopathies occur but are even less common.

HETEROZYGOUS HEMOGLOBINOPATHIES

A number of amino acid substitutions occur in the heme pocket where they either increase the stability of the methemoglobin form (Hb M) or alter the affinity of the heme for oxygen; the latter usually alters the stability of the molecule as well.

Other substitutions affect the αβ contact sites; these also can change stability and oxygen affinity of the molecule (Perutz, 1968).

These functionally significant hemoglobinopathies are heterozygous; usually the concentration of the abnormal hemoglobin is less than 50 per cent. Generally, the hemoglobins with abnormal alpha chains form a smaller proportion of the total (10 to 25 per cent) than do those with abnormal beta chains (35 to 50 per cent) (Bunn, 1977).

Hemoglobins Associated with Methemoglobinemia and Cyanosis

Hemoglobin M. Five abnormal hemoglobins are associated with clinical methemoglobinemia and cyanosis which do not respond to methylene blue (Table 29–3). The common feature is that all have an amino acid substitution at or near the heme group so that methemoglobin is unusually stable, and reduction to ferrous heme and hence reversible binding of oxygen are prevented.

Cyanosis from birth is seen in hemoglobin M disease with alpha chain abnormalities, but does not appear for two to four months if the abnormality is in the beta chain—that is, until beta chain production approaches adult levels. The cyanosis is, of course, not associated with enzyme abnormalities in the red cell, toxic drugs, or cyanotic heart disease, conditions which must be considered in the differential diagnosis.

All Hb M disorders thus far discovered are heterozygotes. Some types of Hb M will not separate from Hb A on alkaline electrophoresis. If the hemolysate is first converted to methemoglobin, the Hb M will migrate differently from normal methemoglobin at pH 7.1. The absorption spectra of the eluted Hb M, which may be distinctive, can be compared with that of normal methemoglobin (Bunn, 1977). Amino acid analysis of peptide maps of tryptic digests of the abnormal hemoglobin will enable identification of the Hb M. This may be performed at a reference laboratory.

Hemoglobins Associated with Altered Oxygen Affinity

Increased Affinity and Polycythemia. Over 50 alpha and beta chain abnormalities have been described (Winslow, 1983). Some are listed in Table 29–3. The oxygen dissociation curve is shifted to the left. The P_{50}, the partial pressure of oxygen at which hemoglobin is 50 per cent saturated, is decreased. Under physiologic conditions, the normal P_{50} of whole blood is 26 mm Hg; in this disorder it has ranged from 5 to 23 mm Hg. Since the hemoglobin has high affinity for oxygen, the tissues are relatively hypoxic at any given Po_2, resulting in increased erythropoietin production and polycythemia. Since the amino acid substitution is inside the molecule, usually the abnormal hemoglobin is indistinguishable from Hb A on electrophoresis (Stamatoyannopoulos, 1971).

Hemoglobin Chesapeake. An alpha chain abnormality associated with mild asymptomatic polycythemia in a Caucasian family was the first described (Charache, 1966). The features were similar to those of benign familial polycythemia. The abnormal hemoglobin, accounting for about 30 per cent of the total, had an increased affinity for oxygen which resulted in significantly elevated hematocrit levels. The abnormal hemoglobin could be detected by starch block or starch gel electrophoresis.

These disorders are autosomal dominant; only heterozygotes have been described. The hemoglobin concentration has ranged from 15 to 23.8 g/dl. Only about half of these abnormal hemoglobins can be separated from Hb A by starch gel or cellulose acetate electrophoresis at pH 8.6. Measurement of oxygen affinity is required to establish the diagnosis (Bunn, 1977).

Decreased Affinity and Cyanosis. Six abnormal hemoglobins are stable and have decreased oxygen affinity (Table 29–3; Bunn, 1977). The oxygen dissociation curve is shifted to the right, and the P_{50} is increased. Two of these are associated with cyanosis. The hemoglobin level may be somewhat low on the basis of the high P_{50}.

Hemoglobin Kansas. This hemoglobin, described in a Caucasian boy, had just the opposite property from Hb Chesapeake, an abnormally low affinity for oxygen. The clinical features were cyanosis since infancy, normal arterial oxygen tension, and reduced oxygen saturation. Electrophoresis after conversion to methemoglobin allowed separation from Hb A (Reissman, 1961).

UNSTABLE HEMOGLOBINS (White, 1971; Winslow, 1983)

Over 70 variants have been described in which the hemoglobin precipitates within the red cell as Heinz bodies. Some are listed in Table 29–3. Most of the abnormalities are beta chain; some are alpha. Amino acid substitution or deletion renders the Hb molecule unstable through molecular mechanisms discussed in the references cited. Precipitated Hb attaches to the cell membrane and shortens its survival; the cells are inflexible; Heinz bodies are removed by the spleen; the further damaged cells have a shortened survival. The oxygen affinity is usually abnormal and may be increased or decreased. Some of these unstable hemoglobins have been defined as the cause of what were originally called "congenital Heinz body hemolytic anemias."

All patients have been heterozygous. The clinical features have shown considerable variation, from severe hemolytic anemia in the first year of life (e.g., Hb Hammersmith, Hb Bristol) to a very mild chronic hemolytic anemia (e.g., Hb Louisville, Hb Hasharon) which may be exacerbated by drugs (e.g., Hb Zurich). A few unstable hemoglobins have been discovered incidentally in clinically normal individuals (e.g., Hb Tacoma, Hb Sogn).

Jaundice and splenomegaly are common, as in other hemolytic anemias. More distinctive in some cases is the excretion of darkly pigmented urine (only during hemolytic crises in mild variants). The urine pigment appears to be a dipyrrole, probably a breakdown product of denatured hemoglobin. Cyanosis is present in some patients and is due to met- and sulfhemoglobinemia or to low oxygen affinity.

The anemia is normocytic and normochromic to hypochromic, the latter because of the loss of hemoglobin from the cells (in the form of Heinz bodies) in the reticuloendothelial organs. Patients with relatively high hemoglobin concentrations in the steady state usually have hemoglobin variants with a high oxygen affinity and an unexpectedly high reticulocyte count (e.g., Hb Köln, Hb Gun Hill). On the other hand, patients with rather low hemoglobin concentrations may be relatively asymptomatic if their hemoglobin has a low oxygen affinity; their reticulocyte counts are unexpectedly low for the hemoglobin concentration (e.g., Hb Hammersmith). Heinz bodies are rarely seen in circulating red cells before splenectomy, though sometimes they may be generated by incubating the red cells with brilliant cresyl blue or new methylene blue. After splenectomy, Heinz bodies are readily demonstrable in a large proportion of cells; blood film shows irregularly contracted cells and basophilic stippling which may be pronounced.

In splenectomized patients, the Heinz bodies may interfere with hemoglobin determinations and with electronic platelet and white cell counts. Before measuring the absorbance of the hemolysate it should be centrifuged to remove the Heinz bodies. Platelet and leukocyte counts should be performed by visual methods.

Hemoglobin electrophoresis is normal in about one fourth of patients. Hb A_2 may be elevated in β-chain variants because of the loss of the abnormal hemoglobin from the cells. Hb F may be increased to a level of 10 to 15 per cent. The key laboratory determinations are the heat instability and isopropanol precipitation tests.

Heat Instability Test. Most unstable hemoglobins precipitate more rapidly than normal hemoglobins when incubated at 50°C. (Dacie, 1975). Both normal and unstable hemoglobins precipitate more rapidly in Tris-buffer than in phosphate buffers. In a hemolysate in Tris-buffer, an easily visible precipitate forms within an hour if an unstable hemoglobin is present; the control sample is clear or slightly cloudy. Slight precipitation is equivocal; the test should be repeated and the isopropanol precipitation test performed as well. Precipitates accounting for 10 to 40 per cent of the total Hb are found in unstable hemoglobin disorders.

Isopropanol Precipitation Test (Carrell, 1972). A relatively nonpolar solvent weakens the internal bonds of hemoglobin and decreases its stability. An unstable hemoglobin precipitates within 20 minutes in the nonpolar solvent isopropanol, whereas a normal hemolysate remains clear for 30 to 40 minutes. False positive results occur with high levels of Hb F.

Thalassemias

Thalassemias comprise a heterogeneous group of hereditary disorders of hemoglobin synthesis in persons of Mediterranean, African, and Asian ancestry.

The common characteristic of these disorders is impaired production of polypeptide chains of hemoglobin; that is, the *rate* of synthesis is diminished but the chain formed is, in most cases, structurally normal. In β thalassemias, β chain production is decreased. Alpha thalassemia, δβ, δ, and σδβ thalassemias have decreased synthesis of the respective polypeptide chains. These various conditions constitute the "thalassemia syndromes" (Weatherall, 1981). Orkin (1976), Kan (1983), and Weatherall (1983b) have summarized evidence for the genetic defects in these syndromes, which, in the majority of cases, result in a quantitative deficiency of messenger RNA (mRNA).

MOLECULAR DEFECTS

Information about the molecular abnormalities has been derived from studies employing techniques previously mentioned (p. 675) and summarized by Phillips (1981) and Weatherall (1982).

In β^0 thalassemia, β-chain synthesis is absent. The β globin genes are intact; only very rarely is the gene deleted. In some cases mRNA is absent, in other cases mRNA is present but non-functional. There is considerable heterogeneity in the molecular defects; most are as yet undetermined.

In β^+ thalassemia, β-chain synthesis is reduced. Several types of defects in transcription and processing of mRNA result in decreased amounts of β-chain mRNA.

In δβ thalassemias different deletions involving both the δ- and the β-genes have been described. In γδβ thalassemia a long deletion including the γ-genes and the δ-gene stops short of the β-gene, but the output of the latter is greatly reduced. Lepore hemoglobins have normal α-chains and abnormal δβ-chains. The latter are produced by δβ-fusion genes which are the result of unequal crossover between δ- and β-globin genes during meiosis.

The α thalassemias are generally due to gene deletions of various lengths. The α^0 thalassemia determinant (α thalassemia 1) results from deletion of both α-globin genes on the chromosome, which therefore directs no α-chain synthesis. The α^+ thalassemia determinant (α thalassemia 2) is due either to various sized *deletions* which result in the absence of one of the two α-globin genes on chromosome 16 or to *nondeletion defects* which reduce the output of mRNA.

Hb Constant Spring is due to an abnormal termination codon in an α-globin gene which results in an elongated α-chain with 31 extra amino acids. For unknown reasons, the chain synthesis is slow, resulting in the clinical findings of α thalassemia.

BETA THALASSEMIA

The clinical and hemoglobin findings in the β thalassemias are summarized in Table 29–4. The disorders are very heterogeneous, phenotypically as well as at the level of the molecular defects. The terms *thalassemia major*, *thalassemia intermedia*, and *thalassemia minor* refer to clinical severity and are not genetic designations.

Homozygous β Thalassemia (Thalassemia Major; Cooley's Anemia). With an absence (β^0) or a marked decrease (β^+) in β-chain production, γ-chain production remains high (Hb F is elevated), and there is an excess of α-chains. Aggregates of α-chains (α_4) are unstable and precipitate in the normoblast or red cell and damage the cells. Precipitates and cells are removed, causing ineffective erythropoiesis and a severe hemolytic anemia.

Clinical findings include jaundice and splenomegaly, which become evident early in childhood. Prominent frontal bones, cheek bones, and jaws impart a mongoloid appearance. These changes and the roentgenographic findings of thinned cortex of the long and flat bones and thickening of the skull with osteoporosis ("hair-on-end" appearance) reflect the extreme bone marrow hyperplasia in response to the hemolytic process. Growth is stunted and puberty is delayed. Most patients require regular transfusions, and develop problems due to iron loading. Hemochromatosis commonly develops, and the major cause of death is cardiac failure due to myocardial siderosis by the end of the third decade.

Blood. Unlike most hemolytic diseases, the anemia is hypochromic and microcytic. This is probably due to the defect in hemoglobin synthesis. Extreme poikilocytosis with bizarre shapes, target cells, ovalocytosis, Cabot rings, Howell-Jolly bodies, nuclear fragments, siderocytes, anisochromia, anisocytosis, and often extreme normoblastosis are present. Poikilocy-

Table 29–4. BETA THALASSEMIAS*

Syndrome	Genotype	Hemoglobin Pattern	Clinical Features
Homozygous states:			
β^+ thalassemia	β^+/β^+	Thalassemia major; or thalassemia intermedia	↓ Hb A, ↑ Hb F, variable Hb A_2
β^0 thalassemia	β^0/β^0	Thalassemia major	0 Hb A, variable Hb A_2, residual Hb F
$\delta\beta^0$/thalassemia	$\delta\beta^0/\delta\beta^0$	Thalassemia intermedia	0 Hb A and Hb A_2, 100% Hb F
Hb Lepore	Lepore/Lepore	Thalassemia major	0 Hb A, Hb A_2; 75% Hb F, 25% Hb Lepore
Heterozygous states:			
β^+ thalassemia	β^+/β	Thalassemia minor	↑ Hb A_2, slight ↑ Hb F
β^0 thalassemia	β^0/β	Thalassemia minor	↑ Hb A_2, slight ↑ Hb F
$\delta\beta^0$ thalassemia	$\delta\beta^0/\delta\beta$	Thalassemia minor	5–20% Hb F
Hb Lepore	Hb Lepore/β	Thalassemia minor	↑ Hb F, ↓ Hb A_2, 5–15% Hb Lepore

*Modified from Orkin, S. H., and Nathan, D. G.: N. Engl. J. Med. *307*:32, 1982.

tosis is more striking in patients with intact spleens; normoblastosis is more severe after splenectomy. Normoblasts have hypochromic cytoplasm and, especially after splenectomy, aggregates of densely staining hemoglobin (Plate 29-2*F*), which probably represent precipitated alpha chains (with heme attached). Incubation of the blood with methyl violet (as for Heinz bodies, p. 689) stains these precipitates in both red cells and normoblasts. The reticuloycte count is less elevated than expected for the degree of anemia because of destruction of erythroid precursors in the marrow. Osmotic resistance of the red cells, serum iron, and indirect-reacting bilirubin are increased.

Marrow. Marked normoblastic hyperplasia is present. Many late normoblasts show inclusion bodies as in the blood. Intramedullary destruction of hemoglobin (ineffective erythropoiesis) is markedly increased in thalassemia major. Storage iron and sideroblasts are increased.

Hemoglobin Studies. In β^0 thalassemia, Hb A is absent, Hb F is as high as 98 per cent. and Hb A_2 is about 2 per cent. In β^+ thalassemias (Mediterranean), Hb F is 60 to 95 per cent, with Hb A present. Although Hb A_2 may or may not be increased, the ratio of A_2 to A is always increased. In blacks with β^+ thalassemia (Negro), the clinical features are less severe ("thalassemia intermedia") and transfusion is usually unnecessary; Hb F is 20 to 40 per cent, Hb A_2 is 2 to 5 per cent, and Hb A levels are higher.

Heterozygous β Thalassemia (Thalassemia Minor; Cooley's Trait). Clinical findings are as follows: The features in heterozygous β thalassemia vary from moderately severe anemia (thalassemia intermedia) to completely normal clinical findings. The severe intermediate forms of heterozygous thalassemia are rare and are found in Mediterranean individuals but not in blacks; in the latter, heterozygous thalassemia is uniformly mild. In many persons, there is a mild hypochromic, microcytic anemia with slight hemolytic jaundice and splenomegaly. Most individuals with thalassemia minor, however, have no symptoms or abnormal physical signs.

Blood. Usually there is no anemia. Characteristically, the red cell count is elevated and the hemoglobin and hematocrit are reduced. The MCH is low, usually less than 22 pg; and the MCV is low, between 50 and 70 fl. The MCHC is sometimes low but often normal. On stained films, the cells have a moderate degree of microcytosis and poikilocytosis; target cells and basophilic stippling are often present. Osmotic fragility is decreased. The serum iron is normal or high and the serum ferritin is normal.

Marrow. Normoblastic hyperplasia and elevated storage iron may be found.

Hemoglobin Studies. Hb A_2 is elevated in the 3.5 to 7 per cent range. Hb F is slightly elevated (1 to 2 per cent) in about half of the cases. If the Hb F exceeds 5 per cent, it is likely that a gene for hereditary persistence of fetal hemoglobin (HPFH) is also present.

In some cases of heterozygous β thalassemia, the Hb A_2 is normal. One form, designated *Type 1 normal Hb A_2 β thalassemia*, has a normal hemoglobin pattern and minimal hematologic changes (the "silent" β thalassemia gene). The other, *Type 2 normal Hb A_2 β thalassemia*, has typical thalassemic red cell changes. Globin synthesis studies are necessary to identify Type 1, and to distinguish Type 2 from α thalassemia minor (Weatherall, 1983a).

δβ Thalassemias. In the homozygous state, these are characterized by thalassemia intermedia and absence of both Hb A and Hb A_2. Heterozygotes have thalassemia minor, with 5 to 20 per cent Hb F and normal Hb A_2.

Hemoglobin Lepore Syndromes. Hb Lepore is an abnormal hemoglobin that has a normal α-chain combined with a composite δβ-chain (Weatherall, 1981). It probably occurred due to chromosome misalignment with crossing-over and fusion of genetic material at the δβ-gene complex. Different Hb Lepores have been described, depending on the point of fusion. Because the composite δβ-chain is synthesized at a slow rate, it results in a hypochromic microcytic red cell picture resembling the thalassemias (Table

29–4). Lepore migrates similarly to Hb S on alkaline electrophoresis.

DOUBLE HETEROZYGOSITY FOR BETA THALASSEMIA AND BETA HEMOGLOBINOPATHY

Patients doubly heterozygous for β thalassemia and a β-chain hemoglobin variant have levels of Hb A which are *less* than the level of the variant hemoglobin. In the simple sickle cell trait, for example, the level of Hb A always exceeds that of Hb S.

Sickle Cell–Thalassemia (Hb S/β Thalassemia). Hb S/β^0 thalassemia is more severe than Hb S/β^+ thalassemia. The anemia and clinical findings vary from slight to severe, with manifestations similar to those in sickle cell anemia (Hb SS). In contrast to Hb SS, the spleen in Hb S/β thalassemia remains enlarged after childhood and into adult life.

Blood. Pronounced microcytosis, variable hypochromia, and many target cells are present. Sickled cells are uncommon. The MCV and MCH are low.

Hemoglobin Studies. The solubility test and sickling test are of course positive. In Hb S/β^+ thalassemia, Hb A = 15 to 30 per cent, Hb S = over 50 per cent, Hb F = 1 to 20 per cent, and Hb A_2 is increased, usually over 4.5 per cent. Though these individuals clinically may resemble sickle trait (Hb AS), in S/β^+ thalassemia the amount of Hb S always exceeds Hb A; in Hb AS, Hb A always exceeds Hb S.

In Hb S/β^0 thalassemia, Hb A is absent, Hb S is 75 to 90 per cent, Hb F is 5 to 20 per cent, and Hb A_2 is usually increased, over 4.5 per cent. This disorder clinically and hematologically resembles sickle cell disease. The main difference is that in Hb S/β^0 thalassemia, the MCV and MCH are lower and the Hb A_2 is increased. Family study is often necessary for a clear distinction (Lehmann, 1977; Wrightstone, 1974).

Hemoglobin C–Thalassemia. This occurs mainly in blacks, in whom it tends to result in little disability. Patients of Mediterranean extraction usually have moderately severe hemolytic anemia.

Blood. The MCH and MCV are reduced. On the blood film are hypochromic target cells, fragmented red cells, and microspherocytes, many of which have a folded appearance.

Hemoglobin Studies. In Hb C β^0 thalassemia, Hb C is 90 to 95 per cent, Hb F is 5 to 10 per cent, and Hb A is absent. In Hb C β^+ thalassemia, Hb A is 20 to 30 per cent, and Hb C 70 to 80 per cent. Hb A_2 levels cannot be studied when Hb C is present, as there are no satisfactory methods for separating the two.

Hemoglobin E–Thalassemia. In this Southeast Asian disorder, a clinical and hematologic picture similar to thalassemia major is usual.

Hemoglobin Studies. Hb E, 15 to 95 per cent; Hb F, 5 to 85 per cent. It is of interest that Hb A is nearly always absent. This emphasizes the fact that absence of Hb A cannot be taken as proof of homozygosity; it must be supported by family studies.

ALPHA THALASSEMIAS

Whereas there is one β-globin gene per haploid genotype, there are two α-globin genes. The normal haplotype is designated $\alpha\alpha/$. The mild α thalassemia determinant ($-\alpha/$) is α^+ thalassemia, formerly called α thalassemia 2, a deletion of one gene. The severe α thalassemia determinant ($- -/$) is α^0 thalassemia, formerly called α thalassemia 1, a deletion of two genes. The main forms of α thalassemias are outlined in Table 29–5.

Hydrops Fetalis with Hb Bart's. Complete absence of α-chains is incompatible with life. Infants are stillborn with severe edema, marked anemia, and marked hepatosplenomegaly. The blood shows marked anisocytosis, poikilocytosis, microcytosis, and erythroblastosis. ABO or Rh incompatibility is absent. Because of the absence of α-chains, no Hb A ($\alpha_2\beta_2$)

Table 29–5. ALPHA THALASSEMIAS*

Syndrome	Genotype	Clinical Features	Hemoglobin Pattern	
			Newborn	***After First Year***
Hydrops fetalis	$- -/- -$	Fetal or neonatal death with severe anemia	Hb Bart's >80% Hb H, Hb Portland	—
Hb H disease	$- -/- \alpha$ $(- -/\alpha\alpha^{cs})$	Chronic hemolytic anemia	Hb Bart's 20–40% (Hb CS present)	Hb H 5–30% Hb Bart's ± trace (Hb CS 2–3%)
Thalassemia minor	$- -/\alpha\alpha$ $-\alpha/-\alpha$ $\alpha\boxed{\alpha}/\alpha\boxed{\alpha}$	Little or no anemia; thalassemic RBC	Hb Bart's 2–10%	None
Silent carrier	$-\alpha/\alpha\alpha$ $(\alpha\alpha/\alpha\alpha^{cs})$	No clinical or hematologic abnormality	Hb Bart's 1–2% (Hb CS present)	None (Hb CS 1%)
Normal	$\alpha\alpha/\alpha\alpha$	No clinical or hematologic abnormality	Hb Bart's 0-trace	None

α^{cs} = α-structural gene for Hb Constant Spring; $\boxed{\alpha}$ = nondeletion α-thalassemia gene.

*Modified from Wintrobe, M. M., Lee, G. R., Boggs, D. R., Bithell, T. C., Foerster, J., Athens, J. W., and Lukens, J. N.: Clinical Hematology. 8th ed. Philadelphia, Lea and Febiger, 1981.

or Hb F ($\alpha_2\gamma_2$) is present. Large quantities of Hb Bart's (γ_4) and some Hb H (β_4) are present; both of these migrate faster than Hb A on alkaline electrophoresis.

Hemoglobin H Disease. Three of the four α-genes are absent. A chronic anemia with the clinical picture of thalassemia intermedia is usual, though the severity varies. Hb H disease has been described in almost all racial groups, especially in Southeast Asia, Greece, and parts of the Middle East; it is very rare, however, in blacks.

Blood. The MCV and MCH are decreased. The blood film shows hypochromia, target cells, and anisopoikilocytosis (Plate 29-2*G*). Reticulocytes are usually 4 to 5 per cent. Vital staining of the blood with an oxidizing dye such as brilliant cresyl blue induces pale blue inclusion bodies (Hb H precipitates) in many of the red cells, which contrast with the deep blue precipitates of RNA in reticulocytes (Plate 29-2*H*, p. 670). After splenectomy, single large Heinz bodies are seen.

Hemoglobin Studies. Hemoglobin electrophoresis shows a rapidly migrating band of Hb H (β_4) accounting for 4 to 30 per cent of the hemoglobin, and traces of the slightly less rapidly migrating Hb Bart's (γ_4). Hb H can be precipitated *in vitro* and lost from the hemolysate by careless handling or prolonged storage. Hb Bart's is alkali resistant and may be measured with Hb F (which is not increased in Hb H disease). The percentage of Hb Bart's is 20 to 40 per cent at birth; it gradually falls thereafter, but the level in adults is quite variable.

Hemoglobin H Preparation. During incubation of two parts of blood in one of 1 per cent brilliant cresyl blue stain, the unstable Hb H (β_4) gradually precipitates as multiple small pale blue inclusions uniformly distributed on the red cell membrane (Plate 29-2*H* and *I*). Hb H inclusions must be distinguished from (1) the granules and reticular networks in reticulocytes, which are darker blue in color, and (2) preformed Heinz bodies, which are larger, also darker blue, and often attached to the membrane. After 10 to 20 minutes of incubation at room temperature, Hb H inclusions are present in at least half of the red cells in Hb H disease, and in a very rare red cell in α thalassemia minor. The larger Heinz bodies may be found after splenectomy in Hb H disease.

Thalassemia Minor (Heterozygous α^0 Thalassemia or Homozygous α^+ Thalassemia). Absence of two α-genes results in a clinical picture similar to β-thalassemia minor with very mild anemia, microcytosis, a normal serum iron, normal serum ferritin, and normal red cell protoporphyrin.

Hemoglobin Studies. Diagnosis is best made by finding 5 to 6 per cent Hb Bart's in cord blood; normally, only trace amounts (<0.5 per cent) are found. In adults Hb H inclusion bodies in some cases can be found in a very small percentage of red cells (perhaps 1 in 10^5), if *exhaustively sought after* (Wasi, 1974). Otherwise no evidence of hemoglobin imbalance is detectable by standard techniques, and the diagnosis is one of excluding iron deficiency and β thalassemia or demonstrating a decreased α-chain/β-chain synthesis ratio (~0.6).

Silent Carrier of α Thalassemia (Heterozygous α^+ Thalassemia). One of four α-globin genes is absent. No hematologic abnormality is detectable in adults; MCV, blood film, and hemoglobin studies are normal. In infants, Hb Bart's accounts for 1 to 2 per cent of the cord blood hemoglobin. The diagnosis cannot be made reliably in the adult.

Hemoglobin Constant Spring. Hb Constant Spring (Hb $\overline{CS}$) is an α-chain variant with 31 extra amino acids. It is synthesized slowly and results in a thalassemia-like picture (Table 29–5). The homozygous state appears as a mild thalassemia with microcytosis and 5 to 6 per cent Hb $\overline{CS}$, normal Hb A_2, trace amounts of Hb Bart's, and the rest Hb A (Weatherall, 1981). The heterozygous state shows no hematologic abnormality: normal Hb A and A_2 and about 1 per cent Hb $\overline{CS}$. The abnormal Hb migrates more slowly than Hb A_2 at alkaline pH and is easily missed. The gene behaves similarly to that in a silent carrier (α^+ thalassemia trait) and is found in about 40 per cent of cases of Hb H disease in Southeast Asia (see Table 29–5).

HEREDITARY PERSISTENCE OF FETAL HEMOGLOBIN F (HPFH)

A group of conditions with Hb F production persisting beyond infancy without significant hematologic abnormalities is known as HPFH. It is found in about 0.1 per cent of American blacks; there are also a Greek form and other variants.

In blacks, the homozygote has slightly microcytic, hypochromic red cells without anemia. Hb F = 100 per cent; no Hb A or Hb A_2 is present. This lack of β- and δ-chain synthesis has been shown to be due to deletion of the δβ-gene complex (Weatherall, 1981).

In the heterozygote, no hematologic abnormalities are found. Hb F = 20 to 30 per cent, Hb A_2 = 1 to 2.1 per cent, with the remainder Hb A. With the acid elution technique, the Hb F is homogeneously distributed among the red cells in the Negro or *pancellular* type of HPFH. This is in contrast to β thalassemia, in which the distribution is heterogeneous.

The most common *heterocellular* HPFH is the Swiss type. There are no hematologic changes and 1 to 3 per cent Hb F, which is heterogeneously distributed among the red cells. It is difficult to define because it overlaps the normal. When inherited with a β thalassemia gene the result is a higher Hb F than is found in a heterozygous β thalassemia alone (Weatherall, 1981).

PRENATAL DIAGNOSIS OF HEMOGLOBIN DISORDERS (Kan, 1983; Weatherall, 1983b)

Prevention of the occurrence of severe forms of thalassemia and of sickle cell anemia is possible through (1) genetic counseling of prospective parents and (2), if both parents are carriers, prenatal diagnosis and the option of therapeutic abortion.

Since 1974, the technique of sampling fetal blood at 15 to 20 weeks' gestation by placental aspiration or direct vision fetoscopy has been employed for the diagnosis of thalassemia major. The blood is incubated with labeled amino acids, and synthetic rates of α, β, and γ globin chains are determined. A β/γ ratio of less than 0.02 indicates homozygous β thalassemia; the normal β/γ ratio is 0.08 to 0.10 at this age. Although the fetal mortality of the procedure is 5 to 10 per cent, this procedure has been well accepted in some populations and has reduced the number of homozygotes born.

Utilizing amniocentesis (which has considerably less morbidity), it is possible to obtain fetal cells, isolate the DNA, and detect genetic abnormalities.

1. For each restriction endonuclease DNA is cleaved in many specific sites. A base substitution in DNA can eliminate (or create) a restriction recognition site. When these are in the vicinity of β globin genes, analysis of the sizes of the DNA fragments which contain the β globin gene will (in populations with certain polymorphisms) show linkage with either the thalassemia gene or the sickle gene. By studying both parents it will be possible to determine whether the findings in the fetal DNA will be decisive or not.

2. More direct analysis by restriction endonuclease gene mapping is possible for the thalassemias that show gene deletion (α thalassemias and a very few β thalassemias), but this is not useful for thalassemia major.

3. Certain restriction endonucleases (Dde I, Mst II) cleave normal DNA at the $\beta^{5,6,7}$ globin gene site; and the sickle mutation at β^{6} abolishes the cleavage site. The resulting patterns of DNA fragments which contain the β globin gene allow distinction among normal DNA, heterozygous β^{S}-DNA, and homozygous β^{S}-DNA. This, therefore, can provide accurate prenatal diagnosis of sickle cell anemia by amniocentesis (Chang, 1982; Orkin, 1982).

Hemolysis—Metabolic Disorders

Deficient enzyme activity in the erythrocyte may result in abnormalities that lead to premature destruction and hemolytic anemia; these disorders are usually inherited. Interference with or oxidative stress on erythrocyte metabolism, however, can sometimes result in hemolysis in individuals who have normal erythrocytes (see Table 14–19, p. 278).

Erythrocyte Metabolism. The mature red cell lacks mitochondria and, therefore, oxidative phosphorylation and Krebs' cycle activity. Energy production is mainly glycolytic, 90 per cent of which occurs through the Embden-Meyerhof pathway, as glucose goes to lactic acid with the net production of two moles of ATP (Fig. 29–15). ATP is needed for the energy-requiring reactions in the cell: for active cation trans-

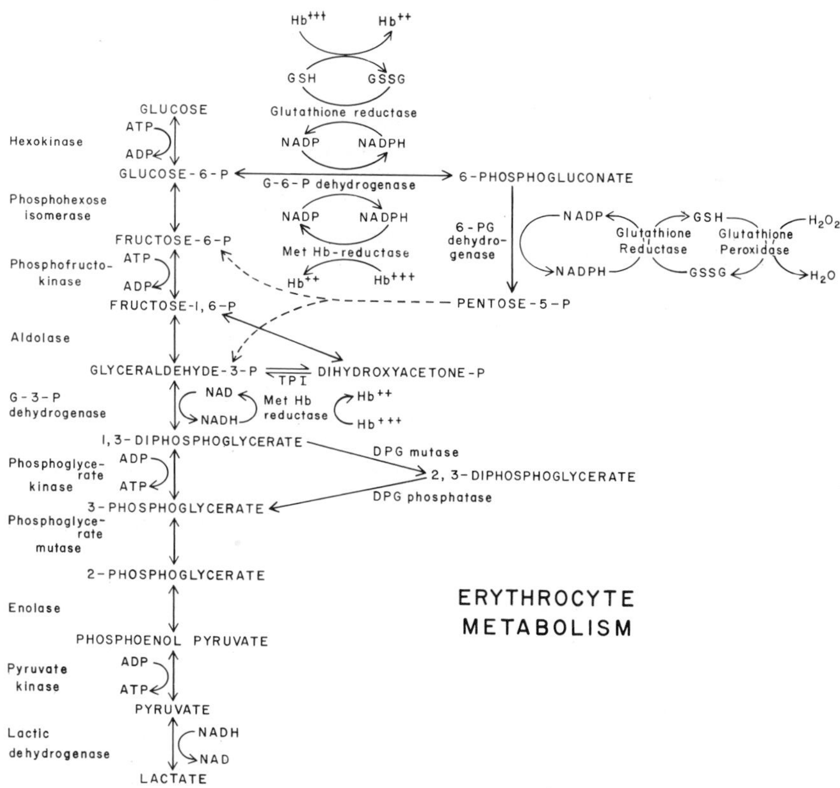

Figure 29–15. Erythrocyte metabolism is discussed in the text. Normally most hemoglobin (methemoglobin, Hb^{+++}) is reduced to hemoglobin (Hb^{++}) by nicotinamide adenine dinucleotide–linked methemoglobin reductase (NAD, Met Hb reductase). NADP-linked methemoglobin reductase requires methylene blue for activation and is more effective in drug-induced methemoglobinemia than the normal cell mechanism. GSH = reduced glutathione; GSSG = oxidized glutathione.

port across the membrane, for maintaining membrane deformability, and for preserving the cell's biconcave shape. Most of the hemiglobin (methemoglobin) produced in the normal cell (about 3 per cent of the total per day) is reduced by NAD-linked Met Hb reductase. The pentose phosphate pathway (hexose monophosphate shunt) generates NADPH in the first two steps, through the enzymes glucose-6-phosphate dehydrogenase (G6PD) and 6-phosphogluconate. NADPH production is linked to glutathione reduction and, through this mechanism, to preservation of vital enzymes and hemoglobin from oxidation. Small amounts of oxidized hemoglobin (methemoglobin) are reduced by GSH (glutathione). Activity of the pentose phosphate pathway increases when the cell is exposed to an oxidant drug, probably as a result of increased NADP production. If an enzyme in this pathway lacks activity, GSH cannot be produced and hemoglobin will be oxidized by the oxidant stress. Oxidation in the red cells is mediated by high energy derivatives of oxygen referred to collectively as activated oxygen (Carrell, 1975). Oxidized Hb denatures and precipitates as Heinz bodies which adhere to the membrane, inducing rigidity and a tendency to lysis. Moderate enzyme deficiencies in this pathway (e.g., G6PD) may not be associated with anemia; however, an acute hemolytic episode occurs if the cells are challenged by oxidant stress (e.g., drugs, infection).

Deficiencies in the Embden-Meyerhof pathway result in impaired ATP generation and a chronic hemolytic anemia. The mechanism of the red cell destruction here is less clear. Heinz bodies are not formed. It appears that lack of cell deformability and impaired cation pumping may be important in the hemolytic process (LaCelle, 1971).

The Rapoport-Luebering shunt provides for the conversion of 1,3-diphosphoglycerate (1,3-DPG) to 2,3-diphosphoglycerate (2,3-DPG) instead of directly to 3-phosphoglycerate (3-PG) (Fig. 29–15). If this shunt is operating, generation of two moles of ATP (per mole of glucose) is bypassed; the result is no net energy production in glycolysis. However, 2,3-DPG combines with the β-chain of hemoglobin and decreases the affinity of hemoglobin for oxygen. At a given partial pressure of oxygen, therefore, increased 2,3-DPG allows more oxygen to leave hemoglobin and go to the tissues; the oxygen dissociation curve is shifted to the right (p. 632, Fig. 28–2). Increased activity of this shunt is apparently stimulated by hypoxia.

Glucose-6-Phosphate Dehydrogenase (G6PD) Deficiency (Beutler, 1978). About 10 per cent of male American blacks who were given the anti-malarial drug primaquine during the Korean War developed a self-limited, acute hemolytic anemia. Only the older red cells were destroyed, and it was found that the deficiency in the susceptible red cells was in G6PD.

It has since been found that G6PD deficiency is widespread throughout the world. Among Caucasians, the highest incidence is in Kurdish Jews; the deficiency is also found in blacks and in Orientals.

Since G6PD is determined by a gene on the X chromosome, full expression of the deficiency is found in the male hemizygote. Partial expression may be found in the heterozygous female who has two populations of red cells, one normal and one deficient. The deficiency of G6PD limits the regeneration of NADPH, which renders the cell vulnerable to oxidative denaturation of hemoglobin. Since, normally, G6PD is highest in young cells and decreases as the cell ages, in persons with G6PD deficiency the older cells are preferentially destroyed.

Hemolytic susceptibility in affected persons can increase greatly during intercurrent illness or upon exposure to various drugs which have oxidant properties (Table 29–6).

The genetic heterogeneity is great and is expressed as variation in the stability and the electrophoretic and catalytic properties of the enzymes, in the degree of deficiency, in the types of cells in the body affected, in the types of drugs which will produce hemolysis, and in the susceptibility to chronic hemolysis or to neonatal jaundice (Oski, 1972). The most common ("normal") G6PD isozyme in all population groups is designated as B. In blacks, an electrophoretically more rapid variant, A, is prevalent and has almost the same activity; 20 per cent of black males have this variant. Eleven per cent of black males have the A-type of G6PD, which has only 5 to 15 per cent of the normal enzyme activity; it is these individuals who are susceptible to hemolysis after ingesting oxidant drugs or during infection. The most common variant in Caucasians is G6PD-Mediterranean, found in Mediterranean populations; the level of enzyme activity in affected males is low, often less than 1 per cent. These individuals usually are not anemic, but may have somewhat more severe and non–self-limited hemolytic anemia with infections, and with a wider variety of drugs than the black variant (Beutler, 1978). In a subgroup of G6PD deficient subjects, severe hemolysis may occur within hours after eating fava beans ("favism"). Although the vast majority of G6PD-deficient subjects worldwide are not anemic, a small proportion of persons with G6PD-Mediterranean (and persons with some rarer variants) have a chronic non-spherocytic hemolytic anemia.

The laboratory findings during active hemolysis are

Table 29–6. DRUGS AND CHEMICALS WHICH HAVE CLEARLY BEEN SHOWN TO CAUSE CLINICALLY SIGNIFICANT HEMOLYTIC ANEMIA IN G-6-PD DEFICIENCY*

Acetanilid	Pentaquine
Methylene blue	Phenylhydrazine
Nalidixic acid (Negram)	Primaquine
	Sulfacetamide
Naphthalene	Sulfanilamide
Niridazole (Ambilhar)	Sulfamethoxazole (Gantanol)
	Sulfapyridine
Nitrofurantoin (Furadantin)	Thiazolesulfone
	Toluidine blue
Pamaquine	Trinitrotoluene (TNT)

*From Beutler, E.: Hemolytic Anemia in Disorders of Red Cell Metabolism. New York, Plenum Medical Book Company, 1978.

those of hemolytic anemia in general. In the blood film, one finds poikilocytes, some spherocytes, and irregularly contracted cells which stain densely and have contraction of Hb from a part of the cell membrane. These probably are cells from which Heinz bodies have been removed by the spleen. After supravital staining with methyl violet, Heinz bodies may be present early in an acute hemolytic episode. G6PD deficiency may be detected by one of the screening tests: the dye reduction test, the ascorbate cyanide test, or a fluorescent spot test. Confirmation is made with a quantitative assay.

Heinz Bodies (Dacie, 1975). When hemoglobin denatures, it forms precipitates which are known as Heinz bodies. These precipitates cannot be detected in Romanowsky stained, air-dried blood films, but after vital staining with methyl violet or crystal violet, Heinz bodies stain deep purple. They vary from 1 to 4 μm in diameter and often attach to the red cell membrane. They also stain, but less intensely, as pale blue inclusions in reticulocyte stains, e.g., new methylene blue.

The presence of Heinz bodies in freshly drawn blood indicates that (1) an oxidizing drug or chemical (e.g., phenylhydrazine, chlorate, naphthalene, dapsone) has been ingested in sufficient amount to overwhelm the normal protective mechanisms of the red cell and denature hemoglobin; (2) a drug such as primaquine (Table 29–6) has been ingested by an individual with G6PD deficiency (or another defect resulting in a deficiency of reduced glutathione) so that hemoglobin is not protected from oxidative denaturation; or (3) the subject has an unstable hemoglobin or thalassemia.

Dye Reduction Test of Motulsky (Dacie, 1975). This test is conveniently performed using commercially available kits. In principle, a mixture of glucose-6-phosphate, NADP, and brilliant cresyl blue dye in buffer is incubated with hemolysate. If G6PD is present, the NADP will be reduced to NADPH (Fig. 29–15), which, in turn, will reduce the blue dye to its colorless form. The time needed for this reduction to take place is noted for the patient's blood and for that of a normal control with an identical hemoglobin concentration (adjusted if necessary). This time is inversely proportional to the amount of G6PD present and is prolonged in G6PD-deficient subjects.

The dye reduction test is specific and can be performed on stored blood. It has the advantage that it can be performed on microsamples, but is likely to give false negative results in heterozygotes and black males with G6PD deficiency during a hemolytic episode (Fairbanks, 1969).

Ascorbate Cyanide Test (Jacob, 1966). When blood is incubated with a solution of sodium cyanide and sodium ascorbate, hydrogen peroxide is generated from the coupled oxidation of ascorbate and hemoglobin. Cyanide inhibits catalase, hydrogen peroxide is available to oxidize hemoglobin, and the brown color of methemoglobin is discernible. This occurs more rapidly in G6PD-deficient cells than in normal cells.

The ascorbate cyanide test is not specific, in that pyruvate kinase deficiency, paroxysmal nocturnal hemoglobinuria, and unstable hemoglobins will give a positive result. It is the most sensitive of the screening tests, in that it uses intact cells and will detect the deficiency in black males during hemolytic episodes and in heterozygotes (Fairbanks, 1969).

Fluorescent Spot Test. Whole blood is added to a mixture of glucose-6-phosphate (G6P), NADP, saponin, and buffer, and a spot of this mixture is placed on filter paper and observed for fluorescence with ultraviolet light. If G6PD is present, NADP is converted to NADPH. Since phosphogluconate dehydrogenase is present in most hemolysates, further NADP is converted to NADPH (Fig. 29–15). NADPH fluoresces but NADP does not. The normal control sample fluoresces brightly, and lack of fluorescence indicates G6PD deficiency. By reoxidizing any small amounts of NADPH formed, oxidized glutathione (GSSG) enhances the ability of the test to detect mild G6PD deficiency. This is the recommended screening test for G6PD deficiency (Beutler, 1979b).

Quantitative Assay of G6PD (Beutler, 1975). For G6PD, most assays are based on the rate of reduction of NADP to NADPH, measured spectrometrically at 340 nm, when a hemolysate is incubated with G6P.

In heterozygotes or in acute hemolysis in black subjects with G6PD deficiency, the diagnosis may be obscured even with the assay because of the increased level of G6PD in reticulocytes and younger erythrocytes. Usually, however, the ascorbate cyanide screening test will be positive in these instances.

Pyruvate Kinase Deficiency (Tanaka, 1962). The most common red cell enzyme deficiency involving the Embden-Meyerhof glycolytic pathway, PK deficiency results in a mild to moderately severe hemolytic anemia with splenomegaly. The anemia may be detected in infancy, or not until adult life in milder cases. Patients tolerate the anemia rather well because of high levels of 2,3-DPG, which occur as a result of the block in glycolysis. The blood film may show no notable red cell abnormalities until after splenectomy, when echinocytes, irregularly contracted cells, and crenated red cells may be prominent. Reticulocyte counts are elevated, and increase further after splenectomy.

Inheritance is autosomal recessive, but this is probably true only in consanguineous families. PK mutants are numerous and are not detected in phenotypically normal heterozygotes who have one half the normal PK activity. Most PK deficient hemolytic anemias are therefore probably double heterozygotes for two mutant genes (Valentine, 1979). Acquired PK deficiency occurs occasionally in myelodysplastic disorders and leukemias (Valentine, 1979; Miwa, 1981).

The autohemolysis test gives variable results. Some patients show only a mild increase in autohemolysis that is partially prevented by glucose (Type I), and others have a greater increase that is not prevented by glucose (Type II). Heinz bodies are not found. The diagnosis is made by a specific screening test or enzyme assay.

Splenectomy is indicated in cases requiring transfusions. After splenectomy, the hemoglobin usually increases by 1 to 2 g/dl, and the reticulocytes increase sharply, although hemolysis persists (Miwa, 1981).

Fluorescent Spot Test (Beutler, 1975). Pyruvate kinase catalyzes the phosphorylation of ADP to ATP by phosphoenolypyruvate (PEP) with the formation of pyruvate. Pyruvate then reduces any NADH present to NAD with the formation of lactate (see Fig. 29–15). Loss of fluorescence of NADH under ultraviolet light is observed as evidence of the presence of PK.

Leukocytes must be removed from the sample because normally they contain about 300 times as much PK as do red cells, and in PK deficiency the red cells but not the leukocytes are deficient.

Quantitative Assay of PK. The same principle is employed as in the screening test, but the rate of decrease of O.D. at 340 nm is measured. A negative screening test or a normal PK assay (using the standard high substrate [PEP] concentrations) does not rule out PK-deficient hemolytic anemia. Since mutant PK enzymes may have normal activity at high PEP concentrations and decreased activity at low PEP concentrations, it is necessary to perform the assay in both ways (Beutler, 1975).

Other Glycolytic Enzyme Deficiencies (Valentine, 1979; Keitt, 1981). Other enzyme deficiencies in the *Embden-Meyerhof pathway* are rarer. When severe, they produce hemolytic anemias, with two exceptions: (1) Lactate dehydrogenase deficiency has no clinical manifestations. (2) Deficiencies of 2,3-DPG mutase and 2,3-DPG phosphatase activities occur together and result in erythrocytosis as a result of lack of 2,3-DPG, shifting the oxygen dissociation curve of Hb to the left.

Other enzyme deficiencies in the *hexose monophosphate* shunt are quite rare. They include the two enzymes involved in glutathione synthesis: γ-glutamyl cysteine synthetase and glutathione synthetase. As in G6PD deficiency, hemolysis increases with oxidant drug exposure or infection.

There is no good evidence, however, for the causation of chronic hemolytic anemia by 6-phosphogluconate deficiency, glutathione reductase (GR) deficiency, or glutathione peroxidase (GP_x) deficiency (Beutler, 1979a). GR contains flavine-adenine dinucleotide and is often partially deficient because of dietary riboflavin deficiency. GP_x is one half normal in about 30 per cent of the Jewish population due to homozygosity for a gene for low GP_x activity; in addition, GP_x activity is dependent on selenium intake in the diet. In neither case is there an association with a hematologic disorder.

Pyrimidine-5′-Nucleotidase (PN) Deficiency (Paglia, 1981). When RNA is degraded in the reticulocyte, pyrimidine nucleotides must be dephosphorylated by PN in order to cross the red cell membrane. Autosomal recessive PN deficiency results in accumulation of pyrimidines, and the impaired degradation of RNA results in pronounced basophilic stippling in red cells on the blood film. This is probably one of the more common enzyme deficiencies responsible for hereditary hemolytic anemia (Beutler, 1979a).

The disorder is characterized by mild to moderate chronic hemolysis, reticulocytosis (~10 per cent), marked basophilic stippling, and splenomegaly without notable improvement after splenectomy. A screening test employs measurement of the U.V. absorption spectrum of deproteinized extracts of red cells. In PN deficiency the major absorption peak is shifted from the normal 258 nm to 270 to 280 nm, due to the residual pyrimidine nucleotides UDP and CDP. Diagnosis requires demonstration of decreased nucleosidase activities.

Acquired PN deficiency occurs in lead poisoning and is probably responsible for the basophilic stippling in that condition.

Hemolysis—Acquired; Extrinsic

CHEMICAL AGENTS

Agents Hemolytic to Normal Cells. The action of chemical agents depends on the dose and on other factors, many of which are known only vaguely. They range from simple substances, such as water, to some that are highly complex.

When used as irrigating fluid, distilled water was found responsible for acute hemolytic anemia as a result of entry into venous channels during transurethral resection.

In addition to anemia some chemicals produce methemoglobinemia, and some are responsible for cyanosis (toluene, trinitrotoluene, nitrobenzene, acetanilid, and phenacetin). Some may lead to aplastic anemia (toluene and trinitrotoluene). Promin, a sulfone derivative, makes blood turn chocolate brown.

Lead toxicity may produce progressive anemia, with basophilic stippling, reticulocytosis, normoblastemia, Cabot's rings, Howell-Jolly bodies, and leukocytosis. Lead not only causes damage to the red cell and hemolysis, but also produces defects in the heme synthetic pathway. In cases of chronic exposure to lead, basophilic stippling, more in the marrow than in the peripheral blood, and coproporphyrinuria are the characteristic findings. These changes produce defective erythrocytes, which are removed by the spleen.

Agents Hemolytic to Abnormal Cells. Certain drugs and chemicals which have oxidizing activity (Table 29–6) may produce hemolytic anemia in individuals with G6PD deficiency or other defects resulting in glutathione deficiency. In addition, unstable hemoglobins such as Hb Zürich have a propensity for drug-induced hemolytic anemia. Premature infants, although they have high levels of G6PD, have glutathione instability and low levels of glutathione and may develop hemolytic anemia when given large doses of synthetic water-soluble analogues of vitamin K.

It must be remembered that, if the exposure to these oxidant substances is great enough, acute hemolytic anemia may be produced in normal individuals.

During the acute hemolytic episode, Heinz bodies can frequently be demonstrated by direct vital staining of blood with methyl violet. Red cells with Heinz bodies are removed from the circulation by the spleen, or the Heinz bodies are extracted from the red cells by splenic action. Therefore, Heinz bodies may not be found in the blood if the spleen is effectively removing them or after the acute hemolytic process has abated.

Tests for G6PD deficiency, the most common underlying cause of drug-sensitive hemolytic anemia, are described on page 689.

PHYSICAL AGENTS

Heat. Extensive burns produce hemolytic anemia, probably because of direct damage to red cells. The blood film may show remarkable morphologic abnormalities of the red cells, including budding fragmentation of the membrane and microspherocytosis. The most severe abnormalities are often found immediately after extensive burns before a reticulocyte response has had time to develop (Fig. 27–24). The badly damaged cells are rapidly removed from the circulation.

Traumatic Hemolysis. Hemolytic anemia characterized by striking morphologic abnormalities of the red cells, which include fragments (schistocytes) and irregularly contracted cells (triangular cells, helmet cells), has been attributed to physical trauma to the red cells (Fig. 27–29; Plate 29–2*L*). The basis of the hemolytic process is probably damage to the red cells in their contact with loose fibrin meshworks (intravascular coagulation) or with pathologic vascular lesions. Fragmentation of the cells results with or without intravascular lysis. Two general categories are recognized in this group of disorders, aptly termed the "red cell fragmentation syndrome."

Cardiac Valvular Disease and Prostheses. Chronic intravascular hemolysis associated with low serum haptoglobin, hemosiderinuria, reticulocytosis, and red cell abnormalities (e.g., schistocytes and irregularly contracted cells) may occur after surgical replacement of a diseased heart valve with a prosthesis or after surgical repair of a septal defect with a plastic patch (Marsh, 1969). This has been attributed to mechanical damage of red cells in the turbulent environment of a leaky valve or of a roughened surface uncovered by endothelial cells. Repair of the valve or coverage of the patch by endothelium has improved the hemolytic process. Other studies have shown that some patients with cardiac valvular disease have a hemolytic process which may be altered by surgery. The chronic intravascular hemolysis may lead to iron deficiency.

Microangiopathic Hemolytic Anemia. Hemolytic anemia with red cell fragmentation (e.g., schistocytes and irregularly contracted cells) has been described in malignant hypertension, thrombotic thrombocytopenic purpura, and disseminated carcinoma, in which a common factor was the presence of pathologic lesions involving small blood vessels. The hypothesis was advanced that the hemolytic anemia in these conditions may be an expression of mechanical or perhaps chemical effects of the vascular lesions on the red cells, and the process was designated "microangiopathic" (Brain, 1962). The role of disseminated or local intravascular coagulation has been recognized as an important factor (though not necessarily the inciting factor) in the pathogenesis of microangiopathy and the resultant hemolysis (Brain, 1972).

A rather distinct clinical state that probably belongs in the latter group as far as the hemolytic mechanism is concerned is the *hemolytic-uremic syndrome (HUS).* It occurs most commonly in infants less than two years of age and is often preceded by a viral infection. Hemolytic anemia with bizarre red cells, variable thrombocytopenia, and uremia are the cardinal features. Death formerly occurred in almost half the cases; the renal pathology has included acute glomerulonephritis and thrombotic and necrotic vascular lesions associated with patchy, bilateral renal cortical necrosis. With supportive therapy, including transfusions and dialysis, some have reported mortality reduced to 5 to 15 per cent (Aster, 1983).

The HUS appears in some way to be related to *thrombotic thrombocytopenic purpura (TTP).* TTP occurs in young adults, more often female than male, and manifests neurologic symptoms in addition to fever, microangiopathic hemolytic anemia, severe thrombocytopenia, and uremia. There is more widespread distribution of microvascular occlusive lesions with hyaline thrombi and endothelial proliferation. The etiology is unknown, but evidence has been presented for plasma-mediated immune endothelial injury and spontaneous platelet aggregation as well as impaired prostacyclin production by endothelium. With the empiric therapy of glucocorticoids, platelet inhibitors, and plasmapheresis or plasma transfusion, the remission rate seems to have improved from about 30 per cent to about 70 per cent (Bukowski, 1982; Aster, 1983).

VEGETABLE AND ANIMAL POISONS

Inhalation of pollens of the fava bean plant or ingestion of the bean itself may be followed by a fulminant hemolytic anemia in sensitive persons, mainly of Mediterranean origin. Glucose-6-phosphate dehydrogenase (G6PD) deficiency of the red cells plus some undefined, possibly separately inherited factor makes the individual sensitive to the fava bean. G6PD-deficient persons with and without the sensitivity to the fava bean may be found in the same family. Some insect and snake venoms may be associated with hemolysis.

INFECTIOUS AGENTS

Destruction of erythrocytes by plasmodia is responsible for the anemia in malaria. This is supported by the observation that the osmotic and mechanical fragility of parasitized erythrocytes is increased. Inhibition of marrow activity may be an additional factor. Fulminant hemoglobinuria (blackwater fever) is a complication of *P. falciparum* malaria. Its frequency after quinine therapy suggests an autoimmune mechanism mediated by the drug.

Oroya fever, a frequently fatal disease that occurs in Peru, is characterized by a hemolytic anemia and leukocytosis. *Bartonella bacilliformis* is the responsible agent.

Babesiosis, a protozoan infection transmitted by ticks from rodents or cattle, is associated with hemolysis; parasites may be seen in red cells on Romanowsky-stained blood films.

Hemolytic anemia with cold agglutinins may complicate mycoplasma pneumonia and infectious mononucleosis. This is due to the effect of antibody on the red cells.

Hemolytic anemia of varying severity is frequent in some bacterial infections. A notable example is *Clostridium welchii* septicemia following septic abortion or biliary tract surgery, which may be accompanied by a dramatic and life-threatening hemolytic crisis.

IMMUNE HEMOLYTIC ANEMIAS

Immune hemolytic anemias are disorders in which erythrocyte survival is reduced because of the deposition of immunoglobulin and/or complement on the red cell membrane. The immune hemolytic anemias can be grouped according to the presence of autoantibodies, isoantibodies, or drug-related antibodies (Table 29–7).

Table 29–7. CLASSIFICATION OF IMMUNE HEMOLYTIC ANEMIAS

Autoimmune hemolytic anemias
Associated with warm antibodies
Associated with cold antibodies
Isoimmune hemolytic anemia
Hemolytic disease of newborn
Rh incompatibility
ABO incompatibility
Drug-induced hemolytic anemia
Adsorption of immune complexes to red cell membrane
Adsorption of drug to red cell membrane
Induction of autoantibody by drugs
Non-immunologic adsorption of immunoglobulin to red cell membrane

Autoimmune Hemolytic Anemia (AIHA). The autoimmune hemolytic anemias are due to an altered immune response resulting in the production of antibody against the host's own erythrocytes, with subsequent hemolysis. The AIHA's can be classified according to serologic or clinical characteristics (Table 29–8). Some AIHA's are mediated by antibodies with maximum binding affinity at 37°C., and other AIHA's are mediated by antibodies with their maximum binding affinity at 4°C. In addition, AIHA's could be viewed according to their association with other disorders. Twenty to 80 per cent of the cases of AIHA have been associated with some underlying disorder, and the remainder are idiopathic (Dausset, 1950; Pirofsky, 1975).

Etiology and Pathophysiology. The cause of the production of autoantibody in patients with AIHA is unknown. However, several mechanisms have been suggested. Autoimmune antibodies are sometimes produced following an infection. This is typically seen with the elaboration of anti-I in patients with *Mycoplasma pneumoniae* infections. It has been hypothesized that the autoantibody may be a response to sensitization from a breakdown component of the *Mycoplasma pneumoniae* organism (Weens, 1974). In infectious mononucleosis, anti-i antibody is present in the serum of patients and it occasionally results in AIHA. Since the i-antigen is normally on the lymphocyte membrane, perhaps in this disorder the production of anti-i is part of an effort to remove host-infected B cells.

The development of AIHA in patients with lymphoproliferative disorders or with autoimmune disorders may relate to some abnormality with B cells, T cells, macrophages, or the interaction among these cells. Perhaps loss of T cell suppressor function could result in unrestrained production of red cell antibody by B cells (Weens, 1974). This hypothesis is strengthened by the observation that alpha-methyldopa, a drug known to cause the development of anti–red cell antibodies, inhibits the activation of suppressor T lymphocytes (Kirtland, 1980).

In AIHA associated with warm type antibody, there is IgG coating of erythrocytes with or without complement fixation. Clearance of red cells occurs mostly in the spleen. In the absence of complement fixation, it appears that the Fc portion of the red cell–bound IgG immunoglobulin interacts with the Fc receptor present on the membrane of splenic macrophages located along the cords of Billroth. Thus sensitized erythrocytes are either retained, phagocytosed, or fragmented by splenic macrophages during their passage through the spleen (Frank, 1977).

In AIHA associated with the production of cold type autoantibody, the erythrocytes are usually coated with IgM immunoglobulin. Under these circumstances, the fixation of complement frequently occurs. In paroxysmal cold hemoglobinuria, the offending antibody is an IgG immunoglobulin which fixes complement. If the entire complement sequence is activated, there may be intravascular hemolysis. This phenomenon may occur in cases of cold hemagglutinin disease as well as paroxysmal cold hemoglobinuria. If complement activation fails to proceed to completion but is halted at an intermediate stage, intravascular lysis of the erythrocytes may not occur. However, extravascular hemolysis can still continue. In this situation, sensitized cells with C3b on the membrane are bound

Table 29–8. AUTOIMMUNE HEMOLYTIC ANEMIA*

Associated with Warm Antibodies		Associated with Cold Antibodies	
Associated Disorder	***Percentage of Patients***	***Associated Disorder***	***Percentage of Patients***
Idiopathic	41	Idiopathic cold hemagglutinin disease	13
Lymphomas	13	*Mycoplasma pneumoniae*	8
Systemic lupus erythematosus	5	Infectious mononucleosis	1
Other autoimmune disorders	7	Lymphomas	2
Miscellaneous	5	Paroxysmal cold hemoglobinuria	5
Total	71		29

*Modified from Dacie, J. V., and Worlledge, S. M.: Prog. Hematol., *6*:82, 1969.

in the liver by the interaction of C3b and its receptors on Kupffer cells (Frank, 1977). Erythrocytes may be phagocytosed entirely or portions of the cells may be removed, resulting in fragmentation and spherocyte formation.

AIHA Associated with Warm Antibody. The warm antibody type of AIHA is slightly more frequent in females than males and most likely to occur in individuals 40 years or older. The clinical signs and symptoms frequently are those of an underlying disorder. However, in individuals with idiopathic AIHA, the patient may have noted the presence of a mild upper respiratory tract infection just prior to the onset of hemolysis. As the disorder progresses, there may be weakness, dizziness, and fever. Jaundice can be a presenting complaint.

Laboratory findings include the presence of a moderate to severe anemia. The neutrophil count may be increased. In a small proportion of cases thrombocytopenia can exist. The peripheral film frequently shows spherocytosis, red cell fragmentation, polychromasia, and a few normoblasts (see Fig. 27–23). Reticulocyte percentage is high in approximately 50 per cent of patients. The lack of reticulocytosis should not keep one from making a diagnosis of autoimmune hemolytic anemia (Pirofsky, 1975). The bone marrow exhibits normoblastic erythroid hyperplasia, sometimes with mild megaloblastic changes.

There is usually a decrease in serum haptoglobin and an increase in unconjugated bilirubin. The osmotic fragility and autohemolysis test can be either normal or abnormal.

The direct and indirect antiglobulin tests indicate the presence of erythrocyte antibodies. The specificity of the autoantibody is usually directed against antigens of the Rh system. However, activity against U, LW, Kell, jk^a, and Fy^a antigens may also occur. The warm antibody is most likely an IgG immunoglobulin with subclass IgG1 and less frequently with IgG3. When either IgG2 or IgG4 is present on the red cells alone, there is no associated hemolytic reaction (Petz, 1980). Occasionally the antibody may be an IgA immunoglobulin and rarely an IgM immunoglobulin. Complement may be detected on the erythrocyte membrane in slightly over half of the cases.

In some cases sensitized red cells contain less immunoglobulin than can be detected using commercially prepared antiglobulins, which are normally sensitive to 250 to 500 molecules of IgG/red cell (Gilliland, 1976). Under these circumstances the autoantibody can at times be detected with an antiglobulin consumption test (Rosse, 1974).

The clinical course of AIHA associated with warm antibody is characterized by periods of remissions and relapse. In secondary AIHA, the course and prognosis is related to the nature of the underlying disorder. In idiopathic AIHA, the complications of the hemolytic disorder may be severe and lead to the demise of the patient. The overall prognosis of this disorder is difficult to determine. Pirofsky (1975) observed a 40 per cent mortality rate, whereas Worlledge (1974) noted only a 14 per cent mortality rate in 85 patients observed for a period of three months to seven years.

AIHA Associated with Cold Antibody. AIHA associated with cold antibody can be mediated by an IgM immunoglobulin and less frequently by an IgG immunoglobulin. The IgM autoantibody is associated with a syndrome known as cold hemagglutinin disease, whereas the IgG autoantibody is seen with paroxysmal cold hemoglobinuria (Brown, 1977).

Cold Hemagglutinin Disease. Cold hemagglutinin disease occurs in individuals usually over the age of 50 years and in females more often than in males. In some cases cold hemagglutinin disease is associated with a lymphoreticular malignancy or autoimmune disorder. Other cases appear as a complication of infection (especially *Mycoplasma pneumoniae*). Cases unassociated with an underlying disorder are listed as idiopathic.

Symptoms and signs vary widely. Some individuals may complain of acrocyanosis or Raynaud's phenomenon. Others will have episodes of hemolysis following exposure to cold (Swisher, 1977).

The laboratory findings usually indicate an anemia. Spherocytes and polychromatophilic erythrocytes are present to a variable degree in the blood film. There may be marked red cell agglutination which should be differentiated from rouleau formation (see Figs. 27–35 and 27–36). A mild leukocytosis can exist.

The cold antibody is usually an IgM immunoglobulin with anti-I, or less frequently anti-i, specificity. Rarely do other specificities exist. In the chronic idiopathic form of cold hemagglutinin disease, the antibody tends to be monoclonal IgM, *k* with anti-I specificity or IgM, λ with anti-i specificity (Petz, 1980). The autoantibody is also capable of fixing complement. When the titer of cold antibody is very high, the thermal range of antibody activity may extend up to 37°C. The direct antiglobulin test is positive only if the reagents contain anti-complement activity. Thus one usually observes a positive antiglobulin reaction with the broad spectrum and nongamma reagents but no agglutination with only the gamma reagent.

Paroxysmal Cold Hemoglobinuria. Paroxysmal cold hemoglobinuria is a very rare disorder that can occur in an individual of any age. Females are as frequently involved as males. Patients have symptoms of acute hemolysis following exposure to the cold. There are chills, fever, pain in the back and legs, and hemoglobinuria. The acute form may follow an acute viral illness, but the chronic form is associated with congenital syphilis.

The laboratory features consist of anemia, elevated reticulocyte count, increased concentration of indirect bilirubin, and the presence of hemoglobin in the urine.

The serum contains a cold hemolysin with biphasic activity. This antibody, first described by Donath and Landsteiner (1904), is an IgG immunoglobulin which fixes the first components of complement (C1–C4) in the cold (4°C.). As the temperature rises to 25 to 37°C., the remainder of the complement proteins are activated and erythrocyte lysis results. The specificity of the antibody is directed against the P antigen. In general the prognosis is good.

4

Isoimmune Hemolytic Anemia. Isoimmune hemolytic anemia usually occurs in newborns following the transplacental passage of maternal anti-fetal red cell antibody. Isoimmune hemolytic disease of the newborn most frequently results from incompatibility in Rh and ABO erythrocyte antigens between mother and fetus. In rare cases some other red cell antigen may be responsible for this disorder. (See Chapter 43).

In isoimmune hemolytic disease of the newborn due to *Rh incompatibility,* prior sensitization is necessary to initiate the disease process. This sensitization usually occurs during pregnancy when Rh(D) fetal red cells cross the placenta and enter the circulation of a mother with Rh negative cells. Maternal sensitization can also occur by a previous incompatible transfusion. Under either of these circumstances, maternal IgG antibodies are produced against the fetal cells. If a subsequent pregnancy occurs in a sensitized mother, fetal erythrocytes again reach the maternal circulation and restimulate an antibody response resulting in transfer of anti-Rh(D) antibody across the placenta and reduced fetal red cell survival.

In the *ABO system* anti-A or anti-B antibodies of the IgG class may arise spontaneously in the mother; their presence does not require prior transfusion or pregnancy. As a result, first-born children may suffer from isoimmune hemolytic disease when ABO incompatibility exists.

The clinical features of *isoimmune hemolytic disease of the newborn due to Rh incompatibility* vary greatly. Some newborns experience only mild jaundice. Others initially appear markedly pale and then develop jaundice. They can have prominent hepatosplenomegaly. The disease may be complicated by a bleeding diathesis, marked acid-base abnormalities, and kernicterus. In very severe cases, patients can present with hydrops fetalis (Zipursky, 1974).

Early examination of the blood usually reveals an increase of nucleated erythrocytes, which may include forms as immature as pronormoblasts. Although this finding gave the disease its name, *erythroblastosis fetalis,* erythroblastosis is not always present, especially if the examination is not done immediately after birth.

Up to 2.0×10^9 nucleated red cells/L in term infants and up to 5.0×10^9/L in premature infants are commonly seen in this disorder. Normally, nucleated red cells average 0.5×10^9/L in term infants and 1.0 to 1.5×10^9/L in premature infants. Blood from the umbilical vein for early examination is more reliable than peripheral (capillary) blood because the erythrocyte count and the hemoglobin may be significantly altered between birth and ligation of the cord.

Generally there are a macrocytic anemia of varying severity and an increase in reticulocytes. Occasionally anemia may develop suddenly on the second or third day. The leukocyte count is frequently elevated, with immature leukocytes. There is pronounced normoblastic hyperplasia of the marrow.

In severely affected infants, there may be thrombocytopenia, depression of the prothrombin complex procoagulants, or diffuse intravascular coagulation.

A direct antiglobulin test on fetal erythrocytes indicates the presence of an IgG antibody. When the maternal serum and an eluate from the fetal erythrocytes are incubated separately with a panel of O cells, one can usually demonstrate the presence of antibody with Rh(D) specificity. In Rh negative pregnant women known to be sensitized to Rh(D), the titer of antiRh(D) antibody is measured periodically during pregnancy to serve as a guide for performing amniocentesis (see p. 1053).

Isoimmune hemolytic disease of the newborn associated with ABO incompatibility is less severe than that observed with Rh incompatibility. Occasionally the diagnosis is suggested by the presence of unexplained hyperbilirubinemia in a group A or B newborn infant from a group O mother.

Laboratory findings usually show a mild anemia and modest reticulocytosis. In contrast to Rh isoimmune disease, spherocytosis in ABO isoimmune disease may be prominent. However, there may be no anemia. The fetal cells are usually weakly positive with the antiglobulin reagents. Serum from the newborn and eluates from the cells should contain anti-A or anti-B antibody. In addition, the maternal serum should contain high titers of anti-A or anti-B antibodies of the IgG subclass.

Drug-Induced Immune Hemolytic Anemia. Immune hemolytic anemia may occur following the administration of drugs. Four mechanisms appear to mediate the immune hemolysis (Petz, 1975).

Adsorption of Immune Complexes to Red Cell Membrane. Numerous drugs are known to provoke an antibody response with subsequent adsorption of immune complexes to the erythrocyte membrane (Table 29–9). The drug-induced antibody is usually IgM and tends to fix complement, resulting in lysis of cells.

Patients present with acute intravascular hemolysis, hemoglobinemia, and hemoglobinuria. The direct antiglobulin reaction is positive if the reagents contain

Table 29–9. DRUGS ACCEPTED AS CAUSING IMMUNE HEMOLYTIC ANEMIA BY THE ADSORPTION OF IMMUNE COMPLEXES TO RED CELLS*

Stibophen
Quinidine
Para-aminosalicylic acid
Quinine
Phenacetin
Chlorinated hydrocarbon-containing insecticides
Antihistamines
Sulfonamides
Isonicotinic acid hydrazine
Chlorpromazine
Aminopyrine
Dipyrone
Melphalan
Mefanamic acid
Sulfonylureas
Insulin
Rifampin

*Modified from Petz, L. D., and Garratty, G.: Clin. Haematol., *4*:181, 1975.

anti-complement activity. The reaction usually is negative with the gamma reagent because it contains little anti-IgM or complement specificity.

The diagnosis can be determined by incubating the patient's serum with the offending drug in the presence of target erythrocytes, and observing agglutination, lysis, or sensitization of the erythrocytes.

Adsorption of Drug to Red Cell Membrane. Penicillin and cephalosporin combine with protein normally present on the erythrocyte membrane. These drugs, once bound to the red cell membrane, form haptenic groups and provoke an immune response. Both IgM and IgG antibodies are made, but only the IgG antibodies are associated with the immune hemolysis. Complement is not involved. The erythrocytes, coated with IgG antibody, are presumably removed via the Fc receptors on macrophages in the spleen.

The direct antiglobulin test is strongly positive. Antibody eluted from patient's erythrocytes will react only with red cells previously treated with penicillin or cephalosporins.

Induction of Autoantibody by Drugs. In approximately 15 per cent of patients using the antihypertensive drug alpha-methyldopa, a positive direct antiglobulin reaction is present. The antibody is of the IgG class and in some studies appears to have Rh specificity (Croft, 1968). However, other studies indicate that there may be non-specific erythrocyte adsorption of γ-globulin altered by exposure to alpha-methyldopa (Gottlieb, 1974). Kirtland (1980) demonstrated that alpha-methyldopa caused an elevation of intracellular lymphocyte cyclic AMP and an inhibition of T lymphocyte suppressor activity. These investigators postulated that these effects may lead to unregulated autoantibody production by B cells in some patients.

The development of the positive antiglobulin reaction is dose-dependent. Thirty-six per cent of patients have a positive antiglobulin reaction when consuming 2 g or more of alpha-methyldopa per day, and 11 per cent have a positive reaction when taking only 1 g daily. An immune hemolytic anemia occurs in less than 1 per cent of patients (Petz, 1975). L-Dopa and mefenamic acid are two additional drugs which have been reported to cause an autoimmune hemolytic anemia in a fashion similar to alpha-methyldopa.

Non-Immunologic Adsorption of Immunoglobulin to Red Cell Membrane. Cephalosporins appear to alter the erythrocyte membrane, resulting in the non-specific adsorption of plasma proteins to its surface. As a result, IgG and IgM immunoglobulin may be loosely bound to red cell membrane. This phenomenon can then cause a positive direct antiglobulin reaction (Petz, 1980).

Laboratory Diagnosis of Anemia

This section is based on the useful approach given by Wheby (1966). The diagnosis and study of anemia require the proper use and interpretation of laboratory measurements. Prerequisite for the efficient use of the laboratory are a careful history and physical examination, both of which lead to the initial laboratory measurements and provide important guidance in determining the nature of the anemia.

Whether the patient is anemic and can be ascertained by determining whether the hemoglobin, hematocrit, or erythrocyte count lies below the reference intervals for age and sex. Then the task is to define the underlying cause or mechanism for the anemia.

Usually the CBC (WBC, RBC, Hb, Hct, MCV, MCH, MCHC) and examination of a Wright's stained film are parts of the routine examination of the blood. It is possible that all these values could be normal in the presence of a mild macrocytic anemia, in which the RBC does not fall below the normal range, and the macrocytes present (and detectable on the blood film) do not elevate the MCV above the normal range.

Once anemia is discovered, the basic examination of the blood should include the following: (1) hemoglobin, hematocrit, and RBC count, for calculation of *indices* (if not already available with multichannel instrument); (2) blood film examination; (3) leukocyte count; (4) platelet count (if apparently abnormal on examination of the film or if suspected to be abnormal on clinical grounds); and (5) reticulocyte count.

With current multichannel instruments, all red cell values and the indices have comparable precision. Indices are *mean* values, however, and will not detect different populations of cells which balance each other. For example, combined deficiencies of folate and iron may give rise to populations of macrocytic and hypochromic microcytic cells, which could yield normal indices. Careful examination of the blood film is essential, and cell volume distribution curves (p. 598) are very useful in defining these mixtures.

4

Examination of the blood film will determine the *morphologic type* of anemia. In addition, certain changes or combinations of findings will suggest the mechanism involved.

Increased numbers of *polychromatic* macrocytes, with or without normoblasts, suggest increased erythropoiesis, and in the untreated patient this is usually due to hemorrhage or hemolysis. Here, the history (of blood loss) or physical examination (jaundice or splenomegaly) will help.

Findings suggestive of hemolysis are *poikilocytes* (abnormally shaped cells), *sickle cells, irregularly contracted forms* (including red cell fragments or schistocytes), and *spherocytes*. Sometimes it is difficult to detect spherocytes in hereditary spherocytosis because of minimal anisocytosis. The two findings in the red cells that are helpful here are the presence of a low MCD (mean cell diameter) between 6.0 and 6.5 μm (normal = 7.0 to 7.4) and spheroidocytes with eccentric pallor.

Target cells may be found in hemoglobinopathies, especially in homozygous states for Hb C, Hb D, and Hb E, and in thalassemia. They may be present in any *hypochromic* anemia, though usually in smaller numbers. Target cells without microcytosis are also found in liver disease and in the absence of a spleen.

Fine *basophilic stippling* (which is due to precipitation

of RNA) may be found in polychromatic red cells associated with a significant increase in the generation of erythrocytes, as in response to hemorrhage or hemolysis. Coarse basophilic stippling suggests an abnormality in hemoglobin synthesis. It is found in megaloblastic anemias, thalassemias, refractory anemias, and lead poisoning. In particular, hypochromasia or microcytosis with stippling is against the diagnosis of iron deficiency anemia and more suggestive of thalassemia or lead poisoning.

The combination of *oval macrocytes* (especially egg-shaped macrocytes) and *hypersegmented neutrophils* indicates the very likely existence of megaloblastic anemia.

Finally, examination of the blood film allows the evaluation of *qualitative abnormalities in leukocytes and platelets* as well as an estimate of their numbers. Blood diseases that may be first suspected or detected in this manner are many and include chronic lymphocytic leukemia, compensated hemolytic anemia, early megaloblastic anemia, and anomalies of red cells, such as hereditary elliptocytosis, or of leukocytes, such as the Pelger-Huët anomaly.

After the basic studies just mentioned the choice of further procedures depends upon the morphologic type of the anemia as determined by the indices and the blood film.

MACROCYTIC ANEMIA (MCV GREATER THAN 96 FL)

These anemias are normochromic, as determined by appearance on the film and by the MCHC. The first step is to ascertain whether the anemia is megaloblastic. The clues from the film have been mentioned. A *bone marrow aspiration* should be done to confirm the presence of megaloblastosis.

Megaloblastic Marrow. If the marrow is *megaloblastic,* with characteristic changes in both red cell and white cell precursors, the anemia in all likelihood is due to folate or vitamin B_{12} deficiency.

See sections on diagnosis of vitamin B_{12} deficiency (p. 659) and of folate deficiency (p. 661). Once the *type* of deficiency is defined, the *cause* must be determined.

Non-megaloblastic Marrow. If the marrow is *not megaloblastic,* conditions which can be associated with macrocytosis should be investigated. These include liver disease, hemolytic anemias, hypothyroidism, alcoholism, and refractory or hypoplastic anemia. Anemias associated with these disorders, though they *may* be macrocytic, are more usually normocytic and thus are considered with the normocytic anemias.

MICROCYTIC AND HYPOCHROMIC ANEMIAS (MCV < 80 FL; MCH < 27 PG)

If the counts are performed on a Coulter Counter Model S, the MCHC is likely to be in the normal range, with slight to moderate degrees of hypochromia. Consequently the MCV has assumed the leading role in the detection of microcytic hypochromic anemias.

These anemias reflect a quantitative defect in hemoglobin synthesis.

1. *Iron deficiency anemias* are due to increased requirement or blood loss not balanced by intake.
2. *Anemia of chronic disorders,* otherwise known as "sideropenic anemia associated with reticuloendothelial siderosis," or "simple chronic anemia," is associated with infection, neoplasia, or collagen disease. This anemia may be normochromic and normocytic but in longstanding disease is often hypochromic and microcytic.
3. *Thalassemia* is a genetically determined impairment in the rate of globin synthesis.
4. *Sideroblastic anemia* is that group of refractory anemias with erythroid hyperplasia of the marrow in which a defect in hemoglobin synthesis creates a population of hypochromic microcytic cells. The picture is dimorphic, and macrocytes may prevail, making the MCV normal or high.

Since *iron deficiency* is the most common, the first step is to determine whether the body lacks iron.

When blood loss cannot be documented, serum ferritin, serum iron and iron-binding capacity, or bone marrow study for iron should be performed. These will usually discriminate between the two most common anemias in this category, iron deficiency and simple chronic anemia associated with some other disease—frequently chronic infection or cancer. In

Table 29–10. LABORATORY FEATURES IN MICROCYTIC HYPOCHROMIC ANEMIAS

	Serum Iron	Serum TIBC	% Saturation	Marrow: % *Sideroblasts*	Marrow: *Iron Stores*	Serum Ferritin	FEP	Hb A_2	Hb F
Iron deficiency	↓	↑	↓	↓	↓	↓	↑	N-↓	N
β-Thalassemia trait	N (↑)	N	N	N	N-↑	N-↑	N	↑	N-↑
Anemia of chronic disease	↓	N-↓	↓	↓	N-↑	N-↑	↑	N	N
Sideroblastic anemia	↑	↓	↑	↑	↑	↑	↑(↓)	N	N-↑

TIBC = total iron binding capacity; FEP = Free erythrocyte porphyrins; ↓ = decreased; N = normal; ↑ = increased.

both, the serum iron is low, but in iron deficiency the total iron-binding capacity is elevated, whereas in simple chronic anemia it is normal or decreased. Storage iron in the marrow is depleted in iron deficiency but is normal or elevated in simple chronic anemia. Iron deficiency anemia in an adult male almost always means chronic blood loss; the source must be found and corrected, if necessary.

Hypochromic anemias (or erythrocytoses) with basophilic stippling and normal or increased serum iron are most likely *thalassemias,* and the next examinations to perform are hemoglobin electrophoresis and determination of Hb A_2 and Hb F. Family studies are often necessary.

Least common in this group are the *sideroblastic anemias.* In addition to refractory sideroblastic anemia already discussed, a very similar picture may occur after therapy with certain drugs (e.g., isoniazid) and in chronic lead poisoning. Basophilic stippling is common in this group of anemias.

Table 29–10 summarizes the laboratory distinctions in hypochromic anemias.

NORMOCYTIC AND NORMOCHROMIC ANEMIAS (MCV 80-96 FL)

This large group of anemias has many causes. A useful approach is evaluation of the erythrokinetics in a given patient (p. 635). Often a reticulocyte production index (RPI) or absolute reticulocyte count and evaluation of a bone marrow aspirate will suffice. The reticulocyte count is the simplest measure of effective erythropoiesis.

Optimal Marrow Response: Reticulocyte Production Index over Two. If the output of reticulocytes has exceeded two times normal, as determined by the absolute reticulocyte count or RPI, it can be assumed that the marrow has reached an optimal response. The cause for the anemia is then either *acute blood loss* or *hemolysis.* If blood loss cannot be proved, evidence that hemolysis is in fact present must be sought.

Erythroid hyperplasia of the marrow, serum bilirubin, urine or fecal urobilinogen will indicate whether erythropoietic activity and destruction are increased. Red cell survival determination may be needed to prove hemolysis in some cases. Low serum haptoglobin points to hemolysis, but a normal level does not exclude it. None of these measurements will specify whether hemolysis is intravascular or extravascular, but elevated plasma hemoglobin, hemoglobinuria, and hemosiderinuria indicate intravascular hemolysis.

Once it is determined that excessive hemolysis is occurring, the type of hemolytic mechanism must be ascertained.

The *direct antiglobulin (Coombs) test* is a useful guide to further study.

If the direct antiglobulin (Coombs) test is *positive,* tests to determine the type and specificity of the antibody should be undertaken. If the antibody is non-specific, tests such as cold agglutinins, the Donath-Landsteiner test, and serum protein electrophoresis may help to define the process.

If the direct antiglobulin (Coombs) test is *negative,* what examinations are performed next will depend upon the clinical findings and the results of the measurements already made.

If hereditary spherocytosis is suspected, osmotic fragility before and after 24-hour incubation at 37°C. and family studies will be necessary.

If a non-spherocytic congenital hemolytic anemia is suspected, screening for glucose-6-phosphate dehydrogenase and pyruvate kinase deficiencies, hemoglobin electrophoresis, and a sickle cell test will be helpful. If these are negative, the heat instability test, isopropanol solubility test, and autohemolysis test should be considered.

If thalassemia seems likely, determinations of HbA_2 and Hb F are appropriate. Thalassemia is unique in that it is both hypochromic and hemolytic. Again, family studies are often helpful.

If drug-induced hemolysis is suspected, a test for Heinz bodies, screening test for glucose-6-phosphate dehydrogenase and, if possible, tests for a drug-dependent autoantibody are indicated.

If the nature of the hemolytic anemia is obscure, a sugar-water test for paroxysmal noctural hemoglobinuria should be performed.

Inadequate Marrow Response: Reticulocyte Production Index under Two. The mechanism of the anemia may be ineffective erythropoiesis. Conditions with the greatest degree of ineffective erythropoiesis appear in other categories (e.g., megaloblastic anemia and thalassemia), but some idiopathic refractory anemias have a hyperplastic bone marrow and impaired delivery of the cells to the blood. In some of these, abnormalities in erythroid precursors suggestive of megaloblastic change may be present, but the granulocytic and megakaryocytic changes usually seen in megaloblastic anemia are lacking.

A low reticulocyte count may indicate decreased production caused by inadequate stimulation of the marrow. Chronic renal disease may result in impaired production of erythropoietin. Certain endocrinopathies, such as hypopituitarism or hypothyroidism, may result in regulation of hemoglobin production at a lower level due to decreased tissue need for oxygen.

A large group of normochromic anemias associated with various chronic diseases form a heterogeneous group characterized by failure of the marrow to meet the need of a slightly decreased red cell survival. Some of these are anemia of chronic disorders associated with infection, cancer, or rheumatoid arthritis and have the defect in iron metabolism noted above under the hypochromic microcytic anemias. The reasons for inadequate stimulation or response of the marrow are sometimes not well understood.

Inability of the marrow to respond to erythropoietin may be due to damage to the marrow by drugs or toxic chemicals, to unknown causes, or to infiltration of the marrow by neoplastic cells or fibrous tissue.

In these conditions with low reticulocyte counts in which the marrow is not effectively producing erythrocytes, it is usually helpful to examine the bone marrow. Other studies to determine the underlying disease process can then proceed according to the marrow picture, the assessment of erythrokinetics, and the clinical findings.

Table 29–11. CLASSIFICATION OF POLYCYTHEMIA*

Relative polycythemia
1. Diminished plasma volume: dehydration; shock
2. Spurious polycythemia (stress polycythemia; Gaisböck's syndrome)

Absolute polycythemia
1. Secondary polycythemia (increased erythropoietin)
   a. Appropriate erythropoietin production: hypoxia
      1. Arterial oxygen unsaturation: high altitude; pulmonary disease; cyanotic heart disease; smoker's polycythemia; methemoglobinemia; Hb M
      2. High oxygen affinity hemoglobinopathy
   b. Inappropriate erythropoietin production
      1. Neoplasms: renal carcinoma; cerebellar hemangioma; hepatoma; uterine fibroids; adrenal cortical neoplasms
      2. Renal pathology: cysts; hydronephrosis; transplantation
   c. Familial polycythemia
2. Polycythemia vera

*Modified from Berlin, N. I.: Semin. Hematol., *12*:339, 1975.

POLYCYTHEMIA

Polycythemia is an increased concentration of erythrocytes in the blood that is above the normal for age and sex. Usually, but not always, the hematocrit and hemoglobin are also elevated.

Absolute polycythemia refers to an increase in the total red cell mass in the body; in *relative polycythemia,* the total red cell mass is normal, but the hematocrit is elevated because the plasma volume is decreased. Polycythemia may be classified as in Table 29–11.

Relative Polycythemia

Relative polycythemia refers to an increase in hematocrit or red cell count due to decreased plasma volume; total red cell mass is not increased. This occurs in acute dehydration, e.g., in severe diarrhea or burns, and in patients on diuretic therapy.

In spurious polycythemia (Gaisböck's syndrome), the red cell mass is often high normal and the plasma volume is low normal; these patients have been regarded as an extreme of the normal physiologic state. Almost all are men, have a high incidence of tobacco smoking, and tend to be obese and to have hypertension. Weinreb (1975) compared a group of these patients with a second group, similar except that the elevated hematocrit was due primarily to decreased plasma volume. The latter group had a greater tendency to hypertension and hypercholesterolemia, and had a poorer survival.

Smoking as a cause of polycythemia has been stressed (Smith, 1978); it is likely that smoking is an important factor in some cases of "spurious polycythemia."

Absolute Polycythemia

APPROPRIATE ERYTHROPOIETIN PRODUCTION DUE TO HYPOXIA

Arterial Oxygen Unsaturation. Lack of oxygen reaching the blood for whatever reason results in arterial unsaturation, impaired oxygen delivery to the tissues, increased production of erythropoietin, erythroid hyperplasia in the marrow, and resultant erythrocytosis (Balcerzak, 1975). The red cell mass is increased. As a response to the hypoxia, the red cell 2,3-DPG and the P_{50} are increased. In contrast to polycythemia vera, there is usually no leukocytosis or thrombocytosis, and the neutrophil alkaline phosphatase is normal. Arterial oxygen unsaturation may be the cause of polycythemia in persons living at high altitudes, in patients with chronic pulmonary disease and a block in diffusion of oxygen into the blood, in cyanotic heart disease in which there is right to left shunt, in cigarette smokers (Smith, 1978), and in methemoglobinemia whether due to enzyme deficiency (p. 583), chronic drug effect, or a structurally abnormal hemoglobin (Hb M) (p. 681).

High Oxygen Affinity Hemoglobinopathy. Another cause of tissue hypoxia is the presence of a structurally abnormal hemoglobin which has a high affinity for oxygen (p. 682; Adamson, 1975). As in other functional hemoglobinopathies, the disorder occurs in the heterozygote. The abnormal hemoglobin releases less oxygen to the tissues than does normal hemoglobin at the same Po_2; the oxygen dissociation curve is shifted to the left and the P_{50} is decreased. The red cell 2,3-DPG is not increased. As in arterial oxygen unsaturation, there is increased erythropoietin production and erythrocytosis. It must be emphasized that routine hemoglobin electrophoresis often does not detect these hemoglobin variants because the amino acid substitution is at one of the $\alpha\beta$ contact sites or near the heme pocket. A low P_{50} therefore is presumptive evidence for a hemoglobinopathy. The heat instability test for unstable hemoglobin should be done, since some hemoglobins with high affinity and polycythemia are unstable.

INAPPROPRIATE ERYTHROPOIETIN PRODUCTION

Neoplasms. Neoplasms, either benign or malignant, have been associated with polycythemia (Balcerzak, 1975). Renal neoplasms account for the majority. In almost all cases, erythrocytosis has disappeared after resection of the tumor. The mechanism is not clear. Some of these neoplasms have been shown to contain, and presumably produce, erythropoietin (e.g., cerebellar hemangioma, hypernephroma, some hepatomas).

Renal Disorders. In other neoplasms or growths (e.g., renal cysts, hydronephrosis, ovarian carcinoma, some hepatomas) it appears that the mass impinging on the kidney induces increased renal production of ESF due to increased pressure or local hypoxia within the kidney. Renal ischemia (and hypoxia) due to arterial occlusion also is the probable mechanism for erythrocytosis in patients with renal transplants; narrowing of small arteries occurs during the rejection reaction.

Familial Polycythemia. In certain families erythrocytosis occurs in siblings but not in parents, and analysis has supported an autosomal recessive inheritance (Adamson, 1975). These individuals have no abnormalities in hemoglobin function nor do they have detectable renovascular or cardiopulmonary defects. Studies have shown increased erythropoietin production unrelated to hemoglobin concentration, and have suggested a *defect in the regulation of erythropoietin production.* Individuals with this disorder are involved earlier in life, have higher Hb and Hct levels, and more often have splenomegaly than do persons with polycythemia due to a *high oxygen affinity hemoglobinopathy,* which has autosomal dominant inheritance, and has been discussed on p. 698.

Marked decrease in red cell 2,3-DPG associated with *deficiency of 2,3-DPG mutase and 2,3-DPG phosphatase* activities results in polycythemia and appears to be inherited as an autosomal recessive condition (Rosa, 1978).

What is not clear at the present time is whether different pathophysiologic mechanisms may be operative in other patients with "benign familial erythrocytosis," since many of the patients reported have not been studied with currently available techniques.

POLYCYTHEMIA VERA (PV)

Polycythemia vera is a panmyelosis, that is, a condition in which excessive proliferation occurs in megakaryocytes and granulocytes as well as in erythrocytes. It is manifested by erythrocytosis, leukocytosis, and thrombocytosis of varying degree. The etiology is unknown. PV is discussed with the myeloproliferative disorders (p. 727).

Measurement of Erythrocyte and Plasma Volume

The diagnosis of absolute polycythemia depends on reliable measurements of erythrocyte and plasma volumes. The erythrocyte and plasma volumes are measured by the use of radioactive isotopic tracers and the dilution principle. The most commonly employed tracers are ^{51}Cr in the form of sodium chromate bound to erythrocytes for measurement of erythrocyte volume. Iodine-125 or iodine-131 is bound to albumin and can be used to measure plasma volume.

For detailed description of measurement of red cell and plasma volume, see the report of the International Committee for Standardization in Hematology (1980b).

Erythrocyte Volume. In brief, blood is collected from the patient and the erythrocytes are labeled with ^{51}Cr. The chromated erythrocytes are washed in saline. An aliquot of the ^{51}Cr erythrocytes diluted in saline is injected intravenously into the patient. After a period of equilibration, usually 10 to 20 minutes, a sample of blood is withdrawn from the opposite arm. In cases where the equilibration time is likely to be prolonged (as in splenomegaly, heart failure, or shock) another sample should be withdrawn 60 minutes after injection.

Radioactivity of each sample is recorded by a scintillation counter. The erythrocyte volume (EV) is calculated using the formula:

$$\text{EV (ml)} = \frac{\text{I(cpm)}}{\text{C(cpm/ml)}}$$

where I = total injected radioactivity (counts per minute)
C = radioactivity in erythrocytes after mixing is complete (counts per minute per milliliter of erythrocytes).

Table 29–12. CLINICAL EFFECT OF VARIABLE RELATIONSHIP BETWEEN RED-CELL VOLUME AND PLASMA VOLUME*

Red-Cell Volume	Plasma Volume	Cause	Effect
Normal	High	Pregnancy Cirrhosis Nephritis Congestive cardiac failure	Pseudoanemia
Normal	Low	Stress Peripheral circulatory failure Dehydration Edema Prolonged bed rest	Pseudopolycythemia
Low	Normal	Anemia	Accurate reflection of degree of anemia
Low	High	Anemia	Anemia less severe than indicated by blood count
Low	Low	Hemorrhage Severe anemia (when PCV below 0.2)	Anemia more severe than indicated by blood count
High	Normal to low	Polycythemia	Accurate reflection of polycythemia or polycythemia less severe than apparent
High	High	Polycythemia (when PCV > 0.5)	Polycythemia more severe than apparent
Normal or even high	High	Marked splenomegaly	Pseudoanemia

*From Dacie, J. V., and Lewis, S. M.: Practical Haematology. 5th ed. Edinburgh, Churchill Livingstone, 1975.

4

Plasma Volume. Approximately 20 ml of blood is withdrawn from a patient. After centrifugation, the plasma is removed and radioiodine-labeled albumin is added. After mixing, the labeled plasma is injected intravenously into the patient. At 10, 20, and 30 minutes following the injection, 5 ml of blood is removed and the radioactivity is counted in a well-type scintillation counter. The radioactivity at zero time (P_0) is determined by plotting the three points on semilogarithmic graph paper and extrapolating to zero time. A standard is prepared by diluting an aliquot of the radioiodine-labeled albumin with saline containing a small amount of detergent.

The plasma volume (PV) is calculated using the formula

$$\text{PV (ml)} = \frac{\text{S(cpm/ml)} \times \text{D} \times \text{V(ml)}}{\text{P}_0 \text{ (cpm/ml)}}$$

where S = counting rate of standard (counts per minute/ml)
D = dilution of diluted standard solution
V = volume of radioiodine-labeled albumin solution injected
P_0 = counting rate of plasma sample corrected to zero time (counts/minute/ml).

Interpretation. The normal erythrocyte volume for men is 20 to 36 ml/kg, and for women it is 19 to 31 ml/kg. The plasma volume for men is 25 to 43 ml/kg and for women is 28 to 45 ml/kg. In newborns and premature infants the red cell volume and plasma volume in ml/kg are higher than in adults.

Patients with polycythemia have red cell volumes exceeding 36 ml/kg for men and 32 ml/kg for women. Changes in erythrocyte volume and plasma volume in a variety of conditions are recorded in Table 29–12.

Adamson, J. W.: Familial polycythemia. Semin. Hematol., *12*:383, 1975.

Alter, B. P., Potter, N. U., and Li, F. P.: Classification and aetiology of the aplastic anemias. Clin. Haematol., 7:431, 1978.

Alter, B. P., Rappaport, J. M., and Parkman, R.: The bone marrow failure syndromes. *In* Nathan, D. G., and Oski, F. A. (eds.): Hematology of Infancy and Childhood. 2nd ed. Philadelphia, W. B. Saunders Company, 1981, p. 168.

Aoki, Y.: Multiple enzymatic defects in mitochondrion hematological cells of patients with primary sideroblastic anemia. J. Clin. Invest., 66:43, 1980.

Aster, R. H.: Thrombocytopenia due to enhanced platelet destruction. *In* Williams, W. J., Beutler, E., Erslev, A. J., and Lichtman, M. A.: Hematology. 3rd ed. New York, McGraw-Hill Book Company, 1983, p. 1298.

Balcerzak, S. P., and Bromberg, P. A.: Secondary polycythemia. Semin. Hematol., *12*:353, 1975.

Bauman, A. W., and Swisher, S. N.: Hyporegenerative processes in hemolytic anemia. Semin. Hematol., *4*:265, 1967.

Beck, W. S. (ed.): Hematology. 3rd ed. Cambridge, Mass., MIT Press, 1981.

Bentley, S. A.: Red cell survival studies reinterpreted. Clin. Haematol., 6:601, 1977.

Berlin, N. I.: Diagnosis and classification of the polycythemias. Semin. Hematol., *12*:339, 1975.

Betke, K., Marti, H. R., and Schlict, I.: Estimation of small percentages of foetal haemoglobin. Nature, *184*:1877, 1959.

Beutler, E.: Hemolytic Anemia in Disorders of Red Cell Metabolism. New York, Plenum Medical Book Company, 1978.

Beutler, E.: Red cell enzyme defects as nondiseases and as diseases. Blood, *54*:1, 1979a.

Beutler, E.: Red Cell Metabolism. A Manual of Biochemical Methods. 2nd ed. New York, Grune & Stratton, Inc., 1975.

Beutler, E., Glumbe, K. G., Kaplan, J. C., Lohr, G. W., Ramot, B., and Valentine, W. N.: International Committee for Standardization in Haematology: Recommended screening test for glucose-6-phosphate dehydrogenase (G-6-PD) deficiency. Br. J. Haematol., *43*:469, 1979b.

Bottomley, S.: Sideroblastic anemia. Clin. Haematol., 11:389, 1982.

Brain, M. C.: Microangiopathic haemolytic anaemia (MHA). Br. J. Haematol., *23*(Suppl.):45, 1972.

Brain, M. C., Dacie, J. V., and Hourihane, D. O'B.: Microangiopathic haemolytic anaemia; the possible role of vascular lesions in pathogenesis. Br. J. Haematol., *8*:358, 1962.

Briere, R., Golias, T., and Batsakis, J. G.: Rapid qualitative and quantitative hemoglobin fractionation, cellulose acetate electrophoresis. Am. J. Clin. Path., *44*:695, 1965.

Brown, D. L: Haematological disorders. *In* Holborow, E. J., and Reeves, W. G. (eds.): Immunology in Medicine. New York, Grune & Stratton, Inc., 1977, p. 911.

Bukowski, R. M.: Thrombotic thrombocytopenic purpura: A review. Progr. Hemost. Thromb., *6*:287, 1982.

Bunn, H. F., Forget, B. G., and Ranney, H. M.: Human Hemoglobins. Philadelphia, W. B. Saunders Company, 1977.

Camitta, B. M., Strob, R., and Thomas, E. D.: Aplastic anemia: Pathogenesis, diagnosis, treatment and prognosis. N. Engl. J. Med., *306*:645, 712, 1982.

Camitta, B. M., Thomas, E. D., Nathan, D. G., Gale, R. P., Kopeckly, K. J., Rappeport, J. M., Santos, G., Gordon-Smith, E. C., and Storb, R.: A prospective study of androgens and bone marrow transplantation for treatment of severe aplastic anemia. Blood, *53*:504, 1979.

Carrell, R. W., and Kay, R.: A simple method for the detection of unstable hemoglobins. Br. J. Haematol., *23*:615, 1972.

Carrell, R. W., Winterbourn, C. C., and Rachmilewitz, E. A.: Activated oxygen and hemolysis. Br. J. Haematol., *30*:259, 1975.

Cartwright, G. E.: The anemia of chronic disorders. Semin. Hematol., *3*:351, 1966.

Cartwright, G. E., and Lee, G. R.: The anemia of chronic disorders. Br. J. Haematol., *21*:147, 1971.

Chanarin, I.: Investigation and management of megaloblastic anaemia. Clin. Haematol., 5:747, 1976.

Chanarin, I.: The Megaloblastic Anaemias. 2nd ed. Oxford, Blackwell Scientific Publications, Ltd., 1979.

Chanarin, I., Barkhan, P., Peacock, M., and Stamp, T. C. B.: Acute arrest of haemopoiesis. Br. J. Haematol., *10*:43, 1964.

Chang, J. C., and Kan, Y. W.: A sensitive new prenatal test for sickle-cell anemia. N. Engl. J. Med., *307*:30, 1982.

Charache, S., Weatherall, D. J., and Clegg, J. B.: Polycythemia associated with a hemoglobinopathy. J. Clin. Invest., *45*:813, 1966.

Chernoff, A. I., and Singer, K.: Studies on abnormal hemoglobins. IV. Persistence of fetal hemoglobin in the erythrocytes of normal children. Pediatrics, *9*:469, 1952.

Conley, C. L., and Charache, S.: Mechanisms by which some abnormal hemoglobins produce clinical manifestations. Semin. Hematol., *4*:53, 1967.

Cooper, B. A.: Megaloblastic anaemia and disorders affecting utilization of vitamin B_{12} and folate in childhood. Clin. Haematol., 5:631, 1976.

Cooper, R. A.: Destruction of erythrocytes. *In* Williams, W. J., Beutler, E., Erslev, A. J., and Rundles, R. W. (eds.): Hematology. 2nd ed. New York, McGraw-Hill Book Co., 1977a, p. 216.

Cooper, R. A., and Jandl, J. H.: Acanthocytosis. *In* Williams, W. J., Beutler, E., Erslev, A. J., and Rundles, R. W. (eds.): Hematology. 2nd ed. New York, McGraw-Hill Book Co., 1977b, p. 461.

Croft, J. D., Jr., Swisher, S. N., Gilliland, B. C., Bakermeier, R. F., Leddy, J. P., and Weed, R. I.: Coombs' test positivity induced by drugs: Mechanisms of immunologic reactions and red cell destruction. Ann. Intern. Med., *68*:176, 1968.

Dacie, J. V.: Autoimmune hemolytic anemia. Arch. Intern. Med., *135*:1293, 1975.

Dacie, J. V.: Paroxysmal nocturnal haemoglobinuria. The Scientific Basis of Medicine: Annual Reviews. London, The Athlone Press, 1972.

Dacie, J. V., and Lewis, S. M.: Practical Haematology. 5th ed. Edinburgh, Churchill Livingstone, 1975.

Dausset, J., and Colombani, J.: The serology and the prognosis of 128 cases of autoimmune hemolytic anemia. Blood, *14*:1280, 1950.

Diamond, L. K., Wang, W. C., and Alter, B. P.: Congenital hypoplastic anemia. Adv. Pediatr., *22*:349, 1976.

Diggs, L. W.: Sickle cell crises. Am. J. Clin. Path., *44*:1, 1965.

Efremov, C. D., Huisman, T. H. J., Bowman, K., Wrightstone, R. N., and Schroeder, W. A.: Microchromatography of hemoglobins. II. A rapid method for determination of hemoglobin A_2. J. Lab. Clin. Med., *83*:657, 1974.

Erslev, A. J.: Anemia of chronic renal failure. *In* Williams, W. J., Beutler, E., Erslev, A. J., and Rundles, R. W. (eds.): Hematology. 2nd ed. New York, McGraw-Hill Book Co., 1977a, p. 288.

Erslev, A. J.: Anemia of endocrine disorders. *In* Williams, W. J., Beutler, E., Erslev, A. J., and Rundles, R. W. (eds.): Hematology. 2nd ed. New York, McGraw-Hill Book Co., 1977b, p. 295.

Fairbanks, V. F., Fahey, J. L., and Beutler, E.: Clinical Disorders of Iron Metabolism. 2nd ed. New York, Grune & Stratton, 1971.

Fairbanks, V. F., and Fernandez, M. N.: The identification of metabolic errors associated with hemolytic anemia. J.A.M.A., *208*:316, 1969.

Finch, C. A., Cook, J. D., Labbe, R. F., and Culala, M.: Effect of blood donation on iron stores as evaluated by serum ferritin. Blood, *50*:441, 1977.

Fleming, A. F.: Hypoplastic anaemia of pregnancy. Clin. Haematol., *2*:477, 1973.

Frank, M. M., Schreiber, A. D., Atkinson, J. P., and Jaffe, C. L.: Pathophysiology of immune hemolytic anemia. Ann. Intern. Med., *87*:210, 1977.

Fukagawa, N., Friedman, S., Gill, F. M., Schwartz, E., and Shaller, C.: Hereditary spherocytosis with normal osmotic fragility after incubation. Is the autohemolysis test really obsolete? J.A.M.A., *242*:63, 1979.

Gilliland, B. C.: Coombs-negative immune hemolytic anemia. Semin. Hematol., *13*:267, 1976.

Good, R. A.: Aplastic anemia—suppressor lymphocytes and hematopoiesis. N. Engl. J. Med., *296*:41, 1977.

Gottlieb, A. J., and Wurzel, H. A.: Protein-quinone interaction: *In vitro* induction of indirect antiglobulin reactions with methyldopa. Blood, *43*:85, 1974.

Götze, O., and Müller-Eberhard, H. J.: Paroxysmal nocturnal haemoglobinuria: Hemolysis initiated by the C3 activator system. N. Engl. J. Med., *286*:180, 1972.

Gralnick, H. R., Galton, D. A. G., Catovsky, D., Sultan, C., and Bennett, J. M.: Classification of acute leukemia (N.I.H. conference). Ann. Intern. Med., *87*:740, 1977.

Hagler, L., Pastore, R. E., and Bergin, J. J.: Aplastic anemia following viral hepatitis: Report of two fatal cases and literature review. Medicine (Baltimore), *54*:139, 1975.

Hall, C. A.: Transcobalamins I and II as natural transport proteins of vitamin B_{12}. J. Clin. Invest., *56*:1125, 1975.

Ham, T. H.: Studies on the destruction of red blood cells. I. Chronic hemolytic anemia with paroxysmal nocturnal hemoglobinuria: An investigation of the mechanism of hemolysis, with observations on five cases. Arch. Intern. Med., *64*:1271, 1939.

Harris, J. W., and Kellermeyer, R. W.: The Red Cell: Production, Metabolism, Destruction: Normal and Abnormal. Rev. Ed. Cambridge, Mass., Harvard University Press, 1970.

Hartmann, R. C., Jenkins, D. E., Jr., and Arnold, A. B.: Diagnostic specificity of sucrose hemolysis test for paroxysmal nocturnal hemoglobinuria. Blood, *35*:462, 1970.

Herbert, V.: Experimental nutritional folate deficiency in man. Trans. Assoc. Am. Physicians, *75*:307, 1962.

Herbert, V.: Megaloblastic anemias. *In* Beeson, P., and McDermott, W. (eds.): Textbook of Medicine. 14th ed. Philadelphia, W. B. Saunders Company, 1975.

Hillman, R. S., and Finch, C. A.: Red Cell Manual. 4th ed. Philadelphia, F. A. Davis Co., 1974.

Hirst, E., and Robertson, T. I.: The syndrome of thymoma and erythroblastopenia anemia. Medicine, *46*:225, 1967.

Hoffbrand, A. V.: Megaloblastic Anaemia. *In* Hoffbrand, A. B., and Lewis, S. M. (eds.): Postgraduate Haematology. 2nd ed. New York, Appleton-Century-Crofts, 1981.

Huisman, T. H. J., and Jonxis, J. H. P.: The Hemoglobinopathies. Techniques of Identification. New York, Marcel Dekker, Inc., 1977.

Huisman, T. H. J., Schroeder, W. A., Brodie, A. N., Mayson, S. M., and Jakway, J.: Microchromatography of hemoglobins. III. A simplified procedure for the determination of hemoglobin A_2. J. Lab. Clin. Med., *86*:700, 1975.

International Committee for Standardization in Haematology: Recommended method for radioisotope red-cell survival studies. Br. J. Haematol., *45*:659, 1980a.

International Committee for Standardization in Haematology: Recommended methods for measurement of red-cell and plasma volume. J. Nucl. Med., *21*:793, 1980b.

Jacob, H. S., and Jandl, J. H.: A simple visual screening test for glucose-6-phosphate dehydrogenase deficiency employing ascorbate and cyanide. N. Engl. J. Med., *274*:1162, 1966.

Jacobs, A.: Erythropoiesis and iron deficiency anemia. *In* Jacobs, A., and Worwood, M.: Iron in Biochemistry and Medicine. New York, Academic Press, 1974, p. 405.

Jacobs, A., and Worwood, M.: The biochemistry of ferritin and its clinical implications. Prog. Hematol., *9*:1, 1975.

Jandle, J. H.: Hereditary spherocytosis. *In* Beutler, E. (ed.): Hereditary Disorders of Erythrocyte Metabolism. New York, Grune & Stratton, Inc., 1968.

Kan, Y. W.: The Thalassemias. *In* Stanbury, J. S., Wyngaarden, J. B., Fredrickson, S. S., Goldstein, J. L., and Brown, M. S.: The Metabolic Basis of Inherited Disease. 5th ed. New York, McGraw-Hill Book Company, 1983, p. 1711.

Keitt, A. S.: Diagnostic strategy in a suspected red cell enzymopathy. Clin. Haematol., *10*:3, 1981.

Kern, P., Heimpel, H., Heit, W., and Kubanek, B.: Granulocytic progenitor cells in aplastic anaemia. Br. J. Haematol., *35*:613, 1977.

Kirtland, H. H., Mohler, D. N., and Horwitz, D. A.: Methyldopa inhibition of suppressor-lymphocyte function. A proposed cause of autoimmune hemolytic anemia. N. Engl. J. Med., *302*:825, 1980.

Krantz, S. B.: Pure red-cell aplasia. N. Engl. J. Med., *291*:345, 1974.

Kreig, A. F., and Henry, J. B.: Hemoglobin electrophoresis. Clinical pathology correlations of hemoglobinopathies and thalassemias. N.Y. State J. Med., *67*:1275, 1967.

Kunkel, H. G., Ceppellini, R., Müller-Eberhard, U., and Wolf, J.: Observations on the minor basic hemoglobin component in blood of normal individuals and patients with thalassemia. J. Clin. Invest., *36*:1615, 1957.

LaCelle, P. L., and Weed, R. I.: The contribution of normal and pathologic erythrocytes to blood rheology. Prog. Hematol., *7*:1, 1971.

Lehmann, H., Huntsman, R. G., Casey, R., et al.: Erythrocyte disorders—anemias related to abnormal globin. *In* Williams, W. J., Beutler, E., Erslev, A. J., and Rundles, R. W. (eds.): Hematology. 2nd ed. New York, McGraw-Hill Book Co., 1977, p. 494 ff.

Lewis, S. M., and Dacie, J. V.: The aplastic anaemia–paroxysmal nocturnal haemoglobinuria syndrome. Br. J. Haematol., *13*:236, 1967.

Lewis, S. M., and Verwilghen, R. L.: Dyserythropoiesis and dyserythropoietic anemias. Prog. Hematol., *8*:99, 1973.

Lux, S. E.: Hemolytic anemias. III. Membrane disorders. *In* Beck, W. S. (ed.): Hematology. 3rd ed. Cambridge, Mass., MIT Press, 1981, p. 197.

Lynch, R. E., Williams, D. M., Reading, J. C., and Cartwright, G. E. The prognosis in aplastic anemia. Blood, *45*:517, 1975.

Marengo-Rowe, A. J.: Rapid electrophoresis and quantitation of haemoglobins on cellulose acetate. J. Clin. Path., *18*:790, 1965.

Marsh, G. W., and Lewis, S. M.: Cardiac haemolytic anaemia. Semin. Hematol., *6*:133, 1969.

Maslow, W. C., Beutler, E., Bell, C. A., Hougie, C., and Kjeldsberg, C. R.: Practical Diagnosis: Hematologic Disease. Boston, Houghton Mifflin Professional Publishers, 1980.

Mauer, A. M.: Pediatric Hematology. New York, McGraw-Hill Book Co., 1969.

Milner, P. F., and Gooden, H.: Rapid citrate-agar electrophoresis in routine screening for hemoglobinopathies using a simple hemolysate. Am. J. Clin. Path., *64*:58, 1975.

Miwa, S.: Pyruvate kinase deficiency and other enzymopathies of the Embden-Meyerhof pathway. Clin. Haematol., *10*:57, 1981.

Mollin, D. L., Anderson, B. B., and Burman, J. F.: The serum vitamin B_{12} level: Its assay and significance. Clin. Haematol., *5*:521, 1976.

Nathan, D. G.: The thalassemias. *In* Beck, W. S. (ed.): Hematology. 3rd ed. Cambridge, Mass., MIT Press, 1981, p. 157.

Nathan, D. G., and Oski, F. A. (ed.): Hematology of Infancy and Childhood. 2nd ed. Philadelphia, W. B. Saunders Company, 1981.

O'Gorman Hughes, D. W.: Aplastic anemia in childhood. III. Constitutional aplastic anemia and related cytopenias. Med. J. Aust., *2*:519, 1974.

Orkin, S. H., Little, P. F. R., Kazazian, H. H., Jr., and Boehm, C. D.: Improved detection of the sickle mutation by DNA analysis. Application to prenatal diagnosis. N. Engl. J. Med., *307*:32, 1982.

Orkin, S. H., and Nathan, D. G.: The thalassemias. N. Engl. J. Med., *295*:710, 1976.

Oski, F. A., and Naiman, J. L: Hematologic Problems in the Newborn. 2nd ed. Philadelphia, W. B. Saunders Company, 1972.

Paglia, D. E., and Valentine, W. N.: Haemolytic anaemia associated with disorders of the purine and pyrimidine salvage pathways. Clin. Haematol., *10*:81, 1981.

Palek, J., and Lux, S. E.: Red cell membrane skeletal defects in hereditary and acquired hemolytic anemias. Semin. Hematol., *20*:189, 1983.

Pearson, H. A., Spencer, R. P., and Cornelius, E. A.: Functional asplenia in sickle cell anemia. N. Engl. J. Med., *281*:923, 1969.

Perutz, M. F., and Lehmann, H.: Molecular pathology of human hemoglobin. Nature (London), *219*:902, 1968.

Petz, L. D. and Garraty, G.: Acquired Immune Hemolytic Anemias. New York, Churchill Livingstone, 1980.

Petz, L. D., and Garratty, G.: Drug-induced haemolytic anemia. Clin. Haematol., *4*:181, 1975.

Phillips, J. A., III, and Kazazian, H. H., Jr.: Globin gene analysis by restriction endonuclease mapping. *In* Fairbanks, V. F. (ed.): Current Hematology, Vol. 1. New York, John Wiley & Sons, 1981, p. 1.

Piomelli, S.: A micromethod for free erythrocyte porphyrins: The FEP test. J. Lab. Clin. Med., *81*:932, 1973.

Pirofsky, B.: Immune hemolytic disease: The autoimmune hemolytic anaemias. Clin. Haematol., *4*:167, 1975.

Prchal, J. T., Throckmorton, D. W., Carroll, A. J., III, Fuson, E. W., and Gams, P. A.: A common progenitor for human myeloid and lymphoid cells. Nature, *274*:590, 1978.

Reissman, K. R., Ruth, W. E., and Nomura, T. A.: A human hemoglobin with lowered oxygen affinity and impaired heme-heme interactions. J. Clin. Invest., *40*:1826, 1961.

Rosse, W. F.: The detection of small amounts of antibody on the red cell in autoimmune hemolytic anaemia. Ser. Haematol., 7:358, 1974.

Rosse, W. F.: Paroxysmal nocturnal hemoglobinuria. *In* Williams, W. J., Beutler, E., Erslev, A. J., and Rundles, R. W. (eds.): Hematology. 2nd ed. New York, McGraw-Hill Book Co., 1977, p. 560.

Rudzki, Z., Nazaruk, M., and Kimber, R. J.: The clinical value of the radioassay of serum folate. J. Lab. Clin. Med., *87*:859, 1976.

Saarinen, U. M., and Siimes, M. A.: Developmental changes in serum iron, total iron-binding capacity, and transferrin saturation in infancy. J. Pediatr., *91*:875, 1977.

Schleider, C. T. H., Mayson, S. M., and Huisman, T. H. J.: Further modification of the microchromatographic determination of hemoglobin A_2. Hemoglobin, *1*:503, 1977.

Schmidt, R. M.: Laboratory diagnosis of hemoglobinopathies. J.A.M.A., *224*:1276, 1973.

Schmidt, R. M., and Brosious, E. F.: Basic Laboratory Methods of Hemoglobinopathy Detection. 6th ed. Atlanta, U.S. Dept. Health, Education and Welfare, Center for Disease Control, 1976. [HEW Publ. No. (CDC) 77–8266]

Schmidt, R. M., Rucknagel, D. L., and Necheles, T. F.: Comparison of methodologies for thalassemia screening by HbA_2 quantitation. J. Lab. Clin. Med., *86*:873, 1975.

Schneider, R. G., Hightower, B., Hosty, T. S., Ryder, H., Tomlin, G., Atkins, R., Brimhall, B., and Jones, R. T.: Abnormal hemoglobins in a quarter million people. Blood, *48*:629, 1976.

Shepard, M. K., Weatherall, D. J., and Conley, C. L.: Semi-quantitative estimation of the distribution of fetal hemoglobin in red cell populations. Bull. Johns Hopkins Hosp., *110*:293, 1962.

Siimes, M. A., Addiego, J. E., and Dallman, P. R.: Ferritin in serum: diagnosis of iron deficiency and iron overload in infants and children. Blood, *43*:581, 1974a.

Siimes, M. A., and Dallman, P. R.: New kinetic role for serum ferritin in iron metabolism. Br. J. Haematol., *28*:7, 1974b.

Singer, K., Chernoff, A. I., and Singer, L.: Studies on abnormal hemoglobins. I. Their demonstration in sickle cell anemia and other hematologic disorders by means of alkali denaturation. Blood, 6:413, 1951.

Sleisenger, M. H.: Malabsorption: Management. *In* Wyngaarden, J. B., and Smith, L. H., Jr. (eds.): Cecil Textbook of Medicine. 16th ed. Philadelphia, W. B. Saunders Company, 1982, p. 690.

Smith, J. R., and Landaw, S. A.: Smoker's polycythemia. N. Engl. J. Med., *298*:6, 1978.

Stamatoyannopoulos, G., Bellingham, A. J., Lenfant, C., and Finch, C. A.: Abnormal hemoglobins with high and low oxygen affinity. Ann. Rev. Med., *22*:221, 1971.

Stebbins, R., and Bertino, J. R.: Megaloblastic anaemia produced by drugs. Clin. Haematol., *5*:619, 1976.

Stenman, U-H: Intrinsic factor and the vitamin B_{12} binding proteins. Clin. Haematol., *5*:473, 1976.

Stockman, J. A., Weiner, L. S., Simon, G. E., Stuart, M. J., and Oski, F. A.: The measurement of free erythrocyte porphyrin (FEP) as a simple means of distinguishing iron deficiency from beta-thalassemia trait in subjects with microcytosis. J. Lab. Clin. Med., *85*:113, 1975.

Swisher, S. N., and Burka, E. R.: Cryopathic hemolytic syndrome. *In* Williams, W. J., Beutler, E., Erslev, A. J., Rundles, R. W. (eds.): Hematology. 2nd ed. New York, McGraw-Hill Book Co., 1977, p. 596.

Tanaka, K. R., Valentine, W. N., and Miwa, S.: Pyruvate kinase (PK) deficiency hereditary non-spherocytic hemolytic anemia. Blood, *19*:267, 1962.

Tietz, N. W. (ed.): Clinical Guide to Laboratory Tests. Philadelphia, W. B. Saunders Company, 1983.

Valentine, W. N.: Hemolytic anemia and inborn errors of metabolism. Blood, *54*:549, 1979.

Wang, W. C., and Mentzer, W. C.: Differentiation of transient erythroblastopenia of childhood from congenital hypoplastic anemia. J. Pediatr., *88*:784, 1976.

Wasi, P., Na-Nakorn, S., and Pootrakul, S-N.: The alpha-thalassemias. Clin. Haematol., *3*:383, 1974.

Weatherall, D. J.: The diagnostic features of the different forms of thalassemia. *In* Weatherall, D. J. (ed.): Methods in Hematology, 6. Edinburgh, Churchill Livingstone, 1983a, p. 1.

Weatherall, D. J.: The molecular genetics of haemoglobin—the thalassaemias. *In* Hoffbrand, A. V. (ed.): Recent Advances in Haematology. 3rd ed. Edinburgh, Churchill Livingstone, 1982, p. 45.

Weatherall, D. J.: The Thalassemias. *In* Williams, W. J., Beutler, E., Erslev, A. J., and Lichtman, M. A.: Hematology. 3rd ed. New York, McGraw-Hill Book Company, 1983b, p. 493.

Weatherall, D. J., and Clegg, J. B.: The Thalassamia Syndromes. 3rd ed. Oxford, Blackwell Scientific Publications, 1981.

Weens, J. H., and Schwartz, R. S.: Etiologic factors in autoimmune hemolytic anemia. Ser. Hematol., 7:303, 1974.

Weinreb, N. J., and Shih, C-F.: Spurious polycythemia. Semin. Hematol., *12*:397, 1975.

Wheby, M. S.: Using a clinical laboratory in the diagnosis of anemia. Med. Clin. North Am., *50*:1689, 1966.

White, J. M., and Dacie, J. V.: The unstable hemoglobins—molecular and clinical features. Prog. Hematol., 7:69, 1971.

WHO Tech. Rep. Ser. 503, 1972. Nutritional Anemias: Report of a WHO group of experts.

Wiley, J. S., Ellory, J. C., Shuman, M. A., Shaller, C. C., and Cooper, R. A.: Characteristics of the membrane defect in the hereditary stomatocytosis syndrome. Blood, *46*:337, 1975.

Williams, D. M., Lynch, R. E., and Cartwright, G. E.: Prognostic factors in aplastic anemia. Clin. Haematol., *12*:467, 1978.

Winslow, R. M., and Anderson, W. F.: The Hemoglobinopathies. *In* Stanbury, J. B., Wyngaarden, J. B., Fredrickson, D. S., Goldstein, J. L., and Brown, M. S. (eds.): The Metabolic Basis of Inherited Disease. 5th ed. New York, McGraw-Hill Book Company, 1983, Chap. 76.

Wintrobe, M. M., Lee, G. R., Boggs, D. R., Bithell, T. C.,

Foerster, J., Athens, J. W., and Lukens, J. N.: Clinical Hematology. 8th ed. Philadelphia, Lea and Febiger, 1981.
Worlledge, S.: Immune haemalytic anaemias. *In* Hardisty, R. M., and Weatherall, D. J. (eds.): Blood and Its Disorders. Oxford, Blackwell Scientific, 1974, p. 714.
Worwood, M.: Serum ferritin. *In* Cook, J. D. (ed.): Iron. Edinburgh, Churchill Livingtone, 1980, p. 59.
Wrightstone, R. N., and Huisman, T. H. J.: On the levels of hemoglobins F and A_2 in sickle-cell anemia and related disorders. Am. J. Clin. Path., *61*:375, 1974.
Young, N.: Aplastic anemia. Research themes and clinical issues. Prog. Hematol., *12*:227, 1981.
Yunis, A. A., and Bloomberg, G. R.: Chloramphenicol toxicity: Clinical features and pathogenesis. Prog. Hematol., *4*:138, 1964.
Zarkowsky, H. S.: Heat-induced erythrocyte fragmentation in neonatal elliptocytosis. Br. J. Haematol., *41*:515, 1979.
Zipursky, A.: Hemolytic disease of the newborn. *In* Nathan, D. G., and Oski, F. A. (eds.): Hematology of Infancy and Childhood. Philadelphia, W. B. Saunders Company, 1974, p. 280.

30

LEUKOCYTIC DISORDERS

FREDERICK R. DAVEY, M.D., and DOUGLAS A. NELSON, M.D.

NON-NEOPLASTIC DISORDERS

Quantitative study of leukocytes includes the concentration of all the white cells, the total leukocyte count (white blood cell count; WBC) and the relative and absolute concentrations of the various forms of white cells. The term *leukocytosis* refers to an increase in the total WBC above the upper limit of normal for age and sex. *Leukopenia* is a total WBC below normal. Although all leukocytes act in defending the body, their functions differ and it is best to regard them as separate systems. An increase or decrease in the absolute concentration of cells in each series is termed *neutrophilia* (neutrophilic leukocytosis) and *neu-*

tropenia; eosinophilia (eosinophilic leukocytosis) and *eosinopenia; basophilia* (basophilic leukocytosis) and *basopenia; lymphocytosis* and *lymphocytopenia; monocytosis* and *monocytopenia.* Qualitative study of leukocytes includes structural abnormalities in cytoplasm and nucleus and, to an increasing extent, functional abnormalities as well.

One purpose of the study of leukocytes is to help in establishing a diagnosis. Occasionally the examination alone may furnish a positive specific diagnosis, for example, in leukemia. More frequently it may be diagnostically helpful together with other clinical or laboratory data, for example, in acute appendicitis or infectious mononucleosis. Another purpose is to help in establishing a prognosis. For example, leukopenia in acute appendicitis or pneumonia is considered prognostically unfavorable.

Finally, study of the leukocytes is helpful in following the course of disease. For example, toxic effects of radiotherapy and chemotherapy may be recognized, and recovery monitored, by examination of leukocytes.

For these reasons the leukocyte count is performed for almost every patient admitted to the hospital regardless of disease.

Granulocytic and Monocytic Disorders

NEUTROPHILIA

Neutrophilic leukocytosis or neutrophilia refers to an absolute concentration of neutrophils in the blood above normal for age. Reference intervals are given in Table 27–5; age variations are discussed on page 621.

Mechanisms (Boggs, 1983; Finch, 1977). The primary factors influencing the neutrophil count are (1) the rate of inflow of cells from the bone marrow; (2) the proportion of neutrophils in the marginal granulocyte pool (MGP) and the circulating granulocyte pool (CGP); and (3) the rate of outflow of neutrophils from the blood (see p. 638).

Physiologic leukocytosis is produced by factors or situations that do not involve tissue damage. Severe exercise, hypoxia, stress, or the injection of epinephrine will result in a decrease in the MGP and a corresponding increase in the CGP, resulting in a pseudoneutrophilia. This is a simple redistribution of cells between the CGP and MGP.

Stress of greater severity or injection of endotoxin, corticosteroids, or etiocholanolone results in an increased inflow of cells to the blood from the marrow storage pool. As a result, the maturation and storage pool in the marrow is diminished, and both MGP and CGP are enlarged. A greater neutrophilia is possible here because of the much larger size of the storage pool than the CGP and MGP. Band neutrophils and metamyelocytes are likely to be present.

In both of the above an acute neutrophilia occurs as a result of redistribution of cells, without input from increased production. Chronic neutrophilia may be produced by corticosteroids, which decrease the egress of neutrophils from the blood and result in increased CGP and MGP without necessarily increasing the production of neutrophils.

In contrast to the above, *pathologic leukocytosis* is an increased WBC which occurs as a result of disease, and usually is a response to tissue damage (Table 30–1). This leukocytosis is most often a neutrophilia.

In addition to the random loss of neutrophils from the circulation in various body secretions, neutrophils leave the blood by ameboid movement when attracted to a focus of inflammation in tissues, presumably by chemotactic substances. It is from the marginal granulocyte pool (MGP) that the neutrophils leave the blood, pass between capillary endothelial cells, and reach the tissues.

In acute infection, increased margination of neutrophils and outflow from blood to tissues would lead to neutropenia were there not a flow of neutrophils from the marrow storage compartment into the blood. Since the latter overcompensates, the result is a neutrophilia. Usually production and storage compartments then increase in the marrow and are able to sustain the increased CGP (neutrophilia) and MGP in the face of the increased flow of neutrophils from the blood into the inflammatory site. In these instances, the marrow will show granulocytic hyperplasia (decreased E/G ratio and increased cellularity), with maturation intact.

If the demand for neutrophils is extremely great, as in severe infection, there may be depletion of the marrow storage pool and a decreased CGP (neutropenia) and MGP, because the supply of cells is insufficient for the demand. In these instances, the marrow will show increased numbers of early neutrophil precursors, through the myelocyte stage, but decreased numbers of metamyelocytes, bands, and neutrophils.

Causes

Infection. Systemic infections due to various bacteria, fungi, spirochetes, and viruses may cause neutrophilia. In some, this may be preceded by a transient neutropenia, especially if the infection is severe. Some bacterial infections result in persistent neutropenia, such as typhoid fever, paratyphoid fever, and brucellosis. Whether this is due to the mechanism cited above for severe infection, or to a toxic depression of the marrow, or to a combination, is not clear.

Appendicitis, salpingitis, otitis media, and other localized infections caused by pyogenic organisms usually result in neutrophilia.

A characteristic pattern of response to infection includes progressive neutrophilic leukocytosis, increase of young forms (shift to the left), and fall in eosinophils. When the infection begins to subside and the fever drops, a gradual transformation in the blood picture occurs: the total number of leukocytes goes down, and the number of monocytes increases. This monocytic phase is gradually replaced by a relative or slight absolute lymphocytosis and eosinophilia as recovery proceeds.

Other disorders associated with neutrophilia are listed below. In some of them, one or more of the mechanisms described above are operating; in others, the mechanism is unclear.

Toxic

Metabolic. Uremia, eclampsia, gout, diabetic acidosis.

Drugs and Chemicals. Lead, mercury, potassium

4

Table 30–1. PATHOLOGIC LEUKOCYTOSIS

Cause	Cell Type
Allergy	Eosinophil
Brucellosis	Lymphocyte, monocyte
Convulsions	Neutrophil or lymphocyte
Drugs and poisons	
ACTH	Neutrophil
Adrenaline	
Camphor	Neutrophil and eosinophil
Copper sulfate, phosphorus, carpine	Eosinophil
Tetrachlorethane, Adrenaline	Monocyte, neutrophil, and lymphocyte
Other (acetanilid, arsenicals, benzene, CO, digitalis, lead, phenacetin, turpentine, venoms)	Neutrophil
Hemolysis	Neutrophil
Hemorrhage	Neutrophil
Hodgkin's disease	Neutrophil, eosinophil, and monocyte
Infectious lymphocytosis	Lymphocyte
Infectious mononucleosis	Lymphocyte, atypical changes
Leukemia	Granulocyte, lymphocyte, or monocyte
Loeffler's syndrome, periarteritis nodosa, pernicious anemia	Eosinophil
Polycythemia vera	Neutrophil, eosinophil, basophil
Toxemias: diabetic acidosis, eclampsia, gout, uremia	Neutrophil
Tuberculosis	Neutrophil, eosinophil, lymphocyte, monocyte
Tumors involving	
Marrow and serous cavities	Neutrophil and eosinophil
Ovary	Eosinophil
GI tract and liver	Neutrophil
Typhoid fever	Lymphocyte

chlorate, digitalis, epinephrine, corticosteroids, turpentine, ethylene glycol, benzene.

Physical and Emotional Stimuli. Heat, cold, muscular activity, anoxia, pain, fear, anger.

Tissue Destruction or Necrosis. Myocardial infarction, burns, surgical operations, crush injuries, fractures, neoplastic disease (especially with extensive necrosis).

Hemorrhage. Especially if bleeding has occurred within a serous cavity (peritoneal, pleural, joint, subdural).

Hemolysis. Especially with rapid hemolysis, as in hemolytic crises or hemolytic transfusion reactions.

Hematologic Disorders. Myeloproliferative disorders, myelogenous leukemia, postsplenectomy state.

Determinants. Certain host factors modify the degree of neutrophilic response. Children respond more intensely than adults. The degree of neutrophilia produced may be impaired by the same factors that impair erythrocyte production (iron lack, folate or vitamin B_{12} deficiency) or by marrow failure due to other causes. Imperfectly defined factors which enable the body to localize an infection may play a role: the more localized the process, the more pronounced the neutrophilia.

Other factors modifying the neutrophilic response are due more to the microorganism than to the host. Pyogenic bacteria, especially, induce neutrophilia. Within limits the more virulent the agent, the higher the neutrophil count. When the infection is overwhelming, however, there is apt to be a neutropenia and greater shift to the left due to the mechanism described above.

Therapy of infections with antibiotic agents may modify the leukocytic response to infection. Steroid therapy, though causing neutrophilia, tends to impair the host response to infection, probably because of diminished movement of neutrophils into the tissues and increased lysosomal stability.

NEUTROPENIA

Neutropenia is a reduction of the absolute neutrophil count below 2×10^9/L for whites and below 1.3×10^9/L for blacks. The term *agranulocytosis* has been used for severe neutropenia; this is almost always associated with depletion of eosinophils and basophils as well. If the neutrophil count is less than 1×10^9/L, the risk of infection is considerably increased over normal, and if there are less than 0.5×10^9 neutrophils per liter, the risk of infection is great.

The mechanisms by which neutropenia occur include (1) decreased flow of neutrophils from marrow into blood due to either lack of production or ineffective production; (2) increased removal of neutrophils from the blood; (3) altered distribution between circulating granulocyte pool (CGP) and marginal granulocyte pool (MGP); or (4) combinations of these. Neutropenias are not so neatly classified as anemias. In recent years, however, a sound approach has been made, using data from radioisotopic measurements of proliferative activity, maturation time, survival in the circulation, and measurement of MGP and CGP in addition to the usual bone marrow and peripheral blood studies (Finch, 1977). A classification is given in Table 30–2. It should be noted that drugs induce neutropenia through several mechanisms and are a

Table 30–2. CLASSIFICATION OF NEUTROPENIA*

I. *Myeloid hypoplasia*
   A. Infantile genetic agranulocytosis (Kostman); familial neutropenia; cyclic neutropenia; chronic (hypoplastic) neutropenia; neutropenias associated with lymphocytic disorders; myelophthisic neutropenia.
   B. Drug induced:
      1. Cytolytic:
         a. Alkylating agents (nitrogen mustard, cyclophosphamide, chlorambucil, busulfan).
         b. Ionizing radiation.
         c. Mitosis inhibitors (colchicine, vinblastine, vincristine).
         d. DNA depolymerization (procarbazine).
      2. Metabolic interference with DNA synthesis:
         a. Purine and pyrimidine antagonists (cytosine arabinoside,† methotrexate,† 6-mercaptopurine, azathioprine, hydroxyurea).
         b. Phenothiazine type (phenothiazines, dibenzazepine compounds, antithyroid compounds,† sulfonamides,† antibiotics, anticonvulsants).
         c. Others (chloramphenicol,† benzene†).
      3. Idiosyncratic:
         a. Acute, days to weeks (quinine, quinidine, indomethacin, procainamide, thiazides, sulfonamides,† phenylbutazone,† antithyroids†).
         b. Chronic, months to years (chloramphenicol,† phenylbutazone,† benzene,† gold salts†).

II. *Marrow hyperplasia with ineffective granulocytopoiesis*
   A. Chédiak-Higashi syndrome; megaloblastic anemia; myeloproliferative disorders (these may belong in IV).
   B. Drug induced:
      1. Impaired nucleic acid synthesis (cytosine arabinoside,† methotrexate,† phenytoin).
      2. Others (alcohol, chloramphenicol†).

III. *Decreased survival in circulation* due to increased utilization or increased destruction.
   A. Bacterial infections; viral infections; protozoal infections; chronic benign neutropenia of childhood; chronic idiopathic neutropenia in adults; splenic neutropenia; neonatal isoimmunization neutropenia; acquired immunoneutropenia.
   B. Drug induced (immunologic mechanism):
      Aminopyrine, amidopyrine, phenylbutazone,† sulfapyridine.†

IV. *Combination of impaired production (I or II) and decreased survival (III)*
   A. Megaloblastic anemia; severe bacterial infections; mycobacterial infections; chronic idiopathic myelokathexis.
   B. Drug induced (very likely):
      Alcohol, purine and pyrimidine inhibitors, aminopyrine.

V. *Pseudoneutropenia (shift from CGP to MGP)*
   A. Endotoxin.
   B. Drug induced: (?) anesthetic agents, ether, pentobarbital.

*Adapted from Finch, S. C.: *In* Williams, W. J., Beutler, E., Erslev, A. J., and Lichtman, M. A. (eds.): Hematology. 3rd ed. New York, McGraw-Hill Book Co., Inc., 1983.

†Drugs cited for more than one mechanism.

very important consideration in any differential diagnosis of leukopenia.

Myeloid Hypoplasia. Kostman's infantile genetic agranulocytosis is a rare autosomal recessive condition appearing in early infancy. The marrow usually shows increased early granulocytes but few maturing forms, and the neutrophil survival is normal. A soluble factor necessary for granulocyte maturation appears to be lacking (Barak, 1971).

Chronic familial neutropenia and cyclic neutropenia appear to be autosomal dominant conditions. The latter usually has a period of about 21 days, and appears to be due to periodic stem cell failure. Neutrophil precursors disappear prior to the fall in circulating neutrophils and reappear during the neutropenic phase. Other congenital and familial neutropenias have been described.

Patients with dysfunctional lymphocytes frequently exhibit some degree of neutropenia. Males with X-linked agammaglobulinemia are often neutropenic.

Isolated neutropenia or agranulocytosis is uncommon in adults. When the marrow is damaged, by a myelophthisic process such as metastatic carcinoma or Gaucher's disease replacing the marrow, or by drugs, usually the damage is not limited to granulopoiesis but affects normoblasts and megakaryocytes as well. Because of the short life span of granulocytes, however, neutropenia is the earliest recognizable effect in the blood. It takes weeks before damage to the erythropoietic tissue becomes manifest because of the long life span of erythrocytes. Platelets have a rather short life span but, on the other hand, megakaryocytes are more resistant to damage.

Drugs are an important cause of neutropenia, and, as outlined in Table 30–2, may act in different ways. Drugs that have the effect of destroying or interfering with mitosis of the proliferating cells are frequently used in the therapy of malignant disease. Important and limiting side effects of such chemotherapy are severe neutropenia with its risk of infection, and severe thrombocytopenia with risk of bleeding; anemia is more readily controlled with transfusion.

Idiosyncratic drug effects refer to those in which host susceptibility factors predominate; that is, there is little relationship with dose and duration of drug therapy.

Ineffective Granulocytopoiesis. Neutropenia due to increased ineffective granulocytopoiesis occurs in megaloblastic anemias as a result of drugs that have an antifolate effect. Of course, anemia is usually present if therapy is prolonged, and often thrombocytopenia as well. The marrow is usually hyperplastic. In addition to increased destruction of cells in the marrow there is some evidence that circulating neutrophils have a shortened survival. Indirect evidence for increased granulocyte turnover in this group of neutropenias with hypercellular marrow is an increased serum muramidase (lysozyme) (Catovsky, 1971).

Decreased Survival. Transient neutropenia may occur early in some infections, followed by leukocytosis once the marrow production catches up with the demand. As previously noted, in severe, extensive bacterial infection, neutropenia with a shift to the left may be due to inability of marrow production to keep up with the peripheral utilization. Some bacterial infections, notably brucellosis and Salmonella infections, are prone to be associated with neutropenia; they may have some depressing effect on the marrow as well. Viral infections such as measles and rubella have neutropenia for several days after appearance of the rash; this is probably due in part to increased utilization. Lymphocytosis is present and persists after the neutropenia subsides.

The neutropenia of hypersplenism has been attributed to selective removal of neutrophils by the spleen. It is associated with neutrophilic hyperplasia of the marrow and is corrected by splenectomy. Splenomegaly due to many causes may have shortened neutrophil survival and neutropenia; these include congestive splenomegaly, Felty's syndrome, Gaucher's disease, and lymphoma. In some cases of Felty's syndrome (neutropenia and splenomegaly in rheumatoid arthritis), there may be a neutrophil-specific antibody involved.

Evidence has been accumulating that there are antibodies capable of clumping leukocytes of all varieties under proper experimental conditions (leukoagglutinins). Leukopenia in the newborn may be produced by leukoagglutinins coming from the mother. Studies have demonstrated that autoantibodies also may be responsible for immune neutropenia or immune panleukopenia. Several antibodies with agglutinating or cytotoxic activity against specific neutrophilic antigens have been considered responsible for neutropenia (Lalezari, 1975; Thompson, 1980). An autoantibody with cytotoxic activity against mature granulocytes, monocytes, and lymphocytes as well as primitive myeloid cells has been shown to result in episodic autoimmune panleukopenia (Cline, 1976).

Drug-induced neutropenia due to immune mechanisms has been well described for aminopyrine. In about 1 per cent of persons, seven to ten days after first taking the drug, chills, headache, fever, and neutropenia with a shift to the left occur. Slight granulocytic hyperplasia is noted in the marrow. If the drug is continued, mucosal ulceration and sepsis may occur, and granulocytic precursors may disappear from the marrow. If, on the other hand, the drug is discontinued, the neutrophil count returns to normal levels in a week. An antibody develops in these patients which, in the presence of the drug, causes enhanced destruction of neutrophils. Of the possible mechanisms involved, a drug–plasma protein complex is probably the antigen; the antigen-antibody complex non-specifically adsorbs on the cells and leads to their destruction (Finch, 1977).

Combinations. As indicated, some of the conditions discussed above are probably combinations of increased destruction and impaired effective production.

Pseudoneutropenia. Small doses of endotoxin will cause a shift of neutrophils into the MGP from the CGP, giving an apparent neutropenia, prior to causing a leukocytosis. In animals, anesthetic agents such as ether will cause the same kind of pseudoneutropenia (Boggs, 1983).

MORPHOLOGIC ALTERATIONS IN NEUTROPHILS

In addition to quantitative changes, qualitative morphologic alterations also occur in neutrophils. Some of these, such as toxic granules or cytoplasmic vacuoles, are acquired and disappear after the stimulus which provoked them is gone. Others are hereditary and persist through life, with or without functional impairment. These are well illustrated and reviewed by Brunning (1970).

It should be noted that disorders of leukocyte function may exist without any structural abnormality detectable with the usual modes of morphologic examination. These are discussed on page 710 and in Chapter 35.

Toxic Granulation. Toxic granules are dark blue to purple cytoplasmic granules in the metamyelocyte, band, or neutrophil stage. They are peroxidase positive and may be numerous or few in number; there may be less peroxidase activity in toxic than in normal neutrophils. Toxic granulation is found in severe infections or other toxic conditions (Plate 30–1*A*).

Normally neutrophil granules are tan to pink in color in neutrophil metamyelocytes, bands, and mature forms. Even the non-specific or azurophil granules which are dark blue on the promyelocyte stage normally lose their basophilia in the mature neutrophil, where they constitute about one third of the granules in the human. Toxic granules are azurophil granules that have retained their basophilic staining reaction by lack of maturation, or that have developed increased basophilia in the mature neutrophil. In addition, perhaps skipped divisions during the development of the neutrophil may result in a greater proportion of the granules being of the azurophil type. Increased basophilia of azurophil granules simulating toxic granules may occur in normal cells with prolonged staining time or decreased pH of the staining reaction (McCall, 1969).

Irregular basophilia of the cytoplasm is also common in toxic conditions and appears to reflect impaired cytoplasmic maturation. If discrete, this focal basophilia is known as a Döhle inclusion body (see below).

Cytoplasmic vacuoles are also signs of toxic change if the possibility of degeneration artefacts can be eliminated by making films from fresh blood free of anticoagulant. Vacuoles or irregular depletion of granules implies that phagocytosis has occurred (Plate 30–1*B*).

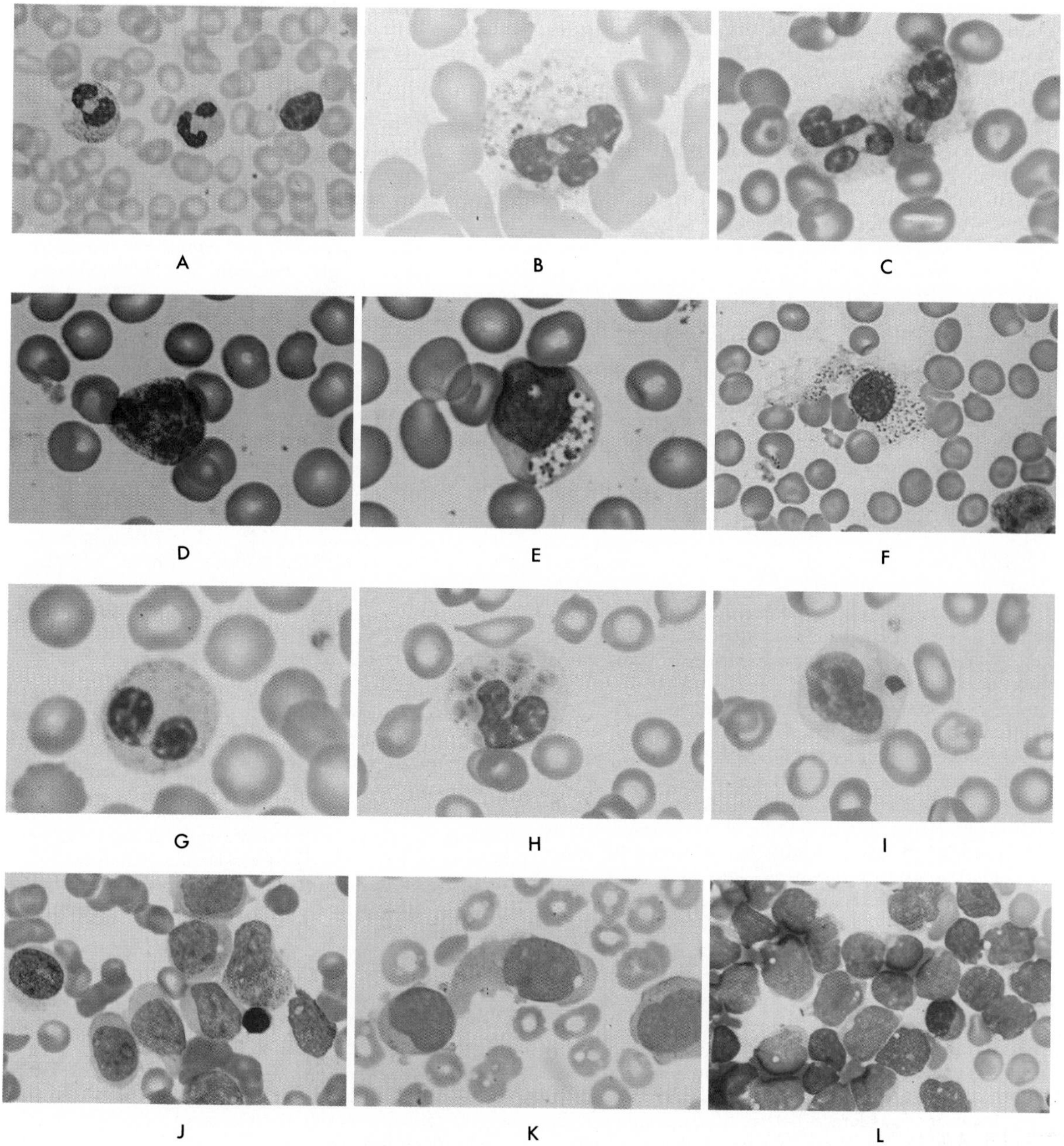

A B C

D E F

G H I

J K L

Plate 30–1. *A,* Toxic neutrophil, *left,* with cytoplasmic vacuoles and heavy azurophilic granules. Normal neutrophil, *center.* Lymphocyte, *right. B,* Toxic neutrophil. Partial degranulation, fusion of granules, vacuoles, and phagocytized diplococcus. Blood film from a patient with meningococcemia. *C,* May-Hegglin anomaly. Note the large pale blue inclusions at the outer margins of each neutrophil. *D,* Alder-Reilly anomaly, Hurler's syndrome. Deeply staining azurophilic granules almost obscure the nucleus of the neutrophil. The Alder-Reilly anomaly may be found in some cases of mucopolysaccharidosis (in which case the granules are usually metachromatic), or it may be found as a hereditary anomaly in apparently healthy persons. These cells resemble neutrophils with intense toxic granulation. *E,* Lymphocyte with basophilic inclusions surrounded by halos, characteristic of mucopolysaccharidosis. These inclusions are metachromatic. Peripheral blood film, Hurler's syndrome. *F,* Histiocyte or macrophage with numerous basophilic inclusions which are surrounded by clear spaces or halos. These granules are metachromatic and characteristic of mucopolysaccharidosis. Bone marrow film, Hurler's syndrome. *G,* Pelger-Huët anomaly, neutrophil. *H,* Chédiak-Higashi anomaly, band neutrophil. Neutrophil granules have fused into irregular masses which stain gray rather than tan. *I,* Chédiak-Higashi anomaly, lymphocyte. Azurophilic inclusions are much larger than azurophilic granules in lymphocytes of normal persons. *J,* Acute myelogenous leukemia. Several myeloblasts and one abnormal neutrophil myelocyte. *K,* Acute myelomonocytic leukemia. Blast, *left;* immature monocytes, *center* and *right. L,* Acute lymphoblastic leukemia. The lymphoblasts have more nuclear irregularity and a higher nuclear to cytoplasmic ratio than myeloblasts.

Another toxic change in the neutrophil is the occasional appearance of several sharp or blunt spicules extending out from the nucleus (see Plate 27–1*A*).

Döhle Inclusion Bodies. These are small, oval inclusions in the peripheral cytoplasm of polymorphonuclear neutrophils, which stain pale blue with Wright's stain. They are remnants of free ribosomes or rough surfaced endoplasmic reticulum persisting from an earlier stage of development. Originally Döhle bodies were described as being especially prominent in scarlet fever, but they are seen in many other infectious diseases, in burns, in aplastic anemia, and following administration of toxic agents. They frequently accompany toxic granulation in the neutrophil. With the light microscope, Döhle bodies resemble the inclusions seen in the May-Hegglin anomaly (Plate 30–1*C*).

May-Hegglin Anomaly. This is a rare autosomal dominant condition characterized by the presence of pale blue inclusions resembling Döhle bodies in neutrophils, giant platelets, and, in some persons, thrombocytopenia. The inclusions are larger and more prominent than the Döhle bodies found in infections (Plate 30–1*C*). They have been described in eosinophils, basophils, and monocytes as well as in neutrophils (Brunning, 1970). The blue staining of the inclusions can be abolished by prior treatment of the cells with ribonuclease. With electron microscopy, the appearance of the inclusions differs from that of Döhle bodies, suggesting structural alterations in RNA (Jenis, 1971).

Alder-Reilly Anomaly. Dense azurophilic granulation in all white blood cells was described by Alder in 1939 (Plate 30–1*D*). In neutrophils it may resemble toxic granulation, but is unrelated to infection and is not transient. In 1941, Reilly described similar granulocytes in some but not all patients with gargoylism (the Hurler syndrome or, more generally, the genetic mucopolysaccharidoses). Other observations have shown that the heavy granulation in neutrophils can occur either as a feature of the genetic mucopolysaccharidoses or independently in otherwise healthy persons (Brunning, 1970).

Occurring more often than the Alder-Reilly anomaly in the genetic mucopolysaccharidoses is a metachromatic inclusion in the lymphocytes surrounded by a clear space (Plate 30–1*E*). Macrophages in the marrow frequently contain similar granulation (Plate 30–1*F*). This group of disorders is inherited and is characterized by deficiencies or derangement in various lysosomal enzymes required for degrading mucopolysaccharides. The result is abnormal deposition and storage of mucopolysaccharides in multiple organs. Skeletal abnormalities are prominent (Groover, 1972; McKusick, 1983).

Pelger-Huët Anomaly. This hereditary, autosomal dominant condition involves failure of normal segmentation of granulocytic nuclei. Most nuclei are band shaped or have two segments but no more (Plate 30–1*G*). The chromatin is quite coarse, and these are not normal young band forms. When a large number of band neutrophils appear in the differential count in a patient without infection or other cause, careful analysis of the blood films of the patient and of family members will occasionally establish the presence of the Pelger-Huët anomaly.

A similar appearing, acquired disorder of nuclear segmentation in granulocytes may occasionally be found in cases of granulocytic leukemia, myeloproliferative disorders, some infections, and after exposure to certain drugs (Brunning, 1970); this is sometimes called the pseudo-Pelger anomaly. In addition to the band forms and neutrophils with only two segments, mature cells with round non-segmented nuclei and coarse chromatin are common, in contrast to the congenital Pelger-Huët anomaly.

Chédiak-Higashi Syndrome. This rare, autosomal recessive disorder is characterized by partial albinism, photophobia, abnormally large granules in leukocytes and other granule-containing cells, and frequent pyogenic infections. An accelerated lymphoma-like phase occurs, with lymphadenopathy, hepatosplenomegaly, and pancytopenia; lymphoid infiltrates are widespread and death ensues at an early age (Blume, 1972). Granulocytes, monocytes, and lymphocytes contain giant granules (Plate 30–1*H* and *I*) which appear to be abnormal lysosomes (White, 1967). Leukocyte functional abnormalities exist (Stossel, 1977).

FUNCTIONAL DISORDERS OF NEUTROPHILS

Inherited and acquired disorders affecting leukocytes may result in abnormal function and consequent susceptibility to infections (Stossel, 1977). Often, the leukocytes are normal in number and in morphologic appearance.

Deficiencies of humoral factors (antibodies, components of complement) may result in defective chemotaxis or opsonization. Cellular abnormalities (contractile protein dysfunction, enzyme deficiencies) may result in defects in motility, phagocytosis, or microbial killing (Miller, 1977).

These disorders are discussed in Chapter 35.

EOSINOPHILIA

Eosinophilia exists if blood eosinophils exceed 0.35 $\times$ 10^9/L when direct chamber counts are used, or 0.5 $\times$ 10^9/L when the count is calculated from the 100 or 200 cell differential and the total leukocyte count.

Allergic Diseases. Allergic and atopic conditions such as bronchial asthma and seasonal rhinitis (hay fever) are characterized by eosinophilia. These immune reactions are mediated by IgE, which results in mast cell and basophil degranulation with the release of a chemotactic factor for eosinophils. Eosinophils are found in the blood, marrow, sputum (in bronchial asthma), and in nasal and conjunctival discharges (in hay fever). Blood eosinophilia is usually only mild or moderate (0.4 to 1.0 $\times$ 10^9/L).

In asthma, absolute eosinophil counts have been useful in management because the level of eosinophils positively correlates with pulmonary performance, indicates the adequacy of steroid therapy, and may indicate the presence of complicating infections (Beeson, 1977).

Skin Disorders. Atopic dermatitis and eczema are often accompanied by blood eosinophilia, especially in children. In pemphigus, eosinophilia is characteristic. Eosinophilia is frequently associated with acute urticarial reactions but is uncommon in chronic urticaria.

Parasitic Infestations. Eosinophilia is more pronounced if tissues are invaded (for example, trichinosis) than when parasites are inhabiting the lumen of a viscus (for example, tapeworm). Eosinophilia disappears in some forms of infestation when encystment occurs (for example, cysticerosis).

In trichinosis eosinophils begin to rise in the blood within days after infection. The peak of the eosinophilia is during the third or fourth week. Eosinophilia may be absent, however, in severe infestation with trichinae.

Leukocytosis and eosinophilia extending over months are seen in visceral larva migrans (dog and cat roundworm) infestation. In this condition pulmonary lesions (Loeffler's syndrome) may be present.

Another parasitic infestation with eosinophilia is creeping eruption caused by larvae of the dog or cat hookworm.

Infectious Diseases. Eosinophilia of various degrees is seen in some infectious diseases. In scarlet fever, eosinophilia is commonly associated with the cutaneous rash, which is probably allergic in nature. Chorea may be associated with eosinophilia, but other forms of rheumatic fever are not.

In conditions characterized by neutrophilia, eosinophilia is uncommon; often this may be due to increased adrenal corticosteroid secretion in disease. For example, when a lesion that is responsible for eosinophilia (such as an echinococcus cyst) becomes infected and suppurates, neutrophilia replaces eosinophilia. The same phenomenon is also observed in acute infections (for example, pneumococcus pneumonia).

Pulmonary Eosinophilias. *Loeffler's syndrome* is characterized by repeated, transient pulmonary exudates accompanied by cough, often producing sputum which contains eosinophils. The syndrome resolves in a few weeks. It may be caused by certain drugs, inhaled antigens, or helminth (roundworm) infestation during periods of dissemination when the parasites pass from the blood into the alveoli of the lung.

The *P.I.E.* syndrome (pulmonary infiltration with eosinophilia) refers to a more severe disorder characterized by a chronic and relapsing fever, cough, dyspnea, and other symptoms. Etiology may be bacterial, viral, or fungal infection, allergic reaction to drugs, or parasitic infestations. The difference from Loeffler's syndrome appears to be one of severity (Wintrobe, 1981).

Tropical pulmonary eosinophilia is a syndrome of paroxysmal cough and bronchospasm associated with marked eosinophilia. It is found mainly in India, Southeast Asia, and the South Pacific. There is a predilection for males and for Indians, among racial groups living in an endemic area. Serum IgE levels are very high. Interestingly, epinephrine induces a rise instead of a fall in blood eosinophils (Beeson, 1977). The disease is probably a hyperimmune reaction caused by microfilariae, which may be found occasionally in lung or lymph node biopsies, but not in blood. The patients have a high titer of filarial complement-fixing antibodies in the blood. Response to the antifilarial drug diethylcarbamazine is curative (Ottesen, 1982).

Hypereosinophilic Syndrome. Persistent high levels of eosinophils for long periods of time, no evidence of known causes of eosinophilia, and signs and symptoms of organ involvement are criteria for inclusion of patients in this syndrome (Chusid, 1975). The organ most consistently affected is the heart, with mural thrombi and endocardial and myocardial fibrosis. Hepatosplenomegaly is common. Most patients have a hypersensitivity reaction of some type; it is an open question whether some patients have a form of eosinophilic leukemia (p. 732). Regardless of cause, large numbers of circulating eosinophils appear to damage the heart by some unknown mechanism.

Reactive eosinophilia can often be differentiated from an eosinophilic leukemia by the use of cytochemical stains (Liso, 1977). Eosinophilic leukemias usually have an increased proportion of myeloblasts and eosinophilic myelocytes. In addition, the presence of an abnormal karyotype in a patient with eosinophilia may suggest the appearance of a leukemic clone.

Blood Diseases. In chronic myelogenous leukemia and, to a lesser extent, in other myeloproliferative disorders eosinophilia is common. Mild eosinophilia may be found in marrow and blood in pernicious anemia.

Other Conditions. Splenectomy is frequently followed by eosinophilia and lymphocytosis. This may last for several months.

There is no satisfactory explanation for occasional instances of moderate and even severe eosinophilia, general or local, in patients with various neoplasms and a variety of other conditions (for example, ovarian cysts). Eosinophilia is seen more frequently in neoplasms involving serous surfaces and bone and in those with necrosis. Eosinophilia associated with malignant tumors often persists until the primary neoplasm is removed or significantly reduced in size. The eosinophils may be hypogranular and vacuolated. In addition, the eosinophil count may exceed 100×10^9/L. In Hodgkin's disease, the majority of patients do not have blood eosinophilia, though when present it is sometimes marked in degree (Beeson, 1977).

Various drugs have been reported to be responsible for eosinophilia: pilocarpine, physostigmine, digitalis, para-aminosalicylic acid, sulfonamides, and others. On the other hand, atropine is supposed to depress the eosinophils.

Hereditary eosinophilia occurs rarely in the absence of other recognized causes of eosinophilia (Naiman, 1964).

EOSINOPENIA

Eosinopenia is a decreased level of circulating eosinophils, below the lowest reference value of 0.04×10^9/L. In order to be detected, large numbers of cells must be counted, using direct hemacytometer counts

(p. 589) or automated counts with an instrument such as the Hemalog D (p. 618).

Eosinopenia occurs in any situation that results in acute stress, due to adrenal glucocorticoid and epinephrine secretion (either causes eosinopenia), and also in acute inflammatory states. A rapid decrease in circulating eosinophils occurs due to margination or migration into inflammatory sites. Release of eosinophils from the marrow is temporarily inhibited, and later eosinophil production is inhibited. Once the acute process subsides, immune stimulation of eosinophil production may occur; this is mediated by T lymphocytes (Beeson, 1977). Eosinopenia of 0 to 0.03 × 10^9/L also may occur in Cushing's syndrome or following the administration of corticosteroids.

BASOPHILIA

Basophilia is an increase of basophils in the blood to a level above 0.2 × 10^9/L if calculated from the differential count and the total leukocyte count, and above 0.08 × 10^9/L if counted directly in a hemacytometer chamber or with the Hemalog D (Gilbert, 1975b).

Basophilia is seen most frequently in allergic reactions, chronic myeloid leukemia, myeloid metaplasia (extramedullary myelopoiesis), and polycythemia vera. Relative basophilia may be transient following irradiation. Basophilia may be present in hypothyroidism and chronic hemolytic anemia and following splenectomy.

BASOPENIA

A decreased basophil count (less than 0.01 × 10^9/L) can be detected only when large numbers of basophils are counted directly. With direct basophil counting, it has been determined that basophils, like eosinophils, show diurnal variation. The level is lowest in the morning and highest during the night. Sustained treatment with adrenal glucocorticoids induces a basopenia. Acute infection or stress results in a fall in basophils. About half of patients with hyperthyroidism have a basopenia (Gilbert, 1975b).

MONOCYTOSIS

Monocytosis is an increase of monocytes above the upper reference value, usually 1.0 × 10^9/L (Table 27–5).

Monocytosis is present during the recovery stage from acute infections and from agranulocytosis, where it is considered a favorable sign. In contrast, an increase of monocytes in tuberculosis is a poor prognostic sign.

Monocytosis may be present in subacute bacterial endocarditis. In this condition monocytes may show phagocytosis of other blood cells, red blood cells, and leukocytes. It may be present in mycotic, rickettsial, protozoal, and viral infections.

Infectious disease, however, is an uncommon cause of monocytosis. Maldonado (1965) reviewed 160 successive cases of absolute monocytosis at the Mayo Clinic. Over half (85) were associated with *hematologic disease:* 20 had monocytic or granulocytic leukemia; 20 had lymphoma (Hodgkin's disease was most frequent); 7 had multiple myeloma; 6 had myeloproliferative disorders; and, in 18, the cause was indeterminate. *Malignant disease* accounted for 13 cases; *connective tissue disorders,* 16; *infectious disease,* 9; *fever of unknown origin,* 7; *ulcerative colitis,* 4; *regional enteritis,* 4; *non-tropical sprue,* 2; and *cirrhosis,* 3 cases. *Miscellaneous* and *indeterminate causes* made up the remaining 17 cases. Among hematopoietic dysplasias, an unexplained monocytosis occasionally seems to precede the development of leukemia by months or years (p. 731).

MONOCYTOPENIA

A decrease in circulating monocytes below the lower reference value of 0.2 × 10^9/L is a monocytopenia. Few studies have dealt with monocytopenia, because of (1) the large number of cells that must be counted in a differential in order to obtain reliable counts; (2) the distributional bias of wedge blood film for monocytes compared with the spinner-made blood film (p. 603); and (3) the unavailability, until recently, of automation allowing large numbers of cells to be counted routinely (Hemalog D, p. 618).

During therapy with prednisone, monocytes fall during the first few hours after the first dose, but return to above original levels by 12 hours (Rinehart, 1975). Monocytopenia has been observed in hairy cell leukemia (Seshadri, 1976).

Lymphocytic and Plasmacytic Disorders

LYMPHOCYTES IN NORMAL INDIVIDUALS (see also Chapters 34 and 36)

In normal individuals the absolute numbers of lymphocytes and T cells are highest at birth (Fig. 30–1). At this time, lymphocytes represent approximately 90 per cent of all leukocytes (Andersen, 1974). During the first three to seven days of life there is a slight decrease in the number of lymphocytes. However, during the second week of life, the lymphocyte count returns to the level observed at birth. Cellular immune function in the newborn is comparable to that in normal adults (Carr, 1974; Ceppellini, 1971).

During the first decade of life, the absolute lymphocyte count and the absolute number of T cells decrease but remain higher than observed in the adult. By the time of adolescence, the absolute lymphocyte count and the absolute number of T cells have leveled off at values observed throughout adulthood. The absolute number of B lymphocytes remains stable during all stages of life (Davey, 1977). In adolescence and adulthood, lymphocytes constitute about 20 to 40 per cent of all leukocytes or 1.5 to 4.0 × 10^9 cells per liter (p. 000).

There is some disagreement regarding the absolute number of lymphocytes and number of T cells in aged individuals. Although some studies (Diaz-Jouanen, 1975; Smith, 1974) indicate that there is a decrease in total lymphocyte count and T cell numbers, other investigators find no significant change in total lymphocytes or T cells in aged individuals (Davey, 1977;

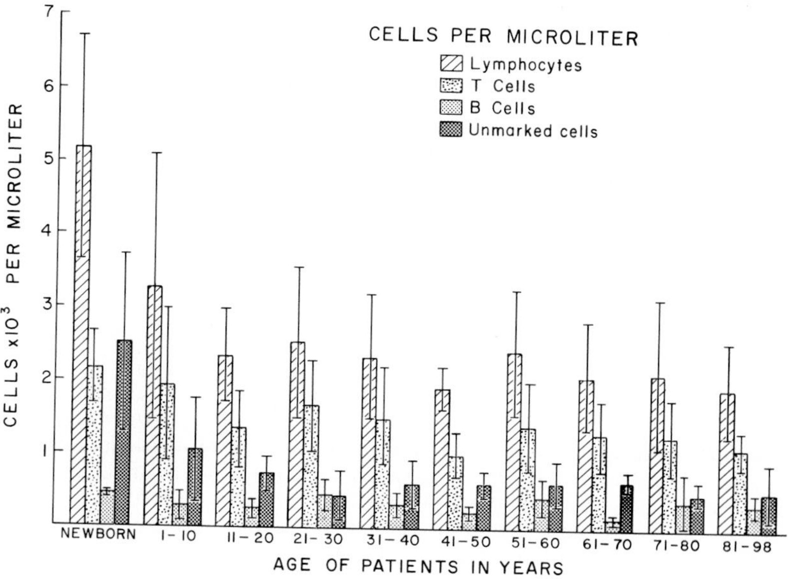

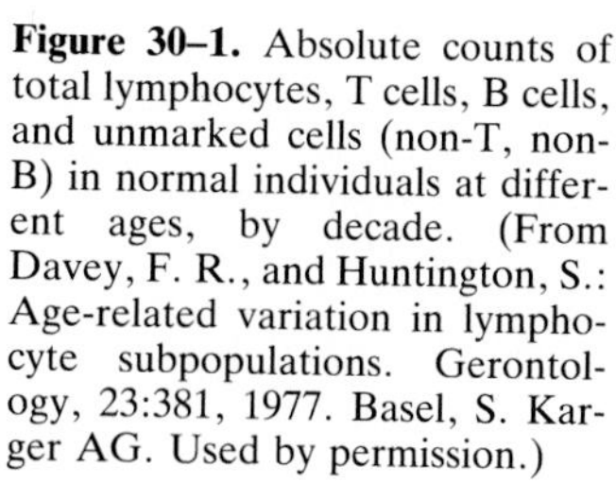
Figure 30–1. Absolute counts of total lymphocytes, T cells, B cells, and unmarked cells (non-T, non-B) in normal individuals at different ages, by decade. (From Davey, F. R., and Huntington, S.: Age-related variation in lymphocyte subpopulations. Gerontology, 23:381, 1977. Basel, S. Karger AG. Used by permission.)

Weksler, 1974). Elderly individuals have depressed delayed skin reactivity (Waldorf, 1968). In addition, lymphocytes from elderly individuals respond poorly to mitogens (Hallgren, 1974) and to allogenic lymphocytes (Weksler, 1974). Serum immunoglobulins, an index of B cell activity, are not reduced in the elderly (p. 872). In fact, aged individuals have a higher frequency of anti–smooth muscle, antimitochondrial, antiparietal cell, antinuclear, rheumatoid, and lymphocytotoxic antibodies (p. 925) (Ooi, 1974; Waldorf, 1968).

LYMPHOCYTOSIS

Lymphocytosis is an increase in the number of lymphocytes in the peripheral blood; the reference intervals are 1.5 to 4.0 × 10^9/L in the adult and 1.5 to 8.8 × 10^9/L in the child. Relative lymphocytosis (an increase in the percentage of lymphocytes) is present in various conditions and is especially prominent in disorders with neutropenia.

Infectious Lymphocytosis. This infectious and contagious disease, described by C. H. Smith (1941), is characterized by lymphocytosis and occurs mainly in children. The incubation period is 12 to 21 days.

Antibody and viral studies have indicated a relationship between infectious lymphocytosis and coxsackievirus A (Horowitz, 1968), coxsackievirus B6 (Nkrumah, 1973), echoviruses (Mandal, 1973) and adenovirus type 12 (Olson, 1964). No association has been noted with Epstein-Barr virus, cytomegalovirus, or herpesvirus (Blacklow, 1970). Although the disease usually has no systemic manifestations, sometimes vomiting, fever, abdominal discomfort, signs suggesting involvement of the nervous system, cutaneous rashes, upper respiratory infections, and diarrhea occur. Leukocytosis (20 to 50 × 10^9/L, sometimes over 100 × 10^9/L) usually precedes the clinical manifestations. From 60 to 95 per cent of blood leukocytes are mature, small lymphocytes. In contrast to infectious mononucleosis, atypical lymphocytes (p. 715) are uncommon. There is usually an eosinophilia. The lymphocytosis usually lasts three to five weeks, sometimes longer. Other blood changes are unusual. The marrow has no characteristic changes; an increased percentage of lymphocytes has been observed but is probably an artifact due to admixture of peripheral blood. Lymph node enlargement is rare and minimal when present. The spleen and liver are rarely if ever enlarged. Lymph node biopsy may show reactive follicular hyperplasia but no characteristic changes.

The tests for infectious mononucleosis (p. 715) are negative. In some cases there has been an increase of white cells in the cerebrospinal fluid, with about 40 per cent lymphocytes. The course is benign.

Another form of infectious lymphocytosis in children has a chronic course. The leukocyte count is 10 to 25 × 10^9/L with 60 to 80 per cent lymphocytes of normal appearance. Slight eosinophilia, monocytosis, and plasmacytosis are also present. As a rule, the children have enlargement of tonsils, lymph nodes, and spleen and a history of recurrent upper respiratory infections. The marrow shows no abnormalities.

Pertussis. Whooping cough (pertussis) occurs during childhood, especially in unimmunized children. The etiologic agent is *Bordetella pertussis* (hemophilus pertussis) which produces an inflammatory reaction of the entire respiratory tract.

The incubation period is approximately two weeks, and the first symptoms are those of a head cold. Later the patient develops paroxysms of coughing productive of thick sputum. There is frequently pain over trachea and bronchi (Brooksaler, 1967).

Patients frequently develop significant lymphocytosis. Counts higher than 30 × 10^9/L have been recorded. The lymphocytes are small and mature. The lymphocyte count is highest during the first three weeks of the illness, then decreases during the fourth and subsequent weeks (Lagergren, 1963). The lymphocytosis is due to the release of lymphocytosis-promoting factor (LPF) from the organism. LPF causes a transient increased mobilization of lymphocytes from lymphoid organs followed by inhibition of recirculation of lymphocytes from blood into the lymph flow. Thus, the lymphocytosis is due to a redistribution of lymphocytes into the peripheral circulation without increased lymphopoiesis (Rai, 1971; Morse, 1970).

Infectious Mononucleosis. Infectious mononucleosis is usually a self-limited infectious disease of the reticuloendothelial tissue produced by an infection with Epstein-Barr virus, a member of the herpes group. The disorder most frequently involves adolescent children and young adults. It has characteristic clinical, hematologic, and pathologic features and specific serologic alterations.

Etiology. Strong serologic and epidemiologic evidence now implicates the Epstein-Barr virus (EBV) as the cause of infectious mononucleosis (IM) (Henle, 1974). The EBV was originally found in cell culture of Burkitt's lymphoma. High titers of antibody to EBV are found in the serum of patients with Burkitt's lymphoma and carcinoma of the postnasal space.

The EBV is apparently spread to susceptible individuals through oral contact. When EBV gets into the mouth of a previously unexposed individual, it infects B lymphocytes in the lymphoid tissue of the oral pharynx. Generalized disease occurs either as a result of a viremia with EBV traveling to B cell sites in other lymphoid tissues or as a result of EBV-infected B cells from the oral pharynx traveling to other lymphoid tissues (Epstein, 1977). During the acute phase of the disease, afflicted individuals develop antibodies to the viral capsid antigen and membrane antigen. Some antibodies appear only transiently, whereas other antibodies remain for life.

Within the first week of the illness the patient develops a lymphocytosis. The atypical lymphocytes are due to changes in both B and T cells. B lymphocytes are transformed early in the disease owing to the direct effects of the EBV (Mangi, 1974). It appears that B cells bear receptors for EBV (Jondal, 1973). Later on, T cells form atypical lymphocytes as a response to neoantigen on the surface of B cells. The EBV induces the formation of a lymphocyte-detected membrane antigen which appears to be recognized by killer T cells (Rickinson, 1977). Thus, the B cell, infected with EBV, is responsible for the generation of activated T cells in the blood and in all the lymphoreticular system, resulting in a lymphocytosis, lymphadenopathy, and splenomegaly. Resolution of the illness is due in part to the elimination of infected B cells by the killer T cells. In addition, virus-neutralizing antibodies and T lymphocytes reduce the number of productively infected cells in the oropharynx. A low level of EBV infection persists for life. The virulence of this infection is controlled by the presence of neutralizing antibodies and by cellular immune responses.

Clinical Features. The disease has been observed in patients from three months to 70 years of age but is most common in adolescents and young adults. The onset is vague, indefinite, and similar to the onset of other infectious diseases. Patients usually have fever, sore throat, and lymphadenopathy (Table 30–3).

The lymph node enlargement is usually moderate in degree. Cervical lymph nodes are most often the first to be enlarged; other regions, including mediastinal and inguinal, are then affected. The lymphadenopathy usually has regressed by three weeks. Splenomegaly is common. The liver is less frequently enlarged. A rash may be observed in 3 to 6 per cent of patients. If ampicillin is administered, 69 to 100 per cent of patients may develop a rash (Karzon, 1976).

Complications. Of the rare anemias associated with infectious mononucleosis, hemolytic anemia is the most common, occurring in 1 to 3 per cent of cases. The cause now appears to be related to the anti-i antibody produced frequently in this disease (Worlledge, 1969).

Mild thrombocytopenia occurs in about half the cases, but the platelet count is not often less than 100×10^9/L. Thrombocytopenic purpura with hemorrhagic complications is exceedingly rare (Sharp, 1969).

Involvement of the liver demonstrable by biopsy is common in infectious mononucleosis. Abnormal liver

Table 30–3. CLINICAL FINDINGS IN 106 CASES OF INFECTIOUS MONONUCLEOSIS

	No. Cases	Per Cent		No. Cases	Per Cent
Lymphadenopathy	101	95.3	Skin rash	5	4.7
Fever	93	87.7	Epistaxis	3	2.8
Pharyngitis	64	60.4	Icterus	3	2.8
Without membrane	50	47.2	Loss of weight	2	1.9
With membrane	14	13.2	Diarrhea	2	1.9
Splenomegaly	51	48.1	Arthritic pains	2	1.9
Headache	26	24.5	Purpura	2	1.9
Hepatomegaly	24	22.6	Gingivitis	2	1.9
Prostration	11	10.4	Convulsions	1	0.9
Emesis	10	9.4	Toothache	1	0.9
Pain in abdomen	8	7.6	Albuminuria	14	13.2
Upper abdomen	6	5.7	Positive test for syphilis	3	2.8
Lower abdomen	2	1.9	Relapses (17 days to 2 months)	7	6.5
Stiffness or pain in neck	6	5.7	Recurrence (1 year)	1	0.9

function tests indicative of hepatitis occur in 85 to 100 per cent of patients. Clinical jaundice is rare, but cases have been reported in which jaundice and acute pharyngitis were the only clinical manifestations of infectious mononucleosis, with positive hematologic and serologic findings. The jaundice is, as a rule, hepatocellular, with elevation of both conjugated and non-conjugated serum bilirubin, bilirubinuria, and elevated urine urobilinogen.

Approximately one third of patients with IM carry beta-hemolytic streptococci in the pharynx. Thus one should give attention to strict clinical, hematologic, and serologic criteria in distinguishing IM from streptococcal pharyngitis.

Hematologic Features. Leukocytes are increased, usually ranging from 12 to 25 $\times$ 10^9/L. Rarely, counts as high as 80 $\times$ 10^9/L have been recorded. The leukocytosis is usually due to lymphocytosis (60 to 90 per cent) composed of a variety of atypical lymphocytes (Wood, 1967). The total leukocyte count, as a rule, returns to normal within three weeks. The atypical lymphocytes have nuclear alterations and an increase in the amount and basophilia of cytoplasm.

Nuclei may have "open" chromatin and deep indentations ("leukocytoid lymphocytes," Downey type I; Plate 30–2*E*). The cytoplasm shows basophilia, an increase of azurophilic granules, and frequently vacuoles. Some cells resemble plasma cells; some resemble monocytes. Cells which have a relatively smooth but still mature nucleus and abundant smooth cytoplasm with patchy peripheral and radial basophilia have been called "stress" lymphocytes or Downey type II (Plate 30–2*A* to *D*, 30–6*I*). They are often the most numerous. Occasionally lymphocytes have transformed into blast-like cells, presumably in response to the viral stimulation. These immature lymphocytes, usually representing only a small percentage of the total lymphocyte count, are large reticular lymphocytes (non-leukemic lymphoblasts) with a coarsely reticular nucleus and abundant deeply basophilic cytoplasm (Downey type III; Plate 30–2*C* and *G*, 30–6*H*, 28–3*J* and *K*). In contrast, lymphoblasts of acute lymphocytic leukemia are usually smaller, with a very fine chromatin pattern and very little cytoplasm (Plate 30–1*L*, 30–2*H*, 30–3*G*) (Downey, 1923).

Often the number of monocytes rises transiently. The term mononucleosis refers to an increase of lymphocytes and not monocytes.

The cytologic alterations are not pathognomonic of IM. Similar cells are found in a variety of disorders including cytomegalovirus mononucleosis, toxoplasmosis, and infectious hepatitis, and usually to a lesser extent in viral pneumonia, varicella, mumps, and viral exanthemas of children.

Neutrophils are relatively and absolutely decreased in most cases during the first week of illness. During this time there may be a shift to the left, with an increase of band cells and metamyelocytes. Toxic granules and Döhle bodies may be seen. The eosinophils are within normal limits.

The bone marrow from patients with IM usually shows an increased cellularity (Boyd, 1968). There is an increased number of lymphocytes, macrophages, plasma cells, megakaryocytes, and erythroid cells. The neutrophilic series appears decreased. About half of the cases may have collections of mononuclear cells forming loose granulomas (Hovde, 1950).

Early in the illness, the histopathology of lymph nodes usually shows a follicular hyperplasia with prominent germinal centers. In addition, there is intense hyperplasia of the interfollicular area. Throughout the follicle and especially at the margin of the germinal centers are large stimulated lymphocytes. Mitoses are frequent. Peripheral sinuses are filled with collections of histiocytes, mononuclear cells, and large stimulated lymphocytes. There may be lymphocytic infiltration of the capsule. The medullary cords are obscured and plasma cell elements do not appear increased. Blood vessels are prominent and endothelial cells are swollen and assume an epithelium-like appearance (Gall, 1940). Reed-Sternberg–like cells may also be present (Lukes, 1969). During later stages, hyperplasia of the follicles and paracortical areas is less pronounced and sinuses are less crowded. Medullary cords appear within normal limits (Carter, 1969).

Serological Findings

Heterophil Antibody. Paul (1932) first described the presence of sheep cell agglutinins in the sera of patients with IM. Unfortunately, the presence of sheep cell agglutinins is not a specific finding for IM and can be present in other disorders.

Davidsohn (1937) demonstrated that the heterophil antibodies in patients with IM are absorbed by beef erythrocytes in contrast to heterophil antibodies present in other disorders. The latter are absorbed by the Forssman antigen such as that found in guinea pig kidney. The differential absorption test (Paul-Bunnell-Davidsohn test) is highly specific for IM.

The spot test for IM (Lee, 1968) is based on the principle that horse erythrocytes are more sensitive than sheep erythrocytes in testing for IM. Serum is mixed with a suspension of finely ground guinea pig kidney on one part of the slide and with a suspension of beef erythrocyte stroma on another. Horse erythrocytes are added to each spot and mixed. A positive test for IM shows agglutination of horse erythrocytes of serum absorbed with guinea pig kidney but not by serum absorbed with beef erythrocyte stroma. The spot test has proved to be a simple, rapid, highly specific, and sensitive test for the heterophil antibodies of IM. False positive tests occur, but are very rare (Horowitz, 1979). False negative tests occur particularly in young children who produce heterophil antibodies (IgM immunoglobulin) in limited amounts. In heterophil negative IM, the diagnosis may be substantiated by assay for antibody to EBV.

Epstein-Barr Virus Antibodies. Several antibodies are produced by the host in response to a variety of EBV antigens (Karzon, 1976) (Table 30–4). Antibody to the viral capsid antigen arises within the first two weeks of the onset. This antibody is measured by an immunofluorescent method and is probably the most widely used assay for determining exposure to EBV. Assaying for the presence of EBV antibody is usually limited to the few cases of heterophil negative IM.

Other Serologic Reactions. In addition to heter-

4

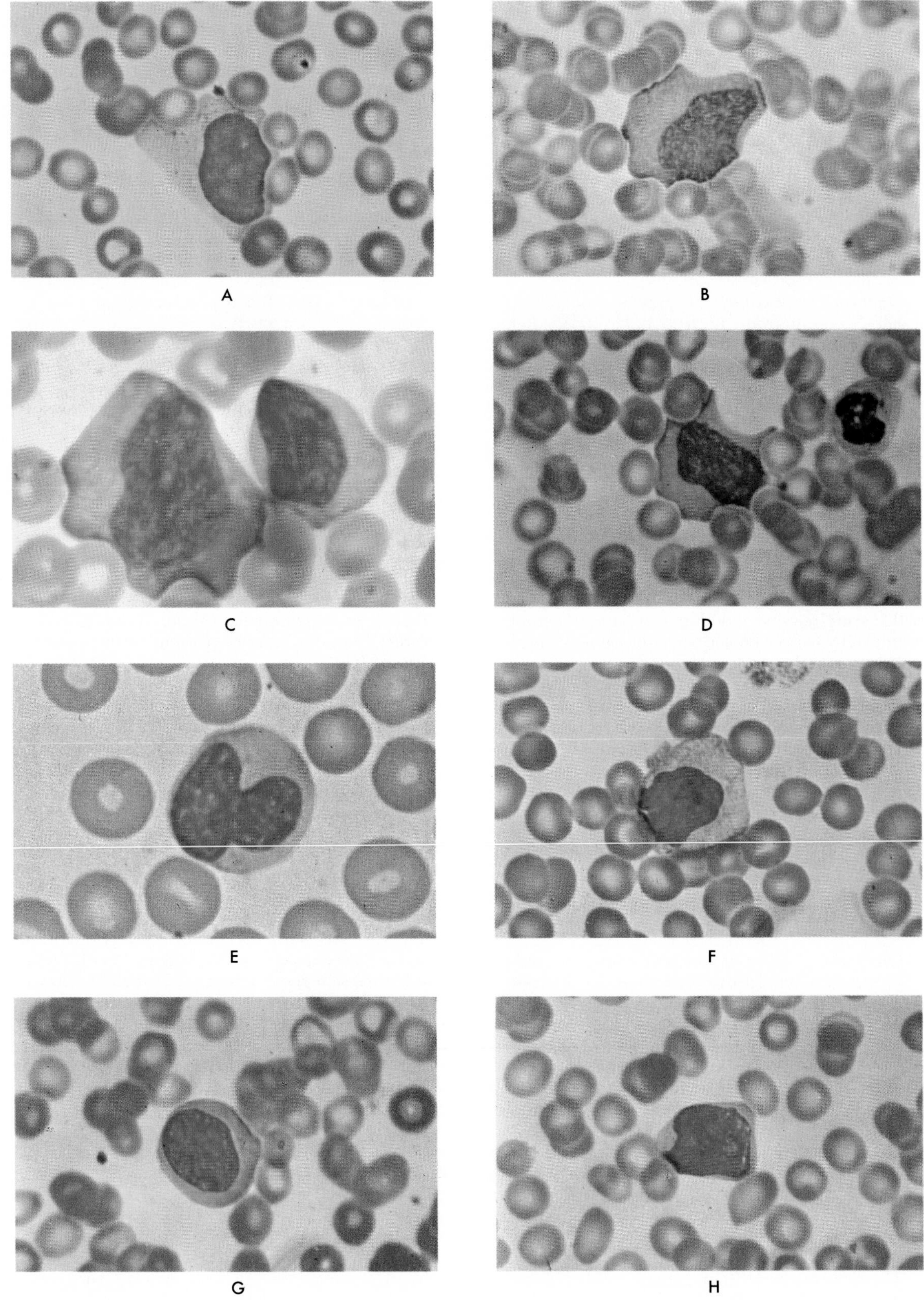
A
B
C
D
E
F
G
H

Table 30–4. MEASUREMENT OF ANTIBODIES TO EBV*

Antigen	Detection System†	Time of Appearance	Persistence
Viral capsid antigens (VCA)	IF	Early	IgM—temporary IgG—life
Early antigen (EA): Diffuse (D)	IF	Early (80–85%)	Temporary
Restricted (R)	IF	Late (rare)	Temporary
Cell membrane antigen (MA)	IF	Intermediate	Life
Nuclear antigen (EBNA)	IF (anti-C′)	Delayed	Life
Neutralizing	Neut.	Intermediate	Life
CF (Soluble or S)	CF	Delayed	Life
(Viral or V)	CF	? Early	? Life

*From Karzon, D. T.: Infectious mononucleosis. *In* Schulman, I., et al. (eds.): Advances in Pediatrics, Vol. 22. Copyright © 1976 by Year Book Medical Publishers, Inc., Chicago. Used by permission.

†IF = immunofluorescence. CF = complement fixation.

ophil and EBV antibodies, patients with IM frequently produce antibodies to a wide variety of antigens. Antibodies against human erythrocytes, leukocytes, and platelets have been described. Patients with IM have an increased frequency of cold agglutinins. Positive tests to rheumatoid factor and antinuclear factor have been reported. There are elevated titers against a variety of organisms including *Proteus, Salmonella, Streptococcus* MG, *Listeria monocytogenes,* and Newcastle disease virus (Davidsohn, 1969).

Differential Diagnosis. The clinical, hematologic, and serologic features of IM permit an accurate diagnosis to be made in over 90 per cent of the cases. When this test is negative, one must consider several possibilities. The patient could still have EBV antibody–positive but heterophil-negative IM. However, cytomegalovirus infection is the most common cause of heterophil-negative mononucleosis. Other possibilities include toxoplasmosis, infectious hepatitis, and ingestion of drugs (*p*-aminosalicylic acid, phenytoin (Dilantin), and diaminodiphenylsulfone).

Course. IM is a benign disorder and complications occur in less than 5 per cent of patients. The disorder usually resolves in three to four weeks. Fatalities are extremely rare, but tend to occur in members of the same family (Purtilo, 1979). Further studies indicate that the affected individuals frequently suffered from sex-linked lymphoproliferative syndrome.

Cytomegalovirus Infection. Some individuals infected with cytomegalovirus develop a syndrome identical to infectious mononucleosis. This disorder can occur following massive blood transfusions (post-transfusion mononucleosis) or spontaneously in previously healthy individuals (cytomegalovirus mononucleosis) (Foster, 1969; Klemola, 1969). The patient has fever, chills, profound malaise, and myalgia. There may be a sore throat (but not exudative pharyngitis) and lymphadenopathy. Occasionally splenomegaly is found, but hepatomegaly does not occur.

Leukocytosis is characteristic with absolute lymphocytosis. Usually 20 per cent or more of the leukocytes are atypical lymphocytes. Bone marrow aspirates have shown an increased number of normal lymphocytes and atypical lymphocytes. Hepatic enzymes are frequently abnormal. In a small percentage of patients, there may be an increased titer of cold agglutinins, rheumatoid factor, and antinuclear antibodies. There is no rise in heterophil, Epstein-Barr virus, or toxoplasma antibodies. The diagnosis is usually made by isolating the cytomegalovirus from urine or demonstrating a rise in antibody by the complement fixation or indirect hemagglutination techniques (Jordan, 1973).

Toxoplasmosis. In children and adults, toxoplasmosis can produce a disorder similar to infectious mononucleosis (Beverley, 1958). Patients present with fever, lymphadenopathy, and an increased number of atypical lymphocytes in the peripheral blood (Siim, 1951). Rarely is there splenomegaly. Pharyngitis and upper respiratory tract infection are usually absent.

Plate 30–2. *A,* Infectious mononucleosis. All the photographs of the lymphocytes of infectious mononucleosis are from patients with characteristic clinical findings and with positive differential tests. The lymphocyte is larger than any normal so-called large lymphocyte. The cytoplasm is abundant, clear, and moderately basophilic, especially close to the edges of the cell; red azure granules are accumulated along the upper periphery. The cytoplasm is delicate, and the surrounding red cells leave an indentation in the cytoplasm, giving it a scalloped appearance. The nucleus is oval, and the chromatin is delicate and less dense than in normal large lymphocytes. Three nucleoli are seen clearly. The two red cells adjacent on the right made indentations, even in the nucleus, suggesting that it is plastic. There is a light perinuclear zone. The characteristic lymphocytes in infectious mononucleosis are called atypical lymphocytes. *B,* Atypical lymphocyte, infectious mononucleosis. Notice sharp separation of nuclear chromatin and parachromatin, and basophilic cytoplasm. *C,* Reticular lymphocyte (non-leukemic lymphoblast), *left;* atypical lymphocyte with greater nuclear maturity, *right.* Infectious mononucleosis. *D,* Atypical lymphocyte, *center;* normal lymphocyte, *right.* Infectious mononucleosis. *E,* Atypical lymphocyte with "leukocytoid" nucleus. Infectious mononucleosis. *F,* Normal monocyte. *G,* Reticular lymphocyte (non-leukemic lymphoblast); infectious mononucleosis. The nuclear chromatin is uniform and granular (or reticular). Nucleoli are conspicuous. The cytoplasm is deeply basophilic. Note the difference between this cell and the lymphoblast of acute leukemia *(H). H,* Lymphoblast, acute lymphoblastic leukemia.

Table 30–5. CAUSES OF LYMPHOCYTOSIS*

Lymphocytosis Associated with Atypical Lymphocytes			**Lymphocytosis Associated with Small Mature Lymphocytes**
Per Cent of White Cells Which Are Atypical Lymphocytes		***Uncommon Causes***	
>20	***<20***		
Infectious mononucleosis Infectious hepatitis "Post-transfusion" syndrome Cytomegalovirus infection *p*-aminosalicylic acid (PAS) hypersensitivity Phenytoin (Dilantin) and mephenytoin (Mesantoin) hypersensitivity	(a) Infections Mumps,† varicella,† rubeola, rubella, atypical pneumonia, herpes simplex, herpes zoster, roseola infantum, influenza,† other viral illnesses, tuberculosis,† rickettsialpox, brucellosis,† toxoplasmosis† (b) Radiation (c) Other Letterer-Siwe disese Agranulocytosis Lead intoxiction Stress Leukemia and lymphoma†	Tertiary syphilis† Congenital syphilis† Smallpox Tetrachlorethane poisoning TNT poisoning Organic arsenical hypersensitivity Severe dermatitis herpetiformis	Infectious lymphocytosis Pertussis

*Modified from Wood, T. A., and Frenkel, E. P.: The atypical lymphocyte. Am. J. Med., *42*:923, 1967.
†Higher counts of atypical lymphocytes occasionally found.

The histopathology of lymph nodes is usually distinctive and correlates closely with elevated toxoplasma antibody titers (Dorfman, 1973). Biopsies of lymph nodes usually show reactive follicular hyperplasia; clusters of epithelioid histiocytes and germinal centers, cortical and paracortical areas; and distention of sinuses by monocytoid cells (Saxén, 1959). Bone marrow biopsies usually have no specific pathologic lesion.

The diagnosis is established by demonstrating an elevation of toxoplasma antibodies by the Sabin-Feldman dye test, fluorescent-antibody, or hemagglutination techniques (Feldman, 1968).

Miscellaneous Causes of Lymphocytosis. Numerous disorders have been associated with lymphocytosis. A partial listing of illnesses associated with relative or absolute lymphocytosis is provided in Table 30–5.

LYMPHOCYTOPENIA

Lymphocytopenia is an absolute lymphocyte count below 1.5×10^9/L in adults and below 3.0×10^9/L in children. A number of immunologic deficiency disorders which are genetically determined have lymphocytopenia along with various other immunologic defects of either humoral or cell-mediated immunity (Hoyer, 1968). Lymphocytopenia in these disorders is due to impaired lymphopoiesis. Increased levels of adrenocortical hormones, the administration of chemotherapeutic drugs, or irradiation will result in lymphocytopenia. Impaired drainage of the intestinal lymphatics with loss of lymphocytes into the intestines due to a number of causes has been implicated as a mechanism for lymphocytopenia. In advanced cases of Hodgkin's disease and terminal cases of carcinoma, lymphocytopenia is often observed.

FUNCTIONAL DISORDERS OF LYMPHOCYTES

Functional disorders of lymphocytes can be inherited or acquired. The immune deficiency may be due to a disorder in monocytes, B cells, T cells, stem cells, suppressor cells, or a combination. The inherited functional disorders are discussed in Chapter 41.

Acquired functional abnormalities of lymphocytes are most frequently observed in lymphoid malignancies. Decreased B cell function is observed in chronic lymphocytic leukemia in which two thirds of the patients have hypogammaglobulinemia. In multiple myeloma there is a diminished synthesis of normal immunoglobulin in the presence of high levels of paraprotein.

Diminished T cell activity has been described in patients with Hodgkin's disease, sarcoidosis, and leprosy. In Hodgkin's disease, the diminished T cell activity may be the result of the suppressive effects of monocytes. In autoimmune diseases, a loss of suppressor T cells has been observed.

In severe malnutrition and in patients with terminal malignancies there is diminished humoral and cell-mediated immunity.

The diagnosis of functional disorders of lymphocytes requires the use of skin tests, enumeration of B and

T cells, measurement of serum immunoglobulin and antibodies, and a variety of *in vitro* lymphocyte assays which record their response to mitogens and antigens (p. 840).

PLASMACYTOSIS

Plasma cells are not normally present in circulating blood. They are increased in a variety of chronic infections, in allergic states, in the presence of neoplasms, and in other conditions in which the serum gamma globulin is elevated. Plasma cells have also been recorded in the blood of patients with viral disorders, including rubella, measles, chickenpox, and mumps. They are moderately increased in cutaneous exanthemas, infectious mononucleosis, syphilis, subacute bacterial endocarditis, sarcoidosis, and collagen diseases. Their increase is usually linked with an increase in lymphocytes, monocytes, and eosinophils.

In the marrow, an average of 1 per cent of plasma cells is present in adults. An increase beyond 4 per cent is significant; lower values are found in children (see Table 28–2). Increases up to 20 per cent of plasma cells may be found in a variety of conditions other than multiple myeloma, including metastatic carcinoma, chronic granulomatous infections, conditions linked with hypersensitivity, and following administration of cytotoxic drugs. They are often increased in aplastic anemia, but this is probably just a relative increase. On the other hand, they are decreased or absent in agammaglobulinemia.

Leukemoid Reactions

A leukemoid reaction is an excessive leukocytic response. It includes leukocytosis of 50×10^9/L or higher with a shift to the left; lower counts, even below normal, with considerable numbers of immature granulocytes; and, similar quantitative or qualitative changes in lymphocytes or monocytes. Depending on the predominant cell, leukemoid reactions may be neutrophilic, eosinophilic, lymphocytic, or monocytic. No explanation for these apparent temporary aberrations in normal regulatory control mechanisms is yet available. The reactions are irregular in degree, even when associated with the same inciting agent.

Neutrophilic Leukemoid Reactions. Excessive neutrophilia may occur in many situations, including hemolysis, hemorrhage, malignancy with bony involvement, Hodgkin's disease, myelofibrosis, infections (especially tuberculosis), severe burns, eclampsia, and certain intoxications.

Examination of the blood is usually more helpful than marrow examination. Leukemoid reactions lack the characteristic differential count that is seen in CML, including the myelocyte "peak," eosinophilia, and basophilia (p. 726). Also, the leukemic hiatus so characteristic of acute leukemia is absent.

Eosinophilic Leukemoid Reactions. Cells as immature as eosinophilic myelocytes rarely appear in the blood in reactive eosinophilia, in which the leukocyte count may exceed 50×10^9/L. Eosinophilic leukemoid reactions usually occur in children and usually are caused by parasitic infections. The hypereosinophilic syndrome in adults is leukemoid (p. 711).

Erythroblastosis. In patients with or without anemia, circulating normoblasts frequently are accompanied by a neutrophilic leukemoid reaction; this, then, is a *leukoerythroblastotic reaction* (p. 611). A moderate anemia with normoblasts in the peripheral blood is fairly common in metastatic carcinoma involving bone marrow.

Lymphocytic Leukemoid Reactions. Extremely high counts of normal-appearing lymphocytes may occur in infectious lymphocytosis and in pertussis (p. 713). When atypical lymphocytes are strikingly increased or immature (which may occur in conditions such as infectious mononucleosis), the distinction from leukemia may be difficult (p. 715). Tuberculosis may be associated with either type of lymphocytosis.

Examination of the marrow often is useful, since lymphocytes are minimally increased, if at all, in most leukemoid reactions in contrast to leukemia.

NEOPLASTIC AND RELATED DISORDERS PRIMARILY INVOLVING LEUKOCYTES

Definition and Classification of Leukemias

Leukemia is a generalized neoplastic proliferation or accumulation of leukopoietic cells with or without involvement of the peripheral blood. Leukocytosis, abnormal circulating cells, and infiltration of nonhematopoietic tissues are frequently but not invariably present.

The *acute leukemias,* if no remission is induced, usually are fatal within three months. The bone marrow is usually packed with primitive cells of the series involved with very little evidence of differentiation.

Subacute leukemias are often categorized with the acute leukemias, but when the term is used it implies a longer natural history of three to 12 months and cells of intermediate differentiation. Patients with *chronic leukemias* usually survive more than one year after the onset of symptoms if no remission occurs. The cell type is more differentiated.

The leukemias are also classified according to cytologic characteristics. There are two major cytologic categories, myeloid and lymphoid, which are further divided depending on the level of differentiation of the predominant cell type. The proliferation in acute myeloid leukemia consists predominantly of myeloblasts, whereas in chronic myeloid (myelogenous) leukemia it consists mostly of more differentiated cells (myelocytes, metamyelocytes, neutrophils) and relatively few myeloblasts. In acute lymphoid leukemia the proliferation is of lymphoblasts. In contrast, in chronic lymphoid leukemia it is composed of small mature lymphoid cells.

CYTOCHEMICAL STAINS USEFUL IN THE DIAGNOSIS OF LEUKEMIA

It is often difficult to differentiate the leukemic blasts of acute myeloid leukemia from those of acute

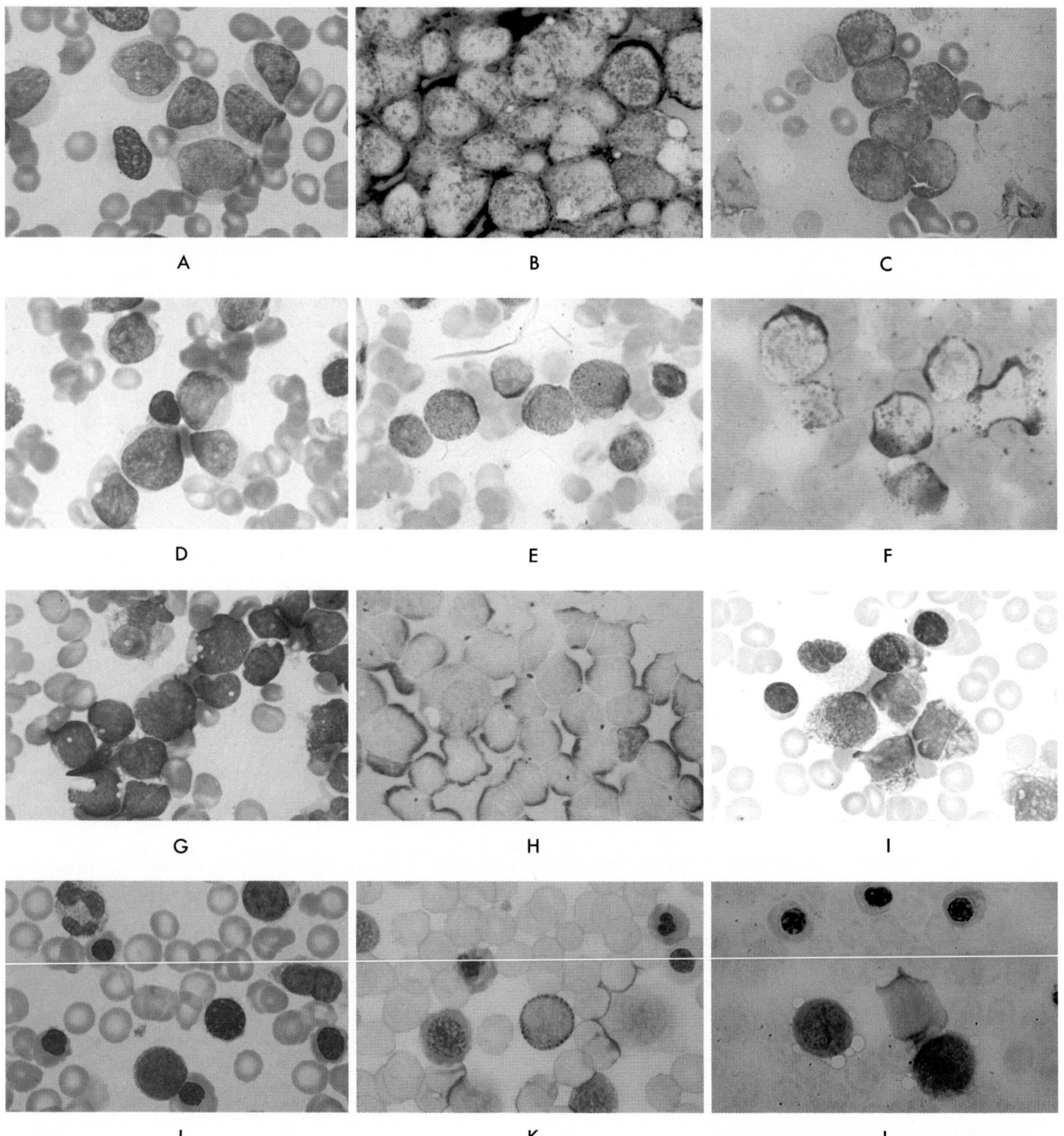

Plate 30–3. *A,* Acute myelogenous leukemia (AML), Wright-Giemsa stain. No maturation is evident. This corresponds to the M_1 category of the French-American-British (FAB) classification (Table 30–8). *B,* AML, Sudan black B reaction. Same case as *A.* Though granules are not visible with the Wright-Giemsa stain, all of the blasts contain sudanophilic material (brown granules). The peroxidase reaction was similarly positive. *C,* Acute myelogenous leukemia with partial maturation (M_2). Naphthol AS-D chloroacetate esterase reaction. All stages of developing neutrophils have a positive reaction. *D,* Acute myelomonocytic leukemia (AMML), Wright-Giemsa stain. No cytoplasmic maturation is evident. This stain alone does not allow a definitive diagnosis. *E,* AMML, Sudan black B reaction. Same case as *D.* A moderate proportion of the blasts contains sudanophilic material. *F,* AMML, alpha naphthyl acetate esterase reaction. Same case as *D.* Most of the blasts contain non-specific esterase (which is fluoride-sensitive). Cytochemical reactions, therefore, lead to the diagnosis of myelomonocytic leukemia. *G,* Acute lymphoblastic leukemia (ALL), Wright-Giemsa stain. Most of the blasts are small and the cytoplasm is scanty. This corresponds to the L_1 category of the FAB classification (Table 30–11). *H,* ALL, periodic acid-Schiff (PAS) reaction. Same case as *G.* A moderate proportion of the blasts contains one or more large granules or "blocks" of PAS-positive material. *I,* Acute promyelocytic leukemia, Wright-Giemsa stain. The majority of cells have abundant azurophil granules, often large. Usually, some cells contain multiple Auer rods, as in the cell at the right. The nuclei are irregularly shaped or indented (Rieder forms). This is the hypergranular promyelocytic category M3 of the FAB classification.

Legend continued on opposite page

Table 30–6. CYTOCHEMICAL REACTIONS IN NORMAL CELLS AND IN BLASTS AND IMMATURE CELLS OF ACUTE LEUKEMIAS*

	Sudan Black B Peroxidase	Chloroacetate Esterase	Non-specific Esterase	PAS
Cells				
Promyelocyte	+	+ (a)	−	±
Neutrophil	+ +	+ + (a)	−	+ + +
Monocyte	±	−	+ + +	±
Lymphocyte	−	−	−/± (b)	−/+
Normoblast	−	−	− (c)	− (d)
Megakaryocyte	−	−	+ +	+ + +
Leukemias				
ALL	−	−	± (e)	+ + (f)
AML	+ +	+ + (a)	−	±
APL	+ + +	+ + +	−	±
AMML	±	±	+ + +	+
AUL	−	−	−	−

Key:
− negative
± weakly positive or few positive cells
+ moderately positive
+ + moderately to strongly positive
+ + + strongly positive (most cells)

ALL = acute lymphoid leukemia
AML = acute myeloid leukemia
APL = acute promyelocytic leukemia
AMML = acute myelomonocytic leukemia
AUL = acute unclassified leukemia

Comments: (a) Chloroacetate esterase is less consistently positive than SBB or PX.
(b) Some normal lymphocytes have *focal* positivity.
(c) Strong non-specific esterase activity is present in some cases of erythroleukemia and dyserythropoiesis.
(d) Positive in erythroleukemia, to a lesser degree in some cases of iron deficiency and thalassemia.
(e) Some cases of ALL have *focal* positivity.
(f) Some cases of ALL; coarse granules ± blocks.

*Modified from Nelson, D. A., and Davey, F. R.: Leukocyte esterase. *In* Williams, W. J., Beutler, E., Erslev, A. J., and Lichtman, M. A. (eds.): Hematology. 3rd ed. New York, McGraw-Hill Book Co., 1983, p. 1653.

lymphoid leukemia using Romanowsky-stained films alone. However, several cytochemical staining procedures are very helpful in making this distinction. When the results of appropriate cytochemical reactions are used together with the morphologic observations derived from the Wright-Giemsa–stained films, a precise diagnosis can be made in over 95 per cent of cases. The following cytochemical reactions have proved helpful in the differential diagnosis of acute leukemia.

Sudan Black B Stain and Peroxidase (Myeloperoxidase). Sudan black B stains phospholipids and sterols. It appears to stain both azurophilic and specific granules in neutrophils, whereas the peroxidase is found only in azurophilic granules (Sheehan, 1947). Cytoplasmic granules stain faintly in neutrophil precursors and strongly in mature neutrophils with Sudan black B. Eosinophilic granules are also positive, but often show a central pallor. Monocytes may be unstained or may contain a few positive granules. Lymphocytes and lymphoblasts are negative, but at least some myeloblasts contain Sudan black–positive granules (Plate 30–3*B* and *E*).

The peroxidase reaction is based on the principle that in the presence of hydrogen peroxide, myeloperoxidase in leukocyte granules oxidizes benzidine dihydrochloride from a colorless form to a blue or brown derivative which is localized at the site of the enzyme (Kaplow, 1965). Myeloperoxidase activity is present at all stages of neutrophil development and is localized in the azurophilic (nonspecific) granules. Eosinophils show an intense reaction. Lymphocytes, mature basophils, and erythroid forms do not stain. Monocytes stain less intensely than do neutrophils, and the granular precipitates are smaller. Using 3,3′-diaminobenzidine-HCl (DAB) as a substrate for the peroxidase reaction instead of benzidine-HCl results in a greater proportion of positive blast cells in acute myeloid leukemia (Cardullo, 1981). DAB demonstrates catalase as well as myeloperoxidase, and the cytochemical reaction has been called hydroperoxidase.

The Sudan black B and the peroxidase reactions show roughly similar patterns in the various cell types (Table 30–6) (Hayhoe, 1964). The Sudan black B and the hydroperoxidase reaction are somewhat more sensitive than the myeloperoxidase reaction in our expe-

4

Plate 30–3 *Continued. J,* Erythroleukemia, Wright-Giemsa stain. One primitive blast (*lower center*), one abnormal monocyte (*upper right*), one neutrophil, and five nucleated erythroid cells are present. Most of the latter are abnormal. *K,* Erythroleukemia, PAS reaction. Same case as *J.* Of the six nucleated erythroid cells in this field, five are PAS-positive: in the most immature the reactive material is granular (*lower center*); in the others it is diffuse. A monocyte and a blast are PAS-negative; a neutrophil is PAS-positive. *L,* Erythroleukemia, alpha-naphthyl butyrate reaction. Same case as *J.* Monocytes are strongly positive for this non-specific esterase reaction; they were increased in number and morphologically abnormal and part of the leukemic process. Erythroid, granulocytic, and monocytic cell lines are demonstrably involved in this case.

rience. These techniques are most useful in distinguishing acute myeloid from acute lymphoid leukemia.

Peroxidase activity may be absent in some toxic neutrophils from patients with infection, acute myeloid or myelomonocytic leukemia, and the rare congenital myeloperoxidase deficiency.

Esterases. The leukocyte esterases hydrolyze an ester which is a derivative of naphthalene (Yam, 1971b). A naphthol (or naphthyl) compound is liberated and rapidly couples with a diazonium salt present in the mixture resulting in a brightly colored precipitate at or near the site of the enzyme activity.

The cytochemical reactions for esterases are positive in many cell types. The chloroacetate esterase reaction, using naphthol-AS-D-chloroacetate as a substrate, is positive in neutrophils and precursors and weak or negative in monocytes and precursors and in other blood cells (Plate 30–3*C*). The reactions of chloroacetate esterase are similar to those of Sudan black B and peroxidase in the acute leukemias, but they are more specific for the neutrophil series. Whereas chloroacetate esterase is more consistently negative in monocytes than Sudan black B or peroxidase, it is also less sensitive than the latter two staining reactions in the cells of the granulocytic series.

The non-specific esterases, using α-naphthyl acetate or α-naphthyl butyrate as substrates, are strongly positive in monocytes but weak or negative in granulocytes (Plate 30–3*F* and *L*). Megakaryocytes and tissue macrophages are strongly positive. Alpha-naphthyl acetate esterase is also positive in basophils and plasma cells, focally positive in resting T lymphocytes, and weakly positive in the normoblasts of some normal individuals. Sodium fluoride inhibits the reaction in monocytes, megakaryocytes, platelets, and plasma cells but not that in neutrophils or lymphocytes (Li, 1973). When the reaction is performed at a pH of 8, α-naphthyl butyrate esterase can be used to differentiate subpopulations of T lymphocytes, B lymphocytes, null cells, and monocytes (Higgy, 1977).

Alpha-naphthyl acetate esterase and α-naphthyl butyrate esterase are useful in distinguishing neutrophil precursors from monocytes and precursors in the acute leukemias (Table 30–6). The α-naphthyl acetate esterase reaction is focally positive in the blasts of a small proportion of patients with acute lymphoid leukemia. In some cases, this focal activity is associated with neoplastic T lymphocytes. In addition, a positive reaction may be also observed in the leukemic cells of megakaryocytic, eosinophilic, and basophilic leukemias, and in the erythroblasts of erythroleukemia.

Periodic Acid–Schiff (PAS) Reaction. The PAS reaction is based on the principle that periodic acid (HIO_4) is an oxidizing agent that converts hydroxy groups on adjacent carbon atoms to aldehydes (Hayhoe, 1964). The resulting dialdehydes are combined with Schiff's reagent to give a red-colored product. A positive reaction is therefore seen with polysaccharides, mucopolysaccharides, and glycoproteins.

In blood cells a positive PAS reaction usually indicates the presence of glycogen. This is demonstrated by digestion with amylase and consequent loss of staining. Neutrophils react at all stages of development, the most strongly in the mature stage. The same is true of eosinophils. The glycogen is not in the granules, but in background cytoplasm. Myeloblasts contain a few small PAS-positive granules. Monocytes have a faint staining reaction in the form of fine granules. Lymphocytes may contain a few small or large granules. Normoblasts are normally PAS negative.

In erythroleukemia (Plate 30–3*K*) and in thalassemia some of the erythroid precursors are PAS positive. This is true to a lesser extent in iron-deficiency anemia and sideroblastic anemias. In acute lymphocytic leukemia the lymphoblasts often contain large coarse clumps of PAS-positive material (Plate 30–3*H*). In chronic lymphocytic leukemia and lymphomas as well as in infectious mononucleosis the lymphocytes may have increased numbers of PAS-positive granules.

Acid Phosphatase (Katayama, 1977). Acid phosphatase in the cells hydrolyzes the substrate, naphthol AS-BI phosphoric acid. The naphthol released is insoluble and couples with "hexazotized" pararosanilin. The colored precipitate in the cytoplasm of the cells indicates acid phosphatase activity. If L(+) tartaric acid is in the solution, it inhibits the isoenzymes of acid phosphatase that are present in most cells, but not that of the cells of hairy cell leukemia (leukemic reticuloendotheliosis).

Red granules in the cytoplasm indicate acid phosphatase activity. The reaction is positive to varying degrees in most normal (and abnormal) leukocytes. Monocytes stain more intensely than neutrophils and precursors. Lymphocytes normally contain little activity; T cells appear to react positively; B cells are usually negative (Tamaoki, 1969).

The acid phosphatase reaction is useful in two areas. First, one of the elements in confirming a diagnosis of *hairy cell leukemia* (p. 736) is the presence of tartrate-resistant acid phosphatase in the abnormal cells. It must be realized, however, that a small fraction of cases of hairy cell leukemia do not show this reaction (Katayama, 1977). Second, in the subclassification of *acute lymphocytic leukemia,* definite focal positivity for acid phosphatase in the blasts is evidence in favor of T cell origin (Catovsky, 1978). A diffusely positive reaction product is not specific for T lymphocytes.

Neutrophil Alkaline Phosphatase. The enzyme is located in neutrophils from the metamyelocyte to the segmented stage, probably in a "tertiary" granular fraction. It can be detected by exposure to the substrate (a naphthol phosphate) in the presence of a diazonium salt (fast blue or fast violet) at an alkaline pH 9.5 (Kaplow, 1963). The substrate is hydrolyzed by the enzyme, releasing a phosphate and an aryl-naphtholamide. The latter is immediately coupled to the diazonium salt, forming an azo dye. After counterstaining, one hundred mature neutrophils are scored (0 to 4) according to the intensity of the staining reaction, from negative to the most intense. Adding the scores for the 100 neutrophils will give a total score with a possible range of 0 to 400. Reference values must be determined for each laboratory, and usually are about 20 to 100.

Increased activity occurs in infections, polycythemia vera, Hodgkin's disease, and in some cases of myelofibrosis with myeloid metaplasia. Decreased activity is found in chronic myeloid leukemia, acute myeloid leukemias, paroxysmal nocturnal hemoglobinuria, aplastic anemia, hereditary hypophosphatasia, and some viral infections, especially infectious mononucleosis.

Myeloproliferative Disorders

The myeloproliferative disorders comprise a group of closely related syndromes characterized by self-perpetuating proliferation of bone marrow cells: erythroid precursors; granulocytes and monocytes; and megakaryocytes. The proliferation is abnormal, and the cause is unknown (Gunz, 1974). Marrow, spleen, liver, and lymph nodes may be involved; these are the organs that normally participate in fetal hematopoiesis. All cell lines may be involved in the proliferative process (panmyelosis), or a single cell line may predominate.

The acute myeloproliferative disorders include the subgroups of acute myeloid leukemia: myeloblastic, promyelocytic, myelomonocytic, and the Di Guglielmo syndrome (erythremic myelosis and erythroleukemia).

The chronic myeloproliferative disorders include polycythemia vera (PV), myelofibrosis with myeloid metaplasia (MMM), thrombocythemia, and chronic myelogenous leukemia (CML). A related group of disorders are the myelodysplastic or dysmyelopoietic syndromes (p. 730).

It is known that erythroid, granulocytic-monocytic, and megakaryocytic cell lines are derived from a common hematopoietic stem cell (p. 626; see Fig. 28–1). Studies in individuals with a myeloproliferative disorder who were heterozygous for glucose 6-phosphate dehydrogenase (G6-PD) isoenzymes have shown that only one isoenzyme was present in erythrocytes, granulocytes (and monocytes), and platelets, whereas both isoenzymes were found in other tissues of these patients. This has been demonstrated in CML (Fialkow, 1977), in PV (Adamson, 1976), and in MMM (Jacobson, 1978). Such evidence strongly supports the concept that myeloproliferative disorders are clonal in nature (and, by implication, neoplastic), having arisen from a single pluripotential hematopoietic stem cell. The fibrosis that may occur in the marrow in all of these conditions is not monoclonal and hence is likely to be reactive (Adamson, 1978).

The new clone appears to have a proliferative advantage over normal cells which it gradually replaces. Also, it has a variable degree of genetic instability and is predisposed to generate additional clones leading to an enhanced probability for acute leukemia to develop (Galton, 1977; Nowell, 1977). This increased probability of acute leukemia is greatest in CML, but is present in most of the myeloproliferative disorders.

Self-limited proliferative reactions of the marrow to known stimuli are not considered here to be among the myeloproliferative disorders.

ACUTE MYELOID LEUKEMIA (AML)

Acute myeloblastic leukemia, promyelocytic leukemia, myelomonocytic leukemia, and erythroleukemia share certain features.

Clinical Features. Acute myeloid leukemia (AML) is the most common form of acute leukemia during the first few months of life. During childhood and adolescence it is relatively rare. However, during the middle and later years of life it becomes the most frequently observed form of acute leukemia.

The onset of AML often resembles an acute infection or even a septic condition. Other changes include thrombocytopenia, rapidly developing anemia, and signs of granulocytic insufficiency, with ulcerations of mucous membranes (especially of the mouth and throat) and fever. Enlargement of lymph nodes, spleen, and liver is not pronounced. Marked prostration and general malaise may be present. The course is rapidly progressive.

FAB Classification. A French-American-British (FAB) cooperative group has published proposals for the classification of acute leukemias (Bennett, 1976). The classification is based on morphology of cells in Romanowsky-stained blood and marrow films and certain supplemental cytochemical reactions (Tables 30–6 and 30–7). They emphasized the need for excellent technical preparations of blood and marrow films and the need for caution before diagnosing leukemia from hypocellular specimens.

In a revision of the criteria (Bennett, 1982) the FAB group characterizes two types of blast cells: both have central nuclei with fine, uncondensed chromatin and prominent nucleoli (usually three to five); Type I blasts lack cytoplasmic granules, but Type II blasts have small numbers of primary (azurophilic) granules. Promyelocytes with relatively normal features are excluded. According to these criteria, over 30 per cent blasts in the marrow suffice for the diagnosis of AML in any of the six categories (M1 to M6).

Acute Myeloblastic Leukemia (M1 and M2). In M1, myeloblasts usually predominate in the marrow, and granulocytic maturation is lacking (Plate 30–1*J*, 30–3*A*). Since M1 can be confused with acute lymphoid leukemia, cytochemical staining reactions are helpful in making the correct diagnosis. M2 can be distinguished from M1 by the maturation of the neoplastic cells beyond the myeloblastic and promyelocytic stages. More than 30 per cent of the marrow cells are blasts (Type I and Type II). If many myelocytes and metamyelocytes and increased basophils are present, consideration should be given to the possibility of a blastic transformation of chronic granulocytic leukemia rather than *de novo* AML. Abnormalities of maturation such as deficient granulation in mature neutrophils and hyposegmentation of nuclei (pseudo–Pelger-Huët anomaly) are often present in AML.

With Romanowsky stains, *Auer rods* are linear or spindle-shaped red-purple inclusions in blasts or promyelocytes (Plate 30–3*I*). Less commonly they may

Table 30–7. FRENCH-AMERICAN-BRITISH (FAB) CLASSIFICATION OF THE ACUTE MYELOID LEUKEMIAS (M)*

A. Granulocytic component predominant
  M1: Myeloblastic without maturation
    (>3% blasts peroxidase positive, or azure granules ± Auer rods)
  M2: Myeloblastic with maturation
    (>30 cells = Blasts, Types I and II; maturation beyond promyelocytes present)
  M3: Hypergranular Promyelocytic
    (Majority of cells abnormal promyelocytes; Auer rods usual)
B. Monocytic component predominant
  M4: Myelomonocytic
    (>20% promonocytes and monocytes; >20% blasts and abnormal granulocytic precursors
  M5: Monocytic
    (Poorly differentiated or differentiated; <20% abnormal granulocytic precursors)
C. Erythropoietic Component Predominant
  M6: Erythroleukemia
    (>50% cells = erythroid, abnormal; or >30% cells erythroid + 10% bizarre erythroid cells + >30% blasts Types I and II; ± Auer rods ± abnormal megakaryocytes)

*Modified from Bennett, J. M., et al.: Br. J. Haematol., *33*:451, 1976, and *51*:189, 1982.

be seen in more mature neutrophils. Auer rods are derivatives of azurophilic granules and stain positively for Sudan black B, myeloperoxidase, chloroacetate esterase, and acid phosphatase. Auer rods can be found in any of the varieties of AML (M1 to M6, but especially in M1 to M3). They are almost never found in any other condition, including CML.

Some cases of M2 are associated with a chromosomal translocation, t(8;21), an abnormality not yet found in other disorders (Catovsky, 1981).

Acute Promyelocytic Leukemia (M3). Promyelocytes instead of myeloblasts predominate in the marrow in hypergranular promyelocytic leukemia (M3). Azurophilic granules are abundant and intensely stained. Auer rods are found in almost all cases, and frequently are multiple in a given cell (Plate 30–3*I*). The disorder usually has a fulminant course, punctuated by bleeding which is more severe than would be expected from the degree of thrombocytopenia. This is attributed to intravascular coagulation that is apparently initiated by the procoagulant material from the granules of the abnormal cells.

A variant of M3 is hypogranular or microgranular promyelocytic leukemia, in which cytoplasmic granules appear sparse with light microscopy but are numerous but smaller with electron microscopy (Golomb, 1980). The cytochemical staining reactions are often equally as strong as in hypergranular M3. In microgranular M3, cells with Auer rods and hypergranular promyelocytes are found only in small numbers. Nuclei of most leukemic cells are bilobed or reniform, and confusion with an atypical monocytic leukemia is frequent.. The clinical course is similar to that of hypergranular M3.

In almost 50 per cent of patients with M3 a specific chromosomal translocation, t(15;17), has been observed (Testa, 1978).

Cytochemistry (M1, M2, and M3). According to the defining criteria of Hayhoe (1972), over 5 per cent of the cells (and usually more than 85 per cent) have positive granular staining with Sudan black B (Plate 30–3*B*). More than 5 per cent of the cells are also peroxidase positive. Staining of the blasts or early promyelocytes is the important criterion; occasionally the blasts fail to show these reactions if they have failed to show any development of azurophilic granules; on the other hand, sometimes no granules can be seen with Wright's stain, and yet the blasts are peroxidase and Sudan black B positive. Almost always these two stains react in parallel. Auer rods are positive with these staining reactions. Naphthol AS-D chloroacetate esterase is positive in developing granulocytes also, but alpha-naphthyl acetate esterase is usually negative. In promyelocytic leukemia (M3), these reactions are more intensely positive than in M1 and M2. The PAS stain shows faint diffuse or granular staining in some blasts or early promyelocytes.

The neutrophil alkaline phosphatase score is usually low, suggesting that these neutrophils are derived from the leukemic blasts.

Acute Myelomonocytic Leukemia (AMML; M4 and M5). Monocytes originate in the bone marrow from a stem cell common to granulocytes, erythroid cells, and megakaryocytes. In the monocytic leukemias there is a spectrum, from cases with slight monocytic and strong myeloblastic components to those that are almost purely monocytic (Hayhoe, 1964, 1972). When both components are present (to an extent of at least 20 per cent of the total cellular elements each), the FAB category is myelomonocytic (M4); pure or relatively pure monocytic leukemia is designated M5 (Table 30–7).

Two subtypes are recognized in the M5 form of AML: the poorly differentiated (monoblastic) subtype is characterized by large blasts in the bone marrow and peripheral blood (Plate 30–3*D* to *F*); the differentiated type has monoblasts, promonocytes, and monocytes (Plate 30–1*K*), but the blood has a higher proportion of monocytes than observed in the bone marrow, in which the most common cell is the promonocyte (Bennett, 1976). Esterase cytochemistry is helpful in distinguishing M2 from M4, M4 from M5, and M1 from M5.

The nuclei of promonocytes and abnormal monocytes in AMML have delicate reticular chromatin and several (three to five) nucleoli. The nuclei are folded, indented, and frequently twisted or even coarsely segmented. There is usually abundant cytoplasm (the nuclear-cytoplasmic ratio is low) and often many fine azurophilic granules (Plate 30–1*K*). Phagocytosis of red cells or cell debris may be seen. Auer rods may be present in the abnormal monocytes as well as in the blasts. Neutrophils may have diminished granules; the pseudo-Pelger anomaly may be present; and eosinophils may be abnormal.

Monocytes constitute over 1 per cent of the circulating leukocytes. Normoblasts are not usually found in the blood, nor do they predominate in the marrow. Megakaryocytes are less likely to be depleted in the marrow in this form of acute leukemia, and thrombocytopenia is less frequent.

Cytochemistry (M4 and M5) (Table 30–6). Sudan black B positivity is often present in the monocytes and is finer than that seen in granulocyte precursors. The peroxidase reaction also tends to be less strong, and usually is negative in the younger cells (Plate 30–3*E*). The alpha-naphthyl acetate and alpha-naphthyl butyrate esterase reactions are positive in the monocytes and monoblasts (Plate 30–3*F, L*), and the naphthol AS-D chloroacetate esterase is negative, the reverse of the findings in the granulocyte precursors in M1 and M2. This makes these esterase reactions particularly valuable in the diagnosis of myelomonocytic leukemia. The PAS reaction may be negative or show granular positivity, especially in M5.

Patients with myelomonocytic leukemia characteristically have markedly increased levels of muramidase (lysozyme) in the serum and urine (Osserman, 1966). If the cells are poorly differentiated or significantly abnormal morphologically they may not produce muramidase (Catovsky, 1971).

Di Guglielmo Syndrome (Erythroleukemia, M6). Another variant of AML is erythroleukemia, which refers to an abnormal proliferation of both erythroid precursors and granulocytic precursors (Table 30–7). Morphologic abnormalities are usually pronounced.

Very rarely there is virtually no granulocytic involvement in the neoplastic process and primitive erythroblasts predominate, in which case the condition is called *erythremic myelosis.* This disease has a rapid course resembling that of acute leukemia.

Usually there is a mixture of variable proportions of erythroid precursors and myeloblasts, *erythroleukemia,* which may include abnormal megakaryocytic and monocytic proliferations in addition. This also usually has a rapid course, but is more variable and sometimes may be subacute or even chronic.

When the abnormal erythroid proliferation is minimal and the myeloblastic proliferation predominates, the picture of *acute myeloblastic leukemia* is seen.

Although each disorder may occur *de novo,* occasionally one sees progression from an initial erythremic myelosis to erythroleukemia to a final termination in acute myelogenous leukemia in a single patient. This group of disorders has been designated the *Di Guglielmo syndrome* (Gunz, 1974).

Erythroid precursors are abnormal, predominate in the hyperplastic marrow, and usually are present in the blood (Plate 30–3*J*). They are irregular in outline, often with pseudopods. The nuclear:cytoplasmic ratio is not high. Nuclear shape is often bizarre, with atypical megaloblastic features. Nucleoli tend to be large. Mitoses and multinucleated giant forms are numerous. Vacuolation of cytoplasm in pro- and basophilic erythroblasts is often present. In erythremic myelosis and the more acute forms of erythroleukemia, there is an apparent arrest of maturation and fewer polychromatic and orthochromatic forms are present. In chronic forms of erythroleukemia, later normoblasts are present in larger numbers. Myeloblasts are increased in erythroleukemia, and Auer rods may be found in them or in promyelocytes. Abnormalities in neutrophils and eosinophils may be seen. Monocytic proliferation may be a part of the process. Abnormal megakaryocytes are often prominent and include giant forms with bizarre nuclear fragmentation and small fragmented megakaryocytes with one or two apparently diploid nuclei. Atypical platelets may be found in the blood (Plate 30–4*F* and *G*).

Cytochemistry (M6). Some of the erythroid precursors at all stages of maturation show strong cytoplasmic PAS positivity. This is granular in early erythroid precursors and diffuse in later stages (Plate 30–3*K*). Erythroid precursors are PAS negative in normal individuals and in most diseases, including nutritional megaloblastic anemia. They are sometimes positive, however, in iron deficiency anemia and thalassemia and in refractory sideroblastic anemia or refractory anemia with dyshematopoiesis (Hayhoe, 1964). In erythroleukemia increased numbers of primitive cells showing Sudan black and peroxidase positivity (myeloblasts) are found. A non-specific esterase-positive monocytic component is often evident (Plate 30–3*L*). Neoplastic erythroid precursors are also sometimes positive for the alpha-naphthyl acetate esterase reaction (Hayhoe, 1972).

Course. Table 30–8 shows the distribution of cases according to the FAB classification (Sultan, 1981). Current data suggest that a smaller proportion of patients with M4 and M5 variants enter a complete remission. In addition, patients with erythroleukemia may have a very poor prognosis (Roggli, 1981).

CHRONIC MYELOID LEUKEMIA (CML)

Clinical Features. CML occurs primarily in young and middle-aged adults. The onset is insidious and the disorder may be discovered accidentally on a routine blood test. The patient may have symptoms of anemia and weight loss or simply may complain of malaise. The spleen enlarges progressively, and the patient begins to lose weight and have fever and night sweats associated with increased metabolism due to granulocyte turnover. The discomfort associated with an enlarged spleen may bring the patient to the doctor. Infarcts in the spleen may produce left upper quadrant pain. Excessive bleeding or bruising may occur in the later stages of the disease. Lymphadenopathy, though often present, is rarely prominent.

Laboratory Features

Blood. The leukocyte count is usually over 50×10^9/L and may exceed 300×10^9/L. The differential

Table 30–8. CLINICAL FEATURES OF AML ACCORDING TO THE FAB CLASSIFICATION (M1–M6)*

Variant	Percentage of Cases	Male/Female Ratio	Mean Age (Years)	Percentage in Complete Remission
M1	21	1.3	51	59
M2	32	1.0	48	60
M3	16	0.9	41	63
M4	16	0.7	52	38
M5	12	0.8	52	36
M6	3	—	—	—

*Modified from Sultan, C., et al.: Br. J. Haematol., *47*:545, 1981. Blackwell Scientific Publications, Ltd., Oxford. Percentages in complete remission are based on 100 cases.

count is characteristic. There is a complete spectrum of granulocytic cells, from a few myeloblasts to mature neutrophils. Myeloblasts are less than 10 per cent of the cells. Myelocytes and neutrophils both exceed the other cell types. This bimodal distribution helps to exclude other myeloproliferative disorders and reactive leukocytoses (Spiers, 1977). The relative percentage of neutrophil myelocytes increases as the total leukocyte count increases. Basophilia is consistently present. Eosinophilia is almost always noted, along with the presence of eosinophil myelocytes. Monocytes are also absolutely increased in most patients.

Anemia is present in the majority of patients at the time of diagnosis. In others it appears during the course of the disease as a result of decreased RBC production. Erythrocytes are normochromic and normocytic. A few normoblasts can usually be found.

Thrombocytosis is present at the time of diagnosis in over half of patients. Less than 15 per cent of patients have a thrombocytopenia.

Marrow. The marrow is markedly hypercellular due primarily to granulocytic proliferation, with all stages represented. Eosinophil and basophil precursors are often increased. Normoblasts tend to be decreased. Frequently the marrow cannot be aspirated because of the density of cells packed together or (especially later in the disease) because of increased reticulin, which can be demonstrated on marrow biopsy. In a minority of patients are found macrophages laden with blue pigment (sea-blue histiocytes) or macrophages indistinguishable from Gaucher cells.

It is well to remember that even a typical bone marrow is not diagnostic of CML. On the other hand, the diagnosis can be made from the peripheral blood film in most cases.

Neutrophil Alkaline Phosphatase. The neutrophil alkaline phosphatase (NAP) is greatly reduced or absent in over 90 per cent of patients with CML. It is greatly elevated in polycythemia vera; elevated, normal, or low in myelofibrosis with myeloid metaplasia; and normal or elevated in leukemoid reactions (Gunz, 1974). During remission of CML with a normal appearing blood picture, in most cases, the NAP continues to be low; in about one third of patients it returns to normal (Rosner, 1972). The NAP increases in the accelerated and blastic phases of the disease. It may also increase in response to infection as it does in normal individuals.

Cytogenetic Abnormalities. In direct bone marrow preparations and in metaphases of cultured peripheral blood, 90 to 95 per cent of patients with hematologically typical CML have an abnormally small acrocentric chromosome. With banding techniques this has been shown to be chromosome 22; part of the long arm has been translocated to another chromosome, usually chromosome 9. The abnormal small chromosome was first detected in 1960 by Nowell and Hungerford and is called the Philadelphia (Ph^1) chromosome. The Ph^1 chromosome is present in blood and marrow cells during relapse and is demonstrable in the marrow also during remission. It appears that the Ph^1 chromosome is present in precursors of granulocytes, in normoblasts and megakaryocytes, in lymphocytes only in some cases, but not in skin cells.

The small proportion of patients with CML who lack the Ph^1 chromosome are characteristic in most other respects: average age, spleen size, marrow and blood picture, and NAP values. On the average, however, the patients in this Ph^1-negative group have less elevated white blood cell counts, have lower platelet counts, include a larger proportion of children, respond less well to therapy, and have a shorter survival (Tjio, 1966). Children with Ph^1-negative CML ("juvenile CML") are usually one to two years old; their erythrocytes contain 30 to 70 per cent Hb F and also show other fetal characteristics (Mauer, 1974).

Other Findings. Serum vitamin B_{12} and vitamin B_{12}–binding proteins are usually increased considerably, as a result of increased transcobalamin I, and are thought to reflect the size of the total blood granulocyte pool. The serum muramidase is also increased.

Course. Treatment with busulfan usually controls the disease in the chronic phase. After a median period of about three years, the disease changes into a more aggressive or accelerated phase. This is characterized by one or more features of progressive myeloproliferation: basophilia, thrombocytosis, leukocytosis, increasing splenomegaly, anemia, and reticulin myelofibrosis. These features become refractory to chemotherapy (Canellos, 1976). Preceding these changes, new clones of cells with cytogenetic abnormalities may be demonstrated, and, frequently, a change occurs in the *in vitro* growth characteristics of the committed progenitor cells in soft agar cultures (Metcalf, 1977).

In about one third of cases, the accelerated phase

is characterized by a progressive increase in blasts and promyelocytes; when they exceed 30 per cent of cells in blood or marrow, it is regarded as the blastic phase of the disease. In the majority of cases, the blastic phase follows the accelerated phase by a few months; in a small proportion of cases, the blastic phase may be the first presentation of the disease (Peterson, 1976). These patients usually have the Ph^1 chromosome, with or without morphologic evidence of CML, such as basophilia. The NAP becomes normal or high in most patients in the blastic phase.

The morphologic patterns in the blastic phase of CML resemble acute myeloblastic leukemia in the majority of cases, although Auer rods are found but rarely. In approximately one third of cases, however, the appearance is that of acute lymphoblastic leukemia (ALL) (Rosenthal, 1977). In many of these latter cases, the blasts are positive for terminal deoxynucleotidyl transferase (Marks, 1978). The distinction is useful because the latter (ALL) may respond to ALL-oriented therapy but the former (AML) do not (Peterson, 1976).

Median survival after onset of the blastic phase of CML is about two months overall and about ten months in patients who respond by going into remission (Canellos, 1976).

POLYCYTHEMIA VERA (ERYTHREMIA, PRIMARY POLYCYTHEMIA)

Polycythemia vera is characterized by excessive proliferation of erythroid, granulocytic, and megakaryocytic elements in the marrow (panmyelosis). This is reflected in the blood in an absolute increase in the red cell mass, leukocytosis, and thrombocytosis. Erythropoietin excretion in the urine is decreased. The production of erythrocytes appears to be autonomous, but it does respond to erythropoietin when the patient has become anemic through blood loss. The cause of this panmyelosis and pancytosis is unknown.

Clinical Features. The disease is more frequent in men than in women. It usually begins in middle age. Affected patients exhibit ruddy cyanosis. Splenomegaly is present in two thirds of patients. Thrombotic or hemorrhagic phenomena occur in about half of patients. Myocardial infarction, cerebral thrombosis, splenic infarction, pulmonary infarcts, and thrombophlebitis account for the most frequent thrombotic episodes; upper gastrointestinal bleeding, often from peptic ulcer, is the most common bleeding problem (Wasserman, 1966). Pruritus, especially after bathing, is common.

Blood. The erythrocytes number 6 to 12 $\times$ 10^{12}/L, and the hemoglobin is 18 to 24 g/dl. The MCV, MCH, and MCHC are normal or low. The erythrocytes are hypochromic and microcytic if chronic blood loss has occurred. Macrocytes, polychromatic cells, and normoblasts may be found but are not a prominent feature of the disease. Red cell production is increased. Red cell destruction is normal during the period of erythrocytosis; later in the disease, as splenomegaly develops, the red cell survival diminishes. The total blood volume is increased, primarily because of the increased red cell mass, though the plasma volume may also be elevated to a lesser degree. Blood viscosity is high, and it may be difficult to prepare good blood films. The ESR is reduced.

The platelet count is increased in about two thirds of patients, often to levels exceeding 1000 $\times$ 10^9/L. In 80 per cent of untreated patients, functional platelet abnormalities can be detected by platelet aggregation studies (Gilbert, 1975a). Decreased aggregation in response to epinephrine is most common, but may be found in response to other reagents as well. No consistent clotting defect has been found in polycythemia vera.

Moderate neutrophilic leukocytosis in the range of 10 to 30 $\times$ 10^9/L is common. Immature granulocytes are seen in about one half of cases and basophils are often absolutely increased. The neutrophil alkaline phosphatase is markedly elevated in 80 per cent of patients. Serum vitamin B_{12} binding capacity and serum muramidase are usually elevated.

The arterial oxygen saturation is normal. Hyperuricemia appears in many patients with polycythemia vera due to the increased nucleic acid metabolism, and in some patients, secondary gout or renal uric acid stones occur.

Soft agar culture of blood cells reveals normal to increased numbers of colonies (GM-CFC; p. 627). The colony stimulating activity (GM-CSF) in the blood is usually increased (Metcalf, 1977).

Marrow. The marrow is characteristically hypercellular, with all the elements (erythroid, granulocytic, and megakaryocytic) sharing the hyperplasia; fat is decreased (Plate 30–4*A*). In a study of patients of the Polycythemia Vera Study Group (PVSG) 90 per cent had moderate or marked hypercellularity; only 6 per cent were normocellular and none hypocellular (Ellis, 1975). Increased reticulin is often present and correlates positively with the cellularity. Storage iron is decreased or absent in 95 per cent of cases.

In vitro culture of marrow cells results in the growth of substantial numbers of erythroid colonies without added erythropoietin (EP); this suggests that the clone is EP independent or abnormally sensitive to EP (Prchal, 1974).

Diagnosis. Criteria of the PVSG for the diagnosis of PV are as follows (Berlin, 1975):

1. Increased total erythrocyte volume (males, ≥36 ml/kg; females, ≥32 ml/kg).

2. Normal arterial oxygen saturation (≥92 per cent).

3. Either splenomegaly, or two of the following: (a) thrombocytosis (>400 $\times$ 10^9/L); (b) leukocytosis (>12 $\times$ 10^9/L); (c) increased neutrophil alkaline phosphatase; (d) increased serum vitamin B_{12} (>900 μg/L) or unsaturated B_{12} binding capacity (>2200 μg/L).

If doubt remains about the diagnosis of polycythemia vera, a search for other causes of polycythemia should be made.

Course. Polycythemia vera is a chronic disease; patients usually live 10 to 20 years under good control. Phlebotomy, chlorambucil, and ^{32}P have been used to control the manifestations of the disease. Because of the high incidence of complications in untreated cases, surgery should not be undertaken unless the hemato-

4

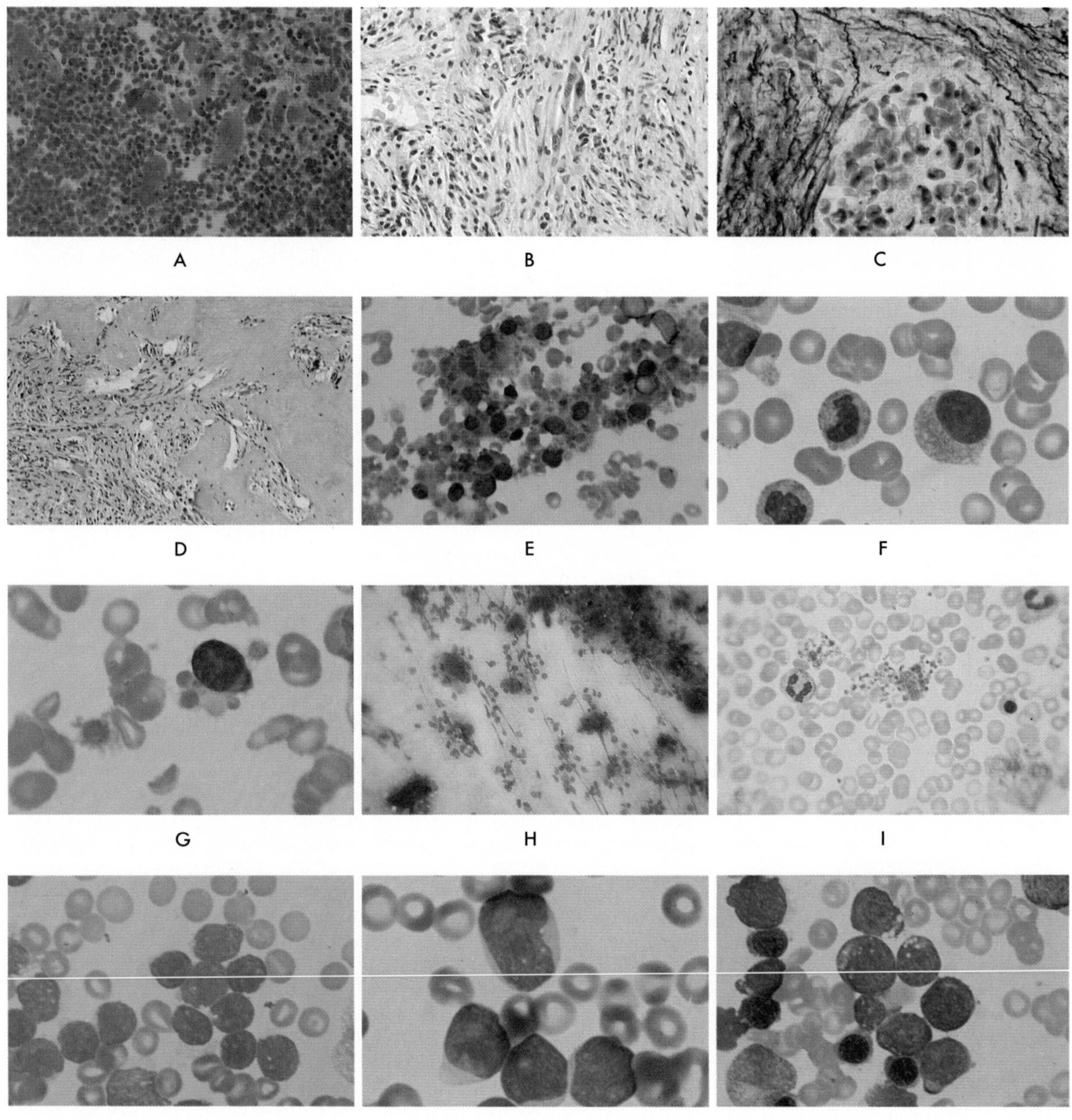

Plate 30–4. The stain is Wright's or Wright-Giemsa unless otherwise noted. *A,* Polycythemia vera, bone marrow biopsy. Hematoxylin and eosin. Solidly cellular marrow with panmyelosis, i.e., the hypercellularity is due to increased erythroid, granulocytic, and megakaryocytic proliferation. *B,* Myelofibrosis with myeloid metaplasia (MMM), bone marrow biopsy, H & E. Reticulin and collagen fibrosis accounts for the increased intercellular material; note the distortion of the megakaryocytes (*right center*). This marrow is considerably less cellular than *A. C,* MMM, bone marrow biopsy, reticulin stain. Reticulin fibers are coated with silver in this reaction and appear dark. They are the major component of the myelofibrosis in the early phases of MMM: only later does the collagen staining reaction appear. Note the large vascular space; these are often present in the marrow in MMM. *D,* MMM with osteosclerosis, bone marrow biopsy, H & E stain. Note the irregular new bone formation and apparent continuity of fibers from the marrow with those in the bone (*upper center*). *E,* MMM, touch preparation of marrow biopsy. A mass of abnormal platelets, most with diminished granules, and many separate, small megakaryocytic nuclei (each the size of a small lymphocyte). These abnormal micro megakaryocytes and masses of atypical platelets can often be found on touch preparations of marrow biopsies in MMM. Usually aspiration of marrow tissue is impossible. *F,* MMM, blood film. To the right of the neutrophil near the center is a micromegakaryocyte; note the intensely staining nuclear chromatin and fine azure granules in the cytoplasm. Often the cytoplasm is less abundant in these cells. *G,* MMM, blood film. The nucleated cell is a micromegakaryoblast. Cells such as this are frequently mistaken for lymphocytes. Adjacent to it are three large poorly granular platelets; another is seen to the left in the field.

Legend continued on following page

crit has been reduced to normal levels (Wasserman, 1964).

In about 20 to 40 per cent of patients, progressive anemia, gradual splenic enlargement, and further elevation of the leukocyte count, with more immature granulocytes and more circulating nucleated red cells, may occur. Many erythrocytes become oval; teardrop-shaped cells (dacrocytes) become prominent; and poikilocytic red cells increase in number (see Figs. 27–26 and 27–27). Bone marrow aspiration becomes impossible because of myelofibrosis, and splenomegaly increases owing to extramedullary hematopoiesis. The manifestations at this stage of the disease are indistinguishable from myelofibrosis with myeloid metaplasia (Plate 30–4*B* to *G*).

Another late complication of polycythemia vera is acute leukemia (Landaw, 1975). An increased risk of developing acute leukemia is associated with PV itself (phlebotomy treatment alone). To this is added the leukemogenic potential contributed by the effective myelosuppressive agents; of these, the risk with chlorambucil exceeds that with ^{32}P (Silverstein, 1981). It does appear, however, that treatment with phlebotomy alone results in shorter survival than treatment with myelosuppressive agents.

MYELOFIBROSIS WITH MYELOID METAPLASIA

Synonyms for what is probably the same basic disease process include myelosclerosis with myeloid metaplasia, myeloid megakaryocytic hepatosplenomegaly, aleukemic myelosis, agnogenic myeloid metaplasia, and many others.

Definition. This is a chronic, progressive panmyelosis characterized by a triad of findings: varying degrees of fibrosis of the marrow, massive splenomegaly due to extramedullary hematopoiesis, and a leukoerythroblastic anemia with marked red cell abnormalities, circulating normoblasts, immature granulocytes, and atypical platelets (Gunz, 1974; Ward, 1971).

Clinical Features. The disorder occurs typically in persons over the age of 50 and has an insidious onset, with weight loss, anemia, and abdominal discomfort due to the large spleen. Often the liver is enlarged as well, and the patient may be slightly jaundiced. On x-ray, diffuse or patchy osteosclerosis may appear in one third to one half of patients; osteoporosis may be seen also.

Blood. A moderate normochromic, normocytic anemia (frequently with some hypochromic cells and basophilic stippling), moderate anisocytosis, and marked poikilocytosis, including prominent teardrop forms (dacrocytes) and elliptocytes, are characteristic (see Figs. 27–26 and 27–27). Normoblasts are often present in numbers out of proportion to the degree of anemia, and a slight reticulocytosis is frequently found. The anemia may have a complicated origin, with components of marrow failure, ineffective erythropoiesis, and hemolysis. The leukocyte count is normal or, more commonly, moderately increased; immature neutrophils and occasionally even myeloblasts are present. The NAP is most often elevated, but occasionally may be normal or decreased (Takácsi-Nagy, 1975). Chromosomal studies have not shown the presence of the Philadelphia (Ph^1) chromosome, which is so characteristic of CML. Basophils are often increased in number. Platelets are normal or decreased in number (rarely increased) and often are atypical, with distinct "zones": a clear hyaloplasm and a central pale chromomere which lacks the usual concentration of azurophilic granules (Plate 30–4*E* to *G*). Micromegakaryocytes the size of lymphocytes with both nucleus and cytoplasm or small megakaryoblasts may usually be found if searched for; on rare occasions, they are present in considerable numbers (Plate 30–4*E* to *G*; see also Plate 28–3*H*).

In vitro culture studies of blood cells have generally shown considerably increased colonies (GM-CFC) and clusters, which are similar to the pattern in CML. The serum colony stimulating activity (GM-CSF) appears to be very high (Metcalf, 1977).

Serum uric acid is frequently increased. Serum vitamin B_{12} and unsaturated B_{12} binding globulin are normal or elevated.

Marrow. It is usually impossible to aspirate marrow, and a needle biopsy or a surgical biopsy is necessary; this is especially true later in the course of the disease. Early in the disease, the marrow may be hypercellular, with panmyelosis and prominently increased megakaryocytes which are frequently abnormal. On histologic sections there is a diffuse increase in reticulin fibers which is demonstrable with silver stains (Rappaport, 1966); patchy fibrosis may be present.

Later the marrow becomes more fibrotic, with residual islands of atypical megakaryocytes, erythroid, and granulocytic precursors. The fibrosis is of loose connective tissue with scanty collagen, but reticulin fibers are abundant. Foci of osteoid may be found, and the bony trabeculae are sometimes irregularly thickened (myelosclerosis). The marrow may show a mixture of hyperplasia and fibrosis in one sample or may differ in different sites of the body (Plate 30–4*A* to *E*).

Course. A significant proportion of cases of myelofibrosis with myeloid metaplasia represent a late

Plate 30–4 *Continued. H*, Thrombocythemia, bone marrow film, low power. An abundance of megakaryocytes dominates the marrow films from most aspirations in thrombocythemia. *I*, Thrombocythemia, blood film. Individual platelets usually appear normal, except that they are frequently large. The features of the blood film are considerably increased numbers of platelets, neutrophilia, and often hypochromic microcytic red cells as a result of chronic blood loss. *J*, ALL, FAB-L1, marrow film. the blast are small and have high N/C ratios, inconspicuous nucleoli, regular nuclear outline (× 400). *K*, ALL, FAB-L2, blood film. The blasts are large and have lower N/C ratios, prominent nucleoli, and often irregular nuclear outlines (× 800). *L*, ALL, FAB-L3, marrow film. The blasts are moderately large and uniform in size and have a moderate amount of intensely basophilic cytoplasm which often contains vacuoles (× 400).

stage, after many years' progression, of typical polycythemia vera. The usual course of MMM is one of progressive anemia and enlargement of the spleen; hemolysis frequently becomes an increasing element in the anemia. Infections may be a serious problem. Portal hypertension occurs in 10 to 20 per cent of cases and may result in bleeding esophageal varices. It may be due to portal vein thrombosis or intrahepatic obstruction due to myeloid metaplasia coupled with increased portal blood flow (Laszlo, 1975).

The median survival is about 5 years, slightly longer than that of chronic granulocytic leukemia, but considerably less than that of polycythemia vera; however, patients may occasionally live as long as 10 to 15 years. In patients with longer survival, frequently the terminal event is an acute leukemia.

THROMBOCYTHEMIA

As distinguished from *thrombocytosis,* the term *thrombocythemia* should probably be confined to situations in which the platelet count is persistently elevated to levels at least three times normal (Gunz, 1974). Thrombocythemia, thus defined, will usually be part of the general picture of other myeloproliferative disorders: polycythemia vera, chronic myelogenous leukemia, and, rarely, myelofibrosis with myeloid metaplasia.

Occasionally, however, thrombocythemia may be the predominant feature of the hematologic picture, and in these cases it is commonly associated with bleeding problems. Gunz (1960) regards hemorrhagic thrombocythemia as a clinical syndrome; the pathologic features cannot be separated from those of the other myeloproliferative disorders. It is probably most closely related to polycythemia vera.

Clinical Features. Characteristic are recurrent, spontaneous hemorrhages, which are most commonly gastrointestinal. Hemorrhages are occasionally preceded or accompanied by thrombosis in superficial or deep veins. Purpura has not been described. Slight splenomegaly as measured with radioisotopic techniques occurs in 50 per cent of cases.

Blood (Plate 30–4*I*). The most striking feature is the marked increase in platelets (maximum values: 0.9 to 14.0 $\times$ 10^{12}/L), often with abnormal and giant forms and usually accompanied by fragments of megakaryocytes. Neutrophilic leukocytosis is almost always present, and the NAP is usually normal. Hypochromic microcytic anemia due to chronic blood loss is present in many cases; at other times, erythrocytosis may be evident. Platelet function defects in myeloproliferative diseases, especially thrombocythemia, are frequently demonstrable. The most typical finding is decreased aggregation in response to epinephrine (Spaet, 1969).

Marrow (Plate 30–4*H*). The marrow shows a panmyelosis with increased megakaryocytes. Splenic extramedullary hematopoiesis may be present.

Diagnosis. Criteria of the PVSG for the diagnosis of thrombocythemia are (Laszlo, 1975):

1. Platelet count exceeding 1000 $\times$ 10^9/L on at least two occasions.
2. Megakaryocytic hyperplasia and sufficiency of iron stores in marrow.
3. Normal red cell mass.
4. No prior splenectomy.
5. No identifiable cause for thrombocytosis.

Course. Most cases are stable for many years, but a small proportion may merge into other myeloproliferative disorders or, rarely, develop into acute leukemia (Silverstein, 1981).

MYELODYSPLASTIC SYNDROMES

Myelodysplastic syndromes (MDS) occur primarily in persons over age 50 and usually present as an anemia refractory to hematinics, with or without neutropenia and thrombocytopenia. Liver, spleen, or lymph nodes are not usually enlarged. The marrow is hypercellular and maturation is abnormal in one or more of the three hematopoietic cell lines, and blast cells are often increased. This group of disorders has been called "preleukemias" (Saarni, 1973) or dysmyelopoietic syndromes because of the high proportion of cases which ultimately progress to overt acute leukemia (Gralnick, 1977). The FAB Cooperative Group (Bennett, 1976, 1982) has described and classified these disorders.

Types of Abnormal Cellular Maturation. *Dyserythropoiesis* includes nuclear fragmentation or karyorrhexis, multinuclearity, irregularly staining cytoplasm, basophilic stippling, and ring sideroblasts. Erythroid cells may be decreased or increased in number. Erythrocytic abnormalities in the blood film include oval macrocytes, anisochromia, basophilic stippling, dacrocytes, and reticulocytopenia.

Dysgranulopoiesis includes retarded nuclear maturation and distorted cytoplasmic maturation, with azurophilic granules either unstained or abnormally large and decreased numbers of specific granules. In the blood film one may see nuclear hyposegmentation (pseudo–Pelger-Huët anomaly) or bizarre hypersegmentation, and irregular retention of cytoplasmic basophilia or lack of cytoplasmic granules.

Dysmegakaryocytopoiesis includes large megakaryocytes with unsegmented nuclei, micromegakaryocytes, and megakaryocytes with two or more small unconnected nuclei. Megakaryocytes may be decreased in number. In the blood film giant hypogranular platelets are frequent and micromegakaryocytes are seen rarely.

Blood and Marrow Findings. Five types of myelodysplastic syndromes have been defined by the FAB Cooperative Group (Bennett, 1982). Agranular blast cells and blast cells with a few azurophilic granules are included as "blasts"; promyelocytes are excluded.

Refractory Anemia (RA). Anemia with reticulocytopenia and abnormal erythrocytes are the presenting findings. Abnormal granulocytes are rare, and blasts are less than 1 per cent in the blood. The marrow is normocellular to hypercellular with erythroid hyperplasia and/or dyserythropoiesis and fewer than 5 per cent blasts.

Refractory Anemia with Ring Sideroblasts. In addition to the findings of RA, ring sideroblasts are present and exceed 15 per cent of all marrow cells. Defective cytoplasmic maturation and anisochromic erythrocytes are associated abnormalities.

Refractory Anemia with Excess Blasts (RAEB).

The blood shows cytopenia in two or three of the cell lines, and less than 5 per cent circulating blasts. The marrow is hypercellular, with variable erythroid or granulocytic hyperplasia. Dyspoietic changes are present in all three cell lines, and 5 to 20 per cent of the marrow cells are blasts.

Chronic Myelomonocytic Leukemia (CMML). In the blood are a persistent monocytosis ($>1 \times 10^9$/L), frequently neutrophilia with morphologic abnormalities, and less than 5 per cent blasts. The marrow is similar to that in RAEB but often has increased promonocytes. These may be distinguished from the abnormal myelocytes by nonspecific esterase staining.

RAEB in Transformation. The findings are similar to those in RAEB with the addition of any of the following: (1) greater than 5 per cent blasts in the blood, (2) 20 to 30 per cent blasts in the marrow, or (3) the presence of Auer rods. In this group are patients with cytopenias and symptoms of short duration which do not fit into the other categories of MDS or of AML. A minimum of 30 per cent blasts is required for the diagnosis of AML (M1 through M6).

OTHER FORMS OF LEUKEMIA

Acute Undifferentiated (Stem Cell) Leukemia. This is a variety of acute leukemia in which the predominant cells are blast forms that cannot be classified using cytochemical or immunologic methods. We believe that it occurs, that it is very rare, and that it might better be designated "unclassifiable leukemia."

Chloroma. Rarely in AML there is formation of tumors originating from periosteum, especially of skull, orbits, nasal sinuses, ribs, and vertebrae. Exophthalmos with disturbances of vision may occur. The sectioned surface of the tumor shows a green color, and the tumor contains large amounts of verdoperoxidase and protoporphyrin. The color fades on exposure and can be restored with hydrogen peroxide and preserved by glycerin. There are aleukemic and leukemic forms, the latter with myeloblasts in the blood. Clinically the latter cases are identical with AML.

Granulocytic Sarcoma (Myeloblastic Sarcoma). This localized tumor of myeloblasts differs from chloroma only by absence of pigment. Like chloroma it is rare, since the tissue involvement in AML is usually a diffuse infiltrative process.

Patients with granulocytic sarcomas range in age from 2 to 81 years. Three clinical settings are found: (1) no known disease, (2) a known myeloproliferative disorder, and (3) acute myeloid leukemia (Neiman, 1981). Myeloblastoma may occur preceding or at the time of the blastic phase of CML in skin, lymph nodes, and extradural masses or in localized, lytic bone lesions (Rosenthal, 1977). Diagnosis depends upon recognizing the nature of the primitive cells. This is facilitated by making touch imprint preparations of cut sections of the tumor and staining them with Romanowsky stains and cytochemical reactions. In formalin-fixed, embedded tissue, the naphthol AS-D chloroacetate esterase reaction and the antilysozyme immunoperoxidase technique may be helpful, since the enzymes resist destruction during tissue processing (Leder, 1964; Neiman, 1981).

Eosinophilic Leukemia. This occurs but is extremely rare. Acute and chronic forms have been described; the cells infiltrating the tissues are immature eosinophils. It is generally regarded to be a variant of AML or CML, as the case may be, since other myeloid elements are usually involved, but to a lesser degree. It may be difficult or impossible to differentiate this lesion from the hypereosinophilic syndrome. Leukocytosis and eosinophilia, no matter how high, are not sufficient to establish the diagnosis of leukemia; both can be seen in parasitic infestation. But the diagnosis can be made when there is, in addition, persistent eosinophilia associated with immature forms in the blood as well as marrow; significantly increased blasts in the marrow (>5 per cent); a positive chloroacetate esterase reaction in the eosinophilic precursors; tissue infiltration by immature eosinophils; and an acute course associated with anemia, thrombocytopenia, or increased susceptibility to infection (Rickles, 1972; Liso, 1977).

Basophilic Leukemia. Extremely high basophil counts overshadowing other myeloid involvement are seen occasionally in myeloid leukemia, especially CML. A basophilic phase of CML is sometimes seen as part of the accelerated phase of the disease. It should be kept in mind that mast cells that resemble basophilic granulocytes are present in large numbers in the skin and marrow in urticaria pigmentosa.

Neutrophilic Leukemia. This is similar to eosinophilic and basophilic leukemia, but the cell type is the segmented granulocyte with very few immature forms. It is extremely rare.

Megakaryoblastic Leukemia (Acute Myelofibrosis). A rare form of acute leukemia is characterized by a predominance of megakaryocytes or megakaryoblasts in the bone marrow, accompanied by an increase in reticulum fibers. The disorder usually occurs in the middle to late years of life, and males are more often affected than females. At the time of presentation, the patients typically have pancytopenia without organomegaly or lymphadenopathy. The bone marrow is both cellular and fibrotic, with immaturity and atypia in all three cell lines; megakaryocytes and their precursors usually predominate. The blasts have a high nuclear to cytoplasmic ratio and multiple nucleoli; a minority of them are large and contain multilobed nuclei. With cytochemistry, blasts are positive for PAS and alpha-naphthyl acetate esterase (partially inhibited by sodium fluoride) and negative for alpha-naphthyl butyrate esterase. Ultrastructural demonstration of platelet peroxidase in the blasts is helpful in confirming their megakaryocytic nature. The prognosis of acute megakaryoblastic leukemia is very poor. Terminally the patients have leukocytosis and hepatosplenomegaly (den Ottolander, 1979; Bearman, 1979).

CELL CULTURE STUDIES

In vitro, GM-CFC cultures in semisolid agar with blood leukocyte feeder layers provide a means of studying disorders of granulopoiesis (Metcalf, 1977). In AML and myelodysplastic syndromes (especially RAEB), patients with "nonleukemic" *in vitro* growth patterns (reduced GM-CFC colony growth or no growth) seem to have a better prognosis than patients with "leukemic" *in vitro* growth patterns (abortive cluster growth predominating). In CMML and in CML and other myeloproliferative disorders, marrow GM-CFC growth is usually increased; but when the aggressive phase of CML or acute leukemia occurs, colonies decrease and abnormal cluster growth predominates (Sultan, 1977; Greenberg, 1981).

In vitro clonogenic culture systems are beginning to provide insight into mechanisms involved in disorders of granulocytopoiesis, but they also may provide some prognostic information (e.g., in AML). They are not yet readily available, however, in clinical laboratories.

Lymphoproliferative Disorders

The lymphoproliferative disorders represent a group of neoplastic conditions originating from cells of the lymphoreticular system. When neoplastic cells involve predominantly the blood and bone marrow, the condition is called a leukemia. However, when the condition is predominantly limited to lymph nodes and/or organs, the disorder usually is called lymphoma. Occasionally, lymphomas may develop into leukemia; for example, a diffuse well differentiated lymphocytic lymphoma may in time involve the blood and thus be indistinguishable from chronic lymphocytic leukemia. Lymphocytic leukemias and lymphomas arise from cells of a common lineage.

Our understanding of the lymphoproliferative disorders has been greatly enhanced by the detection of lymphocyte markers. These assays have been helpful in the diagnosis of the lymphoproliferative disorders and, increasingly, in their treatment.

IMMUNOLOGIC CELL MARKERS

During the past decade, there has been a great increase in the knowledge of lymphocyte subpopulations, lymphocyte interaction, and lymphocyte differentiation. A partial list of cell marker assays for lymphocytic membrane receptors, surface antigens, and enzymes is given in Table 30–9.

Thymic dependent lymphocytes (T cells) are characterized by their ability to form spontaneous rosettes with sheep erythrocytes (ER) and by distinct T cell antigens. B lymphocytes can be determined by the presence of surface membrane immunoglobulin and B cell specific antigens. In addition, a population of B cells in the early to mid stages of differentiation form spontaneous rosettes with mouse erythrocytes. Monocytes adhere to plastic dishes, phagocytize microorganisms and inert substances, and stain diffusely for nonspecific esterases. A fourth population (null cell group) is characterized by an absence of mononuclear cell markers but, nevertheless, is rich in granulocyte colony forming cells. Ia antigens, receptors for the Fc portion of immunoglobulin, and receptors for complement are present in subpopulations of B cells and T cells, but are predominantly associated with peripheral blood B cells.

Several monoclonal antibodies define various stages of the differentiation of T cells (Table 30–10) and B cells. B_1 monoclonal antibody defines mature and immature B cells excluding plasma cells, and B_2 antibody defines a cell in the early to mid-stages of B cell differentiation (Fig. 30–2). Many of these monoclonal antibodies are commercially available and permit the detection of lymphocyte antigens by way of direct or indirect fluorescence microscopy. These assays are reproducible and relatively easy to perform. An excellent review of monoclonal antibodies and their use in human leukemias and lymphomas is that of Nadler (1981).

ACUTE LYMPHOID LEUKEMIA (ALL)

Clinical Features. This disorder occurs primarily in children between two and ten years of age. However, a second peak in the frequency of ALL occurs in middle-aged and elderly adults. Individuals with this disorder often present with symptoms of fatigue, fever, and bleeding. Generalized lymphadenopathy, splenomegaly, and hepatomegaly are common findings. Since the leukemic cells infiltrate many tissues of the body, other symptoms may occur. Leg pain can be associated with periosteal infiltrates; and headaches, nausea, and vomiting with meningeal leukemia. The

Table 30–9. CLASSIFICATION OF LYMPHOCYTE SUBSETS*

Lymphocyte Subsets	E Rosettes†	HuThy Antigen‡	"Ia-like" Antigen	SMIg§	CIg¶	TdT**
Prelymphocyte	−	−	+	−	−	+
Thymocyte	+	+	−	−	−	+
T lymphocyte	+	+	−	−	−	−
Pre-B cell	−	−	+	−	+	±
B lymphocyte	−	−	+	+	−	−
Plasma cell	−	−	−	−	+	−

*From Kurec, A. S., and Davey, F. R.: Hum. Path., *12*:867, 1981.
†Rosette forming cells with sheep erythrocytes.
‡Human thymus antigen.
§Surface membrane immunoglobulin.
¶Cytoplasmic immunoglobulin.
**Terminal deoxynucleotidyl transferase.

Table 30–10. CELL SURFACE ANTIGENS EXPRESSED ON T CELL–DERIVED HUMAN LEUKEMIAS AND LYMPHOMAS*

T Cell Differentiation	T Cell Antigens By Stage	T Cell Malignancies
Stage I—prothymocyte	T9, T10 or T10	Majority of T-ALL
Stage II—thymocyte	T6, T4, T5/8, T10	Majority of T-LL
Stage III—thymocyte	T4, T5/8, T10, T1, T3	Minority of T-LL Rare T-ALL
Mature T—inducer	T1, T3, T4	All Sézary and mycosis fungoides; majority of T-CLL
Mature T—cytotoxic supressor	T1, T3, T5/8	Rare T-CLL

*From Nadler, L. M., Ritz, J., Griffin, J. D., Todd, R. F., III, Reinherz, E. L., and Schlossman, S. F.: Diagnosis and treatment of human leukemias and lymphomas utilizing monoclonal antibodies. *In* Progress in Hematology, *12*:187–225, 1981, E. B. Brown (ed.). New York, Grune & Stratton. By permission.

ALL = acute lymphoblastic leukemia; LL = lymphoblastic lymphoma; CLL = chronic lymphocytic leukemia.

rapid onset of unconsciousness usually indicates subarachnoid hemorrhage.

Blood. Anemia is present if clinical manifestations are fully developed. It is usually normocytic. Frequently, nucleated red cells are present. Thrombocytopenia of moderate to marked degree is the rule. The leukocyte count is occasionally very high (over 100 $\times$ 10^9/L), often is slightly elevated, but is perhaps most frequently normal or decreased. The predominant cell is the lymphoblast or immature lymphocyte (Plate 30–2*H*). Pancytopenia is a common finding in acute leukemia.

Marrow. By the time the patient is symptomatic, the hematopoietic cells and fat are usually replaced by diffuse infiltration of lymphoblasts.

In the L1 type according to the FAB classification (Table 30–11), the lymphoblast has a high nuclear-cytoplasmic ratio. The nuclei are regular and not indented or twisted. The chromatin pattern is fine and uniform. Usually only one or two nucleoli are present. The cytoplasm is scanty in amount, pale blue, and homogeneous, usually without granules (Plate 30–1*L*, 30–3*G*, and 30–4*J*). The L1 type is homogeneous in these characteristics and is the type

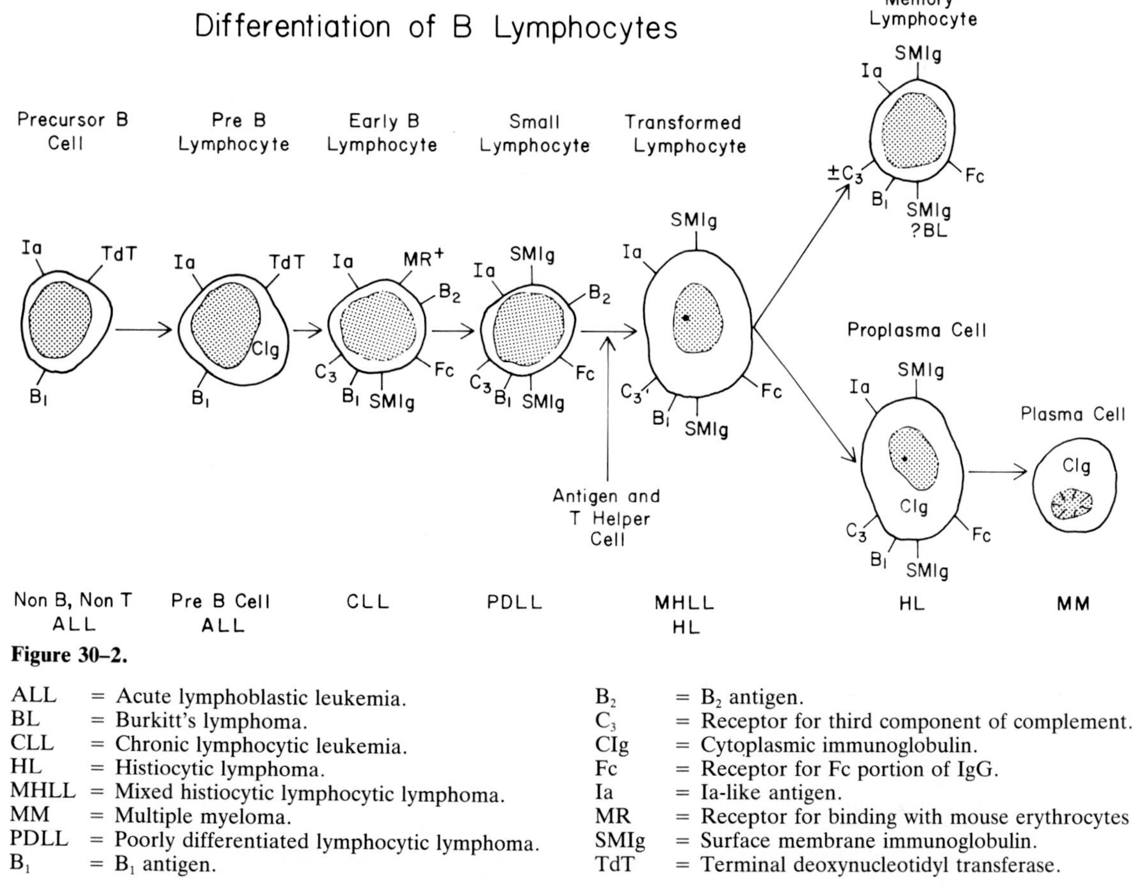

Figure 30–2.

ALL = Acute lymphoblastic leukemia.
BL = Burkitt's lymphoma.
CLL = Chronic lymphocytic leukemia.
HL = Histiocytic lymphoma.
MHLL = Mixed histiocytic lymphocytic lymphoma.
MM = Multiple myeloma.
PDLL = Poorly differentiated lymphocytic lymphoma.
B_1 = B_1 antigen.
B_2 = B_2 antigen.
C_3 = Receptor for third component of complement.
CIg = Cytoplasmic immunoglobulin.
Fc = Receptor for Fc portion of IgG.
Ia = Ia-like antigen.
MR = Receptor for binding with mouse erythrocytes
SMIg = Surface membrane immunoglobulin.
TdT = Terminal deoxynucleotidyl transferase.

Table 30–11. FRENCH-AMERICAN-BRITISH (FAB) CLASSIFICATION OF THE ACUTE LYMPHOBLASTIC LEUKEMIAS (L)*

Cytology	L1	L2	L3
Size	Small	Large	Large and homogeneous
Chromatin	Homogeneous	Variable	Finely stippled
Shape	Regular	Irregular	Oval to round
Nucleoli	Rare	Present	1–3
Cytoplasm	Scanty	Moderate	Moderate
Basophilia	Moderate	Variable	Intense

*From Bennett, J. M., et al.: Br. J. Haematol., *33*:451, 1976. Blackwell Scientific Publications, Ltd., Oxford.

of leukemia that is common in children. In L2 a larger cell type prevails (Plate 30–2*H*) and 30–4*K*) and usually there is more variation in cytologic features within and between cases. It is less common in children and is the usual adult type of ALL. L3 represents the Burkitt type of ALL (see Plate 30–4*L* and 30–5*H*). The cells are large and uniform; they have a round or oval nucleus with prominent nucleoli and deeply basophilic cytoplasm which usually contains vacuoles.

The precision of the diagnosis of the L1 and L2 variants has been improved by employing a scoring system (Bennett, 1981; Table 30–12). In this system, the nuclear to cytoplasmic ratio, number and prominence of nucleoli, nuclear shape, and cell size are the features which distinguish between L1 and L2 variants.

Table 30–12. FAB SCORING SYSTEM FOR L1 AND L2 VARIANTS*

Criteria†	Score
High N/C ratio ≥ 75% of cells	+
Low N/C ratio ≥ 25% of cells	–
Nucleoli: 0–1 (small) ≥ 75% of cells	+
Nucleoli: 1 or more (prominent) ≥ 25% of cells	–
Irregular nuclear membrane ≥ 25% of cells	–
Large cells > 50% of cells	–

*From Bennett, J. M., et al.: Br. J. Haematol., *47*:553, 1981. Blackwell Scientific Publications, Ltd., Oxford.

†Criteria which are not met (or intermediate results) result in no score. The possible total score for a case ranges from −4 to +2. A score of 0 to +2 results in a diagnosis of L1 and a score of −1 to −4 in a diagnosis of L2.

Approximately 71 per cent of cases of childhood ALL are L1, 27 per cent L2, and 2 per cent L3 variants. In adult patients with ALL, however, L2 is the most commonly observed cytologic variant. In addition, it appears that more children with the L1 variant remain in hematologic remission at one year than children with L2 morphology (Viana, 1980). The prognostic significance of the FAB classification in adults is not yet clear, but more patients with L1 morphology may obtain a complete remission than patients with the L2 variant.

Cytochemistry (Table 30–6). The blasts are negative for Sudan black B, peroxidase, and naphthol AS-D chloroacetate esterase. The diagnosis of ALL cannot be made with certainty until the Sudan black B or peroxidase reaction has been performed to show that the blasts are negative. In a few cases of L2, azurophilic granules may be present, but they are Sudan black B and peroxidase negative. The acid phosphatase reaction is moderately or strongly positive in the blasts in about 20 per cent of cases of ALL. Most of these appear to be T cell leukemias (Catovsky, 1978). The PAS stain usually shows coarse blocks of material in at least some lymphoblasts (Plate 30–3*H*).

Immunologic Cell Markers. ALL can be divided into five subtypes, depending on the reaction of blasts with lymphocyte cell marker assays (Table 30–13). T

Table 30–13. CLASSIFICATION OF ACUTE LYMPHOBLASTIC LEUKEMIA

Subtypes of Acute Lymphoblastic Leukemia	E Rosettes*	HuThy† Antigen OKT 10 Antigen‡	C-ALL§ Antigen	Ia-Like Antigen	SMIg¶	CIg**	TdT††	Approximate Per Cent of Population
T cell	+	+	–	–	–	–	+	10–20
Common cell	–	–	+	+	–	–	+	60–70
Null cell	–	–	–	+	–	–	+	3–6
Pre-B cell	–	–	–	+	–	+	±	13–17
B cell	–	–	–	+	+	–	–	2–4

*Rosette forming cell with sheep erythrocytes.
†Human thymus antigen.
‡Human thymus antigen of the OKT series.
§Common ALL antigen.
¶Surface membrane immunoglobulin.
**Cytoplasmic immunoglobulin.
††Terminal deoxynucleotidyl transferase.

cell leukemias, which account for 10 to 20 per cent of cases of ALL, occur predominantly in boys who tend to be slightly older than children with the common ALL (see below). T cell ALL usually has a high leukocyte count and a widening of the mediastinum by X-ray. The prognosis in T cell ALL is usually worse than in the common ALL.

The most frequent form of ALL in children is the common ALL. The diagnosis can be made with certainty only when antisera specific for the common ALL antigen react with the patient's blasts. The diagnosis of pre–B cell ALL rests upon the demonstration of IgM within the cytoplasm of the blasts. Patients with common ALL and pre–B cell ALL have similar laboratory and clinical features (Vogler, 1981) as well as a relatively good prognosis.

In the B cell type of ALL, lymphoblasts have surface immunoglobulin restricted to one light chain and usually correspond to the L3 variant of the FAB classification. In contrast, the other immunologic subtypes of ALL show no distinctive correlation with the FAB classification. The B cell type is the rarest subgroup of ALL and has a poor prognosis. It may represent a more advanced phase of non-African Burkitt's lymphoma.

Terminal Deoxynucleotidyl Transferase. Terminal deoxynucleotidyl transferase (TdT) is an intracellular DNA polymerase that is present in immature cells of the T and B cell series. A small percentage of pre-B cells and 60 to 85 per cent of thymocytes are positive for this enzyme. In contrast, peripheral blood T cells and mature B cells lack TdT activity.

The most commonly used method for measuring TdT is the immunofluorescence assay which employs a specific antibody, prepared in rabbits, against purified TdT from calf thymus. Since the primary antibody cross-reacts with human TdT, the enzyme can be detected by incubating the cell preparation with fluorescein isothiocyanate conjugated goat anti-rabbit IgG. This method is easy to perform and gives reliable results (Stass, 1979).

The TdT assay has utility in the diagnosis of acute lymphoid leukemia, lymphoblastic lymphoma, and blastic crisis of CML. Lymphoblasts in over 90 per cent of cases of ALL are positive for TdT, whereas blasts from less than 5 per cent of acute non-lymphocytic leukemia contain TdT. In over 90 per cent of lymphoblastic lymphomas, neoplastic cells contain TdT activity. In contrast, the other non-Hodgkin's lymphomas are negative for TdT. In some cases of CML in blast crisis, the blasts are positive for TdT. Many of these patients often respond to drugs considered successful in treating ALL.

Prognostic Factors. Good prognostic factors in patients with ALL are usually identified as female gender, less than eight years of age, leukocyte counts of less than 100 × 10⁹/L, L1 FAB morphology, and common ALL and pre-B cell subtypes. Only the first four factors have been shown to be independent prognostic characteristics.

CHRONIC LYMPHOCYTIC LEUKEMIA (CLL)

Clinical Features. CLL is rare under the age of 40; most cases occur over the age of 60. It is more than twice as common in men as in women. The onset is insidious and the disease is commonly discovered by chance during the investigation of another problem. Lymphadenopathy, asymptomatic or associated with symptoms such as weakness, fatigue, anorexia, and weight loss, may cause the patient to come to the physician. Enlarged lymph nodes are usually evident, and frequently hepatosplenomegaly is also found (Table 30–14).

Blood. The leukocyte count is usually between 30 and 200 × 10^9/L, and 80 to 90 per cent of these are small lymphocytes which are monotonously similar in appearance and usually look normal. Nuclear chromatin may be coarsely condensed and more sharply separated by parachromatin than in normal lymphocytes or, in some cases, the chromatin is less condensed than normal. Sometimes nucleoli are evident in many

Table 30–14. COMPARISON OF CHRONIC LYMPHOCYTIC LEUKEMIA (CLL), PROLYMPHOCYTIC LEUKEMIA (PL), LYMPHOSARCOMA CELL LEUKEMIA (LSL), AND HAIRY CELL LEUKEMIA (HCL)*

	CLL	PL	LSL	HCL
Mean age	55	65	60	50
Male/female	2:1	6.5:1	2.5:1	4:1
Initial mean lymphocytic count (× 10^9/L)	90	350	40	Usually pancytopenia
Lymphadenopathy	Moderate	Mild	Moderate	Mild
Splenomegaly	Moderate	Frequently massive	Moderate	Frequently massive
Hepatomegaly	Moderate	Moderate to massive	Moderate	Mild
Morphology of neoplastic cell	Small lymphocyte (T cell variant clover leaf nuclei)	Prolymphocyte	Small cleaved	Hairy cell
Lineage of neoplastic cells	≃ 95% B cell ≃ 5% T cell	≃ 95% B cell ≃ 5% T cell	Virtually all B cell	Virtually all B cell
Response to therapy	Good	Poor	Fair	Good
Mean survival (years)	6–7	1	4–5	5–6

*Adapted from Galton, D. A. G., Goldman, J. M., Wiltshaw, E., Catovsky, D., Henry K., and Goldenberg, G. J.: Br. J. Haematol., *27*:7, 1974. Oxford, Blackwell Scientific Publications.

of the lymphocytes. Size variation is minimal. Cytoplasm is of small to moderate amount. In a minority of patients a small proportion of the lymphocytes is immature. Usually these are prolymphocytes or reticular lymphocytes (transformed lymphocytes).

Often there is neither anemia nor thrombocytopenia at the time of diagnosis. Anemia due to impaired production does develop as the marrow is replaced by leukemic cells. In addition, erythrocyte life span in some patients with CLL may be reduced. This is especially true when there is marked splenomegaly. Autoimmune hemolytic anemia develops in about 10 per cent of patients. Thrombocytopenia is often slight and occasionally becomes severe as the disease progresses, so that hemorrhagic manifestations appear. Thrombocytopenia is usually due to hypoproliferation but may also be secondary to an immune process or splenic sequestration.

Marrow. The usual early finding is the presence of slight to moderate lymphocytosis. Since the lymphocytes are morphologically normal, examination of marrow films may be equivocal. Histologic sections of aspirated particles or biopsy material are very helpful. Small to medium-sized areas of lymphocytes are present and have indistinct margins; lymphocytes are infiltrating into adjacent hematopoietic tissue. If an autoimmune hemolytic anemia is present, erythropoiesis becomes prominent. Later in the disease, lymphocytes overrun the marrow, largely replacing hematopoietic tissue.

Differential Diagnosis. Persistent lymphocytosis in excess of $15 \times 10^9/L$ over a period of several weeks or months in an adult over 40 years of age is good evidence for CLL. Marrow examination, especially histologic sections, should confirm this diagnosis. In children lymphocyte counts in excess of $100 \times 10^9/L$, morphologically mimicking CLL, may be found transiently in infectious lymphocytosis or pertussis.

In contrast to CLL with normal-appearing lymphocytes is a somewhat less common variant, *lymphosarcoma cell leukemia* (Plate 30–6G). In the latter the cells have variably condensed chromatin, usually less than in CLL, and oval or notched nuclei (Table 30–14). Deep clefts in the nuclei are characteristic. This type of lymphocytic leukemia is associated with poorly differentiated lymphocytic lymphoma, which is almost always nodular in its histologic pattern. In CLL, on the other hand, the histologic pattern of the involved lymph node is a diffuse, well-differentiated lymphocytic lymphoma.

Prolymphocytic leukemia is another variant of CLL (Galton, 1974). The disorder is characterized by a very marked lymphocytosis (mean $355 \times 10^9/L$), massive splenomegaly, moderate hepatomegaly, and inconspicuous lymphadenopathy. The malignant lymphoid cells have a large vesicular nucleolus, condensed nuclear chromatin, and moderate amount of cytoplasm.

Immunologic Cell Markers. Most cases of CLL, lymphosarcoma cell leukemia, and prolymphocytic leukemia are of B cell lineage. Neoplastic cells from these disorders contain surface-bound immunoglobulin usually restricted to IgM and to a single light chain, supporting the clonal origin of the leukemic cells. However, lymphosarcoma cells and prolymphocytic leukemia cells have greater concentrations of membrane-bound immunoglobulin than cells from patients with CLL.

In virtually all cases of B cell CLL, 25 to 90 per cent of neoplastic cells form spontaneous rosettes with mouse erythrocytes. In approximately 40 per cent of cases of hairy cell leukemia, neoplastic cells will also form rosettes with mouse erythrocytes. However, leukemic cells from other B cell malignancies rarely form rosettes with mouse erythrocytes. Since CLL cells may express only small concentrations of membrane-bound immunoglobulin, the mouse rosette assay may be helpful in confirming the diagnosis of CLL (Catovsky, 1981).

Immunologic phenotyping of neoplastic cells from patients with CLL and prolymphocytic leukemia has also indicated that a small percentage of cases are derived from T cells. The predominant cells in T cell CLL often contain a cloverleaf-shaped nucleus with clumped chromatin (Uchiyama, 1977). Skin involvement occurs in 60 per cent of these cases. A human T cell leukemia virus (HTLV) has been associated with T cell CLL and other cutaneous T cell lymphomas (Poiesz, 1980).

Course. A staging classification of cases of CLL has been offered by an international workshop (Binet, 1981). The prognosis of patients with CLL correlated with the size of the total body lymphocyte pool and presence of anemia or thrombocytopenia. The median survival for B cell CLL is about six years, whereas it is one year for T cell CLL.

Prolymphocytic leukemia is usually less responsive to treatment than CLL in general, and has a poorer prognosis.

HAIRY CELL LEUKEMIA (HCL, LEUKEMIC RETICULOENDOTHELIOSIS)

Bouroncle (1958) described this rare disorder which is clinically variable in its manifestations. It occurs more frequently in males than in females. The mean age of afflicted patients is 50 years. It has an insidious onset and is characterized by proliferation of the abnormal cells in the reticuloendothelial organs and blood. Splenomegaly is the predominant physical finding (Table 30–14).

Pancytopenia or depression of only two cell lines is the usual finding, with variable numbers of hairy cells. In the majority of cases bone marrow aspiration is difficult. Marrow biopsy shows a marrow that varies in cellularity, often having both hypocellular and hypercellular areas and reticulin fibrosis. Hairy cells are considerably increased in number.

Morphologically the cells are medium sized (10 to 20 μm diameter), with round to oval nuclei, though many are notched or dumbbell shaped. The chromatin pattern is usually uniformly reticular, and nucleoli are small and inconspicuous. In some cells chromatin is more condensed, resembling that of a lymphocyte. The cytoplasm is moderate in amount, often has

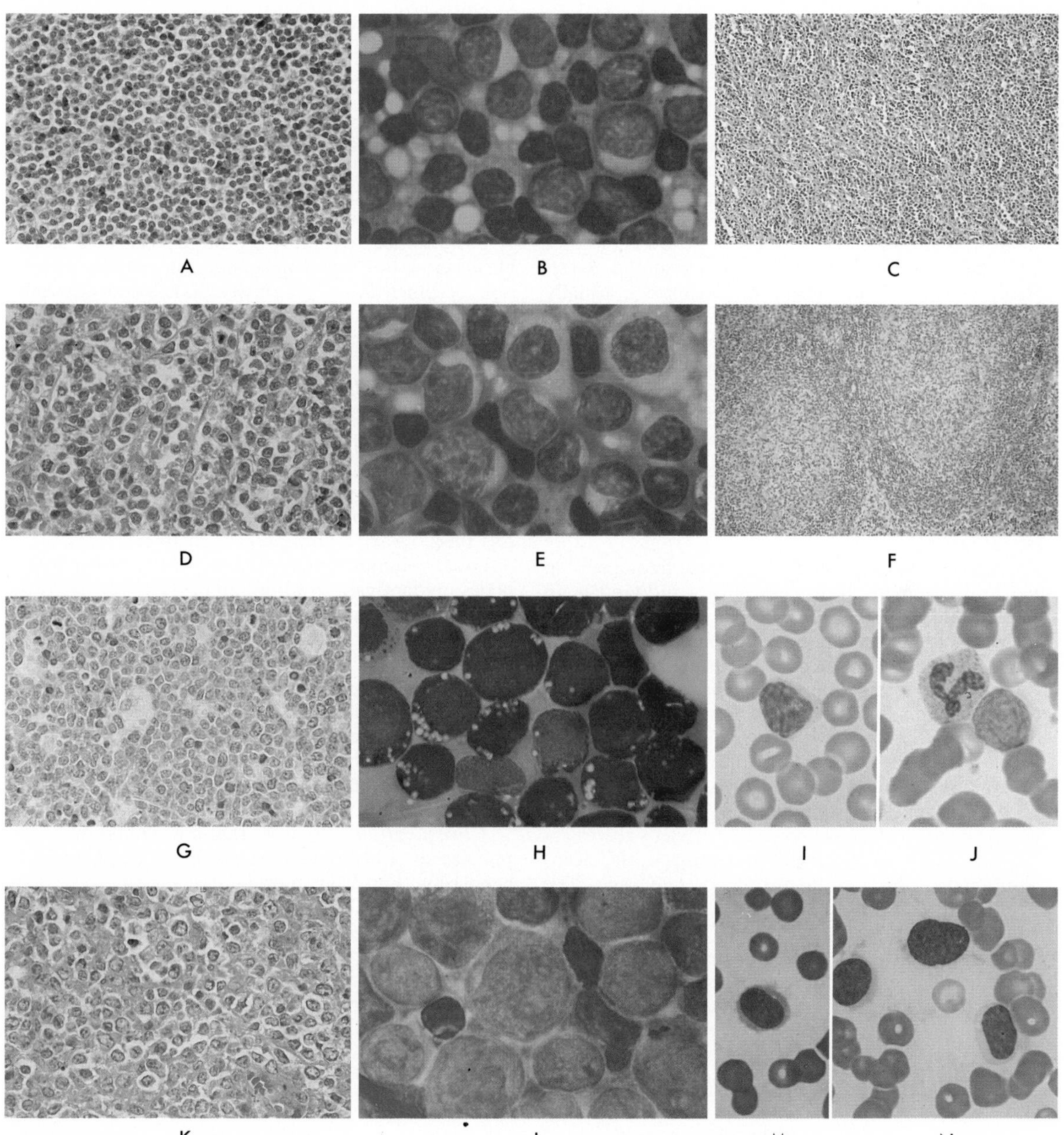

Plate 30–5. *A,* Well-differentiated lymphocytic lymphoma. The lymph node is infiltrated by small lymphocytes. Hematoxylin and eosin (H & E), × 400. *B,* Touch preparation of well-differentiated lymphocytic lymphoma. The majority of lymphocytes are small lymphocytes; however, occasional stimulated lymphocytes are present. Wright-Giemsa, ×900. *C,* Non-Hodgkin's lymphoma with diffuse pattern. Compare with *F.* H & E, ×100. *D,* Poorly differentiated lymphocytic lymphoma. Note the presence of lymphoid cells with angulated and clefted nuclei, occasional nucleoli, and scant cytoplasm. Mitotic figures are more frequent than in *A.* H & E, ×400. *E,* Touch preparation of poorly differentiated lymphocytic lymphoma. The majority of cells are stimulated lymphocytes with occasional mature lymphocytes. Wright-Giemsa, ×900. *F,* Non-Hodgkin's lymphoma with follicular pattern. Compare with *C.* H & E, ×100. *G,* Burkitt's lymphoma. Large primitive lymphoid cells are positioned around tissue macrophages (H & E, ×400). *H,* Touch preparation of Burkitt's lymphoma. Neoplastic cells contain fine reticular chromatin. Cytoplasm is intensely basophilic and frequently contains multiple vacuoles. Wright-Giemsa, ×900. *I, J,* Sézary cells, blood film, from a patient with mycosis fungoides. Wright-Giemsa stain, ×400. These are mononuclear cells with scanty cytoplasm and a deeply indented or convuluted nucleus. The cell on the left has more chromatin condensation than the cell adjacent to the neutrophil on the right. *K,* Histiocytic lymphoma. Large lymphoid cells with prominent nuclei, thickened nuclear membrane, conspicuous nucleoli, and more abundant cytoplasm. H & E, ×400. *L,* Touch preparation of histiocytic lymphoma. Neoplastic cells are large, measuring approximately 20 μm in diameter. The nuclear chromatin is fine and reticular; nucleoli are prominent. Wright-Giemsa, ×900. *M, N,* Leukemic reticuloendotheliosis (hairy cell leukemia), blood film, Wright-Giemsa stain, ×400. The two left-most cells are "hairy cells." They have less condensed but more intensely staining chromatin and more irregular cytoplasmic margins than normal lymphocytes (cell at farthest right).

numerous hair-like projections and frayed borders, and stains gray with Wright's stain (Plate 30–5*M* and *N*).

Cytochemically these cells contain acid phosphatase, which is resistant to inhibition by tartrate; this is in contrast to the isozymes of acid phosphatase present in other hemic cells (Yam, 1971a). The cells are usually subtypes of B lymphocytes, since in some cases the cells appear to synthesize surface immunoglobulin (Catovsky, 1977). However, other studies show that the cells have both phagocytic and B cell properties (Fu, 1974). The clinical course is usually chronic, but may be acute or subacute. The median survival is between five and six years. Splenectomy appears to be of significant benefit to many patients.

MYCOSIS FUNGOIDES AND SÉZARY'S SYNDROME

Mycosis fungoides is a lymphoreticular neoplasm primarily involving the skin. As the disorder evolves, neoplastic cells infiltrate the lymph nodes and other visceral organs.

Mycosis fungoides occurs twice as frequently in men as in women. It usually affects individuals in their middle to late years.

The disorder first appears as an eczematoid, psoriaform, or nonspecific exfoliative dermatitis. The lesions tend to form plaques and then tumors which often ulcerate. Some patients develop generalized erythroderma.

Biopsies of the skin reveal lymphocytic and mononuclear cell infiltrates in the dermis. Neoplastic cells and normal-appearing lymphocytes infiltrate the epidermis and form clusters known as Pautrier's abscesses. This is usually accompanied by parakeratosis, acanthosis, spongiosis, and elongation of rete pegs. The nuclei of the neoplastic cells frequently have a cerebriform appearance.

In advanced stages of the disease, neoplastic cells infiltrate the lymph nodes, liver, spleen, and other organs (Rappaport, 1974).

Occasionally atypical mononuclear cells with cerebriform nuclei are present in the peripheral blood (Plate 30–5*I* and *J*). In addition, when lymphocytosis exists (especially in the erythremic patient) the disorder is called *Sézary's syndrome.* Neoplastic cells from patients with mycosis fungoides and Sézary's syndrome appear to be T lymphocytes (Flandrin, 1974); in approximately 50 per cent of cases the cells demonstrate helper activity (Table 30–10).

The disorder may follow a prolonged chronic course. However, following lymph node infiltration, the disease becomes more progressive, and death, usually due to infection, occurs within two years (Van Scott, 1977).

MALIGNANT LYMPHOMA

Malignant lymphoma is a neoplastic proliferation of one of the cell types of the lymphopoietic-reticular tissue. If a mixture of more than one cell type appears to be present, it probably represents a variation in the size, configuration, or degree of differentiation of one cell type, rather than separate cell lines.

Usually lymphoma begins in and involves lymph nodes predominantly, although other sites such as the spleen and the gastrointestinal tract are frequent areas of origin as well. As the disease progresses, proliferation spreads to lymphoid tissue beyond the site of origin. In advanced disease, infiltrations of neoplastic cells are found in many organs throughout the body. When lymphoma originates in extranodal tissue, e.g., the stomach or lung, the course is likely to be more benign than otherwise.

Non-Hodgkin's Lymphomas

Classification. Because the non-Hodgkin's lymphomas are a heterogeneous group of lymphoreticular neoplasms, numerous morphologic classifications have been presented. The classification of Rappaport (1966) has gained wide use in the United States (Table 30–15). Studies have shown that this classification gives a good correlation between histopathology and clinical presentation, survival, and response to therapy. It is

Table 30–15. REVISED RAPPAPORT CLASSIFICATION FOR NON-HODGKIN'S LYMPHOMA*

Histiocytic Subgroups	Relative Incidence (%)	Five Year Survival (%)
Nodular pattern		
Lymphocytic, well differentiated	1–2	75
Lymphocytic, poorly differentiated	15–20	70
Mixed lymphocytic-histiocytic	15–20	50
Histiocytic	4–7	70
Diffuse pattern		
Lymphocytic, well differentiated (with or without plasmacytoid features)	2–3	65
Lymphocytic, poorly differentiated (with or without plasmacytoid features)	8–15	40
Mixed lymphocytic-histiocytic	8–12	35
Histiocytic (with or without sclerosis)	28–35	40
Undifferentiated	1–2	<10
Burkitt's tumor	1–2	<5
Lymphoblastic (with or without convoluted cells)	2–3	30
Unclassified		

*From Golomb, H., Gams, R., Hoppe, R.: Hematology, 1981. Education Program, American Society of Hematology.

now recognized, however, that the large cells, designated "histiocytes" in the Rappaport classification, in most instances are actually of lymphocytic origin, and that true histiocytic lymphomas are rare. Because of the problems with the terminology, other classifications have been proposed and demonstrated to be clinically relevant. These newer classifications have led to revisions of the Rappaport classification which include newly described clinicopathologic entities. Multiple classifications have resulted in confusion and controversy regarding the appropriate terminology for the non-Hodgkin's lymphomas. As a result, the National Cancer Institute initiated a multi-institutional study including a panel of expert hematopathologists to review over 1000 cases of non-Hodgkin's lymphomas. This study resulted in a classification known as the "Working Formulation of Non-Hodgkin's Lymphoma for Clinical Usage" (Non-Hodgkin's Lymphoma Pathologic Classification Project, 1982). The formulation is proposed not as a new classification but as a means of translation among the various systems and to facilitate clinical comparisons of therapeutic trials. Accordingly, we use the Working Formulation in conjunction with the revised Rappaport classification.

The Rappaport classification first divides the non-Hodgkin's lymphomas into two major categories, nodular and diffuse. In the former, neoplastic cells are arranged throughout the lymph node in a nodular pattern (Plate 30–5*F*). The normal architecture of the lymph node (including normal germinal centers) is lost in the proliferation, neoplastic cells infiltrate the capsule, and there is cellular atypia. In the diffuse lymphomas, no nodularity is apparent in the specimen. Instead, the involved lymph node is composed of neoplastic lymphoid cells infiltrating the tissue in an even distribution (Plate 30–5*C*). The second requirement of the Rappaport classification is proper identification of the neoplastic cells according to cytologic types (Table 30–15).

The Working Formulation confirms the significance of differentiating the nodular from the diffuse pattern. However, it replaces the term "nodular" with "follicular." Independent of cell type, the follicular pattern has a more favorable survival.

Working Formulation of Non-Hodgkin's Lymphomas

Low Grade Malignancy

Malignant Lymphoma, Small Lymphocytic (SL) (Rappaport; Lymphocytic Well Differentiated) (Plate 30–5*A* to *C*). The cell type is the small lymphocyte, with clumped chromatin indistinguishable from the normal lymphocyte. Mitoses are rarely seen. The pattern of node and marrow involvement is characteristically diffuse. Though it may begin in lymph nodes, the accumulative process involves the bone marrow quite early in its course, and the blood lymphocyte count is then elevated. The usual diagnosis, therefore, is chronic lymphatic leukemia rather than well differentiated lymphocytic lymphoma. It is essentially the same disease.

Plasmacytoid lymphocytes may be prominent in patients with gammopathies, although plasma cells may be numerous without evidence of a paraproteinemia.

Malignant Lymphoma, Follicular, Predominantly Small Cleaved Cell (FSC) (Rappaport; Nodular, Poorly Differentiated Lymphocytic) (Plate 30–5*D* to *F*). There is predominantly a follicular pattern. The proliferating cell is a lymphocyte with a nucleus which has less condensation of chromatin than the normal circulating lymphocyte; an irregular, cleft, or indented nuclear shape; and small, inconspicuous nucleoli. The cytoplasm is scant in amount.

Malignant Lymphoma, Follicular, Mixed Small Cleaved and Large Cell (FM) (Rappaport; Nodular, Mixed Lymphocytic-Histiocytic). The pattern is follicular and the lymphoma is composed of an equal portion of large and small cleaved lymphocytes. Large non-cleaved cells are present and contain prominent nucleoli.

Intermediate Grade Malignancy

Malignant Lymphoma, Follicular, Predominantly Large Cell (FL) (Rappaport; Nodular Histiocytic) (Plate 30–5*K* and *L*). Large cleaved and non-cleaved cells are observed in a follicular pattern. The large cleaved cells are usually more numerous. Many mitotic figures are present within the tumor.

Malignant Lymphoma, Diffuse Small Cleaved Cell (DSC) (Rappaport; Diffuse Lymphocytic, Poorly Differentiated). This tumor is composed of small lymphocytes with scanty cytoplasm. The nuclear membrane is irregular, angulated, and often cleaved. There is no evidence of a nodular pattern. A small number of large cleaved cells may be present.

Malignant Lymphoma, Diffuse, Mixed Small and Large Cell (DM) (Rappaport; Diffuse Mixed Lymphocytic-Histiocytic). Some of these lymphomas represent the diffuse counterpart of follicular mixed lymphomas. However, some may be composed of lymphocytes containing irregular and lobated nuclei and represent a T cell neoplasm.

Malignant Lymphoma, Diffuse, Large Cell (DL) (Rappaport; Diffuse Histiocytic). (Plate 30–5*K* and *L*). The tumor is composed predominantly of large cleaved and non-cleaved cells. The nucleus has reticular chromatin and a large prominent nucleolus. The cytoplasm is moderately abundant. Small lymphocytes are occasionally present. There is no evidence of a follicular pattern.

High Grade Malignancy

Malignant Lymphoma, Large Cell, Immunoblastic (IBL) (Rappaport; Diffuse Histiocytic). This lymphoma is composed of large cells with oval vesicular nuclei and one or more prominent nucleoli. In some cases the nuclei appear to be eccentrically placed with abundant cytoplasm suggesting plasmacytic differentiation. In other cases, the nuclei are placed centrally and the cytoplasm has a clear appearance. A third variant is more polymorphous and contains a mixture of small lymphocytes with twisted nuclei and larger lymphocytes with clear cytoplasm. These large cells may have hyperlobated nuclei simulating Reed-Sternberg cells.

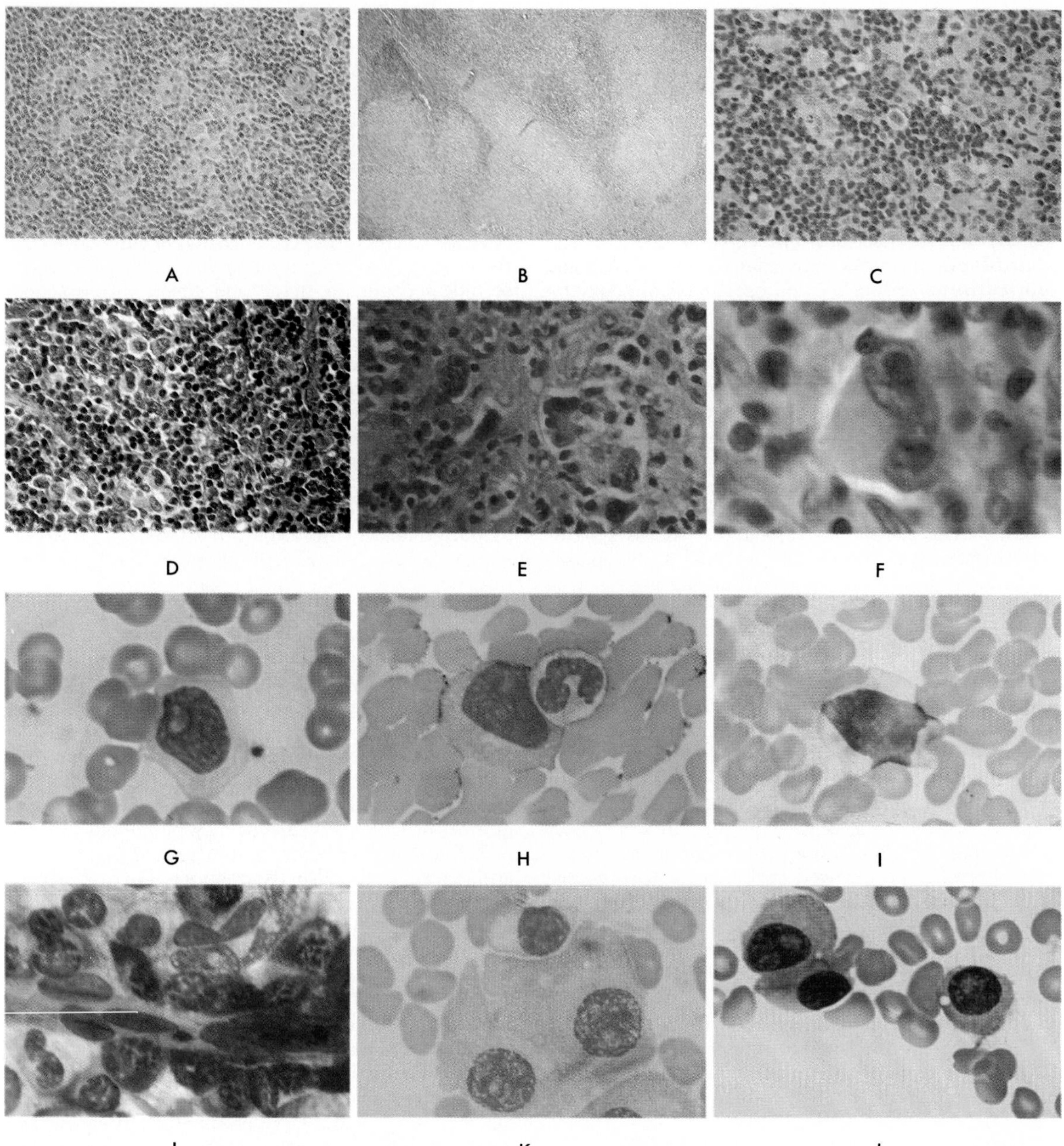

Plate 30–6. *A*, Hodgkin's disease, lymphocyte predominance type. The mature lymphocyte is the most common cell. Histiocytes are frequently present. Reed-Sternberg cells are rare. Eosinophils and plasma cells are infrequent. Hematoxylin and eosin (H & E), ×250. *B*, Hodgkin's disease, nodular sclerosis type. Broad bands of collagen course through the lymph node, forming nodules of lymphoid tissue. H & E, ×100. *C*, Hodgkin's disease, nodular sclerosis type. Note presence of "lacunar" Reed-Sternberg cells with multinuclei and pale cytoplasm. H & E, ×400. *D*, Hodgkin's disease, mixed type. There are numerous Reed-Sternberg cells and histiocytes. Eosinophils and plasma cells are characteristically present. H & E, ×400. *E*, Hodgkin's disease, lymphocyte depletion type. There are several multinucleated Reed-Sternberg cells and many abnormal mononuclear cells. Lymphocytes are less prominent. There is a background of proteinaceous material and disorderly fibrosis. H & E ×400. *F*, Reed-Sternberg cell, in Hodgkin's disease, mixed type. *G*, Poorly differentiated lymphocytic lymphoma, leukemic phase. Blasts, such as this cell, and cells with more chromatin condensation and notched nuclei (as in Plate 30–5E) are found in the blood in a minority of patients with PDLL, usually late in the disease. *H*, Lymphocytic reaction. This reticular lymphocyte in the blood of a patient with a viral infection resembles the malignant blast in *G*. This type of reactive blast form ("non-leukemic lymphoblast") usually has more deeply basophilic cytoplasm and is associated with numerous characteristic atypical lymphocytes, as in *I*. *I*, Atypical lymphocyte, blood film. *J*, Plasma cells adjacent to the endothelial cells lining a blood vessel in bone marrow film from a patient with rheumatoid arthritis. In mature plasma cells the nuclear chromatin is coarsely clumped and the cytoplasm is deeply basophilic. *K*, Multiple myeloma, bone marrow film. The abnormal plasma cells have abundant cytoplasm and eccentric nuclei. In contrast to normal plasma cells, however, the cytoplasm is less deeply basophilic, the chromatin is not coarsely clumped, and nucleoli are prominent. *L*, Multiple myeloma, bone marrow film. The dissociation between advanced cytoplasmic maturation (abundant, usually basophilic cytoplsm with a prominent Golgi zone) and delayed nuclear maturation (prominent nucleolus, less chromatin condensation) is the most useful feature in distinguishing the abnormal plasma cells in myeloma from normal plasma cells.

Malignant Lymphoma, Lymphoblastic (LBL) (Rappaport; Lymphoblastic Convoluted/Non-convoluted). These tumors typically have a diffuse pattern. The neoplastic cells have scanty cytoplasm. In approximately 50 per cent of the cases, the nuclear contour is convoluted. In the remaining cases the nuclei are round. Mitoses are numerous. On touch preparations the cells simulate lymphoblasts of ALL.

Malignant Lymphoma, Small Non-Cleaved Cell (SNC) (Rappaport; Undifferentiated, Burkitt's and Non-Burkitt's) (Plate 30–5*G* and *H*). The cells are homogeneous with round to oval nuclei, reticular chromatin, small nucleoli, and slight to moderate cytoplasm. The cells grow as a syncytium, macrophages with abundant cytoplasm interspersed among the tumor cells giving a "starry sky" histologic appearance. Touch preparations reveal cells similar to the morphology of L3 ALL.

Miscellaneous. This group includes composite lymphoma, mycosis fungoides, true histiocytic lymphoma, extramedullary plasmacytoma, and otherwise unclassifiable lymphomas.

A summary of the major clinical features of the subtypes of the working formulation of non-Hodgkin's lymphomas can be found in Table 30–16.

Immunologic Classification of Non-Hodgkin's Lymphomas. Utilizing a variety of immunologic techniques, one can categorize a malignant lymphoid proliferation according to cells of origin and level of differentiation (Tables 30–10 and 30–13; Fig. 30–2). It now appears that the lymphoproliferative disorders are neoplastic tumors which are blocked at certain stages of differentiation. Thus most cases of ALL represent proliferation of cells at the earliest stage of B cell differentiation, whereas CLL and poorly differentiated lymphocytic lymphoma are blocked at the early to middle stages of differentiation. Multiple myeloma represents a B cell neoplasm which can fully differentiate.

Hodgkin's Disease. The current classification of Hodgkin's disease is that of the Rye conference (Lukes, 1966). Hodgkin's disease is generally regarded as a malignant lymphoma, but has different histology in that the cells reacting to the neoplasm usually predominate rather than the neoplastic cells themselves. The hallmark of Hodgkin's disease is the Reed-Sternberg cell (Plate 30–6*F*), which is a large binucleated or multinucleated cell with each nucleus bearing a very large nucleolus.

Hodgkin's disease may occur from early childhood to old age. Increased frequency is noted between 15 and 35 years and after age 50. Males predominate, especially in childhood; disease in females under age 30 is usually nodular sclerosis in type.

Classification. Diagnosis is made histologically, usually from a lymph node biopsy (Table 30–17).

The lymphocytic predominance group shows numerous lymphocytes with a variable degree of histiocytic proliferation without necrosis or fibrosis and few Reed-Sternberg cells (Plate 30–6*A*). Prognosis is best in this group, which tends to be localized to the cervical nodes and occurs most frequently in young males.

Nodular sclerosis is characterized by broad bands of collagen separating nodules of lymphoid tissue and the presence of "lacunar cells," which are large atypical histiocytes with abundant pale cytoplasm. Classic Reed-Sternberg cells are difficult to find (Plate 30–6*B* and *C*). This variety of Hodgkin's disease is common and often is first discovered as a mediastinal mass in a young woman.

The *mixed type* has a variety of cell types: lymphocytes, plasma cells, eosinophils, histiocytes, and Reed-

Table 30–16. CLINICAL CHARACTERISTICS OF 1014 PATIENTS IN THE TEN SUBTYPES OF THE WORKING FORMULATION OF NON-HODGKIN'S LYMPHOMAS FOR CLINICAL USAGE*

Prognostic Group	Low Grade			Intermediate Grade				High Grade		
Subtype	SL	FSC	FM	FL	DSC	DM	DL	IBL	LBL	SNC
Per cent	3.6	22.5	7.7	3.8	6.9	6.7	19.7	7.9	4.2	5.0
Age range (years)	26–79	3–87	26–99	16–82	10–91	22–90	10–88	10–81	11–90	3–90
Median	60.5	54.3	56.1	55.4	57.9	58.0	56.8	51.3	16.9	29.8
Sex ratio (M:F)	1.2	1.3	0.8	1.8	2.0	1.1	1.0	1.5	1.9	2.6
Pathologic stage (%)										
I	3	8	15	15	9	19	16	23	7	13
II	8	10	12	12	19	26	30	29	20	21
III	8	16	28	15	12	13	10	16	2	9
IV	81	66	46	58	60	42	44	33	72	57
Bone marrow involved†	71	51	30	34	32	14	10	12	50	14
Survival										
Median (years)	5.8	7.2	5.1	3.0	3.4	2.7	1.5	1.3	2.0	0.7
5-year (%)	59.0	70.0	50.0	45.0	33.0	38.0	35.0	32.0	26.0	23.0
Complete remission (%)	61	73	65	61	56	69	59	53	69	48
Median time to relapse (years)	>5.4	5.0	5.2	>8.0	2.1	4.3	>8.4	3.5	1.1	>7.7

*Non-Hodgkin's lymphoma pathologic classification project. Rosenberg, S. A., Chairman, Writing Committee. From National Cancer Institute–sponsored study of classifications of non-Hodgkin's lymphomas. Summary and description of a working formulation for clinical use. Cancer, *49*:2112, 1982.

†At initial evaluation.

Table 30–17. HISTOLOGIC CLASSIFICATION OF HODGKIN'S DISEASE

Subtype	Major Morphologic Alteration	Percentage of Cases
Lymphocyte predominant	Usually diffuse, sometimes vaguely nodular pattern, abundant lymphocytes, few Reed-Sternberg cells, no fibrosis	7
Nodular sclerosis	Nodular pattern formed by birefringent collagen bands; moderate number of lymphocytes, eosinophils, plasma cells; Lacunar variant of Reed-Sternberg cells	68
Mixed cellularity	Diffuse involvement, numerous Reed-Sternberg cells, moderate number of lymphocytes, eosinophils, plasma cells	23
Lymphocyte depletion	Diffuse involvement, decreased cellularity, occasionally numerous bizarre-shaped Reed-Sternberg cells	2

Sternberg cells, which are often quite numerous. Necrosis and disorderly fibrosis may be present (Plate 30–6*D*).

The rare *lymphocyte depletion* type (Plate 30–6*E*) is more often diffuse fibrosis than reticular. It is sometimes associated with an acute febrile illness accompanied by pancytopenia and lymphocytopenia. There may be a paucity of peripheral lymphadenopathy, though some cases have a generalized enlargement of lymph nodes. The lack of leukocytosis and thrombocytosis and more frequent involvement of the bone marrow contrast with other forms of Hodgkin's disease (Neiman, 1973).

Blood. Normocytic, sometimes severe, anemia is seen in about 50 per cent of cases.

The leukocyte count may be elevated, normal, or reduced. The differential count shows neutrophilia, lymphocytopenia, monocytosis, and eosinophilia. Either all or any combination of these may be present.

Neutrophilic leukocytosis is seen, especially when lymph nodes are involved, and neutropenia, when bone marrow is involved. The blood changes seem to depend on the stage of the disease and on some poorly understood mechanisms. The neutrophil alkaline phosphatase is elevated during activity of the disease; it returns to normal during remissions.

The most frequent finding is a moderate leukocytosis, with white cell counts ranging from 12 to 25 $\times$ 10^9/L and a relative and even absolute lymphopenia. A slight shift to the left may be present in the neutrophils. As a rule, lymphopenia is prognostically a poor omen.

Monocytosis is frequent. Eosinophilia has been described in about 20 per cent of patients and may be extreme. The platelet count may be increased, normal, or decreased, the latter especially with marrow involvement.

Both the histologic changes noted above and the blood and marrow findings appear to be manifestations of different host responses to the disease.

Marrow. Frequently there is a granulocytic hyperplasia with a shift to the left, slight monocytosis, and eosinophilia.

If marrow biopsy is performed in patients with systemic symptoms or with clinical Stage III or Stage IV disease, it will be positive in about 10 per cent of patients (Rosenberg, 1971). Positive biopsy is interpreted as (1) the presence of Reed-Sternberg cells in an appropriate pleomorphic cellular stroma; or, less commonly, (2) abnormal infiltration of lymphocytes, histiocytes, and fibrosis without classic Reed-Sternberg cells, but with abnormal mononuclear cells and documented Hodgkin's disease in other sites.

In the rare lymphocyte depletion type of Hodgkin's disease, dissemination is widespread and bone marrow is involved in most cases.

Clinical Staging. Clinical staging is currently employed to determine the extent of the disease at the time of diagnosis. Besides history and physical examination, extensive radiographic studies, radioisotope scans, CBC, platelet count, erythrocyte sedimentation rate, neutrophil alkaline phosphatase, bone marrow biopsy, liver function studies, urinalysis, and skin tests for delayed hypersensitivity are performed. *Stage I disease* is limited to lymph nodes in one anatomic region or two contiguous regions on one side of the diaphragm. *Stage II disease* involves more than two contiguous regions or two non-contiguous regions on one side of the diaphragm. *Stage III disease* is present on both sides of the diaphragm but is confined to lymphoid tissue. *Stage IV disease* involves bone marrow or any other organ, in addition to lymphoid tissue. All stages are additionally classified as A if systemic symptoms are absent, B if they are present. This extensive diagnostic approach is to define areas of involvement and facilitate radiation therapy, which is combined with chemotherapy. It is part of the current aggressive approach to the management of Hodgkin's disease, which is resulting in longer survival and even apparent cure in some patients.

Immunologic studies in Hodgkin's disease have shown that cell-mediated immunity is defective when extensive disease is present.

Plasma Cell Dyscrasias and Lymphoreticular Malignancies Associated with Abnormal Immunoglobulin Synthesis

Immunoglobulins are discussed in Chapter 36.

Polyclonal gammopathy refers to an increase in the serum of several different immunoglobulins which are the products of many different clones of plasma cells. This is usually a response to antigenic stimulation.

Monoclonal gammopathy refers to an increase in the serum of one specific class, subclass, and type of immunoglobulin molecule (or fragment thereof); this is the product of plasma cells or lymphocytes which originated from a single cell or clone. Monoclonal gammopathy is found in multiple myeloma, some lymphomas (including Waldenström's macroglobulinemia and heavy chain diseases), some patients with primary amyloidosis, a few patients with carcinoma, and some individuals with no known underlying disease *(benign monoclonal gammopathy)*. The latter group may constitute up to one third of all monoclonal gammopathies (Ritzmann, 1972); it includes primarily elderly individuals who have a lower concentration of the homogeneous immunoglobulin (less than 2 g/dl) which does not change for long periods of time.

MULTIPLE MYELOMA

This is a neoplastic proliferation of plasma cells or morphologically abnormal plasma cells (myeloma cells), primarily occurring in the bone marrow either in nodules or diffusely. Though plasma cells also proliferate in lymph nodes and spleen, these organs are rarely enlarged.

Clinical. Multiple myeloma is rare under age 40. The mean age at the time of diagnosis is 62 years. The incidence of this disease is equal in men and women. Bone pain is the most common symptom, and pathologic fractures are frequent. Neurologic symptoms may be prominent from encroachment of tumor which has broken through the bony cortex on spinal nerves or spinal cord. Bone destruction leads to calcium mobilization, with increase of calcium in the serum and metastatic calcification. The growth of myeloma cells in the marrow produces multiple tumors, which appear on x-ray as multiple punched-out osteoporotic lesions; occasionally the growth is diffuse and appears as diffuse osteoporosis. An unusual propensity to infection is common because of impaired production of antibodies.

Blood. There is usually a normochromic normocytic anemia; normoblasts may be present in the blood. The leukocyte count is slightly decreased, normal, or slightly increased. Occasionally young neutrophils or even myeloblasts may be found. The platelet count is usually normal, but may be decreased. The most striking feature of the blood film is the marked degree of rouleau formation, which may make cell counting difficult (see Fig. 27–35).

Marrow. The bone marrow shows the presence of plasma cells or myeloma cells, varying from less than 1 per cent to over 90 per cent, depending upon the degree of involvement in the site of marrow aspirated. Cytologically the cells may be indistinguishable from normal plasma cells, but they usually show abnormalities, such as less clumping of nuclear chromatin, large nucleoli, lack of a perinuclear clear zone, lighter blue cytoplasm, or varying degrees of anaplasia (Plate 30–6*K* and *L*). The dissociation of nuclear and cytoplasmic maturation is a distinctive feature of the myeloma cells (Bernier, 1976).

Immunoglobulins (see also p. 860). Serum globulin is usually increased, often strikingly so. This increase is responsible for the tendency toward rouleau formation and an elevated erythrocyte sedimentation rate (ESR). Serum protein electrophoresis usually shows an M-spot, a homogeneous band in the gamma or beta region; less commonly there is hypogammaglobulinemia (when only light chains are produced by the neoplastic plasma cells). Immunoelectrophoresis indicates that the monoclonal protein is IgG in over half the cases of multiple myeloma, IgA in about one fifth, IgD in less than 1 per cent, and IgE very rarely. In each of these groups of myeloma, some patients secrete Bence Jones protein (light chains, kappa *or* lambda) in addition to the whole immunoglobulin molecule. In about one quarter of patients with multiple myeloma, only light chains (Bence Jones protein) are produced by the abnormal plasma cells. Hypogammaglobulinemia is found in the latter group because light chains are filtered through the renal glomerulus, leaving little or none in the serum, in addition to the fact that immunoglobulin production by the non-malignant plasma cells is greatly reduced in all patients with multiple myeloma.

Roughly 5 per cent of myeloma proteins are cryoglobulins, that is, proteins which precipitate from cooled serum and redissolve on warming.

Proteinuria is frequently present in multiple myeloma. In somewhat over 50 per cent of patients Bence Jones protein is present. This may be detected by its property of precipitating from acidified urine heated to 50°C. and redissolving when the urine is boiled, or by electrophoresis of a concentrate of urine on which it migrates as a narrow band in the gamma globulin region. If renal damage has occurred, albumin and whole immunoglobulin molecules are also found in the urine. Excretion of Bence Jones protein often results in obstruction and elimination of nephrons, and the so-called myeloma kidney. Renal insufficiency is common and is the presenting feature of multiple myeloma in some cases.

Amyloidosis, which is present in about 10 to 15 per cent of cases of multiple myeloma, may be a factor in the renal failure. Amyloid fibrils in cases of myeloma appear to have as the major protein component of their fibrils the light chains of immunoglobulin molecules (Glenner, 1973).

The diagnosis of multiple myeloma is secure if the marrow contains large numbers of morphologically bizarre, malignant-appearing plasma cells. If large numbers of normal-appearing plasma cells and plasma-cell precursors are present in the marrow, the diagnosis is not established unless punched-out, lytic bone lesions are demonstrated by x-ray, or Bence Jones proteinuria or a monoclonal gammopathy is also present.

The prognostic importance of several different laboratory measurements and clinical features has been demonstrated. These clinicopathologic features have been correlated with the total body tumor cell mass and used as a basis for a clinical staging system (Table 30–18) (Durie, 1975; Woodruff, 1979).

Median survival after diagnosis is approximately three years. In almost 5 per cent of patients, acute leukemia develops (usually myelomonocytic) (Rosner, 1974). This may be preceded by sideroblastic anemia (Khaleeli, 1973).

Table 30–18. MYELOMA CLINICAL STAGING SYSTEM*

			Median Survival
Stage I		Low myeloma cell mass (<0.6 × 10^{12} cells/M^2)	
	Criteria:	All of the following Hgb >100 g/L Serum calcium <3.0 mmol/L X-ray: normal bone structure or one lesion only M-component production rates IgG value <50 g/L IgA value <30 g/L Urine light chain excretion <4 g/24 hr	64 mo
Stage II		Intermediate myeloma cell mass (0.6–1.2 × 10^{12} cells/M^2)	
	Criteria:	Fitting neither Stage I nor Stage II	32 mo
Stage III		High myeloma cell mass (>1.2 × 10^{12} cells/M^2)	
	Criteria:	Any of the following Hgb <85 g/L Serum calcium >3.0 mmol/L Advanced lytic bone lesions M-component production rates IgG value >70 g/L IgA value >50 g/L Urine light chain excretion >12 g/24 hr	6 mo
Subclassification		A = Serum creatinine value <20 mg/L B = Serum creatinine value >20 mg/L	

*From Durie, B. G., and Salmon, S. E.: Cancer, *36*:842, 1975.

Plasma Cell Leukemia. Often in multiple myeloma a few plasma cells are found in the peripheral blood. Only in the rare instances of myeloma in which large numbers of plasma cells circulate is the term plasma cell leukemia used. Patients with plasma cell leukemia tend to have tissue infiltration, advanced stage disease, and poor survival.

WALDENSTRÖM'S MACROGLOBULINEMIA

Macroglobulins (IgM immunoglobulns) constitute 3 to 10 per cent of serum proteins. They have a high molecular weight (10^6 daltons), a sedimentation constant of 18 to 20 Svedberg units, and a high carbohydrate content and are characterized by a mu heavy chain and either kappa or lambda light chains. Increases of serum macroglobulins which are polyclonal may be seen in chronic infections or in collagen diseases. Monoclonal macroglobulinemia is found in a few individuals without detectable disease, in some cases of malignant lymphoma, and in chronic lymphocytic leukemia. It appears that Waldenström's macroglobulinemia is a variant of CLL (or well-differentiated lymphocytic lymphoma) in which there is a greater degree of maturation of the B lymphocytes into plasma cells (Preud'homme, 1972).

Clinical. Waldenström's macroglobulinemia is found in individuals over the age of 40, with a peak incidence between ages 60 and 70. It is characterized by a general proliferation of lymphocytes (and plasma cells) and the presence of at least 1 g/dl of monoclonal IgM in the serum, amounting to at least 15 per cent of the total serum protein.

The clinical features of the disease are effects of the increased serum macroglobulins, which commonly cause symptoms due to increased viscosity, and the cell proliferation itself, which accounts for hepatosplenomegaly and some degree of lymphadenopathy. In contrast to multiple myeloma, bone pain and osteolytic lesions on x-ray are rare. Hyperviscosity and sludging of blood may lead to visual disturbances, neurologic symptoms, impaired kidney function, and right-sided congestive heart failure. Hemorrhagic phenomena may be caused by the macroglobulins adhering to platelets, which interferes with their function, and forming complexes with plasma clotting factors, which impairs their activity. Cryoglobulinemia occurs somewhat more frequently than with myeloma and may be responsible for sensitivity to cold and Raynaud's phenomenon.

Blood. Normochromic, normocytic anemia is sometimes associated with thrombocytopenia or pancytopenia. Relative or slight absolute lymphocytosis is usually found. Marked rouleau formation is present on the blood film, and the sedimentation rate is usually extremely rapid, although it may be low if macrocryoglobulins are present and the test is carried out at a lower temperature. The anemia is occasionally hemolytic with a positive Coombs' test.

Marrow. Often the marrow cannot be aspirated readily. Lymphoid cells are increased in number.

These usually resemble normal small lymphocytes, but sometimes plasmacytoid cells are present and plasma cells may be increased in number. PAS-positive inclusions are often seen in the cytoplasm and nucleus of the lymphoid cells. Tissue mast cells are increased in number.

Immunoglobulins (see also p. 860). Serum globulin is usually markedly increased.

The *relative serum viscosity* may be simply measured using an Ostwald viscometer. The average time for descent of the serum at room temperature is expressed as a ratio to that of distilled water. The normal range is 1.4 to 1.8. It is considerably elevated in most patients with macroglobulinemia. Symptoms of hyperviscosity appear in most patients when the relative serum viscosity is between 6 and 8, though the threshold varies among patients (MacKenzie, 1972).

The identification of the paraprotein is achieved by *immunoelectrophoresis*. Together with the mu heavy chains, only one type of light chain is found. The total monoclonal IgM exceeds 10 mg/ml (1 g/dl).

Bence Jones proteinuria occurs in about 10 per cent of patients.

HEAVY CHAIN DISEASE

A small number of patients produce and excrete heavy chain fragments without associated light chains (see also p. 861). Some of these proteins show structural mutations (Frangione, 1973).

Gamma Heavy Chain Disease (γ-HCD). This disorder clinically resembles malignant lymphoma rather than myeloma, with lymphadenopathy, hepatosplenomegaly, fever, and propensity to infections. Anemia is constantly present, often with leukopenia and thrombocytopenia. Atypical lymphocytes or plasma cells are frequently present in the blood, and two cases have terminated in plasma cell leukemia. The marrow is usually abnormal, with increased plasma cells and lymphocytes and eosinophils, but is not diagnostic. Usually, but not always, the histology of lymphoid tissue indicates a malignant lymphoproliferative disease. A rather broad serum protein "spike" has been found in the beta-gamma region in most patients, accompanied by hypogammaglobulinemia. The diagnosis is made by showing that the protein reacts on immunoelectrophoresis with antisera to γ-chains but not to light chains. The protein is also found in the urine in varying amounts, though concentration techniques may be necessary to demonstrate it.

Alpha Heavy Chain Disease (α-HCD). This disorder appears to be more common than γ-HCD, and involves a younger age group. The uniform clinical pattern in most patients is malabsorption and diarrhea accompanying a massive lymphoplasmacytic infiltration of intestinal mucosa, or a histiocytic lymphoma of the intestine. In a few patients, the respiratory tract has been involved instead. Bone marrow and other lymphoid organs have not been involved. Usually routine protein electrophoresis is negative, but small amounts of alpha chain may be detected in the serum and sometimes in the urine with immunoelectrophoresis. The abnormal protein does not contain light chains (Seligmann, 1975).

Mu Heavy Chain Disease (μ-HCD). The few patients who have been described have had chronic lymphocytic leukemia with vacuolated plasma cells in the marrow. Routine serum electrophoresis showed only hypogammaglobulinemia. The μ heavy chain was detected by serum immunoelectrophoresis; it was not found in the urine. In most patients, however, the urine contained light chains (κ) in large amounts (Franklin, 1975).

Adamson, J. W., and Fialkow, P. J.: The pathogenesis of myeloproliferative syndromes. Br. J. Haematol., *38*:299, 1978.

Adamson, J. W., Fialkow, P. J., Murphy, S., Prchal, J. F., and Steinman, L.: Polycythemia vera: Stem-cell and probable clonal origin of the disease. N. Engl. J. Med., *295*:913, 1976.

Alder, A.: Über konstitutionell bedingte Granulationsveränderungen der Leukocyten. Deutsch. Arch. Klin. Med., *183*:372, 1939.

Andersen, V., and Andersen, E.: Changes in blood lymphocytes during the neonatal period. Acta Paediatr. Scand., *63*:266, 1974.

Barak, Y., Paran, M., Levin, S., and Sachs, L.: *In vitro* induction of myeloid proliferation and maturation in infantile genetic agranulocytosis. Blood, *38*:74, 1971.

Bearman, R. M., Pangalis, G. A., and Rappaport, H.: Acute ('malignant') myelosclerosis. Cancer, *43*:279, 1979.

Beeson, P. B., and Bass, D. A.: The Eosinophil. Vol. XIV in the series Major Problems in Internal Medicine, Smith, L. H., Jr. (ed.). Philadelphia, W. B. Saunders Company, 1977.

Bennett, J. M., Catovsky, D., Daniel, M-Th., Flandrin, G., Galton, D. A. G., Gralnick, H. R., and Sultan, C.: Proposals for the classification of the acute leukaemias. French-American-British (FAB) Co-operative Group. Br. J. Haematol., *33*:451, 1976.

Bennett, J. M., Catovsky, D., Daniel, M-Th., Flandrin, G., Galton, D. A. G., Gralnick, H. R., and Sultan, C.: A variant form of hypergranular promyelocytic leukemia (M3). Br. J. Haematol., *44*:169, 1980.

Bennett, J. M., Catovsky, D., Daniel, M-Th., Flandrin, G., Galton, D. A. G., Gralnick, H. R., and Sultan, C.: The French-American-British (FAB) Co-operative Group: The morphological classification of acute lymphoblastic leukaemia: Concordance among observers and clinical correlations. Br. J. Haematol., *47*:553, 1981.

Bennett, J. M., Catovsky, D., Daniel, M-Th., Flandrin, G., Galton, D. A. G., Gralnick, H. R., and Sultan, C.: The French-American-British (FAB) Cooperative Group: Proposals for the classification of the myelodysplastic syndromes. Br. J. Haematol., *51*:189, 1982.

Berard, C. W., and Dorfman, R. F.: Histopathology of malignant lymphomas. Clin. Haematol., *3*:39, 1974.

Berlin, N. J.: Diagnosis and classification of the polycythemias. Semin. Hematol., *12*:339, 1975.

Bernier, G. M., and Graham, R. C., Jr.: Plasma cell asynchrony in myeloma: Correlation of light and electron microscopy. Semin. Hematol., *13*:239, 1976.

Beverley, J. K. A., and Beattie, C. P.: Glandular toxoplasmosis. A survey of 30 cases. Lancet, *2*:379, 1958.

Binet, J. L., Catovsky, D., Chandra, P., Dighiero, G., Montserrat, E., Rai, E. R., and Sawitsky, A.: Chronic lymphocytic leukemia: Proposal for a revised prognostic staging system. Br. J. Haematol., *48*:365, 1981.

Blacklow, N. R., and Kapikian, A. Z.: Serological studies with E B virus in infectious lymphocytosis. Nature, *226*:647, 1970.

Blume, R. S., and Wolff, S. M.: The Chédiak-Higashi syndrome: Studies in four patients and a review of the literature. Medicine (Baltimore), *51*:247, 1972.

Boggs, D. R., and Winkelstein, A.: White Cell Manual. 4th ed. Philadelphia, F. A. Davis Co., 1983.

Bouroncle, B. A., Wiseman, B. K., and Doan, C. A.: Leukemic reticuloendotheliosis. Blood, *13*:609, 1958.

Boyd, J. F., and Reid, D.: Bone marrow in nine cases of clinical glandular fever and a review of the literature. J. Clin. Path., *21*:638, 1968.

4

Brooksaler, F., and Nelson, J. D.: Pertussis. A reappraisal and report of 190 confirmed cases. Am. J. Dis. Child., *114*:389, 1967.

Brunning, R. D.: Morphologic alterations in nucleated blood and marrow cells in genetic disorders. Hum. Path., *1*:99, 1970.

Canellos, G. P.: Chronic granulocytic leukemia. Med. Clin. North Am., *60*:1001, 1976.

Cardullo, L. D., Morilla, R., and Catovsky, D.: Significance of Phi bodies in acute leukemia. J. Clin. Path., *34*:153, 1981.

Carr, M. C., Stites, D. P., and Fudenberg, H. H.: Cellular immune aspects of the human fetal-maternal relationship. III. Mixed lymphocyte reactivity between related maternal and cord blood lymphocytes. Cell. Immunol., *11*:332, 1974.

Carter, R. L., and Penman, H. G.: Histopathology of infectious mononucleosis. *In* Carter, R. L., and Penman, H. G. (eds.): Infectious Mononucleosis. Oxford, Blackwell Scientific Publications, 1969.

Catovsky, D.: Hairy-cell leukaemia and prolymphocytic leukaemia. Clin. Haematol., *6*:245, 1977.

Catovsky, D. (ed.): The Leukemic Cell. Edinburgh, Churchill Livingstone, 1981.

Catovsky, D., Cherchi, M., Greaves, M. F., Janossy, G., Pain, C., and Kay, H. E. M.: Acid-phosphatase reaction in acute lymphoblastic leukaemia. Lancet, *1*:749, 1978.

Catovsky, D., Galton, D. A. G., Griffin, C., Hoffbrand, A. V., and Szur, L.: Serum lysozyme and vitamin B_{12} binding capacity in myeloproliferative disorders. Br. J. Haematol., *21*:661, 1971a.

Catovsky, D., Galton, D. A. G., and Griffin, C.: Significance of lysozyme estimations in acute myeloid and chronic monocytic leukaemia. Br. J. Haematol., *21*:565, 1971b.

Ceppellini, R., Bonnard, G. D., Coppo, F., Miggiano, C., Pospisil, M., Curtoni, E. S., and Pellegrino, M.: Mixed leukocyte cultures and HL-A antigens. I. Reactivity of young fetuses, newborns, mothers at delivery. Transplant. Proc., *3*:58, 1971.

Chusid, M. J., Dale, D. C., West, B. C., and Wolff, S. M.: The hypereosinophilic syndrome. Medicine (Baltimore), *54*:1, 1975.

Cline, M. J., Opelz, G., Saxon, A., Fahey, J. L., and Golde, D. W.: Autoimmune panleukopenia. N. Engl. J. Med., *295*:1489, 1976.

Davey, F. R., and Huntington, S.: Age-related variation in lymphocyte subpopulations. Gerontology, *23*:381, 1977.

Davidsohn, I.: Serologic diagnosis of infectious mononucleosis. J.A.M.A., *108*:289, 1937.

Davidsohn, I., and Lee, C. L.: The clinical serology of infectious mononucleosis. *In* Carter, R. L., and Penman, H. G. (eds.): Infectious Mononucleosis. Oxford, Blackwell Scientific Publications, 1969.

Davidsohn, I., and Nelson, D. A.: The Blood. *In* Davidsohn, I., and Henry, J. B. (eds.): Clinical Diagnosis by Laboratory Methods. 15th ed. Philadelphia, W. B. Saunders Company, 1974, p. 262.

Diaz-Jouanen, E., Strickland, R. G., and Williams, R. C.: Studies of human lymphocytes in the newborn and the aged. Am. J. Med., *58*:620, 1975.

Dorfman, R. F., and Remington, J. S.: Value of lymph-node biopsy in the diagnosis of acute acquired toxoplasmosis. N. Engl. J. Med., *289*:878, 1973.

Downey, H., and McKinlay, C. A.: Acute lymphadenosis compared with acute lymphatic leukemia. Arch. Intern. Med., *32*:82, 1923.

Durie, B. G. M., and Salmon, S. E.: A clinical staging system for multiple myeloma: Correlation of measured myeloma cell mass with presenting clinical features, response to treatment and survival. Cancer, *36*:842, 1975.

Ellis, J. T., Silver, R. T., Coleman, M., and Geller, S. A.: The bone marrow in polycythemia vera. Semin. Hematol., *12*:433, 1975.

Epstein, M. A., and Achong, B. G.: Pathogenesis of infectious mononucleosis. Lancet, *2*:1270, 1977.

Feldman, H. A.: Toxoplasmosis. N. Engl. J. Med., *279*:1370, 1431, 1968.

Fialkow, P. J., Jacobson, R. J., and Papayannopoulou, T.: Chronic myelocytic leukemia: Clonal origin in a stem cell common to the granulocyte, erythrocyte, platelet and monocyte/macrophage. Am. J. Med., *63*:125, 1977.

Finch, S. C.: Granulocytopenia (Chapter 83) and Granulocytosis (Chapter 84). *In* Williams, W. J., Beutler, E., Erslev, A. J., and Rundles, R. W. (eds.): Hematology. 2nd ed. New York, McGraw-Hill Book Co., Inc., 1977.

Flandrin, G., and Brouet, J-C.: The Sézary cell: Cytologic, cytochemical and immunologic studies. Mayo Clin. Proc., *49*:575, 1974.

Foster, K. M., and Jack, I.: A prospective study of the role of cytomegalovirus in post-transfusion mononucleosis. N. Engl. J. Med., *280*:1311, 1969.

Frangione, B., and Franklin, E. C.: Heavy chain diseases: Clinical features and molecular significance of the disordered immunoglobulin structure. Semin. Hematol., *10*:53, 1973.

Franklin, E. C.: μ-Chain disease. Arch. Intern. Med., *135*:71, 1975.

Fu, S. M., Winchester, R. J., Rai, K. R., and Kunkel, H. G: Hairy cell leukemia: Proliferation of a cell with phagocytic and B-lymphocyte properties. Scand. J. Immunol., *3*:847, 1974.

Gall, E. A., and Stout, H. A.: The histological lesion in lymph nodes in infectious mononucleosis. Am. J. Path., *16*:433, 1940.

Galton, D. A. G.: The chronic leukaemias. *In* Hoffbrand, A. V., Brain, M. C., and Hirsh, J. (eds.): Recent Advances in Haematology. 2nd ed. Edinburgh, Churchill Livingstone, 1977.

Galton, D. A. G., Goldman, J. M., Wiltshaw, E., Catovsky, D., Henry, K., and Goldenberg, G. J.: Prolymphocytic leukaemia. Br. J. Haematol., *27*:7, 1974.

Gerber, P., Walsh, J. H., Rosenblum, E. N., and Purcell, R. H.: Association of EB-virus infection with the postperfusion syndrome. Lancet, *1*:593, 1969.

Gilbert, H. S.: Definition, clinical features and diagnosis of polycythaemia vera. Clin. Haematol., *4*:263, 1975a.

Gilbert, H. S., and Ornstein, L.: Basophil counting with a new staining method using Alcian blue. Blood, *46*:279, 1975b.

Glenner, G. G., Terry, W. D., and Isersky, C.: Amyloidosis: Its nature and pathogenesis. Semin. Hematol., *10*:65, 1973.

Golomb, H. M., Rowley, J. D., Vardiman, J. W., Testa, J. R., and Butler, A.: "Microgranular" acute promyelocytic leukemia: A distinct clinical, ultrastructural, and cytogenetic entity. Blood, *55*:253, 1980.

Gralnick, H. R., Galton, D. A. G., Catovsky, D., Sultan, C., and Bennett, J. W.: Classification of acute leukemia. Ann. Intern. Med., *87*:740, 1977.

Greenberg, P. L.: Granulocytopoiesis in vitro: Regulatory and clinical implications. *In* Fairbanks, V. F. (ed.): Current Hematology, Vol. 1. New York, John Wiley & Sons, 1981, p. 219.

Groover, R. V., Burke, E. C., Gordon, H., and Berdon, W. E.: The genetic mucopolysaccharidoses. Semin. Hematol., *9*:371, 1972.

Gunz, F. W.: Hemorrhagic thrombocythemia: A critical review. Blood, *15*:706, 1960.

Gunz, F., and Baikie, A. G.: Leukemia. 3rd ed. New York, Grune & Stratton, Inc., 1974.

Hallgren, H. M., Kersey, J. H., Gajl-Peczalska, K. J., Greenberg, L. J., and Yunis, E. J.: T and B cells in aging humans. Fed. Proc., *33*:646, 1974.

Hayhoe, F. G. J., and Cawley, J. C.: Acute leukaemia: Cellular morphology, cytochemistry and fine structure. Clin. Haematol., *1*:49, 1972.

Hayhoe, F. G. J., and Quaglino, D.: Haematological Cytochemistry. Edinburgh, Churchill Livingstone, 1980.

Hayhoe, F. G. J., Quaglino, D., and Doll, R.: The Cytology and Cytochemistry of Acute Leukaemias. London, Her Majesty's Stationery Office, 1964.

Henle, W., Henle, G. E., and Horwitz, C. A.: Epstein-Barr virus specific diagnostic tests in infectious mononucleosis. Hum. Path., *5*:551, 1974.

Higgy, K. E., Burns, G. F., and Hayhoe, F. G. J.: Discrimination of B, T and null lymphocytes by esterase cytochemistry. Scand. J. Haematol., *18*:437, 1977.

Horowitz, C. A.: Persistently falsely positive rapid tests for infectious mononucleosis. Am. J. Clin. Path., *72*:807, 1979.

Horowitz, M. S., and Moore, G. T.: Acute infectious lymphocytosis. An etiologic and epidemiologic study of an outbreak. N. Engl. J. Med., *279*:399, 1968.

Hovde, R. F., and Sundberg, R. D.: Granulomatous lesions in the bone marrow in infectious mononucleosis. Blood, *5*:209, 1950.

Hoyer, J. R., Cooper, M. D., Gabrielsen, A. E., and Good, R. A.: Lymphopenic forms of congenital immunologic deficiency diseases. Medicine (Baltimore), *47*:201, 1968.

Jacobson, R. J., Salo, A., and Fialkow, P. J.: Agnogenic myeloid metaplasia: A clonal proliferation of hematopoietic stem cells with secondary myelofibrosis. Blood, *51*:189, 1978.

Jenis, E. H., Takeuchi, A., Dillon, D. E., Ruymann, F. B., and

Rivkin, S.: The May-Hegglin anomaly: Ultrastructure of the granulocytic inclusion. Am. J. Clin. Path., *55*:187, 1971.

Jondal, M., and Klein, G.: Surface markers on human B and T lymphocytes. II. Presence of Epstein-Barr virus receptors on B lymphocytes. J. Exp. Med., *138*:1365, 1973.

Jordan, M. C., Rousseau, W. E., Stewart, J. A., Noble, G. R., and Chin, T. D. Y.: Spontaneous cytomegalovirus mononucleosis: Clinical and laboratory observations in nine cases. Ann. Intern. Med., *79*:153, 1973.

Kaplow, L. S.: Cytochemistry of leukocyte alkaline phosphatase. Am. J. Clin. Path., *39*:439, 1963.

Kaplow, L. S.: Simplified myeloperoxidase stain using benzidine dihydrochloride. Blood, *26*:215, 1965.

Kaplow, L. S.: Substitute for benzidine in myeloperoxidase stains. Am. J. Clin. Path., *63*:451, 1975.

Karzon, D. T.: Infectious mononucleosis. Adv. Pediatr., *22*:231, 1976.

Katayama, I., and Yang, J. P. S.: Reassessment of a cytochemical test for differential diagnosis of leukemic reticuloendotheliosis. Am. J. Clin. Path., *68*:268, 1977.

Khaleeli, M., Keane, W. M., and Lee, G. R.: Sideroblastic anemia in multiple myeloma: A preleukemic change. Blood, *41*:17, 1973.

Klemola, E., von Essen, R., Wager, O., Haltia, K., Koivuniemi, A., and Salmi, I.: Cytomegalovirus mononucleosis in previously healthy individuals. Ann. Intern. Med., *71*:11, 1969.

Lagergren, J.: The white blood cell count and the erythrocyte sedimentation rate in pertussis. Acta Paediatr., *52*:405, 1963.

Lalezari, P., Jiang, A-F., Yegen, L., and Santorineou, M.: Chronic autoimmune neutropenia due to anti-NA2 antibody. N. Engl. J. Med., *293*:744, 1975.

Landaw, S. A.: Acute leukemia in polycythemia vera. Semin. Hematol., *13*:33, 1975.

Laszlo, J.: Myeloproliferative disorders (MPD): Myelofibrosis, myelosclerosis, extramedullary hematopoiesis, undifferentiated MPD, and hemorrhagic thrombocythemia. Semin. Hematol., *12*:409, 1975.

Leder, L. D.: The selective enzymochemical demonstration of neutrophilic myeloid cells and tissue mast cells in paraffin sections. Klin. Wochenschr., *42*:533, 1964.

Lee, C. L., Davidsohn, I., and Panczyszyn, O.: Horse agglutinins in infectious mononucleosis. II. The spot test. Am. J. Clin. Path., *49*:12, 1968.

Li, C. Y., Lam, K. W., and Yam, L. T.: Esterases in human leukocytes. J. Histochem. Cytochem., *21*:1, 1973.

Liso, V., Troccoli, G., Specchia, G., and Magno, M.: Cytochemical "normal" and "abnormal" eosinophils in acute leukemias. Am. J. Hematol., *2*:123, 1977.

Lukes, R. J., Craver, L. L., Hall, T. C., Rappaport, H., and Rubin, P.: Hodgkin's disease, report of Nomenclature Committee. Cancer Res., *26*:1311, 1966.

Lukes, R. J., Tindle, B. H., and Parker, J. W.: Reed-Sternberg–like cells in infectious mononucleosis. Lancet, *2*:1003, 1969.

MacKenzie, M. R., and Fudenberg, H. H.: Macroglobulinemia: An analysis of forty patients. Blood, *39*:874, 1972.

Maldonado, J. E., and Hanlon, D. G.: Monocytosis: A current appraisal. Mayo Clin. Proc., *40*:248, 1965.

Mandal, B. K., and Stokes, K. J.: Acute infectious lymphocytosis and enteroviruses. Lancet, *2*:1392, 1973.

Mangi, R. J., Niederman, J. C., Keleher, J. E., Dwyer, J. M., Evans, A. S., and Kantor, F. S.: Depression of cell-mediated immunity during acute infectious mononucleosis. N. Engl. J. Med., *291*:1149, 1974.

Marks, S. M., Baltimore, D., and McCaffrey, R.: Terminal transferase as a predictor of initial responsiveness to vincristine and prednisone in blastic chronic myelogenous leukemia. N. Engl. J. Med., *298*:812, 1978.

Mauer, A. M., Lampkin, B. C., and McWilliams, N. B.: The leukemias and reticuloendothelioses. *In* Nathan, D. G., and Oski, F. A. (eds.): Hematology of Infancy and Childhood. Philadelphia, W. B. Saunders Company, 1974, p. 665.

McCall, C. E., Katayama, I., Cotran, R. S., and Finland, M.: Lysosomal and ultrastructural changes in human "toxic" neutrophils during bacterial infection. J. Exp. Med., *129*:267, 1969.

McKusick, V. A., and Neufeld, E. F.: The mucopolysaccharide storage diseases. *In* Stanbury, J. B., Wyngaarden, J. B., Fredrickson, D. S., Goldstein, J. L., and Brown, M. S. (eds.): The Metabolic Basis of Inherited Disease. New York, McGraw-Hill Book Co., 1983, p. 751.

Metcalf, D.: Hemopoietic Colonies. *In vitro* cloning of normal and leukemic cells. Recent Results in Cancer Research, Vol. 61. New York, Springer-Verlag, Inc., 1977.

Miescher, P. A., and Farquet, J. J.: Chronic myelomonocytic leukemia in adults. Semin. Hematol., *11*:129, 1974.

Miller, M. E.: Disorders of neutrophil function. Am. J. Hematol., *3*:257, 1977.

Morse, S. I., and Barron, B. A.: Studies on the leukocytosis and lymphocytosis induced by *Bordetella pertussis*. III. The distribution of transfused lymphocytes in pertussis-treated and normal mice. J. Exp. Med., *132*:663, 1970.

Nadler, L. M., Ritz, J., Griffin, J. D., Todd, R. F., III, Reinherz, E. L., and Schlossman, S. F.: Diagnosis and treatment of human leukemias and lymphomas utilizing monoclonal antibodies. Progr. Hematol., *12*:187, 1981.

Naiman, J. L., Oski, F. A., Allen, F. H., and Diamond, L. K.: Hereditary eosinophilia: Report of a family and review of the literature. Am. J. Hum. Genet., *16*:195, 1964.

Neiman, R. S., Barcos, M., et al.: Granulocytic sarcoma: A clinicopathologic study of 61 biopsied cases. Cancer, *48*:1426, 1981.

Neiman, R. S., Rosen, P. J., and Lukes, R. J.: Lymphocyte-depletion Hodgkin's disease. N. Engl. J. Med., *288*:751, 1973.

Nelson, D. A., and Davey, F. R.: Leukocyte esterases. *In* Williams, W. J., Beutler, E., Erslev, A. J., and Rundles, R. W. (eds.): Hematology, 2nd ed. New York, McGraw-Hill Book Co., 1977, p. 1633.

Nkrumah, F. K., and Addy, P. A. K.: Acute infectious lymphocytosis. Lancet, *1*:1257, 1973.

Nowell, P. C.: Preleukemia: Cytogenetic clues in some confusing disorders. Am. J. Path., *89*:459, 1977.

Non-Hodgkin's Lymphoma Pathologic Classification Project: National Cancer Institute sponsored study of classifications of Non-Hodgkin's lymphoma. Cancer, *49*:2112, 1982.

Nowell, P. C., and Hungerford, D. A.: A minute chromosome in human chronic granulocytic leukemia. Science, *132*:1497, 1960.

Olson, L. C., Miller, G., and Hanshaw, J. B.: Acute infectious lymphocytosis presenting as a pertussis-like illness: Its association with adenovirus type 12. Lancet, *1*:200, 1964.

Ooi, B. S., Orlina, A. R., Masaitis, L., First, M. R., and Pollak, V. E.: Lymphocytotoxins in aging. Transplantation, *18*:190, 1974.

Osserman, E. F., and Lawlor, D. P.: Serum and urinary lysozyme (muramidase) in monocytic and monomyelocytic leukemia. J. Exp. Med., *124*:921, 1966.

Ottensen, E. A.: Tropical eosinophilia. *In* Wyngaarden, J. B., and Smith, L. H. Jr.: Cecil Textbook of Medicine. 16th ed. Philadelphia, W. B. Saunders Company, 1982, p. 1776.

den Ottolander, G. J., te Velde, J., Brederoo, P., Geraedts, J. P. M., Slee, P. H. T., Villemze, R., Zwaan, F. E., Haak, H. L., Muller, H. P., and Bieger, R.: Megakaryoblastic leukaemia (acute myelofibrosis): A report of three cases. Br. J. Haematol., *42*:9, 1979.

Paul, J. R., and Bunnell, W. W.: The presence of heterophile antibodies in infectious mononucleosis. Am. J. Med. Sci., *183*:90, 1932.

Peterson, L. C., Bloomfield, C. D., and Brunning, R. D.: Blast crisis as an initial or terminal manifestation of chronic myeloid leukemia. A study of 28 patients. Am. J. Med., *60*:209, 1976.

Pierre, R. V.: Preleukemic states. Semin. Hematol., *11*:73, 1974.

Poiesz, B. J., Ruscetti, F. W., Gazdar, A. F., Bunn, P. A., Minna, J. D., and Gallo, R. C.: Detection and isolation of type C retrovirus particles from fresh and cultured lymphocytes of a patient with cutaneous T-cell lymphoma. Proc. Natl. Acad. Sci., *77*:7415, 1980.

Prchal, J. F., and Axelrod, A. A.: Bone marrow responses in polycythemia vera. N. Engl. J. Med., *290*:1382, 1974.

Preud'homme, J. L., and Seligmann, M.: Surface bound immunoglobulins as a cell marker in human lymphoproliferative diseases. Blood, *40*:777, 1972.

Purtilo, D., Paquin, L., DeFlorio, D., Virzi, F., and Sakhuja, R.: Immunodiagnosis and immunopathogenesis of the X-linked recessive lymphoproliferative syndrome. Semin. Hematol., *16*:309, 1979.

Rai, K. R., Chanana, A. W., Cronkite, E. P., Joel, D. D., and Stevens, J. B.: Studies on lymphocytes. XVIII. Mechanisms of lymphocytosis induced by supernatant fluids of *Bordetella pertussis* cultures. Blood, *38*:49, 1971.

Rai, K. R., Sawitsky, A., Cronkite, E. P., Chanana, A. D., Levy,

4

R. N., and Pasternack, B. S.: Clinical staging of chronic lymphocytic leukemia. Blood, *46*:219, 1975.

Rappaport, H.: Tumors of the hematopoietic system. *In* Atlas of Tumor Pathology. Washington, D.C., Armed Forces Institute of Pathology, Section III, Fascicle 88, 1966.

Rappaport, H., and Thomas, L. B.: Mycosis fungoides: The pathology of extracutaneous involvement. Cancer, *34*:1198, 1974.

Reilly, W. A.: The granules in the leukocytes in gargoylism. Am. J. Dis. Child., *62*:489, 1941.

Rickinson, A. B., Crawford, D., and Epstein, M. A.: Inhibition of the *in vitro* outgrowth of Epstein-Barr virus–transformed lymphocytes by thymus-dependent lymphocytes from infectious mononucleosis patients. Clin. Exp. Immunol., *28*:72, 1977.

Rickles, F. R., and Miller, D. R.: Eosinophilic leukemoid reaction. J. Pediatr., *80*:418, 1972.

Rinehart, J. J., Sagone, A. L., Balcerzak, S. P., Ackerman, G. A., and LoBuglio, A. F.: Effects of corticosteroid therapy on human monocyte function. N. Engl. J. Med., *292*:236, 1975.

Ritzmann, S. E., Daniels, J. C., Lawrence, M. C., Beathard, G. A., and Levin, W. C.: Monoclonal gammopathies, present status. Texas Med., *68*:91, 1972.

Roggli, V. L., Surback, J., and Saleem, A.: Prognostic factors and treatment effects on survival in erythroleukemia: A retrospective study of 134 cases. Cancer, *48*:1101, 1981.

Rosenberg, S. A.: Hodgkin's disease of the bone marrow. Cancer Res., *31*:1733, 1971.

Rosenthal, S., Canellos, G. P., DeVita, V. T., Jr., and Gralnick, H. R.: Characteristics of blast crisis in chronic granulocytic leukemia. Blood, *49*:705, 1977.

Rosner, F., and Grunwald, H.: Multiple myeloma terminating in acute leukemia. Report of 12 cases and review of the literature. Am. J. Med., *57*:927, 1974.

Rosner, F., Schreiber, Z. R., and Parise, F.: Leukocyte alkaline phosphatase. Fluctuations with disease status in chronic granulocytic leukemia. Arch. Intern. Med., *130*:892, 1972.

Saarni, M. I., and Linman, J. W.: Preleukemia. The hematologic syndrome preceding acute leukemia. Am. J. Med., *55*:38, 1973.

Saxén, E., and Saxén, L.: The histological diagnosis of glandular toxoplasmosis. Lab. Invest., *8*:386, 1959.

Seligmann, M.: Immunochemical, clinical and pathological features of α-chain disease. Arch. Intern. Med., *135*:78, 1975.

Seshadri, R. S., Brown, E. J., and Zipursky, A.: Leukemic reticuloendotheliosis. A failure of monocyte production. N. Engl. J. Med., *295*:181, 1976.

Sharp, A. A.: Platelets, bleeding and haemostasis in infectious mononucleosis. *In* Carter, R. L., and Penman, H. G. (eds.): Infectious Mononucleosis. Oxford, Blackwell Scientific Publications, 1969.

Sheehan, H. L., and Storey, G. W.: An improved method of staining leukocyte granules with Sudan black B. J. Path. Bacteriol., *59*:336, 1947.

Siim, J. C.: Acquired toxoplasmosis. Report of seven cases with strongly positive reactions. J.A.M.A., *147*:1641, 1951.

Silverstein, M. N.: Myeloproliferative diseases. *In* Fairbanks, V. F. (ed.): Current Hematology, Vol. 1. New York, John Wiley & Sons, 1981, p. 246.

Smith, C. H.: Infectious lymphocytosis. Am. J. Dis. Child., *62*:231, 1941.

Smith, E., Kochwa, S., and Wasserman, L. R.: Aggregation of IgG globulin *in vivo*. Am. J. Med., *39*:35, 1965.

Smith, M. A., Evans, J., and Steel, C. M.: Age-related variation in proportion of circulating T cells. Lancet, *2*:922, 1974.

Spaet, T. H., Lejnieks, I., Gaynor, E., and Goldstein, M. L.: Defective platelets in essential thrombocythemia. Arch. Intern. Med., *124*:135, 1969.

Spiers, A. S. D., Bain, B. J., and Turner, J. E.: The peripheral blood in chronic granulocytic leukemia. Study of 50 untreated Philadelphia-positive cases. Scand. J. Haematol., *18*:25, 1977.

Stass, S. A., Schumacher, H. R., Kenelis, T. P., and Bollum, F. J.: Terminal deoxynucleotidyl transferase immunofluorescence of bone marrow smears. Am. J. Clin. Path., *72*:898, 1979.

Stossel, T. P., and Boxer, L. A.: Qualitative abnormalities of granulocytes. *In* Williams, W. J., Beutler, E., Erslev, A. J., and Rundles, R. W. (eds.): Hematology. 2nd ed. New York, McGraw-Hill Book Co., 1977, p. 756.

Sultan, C., Deregnaucourt, J., Ko, Y. W., Imbert, M., Ricard D'Agay, M. F., Gouault-Heilmann, M., and Brun, B.: Distribution of 250 cases of acute myeloid leukemia (AML) according to the FAB classification and response to therapy. Br. J. Haematol., *47*:545, 1981.

Sultan, C., Imbert, M., Riard, M. F., and Marquet, M.: Myelodysplastic syndromes. *In* Lewis, S. M., and Verwilghen, R. L. (eds.): Dyserythropoiesis. London, Academic Press, 1977.

Takácsi-Nagy, L., and Graf, E.: Definition, clinical features and diagnosis of myelofibrosis. Clin. Haematol., *4*:291, 1975.

Tamaoki, N., and Essner, E.: Distribution of acid phosphatase, β-glucuronidase, and N-acetyl-β-glucuronidase activities in lymphocytes of lymphatic tissues of man and rodents. J. Histochem. Cytochem., *17*:238, 1969.

Testa, J. R., Golomb, H. M., Rowley, J. D., Vardiman, J. M., and Sweet, D. L.: Hypergranular promyelocytic leukemia (APL): Cytogenetic and ultrastructural specificity. Blood, *52*:272, 1978.

Thompson, J. S., and Severson, C. D.: Granulocyte antigens. *In* Bell, C. A. (ed.): A seminar in antigens in blood cells and body fluids. Washington, D.C., American Association of Blood Banks, 1980, p. 151.

Tijio, J. H., Carbone, P. P., Whang, J., and Frei, E.: The Philadelphia chromosome and chronic myelogenous leukemia. J. Natl. Cancer Inst., *36*:567, 1966.

Uchiyama, T., Yodoi, J., Sagawa, K., Takatuski, K., and Uchino, H.: Adult T-cell leukemia: Clinical and hematologic features of 16 cases. Blood, *50*:481, 1977.

Van Scott, E. J., and Vonderheld, E. C.: Mycosis fungoides and Sézary syndrome. *In* Williams, W. J., Beutler, E., Erslev, A. J., and Rundles, R. D. (eds.): Hematology. 2nd ed. New York, McGraw-Hill Book Co., 1977.

Viana, M. B., Maurer, H. S., and Ferenc, C.: Subclassification of acute lymphocytic leukemia in children: Analysis of the reproducibility of morphological criteria and prognostic implications. Br. J. Haematol., *44*:383, 1980.

Vogler, L. B., Crist, W. M., Sarrif, A. M., Pullen, D. J., Bartolucci, A. A., Falletta, J. M., Dowell, B., Humphrey, G. B., Blackstock, R., Van Eys, J., Metzgar, R. S., and Cooper, M. D.: An analysis of clinical and laboratory features of acute lymphocytic leukemias with emphasis on 35 children with pre-B leukemia. Blood, *58*:135, 1981.

Waldorf, D. S., Willkens, R. E., and Decker, J. L.: Impaired delayed hypersensitivity in an aging population. Association with antinuclear reactivity and rheumatoid factor. J.A.M.A., *203*:831, 1968.

Ward, H. P., and Block, M. H.: The natural history of agnogenic myeloid metaplasia (AMM) and a critical evaluation of its relationship with the myeloproliferative syndrome. Medicine (Baltimore), *50*:357, 1971.

Wasserman, L. R., and Gilbert, H. S.: Surgical bleeding in polycythemia vera. Ann. N.Y. Acad. Sci., *115*:122, 1964.

Wasserman, L. R., and Gilbert, H. S.: Complications of polycythemia vera. Semin. Hematol., *3*:199, 1966.

Weksler, M. E., and Hütteroth, T. H.: Impaired lymphocyte function in aged humans. J. Clin. Invest., *53*:99, 1974.

White, J. C.: The Chédiak-Higashi syndrome: Cytoplasmic sequestration in circulating leukocytes. Blood, *29*:435, 1967.

Wintrobe, M. M., Lee, G. R., Boggs, D. R., Bithell, T. C., Foerster, J., Athens, J. W., and Lukens, J. N.: Clinical Hematology. 8th ed. Philadelphia, Lea & Febiger, 1981.

Wood, T. A., and Frenkel, E. P.: The atypical lymphocyte. Am. J. Med., *42*:923, 1967.

Woodruff, R. K., Wadsworth, J., Malpas, J. S., and Tobias, J. S.: Clinical staging in multiple myeloma. Br. J. Haematol., *42*:199, 1979.

Worlledge, S. M., and Dacie, J. V.: Hemolytic and other anaemias in infectious mononucleosis. *In* Carter, R. L., and Penman, H. G. (eds.): Infectious Mononucleosis. Oxford, Blackwell Scientific Publications, 1969.

Yam, L. T., Li, C. Y., and Lam, K. W.: Tartrate-resistant acid phosphatase isoenzyme in the reticulum cells of leukemic reticuloendotheliosis. N. Engl. J. Med., *284*:357, 1971a.

Yam, L. T., Li, C. Y., and Crosby, W. H.: Cytochemical identification of monocytes and granulocytes. Am. J. Clin. Pathol., *55*:283, 1971b.

31

BLOOD PLATELETS

JONATHAN L. MILLER, M.D., PH.D.

PLATELET FUNCTIONAL ANATOMY

A well-prepared peripheral blood film (Plate 27–1, p. 613) offers the opportunity for evaluation of platelet numbers, size, distribution, and light microscopic structure. Although subtle abnormalities of platelet structure usually require electron microscopic analysis, gross absence or asymmetry of granulation and grossly aberrant platelet surfaces may be evident. In films from non-anticoagulated finger-stick specimens, some platelet clumping is an expected feature. In instances of observed abnormalities, artifacts resulting from improper specimen collection or handling should always be considered, and a repeat specimen obtained if a satisfactory explanation for the abnormality is not apparent.

In cases of suspected platelet structural abnormalities, electron microscopy allows much more precise characterization of the defect. Preparative methods optimal for the study of platelet ultrastructure have been described (Gerrard, 1979), and it is essential that meticulous care be given to the collection and processing of such specimens.

Normal features of the platelet that may be visualized ultrastructurally are shown in Figure 31–1. The outer surface of the platelet, the *glycocalyx,* is rich in glycoproteins—both those adsorbed from the plasma and those integral to the platelet membrane. A submembranous band of *microtubules,* composed of the protein tubulin, provides structural support for the normally discoid cell. Contractile *microfilaments* (in the platelet also referred to as *thrombasthenin*) may also be seen. These are composed principally of platelet actin and platelet myosin. An extensive *open canalicular system* within the platelet has been demonstrated by a variety of methods to be in direct communication with the extracellular environment. Often seen in close proximity to the open canalicular system is the *dense tubular system.* This system, apparently derived from the smooth endoplasmic reticulum, shows positive staining for platelet peroxidase activity (Breton-Gorius, 1972), in accord with its role as a site for arachidonic acid metabolism within the platelet. The dense tubular system is also believed to function as a calcium-sequestering pump, providing low levels of cytoplasmic calcium in the resting platelet (Statland, 1969).

A variety of inclusions may be recognized within the platelet cytoplasm. Both *mitochondria* and *glycogen* may be identified. Lighter staining *alpha granules,* less frequent *dense core* (or "bull's eye") *granules, lysosomes,* and *peroxisomes* may also be seen. The alpha granules contain a number of different proteins, including platelet fibrinogen, the platelet-derived growth factor (PDGF), von Willebrand factor (vWF), beta-thromboglobulin (βTG), and the heparin-neutralizing platelet factor 4 (PF4). The dense core granules are known to be the locus of stored, non-metabolic pools of adenosine diphosphate (ADP), adenosine triphosphate (ATP), 5-hydroxytryptamine (5-HT), and calcium. For further description of the platelet's subcellular structures, the interested reader is referred to several excellent reviews (White, 1981, 1982; Zucker-Franklin, 1981).

In recent years detailed study of the platelet *membrane glycoproteins* has led to an improved understanding of platelet function. Through radioactive labeling of surface glycoprotein amino acid or sugar residues, solubilization of the platelet membranes, electrophoretic separation of the solubilized proteins on polyacrylamide gels, and autoradiography of the gels, the different platelet membrane glycoproteins may be identified (Phillips, 1980). A numbering system for these glycoproteins based upon electrophoretic migration has emerged (Berndt, 1981). Although over 30 bands may be seen, only a handful have been associated with specific functions. These are shown diagrammatically in Figure 31–2.

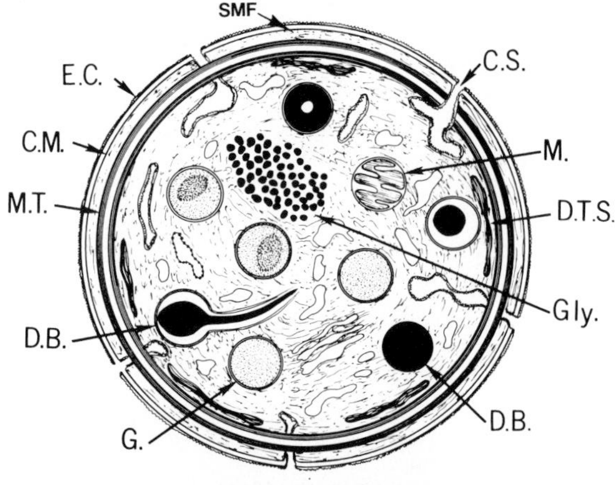

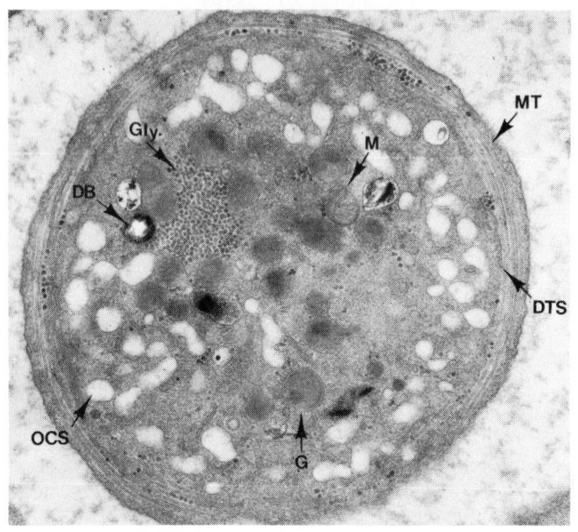

Figure 31–1. Platelet ultrastructure. The diagram summarizes ultrastructural features observed in thin sections of discoid platelets cut in the equatorial plane. Components of the peripheral zone include the exterior coat (EC), trilaminar unit membrane (CM), and submembrane area containing specialized filaments (SMF) which form the wall of the platelet and line channels of the surface-connected open canalicular system (CS). The matrix of the platelet interior is the sol-gel zone containing actin microfilaments, structural filaments, the circumferential band of microtubules (MT), and glycogen (Gly). Formed elements embedded in the sol-gel zone include mitochondria (M), granules (G), and dense bodies (DB). Collectively they constitute the organelle zone. The membrane systems include the surface-connected open canalicular system (OCS) and the dense tubular system (DTS) which serve as the platelet sarcoplasmic reticulum. The electron micrograph shows a platelet sectioned in the equatorial plane which reveals most of the structures indicated on the diagram. (From White, J. G., et al.: *In* Bloom, A. L., and Thomas, D. P. [eds.] Haemostasis and Thrombosis. New York, Churchill Livingstone, 1981.)

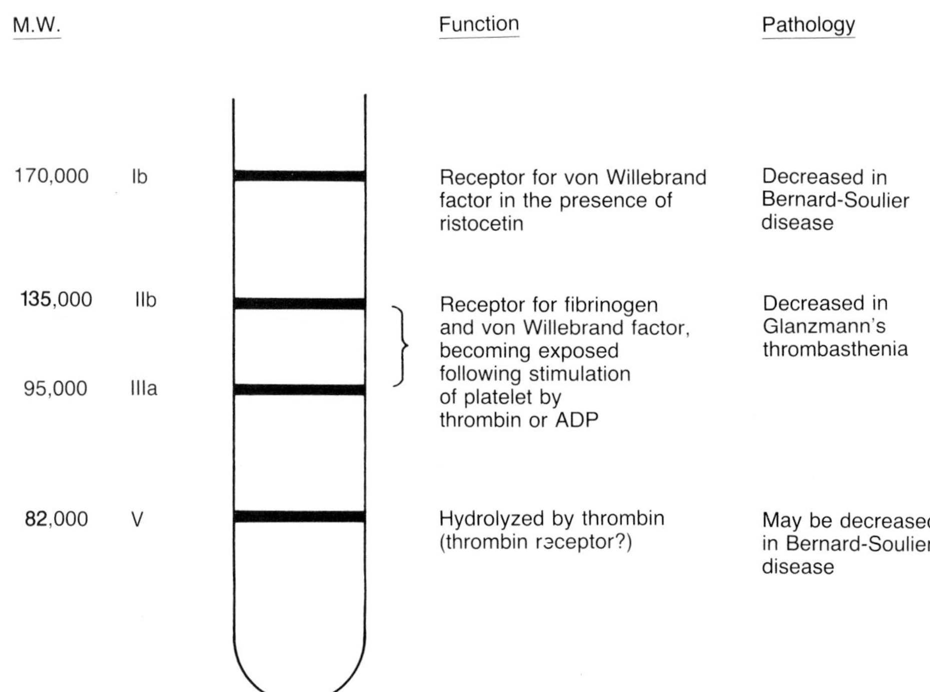

Figure 31–2. Platelet surface membrane glycoproteins. Diagram of major glycoproteins detectable by SDS polyacrylamide gel electrophoresis.

Platelet Activities in Hemostasis and Their Laboratory Measurements

Following vascular injury, blood platelets rapidly *adhere* to the exposed subendothelium. Collagen and most likely several other subendothelial structures serve as effective platelet stimuli. Although a number of *in vitro* laboratory tests have been used to assess the adhesion properties of platelets, most have now been abandoned due to poor reproducibility. Several newer methods utilizing perfusion of blood samples through arterial strips are currently under research study.

Through activation of the coagulation system (Chap. 32) thrombin is produced, and may serve as another very potent stimulus for platelet activation. Upon stimulation by thrombin, collagen, or various other agents, platelets change in shape from discoid to spherical, extend pseudopods, undergo internal contraction resulting in centralization of their alpha granules and dense core granules, and ultimately release from the cell the contents of these granules. Depending upon the strength of the stimulus, the contents of the alpha, dense core, or even lysosomal granules may be released (Fig. 31–3). During the activation process, alterations in membrane glycoproteins also occur, resulting in the formation of receptors for plasma glycoproteins including fibrinogen (Bennett, 1979) and von Willebrand factor (Fujimoto, 1982a, b). Presumably through bridging provided by these glycoproteins, in the presence of calcium, platelets now show a stickiness not only toward subendothelial surfaces but toward each other, resulting in *platelet aggregation. In vivo,* aggregates of platelets reinforced by fibrin are termed *thrombi.*

The initial laboratory evaluation of platelets includes a *platelet count.* This measurement has now become a routine component of the CBC in an era of electronic particle counting instrumentation. Evaluation of the peripheral blood film should permit at least a rough corroboration of the measured count. In cases of severe thrombocytopenia, or whenever cellular fragments may be spuriously affecting the automated count, a manual phase contrast count with a hemocytometer chamber should be performed (Brecher, 1950). The reference interval for the platelet count is approximately 150 to 400 × 10^9/L.

No currently available laboratory test faithfully reflects the platelets' ability to accomplish their enormously complex series of functions in a manner consistent with normal hemostasis. A carefully performed template *bleeding time* test using either a standardized template (Mielke, 1969) or a disposable, spring-loaded blade (described in detail by Hoyer, 1982) is probably the best overall screening test yet available. In these tests a blood pressure cuff is placed around the upper arm and is inflated to maintain a constant pressure of 40 mm Hg. A standardized cut is then made on the volar surface of the forearm, a timer is started, and at 30-second intervals the resulting drops of blood are blotted with filter paper (with care that the paper does not directly touch the wound edge itself). When blood no longer stains the filter paper, the timer is stopped. Above platelet counts of 100 × 10^9/L, bleeding times should fall within the laboratory's established reference interval (Thompson, 1983). Prolonged bleeding times in such cases are most frequently associated with the prior ingestion of drugs having an anti-platelet action (e.g., aspirin), von Willebrand's disease, or congenital platelet abnormalities.

Further evaluation of a suspected defect of platelet function can be obtained through laboratory study of *platelet aggregation and secretion* in response to a battery of platelet stimulating agents. When citrated platelet-rich plasma is continuously stirred in a *platelet aggregometer* and a light beam passed through the suspension, platelet aggregation in response to an added chemical stimulus can be monitored by changes in light transmittance (Born, 1962). Discoid to spheroid shape change is seen as an initial decrease in transmittance, whereas the subsequent formation of platelet clumps allows more light to pass through the suspension to the photodetector and is recorded as an increase in light transmittance. In instruments equipped with a second channel for monitoring secretion, the release of ATP from platelet dense granules is simultaneously measured. This is accomplished by adding the firefly luminescence substrate and enzyme, luciferin and luciferase, to the platelet-rich plasma; released ATP then functions as a cofactor in the light-producing luciferin-luciferase reaction, and light emission is recorded with a second photodetector. Because of separation of wavelengths, the aggregation and release channels can be monitored independently (Fig. 31–4). The release of ATP in most cases may be assumed to reflect the release of the other constituents of dense granules, which are less easily measured (i.e., ADP, serotonin, calcium). Currently utilized platelet stimuli include various concentrations of collagen, epinephrine, ADP, ristocetin, and the calcium ionophore A23187 (Fig. 31–5). Arachidonic acid or cryoprecipitate may also serve as useful stimuli in appropriate

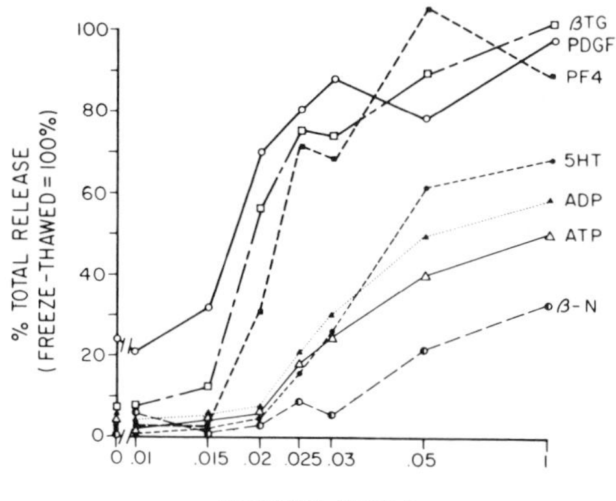

Figure 31–3. Platelet release reaction as a function of stimulus strength. With increasing thrombin concentrations, constituents of the alpha granules (platelet factor 4, PF4; platelet-derived growth factor, PDGF; β-thromboglobulin, βTG), dense granules (ATP; ADP; serotonin, 5HT), and lysosomal granules (β-N-acetylglycosaminidase, β-N) are released. (From Witte, L.D., et al.: Circ. Res., *42*:402, 1978.)

4

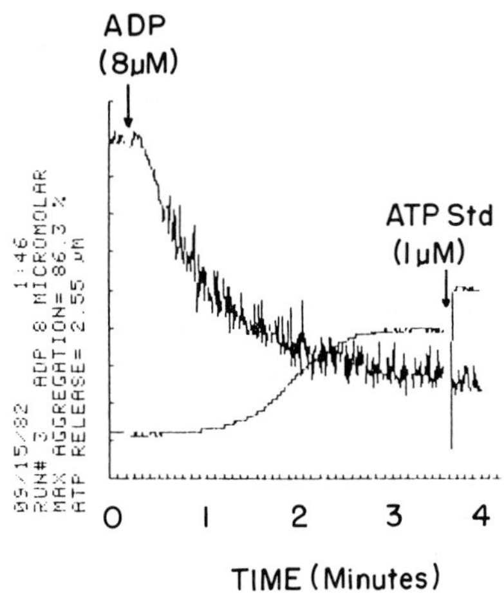

Figure 31–4. Simultaneously measured platelet aggregation and secretion of ATP. Upper trace: Platelet aggregation. Increasing aggregation shown as downward deflection, with platelet-rich plasma initially set at 90 per cent full vertical scale and platelet-poor plasma at 10 per cent. Lower trace: Platelet secretion. Increasing secretion of ATP shown as upward deflection. As indicated by right arrow, ATP was added following the secretory response as an internal calibration standard. Data corresponding to the measurements are indicated to the left of the traces. (From Miller, J. L.: Am. J. Clin. Path., *81*:471, 1984.

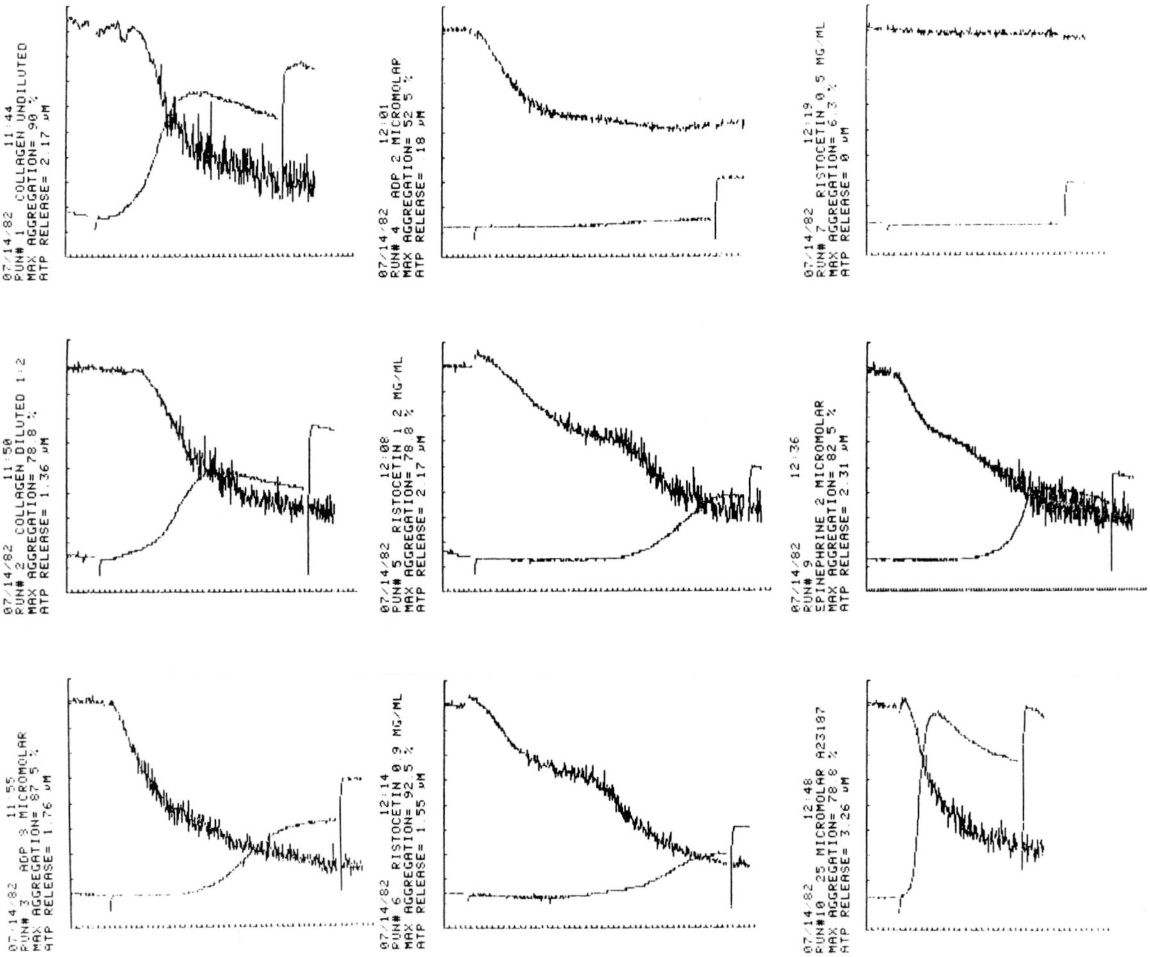

Figure 31–5. Composite of normal platelet aggregation and ATP secretion tracings in response to a series of platelet stimulatory agents. All tracings represent a full-scale time-base of 5 minutes except for run No. 9 (2 μM epinephrine) which represents 10 minutes. (From Miller, J. L.: Am. J. Clin. Path., *81*: in press, 1984.

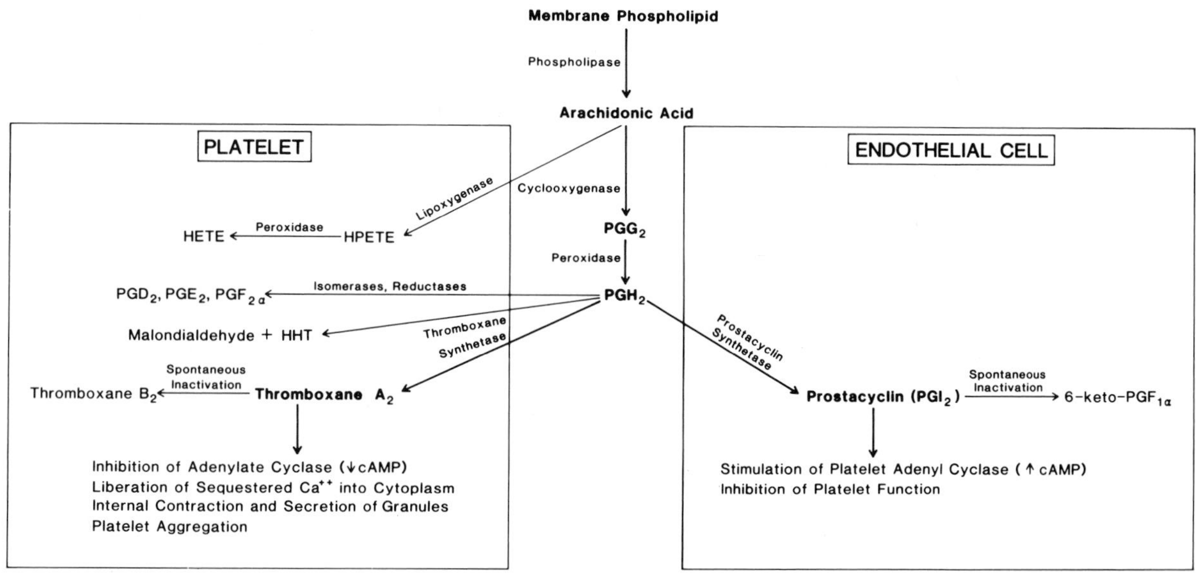

Figure 31–6. Pathways of arachidonic acid metabolism in platelets and endothelial cells. Thrombin or other stimuli promote the liberation of arachidonic acid from membrane phospholipid through the action of phospholipases.

circumstances. Although clearly of paramount importance as a platelet stimulus *in vivo,* thrombin is difficult to employ with platelet-rich plasma, due to interference from the formation of fibrin. The partially trypsinized γ-thrombin, however, retains platelet stimulating activity but largely lacks clotting activity and may prove useful (Charo, 1977). Approaches for testing platelet aggregation may be found in Coller (1979) and Triplett (1978) and for the simultaneous testing of platelet aggregation and ATP secretion in Miller (1984).

The contractile abilities of activated platelets also result in contraction (or "retraction") of formed clots. In the test tube, *clot retraction* may be quantitatively assessed (Owen, 1969). In thrombocytopenia or in Glanzmann's thrombasthenia, clot retraction is delayed or incomplete.

Not only do platelets serve as the key mediators of primary hemostasis, but also in a number of activation steps of coagulation factors. Platelets have been shown to have a role in the activation of "contact factors" XII and XI (Walsh, 1972a and b; Ogston, 1981), to provide highly ordered phospholipoprotein surfaces for the activation of factors IX, X, and prothrombin (Table 32–2), and to contain endogenous factor V which appears to play a key role in the formation of a receptor on the platelet surface for activated factor X (Miletich, 1978). Study of these various procoagulant activities of patient platelets is not currently standard in most laboratories, but may be indicated in individual situations.

Pathways of Platelet Activation by Platelet Stimuli

Despite a great amount of research upon platelet physiology and pharmacology, a clear understanding of the actual sequence of reactions following initial platelet stimulation has not yet been achieved. Rather, a number of events are known to occur, and interruption of the events by either acquired or congenital abnormalities has been shown to have varying detrimental effects, depending upon the stimulus being employed. In particular, the mobilization of arachidonic acid from membrane phospholipids, and its metabolism through the cyclooxygenase pathway to the potent pro-aggregatory agent thromboxane A_2 (Fig. 31–6), is now a well-defined intermediary mechanism occurring in response to a variety of platelet stimuli. However, even after potent cyclooxygenase-inhibiting agents such as acetylsalicylic acid (aspirin) have fully blocked this pathway, strong stimuli such as thrombin, high concentrations of collagen, and A23187 remain capable of producing full aggregatory responses. This suggests that at least one pathway, and possibly still others, exist within the platelet and remain to be elucidated.

Except in the case of simple cell agglutination, such as is induced by ristocetin, all platelet aggregating agents require the presence of free calcium ions. The roles of calcium in platelet function appear multiple, including promotion of platelet contractile and secretory phenomena and of the formation (or unmasking) of membrane receptors. Agents which interfere with intra-platelet calcium fluxes (e.g., local anesthetics), calcium-binding proteins (e.g., phenothiazines), or extracellular free calcium (e.g., chelating agents) may accordingly be expected to produce inhibitory results when platelet function is tested (Feinstein, 1981).

QUANTITATIVE PLATELET DISORDERS

Thrombocytopenia

Decreased numbers of circulating platelets can result from a wide variety of causes (Table 31–1), and

4

Table 31–1. MECHANISMS UNDERLYING THROMBOCYTOPENIA*

A. Disorders of production
   1. Decreased megakaryocytopoiesis
      a. Congenital disorders (Fanconi's anemia, TAR syndrome, intrauterine drugs or infection, etc.)
      b. Acquired hypoplasia (radiation, chemicals, alcohol, insecticides, drugs such as thiazides, chloramphenicol, or cancer chemotherapy, infections, lupus erythematosus, idiopathic, etc.)
      c. Marrow replacement (metastatic carcinoma, myeloma, leukemia, lymphoma, myelofibrosis, etc.)
   2. Ineffective platelet production
      a. Hereditary thrombocytopenia (autosomal dominant, May-Hegglin anomaly, Wiskott-Aldrich syndrome, etc.)
      b. B_{12} or folate deficiency
      c. Other (di Guglielmo's syndrome, paroxysmal nocturnal hemoglobinuria, preleukemia, etc.)

B. Disorders of distribution and dilution
   1. Splenic pooling (congestive, infiltrative, inflammatory, infectious, hyperplastic, neoplastic etc.)
   2. Hypothermia
   3. Dilution by transfused stored blood

C. Disorders of destruction
   1. Combined consumption
      a. Snake venoms
      b. Tissue injury (surgical, trauma, anoxia, toxic necrosis, etc.)
      c. Obstetrical complications (abruptio placentae, retained dead fetus, amniotic fluid embolism, toxemia, etc.)
      d. Neoplasms (promyelocytic leukemia, carcinoma, hemangioma, etc.)
      e. Infection (bacterial, viral, rickettsial, etc.)
      f. Intravascular hemolysis
   2. Isolated platelet consumption
      a. Thrombotic thrombocytopenic purpura
      b. Hemolytic-uremic syndrome
      c. Vasculitis (disseminated lupus erythematosus, other collagen vascular disease, bacteremia, etc.)
      d. Cardiopulmonary prostheses
   3. Immune destruction
      a. Autoimmune (acute, chronic, transplacental, secondary, etc.)
      b. Post-transfusion purpura
      c. Isoimmune neonatal purpura
      d. Drug-induced antibodies (gold, quinine, quinidine, sulfonamide derivatives, etc.)
      e. Others

D. Combination thrombocytopenia
      a. Alcoholic liver disease
      b. Lymphoproliferative disorders
      c. Cardiopulmonary bypass
      d. Others (malignancies, infection, etc.)

*From Burstein, S. A., and Harker, L. A.: *In* Bloom, A. L., and Thomas, D. P. (eds.): Haemostasis and Thrombosis. Edinburgh, Churchill Livingstone, 1981.

Table 31–2. FEATURES OF ACUTE AND CHRONIC ITP*

	Acute	Chronic
Peak age incidence	Children 2–6 years of age	Adults, 20–40 years of age
Sex predilection	None	3:1 ratio of female to male patients
Antecedent infection	Common 1–3 weeks prior to onset	Unusual
Onset of bleeding	Abrupt	Insidious
Hemorrhagic bullae in mouth	Present in severe cases	Usually absent
Platelet count	$<20 \times 10^9$/L	30–80 $\times 10^9$/L
Eosinophilia and lymphocytosis	Common	Rare
Duration	2–6 weeks; rarely longer	Months or years
Spontaneous remissions	Occur in 80% of cases	Uncommon; fluctuating course common

*From Bithell, T. C.: Thrombocytopenia. *In* Wintrobe, M. M., et al. (eds.): Clinical Hematology. 8th ed. Philadelphia, Lea and Febiger, 1981, Chapter 47.

the resulting bleeding tendency may be the first sign of an underlying disease process. Usually the clinical history will permit differentiation between an acquired and a congenital process, although some congenital thrombocytopenias (e.g., those associated with Fanconi's anemia) are typically delayed three to ten years in onset.

Acquired aplastic anemias involving the erythroid and granulocytic lines as well as the megakaryocytic line are seen more commonly than are pure megakaryocytic aplasias. Toxic chemical exposures, viral illnesses, and, frequently, unexplained causes may underlie the aplasia.

Study of the bone marrow is usually required in order to assess whether the thrombocytopenia is due at least in part to a failure of platelet production. Bone marrow aspirates are often less reliable than bone marrow biopsies for ascertaining actual numbers of megakaryocytes present. In some instances abnormalities in megakaryocyte structure may be found, although the mere presence of an increased proportion of the more immature, basophilic megakaryocytic forms must not be taken as evidence of a qualitative megakaryocytic disorder.

In contrast to estimations of megakaryocyte numbers, it is usually difficult to assess abnormalities in megakaryocyte size or lobulation pattern from biopsy or clot sections. This is due to the fact that one section may sample only a small portion of the relatively large megakaryocyte cell. For such purposes a well prepared Romanowsky stain on an aspirate smear or on a biopsy touch preparation is typically most helpful.

Decreased numbers of circulating platelets may be seen with *splenomegaly* of any cause, due to the resulting increase in *sequestration of platelets* by the spleen. A compensatory increase in platelet production is usually seen (Thompson, 1983).

One of the most important and frequently encountered forms of enhanced consumption of platelets is in the acquired disorder *immunologic thrombocytopenic purpura* (ITP). The clinical history will usually be most helpful in arriving at a tentative diagnosis, and in particular in distinguishing between the acute and chronic forms of ITP (Table 31–2). The study of platelet-associated immunoglobulins in patients suspected of having ITP has been widely employed in recent years in an effort to identify immune-mediated processes. However, more recent investigations have cast serious doubt upon the predictive value of positive findings in such cases, due to increasing awareness that immunoglobulin not influencing platelet survival or function may be associated with platelets in a wide variety of clinical settings (Kelton, 1982). Such problems in interpretation would probably not apply, however, to the demonstration of anti-platelet antibodies in patient serum that can be demonstrated to bind to platelets only in the presence of specific drugs (e.g., quinidine). A variety of different techniques are available for the demonstration of platelet-associated immunoglobulins (e.g., von dem Borne, 1980; Dixon, 1975; Cines, 1979; Faig, 1982).

More definitive assessment of platelet survival may be accomplished by labeling either the patient's own or heterologous platelets with a radioactive isotope and following the survival of the reinfused platelets (Shulman, 1982a). The ^{51}chromium and DF ^{32}P labels used in the past provide a number of methodological problems, and have been increasingly supplanted by ^{111}indium. The radiation exposure and requirement for technical proficiency in performing these studies have tended to restrict their frequent application in most centers. A non-isotopic method based upon the recovery of malondialdehyde formation in platelets newly released from the marrow following aspirin ingestion is also available (Stuart, 1975).

It must be emphasized that other routine studies may provide very helpful correlative data for elucidating the cause of a thrombocytopenia. The blood film will frequently reveal fragmented erythrocytes in *thrombotic thrombocytopenic purpura* (TTP) or the *hemolytic-uremic syndrome* (HUS). In the acute phase of *disseminated intravascular coagulation* (DIC) there will often be an associated hypofibrinogenemia and an increase of fibrin(ogen) degradation products (see Chap. 32). Isoimmune neonatal thrombocytopenia (Shulman, 1982b) should be suspected when thrombocytopenia occurs in the newborn period.

Thrombocytosis

Increased platelet counts, or thrombocytosis, may be seen both as a benign, reactive process and as a manifestation of a myeloproliferative disorder (Table 31–3; see also Chap. 30). The blood film should confirm an electronic cell count, showing that the increased particles in fact correspond to platelets and not to cell fragments or other entities. The smear also affords an opportunity to assess deviations in platelet size, morphological appearance, and clumping tendencies. In autonomous thrombocytoses which are part

4

Table 31–3. CAUSES OF THROMBOCYTOSIS*

A. Autonomous thrombocytosis
   1. Essential thrombocytosis (thrombocythemia)
   2. Myeloproliferative disorders (polycythemia vera, myelofibrosis, chronic myelogenous leukemia)
B. Reactive thrombocytosis
   1. Iron deficiency
   2. Inflammatory disease
   3. Malignancy
   4. Splenectomy
   5. Drugs
   6. Redistribution of platelets
   7. Rebound thrombocytosis
   8. Other pathological conditions
C. Other forms (dyshematopoiesis, etc.)

*From Burstein, S. A., and Harker, L. A.: *In* Bloom, A. L., and Thomas, D. P. (eds.): Haemostasis and Thrombosis. Edinburgh, Churchill Livingstone, 1981.

of myeloproliferative syndromes, large hypogranular platelets may sometimes be seen.

It has been stated that reactive processes typically do not produce platelet counts over 1000×10^9/L but that myeloproliferative processes frequently do; nonetheless, this criterion is reliable neither for diagnosis nor for the decision whether to institute antiplatelet therapy. Particularly in the case of myeloproliferative syndromes, the individual patient may be asymptomatic, have a tendency to bleed, or have a tendency to thrombose; at present, the most appropriate clinical approach appears to be a response to such tendencies once they become evident. In documented cases of myeloproliferative syndromes there have been reports of abnormalities in platelet and megakaryocyte structure, platelet surface membrane receptors, platelet aggregation patterns, platelet coagulant activity, and arachidonic acid metabolism (see review by Murphy, 1983). However, no unified set of diagnostic criteria has yet emerged in this field.

INHERITED DISORDERS OF PLATELET FUNCTION (Table 31–4)

Surface Membrane Abnormalities

Our understanding of qualitative platelet disorders in molecular terms has perhaps made the greatest advance in two disorders involving abnormalities of surface membrane glycoproteins, Glanzmann's thrombasthenia and Bernard-Soulier disease. Laboratory evaluation of these disorders is correspondingly well developed.

In non-anticoagulated blood films prepared from patients with *Glanzmann's thrombasthenia,* platelets typically are present in normal number and individually normal in appearance, but show a characteristic tendency to remain isolated, without the platelet-platelet clumping seen in normal blood films. In the aggregometer, platelets show a striking failure to aggregate in response to all aggregating agents. Ristocetin does induce an initial agglutination and a normal degree of release, but disagglutination then follows rather than a secondary wave corresponding to true aggregation. The platelet release reaction also usually proceeds normally with strong stimuli such as calcium ionophore or thrombin, but may be diminished with collagen or the weaker stimuli, ADP and epinephrine. Clot retraction is decreased, mildly to severely.

A rather wide variety of additional cellular abnormalities were described in the earlier literature on Glanzmann's thrombasthenia. However, a unifying concept of this disease emerged from the studies by Nurden and Caen (1974) and by Phillips and coworkers (1975, 1977) that *all* patients with Glanzmann's thrombasthenia shared a decrease in content of surface membrane glycoproteins IIb and IIIa. Studies of platelet surface antigens have also revealed a significant decrease of both the Zw^a (Pl^{A1}) and Zw^b antigens in these patients, thus providing an additional, apparently fairly specific test for this entity (Kunicki, 1978a; van Leeuwen, 1981). Recently, a monoclonal antibody assay for platelet membrane glycoproteins has been reported for the diagnosis of Glanzmann's thrombasthenia, as well as of Bernard-Soulier disease (see below), requiring only small volumes of whole blood for the assay (Montgomery, 1983).

Very likely as a consequence of their abnormality of glycoproteins IIb and IIIa, platelets from patients with Glanzmann's thrombasthenia fail to bind ^{125}I-fibrinogen following stimulation with ADP or epinephrine (Bennett, 1979; Mustard, 1979). This lack of the normally inducible fibrinogen-binding sites appears a likely candidate for the dominant pathological lesion in Glanzmann's thrombasthenia. Decreases in α-actinin and internal platelet fibrinogen have also been reported in some patients with Glanzmann's thrombasthenia, but their role in the etiology of the platelet dysfunction is presently less clear.

The blood film from a patient with *Bernard-Soulier disease* may resemble that from some patients with immunologic thrombocytopenic purpura (ITP) in that the platelets tend to be larger than normal, and there is a mild to moderate thrombocytopenia. Findings in the aggregometer are almost the reciprocal of those in Glanzmann's thrombasthenia: aggregation and release are normal with all agents *except* ristocetin. In addition, the release reaction induced by thrombin may be decreased.

Unlike von Willebrand's disease (vWD), in which there is also diminished platelet agglutination in response to ristocetin, in Bernard-Soulier disease the addition of exogenous vWF (present in plasma cryoprecipitate fractions) does not restore ristocetin-induced agglutination of platelets. This important difference is attributable to the finding that whereas in vWD there is a deficiency in plasma von Willebrand factor, in Bernard-Soulier disease the deficiency is in the platelet membrane receptor to which the von Willebrand factor must bind for normal hemostasis.

When platelet surface membrane glycoproteins from patients with Bernard-Soulier disease are analyzed, glycoproteins Ib, Is, and, more recently (Nurden, 1981; Clemetson, 1982), V have been found to be decreased. Although direct proof is still lacking, the failure of von Willebrand factor to agglutinate Bernard-Soulier platelets in the presence of ristocetin is widely believed to be attributable to the deficiency of glycoprotein Ib (Phillips, 1980). Additionally, diminished responsiveness of these platelets to thrombin may be due to the abnormality in glycoprotein V. As with Glanzmann's platelets, a distinct antigenic abnormality may also be detected in Bernard-Soulier platelets: whereas virtually all normal platelets possess an antigenic site for antiplatelet antibodies arising in patients with a hypersensitivity to quinidine or to quinine, platelets from patients with Bernard-Soulier disease do not appear to have this receptor (Kunicki, 1978b). Absence of this normal platelet antigenic moiety may also be attributable to the abnormal glycoproteins in this disorder.

An autosomal dominant bleeding disorder termed

platelet-type von Willebrand's disease (Miller, 1982) has recently been described in which patients characteristically have low-normal platelet counts, normal factor VIII coagulant activity and VIII-related antigen, and decreased ristocetin cofactor activity (see discussion of von Willebrand's disease in Chap. 32, p. 775). An apparently similar disorder in a family studied by Weiss (1982b) has been termed pseudo–von Willebrand's disease. On agarose gel electrophoresis of plasma there is a selective decrease of the higher molecular weight multimers, similar to that seen in Type II von Willebrand's disease. However, unlike platelets from patients with Type II von Willebrand's disease, platelets from patients with platelet-type von Willebrand's disease show an increased ability to bind normal von Willebrand factor (Miller, 1983). In the diagnostic laboratory this increased binding is reflected by the ability of unusually low concentrations of ristocetin (0.3 to 0.5 mg/ml) to produce strong aggregation of platelets in this disorder, a finding also observed in Type IIB von Willebrand's disease (Ruggeri, 1980). Cryoprecipitate, however, when added to platelet-type vWD platelets without additional aggregating agents, is capable of inducing aggregation; cryoprecipitate added to normal or to Type IIB vWD platelets, in contrast, does not produce aggregation (Fig. 31–7).

Storage Granule Abnormalities

A variety of platelet disorders have been described that involve as their primary abnormality a deficiency of one or more types of storage granules. Several syndromes involving the dense storage granules in particular are now recognized, all of which are associated with additional clinical abnormalities distinct from those of the platelets themselves (see review by Nichols, 1981).

In the *Hermansky-Pudlak* syndrome (Hermansky, 1959) patients have a deficiency of dense granules. They characteristically manifest an oculocutaneous albinism, and macrophages of their reticuloendothelial system contain ceroid-like deposits. Patients with the *Chédiak-Higashi* syndrome may also be partially albino and appear prone to frequent infections. As in granulocytes from patients with this disorder, giant inclusion granules may be found in the platelet cytoplasm. Patients with the Chédiak-Higashi syndrome as well as those with the *Wiskott-Aldrich* syndrome (Grottum, 1969) and the *thrombocytopenia with absent radii (TAR)* syndrome (Day, 1972) have a decreased platelet count in addition to deficiencies in dense granule content. Unlike the other syndromes, which show autosomal recessive patterns of inheritance, Wiskott-Aldrich syndrome is sex-linked.

Patients with disorders involving the dense granules characteristically show diminished platelet aggregation, particularly of the second phase, with the weaker agents (ADP, epinephrine, low concentrations of collagen). However, arachidonic acid and higher concentrations of the weaker agents, as well as the stronger agents (calcium ionophore, thrombin), may produce a relatively normal degree of aggregation. Since the release of dense granule materials (ADP, ATP, serotonin, calcium) is decreased in such patients, these findings provide additional support for the emerging concept that the stronger agents induce aggregation by *multiple pathways,* including mechanisms largely or wholly independent of the release of intracellular ADP (Huang, 1980). In storage granule abnormalities, assay of *total* cellular content of ATP and ADP reveals a characteristic increase in the ratio of ATP to ADP, reflecting decreased nucleotides in the dense granular storage pool. This is due to the lower ATP:ADP ratio (2:3) in the storage pool compared to a much higher ratio (8:1 to 10:1) in the cytoplasmic metabolic pool (Weiss, 1982a). Finally, though patients with *Down's* syndrome appear to have a normal content of platelet dense granules, an abnormality of serotonin uptake into these dense granules has been reported (McCoy, 1978).

Patients possessing an absence of the *alpha granules* have also been described. Because of the pale gray color of these large platelets on Romanowsky-stained blood films, this disorder has been named the *gray platelet* syndrome (Raccuglia, 1971). By electron microscopy there appears to be a selective decrease of the alpha granules (White, 1979), and biochemical analyses have confirmed associated decreases in cellular content of platelet fibrinogen, platelet factor 4, beta-thromboglobulin, and platelet-derived growth factor. Both aggregation and the platelet release reaction have been reported to be characteristically decreased in these patients.

In addition to patients showing a selective decrease of either alpha or dense granules, a growing number of cases have now been reported in which a combined deficiency of alpha and dense granules appears to exist. These cases presently appear heterogeneous and await more detailed characterization.

Finally, a number of patients with varying degrees of clinical bleeding appear to have a normal complement of storage granules, but secretion by their platelets is somehow impaired. Although the mechanism(s) for such impairment remains largely unknown, possible abnormalities in calcium mobilization, cyclic nucleotide metabolism, and cytoskeletal proteins are currently under investigation.

Deficiencies of Thromboxane Generation

Several patients have now been reported whose platelets fail to respond to arachidonic acid but show a normal aggregation and release pattern in response to the endoperoxide PGG_2. In those cases in which the possibility of drug ingestion can be absolutely eliminated, patients with this "aspirin-like" defect appear to have a deficiency of the cyclooxygenase enzyme (Nichols, 1981). The possibility of a deficiency of thromboxane synthetase has also been considered in several patients, but the definite existence of such a clinical entity still remains to be established.

Table 31–4. DIAGNOSTIC CRITERIA FOR INHERITED DISORDERS OF PLATELET FUNCTION*

Major Categories	Aggregation Pattern in Platelet-Rich Plasma	Release of ATP and Serotonin	Inheritance	Other Characteristic Abnormalities
I. Surface membrane defects				
Glanzmann's thrombasthenia	Markedly decreased with all agents except ristocetin (which may show a reversible single phase)	Normal with thrombin, calcium ionophore, and ristocetin; may be decreased with collagen, ADP, and epinephrine	Autosomal recessive	Decreased clot retraction; decreased platelet clumping on blood smear; glycoproteins IIb and IIIa decreased or absent; fibrinogen receptor, $Zw^a(Pl^{a1})$ and Zw^b antigens, and α-actinin decreased; internal platelet fibrinogen may be decreased
Bernard-Soulier disease	Markedly decreased with ristocetin, without correction by von Willebrand factor; decreased with thrombin; normal response to other agents	Decreased with ristocetin	Autosomal	Platelets appear large on blood smear and are frequently decreased in number; glycoproteins Ib, Is, and possibly V decreased; decreased receptor for quinidine-dependent antibodies; decreased adhesiveness to glass beads or to subendothelium
II. Platelet-type von Willebrand's disease	Increased at low ristocetin concentrations; addition of cryoprecipitate by itself produces aggregation; normal response to other agents	Cryoprecipitate by itself produces release; normal with other agents	Autosomal	Borderline thrombocytopenia; selective decrease of higher molecular weight von Willebrand factor multimers in plasma; increased platelet binding of normal von Willebrand factor
III. Granule defects				
Dense granule deficiencies (Hermansky-Pudlak, Chédiak-Higashi, Wiskott-Aldrich, and thrombocytopenia with absent radii syndromes, or as an isolated abnormality)	Decreased aggregation, particularly of second phase, with weak agents; usually normal response to arachidonic acid, calcium ionophore, and high concentrations of weaker agents	Decreased	Autosomal (except for Wiskott-Aldrich syndrome, which is sex-linked)	Decreased dense granule content of ADP, ATP, 5-HT, and calcium; increased total platelet ATP:ADP ratio; oculocutaneous albinism and reticuloendothelial ceroid deposition in Hermansky-Pudlak; thrombocytopenia associated with Chédiak-Higashi, Wiskott-Aldrich, and thrombocytopenia with absent radii; decreased autologous platelet survival and an increase in platelet-associated IgG is seen in Wiskott-Aldrich syndrome

Alpha granule deficiencies (gray platelet syndrome)	Decreased with all agents	Decreased with all agents	Autosomal	Large, pale-appearing platelets on blood smear, accompanied by thrombocytopenia; decreased alpha granules by electron microscopy; decreased cellular content of platelet fibrinogen, platelet factor 4, β-thromboglobulin, and platelet-derived growth factor
Combined dense and alpha granule deficiency	Decreased	Decreased		Heterogeneity of granule deficiencies reported
IV. Defects in platelet arachidonic acid metabolism (platelet cyclooxygenase deficiency)	Decreased with weak agents; unresponsive to arachidonic acid but normal response to platelet endoperoxides	Decreased with weak agents; normal response to platelet endoperoxides		Formation of lipoxygenase products from exogenous ^{14}C-arachidonic acid appears to be normal
V. Miscellaneous Isolated disorders of aggregation and/or release; as a concomitant finding in a variety of pathologic states including Epstein syndrome, the May-Hegglin anomaly, inherited disorders of connective tissue, glycogen storage disease type I, fructose 1:6-diphosphatase deficiency, Down's syndrome, and congenital (cyanotic and acyanotic) heart disease	Variable	Variable		Heterogeneity of defects

*Modified from Stuart, M. J., and Miller, J. L.: *In* Brain, M. C., and McColloch, P. B. (eds.): Current Therapy in Hematology-Oncology 1983–84. Philadelphia, B. C. Decker, Inc., 1983.

4

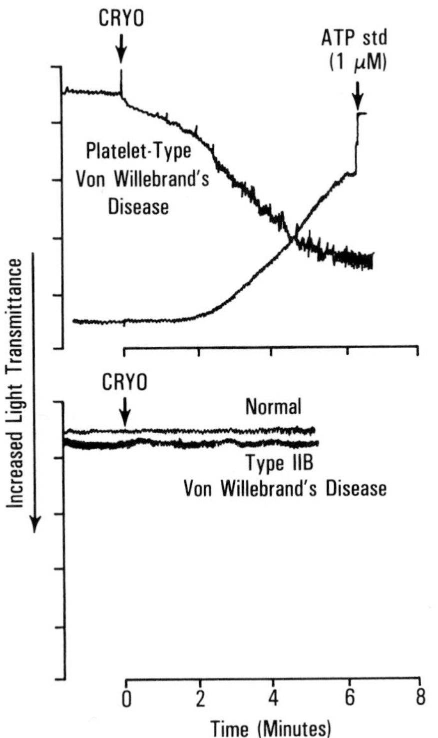

Figure 31–7. Differentiation of platelet-type vWD from Type IIB vWD. Addition of cryoprecipitate alone to platelet-rich plasma of patients with platelet-type vWD produces aggregation and ATP secretion, but is without effect in normal individuals or in patients with Type IIB vWD. (Reproduced from Miller, J. L., et al.: J. Clin. Invest., *72:* 1532, 1983, by copyright permission of the American Society for Clinical Investigation.)

ACQUIRED DISORDERS OF PLATELET FUNCTION

Patients with previously normal hemostasis may acquire a variety of disorders of platelet function. The most frequent cause is ingestion of drugs having inhibitory effects upon platelets (see below), but a number of other disease states may also adversely affect platelet function.

Patients with *myeloproliferative disorders* may present not only with abnormalities of platelet numbers (see above) but also with qualitative platelet abnormalities. These abnormalities may be at the level of platelet membrane glycoproteins (Bolin, 1977), membrane receptors for platelet agonists or antagonists (Kaywin, 1978; Ganguly, 1978; Cooper, 1978), platelet coagulant activity (Walsh, 1977), adenine nucleotide content (Cowan, 1975; Rendu, 1979), or prostaglandin synthesis (Keenan, 1977; Schafer, 1982; Jubelirer, 1980; Pareti, 1982). Studies of platelet aggregation may be helpful, most frequently revealing decreased responsiveness to epinephrine (Spaet, 1969) or to other platelet stimuli. Structural abnormalities have been identified not only in the platelets (Maldonado, 1974b) but also in the megakaryocytes (Maldonado, 1974a) in a number of patients with myeloproliferative disorders. Demonstration of platelet peroxidase activity through ultrastructural cytochemistry, moreover, may permit the identification of megakaryocytic lineage in blast crises of CML (Breton-Gorius, 1978) or in other hematologic neoplasms.

Patients with myeloma or lymphoproliferative disorders associated with *paraproteins* frequently have been observed to have prolonged bleeding times and abnormal platelet function (Perkins, 1970; Penny, 1971; Lackner, 1973). It has been proposed that coating of the platelet by immunoglobulin may be responsible for impaired aggregation (Bang, 1972), but other mechanisms may also be involved.

Open heart surgery utilizing *cardiopulmonary bypass* is typically associated both with a decrease in the number of circulating platelets and with the development of platelet functional defects (McKenna, 1975). Depletion of platelet α-granules (Harker, 1980) following bypass has been reported. The infusion of prostacyclin during bypass surgery in experimental animals at doses too low to prevent the release of granule proteins did, nevertheless, prevent prolongation of bleeding times (Malpass, 1981). This finding underscores the complexities involved in elucidating mechanisms underlying hemostatic impairment in such procedures. Additionally, activation of both the coagulation and fibrinolytic systems, anticoagulation with heparin, and neutralization of heparin with protamine—events that typically accompany open heart surgery—clearly may contribute to the development of a hemostatic imbalance.

Acquired storage pool deficiency has been reported in patients with systemic lupus erythematosus and other autoimmune disorders (Regan, 1974; Zahavi, 1974; Weiss, 1980), chronic ITP (Clancy, 1972), disseminated intravascular coagulation (Pareti, 1976), and a variety of other hematologic or non-hematologic disorders. The mechanisms leading to deficiencies appear to be varied. Deficiencies of platelet dense granules have been demonstrated in isolated platelets both by means of altered ATP:ADP ratios (see above) and by abnormalities of serotonin uptake (Pareti, 1980).

Patients with *uremia* have long been known to suffer impairment of primary hemostasis. The increased blood levels of guanidinosuccinic acid (Horowitz, 1970) and phenolic acids (Rabiner, 1970) that may be found in uremic patients have been shown capable of inducing dysfunction of normal platelets *in vitro.* Recently, moreover, increased vascular prostacyclin production (Remuzzi, 1977) and decreased platelet thromboxane production (Smith, 1981) have been reported in uremic patients, both of which alterations would be expected to contribute to impaired hemostasis. Finally, though the mechanism of action remains unclear, patients with uremia have been reported recently to have experienced significant hemostatic improvement following transfusion of cryoprecipitate (Janson, 1980).

Platelet function is inhibited both *in vivo* and *in vitro* by a great number of *drugs.* Some of the major

Table 31–5. DRUGS CAPABLE OF INHIBITING PLATELET FUNCTION*

Agents that affect prostanoid synthesis:
- Aspirin
  - Corticosteroids
  - Others (e.g., indomethacin, phenylbutazone, ibuprofen, fenprofen, naproxen, sulfinpyrazone, furosemide, vitamin E)

Adenylate cyclase activators:
- Prostanoids (e.g., prostacyclin, PGE_1, PGD_2)
- Others (e.g., isoprenaline, adenosine)

Phosphodiesterase inhibitors:
- Pyrimidopyrimidines (e.g., dipyridamole)
- Methyl xanthines (e.g., caffeine, theophylline, aminophylline, papaverine)

Antimicrobial agents:
- Penicillins and cephalothins (e.g., carbenicillin, penicillin G, ticarcillin, ampicillin, cephalothin)
- Others (e.g., nitrofurantoin, ristocetin, hydroxychloroquin)

Membrane stabilizing agents:
- Local anesthetics (e.g., procaine, Xylocaine)
- Antihistamines (e.g., diphenhydramine, promethazine)
- Tricyclic antidepressants (e.g, imipramine, nortriptyline)

Sympathic blocking agents:
- Alpha-antagonists (e.g., phentolamine)
- Beta-antagonists (e.g., propranolol)

Miscellaneous drugs
- Heparin
- Dextrans
- Ethanol
- Other (phenothiazines, clofibrate, halofenate, reserpine, methysergide)

*From Rao, A. K., and Walsh, P. N.: Clin. Haematol., *12*:201, 1983.

drugs known to impair platelet function are listed according to their mechanism of action upon platelets in Table 31–5. Interpretation of bleeding times or of platelet function tests is complicated considerably when the patient has recently taken one or more such agents. In the case of a drug such as aspirin, which irreversibly acetylates the platelet's cyclooxygenase enzyme, up to ten days must elapse before the affected circulating platelets are fully replaced by new platelets. Elective studies of platelet function should accordingly be planned so as to minimize recent drug exposure, to the extent that abstinence from medications would be unlikely to compromise significantly the health or well-being of the patient.

EVALUATION OF PATIENTS WITH SUSPECTED PLATELET DISORDERS

The evaluation of patients with a clinical history or symptoms suggesting a bleeding tendency involves consideration of the coagulation and fibrinolytic systems (see Chap. 32) as well as of the blood platelets. An approach to such evaluation is outlined in Table 31–6. A carefully conducted history can be the single most important factor leading to a diagnosis in many patients. Determination of whether the disorder is likely to be congenital or acquired is most important. A platelet count in conjunction with a prolonged

Table 31–6. EVALUATION OF PATIENTS WITH SUSPECTED PLATELET DISORDERS*

History and physical examination.
- Detailed evaluation of bleeding tendencies—onset, frequency, duration and severity, transfusion requirement, and characteristic sites of involvement
- Bleeding associated with surgery or trauma—tonsillectomy, tooth extractions, and circumcision
- Drug history—including multi-ingredient formulations that may contain aspirin or other known antiplatelet agents.
- Family history—inheritance pattern and severity of bleeding
- Complete physical examination—including signs of recent bleeding (petechiae, ecchymoses, purpura, etc.), restricted joint mobility, and findings associated with particular congenital abnormalities (absent radii, albinism, telangiectasia, and inherited connective tissue disorders

Coagulation and fibrinolytic system testing
- Screening (and, if indicated, more definitive) tests in order to detect abnormalities not related to platelets

Bleeding time
- Characteristically prolonged in von Willebrand's disease, thrombocytopenia, and functional platelet disorders

Laboratory evaluation of platelets

Basic studies
- Peripheral blood smear—numbers, size, appearance, clumping tendency
- Electronic platelet count—including platelet sizing
- Platelet aggregation (and simultaneous ATP release when firefly luciferin-luciferase reaction utilized) on platelet-rich plasma in response to collagen, ADP, epinephrine, ristocetin, arachidonic acid, and calcium ionophore (A23187)
- Clot retraction

Specialized studies
- Membrane related:
  - Surface membrane glycoprotein characterization
  - Platelet surface antigen assays—$Zw^a(Pl^{A1})$, Zw^b, receptor for quinidine-associated antibody
  - Platelet-ligand binding studies—fibrinogen, thrombin, and von Willebrand factor
  - Platelet adhesiveness studies
  - Studies of uptake and release of radioactive serotonin
- Granule related:
  - Analysis of intracellular constituents—ATP, ADP, serotonin, platelet fibrinogen, platelet factor 4, β-thromboglobulin, platelet-derived growth factor, α-actinin, and lysosomal enzymes
- Miscellaneous:
  - Evaluation of platelet morphology by electron microscopy
  - Evaluation of arachidonic acid metabolism through the cyclooxygenase and lipoxygenase pathways, and evaluation of endoperoxide-induced aggregation
  - Platelet survival
  - Platelet-associated antibody determination
  - Evaluation of platelet coagulant activities

*From Stuart, M. J., and Miller, J. L.: *In* Brain, M. C., and McColloch, P. B. (eds.): Current Therapy in Hematology-Oncology 1983–84. Philadelphia, B. C. Decker, Inc., 1983.

bleeding time will help determine whether the bleeding tendency is explainable by decreased platelet numbers alone, or whether another abnormality is present. Since von Willebrand's disease is far more common than congenital disorders of platelet function, an evaluation of disordered primary hemostasis will frequently necessitate analysis of the factor VIII/von Willebrand factor complex, as discussed in Chapter 32. Finally, although many patients will be adequately diagnosed through the application of basic studies, a number of patients will require one or more of the specialized studies indicated in Table 31–6 in order for a definitive diagnosis to be reached.

Bang, N. U., Heidenreich, R. O., and Trygstad, C. W.: Plasma protein requirements for human platelet aggregation. Ann. N.Y. Acad. Sci., *201*:280, 1972.

Bennett, J. S., and Vilaire, G.: Exposure of platelet fibrinogen receptors by ADP and epinephrine. J. Clin. Invest., *64*:1393, 1979.

Berndt, M. C., and Phillips, D. R.: Platelet membrane proteins: Composition and receptor function. *In* Gordon, J. L. (ed.): Platelets in Biology and Pathology—2. New York, Elsevier/North-Holland Biomedical Press, 1981, pp. 43–75.

Bolin, R. B., Ikumura, T., and Jamieson, G. A.: Changes in distribution of platelet membrane glycoproteins in patients with myeloproliferative disorders. Am. J. Hematol., *3*:63, 1977.

Born, G. V. R.: Aggregation of blood platelets by adenosine diphosphate and its reversal. Nature, *194*:927, 1962.

Brecher, G., and Cronkite, E. P.: Morphology and enumeration of human blood platelets. J. Appl. Physiol., *3*:365, 1950.

Breton-Gorius, J., and Guichard, J.: Ultrastructural localization of peroxidase activity in human platelets and megakaryocytes. Am. J. Path., *66*:277, 1972.

Breton-Gorius, J., Reyes, F., Vernant, J. P., Tulliez, M., and Dreyfus, B.: The blast crisis of chronic granulocytic leukaemia: Megakaryoblastic nature of cells as revealed by the presence of platelet peroxidase: A cytochemical ultrastructural study. Br. J. Haematol., *39*:295, 1978.

Burstein, S. A., and Harker, L. A.: Quantitative platelet disorders. *In* Bloom, A. L., and Thomas, D. P. (eds.): Haemostasis and Thrombosis. Edinburgh, Churchill Livingstone, 1981, pp. 279–300.

Charo, I. F., Feinman, R. D., and Detwiler, T. C.: Interrelations of platelet aggregation and secretion. J. Clin. Invest., *60*:866, 1977.

Cines, D. B., and Schreiber, A. D.: Immune thrombocytopenia: Use of a Coombs antiglobulin test to detect IgG and C3 on platelets. N. Engl. J. Med., *300*:106, 1979.

Clancy, R., Jenkins, E., and Firkin, B.: Qualitative platelet abnormalities in idiopathic thrombocytopenic purpura. N. Engl. J. Med., *286*:622, 1972.

Clemetson, K., McGregor, J. L., James, E., Dechavanne, M., and Lüscher, E. F.: Characterization of the platelet membrane glycoprotein abnormalities in Bernard-Soulier syndrome and comparison with normal by surface-labeling techniques and high-resolution two-dimensional gel electrophoresis. J. Clin. Invest., *70*:304, 1982.

Coller, B. S.: Platelet aggregation by ADP, collagen and ristocetin: A critical review of methodology and analysis. *In* Seligson, D., and Schmidt, R. M. (eds.): CRC Handbook Series in Clinical Laboratory Science, Section I: Hematology, Volume I. Boca Raton, CRC Press, Inc., 1979, pp. 381–396.

Cooper, B., Schafter, A. I., Puchalsky, D., and Handin, R. I.: Platelet resistance to prostaglandin D_2 in patients with myeloproliferative disorders. Blood, *52*:618, 1978.

Cowan, D. H., Graham, R. C., Jr., and Baunach, D.: The platelet defect in leukemia: Platelet ultrastructure, adenine nucleotide metabolism, and the release reaction. J. Clin. Invest., *56*:188, 1975.

Day, H. J., and Holmsen, H.: Platelet adenine nucleotide 'storage pool deficiency' in thrombocytopenic absent radii syndrome. J.A.M.A., *221*:1053, 1972.

Dixon, R., Rosse, W., and Ebbert, L.: Quantitative determination of antibody in idiopathic thrombocytopenic purpura. N. Engl. J. Med., *292*:230, 1975.

Faig, D., and Karpatkin, S.: Cumulative experience with a simplified solid-phase radioimmunoassay for the detection of bound antiplatelet IgG, serum auto-, allo-, and drug-dependent antibodies. Blood, *60*:807, 1982.

Feinstein, M. B., Rodan, G. A., and Cutler, L. S.: Cyclic AMP and calcium in platelet function. *In* Gordon, J. L. (ed.): Platelets in Biology and Pathology—2. New York, Elsevier/North-Holland Biomedical Press, 1981, pp. 437–472.

Fujimoto, T., and Hawiger, J.: Adenosine diphosphate induces binding of von Willebrand factor to human platelets. Nature, *297*:154, 1982a.

Fujimoto, T., Ohara, S., and Hawiger, J.: Thrombin-induced exposure and prostacyclin inhibition of the receptor for factor VIII/von Willebrand factor on human platelets. J. Clin. Invest., *69*:1212, 1982b.

Ganguly, P., Sutherland, S. B., and Bradford, H. R.: Defective binding of thrombin to platelets in myeloid leukemia. Br. J. Haematol., *39*:599, 1978.

Gerrard, J. M., Kindom, S. E., Peterson, D. A., Peller, J., Krantz, K. E., and White, J. G.: Lysophosphatidic acids: Influence on platelet aggregation and intracellular calcium flux. Am. J. Path., *96*:423, 1979.

Grottum, K. A., Hovig, T., Holmsen, H., Abrahamsen, A. F., Jeremic, M., and Seip, M.: Wiskott-Aldrich syndrome: Qualitative platelet defects and short platelet survival. Br. J. Haematol., *17*:373, 1969.

Harker, L. A., Malpass, T. W., Branson, H. E., Hessel, E. A., and Slichter, S. J.: Mechanism of abnormal bleeding in patients undergoing cardiopulmonary bypass: Acquired transient platelet dysfunction associated with selective alpha granule release. Blood, *56*:824, 1980.

Hermansky, F., and Pudlak, P.: Albinism associated with hemorrhagic diathesis and unusual pigmented reticular cells in the bone marrow: Report of two cases with histochemical studies. Blood, *14*:162, 1959.

Horowitz, H. I., Stein, I. M., Cohen, B. D., and White, J. G.: Further studies on the platelet inhibitor effect of guanidinosuccinic acid: Its role in uremic bleeding. Am. J. Med., *49*:336, 1970.

Hoyer, L. W.: The assessment of von Willebrand's disease. *In* Bloom, A. L. (ed.): Methods of Hematology, Vol. 5: The Hemophilias. New York, Churchill-Livingstone, 1982, pp. 106–121.

Huang, E. M., and Detwiler, T. C.: Reassessment of the evidence for the role of secreted ADP in biphasic platelet aggregation: Mechanism of inhibition by creatine phosphate plus creatine phosphokinase. J. Lab. Clin. Med., *95*:59, 1980.

Janson, P. A., Jubelirer, S. J., Weinstein, M. G., and Deykin, D.: Treatment of the bleeding tendency in uremia with cryoprecipitate. N. Engl. J. Med., *303*:1318, 1980.

Jubelirer, S. J., Russell, F., Vaillancourt, R., and Deykin, D.: Platelet arachidonic acid metabolism and platelet function in ten patients with chronic myelogenous leukemia. Blood, *56*:728, 1980.

Kaywin, P., McDonough, M., Insel, P. A., and Shattil, S. J.: Platelet function in essential thrombocythemia: Decreased epinephrine responsiveness associated with a deficiency of platelet α-adrenergic receptors. N. Engl. J. Med., *299*:505, 1978.

Keenan, J. P., Wharton, J., Shepherd, A. J. N., and Bellingham, A. J.: Defective platelet lipid peroxidation in myeloproliferative disorders: A possible defect of prostaglandin synthesis. Br. J. Haematol., *35*:275, 1977.

Kelton, J. G., Powers, P. J., and Carter, C. J.: A prospective study of the usefulness of the measurement of platelet-associated IgG for the diagnosis of idiopathic thrombocytopenic purpura. Blood, *60*:1050, 1982.

Kunicki, T. J., and Aster, R. H.: Deletion of the platelet-specific alloantigen Pl^{A1} from platelets in Glanzmann's thrombasthenia. J. Clin. Invest., *61*:1225, 1978a.

Kunicki, T. J., Johnson, M. M., and Aster, R. H.: Absence of the platelet receptor for drug-dependent antibodies in the Bernard-Soulier syndrome. J. Clin. Invest., *62*:716, 1978b.

Lackner, H.: Hemostatic abnormalities associated with dysproteinemias. Semin. Hematol., *10*:125, 1973.

Maldonado, J. E.: Dysplastic platelets and circulating megakaryocytes in chronic myeloproliferative disease. Blood, *43*:811, 1974a.

Maldonado, J. E., Pintado, T., and Pierre, R. V.: Dysplastic platelets and circulating megakaryocytes in chronic myeloproliferative disease. I. The platelets: Ultrastructure and peroxidase reaction. Blood, *43*:797, 1974b.

Malpass, T. W., Hanson, S. R., Savage, B., Hessel, E. A., and Harker, L. A.: Prevention of acquired transient defect in platelet plug formation by infused prostacyclin. Blood, *57*:736, 1981.

McCoy, E. E., and Enns, L.: Sodium transport, ouabain binding, and (Na^+/K^+)-ATPase activity in Down's syndrome platelets. Pediatr. Res., *12*:685, 1978.

McKenna, R., Bachmann, F., Whittaker, B., Gilson, J. R., and Weinberg, M.: The hemostatic mechanism after open-heart surgery. II. Frequency of abnormal platelet functions during and after extracorporeal circulation. J. Thorac. Cardiovasc. Surg., *70*:298, 1975.

Mielke, C. H., Jr., Kaneshiro, M. M., Maher, I. A., Wiener, J. M., and Rapaport, S. I.: The standardized normal Ivy bleeding time and its prolongation by aspirin. Blood, *34*:204, 1969.

Miletich, J. P., Jackson, C. M., and Majerus, P. W.: Properties of the factor Xa binding site on human platelets. J. Biol. Chem., *253*:6908, 1978.

Miller, J. L.: Platelet function testing: An improved approach utilizing lumi-aggregation and an interactive computer system. Am. J. Clin. Path., *81*:471, 1984.

Miller, J. L., and Castella, A.: Platelet-type von Willebrand's disease: Characterization of a new bleeding disorder. Blood, *60*:790, 1982.

Miller, J. L., Kupinski, J. M., Castella, A., and Ruggeri, Z. M.: von Willebrand factor binds to platelets and induces aggregation in platelet-type but not Type IIB von Willebrand disease. J. Clin. Invest., *72*:1532, 1983.

Montgomery, R. R., Kunicki, T. J., Taves, C., Pidard, D., and Corcoran, M.: Diagnosis of Bernard-Soulier syndrome and Glanzmann's thrombasthenia with a monoclonal assay on whole blood. J. Clin. Invest., *71*:385, 1983.

Murphy, S.: Thrombocytosis and thrombocythaemia. Clin. Haematol., *12*:89, 1983.

Mustard, J. F., Kinlough-Rathbone, R. L., Packham, M. A., Perry, D. W., Harfenist, E. J., and Pai, K. R. M.: Comparison of fibrinogen association with normal and thrombasthenic platelets on exposure to ADP or chymotrypsin. Blood, *54*:987, 1979.

Nichols, W. L., Didisheim, P., and Gerrard, J. M.: Qualitative platelet disorders. *In* Poller, L. (ed.): Recent Advances in Blood Coagulation—3. New York, Churchill Livingstone, 1981, pp. 41–80.

Nurden, A. T., and Caen, J. P.: An abnormal platelet glycoprotein pattern in three cases of Glanzmann's thrombasthenia. Br. J. Haematol., *28*:253, 1974.

Nurden, A. T., and Dupuis, D.: The reduced aggregation response of Bernard-Soulier platelets to thrombin may be related to abnormal glycoprotein V. Thrombos. Haemostas., *46*:22, 1981.

Ogston, D.: Contact activation of blood coagulation. *In* Poller, L. (ed.): Recent Advances in Blood Coagulation—3. New York, Churchill Livingstone, 1981, pp. 109–123.

Owen, C. A., Jr., Bowie, E. J. W., Didisheim, P., and Thompson, J. H.: The Diagnosis of Bleeding Disorders. Boston, Little, Brown and Company, 1969.

Pareti, F. I., Capitanio, A., Mannucci, L., Ponticelli, C., and Mannucci, P. M.: Acquired dysfunction due to the circulation of "exhausted" platelets. Am. J. Med., *69*:235, 1980.

Pareti, F. I., Capitanio, A., and Mannucci, P. M.: Acquired storage pool disease in platelets during disseminated intravascular coagulation. Blood, *48*:511, 1976.

Pareti, F. I., Gugliotta, L., Mannucci, L., Guarini, A., and Mannucci, P. M.: Biochemical and metabolic aspects of platelet dysfunction in myeloproliferative disorders. Thrombos. Haemostas., *47*:84, 1982.

Penny, R., Castaldi, P. A., and Whitsed, H. M.: Inflammation and haemostasis in paraproteinaemias. Br. J. Haematol., *20*:35, 1971.

Perkins, H. A., and McKenzie, M. R., and Fudenberg, H. H.: Hemostatic defects in dysproteinemias. Blood, *35*:695, 1970.

Phillips, D. R.: An evaluation of membrane glycoproteins in platelet adhesion and aggregation. Prog. Hemostas. Thromb., *5*:81, 1980.

Phillips, D. R., and Agin, P. P.: Platelet membrane defects in Glanzmann's thrombasthenia. Evidence for decreased amounts of two major glycoproteins. J. Clin. Invest., *60*:535, 1977.

Phillips, D. R., Jenkins, C. S. P., Lüscher, E. F., and Larrieu, M. J.: Molecular differences of exposed surface proteins on thrombasthenic platelet plasma membranes. Nature, *257*:599, 1975.

Rabiner, S. F., and Molinas, F.: The role of phenol and phenolic acids on the thrombocytopathy and defective platelet aggregation of patients with renal failure. Am. J. Med., *49*:346, 1970.

Raccuglia, G.: Gray platelet syndrome: A variety of qualitative platelet disorder. Am. J. Med., *51*:818, 1971.

Rao, A. K., and Walsh, P. N.: Acquired quantitative platelet disorders. Clin. Haematol., *12*:201, 1983.

Regan, M. G., Lackner, H., and Karpatkin, S.: Platelet function and coagulation profile in lupus erythematosus. Ann. Intern. Med., *81*:462, 1974.

Remuzzi, G., Cavenaghi, A. E., Mecca, G., Donati, M. B., and De Gaetano, G.: Prostacyclin-like activity and bleeding in renal failure. Lancet, *2*:1195, 1977.

Rendu, R., Lebret, M., Nurden, A., and Caen, J. P.: Detection of an acquired platelet storage pool disease in three patients with a myeloproliferative disorder. Thrombos. Haemostas., *42*:794, 1979.

Ruggeri, Z. M., Pareti, F. I., Mannucci, P. M., Ciavarella, N., and Zimmerman, T. S.: Heightened interaction between platelets and factor VIII/von Willebrand factor in a new subtype of von Willebrand's disease. N. Engl. J. Med., *302*:1047, 1980.

Schafer, A. I.: Deficiency of platelet lipoxygenase activity in myeloproliferative disorders. N. Engl. J. Med., *306*:381, 1982.

Shulman, N. R., and Jordan, J. V., Jr.: Platelet dynamics. *In* Colman, R. W., Hirsh, J., Marder, V. J., and Salzman, E. W. (eds.): Hemostasis and Thrombosis. Philadelphia, J. B. Lippincott, 1982a, pp. 237–258.

Shulman, N. R., and Jordan, J. V., Jr.: Platelet immunology. *In* Colman, R. W., Hirsh, J., Marder, V. J., and Salzman, E. W. (eds.): Hemostasis and Thrombosis. Philadelphia, J. B. Lippincott, 1982b, pp. 274–342.

Smith, M. C., and Dunn, M.: Impaired thromboxane production in renal failure. Nephron, *29*:133, 1981.

Spaet, T. H., Lejnieks, F., Gaynor, E., and Goldstein, M. L.: Defective platelets in essential thrombocythemia. Arch. Intern. Med., *124*:135, 1969.

Statland, B. E., Heagan, B. M., and White, J. G.: Uptake of calcium by platelet relaxing factor. Nature, *223*:521, 1969.

Stuart, M. J., and Miller, J. L.: Congenital disorders of platelet function. *In* Brain, M. C., and McColloch, P. B. (eds.): Current Therapy in Hematology-Oncology 1983–1984. Philadelphia, B. C. Decker, Inc., 1983, pp. 182–188.

Stuart, M. J., Murphy, S., and Oski, F. A.: A simple nonradioisotope technic for the determination of platelet life-span. N. Engl. J. Med., *292*:1310, 1975.

Thompson, A. R., and Harker, L. A.: Manual of Hemostasis and Thrombosis. 3rd ed. Philadelphia, F. A. Davis Company, 1983.

Triplett, D. A. (ed.): Platelet Function: Laboratory Evaluation and Clinical Application. Chicago, American Society of Clinical Pathologists, 1978.

van Leeuwen, E. F., von dem Borne, A. E. G., Jr., von Riesz, L. E., Nijenhuis, L. E., and Engelfriet, C. P.: Absence of platelet-specific alloantigens in Glanzmann's thrombasthenia. Blood, *57*:49, 1981.

von dem Borne, A. E. G., Helmerhorst, F. M., van Leeuwen, E. F., Pegels, H. G., von Riesz, E., and Engelfriet, C. P.: Autoimmune thrombocytopenia: Detection of platelet autoantibodies with the suspension immunofluorescence test. Br. J. Haematol., *45*:319, 1980.

Walsh, P. N.: The role of platelets in the contact phase of blood coagulation. Br. J. Haematol., *22*:237, 1972a.

Walsh, P. N.: The effects of collagen and kaolin on the intrinsic coagulant activity of platelets. Evidence for an alternative pathway in intrinsic coagulation not requiring factor XII. Br. J. Haematol., *22*:393, 1972b.

Walsh, P. N., Murphy, S., and Barry, W. E.: The role of platelets in the pathogenesis of thrombosis and hemorrhage in patients with thrombocytosis. Thrombos. Haemostas., *38*:1085, 1977.

Weiss, H. J.: Inherited disorders of platelet secretion. *In* Colman, R. W., Hirsh, J., Marder, V. J., and Salzman, E. W. (eds.): Hemostasis and Thrombosis. Philadelphia, J. B. Lippincott, 1982a, pp. 507–515.

Weiss, H. J., Meyer, D., Rabinowitz, R., Pietu, G., Girma, J. P., Vicic, W. J., and Rogers, J.: Pseudo von Willebrand's disease: An intrinsic platelet defect with aggregation by unmodified human factor VIII/von Willebrand factor and enhanced adsorption of its high molecular weight multimers. N. Engl. J. Med., *306*:326, 1982b.

Weiss, H. J., Rosove, M. H., Lages, B. A., and Kaplan, K. L.: Acquired storage pool deficiency with increased platelet-associated IgG. Report of five cases. Am. J. Med., *69*:711, 1980.

4

White, J. G.: Ultrastructural studies of the gray platelet syndrome. Am. J. Path., *95*:445, 1979.

White, J. G., Clawson, C. C., and Gerrard, J. M.: Platelet ultrastructure. *In* Bloom, A. L., and Thomas, D. P. (eds.): Haemostasis and Thrombosis. New York, Churchill Livingstone, 1981, pp. 22–49.

White, J. G., and Gerrard, J. M.: Anatomy and structural organization of the platelet. *In* Colman, R. W., Hirsh, J., Marder, V. J., and Salzman, E. W. (eds.): Hemostasis and Thrombosis. Philadelphia, J. B. Lippincott, 1982, pp. 343–363.

Wintrobe, M. M., Lee, G. R., Boggs, D. R., Bithell, T. C., Foerster, J., Athens, J. W., and Lukens, J. N.: Clinical Hematology. 8th ed. Philadelphia, Lea & Febiger, 1981.

Witte, L. D., Kaplan, K. L., Nossel, H. L., Lages, B. A., Weiss, H. J., and Goodman, D. S.: Studies of the release from human platelets of the growth factor for cultured human arterial smooth muscle cells. Circ. Res., *42*:402, 1978.

Zahavi, J., and Marder, V. J.: Acquired 'storage pool disease' of platelets associated with circulating anti-platelet antibodies. Am. J. Med., *56*:883, 1974.

Zucker-Franklin, D.: Megakaryocytes and platelets. *In* Atlas of Blood Cells: Function and Pathology. Zucker-Franklin, D., Greaves, M. F., Grossi, G. E., and Marmont, A. M. (eds.): Philadelphia, Lea & Febiger, 1981, pp. 557–602.

32

BLOOD COAGULATION AND FIBRINOLYSIS

JONATHAN L. MILLER, M.D., PH.D.

NORMAL COAGULATION MECHANISMS

The arrest of bleeding depends upon primary platelet plug formation in conjunction with the elaboration of a stable fibrin clot. The formation of this clot involves the sequential interaction of a series of plasma proteins in a highly ordered and complex fashion, as well as interaction of these complexes both with blood platelets and with materials released from tissues. In recent years there has been intensive investigation of all aspects of the blood coagulation system. With increased availability of purified coagulation factors for research, it has been possible to study the interactions (and conditions for interactions) among individual factors directly. In many cases this has led to understanding at greater depth the interactions that had been defined in previous decades by means of "experiments of nature," in which patients with bleeding disorders were found to be deficient in a specific factor. In other instances, however, new interactions have now been established, including apparent "crossover reactions" connecting the classically formulated "intrinsic" and "extrinsic" systems, as well as important positive and negative feedback loops occurring at multiple levels of the cascade. Improved diagnosis and treatment of bleeding syndromes are the primary clinical beneficiaries of the new knowledge, and these bleeding diatheses are now being reassessed in the light of this new knowledge (Nemerson, 1981).

Of major conceptual importance is how to approach and understand the many chemical reactions that subserve hemostasis from the initial bleeding stimulus to final formation of a stable clot. To accomplish this task it is necessary to understand first the normal series of reactions, and then how to localize an abnormality to the specific factor or factors responsible. An overview of the participants currently believed to play critical roles in the normal hemostatic mechanism is first presented (Table 32–1 and Fig. 32–1). Laboratory methods to localize hemostatic abnormalities are then considered. In the latter process, portions of the normal coagulation cascade are artificially broken up into smaller, incomplete segments that lend themselves to laboratory localization of factor defects. It must be emphasized, however, that tests (p. 769) such as the activated partial thromboplastin time (aPTT), prothrombin time (PT), or thrombin time (TT) are merely convenient laboratory aids to diagnosis. The "intrinsic pathway," "extrinsic pathway," and other segments that these tests appear to define should accordingly not be thought of as actual physiologic pathways of hemostasis.

INITIATING REACTIONS

The coagulation system appears to be initiated by activation of *factor XII* (Hageman factor) and/or *factor VII*. It is still unclear what the initial stimuli for activation of these factors are *in vivo*. Once formed, activated factor XII (XIIa) participates in a positive feedback loop involving *prekallikrein* and *high molecular weight kininogen (HMWK)* to generate still more XIIa. Whether traces of XIIa participate in the initial activation of XII is not yet known. Of prime importance, however, is the presence of negatively charged surfaces, upon which the rate of these reactions is greatly enhanced. Injury to a blood vessel may provide

Table 32–1. PLASMA COAGULATION FACTORS*

Factor	(Synonym)	Probable Site of Synthesis	Vitamin K Dependent	Half-Life of Activity (Hours)	Molecular Weight (Chain Structure)	Function of Active Form
Fibrinogen	(Factor I)	Liver	No	70–120	340,000 ($\alpha_2\beta_2\gamma_2$)	Clot structural protein
Prothrombin	(Factor II)	Liver	Yes	70–110	72,000	Serine protease
Factor V	(Proaccelerin)	Liver	No	12–36	350,000	Cofactor
Factor VII	(Proconvertin)	Liver	Yes	4–6	48,000	Serine protease
Factor VIII:C	(Antihemophilic factor)	Liver	No	10–14	150,000	Cofactor
von Willebrand factor	(Factor VIIIR)	Endothelium	No	22–40	>10,000,000 (multimers of 200,000 M.W. subunits)	Cofactor for platelets
Factor IX	(Christmas factor)	Liver	Yes	8–24	57,000	Serine protease
Factor X	(Stuart-Prower factor)	Liver	Yes	24–60	59,000 (dimer)	Serine protease
Factor XI	(Plasma thromboplastin antecedent)	Liver	No	50–80	160,000 (dimer)	Serine protease
Factor XII	(Hageman factor)	?Liver	No	50–60	80,000	Serine protease
Factor XIII	(Fibrin stabilizing factor)	Liver	No	10–14 days	320,000 ($\alpha_2\beta_2$)	Transamidase
Prekallikrein	(Fletcher factor)	?Liver	No	?	85,000	Serine protease
HMW kininogen	(Fitzgerald factor)	?Liver	No	?	110,000	Cofactor

*Data compiled from multiple sources, including Wintrobe (1981) and Thompson (1983).

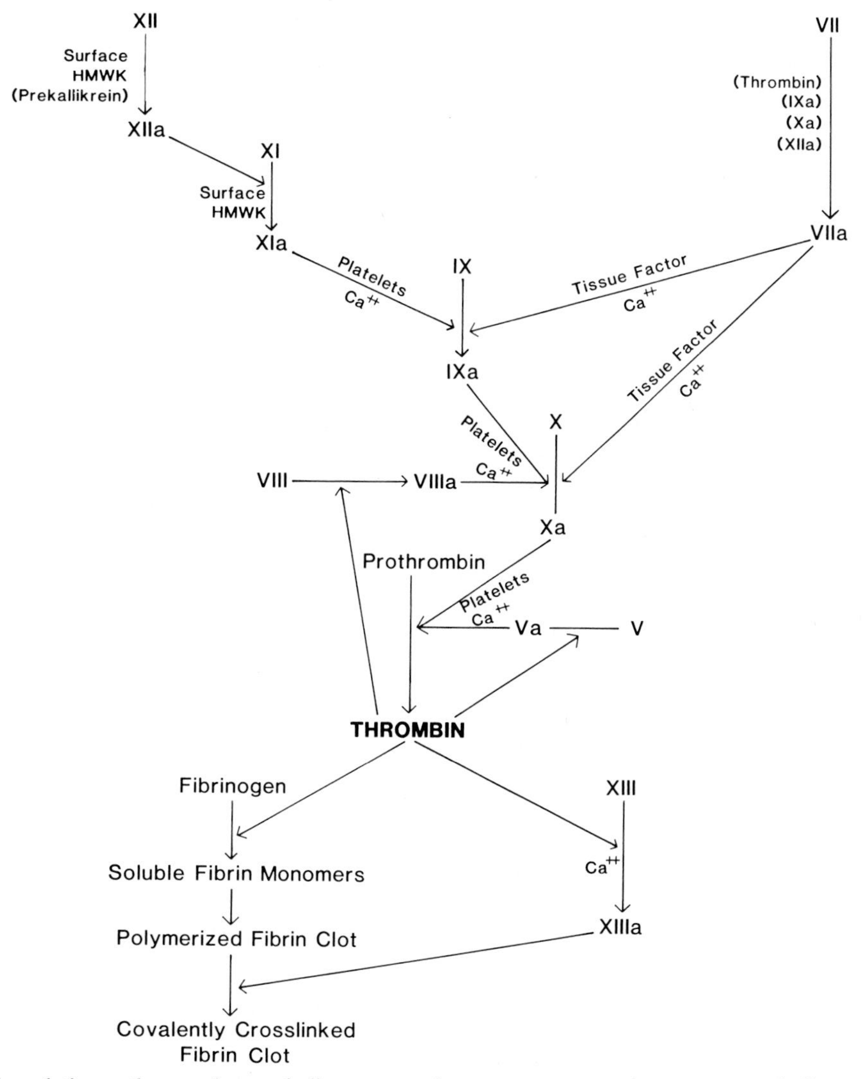

Figure 32–1. Coagulation pathways. Arrows indicate steps where precursor proteins are enzymatically converted to their active forms. These active forms in turn possess enzymatic activity, except for factors VIIIa and Va, which function as cofactors, and fibrin monomers, which serve as the structural building blocks for the fibrin clot. Required cofactors are indicated along the arrows of the individual activation reactions. Exogenous phospholipid may be utilized in place of platelets. Agents not unequivocally required but capable of enhancing particular reactions are shown in parentheses.

such surfaces in the course of normal hemostasis. Surface contact and the presence of HMWK also greatly facilitate the activation of factor XI by XIIa. In the absence of prekallikrein, factor XIIa is generated more slowly, as are factor XIa and the subsequently formed activated factors.

Recent laboratory studies have indicated that factor VII can be transformed to its active, enzymatic form following proteolytic attack by factors XIIa, Xa, IXa, or thrombin (Zur, 1981). Which, if any, of these potential activators is primarily responsible for achieving activation of factor VII *in vivo* is presently unknown.

INTERMEDIATE REACTIONS

Once activated, VIIa is a potent serine protease capable of activating *factor IX* or *factor X* in the presence of lipoprotein, termed *"tissue factor,"* and ionized calcium (Fig. 32–1). Tissue factor is produced in many tissues, and has been demonstrated in cultured human endothelial cells, smooth muscle cells, and fibroblasts (Maynard, 1977). Circulating blood monocytes are also capable of developing tissue factor activity (Edwards, 1981).

In addition to the VIIa/tissue factor "pathway" of activation, factor IX can also be activated by *factor XIa.* This reaction does not require the presence of tissue factor lipoprotein, but it does require negatively charged phospholipids, as well as ionized calcium. *In vivo,* blood platelets are presumed to be the primary source of these phospholipids. In the resting state a limited amount of utilizable phospholipid is probably present on the platelet surface, but during platelet activation in the course of hemostasis (see Chap. 31)

4

there appears to be a "flip-flop" of phosphatidylserine and phosphatidylethanolamine from the cytoplasmic surface to the outer surface of the platelet membrane (Bevers, 1982). This shift of phospholipids probably is instrumental in providing an optimal surface for facilitating coagulant activation reactions. In the laboratory, phospholipid extracts ("partial thromboplastins") added to platelet-free plasma will replace platelet phospholipid in supporting the activation of IX by XIa, as well as in the subsequent steps shown in Figure 32–1 where platelets are indicated as cofactors.

Factor X can be activated directly by VIIa in the presence of tissue factor and calcium (Fig. 32–1). It can also be thought of as being *indirectly* activated by factor VIIa, since following the activation of factor IX by VIIa/tissue factor, IXa will form a complex with phospholipid and activated factor VIII which, in the presence of calcium, activates factor X. Recent biochemical studies measuring kinetics of the individual activation reactions with purified factors suggest that the formation of Xa by this indirect route may proceed at a rate equal to or greater than that of activation of X by VIIa/tissue factor (the classic "extrinsic pathway"). Additionally, this route may be at least as significant a one as the activation of IX by XIa/phospholipid and subsequent activation of X by IXa/phospholipid/VIIIa (the classic "intrinsic pathway"). If this emerging concept is upheld by *in vivo* studies, it would help explain why deficiencies of the *contact factors* of the "intrinsic pathway" are in most cases not associated with a clinical bleeding tendency, whereas deficiencies of factors VIII and IX are associated with serious bleeding tendencies which are not circumvented by the existence of an unimpaired "extrinsic pathway" (Nemerson, 1981).

Once formed, factor Xa in turn becomes the activator of the zymogen *prothrombin* (factor II). *In vivo,* this reaction is thought to proceed on the surface of platelets, where activated *factor V* (of plasma or platelet origin) in the presence of calcium forms a receptor for Xa, and the potent "prothrombinase" thereby formed catalyzes the conversion of prothrombin to the active enzyme thrombin. The importance of each of these cofactors to the production of thrombin, as well as the dramatic contrast of reaction rates when simple phospholipids are substituted for platelets in this process, is evident in Table 32–2.

Table 32–2. EFFECTS OF COFACTORS UPON RATE OF THROMBIN FORMATION FROM PROTHROMBIN*

Cofactors	Relative Rate
Factor Xa, Ca^{++}	1
Factor Xa, Phospholipid, Ca^{++}	50
Factor Xa, Phospholipid, Factor Va, Ca^{++}	20,000
Factor Xa, Platelets, Ca^{++}	300,000

*From Miletich, J. P., et al.: J. Biol. Chem., *253*:6908, 1978.

CLOT FORMATION

Thrombin formation marks a critical event in the hemostatic process. Thrombin directly cleaves peptide fragments from the α and β chains of fibrinogen (fibrinopeptides A and B, respectively) to create fibrin monomers that subsequently assemble into a highly ordered, polymeric fibrin clot. Thrombin also functions as an extremely potent physiological stimulus of platelet activation (Chap. 31). Thrombin proteolysis of native factors VIII and V produces activated forms of these molecules (Fig. 32–1), providing amplification for the activation of factor X and prothrombin, respectively.

Formation of fibrin polymer is the endpoint that is detected in virtually all clotting time tests of the coagulation system (aPTT, PT, TT, etc.). This clot, however, is still rather loose, being held together principally by electrostatic interactions between neighboring molecules of fibrin monomer. Final stabilization of the clot is achieved by the formation of covalent lysine to glutamine linkages between γ chains of adjacent fibrin molecules, as well as between adjacent α chains, through the activation of *factor XIIIa (fibrin stabilizing factor).* This transglutaminase enzyme is formed from its inactive zymogen (factor XIII) by the proteolytic action of thrombin. Not only is calcium required for XIII activation, but recent studies have also demonstrated that fibrinogen itself may serve as a cofactor in this reaction. Factor XIIIa additionally covalently cross-links the physiologic inhibitor of fibrinolysis, α_2-antiplasmin inhibitor, to the fibrin clot, making the clot less susceptible to lysis by plasmin.

When platelets are present during clot formation, there is eventual contraction of the formed clot, which is thought to be mediated by the platelet contractile protein, thrombosthenin. The precise *in vivo* correlate of this "clot retraction" observable in the test tube is not fully understood.

NATURAL INHIBITORS OF COAGULATION

The regulation of coagulation reactions is extremely complex, as might be anticipated from the number of different factors and cofactors involved in the hemostatic process. Conditions which promote the cascading reactions, as opposed to those which inhibit the process, are poorly understood, although they usually are associated with tissue injury.

Of the known natural inhibitors of coagulation, *antithrombin III* appears to be the most important. Antithrombin III is the principal physiologic inhibitor of thrombin and of factor Xa. It has also been shown to possess inhibitor activity against factors XIIa, XIa, and IXa. Antithrombin III and thrombin appear to form a 1:1 complex which is enzymatically inactive, and which can be detected by specific antibodies raised against this complex. It has been suggested that monitoring the titer of this antigenic complex might be one means of assessing the extent of *in vivo* coagulation (Collen, 1977, 1981). In the presence of heparin, the anticoagulant activity of antithrombin

III is greatly enhanced, and this enhancement is in fact believed to constitute the primary mechanism of heparin's anticoagulant effects. For example, the rate constant for the reaction between thrombin and antithrombin III is increased over two thousand times in the presence of a highly active, low molecular weight heparin fraction (Collen, 1981).

Thrombin activity is also inhibited by the glycoprotein *α_2-macroglobulin* (MW, 725,000 daltons). With the exception of kallikrein, none of the other coagulant enzymes is significantly inhibited by α_2-macroglobulin. Thrombin interacts with α_2-macroglobulin in such a fashion that while the thrombin-α_2-macroglobulin complex still retains enzymatic activity against small, synthetic substrates, its actions on large, natural substrates are effectively inhibited, most likely due to steric hindrance. It has been estimated that in the circulation approximately 75 per cent of the thrombin formed is inactivated by antithrombin III, and the remaining 25 per cent by α_2-macroglobulin.

The plasma inhibitor of the first component of complement, *$C\bar{1}$ inhibitor,* has been shown also to possess inhibitory activity against factor XIIa, factor XIa, and kallikrein. The physiological importance of these reactions is presently unknown. Similarly, though α_1-antitrypsin can be demonstrated *in vitro* to show inhibitory activity against thrombin, kallikrein, and factor XIa, there is little clinical evidence to support a significant role for α_1-antitrypsin in coagulation *in vivo.*

Protein C (MW, 62,000 daltons) is a natural inhibitor of coagulation whose synthesis is dependent upon vitamin K. Protein C circulates in its inactive zymogen form and is activated by thrombin (Kisiel, 1977) in the presence of the endothelial cell–associated cofactor thrombomodulin (Esmon, 1981). Activated protein C proteolytically cleaves activated factors VIII and V, bringing about the inactivation of these important coagulant factors. It is believed that a natural inactivator of protein C also exists, and the absence of such an inactivator has been postulated to explain cases of rare, apparent combined "deficiencies" of factors V and VIII (see below). Additionally, decreased levels of protein C have been reported in familial thrombotic disease (Griffin, 1981) and in some patients with intravascular coagulation (Griffin, 1982).

LABORATORY SCREENING TESTS OF COAGULATION

All coagulation testing is critically dependent upon the quality of the plasma specimen obtained. A clean venipuncture with a minimum of trauma to tissues is required. Often a two-syringe technique is used, in which a few milliliters of blood obtained in the first syringe either is utilized for purposes other than coagulation testing or is discarded. Citrate is the anticoagulant routinely used for coagulation screening tests, as well as for many of the more specialized coagulation tests. Citrated plasma essentially free of platelets is prepared by standard centrifugation procedures.

The *prothrombin time* (PT) is performed by adding a source of tissue extract (typically from brain or lung) to citrated plasma, adding an excess of calcium, and measuring the time for clot formation. Prolongations of the PT may be associated with deficiencies of factors comprising the classic "extrinsic pathway"—factors VII, X, V, II, and fibrinogen, a combination of these factors, or the presence of an inhibitor.

The *activated partial thromboplastin time* (aPTT, or simply PTT) is performed upon citrated plasma by activating the contact factors (e.g., with kaolin, ellagic acid, or celite), adding a standardized phospholipid preparation as a platelet substitute, and then measuring the time for clot formation following the addition of an excess of calcium. The aPTT will be prolonged by a deficiency in factors comprising the classic "intrinsic pathway"—prekallikrein, HMWK, factors XII, XI, IX, VIII, X, V, II, and fibrinogen, or by inhibitors directed against the involved factors or complexes. Shortening of the aPTT may be seen in conjunction with an activated coagulation system, for instance in a compensated, low-grade consumptive coagulopathy.

The *thrombin time* (TT) is performed by adding exogenous thrombin to citrated plasma and measuring the time to clot formation. A deficiency (or abnormality) of fibrinogen and the presence of heparin or fibrin(ogen) degradation products are the most common causes of a prolonged TT.

NORMAL FIBRINOLYSIS

Clot formation serves to interrupt blood loss from damaged vessels, but ultimately the clot must be removed if blood flow is to resume. This latter condition is achieved through dissolution of the clot by the *fibrinolytic system* (Table 32–3). The enzyme *plasmin* sequentially cleaves a series of bonds in the fibrin molecules, releasing peptidic *fibrin degradation products* (FDP), and producing clot lysis.

Several mechanisms leading to the formation of active plasmin have been elucidated (Fig. 32–2). Activation of the contact factors of coagulation is associated with conversion of the inactive zymogen, *plasminogen,* to the active enzyme plasmin. Factor XIIa, kallikrein, and high molecular weight kininogen all appear to play roles in this process, although the precise mechanisms are still under investigation. Native plasminogen, having a molecular weight of about 90,000 daltons and an amino-terminal glutamic acid ("glu-plasminogen"), undergoes limited proteolytic cleavage of the amino-terminal region by plasmin molecules to produce "lys-plasminogen." Lys-plasminogen then undergoes cleavage of a single arginine-valine bond to produce active plasmin ("lys-plasmin"). Activation of plasminogen by either the "extrinsic" or "exogenous" pathways (see below) proceeds via cleavage of the same arginine-valine bond. Although glu-plasminogen can also undergo this arginine-valine bond cleavage, activation proceeds at a much faster rate if glu-plasminogen is first converted to lys-plasminogen.

Table 32–3. MOLECULAR COMPONENTS OF THE PLASMA FIBRINOLYTIC SYSTEM*

Name	Molecular Weight	Baseline Plasma Concentration	Plasma Half-life	Functional Properties
Plasminogen	Single chain M.W. 88,000 (glu_1 form) M.W. 80,000 (lys_{77} form)	2.4 μM (21 mg/dl)	2.2 days 0.8 days	Zymogen; lysine binding sites to fibrin on "kringle" portions; activator-sensitive site at arg_{560}-val
Plasmin	Two chains M.W. 85,000 (glu_1 form) M.W. 77,000 (lys_{77} form) M.W. 38,000 (val_{442} form)	0	0.1 second	Serine protease; active site on light chain (M.W. 26,000); variable size of heavy chain containing "kringle" structures
α_2 Plasmin inhibitor	Single chain M.W. 67,000	1.0 μM (7 mg/dl)	2.6 days	Inhibits fibrinogen lysis by 1:1 complex with plasmin light chain; prevents binding of plasmin to fibrin; is itself bound to fibrin by factor XIIIa
Plasminogen activators				
Extrinsic (tissue, vascular)	One or two chains M.W. 60,000–70,000	Trace	15 minutes	Vascular type derived from endothelial cells and secreted into blood; high affinity for fibrin; cleave arg_{560}-val site on plasminogen
Exogenous				
Streptokinase	Single chain M.W. 48,000	—		Non-enzymatic, indirect action via 1:1 activator complex with plasminogen
Urokinase	Two chains M.W. 55,000 M.W. 32,000	—	10 minutes	Serine protease; direct action on arg_{560}-val bond of plasminogen

*From Francis, C. W., and Marder, V. J.: *In* Williams, W. J., et al. (eds.): Hematology. 3rd ed. New York, McGraw-Hill, 1983, with permission.

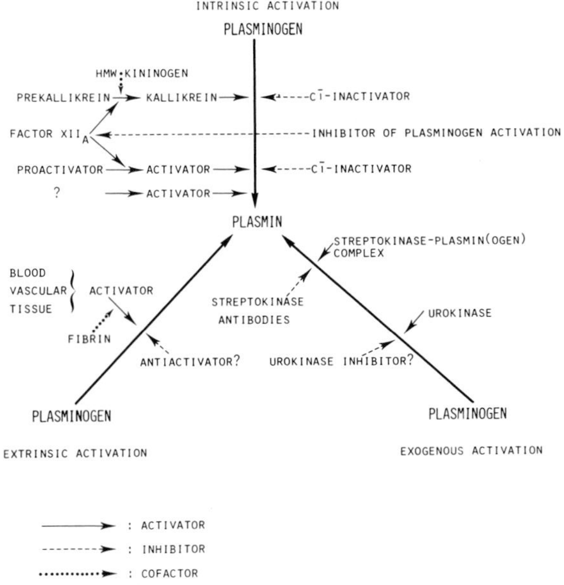

Figure 32–2. Pathways of plasminogen activation. (From Collen, D.: Thrombos. Haemostas., *43*:77, 1980.)

A proteolytic enzyme(s) with molecular weight of about 60,000 daltons, produced in vascular and other tissues, possesses *plasminogen activator* activity. Binding of activator to fibrin greatly enhances its activity. Additionally, plasminogen activators have been described in a variety of tumors.

Urokinase is a potent plasminogen activator that has been identified in human urine, as well as in human embryonic kidney cultures. It appears to be structurally different from tissue plasminogen activator. Purified urokinase, although still quite expensive, is utilized clinically in thrombolytic therapy.

The bacterial protein *streptokinase* also possesses plasminogen activator activity and is used in thrombolytic therapy. Streptokinase differs from the previously described plasminogen activators in that it is not an enzyme. Instead, streptokinase binds to plasminogen (or to plasmin), whereupon the streptokinase-plasmin(ogen) complex then develops plasminogen activator activity. Antigenicity of streptokinase has been a limiting feature, and work is currently in progress to try to identify functional portions of the streptokinase molecule that might possess much lower antigenic activity.

Plasmin once formed is capable of degrading not only fibrin clots but native fibrinogen as well. The sequence of proteolytic steps by which this latter process occurs has been intensively studied, and an increasingly complex nomenclature of degradation products has resulted. A simplified, schematic diagram of these steps is presented in Figure 32–3. The earliest proteolytic activity results in the still-clottable X fragment, which is subsequently degraded to the unclottable Y and D fragments. The Y fragment, consisting of D plus E portions, is then itself split into these components. Small peptides are also produced at a number of the proteolytic cleavages.

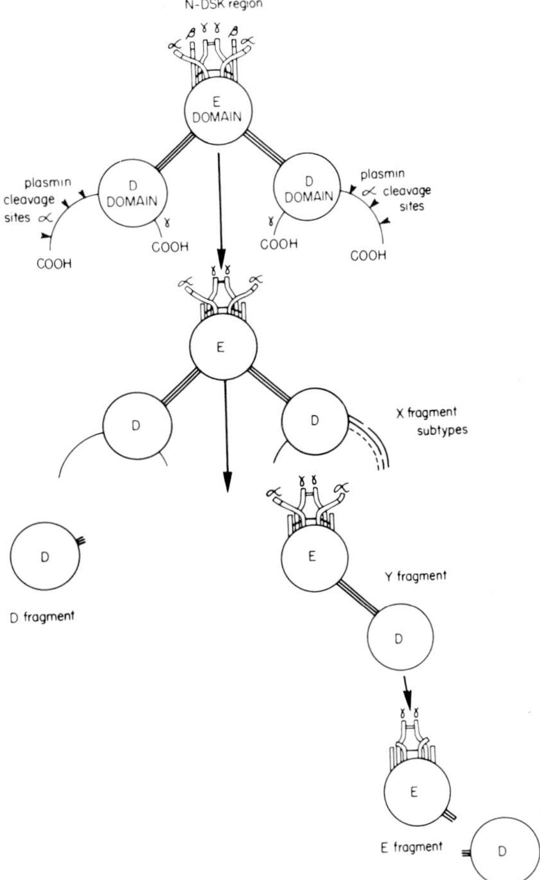

Figure 32–3. Degradation of fibrinogen by plasmin. (From Rosenberg, R. D.: *In* Beck, W. S. [ed.]: Hematology. 3rd ed. Cambridge, Mass., MIT Press, 1981.)

When a normally cross-linked fibrin clot is dissolved by plasmin, isolated D and E fragments are not the characteristic end-stage fragments. Rather, a variety of complexes are found, most characteristically one composed of two D and one E moieties ("D_2E" fragment). The degradation of cross-linked fibrin is shown schematically in Figure 32–4.

By rendering fibrinogen unclottable and lysing fibrin clots, plasmin directly counterbalances the tendency toward coagulation. Direct effects of plasmin against the aggregation of platelets induced by thrombin have also been demonstrated (Miller, 1975). Plasmin additionally exerts proteolytic attack upon activated factors VIII:C and V, hastening their inactivation. Finally, the FDP produced in fibrinolysis themselves possess anticoagulant effects, inhibiting fibrin polymerization and enzymatic activity of some coagulant enzymes, most notably thrombin. FDP at concentrations achievable during *in vivo* fibrinolysis do not appear to exert significant effects upon platelet aggregation (Miller, 1975; Solum, 1973).

The primary inactivator of plasmin is a protein of 70,000 daltons known as α_2-antiplasmin. α_2-Antiplasmin quickly forms a 1:1 stoichiometric complex with plasmin, and the assay of this complex may serve

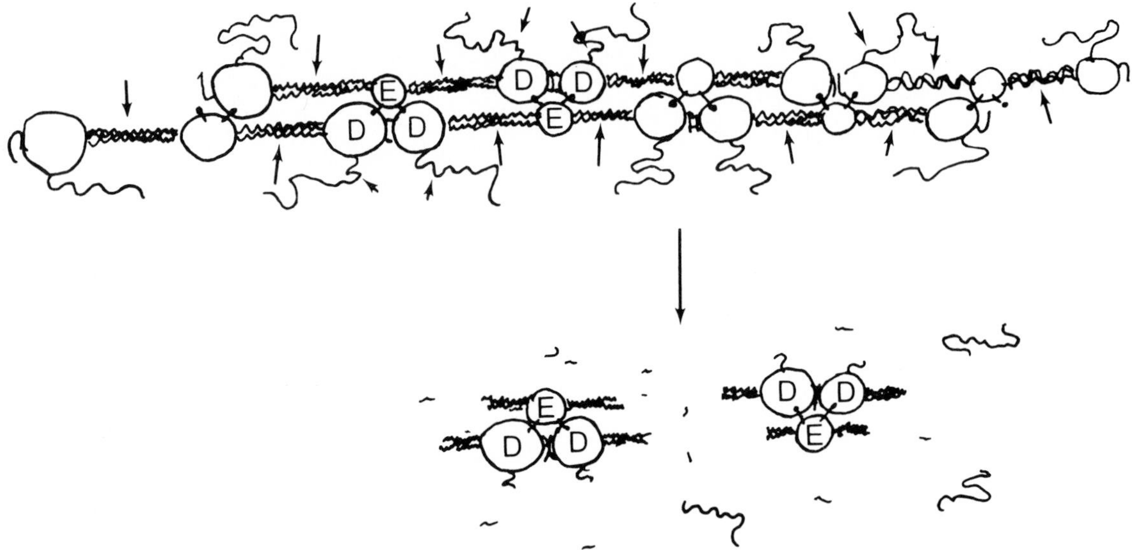

Figure 32–4. Degradation of a cross-linked fibrin clot by plasmin. (From Doolittle, R. F.: *In* Bloom, A. L., and Thomas, D. P. [eds.]: Haemostasis and Thrombosis. Edinburgh, Churchill Livingstone, 1981.)

as a useful indicator of *in vivo* fibrinolysis (Collen, 1980). α_2-Macroglobulin can also be demonstrated to have antiplasmin activity, but it is slower acting and probably of only minor importance in normal hemostasis.

Except in instances such as disseminated intravascular coagulation, it is unusual to have actual *fibrinogenolysis in vivo.* Even in the rare patient with a congenital absence of α_2-antiplasmin, significant fibrinogenolysis is not observed. Within the gel-phase of a clot, however, conditions are quite different. Despite the presence of α_2-antiplasmin cross-linked to polymerizing fibrin by factor XIIIa, plasmin present within the clot is somehow able to bring about eventual *fibrin* dissolution. The precise mechanisms whereby fibrinolytic activators and inactivators actually reach a balance favoring or hindering fibrinolysis are complex, and are still being elucidated.

LABORATORY TESTS OF FIBRINOLYSIS

FDP produced during fibrinolysis *in vivo* may bind to fibrinogen or remain freely circulating. Only the latter fraction is measured when patient serum is assayed for FDP, so that falsely negative values constitute a potential problem for this test. In the tanned red cell hemagglutination inhibition immunoassay, FDP present in the patient's serum neutralize antifibrinogen antiserum, thereby preventing the antiserum from agglutinating fibrinogen-coated erythrocytes. A more rapid, semi-quantitative method is also available in which FDP present in patient serum directly agglutinate latex beads coated with antifibrinogen antibody.

The *whole blood clot lysis time* is a simple screening test in which a tube of whole blood is allowed to clot and dissolution of the clot is subsequently examined. In normal individuals the clot remains undissolved even 24 hours after clot formation. In the absence of normal anti-plasmin activity or in some fibrinolytic states, lysis may be observed after several hours. Plasma can also be admixed with dilute acid to precipitate a fraction relatively rich in plasminogen activator, plasminogen, and fibrinogen, but relatively poor in anti-plasmins. This "euglobulin" fraction can subsequently be redissolved in buffer and clotted by recalcification, and the time for clot lysis measured. Such *euglobulin clot lysis* is normally complete in two to four hours, but may be shortened with increased fibrinolysis, particularly in association with increased plasminogen activator activity.

Both *plasminogen* and *α_2-antiplasmin* may be measured antigenically in patient plasma. Functional plasminogen and antiplasmin assays have recently also become available that utilize synthetic substrates in either spectrophotometric or fluorometric measuring systems.

CONGENITAL DEFICIENCIES OF HEMOSTATIC FACTORS

HEMOPHILIA A

Hemophilia A is the most common congenital disorder of the coagulation factors, affecting approximately one in 10,000 persons in the whole population (Levine, 1982). This deficiency of normal factor VIII:C is determined by a defect on the X chromosome, with the result that hemizygous males are primarily affected. Although female carriers ordinarily do not have a bleeding diathesis, there are a number of conditions in which females may also experience clinical hemophilia (Bloom, 1981). These genetic abnormalities in phenotypic females include a single functional X chromosome bearing the hemophilia gene, extreme lyonization in a heterozygote, and true homozygosity for the hemophilia gene. In approximately one third of newly diagnosed cases of hemophilia no antecedent family history of bleeding can be obtained, suggesting either several generations of silent carriers or a recent mutation.

"Spontaneous" hemorrhages may be seen frequently in patients having <0.01 U/ml of factor VIII:C. (Factor activities are expressed as arbitrary units (U) per milliliter, where 1 U/ml corresponds to the amount of activity present in 1 ml of a normal plasma pool.) Patients with such levels are considered *severe* hemophiliacs. Levels of factor VIII:C up to 0.05 U/ml are usually associated with *moderate* clinical severity, whereas patients with values between 0.05 and 0.30 U/ml are considered *mild* hemophiliacs and typically will bleed excessively only in association with trauma or surgical procedures.

Bleeding histories in patients with hemophilia typically indicate bleeding into joints or muscles, excessive postoperative hemorrhage, and generally easy bruising. Bleeding at mucous membrane or skin sites is not as pronounced as in von Willebrand's disease or in platelet disorders. Intracranial hemorrhage remains a major cause of death in hemophiliacs (Levine, 1982; Bloom, 1981).

Although the bleeding time in patients with hemophilia has traditionally been thought to be normal, recent studies (Buchanan, 1980; Eyster, 1981) suggest that some patients with hemophilia may in fact show a prolongation of the template bleeding time (Chap. 31, p. 751). The prothrombin time and the thrombin time are characteristically normal. Tests which screen for the "intrinsic pathway" will be abnormal if they are of adequate sensitivity. The aPTT should be prolonged if factor VIII:C levels are below 0.4 U/ml, and this has proved an acceptable screening test in most cases. It is important to emphasize, however, that when a hemophiliac is being treated, in particular postoperatively, the aPTT does not provide an acceptable substitute for specific factor VIII:C assays. Both overestimation and underestimation of actual VIII:C levels may result from attempts to interpret aPTT values in patients undergoing VIII:C replacement therapy, and may lead to inappropriate subsequent therapy.

Factor VIII:C activity may be assayed by either one-stage techniques based upon the aPTT (Hardisty, 1962), or two-stage techniques based upon the thromboplastin generation test (Denson, 1976). In either case, patient plasma is assessed for its ability to shorten the time to clot formation of plasma from a severe hemophiliac devoid of factor VIII:C activity.

Human alloantibodies to the factor VIII coagulant moiety are produced in a minority of severe hemophiliac patients who receive factor VIII replacement therapy (see below). These antibodies typically do not produce precipitin reactions. Utilized earlier in antibody neutralization studies, these alloantibodies identified "cross-reacting material" in the plasma of some patients with mild-moderate hemophilia (so-called "CRM+" patients). Quantitative, more reproducible studies have utilized such antibodies in immunoradiometric assays of factor VIII coagulant antigen (VIII:CAg) (Lazarchick, 1978). In normal individuals correlation between plasma VIII:C (activity) and VIII:CAg is excellent. Although VIII:C activity is not found in *serum*, VIII:CAg remains detectable in serum, usually at 60 to 85 per cent of the plasma level (Hoyer, 1982). Levels of VIII:CAg are very low or undetectable in most severe hemophiliacs. In patients with mild-moderate hemophilia, VIII:CAg levels usually are equal to or slightly greater than VIII:C. In those few hemophiliacs in whom VIII:CAg levels remain normal, there is likely to be a qualitative abnormality of their VIII:C molecules.

On the average, maternal carriers have 0.5 U/ml VIII:C activity, yet individual variation in levels is too great to allow carrier detection from VIII:C assays alone in individual women. Predictive value is greatly increased, however, if in addition to VIII:C values, measurement is also made of the von Willebrand factor (vWF) portion of the factor VIII complex. Zimmerman (1971) showed that antibodies produced in rabbits to the human factor VIII complex detect a factor VIII-related antigen (so-called VIIIR:Ag or vWF antigen) that is associated with circulating VIII:C, but that is synthesized independently under autosomal control, presumably by endothelial cells (Jaffe, 1974). When patient plasma is electrophoresed through agarose containing such a rabbit antiserum, immunoprecipitin lines resembling rockets result (Fig. 32–5). The height of the rocket is proportional to the

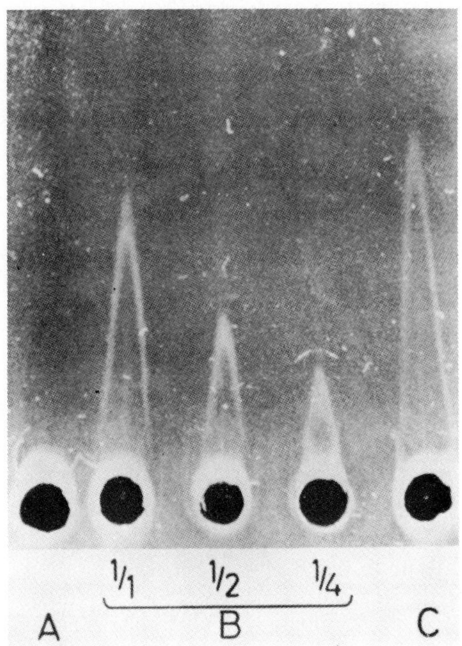

Figure 32–5. Laurell immunoelectrophoresis assay of von Willebrand factor. *A*, Plasma from patient with von Willebrand's disease. *B*, Doubling dilutions of normal plasma. *C*, Plasma from a patient with hemophilia A. (From Rizza, C. R.: *In* Biggs, R. [ed.]: The Treatment of Haemophilia A and B and von Willebrand's Disease. Oxford, Blackwell Scientific Publications, 1978.)

4

concentration of vWF present in the plasma. In normal individuals the ratio of vWF to VIII:C approaches unity. Like VIII:C, vWF appears to have characteristics of an acute phase reactant, so that transient elevations in VIII:C are generally accompanied by similar elevations in vWF. In carriers of hemophilia A, vWF levels are normal, with VIII:C levels frequently one half or less as great, resulting in characteristically decreased VIII:C/vWF ratios. As Graham (1979) has emphasized, however, carrier identification based solely on a comparison between patient ratios and those obtained in normal individuals may lead to serious errors. Graham has proposed that laboratories establish a discriminant analysis based on pools of both obligate carriers and normal individuals, and that the resulting patient discriminant value be combined with pedigree analysis of the patient's family to obtain a final estimate of carrier likelihood. Finally, although theoretically promising, studies employing measurements of VIII:CAg in addition to VIII:C and vWF have not yet significantly improved accuracy of carrier detection in hemophilia.

Pre-natal diagnosis of hemophilia has also recently become available following the development of VIII:CAg assays (Firshein, 1979). Samples of blood obtained from unaffected fetuses at 18 to 20 weeks' gestation may be expected to show detectable levels of VIII:CAg, as well as ratios of VIII:CAg to vWF appropriate for fetal age. Although such studies are presently confined to specialized centers, wider application of these techniques may be expected with increasing experience.

Hemophilia is treated principally by factor VIII replacement therapy, either as cryoprecipitate or as factor VIII concentrates. In approximately 11 to 15 per cent of patients with severe hemophilia, antibodies develop which inhibit VIII:C (Shapiro, 1979). Since the degree of anamnestic response and the antibody titer greatly affect the therapeutic approach in individual patients, it is important that laboratories be able to provide reproducible inhibitor level measurements. The two-hour "Bethesda" method (Kasper, 1975, 1982) has achieved wide acceptance, and inhibitors are generally expressed in Bethesda units. One Bethesda unit corresponds to the ability of patient plasma to inactivate 50 per cent of the VIII:C activity of an equal volume of normal plasma following a two-hour incubation at 37°C. Inhibitor assays based upon the aPTT have also shown promise, and are the subject of continuing studies (Lossing, 1977; Ewing, 1982).

Current modes of therapy for patients with inhibitors include the use of higher doses of factor VIII replacement therapy in patients with low-titered inhibitors. In cases of high-titered inhibitors, nonactivated or activated factor IX concentrates may be used in an attempt to "bypass" the factor VIII inhibitory activity. There is currently no accepted laboratory test for monitoring such "bypass" therapy; response must be assessed clinically. Recently, some hemophilia A patients with inhibitors have been treated successfully with purified factor VIII:C concentrates obtained from porcine plasma. Finally, studies are continuing to assess the ablation of the antibodies, either by chemotherapeutic approaches or by production of immune tolerance following the prolonged infusion of large amounts of factor VIII concentrate.

Rarely, patients have been encountered who appear to have a combined deficiency of factor VIII:C and factor V. Transmission is autosomal, and at least 0.01 to 0.05 U/ml of each factor is characteristically measurable. It has been proposed that at least some of these cases may represent a deficiency of inactivator of protein C (p. 769). Activated protein C would accordingly provide enhanced proteolysis of activated factors VIII:C and V, as well as of the unactivated forms of these molecules.

HEMOPHILIA B

Congenital deficiency of factor IX, or hemophilia B, is also an X chromosome–linked disorder, occurring approximately one fifth as frequently as hemophilia A. The clinical manifestations of hemophilia B are virtually indistinguishable from those of hemophilia A. Since replacement therapy is entirely different, consisting primarily of plasma fractions enriched in factor IX rather than factor VIII, it falls upon the laboratory to differentiate these two disorders.

As in hemophilia A, patients with hemophilia B typically have a prolonged aPTT, normal thrombin time, and normal bleeding time. Although most also have a normal prothrombin time, one subgroup of patients (the B_m variant) has a prolonged prothrombin time when ox-brain thromboplastin is employed, presumably due to inhibition of the thromboplastin by the abnormal factor IX (Kidd, 1963; Hougie, 1967). In rare kindreds, the factor IX level appears to increase as the individual matures (Leyden variant) (Veltkamp, 1970).

With clinical suspicion of hemophilia, a prolonged aPTT, and a normal factor VIII:C level, a specific assay for factor IX activity should be performed. As with VIII:C assays, either a one-stage or a two-stage assay may be performed, utilizing substrates severely deficient in factor IX. Levels of circulating factor IX activity usually correlate with clinical severity, as described above for factor VIII.

A number of variants have been described in hemophilia B, which appear to reflect different functional abnormalities of altered factor IX molecules, and are reviewed by Bloom (1981). Carrier detection in hemophilia B has proved more complicated than in hemophilia A, with varying opinions as to the role of determinations of factor IX antigenic levels in the different variants (Graham, 1979; Kasper, 1977; Pechet, 1978; Thompson, 1977).

Inhibitors to factor IX develop in about 3 per cent of hemophilia B patients overall, and in approximately 7 to 10 per cent of those with severe disease (Shapiro, 1979). These are usually immediately-acting antibodies, as opposed to the time-dependent antibodies characteristic of hemophilia A, and titers tend to fall more rapidly upon the termination of factor IX exposure than is often seen in the case of inhibitors to factor VIII.

VON WILLEBRAND'S DISEASE

Although hemophilia A has traditionally been considered the most frequently occurring congenital bleeding disorder, increasing identification of patients with milder forms of von Willebrand's disease (vWD) suggests that the overall incidence of vWD may be equal or even greater. Transmission of vWD is usually autosomal dominant. A small number of cases have been described, however, in which transmission appears to be autosomal recessive.

Patients with vWD characteristically bleed from mucous membranes and cutaneous sites. Easy bruising, epistaxis, gastrointestinal bleeding, and excessive bleeding following tonsillectomy or dental extractions may be prominent. Menorrhagia may be pronounced. Hemarthroses and deep muscle hematomas, in contrast, are not usually characteristic of vWD, except in the most severe cases which have a concomitant severe decrease of VIII:C (see below).

An autosomal chromosome determines the synthesis of the von Willebrand factor (vWF) molecule, whereas the X chromosome determines the synthesis of the VIII:C molecule. The two proteins circulate in the blood as a noncovalently linked complex (VIII/vWF complex). vWF is synthesized by endothelial cells (Jaffe, 1973, 1974) and by megakaryocytes (Nachman, 1977). Indirect evidence has suggested that VIII:C synthesized in the liver (possibly by hepatic reticuloendothelial cells) binds to vWF that enters the hepatic circulation and that the VIII/vWF complex then passes into the general circulation (Owen, 1979, 1981).

In contrast to the relatively small VIII:C molecule of molecular weight approximately 150,000 daltons, the molecular weight of vWF has been estimated in excess of 20 million daltons. The vWF molecule appears to consist of a basic monomeric form (of approximately 200,000 daltons) that combines with additional monomers to produce a series of multimers of increasing size. The largest multimers, in particular, appear to possess functional activities contributing to platelet-mediated hemostatic events (Zimmerman, 1982).

A central role of vWF appears to be in the adhesion of platelets to subendothelial surfaces following vessel injury. Demonstration of prolonged template bleeding times (Chap. 31) in patients with vWD is accordingly of primary diagnostic importance. The aPTT in some patients will additionally be prolonged if there is a sufficiently decreased VIII:C activity. The prothrombin time and thrombin times are normal. Although tests of platelet adhesiveness in glass bead columns show decreased adhesiveness in patients with vWD, difficulties in reproducibility have prompted the abandonment of this test in most laboratories.

Measurement of the different component activities of the factor VIII/vWF complex is necessary for a more specific diagnosis. The Laurell "rocket" immunoelectrophoresis technique (Fig. 32–5) is still the most commonly utilized quantitative method to detect total vWF antigenically. Immunoradiometric techniques (Hoyer, 1972; Girma, 1979) offer the advantage of sensitivity, and may be utilized more frequently in coming years. The ability of vWF to interact with platelets may be assayed in the vWF's *ristocetin cofactor* activity. This test is performed by quantitating the ability of patient plasma (the source of vWF ristocetin cofactor activity) to support ristocetin-induced agglutination of either freshly washed (Weiss, 1973) or formalin-fixed (Macfarlane, 1975) normal platelets by the antibiotic ristocetin. This test is generally considered a more sensitive assay of decreases in vWF functional activity than are aggregation studies based upon the direct addition of ristocetin to the patient's own platelet-rich plasma (Meyer, 1982). Measurement of VIII:C activity is performed as described in the evaluation of hemophilia A.

In order to detect qualitative abnormalities of vWF multimeric structure, agarose gel multimeric analysis, crossed immunoelectrophoresis (CIE), or CIE utilizing radiolabeled antibody is performed. In the first-named method, patient plasma is electrophoresed on sodium dodecyl sulfate (SDS) agarose gels, and radiolabeled antibody specific for human vWF then is incubated with the gels. Radioautographs then are made, which reveal the different molecular weight multimers of vWF present in the patient's plasma (Fig. 32–6). CIE (with or without radiolabeled antibody) affords similar qualitative information, but without resolution of the multimeric bands.

vWD now appears to comprise a heterogeneous group of disorders, in which qualitative and/or quantitative abnormalities of vWF are present (Table 32–4). The more common autosomal dominant types of vWD may be further classified on the basis of laboratory testing. *Type I* constitutes "classic vWD," in which levels of vWF antigen, ristocetin cofactor, and VIII:C are decreased in generally equivalent fashion. Multimeric analysis shows a partial decrease of all multimers, without a selective loss of the higher molecular weight multimers. Platelet vWF is present in normal amount and has a normal multimeric composition. Clinical expression in the Type I patients may be highly variable. In fact, in the milder cases vWF may be within normal limits at the time of the initial study, necessitating repeated studies in order to reach a diagnosis (Zimmerman, 1983).

The Type II variants of vWD are recognized by a selective absence of the higher molecular weight multimers of vWF. In *Type IIA*, concentrations of ristocetin more than adequate to promote platelet aggregation in platelet-rich plasma (PRP) from normal individuals (>2 mg/ml) are unable to produce significant aggregation in patient PRP. Conversely, in *Type IIB*, not only do standard concentrations of ristocetin (0.9 to 1.2 mg/ml) produce aggregation, but in fact aggregation is typically produced by ristocetin concentrations even lower than those required to produce aggregation in normal PRP (0.3 to 0.5 mg/ml). Levels of ristocetin cofactor also appear to distinguish Types IIA and IIB fairly well; patients with IIA disease have undetectable or barely detectable ristocetin cofactor activity, whereas patients with IIB disease typically have either mildly to moderately decreased or normal levels (Ruggeri, 1980a). vWF antigen and VIII:C

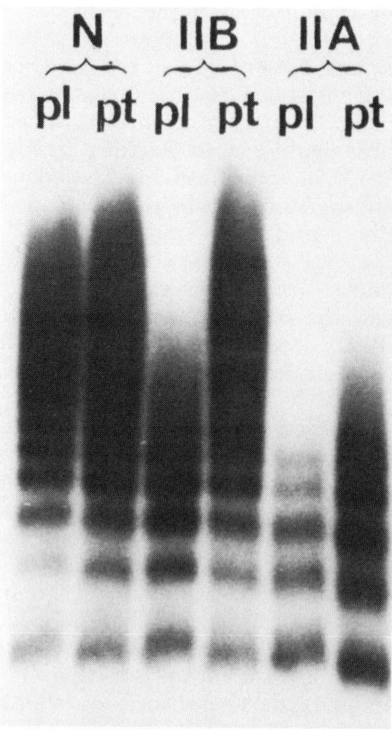

Figure 32–6. Multimeric composition of plasma (pl) and platelet (pt) von Willebrand factor. SDS-agarose gel electrophoresis of samples, followed by incubation of gels with ^{125}I-anti-vWF and subsequent autoradiography. Both Type IIA and IIB plasmas lack the highest molecular weight multimers seen in normal (N) plasmas, but only the IIA platelets lack the highest molecular weight multimers. In Type I vWD all of the multimers are usually present in normal proportion, but all are decreased in quantity (not shown in figure). (Reproduced from Ruggeri, Z. M., and Zimmerman, T. S.: J. Clin. Invest., *65*:1318, 1980, by copyright permission of the American Society of Clinical Investigation.)

levels are characteristically either normal or only mildly decreased in both subtypes.

Platelet vWF multimer patterns appear relatively normal in Type IIB, but there is a significant reduction of the larger multimers in platelet extracts from Type IIA patients. These findings have been interpreted to suggest that in Type IIA there is an error of vWF synthesis resulting in an absence of production of the higher molecular weight multimers. In Type IIB patients these multimers would be produced, but due to their abnormally heightened ability to bind to platelets, they would appear decreased in plasma samples yet present in at least normal amount in platelets. Studies of the binding properties of Type IIB vWF to normal platelets appear to support these findings (Ruggeri, 1980a, 1982a).

A third Type II variant, characterized by absence of the larger vWF multimers in both plasma and platelets, and an abnormality of repeating multimeric units on agarose electrophoresis, has been termed *Type IIC* by Ruggeri (1982b). This vWD variant is further notable in that inheritance appears to be autosomal recessive. A family with similar findings has also recently been reported by Mannucci (1983).

An additional disorder showing selective absence of the higher molecular weight multimers of plasma vWF has been termed *platelet-type vWD* (Miller, 1982). Patients with platelet-type vWD share many similarities with Type IIB patients, including a heightened aggregation response when low concentrations of ristocetin are added to patient PRP. These patients additionally tend to have borderline thrombocytopenia, bleeding times near the upper limit of normal, and an abnormally enhanced ability of their *platelets* to bind circulating vWF. An apparently similar disorder in a family studied by Weiss (1982) has been termed pseudo-vWD. The ability of cryoprecipitate without the addition of ristocetin to produce aggregation in PRP appears to be an additional and quite simple method for distinguishing platelet-type vWD from Type IIB vWD (Miller, 1983; see also Chapter 31).

The most severely affected patients with vWD typically have an autosomal recessive disorder that has been termed *Type III vWD*. Inheritance patterns are either truly homozygous or doubly heterozygous. vWF antigen is nearly undetectable, ristocetin cofactor activity markedly reduced or absent, and VIII:C activity moderately to severely reduced but always present (0.01 to 0.05 U/ml). In some patients a selective loss of the larger multimeric forms of vWF (less anodic forms on CIE) has also been found (Zimmerman, 1979).

OTHER CONGENITAL DEFICIENCIES

In comparison with hemophilia A and B (and with vWD), congenital deficiencies of the other coagulation factors are quite rare (Table 32–5). Additionally, inheritance of these latter disorders is autosomal, and in most instances recessive.

Deficiencies of Factor XII, HMWK, or prekallikrein have not been associated with clinical bleeding tendencies. In most cases of *factor XI deficiency* (of which the highest incidence appears to be in Ashkenazi Jews) only mild bleeding is observed. Even in cases in which factor XI is virtually undetectable, severe bleeding resembling hemophilia is not frequently observed (Rapaport, 1981). These clinical observations, in conjunction with laboratory studies utilizing highly purified factor preparations, have led to the view that activation of factor IX by the tissue factor pathway (Fig. 32–1) may be of considerable importance *in vivo* (Rapaport, 1981; Nemerson, 1981).

Patients with a deficiency of one of the above factors typically have a prolonged aPTT and normal prothrombin and thrombin times. If the aPTT corrects when mixed 1:1 with normal plasma, and factors VIII:C and IX assay within normal limits, the abnormality may be presumed to be localized to the contact factors. Normalization of the aPTT following prolonged incubation of plasma with the activating agent (e.g., kaolin) suggests that the deficiency may be in prekallikrein. Substrate plasmas deficient in factors

Table 32–4. LABORATORY DIAGNOSIS OF CLASSIC VON WILLEBRAND'S DISEASE (TYPE I) AND VARIANTS*

	Autosomal Dominant				Autosomal Recessive	
	Type I	***Type IIA***	***Type IIB***	***Platelet-type***	***Type IIC***	***Type III***
Bleeding time	Increased or normal	Increased	Increased	Increased	Increased	Increased
Platelet count	Normal	Normal	Normal or decreased	Low normal or decreased	Normal	Normal
VIII:C	Decreased	Normal or decreased	Normal or decreased	Normal or decreased	Normal	Markedly decreased
VIIIR:Ag	Decreased	Decreased or normal	Decreased or normal	Normal or decreased	Decreased or normal	Markedly decreased
VIIIR:RCo	Decreased	Markedly decreased	Decreased or normal	Decreased or normal	Decreased	Markedly decreased
Crossed immunoelectrophoresis of plasma vWF	Normal	Abnormal	Abnormal	Abnormal	Abnormal	Variable
Multimeric structure of vWF						
Plasma	Normal	Absence of largest and intermediate multimers	Absence of largest multimers	Absence of largest multimers	Absence of largest multimers and abnormal band structure	Variable
Platelets	Normal	Absence of largest and intermediate multimers	Normal	Normal	Absence of largest multimers and abnormal band structure	Variable
Ristocetin-induced platelet aggregation in patient PRP	Decreased or normal	Markedly decreased	Increased	Increased	Decreased	Markedly decreased
Ristocetin-induced binding of vWF to platelets						
Patient plasma + normal platelets		Decreased	Increased	Normal or decreased		
Normal plasma + patient platelets		Normal	Normal	Increased		
vWF-induced aggregation of unstimulated patient platelets in PRP			Absent	Present		

*Data compiled from multiple sources, including Zimmerman and Ruggeri (1983), Holmberg et al. (1983), and Miller et al. (1983).

Abbreviations: VIII:C, factor VIII coagulant activity; vWF, von Willebrand factor; VIIIR:Ag, factor VIII–related antigen (vWF antigen); VIIIR:RCo, ristocetin cofactor activity; PRP, platelet-rich plasma.

4

Table 32–5. FREQUENCY AND MODE OF TRANSMISSION OF INHERITED DISORDERS OF BLOOD COAGULATION*

Deficiency	Frequency	Inheritance
Fibrinogen:		
Afibrinogenemia	Rare (more than 100 cases)	Autosomal recessive
Hypofibrinogenemia	Rare (more than 100 cases)	Autosomal recessive
Dysfibrinogenemia	Rare (less than 100 cases)	Autosomal recessive or autosomal dominant
Prothrombin	Rare (8 cases)	Probably autosomal recessive
Factor V	Rare (52 cases)	Autosomal recessive
Factor VII	Rare (less than 100 cases)	Autosomal recessive (incomplete)
Factor VIII	Most common hemophilia (~1/5000 males)	X-linked recessive
Factor IX	Less common hemophilia (~1/25,000 males)	X-linked recessive
Factor X	Rare (20 cases)	Autosomal recessive (incomplete)
Factor XI	Uncommon	Autosomal recessive (primarily in Jews)
Factor XII	Rare (more than 100 cases)	Autosomal recessive
Factor XIII	Rare	Autosomal recessive
Fletcher factor (prekallikrein)	Rare (less than 10 cases)	Autosomal recessive
High-molecular-weight kininogen	Rare (less than 10 cases)	?

*Modified from Abildgard, C. F.: *In* Nathan, D. G., and Oski, F. A. (eds.): Hematology of Infancy and Childhood. Philadelphia, W. B. Saunders, 1981.

XI, XII, HMWK, or prekallikrein are now commercially available for the performance of specific assays.

Factor VII deficiency may be associated with serious bleeding tendencies. Levels of 0.03 to 0.10 U/ml factor VII are frequently adequate to prevent serious bleeding, but the presence of only trace levels has been associated with major hemorrhages (Rapaport, 1981). Onset of hemorrhagic symptoms may be either early in life or delayed until adolescence or even later (Bloom, 1981). Laboratory studies show a prolonged prothrombin time but a normal aPTT and thrombin time. In this setting, a normal Russell's viper venom (RVV) time suggests a deficiency of factor VII activity, and a specific assay for factor VII should be employed to confirm this diagnosis.

Deficiency of factor X activity appears to derive from a variety of qualitative as well as quantitative abnormalities of the factor X molecule, and is variable in its clinical severity. In most (but not all) cases both the aPTT and the prothrombin time will be prolonged. Although in the originally reported kindreds the RVV time was abnormal, variants with normal or only slightly prolonged RVV times have been reported (Table 32–6) (Roberts, 1981).

Congenital deficiency of factor V is quite rare. Moreover, the level of plasma factor V does not show a good correlation with clinical severity. Recent studies of patients with congenital factor V deficiency have suggested a correlation between severity of bleeding and the inability of patient platelets to bind factor Xa and increase the rate of thrombin formation at the platelet surface (Miletich, 1978b). Since the platelet surface likely serves as the key site for activation of the coagulation proteins *in vivo,* this explanation is appealing and might even apply to deficiencies of other factors. Additionally, about one third of patients with factor V deficiency have had a prolongation of their bleeding time, again possibly attributable to an abnormality of their platelet-associated factor V (Bloom, 1981). Detection of decreased plasma levels

Table 32–6. GENETIC VARIANTS OF FACTOR X*

	Clotting Assays				
Variants	***Partial Thromboplastin Time***	***Prothrombin Time***	***Russell's Viper Venom Time***	**Factor X Antibody Neutralization**	**CRM†**
Prower	Abnormal	Abnormal	Abnormal	+ + +	CRM^+
Stuart	Abnormal	Abnormal	Abnormal	–	CRM^-
Factor X Friuli	Abnormal	Abnormal	Normal	+ + +	CRM^+
Patient R.E.D.	Slightly abnormal	Abnormal	Slightly abnormal	+	$CRM^{partial}$‡
Patient G. S.	Abnormal	Slightly abnormal	Slightly abnormal	–	CRM^-
Patient G. F.	Abnormal	Normal	Normal	+ + +	CRM^+

*Modified from Roberts, H. R., et al.: *In* Menache, D., Surgenor, D. M., and Anderson, H. (eds.): Hemophilia and Hemostasis. New York, Atan R. Liss, 1981.

†CRM = cross-reacting material indicating factor X antigen.

‡Indicates a group demonstrating partial neutralization of the antibody.

Table 32–7. CHARACTERISTIC FEATURES AND DIFFERENTIAL DIAGNOSIS OF INHERITED AND ACQUIRED DISORDERS OF FIBRIN FORMATION AND STABILIZATION*

Congenital Disorder	Mode of Inheritance	Leading Symptoms/Predominant Localization of Hemorrhage	Disorder to be Excluded
Afibrinogenemia	Autosomal recessive	Severe hemorrhage Umbilical Mucosal Gastrointestinal Intracranial	—
Hypofibrinogenemia	Dominant	Moderate bleeding: mucosal Frequently asymptomatic	Intravascular coagulation Liver failure (Hypodysfibrinogenemia)
Dysfibrinogenemia	Dominant	Frequently asymptomatic Bleeding moderate to severe Mucosal Post-traumatic Postoperative Thromboembolism Wound dehiscence	Intravascular coagulation Plasma proteolysis (fibrinolysis) Liver failure Hepatoma Myeloma (Factor XIII deficiency) (Hypofibrinogenemia)
Factor XIII deficiency	Autosomal recessive	Bleeding moderate to severe (delay after trauma) Umbilical Mucosal Intracranial Delayed wound healing	Acquired factor XIII deficiency Autoimmune antibody Antituberculous drugs (Dysfibrinogenemia with abnormal fibrin cross-linking)

*From Beck, E. A.: *In* Colman, R. W., et al. (eds.): Hemostasis and Thrombosis. Philadelphia, J. B. Lippincott, 1982.

of factor V is based upon prolonged aPTT and prothrombin time, but normal thrombin time, in the absence of an inhibitor; specific assay of factor V may then be performed by a modified prothrombin time test, utilizing as substrate normal plasma that has been depleted of factor V.

Although quite rare, *hereditary prothrombin disorders* representing a variety of qualitative abnormalities (dysprothrombinemias) have been reported, as well as true hypoprothrombinemias. The prothrombin time and usually also the aPTT are prolonged, and factors VII, X, and V and fibrinogen are usually normal. A variety of different functional and immunologic assays are available for definitive study of the patient's prothrombin, as recently reviewed by Roberts (1981) and by Bloom (1981).

Inherited disorders of fibrin formation and stabilization comprise both quantitative deficiencies and qualitative abnormalities of fibrinogen, as well as deficiencies of the fibrin cross-linking enzyme, factor XIII. The major clinical characteristics distinguishing these disorders are summarized in Table 32–7 (Beck, 1982).

Since any test utilizing coagulation of the patient's own plasma is dependent upon the level of functional fibrinogen present, the aPTT, prothrombin time, and, particularly, the thrombin time test usually are prolonged in fibrinogen disorders. In contrast, these tests are normal in cases of factor XIII deficiency. Solubility of a formed clot in 5 molar urea reflects the lack of covalent fibrin-fibrin cross-linkages in severe factor XIII deficiency. In less severe deficiencies of factor XIII, diagnosis of the abnormality may require demonstrating decreased ability of patient plasma to catalyze incorporation into casein of the fluorescent probe monodansylcadaverine (Lorand, 1969), or of the radioactive probe ^{14}C-putrescine (Dvilansky, 1970).

A variety of chemical, functional, and immunological assays are available to measure the level of fibrinogen in plasma. Measurement of total clottable protein by the method of Ratnoff and Menzie (1951) is widely employed as a reference method. However, in cases of dysfibrinogenemia, measurement of fibrinogen utilizing the *rate* of clot formation by the method of Clauss (1957) or one of the several variations of this method may prove significantly more sensitive in detection of the abnormality (Beck, 1979, 1982). Immunological measurement of fibrinogen will typically agree fairly closely with functional assays in true hypofibrinogenemias, but may give significantly higher values in the dysfibrinogenemias.

The individual dysfibrinogenemias have traditionally been named according to the city in which they were discovered (e.g., "fibrinogen Detroit"). Structural defects of the molecule are associated with abnormalities in the release of fibrinopeptides A and B, polymerization of fibrin monomers, cross-linking by factor XIII, and eventual lysis by plasmin. Specific features of the individual dysfibrinogenemias are detailed in several excellent reviews (Beck, 1982; Menache, 1981; Bloom, 1981).

ACQUIRED DISORDERS OF COAGULATION

FACTOR VIII/VON WILLEBRAND FACTOR

Inhibitors arising in patients with congenital deficiencies of factor VIII:C have been discussed above.

Inhibitors to factor VIII:C arise rarely in previously healthy individuals, and most notably occasionally in women subsequent to childbirth. Although variable in severity, most inhibitors eventually disappear over a period of months, but occasionally only after several years. Unlike inhibitors developing in some patients with hemophilia A, these inhibitors characteristically do not show an anamnestic response following factor VIII therapy. In addition, the antibody may react with the VIII:C moiety in such a way that the inhibitor–VIII:C complex found retains significant VIII:C activity (Biggs, 1972; Gawyrl, 1982).

A number of cases of acquired von Willebrand's disease have now also been seen in patients with autoimmune disease and with lymphoproliferative or, rarely, other neoplastic disorders. Antibodies to von Willebrand factor associated with the tumor have been identified in several cases, and are generally presumed to be responsible for such bleeding disorders. In some cases it is possible that the neoplastic cells might act by binding more of the higher molecular weight multimers of von Willebrand factor (Joist, 1978).

FACTOR IX

Inhibitors arising in patients with congenital deficiencies of factor IX have been discussed above. Inhibitors in non-hemophiliacs are very rare, but have occurred in a small number of postpartum women, and a small number of patients with autoimmune disorders or the nephrotic syndrome (Shapiro, 1979).

OTHER COAGULATION FACTORS

Isolated inhibitors to these factors are quite rare, and few generalizations can be made. Occasional patients with autoimmune or neoplastic disorders are found to produce antibodies that appear specific for individual factors. Development of inhibitors to factor XIII has occurred following drug ingestion, most notably isoniazid. Inhibitors to factor V have also been attributed to antibiotic therapy in rare patients, or have appeared to commence following major surgery. Finally, deficiencies of factor X occasionally arise in association with amyloidosis, possibly due to binding of the factor X by amyloid (Shapiro, 1979).

LUPUS-LIKE ANTICOAGULANT

About 5 to 10 per cent of patients with systemic lupus erythematosus, a significant number of patients on phenothiazine therapy, patients taking a variety of other drugs, occasional patients with lymphoproliferative disorders, and occasional patients in whom neither an underlying disease nor a drug can be identified develop inhibitors known as "lupus-like anticoagulants." These inhibitors are heterogeneous, but have in common being IgG or IgM antibodies that appear to be directed at phospholipid or phospholipoprotein components involved in the activation of coagulation factors. The outstanding feature of these anticoagulants is that, unless there is an additional hemostatic abnormality (most often thrombocytopenia, for example, in the case of systemic lupus), *presence of a lupus-like anticoagulant is not associated with a clinical bleeding tendency.*

A lupus-like anticoagulant usually comes to attention first from a prolonged aPTT. The prothrombin time is either normal or mildly prolonged, and the thrombin time is normal. Since the need to diagnose a lupus-like anticoagulant often comes about as part of a preoperative patient workup, further testing usually is required in order to eliminate the possibility of a clinically significant coagulation inhibitor. Unfortunately, there is currently no single test specific for identification of a lupus-like anticoagulant (see review by Shapiro, 1982). The following criteria have been suggested by Mueh (1980):

1. For patients whose aPTT is at least five seconds above the upper limit of the normal range, one part of patient plasma is mixed with one part of normal plasma, and an aPTT then performed (i.e., without prior incubation of the plasma mixture). The aPTT of the mixture remains prolonged at least five seconds beyond that of the same normal plasma run in parallel.
2. At least two specific one-stage assays for factors of the intrinsic system (i.e., VIII, IX, XI, XII) reveal apparent factor deficiencies of less than 50 per cent of normal.
3. As the patient plasma is increasingly *diluted* in the above assays (i.e., beyond the 1:5 or 1:10 dilution normally utilized in a factor assay), the measured activity of one or more of these factors appears to increase.
4. No other apparent causes of the abnormal coagulation studies can be identified.

Similar criteria have recently been recommended in an international cooperative study (Green, 1983).

The tissue thromboplastin inhibition test (Schleider, 1976) is also widely used to identify a lupus-like anticoagulant. In this test the thromboplastin source used in prothrombin determinations is diluted in order to increase its sensitivity to inhibitors. Despite its sensitivity, this test should not be considered specific for lupus-like inhibitors.

In several cases substitutions of resting or activated platelets for exogenous phospholipid in the aPTT or RVV time tests have been shown to correct the abnormality associated with a lupus-like anticoagulant (Thiagarajan, 1980; Shapiro, 1981). The extent to which such assays may become generally useful is at present unknown.

Occasionally a lupus-like anticoagulant may be present in a patient for whom assay of a specific intrinsic system coagulation factor is required. In such cases a two-stage assay may be desirable, since the lupus-like anticoagulant appears to have less effect upon these assays (Green, 1983).

In summary, the lupus-like anticoagulants appear to represent antibodies with immediately-acting inhibitory activities directed against components required for performance of certain *in vitro* coagulation tests. *In vivo,* platelets serve as the source of highly specific, oriented phospholipoproteins subserving coagulation reactions. It is likely that the lupus-like anticoagulant bears little or no clinical significance because it does not direct appreciable inhibitory activity against platelet-mediated coagulant activation *in vivo.* In fact, there have been several reports suggesting that this group of patients may actually bear an increased risk for *thrombotic* disorders (Mueh, 1980; Shapiro, 1982).

LIVER DISEASE

Hemostasis in liver disease is complex, due to the many different roles of the liver in the synthesis of coagulation and fibrinolysis factors, the breakdown or removal of factor complexes, and its poorly understood influences upon platelet production and function. Decreases in the vitamin K–dependent factors (II, VII, IX, X) are the earliest changes usually encountered in liver disease, resulting in a prolonged prothrombin time and possibly also aPTT. Fibrinogen levels may be decreased or increased, depending upon the type of liver disease. Even in chronic liver disease accompanied by high fibrinogen levels, however, the thrombin time may be prolonged; in at least some cases this appears attributable to disordered fibrinogen synthesis resulting in functionally abnormal fibrinogen molecules.

Factor VIII:C, vWF antigen, and ristocetin cofactor activities are frequently elevated in acute hepatic failure and in chronic liver disease. Such elevations would not be inconsistent with severe hepatocellular damage, on the basis of our current knowledge that von Willebrand factor is synthesized by endothelial cells and megakaryocytes, and that VIII:C produced from hepatic synthesis more likely derives from hepatic reticuloendothelial cells than from hepatocytes themselves.

Patterns of screening tests and specific assay results typically found in different types of liver disease are shown in Tables 32–8 and 32–9. An assessment of bleeding risk in patients with liver disease can, in most instances, be made based upon the results of the routine coagulation screening tests, together with a platelet count and bleeding time.

VITAMIN K DEFICIENCY

Inadequate vitamin K levels lead to an impairment in the synthesis of coagulation factors VII, IX, and X and prothrombin. This fat-soluble vitamin promotes the post-ribosomal addition of a second carboxyl group to glutamic acid in the zymogen molecules, producing gamma carboxyglutamic acid (or "Gla") forms of these molecules. The highly negatively charged Gla regions are thought to be responsible for binding of the molecules to negatively charged phospholipids (e.g., at the surfaces of activated platelets) through a bridging action of the positively charged, divalent calcium ions (Jackson, 1981).

In vitamin K deficiency the prothrombin time typically is prolonged, and the aPTT may be also. Since fibrinogen synthesis is not vitamin K dependent, the thrombin time remains normal. The recently described inhibitory coagulation factor protein C (see above) is also vitamin K dependent, and its functions may be impaired during vitamin K deficiency.

Vitamin K is normally obtained both through the dietary intake of vitamin K_1 produced by plants and from the production of vitamin K_2 by intestinal bacteria. Inadequate diet, biliary obstruction, intestinal malabsorption, and gut sterilization by antibiotics are among the contributing causes of clinical vitamin K deficiency. Vitamin K deficiency in the neonatal period may also predispose to hemorrhagic disease of the newborn. Parenteral administration of vitamin K_1 will correct the associated coagulation abnormalities within 6 to 24 hours.

Intentional induction of a vitamin K deficiency–like state forms the basis for therapeutic anticoagulation by *coumarin* or its derivatives. These pharmacological antagonists of vitamin K can be taken orally, resulting in the development of a full anticoagulant effect in several days. Maintenance of the prothrombin time at 1½ to 2½ times basal levels is the most commonly employed method for monitoring coumarin therapy; however, as discussed by Poller (1981), there is a considerable range of apparent therapeutic ratios, depending upon the reagents and the methodology employed. Efforts to realize greater standardization in such testing are currently in progress (Triplett, 1982).

HEPARIN

Heparin is a sulfated mucopolysaccharide capable of binding to antithrombin III, thereby greatly increasing the anticoagulant activity of the antithrombin III molecule (Barrowcliffe, 1981). Administration of heparin provides a potent form of anticoagulation, rapidly inhibiting the activities of thrombin, factor Xa, and the other serine protease coagulation factors (Table 32–1). Although heparin is commonly utilized in the treatment of thrombosis, there is still no general consensus as to the optimal method of monitoring heparin therapy. Indeed, it is uncertain whether the most appropriate test is one that measures the coagulability of plasma, such as the aPTT, as opposed to one that more directly provides an estimate of the plasma heparin concentration itself (Edson, 1982). Currently, nevertheless, the aPTT remains the test most commonly employed for this purpose. It should be emphasized that standardization of aPTT reagents in the individual laboratory for heparin monitoring is of considerable importance in the development of an aPTT therapeutic range (Thomson, 1982; Ingram, 1982).

Plasma samples obtained for coagulation testing occasionally show striking prolongations in the thrombin time, together with variable prolongations of the aPTT, and occasionally also of the prothrombin time. When no other cause is apparent, the presence of heparin, arising in the patient, in an infusion line, or in the blood processing itself must be considered. In particular, whenever all three of the above tests are prolonged over 90 seconds, the possibility of the presence of heparin should be considered foremost. Commercially available anion-exchange resins now allow rapid removal of even full therapeutic doses of heparin from plasma; following this, most coagulation tests approach pre-heparin values (Cowan, 1981). Alternatively, the presence of heparin may be established if the addition of protamine sulfate or polybrene normalizes the test values (Hoffman, 1980). These positively charged substances neutralize the negatively charged heparin molecule.

Table 32–8. COAGULATION TESTS IN LIVER DISEASE*

Condition	One-Stage Prothrombin Time	Partial Thromboplastin Time	Thrombin Time	Fibrinogen	Platelet Count
Acute viral hepatitis	N or ↑	N or ↑	N or ↑	N or ↑	N
Acute liver failure	↑ ↑	↑ ↑	↑ ↑	↓	↓
Cirrhosis Wilson's disease Hemochromatosis	↑ or N	↑, ↓ or N	↑ or N	N, ↑ or ↓	↓
Obstructive jaundice	↑ ↑	↑ or N	N or ↑	↑	N
Biliary cirrhosis	↑ ↑	↑	↑	↑	↓
Post partial hepatectomy	↑	↑	↑	↓	↓
Hepatoma Secondary deposits in the liver	↑	↑	↑ ↑	↑, N or ↓	↑, N or ↓

↑ = Prolonged or raised. ↓ = Shortened or reduced. N = Normal.
*From Brozovic, M.: *In* Bloom, A. L., and Thomas, D. P. (eds.): Haemostasis and Thrombosis. Edinburgh, Churchill Livingstone, 1981.

Table 32–9. HEMOSTATIC FACTORS IN DIFFERENT FORMS OF LIVER DISEASE*

Condition	II	VII	IX	X	V	VIII:C	VIIIR:Ag	XIII	AT III	Plasminogen	Clot Lysis Times
Viral hepatitis	↓	↓	N	↓	↓	N	↑	N or ↓	N or ↓	N	N or ↑
Acute liver failure	↓	↓	↓	↓	↓	↑↑	↑↑	↓	↓↓	↓	N, ↑, ↓
Cirrhosis Wilson's disease Hemochromatosis	↓	↓	↓	↓	↓	↑	↑	↓	↓	↓	↓
Obstructive jaundice	↓↓	↓↓	↓↓	↓↓	N or ↑	↑	↑↑	↑	↑	N	N
Biliary cirrhosis	↓↓	↓↓	↓↓	↓↓	↓	↑	↑↑	↓	↓	↓	↓
Post partial hepatectomy	↓	↓	↓	↓	↓	↑	↑	↓	↓	↓	↓
Hepatoma carcinoma	↓	↓	↓	↓	↓	↑	↑↑	↓	↓	↓	↓, N or ↑

↑ = Prolonged or raised. ↓ = Shortened or reduced. N = Normal.
*From Brozovic, M.: *In* Bloom, A. L., and Thomas, D. P. (eds.): Haemostasis and Thrombosis. Edinburgh, Churchill Livingstone, 1981.

Table 32–10. CLINICAL CONDITIONS ASSOCIATED WITH CONSUMPTIVE THROMBOHEMORRHAGIC DISORDERS*

Underlying Disease	Predominant Form of Consumptive Disorder
Sepsis	DIC, variable severity
Neoplasm	DIC, often chronic, but heterogeneous clinical manifestations and rare systemic fibrinolysis
Obstetric	Localized and/or disseminated; wide variation in clinical severity
Hepatic disease	Variable; hyperfibrinolysis more likely than DIC
TTP/HUS	Systemic; predominant platelet involvement
Giant cavernous hemangioma	Localized, intravascular
Arterial aneurysm	Localized, intravascular
Snake bite	DIC, variable thrombocytopenia
Massive hemolysis	DIC
Trauma/surgery/hyperthermia	DIC; occasional fibrinolysis that may mask an underlying DIC
Streptokinase/urokinase	Systemic fibrinolysis
Menorrhagia/hemorrhagic cystitis	Localized fibrinolysis

*From Marder, V. J., et al.: *In* Colman, R. W., et al. (eds.): Hemostasis and Thrombosis. Philadelphia, J. B. Lippincott, 1982.

CONSUMPTIVE THROMBOHEMORRHAGIC DISORDERS

A wide variety of systemic and localized pathologic processes may lead to activation of the coagulation and/or fibrinolytic systems (Table 32–10). Depending upon the balance struck between these two systems in the individual case, the immediate clinical result may be thrombosis, bleeding, or even a combination of the two.

The release of thromboplastic material into the circulation will lead to a triggering of the coagulation system, with subsequent activation of the fibrinolytic system. Such an event has been termed *consumptive coagulopathy,* or *disseminated intravascular coagulation (DIC).* A wide variety of underlying causes may predispose to DIC, and it is imperative that the underlying condition be detected so that therapy specific for the disorder may be instituted. Clinically suspected acute DIC may be verified by laboratory testing. Typically the patient's platelet count will drop, and the aPTT, prothrombin time, and thrombin time will be prolonged. FDP will be elevated, and the patient's fibrinogen level will have decreased from its previous value. Paracoagulation tests for circulating fibrin monomers such as the *ethanol gelation test* or the *serial dilution protamine sulfate test* (Niewiarowski, 1971) may be positive. Radioimmunoassay for *fibrinopeptide A* released from fibrinogen by thrombin is a more reliable test for *in vivo* thrombin activity, and nearly always shows increased values (Nossel, 1974). Should the initiating process persist, the DIC may progress from an acute to a more chronic form. Chronic DIC may be encountered, for example, in patients with malignancies or autoimmune disorders (Marder, 1982). In some instances in which the rate of consumption of individual hemostatic components is not excessive, a compensatory increase in their production may lead to a normalization, or even an increase, of their circulating levels.

The initiation of *systemic hyperfibrinolysis* without a prominent, accompanying DIC is a decidedly less common occurrence. Among disorders in which it may be encountered occasionally are liver disease (Fletcher, 1964) and certain tumors that appear to produce plasminogen activators (Donati, 1981). Antithrombotic therapy with streptokinase or urokinase also may lead to a systemic hyperfibrinolytic state. Decreased fibrinogen (due to active plasmin in the circulation), increased FDP, and shortened whole blood or euglobulin clot lysis times are typical findings. Finally, the recent development of a radioimmunoassay for *fibrinopeptide* $B\beta 1{-}42$ may prove useful as a specific measure of early plasmin proteolysis of the fibrinogen molecule (Nossel, 1982).

Localized renal thrombi or multi-organ thrombus formation is associated with the *hemolytic-uremic syndrome* (HUS) and *thrombotic thrombocytopenic purpura* (TTP), respectively. Although the etiology of this family of disorders remains unclear, involvement of platelets in intraluminal arteriolar thrombi is the characteristic pathological finding (Marder, 1982). Laboratory findings typically include thrombocytopenia and microangiopathic hemolytic anemia. Although the thrombin time may be prolonged and the level of FDP increased, convincing evidence of DIC is usually not present in most cases. When laboratory evidence of DIC is found, it is believed likely to be secondary to the severe hemolysis and subsequent release of red cell fragments that may occur in HUS and TTP (Bukowski, 1982).

4

APPROACH TO THE PATIENT

Hemostatic evaluation in the individual patient begins first and foremost with a thorough clinical history and physical examination. It is critical to determine whether the degree of bleeding appears disproportionate to the inciting incident(s). Tracing the onset of an apparent bleeding tendency can help determine if the abnormality is inherited or acquired. A careful systems review and questioning concerning previous surgery, dental procedures, trauma, and blood transfusions may reveal important clues of a disorder or may reinforce a clinical impression of hemostatic normality. A detailed family history may give important information regarding the mode of transmission of inherited disorders, or reinforce the impression that a particular disorder is acquired.

The pattern of bleeding in primary hemostatic (platelet or von Willebrand factor) disorders tends to be different from that in secondary hemostatic (coagulation) disorders (Table 32–11), although some degree of overlap of these features is to be expected. In disorders of primary hemostasis, the bleeding time typically will be prolonged. If the platelet count is normal and no history can be elicited of ingestion of drugs that could have a detrimental effect upon

Table 32–11. NATURE OF BLEEDING IN PRIMARY AND SECONDARY HEMOSTATIC DISORDERS*

Parameter	Primary Hemostatic Disorders	Secondary Hemostatic Disorders
Bleeding source	Usually capillary	Usually small artery
Lesion	Cutaneous and mucosal petechiae and/or ecchymoses	Often intramuscular and deep hematomas
Preceding trauma	Unusual	Frequent, but delayed onset of bleeding
Complications of venipuncture	Superficial ecchymoses around venipuncture site	No superficial ecchymoses, but hemorrhage may occur if firm external pressure not maintained long enough

*From Handin, R. I., and Rosenberg, R. D.: *In* Beck, W. S. (ed.): Hematology. Cambridge, Mass., MIT Press, 1981.

platelet function, the possibility of von Willebrand's disease should be considered. Measurement of vWF antigen and of ristocetin cofactor activity should be performed and, if the levels are decreased, further characterization by means of multimeric analysis of von Willebrand factor may be undertaken. Normal values of vWF antigen and ristocetin cofactor activity raise the possibility of a qualitative platelet defect, either congenital or acquired. Platelet aggregation (or lumi-aggregation) and measurement of clot retraction, together with evaluation of platelet morphology on a peripheral blood smear, may suggest a recognizable platelet defect. More specialized platelet studies (Table 31–6, p. 761) may be of additional help in reaching a diagnosis. Repeated study of the patient, together with studies on members of the patient's family, may be necessary before a definitive diagnosis can be reached in some cases.

Disorders of secondary hemostasis usually do not present with a prolonged bleeding time. The whole blood clot lysis test, or a variant of this test, can serve as a screening test (albeit not very sensitive) for enhanced fibrinolysis. Should an abnormality in fibrinolysis be suspected, measurement of FDP in serum, euglobulin clot lysis time, or more specialized tests may be undertaken.

The routine use of the prothrombin time, the aPTT, and the thrombin time will greatly help narrow the diagnostic possibilities in most cases of secondary hemostatic disorders. Although there is no one single approach, some form of progression from the simpler, screening types of tests to specific assays for only a small number of different factors is necessary. Figures 32–7 and 32–8 represent such an approach to the diagnosis of both inherited and acquired disorders of secondary hemostasis.

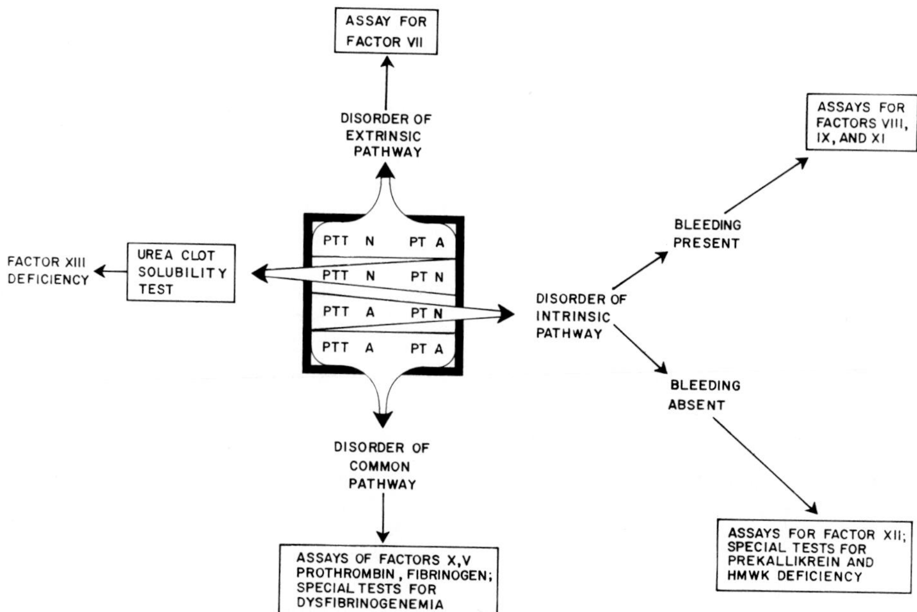

Figure 32–7. Laboratory diagnosis of hereditary coagulation disorders. HMWK = high molecular weight kininogen; PTT = partial thromboplastin time; PT = prothrombin time; N = normal; A = abnormal. (From Bithell, T. C.: The diagnostic approach to the bleeding disorders. *In* Wintrobe, M. M., et al. [eds.]: Clinical Hematology. 8th ed. Philadelphia, Lea and Febiger, 1981, Chapter 45.)

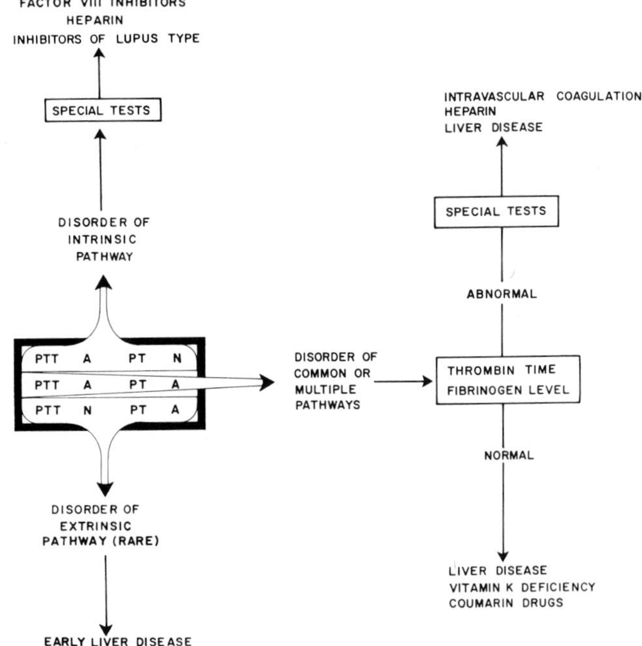

Figure 32–8. Laboratory diagnosis of acquired coagulation disorders. (From Bithell, T. C.: The diagnostic approach to the bleeding disorders. *In* Wintrobe, M. M., et al. [eds.]: Clinical Hematology. 8th ed. Philadelphia, Lea and Febiger, 1981, Chapter 45.)

Abildgaard, C. F.: Diseases of coagulation: The fluid phase. *In* Nathan, D. G., and Oski, F. A. (eds.): Hematology of Infancy and Childhood. Philadelphia, W. B. Saunders, 1981, pp. 1189–1233.

Barrowcliffe, T. W., and Thomas, D. P.: Antithrombin III and heparin. *In* Bloom, A. L., and Thomas, D. P. (eds.): Haemostasis and Thrombosis. Edinburgh, Churchill Livingstone, 1981, pp. 712–724.

Beck, E. A.: Congenital abnormalities of fibrinogen. Clin. Haematol., *8*:169, 1979.

Beck, E. A.: Congenital disorders of fibrin formation and stabilization. *In* Colman, R. W., Hirsh, J., Marder, V. J., and Salzman, E. W. (eds.): Hemostasis and Thrombosis. Philadelphia, J. B. Lippincott, 1982, pp. 185–209.

Bevers, E. M., Comfurius, P., van Rijn, J. L., Hemker, H. C., and Zwaal, R. F.: Generation of prothrombin-converting activity and the exposure of phosphatidylserine at the outer surface of platelets. Eur. J. Biochem., *122*:429, 1982.

Biggs, R., Austen, D. E. G., Denson, K. W. E., Borrett, R., and Rizza, C. R.: The mode of action of antibodies which destroy factor VIII. II. Antibodies which give complex concentration graphs. Br. J. Haematol., *23*:137, 1972.

Bloom, A. L.: Inherited disorders of blood coagulation. *In* Bloom, A. L. and Thomas, D. P. (eds.): Haemostasis and Thrombosis. Edinburgh, Churchill Livingstone, 1981, pp. 321–370.

Brozovic, M.: Acquired disorders of blood coagulation. *In* Bloom, A. L., and Thomas, D. P. (eds.): Haemostasis and Thrombosis. Edinburgh, Churchill Livingstone, 1981, pp. 411–438.

Buchanan, G. P., and Holtkamp, C. A.: Prolonged bleeding time in children and young adults with hemophilia. Pediatrics, *66*:951, 1980.

Bukowski, R. M.: Thrombotic thrombocytopenic purpura: A review. *In* Spaet, T. H. (ed.): Progress in Hemostasis and Thrombosis, Vol. 6. New York, Grune & Stratton, 1982, pp. 287–337.

Clauss, A., Gerinnungsphysiologische Schnellmethode zur Bestimmung des Fibrinogens. Acta Haemat., *17*:237, 1957.

Collen, D.: On the regulation and control of fibrinolysis. Thrombos. Haemostas., *43*:77, 1980.

Collen, D.: Natural inhibitors of haemostasis, with particular reference to fibrinolysis. *In* Bloom, A. L., and Thomas, D. P. (eds.): Haemostasis and Thrombosis. Edinburgh, Churchill Livingstone, 1981, pp. 225–235.

Collen, D., De Cock, F., and Verstraete, M.: Quantitation of thrombin–antithrombin III complexes in human blood. Eur. J. Clin. Invest., *7*:407, 1977.

Cowan, J. F., Khan, M. B., Vargo, J., and Joist, J. H.: An improved method for evaluation of blood coagulation in heparinized blood. Am. J. Clin. Path., *75*:60, 1981.

Denson, K. W. E.: The simplified two-stage assay for factor VIII. *In* Biggs, R. (ed.): Human Blood Coagulation, Haemostasis and Thrombosis. 2nd ed. Oxford, Blackwell Scientific Publications, 1976, p. 688.

Donati, M. B., Poggi, A., and Semeraro, N.: Coagulation and malignancy. *In* Poller, L. (ed.): Recent Advances in Blood Coagulation. New York, Churchill Livingstone, 1981, pp. 227–259.

Doolittle, R. F.: Fibrinogen and fibrin. *In* Bloom, A. L., and Thomas, D. P. (eds.): Haemostasis and Thrombosis. Edinburgh, Churchill Livingstone, 1981, pp. 163–191.

Dvilansky, A., Britten, A. H. F., and Loewy, A. G.: Factor XIII assay by an isotope method. I. Factor XIII (transamidase) in plasma, serum leukocytes, erythrocytes and platelets and evaluation of screening tests of clot solubility. Br. J. Haematol., *18*:399, 1970.

Edson, J. R.: Discussion of the control of heparin therapy by the activated partial thromboplastin time: Sensitivity of various thromboplastins to heparin. *In* Triplett, D. A. (ed.): Standardization of Coagulation Assays: An Overview. Skokie, Ill., College of American Pathologists, 1982, pp. 204–205.

Edwards, R. L., Rickles, F. R., and Cronlund, M.: Abnormalities of blood coagulation in patients with cancer: Mononuclear cell tissue factor generation. J. Lab. Clin. Med., *98*:917, 1981.

Esmon, C. T., and Owen, W. G.: Identification of an endothelial cell cofactor for thrombin-catalyzed activation of protein C. Proc. Natl. Acad. Sci. U.S.A., *78*:2249, 1981.

Ewing, N. P., and Kasper, C. K.: In vitro detection of mild inhibitors to factor VIII in hemophilia. Am. J. Clin. Path., *77*:749, 1982.

Eyster, M. E., Gordon, R. A., and Ballard, J. O.: The bleeding time is longer than normal in hemophilia. Blood, *58*:719, 1981.

Firshein, S. I., Hoyer, L. W., Lazarchick, J., et al.: Prenatal diagnosis of classic haemophilia. N. Engl. J. Med., *300*:937, 1979.

Fletcher, A. P., Biederman, O., Moore, D., et al.: Abnormal plasminogen-plasmin system activity (fibrinolysis) in patients

4

with hepatic cirrhosis: Its cause and consequences. J. Clin. Invest., *43*:681, 1964.

Francis, C. W., and Marder, V. J.: Mechanisms of fibrinolysis. *In* Williams, W. J., Beutler, E., Erslev, A. J., and Lichtman, M. A. (eds.): Hematology. 3rd ed. New York, McGraw-Hill, 1983, pp. 1266–1276.

Gawyrl, M. S., and Hoyer, L. W.: Inactivation of factor VIII coagulant activity by two different types of human antibodies. Blood, *60*:1103, 1982.

Girma, J. P., Ardaillore, N., Meyer, D., Lavergne, J. M., and Larrieu, M. J.: Fluid-phase immunoradiometric assay for the detection of qualitative abnormalities of factor VIII/von Willebrand factor in variants of von Willebrand's disease. J. Lab. Clin. Med., *93*:926, 1979.

Graham, J. B.: Genotype assignment (carrier detection) in the haemophilias. Clin. Haematol., *8*:115, 1979.

Green, D., Hougie, C., Kazmier, F. J., Lechner, K., Mannucci, P. M., Rizza, C. R., and Sultan, Y.: Report of the working party on acquired inhibitors of coagulation: Studies of the "lupus" anticoagulant. Thrombos. Haemostas., *49*:144, 1983.

Griffin, J. H., Evatt, B., Zimmerman, T. S., Kleiss, A. J., and Wideman, C.: Deficiency of protein C in congenital thrombotic disease. J. Clin. Invest., *68*:1370, 1981.

Griffin, J. H., Mosher, D. F., Zimmerman, T. S., and Kleiss, A. J.: Protein C, an antithrombotic protein, is reduced in hospitalized patients with intravascular coagulation. Blood, *60*:261, 1982.

Handin, R. I., and Rosenberg, R. D.: Hemorrhagic disorders. III. Disorders of primary and secondary hemostasis. *In* Beck, W. S. (ed.): Hematology. 3rd ed. Cambridge, Mass., MIT Press, 1981, pp. 425–439.

Hardisty, R. M., and Macphorson, J. C.: A one-stage factor VIII (anti-haemophilic globulin) assay and its use on venous and capillary plasma. Thromb. Diath. Haemorrh., *7*:215, 1962.

Hoffman, J. J. M. L., and Meulendijk, P. N.: Evaluation of a heparin neutralizer. Thrombos. Res., *18*:897, 1980.

Hougie, C., and Twomey, J. J.: Haemophilia B_M: A new type of factor IX deficiency. Lancet, *1*:698, 1967.

Hoyer, L. W.: Immunologic studies of antihemophilic factor (AHF, factor VIII). IV. Radioimmunoassay of AHF antigen. J. Lab. Clin. Med., *80*:822, 1972.

Hoyer, L. W.: Biochemistry of factor VIII. *In* Colman, R. W., Hirsh, J., Marder, V. J., and Salzman, E. W. (eds.): Hemostasis and Thrombosis. Philadelphia, J. B. Lippincott, 1982, pp. 39–53.

Ingram, G. I. C., Brozovic, M., and Slater, N. G. P.: Bleeding Disorders: Investigation and Management. 2nd ed. Oxford, Blackwell Scientific Publications, 1982, p. 326.

Jackson, C. M., and Brenckle, G. M.: Biochemistry of prothrombin activation. *In* Bloom, A. L., and Thomas, D. P. (eds.): Haemostasis and Thrombosis. Edinburgh, Churchill Livingstone, 1981, pp. 140–162.

Jaffe, E. A., Hoyer, L. W., and Nachman, R. L.: Synthesis of antihemophilic factor antigen by cultured human endothelial cells. J. Clin. Invest., *52*:2757, 1973.

Jaffe, E. A., Hoyer, L. W., and Nachman, R. L.: Synthesis of von Willebrand factor by cultured human endothelial cells. Proc. Natl. Acad. Sci., U.S.A., *71*:1906, 1974.

Joist, J. H., Cowan, J. F., and Zimmerman, T. S.: Acquired von Willebrand's disease. Evidence for a quantitative and qualitative factor VIII disorder. N. Engl. J. Med., *298*:988, 1978.

Kasper, C. K., Aledort, L. M., Counts, R. B., et al.: A more uniform measurement of factor VIII inhibitors. Thrombos. Diath. Haemorrh., *34*:869, 1975.

Kasper, C. K., and Ewing, N. P.: Measurement of inhibitor to factor VIII C (and IX C). *In* Bloom, A. L. (ed.): The Hemophilias. Edinburgh, Churchill Livingstone, 1982, pp. 39–50.

Kasper, C. K., Osterud, B., Minami, J. Y., Shonick, W., and Rapaport, S. I.: Hemophilia B: Characterization of genetic variants and detection of carriers. Blood, *50*:351, 1977.

Kidd, P., Denson, K. W. E., and Biggs, R.: The thrombotest reagent and Christmas disease. Lancet, *2*:522, 1963.

Kisiel, W., Canfield, W., Erisson, L., and Davie, E. W.: Anticoagulant properties of bovine plasma protein C following activation by thrombin. Biochemistry, *16*:5824, 1977.

Lazerchick, J., and Hoyer, L. W.: Immunoradiometric measurement of the factor VIII procoagulant antigen. J. Clin. Invest., *55*:1048, 1978.

Levine, P. H.: The clinical manifestations and therapy of hemophilias A and B. *In* Colman, R. W., Hirsh, J., Marder, V. J., and Salzman, E. W. (eds.): Hemostasis and Thrombosis. Philadelphia, J. B. Lippincott, 1982, pp. 75–90.

Lorand, L., Urayama, T., de Kiewiet, J. W. C., and Nossel, H. L.: Diagnostic and genetic studies of fibrin-stabilizing factor with a new assay based on amine incorporation. J. Clin. Invest., *48*:1054, 1969.

Lossing, T. S., Kasper, C. K., and Feinstein, D. I.: Detection of factor VIII inhibitors with the partial thromboplastin time. Blood, *49*:793, 1977.

Macfarlane, D. E., Stibbe, J., Kirby, E. P., Zucker, M. B., Grant, R. A., and McPherson, J.: A method for assaying von Willebrand factor (ristocetin cofactor). Thromb. Diath. Haemorrh., *34*:306, 1975.

Mannucci, P. M., Lombardi, R., Pareti, F. I., Solinas, S., Mazzucconi, M. G., and Mariani, G.: A variant of von Willebrand's disease characterized by recessive inheritance and missing triplet structure of von Willebrand factor multimers. Blood, *62*:1000, 1983.

Marder, V. J., Martin, S. E., and Colman, R. W.: Clinical aspects of consumptive thrombohemorrhagic disorders. *In* Colman, R. W., Hirsh, J., Marder, V. J., and Salzman, E. W. (eds.): Hemostasis and Thrombosis. Philadelphia, J. B. Lippincott, 1982, pp. 664–693.

Maynard, J. R., Fintel, D. J., Pitlick, F. A., et al.: Tissue factor coagulant activity of cultured human endothelial and smooth muscle cells and fibroblasts. Blood, *50*:387, 1977.

Menache, D.: Congenital abnormal fibrinogens. *In* Menache, D., Surgenor, D. M., and Anderson, H. (eds.): Hemophilia and Hemostasis. New York, Alan R. Liss, 1981, pp. 205–220.

Meyer, D., and Zimmerman, T. S.: von Willebrand's disease. *In* Colman, R. W., Hirsh, J., Marder, V. J., and Salzman, E. W. (eds.): Hemostasis and Thrombosis. Philadelphia, J. B. Lippincott, 1982, pp. 64–74.

Miletich, J. P., Jackson, C. M., and Majerus, P. W.: Properties of the factor Xa binding site on human platelets. J. Biol. Chem., *253*:6908, 1978a.

Miletich, J. P., Majerus, D. W., and Majerus, P. W.: Patients with congenital factor V deficiency have decreased factor Xa binding sites on their platelets. J. Clin. Invest., *62*:824, 1978b.

Miller, J. L., and Castella, A.: Platelet-type von Willebrand's disease: Characterization of a new bleeding disorder. Blood, *60*:790, 1982.

Miller, J. L., Katz, A. J., and Feinstein, M. B.: Plasmin inhibition of thrombin-induced platelet aggregation. Thrombos. Diath. Haemorrh., *33*:286, 1975.

Miller, J. L., Kupinski, J. M., Castella, A., and Ruggeri, Z. M.: von Willebrand factor binds to platelets and induces aggregation in platelet-type but not type IIB von Willebrand disease. J. Clin. Invest., *72*:1532, 1983.

Mueh, J. R., Herbst, K. D., and Rapaport, S. I.: Thrombosis in patients with the lupus anticoagulant. Ann. Intern. Med., *92*:156, 1980.

Nachman, R., Levine, R., and Jaffe, E. A.: Synthesis of factor VIII antigen by cultured guinea pig megakaryocytes. J. Clin. Invest., *60*:914, 1977.

Nemerson, Y., and Zur, M.: Is hemophilia a disease of the tissue factor pathway of coagulation? *In* Menache, D., Surgenor, D. M., and Anderson, H. (eds.): Hemophilia and Hemostasis. New York, Alan R. Liss, 1981, pp. 77–83.

Niewiarowski, S., and Gurewick, V.: Laboratory identification of intravascular coagulation: The serial dilution protamine sulfate test for the detection of fibrin monomer and fibrin degradation products. J. Lab. Clin. Med., *77*:665, 1971.

Nossel, H. L.: Coagulant proteins in thrombosis. *In* Colman, R. W., Hirsh, J., Marder, V. J., and Salzman, E. W. (eds.): Hemostasis and Thrombosis. Philadelphia, J. B. Lippincott, 1982, pp. 726–737.

Nossel, H. L., Yudelman, I., Canfield, R. E., et al.: Measurement of fibrinopeptide A in human blood. J. Clin. Invest., *54*:43, 1974.

Owen, C. A., and Bowie, E. V. W.: Generation of plasmatic coagulation factors by the isolated rat liver perfused with completely synthetic blood substitute. Thrombos. Res., *22*:259, 1981.

Owen, C. A., Bowie, E. V. W., and Fass, D. N.: Generation of factor VIII coagulant activity by isolated, perfused neonatal pig liver and adult rat livers. Br. J. Haematol., *43*:307, 1979.

Pechet, L., Tiarks, C. Y., Stevens, J., Sudhindra, R. R., and Lipworth, L.: Relationship of factor IX antigen and coagulant in hemophilia B patients and carriers. Thrombos. Haemostas., *40*:465, 1978.

Poller, L.: Oral anticoagulant therapy. *In* Bloom, A. L., and Thomas, D. P. (eds.): Haemostasis and Thrombosis. Edinburgh, Churchill Livingstone, 1981, pp. 725–736.

Rapaport, S. I.: The activation of factor IX by the tissue factor pathway. *In* Menache, D., Surgenor, D. M., and Anderson, H. (eds.): Hemophilia and Hemostasis. New York, Alan R. Liss, 1981, pp. 57–76.

Ratnoff, O. D., and Menzie, C.: A new method for the determination of fibrinogen in small samples on plasma. J. Lab. Clin. Med., *37*:316, 1951.

Rizza, C. R.: von Willebrand's disease. *In* Biggs, R. (ed.): The Treatment of Haemophilia A and B and von Willebrand's Disease. Oxford, Blackwell Scientific Publications, 1978, pp. 172–180.

Roberts, H. R., Griffith, M. J., Braunstein, K. M., and Lundblad, R. L.: Structural abnormalities of the vitamin K–dependent clotting factors. *In* Menache, D., Surgenor, D. M., and Anderson, H. (eds.): Hemophilia and Hemostasis. New York, Alan R. Liss, 1981, pp. 85–102.

Rosenberg, R. D.: Hemorrhagic disorders. Protein interactions in the clotting mechanism. *In* Beck W. S. (ed.): Hematology. Cambridge, Mass., MIT Press, 1981, pp. 373–400.

Ruggeri, Z. M., Lombardi, R., Gatti, L., Bader, R., Valsecchi, C., and Zimmerman, T. S.: Type IIB von Willebrand's disease: Differential clearance of endogenous versus transfused large multimer von Willebrand factor. Blood, *60*:1453, 1982a.

Ruggeri, Z. M., Nilsson, I. M., Lombardi, R., Holmberg, L., and Zimmerman, T. S.: Aberrant structure of von Willebrand factor in a new variant of von Willebrand's disease (Type IIC). J. Clin. Invest., *70*:1124, 1982b.

Ruggeri, Z. M., Pareti, F. I., Mannucci, P. M., Ciavarella, N., and Zimmerman, T. S.: Heightened interaction between platelets and factor VIII/von Willebrand factor in a new subtype of von Willebrand's disease. N. Engl. J. Med., *302*:1047, 1980a.

Ruggeri, Z. M., and Zimmerman, T. S.: Variant von Willebrand's disease: Characterization of two subtypes by analysis of multimeric composition of factor VIII/von Willebrand factor in plasma and platelets. J. Clin. Invest., *65*:1318, 1980b.

Schleider, M. A., Nachman, R. L., Jaffe, E. A., et al.: A clinical study of the lupus anticoagulant. Blood, *48*:499, 1976.

Shapiro, S. S.: Antibodies to blood coagulation factors. Clin. Haematol., *8*:207, 1979.

Shapiro, S. S., and Thiagarajan, P.: Lupus anticoagulants. *In* Spaet, T. H. (ed.): Progress in Hemostasis and Thrombosis, Vol. 6. New York, Grune & Stratton, 1982, pp. 263–285.

Shapiro, S. S., Thiagarajan, P., and De Marco, L.: Mechanism of action of the lupus anticoagulant. Ann. N.Y. Acad. Sci., *370*:359, 1981.

Solum, N. O., Rigollot, C., Budzynski, A. Z., et al.: A qualitative evaluation of the inhibition of platelet aggregation by low molecular weight degradation products of fibrinogen. Br. J. Haematol., *24*:419, 1973.

Thiagarajan, P., Shapiro, S. S., and De Marco, L.: Monoclonal immunoglobulin M lambda coagulation inhibitor with phospholipid specificity. Mechanism of a lupus anticoagulant. J. Clin. Invest., *66*:397, 1980.

Thompson, A. R.: Factor IX antigen by radioimmunoassay in heterozygotes for hemophilia B. Thrombos. Res., *11*:193, 1977.

Thompson, A. R., and Harker, L. A.: Manual of Hemostasis and Thrombosis. 3rd ed. Philadelphiia, F. A. Davis, 1983.

Thomson, J. M.: The control of heparin therapy by the activated partial thromboplastin time: Sensitivity of various thromboplastins to heparin. *In* Triplett, D. A., (ed.): Standardization of Coagulation Assays: An Overview. Skokie, Ill., College of American Pathologists, 1982, pp. 195–203.

Triplett, D. A. (ed.): Standardization of Coagulation Assays: An Overview. Skokie, Ill., College of American Pathologists, 1982.

Veltkamp, J. J., Meilof, J., Remmelts, H. G., van der Vlerk, D., and Loeliger, E. A.: Another genetic variant of haemophilia B: Haemophilia B Leyden. Scand. J. Haematol., *7*:82, 1970.

Weiss, H. J., Hoyer, L. W., Rickles, F. R., Varma, A., and Rogers, J.: Quantitative assay of a plasma factor deficient in von Willebrand's disease that is necessary for platelet aggregation. Relationship to factor VIII procoagulant activity and antigen content. J. Clin. Invest., *52*:2708, 1973.

Weiss, H. J., Meyer, D., Rabinowitz, R., Pietu, G., Girma, J. P., Vicic, W. J., and Rogers, J.: Pseudo–von Willebrand's disease: An intrinsic platelet defect with aggregation by unmodified human factor VIII/von Willebrand factor and enhanced adsorption of its high-molecular-weight multimers. N. Engl. J. Med., *306*:326, 1982.

Wintrobe, M. M., Lee, G. R., Boggs, D. R., et al. (eds.): Clinical Hematology. 8th ed. Philadelphia, Lea & Febiger, 1981.

Zimmerman, T. S., Abildgaard, C. F., and Meyer, D.: The factor VIII abnormality in severe von Willebrand's disease. N. Engl. J. Med., *301*:1307, 1979.

Zimmerman, T. S., Ratnoff, O. D., and Powell, A. E.: Immunologic differentiation of classic hemophilia (factor VIII deficiency) and von Willebrand's disease, with observations on combined deficiencies of antihemophilic factor and proaccelerin (factor V) and on an acquired circulating anticoagulant against antihemophilic factor. J. Clin. Invest., *50*:244, 1971.

Zimmerman, T. S., and Ruggeri, Z. M.: von Willebrand's disease. *In* Spaet, T. H. (ed.): Progress in Hemostasis and Thrombosis, Vol. 6. New York, Grune & Stratton, 1982, pp. 203–236.

Zimmerman, T. S., and Ruggeri, Z. M.: von Willebrand's disease. Clin. Haematol., *12*:175, 1983.

Zur, M., and Nemerson, Y.: Tissue factor pathways of blood coagulation. *In* Bloom, A. L., and Thomas, D. P. (eds.): Haemostasis and Thrombosis. Edinburgh, Churchill Livingstone, 1981, pp. 124–139.

Part V

IMMUNOLOGY AND IMMUNOPATHOLOGY

EDITED BY RUSSELL H. TOMAR, M.D., JOHN BERNARD HENRY, M.D., and JOSEF V. KADLEC, S.J., M.D., Ph.D.

33

HLA: THE MAJOR HISTOCOMPATIBILITY COMPLEX

IMMUNOGENETICS OF HLA ANTIGENS

Armead H. Johnson, Ph.D.,
Robert J. Hartzman, M.D.,
and Mary Ann Robinson, Ph.D.

INTRODUCTION

The survival of an individual is dependent upon the ability to recognize foreign substances (antigens) and to respond to them. Although this defense mechanism is basic to one's survival in a hostile world of microorganisms, this same defense system becomes a major obstacle when we attempt to transplant tissues from one individual to another, since antigens present on cell surfaces act as foreign antigens and evoke the initiation of an immune response by the host. These cell surface antigens that are capable of eliciting an immune response when transplanted into another individual are called histocompatibility antigens. All mammals have many histocompatibility systems or complexes; however, in each species there is only one major histocompatibility complex (MHC), which represents the primary obstacle to transplantation of foreign tissue. Not only mammals but also certain birds, amphibians, and fishes have an MHC. In man the major histocompatibility complex is called HLA. The MHCs from different species are remarkably similar in both structure and function and are composed of a cluster or complex of genes. Why has such a gene complex been conserved throughout speciation? One hypothesis is that the genes within the MHC are essential to survival of the species.

Although antigens within the MHC were defined by transplantation of normal tissues and tumors, the ability to elicit graft rejection is an artificially imposed function. The normal functions of genes and gene products within the MHC are only now beginning to be uncovered. It has become clear that cells involved in the immune response (responder, helper, suppressor, and effector) are under the control of the genes within the MHC. Currently a great effort is being made to gain a better understanding of the control of the immune response, especially as it applies to transplantation, cancer, and disease susceptibility. Once the mechanisms of control of the immune response are understood, then therapeutic and preventive intervention can be implemented. Appreciation of the basic concepts of the immunogenetics of the human MHC, then, is essential to developing a proper understanding of the etiology, pathogenesis, and possible therapy of human disease states which have an immunologic component.

On the basis of structure, genetic origin, and function, products of the MHC have been grouped into three classes: Class I, Class II, and Class III. Human Class I includes HLA-ABC antigens; Class II includes HLA-DR/D, MB/DC, and SB antigens; and Class III includes MHC-linked complement components. The genetics, nomenclature, techniques of detection, structure, and function of Class I and Class II antigens will be discussed in this section. Class III MHC-linked complement products are discussed in the following section of this chapter.

PRINCIPLES OF IMMUNOGENETICS APPLIED TO THE MAJOR HISTOCOMPATIBILITY COMPLEX

Genetics

Basic Genetics. Mendel's first law, the Law of Segregation, is based on the principle that hereditary characteristics are determined by factors which are distributed to progeny. In any one individual these factors, or genes as they are now called, are present in pairs. During meiosis, the genes segregate randomly during formation of the gametes so that only one of the pair or haploid number is transmitted by any given gamete. The double or diploid number is restored when the male and female gametes fuse to form the zygote. Thus for a trait determined by one gene, there will always be four possible genetic combinations, each with an equal probability of occurrence. These laws of segregation and random assortment apply to the genes of the HLA system. Suggestions for a review of basic genetics are given in the References. Definitions are given below for genetic terms which will be used in this chapter (Crow, 1976).

Gene: the unit factor of inheritance.

Locus: the position of a gene on a chromosome.

Allele: an alternate form of a gene expressed at a single locus.

Homozygous: having identical or indistinguishable alleles at the locus or loci in question.

Heterozygous: having different alleles at the locus or loci in question.

Co-dominance: the state where each gene expresses its characteristic effect equally in the heterozygote.

Polymorphic: having two or more distinct phenotypes maintained in a population.

Genotype: the genetic constitution of an organism or individual.

Phenotype: the observable characters produced by the genes.

Homologous chromosomes: the two members of a chromosome pair which have corresponding gene loci, one derived from each parent.

Crossing-over: the exchange of segments between homologous chromosomes.

Recombination: reassortment of genes so that the gamete contains genes of both paternal and maternal origin. (When the genes are linked, this is accomplished by crossing-over.)

Allo-(antigen, graft): refers to those antigenic differences between individuals of a single species.

Centimorgan: the frequency of recombination between two linked loci expressed as a per cent which reflects the distance between the two loci.

Genetics of HLA. The major histocompatibility complex in man, HLA, is located on the short arm of chromosome 6. It spans approximately 3.0 centimorgans, an area which contains enough genetic material to encode numerous proteins. The HLA complex is divided into six regions: HLA-A, HLA-C, HLA-B, HLA-D/DR, MB/DC, and SB (Fig. 33–1). Each region encodes a minimum of one cell surface glycoprotein. These HLA antigens, which are an integral part of the cell membrane, are highly polymorphic both serologically and structurally. Indeed, they are the most polymorphic system yet known in man. Such polymorphism is thought to be maintained by and essential for the function of these molecules which, as experimental evidence suggests, is to allow cells of the immune system to discriminate between self and non-self or altered self. Other molecules included in the MHC include four proteins of the complement cascade (C2, C4A, C4B, BF) and glyoxylase-1 enzyme. These components will be covered subsequently.

For comparative purposes a brief description of H-2 in the mouse MHC is included here. The murine H-2 complex is perhaps the most extensively studied and understood MHC, both structurally and functionally.

MOUSE CHROMOSOME 17

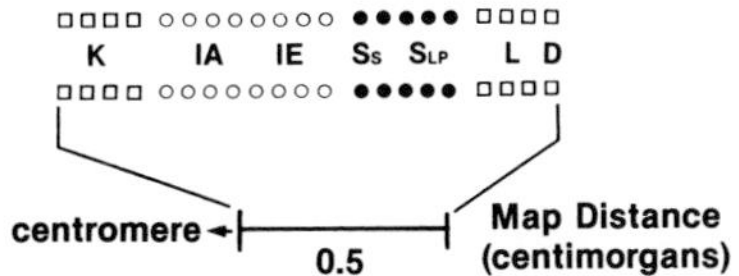

HUMAN CHROMOSOME 6

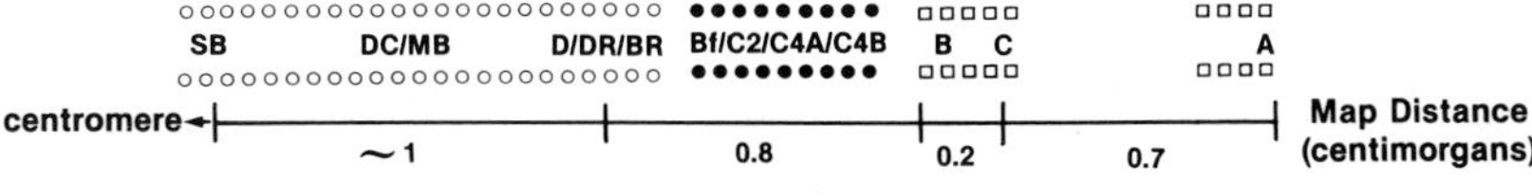

Molecules: Class I (□□□) Class II (○○○) Class III (●●●) /= Unknown Map Order

Figure 33–1. Schematic diagram comparing mouse and human MHC region.

ally, due to the existence of inbred and congenic strains of mice (strains that differ only at discrete genetic regions) which permit elegant experimental designs. Parallels between H-2 and homologous HLA products will be drawn in this chapter for various regions, genes, and functions. Figure 33–1 shows the comparison of the MHC of mouse and man. H-2 is located on chromosome 17 of the mouse. It is divided into five major regions: K, I, S, L, and D. H2-K, L, and D are Class I antigens and are homologous to HLA-B, C, and A, respectively. There is an additional group of Class I antigens on chromosome 17 of the mouse called TLa/Qa. Possible human equivalents of TLa and Qa have been recently identified but will not be discussed in this chapter. The S region encodes for complement components. The I region encodes Class II or Ia (immune response associated) antigens which are associated with certain immune responses (IR genes). The murine I region is composed of several subdivisions: IA, IB, IJ, IC, and IE. The D/DR region in man is similar in both structure and function to the murine I region except for its location relative to the Class I antigens.

Inheritance. The HLA loci are closely linked, that is, they segregate en bloc to the offspring. The complex of linked genes which reside on one of the pair of homologous chromosomes and which segregate en bloc to the offspring is termed a "haplotype." Each individual inherits two HLA haplotypes, one from each parent, and thus has two alleles from each of the loci.

The inheritance of HLA follows the rules of segregation set down by Mendel. Within a family each child inherits one HLA haplotype from the mother and one from the father. By convention the paternal haplotypes are always designated a and b and the maternal haplotypes c and d. Thus, there are four possible HLA genotypes in the offspring: ac, ad, bc, and bd. Since the chances of inheriting a given genotype are random, then the probability of occurrence of each genotype is 1 in 4. In a family with five children, at least two of the children will be HLA identical (assuming no recombination). An example of a mating and its four possible genotypes is given in Figure 33–2.

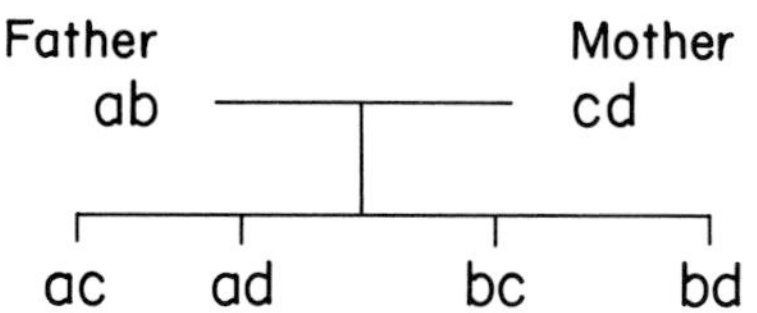

Figure 33–2. Segregation of alleles at a single locus.

Although the genes of the HLA-A, B, C, D/DR, and SB series are closely linked, a number of families have been reported in which a crossover has occurred (Fig. 33–3). The frequency of crossing over between two linked loci is proportional to the distance separating those loci. The genetic map distances calculated from the frequency of recombination are shown in Figure 33–1. The map order is HLA-A, C, B, D/DR, DC/MB, SB, with HLA-A being distal to the centromere. The frequency of recombination between HLA-A and B is 0.0087, expressed as 0.87 centimorgan. The HLA-C locus maps between HLA-A and B and is 0.7 centimorgan from HLA-A and 0.2 centimorgan from HLA-B. HLA-D/DR maps 0.8 centimorgan centromeric to HLA-B. DC/MB has been mapped between HLA-D/DR and SB by irradiation induced HLA loss mutants. The map distance is not known. SB maps approximately 1.0 centimorgan centromeric to HLA-D/DR. The map distance between HLA-D and SB is a best estimate since only a limited number of families have been typed for SB to date.

Linkage Disequilibrium. The tendency for certain alleles at two loci to occur significantly more frequently in the same haplotype than would be expected on the basis of chance alone is called linkage disequilibrium. Linkage disequilibrium is a hallmark of the HLA system and extends from HLA-A through the HLA-D/DR region, including the genes controlling serum complement components. The significance of linkage disequilibrium as it applies to immune competence and disease is discussed in the second section of this chapter. The best known example of linkage disequilibrium is the A1, Cw7, B8, DR3, Dw3, MB2, MT2 haplotype in Caucasoids which occurs approximately four times more frequently than would

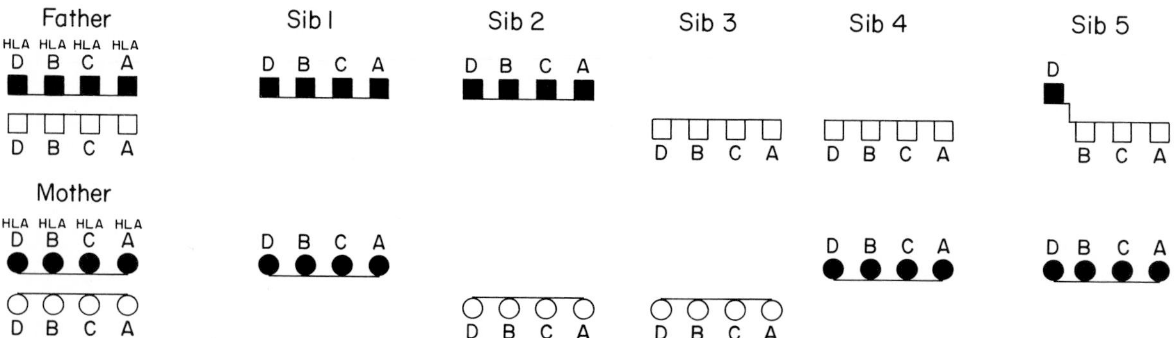

Figure 33–3. HLA haplotype segregation within a family. Sibling 5 is a recombinant between the paternal HLA-B and HLA-D loci. This means that sibling 5 is HLA-A, HLA-B, and HLA-C identical to sibling 4, yet they are reactive to each other in MLC because of non-identity at the HLA-D locus as a result of recombination.

be expected by chance. Linkage disequilibrium will be discussed in more detail in the next section of this chapter.

Ethnic Variation. HLA typing of the human population groups of the world was undertaken between June 1970 and June 1972 as the purpose of the 1972 International Histocompatibility Workshop. The accumulated data from the 80 population groups investigated, as well as from many subsequent studies, have provided several conclusions: (1) frequencies of HLA antigens differ significantly between ethnic subpopulations; (2) some HLA antigens are either confined to or found at a much greater frequency in one ethnic subpopulation compared with another; and (3) haplotypes and linkage disequilibrium differ between races.

Nomenclature

HLA terminology is designated by a World Health Organization (WHO) Committee for HLA Nomenclature. The current nomenclature was adopted in 1975. Each locus within the HLA complex is designated by one or more letters following HLA (HLA-A, HLA-B, HLA-C, HLA-D/DR). Each new locus identified within the system will be assigned the next letter in the alphabet. International exchanges of typing reagents are organized every two to four years (International Histocompatibility Workshops) and the results published. Provisional workshop assignments are designated by a "w" preceding the number.

Table 33–1 shows the currently established HLA and workshop, "w," specificities. Alleles within the HLA-A and B loci are not numbered consecutively for historic reasons. Although some C locus specificities are considered well defined, the "w" designation has not been dropped because the notation would then be similar to that for the complement system. All of the HLA-D specificities retain the "w" designation since these specificities are not considered well defined for reasons which are discussed in the subsequent section. Following each workshop, several old specificities are "split" as the definition becomes more refined until ultimately the unique epitope on the molecule is identified. The most narrow definition of the specificity is called the subtypic specificity. The broader, shared specificities are called supertypic specificities. For example, Bw44 and Bw45 are subtypic specificities of the supertypic specificity B12. Thus a cell which is either Bw44 or Bw45 must also be positive for B12.

Notice that there is not 4 or 6 in either the A or the B allelic series. These numbers were reserved for the 4a,4b leukocyte system which was being investigated at the time the original nomenclature system was developed in 1967. Only in 1977 were experiments reported that showed that the 4a (now Bw4) and 4b (now Bw6) specificities reside on the same molecule but at a different site from the B locus subtypic specificities. Bw4 and Bw6 are a diallelic system, and all B locus specificities are characteristically either w4 or w6.

Table 33–1. NOMENCLATURE FOR FACTORS OF THE HLA SYSTEM

Locus A	Locus B	Locus D
A1	B5*	Dw1
A2	B7^{+}	Dw2
A3	B8^{+}	Dw3
A9	B12^{*+}	Dw4
A10	B13*	Dw5
A11	B14^{+}	Dw6
A25 (10)	B15^{*+}	Dw7
A26 (10)	B17*	Dw8
A28	B18^{+}	Dw9
A29 (19)	B27*	Dw10
Aw19	B37*	Dw11
Aw23 (9)	B40^{+}	Dw12
Aw24 (9)	B16*	
Aw30 (19)	Bw21^{*+}	**Locus DR**
Aw31 (19)	Bw22^{+}	DR1
Aw32 (19)	Bw35^{+}	DR2
Aw33 (19)	Bw38*(16)	DR3
Aw34	Bw39^{+}(16)	DR4
Aw36	Bw41^{+}	DR5
Aw43	Bw42^{+}	DR6
	Bw44*(12)	DRw7
Locus C	Bw45^{+}(12)	DRw8
Cw1	Bw46^{+}	DRw9
Cw2	Bw47^{+}	DRw10
Cw3	Bw48^{+}	
Cw4	Bw49*(21)	
Cw5	Bw50^{+}(21)	
Cw6	Bw51*(5)	
Cw7	Bw52*(5)	
Cw8	Bw53*	
	Bw54^{+}(22)	
	Bw55^{+}(22)	
	Bw56^{+}(22)	
	Bw57^{+}(17)	
	Bw58^{+}(17)	
	Bw59*(8)	
	Bw60^{+}(40)	
	Bw61^{+}(40)	
	Bw62^{+}(15)	
	Bw63*(15)	

The numbers in parentheses represent previous assignments (supertypic specificity). HLA-B locus antigens can be further typed by their reactivity with HLA-Bw4 and HLA-Bw6 antisera indicated by * or $^{+}$.

Currently there are 20 A locus alleles, 40 B locus alleles, and 8 C locus alleles, which have been given WHO Nomenclature Committee assignments. HLA-D is identified by cellular techniques, whereas HLA-DR, which stands for HLA-D related, is identified by serologic techniques. There are 12 HLA-D specificities and 10 HLA-DR specificities. The relationship between HLA-D and DR specificities is not fully understood and is discussed later.

HLA-A, B, C Regions—Class I Molecules

The HLA-A and B locus alleles were the first to be described. Anti-leukocyte antibodies in man were observed as early as the 1920's, but it was not until the 1950's that a systematic study began. Jean Dausset was the first (1952) to convincingly demonstrate antileukocyte antibodies (leukoagglutinins) in the blood of leukopenic patients and to suggest that these leukoagglutinins were probably alloantibodies since they did not react with leukocytes from the antibody producer but did react with a percentage of leukocytes from red cell group O unrelated individuals (1954). Shortly thereafter Rose Payne in Los Angeles reported that serum from patients with febrile non-hemolytic blood transfusion reactions frequently contained leukoagglutinins which demonstrated allospecificity. In 1958, Dausset described the first HLA alloantigen MAC (now A2 + A28) and showed it to be genetically determined using family studies. Originally all the leukocyte specificities were thought to be the product of a single locus. However, in 1964, Dausset proposed a 2 gene model each with multiple allèles which he called HL-1. The 2 gene model was substantiated by the identification of a recombinational event that separated the two allelic series. These two allelic series were called the First or LA (now HLA-A) and the Second or Four series (now HLA-B). These names derived from the fact that the LA 1,2,3 allelic series was described by Payne in 1967 and the 4a,4b allelic series was described by van Rood in 1969. A third locus was first proposed in 1970; however, it was not confirmed by recombination until 1975. This third locus was designated HLA-C following the 1975 International Histocompatibility Workshop. The C locus gene product is apparently less immunogenic since Ferrara and colleagues attempted to identify new C locus alleles by planned immunizations using lymphocytes from donors mismatched with the recipient only for a "blank" at the C locus. No new antisera which identified a new C locus allele were obtained from 50 planned hyperimmunizations.

Structure of Class I Molecules. HLA-ABC (Class I) antigens consist of a transmembrane glycoprotein heavy chain non-covalently associated with β_2-microglobulin, with the stoichiometry of the subunits being 1:1 (Fig. 33–4). The heavy chain has a molecular weight of 44,000, and β_2-microglobulin has a molecular weight of 11,600 daltons. The heavy chains are encoded within the HLA complex and are highly polymorphic, whereas β_2-microglobulin is encoded on chromosome 15 and has not been found to be polymorphic in humans. The presence of β_2-microglobulin has been shown to be essential for the expression of HLA-ABC antigens on the cell surface.

Primary structural information has been reported for the papain-derived fragments of HLA-A2, A28, a pool of HLA Class I molecules, and the entire HLA-B7 molecule. HLA-C molecules have proved to be difficult to isolate and may be more readily degraded than are HLA-A and B molecules. However, HLA-C is thought to have a structure similar to those of HLA-A and B. From these complete or virtually complete amino acid sequences as well as sequences obtained for murine Class I antigens, several conclusions may be drawn regarding the structure of Class I molecules.

Class I molecules are oriented with the amino terminus extracellular and the carboxyl terminus in-

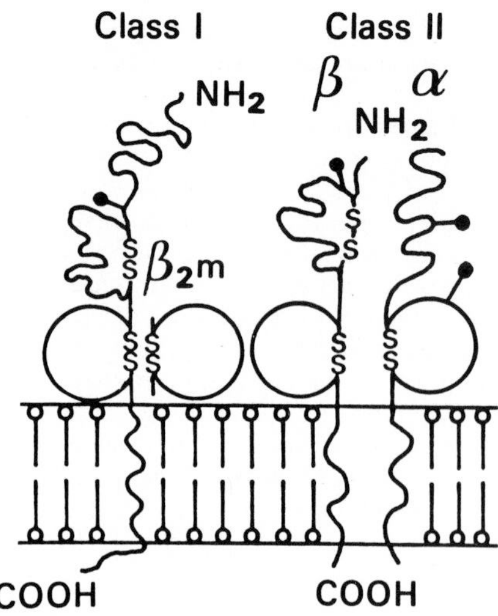

Figure 33–4. A schematic model of Class I and Class II molecules.

tracellular and are divided into five domains or segments. The extracellular segment of the Class I heavy chain is divided into three domains designated α1, α2, and α3, each consisting of about 90 amino acid residues. The amino terminal α1 domain contains a glycosylation site at the asparagine residue in position 86. The α2 and α3 domains each contain disulfide loops of 63 and 86 amino acids, respectively. Carboxyl to the α3 domain, the transmembrane segment, consists of approximately 24 amino acids which are mostly hydrophobic residues. The intracellular segment of the molecule to the carboxyl terminus consists mainly of hydrophilic residues with a cluster of basic residues adjacent to the cytoplasmic surface of the cell membrane. Other membrane-bound molecules have been found to have similar clustering of basic residues which are thought to anchor the molecule in the membrane by charge interaction with the negatively charged membrane. The cytoplasmic portion of the molecule may be phosphorylated at certain serine residues which theoretically could transmit signals during an immune response.

Comparison of the amino acid sequences of the various HLA-A and B molecules reveals that there is a high degree of homology among these glycoproteins. The overall homology between B7 and HLA-A2 is 86 per cent. The majority of the sequence differences are located between residues 43 and 195 (variable region), which has three main areas where the amino acid substitutions cluster (hypervariable regions): residues 65 to 80, 105 to 116, and 177 to 194. Data suggest that the three hypervariable regions may be responsible for the antigenic diversity observed with human Class I antigens. As further sequence information becomes available for other antigens, detailed comparisons can be made to search for molecular areas responsible for alloantigenicity as well as functionally active sites that may not be recognized by antibodies.

Function of Class I Molecules. Class I molecules are involved in the effector arm of the immune response and have been hypothesized to be involved in differentiation during embryogenesis. One central function is the recognition and elimination of virally infected cells. Viral antigens are expressed on the cell surface in association with Class I antigens. Cytotoxic T lymphocytes (CTL) are directed against the priming virus in conjunction with the Class I antigens.

In the experimental system used to dissect this mechanism, cytotoxic lymphocytes (CTL) are raised by *in vitro* stimulation with virally infected autologous cells. The recognition and lysis of target cells is doubly restricted to the priming virus strains and to certain HLA-A and B antigens present on the responder cell. Thus, only target cells sharing the appropriate HLA-A or B antigens with the responder and infected with the appropriate virus strain will be lysed.

HLA-D/DR, DC/MB, SB Subregions—Class II Molecules

Gene products within this region are different structurally and functionally from the HLA-A, B, and C antigens and also promise to be more complex. These antigens are on Class II molecules (Figs. 33–1 and 33–4) and are the human equivalent of murine I region antigens. If antigens within this region do indeed represent the products of immune response (IR) genes, then they must be able to generate extreme diversity not unlike the diversity of immunoglobulins. Antigens in this region were initially identified using cellular techniques directed at determining the antigens responsible for stimulation in leukocyte culture between allogeneic cells.

Cellular Definition of Antigens in the HLA-D/DR Region. In proliferative responses, one cell recognizes antigenic differences and begins to replicate in response to these differences. These antigens could be from foreign molecules previously experienced by the organism, for example, influenza antigen, or from antigens on the surface of cells from another individual, allogeneic cells. When cells from two individuals are put together in culture, proliferation to alloantigens results. This response is called the mixed leukocyte culture (MLC) or mixed leukocyte reaction (MLR). Bach and Amos (1967) found by serotyping for the HLA-A and HLA-B specificities that cells from siblings who were HLA identical failed to respond to each other in MLC. Since antibodies were frequently found in response to HLA-A and B following *in vivo* stimulation (pregnancy, transplantation of blood and organs) it seemed logical to conclude that these same antigens would also cause a hardy proliferation response *in vitro*. However, this hypothesis of HLA-A and B as the stimulating determinants was soon challenged. In 1971, Yunis and Amos analyzed several families with unexplained reactivity in a family MLC and proposed that stimulation in MLC is controlled by a gene separate from HLA-A and B. This hypothesis was confirmed in 1972 by Eijsvoogel in a family study. Further, Thorsby showed that cells from unrelated individuals who typed identically for HLA-A and B specificities usually responded to each other in MLC. Thus the stimulating alloantigens in MLC are genetically linked to HLA-A and B yet separable from them by recombination. These stimulating determinants are now collectively known as HLA-D (Figs. 33–1 and 33–4 and Table 33–1).

Definition of HLA-D Using Homozygous Typing Cells. Homozygous typing cells (HTC) are cells from individuals who have two copies of the same HLA-D specificity (i.e., are homozygous). In the early 1970's it was hypothesized that if the stimulator (irradiated or mitomycin C treated cells) had two identical copies of the same MLC stimulating determinant (was homozygous), a heterozygous responder cell which shared one copy of this MLC stimulating determinant would not see any foreign antigens on the stimulator cell. Thus the heterozygous responder would not detect any alloantigen different from self on the homozygous stimulator and would not proliferate. The most likely source of homozygous cells was proposed to be offspring of first cousin marriages since offspring of first cousin marriages have a 1 in 16 chance of carrying two copies of any particular gene inherited from one grandparent. As expected, offspring of first cousin marriages preselected to be homozygous for HLA-A and B failed to stimulate either heterozygous parent or haploidentical siblings. Further, cells from these homozygous individuals responded normally to their parents' cells and heterozygous siblings' cells in MLR. These homozygous cells also failed to stimulate the lymphocytes of some unrelated heterozygous individuals. Thus, homozygous cells could be and are used to "type" for the MLC stimulating determinants. By 1975, a variety of HTC had been identified and exchanged during the sixth International Histocompatibility Workshop. Twelve HLA-Dw specificities are currently accepted.

It should be kept in mind that the reactivities expressed here could be caused by either the product of one gene or the products of multiple closely linked genes in linkage disequilibrium.

Definition of HLA-D/DR Using Primed Lymphocyte Typing (Primed Lymphocyte Test, PLT). Cells which have been stimulated *in vitro* first undergo proliferation and then revert to a resting state. Although these cells are relatively quiescent, they retain the "memory" of the stimulation, that is, they have become primed. Cells primed to alloantigens *in vitro* can undergo specific rapid secondary responses to alloantigens which are similar to or the same as HLA-D. Initially it was felt that PLT was simply a more rapid method of detecting the alloantigens recognized by HTC typing, with one important additional advantage: reagents could be created *in vitro*. One no longer had to wait for a homozygous individual to be identified. Priming could be performed between cells from any two individuals who shared one HLA-D type.

Several problems became evident immediately. First, when primed cells were generated between two family members matched for one haplotype, up to 75 per cent of primed reagents created were far more broadly reactive in secondary test culture than expected. Second, it was not clear whether HLA-D or the serologically defined B cell specificities HLA-DR were recognized. (Further discussion of DR is reviewed subsequently.) Correlation between HLA-DR and PLT (primed lymphocyte typing) specificity was higher than correlation between HLA-D and PLT specificity. Experiments demonstrated that both HLA-D and HLA-DR could be individually defined by carefully selecting the priming combinations. Thus, a cell which expressed DR2/Dw12 could be stimulated with a DR2/Dw2 cell to generate a PLT specific for Dw2 and fail to recognize DR2, and also cells which recognize both DR2 and Dw12 could be generated.

Serological Definition of Specificities Within the D/DR Region

Definition of HLA-DR. Because mixed lymphocyte cultures require seven days to perform, a rapid, serological detection of HLA-D was sought. Since the predominant gene products which cause primary MLC activity in the mouse had been shown to be the I region antigens with a restricted tissue distribution, investigators began to look at lymphocyte subpopulations for such determinants in man (Fig. 33–1). Allospecificities which were present on B lymphocytes but not on T lymphocytes were described in the mid 1970's. During the seventh International Histocompatibility Testing Workshop (1977), a large number of B cell reactive antisera were tested against a panel of HLA-D typed lymphocytes. The resulting antiserum clusters based on the antiserum reactivity against a panel of HLA-D typed individuals were associated with but not identical to the HLA-D "antigen" definition. The WHO Nomenclature Committee decided (following much debate) that there was a reasonable doubt that these serologically defined specificities were either the same as or different from the HLA-D locus specificities. Therefore the B cell antigen allelic series was called HLA-DR for D-related. B cell "specificities," termed HLA-DR, were assigned sequential numbers which corresponded with the associated HLA-D alleles. At this time only eight HLA-DR alleles could be defined. In the 1980 International Histocompatibility Testing Workshop, an additional two DR alleles were clearly defined; however, they had no corresponding HLA-D type. The WHO HLA Nomenclature Committee decided to assign them the next sequential numbers, namely DRw9 and DRw10, even though the D locus specificities Dw9 and Dw10 showed no association with DRw9 and DRw10. Therefore, from this point on, HLA-DR no longer has a one-to-one relationship with the HLA-D specificities (Table 33–1).

One of the interesting relationships between HLA-D and HLA-DR specificities is the appearance that HLA-DR is less polymorphic than HLA-D. For example, cells carrying any one of three different HLA-D types, Dw2, Dw12, or TB-24, all type serologically as DR2. Using appropriate combinations, primed lymphocytes could be generated against DR2, Dw2, Dw12, and TB-24. Although this conclusively proved that HLA-D and DR were different, it did not conclusively differentiate the two genetic possibilities: two (or more) distinct gene products or microheterogeneity (the DR2 gene product could carry minor components corresponding to Dw2, 12, or TB-24). DR4 is also associated with any one of five different HLA-D types—Dw4, Dw10, DB3, DYT, and LD40. The relationship between HLA-D and HLA-DR is still not totally understood; evidence from molecular genetic techniques and from T cell cloning indicates that both D and DR are complex and related in an as yet undetermined manner.

Definition of "Other" B Cell Antigens. Considerable confusion has existed until very recently about these "other" B cell specificities, their relationship to each other, and their relationship to HLA-DR (Fig. 33–1 and Table 33–1). There are several primary reasons for this confusion: (1) because of extreme linkage disequilibrium and/or close map distance they are strongly associated with DR specificities; (2) frequently antisera against these other B cell specificities also contain antibodies against HLA-DR; and (3) MT specificities are not one allelic series. Immunochemistry and molecular genetics together have begun to unravel what promises to be a complicated puzzle. This section will discuss these findings in reference to the serology. A description of the immunochemistry and molecular genetics follows.

The first undisputed demonstration of a second B cell molecule was by Tosi and colleagues (1978) combining serologic, genetic, and immunochemical techniques. This "antigen" was called DC-1. Subsequently several other B cell specificities were described during 1980: MB, BR, and MT. Table 33–2 gives the DR associations of each of the other B cell antigen series.

The DC/MB antigens are expressed on a Class II molecule distinctly different from DR. The DC/MB molecule is the human equivalent of the mouse I-A region product, while HLA-DR is the human equivalent of the mouse I-E region product. Notice that the specificities DC-1, MB-1, and MT-1 are all associated with DR1, 2, w6, w10. Recently investigations utilizing immunochemical techniques have demonstrated that DC-1, MB-1, and MT-1 are identical. MB2 (associated primarily with DR3 and DR7) has been shown to be structurally similar to the DC-1 or MB-1 molecule and behaves as an allelic product in both population and family studies. MB3 (associated primarily with DR4, DR5, and DRw8) has not been immunochemically characterized to date but does behave as an allele of MB1 and MB2 in population and family studies.

Still a third human Class II molecule has been conclusively demonstrated. The prototype of this molecule is BR4×7, originally described in 1980, and is similar to and probably identical to MT3. Both BR4×7 and MT3 are associated primarily with DR4, DR7, and DRw9. Although different from DR, the BR4×7 molecule is more structurally similar to the DR molecules than to the MB/DC molecule. (Further details are presented subsequently.)

In conclusion, at least three allelic series within the D/DR region have been described serologically. These are (1) HLA-DR, (2) DC/MB, and (3) BR. The MT specificities are part of both the DC/MB and the BR

Table 33–2. B CELL ANTIGENIC SPECIFICITIES IN ADDITION TO HLA-DR*

Additional B Cell Specificities	DR1,2,6,10	DR3,7	DR4,5,(8)(6)(9)	DR3,5,6,8	DR4,7,(9)
DC	DC-1	DC-3	DC-4		
BR				BR-3	BR-4
MB	MB-1	MB-2	MB-3		
MT	MT-1		MT-4	MT-2	MT-3

*The numbers in parentheses indicate that the association with that DR antigen is not as strong.

allelic series. Immunochemical analyses have demonstrated that antisera which define the MT2 specificity contain antibodies against two species of Ia molecules. The antisera react with a DR-like molecule and thus appear to contain antibodies against a truly supertypic specificity. In addition, the same MT2 antisera also react with a BR-like molecule. Several investigators have reported recombinations between HLA-DR and DC/MB, although none of these have been unequivocally accepted. Irradiation-induced lymphoblastoid cell line mutants have been isolated which have lost the expression of HLA-A, B, C, and DR but retained the expression of DC/MB, substantiating that DR and DC/MB are under different genetic control (Fig. 33–1).

Definition of SB Antigens. SB (secondary B cell) antigens are defined by primed lymphocytes (PLT). These antigens are weak and usually undetectable stimulating determinants in primary MLC, although they cause very strong stimulation in secondary culture. During the late 1970's, several investigators demonstrated that cells could be primed for antigens other than HLA-D. Termijtelen generated a particularly interesting primed cell (PL 3A) by priming two Dw3 homozygous typing cells against each other. Activity in secondary test culture was not associated with any known HLA specificity. In 1979, Mawas and Charmot showed that a primed reagent could be generated between two siblings who were identical for HLA-A, B, C, D, and DR but where one sibling expressed a recombination somewhere between HLA-D and the glyoxylase locus five recombinant units centromeric to HLA-D. Concomitantly during 1979, Shaw developed a logical allelic system. He primed lymphocytes from unrelated donor pairs who were identifical for HLA-A, B, C, and DR and was able to define five specificities which behaved as part of a single segregant series. He called these determinants SB for secondary B cell antigens.

Two recombinants between HLA-D/DR and SB have subsequently been identified. This segregant series is located approximately 1 centimorgan centromeric to HLA-D/DR (Fig. 33–1). Studies with irradiation-induced HLA loss mutant cell lines have confirmed that SB is a separate gene product. SB determinants are on Class II molecules; they are expressed on B cells and monocytes but not resting T lymphocytes; they have very different gene frequencies in different ethnic populations; and they act as restricting determinants for antigen presentation between monocytes and T cells. Recently SB antigens have been identified with both monoclonal antibodies and alloantisera.

T Cell Cloning. In the 1970's it was hypothesized that the complex reaction patterns identified, using both cellular and serologic typing methods, were probably due to as yet undefined MHC antigenic determinants. Were these additional determinants due to slight variations of one molecule, for example, HLA-D, or were these complex reaction patterns due to additional molecules encoded by additional MHC genes? The ultimate cellular technique which might define the smallest differences between cells is the use of cloned primed lymphocytes. Using cloning techniques, one can identify those antigens which stimulate a single primed lymphocyte. As the reactivity of lymphocytes is precommitted to recognize discrete antigenic determinants during embryogenesis, T cell cloning also is valuable in determining the variety and frequency of cells committed to certain antigens. Thus a panel of cloned T cells which are derived from a PLT directed against alloantigens should tell us about the number of different MHC determinants present on stimulating lymphocytes. Analysis of T cell clone typing has already produced a large body of information about MHC antigens using classic genetic techniques such as typing of families and unrelated HLA typed individuals. As expected, the reaction patterns are very complex, but some general conclusions can be drawn. The majority of the clones derived from alloreactive PLT's recognize Class II MHC gene products. Most of these clones recognize antigens similar to HLA-D or DR, a smaller percentage recognize SB-like determinants, and rarely clones recognize MB/MT-like antigens. There have been a few reports of clones which recognize Class I MHC products, but these clones are of the cytotoxic variety and not of the helper T cell variety like most clones that recognize Class II molecules. Clones which recognize antigens that do not appear to be encoded within the MHC have been reported, but the exact nature of these non-MHC encoded stimulating antigens is unknown. Very few of the clones give reaction patterns which correlate precisely with any classic specificity. For example, one clone may recognize two thirds of the HLA-DR1 stimulating cells, and another clone derived from the same priming may recognize two thirds of the HLA-DR1 stimulating cells, but with only partial concordance between the reaction patterns of the first versus second clone. Does this mean that there are two very similar molecules which together make the classic DR1 antigen, or does this mean that there are small differences between DR1 molecules from different individuals? Classic family and population studies cannot differentiate these two possibilities. As we now know that Class II genes are composed of alpha and beta chains (see subsequent section for details) which are not necessarily adjacent and that some of these gene sequences are probably less than 0.1 recombinant unit apart, the classic method of identifying a naturally occurring recombinant family would be unlikely to produce results in a reasonable length of time. Thus we must rely on several evolving techniques such as DNA hybridization, molecular studies of MHC gene products, and stimulation of clones with induced mutations of lymphoblastoid cell lines to resolve these issues.

A second major question being addressed with T cell clones is the regulation of immune responses by Class II MHC antigens. As primed lymphocytes can be generated against alloantigens, primed lymphocytes can be also generated against other antigens such as viruses. Peripheral blood lymphocytes stimulated with these antigens can be cloned. These antigen-reactive T cell clones replicate in response to the stimulating antigen only in the presence of a second "antigen presenting cell" such as a macrophage, a B cell, or B-lymphoblastoid cell line. However, not all antigen presenting cells are capable of functioning in conjunction with any one cloned T cell. The interaction between clone and presenting cell is limited to ("restricted" by) MHC Class II antigens. Thus most antigen-reactive (e.g., influenza) T cell clones generated from a DR1 positive cell donor respond to the antigen in the presence of most (but not all) antigen presenting cells which are also DR1 positive. The range of restriction appears to be as varied as the range of stimulation of alloreactive T lymphocyte clones. Thus the analysis of response to antigen restriction is used in conjunction with other methods of analysis to determine the expression of MHC gene products and, of great importance, allows one to look at the function of these MHC products in immunologic responses.

Structure of Class II Molecules. Class II molecules consist of two integral membrane glycoprotein chains designated alpha and beta with apparent molecular weights of 33,000 to 34,000 and 27,000 to 30,000, respectively (Fig. 33–4). Studies using chemical cross-linking agents indicate that the stoichiometry of subunits is 1:1. Alpha and beta chains are noncovalently associated but extremely stable and can be separated in the presence of sodium dodecyl sulfate (SDS) only when heated to 80°C. Both chains are encoded within the MHC.

Isolation and amino acid sequences have been recently published for both the DR alpha and beta chains. The DR molecule has amino acid sequence homology with the murine I-E molecule (Fig. 33–1). Class II molecules, like Class I, are oriented with the amino terminus extracellular and the carboxyl terminus intracellular with the molecule divided into domains. The extracellular segment of the DR beta chain consists of two domains each containing an intrachain disulfide bridge and in this respect resembles Class I MHC molecules as well as immunoglobulins. Also as in Class I molecules, there seems to be a major variable region which is localized between positions 60 and 69. The majority of the amino acid differences found in this segment can be accounted for by single nucleotide interchanges. The extracellular segment of the DR alpha chain also consists of two domains. The carboxyl terminal domain contains an intrachain disulfide bridge and shows sequence homology to the corresponding domain of the beta chain, Class I molecules, and the CH_3 domain of immunoglobulin molecules. To a lesser extent the amino terminal domain shows sequence homology to the amino terminal domain of beta chains.

The DNA corresponding to both DR alpha and beta chains have been cloned and completely sequenced. The three cDNA alpha chain sequences reported are identical to one another with the exception of a single nucleotide difference found in the cytoplasmic domain of one clone. The data indicate that there is a single DR alpha chain gene per haplotype and at least two nonallelic DR beta chain genes. Additional DR beta chain genes may exist, but it is not yet known if they are all expressed. Recently microfingerprinting (peptide digest maps) has indicated that the DR and BR alpha chains could not be readily distinguished from one another, yet were clearly different from the DC alpha chain. However, the beta chains for all three specificities (DR, BR, DC) differ markedly from each other. Thus the DR and BR subsets most likely share an alpha chain but consist of different beta chains and represent the two "DR-like," $\alpha_1\beta_1$, $\alpha_1\beta_2$ molecules.

A second Class II molecule, DC or MB, has been unequivocally shown to be different from HLA-DR. Both the alpha and beta chains precipitated by DC-1 antibodies have been shown to be different from the alpha and beta chains precipitated by DR antisera using 2D gels, peptide mapping, and amino terminal sequence analysis. Furthermore cDNA corresponding to DC alpha and beta chains have been isolated and characterized as different from the DR alpha and beta cDNA clones. Complete amino acid sequences of both DC alpha and beta chains can be discerned from the DNA sequence of the cDNA clones and have been shown to be homologous to murine I-A antigens.

Experimental evidence indicates that there is a third Class II molecule, SB, which is composed of unique alpha and beta chains (Fig. 33–1). The SB alpha and beta chain genes are different from both DR (I-E like) and DC (I-A like) molecules, although recent DNA sequencing data indicate that the SB molecule contains sequences homologous to both DR and DC in a patchwork-like arrangement. A counterpart for SB has not been found in the mouse.

Thus the human "I region" equivalent appears to be more complex than its murine counterpart (i.e., a larger number of α chains and of β chains). Data from immunochemical, molecular genetic, and immunogenetic techniques indicate that there is a minimum of three distinct subsets of human Class II molecules (I-A like, I-E like, and unique). The genes for the human alpha and beta chains have not been mapped in man. However, data from several different laboratories indicate that there is a minimum of three distinct α chains and seven distinct β chains. Due to the availability of recombinant mouse strains, it has been possible to map the similar Class II genes in the mouse. Genes for both α and β chains of I-A subregion products map to the I-A subregion. I-E molecules consist of an α chain encoded in the I-E subregion and a β chain encoded in the I-A subregion. Although the I region in the mouse contains several subregions defined by classic immunogenetic methods, structural genes have been identified for only two of these subregions (Fig. 33–1).

Techniques for Detecting HLA Antigens

Histocompatibility testing or HLA typing is performed in a limited number of laboratories because it uses specialized complex procedures and reagents. In addition, interpretation and translation of the results requires considerable expertise. However, histocompatibility laboratories are found in medical centers which have organ transplantation programs and/or as parts of large blood banks and transfusion services. For specific techniques the reader should refer to the AACHT (American Association for Clinical Histocompatibility Testing) Manual and the National Institute of Allergy and Infectious Diseases Hand Book.

Serologic Techniques. Originally leukoagglutination was used; however, this technique is notorious for giving non-reproducible reactions. Lymphocytotoxicity testing, which was originally utilized in the mouse system by Gorer and Amos, was modified by Terasaki and McClelland for use in the human system. This assay represented a tremendous technical advance since reproducibility is greater than 98 per cent under controlled, standardized conditions.

Lymphocyte Preparation. Lymphocytes are employed routinely in HLA typing assays and are readily obtained from peripheral whole blood by layering onto a Ficoll-Hypaque gradient which separates blood cells according to density. Following centrifugation, one obtains a layer at the serum-Ficoll-Hypaque interface which is 99 per cent mononuclear cells. These separated peripheral blood lymphocytes (PBL) can be used for HLA-ABC typing.

An additional separation step is necessary before typing for HLA-D/DR region antigens. To test for these antigens it is necessary to enrich for B lymphocytes or to use a special two-color fluorescent technique. Three enrichment procedures are in general use for the separation of the B lymphocyte subset: (1) Nylon wool adherence. B cells and monocytes preferentially adhere when a Ficoll-Hypaque separated lymphocyte preparation is incubated on a nylon wool column. T lymphocytes are easily washed off since they are relatively non-adherent. Once the T cells have been washed off, the B cells can be removed following vigorous agitation while monocytes remain adhered. Although technique dependent, under appropriate conditions good enrichment of B cells can be obtained. This technique is the one of choice of many clinical histocompatibility laboratories because it is relatively rapid and does not require specialized equipment or reagents. (2) E rosette depletion of T cells. T lymphocytes have a cell surface receptor which weakly binds sheep red blood cells (SRBC) forming a rosette with the T cell in the center. The rosetted T cells can then be separated on a Ficoll-Hypaque gradient, leaving the B cells and monocytes at the gradient interface. Since the bond between the E rosette receptor on the T cell and the SRBC is weak, the shear forces during centrifugation can break up the rosette, releasing the trapped T lymphocyte and decreasing the B cell purity. (3) Immunoadsorption of B cells to plastic dishes or flasks coated with an affinity purified anti-human immunoglobulin ("panning"). Affinity purified anti-human immunoglobulin will bind to plastic by adherence. When a mononuclear cell suspension is placed in the flask or dish, B lymphocytes bind to the antibody coated surface by their immunoglobulin receptors. The unbound T lymphocytes are easily washed off. The immunoglobulin positive cells (B cells) are recovered by competition using elution media which contains an excess of immunoglobulin. Although B cell purity is excellent and a uniform population is reproducibly obtained because of the positive selection, this technique is used primarily in specialized research laboratories. It requires special reagents and is more expensive and slightly more time consuming than the nylon adherence technique or SRBC rosetting technique.

HLA-Typing Sera. The major source of HLA antisera is from multipara. During pregnancy the woman will mount an immune response to the paternal antigens present on the fetus. Other sources of antisera are from transplant recipients, multi-transfused patients, and planned immunizations of humans and of other primates. Sera from these sources are tested against panels of lymphocytes of known HLA type (screened) for the presence of useful antisera. Thus large screening programs must be maintained to identify reagents for one's own use and for exchange with colleagues since these antisera have not been commercially available in the past. Recently both bulk antisera and HLA-typing trays have become commercially available. For most clinical typing these are adequate; but they are not yet adequate for research since the source of identification of new specificities and even alleleic systems is through characterization of sera with new and unexplained reactivity patterns.

Because of the extreme antigenic complexity of HLA antigens, several antisera must be used to define each specificity. Frequently from 120 to 210 antisera are used to define the HLA-A, B, C specificities and from 60 to 140 are used to define the B cell specificities. Since many antisera have multiple antibodies and specificities are assigned by reactivity patterns, the reactivity of each antiserum should be thoroughly known by the individual interpreting the results. Most antisera tend to have false positive and false negative reactions and some rarer antigens are defined by reactivity patterns of multispecific antisera.

Lymphocyte Microcytotoxicity Assay. HLA typing for the HLA-A, B, C, DR, MB, MT, DC, BR antigens is conventionally performed by a microcytotoxicity assay. The HLA antigen profile is determined by testing the whole lymphocyte preparation (PBL) or T lymphocytes (for ABC) or the enriched B lymphocytes (for DR, MB, MT, DC) against a panel of well characterized antisera. The assay is a two stage test which uses only 1 μl of antiserum and 1 μl containing 2000 lymphocytes. During the sensitization stage, the lymphocytes are incubated with the antisera generally for 30 minutes at 22 to 24°C. Carefully prescreened and standardized rabbit serum as a source of complement is added in excess and the mixture incubated for an additional 60 minutes. Frequently the incubation times are extended to 60/60 or 60/120 minutes respectively for B cell typing. If the lymphocytes carry a cell surface antigen recognized by complement fixing antibodies in the serum, the antibodies bind to the cells and the cells are subsequently killed following addition of complement. Complement mediated lysis results in changes in the permeability of the cell membrane that can be easily judged microscopically by the penetration of vital dyes. The assay is terminated by addition of eosin and formalin or trypan blue with EDTA. Reactions are read microscopically for per cent lysis and numerically graded. Greater than 40 per cent lysis is considered a weak positive, and greater than 60 per cent lysis is considered positive. Less than 20 per cent reflects a negative reaction. From 20 to 40 per cent lysis is considered questionably positive.

All lymphocytotoxicity procedures involve complement fixation which can introduce a potential source of error and major variability in laboratory diagnosis. The source of complement is rabbit serum, but there are no standards on age, pool size, or potency. Therefore, meticulous quality control procedures by individual laboratories are of primary importance in the selection of rabbit serum for the lymphomicrocytotoxicity assay. Each complement lot must be pretested for inherent cytotoxicity and for activity. The method recommended is to perform crosshatch titrations of antiserum and complement against cells from several individuals with appropriate positive and negative antisera. The same antisera and cells should always be used. In addition, a panel of lymphocytes should be HLA typed using the new lot of complement in parallel with the old lot of complement.

Cross-Reactivity. The problem of extensive cross-reactivity has affected HLA typing and research from the beginning. Cross-reactivity combined with polyspecificity is responsible for the complex reactivity patterns of the antisera. Cross-reactivity is also one of the major causes for the practice of "splitting" HLA antigens. Cross-reactivity between alleles at the A and B loci has been extensively studied and classified into cross-reactivity groups (CREG). A diagram of cross-reactivity at the A locus and at the B locus is given in Figures 33–5 and 33–6. Fuller has presented a detailed discussion of serologic cross-reactivity at the A and B loci (Miller, 1981). The molecular basis for cross-reactivity is not known but will be elucidated by DNA sequencing of HLA alleles in the near future. It is already evident that there are conserved sequences as well as highly variable sequences in the amino acid chains which make up the molecules. There are several obvious models for cross-reactivity which are probably all operable either alone or combined. For a detailed discussion of models, refer to Tanagaki (1982).

Cellular Techniques. Cellular replication can be used as an indirect measure of recognition of alloantigens. Although replication of lymphocytes frequently accompanies recognition of antigens, other cellular activities that do not necessarily require replication may follow recognition, such as antibody production or lymphocyte mediated cytotoxicity. In addition, Class I MHC alloantigens do not cause adequate replication to be detected in our usual tests (or result in no replication), but recognition of some Class II alloantigens results in marked replication by as many as 3 per cent of cells in culture. Some Class II alloantigens stimulate measurable replication in primary culture, while some require stimulation of previously primed cells for detection.

Mixed Leukocyte Culture (MLC). The basic miniaturized MLC culture and leukocyte culture harvesting techniques used today were developed in 1969 by Hartzman. Peripheral blood mononuclear cells relatively free of platelets and erythrocytes are obtained by using a Ficoll-Hypaque gradient technique of Boyum. This lymphocyte separation method is particularly important as it removes most granulocytes which can non-specifically suppress *in vitro* replication if substantial numbers are present. Mononuclear cells to be used as stimulator cells are irradiated (generally 2000R ^{37}Ci) or treated with mitomycin C (generally 25 to 50 μg/ml). Responder and stimulator cells are

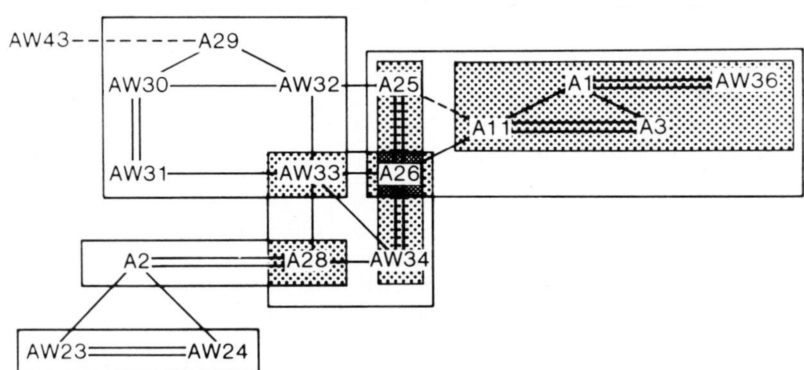

Figure 33–5. HLA-A cross-reactivity. An updated diagram of the cross-reactive antigens of the HLA-A locus. This schema was developed from studies by Rodey and Fuller using a large battery of alloantisera and platelet absorption/elution and antiglobulin techniques. Strong cross-reactivity is indicated by double bars and overlapping cross-reactivity by stippling. (Reproduced with permission from Miller, W. V., and Rodey, G.: HLA Without Tears. Chicago, American Scoeity of Clinical Pathologists, 1981.)

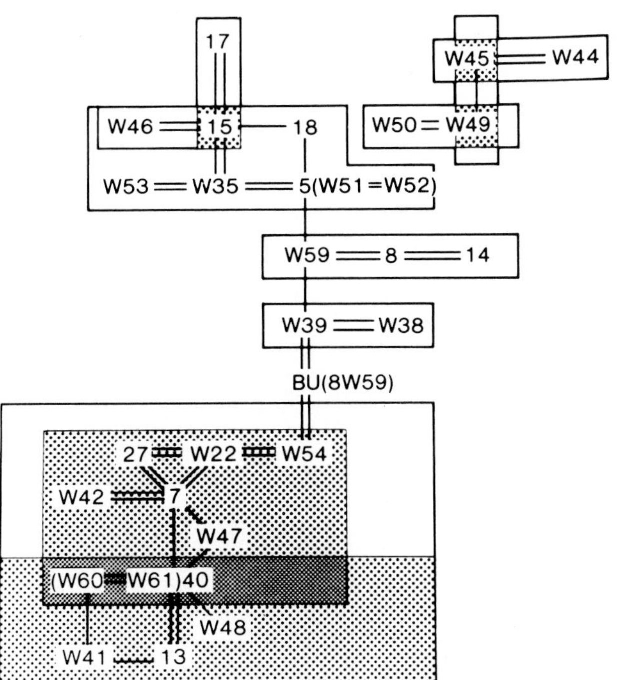

Figure 33–6. HLA-B cross-reactivity. An updated diagram of the cross-reactive antigens of the HLA-B locus. This schema was developed from studies by Rodey and Fuller using a large battery of alloantisera and platelet absorption/elution and antiglobulin techniques. Strong cross-reactivity is indicated by double bars and overlapping cross-reactivity by stippling. (Reproduced with permission from Miller, W. V., and Rodey, G.: HLA Without Tears. Chicago, American Society of Clinical Pathologists, 1981.)

then added to tissue culture plates (usually a 96 well/round bottom well plate with 300 to 400 μl maximum capacity) in a total volume of 50 to 200 μl of tissue culture media containing several supplements, including serum and antibiotics. Cells are incubated five to six days, at which time 1 to 2 μCi ^{3}H-thymidine (2 to 20 Ci/mM) is added to each well followed by 6 to 18 hours of additional incubation to permit uptake and incorporation of thymidine. Then cells are washed free of unincorporated thymidine onto small fiberglass filters using a semi-automated harvester. The amount of ^{3}H-thymidine remaining on the filter and thus the amount of thymidine incorporation is assayed with a scintillation spectrometer.

In culture, cells undergo the process of recognition and then begin to react. Under usual conditions, no thymidine incorporation can be detected for 48 to 72 hours, although glucose metabolism can be detected within one hour and insulin and transferrin receptor changes can be identified within several hours. After the initial "latent" phase, replication begins and continues at a rapid pace up to the sixth to eighth day of culture, depending on the "strength" of the stimulus. Greater cellular activation results in earlier peak responses. During this time, many large blast lymphocytes can be seen in the culture, the number being proportional to the uptake of thymidine.

Primed Lymphocyte Test (PLT). After reaching their peak, many of the replicating cells revert to the appearance of small quiescent lymphocytes and no longer incorporate large amounts of thymidine. These resting cells remain stable in tissue culture, if adequate nutrients are provided, for another 5 to 30 days. The return to quiescence and stability of these stimulated cells is of central importance to a number of other tests of cellular recognition. Each lymphocyte is precommitted to react to a single antigenic determinant; thus replication in primary culture increases the number of cells capable of recognizing a given stimulating determinant. As there are many cells and many antigenic determinants in any one "bulk" leukocyte culture, many clones of cells reactive to each of the many antigenic determinants present proliferate. Thus at the end of a 10-day stimulation period, most of the cells present in the culture are the daughter cells of single cells which have divided and reverted to a resting stage. A second property of these cells which have been in culture is the very brief "latent" phase when restimulated *in vitro*. This process of stimulating the lymphocytes *in vitro* for use in subsequent tests is called priming.

In the PLT (primed lymphocyte test), lymphocytes which have been primed to the desired antigens are cryopreserved in a way which maintains viability. To maintain viability cells are frozen in the cryoprotective agent dimethylsulfoxide, which acts to stabilize membranes and alter transport of ions. Cells can be frozen in discrete stages or controlled rate (−1°C./min) frozen and stored at low temperature (generally the vapor phase of liquid nitrogen), keeping in mind that warming to −30°C. for even brief periods and recooling results in severe damage to the functional capacity of the cell. In the test phase of the PLT, cryopreserved primed lymphocytes are thawed and washed free of the dimethylsulfoxide, or freshly primed lymphocytes can be used. Primed cells are stimulated with a test panel of peripheral blood mononuclear cells using techniques similar to the primary mixed leukocyte reaction. The tissue culture is incubated for 48 to 80 hours, labeled with ^{3}H-thymidine, and harvested after an additional 6 to 18 hours and radioactive incorporation assessed.

T Cell Cloning. Using a modification of the PLT technology, primed cells can be restimulated in limiting dilution cultures so that large numbers of cells can be derived from a single primed lymphocyte. Essentially primed cells are diluted and distributed into microtest (10 to 20 μl/well) plates along with the irradiated specific stimulator cell in high excess (10,000 cells per well) so that the stimulator cell also acts as a feeder cell along with T cell growth factor (the supernatant media from stimulated lymphocytes containing interleukin-2 [IL-2]). After five to ten days of incubation, replicating lymphocytes can be detected in some wells. Cells from "positive" wells are transferred to larger wells along with additional feeder cells and IL-2. A modest variation of this procedure allows one to generate clones of T lymphocytes directed against non-cellular antigens such as viruses. These antigen specific clones are developed by priming with the desired antigen followed by cloning in the presence of feeder cells which share Class II major histocompatibility specificity with the responder cell. Once either allospecific clones or antigen specific clones are generated, very large numbers of these cells (10^{10}) can be produced and cryopreserved for extended analysis of specificity, genetic restriction, protein and nucleic acid analysis, and functional studies.

ORGAN TRANSPLANTATION

Organ transplantation represents one of the largest challenges still open to medical science. Renal transplantation is a routine procedure in more than 150 major North American medical centers as therapy for end-stage kidney disease (Terasaki, 1983). More recently bone marrow, heart, liver, and pancreas transplants are gaining wide acceptance as therapeutic procedures. The major obstacle to transplantation is immunologically mediated rejection of the graft. Such rejection is a manifestation of the uniqueness of the individual and is fundamental since the survival of an individual is dependent upon the ability to recognize foreign antigens (be it a viral or bacterial pathogen, tumor, or unfortunately allogeneic cells) and to respond to them. Therefore the success of transplants relies on the ability to circumvent the immune reaction, which is accomplished largely by immunosuppressive therapy but also depends on the degree of histocompatibility between the donor and the recipient. Cytotoxic and immunosuppressive agents such as azathioprine and prednisone have been used with moderate success over a number of years. Several therapies more specific to transplant rejection are being developed. Cyclosporine A has recently become available, and experimental trials have shown it to be a powerful immunosuppressive agent (Abramowicz, 1983). As extended (five years) trials have not been completed, the full impact of the drug on the importance of histocompatibility testing has not been thoroughly analyzed.

In addition, other modulators of the immune response, for example, monoclonal antibodies against the T cell surface antigen T-12, are being vigorously pursued. The following is a discussion of histocompatibility in transplantation.

History

The genetic basis of transplantation was first determined in mice as a result of tumor transplantation experiments in 1916 by Little and Tyzzer and subsequently extended to transplants of normal tissue. Little demonstrated that skin grafts within inbred strains (autografts) were successful, while grafts between inbred strains (allografts) were not; grafts from either parent inbred strain to first generation (F_1) hybrids survived in all animals, whereas grafts from F_1 hybrid offspring to either parent did not survive. In addition, skin from second generation (F_2) animals or subsequent generations survived on F_1 animals. The foregoing observations established the laws of transplantation. In 1948 Snell named the factors or genes determining the fate of allografts "histocompatibility" or "H" genes. Also in 1948 the major histocompatibility locus in the mouse, H-2, was defined by Gorer, who had first described the alloantigens in 1937. There are other histocompatibility or H systems in the mouse, but these have a relatively minor effect on the outcome of grafting and can be overcome by immunosuppression much more easily.

Renal Transplantation

Renal transplantation was implemented in the early 1960's. Since convincing evidence already existed in experimental animals that antigens of the MHC represent the major barriers to successful allografting, HLA typing was used to determine compatibility between donor and recipient.

The Significance of Matching for HLA in Living-Related Transplants. Initially, the influence of MHC antigens on grafting was investigated through skin grafting between family members. Skin grafts from MHC or HLA identical siblings survived significantly longer than grafts between one haplotype matched siblings, parents, or unrelated donors. These observations were extended to and confirmed in renal transplantation during the 1970's.

Within a family, each child inherits one HLA haplotype from each parent in a random fashion; thus there are only four HLA genotypes possible in a sibship (Fig. 33–2). The probability of occurrence of each genotype is thus 1 in 4. Therefore, approximately 25 per cent of all siblings will inherit the same parental HLA haplotypes and are termed "HLA-identical." Fifty per cent of the siblings will share one HLA haplotype and are termed "haploidentical," while 25 per cent will share no HLA haplotype and are called "haplodistinct." Since offspring inherit one HLA haplotype from each parent, it follows that the parent-child combination will always be haploidentical. Figure 33–7 shows survival results of a series of

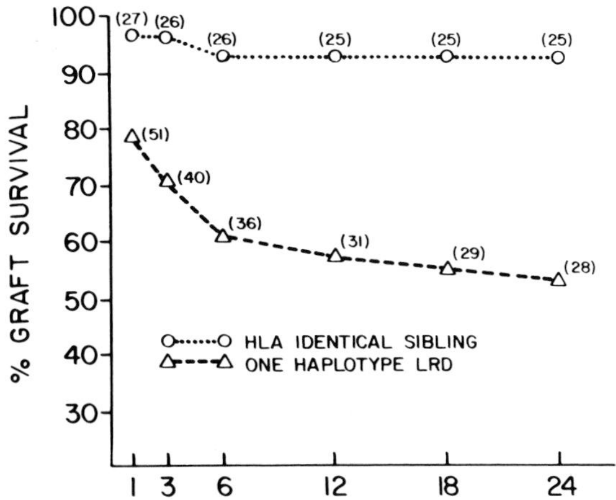

Figure 33–7. Renal allograft survival in living related donor (LRD) transplants. (Modified from Anderson, C. B., Sicard, G. A., Rodey, G. E., Anderman, C. K., and Etheredge, E. E.: Transplant. Proc., *15*:941, 1983.)

living-related donor renal allografts. Overall survival of HLA-identical sibling transplants at two years (and even up to ten years) is approximately 90 per cent. Haploidentical and haplodistinct grafts survive less well. Thus, provided medical reasons permit, the order of priorities in living-related allograft donor selection is based on decreasing order of histocompatibility: (1) monozygotic twin; (2) HLA-identical siblings; (3) HLA-haploidentical siblings; (4) HLA-haploidentical child or parent; and (5) first order relatives, grandparents, aunts, uncles, or cousins, preferably haploidentical. Note that a monozygotic twin would also share the other minor histocompatibility antigens and be the ultimate match equal to an autograft.

The dogma that organ transplants from HLA-identical (and ABO compatible) siblings survive very well and significantly better than organs transplanted between HLA-mismatched siblings or parents has been consistently verified. These data comparing HLA matched and mismatched sibling donors leave no room for doubt that the HLA complex represents a major barrier to successful renal transplantation and is indeed the major histocompatibility complex in man.

The Significance of Matching for HLA in Unrelated Cadaver Transplants. Compared with results obtained with living-related transplants, the results of matching for HLA in cadaver (unrelated) transplants are not as clear. Initial encouraging studies reported that recipients of cadaver transplants which were matched for HLA antigens (then only A and B loci) had a better outcome than those with HLA-A and B mismatched transplants. Organ sharing groups were set up on a regional basis in order to have a large enough recipient pool to be able to obtain a good HLA-A, B match. Now it is generally accepted that the effect of matching for A and B locus antigens in cadaver transplants is minor. Overall one-year survival of HLA-A, B identical cadaver kidneys is only 60 to 70 per cent compared with the approximately 90 per cent one-year survival of kidneys from HLA identical siblings. Why is there such a large (20 to 30 per cent) difference in graft survival between HLA-A, B identical sibling versus unrelated transplants? There must be other factors, mainly in the MHC, which exert a major influence on graft survival. Antigens in the D/DR region are very likely candidates. There are theoretical reasons why these antigens may be a major factor in matching for allografting. One of the first steps in allosensitization is activation of T helper cells which occurs via antigens in the D/DR region; thus matching for D/DR would influence the inductive phase of the response. If initiation of the anti-allograft response can be prevented or reduced by matching, one would expect improved graft acceptance. On the other hand, matching for HLA-A, B antigens is directed at the effector end of the response since the A and B locus antigens are primarily targets for attack by lymphocytes and antibody. Thus they are more important after sensitization. (HLA-DR can also be a target antigen for antibody and cytotoxic killers.)

The earliest studies to evaluate the effect of antigens in the D/DR region were conducted between 1975 and 1977. Since the D/DR antigens are the major stimulating determinants in the MLR, these early studies attempted to determine the role of the MLR in predicting the outcome of human cadaveric renal transplantation. Most studies of MLR suggested that low responses between the recipient and donor were good predictors of increased graft survival. Since the MLR test requires seven days, this assay could not be used as a practical predictor for cadaver renal transplantation. As mentioned previously, a serological definition of HLA-D was being sought. By 1977, typing for HLA-DR was possible. Ting and Morris immediately DR typed cadaver donors and recipients transplanted between 1975 and 1977 using frozen lymphocytes in a retrospective study. The results suggested that matching for DR might influence graft survival. Reports from several independent groups confirmed these findings. Unlike the ultimately disappointing graft survival results obtained with HLA-A, B antigen matching in cadaver transplant, graft survival analyzed on the basis of DR matching has not only remained encouraging over the past five years but improved. As can be seen in Figure 33–8, 18-month graft survival with a two HLA-DR match is 92 per cent from one center. Currently, almost all transplant centers that use DR matching as a first priority in selection of a recipient for a cadaveric kidney find that matching for DR increases graft survival (range 80 to 94 per cent). Several questions about matching for HLA in renal allografting remain unanswered. Do zero DR mismatched grafts do as well as two DR matched? Do one DR matched or mismatched grafts do better than zero DR matched? Does matching for HLA-A, B, C antigens in addition to HLA-DR increase graft survival? What is the long term (five- to ten-year) effect in DR matched compared with non-DR matched patients? As prior transfusions and certain immunosuppressive regimens improve transplant survival, all of these questions must be asked in the transfused versus the non-transfused patient along with the effect of immunosuppression for both short term and long term (five to ten years) effect in DR matching.

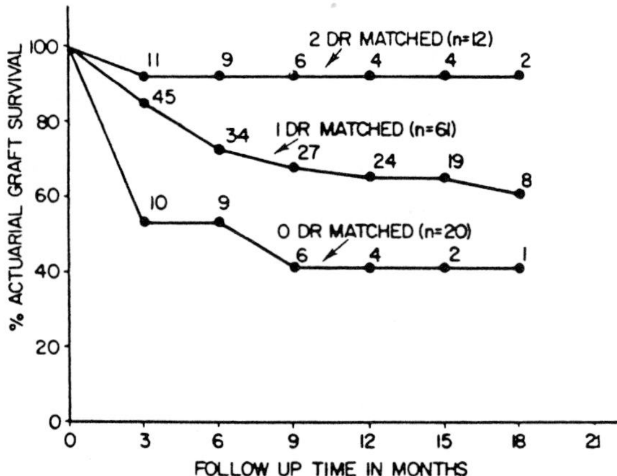

Figure 33–8. Actuarial graft survival of renal allografts prospectively matched for two, one, or zero HLA-DR antigens. Number at each point is the number of patients at risk. Numbers in parentheses, total number of patients entered (two DR versus one DR, $0.10 < P < 0.25$; two DR versus zero DR, $0.01 < P < 0.05$; one DR, versus zero DR, $0.05 < P < 0.10$). (Reproduced from Goeken, N. E., Thompson, J. S., and Corry, R. J.: Transplantation, *32*:523, 1981.)

The Significance of the Lymphocyte Crossmatch. The crossmatch test measures the state of presensitization, if any, in the potential recipient against a specific donor. There are numerous serologic and cellular methods for analyzing the donor-specific presensitization state; however, complement mediated lymphocytotoxicity is used conventionally in all histocompatibility (HLA) laboratories. This assay tests for the presence of cytotoxic antibodies in the serum of the potential recipient which react with lymphocytes of the specific donor and is probably the most important contribution of the HLA tissue typing laboratory to clinical renal transplantation.

The first report of a positive crossmatch in a patient who hyperacutely rejected the graft was from Terasaki and colleagues. This report was confirmed by numerous laboratories during the next several years. A positive crossmatch between donor lymphocytes and recipient serum became contraindicative to performing the transplant. The high correlation between a positive lymphocyte crossmatch and hyperacute allograft rejection is not surprising since HLA antigens are found in large amounts in the kidney.

With the identification of B cell alloantigens in the mid-1970's, a re-evaluation of the crossmatch occurred. Many of the weakly positive crossmatches (20 per cent lysis) could be directed against B cell alloantigens since B cells constitute 10 per cent (3 to 21 per cent) of peripheral blood lymphocytes. Were antibodies against HLA-DR antigens also contraindicative to transplantation (i.e., B cell positive, T cell negative crossmatch)? This question has not yet been answered. Antibodies detected in the B cell crossmatch are not always against HLA-DR, and the distinction can be hard to make. Antibodies detected in the B cell crossmatch can be (1) anti-HLA-DR, (2) weak anti-ABC antibodies since B cells are more sensitive to complement dependent assays than are T cells, (3) non-DR antibodies both cold and warm reacting, or (4) non-DR antibodies such as anti-Lewis.

Therefore, currently the only unequivocal statement that can be made is that a positive T cell crossmatch detected by conventional lymphocytotoxicity technique with sera which are negative with autologous lymphocytes is contraindicative to transplantation. Antibodies detected by such methods are for the majority against HLA-A, B, C antigens. B cell crossmatches should be performed when possible and the data collected, but not used to indicate whether a transplant should be performed. Care must be taken to include controls and other procedures (absorption with platelets, incubation at 5°C. [cold] and 37°C. [warm]) for retrospective analysis.

The sensitivity of the lymphocytotoxicity test used to detect a preformed antibody against HLA-A, B, C is also currently being evaluated. Until very recently, the dogma was the more sensitive the crossmatch test, the better. In many laboratories, extended incubations were used to increase the sensitivity of the crossmatch test as well as an antiglobulin cytotoxicity test. However, the extended incubation assay has been questioned. Jeannet and colleagues have reported the successful outcome in 14 of 15 grafts performed with a negative room temperature T cell and B cell crossmatch and a complement incubation time of 60 minutes but a positive crossmatch when this complement incubation time was increased to 120 minutes. Since this activity can be removed by absorption with platelets, the activity detected with the extended incubation times is probably weak antibodies to HLA-A, B, C. Another technique which dramatically increased the sensitivity of the lymphocytotoxicity assay employs the addition of an antiglobulin reagent prior to the addition of complement. This technique was developed by Johnson in 1971 and is currently used as an adjunct crossmatch technique in many centers. The antiglobulin test not only detects low levels of cytotoxic antibodies (as with extended incubation times and addition of antithymocyte globulin) but also detects inherently non-complement fixing antibodies. Several retrospective studies have indicated that the antibodies detected by the antiglobulin test are clinically relevant and are predictive of a poor post-transplant course. For further review of the crossmatch the excellent overview of Ting (1983) should be consulted.

An important consideration in the crossmatch is which serum samples should be used for testing. After immunization in a patient who develops lymphocytotoxic antibodies, the cytotoxic antibody may disappear from the serum or react with less frequency as time passes. Hence the importance of at least monthly blood serum collections from patients awaiting transplantation to ascertain PRA or per cent reactive antibody and subsequent freezing of serum aliquots for crossmatch at the time of impending renal transplantation. The most highly reactive serum is the peak serum. Peak (PRA) and current serum samples for crossmatching are standard operating procedure in virtually all HLA tissue typing laboratories. This allows identification of a patient with a negative

Table 33–3. PROGNOSTIC VARIABLES OF INTEREST IN CADAVER (CAD) RENAL TRANSPLANTATION

1. ABO blood type and anti A_1 and anti Le^a when appropriate
2. HLA-A, B histocompatibility
3. DR histocompatibility
4. Preformed cytotoxic antibody (PRA or percent reactive antibody)
5. Crossmatch (T cell and B cell warm/cold) current and peak sera
6. Prior transplantation
7. Pretransplant blood transfusions
8. Prior nephrectomy of native kidney
9. Recipient race
10. Diabetes mellitus
11. Acute tubular necrosis
12. Antilymphocyte serum
13. Cyclosporine A
14. Donor race
15. Splenectomy pretransplant
16. Total kidney preservation time (ice versus perfusion)
17. Recipient age

current crossmatch (antibody no longer present after prior sensitization and persisting memory for the antigen) but a positive crossmatch with peak serum specimen to avoid a potential second set renal allograft rejection. However, the clinical relevance of the positive peak sera crossmatch from sera specimens at least a year old is being questioned when the current specimen is negative. Other important factors include strength of antibody (PRA) and rate of decline and whether patients should be transfused after reaching peak response or whether antibody level should be left to fall by itself. (Ting, 1983). As stated, the PRA (per cent reactive antibody) sera specimens provide helpful information to ascertain prior immunization status of a potential renal transplant recipient. With PRAs in excess of 60 to 90 per cent, the decreased likelihood of a negative crossmatch with a current serum specimen is probable. SEOPF (Southeast Organ Procurement Foundation) trays which contain sera samples from registered patient recipients who have high PRAs, i.e., 60 per cent of lymphocyte cells reacting with patient sera, are distributed to collaborating laboratories. This permits identification of more favorable recipient candidates among the most difficult to crossmatch patients (high PRAs least likely to be transplanted) and ensures alternative use of kidney for the best match (e.g., two DR match for cadaveric donors and negative crossmatch). With the availability of more expeditious information processing (computer), the relative prognostic importance of several variables of interest in cadaver renal transplants may be assessed to improve further renal transplant outcome (Table 33–3). This should permit evolution of decision tree analyses for cadaveric donor matching.

Allogeneic Bone Marrow Transplantation

Most bone marrow transplants are currently performed for one of three diseases: (1) aplastic anemia, (2) leukemia, or (3) severe combined immunodeficiency (SCID). These transplants are among the most difficult of all clinical procedures for several reasons. First, at the time of transplantation the recipients are nearly totally immunodeficient, either because of inherited deficiency (SCID) or because of the pretransplant therapy of aplastic or leukemic patients (cytotoxic chemotherapy and irradiation) which prevents the immune system of the recipient from rejecting the donor marrow that is infused several days after recipient pretreatment. The amount of cytotoxic pretreatment is high enough to eliminate circulating leukocytes, nearly eliminate platelets, and abrogate production of new erythrocytes. Thus the recipient is profoundly susceptible to all types of infection and would certainly die if not rescued by extraordinary medical care and the allogeneic bone marrow. The second profound risk is the potential of immunologic attack of the recipient by the transplanted marrow—graft versus host disease (GVH). GVH has several forms and is frequently fatal. Antigens of the major histocompatibility complex can act as initiators as well as attack sites for GVH. In spite of these difficulties a number of transplant centers have demonstrated extraordinary success. Recent reports from the largest transplant center (The Fred Hutchinson Cancer Center in Seattle) demonstrate extraordinary success with allogeneic transplant for aplastic anemia (75 per cent survival) and good success for leukemic patients transplanted during their first remission of the disease. Until recently, it has been generally accepted that only HLA identical sibling donors were acceptable bone marrow donors. Over the past several years, transplants with donors who are slightly mismatched for HLA antigens have been performed primarily by the group at Seattle. Donors have been family members (usually parents or siblings) who differ with the recipient by only one or two antigens (HLA-ABC or HLA-DR) on one haplotype and are identical for the second haplotype. In one instance an HLA identical but unrelated donor was used. Success with these slightly mismatched donors has been nearly identical to success with HLA identical sibling donors for transplantation of leukemic patients.

There are a number of questions which lie ahead for the use of HLA mismatched marrow donation. Will the use of mismatched donors be successful for the treatment of aplastic anemia? How much mismatching can be tolerated? Will extensive mismatching lead to failure of the immune system (immunologic reconstitution) after transplantation? Can mismatched T and B cells of the donor immunologically cooperate with macrophages and other cells of the recipient? Can the transplanter treat donor marrow and/or the recipient to prevent GVH? Can the transplanters obtain pure "stem cells" for transplantation, and how would stem cells function both hematologically and immunologically? If the problems surrounding this most difficult procedure are overcome, bone marrow transplantation may become one of the most widely used methods for the treatment of a variety of diseases.

Review of General Genetics

Crow, J. F.: Genetics Notes. Minneapolis, Burgess Publishing Co., 1976.

Strickberger, M. W.: Genetics. New York, Macmillan, 1968.

Histocompatibility Testing Methods

NIAID Manual of Tissue Typing Techniques 1979–1980. NIH Publication number 80–545. Bethesda, Md., 1979.

Terasaki, P. I.: Histocompatibility Testing 1980. Los Angeles, UCLA Tissue Typing Laboratory Publishing, 1980.

Zachary, A. A., and Braun, W. E. (eds.): The AACHT Laboratory Manual. New York, The American Association for Clinical Histocompatibility Testing Publishing, 1981.

Immunogenetics Reviews

Miller, W. V., and Rodey, G.: HLA Without Tears. Chicago, American Society of Clinical Pathologists, 1981.

Moller, G.: Structure and Function of HLA-DR. Immunol. Rev., *66*:187, 1982.

Paul, W. E. (ed.): Fundamental Immunology. New York, Raven Press, 1983.

Zaleski, M. B., Dubiski, S., Niles, E., and Cunningham, R. K.: Immunogenetics. Boston, Pitman, 1983.

Immunochemistry Reviews

Hood, L., Steinmetz, M., and Malissen, B.: Genes of the major histocompatibility complex of the mouse. Ann. Rev. Immunol., *1*:529, 1983.

Lee, J., and Trowsdale, J.: Molecular biology of the major histocompatibility complex. Nature *304*:214, 1983.

Shackelford, D. A., Kaufman, J. F., Korman, A. J., and Strominger, J. L.: HLA-DR antigens: Structure, separation of subpopulations, gene cloning and function. Immunol. Rev., *66*:133, 1982.

Strominger, J. L., Engelhard, V. H., Fuks, A., Guild, B. C., Hyafil, F., Kaufman, J. F., Korman, A. J., Kostyk, T. G., Krangel, M. S., Lancet, D., Lopez de Castro, J. A., Mann, D. L., Orr, H. T., Parham, P. R., Parker, K. C., Ploegh, H. L., Pober, J. S., Robb, R. J., and Shackelford, D. A.: Biochemical analysis of products of the MHC. *In* Dorf, M. E. (ed.): The Role of the Major Histocompatibility Complex in Immunobiology. New York, Garland STPM Press, 1981, pp. 115–172.

Tanigaki, N., Tosi, R., Duquesnoy, R. J., and Ferrara, G. B.: Three Ia species with different structures and alloantigenic determinants in an HLA-homozygous cell line. J. Exp. Med., *157*:231, 1983.

General Literature

Abramowicz, M. (ed.): Cyclosporine—a new immunosuppressive agent. Med. Letter, *25*:77, 1983.

Benacerraf, B.: Role of MHC gene products in immune regulation. Science, *212*:1229, 1981.

Bradley, B., Oliver, R. T. D., Mendell, N., and Stevens, A.: The Primed Lymphocyte (PL) Exchange Histocompatibility Testing 1977. Bodmer, W. F. (ed.). Copenhagen, Munksgaard, 1978, pp. 142–152.

Dausset, J.: The major histocompatibility in man. Science, *213*:1469, 1981.

Heise, G., Johnson, A., Fuller, A., and Ward, F. E. (eds.): Cellular Immunology, 1983. New York, AACHT, 1983.

Snell, G. D.: Studies in histocompatibility. Science, *213*:172, 1981.

Tanigaki, N., and Tosi, R.: The genetic control of human Ia alloantigens: A three-loci model derived from the immunochemical analysis of 'supertypic' specificities. Immunol. Rev., *66*:5, 1982.

Terasaki, P. I., Perdue, S., Sasaki, N., Mickey, M. R., and Whitby, L.: Improving success rates of kidney transplantation. J.A.M.A., *250*:1065, 1983.

Ting, A.: The lymphocytotoxic crossmatch test in clinical renal transplantation. Transplantation, *35*:403, 1983.

Tosi, R., Tanigaki, N., Centis, D., Ferrara, G. B., and Pressman, D.: Immunological dissection of human Ia molecules. J. Exp. Med., *148*:1592, 1978.

HLA and Disease—General

Braun, W. A.: HLA and Disease: A Comprehensive Review. Boca Raton, Fla., CRC Press, Inc., 1979.

Dausset, J., and Svejgaard, A. (eds.): HLA and Disease. Copenhagen, Munksgaard, 1977.

Schaller, J. G., and Hansen, J. A.: HLA relationships to disease. Hosp. Pract., *16*:41, 1981.

Journals of Special Interest

Human Immunology
Immunogenetics
Tissue Antigens
Transplantation
Transplantation Proceedings

THE MHC (MAJOR HISTOCOMPATIBILITY COMPLEX) AND DISEASE

E. J. Yunis, M.D.,
Z. Adweh, Ph.D.,
D. Raum, M.D.,
S. Y. Yang, Ph.D.,
and C. A. Alper, M.D.

THE IMMUNE RESPONSE

The immune system of animals is composed of a number of helper and suppressor functions, working in an integrated fashion to produce a response in the presence of an antigen. The integration of these opposing functions—suppression and help—is responsible for regulating the immunologic balance. The immune response is controlled at several genetic levels, the most important of which is the major histocompatibility complex (MHC). In the mouse and guinea pig, and probably in man, the immune system is regulated by molecules coded by genes within the MHC. These genes are located within the H-2 region of chromosome 17 of the mouse, and within the HLA region of the sixth chromosome in humans (Shreffler, 1975; Klein, 1975, 1978, 1981; Benacerraf, 1977; Yunis, 1981; Amos, 1979).

The products of the histocompatibility genes control antigenic recognition, production of antibodies, lymphocytic proliferation, cytotoxicity, and the suppression of the immune response. Regulation of the immune system is mediated by three types of cells: T lymphocytes and B lymphocytes, and macrophages.

Cellular immunity is based on the function of T cells, whereas humoral immunity results from the differentiation of B cells. The Ia glycoproteins, important molecules which are involved in the control of the immune response, are coded by the MHC. Specifically, in man, the Ia (immune response associated) molecules are encoded by the HLA-D region within the short arm of chromosome 6 and are called HLA-DR (HLA-D related). The macrophage or activated B lymphocyte presents antigens through these HLA-DR molecules to the T or B cells. In the case of T cells, presentation of the antigen is to a T cell subset either of helper cells or of suppressor cells. Such interactions may produce cellular immunity (cytotoxic effectors or delayed hypersensitivity reactions) and/or antibody response.

"Class I" molecules are coded by three loci of chromosome 6, the HLA-A, B, C regions which are expressed on most nucleated cells of the body and also on platelets. Molecules of "Class II" are the Ia molecules and expressed on macrophages, on B lymphocytes, and on activated T lymphocytes, but not on resting T lymphocytes. Other molecules encoded by the MHC include proteins of the complement cascade (C2, C4, and factor B) and GLO-I (Fig. 33–9). Interaction of macrophages and B cells produces specific antibodies expressed in five types of immunoglobulin: IgG, IgM, IgA, IgD, and IgE. B and T cells can be identified in both the lymphoid organs of man and animals and in the peripheral blood (55 to 75 per cent T lymphocytes, 15 to 20 per cent B lymphocytes, and 5 to 30 per cent null cells and monocytes).

Two main types of T cells circulate in the blood. These are identifiable according to the presence of certain antigens, which can be recognized by monoclonal antibodies. T4 or Leu3 antigens characterize helper cells, and are found on 60 to 70 per cent of the T lymphocytes in blood and in most thymocytes. T8 or Leu4 antigens identify suppressor and cytotoxic cells, which constitute 30 per cent of peripheral blood T cells. Regulation of the latter cell types is affected in many autoimmune diseases. For instance, a T8 cell disorder is found in some individuals with systemic lupus erythematosus (Rheinherz, 1980).

The main function of the T cell subsets in the immune response to antigens is restricted by the products of the MHC: the helper cells proliferate in the presence of Class II histocompatibility antigens as compared with the cytotoxic T lymphocytes whose targets are primarily Class I histocompatibility restricted.

Immune imbalance may be important in the pathogenesis of certain diseases, including lupus erythematosus, rheumatoid arthritis, multiple sclerosis, Addison's disease, and Kaposi's sarcoma, all of which have demonstrable immunological manifestations (Yunis, 1981; Amos, 1979; Raum, 1981). Diseases characterized by immunological imbalances or distur-

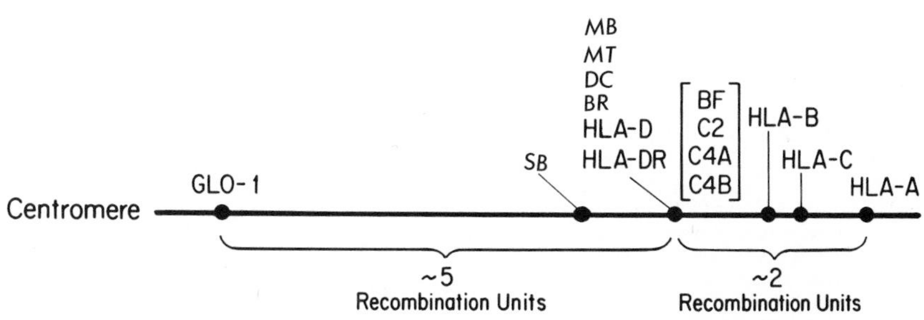

Figure 33–9. Genetic mapping of the midportion of the short arm of chromosome 6.

bances of immune regulation, as well as many others without known immunological abnormalities (e.g., idiopathic hemochromatosis, ankylosing spondylitis), have been described as diseases with a genetic component which involves the MHC. Therefore, the alleles of MHC origin are important not only in studies of the control of the immune responses, but also of abnormalities of the immune responses associated with diseases.

The following discussion will consider only the association or linkage of diseases to the MHC. It will not deal with other genetic systems that control the immune responses or with other markers for disease susceptibility, such as those of the immunoglobulins.

GENETICS OF THE MAJOR HISTOCOMPATIBILITY COMPLEX (MHC)

The MHC on Chromosome 6—Chromosomal Locations of GLO and PGM3. GLO and PGM3 are two enzymes, the genes for which are important markers of human chromosome 6. PGM3 (phosphoglucomutase 3) is an intracellular enzyme, usually studied in leukocytes, which is important in anaerobic glucose metabolism. (It translocates a phosphate group from the carbon 1 to the carbon 6 position of glucose.) GLO-I (glyoxalase I) is an intracellular enzyme usually studied in erythrocytes which catalyzes the conversion of methylglyoxal and glutathione to S-lactoyl-glutathione.

Chromosome 6 is thought to be about 150 centimorgans long. The HLA loci were assigned to this chromosome on the basis of study of a family in which the long and short arms of the chromosome were inverted about its centromere. The loci were also so assigned by study of cultures of fibroblasts containing a balanced reciprocal translocation between the short arms of chromosome 1 and chromosome 6 fused with an established line of Chinese hamster cells, and by the study of chromosome 6 in teratomas. Linkage of HLA and PGM3 has been established by family studies. The locus for glyoxalase I (GLO) is also linked to the MHC. GLO is probably located beyond HLA-D, about 10 centimorgans from HLA-B. PGM3 is about 15 centimorgans from HLA-B in males, while the recombination rate in females is 3.6 times that of males. The distance between the HLA-A and HLA-B loci is thought to be about 1 centimorgan, while there is less than 1 centimorgan between HLA-B and HLA-D. In further studies of the order of genes, the possibility that PGM3 is on the HLA-A side of the HLA complex has been proposed (Raum, 1981; Francke, 1977; Lamm, 1971, 1974; Ott, 1976; Jongsma, 1973; Bender, 1976; Reinsmoen, 1977).

Chromosomal Positions of C2, BF, C4A, and C4B.* These proteins of the complement system areencoded in chromosome 6 by four genes (Fig. 33–10). The structural locus for BF is closely linked to HLA in man. In the initial family studies, no crossovers were observed; however, subsequent studies have identified some HLA-BF crossovers. The structural locus for C2, including a deficient allele, is also known to be linked to the HLA region. No crossover has yet been observed between *C2* and *BF*. These two loci—*C2* and *BF*—are thought to be products of a tandem gene duplication. This view is also supported by family studies and by partial amino acid sequence analysis of these proteins; purified C2 has an amino acid composition very similar to that of B. Close linkage has been confirmed in the mouse for H-2-BF and H-2-GLO, in the guinea pig for C2-C4-BF-GPLA, in the rhesus monkey for RhLA-BF, and in the chimpanzee for ChLA-BF-C2. Mouse C4 is known to be polymorphic and identical with Ss, and coded within the H-2. The S region in the mouse has been precisely located between the H-2I-C and H-2D regions. It is also known that there are two loci in the H-2S region: Ss, which codes for functional C4, and another locus, Slp, which codes for a C4-like molecule that does not possess C4 hemolytic activity. Structural polymorphism has been detected in mouse Ss. There is also structural polymorphism in Slp. Genetic polymorphism of C4-binding protein has been described in the mouse and is also H-2 linked. (References for this section are listed in Raum [1981].)

The linkage of the C4 loci to HLA was inferred from the study of C4 deficient families. However, C4 deficiency in the heterozygote is difficult to detect. The two C4 loci are closely linked to HLA and produce the "red blood cell" antigens, Rodgers and Chido. After desialation and cross-immunoelectrophoresis, half-null haplotypes for C4 can be identified. Immunofixation electrophoresis with anti-C4 of desialated samples reveals extensive polymorphism of C4A and C4B. There were six confirmed crossovers between HLA-A and HLA-B or HLA-A and HLA-C. In each case, C2, C4A, C4B, BF, and GLO segregated with HLA-B, D and DR. There were five HLA-B, HLA-D/DR crossovers, and in each case C2, C4A, C4B, BF, and GLO segregated with HLA-D/DR rather than with HLA-B. Other studies have described the mapping of these genes between HLA-B and D/DR. The finding of C2-deficient homozygotes who are heterozygous for HLA-DR but HLA-B18 homozygous also argues for the location of complement loci between HLA-B and HLA-DR.

Although C2, C4A, C4B, and BF are all polymorphic and alleles are expressed as co-dominant traits, the C2 is the least informative and the C4 loci (A and B) are the most informative (Figs. 33–10 and 33–11). The identification of the C4 haplotypes or complotypes (see below) will require family studies.

The Complotypes.* The loci for complement proteins C2 and BF and the two loci for C4 are closely linked to one another. In many informative meioses no crossover has been detected between these four loci, suggesting that specific BF, C2, C4A, and C4B haplotypes are inherited as single genetic units. In addition, the alleles of these four loci in populations

*The nomenclature for genetic polymorphism of factor B, C2, and the duplicated loci for C4, C4A, and C4B conforms with the International System for Human Gene Nomenclature. Null alleles and null variants are designated "QO." Specific BF, C2, C4A, and C4B alleles form haplotypes (complotypes) that are inherited as gametic units. Complotypes are given in arbitrary order as BF, C2, C4A–C4B types. Thus SC01 represents *BF*S, C2*C, C4A*QO, C4B*1*.

*See previous footnote.

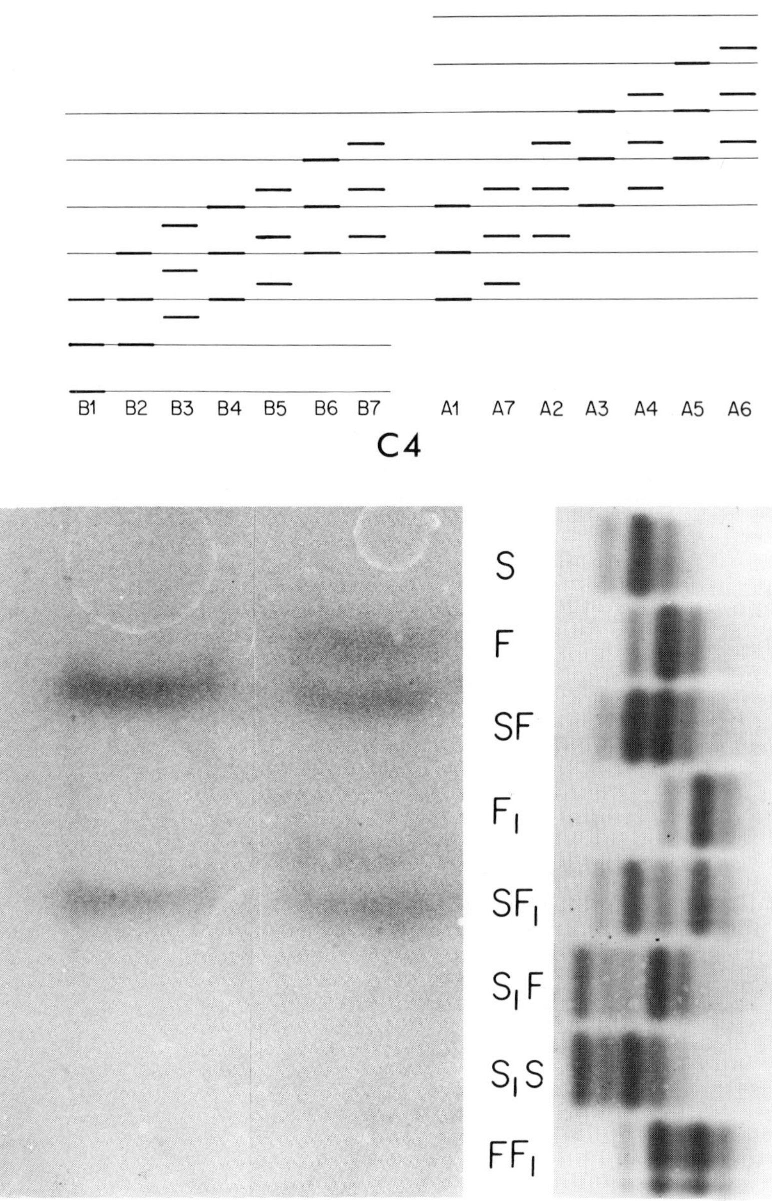

Figure 33–10. Electrophoresis positions of C4 variants relative to one another (diagram). The variants at the C4B (Chido) locus are shown at the left and those at the C4A (Rodgers) locus are shown at the right. Each gene product consists of three bands. It will be noted that some of the C4B variants correspond closely in position to C4A variants (B7 and A2, for example). The distinction between them is made by use of a C4 sensitive overlay agarose gel in which only C4B variants have appreciable C4 hemolytic activity (Awdeh, 1980). The BQO and AQO (null genes) show no bands.

In the lower portion (left side) of the figure, examples of the common C2 type (C) and a heterozygote BC are shown using isoelectric focusing in polyacrylamide gel using agarose gel overlay, containing antibody-sensitized sheep erythrocytes and a 1/90 dilution of normal human serum (Alper, 1976).

In the lower portion (right side) of the figure, examples are shown of electrophoretic patterns of BF variants after agarose gel electrophoresis and immunofixation with anti BF antisera. Each gene product consists of one main band and two minor ones. The anode was at the right.

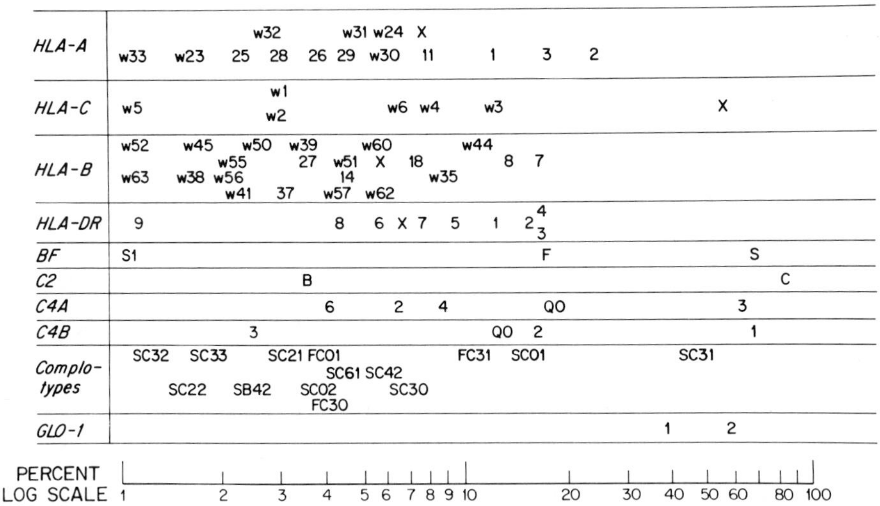

HLA-A	w33 w23 25 w32 28 26 29 w31 w30 w24 11 X 1 3 2
HLA-C	w5 w1 w2 w6 w4 w3 X
HLA-B	w52 w63 w45 w38 w55 w56 w50 w41 w39 37 27 w51 14 w57 w60 X w62 18 w35 w44 8 7
HLA-DR	9 8 6 X 7 5 1 2 4 3
BF	S1 F S
C2	B C
C4A	6 2 4 QO 3
C4B	3 QO 2 1
Complo-types	SC32 SC22 SC33 SB42 SC21 FC01 SC02 FC30 SC61 SC42 SC30 FC31 SC01 SC31
GLO-1	1 2

PERCENT LOG SCALE 1 2 3 4 5 6 7 8 9 10 20 30 40 50 60 80 100

Figure 33–11. Approximate gene frequencies of alleles of the human MHC among Caucasians of Boston, Massachusetts.

occur in much the same manner as alleles of the Rh and MNS systems, in specific combinations not predicted by their gene frequencies. These units are termed "complotypes." We have found 14 complotypes with frequencies in excess of 1 per cent (Table 33–4) in normal Caucasian families. Although no recombinations have been observed among the different complement loci and HLA-DR, it is predicted that when such recombinations are found, they will serve to map the order of complement loci (Alper, 1983).

Extended Haplotypes—Linkage Disequilibrium and the MHC. In certain populations, alleles of MHC genes occur in association with certain other alleles more frequently than expected from the allele frequencies alone. Family studies have suggested that they occur together on the same chromosome and are therefore inherited together (Alper, 1982, 1983; Awdeh, 1983). Otherwise stated, alleles in linkage disequilibrium occur on the same chromosome with a frequency different from that predicted by their overall gene frequencies. Linkage disequilibrium can be introduced by intermixture of two populations with initially different gene frequencies or may have originated by inbreeding, random drift, or sampling bias. However, at the chromosomal distances separating HLA-A, B and D, DR, it is unlikely that any of these mechanisms could have operated on a given pair for more than several thousand years; hence, they are not plausible explanations for most of the linkage disequilibria observed in the major ethnic groups of man. Table 33–5 lists some of the pairs of alleles which are non-randomly associated (Alper, 1982). It will be noted that most of these pairs share common alleles; for example, HLA-A1, B8 and HLA-B8, DW3/DR3 share HLA-B8.

We have recently observed that non-random association of MHC alleles can also include the complotypes and, in some cases, the GLO alleles. The chromosomal distribution of HLA-A, B, C, and DR and the serum complement protein alleles (complotypes) was studied in normal Caucasian families. Eight combinations were found to occur at frequencies significantly higher than expected (Table 33–6). In such combinations, the variation of HLA-A was limited.

Two mechanisms seem likely to account for long term maintenance of linkage disequilibrium: selection and crossover suppression. Selection, which has often been considered in relation to this problem, has usually been assumed to operate either via immune response genes, which are suspected from animal studies to be located close to HLA-D, DR in man or, alternatively, via interactions of HLA gene products with agents in the environment. Crossover suppression

Table 33–4. COMPLOTYPE FREQUENCIES AND LINKAGE DISEQUILIBRIA AMONG 623 RANDOM NORMAL CHROMOSOMES FROM CAUCASIANS*

Complotype	Frequency
SC31	0.43
SC01	0.127
FC31	0.096
SC30	0.053
SC42	0.040
SC61	0.034
FC30	0.031
FC01	0.029
SC02	0.029
SC21	0.022
SB42	0.019
SC33	0.014
SC22	0.013
SC32	0.011

*Complotypes are given as abbreviated letters and numbers in arbitrary order: BF, C2, C4A, and C4B.

Table 33–5. HAPLOTYPE PAIRS IN LINKAGE DISEQUILIBRIUM*

Haplotype	Δ/1000†	HF/1000‡	Haplotype	Δ/1000	HF/1000
A2,B12	27.2	64.5	B12,DR7	26.7	41.3
A1,B8	57.2	64.1	B8,DR3	62.3	70.1
A29,B12	27.3	33.1	B12,DW2	18.4	30.3
A3,B7	18.5	28.3	B7,DR2	37.6	46.2
A1,B17	16.0	22.4	B17,DR7	22.8	29.4
A1,B5	13.7	20.6			
AW23,B12	17.6	19.3	B12,DW4	15.3	22.6
AW30,B18	16.6	17.0	B18,DR3	12.9	18.2

*Data from Bodmer, W. F., and Bodmer, J. G.: Br. Med. Bull., *34*:309, 1978.
†Δ = observed haplotype (PQ) frequency − (frequency of P × frequency of Q).
‡HF = haplotype frequency.

that selectively affects that region of the sixth human chromosome which includes the major histocompatibility complex could also maintain linkage disequilibrium. Thus, if on certain sixth chromosomes, crossing over at meiosis in this region occurred at a substantially lower rate than on other sixth chromosomes, the HLA and other MHC alleles of these chromosomes would remain together through more generations than predicted from the general crossover rate. The mouse T/t locus appears to provide examples both of selective crossover suppression and of selection at the gametic level, the apparent result of non-mendelian inheritance (i.e., male transmission bias) with non-random association of alleles. Likewise, one human 6p haplotype, HLA-B8, DR3, SCO1, GLO2, was found to be transmitted from males to 83 per cent of their offspring. The same haplotype with GLO 1 had no transmission bias. It was suggested that this GLO2-marked chromosome may be a human analogue of a murine t mutant (Awdeh, 1983).

ATTEMPTS TO LOCATE IMMUNE RESPONSE GENES IN MAN

Much of what is known about the genetic control of the immune responses comes from the study in laboratory animals, particularly the mouse and guinea pig, of the antibody response to antigens, such as synthetic polypeptides, with restricted antigenic determinants.

Attempts to study the human antibody response to very similar antigens (polypeptides of three amino acids) have been difficult for several reasons. Many individuals have a delayed skin response to these polymers, even when there has been no known prior exposure. Furthermore, there is no correlation between the skin reaction and the proliferative response of lymphocytes from the same individual on exposure *in vitro* to the polymer. The lymphocytes of nearly all persons who have not been exposed exhibit a proliferative response *in vitro*, but these responses are not correlated with HLA types. In one study of immune responses to synthetic polypeptides, however, subjects could be classified into high, intermediate, and non-responder phenotypes. Family studies indicated that high responses were inherited as a dominant HLA-linked trait.

A more propitious approach examined the antibody response to porcine and bovine insulin, which is known to be under genetic control in mice. In patients with diabetes mellitus, all of whom had been exposed to insulin over a long period, there was an association between high antibody response and HLA-B15, and with lack of response and HLA-B8.

Studies of total IgE level and antibody titers to the minor ragweed allergen, Ra3, in both allergic and non-allergic populations at first appeared to reveal polygenic control. Some authors proposed that high levels of IgE are determined by two recessive alleles. Others found polygenic heritability, with evidence for a major regulatory locus at which a recessive homozygote maintains high levels of IgE. Reanalysis of the data by another method did not confirm this finding, however. Analysis of IgE levels in families suggested heterogeneity among the families. Hence, it appears that inheritance of regulation of IgE basal level is not HLA-linked and may be polygenic. Comprehensive HLA association with such allergic diseases as asthma, hay fever, urticaria, and eczema has been sought, but has not been found. This does not mean, however, that HLA-linked genes are not involved in the pathogenesis of these diseases. Allergic diseases seem to be natural candidates for association with "susceptibility genes." Immune response studies with purified aeroantigens, such as ragweed antigen E, Ra3, and Ra5, have included a population study of IgE response to the low-molecular-weight allergen, Ra5, in which an association with HLA-B7 cross-reacting groups was shown. A significant positive association was found between Ra3 response and total serum IgE and the presence of A2 and A28, with negative association with A3 and A11. The individuals studied were all highly allergic, clinically, to ragweed, grass pollens, or both. Nevertheless, these findings were not con-

Table 33–6. EXTENDED HAPLOTYPES

Haplotype	Frequency
B8,DR3, SC01	0.093
B7,DR2,SC31	0.059
B12,DR7,FC31	0.037
B17,DR7,SC61	0.034
B12,DR4,SC30	0.028
B14,DR1,SC22	0.011
B40,DRw6,SC02	0.011
B15,DR4,SC33	0.009

5

firmed by other investigators. There appeared to be an association of ragweed hay fever, intense skin reactivity to antigen E, and HLA haplotypes in some families with ragweed hay fever. Two other families showed linkage of HLA haplotype and sensitivity to antigen E. Other factors may be influential (e.g., environmental factors or epistatic interaction of other genes). No linkage with HLA was found in other families. Hence, it appears that there may be a gene for ragweed sensitivity linked to HLA in some families, while IgE levels are controlled by a second, non-HLA-linked locus (or loci). In other reports, atopic patients showed an association to HLA-DR2. It appears that this association prognosticates response to allergen immunotherapy. No linkage studies of Ra5 responses to HLA have been documented, however.

The response to streptokinase/streptodornase of human lymphocytes revealed a significant association with HLA-B5, and there was also an association between HLA-Cw3 and a low *in vitro* response to vaccinia virus. Reports of the antigen-specific T cell proliferative response *in vitro* to streptococcal cell wall antigen and to schistosomal antigen demonstrated that low response was dominant, and that low response to schistosomal antigen is associated with the HLA haplotype HLA-Bw52, Dw12, DR2 in Japanese. Also, that the expression of low responsiveness was controlled by an immune suppressor gene Is-Scw (streptococcal cell wall antigen), which is HLA-linked and controls the generation of antigen-specific suppressor T cells (Sasazuki, 1981).

A highly significant ($P<0.0001$) association was noted between HLA-DR3 and the presence of antibodies to native DNA, not only in patients with systemic lupus erythematosus but also in non-lupus individuals. HLA-DR3 and anti-DNA antibody may distinguish a clinical subgroup of systemic lupus erythematosus from another subgroup with HLA-DR2 and anti-SM antibody. Japanese patients with high titers of anti-DNA antibody showed a strong association with HLA-Bw35, although SLE patients as a whole do not.

The HLA markers have been useful in the investigation of virus-host interactions in two general ways: (1) restriction phenomenon by allele modification and (2) the study of the genetics of the immune response. For example, HLA restriction was found in the target-effector cell lysis of influenza virus–infected cells. On the other hand, in studies of both monozygotic and dizygotic twins, the antibody response to measles vaccine and diphtheria toxoid correlated directly with the number of shared HLA haplotypes. The antibody response to a live, attenuated intranasal influenza A vaccine was poorest in HLA-Bw16 individuals. On intramuscular injection of an influenza vaccine, however, no association between antibody response and HLA-Bw16 was noted, but the antibody response *in vitro* was lowest in carriers of HLA-Bw35. Among Japanese, there was a possible association between HLA-B15 and a high antibody response to rubella virus, as well as between B5 and Bw22 and a low response. The same study revealed an increased HLA-B15 and a decreased Bw22 among mothers of babies with congenital rubella syndrome.

More important for this discussion is the fact that IgA deficiency (it occurs in about one in 700 apparently healthy blood donors) was associated with B8 and DR3. Recently, also, an association between HLA-B8 and immunization against the platelet specific antigen, Zw^a, was found. (For references for this section, see Raum [1981] and Svejgaard [1983].)

Possible associations of the HLA system with adverse reactions to drugs have seldom been explored. Recently, however, gold and D-penicillamine nephropathy have been associated with HLA-B8 and HLA-DR3 and hydralazine SLE with HLA-DR4 (Svejgaard, 1983), thus suggesting that HLA plays an important role in drug-induced autoimmune disease. Also, the frequency of HLA-Bw44 was significantly increased among psychiatric patients who developed autoantibodies after chronic treatment with chlorpromazine (Canoso, 1982).

MHC AND DISEASE

Methods of Detecting Association or Linkage of Disease with Genetic Markers

The Strength of an Association. Several methods have been devised for detecting the degree of association of genetic markers to hypothesized genes for disease susceptibility. One is to compute the risk of disease among individuals carrying a specific allele of a polymorphic system (Yunis, 1981; Amos, 1979; Svejgaard, 1983). Here, relative risk (RR) calculates the risk of carrying a marker in a population of diseased individuals compared with a control population. More interesting is an estimate of the risk of having disease in an individual carrying the marker (Tables 33–7 and 33–8).

This strength of association is the δ of Bergston and Thomson (Svejgaard, 1983), which is the same as the etiologic fraction (EF) of Miettinen (1976).

$$\text{Relative risk RR} = \frac{a \times d}{b \times c}$$

$$\text{Etiologic fraction EF} = \left(\frac{RR - 1}{RR}\right)\left(\frac{a}{a + b}\right)$$

$$= \left(\frac{RR - 1}{RR}\right)(hp)$$

	NUMBER OF INDIVIDUALS	
	Character Positive	*Character Negative*
Patients	a	b
Control	c	d

Frequency of character in patients (hp)

$$hp = \frac{a}{a + b}$$

Similarly, in decreased risks, for which the RR is less than 1, the PF (preventive factor) can be used.

$$PF = \frac{(1 - RR)(hp)}{RR(1 - hp) + hp}$$

Table 33–7. EXAMPLES OF ASSOCIATION BETWEEN HLA AND DISEASE

Disease	HLA Antigen	Relative Risk (RR)*	Etiologic Fraction (EF)†
Arthropathies			
Ankylosing spondylitis	B27	87.4	0.89
Reiter's syndrome	B27	37.0	0.77
Rheumatoid arthritis	DR4	4.2	0.38
Endocrine diseases			
Juvenile and/or insulin-dependent diabetes	D/DR3	3.3	0.39
	D/DR4	6.4	0.63
	D/DR2	0.2	
Graves' disease	D/DR3	3.7	0.42
Idiopathic Addison's disease	D/DR3	6.3	0.58
Eye diseases			
Acute anterior uveitis	B27	10.4	0.47
Optic neuritis	D/DR2	2.4	0.27
Inflammatory disease			
Subacute thyroiditis	B35	13.7	0.65
Intestinal disease			
Celiac disease	D/DR3	10.8	0.72
Liver disease			
Chronic autoimmune hepatitis	B8	9.0	
Neurological disease			
Multiple sclerosis	D/DR2	4.1	0.45
Skin diseases			
Psoriasis vulgaris	Cw6	13.3	0.81
Pemphigus (Jews)	D/DR4	14.4	0.81
Dermatitis herpetiformis	D/DR3	15.4	0.80
Behçet's disease	B5	6.3	0.34
Systemic diseases			
Myasthenia gravis	D/DR3	2.5	0.30
	B8	2.7	0.30
Sicca syndrome	D/DR3	9.7	0.70
Systemic lupus erythematosus	D/DR3	5.8	0.58
Idiopathic hemochromatosis	A3	8.2	0.67
	B14	4.7	0.13
Goodpasture's syndrome	D/DR2	15.9	0.82
Idiopathic membranous nephropathy	D/DR3	12.0	0.69

*RR = relative risk. Calculated by $\frac{a \times d}{b \times c}$, where a and b are the number of individuals with character present or absent in the patients and c and d the characters present or absent in the control population.

†EF = etiologic fraction $= \frac{(RR-1)}{(RR)} \frac{(a)}{(a+b)} = \frac{(RR-1)}{(RR)} (hp)$

Table 33–8. RISKS (RR)* FOR MHC ALLELES IN SEVERAL DISEASES

5

Disease	HLA-A Allele	HLA-A RR	HLA-B Allele	HLA-B RR	HLA-DR Allele	HLA-DR RR	BF Allele	BF RR
Juvenile onset insulin-dependent	A1	1.6	B8	2.5	DR3	4.5		
diabetes mellitus			B15	2.5	DR4	4.5		
			B18	2.5			BFF1	8
			B7	0.1				
			B7	0.1	DR2	0.1		
Multiple sclerosis	A3	1.8	B7	2.5	DR2	4.2		
Gluten enteropathy	A1	1.8	B8	8.0	DR3	17		
Chronic active hepatitis	A1	1.7	B8	3.0	DR3	2.2		
Idiopathic membranous			B8	2.3	DR3	4.4		
glomerulonephritis			B18	2.3			BFF1	16
Idiopathic hemochromatosis	A3	4.8	B7	1.9			BFF	2.0
	A1	2.0	B14	4.9	DRW6	3.1		
			B15	3.5	DR4	2.9		

$$*RR = \frac{\text{patients with marker}}{\text{patients without marker}} \times \frac{\text{controls without marker}}{\text{controls with marker}}$$

The EF and PF fractions can vary between 0 (no association) and 1.0 (maximal association).

Sib Pair Analysis. This method was introduced to overcome the problems of incomplete penetrance of diseases and variations in age of onset. The method is based on the assumption that if HLA and/or genes closely linked to HLA have no influence on the development of a disease, then the affected sib pairs will share HLA haplotypes with a normal frequency: 25 per cent will share both, 50 per cent will share one, and 25 per cent will share no haplotypes. Thus, observed and expected distributions of haplotype sharing are compared (Penrose, 1935; Thomson, 1977). Once the mode of inheritance has been established, the "disease" gene frequency and penetrance can be established (Thomson, 1977).

Analysis of Mode of Inheritance Based on Population Studies. Thomson and Bodmer (1979) have devised a method for analyzing population data for markers closely linked to susceptibility loci for diseases with incomplete penetrance. In essence, this method predicts the proportion of homozygotes, heterozygotes, and non-carriers for the linked marker expected in the cases of dominant and of recessive inheritance. The greatest difference between the two modes of inheritance is obtained in the proportion of individuals who are homozygotes for the marker. Application of this method to HLA-B27 and ankylosing spondylitis led on statistical grounds to rejection of a recessive mechanism. Thus, it was concluded that susceptibility to ankylosing spondylitis is inherited as a dominant trait.

We have applied the same method of analysis to the distribution of *BF*F1* among 1107 patients with insulin-dependent diabetes mellitus (IDDM). For dominant inheritance 1.89 homozygotes were predicted, and for recessive inheritance 6.2. Seven *BF*F1* homozygotes were found, a result consistent only with recessive inheritance. Other modes of inheritance that could be rejected by these observations include simple dominant, epistatic (disease resulting from the presence of non-allelic genes), or overdominant (disease with greater penetrance when two specific alleles are present than when other combinations, including homozygosity for each of the specific alleles, occur). Although a mixed model with different penetrances for homozygotes and heterozygotes could not be completely ruled out, other considerations make such a model unsatisfactory. In particular, the IDDM susceptibility gene would have to be at some appreciable distance (more than 2 cM) from the BF locus: IDDM is known to be an ancient disease, and it is difficult to imagine linkage disequilibrium being preserved for any significant number of generations at this distance.

Lod Score Method. This is a statistical measure of linkage: (1) The Z value is the ratio of the maximum likelihood of finding linkage (less than 0.5) to that of no linkage (0.5) at a particular recombination value; and (2) the θ value or recombination frequency which is a measure of distance from a given locus corresponding to maximum Z value. The lod score expresses the probability that alleles at two loci will segregate together, in terms of the ratio between the observed recombination frequency θ, and 0.50, the recombination frequency for alleles which assort independently. Various values of θ from 0 to 0.5 are substituted in the equation

$$P(F_1/\theta) = 1/2\,[\theta^r(1-\theta)^{n-r} + \theta^{n-r}(1-\theta)^r]$$

where n = the number of children and r = the number of recombinants. The probability of obtaining a pedigree for a given value of θ is expressed as the ratio of $P(F_1/\theta)$ to $P(F_1/0.5)$ and then converted to the lod score (z) where

$$z = \log \frac{P(F_1/\theta)}{P(F_1/\theta = 0.5)}$$

and Z = Σ of all z. Values of z greater than zero favor linkage and those less than zero are against linkage. In general, a Z value greater than 3 (for some values of θ less than 0.5) means that the odds in favor of linkage are 1000 to 1 (probability 1/1000, as opposed to no linkage or independence). It is easier to calculate linkage for codominant traits, i.e., HLA and GLO, than for recessive traits. In studies of linkage of HLA and disease, the parents may have recessive susceptibility or a dominantly expressed impenetrant susceptibility gene. In such cases, the presence of the disease in the children may determine the likelihood of transmission by the father or mother (dominant) or both (recessive) (Sutton, 1980).

The Disease Susceptibility Gene as a Marker for MHC

C2 Deficiency. C2 deficiency is perhaps the most common complement deficiency in Caucasians. The normal range of serum levels of C2 (mean ± 2 SD) is narrow enough that half-normal levels lie outside the normal range. This has made possible the detection of heterozygous C2-deficient individuals. The incidence of C2 deficiency in the general Caucasian population approaches one homozygous deficient individual per 10,000 blood donors. In another study, 1.2 per cent of random individuals were found to be heterozygous C2 deficient. First discovered in healthy individuals, homozygous C2 deficiency was later described in association with systemic lupus erythematosus, Henoch-Schönlein purpura, and polymyositis.

C2 deficiency is due to a null allele at the structural locus. This deficiency has been found in association with the HLA haplotype HLA-A25, HLA-B18, HLA-DR2 and closely linked to HLA-DR in family studies. The deficiency allele (*C2*QO*) is almost always part of the complotype BFS, C2QO, C4A4, C4B2 (Raum, 1981).

C4 Deficiency. Genetic analysis of C4 polymorphism in the family of a child with homozygous C4 deficiency demonstrated that several family members, including the child's parents, carried a C4 haplotype, *C4A*QO, C4B*QO*, which produced no detectable protein at either the Chido (C4B) or Rodgers (C4A) locus and that the C4 deficiency was linked to HLA.

Numerous observations have been made of associations between inherited complement component deficiency states and immunological diseases. Whether this association is causative or fortuitous is not clear, however. Many patients with rheumatic disease have been screened for complement abnormalities, in part because acquired abnormalities of complement are used to diagnose and monitor some of these disease states. Whereas patients with homozygous deficiency states are rare, those with heterozygous states are necessarily much more common. For C2 deficiency, the incidence predicted in the general population, from homozygous deficiency and from screening random blood donors for heterozygous deficiency, is about one in 50 to one in 100. If this is correct, then systemic lupus erythematosus (SLE) occurs two to three times more frequently among heterozygous C2-deficient individuals than in the normal population. In 38 reported homozygous C2-deficient individuals, 23 had autoimmune diseases and 14 of these had SLE or discoid lupus. Nearly one third had no illness, however. Whether the predisposition to lupus in C2-deficient individuals is secondary to an abnormal function of the complement system is not clear. Partial resolution of this problem awaits complete MHC typing of individuals with immune complex disease who are heterozygous for C2 or C4 deficiency. While C2 deficiency per se may be instrumental in the development of SLE or of immune complex disease in patients homozygous for these deficits, homozygous C2-deficient relatives of propositi have a lower incidence of autoimmune disease. Additionally, several patients with C1 inhibitor deficiency have also been reported to have systemic or discoid lupus erythematosus, and all four patients with reported homozygous C4 deficiency have had lupus or a lupus-like syndrome (Raum, 1981).

21-Hydroxylase Deficiency. One form of congenital adrenal hyperplasia results from a deficiency or a dysfunctional allele for 21-hydroxylase, an enzyme of cortisol metabolism. Deficiency of the enzyme results in virilization, or virilization and salt-wasting. In family studies, these syndromes have been shown to be inherited as simple autosomal recessive traits linked to the MHC. Attempts to localize the 21-OH gene have been inconclusive; however, the disease was found to be associated with the extended haplotype HLA-Bw47, DR7 and the complotype FCO, 31 (Dupont, 1980; Fleishnick, 1983).

HLA-Linked Diseases—The Disease Susceptibility Gene as One Marker of a Polygenic Disease

There are diseases in which at least one important genetic factor is HLA linked. Disorders such as multiple sclerosis, juvenile diabetes mellitus, Graves' disease, psoriasis, and celiac disease, for example, have previously been known to have a major genetic component, and now it is recognized that one of the genetic factors in each of these diseases is HLA linked. In some diseases the HLA-region has served as a genetic marker for recessive or dominantly inherited disease susceptibility genes.

At present, dominantly inherited diseases have been studied in which genetic linkage to HLA has either been suggested (Paget's disease of the bone and hereditary hemorrhagic telangiectasia [Osler-Weber-Rendu disease]) or established (spinocerebellar ataxia and ankylosing spondylitis).

Another disease which has been studied for linkage to HLA is idiopathic hemochromatosis. In the past, this condition was thought to be inherited as an autosomal dominant trait, with incomplete penetrance in females because of excessive loss of blood during menstruation and pregnancy. Now, however, it is established that the disease is inherited as an autosomal recessive trait. Studies of linkage to HLA, in families with this disorder, indicate that two HLA-linked genes are probably involved in development of the disease but that the disease might be a simple autosomal recessive trait, with the disease gene located 10 to 15 centimorgans outside the HLA complex. In either case, the studies demonstrate that a gene or genes of importance in iron metabolism are located close to the HLA complex. It has also been shown that in idiopathic hemochromatosis the disease gene is in genetic linkage disequilibrium with the HLA determinants A3 and B14 (Amos, 1977; Cartwright, 1979).

Genetic studies in patients with juvenile insulin-dependent diabetes mellitus (IDDM) have been controversial for many years, but the use of HLA as a genetic marker system in this disease has provided new insights into the genetic factors involved. Linkage analysis of IDDM is complicated by problems of variability in age of onset and the degree of genetic penetrance. Some studies suggested that IDDM is a recessively inherited disease with 50 per cent penetrance. Data consistent with recessive inheritance and inconsistent with dominant inheritance were obtained by analyzing BF types in more than 1000 IDDM patients (Raum, 1981).

During the Eighth International Workshop, the HLA haplotype sharing observed among affected sib pairs showed that susceptibility to IDDM cannot be dominant (with incomplete penetrance). These studies also questioned the recessive model of inheritance (with incomplete penetrance) because the frequency of the susceptibility gene consistent with the data would be so high as to be associated with a penetrance too low to be consistent with the known frequency of IDDM among all siblings of IDDM propositi. An intermediate model has been suggested which assumes a gene dose effect such that there is higher penetrance for those individuals who are homozygous for susceptibility. However, the higher incidence of diabetes in HLA-DR3/DR4 heterozygotes than in DR3 or DR4 homozygotes questions the power of that interpretation to serve as the sole model for explaining the genetics of IDDM (Terasaki, 1980).

MHC and Disease Association

The majority of studies of HLA and disease have been performed on a population basis, involving diseases that generally do not occur in several members of a family. A detailed description of these conditions has been given (Ryder, 1979). A summary is presented in Table 33–7. Most of the studies are, therefore, reports of HLA and disease associations based on comparisons of phenotype frequencies in a patient group and a normal control population. The majority of the RR (relative risk) factors for HLA and disease range from 3 to 15. For example, a relative risk of 5.5 for HLA-B8 positive individuals for developing a particular disease would indicate that such a person has a 5.5-fold higher risk for developing that disease than does a HLA-B8 negative individual. Genetic markers of MHC-associated disease and other HLA associations not listed in Table 33–7 are discussed below and have been referenced previously (Raum, 1981).

Rheumatoid arthritis (RA) with onset in adulthood differs clinically from juvenile rheumatoid arthritis (JRA). In recent years, attempts have been made to classify JRA into several distinct syndromes based on the mode of onset. Three main groups are (a) systemic with daily intermittent fever, (b) polyarticular arthritis, and (c) pauciarticular. The pauciarticular group is further subdivided into (1) persistent pauciarticular, (2) conversion to polyarticular, (1a) males with onset over the age of eight, and (1b) a form with iritis. The soundness of this clinical classification has been borne out by studies of HLA associations and by long-term follow-up. It has been shown that HLA-DR4 is strongly associated with RA in white adults (relative risk [RR] = 6), whereas relative to controls this antigen is not increased in JRA patients. Furthermore, other HLA-D and HLA-DR associations vary with clinical grouping within the JRA population: male JRA patients with onset after eight years have a markedly increased incidence of HLA-B27. Early-onset pauciarticular JRA and iritis are associated with HLA-DR5. Two other diseases (renal carcinoma and acquired immunodeficiency syndrome [AIDS]) have also been found to be associated with HLA-DR5. The systemic form of JRA is particularly suspect of viral origin because of clinical manifestations such as high fever and rash. Recently, a mathematical model has been developed on the assumption that the JRA susceptibility gene is inherited in a dominant fashion. From the study of four families, it was concluded that the postulated gene is very near the MHC.

A study of complotypes in 45 JRA patients with early onset of pauciarticular disease revealed an increased frequency of C4A*3, B*1, BF*S and of a unique haplotype, C4A*3, B*2, BF*S. In 32 patients with onset of pauciarticular disease after eight years of age there was a marked increase in C4A*4, B*2, BF*S. Among 15 patients with later onset of polyarticular JRA, the frequency of C4A*QO, B*1, BF*S was 33 per cent compared with 10 per cent in normals. This was also increased (29 per cent) in 14 patients with sudden onset of JRA in whom a unique complotype, C4A*4, B*1, BF*S, occurred with a frequency of 7 per cent.

Systemic lupus erythematosus (SLE) is also a heterogeneous disorder with protean manifestations. From the clinical point of view, the most striking difference among patients is that some are barely affected while others are severely affected, developing dermatitis, glomerulonephritis, or vasculitis. HLA studies of SLE patients as a group reveal a weak association with HLA-B8 and stronger associations with HLA-DW2 (RR = 3.25) and with HLA-DW3 (RR = 2.81).

In New York and Bogota, a novel B cell alloantigen has been found in association with 70 to 75 per cent of rheumatic fever patients, as compared with 17 per cent of controls. Myasthenia gravis has been shown to be mediated by antiacetylcholine receptor antibodies and has been associated with HLA-A1, B8 and DR3 and Gm type 1, 4, 12 in Caucasians but not in Japanese patients.

Celiac disease in Caucasians is strongly associated with DR3 and to a lesser extent with DR7, with a highly significant increase among patients in DR3, 7 heterozygotes. Examination of 13 multiple case families was consistent with recessive inheritance. These data suggest a susceptibility gene frequency of 0.35 and a low penetrance and argue that environmental factors may play a large role in the pathogenesis of celiac disease. Celiac disease is also associated with a gliadin receptor, the occurrence of which does not appear to be HLA-linked.

A number of causes of renal failure are mediated by immunological injury. Antiglomerular basement membrane antibody disease or Goodpasture's syndrome is associated with HLA-DR2; systemic lupus erythematosus with DR2 and DR3; poststreptococcal glomerulonephritis with a unique allele; non-poststreptococcal glomerulonephritis and Henoch-Schönlein purpura with HLA-BW35. Idiopathic membranous glomerulonephritis has been shown to be associated with DR3, BFF1, and MB2 in western Europe and with MT2 in the United States. HLA-DR4 frequencies were increased in 45 patients with IgA nephropathy (49 per cent compared with 20 per cent in controls).

In chronic active hepatitis associated with antinuclear antibodies, anti–smooth muscle antibodies, and antimitochondrial antibodies, there was an association with HLA-A1, B8, DR3, but in patients with HB_sAg (hepatitis B antigen) no HLA association was found. In another well-studied example, among Caucasians with juvenile onset diabetes mellitus (IDDM), there is an increased frequency of HLA-B8, B15, and B18, each with relative risk, or RR, of about 2.5 and a decreased frequency of HLA-B7. In this same group there is an increased incidence of HLA-DW3 and of HLA-DW4 (RR = 4.5), and a markedly increased incidence of the complement marker BFF1 (RR = 7.5) and of several unassigned antisera lacking DR specificity and having low reactivity against T lymphocytes (RR = 6.08, 9.55, 5.55, and 28).

Twenty-four of 106 IDDM white patients in Boston were found to carry the BF*F1 allele, the gene frequency of which is less than 1 per cent. Whereas the RR (relative risk) of BFF1 for prediction of IDDM is higher than that of DR3, the EF (etiologic fraction) is higher for DR3 than BFF1 (0.35 vs. 0.21); but in other diseases the relative risk and etiologic fraction are both high (e.g., in ankylosing spondylitis and psoriasis vulgaris).

The association of BFF1 with IDDM has been confirmed in several other Caucasian populations. Review of these data suggests that differences in *BF*F1* frequency between the populations studied are due to the heterogeneity of IDDM patients as well as to ethnic differences. Further heterogeneity is related to age of onset. Indeed, the data confirmed a difference in HLA-DR associations in patients with onset of IDDM above and below 20 years of age, suggesting that patients with IDDM with onset under 20 years of age form the most homogeneous population so far defined. Further evidence of heterogeneity within IDDM has been reported in several studies. In IDDM with onset under 16 years of age, there is a preponderance of males, whereas in patients with onset over age 40, there is a preponderance of females. Among patients with early onset IDDM, most have islet cell antibodies at diagnosis, but these are usually transient. Another group of patients showed persistent antibodies, female preponderance, and late onset.

An excess of HLA-DR2 homozygotes has been found in tuberculoid leprosy, suggesting that inheritance of susceptibility is recessive; also, there was an excess of identical HLA haplotypes among siblings affected with this disease.

The Association of Disease with Extended Haplotypes

The literature is rich with studies of associations between MHC alleles and a variety of diseases. These have established that certain HLA-A, B, C, D, DR, C2, C4, or BF alleles occur more frequently in patients (i.e., have a significant positive relative risk) than in healthy control populations, whereas other such genes may be reduced in frequency among patients (have negative relative risk). Table 33–6 gives an abbreviated list of such "markers" in a number of diseases. The relative risks of each of these have been assumed, when positive, to provide some information concerning the chromosomal location of postulated MHC-linked susceptibility genes. For most of the diseases studied, the relative risks are highest for HLA-D, DR, or one or more complement genes (Table 33–4). Genes with reduced relative risk are thought to be "protective."

An examination of the data of Tables 33–5 and 33–8 suggests a number of possible extended haplotypes. The most striking set of types that occur together as a marker for disease is HLA-A1, B8, Dw3/DR3. The frequency of this set is increased among patients with, among other conditions, juvenile onset IDDM, gluten enteropathy, Graves' disease, dermatitis herpetiformis, and chronic active hepatitis. An additional candidate is HLA-B18, DW3, DR3, BFF1, found in IDDM and membranous nephropathy. Still another is HLA-A3, B7, DW2/DR2, which is increased in patients with multiple sclerosis but decreased in association with IDDM and gluten enteropathy. Rare combinations in normal populations may also mark extended haplotypes which are difficult to detect in such populations. If a disease susceptibility gene is trapped on more than one extended haplotype in a given population, an increase in the frequency of the MHC markers on those chromosomes can be expected among patients. That effect would explain the observed increases in HLA-B8, B15, B18, and HLA-DR3 and DR4 in Caucasians with IDDM. These associations are strengthened by the presence of two DR3 extended haplotypes associated with IDDM:B8, DR3, SC01 and B18, DR3, F1C30 and one DR4 extended haplotype, B15, DR4, SC33. In addition, one extended haplotype, B7/DR2, SC31, has been found to be protective (Alper, 1982), suggesting the absence of a susceptibility gene on this extended haplotype.

One of the four extended haplotypes associated with IDDM, the B8, DR3, SC01, is found almost exclusively in association with GLO-2. A second example of a disease associated with an extended haplotype and GLO-1 is 21-hydroxylase deficiency (congenital adrenal hyperplasia), in which 13 out of 15 haplotypes HLA-Bw47, DR7, FCO,31 were GLO-1 as compared with a frequency of GLO-1 haplotypes among all normal chromosomes of about 40 per cent.

It is likely that some extended MHC haplotypes arose by mechanisms other than suppression of recombination or male transmission preference. In the case of a rare MHC-linked mutation or allele restricted to one ethnic group, recent origin may be the most likely explanation for an extended haplotype. The C2 deficiency haplotype, HLA-A25, B18, DW2, DR2, BFS, C2QO, C4A4, B2 may be an example of the product of this mechanism (founder effect). Hereditary homozygous C2 deficiency (C2QO/C2QO) has been reported in North American Caucasian and Northern and Central European families only, an observation consistent with recent evolutionary origin as a single mutation on an individual chromosome 6 with that type. Also consistent with this view is that among C2QO-bearing chromosomes about 50 per cent carry HLA-A25, 60 per cent carry HLA-B18, and most, but not all, carry HLA-DW2, DR2. On almost all, C2QO is part of the complotype BFS, C2QO, C4A4, C4B2 (Alper, 1982). While 50 per cent of *C2*QO*-bearing chromosomes carry HLA-A25, the remaining 50 per cent carry a random assortment of HLA-types. The same is true for each of the MHC loci, suggesting that crossover suppression is *not* operating. Other rare extended haplotypes which may also be markers for disease susceptibility are HLA-Aw30, B18, DR3, F1C30 in IDDM, and HLA-A3, Bw47, DR7, FCO,31, GLO1 in 21-hydroxylase deficiency (Alper, 1982; Fleishnick, 1983). In these cases a mutation of recent origin may have been restricted to one ethnic group and the extended haplotype introduced in a new population may carry the disease as a "founder effect."

POSSIBLE MECHANISMS FOR MHC AND DISEASE ASSOCIATION

There are a number of diseases in which specific alleles of various MHC loci occur at higher frequencies in patients than in normal control populations. These associations may have arisen in several ways: inbreeding, population stratification, or linkage. The Fifth International Histocompatibility Workshop in 1972 demonstrated that most antigens of the HLA system vary considerably in frequency at different geographical locations. These results emphasize the necessity of selecting control populations carefully for comparison with the gene frequencies observed in the disease populations. It appears, however, that at least some of the observed associations do represent linkage of a disease susceptibility locus to the MHC or else arise from an interaction of MHC antigens with environmental factors, initiating a pathological process. A number of possible mechanisms for such effects have been suggested, many of which derive from experimental study of the mouse. Because the number of associations already detected is large, it seems probable that more than one of the proposed mechanisms is operative. The traditional mechanisms postulated are as follows:

Altered Self-Antigens. As previously discussed, it appears that T cells demonstrate commitment to the MHC and that H-2 and HLA antigens probably play a role in immune surveillance. Jerne (1971) and Benacerraf (1978) have proposed that functionally mature T cells have low reactivity for autologous MHC antigens and concomitantly high affinity for allogeneic antigens. This model predicts that clones of T cells induced by xenogeneic MHC antigens should be highly cross-reactive with allogeneic MHC antigens, and alloreactive T cells should be highly cross-reactive with modified syngeneic cells. Both predictions have been confirmed, and the reactivities shown to be dependent on the H-2D and H2-K type of the host. Similarly, Zinkernagel and Doherty (1974) have demonstrated that the immune response to virus-infected cells is restricted to cells bearing the same altered H-2D or H2-K molecules. In a family study in man, cytotoxic T cell responses to influenza virus–infected autologous cells *in vitro* showed T cell recognition of influenza virus (by cytotoxicity) which was dependent upon HLA type (McMichael, 1977). This restriction can be demonstrated with isolated HLA antigens reconstituted into phospholipid vesicles (Engelhard, 1980). Accordingly, a factor has been identified in *Klebsiella pneumoniae* culture filtrates which modifies either an HLA-B27 or a closely associated cell surface component (Geczy, 1981). This modified HLA-B27 induces effector cells capable of injuring specific target tissues (e.g., synovia and cartilage) bearing "altered self" determinants. The destruction of appropriate target cells may trigger a complex chain of events leading to ankylosing spondylitis or uveitis. Reactive arthritis may also follow *Yersinia* or *Shigella* infection, but these organisms have not been shown to alter antigen specificities. Among patients with ankylosing spondylitis, reactive arthropathies, and acute anterior uveitis, about 90 per cent of Caucasian patients, as compared with 5 to 10 per cent of healthy controls, have B27. This susceptibility appears to be inherited as a simple dominant trait. The association of B27 with these syndromes in four racial groups (Caucasians, Blacks, Japanese, American Indians) suggests that B27 itself or a gene closely linked to B27 is involved in the pathogenesis of these diseases.

Another example of MHC and disease association which may be explained by some interaction between an HLA antigen and an etiologic agent is gluten-sensitive enteropathy. Organ cultures in patients with active gluten-sensitive enteropathy demonstrated that gluten exerts a toxic effect on intestinal mucosa, inhibiting the epithelial cell maturation. This effect was seen more frequently in HLA-B8 positive patients with active gluten-sensitive enteropathy than in HLA-B8 negative patients (Falchuk, 1980).

Molecular Mimicry. It is postulated that in certain cases HLA gene products may resemble or be closely related in structure to an antigen of an infective agent, hence rendering the system unresponsive because of cross-tolerance. This mechanism has been invoked to explain both the HLA-B27–associated diseases and certain other diseases with strong HLA-B associations: Behçet's disease (HLA-B5) and de Quervain's subacute thyroiditis (HLA-BW35). A number of bacterial antigens have been examined for cross-reactivity with human HLA antigens, but few positive findings have been reported.

Immune Response and Immune Suppression Genes. Such genes, which have been demonstrated in mouse and guinea pig, form the basis for assumptions that at least some HLA-D/DR–associated diseases are due to altered or suppressed immune responses. In keeping with this concept, a number of diseases involving autoimmunity, or suspected to have autoimmune components, have shown a stronger association with HLA-D/DR. Juvenile onset IDDM, Graves' disease, idiopathic Addison's disease, myasthenia gravis, dermatitis herpetiformis, celiac disease, chronic active hepatitis (lupoid type), Sjögren's syndrome, and systemic lupus erythematosus all have a significant association with Dw3 and DR3 in Caucasians. This type of association also seems relevant in multiple sclerosis and tuberculoid leprosy (DR2-associated). The Eighth International Histocompatibility Workshop (1980) has demonstrated IDDM to be associated with DR4 in all populations and with DR3 in most (Terasaki, 1980). Recently, cytotoxic antibodies to beta cells in the serum of patients with IDDM have been demonstrated, though these antibodies were also found in the serum of 25 per cent of first-degree relatives.

Interestingly, in Japanese the haplotype HLA-Bw52, HLA-Dw12, HLA-DR2 is associated with low responses to antigens (streptococcal wall antigen, tetanus toxoid, *Schistosoma japonicum* antigen, and cedar pollen antigen) and with resistance to IDDM and adult rheumatoid arthritis. In contrast, the haplotype Bw54, DYT, DR4 was associated with high immune response to the same antigens and with susceptibility to IDDM and adult rheumatoid arthritis. It has also been suggested that an important mechanism of HLA association is the deficiency of T cell specific suppressor cells which are HLA restricted (Sasazuki, 1981). For example, absence of dominant suppressor genes may result in predisposition to autoimmune diseases.

Receptor. It has been hypothesized that HLA antigens serve as receptors for pathogens. For instance, the Duffy red cell antigen acts as a receptor for malarial parasites and Duffy-negative individuals show correspondingly high resistance to malaria (Miller, 1975); in this case, susceptibility should be dominant. The HLA-A and HLA-B antigens have likewise been identified as receptors for Semliki Forest virus (Helenius, 1978), as well as other viruses.

Accidental. Some diseases show association for defective or absent proteins also coded for in the HLA region. Idiopathic hemochromatosis shows an association with HLA-A3. Partial biochemical expression is seen in heterozygous carriers, though progressive accumulation of iron in the liver occurs only in homozygotes (Amos, 1977; Cartwright, 1979). In a large collaborative study of hemochromatosis, a considerable excess of diseased sibs HLA identical with the proband supported a recessive mode of inheritance of a single gene.

HLA-Linked Genes. Defects in HLA-linked genes related to the complement system might be responsible for some HLA-related disease susceptibilities. Genetic linkage disequilibrium has been used to study chromosome segments as markers for diseases. For example the association of C2 deficiency with the extended haplotype HLA-A25, HLA-B18, HLA-DR2, BFS, C4A4B2.

We have mentioned previously that the C2 deficiency associated with HLA haplotypes probably arose as a recent mutation in the C2 gene and that HLA association is probably the result of population stratification (founder effect). In cases where mutations may occur on an extended haplotype with male transmission preference (Alper, 1982; Awdeh, 1983), we have postulated that it would be likely to function as a genetic sink, accumulating deleterious mutations, including those for some diseases.

HLA as a Marker for Abnormal Differentiation Antigens. Studies of H-2 have revealed a closely linked region which controls differentiation in the mouse (DeWolf, 1979). It is conceivable that certain HLA associations arise by linkage disequilibrium with abnormal alleles of human differentiation genes. For instance, human testicular teratocarcinoma is associated with DW7.

It appears that more than one of the mechanisms just described may play a role in the pathogenesis of different diseases. For example, diseases with high relative risk for alleles of the HLA-B locus may be explained either by the altered self mimicry or by the receptor hypothesis, whereas other diseases may involve HLA-linked genes that are directly or indirectly involved in regulation of the immune response. The finding that the 21-hydroxylase gene of the steroid-hormone pathway is located within HLA also implies that impairment of some non-immunologic regulatory functions might produce HLA-associated disease.

DISCUSSION

It can be seen that MHC disease associations can be conveniently divided into a group due to coincidentally linked genes, for example, enzyme deficiencies for which the biochemical basis is not understood, and a group arising from abnormalities in immune recognition or regulation (Amos, 1979; Sasazuki, 1981). Some of the latter may be due to abnormalities of cytotoxic T cell regulation, resulting in T cell autoaggression, as in ankylosing spondylitis, and presumably mediated by HLA-A and B interactions with T cells. On the other hand, some HLA-D/DR associations may be due to linked immune response genes, perhaps explaining abnormal antibody production, as in myasthenia gravis. HLA-D/DR associations may also be primary, since these antigens participate in T cell, B cell, and macrophage interactions. For instance, different HLA-D/DR antigens may mediate presentation of antigen with different efficiency. In the case of HLA-DW2/DR2 associations, many of the diseases are thought to show abnormalities of suppressor T cell function, which may implicate an immune response (or suppressor) gene closely linked to HLA-D/DR, possibly via a suppressor cell. Alternatively, a non–T cell stimulator defect resulting in reduced or absent autologous mixed lymphocyte reaction has been described in systemic lupus erythematosus. A number of the diseases associated with HLA-DW4/DR4 show abnormalities of humoral response, possibly implicating abnormalities of control of humoral response in some cases. When more than one gene participates in susceptibility, only one of which is HLA-linked, the outbred nature of the human population may conceal the association.

The pathologist and the physician in general should be aware that the knowledge presented in this chapter may be useful to illustrate how the MHC may help nosologic classification of diseases. Nosologic classification is based partly on the knowledge of the consequences of etiologic factors and partly upon grouping clinical signs and symptoms into syndromes. Additional information concerning clinical aspects of a disease, such as differences in age of onset, differing prognosis, and new subgrouping of symptoms, can lead to new subdivisions of diseases (splitting), as in the separation of juvenile onset and mature onset as two distinct forms of diabetes. Increase in knowledge of etiology might also lead to the inclusion in one disease of several conditions of varying clinical manifestations (lumping).

From the point of view of susceptibility, diseases result from many factors, primarily interactions of genetic factors with the environment. Genetically speaking, diseases may also be caused by a single point mutation that affects several organs and presents several manifestations (pleiotropism); however, a single clinical manifestation may result from different mutations at the same or different points in the genome (genetic heterogeneity or polygenic factors in diseases). Of course, since environmental factors are important in most diseases and since few diseases show complete expression even in monozygotic twins, it is expected that not all individuals who inherit abnormal genes will be affected (penetrance).

We have described a new approach to the study of disease susceptibility at the population level. Utilizing other genetic markers, such as the complotypes, which are non-randomly associated to HLA or may be randomly associated to HLA, it is possible to investigate both recent and ancient mutations within or near the HLA loci. We believe that if a mutation is recent, the corresponding disease may be found in excess in a particular population, perhaps because the haplotype carrying the susceptibility gene originated in a population where that haplotype occurred with different frequency than in the population into which the affected individual(s) migrated (founder effect). Conversely, if the mutations occur in a haplotype (extended haplotype) which has been maintained by non-random association (linkage disequilibrium), then the disease or several diseases may be marked by that haplotype. In this regard, many clinicians believe that there is a link between such conditions as Graves' disease and Addison's as a polyglandular disease, possibly with common etiology. The transmission of extended haplotypes might, after a single mutation within the haplotype, result in the production of disease after interactions of the haplotype both with other susceptibility genes on other chromosomes and with environmental factors. Alternatively mutiple mutations within the extended haplotype might lead to disease upon interactions with the environment. Since several diseases are associated with different alleles of the MHC, it is obvious, however, that the mechanisms involved in MHC associations are complex.

SUMMARY

We have presented a summary of the immune response, pointing out that it is possible to identify diseases associated with a disturbance of immune regulation, as demonstrated by partial cellular subset defects. Since the immune response is controlled by several genes, it is obvious that such diseases may be caused by disturbances of any of the theoretically involved genes. We have described only the relevance of genes in the MHC to the study of diseases. In some diseases, the susceptibility gene located within the MHC is solely responsible for the disease, for example, in complement deficiencies and 21-hydroxylase deficiency. In other diseases, the susceptibility gene appears to interact both with other genes and with the environment to cause a disease. The susceptibility gene may be dominant, as in the case of cerebellar ataxia, or recessive, as in the case of idiopathic hemochromatosis or IDDM. In these examples, the disease susceptibility gene is said to be linked to HLA or the MHC, or may be located within the MHC.

Apart from autoimmune disease, MHC alleles have been shown to be associated with diseases of different specialties of medicine: neurology, psychiatry, infectious diseases, rheumatology, orthopedic surgery, hematology, endocrinology, oncology, dermatology, and cardiology. The strongest association, however, is with the autoimmune diseases, which explains why the mechanisms most likely to explain disease associations are perhaps related to self-altered antigen and disturbances in the function of macrophage and B and T lymphocytes, producing alterations of MHC functions resulting in altered interactions between the host and the environment.

Alper, C. A.: Inherited structural polymorphism in human C2: Evidence for genetic linkage between C2 and Bf. J. Exp. Med., *144*:1111, 1976.

Alper, C. A., Awdeh, Z. L., Raum, D., and Yunis, E. J.: Extended major histocompatibility complex haplotypes in man: Role of alleles analogous to murine t mutants. Clin. Immunol. Immunopathol., *24*:276, 1982.

Alper, C. A., Raum, D., Karp, S., Awdeh, Z. L., and Yunis, E. J.: Serum complement "supergenes" of the major histocompatibility complex in man (complotypes). Vox Sang., *45*:62, 1983.

Amos, D. B., Johnson, A. H., Cartwright, G., Edwards, C., and Skolnick, M.: HLA and B cell antigens in hemochromatosis. Tissue Antigens, *10*:206, 1977.

Amos, D. B., and Yunis, E. J.: An introduction to HLA and disease surveillance. *In:* Amos, D. B., Schwartz, R. S., and Janicki, B. W. (eds.): The Immune Mechanisms and Disease. New York, Academic Press, 1979, p. 139.

Awdeh, Z. L., and Alper, C. A.: Inherited structural polymorphism of the fourth component of complement (C4). Proc. Natl. Acad. Sci., *77*:3576, 1980.

Awdeh, Z. L., Raum, D., Yunis, E. J., and Alper, C. A.: Extended HLA-complement allele haplotypes: Evidence for T/t-like complex in man. Proc. Natl. Acad. Sci. U.S.A., *80*:259, 1983.

Benacerraf, B.: A hypothesis to relate the specificity of lymphocytes and the activity of I region-specific Ir genes in macrophages and B lymphocytes. J. Immunol., *120*:1809, 1978.

Benacerraf, B.: Role of major histocompatibility complex in genetic regulation of immunologic responsiveness. Transplant Proc., *8*:825, 1977.

Bender, K. N., and Grzeschik, K. H.: Possible assignment for the glyoxalase 1 gene to chromosome 6 using man-mouse somatic cell hybrids. Human Genet., *31*:341, 1976.

Canoso, R. T., Lewis, M. E., and Yunis, E. J.: Association of HLA-Bw44 with chlorpromazine-induced antibodies. Clin. Immunol. Immunopathol., *25*:278, 1982.

Cartwright, G. E., Edwards, C. Q., Kravitz, K., Skolnick, M., Amos, D. B., Johnson, A., and Buskaajaer, L.: Hereditary hemochromatosis, phenotypic expression of the disease. N. Engl. J. Med., *301*:175, 1979.

DeWolf, W. C., Lange, P. H., Einarson, M. E., and Yunis, E.: HLA and testicular cancer. Nature, *277*:216, 1979.

Dupont, B., Pollack, M. S., Levine, L. S., O'Neil, G. J., Hawkins, B. R., and New, M. I.: Joint Report. Congenital adrenal hyperplasia. *In:* Terasaki, P. I. (ed.): Histocompatibility Testing 1980. Los Angeles, UCLA Tissue Typing Laboratory, 1980.

Engelhard, V. H., Kaufman, J. F., Strominger, J. L., and Burakoff, S.: Specificity of mouse cytotoxic T-lymphocytes stimulated with either HLA-A and -B or HLA-DR antigens reconstituted into phospholipid vesicles. J. Exp. Med., *152*:54s, 1980.

Falchuk, Z. M., Nelson, D. L., Katz, A. J., Bernardin, J. E., Kasarda, D. D., Hauge, N. E., and Strober, W.: Gluten-sensitive enteropathy. Influence of histocompatibility type on gluten sensitivity in vitro. J. Clin. Invest., *66*:227, 1980.

Fleishnick, E., Awdeh, Z. L., Raum, D., Granados, J., Alosco, S. M., Crigler, J. F., Jr., Gerald, P. S., Giles, C. M., Yunis, E. J., and Alper, C. A.: Extended MHC haplotype in 21-hydroxylase deficiency congenital adrenal hyperplasia: Shared genotypes in unrelated patients. Lancet, *1*:152, 1983.

Francke, U., and Pellegrino, M. A.: Assignment of the major histocompatibility complex to a region of the short arm of chromosome 6. Proc. Natl. Acad. Sci. U.S.A., *74*:1147, 1977.

Geczy, A. F., Alexander, K., Bashir, H. V., Edmonds, J. P., Upfold, L., and Sullivan, J.: HLA-B27, Klebsiella and ankylosing spondylitis: Biological and chemical studies. *In:* Moller, G. (ed.): Immunological Reviews. Copenhagen, Munksgaard, 1981, Vol. 70, pp. 23–50.

Helenius, A., Morein, B., Fries, E., Simons, K., Robinson, P., Schirrmacher, V., Terhorst, C., and Strominger, J. C.: Human (HLA-A and HLA-B) and murine (H-2K and H-2D) histocompatibility antigens are cell surface receptors for Semliki Forest virus. Proc. Natl. Acad. Sci. U.S.A., *75*:3846, 1978.

Jerne, N. K.: The somatic generation of immune recognition. Eur. J. Immunol., *1*:1, 1971.

Jongsma, A. N., van Someren, H., Westerveld, A., Hagemeier, A., and Peerson, P.: Localization of the genes on human chromosomes by studies of human–Chinese hamster somatic cell hybrids. Assignment of PGM3 to chromosome C6 and regional mapping of the PGD, PGM, and pep-C genes on chromosome A1. Humangenetik, *20*:195, 1973.

Klein, J.: Biology of the Mouse Histocompatibility-2 Complex. New York, Heidelberg, Berlin, Springer-Verlag, 1975.

Klein, J.: Demystifying the major histocompatibility complex. Immunol. Today, *2*:166, 1981.

Klein, J., Flaherty, L., Van de Berg, J. L., and Shreffler, D. C.: H-2 haplotypes, genes, regions, and antigens: First listing. Immunogenetics, *6*:489, 1978.

Lamm, L. U., Friedrich, U., Petersen, G. B., Jorgensen, J., Nielson, J., Therkelsen, A. J., and Kissmeyer-Nielsen, F.: Assignment of the major histocompatibility complex to chromosome 6 in a family with a pericentric inversion. Human Hered., *24*:273, 1974.

Lamm, L. U., Svejgaard, A., and Kissmeyer-Nielsen, F.: PGM3:HLA is another linkage in man. Nature, *231*:109, 1971.

McMichael, A. J., Ting, A., Sweerink, H. J., and Askonas, B. A.: HLA restriction of cell-mediated lysis of influenza virus–infected human cells. Nature, *270*:524, 1977.

Miettinen, O. S.: Estimability and estimation in case-referent studies. Am. J. Epidemiol., *103*:226, 1976.

Miller, L. H., Mason, S. J., Dvorak, J. A., McGinniss, M. H., and Rothman, I. K.: Erythrocyte receptors for *(Plasmodium knowlesi)* malaria: Duffy group determinants. Science, *189*:561, 1975.

Ott, J., Linder, D., McGaw, B. K., Lovrien, E. W., and Hecht, F.: Estimating distances from the centromere by means of benign ovarian teratomas in man. Ann. Human Genet., *40*:191, 1976.

Penrose, L. S.: The detection of autosomal linkage in pairs of brothers and sisters of unspecified parentage. Ann. Eugen., *6*:133, 1935.

Raum, D., Awdeh, Z., Yunis, E. J., and Alper, C. A.: Major histocompatibility markers in disease. Clin. Immunol. Allergy, *1*:305, 1981.

Reinsmoen, N. L., Friend, P. S., Miller, W. V., Burgdorf, A., Giblett, E. R., and Yunis, E. J.: Inheritance of recombinant HLA-GLO haplotype suggesting the gene sequence. Nature, *267*:276, 1977.

Rheinherz, E. L., and Schlossman, S. F.: The differentiation and function of human T lymphocytes. Cell, *19*:821, 1980.

Ryder, L. P., Andersen, E., and Svejgaard, A. (eds.): HLA and Disease Registry. Third Report. Copenhagen, Munksgaard, 1979, pp. 1–61.

Sasazuki, T., Nishimura, Y., Muto, M., and Ohta, N.: HLA-linked genes controlling immune response and disease susceptibility. *In:* Moller, G. (ed.): Immunological Reviews. Copenhagen, Munksgaard, 1981, Vol. 70, pp. 51–75.

Shreffler, D. C., and David, C. S.: The H-2 major histocompatibility complex and the I immune response region: Genetic variation, function, and organization. Adv. Immunol., *20*:125, 1975.

Sutton, H. E.: An Introduction to Human Genetics. 3rd ed. Philadelphia, W. B. Saunders Company, 1980, pp. 415–425.

Svejgaard, A., Platz, P., and Ryder, L. P.: HLA and disease 1982—a survey. *In:* Moller, G. (ed.): Immunological Reviews. Copenhagen, Munksgaard, 1983, Vol. 70, pp. 193–218.

Terasaki, P. I. (ed.): Histocompatibility Testing 1980. Los Angeles, UCLA Tissue Typing Laboratory, 1980.

Thomson, G., and Bodmer, W.: The genetic analysis of HLA and disease association. *In:* Dausset, J., and Svejgaard, A. (eds.): HLA and Disease. Copenhagen, Munksgaard, 1977.

Thomson, G., and Bodmer, W.: HLA haplotype associations with disease. Tissue Antigens, *13*:91, 1979.

Yunis, E. J., and Dupont, B.: The HLA system. *In:* Nathan, D. G., and Oski, F. A. (eds.): Hematology of Infancy and Childhood, Vol. II. Philadelphia, W. B. Saunders Company, 1981, p. 1438.

Zinkernagel, R. M., and Doherty, P. C.: Immunological surveillance against altered self components by sensitized T lymphocytes in lymphocytic choriomeningitis. Nature, *251*:547, 1974.

34

CELLS OF THE IMMUNE SYSTEM

DAVID T. ROWLANDS, JR., M.D., THERESA L. WHITESIDE, PH.D., and RONALD P. DANIELE, M.D.

LYMPHOCYTES

Lymphocytes localized to tissues or circulating in blood or lymph make up the cellular system principally responsible for immunity in vertebrates. The tissues where lymphocytes are found may be divided into *primary lymphoid organs* (the thymus and bone marrow), in which antigen-independent processes of division and differentiation create new lymphoid cells, and *secondary lymphoid organs* (lymph nodes, spleen, and portions of the gastrointestinal tract), in which antigen-driven antibody production and generation of effector cells take place. Maximal expression of immune responses by lymphocytes usually requires interactions with macrophages or their products.

Structure of Lymphocytes

General Characteristics. Lymphocytes, stained by conventional methods and seen through the light microscope, have deceptively homogeneous appearances. The two major functional divisions (T and B cells) cannot be distinguished from each other morphologically, although an experienced observer may recognize certain subtle differences between B and T cells. Lymphocytes are approximately the same size as other leukocytes (8 to 12 μm), and their distinctly defined cellular membranes have rounded and regular contours (Chap. 27, p. 615). Their nuclei are equally uniform, having dense nuclear chromatin which on detailed examination appears clumped. The lack of staining of the cytoplasm led early students of lymphocytes to believe that these cells had little functional activity. The cytoplasm of lymphocytes has a bland appearance due to the paucity of cellular organelles. Today, large lymphocytes are thought to be "activated" cells involved in a distinct functional activity. Lymphoblasts are larger by at least two-fold than their mature counterparts, have large nucleoli, and have large cytoplasmic volumes with numerous polyribosomes and well-developed Golgi zones.

The electron microscope highlights the clumped appearance of the nuclear chromatin in lymphocytes. As might be expected from light microscopy, their cytoplasm contains a few lysosomes, sparse mitochondria, a small Golgi zone, and poorly formed aggregates of RNA. The plasma membrane of a lymphocyte is a typical unit membrane.

Plasma Cells. Plasma cells are derived from lymphocytes and clearly represent cells designed for the synthesis of immunoglobulins. They are of about the same size as lymphoblasts and have equally sharply defined cell walls (p. 615). Their nuclei are eccentrically placed within the cell and, except for a small indentation, are round in appearance. The nuclear chromatin is as intensely stained as that of lymphocytes, but is distributed more regularly in a pattern resembling the spokes of a wheel ("cartwheel nucleus"). The cytoplasm, except for one small area, stains intensely with pyronin, reflecting the large quantities of RNA available in the cellular cytoplasm. The unstained zone in the cytoplasm corresponds to the indented portion of the nucleus and is the site of the well-developed Golgi apparatus. As might be anticipated by its pronounced pyroninophilia, abundant and highly organized ribosomes are found in the cytoplasm of plasma cells. Well-developed plasma cells may contain small granules or bodies which stain with eosin or other acidic dyes and are called Russell bodies. These consist of large cisternae within the endoplasmic reticulum. Unusually large amounts of immunoglobulins lie within these cisternae. Plasma cells not only produce antibodies but actively release or secrete them.

Cell Surfaces. The structural features of lymphoid cells are significant with regard to their performance as synthesizers of highly specialized products such as immunoglobulins and lymphokines. Clearly, receipt of appropriate signals and the transmission of the external message to the internal portions of these cells are of great importance. In recent years, it has become clear that recognition of stimuli occurs at the cell surfaces of lymphocytes and involves specialized surface receptors. The surface properties are of paramount importance in the cell biology of lymphocytes. The presence of these receptors permits identification and enumeration of subsets of lymphocytes and allows for some understanding of the roles these cells play in normal and disease processes.

The cell surface of lymphocytes is regarded as a fluid mosaic permitting extensive rearrangement of surface molecules (Singer, 1974). Recent evidence suggests, however, that these molecules are also under variable degrees of restriction and modulation by a submembranous apparatus consisting of microfilaments and microtubules. Modulation of surface antigens affords a means for controlled interactions between cells and their milieu. The dynamic nature of the lymphocyte membrane is best illustrated in a phenomenon of "capping" (Schreiber, 1976). In several animal species and man, immunoglobulin (Ig) molecules are evenly distributed over the surfaces of certain lymphocytes (B cells), as determined by using fluorescein-labeled anti-Ig. Upon reaction with the antibody, microclusters of Ig–anti-Ig begin to flow rapidly to one pole of the cell in an energy-requiring process which results in the formation of a polar cap. The cytoplasm underneath the cap contracts, leading to the formation of a uropod at the opposite pole and a flow of cytoplasm away from the cap. The result is a transient motion of the lymphocyte, accompanied by endocytosis or internalization of the surface Ig–anti-Ig complexes. Capping in lymphocytes is thought to be dependent on the membrane-cytoplasm interaction because myosin—a component of microfilaments which form a cytoskeleton—shifts in close apposition to the Ig–anti-Ig microclusters. Nucleotides and calcium appear to share in this modulation.

Surface receptors are not constant features of lymphoid cells. Qualitative and/or quantitative changes in receptors may occur as a reflection of cellular development or antigen-driven differentiation and reflect functional characteristics of lymphocytes. Murine lymphocytes have been most extensively studied in this regard. Immunologically immature murine T lymphocytes express several surface receptors (G_{1x}, TL, Thy_1, Ly_1, $Ly_{2.3}$, Lys, H_2) (Cantor, 1975), and murine B cells go through a well-defined sequence of maturation steps reflected by surface Igs (Niewenhuis, 1981). Similar events have now been described in the development of human T and B lymphocytes (Reinherz, 1980; Kuritani, 1982).

Antibody- or ligand-mediated redistributions of surface molecules may lead to a reversible removal of these molecules from membranes. The removal may be accomplished by either or both of the following mechanisms. As a result of surface membrane turnover, some surface constituents are continually shed to the outside of the cell, a process known as exocytosis (Schreiber, 1976). In contrast, pinocytosis involves the internalization and perhaps reutilization of the molecules being removed from the surface. Little is known about the mechanisms and significance of these processes in lymphoid cells. They are energy dependent, for metabolically inhibited cells do not undergo pinocytosis. It may be speculated that continual removal of the "used-up" receptors, enzymes, and other membrane constituents keep the cell surface in a virgin state, freed from all the complexes formed between surface sites and environmental factors, free to accept new stimuli or messages.

Lymphocytes are the key cells of the immune system. By virtue of their surface receptors, they are responsible for recognition of antigens and for the appropriate response to these antigens. They are qualified not only to initiate specific antibody-mediated immune responses but also to gear their cellular machinery to elaborate and release a variety of other factors that are capable of acting as effector molecules. These effector molecules, in turn, may in a specific or non-specific way affect or be affected by other lymphocytes, other leukocytes (e.g., monocytes), and other tissue cells. Lymphocytes are capable of and required to establish an effective cooperation with other cells of the reticuloendothelial system for the immune response to take place. In order for the immune system to function efficiently, a high degree of regulation must be built in and/or responsible for this regulation. Finally, lymphocytes must be responsible for maintaining immunologic memory.

Heterogeneity of Lymphocytes

The immune response comprises a complex and not yet fully understood series of events which are antigen driven and which result in synthesis and secretion of antibodies ("humoral immunity") and/or delayed-type hypersensitivity reactions broadly referred to as "cell-mediated immunity." Lymphocytes mediate all phases of the immune response; however, not *all* lymphocytes participate in *all* stages of this response at *all* times.

The broadest separation of lymphocyte compartments can be made by designating one portion as T cell (thymus-dependent) and the other portion as B cell (bursal or bone marrow derived). It was shown in the early 1960's that surgical removal of thymuses in very young animals resulted in the failure of development of lymphoid tissues located in lymph nodes and spleen and in defective immune responses. The classic experimental work of Glick (reviewed in Cooper, 1974), indicated that removal of the bursa of Fabricius in chickens resulted in a loss of certain B lymphocyte–dependent functions. Similarly, Claman (1966) showed that B cell functions in mammals could be supplied by cells of the bone marrow. These studies also led to a concept that will be enlarged upon later—namely, that cellular interactions between T and B cells were required for complete expression of the immune response.

Today, it is well established that T and B lymphocytes are heterogeneous not only in their functional activities (Table 34–1) but also in their origins, life spans, migration patterns, anatomical distribution, and surface characteristics.

B Lymphocytes. These cells are precursors of plasma cells which synthesize and release immunoglobulins. It is generally accepted that B lymphocytes have easily detectable immunoglobulin (Ig) on cell membranes. There is diversity within the B lymphocytes such that individual B cells are restricted in the types of antibodies which they can synthesize and release. In man, there are four subclasses of IgG and two of IgA and two types of light chains. Therefore, if a given mature B lymphocyte or plasma cell is capable of producing only one class (isotope) of immunoglobulin, there must be at least 18 different types of B lymphocytes in the normal human adult. The situation is further complicated by the fact that each type of B lymphocyte probably produces Ig receptors with a single and unique antigen specificity. Thus, there are many types of B lymphocytes, each capable of recognizing a unique antigen through idiotypic determinants of their Ig receptors. Approximately 10 to 15 per cent of circulating blood lymphocytes are immunoglobulin-bearing cells, and the immunoglobulins most frequently seen on these cells are IgM and IgD (Rowe, 1973). IgG- and IgM-positive lymphocytes are found primarily in organized lymphoid tissues, while at sites of external immunoglobulin secretion (e.g., in the gastrointestinal and respiratory tracts), IgA- and IgE-bearing cells predominate.

B cells also have receptors on their surfaces which recognize the Fc portion of immunoglobulins (Fc receptors), as well as receptors which recognize and react with components of the complement system (C3 receptors; Ross, 1973). Although these receptors can be found on cells other than B lymphocytes, there is evidence that C3 receptors, immunoglublins, and Fc receptors are found on most B lymphocytes (Ehlenberger, 1976). However some SIg-positive B lymphocytes may not express C3 receptors and/or Fc receptors. It appears then that the B cell compartment is actually made up of various populations of cells having one or more of the surface markers described above. B lymphocytes also bear receptors not found on other cells, namely, B specific antigens and receptors for Epstein-Barr virus (Table 34–2).

Proliferation on exposure of B cells to antigens *in vitro* is limited so that activation of more than 2 to 3 per cent of the B cells to a particular antigen is uncommon. Considering the vast array of antigens to which an animal can respond *in vivo,* such responsiveness to individual antigens implies that recognition is relatively rather than rigidly specific for the antigens in question. Antigen recognition is through surface immunoglobulins.

Human B cells differ from those of other species in being generally unresponsive to polyclonal mitogens.

Table 34–1. BIOLOGIC REACTIONS MEDIATED BY LYMPHOCYTES

Reaction	B-Lymphocyte Antibodies	T-Lymphocyte Sensitized Cells
Protection against infection	Encapsulated bacteria (streptococci, meningococci, *H. influenzae,* etc.)	Intracellular pathogens (viruses, bacteria, fungi, protozoa)
Transplant rejection	Major cause of hyperacute rejections; also important in acute and chronic rejections—may be protective of the graft	Major mechanism for chronic rejection
Graft versus host reaction	Not involved	Involved
Tumor immunity	May enhance tumor growth; antibody-dependent cellular cytotoxicity	Major mechanism for eliminating tumor cells
Autoimmunity	Mediate "immune-complex" disease and autoimmune disease of blood	Involved in pathogenesis of solid organ disease (thyroiditis, adrenalitis)
Tolerance	May participate through feedback and/or immune complex inhibition	Generation of suppressor lymphocytes

Table 34–2. MARKERS USEFUL FOR DETECTION OF HUMAN T AND B LYMPHOCYTES

T lymphocytes
E antigen (E rosettes)
T-cell specific antigens (see Table 34–3)
Ia-like antigens (activated T cells)
Enzymes:
Terminal deoxynucleotidyl transferase (Tdt)
Alpha naphthyl acetate esterase (ANAE)
Purine nucleoside phosphorylase (PNP)
Adenosine deaminase (ADN)
Beta glucoronidase (BG)
Acid phosphatase (AP)
B lymphocytes
Surface Ig*
B-cell specific antigens (see Table 34–3)
Ia-like antigens*
Receptors for C3*
Receptors for EB virus
Receptors for the Fc portions of IgG*
Enzymes: 5′ nucleotidase (5′NT)

*These markers are not specific for B lymphocytes and may be present on monocytes, granulocytes, tissue cells, and some T lymphocytes.

Although PHA is a general mitogen for T cells, it can also stimulate B cells when insolubilized. Pokeweed mitogen (PWM), originally believed to be a B cell mitogen, has been shown to act on both B and T cells in man (Greaves, 1972b).

As indicated earlier, plasma cells represent the extreme maturation form of B lymphocytes. They are fully equipped for massive protein synthesis and are restricted with regard to the class and specificity of the immunoglobulins which they synthesize and secrete. Plasma cells differ significantly from their progenitor lymphocytes in having little in the way of immunoglobulin, Fc, or complement surface receptors. Further, a plasma cell antigen (PC1) is found only on antibody-secreting cells and not on B cell precursors.

T Lymphocytes. These cells are responsible for reactions of cellular immunity, are important modulators of humoral immunity, and serve with macrophages in the proper presentation of antigens to B cells. Because cell-mediated immunity is antigen directed, T cells must have surface receptors which recognize antigens exercising a degree of specificity similar to that of B cells. Immunoglobulins on surfaces of T cells may function as receptors but are not easily detected by conventional procedures, perhaps because they are buried in the membrane, are sparse, or are present as monomers or polypeptide chains.

An important surface property of human T lymphocytes from the standpoint of clinical medicine is the receptor for sheep erythrocytes (Table 34–2). This surface receptor is selective for human T lymphocytes, but its detection is temperature dependent. Fc receptors are not abundant, but T lymphocytes may express them. T lymphocytes proliferate in response to appropriate concentrations of PHA or concanavalin A (Con A). Interestingly, B cells and other lymphoid cells also express receptors for these mitrogens, but, as mentioned above, their proliferative response may be negligible or nil. T cells respond by proliferation to alloantigens related to the major histocompatibility complex and expressed on allogeneic cells, including B cells. Finally, some T lymphocytes may express specific differentiation antigens, such as theta antigen in the mouse, antigens identifiable with anti-thymocyte or anti-brain sera in man (Cantor, 1976), and an increasing array of monoclonal reagents listed in Table 34–3 for use in man.

Human Immunoregulatory T Lymphocyte Subpopulations. Until recently, the elucidation of cell-to-cell interactions in the regulation of the immune response in humans has been hindered by the inability to identify participating lymphocyte subpopulations. With the development of monoclonal antibodies, stable glycoprotein markers (differentiation antigens) have been detected on the surfaces of human lymphocytes (Terhorst, 1980).

Mature immunologically competent T lymphocytes in the circulation and peripheral lymphoid tissue can be segregated into two subpopulations on the basis of the differentiation antigens they express (Table 34–4). Monoclonal antibodies allow us to recognize the $T1^+$ $T3^+$ $T4^+$ and $T1^+$ $T3^+$ $T5/T8^+$ subpopulations. These represent helper/inducer and cytotoxic/suppressor subpopulations, respectively. All circulating peripheral T cells are strongly positive for the T1 and T3 antigens, whereas the T4 antigen is expressed on about 50 to 65 per cent of the peripheral T cells and the T5/T8 antigen is present on 20 to 30 per cent of the T cells. The T4 and T5/T8 antigens identify phenotypically mutually exclusive subsets and seem to represent functionally distinct T cell subpopulations.

Functionally, the T4 subpopulations respond to soluble antigen and proliferate maximally to cell surface antigens, alloantigens (mixed lymphocyte reaction), and phytohemagglutinin. In contrast, the T5/T8 subpopulation contains cytotoxic effector T cells and responds less to phytohemagglutinin than does T4. Both subpopulations, however, respond equivalently to concanavalin A.

The most important difference between these subsets involves their regulatory role in the immune response. The T4 subset provides necessary help for B cells to proliferate and differentiate into antibody-producing cells. In contrast, the T5/T8 subset exerts a suppressive or regulatory function in the immune system.

Other Lymphocytes. Cells which cannot be labeled as T or B cells on the basis of their surface properties constitute a "third lymphocyte population." The existence of this third population has been deduced from lymphocyte enumeration studies, where the sums of identifiable T and B lymphocytes seldom exceed the figure of 90 per cent. Indeed, more careful search resulted in the discovery of lymphocytic cells which could not be "tagged" by any of the available reagents. These are referred to as "null" cells. The name should not be taken to mean that at a given time null cells do not bear any receptors recognizable by the methods

Table 34–3. A PARTIAL LIST OF COMMERCIALLY AVAILABLE MONOCLONAL ANTIBODIES TO HUMAN LYMPHOCYTE AND MONOCYTE SURFACE ANTIGENS (1983)

Mononuclear Cells Active with Antibody	Antigenic Specificity	Trade Designations*
T lymphocytes	Total, "pan" T cell population	OKT 1, OKT3, Leu-1, T101
	T cells forming E rosettes	OKT11, T 11, Leu-5
	Helper/inducer T cells	OKT 4, T 4, Leu-3a, Leu-3b
	Suppressor/cytotoxic T cells	OKT8, T 8, Leu-2a, Leu-2b, OKT 5
	Subpopulations of thymocytes	OKT 4, OKT 5, OKT 6, OKT 8, OKT 9, OKT 10
	Activated T cells	OKTIal, HLA-DR, I-2, OKT 9, 5E9, B3/25
B lymphocytes	Ig^+ cells, plasma cells	Monoclonal antibodies to human Igs
	Total B cells	B-1, Leu-10, BA-1
	B cells expressing Ia antigens	OKIal, HLA-DR, I-2
NK/K cells	Large granular lymphocytes	Leu-7
Monocytes/macrophages	Adherent cells	OKIa, I-2, MAC-1, Mo2
	Non-adherent cells	OKIa, I-2, MAC-1
	Dendritic (Langerhans cells)	OKT 6
Abnormal lymphocytes	Common ALL antigen (CALLA)	J5, BA-3
	Leukemia-associated antigen p24	BA-2

*OK designations are available through Ortho Pharmaceuticals, Raritan, N.J. Leu designations are available through Becton-Dickinson, Mountain View, Cal. 5E9 is available through NIAID monoclonal antibody serum bank, Bethesda, Md. Other monoclonal antibodies listed can be obtained from Coulter Electronics, Inc., Hialeah, Fla., and Hybritec Inc., San Diego, Cal.

at hand. Whether null cells represent undifferentiated stem cells, immature T or B cells, or those lymphocytes that have lost recognizable surface receptors remains to be discovered. There is some evidence, for example, that about half of human lymphocytes that lack identifiable markers for T or B cells will eventually synthesize demonstrable surface Ig when cultured *in vitro* for seven days (Chess, 1975).

A second type of lymphocyte, which fits with neither T nor B cells, has been identified in human peripheral blood. These are *"L cells,"* so named because of the labile surface IgG they bear (Lobo, 1975, 1976). They have high-affinity Fc receptors, which differ from those on B cells by being resistant to digestion with trypsin. L cells do not have surface receptors for C3, and they fail to adhere to nylon wool columns. They are non-phagocytic, non-adherent to glass, and negative for non-specific esterases, making it unlikely that they are monocytes. The functional properties of L lymphocytes are unlike those of T cells, B cells, or monocytes. They do not proliferate in response to mitogens or soluble antigens, but are capable of enhancing *in vitro* responses of T lymphocytes supplemented with monocytes. L lymphocytes have a cytotoxic potential but cannot develop into antibody-producing cells. The site of origin and role of L lymphocytes in the immune response are unknown.

A third type of non-T, non-B lymphocyte is large granular lymphocytes (LGL). LGL includes natural killer (NK) cells as well as killer (K) lymphocytes which mediate antibody-dependent cytotoxicity (ADCC). Nearly all of the LGL have Fc receptors and bear a unique surface antigen recognized with a

Table 34–4. MONOCLONAL ANTIBODIES TO HUMAN T CELL SURFACE ANTIGENS*

Monoclonal Antibodies	Cell Surface Expression (% Reactivity with Antibodies)		Commercial Designations†
	Thymocytes	*T Cells*	
Anti-T1	10	100	OKT1, Leu1
Anti-T3	10	>90	OKT3, Leu4
Anti-T4	75	60	OKT4, Leu3a/Leu3b
Anti-T5	80	25	OKT5
Anti-T8	80	30	OKT8, Leu2a, Leu2b
Anti-T6	70	0	NAI/34, OKT6
Anti-T9	10	0	OKT9, 5E9
Anti-T10	95	5	OKT10

*Modified from Reinherz (1980).

†OK designations are available through Ortho Pharmaceuticals, Raritan, N.J. Leu designations are available through Becton-Dickinson, Mountain View, Cal. 5E9 is available throuth NIAID monoclonal antibody serum bank, Bethesda, Md. NAI/34 is available through Accurate Chemical, N.J. Coulter antisera are similar to OK or Ortho but designated cc for Coulter Clone.

monoclonal antibody HNK-1 (Abo, 1981) or anti Leu-7. The LGL are heterogeneous, comprising several subsets, some of which express low affinity receptors for sheep red blood cells (SRBC). Functionally, NK cells can be distinguished from other types of cytotoxic cells (i.e., killer and cytotoxic T lymphocytes) because they mediate cytotoxic reactions without prior sensitization. They have been implicated in defensive mechanisms against tumors and against virally transformed cells (Herberman, 1981).

It can be clearly seen, then, that the division of lymphocytes into two separate compartments—T cells and B cells—is an oversimplification. While emphasizing the differences between the two major lymphocyte populations, this simplistic representation of compartmentalization fails to stress the enormous heterogeneity seen within each class, as well as the fact that the T and B cells have a common origin, intimately interact with each other, and inhabit the same lymphoid organs.

RELATIONSHIP OF LYMPHOCYTES TO IMMUNE RESPONSES

The essence of the immune response is that "antigens" are recognized by appropriate cells in the lymphoreticular system. Recognition is followed by an intricate series of cell-to-cell and intracellular events culminating in the synthesis and release of effector molecules involving T cells, B cells, and macrophages.

T Cell Help. The precise mechanism of *T cell help* is not fully understood (Feldmann, 1974; Gershon, 1974). In lower animals, it has been demonstrated that certain antigens can induce antibody synthesis without the cooperation of T lymphocytes ("T-independent"), while other antigens require T cell help for the successful generation of an immune response ("T-dependent"). Studies of immune responses to hapten-carrier conjugates indicated that most antigens are "T-dependent" and contain two types of determinants: carrier determinants, which are recognized by helper T cells, and haptenic determinants, with which antibody-producing cells (B cells) react directly. For an immune response to occur, T-B cooperation is necessary. It requires (1) the presence of T and B cells and (2) physical linkage of the carrier and hapten. If an animal can produce B cells capable of recognizing the haptenic determinants but for some reason cannot produce T cells capable of recognizing the carrier determinant, only a limited antibody response will ensue. The antibody produced in this situation is hapten-specific IgM. On the other hand, if the responding animal's T cells are competent to recognize and react with the carrier determinant, a full-strength antihapten IgG response takes place. Thus, it appears that a main consequence of a T cell–B cell interaction is to provide a mechanism for regulating the magnitude and quality of the immune response. We do not know why certain antigens are "T-dependent" and others are "T-independent," but the repetitive subunit structure of all T-independent antigens (such as pneumococcal polysaccharides) suggests that the spatial orientation and/or molecular conformation of the antigen may be important for B cell recognition.

No firm conclusions can be drawn at present regarding the manner in which T and B cells cooperate in the immune response. Helper cells may influence effector cells by one or several soluble factors and/or cell-to-cell interactions.

Suppressor T Cells. It is thought that these cells are involved in the control of both cellular immunity and antibody synthesis through soluble factors they elaborate. There is evidence that, in the mouse, suppressor T cells are a distinct subpopulation of T lymphocytes with unique surface determinants (Ly 2, 3 antigens) (Cantor, 1975). A similar cell population defined by surface antigens has been recognized in man (Reinherz, 1980).

B Cells. When B lymphocytes are stimulated by an antigen, two events take place: (1) proliferation resulting in clonal expansion and (2) the differentiation of clones to antibody secreting cells. It is currently believed that at least two activating signals must be received by a B cell to undergo differentiation. The B cell–antigen interaction involving surface immunoglobulin receptors is an obligatory activation signal required of all B cells. This interaction may result in functional tolerance unless a second signal for activation is received by the B cell via a specific non-immunoglobulin receptor. The nature of this receptor or receptors is not known, but it appears that the second signal necessary for differentiation is derived from T helper lymphocytes. This T helper–B interaction is major histocompatibility complex (MHC)–restricted, i.e., is dependent on the expression of the appropriate MHC-encoded determinants on the interacting cells. It is also possible that macrophage-derived products function as amplifiers of B cell differentiation.

Macrophages. Macrophages as well as lymphocytes participate in both "T-dependent" and "T-independent" immune responses. Macrophages are phagocytic, adhere to glass, and are found fixed in tissues or free in peritoneal exudates and vascular circulations of all known multicellular species of animals. Efficient phagocytosis of bacteria by macrophages depends upon antibody molecules (opsonins), which can coat these bacteria. The bacterial antigen-antibody complexes are recognized by the Fc receptors for IgG on the cell surfaces of macrophages, taken up, and processed intracellularly. The C3 receptors have an evident physiologic role enhancing phagocytosis by macrophages. A major portion of antigen taken up by the phagocyte is digested. However, approximately 1 per cent of antigen presented to macrophages remains on the surface of the cell, serving as an available site for stimulating lymphocytes, which are capable of recognizing (i.e., equipped with appropriate surface receptors) this antigen (Unanue, 1982). Only a minority of macrophages can present antigen to T cells; these must express Ia antigens. While specificity in the immune response depends on lymphocytes, the macrophage is essential in antigen processing, cell interactions, and optimal functioning of lymphocytes; however, macrophages appear not to be antigen specific. Macrophages are also essential for *in vitro* antibody production and mitogen responses. In most instances, interactions between macrophages and lymphocytes are genetically restricted, depending on the MHC and the MHC-related antigen determinants.

Cellular Interactions in the Generation of the Immune Response. No definite conclusion can be drawn at present regarding the mechanism of T-B cell cooperation. A current model depicting the cellular interactions involved in T cell stimulation by antigen or mitogen is shown in Figure 34–1. By this scheme, the first step involves macrophages which are necessary for both mitogen and antigen stimulation of T cells. It is now apparent that after interaction with antigen or lectin, macrophages are activated to produce a soluble product called lymphocyte activating factor (previously designated LAF) and now termed interleukin-1 (IL-1). This factor is required for initiation of the second step in T cell activation, which induces a subpopulation of T cells to express specific receptors for another soluble factor called T cell growth factor (TCGF) or interleukin-2 (IL-2). The combination of antigen or lectin with IL-1 or macrophage-derived LAF induces a subset of T cells to produce T cell growth factor or IL-2. Recent studies suggest that the helper/inducer or T4 subset is activated by antigen/mitogen plus LAF to differentiate both to produce and to acquire receptors for IL-2. The binding of IL-2 molecules to the specific receptor sites on T cells induces cell proliferation. The mitogenic effect of IL-2 results in a clonal expansion of T cells which is dependent on the concentration of IL-2. Il-2 is specific for T cells in that it is not mitogenic for unstimulated lymphocytes, activated B cells, or cells of other lineages.

While the model depicts a similar pathway for both mitogens and antigens, important differences exist. For example, in order for T cells to respond to antigens, macrophages appear necessary because of their ability to produce IL-1, but also because of their role in presenting antigens to T cells in an MHC-restricted fashion. It is still unsettled as to whether macrophages are physically required for this MHC-restricted presentation for all antigens. It is also unclear as to whether macrophages produce other soluble mediators (besides IL-1) which may contain MHC products in association with antigen.

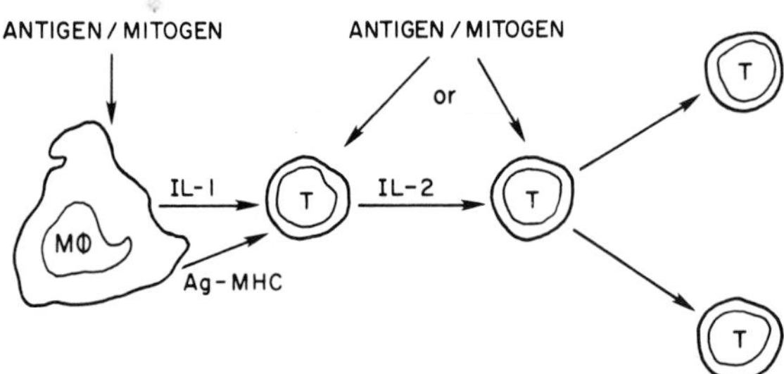

Figure 34–1. Schema of cellular interactions in the lymphocyte response to antigens or mitogens. Macrophages (Mϕ) or their soluble product interleukin-1 (IL-1) is required for T cells to produce and respond to interleukin-2 (IL-2); IL-2 is specifically mitogenic for lymphocytes. For antigen stimulation, antigen (Ag) in combination with Mϕ products of the MHC locus is physically presented to responsive lymphocytes.

Of considerable theoretical and practical importance has been the observation that once T cells acquire the receptor for IL-2, they no longer require the presence of antigen or mitogen for continued proliferation. The periodic addition of appropriate concentrations of IL-2 has permitted long-term clonal growth of T cells. When the initial stimulus is an antigen, continuously dividing T cells (CTCs) retain specificity for the original antigen. Cloning of antigen-specific T cells and their long-term growth *in vitro* provide a means for characterization of antigen-specific soluble factors and of cell-cell interactions in the immune response.

DIFFERENTIATION OF THE LYMPHOID SYSTEM

Experimental studies with thymectomized mammals and bursectomized birds, as well as observations on patients with various immunodeficiency disorders, indicate that, from a developmental viewpoint, the lymphoid system can be divided into three compartments. The first, the pool of undifferentiated stem cells, is a source of ancestral lymphoid cells capable of extensive proliferation and maturation into functionally competent cells. The second, the central or "primary" lymphoid tissues (thymus and bursa or bursa-equivalent in mammals), controls the development of lymphoid cells and is the site of intense, antigen-independent lymphopoiesis. The third compartment encompasses peripheral or "secondary" lymphoid organs (spleen, lymph nodes, gut-associate lymphoid tissue) and is made up of mixed populations of functionally differentiated T and B cells. T and B cells have distinct anatomic locations in the peripheral lymphoid organs. In lymph nodes, for example, B cells populate follicular areas, while T cells are found in paracortical regions. It must be emphasized that at any given time a great majority of lymphocytes (80 per cent or more) exist outside the lymphoid tissues, i.e., in the blood and tissues.

Embryonic Origin of Lymphocytes. Lymphoid cells make their first appearance in the yolk sac of fetal liver, along with other hematopoietic stem cells (Cooper, 1974). All lymphocytes are derived from a primitive pluripotential stem cell to be found in the blood islets of the yolk sac. In fetal life, the liver is a source of stem cells and later, in postnatal life, bone marrow becomes a pool of pluripotential stem cells. There are two distinct pluripotential stem cells. One, capable of forming colonies *in vivo* (CFU-S) and at a later stage of development *in vitro* (CFU-C), is a progenitor of myeloid and erythroid elements. The other, unable to grow *in vitro* under any known conditions, is an ancestral cell for lymphocytes. Both stem cells are derived from a more primitive cell (Abramson, 1977). Lymphoid cells capable of producing immunoglobulins can be detected around the eighth week of human embryonic life. In the mouse fetal liver, the first sign of B cells is glimpsed through the appearance of cells with IgM in their cytoplasm and, a bit later, on their surfaces. Similar cells are detectable in human bone marrow. This suggests that the commitment to B cell differentiation takes place before developing lymphoid cells reach these final microenvironments. Migration from fetal liver or adult bone marrow to primary lymphoid tissues must occur via the bloodstream. Once there, the progenitor cells come under inductive influences thought to be mediated by epithelial elements of the lymphoid tissue and become committed to the lymphoid pathway of differentiation. Little is known about the properties of these inductive factors, but it is possible that humoral factors, such as erythropoietin in the marrow and thymosin in the thymus, play important roles.

The first organs to become inhabited by lymphocytes during development are the thymus, fetal liver, and bursa-like tissue. In the thymus and bursa in the chicken, a very high mitotic index can be observed even before the fetus is born. A similar phenomenon is seen in germ-free animals. These observations have been taken as evidence that lymphopoiesis is dependent on a supply of stem cells. When the thymus is depleted of lymphocytes by irradiation or cortisone treatment, the influx of new stem cells results in repopulation with lymphocytes and further development of immune responsiveness. Mature B lymphocytes or even thymocytes cannot effectively repopulate the thymus. Removal of primary lymphoid organs early in development results in absent or defective immune responses. Removal of these organs in an adult does not influence immune competence unless the pool of immunocompetent lymphocytes is simultaneously depleted by irradiation or other measures. In such cases, repair of the immune system is dependent on the supply of stem cells and the presence of primary lymphoid organs. Thus, central lymphoid tissues are needed for the development of immunologic competence but not for maintaining such competence.

The presence of epithelial cells in the primordial thymus and persistence of epithelial cells into adult life suggests that epithelial cells serve as a hormonal source acting locally to induce maturation of lymphocytes from appropriate mesenchyme. When thymus epithelial cells are separated *in vitro* by a cell-impermeable Millipore filter from appropriate mesenchymal cells, maturation of lymphocytes from mesenchymal cells is readily demonstrated. It has been observed that transplants of thymic epithelial cells into thymectomized animals are sufficient for development of normal thymic function required for lymphocyte maturation. Also a hormone-like substance, "thymosin," restores thymus dependent activity in otherwise thymus-free animals (Bach, 1971). More recently, preparations of thymosin have been used successfully in the treatment of some children with congenital thymic deficiencies. The epithelial elements constitute a microenvironment of the thymus needed for development of functionally competent lymphocytes.

Experimental studies in bursectomized and thymectomized chickens, as well as studies of immunologically defective humans, made it clear that sites other than the thymus were important in the maturation of the B lymphocytes. Following this demonstration, an extensive search for the bursal equivalent in mammals was made. As might be supposed, lymphoid masses with associated epithelial cells became prime candidates, since similar cellular relationships were recognized in both the thymus and the bursa of Fabricius. Various tissues along the gastrointestinal tract (e.g., tonsils and Peyer's patches) suited this theory. None of these, however, have been shown conclusively to be bursal equivalents in mammals. It now seems that the bone marrow is the most likely source of B cell precursors, with the liver producing such cells quite early in development.

Development of Lymphocytes. Production of new immunocompetent T and B lymphocytes continues throughout life, although the rate slows down in older animals (Cooper, 1974). As Figure 34–2 illustrates,

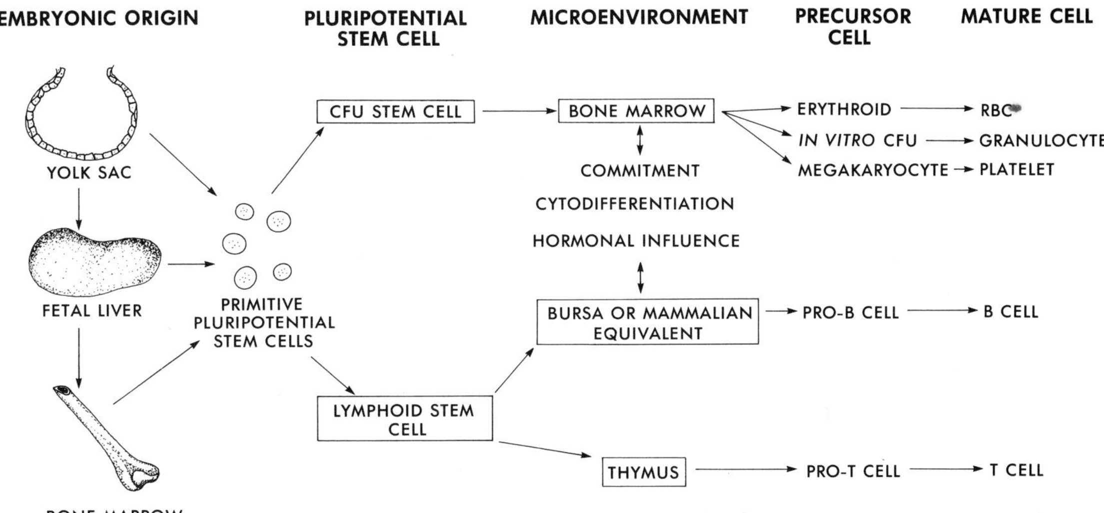

Figure 34–2. Illustration of the relationships between sources of stem cells and the sites of maturation of hematopoietic cells and lymphocytes.

5

pro-T and pro-B cells migrate to the thymus and the bursa-like lymphoid tissue, respectively, where cytodifferentiation commences. This differentiation involves many steps, alterations in surface markers, and changes in functional properties of maturing lymphocytes. Through the use of monoclonal antibodies specific for differentiation antigens on maturing cells, it has been possible to identify and actually isolate lymphocytes at distinct stages of their maturation.

The phenotype of maturing murine T cells undergoes continual changes as it develops from a primitive prothymocyte into a functionally specialized circulating T cell. The first antigen to be identified as characteristic of thymic lymphocytes was the A or Thy-1 antigen in the mouse. This antigen is carried by thymic lymphocytes into peripheral lymphocyte pools such as the spleen and lymph nodes. Its presence on the surface of a cell is used to distinguish thymus-derived from other lymphocytes. The Thy-1 antigen is expressed in large quantities on thymocytes but in much decreased quantities on T cells in peripheral lymphoid tissues. The Lyt series of differentiation antigens is also demonstrable on T cells. The presence of certain Lyt antigens can be correlated with distinct functional subpopulations of T cells. T cells with Lyt 1^+ 2, 3^- phenotype control delayed hypersensitivity, are involved in responses to the MHC antigens (mixed lymphocyte-reactive cells), and serve as helper cells (T_H) in immune responses to T-dependent antigens. The Lyt 1^-, 2, 3^+ cells appear to effect cell-mediated lympholysis and include a population of suppressor cells (Ts) (Cantor, 1975). The T cells carrying all three Lyt antigens (Lyt 1^+, 2, 3^+) may represent precursor cells. The constancy of Lyt antigen expression by T cells has been questioned (Thomas, 1982). The observed inconsistencies in the relationships between the Lyt phenotype and function of T cells appears to reflect at least in part a previously unrecognized complexity of T cell functions. For example, Ts cells may be Lyt 1^-, 2, 3^+, Lyt 1^+, 2, 3^+, or Lyt 1^+, 2, 3^-, and the expression of one of these phenotypes may depend on the state of their activation and the role they play in the immunoregulatory circuit (Thomas, 1982). Thus, not one but many Ts subpopulations exist. It should be remembered that the Lyt phenotype expressed by a functionally differentiated T cell is not immutable and may change during activation by an antigen. Certain other antigens on murine T cells appear to be more stable. The thymus leukemia (TL) antigen is a classic differentiation antigen and is expressed exclusively on thymocytes and not on circulating T cells. In the mouse, T cell differentiation involves a thymus-sponsored conversion of Ia^+ prothymocytes into thymocytes bearing a full complement of the T cell markers and eventually into at least three sets of T cells, each programmed for a different function and each bearing at least one, often more, distinct surface antigens.

Human T cell differentiation from the precommitted stem cell in a bone marrow to a mature, circulating T lymphocyte also involves a series of phenotype changes which can be identified with monoclonal reagents and related to the functional repertoire of each differentiating cell. During the differentiation, surface and cytoplasmic antigens change qualitatively as well as quantitatively. Thus, an early cortical thymocyte has relatively few "markers": Ia-like antigens, receptors for peanut agglutinin (PNA), and a cytoplasmic enzyme, terminal deoxynucleotidyl transferase (Tdt). In contrast, a thymocyte departing from medulla for peripheral lymphoid tissues is no longer responsive to PNA or Tdt-positive but instead is enriched in Ia-like antigens, can form rosettes with sheep erythrocytes, and expresses a full array of T cell-specific antigens such as T1, T11, T10, T6, T3, T4, and T8. Mature T lymphocytes can be phenotypically and functionally divided into T4 (inducer-helper) and T8 (suppressor-cytotoxic) populations (Reinherz, 1980).

Present concepts of the maturation of B cells also include a pre-B cell which arises from the stem cell in the marrow or fetal liver. It is thought that the pre-B cell, like pre-thymocyte, has no detectable surface markers (is "null") (Vogler, 1976). The first marker to appear on maturing B cells is immunoglobulin M in the cell cytoplasm (Raff, 1978). Immunoglobulin D appears on these IgM-positive cells at a somewhat later time in both the mouse and man. These precursors of antibody-producing cells have been most extensively studied in the mouse. The ability of these cells to recognize antigens probably precedes their abilities to synthesize antibodies. It has been hypothesized that IgD may be the "early" cell surface receptor for antigens (Rowe, 1973). The sequence for development of B-lymphocyte surface receptors appears to be surface immunoglobulin (IgM + IgD) → receptors for the Fc portion of immunoglobulin → receptors for C3 → Ia antigens. The B cell emerges from the maturation process bearing receptors for an antigen, which in fact are antibody molecules inserted into the surface membrane.

During cell maturation, "switchover" of membrane immunoglobulin may occur, so that B cells which initially express only IgM or IgD on their surfaces switch to an IgG or IgA phenotype. During the switchover, there may be brief periods when immunoglobulins with two different isotypes are expressed on the cell. It has been suggested that the immunoglobulin class on a lymphocyte reflects the extent of differentiation of B cells. Molecular mechanisms and experimental evidence for the immunoglobulin class switchover are now being elucidated by molecular cloning and nucleotide sequence analysis (Davis, 1980). The approach has been to isolate and compare the structure of the expressed (adult) Ig genes coding for the heavy (H) Ig chains with that of germline H chain genes. Such studies have led to a proposal that a complete H chain gene is created by at least two types of DNA rearrangements that occur during differentiation of B lymphocytes.

Other surface receptors that characterize the B cell line include plasma cell antigen (PC1) found on antibody-secreting cells but not on B cell precursors and several glycoprotein antigens found selectively on surfaces of human B cells, and reactive with monoclonal antibodies (Table 34–3).

Maturation and differentiation of lymphocytes are not completely understood. They involve a complex series of progressive and regressive changes in surface receptors under genetic control and influences of an hematopoiesis-inducing microenvironment. The many unanswered questions about differentiation focus on the nature, properties, and responses of prolymphocytes, the commitment process, the signals necessary for differentiation influences exerted on developing cells by their microenvironments, the role of antigens in the differentiation process, and synchronization of surface properties with functional maturation of developing lymphocytes.

Recirculation of Lymphocytes. Lymphocytes are not permanent residents of any one lymphoid tissue (Sprent, 1977). Rather they briskly move throughout all tissues of the body. As many as 80 per cent of small lymphocytes in the blood of adult animals are long-lived cells capable of extensive and long-term recirculation. Both small T and B lymphocytes recirculate. The pathway of recirculating lymphocytes takes them from the bloodstream to the extravascular connective tissue spaces and peripheral blood via the lymphatic vessels and back to the blood via the lymphatic system (Fig. 34–3).

Blood-borne cells extravasate from blood within lymph nodes so that small lymphocytes are continually added to the lymph; about 10 per cent of lymphocytes which enter a node in the arterial blood do not exit via the venous route but instead extravasate to the lymph (DeSousa, 1981). This passage from blood to lymph is initiated at the special segments of postcapillary venules with a high cuboidal epithelium (HEPCV = high epithelium postcapillary venules) shortly after blood-borne cells enter the node (i.e., near the cortico-paracortical junction). Migrations through the node occur via one of three routes: (1) a paracortical sinus route where the cells enter a subfollicular sinus, pass through sinuses in paracortex and medulla, and leave the node via the efferent lymphatic; (2) a paracortical cord route, which takes longer than the sinus route and is principally taken by T cells; most of these cells leave the cords at the paracortex-medulla junction to enter the medullary sinuses and reach the efferent lymphatic; or (3) the perifollicular route, followed mainly by B cells which pass through a series of perifollicular capillaries and eventually end up in the subfollicular sinuses (Kelly, 1975). The minimum transit time of a population of labeled small lymphocytes from blood to lymph is about two to four hours in the rat.

In the spleen, the migrating small lymphocytes pass through the pores of the marginal sinus to enter periarteriolar lymphocyte sheaths. From there they exit, probably via the marginal zone channels. During the two- to four-hour passage through the spleen, there are ample opportunities for lymphocytes to extravasate into the splenic tissue in much the same way as in the lymph nodes. In the gut lymphoid tissue, the cells migrate from the blood via postcapillary venules into interfollicular lymphoid tissue and out via the lacteals. It is of interest that in the lymph nodes, spleen, or gut-associate lymphoid tissue, recirculating lymphocytes do not migrate through the follicle or germinal centers.

It appears that the single most important factor determining which lymphocytes recirculate lies in the cell surface characteristics. Experiments in which treatments with trypsin or neuraminidase were shown to radically alter the migration patterns of lymphocytes support this view. Exposure to viruses, bacteria, other microorganisms, and antigens also alter cell surface characteristics of lymphocytes and, thus, play important roles in modifying their migration patterns through lymphoid tissues.

Responses to Antigenic Stimulation. Introduction of antigen into an intact animal produces profound changes in peripheral but little change in central

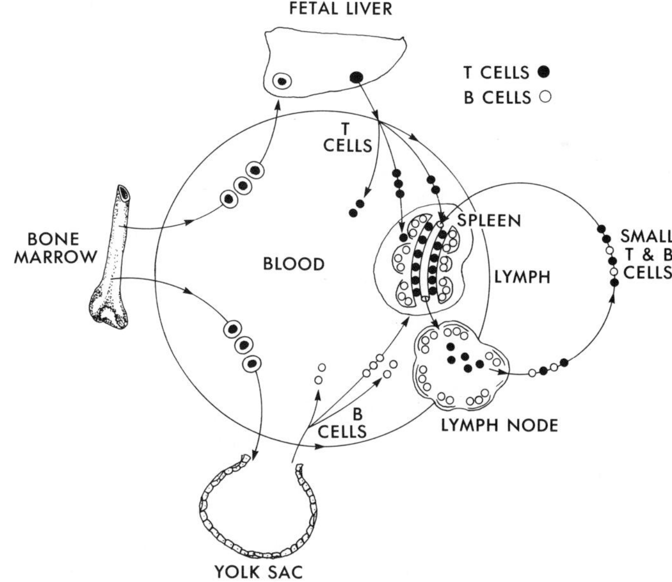

Figure 34–3. Recirculation of lymphocytes showing the interrelationships of T and B cells with various lymphoid tissues.

5

lymphoid tissues. The sites of maximal alterations of the peripheral lymphoid tissues after injection of antigens are determined in large measure by the route of injection of antigen. If the injection is subcutaneous, regional lymph nodes are most extensively modified, while an intravenous injection of antigen causes profound alterations of the splenic lymphoid follicles. Other factors, such as the nature of the antigens, its speed of degradation within macrophages, and whether there is a pre-existing antibody determine where and for how long the antigen is retained in the lymphoid tissues.

Antigens injected subcutaneously enter regional lymph nodes through afferent lymphatics. Much of the antigen uptake in the node is by the sinus-lining macrophages. They degrade a major portion of the antigen, although some antigen remains in a surface-associated, native form. Antigen which passes through the first node remains in the circulation until specific antibodies appear.

Within two to three days after subcutaneous administration of an antigen, the draining lymph node is characterized by enlarged paracortical cords and the presence of many blast cells. This is followed by the formation of active germinal centers and the appearance of plasma cells in the medulla. The sequence of events may be reconstructed as follows. First, the draining lymph node swells visibly owing to a reduction in the number of cells exiting via the efferent lymph. "Sinus plugging," which refers to filling up of the sinuses in the paracortex with aggregates of lymphocytes, also contributes to the node swelling. The traffic through the sinuses becomes very sluggish because of stickiness and enlargement of macrophages lining the sinuses in the paracorticomedullary junction. Next, the paracortical cords begin to fill uniformly with lymphocytes and swell until the entire paracortex becomes spherical. The lymphocytes stacked up in the paracortical cords undergo extensive mitotic activity. Both T and B lymphocytes divide, although the peak of mitotic activity of B cells lags behind that of T cells. Shortly after the onset of mitoses, plasmablasts may be seen at or near the paracorticomedullary junction. Some of these blast cells leave the node through medullary sinuses emptying into efferent lymphatics, but the majority differentiate into sessile plasma cells within the medulla.

The magnitude and length of "lymphocyte trapping" by the activated node depend on the amount and physical characteristics of antigen and are self-limiting. On day four or five, the trapping ends and cells from congested paracortical sinuses pour into medullary sinuses and out of the node so that its lymphocyte output rises to 5 to 10 times normal. Paracortical cords decrease in size, and a week or 10 days after antigenic stimulation the number of cells in the efferent lymph has returned to normal. Although both proliferation and differentiation of lymphocytes may be observed in nodes within 24 to 48 hours of injection of an immunizing dose of antigen, antibody formation is not detected until the second to fourth day when it is seen in the deep paracortex or medulla. Germinal centers do not appear until after five to seven days in primary and four to six days in secondary immune responses. This means that germinal centers are not significantly involved in the initiation of antibody synthesis. Once synthesis starts, immune complexes composed of specific antibody and eliciting antigen localize on surfaces of dendritic cells within follicles. This is followed by the accumulation of large pyroninophilic dividing cells at that site. They are surrounded by a cuff of medium and small lymphocytes. It is uncertain what happens to the progeny of the dividing cells in germinal centers. They probably pass slowly into the follicular paracortex. They may be memory B lymphocytes, since elimination of germinal centers results in normal antibody production but a failure to develop immunologic memory.

PROPERTIES USEFUL FOR STUDIES OF LYMPHOCYTES

Analysis of subpopulations of lymphocytes is ordinarily a two-step process. The first is separation of lymphoid cells from others. This step depends upon physical characteristics of the cells (e.g., size or density) or cell surface properties which determine their differential adherence to substrates such as glass or to specific ligands such as immunoglobulins. The conditions chosen for such separations are of critical importance and should be selected with an eye to the purpose of the study. Some methods of separation may provide a good cell recovery, while others may be more effective in preserving the metabolic qualities of the purified cells.

The second process in analysis of subpopulations of lymphocytes is quantitation. Quantitation depends on the presence of receptors located on cell surfaces. It must be remembered that mononuclear cells other than lymphocytes may express the same receptors as lymphocytes. This is particularly important with respect to monocytes and macrophages. Therefore, it is important to remove such cells prior to the study of lymphocytes, or to identify the non-lymphocytes as contaminants of a given lymphocyte population. The receptors which permit enumeration of lymphocytes include surface immunoglobulins (SIg), B and T cell specific antigens, and receptors for complement components, for IgG or IgM immunoglobulins (FcR), and for sheep erythrocytes (E) (Aiuti, 1974). Only some of these are specific for lymphocytes (Table 34–2). Surface immunoglobulins, although synthesized exclusively by lymphocytes, may be absorbed to surfaces of other cells (e.g., monocytes). The receptor of E, thought to be specific for human T cells, has been detected on a variety of human tissue cells, although not on other mononuclear cells (Woda, 1977). The FcR may be expressed on all mononuclear cells. Lymphocyte subpopulations may now be enumerated in suspension, in cytocentrifuge smears, and in tissue sections.

Functional properties of lymphoid cells have been used only sparingly in enumerating the enriched cell populations of lymphocytes. Stimulation of lymphocytes with mitogens, such as PHA, Con A, or pokeweed, have been used to identify responsive T or B cells, and only in the case of PHA have these methods been modified to permit actual enumeration of T cells based on their responsiveness to PHA (Rowlands, 1974). Similarly, mixed lymphocyte cultures have been used in a semiquantitative manner to determine the capacities of lymphocytes to stimulate the proliferation of other lymphocytes or to respond to other lymphocytes. Recently, measurement of synthetic properties of lymphocytes (i.e., production of immunoglobulins or lymphokines) have been frequently used in defining abnormalities in lymphocyte subpopulations in disease states. Other functional properties, such as antibody-dependent or antibody-independent cytotoxicity, have also served as a guide for characterizing the T or B cell components of lymphocytes.

The desirability of identifying subpopulations of lymphocytes in solid tissues is obvious, especially where it relates to involvement of these cells in tissue damage and to diagnosis of lymphomas. Methods for such studies are now available and include immunomicroscopy with labeled antisera specific for T and B cells and rosetting techniques.

Techniques Useful in the Clinical Laboratory

Isolation of Lymphocytes. Lymphocytes can be separated from other formed elements of the blood by velocity sedimentation or by density-gradient centrifugation. Velocity sedimentation uses gradients of protein such as albumin, dextran, or fetal calf serum, and the separation is a function of the radius of the cellular elements. Whether the separation is carried out by gravity or under the influence of centrifugation, the end result is an enrichment of the upper layers with mononuclear cells, especially T and B cells. The second method, density gradient centrifugation, depends upon the specific gravity of a gradient (either linear or discontinuous), made up by solutions such as albumin or Ficoll. The lighter cells (those with the greatest nucleus/cytoplasm ratio) band nearest the top of the gradient, with each cell population seeking that specific gravity that corresponds to its own in the gradient.

Among the various methods available for separation of lymphocytes, the Ficoll-Hypaque technique of Boyum (1968, 1974) has been used with greatest apparent success. For the Ficoll-Hypaque (F/H) technique (Fig. 34–4), bloods should be collected in heparin free of preservative, diluted (1:3) with a balanced salt solution, layered onto a Ficoll–sodium metrizoate gradient with a density of 1.077 g/ml, and centrifuged at 400 g for 30 minutes at 22 to 25°C. It is important to ensure that centrifugation of blood preparations occurs at the same temperature at which the specific gravity of the Ficoll-Hypaque gradient has been established.

Separated lymphoid cells are collected from the interface by means of a Pasteur pipette and washed three times, using calcium-free saline to minimize clumping. In certain cases it may be necessary to incubate the cells collected at the interface at 37°C. for periods between 2 and 24 hours. This facilitates removal of exogenous immunoglobulins from the surface of lymphocytes and monocytes. To ensure good viability, at least 2 per cent of serum or a protein (e.g., BSA) should be included in the washing medium. Surface immunoglobulin may be acquired factitiously by two mechanisms: (1) the absorption of either immunoglobulin or antigen/antibody complexes via the Fc receptor, or (2) the directing of antibodies toward determinants of the mononuclear cells (Lobo, 1975; Daniele, 1976).

The shape or dimensions of the tube used to form the gradient do not affect the results of cell separation. If the conditions of separation are adhered to rigorously, recovery of nearly 90 per cent of the cells applied to the gradient can be anticipated. Losses of as many as 30 per cent of the cells may occur, usually owing to poor initial recovery at the interface or to improper washing procedures. Yields of less than 60 per cent are unacceptable and may lead to distortions in the T and B cell ratios of the final preparation.

It should be pointed out that procedures for separation have been developed largely using peripheral blood from normal subjects. Separations of lymphocytes from patients with lymphoproliferative or other disorders may require modifications. In those circumstances, the physical characteristics of lymphocytes may be altered and careful adjustment of the purification procedure may be necessary.

Monocyte contamination of lymphocyte preparations may represent another serious problem, since monocytes may account for as many as 40 per cent of the mononuclear cells isolated from peripheral blood using the Ficoll-Hypaque technique (Zucker-Franklin, 1974). These cells are especially significant, since they carry certain surface receptors also seen on B cells. Thus, a quantitative assay (e.g., for C3 receptors) could result in an overestimation of the B cell population if significant contamination with monocytes is present. Normally, monocytes can be easily distinguished from lymphocytes on morphologic or histochemical grounds, e.g., by their ability to phagocytize and by the high concentrations of hydrolytic enzymes. However, identification of these cells may be more difficult in the disease state.

Techniques for Separation of Monocytes from Lymphocytes. One of the methods commonly used depends on phagocytic properties of monocytes. The preparation of mononuclear cells is incubated at 37°C. with iron particles coated with poly-L-lysine or with uniformly sized (0.8 mm in diameter) latex particles coated with IgG for a period of

5

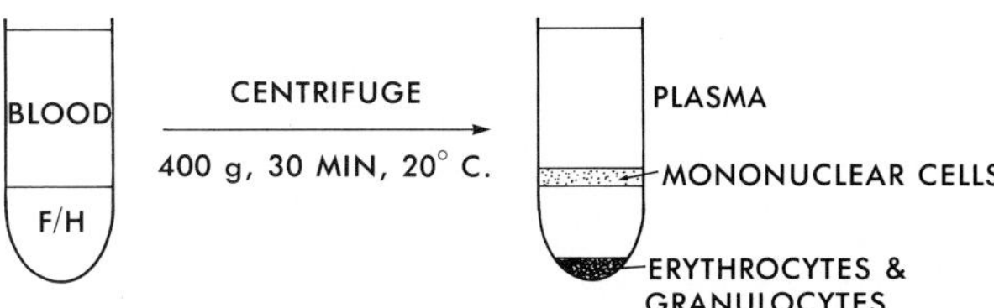

Figure 34–4. Blood collected in preservative-free heparin is layered on Ficoll-Hypaque. After centrifugation, the mononuclear cells appear as a discrete layer.

time sufficient for phagocytosis (30 to 60 minutes). The monocytes are then separated from the lymphocytes either by centrifugation or by the passage of cells over a strong magnet.

The second method depends on the adherence of monocytes to glass surfaces. It is best done before gradient centrifugation using leukocyte-rich plasma or whole peripheral blood. A suitable adherent surface may be provided by Petri dishes, glass slides, or a flask with a flat surface. The cells are incubated in a Petri dish or glass flask (flat-bottom) for 45 to 60 minutes at 37°C. The addition of human or fetal calf serum aids in monocyte adherence. Non-adherent cells (lymphocytes) are gently washed away from the glass or plastic surfaces. To isolate monocytes, cells adhering to such surfaces are teased off with a rubber policeman. The removal of adherent cells may be facilitated by prior incubation in the cold with 5mM EDTA or 12mM lidocaine.

The third method for removal of monocytes from mononuclear cell preparations utilizes G-10 gels (Jerrells, 1980). The cells in a serum-containing medium are poured onto small columns of Sephadex G-10 and incubated at 37°C. for 15 minutes. Monocytes adhere to the gel, while most of the lymphocytes are recovered by washing with media at room temperature. Preparations containing less than 1 per cent of monocytes can be obtained using this simple technique.

These methods yield lymphocyte preparations of high purity (90+ per cent) but have a disadvantage of large lymphocyte losses (up to 50 or 60 per cent) with reference to the starting material. Losses of lymphocytes are greatest in the methods relying on phagocytosis and are due to non-specific adherence of the foreign particles (latex, iron) to the surfaces of lymphocytes. These losses are especially significant in preparations containing activated lymphocytes. The purification method based on adherence of monocytes to glass surfaces causes less non-specific loss of lymphocytes but is cumbersome when large volumes of cells are to be processed. The method utilizing a Sephadex G-10 column is the most reliable and is recommended for peripheral bloods. To remove monocytes from other body fluids, adherence methods are generally used.

The one general method of correcting for contamination of suspensions or tissues with monocytes uses histochemical procedures (i.e., peroxidase stain) (Zucker-Franklin, 1974). The other corrective method depends on conventional light microscopy but can be done with greater certainty when various monocyte markers are provided to aid the morphologist. In general, this can be done by permitting monocytes to phagocytize particles, such as latex, carbonyl iron, or IgG-coated red blood cells, before doing differential counts. Errors may occur due to non-specific attachment of latex particles or iron to the surfaces of lymphocytes. Antibody-coated red blood cells are superior to latex for this purpose, since extracellular red blood cells may be eliminated by osmotic lysis before differential counts are done. Monoclonal antibodies to surface antigens on monocytes may be used either to deplete monocytes in the presence of complement or to identify them in acetone-fixed smears by immunoperoxidase techniques.

Enumeration of Lymphocytes. Cell surface markers have provided the basis for enumerating subpopulations of T and B lymphocytes. In applying techniques based on these characteristics to quantitation of lymphocytes and in interpreting the results so achieved, it is necessary to understand that the expression of surface markers is subject to continual changes, as it depends on metabolic activities of the cells. Therefore, these techniques are not foolproof and, in fact, much variability may be seen among different laboratories engaged in lymphocyte quantitation using the same protocols.

Enumeration of B Cells. The markers used to detect B cells are surface immunoglobulins, receptors for Fc portions of IgG, receptors for the activated third component of complement, and B-cell specific antigens (Table 34–2). The methodology for each of these assays is currently subject to considerable refinement, so that it is difficult to select one general method applicable to all laboratories and all clinical situations. With this in mind, the methods outlined below will include brief descriptions of those assays that are most reliable and most widely used.

Detection of Surface Immunoglobulins. The principle of this method is based on quantitative detection of immunoglobulins on the cell surface of B cells other than mature plasma cells using antisera specific for the heavy chain or the light chain classes of human immunoglobulins. Quantitation is possible by labeling these antisera with compounds such as fluorescein or rhodamine and counting positively stained lymphocytes (Fig. 34–5).

Clearly, it is necessary that the antisera be highly specific and that they be adequately labeled. When commercial reagents are used, it is essential that the specificity of antisera be checked against reliable standards, as described on page 000. Such standards include myeloma cells or beads to which are coupled well characterized myeloma proteins. Specificity can then be ascertained by agglutination of erythrocytes coated with the immunoglobulin, staining of coated beads, or inhibition of staining of lymphocyte surface (Aiuti, 1974).

Precautions must be taken to wash the cells adequately so as to remove serum components adsorbed to their cell surfaces by virtue of the Fc receptors. Several methods have been proposed to determine which cells truly synthesize surface Ig and, therefore, by definition are B cells. Cells may be incubated overnight after controlled trypsinization of the cell to remove all surface immunoglobulins without injury to the cell. The cells are allowed to incubate in serum-free medium for periods of 6 to 24 hours to permit resynthesis of surface immunoglobulins (Rowlands, 1974; Lobo, 1975).

Immunofluorescent assay involves incubation of washed

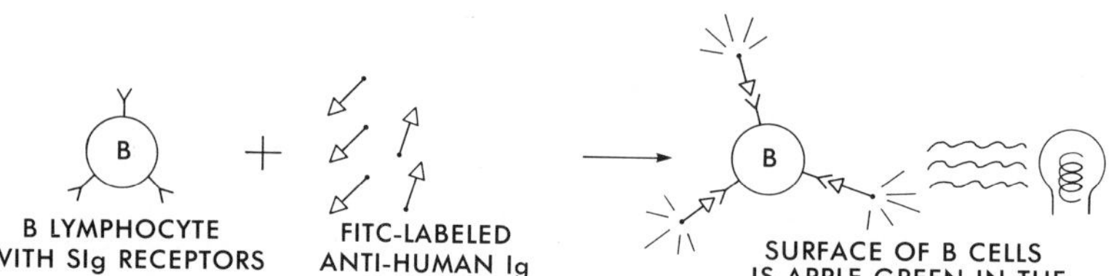

Figure 34–5. Appropriately labeled antibodies to human immunoglobulins can react with surfaces of B lymphocytes and are then detected by fluorescence.

Table 34–5. DISTRIBUTION OF SURFACE MARKERS ON LYMPHOCYTES ISOLATED FROM NORMAL CONTROLS AND PATIENTS WITH LYMPHOPROLIFERATIVE DISEASES*

Surface Marker	Normal Blood	Normal Lymph Node	Leukemia (CLL)	Malignant Node (PDLL-N)
IgG	3	12	2	54
A	2	8	1	4
M	12	16	80	60
D	10	14	75	10
K	8	20	83	63
λ	5	11	1	2
E	68	70	10	34
EAC	25	30	30	50
EA	14	16	12	4

*Data from representative cases. Monocytes were not removed from the peripheral blood. Figures are expressed as % of positive cells.

and/or trypsinized lymphocytes with fluoresceinated monospecific antisera at 4°C. for 30 minutes (sodium azide may aid in preventing capping). A fluorescence microscope with epi-illumination is necessary to enumeration of the stained lymphocytes. It is recommended that monospecific antibodies to the various heavy and light chains rather than a polyvalent serum be used for quantitations. This allows for enumeration of B cells bearing different immunoglobulin classes and of lambda- and kappa-positive cells. Since the proportions of cells expressing different immunoglobulins may deviate from normal in disease, such enumeration may be clinically important. It has been suggested that the fluoresceinated F(ab')$_2$ fragments of monospecific antisera be used to avoid binding of these reagents to B cells through the Fc portions of their heavy chains (Winchester, 1975). This precaution seems to be particularly necessary when cells obtained from neoplasma are evaluated. All antisera used for enumerations of B cells must be checked for monospecificity by established immunologic procedures and must be centrifugated (100,000 g) immediately prior to staining to remove aggregates that may have high binding affinity for the Fc receptors. Conventional and especially monoclonal anti-Ig sera must be titered with normal human lymphocytes to avoid nonspecific staining. Table 34–5 shows the distribution of normal immunoglobulin-bearing (SIg$^+$) cells in human blood and selected lymphoid tissues.

There seems to be considerable variation in the literature with regard to the relative proportion of SIg$^+$ cells detected in the human peripheral blood (range 10 to 20 per cent or more). In more recent studies, fewer SIg$^+$ cells are detected, undoubtedly reflecting the increased specificity of commercially available antisera and improved measures of eliminating exogenous Ig. It is essential that individual laboratories establish their own lymphocyte panels to serve as normal controls. When peripheral blood lymphocytes are studied with regard to SIg, each of the major immunoglobulin classes can be identified on these cells. However, the dominant classes of immunoglobulins are likely to be IgM and IgD, and the normal ratio of k+/λ+ cells is 2/1. In disease states, these proportions may change (Table 34–5).

Detection of Fc Receptors. The receptors for Fc portions of immunoglobulins can be detected using immunomicroscopy or rosetting techniques. The former is an exact duplicate of the method outlined above, except that labeled aggregated human IgG is used in place of anti-immunoglobulin. There are several rosetting techniques available for detection of Fc receptors, all based on the principle that antibodies of the IgG class, when placed on the surface of an erythrocyte, present their altered Fc portions to those cells that carry appropriate receptors. These cells bind to the antibody-coated erythrocytes (Fig. 34–6), forming easily recognizable rosettes. The number of EA rosettes formed by lymphoid cells depends on many factors, such as purity of the antibody used to coat the erythrocytes. The spatial orientation and concentration of Fc receptors for IgG vary among lymphoid cells. For example, as mentioned previously, a subpopulation of lymphocytes (L cells) with Fc receptors that are resistant to digestion with trypsin and that have a high affinity for altered Ig has been identified in the human peripheral blood (Fig. 34–7). These L cells apparently do not synthesize immunoglobulin, do not have the E receptor for sheep erythrocytes, and are non-adherent and non-phagocytic. The precise functional role of these cells remains to be determined (Lobo, 1976). They may interfere with assays for SIg$^+$ cells, giving spuriously high values unless the precautions described earlier (i.e., incubation in the absence of autologous serum or controlled trypsinization) are employed.

It is apparent that the Fc receptors for Ig are not specific for B cells. For example, a subpopulation of T lymphocytes (TG or T$_\gamma$ cells) is known to express the Fc receptors for IgG under normal circumstances. Another subpopulation of

5

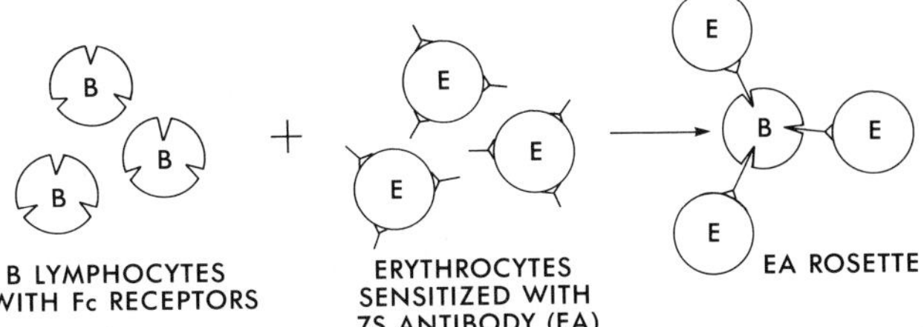

Figure 34–6. B cells when mixed with antibody-coated erythrocytes form rosettes.

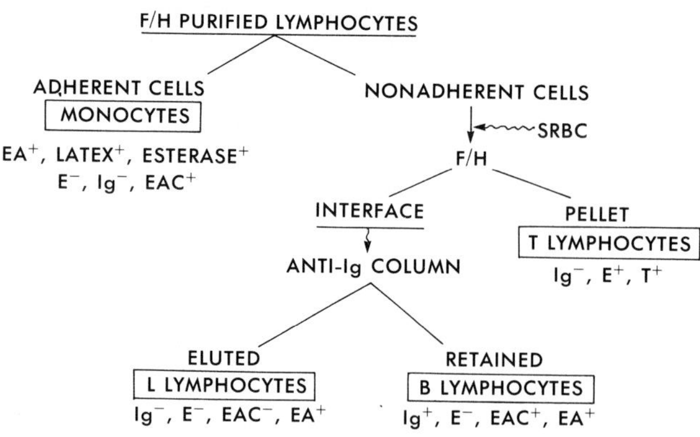

Figure 34–7. The diagram represents the ways in which cell surface properties may be used to separate and categorize subsets of human B and T lymphocytes.

T lymphocytes has surface receptors for IgM (Tm or Tμ cells). Activated T lymphocytes acquire the ability to bind IgG on their surface (Mingari, 1982). The Fc receptors for IgG also occur on a variety of non-lymphoid cells, including many tissue cells.

Detection of Complement Receptors. Complement receptors are detectable on many different cell types, including lymphocytes and monocytes. Those on B cells may be of at least two types. One recognizes the C3d and the other the C3b fragment of C3. A rosetting method employing sheep erythrocytes sensitized with subagglutinating amounts of anti-SRBC antibody and with components of complement (EAC) is used for detection of cells bearing receptors for C3 (Fig. 34–8).

Two systems have been used to detect B lymphocytes with complement receptors (Ross, 1973). In one, mouse complement is used. This has the advantage of detecting both C3d and C3b. An alternative technique using human complement requires multiple incubation steps for the preparation of indicator cells. These are prepared by coating sheep red blood cells first with subagglutinating concentrations of anti-SRBC serum, followed by incubation with purified human C1, C4, C2, and C3 in that order.

The mean value for EAC-positive lymphocytes in the circulation of healthy adults is 15 per cent (range of 10 to 19 per cent), but this figure varies among laboratories, and it is essential for each laboratory to establish its own normal mean and range.

Certain general requirements apply to this and other rosetting techniques. Thus, a lymphocyte reacting with three or more indicator cells forms a rosette; at least 200 lymphocytes must be counted to determine a proportion of rosetting cells; since cells other than lymphocytes have C3 and Fc receptors, lymphocytes must be purified prior to rosetting; trypsinization of SRBC prior to sensitization is recommended to avoid errors due to spontaneous rosette formation; a subagglutinating dose must be determined for each batch of antierythrocyte serum; controls with E and EA coated with 7S and 19S antibody are required. The foregoing serves to emphasize that rosetting techniques, although simple in principle, are technically demanding.

Detection of B-Cell Antigens. Although heteroantisera to human B cell antigens have been prepared for research purposes in several laboratories, the recent commercial availability of murine monoclonal antibodies makes this technique well suited for clinical purposes. Table 34–3 lists several of these antibodies. They can be obtained labeled with fluorescein for direct immunofluorescence or unlabeled for more sensitive two-step procedures. Like all monoclonal reagents, these have to be titered for optimal staining. The details of a staining procedure are the same for T and B cells and the enumeration of cells reactive with the antibody can be done using a fluorescent microscope or a laser cytofluorometer. Malignant B lymphocytes may express different surface antigens than normal B cells.

Enumeration of T Cells. Like B cells, human T lympho-

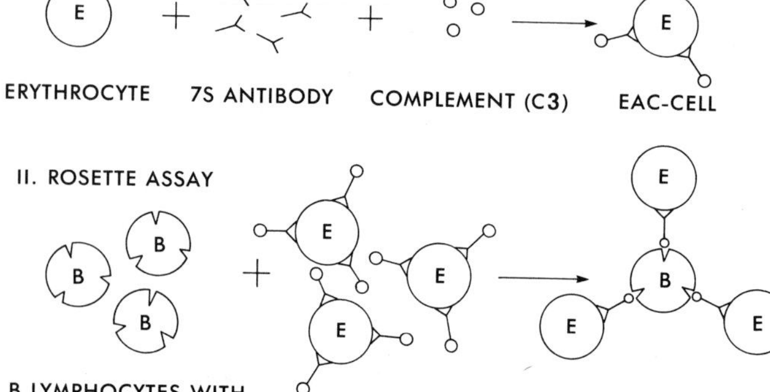

Figure 34–8. B cells can be detected by rosette formation using sheep erythrocytes which have been treated with appropriate antibody and complement.

cytes can be identified and counted in suspensions of mononuclear cells by virtue of certain surface receptors (Table 34–2).

E Rosette Formation. T cells are capable of forming spontaneous rosettes with unmodified sheep erythrocytes (E). The T-rosette assay is simple and thus accessible to all clinical laboratories. It calls for washed lymphocytes and washed SRBC (E) in a 1 per cent suspension to be mixed and centrifuged briefly (Fig. 34–9). The critical factor in this assay is the ratio of sheep cells to lymphocytes. It has been recommended that a ratio of 50:1 or 100:1 be used for optimal results (Aiuti, 1974). The tube is then placed in a refrigerator (4°C.) for at least 16 hours. Resuspended cells are then examined in a hemocytometer to determine the proportion of rosetting cells.

The E rosette assay is reproducible only if performed under carefully controlled conditions, as many factors may affect E rosette formation. The percentages of E rosettes in normal human peripheral blood range from 60 to 80 per cent, depending on the laboratory. Normal controls must always be included. Modifications that have been described undoubtedly measure different subpopulations of T lymphocytes. The best known modification consists of mixing SRBC with lymphocytes only for a brief period during centrifugation and measures "active E rosettes." The latter are formed by subpopulations of T cells which have "high affinity" receptors for SRBC and which may be altered in number or in their capacity to rosette with SRBC in disease states. Thus, both the determination of total T rosettes (long-term incubation 4°C.) and active E rosettes (brief incubation) may be clinically significant. Approximately 25 per cent of human blood lymphocytes form active E rosettes. It has been suggested that enumeration of active E rosettes is more sensitive in detecting defects in T cell function than is measurement of total T cells.

Little is known about the nature of the T rosette phenomenon. Recent experiments indicate that the binding of SRBC to human T cells represents a receptor-ligand interaction rather than a non-specific electrical charge event. The receptor for SRBC appears to be a protein which can be isolated by controlled enzymatic proteolysis from the surfaces of T lymphocytes.

Detection of T-Cell Specific Antigens. With monoclonal antibodies directed to individual glycoproteins in surfaces of T lymphocytes, it is now possible to distinguish T lymphocyte subpopulations which bear unique T cell determinants. Table 34–3 provides a partial list of murine monoclonal antibodies useful in enumerating T cells and their subpopulations. These reagents must be titered for optimal activity, with dilutions of 1:50 usually being satisfactory. Appropriately diluted fluoresceinated antibodies (50 μl) can then be incubated with 50 μl of lymphocytes (5×10^6 cells/ml) for 30 minutes at 4°C. The antibody-treated cells are then washed ×2 in PBS and analyzed. In indirect immunofluorescence, fluoresceinated antibody against mouse immunoglobulin is used as second reagent at a predetermined dilution. This reagent should be centrifuged immediately prior to use. Incubation is carried out for 30 minutes at 4°C. and is followed by two washes in PBS at 4°C. Cells are resuspended in 0.5 ml of PBS and examined. Although the usual fluorescent microscope may be used for analysis, automated laser flow cytometers generally yield better and more consistent results. This is largely a reflection of their capability to detect low levels of fluorescence and to screen many hundreds of thousands of cells in a very short time.

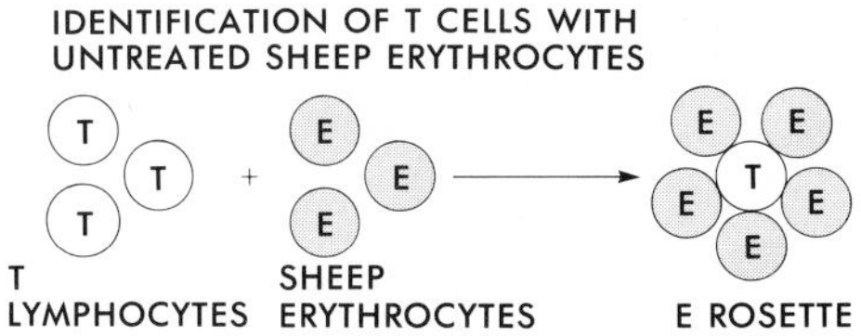

IDENTIFICATION OF T CELLS WITH UNTREATED SHEEP ERYTHROCYTES

T LYMPHOCYTES + SHEEP ERYTHROCYTES → E ROSETTE

Figure 34–9. Human T cells can be detected by rosette formation using untreated sheep erythrocytes.

Determination of Ia-Like Antigens on Lymphocytes. Detailed analysis of the major histocompatibility locus in mice shows a distinct and now well-defined association with Ia (immune associated) antigens. A similar association has been defined in man. Monoclonal antibodies (see above) may be used for their detection. Ia-like antigens are expressed on human B cells, activated T cells, some NK cells, and certain non-lymphoid cells—namely, monocytes and endothelial cells.

Determination of Lymphocytes in Tissue Sections. Immunologic techniques that have been used in recent years for studies of lymphocytes *in situ* included immunofluorescence and immunoperoxidase with conventional antibodies to cell surface antigens (immunomicroscopy) and rosetting in tissue using untreated or antibody-coated indicator cells. Recent development of highly sensitive immunohistologic techniques allows for phenotyping of lymphocytes in tissue with monoclonal antibodies on frozen sections. The commercial availability of monoclonal antibodies to surface and intracellular antigens on lymphoid cells and introduction of avidin-biotin–amplified enzyme staining provide a highly sensitive and simple way of characterizing lymphocytes in tissues and of determining their localization and interrelationships with other cells. In addition, this approach allows for maximal preservation of architectural integrity of tissues.

Immunomicroscopy. To detect and subtype T and B lymphocytes in tissues by immunomicroscopy, a requirement for specific reagents must be met. Generally, it is not enough to use one monoclonal antibody, especially with pathologic specimens. It is advisable to use a carefully chosen panel of reagents in which different antigenic specificities are represented by two or three monoclonal antibodies. The second requirement is for tissue preparation such that it does not destroy or denature those antigens on the surfaces of lymphocytes that are recognized by monoclonal antibodies used for typing. Most cell surface antigens on lymphocytes do not survive routine fixation and embedding that are needed for the immunoperoxidase method. Frozen sections, on the other hand, offer good preservation of both surface and intracytoplasmic lymphocyte antigens. The third requirement for successful phenotyping is for freshly harvested or appropriately preserved biopsy material. Tissues must be embedded in OCT media and frozen in a cryostat immediately after surgery, or they may be stored frozen in liquid nitrogen.

The ABC or avidin-biotin-peroxidase complex method uses avidin to bridge antibody labeled with biotin and biotinylated enzyme (e.g., peroxidase), as illustrated in Figures 34–10 and 34–11. Avidin, an egg-white protein, has a very high affinity for biotin, and it amplifies the immunologic reaction to achieve the sensitivity necessary for detection of sparse surface antigens.

The procedure, performed on frozen, air-dried, and acetone-fixed sections, involves sequential incubations with (1) primary antibody, which is either monoclonal or conventional and specific for an antigen in tissue; (2) secondary antibody labeled with biotin; (3) avidin-biotin-peroxidase complex; (4) chromogen to develop enzymatic reaction; and (5) hematoxylin to counterstain the tissue (Hsu, 1981). Immunostained cells develop a red-brown color corresponding to the reaction product on their cell membranes. Staining can be completed in two hours, and all reagents

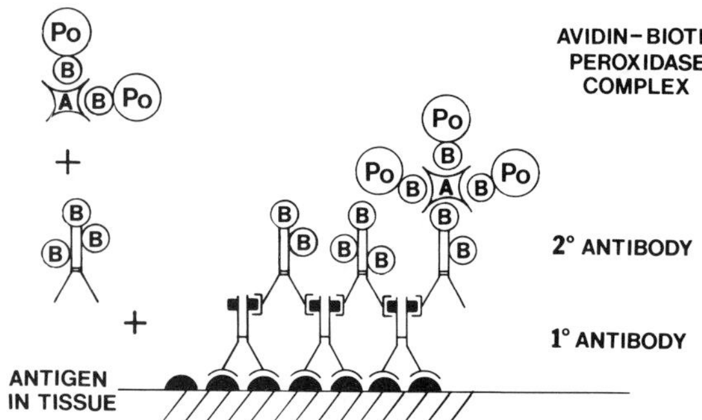

Figure 34–10. The avidin-biotin-peroxidase complex technique. The primary antibody is specific for the antigen in tissue. The secondary antibody is labeled with biotin. The complex of avidin–biotin–horseradish peroxidase is commercially available.

are commercially available. Embedded tissues or sections can be stored in a freezer for months and stained when convenient. Different chromogens may be used to develop the color. Endogenous avidin-binding activity that exists in tissues such as liver, kidney, breast, and adipose tissues, all of which are rich in biotin, can be blocked by incubating the sections with avidin, then flushing them with biotin prior to treatment with a primary antibody. Lymphoid tissues have little endogenous biotin and do not require blocking.

Rosetting Methods. Rosetting techniques used for detection of T and B lymphocytes can be performed on cryostat tissue sections as well as in cellular suspensions (Fig. 34–12). Rosetting in tissue is laborious and has largely been superseded by the IF or ABC techniques utilizing monoclonal antibodies. Indicator cells (E, EA, and EAC) prepared for the enumeration of lymphocytes in suspensions may be used on air-dried, unfixed tissue sections under carefully controlled conditions.

The methods for enumerations of T and B lymphocytes that we chose to present here can, at this time, be applied in a clinical laboratory with a fair degree of success. It is essential to bear in mind, however, that there is much we do not understand about surface properties of lymphocytes, that there may be overlaps in surface markers between T and B lymphocytes or lymphocytes and other mononuclear

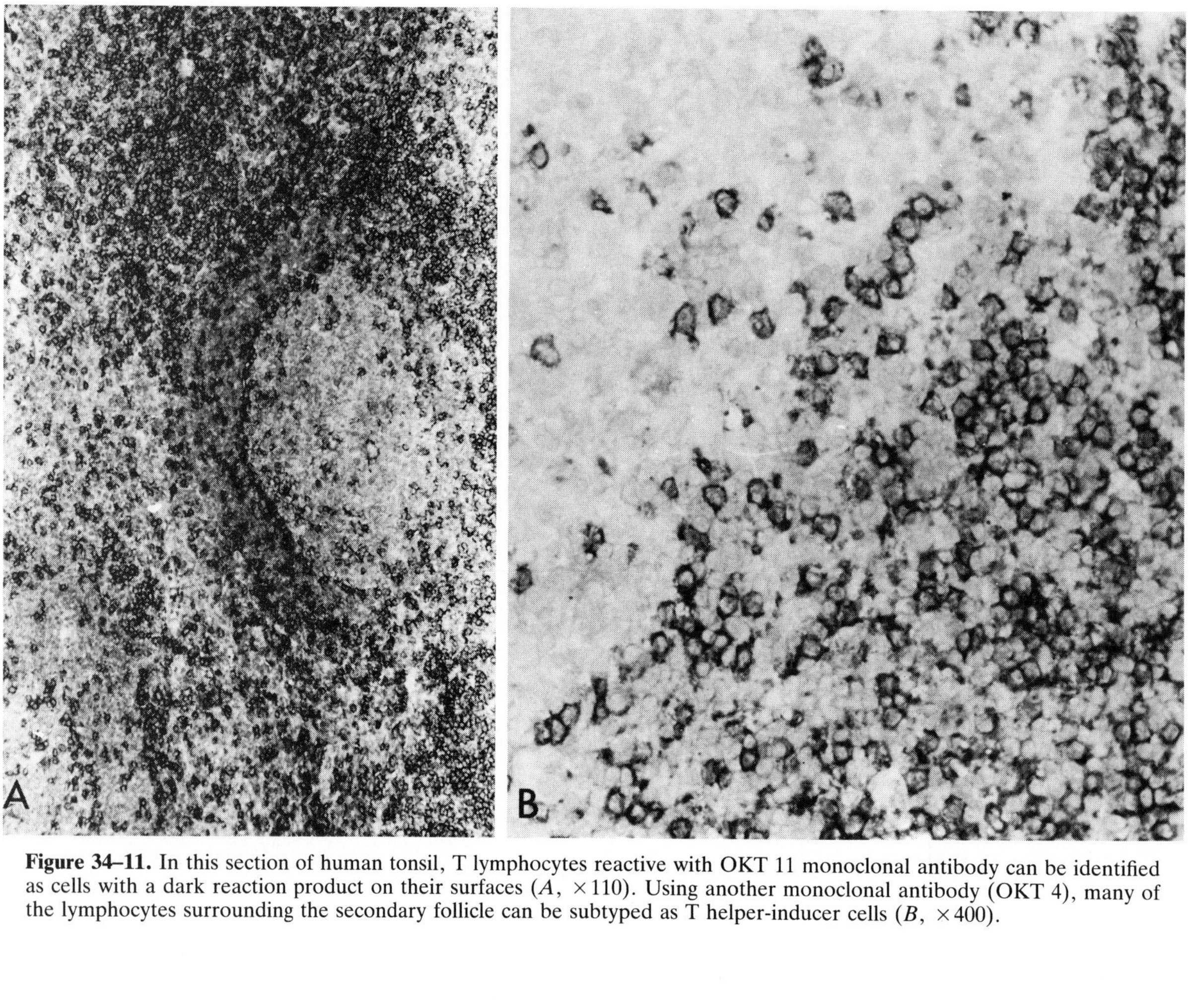

Figure 34–11. In this section of human tonsil, T lymphocytes reactive with OKT 11 monoclonal antibody can be identified as cells with a dark reaction product on their surfaces (*A*, ×110). Using another monoclonal antibody (OKT 4), many of the lymphocytes surrounding the secondary follicle can be subtyped as T helper-inducer cells (*B*, ×400).

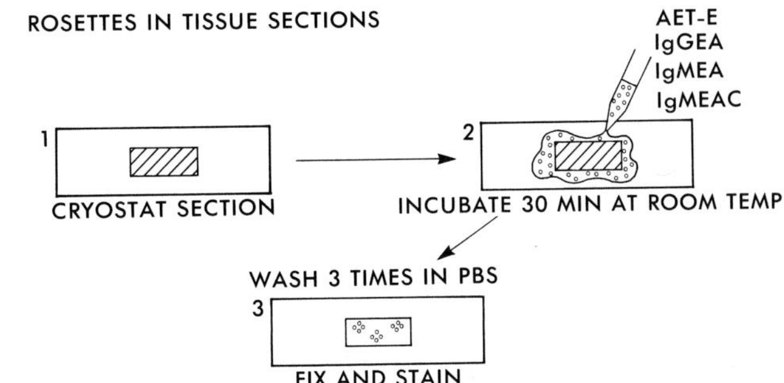

Figure 34–12. Cryostat tissue sections when incubated with various erythrocyte preparations show rosette formation.

cells, and that a judicious interpretation of results requires proper controls, must be performed in the light of clinical facts, and calls for a highly trained and experienced interpreter.

Methods for Separation of Lymphocyte Populations

Adaptations of nearly all of the techniques described so far can be applied to separations and isolations of individual subpopulations of lymphocytes. For example, using rosetting and Ficoll-Hypaque gradients, E-positive lymphocytes can be centrifuged and recovered in a pellet, leaving the non-E rosetting population at the gradient interface. This latter population can in turn be rosetted with EA or EAC indicator cells, so that EA- or EAC-positive lymphoid cells, respectively, are recovered following gradient centrifugation. Other techniques frequently utilize differential adherence of lymphocytes to various solid surfaces coated with antibodies or to appropriately charged columns as well as cytotoxic potentials of selective antilymphocyte sera in the presence of complement. Table 34–6 lists those separation techniques that have been most widely used. It is essential to monitor cells undergoing separation procedures for their surface characteristics in order to quantitate the recovered subpopulations and estimate their purity. Figure 34–7 further illustrates how surface properties of lymphocytes may be used for the separation of different lymphocyte subpopulations.

Newer technology utilizing lasers and monoclonal antibodies permits separation of specific subpopulations of mononuclear cells. This cell sorting technology is largely suitable for analytical purposes rather than preparative needs and is, at present, not likely to be available in the average clinical laboratory. A more widely adaptable technique for preparing lymphocyte subpopulations is the so-called "panning." It utilizes monoclonal reagents adsorbed to a plastic plate for selective removal of cells reactive with the monoclonal reagents.

Measurement of Functional Capacities of Lymphocytes

Functional properties of lymphocytes, such as *in vitro* responsiveness to mitogens, soluble antigens, allogeneic cells, and abilities to produce immunoglob-

Table 34–6. METHODS FOR SEPARATION OF HUMAN LYMPHOCYTE SUBPOPULATIONS ON THE BASIS OF CELL SURFACE PROPERTIES

Method of Separation	Way of Recovery	Lymphocyte Subpopulation
I. Rosetting followed by gradient centrifugation*	In the pellet	E EA EAC
	In the interface	Unrosetted cells
II. Immunoadsorbent column charged with		
(a) anti-Ig	Retained	SIg^+
	Eluted	SIg^-
(b) anti-T cell	Retained	T cells
	Eluted	B, L, null cells
III. "Panning" on plates coated with		
(a) anti-Ig or anti-B cell	On the plate	B cells
	In suspension	T and L cells
(b) anti-T cell	On the plate	T cells
	In suspension	B and L cells
IV. Adherence to glass, nylon, wool, etc.	Adherent	B cells
	Nonadherent	T and L cells
V. Cytotoxicity with anti-lymphocyte sera and complement:		
(a) anti-B cell	Not killed	T, null, L cells
(b) anti-T cell	Not killed	B, null, L cells
(c) anti-null cell	Not killed	T, B, L cells

*The unrosetted cells from the interface of Ficoll-Hypaque gradients can be rosetted again and separated further on another gradient.

Table 34–7. FUNCTIONAL PROPERTIES OF THE LYMPHOCYTE SUBPOPULATIONS ISOLATED FROM HUMAN PERIPHERAL BLOOD

	T cells	B cells	L cells*	T+B	T+L
In vitro proliferation:					
Mitogen					
PHA	+++	+	−	++++	++++
Con A	++	+	−	++++	++++
PWM	+	++	−	++++	+
MLC					
Stimulator	+	++++	+		
Responder	++++	+	−		
Antigens	++	+	−	++++	++++
PWM-induced Ig synthesis	−	+	−	++++	−
Antibody-dependent cytotoxicity	−	+	++++		

*Some investigators designate these as K cells.

ulins or lymphokines and to effect cell mediated or antibody-dependent cytotoxicity, may be used for identification and, to a certain extent, for quantitative purposes. Some of these *in vitro* assays require unusually sophisticated equipment and thus are not accessible to a majority of clinical laboratories. Still, these assays are necessary for an accurate appraisal of the immune status in man, because it is the functional competence of lymphocytes, not their number, that ultimately determines immune responsiveness. We wish to emphasize, however, that the functional *in vitro* assays may not always reflect the *in vivo* situation at hand. For example, a normal *in vitro* response to an antigen (e.g., mumps) does not necessarily mean that the responsive lymphocytes are immunologically competent *in vivo*. Many factors in the body (serum components, cellular products, enzymes, inhibitors, hormones) may influence functional capabilities of lymphocytes. Until better correlations are established between various *in vitro* assays and *in vivo* responsiveness, their clinical significance must remain limited. None of the *in vitro* assays mentioned earlier can, at this time, be recommended as the best functional assay; we do not know whether lymphocytes secreting lymphokines or effecting cell-mediated cytotoxicity *in vitro* can do the same *in vivo* and how important these functions may be in any one biologic reaction mediated by lymphocytes *in vivo*. Functional properties of lymphocyte subpopulations isolated from normal peripheral blood may be tested by procedures similar to those listed in Table 34–7.

Lymphocyte Proliferation. Responses to soluble plant lectins—in particular phytohemagglutinin (PHA) and concanavalin A (Con A)—are thought to measure a functional potential of human T cells and have been widely used. These mitogens can be particularly useful probes of T cell function, since T cells which respond to antigens may represent less than 1 per cent of the T cells employed in the *in vitro* culture, whereas as many as 50 to 60 per cent of the T cells will respond to PHA and Con A. Furthermore, a number of *in vitro* studies have established that mitogen responsiveness is fundamentally similar to antigen responses and may be used as a model of antigen stimulation (Greaves, 1972).

The principle of mitogenic stimulations is illustrated in Figure 34–13. The stimulation index gives a semi-quantitative measure of the response. Normal controls must be run simultaneously with a patient's lymphocytes. It is necessary to stimulate lymphocytes at several different concentrations of PHA, because optimal response is often concentration dependent. Three- and seven-day incubations

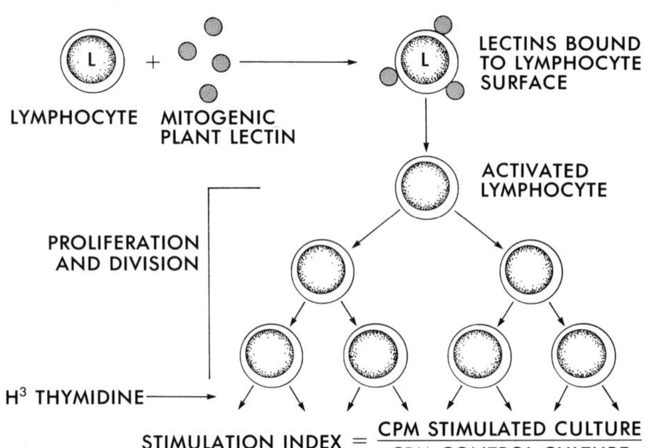

Figure 34–13. Lymphocytes may be stimulated into proliferation by antigens, allogeneic lymphocytes, or nonspecific lectins. The response to allogeneic lymphocytes is called the mixed lymphocyte culture (MLC).

are necessary because normal cells respond optimally on day 3, while the peak response may be delayed in disease. Extreme care must be taken in evaluating these responses to avoid misinterpretation of dilutional effects. For example, when cells from patients with CLL were stimulated with PHA, delayed responses were observed and thought to be caused by defective T cells in these patients. However, when the technique was modified to measure the number of cells going into mitosis as a function of time by adding colchicine at the start of the culture and H^3 thymidine two hours before its termination, it appeared that the T cells from CLL patients were functionally normal (Rowlands, 1974). Thus, the poor proliferative response to T cell mitogens in patients with CLL appears to be due to a reduction in the number of responsive T cells and concomitant increase in neoplastic B cells.

The example of PHA stimulation illustrates the difficulties inherent in all assays of functional properties of lymphocytes, interpretation being the key. To complicate matters, it now appears that certain B cells, in addition to subpopulations of T cells, are responsive to PHA and Con A. It is noteworthy, however, that when lymphocyte responses are measured at their peak, for example, at three or four days, the responding lymphocytes are almost entirely T cells (Greaves, 1972). Significant B cell proliferation appears to occur later in the proliferative response, at some time between five and seven days. Con A probably stimulates a different subpopulation of T lymphocytes than does PHA, and pokeweed mitogen (PWM), formerly considered primarily a B cell mitogen, activates both T and B cells. Human lymphocytes do not proliferate in response to endotoxin or antihuman Fab. It is now held that T lymphocytes are primarily responsible for specific antigen-mediated proliferations. Fractionations of lymphocytes and removal of different lymphocytic and monocytic subpopulations seem to affect *in vitro* responses to mitogens and/or antigens, and contributions of the different fractions to full-scale *in vitro* responses are now being evaluated. For example, optimal responses to both mitogens and antigens may require the presence of monocytes or factors produced by monocytes.

Allogeneic stimulation, also known as mixed lymphocyte culture (MLC), has been widely employed in clinical laboratories in histocompatibility testing preceding transplantations (Chap. 33). If lymphocytes from two individuals differ at the genetically determined HLA-D locus, they will stimulate each other into proliferation under optimal culture conditions. By preventing one set of lymphocytes from division by irradiation or treatment with mitomycin C, it may be determined whether they act as stimulators or responders in this system. When the kidney recipient's lymphocytes respond by proliferation to the donor's lymphocytes, chronic rejection of the kidney graft may be anticipated. In contrast, in bone marrow transplantations, where graft versus host rejections are the danger, proliferation of the donor's lymphocytes in response to the recipient's indicates poor prognosis. The lack of response in MLC indicates compatibility at the D locus.

Cytotoxicity. Cytotoxicity assays measure the capabilities of lymphocytes to kill target cells in reactions not involving complement. Three types of lymphocytotoxicity are recognized: (1) Cell-mediated lympholysis (CML), in which cytotoxic, specifically sensitized T lymphocytes may be shown to release radioactive chromium from the labeled target tissue (Cerottini, 1974). CML is an energy-dependent process which requires direct contact between a target cell and cytotoxic T lymphocytes (Fig. 34–14). (2) Antibody-dependent lympholysis mediated by cells with high-avidity Fc receptors called K (killer) cells (Cerottini, 1974; Perlmann, 1975). The K cell recognizes and reacts with antibody coating the target cell, so that the specificity of this cytotoxic reaction is determined by the anti-target antibody (Fig. 34–15). (3) Cytotoxicity mediated not by cells but by cellular products of these cells. A variety of such products are known to be released by activated lymphocytes, and they are collectively labeled as lymphocytotoxins because of their injurious effects on cells. The biologic importance of these cytotoxic reactions is not clear, although there is some

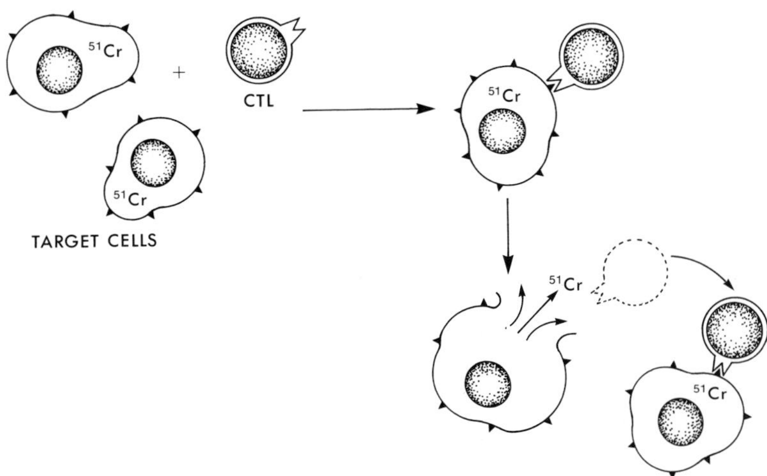
CELL-MEDIATED CYTOLYSIS IN WHICH SPECIFICALLY IMMUNIZED CYTOTOXIC T LYMPHOCYTES (CTL) INTERACT DIRECTLY WITH TARGET CELLS. THE QUANTITATIVE ASSAY MEASURES ⁵¹Cr RELEASE FROM ⁵¹Cr-LABELED TARGET CELLS FOLLOWING THE INCUBATION OF TARGET CELLS WITH THE APPROPRIATE NUMBER OF CTL'S. ONE CTL MAY KILL MORE THAN ONE TARGET CELL.
51Cr
+
CTL
51Cr
51Cr
TARGET CELLS
51Cr
51Cr

Figure 34–14. Cell-mediated cytolysis is produced when cytotoxic T cells interact with appropriate target cells. Cytotoxicity is evidenced by release of ^{51}Cr from labeled target cells.

5

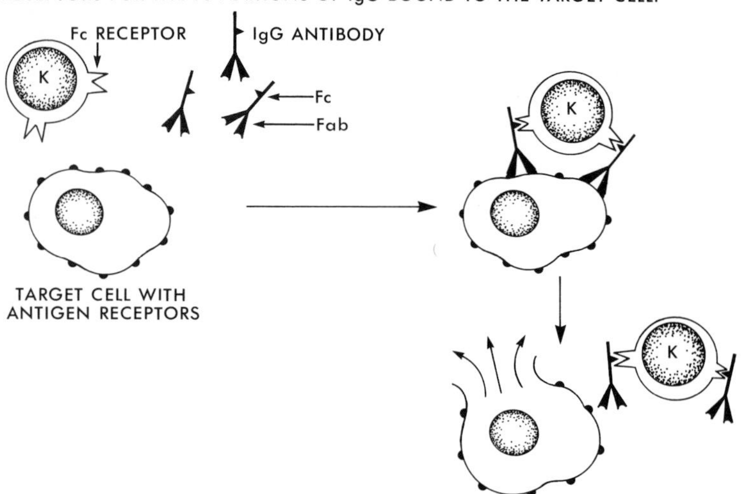
ANTIBODY-DEPENDENT CYTOLYSIS. INTERACTION BETWEEN THE K CELL AND TARGET CELL IS MEDIATED BY THE IgG ANTIBODY WITH SPECIFICITY DIRECTED TO AN ANTIGEN ON THE TARGET CELL SURFACE. K CELL HAS HIGH-AFFINITY RECEPTORS FOR THE Fc PORTIONS OF IgG BOUND TO THE TARGET CELL.
Fc RECEPTOR
IgG ANTIBODY
K
Fc
Fab
TARGET CELL WITH ANTIGEN RECEPTORS

Figure 34–15. Antibody-dependent cytolysis results when a K cell having high affinity receptors for Fc portions of Ig binds to target cells through associated IgG antibodies.

evidence that CML may play particularly significant roles in allogeneic transplant systems and in viral infections. The presence of naturally occurring cytotoxic cells has been correlated with defense against syngeneic tumors in the mouse. These so-called natural killer cells are similar to K or L cells.

Lymphocyte Products. Lymphocytes activated by mitogens or antigens release a variety of substances (Table 34–8), some of which are antigen specific. Quantitative *in vitro* assays for synthesis of immunoglobulins by isolated human lymphocytes have been developed (Choi, 1977; Hannam-Harris, 1980). Human B and T cells are cultured in a medium containing labeled amino acids and the stimulator concentration of PWM. The B cells which differentiate into immunoglobulin-synthesizing plasma cells can be estimated morphologically, and/or labeled immunoglobulins in the culture supernatant can be quantitated using immunoprecipitation with anti-Ig sera. If radiolabeling is not convenient, other techniques, including a solid phase radioimmunoassay or a reverse hemolytic plaque assay (Gronowicz, 1976), are available for quantitating the number of Ig secreting cells. The T cells play a regulatory role in this system by either helping the B cells in carrying on Ig synthesis or, under certain conditions, suppressing this synthesis.

Table 34–8. A PARTIAL LISTING OF SOLUBLE FACTORS RELEASED BY ACTIVATED LYMPHOCYTES

MIF	Macrophage inhibition factor
MAF	Macrophage activating factor
MCF	Macrophage chemotactic factor
BF	Blastogenic factor
TF	Transfer factor
PF	Permeability factor
ECF	Eosinophil chemotactic factor
LTF	Lymphocytotoxic factor
NCF	Neutrophil chemotactic factor
LIF	Leukocyte inhibition factor
CIF	Cloning inhibition factor
I	Interferon
SRF	Skin reactive factor
TCGF	T cell growth factor or IL-2

The production of lymphokines affords another way of estimating responsiveness of lymphocytes to external stimuli. As illustrated in Figure 34–16, only lymphocytes presensitized to an antigen are capable of elaborating the soluble factors when exposed to this antigen *in vitro*. Lymphokines are recognized by their effect on other cells, e.g., macrophages, whose migration they inhibit. The quantitative *in vitro* assay (migration inhibition factor [MIF] assay, Fig. 34–16) was developed to measure the release of certain lymphokines by lymphocytes isolated from the peripheral blood. The assay is laborious, technically demanding, and time consuming. As such, it does not lend itself to clinical situations, and various simplified versions, such as the leukocyte migration inhibition microdroplet technique, are used instead. Recently, attempts have been made to standardize this assay for clinical use, and to make available a standard lymphokine preparation so that "quantitative" LIF can be performed (Hamblin, 1982). Studies indicate that in certain diseases neither the LIF assay nor its modifications correlate with other *in vitro* assays of cell-mediated immunity, with *in vivo* skin tests, or with clinical observations. It has been established that B cells, as well as T cells, are capable of producing MIF after stimulation with antigens and mitogens (Rocklin, 1974).

Skin Tests. These assay the ability of the patient's lymphocytes to recognize and respond *in vivo* to an antigen. Unlike the *in vitro* procedures discussed earlier, intradermal skin tests offer an opportunity to determine a delayed hypersensitivity response in the presence of all inhibitory or stimulatory factors that are present in the body but not in a test tube. Delayed hypersensitivity skin tests are valuable in the overall assessment of immunocompetence. Delayed hypersensitivity skin tests should be the first assay performed when cell-mediated immunity is being assessed. Inability of the skin to react to a battery of common antigens to which the subject could have been expected to be exposed is termed anergy. Antigens included in such a battery may vary and should include at least five antigens, e.g., PPD, Candida, mumps, streptokinase-streptodornase, Trichophyton. A skin's response to antigens to which lymphocytes in

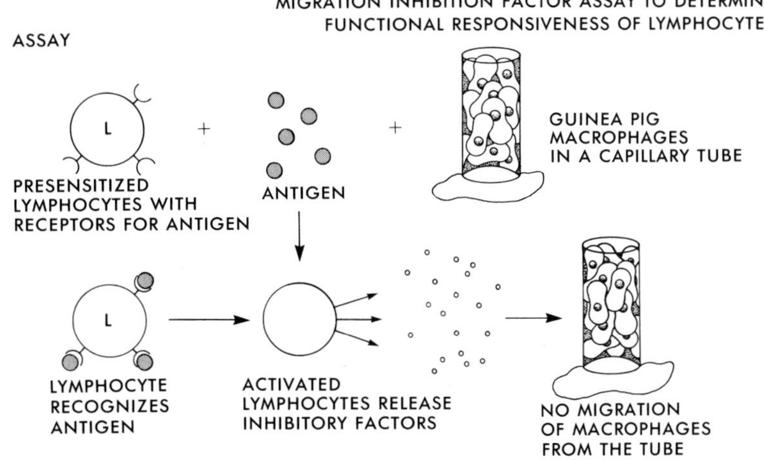

Figure 34–16. Interaction of appropriate antigen and lymphocytes causes release of MIF, which alters the migration of macrophages from a capillary tube.

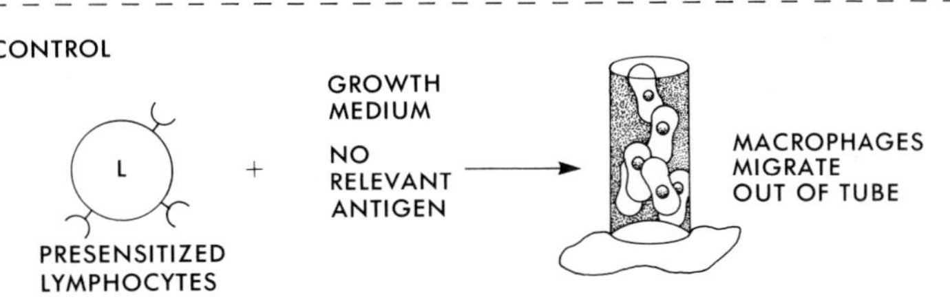

$$\text{PER CENT MIGRATION INHIBITION} = 1 - \frac{\text{MIGRATION AREA WITH ANTIGEN}}{\text{MIGRATION AREA OF CONTROL}} \times 100$$

a healthy adult are likely to be sensitized must be distinguished from a response to new antigens such as DNCB (dinitrochlorobenzene). The former skin test estimates immunologic memory and the ability to mount an immune response, while the latter measures the ability to mount an immune response following sensitization with a new antigen. Skin tests with DNCB appear to give a better estimate of immunocompetence than those with recall antigens. The DNCB skin test requires local sensitization with the chemical, followed 10 to 14 days later by a challenge dose applied to the skin surface.

Delayed hypersensitivity skin tests are read 24 to 48 hours following intradermal injection of the antigens. The diameter of an area of induration is an index of cutaneous hypersensitivity, and it must equal or exceed 5 mm for the test to be positive. Negative response to a preliminary (low) dose of an antigen should always be confirmed by testing with higher concentrations of the same antigen. Also, negative responses indicate anergy only if the patient's inflammatory response (which is a component of a delayed hypersensitivity reaction) is unimpaired. Rebuck's skin-window technique or local irritants, such as croton oil, may be used to assess patient's inflammatory responses. Skin tests with recall antigens are of no value in establishing the diagnosis of defective cell-mediated immunity during the first year of life. Infants may fail to react because of lack of previous contact with a given antigen. Occasional patients may develop marked local reactions to skin tests. Topical corticosteroids may be used to relieve these local symptoms. Skin test results may or may not correspond to results of other *in vitro* functional assays. Skin tests are also discussed in Chapter 41 (p. 967).

There are many assays available today for enumeration and functional assessment of lymphocytes. Only some of these assays were discussed here. We wish to emphasize that there are many components to cell-mediated and humoral immunity. Because of poor correlations observed between various *in vitro* assays, *in vivo* skin tests, and clinical data, it may be that each test measures only one component or a limited number of components. Our ability to assess immunocompetence is thus limited. Our understanding of how the various components influence each other or are affected by other factors *in vivo* is also limited. Therefore, while enumerating lymphocytes or determining their functional responses in patients, it is necessary to remember these limitations and to use judgment in applying the obtained data to diagnostic or prognostic considerations. These assays and their uses are also discussed in Chapters 33 and 38.

APPLICATION OF IMMUNOLOGIC METHODS TO HUMAN DISEASES

It is apparent, even at this early stage, that immunologic techniques, such as those described, have contributed to an increased understanding of the role of the immune processes in human diseases. In some instances, these techniques have also provided a rationale for therapy. The effectiveness of immunologic methods in studying disease can best be illustrated in three groups of diseases: immunodeficiency states, lymphoproliferative malignancies, and autoimmune phenomena.

Immunodeficiency Diseases. Although the first description of immunodeficiency was made only 25 years ago, present-day clinicians are able to recognize and diagnose a wide spectrum of syndromes having distinct clinical features, unique immunologic defects, and characteristic biochemical abnormalities. Further corrective measures have become available for many of these diseases. It is through the study of immunodeficiencies in humans and in animals that the first glimpse of functional divisions within the lymphoid system was obtained. Today, immunodeficiencies are known to be a result of derangements in differentiation and functional diversification of T and/or B lymphocytes. These derangements or "blocks" in lymphoid cell differentiation may be genetically determined, induced by external factors, or secondary to a physiologic imbalance of the normally differentiated lymphoid system. Evaluation of patients with immunodeficiency is discussed in Chapter 41 (p. 964).

Lymphoproliferative Diseases. This group of diseases has been extensively studied by immunologic methods (Aiuti, 1974; Ross, 1973). In some instances these methods are an important diagnostic tool; in the majority of lymphoproliferative malignancies, they are helpful in characterization of malignant subpopulations and in shedding some light on their nature and derivation. For the purpose of this discussion, we have selected a few diseases that illustrate the usefulness of the procedures available to the clinician.

It is reasonable to think of lymphoproliferative diseases as representing monoclonal proliferations of lymphoid cells at one particular stage of normal differentiation. In this context, a tremendous heterogeneity in properties of lymphoid cells in different cases of the same disease can be conveniently explained in terms of errors at different stages of differentiation.

Multiple myeloma (MM), Waldenström's macroglobulinemia (WM), and heavy chain diseases are the three instances in which the contribution of immunologic techniques to diagnosis cannot be overemphasized. All three represent proliferations of cells in the B cell lineage, with the plasmacytoid lymphocytes in WM being less differentiated than neoplastic plasma cells in MM. While the clinical features and histopathology of all three diseases are characteristic, serum protein electrophoresis, immunoelectrophoresis, and immunofluorescence studies of bone marrow biopsies are virtually diagnostic. Even a small number of plasma cells in the bone marrow biopsies indicates MM, if all contain the same homogeneous protein demonstrated in the patient's serum.

In applying immunologic techniques to studies of leukemias and lymphomas, it is necessary to be aware of certain difficulties: (1) The performance of the E rosette test requires special attention, since a minor technical modification may cause major variations in the results. The temperature, quantity of SRBC, incubation time, and addition to decomplemented and SRBC-adsorbed human serum may all alter the results. For example, there are leukemic ALL blasts that express the receptor for SRBC and form E rosettes at 37°C., while a majority of normal human T cells do not. (2) If monoclonal antibodies are used for T cell studies, it is essential to employ *panels* of well-characterized reagents because patterns of reactivity of malignant cells may differ from those of normal T lymphocytes. The detection of SIg on a lymphocyte does not mean that it synthesizes that SIg. A possibility of surface adherence by free Ig, aggregated Ig, or antigen-antibody complexes through the Fc receptors must be considered. The adhering products may originate in the patient's serum or may be introduced with the antisera used for immunofluorescence. Thus, a proof of synthesis (i.e., presence of intracellular Ig, ability to resynthesize the SIg after trypsin treatment) is necessary for interpretation of immunofluorescence tests in these cases. (3) Applications of techniques used for normal circulating cells to neoplastic tissues must be done cautiously. There is always a possibility of a selective loss during purification procedures, as cellular characteristics of malignant mononuclear cells may be different from those of normal cells. Also, the presence of both normal and tumor cells requires careful morphologic controls when cell markers are studied to ascertain which cells express the marker. (4) Results of cell marker studies should be correlated to other diagnostic methods such as histology, clinical picture, and conventional and scanning electron microscopy. These points emphasize the necessity for a battery of immunologic tests, rather than any single one when evaluating neoplastic lymphoid cells.

When chronic lymphocytic leukemia (CLL) is studied by immunologic techniques, a majority of cases fall into a B cell category because the membrane phenotype of these neoplastic cells is $SIg^+FcR^+C3R^+E^-$. The majority of the SIg^+ cells have monoclonal IgM on their surface, and this IgM is often associated with IgD having the same light chain. The quantities of SIg on CLL cells are low compared with normal cells. All SIg^+ CLL cells do not necessarily have the Fc receptors and C3 receptor. In fact, subgroups of CLL have been described with $SIg^+FcR^+C3R^-E^-$ and $SIg^+FcR^-C3R^+E^-$ phenotypes. Also, a small proportion of CLLs have cells with the SIg^- $FcR^+C3R^+E^-$ phenotype. To make things even more complicated, rare CLL cases appear to be T cell neoplasms, because their neoplastic lymphocytes express E rosette markers rather than SIg. On the basis of the foregoing, it appears that chronic lymphocytic leukemia, although classified as a B cell neoplasm, represents a mixed immunologic entity.

Acute lymphocytic leukemias (ALL) are as heterogeneous as the chronic leukemias. The majority of ALLs (80 per cent) fall into the category of the "null"-cell diseases, with the membrane phenotype: $SIg^-FcR^-C3R^-E^-$. This does not imply that these neoplastic cells are devoid of all immunologic markers. In fact, various leukemia-associated antigens as well as Ia-like antigens may be detected on these cells with appropriate immunologic reagents. Thus, "common" ALL with blasts expressing CALLA (common ALL antigen) constitutes the majority of "non-T, non-B" ALL and has the best prognosis. Most of the "null"-cell ALLs appear to belong to the B cell lineage because the genes coding for expression of immunoglobulin are "activated" (see Chap. 36). The second group of patients with ALL (20 per cent) have what appears to be a T-cell malignancy, and the cellular phenotype is $SIg^-FcR^-C3R^-E^+$. Also, a small proportion of ALL cases have been described with neoplastic cells of the B cell types (SIg^+). Correlations between immunologically defined subgroups and prognosis have been conflicting. Markers characteristic for both T and B lymphocytes are occasionally seen on the cells of patients with lymphocytic leukemias.

Sézary's syndrome is a T cell cutaneous lymphoma characterized by progressive infiltrations of skin, lymphoid tissues, and visceral organs by malignant lymphocytes exhibiting surface characteristics of T cells: the absence of SIg, complement, and Fc receptors and the ability to form E rosettes (Haynes, 1980). *In vitro* studies of isolated Sézary cells show them to be defective in proliferative responses to plant mitogens or in mixed lymphocyte culture as well as in killing of target cells in the cytotoxicity assays. These cells spontaneously release a lymphokine resembling MIF, so that some patients may have detectable circulating levels of this factor. Recently, using the *in vitro* system for studies of Ig synthesis in the presence of PWM, it was possible to show that the T lymphocytes from these patients fail to regulate *in vitro* synthesis of Ig in a normal manner. Isolated Sézary cells continued exercising helper activity even at such high lymphocyte concentrations as are suppressive in normal controls. This led to a theory that Sézary's syndrome represents a malignant proliferation of helper cells. Presumably, these abnormal helper cells are also responsible for excessive lymphokine production. Furthermore, these malignant cells are T4+. Sometimes these cells are suppressive in *in vitro* assays (Hopper, 1980). Cutaneous T cell lymphomas appear to be related to the subacute T-cell leukemias described in southern Japan. Both involve T4+ lymphocytes and have been associated with the human T cell leukemia virus.

Cutaneous T cell lymphomas may at times be difficult to differentiate from non-malignant exfoliative erythrodermas and other skin diseases. The application of the rosetting and immunofluorescence techniques to cryostat sections may be helpful in the positive identification of malignant T cells in cutaneous lymphoid infiltrates.

There is little doubt that application of immunologic techniques to studies of lymphoproliferative diseases, as in immunodeficiencies, has been most successful in identifying and partially characterizing abnormal lymphoid populations. We have tried to show the reader how such identification can be achieved and interpreted. It is also obvious that there are many uncertainties as to the clinical significance of such analysis. On the positive side is the fact that immunologic characteristics of neoplastic lymphocytes may be indicative of prognosis. In ALL, the 70 per cent or so of patients with blasts expressing CALLA have a much better prognosis and response to chemotherapy than the 30 per cent of patients with the T cell, B cell, or "null"-cell leukemia who require more intensive therapy. Lymphoproliferative diseases are also discussed in Chapter 30.

Autoimmune Diseases. Immunologic evaluation of patients for autoimmune diseases begins with the search for the humoral or cellular immune component that is directed against the patients' own tissues. Traditionally, the demonstration of high titers of autoantibodies to the affected organ has been a hallmark and the diagnostic feature of autoimmune disease. High levels of antithyroid antibodies in Hashimoto's thyroiditis or of antierythrocyte antibodies in autoimmune hemolytic anemia (AIHA) illustrate the point. Both serologic and immunofluorescence techniques are available for the detection of autoantibodies. However, it has become apparent recently that autoantibodies to multiple organs are often detectable in patients with autoimmune diseases and that these autoantibodies may not be pathogenic. Thus, the presence of autoantibody does not necessarily mean that a relevant lesion exists. For example, in patients who recovered from an infection with *Mycoplasma pneumoniae,* cold agglutinins reactive with autologous red cells are detectable, but hemolytic anemia is an infrequent complication. Healthy elderly individuals often have serum autoantibodies (rheumatoid factors, antinuclear antibodies). Patients with chronic liver diseases often have antibodies to smooth muscle, mitochondria, and nuclear antigens. Antinuclear antibodies have been detected in patients treated with certain drugs who do not have any sign of SLE. Finally, healthy relatives of patients with SLE frequently produce antinuclear antibodies. This means that autoantibodies may be a result of infections, drugs, aging, or genetic susceptibility and are not a sufficient reason to diagnose autoimmune disease.

Many autoimmune disorders are now believed to be mediated by cellular immune mechanisms rather than humoral immunity. Several well-studied animal models, such as allergic encephalitis or the NZB/NZW mouse model, support this concept.

The *in vitro* techniques we discussed can now be applied to the evaluation of cell-mediated immunity in patients with autoimmune diseases. It may be expected that lymphocytes which become sensitized to autoantigens as a result of a traumatic event (e.g., infection or other tissue damage) can inflict an injury to the relevant tissue or organ. Indeed, such autosensitized lymphocytes have been demonstrated in patients with pernicious anemia, thyroiditis, diabetes mellitus, and others. For example, lymphocytes from patients with pernicious anemia respond *in vitro* to intrinsic factors, to other gastric antigens, or to both, as assessed by the release of MIF or by proliferation in culture. Lymphocyte transformation in response to thyroglobulin has been described in patients with thyroiditis. The leukocyte migration inhibition tests are generally positive when thyroid extracts or thyroid microsomes are used to stimulate cells from patients with Hashimoto's disease, primary myxedema, or thyrotoxicosis. Leukocytes from these patients were also reported to exercise a direct cytotoxic effect on thyroid cells in monolayer cultures. The leukocyte migration inhibition tests and lymphocyte transformation to pancreatic antigens appear to be positive in a majority of patients with diabetes mellitus. The presence of autosensitization of lymphocytes demonstrable *in vitro* in patients with autoimmune disorders implies their involvement in tissue-damaging processes, but it does not implicate them in the pathogenesis of the disease. It is not clear whether the autosensitization is secondary to the pathogenic event.

A characteristic feature of many autoimmune diseases is their well-documented association with malignancies and with immunodeficiencies: AIHA with chronic lymphocytic leukemia, Sjögren's syndrome with its numerous serologic abnormalities and its tendency toward malignant deterioration, and autoimmune polyendocrine deficiencies with immunoglobulin abnormalities provide well-known examples of this thesis. Also, every autoimmune disease is characterized by an association with multiple autoantibodies. Clinical observations show that all autoimmune diseases form clusters of related syndromes: polyendocrinopathies, sequential AIHA and immune thrombocytopenia, Hashimoto's thyroiditis together with Graves' disease, and others. These features indicate that a fundamental disturbance in the regulation of the immune response may be a basic abnormality in autoimmune diseases.

Through the use of immunologic methods, the nature of abnormal immunoregulation in autoimmune individuals is beginning to be elucidated. It appears that a selective absence of one subpopulation of T lymphocytes, the suppressor cells, may account for the spectrum of abnormalities listed above. This has been demonstrated in the New Zealand mouse model as well as in patients with SLE. In the latter, the selective loss of a suppressor T cell may be due to anti-T cell antibodies in the circulation. It is not known what leads to the loss or decrease in the suppressor T cell population in other autoimmune diseases. In all, the result is deranged immune responsiveness to auto- as well as exogenous antigens. This view of autoimmune phenomena, brought about by recent developments in immunology, may functionally alter our treatment of this group of diseases. Immunosuppression, currently a standard therapeutic modality in autoimmune disease, may have to be replaced by controlled and preferably selective immunostimulation with the hope of activating T lymphocytes that are not doing their job. Autoimmunity is discussed further in Chapter 39.

Abo, T., and Balch, C. M.: A differentiation antigen of human NK and K cells identified by monoclonal antibody (HNK-1). J. Immunol., *127*:1024, 1981.

Abramson, S., Miller, R. G., and Phillips, R. A.: The identification in adult bone marrow of pluripotent and restricted stem cells of the myeloid and lymphoid systems. J. Exp. Med., *145*:1567, 1977.

Aiuti, F., Cerrottini, J. C., Coombs, R. R. A., Cooper, M., Dickler, H. B., Froland, S. S., Fudenberg, H. H., Graves, M. F., Grey, H. M., Kunkel, H. G., Natvig, J. B., Preud'homme, J. L., Rabellino, E., Ritts, R. E., Rowe, D. S., Seligman, M., Siegal, F. P., Stjernsward, J., Terry, W. D., and Wybrand, J.: Identification, enumeration, and isolation of B and T lymphocytes from human peripheral blood. Scand. J. Immunol., *3*:521, 1974.

Bach, J. F., Dardenne, M., Goldstein, A., Guka, A., and White, A.: Appearance of T cell markers in bone marrow rosette forming cells after incubation with thymosin, a thymic hormone. Proc. Nat. Acad. Sci. (Wash.), *68*:2734, 1971.

Boyum, A.: Separation of blood leucocytes from blood and bone marrow: Introduction. Scand. J. Clin. Lab. Invest., *21*(Suppl. 97):77, 1968.

Boyum, A.: Separation of blood leucocytes, granulocytes and lymphocytes. Tissue Antigens, *4*:269, 1974.

Cantor, H., and Boyse, E. A.: Functional subclasses of T lymphocytes bearing different Ly antigens. II. Cooperation between subclasses of Ly cells in the generation of killer cell activity. J. Exp. Med., *141*:1390, 1975.

Cantor, H., and Weissman, I.: Development and function of subpopulations of thymocytes and T lymphocytes. Prog. Allergy, *20*:1, 1976.

Cerottini, J. C., and Brunner, K. T.: Cell-mediated cytotoxicity, allograft rejection and tumor immunity. Adv. Immunol., *18*:67, 1974.

Chess, L., MacDermott, R. P., and Schlossman, S. F.: Immunologic functions of isolated human lymphocyte subpopulations. VI. Further characterization of the surface Ig negative, E rosette negative (null cell) subset. J. Immunol., *115*:483, 1975.

Choi, T. S.: Serological precipitation method for studying biosynthesis and secretion of immunoglobulin by human peripheral blood lymphocytes. J. Immunol. Methods, *14*:37, 1977.

Claman, H. N., Chaperon, E. A., and Triplett, R. F.: Immunocompetence of transferred thymus–marrow cell combinations. J. Immunol., *97*:928, 1966.

Cooper, M. D., and Lawton, A. R.: The development of the immune system. Sci. Am., *231*:559, 1974.

Daniele, R. P., and Rowlands, D. T., Jr.: Lymphocyte subpopulations in sarcoidosis: Correlation with disease activity and duration. Ann. Intern. Med., *85*:593, 1976.

Davis, M. M., Kim, S. K., and Hood, L.: Immunoglobulin class switching: Developmentally regulated DNA rearrangements during differentiation. Cell, *22*:1, 1980.

DeSousa, M.: Lymphocyte Circulation. Experimental and Clinical Aspects. New York, John Wiley & Sons, 1981.

Ehlenberger, A. G., McWilliams, M., Phillips-Quagliata, J. M., Lamm, M. E., and Nussensweig, V.: Immunoglobulin-bearing and complement-receptor lymphocytes constitute the same population in human peripheral blood. J. Clin. Invest., *57*:53, 1976.

Feldman, M.: Antigen-specific T cell factors and their role in the regulation of T-B interaction. *In* Sercarz, E., Williamson, A. R., and Fox, C. R. (eds.): The Immune System: Genes, Receptors, Signals. New York, Academic Press, 1974, p. 497.

Gershon, R. H.: T cell control of antibody production. Contemp. Top. Immunobiol., *3*:1, 1974.

Greaves, M. F., and Baunninger, J.: Activation of T and B lymphocytes by insoluble phytomitogens. Nature (New Biol.), *235*:67, 1972a.

Greaves, M. F., and Janossy, G.: Elicitation of selective T and B lymphocyte responses by cell surface ligands. Transplant. Rev., *11*:87, 1972b.

Gronowicz, E., Coutinho, A., and Melchers, F.: A plaque assay for all cells secreting Ig of a given type or class. Eur. J. Immunol., *6*:588, 1976.

Hamblin, A. S., Zawisza, B., Shipton, U., Dumonde, D. C., DenHollander, F. C., and Verheul, H.: The use of human lymphoid cell line lymphokine preparations (LCL-LK) as working standards in the bioassay of human leukocyte migration inhibition factor (LIF). J. Immunol. Methods, *54*:317, 1982.

Hannam-Harris, A. C., Gordon, J., and Smith, J. L.: Immunoglobulin synthesis by neoplastic B lymphocytes: Free light chain synthesis as a marker of B cell differentiation. J. Immunol., *125*:2177, 1980.

Haynes, B. F., Bunn, P., Mann, D., Thomas, C., Eisenbarth, G. S., Minna, J., and Fauci, A. S.: Cell surface differentiation antigens of the malignant T cell in Sézary syndrome and mycosis fungoides. J. Clin. Invest., *67*:523, 1980.

Herberman, R. B., and Ortaldo, J. R.: Natural killer cells: Their role in defense against disease. Science, *214*:24, 1981.

Hopper, J. E., and Haren, J. M.: Studies on a Sézary lymphocyte population with T-suppressor activity. J. Clin. Immunol. Immunopathol., *17*:43, 1980.

Hsu, S. M., Raine, L., and Fanger, H.: Use of avidin-biotin-peroxidase complex (ABC) in immunoperoxidase techniques: A comparison between ABC and unlabeled antibody (PAP) procedures. J. Histochem. Cytochem., *29*:577, 1981.

Jerrells, T. R., Dean, J. H., Richardson, G. L., and Herberman, R. B.: Depletion of monocytes from human peripheral blood mononuclear leukocytes: Comparison of the Sephadex G-10 column method with other commonly used techniques. J. Immunol. Methods, *32*:11, 1980.

Kelly, R. G.: Functional anatomy of lymph nodes. I. The paracortical cords. Int. Arch. Allergy Appl. Immunol., *48*:836, 1975.

Kuritani, T., and Cooper, M. D.: Human B-cell differentiation. III. Enhancing effect of monoclonal anti-immunoglobulin D antibody on pokeweed mitogen–induced plasma cell differentiation. J. Immunol., *129*:2490, 1982.

Lobo, P. I., and Horwitz, D. A.: An appraisal of Fc receptors on human peripheral blood B and L lymphocytes. J. Immunol., *117*:939, 1976.

Lobo, P. I., Westervelt, F. B., and Horwitz, D. A.: Identification of two populations of immunoglobulin-bearing lymphocytes in man. J. Immunol., *114*:116, 1975.

Mingari, M. C., Moretta, A., Pantaleo, G., and Moretta, L.: Surface markers of resting and activated human T cells. Functional implications and experimental limits. Springer Semin. Immunopath., *5*:477, 1982.

Nieuwenhuis, P., B-cell differentiation *in vivo*. Immunology Today, *2*:104, 1981.

Perlmann, P., Perlmann, H., Larsson, A., and Wahlin, B.: Antibody-dependent cytolytic effector lymphocytes (K cells) in human blood. J. Reticuloendothel. Soc., *17*:241, 1975.

Raff, M. C., Megson, M., Owen, J. J. T., and Cooper, M. D.: Early production of intracellular IgM by B-lymphocyte precursors in mouse. Nature, *259*:224, 1978.

Reinherz, E. L., and Schlossman, S. F.: The differentiation and function of human T lymphocytes. Cell, *19*:821, 1980.

Rocklin, R. E., MacDermoth, R. P., Chess, L., Schlossman, S. F., and David, J. R.: Studies on mediator production by highly purified human T and B lymphocytes. J. Exp. Med., *140*:1303, 1974.

Ross, G. D., Rabellino, E. M., Polley, M. J., and Grey, H. M.: Combined studies of complement receptor and surface immunoglobulin-bearing cells and sheep erythrocyte rosette-forming cells in normal and leukemic human lymphocytes. J. Clin. Invest., *52*:377, 1973.

Rowe, D. S., Hug, K., Forni, L., and Pernis, B.: Immunoglobulin D as a lymphocyte receptor. J. Exp. Med., *138*:965, 1973.

Rowlands, D. T., Daniele, R. P., Nowell, P. C., and Wurzel, H. A.: Characterization of lymphocyte subpopulations in chronic lymphocytic leukemia. Cancer, *34*:1962, 1974.

Schreiber, G. F., and Unanue, E. E. R.: Membrane and cytoplasmic changes in B lymphocytes induced by ligand-surface immunoglobulin interaction. Adv. Immunol., *24*:37, 1976.

Singer, S. J.: Molecular biology of cellular membranes with applications to immunology. Adv. Immunol., *19*:1, 1974.

Sprent, J.: Recirculating lymphocytes. *In* Marchalonis, J. J. (ed.): The Lymphocyte: Structure and Function. New York, Marcel Dekker, 1977.

Terhorst, C., VanAgthoven, A., Reinherz, E., and Schlossman, S.: Biochemical analysis of human T lymphocyte differentiation antigens T4 and T5. Science, *209*:520, 1980.

Thomas, D. B., and Calderon, R. A.: T helper cells change their Lyt-1,2 phenotype during an immune response. Europ. J. Immunol., *12*:16, 1982.

Unanue, E. R.: The regulatory role of macrophages in antigenic stimulation. Adv. Immunol., *15*:45, 1972.

Vogler, L. B., Pearl, E. R., Gathings, W. E., Lawton, A. R., and Cooper, M. D.: B lymphocyte precursors in bone marrow in immunodeficiency state. Lancet, *2*:376, 1976.

Whiteside, T. L., Kumagai, Y., Medsger, T. A., and Rodnan, G. P.: Discrepancies between *in vivo* and *in vitro* responses to Candida antigen in patients with progressive systemic sclerosis (PSS; scleroderma). J. Clin. Immunol., *1*:250, 1981.

Whiteside, T. L., and Rabin, B. S.: Surface immunoglobulin on activated human peripheral blood thymus-derived cells. J. Clin. Invest., *57*:762, 1976.

Winchester, R. J., Fu, S. M., Hoffman, T., and Kunkel, H. G.: IgG on lymphocyte surfaces; technical problems and the significance of a third cell population. J. Immunol., *114*:1210, 1975.

Woda, B. A., Fenoglio, C. M., Nette, E. G., and King, D. W.: The lack of specificity of the sheep erythrocyte–T lymphocyte rosetting phenomenon. Am. J. Path., *88*:69, 1977.

Zucker-Franklin, D.: The percentage of monocytes among "mononuclear" cell fractions obtained from normal human blood. J. Immunol., *112*:234, 1974.

35

PHAGOCYTIC CELLS: POLYMORPHONUCLEAR CELLS AND MONOCYTES

EUFRONIO G. MADERAZO, M.D., and PETER A. WARD, M.D.

As the name implies, phagocytes are cells that are endowed with the ability to engulf particles. In general these include the polymorphonuclear granulocytes (neutrophils and eosinophils), the monocytes of the blood, and, at the tissue level, the macrophages. Although other cells such as certain endothelial cells and the alveolar lining cells are also known to internalize particles, we will concern ourselves only with the blood-associated phagocyte cells: neutrophils and monocytes.

PHYSIOLOGY OF PHAGOCYTES

Although evidence is fragmentary, it is generally believed that monovalent and divalent cations, metabolic fuels such as ATP and GTP, cyclic nucleotides, and microtubules and microfilaments are responsible for the translation of chemical and electrical energy into mechanical work. The precise role of these various factors and their interplay are poorly understood.

Both *microtubules* and *microfilaments* are filamentous cytoplasmic structures that are currently believed to play important roles in cellular functions. Microtubules are hollow filaments made up of polymers of a well-known protein, tubulin. The interaction of microtubules with membranes controls the movement and distribution of membrane transport proteins and cell surface receptors. These effects suggest their importance as regulators in the movement of substances through the cell membrane and in membrane-membrane or membrane-substrate interactions in cell adherence and locomotion (both random and chemotactic). In addition, microtubules also direct the traffic of cytoplasmic inclusions and thereby influence the release of intracytoplasmic substances, particularly lysosomal granule contents (Goldstein, 1973). The effects of microtubule disturbance on cell function are seen in Chédiak-Higashi cells (Oliver, 1976) and in cells treated with the antitubulin drug, colchicine (Rinehart, 1977).

Microfilaments are smaller in diameter than the microtubules and are made up of actin polymers. These structures are arranged randomly or oriented in subplasmalemmal bundles. It is hypothesized that cell-substrate contact activates actin-binding protein and myosin which gels and contracts the actin filaments (Stossel, 1978). The importance of microfilament in cell adherence, locomotion, phagocytosis, and degranulation has been shown in cells treated with low concentrations of cytochalasin B (Rinehart, 1977), which dissolves actin gels, and in cells from a child with dysfunctional leukocytic actin (Boxer, 1974).

To facilitate engulfment, the phagocytes have to be brought in close proximity to their target particles. This requires leukocytic mobilization, a phenomenon that involves two events, adherence to endothelial surfaces and locomotion. Adherence to endothelial cells allows the phagocyte to gain a foothold in the vascular network. This is an important prerequisite to the mobilization of leukocytes into extravascular sites. Adherence to endothelial cells is also important for locomotion itself, since the phagocyte moves in a "head over heels" fashion, which requires that a part of the cell be firmly anchored. The regulatory mechanism of adherence is at present mostly unknown.

Cell locomotion is either "random" or "chemotactic." Random locomotion is similar to the movements of a blind man left in the middle of an open field. The probability of his moving in one direction would be equal to the probability of his going in any other direction. Chemotaxis is the unidirectional response to a concentration gradient of a chemical attractant. This is similar to the same blind man going in the direction of the sound he hears. Random locomotion is either non-stimulated or stimulated (chemokinetic or a non-oriented response to the presence of chemotactic or other chemical substances). To differentiate these responses of leukocytes from responses of other cells such as bacteria and amebae, the terms leukotaxis and leukokinesis were introduced. The most important source of chemotactic factors is the complement system from which is derived the chemotactic fragment of C5. Cell-derived chemotactic factors such as those from lymphocytes, granulocytes, and macrophages have also been described (Ward, 1974). The humoral regulation of leukocyte locomotion has been studied more extensively than regulators of other leukocyte functions, such as phagocytosis. These regulators include the chemotactic factor inactivator (CFI) (Ward, 1974), the cell-directed inhibitor of leukotaxis (CDI) (Maderazo, 1977), and the leukokinesis-enhancing factor (LEF) (Maderazo, 1979), also called "chemokinetic factor."

CFI acts directly on chemotactic factors to bring about their inactivation. Two types of inactivators have been identified, both of which are heat-labile and non-dialyzable, one being an α-globulin and the other a β-globulin. Elevations of serum CFI have been associated with chemotactic defects and have been observed in patients with Hodgkin's disease, sarcoidosis, and lepromatous leprosy.

The cell-directed inhibitor (CDI) is another regulator of cell locomotion which is present in normal serum. It acts directly on both polymorphonuclears and monocytes to inhibit locomotion and phagocytosis. Both IgG and IgA have CDI activity; however, their concentration in serum does not correlate with serum CDI activity. This suggests that only certain forms of these immunoglobulins are inhibitory or that other nonimmunoglobulin factors are reponsible for abnormally high serum CDI activity (Woronick, 1981). Elevations of CDI in serum have been associated with abnormal leukocytic locomotion and have been observed in patients with anergy, cirrhosis, cancer, and recalcitrant adult periodontitis. Other lower molecular weight cell-directed inhibitors have been described but were not more thoroughly characterized.

Phagocytosis is initiated by attachment of a particle to the surface of the phagocyte, followed by invagination of the particle along with a portion of the cell membrane. Two major enhancers of phagocytosis have been described: the opsonins which coat the target particles to render them palatable to the phagocyte (Winkelstein, 1973) and tuftsin, which acts directly on the cell to stimulate its phagocytic activity (Najjar, 1975). The heat-stable specific opsonin is specific antibody acting alone or in combination with complement activated via the classic pathway. The heat-labile opsonin includes the complement system and its C3b and C5b products which are generated via activation of the classic or alternative complement pathways. It is not clear how opsonins enhance phagocytosis, but it appears that immunoglobulin can act as a ligand that attaches to the bacterial surface antigen via its $F(ab)_2$ portion and to specific receptor sites on the phagocyte cell surface via the Fc portion of the Ig molecule. Presumably, C3b can also act as a ligand, since both neutrophils and monocytes have receptors for C3b. Opsonic deficiencies have been described in newborn infants, in sickle cell disease, and in deficiency states of C3 and C5 components of complement.

Once the microbe is phagocytosed a series of events within the neutrophil leads to the eventual *killing* and *digestion* of the microbe (Spitznagel, 1977). First, the phagosomal membrane will fuse with the lysosomal granule membrane forming the phagolysosome, resulting in the release of lysosomal granule contents into the phagocytic vacuole. This is followed by a burst of metabolic activity leading to killing and digestion of the microbe. For simplicity, this microbicidal mechanism can be categorized under oxygen-dependent and oxygen-independent systems. The former consists of myeloperoxidase and cofactors (halides, thiocyanate, thyroxine, and triiodothyronine), hydrogen peroxide, superoxide anions, hydroxyl radicals, and singlet oxygen. This system, by a series of powerful oxidation-reduction reactions, is assumed to destroy and digest phagocytosed microbes. The oxygen-independent system includes low pH, lysozyme, lactoferrin, and cationic proteins. These factors are microbicidal or microbistatic per se. For example, acid-sensitive organisms may be killed by the low pH achieved in the phagocyte vacuole, lysozyme lyses bacterial cell wall, lactoferrin binds iron and deprives the organism of an essential nutrient, and cationic proteins may interfere with microbial metabolism by binding to acidic groups of the microbial surface. Various disorders have been found to be associated with an abnormality of microbial killing function by phagocytes, but the prototype is chronic granulomatous disease of childhood (Quie, 1975).

Since the same factors and resources of the cells often subserve various cell functions, it is common to observe multiple dysfunctions resulting from a single subcellular abnormality. For example, a patient with leukocytic actin dysfunction (Boxer, 1974) had problems in granulocyte locomotion, phagocytosis, and degranulation, since all these functions require normal microfilament activity. Leukocyte adherence studies were not reported, but that too would be expected to be affected, since adherence also requires microfilament activity. Chédiak-Higashi cells have dysfunctions of chemotaxis and microbial killing owing to an abnormality of microtubule assembly. The defective chemotaxis reflects the importance of microtubule function in membrane and membrane-substrate activities and in sensing chemotactic stimuli, whereas the defective microbial killing function reflects the requirement of microtubules for the control of cytoplasmic granule traffic, lysosomal granule and phagosome membrane fusion, and lysosomal enzyme release. Because of the cell surface activity of microtubules, Chédiak-Higashi cells may also be expected to have decreased adherence.

RELATIONSHIPS BETWEEN THE HOST AND THE MICROBES

The diagram shown in Figure 35–1 shows a balance in which microbial factors are on one side and the host factors are on the other side. The microbial factors include microbial virulence and microbial quantity. Virulence includes all the factors that make the microbe detrimental to the host, such as toxins, enzymes that may increase invasiveness of microbes, substances that may neutralize the host defenses, and others. On the other side of the balance are the host factors consisting of local, humoral, and cellular defenses. Under normal conditions this balance is tilted in favor of the host, and the degree of the tilt is a measure of host reserve favoring host defense over microbial factors. In a normal host, infection can occur in one of several conditions. The quantity of the microbes can be increased to overwhelm a normal host. For instance, in one of the "Earth Day" celebrations (Fass, 1971) epidemic histoplasmosis occurred in a large group of young, apparently normal individuals who were exposed to high concentrations of dust contaminated with bird droppings. Because of increased virulence, infections can also occur in the normal host even if the amount of exposure is not overwhelming. For example, most normal individuals exposed to *Neisseria gonorrhoeae, Shigella,* or *Vibrio cholerae* will be infected.

The epithelial cover, together with the antimicrobial substances in secretions and the phagocytes and lymphocytes in the subepithelial mucosal regions, provides local defenses against penetration by microbes. The importance of this first line of defense is shown by infections that occur when the skin is broken, such as in wounds and burns, abnormalities of drainage due to obstruction, and ciliary immobility in the upper airways.

The major components of the humoral defenses are the immunoglobulins (antibodies) and the complement system. The immunoglobulins function mainly as a trigger for complement activation and as a potentiator of cellular function, particularly phagocytosis, by opsonization of target particles. Antibody can also inactivate microbial toxins by its neutralizing or antitoxin activity. The complement system, like the antibodies, also functions mainly by regulating or potentiating cell function by generation of the complement-derived chemotactic factors and the phagocytosis-enhancing factors. But by itself complement can also directly lyse bacteria, which is probably important for the defense against gram-negative organisms, particularly against the *Neisseria* species.

The cellular factors are made up of the polymorphonuclear cells, monocytes and macrophages, and lymphocytes. The lymphocytes function mainly by their ability to secrete a wide variety of substances (lymphokines and immunoglobulins) with a broad spectrum of activities. Lymphocytes also contain immunologic memory and probably represent the principal cells involved in identifying a foreign material as "non-self." Lymphocytes also have profound influences on the activities of other cells such as monocytes and macrophages and even other lymphocytes. Together with other cells, particularly the macrophages, lymphocytes are the main cells involved in cell-mediated immunity, which is expressed in cutaneous delayed hypersensitivity reaction, protection against extracellular organisms, protection against neoplasms, and graft rejection.

As can be seen from the above organization of the host defense system, the various host factors do not act independently, but rather act in concert with one another.

CLINICAL MANIFESTATIONS OF PHAGOCYTE ABNORMALITIES

Table 35–1 shows that the infecting organism often indicates abnormalities in host defense mechanisms. In general, recurrent infections owing to extracellular organisms are manifestations of abnormalities of immunoglobulins, complement, or polymorphonuclear cells. Infections owing to intracellular organisms suggest disorders of monocytes, macrophages, and lymphocytes, and also immunoglobulins and complement. Therefore, any recurrent infection should require the evaluation of phagocytes (either polymorphonuclear

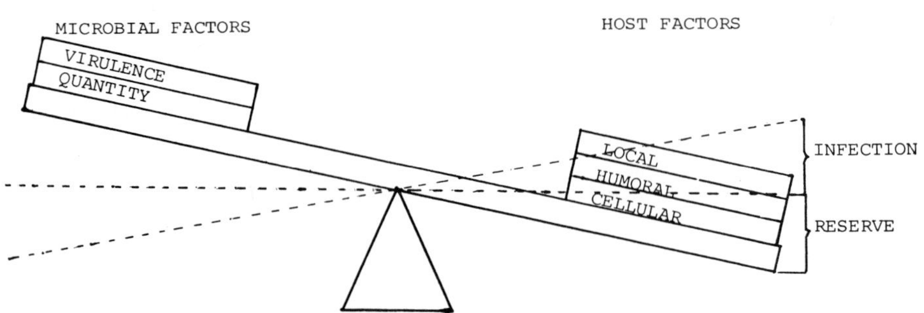

Figure 35–1. Diagram showing the preferable relationship between the host and the microbial factors—the host factors exceed the microbial factors. Changes from this relationship that favor the microbe will tilt the see-saw in the opposite direction, resulting in infection.

Table 35–1. PATHOGENIC AGENTS THAT MAY SIGNAL UNDERLYING HOST DEFENSE DISORDER

Observed Pathogen	Suspected Disorder
Extracellular bacteria *Staphylococcus* *Streptococcus* *Hemophilus* *Meningococcus* *Enterobacter* *Pseudomonas* *Serratia* Others	Serum: antibody, complement Cells: granulocytes
Intracellular agents Bacteria: *Salmonella, Brucella, Listeria, Nocardia, Actinomyces, Mycobacteria* Viruses: *Herpes, CMV, Vaccinia, Influenza,* etc. Fungi: *Cryptococcus, Aspergillus, Histoplasma, Candida,* etc. Protozoa: *Toxoplasma, Pneumocystis,* etc.	Serum: antibody, complement Cells: macrophage, monocyte, and lymphocyte

cells, monocytes, or both), immunoglobulins, and the complement system.

Aside from the signs and symptoms specifically attributable to the primary disease associated with phagocyte abnormalities, certain manifestations signal the presence of a phagocyte dysfunction.

Recurrent or frequent infections are the most common manifestation that results in referral for phagocyte function testing. The most common site of the infection is the skin and adjacent soft tissues, and the most frequent pathogens are *Staphylococcus aureus* and hemolytic streptococci. The next most frequent site of involvement is the upper and lower respiratory tract, followed by infections in other locations, including the blood stream.

Any severe or life-threatening infection, especially if no apparent increase in the microbial factors (virulence and quantity) is present and no obvious breaks in the local defenses (epithelial linings, secretory immunoglobulin) are evident. Contrary to some reports, patients who develop *Listeria* meningitis, for example, should be considered abnormal.

Inappropriate response to infections in patients with serious bacterial infections. Absence of fever and other signs of infection in a patient with systemic infection can indicate a host disorder.

Low white blood cell count in acutely infected body fluids. This should be considered an obvious sign of abnormal host cell mobilization. The low white cell count in ascitic fluid of cirrhotics with spontaneous peritonitis is one example.

Infections that do not respond to seemingly appropriate therapy such as bacteremic *Pseudomonas* pneumonia. One series showed a mortality of 100 per cent regardless of antibiotic therapy (Iannini, 1974). Many (30 per cent) patients were leukopenic and some had diseases associated with granulocyte dysfunctions. If the white cell count is normal in a non-responsive patient, a qualitative defect of phagocytes should be suspected.

"Cold" abscess owing to organisms that ordinarily cause "hot" abscesses, such as "cold" abscess formation due to staphylococci in patients with chronic granulomatous disease of childhood, and in some patients with the syndrome of eczema, hyperimmunoglobulinemia E, and leukotactic abnormality (Hill, 1975).

Granulomatous reaction to a non-granulomatous infection suggests a host defect. Analyses of factors that lead to granuloma formation indicate that such a reaction occurs if one of two conditions exists: (1) the phagocytosed particle is resistant to intracellular enzymes and is not effectively destroyed, or (2) the phagocytes have an abnormal digestive mechanism. Thus, granuloma formation occurs as a response to mycobacterial infections or peritoneal contamination with glove powder, since these particles are difficult for phagocytes to digest. On the other hand, easily digestible organisms, such as staphylococci and *Escherichia coli,* can cause granuloma formation in the presence of phagocytes with bactericidal disorders, such as those in patients with chronic granulomatous disease of childhood and in malakoplakia.

PHAGOCYTE FUNCTION TESTS

The preceding section tells us when to suspect the presence of a phagocyte abnormality and for whom (most likely patients) to request specific determinations. The next step is to decide what measurements and examinations are needed. To this end, several manifestations are important, since they allow immediate focus on certain dysfunctions: for example, a patient who develops a granulomatous reaction as a result of infection from non–granuloma-forming bacteria will require tests for microbial killing; a patient with "cold" abscesses owing to staphylococci or streptococci should be tested for phagocyte leukotaxis and microbial killing; a patient with acute bacterial meningitis with inappropriately low granulocyte count in the cerebrospinal fluid not due to a parameningeal focus may have a granulocyte mobilization defect and requires testing for leukotaxis; the same is true in acute bacterial peritonitis with low cell counts in ascitic fluid. Most other manifestations do not allow the pinpointing of specific dysfunctions and, therefore, will require screening procedures for all four major phagocyte functions (adherence, locomotion, phagocytosis, and microbial killing). Granulocytes are tested if the organisms responsible for the infectious problem are "extracellular bacteria," whereas monocytes are best tested first if the pathogens are "intracellular agents" (Table 35–1).

All tests to be discussed are bioassays with great variability. Consequently, adequate controls are needed and interpretation of the results must be conservative.

Preparations of Human Leukocytes

Polymorphonuclear Cells. Venous blood is collected into a plastic syringe containing 50 units of preservative-free heparin (sodium) per milliliter of blood. The syringe is stood on its plunger to allow the red cells to sediment by gravity for 30 to 60 minutes. The leukocyte-rich plasma is then collected into a plastic 40 ml test tube, using a bent needle (or a polyethylene catheter attached to the tip of the syringe needle), and centrifuged at low speed (500 g) for 10 minutes. The cell button is resuspended in Medium 199 (pH 7.4) and the concentration is adjusted to 5×10^6 cells/ml.

In some subjects (frequently males) in whom erythrocytes sediment very slowly or not at all, rapid sedimentation can be achieved by adding 6 per cent hetastarch in saline at a ratio of 1:2 to the heparinized blood sample.

Monocytes. Monocytes are prepared by density gradient centrifugation in Ficoll-Hypaque, as described on p. 799.

Leukocyte Adherence Assay

Various methods of determining leukocyte adherence are known; among these are *in vivo* procedures such as determinations of the marginating pool of granulocytes using injected epinephrine (Athens, 1961), and *in vitro* methods using glass beads. The easiest and most reproducible assay, however, is that using scrubbed nylon fibers (MacGregor, 1974). A modification of this technique is used in our laboratory. In this method, when washed leukocyte samples as described above and 40 mg of nylon fibers are used, most normal individuals have a 90 per cent or greater adherence.

This assay system is highly reproducible if several variables are closely monitored. First, washing of cells will increase adherence by approximately 10 to 20 per cent. Therefore, if one uses heparinized whole blood or leukocyte-rich plasma in which the cells are not washed, the normal values have to be correspondingly lowered or, preferably, determined in each laboratory beforehand. Second, the amount of nylon fibers used should be weighed as accurately as possible. In experiments using various amounts of fibers, it was shown that adherence increases directly with the weight of fibers used, peaks at approximately 50 mg, and plateaus thereafter. The use of 40 mg of fibers is therefore sensitive in detecting decreased adherence values, but insensitive to increases in adherence. To detect adherence greater than normal, lesser amounts of fibers (e.g., 20 mg) should be used. Another critical factor to control is the length of the packed fiber column, since the shorter the column, the greater the adherence, and vice versa.

Materials

1. Leukocyte preparations from the patient and normal individual.
2. Plastic tuberculin or insulin syringes (Pharmaseal).
3. Scrubbed nylon fibers (Fenwall).
4. TC Medium 199, pH 7.4 (Difco).
5. Counting chamber.
6. Micropipette counting system (Unopette, B-D).

Method. Scrubbed nylon fibers (40 mg) are packed into plastic tuberculin (or insulin) syringes, and the packed column adjusted to 15 mm in length. The leukocyte preparation (0.5 ml) with a known granulocyte count is then applied to the top of the column and allowed to filter through. The filtrate is collected and recounted. This can be accomplished in a two- to three-minute period. The per cent adherence is then calculated as follows:

$$\text{Per cent adherence} = \frac{\text{Granulocyte count of original sample} - \text{Granulocyte count of filtrate}}{\text{Granulocyte count of original sample}} \times 100$$

Leukotaxis Assay

The easiest and the most available *in vivo* assay for leukocyte mobilization appears to be the delayed cutaneous hypersensitivity reaction. Another *in vivo* method is the Rebuck skin window technique (Rebuck, 1955). The chief problems with these procedures include their non-specificity, the difficulty in standardization and reproducibility, and their inconvenience.

Various *in vitro* procedures are available, the most popular being the Boyden micropore filter technique because of its relative simplicity, convenience, and applicability to performance of many experiments in one day. This method uses a chamber which is divided by a micropore filter into an upper (or cell) and a lower (or chemotactic factor) compartment. The cells are placed in the upper compartment and allowed to migrate from the proximal to the distal surface of the filter. Three methods have been used to evaluate polymorphonuclear cell locomotion into the micropore filter (summarized in Table 35–2). The first method involves the enumeration of the number of cells that have reached a predetermined distance. The second method measures the distance reached by the fastest or the deeper-most cells. The third method incorporates both the *number* of cells and the *distance* of

Table 35–2. METHODS OF MICROPORE FILTER LEUKOTACTIC ASSAY

	Method 1	**Method 2**	**Method 3**
Mechanics	*Number* of cells that have reached a predetermined distance	*Distance* migrated by the fastest cells	Average distance migrated per cell
Examples	1. Distal surface cell count (Boyden, 1962) 2. Radioassay-double filter technique (Gallin, 1973) 3. Cell count distal to cell monolayer (Ward, 1968) 4. Distal surface cell count with correction for detached cells (Keller, 1972; Frei, 1974)	"Leading front technique" (Zigmond, 1973)	"Distance per cell on microsectioning technique" (Maderazo, 1978)
Problems due to:			
1. Cell detachment from distal filter surface	Yes (Method 1, Example 1)	No	No
2. Magnification and minification of defects	Yes	No	No
3. Large variability	Yes	No	No
4. Susceptibility to bias	More	Less	Least
5. Inability to detect defects of mass migration	No	Yes	No
6. Laboriousness	Less	Less	More

migration. An example of the first is the original method described by Boyden in which cells are allowed to migrate completely through the filter. Those cells that have reached the distal surface are then counted. Modifications of the first method include counting of all cells that have moved distal to the cell monolayer, the radioassay double-filter technique using radioactive chromium-labeled granulocytes, and the distal filter surface counts with corrections for detached cells (which is done by using a second filter to catch cells that have detached from the distal surface of the upper filter or by cell counts in the fluid in the lower compartment). The second method, known as the "leading front" technique, was described by Zigmond (1973). In this method the cells are not allowed to penetrate completely the thickness of the filter. The distance migrated by the fastest cells is recorded and used as the measure of locomotion.

There are problems with these methods. With the first method the most widely known problem is cell detachment from the distal filter surface. This detachment is variable, increases with time of incubation, and is probably indirectly related to leukocyte adherence. The second problem is the magnification or minification of leukotactic defects. Magnification occurs because only those cells that have reached the distal surface are counted and are given a grade of 100 per cent migration, whereas those cells that do not reach the distal surface are not counted and are given a grade of 0 per cent migration regardless of how close to the distal surface they have migrated. In our experience this has led to the clinical laboratory discrepancy in which a relatively well patient has a greater than 90 per cent inhibition of leukotaxis. This has resulted in some individuals questioning the relevance of leukotaxis assays, because many patients with chemotactic inhibition approaching 100 per cent did not die when they had serious infections. In addition to magnification of abnormalities, errors are also magnified. Reduction to the point that a previously obvious defect is not detected has been observed less frequently. This occurs on prolonged incubation of chambers, where the slowly moving (abnormal) cells are allowed enough time to reach the distal surface, at the same time that an increasing number of normal cells on the distal surface are detaching. The third problem of this method is the error created by non-uniformity of the cell distribution on the filter. Unless the total area of the filter is counted, representative areas of low or high counts could be selected for counting depending upon the bias of the reader. Yet if fields are not selected the variation often becomes so great that in many instances the data cannot be evaluated. The radioassay double filter technique will correct this problem because the total number of radiolabeled cells detached from the distal surface of the upper filter is counted.

The second method ("leading front" technique) depends on accepting the concept that the cell population is homogeneous in its migration characteristics through the micropore filter, and that, therefore, the fastest migrating cells represent the total cell population. We have found that this concept is not true, since at least two types of cells with different behaviors

5

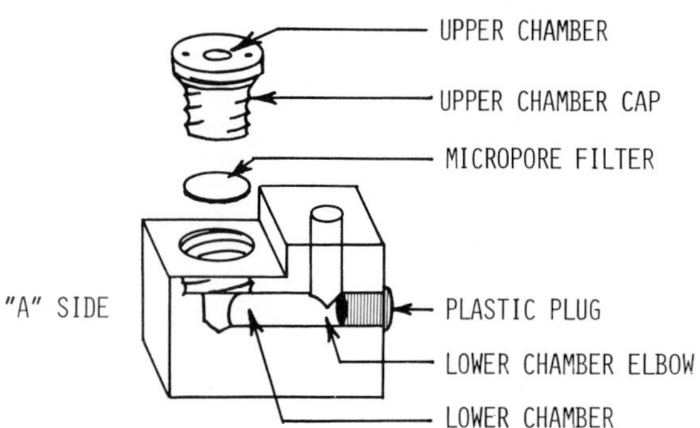

Figure 35–2. Clear acrylic leukotactic chamber (Ahlco Corporation, Southington, Ct.).

of migration in micropore filters exist. In addition, since it is mainly a measure of distance migrated by a few representative cells, it may not detect disorders of mass migration.

The method presented will incorporate measurements of both the cell number and the distance migrated by the cells.

Materials

1. Leukocyte and serums from the patient and normal control.
2. Leukotactic chambers (Ahlco Corporation, Southington, Ct.) (Fig. 35–2).
3. Micropore filters, 13 mm diameter and 5 μm pore size (Sartorius).
4. Sodium heparin, preservative-free.
5. TC Medium 199, pH 7.4 (Difco).
6. Staining cassettes for micropore filters (Ahlco Corporation, Southington, Ct.) (Fig. 35–3).
7. Staining chemicals: (a) 100% isopropyl alcohol. (b) Acid hematoxylin (4 ml concentrated acetic acid/100 ml Gill formulation hematoxylin). (c) Acid alcohol (3 drops HCl/200 ml 70% isopropyl alcohol). (d) Xylene.
8. Preparation of chemotactic factors: (a) Bacterial chemotactic factor: *Escherichia coli* is incubated in Medium 199 at 37° C. for 24 to 48 hours. After incubation the bacteria are removed by ultracentrifugation at 20,000 rpm for 20 minutes. The filtrate is then saved and tested for chemotactic activity. The least amount producing the most activity is used in subsequent experiments. (b) Activated serum: Normal serum is activated by incubation with zymosan (1 ml serum and 5 mg zymosan) at 37° C. for five minutes. This procedure will generate complement-derived chemotactic factors in the serum. A 3 per cent concentration of this material is used in the lower compartment to test chemotactic function. Besides zymosan, other substances have been used to activate serum, such as endotoxin and immune complexes.

Method. A micropore filter is placed on the floor of the upper chamber compartment and the upper chamber cap is placed and tightened slightly. (Excessive tightening may produce corrugations of the filter which result in irregular deposition of cells). The lower compartment is filled with the properly diluted chemotactic factor such as zymosan-activated serum or *Escherichia coli* supernate up to the elbow; 0.1 ml of the cell suspension containing 5 × 10^6 cells/ml is added to the upper compartment, which is then filled completely with Medium 199. Following this, the lower compartment is filled similarly with Medium 199. (Filling

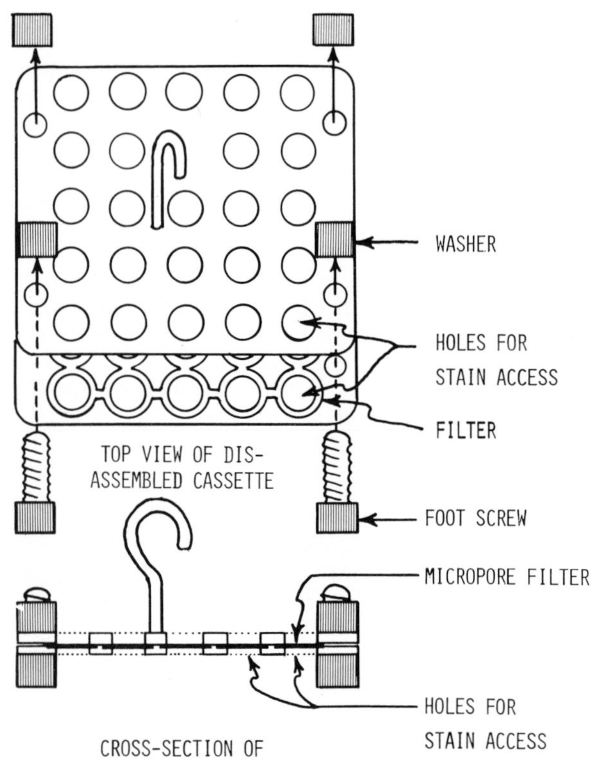

Figure 35–3. Staining cassette for 13 mm micropore filters (Ahlco Corporation, Southington, Ct.).

Table 35–3. PROTOCOL FOR PHAGOCYTE LOCOMOTION WORK-UP

Upper Compartment (Cells + Serum)		Lower Compartment (Factor)	To Test or Screen for:
Normal	+ No	No	Nonstimulated locomotion
Patient's	+ No	No	
Patient's	+ No	Activated* normal serum	Chemotaxis, complement-derived chemotactic factor, and chemotactic factor inactivator
Normal	+ No	Activated* normal serum	
Normal	+ No	Activated* patient's serum	
Normal	+ Normal	No	Cell-directed inhibitor of leukotaxis and leukokinesis-enhancing factor
Normal	+ Patient's	No	
Patient's	+ Normal	No	

*See p. 854 for serum "activation" by zymosan.

the lower compartment completely before the upper compartment is filled will lead to seepage of the chemotactic factor through the filter into the upper compartment.) The prepared chambers are incubated in air at 37° C.

The optimal incubation time is one that will allow the fastest migrating cells to reach at least halfway, but not completely penetrate the thickness of the filter. Periods that do not allow sufficient penetration into the depths of the filter are insensitive in detecting defects, except for the more severe ones. Table 35–3 shows the usual protocol for polymorphonuclear cell migration. In our laboratory, cells tested in the absence of serum or plasma in the upper compartment are incubated for 90 minutes, while cells tested with serum or plasma are tested for 60 minutes. Preventing cells from completely penetrating the filter avoids the variability of cell loss owing to cell detachment from the distal surface.

After incubation, the filters are removed, placed in specially made staining cassettes (Fig. 35–3), and, without being allowed to dry, quickly fixed in 100 per cent isopropyl alcohol for 30 seconds. The filters are then stained in hematoxylin for four minutes, rinsed in water, decolorized in acid alcohol for 30 seconds, rinsed in water again, dehydrated in three successive absolute isopropyl alcohol baths for five minutes each, and finally cleared in xylene for five to ten minutes. The stained filters are mounted on slides with Permount and covered with a thin cover slip.

The cells are counted (using 400 × magnification) at every 10 μm interval from the proximal cell monolayer to the distal surface. The number of cells counted per level is multiplied by the distance of that level to the proximal cell monolayer. Then the products obtained are added and the sum is divided by the total number of cells counted. The number obtained is the locomotion index (LI, which is the average distance [in micrometers] migrated by the cells within the allotted chamber incubation time). Refer to Table 35–4 for sample calculation. Three or more fields are counted and the LI for each duplicate or triplicate filter is calculated.

Evaluation of Results. Because of large day-to-day variability that occurs if the several variables are not stringently controlled, normal controls are performed simultaneously with each experiment. Variability also exists among normal cells and serums. In our laboratory, cell indices less than 64 per cent and serum values below 72 per cent of control values are generally abnormal. It is preferable, however, to retest the patient using a different normal control before making a final interpretation.

Phagocytosis Assay

The methods chosen for discussion here are used in our laboratory because of their relative simplicity, sensitivity, precision, and reproducibility. We do not use methods of quantitation by direct microscopic counting of "phagocytized" particles, despite their greater simplicity, because of difficulty in differentiating between *surface* and *internalized* particles.

The phagocytosis radioassay is quite complex and involved but is included because of its sensitivity and precision. For screening purposes, however, the quantitative nitroblue tetrazolium reduction test is sufficient. The NBT reduction test is simple, rapid, sensitive, and reproducible; it requires fewer cells for testing; it is better known and more widely applied; and it requires equipment that is generally available

Table 35–4. CALCULATION OF LOCOMOTION INDEX (LI)*

Distance from Origin (A) (in μm)	Number of Cells (B)	Cells × Distance (A × B)
0 (monolayer)	15	0
10	37	370
20	12	240
30	10	300
40	13	520
50	7	350
60	8	480
70	9	630
80	4	320
90	6	540
100	0	0
Total excluding monolayer count:	106	3750†
Total including monolayer count‡:	121	

*LI_{10} excluding monolayer = 3750 ÷ 106 = 35.38 μm. LI_0 including monolayer = 3750 ÷ 121 = 30.99 μm.

†This number is the total distance migrated by all the cells in cell-μm.

‡Inclusion of monolayer count in calculation of LI improves sensitivity of the method in assessment of nonstimulated migration and responses to chemotactic factor.

LI_{20} to LI_{90} can also be calculated.

5

in most, if not all, laboratories. Chemiluminescence (CL) assay is an equivalent examination that uses light emission (probably derived from singlet oxygen formation in phagocytizing leukocytes) as the indicator of phagocytic and oxygen-dependent microbicidal activities (Allen, 1972). The CL assay requires more cells to produce optimally detectable light emission; red cell contamination interferes with its measurement, requiring greater cell handling; and finally, a scintillation spectrophotometer, not generally available, is required for measurement of luminescence. Hence, CL will not be discussed further.

PHAGOCYTOSIS RADIOASSAY

In this method iodine-125–labeled bovine serum albumin antigen-antibody (immune complex) precipitate is used as the particles for engulfment (Ward, 1973). This method cannot be used to test opsonizing activity of serum. The most important technical aspect to monitor is the efficiency of removing extracellular immune precipitate from cells containing ingested immune precipitate. Two controls are performed simultaneously to quantitate this efficiency.

Materials

1. Patient's and normal polymorphonuclear leukocytes.
2. Bovine albumin in Cohn Fraction V (Mann Research Laboratory).
3. Crystalline bovine serum albumin (BSA) (Pentex).
4. Deep-well crystal scintillation gamma detector and scaler counter.
5. Ethylenediaminotetraacetic acid (EDTA).
6. TC Medium 199, pH 7.4 (Difco).
7. Phosphate-buffered saline, pH 7.4 (PBS).
8. Preparation of radiolabeled immune precipitate: (a) Antibody to BSA is prepared from rabbits immunized by repeated intradermal injections of 10 mg crystalline BSA. (b) The IgG fraction is obtained by DEAE cellulose fractionation of the hyperimmune serum. (c) With the use of quantitative precipitin analysis, the equivalence point of antigen-antibody binding is determined. (d) Next, BSA (bovine serum albumin) is labeled with iodine-125 by incubation of 1 mg BSA with 0.5 mC of ^{125}I (New England Nuclear). (e) An approximate quantity of labeled and unlabeled BSA is added to the antibody to form a dense precipitate, which is incubated at 37°C. for two hours and then kept at 4°C. overnight. The precipitate is washed and suspended in phosphate-buffered saline (PBS) to give 600 μg antibody nitrogen/ml.

Method

1. Cells (1×10^7/0.25 ml in Medium 199), immune precipitate (0.20 ml containing 20 to 30 μg antibody nitrogen with antigen at equivalence and radioactivity of about 10 to 15 $\times$ 10^3 cpm), and 0.20 ml of PBS are mixed and the initial radioactivity is counted and recorded.
2. The mixture is incubated at 37°C. for 30 minutes in a shaking water bath following which 0.1 ml of 0.2 M EDTA is added to stop the reaction. Then excess BSA (0.1 ml of 400 mg BSA/ml) is added to solubilize extracellular immune precipitate, and the mixture is incubated for another 30 minutes at 37°C. in the water bath. After incubation, the mixture is diluted with 3 ml PBS and centrifuged at 1000 g for 20 minutes. The supernatant fluid is discarded and the residual radioactivity is determined in the deep-well scintillation counter.
3. Both EDTA and BSA controls are used to monitor the efficiency of separating extracellular from intracellular immune complexes. The closer the values to background activity, the greater the efficiency. (a) EDTA is added to the cells prior to incubation with immune precipitate. (b) Excess BSA is added to immune precipitate prior to incubation with cells.
4. For calculation of phagocytosis, the uptake of radiolabeled immune complexes by "normal" (reference) cells is determined in duplicate and the average value obtained. The ratio of the corresponding value derived from patient cells to that value as described above multiplied by 100 gives per cent phagocytosis by patient cells as compared with normal cells.

Thus, per cent phagocytosis can be calculated:

$$\%\ \text{phagocytosis} = \frac{\text{uptake by patient cells}}{\text{uptake by control cells}} \times 100$$

If this assay is properly performed, test-to-test coefficient of variation is less than 1 per cent. The variability of phagocytosis in a normal population using this method has not been determined.

Quantitative Nitroblue Tetrazolium (NBT) Test

The quantitative NBT assay is an indirect test used to screen for disorders of phagocytosis and bacterial killing (oxygen-dependent bactericidal system). Defects of bacterial killing function owing to abnormalities of the oxygen-independent factors will not be detected by this assay. The method is slightly modified from that by Baehner (1968).

Materials

1. Normal and patient's polymorphonuclear cells.
2. Zymosan (Sigma) is opsonized with serum (2 mg zymosan with 0.05 ml serum) by incubation at 37°C. for five minutes.
3. Nitroblue tetrazolium Grade III (Sigma).
4. Potassium cyanide, 0.01 M.
5. Hydrochloric acid, 0.5 N.
6. Pyridine (Fisher Scientific).
7. Spectrophotometer.

Method

1. Polymorphonculear cells (2×10^6 cells in 0.4 ml Medium 199) are mixed with 0.05 ml of opsonized zymosan and 0.1 ml of 0.01 M of potassium cyanide and incubated in a shaking water bath at 37°C. After 10 minutes, 0.1 ml of NBT (2 mg/ml in water) is added and incubation is continued. After 15 minutes, the reaction is stopped with 4 ml of 0.5 N hydrochloric acid.
2. The tubes are centrifuged at 1000 g at 4°C. for 10 minutes, the supernatant fluid is discarded, and the reduced NBT (formazan) is extracted from the cell button with 4 ml of pyridine in a boiling water bath for 10 minutes under an exhaust hood.
3. The absorption of the extract is then determined in a spectrophotometer at 550 nm using pyridine as the blank control.
4. As a control a tube of cells without opsonized zymosan is run simultaneously to correct for spontaneous NBT reduction, which is high in certain conditions (Lace, 1975). The corrected NBT reduction is obtained by subtracting the control value from results obtained in the presence of opsonized zymosan. (For determination of serum opsonizing activity, use a control consisting of cells and unopsonized zymosan.)
5. The per cent decrease of NBT reduction can then be determined as follows:

Per cent decrease of NBT reduction =

$$\frac{\text{Normal NBT} - \text{Patient's NBT}}{\text{Normal NBT}} \times 100$$

where normal NBT = A_{550} of extracted blue formazan in normal cells and patient's NBT = A_{550} of extracted blue formazan in patient's cells. The value in 10 normals is 0.458 ± 0.101 (mean ± S.D.).

Phagocytosis assay using radiolabeled immune precipitate can be combined with NBT assay to differentiate between a defect of phagocytosis and an inability to generate reducing activity for NBT dye. This can be done by replacing 0.05 ml of opsonized zymosan with 0.025 ml of immune complex.

Bacterial Killing Assay

Most methods of quantitating bacterial killing by phagocytes are laborious, expensive, and require practice to obtain reproducible results. The method we use is a modification of a technique described previously (Tan, 1971), which uses *Staphylococcus aureus* as the test organism and lysostaphin to kill extracellular organisms. With this technique it is possible to define separately the engulfment and the bactericidal process. To facilitate understanding of this complicated method, it is illustrated in Table 35–5.

Materials

1. Patient's and control polymorphonuclear leukocytes.
2. Eighteen-hour trypticase soy broth culture of *Staphylococcus aureus*.
3. Mueller-Hinton agar plates. These are used because they are transparent, which allows counting of the colonies through the agar without opening the plates.
4. Sterile plastic tubes with caps.
5. Isotonic saline.
6. TC Medium 199, pH 7.4 (Difco).
7. Lysostaphin, 10 units/ml (Schwarz-Mann, Becton-Dickinson).
8. Trypsin, 2.5%.
9. Distilled water.
10. Sonifer (W-140, Branson Sonic).
11. Spectrophotometer.

Method

1. An 18-hour broth culture of *Staphylococcus aureus* in trypticase soy broth is washed twice with sterile distilled water. The bacterial button is resuspended in 4 ml of distilled water and then sonicated for 15 seconds at 45 watts to disaggregate the bacteria. The solution is then adjusted to an absorbance of 0.75 at 650 nm using a spectrophotometer. This solution should contain 4 × 10^8 bacteria/ml.

Table 35–5. SCHEMATIC ILLUSTRATION OF LEUKOCYTE BACTERICIDAL ASSAY

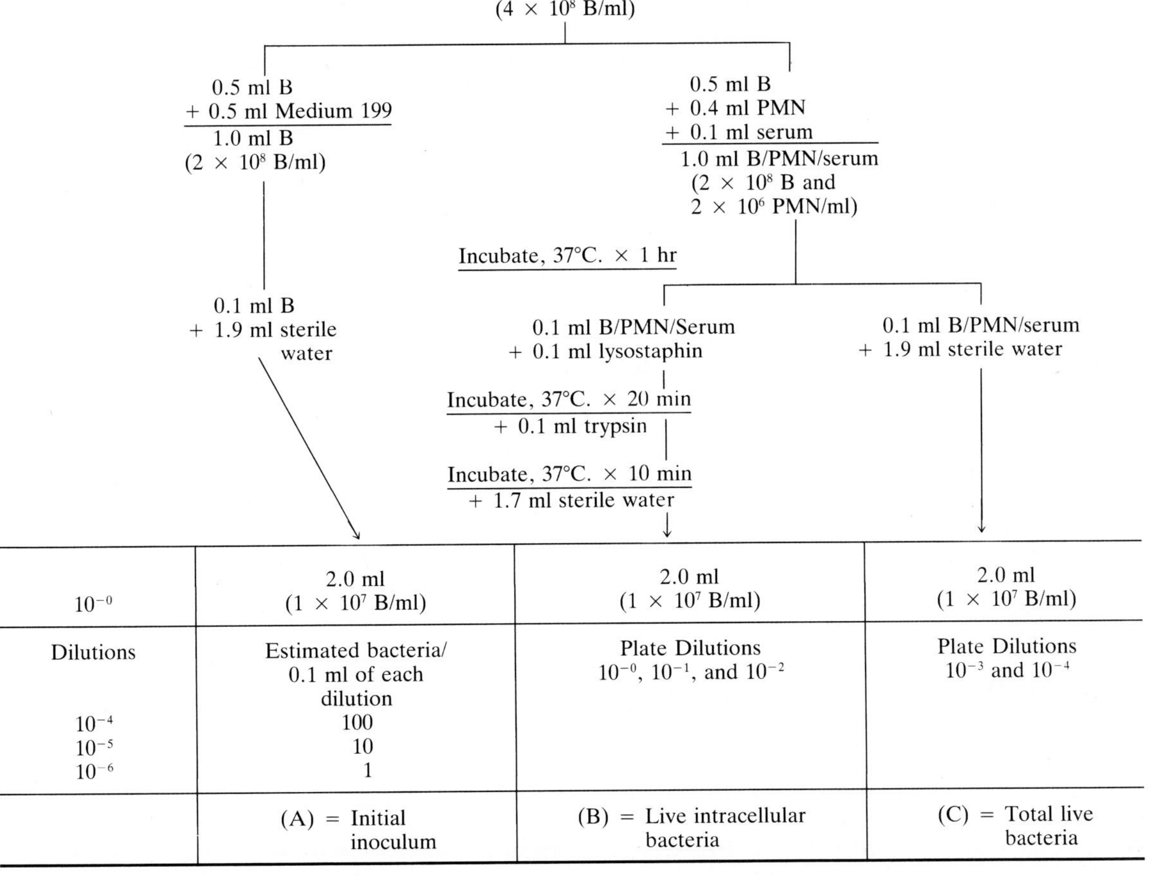

2. To a 0.5 ml aliquot of bacterial suspension in a capped plastic tube, 0.4 ml of PMN solution (containing 5 × 10^6 cells/ml) and 0.1 ml of serum are added and incubated in a shaking water bath at 37°C. for one hour.

3. After incubation, 1.9 ml of distilled water is added to 0.1 ml of the bacteria-PMN-serum mixture. Serial 10-fold dilutions are then carried out with distilled water and 0.1 ml portions from each of the 10^{-3} and 10^{-4} dilutions are plated by spreading evenly over Mueller-Hinton agar plates using a smooth sterile L-shaped glass rod spreader. This will enumerate the *total live bacteria* (live extracellular and intracellular bacteria).

4. Into another 0.1 ml portion of the incubated bacteria-PMN-serum mixture is added 0.1 ml of lysostaphin (10 units/ml) and incubated in the water bath at 37°C. for 20 minutes. After incubation, 0.1 ml of 2.5 per cent trypsin is added to inactivate the lysostaphin and the mixture reincubated at 37°C. for another 10 minutes. Two serial 10-fold dilutions with distilled water are carried out and 0.1 ml of the undiluted and the two 10-fold dilutions are plated. This will enumerate only *live intracellular bacteria,* since lysostaphin will destroy all bacteria not within cells.

5. To determine the number of live bacteria in the *initial inoculum,* 0.5 ml of the bacterial suspension is mixed with 0.5 ml of Medium 199. Serial 10-fold dilutions are made and 0.1 ml portions of the 10^{-4}, 10^{-5}, and 10^{-6} dilutions are plated.

6. The plates are incubated in air at 37°C. for 18 to 24 hours and the number of colonies on each plate is counted. Counts from countable higher dilutions are used. Calculation of killed intracellular (D) and total phagocytosed bacteria (E) can then be made from A (initial inoculum), B (live intracellular bacteria), and C (total live bacteria), thus:

D (killed intracellular bacteria) = A − C
E (phagocytosed bacteria) = B + D

Values that exceed the control by one log or greater are abnormal.

To test for phagocytosis and bacterial killing of gram-negative organisms, antibiotics can be used to eliminate extracellular bacteria. For example, to test for *Escherichia coli* phagocytosis and killing, gentamicin can be used. Antibiotic concentration five times higher than the minimum inhibitory concentration (MIC) for the strain of the organism is used in step 4, so that during the lysis procedure the 1:10 dilution of the mixture (0.2 ml to 2 ml) with distilled water will sufficiently lower the antibiotic concentration below the MIC.

Monocyte Function Test

The preceding paragraphs have discussed testing of polymorphonuclear cell function. With few modifications the same techniques can be applied for monocytes. Monocytes are generally more adherent than polymorphonuclear cells so that testing monocyte adherence requires lowering the amount of nylon fibers, for example, from 40 to 30 mg per column.

For testing monocyte locomotion, these modifications are necessary: (1) use micropore filters of 8 μm porosity, (2) use specific chemotactic factor for monocyte response, since monocytes do not usually respond to most *E. coli*–derived chemotactic factors, and (3) incubate the chamber for three hours. For screening purposes, testing non-stimulated migration and chemotactic responsiveness is all that is necessary.

Increasing the incubation time of the cell-immune precipitate mixture to 60 minutes is the only modification necessary when testing monocyte phagocytosis using the radioassay method, but the values are generally lower than those obtained for polymorphonuclear cells. NBT reduction by monocytes is also lower and slower. The incubation period of the cell-opsonized zymosan mixture is extended to 60 minutes. The amount of formazan extracted is consistently four to six times less than that obtained in the same number of polymorphonuclear cells incubated for the same period of time. Increasing zymosan or NBT dye concentration does not significantly increase NBT reduction.

Comparative studies between the bactericidal powers of monocytes and polymorphonuclear cells have been reported (Steigbigel, 1974). In general, the former is said to be less active than the latter. No modification of the microbicidal assay is necessary when testing monocytes.

Allen, R. C., Stjerholm, R. L., and Steele, R. H.: Evidence for the generation of an electronic excitation state(s) in human polymorphonuclear leukocytes and its participation in bactericidal activity. Biochem. Biophys. Res. Commun., *47*:679, 1972.

Athens, J. W., Raab, S. O., Haab, O. P., Mauer, A. M., Ashenbrucker, H., Cartwright, G. E., and Wintrobe, M. M.: Leukokinetic studies. IV. The total blood, circulating, and marginating granulocyte pools and the granulocyte turnover rate in normal subjects. J. Clin. Invest., *40*:989, 1961.

Baehner, R. L., and Nathan, D. G.: Quantitative nitroblue tetrazolium test in chronic granulomatous disease. N. Engl. J. Med., *278*:971, 1968.

Boxer, L. A., Hedley-Whyte, E. T., and Stossel, T. P.: Neutrophil actin dysfunction and abnormal neutrophil behavior. N. Engl. J. Med., *291*:1093, 1974.

Boyden, S.: The chemotactic effect of mixtures of antibody and antigen on polymorphonuclear leukocytes. J. Exp. Med., *115*:453, 1962.

Fass, R. J., and Saslaw, S.: Earth day histoplasmosis. A new type of urban pollution. Arch. Intern. Med., *128*:588, 1971.

Frei, P. C., Baisero, M. H., and Ochsner, M.: Chemotaxis of human polymorphonuclears *in vitro.* II. Technical study. J. Immunol. Methods, *5*:375, 1974.

Gallin, J. I., Clark, R. A., and Kimball, H. R.: Granulocyte chemotaxis. An improved *in vitro* assay employing ^{51}Cr-labelled granulocytes. J. Immunol., *110*:233, 1973.

Goldstein, I., Hoffstein, S., Gallin, J., and Weissmann, G.: Mechanisms of lysosomal enzyme release from human leukocytes: Microtubule assembly and membrane fusion induced by a component of complement. Proc. Natl. Acad. Sci. U.S.A., *70*:2916, 1973.

Hill, H. R., and Quie, P. G.: Defective neutrophil chemotaxis associated with hyperimmunoglobulinemia E. *In* Bellati, J. A., and Dayton, D. H. (eds.): The Phagocytic Cell in Host Resistance. New York, Raven Press, 1975.

Iannini, P. B., Claffey, T., and Quintiliani, R.: Bacteremic pseudomonas pneumonia. J.A.M.A., *230*:558, 1974.

Keller, H. U., Borel, J. F., Wilkinson, P. C., Hess, M. W., and Cottier, H.: Reassessment of Boyden's technique for measuring chemotaxis. J. Immunol. Methods, *1*:165, 1972.

Lace, J. K., Tan, J. S., and Watanakunakorn, C.: An appraisal of the nitroblue tetrazolium reduction test. Am. J. Med., *58*:685, 1975.

MacGregor, R. R., Spagnuolo, P. J., and Lentnek, A. L.: Inhibition of granulocyte adherence by ethanol, prednisone, and aspirin, measured with an assay system. N. Engl. Med., *291*:642, 1974.

Maderazo, E. G., Ward, P. A., Woronick, C. L., and Quintiliani,

R.: Partial characterization of a cell-directed inhibitor of leukotaxis in human serum. J. Lab. Clin. Med., *89*:190, 1977.

Maderazo, E. G., and Woronick, C. L.: A modified micropore filter assay of human granulocyte leukotaxis. *In* Gallin, J. I., and Quie, P. G. (eds.): Leukocyte Chemotaxis. New York, Raven Press, 1978.

Maderazo, E. G., Woronick, C. L., and Ward, P. A.: Leukokinesis-enhancing factor in human serum: Partial characterization and relationship to disorders of leukocyte migration. Clin. Immunol. Immunopath. *12*:382, 1979.

Najjar, V. A.: Defective phagocytosis due to deficiencies involving the tetrapeptide tuftsin. J. Pediatr., *89*:1121, 1975.

Oliver, J. M.: Impaired microtubule function correctable by cyclic GMP and cholinergic agonists in the Chédiak-Higashi syndrome. Am. J. Path., *85*:395, 1976.

Quie, P. G.: Pathology of bactericidal power of neutrophils. Semin. Hematol., *12*:153, 1975.

Rebuck, J. W., and Crowley, J. H.: Method of studying leukocyte function in vivo. Ann. N.Y. Acad. Sci., *59*:757, 1955.

Rinehart, J. J., and Boulware, T.: Microfilament and microtubule function in human monocytes. J. Lab. Clin. Med., *90*:737, 1977.

Spitznagel, J. K.: Bactericidal mechanisms of the granulocyte. *In* Greenwalt, T. J., and Jamieson, G. A. (eds.): Progress in Clinical and Biological Research, Vol. 13. New York, Alan R. Liss, Inc., 1977.

Steigbigel, R. T., Lambert, L. H., Jr., and Remington, J. S.: Phagocytic and bactericidal properties of normal human monocytes. J. Clin. Invest., *53*:131, 1974.

Tan, J. S., Watanakunakorn, C., and Phair, J. P.: A modified assay of neutrophil function. Use of lysostaphin to differentiate defective phagocytosis from impaired intracellular killing. J. Lab. Clin. Med., *78*:316, 1971.

Ward, P. A.: Leukotaxis and leukotactic disorders. A review. Am. J. Path., *77*:520, 1974.

Ward, P. A., Lepow, I. H., and Newman, L. J.: Bacterial factors chemotactic for polymorphonuclear leukocytes. Am. J. Path., *53*:725, 1968.

Ward, P. A., and Zvaifler, N. J.: Quantitative phagocytosis by neutrophils. I. A method with immune complexes. J. Immunol., *111*:1771, 1973.

Winkelstein, J. A.: Opsonins: Their function, identity and clinical significance. J. Pediatr., *82*:747, 1973.

Woronick, C. L., Malnick, J., and Maderazo, E. G.: Cell-directed inhibitor of human leukocyte locomotion. J. Lab. Clin. Med., *98*:58, 1981.

Zigmond, S. H., and Hirsch, J. G.: Leucocyte locomotion and chemotaxis. New methods for evaluation and demonstration of a cell-derived chemotactic factor. J. Exp. Med., *137*:387, 1973.

5

36

IMMUNOGLOBULINS AND PARAPROTEINS

MANUEL J. RICARDO, JR., PH.D., and RUSSELL H. TOMAR, M.D.

INTRODUCTION

Antibodies are globular proteins which bind antigen. The association of antibody activity with the gamma globulin fraction of serum was first shown by Tiselius (1939), who hyperimmunized rabbits with pneumococcal polysaccharides to produce high titers of circulating antibody. After examining the effect of absorbing the serum with antigen, he noted that only the gamma globulin fraction was significantly reduced on the electrophoretic profile.

We now recognize that heterogeneity exists in the types of molecules that can function as antibodies and that their exquisite antigenic specificity appears to rest solely in the amino acid sequence of their N-terminus. The gamma globulins are now called immunoglobulins. The immunoglobulin molecules are classified into different isotypes based on differences in amino acid sequence of the C-terminus of the molecule. In man, five major isotypes can be distinguished: immunoglobulin M (IgM), IgG, IgA, IgE, and IgD. Molecular genetics has provided insights into the ways by which complete antibody molecules are formed. We now know which chromosome codes for the heavy and light chains and something about the structural function of that piece of genetic material as it relates to antibody formation and antigen specificity.

IMMUNOGLOBULIN STRUCTURAL FEATURES

Electrophoretic Mobility. The classification of immunoglobulins based strictly on electrophoretic mobility is inadequate because antibodies migrate from α^1 to γ^2. For example, purified human IgG displays a broad range of mobilities. This heterogeneity is related somewhat to a further subclassification of immunoglobulins and especially to distinct biologic activities. Thus, unlike other serum proteins such as albumin, immunoglobulins display a broad band upon electrophoresis. When immunoglobulins of identical structure are present, namely monoclonal immunoglobulins, a single sharp band is seen.

Polypeptides. Porter and Edelman described two sizes of polypeptide chains under denaturing and reducing conditions. The 50,000 dalton polypeptide was called heavy (H) chain, and the 23,000 dalton polypeptide was designated light (L) chain. From their studies, the basic structure of an IgG molecule was formulated as 2 H-chains and 2 L-chains based on the amount of both polypeptides recovered from the molar amount of native IgG reduced. Subsequent studies with other human and animal immunoglobulin isotypes have shown that all possess the same fundamental disulfide-linked, four-chain structure and an accessory J polypeptide chain. Secretory dimeric IgA has a

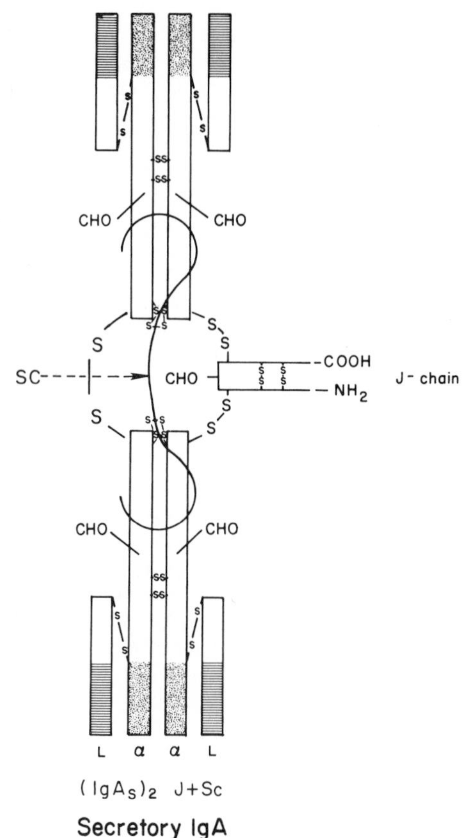

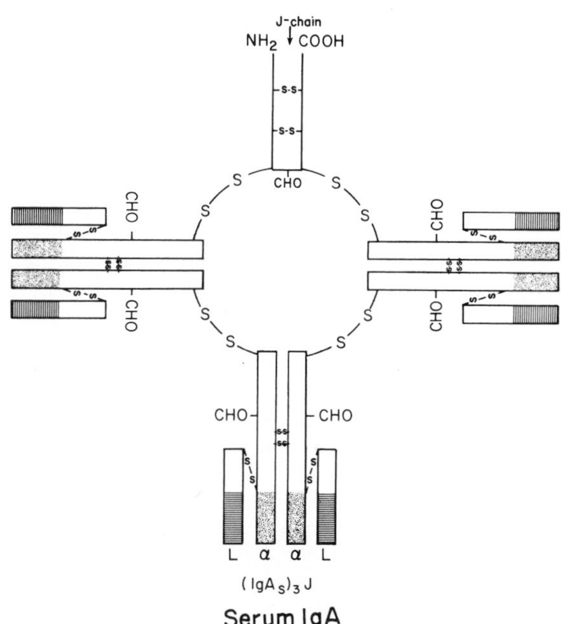

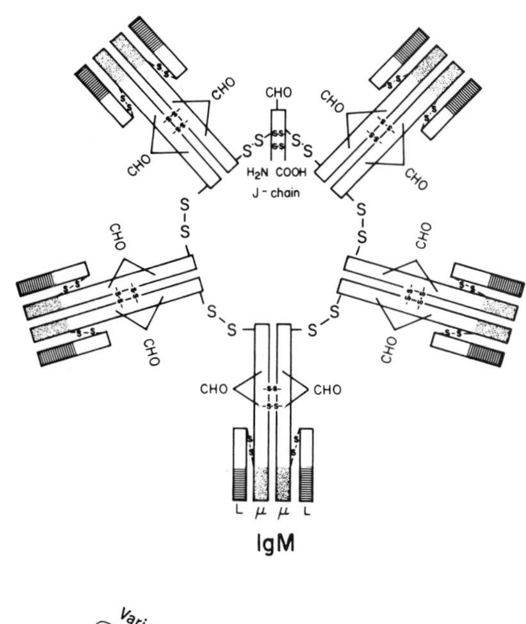

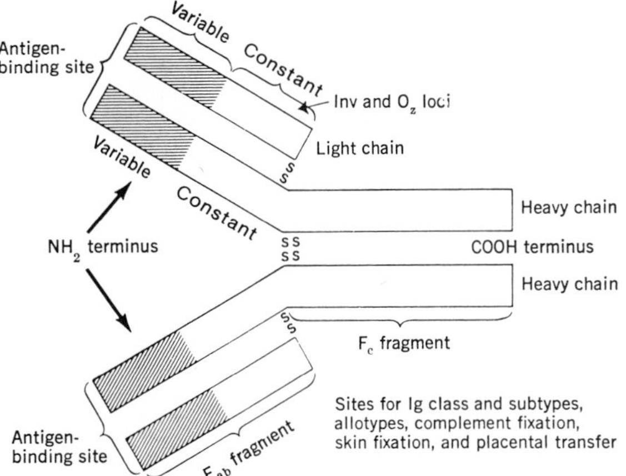

Figure 36–1. Representative structures of the polymeric immunoglobulins (IgA and IgM). The basic immunoglobulin unit consists of two light and two heavy chains. These units may be present in pairs, triads, or pentamers. The accessory J-chain is associated with each of the polymers and is believed to be linked by disulfide bonds to two of the subunits. The secretory component (SC) is found only in secretory dimeric IgA and may or may not be disulfide linked. The linkage shown in the diagram is hypothetical. The positions of the oligosaccharide groups are indicated by CHO. The variable regions of both heavy and light chains are delineated by dots and horizontal lines, respectively. In humans, IgM is always found as a pentamer and IgA as a monomer, dimer, or trimer in serum. *Lower right*, Schematic diagram of an immunoglobulin molecule (From Harnes, D. R.: Postgrad. Med., *48*:66, 1970).

5

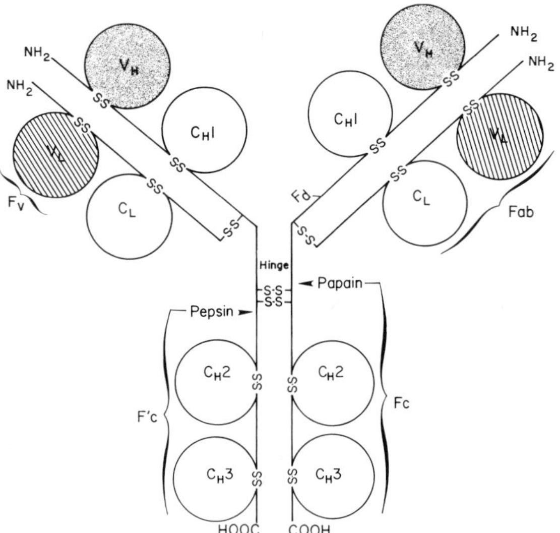

Figure 36–2. Schematic representation of immunoglobulin G molecule. The relative positions of the *interchain* disulfide bonds and the *intrachain* disulfide bonds which form the loop regions are shown. Each of the loops delineates the domain of the light and heavy chain labeled accordingly. The probable sites of enzymatic cleavage in the "hinge" region by papain or pepsin are indicated. The papain fragments are designated Fab and Fc. The pepsin fragments are Fc′ and Fab′2 (two Fab fragments disulfide linked). Digestion of Fab with pepsin under the proper conditions will yield the fragment Fv (V_H and V_L non-convalently associated). The part of the heavy chain which contributes to the Fab fragment is designated Fd. See text, below, for further details.

J chain plus an additional accessory polypeptide, the secretory component. The structure of immunoglobulins is illustrated in Figure 36–1.

Fab, Fc, Fd, Fv. Immunoglobulins can be split by the proteolytic enzyme papain into two major 3.5S components. The fragment capable of combining with antigen to form a soluble complex, which will not precipitate because it is univalent, was designated Fab (fragment antigen binding) by Porter (1959). The other fragment, which lacks binding affinity for antigen, is termed Fc (fragment crystallizable), even though these Fc fragments do not crystallize readily (Fig. 36–2).

Another proteolytic enzyme, pepsin, cleaves the intact IgG molecules above the interheavy chain disulfide bond generating a 5S component consisting of two Fab fragments and designated Fab′2. Fab′2 is bivalent and can still precipitate with antigen (Nisonoff, 1960). Extensive reduction of Fab′2 or Fab with mercaptans yields an Fd′ or Fd fragment (N-terminal half of the heavy chain), respectively, and free light chain. The enzyme-sensitive portion of antibody molecules is designated the "hinge" region. Pepsin cleavage of Fab′2 or Fab fragment can yield an Fv (fragment variable, the N-terminal fragment) fragment under carefully controlled conditions.

Disulfide Bonds. Immunoglobulins possess both interchain H-L and H-H disulfide bonds. The light chain cysteine residue that contributes to the H-L linkage is at the C-terminus of the chain (human κ) or adjacent to it (human λ). This contrasts to the position of the H-L linking cysteine residues in the heavy chain at position 131 or about 214, depending on isotype and animal species. Whereas these disulfide bonds stabilize the structure, they apparently are not essential in every case because some IgA monomers and IgD molecules lack the H-L bonds. On the other hand, the H-H disulfides are critical, along with their high proline content, in giving the "hinge" region of the molecule a degree of inflexibility. This structural feature is important in allowing the Fab arms of the molecule to rotate 180 degrees (segmental flexibility) in solution or on the surface of cells for antigen interaction.

All immunoglobulin proteins have intrachain disulfide bonds that are essential in establishing the domain structure in both polypeptide chains. The polymeric immunoglobulins are characterized by possessing intersubunit disulfide bonds that maintain the polymeric form. In addition, they contain the accessory polypeptide J chain, which is also disulfide linked between two monomer units (Mestecky, 1974). The secretory component (SC) or transport piece found exclusively in dimeric secretory IgA may be disulfide linked to the monomers (Underdown, 1977).

Carbohydrate Moieties. One of the striking differences in the structure of immunoglobulin is the number, sequence, kind, and location of carbohydrate groups. Carbohydrate is found usually in the constant regions of heavy chains and rarely in the variable region or light chain.

Secretory IgA has a higher carbohydrate content than serum IgA because of the carbohydrate in the secretory component. IgM, IgD, and IgE have the largest amounts of oligosaccharide, followed by IgA and then by IgG (Table 36–1).

Although the function of the carbohydrate moiety is not precisely understood, it appears to play a role in the secretion of antibodies by plasma cells and in biologic functions associated with the Fc fragment.

Heavy Chains. There are five major classes of heavy chains (μ, γ, α, δ, and ε) in man. Although all five isotypes have the same basic four-chain structure in the monomeric form, they differ characteristically in the amino acid sequence of their class-specific heavy chain. This difference is restricted to the constant region sequences. Furthermore, the constant region sequences of heavy chains determine such characteristic differences in immunoglobulin class structure as (1) the length of the chain and the number of domains; (2) the number and location of the interchain, intrachain, and intersubunit disulfide bridges; (3) the position, number, and kind of oligosaccharides attached to the heavy chain; and (4) the degree of polymerization of the immunoglobulin molecules.

Antibodies generally exhibit two sets of interlinked functions in which the heavy chain is the major participant: (1) specific binding of antigen at the Fv region of the molecule and (2) biologic or effector activities. The latter functions are localized at the Fc part of the molecule and under physiologic conditions come into effect only after antigen binding.

Light Chains. The light chains (about 214 amino acids) are common to all immunoglobulin isotypes. Structural examination of light chains was made

Table 36–1. PHYSICAL PROPERTIES OF HUMAN IMMUNOGLOBULINS

WHO Designation	**IgM**	**IgG**	**IgA**	**IgD**	**IgE**
Heavy chains	μ	γ	α	δ	ϵ
Heavy chain subclasses	μ_1, μ_2	$\gamma_1, \gamma_2, \gamma_3, \gamma_4$	α_1, α_2	–	–
Light chains	κ or λ	κ or λ	κ or λ	κ or λ	κ or λ
Molecular formula	IgM(κ) $(2\mu 2\kappa)_5$ IgM(λ) $(2\mu 2\lambda)_5$	IgG(κ) $2\gamma 2\kappa$ IgG(λ) $2\gamma 2\lambda$	IgA(κ) $(2\alpha 2\kappa)_{1\text{-}3}$ IgA(λ) $(2\alpha 2\lambda)_{1\text{-}3}$ IgA(κ)$(2\alpha 2\kappa)_2$S† IgA(λ) $(2\alpha 2\lambda)_2$S	IgD(κ) $2\delta 2\kappa$ IgD(λ) $2\delta 2\lambda$	IgE(κ) $2\epsilon 2\kappa$ IgE(λ) $2\epsilon 2\lambda$
Number of 4-chain units per molecule	5	1	1–3	1	1
Heavy chain molecular weight, daltons	70,000	50,000–60,000	55,000	62,000	70,000
Light chain molecular weight, daltons	23,000	23,000	23,000	23,000	23,000
Sedimentation coefficient, S_{20w}	18.0–19.0	6.7–7.0	6.6–14.0	6.9–7.0	7.9–8.0
Molecular weight, daltons	900,000	143,000–160,000	159,000–447,000	177,000–185,000	187,000–200,000
Electrophoretic mobility	γ^1-β^1	γ^2-α^1	γ^2-β^2	γ^1	γ^1
Carbohydrate content, per cent	7–14	2.2–3.5	7.5–9.0	12–13	11–12
Heavy chain allotypes	–	Gm	Am	–	–
Light chain allotypes	Km(κ)*	Km(κ)*	Km(κ)*	Km(κ)*	Km(κ)
Valency for antigen binding	5(10)	2	2,4 (? polymeric forms)	2	2
Number of domains	5	4	4	4	5

*Formerly designated Inv marker.
†Dimer in external secretions carries secretory component -S.

possible by the discovery that some individuals with myeloma disease have in their urine a monoclonal dimeric form of light chains called Bence Jones protein. The dimer polypeptide chain is derived from the light chain pool in the synthesis of the myeloma immunoglobulin protein. Serologic analysis with antisera raised in rabbits against Bence Jones proteins from several patients led to the discovery of two isotypic forms of light chains (κ and λ). The isotypic determinants of κ or λ reside in the respective constant region of the light chain. As one would expect, the parent myeloma protein would react only with either κ or λ antisera, never both. The reaction of normal globulin (normal serum antibodies) with these reagents showed that molecules with κ or λ chains are present. The two isotypic specificities were never found on the same molecule. The ratio of κ:λ in normal serum is 2:1, although this ratio can vary in different species, as well as between different populations of antibodies. Interestingly, the number of reported cases of myeloma protein carrying κ or λ chains is also approximately 2:1, suggesting that the cells producing κ or λ chains are at equal risk for neoplastic conversion.

Accessory Polypeptide Chains. The presence of the J chain in polymeric immunoglobulins and its absence from monomeric immunoglobulins suggest that it may be important in facilitating the polymerization of the IgA and IgM subunits into their appropriate polymeric form (Inman, 1974). In the case of secretory IgA, the presence of J chain is clearly mandatory for the association of the secretory component (SC). The binding site for SC is probably in the Fc structure, the conformation of which is dependent on the presence of J chain (Fig. 36–1).

The J chain is a small glycopeptide with a distinctive acidic property and a fast electrophoretic mobility in alkaline gels. The 15,000 dalton J polypeptide has appreciable amounts of arginine (9 residues), aspartic acid (20 residues), and glutamic acid (13 residues) per molecule and represents less than 5 per cent of the total polymer protein.

The secretory component is preferentially associated with dimeric IgA in external secretions but is not bound to any protein in serum, including serum IgA. The secretory component may exist in free form or bound to secretory IgA by strong non-covalent interactions. The binding does not usually involve covalent bonding, although disulfide bonds have been implicated in a small fraction of human secretory IgA molecules. The secretory component is a single glycopeptide with a high carbohydrate content and an electrophoretic mobility in the fast β range with a molecular weight of 71,000 daltons.

Much of the IgA secreted by the plasma cells in exocrine glands and mucous membranes is dimeric. The secreted IgA passes from the interstitial tissues across the epithelial basement membrane into epithelial layer. At some point before its secretion into the lumen, IgA combines with secretory component made in epithelial cells. Thus, the fully assembled secretory IgA molecule is the synthetic product of two distinct types of cells (plasma cells and epithelial cells), both of which reside locally in the mucous membrane or gland. The exact site where dimeric IgA couples with secretory component is not known but may be either inside the epithelial cell or at its surface.

Immunoglobulin Domain. The domain hypothesis proposed by Edelman (1962) has provided an important conceptual framework upon which to build our

Table 36–2. BIOLOGIC PROPERTIES OF IMMUNOGLOBULIN DOMAINS (IgG)*

Domain	Known or Probable Function
C_H3	1. Cytotrophic reactions involving: (a) Macrophages and monocytes (b) Heterologous mast cells (c) Cytotoxic killer (K) cells (d) B cells 2. Non-covalent assembly of heavy and light chains
C_H2	1. Binding of complement (Clq) 2. Control of catabolic rate
C_H1/C_L	1. Non-covalent assembly of heavy and light chains 2. Covalent assembly of heavy and light chains 3. Spacers between interdomain interactions involving antigen binding and effector functions
V_H/V_L	1. Antigen binding 2. Non-covalent bonding of heavy and light chains

*From Dorrington, K. J., and Painter, R. H.: Biological activities of the constant region of immunoglobulin G. In Mandel, T. E., et al., (eds.): Process in Immunology III. Canberra City, Australian Academy of Science, 1977.

understanding of the structural and functional properties of immunoglobulins and antibodies. Primary sequence data provided the first impetus toward the formulation of a domain concept. Complete amino acid sequences have been determined for κ, λ, γ, μ, α, and ϵ chains of human immunoglobulins. Taken together, these sequences have indicated that both heavy and light chains could be divided into contiguous homology regions. The light chain homologous subunits were designated V_L or variable part of the light chain, and C_L or constant portion of the light chain. The heavy chains have one V_H domain and three or four constant region domains, C_H1 to C_H4 (Fig. 36–2). Reduction of the intrachain disulfide bonds followed by sequence analysis has revealed that each domain segment contains a single disulfide loop which spans 60 to 80 amino acid residues. The average length of each domain segment is approximately 110 residues, which includes the amino acid residues of the disulfide loop. The light chains of human IgG have two loop sections per polypeptide chain, whereas the heavy chains have four or five loop sections. In formulating the domain concept, Edelman proposed that such domain has evolved to perform a specific function(s). Experimental data have lent support to this hypothesis. A summary of the current state of knowledge regarding the functional differentiation of immunoglobulin domains is given in Table 36–2. Although a number of biologic properties of immunoglobulins have not yet been ascribed to a particular domain, it has become evident that the concept of structural-functional domains now stands as one of the basic principles of immunoglobulin biology.

ANTIBODY DIVERSITY

Introduction. It has been estimated that man can produce up to 10^9 different antibodies. Immunologists have debated whether man is born with the ability to make these antibodies (germ-line theory) or if during life we "learn" to make these proteins (somatic or instructional theory). There is little evidence to support a strictly instructional hypothesis such as antigen templates for antibody. Over the past several years, a formulation has been made combining these hypotheses. This formulation is based on data developed genetic probes.

Isotypes, Allotypes, the Antigen Binding Site, and Idiotypes. Most immunoglobulins have three different genetic markers (Table 36–3). *Isotype* refers to the genetic marker that determines the immunoglobulin class and resides in the constant region of the heavy and light chains. There are five known immunoglobulin isotypes, IgG, IgA, IgM, IgD, and IgE, each

Table 36–3. SUMMARY OF IMMUNOGLOBULIN VARIANTS*

Type of Variation	Distribution	Variant	Location	Examples
Isotypic	All variants present in serum of a normal individual	Classes Subclasses Types Subtypes Subgroups	C_H C_H C_L C_L V_L, V_H	IgM, IgE IgA_1, IgA_2 κ, λ $\lambda 0z^+$, $\lambda 0z^-$ $V_{\kappa I}$, $V_{\kappa II}$, V_{HI}, V_{HII}
Allotypic	Allelic forms not present in all individuals	Allotypes	Mainly C_H/C_L Occasionally V_H/V_L	Gm group (human) b_4, b_5, b_6, b_9
Idiotypic	Antigenic individuality specific to each Ig molecule	Idiotypes	V_H/V_L	Determinant identified by antibody specific to an individual immunoglobulin molecule

*Modified from Roitt (1980).

Table 36–4. PHYSIOLOGIC PROPERTIES OF HUMAN IMMUNOGLOBULINS

	IgM	IgG	IgA	IgD	IgE
Normal adult serum concentration mg/ml	1.2–4.0	8.0–16.0	0.4–2.2	0.03	17–450 ng/ml
International units/ml	69–322	92–207	54–268	–	<100
Per cent total immunoglobulin	13	80	6	1	0.002
Intravascular distribution, per cent	41	48	76	75	51
Synthetic rate, mg/kg/d	2.2	35	24	0.4	0.003
Catabolic rate in serum, per cent/d (day)	10.6	6	24	37	90
(or half-life, d)	(5–6)	(18–23)	(5–6.5)	(2.8)	(2.3)

able to combine with κ or λ light chains leading to 10 different immunoglobulin composites that are present in all individuals of a given mammalian species. There are subclasses and subtypes of immunoglobulins (Table 36–1). All variants may be seen in an individual "normal" serum. *Allotypes* are genetically inherited variations in amino acid sequence most commonly localized on the constant portion of the heavy or light chains. These alleleic forms are not present in all individuals but may be used as genetic markers in family or anthropological studies (Table 36–4). The *antibody combining site* of immunoglobulins has been studied in great detail. Amino acid analysis of a number of purified paraproteins and induced antibodies has revealed that, within a given major immunoglobulin isotype, the N-terminal amino acid (N1–N110) portions of both heavy and light chains show considerable variation, whereas the remaining part of the chains is relatively constant in structure. A comparison of light chain sequences has revealed that residues around positions 30, 50, and 90 are *hypervariable.* These "hot spots" on the light chains are designated L_V1, L_V2, and L_V3, respectively. A similar conclusion was reached for the heavy chain after extensive sequence analysis of V_H regions (H_V1, H_V2, and H_V3). An additional segment of hypervariability (positions 86 to 91) has been described for some heavy chains (Fig. 36–3).

Several studies have shown that the proteolytic fragments Fab and Fab′2 obtained from induced antibodies contain the antigen-specific binding sites, thus implicating the variable domains (V_L/V_H) or the constant domains (C_L/C_H1) in antigen recognition.

Further work demonstrated that the V_L/V_H domain was capable of binding antigens. Direct evidence that the variable region on both heavy and light chains contributes to antibody specificity is suggested by experiments in which isolated chains are examined for their antigen-combining potential. Isolated heavy chains demonstrate varying degrees of residual activity, but light chains show relatively little. However, on recombination there is always a significant increase in antigen-binding capacity.

Idiotypes are genetic variants associated with the immunoglobulin antigen-combining sites. Each idiotype is clonally derived, i.e., one B lymphocyte alone expresses one unique idiotype. Idiotypy imparts an antigenic individuality to the immunoglobulin molecule. Such variable region structures or idiotypes, when injected into heterologous species, elicit antibodies (anti-idiotypes). A given idiotype consists of a set of reactivities against epitopes, and both immunoglobulin chains are needed for full idiotypic expression (Natvig, 1973).

Idiotypes, anti-idiotypes, and even anti-anti-idiotypes play a prominent role in Jerne's "network" theory of immune regulation (Bona, 1981).

Gene Activation. The genes coding for the human heavy chain are on chromosome 14; for kappa chain on chromosome 2; and for lambda chain on chromo-

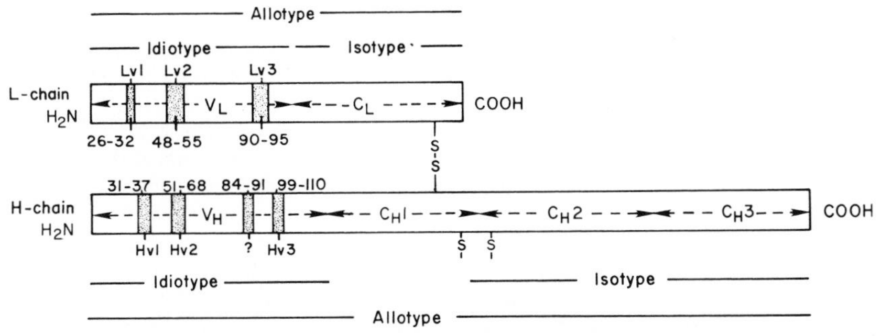

Figure 36–3. The structure of the light and heavy chains showing the positions and lengths of the hypervariable regions in the V_L domain (designated Lv1, Lv2, Lv3) and V_H domain (designated Hv1, Hv2, Hv3). The amino acid residues are numbered starting from the N-terminal. In some heavy chains an additional (?) hypervariable region (N89-N91) has been observed. The diagram also illustrates the region(s) where the major immunoglobulin variants may be found. The idiotypic determinants are found exclusively in the V_L and V_H domains and the isotypic marker in the constant regions of both chains. The allotypic markers can occur throughout the entire length of both chains.

5

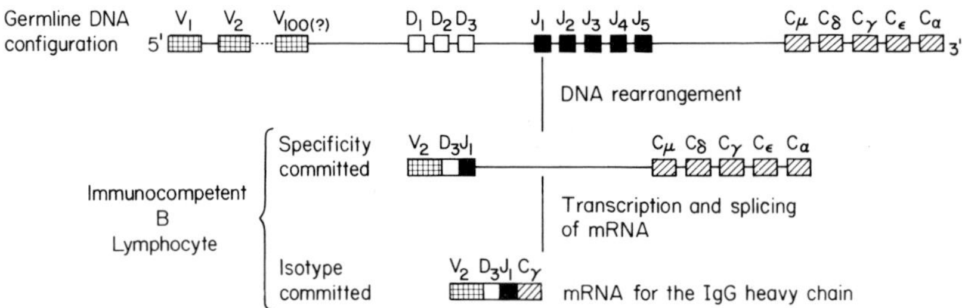

Figure 36–4. Organization and rearrangement of the heavy chain immunoglobulin genes (exons) on the mouse 12 chromosome. Each V_H gene has a leader sequence (not shown) that is required for passage of the polypeptide through the endoplasmic reticulum that subsequently is cleaved. The constant region genes are identified by the heavy isotype, and more than one gene exists for the Cμ, Cγ, and Cα isotypes. The switch sites are located at the 5[1] end of the CH genes (not shown). The solid line represents the intervening sequences (introns) between the genes (Macru, 1982).

some 22. The human major histocompatibility complex is coded for on chromosome 6 (Chap. 33). Thus at least four regions on four different chromosomes are involved in the production and regulation of immune responses.

Mammalian species produce an estimated 10^9 unique antibodies. One goal in molecular immunology is to understand the mechanisms responsible for generation of this vast repertoire. The finding that the variable region of immunoglobulin heavy chains is encoded in three separate DNA segments (exons) separated by intervening nucleotide sequences (introns) has provided insights as to how antibody diversity can be generated. These three distinct structural gene segments have been designated variable (V_H), diversity (D_H, representing the most diverse region), and joining (J_H) (Leder, 1980). The joining segment should not be confused with the J chain polypeptide associated with the polymeric immunoglobulins.

During the differentiation of antibody-producing cells or B cells, the V_H, D_H, and J_H gene segments are joined in a process that results in the loss of the intervening DNA (Fig. 36–4). The rearranged V_H-D_H-J_H gene remains separated, however, from the constant gene (C_H) by the noncoding region of DNA. The V_H-D_H-J_H gene and C_H gene eventually become joined by the splicing out of the intervening sequence during messenger RNA processing. Therefore, the formation of mRNA results from two physically and temporally distinct nucleic acid rearrangements: (a) ligation of the V_H-D_H-J_H gene segments; and (b) removal of the intervening sequence between the V_H-D_H-J_H gene and the constant gene during mRNA processing. The first rearrangement step is responsible for generating antibody diversity at the antigen combining level because multiple genes for V_H (100?), D_H (3), and J_H (5) exist, and any V_H gene segment is capable of recombining with any D_H segment and the V_H-D_H complex with any of the available J_H gene segments. Thus, an enormous amount of antigen-binding diversity can be created by chance recombinatorial joining (minimal number $= 100 \times 3 \times 5 = 1500$ different V_H-D_H-J_H gene complex) employing a small number of germline genes ($100 + 3 + 5 = 108$). If somatic mutations are introduced into the V_H gene pool during evolution, this would increase diversity. The second rearrangement step generates isotypic diversity (class and subclasses of immunoglobulins) because V_H-D_H-J_H gene complexes can combine randomly with any C_H gene segment.

The same general principles apply to the DNA organization and rearrangement of the κ and λ chain genes. However, light chain isotypes lack a D gene segment, and the entire variable region is encoded by only two structural genes (V_κ and J_κ genes or V_λ and J_λ genes). Furthermore, the size of the V_κ and in particular the V_λ gene pools are considerably smaller than that the V_H gene pool. Because the configuration and specificity of the antigen-binding site is affected by both heavy and light chains, combinations of heavy chains with any of the multitude of kappa and lambda light chains also will enhance antibody diversity (Korsmeyer, 1981).

BIOLOGICAL ACTIVITY

Distribution and Concentration of Immunoglobulins in Body Fluids. There is a direct relationship between the concentration of a particular immunoglobulin class or subclass in body fluids and the number of plasma cells secreting that particular isotype. The number of plasma cells forming immunoglobulins differs for each class. The rate of synthesis of a given antibody per plasma cell may also differ but generally is similar for all classes. Therefore, this factor plays a minor role in influencing the concentration of a particular immunoglobulin. On the other hand, the rate of catabolism of a given antibody class plays a major role in determining the concentration of serum immunoglobulins. The constant region of an immunoglobulin heavy chain is involved in this catabolism and, therefore, in regulating the distribution and levels of immunoglobulins in body fluids. Finally, the rate at which immunoglobulin exchange occurs between intra- and extravascular spaces will affect the concentrations of antibody. The rate of exchange between plasma and lymph space depends primarily upon the diffusion coefficient of the immunoglobulin. For example, IgG has a high diffusion coefficient and can predominate in extravascular spaces, whereas IgM has a low diffusion coefficient and is found predominantly in serum. Relatively large amounts of IgD have been reported in the intravascular space, suggesting that it has a low diffusion coefficient. This may well result from asymmetry of the IgD molecule caused by its three oligosaccharide moieties. IgA is relatively more concentrated in lymph than in serum, probably because of the local synthesis of IgA in the intestines and drainage into the thoracic duct.

The external fluids of saliva, tears, bronchial secretions, colostrum, and intestinal secretions all have much lower concentrations of immunoglobulin than does serum. The major class of total immunoglobulin in these secretions is IgA. The average concentration ratios of IgA to IgG secretions is 20:1, compared with 1:5 in serum. IgM is the only other known immunoglobulin that is capable of interacting with secretory component. In some instances, agammaglobulinemic individuals, who lack both IgG and IgA, have a compensatory increase in IgM. IgE immunocytes are found more frequently in lymphoid tissue around secretory glands than in lymph nodes and spleen. Because of this, IgE also may be more concentrated in secretions.

In man, the concentration of immunoglobulin in the cerebrospinal fluid is very small. The IgG concentration in these fluids is about 1/100 of that in serum and makes up approximately 12 per cent of the total cerebrospinal proteins. The levels of both IgA and IgM are equally small, and IgD and IgE apparently are undetectable in these fluids. Immunoglobulin entry into the cerebrospinal fluid may occur by passive diffusion across the blood-brain barrier and/or by direct entry after synthesis by plasma cells in the central nervous tissue.

Man and most animals are unable to form appreciable quantities of antibody until sometime after birth, when they become immunologically mature. Therefore, immune protection is provided to the offspring by the transfer of IgG from the mother to the young. In man and other primates, prenatal transfer of immunoglobulin to the fetus appears to be the major route, and only IgG is transferred. Although human colostrum is rich in IgA, this immunoglobulin is probably not transferred to serum but rather plays an important role in immune function within the gastrointestinal tract. In some animals, such as mice, rabbits, and rats, only IgG is transferred via the yolk sac during pregnancy and additional IgG present in their colostrum is transferred to the young by intestinal absorption in the first 24 postnatal hours (Spiegelberg, 1974).

Metabolism. Immunoglobulins are constantly being synthesized and catabolized in the body. The synthetic rates and average half-life in days of human immunoglobulin are summarized in Tables 36–4 and 36–5. IgG_1 has one of the highest synthetic rates and the longest half-life of the IgG subclasses. IgG_3, however, has a much shorter plasma half-life and a much faster turnover rate. Several studies of IgG_3 myeloma protein have established that the rapid turnover of IgG_3 is a property of this IgG subclass and seems intimately related to the structural difference in the Fc portion of the IgG_3 chain and the number of interheavy disulfide bridges. IgG turnover studies in a number of diseases support the concept of the concentration-catabolism effect, namely, that the catabolic rate of IgG is related directly to its serum concentration. A low fractional turnover rate is seen with reduced serum IgG levels and high fractional turnover rate with high serum IgG levels. In some cases, abnormalities in metabolism can be associated with a normal serum immunoglobulin level. This is seen in patients with various connective tissue diseases, such as systemic lupus erythematosus, rheumatoid arthritis, polmyositis, and various forms of vasculitis. These individuals have increased IgG fractional turnover rates and shortened half-lives, indicating hypercatabolism. However, a simultaneous increase in synthesis may counteract this hypercatabolism and result in elevated serum IgG levels (Waldmann, 1969).

The fractional turnover rate of IgM is independent of the serum concentration and, thus, differs from IgG metabolism. IgM proteins derived from either monoclonal or polyclonal proliferation have similar catabolism rates. However, the fractions of the IgM pool which have cold agglutinin properties generally are catabolized more rapidly. Patients with chronic idiopathic cold agglutinin syndrome synthesize IgM at about 10 times the normal rate. Individuals subjected to repeated malarial infection, characterized by splenic enlargement (tropical splenomegaly syndrome), also display markedly increased IgM synthesis.

IgA_2 molecules are catabolized more rapidly with a shorter plasma half-life than IgA_1. The reported synthetic and catabolic rates for IgA in Table 36–4 are for IgA_1 subclass, since IgA_1 constitutes the majority of the IgA pool in serum.

A distinguishing feature of IgD metabolism is its high fractional turnover rate and short plasma half-life (see Table 36–4). Currently, it remains unclear whether IgD catabolism follows the concentration-catabolism effect.

Immunoglobulin E has the lowest serum concentration of the five classes of antibodies, and its metabolic pool size is approximately 10^5 times smaller than that of IgG. The low level of IgE in plasma is the result of the highest turnover rate, the shortest half-life, and the lowest synthetic rate (1/1000 that of IgG) of the immunoglobulins (see Table 36–4). It is possible that the fixation of IgE to cell surface receptors of various tissues may be involved in the catabolism of IgE. Therefore, saturation of IgE cell surface receptors may lead to prolonged survival of unbound IgE molecules in the serum.

Characteristics of Immunoglobulins

Immunoglobulin G. IgG is the major immunoglobulin class (80 per cent) found in human and animal serum (Table 36–4). There are four subclasses which were first distinguished by antigenic differences in their Fc portion (C-terminus). These subclasses also show distinct peptide and biologic differences, which

Table 36–5. PROPERTIES ASSOCIATED WITH SUBCLASSES OF HUMAN IMMUNOGLOBULIN G

Combined Properties of IgG Subclasses	IgG_1	IgG_2	IgG_3	IgG_4
Per cent distribution of total normal serum IgG	66 ± 8	23 ± 8	7.3 ± 3.8	4.2 ± 2.6
Synthetic rate, mg/kg/d, in serum	25	?	3.4	?
Fractional catabolic rate, per cent/d (day), (half-life, d)	8 (23)	6.9 (23)	16.8 (7)	6.9 (23)
Ratio of κ:λ	1.4–2.4	1.0–1.1	1.1–1.3	5.0–7.0
Allotypic markers (Gm types)	a,z,f,x	n	bo,bi,bz g,st,etc.	?
Complement-fixing capacity	+2	±	+3	–
Heterologous skin-binding capacity	+	–	+	+
Placental transfer to fetus	+	±	+	+
Macrophage receptor	+	–	+	–
Reaction with protein A	+	+	–	+
Dominant antibody activities:				
Antitetanus toxoid	+2	+	+	±
Antidiphtheria toxoid	+2	+	+	±
Antithyroglobulin	+2	+	+	±
Anti-DNA	+2	+2	±	±
Anti-Rh	+2	–	+	±
Anti-Factor VIII	–	–	–	+
Antidextran	–	+	–	–
Antilevan	–	+	–	–
Antiteichoic acid	–	+	–	–
Number of interheavy chain disulfide bonds in hinge region	2	4	5	2
Positiion of light-heavy chain disulfide bond on the heavy chain	N214	N131	N131	N131

are summarized in Table 36–5. The biologic individuality of different immunoglobulin classes, including the IgG subclasses, is dependent on the heavy chain regions, particularly Fc. Nevertheless, the relationship between biologic activity and difference in primary structure is unclear. IgG_1 and IgG_4 molecules differ in their constant region by 14 residues, 11 of which are located in the C_H2 domain. The types of amino acid replacements observed in the Fc fragment of IgG_4 can explain its highly anionic electrophoretic mobility compared with that of the other IgG subclasses, but it is not yet possible to ascribe a particular biologic function to a unique primary sequence.

Complement activation through binding of C1q is most efficient with IgG_1 and IgG_3 antibodies, although IgG_2 is also active. Antibodies of the IgG_4 class generally are not active in binding complement through the classic pathway.

Immunoglobulin G is the only class of antibody that clearly passes through the placenta. The degree of placental transfer of the four IgG subclasses is, however, still a matter of uncertainty. Some reports have shown that IgG_1, IgG_3, and IgG_4 are present in the cord blood in quantities corresponding to those of the mother, while IgG_2 levels generally are lower. The ability of IgG to cross the placenta provides a major line of defense against infection for the first weeks of a child's life. Normally, the human fetus begins to receive significant quantities of maternal IgG transplacentally at around 12 weeks' gestation, although small amounts have been detected in the fetus as early as 8 weeks. The quantity increases steadily until, at birth, cord serum contains a concentration of IgG comparable to or greater than that of maternal serum. Barring any immunologic disorders, adult levels of IgG are reached in the child six or seven years after birth and remain relatively constant throughout life with IgG_1 the dominant isotype.

Immunoglobulin G_3 makes up only about 7 per cent of the total IgG pool in serum but has a number of special properties that appear significant in disease. IgG_3 shows a striking concentration-dependent aggregation that probably is involved in its affinity for C1q. In addition, hyperviscosity of serum may result from relatively low levels of this subclass because of this aggregation. This property of IgG_3 has been implicated in hyperviscosity states. Also, the IgG_3 antibodies apparently are selectively retained in the sera of a number of patients with generalized hypogammaglobulinemia.

IgG antibodies have a high diffusion coefficient, which enables IgG to diffuse into the extravascular body spaces more readily than other immunoglobulin classes. IgG, being the predominant immunoglobulin in these spaces, carries the major burden of neutralizing bacterial toxins and of binding of microorganisms to enhance their phagocytosis. The complexes of bacteria with IgG antibody can adhere to phagocytic cells because these cells (macrophages and neutrophils) have specialized surface receptors for sites on the Fc portion of the IgG molecule. Furthermore, only IgG antibodies coating target cells (e.g., tumor cells) will sensitize them for extracellular killing by specialized K cells (killer cells) that also possess Fc receptors. A summary of the physical and biologic properties of IgG is given in Tables 36–1, 36–2, 36–4, and 36–6.

Immunoglobulin A. Interest in IgA has increased in recent years because it is the principal antibody in most external secretions. It is the main immunoglobulin made by plasma cells in glands and mucous membranes. In the lamina propria of human gastrointestinal tract, there are approximately 20 IgA immunocytes per IgG immunocyte in close contact with the overlying glandular epithelium. By contrast, in peripheral lymph nodes and spleen the ratio is about 1:3 (IgA:IgG). In humans, serum IgA is mostly monomeric (7S) and of the IgA_1 subclass (90 per cent), whereas in other animal species serum IgA tends to be dimeric but lacks secretory component. In the mucosa, secretory IgA, mostly of the IgA_2 heavy chain isotype (60 per cent), apparently plays an important role as the first line of defense to protect the body against both microbial infections and the entrance of other foreign macromolecules. It has been postulated that IgA inhibits the adherence of microorganisms to the surface of mucosal cells, thereby preventing their entry into body tissues. This diminution in absorption may protect the individual against harmful antigens by forming non-absorbable complexes that could be degraded by proteolytic enzymes on the surface of the intestine. Usually, IgA can be found in saliva, tears, and other secretions earlier than in serum. Secretory IgA also reaches adult levels sooner than serum IgA. The IgA system in the intestinal tract of humans, for example, may be fully developed by 2 years of age, while serum IgA levels do not normally reach adult concentrations until 12 years of age. The factor(s) responsible for the slower maturation of the serum IgA system are not understood. Because of this difference in the maturation rate and the unique role of secretory IgA antibodies, some consider the secretory immune system as a separate entity and not merely as an offshoot of the humoral immune system, where IgG predominates.

The biologic properties of human IgA are summarized in Table 36–6. Whether IgA antibodies can mediate any secondary effector functions following the union of their combining sites with antigen remains unclear. More studies are needed to determine if differences exist between IgA_1 and IgA_2 antibodies and between serum and secretory IgA antibodies. IgA immunoglobulins apparently cannot fix complement by the classic pathway. However, a number of reports indicate that if experimentally aggregated, both serum IgA_1 and IgA_2 and secretory IgA are effective activators of the alternative complement pathway. Antiviral activity by IgA antibodies has been demonstrated in individuals given either of the polio vaccines. The oral Sabin vaccine resulted in an appreciable coproantibody response. In rats, secretory IgA is believed to play an important role in preventing dental caries. In the alimentary tract, IgA antibodies are undoubtedly being formed against a myriad of environmental antigens. For example, IgA immunodeficiencies, discussed in Chapter 41, can lead to increased levels and incidence of humoral antibodies directed against antigens derived from food and intestinal organisms. It is believed that these antibodies are formed because the antigens are not being absorbed in the epithelial wall of the intestine by IgA, and penetrate the intestinal lining and enter the circulation. Secretory IgA thus appears particularly suitable for performing this absorption function for two reasons: (1) its dimeric nature allows for greater antigen binding and (2) the presence of secretory component appears to increase the molecule's resistance to proteolysis, which allows it to function in the enzyme-rich milieu of the gastrointestinal tract.

Although the gut-associated lymphoid tissue is probably the major source of polymeric IgA in serum, there are probably other sites of origin. A small number of IgA precursor cells, which can differentiate into cells that synthesize polymeric IgA, have been

Table 36–6. BIOLOGIC PROPERTIES OF HUMAN IMMUNOGLOBULINS

	IgM	IgG	IgA	IgD	IgE
Agglutinating capacity	+4	±	+2	–	–
Complement-fixing capacity	+4	+	–	–	–
Homologous anaphylactic hypersensitivity	–	–	–	–	+4
Heterologous guinea pig anaphylaxis	–	+	–	–	–
Fixation to homologous mast cells and basophils	–	±	–	–	+4
Cytophilic binding to macrophages	–	+	±	–	–
Placental transport to fetus	–	+	–	–	–
Rheumatoid factor-binding activity	–	+	–	–	–
Present in external secretions	±	+	+4	–	+2

Other characteristic properties:

IgM—Produced early in immune response, first effective defense against bacteremia.
IgG—Combats microorganisms and their toxins in extravascular fluids.
IgA—Defends external body surfaces.
IgD—Present on lymphocyte surface of immunocompetent cells, important for B cell activation and/or immunoregulation.
IgE—Raised in parasitic infections, responsible for symptoms of atopic allergy.

localized in peripheral lymph nodes, spleen, and bone marrow cells. In addition, some cells committed to IgA production may migrate to extraintestinal lymphoid tissue from the gut. The serum monomeric IgA may originate from the spleen, lymph node, bone marrow, or gut.

The structure of IgA is similar to that of the other immunoglobulins. However, the IgA_2 immunoglobulin is unique in that it lacks light-heavy disulfide bonds. The light chains are linked to each other by a disulfide bridge. The association of the light and heavy chain dimers is by strong non-covalent interactions. Other important physical properties of the IgA molecule are given in Tables 36–4 and 36–6.

Immunoglobulin M. Structural studies of IgM have been done with proteins obtained from patients suffering from Waldenström's macroglobulinemia. They have served as a model for structural analysis of IgM antibodies, just as myeloma proteins and Bence Jones proteins are models for IgG antibodies and light chains, respectively. Human IgM's are referred to frequently as macroglobulin because they have a molecular weight of about 900,000 daltons. Each molecule can be dissociated into five similar subunits (IgM_s), each having a molecular weight of 180,000 daltons which bears an extra C_H domain. As with IgA, polymerization of the IgM_s subunits appears to be a process involving the addition of J chain and carbohydrate groups immediately before or coinciding with its release from the cell. The monomers are joined through an intersubunit disulfide bond on each μ chain or the J chain to form a pentamer. This circular pentameric arrangement illustrated in Figure 36–1 has been confirmed by electron microscopy studies. The theoretical combining valency of IgM is 10, but this is observed only on interaction with small haptens; with larger antigens the effective valence falls to 5, perhaps because of some form of steric hindrance. Because of their high valence, IgM antibodies are extremely efficient agglutinating and cytolytic antibodies. A summary of the physical and biologic properties associated with IgM is given in Tables 36–4 and 36–6 (Metzger, 1970).

There is evidence that IgM antibodies were the first to evolve, and they are usually the first to appear in ontogeny. In the lower vertebrates, however, IgM antibodies do exist as monomeric subunits and not as a pentamer as in mammals. In humans, IgM constitutes approximately 10 per cent of normal serum immunoglobulins. They appear early in response to infection, and it is likely that they play a role of particular importance in cases of bacteremia. IgM proteins predominate in certain humoral immune responses such as antibodies to blood group antigens (isohemagglutinins), the Wasserman antibodies in syphilis, antibodies to the typhoid 0 antigen, and many antibodies to other microbial antigens.

Approximately six days after birth, the serum concentration of IgM rises sharply. This rise normally continues for about a month, diminishes somewhat, and then continues to rise until adult levels are achieved by about one year of age. Macroglobulins are distributed predominantly in the intravascular pool in both humans and rabbits. Unlike IgG antibodies, no extensive maternal-fetal transport of IgM takes place.

Membrane-bound IgM, which exists as a monomer subunit, is the first immunoglobulin to be detected on the surface of B lymphoid cells. In humans, monomer IgM (with IgD) is the major immunoglobulin expressed on the surface of immunocompetent B lymphocytes. This is discussed in Chapter 34. IgM and IgG antibodies are responsible for most of the specific activities classically associated with antibodies, including precipitation, agglutination, transfusion reactions, hemolysis, and complement fixation. On the surface of cells a single molecule of IgM suffices to fix C1q, whereas two IgG antibody molecules are required for fixation. Differences in C1q activation by IgM and IgG also become apparent when the temperature is varied. The C1q is efficiently activated by IgG at both 4° and 37°C., whereas IgM is very efficient only at the lower temperature.

The plasma cells of patients with macroglobulinemia generally contain intracellular IgM in the 19S polymer form. In most systems studied, the IgM appears in the vascular fluids in its final 19S form; intracellularly it is in the IgM_s (7S) form. However, in human autoimmune disorders, such as systemic lupus erythematosus, the 7S form can be detected in appreciable amounts in serum. Selective IgM deficiency is a rare disorder associated with the absence of IgM and normal levels of other immunoglobulin classes (Chap. 41). The cause of this disorder is unknown.

Immunoglobulin D. Compared with other immunoglobulins, IgD is a relatively minor component in serum (Table 36–4). The normal human population is segregated into three groups. Seventy per cent of the population has an IgD serum concentration of 20 to 50 μg/ml. The other two groups, each of which represents 15 per cent of the population, contain very low levels of IgD (3 μg/ml) or very high levels of IgD (100 to 400 μg/ml). The reason for the large differences in IgD serum concentration, both in children and in adults, is not known. IgD usually is detected in serum at about six months of age. However, analysis of some human cord sera show that it contains IgD, and comparison of the concentrations of maternal vs. cord serum IgA, IgM, and IgD suggests that the fetus is capable of synthesizing IgD.

In disease states, the IgD concentration can vary greatly. In chronic infections, IgD levels increase, as do those of the other immunoglobulins. To date, no specific increase of IgD has been associated with a particular disease. Patients with allergies and autoimmune diseases do not show an abnormal IgD concentration. IgD is usually absent in hypogammaglobulinemic individuals. IgD has not been found in external secretions or body fluids other than serum. Only about 2 per cent of patients suffering from multiple myeloma produce IgD paraproteins, generally with concentration levels lower than those of IgG, IgA, and IgM myeloma proteins. IgD myelomas are usually of lambda (λ) chain isotype (80 to 90 per cent), and almost all patients have considerable Bence Jones protein in their urine.

The lability of IgD to heat and acid resembles IgE and thus differs from IgG, IgA, and IgM. Both IgD and IgE are present in the serum in very low concentrations and are rapidly catabolized. Neither of these isotypes can bind complement. It now appears that cell-bound IgD is biologically far more important than serum IgD.

Antibody activity in IgD has been difficult to demonstrate in spite of its structural similarities to other immunoglobulins. However, IgD activity against insulin, penicillin G, milk protein, diphtheria toxoid, nuclear antigens, bovine gamma globulin, and thyroid antigens has been reported. The biologic function of serum IgD is still unknown (Leslie, 1975).

A large proportion of human, mouse, and monkey B lymphocytes carry both IgM and IgD on their surfaces. These findings have been extended to B lymphocytes in spleen and newborn (cord) blood lymphocytes. In all these cases the number of IgD^+ cells was much greater than would be expected from a consideration of the concentration of IgD in serum. The possibility that IgD on the cells was acquired by passive adsorption was excluded by the demonstration that after proteolytic stripping of membrane-bound IgD, it was regenerated. The finding that both IgD and IgM are simultaneously present on a high proportion of lymphocytes was unexpected. Surface IgD and IgM were both shown to have the same light chain, idiotype, and antibody specificity and variable region sequences. These membrane-bound immunoglobulins are likely to act as distinct receptors for the same antigen. Following exposure to antigen or mitogen, stimulated cells rapidly decrease their surface IgD. Eight days after stimulation, no IgD^+ B lymphocytes can be detected. These findings have caused considerable speculation about the role of surface IgD in the induction of humoral response and tolerance. It has been postulated that immunocompetent B lymphocytes bearing only IgM are susceptible to tolerance upon antigen exposure, while IgM- and IgD-bearing cells upon exposure to antigen lead to B cell differentiation and maturation. The role IgD plays would be viewed as turning on, turning off, or modulating (controlling) B cell division and/or differentiation. The regulatory influence of IgD could be linked to a suppression of surface IgD or to a release or cleavage of the surface IgD during the triggering process. The latter possibility seems attractive, because IgD has a remarkable susceptibility to degradation that may account for its very short half-life in the body (see Table 36–4).

Among the human immunoglobulins, IgD has two unique structural features. In both the intact molecule and the Fc fragment, the globular domains appear to be less compact than in other immunoglobulins. This difference in conformation may account in part for increased susceptibility to proteolysis. The other feature is the presence of only one interheavy chain disulfide bond.

Immunoglobulin E. This class of antibody represents a minor but distinct isotype of proteins in the serum of man and higher primates. IgE was first discovered in the sera of patients with hay fever. It is now firmly established that reaginic hypersensitivity reactions in atopic diseases are mediated by IgE antibody.

Immunoglobulin E levels can be elevated up to 30 times normal in various diseases, among which atopic disorders and parasitic infestations appear to be the most prominent. Elevated amounts of monoclonal IgE have been found in the serum of patients with IgE myeloma. The main physiologic role of IgE is still uncertain. Persistence of the immunoglobulin class through evolution suggests that it might be important in the survival of the individual, but obviously atopic diseases do not seem to promote survival of the species. Perhaps its importance is to be found in the widespread occurrence of IgE-mediated immune reactivity in parasitic (helminthic) infection. It is thought that histamine release resulting from contact of parasite antigens with mast-cell bound IgE antibody in the gut wall facilitates rejection of the intruders.

Only a very small proportion of plasma cells in the body are synthesizing IgE at any given time. In nonatopic individuals, recurrently infected tonsils and adenoids removed by surgery possess a large number of plasma cells which stain with anti-IgE. Bronchial and peritoneal lymph nodes, as well as the gastrointestinal mucosa, contain some IgE-forming plasma cells. By contrast, IgE-forming cells are scarce in human spleen, subcutaneous lymph nodes, and respiratory mucosa.

The role of IgE antibodies in immediate hypersensitivity reactions is due to their attachment to membrane receptors on mast cells and basophilic granulocytes. This cytotropic property has been shown to be located in the Fc fragment. Upon combining with certain specific antigens, called allergens, on the surface of these cells, IgE antibodies trigger the degranulation of mast cells, with the release of pharmacologic mediators (vasoactive amines) responsible for the characteristic wheal and flare skin reactions evoked by the exposure of the skin of allergic individuals to allergens (Type I hypersensitivity). IgE antibodies provide a striking example of the bifunctional nature of antibody molecules. The Fc portion of the molecule binds to the target cells, whereas the Fab portion binds the allergen. Type I hypersensitivity is discussed in Chapter 40.

A comparison of the molecular weight of ϵ-chain to the other isotypes of heavy chain indicates that it is larger by an amount corresponding to one domain. Like IgG and IgD, IgE normally exists only in monomeric form. The physiochemical and biologic properties of IgE are given in Tables 36–4 and 36–6.

Assemblage of Immunoglobulins. Heavy and light chains are coded for and produced independently within plasma cells. Normally, there is a slight excess of light chains produced in relationship to heavy chains.

The synthesis and assembly of immunoglobulins follow the general rules established for proteins exported from the cells. The assembly may follow any of three possible pathways:

(1) $H + L \rightarrow HL + HL \rightarrow H_2L_2$

(2) $H + H \rightarrow H_2 + L \rightarrow H_2L + L \rightarrow H_2L_2$

(3) $H + L \rightarrow HL + H_2L + L \rightarrow H_2L_2$

5

Table 36–7. SERUM IMMUNOGLOBULIN CONCENTRATIONS*

Age (Years)	Mean IgG (mg/ml)		Mean IgA (mg/ml)	
	White Male	*White Female*	*White Male*	*White Female*
5–9	10.28	11.05	1.09	1.10
10–14	10.41	11.13	1.16	1.15
15–19	10.55	11.20	1.23	1.21
20–24	10.69	11.28	1.32	1.28
25–29	10.83	11.35	1.40	1.35
30–34	10.98	11.43	1.50	1.42
35–39	11.12	11.50	1.59	1.49
40–44	11.27	11.58	1.70	1.57
45–49	11.42	11.66	1.81	1.65
50–54	11.57	11.74	1.93	1.74
55–59	11.72	11.81	2.06	1.83
60–64	11.88	11.89	2.20	1.93
65–69	12.04	11.97	2.34	2.03
70–74	12.20	12.05	2.49	2.14
75 +	12.36	12.13	2.66	2.26

*The data were derived from 3213 serum samples collected from an unselected group of subjects from a single health community (Tecumseh, Michigan) (Cassidy, 1974).

There is no single assembly pathway that operates for all cells or all immunoglobulins of any one class. Fully assembled IgG may be secreted 30 to 40 minutes after the initiation of synthesis. Several factors affect the rate of immunoglobulin assembly: (1) the concentration of heavy and light chains at individual sites in the cisternae; (2) the extent of complementarity between the newly synthesized heavy and light chains, particularly their variable regions; (3) the rate of disulfide bond formation; and (4) the rate of glycosylation just before secretion. Assembly is more quickly accomplished if nearly equimolar amounts of complementary heavy and light chains are present in the cisternae (Bevan, 1972).

Serum Immunoglobulin Levels. Valid interpretation of serum immunoglobulin levels requires recognition of biologic variations that exist throughout the life span of the individuals. The most important of these variables are age, sex, and race.

Studies on a large unselected group of healthy white subjects (3213) from a single community (Tecumseh, Michigan) have shown that the mean concentrations of IgG and IgA increase with age, with slight but significant differences between the sexes. Females were reported to have higher serum levels of IgG and lower levels of IgA (Table 36–7). Although these sex differences for IgG and IgA are statistically significant, their biologic meaning is not apparent. The IgM levels in these subjects remained relatively constant with age. However, females had higher mean levels of IgM (1.06 mg/ml) than males (0.77 mg/ml).

Several studies have reported that immunoglobulin levels and more recently specific immunoglobulin levels are higher in persons with pigmented skins. Table 36–8 presents the results obtained in a healthy biracial population in Evans County, Georgia. Blacks had higher levels of the three major immunoglobulins (IgM, IgG, and IgA) than did whites. The most prominent difference was in IgG. No urban-rural difference in immunoglobulin levels was noted in this study. White- and blue-collar workers in Rochester, New York, had serum levels of IgM and IgG similar to those of white subjects in rural Georgia. A triracial study in Durban, Natal, has shown that Bantu male adults have significantly higher levels of IgM (32 per cent more), IgG (40 per cent more), and IgA (32 per cent more) in their sera than comparable whites in this community, born in the same year and having the same ABO blood group. Healthy Asiatic male adults had about 20 per cent more IgG, 23 per cent more IgA, and 7 per cent more IgM than comparable whites. Control groups used in these studies were matched for age, sex, and race, as well as for several environmental factors (Cassidy, 1974; Lichtman, 1967).

HYPERIMMUNOGLOBULINEMIA

Increases in gamma globulin are usually first noted after a serum protein electrophoresis, a measurement of total protein, and/or measurements of albumin and gamma globulin fractions (see Chap. 12). Reference values for the different immunoglobulins vary with age, sex, and race (Tables 36–7 and 36–8). Increases in immunoglobulins are referred to as monoclonal or polyclonal. Monoclonal immunoglobulins from any

Table 36–8. SERUM IgG CONCENTRATION IN A BIRACIAL POPULATION*

Sex	Age (Years)	No. Samples Tested	Whites Mean (± SE) (mg/ml)	No. Samples Tested	Blacks Mean (± SE) (mg/ml)
	15–34	17	11.2 (7.3)	21	13.4 (6.5)
Men	35–54	17	10.8 (5.9)	19	13.5 (9.0)
	55–74	20	10.9 (7.4)	20	13.3 (5.8)
	15–34	19	10.6 (6.3)	18	15.6 (8.0)
Women	35–54	19	12.3 (3.4)	15	15.4 (6.4)
	55–74	20	10.9 (6.1)	16	14.2 (9.6)

*The data are representative of subjects living in Evans County, Georgia (Lichtman, 1967).

one individual are structurally identical and are believed to result from the clonal expansion of a single immunoglobulin-producing lymphoid cell. Polyclonal immunoglobulins in the same individual are structurally different from each other in one or more important ways—by class, as polyclonal IgG, IgA, or IgM; by light chain, κ or λ; or by antigen specificity. Polyclonal immunoglobulins arise from the expansion of several to many different immunoglobulin-producing lymphoid cells.

Polyclonal increases in immunoglobulins have been associated with many disease states (Table 36–9) (Buckley, 1977; Cushman, 1973; Bjorkstein, 1976). Serum protein electrophoresis is often sufficient to establish this condition. Immunoelectrophoresis and/or determination of individual immunoglobulins may be of help at times in order to confirm a polyclonal distribution and/or an increased concentration in one or more immunoglobulin classes. Increases in serum immunoglobulins may result from decreased catabolism and/or increased synthesis. The control mechanisms for these events are not understood. It is likely that in some cases, as with the elevated immunoglobulins in systemic lupus erythematosus, a defect in T cell regulation exists. The implications of elevated immunoglobulins are unknown. Most immunoglobulins appear not to be directed toward a specific or set of specific antigenic determinants. It also should be noted that most autoantibodies are not monoclonal, but polyclonal. In general, polyclonal increases in gamma globulin are thought to be related to antigenic stimulation of a chronic nature.

Monoclonal immunoglobulins or fragments of immunoglobulins have been associated with a number

Table 36–9. POLYCLONAL HYPERIMMUNOGLOBULINEMIAS: SOME ASSOCIATED DISEASE STATES

Condition	**Immunoglobulin Classes**
Immunodeficiency diseases	
Hyperimmunoglobulin E and recurrent infections	IgE
Wiskott-Aldrich syndrome	IgA, IgE
"Dysgammaglobulinemia Type I"	IgM
Hyperimmunoglobulin A and recurrent infections	IgA
Infections	
Congenital infections (syphilis, toxoplasmosis, rubella, cytomegalovirus)	IgM
Infectious mononucleosis	IgM or all
Trypanosomiasis	IgM or all
Intestinal parasitism	All classes
Several helminthic infections	IgE
Visceral larva migrans	All classes
Chronic granulomatous disease of childhood	All classes
Leprosy	All classes
Chronic infection in general	All classes, with a preference for IgG
Liver Diseases	
Chronic active hepatitis	IgG predominates
Acute hepatitis	IgG predominates
Biliary cirrhosis	IgM predominates
Lupoid hepatitis	All classes
Pulmonary disorders	
Pulmonary hypersensitivity syndrome	All classes
Sarcoidosis	All classes
Berylliosis	All classes
"Autoimmune" disorders	
Systemic lupus erythematosus	All classes
Rheumatoid arthritis	IgA or all
Many "autoimmune" states such as thyroiditis	All classes
Scleroderma	All classes
Cold agglutinin disease	IgM
Anaphylactoid purpura	IgA
Miscellaneous	
Down's syndrome	All classes
Amyloidosis	All classes
Narcotic addiction	IgM
Renal tubular disease	All classes

Table 36–10. SELECTED CONDITIONS WHICH HAVE BEEN ASSOCIATED WITH MONOCLONAL IMMUNOGLOBULINS

Multiple myeloma
Macroglobulinemia of Waldenström
Chronic lymphocytic leukemia
Other leukemias
Lymphomas
"Benign" monoclonal gammopathy
Systemic capillary leak syndrome
Amyloidosis
Chronic liver disease such as chronic active hepatitis, primary biliary cirrhosis
Autoimmune disorders, including rheumatoid arthritis, systemic lupus erythematosus, thyroiditis, pernicious anemia, polyarteritis nodosa, Sjögren's syndrome
Gaucher's disease
Malignancies of various types
Hereditary spherocytosis

of disease conditions (Table 36–10) (Atkinson, 1977; Benbassat, 1976; Ko, 1976; Michaux, 1969; Schafer, 1978; Wells, 1974).

The incidence of monoclonal immunoglobulins (M components) in unselected population studies is estimated to be 0.9 per cent (Bachman, 1965; Axelsson, 1968). Of course, a much higher percentage of "positives" will be found in clinical laboratories where the sera to be tested are preselected. Multiple myeloma and macroglobulinemia of Waldenström account for as few as 2 per cent (Axelsson, 1968) and as many as 78 per cent of all subjects with M components. One can expect that at least one half to two thirds of all M components detected will be from patients with these two disorders (Isobe, 1971; Ameis, 1976). In the study by Axelsson (1968), the presence of monoclonal immunoglobulins increased progressively with age: 0.16 per cent of those 25 to 49 years of age; 1.61 per cent of those 50 to 79 years; and 9.2 per cent of those 80 to 89 years of age. In that same study the monoclonal protein was IgG in 61 per cent, IgA in 27 per cent, IgM in 8 per cent, and biclonal in 5 per cent. In other series, light chain myelomas have accounted for up to 25 per cent of all myeloma proteins (Isobe, 1971; Wells, 1974). Multiple myeloma and macroglobulinemia of Waldenström are reviewed in Chapter 30.

Requests to examine sera for the presence of a monoclonal protein are generated by a physician who recognizes that a patient has clinical symptoms and signs of such disorders, or by the laboratory examination of a serum protein electrophoresis that suggests a monoclonal protein. If there indeed is an M component in a serum protein electrophoresis, a quantitative measurement of immunoglobulins by radial immunodiffusion, nephelometry, or another suitable technique can virtually identify the specific immunoglobulin if only one of the major three classes is increased. Of course, this will neither determine the light chain of a monoclonal immunoglobulin nor detect light chain myelomas. There may be confusion in biclonal immunocytopathies. Quantitative immunoglobulins are useful in monitoring the course of the disease and its treatment. Quantitative immunoglobulins may be helpful in separating a benign from a malignant condition. Monoclonal immunoglobulin G levels of 2 g/100 ml (220 IU/ml) or immunoglobulin A levels of 1 g/100 ml (480 IU/ml) (Isobe, 1971) or greater suggest a malignant condition. In many malignant immunocytopathies, the concentration of nonmonoclonal immunoglobulins is reduced. Thus, deficiency of polyclonal immunoglobulins is evidence of malignancy. Waldmann and his associates (1978) have demonstrated that in many cases this decrease in polyclonal immunoglobulins is caused by a macrophage-like suppressor cell. Paradoxically, then, the patient with a malignant immunocytopathy is immunodeficient while possessing large amounts of a "nonsense" immunoglobulin produced by a poorly controlled clone of lymphoid cells.

Immunoelectrophoresis (IEP) (described in Chap. 38) is useful in detecting the specific monoclonal protein or proteins. Thus, in patients with suspicious signs, symptoms, or especially hematopathologic findings in the peripheral blood, bone marrow, or lymph node, an IEP may be diagnostic. Whether or not serum protein electrophoresis should precede an IEP depends on the relative availability of these techniques and the sophistication of each in a laboratory. For example, agarose serum protein electrophoresis is probably as sensitive as IEP at detecting most M components. However, electrophoresis on paper or cellulose acetate is not as sensitive. Another way of selecting sera for IEP is by reviewing serum protein electrophoresis determinations. Table 36–11 and Figure 36–5 describe approaches to the diagnosis and management, respectively, of patients with M components.

Immunoelectrophoresis (IEP) is a sensitive, relatively uncomplicated procedure to detect M components and their heavy and light chain components. IEP allows one to semiquantitate the concentration of the immunoglobulins. Technical details of this procedure can be found in Chapter 38. Patients' sera should be compared with normal sera or a normal pool. For example, we pool 100 to 200 ml of blood from normal individuals, quick freeze 1 ml aliquots with dry ice and acetone, and store at $-70°C$. We do not refreeze the unused control sera but discard after retaining for three days at 4°C. The control sera must be HBsAg negative.

The following antisera should be used: anti-whole human sera; anti-IgG (γ chains), anti-IgM (μ); anti-IgA (α), anti-κ, and anti-λ (Fig. 36–6). It is important to realize that not all antisera are alike in strength and specificity and that it is possible that M component may not be detected with one of the antisera, yet present with a second. Thus, each lot of antisera should be compared for titer, such as by gel diffusion against control sera, and specificity against whole human serum in an IEP. Interpretation of an IEP may take considerable experience, but generally one is searching for a disruption of a normally smooth line, i.e., by bowing, thickening, or changed mobility. Examples of IEP are shown in Figure 36–6. Immunoelectrophoresis is a very useful technique but has

Table 36–11. INTERPRETATION OF SERUM IMMUNOELECTROPHORESIS (IEP)

1. No monoclonal immunoglobulin demonstrated—normal pattern.
2. No monoclonal immunoglobulin demonstrated; quantitative immunoglobulin assays indicate a polyclonal increase in one or more classes.
3. Monoclonal
   a. IgG-κ
      IgG-λ
   b. IgA-κ
      IgA-λ
   c. IgM-κ
      IgM-λ
   with mobility of light chain mirroring that of heavy chain and with normal or decreased quantities of polyclonal immunoglobulins. Examine urine for light chains.
4. Monoclonal light chain only (κ or λ)
   a. IEP with anti-IgE, IgD if possible.
   b. Quantitate IgE, IgD if possible.
   c. No evidence of γ, μ, α, ϵ, σ heavy chains, then light chain M component.
   d. Examine urine for monoclonal light chains.
5. Monoclonal heavy chain only (α, γ, μ)
   a. Check anti-light chain antisera for potency.
   b. Examine urine for presence of same M component (heavy chain).
   c. IgG heavy chain: gel filtration on G-200 or ultracentrifugation, if available (4S protein compared with 7S whole IgG molecule).

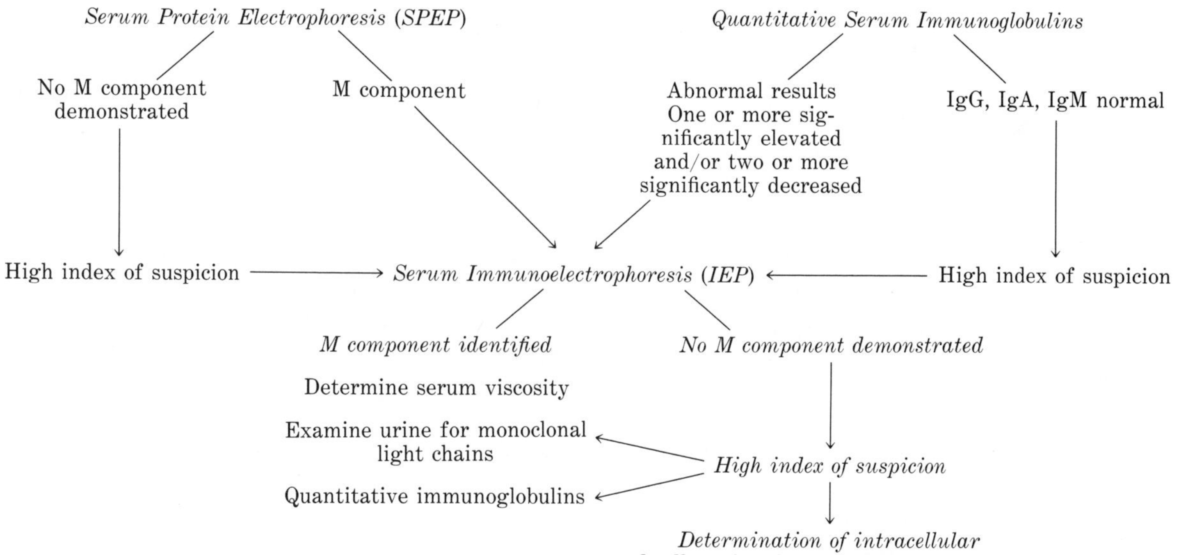

Figure 36–5. Approach to the laboratory evaluation of monoclonal gammopathies. Immunoelectrophoresis should be performed if the serum protein electrophoresis and/or serum immunoglobulin concentrations are abnormal as noted or if there is a high index of suspicion due to the patient's clinical presentation. Quantitative immunoglobulins and serum viscosity are useful measurements for monitoring the patient. Monoclonal light chains in the urine (≥200 mg/24 hours) suggest a malignant condition. This approach supplements hematopathologic and clinical information.

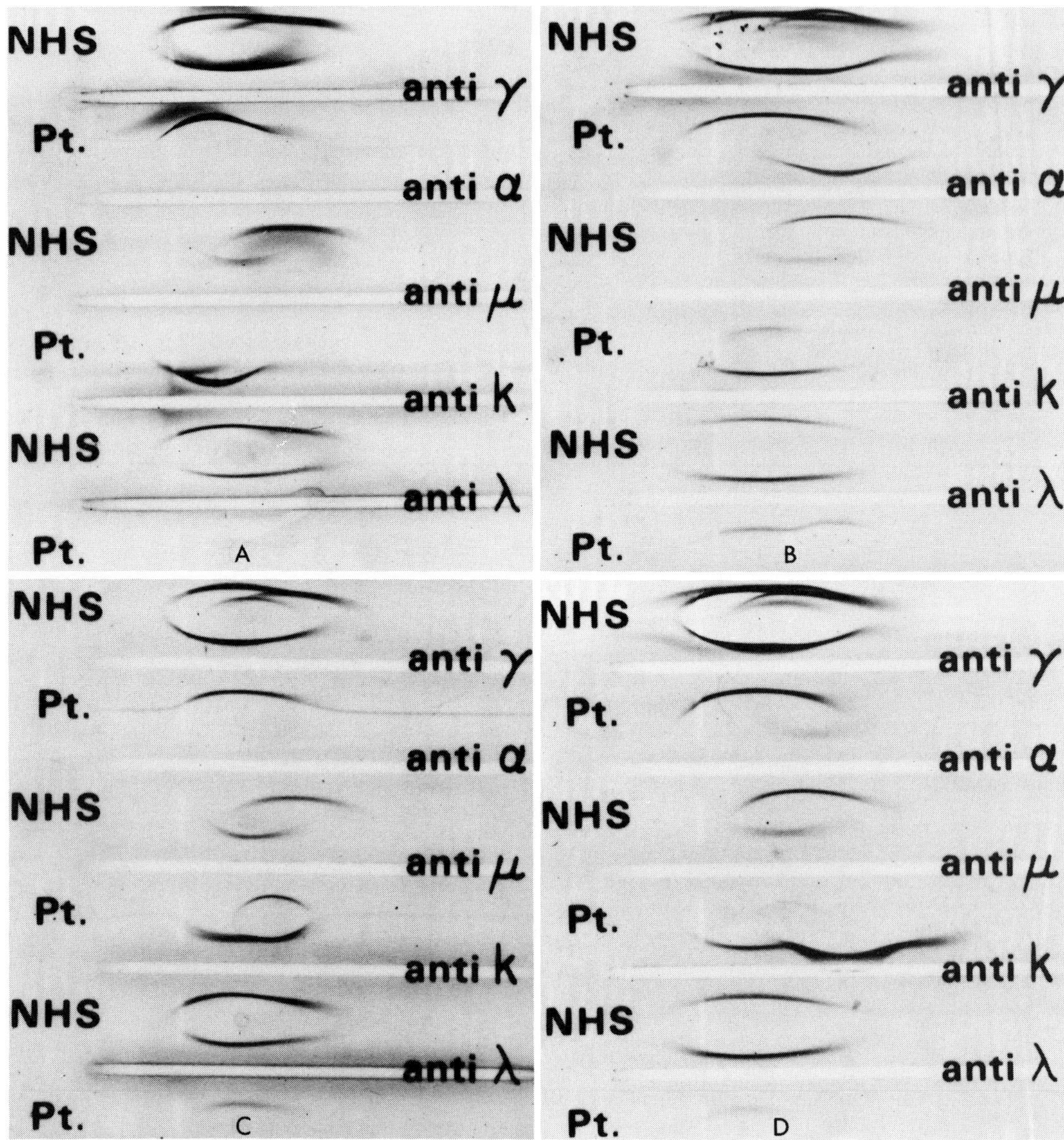

Figure 36–6. Monoclonal immunoglobulins demonstrated by serum immunoelectrophoresis. Aliquots of patient serum and a pool of normal human serum were subjected to electrophoresis on polyacrylamide at pH 8.6 (Poly-E-Film, Pfizer). The separated proteins were reacted overnight with antisera to (1) whole human serum, (2) a combination of IgG, IgA and IgM, (3) γ, (4) α, (5) μ, (6) κ, and (7) λ chains, respectively. The membranes were washed and stained with Amido Black B. *A*, IgG-κ M component. *B*, IgA-λ M component. *C*, IgM-κ M component. *D*, κ light chain M component.

Illustration continued on opposite page

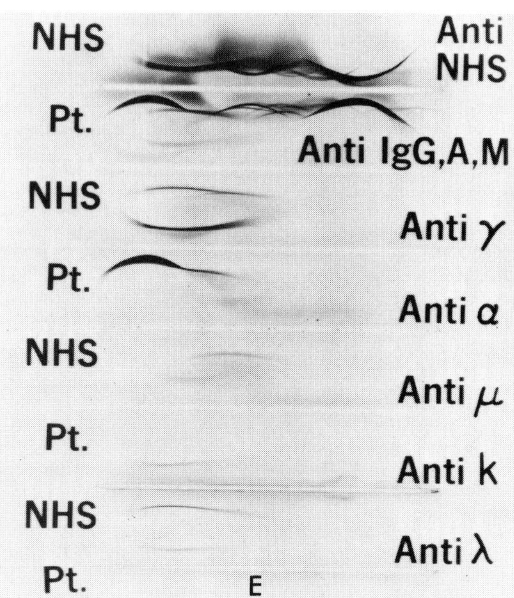

Figure 36–6 *Continued. E*, γ heavy chain M component.

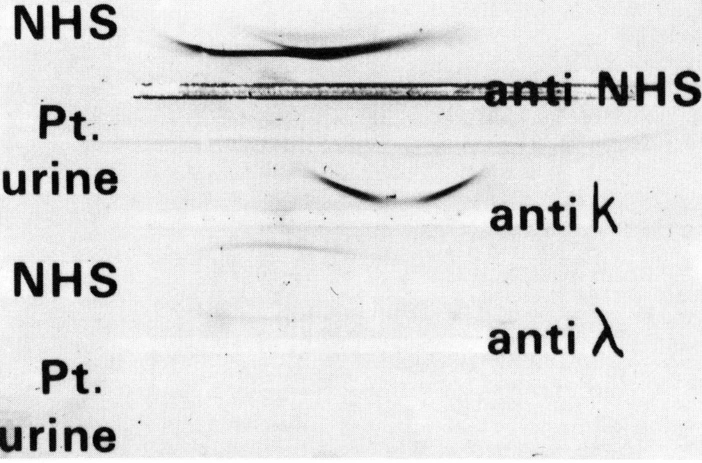

Figure 36–7. Monoclonal light chains detected by urine immunoelectrophoresis. A spot urine sample is concentrated by drying from the frozen state or through a membrane (Minicon, Amicon). The sample is subjected to electrophoresis and allowed to react with antisera to polyvalent IgG, IgA, and IgM, as well as κ and λ chains. Normal human serum (NHS) is used as a reference. This patient has a monoclonal κ light chain in the urine (Bence Jones protein).

5

limitations. IEP may identify the presence of a heavy and a light chain but does not ensure that one indeed has an entire immunoglobulin molecule with the formula of two heavy chains and two light chains.

It is also possible, but unusual, to have monoclonal immunoglobulins present in amounts below the level of detection of the system used. The lower level of detection can be estimated by diluting a known monoclonal immunoglobulin and testing it by IEP. Since monoclonal proteins of IgM, IgA, IgD, and IgE may be present in relatively small quantities compared with IgG, the light chain portion of the whole non-IgG immunoglobulin may not be detected by IEP. The inability to detect light chains of immunoglobulins in lesser concentration in the presence of IgG of greater concentration is referred to as an "umbrella effect." Therefore, other procedures may be required to rule out heavy chain or Franklin's disease. Heavy chain disease is discussed in Chapter 30. It is possible that the serum being tested and the antibody being used are not in the proper concentrations and that the M component may be missed. Finally, it is possible that the antisera being used will not detect the available determinants on a particular M component. If one has a high index of suspicion, it may be useful to use a second antiserum from another source.

Monoclonal light chains in the urine, Bence Jones protein, may be detected in more than half of the patients with multiple myeloma (Isobe, 1971; Wells, 1974). Polyclonal light chains may be detected in other disorders, usually as a part of complete immunoglobulin molecules. The detection of Bence Jones protein by heat is reviewed in Chapter 18. Immunoelectrophoresis of urine is more specific and more sensitive than the heat test. IEP on urine with sufficient protein or concentrated by lyophilization or through selective membranes (Minicon, Amicon) can identify monoclonal light chains. This is illustrated in Figure 36–7. Measurement of serum viscosity is discussed in Chapter 27.

Ameis, A., Ko, H. S., and Pruzanski, W.: M components—a review of 1242 cases. Can. Med. Assoc. J., *144*:889, 1976.

Atkinson, J. P., Waldmann, T. A., Stein, S. F., Gelfand, J. A., MacDonald, W. J., Heck, L. W., Cohen, E. L., Kaplan, A. P., and Frank, M. M.: Systemic capillary leak syndrome and monoclonal IgG gammopathy. Medicine, *56*:225, 1977.

Axelsson, N., and Hellen, J.: Frequency of M components in 6995 sera from an adult population. Br. J. Haematol., *15*:417, 1968.

Bachman, R.: The diagnostic significance of the serum concentration of pathological proteins. Acta Med. Scand., *178*:801, 1965.

Benbassat, J., Fluman, N., and Zlotnick, A.: Monoclonal immunoglobulin disorders: A report of 154 cases. Am. J. Med. Sci., *27*:325, 1976.

Bevan, M. J., Parkhouse, R. M. R., Williamson, A. R., and Askonas, B. A.: Biosynthesis of immunoglobulins. Prog. Biophys. Mol. Biol., *25*:131, 1972.

Bjorkstein, B., and Lundmark, K. M.: Recurrent bacterial infections in four siblings with neutropenia, eosinophilia, hyperimmunoglobulinemia A, and defective neurotrophil chemotaxis. J. Infect. Dis., *133*:63, 1976.

Bona, C., and Hiernaux, J.: Immune response: Idioptype–anti-idiotype network. CRC Crit. Rev. Immunol., *2*:33, 1981.

Buckley, R. H.: *In* Altman, P. L., and Katz, D. D. (eds.): Human Health and Disease II. Bethesda, Md., FASEB, 1977.

Cassidy, J. T., Nordby, G. L., and Dodge, H. J.: Biologic variation of human serum immunoglobulin concentrations: Sex-age specific effects. J. Chron. Dis., *27*:507, 1974.

Cushman, P., and Grieco, M. H.: Hyperimmunoglobulinemia associated with narcotic addiction. Am. J. Med., *54*:320, 1973.

Dorrington, K. J., and Painter, R. H.: Biological activities of the constant region of immunoglobulin G. *In* Mandel, T. E., et al. (eds.): Progress in Immunology III. Canberra City, Australian Academy of Science, 1977.

Edelman, G. M., and Gally, J. A.: *In* Schmitt, F. O. (ed.): Arrangement and Evolution of Eukaryotic Genes. The Neurosciences Second Study Program. New York, Rockefeller University Press, 1970.

Inman, F. P., and Mestecky, J.: The J chain of polymeric immunoglobulins. *In* Ada, G. L. (ed.): Contemporary Topics in Molecular Immunology, Vol. 3. New York, Plenum Press, 1974.

Isobe, T., and Osserman, E. F.: Pathologic conditions associated with plasma cell dyscrasias: A study of 806 cases. Ann. N.Y. Acad. Sci., *190*:507, 1971.

Ko, H. S., and Pruzanski, W.: M components associated with lymphoma: A review of 62 cases. Am. J. Med. Sci., *272*:175, 1976.

Korsmeyer, S. J., Hieter, P. A., Ravetch, J. V., Poplack, D. G., Waldmann, T. A., and Leder, P.: Developmental hierarchy of immunoglobulin gene rearrangements in human leukemia pre-B-cells. Proc. Natl. Acad. Sci., *78*:7096, 1981.

Leder, P. E., Max, J. G., Seidman, S. P., Kwan, M., Scharff, M., Nav, M., and Norman, B.: Recombination events that activate, diversify, and delete immunoglobulin genes. Cold Spring Harbor Symposium, Quant. Biol., *45*:859, 1980.

Leslie, G. A., Correa, R. H. L., and Holmes, J. R.: Structure and biological functions of human IgD. Int. Arch. All. Appl. Immunol., *49*:350, 1975.

Lichtman, M. A., Vaughan, J. H., and Hames, C. G.: The distribution of serum immunoglobulins, anti-γ-G globulins and antinuclear antibodies in White and Negro subjects in Evans County, Georgia. Arthritis Rheum., *10*:204, 1967.

Macru, K. B.: Immunoglobulin heavy-chain constant-region genes. Cell, *29*:719, 1982.

Mestecky, J., Schrohenloher, R. E., Kulhavy, R., Wright, G. P., and Tomana, M.: Site of J chain attachment to human polymeric IgA. Proc. Natl. Acad. Sci., *71*:554, 1974.

Metzger, H.: Structure and function of γ M macroglobulins. Adv. Immunol., *12*:57, 1970.

Michaux, J. L., and Heremans, J. F.: Thirty cases of monoclonal immunoglobulin disorders other than myeloma or macroglobulinemia. Am. J. Med., *46*:562, 1969.

Natvig, J. B., and Kunkel, H. G.: Human immunoglobulins—classes, subclasses, genetic variants and idiotypes. Adv. Immunol., *16*:1, 1973.

Nisonoff, A., Wissler, F. C., Lipman, L. N., and Woernley, D. L.: Separation of univalent fragments from the bivalent rabbit antibody molecule by reduction of disulfide bonds. Arch. Biochem. Biophys., *89*:230, 1960.

Porter, R. R.: The hydrolysis of rabbit γ-globulin and antibodies with crystalline papain. Biochem. J., *73*:119, 1959.

Roitt, I.: Summary of immunoglobulin variants. *In* Essential Immunology. 4th ed. Oxford, Blackwell Scientific Publications, 1980.

Schafer, A. I., Miller, J. B., Lester, E. P., Bowers, T. K., and Jacobs, H. S.: Monoclonal gammopathy in hereditary spherocytosis: A possible pathogenetic relation. Ann. Intern. Med., *88*:45, 1978.

Spiegelberg, H. L.: Biological aspects of immunoglobulins of different classes and subclasses. Adv. Immunol., *19*:259, 1974.

Tiselius, A., and Kabat, E. A.: An electrophoretic study of immune sera and purified antibody preparations. J. Exp. Med., *69*:119, 1939.

Underdown, B. J., DeRose, J., and Plaut, A.: Disulfide bonding of secretory component to a single monomer subunit in human secretory IgA. J. Immunol., *118*:1816, 1977.

Waldmann, T. A., and Strober, W.: Metabolism of immunoglobulins. Prog. Allergy, *13*:1, 1969.

Waldmann, T. A., Blaese, R. M., Broder, S., and Krakaner, R. S.: Disorders of suppressor immunoregulatory cells in the pathogenesis of immunodeficiency and autoimmunity. Ann. Intern. Med., *88*:226, 1978.

Wells, J. V., and Fudenberg, H. H.: Paraproteinemias. DM, February, 1974.

37

COMPLEMENT

THELMA A. GAITHER, B.S., and MICHAEL M. FRANK, M.D.

The complement system is composed of a series of circulating blood proteins which serve as mediators of the inflammatory response. In addition, the complement proteins are important in the opsonization of foreign particulate matter, including bacteria, and in cytotoxic reactions toward cells and microorganisms. Thus, the complement system has evolved as a complex interacting series of proteins designed to mediate host defense reactions and to protect against infections. In general, there are very few individuals deficient in one of these proteins. Furthermore, the absence of a component generally is not overtly responsible for manifestation of a disease state. This is in sharp contrast to inherited defects in the coagulation cascade. The usual role of the complement system in disease is to produce tissue damage. In these situations, the complement system is functioning normally, but it is being activated under abnormal circumstances. For example, circulating immune complexes may be deposited in the kidneys of patients with systemic lupus erythematosus, and these circulating complexes may activate complement in a perfectly normal fashion. This normal activation process may lead to renal inflammation and glomerular damage. In this case, the complement system is functioning normally but, nevertheless, is intimately associated with the development of disease.

STRUCTURE AND FUNCTIONAL RELATIONSHIPS

The proteins in the complement system are given either numerical or letter designations. These proteins circulate as inactive precursors in serum and are activated in a very precise biochemical sequence. In many cases, activation of the proteins is associated with cleavage of the protein component. The larger fragment produced by the protein cleavage is responsible for continuation of the complement sequence. The smaller fragment often has the function of promoting the inflammatory response. There are a number of ways in which complement proteins can be activated. For example, proteolytic enzymes, such as those released from certain bacteria, may cleave a complement protein, leading to the uncovering of the active site and the propagation of the complement sequence. More often, antigen-antibody complexes on microbial or viral surfaces are the inciting agents. The processes which transpire when these agents interact with complement have been examined in detail.

Sequence of Reactions of the Classic Pathway

This pathway is responsible for the lysis of most antibody-sensitized cells. In many of the assays where the classic pathway is studied, the presence of a functionally active component is indicated by the lysis of sheep erythrocytes sensitized with rabbit antibody. Sheep erythrocytes are particularly advantageous for use because, for reasons that are not completely understood, they are much more easily lysed by antibody and complement than are erythrocytes from other species. Sheep erythrocytes have on their surface a potent lipopolysaccharide antigen, the Forssman antigen. This antigen is widely distributed in nature. The critical antigenic grouping in this lipopolysaccharide is a specific sugar linkage which is seen as very foreign in animals that do not have the enzymes to form this linkage. Rabbits are a Forssman-negative species and respond to the injection of sheep erythrocytes by producing enormous amounts of anti-Forssman antibody. Thus, high titer antiserum to the sheep erythrocyte is easily obtainable and sheep erythrocytes themselves, being easily lysed by fresh serum, are sensitive indicator particles for the presence of lytic complement activity.

Activation of the classic complement pathway is initiated by the interaction of antigen with C1-fixing antibody. Not all classes of immunoglobulin activate the classic pathway. IgM and IgG subclasses IgG_1, IgG_2, and IgG_3 are the immunoglobulins that bind and activate C1. This reaction has been studied in detail in several model systems. The precise molecular nature of the antigen-antibody-C1 interaction is not clear, but it is known that C1 binds to the Fc fragment of antibody in the antigen-antibody complex by a non-covalent, easily reversed linkage. C1 itself is a complex protein composed of three subunits, C1q, C1r, and C1s, which are held together in the presence of calcium.

The portion of the C1 molecule which interacts with immunoglobulin is the C1q subcomponent. The ability of C1q to interact with aggregated immunoglobulin has provided the basis for a number of new tests designed to detect the presence of soluble immune complexes in the blood of patients with a variety of diseases. Radiolabeled C1q is added to the serum or plasma sample, and one of a number of techniques is used to differentiate free C1q from that bound to protein components of serum. The presence of bound C1q suggests the presence of immunoglobulin complexes in the serum or plasma sample. These techniques are discussed further on p. 934 (Zubler, 1976).

The binding of C1 to antibody in turn leads to activation of C1. It appears that a single molecule of most IgM antibodies can "fix" and activate one molecule of C1. The activated component in each case is indicated by ($\overline{\ }$); thus, activated C1 is designated as $C\overline{1}$. Although C1 binding by a single IgG molecule has been described, C1 binding usually requires an IgG doublet, two molecules side by side, in most of the experimental models studied.

The fact that the binding of C1 by IgG requires cooperative interaction of several IgG molecules has consequences of clinical importance. Since IgG molecules bind to a cell surface in a random fashion, it may require the attachment of hundreds or thousands of IgG molecules to obtain a C1-fixing site. This is thought to be the explanation for the fact that anti-Rh antibodies of the complement-fixing subclasses do not effectively provide a site for complement fixation when they bind to human erythrocytes. The appropriate Rh antigens are sparsely scattered on the erythrocyte surface, and this precludes the formation of antibody doublets, with subsequent complement fixation. Thus, complement activation is not noted in most anti-Rh mediated hemolytic states, whereas it is noted in hemolytic states mediated by cold agglutinins and anti-A, B, and O blood group substance antibodies.

The activation of C1 leads to the generation of an enzymatic site which in model systems has been shown to have esterase activity. This activation is associated with cleavage of the protein chains in C1r and C1s. The activated antigen-antibody C1 complex now is capable of interacting with the next component in the complement sequence, C4. C4 is cleaved by C1 acting as an enzyme, and two cleavage fragments are formed. The larger fragment is highly reactive for a few moments after its formation and appears to bind to any suitable receptor in the microenvironment. Some of the activated C4 molecules bind to the erythrocyte cell membrane as a cluster around the antigen-antibody-C1 site. Therefore, one antibody site can lead to the deposition of many C4 molecules. The antibody C1-C4 complex can, in turn, bind to and activate the next component in the sequence, C2. Again, this reaction involves cleavage of the component. In this case, C1 esterase in association with C4 and in the presence of Mg^{++} can cleave C2, leading to the formation of a $C\overline{142}$ complex. This complex is unstable. However, in the presence of C3, the hemolytic sequence is continued and C3 is cleaved into two fragments, C3a and C3b. C3a is released and C3b is bound to the erythrocyte membrane. Again, amplification is an important part of the C3 reaction in that hundreds of C3b molecules may be deposited at each complement-fixing site. If C3 is not present, the $C\overline{142}$ complex decays to $C\overline{14}$, releasing an inactivated fragment of C2. Many of the remaining reactions in the complement sequence follow this general formulation. The $C\overline{1423b}$ complex can bind and then cleave C5 into two fragments, C5a and C5b. Again, C5b attaches to the cell membrane and continues the hemolytic sequence, and the C5a fragment is released. This general pattern is continued for C6, C7, C8, and C9; however, the reactions differ in detail. Activation of several of these components does not appear to be accompanied by cleavage. When all of the complement components have reacted with a site on the cell surface, the cell membrane may be damaged in such a way that the cell lyses.

Biologic Functions Associated with Activation

As discussed above, the complement system subserves many functions which do not involve cell lysis. Many of the features of the inflammatory response are promoted by complement fragments, and complement plays a key role in opsonization. Table 37–1 lists the most widely accepted biologic functions of complement components and complement fragments. Most of these biologic properties are self-explanatory. It should be mentioned that anaphylatoxic factors cause

Table 37–1. BIOLOGIC ACTIVITIES OF THE COMPONENTS OF THE COMPLEMENT SYSTEM OF MAN

C1	Increases affinity of some antibodies
C1q	Aggregation of antigen-antibody complexes
C1,4	Viral neutralization
C4b	Immune adherence receptors on lymphocytes, PMN's, macrophages, and primate erythrocytes
C2	Cleavage product may have kinin-like properties
C3a	Anaphylatoxic, immunoregulatory
C3b	Opsonic immune adherence receptors on B-lymphocytes, PMN's, macrophages, and primate erythrocytes
$C3b_i$	Receptor on PMN's, B lymphocytes, primate erythrocytes, and macrophages
C3d	Receptor on lymphocytes and macrophages
C5a	Chemotactic, anaphylatoxic, immunoregulatory
$C\overline{567}$	Chemotactic
C8,9	Lysis

mast cells to degranulate and release their various mediators in the absence of cytotoxicity. The opsonic properties of the complement proteins appear to depend on the presence of specific receptors on the surface of phagocytic cells. Foreign materials with opsonically active fragments on their surface interact with these receptors, leading first to membrane adherence and, as a second step, to phagocytosis.

Many of the biologic properties of these complement fragments are controlled by the presence in serum of specific protein inhibitors. Thus, the enzymatic activity of activated C1 is destroyed by the C1 esterase inhibitor; the integrity of the opsonically active protein C3b may be destroyed by the C3b inactivator; and an inactivator of cell-bound C6 exists. There is also an inactivator of the vasoactive material, anaphylatoxin, which destroys the activity of C3a and, to a lesser extent, C5a. Other regulatory proteins exist which are beyond the scope of this review.

Complement Receptors. Receptors which recognize various fragments of complement components are present on phagocytic cells, lymphoid cells, nonprimate platelets, primate erythrocytes, and cells in other organs. Such receptors have been described for C1q, C4b, C3b, $C3b_i$, C3d, C5, and β1H. The interaction of C3 fragments with specific receptors on phagocytic cells provides the biochemical basis for opsonization (Berger, 1982).

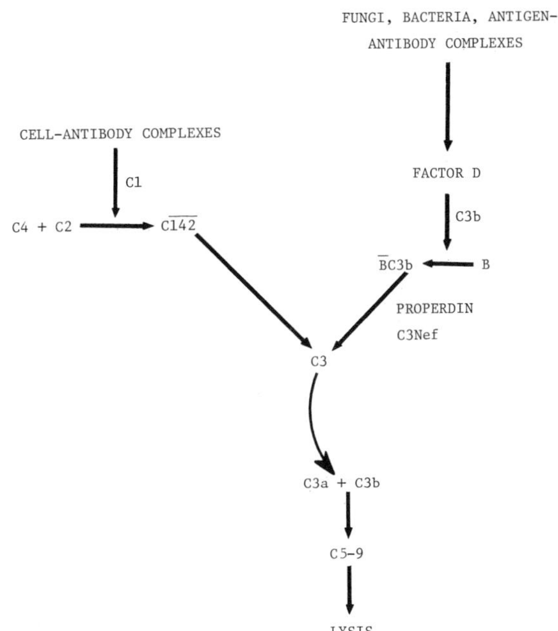

Figure 37–1. Pathways of complement activation. B = Factor B. C3Nef = C3 nephritic factor. The activated complement complex is indicated by the bar above the letter and numbers. The classic pathway of activation utilizes C1, C4, and C2, and the alternative pathway utilizes factors D, B, and C3b.

Alternative Complement Pathway

In recent years, it has become clear that there is another mechanism for the activation of complement which does not utilize the classic complement components, C1, C4, and C2, and which does not have an absolute requirement for antibody. When many microorganisms are exposed to fresh serum, they activate and bind to their surface the opsonically important complement component, C3, as well as the later components in the complement series which mediate bacterial lysis. Further analysis of this mechanism has demonstrated that there exists a pathway of complement activation which is phylogenetically older than the classic pathway and which bypasses the early components of the classic pathway. This pathway is composed of a series of proteins which resemble the classic complement components in their mechanism of action. The details of the protein interactions which make up this pathway are still not completely clear. As shown in Figure 37–1, there are a number of components in the *alternative or properdin pathway* which are analogous to the components of the *classic complement pathway* and which function to form a C3 cleaving enzyme. Properdin factor D is analogous to C1 of the classic complement pathway. It is a DFP (diisofluorophosphate)-inhibitable active enzyme which is heat labile, as is C1. Properdin factor B is analogous to C2. This component of the alternative pathway also is heat labile and forms a non-stable enzyme complex which is important in the cleavage of C3. It appears that a C3 cleavage product, C3b, serves the same role in the alternative pathway that C4 serves in the classic pathway. C3b, in combination with properdin factors B and D, forms an enzyme which is capable of cleaving C3. Thus, if a small amount of cleaved C3 can be generated, a major amplification of C3 cleaving capacity can be achieved via C3b interacting with components of the alternative pathway.

There are at least two regulatory proteins which are important in preventing the C3 cleaving enzyme formed by alternative pathway activation from decaying, thereby increasing the effectiveness of the cleaving enzyme. These two proteins are properdin and so-called C3 nephritic factor. The latter factor derives its name from the fact that it was first discovered in the sera of patients with membranoproliferative glomerulonephritis and low serum C3. When this factor is added to normal fresh serum with intact alternative pathway mechanisms, marked C3 cleavage results, with a dramatic fall in C3 titer. When the C3 nephritic factor was first discovered, it was hoped that this agent would provide an explanation for the low C3 and concomitant nephritis seen in membranoproliferative glomerulonephritis, but it is now clear that this protein simply serves a regulatory role in alternative pathway activation.

The mechanisms for activation of the alternative pathway are under active investigation. Although bacterial and fungal surfaces with repeating polysaccharide subunits are important in activating the alternative complement pathway, aggregated immunoglobulins and, presumably, antigen-antibody complexes of a number of types perform a similar function. Thus, complexes containing IgM, IgG, IgA, and IgE can activate the alternative pathway, although

Table 37–2. A MORE COMPLETE VERSION OF THE CLASSIC AND ALTERNATIVE PATHWAYS

Classic Pathway

$$1.\ \text{EA} + \text{C1qrs} \xrightleftharpoons{\text{Ca}^{++}} \text{EAC1} \rightarrow \text{EAC}\overline{1}$$

$$\Updownarrow \text{Ca}^{++}$$

$$\text{C1q, C1r, C1s}$$

$$2.\ \text{EAC}\overline{1} + \text{C4} \rightarrow \text{EAC}\overline{14b} + \text{C4a}$$

$$3.\ \text{EA}\overline{14} + \text{C2} \xrightarrow{\text{Mg}^{++}} \text{EAC}\overline{142a} + \text{C2b}$$

$$\downarrow$$

$$\text{EAC}\overline{14} + \text{C2a}^{d}$$

$$4.\ \text{EAC}\overline{142} + \text{C3} \rightarrow \text{EAC1423b} + \text{C3a}$$

$$\searrow \text{C2a}^{d}$$

$$\downarrow$$

$$\text{EAC143b (see below for C3b decay)}$$

$$5.\ \text{EAC}\overline{1423} + \text{C5} \rightarrow \text{EAC}\overline{14235}\text{b} + \text{C5a}$$

$$\searrow \text{C2a}^{d} + \text{C5b}^{d}$$

$$\downarrow$$

$$\text{EAC143}$$

$$6.\ \text{EAC}\overline{14235} + \text{C6} \rightarrow \text{EAC}\overline{142356}$$

$$\searrow \text{C2a}^{d}$$

$$\downarrow$$

$$\text{EAC14356} \rightleftharpoons \text{EAC143} + \text{C56}$$

$$7.\ \text{EAC}\overline{142356} + \text{C7} \rightarrow \text{EAC}\overline{1423567}$$

$$8.\ \text{EAC}\overline{1423567} + \text{C8} \rightarrow \text{EAC}\overline{12345678} \rightarrow \text{slow lysis}$$

$$9.\ \text{EAC14235678} + \text{C9} \rightarrow \text{EAC1-9}$$

$$10.\ \text{EAC1-9} \xrightarrow{37^{\circ}\text{C}} \text{E*} \xrightarrow[\text{Inhibited}]{\text{0.09 M EDTA}} \text{Lysis}$$

Subunit and fragment letter designations are used only when they first appear. C2 is required to maintain active enzymatic activity through the C5 step. Superscript "d" indicates a decay product. EAC1-7 is stable with regard to the action of C8 and C9. The build-up of C5–9 on and in the lipid bilayer leads to the development of a transmembrane pore. The bar is over the active enzyme. E* refers to a cell which has reacted with all of the components of complement and which will go on the lysis.

EA = erythrocyte plus antibody
EAC = erythrocyte plus antibody plus complement

in the absence of classic pathway activation rather large amounts of complexes are required. The biochemical interactions which comprise alternative pathway activation and the biologic consequences of this activation are still being defined. However, they appear to be very similar to those which result from classic pathway activation. As will be made clear subsequently, there are a number of diseases which appear to be associated with classic pathway activation and a number of diseases which are more commonly associated with activation of the alternative pathway. It is in identification and definition of these diseases that the clinical pathologist will often be asked to aid the clinician. A more detailed version of complement activation is presented in Table 37–2.

COMPLEMENT IN DISEASE STATES

As mentioned previously (p. 880), in most disease states complement functions normally in producing inflammation and tissue damage. When complement plays a role in the development of a disease, it is often being activated by an abnormal antibody, immune complex, or foreign material. It is frequently of importance to assess the level of one or another component of complement as a means of following the activity of a disease process. Thus, patients with active lupus erythematosus may have depressed levels of C3 and C4, and these component levels may be followed as a rough index of disease activity.

When one determines the levels of a component in serum, it is important to recognize that this represents a static measurement of serum proteins which are turning over rapidly. Even in the normal individual, the fractional catabolic rate of most of the components which have been measured is on the order of 2 per cent per hour. Many of these proteins behave as acute phase reactants, and their levels in serum may rise dramatically in inflammatory states. Their rates of catabolism may increase greatly in various autoimmune diseases. The finding of a decreased level of a

Table 37–2. A MORE COMPLETE VERSION OF THE CLASSIC AND ALTERNATIVE PATHWAYS *(Continued)*

Alternative Pathway

Bacteria, fungi, antigen-antibody complexes, zymosan (Z), inulin, PNH erythrocyte surface initiate; but the mechanism of initiation is still not certain.

Once C3b is generated, the sequence continues as in line 2.

1. $Z + C3 + \overline{D} + B + P \xrightarrow{Mg^{++}}$ small quantity $ZC\overline{3bBb} + C3a + Ba$
2. $ZC3b + B + D + C3 \xrightarrow{Mg^{++}}$ additional sites $Z\overline{3bBb} + Ba + C3a$
3. $ZC\overline{3bBb} \rightarrow ZC3b + Bb$ inactive (decay)
4. $ZC\overline{3bBb} \xrightarrow[\text{Properdin}]{} ZC\overline{3bBb}$ (stabilized)
5. $ZC\overline{3bBb} \xrightarrow[\text{C3NeF}]{} ZC\overline{3bBb}$ (stabilized)
6. $Z\overline{C3bBb} + C5 \rightarrow ZC3bBbC5b + C5a$

The cascade continues

C3NeF, present in some patients with glomerulonephritis, appears to represent IgG anti C3bBb.

C3b Inactivation Sequence

1. $EACl\text{-}3b + H \rightarrow EACl\text{-}3b\ H$
2. $EACl\text{-}3bH + (I) \rightarrow EACl\text{-}_iC3b$
3. $EACl\text{-}3b_i$ + Serum trypsin-like enzyme $\rightarrow EACl\text{-}3d + H + C3c$

Subscript "i" represents partial cleavage with inactivation of site.

β_1H appears to occupy the same site as B on C3b and can displace B.

D = Factor D
B = Factor B
P = Properdin
I = C3b Inactivator
H = Factor H (β_1H)

component may raise suspicion that the complement system is participating in tissue damage but does not prove it. The finding of a normal serum level of a component does not preclude the participation of complement in tissue injury. For example, patients with primary biliary cirrhosis have an increased catabolic rate of C3, and it has been suggested that C3 may play some role in the development of this disease. Nevertheless, the level of C3 in the serum of patients with primary biliary cirrhosis is almost always elevated. In this case, increased synthesis obscures the increased catabolism. It should also be recognized that complement function in various body compartments may differ. Complement activity in the blood of patients with seropositive rheumatoid arthritis may be normal or elevated; however, the complement activity of joint fluid may be severely depressed.

The final general concept to be discussed is that of the "complement profile." Earlier sections have introduced the classic and alternative complement pathways and their mechanisms of action. In recent years, an attempt has been made to determine which pathway of complement activation predominates in mediating tissue damage or depressed component levels in one or another illness. The simplest approach to this problem examines the levels of various components and assumes that decreased levels of a component of one or the other pathway are more likely to occur when that pathway is activated. Therefore, if a patient has depressed levels of C3 and C4 and normal levels of properdin factor B and properdin, the classic pathway is likely to be involved. If a patient has decreased levels of C3 and factor B and/or properdin and normal levels of C4, alternative pathway activation is most likely. In this way, determining the levels of a limited number of components can provide a great deal of information. Except in the case of the genetically controlled complement abnormalities, one never needs to know the levels of all complement components, except for investigational purposes.

There is now considerable interest in the detection of decay products in various body fluids. Thus, C3 decay products have been found in sera of patients with primary biliary cirrhosis, rheumatoid arthritis, and lupus erythematosus.

A detailed discussion of the levels of complement components in various disease states (Frank, 1975) is beyond the scope of this review. Nevertheless, a brief statement as to the role of complement in various groups of illnesses will be provided. It is fair to state that the role of complement in each of these disease groups is under active investigation.

Diagnosis or Assessment of Clinical Activity in Disease

Rheumatologic Diseases. The most straightforward example of a rheumatologic disease mediating many of its effects via complement activation is that of *systemic lupus erythematosus.* Circulating immune complexes activate complement and are deposited in a variety of tissue sites, leading to tissue damage. It has been suggested that determination of levels of C3 and C4 is helpful in following the activity of this disease. Depressed levels of complement in joint fluid have been shown to exist in a number of other rheumatologic conditions, including rheumatoid arthritis.

Normal or elevated serum complement levels are found in juvenile rheumatoid arthritis, most patients with adult onset rheumatoid arthritis, palindromic arthritis, pseudogout, gout, Reiter's syndrome, and gonococcal arthritis.

Depressed CH_{50} and cleavage products of C3 and properdin factor B are thought to represent intra-articular activation in the synovial fluid of almost all patients with seropositive rheumatoid arthritis and many patients with seronegative rheumatoid arthritis, SLE, pseudogout, gout, Reiter's syndrome, and gonococcal arthritis. This is not true of fluids obtained from patients with degenerative arthritis (Hunder, 1977).

Infectious Diseases. As previously discussed, one major function of the complement system is to protect against infection. Patients with gram-negative septicemia and shock are often depleted of C3 and components of the alternative pathway, as are patients with certain fungal diseases, such as cryptococcal septicemia. A major area for future investigation concerns the role of complement in the tissue damage associated with chronic infection. This is an area which is only beginning to be explored. It is known that patients with HB_SAg-positive infectious hepatitis have an early fall in serum C3, which later returns to normal. This may be associated with signs of immune complex disease, e.g., arthralgia. In a similar fashion, complement appears to play an important role in a number of parasitic infections, including malaria. In patients with vivax malaria C1, C4, and C2 may be depressed. In patients with falciparum malaria, C3 may be depressed as well.

Renal Diseases. Complement is thought to be of key importance in glomerular damage in a variety of the glomerulonephritides (Michael, 1974). This is usually demonstrated by the deposition of C3 and/or other components in the vicinity of the glomerular basement membrane (Table 37–3). Many of these patients will show activation of the alternative pathway on serum analysis. The role of complement in interstitial and tubular disease is less clear. However, there are those who believe that complement may have some function in these disorders as well.

Dermatologic Diseases. As in the other groups of diseases listed, complement is thought to play a part in the ongoing tissue damage in a variety of dermatologic illnesses. These include pemphigus vulgaris, bullous pemphigoid, and herpes gestationis. It should be noted that serum complement levels are usually normal or elevated in these chronic inflammatory states, and the importance of complement is suggested by immunofluorescent analysis of tissue biopsies and by studies of blister fluid.

Hematologic Diseases. In many types of autoimmune hemolytic anemia, complement plays an important role in opsonization of erythrocytes, leading to their clearance by cells of the reticuloendothelial system. However, even in those cases in which complement is clearly involved, serum complement levels are often normal. Complement is particularly important in the clearance of cells coated by IgM cold agglutinins antibody with anti-I specificity. Another complement-related hematologic problem is paroxysmal nocturnal hemoglobinuria (PNH). In this illness, the patient's erythrocytes and other blood cell elements develop a membrane defect which renders them exceedingly susceptible to complement-mediated lysis. This acquired cellular defect is associated with hemolysis due to activation of the alternative pathway by the cell membrane.

Table 37–3. COMPLEMENT LEVELS IN SELECTED RENAL DISEASES

	C1	C4	C2	C3	P	B
Acute glomerulonephritis	N	D	D	D	D	N or D
Systemic lupus erythematosus	D	D	D	D	N or D	D
Membranoproliferative glomerulonephritis	N	N	N	D	N or D	N or D
Post-streptococcal glomerulonephritis	Normal in initial sera (<10 days) in some studies					
" Later	D	D slight	D slight	D	D	N or D
Idiopathic nephrotic syndrome	N	N	N	N		D
Anaphylactoid purpura with nephritis	N or D low levels transient	N or D	N	—	N or D	N

Note: The syndrome of partial lipodystrophy may be associated with C3 depression, C3NeF in serum, and membranoproliferative glomerulonephritis.

B = Factor B; D = depressed; N = normal; and P = properdin.

GENETIC DISORDERS

As discussed previously, the number of patients with genetically controlled complement disorders is few, and these patients are of greatest interest because they allow us to determine the role of complement components in various biologic phenomena and in various disease states. In general, the absence of the components follows simple mendelian genetics and is inherited as an autosomal recessive trait. Thus, heterozygous patients tend to have half normal levels or less and homozygous-deficient patients have little or no detectable component activity. As shown in Table 37–4, deficiencies are known for almost every component of the classic pathway. Most of these patients present with one or another manifestation of autoimmune disease, and the role of complement deficiency in the development of these diseases is under active investigation. One interesting hypothesis is that autoimmunity may be a manifestation of chronic viral illness. If complement aids in viral neutralization, an interruption of those pathways of activation may promote chronic viral infection. It is striking that deficiencies other than C3 deficiency are not generally associated with the presence of acute infectious diseases. This is attributed to the fact that the alternative pathway is available for opsonization of microorganisms in most of the deficiency states. C3 is a key component of both pathways and plays a key role in opsonization. Thus, absence of this component is associated with infection with a wide variety of pathogens, especially in childhood before the development of high titer antibodies. Interestingly, deficiency of a number of the late-acting components is associated with a high incidence of disseminated infection with *Neisseria* organisms (Agnello, 1978; Tappeiner, 1982; Peterson, 1979).

A group of patients with Leiner's syndrome has been evaluated, and it is suggested that these patients have abnormal C5 function. The data on which this conclusion rests are based on highly complex assays, and it appears at present that this conclusion is not warranted. The defect in Leiner's disease could reside at another step in the alternative complement pathway.

Table 37–4. INBORN ERRORS OF THE COMPLEMENT SYSTEM OF MAN

C1q:	Partial with thymic alymphoplasia, hypogammaglobulinemia; complete with systemic lupus erythematosus
C1r:	Systemic lupus erythematosus, glomerulonephritis
C1s:	Systemic lupus erythematosus
C4:	Systemic lupus erythematosus
C2:	Most common deficiency—discoid lupus erythematosus, systemic lupus erythematosus, glomerulonephritis, anaphylactoid purpura, dermatomyositis, vasculitis
C3:	Frequent infections—all pyogens—resemble congenital hypogammaglobulinemia
C5:	Systemic lupus erythematosus
C6:	Repeated *Neisseria* infections
C7:	*Neisseria* infections
C8:	*Neisseria* infections, systemic lupus erythematosus
C9:	No clear disease association
H:	Hemolytic-uremic syndrome (Thompson, 1981)

Properdin (partial): Asymptomatic (Davis, 1980)

C1 inhibitor: Hereditary angioedema. *Note:* C1 normal or depressed, C3 always normal. Occasional patients with lymphoid malignancies or autoimmune disease may consume or destroy their C1 esterase inhibitor and develop the clinical picture of hereditary angioedema.

C3 inactivator: Recurrent infections

Deficiencies of C1–9 are associated with CH_{50} of 0. Deficiencies of C1, C4, C2 associated with systemic lupus erythematosus often have negative LE preps. Deficiencies of C3–9 are associated with the absence of bactericidal activity of serum. Deficiency of C3 or C5 is associated with absent or diminished chemotactic activity of serum and may be associated with absent leukocyte response to infection. The genes for C2, C4, and properdin factor B are clearly linked to HLA. All inheritance patterns studied to date are autosomal recessive with the exception of C1 inhibitor deficiencies.

ASSAY OF COMPONENTS

General Principles and Types of Assays

Today, accurate methods are available for measuring each of the nine classic pathway components, most of the alternative pathway components, and several enzymes and inhibitors which regulate the complement system. However, many of these methods are still considered research techniques and are not available on a routine basis. We will confine our attention to techniques which do not require a laboratory skilled in complement research for their performance. In general, two types of techniques are in use: those that measure the complement proteins as antigens in serum and those that measure the functional activity of the components. Both techniques have advantages and disadvantages as research and diagnostic tools, and these will be reviewed.

Methods for antigenic (immunochemical) analysis are generally simpler to perform. These antigenic assays are highly specific and require fewer specialized reagents and considerably less personnel time. Reagents for measuring several proteins of the complement system are commercially available, including C1q, C4, C3, C5, properdin factor B, and C1 inhibitor. In these assays, either serum or plasma can be used, and the commonly available methods of freezer storage (−20°C.) are sufficient. For these reasons, antigenic assays are easily adaptable to a routine laboratory. On the other hand, antigenic assays are less sensitive than functional assays, and they may detect degraded non-functional components.

Functional complement assays are both sensitive and precise tools for providing important information on the activity of a component. Some of these methods may be used to quantitate activity at the molecular level, while others express complement function in arbitrary titration units. Commercial reagents are available for titrating all components of the classic pathway system. However, for the most part, these assays are performed in a limited number of research facilities at this time. Most functional assays involve complex, time-consuming procedures, which require special, relatively highly purified, expensive reagents.

Procedures for Evaluating Functional Activity

HANDLING OF SAMPLES

The proper handling of samples is critical for correct functional analysis. For most functional complement assays, serum rather than plasma is chosen for analysis because both chelators (EDTA) and heparin are anticomplementary. EDTA plasma may be used, however, in some functional tests where the sample is diluted enough (> 1:100) to overcome the chelating effect of EDTA. To obtain serum for functional assays, a fresh blood sample is allowed to clot at room temperature for ½ hour and then in the cold for about one hour. If C1q binding studies are needed, the sample is allowed to clot two hours at room temperature. In this case, complete clot polymerization appears to facilitate accurate assay. If cryoprecipitating antibodies are suspected, clot formation and centrifugation of the specimen should proceed at 37°C., since complement fixation may occur if the specimen aliquot is chilled. To separate serum, the clot is rimmed and usually is centrifuged in the cold. Serum should be stored in multiple aliquots to avoid thawing and refreezing. The serum aliquots should be stored immedately at −40°C. to −70°C. Serum aliquots can be stored for long periods at −70°C. without loss of activity. When sera are to be transported, they should be well sealed before being packed in a container with large quantities of dry ice.

REAGENTS AND EQUIPMENT

Almost all functional analyses can be performed with equipment limited to a spectrophotometer, pH meter, conductivity meter, precision balance, refrigerated centrifuge, and water baths which can be regulated with precision at 37°C. and 30°C. The usual array of calibrated pipettes, graduated beakers, etc., is needed, and it should be mentioned that it is advisable to avoid using mouth pipetting with blood samples from diverse sources. Methods for preparing solutions commonly used in functional complement assays are outlined in Table 37–5. Two basic reagents are required for titrating lytic activity. They are washed and standardized sheep erythrocytes (E) and rabbit antiserum to sheep erythrocyte stroma (A).

Preparation of Sheep Erythrocytes (E). Sheep blood is drawn aseptically into an equal volume of sterile Alsevers solution. This preparation of sheep cells is commercially available. The anticoagulated whole blood is stored for at least one week at 4°C.

Table 37–5. SOLUTIONS COMMONLY USED IN COMPLEMENT ASSAYS

Stock solutions

1. *Veronal-buffered saline (Stock VBS)*
   To prepare 2 L, dissolve 83.0 g NaCl and 10.19 g Na-5,5′ diethyl barbiturate in 1.5 L of distilled water. Mix vigorously while titrating to pH 7.35 ± 0.05 with 1 N HCl. Bring to 2.0 L volumetrically with distilled water. This solution is five times the concentration of an isotonic solution and may be stored at 4°C. for at least one month. It is diluted immediately before use.
2. *0.10 M disodium ethylenediamintetraacetate (Stock EDTA)*
   Dissolve 37.2 g in about 800 ml of distilled water. Adjust the pH to 7.65 ± 0.05 with 2 N NaOH and bring to 1.0 L with distilled water. Store at 4°C. Stock EDTA may be used for at least three weeks.
3. *Dextrose with Ca^{++}, Mg^{++}, and gelatin (D)*
   A 5 per cent solution of dextrose in distilled water (D5W) is obtained from commercial sources. Approximately 1 L is measured volumetrically, 1.0 ml of Stock Solution 6 is added, and the solution brought to 1.0 L. 100 to 200 ml of the mixed solution is added to 1 g of gelatin in an Erlenmeyer flask and heated until all of the gelatin granules have dissolved. After the remaining solution is added, the D is well mixed and stored at 4°C. D may be used for one week.
4. *2.00 M $MgCl_2$ solution*
   Prepare about 200 ml of solution containing $MgCl_2$ at approximately 3 M. Measure the specific gravity of the solution and determine the $MgCl_2$ concentration from the *Handbook of Chemistry and Physics* (conversion tables for concentrated values of aqueous solutions). Adjust the concentration to 2.00 M by adding distilled H_2O.
5. *0.300 M $CaCl_2$ solution*
   About 200 ml of an approximately 0.5 M solution of $CaCl_2$ is prepared. Measure the specific gravity of this solution and determine $CaCl_2$ concentration as described above. Adjust to 0.300 M by adding distilled H_2O.
6. *Stock metals*
   A solution containing 1.0 M $MgCl_2$ and 0.15 $CaCl_2$ is prepared by combining equal volumes of solutions 4 and 5.

Working solutions

1. *Isotonic VBS with gelatin and metals (VBS)*
   To prepare 1 L add 200 ml of Stock Solution 1 to a 1 L volumetric flask. Add 1.0 ml Stock Solution 6 and bring to 1.0 L with distilled H_2O. Add 0.1 per cent gelatin as in Stock Solution 3. VBS should be prepared fresh every three to five days and stored at 4°C.
2. *Isotonic VBS-dextrose of lowered ionic strengths (DVBS)*
   Buffers of varying ionic strengths are prepared by mixing Stock solution 3 with Working Solution 1 in varying proportions. 0.065 μ DVBS is prepared by mixing three parts of the former solution with two parts of the latter. DVBS should be prepared fresh.
3. *Isotonic VBS-EDTA buffer (EDTA)*
   Mix nine parts of Working Solution 1 without metals with one part of Stock Solution 2. This solution is stable for at least one week at 4°C.
4. *C-EDTA*
   Dilute fresh guinea pig serum (titer of at least 170) 1:25 in Working Solution 3. This reagent is stable for one week at 4°C.

before use and may be used for up to six weeks if sterility is maintained. Studies have shown that the age of sheep cells can greatly influence the titers of most complement components (Gaither, 1973), and titers may be falsely low with fresh cells. An appropriate volume of cells is removed for washing under sterile conditions. After centrifugation, the supernatant and buffy coat are removed. Cells are suspended in 0.01 M EDTA buffer and incubated at 37°C. for 10 minutes. The cells are washed in EDTA, followed by three washes in VBS. The washed, packed cells are then diluted about 15-fold in VBS. To determine cell concentration, a small sample of the cells is diluted 1:25 in distilled water. The optical density (O.D.) of the lysate is determined at 541 nm. In general, an O.D. of 0.420 corresponds to a sheep cell concentration of 1×10^9 cells/ml. Cells at this concentration, which are stored in VBS, are designated as "E." E may be stored at 4°C. and utilized for approximately one week. Additional washes immediately before use may be required to remove any lysed cells from the preparation. For some studies, 1.5×10^8 red cells/ml are required. A 1:25 dilution of such cells in distilled water corresponds to an O.D. of 0.560 at 412 nm.

Preparation of Anti-Sheep Erythrocyte Antibody (A). Two types of anti-sheep erythrocyte antibody are in common use: antibody to whole sheep erythrocytes and antibody to the Forssman antigen on the erythrocytes. Either appears to be satisfactory for studies of "whole" complement activity (CH_{50}); however, most workers who report functional titrations of individual components utilize rabbit anti–Forssman antibody. Antibody with a high degree of specificity for the Forssman antigen of sheep erythrocytes can be prepared by immunizing rabbits with boiled sheep erythrocyte stroma. The procedures for preparation of stroma and rabbit immunization are explained fully in Kabat's textbook (1961). For the purpose of the complement studies presented here, the immunization schedule and procedure should be designed to produce antisera in which most of the hemolytic activity is in the IgM fraction. Before use, the complement activity of the antiserum is destroyed by heat inactivation for 30 minutes at 56°C. Antisera with acceptable activity may be diluted, usually to 1:100, in normal saline and stored at −20°C. for many months or at 4°C. for short periods of time.

A 15-minute kinetic assay is used to titrate anti-Forssman antibody (Table 37–6). The unit of hemolytic antibody, AB_{50}, is defined as that amount of antiserum which, under the described conditions, lyses half of the red cells in exactly 15 minutes. A series of accurately prepared dilutions of the antiserum is prepared in VBS. A dilution of pooled guinea pig complement, usually diluted 1:7.5 in VBS, is the complement source. The guinea pig serum complement must be preadsorbed with E to remove natural hemolysin. In the assay, 0.5 ml E (5×10^8/ml) is mixed with 0.5 ml of the appropriate dilutions of antiserum. After 15 minutes at 37°C., 0.25 ml of the diluted guinea pig complement is added, and the mixture is incubated further at 37°C. In this and all other titrations discussed, the cells are mixed frequently to maintain a uniform cell suspension. After exactly 15.0 minutes, the reaction is stopped with the addition of 2.5 ml of ice cold EDTA, mixed, and centrifuged. The supernatants are analyzed photometrically at 541 nm and the titers determined using the Von Krogh equation (see below). Controls include E plus complement (CBC), E with buffer alone (CB), and E lysed 100 per cent in distilled H_2O.

Titration of complement requires sheep E sensitized with an optimal amount of antibody (A). An optimally sensitized preparation contains sufficient antibody so that the complement titer is independent of antibody concentration. To determine the optimal amount of antibody, 0.5 ml of a series of two-fold falling

Table 37–6. PROTOCOL FOR TITRATION OF ANTIBODY AND SAMPLE DETERMINATIONS

	Test Tube					
	1	*2*	*3*	*CB*	*CBC*	*100%*
E (5×10^8 ml)	0.5	0.5	0.5	0.5	0.5	0.5
Hemolysin, 0.5 ml	1:20,000	1:40,000	1:80,000	—	—	—
			Incubate 10.0 minutes 37°C.			
Guinea pig complement, 1:7.5	0.25	0.25	0.25	—	0.25	—
			Incubate 15.0 minutes 37°C.			
EDTA buffer, ml	2.5	2.5	2.5	2.75	2.5	—
H_2O (ml)	—	—	—	—	—	2.75
Absorbance (O.D.) 541 nm	0.454	0.137	0.040	0.003	0.014	0.698
Absorbance (O.D.) Corr.	0.440	0.123	0.026	—	—	0.695
y/1 − y	1.73	0.215	0.039	—	—	—
Titer, AB_{50}	24,000	—	—	—	—	—

E = Sheep erythrocytes.
CB = Sheep erythrocytes with buffer alone.
CBC = Sheep erythrocytes plus complement.
y = Absorbance (corrected) of test sample/absorbance (corrected) of 100% lysed sample.
AB_{50} = Amount of antiserum which under described conditions lyses half of the erythrocytes in exactly 15 minutes.

5

dilutions of antibody is added to an equal volume of E with careful mixing. After incubating the sensitized cells for 10 minutes at 37°C., 5.5 ml VBS and 1.0 ml of a dilution of fresh frozen guinea pig serum complement (1 CH_{50} Unit) are added. After incubating the mixture at 37°C. for one hour, the cells are sedimented, the absorbance (O.D.) of the supernatant is determined at 541 nm, and the percentage of lysed cells determined. The per cent lysis is plotted versus the log of the dilution of the antiserum. A strong antiserum will cause optimal lysis at a dilution of > 1:500. Sheep erythrocytes sensitized with optimal amounts of antibody are designated EA. Sensitization is accomplished using a very standarized procedure. A volume of E is placed in a container which allows for easy mixing. The diluted antiserum is slowly pipetted in a dropwise fashion into an equal volume of cells, with constant swirling of the contents to ensure an even distribution of antibody on the cells. Antibody is always added to E. EA are generally incubated for 15 minutes at 30°C. or 37°C. before use. They remain stable when stored at 4°C. but may require additional washes in VBS if spontaneous cell lysis occurs.

Cellular intermediates in the complement system with membrane-bound components are also used for functional assays. EAC4 have cell-bound C4 and may be used as a reagent for measuring the remaining eight components. There are a number of methods available for forming this intermediate. Each begins with the preparation of EA. Some investigators recommend that twice the optimal concentration of antibody be used. The procedure used in our laboratory is as follows: A 10 ml volume of EA containing 5 × 10^8 cells/ml is chilled to 0°C., and partially purified guinea pig C1 (500 to 1000 C1 effective molecules or sites per ml of suspension) is added (e.g., if the commercially supplied C1 has a titer of 10,000 units, it would be diluted 1:10 to yield 1000 sites/cell). Guinea pig C1 is compatible with the early human components and is generally chosen for preparing both guinea pig and human intermediates. The EAC1 solution is mixed well and held at 0°C. for 15 minutes to form the complement cell intermediate EAC1. A solution containing 2 ml of fresh or fresh frozen human serum complement and 18 ml of EDTA buffer is prepared, heated at 37°C. for 15 minutes to ensure chelation of all calcium and magnesium, and then cooled to 0°C. This ice cold solution is addded to 0°C. EAC1 with vigorous mixing. After 15 minutes, incubation at 0°C., the cells are washed two times in EDTA in the cold and three times in VBS. During the 15 minute incubation, two competing reactions occur. C4 functions in the absence of metals. On the other hand, EAC1 is EDTA sensitive and C1 dissociates from the intermediate in the absence of calcium. Thus, two reactions proceed:

$$\text{EAC1} + \underset{\text{Serum}}{\text{EDTA}} \begin{cases} \nearrow \text{EAC14} \xrightarrow{\text{EDTA}} \text{EAC4} + \text{C1q r \& s} \\ \searrow \text{EA} + \text{C1q r \& s} \end{cases}$$

Under the condition of the procedures, adequate amounts of C4 combine with EAC1 before the C1 is stripped from the cellular intermediate. The EAC4 cells are suspended in VBS to 1.5 × 10^8/ml and stored at 4°C. They retain C4 on their surface indefinitely and can be used as long as the preparation can be washed free of the hemoglobin, which represents non-specific lysis of some of the stored cells. Before use, EAC4 should be tested to determine if the cells have a sufficient number of C4 sites. A simple test in which the remaining eight components are added in excess is sufficient. EAC4 should lyse completely within five minutes. More precise information on the number of EAC14 sites available for interaction with C2 can be obtained from t_{max} determinations (Kabat, 1961; Rapp, 1970). The t_{max} measurement refers to a complex kinetic reaction in which the time for maximum lysis of a specific cell mixture is related to the number of C4 sites/cell. The EAC14 intermediate is prepared by adding partially purified guinea pig C1 to EAC4 suspended in DVBS at an ionic strength of 0.065 μ. EAC4 are prepared as described. To saturate EAC4 with C1, at least 200 to 400 molecules of C1 per cell is added. C1 is allowed to react with EAC4 for 10 minutes at 30°C. To remove free C1 and other contaminating components, the EAC14 cells are then washed with 0.065 μ DVBS. The washed cells are stored in the same buffer, generally at 1.5 × 10^8/ml. EAC14 remains stable when stored at 4°C. under these conditions for days to weeks. It should be noted that it is possible to prepare EAC1, EAC14, and EAC4 and store these cells for prolonged periods of time in liquid nitrogen (Rowe, 1965; Hunsicker, 1975). Such cells are perfectly acceptable for use in functional complement titrations. The EAC4 intermediate may also be prepared by adding partially purified components directly to EA. EA, described above, are suspended in 0.065 μ DVBS to 1.5 × 10^8/ml. Guinea pig C1 is added in excess (500 to 1000 sites/cell), and the mixture is incubated at 30°C. for 15 minutes. After one wash in 0.065 μ DVBS, EAC1 are resuspended in the same buffer. Partially purified human C4 is added at a concentration which yields 100 sites per cell, and the mixture is brought to 37°C. for 30 minutes. EAC14 may be washed in DVBS and used for complement assays where that intermediate is required, or they may be converted to EAC4 cells by removing the C1 with several EDTA washes.

The simplest functional assay of the classic pathway measures total hemolytic complement. The absence of any one of the nine components results in a total hemolytic complement titer (CH_{50}) of zero. However, a normal value does not exclude reduced levels of individual components. When a patient's history and symptoms suggest a possible deficiency, hemolytic titrations of individual components may be required.

The procedure for total complement evaluation is outlined in the sample titration (Table 37–7). The titer is expressed in CH_{50} units (the reciprocal of the dilution of complement which lyses 50 per cent of the EA). In this case, the 50 per cent end point is determined from the Von Krogh transformation. This empirically derived formula converts the S-shaped dose-response curve into a linear curve. Values of y/1 − y are calculated, in which y equals the percentage of red cells lysed in a test dilution. A graph is constructed in which the log of the relative volume of complement is plotted against the log of y/1 − y values. Usually, a straight line is obtained, and the titer is calculated by determining the relative volume of complement at which y/1 − y equals 1.0 (the point where 50 per cent lysis is obtained). That value is divided into the original serum dilution (1:60 for human serum) to calculate the concentration of serum complement which lyses 50 per cent of the cells. The reciprocal of this value is the complement titer. It

Table 37–7. PROTOCOL FOR TITRATION OF WHOLE COMPLEMENT AND SAMPLE DETERMINATIONS

	Test Tube							
	1	*2*	*3*	*4*	*5*	*CB*	*CBC*	*100%*
VBS (ml)	5.5	5.3	5.0	4.5	4.0	6.5	5.5	—
5 × 10^8/ml EA	1.0	1.0	1.0	1.0	1.0	1.0	—	1.0
Serum (1:60)	1.0	1.2	1.5	2.0	2.5	—	2.0	—
H_2O (ml)	—	—	—	—	—	—	—	6.5
				Incubate 1 Hour 37°C.				
Absorbance (O.D.) 412 nm	0.102	0.185	0.322	0.490	0.596	0.008	0.003	0.664
Absorbance (O.D.) Corr.	0.094	0.177	0.314	0.482	0.588	—	—	0.656
y/1 − y	0.167	0.370	0.918	2.77	8.65	—	—	—
Titer, CH_{50}	39.5	—	—	—	—	—	—	—

VBS = Veronal-buffered saline (see Table 37–5).
CB = Sheep erythrocytes with buffer alone.
CBC = Sheep erythrocytes plus complement.
y = Absorbance (corrected) of test sample/absorbance (corrected) of 100% lysis sample.

expresses the number of 50 per cent hemolytic units which are present in 1.0 ml of undiluted serum.

To measure most complement components individually, partially purified components are required. However, C4 is an exception because of the availability of C4-deficient guinea pig serum (C4D). This assay is based on the principle that the deficient serum supplies all other components in excess. The assay for C4 is greatly simplified. The deficient serum must be fresh or frozen fresh to prevent loss of complement activity.

The C4 assay is performed in 0.084 μ DVBS. C4D is diluted 1:75 and kept ice cold until used. A broad range of serum dilutions is prepared—1:1,000, 1:10,000, and several two-fold falling dilutions, starting at 1:50,000. EA are prepared as described and suspended to 1.5 × 10^8/ml. Generally, a 0.2 ml volume of the serum dilution is added to 0.2 ml of EA and 0.2 ml C4D. The mixture is incubated at 37°C. for one hour; 2.0 ml of EDTA is added, the tubes are centrifuged, and the supernatant is analyzed spectrophotometrically at 412 nm. Controls include EA plus C4D, EA plus buffer, and a 100 per cent lysis control. A standard serum should be included each time this assay is performed because several variables may affect the titer on a given day. This method and the procedure for calculating C4 titer are outlined in Table 37–8.

The assay for serum C4 is extremely efficient, yielding titers which are greater than titers obtained by the more complex standard procedure.

Standard procedures for measuring the hemolytic activity of each of the components of the classic pathway are outlined in Table 37–9. The following general methods apply to these assays:

1. Low ionic strength buffer (0.065 μ DVBS) is utilized.
2. The cellular intermediate is suspended to 1.5 × 10^8 cells/ml.
3. All serum and complement dilutions are prepared fresh and held at 0°C. to 4°C.
4. Reaction mixtures are frequently mixed to ensure adequate cell suspensions.
5. When individual components are required in excess, C1 is added at a concentration which yields

Table 37–8. PROTOCOL FOR TITRATION OF C4 BY C4D METHOD AND SAMPLE DETERMINATION

	Test Tube					
	1	*2*	*3*	*CB*	*C4D*	*100%*
EA (1.5 × 10^8/ml)	0.2	0.2	0.2	0.2	0.2	0.2
Serum, 0.2 ml starting with 1:100,000	1:1	1:2	1:4	—	—	—
C4D serum 1:75	0.2	0.2	0.2	—	0.2	—
0.084 μ DVBS	—	—	—	0.4	0.2	—
			Incubate 1 Hour 37° C.			
EDTA	2.0	2.0	2.0	2.0	2.0	—
H_2O (ml)	—	—	—	—	—	2.4
Absorbance (O.D.) 412 nm	0.847	0.559	0.330	0.011	0.024	1.087
Absorbance (O.D.) Corr.	0.823	0.535	0.306	—	—	1.076
Z	1.45	0.688	0.335	—	—	—
Titer	141,380	—	—	—	—	—

EA = Sheep erythrocytes with antibody.
CB = Sheep erythrocytes and buffer alone.
C4D = C4-deficient serum.
Z = Average number of sites damaged by complement per sheep erythrocyte.

5

Table 37–9. STANDARD HEMOLYTIC ASSAYS OF CLASSIC PATHWAY COMPONENTS

Component		Volume (ml)
C1	Test dilution	0.2
	EAC4	0.2
	1 hour 30°C.	
	C2	0.2
	10 min. 30°C.	
	CEDTA 1:25	2.0
	1 hour 37°C.	
C2	Test dilution	0.2
	EAC14	0.2
	30°C. t_{max}	
	CEDTA 1:25	2.0
	1 hour 37°C.	
C5	Test dilution	0.2
	EAC14	0.2
	C367 reagent	0.2
	C2	0.2
	30 min. 30°C.	
	C89 reagent	0.2
	1 hour 37°C.	
	EDTA	2.0
C7	Test dilution	0.2
	EAC14	0.2
	C356	0.2
	C2	0.2
	30 min. 30°C.	
	C89	0.2
	1 hour 37°C.	2.0
	EDTA	
C9	EAC14	0.2
	C2	0.2
	C3567	0.2
	30 min. 30°C.	
	Test dilution	0.2
	C8	0.2
	1 hour 37°C.	
	EDTA	2.0
C4	Test dilution	0.2
	EAC1	0.2
	20 min. 37°C.	
	C2	0.2
	10 min. 30°C.	
	CEDTA 1:25	2.0
	2 hours 37°C.	
C3	Test dilution	0.2
	EAC14	0.2
	C5,6,7 reagent*	0.2
	C2	0.2
	30 min. 30°C.	
	C8,9 reagent	0.2
	1 hour 37°C.	
	EDTA	2.0
C6	Test dilution	0.2
	EAC14	0.2
	C357	0.2
	C2	0.2
	30 min. 30°C.	
	C89	0.2
	1 hour 37°C.	
	EDTA	2.0
C8	EAC14	0.2
	C2	0.2
	C3567	0.2
	30 min. 30°C.	
	Test dilution	0.2
	C9	0.2
	1 hour 37°C.	
	EDTA	2.0

*If each of the components in the mixed reagent has a titer of 1000, 1.0 ml C5, 1.0 ml C6, and 1.0 ml C7 may be mixed and brought to a total volume of 10.0 ml. This reagent contains the recommended 100 sites/cell for each component.

from 500 to 1000 C1 sites/cell, and the remaining eight components are added at concentrations which yield 100 sites/cell. Often, the titers of commercial complement components are expressed as CH_{50} units/ml. The CH_{50} titer is the reciprocal of the dilution yielding 50 per cent lysis, at which point the Z value is approximately 0.70 site per cell (see below).

Immune hemolysis is the result of a complex series of reactions which occur on the cell surface. Photometric measurements show the proportion of cells lysed by this series of reactions. The principle of Poisson distribution is applied to relate the degree of hemolysis to the molecular events which occur on the cell surface. This approach is based on the assumption that the interaction of cell-bound antigen, antibody, and complement occurs in random fashion and that the amount of lysis is the sum of a large number of interactions in which limited quantities of the component being titrated interact with other components which are all in excess. It is well established that one lesion on the erythrocyte surface which has interacted with hemolytic antibody and all of the complement components can cause cell lysis. The Poisson distribution is used to relate the number of lysed cells (cells with one or more lesions) to the concentration of the antibody or complement reactant being titrated. The average number of damaged sites per red cell is expressed as Z. The equation relating this value to lysis is: $Z = -\ln(1 - y)$, where y is the percentage of lysed cells. To calculate the titer of the component being measured, Z values are plotted on the ordinate against serum concentration plotted on the abscissa on an arithmetic or a log-log graph. The titer is the reciprocal of the dilution of serum which corresponds to a Z value of 1.0 or one hit per cell.

Complement Levels by Antigenic Assay

For use in antigenic assays, the specimen should be refrigerated or frozen. Bacterial contamination may cause protein denaturation or fragmentation, while freezing and thawing do not usually have an adverse effect on antigenic levels. For certain complement assays, the specimen is diluted in saline to achieve the correct concentration range for accurate quantitation. When C3 is assayed and precise titrations are desired, using C3c standards, sterile sera should be incubated at 37°C. for several days prior to analysis.

Antigenic analysis of complement proteins makes use of one of several immune precipitin techniques. Single radial immunodiffusion (RID) is the most commonly employed method for specific quantitation of protein. Basically, one of two approaches is used: that of Mancini (1965), or that of Fahey (1965). In both methods, antigen is loaded into wells in a gel containing antibody and rings of precipitation are formed. In the Fahey method, the time at which results are read is critical because the antibodies in the gel matrix are not in excess and, therefore, diffusion end points are not reached. This can lead to inaccurate evaluations of antigenic complement. The technique of Mancini, considered to be both sensitive and accurate, employs the more simplified end point methodology with antibody excess in the gel. The Mancini method is used by most commercial firms in the preparation of immunodiffusion plates. These methods are discussed further in Chapter 38.

Radial immune diffusion kits are commercially available for several complement components, including C3, C4, and factor B. These kits consist of plates which contain a thin layer of 2 per cent agarose containing a monospecific antibody. Protein standard serum, a stabilized pool of normal human serum, is supplied, usually in prediluted solutions. Each standard solution contains a specific amount of the particular protein being measured for use in construction of the reference curve. A delivery device (a microliter syringe or calibrated pipetter), which can accurately measure and deliver lambda quantities of serum, is useful; and a calibrated magnifier, which is accurate to 0.1 mm, is needed.

COMPLEMENT FIXATION TESTS

A detailed consideration of this procedure will not be presented here, since a complete discussion of this topic is available (Kabat, 1961). Nevertheless, complement fixation reactions are of great importance in clinical diagnosis and will be mentioned briefly. The test procedure depends on the ability of fresh serum complement to interact with antigen-antibody complexes. In the first step of the reaction, the complement is incubated with the materials which may contain antigen and antibody. If antigen-antibody complexes are formed, they will interact with complement in much the same way as a complex of antibody and a cell surface antigen interact with complement. The complement is activated, components are fragmented, and the complement is "used up" or "fixed." In the second stage, sensitized sheep cells (EA) are added, and the mixture is incubated at 37°C. for one hour. If the serum contains antibody to the antigen used, complement is fixed and is, therefore, no longer available to lyse the EA. Thus, the absence of lysis indicates a positive reaction, while complete lysis indicates a negative result.

There are two general approaches to complement fixation tests. In the first one, concentrated, fresh serum is the complement source; and the amount of complement fixed is determined by titration of the serum before and after fixation. In the second one, a dilution of serum is used that will provide either just enough complement for lysis of the EA or slightly more than enough (3 to 5 CH_{50} Units). In this case, the sensitized cells are added without further dilution. Incubation of the test materials with complement can take place at 37°C. for one hour or overnight in the cold. In general, cold incubation leads to higher titers.

Complement can be inactivated by a number of agents other than antigen-antibody complexes, such as bacteria, endotoxins, yeast, and aggregated gamma globulins. Therefore, controls are necessary to demonstrate that neither the serum nor the antigen alone will fix complement. The complement fixation test is particularly valuable in that it does not require that antigens or antibodies be present in highly purified form, both soluble and particulate antigens may be utilized, and antigens as well as antibodies may be measured.

Agnello, V.: Complement deficiency states. Medicine, *57*:1, 1978.

Atkinson, J. P., and Frank, M. M.: Complement. *In* Parker, C. W. (ed.): Clinical Immunology. Philadelphia, W. B. Saunders Co., 1980, pp. 219–271.

Berger, M., Gaither, T. A., and Frank, M. M.: Complement receptors. Clin. Immunol. Rev., *1*:471, 1982.

Davis, C. A., and Forristal, J.: Partial properdin deficiency. J. Lab. Clin. Med., *96*:633, 1980.

Fahey, J. L., and McKelvey, E. M.: Quantitative determination of serum immunoglobulins in antibody agar plates. Immunology, *94*:84, 1965.

Frank, M. M.: Complement. *In* Current Concepts. Scope Publication, 1975, pp. 1–48.

Gaither, T. A., and Frank, M. M.: Studies of complement-mediated membrane damage. The influence of erythrocyte storage on susceptibility to cytolysis. J. Immunol., *110*:482–489, 1973.

Hunder, G. G., McDuffie, F. C., and Mullen, B. J.: Activation of C3 and factor B in synovial fluids. J. Lab. Clin. Med., *89*:160, 1977.

Hunsicker, L. G., and Mayes, E. R.: Preservation of antibody and complement bearing sheep erythrocytes (EA and EACH) by glycerol freezing. Fed. Proc., *34*:955, 1975.

Kabat, E. A., and Mayer, M. M.: Experimental Immunochemistry. 2nd ed. Springfield, Ill., Charles C Thomas, Publisher, 1961.

Mancini, G., Carbonara, A. O., and Hermans, J. T.: Immunochemical quantitation of antigens by single radial immunodiffusion. Int. J. Immunochem., *2*:235, 1965.

Michael, A., and McLean, R.: Evidence for activation of the alternate pathway in glomerulonephritis. Adv. Nephrol. *4*:49, 1974.

Peterson, B. H., Lee, T. J., Snyderman, R., and Brooks, G. F.: *Neisseria gonorrhoeae* bacteremia associated with C6, C7 or C8 deficiency. Ann. Intern. Med., *90*:917, 1979.

Rapp, H. J., and Borsos, T.: Molecular Basis of Complement Action. New York, Meredith Corporation, 1970.

Rowe, A. W., and Allen, F. H., Jr.: Freezing of blood droplets in liquid nitrogen for use in blood group studies. Transfusion, *5*:379, 1965.

Tappeiner, G.: Disease states in genetic complement deficiencies. Int. J. Dermatol., *21*:175, 1982.

Thompson, R. A., and Winterborn, M. H.: Hypocomplementaemia due to a genetic deficiency of β1H globulin. Clin. Exp. Immunol., *46*:110, 1981.

Zubler, R. H., and Lambert, P. H.: The ^{125}I-Cq binding test for the detection of soluble immune complexes. *In* Bloom, B. R., and David, J. R. (eds.): In Vitro Methods in Cell-Mediated and Tumor Immunity. New York, Academic Press, 1976, pp. 565–572.

38

ANTIBODY AS REAGENT

ROBERT M. NAKAMURA, M.D., and ERNEST S. TUCKER, III, M.D.

5

GENERAL NATURE AND CHARACTERISTICS OF ANTIBODIES

Nature of Antibodies

All antibodies are globulins that are made up of heavy and light polypeptide chains. They are distinct from other globulins by their capability of complexing with antigenic determinants of complementary combining sites. The immunologic specificity of the antibody refers to its ability to combine with substances bearing a unique physicochemical feature, the corresponding antigenic determinant.

Certain generalizations can be made about antibodies:

1. They are produced in response to antigenic stimulation.

2. There are five classes (isotypes) of immunoglob-

ulins. IgG immunoglobulins are further divided into four subgroups and the IgA and IgM into two subgroups. All known antibody molecules have either kappa or lambda light chains.

3. Antibodies are heterogeneous in structure, in affinity with corresponding antigenic sites, and in their function *in vivo* and *in vitro.*

4. All antibodies have the capacity to bind with their respective antigens.

Antibodies may be classified according to their origin, their host specificity, or the characteristics of the immunologic reactions in which they are involved. Most antibodies are found free and circulating in plasma, but some specific immunoglobulins such as IgE occur as cell-associated or cytophilic antibodies which after being synthesized become associated with other cells through the Fc part of the molecule.

The term *natural antibody* is customarily applied to isohemagglutinins which are hereditary and may reflect bacterial antibodies and which sometimes occur in low concentrations in human and animal sera. The term natural antibodies probably should be limited to those immunoglobulins which, like the isohemagglutinins, are inherited and appear in the serum at certain times in the life of the individual.

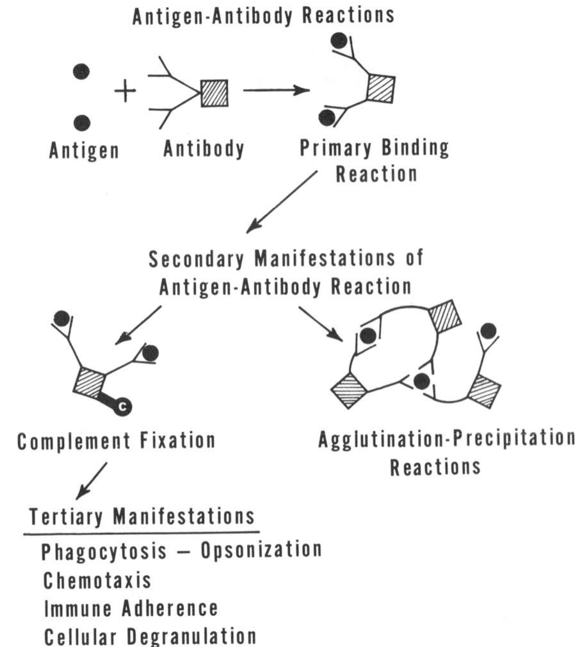

Figure 38–1. Types of immunologic reaction.

Immunologic Reaction

(Weir, 1973)

The binding reaction between antigen and antibody may be represented by the following equation:

$$Ag + Ab \underset{Kd}{\overset{Ka}{\rightleftharpoons}} Ag \cdot Ab$$

Ag represents one of the often multiple antigenic sites on a given molecule, and Ab represents one or two or more antigenic binding sites on a given antibody molecule. Similar to a chemical reaction, there is an association and dissociation constant and the summated effect of the two yields an equilibrium constant. The total concentration of antibody in the sample is the sum of the free and bound antibody sites, and the concentration of the free antibody sites under any given circumstance is governed by the law of mass action, according to the following equation:

$$K = \frac{Ag \cdot Ab}{(Ag) \times (Ab)}$$

The antibody populations with high avidity or affinity are those with high K values, and the antibody populations with relatively low avidity have low K values (Hudson, 1976).

Types of Immunologic Reaction

Antigen-antibody tests may be classified according to whether the test is dependent upon a primary interaction between the antibody and antigen or is based on a secondary manifestation such as precipitation, flocculation, agglutination, complement fixation, etc., following the primary interaction. The tertiary manifestations of antigen-antibody reactions are those that occur as biologic reactions which follow primary and secondary levels of antigen-antibody reactions. The tertiary reactions include many of the biologic effects of complement activation, such as opsonization, phagocytosis, chemotaxis, etc. (Fig. 38–1).

The primary interaction between antigen and antibody is the first step in a series of reactions and biochemical processes which may or may not proceed to a secondary or tertiary reaction discussed below. The primary interaction is the specific recognition and combination of an antigenic determinant with the binding site of its corresponding antibody.

Quantitative tests dependent entirely on primary interaction between antigen and antibody include immunofluorescence, radioimmunoassay, and immunoenzymatic assays. The *primary tests* are more sensitive than the secondary or tertiary tests and are not dependent upon variables which control secondary or tertiary reactions. The primary tests require the following: (1) Either a purified antigen or an antibody preparation for the reaction. (2) A technique to quantitate the antigen or antibody with use of a radioisotope, enzyme, or fluorescent label. (3) A method to separate the antigen-antibody reaction complex from free antigen or antibody in solution. *Secondary manifestations* of antigen-antibody reactions include precipitation in solution or in gel, direct agglutination or agglutination of erythrocyte or other particles coated with antigen or antibody, and complement fixation. *Tertiary manifestations* of antigen-antibody reactions include phagocytosis-opsonization, chemotaxis, immune adherence, and cellular degranulation.

Antibody molecules are capable of recognizing, binding, and complexing with specific antigen. In the case of reaction of specific IgG with a hapten antigen, the complexes are usually $(\text{hapten})_2 - (\text{antibody})_1$. In the case of multivalent protein antigens, complexes of varying size may be formed proportional to the concentrations of the antibody and antigen. Immune complexes of varying size have different degrees of solubility; their ability to localize along vascular basement membrane and fix complement *in vivo* is responsible for a wide range of immune complex–mediated hypersensitivity diseases. Thus, a full understanding of antigen-antibody interaction involves a knowledge first of type, specificity, affinity, and concentration of antibody, then of antigen concentration, and finally of biologic activity.

Sensitivity and Specificity of Immunologic Tests

A wide spectrum of different immunologic methods is currently available. Antibodies differ widely in their specificity and sensitivity. Primary antigen-antibody binding assays can be sensitive in the nanogram to picogram per milliliter range. Variation in standardization and specificity of immunologic methods is a common problem. Antibodies which have a high affinity and are potent may give unwanted cross-reactions while weak antisera may be specific but not sensitive. Cross-reaction refers to immunologic reactivity of two or more antigens with the same antiserum or to the reactivity of two or more sera with one antigen.

Varying levels of sensitivity are well illustrated by the numerous tests available for the detection of hepatitis B associated surface antigen (HBsAg). The agar gel diffusion test may be considered to be a precipitin test with the sensitivity value of one. The cross electrophoretic or electroimmunodiffusion method increases the sensitivity 10 times, whereas the radioimmunoassay procedure for HBsAg will increase the sensitivity 10,000 times.

The sensitivity of the agar gel test for alpha-1-fetoprotein is in the range of 3000 ng/ml. Most of the positive determinations are significant and may be diagnostic for hepatocellular carcinoma or embryonal cell carcinoma. A current radioimmunoassay procedure, however, has a sensitivity to 1 ng/ml but will reveal many more "positive" specimens. The former method will have more false negatives, the latter more false positives.

Relative sensitivity of immunologic tests involving secondary manifestations of antigen-antibody reactions is listed in Table 38–1.

Table 38–1. RELATIVE SENSITIVITY OF IMMUNOLOGIC TESTS INVOLVING SECONDARY MANIFESTATIONS OF ANTIGEN-ANTIBODY REACTIONS*

Immunologic Test	Minimum of Antibody N (μg) Detectable or Needed for Reaction
Precipitation	
Tube precipitation	0.1
Immunodiffusion	0.1–0.3
Agglutination	
Qualitative	0.05
Quantitative	0.02–0.1
Hemagglutination, passive	0.001
Hemagglutination-inhibition	0.001
Coombs' reaction	0.01
Complement fixation	0.05

*Modified from Kwapinski, J. B. G.: Methodology of Immunochemical and Immunological Research. New York, Wiley-Interscience, Inc., 1972.

PRECIPITIN REACTIONS

The precipitin reaction occupies an important position in immunology and occurs when serum from a sensitized animal is mixed with the immunizing antigen. The precipitate that forms represents large complexes of antigen and antibody that have combined to form an insoluble lattice. The first observation of the reaction was reported by Kraus in 1897 when he observed a precipitin reaction on mixing antisera to typhoid bacillus with cell-free filtrates of cultures from typhoid organisms. Many investigators since then have used the precipitin reaction to identify and quantitate immunologic reactions. Some major investigators who have contributed to our knowledge of the precipitin reaction include such prominent individuals as Ehrlich, Heidelberger, Kendall, Pauling, Boyd, Nuttal, and Landsteiner.

The modern refinements of the quantitative precipitin technique as an analytical tool for measurement of antibody were extensively developed by Heidelberger and Kendall. Much of their work, which was carried out during the early 1930s, stands today as a major contribution to the science of immunology and immunochemistry.

Varied applications of the precipitin reaction will be discussed as an important tool in immunochemistry for the identification and quantification of a wide range of antigenic substances. Each of the modes of application of the precipitin technique has a differing advantage of sensitivity, specificity, and simplicity. Immunoprecipitin techniques will no doubt enjoy a continually broadening application in the clinical laboratory. The disadvantages of these techniques are relatively minor compared with other more cumbersome, less direct, and complex techniques for macromolecular analysis. A diversity of specific antisera is critical in the continued growth and application of these techniques. Currently such antisera are available from only a limited number of commercial or research sources and for only a limited number of antigenic substances. Another major problem is availability of stable and well-defined standards. Also lacking are control sera of sufficient stability to compare favorably with those used in other areas of clinical laboratory analysis.

The limitation of the sensitivity of these assays is a

major consideration. Even under the best conditions of enhanced sensitivity afforded by the newer light-scattering techniques, the accuracy and sensitivity of immunoprecipitin assays are not satisfactory below a range of 0.1 to 0.5 mg/dl. This limits certain applications of immunoprecipitin assays, but the techniques appear quite sufficient for quantification of many major serum proteins and a wide range of other biologic molecules of importance in clinical medicine. Some important trace proteins, polypeptides, and endocrine factors cannot be accurately measured by the current methods of immunoprecipitin assay. Their measurement by the more sensitive techniques of radioimmunoassay, enzyme-linked immunoassay, and immunofluorescence will be discussed in other sections of this text.

Principles

The quantitative precipitin reaction, as it is known today, provides a systematic approach to determining the amount of either antibody or antigen by defining the optimal proportions of each reactant in the formation of the immune precipitate. The approach usually followed is to prepare a series of test tubes, each containing a fixed amount of antisera; to each tube in sequence an increasing quantity of the antigen used for immunization is added. Following addition of antigen, an appropriate period of time is allowed for the reaction to occur and precipitate to form. The amount of nitrogen or protein in the precipitate is then determined by measuring the nitrogen, often by the micro Kjeldahl method. In appropriate proportions, all the antigen is precipitated; therefore, the nitrogen of the precipitate due to antigen can be subtracted and a direct determination of antibody nitrogen in the immune sera can be made. As will be noted subsequently, the precipitin reaction forms the basis for many quantitative and qualitative immunochemical techniques now used in the clinical laboratory (Kabat, 1961).

Investigation of factors affecting the precipitin reaction was extensively pursued by Heidelberger and Kendall, who found that, in addition to the relative proportions of reactants, conditions of temperature, pH, ionic strength of the medium, and certain characteristics of antibody known as avidity and affinity are important in formation of the immune precipitate. A graphic illustration of the pattern of precipitin formation when there is sequential addition of increasing quantities of antigen to a fixed quantity of antiserum is shown in Figure 38–2. It can be noted that there occurs a point of maximum, or optimal, precipitation designated as the *point of equivalence.* Continued addition of antigen following the equivalence point results in a solubilizing effect on the precipitate. This is thought to occur because of the formation of small complexes with the excess antigen. These small complexes do not lead to the formation of the lattice structure. In such conditions, it can be seen that the small soluble complexes may have a ratio of two molecules of antigen to a single molecule

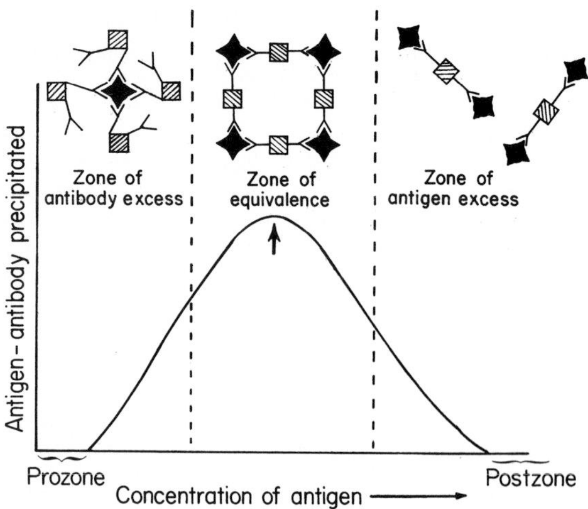

THE QUANTITATIVE PRECIPITIN CURVE

Plot obtained by adding increasing amounts of a soluble antigen to fixed volumes of monospecific antiserum. Maximum precipitate (↑) is formed at optimal ratio of antigen to antibody called the equivalence point.

Figure 38–2.

of antibody. Indeed, antigen excess may sometimes be adjusted to a point where the precipitate completely redissolves, leaving no visible evidence of an antigen/antibody reaction. This zone of solubility in antigen excess is referred to as the *post-zone* phenomenon. By contrast, inspection of Figure 38–2 also shows that early in the course of adding antigen a condition of marked antibody excess exists and there is also a lack of precipitate formation. This is presumably due to formation of highly soluble complexes with abundant antibody so that antibody molecules may exceed six to seven for each molecule of antigen. This area of the precipitin curve in antibody excess where no precipitate is observed is known as the *pro-zone.*

Inspection of the contour of the precipitin curve in Figure 38–2 also reveals that the equivalence point, or point of maximum precipitate, generally occurs over a narrow range of antibody/antigen ratios. The ratios commonly found are in the range of three or four molecules of antibody to one molecule of antigen. It should be emphasized that this relatively narrow zone of equivalence occurs largely with those antigens which are easily soluble and which contain a minimum number of antigen reactive sites in each molecule. By contrast, the precipitin curves for large poorly soluble or particulate antigens exhibit a very broad zone of precipitate and, in such instances, the precipitin reaction does not offer the degree of quantitation that can be obtained with a smaller soluble antigen (Kabat, 1961).

Another circumstance which alters the narrow zone of equivalence in the precipitin curve occurs when a mixture of antibodies is present in the immune serum, and these react with the differing antigens in the immunizing material. Such a multicomponent reactant system will also give a broader zone of equivalence than the singular reactive systems. The zone of equivalence in multicomponent reactions tends to be somewhat rounded in contrast to a sharply narrow zone with the single reactant. The explanation for this is that in the multicomponent system each subgroup of antigen/antibody reactants forms a precipitate with varied ratios of antigen to antibody. Consequently, some begin to precipitate early on addition of the antigen mixture, while increasing additions of antigen precipitate with other antibody populations. As will be noted later, the individual antigen/antibody reactants in such a multicomponent precipitin system can best be separated by using a semisolid supporting medium such as agar gel rather than a liquid medium for the reaction (see Fig. 38–5).

The chemical structure of the precipitate is important in further understanding the nature of the precipitin reaction. As shown in Figure 38–3, the immune complexes formed throughout the range of any precipitin reaction will vary in the composition ratio of antibody to antigen. As discussed in Chapter 36, we know much about the structure and combining sites of various classes of antibody in vertebrates and other animals. These data clearly reveal that each molecule of antibody has a minimum of at least two combining sites for antigen. Classically, two combining sites are described for immunoglobulins of the classes IgG, IgA, and IgE. IgM is known to be composed of multiple subunits which resemble the 7S structure of IgG and generally will possess from 5 to 6 combining sites for antigens. IgA may also occur in the form of a dimer or trimer and exhibit additional combining sites. Antigens, on the other hand, usually exhibit extensive variation in chemical structure and reactive antigenic sites. Knowledge of and characterization of all the possible ranges of antigen configurations are beyond our current scope. However, it can be assumed that, since antigen as well as antibody link together to form a three-dimensional lattice structure, antigen must provide the key link in the lattice. Based on this assumption, antigen sites would of necessity occur in clusters of at least 4 to 5 per molecule in order to link up the bivalent combining antibody in a lattice configuration. As the foregoing discussion indicates, the point of equivalence is taken to represent the maximum linkages between antigen and antibody, and this configuration gives rise to the greatest amount of precipitate. The drawings in Figure 38–3 diagrammatically show the variability in antigen/antibody structure which is presumed to exist at different parts of the precipitin curve. At the point of equivalence the regular lattice structure as shown is expected, while in the conditions of high solubility of an immune complex in antigen excess an increase of antigen could give a ratio of antibody to antigen as low as 0.5. In those circumstances in which the antigen possesses only a single reactive site, linkage and lattice formation would not occur and a precipitate would not be formed (Kabat, 1961).

Factors and Conditions Affecting the Precipitin Reaction

Brief mention has been made of the conditions of temperature, pH, and antibody reactivity which affect the

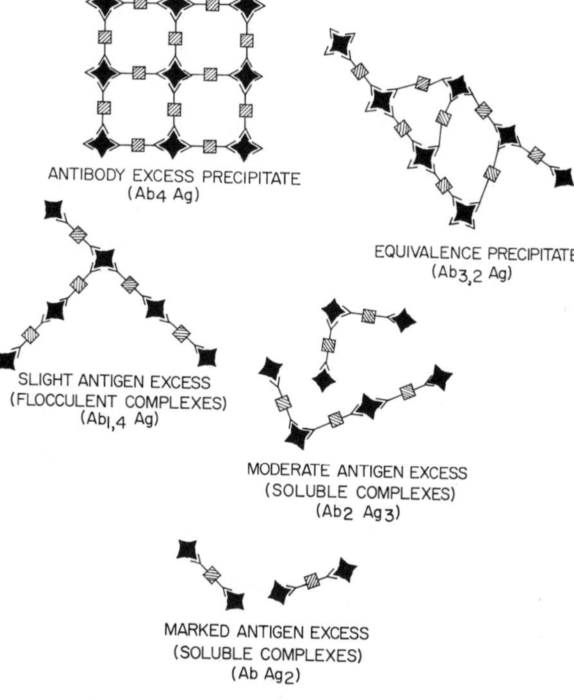

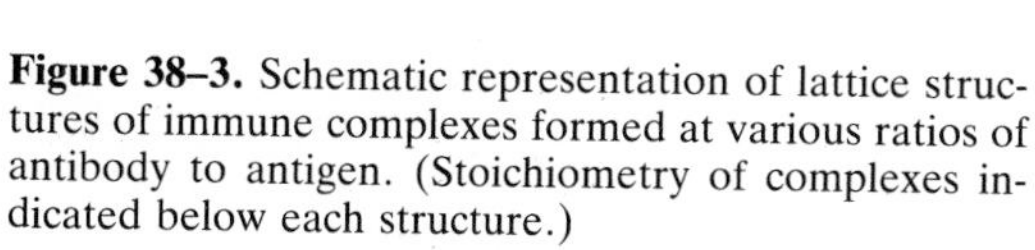

Figure 38–3. Schematic representation of lattice structures of immune complexes formed at various ratios of antibody to antigen. (Stoichiometry of complexes indicated below each structure.)

precipitin reaction. In some reactant conditions the precipitate may form equally well at 0°C. and at 37°C. However, many antisera will be found which exhibit higher specific reactivity at some temperatures than at others. Commonly the conditions of wide ranges of temperature are met by initially allowing incubation to proceed at 37°C. for a few hours, then followed by a period of incubation at 0 to 4°C. The relative amount of precipitate which forms under the different conditions is then determined. pH appears to have an effect in that immune complexes appear to form most abundantly in the neutral range between 6 and 7.5, while higher and lower pH extremes may dissociate or prevent the formation of the complexes (Kabat, 1961).

Salt concentration of the reactant medium, usually as sodium chloride concentration, exhibits a substantial effect on immune complex formation in the precipitin reaction. In general, high quantities of salt appear to increase solubility of the complexes and cause a shift in equilibrium between the reactants so that dissociation occurs in those complexes which have formed, and formation of new complexes is prevented. The increase in salt concentration above 0.15 M brings a striking decrease in the amount of precipitate. However, it has been observed that antisera from birds and other avian species may exhibit increased precipitin reaction in the presence of higher salt concentrations.

Certain characteristics of the antibody itself will have an effect on the precipitin reaction. The specificity and affinity of the antibody for antigenic sites affect the velocity of the reaction. The specificity of an antibody is measured by determining affinity of the antisera for a group of closely related antigens. Usually, when there is high specificity and strong affinity for the antigens, precipitin reaction will readily result with both the immunizing and closely related antigens. In contrast, antibodies with low affinity, even if highly specific, tend to react only with the immunizing antigen and not to any extent with related antigens and to give weak precipitin reactions.

The avidity of the antibody is also important in the precipitin reaction. This characteristic of the antibody determines the degree of stability of the antigen/antibody complex at the antigen binding site. The tendency of complexes to dissociate and dissolve decreases substantially as the avidity of the antiserum increases. Avidity also affects the amount of antibody in the precipitate as well as the contour of the zone of equivalence. With increased avidity there is an increase in the combining stability of the antibody with the antigen.

In addition to the known characteristics of antibodies there are other less well understood factors of molecular structure which affect the ability of antibody to form precipitates that remain stable combined with antigen. Other factors affect the rate of formation and solubilization of the complexes. In general, as was indicated earlier, the precipitates will dissolve or become solubilized with increasing additions of antigen or in the presence of excess antibody. However, instances have been observed in which certain antigen/antibody precipitates do not exhibit this easily reversible solubility. They remain as precipitates for long periods and often appear to undergo reversible solubility at a very slow rate or not at all. Such a phenomenon was described by Danysz in 1902 and the term Danysz phenomenon is now used to designate insolubility of some immune precipitates. In contrast to the poorly soluble precipitates, there also are populations of antibody which are so poorly reactive with antigen that they are non-precipitating. Such non-precipitating antibody can only be detected by special techniques. One technique is known as co-precipitation, in which known precipitating reactants are added to a suspension of non-precipitating antibody to produce a carrier, or co-precipitation, effect on the otherwise non-reacting antibody (Kabat, 1961; Garvey, 1977).

Clinical Laboratory Applications of the Precipitin Reaction

The sensitivity, simplicity, and specificity of the precipitin reaction have provided the basis for its importance as an analytical technique in the clinical laboratory. Adaptation of the precipitin reaction to semisolid media such as agar gel and agarose greatly simplified the routine applications of the technique. Investigators such as Preer, Oakley-Fulthorpe, and Oudin refined the use of precipitin reaction in gel diffusion systems for the quantitative estimate of antibody content of immune sera. These investigators emphasized the quantitative significance of the thickness of the precipitin line formed in gels at the point of equivalence (Fig. 38–4). In the early 1960's, investigators such as Mancini, Carbonara, and Heremans, as well as Fahey and McKelvey, adapted the immunoprecipitin reaction in gels to a highly sensitive and specifically quantitative technique of single radial immunodiffusion which is now in common use. This technique will be covered in detail later in this section. Grabar and Williams combined the techniques of electrophoresis and immunodiffusion in gel media to introduce yet another dimension to identification and quantification of complex macromolecules. All of these techniques are now used in determinations of specific antibody concentration and in the determination of the identity and concentration of a wide variety of antigenic macromolecules. These antigens include a wide range of serum proteins and tissue proteins, as well as complex polysaccharides, nucleic acids, and a variety of synthetic chemical compounds (Crowle, 1961; Mancini, 1965; Fahey, 1965).

In the following sections there will be discussion of particular applications of the immunodiffusion reaction in gels. Many of these applications relate to specific design of the gel chamber and the points of application of antigen and antibody.

Single immunodiffusion involves incorporation of antibody into the agar gel at a temperature sufficiently low to prevent denaturation and yet allow subsequent filling of an appropriate chamber—either small test tubes, Petri dishes, or glass slide surfaces (Fig. 38–5). Direct application of the test antigen is then made either as an overlay in the test tube or by diffusion

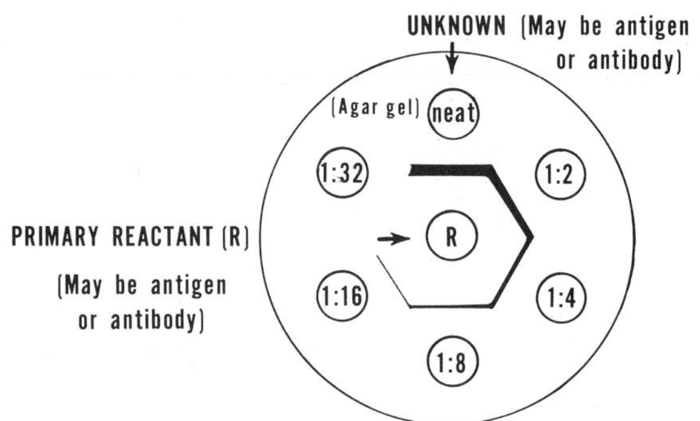

Figure 38–4. Estimate of antigen (or antibody) content using serial dilution of unknown against primary reactant. (Double immunodiffusion Ouchterlony technique.) Note decreasing thickness of precipitin line which disappears at fivefold dilution of unknown.

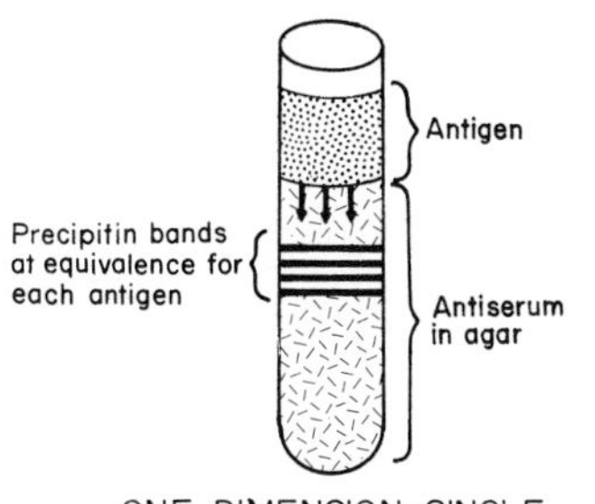

ONE DIMENSION-SINGLE IMMUNODIFFUSION (OUDIN TUBE) (Antigen diffuses from overlay into agar containing antiserum where precipitin lines form at the equivalence points for each separate antigen)

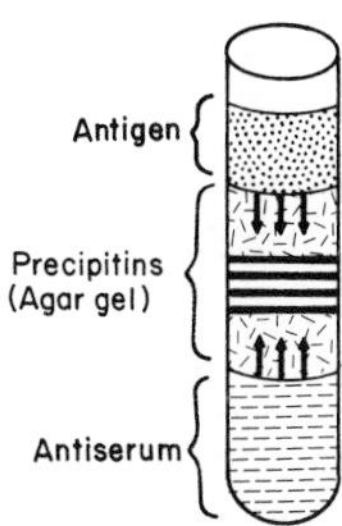

ONE DIMENSION-DOUBLE IMMUNODIFFUSION (Antigen diffuses into agar from overlay while antibody diffuses from below. Precipitin bands form at equivalence points for each separate antigen)

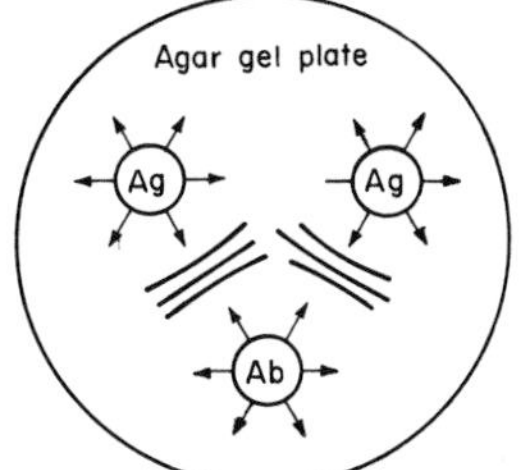

TWO DIMENSION-DOUBLE IMMUNODIFFUSION OUCHTERLONY (Antigens and antibody diffuse radially into agar. Precipitin bands form at equivalence points for each separate antigen. Location and arrangement of wells in agar can vary to compare a variety of antigens and antibodies)

Figure 38–5. Single and double immunodiffusion reactions: Use of immunoprecipitin reactions in gel to determine presence of multiple reactants in antigen and antibody preparations.

from a well punched in the agar plates. After a period of time to allow for diffusion and equilibrium, there occurs formation of precipitin bands in the agar. Visual observation by inspection confirms the presence of a precipitin line in the agar. This line is formed at the point of optimum antigen/antibody ratio, which is the same as the equivalence point earlier described in the precipitin reaction. The distance of the precipitin line from the point of application of antigen has been shown to be directly proportional to the concentration of antigen when using a defined quantity of antiserum in the agar. By a graphic comparison with preparations of antigen standards, the quantity of the unknown antigen can be determined. The principle of the technique is that antigen diffuses through the agar-containing antibody until the point of equivalence is reached and a precipitin line forms (Williams, 1970).

Double immunodiffusion incorporates an agar gel to act as a supporting medium which separates the antigen and antibody (Figs. 38–5 and 38–6). The type of chamber selected for the study can be a test tube, a Petri dish, or a glass slide containing agar. The antigen and antibody are applied at separate points by punching wells in the agar or placing antibody at the base of the test tube separating it from the antigen by a layer of agar gel. After diffusion of the reactants into the agar over a suitable period, usually 18 to 48 hours, the reactants will contact at the interface of diffusion, and at the equivalence point there will be formation of a precipitin line. This method can be used in a semi-quantitative way by inspecting the thickness of the precipitin line and determining the distance of migration from the reactant wells. Comparison is made with a standard antigen of known concentration which has reacted in a companion set-up.

The double immunodiffusion reaction also affords

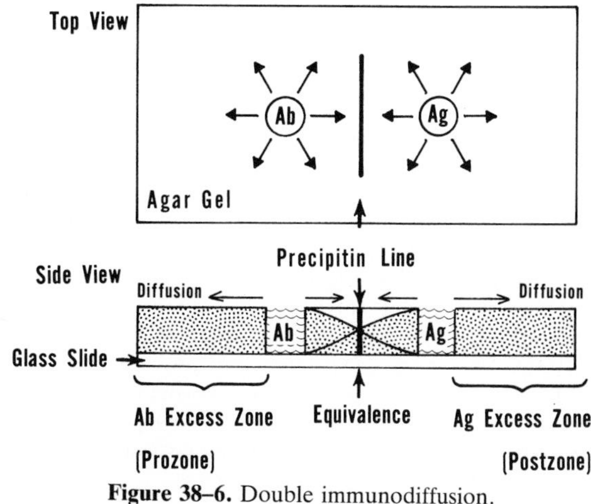

Figure 38–6. Double immunodiffusion.

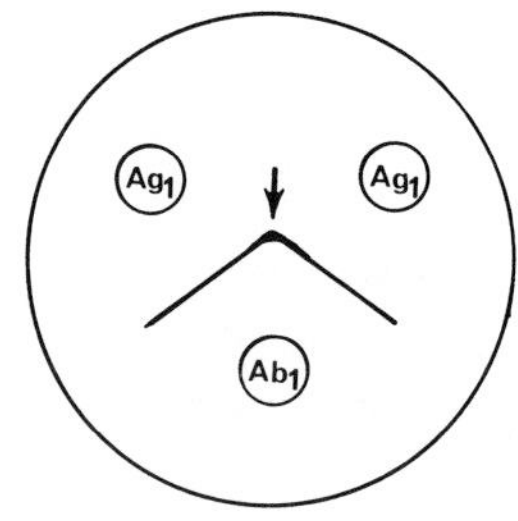

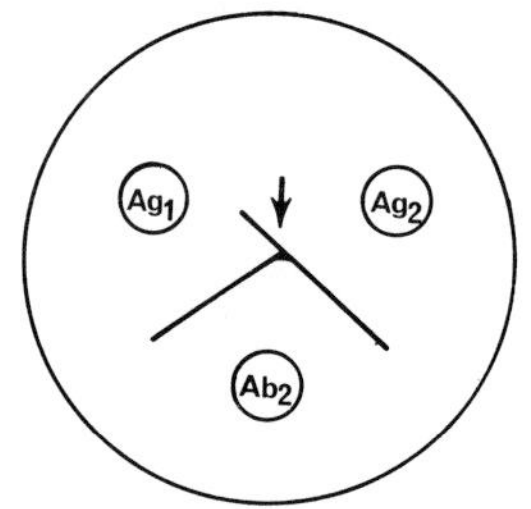

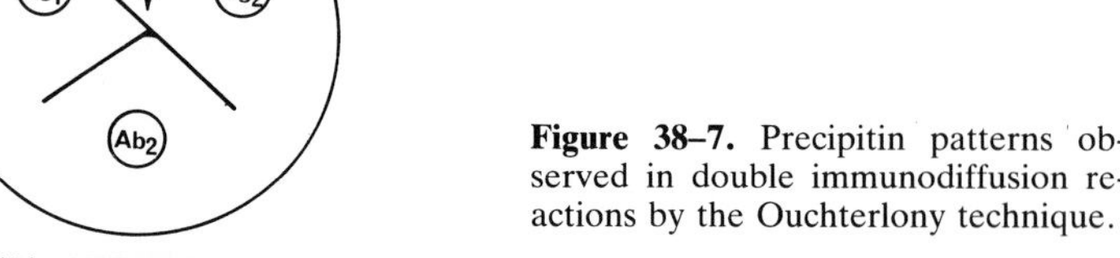

Figure 38–7. Precipitin patterns observed in double immunodiffusion reactions by the Ouchterlony technique.

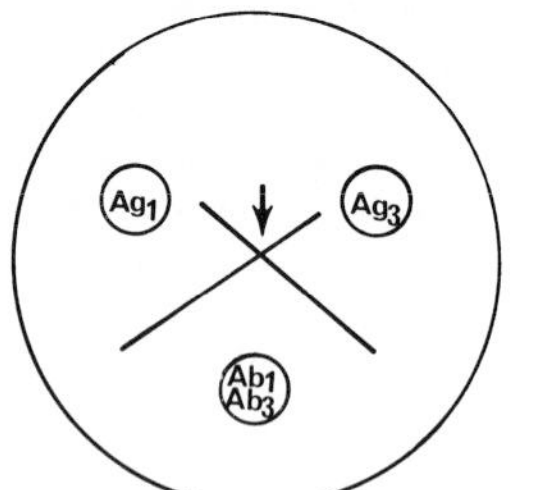

a rapid and simple method of determining relative concentrations of antigen and antibody in different preparations. As shown in Figure 38–6, the diffusion of antigen and antibody from application sites in the wells leads to formation of a precipitin line at some point between the two wells. The precipitin line forms at the point of equivalence. In those situations in which the line forms equidistant from antigen and antibody wells, this finding is direct evidence that the amount of antibody and antigen in each preparation is balanced at the optimal ratio. When a precipitin band forms close to the antigen well, this indicates an excess of antibody over that of antigen. By contrast, when the precipitin band develops near the antibody well, excess antigen is indicated. In some instances a precipitin band may not form. In such a case, the cause could be either antibody excess (pro-zone phenomenon) or antigen excess (post-zone phenomenon). In such instances, alternate serial dilution of each one of the reactants with repeat of the assay will eventually give precipitin formation. The dilutions required and position of the precipitin line reveal the presence of antigen or antibody excess (Garvey, 1977).

Double immunodiffusion in two dimensions is a method described by Ouchterlony which represents a variation of the double immunodiffusion technique. This procedure is usually carried out in a gel medium in a Petri dish or on a glass slide and it is used for comparing different antigens or different antibodies. Figure 38–7 illustrates the appearance of precipitin patterns that may be encountered in this analysis. Molecules that share an identical antigenic structure exhibit a pattern of complete coalescence of the precipitin lines, while those with partial antigenic differences exhibit a spur pattern. Those of complete antigenic difference show crossing of the precipitin bands (Williams, 1970; Garvey, 1977).

The *electroimmunodiffusion reaction* (counter immunoelectrophoresis) is a variation of the double immunodiffusion reaction created by augmenting the diffusion of the reactants in agar gel by use of an electric current. The schematic for this technique is illustrated in Figure 38–8 and is similar to that followed in the usual double immunodiffusion reaction. Antibody is placed in the well favoring its migration in the direction of the cathode, while antigens that tend to be more negatively charged are placed in the well favoring migration to the anode. The electrophoretic

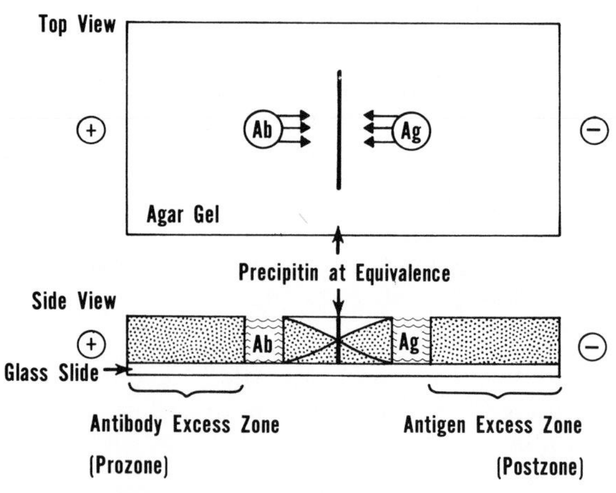

Figure 38–8. Electroimmunodiffusion.

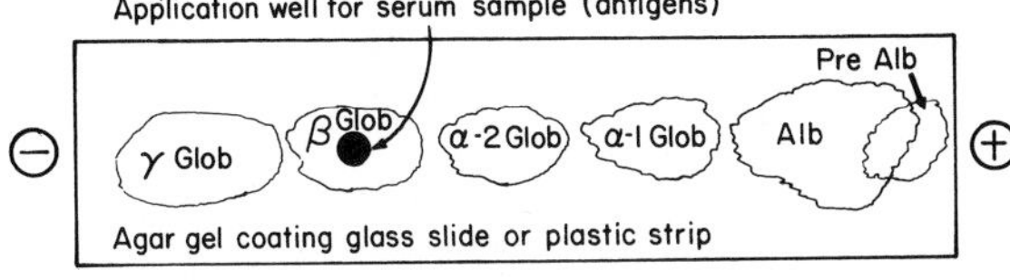

Step I: Separation of serum protein fractions by electrophoresis in agar gel

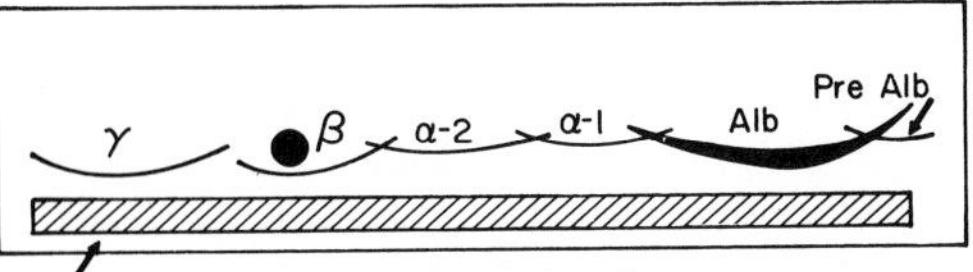

Step 2: Precipitin lines form following two dimensional immunodiffusion reaction in agar after application of specific antiserum in trough. (Incubate in moist chamber overnight)

Figure 38–9. Steps involved in precipitin analysis by the technique of immunoelectrophoresis.

effect enhances mobility of the reactants and speeds up their movement toward each other. A precipitin line which occurs at a point of equivalence thus requires a much shorter time for development owing to the augmentation by electrophoresis. The size and position of the precipitin band provides the same type of information regarding equivalence or antigen/antibody excess as in the simple double immunodiffusion system (Ritzmann, 1975).

Immunoelectrophoresis couples electrophoretic separation with the two-dimensional immunodiffusion reaction and is now used extensively for specific identification and semiquantitative estimation of a wide range of antigens. The steps of the technique are outlined diagrammatically in Figure 38–9. The first step involves application of a macromolecular sample such as human serum for electrophoresis in agar gel on a plastic or glass support. On completion of the electrophoresis, a trough is prepared along one margin of the slide and specific antiserum is applied in the trough. Diffusion is then allowed to proceed. In the diagram of Step 2 in Figure 38–9 there is shown a representative pattern of precipitin lines which form with human serum using a multispecific antiserum to human serum proteins. Notice that the relative thickness of individual bands is proportional to their relative concentrations. Their respective positions in the electrophoretic migration also aid in their identity. By using this method homogeneous populations of macromolecules such as those which occur in monoclonal gammopathies of multiple myeloma or Waldenström's macroglobulinemia exhibit narrow localized areas of thickening of the precipitin bands. Indeed, this approach is the definitive method for identifying such monoclonal immunoglobulins. By using monospecific antisera to different components of immunoglobulins, a differential immunoelectrophoretic study of monoclonal proteins can give a definite identification as to light and heavy chain composition. This technique also finds wide application in other areas of immunologic investigation where separation and identification of different macromolecules are required. It is also quite useful in the study of cleavage or proteolytic breakdown of macromolecules such as those of the serum complement and properdin systems (Rose, 1973; Ritzmann, 1975).

Quantitative Techniques Utilizing Immunoprecipitin Reactions in Gels

Brief mention has already been made of using precipitin reactions in gel to quantify both antigens and antibody. The *radial immunodiffusion* (RID) technique has proved to be a most useful method for immunoglobulin and serum protein quantitation in the clinical laboratory during the past few years. The essential elements of the technique are diagrammed in Figure 38–10. This illustration shows that the RID technique indeed has advantages of operational simplicity as well as sensitivity and specificity. The approach basically represents a variation of the single immunodiffusion technique where antibody has been incorporated into the agar which is poured into a plate or onto a glass slide. Wells are then cut in the agar and test material is placed in the wells. Antigen standards of known amount are placed in some wells along with unknown test material in others. After allowing an adequate time for diffusion and formation of precipitin rings about the wells, a standard curve is graphically drawn by measuring the diameters (or areas) of the precipitin rings for the different concentration standards. These are plotted on orthographic or semilog paper. The diameters of precipitin rings of the unknown (or areas) are then measured and plotted on the standard curve. By direct inspection a determination of the concentration of the unknown test material can be made. The specificity of this reaction quite obviously depends on the quality and monospecificity of the antiserum used as the reagent in the

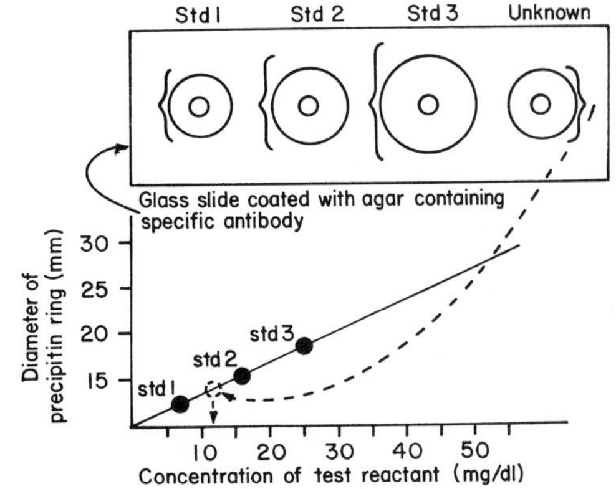

Figure 38–10. Diagram of immunoquantitation by method of single radial immunodiffusion (Techniques of Mancini, Carbonara, and Heremans; and of Fahey and McKelvey).

5

gel. Antisera which lack sharp specificity may give rise to more than one precipitin ring. In some instances deterioration of the unknown test material may result in breakdown fragments that also give rise to artifactual double or triple precipitin ring formation. However, such problems are only infrequently encountered and, in general, the method is the simplest and most direct for quantitation of complex macromolecules (Mancini, 1965; Fahey, 1965).

Single dimension electroimmunodiffusion, developed by Laurell in the 1960's, represents an important variation of the single immunodiffusion reaction. The method involves the use of agar gel with antibody incorporated into the agar as in RID. Sample application is made at one margin of the gel plate into wells followed by electrophoresis of the test samples into the agar. The elements of this technique are diagrammed in Figure 38–11. The effect of electrophoresis is to enhance migration into the agar of the test specimens, which form precipitin lines with the intrinsic antibody in a configuration that resembles a rocket. Indeed, the technique has often been referred to as the "rocket technique" because of the conical shape of the precipitin lines exhibiting an apex at the far point of migration from the application well. The height of the "rocket" or length of the precipitin arc from the application well to the apex has been shown to be directly proportional to the amount of applied antigen. Antigen standards are applied along with the unknown test material in the assay. The heights of the precipitin "rockets" of each standard are plotted graphically to establish a standard curve. The concentration of the unknown is then determined by locating the height of the precipitin "rocket" of the unknown on the standard plot. This method closely parallels that of radial immunodiffusion (RID). It offers the advantage of more rapid completion of the assay owing to the enhanced migration achieved by use of electrophoresis. Commonly, this procedure can be completed in a few hours, whereas the radial immunodiffusion (RID) techniques require from 18 to 48 hours to complete precipitin ring formation. One important limitation of the "rocket" technique is that the relative net charge of macromolecules at the pH used in the test must be accurately estimated. This charge on the molecules will determine the direction of migration to either anode or cathode. Those antigens with positive net charges will migrate to the cathode, while those with negative charge will exhibit anodal migration. This point is of importance to determine actual positioning of the positive and negative electrodes in the electrophoretic assembly. The use of chemical cross-linking of antigens to carriers such as albumin by formaldehyde or glutaraldehyde can be employed to alter the electrophoretic migration of many antigens (Axelsen, 1975).

During the past decade, a number of investigators have developed techniques for *immunoprecipitin analysis by the use of light-scattering devices*. The occurrence of immune complex formation has been related to the amount of such light scattering and used as a basis for antigen quantitation. This approach has been accompanied by the development of sophisticated instruments specifically designed to rapidly measure light scattering, a technique known as nephelometry. The technique of nephelometry, as contrasted to turbidimetric absorbance or emission spectroscopy, is based on scatter reflectance of the transmitted light, which is detected by a photomultiplier tube and not on absorbance of transmitted light as in turbidimetric assays. This approach has proved useful because of its sensitivity and specificity for rapidly detecting immune complex formation. The technique is diagrammed in Figure 38–12. It can be observed in the diagram that filtered light of a certain wavelength enters the analytical cell containing a suspension of reactant material and on striking the immune complexes scatters randomly. The photomultiplier tube located at an angle of 30 to 90 degrees from incident light collects the light scatter as it is reflected from the small particles of the immune complex formations in the test material. The sensitivity of the reflectance system has been further enhanced by using a fluorescent light source. Also, use of enhancing reagents such as polyethylene glycol (PEG) has improved the assay by increasing the speed and sensitivity of immune complex formation so that measurements can be made within seconds to minutes after antigen-antibody mixing, thus affording an extremely rapid approach to immunoquantitation. Within the last few

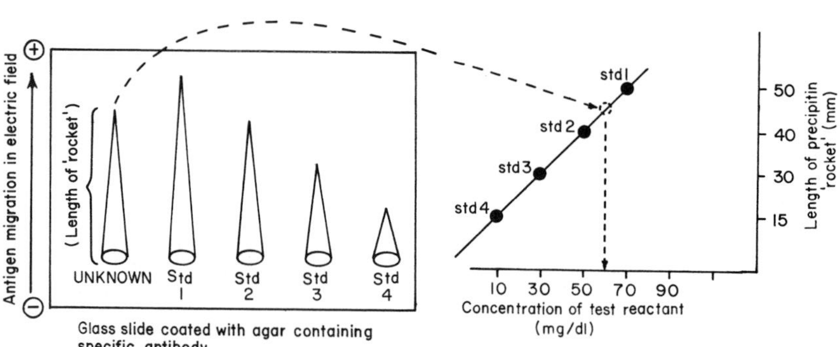

Figure 38–11. Diagram of immunoquantitation by method of single one-dimensional electroimmunodiffusion (Laurell technique of "rocket" electrophoresis).

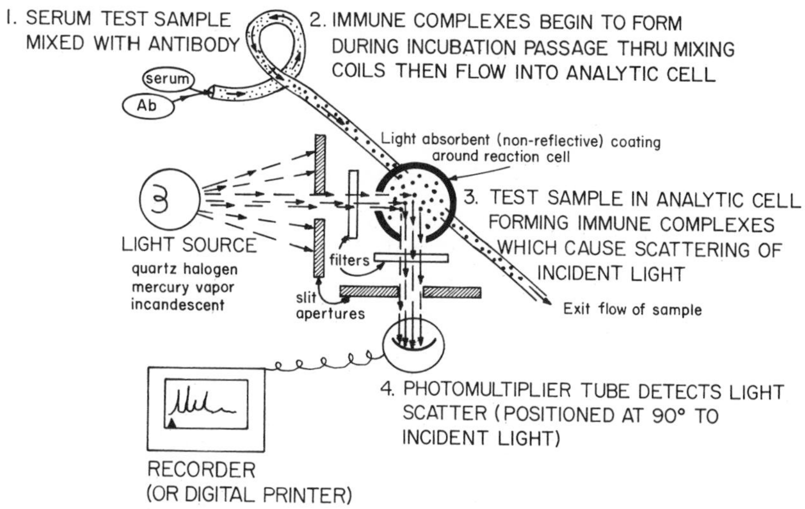

Figure 38–12. Schematic of apparatus for continuous flow nephelometric analysis. Immunoprecipitin reaction is detected by light-scattering effect of immune complexes. Reactants are measured quantitatively by the amount of light scattering.

years, improved instruments utilizing laser and other light sources along with microprocessors to determine rate reactions of precipitin formation have appeared. Such devices offer the promise of even more rapid and sensitive precipitin assays (Larson, 1970).

One limitation of this technique is that the antisera and test specimens must have low levels of intrinsic light scattering activity. The antiserum must have high affinity and monospecificity for the assay antigen. Antiserum exhibiting these properties is referred to as "nephelometric grade." Those nephelometric systems which employ "steady state" conditions require that optimum antigen-antibody ratios be established for use in the assays. This is necessary in order to determine those dilutions of antigen and antibody which are sufficient to produce a light scattering by developing immune complex formation but avoid rapid development of large particulates that cause an uneven distortion of the light-scattering response. Once the ratios have been determined, the antiserum is mixed to the diluted test specimen either individually, in a continuous flow system, or under conditions of constant mixing as in a rotary chemical analyzer. Once "steady state" conditions have developed, light-scattering measurements are made. The peak height of response from the photomultiplier tube is recorded by a recorder on a graphic plot or on a digital printout. Standards that contain known concentrations of the antigen are recorded in order to plot a standard curve using the height of the response that is proportional to the concentration. By plotting the peak response of the test unknown, the concentration can then be determined by direct inspection of the plot of the standards. Alternative methods for determining the unknown concentration are based on use of a microprocessor or programmable calculator. These devices are now commonly employed with the analytical instruments and simplify the reduction of data in an analytical program to determine the amount of the unknown in a given specimen (Larson, 1970; Ritchie, 1978).

AGGLUTINATION TESTS

Agglutination is a classic serologic reaction that involves clumping of a cell suspension by specific antibody. This phenomenon may be observed when particulate antigens such as blood cells or bacteria are exposed to specific antibody under appropriate conditions. Reactions of soluble antigens can be adapted to agglutination tests by the coated or covalent linking of the antigen or specific antibody to a particulate carrier, e.g., red cells, latex particles.

The agglutination reaction takes place in two stages: the antibody first unites with antigen, and then the agglutination occurs. When a given antibody to red cells causes agglutination, the antibody is called "complete." If the antibody unites with specific antigen on the red cells without agglutination, the antibody is called "incomplete." An "incomplete" antibody can be demonstrated by the antiglobulin test. Certain incomplete antibodies do not cause agglutination of red cells in saline, but only when the reaction mixture has a 20 to 30 per cent albumin concentration or the red cells are treated with certain proteolytic enzymes.

The agglutination test is semi-quantitative and the agglutination of either insoluble native antigens or antigen-coated particles can be assessed visually with or without a microscope. Advantages of the agglutination reactions are the high degree of sensitivity and the wide variety of antigens that may be detected with the use of antigen or antibody-coated particles. The simplicity of the reaction is deceiving, since correct interpretation of the reaction requires a strict quality control program with use of well-characterized reagents and knowledge of causes of false positive and false negative results. Major requirements in the agglutination tests are the availability of stable cell or particle suspension, the presence of one or more antigens close to the surface, and the knowledge that the incomplete or non-agglutinating antibodies are not detectable without modification. The IgM anti-

Table 38–2. AGGLUTINATION TESTS

Direct agglutination tests
Simple
High viscosity
Enzyme treated cells
Indirect (passive) agglutination
Antigen coated or covalently linked to particles
Red cells
Inert particles such as latex, bentonite
Antibody-coated or covalently linked to particles (reverse passive)
Antiglobulin tests
Direct Coombs' (red cells)
Indirect Coombs' (red cells)
General antiglobulin tests
Rose-Waaler
Rheumatoid factor

body is about 750 times more efficient than IgG in agglutinations and the presence of IgM antibody will definitely influence the test results.

Agglutination reactions may generally be classified as *direct, indirect (passive),* or *antiglobulin,* as shown in Table 38–2 (Kwapinski, 1972; Singer, 1973–74).

Direct Agglutination Assay

The simple direct agglutination assay is a classic reaction which involves clumping of a cell or insoluble particulate suspension, as bacteria, fungi, and other microbial organisms, by specific antibody. The aggregation is brought about by antibody molecules with two or more combining receptors linking the cells or particles. A reaction is possible with antigens at or close to the cell surface. Special modifications are required to demonstrate incomplete antibodies that may fail to produce agglutination. For example, with Rh blood group antibodies and human bacilli antibodies, the agglutinins are IgM, while the incomplete antibodies are smaller IgG and IgA molecular species. Tests for detection of specific antibody are performed by determination of the dilution of serum that will agglutinate a constant amount of antigen. Because of the inherent variability of the test, a titer of a given serum is not considered significantly different from that of another serum sample value unless there is a four-fold difference.

In many cases, incomplete antibodies may fail to produce agglutination of red cells in saline or dilutions of serum and saline, whereas if this medium is replaced by one with a *higher viscosity*, such as 5 to 30 per cent bovine serum albumin, dextran, or polyvinyl pyrolidine, agglutination may be visible and a more sensitive assay established.

Treatment of human red cells with certain *enzymes* renders them directly agglutinable by some incomplete antibodies such as Rh_0. Many enzymes, such as trypsin, papain, ficin, and bromelin, have been investigated and found to be effective. This procedure has become standard in blood grouping laboratories for detection of many of the incomplete antibodies and is discussed in Chapter 42.

Passive or Indirect Agglutination

This technique has wide and versatile application in the clinical laboratory and involves the agglutination of cells or inert particles coated with soluble antigen or antibody. The cells or inert particles are passive carriers and the antigens may be physically absorbed or covalently coupled to the surface (Fig. 38–13). In the development of passive agglutination tests, cells or particles are needed to which antigens of different chemical nature may be firmly adsorbed or chemically linked. The cell or particle should also form stable and agglutinable suspensions.

Human red cells are often used as agglutinable carriers, but cells of other species may also be used. When erythrocytes are used as the inert particles, the serum samples must first be absorbed with uncoated cells to remove heterophile and other non-specific antibodies that may cause non-specific agglutination. The cells are usually readily available and can often be fixed with formalin, glutaraldehyde or pyruvic aldehyde and stored for prolonged periods.

Many antigens will spontaneously adsorb to red blood cells and form good reagents for antibody detection. Examples are bacterial lipopolysaccharides, purified protein derivative (PPD), penicillin, and many microbial antigens. Since many proteins adsorb poorly to cells, mild treatment of erythrocytes with *tannic acid* or similar reagent may increase the amount of cell-bound antigen or antibody. This test has wide diagnostic application.

Protein antigen may be *chemically coupled* by covalent bonds to the red cell membrane. One common procedure involves cross-linking with bidiazotized benzidine (BDB). The BDB method has had similar applications to the tanned red cell technique. Other coupling agents, such as chromic chloride, glutaraldehyde, cyanuric chloride, and a water-soluble carbodiimide, have also found use.

Inert particles such as bentonite, latex, colloidion, and charcoal have been used to adsorb many classes of antigens, including proteins, carbohydrates, and DNA. Latex is a suspension of spherical polystyrene polymer particles. Proteins or polysaccharides adsorb

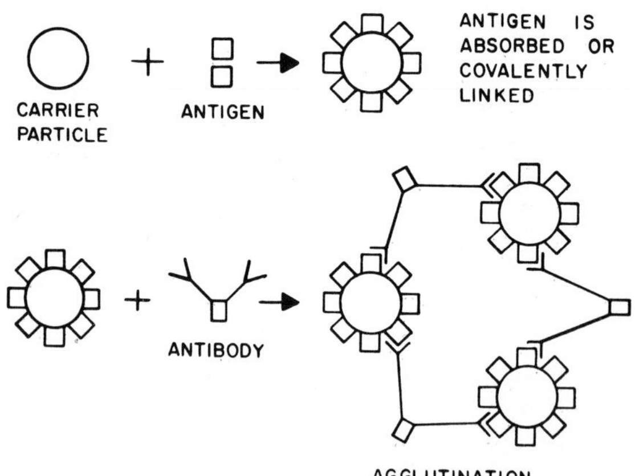

Figure 38–13. Passive agglutination.

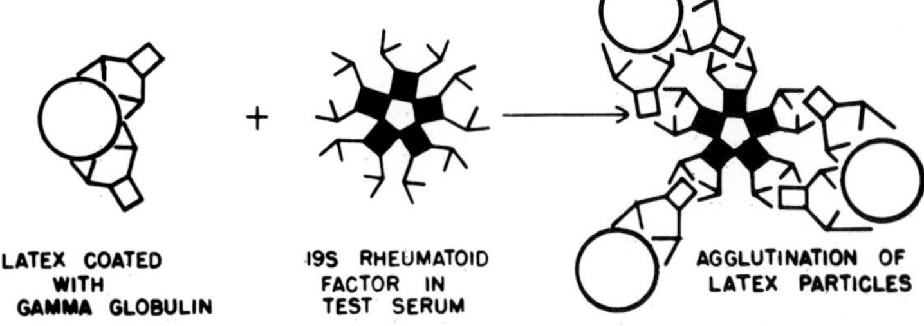

Figure 38–14. Latex agglutination test for rheumatoid factor. (Reproduced with permission from Nakamura, R. M.: Immunopathology: Clinical Laboratory Concepts and Methods. Boston, Little, Brown & Co., 1974.)

to the surface and will encourage particles to be clumped by specific antibody. Latex particles with carboxyl group can be convalently linked to various protein antigens. Examples are latex fixation for detection of rheumatoid factor (Fig. 38–14) and agglutination of DNA-coated red cells for detection of anti-DNA antibody (Singer, 1973–74).

Antiglobulin Test (Coombs' Test)

This ingenious test was first described in 1908 by Moreschi and was rediscovered by Coombs and coworkers in 1945 to demonstrate incomplete antibodies to red cell antigens. "Incomplete" antibodies such as anti–Rh IgG, fail to produce agglutination of a saline suspension of homologous red cells, but nevertheless combine firmly with antigens on the erythrocyte. After washing away other serum proteins, the anti-RH IgG remains on the cell surface. The erythrocytes may then be agglutinated by the addition of rabbit anti-human IgG (Fig. 38–15). The antiglobulin test is a simple serologic method of showing globulins firmly attached to the cell. The *indirect test* assays serum for antibody by allowing it to react with reference cells. The *direct test* assays for antibody already on the patient's erythrocytes. These determinations are discussed in Chapter 42.

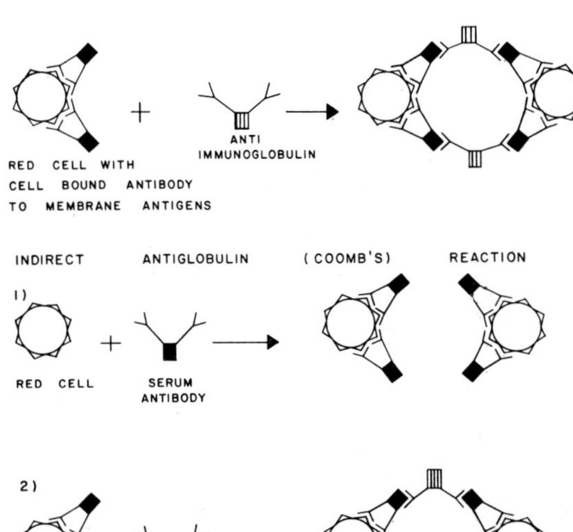

Figure 38–15. Direct and indirect Coombs' reaction.

The reaction between the antiglobulin serum and red cells sensitized with Rh(D) incomplete antibody may be *inhibited* by gamma globulin in solution. The specific nature of this inhibition has been utilized in determining the species specificities of gamma globulin in unknown samples of serum, blood stains, etc. This technique is much more sensitive than the direct precipitin method.

The *Rose-Waaler test* is an antiglobulin test using sheep red cells sensitized with a subagglutinating dose of rabbit anti–sheep erythrocyte IgG. Rheumatoid factor, 19S IgM, will combine with the fixed 7S IgG and produce agglutination.

TISSUE IMMUNOFLUORESCENT ANTIBODY TECHNIQUES

Fluorescent-labeled antibody was first used by Coons and associates in 1941 for studying localization of antigens in tissues. The fluorescent dye was used as a chemically linked marker on the specific antibody and did not alter its immunologic reactivity. The two fluorochromes most widely used today are fluorescein and rhodamine or their stable derivative. Fluorescein has a yellowish green fluorescence with a maximum at about 520 nm, and rhodamine has a reddish orange fluorescence with a maximum at about 620 nm. These compounds have been the fluorochromes of choice because of intensity or efficiency of fluorescence.

The green fluorescence of fluorescein offers two important advantages over the red fluorescence of rhodamine: (1) The human eye is more sensitive to the apple-green color than to the reddish orange color, and (2) red autofluorescence is more common in nature than green autofluorescence. The most popular conjugate used in the clinical laboratory is the fluorescein isothiocyanate conjugated antiserum. The isothiocyanate derivative is stable and is coupled to the free amino groups of the protein to form a carbamido linkage. Tetramethylrhodamine isothiocyanate can be conjugated in a similar manner as fluorescein isothiocyanate for the reddish orange fluorescent reagent (Nakamura, 1974).

Immunohistochemical Methods for Use of Fluorescent Antibody

In the use of fluorescent-labeled antibody, there are various methods that can be used to detect the presence both of unknown antigens and tissues or smears and

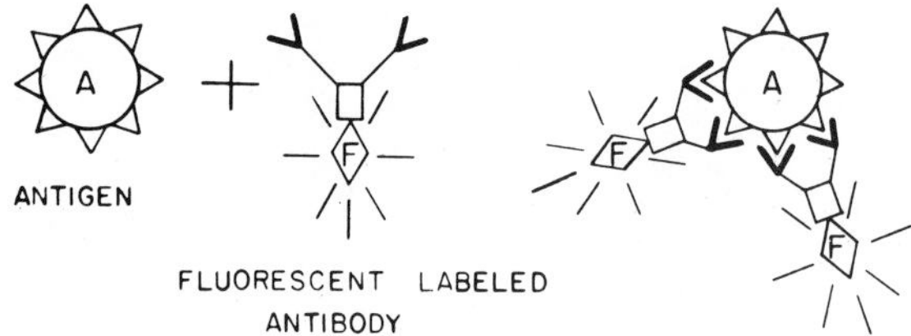

Figure 38–16. Direct method for fluorescent labeled antibody. (Reproduced with permission from Nakamura, R. M.: Immunopathology: Clinical Laboratory Concepts and Methods. Boston, Little, Brown & Co., 1974.)

of unknown antibodies in the patient's serum. The common methods are the direct, indirect, inhibition, and complement staining methods (Kawamura, 1977).

In the *direct method*, the antibody is labeled with fluorescent compound and is used to detect the presence of antigen in tissue fixed to a slide. The fluorescent-labeled antibodies are added to the antigen in its optimal dilution and allowed to react for at least 30 minutes at room temperature or at 37° C. (Fig. 38–16). The preparation is next washed to remove the labeled gamma globulins, which do not react with the antigen. The smear tissue sections are blotted and the preparation mounted with buffered glycerol for examination with the fluorescent microscope.

The *indirect method* is utilized for detection of either unknown antigen in tissue sections or unknown antibody in the patient's serum (Fig. 38–17). The specific antigen-antibody—both unlabeled—reaction may be visualized by addition of labeled antibody directed against the antibody in the primary reaction. The antigen plus antibody globulin plus labeled anti-antibody complex results in fluorescence of the coated antigen. The indirect method has the advantage of utilizing a single-labeled anti-antibody globulin to detect many different specific antigen-antibody reactions occurring within a given species. For example, fluoresceinated rabbit or goat anti-human globulin may be used to detect a wide variety of human antibody-antigen reactions. In the detection of the unknown antigen or antibody the tissue sections or smear is reacted with unlabeled antiserum and allowed to react for 30 to 60 minutes at room temperature or at 37°C. The preparation is thoroughly washed to remove unlabeled antibody unattached to the antigen. Labeled anti-antibody globulin is then incubated with the preparation as in the direct technique.

The *inhibition method* is often employed as a control for testing the specificity of the antibodies in the direct fluorescent procedure. It has also been applied for detection of certain microorganisms such as *Toxoplasma gondii*. Antigen becomes saturated when treated with unlabeled specific antibody. Therefore, upon subsequent exposure to specific labeled antibody, no antigen fluorescence can be detected. Optimal concentrations of both labeled and unlabeled antibodies must be determined.

The *complement staining method* is similar to the indirect technique except that the labeled antibody is directed against complement components, often of guinea pig origin. The method is useful to detect either unknown antigen or antibody in patient's serum. For example, tissue is treated with serum which may contain the antibody in question. This antibody must be able to fix complement. A source of complement is added and finally the antigen-antibody complex is reacted with labeled anticomplement. This results in fluorescence of the complement-binding complexes.

Applications of Fluorescent Antibody Methods

(Cherry, 1980)

Fluorescent-labeled antibody methods are primarily used as a histochemical or cytochemical tool for detection and localization of antigen and antibody reactions. The procedure has been used for the detection

STEP 1

ANTIGEN ANTIBODY

STEP 2

FLUORESCENT ANTI—GLOBULIN

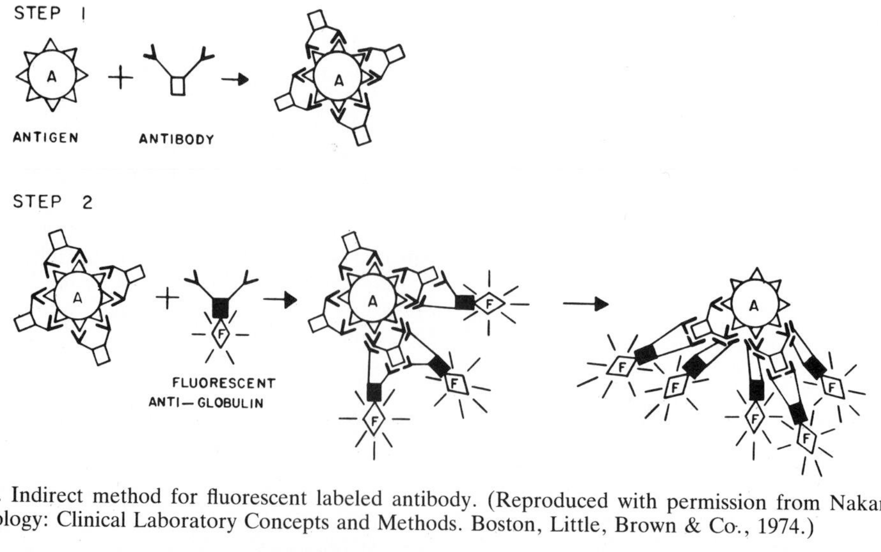

Figure 38–17. Indirect method for fluorescent labeled antibody. (Reproduced with permission from Nakamura, R. M.: Immunopathology: Clinical Laboratory Concepts and Methods. Boston, Little, Brown & Co., 1974.)

tion of specific antibodies in patients' sera; localization of antigen, antibody, complement, and immune complexes on various cells and tissue sections; localization and fate of injected foreign antigens; localization and site of multiplication of infectious agents for use in the rapid diagnosis of microbial infections; and localization of various hormones and enzymes in cells and tissue sections.

More recently, fluorescent-labeled antibody methods are being used to quantitate antigen and antibodies similar to radioimmunoassay methods with comparable levels of sensitivity. The procedures require extensive purification and characterizations of the fluorescent reagents, as well as special instrumentation to decrease non-specific background while increasing specificity and sensitivity.

The immunofluorescent methods may in many instances be replaced by enzyme-labeled antibody methods. The fluorescent antibody methods have been used for a longer period of time and have the advantages of greater availability of well-characterized, standardized reagents and procedures.

Quality Control

Controls in the staining with labeled antibodies, as in any standard laboratory procedure, are a necessary part of the procedure. Control procedures include:

1. Absorption of the antibody from the labeled antiserum by the specific antigen before staining the preparation.

2. Comparison of the fluorescence of the experimentally positive slide with similar tissue material known to be non-reacting, e.g., a tissue exhibiting a different pathologic process.

3. The use of unrelated fluorescent antisera or fluorescent normal globulin on the experimental tissue.

4. Inhibition or the "blocking" of fluorescence by prior application of unlabeled antibody. This method may yield only partial inhibition.

The specificity of the staining reaction should be monitored by blocking the staining reaction by pretreatment with unlabeled homologous antiserum. Complete inhibition can often be achieved by appropriate manipulation of pretreatment and staining times. A pretreatment:staining time ratio of 8:1 is generally recommended. Often the inhibition may not be complete owing to the continuous exchange of conjugate with unlabeled antibody. The specificity may also be checked by blocking the reaction by absorbing the labeled antibody with specific antigen. The antigen should be coupled to a solid phase carrier to avoid formation of soluble immune complexes. Lastly, the labeled antibody may be displaced with unlabeled antibody.

Several causes of non-specific staining are listed in Table 38–3. A common cause is a high dye:protein ratio of the conjugate which is more negatively charged and produces artificial staining reactions. The more highly negatively charged conjugates may be selectively removed by DEAE-cellulose chromatography or by precipitation and after dialysis with buffers in a pH range of 6.0 to 6.2. The non-specific staining may be reduced by means of the classic procedure of absorption of conjugates with tissue homogenates.

Table 38–3. FACTORS IN NON-SPECIFIC IMMUNOFLUORESCENT STAINING REACTIONS

1. Quality of conjugate dye
2. Fraction of antiserum conjugated, i.e., IgG or gamma globulin fraction
3. Titer of specific antibody
4. Specificity of antiserum conjugation procedure
5. Presence of free dye
6. Dye:protein ratio
7. Procedures to remove high dye:protein conjugates
   a. DEAE cellulose chromatography
   b. Tissue powder absorption
8. Counterstains
9. Tissue preparation

Several procedures are required to control fluorescein-labeled conjugates. They may be checked by dialysis for absence of unbound fluorescein and may be separated from unbound fluorescein by gel filtration. Protein concentrations may be determined by the biuret reaction with readings at 560 nm instead of the usual 540 nm to avoid interference from fluorescein absorbency. An alternative method for determination of the protein concentration is measuring absorbance at 280 nm and 495 nm and using the following formula:

$$\text{Protein (mg/ml)} = \frac{\text{O.D. 280 nm} - 0.35\ (\text{O.D. 495 nm})}{1.4}$$

Cellulose acetate or gel electrophoresis may be used to evaluate for the presence of unbound fluorescent material and of protein added to previously conjugated protein. After electrophoresis the strip is examined under a Woods' light (366 nm) for fluorescence of separated proteins. The location and brightness of each band should be noted and sketched. The strip is then stained with an appropriate protein stain such as Ponceau S and scanned by a densitometer. The Ponceau S-stained strip is compared with the sketch of fluorescence made before protein staining. A fluorescent band beyond the albumin position indicates the presence of unreacted fluorescein. A strong fluorescence in the gamma globulin region with no fluorescence in the beta area denotes a high concentration of labeled gamma globulin and indicates that the gamma globulin fraction alone was labeled with fluorescein. The absence of fluorescein in bands stained by Ponceau S as alpha one, alpha two, or albumin indicates that protein has been added to FITC-(fluorescent conjugate) labeled protein.

Immunoelectrophoresis is performed in which the fluoresceinated antisera are reacted against normal whole human sera. A heavy line of precipitation in the IgG region should be obtained. Additional lines with antibodies to serum proteins other than immunoglobulins are often seen in commercial antisera. The extraneous antibodies may not necessarily interfere with the specificity of the immunofluorescent test; however, they contribute to increased non-specific staining. Also, the presence of contaminant antibodies casts doubt on the purity of the antigen used for immunization. Spurs from the IgG line produced by cross-reaction of the anti-IgG conjugate with IgM or IgA in the electrophoresed normal human serum may be expected in the presence of antibodies to the light chain of IgG. The light-chain antibodies may be specifically removed by absorption with purified human IgM or IgA preparations. Cross-reactions of antibodies to the light chain in antisera to IgG with light-chain antibodies of IgM and IgA do not usually occur in immunofluorescent staining, provided that the immunization is carried out with purified IgG and the conjugate is diluted to ¼ unit/ml. Thus at ¼ unit/ml of anti-IgG, no visible immunofluorescent staining occurs with IgA or IgM immunoglobulins in indirect immunofluorescent staining reactions. If a concentration of 1 unit/ml of labeled anti-IgG is used and there are anti–light chain antibodies present, then the IgG antiserum will detect the presence of IgA and IgM immunoglobulins.

The gel diffusion precipitin test is performed with reference antiserum to IgG; and the test conjugate against normal human serum should give precipitin lines of complete identity. Cross-reactions of anti–human IgG conjugate with human IgM and IgA may be detected by the precipitin tests.

Determination of immunologic sensitivity of the conjugate is accomplished by measuring the level of specific precipitating antibodies which can be expressed in units/ml. The units of conjugate are based on the titer of antiglobulin determined in the standard gel diffusion precipitin test using 1 mg IgG/ml antigen and two-fold dilutions of the conjugate. The conjugate is more specific for purified IgG than for normal human serum. However, the units of antibody may be determined with normal human serum diluted to contain 1 mg/ml IgG (normal serum diluted 1:12). Agar gel template, recommended for determining the units of antibodies, is a horizontally placed line of wells 2.8 mm in diameter, placed 7.5 mm apart in a gel with a depth of 1.5 mm. Titration is performed by serial two-fold dilutions of the conjugates, which are placed opposite the wells containing the antigen test in a concentration of 1 mg/ml. Pipets are changed with each dilution and plates are incubated at room temperature for 24 hours and read for the highest dilution which gives a visible line of precipitation. This titer is the unitage. A linear pattern agar gel template for gel diffusion should be used instead of one with a circular pattern. Acceptable conjugates should have at least 4 units/1 per cent protein when the unitage assay is employed. This is approximately equivalent to 1 mg precipitating antibody/10 mg protein. Conjugates with lower antibody levels are not recommended for use.

Expressing a fluorescein:protein (F:P) ratio as the ratio of absorbance at 495 nm to that at 280 nm can be recommended only for screening purposes, since the absolute levels of FITC, as well as the F:P ratio, influence nonspecific staining. Also, aromatic compounds having a high absorbance at 280 nm are sometimes added to commercial conjugates as preservatives. F:P ratios may be expressed as micrograms of bound FITC per milligram of protein.

To obtain F:P molar ratios, the weight ratios are multiplied by a factor of 0.411. The conversion formula is derived as follows:

$$\frac{160{,}000}{389 \times 10^3} = 0.411$$

The average molecular weight of immunoglobulin is 160,000 and 389 is the molecular weight of FITC; 10^3 converts milligrams to micrograms. The F:P ratio must be determined before the conjugate is diluted with a protein carrier such as albumin. In an indirect antinuclear antibody test utilizing mouse liver, a molar F:P ratio of approximately 3:1 was found to be optimal for conjugates with 4 units antibody/ml. However, a different molar F:P ratio may be optimal for other systems.

Determination of Working Dilution of Conjugates

Fluoresceinated immunoglobulin can be evaluated in the indirect antinuclear antibody tests with substrate. Chessboard titrations should be carried out with different unit dilutions of fluoresceinated antisera against different high and lower titered sera known to contain antinuclear antibodies. With good fluoresceinated antisera, a plateau end point of 1/6 or 1/64 units may be seen when reacted against high-titered sera. A working dilution of the fluorescein conjugate should be ¼ to ⅛ unit/ml. In the antinuclear antibody test, a working dilution of ¼ unit/ml is recommended, provided the F:P ratio is approximately 3 to 5. This provides for a satisfactory background and will ensure detection of the low-titered sera containing antinuclear antibodies. Also, reproducible titers can be obtained on the same serum containing antinuclear antibodies when tested with a different source of conjugated antisera.

Usually the working dilutions of the anti-IgA and anti-IgM conjugate used should be at least 1 unit/ml. Polyvalent anti-immunoglobulin conjugate should be used at the dilution of 1 unit/ml. In fluorescent kidney biopsy studies, anti-IgM and anti-IgA are recommended for use at a concentration of 1 unit/ml.

When conjugated anti-β_{1C} is used, a working dilution of ½ unit/ml is satisfactory for kidney biopsies. A chessboard titration may be performed in a test system and if a plateau end point of 1/16 unit/ml is seen, then a working dilution of ¼ unit may be used. Criteria for evaluation of anti-β_{1C} conjugates are the same as above. The conjugates should also have 4 units antibody/1 per cent protein/ml.

Conjugates should be stored sterile after membrane filtration, and precautions should be taken to avoid aggregation. Protein concentration for storage should be 2 mg/ml or greater (other proteins such as albumin may be helpful). The conjugates should be divided into small aliquots and thawed only once before use. They should be ultracentrifuged (150,000 g for 30 minutes) before storage and subjected to high-speed centrifugation before use.

Tissue Processing

In tissue immunofluorescence work, it is essential that the tissue be processed so as to preserve antigenic reactivity and general structural morphology. Many antigens are rendered inactive after treatment with the usual fixatives employed for non-immunologic studies.

Substrate and biopsy tissue specimens should be "snap" frozen in liquid nitrogen, liquid nitrogen-isopentane, or dry ice–acetone mixture. The tissue is kept frozen in a non–frost-free freezer, preferably at −70°C., in a sealed container to prevent drying by evaporation. The material can be shipped in dry ice to a reference laboratory if necessary.

Fresh substrate tissue to be frozen is cut into small cubes approximately 3 mm in dimension. The blocks are placed on aluminum foil and covered with optimal cutting temperature compound (OCT, Ames Co., Elkhart, Indiana) and snap frozen by immersion in liquid nitrogen or dry ice and acetone. Then they are wrapped in aluminum foil and placed in a precooled screw cap bottle for storage in a −70°C. freezer. Composite blocks containing several tissues are prepared by placing small folds and pieces of tissue close together on one plate. The frozen section wrapped in aluminum foil is best stored in a tightly sealed bottle with a screw cap at −70°C. The chuck and tissue sections can be carried from the freezer to the cryostat in pressed polystyrene boxes containing solid carbon dioxide. The tissue should not be allowed to thaw before sectioning, since the slightest degree of thawing would allow sections to become unrecognizable. Alternatively, the tissue may be placed in a test tube or small bottle containing isopentane and frozen by immersion into liquid nitrogen or dry ice and acetone. A few minutes should be sufficient for freezing. The tissue should not be left in the solvent for a long period of time, as it dries out and becomes very difficult to section. After the tissue is completely frozen it is removed from the test tube with forceps and placed in another test tube, sealed, and stored in a freezer, preferably at −70°C. Tissue may be stored in a regular freezer at −20°C. or below but should not be stored in an automatic frost-free freezer.

PREPARATION OF NEEDLE BIOPSY TISSUE

Small needle biopsies of kidney, thyroid, or other excisional biopsies of the skin can be collected directly from the operation and carried to the laboratory and mounted upon a section of tongue blade or small sponge (Onkosponge No. 1, Histo-Med, Inc., Paterson, N.J.) with the optimal cutting temperature compound (OCT) and quickly frozen by immersion in liquid nitrogen. The OCT has not been found to interfere with the immunochemical studies.

The sections are cut from 4 to 6 μ on a standard cryostat. The optimal temperature for cutting most tissues depends on the amount of fatty tissue and may vary from −22°C. to lower than −30°C. for tissue with a large amount of lipids. Cleaned microscopic slides should be used. The sections are placed on the slide after drying and may be stored in a −70°C. cabinet.

In order to prevent the loss of water-soluble antigens or antibodies, the tissue or other material on the microscope slide is placed in a mild fixative. One may employ an equal mixture of absolute ethyl alcohol and ethyl ether at room temperature for 10 minutes, followed by 95 per cent ethyl alcohol at room temperature for 10 minutes. However, other agents such as acetone and methyl alcohol have been used. In certain studies, fixatives are not used, as they may destroy the immunologic reactivity of the antigen.

Equipment for Fluorescent Microscopy

The fluorescence microscope can be designed in many ways, and in choosing the type of equipment desired the various factors described below should be considered. Two principles are used in the construction of fluorescence microscopes: transmitted illumination and incident or epi-illumination.

For *transmitted illumination* (Fig. 38–18) two condenser systems are available: the brightfield condenser used in ordinary light microscopy and the darkfield condenser. The brightfield condenser will produce a satisfactory excitation, i.e., a good signal, but the problem of filtering away light of unwanted wavelengths, i.e., optical noise, has not been satisfactorily solved, and brightfield condensers are not recommended for routine fluorescent work. *Darkfield condensers* (oil immersion) are to be preferred. They will give an optimal signal by concentrating the excitation light in a narrow area, but at the same time most of the excitation light will be directed away from the objective front lens, so that the optical noise is significantly decreased.

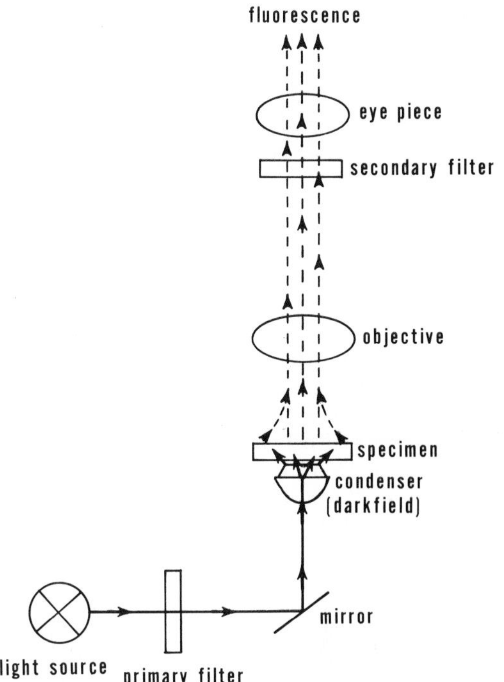

Figure 38–18. Transmitted darkfield immunofluorescence.

For *incident or epi-illumination* (Fig. 38–19) no condenser problems exist, in that the microscope objective itself functions as a condenser. The excitation light is admitted to the microscope tube at a right angle,

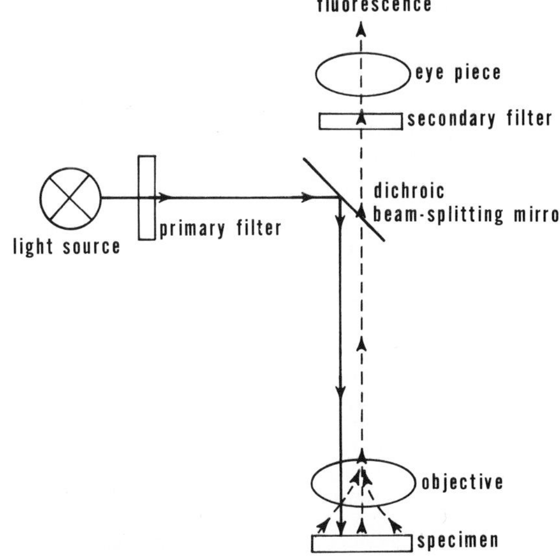

Figure 38–19. Incident immunofluorescence.

5

reflected to the fluorescent specimen by means of a dichroic mirror (i.e., an interference filter), and the fluorescence observed through the dichroic mirror.

The two most effective systems for fluorescence microscopy are transmitted light illumination with a darkfield condenser system and the brightfield incident or epi-illumination.

A conventional microscope can be usually converted to a fluorescence microscope by adding a darkfield condenser and suitable filter systems with a low voltage tungsten or halogen light source. The level of fluorescence produced is suitable for most procedures in the clinical laboratory.

The Ploem type vertical illuminator can be attached to a research type microscope stand. The illuminator is equipped with an interference dividing plate (dichroic mirror) which is mounted above the objective at an angle of 45 degrees to the illuminating beam. The dichroic mirror is matched for excitation and transmission to the fluorochrome. The objective acts as the condenser. A major advantage of epi-illumination is that a narrow band excitation beam may be employed with interchangeable filter systems to detect the two different fluorochromes. Another advantage of epi-illumination is that it can be combined with transmitted illumination, such as phase contrast or polarized light microscopy.

The *light source* must give ample energy in the wavelength range corresponding to the absorption maximum of the fluorochrome used.

High-pressure arc lamps (mercury, xenon, cesium) are traditional light sources for fluorescence microscopy. Their wavelength spectrum extends from the ultraviolet through the visible to the infrared part, consisting of a light continuum and a line spectrum. Subsequent primary filtration is necessary. The ultraviolet component may give rise to fluorescence of tissue proteins and nucleoproteins, the so-called *autofluorescence,* unless suitable filtration is provided.

Halogen lamps (e.g., iodine-quartz lamps) can be operated at very high temperatures, thanks to the quartz bulb and the halogen filling of the bulb. They are cheap, are easy to run, and will provide enough excitation energy for most purposes when used in connection with a suitable primary filter system.

Lasers such as the argon ion laser, helium-cadmium laser, and pulsed organic dye laser are ideal light sources that can provide a very high energy excitation of the two fluorochromes most commonly used: FITC and TRITC. Laser excitation studies have given extremely promising results, but so far laser excitation has been used only in highly specialized laboratories. The availability of relatively cheap, reliable lasers will lead to more widespread use in the future. No filtration of the laser light is needed because of the monochromatic nature of the laser light.

There are generally two types of *primary filters:* (1) the absorption filter, which absorbs light of a certain wavelength and allows light of another wavelength to pass, and (2) the interference filter, which selects the desired band of light by reflection and dispersion of the undesired light. The advantage of the interference filter is that the light passed has a higher intensity than the light passed by the absorption filters.

The primary absorption filters traditionally used were glass or gelatin filters. Their transmission curves must be characterized as far from ideal in most cases, but still such filters have given excellent results when used in combination with high-energy light sources, e.g., high-pressure mercury arc lamps or xenon lamps.

When fluorescein is used as the fluorescent label the common absorption filters used are the Schott BG-12 (2 to 4 mm thick) or No. 5040 Corning filter. The transmission maximum for these filters is frequently in the 366 nm region near ultraviolet. Another set of primary absorption filters looks dark blue and is used for a blue light excitation. Their transmission includes the blue portion of the visible spectrum from 420 to 450 nm. Blue light excitation filters are used in conjunction with secondary filters of a yellow-orange color.

A UG-1 filter with a mercury arc vapor lamp will pass light from 300 to 400 nm and utilizes a moderate absorption band of FITC found between 300 and 400 nm. With use of a UG-1 filter, there is good contrast although the intensity is reduced. The UG-1 filter is useful for immunofluorescence work with liver biopsies for hepatitis B antigen localization. The liver tissue has many autofluorescent tissue substances.

Special fluorescein isothiocyanate (FITC) primary interference filters are now available and recommended for most of the fluorescent work using FITC.

In addition to the above primary exciter filters and heat absorbing filter, one can use a skyblue Schott BG-38 filter. The BG-38 suppresses the transmission in the far red spectrum given by many primary filters. The purpose of the BG-38 is to make the background in the field of view completely black.

A 480 nm yellow filter can be used to reduce tissue autofluorescence associated with excitation by primary BG-12 or FITC interference filters.

The purpose of the *secondary filter* is to transmit all the fluorescence wavelengths and stop all the excitation wavelengths. The secondary filters are inserted in the body of the tube or the eye pieces, or a variety of filters can be utilized in the rotating device in the body of the microscope. The secondary filters serve to remove remnants of exciting light so that only the fluorescent light reaches the observer's eyes. They are inserted between the objective and the observer's eyes, either above the nose piece or in the rotating disk in the stands. Various filters are complementary to the primary filters. For use with FITC labeled compounds, the secondary filter can be a Zeiss 53, which has a peak cut-off point near the maximal emission peak of FITC at 525 nm.

In general, high numerical aperture objectives are to be recommended to increase the *optical signal* at this level also. Fluorite objectives give very satisfactory results in fluorescence microscopy. Dry lenses are easier to handle than oil immersion lenses. For very high aperture objectives an objective diaphragm may be necessary to exclude optical noise.

ANALYTICAL FLUORESCENCE IMMUNOASSAYS

Background and Classification of Fluorescence Immunoassays

The initial development of analytical fluorescent immunoassays was hindered by decreased sensitivity due to background fluorescence of biological samples. Today, the sensitivity of fluorimetric methods can be refined to detect analytes at concentrations of 10^{-15} M. Advances have been made possible by improvements in instrumentation and employment of unique substrates with various immunochemical and enzymatic reactions.

Table 38–4. CLASSIFICATION OF FLUORESCENCE IMMUNOASSAYS

A. Heterogeneous
   1. Solid phase antigen assay
   2. Solid phase antibody assay
B. Homogeneous assays performed with standard instrumentation (endpoint or kinetic measurements)
   1. Increase or decrease of hapten fluorescence by antibody
   2. Fluorescence excitation transfer immunoassay
      a. Direct antigen label
      b. Indirect antigen label
   3. Fluorescence protection immunoassay
   4. Substrate labeled fluorescence immunoassay (SLFIA)
C. Homogeneous assays performed with special instrumentation
   1. Fluorescence polarization
   2. Fluorescence correlation immunoassay with fluorescence-fluctuation spectrometer

The selection of the fluorochrome label is important and should be stable, demonstrate high absorptivity and quantum yield, emit at appropriate wavelengths, and not interfere with the ligand-antibody reaction. The various FIA may be classified as follows: (1) heterogeneous or homogeneous, (2) ligand or antibody labeled, (3) competitive or non-competitive, and (4) solid or non-solid phase.

Table 38–4 represents a working classification of fluorescence immunoassays. Heterogeneous and homogeneous assays and available special instrumentation will be discussed.

Heterogeneous Fluorescence Immunoassays
(Maggio, 1980, 1981)

Most of the available heterogeneous assays, heterogeneous in that the sample requires separation of labeled and unlabeled species, utilize a solid phase antigen or antibody system. In this assay, the label is separated from endogenous interference by attachment to a solid surface, particle, or matrix. These are similar to radioimmunoassays with the substitution of fluorophore label for isotope.

The assay can be either competitive or non-competitive. The method selection is often dependent on the degree of sensitivity and specificity desired. Current assays use a conventional fluorimeter, and the sensitivity of the methods without special instrumentation is often limited to about 10^{-9} to 10^{-10} molar.

Homogeneous Fluorescence Immunoassays
(Nakamura, 1980)

By definition, these immunoassays are performed on homogeneous samples; the methods do not require the separation of bound from free unknown and are usually not sensitive to background sources in the sample.

The homogeneous assays have the advantages of speed and avoidance of the separation step. However, when compared with heterogeneous assays, the homogeneous fluorescence immunoassays have certain disadvantages. The current homogeneous fluorescence immunoassays have a limited sensitivity near 10^{-10} molar of analyte per liter with standard instrumentation. Labeled impurities in the sample may increase background interference. The assays require relatively pure labeled antigen or specific antibody. They also require special instrumentation in order to achieve greater sensitivity.

INCREASE OR DECREASE OF HAPTEN FLUORESCENCE BY ANTIBODY
(Smith, 1977)

In the fluorescence quenching method, the binding of a chromophoric hapten by antibody causes a marked decrease of antibody tryptophan fluorescence. The hapten should absorb in the region of protein fluorescence emission, approximately 300 to 360 nm. Smith has described an enhancement fluoroimmunoassay. A fluorescent derivative of thyroxine (T_4), whose fluorescence was enhanced when bound to anti-T_4 serum, was used in the assay method. The assay involves a short incubation step following the mixing of the sample, labeled T_4, and specific antiserum with subsequent measurement of the fluorescence enhancement (Smith, 1977). An Aminco Bowman SPF fluorimeter was used to measure the degree of fluorescence. With use of a conventional fluorimeter, the technique as published is less sensitive than standard radioimmunoassay methods for T_4; however, removal of the variable background serum sample fluorescence would allow sufficient sensitivity to measure total T_4 levels in clinical patients.

FLUORESCENCE EXCITATION TRANSFER IMMUNOASSAY (Ullman, 1976)

The fluorescence excitation transfer method uses two labels, fluorescein as donor fluorescer and rhodamine as acceptor or quencher. Fluorescein isothiocyanate has a maximum emission of 525 nm and tetramethyl or tetraethyl rhodamine has a strong absorption peak at 525 nm. Therefore, when FITC labeled antigen and rhodamine labeled antibody bind, there is a *quenching* of FITC fluorescence.

This phenomenon involves a dipole-dipole coupled energy transfer from an electronically excited fluorescent dye to an acceptor dye. The rate of energy transfer is inversely proportional to the sixth power of the distance between the donor and acceptor molecules. For adequate reduction of fluorescence with quenching, the donor-acceptor distance between the labels should be about 50 to 70 Angstroms.

There are two types of reactions: (1) direct antigen labeling and (2) indirect antigen labeling. In the first, the antigen (Ag) is labeled with fluorescein (F) and the antibody (Ab) labeled with rhodamine (R) (Fig. 38–20). The second method is similar to the first except that the antigen is labeled *indirectly* by em-

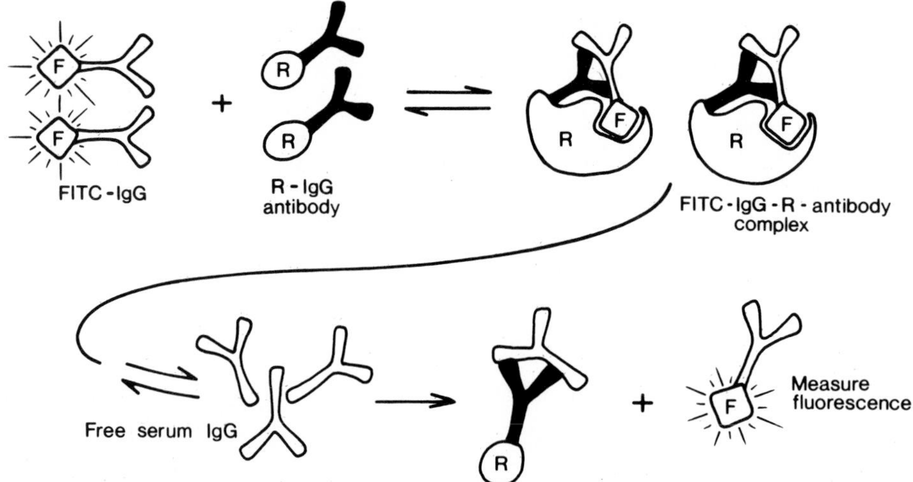

Figure 38–20. Direct antigen labeled fluorescence excitation transfer immunoassay. The antigen is labeled with fluorescein (F), and the antibody is labeled with rhodamine (R). When the fluorescein-labeled antigen and rhodamine-labeled antibody bind, there is a quenching of fluorescein. Then the serum sample containing free IgG is added and the degree of fluorescence measured is proportional to the concentration of serum IgG.

ploying a fluorescein labeled antibody (Fig. 38–21). This method is useful for assay of antigen with multivalent antigenic determinants. Separate portions of specific antibody are labeled with fluorescein and rhodamine, respectively. The admixture of differently labeled fluorescein-tagged antibody and rhodamine-labeled antibody reduces intensity of the fluorescer by adjusting the ratio and amount of donor and acceptor so that they react in close proximity to permit energy transfer. A definite disadvantage of the indirect labeling method is that immunochemically purified antibodies are required so as to avoid excessive fluorescence background due to non-specific fluorescer labeled proteins. These assays have potential sensitivity to the 100 picomole range. The advantages over heterogeneous assays include speed, avoidance of the separation step, and stability of reagents.

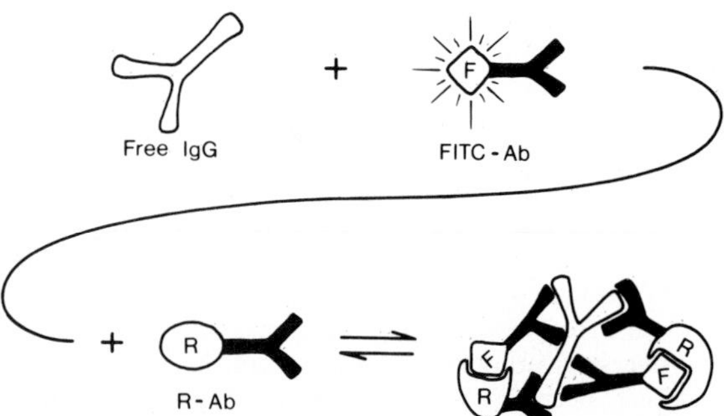

Figure 38–21. Indirect antigen-labeled fluorescence excitation transfer immunoassay. The IgG protein antigen is labeled indirectly with use of purified fluorescein-labeled antibody. The ratio of fluorescein-labeled antibody and rhodamine-labeled antibody is adjusted such that fluorescein is quenched. Addition of serum containing free IgG will result in liberation of fluorescein-labeled antibody, and the degree of fluorescence is proportional to the concentration of serum IgG.

FLUORESCENCE PROTECTION IMMUNOASSAY (Zuk, 1979; Ullman, 1980)

In this assay, the protein antigen is labeled with fluorescein and then reacted with specific antibody to the antigen. The antigen-specific antibody will sterically inhibit the reaction of a second antibody specific for fluorescein which, in turn, will quench the fluorescence of fluorescein when it binds to the fluorophore. The specific anti-fluorescein antibody may be increased in size, which will decrease its ability to interact with the fluorescein coupled to the surface of the antigen within a small space. The procedure may be used to assay for antibody to the antigen or the antigen concentration in a homogeneous system.

The fluorescence protection immunoassay has been used to assay for serum levels of T_4, anticardiolipin antibodies (Fig. 38–22), and human IgG, albumin, and human placental lactogen.

SUBSTRATE-LABELED FLUORESCENCE IMMUNOASSAY (SLFIA)

(Burd, 1977; Boguslaski, 1980)

A homogeneous substrate-labeled fluorescence immunoassay (SLFIA) is usually used for assay of therapeutic drugs and proteins such as IgG and IgM. In the assay, a fluorogenic substrate of β-galactosidase is covalently linked to purified haptenic or protein antigens. The substrate is hydrolyzed into a fluorescent substrate product with cleavage of the galactose moiety (Fig. 38–23).

A typical SLFIA is illustrated by an assay for gentamicin. Gentamicin is coupled to β-galactosyl umbelliferone to form a non-fluorescent substrate. The β-galactosidase cleaves the substrate to release a fluorescent product. However, when the β-galactosyl umbelliferone–gentamicin is combined with specific antibody, cleavage will not occur due to steric hindrance. The procedure *does not* require a *separation step*

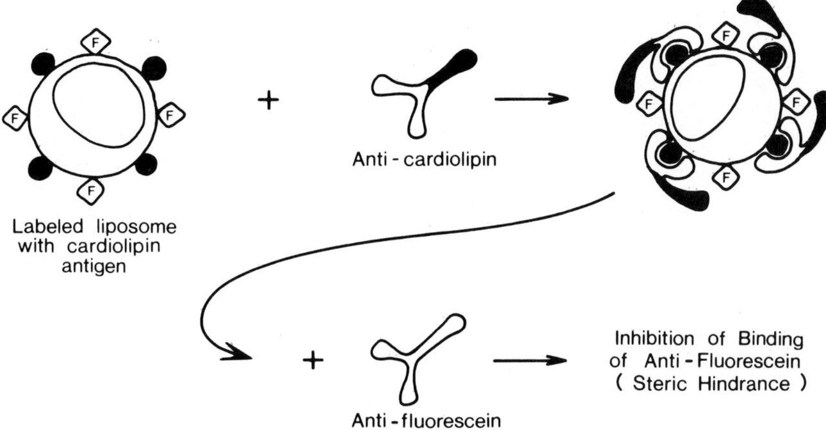

Figure 38–22. Fluorescence protection assay for anti-cardiolipin antibody. The protein antigen is labeled with fluorescein. Antibody specific for fluorescein will quench the fluorescence upon binding to the fluorophore-labeled antigen. The cardiolipin-specific antibody will sterically inhibit the reaction of the antibody specific for fluorescein. The degree of fluorescence measured is proportional to the concentration of cardiolipin-specific antibody.

and is a sensitive homogeneous assay. The rate of production of fluorescence is proportional to gentamicin concentration, and the fluorescent assay yielded values comparable to radioimmunoassay. The fluorescent assay requires 1 μl of serum and detects levels of gentamicin of less than 1 μg/ml. The assay procedure is completed in two to three minutes, and the fluorescence rate reaction is measured with an Aminco-Bowman spectrophotofluorometer equipped with temperature control for the sample compartment.

The SLFIA has been reported for measuring of 12 or more therapeutic drugs. In the case of large molecular weight proteins such as IgM, the SLFIA method has a working range of 0.5 and 5.0 g of IgM per liter when a 50-fold dilution of sera was used.

Special Instrumentation for Homogeneous Fluorescence Immunoassay Systems

Special methods and instrumentations have been developed to eliminate a separation step in fluorescence immunoassays. These include the fluorescence polarization immunoassay and the fluorescence correlation immunoassay with fluorescence-fluctuation spectrometer.

FLUORESCENCE POLARIZATION IMMUNOASSAY

A polarizing lens or prism can resolve light into rays in a single plane. When viewed at right angles to exciting beams of vertically polarized or natural light, fluorescent solutions emit partially polarized fluorescence. The fluorescence polarization principle was first applied to immunoassay procedures by Dandliker and colleagues (1970, 1973). The fluorescence polarization of a small fluorescent-labeled molecule tumbling freely in solution is very low. When the labeled molecule is complexed with antibody, the molecular motion is slowed and the fluorescence polarization is increased. These modulating changes of the fluorescence polarization may be measured to distinguish between free and antibody-bound fluorescent-labeled antigens.

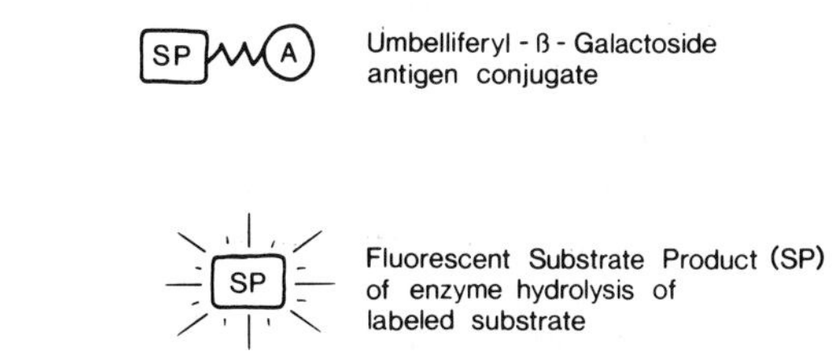

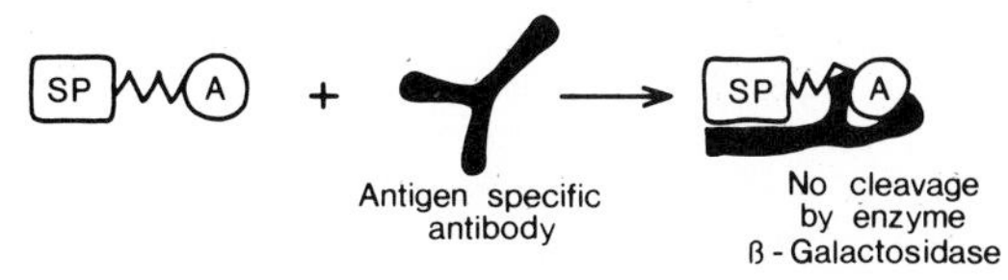

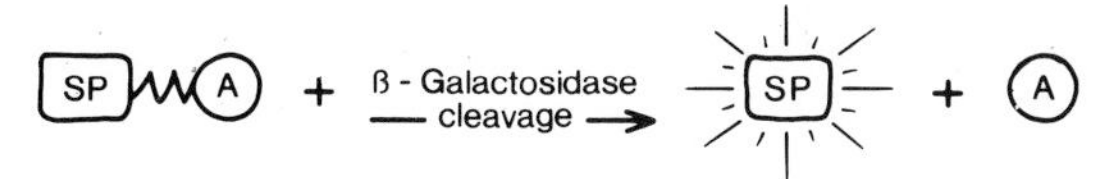

Figure 38–23. Principle of substrate labeled homogeneous fluorescence and enzyme immunoassay. The substrate umbelliferyl-β-galactoside is labeled with antigen. The substrate may be cleaved with formation of a fluorescent product by the enzyme β-galactosidase. When the substrate-labeled antigen is reacted with the antigen-specific antibody there is inhibition of cleavage by the enzyme β-galactosidase. In the assay system, the concentration of the free analyte is proportional to the amount of fluorescent product generated. This assay is applicable for haptens as well as complex protein antigens.

The method is useful for measurement of small fluorescent haptens, when such fluorescent protein antigens combine with antibody. Currently, it has been primarily used in the clinical laboratory to assay for drugs such as gentamicin. Its sensitivity is dependent upon the binding affinity of the antibody, but measures concentrations below 1 ng/ml of human chorionic gonadotropin.

Studies with labeled antibody or antibody fragments showed *no change* in polarization upon mixing antigen and labeled antibody even though there was other evidence that a reaction had occurred.

In the past, the clinical applications of fluorescence polarization have been limited by the high cost and lack of simple and reliable instruments. Recently, suitable instruments have been developed for fluorescence polarization with clinical laboratory immunoassays.

FLUORESCENCE CORRELATION IMMUNOASSAY WITH FLUORESCENCE-FLUCTUATION SPECTROMETER
(Nicoli, 1980; Briggs, 1981)

This method is based on correlations of fluctuation in particle number and measures fluorescent-labeled, antigen-bound microbeads. The assay system does not require a separation step since the instrumentation is programmed to be insensitive to background sources of fluorescence. The complete assay can detect 1 ng of gentamicin/ml in sample volume of 10 μl.

It is a modification of a method to determine the molecular weight of DNA using fluorescent dye binding. The technique is based on two physical phenomena: the number of *fluctuations* of particles with a fixed solution volume due to random Brownian motion, and the diffusion of particles in which the diffusion coefficient is inversely related to particle size.

The immunological reaction must take place on the surfaces of micrometer carrier particles such as latex or acrylamide beads. An instrument is designed to measure the concentration of labeled antigen-antibody complexes while ignoring background unbound fluorescent molecules. This is done by correlating rapid fluctuations in fluorescence with smaller unbound molecules and slower fluctuations with the larger antigen-antibody complexes.

A photomultiplier can detect fluorescence in a volume as small as 10^{-6} ml. A microprocessor is required to calculate and interpret the fluctuating signals.

Other Special Instrumentation for Fluorescence Immunoassays to Increase Sensitivity

Certain innovative instrumentations have been designed to increase sensitivity of the fluorescence immunoassays. The most promising method involves time-resolved fluorimetry.

TIME-RESOLVED FLUORIMETRY
(Soini, 1979, 1983)

This method involves use of fluorescent labels with relatively long half-lives and a pulsed source for exciting fluorescence with a time-resolved fluorometer for eliminating unwanted background fluorescence which usually has a short decay period. The fluorophores which have been used are the pyrene-duty rate derivatives with a decay time of almost 100 nanoseconds, and rare earth metal chelate labels which have a very long decay time of almost 50 to 1000 microseconds.

In time-resolved fluorometers a fast light pulse which excites the fluorophores is used and the fluorescence is measured after a certain time has elapsed from the moment of excitation. With fluorescent probes with a long decay time of over 100 nanoseconds, direct scattering can be removed as well as the nonspecific background fluorescence. The background fluorescent decay times are usually less than 10 nanoseconds. Thus, time-resolved fluorimetry is a suitable way to improve sensitivity over conventional methods of measurements.

Further investigation is needed to determine the use of the rare earth metal chelates as fluorescence probes in immunoassays. The metal chelate label must not alter the standard kinetics of an antigen-antibody and not denature the binding protein. Further, it should be able to fluoresce in an aqueous solution.

Summary of Analytical FIA

Immunofluorescent assays currently being developed have great potential. The fluorescent assay can be developed to have equal or greater sensitivity than current radioimmunoassay procedures. The advantages of immunofluorescent assays are stability of reagents, high sensitivity and speed of measurement, adaptability to automation, sensitive homogeneous systems which do not require separation, and systems which assay multiple constituents in one single assay procedure on the same specimen sample.

The disadvantages of the immunofluorescent procedures are special expensive instrumentation to obtain sensitive assays, and special immunochemically purified, labeled antibody reagents and fluorophore labels to reduce background fluorescence.

ENZYME IMMUNOASSAYS

Background and Classification

The use of enzymes as immunochemical labels in place of radionuclides for use in competitive binding assays was reported in 1971 (Avrameas, 1971).

The most widely used names are ELISA—enzyme-linked immunosorbent assay; EIA—enzyme immunoassay; and EMIT—enzyme-multiplied immunoassay technique (registered trade name of Syva Corp., Palo Alto, California).

The EIA are capable of detecting extremely small quantities of immune reactants. The advantages and disadvantages of EIA are listed in Table 38–5. EIA

Table 38–5. ENZYME IMMUNOASSAYS (EIA): ADVANTAGES AND DISADVANTAGES*

A. Advantages:
   1. Sensitive assays can be developed by the amplification effect of enzymes
   2. Reagents are relatively cheap and can have a long shelf life
   3. Multiple simultaneous assays can be developed
   4. A wide variety of assay configurations can be developed
   5. Equipment can be inexpensive and is widely available
   6. No radiation hazards occur during labeling or disposal of wastes
   7. Rapid simple EIA adaptable to automation can be developed
   8. Homogeneous EIA can be developed for haptens and proteins

B. Disadvantages
   1. Measurement of enzyme activity can be more complex than measurement of the activity of some types of radioisotopes
   2. Enzyme activity may be affected by plasma constituents
   3. Homogeneous assays at the present time have the sensitivity of 10^{-9} M and are not as sensitive as radioimmunoassays
   4. Homogeneous EIA for large protein molecules have been developed but require complex immunochemical reagents

*From O'Sullivan, M. J., et al.: Ann. Clin. Biochem., *16*:221, 1979.

may be classified by (1) which reactant is determined, i.e., antigen or antibody; (2) which reactant is labeled; (3) competitive or non-competitive assay; and (4) method of separation of bound and free reactants. There are several important criteria in the selection of a particular enzyme label, including (1) turnover number—number of substrate molecules converted to product per enzyme site/unit of time; (2) purity; (3) sensitivity; (4) ease and speed of detection; (5) absence of interfering factors in test fluid; (6) potential reactive groups; (7) stability; and (8) suitability for homogeneous EIA. Table 38–6 lists the commonly used enzymes in heterogeneous and homogeneous assays.

There are two major types of EIA—heterogeneous and homogeneous. In the heterogeneous system, the antigen-antibody reaction does not affect the activity of the enzyme label. In homogeneous EIA, the antigen-antibody interaction modulates the activity of the enzyme. Modulation of enzyme activity eliminates the need for a separation step.

The term ELISA (enzyme-linked immunosorbent assay) was first used by Engvall and Perlmann (1971) and identifies a heterogeneous enzyme assay differentiating it from enzyme linked antibody conjugates used in microscopic immunohistochemical staining reactions. ELISA may be developed in several different configurations, and one of the reactants is immobilized onto a solid phase matrix (Voller, 1978).

Table 38–6. ENZYMES COMMONLY USED IN VARIOUS EIA

Enzymes used in heterogeneous EIA
- Horseradish peroxidase
- Alkaline phosphatase
- β-D galactosidase
- Glucose oxidase
- Glucoamylase
- Carbonic anhydrase
- Acetylcholinesterase
- Catalase

Enzymes used in homogeneous EIA
- Lysozyme
- Malate dehydrogenase
- Glucose-6-phosphate dehydrogenase
- Phospholipase-C
- β-D galactosidase

Heterogeneous EIA

The principles involved in heterogeneous EIA are similar to those for radioimmunoassays except that enzyme activity is measured instead of radioactivity. The choice of the separation phase in heterogeneous EIA is limited by the large size of the enzyme label. Acceptable methods include double antibody precipitation, use of solid phase antigen or antibody, or use of beads such as agarose or polyacrylamide. Some investigators have utilized magnetic beads for an ingenious separation system (Guesdon, 1978). The commonly employed heterogeneous EIA are (1) competitive EIA for antigen, (2) immunoenzymometric assay, (3) two site immunoenzymometric assay, (4) sandwich assay for antibody detection, and (5) double antibody immunoenzymometric assay for antigen determination.

COMPETITIVE EIA FOR ANTIGEN (OR HAPTEN)

This method is similar to the classic antigen-labeled RIA. It is a competitive EIA between the unlabeled antigen and enzyme labeled antigen which are competing for a limited amount of specific antibody binding sites. The amount of enzyme-labeled antigen bound by antibody is inversely proportional to the concentration of the unlabeled antigen.

The disadvantage of this method is that significant amounts of pure antigen must be isolated to label with enzyme.

IMMUNOENZYMOMETRIC ASSAY (Maiolini, 1975)

In this EIA, the reactants are in stoichiometric excess. The enzyme-labeled antibody is first reacted

5

with antigen, and excess solid phase antigen is then added to remove unreacted enzyme labeled antibody. The enzyme activity bound to the solid phase is inversely proportional to the concentration of the free antigen.

This configuration may be used to assay for small hapten molecules which cannot be easily assayed by the two-site immunoenzymometric assay (sandwich assay method for antigens). As long as the enzyme-labeled antibody is specific, the antigen does not have to be isolated in pure form.

TWO-SITE IMMUNOENZYMOMETRIC ASSAY (SANDWICH ASSAY FOR ANTIGEN)

A solid phase antibody is first incubated with the antigen to be measured. After washing, enzyme-labeled antibody is then added. The enzyme activity bound to the solid phase is proportional to the concentration of the antigen present. This method is useful for measuring complex antigens and can be used only for antigens which are able to bind at least two antibodies. Monoclonal antibodies reactive at different antigenic sites, one labeled and the second unlabeled solid phase, may be incubated with the unknown antigen simultaneously.

SANDWICH ASSAY FOR ANTIBODY DETECTION (Engvall, 1972)

The solid phase antigen is incubated with a sample containing the antibody to be detected. After the reaction and appropriate washing, the enzyme-labeled second antibody is added. The second antibody is reactive against the first antibody. The amount of enzyme activity found bound to the solid phase is directly proportional to the amount of antigen-specific antibody. This assay is analogous to the radioallergosorbent method.

DOUBLE ANTIBODY IMMUNOENZYMOMETRIC ASSAY FOR ANTIGEN DETERMINATION

This method employs a solid phase antigen. Free antigen prevents antigen-specific antibody from binding to the solid phase. The solid phase is then washed and reacted with enzyme labeled second antibody reactive against the first antibody. The amount of enzyme labeled second antibody bound to the solid phase is inversely proportional to the quantity of the free antigen in the sample (Gnemmi, 1978).

The advantage of this method is that one enzyme labeled antibody can measure many different antigens.

Homogeneous Enzyme Immunoassays

The term homogeneous immunoassay may be applied to any antigen-antibody reaction system in which the measurement of the degree of immune reaction is carried out without a separation of the "free" and the antibody-bound components. Homogeneous enzyme immunoassays have been used for assay of drugs and hormones in the clinical laboratory since the report of Rubenstein (1972). At present, homogeneous enzyme immunoassays are generally less sensitive than heterogeneous enzyme immunoassays. The heterogeneous enzyme immunoassays have equalled the sensitivity of RIA in many applications, whereas the homogeneous enzyme immunoassays may be of one or two orders of magnitude less sensitive than RIA. Homogeneous enzyme immunoassays may require complex immunochemical reagents; however, the systems are rapid, simple, and adaptable to automation. Currently, the chief application of homogeneous enzyme immunoassays is in the determination of low molecular weight analytes such as hormones and drugs. More recently, homogeneous enzyme immunoassay methods have been developed for complex higher molecular weight protein antigens such as IgG (Gibbons, 1980).

There are various types of homogeneous enzyme immunoassays. In each of these assays, the antigen-antibody interaction modulates the activity of the enzyme or enzyme label in the presence of substrate. The modulation of the enzyme activity reflects the degree of the immunochemical reaction. The types of labeled homogeneous enzyme immunoassays are listed in Table 38–7.

ENZYME LABEL

The analyte is covalently labeled with enzyme, and antibody to analyte modulates the activity of the enzyme. The Syva Company, Palo Alto, California, has developed this type of EIA under the trademark EMIT (enzyme multiplied immunoassay technique) for the major antiepileptic, cardioactive, antiasthmatic, antineoplastic, and "abuse" drugs. The EMIT assay system is diagrammed in Figure 38–24. Conjugation of the enzyme to the hapten does not destroy the enzyme activity. However, binding of hapten-specific antibody to the hapten results in inhibition of enzyme activity. Free hapten in the standards or samples relieves this inhibition by competing for antibody. Thus, in the presence of antibody, the enzyme activity is proportional to the concentration of the free hapten. In the usual case, the antibody probably inhibits the enzyme by inducing or preventing conformational changes necessary for enzyme activity (Rowley, 1975).

The exception to the inhibition mechanism is the EMIT thyroxine assay with use of the malate dehydrogenase enzyme. In this instance, the thyroxine–malate dehydrogenase conjugate is enzymatically inactive but activated when bound by thyroxine antibodies (Ullman, 1975). It is believed that the conjugated thyroxine inhibits the enzyme by binding to

Table 38–7. TYPES OF LABELED HOMOGENEOUS ENZYME IMMUNOASSAYS

1. Enzyme
2. Substrate
3. Cofactor
4. Prosthetic group
5. Enzyme modulator
6. Enzyme labeled antibody

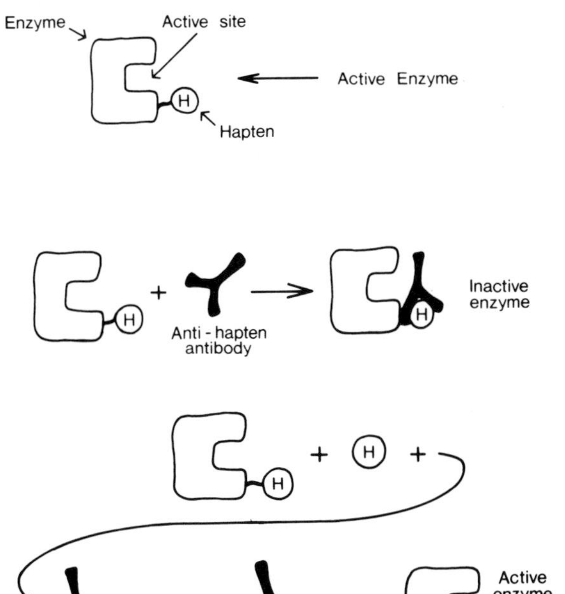

Figure 38–24. Principle of EMIT homogeneous enzyme immunoassay. EMIT (enzyme multiplied immunoassay technique) is useful for assay of haptens and drug molecules. The enzyme is covalently linked with the analyte, and specific antibody to the analyte may increase or decrease the enzyme activity. In this figure the specific antibody to the hapten analyte induces inhibition of the enzyme activity. In the assay, the free hapten analyte will compete for the antibody and the enzyme activity is proportional to the concentration of the free hapten.

the active site, so increasing the "apparent" Km of the substrate. The antibody reactivates the enzyme by "pulling" the thyroxine out from the active site (Fig. 38–25).

In the EMIT assay system, malate dehydrogenase and glucose-6-phosphate dehydrogenase were found to be most useful because they were less likely affected by constituents of serum. These assays generally measure drug in the concentration of mg/liter. However, the digoxin assay has a much lower limit of sensitivity, in the range of 1 μg/liter.

SUBSTRATE LABEL

An enzyme substrate is covalently labeled with an analyte so that binding of the substrate by antibody sterically inhibits enzyme from acting on its substrate. This novel homogeneous substrate labeled fluorescent immunoassay (SLFIA) has been described above in the section on Analytical Fluorescence Immunoassays. It can be used to assay not only drugs and haptens but protein ligands such as IgG and IgM.

A disadvantage of this method is that the amplification properties of the enzyme are not utilized, and thus the assay system has limited sensitivity in the range of 10^{-9} to 10^{-10} molar concentration of the analyte.

COFACTOR

An antigen or analyte is covalently bound to an enzyme cofactor, and the specific antibody to the analyte prevents the cofactor from combining with an appropriate apo-enzyme (Boguslaski, 1982). A number of enzyme cofactor-analyte conjugates have been used to monitor homogeneous enzyme immunoassays. Nicotinamide adenine denucleotide (NAD) has been desensitized and covalently coupled to biotin or 2,4-dinitrophenol (DNP) to form conjugates. NAD is a cofactor involved in the lactic dehydrogenase and diaphorase enzyme reactions. The activity of the cofactor conjugate could be inhibited by the addition of a specific binding protein. For example, coenzyme cycling reaction for estriol measurement has been reported (Kohen, 1978). An estriol-NAD conjugate was cycled using malic and alcoholic dehydrogenases, and the amount of NADPH formed was measured fluorometrically. The cycling was inhibited by IgG antibody to estriol. The assay sensitivity was 2 nanomoles and was sufficient to measure estriol from plasma samples. The disadvantage of this type of assay is that endogenous cofactors and degrading enzymes

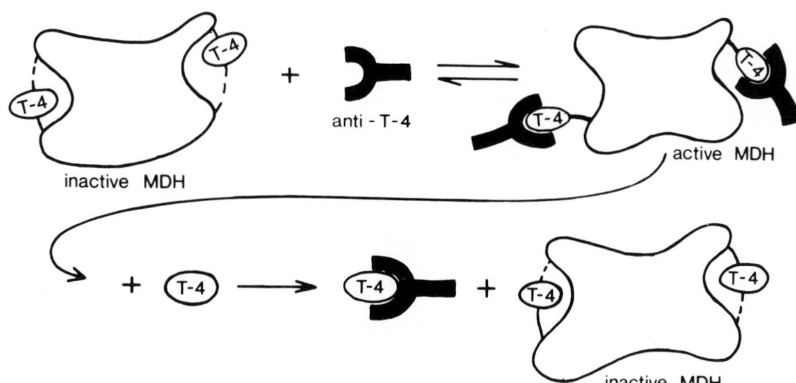

Figure 38–25. Homogeneous EMIT assay for thyroxine (T-4). The EMIT assay for thyroxine utilizes the enzyme malate dehydrogenase (MDH). In this assay the malate dehydrogenase–thyroxine conjugate is enzymatically inactive and binding of specific anti-thyroxine antibodies to the conjugate *increases* the enzyme activity. The concentration of thyroxine in the sample to be measured is inversely proportional to the activity of malate dehydrogenase measured.

in biological samples may interfere with the immunochemical reaction.

PROSTHETIC GROUP LABEL

Similar to cofactor labels, prosthetic groups such as flavin adenine dinucleotide (FAD) can serve as labels in homogeneous enzyme immunoassays (Fig. 38–26). The analyte and a constant amount of analyte-FAD compete for a limited amount of specific antibody binding sites. At equilibrium, the level of free conjugate is proportional to the amount of analyte in the specimen sample and can be determined by the addition of apoglucose oxidase to the reaction mixture. The apoenzyme combines with the free but not the antibody-bound form of the conjugate to generate glucose oxidase in proportion to the amount of free conjugate in the mixture. The active enzyme is generated in the procedure, and an amplification mechanism is also built into this assay. The procedure has been used to assay for theophylline and IgG (Boguslaski, 1982).

ENZYME MODULATOR LABEL

Ngo and Lenhoff (1980) have reported on the enzyme modulator approach to homogeneous enzyme immunoassays. An enzyme modulator may be an antibody, inhibitor, or receptor to the indicator enzyme. The modulator is covalently linked to a ligand that is similar to the analyte so that the amount of modulator free to modify the available indicator enzyme is dependent upon the amount of analyte to be determined. This approach provides built-in amplifying power because the inhibited enzyme can continuously generate products.

ENZYME LABELED ANTIBODY

Phospholipase C has been conjugated to rabbit anti-human IgG. The enzyme activity of the conjugate was inhibited by human IgG but not by rabbit or goat IgG. The substrates used for the enzyme were phospholipids, which formed part of the membrane of erythrocytes (Wei, 1977). Human IgG sterically prevents access of the enzyme label to the substrate which is probably immobilized in the membrane. The appropriate attachment of the substrate to solid matrices may be effective for inhibiting the enzyme activity of the labeled antibody. Because of the mechanism of steric hindrance, large molecular weight antigens are more likely to yield homogeneous assays in this system.

Summary

EIA can be applied to all antigen-antibody systems and include serum proteins, hormones, drugs, and a wide variety of other antigens and antibodies directed against them.

The EIA are affected by certain factors other than those which influence RIA systems: (1) The measurement of enzyme activity requires the addition of substrate and usually a timed addition of reagent to terminate the reaction. This additional step decreases the precision of the EIA when compared to RIA. (2) In EIA, certain compounds and constituents in biological samples may affect the specific enzyme activity and introduce an error. This may be a special problem in some of the homogeneous EIA where one desires a high degree of sensitivity and precision.

EIA methods have been developed with comparable sensitivity to those of RIA. The EIA have become established in many clinical laboratories and are generally being employed for (1) homogeneous assay of low molecular weight compounds such as drugs and antibiotics present in biological samples at relatively high concentrations; (2) qualitative and semiquantitative assays for viral, bacterial, fungal, and parasitic antigens and antibodies; (3) tissue immunohistochemical localization of antigens and antibodies; and (4) alternatives to RIA in smaller laboratories.

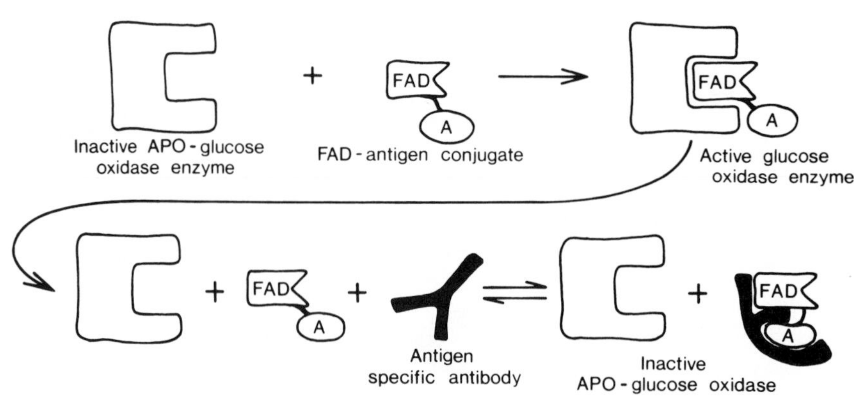

Figure 38–26. Prosthetic group–labeled antigen (ligand)–homogeneous enzyme immunoassay. The prosthetic group flavin adenine dinucleotide (FAD) is conjugated to the analyte (A). FAD is necessary for the glucose oxidase enzyme activity. Specific antibody to the analyte which reacts with FAD-analyte conjugate will inhibit the generation of an active glucose oxidase enzyme. In the assay the concentration of analyte is proportional to the enzyme activity generated. The assay has been used to measure theophylline and IgG.

PRODUCTION AND APPLICATION OF MONOCLONAL ANTIBODIES

Monoclonal antibodies are homogeneous immunoglobulins directed at a single epitope or antigenic determinant and therefore are uniform chemical reagents (Kennett, 1980). The production of monospecific antibodies by monoclonal cell lines derived from a hybridization of myeloma cells and sensitized lymphocytes was launched by Kohler and Milstein in 1975. Monoclonal antibodies are theoretically ideal reagents since all the antibody molecules are identical, are produced continuously from the same cell clone, and thus can be readily standardized.

Conventional and Monoclonal Antisera: Advantages and Disadvantages

Conventional antisera so far used in the diagnostic clinical laboratory are from two sources: (1) heteroantisera, produced by immunizing lower animal species; and (2) alloantisera, produced by cross-immunizing individuals within a species (e.g., sera of multiparous women containing anti-HLA antibodies). Heteroantisera and alloantisera have drawbacks: (1) Batches of antisera may differ with respect to the antibody affinity and specificity since each antiserum is an uncontrolled mixture of polyclonal antibodies. Conventional antisera will contain a broad variety of antibodies with different affinities and Ig classes even for each individual antigenic site. (2) Conventional antisera are limited by quantities and by titer.

Monoclonal antibodies have several unique properties: (1) A monoclonal antibody is derived from one isolated clone and is a well defined reagent, homogeneous in structure, and therefore in immunoreactivity. (2) The methodology for production of monoclonal antibodies allows for production of homogeneous reagents in virtually unlimited quantities. (3) The method is suitable for preparation and isolation of pure monoclonal antibodies with use of non-purified antigens.

There has been considerable experience with murine monoclonal antibodies. Certain disadvantages have been reported: fixed affinity which, if low, may make the antibody unsuitable for use in a very sensitive assay system; limited biological activity; lack of precipitating or agglutinating properties; and unusual sensitivity to changes in pH or salt concentration.

Thus, it is possible that monoclonal antibodies may be inferior to existing conventional antibodies in certain assay systems. Furthermore, polyclonal antibodies may be of particular value in specific applications in providing a "fingerprint" of the multiple determinants of a single antigen.

Methods for Production of Monoclonal Antibodies

Monoclonal antibodies can be produced by use of several different methods. The most common method involves use of the hybridoma technology initiated by Kohler and Milstein (1975). This technology consists of fusing B lymphocytes to murine myeloma cells to form hybrid (hybridoma) cells that will grow in continuous cell culture and produce monospecific "monoclonal" antibodies. This is made possible by use of an appropriately enzyme deficient myeloma cell (such as HGPRT deficiency) and selective media. The enzyme-deficient myeloma cells which have not undergone fusion fail to grow in selective media. The hybrid cells gain the critical enzyme from the immune B cells and thus grow. By limiting-dilution cloning and appropriate assays, the progeny of a single clone making antibody of a single class and specificity may be isolated.

Hybridoma cells can be frozen and stored indefinitely, and can be easily distributed to different hospitals and laboratories. The antibodies can be produced by growth of the specific hybridoma in tissue culture or produced *in vivo* in mouse ascites.

Besides the hybridoma methods, two other methods have been used for production of monoclonal antibodies. They are (1) *in vitro* viral transformation of sensitized lymphocytes to form continuous antibody producing cells (Steinitz, 1978), and (2) hybrid fusion of sensitized lymphocytes and a continuous B lymphocytic cell line (Lundak, 1983).

HYBRIDOMA METHODOLOGY

The hybridoma is an artificially created cell formed by fusing an antibody secreting lymphocyte and myeloma cell. The following hybridomas have been developed for production of monoclonal antibodies: (1) mouse lymphocyte—mouse myeloma; (2) rat lymphocyte—mouse myeloma; (3) human lymphocyte—mouse myeloma; (4) rat lymphocyte—rat myeloma; and (5) human lymphocyte—human myeloma.

The murine myeloma cells have been the most successful and now most widely used. The human lymphocyte–mouse myeloma cells which produce human antibody show preferential loss of human chromosomes, often undergoing a mutation resulting in loss of production of the specific antibody.

Many murine myeloma cell lines are available for production of hybridomas, and the commonly used ones are listed in Table 38–8. The myeloma may be of the secreting or non-secreting variety. The cell lines are selected so that they have drug markers and are resistant to the azoguanine drugs. Because these cell lines lack the enzyme hypoxanthine guanine phosphoribosyl transferase (HGPRT), they cannot synthesize nucleotides when grown in a medium containing hypoxanthine, aminopterin, and thymidine (HAT). HGPRT negative cells cannot divide because the main pathway is blocked by the presence of aminopterin and the salvage pathway is partially blocked by the lack of HGPRT.

A significant breakthrough in technology resulted from the selection of special murine myeloma cell lines. First, a non-secreting myeloma cell line which would produce the immunoglobulin of the fused-sensitized lymphocyte was developed. Next, murine cell lines which had drug markers and were deficient

Table 38–8. CHARACTERISTICS OF HAT-SENSITIVE MOUSE MYELOMA CELL LINES COMMONLY USED FOR SOMATIC CELL HYBRIDIZATION

Short Name	Complete Name	IgG Secretion
X63	P3-X63-Ag8	IgG1, κ
NS-I	Pe-NSI/1-Ag4-1	Intracellular, κ
Sp2/0	Sp2/0 Ag14	Nonsecreting, κ
—	X63-Ag8.653	Nonsecreting, κ
X45	MPC 11-X45-6TG	IgG2b, κ

in certain enzymes were developed. These enzyme deficient cell lines have allowed selective growth in special media of hybrid cells over the parental myeloma cells.

MONOCLONAL ANTIBODIES BY *IN VITRO* TRANSFORMATION OF SENSITIZED LYMPHOCYTES

This method consists of the transformation of a specifically sensitized immune lymphocyte to a continuous lymphoblastoid cell line which produces a monoclonal antibody. Several investigators have reported production of human monoclonal antibodies by transforming sensitized lymphocytes bearing Epstein-Barr virus (EBV) receptors with continuous antibody-secreting human B cell lines.

In principle, immune lymphocytes isolated from a donor or lymphocytes sensitized *in vitro* may be fractionated first to yield an enriched antigen-bearing subpopulation. These antigen-bearing lymphocytes are then infected with supernatants of mycoplasma-free marmoset cell line B95-8 derived EBV. Established cell lines are then tested for antibody secretion and/or antigen-bearing cells. The antibody-secreting population may be enriched by selection for antigen-bearing cells. However, since EBV-transformed B cell lines remain polyclonal for a long time after establishment, the cell lines have to be cloned either by limiting dilution or on soft agar with feeder cells.

Zurawski (1980) has developed human lymphoblastoid cell lines to produce specific monoclonal antibodies by transforming sensitized human lymphocytes with EBV. By this technique, specific human monoclonal antibodies to NNP (4-OH-3,5 dinitrophenoacetic acid) and tetanus toxoid have been produced. Steinitz (1978) has reported that the monoclonal anti-NNP antibodies secreted by three preselected lines were of the IgM kappa type, which was in contrast to the Ig classes of the donor sera which contained both IgM and IgG antibodies.

MONOCLONAL ANTIBODY PRODUCTION BY HYBRID FUSION OF SENSITIZED LYMPHOCYTE AND CONTINUOUS B-LYMPHOCYTIC CELL LINE

Human tonsillar lymphocytes were sensitized *in vitro* with sheep erythrocytes and fused with a Wil-2 lymphoblastoid cell line. The Wil-2 lymphoblastoid cell line is a continuous human B lymphocyte cell line which has been "immortalized" or transformed using the Epstein-Barr (EB) virus. The EB viral genome has been incorporated into the nuclear DNA of the Wil-2 cell.

In this method, the Wil-2 cells were cultured and a mutant cell line was selected for a drug resistant marker with deficiency of the HGPRT enzyme. The mutant cell line was further cloned for high fusion efficiency.

In the formation of antibody producing hybrid cells, the drug resistant lymphoblastoid cell line was then fused with the immune lymphocytes in the presence of polyethylene glycol (PEG). The resulting hybridomas were first screened for antibody secretion and then cloned either by limiting-dilution or on soft agar with feeder cells.

Lundak and Malachowski (1983) have developed several continuous hybrid cell lines which produce monoclonal antibodies specific for sheep erythrocyte antigen. Seventeen of the 22 hybrid cell lines secreted human immunoglobulin, and six of these secreted monoclonal antibodies to drugs (gentamicin, phenytoin, tobramycin, and theophylline), human antigens (C1q receptor, factor VIII, factor VIII-C, melanoma-associated antigens), and mouse cytomegalovirus, DNA, ribonucleoprotein, and mouse histocompatibility antigens.

The general method of production of mouse monoclonal antibodies is illustrated in Figure 38–27. The various steps involved in the production of the monoclonal antibody are outlined in Table 38–9. After fusion, one transfers small aliquots of the cells to a larger number of cells in a tissue culture plate and, after several days, inspects the cells to see if they contain growing colonies. The next major step is to screen the cell supernatant fluids in such cells for the presence of the desired monoclonal antibody. Since the concentration of the monoclonal antibody is in the order of micrograms per milliliter, screening is often carried out by a radioimmunoassay or by enzyme immunoassay.

Because a well containing fused cells may contain more than one hybridoma, the next step is to "clone" the cells. This is often done by the limiting dilution method with use of feeder cells. The separate hybridoma colonies then may be products of one or a very small number of cells. Such individual colonies may be recloned to establish a single homogeneous cell line producing the desired monoclonal antibody. The hybridoma cell line producing the desired antibody may be expanded by *in vitro* culturing methods or by *in vivo* passage by injection into the peritoneal cavity of the mouse. The ascitic fluid obtained from the

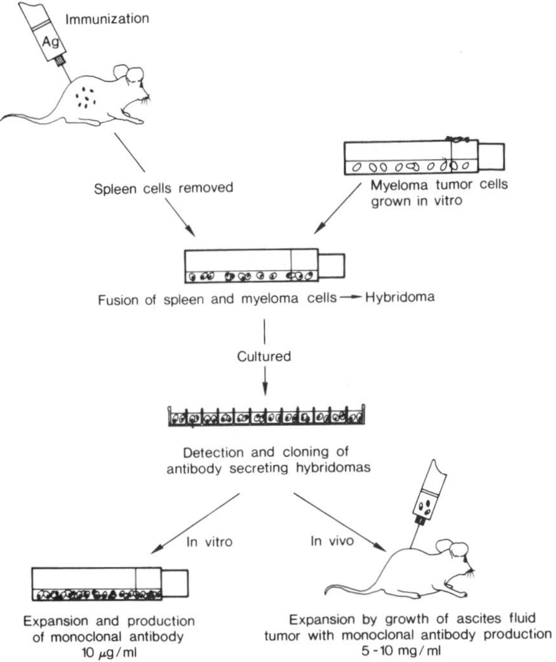

Figure 38–27. General method of production of mouse monoclonal antibody from mouse-mouse hybridomas. The figure shows the various steps such as immunization, fusion of spleen and myeloma cells, detection and cloning of antibody secreting hybridomas, and *in vitro* and *in vivo* expansion of the specific hybridoma.

hybridoma cells may contain 1 to 10 ng/ml of specific monoclonal antibody.

Characterization of the Monoclonal Antibody

Hybridomas and monoclonal antibodies should be characterized in a number of ways: (1) Fusion partners—a description of myeloma cell, antibody producing cells, culture media, passage level, and cloning. (2) Immunogen used and schedule of immunization. (3) Antibody type—Ig type, including isotype and idiotype when applicable. (4) Specificity of antibody—characterization includes antigenic determinant reactivity, affinity constants for a series of defined antigens, yields and titers of antibody produced, *in vitro* or *in vivo*.

Table 38–9. STEPS IN PRODUCTION AND STORAGE OF MOUSE MONOCLONAL ANTIBODY BY THE HYBRIDOMA METHODOLOGY

1. Selection of mouse myeloma line
2. Immunization of mouse with specific antigen for production of sensitized spleen cells
   a. Preparation of spleen cells for fusion
3. Hybridization
4. Assay for specific antibody production by hybridomas
5. Cloning hybridomas by limiting dilution
6. Characterization of monoclonal antibody
7. Mass production
   a. *In vitro* expansion
   b. *In vivo* expansion
8. Freezing and storing hybridomas
   a. Reconstitution

Specific Applications of Monoclonal Antibodies (Nakamura, 1983)

There are several areas of application in which monoclonal antibodies are uniquely suited. In many basic research and clinical applications it has been extremely difficult to characterize specific antigenic determinants with use of the conventional polyclonal antisera. Areas in which monoclonal antibodies are most useful include (1) immunogenic histocompatibility or differentiation antigens; (2) differentiation, tumor, or cell surface antigens that lack polymorphism and are not immunogenic in allogeneic systems but are recognized in xenogenic immunization; (3) viral and bacterial antigens; and (4) single antigenic determinants in a wide variety of proteins, nucleic acids, polysaccharides, etc.

The technique of generating monoclonal antibodies is revolutionizing the isolation and characterization of cell surface histocompatibility markers as well as the identification of specific bacterial and viral proteins. A significant advantage of hybridoma technology is the ability to produce a pure antibody with use of an impure antigen. Monoclonal methodology enables researchers to identify and purify substances with rare specificity such as cellular differentiation antigens, tumor antigens, and hormone receptors.

Within the next several years, monoclonal antibodies should play a significant role in advancing the fundamental knowledge of malignant processes. Monoclonal antibodies have been developed to carcinoembryonic antigens, alpha fetoprotein, and human tumor specific antigens such as colorectal carcinoma antigen, human melanoma, and human breast carcinoma antigens.

In the future, one may perhaps use a panel of monoclonal antibodies to identify specific tumor cell types. Since monoclonal antibodies appear to react to well defined epitopes, a monoclonal antibody found to recognize a human tumor antigen could be used to isolate the specific tumor associated antigen in order to produce more monoclonal antibodies. The various specific monoclonal antibodies to different epitopes on the specific molecule could perhaps be used in combination to confirm the presence of a specific molecule. Thus, it is possible that a panel of specific monoclonal antibodies may be used to identify organ specific tumor-associated antigens.

Many potential commercial applications of monoclonal antibodies have been described. Some applications follow.

1. Provision of specific reproducible diagnostic immunoassays for current laboratory tests (e.g., steroid hormone, polypeptide and protein hormone, immunohematology, hepatitis associated antigens, cancer

assays [CEA, AFP], therapeutic drug monitoring assays, abused drug monitoring).

2. Provision of new diagnostic tests for antigenic determinants not currently distinguished by conventional antisera. Monoclonal antibodies are specific for species and subspecies cell surface and cytoplasmic antigens.

3. Typing of genetic variants of viruses, proteins, and enzymes.

4. Specific and reproducible tissue typing reagents for HLA antigens and other histocompatibility antigens.

5. Immunoadsorbent reagents for specific isolation of antigens, such as estrogen and progesterone receptors.

6. Identification and isolation of cell receptors such as estrogen, progesterone, thyroid stimulating hormone, and acetylcholine receptors.

7. Identification of gene protein products in recombinant DNA experiments.

8. Identification of single antigenic determinants on a wide variety of proteins, nucleic acids, polysaccharides, etc.

9. *In vivo* diagnosis and therapeutic applications for cancer and other diseases involving infection by foreign antigens. Therapeutic applications include immunotherapy and use of antibodies as therapeutic carriers of drugs or cytotoxic agents to a specific antigenic site.

Human Monoclonal Antibody Production

Human monoclonal antibodies to specific antigens will be ideal reagents for *in vivo* diagnosis as well as for *in vivo* therapy. In contrast to a xenogenic source of monoclonal antibody, the human monoclonal antibody will not elicit a host immune response and will avoid the risk of anaphylactic reactions, including serum sickness.

Xenogenic antibodies have already been used for *in vivo* localization of tumors through radioimmunoscintigraphy, localization of myocardial infarction with radiolabeled anti-cardiac myosin antibodies, and neutralization of digoxin toxicity.

Human monoclonal antibodies may be used *in vivo* for passive immunization to toxins and infectious agents; in modulation of immunity of transplant antigens; for detection of idiotypic sites on other antibody and cell surface receptors; as specific tumor antibodies in treatment and localization through radioimmunoscintigraphy; and in modulation or neutralization of drugs and hormones.

There are currently several different methods for production of human monoclonal antibodies. Further work needs to be performed on the technology of *in vitro* sensitization of human lymphoid cells in addition to finding stable and suitable human myeloma cell lines for fusion. In the future, rapid advances will undoubtedly be made in the diagnosis and therapy of tumors and infectious diseases, and in solving problems in many other disciplines of clinical medicine.

Avrameas, S., and Guilbert, B.: Dosage enzymo-immunologiaue de protéines à l'aide d'immunoabsorbants et d'antigènes marqués aux enzymes. C. R. Acad. Sci. Ser. D.:*273*:2705, 1971.

Axelsen, N. H. (ed.): Quantitative immunoelectrophoresis: New developments and applications. Scand. J. Immunol. (Suppl. 2), 1975.

Boguslaski, R. C., and Li, T. M.: Homogeneous immunoassays. Appl. Biochem. Biotechnology, 7:401, 1982.

Boguslaski, R. C., Li, T. M., Benovic, J. L., et al.: Substrate labeled homogeneous fluorescent immunoassays for haptens and proteins. *In* Nakamura, R. M., Dito, W. R., and Tucker, E. S. (eds.): Immunoassays: Clinical Laboratory Techniques for the 1980s. New York, Alan R. Liss, Inc., 1980, pp. 45–64.

Briggs, J., Elings, V. B., and Nicoli, D. F.: Homogeneous fluorescent immunoassay. Science, *212*:1266, 1981.

Burd, J. F., Wong, R. C., Feeney, J. E., Carrico, R. J., and Boguslaski, R. C.: Homogeneous reactant-labeled fluorescent immunoassay for therapeutic drugs exemplified by gentamicin determination in human serum. Clin. Chem., *23*:1402, 1977.

Cherry, W. B.: Immunofluorescence techniques. *In* Lennette, E. H., Balows, A., Hausler, W. J., and Truant, J. P. (eds.): Manual of Clinical Microbiology. 3rd ed. Washington, D.C., American Society of Microbiology, 1980.

Crowle, A. J.: Immunodiffusion. New York, Academic Press, 1961.

Dandliker, W. B., and de Saussure, V. A.: Fluorescence polarization in immunochemistry. Immunochemistry, *7*:799, 1970.

Dandliker, W. B., Kelly, R. J., Dandliker, J., et al.: Fluorescence polarization immunoassay. Theory and experimental method. Immunochemistry, *10*:219, 1973.

Engvall, E., and Perlmann, P.: Enzyme linked immunosorbent assay (ELISA). Quantitative assay of immunoglobulin G. Immunochemistry, *8*:871, 1971.

Engvall, E., and Perlmann, P.: Quantitation of specific antibodies by enzyme-labelled anti-immunoglobulin in antigen-coated tubes. J. Immunol., *109*:129, 1972.

Fahey, J. L., and McKelvey, E. M.: Quantitative determination of serum immunoglobulins in antibody-agar plates. J. Immunol., *94*:84, 1965.

Garvey, J. S., Cremer, N. E., and Sussdorf, D. H.: Methods in Immunology. 3rd ed. Reading, Mass., W. A. Benjamin, 1977, pp. 273–327.

Gibbons, I., Skold, C., Rowley, G. L., and Ullman, E. F.: Homogeneous enzyme immunoassay for proteins employing β-galactosidase. Anal. Biochem., *102*:167, 1980.

Gnemmi, E., O'Sullivan, M. J., Chieregatti, G., Simmons, M., Simmonds, A., Bridges, J. W., and Marks, V.: A sensitive immunoenzymometric assay (IEMA) to quantitate hormones and drugs. *In* Pal, S. B. (ed.): Enzyme-Linked Immunoassay of Hormones and Drugs. Berlin and New York, Walter de Gruyter, 1978, pp. 29–41.

Guesdon, J., Thierry, R., and Avrameas, S.: Magnetic EIA for measuring human IgE. J. Allerg. Clin. Immunol., *61*:23, 1978.

Hudson, L., and Hay, F. C.: Practical Immunology. London, Blackwell Scientific Publications, 1976.

Kabat, E. A.: Kabat and Mayer's Experimental Immunochemistry. 2nd ed. Springfield, Ill., Charles C Thomas, Publisher, 1961.

Kawamura, A., Jr.: Fluorescent Antibody Techniques and Their Applications. Baltimore, University Park Press, 1977.

Kennett, R. H., McKearn, T. J., and Bechtol, K. B.: Monoclonal Antibodies. Hybridomas: A New Dimension in Biological Analyses. New York, Plenum Press, 1980.

Kohen, F., Hollander, Z., Yeager, F. M., Carrico, R. J., and Boguslaski, R. C.: A homogeneous EIA for oestriol monitored by co-enzymatic cycling reactions. *In* Pal, S. B. (ed.): Enzyme-Linked Immunoassay of Hormones and Drugs. Berlin and New York, Walter de Gruyter, 1978, pp. 67–79.

Kohler, G., and Milstein, C.: Continuous cultures of fused cells secreting antibody of predefined specificity. Nature, *256*:495, 1975.

Kwapinski, J. B. G.: Methodology of Immunochemical and Immunological Research. New York, Wiley-Interscience, Inc., 1972.

Larson, C., Orenstein, B., and Ritchie, R. F.: An automated method for quantitation of proteins in body fluids. *In* Advances in Automated Analysis, Vol. 1. Technicon International Congress. Miami, Thurman Associates, 1970, pp. 101–104.

Lundak, R. L., and Malachowski, R. M.: Production of human-

human hybridomas secreting specific antibody following in vitro immunization. Proc. Nat. Acad. Sci., in press, 1983.

Maggio, E. T.: Recent advances in heterogeneous fluorescence immunoassays. *In* Nakamura, R. M., Dito, W. R., and Tucker, E. S. (eds.): Immunoassays: Clinical Laboratory Techniques for the 1980s. New York, Alan R. Liss, Inc., 1980, pp. 1–10.

Maggio, E. T., and Nakamura, R. M.: Immunology: Current and future technology assessment. Clin. Lab. Med., *1*:77, 1981.

Maiolini, B., Ferrua, B., and Masseyeff, R.: Enzyme immunoassay of human alphafoetoprotein. J. Immunol. Method., *6*:355, 1975.

Mancini, G., Carbonara, A. O., and Heremans, J. F.: Immunochemical quantitation of antigens by single radial immunodiffusion. Immunochemistry, *2*:235, 1965.

Milstein, C., and Lennox, E.: The use of monoclonal antibody techniques in the study of developing cell surfaces. Curr. Topics Devel. Biol., *14*:1, 1980.

Nakamura, R. M.: Immunopathology: Clinical Laboratory Concepts and Methods. Boston, Little, Brown and Co., 1974.

Nakamura, R. M.: Future trends and applications of immunofluorescent techniques. *In* Keitges, P. W., and Nakamura, R. M. (eds.): Diagnostic Immunology: Current and Future Trends. Skokie, Ill., College of American Pathologists, 1980, Chap. 3, p. 111.

Nakamura, R. M., Maggio, E. T., and Ott, R.: Monoclonal antibodies: methods of production and applications in the clinical laboratory. *In* Batsakis, J., and Homburger, H. A. (eds.): Clinical Laboratory Annual., Vol. 2. New York, Appleton-Century-Crofts, 1982, pp. 57–79.

Ngo, T. T., and Lenhoff, H. M.: Enzyme modulators as tools for the development of the homogeneous enzyme immunoassays. FEBS Letters, *116*:285, 1980.

Nicoli, D. F., Briggs, J., and Elings, V. B.: Fluorescence immunoassay based on long time correlations of number fluctuations. Proc. Natl. Acad. Sci. USA, 77:4904, 1980.

O'Sullivan, M. J., Bridges, J. W., and Marks, V.: Enzyme immunoassay: A review. Ann. Clin. Biochem., *16*:221, 1979.

Ritchie, R.: Automated Immunoanalysis, Part I & Part II. New York, Marcel Dekker, Inc., 1978.

Ritzmann, S. E., and Daniels, J. C. (eds.): Serum Protein Abnormalities—Diagnostic and Clinical Aspects. Boston, Little, Brown and Co., 1975.

Rose, N. R., and Bigazzi, P. E. (eds.): Methods in Immunodiagnosis. New York, John Wiley & Sons, 1973, pp. 1–30.

Rowley, G. L., Rubenstein, J. E., Huisjen, J., and Ullman, E. F.: Mechanism by which antibodies inhibit hapten-malate dehydrogenase conjugates. J. Biol. Chem., *250*:3759, 1975.

Rubenstein, K. E., Schneider, R. S., and Ullman, E. F.: 'Homogeneous' enzyme immunoassay. A new immunological technique. Biochim. Biophys. Res. Commun., *47*:846, 1972.

Singer, J. M.: Standardization of the latex test for rheumatoid arthritis serology. Bull. Rheum. Dis., *24*:762, 1973–74.

Smith, D. S.: Enhancement fluoroimmunoassay of thyroxine. FEBS Letters, 77:25, 1977.

Soini, E., and Hemmila, I.: Fluoroimmunoassay: Present status and key problems. Clin. Chem., *25*(3):353, 1979.

Soini, E., and Kojola, H.: Time-resolved fluorometer for lanthanide chelates—a new generation of non-isotopic immunoassays. Clin. Chem., *29*:65, 1983.

Steinitz, M., Koskimies, S., Klein, G., and Makela, O.: Establishment of specific antibody producing human lines by antigen preselection and EBV-transformation. *In* Melchers, F., Potter, M., and Warner, N. (eds.): Lymphocyte Hybridomas. New York, Springer-Verlag, 1978, pp. 156–163.

Ullman, E. F., Bellet, M. F., Brinkley, J. M., and Zuk, R. F.: Homogeneous fluorescence immunoassays. *In* Nakamura, R. M., Dito, W. R., and Tucker, E. S. (eds.): Immunoassays: Clinical Laboratory Techniques for the 1980s. New York, Alan R. Liss, Inc., 1980, pp. 13–41.

Ullman, E. F., Blakemore, J., Leute, R. K., Eimstad, W., and Jaklitsch, A.: Homogeneous enzyme immunoassay for thyroxine. Clin. Chem., *21*:1011, 1975.

Ullman, E. F., Schwartzberg, M., and Rubenstein, K. D.: Fluorescent excitation transfer assay—a general method for determination of antigen. J. Biol. Chem., *251*:4172, 1976.

Voller, A., Bartlett, A., and Bidwell, D. E.: Enzyme immunoassays with special references to ELISA techniques. J. Clin. Path., *31*:507, 1978.

Wei, R., and Reibe, S.: Preparation of a phospholipase C–antihuman IgG conjugate and inhibition of its enzymatic activity by human IgG. Clin. Chem., *23*:1386, 1977.

Weir, D. M.: Immunochemistry. *In* Handbook of Experimental Immunology, Vol. 7. 2nd ed. London, Blackwell Scientific Publications, 1973.

Williams, C. A., and Chase, M. W. (eds.): Methods in Immunology and Immunochemistry, Vol. III. New York, Academic Press, Inc., 1970.

Zuk, R. F., Rowley, G. L., and Ullman, E. F.: Fluorescence protection immunoassay: A new homogeneous assay technique. Clin. Chem., *25*:1554, 1979.

Zurawski, V. R., Jr., Black, P. H., and Haber, E.: Continuously proliferating human cell lines synthesizing antibody of predetermined specificity. *In* Kennett, R. H., McKearn, T. J., and Bechtol, K. B. (eds.): Monoclonal Antibodies. Hybridomas: A New Dimension in Biological Analyses. New York, Plenum Press, 1980, Chap. 2, p. 19.

5

39

AUTOANTIBODIES: AUTOIMMUNITY AND IMMUNE COMPLEXES

BURTON ZWEIMAN, M.D., and ROBERT P. LISAK, M.D.

CURRENT CONCEPTS

An understanding of current concepts of autoimmunity and its pathogenic mechanisms requires a brief discussion of the regulation of immune responses. The latter depends on a highly complex set of interactions among antigen, antibody, immune complexes, complement, macrophages, and one or more subpopulations of lymphocytes (Fauci, 1980). Components include (1) genetic control through immune response genes linked directly or indirectly to the histocompatibility complex; (2) cellular cooperation between macrophages and lymphocytes and between T and B lymphocytes themselves (Cantor, 1979); and (3) a primary regulatory role of T lymphocytes in both the initiation (helper T cell function) and prevention/termination (suppressor T cell function) of a particular immune function. This important regulatory function determines the degree of antibody formation by B cells or conversion of such cells to plasma cells, the normal switch from IgM to IgG antibody production against a particular antigen, and the degree of direct T cell–mediated reactivity, among other functions. The end result of an effective functioning immune response would be the harmonious appearance of normal immune reactivity expressed appropriately with self/non-self discrimination (Miller, 1982).

Autoimmunity represents a breakdown of such self/non-self discrimination which may or may not result in adverse effects in the host (Theofilopoulos, 1982). Some consider it a termination of the natural unresponsive (tolerant) state. Currently, many investigators believe that such tolerance is induced by at least two mechanisms involving contact between antigen and immunocompetent cells: (1) elimination of the small clone of immunocompetent cells "programmed" to react with the antigen (Burnet's clonal selection theory), and (2) induction of unresponsiveness in the immunocompetent cells through excessive antigen binding to them and/or through triggering of a suppressor mechanism. Recent evidence (Miller, 1982) suggests that normal immune responses are modulated by both antigen-specific and non-specific suppressor cell activity as part of an immunologic network. A major mechanism in antigen-specific suppression of humoral immune responses appears related to an anti-idiotypic immune response induced by the antigen binding site (idiotype) unique for a particular antibody (Jerne, 1975; Miller, 1982). In the converse situation, prolonged antigenic stimulation such as that occurring in certain chronic infections leads to polyclonal activation of B cell responses with resultant polyclonal hypergammaglobulinemia.

There is increasing evidence that much of tolerance to tissue antigens is an active process involving T cells. B cells with surface receptors for DNA and other tissue components are present in small numbers in the normal circulation. The reason why immune responses to such substances develop weakly or belatedly in normals may relate to the experimental observation that tolerance in the T cell population is achieved much more readily than in B cells with the low concentrations of antigen that would be released from tissues in normal catabolism (Howard, 1975; Allison, 1974). In this "T cell tolerance," (1) the "helper" T cell function to concentrate antigens more effectively for presentation to the B cell may be depressed; (2) suppressor T cells may reduce the helper T cell function that does persist; and (3) there is lack of conversion of IgM to IgG antibody synthesis by those B cells which may be activated directly by certain antigens.

It is also apparent that tolerance is terminated more readily, as well as induced with more difficulty, in B lymphocytes (Theofilopoulos, 1982). Therefore, in many cases, B cells are ready to produce autoantibodies at any time, and frequently do this weakly in normals, especially with increasing age. However, such autoimmune reactivity increases markedly and prematurely when helper T cells are made responsive (or lose tolerance) to autoantigens. Conditions which may lead to such T cell responsiveness include (1) exogenous alterations of normal host components by agents such as the type C viruses which incorporate membrane components as they bud from the infected cell; (2) haptens which may complex to tissue proteins acting as a carrier; (3) tolerance to tissue components which may also be lost when immune responses are induced to a foreign antigen, which cross-reacts with normal tissue components; and (4) non-specific stimulation of helper T cells by adjuvants or depression of the regulating suppressor T cell activity (Miller, 1982).

The lack of normal regulation of immune responses may play a role in the increased production of autoantibodies by mutant lymphoid clones in lymphoproliferative and immune deficiency states. In this regard, clinical autoimmune disease may commonly reflect a form of immunologic deficiency. Because of absent or defective lymphocytes, invading microorganisms may not be handled normally, persisting in and altering tissue cells with resultant uncovering of previously sequestered antigenic sites or formation of "neo-antigens." It is of note that in selective IgA deficiency, a particularly high prevalence of autoimmune disorders is seen (Wells, 1975). This may relate to a defective barrier to entry of foreign substances at mucosal surfaces associated with the IgA deficiency.

Although most agree that the T and B cell populations are generally exposed to only low levels of tissue components during development, the previous concept that elements of organs such as the brain, thyroid, adrenal, and testis are sequestered from contact with the immune apparatus has been questioned by evidence of the normal circulation of such components even in the adult stage (Volpe, 1981). It is evident that the capacity for autoimmune reactivity is constantly present in normal individuals (Allison, 1974). Expression (or lack of it) appears to be modulated by a complex set of interacting factors such as (1) *sex*: autoimmune responses are more common in the female and certain hormones affect autoantibody formation; (2) *genetics:* there is an increased evidence of autoimmune antibodies in the sera of near relatives of those with certain autoimmune diseases (DeHoratius, 1975); (3) *age:* many autoantibodies (e.g., rheumatoid factor, antinuclear antibodies, antithyroglobulin antibodies) are found more commonly in asymptomatic aged than in young individuals; (4) *thymic control:* evidence that thymus plays a role in autoimmunity includes the observations that (a) the onset in life of naturally occurring autoimmune disease and immunodeficiency in NZB/W mice is accelerated by neonatal thymectomy (Decker, 1979), and (b) thymic hyperplasia is seen in at least some clinical autoimmune states (Burnet, 1972); (5) *exogenous factors:* (sunlight, drugs, or certain virus infections may "trigger" a prominent autoimmune response by T cell activation or some other mechanisms (Phillips, 1975).

Autoimmune responses do not necessarily result in disease. Several investigators have adapted Koch's postulates in an attempt to relate autoimmunity to disease. These might include:

1. Demonstration of an immune response (humoral and/or cellular) to a well-defined tissue antigen alone or complexed to a foreign agent.
2. Induction of an immune response to that antigen in experimental animals, resulting in lesions similar to those seen in disease.
3. Transfer of the disease to normal recipients with products of the experimental autoimmune response.

It has been difficult to meet all these criteria in suspect human diseases. Therefore, some have postulated that an autoimmune mechanism is likely when several clinical manifestations are present. Some of these are listed in Table 39–1 with the understanding that no one criterion specifically identifies autoimmunity.

The immunogenic stimulus in autoimmunity may be (1) foreign substance which induces an immune response that cross-reacts against tissue components; (2) a complex of the foreign substance with the tissue, sometimes in a hapten-carrier relationship; (3) an endogenous material, sometimes restricted to one organ; or (4) no obvious antigen defined. To a major degree, the nature and locale of this immunogenic stimulus will determine whether the disease manifestations are localized or systemic. Those localized predominantly to one organ system include endocrine (Hashimoto's thyroiditis, Addison's disease), gastrointestinal tract (pernicious anemia, autoimmune liver disease), and neuromuscular system (certain demyelinating diseases, myasthenia gravis). However, although the autoantibodies are organ- (and sometimes species-) specific, it is not unusual to find other antitissue antibodies in the serum of patients with disease manifestations in only one organ system (Irvine,

Table 39–1. PRESUMPTIVE CLINICAL EVIDENCE SUGGESTING AN AUTOIMMUNE MECHANISM IN A HUMAN DISEASE

1. Pathologic picture similar to that in experimental autoimmune states
2. Presence of humoral or cell-mediated immune response to tissue antigens
3. Decrease in serum complement component(s)
4. Presence of other possible autoimmune disease
5. Familial prevalence of the same or other putative autoimmune disease
6. Clinical improvement following steroid or cytotoxic ("immunosuppressive") therapy

1975b). For example, antithyroglobulin antibodies are more commonly found in the sera of those with pernicious anemia and myasthenia gravis; however, only a minority of such patients develop concomitant thyroiditis. In addition, there is an increased familial prevalence not only of the particular organ-associated autoimmune disease, but also of the antibodies against components of other organs.

What mechanism underlies this association of anti-organ antibodies in these patients or their near relatives? The answer is not clear. However, based on our foregoing discussion of T and B lymphocyte activities, it is conceivable that genetically controlled B cell hyperactivity against certain organ components characterizes this patient population, with resultant modest increase in T cell responses against one particular organ. This may result in marked increases in humoral (and possibly cell-mediated) immune responses that are associated with disease induction. The role of cell-mediated immunity in human autoimmune disease states is not well-defined (Stiller, 1975).

In a second group of diseases, the autoimmune response is not directed against organ- or species-specific antigens (DNA and other nuclear antigens, mitochondria). Rather, they seem to reflect a generalized abnormal humoral hyper-reactivity, possibly because of defective suppressor T cell function. The lesions are likely due at least in part to deposition of immune complexes containing tissue components, often with complement, with involvement of multiple organs. Therefore, it is not surprising that there is significant overlap in the clinical manifestation of this collagen-vascular disease group (e.g., SLE, rheumatoid arthritis).

However, these distinctions are by no means clear cut. There are instances in which autoimmunity appears primarily organ-directed, but is also expressed as multiple antibodies against organ non-specific antigens. Examples of this are biliary cirrhosis and Sjögren's syndrome. In addition, tissue components may be released from an organ damaged by an organ-specific autoimmune reaction; these components may also combine with preformed antibodies to form a pathogenic immune complex damaging formed elements (e.g., hemolytic anemias) or the glomerulus.

AUTOIMMUNITY AND COLLAGEN-VASCULAR DISORDERS

The term collagen-vascular disorders has been commonly applied to a group of disorders with multisystemic manifestations even though prominent blood vessel involvement is only sometimes seen, and primary involvement of collagen rarely. Most observers would include systemic lupus erythematosus, rheumatoid arthritis, periarteritis nodosa, and probably scleroderma. Common features are inflammatory reactions, a potential for involvement of any organ system, and an understandable merging of one clinical presentation into another. These considerations should be kept in mind when evaluating the diagnostic and prognostic significance of one or more of the immunologic findings present in these disorders. The observer will then be more understanding of the overlap in prevalence of immunologic as well as clinical findings. In this regard, it should be emphasized that the result of any one laboratory determination is still only partial evidence to confirm a clinical impression and not diagnostic by itself. Because of the chronic inflammatory reactivity, likely owing at least in part to antigenic stimulation, it is not surprising to find elevated sedimentation rates and polyclonal increases in serum gamma globulins detected by one or more methods. It is to some of the antibody activities in these gamma globulins that we will first direct our attention.

Antinuclear Antibodies (ANA)

Antibodies directed against a large number of tissue components have been found in systemic lupus erythematosus (SLE). Of these, the antinuclear antibodies have been the center of most interest because of their diagnostic usefulness and pathogenic implications. Since the discovery of the L.E. cell (Hargraves, 1948), an ever-increasing number of nuclear components have been isolated which react to varying degrees with lupus sera, utilizing techniques that presumably measure antigen-antibody activity. A list of the currently described major nuclear "antigens" is shown in Table 39–2. Because of their widespread clinical use, immunofluorescence techniques for detection of ANA will be discussed first and in greater detail.

IMMUNOFLUORESCENT METHOD

Binding of gamma globulins to a variety of cell nuclear substrates has been demonstrated with considerable utility in many laboratories using immunofluorescent techniques. Immunofluorescence is a histochemical method for detecting antigens in tissue (direct technique) or antibodies which bind *in vitro* to tissue antigens (indirect technique). The mechanisms underlying this technique are discussed in Chapter 38. However, a common approach for detecting ANA includes:

Mammalian cells—fixed gently
↓ washed with buffered saline
Incubation with test or control serum
↓ washed with buffered saline
Incubation with fluorescein-conjugated antihuman immunoglobulins (previously absorbed with tissue powder)
↓ washed with buffered saline
Counterstain with diluted Evans blue or rhodamine (optional)
↓ washed with buffered saline
Mount cover slip with buffered glycerol and read in microscope adapted for fluorescence.

This technique is relatively simple; with the development of interference filters, availability of an ultraviolet light source is no longer required but may still be preferable. There are many minor variations and adaptations of this technique, with no one uniformly superior to the rest (Rothfield, 1976). However, several *technical factors* and *potential pitfalls* must be kept in mind. There can be considerable interlaboratory variation in the results obtained in analysis of the same specimen (Feigenbaum, 1982). Nuclear substrates from a variety of cell cultures, blood smears, tissue imprints, and tissue sections have been used.

Table 39–2. NUCLEAR ANTIGENS DETECTED BY IMMUNOFLUORESCENCE ANTI-NUCLEAR ANTIBODY TESTING

Particular or soluble nucleoprotein
DNA
Sm antigen
Nuclear ribonucleoprotein
Low molecular weight RNA (4–6S)
Histones
Others?

Recent evidence suggests that certain cultured cells provide a more sensitive substrate and may be preferable in exhibiting certain fluorescence patterns. However, this may be associated with more reactivity (generally in low titer) in normal sera. Leukocyte specific preferential ANA have been reported, particularly in rheumatoid arthritis and Felty's syndrome (Wiik, 1980). Mild fixation (e.g., acetone for 10 minutes) retards "leaking out" of aqueous-extractable nuclear antigens during the washing procedures. Some commercially prepared antisera tend to be heavily conjugated with high fluorescein:protein ratios and will therefore bind more non-specifically to the tissue substrate. This may make interpretation of nuclear staining more difficult. Use of gamma globulin fraction of the antiserum which has been extensively dialyzed and affinity column fractionated will reduce the non-specific effects. Each lot of fluoresceinated antiserum should be standardized using a chess board technique (Hale, 1971).

Advantages of the immunofluorescent detection of ANA (Rothfield, 1976) are several. It is a very sensitive screening test. Tests are positive in significant titer in greater than 95 per cent of patients with active untreated SLE. A persistently negative ANA by this method effectively rules out this diagnosis (Tan, 1982). Patients with "ANA-negative" SLE have been reported to exhibit a high incidence of malar rash and photosensitivity, decreased incidence of nephritis, and presence of antibodies against other cellular components (Maddison, 1981). The ANA present against all nuclear components can be semiquantitated using serum dilution titers. Relatively large numbers of sera can be tested at one time and, where needed, immunofluorescence tests for other anti-tissue antibodies (discussed later) can be performed with the appropriate substrates at the same time, at considerable saving in technician time.

However, there are *disadvantages* of the immunofluorescent ANA technique. It is not very specific for SLE. After one has determined a minimal dilution (varying with the techniques used locally) at which an acceptably low percentage of normal serums react, positive responses are seen in a sizable number of disease states other than SLE and in up to 10 per cent of elderly "normal" individuals (Table 39–3). Sera from many patients treated with hydralazine and procainamide, and to a lesser extent with several other drugs, will also be positive (Alarcon-Segovia, 1976). Detection of all ANA by immunofluorescence, while advantageous in screening, does not allow a consistent distinction of antibodies against individual nuclear components. Finally, the very sensitivity of the immunofluorescent technique contributes to its inconsistency as a parameter to follow activity of the disease and effects of therapy (Rothfield, 1976; Weitzman, 1977).

Table 39–3. PREVALENCE OF POSITIVE* ANA TESTS BY IMMUNOFLUORESCENCE IN SOME CLINICAL STATES

Systemic lupus erythematosus	>95%
Rheumatoid arthritis	25–30%
Juvenile rheumatoid arthritis	20%
Sjögren's syndrome	50–60%
Progressive systemic sclerosis	60–70%
Dermatomyositis/polymyositis	<10%†
Periarteritis nodosa (typical)	<10%
Myasthenia gravis and/or thymoma	30–50%
Drug-induced states‡	
Hydralazine	35–50%
Procainamide	50–70%
Anticonvulsants	8–15%
Normals	<5%
Normals, elderly (>70 yrs.)	10%

*Positive in at least 1:10 serum dilution.

†High incidence of an apparently unique ANA in one report (see text).

‡Results vary considerably in reports which may reflect, in part, population treated and duration of treatment.

Attempts have been made to improve the diagnostic specificity of immunofluorescent ANA determinations by the use of serial dilution titers. It is true that higher ANA titers (often >1:160) are found in active SLE compared with other conditions (Ritchie, 1967), but there is considerable overlap, particularly in "highly expressed" rheumatoid arthritis and Sjögren's syndrome. There is also no precise correlation between ANA titers and anti-DNA antibody levels in SLE (Weitzman, 1977). Certain patterns of fluorescent staining of the nucleus have been found to correspond fairly well, but not uniformly, to certain nuclear components (Nakamura, 1978; Rothfield, 1976) (Table 39–4 and Fig. 39–1). The "peripheral rim" or "shaggy" pattern has been more commonly but not

Table 39–4. NUCLEAR ANTIGENS AND IMMUNOFLUORESCENCE PATTERNS IN SOME CLINICAL STATES

Immunofluorescence Pattern	Antigen	Clinical States*
Diffuse or homogeneous	Nucleoprotein Others?	SLE, RA, SS, Sj, drug-induced
Rim (shaggy)	DNA Nucleoprotein	SLE, occasionally others
Speckled	Nuclear RNA-protein Sm Histone Others	SLE, MCTD, SS, Sj, RA, drug-induced

*SLE = systemic lupus erythematosus; RA = rheumatoid arthritis; SS = progressive systemic sclerosis; Sj = Sjögren's syndrome; MCTD = mixed connective tissue disease.

5

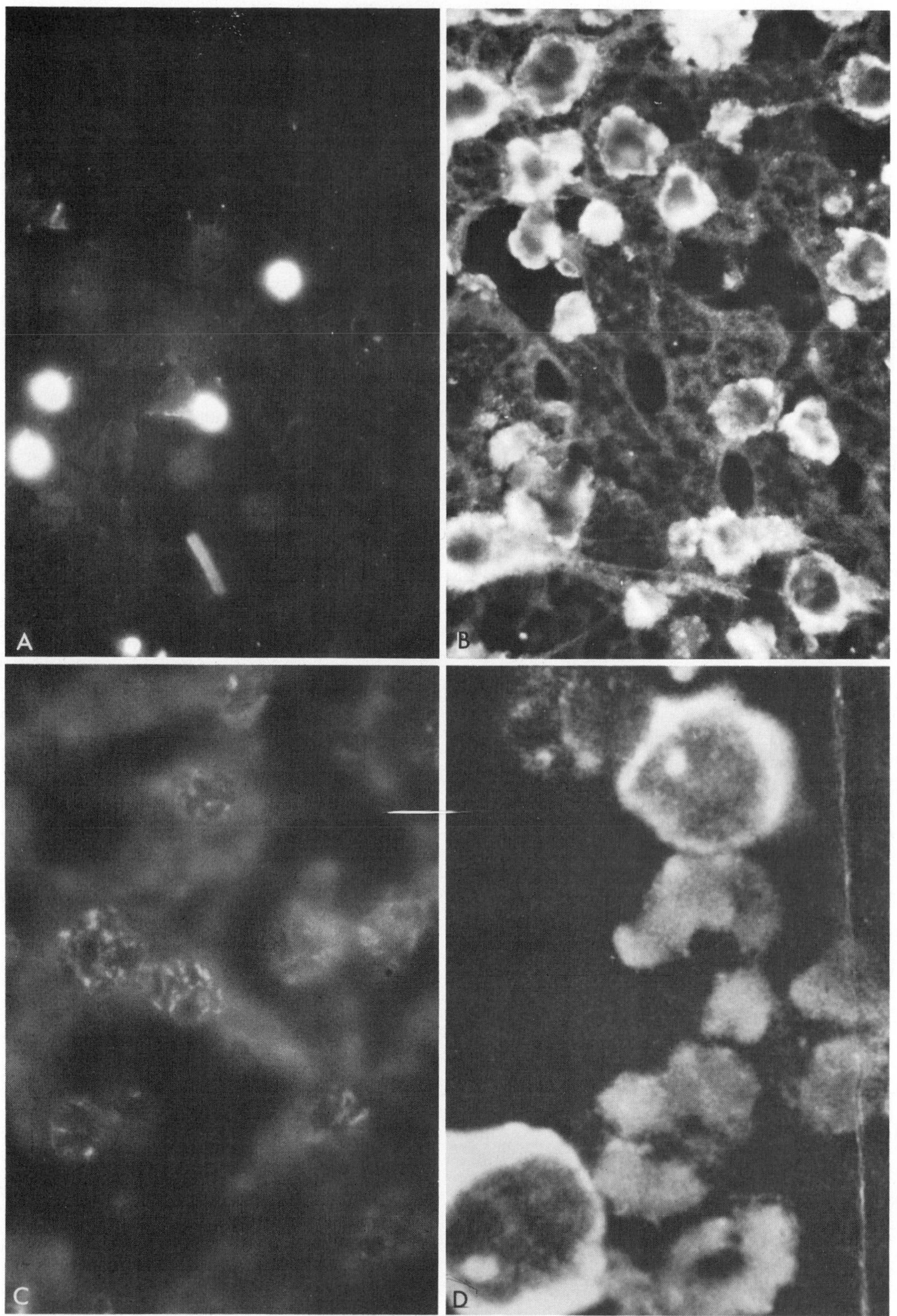

Figure 39–1. Immunofluorescence patterns due to binding of antinuclear antibodies, all at 600× magnification. *A*, Inverse diffuse fluorescence. *B*, Peripheral rim pattern. *C*, Speckled pattern. *D*, Nucleolar and cytoplasmic fluorescence.

uniformly associated with anti-DNA antibodies found in active SLE. However, the frequent concomitant presence of antinucleoprotein antibodies may also give rim patterns at times; it also may result in an intense diffuse fluorescence, making the rim pattern difficult to see. The nucleolar staining pattern seen with binding of certain sera from scleroderma and SLE patients may also be masked by intense diffuse nuclear staining.

The L. E. cell phenomenon bears special mention because of its original role in expanding immunologic knowledge about SLE and the continued widespread use of the L.E. phenomenon (Zweiman, 1976). This is essentially an *in vitro* phenomenon; L.E. cells are rarely found *in vivo* except in bone marrow or in inflammatory exudates. In a commonly used technique, heparinized blood is agitated with glass beads or by other mechanical means so that nuclei are released from disrupted leukocytes. When these nuclei interact with antinucleoprotein antibodies in the serum, they are altered, with loss of chromatin pattern and a resultant homogeneous appearance (hematoxylin bodies). The hematoxylin bodies are phagocytized by remaining viable leukocytes in a complement-dependent reaction resulting in blood granulocytes with cytoplasm stretched and nucleus displaced by a homogeneous inclusion which is stained light blue by Wright's stain.

A positive L.E. cell test (generally considered when at least four typical L.E. cells are found in a 20 minute search) is found in about 50 to 80 per cent of SLE patients and is therefore a much less sensitive screening test. L.E. cell tests also become negative more readily than immunofluorescent ANA tests in steroid-treated individuals. Other disadvantages include the relatively time-consuming nature of the tests performed in large numbers of patients, including the tedious reading period (for at least 20 minutes) and sometimes subjective elements in visual interpretation. Positive L.E. cells tests are more specific for SLE but are also found in about 5 per cent of rheumatoid arthritics, in some scleroderma patients (particularly those with vasculitis), and in some with drug-induced reactions (Zweiman, 1976). Therefore the diagnostic usefulness of the L.E. cell test has generally been surpassed by other tests. Indeed, positive ANA tests have been included in the recently revised American Rheumatism Association criteria for the diagnosis of SLE (Tan, 1982).

SEROLOGIC TESTS FOR NUCLEAR ANTIGENS

Major recent advances in diagnostic specificity have come from attempts to quantitate antibodies against individual nuclear components.

Antibodies against native double-stranded DNA (anti-nDNA) are thought by most investigators to be present in significant amounts, predominantly in those with active SLE (Griffiths, 1979). Although it is currently debated whether such reactivity is directed partially against small amounts of contaminating single-stranded DNA (ss-DNA), the observation of presumptive anti-DNA antibodies has been used pragmatically to help diagnose and follow the activity of SLE. There is some debate as to how often anti-nDNA antibodies in significant quantity are found in the sera of those with diseases other than active SLE. Different results may reflect technical variables described below.

In *DNA binding assays,* attempts have been made to demonstrate by immunofluorescence binding of human gamma globulins to either purified DNA solutions ("DNA spot test") or DNA-rich microorganisms. However, for a variety of reasons, binding of putative antibodies in sera to radiolabeled (^{3}H or ^{14}C) DNA has been used most extensively in both research and clinical studies in recent years. In most assays, radiolabeled DNA is incubated at 37°C. and then at 4°C. with test and control sera. Any resultant DNA–gamma globulin complex is separated from the free DNA by either precipitating DNA–gamma globulin complex with 50 per cent saturated ammonium sulfate (Farr technique; Pincus, 1969) or by trapping the DNA–gamma globulin complex on cellulose filters during gentle vacuum filtration (Talal, 1976).

In either method, the radiolabeled bound DNA (in the precipitate or on the filter) is counted in a scintillation counter and generally expressed as a percentage of the labeled DNA added to the serum.

Although each method has intrinsic advantages and disadvantages, the major overall *advantages* of the binding assay are several. It measures presumptive antigen-antibody interaction directly without requirement for a secondary reaction (hemagglutination, complement fixation, etc.) that may add technical and biologic variables. Radiolabeled or DNA preparations (now commercially available) are stable at −20°C. and can be used almost immediately in the test. Semiquantitation is feasible and inhibition studies with "cold" DNA (or with a test serum presumably containing DNA) can be performed.

However, several *disadvantages and pitfalls* of the binding techniques should be kept in mind. First, the selectivity of the test for SLE requires that the antigen preparation contain little contaminating single-strand DNA (ss-DNA); there is considerable binding to ss-DNA of sera in a number of disease and drug-induced states, and in some normals as well (Griffiths, 1979). There is some debate as to the degree of contamination of "native" DNA preparations with ss-DNA, and whether the activity we call "anti-DNA" is really directed against such contaminants. However, in experienced hands, this technique is pragmatically useful, provided that each new lot of labeled DNA is calibrated. Second, DNA binds to serum components other than gamma globulins (Aarden, 1976). Prior 56°C. incubation of sera should be done to inactivate the first component of complement, a major nonimmunologic binder of DNA. Low degrees of binding occur when the technique is carried out effectively; normal sera should bind <10 per cent of the added labeled DNA. Binding of >20 per cent is generally positive in most laboratories. In Table 39–5, the prevalence of such binding in different disease states is listed, with the understanding that variable results have been reported by different groups, possibly because of technique variables. These sometimes

5

Table 39–5. PREVALENCE OF ELEVATED ANTI-DNA ANTIBODY IN SOME CLINICAL STATES*

	Percentage of Sera with Elevated Binding of nDNA
Active SLE	65–80%
Questionable SLE	30%
Discoid LE	15–20%
Rheumatoid arthritis	10%
Other collagen vascular diseases	5–15%
Drug-induced positive ANA	10%
Normals	0–2%

*Modified from Pincus, T., Schur, P. H., Rose, J. A., Decker, J. K., and Talal, N.: N. Engl. J. Med., *281*:701, 1969, and Talal, N.: Med. Clin. North Am., *61*:205, 1977.

result in considerable inter- and intralaboratory variability (Feigenbaum, 1982; Adams, 1982). Although DNA binding can be quantitated, the pattern is nonlinear. Some (Pincus, 1969) recommend comparing DNA binding by a positive control serum. For individual patients, it may be preferable to establish ranges of binding percentages which are then indicated as strong, moderate, weak (but definite), equivocal, and negative. In SLE, strongly positive binding is found particularly in the sera of those with active renal or central nervous system manifestations.

Some groups (Ballou, 1979) have found the immunofluorescent binding of serum Ig to nDNA in the kinetoplast of the hemoflagellate *Crithidia luciliae* to be a specific and semi-quantitative measurement of anti-DNA antibodies. Although this assay offers the advantage of being performed in serial dilution along with other immunofluorescence tests, some investigators do not find it as sensitive as the radioimmunoassay.

Occasionally, anti-DNA tests will be negative in sera obtained at the peak of an acute exacerbation of SLE. Robitallie (1973) has shown free circulating DNA (antigen excess) in some such situations. He has modified immunodiffusion and hemagglutination techniques utilizing patient sera with high anti-DNA titers as a reagent to detect DNA present in at least moderate amounts. Others recommend assaying the increased capacity of serum treated with DNAse to bind radiolabeled DNA as a measure of complexes containing DNA (Bardana, 1975). In addition to use in diagnosis, measurement of anti-DNA antibodies have been employed to predict the future course and response to therapy in SLE. As reviewed by Ludovicio (1980), the predictive value of a single anti-DNA determination at the time of initial evaluation has varied in different studies. Adler (1975) has found that a lack of decrease in serum anti-DNA activity following therapy for several months was associated with progressive clinical deterioration. Although levels of all anti-nDNA antibodies do not always correlate with clinical severity in SLE, some have found that anti-DNA of the IgG class (Ross, 1978) or altered avidity (Winfield, 1977a) is associated with more active nephritis.

As mentioned earlier, speckled patterns in the immunofluorescent ANA test have been found in a variety of disease and drug-induced states, and likely reflected binding to one or more nuclear components which were at least partially extracted by aqueous solvents, the so-called extractable nuclear antigens (ENA). More recently, the nature and diagnostic significance of at least two of these components have been better defined (Tan, 1976b; Maddison, 1977). The *Sm antigen* is a non-histone, nuclear protein, devoid of nucleic acids against which antibodies are found predominantly, if not exclusively, in active SLE, particularly when there is renal involvement present. Antibodies against nuclear *ribonucleoprotein (RNP)* are found in sera of some SLE patients, generally with milder disease (Sharp, 1976). However, these antibodies are also found in other collagen-vascular diseases, including a high percentage of those with an overlapping clinical picture consisting of some manifestations of scleroderma, polymyositis, and SLE without a typical clinical pattern for any of these more defined syndromes. In this disorder, called the "mixed connective disease syndrome" by some (Sharp, 1976), major renal involvement is unusual and the clinical response to relatively low doses of corticosteroids is good.

Detection of antibodies against both the Sm and RNP is generally carried out using a hemagglutination assay involving tanned sheep erythrocytes (RBC) coated with the reactant. For screening purposes, Tan (1976b) extracts a relatively impure saline-soluble extract of rabbit thymus; portions of this extract are pretreated with RNAse (to inactivate the RNP). Although other components are likely present, Tan believes that almost all of the antibody reactivity against the extract is directed to Sm and/or RNP.

In this assay (assuming negative control tests with extract coated sheep erythrocytes in buffer and with uncoated sheep erythrocytes in test serum), agglutination by a serum of extract-coated sheep erythrocytes indicates antibodies against the Sm and/or RNP components.

Agglutination by the same serum titer of sheep red blood cells coated with RNAse treated extract indicates that the antibody is directed against the Sm antigen. A titer lower than that against the untreated antigen indicates the presence of antibody activity against both Sm and RNP. No agglutination by the same serum of sheep erythrocytes coated with RNAse treated extract indicates antibodies against only RNP.

The major *advantages* of this assay are the use of relatively defined nuclear components rather than an immunofluorescence pattern, relative ease of performance without specialized equipment, and semiquantitation by serum serial dilution. *Disadvantages and possible pitfalls* include variables in any hemagglutination technique and the need to adjust pH very carefully for consistent binding of the extract to the erythrocytes and for RNAse inactivation. For this reason, counter-immunoelectrophoresis and ELISA techniques are being utilized to measure anti ENA antibodies. In addition, the lack of standardized, commercially prepared "antigen" components has generally limited the use of this technique to date to a few research-oriented laboratories. There has been increasing interest in the measurement of antibodies against other nuclear and cytoplasmic components (Alspaugh, 1979). Antibodies against the cytoplasmic antigen Ro (or SS-A) are found in about 25 per cent of SLE and 40 per cent of Sjögren's syndrome patients; anti-La (or SS-B) is sometimes found along with anti-Ro in those SLE patients with less severe disease and lower anti-DNA antibodies (Wasicek, 1982). Cutaneous manifestations, including prominent photosensitivity, are also common in such patients (Alexander, 1981). Counterimmunoelectrophoresis has also been suggested as a technique to detect these antibodies. These techniques hold promise in the continuing search for assays which will increase the specificity of diagnosis of collagen-vascular disorders and/or provide laboratory guidelines for prognosis and treatment. Examples of the latter appear to be the improved prognosis in SLE generally associated with the presence of anti-RNP antibodies and the absence of anti-Sm activity. Also, Sharp (1976) reported that lupus nephritis associated with anti-RNP as well as anti-DNA antibodies is more likely to respond to treatment than when anti-DNA antibodies are persistent and anti-RNP are absent.

USE OF ANA DETERMINATION IN THE DIFFERENTIAL DIAGNOSIS OF SLE

Screening for the diagnosis of SLE—perform immunofluorescent ANA test first:

1. Consistently *negative* test—strong evidence against the diagnosis of active, untreated SLE.
2. *Borderline* postive suggests:
   a. SLE—inactive and/or under treatment with steroid and/or cytotoxic therapy.
   b. Certain other diseases or drug-induced states. If this test becomes negative after drug withdrawn (may take months), suspect drug-induced reaction, especially if anti-nDNA tests are negative. Otherwise, suspect underlying SLE.
3. *Strong positive*—SLE or (less likely) other conditions.
   a. Check titer—the higher the titer, the more likely the patient has SLE (but consider highly expressed rheumatoid arthritis, Sjögren's syndrome).
   b. Perform anti-DNA antibody—if >20 per cent by binding assay, strongly suggests diagnosis of SLE. If binding is <20 per cent, this suggests (1) SLE inactive or (sometimes) activity limited to skin or musculoskeletal system; (2) SLE being treated with large doses of steroids; (3) SLE in some major acute flare-ups—anti-DNA antibodies complexed *in vivo* with DNA; search for circulating DNA; (4) Other disease states—assay for rheumatoid factor and anti-Sm, anti-RNP, anti-Ro, anti-La (if available).

Rheumatoid Factors and Rheumatoid Arthritis

Gamma globulins with demonstrable anti–gamma globulin activity have long been called rheumatoid factors (RF) because of their occurrence in sera of over 80 per cent of patients with rheumatoid arthritis (RA). However, they are commonly found in significant amounts in a number of other diseases frequently characterized by hypergammaglobulinemia, as well as in a sizable percentage of asymptomatic elderly individuals (Vaughn, 1969) (Table 39–6). It should be emphasized that the diagnosis of RA, like that of SLE, is based on a constellation of clinical manifestations with laboratory studies confirming clinical impressions.

First, we must define exactly what we mean by rheumatoid factors. Highly purified immunoglobulins are only weakly immunogenic, particularly in the same species. The observations that the serum of many RA patients agglutinated sheep erythrocytes coated with rabbit anti-sheep red blood cell antibody (Rose-Waaler test) led to the finding that similar binding by RA serum to heat-aggregated human gamma globulin coated on inert particles such as latex beads or bentonite resulted in the agglutination or flocculation (respectively) of the latter. The responsible serum factor was found to be an IgM gamma globulin, which could be quantitated by serial dilution of the test serum. Earlier, observers thought that rheumatoid factors reacted with unique antigenic determinants uncovered or formed when normal gamma globulins were altered by exogenous factors, possibly an infection. A form of autoimmunity would then result. More recent findings have suggested that the situation is much more complex.

Although RF production may be induced by exogenously altered autologous gamma globulin, the usual rheumatoid factors react with determinants found in both aggregated and native IgG. Reactivity with the aggregated form is more likely because of the multivalent antigenic sites achieved during the process of aggregation. Indeed, the presence of normal (unaggregated) IgG in the test serum may competitively inhibit to some degree the *in vitro* binding of the aggregated IgG reagent to IgM rheumatoid factors in the same specimen (Winchester, 1976).

RF can be of any immunoglobulin class; most of the clinically applied methods reflect the amount of IgM RF

Table 39–6. RHEUMATOID FACTOR–POSITIVE LATEX FIXATION TESTS IN VARIOUS CLINICAL STATES

Clinical States	Percentage Positive (≥1:160 Dilution)
Rheumatoid arthritis	80%
Juvenile rheumatoid arthritis	20%
Ankylosing spondylitis	<15%
Infections	
SBE	48%
Viral disease, non-specific	15%
Infectious hepatitis	24%
Tuberculosis	11%
Leprosy	24%
Lung diseases	
Bronchitis	62%
Asthma	17%
Silicosis	15%
Idiopathic pulmonary fibrosis	32%
Miscellaneous disease	
Sarcoid	17%
Cirrhosis of liver	36%
Sjögren's syndrome	>90%
Myocardial infarction	12%

because of the greater efficacy of pentavalent IgM molecules in agglutination reactions (Winchester, 1976). RF of the IgG, IgA, and IgE classes are more difficult to assay and are still of uncertain diagnostic significance (Wernick, 1981).

RF found in RA and chronic infectious/inflammatory states is generally polyclonal. However, monoclonal (paraprotein) rheumatoid factors may be found in paraproteins formed in multiple myeloma, Waldenström's macroglobulinemia, purpura hyperglobulinemia, and certain other lymphoproliferative states (Block, 1982). A cold-reactive RF forms mixed cryoprecipitates with native IgG. It is seen in some patients with SLE, Sjögren's syndrome, and infectious mononucleosis, and in the "mixed cryoglobulinemia" syndrome (see later section) presenting with vasculitis, arthritis, and frequently progressive glomerulonephritis.

RF is produced actively in the synovium of involved joints (Johnson, 1975). It is present, along with IgG, in the neutrophils, and sometimes in cryoprecipitable complexes, in the inflammatory joint fluid. RF here are generally IgM but may be IgG or IgA as well.

The complexes of RF and "substrate" IgG found in the serum appear to differ in several respects from those in the joint fluid (possibly involving antigen-IgG immune complexes or self-associating IgG rheumatoid factors as well) and generally do not bind C1q well. The latter probably at least partially explains why depressed serum complement levels and glomerulonephritis are so much less common in RA than in SLE.

The pathogenic significance of RF is still debated. Some have speculated that RF may exert a protective role in promoting phagocytic clearance of circulating immune complexes (Tesor, 1970). Some RF react with nuclear components as well as IgG (Karsh, 1982). Serum RF levels are normal in some patients with classic RA (Winchester, 1976). Some have suggested that RF may be an abortive protective mechanism and that the high (sometimes extremely high) RF levels found in highly expressed RA with a worse prognosis reflects a very potent pathogenic process to which RF production is a response. However, it is conceivable that in such patients the large IgG-IgM complexes are pathogenic (since depressed serum complement levels are more common then). Indeed, therapeutic attempts have been made to reduce the levels of RF, and presumably the toxic complexes, with penicillamine, or plasmapheresis.

CLINICAL APPLICATION OF RHEUMATOID FACTOR DETERMINATIONS

The major reason for looking for RF is when RA is suspected. In this regard RF determination should be considered only in light of the clinical picture, evidence of inflammatory reaction (sedimentation rate, possibly serum protein electrophoresis), appropriate joint x-rays, and examination of the joint fluid for appearance, cell count, crystals, mucin clot and protein levels, complement levels, and culture where appropriate. Several technical approaches to measure RF are used, some of which will be discussed here.

Although RIA and ELISA techniques have been developed (Wernick, 1981; Karsh, 1982), the latex fixation test of Singer (1975) is still used in most clinical laboratories for RF determinations. *Advantages* are the relative simplicity and speed of performance. *Disadvantages and possible pitfalls* include the following: (1) It generally detects mainly IgM RF. (2) Low levels are present in normals, particularly with increasing age. These may be a heterogeneous group of antigammaglobulins (Singer, 1975). Therefore, normal ranges have to be established for each laboratory. (3) A titer of $\geq$1:60 is a reasonable starting point; some observers feel that the extensively marketed and commonly used "slide latex" tests are less sensitive and reproducible than the tube latex test. (4) False positive RF tests may be seen in sera which are hyperlipidemic or contain bulky cryoglobulins, or in which the first component of complement has not been inactivated.

True "positive" RF tests are found, generally less frequently and in lower titer, in a number of inflammatory conditions other than RA, such as subacute bacterial endocarditis, sarcoidosis, infectious mononucleosis, and SLE (Table 39–6). However, most of these conditions are characterized by prominent hypergammaglobulinemia, in helpful distinction to the normal or slightly elevated levels seen in typical RA. The highly expressed RA patients with nodules in subcutaneous areas, vasculitis, and sometimes involvement of the heart, lungs, and eyes, are generally not difficult to distinguish clinically; serum RF levels are often very high here. The distinction between RA and SLE on clinical grounds is sometimes difficult, especially in the early stages. A helpful point is that almost all the 20 to 25 per cent of RA patients whose serum is ANA positive also have prominently elevated serum RF levels as well; by contrast, RF appears in only about 20 per cent of SLE patients (generally in modest titer), almost all of whom have positive ANA tests, often with hypergammaglobulinemia.

A number of clinical pictures considered in the diagnosis of RA may present with negative RF determination:

1. *Early RA*—significantly elevated RF titers may not be seen in the serum for the first several months; RF may be found in the inflammatory joint fluid before it is seen in the serum.

2. *Juvenile RA*—positive latex RF tests are found in a minority of typical cases. There is some debate as to whether RF or other IgG classes are increased (Wernick, 1981). RF are seen more commonly with (a) onset past age 10 or (b) fever, subcutaneous nodules, and ANA. The latter are found more commonly when iridocyclitis is present. Evidence of currently or recently antecedent streptococcal infection should be looked for where appropriate.

3. *Arthritis associated with certain systemic diseases* such as Marie-Strümpell ankylosing spondylitis, Reiter's syndrome, colitic arthropathy, and psoriatic arthritis. The initiating events likely differ in these individuals, but spondylitis, sacroileitis, ocular involvement, and increased incidence of histocompatibility type B 27 are seen in most. RF levels and complement levels in both serum and joint fluids are usually normal.

4. In some "definite" and a few "classic" RA cases defined by clinical criteria (Ropes, 1956), RF levels are consistently negative.

Cryoglobulins

Cryoglobulins are immunoglobulins (Ig) of a single class, or complexes consisting of more than one Ig class, which are altered by some process which makes them insoluble to varying degrees at temperatures below 37°C. (Block, 1982). This alteration may involve binding with presumptive antigens and/or complement components either prior to or during the process of cryoprecipitation. Although such precipitation generally is most striking at 4°C., some degree of it occurs at temperatures of 30 to 31°C. reached in some distal small vessels—of obvious biologic significance. Cryoglobulins are heterogeneous in type and formation and may play important roles in vasculitis and nephritis associated with systemic disease. Cryoglobulins may be classified as follows:

Single monoclonal immunoglobulin (cryoglobulin 1)—these are paraproteins most commonly IgG (in multiple myeloma) and IgM (in macroglobulinemia, some lymphomas), but IgA and "Bence Jones" types have been described. Such cryoglobulins are also sometimes seen in "benign" monoclonal gammopathy, which may or may not be followed by overt lymphoproliferative malignancy years later. Single monoclonal cryoglobulins are generally present in high (>5 mg/ml) concentration in the serum.

Mixed polyclonal-monoclonal (cryoglobulin 2)—these are complexes of a polyclonal "antigen" (generally IgG) and monoclonal IgM with anti-IgG (rheumatoid factor activity). The monoclonal anti-IgG may occasionally be in the IgG or IgA class. This polyclonal-monoclonal complex is often associated with IgM lymphoproliferative states, with certain IgM antibody activities (cold agglutinins, heterophil antibody) also present in the complex. This type of cryoglobulin is present in moderate to high (>1 mg/ml) levels in the serum.

Mixed polyclonal-polyclonal (cryoglobulin 3)—in this complex, both components are polyclonal (most commonly IgG-IgM, occasionally IgG-IgM-IgA). Complement components are frequently present (particularly C1q), and various antigenic and antibody activities in the cryoprecipitate have been described. These cryoglobulins are present in low (<1 mg/ml) levels in the serum and constitute over half the cases of cryoglobulinemia. Very low levels (<80 μg/ml) are found in up to 50 per cent of normal sera. The exact constituents of cryoprecipitate vary not only between conditions but also among individual patients with the same condition. It has now been appreciated that the Ig components with rheumatoid factor activity may be binding to the Fc portion of another Ig molecule which is also bound in an immune complex.

Mixed cryoglobulins may be found in certain infections such as HBs antigen–positive hepatitis, cytomegalovirus, infectious mononucleosis, and lepromatous leprosy. Antigenic determinants of the infectious organism may be found in some cases when dissociation of the complex is feasible. The immunoglobulin (Ig) here is frequently IgM, especially in certain viral infections.

Cryoprecipitates commonly encountered in sera of SLE patients have been found to contain different component patterns in different studies. IgG-C1q complexes without other complement components and antilymphocyte as well as anti-IgG in IgM components of mixed cryoglobulins have been found. The IgM with rheumatoid factor activity appears to be deposited in tissue lesions as part of the complex. Opinions vary as to the frequency with which DNA–anti-DNA complexes are present (Winfield, 1977b).

MECHANISMS AND CLINICAL MANIFESTATIONS ASSOCIATED WITH CRYOGLOBULINEMIA

Cryoglobulins, types 1 and 2, occur mainly in immunoproliferative disorders (about 5 per cent of those with multiple myeloma, and an even higher percentage of patients with macroglobulinemia, lymphomas, and lymphocytic leukemias). Type 2 and 3 cryoglobulins are generally associated with conditions in which prominently elevated rheumatoid factor levels are seen, including certain acute and chronic infections and autoimmune disorders. However, in at least one third of cases, cryoglobulins appear in the absence of overt associated disease and are called "essential." Symptoms which occur depending on the nature of the cryoglobulin generally are due to the *precipitability* in cooler parts of the body. These include Raynaud's phenomenon and acrocyanosis; in more severe cases with high levels of cryoglobulins (or exposure to very cold temperatures) digital necrosis with gangrene can occur. Cryoglobulins may be found in up to 20 per cent of patients with cold-induced urticaria. Purpura in the lower extremities is common because of cooler skin temperatures and effects of stasis. *Hyperviscosity* may lead to sludging in certain vessels (most readily observed in the retinal and conjunctival areas) and may contribute to the ischemic changes, including those in the nervous system. *Immune complexes* may also contribute to symptoms. Twenty per cent of patients with cryoglobulins (not including those with SLE) may have renal disease, most commonly a diffuse glomerulonephritis. In these cases immunoglobulin and complement are found in a granular pattern in the glomerulus. This is most commonly seen in type 2 cryoglobulins, without any correlation between the type of cryoglobulin and precise pattern of renal histopathology. Immune complex patterns of manifestation may include joint symptoms with mixed cryoglobulins, especially type 3, and intra-abdominal vascular involvement.

Thus one can find manifestations that appear to be due to the cryoglobulins per se without associated defined collagen-vascular or "autoimmune disease." This is best exemplified in the "mixed cryoglobulin" syndrome originally described by Meltzer (1967), with joint and skin involvement and sometimes progressive glomerulonephritis. On the other hand, there is increasing evidence for the role of cryoglobulins, not only in collagen-vascular lymphoproliferative disorders but also in other putative "immune-complex" mediated diseases, such as acute post-streptococcal glomerulonephritis (McIntosh, 1975). In the latter, the cryoprecipitates may contain Ig with anti-streptococcal antibody, and their presence seems to correlate with active or persistent disease.

The *techniques* for detection of cryoglobulins will be more reliable and provided that certain simple precautions are observed (Stites, 1980): (1) The blood should be allowed both to clot and to be transported at as close to body temperature as feasible to avoid losing small amounts of cryoglobulin, which occurs when clotting takes place at cool temperatures; (2) for the same reason, serum separation should be carried out in a warm environment; (3) serum then stored at 4°C. should be observed for at least four days before a negative report is submitted; (4) to be definitely identified as a typical cryoprecipitate, the cold-precipitable material must be in a clear serum specimen obtained by complete clotting and should redissolve completely on warming of the chilled specimen. A gross screening method has been the "cryocrit" determination in which the serum is cold-incubated in a hematocrit tube, which is then centrifuged in the cold after maximal cryoprecipitation has occurred. The relative volume occupied by the cryoprecipitate is then expressed on a percentage basis. More quantitative assessments have been reported by determining the protein content of the cryoprecipitate or by laser nephelometry.

Immune Complexes and Their Measurement in Disease States

INTRODUCTION

With increasing interest in the possible role of immune complexes in causing tissue damage or affecting immunoregulation, great efforts have been made to develop methods to measure circulating immune complexes. Efforts to date are limited by several considerations: (1) clinically applicable techniques measure putative complexes by indirect means; (2) many of the techniques involve biologic assays with the intrinsic variability of such assays; (3) immune complexes vary widely in the nature of components and biologic properties, and one technique may not accurately measure all types of immune complexes; (4) physically, aggregated gamma globulins, the usual standard in most assays, may mimic the aggregation of Ig that occurs *in vivo* during immune complex formation, but may not be a valid standard for analysis of all types of immune complexes.

Many assays have been described (Johnson, 1982) (Table 39–7), but the discussion here will emphasize those most widely employed in the United States.

Table 39–7. SOME APPROACHES TO THE MEASUREMENT OF CIRCULATING IMMUNE COMPLEXES

- A. Physical properties of the complex
  1. Ultracentrifugation
  2. Differential precipitation
- B. Chemical biologic properties of the antibody and complement fractions
  1. Reaction with circulating free molecules
     - a. Complement consumption
     - b. Tests involving first component of complement (C1)
       - (i) C1q precipitin assay
       - (ii) ^{125}I-C1q binding assay
       - (iii) Solid phase radioimmunoassay
  2. Reaction with membrane receptors
     - a. Receptors for Fc fragment
       - (i) Platelet aggregation
       - (ii) Inhibition of EA rosette
       - (iii) Inhibition of antibody-dependent cellular cytotoxicity
     - b. Receptors for complement
       - (i) Raji cell radioimmunoassay
       - (ii) Raji cell immunofluorescence
- C. Capacity of foreign factors to react with complexes
  1. Soluble factors
     - a. Inhibition of RF to aggregated IgG
     - b. Inhibition by RF of IgG-coated latex particles
     - c. Bovine conglutinin assays
  2. Non-soluble factors
     - a. Competitive inhibition of phagocytosis

COMPLEMENT-RELATED ASSAYS

The C1q Precipitin Assay. The C1q molecule, a subunit of the first component of complement, binds with monomeric IgG (in the IgG_1, IgG_2, IgG_3 sub-classes) and IgM. The binding of C1q is markedly increased if the IgG is aggregated, even when (in certain situations) the aggregated Ig is soluble. When large amounts of C1q binding aggregated Ig are present, a precipitin reaction by immunodiffusion technique can be observed. However, the relative insensitivity of this technique has limited its diagnostic applicability to conditions such as SLE in which large amounts of circulating complexes are present.

Complement-Binding Assays. This modification employs the binding of radiolabeled C1q to a test serum in comparison with binding of this labeled reagent to a standardized soluble preparation of aggregated IgG (Nydegger, 1974; Hay, 1976). Because such interaction generally does not result in an insoluble reaction product, separation of the bound C1q has been accomplished by means such as the addition of appropriate concentrations of polyethylene glycol (PEG). This addition results in precipitation of complexes (including bound C1q) over 200,000 dalton m.w., whereas the unbound C1q (<200,000 m.w.) remains in the supernatant. Normal sera generally bind up to 11 per cent of added C1q. This technique (Woodrofe, 1977) is more sensitive than the precipitin assay; however, *disadvantages* and *potential pitfalls* must be considered: (1) C1q may be bound by Ig molecules which are physically aggregated (such as occurs sometimes during storage). Freshly obtained sera or sera stored at −70°C. should be used whenever possible (Woodrofe, 1977). (2) Substances other than Ig complexes may bind C1q. For example, double-stranded and single-stranded DNA (which may be found in serum and pathologic fluids) bind C1q, as do certain other polyribonucleotides, heparin, and endotoxins. Prior heat inactivation of the serum will eliminate some of this non-immunologic binding of C1q. However, it also reduces the binding of the aggregated IgG, decreasing the sensitivity of the test (Zubler, 1976). A solid phase radioimmunoassay has been developed which detects binding of Ig or aggregated Ig (Theofilopoulos, 1980).

METHODS INVOLVING RHEUMATOID FACTORS

The principle underlying these techniques is that rheumatoid factors (particularly monoclonal ones occurring in macroglobulinemia or as components of certain cryoglobulins described above) will bind to immune complexes. In a situation analogous to that seen with C1q, a precipitin-in-agar reaction can be observed if the high levels of immune complexes are present (Winchester, 1971). However, more recently, a binding inhibition approach has been tried, using one of two modifications.

A solid-phase radioimmunoassay (Luthra, 1975) utilizes monoclonal rheumatoid factor bound to an insoluble support such as polystyrene tube or microcrystalline cellulose. The ability of the test serum when first applied to block the subsequent binding of a standardized ^{125}I-labeled aggregated gamma globulin is measured in comparison with the blocking ability of unlabeled aggregated gamma globulin. The latter is used in several concentrations so that a standard curve can be derived. By plotting the degree of binding-inhibition which results from use of the test serum against the standard curve, one can estimate the activity equivalent to a certain amount of soluble aggregated Ig complexes.

In a second modification, single latex particles of a particular size are coated with soluble aggregated IgG (Levinsky, 1977). Such particles would ordinarily be aggregated by addition of a rheumatoid factor. If the test serum is incubated with the rheumatoid factor (RF) in advance, the binding of the RF to any immune complexes in the serum will reduce the aggregation of the coated latex particles subsequently added to the mixture. The number of non-agglutinated particles is counted.

These RF binding techniques are very sensitive but have major *limitations* and *potential pitfalls:* (1) They do not measure immune complexes directly; as with C1q, physically aggregated and monomeric IgG elements in the serum may prevent subsequent binding of the RF to either the labeled aggregated IgG or IgG-coated latex particles. (2) The use of aggregated IgG (either labeled or on latex particles) to simulate an immune complex may not always be valid, depending on the nature of the immune complex. (3) Different RF do vary in the degree of affinity for complexed IgG and aggregated IgG. The greater the affinity; the more sensitive the assay. In most cases, it appears that monoclonal RF without cryoglobulin properties seem to work most effectively with good sensitivity. This variance may present a major problem because of the limited amount of monoclonal RF from a single patient donor available for long-term use. Use of the more readily available polyclonal RF will result in a sensitive assay; however, polyclonal RF which may be present in test sera will affect the determination. (4) Methods utilizing RF reagents may preferentially detect smaller circulating immune complexes not picked up by other techniques. This may result in the more common reporting of positive results in rheumatoid arthritis sera which seem to contain disproportionately more of these smaller complexes.

PLATELET AGGREGATION TESTS (Myllyla, 1973)

Since immune complexes tend to aggregate platelets, aliquots of pooled washed platelets from normal donors may be incubated with serial dilutions of test and positive control (immune complex–containing) sera overnight, generally at 37°C. Although sensitive, this assay is sometimes quite variable from day to day, possibly relating to platelet sources used, among other factors.

THE RAJI CELL ASSAY

Principle of the Raji Cell Assay (Theofilopoulos, 1976). Different B lymphoblastoid cells maintained in culture retain varying densities of the surface membrane Ig (SIg) receptors for the Fc portion of IgG and for C3. The Raji line cells have no SIg, low avidity Fc receptors, and high density of receptors for C3. These characteristics have been used to determine the amount of gamma globulin from a test or control serum which binds to a prescribed number of Raji cells, detected by the subsequent attachment of radiolabeled anti-human IgG. The principle underlying this assay is that the relatively weak binding of circulating Ig to the Fc receptor serves as a fair estimate of the "background" binding of monomeric Ig when there is little or no immune complex alteration of the Ig. More IgG which is part of a circulating immune complex with antigen and complement binds to the Raji cells than does monomeric IgG, because the complex binds not only to the weaker Fc receptor but also to the strong C3 receptor. In this way, the binding of test sera can be compared with a standard curve derived from the binding of measured amounts of aggregated IgG (with bound complement).

The major *advantages* of the Raji cell assay are as follows (Woodrofe, 1977): (1) It is very sensitive. As little as 5 μg of bound aggregated IgG can be detected. In comparison, the usual sensitivity of C1q binding assays and monoclonal RF assays are to levels of 50 and 25 μg, respectively. (2) Determinations are not altered in sera which is heated to 56°C., stored in the frozen state, or to which is added heparin, DNA, or endotoxin. (3) No unique reagents such as highly purified C1q or monoclonal RF are required. ^{125}I anti-IgG is needed, but the capacity for preparation of this reagent is more readily available with likelihood that it can be supplied to clinical laboratories.

Disadvantages and potential pitfalls (Woodrofe, 1977) of this technique include the following: (1) There is a need to maintain a lymphoblastoid cell line in continuous culture. This is technically not too difficult. However, the varying results obtained in different laboratories using this technique may be due in part to different cell receptor characteristics which developed when aliquots of what was originally one cell line have been maintained by different groups. (2) The great sensitivity of the technique is accomplished by higher binding of normal IgG than is seen with other techniques. (3) More day-to-day variation in the binding equivalents requires establishing a standard curve with each test run (Woodrofe, 1977). (4) Antilymphocyte antibodies may bind to or cause lysis of the cultured cells. (5) Antigens liberated from dead Raji cells may combine with the free complexes. A Raji cell assay employing immunofluorescence (Theofilopoulos, 1980) is more specific since it detects binding only to living cells, but is not as readily performed on a large number of samples as is the assay using ^{125}I-anti-IgG.

A VIEW OF THE CURRENT SIGNIFICANCE OF ASSAYS FOR IMMUNE COMPLEXES

This field is one characterized by rapid change, with findings of uncertain significance. There appears to be little question that serum of many patients with active SLE contains putative immune complexes by almost any technique employed; estimation of such levels may help in determining prognosis and response to therapy. Consistent findings seem to be present in some stages of hepatitis, "essential mixed cryoglobulinemia," and certain other vasculitis patterns. However, there have been increasing, and sometimes bewildering and contradictory, reports of presumptive circulating immune complexes detected by one technique or another. These include a variety of infections, malignancy, and childhood nephrotic syndrome to name a few. It is certainly conceivable that circulating immune complexes do occur quite commonly in disease and may be of varying degrees of pathogenic importance. It is also likely that optimal immune complex detection may require concomitant use of several techniques, each with its own intrinsic advantages and disadvantages. For example, the Raji cell assay is very sensitive for detecting the presence of relatively large complexes with bound C3. By comparison, monoclonal RF techniques are better for detecting smaller complexes, and the C1q binding assays are sensitive for complexes which effectively bind that complement component.

ORGAN-DIRECTED AUTOIMMUNE STATES

Autoimmunity in Endocrine Disorders

THYROID

Introduction. The thyroid appears to be one of the best examples of how a postulated autoimmune pathogenesis might cause organ-directed disease (reviewed by Volpe, 1981). Although there is much still to be learned about the exact mechanisms involved, current theories suggest that normal thyroglobulin (presumably released from the thyroid) circulates systemically in very low amounts. This may be sufficient to induce a "low-zone" (low dose) T lymphocyte tolerance in normals, with weak production of antithyroglobulin by those B cells with receptors for thyroglobulin, increasing gradually (particularly in females) with age. Likely because of some alteration of the thyroid by infections or chemical or other factors, there is induced in the (genetically?) predisposed individual immune responses to one or more thyroid components. These immune responses may or may not cause tissue destruction, but are frequently valuable as diagnostic markers (Tanner, 1982). It is uncertain whether there are defects in specific or non-specific suppressor cell activity in those with presumed autoimmune thyroid disease (Miller, 1982).

Some consideration of the major thyroid disorders in which immunologic study is of assistance will be helpful before considering the individual tests. Hashimoto's thyroiditis is an inflammatory condition occurring in about 1 to 2 per cent of the population, mainly in middle-aged women and characterized by gland enlargement due to marked lymphocytic inflammatory changes (Volpe, 1981). The latter may consist of lymphoid follicles with active germinal centers, in which much of the antithyroglobulin antibody appears to be synthesized. Normal thyroid glandular structures are adversely altered, and in prominent cases progressive disease may lead to thyroid atrophy and myxedema. In *thyrotoxicosis,* the thyroid may contain small areas of lymphoid infiltration as well as evidence of the typical glandular hyperactivity. Graves' disease is a multisystemic disorder, particularly in young to middle-aged females, consisting (to varying degrees) of (1) hyperthyroidism with diffuse hyperplasia of the thyroid (the most common pattern seen with diffuse toxic goiter); (2) a myopathy; (3) an infiltrative ophthalmopathy, frequently leading to exophthalmos; and (4) presence of long-acting thyroid stimulator (LATS).

As with all the organ-oriented diseases associated with autoantibody production, it is very important to determine when the antibodies under discussion are pathogenic or are epiphenomena, reacting to antigens liberated as a result of tissue damage owing to non-immune causes. A third possibility is that the immune reactivity is not the primary pathogenic event but, once present, causes further tissue damage. Evidence against a primary pathogenic role for thyroid autoantibodies in Hashimoto's and Graves' diseases is (1) the lack of correlation between the level of autoantibody and the severity of disease in individual cases, and (2) the lack of development of thyroid disease in infants born with high levels of antithyroid antibodies because of placental transfer. The failure to transfer disease when antibodies are present in the serum may mean that the pathogenic antibodies had been bound by thyroid tissue in the serum donor.

Specific Laboratory Determinations. In terms of laboratory evaluation, the best *screening* test for all antithyroid antibodies appears to be immunofluorescence using frozen section of primate thyroid tissue, preferably obtained from thyrotoxic glands of blood group O humans (Tung, 1974). This technique can detect with reasonable sensitivity antibodies to thyroglobulin, with a floccular pattern seen in the colloid, the "second colloid antigen" (CA-2) resulting in a diffuse staining, and microsomal antigens of thyroid epithelial cells leading to cytoplasmic (but not nuclear) staining of these cells but not of epithelial cells of other organs such as the kidneys.

The technique employed is similar to that used in other indirect immunofluorescent techniques with the understanding that use of methanol-fixed (for colloid antigens) and unfixed (for epithelial antigens) sections of primate thyroid tissue is essential, and specificity for thyroid cells must be demonstrated.

Positive binding is seen in low dilutions of normal sera, possibly related to asymptomatic focal lymphocytic thyroiditis. Positive tests are found in up to 90 per cent of those with active Hashimoto's thyroiditis, and a persistently negative test mitigates strongly against this diagnosis, in comparison with the weakly positive or negative reactions seen commonly in other types of non-toxic goiter and thyroid tumors. Positive staining is seen with a majority of sera from those with idiopathic myxedema (although more sensitive techniques may sometimes be required). On the other hand, the immunofluorescence technique is the only current method available for detection of antibodies to the CA-2 antigen of colloid. The latter antibodies are still of uncertain significance; however, some report their presence in 5 to 8 per cent of thyroiditis patients in the absence of other demonstrable anti-thyroid antibodies (Bigazzi, 1976). However, positive CA-2 reactions are also seen with sera of 30 to 50 per cent of those with de Quervain's thyroiditis, Graves' disease, and thyroid cancer.

However, strongly positive binding of serum antibodies specific for colloid or epithelial cells does not make a diagnosis of lymphocytic thyroiditis and/or idiopathic myxedema. One or more antithyroid antibodies (particularly those directed against thyroid epithelial cells) are found in a minority of those with other thyroid disorders, other "antitissue" autoimmune states like pernicious anemia, myasthenia gravis, SLE, and highly expressed rheumatoid arthritis (Bigazzi, 1976).

Antithyroglobulin Serologic Tests. Measurement of *antithyroglobulin antibodies* by the tanned cell *hemagglutination* test is used extensively. Its major *advantages* are (1) the specificity of the reaction for a particular antigenic group, and (2) its great sensitivity (greater than immunofluorescence). A very high antibody titer (>1:1000) suggests a diagnosis of Hashimoto's thyroiditis or "primary" myxedema, rather than other thyroid or non-thyroid conditions. *Disadvantages* of this technique are as follows: (1) The requirement for relatively pure thyroglobulin. However, this need appears to be currently met from commercial sources, including some kits which have been used with good results. (2) The need to consider heterophil antibodies against the carrier cells. However, this is generally not a major problem, since diagnostic titers of antithyroid antibodies are generally present at much greater serum dilution than is the case for the heterophil antibodies. (3) Like screening immunofluorescence, it is not too specific. Some reactivity is seen with sera of normals, especially in older females, possibly reflecting "silent" thyroiditis. Once upper limits of normal have been established in each laboratory, positive responses are seen in 75 per cent of those with Hashimoto's disease and idiopathic myxedema and in 40 per cent of those with Graves' disease and thyroid tumors (Table 39–8). However, titer differences noted above may help in the differential diagnosis, since very high titers are unlikely in any disease except Hashimoto's thyroiditis or Graves' disease (Scherbaum, 1982).

Antithyroglobulin antibodies have also been measured by the precipitin and latex agglutination technique. Both of these are insufficiently sensitive for diagnostic screening purposes; however, positive responses in significant titer are more specific for Hashimoto's thyroiditis and idiopathic myxedema.

Measurement of Antithyroid Microsomal Antibody. The screening immunofluorescence test is currently the most sensitive method for detecting antigens from lipoprotein membranes of microsomes in the cytoplasm of thyroid epithelial cells (from an unfixed thyrotoxic gland (Bigazzi, 1976; Scherbaum, 1982) in the measurement of *antithyroid microsomal antibody*. The apical staining in the epithelial cells can generally be distinguished readily from the colloid staining noted above and from the cytoplasmic staining due to antimitochondrial antibodies. It is positive in 70 to 90 per cent of those with active thyroiditis, 65 per cent of those with idiopathic hypothyroidism, 50 per cent of those with thyrotoxicosis, and about 17 per cent of those with thyroid tumors (Table 39–8). The complement fixation assay is less sensitive, but more specific, generally being positive only in those with active thyroiditis. A useful hemagglutination assay is also now commercially available.

Measurement of Long-Acting Thyroid Stimulator (LATS). Long-acting thyroid stimulator (LATS) is a polyclonal gamma globulin which appears to bind to a receptor on thyroid cells with a pattern similar to any antigen-antibody reaction (Volpe, 1981). It stimulates thyroid activity and is assayed by measuring the release of radioactive iodine from mouse thyroid at 8 to 24 hours (compared to the two-hour release period for TSH). It is present in the sera of about 50 per cent of those with Graves' disease where it is thought by some to be involved in its pathogenesis without feedback inhibition of its synthesis by thyroid hormone. LATS is absent or present only in small amounts in patients with nodular toxic goiter or other thyroid disorders. However, there are several other Igs in the serum of Graves' disease patients that may (1) stimulate the thyroid directly, (2) increase thyroid adenylcyclase, or (3) protect LATS from being absorbed (reviewed by Volpe, 1981).

SUMMARY

Immunofluorescence Screening Test. Negative

Table 39–8. PREVALENCE OF ANTI-THYROID ANTIBODIES IN SOME DISEASES*

	Antibodies		
Clinical State	***Thyroglobulin***	***CA-2*†**	***Thyroid Epithelial***
Hashimoto's	75–95%	40–70%	70–90%
Idiopathic myxedema	75%	40%	65%
Graves'	40%	5–10%	50%
Non-toxic goiter	20–30%	–	20%
Thyroid cancer	40%	10%	15%
Pernicious anemia	25%	–	10%
Normals	10%	–	10%
Normals > 70 years old	20% +	–	20% +

*Modified from Bigazzi, P. L., and Rose, N. R.: *In* Rose, N. R., and Friedman, H. (eds.): Manual of Clinical Immunology. Washington, D.C., American Society of Microbiology, 1976; Tung, K. S. K., Ramos, C. V., and Deodhar, S. D.: Am. J. Clin. Path., *61*:549, 1974; and Doniach, D.: *In* Bastenie, V. A., and Gepts, W. (eds.): Immunology and Autoimmunity in Diabetes Mellitus. Amsterdam, Excerpta Medica, 1974.

†CA-2 = colloid antigen, or "second antigen of the colloid."

5

staining of colloid and epithelial cytoplasm is strong evidence against diagnosis of active Hashimoto's thyroiditis or primary myxedema, in comparison with other types of thyroiditis, nodules, or tumors. Positive response, not diagnostic for thyroiditis, is seen in other thyroid disorders and other autoimmune states.

Thyroglobulin Hemagglutinin Test. This is not specific, but high (>1:1000) titers are unusual except in Hashimoto's thyroiditis, Graves' disease, and some cases of "idiopathic" hypothyroiditis.

Tests for Microsomal Antigen. When positive, these tests strongly suggest active Hashimoto's thyroiditis or Graves' disease.

ADRENAL

More than two thirds of cases of Addison's disease are idiopathic; evidence suggests that many of these are autoimmune in etiology, analogous to Hashimoto's thyroiditis (Doniach, 1981). In about 40 to 70 per cent of those with Addison's disease, the serum contains antibodies (generally in <1:100 titer) against cortical elements, probably microsomal, as detected by immunofluorescence (Doniach, 1981; Bigazzi, 1976) and other techniques. In some cases antibodies against adrenal cell surfaces have been noted (Doniach, 1981). These antibodies, generally present in low titer, are not a simple reflection of adrenal cell damage, since they are present in only 7 to 18 per cent of those with adrenals markedly involved by tuberculosis, and in only 1 per cent of normals (Bigazzi, 1976). These antibodies generally bind to components in the whole adrenal cortex, but may occasionally involve only individual zones.

There is a striking incidence (over 40 per cent) of putative autoimmune involvement of other endocrine glands in patients with Addison's disease (Doniach, 1981; Neufeld, 1981): (1) Thyroid (Hashimoto's and Graves' diseases, asymptomatic antithyroid antibodies). (2) Ovary with antibodies reacting with steroid-producing cells in the theca interna. These cells may contain antigens that cross-react with antigens in the adrenal cortex. (3) Pernicious anemia. (4) Diabetes. (5) Hypoparathyroidism. Chronic hepatitis, vitiligo, and pernicious anemia are associated with idiopathic adrenal insufficiency. Some (Neufeld, 1981) feel that such polyglandular autoimmune syndromes can be divided into two subgroups. It is of interest that the converse situation is not the case; anti-adrenal antibodies are unusual in other autoimmune disorders unless there is associated adrenal gland involvement.

OVARY AND TESTIS

Antibodies against cytoplasmic components of different cells of the ovary have been described in Addison's disease and in premature ovarian failure (Sotsiou, 1980). These techniques are generally still limited to research laboratories and are not standardized for clinical use.

Antisperm antibodies have been investigated in the sera of infertile couples by a variety of techniques (Rumke, 1978; Rose, 1976). Several agglutination techniques utilize semen of either the patient or a homologous male (if enough sperm of adequate motility are not available from the former). In studies from several laboratories, appropriately diluted (generally >1:8) sera of about 18 per cent and 9 per cent of infertile males and females, respectively, agglutinate test sperm, provided that several approaches are used and borderline response tests are repeated. By contrast, such reactivity is found in only 3 per cent of normal sera (Witkin, 1982). Elevated serum antisperm antibody levels are found after vasectomy, but only occasionally in males with primary testicular agenesis. Sperm immobilization and spermatotoxicity tests have been used less extensively, with need for more comparative studies in large patient groups. Seminal fluid (Witkin, 1982) may contain antisperm antibody of IgA class, as detected by ELISA. It appears that extensive experience with these techniques is required to make valid interpretations of the sometimes subjective findings.

DIABETES MELLITUS

Because of the relatively high incidence of autoimmune disorders in those with diabetes, an immunologic basis for this common condition has been sought (de Winkel, 1982). Antibodies reacting with all cells of the islets have been found in those patients with diabetes accompanying "autoimmune endocrine" disorders. There appears to be a higher incidence of these anti–islet cell antibodies in groups of patients with insulin-dependent diabetes. Indeed, some feel the presence of these antibodies is a marker of insulin dependency (Irvine, 1977). In addition to the common appearance of anti-insulin antibodies in insulin-treated subjects, the same antibodies have also been found in sera of some untreated diabetics. Such antibodies have also been found in sera of a small group of patients with normal fasting blood sugar and postprandial hypoglycemia. An immunoglobulin in the sera of insulin-resistant diabetics appears to bind to a tissue receptor for insulin, preventing some of the insulin biologic effects (Flier, 1976). More recently, antibodies which bind to and possibly kill pancreatic islet cells have been found in the majority of young insulin-dependent diabetics (reviewed by de Winkel, 1982). These techniques are still in the research stage.

Autoimmunity in Gastrointestinal Disorders

PERNICIOUS ANEMIA AND ATROPHIC GASTRITIS

The histopathologic picture in atrophic gastritis that almost always accompanies pernicious anemia is characterized by lymphocytic infiltrate and absence of parietal and chief cells (Irvine, 1975a). Associated with the lesion is decreased synthesis of gastric acid and intrinsic factor. The latter normally binds ingested vitamin B_{12} at one site and binds to receptors in the distal ileum at another of its sites. In this manner, vitamin B_{12} transport across the ileum is affected.

Besides the histologic picture, several other immunologic findings suggest an autoimmune pathogenesis of pernicious anemia (McGuigan, 1980). Antibodies against a lipoprotein cytoplasmic component of gastric parietal cells are detected by immunofluorescence in up to 90 per cent of those with pernicious anemia, in a lower percentage (about 60 per cent) of those with atrophic gastritis without hematologic abnormalities, and in those with other autoimmune diseases such as thyroiditis. These antibodies, like certain other antitissue antibodies, are unusual in young normals but are found with increasing frequency in the asymptomatic older age group (15 per cent in those >60 years old).

Autoantibodies to intrinsic factor are found less commonly (40 to 60 per cent) in pernicious anemia, but appear more specific for this disorder (Strickland, 1971). A radioimmunoassay technique is required. The antibody may well be pathogenic and not just a result of gastric mucosal damage, since transplacental transfer of anti–intrinsic factor antibody can result in defective vitamin B_{12} absorption in the infant without any atrophic gastritis. These antibodies may bind to either the binding site for vitamin B_{12} or another site. These antibodies may also affect intrinsic factor production. There is an increased association of atrophic gastritis and pernicious anemia with other putative autoimmune diseases.

AUTOIMMUNE LIVER DISEASE

Autoimmune responses as a possible cause of chronic liver disease remain a fascinating enigma (Kohler, 1982; Taylor, 1982). Several commonly occurring manifestations suggest an organ-localized autoimmune pathogenesis, based on the criteria listed earlier in this chapter, e.g., hypergammaglobulinemia, prominent lymphocyte and plasma cell inflammatory responses occurring mainly in the liver, familial occurrence, one or more circulating antitissue antibodies, and response (sometimes) to therapies effective against experimental autoimmune disorders. Yet most of the autoantibodies are neither liver- nor species-specific; indeed, they react less with liver tissue than with some other tissue sources. Therefore, the pathogenetic significance of these antibodies is uncertain; however, they are of certain pragmatic value in the diagnosis and prognosis of certain conditions noted here.

Chronic active hepatitis is an inflammatory condition that may occur at any age, but most commonly in young women (Czaja, 1981). It is characterized by prominent lymphocyte and plasma cell inflammatory changes which start in the portal tracts. In the more benign ("persistent hepatitis") form, it is limited to those areas. In the more aggressive form, both acute and chronic inflammatory changes (with histiocytes and ductal proliferation) disrupt the limiting plate with resultant "piecemeal necrosis" of adjacent liver parenchyma. Associated with this are clinical and laboratory signs of continued liver inflammation and dysfunction. In some cases, this condition is a result of chronic viral infection or inflammation. In other cases, there are a number of immunologic abnormalities present to varying degrees, in addition to the commonly occurring hypergammaglobulinemia and increased sedimentation rate. Defects in immunoregulation are commonly found, possibly leading to unrestrained Ig production. In some patients, joint, skin, and serosal manifestations may appear, along with serologic findings such as positive ANA and L.E. cell tests, suggestive of SLE. This pattern, occurring predominantly in young women, has been called "lupoid hepatitis" (Mackay, 1956). Overall, the prognosis in aggressive chronic active hepatitis is not good, with significant mortality reported at five years.

Idiopathic biliary cirrhosis (Taylor, 1982; Kohler, 1982) is a slowly progressive condition starting with apparently non-infectious inflammation in the bile ducts of young to middle-aged women and manifested initially as painless jaundice with itching. There is progressive ductal occlusion and resultant cirrhosis which may progress to end-stage liver failure. Lesions may occur in salivary and pancreatic tissue. Familial incidence, increased serum IgM, depression of cellular immunity, and associated "autoimmune disorders" are all increased in frequency in this syndrome. Prominent decreases in suppressor T cells are common, leading to the theory that the tissue damage results from an unmodulated attack against host tissue antigens. A major differential diagnosis is biliary cirrhosis secondary to extrahepatic obstruction.

Idiopathic cirrhosis (Husby, 1977) is an ill-defined entity that may actually represent a collection of disorders characterized by the gradual onset of hepatic dysfunction with varying degrees of jaundice. There is no past history of definite antecedent hepatitis, alcoholic abuse, or other toxic or nutritional factors. An autoimmune basis has been postulated for certain *drug-induced hepatotoxicity* (Taylor, 1982) reactions such as those associated with repeated halothane use. However, the evidence is still quite indirect and circumstantial.

Four types of antibody determinations, all nonspecific for liver disease, have been found to be of some prognostic value (Table 39–9).

1. *Anti-smooth muscle antibodies* (Whittingham, 1966) are of IgM or IgG class, are non–organ- and non–species-specific, and are assayed most commonly by immunofluorescence using unfixed frozen section of either rat stomach wall or renal vessels. A uniform diffuse fluorescence of the muscle fibers is seen with sera diluted at least 1:10 in <5 per cent of normals but up to 90 per cent of those with chronic active hepatitis and 25 to 40 per cent of those with biliary cirrhosis and idiopathic cirrhosis. Serum anti–smooth muscle antibodies are also found transiently in many (as high as 80 per cent) cases of viral hepatitis without any temporal or immunologic relationship to known viral antigens. Anti–smooth muscle antibodies are also common in infectious mononucleosis (up to 80 per cent of those with high titer heterophil antibodies), certain malignant tumors, and perhaps intrinsic asthma (Holborow, 1972). However, titers of ≥1:100 suggest progressive chronic active hepatitis (Husby, 1977). By contrast, sera of SLE patients with strong antinuclear antibody reactivity are rarely positive for anti–smooth muscle antibody. *Possible pitfalls* of this technique include false negative results when insufficiently fresh or fixed tissue substrates are used.

Table 39–9. PREVALENCE OF AUTOANTIBODIES IN LIVER DISEASE*

Disease	Anti-Smooth Muscle	Antimitochondrial	ANA
Chronic active hepatitis	70–90%	30–60%	60%
Chronic persistent hepatitis	45%	15–20%	15–30%
Acute viral hepatitis	10–30%	5–20%	20%
Acute alcoholic hepatitis	0	0	0
Biliary cirrhosis	30%	60–70%	5%
Cryptogenic cirrhosis	15%	30%	0
Alcoholic (Laennec's) cirrhosis	0	0	5%
Extrahepatic biliary obstruction	5–10%	5–10%	5%

*Modified from Whittingham, M. B., Irwin, J., Mackay, I. R., and Smalley, M.: Gastroenterology, *51*:499, 1966; and Husby, G., Skrede, J., and Blomhoff, J. P.: Scand. J. Gastroenterol., *12*:297, 1977.

Antimitochondrial antibodies may be IgG, IgM, or IgA and are also not specific for organ or species source. The antigen appears to be a lipoprotein component on the inner mitochondrial membrane. Fresh unfixed sections of rat kidney are used most commonly as substrates in a standard immunofluorescence technique with intense diffuse staining of the cytoplasm of ductal tubules at serum dilutions of at least 1:10 considered positive. Such positive reactions are seen in <1 per cent of normals but in up to 94 per cent of those with biliary cirrhosis, and 25 per cent of those with chronic active hepatic or idiopathic cirrhosis. Titers of >1:160 are generally found only in biliary cirrhosis. A very helpful distinguishing point in the differential diagnosis of obstructive jaundice is that antimitochondrial antibodies are absent in early infectious hepatitis, alcoholic cirrhosis, or extrahepatic biliary obstruction.

3. *Antinuclear antibodies* (ANA) are commonly found in the three liver conditions described but are unusual in viral hepatitis or alcoholic cirrhosis. A helpful distinguishing point is that ANA in liver diseases is generally accompanied by positive anti–smooth muscle and negative anti-DNA tests, whereas the ANA in SLE is commonly accompanied by anti-DNA antibodies, while anti–smooth muscle antibodies are infrequent. Several kits recently marketed offer the potential advantage of detecting three antibodies with one substrate (rat kidney).

One of the perplexing aspects of putative autoimmune liver disease is that it has been very difficult to demonstrate antibodies specific for liver cells in the sera of such patients, which frequently contain one or more non–tissue-specific autoantibodies.

4. More recently, *antibodies directed against one or more liver antigens* have been described with the additional finding that the serum of chronic active hepatitis patients may initiate antibody dependent cellular cytotoxicity against target hepatocytes (Kohler, 1982; Taylor, 1982).

Summary

1. Anti–smooth muscle antibody determinations help distinguish lupoid hepatitis from SLE; when present in high titer, the antibodies may indicate progressive liver disease. There is no evidence that this antibody is pathogenic, but may reflect "uncovering" of antigenic sites in the small amount of muscle elements in liver cells damaged by inflammation.

2. Antimitochondrial antibodies help distinguish biliary cirrhosis from extrahepatic obstruction, viral hepatitis, and alcoholic cirrhosis.

3. ANA are positive in several liver diseases as well as in SLE. Anti-DNA are generally negative, whereas anti–smooth muscle and/or antimitochondrial antibodies are positive in liver disease.

4. Anti–liver antigen antibodies may play a pathogenic role by direct action, by arming cytotoxic cells, or as components in immune complexes.

AUTOIMMUNITY AND INFLAMMATORY BOWEL DISEASE

In reviews of this field, McGuigan (1980) and Taylor (1982) pointed out that antibodies reacting with colon components are commonly found in the sera of patients with chronic ulcerative colitis, Crohn's disease of the colon, and in some cases of regional ileitis. The antigenic determinant in at least some of the cases is a mucopolysaccharide localized in the cytoplasm of the epithelial cells of the mucosa. These determinants may cross-react with lipopolysaccharides in *Escherichia coli,* which is commonly found in the bacterial flora of the gut. There is an increased incidence of circulating immune complexes in the sera of these patients.

However, such anticolon antibodies by themselves are not cytotoxic for human fetal colon tissue; nor do their titers correlate well with the severity, duration, course, or extent of disease; therefore, their clinical usefulness is limited at present. There is more evidence that lymphocytes from some patients with inflammatory bowel disease are cytotoxic for human fetal colon tissue. It is not clear whether antibody-dependent cellular cytotoxicity plays a role. A finding of uncertain significance is the presence of circulating immune complexes and the depressed capacity to express delayed hypersensitivity (anergy) which occurs commonly, but not uniformly, in inflammatory bowel disease.

Skin Disorders

INTRODUCTION

The skin may be involved in autoimmune reactions in at least three ways: first, inflammatory involvement of cutaneous vessels with secondary effects such as

Table 39–10. AUTOIMMUNITY AND THE SKIN

Disorder	Pattern on Direct Immunofluorescent Staining	Serum Antibody Activity
Systemic lupus erythematosus	Ig* and complement at dermal-epidermal junction in affected, sometimes normal skin	Immune complexes, some nuclear antigens
Discoid lupus	As in SLE, but only in affected skin	? Probably same as SLE
Bullous pemphigoid	Linear deposition Ig and complement in basement membrane of lesions	Anti-basement membrane
Pemphigus group	Ig and complement deposited in intercellular spaces of epidermis (varying patterns)	Against 1 or more epidermal components (keratinocytes, bridges)
Dermatitis herpetiformis	Granular deposition IgA and alternative complement pathway components	? Related to jejunal antigens?

*Ig = Immunoglobulin.

some lesions in SLE, hypersensitivity angiitis, and the syndrome of urticaria and "palpable purpura" with or without mixed cryoglobulinemia (Sofer, 1976) already referred to; second, deposition of putative circulating immune complexes in the skin as may occur in SLE; and third, localized autoreactivity against skin components, as may be seen in certain primary skin disorders. Patterns of response are summarized in Table 39–10.

In the majority of both systemic (SLE) and discoid (DLE) forms of lupus erythematosus, deposition of immunoglobulin (mainly IgG) and complement can be demonstrated by immunofluorescence in a granular pattern just beneath the dermal-epidermal junction of involved skin corresponding to the area of histologic involvement (Wertheimer, 1976) (Fig. 39–2). A fascinating finding of diagnostic and likely great pathogenetic importance is that similar deposition patterns can be found in uninvolved skin in 50 to 60 per cent of SLE patients but not in patients with DLE or other skin disorders. The latter deposition pattern is seen more commonly in those with active systemic disease; it is currently debated whether it correlates well with prominent renal involvement (Gilliam, 1974). A major portion of the immunoglobulin deposited appears to have antinuclear (and possibly anti-DNA) activity, suggesting the presence of immune complexes deposited from the circulation or formed locally. Immunoglobulin in the serum from such patients does *not* bind *in vitro* to the dermal-epidermal junction of normal skin (Tan, 1976a).

Bullous pemphigoid is a chronic, relatively benign disorder (Ahmed, 1977). It is characterized by numerous subepidermal bullae forming at the dermal-epidermal junction. Lesions may be isolated to one part of the body, but mucosal lesions are uncommon. Immunofluorescence study shows deposition of IgG, complement components, and fibrin in a *linear* pattern along the basement membrane, unlike the granular, or "lumpy," pattern seen in SLE (Landry, 1973). The blister fluid contains several chemotactic factors and decreased complement levels, suggesting local activation. In contrast to the situation in SLE, serum IgG and complement from most bullous pemphigoid patients will bind *in vitro* to the dermal-epidermal junction of skin from a variety of species (Landry, 1973); they will also bind *in vivo* when the serum is transferred to normal subhuman primates, but no lesions have been observed at these sites. However, they will induce a bullous pemphigoid–type disease when injected into the rabbit cornea. The inconsistent correlation between titer of anti–basement membrane antibody and extent of disease have suggested to some that these humoral responses are secondary events, possibly to virus-induced tissue damage. The normal serum complement profiles also suggest a local activation process. The increased incidence of malignant tumors in those with bullous pemphigoid has been noted, but searches for cross-reacting antigens in skin components and tumors have not turned up impressive findings to date.

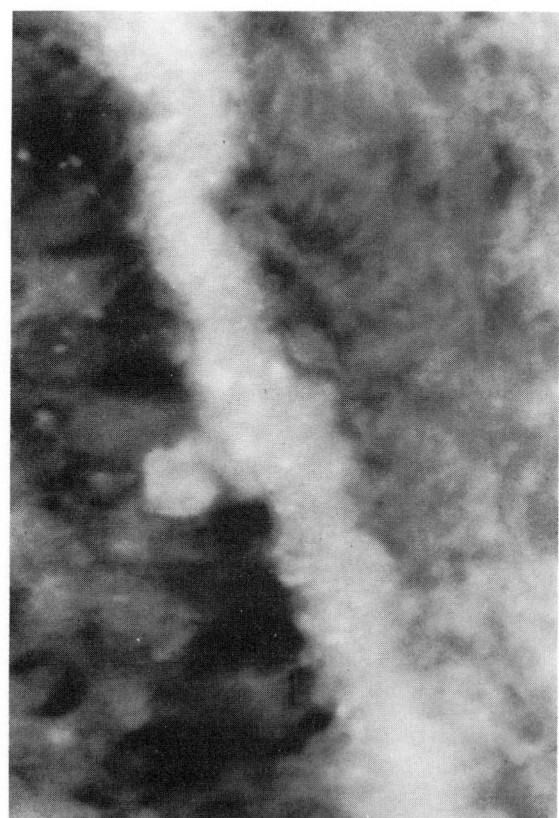

Figure 39–2. Immunofluorescence study of SLE skin lesion. Deposition of IgG in an irregular fashion along dermal-epidermal junction (×600).

Pemphigus represents a group of disorders of varying grades of severity (Jordan, 1981), including pemphigus vulgaris, pemphigus vegetans, and pemphigus foliaceus (Brazilian and erythematous forms) characterized by intraepidermal bullae likely due to loss of integrity of the prickle cell layer (acantholysis) of the epidermis. Immunofluorescence study shows deposition in 90 per cent of patients of Ig (mainly IgG) and complement components on the surface of epidermal cells. There is evidence of local complement activation in the blister fluid. The sera of a large majority of such patients contain immunoglobulin which reacts with intercellular substances of the prickle cell layer, possibly the glycocalyx of the keratinocytes. Some studies (Criswell, 1981) suggest that a diverse pattern of specificity for antigen localization and species of the substrate skin may be seen with the use of sera from patients with different pemphigus subtypes. These antibodies may be pathogenetic, since the titer correlates with activity of the disease, immunoglobulin deposition is frequently seen in the epidermis of skin with little or no inflammatory involvement, the depth within the epidermis of the *in vitro* binding of the serum immunoglobulin appears to correlate with the primary locus of the lesion in the serum donor, and high-titered sera can transfer to rabbits or monkeys a predisposition to the formation of pemphigus-like lesions. Pemphigus antibody may cause local release of proteases, with subsequent disruption of epidermal cell to cell adhesion.

Dermatitis herpetiformis is a chronic disease (Katz, 1980) characterized by intense pruritic and subepidermal bullae similar to those seen in bullous pemphigoid, but occurring more on extensor surfaces in younger individuals. Immunofluorescence also shows deposition of immunoglobulins and complement at the dermal-epidermal junction, most prominently at the tips of the dermal papillae where microabscesses are common. However, several differences from the findings in bullous pemphigoid have been observed: (1) The deposition pattern is granular, suggesting an immune complex rather than anti–basement membrane activity. A circulating 10S putative immune complex has been described. (2) The predominant immunoglobulin detected has been IgA, with evidence of activation of the alternative complement pathways. This unusual pattern has strengthened the association of this apparently localized skin condition to gluten-sensitive enteropathy (Katz, 1980). Elevated serum IgA and antigluten levels are common, and similar jejunal lesions are seen commonly in both conditions, although clinical intestinal manifestations are unusual in the skin disorder. (3) The serum of dermatitis herpetiformis patients does not bind to the basement membrane; in a minority of cases an antireticulin antibody has been described. There is an increased incidence of elevated antinuclear, antithyroglobulin, and antimicrososomal antibodies. There is also evidence of circulating immune complexes, but serum complement levels are usually normal. Many patients have HLA antigens B_8 and DW3 and associated atrophic gastritis.

Finally, we will consider *other skin or mucosal disorders*. In recurrent aphthous stomatitis and the possibly related Behçet's syndrome, ulcerative lesions of the mucosa and skin are characterized by non-specific inflammation and severe patterns of immune reactivity directed against cells of skin and mucosa from a variety of sources. No diagnostic or pathogenic significance of such responses has been definitely shown. The same conclusion may be drawn about a cytotoxic antibody against the superficial epidermis of homologous skin, which is found in the serum of many patients with generalized eczema and exfoliative dermatitis.

CLINICAL IMMUNOLOGIC APPROACH TO SKIN DISEASE

Skin Biopsy for Histopathologic Changes with Immunofluorescence

1. Deposition of immunoglobulin along dermal-epidermal junction.
   a. In lesions—seen in several diseases.
   b. Granular deposition of IgG and other immunoglobulins, complement in lesions, and sometimes in uninvolved skin—suspect SLE.
   c. Granular deposition of IgA close to epidermal-dermal junction in and near involved skin at tips of papillae—suspect dermatitis herpetiformis.
   d. Linear deposition of Ig and complement—suspect bullous pemphigoid.
2. IgG deposition in intercellular areas (intracellular bridges, other loci) within epidermis—suspect pemphigus.

Serum Studies

1. Ig binding to epidermal cell areas—positive in bullous pemphigoid, negative in SLE and dermatitis herpetiformis.
2. Ig binding to intercellular areas—suspect pemphigus.
3. Search for ANA—positive in SLE, less commonly in herpetiformis and bullous pemphigoid—anti-DNA points to SLE.
4. Rheumatoid factor—frequently positive in pemphigus, bullous pemphigoid.
5. Complement profile—prominent decreases suggest immune complex deposition pattern associated with vasculitis, palpable purpura, SLE.

Technical Factors and Possible Pitfalls

1. Choice of fresh skin lesions without extensive destructive changes, including normal skin, will lead to more likely detection by immunofluorescence.
2. Non-specific binding of fluorescein to damaged skin requires careful control.
3. Indirect (serum) assays may detect high titer anti–blood group antibodies or ANA localized on skin cells that may make interpretation to this point difficult unless adequate controls are carried out.

Renal Disease

The kidney has long been suspected as a locus of human immune disease (Wilson, 1981). These impressions have been based mainly on the extrapolation from impressive experimental animal findings, and more limited findings in a few human diseases. However, much of the evidence is circumstantial, based on the findings by immunohistochemical techniques of the deposition of immunoglobulins and complement components in the glomerulus. Therefore, it must first be determined that such localization does not simply reflect just the deposition of any serum protein in a highly vascular tissue damaged by non-immune mechanisms. A test of whether immunoglobulins found in the kidney glomerulus (or any inflamed tissue area, for that matter) could consist of these sequential steps:

1. Determination that immunoglobulins and/or complement components are present in higher concentration than a serum protein such as albumin thought to be uninvolved in immune reactions. Evidence of fibrinogen deposition is less helpful in this regard, since it probably can be seen in both immune and non-immune responses.
2. Determination that immunoglobulins eluted from involved tissues have antibody activity *in vitro*. If the antibody activity per milligram of gamma globulin in the tissue eluates is greater than seen in the serum obtained concomitantly from the patient, preferential tissue localization of the antibody is suggested.
3. Identification of the antigen in the lesion.
4. If the antibody isolated is detected against a component of kidney tissue, such activity should be demonstrated *in vitro* (by immunohistochemical or serologic study), or by passive transfer to animals.

Unfortunately, logistic and ethical considerations in human disease frequently limit demonstration to only the first steps, resulting in the circumstantial nature of the evidence. Comparisons with the experimental autoimmune kidney disease models have led to exciting hypotheses.

It is generally accepted (Wilson, 1981) that most immunologically mediated renal diseases fall into several categories (Table 39–11). In the *first*, antibodies are induced *in vivo* against the basement membrane (BM) of the glomerulus (and possibly the renal tubule or lung basement membrane). The factors making such membranes autoantigenic in humans are not well defined. However, it appears likely that binding of drugs such as methicillin, certain infectious agents, and even the renal damage caused by other immune mechanisms may lead to such responses. The end result may be direct damage to the BM with or without complement activation. The production of anti-BM antibodies appears to be self-limited, lasting weeks to months after removal of the inciting agent with nephrectomy. This characteristic may be of practical importance, to be discussed later.

Table 39–11. CATEGORIES OF "IMMUNOLOGIC" RENAL DISEASE

Associated anti–glomerular basement membrane antibody
Most cases of Goodpasture's syndrome
Some rapidly progressive glomerulonephritis
Altered membrane by virus? drugs?
Associated with circulating immune complex
SLE
Certain other vasculitis
Certain infections—bacteria. treponemal viral, parasitic
Tumors?
Ig/anti-Ig
Membranoproliferative glomerulonephritis
Alternative complement activation
? Genetic factors
Tubulo/interstitial nephritis
Drugs, infection?
Associated with immune complex–mediated disease
Involvement of transplanted kidneys

In the *second* category, immune complexes composed of non-renal antigens and corresponding antibodies are deposited in one or more of several loci in the glomerulus, possibly dependent on the size and other characteristics of the complex. For example, immune complex deposits localized in the mesangium should be relatively large and cleared readily with mild disease. Complexes localized in the subepithelial area would be larger but still not as damaging as those trapped on the subendothelial side of the GBM where inflammatory responses are most prominent. Recent evidence suggests that potentially damaging immune complexes may be formed *in situ* involving antigens already present or fixed in the glomerulus (Couser, 1980).

Immune complex activation of complement in glomerular basement membrane (GBM) may be augmented by the presence of cells with receptors for C3 located in that area. The result of this activation likely involves release of biologically active products, including those which attract granulocytes to the site. The end result of this chain of events is an inflammatory response type of tissue injury.

There is increasing evidence that nonimmunologically activated complement may cause another category of glomerular disease. In these cases, activation of the alternative complement pathway (Chap. 37) appears to be the mechanism involved, analogous to the *in vitro* activation of C3 by certain bacterial products and polysaccharides.

However, it should be stressed that current knowledge indicates that the term "glomerulonephritis" is non-specific insofar as pathogenesis, with inclusion of a variety of glomerular disorders. We will now look at a few such disorders.

DISORDERS WITH ANTI–GLOMERULAR BASEMENT MEMBRANE (GBM) ANTIBODY

These likely represent less than 5 per cent of glomerular disorders (Wilson, 1977). They are characterized by a *linear* deposition of immunoglobulin and sometimes complement along the GBM (Wilson, 1981) (Fig. 39–3). Histologically, prominent epithelial cell proliferation around the capillary loop frequently leads to a rapidly progressive proliferative glomerulonephritis with marked crescent formation.

Goodpasture's syndrome is an uncommon disease which shows involvement of alveolar and glomerular basement membranes such as anti–GBM antibody leading to alveolar hemorrhage and almost invariably fatal glomerulonephritis if untreated. Milder forms of the disease have been recognized. However, it must be noted that Ig linear deposition patterns by immunofluorescence may not always be diagnostic in anti–GBM disease. (1) Finely granular deposits may

5

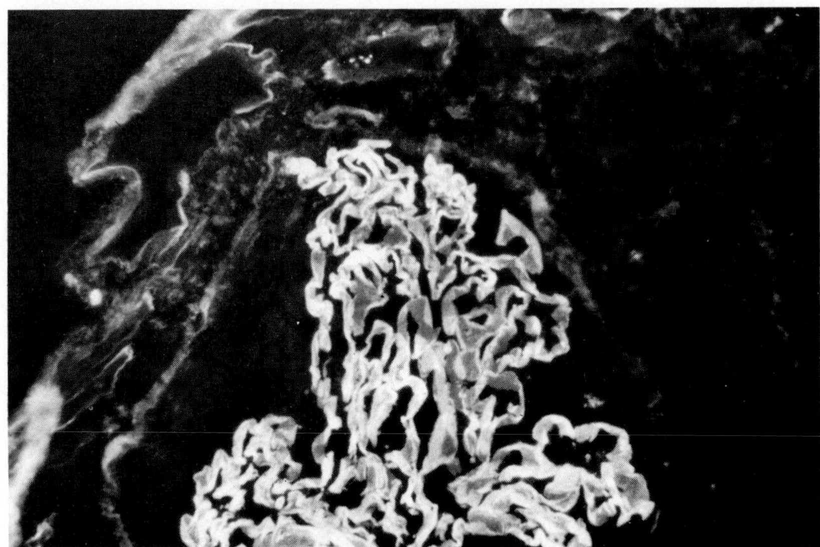

Figure 39–3. Immunofluorescence study of a renal biopsy in Goodpasture's syndrome. Deposition of IgG in a smooth linear pattern along the glomerular basement membrane (×600).

look linear unless high magnification is employed. (2) Linear patterns may occasionally be due to deposition of Ig which have no anti–GBM activity, such as in early SLE. (3) In later stages of Goodpasture's syndrome, glomerular damage may mask the typical linear pattern with a more lumpy appearance on immunofluorescence. In occasional patients, Goodpasture's syndrome appears to be associated with immune complex deposition (Wilson, 1977).

More recently, passive hemagglutination and radioimmunoassays have been used to determine serum anti–GBM antibody. The sensitivity of such techniques and the correlation of antibody titers obtained with the severity of disease has varied among investigators. Wilson (1977) has reported what appears to be a highly sensitive and specific radioimmunoassay for antibodies to the non-collagenous protein of the GBM. Positive results were seen in sera from 76 of 78 patients with Goodpasture's syndrome and 43 of 52 patients with other forms of anti–GBM nephritis. In contrast, only a low incidence was seen in those with either immune-complex type (2 of 393) or negative (1 of 222) immunoglobulin deposition patterns in the GBM.

Measurement of the anti–GBM antibodies may turn out to be of considerable assistance not only in diagnosis but also in monitoring a new therapeutic approach (plasmapheresis to remove anti–GBM antibodies), which has been shown experimentally to cause the glomerular damage (Lang, 1977).

IMMUNE COMPLEX–MEDIATED GLOMERULONEPHRITIS

The characteristic finding in this category is the immunofluorescent demonstration of Ig and C3 deposited in and near the GBM in an irregular pattern varying from granular to large globular accumulations. It has been estimated (Wilson, 1976) that such patterns are seen in 70 to 80 per cent of those with human glomerulonephritis. In about one third of those with "immune complex type" immunofluorescent immunoglobulin (Ig) deposition patterns, a putative circulating immune complex was detected by one or another of the techniques described earlier in this chapter.

The strongest evidence for immune complex pathogenesis comes in *SLE*, in which irregular deposits of Ig and complement components are found in almost all cases with glomerular involvement (Fig. 39–4). Eluted Ig has been shown in some cases to exhibit strong antibody activity against ribosomes and a variety of nuclear antigens, including DNA (Winfield, 1975). There is also at least indirect evidence that DNA is present in involved areas of the capillary as well. Although a linear deposition may be seen in the GBM of early lupus nephritis, anti–GBM activity in either the tissue eluates or serum of such patients is unusual (Wilson, 1977).

Several histologic patterns have been described with the understanding that progression from less prominent to more severe involvement may occur in individual patients (Baldwin, 1982). In *focal* glomerulonephritis, mesangeal and endothelial cell proliferation occurs in isolated capillary loops of some glomeruli. Immunoglobulin (Ig) and C3 deposition is generally limited to the mesangium. The clinical presentation is variable with modest urinary abnormalities and a stable course in some but progressive renal disease in others. In the uncommon *membranous glomerulonephritis* presentation, there is a diffuse hypertrophy of the basement membrane with little cellular proliferation. A diffuse, finely granular deposition of IgG and complement is seen throughout the glomeruli with electron-dense deposits on the epithelial aspects of the

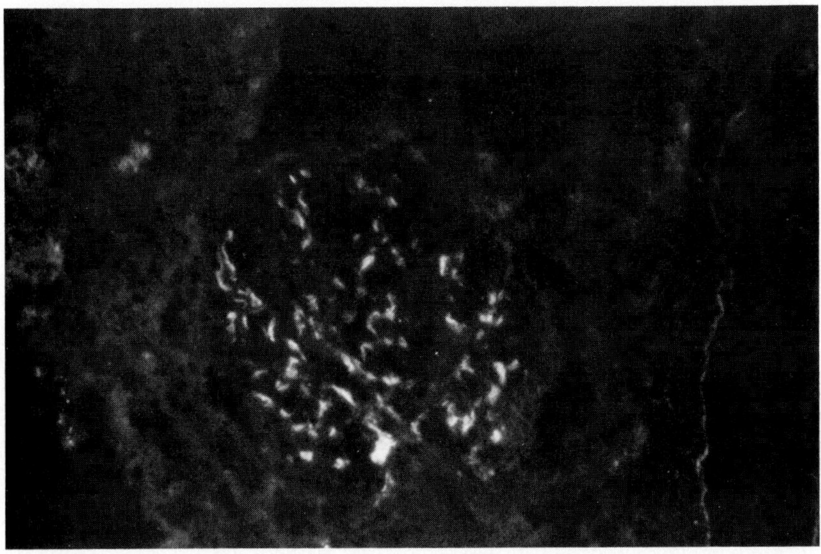

Figure 39–4. Immunofluorescence study of a renal biopsy in systemic lupus erythematosus. Deposition of IgG in an irregular, granular pattern along the glomerular basement membrane (×600).

membrane. The nephrotic syndrome with a slowly progressive course is the usual presentation.

The *diffuse proliferative glomerulonephritis* picture is the most abnormal with the worst prognosis. Almost all glomeruli are involved with irregular proliferation of both mesangial and endothelial cells. Irregular thickenings in the basement membrane may result in the "wire loop" appearance of the clinically described lesion. There is heavy irregular deposition of Ig and of components of both the classic and alternative pathways. Large electron-dense deposits starting in the subendothelial area may also be found in the basement membrane itself. The clinical picture is that of severe renal disease, often progressing to end-stage renal failure within a period of months to several years.

OTHER EXAMPLES OF IMMUNE COMPLEX–MEDIATED DISEASE

Putative immunohistochemical evidence of immune complex deposition in the kidney has been reported in at least some patients with systemic disorders with or without evidence of joint, skin, or vessel inflammation (Wilson, 1977). Examples include the following: (1) HB_s antigen–positive hepatitis, sometimes also with urticaria, joint symptoms, or evidence of vasculitis elsewhere. These extrahepatic manifestations may be most prominent during the time period before obvious clinical signs of hepatic inflammation become obvious. (2) Infections with beta-streptococci, spirochetes, *Plasmodium malariae, Salmonella typhosa, Mycobacterium leprae, Schistosoma mansoni, Toxoplasma* (Gamble, 1975; Ward, 1969; Tesor, 1970), and certain viruses such as lymphocytic choriomeningitis and Epstein-Barr. (3) Chronic infections of heart valves or shunts with *Staphylococcus, Corynebacterium bovis* or *Enterococcus* (Strife, 1976). (4) Thyroglobulin and possibly other tissue antigens to which prominent antibody responses occur in autoimmune diseases. Tumor-antitumor antibody has also led to deposition of complexes (Lewis, 1971). This list will undoubtedly increase as intensive studies are carried out in a wide variety of disease states. It may even be that the transient "febrile proteinuria," long noted in association with certain infectious diseases, may reflect in part a self-limited glomerular inflammatory reaction due to circulating complexes.

A similar deposition pattern is seen in kidneys from some patients with *idiopathic glomerulonephritis.* It is not clear whether immunologic mechanisms play a role in the latter situation. In *acute post-streptococcal glomerulonephritis,* deposition of C3 and properdin, and only sometimes IgG, is seen. In the severe and often rapidly fatal *rapidly progressive glomerulonephritis,* fibrinogen deposition is especially heavy, along with IgG, C3, and prominent epithelial crescents.

Membranoproliferative Glomerulonephritis. In about 10 per cent of kidneys examined by immunofluorescence, deposits of complement components in the absence of Ig are found in the glomeruli. Some of these cases appear to be examples of advanced stages of immune-complex–induced nephritis with possible activation of the alternative complement pathway by previously damaged GBM (Wilson, 1977). There appears to be a subgroup of patients described originally by West and his colleagues (1966) with a membranoproliferative glomerulitis, "tram track" changes of the GBM seen in ultramicroscopy, and markedly decreased levels of the later complement components. In at least some of these patients, a circulating gamma globulin ("C3 nephritic factor") appears to activate C3 by the alternative pathway (see Chap. 37). However, the ultimate result of this activation is progressive glomerular damage with subsequent renal insufficiency.

Immune Tubulointerstitial Disease. An experimental autoimmune inflammatory disease in the renal tubules can be induced by appropriate sensitization to renal tubule BM (TBM), analogous to that seen with GBM. In some instances, there is cross-reactivity between GBM and TBM in these experimental models. Likewise, anti-TBM antibodies are found in about 70 per cent of those with Goodpasture's syndrome and more commonly than anti-GBM in renal transplant recipients (Wilson, 1977). Linear deposits of Ig are found in the renal tubules. Such deposits are also found in some patients with methicillin-induced tubular disease. Anti-TBM antibodies without anti-GBM antibodies are found in some patients with immune complex–induced glomerulonephritis and may play a role in the peritubular and interstitial inflammatory cell responses seen in some cases of SLE and certain other disorders. In some cases such interstitial disease may be the major component in detectable renal disease, with granular deposits along tubule walls.

CLINICAL LABORATORY APPROACH TO THE STUDY OF SUSPECTED AUTOIMMUNE RENAL DISEASE

Direct immunofluorescence studies of renal tissue from patients constitute the main approach available. Proper processing of specimens for frozen section preparation is critical here. Only a limited number of glomeruli are available in many needle biopsy specimens and all are needed for study when the disease involvement is focal. Mild fixation (95 per cent alcohol or acetone for short periods) is generally helpful, but excessive fixation must be avoided. One should look for deposition of "non-immunologic" serum proteins such as albumin, using similar immunofluorescent techniques. As in any immunofluorescent method, the quality of the fluorescein-conjugated antiserum (preferably the Ig fraction of the latter) is an important determinant of both sensitivity and selectivity. One must determine periodically that the reagents used do not bind non-specifically to kidney tissue which is normal or damaged by non-immune mechanisms. Fluorescein-antibody techniques are discussed in Chapter 38.

Measurement of anti–GBM antibodies is also performed. The only technique readily available is that of indirect immunofluorescence. Acetone-fixed frozen sections of normal kidney are incubated with test and control sera; after appropriate washes, the section is incubated with fluorescein-conjugated antiserum to one or more human Ig components. Although serial dilution studies have been reported, it is not clear how quantitative this technique is for anti–GBM antibodies. Some (Evans, 1975) have pointed out that a non-specific faint linear fluorescein pattern may result from the binding of normal serum components to the GBM of normal human kidneys. They have suggested the use of normal monkey kidney tissue to obviate this problem.

Passive hemagglutination tests and radioimmunoassays for anti–GBM antibody depend upon the nature and quality of the GBM component used as the antigen. Findings with use of one preparation by Wilson (1977) have already been described. Others (Evans, 1975) have noted that such serologic assays may be more sensitive than indirect immunofluorescent approaches, but there may be real technical problems with breakdown of GBM components used in the assays.*

Cardiac Disorders

An immunologic basis for *rheumatic heart disease* (RHD) has been suspected for a long time. The sera of many patients with RHD contain antibodies which bind *in vitro* to foci in the myocardium and heart valves (Kaplan, 1969). Antimyocardial antibodies may be responsible for the deposition of immunoglobulin and complement components found in the same area of RHD tissues at autopsy. These antibodies appear to be strongly cross-reactive with streptococcal antigens and are not toxic to heart tissue unless the latter is damaged previously by some other cause. Because antiheart antibodies are commonly found in those with recent streptococcal infection without cardiac sequelae, detection of such antibodies has not been a particularly useful diagnostic test.

About 3 per cent of those with a recent myocardial infarction will manifest a clinical syndrome including fever and chest pain, often with signs of pleuritis and pericarditis and musculoskeletal symptoms (Kaplan, 1969). Antiheart antibodies, not cross-reacting with streptococci, are found in the sera of about 30 per cent of such individuals. A similar picture may be seen in some individuals who had undergone recent surgical procedures on the heart. The pathologic or diagnostic significance of such antibodies has not been demonstrated.

Neuromuscular System

There are several important neurologic diseases in which the immune system may play an important role in the pathogenesis and/or etiology. There have been a number of investigations of serologic and cellular immune abnormalities in these entities. In some instances these findings are helpful in confirming the clinical diagnosis; in others, the immunologic phenomena are primarily investigative at this time. In one disorder, myasthenia gravis, there is an assay for an autoantibody which has become part of the diagnostic armamentarium.

MULTIPLE SCLEROSIS

Multiple sclerosis is a common demyelinating disease of the central nervous system. Important pathologic changes consist of (1) perivenous cuffs of mononuclear inflammatory cells; (2) perivascular and periventricular confluent areas of myelin loss called plaques, with

*Complement components in renal diseases are discussed in Chapter 37.

Table 39–12. EVIDENCE FOR AUTOIMMUNITY IN MULTIPLE SCLEROSIS

1. Antibodies to myelin and myelin constituents
2. Antibodies to oligodendroglia
3. *In vitro* myelinotoxicity and glial toxicity of serum and CSF (cerebrospinal fluid)
4. Oligoclonal increase in CSF Ig
5. *In vitro* cell-mediated immunity by blood and CSF cells to myelin components
6. Similarity of MS and experimental allergic encephalomyelitis
7. Increase in certain HL-A and Ia antigens (HL-A A3, B7, DW2, and DRW2)

relative preservation of neurons and axons; and (3) astrocytic proliferation (Adams, 1977). Current research into the etiology and pathogenesis of multiple sclerosis relates to viral factors (Lisak, 1980) and abnormalities of immune regulation (Weiner, 1982).

There is much evidence, largely indirect, that viruses may be etiologic agents in multiple sclerosis. However, there is considerable controversy in the literature related to this evidence as regards reproducibility and interpretation of the findings. An equally large and indirect body of experimental evidence suggests an autoimmune pathogenesis (Table 39–12). However, the lack of reproducible findings has made for varying interpretations concerning the cause of multiple sclerosis. The lack of specificity of many of these viral and immune-related abnormalities limits the diagnostic and prognostic usefulness of most of these assays.

Various theories have been advanced to tie the seemingly conflicting data related to viruses, autoimmunity, and immunogenetics together. These include (1) shared antigenicity between viruses and myelin constituents; (2) release of a hidden antigen by a subclinical infection; (3) attempts by the immune system to destroy a virus within a nervous system cell; (4) molecular mimicry between virus and an HLA or Ia antigen; (5) virus combining with or directing the synthetic apparatus of host cells to form or produce a neoantigen; (6) virus acting as a hapten and triggering a response against the self tissue, the carrier molecule; and (7) increase in autoimmune reaction owing to failure of normal immunologic control mechanisms, more likely to occur in genetically susceptible subjects.

Laboratory Measurements in the Diagnosis of Multiple Sclerosis (MS)

Protein Studies in the Cerebrospinal Fluid (CSF). The laboratory measurement of current greatest diagnostic use is analysis of CSF for the percentage of immunoglobulin (Ig), as well as the Ig pattern in the CSF protein. It has been found that spinal fluid Ig is increased (>13 per cent of total protein) in the CSF of 65 to 75 per cent of MS patients at some time during the course of the disease (Tourtellotte, 1971). In addition, various formulas have been proposed which employ measurements of serum and CSF IgG and albumin to derive a CSF index and other formulas which estimate daily CSF IgG synthesis. Various methods have been used to characterize the immunoglobulin in CSF. Of these, electrophoresis in agarose currently seems to be the most useful technique (Link, 1971; Johnson, 1977). A picture of a typical CSF pattern in MS is shown in Figure 39–5. *Advantages* of this technique include (1) use of commercially available prepoured agarose plates and simple, relatively inexpensive electrophoretic apparatus; (2) the ability to determine the total protein, percentage, and amount of Ig using a gel scanner and the presence of an oligoclonal pattern in a single assay; (3) the high sensitivity of the technique, being positive in 80 to 95 per cent of patients with multiple sclerosis and in about 50 to 60 per cent with the first attack; (4) treatment of the agarose slide with anti–human immunoglobulin prior to staining for protein, which may further enhance demonstration of the bands (Cawley, 1976); (5) electrophoresis in agarose is more sensitive than that in agar or on cellulose acetate in demonstrating oligoclonal bands when the total Ig percentage is normal; (6) the utility in demonstrating protein patterns not feasible with techniques such as radial immunodiffusion, tube precipitin reactions, and electroimmunodiffusion; and (7) less technical difficulty, less expense, and more diagnostic usefulness than isoelectric focusing, acrylamide gel electrophoresis, and isotachyphoresis. A radioimmunoassay has recently been described which allows the demonstration of IgM and IgA as well as IgG elevations (Mingioli, 1978), but these techniques are not yet adapted to clinical use.

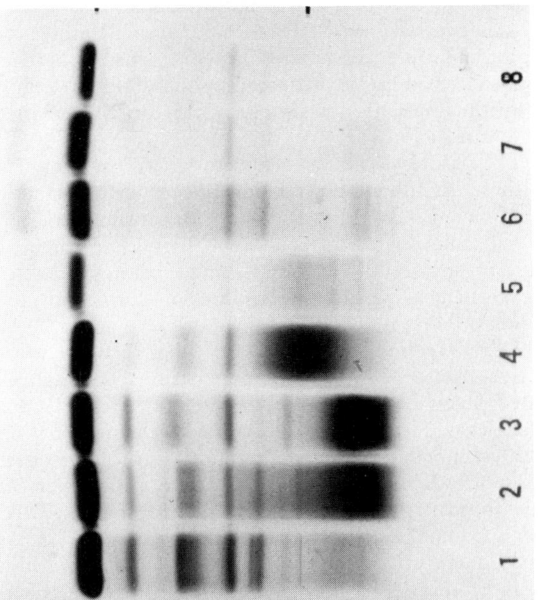

Figure 39–5. Agarose electrophoresis of serum (Gels No. 1 to 4) and cerebrospinal fluid (Gels 5 to 8). Left is anode. The dense band seen on the right of Nos. 1 to 4 is gammaglobulin. No. 8 shows no bands in that region, but Nos. 5, 6, and 7 demonstrate oligoclonal bands characteristic of multiple sclerosis. (Courtesy of Doctor Dean Arvan.)

Table 39–13. CONDITIONS ASSOCIATED WITH OLIGOCLONAL CEREBROSPINAL FLUID (CSF) GAMMA GLOBULINS

1. Multiple sclerosis
2. Neurosyphilis
3. Subacute sclerosing panencephalitis
4. Chronic mycobacterial and fungal meningitis
5. Chronic viral meningitis and meningoencephalitis (uncommon)
6. Acute viral meningitis (uncommon)
7. Optic neuritis
8. Acute disseminated encephalomyelitis (?)

The major *disadvantage* of agarose electrophoresis is the need to concentrate CSF prior to use. Newer apparatus are available which greatly simplify this procedure, and the substitution of silver nitrate for standard protein stains will likely allow examination of very small amounts of CSF without the need for concentration of the specimen. In addition, all assays for oligoclonal CSF proteins should be interpreted with the understanding that such CSF paraproteins are not found exclusively in MS (Table 39–13). However, the combination of clinical manifestations and evidence of infection with either syphilis or other infectious agents may be of aid in distinguishing these other diseases from MS. Oligoclonal bands have been shown to be present in the spinal fluid of patients with optic neuritis (Sandberg-Wollheim, 1975). Some of these patients have gone on to develop multiple sclerosis, but only after 5 to 20 years will we know if all optic neuritis patients with oligoclonal bands are destined to develop clinical multiple sclerosis.

It is necessary with all of the above techniques to perform simultaneous assays on sera to ensure that the abnormal pattern or increased spinal fluid immunoglobulin levels do not simply mirror an abnormality of serum globulins.

The nature of the antigen(s) to which the majority of these immunoglobulin bands of presumed antibody are directed is not known. This is in contradistinction to subacute sclerosing panencephalitis where incubation of spinal fluid with cell lines bearing measles virus antigens results in absorption of most of the bands (Mehta, 1976).

CSF Myelin Basic Protein. The CSF of most patients with MS in acute exacerbation contains elevated levels of myelin basic protein (Cohen, 1976). The elevated levels seem to reflect active demyelination or myelin destruction and are found in disorders other than MS (Whitaker, 1980). Since normal levels of myelin basic protein do not exclude MS and elevated levels do not confirm the presence of MS, the test has little diagnostic value. Serial studies of CSF myelin basic protein levels may prove of use in future therapeutic studies as an index of disease activity.

Serum Autoantibodies in MS. Several *serum autoantibodies* have been reported to occur frequently in MS (Lisak, 1980). The diagnostic usefulness of binding to myelin and/or oligodendrocytes in monolayer or suspension cultures is limited because serum from normal subjects or patients with other neurological diseases may also bind. Assessment of binding of MS serum or CSF to myelin, myelin components, or oligodendrocytes should be considered research tests.

Measles-Lymphocyte Studies. It has been reported by some that the peripheral blood lymphocytes of patients with multiple sclerosis form a greater number of rosettes with a cell line containing measles virus, when compared with normals or patients with other neurologic diseases (Levy, 1976). However, others have found considerable overlap between MS patients and normals (Dore-Duffy, 1979). The reported differences between MS patients and controls is due to adherence properties of the lymphocytes which may relate to prostaglandin synthesis by the blood cells.

GUILLAIN-BARRÉ SYNDROME

Guillain-Barré syndrome is an acquired disease of peripheral nerve and roots often associated with recent viral illness or immunizations or, rarely, with surgery, systemic lupus erythematosus, lymphoma, or pregnancy (Asbury, 1969; Arnason, 1971). The pathologic features include an inflammatory perivascular infiltrate consisting of lymphocytes, monocyte-macrophages, and segmental demyelination. The lesions are virtually identical with those seen in experimental allergic neuritis, a disease induced in animals by sensitization with peripheral nerve, peripheral myelin, or certain myelin components in Freund's complete adjuvant. Considerable controversy exists over the nature of the peripheral nerve myelin constituent responsible for induction of the experimental disease and the relative roles of cell-mediated and humoral immune responses. A similar situation pertains in Guillain-Barré syndrome; various investigators have reported antibodies and cell-mediated immunity to myelin or components of myelin. Currently, there is no specific immunologic diagnostic test for Guillain-Barré syndrome. The diagnosis is still based on the clinical picture and supported by an increase in cerebrospinal fluid total protein with an absence of pleocytosis and evidence for peripheral nervous system demyelination on electrophysiologic testing. There is a group of patients who present with progressive acquired or sometimes relapsing demyelinative neuropathy. In some of these patients a monoclonal gammopathy (IgG or IgM) can be demonstrated in the absence of amyloidosis, multiple myeloma, solitary plasmacytoma, or Waldenström's macroglobulinemia (Kelly, 1982b; Smith, 1983). In patients with these clinical syndromes, analysis of the serum using agarose electrophoresis with or without immunofixation may prove helpful. In the instance of demyelinating neuropathy with IgM_K paraproteinemia, the IgM seems to be antibody to myelin or Schwann cell; in many cases, myelin-associated glycoprotein seems to be the antigen (Braun, 1982). Whether this antibody is pathogenic is not as yet known (Asbury, 1981).

MYASTHENIA GRAVIS

Myasthenia gravis (MG) is a disorder of the neuromuscular junction characterized by neurophysiologic and immunologic abnormalities (Lisak, 1982; Linstrom, 1977). It has been demonstrated that there is a decrease in available receptor for acetylcholine (Frambrough, 1973) and frequently anatomic defects in the neuromuscular junction muscle endplate, leading to a post-synaptic defect. In acquired MG the post-synaptic abnormalities seem to be the result of antibodies to acetylcholine receptor. The various congenital forms of MG are due to abnormalities at the neuromuscular junction, including decreased receptor in some forms, but not secondary to antibodies. Clinical manifestations of MG include motor weakness, especially on repetitive stimulation or sustained effort.

While it is clear that antibodies to acetylcholine receptor are important in producing the neuromuscular block, it is not clear which immunopathogenic mechanisms are involved. The motor endplate is often abnormal in appearance and IgG and C3 and C9 are found at the junction, suggesting that complement-mediated antibody determined damage is an important mechanism (Engel, 1977). Other endplates appear to show no evidence of damage, and it has been shown that antibodies to acetylcholine "receptor" are capable of increasing the normal rate of degradation resulting in less available receptor (Drachman, 1978). In addition, a small amount of antibody seems to be directed to the ligand (bungarotoxin or acetylcholine) binding portion of the receptor. The absolute titer of antibodies to receptor does not correlate with the degree of clinical severity; however, the latter may correlate with the amount and biologic activity of different antiacetylcholine receptor antibodies.

Several lines of evidence suggest that more broad-based autoimmunity and defects in immunoregulation are present in patients with MG (Table 39–14). Histologic abnormalities are found in the thymus, and there is an increase in other autoimmune diseases and autoantibodies. Early immunofluorescence studies showed antibodies to one or more structural components of normal muscle in greater than 1:60 titer in about 30 per cent of the myasthenics, 90 per cent of those with MG plus thymoma, and 30 per cent of those with thymoma alone (Fig. 39–6). The last-named finding is likely related to the observation that the antimuscle antibodies bind to the thymic myoid cells. Some have postulated that the thymus is the site of the primary immune stimulus for the production of such antibodies and perhaps for antiacetylcholine receptor antibodies as well. The antimuscle antibodies do not appear to be pathogenic and are not useful in the diagnosis of MG. It has been suggested

Table 39–14. IMMUNOPATHOGENESIS OF MYASTHENIA GRAVIS

1. Thymic hyperplasia with germinal follicles (70%)
2. Thymoma (10–15%)
3. Antibodies to acetylcholine receptor and muscle
4. Transfer of neuromuscular block to mice with myasthenic Ig
5. Other (non-neuromuscular) antibodies
6. Associated with other "autoimmune" diseases
7. Cell-mediated immunity to muscle and acetylcholine receptor
8. Increase in thymic B cells
9. Autologous mixed leukocyte reaction between thymus and blood cells
10. Increase in HLA-A1, A3, B8, and DW3

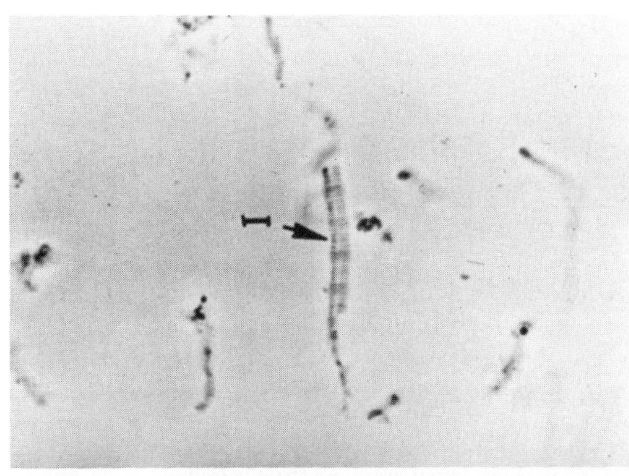

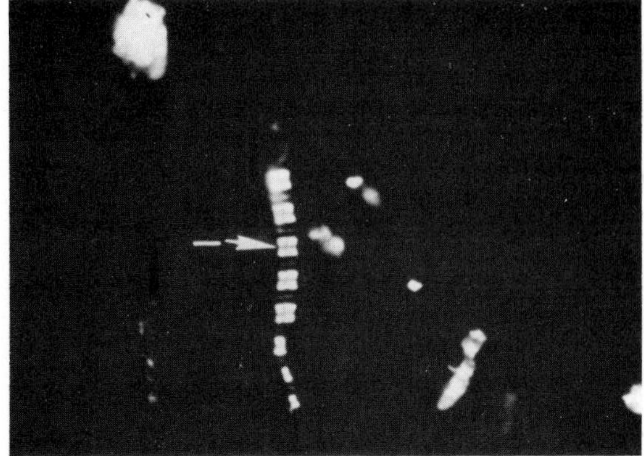

Figure 39–6. Binding of IgG from serum of myasthenia gravis patient to muscle structural bands (arrow); immunofluorescence (bottom) and phase (top) study (×400). (Courtesy of Doctor Donald Schotland.)

that the absence of antimuscle antibodies is strong evidence against the presence of a thymoma in a patient with MG.

Laboratory Diagnosis of Myasthenia Gravis. The diagnosis of myasthenia gravis is based on the clinical picture and confirmed by certain pharmacologic and clinical electrophysiologic tests (Lisak, 1982). Demonstration of elevated titers to human acetylcholine receptor can be demonstrated in 80 to 90 per cent of patients with acquired generalized myasthenia (Linstrom, 1977; Lisak, 1982; Kelly, 1982a); but perhaps only 20 to 30 per cent of patients with acquired ocular myasthenia have elevated levels of such antibodies. Patients with congenital MG never have increased serum antibodies to acetylcholine receptor.

Detection of serum antibodies to acetylcholine receptor may be very helpful in establishing the diagnosis of MG, especially in a difficult case; but the failure to demonstrate such antibodies clearly does not rule out the diagnosis. The most widely employed assay is a radioimmunoassay (RIA) in which acetylcholine receptor-rich material obtained from human muscle is reacted with ^{125}I-labeled alpha-bungarotoxin (available commercially) which binds to the acetylcholine binding site on the receptor molecule. This receptor/^{125}I-alpha-bungarotoxin is then incubated with the test human serum. Immune complexes con-

5

sisting of serum antiacetylcholine receptor antibodies plus acetylcholine receptor/^{125}I-alpha-bungarotoxin are precipitated, using anti-human IgG or staphylococcal protein A. Preparations of human acetylcholine receptor vary widely in bungarotoxin binding and antibody binding capacity; known standard positive and negative serum controls must be included in all determinations. Since ^{125}I-alpha-bungarotoxin binds to the acetylcholine binding site of the receptor, antibodies directed at that site will be underestimated. In order to obviate that problem, other assays have been used, including a RIA in which ^{125}I-alpha-bungarotoxin sites are not fully saturated. Since all of these assays involve extraction procedures to obtain the receptor preparation, antibodies directed at antigenic sites that are hidden or denatured by the extraction will not be detected.

DERMATOMYOSITIS AND POLYMYOSITIS

Polymyositis and dermatomyositis are acquired inflammatory myopathies of unknown etiology (Bohan, 1975). Although often considered together, each almost certainly represents several distinct albeit related syndromes. Dermatomyositis includes (1) childhood dermatomyositis, a disease in which pathologic evidence for vasculitis is quite prominent, and (2) adult dermatomyositis with or without associated neoplasm. It is not clear that the presence or absence of associated solid tumor implies a different pathogenesis. Polymyositis is a syndrome which can be either idiopathic, not associated with any other disease, or associated with clinical and/or serologic evidence of other "collagen-vascular" or "autoimmune" diseases, including scleroderma, rheumatoid arthritis, systemic lupus erythematosus, and Sjögren's syndrome. There is little evidence for any association of polymyositis with neoplasm. Polymyopathy is a term best applied to acquired myopathies, including polymyositis, as well as other acquired myopathies such as sarcoid, metabolic, endocrine, and non-inflammatory carcinomatous myopathies.

The prominent vasculitis noted in childhood dermatomyositis in muscle and other organ systems strongly suggests that immune complexes may be involved in the pathogenesis of this disease. The demonstration of immunoglobulin and complement in the vessels of such patients (Whitaker, 1972) lends support to this hypothesis. Vasculitis is not generally a prominent feature of adult dermatomyositis. Although vasculitis is seen in some muscle biopsies of patients with idiopathic polymyositis and polymyositis associated with other collagen-vascular diseases, it is not common or usually prominent. Serum antibodies to muscle are not found in dermatomyositis and polymyositis.

Patients with dermatomyositis and polymyositis with or without associated neoplasm or other collagen-vascular diseases often have serologic abnormalities, including increased erythrocyte sedimentation rate, increased serum immunoglobulins, and increased antinuclear antibodies. Depression of serum complement is not usually seen unless associated with the accompanying collagen-vascular disease, even in childhood dermatomyositis. It has been reported that sera of about 50 per cent of patients with dermatomyositis and polymyositis react with nuclear material extracted from calf thymus which is not RNA or DNA (Reichlin, 1976; Wolfe, 1977).

To date, other diseases associated with antinuclear antibodies do not seem to react with this antigen unless myositis is part of the clinical picture in the patient. If the presence of this antibody can be confirmed by other groups, it will be of aid in helping to distinguish polymyositis from the larger spectrum of acquired myopathies. Currently, the diagnosis of dermatomyositis and polymyositis is based on the clinical picture and confirmed by (1) elevation of serum enzymes, especially creatinine phosphokinase; (2) myopathic and "irritative" patterns on electromyography; and (3) inflammatory myopathic muscle biopsy with or without vasculitis.

Lymphocytes

ANTILYMPHOCYTE ANTIBODIES

Circulating antibodies of the IgG type which react with lymphocytes have long been detected in the sera of some polytransfused subjects and multiparous females. The antibodies appear to be directed against HLA (histocompatibility locus antigen) components in the donor cells, and react best at room temperature or at 37°C. In addition, a different type of antilymphocyte antibody of the IgM type exerts cytotoxic effects on human lymphocytes most strongly at 15°C. (Kunkel, 1975). The latter antibodies react predominantly with T lymphocytes, but anti–B lymphocyte activity may be seen in some sera. Lymphocytes of different normal donors show varying susceptibility to the cytotoxic effects of these cold-reactive antibodies, not based on the usual HLA specificities. Cold-reactive antibodies have been found in SLE patients and close household contacts of such individuals (De Horatius, 1975), in rheumatoid arthritis, scleroderma, MG, MS, Hodgkin's disease, and solid tumors, and in normal subjects with recent viral infection or immunizations. In some cases (e.g., SLE) IgG warm-reactive antilymphocyte antibodies are found as well. Serum of some patients with juvenile rheumatoid arthritis (JRA) contains an IgG antibody that reacts with a subpopulation of putative helper lymphocytes.

The biologic significance of such antibodies is not well defined. Some evidence suggests correlation of levels of such antibodies to various lymphocyte populations and subpopulations with the degree of "autoimmune" disease activity and/or depression of cell-mediated immunity. Antilymphocyte antibodies could exert an *in vivo* effect by (1) direct lysis; (2) changing trafficking patterns; (3) altering natural cell turnover, perhaps through the action of cells of the reticular activating system; or (4) modulating the membrane of lymphocytes and altering function.

MIXED LYMPHOCYTE REACTIONS (MLR)

When lymphocytes from two histoincompatible humans are cultured together, the cells of one or both individuals will proliferate as a manifestation of immune reactivity of the T lymphocytes to histocompatibility antigens on cells of the other subject (Bach, 1976). This reactivity is discussed in Chapters 33 and 34. Pertinent to our discussion are observations that these antigens (at the "D" locus) are contained on B and likely on T lymphocytes. Such MLR are valuable indicators of tissue "self" and "non-self" insofar as organ transplantation is concerned. Therefore, it is noteworthy that positive MLR responses have occasionally been seen when human blood lymphocytes obtained during acute exacerbations of leukemia or viral infections (and then freeze-stored in the viable state) react with cells of the same individual obtained during remission.

It is not clear whether such autoreactivity is directed against "neoantigen" that may be formed in virus-altered blood lymphocytes, or whether "hidden" (e.g., fetal) antigens are expressed in the abnormal cells. Positive MLR responses have been reported in at least two of the putative autoimmune disorders discussed here. MLR responses between autologous synovial fluid and blood lymphocytes of some rheumatoid arthritis patients have been reported (Griffiths, 1974). Also, the hyperplastic thymic cells of some myasthenic patients will stimulate blood lymphocytes of the same individuals in a positive MLR (Abdou, 1974). Again, the mechanisms involved are not well defined. However, the MLR may not reflect only allogeneic histoincompatibility in normals. Furthermore, reactivity is induced in T lymphocytes of normals by B cell–enriched fractions of the same blood. Defects in the autologous mixed lymphocyte reaction (AMLR) have been noted in several of the diseases discussed in this chapter.

In summary, techniques for measuring antilymphocyte antibodies and MLR are frequently available in clinical laboratories, at least on a regional basis, related to organ transplantation programs. However, the diagnostic usefulness of the findings in autoimmune disease is not defined sufficiently to recommend application at present.

SOME OTHER CONSIDERATIONS IN THE APPROACH TO AUTOIMMUNE DISEASES

The emphasis in this chapter has been predominantly on assays for humoral autoimmune reactivity detected in the test tube or in tissue. However, findings in experimental autoimmunity models suggest that cell-mediated immune responses may play a major pathogenetic role in some of the conditions already discussed here. At least part of the reason for the emphasis on humoral immunity assays is that the techniques involved have been available for a longer period of time and can be performed relatively easily and reproducibly in the sizable numbers of cases seen in clinical situations. Yet it is conceivable that at least some of these humoral responses to tissue antigens are epiphenomena or occur secondary to tissue damage due to non-immune causes.

Detection of human cell-mediated immune (CMI) responses to the same tissue antigen has been explored in any depth only in recent years. First, one must know whether the individual can manifest CMI responses to exogenous antigens. The most straightforward approach has been the determination of whether subjects with a particular disease manifest less recall-delayed hypersensitivity skin test responses to a panel of ubiquitous antigens as compared with an age-matched control population. Depressed responses (Kantor, 1975), called anergy, are seen in some putative autoimmune disease states, but not commonly enough to be of real diagnostic value. Testing for primary sensitization to contact-sensitizing agents such as dinitrochlorobenzene (Chretien, 1973) are still research procedures. Determinations of the relative and absolute numbers of lymphocyte subpopulations and assays of the *in vitro* functional capabilities of such cells are discussed in another chapter in this section and will not be dealt with here. Suffice it to say that any abnormalities detected in human autoimmune disease have not yet been of sufficient diagnostic value to warrant inclusion of these more time-consuming techniques in a clinical laboratory approach. It should be mentioned that evidence by one or another techniques of *in vitro* blood leukocyte reactivity to components of glomeruli, liver, and colon (in certain types of glomerulonephritis, hepatic disease, and ulcerative colitis, respectively) have been impressive at times. These *in vitro* reactions may reflect pathogenetically important *in vivo* events. However, these assays do not seem to be at the level where they can be applied reproducibly in clinical diagnosis.

Alterations in the complement system have also not been discussed in detail, since this is the subject of Chapter 37. However, it should be stressed that complement activation appears to be involved in a number of the autoimmune reactions described here.

Aarden, L. A., Lakmaker, F., and Fetkamp, T. E. W.: Immunology of DNA. I. The influence of reaction conditions in the Farr assay as used for the detection of anti-ds DNA. J. Immunol. Meth., *10*:27, 1976.

Abdou, N. I., Lisak, R. P., Zweiman, B., Abrahamsohn, I., and Penn, A. S.: The thymus in myasthenia gravis. Evidence for altered cell populations. N. Engl. J. Med., *291*:1271, 1974.

Adams, C. W. M.: Pathology of multiple sclerosis: Progression of the lesion. Br. Med. Bull., *33*:13, 1977.

Adams, I. E., Grant, K. D., and Hess, E. V.: An evaluation of commercial kits for the detection of antibodies to double stranded ANA. Am. J. Clin. Path., 77:54, 1982.

Adler, M. K., Baumgarten, A., Hecht, B., and Siegel, N. J.: Prognostic significance of DNA binding capacity in patients with lupus nephritis. Ann. Rheum. Dis., *34*:344, 1975.

Ahmed, A. R., Maize, J. C., and Provost, T. T.: Bullous pemphigoid. Arch. Dermatol., *113*:1043, 1977.

Alarcon-Segovia, D.: Drug induced antinuclear antibodies and lupus syndrome. Drugs, *12*:69, 1976.

Alexander, E. L., and Provost, T. T.: Anti-Ro and anti-Ca antibodies. Springer Sem. Immunol., *4*:253, 1981.

Allison, A. C.: *In* Katz D. H., and Benacceraf, B. (eds.): Immunologic Tolerance. New York, Academic Press, 1974.

Alspaugh, M., and Maddison, P. J.: Resolution of the identity of certain antigen antibody systems in SLE and Sjögren's syndrome. Arth. Rheum., *22*:796, 1979.

Arnason, B. G. W.: Idiopathic polyneuritis (Landry-Guillain-Barré-Strohl syndrome) and experimental allergic neuritis: A comparison. Res. Publ. Assoc. Res. Nerv. Ment. Dis., *49*:156, 1971.

5

Asbury, A. K., Arnason, B. G. W., and Adams, R. W.: The inflammatory lesion in idiopathic polyneuritis: Its role in pathogenesis. Medicine, *48*:173, 1969.

Asbury, A. K., and Lisak, R. P.: Demyelinative neuropathy and myelin antibodies. N. Engl. J. Med., *303*:638, 1981.

Bach, F. H.: Mixed leukocyte cultures: A cellular approach to histocompatability testing. *In* Bach, F. H., and Good, R. A. (eds.): Clinical Immunology, Vol. 3. New York, Academic Press, 1976, p. 273.

Baldwin, D. S.: Clinical usefulness of the morphological classification of lupus nephritis. Am. J. Kidney Dis., *2*:(Suppl. 1)142, 1982.

Ballou, S. P., and Kushner, I.: Anti-native DNA detection by the *Crithidia luciliae* method. Arth. Rheum., *22*:321, 1979.

Bardana, E., Harbeck, R. J., Hoffman, A. A., Pirofsky, B., and Carr, R. I.: The prognostic and therapeutic implications of DNA: Anti-DNA immune complexes in SLE. Am. J. Med., *59*:515, 1975.

Bigazzi, P. E., and Rose, N. R.: Tests for antibodies to tissue-specific antigens. *In* Rose, M. R., and Friedman, H. (eds.): Manual of Clinical Immunology. Washington, D.C., American Society of Microbiology, 1976.

Block, K. J., and Franklin, E.: Plasma cell dyscrasias and cryoglobulins. J.A.M.A., *248*:2670, 1982.

Bohan, A., and Peters, J. B.: Polymyositis and dermatomyositis. N. Engl. J. Med., *292*:344, 403, 1975.

Braun, P. E., Frail, D. E., and Latov, N.: Myelin-associated glycoprotein is the antigen for a monoclonal IgM in polyneuropathy. J. Neurochem., *39*:1261, 1982.

Burnet, M.: Autoimmunity and autoimmune disease. Philadelphia, F. A. Davis, 1972.

Cantor, H., and Gershon, R. K.: Immunological circuits. Fed. Proc., *38*:2058, 1979.

Cawley, L. P., Minard, B. J., Tourtellotte, W. W., et al.: Immunofixation electrophoretic techniques applied to identification of proteins in serum and cerebrospinal fluid. Clin. Chem., *22*:1262, 1976.

Chretien, P. B., Twomey, P. L., Trahan, E. E., and Catalana, W. J.: Quantitative dinitrochlorbenzene contact sensitivity in pre-operative and cured cancer patient. Natl. Cancer Inst. Monog., *39*:263, 1973.

Cohen, S. R., Herndon, R. M., and McKhann, G. M.: Radioimmunoassay of myelin basic protein in spinal fluid: An index of active demyelination. N. Engl. J. Med., *295*:1455, 1976.

Couser, W. G., and Salant, D. J.: In situ immune complex formation and glomerular injury. Kidney Int., *17*:1, 1980.

Criswell, S. N.: Correlation of circulating intercell antibody titres in pemphigus with disease activity. Clin. Exp. Dermatol., *6*:477, 1981.

Czaja, A. J.: Current problems in the diagnosis and management of chronic active hepatitis. Mayo Clin. Proc., *56*:311, 1981.

Decker, J. L., Steinberg, A. D., Reinertsen, J. L., et al.: SLE: Evolving concepts. Ann. Intern Med., *91*:587, 1979.

De Horatius, R. J., and Messner, R. P.: Lymphocytotoxic antibodies in family members of patients with systemic lupus erythematosus. J. Clin. Invest., *55*:1254, 1975.

de Winkel, M. V., Smets, G., and Gepts, W.: Islet cell antibodies from insulin dependent diabetes. J. Clin. Invest., *70*:41, 1982.

Doniach, D.: *In* Bastenie, V. A., and Gepts, W. (eds.): Immunology and Autoimmunity in Diabetes Mellitus. Amsterdam, Excerpta Medica, 1974.

Doniach, D., and Bottazzo, G. F.: Polyendocrine immunity. *In* Franklin, E. C. (ed.): Clinical Immunology Update. New York, Elsevier, 1981, p. 95.

Dore-Duffy, P., and Zurier, R. B.: Lymphocyte adherence to measles infected cells. Effect of aspirin. J. Clin. Invest., *63*:154, 1979.

Drachman, D. B., Angus, C. W., Adams, R. N., et al.: Myasthenic antibodies cross-link AChR. N. Engl. J. Med., *298*:1116, 1978.

Engel, A. G., Lambert, E. H., and Howard, F. M.: Immune complexes (IgG and C3) at the motor end-plate in myasthenia gravis. Ultrastructural and light microscopic localization and electrophysiologic correlations. Mayo Clin. Proc., *52*:167, 1977.

Evans, D. J., and Mangenalla, P.: Demonstration of circulating antibodies to glomerular basement membrane. Ann. N.Y. Acad. Sci., *254*:600, 1975.

Fauci, A. S.: Immunoregulation in autoimmunity. J. Allergy Clin. Immunol., *66*:5, 1980.

Feigenbaum, P., Medsger, T. A., Kraines, G., and Fries, J. F.: The variability of immunologic tests. J. Rheumatol., *9*:408, 1982.

Flier, J. S., Kahn, C. R., Jarrell, D. B., et al.: The immunology of the insulin receptor. Immunol. Commun., *5*:361, 1976.

Frambrough, D. M., Drachman, D. B., and Satuamarti, S.: Neuromuscular function in myasthenia gravis: Decreased acetylcholine receptors. Science, *182*:293, 1973.

Gamble, C. N., and Reardan, J. B.: Immunopathogenesis of syphilitic glomerulonephritis. N. Engl. J. Med., *292*:449, 1975.

Gilliam, J. N., Cheatum, D. E., Hurd, E. R., et al.: Immunoglobulin in clinically uninvolved skin in SLE. Association with renal disease. J. Clin. Invest., *53*:1434, 1974.

Griffiths, I. D., and Dick, W. C.: Antibodies to DNA antigens: Their specificity and clinical relevance. Europ. J. Clin. Invest., *9*:243, 1979.

Griffiths, M. M., and Williams, R. C.: In vitro peripheral blood and synovial fluid lymphocyte interactions. Arth. Rheum., *17*:111, 1974.

Hale, W. L., and Bergquist, D. N.: Chessboard analyses with anti-nuclear antibodies. Ann. N.Y. Acad. Sci., *177*:354, 1971.

Hargraves, M. M., Richmond, H., and Morton, R.: Presentation of two bone marrow elements: The "tart" cell and the "L. E." cell. Proc. Staff Meet. Mayo Clin., *23*:25, 1948.

Hay, F. C., Ninehan, L. J., and Roitt, I. M.: Routine assay for the detection of immune complexes of known Ig class using solid phase C1q. Clin. Exp. Immunol., *24*:396, 1976.

Holborow, E. J.: Smooth-muscle antibodies, viral infections, and malignant disease. Proc. R. Soc. Med., *65*:481, 1972.

Holborow, E. J.: Standardization. *In* Immunofluorescence. Oxford, Blackwell Scientific Publications, 1970.

Howard, J. G., and Mitchison, N. A.: Immunological tolerance. Prog. Allergy, *18*:43, 1975.

Husby, G., Skrede, J., and Blomhoff, J. P.: Serum Ig and organ non-specific antibodies in diseases of the liver. Scand. J. Gastroenterol., *12*:297, 1977.

Irvine, W. J.: The association of atrophic gastritis with autoimmune thyroid disease. Clin. Endocrinol. Metab., *4*:351, 1975a.

Irvine, W. J., and Barnes, E. W.: Addison's disease, ovarian failure and hypoparathyroidism. Clin. Endocrinol. Metab., *4*:379, 1975b.

Irvine, W. J., McCallum, C. J., Gray, R. S., Campbell, C. J., Duncan, L. J. P., Forquhar, J. W., Vaughan, H., and Morris, P. J.: Pancreatic islet cell antibodies in diabetes mellitus correlated with duration and type of diabetes, coexistent autoimmune diseases and HLA type. Diabetes, *26*:138, 1977.

Jerne, N. K.: The immune system. A web of V-domains. Harvey Lect., *70*:93, 1975.

Johnson, A. H., Mowbray, J. F., and Porter, K. A.: Detection of circulating immune complexes in pathological human sera. Lancet, *1*:762, 1975.

Johnson, K. J., and Ward, P. A.: Biology of disease: New concepts in the pathogenesis of immune complex mediated tissue injury. Lab. Invest., *47*:218, 1982.

Johnson, K. P., Arrigo, S. C., Nelson, B. J., and Ginsberg, A.: Agarose electrophoresis of cerebrospinal fluid in multiple sclerosis. A simplified method for demonstrating cerebrospinal fluid oligoclonal immunoglobulin bands. Neurology, *27*:273, 1977.

Jordan, R. E., and Provost, T. T.: Vesiculobullous diseases. *In* Safai, B., and Good, R. A., (eds.): Immunodermatology. New York, Plenum Press, 1981.

Kantor, F. S.: Infection, anergy and cell mediated immunity. N. Engl. J. Med., *292*:629, 1975.

Kaplan, M. H., and Frengley, J. D.: Autoimmunity to the heart in cardiac disease. Am. J. Cardiol., *24*:459, 1969.

Karsh, J., Halbert, S. P., Anken, M., et al.: Anti-DNA anti-desoxyribonucleoprotein and RF measured by ELISA. Int. Arch. Allergy, *68*:60, 1982.

Katz, S. I., Hall, R. P., Lawley, T. S., et al.: Dermatitis herpetiformis: The skin and the gut. Ann. Intern. Med., *93*:857, 1980.

Kelly, J. J., Dauber, J. R., Lennon, V. A., et al.: The laboratory diagnosis of mild myasthenia gravis. Neurology, *12*:238, 1982.

Kelly, J. J., Kyle, R. A., and O'Brien, R. C.: Presence of monoclonal protein in peripheral neuropathy. Neurology, *31*:1480, 1982b.

Kohler, P. F., and Brown, W. R.: Immunologic aspects of hepatic and gastrointestinal disease. J.A.M.A., *248*:2704, 1982.

Kunkel, H. G., Winfield, J. B., Winchester, R. J., and Wernet, P.: Antibodies to lymphocytes in human sera. *In* Williams, R. W. (ed.): Lymphocytes and Their Interactions. New York, Raven Press, 1975, pp. 183–191.

Landry, M., Sams, W. M., and Jordon, R. E.: Bullous pemphigoid: Elution of in vivo fixed antibody. J. Invest. Dermatol., *61*:348, 1973.

Lang, C. H., Brown, D. C., Stanley, N., et al.: Goodpasture syndrome treated with immunosuppression and plasma exchange. Arch. Intern. Med., *137*:1076, 1977.

Levinsky, R. J., Cameron, J. S., and Soothill, J. F.: Serum immune complexes and disease activity in lupus nephritis. Lancet, *1*:564, 1977.

Levy, N. L., Auerbach, P. S., and Hayes, E. C.: A blood test for multiple sclerosis based on the adherence of lymphocytes to measles infected cells. N. Engl. J. Med., *294*:1423, 1976.

Lewis, M. D., Loughridge, L. W., and Phillips, T. M.: Immunological shades in nephrotic syndrome associated with extrarenal malignant disease. Lancet, *2*:134, 1971.

Link, H., and Muller, R.: Immunoglobulins in multiple sclerosis and infections of the nervous system. Arch. Neurol., *25*:324, 1971.

Linstrom, J. M.: An assay for antibodies to human acetylcholine receptor in serum from patients with myasthenia gravis. J. Immunol. Immunopath., *7*:36, 1977.

Lisak, R. P.: Multiple sclerosis: Evidence for immunopathogenesis. Neurology, *30*:99, 1980.

Lisak, R. P., and Barchi, R. L.: Myasthenia Gravis. Philadelphia, W. B. Saunders, 1982.

Ludovicio, C. L., Zweiman, B., Myers, A. R., Hebert, J., and Green, P. A.: Predictive value of anti-DNA antibody and selected laboratory studies in SLE. J. Rheumatol., 7:843, 1980.

Luthra, H. S., McDuffied, F. C., Hunder, G. G., et al.: Immune complexes in sera and synovial fluids of patients with rheumatoid arthritis: Radioimmunoassay with monoclonal rheumatoid factor. J. Clin. Invest., *56*:458, 1975.

Mackay, I. R., Taft, C. I., and Cowling, D. C.: Lupoid hepatitis. Lancet, *2*:1323, 1956.

Maddison, P. J., Provost, T. T., and Reichlin, M.: Serological findings in patients with "ANA-negative" SLE. Medicine, *60*:87, 1981.

Maddison, P. J., and Reichlin, M.: Quantitation of precipitating antibodies to certain soluble nuclear antigens in SLE. Arth. Rheum., *20*:819, 1977.

McGuigan, J. E., and Leibach, J.: Immunology and disease of the gastrointestinal tract. *In* Parker, C. W. (ed.): Clinical Immunology. Philadelphia, W. B. Saunders, 1980, p. 867.

McIntosh, R. M.: Cryoglobulins III. Quart. J. Med., *44*:285, 1975.

Mehta, P. D., Kane, A., and Thomas, H.: Relationship between homogeneous IgG fractions and measles virus antibody activities in subacute sclerosing panencephalitis brain. J. Immunol., *117*:2053, 1976.

Meltzer, M., and Franklin, E. C.: Cryoglobulins, rheumatoid factors and connective tissue disorders. Arth. Rheum., *10*:489, 1967.

Miller, K. B., and Schwartz, R. S.: Autoimmunity and suppressor T lymphocytes. Adv. Intern. Med., *27*:281, 1982.

Mingioli, E. S., Strober, W., Tourtellotte, W. W., Whitaker, J. N., and McFarlin, D. E.: Quantitation of IgG, IgA, and IgM in the CSF by radioimmunoassay. Neurology, *28*:991, 1978.

Myllyla, G.: Aggregation of human blood platelets by immune complexes in the sedimentation pattern test. Scand. J. Haematol., *19*(Suppl): 1, 1973.

Nakamura, R. M., and Tan, E. M.: Recent progress in the study of autoantibodies to nuclear antigens. Hum. Path., *9*:85, 1978.

Neufeld, M., MacLaren, N. K., and Blizzard, R. M.: Two types of autoimmune Addison's disease associated with different polyglandular autoimmune (PGA) syndromes. Medicine, *60*:355, 1981.

Nydegger, V. E., Lambert, P. H., Gerber, H., and Miescher, P. A.: Circulating immune complexes in the serum in systemic lupus erythematosus and carriers of hepatitis B antigen. Quantitation by binding to radiolabeled C1q. J. Clin. Invest., *54*:297, 1974.

Phillips, P. E.: The virus hypothesis in systemic lupus erythematosus. Ann. Intern. Med., *83*:709, 1975.

Pincus, T., Schur, P. H., Rose, J. A., Decker, J. K., and Talal, N.: Measurement of DNA-binding activity in SLE. N. Engl. J. Med., *281*:701, 1969.

Reichlin, M., and Mattioli, M.: Description of a serological reaction characteristic of polymyositis. Clin. Immunol. Immunopath., *5*:12, 1976.

Ritchie, R. F.: The clinical significance of titered antinuclear antibodies. Arth. Rheum., *10*:544, 1967.

Robitallie, P., and Tan, E. M.: Relationship between deoxyribonucleoprotein and deoxyribonucleic acid antibodies in systemic lupus erythematosus. J. Clin. Invest., *52*:316, 1973.

Ropes, M. W., et al.: Proposed diagnostic criteria for rheumatoid arthritis. Bull. Rheumat. Dis., 7:121, 1956.

Rose, N. R., Hjort, T., Rumke, P. H., et al.: Techniques for the detection of iso- and autoantibodies to human sperm. Clin. Exp. Immunol., *23*:175, 1976.

Ross, G. L., Barland, P., and Grayzel, A. I.: The Ig class of anti-DNA antibodies. J. Rheumatol., *5*:373, 1978.

Rothfield, N. F.: Detection of antibodies to nuclear antigens by immunofluorescence. *In* Rose, N. R., and Friedman, H.: Manual of Clinical Immunology. Washington, D.C., American Society for Microbiology, 1976.

Rumke, P. H.: Autoantibodies against sperm. *In* Cohen, J., and Hendry, W. F. (eds.): Spermatozoa, Antibodies and Infertility. Oxford, Blackwell, 1978, p. 67.

Sandberg-Wollheim, M.: Optic neuritis: Studies on the cerebrospinal fluid in relation to clinical course in 61 patients. Acta Neurol. Scand., *52*:167, 1975.

Scherbaum, W. A., Stockle, G., and Wichmann, J.: Immunologic and clinical characterization of patients with euthyroid and hypothyroid thyroiditis. Acta Endocrinol., *100*:373, 1982.

Sharp, G. C., Irvin, W. S., May, C. M., et al.: Association of antibodies to ribonucleoprotein and Sm antigens with mixed connective tissue disease, SLE and other rheumatic diseases. N. Engl. J. Med., *295*:1149, 1976.

Singer, J.: On standardization of the latex fixation. Bull. Rheum. Dis., *26*:868, 1975.

Smith, I. S., Kahn, S. N., Lacy, B. N., et al.: Chronic demyelinating neuropathy associated with IgM paraproteinemia. Brain, *106*:169, 1983.

Sofer, N. A.: Clinical presentations and mechanisms of necrotizing angiitis of the skin. J. Invest. Dermatol., *67*:354, 1976.

Sotsiou, F., Bottazzo, G. F., and Doniach, D.: Immunofluorescence studies on autoantibodies to steroid producing cells. Clin. Exp. Immunol., *39*:97, 1980.

Stiller, C. R., Russell, A. S., and Dosseter, J. B.: Autoimmunity, present concepts. Ann. Intern. Med., *82*:405, 1975.

Stites, D. P.: Clinical laboratory methods for detection of antigens and antibodies. *In* Fudenberg, H. H., Stites, D. P., Caldwell, J. C., and Wells, J. V. (eds.): Basic and Clinical Immunology. Los Altos, Cal., Lange Medical Publications, 1980.

Strickland, R. G., Baur, S., Ashworth, L. A., E., et al.: A correlative study of immunological phenomena in pernicious anemia. Clin. Exp. Immunol., *8*:25, 1971.

Strife, C. F., McDonald, B. M., Reiley, E. J., et al.: Shunt nephritis. J. Pediatr., *88*:403, 1976.

Talal, N.: Immunologic and viral factors in autoimmune disease. Med. Clin. North Am., *61*:205, 1977.

Talal, N., and Pillarisetty, R.: Radioimmunoassay for antibodies to deoxyribonucleic acid. *In* Rose, N. R., and Friedman, H. (eds.): Manual of Clinical Immunology. Washington, D.C., American Society of Microbiology, 1976.

Tan, E. M.: Immunopathology and pathogenesis of cutaneous involvement in SLE. J. Invest. Derm., *67*:360, 1976a.

Tan, E. M., Cohen, A. S., Fries, J. F., et al.: The 1982 revised criteria for the classification of SLE. Arth. Rheum., *25*:1271, 1982.

Tan, E. M., and Peebles, C.: Quantitation of antibodies to Sm antigen and nuclear ribonucleoprotein by hemagglutination. *In* Rose, N. R., and Friedman, H. (eds.): Manual of Clinical Immunology. Washington, D.C., American Society of Microbiology, 1976b.

Tanner, A. R., Scott Morgan, A. R., Mandell, R., et al.: The incidence of occult thyroid disease associated with thyroid autoantibodies. Acta Endocrinol., *100*:31, 1982.

Taylor, K. B., and Thomas, H. C.: Gastrointestinal and liver diseases. *In* Stiles, D. (ed.): Basic and Clinical Immunology. 4th ed. Los Altos, Cal., Lange Medical Publications, 1982.

Tesor, J., and Schmid, F.: Conversion of soluble immune complexes into complement fixing aggregates by rheumatoid factor. J. Immunol., *105*:1206, 1970.

Theofilopoulos, A. N.: Evaluation and clinical significance of circulating immune complexes. Progr. Clin. Immunol., *4*:63, 1980.

Theofilopoulos, A. N., and Dixon, F. J.: Autoimmune disease, immunopathology and etiopathogenesis. Am. J. Path., *108*:319, 1982.

Theofilopoulos, A. N., Wilson, C. B., and Dixon, F. J.: The Raji cell radioimmunoassay for detecting immune complexes in human sera. J. Clin. Invest., *57*:169, 1976.

Tourtellotte, W. W.: Cerebrospinal fluid immunoglobulins and the central nervous system as an immunological organ particularly in multiple sclerosis and subacute sclerosing penencephalitis. Res. Publ. Assoc. Res. Nerv. Ment. Dis., *49*:112, 1971.

Tung, K. S. K., Ramos, C. V., and Deodhar, S. D.: Anti-thyroid antibodies in juvenile lymphocytic thyroiditis. Am. J. Clin. Path., *61*:549, 1974.

Vaughn, J. H.: Summary: Rheumatoid factors and their biological significance. Ann. N.Y. Acad. Sci., *168*:204, 1969.

Volpe, R.: Immunological aspects of autoimmune thyroid disease. Progr. Clin. Biol. Res., *74*:1, 1981.

Ward, P. A., and Kibukamusoke, I. W.: Evidence for soluble immune complexes in the pathogenesis of the glomerulonephritis of quartan malaria. Lancet, *1*:283, 1969.

Wasicek, C. A., and Reichlin, M.: Clinical and serological differences between SLE patients with antibodies to Ro versus patients with antibodies to Ro and La. J. Clin. Invest., *69*:835, 1982.

Weiner, H. L., and Hauser, S. C.: Neuroimmunology. I. Immunoregulation in neurological disease. Ann. Neurol., *11*:437, 1982.

Weitzman, R. J., and Walker, S. E.: Relation of titered peripheral pattern ANA to anti-DNA and disease activity in SLE. Ann. Rheum. Dis., *36*:44, 1977.

Wells, J. V., Michaeli, D., and Fudenberg, H. H.: Autoimmunity in selective IgA deficiency. Birth Defects, *11*:144, 1975.

Wernick, R.: Serum IgG and IgM rheumatoid factor by solid phase radioimmunoassay. Arth. Rheum., *24*:1501, 1981.

Wertheimer, D., and Barland, P.: Clinical significance of immune deposits in the skin in SLE. Arth. Rheum., *19*:1249, 1976.

West, C. D., Davis, N. C., Forestal, J., Herbst, J., and Spitzer, R.: Antigenic determinants of human B1c and B1q globulins. J. Immunol., *96*:650, 1966.

Whitaker, J. N., and Engel, W. K.: Vascular deposits of immunoglobulin and complement in idiopathic inflammatory myopathy. N. Engl. J. Med., *286*:333, 1972.

Whitaker, J. N., Lisak, R. P., Bashir, R. M., et al.: Immunoreactive myelin basic protein in the cerebrospinal fluid in neurological disorders. Ann. Neurol., 7:58, 1980.

Whittingham, M. B., Irwin, J., Mackay, I. R., and Smalley, M.: Smooth muscle autoantibody in "autoimmune" hepatitis. Gastroenterology, *51*:499, 1966.

Wilk, A.: Granulocyte specific antinuclear antibodies. Allergy, *35*:263, 1980.

Wilson, C. B.: Nephritogen antibody mechanisms involving antigens within the glomerulus. Immunol. Rev., *55*:257, 1981.

Wilson, C. B.: Recent advances in the immunological aspects of renal disease. Fed. Proc., *36*:2171, 1977.

Wilson, C. B., and Dixon, F. J.: The renal response to immunologic injury. *In* Brenner, B. M., and Rector, F. C., Jr. (eds.): The Kidney. Philadelphia, W. B. Saunders Company, 1976.

Winchester, R. J.: Tests for detection of rheumatoid factors. *In* Rose, N. R., and Friedman, H. (eds.): Manual for Clinical Immunology. Washington, D.C., American Society of Microbiology, 1976.

Winchester, R. J., Kunkel, H. G., and Agnello, V.: Occurrence of gamma globulin complexes in serum and joint fluid of rheumatoid arthritis patients. J. Exp. Med., *134*:2865, 1971.

Winfield, J. B., Faiferman, I., and Koffler, D.: Avidity of anti-DNA antibodies in serum and IgG glomerular eluates from patients with SLE. J. Clin. Invest., *59*:90, 1977a.

Winfield, J. B., Koffler, D., and Kunkel, H. G.: Specific concentration of polynucleotide immune complexes in the cryoprecipitates of patients with systemic lupus erythematosus. J. Clin. Invest., *56*:563, 1975.

Winfield, J. B., Winchester, R. J., Wernet, P., and Kunkel, H. G.: Specific concentration of anti-lymphocyte antibody in serum cryopathies of SLE. Clin. Exp. Immunol., *19*:44, 1977b.

Witkin, S. S., Zelikovsky, G., Bongiovanni, A. M., et al.: Sperm related antigen antibodies and CIC in sera of recently vasectomized men. J. Clin. Invest., *70*:33, 1982.

Wolfe, J. F., Adelstein, E., and Sharp, G. C.: Antinuclear antibody with distinct specificity for polymyositis. J. Clin. Invest., *59*:176, 1977.

Woodrofe, A. J., Borden, W. A., Theofilopoulos, A. N., et al.: Detection of circulating immune complexes in patients with glomerulonephritis. Kidney Int., *12*:268, 1977.

Zubler, R. H., Lange, G., Lambert, P. H., et al.: Detection of immune complexes in unheated sera by a modified ^{125}I-C1q binding test: Effect of heating on the binding of C1q by immune complexes and the application of the test to SLE. J. Immunol., *116*:232, 1976.

Zweiman, B., and Hebert, J.: The L. E. cell phenomenon: Mechanisms and significance. Int. J. Dermatol., *15*:121, 1976.

40

HYPERSENSITIVITY REACTIONS

RUSSELL H. TOMAR, M.D.

INTRODUCTION

Immune responses defend the body against a multitude of foreign invaders. Some of these "foreigners" closely resemble our own body constituents. Thus, two extraordinary characteristics of immune responses are their diversity and their specificity, particularly in regard to reacting against "non-self" rather than "self." This distinction between "self" and "non-self" is an active process and the result of a complex set of controls and cellular interactions (described in Chaps. 34 and 39). Unfortunately in spite of many fail-safe systems, these mechanisms can lead to harmful processes rather than protective ones. These harmful processes have been called hypersensitivity or immunological injury reactions and have been grouped into four distinct classes by Gell and Coombs (Roitt, 1980). This classification is an oversimplification and several reactions do not fit neatly into the original package. Nonetheless, it is much easier to learn and teach hypersensitivity reactions using some classifications for guidance (Table 40–1).

TYPE I HYPERSENSITIVITY REACTIONS—IMMEDIATE HYPERSENSITIVITY

Antibody of class IgE may be formed in response to antigenic stimulation. IgE is cytophilic and binds to basophils and mast cells via its Fc portion. When antigen (allergen) contacts two or more cell-bound IgE molecules, a sequence of events occurs which results in the release of a number of biologically active substances (Table 40–2) (Johansson, 1972). Cyclic AMP and perhaps cyclic GMP play roles in modulating this process (Fig. 40–1) (Lichtenstein, 1972; Townley, 1975). Vasoactive amines such as the leukotrienes or SRS-A (slow reacting substance of anaphylaxis) and histamine cause the flow of fluids into the extravascular compartment and contract the smooth muscles. ECF-A (eosinophilic chemotactic factor of anaphylaxis) attracts eosinophils. The effect on the host depends on the site and the extent of damage. These events in the bronchial tree may lead to asthma; in the nasal passages and sinuses, to rhinorrhea or congestion (Frick, 1976). There are three basic methods of detecting anti-allergen IgE: skin testing, either directly or by the passive cutaneous anaphylaxis method (Prausnitz-Küstner); release of histamine from leukocytes; and radioimmunoassay, called the radioallergosorbent test (RAST). These methods are compared in Table 40–3. RAST is safer, less sensitive, but perhaps more specific than skin testing. In several studies it has proved to have a high correlation with bronchial provocative testing using the same antigen (Berg, 1974). A large number of allergens are now commercially available (Pharmacia). Principles of RAST are described in Figure 40–2.

Table 40–1. TYPES OF IMMUNOLOGIC INJURY*

I.	Immediate—mediated by IgE
II.	Cytotoxic—mediated by IgG, IgM, ± complement
III.	Immune complex—mediated by IgG, IgM, complement
IV.	Delayed type hypersensitivity—mediated by mononuclear cells

*After Gell and Coombs.

Most radioallergosorbent assays use allergens covalently bound to cyanogen bromide–activated paper disks. Two methods are commonly used to "score" reactions. The first is based on a reference curve generated with four or five dilutions of pooled human serum with high titers against birch pollen, using birch allergen on the disk. Five reference points are developed and zones of 0, 1, 2, 3, and 4+ reactions are produced, the higher numbers being the most reactive. The second method (suggested by Nalebuff and Fadal (reviewed in Adkinson, 1981) uses a total IgE standard of 25 IU/ml. All samples are related to

5

Table 40–2. VASOACTIVE MEDIATORS DERIVED FROM HUMAN BASOPHILS*

Mediator	Structure	Activity
Histamine	β-Imidazolethylamine	Contracts smooth muscle and increases vascular permeability; stimulates arachidonate metabolism; effects leukocyte migration
Arachidonate metabolites Prostaglandins: D2, E2, F2α, I2 (prostacyclin)	Polyunsaturated C-20 fatty acids	Contract smooth muscle; modulate smooth muscle tone and vascular permeability; effect leukocyte function; inhibit platelet aggregation
Thromboxane A2	Polyunsaturated C-20 fatty acids with oxane ring	Contracts smooth muscle; stimulates platelet aggregation
Slow reacting substance of anaphylaxis (SRS-A)	Leukotrienes C4, D4, E4; polyunsaturated C-20 substituted fatty acids	Contracts respiratory smooth muscle; alters vascular permeability
5-Hydroxyeicosatetraenoic		Directs migration of eosinophils and neutrophils
11-Hydroxyeicosatetraenoic 12-Hydroxyeicosatetraenoic	L-Hydroxyeicosatetraenoic acid	
Eosinophilic chemotactic factor of anaphylaxis (ECF-A)	Val/Ala-Gly-Ser-Glu	Directs migration of eosinophils; modulates surface receptors
Neutrophil chemotactic factor	Neutral protein (>750,000 daltons)	Directs migration of neutrophils

*Modified from Lichtenstein, L.: *In* Bach, F. H., and Good, R. A. (eds.): Clinical Immunology 1. New York, Academic Press, 1972; Orange, R. P., and Austen, K. F.: *In* Ishizaka, K., and Dayton, D. H., Jr. (eds.): Biological Role of the Immunoglobulin E System. Washington, D.C., U.S. Government Printing Office, 1972; and Samuelsson, B.: Science, *220*:568, 1983.

Table 40–3. COMPARISON OF METHODS USED TO MEASURE ANTIALLERGEN IgE*

Assay	Within-Run Variation	Day-to-Day Variation	Sensitivity	Correlation with Bronchial Provocation
Direct intradermal skin test	± two-fold	± three-fold	Excellent	63%
Peripheral leukocyte histamine release	± 10%	± two-fold	Excellent	Good
Radioallergosorbent test	± 15%	± 25%	Good to excellent	90%

*Modified from Berg, T. L. O., and Johansson, S. G. O.: J. Allergy Clin. Immunol., *54*:209, 1974; Yunginger, J. W., and Gleich, G. J.: Pediatr. Clin. North Am., *22*:3, 1975; and Evans, R., III (ed.): Advances in Diagnosis of Allergy: RAST. Miami, Symposia Specialist, 1975.

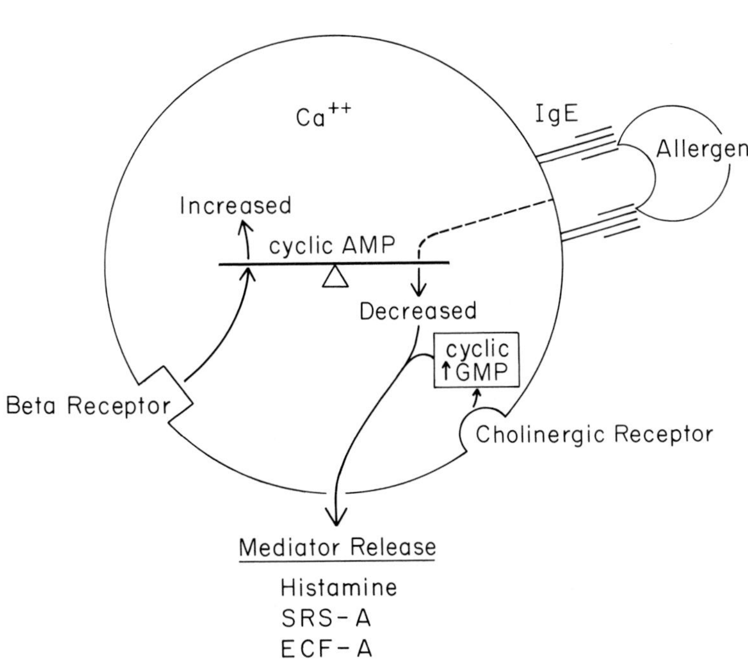

Figure 40–1. Mediator release from cells by allergen-IgE reaction. Two or more cytophilic IgE molecules bind one antigen (allergen) molecule to produce a decrease in intracellular cyclic AMP. This, in turn, incites the release of vasoactive mediators which cause edema, spasm, and eosinophilia in the target tissues. Cholinergic agents, possibly by increasing cyclic GMP levels, may also result in mediator release. β-Adrenergic agents decrease cyclic AMP, thereby reducing mediator release. SRS-A = slow reacting substance of anaphylaxis; ECF-A = eosinophil chemotactic factor of anaphylaxis.

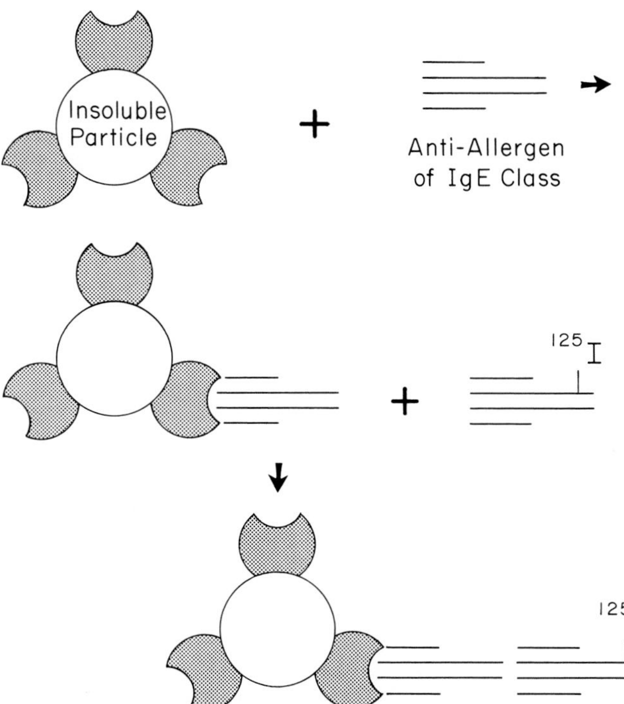

Figure 40–2. The radioallergosorbent test (RAST). The allergen (antigen) is bound to an insoluble material. The patient's serum is reacted with this conjugate. If the serum contains antibody to the allergen, it will be complexed to the conjugate. Radiolabeled anti-IgE is then reacted in the system. If the anti-allergen antibody is of class IgE, the radiolabeled anti-IgE will be added to the conjugate. After appropriate washes, and with proper standards, the amount of antigen-allergen IgE in the patient's serum may be determined.

5

the time required for a preset number of disintegrations per minute (in practice, 25,000 counts per minute). A negative control is also counted and a log/log graph developed relating the number of IgE units to time of accumulating 25,000 counts per minute. Theoretical five-fold dilutions are demarcated and the time required for unknowns to develop 25,000 counts related to the zones. This alternative method is believed to be more sensitive.

RAST is useful in detecting allergy to the common pollen such as ragweed, grasses, trees, and molds. It may also be useful for some animal dander allergies and allergy to milk and egg albumin. It is of little use in most other food sensitivities or drug allergies, including penicillin. It is not totally reliable in insect sting allergy, possibly because of its relative insensitivity. RAST rarely gives false positive results. Its sensitivity may be such to give false negative results, however. Blocking antibodies of IgG isotype may compete and thus interfere with specific IgE antiallergen antibodies.

The major advantages of RAST are that it is safer by not requiring potentially dangerous skin testing and that it is easier to do on an uncooperative patient, such as the very young (Evans, 1975).

Serum IgE may be measured as a screen for atopy. About two thirds of non-atopic adults have IgE levels of less than 20 IU/ml; only 1 in 50 has a level greater than 100 IU/ml. This contrasts sharply to atopic adults, virtually none of whom have values of less than 20 IU/ml. Two thirds of adults with allergies have IgE levels of greater than 100 IU/ml. Thus, a serum IgE level of less than 20 IU/ml practically rules out atopy, while one above 100 IU/ml increases the likelihood of this diagnosis some 30-fold (1 IU ≅ 2 ng) (Yuninger, 1975). Immunotherapy or desensitization initially leads to an increase in serum IgE, but later IgE declines and blocking antibody of isotype IgG may be found (Lichtenstein, 1973). Not all diseases called "allergic" are mediated through IgE. For example, urticaria and systemic anaphylaxis to penicillin caused by anti-penicilloyl antibodies may be mediated by anti-penicilloyl IgE, but hemolytic anemia is mediated by IgG (cytotoxic antibody—Type II). Serum IgE concentration in a number of disease states is shown in Table 40–4. Allergy, at least to ragweed antigen, appears to be inherited, and familial haplotypes with a predisposition to the development of atopy have been described (Levine, 1972). Some characteristics of Type I reactions are given in Table 40–5.

Table 40–4. SERUM IgE LEVELS IN SELECTED CONDITIONS*

Elevated
Atopic dermatitis
IgE myeloma
Hyper-IgE and recurrent infections
Wiskott-Aldrich syndrome
Hodgkin's disease (especially late stages)
Bronchopulmonary aspergillosis
Pemphigoid
Parasites (such as ascariasis)
Leprosy
Elevated to normal
Allergic rhinitis
Allergic asthma
Extrinsic allergic alveolitis
Cystic fibrosis
Aspergilloma
Drug allergies
Severe liver disease
Allergic urticaria
Kawasaki's disease
Periarteritis nodosa
Normal
Intestinal lymphangiectasia
Bronchiolitis
Pemphigus
Thyroiditis
Chronic renal failure
Normal to decreased
Leukemias
Multiple myeloma
Isolated IgA deficiency
Decreased
Ataxia-telangiectasia
Sex-linked hypogammaglobulinemia
Congenital hypogammaglobulinemia
Acquired hypogammaglobulinemia
IgE deficiency

*Modified from Waldmann, T. A., Strober, W., Polmer, S. H., and Terry, W. D.: *In* Ishizaka, K., and Dayton, D. H., Jr. (eds.): The Biological Role of the Immunoglobulin E System. Washington, D.C., U.S. Government Printing Office, 1975; and Arbesman, C. A.: *In* Ishizaka, K., and Dayton, D. H., Jr. (eds.): The Biological Role of the Immunoglobulin E System. Washington, D.C., U.S. Government Printing Office, 1975.

TYPE II HYPERSENSITIVITY REACTIONS—CYTOTOXIC ANTIBODIES

Cytotoxic antibodies are usually of isotypes IgG and/or IgM. Complement is often involved in the mediation of hypersensitivity by this mechanism, either by direct lysis or by attachment to a complement receptor on a phagocytic cell. Cytotoxic antibodies mediate diseases such as autoimmune hemolytic anemia, autoimmune thrombocytopenic purpura, and autoimmune neutropenia, discussed in Chapters 29, 32 and 30, respectively. Antibody-dependent cellular cytotoxicity (ADCC), discussed in Chapter 34, might also be considered a Type II mechanism. Lymphocytotoxic antibodies have been demonstrated in a number of disorders such as systemic lupus erythematosus, rheumatoid arthritis, and malignancies. Their role in the pathogenesis of disease is unclear and is discussed in Chapter 39 (p. 950). Some characteristics of Type II reactions are given in Table 40–6.

TYPE III HYPERSENSITIVITY REACTIONS—IMMUNE COMPLEX DISEASES

Complexes of antigen with antibody of isotypes IgG1, 2, 3, or IgM can fix the first component of

Table 40–5. TYPE I HYPERSENSITIVITY REACTIONS: IMMEDIATE

1. Occur within minutes
2. May result in edema, vasodilation, bronchoconstriction in the target organ
3. Examples: Allergic rhinitis, allergic asthma, atopic dermatitis, some drug reactions, "allergic" urticaria
4. Cells involved: Basophils and mast cells directly; secondary involvement by eosinophils; modulated by thymic-derived lymphocytes
5. Response is probably under genetic control

complement and activate the complement cascade. As noted in Chapter 37 (p. 879), activation of this cascade can lead to tissue injury both directly and through the enzymes of the emigrating leukocytes. The Arthus phenomenon, with appearance of erythema and induration at a skin test site two to eight hours after intradermal injection of antigen, results from the injected antigen's binding locally in tissue to antibody and fixing complement. Not only can localized immune complexes bind complement, but also soluble circulating immune complexes may activate complement. Thus, wherever immune complexes locate, determined by their size, shape, and chemical nature, complement is activated and tissue damage may occur (Cochrane, 1973). Immune complexes are soluble only when antigen and antibody are present in certain ratios, as described in Chapter 39 (p. 934)—generally in modest antigen excess. Von Pirquet and Schick, in their classic study of serum sickness, described the human syndrome of serum sickness produced by injection of horse serum. They noted that precipitating antibody to horse serum is often detectable at the conclusion of these clinical syndromes (von Pirquet, 1951). Dixon and colleagues clearly demonstrated that precipitating antibody cannot be detected because the available antibody is attached to antigen in a soluble complex (Dixon, 1971). Theoretically, all antibody-producing immunogens introduced to a host can result in at least a transient appearance of immune complexes. Rarely does this result in overt disease, probably because of the quantity and quality of these complexes. Immune complex disease is discussed further in Chapter 39. Some characteristics of Type III reactions are given in Table 40–7.

Table 40–6. TYPE II HYPERSENSITIVITY REACTIONS: CYTOTOXIC

1. Occur within minutes to hours
2. Result in destruction of target cell either by direct lysis or ingestion by reticuloendothelial cells; in solid organs, destruction may result in fibrosis
3. Examples: Autoimmune hemolytic anemia, autoimmune (idiopathic) thrombocytopenic purpura, perhaps autoimmune thyroiditis (Hashimoto's) and autoimmune adrenalitis (Addison's)
4. Cells involved: Depends on mechanism but antibody to target requires B lymphocyte or plasma cell
5. Chronic forms (at least) are under genetic control

Table 40–7. TYPE III HYPERSENSITIVITY REACTIONS: IMMUNE COMPLEX

1. Occur within hours
2. Result in edema and accumulation of polymorphonuclear cells at target site and release of lysozymal enzymes; site of injury depends on eventual deposition of immune complexes
3. Examples: Serum sickness, systemic lupus erythematosus, rheumatoid arthritis, some forms of cryoglobulinemia
4. Lymphocytes involved: none directly but B lymphocyte or plasma cells produce antibody under control of T lymphocytes
5. Chronic forms are probably under genetic control

TYPE IV HYPERSENSITIVITY REACTIONS—DELAYED TYPE HYPERSENSITIVITY

Delayed type hypersensitivity (DTH) is most convincingly involved in tissue damage following certain infections, and especially those caused by mycobacteria. The caseous necrosis and cavity seen in tuberculosis are not due to the microorganism proper but to the delayed hypersensitivity response of the host to the mycobacteria. DTH has been implicated in organ-specific autoimmune diseases, in contact dermatitis, and of course in tumor immunity. A description and methods for evaluation of cell-mediated immunity are found in Chapter 34 (p. 839). Characteristics of Type IV reactions are given in Table 40–8.

INHIBITORS TO THERAPEUTIC AGENTS

Because selected therapeutic agents, such as insulin and coagulation factor VIII, are also immunogenic and may appear as "foreign," it is not surprising that they elicit specific antibodies. At times these antibodies may interfere with biologic activity. Maneuvers such as changing the origin of insulin (as from porcine to bovine or fish), using more purified material, and/or using immunosuppressive agents may be required (Mattson, 1975).

ANTIBODIES TO CELL RECEPTORS

Another concept of the pathogenesis of autoimmune disorders involves the presence of antibodies to exposed

Table 40–8. TYPE IV HYPERSENSITIVITY REACTIONS: DELAYED HYPERSENSITIVITY

1. Occur within hours to days
2. Result in the accumulation of mononuclear cells and fibrin and the formation of granulomata
3. Examples: lepromatous leprosy, caseous necrosis of tuberculosis
4. Cells involved: monocyte system and thymic-derived lymphocytes; perhaps basophils in some forms
5. Under genetic control in animal models and possibly man
6. Important in resisting intracellular infections

Table 40–9. EXTRINSIC ALLERGIC ALVEOLITIS*

Disease	Source of Antigen	Precipitins Against
Thermophilic actinomycete spores		
Farmer's lung	Moldy hay and produce	*Micropolyspora faeni*†
Ventilation pneumonitis	Growth in humidified hot-air ventilation system	*Thermoactinomyces candidus*
Fog fever in cattle	Moldy hay	*Thermoactinomyces viridis*
Bagassosis	Moldy sugar cane bagasse	*Thermoactinomyces sacchari*
Mushroom worker's lung	Mushroom compost	*Thermoactinomyces vulgaris*
Fungic spores		
Maple-bark pneumonitis	Moldy maple bark	*Cryptostroma corticale*
Malt worker's lung	Moldy barley or malt dust	*Aspergillus clavatus* *Aspergillus fumigatus*†
Cheese worker's lung	Mold on cheese	*Penicillium caseii*
Suberosis	Moldy cork bark	*Penicillium frequentans*
Sequoiosis	Moldy redwood sawdust	*Graphium* species, *Aureobasidium pullulans*
Paprika-splitter's lung	Paprika dust	*Mucor stolonifer*
Wood-pulp worker's disease	Contaminated logs	*Alternaria* species†
B-P mycosis (BP aspergillosis)	Colonization by fungus in respiratory tract	Antigen from *Aspergillus fumigatus, Penicillium,* etc.†
Animal proteins		
Bird fancier's lung	Bird (pigeon, parrot, hen, budgerigar) droppings, dust	Antigens in serum, droppings†
Pituitary snufftaker's lung	Porcine and bovine posterior pituitary powder	Serum protein and pituitary antigen
Fish meal worker's lung	Fish meal	Fish meal extracts
Insect antigen		
Wheat weevil	Infested wheat flour	*Sitophilus granarius*
Laundry worker's "detergent" lung	Enzymes in detergent	*Bacillus subtilis*
Furrier's lung	Uncertain	Uncertain
Coffee worker's lung	Coffee beans?	Antigen in coffee bean?
Byssinosis	Cotton	Antigens in cotton
Miller's lung	Contaminated grain	*Sitophilus granarius*
Chemicals and drugs		
Toluene diisocyanate	Urethane foaming	
Nitrofurantoin	Iatrogenic	

*Modified from Pepys, J., and Warwick, M. T.: *In* Gell, P. G. H., Coombs, R. R. A., and Lachman, P. J. (eds.): Clinical Aspects of Immunology. 3rd ed. London, Blackwell Scientific Publications, 1975; Fink, J. W.: N.Y. State J. Med., *72*:1834, 1972; and Salvaggio, J. E.: Hosp. Pract., *15*:93, 1980.

†Commercially available (Hollister-Stier or Greer Laboratories).

antigens on cell surfaces. These may be inhibitory, as with anti–insulin receptor or anti–acetylcholine receptor antibodies (myasthenia gravis), or stimulatory, as may be the case with LATS (Graves' disease) (see Chap. 39).

HYPERSENSITIVITY REACTIONS OF MIXED TYPE

Extrinsic Allergic Alveolitis

Fibrosing alveolitis may be divided into two categories: cryptogenic fibrosing alveolitis and extrinsic allergic alveolitis. Cryptogenic fibrosing alveolitis may be characterized by the absence of both granulomata and giant cells on biopsy of the lung; and the presence of non–organ-specific autoantibodies such as ANA or rheumatoid factor (about 60 per cent) and at times circulating immune complexes. This set of disorders is characterized by alveolar wall infiltration and desquamative pneumonia. It is often a diagnosis of exclusion and a similar disease has been associated with a number of other systemic diseases of unknown etiology, such as rheumatoid arthritis, Sjögren's syndrome, dermatomyositis, scleroderma, chronic active hepatitis, and renal tubular acidosis.

Extrinsic allergic alveolitis is characterized by the presence of granulomata, giant cells, mononuclear cells, and plasma cells in the alveoli and interstitium and the absence of desquamative pneumonia. Specific precipitants against an antigen can often be detected. The peripheral airways are most commonly involved. Rarely, as in the case of sarcoidosis, is there systemic involvement. Serum IgG, IgM, and IgA may be increased but IgE is usually not affected. The prevalence of extrinsic allergic alveolitis is uncertain, but 6 to 10 per cent of pigeon breeders and 4 per cent of farmers are affected with forms of the disorder (Reed, 1982). The steps leading to development of this set of disorders may be as follows: exposure to an immunogenic material, such as the spores of *Micropolyspora faeni* in moldy hay (farmer's lung), followed by the formation of 7S serum antibodies. Upon re-exposure, an Arthus-type reaction occurs, leading to extravasation of fluid, emigration of leukocytes, and tissue destruction. This episode is acute and not repeated until re-exposure to the antigen. When the antigen is contained within the body, as in colonization of the respiratory tree with *Aspergillus fumigatus* (bronchopulmonary aspergillosis), the reaction may be continuous and the disease either subacute or chronic. Early and intermediate histopathology shows epithelioid granulomata, suggesting that the response may be in part type IV rather than type III. In addition, at least 10 per cent of afflicted patients will show a type I or an immediate wheal and flare response to skin testing with the appropriate antigen. Individuals with an immediate response are more likely to have bronchospastic episodes in addition to the more commonly seen symptoms of shortness of breath and malaise. Chronic disease can lead to restrictive pulmonary function, and up to 30 per cent of individuals after an exposure have some remaining symptoms (Pepys, 1975; Nicholson, 1972; Lancet, 1971). The role of precipitating antibody in the pathogenesis of hypersensitivity pneumonitis is uncertain, since some individuals with this syndrome have no detectable antibody and many healthy "controls" have detectable antibody. This syndrome can be caused by many antigens, some of which are listed in Table 40–9. Workers in certain industries are particularly prone to these disorders. The economic implications extend beyond this, since cattle and possibly horses may also be affected. Some antigens are available for testing either a skin response or serum precipitins. It appears at this time that the most reliable assay for precipitins commonly available is the microimmunodiffusion test (Flaherty, 1974). The major difficulty in diagnosis is identification of appropriate antigens and the relatively poor sensitivity of the assay systems. The antigenic determinants appear to vary from group to group of microorganisms. Therefore, it is well to use either the specific material to which an individual has been exposed or a pool of materials which are more likely to contain the involved antigens.

More sensitive techniques such as ELISA have also been used. While detection of the antibody is a useful confirmatory procedure, it is not a diagnostic assay. For example, in one study 40 farmers were found to have serum antibodies to the organisms associated with farmer's lung; none of these farmers were ill or had signs of pulmonary dysfunction. Of 1000 healthy controls, 9 per cent have antibody to aspergillus (reviewed in Burrell, 1983). Bronchoalveolar washings reveal an increased number of T lymphocytes in contrast to patients with sarcoidosis (Godard, 1981). Some antigens and kits are commercially available. Caution must be exercised in interpreting results using these systems, since some of the antigens—especially "moldy hay"—contain lipid which appears as a thick, somewhat hazy, precipitant line on a gel diffusion plate. As the antigen is diluted, so is the line giving the appearance of decreasing titers with increasing antigen dilutions. Some *Aspergillus* antigens contain materials which bind to C-reactive protein (CRP) and form a precipitate resembling an Ag-Ab reaction. Patients with high serum CRP levels may appear to have antibody to *Aspergillus* antigens. This *Aspergillus*-CRP reaction requires divalent cations for precipitation to occur. Therefore, solutions containing citrate can prevent or remove such "false positives" (Fink, 1976). Lastly, IgE anti-*Aspergillus* antibody, seen in bronchopulmonary aspergillosis, can be detected through the use of the RAST procedure.

5

Adkinson, N. F., Jr.: The radioallergosorbent test in 1981—limitations and refinements. J. Allergy Clin. Immunol., 67:87, 1981.

Arbesman, C. A.: Clinical implications and metabolism. *In* Ishizaka, K., and Dayton, D. H. (eds.): The Biological Role of the Immunoglobulin E System. Washington, D.C., U.S. Government Printing Office, 1975.

Berg, T. L. O., and Johansson, S. G. O.: Allergy diagnoses and the radioallergosorbent test. J. Allergy Clin. Immunol., 54:209, 1974.

Burrell, R., and Rylander, R.: A critical review of the role of precipitins in hypersensitivity pneumonitis. Eur. J. Resp. Dis., *62*:332, 1983.

Cochrane, C. G., and Koffler, D.: Immune complex disease in experimental animals and man. Adv. Immunol., *16*:185, 1973.

Dixon, F. J.: Experimental serum sickness. *In* Samter, M.: Immunological Diseases. 2nd ed. Boston, Little, Brown and Company, 1971.

Evans, R., III: The radioallergosorbent test (RAST) as a research tool. *In* Evans, R., III (ed.): Advances in the Diagnosis of Allergy: RAST. Symposia Specialists, 1975.

Fink, J. N.: Hypersensitivity pneumonitis due to organic dust inhalation. N.Y. State J. Med., *72*:1834, 1972.

Fink, J. N.: Diseases of the Lung. *In* Rose, N. R., and Friedman, H. (eds.): Manual of Clinical Immunology. Washington, D.C., American Society of Microbiology, 1976.

Flaherty, D. K., Barboriak, J., Emanuel, D., Fink, J., Marx, J., Moore, V., Reed, C. E., and Roberts, R.: Multilaboratory comparison of three immunodiffusion methods used for the detection of precipitating antibodies in hypersensitivity pneumonitis. J. Lab. Clin. Med., *84*:298, 1974.

Frick, O. L.: Immediate hypersensitivity. *In* Fudenberg, H. H., Stites, D. P., Caldwell, J., and Wells, J. V. (eds.): Basic and Clinical Immunology. Los Altos, Cal., Lange Medical Publishers, 1976.

Godard, P., Clot, J., Bousquet, J., and Michel, F. B.: Lymphocyte subpopulations in bronchoalveolar lavages of patients with sarcoidosis and hypersensitivity pneumonitis. Chest, *4*:447, 1981.

Johansson, S. G. O., Bennich, H. H., and Berg, T.: The Clinical Significance of IgE. *In* Schwartz, R. S. (ed.): Progress in Clinical Immunology I. New York, Grune and Stratton, Inc., 1972.

Lancet (editorial): Fibrosing alveolitis. *1*:999, 1971.

Levine, B. B., Stember, R. H., and Fotino, M.: Ragweed hay fever: Genetic control and linkage to HLA haplotypes. Science, *178*:1201, 1972.

Lichtenstein, L. M.: Allergy. *In* Bach, F. H., and Good, R. A. (eds.): Clinical Immunology, Vol. I. New York, Academic Press, Inc., 1972.

Lichtenstein, L. M., Ishizaka, K., Norman, P. S., Sobotka, A. K., and Hill, B. M.: IgE antibody measurement in ragweed hay fever. Relationship to clinical severity and the results of immunotherapy. J. Clin. Invest., *52*:472, 1973.

Mattson, J., Patterson, R., and Roberts, M.: Insulin therapy in patients with systemic insulin allergy. Arch. Intern. Med., *135*:818, 1975.

Nicholson, D. P.: Extrinsic allergic pneumonias. Am. J. Med., *53*:131, 1972.

Orange, R. P., and Austen, K. F.: Immunologic and pharmacologic receptor control of the release of chemical mediators from human lung. *In* Ishizaka, K., and Dayton, D. H. (eds.): The Biological Role of the Immunoglobulin E System. Washington, D.C., U.S. Government Printing Office, 1975.

Pepys, J., and Warwick, M. T.: The lung in allergic disease. *In* Gell, P. G. H., Coombs, R. R. A., and Lachman, P. J. (eds.): Clinical Aspects of Immunity. 3rd ed. London, Blackwell Scientific Publications, 1975.

Reed, C. E., and deShazo, R.: Immunologic aspects of granulomatous and interstitial lung disease. J.A.M.A., *248*:2683, 1982.

Roitt, I.: Essential Immunology. 4th ed. Boston, Blackwell Scientific Publications, 1980.

Salvaggio, J. E.: Immunological mechanisms in pulmonary disease. Clin. Allergy, *9*:659, 1979.

Samuelsson, B.: Leukotrienes: Mediators of immediate hypersensitivity reactions and inflammation. Science, *220*:568, 1983.

Townley, R. G.: Pharmacologic blocks to mediator release: Clinical applications. *In* Adv. Asthma Allergy, *2*:7, 1975.

vonPirquet, C. F. R. H., and Schick, B.: Serum Sickness. Baltimore, Williams and Wilkins Co., 1951.

Waldmann, T. A., Strober, W., Polmar, S., and Terry, W. D.: IgE levels and metabolism in immune deficiency disease. *In* Ishizaka, K., and Dayton, D. H. (eds.): The Biological Role of the Immunoglobulin E System. Washington, D.C., U.S. Government Printing Office, 1975.

Yunginger, J. W., and Gleich, G. H.: The impact of the discovery of IgE on the practice of allergy. Pediatr. Clin. North Am., *22*:3, 1975.

41

IMMUNODEFICIENCY DISEASES

RUSSELL H. TOMAR, M.D., JOSEPH A. BELLANTI, M.D., and JOSEF V. KADLEC, S.J., M.D., PH.D.

Our immune system is very discerning. It develops a visible response to "foreign" substances but not to "self," even when the antigenic structures are quite similar. This "fine tuning" of responses results from the homeostatic interaction of B lymphocytes, macrophages, and, most significantly, the multiple subsets of T lymphocytes (see Chap. 34). It is not surprising that sometimes things run amuck. When one or more components of the immune system are absent or misfire and the fail-safe plan itself fails, autoimmune disease (see Chap. 39) or immunodeficiency states may develop. The failure of an appropriate immunological response may also lead to neoplastic or infectious diseases. Human studies defining the role of immunodeficiency in tumor development have been somewhat disappointing, perhaps because of the subtlety of the deficiency. Thus while tumors do develop in immunodeficient subjects, we have not defined what type of imunodeficiency allows for neoplastic growth. Furthermore, while immunodeficiency states secondary to other conditions—namely, tumors (such as Hodgkin's disease or chronic lymphocytic leukemia), viral infections (such as infectious mononucleosis or cytomegalovirus infection), or the use of drugs (such as cyclophosphamide or azathioprine)—are not uncommon, the level of our understanding is less than for the so-called primary immunological deficiency diseases. For this reason we shall emphasize the latter, particularly as we view the patient who presents with repeated infections.

EVALUATION OF THE PATIENT WITH REPEATED INFECTION

The first question to be answered is whether or not the patient truly suffers from an unusual number of infections. This issue can be difficult to resolve since the average young child may have six viral infections per year. If a reliable history is unavailable, then a period of observation should help to determine to what extent the patient is to be investigated. Moreover, the type or types of microorganisms involved may help in pointing to the direction of the immune injury. Since polymorphonuclear cells, antibodies, and complement are important in destroying bacteria, repeated bacterial infections suggest a defect in one of these mechanisms of antibacterial defense. On the other hand, T lymphocytes are more important in combating intracellular microorganisms such as many viruses, fungi, and some bacteria.

Polymorphonuclear Cell Defects. Patients with polymorphonuclear cell defects generally suffer from pyogenic bacterial infections. Individuals with chronic granulomatous disease of childhood, however, tend to have difficulty with a more select group of bacteria, i.e., those which are catalase-positive such as staphylococci and *Escherichia coli.* This and other phagocytic cell defects are discussed in Chapter 35.

Complement Defects. Complement defects may result in bacterial infections. C3 is critical for optimal phagocytosis. Absence of C3 or of C3 inactivator, which results in decreased C3, leads to syndromes characterized by multiple bacterial infections. Patients who lack C5, C6, C7, and C8 suffer from neisserial infections. Complement, including methods of assay, is discussed in Chapter 37.

Stem Cell Defects. Since all of the cellular elements of the blood stream are thought to derive from a primordial stem cell, it is not surprising that deficiencies in lymphoid cells have been associated with deficiencies of other blood elements, such as polymorphonuclear cells. Virtual absence of these cells has been reported (reticular dysgenesis or DeVaal's syndrome) (Ammann, 1980b). Infants with these conditions have not survived beyond a few weeks of life. Such defects represent the most severe manifestations of the close association between lymphoid cells and hematopoietic tissue (Cline, 1978).

METHODS OF EVALUATING PATIENTS WITH IMMUNODEFICIENCIES

General Considerations. Clinical history should guide the physician in determining the extent and direction of the evaluation. Physical examination may provide further diagnostic clues such as telangiectasia in the ataxia-telangiectasia syndrome, or small stature, hands, and feet in hypogammaglobulinemia with short-limbed dwarfism. Nonimmunological laboratory studies should include a complete blood count with a differential, imunoglobulin levels, blood glucose, BUN or serum creatinine, and assays which consider cystic fibrosis (sweat chloride) or alpha-1-antitrypsin deficiency or tumors if appropriate. A classification of primary immunological diseases is provided in Table 41–1.

METHODS OF EVALUATING PATIENTS WITH HYPOGAMMAGLOBULINEMIA

Immunoglobulins. The essential determination is quantitation of serum immunoglobulins by a routine procedure (see Chap. 36); age-matched reference values should always be given (see p. 872). Immunoelectrophoresis provides only a rough estimate. Serum protein electrophoresis may be valuable if rapid diagnosis is required, e.g., when the individual has a very low serum IgG level and no other rapid procedure is available. Secretions can be examined for the presence of IgA by gel diffusion, using anti-alpha chain antibody. Saliva may be induced by allowing the subject to chew on paraffin. Secretory component (SC) can be measured in the same way, using anti-SC antibody. Determinations of serum IgE and IgD require more sensitive techniques (see Chaps. 36 and 38). Determination of serum IgE may be useful in evaluation of patients with atopic disease and repeated infection. Determination of the quantity of IgG in each of its four subclasses may be relevant but at this time can be done only in a few specialized laboratories.

Antibodies. While we conveniently screen with immunoglobulin determinations, the presence or absence of antibody is far more pertinent information, especially in patients with borderline immunoglobulins. Most laboratories can measure isohemagglutinins as part of their reverse ABO erythrocyte typing

Table 41–1. CLASSIFICATION OF PRIMARY IMMUNODEFICIENCIES

Condition	Dysfunction: *Antibody*	Dysfunction: *T cell*	Comments
Reticular dysgenesis	+	+	Generalized hematopoietic hypoplasia (De Vaal)
Severe combined immunodeficiency (SCID)	+	+	There are at least four types: (1) Congenital X-linked (Swiss). (2) Autosomal inheritance. (3) Associated with absence of the enzyme adenosine deaminase (ADA). Autosomal inheritance. (4) B cells present (SCID with B cells).
Congenital X-linked hypogammaglobulinemia	+	–	There is an absence of B cells and/or precursor B cells (Bruton's).
Transient hypogammaglobulinemia of infancy	+	–	This syndrome occurs at 2–6 months of age and may require temporary treatment with gamma globulin.
Antibody deficiency with normal or increased immunoglobulin	+	+	The ability to develop antibody may be due to a myriad of factors. Some may be due to subclass deficiency as IgG-2 for antibody to *H. influenzae* polysaccharide or inability to "process" certain antigen classes such as polysaccharides.
Common variable hypogammaglobulinemia	+	+	These are largely unclassified (see Table 41–3 for mechanisms). Some recognizable groups are as follows: (1) Dysgammaglobulinemia I—decreased or absent IgG and IgA with normal or increased IgM. Presumed to be due to a failure to switch from IgM to other isotypes. (2) Dysgammaglobulinemia II—decreased or absent IgM and IgA with normal or increased IgG. (3) Selective immunoglobulin deficiency. IgA is the most common, affecting about 1/500 Caucasians born in North America. Associated with gluten-sensitive enteropathy, allergies, or arthritis. Deficiencies of IgM may be associated with tumors in adults. (4) Some common variable hypogammaglobulinemias are associated with deficiency of 5 ecto-nucleotidase on the surface of B cells.

Table 41–1. CLASSIFICATION OF PRIMARY IMMUNODEFICIENCIES (*Continued*)

Condition	Dysfunction		Comments
	Antibody	***T cell***	
T-cell defects	(−)	+	There are many variations. Some have been categorized: (1) Di George's syndrome is associated with dysembryogenesis of the third and fourth brachial pouches, often leading to cardiac abnormalities and failure of the parathyroids as well as the thymus to develop. Antibody production to T-dependent antigens may be impaired. (2) Nezeloff's syndrome—T cell defect associated with normal or elevated gamma globulin. No other physical defects noted. (3) T cell defects associated with absence of the enzyme inosine phosphorylase.
Combined deficiencies	+	+	Several syndromes are recognized: (1) Ataxia-telangiectasia—associated with cerebellar malfunction and skin lesions, IgA (70%) and IgE deficiencies. Abnormal T cell function: T cells cannot be instructed to kill virally infected cells. (2) Wiskott-Aldrich syndrome—a triad of thrombocytopenia, eczema, and repeated infections. Deficiencies of one or more immunoglobulin isotypes may be seen. Abnormal T cell function manifested by the inability to instruct T cells to kill virally infected cells. (3) Immunodeficiency with thymoma associated with autoimmune disorders and aplastic anemia. (4) Immunodeficiency with short-limbed dwarfism, usually has immunoglobulin deficiencies and may also be associated with deficiencies in cell-mediated immunity. (5) Hyper IgE (Job-Buckley syndrome)—probably due to production of IgE antistaphylococcal antibody rather than IgG or IgM.
Acquired immune deficiency syndrome (AIDS)	−	+	The newest of the recognizable immunodeficiency syndromes. The cause of AIDS is unknown. Lymphopenia, especially of so-called T_4, helper/inducer lymphocytes. Occurs in homosexual males, drug addicts, hemophiliacs, Haitians. Associated with Kaposi's sarcoma and opportunistic infections, especially *Pneumocystis carinii pneumonia.*

procedure. Isohemagglutinins usually are not present until about 9 to 12 months of age. The natural anti-A and anti-B are mainly of the IgM class; the immune anti-A and anti-B are of the IgG class. Isohemagglutinins are described in Chapter 42. Antistreptococcal antibodies (e.g., ASO) are often convenient to determine. Since most children in this country are immunized against diphtheria and tetanus, measurement of antibody to these agents is often useful. Thus either primary immunization (unimmunized individual or no boosters within the preceding ten years) or booster injections should lead to the development of anti-tetanus and anti-diphtheria antibodies. One should collect serum prior to and two to three weeks after the booster injection and determine antibody on both samples simultaneously. Pneumococcal polysaccharide can also be used to assess antibody-forming capacity. For many laboratories it is more convenient to use typhoid vaccines, since *Salmonella* agglutinins (as part of "febrile agglutinins") are commonly available. Side effects such as fever, leukocytosis, and pain at injection site are sometimes observed with this vaccine. At least two doses, approximately two to three weeks apart, may be required to elicit antibody formation. Serum specimens should be collected before and two or three weeks after each injection for simultaneous measurements. In general, if serum is collected and frozen in divided aliquots, one specimen may be tested on several different occasions. *Material with living organisms such as oral polio vaccine should never be used in subjects suspected of having an immunologic deficiency syndrome.*

Enumeration of B Lymphocytes. Markers of B cells change during maturation (Chap. 34). Thus no single

5

marker includes all cells destined to become B lymphocytes. Surface Ig, particularly IgM and IgD, is generally accepted as the most reliable B cell marker. Other procedures which may be useful include measurement of complement (EAC) or Fc receptors. These may be technically less time consuming but will identify some non-B cells (Chap. 34). Some of the monoclonal reagents (B-1 Coulter, BA-1 Hybritech) may prove to be as useful as or more useful than surface immunoglobulin. Determination of cytoplasmic IgM may detect an early phase of B cell maturation. Tissue such as lymph nodes may be evaluated by processing and labeling single cell suspensions or by studying histological preparations with appropriate immunofluorescent or immunoenzyme reagents (Chaps. 34 and 38). It has been surprising to find B cells in most patients with decreased immunoglobulins, but it is now apparent that normal B cells often require other cells to function properly (Waldmann, 1982). Patients with congenital X-linked agammaglobulinemia usually have no circulating surface immunoglobulin positive cells; patients with severe combined immunodeficiency (SCID) may have circulating surface immunoglobulin positive cells (WHO Scientific Group, 1978).

Enumeration of T Lymphocyte Subsets. Enumeration of T lymphocytes by their ability to rosette with sheep erythrocytes has not proved particularly helpful in dissecting the hypogammaglobulinemic states. However, the ability to determine surface markers on T lymphocytes with monoclonal antibodies may add new insights. Thus far, the only consistent pattern is that the usual ratio of "helper/inducer" to "suppressor/cytotoxic" cells is often abnormal (Table 41–2) (Pandolfi, 1982).

Functional Assays. Circulating B cells may be examined for their ability to produce antibody *in vitro.* One method detects the number of cells producing Ig by plating lymphocytes in a semi-solid medium with a target susceptible to lysis by immunoglobulin. For example, staphylococcal protein A (SPA) may be coupled to bovine erythrocytes, and subsequently anti-IgG, IgA, or IgM (of animal IgG) may be bound to the SPA-RBC. This mixture is plated in an agarose matrix along with patient cells from a Ficoll-Hypaque interface. The lymphocyte-SPA/erythrocyte mixture is then incubated at 37°C. in a 5 per cent CO_2 incubator for an appropriate period of time. As immunoglobulin is produced, it couples to the anti-Ig–SPA on the bovine erythrocytes. Complement is then added to the plate, causing lysis of erythrocytes and thereby producing visible plaques. The number of plaques is directly related to the number of cells producing that isotype of Ig. If one knows the number of cells plated, then one can determine the percentage of Ig producing cells in the original Ficoll-Hypaque preparation (Pryjma, 1980). The second method involves stimulating cells with a mitogen such as pokeweed mitogen or an antigen such as tetanus or influenza to produce immunoglobulin *in vitro.* The supernatant is collected and immunoglobulin measured by radioimmunoassay or enzyme-linked immunoassay. The cells may be examined for the presence of intracytoplasmic immunoglobulin (Waldmann, 1982). By separating B and T cells and later T cells into subsets, the interplay of these cell populations may be studied. This technique has proved very useful in determining mechanisms involved in immunoglobulin production in "normals" and patients and has provided us with much of our current information about immunodeficiency states (Waldmann, 1982).

Other Determinations. Since anemia, neutropenia, and platelet dysfunctions have been associated with hypogammaglobulinemia, a blood count and micro-

Table 41–2. LYMPHOCYTE SUBSETS IN IMMUNOLOGIC DEFICIENCY DISORDERS

	T Cell Markers (%)					*B Cell Markers (%)*
Condition	***ERL***	T_3	T_4	T_8	T_4/T_8	***SIg***
Severe combined immunodeficiency	0–↓↓	↓↓	↓↓	↓↓		↓↓
Severe combined immunodeficiency with B cells	0–↓↓	↓↓	↓↓	↓↓		N1 to ↑
Congenital X-linked agammaglobulinemia	N1	N1	↓–N1	N1	N1	0–↓↓
DiGeorge's syndrome	0–↓↓					↑
Common variable immunodeficiency	N1–↑	↓–N1	↓–N1–↑	↓–N1–↑	~25% ↓ ~15% ↑	↓–N1
Ataxia-telangiectasia	N1					N1
Wiskott-Aldrich syndrome	↓					N1
Selective IgA deficiency	N1	N1	↓–N1	N1–↑	~20% ↑ ~10% ↓	(N1)
Acquired immune deficiency syndrome (AIDS)	N1–↓↓	N1	↓↓	N1–↑	↓↓	N1–↓

ERL = sheep-erythrocyte rosetting lymphocytes. SIg = surface immunoglobulins.
(Pandolfi, 1982; WHO Scientific Group, 1978.)

Table 41–3. IMMUNE PATHOGENESIS OF HYPOGAMMAGLOBULINEMIA

Absence of stem cells	Reticular dysgenesis
Absence of lymphoid cells	Severe combined immunodeficiency
Absence of B cells or precursor B cells	Congenital X-linked agammaglobulinemia
Absence or diminished T helper cells or factors	Common variable hypogammaglobulinemia
Presence of excess T suppressor cells	Common variable hypogammaglobulinemia
Presence of excess macrophage suppressor cells	Multiple myeloma (polyclonal immunoglobulins)
Presence of antibody to lymphoid tissue	Common variable hypogammaglobulinemia
Dysfunction of B cells	Common variable hypogammaglobulinemia

scopic review with differential should be performed. Autoantibodies such as antinuclear antibodies (ANA) and rheumatoid factor or antireticulin antibodies have been described in patients with immunoglobulin deficiency. Patients deficient in IgA often have 7S IgM (10 per cent), anti-IgA antibodies (40 per cent), and/or antibodies against proteins in food, especially bovine milk (50 to 60 per cent) or gamma globulin (40 to 70 per cent) (Ammann, 1971, 1980a).

Mechanisms Leading to Hypogammaglobulinemia. While some mechanisms leading to decreased Ig are obvious, namely, absence of B cells or B cell precursors, others are more subtle such as imbalances of T helper or T suppressor cells (Table 41-2). Mechanisms which lead to hypogammaglobulinemia are given in Tables 41-3 and 41-4.

Management of Hypogammaglobulinemia. For uncomplicated agamma- or hypogammaglobulinemia, the treatment is to provide adequate immunoglobulin, usually in the form of intramuscular or intravenous gamma globulin. Intravenous plasma may also be used but carries a risk of hepatitis. While local reactions to intramuscular gamma globulin are not uncommon, more severe ones are less likely except in the individual who is deficient in a particular isotype, particularly IgA. This is most often seen in IgA-deficient patients who incidentally receive IgA in plasma when they are hospitalized for purposes such as surgery. *Therefore, if possible, IgA negative plasma should be available within the region, and, for planned procedures, the patient's blood and plasma should be stored ahead of time.* Laboratory measurements are required for determination of the efficiency of therapy. This is generally taken to mean reaching a level of greater than 200 to 300 mg/dl (20 to 30 IU/ml) IgG. Measuring IgG periodically will help to predict the amount of gamma globulin and interval between injections required to achieve that goal.

Table 41–4. CONDITIONS ASSOCIATED WITH SECONDARY HYPOGAMMAGLOBULINEMIA

- Protein losing
  - Nephrotic syndromes
  - Enteropathies
  - Malnutrition
- Reticuloendothelial malignancies
  - Multiple myeloma
  - Macroglobulinemia of Waldenström
  - Chronic lymphocytic leukemia
  - Other leukemias
  - Lymphoma
  - Heavy chain disease
- Autoimmune diseases
  - Rheumatoid arthritis
  - Lupus erythematosus
  - Autoimmune thrombocytopenic purpura
  - Myasthenia gravis
  - Pernicious anemia
- Miscellaneous
  - Amyloidosis
  - Sarcoidosis
  - Hyperlipoproteinemias

METHODS OF EVALUATION OF CELL-MEDIATED IMMUNITY

Skin Tests

The most convenient way of screening for intact delayed-type hypersensitivity is skin testing with recall antigens. These should be antigens to which a large percentage of the population react. Thus, in this country, PPD is of little value. Trichophyton and mumps antigens have been used by several investigators. Probably the two most commonly used agents are Candida antigen (determatophytin "O," Hollister-Stier or Greer Laboratories) and streptokinase-streptodornase (SK-SD, Varidase-Lederle). SK-SD may be used at an initial dilution of 100/25 U/ml with 0.1 ml injected intradermally. If this is negative, some workers have then tested with 400/U/ml. The strength of Candida antigens varies greatly from manufacturer to manufacturer and from lot to lot. Dilutions of 1:50 or 1:100 have most commonly been suggested as initial screening concentrations. SK-SD will soon no longer be available commercially. Other candidate antigens include tetanus and mumps. Children and the elderly are most likely to be non-responsive. Since a skin test requires many steps, such as antigen recognition, inflammatory response, and migration of cells, it is not clear where the defect lies if an individual is unable to respond, i.e., when he is anergic. We tend to believe that a positive skin test rules out a major defect in cell-mediated immunity; however, there may be defects in other T-lymphocyte functions, such as immunoglobulin production help or suppression.

Techniques are avaiable to test the ability of patients to develop a delayed response to a new antigen. BCG immunization for prevention of tuberculosis leading to a positive PPD (purified protein derivative) is of historical interest but should not be used in immune-deficient patients because BCG contains live acid-fast organisms that may cause a potentially fatal disease called BCGosis. The materials most widely used for sensitization are dinitrochlorobenzene (DNCB) and

5

dinitrofluorobenzene (DNFB). Most individuals will not react with a contact dermatitis to low concentrations of these substances. However, a subject may be sensitized in about three weeks by one application of a high concentration of material to the skin, usually on the volar aspect of the forearm. The individual can then be retested with a lesser amount of material, or a reaction will spontaneously reappear at the site of initial sensitization. Precautions must be taken not to apply too much material, since a burnlike reaction often occurs, and not to sensitize oneself. Therefore, gloves, mask, and perhaps gown should be used by the person making up and applying these agents (Spitler, 1980). Virtually all normals can be sensitized with DNCB or DNFB.

Another *in vivo* method of evaluating cell-mediated immunity has been through the use of skin grafts. If a graft from an unrelated donor is applied, it should be rejected within one to two weeks. Because of difficulties of standardization and potential problems of graft-vs-host disease and because other techniques are readily available, skin grafting is rarely necessary.

Enumeration of T Lymphocytes

Human T lymphocytes are most often identified by their ability to rosette with sheep erythrocytes (E rosettes). There are many variations to this simple assay. However, most variations result in a greater or lesser percentage of E rosetting cells. The larger figure, generally 60 to 80 per cent of mononuclear cells, has been called the total T lymphocyte count. The lesser figure, which varies greatly by technique, has been called the active or more avid fraction (Wybran, 1973). The total T lymphocyte figure generally requires fetal calf serum, heating at 37°C. for at least 30 minutes, a high sheep red blood cell/lymphocyte ratio, and overnight incubation at 4°C. The significance of these groups of T cells is not clear, but in several disorders the lesser figure (active T cells) changes with therapy while the total T lymphocyte count remains relatively constant (Wybran, 1975). Human T cells also have receptors for the Fc portions of IgG and IgM. Variations in T_G and T_M have been described in some immunodeficiency states. Monoclonal antibodies against cell membrane antigens present the most useful tool in enumerating T lymphocytes and their subsets (see Chap. 34). The impact of this new information is yet to be appreciated; however, imbalances in T cell subsets will be recognized for the first time and catalogued (Table 41-2). At this writing, the most commonly used antibodies are those marking "pan T cells' (T_3 or Leu_1), sheep erythrocyte rosette receptors (T_{11} or Leu_5), "helper/inducer" cells (T_4 or Leu_{3a}), and the "cytotoxic/suppressor" cells (T_8 or Leu_{2a}). Other antibodies are being made available, and undoubtedly new insights will be gained (Reinherz, 1982).

Functional Assays

LYMPHOCYTE PROLIFERATION

Mitogens. Mitogenic stimulation of lymphocytes is not truly an immunologic phenomenon. The mitogen, often a plant lectin, binds to a material on the cell surface, often a sugar, and induces the cell to divide. There is no prior sensitization. Phytohemagglutinin (PHA) stimulates T helper and T suppressor lymphocytes and B cells to a lesser extent. PHA stimulation has become one of the common ways of screeening for a human T cell defect.

Pokeweed mitogen (PWM) stimulates primarily B cells. B cells will produce immunoglobulins in response to PWM in the presence of T cells and macrophages. Concanavalin A (Con A) stimulates human T and B cells but T cells more vigorously. There appear to be differences in the ability of subsets of T cells to respond to Con A. Cells treated with Con A prior to reculture with another set of cells often act as "suppressor" to further proliferation, the so-called Con A suppressor cell assay (Fauci, 1980).

Antigens. T cells proliferate in response to many antigens. Proliferation to antigens, however, is less intensive and takes longer than proliferation to mitogens. The most commonly used asoluble antigens are PPD, Candida, tetanus, and SK-SD. The mixed lymphocyte response (MLC) is described in Chapters 33 and 34 and is another way of assaying T cell function since the T lymphocyte is the responding proliferating cell in this reaction. The autologous mixed lymphocyte reaction may also be used to evaluate aspects of T cell function (Weksler, 1981).

LYMPHOKINES

Lymphokines are biologically active products of lymphocytes. Many have been described. There are two general procedures for assaying lymphokines. In the first method, the patient's cells are incubated in the test system directly. In the indirect procedure, the patient's lymphocytes are first stimulated by a mitogen such as PHA or an antigen for 24 to 48 hours. The supernate containing the lymphokines is then examined in the test system. The leukocyte inhibition factor assay (LIF) is a direct test wherein human buffy coat leukocytes are incubated in capillary tubes in the presence of antigen. Migration at 37°C. is observed after 18 hours. The guinea pig migration inhibition factor assay (MIF) is an example of an indirect procedure whereby the lymphokines produced by human lymphocytes are collected, concentrated—often by lyophilization—and tested for their ability to inhibit the migration of guinea pig peritoneal macrophages from capillary tube. Presently the best defined of the lymphokines is interleukin II or T-cell growth factor (TCGF) (see Chap. 34). This protein is produced by T cells in response to interleukin I or lymphocyte activating factor (LAF) made by macrophages. Surely some of the defects in CMI result from failure to produce or respond to one or both of these proteins. Interferon (IF), particularly gamma interferon, represents another class of lymphokines. Gamma IF is produced by lymphocytes and has multiple effects on lymphocyte function. Again, it is likely that defects in the production of or response to IF will be found (Oppenheim, 1981).

CYTOTOXICITY

Conceivably defects might exist in the "induction phase," i.e., converting pre-cytotoxic cells to cytotoxic cells, or "effector phase," namely, the actual interaction of killer cells with target resulting in cytoxicity. Other sets of cytotoxic lymphocytes include K cells, which mediate antibody dependent cellular cytotoxicity (ADCC) (Chapter 34), and NK cells, which are responsible for spontaneous cell mediated cytotoxicity (Wahlin, 1976; Herberman, 1981). The biological role of these cells is unclear at this time.

Mechanisms of CMI Defects

These are even less well understood than those for the hypogammaglobulinemias. Clearly the absence of precursor or T lymphocytes (SCID, DiGeorge's syndrome) leads to the absence of CMI. However, most CMI defects are more subtle. With the advent of consistent, convenient methods of enumerating T subsets, we can expect greater insights into these disorders.

Management

Unfortuantely there is no simple equivalent to giving gamma globulin. In general, more dramatic, riskier procedures must be taken. Thus the diagnosis and level of danger to the patient by the disease must be carefully assessed and weighed against the risk of therapy. Treatments such as thymosin, transfer factor, bone marrow transplants, and thymus transplants have had variable success. The patient with SCID will require a bone marrow transplant; little is clear beyond that except that no single therapy is in general use. *Patients who lack CMI function are a risk for graft-vs-host disease, and therefore blood cell products should be irradiated prior to transfusion.*

PROCEEDING WITH THE EVALUATION

A large array of determinations might be performed in evaluating immunodeficiencies. The investigator should use some "horse sense" before getting too deeply involved with such an evaluation. One must define whether there is sufficient evidence of an immunological deficiency for a detailed evaluation. If there is, one should determine whether this evaluation should be done locally, and, if not, where the patient should be sent. It may be fruitless to begin a detailed evaluation if the patient will be re-evaluated elsewhere. Finally, one must estimate the likelihood of helping the subject even after a lengthy and expensive evaluation. Having gone through this philosophical self-examination, one should settle on a course of action. In addition to a complete blood count and differential, immunoglobulin levels and delayed skin responses to recall antigens are generally available screening procedures. Determining if the subject can make antibody is also a valuable procedure available to most laboratories. Enumeration of lymphocyte subsets is becoming available and more valuable as information is gained. Finally, functional assays are more difficult to perform and much more difficult to interpet unless the laboratory has a wide experience in this area. Of course the information gained from these kinds of assays may be the most important in the workup. One method of proceeding is suggested in Table 41-5.

Table 41–5. STAGES IN EVALUATION OF IMMUNOLOGICAL DEFICIENCY STATES

History and physical examination
General laboratory determination: complete blood count with differential; blood glucose, blood urea nitrogen; other determinations as appropriate
Screening studies: serum immunoglobulin levels; delayed type responses to recall antigens
Enumeration of lymphocyte subsets
Antibody production as to diphtheria and/or tetanus toxoids
Lymph node biopsy
In vitro functional assays: proliferative assays to mitogens and/or antigens, including alloantigens; induction and expression of cytotoxicity by T lymphocytes; regulation of immunoglobulin production

Ammann, A. J., and Hong, R.: Selective IgA deficiency: Presentation of 30 cases and a review of the literature. Medicine, *50*:223, 1971.

Ammann, A. J., and Hong, R.: Disorders of the IgA system. *In* Stiehm, E. R., and Fulginiti, V. A. (eds): Immunologic Disorders in Infants and Children. Philadelphia, W. B. Saunders Company, 1980a.

Ammann, A. J., and Hong, R.: Disorders of the T-cell system. *In* Stiehm, E. R., and Fulginiti, V. A. (eds): Immunologic Disorders in Infants and Children. Philadelphia, W. B. Saunders Company, 1980b.

Cline, M. J., and Golde, D. W.: Immune suppression of hematopoiesis. Am. J. Med., *64*:301, 1978.

Fauci, A. S.: Assays for suppressor cells. *In* Rose, N. R., and Friedman, H. (eds.): Manual of Clinical Microbiology. 2nd ed. Washington, D.C., American Society of Microbiology, 1980.

Herberman, R. B., and Ortaldo, J. R.: Natural killer cells: Their role in defenses against disease. Science, *214*:24, 1981.

Oppenheim, J. J.: Lymphokines. *In* Oppenheim, J. J., Rosenstreich, D. C., and Potter, M. (eds.): Cellular Functions in Immunity and Inflammation. New York, Elsevier/North Holland, 1981.

Pandolfi, F., Quinti, I., Frielingidorf, A., Goldstein, G., Businco, L., and Aiuti, F.: Abnormalities of regualtory T-cell subpopulations in patients with primary immunoglobulin deficiencies. Clin. Immunol. Immunopath., *22*:323, 1982.

Pryjma, J., Monoz, J., Virella, G., and Fudenberg, H. H.: Evaluation of IgM, IgG, IgA, and IgE secretion by human PBL in cultures stimulated with PWM and *Staphylococcus aureus* Cowan I. Cell. Immunol., *509*:115, 1980.

Reinherz, E., and Schlossman, S.: Human T-lymphocyte differentiation. Immunol. Today, *3*:239a, 1982.

Spitler, L. E.: Delayed hypersensitivity skin testing. *In* Rose, N. R., and Friedman, H. (eds): Manual of Clinical Immunology. 2nd ed. Washington, D.C., American Society of Microbiology, 1980.

Wahlin, B., Perlmann, H., and Perlmann, P.: Analysis by a plaque assay of IgG- or IgM-dependent cytolytic lymphocytes in human blood. J. Exp. Med., *144*:1375, 1976.

Waldmann, T. A., and Broder, S.: Polyclonal B-cell activators in the study of the regulation of immunoglobulin synthesis in the human system. Adv. Immunol., *32*:1, 1982.

Weksler, M., Moody C. E., Jr., and Kozak, R. W.: The autologous mixed lymphocyte reaction. Adv. Immunol. *31*:271, 1981.

WHO Scientific Group: Immunodeficiency. WHO Technical Report Series #630, 1978.

Wybran, J., and Fudenberg, H. H.: Thymus-derived rosette-forming cells in various disease states: Cancer, lymphomas, bacterial and viral infections, and other diseases. J. Clin. Invest., *52*:1026, 1973.

Wybran, J., and Fudenberg, H. H.: Human thymus-derived rosette-forming cells and immunologic disease. *In* Bergsma, D. (ed.): Immunodeficiency in Man and Animals. Sunderland, Mass., Sinauer Associates, Inc., 1975.

42

IMMUNOHEMATOLOGY

CHANG LING LEE, M.D., and JOHN BERNARD HENRY, M.D.

The term *immunohematology* refers to immunologic reactions involving blood components. Although the term immunohematology had been used by a few investigators for many years, it was neither well defined nor generally accepted until 1954, when Dr. Israel Davidsohn presented "Immunohematology, A New Branch of Clinical Pathology," in his Presidential inaugural address to the American Society of Clinical Pathologists.

Blood elements have been studied intensively. Along with recent advances in immunologic concepts and technology, basic understanding of immunohematology has increased very rapidly. Prior to 1960, major emphasis had been on erythrocytes, whereas since then the immunology of leukocytes, platelets, and plasma components has been the focus of much investigation. The development of new techniques in biochemistry and cytogenetics in the past two decades has also added greatly to the progress of immunohematology.

While the basic sciences were progressing, applications were developing concurrently. The first and most important application of immunohematology is in safe blood transfusion. The second application is understanding of the pathogenesis, diagnosis, and prevention of Rh immunization (sensitization) associated with pregnancy. In addition, plasma and its derivatives have been used in a number of clinical disorders, and platelet and granulocyte transfusions have saved the lives of many patients. While the precise role of immunohematology in organ transplantation remains unclear, its importance cannot be denied.

In addition to clinical medicine, immunohematology has made important contributions in the areas of human genetics, anthropology, criminology, and, recently, in the resolution of disputed parentage problems. The emphasis of this chapter has been placed on essential basic information as well as important applications pertinent to the practice of laboratory medicine.

BASIC IMMUNOHEMATOLOGY

Blood Group Antigens

The term *blood group* used in this chapter refers not only to groups of erythrocyte antigens but also to other blood components, including leukocytes, platelets, and plasma. The term *antigen* refers to a substance that can initiate an immune response and react with reduced antibodies or sensitized lymphocytes. Hence, antigens are also known as immunogens. The term *specificity* refers to the appearance of a substance that can be recognized by immunologic techniques and is commonly used in reference to leukocyte antigens; it may indicate a complex antigen or a fraction of an antigen. The term *factor* has been used to include classic antigens as well as those recognized by immunologic methods not utilizing a specific antibody, e.g., A_2 or A_3. The majority of established antigens or specificities are inherited, follow the rules of inheritance, and serve as useful genetic markers. Those antigens or specificities of blood components that are inherited as a group are referred to as a blood group system. The relationship of genetic markers within HLA, the major histocompatibility complex group, is reviewed in Chapter 33.

BIOLOGIC PROPERTIES

Antigen. Complete antigens are substances which can induce, in an animal host, either a humoral or a cellular immune response, or both; they can react with the elicited antibodies or sensitized lymphocytes. An incomplete antigen, which is known as a *hapten,* cannot elicit an immune response by itself but can react with a specific antibody or block a specific antigen-antibody reaction. Haptens, which may be very simple chemicals, have contributed greatly to the study of antigenic determinants.

Antigenicity. The property of an antigen which induces an immune response is known as antigenicity. Antigenicity varies not only with the type of antigen but also with the immunized host. The species and individual condition of an animal host, as well as the route and frequency of immunization, affect the degree of immune response. In general, the host must lack the injected antigen; otherwise, no immune response can be elicited. Blood group antigens are usually far less antigenic than microorganisms, although erythrocyte antigens seem more antigenic than antigens on leukocytes or platelets or in plasma, as evidenced by the occurrence of strongly reactive erythrocyte antibodies in plasma of transfused patients.

Antigens A and B in the ABO system are by far the most antigenic, since individuals who lack either or both antigens almost always have the antibody(ies). The next most potent antigen is perhaps the $Rh_0(D)$ antigen; two thirds of all $Rh_0(D)$ negative persons will develop $Rh_0(D)$ antibodies after sufficient dosage and frequency exposure to the D antigen (Mollison, 1983). Thus, from a clinical standpoint, these three antigens are by far the most important. However, there are many other erythrocyte antigens that are highly antigenic. The relative potency of some clinically important erythrocyte antigens is listed in Table 42–1.

Antigenic Specificity. Besides antigenicity, specificity is also a very important property of an antigen. The basis of dividing human individuals into four basic erythrocyte groups—A, B, AB, and O—is their reactivity with two antisera containing anti-A or anti-B. Erythrocytes of a group A person will be agglutinated by anti-A but not by anti-B, those of group B, by anti-B but not anti-A, those of group AB by both antisera, while those of group O will be agglutinated by neither of them. This type of clear-cut specificity is reflected by most of the established erythrocyte groups and to some extent by the serum protein groups; however, such specificity is less evident in leukocyte antigens. While cross-reactions are common in leukocyte antigens, certain specificities can, nevertheless, be established through cross-absorption. Uncertainties as to the specificity of an antigen-antibody reaction may arise from questionable technical procedures and/or impure reagents. Therefore, it is of the utmost importance to take all precautions before considering the specificity of either an antigen or an antibody.

PHYSICAL AND CHEMICAL PROPERTIES

Site of Antigen. Biologic differences of various antigens are derived from the differences in their physical and chemical structures; the size, shape, number of available sites, and chemical composition of an antigen are important contributing factors. The smallest *size* of a complete antigen has been shown to have a molecular weight near 4000, while an incomplete antigen can be very small, such as a simple sugar or a benzene ring. Although the shape of blood group antigens remains to be determined, their relationship to the cytoplasmic membrane has been shown to be critical with regard to their activity. For instance, there is an absence of ABO antigen reactivity in the Bombay type of erythrocyte, but the integrity of the red cell membrane seems unaffected. On the other hand, there is evidence indicating the presence of a defective membrane in Rh_{null} individuals who lack all Rh antigens. From these findings, one may assume that the ABO antigens are likely to be extramembranous, whereas the Rh antigens are likely to be intramembranous. These differences may be responsible, at least in part, for the wide differences in the characteristics between the ABO and the Rh antigens.

Table 42–1. RELATIVE ANTIGENICITY OF SEVERAL CLINICALLY IMPORTANT BLOOD GROUP FACTORS*

Antigen	Relative Potency	Antigen	Relative Potency
D	0.70	K	0.10
c	0.041	E	0.0338
k	0.030	e	0.0112
Fy^a	0.0046	C	0.0022
Jk^a	0.0014	S	0.0008
Jk^b	0.0006	s	0.0006

*These figures represent the approximate percentage of persons who are negative for a specific antigen but receive one unit of corresponding antigen-positive blood and develop antibodies to the specific antigen. When relative potency of K antigen is 0.1 as estimated by Kornstad (1957), the relative potency of other blood groups can be estimated as shown by Mollison (1983).

5

Table 42–2. NUMBER OF ANTIGENIC SITES ON EACH ERYTHROCYTE ESTIMATED BY RADIOACTIVE ANTIBODIES*

Site for Antigen	Phenotypes	Number of Antigenic Sites	Site for Antigen	Phenotypes	Number of Antigenic Sites
A	A_1 adult	810–1170 × 10^3	D	DCce	9.9–14.6 × 10^3
	newborn	250–370 × 10^3		Dce	12–20 × 10^3
	A_2 adult	240–290 × 10^3		DcEe	14–16.6 × 10^3
	newborn	140 × 10^3			14.5–19.3 × 10^3
	A_1B adult	460–850 × 10^3		DcE	15.8–33.3 × 10^3
	newborn	220 × 10^3		DCcEe	23–31 × 10^3
	A_2B adult	120 × 10^3		D--	110–202 × 10^3
B	B adult	750 × 10^3		D^u	0.8–3 × 10^3
	A_1B adult	430 × 10^3	c	c+C−	70–85 × 10^3
I	I+	500 × 10^3		c+C+	37–53 × 10^3
Le^a	Le(a+)	4.5–8 × 10^3	e	e+E−	18.2–24.4 × 10^3
K	K+k−	6.1 × 10^3		e+E+	13.4–14.5 × 10^3
	K+k+	3.5 × 10^3	E	e−E+	0.45–25.6 × 10^3

*Figures are taken from Mollison (1983).

Number of Antigenic Sites. The number of antigenic sites on erythrocytes for some antigens is known. Using antibodies labeled with radioactive isotopes such as ^{125}I, it is possible to estimate the number of antigenic sites by the number of radioactive antibodies attached to the erythrocytes. Table 42–2 shows some of the estimated antigenic sites on each erythrocyte. The wide variation in the number of sites can explain the diversity of serologic behavior of these antigens. It is also possible to use antibodies labeled with electron-dense particles such as ferritin to count from an electron micrograph the number of antibodies attached to the erythrocyte surface. With immunoelectron microscopy the findings obtained with radioisotopes have been confirmed (Masouredis, 1973). In addition, the ABO antigens have been shown to cluster, while the Rh antigens remain rather isolated, another contributing factor to their reactivity.

Chemical Composition. The chemical composition of an antigen determines most of its physical and biologic properties. Many of the known complete antigens are proteins, glycoproteins, or lipoproteins. Pure carbohydrate can elicit immune response only in certain animal species, such as man and mouse, whereas pure lipids or free DNA are not antigenic, although they can serve as haptens.

In studies of synthetic peptide chains, the polymers of one type of amino acid may be less antigenic than polymers of different types of amino acids. The presence of specific amino acids, such as glutamic acid, tyrosine, tryptophan, phenylalanine, cystine, and alanine, appears to increase the antigenic effect. In general, glycoproteins or lipoproteins are more immunogenic than pure proteins.

While the antigenicity of an antigen depends a great deal on its size as well as other factors, the specificity is determined by the presence of one or a few simple chemicals such as radicals, amino acids, simple sugars, and fatty acids. These simple but critical chemicals are known as antigenic determinants or epitopes.

Antigenic Determinants. Antigenic determinants were demonstrated by Landsteiner (1929), the father of immunohematology. Using isomers of tartaric acid (TA) as the haptenic components to produce antibodies in rabbits, Landsteiner clearly demonstrated the specificity and sensitivity of immunologic methods (Table 42–3). Anti-l-TA isomers reacted strongly with l-TA but very weakly with d-TA and m-TA. Anti-d-TA reacted strongly only with d-TA isomers, whereas anti-m-TA reacted strongly with m-TA isomers. The change of position between H and OH radicals attached to the second and third carbons was clearly reflected in the immunologic reactions.

The importance of amino acids as determinants for specificity was beautifully demonstrated for immunoglobulins. The fundamental chemical differences among certain allotypes have been worked out (see Chap. 36). For instance, if the amino acid at No. 153 and No. 191 positions of the kappa light peptide chain are alanine and valine, the specificity of this light chain would be Km(3+); if they are valine and leucine, it would be Km(3−). If the amino acid at No. 214 position of the IgG heavy chain is arginine, the specificity would be Glm(a+); if it is lysine, it would be Glm(a−).

The antigenic determinants of some erythrocyte antigens have also been identified recently. Owing to the difficulty of isolating antigens from the erythrocyte's membrane, most of the work has been done with soluble antigens that share the same specificity as those found on the erythrocytes. These soluble antigens are present in saliva, serum, urine, or other tissue fluids. A summary of these soluble antigens is listed in Table 42–4.

After extensive studies of secretions and RBC membrane extracts, the determinants for H, A, B, Le^a, Le^b, P_1, I, and i have been worked out and are summarized in Figure 42–

Table 42–3. SEROLOGIC SPECIFICITY OF ANTIBODIES AGAINST ISOMERS* OF TARTARIC ACID (TA)

Hapten	Antibodies Against Isomers of TA		
	l–TA	d–TA	m–TA
l–TA	+++	+/−	+/−
d–TA	−	+++	+/−
m–TA	+/−	−	+++

*l–TA = COOH–HOCH–HCOH–COOH; d–TA = COOH–HCOH–HOCH–COOH; m–TA = COOH–HCOH–HCOH–COOH

After Landsteiner (1929).

+ and +++ indicate strength of reaction. − indicates absence of reaction.

Table 42–4. DISTRIBUTION OF ERYTHROCYTE ANTIGENS

Antigens	Erythrocytes	Plasma	Secretions	Comments
A,B,H	+	+	+ (Secretors)	Tissues
Lewis	+	+	+	Kidney?
Sd^{a}	+	+	+	Urine
I,i	+	−,+	+	Milk
P	+	+	−	Hydatid cyst
Yk^{a},Cs^{a}*	+	+	−	
Rg^{a},Ch^{a}*	+	+	−	C4F,C4S
Bg^{a}*	+	+	−	HLA-B7
Bg^{b}*	+	+	−	HLA-B17
Bg^{c}*	+	+	−	HLA-A28
Others	+	−	−	

*Antibodies for these antigens often have high titer but weak reaction (low avidity), known as HTLA antibodies.

1. The precursor substance of these determinants consists of D-galactose, N-acetyl-D-glucosamine, another D-galactose, and D-glucose ceramide. With the addition of L-fucose to the precursor substance through the action of a fucosyltransferase, H substance is formed. Substance A is formed by the further addition of an N-acetyl-galactosamine, and B substance is formed by the addition of a D-galactose to the H substance through the appropriate transferases. Similarly, Le^{a} substance is formed by adding L-fucose to the subterminal sugar of the precursor substance, and Le^{b} substance is formed by adding L-fucose to both terminal and subterminal sugars. Likewise, D-galactose is added to the precursor substance to form P$_1$ substance, and D-galactose and N-acetyl-D-glucosamine are added to form i and I substances (with side chains). For details, reviews by Hakomori (1981) and Marcus (1981) should be consulted.

Since the transferases are under genetic control, the presence or absence of a specific transferase has been used to ascertain ABO subgroups. Experimentally, group B erythrocytes have been successfully converted into group O cells with the aid of alpha-galactosidase. The converted O cells have a normal survival time in group A, B, or O individuals and can tolerate the freeze-washing process (Lenny, 1982). The difference between group A and group B is a matter of one sugar, acetyl-galactosamine versus galactose. The presence of a deacetylase in certain lower gastrointestinal pathologies may render group A to appear like group B. This is one of the most attractive explanations for the formation of acquired B.

Chido and Rodgers antigens have been shown to be components of C4. All C4F (fast) individuals lacking the C4S (slow) bands were found to lack the Ch^{a} antigen, whereas all C4S individuals lacking the C4F band were negative for the Rg^{a} antigen. All C4FS individuals were Ch(a+), Rg(a+). Individuals who were negative for Rg^{a} and Ch^{a} were also deficient for C4. The agglutinability of C4-coated red cells in a saline system and the ability of most random serum to neutralize the reactivity of anti-Ch^{a} and anti-Rg^{a} have been used as an aid to the identification of these antibodies. This topic has been reviewed by O'Neill (1981).

The MNSs system presents an entirely different problem since no soluble antigens are available for such studies. Four different types of peptide chains—alpha, beta, gamma, and delta—have been isolated from red blood cell membranes and are known as sialoglycoproteins. The alpha chains (glycophorin A) probably contain the MN specificity and are absent in individuals of the En(a−) phenotype (=M−N−). The delta chains (glycophorin B) contain the Ss specificities and are absent in individuals of S-s-U+/- phenotypes. The determinants of M and N as well as T and Tn antigens have been worked out and are shown in Figure 42–2. The M antigen has more sialic acid than the N antigen. Also, the M antigen has serine and glycine instead of leucine and glutamine at positions 1 and 5 in the peptide portion. The presence of sialic acids as the determinants may explain why M and N antigens may be destroyed by the action of enzymes and why they sometimes cross-react. One can also readily understand why T and Tn are crypto-antigens that may be transiently exposed on human erythrocytes, platelets, and leukocytes by the action of bacterial or viral neuraminidase. Exposure *in vivo* of the T antigen on erythrocytes may be associated with a hemolytic process and occasionally, in infants, with thrombocytopenia and

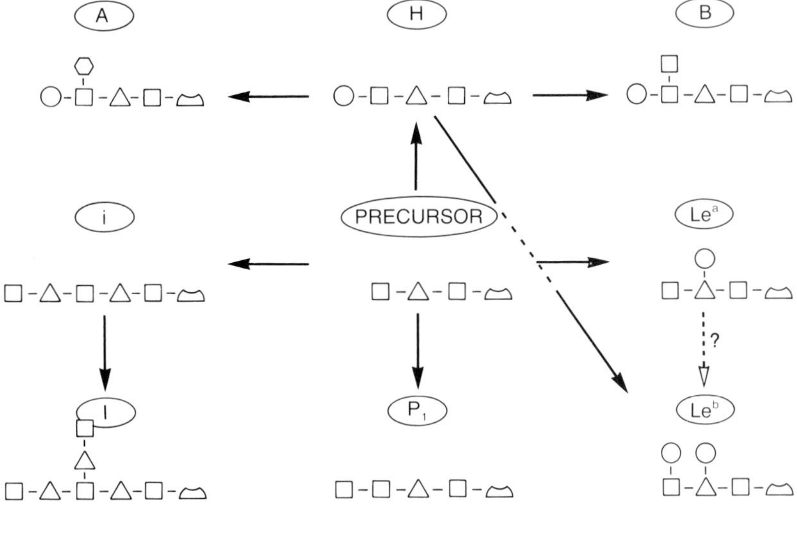

Figure 42–1. Some known erythrocyte antigenic determinants.

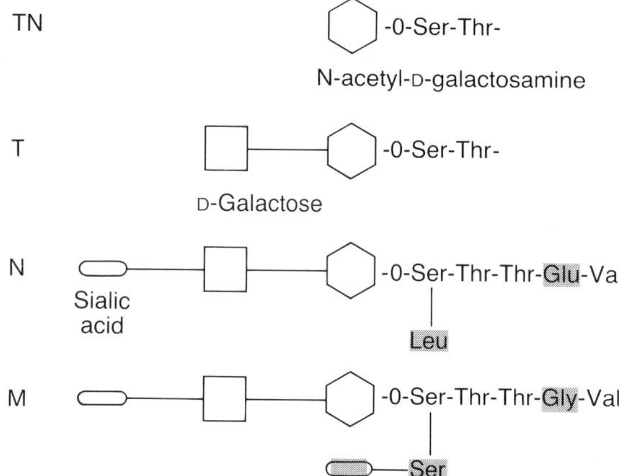

Figure 42–2. Determinants of Tn, T, M, and N antigens.

acute renal failure (Klein, 1977). These clinical manifestations have been attributed to the presence of the patients' own natural anti-T antibodies or to anti-T in the transfused blood. (The T antigen can be exposed on kidney tissue by neuraminidase.) In view of these findings, it is clearly important to transfuse washed cells to patients whose own cells are T exposed (Anstee, 1981).

While the determinants of the HLA antigens remain unknown, their chemical composition has been partly elucidated (Chap. 33). HLA-A, -B, and -C antigens, which are on virtually every human cell, consist of two peptide chains (glycoprotein): a large one about 44,000 MW, anchored in the cell membrane and a smaller one, about 12,000 MW (beta 2-microglobulin), attached in non-covalent association with the larger chain. HLA-D and -DR antigens, which are found chiefly on the surface of immunocompetent cells, consist also of two peptide chains of glycoprotein, MW 34,000 and 29,000, anchored in the cell membrane (Schwartz, 1982).

Ceramide is not the only lipid that has been shown to be an antigenic determinant related to immunohematology. Caprylate, an octanoic acid derivative, has been shown to be responsible for the so-called "albumin agglutination phenomenon," in which human antibodies agglutinate all human erythrocytes in the presence of bovine albumin. At first albumin was thought to be the responsible antigen; however, an additive used as a preservative for albumin, sodium caprylate, was found to be the determinant (McGinniss, 1972). Anticaprylate antibodies are uncommon but have been observed repeatedly among persons without any known stimulation.

GENETICS

The chemical structure of blood group antigens is determined by inheritance. Each antigen is governed by at least a pair of allelic genes, one from the father and the other from the mother. When the pair of genes is identical, it is known as a homozygote; when different, as a heterozygote. If only two alternate allelic genes (*P* and *Q*) are responsible for one pair of antigens, three types of zygotes are normally found, *P/P*, *Q/Q*, and *P/Q*; they are known as genotypes. Their corresponding phenotypes would be P+Q−, P−Q+, and P+Q+, which are identifiable serologically. Results of phenotyping a population can be used to predict the phenotypes of children in families. When such predictions are confirmed by actual observation, the allelic relationship of *P* and *Q* can be assumed and a blood group system can be assigned.

Population Studies. If a monospecific anti-P serum reacts with erythrocytes of 64 per cent of the population, in the absence of an anti-Q serum, one may assume that the remaining 36 per cent would have the frequency of homozygotes of genotype *Q/Q*. The frequency of *Q* (normally represented by q) would be $0.36^{1/2} = 0.6$. Its allelic gene frequency (normally represented by p) would be $1 - 0.6 = 0.4$, since $p + q = 1.0$. These two values may not be the true values, but they can be used as the working parameters to estimate the genotype frequencies:

Frequency of
P/P $= p \times p = 0.4 \times 0.4 = 0.16$ or 16%
Q/Q $= q \times q = 0.6 \times 0.6 = 0.36$ or 36%
P/Q $= 2pq = 2 \times 0.4 \times 0.6 = 0.48$ or 48%

Phenotype frequency of:
P+ $= p \times p + 2pq = 0.16 + 0.48 = 0.64$ or 64%
Q+ $= q \times q + 2pq = 0.36 + 0.48 = 0.84$ or 84%

Since only 50 per cent of the children of a heterozygote (*P/Q*) are expected to be P + or Q+, children of a P+ parent are expected to be:
P+ $= (0.16 \times 100\% + 0.48 \times 50\%)/(0.16 + 0.48) = 62.5\%$
P− $= 1 - 0.625 = 0.375$ or 37.5%

Similarly, children of a Q+ parent:
Q+ $= (0.36 \times 100\% + 0.48 \times 50\%)/(0.36 + 0.48) = 71.5\%$
Q− $= 1 - 0.715 = 0.285$ or 28.5%

Hence, phenotypes of children of different matings can be expected as follows:

MATING	CHILDREN EXPECTED	
	P−	P+
P− × P−	100%	0%
P− × P+	37.5%	62.5%
P+ × P+	0.375^2 = 14%	1 − 14% = 86%

MATING	CHILDREN EXPECTED	
	Q−	Q+
Q− × Q−	100%	0%
Q− × Q+	28.5%	71.5%
Q+ × Q+	0.285^2 = 8%	1 − 8% = 92%

Family Studies. All of the above values are estimates based on the assumption that *P* and *Q* are allelic genes. This assumption should be verified by studying the members of many families. Owing to sampling problems, the observed values are rarely the same as the expected values, but the validity can be evaluated statistically. If the values obtained from family studies are in agreement with predicted values, the gene frequency of 0.4 for the p and 0.6 for the q can be accepted. Then, one should check other gene frequency values close to 0.4 to 0.6 of known antigens and attempt to establish non-identity. A similar study should be done when and if anti-Q serum is found. Should values from anti-P and anti-Q be in agreement with what was expected, *P* and *Q* are likely to be allelic and can be assigned to one blood group system. This is, of course, an oversimplified procedure for the assignment of blood group antigens to one blood group system.

Based on the results of genetic studies of various erythrocyte antigens, Race and Sanger have assigned them into 21 major blood group systems and two groups for the so-called "public" and "private" antigens (Table 42–5). These systems, especially those of clinical importance, will be discussed subsequently under erythrocyte blood group systems.

Table 42–5. TIME AND RECOGNITION OF MAJOR HUMAN ERYTHROCYTE SYSTEMS AND ANTIGENS*

Time Recognized	Major Systems	Public Antigens	Private Antigens
1901	ABO		
1902–1925			
1926–1930	MN, P		
1931–1935	Se		
1936–1940	Rh		
1941–1945	Lu		
1946–1950	K, Fy		1
1951–1955	Jk, Le, Di	1	3
1956–1960	Yt	2	2
1961–1965	Au, Xg, Do, Sc, Cs	2	8
1966–1970	Co, Sd, Bg, Ch	6	7
1971–1975		2	7

*Adapted from Race (1975b).

Immune Response Relating to Blood Banking

Immune response is negligible in the unborn and is lacking in germ-free animals; therefore, it is considered developed only after antigenic stimulation. The term *naturally occurring antibodies* does not mean there has been no antigenic stimulation, but rather that it is not identified.

A human host may respond to three types of antigenic stimulation: (1) heterologous antigens, from other species such as microorganisms; (2) isologous antigens, from the same species such as blood components of other individuals; (3) autologous antigens, from the same individual, probably slightly modified by medication or viruses and no longer recognizable as one's own antigen.

Immune responses can be divided into two stages, the primary and the secondary. In primary immune response, the host is exposed to the antigen for the first time. It is usually detectable within 7 to 14 days or longer, and antibodies are of the IgM class in low titer. In the secondary immune response, the host is re-exposed to the same antigen. It is usually detectable within a week and antibodies are predominantly of the IgG class in high titer.

There are two major types of immune responses: the humoral immune response, the production of antibodies, and the cellular immune response, the formation of sensitized lymphocytes. Cells responsible for both types of immune response originate from the stem cells in the bone marrow, but they differentiate under the influence of two different types of lymphoid tissue into two populations of lymphocytes, known as B-lymphocytes or B cells and T-lymphocytes or T cells.

Macrophages are also known to be involved in immune response. Since all three types of cells have been extensively reviewed in Chapters 34 and 35, one table (Table 42–6) and one illustration (Fig. 42–3) are presented here for a brief review.

IMMUNOLOGIC TOLERANCE AND ENHANCEMENT

Although a host may be unresponsive to a normal antigen for many reasons, only three will be mentioned. First, a person may be a non-responder. It has been shown that about one third of Rh_0-negative women are believed to be non-responders and will not develop anti-D despite repeated immunization. Second, when a fetus is injected with a soluble or particulate antigen, the infant will not form antibodies against the specific antigen. Third, a similar type of immunologic tolerance can also be induced in adults. Using the same antigen, tolerance can be induced with a low dose or a high dose, while a very low dose or medium dose would sensitize the host. It is possible that with the high dose level, both the T and B cells are rendered unresponsive. The greater difficulty encountered in making B-lymphocytes tolerant might be related to the high density of surface receptors which require a large number of antigen molecules to become saturated. Cyclophosphamide, a cytotoxic agent for dividing B-lymphocytes, has been shown to facilitate the induction of tolerance. In general, soluble

Table 42–6. CHARACTERISTICS OF LYMPHOCYTES AND MACROPHAGES

Characteristics	T Lymphocyte	B Lymphocyte	Macrophage
Differentiation	Thymus	Bone marrow	Bone marrow
Immune response	Cellular	Humoral	Both
Distribution:			
Lymph node	Cortex	Germinal center	Sinuses
Lymph, thymus	85%	15%	+
Blood*	80–90%	5–10%	+
Spleen, tonsil	50%	50%	+
Bone marrow	25%	75%	+
Surface markers:			
SIg (IgM, IgD)	to 10^3	to 10^5	–
Fc receptor (IgG)	+/–	+	+ (not IgG 4)
C3b receptor	–	+	some
HLA-A, B, C	+	+	+
DRw	–	+	+
RBC receptor	Sheep	Mouse	
Sensitivity to:			
Concanavalin A	+	?	–
Lipopolysaccharides	–	+	–
X-ray	+	+ + + +	–
Corticosteroids	+	+ +	–
Anti-lymphocyte serum	+ + + +	+	±

*"Null" lymphocytes (5–10%): K (=killer) cells kill IgG coated target cells. Lymphocytes with labile IgG, rapidly lost in culture. Both with strong Fc receptor for IgG.

5

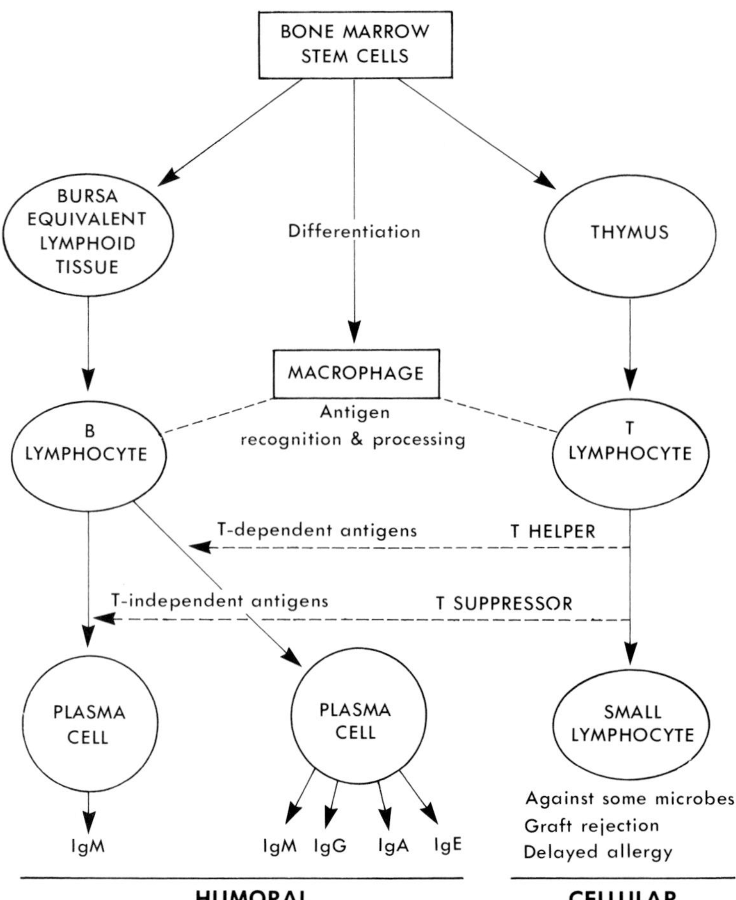

Figure 42–3. Interrelationship among different types of cells involved in humoral and cellular immune response. Bursa equivalent and thymus lymphoid tissues are responsible for the differentiation of stem cells into B and T cells, respectively. Macrophages may play a part in the recognition and processing of antigens, while the plasma cells and small lymphocytes are the effectors in the production of antibodies and in cellular response, respectively.

antigens are more effective in inducing tolerance than are particulate antigens; this may be related to the fact that the latter are readily taken up by macrophages and become more antigenic. Immunologic tolerance can be terminated by the injection of specific antibodies or closely reacting antigens.

Although vaccinations against infectious diseases have been very successful, vaccination against tumor cells often results in early death. This phenomenon is known as immunologic enhancement. Many theories have been proposed, but none has been generally accepted.

Blood Group Antibodies

IMMUNOGLOBULINS AND ANTIGEN BINDING SITES

All proteins with antibody activity and proteins having a structure similar to those of antibodies are designated as immunoglobulins (Ig). While Ig's are normal plasma components, antibody activity develops only in response to antigen stimulation. In order to understand antibodies, one must first be familiar with immunoglobulins, which are reviewed in Chapter 36. Information on immunoglobulins that is essential to blood banking is summarized in Tables 42–7, 42–8, and 42–9.

The specificity of an antibody is related to the hypervariable regions of an immunoglobulin. There are four hypervariable regions in heavy chains and three in light chains, as shown in Figure 36–1 (p. 861). The substitution of amino acids, a modification of the configuration of the peptide chains, or a combination of both determines the specificity of a particular antibody. It is believed that about 20 amino acids are actually in contact with antigens, while only one tetra-peptide may be responsible for the specificity known also as paratopes.

An isolated heavy chain from an antibody can bind the corresponding antigen but will do so less strongly than the original molecule. The isolated light chain binds far less well. A recombined light and heavy chain has a much greater affinity to the antigen than either of the isolated chains.

Since one basic 4-peptide unit of Ig contains 2 Fab portions, all untreated antibodies should be bivalent. The valence of polymers would be multiples of 2, such as $5 \times 2 = 10$ for an IgM antibody. Thus, there is no natural univalent antibody.

ALLOANTIBODIES

The possible presence of alloantibodies to erythrocytes demands the selection of compatible blood. This is the central issue of blood banking. Alloantibodies to erythrocytes can be (1) naturally occurring; i.e., the antigenic stimuli are unknown; (2) a result of immunization through transfusion; or (3) induced by fetal erythrocytes either during pregnancy or at the time of delivery.

Some naturally occurring antibodies appear regu-

Table 42–7. IMPORTANT PROPERTIES OF FIVE CLASSES OF HUMAN IMMUNOGLOBULIN (Ig)

Classes of Ig	IgG	IgM	IgA	IgD	IgE
Heavy chains	γ	μ	α	δ	ξ
Light chains	κ, λ	κ, λ	κ, λ	κ, λ	κ, λ
Special chains		J	J, Sc		
No. of 4-peptide units	1	5	1–3	1	1
CHO content (%)	3	12	8	13	12
Mol. wt. (monomer)	150,000	900,000	160,000	185,000	200,000
Sedimentation coefficient	7S	19S	7–11S	7S	8S
Inactivated by SH- or heat	+/−	++++	++		+++
Development in immune response	Late secondary	Early primary			
Half life *in vivo*	22 days	5 days	6 days	3 days	2.5 days
Concentration: mg/ml	8–16	0.5–2	1.4–4	0–0.4	Trace
(%)	(80)	(6)	(13)	(1)	
Distribution other than intravascular	Tissue fluids		Secretions		Secretions
Cross placenta	Yes	No	No	No	No
Induce agglutination	+	++++	++		
Fix complement pathway	Classic, alternate?	Classic	Alternate possible		Alternate possible

larly in persons who lack the corresponding antigen such as anti-A in group B, anti-B in group A, anti-A,B in group O, or anti-PP_1P^k in p persons. It is obvious that these antibodies are of utmost importance for safe blood transfusion therapy. One cannot and must not ignore the presence of these antibodies.

Naturally occurring antibodies may appear only in a certain percentage of the population who lack the respective antigen. For example, 5 to 20 per cent Le(a—b—) persons have anti-Le^a. Other incidences include: 3 per cent with anti-M^g, 2 per cent with anti-Vw, about 1 per cent with anti-Le^b or anti-Wr^a or anti-P_1, and about 0.1 per cent with anti-E, about 0.02 per cent with anti-M or anti-N or anti-S (Mollison, 1983). These groups of alloantibodies are usually of low titer with equivocal clinical significance.

Routine compatibility testing (the crossmatch) indicates that there is no detectable incompatibility and usually a match in terms of ABO and Rh_0(D) type specificity. Blood transfusion may introduce erythrocytes containing a number of antigens which the recipient lacks. Some of these antigens may be highly antigenic and may induce the production of specific antibodies in the recipient; the clinical significance of these antibodies varies. For a ready reference, Table 42–10 lists the Ig class, optimal reacting conditions, clinical implication, and the chance of finding compatible donors for each antibody. Additional comments can be found in the discussion of each blood group system subsequently.

Alloantibodies to leukocytes or platelets are reviewed elsewhere (pp. 708 and 754).

Table 42–8. SOME KNOWN PROPERTIES OF THE FOUR SUBCLASSES OF IMMUNOGLOBULIN G*

Subclasses of IgG	IgG1	IgG2	IgG3	IgG4
Heavy peptide chain	r1	r2	r3	r4
κ/λ ratio	2.4	1.1	1.4	8.0
Genetic markers	a, x, f, z	n	b0, b1, b3, b4 b5, c3, c5, g, s. t, u, v	4a, 4b
Half life *in vivo* in days	22	22	9	22
Relative serum concentration	64–70%	23–28%	4–7%	3–4%
Cross placenta	+	+/−	+	+
Fix complement	++	+	+++	+/−
Bind to macrophage	+++	++	+++	+/−
Combine with staph protein A	+++	+++	−	+++
Induce rosette	+		+++	
Cryoprecipitation	+	+/−	+++	+/−
Spontaneous aggregation	−	−	+++	−
Dominant antibodies	Immune anti-A, anti-Rh	Anti-dextrans	Anti-Rh	Anti-AHF

*Modified from Roitt (1974, p. 40).

5

Table 42–9. VARIANTS OF HUMAN IMMUNOGLOBULINS*

Designation	Meaning	Subvariants	Determinant Location	Examples
Isotypes	Present in all normal human individuals	Classes	C_H	IgG, IgM, IgA, IgD, IgE
		Subclasses	C_H	IgG1, IgG2, IgG3, IgG4, IgA1, IgA2
		Types	C_L	κ, λ
Allotypes	Genetic markers present in some individuals but not in others	IgG1	C_H	G1m(a), (x), (f), (z)
		IgG2	C_H	G2m(n), G2m(−n)
		IgG3	C_{H3}	G3m(b), (c), (g) . . .
		κ chain	C_L	Km(1), (2), (3)
Idiotypes	Specificity of each immunoglobulin		V_H or V_L	Determinant of individual myeloma protein

*Modified from Roitt (1980, p. 46).

AUTOANTIBODIES

The term *autoantibody* is used for any antibody that reacts with an antigen of the same subject producing the antibody. It also reacts often with the same antigen of other normal persons. Results from the reaction may induce hemolytic anemia, leukopenia, or thrombocytopenia, but frequently autoantibodies produce no demonstrable signs except laboratory findings. When proper reagents are used, the direct antiglobulin tests are often positive, while the indirect antiglobulin test may or may not be positive. Based upon the optimal reacting temperature, autoantibodies are classified into two general categories: cold (usually IgM) and warm (usually IgG). Among those autoantibodies producing anemias, about 15 per cent are of the cold variety and the remaining 85 per cent are of the warm variety. Autoantibodies to erythrocytes have been well studied and will be the next subject of discussion (Fig. 42–4). Autoimmune hemolytic anemia is reviewed in Chapter 29.

Cold Autoantibodies. The majority of cold autoantibodies are agglutinins and agglutinate erythrocytes strongly at 4°C., weakly at 24°C., and either very weakly or negatively at 37°C. Cold autoagglutinins can be detected in many normal persons; only a small percentage of them are associated with disease states. However, their clinical significance should not be neglected; cold autoagglutinins often interfere with proper typing and crossmatching. In some cases, it is difficult to establish their specificities; nevertheless, the following specificities can often be identified.

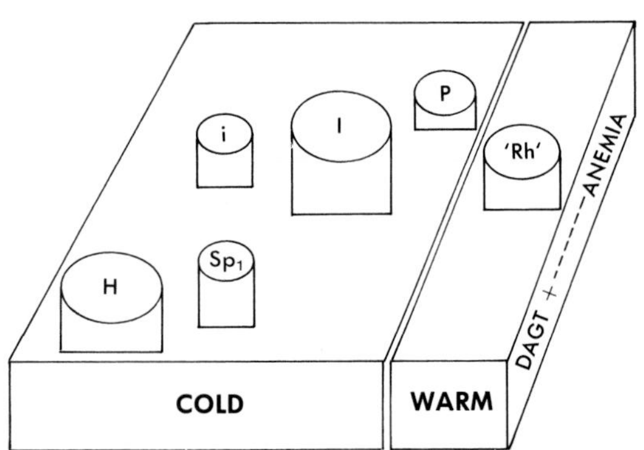

Figure 42–4. Specificity of common cold and warm autoagglutinins which can induce from only a positive direct antiglobulin test (DAGT) to severe anemia in patients. Specificity of autoantibody is indicated in i, I, P, H, Sp_1, and Rh (usually e). (Adapted from Mollison, 1983.)

Anti-H. Low titer anti-H can be demonstrated in many normal persons. These agglutinins clump group O or A_2 erythrocytes strongly but react weakly or negatively with A_1 or A_1B cells, and not at all with O_h cells. They can be neutralized by saliva containing H substance, the exception being the anti-H produced in an O_h individual. There is evidence to indicate that these agglutinins are not immunoglobulins but act very much like properdin, which is an important factor in the alternative pathway of complement activation (Mollison, 1983).

Anti-I. Anti-I is normally an IgM antibody. Those found in normal persons or in cord blood are of low titer and those associated with mycoplasma pneumonia infections are usually of high titer. Anti-I antibodies are separable from antibodies to mycoplasma pneumonia and cannot be absorbed out by mycoplasma pneumonia organisms. Anti-I antibodies react positively with erythrocytes that have I antigens but negatively with those containing only i antigens, including some cord cells. The antibody can sometimes be neutralized with fluids containing I substance, such as milk and saliva. Reactivity of anti-I may be enhanced in the presence of enzyme in the medium or by bovine albumin. The former is a useful criterion for distinguishing anti-I from anti-Sp_1, which is usually inactive after enzyme treatment. Anti-Sp_1 is a very rare antibody and is probably identical to anti-Pr_1 and Pr_2.

Anti-i. Anti-i is normally an IgM antibody but may be IgG or both. Anti-i is often associated with infectious mononucleosis or other types of reticulosis, with or without hemolytic anemia (low incidence). Anti-i antibodies are separable from antibodies specific for infectious mononucleosis.

Serologic differentiation of anti-H, anti-HI, auto anti-I, anti-i, and anti-Sp_1 is summarized in Table 42–11.

Table 42–10. SELECTED ERYTHROCYTE ALLOANTIBODIES:
Immunoglobulin class, optimal reaction phase, clinical implications, and chance of finding a compatible donor

	Immunoglobulin			Optimal Reaction				Hemolysis in			Compatible Donor*		
Anti-	*IgM*	*IgG*	*IgA*	*Sal*	*Alb*	*AGT*	*Enz*	*Vitro*	*Recipient*	*Newborn*	*Type*	*White (%)*	*Black (%)*
B	3	1	1	4				2	4	2	A,O	85	76
A_1	4			4							A_2,O	48	52
A	3	1	1	4				2	4	2	B,O	56	69
A,B	1	3		4				1	4		O	45	49
H†	4			4				3		0	O_h	Very rare	
I	3	1		3			3			0	I−	Very rare	
i	3	2	3							0			
P_1	3			3				1	2	0	P_1−	21	6
P		2	2										
PP_1P^k (Tj^a)	3	1		3				4	1	1		Very rare	
Le^a	3	1		3		2	3	2	1	0	Le(a−)	78	77
Le^b	4			4		3	3	1	1	0	Le(b−)	28	45
Lu^a	3	1		3				0		1	Lu(a−)	92	96
Lu^b	3	1	1	3				0	1		Lu(b−)	<0.1	<0.1
M	3	1		3		1	0	0	1	1	M−	22	30
N	3	1		3			0	0	0‡	0‡	N−	28	26
S	2	2		3		1		0	1	1	S−	45	69
s	1	3				3		0	2	1	s−	11	3
U		3				4		0	2	1	U−	None	1
D	1	3	1	1	3	3	3	0‡	3	4	D−	15	8
C	1	3		1	3	3	3	0	2	1	C−	30	68
DC	1	3		1	3	3	3	0	1	1	DC−	13	7
C^w	2	2		1	3	3	3	0	1	1	C^w−	99	100
c		3			3	3	3	0	2	2	c−	20	1
E	1	3		1	3	3	3	0	2	2	E−	70	98
e		3			3	3	3	0	1	1	e−	2	2
K	1	3		1		3	3	0	2	2	K−	91	97
k		4				3	3	0	1	1	k−	0.2	0.1
Kp^a		4				3	3	0	1	1	Kp(a−)	98	99.9
Kp^b		4				3	3	0	1	1	Kp(b−)	<0.1	0.1
Js^a		4				3	3	0	1	1	Js(a−)	>99.9	81
Js^b		4				3	3	0	1	1	Js(b−)	<0.1	1
Jk^a		4				3	3	0	1	1	Jk(a−)	23	9
Jk^b		4				3	3	0	1	1	Jk(b−)	28	57
Fy^a	1	4		1	3	3	1/0	0	1	1	Fy(a−)	34	90
Fy^b		4			3	3	1/0	0	1		Fy(b−)	17	77
Ch^a	3					3		0			Least incompatible		
Sd^a	3			3		2		0	1	0	Least incompatible		
Yt^a	2	2		3		2		0	1	?	Yt(a−)	<0.1	
Vel	3					3	2	2	0		Vel−	<0.1	
Wr^a	3			3				0	1	1	(Wr(a−)	>99.9	

4 = almost all 3 = most 2 = some 1 = few 0 = none

*Approximate values, mostly based on the frequencies in the AABB Technical Manual (1981).

†In Bombay individuals.

‡Only one case reported.

5

Anti-P. Anti-P has been observed primarily in patients with paroxysmal cold hemoglobinuria, a syndrome often associated with syphilis, mumps, or measles, and is known as the DL (Donath-Landsteiner) antibody. These antibodies are IgG and are capable of fixing complement on erythrocytes at 4°C. These complement-coated erythrocytes then hemolyze at 37°C.; hence, DL antibody is referred to as an autohemolysin or biphasic hemolysin.

Warm Autoantibodies. Patients with warm autoantibodies usually have a positive direct antiglobulin test (DAT) and a shortened red blood cell survival, although such patients may not have anemia. Warm autoantibodies can be primary or secondary. Primary means the etiology is unknown, while secondary is attributed to the presence of other disease conditions. With improvement in the diagnostic procedures, the ratio between primary and secondary has changed from 7:3 to 3:7. Since viruses and medications have been implicated in a number of cases of warm autoantibodies, a similar association may be expected in the remaining so-called "idiopathic" or "primary" warm autoantibodies. It should be remembered that not all hemolytic anemias are due to the presence of

Table 42–11. DIFFERENTIATION OF SPECIFIC COLD AGGLUTININS

Test Erythrocytes		Cold Agglutinins				
	Antigens					
Types	*H I i*	*Anti-H**	*Anti-HI*†	*Anti-I*‡	*Anti-i*§	*Anti-Sp_1*¶
A_1i	− − +	−	−	−	3+	3+
Oi	+ − +	3+	−	−	3+	3+
O_{cord}	+ − +	3+	−	+, −	3+	3+
OI	+ + −	3+	3+	3+	−	3+
A_2	+ + −	1+	2+	3+	−	3+
A_1I	− + −	−	−	3+	−	3+
O_h	− + −	−	−	3+	−	3+

*Neutralized by H substance.
†Neutralized by H substance only in rare types of anti-H-(-i).
‡Common in mycoplasma pneumoniae infection, some neutralized by I substance.
§Common in infectious mononucleosis and other forms of reticulosis.
¶? = Anti-Pr_1, Pr_2: receptors on RBC's are destroyed by proteases.

autoantibodies; alloantibodies and many other nonimmunologic factors can also be the cause (see Chap. 29).

The majority of warm autoantibodies (from 56 to 100 per cent in various reports) can be demonstrated with the direct antiglobulin test using anti-IgG serum, from 31 to 51 per cent by anti-complement serum as well, and from 11 to 45 per cent by anticomplement serum alone. Although a few examples are detected by anti-IgA alone or concurrently with anti-IgG or anti-complement, a few others are also positive with anti-IgM serum. The eluate from the erythrocytes and antibodies present in the serum of the same patient usually reacts best at 37°C. by the antiglobulin test. Those antibodies demonstrable with anti-IgG serum are either IgG1 or IgG3. IgG3 antibodies are often associated with overt hemolysis. Anti-complement serum containing anti-C3d has been found most useful.

Usually, the strength of the direct antiglobulin reaction shows no correlation with the degree of anemia. In many cases, the specificity of warm autoantibodies cannot be established. In some cases, autoantibodies may react selectively more strongly with cells that have certain Rh or LW antigens, especially hr″(e) antigens. According to their reactivity, autoantibodies have been designated as anti-nl, anti-pdl, and anti-dl. Anti-nl does not react with Rh deletions (Dc—,D—,DC^w—) or Rh_{null} cells; anti-pdl reacts with Rh deletion cells but not Rh_{null} cells, and anti-dl reacts with all cells (Wiener, 1963).

Although many investigators have evaluated this problem with different techniques, the clinical implication of their results remains uncertain. Although one usually tries to avoid transfusing patients with warm autoimmune hemolytic anemia, the use of the least incompatible blood for transfusion of these patients is being generally accepted; however, before such a decision is made, one *must exclude* the possibility of the concurrent presence of alloantibodies.

Autoantibodies against Leukocytes and Platelets. Both cold and warm autoantibodies against leukocytes and platelets are encountered and will be discussed elsewhere (p. 708 and p. 754). Cold lymphocytotoxins are quite common if one tests for them, especially with B-lymphocytes (Terasaki, 1978).

GLOBULINS ON ERYTHROCYTES INDUCED BY MEDICATION

Many drugs are known to induce a positive direct antiglobulin test (DAT) and can be classified into the following four categories (Fig. 42–5):

Autoantibodies on Erythrocytes. About 15 per cent of hypertensive patients who receive methyldopa (Aldomet) for three to six months or longer have been found to have a positive DAT and about 0.8 per cent of them to have hemolytic anemia. The positive DAT becomes negative gradually after the termination of methyldopa treatment; it may take from a few months to two years. Serologically, antibodies found on erythrocytes or in serum are indistinguishable from those autoantibodies found in patients with idiopathic autoimmune hemolytic anemia. Antibodies are usually

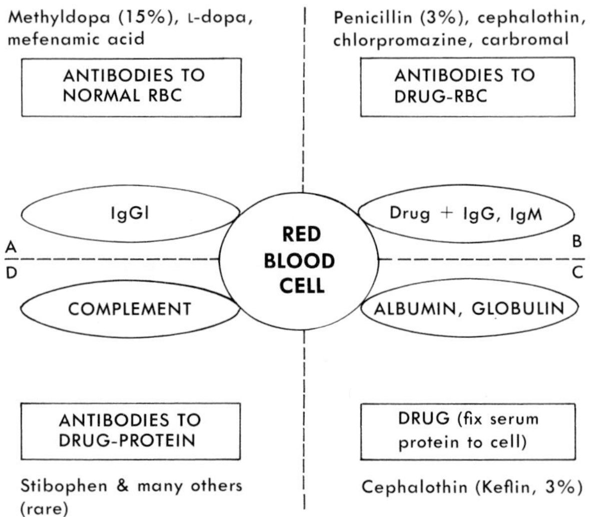

Figure 42–5. Four possible mechanisms for drug-induced positive direct antiglobulin test. Reactive agents on erythrocytes are in ovals; reactive agents in serum are in rectangles. Examples of drugs in each category are given.

of the IgG subclass with both kappa and lambda light chains and may have Rh or LW specificity. Although several hypotheses have been proposed for the development of these antibodies, none has been generally accepted. About 10 per cent of parkinsonian patients receiving L-dopa, closely related to methyldopa, develop a positive DAT, but there has been no report of overt hemolysis in these patients. Although several cases of autoimmune hemolytic anemia have been reported in patients receiving mefenamic acid, an analgesic, a positive DAT among patients taking this drug is uncommon.

Antibodies on Erythrocytes. About 3 per cent of those patients receiving large doses (for example, 10 million units daily for at least a week) of penicillin intravenously have been found to have a positive DAT, while only a few of them are found to have hemolytic anemia. The positive DAT disappears soon after the penicillin is stopped. Cephalothin (Keflin), carbromal, chlorpromazine, and methadone may behave like penicillin. These drugs bind firmly to the red blood cells and react chemically with certain protein groups to form haptenic determinants such as benzylpenicilloyl (BPO). Antibodies are formed against the BPO which are detectable on the erythrocytes and in the serum when penicillin-coated cells are used. Penicillin antibodies may be IgM or IgG. The IgM type may be very common if a very sensitive method is used for detection. This is likely due to exposure to penicillin in many foods. The IgG type may be associated with the IgM type or by itself. Penicillin antibodies usually do not fix complement; intravascular hemolysis has been seen but is rare. There is no evidence to indicate that IgG penicillin antibodies are associated with the allergic state to penicillin which a patient may have.

Serum Proteins on Erythrocytes. Cephalothin may also fix serum proteins (albumin, globulins including complement components) on erythrocytes non-immunologically. About 3 per cent of those patients receiving about 6 g/day are found to have a positive DAT. Only two cases of hemolytic anemia have been reported; these were probably due to direct attachment of cephalothin to erythrocytes and subsequent antibody production. Loridine (cephaloridine) as well as other drugs within the cephalothin family may react similarly. Antiglobulin sera of different specificity, including anti-albumin, can give a positive DAT. Anti-cephalothin (antibodies) in the serum can be detected with cephalothin-coated erythrocytes.

Complement Components on Erythrocytes. Many drugs can form a complex with serum proteins, and antibodies may develop against these drug-protein complexes. As a result of this antibody-drug-protein reaction, complement components, especially C3, are fixed to the erythrocytes through their C3b receptors. Only anti-C3 antiglobulin serum will detect this type of coating on erythrocytes. Antibodies in the serum can be detected only in the presence of the drug-protein complex. The following medications have been reported to give this type of reaction (all are very rare): acetaminophen, aminopyrine (Pyramidon), chloramphenicol, antihistamines, insecticides, dipyrone, insulin, isoniazid, melphalan, *p*-aminosalicylic acid, phenacetin, quinine, quinidine, rifampin, stibophene (Fuadin), sulfa drugs, sulfonylurea derivatives, methadone,* streptomycin,* and tetracycline.*

Many drugs have also been incriminated in cases of leukopenia or thrombocytopenia. There is no doubt that mechanisms similar to those for erythrocytes may be involved; however, tests are not yet available at the routine laboratory level.

LECTINS

Lectins are specific receptor proteins present in plants (usually their seeds), invertebrate animals (snails, crabs, etc.), and lower vertebrates (fish ova). Although many lectins have been reported (Bird, 1977), only several of them have been found useful in blood banking and are listed in Table 42–12.

The anti-H lectin of *Ulex europaeus* strongly agglutinates group O erythrocytes. It reacts weakly with A_2 cells and very weakly with A_1 or B cells. It is readily inhibited by H substance; some are inhibited by L-fucose and the others by N-acetyl-D-glucosamine. Since the potency of the lectin varies with the source of *Ulex europaeus,* each preparation should be standardized before use. Anti-H lectin is most useful in the study of secretors; saliva of a secretor contains H substances.

The anti-A_1 lectin of *Dolichos biflorus* agglutinates A_1 erythrocytes, an activity which can be inhibited by A substance of N-acetyl-D-galactosamine. Anti-A_1 lectin has been widely used to group A cells and to separate a minor population of A_1 cells from cells of other groups.

*Mechanism for these drugs is not yet certain.

5

Table 42–12. LECTINS USEFUL IN BLOOD BANKING

Lectin	Activity Inhibited by	Serological Specificity
Ulex europaeus	L-fucose N-acetyl-D-glucosamine	Anti-H
Lotus tetragonolobus	L-fucose	Anti-H
Vicia graminea	β-D-galactose	Anti-N
Arachis hypogaea	β-D-galactose	Anti-T, anti-Tk
Dolichos biflorus	α-N-acetyl-D-galactosamine	Anti-A, anti-Tn, anti-Cad
Salvia sclarea	α-N-acetyl-D-galactosamine	Anti-Tn
Salvia horminum	α-N-acetyl-D-galactosamine	Anti-Tn, anti-Cad(separable)
Bandeiraea simplicifolia	α-D-galactose (BS-I) N-acetyl-D-glucosamine (BS-II)	Anti-B Anti-Tk
Helix pomatia	α or β-N-acetyl-D-galactosamine	Anti-A, -TN, -Cad
Glycine soja	N-acetyl-D-galactosamine	Anti-T, -Tn, -Cad

The anti-N lectin of *Vicia graminea* agglutinates type N erythrocytes and its activity is inhibited by D-galactose. In addition to typing erythrocytes, anti-N lectin has been useful in elucidating the chemical composition of the M and N antigens.

The anti-T lectin of *Arachis hypogaea* (peanut), anti-Tn of *Salvia sclarea,* and the separable anti-Tn + anti-Cad lectin of *Salvia horminum* are very useful in the study of erythrocyte polyagglutination.

Recently, receptors for peanut agglutinin (PNA) have been demonstrated in lymphoblasts of acute lymphocytic leukemia children. Eight out of 12 patients having more than 15 per cent PNA-positive lymphoblasts had relapse, while none of 12 patients having less than 15 per cent PNA-positive lymphoblasts had relapse. (Levin et al., 1980).

MONOCLONAL ANTIBODIES

Monoclonal antibodies are synthesized by lymphocyte hybridomas. Hybridomas are produced by the fusion of antibody-producing cells from immunized animals and myeloma cells by the addition of polyethylene glycol. Some of the hybridoma cells can grow continuously in the selected culture medium and produce antibodies against the immunizing antigens. Each cell, which can produce only one type of antibody, can then be isolated and subcultured to produce a large amount of antibody of the same specificity. These hybridoma cells can also be maintained in a frozen state or reinjected into animals (usually mice) to produce ascites tumors with high concentrations of antibodies in the fluid. In other words, immortal cells from a single clone are available to produce antibodies against a specific antigen.

Monoclonal antibodies differ from conventional antibodies in three aspects: (1) Specificity: they react with one instead of multiple antigenic determinants. (2) Purity: all not just a fraction of the immunoglobulins are antibodies. (3) Reproducibility: the same specificity is expected from every subculture of a single clone.

Because of these unique properties, the following applications are expected: (1) A standard or reference antibody of each specificity will be available. (2) Antibodies against intact membranous antigens can be produced. Antibodies to differentiate the types of lymphocytes are already available and so are antibodies for some red and white blood cells, as well as hepatitis B surface antigens. Of course they are monospecific. (3) Antibodies against specific tumor antigens can and have been produced for *in vitro* specific diagnoses. When human hybridomas become practical, such antibodies can be used unlabeled or labeled with radioactive isotopes or cytotoxic agents to reach selectively the tumor cells. (4) The current labeling technology (radioactive isotopes, enzymes, ferritin, fluorochrome, latex particles, and others) can be greatly improved with the use of pure antibodies to reduce much of the background. (5) Monoclonal antibodies have been used to purify antigens. For instance, interferon has been concentrated 5000 times through the use of monoclonal anti-interferon antibodies.

Monoclonal antibodies to T lymphocytes, carcinoembryonic antigen, hepatitis B antigen, C3d, IgE, and prostatic acid phosphatase are available in the United States, and those to the A and B antigens of the ABO red blood cell system in England. An excellent review is found in Milstein (1980).

Complement and Blood Banking

Complement concerns blood bankers in two major areas: its involvement in the sensitization of erythrocytes, leukocytes, and platelets *in vivo* and its involvement in the detection of an antigen-antibody and related reactions *in vitro.* Since a detailed description of complement components, their detection and quantitation, and their changes in various diseases is presented in Chapter 37, only a brief outline of complement components that are pertinent to our two subjects will be presented.

ROLE OF COMPLEMENT IN THE DESTRUCTION OF ERYTHROCYTES IN VIVO

Antibodies against erythrocyte antigens, either allo- or auto-, are the most common causes for binding complement on erythrocytes *in vivo.* Complement may also be fixed on erythrocytes through an antigen-antibody reaction which may be only partly related to erythrocytes, such as antibodies against penicillin-erythrocyte complexes, or completely unrelated, such as antibodies to a chemical-protein complex. Leukocytes and platelets coated with antibodies may also fix complement but have not been well studied.

Intravascular Hemolysis. Intravascular hemolysis is the usual outcome of sensitization of erythrocytes with complement. Lysis of erythrocytes normally occurs through the classic pathway. Erythrocyte stromata which resemble the endotoxins may also initiate an activation through the alternative pathway, which may amplify the reactions of both pathways. This is typical for ABO incompatibility transfusion reactions. Other IgM antibodies, as well as some IgG antibodies (which are able to fix complement), can also induce an intravascular hemolysis.

Extravascular Hemolysis. Extravascular destruction of erythrocytes usually happens through phagocytosis. As shown in Table 42–13, macrophages, monocytes, and granulocytes all have receptors for C3b and C4b. Erythrocytes with bound complement can thus attach to these cells. Those erythrocytes coated with Ig can also attach to these cells through their Fc receptors. Erythrocytes immobilized by macrophages can be completely engulfed or partly engulfed or escape from phagocytosis with the help of serum C3bINA, which splits the C3b and frees the erythrocytes (Fig. 42–6). The incomplete erythrocytes that have escaped from partial phagocytosis may circulate again as spherocytes. Although phagocytosis is not entirely complement-dependent, Mollison (1983) has demonstrated that erythrocytes

Table 42–13. COMPLEMENT RECEPTORS ON HUMAN CELLS

Human Cells	Complement Receptors	
	C3b, C4b	***C3d***
Macrophages/monocytes	+	–?
Granulocytes	+	–
Erythrocytes	+	–
B lymphocytes	+	+

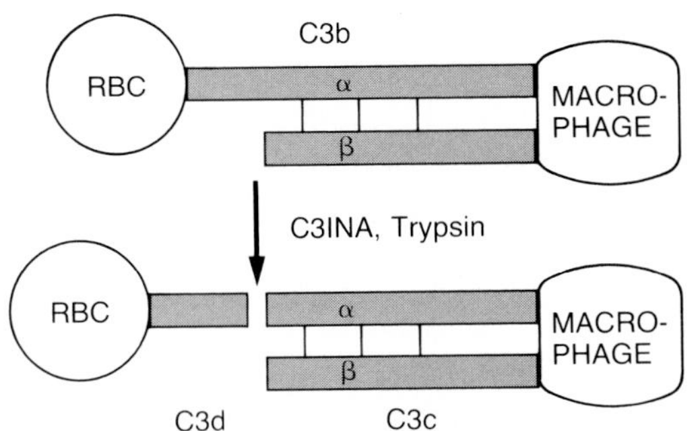

Figure 42–6. When C3 is activated, C3a and C3b are formed. C3b has RBC receptor on one end and macrophage receptor on the other side to facilitate erythrophagocytosis. When C3b is activated by C3INA *in vivo* or trypsin *in vitro*, C3c and C3d are formed. C3d remains on the RBC which can be detected by anti-C3d.

coated with antibodies and complement tend to be destroyed in the liver within a short time, whereas those coated only with antibodies tend to be destroyed more slowly in the spleen. It is generally believed that in the presence of complement, phagocytic activity is enhanced.

The presence of receptors for C3b and C3d on B-lymphocytes and for C3b on other kinds of leukocytes may indicate that complement also plays an important role in the fate of leukocytes.

ROLE OF COMPLEMENT IN BLOOD BANKING TEST PROCEDURES

Hemolysins. To demonstrate the presence of immune anti-A or anti-B or the so-called Donath-Landsteiner antibody (anti-P, IgG, fixes complement at 4°C. and lyses the erythrocytes at 37°C.), complement is required. The blood specimen for these tests should not be drawn in tubes containing citrate or EDTA, or be inactivated at 56°C. for 30 minutes. The tests should be done with a fresh specimen. Complement is relatively unstable and deteriorates on storage. More than 50 per cent of its activity is lost in one day at 37°C., in two days at room temperature, or in three weeks at 4°C.; more than 90 per cent activity remains after four weeks at −20°C. and after 12 weeks at −55°C. (Garratty, 1970.)

Detection of Autoantibodies. There is no question about the value of complement in the study of autoantibodies. A certain percentage of autoantibodies can be detected only by anti-C antiglobulin serum; other portions can be detected by anti-C and anti-IgG, and the remaining by IgG only. However, the pattern of direct antiglobulin reaction in general has diagnostic value only in a negative sense; a positive reaction with anti-C is usually not found in patients treated with methyldopa, while a negative reaction is in general against the diagnosis of systemic lupus erythematosus. Various reports have also shown that anti-C3d is the most important component for this purpose. The use of anti-C4d has not been helpful in detecting additional antibodies, but it may pick up some non-specific coating from cold agglutinins after the blood specimen has been drawn from the patient. It is recommended that to detect a true *in vivo* coating of Ig and complement, the blood specimen should be drawn in EDTA tubes to avoid *in vitro* coating. Although so-called broad-spectrum antiglobulin serum, which has an undefined content, is suitable for routine purposes, it should not be used for critical investigative studies.

Detection of Alloantibodies. The role of complement has not been uniformly agreed upon. Few well-documented alloantibodies have been detected with only anti-C serum where other techniques without the use of complement failed to do so. On the other hand, all antibodies detectable in serum could also be detected in citrate and EDTA plasma (Myhre, 1972; Kitagawa, 1978) with equal or higher scores.

In typing erythrocytes, the strength of the antiserum is known and its specificity is defined by recommended techniques. The use of anti-C serum in this test system is superfluous and is generally not recommended, since it may detect some undesirable antigen-antibody reactions. The value of complement in crossmatching has not been generally agreed upon.

HLA Typing. Complement is required for lymphocytoxicity testing and for complement fixation tests using platelets. Recent demonstration of receptors for C4, factor B on lymphocyte membranes and of the syntenic location of genes for C2, C4, and factor B with the HLA loci is most interesting (Chap. 33).

Hepatitis Testing. Complement fixation has been used in a number of laboratories for studying hepatitis, while the immune adherence test is currently being used in some laboratories for testing HAsAg.

Immunologic Reactions Involving Erythrocytes

Hemagglutination, hemagglutination inhibition, and hemolysis, which are the observed phenomena and main concerns of routine blood bank personnel, will be discussed here and the remaining immunologic reactions will be reviewed under each appropriate subject.

FACTORS AFFECTING HEMAGGLUTINATION

Specific hemagglutination is the single most important reaction in blood banking. There are four groups of factors that can influence the outcome of the reaction: These include (1) the erythrocyte, (2) the serum, (3) the medium, and (4) the physical conditions under which the reaction takes place.

Erythrocytes. The importance of the type, number, and location of antigens on the erythrocytes is illustrated by the ABO and Rh antigens. The number of ABO sites may be close to one million per cell, and they are considered to be extramembranous; thus, erythrocytes are easily agglutinated with the appropriate antibodies. On the other hand, the Rh antigens have only about 10,000 to 30,000 sites per cell and are considered to be intramembranous; thus, they are less easily agglutinated by the appropriate antibodies.

Antibodies. IgG class antibodies often require antiglobulin serum for their demonstration, while IgM antibodies do not. The presence of complement may be required for some reactions. A high concentration of serum globulin or fibrinogen may create rouleaux formation.

Medium. Low pH and low ionic strength medium, such as acidified glucose, accelerate the binding of antibodies onto red blood cells. After 10 years, there has been a resurgence of interest in low ionic strength salt solution (LISS) in antibody screening and crossmatching (Hughes-Jones, 1964; Löw, 1974). Various enzymes, as well as macromolecules, are also used to enhance agglutination.

Physical Conditions. Physical conditions, such as the incubation temperature and time, as well as the duration and speed of centrifugation, markedly affect the agglutination reaction.

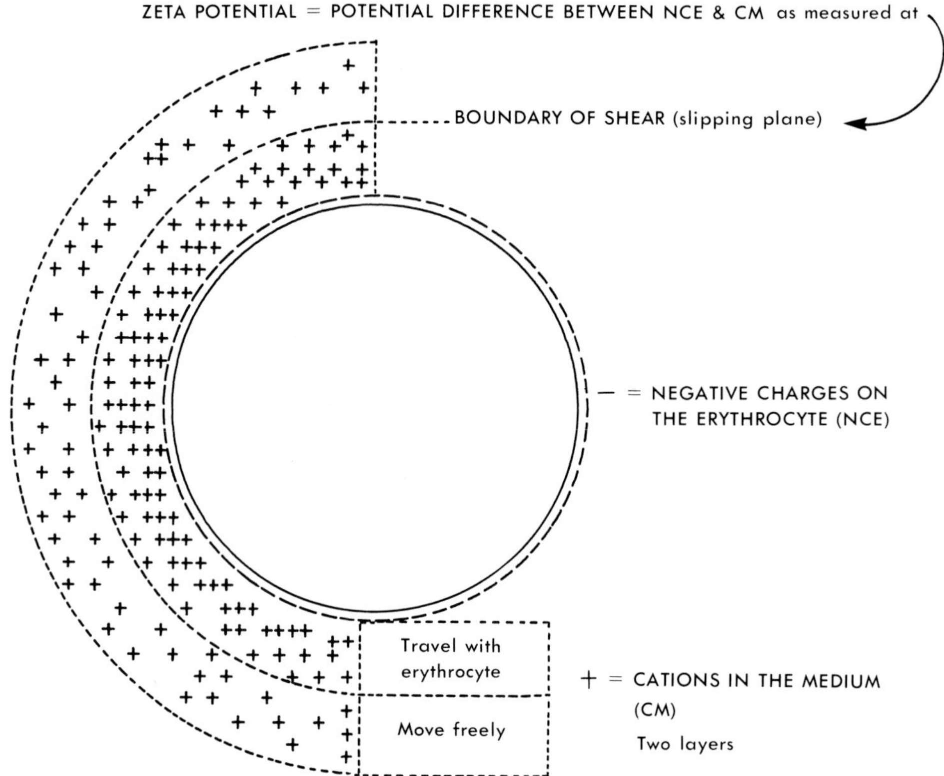

Figure 42–7. Diagrammatic presentation on the measurement of zeta potential of erythrocytes.

The above-mentioned factors may influence hemagglutination through their effect on a basic property of erythrocytes, the presence of negative charges on their surface.

Negative Charges. Under normal conditions, erythrocytes remain apart at a distance of approximately 25 nm. This is attributed to the repelling force of negative charges that are present on the surface of the erythrocyte. The presence of these negative charges can be demonstrated by placing the red blood cells in an electrical field and observing their migration toward the positive pole. This migration can be abolished if the cells are treated with certain enzymes capable of degrading sialic acid. Thus, the negative charges on the erythrocyte can be attributed to sialic acid content.

Zeta Potential. The degree of negative charge on an erythrocyte has been expressed by "zeta potential," a term meaning the potential difference between the negative charges on erythrocytes and the cations in the medium. Cations in the medium can be divided into two groups, those which attach firmly to erythrocytes and move together with the erythrocytes and those which move freely in the medium. The boundary between these two layers of cations is known as "boundary of shear" or "slipping plane." It is at this point that the zeta potential is determined and expressed in −mV (Fig. 42–7). The optimal range for IgM antibodies is −22 to −17mV, and for IgG, −11 to −4.5mV. The smaller the absolute values of zeta potential, the shorter the distance between the two erythrocytes (Pollack, 1970).

INDUCING HEMAGGLUTINATION

Hemagglutination can be induced in two ways, either by reducing the distance between the erythrocytes or by providing bridges between two short antibodies (Fig. 42–8). In terms of the former, treatment of erythrocytes with enzymes such as neuraminidase, trypsin, papain, bromelin, or ficin irreversibly reduces the sialic acid content and lowers the zeta potential values. Thus, treated cells are readily agglutinated by appropriate antibodies. Since sialic acid is known to be one of the determinants for M and N antigens, enzyme treatment of these cells may destroy these antigens.

The exact mechanism of albumin enhancement in the reaction of certain antibodies is not yet known. One theory is that albumin behaves like electric condensors and has its positive charges neutralizing the negative charges on erythrocytes.

Polybrene and protamine, which are used in AutoAnalyzer systems (Technicon Corporation), provide an excess number of cations which neutralize the negative charges on the erythrocyte and produce non-specific aggregates. Short specific antibodies would then have the chance to touch more than one cell and produce specific agglutination. The addition of certain electrolytes, which counteract the effect of polybrene or protamine, would disperse the non-specific aggregates but not the specific aggregates. In this way, it is possible to detect and identify either the specific antigens or antibodies.

Centrifugation forces the erythrocytes to come closer together and facilitates hemagglutination.

In terms of inducing hemagglutination by providing bridges between antibodies (Fig. 42–8). IgM antibodies with dimensions greater than 35 nm are able to reach more than one erythrocyte to form aggregates and are known as "complete" antibodies.

IgG antibodies with dimensions usually less than 25 nm can agglutinate only those red blood cells having intracel-

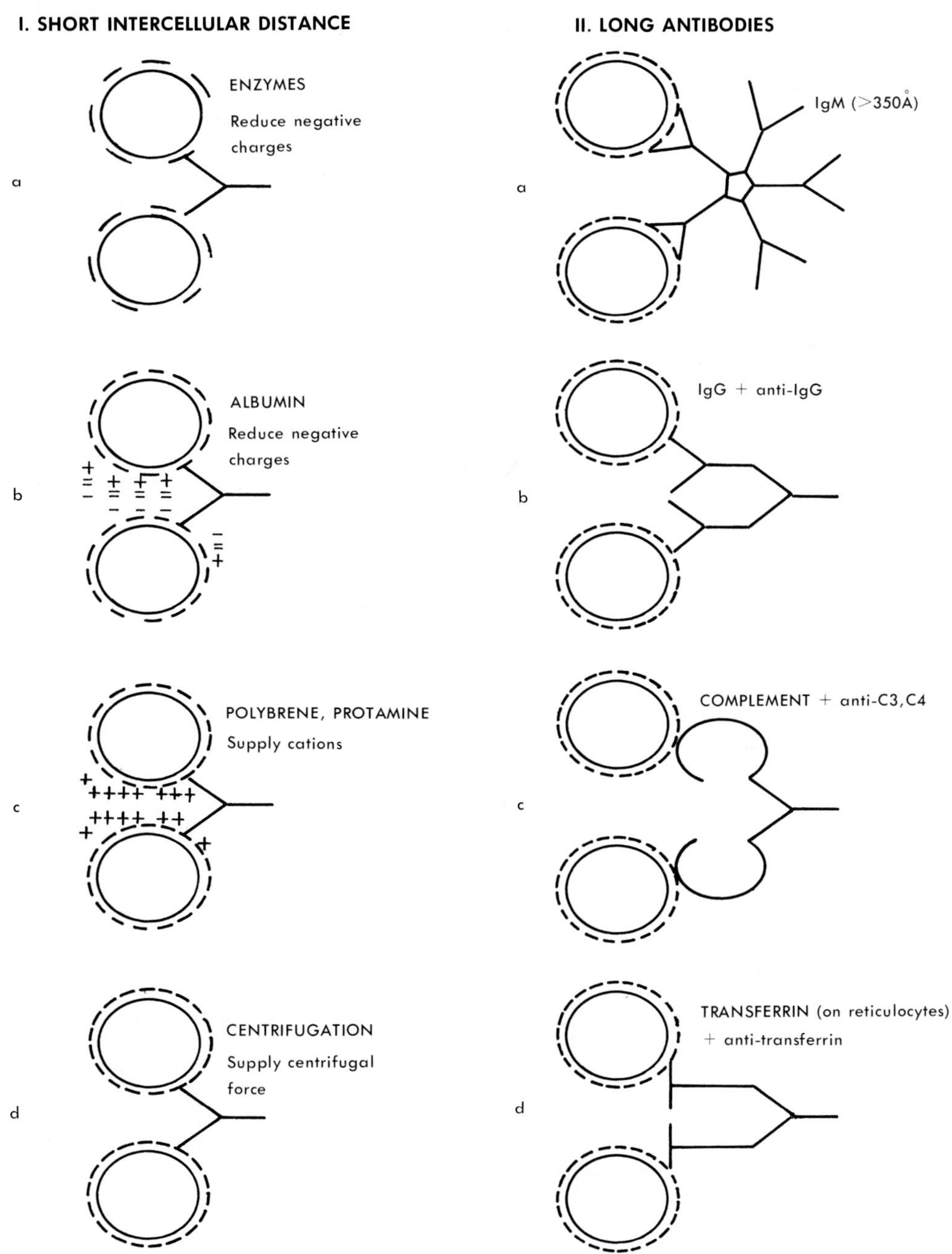

Figure 42–8. Two basic mechanisms of inducing hemagglutination.

5

lular distances of less than 25 nm. This may be achieved by any of the previously mentioned factors. Anti-human globulin or anti-complement antibodies may serve as bridges between those antibodies or complement components already attached to individual erythrocytes.

Reticulocytes retain transferrin on their surface in order to transport iron compounds into the erythrocytes to form additional hemoglobin. If the antiglobulin serum also contains anti-transferrin, these antibodies would also serve as bridges to form aggregates of reticulocytes. This reaction may lead to false-positive antiglobulin tests in cases with high reticulocyte counts. However, this is unlikely at the present time owing to improvement in the specificity of anti-human globulin serum.

Non-immune Aggregates. In addition to the non-specific aggregates formed by polybrene and protamine, many other chemicals may induce hemagglutination. A common phenomenon in blood banks is rouleaux formation. Rouleaux are usually induced by a high concentration of dextran, PVP, fibrinogen, or globulin and can be differentiated from true agglutination, either by microscopic appearance or by dispersion upon the replacement of serum with saline.

Non-specific aggregates induced by a high concentration of dextrose have been useful in deglycerolyzing frozen red blood cells.

A third type of non-specific agglutination may be found in cord blood contaminated by Wharton's jelly. The presence of hyaluronic acid, together with albumin, has been shown to be responsible and is usually solved by the addition of hyaluronidase.

In conclusion, in any attempt to use hemagglutination reactions to detect antigens or antibodies, appropriate controls must be used to assure the specificity of the reaction.

HEMAGGLUTINATION INHIBITION

This reaction is used to detect the presence of soluble antigens such as ABH, Le^a, I, P, Sd^a, and Ch^a in saliva, serum, or other fluids. The use of soluble antigen to neutralize a specific antibody for its identification is in fact a two-stage hemagglutination inhibition. These soluble antigens share the same antigenic specificity as found on the erythrocytes and are capable of neutralizing the corresponding antibodies in the serum. The neutralized serum will then no longer agglutinate the erythrocytes. Consequently, the absence of agglutination in hemagglutination inhibition indicates a positive test and signifies the presence of a specific antigen in the fluid tested. The strength of the antibody used in the test must be adjusted to give not more than a 2+ reaction with the indicator cells. The concentration of the soluble antigen can be determined by titration. Examples are the use of saliva in determining the secretor status and plasma for Gm typing.

HEMOLYSIS

This is also a very useful reaction in blood banking. It indicates the presence of immune anti-A or anti-B in reverse serum grouping and helps to identify certain antibodies such as anti-P_1, anti-P, anti-PP_1P^k, anti-Jk^a, anti-Le^a, and, sometimes, anti-Le^b and anti-Vel. It may help to exclude Rh antibodies which are generally non-hemolytic. When a 50 per cent end point is used, hemolysis can quantitate soluble A substance with great accuracy. Since complement is required for this reaction, inactivated serum or plasma cannot be used for this purpose. Incubation at 37°C. facilitates this reaction. Precautions must be taken to avoid hemolysis due to non-immunologic factors such as water or chemicals.

ERYTHROCYTE ANTIGENS AND ANTIBODIES

The ABO System

SPECIAL CHARACTERISTICS

The ABO system has two unique features which are not found in any other blood group system (Table 42–14): (1) the usual presence of strongly reactive agglutinins in the serum of those who lack the corresponding antigen(s), and (2) the regular presence of ABH antigens on many tissue cells and ABH substances in the secretions of secretors. These two unique characteristics make the ABO system by far the most important blood group system in blood transfusion and organ transplantation.

The regular presence of strong anti-A and/or anti-B (antibodies) in the serum renders the demonstration of A and B antigens on erythrocytes a much easier task. This may be the reason that ABO was the first blood group system to be discovered. It is the only blood group system in which examination of the serum (reverse grouping) can be used reliably to confirm the results of forward grouping of erythrocytes.

ANTIBODIES AND AGGLUTININS (Table 42–15)

Human antibodies are readily available, although those from animals and agglutinins from plants are also used in the study of ABO antigens. Human antibodies can roughly be divided into two categories: "natural" and "immune." Both types are the result of immunization. The immunogens of the *"natural" type* are probably bacterial in origin, as some bacteria share A or B antigens. This is demonstrated by the fact that anti-A or anti-B antibodies, if any, are of low titer in infants and expected agglutinins are absent in germ-free animals. "Natural" anti-A or anti-B is usually of the IgM class and is readily neutralized by soluble A or B group substances. "Natural anti-A,B"

Table 42–14. TWO PREDICTABLE SPECIAL FEATURES OF THE ABO SYSTEM

Blood Group	Agglutinins in Serum	Antigens on Certain Tissue Cells (Soluble Substances in Secretors)
O	Anti-A, anti-B	H(O)
A	Anti-B	H, A
B	Anti-A	H, B
AB	None	H, A, B

Table 42–15. ABO ANTIBODIES AND AGGLUTININS

	Serum			
Specificity	***Group***	***Incidence***	***Characteristics***	***Other Sources***
Anti-B	A	All	Usually IgM Titer 1:8-512 Average 1:64	Colostrum (IgA) Salica (IgA) Tears Ascitic fluid Anti-A also found in snails and fish roe
Anti-A,B	O, O_h	All	Usually IgG Reacts with A_x, A_3	
Anti-A	B	All	Usually IgM Titer 1:32-2048 Average 1:256	
Anti-A_1	A_2B A_2 A_x	22-35% 1-8% Most	Few transfusion reactions reported	Anti-A absorbed with A_2 cells *Dolichos biflorus*
Anti-H	O_h Not O_h	All Some	Inhibited by H substance	*Ulex europaeus,* eel, immunized chicken

in group O persons is usually of the IgG class and less readily neutralized by A and B substances.

When group O (anti-A,B) serum is absorbed with group A or B cells, the eluate from such cells usually contains anti-A and anti-B. In addition, group O serum often reacts with subgroups of A (A_x) which may be non-reactive with anti-A. Several theories have been proposed to explain these findings, but none has been generally accepted.

Immune anti-A or anti-B is of the IgG class and is usually the result of immunization through fetal-maternal hemorrhage. Likewise, injection of A or B blood group substances for reagent antiserum production usually results in high titers of immune anti-A or anti-B.

Anti-A_1 reacts with A_1 cells but not with A_2 cells. The antibodies can be derived from human anti-A serum absorbed with A_2 cells or from persons of group A_2B,A_2, or A_x who have anti-A_1 in their sera; however, such anti-A_1 (antibodies) are usually weak and unsuitable for reagent purposes. Anti-A_1 (lectin) properly prepared from *Dolichos biflorus* is a very useful reagent for grouping purposes. Transfusion reactions have been reported on occasion in patients whose blood plasma contained anti-A_1 while receiving A_1 erythrocytes (Mollison, 1983).

Anti-H strongly agglutinates O cells; however, the reactions are weaker with A_2 or A_3 cells, and weakest or negligible with A_1 or A_1B cells. This antibody can usually be neutralized by H substance. The anti-H found in the serum of persons with the O_h (Bombay) phenotype normally agglutinates and sometimes hemolyzes O cells, while that found in non-O_h persons is usually weak and non-hemolytic.

Anti-H prepared from *Ulex europaeus* provides an excellent reagent for determining secretor status and detecting H antigens on certain tissue cells. This lectin is stronger than human anti-H, and it will react with A or B cells; however, this reagent is usually diluted so that it is non-reactive with A_1 cells.

COMMON ABO ANTIGENS

Although many variants of ABO antigens have been described, only A_1, A_2, and B are of practical importance; A_3, A_m, A_x, B_3, and O_h are seen occasionally, while other subgroups are very rare. Only the first two categories are listed in Table 42–16 and will be reviewed.

Genetics. The ABO system is controlled by at least three sets of genes: *H* and *h;* A_1, A_2,*B,* and *O;* and *Se* and *se.* Each set is independent of the others and it can be assumed that each has its own locus. Only the ABO locus has been shown to be on chromosome No. 9 (Westerveld, 1976); the two others remain unassigned.

The product of the H gene is fucosyltransferase, which converts the precursor substance to H substance (Figs. 42–1 and 42–9). In the absence of *H* gene (designated as *hh*), the precursor substance remains unconverted and O_h or Bombay type results. In this case, despite the presence of ABO genes, A or B antigen will not be formed because H substance, the precursor of the A and B antigens, is absent.

There are at least two forms of ABH antigens: soluble glycoproteins found in secretions and plasma and structural lipoproteins which are part of the erythrocyte membrane as well as some epithelial and endothelial cells. Both forms have the same specificity with respect to their reactions with anti-A, anti-B, or anti-H. Soluble ABH antigens can be demonstrated in the secretions of about 80 per cent of the population; these individuals are known as secretors. The secretor status is controlled by a pair of genes *Se* and *se.* In the absence of the *Se* gene (se/se), ABH antigens are not present in the secretions, and these individuals are known as non-secretors (Fig. 42–9).

Since ABH and Lewis antigens share a common precursor (see Fig. 42–1), it is not surprising that the Lewis gene *(Le, le)* is related to the production of ABH antigens. ABH secretors are found to be Le(a−b+) or Le(a−b−), while ABH non-secretors are Le(a+b−) or Le(a−b−) (Table 42–17). In the absence of the H gene, Le^b antigen or substance cannot be formed. This hypothesis is supported by the fact that Le(a−b+) has never been found in a Bombay phenotype (O_h).

Development. Although ABH antigens can be detected on erythrocytes in a six-week-old fetus, they

Table 42–16. DIFFERENTIATION OF COMMON ABO GROUPS

	Erythrocytes + Anti-					Serum + Erythrocytes				Eluate	Substance in Saliva
Phenotype	***A***	***A_1***	***B***	***A,B***	***H***	***A_1***	***A_2***	***B***	***O***	**Anti‡**	**of Secretor**
A_1	4+	4+	–	4+	–	–	–	4+	–	A	H,A
A_{Int}	4+	2+	–	4+	2+	–	–	4+	–	A	H,A
A_2	4+	–	–	4+	2+	†	–	4+	–	A	H,A
A_3	2+*	–	–	2+*	3+	†	–	4+	–	A	H,A
A_m	–/+	–	–	–/+	4+	–	–	4+	–	A	H,A
A_x	–/+	–		1–2+	4+	1+ (Usually)	–	4+	–	A	H
B_1	–		4+	4+	4+	4+		–	–	B	H,B
B_3	–		2+*	2+*	4+	4+		–	–	B	H,B
O	–		–	–	4+	4+	4+	4+	–	H	H
O_h	–		–	–	–	4+	4+	4+	4+	–	–

*Minor population of agglutinates.
†May have anti-A_1.
‡Eluate from cells sensitized with anti-A, anti-B, or anti-H should have the specificity of anti-A, anti-B, or anti-H, respectively.

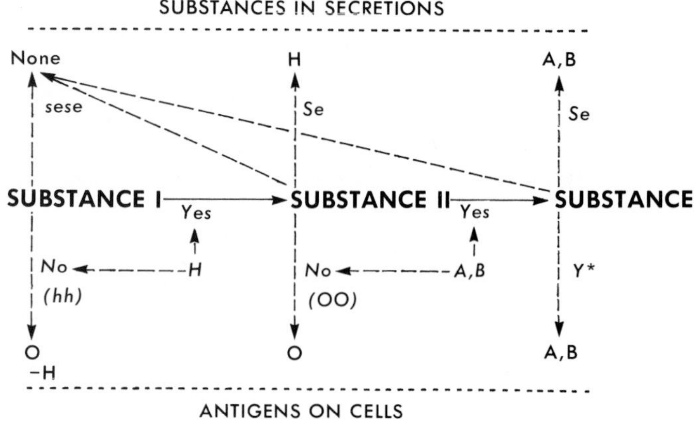

Figure 42–9. Possible genetic pathways in the biosynthesis of ABO antigens and ABH substances. *In the absence of a Y gene, one may have A substance in secretions but no A antigens on erythrocytes.

Table 42–17. ABO SECRETORS AND LEWIS PHENOTYPES

Secretion Status	Secretor		Non-Secretor	
Frequency	80%		20%	
ABH substance	Present		Absent	
Controlling gene	Se		sese	
Lewis gene	Le	lele	Le	lele
Lewis substance	Le^b + Le^a	None	Le^a	None
Lewis phenotype Le	a–b+	a–b–	a+b–	a–b–

Table 42–18. ROUTINE ABO GROUPING OF ERYTHROCYTES

Cells Against Serum with		Serum Against Cells of Group				Frequency (%) in Major U.S. Population*			
Anti-A	*Anti-B*	*A*	*B*	*O*	Interpretation	*Whites*	*Blacks*	*American Indians*	*Orientals*
−	−	+	+	−	O	45	49	79	40
+	−	−	+	−	A	40	27	16	28
−	+	+	−	−	B	11	20	4	27
+	+	−	−	−	AB	4	4	<1	5

*Composite figures, calculated from Mourant, 1976.

are not fully expressed until a child is 6 to 18 months old. An infant who initially was typed as A_2 may later type as A_1.

Distribution. ABH antigens have been found not only in bacteria but also in some animals. Pig A^P cells have been used to differentiate "immune" and "natural" anti-A; only immune anti-A agglutinins are readily absorbed by A^P cells.

In addition to saliva, ABH substances can also be found in secretions of the upper gastrointestinal tract, ovarian cyst fluid, seminal fluid, and amniotic fluid. With the specific red cell adherence technique, ABH antigens can be found on some epithelial cells as well as on all blood vessel endothelium. The presence of ABH antigens on white blood cells (Gurner, 1958) and platelets (Coombs, 1955) has been reported, but controversy exists in this matter.

ABO GROUPING

Routine ABO grouping (Table 42–18): Minimum titers of 1:256 are required for anti-A and anti-B reagents used for the forward grouping (cell grouping.) Anti-A,B from a group O person is a useful reagent for detecting subgroups of A or B. When a differentiation of A_1 and A_2 is required, anti-A_1 is used (Tables 42–16 and 42–19). Meticulous adherence to manufacturers' directions for use of all reagents is essential for accurate and reproducible results. Further discussion of testing for erythrocyte antigens and antibodies is presented subsequently (p. 1002).

In the reverse grouping (serum grouping) cells of groups A_1, B and O are normally used. O cells serve as a control for unexpected antibodies. A_2 cells should be used when one suspects the presence of anti-A_1.

Interpretation of ABO grouping results is usually straightforward. Table 42–16 lists the major characteristics. The observation of a minor population of agglutinates (also known as mixed field) to identify A_3 is very helpful. The ability of test cells to adsorb anti-A or anti-B, as well as secretor status studies, may be of great help in the identification of A_m or A_x (Table 42–16). If feasible, the demonstration of acetyl-galactosaminyltransferase, galactosyltransferase, or fucosyltransferase is useful in confirming the presence of *A, B,* and *H* genes, respectively.

Some Discrepancies in ABO Grouping

1. Unexpected/additional reactions in cell grouping: (a) Cells modified by bacterial enzymes such as those found in patients with acquired B. (b) Abnormal inheritance such as Cis-AB. (In both cases, the cells appear to be group AB with an anti-B component in their serum. See Table 42–20.) (c) Cells modified by chemicals such as hyaluronic acid found in Wharton's jelly: cord cells agglutinate non-specifically; however, the aggregates will disperse with the addition of hyaluronidase. (d) Minor population of cells derived from a chimeric twin or a recent non-group specific transfusion. (e) Cells coated with antibodies with subsequent formation of aggregates in the presence of a high-protein medium. (f) Different types of polyagglutinable cells (Table 42–21).

2. Unexpected additional reactions in serum grouping: (a) The presence of either cold or warm autoagglutinins reacting at room temperature. (b) The presence of alloantibodies such as anti-A_1, anti-H, anti-I, anti-M, anti-Le_a, anti-P_1, and other room temperature-reacting antibodies. (c) The presence of a high concentration of polymers such as gamma globulin, fibrinogen, dextran, or PVP in serum which can induce rouleaux formation. (Microscopic examination and/or saline replacement resolves this problem.) (d) The presence of antibodies directed against (1) lactose or antibiotics such as neomycin or chloramphenicol, which may be present in the reagent red cell preservation solution; (2) caprylate, which is used as a stabilizer for bovine albumin

5

Table 42–19. DIFFERENTIATION BETWEEN A_1 AND A_2 ERYTHROCYTES

Group	A_1	A_2
Quantitative		
Anti-A (weak or diluted)	4+	2+
Antigenic sites: Adult	1,000,000	250,000
Newborn	310,000	14,000
Qualitative		
Reaction with anti-A_1	Positive	Negative
Anti-A_1 in serum	No	Maybe
Antigenic determinant	Type I and II chains A^a, A^b, A^c, A^d	Type II chains only A^a, A^b
N-acetyl-galactosaminyl-transferase activity	Max. at pH 6 More active	Max. at pH 7 Less active

Table 42–20. AN AB PERSON WITH ANTI-B

Possible cause	"CIS-AB"	"Acquired B"
Etiology	Inherited	Action of bacteria*
Person (usually)	Healthy	Lower abdominal pathology
Subgroup (usually)	A_2	A_1
Anti-B (usually)	Weak	Strong
Substance in secretors	A + B	A
Children	A_2B or O	A_1 or O

*Bacterial deacetylase is the most attractive explanation.

preparations; or (3) acriflavin, which is the dye used in preparations of anti-B reagents.

3. Weakened or missing reactions in cell grouping: (a) Subgroups of A or B (see Table 42–16). (Many other variants have been reported, but they are very rare and of little clinical importance.) (b) Weakened antigens, A_g or B_g, in certain disease states such as leukemia. (c) High concentrations of A or B soluble substances in the sera of patients with adenocarcinoma of the stomach. These substances can neutralize the typing serum and give very weak or negative reactions.

4. Weakened or missing expected agglutinins: (a) Hypogammaglobulinemia or agammaglobulinemia. (b) Low titered or absent isoagglutinins, e.g., infants less than six months old or elderly persons.

The Rh System

The Rh system is perhaps the most complex erythrocyte system in terms of the number of antigens reported, the relationship among these antigens, and the nomenclature proposed by different investigators. Our effort will be to present only essential information. Readers who are interested in more detail should consult Race (1975b) and Issitt (1975, 1979).

THE BASIC Rh SYSTEM

The basic information has been derived from five antisera: anti-Rh_0(D), anti-rh′(C), anti-rh″(E), anti-hr′(c), and anti-hr″(e) (Table 42–22). Antigens C and c, as well as E and e, are antithetical; however, the antibody for the antithetical antigen for D has never been found. The term antithetical indicates that the two antigens are controlled by a pair of allelic genes; that is, a person can be *C/C* or *C/c* or *c/c*. A similar condition has been found for the genes *E* and *e*. For convenience of expression, the gene allelic to *D* has been assigned *"d"*. Thus, from serologic evidence, the Rh system can be assigned to three loci of genes, and this is basically the proposal of Fisher and Race (Race, 1975b, p. 179).

From population and family studies, these three loci are close to each other and inherited as a unit; well-documented crossing-over has not been observed. Therefore, Wiener proposed a one-locus theory: the gene complex (haplotype, or genetic endowment of one of a pair of chromosomes) is really one gene with a product of more than one specificity as determined by different antisera. The serologic factors (antigen expression) were named by Wiener as Rh_0, rh′, rh″, hr′, and hr″ respectively for D, C, E, c, and e. To reflect serologic factors from one gene, he used the term agglutinogen; e.g., Rh_z for the three-antigen complex Rh_0, rh′, and rh″; or rh for the two-antigen complex hr′ and hr″. The gene for Rh_z is designated as R^z; that for rh is *r*. Thus, three closely linked subloci for the Rh gene complex can explain the serologic reactions of blood group factors and genetic endowment of an individual or a population; e.g., gene complex (haplotype)→antigen complex (agglutinogen with multiple specificities). Both types of notations are two different interpretations of the same serologic findings in families and in populations. However, many people find the Fisher-Race notation easier to understand and use. Since the number of Rh antigens is increasing, alphabetical notation is no longer practical; Rosenfield proposed a numerical system—Rh1, Rh2, Rh3, Rh4, and Rh5—to represent the five basic antigens. At the present time, both Wiener (Rh) and Fisher-Race (DCE) notations are

Table 42–21. DIFFERENTIATION OF ERYTHROCYTE POLYAGGLUTINATIONS

Reagents	T*	Tk†	Th	Tn‡	Cad
Adult AB serum	+	+	+	+	±
Cord serum	0	0	0	0	0
Polybrene	0	+	+	0	+
Arachis hypogaea	+	+	+	0	0
Arachis hypogaea (papainized RBCs)	+	+ ↑	+ ↓	0	0
Glycine soja	+	0	0	+	+
Dolichos biflorus	0	+		+	+
Salvia sclaera	0	0	0	+	0
Salvia horminum	0	0	0	+	+
Bandeiraea simplicifolia II	0	+	0	0	0

*Using antisera absorbed with T exposed RBCs for correct typing of cells.
†Often associated with acquired B.
‡Using papain treated RBCs for correct typing of cells, often present with mixed field agglutination.

Table 42–22. EXAMPLES OF DIFFERENCES IN CONCEPT AND NOTATION OF THE Rh SYSTEM BY DIFFERENT INVESTIGATORS

Proposed for	by	Concept	Chromosome 1a*	Chromosome 1b*
Haplotype	Wiener	1 locus	R^z	r
	Fisher-Race	3 subbloci	DCE	dce
Antigens produced by the haplotype	Wiener	1 agglutinogen 2-3 factors	Rh_z Rh_o, rh′, rh″	rh hr′, hr″
	Fisher-Race	2-3 antigens	D, C, E	c, e
	Rosenfield et al.	Numerical	Rh1, Rh2, Rh3	Rh4, Rh5

*A pair of chromosomes.

Table 42–23. EIGHT GENE COMPLEXES (HAPLOTYPES) OF THE Rh SYSTEM*

Haplotypes		Antigen Complex†	Frequencies of U.S. Population			
Fisher-Race	*Wiener*	*(Agglutinogen, Wiener)*	*Whites*	*Blacks*	*American Indians*	*Orientals*
Dce	R^0	Rh_0(Rh_0, hr′hr″)	0.04	0.44	0.02	0.03
DCe	R^1	Rh_1(Rh_0, rh′hr″)	0.42	0.17	0.44	0.70
DcE	R^2	Rh_2(Rh_0, hr′rh″)	0.14	0.11	0.34	0.21
DCE	R^z	Rh_2(Rh_0, rh′rh″)			0.06	0.01
dce	r	rh(hr′hr″)	0.37	0.26	0.11	0.03
dCe	r'	rh′(rh′hr″)	0.02	0.02	0.02	0.02
dcE	r''	rh″(hr′rh″)	0.01		0.01	
dCE	r^y	rh_y(rh′rh″)				

*Composite figures, calculated from Mourant et al. (1976).
‡In Fischer-Race nomenclature, antigens are indicated by the letters except 'd.'

Table 42–24. FREQUENCIES OF COMMON Rh PHENOTYPES*

Reaction with Anti-†					Phenotype		Genotype		Frequencies‡			
D	*C*	*c*	*E*	*e*	*Rh*	*DCE*	*Rh*	*DCE*	*Whites*	*Blacks*	*American Indians*	*Orientals*
+	+	+	+	+	Rh_zrh	DCcEe	R^1R^2	*DCe/DcE*	0.1176 (89%)	0.0374 (100%)	0.2992 (89%)	0.294 (97%)
							R^1r''	*DCe/dcE*	0.0084 (6%)		0.0088 (3%)	
							$r'R''$	*dCe/DcE*	0.0056 (5%)		0.0135 (4%)	0.0084 (2.8%)
							rR^z	*dce/DCE*			0.0132 (4%)	0.0006 (0.2%)
+	+	+	−	+	Rh_1rh	DCee	R^1R^0	*DCe/Dce*	0.0168 (5%)	0.1495 (63%)	0.0176 (15%)	0.042 (50%)
							R^1r	*DCe/dce*	0.3108 (95%)	0.0884 (37%)	0.0968 (85%)	0.042 (50%)
+	−	+	+	+	Rh_2rh	DcEe	R^2R^0	*DcE/Dce*	0.0112 (10%)	0.0968 (63%)	0.0136 (15%)	0.0126 (50%)
							R^2r	*DcE/dce*	0.1035 (90%)	0.0572 (37%)	0.0748 (85%)	0.0126 (50%)
+	+	−	−	+	Rh_1Rh_1	DCe	R^1R^1	*DCe/DCe*	0.176 (91%)	0.029 (81%)	0.194 (92%)	0.490 (93%)
							R^1r'	*DCe/dCe*	0.017 (9%)	0.007 (19%)	0.017 (8%)	0.028 (7%)
+	+	−	+	+	Rh_1Rh_z	DCEe	R^1R^z	*DcE/DcE*			0.053 (100%)	
+	−	+	+	−	Rh_2Rh_2	DcE	R^2R^2	*DcE/DcE*	0.02 (88%)	0.012 (100%)	0.116 (94%)	0.044 (100%)
							R^2r''	*DcE/dcE*	0.003 (12%)		0.007 (6%)	
+	+	+	+	−	Rh_2Rh_z	DCcE	R^2R^z	*DcE/DCE*			0.041 (100%)	
+	−	+	−	+	Rh_o	Dce	R^0R^0	*Dce/Dce*	0.0016 (5%)	0.1936 (46%)	0.0004 (8%)	0.0009 (33%)
							R^0r	*Dce/dce*	0.0296 (95%)	0.2286 (54%)	0.0044 (92%)	0.0018 (67%)
−	−	+	−	+	rh	dce	rr	*dce/dce*	0.1369 (100%)	0.0676 (100%)	0.0121 (100%)	0.0009 (100%)
−	+	+	−	+	rh′rh	dCce	rr'	*dce/dCe*	0.0055 (100%)	0.0014 (100%)	0.0044 (100%)	0.0012 (100%)
−	−	+	+	+	rh″rh	dcEe	rr''	*dce/dcE*	0.0028 (100%)		0.0022 (100%)	

Estimated from haplotype frequencies (p,q from Table 42–23) using p^2 for homozygotes and 2pq for heterozygotes.
†+ = positive; − = negative.
‡(%) = per cent of genotypes within a given phenotype.

commonly used. One should be familiar with both designations.

With the help of the five basic antisera, eight antigen complexes (agglutinogens) are possible (Table 42–23). Each can be assigned to a gene complex or haplotype. The corresponding frequencies of four major American populations are listed. The frequency of dCE is extremely low.

Table 42–24 lists the frequencies of 11 common Rh phenotypes (out of 18 possible phenotypes) as detected by the basic five antisera. Common genotypes within each phenotype and the frequency of each genotype are also listed. The zygosity percentage with respect to Rh_0 is important in determining the chance of immunization of pregnant mothers by the father.

Table 42–25. REACTIONS OF FOUR COMPOUND Rh ANTIBODIES WITH ANTIGENS OF EIGHT Rh HAPLOTYPES

Haplotypes	Anti-			
	CE	*Ce*	*cE*	*ce(f)*
R^z(*DCE*) r^y(*dCE*)	+	−	−	−
R^1(*DCe*) *r′*(*dCe*)	−	+	−	−
R^2(*DcE*) *r″*(*dcE*)	−	−	+	+
R^0(*Dce*) *r*(*dce*)	−	−	−	+

THE Rh ANTIBODIES

Antibodies in the Rh system differ from those in the ABO system. With few exceptions (anti-C^w and anti-E), they are immune in origin and usually IgG. IgM and IgA Rh antibodies are very rare. With only one known exception, Rh antibodies do not hemolyze erythrocytes (Mollison, 1983: p. 655). Although saline-reacting Rh antibodies are available, most of them react best by albumin, enzyme, or antigobulin technique. Because of this lack of "naturally occurring" agglutinins, Rh antibodies were not discovered until almost 40 years after the demonstration of ABO antibodies.

Rh_0 antibodies usually develop after fetal-maternal hemorrhage and rarely as a result of transfusion with current blood bank technology (routine Rh_0 typing of all recipients); however, this may occur when platelet or granulocyte concentrates containing Rh_0-positive erythrocytes are transfused to an Rh_0-negative recipient. Once immunized, antibodies may last for many years and the host responds to secondary exposure very vigorously and promptly.

Zygosity or dosage of D antigen usually cannot be revealed by anti-D titration, whereas certain anti-C, anti-c, or anti-E and anti-e will often show dosage when proper techniques are used. Potent anti-D, anti-E, and anti-c are readily available. Good anti-C and anti-e are less readily available and pure anti-C without anti-C^w is rare.

Quite often, Rh antibodies demonstrate multiple specificities as well as single specificity. Some Rh antibodies react only with antigen complexes such as ce (Rh6,f) CE (Rh22), Ce (Rh7), cE (Rh27), and ce^s (Rh10, V) or CcEe complexes such as Rh17, Rh18, Rh34, and Rh38; or all the Rh antigens such as Rh29 and Rh39 (Table 42–25 and Fig. 42–10). Figure 42–10 also shows all other Rh antigens which have been assigned to the Rh system. Each of them has been discovered by the finding of a specific antibody.

Anti-Rh_0(D) not only serves as a blood typing reagent but may also be used in the prevention of Rh_0 immunization. Rh_0 immune globulin (RhIg) may be administered to an Rh_0-negative person receiving Rh-positive erythrocytes through either pregnancy or accidental blood transfusion. One vial (about 300 μg antibody protein) has been recommended for every 15 ml of Rh_0-positive red blood cells (not whole blood). For instance, if a recipient is estimated to have received 100 ml of red blood cells, 7 vials of Rh_0 immune globulin should be given as soon as possible, although satisfactory prevention of immunization has been observed as late as 48 hours after accidental transfusions. When many vials of Rh_0 were given to patients receiving large volumes of Rh_0-positive erythrocytes, no harmful side effects were observed (Mollison, 1983).

THE Rh ANTIGENS

Antigen Rh_0 and Its Subunits. Rh_0 antigen was established through careful clinical observation and animal experimentation. The first anti-Rh_0 serum was produced in rabbits by injecting Rhesus monkey erythrocytes. With this serum, Landsteiner and Wiener found that erythrocytes of 85 per cent of the population react positively and 15 per cent react negatively. The term "Rh" was used to define the antigen discovered.

After A and B antigens, Rh_0(D) is the most antigenic. About two thirds of Rh_0(D) negative (−) persons receiving Rh_0(D) positive (+) blood are likely to develop anti-Rh_0(D). It is for this reason that every blood donor and recipient is typed for Rh_0(D) antigen in addition to the A and B antigens.

Results of D typing are not always clear-cut; some D antigens can be detected only by the antiglobulin test and are designated as D^u ($\mathcal{R}h_0$ Rhw1). There are three types of D^u's: those due to gene interaction, those with an incomplete D, and those due to another type of inheritance.

The first type of D^u is due to the presence of a "C" in the trans position (on the opposite chromosome) such as in the *Dce*/*dCe* genotype. This person may type as D^u, while her children whose genotype is *Dce*/*dce* would be typed as a regular D. This type of D^u is fairly common among blacks owing to the high frequency of the *Dce* haplotype. People with this type of D^u are unlikely to form anti-D when D+ erythrocytes are transfused.

The second type of D^u has been shown to be an incomplete D antigen. Evidence indicates that Rh^o(D) antigen consists of a mosaic with at least four subunits: Rh^A, Rh^B, Rh^C, and Rh^D (Fig. 42–10). When one or more of these sub-units is missing, the D

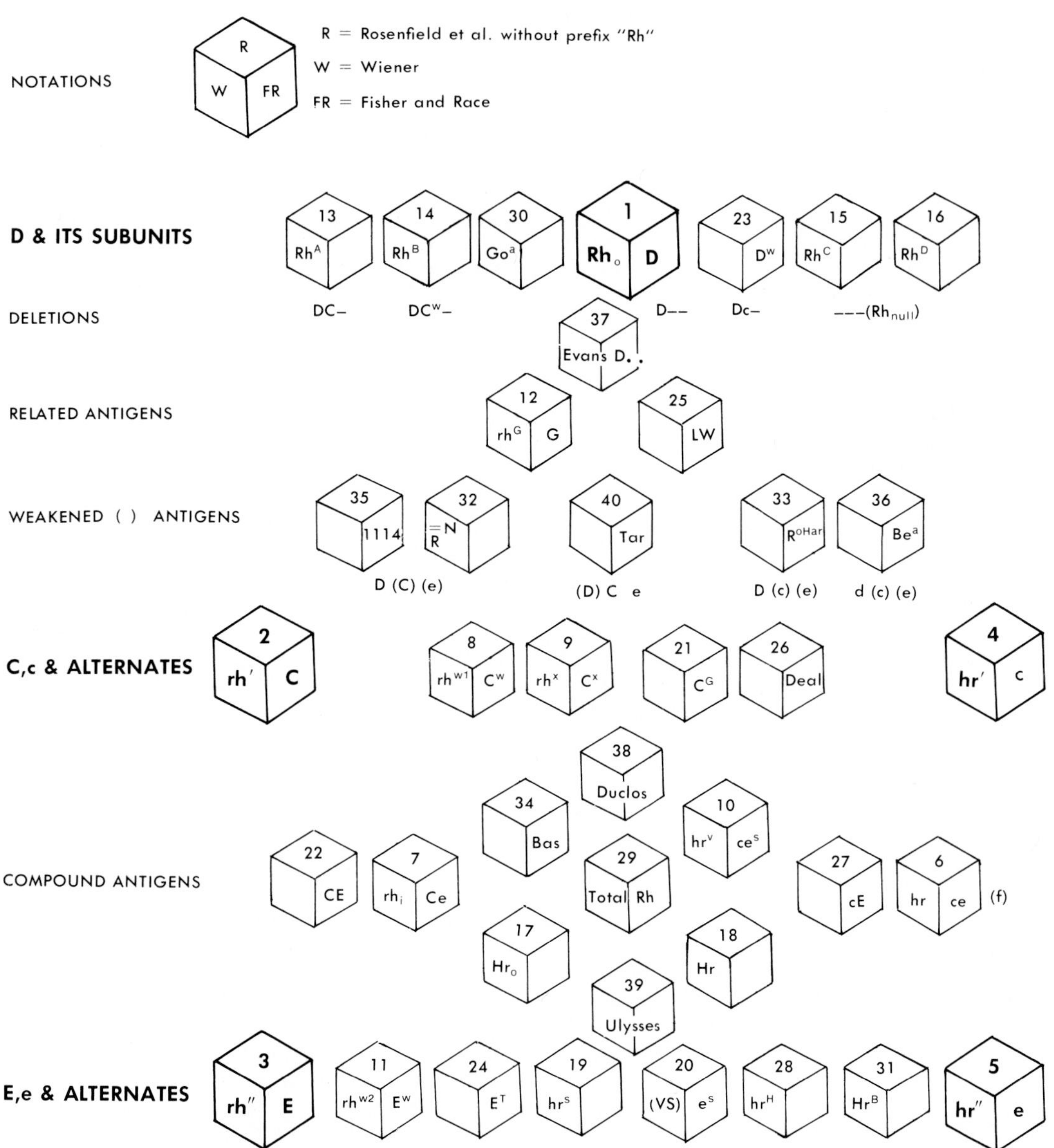

Figure 42–10. Relationships among various Rh antigens with respect to the five specificities.

5

antigen reacts as a D^u. In fact, those with a missing unit (such as $Rh^B = Rh^{ACD}$) may develop antibodies against the missing unit (Rh^B). This can explain why a D+ person may develop an alloanti-D.

There are some D^u's that do not belong to either of these two categories and are called "genetic D^u's" (a poor term, since the other two types are also under genetic control).

A slightly stronger D antigen has been observed in the presence of Rh32 antigen, whereas a moderately strong D antigen occurs with Rh30, Rh35, DC−, DC^w−, and a greatly enhanced D antigen is seen in D−−.

Antigens C and c and E and e. A person will normally type as C+c+, C−c+, or C+c−; similar reactions are found with E and e. Rare exceptions are produced by the gene complex *DC*−, where E and e antigens are absent. Since DCe and DcE are common phenotypes, anti-CE and anti-Ce are common antibodies formed by the person who has the opposite phenotype. In practice, anti-e and anti-C are often weak and less readily demonstrable. From serologic evidence, one can assume that genes controlling the E and e antigen are close to the genes for C and c antigens rather than to the gene for the D antigen. The logical expression of the gene complex would then be *DCE* instead of *CDE*.

Among the alternate antigens for C and c, C^w can be demonstrated in slightly more than 1 per cent of the white population. Since only a few persons have C^w without C antigen on their erythrocytes and few serums have anti-C without anti-C^w, the exact relationship between C and C^w is not clear.

The antigen G that is often associated with either D or C antigens is not a DC complex. Some persons with D or C antigen may not have the G antigen, while some persons have G antigen without the D or C antigen (r^G). However, many anti-D and anti-C serums also contain anti-G. This explains why mothers immunized only to C antigens produce antibodies reacting with D+ cells as well. Hence, anti-G has been referred to as anti-D and anti-C in some earlier literature.

Among the alternates to E and e antigens (Fig. 42–10), e^s (Rh20, VS) is rare in whites but present in 25 per cent of blacks. Other E or e variants are very rare. Compound antigens were discussed under Rh antibodies.

Rare weak variants similar to D^u have been reported for C, c, E, and e and are designated as C^u, c^v, E^u, and e^i, respectively. Weakened antigens in a complex (expressed in parentheses) have been encountered. Examples include Rh35 or D(C)(e) (whites), Rh 32 or D(c)(e) (blacks, $\overline{\overline{R}}^N$), Rh 33 or D(c)(e), ($R^{oHar}$), and Rh36 or d(c)(e)($Be^a$) (Fig. 42–10). Partial deletion of Rh antigens, such as Dc−, DC^w−, D−−and D.. (Rh37,Evans), and LW−, as well as complete deletion Rh_{null}, have been reported. For detailed description of Rh variants, Race (1975b) and Issitt (1975, 1979) give excellent accounts.

Rh Null Syndrome. Erythrocytes lacking all Rh antigens have been found in at least 22 persons in 14 families (Race, 1975b). Most Rh_{null} individuals studied presented with a compensated hemolytic anemia and a defect in the erythrocyte (stomatocytes) with shortened red blood cell survival. Rh antibodies with multiple specificities (anti-C, anti-e, anti-Rh29, etc.) may be present in their serum. Anti-Rh29 reacts with erythrocytes of all types except Rh_{null}. The M, N, En^a, and i antigens may be enhanced, while S, s, U antigens may be depressed in Rh_{null} people.

Possible genetic pathways in the biosynthesis of Rh and LW antigens are illustrated in Figure 42–11 to explain the two types of Rh_{null} phenotypes. A regulator gene is required to convert substance I to substance II and a *"DCE"* gene complex is required to convert substance II to DCE antigens. In the absence of a regulator gene X^1 (expressed by some as X^oX^o), no substance II is produced and the DCE antigens cannot be formed in spite of the existing *DCE* gene. This is known as the "regulator" type of Rh_{null}, who may transmit the *DCE* gene to their children. In the absence of a *DCE* gene (---) from both parents, the children may then be ---/--- (expressed by some as $\overline{r}\overline{r}$) and unable to convert substance II to DCE antigens. In this type of Rh_{null}, which is known as "amorph" type, the parents and children have antigens from only one haplotype such as *DCe*/--- or *dce*/---.

The LW Antigen. Accumulated data indicate that rabbit anti-Rh_o(D) serum is not identical to the anti-Rh_o(D) found in human serum. With proper techniques, antibodies to erythrocytes of the rhesus monkey will react with both D+ and D− cells (adult cells only, not true with cord cells). Human sera with similar specificity have been found; thus, they react strongly with D+, weakly with D−, and not at all with the patient's own cells. Results of family studies indicate that the antigen detected by these sera is inherited independently from the DCE antigens. This antigen is, in fact, similar to the Rhesus antigen. Since the term Rh has been widely used for D antigen, a term LW was proposed by Levine to honor Landsteiner and Wiener. So far, all Rh_{null} people are LW− also; thus, both antigens must be related. A possible

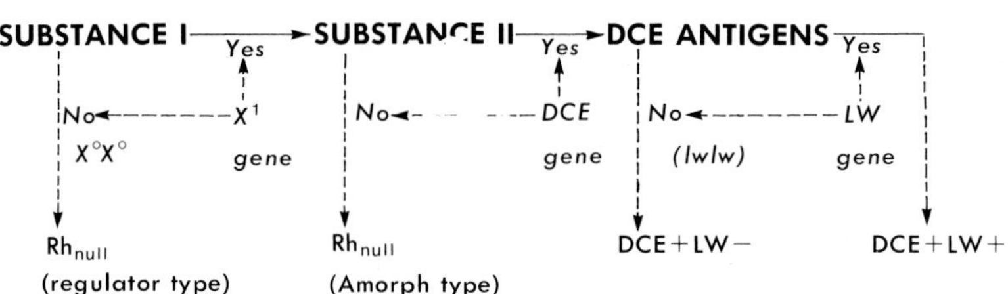

Figure 42–11. Possible genetic pathways in the biosynthesis of Rh and LW antigens. (Modified from Race, 1975b.)

relationship between Rh and LW antigens is illustrated in Figure 42–11.

Anti-LW has been found in LW+ people. In addition, a transient form of LW− has also been observed. There is some evidence to indicate that the LW antigen may be like the D antigen and contain subunits. Four phenotypes, LW1, LW2, LW3 and LW4, have been proposed by their decreasing strength of LW antigen. LW1 is LW positive and D positive; LW2 is LW positive and D negative; LW3 and LW4 could be either D positive or D negative. Anti-LW formed by LW3 individuals will react with RBCs of LW1 and LW2 but not with LW3 or LW4. Anti-LW formed by LW4 individuals will also react with LW3 RBCs. LW3 is the most common phenotype. One must be aware that a person may type as LW-negative by one antiserum and LW-positive by another antiserum. The LW typing serum used in each case, therefore, must be specified.

Rh TYPING

Routine Rh typing for blood donors and recipients involves only the antigen $Rh_o(D)$. Tests for D^u in D− specimens should be done every time. The term Rh_o-positive or Rh_o-negative refers to D+ or D−. To avoid ambiguity, Rh_o-positive or Rh_o-negative should be used; for simplicity, D+ or D− may serve the same purpose. Erythrocytes with C or E antigen should not be classified as Rh-positive. Meticulous adherence to manufacturers' directions for reagents, including sera, is crucial for accurate and specific Rh erythrocyte typing.

To determine the probable Rh genotype or in the case of antibody problems, tests for C, c, E, and e antigens are usually done. Only human antisera are used for clinical purposes. Saline-reacting antisera are available but are difficult to obtain. Potentiating medium which is usually added to Rh antisera to enhance reactivity may cause nonspecific reactions; controls should be included each time. Albumin control, which is still being used in some laboratories, is not identical to diluent control.

Although most Rh antisera react more strongly in the presence of a high-protein medium or enzyme or by antiglobulin test, each serum should be used according to the manufacturer's instructions. A more sensitive method may detect some unwanted weak antibodies.

Other Erythrocyte Antigens and Antibodies

There are about 400 erythrocyte antigens reported in the literature. Race (1975b) groups them into 21 blood group systems with separate groups for "public" and "private" antigens (see Table 42–5). Many of these antigens are of academic interest only, at least at the present time. ABO and Rh are by far the most important systems. Other important ones will be described subsequently.

THE LEWIS SYSTEM

The ABH and Lewis substances are closely related, as evidenced by the following points: (1) Lewis substances share the same precursor substance as ABH substances (see Fig. 42–1). Since H substance is not detectable in the Le(a+b−) phenotype (non-secretor), competition seems the logical explanation. (2) Le^b substance is probably derived from the H substance rather than from Le^a substance. The fact that no O_h phenotype has ever been observed with an Le(a−b+) phenotype tends to support this view. (3) Some Le^b antibodies react better with group O or A_2 cells (with more H antigen) and are designated as anti-Le^{bH}, whereas others react better with A_1 or A_1B cells and are designated as anti-Le^{bL}.

Since Le(a−b−) cells can be converted to Le(a+b−) or Le(a−b+) cells with the addition of plasma containing the appropriate Lewis substance, Lewis antigens on erythrocytes are thought to be the result of adsorption of soluble antigen in the plasma by the red blood cell.

It should be stressed that there is only one *Le* gene. Its silent allele is *le*, and there is no Le^a or Le^b gene, as the name of the antigen implies. Consequently, Le^a and Le^b are *not* antithetical antigens.

The possible biochemical relationships among Le^a, Le^c, Le^b, and Le^d are shown in Figure 42–1. No clinical significance is yet known for Le^c and Le^d antigens.

Both anti-Le^a and Le^b are usually "natural" in origin and of the IgM class. These antibodies may react from 4°C. to 37° C., in different types of media, and by various techniques. Quite often anti-Le^a and occasionally anti-Le^b cause hemolysis *in vitro*. Both anti-Le^a and Le^b are unstable at 4°C. or −18°C. Goat anti-Le^a and anti-Le^b have been found satisfactory as typing reagents. Anti-Le^c, anti-Le^d, and anti-Le^x are very rare and of no clinical importance.

The presence of abundant Lewis substance in the serum may neutralize the antibodies *in vitro* during typing or *in vivo* during transfusion. For the former, washed erythrocytes are recommended for typing; for the latter, the Lewis substance may reduce the effect of antibodies on erythrocytes and, thus, benefit the recipient. The infusion of plasma containing Lewis substance has been advocated by some before the transfusion of Le(a+) or Le(b+) erythrocytes to patients with Lewis antibodies (Mollison, 1983: p. 611).

Hemolytic transfusion reactions due to anti-Le^a have been observed, while those due to anti-Le^b have not been documented. In emergency situations, a number of patients with anti-Le^a have been transfused with Le(a+b−) cells without untoward reactions. Some hospitals do not screen for Le(a−b−) blood for transfusion to patients with anti-Le^b. Perhaps a logical approach would be based on the strength of antibodies. If they are hemolytic or clearly react by the antiglobulin test, compatible blood would seem to be the first choice.

Since Lewis antigens are poorly developed at birth and Lewis antibodies are IgM (i.e., unable to cross the placenta), Lewis antibodies have not been implicated in hemolytic disease of the newborn.

Common phenotypes of the Lewis system are listed in Table 42–26.

THE I AND i ANTIGENS

Since there are very few I-negative adults in the population, the genetics of these antigens have not been well studied; hence, I and i antigens have not

Table 42–26. PHENOTYPES OF THE LEWIS SYSTEM

Phenotypes	Reactions with Anti-		Frequency (%) of U.S. Adults	
	Le^a	***Le***^{b}	***Whites***	***Blacks***
Le(a+b−)	+	−	22	23
Le(a−b+)	−	+	72	55
Le(a−b−)	−	−	6	22
Le(a+b+)*	+	+		

*Encountered occasionally in infants or young children who subsequently become Le(a−b+).

been assigned to a system (Table 42–27). I antigen has also been found in soluble form in saliva, milk, urine, amniotic fluid, ovarian cyst fluid, and hydatid cyst fluid. The antigenic determinant has been shown to contain D-galactose and N-acetyl-D-glucosamine (see Fig. 42–1). Both I and i antigens have been demonstrated on lymphocytes.

Anti-I can be an auto- or alloantibody. Since the frequency of I-negative people is very low, allo anti-I is relatively rare and is found in every *ii* person as a "natural" antibody. Anti-I is usually of low titer but can be very potent. Auto anti-I is very common and is found in many normal persons as well as in those with acquired hemolytic anemia of the cold antibody type. High titered anti-I is usually associated with mycoplasma pneumonia infection.

Anti-i is relatively uncommon but is found in up to 80 per cent of patients with infectious mononucleosis. It may be present in other conditions where the bone marrow is under stress, resulting in premature circulation of erythrocytes. Both anti-I and anti-i are usually IgM but may be IgG. Enzymes usually enhance their reactions with erythrocytes, and both usually react best at 4°C. Strong anti-i may be hemolytic.

Antibodies against a complex of antigens involving I or i antigens have been reported, e.g., IA, IB, IH, IP_1, iH, and iP_1. These antibodies react only when both antigens are present on the cell; they are not a mixture of two antibodies. I antigens are poorly developed at birth, as cord cells usually type as I-negative while adult cells (except those of *ii* people) are I-positive (Table 42–27).

THE P SYSTEM

Biochemically antigens in the P system are related to ABH antigens. The antigenic determinants are composed of three sugars: galactose, N-acetyl-galactosamine, and N-acetyl-glucosamine (see Fig. 42–2). Hydatid cyst fluid can neutralize anti-P_1 and anti-I antibodies. Other similarities between the ABO and P systems are listed in Table 42–28.

Table 42–27. I-i ANTIGENS

Strength of Antigen	Found in Erythrocytes	Incidence
I ↓ i ↑		
i_1	White	Rare
i_2	Blacks	Rare
i_{cord}	Cord	All
I_{int}	Adult (Ii)	Few
I	Adult	Almost all

Phenotypes p, P^k, P_2, and P_1 in the P system have been likened to O_h, O, A_2, and A_1 in the ABO system, respectively. Both p and O_h are very rare and are considered the precursors of each system; each has "natural" antibodies against other antigens of the same system. P^k people produce anti-P just as group O people produce anti-A; similarly, P_2 people produce anti-P_1, and A_2 people produce anti-A_1.

Anti-P_1 is often found in P_2 persons. It is usually IgM, sometimes hemolytic, and may react at different temperatures and by different methods. Anti-P_1 reacts positively with erythrocytes of 79 per cent of whites and 94 per cent of blacks (Widmann, 1981, p. 150). Auto anti-P found in patients with paroxysmal cold hemoglobinuria is usually IgG and fixes complement at 4°C. with lysis of cells at 37°C. This is known as biphasic hemolysis. Anti-PP_1P^k (Tj^a) from p people is almost always hemolytic. Anti-P^k is prepared by absorption of anti-PP_1P^k with P_1+, P^k− cells. None of these antibodies has been known to cause hemolytic disease of the newborn; however, a strong anti-P_1 may cause a hemolytic transfusion reaction.

The phenotypes p and P^k are usually very rare; however, p is not uncommon in northern Sweden, whereas cases of P^k have been reported among Finns. The demonstration of P^k antigen on fibroblast cultures of all but p people tends to support strongly the hypothesis that p is the precursor substance of the P antigen.

THE MNSs SYSTEM

Like the P system, M and N antigens were first identified with animal antisera (Table 42–29); these still remain the most useful reagents for M and N typing. Simple sugars, D-galactose, N-acetyl-galactosamine, and sialic acid are the antigenic determinants (see Fig. 42–2). The main difference between M and N antigens is the number of sialic acid residues; M antigen has a greater number of sialic acid residues than the N antigen. This may explain why some anti-M sera also react with N cells and also why enzymes which degrade sialic acid residues destroy the reactivity of M and N antigens.

Anti-M and anti-N are rarely the cause of hemolytic transfusion reactions or hemolytic disease of the newborn. Anti-N-like antibodies have been demonstrated in some patients undergoing renal dialysis (Howell, 1972). Failure of some kidney grafts has been attributed to the presence of anti-N agglutinins when a cold kidney is transplanted (Belzer, 1971). The addition of anti-S, anti-s, and anti-U to this system changes that situation somewhat. Both transfusion reactions and hemolytic disease of the newborn have been implicated with all three antibodies.

Genes for S and s appear to be closely linked to *M* and *N* genes, although recombination has been observed (Table 42–29). All U− cells are also S−s− (except Rh_{null} cells). However, about 16 per cent of

Table 42–28. SIMILARITY BETWEEN THE ABO AND THE P SYSTEMS

ABO		P	
Phenotype of Erythrocyte	***Antibodies in Serum***	***Phenotype of Erythrocyte***	***Antibodies in Serum***
O_h	Anti-H,-A,-B	p	Anti-PP_1P^k(Tj^a)
O	Anti-A(A + A_1); B	P^k	Anti-P(P + P_1)
A_2	Anti-A_1	P_2	Anti-P_1
A_1	None for A antigen	P_1	None

S− and s− cells are U+. Thus, U antigen is not equal to S plus s, as was formerly believed. The phenotype S−s−U− has been found exclusively in blacks; the gene responsible for this phenotype S−s− is assigned as S^u. Three other antigens, M_1, Hu, and He, are also predominantly found in blacks (24 per cent, 7 per cent, and 3 per cent, respectively) (Race, 1975b: p. 107).

Most human anti-M and anti-N are naturally occurring and IgM, while most anti-S and anti-s are IgG and anti-U is always IgG. Anti-M and anti-N may react better in an acid medium. While anti-s and anti-U behave as typical IgG antibodies, anti-S usually shows decreased reactivity with enzyme-treated S+ cells, just as anti-M and anti-N show decreased reactivity with enzyme-treated M and N cells. There is evidence to suggest that the optimal reacting temperature for IgG anti-s and anti-U is below 37°C. Lectins with anti-M or anti-N specificity are commercially available. By using proper agglutinins, the dosage of M and N and of S and s can often be revealed. The MNSs system is important in disputed parentage examinations. This system is extensively reviewed by Issitt (1981).

THE LUTHERAN SYSTEM

Genetically, the Lutheran gene has been shown to be linked to the secretor gene providing the first autosomal linkage in blood groups. Lutheran is, so far, the only system in which a dominant gene produces a minus-minus phenotype Lu(a−b−) in addition to an amorphic type of Lu(a−b−).

Clinically, Lutheran antibodies produce very few transfusion reactions or hemolytic diseases of the newborn. Anti-Lu^a may be found after incompatible transfusion, but it is usually transient and weak. Anti-Lu^b is very rare. Both antibodies can be IgG, IgM, or IgA. Some are saline-reactive, while others react after enzyme treatment or in the antiglobulin test. Minor population of agglutinates, which were often described in the literature as a characteristic of anti-Lu^a, has not been observed in our laboratories.

Although at least 10 more Lutheran antigens (Lu^3 to Lu^{12}) have been proposed, they have not been well studied, nor are they of any clinical importance. The common phenotypes are listed in Table 42–30.

THE KELL SYSTEM

Like the Rh system, the Kell system has become a complex one. Table 42–31 compares the similarity between these two systems. There are six antisera to define three pairs of antithetical antigens—K and k, Kp^a and Kp^b, and Js^a and Js^b. These antigens are assumed to be controlled by a pair of genes and gene complexes as in the Rh system. The lack of Kell antigens (K_{null}, K_o) or poorly developed Kell antigens (McLeod type) similar to Rh_{null} and Rh_{mod} have been described. However, four of the eight possible haplotypes have not been observed. This fact favors the theory that there may be one basic haplotype and other haplotypes are the result of mutations. Thus far, a change in only one of the three genes has occurred in the Kell system, whereas this is not true with the Rh system.

Eighteen Kell antigens have been described; they are either of high incidence or of low incidence (Table 42–32). Only anti-K (9 per cent K+ in whites) and anti-Js^a (20 per cent Js(a+) in blacks) are relatively

5

Table 42–29. PHENOTYPES OF THE MNSs SYSTEM

Reactions with Anti-						Possible	Frequencies(%) in U.S.A.	
M	***N***	***S***	***s***	***U***	**Phenotype**	**Genotype**	***White***	***Blacks***
+	−				M	*MM*	28	26
+	+				MN	*MN*	50	44
−	+				N	*NN*	22	30
		+	−	+	SU	*SSU*	11	2.7 } 6.8
						SS^uU		4.1
		+	+	+	SsU	*SsU*	44	23.5
		−	+	+	sU	*ssU*	45	50.7 } 68.2
						sS^uU		17.5
		−	−	−	S−s−U−	S^uS^uU-		1.3 } 1.5
		−	−	+	S−s−U+	S^uS^uU+		0.2

Modified from Miller (1977), p. 124, and Race, (1975), p. 101.

Table 42–30. PHENOTYPES OF THE LUTHERAN SYSTEM

Phenotypes	Reactions with Anti-		Frequencies(%) in U.S.A.	
	*Lu*ᵃ	*Lu*ᵇ	*White*	*Black*
Lu(a+b−)	+	−	0.1	0.1
Lu(a+b+)	+	+	6.7	5.2
Lu(a−b+)	−	+	93.2	94.7
Lu(a−b−)	−	−	Very rare	

common, while the other antibodies are relatively rare.

The antigen K_x, which is also found on neutrophils and monocytes, is probably the precursor substance of other Kell antigens. An X-linked gene (X^1k) is required for its conversion; in its absence, K_x would behave as K_{null} (K_o). If X^1k is replaced by X^2k, the McLeod type (weak k, Kp^b, and Js^b) may be formed. With rare exception, the McLeod phenotype occurs in boys with chronic granulomatous disease (CGD) in whom K_x antigen is no longer demonstrable. Neutrophils of McLeod type without CGD have large amounts of K_x antigen. Thus, the lack of K_x antigen may be related to leukocyte dysfunction (Marsh, 1976).

With few exceptions, Kell antibodies are detectable by antiglobulin test and are not hemolytic or enhanced by enzyme. Numerous hemolytic transfusion reactions (extravascular) and a number of cases of hemolytic disease of the newborn have been attributed to Kell antibodies. Kell antigen is strongly antigenic and ranks second to D antigen in antigenicity when A and B antigens are excluded. The demonstration of transient k, Js^b and Kp^b antigens in the culture of erythroid precursor cells (McGinniss, 1982) and the selective inactivation of Kell antigens by the sulfhydro compounds (Branch, 1982) indicate that Kell antigens may be quite different from antigens of other blood group systems.

THE DUFFY SYSTEM

The incidence of Duffy antigens shows marked differences between whites and blacks. Among whites, two allelic Fy^a and Fy^b genes can explain the serologic findings. In blacks, at least three allelic genes, Fy^a, Fy^b, and Fy^4, have to be assumed. Phenotypes and possible genotypes for both populations in the United States are listed in Table 42–33.

Anti-Fy^a and anti-Fy^b are usually immune in origin and of the IgG class. Antiglobulin test is normally required for their detection. Enzymes may reduce the reactivity of anti-Fy^a and anti-Fy^b but will enhance the reactivity of anti-Fy^3, Fy^4, and Fy^5. Anti-Fy^3 reacts with all cells with Fy^a or Fy^b but does not react with Fy(a−b−) cells. The one anti-Fy^5 reported gave results similar to those of anti-Fy^3 except that it also reacted with the cells of the original anti-Fy^3 donor but did not react with Rh_{null} cells. Only one or two anti-Fy^3, anti-Fy^4, and anti-Fy^5 sera have been found thus far (Behzad, 1973; Race, 1975b: p. 358).

The Duffy genes have been assigned to chromosome No. 1 (Donahue, 1968). They are syntenic but not linked to the Rh genes. Erythrocytes of persons with the phenotype Fy(a−b−) appear to resist *Plasmodium vivax* invasion *in vivo* (Miller, 1975). Thus, Duffy determinants "a" or "b" on the erythrocyte membrane seem essential for the invasion of these malarial parasites.

THE KIDD SYSTEM

Thus far, the Kidd system remains simple. Only two allelic genes, Jk^a and Jk^b, are required to explain the serologic findings. Phenotype Jk(a−b−) has been described in certain populations but is very rare (Race, 1975b: p. 366) (Table 42–34).

Anti-Jk^a and anti-Jk^b are usually IgG and detectable usually by the antiglobulin test. Their activities are enhanced by enzymes or by the presence of complement. Although these antibodies may be hemolytic, they are usually weak and accompanied by other antibodies. Hemolytic transfusion reactions and hemolytic disease of the newborn due to Kidd antibodies are not uncommon. These antibodies have also been incriminated in delayed transfusion reactions (Mollison, 1983).

OTHER SYSTEMS

Other systems with two antithetical antigens and systems with abundant soluble antigen, as well as the "public" and "private" antigens, are summarized in Tables 42–35 and 42–36, respectively.

Testing for Erythrocyte Antigens and Antibodies

GENERAL CONSIDERATIONS

Identification. Proper identification of blood specimens or samples, reagents, and containers is absolutely essential

Table 42–31. SIMILARITY IN THE POSSIBLE GENETIC REGULATION OF THE BIOSYNTHESIS OF Rh AND KELL ANTIGENS

		Rh	Kell
Precursor, unconverted		Rh_{null}	$Kell_{null}$ (K_o, K_x)
Precursor, partially converted		Rh_{mod}	McLeod type*
Original basic haplotype		*Dce*	kKp^bJs^b (most common)
Number of genes modified within a haplotype	1	*dce, DCe, DcE* (common)	KKp^bJs^b, kKp^aJs^b, kKp^bJs^a (rare)
	2	*dCe, dcE, DCE* (rare)	KKp^aJs^b, KKp^bJs^a, kKp^aJs^a (not reported)
	3	*dCE* (very rare)	KKp^aJs^a (not reported)

*Strong association with X-linked chronic granulomatous disease of boys.

Table 42–32. PHENOTYPE FREQUENCIES OF KELL ANTIGENS

Relationship	High Incidence Group			Low Incidence Group		
	Antigen	***Whites***	***Blacks***	***Antigen***	***Whites***	***Blacks***
Antithetical:	kk (K2)	99.8%	99.9%	K (K1)	9%	3.5%
	Kp^b (K4)	>99.9%	>99.9%	Kp^a (K3)	2%	<0.1%
	Js^b (K7)	>99.9%	98.9%	Js^a (K6)	<0.1%	19.5%
	Côté (K11)	>99.9%		Wk^a (K17)	0.3%	
Unknown:	Ku (K5)			Ul^a (K10)	2.6%*	
	KL (K9)	>99.9%		K^w (K8)	5%	18%
	K12-K16					
	K18					

*Finnish population.
Modified from Widmann, 1981, p. 151.

in blood banking. Either the name or the code number of the blood donor must be marked clearly with permanent ink. A printed label must be securely attached to the blood sample. It is forbidden in blood banking to work with unlabeled or improperly marked blood samples. The recipient's blood sample label should include the patient's full name and specimen collection date. During testing, all tubes or other types of containers must also be properly identified.

Reagents. Whenever feasible, licensed reagents or those of equivalent quality should be used. Positive and negative controls should be performed on a daily basis. In selected instances, autocontrols and diluent controls should be performed. Reagents should be stored according to manufacturers' instructions, as frozen storage is not always preferable. In addition, the method of testing recommended by the manufacturer must be carefully followed; the use of an antiglobulin test when it is not recommended may detect other unwanted specificities, resulting in a false-positive test.

Erythrocyte Suspension. With possible exception of ABO and Rh typing (depending on reagents used), 2 to 5 per cent saline suspensions of erythrocytes are usually prepared. Usually one drop of a 4 to 5 per cent or 2 drops of a 2 per cent suspension are used for each test. The minimum serum-to-cell ratio is 1, but a larger ratio is preferable, especially for weak antibodies. Repeated exposure of the same cells to additional serum may enhance the reactivity. For critical typings of ABO, Lewis, Chido, Bg, Yt^a, and Sd^a, washed erythrocytes are preferable, as the presence of the antigen in the plasma may neutralize antibodies in the typing serum.

Procedures. Testing for erythrocyte antigens or antibodies can be done on slides or plastic plates with wells (known as microtiter plates). Similarly, test tubes, capillary tubes, or automated machinery may also be used. Currently, test tubes are the most widely used in blood banks. While microtiter plates are becoming increasingly popular, slide testing has become virtually obsolete (Lapinski, 1978). Unless specified, tests referred to in this chapter are tube tests. Other specific procedures will be mentioned under the specific subjects. Since there are many variations of each type of test, one should use that technique which is most familiar. The AABB Technical Manual (Widmann, 1981) serves as a general reference for various common procedures and alternative techniques.

Incubation. Many tests require a period of incubation to allow the antigen-antibody reaction to occur. Three temperatures are normally used: 4°C., 24°C., and 37°C. When a short incubation period is used, the tubes should be placed in a dry bath or water bath to speed up the equilibrium to the desired temperature (conductivity of air is very poor). Prolonged incubation of enzyme-treated cells should be avoided, as non-specific agglutination may occur.

Enzyme Treatment. Bromelin, papain, trypsin, and ficin are widely used to treat erythrocytes in order to obtain stronger reactions or to provide more effective adsorption of antibodies. Bromelin (0.5 per cent at pH 5.5) or cystein papain (0.1 per cent at pH 6.5) can be used together with serum and cells (one-stage enzyme test). A 0.1 per cent solution of papain, trypsin, or ficin at pH 7.3 may be used to pretreat erythrocytes. Erythrocytes then are washed, resuspended, and tested with the appropriate serum; this is known as the two-stage enzyme test. The two-stage test is much more sensitive than the one-stage test, but it is impractical for crossmatching purposes. In addition, owing

Table 42–33. PHENOTYPE FREQUENCIES OF DUFFY ANTIGENS

Reactions with Anti-				Phenotype	Probable Genotype	Frequency(%) in U.S.A.	
Fy^a	Fy^b	Fy^{3*}	Fy^4			***Whites***	***Blacks***
+	−	+	+/−	Fy(a+b−)	Fy^aFy^a Fy^aFy^4	17	.03 8.97 } 9
+	+	+	−	Fy(a+b+)	Fy^aFy^b	49	1
−	+	+	+/−	Fy(a−b+)	Fy^bFy^b Fy^bFy^4	34	1.36 20.64 } 22
−	−	−	+	Fy(a−b−)	Fy^4Fy^4 (or Fy^4Fy)	Extremely rare	68

*Anti-Fy^5 reacts like anti-Fy^3, but it also reacts with cells of the original anti-Fy donor and does not react with Rh_{null} cells.

Adapted from Widmann (1981), p. 154, and Race (1975b), p. 355.

Table 42–34. PHENOTYPES OF THE KIDD SYSTEM

Phenotype	Reactions with Anti-			Frequency (%) in U.S.A.	
	Jk^a	Jk^b	$Jk^{ab}(3)$	*Whites*	*Blacks*
Jk(a+b−)	+	−	+	28	57
Jk(a+b+)	+	+	+	49	34
Jk(a−b+)	−	+	+	23	9
Jk(a−b−)	−	−	−	Very rare	

to sensitivity of the two-stage test, no centrifugation is required before reading results. A high incidence of false positive reactions, especially when followed by an antiglobulin test, may occur if the test is performed improperly.

Enzymes enhance the reactivity of erythrocytes with certain antibodies, such as those of the Rh, Kidd, Lewis, and P systems. Rare examples of Rh and Kidd antibodies can be detected only with enzyme-treated cells. On the other hand, enzyme treatment may reduce reactivity of M, N, Fy^a, Fy^b, and possibly S antigens; apparently, enzymes affect the antigenic determinants of these antigens.

High-Protein Medium. Bovine albumin (22 per cent) has been widely used to potentiate the reactivity of Rh antigens. There is some evidence to indicate that highly polymerized albumin may be more effective. Other polymers such as polyvinyl-pyrrolidone (PVP) and polybrene have also been used to induce rouleaux or non-specific agglutination in special applications.

Other Enhancing Media. In recent years, numerous media for enhancing hemagglutination have become available. Some of these are strictly low ionic strength media (LISS), such as dextrose and glycine, while others also contain polymers of macromolecules (rouleauxing agents). Their effectiveness varies widely, but none are dramatic. In 1974, Lee and Ho developed a manual LISS-polybrene technique which offers greater sensitivity and speed while greatly reducing the use of antiglobulin serum. Similar techniques were subsequently reported by Lalezari (1980), Rosenfield (1979), and Fruitstone (1982). When this technology is perfected, blood bankers may indeed have a better system of detecting hemagglutination.

Centrifugation. In the majority of tests, centrifugation is required to reduce the time of incubation and to facilitate reading of results. The time and speed of each centrifuge should be calibrated by using appropriate controls. To avoid breakage of tubes, the number of tubes and the content in each should be balanced within the tolerance of the centrifuge.

Reading of Results. The presence of hemolysis is an indication of a strong reaction and should be recorded. The tube should be tapped gently until the cell button dislodges from the tube before a reading is taken. Proper illumination with a concave mirror is an invaluable aid for macroscopic reading. By placing the tube about 2.5 inches above a 3-inch concave mirror, aggregates can be differentiated easily from the free cells by looking at the mirror (not at the tube). The strength of the reaction can be recorded as follows with score in parentheses:

H	Hemolysis, presence of free hemoglobin	(10)
4+	One solid aggregate	(10)
3+	One solid aggregate and many small aggregates	(8)
2+	Small aggregates with a clear background	(5)
1+	Small aggregates with a turbid background	(3)

Table 42–35. SOME ERYTHROCYTE SYSTEMS WITH TWO KNOWN ANTITHETICAL ANTIGENS

System	Phenotypes			Optimal Reaction	Implicated in	
	Designated	*Frequency (%) Whites*	*Blacks*		*Hemolytic Transfusion Reaction*	*Hemolytic Disease of the Newborn*
Colton	Co(a+b−)	89.3	100	AGT with enzyme treated cells		Mild
	Co(a+b+)	10.4				
	Co(a−b+)	0.3	<0.1			
	Co(a−b−)	<0.1				
Dombrock	Do(a+b−)	17.2	9.4	AGT with enzyme treated cells		Mild
	Do(a+b+)	49.5	42.5			
	Do(a−b+)	33.3	48.1			
Diego	Di(a+b−)	<0.1*	<0.1	AGT		Yes
	Di(a+b+)	<0.1	0.5			
	Di(a−b+)	>99.9	99.5			
Scianna (Sm-Burrell)	Sc:1,2	<0.1		Some AGT Some saline	Yes	Yes
	Sc:−1,2	0.3				
	Sc:1,−2	99.7	100			
	Sc:−1,−2	<0.1				
Wright	Wr(a+b−)	<0.1	0	Many saline All temperatures Some AGT		
	Wr(a+b+)	<0.1	0			
	Wr(a−b+)	>99.9	100			
	Wr(a−b−)	<0.1				
Cartwright	Yt(a+b−)	91.9	91.6	AGT, 37°C.	Yes	
	Yt(a+b+)	7.8	8.2			
	Yt(a−b+)	0.3	0.2			

*2.5% Chinese, 16% Japanese, 11% Chippewa Indian, 36% Carith Indians.
Modified from Widmann, 1981, p. 156.

Table 42–36. SOME ERYTHROCYTE ANTIGENS WITH AN ABUNDANCE OF SOLUBLE FORM*

Antigen	Incidence in Whites	Remarks
Sd^a	98%	Abundant in urine One case of hemolytic transfusion reaction by Sd(a++) cells
Chido (Ch^a)	98%	Abundant in plasma Ch^a syntenic with HLA locus on chromosome No. 6†
Yk^a or Cs^a	88–97%	Present in plasma May be related to leukocyte antigens
Bg^a	29%	Undiluted high titer sera give weak reactions

*From Issitt, 1975, p. 255.
†Antithetical to Rodgers, likely to be identical to C4 (O'Neill, 1977).
Kn^a and McC^a may be antithetical; antibodies for both are high titer low-avidity types.

All negative reactions when they are required by the procedure should be read under a microscope and recorded as follows:

+W	Presence of aggregates (1)
–	Absence of aggregates (0)
M	Presence of minor population of aggregates (also known as mixed field agglutination mf)
R	Rouleaux, like a stack of coins, disappear with washing

Scores are useful when comparison of strengths of two antisera is made.

Records. Information concerning the donor of the blood sample and results of tests should be entered directly onto a laboratory form, preferably in a book. Ink, not pencil, should be used. The date, the time of testing (if known), and the initials of the technologist should also be recorded. Anyone who makes any change in results must put his or her initials next to the change.

Safety. All safety precautions for a clinical laboratory should be observed. Pipetting of blood components by mouth is not acceptable; a mechanical device should be used instead. All blood components are potentially infectious for viral hepatitis and should be treated with respect even though the HB_sAg test may be negative. Whenever feasible, discarded samples of blood components should be autoclaved before final disposal.

ANTIGLOBULIN TEST

Antiglobulin test (AGT) is also known as the Coombs test in honor of one of the investigators who made the test practical (Coombs, 1945). AGT is based on the principle that anti-human globulin antibodies induce agglutination of erythrocytes coated with globulins. AGT has become a powerful tool in the detection of antigens and antibodies undetectable by other techniques. When AGT is used to detect antibodies bound to erythrocytes *in vivo,* it is known as the direct antiglobulin test (DAT). When AGT is used to detect antibodies in sera by sensitizing erythrocytes *in vitro,* it is known as the indirect antiglobulin test (IAT).

Antiglobulin Sera (AGS). Antiglobulin sera are usually produced in rabbits by immunization. Owing to the different serum components used as immunogens, several types of AGS are available. Polyspecific AGS contain antibodies against human immunoglobulins (mainly IgG) and complement components (mainly C3); the activity against each component varies widely among different manufacturers and different lots of the same manufacturer. Monospecific anti-IgG, anti-IgM, and anti-IgA, as well as anti-C3+C4, anti-C3b, anti-C3d, anti-C-4b, and anti-C4d are commercially available. Because some rabbits may have antibodies against human erythrocytes or human serum protein, only selected rabbits should be used for immunization. Quite often, rabbit anti-human globulin sera require dilution or absorption or both to achieve required specificity and sensitivity.

Erythrocytes Coated with Globulins. In order to standardize antiglobulin sera and to confirm true negative antiglobulin reactions, two types of coated cells are normally used: those coated with IgG and those coated with C3b or C3d. To sensitize erythrocytes with IgG, Rh antibodies are usually used. To prepare cells coated with C3b, anti-Le^a or anti-I and fresh serum are often employed; additional incubation with fresh serum or trypsin to split C3b will leave cells coated with only C3d. In both cases, an appropriate concentration of antibody must be used to give about a 2+ reaction *only* after the addition of anti-IgG or anti-C3b or C3d, respectively.

Procedure. For the direct AGT, blood samples should be drawn in EDTA to prevent sensitization of cells *in vitro* through the activation of complement beyond C1q. For the indirect AGT, erythrocytes should be incubated with appropriate sera or plasma, usually at 37°C. for 15 to 30 minutes. In both cases, erythrocytes should be washed at least four times to remove all unbound free globulins. The time and speed of centrifugation should be standardized using positive and negative controls. All negative tests should be confirmed by (1) reading under the microscope and (2) positive reaction with control cells coated with immunoglobulin or complement.

False Negative Antiglobulin Test (AGT). False negative reactions are usually derived from improper procedures or poor technique, which can be detected by the use of positive and negative controls as well as use of coated erythrocytes in all negative reactions. Common causes are (1) inadequate washing, (2) contamination with serum protein through dirty glassware or fingers, (3) failure to add AGS, (4) inadequate incubation or centrifugation, (5) elution of antibodies through excessive washing or high temperature, especially IgM antibodies, and (6) insufficient amount of serum for sensitization.

False Positive AGT. Common causes include (1) agglutination before the addition of AGS owing to strong cold agglutinins, polyagglutinable cells, prolonged incubation with enzyme treated cells, presence of metallic ions, polybrene, protamine, and use of a low ionic strength medium, which may induce non-specific agglutination; (2) presence of unexpected antibodies in AGS such as anti-species or anti-transferrin; and (3) overcentrifugation.

Sensitivity of AGT. Although the AGT is extremely sensitive, a negative test by no means excludes the presence

5

of antibodies on erythrocytes. It is estimated that 100 to 500 IgG molecules bound on erythrocytes are required for detection by anti-globulin antibodies; a smaller number of IgG's bound on erythrocytes would give a negative reaction. AGS may be more potent against one or two subclasses of IgG but less potent for others; consequently, some antiglobulin sera may not be able to detect certain subclasses of antibodies on erythrocytes.

Applications of DAT. ***Investigation of Autoantibodies.*** The majority of warm autoantibodies are detectable by anti-IgG, while a small percentage are detected only with anti-C3d. Cold autoagglutinins are usually detectable by anti-C3d and rarely by anti-IgM.

Antibodies Induced by Medication. Most are detectable by anti-IgG. Antibodies against a drug-protein complex usually fix complement on erythrocytes, which can then be detected by anti-C3b or anti-C3d.

Hemolytic Disease of the Newborn. Only anti-IgG is needed.

Investigation of a Transfusion Reaction. Polyspecific AGS is recommended.

Applications of IAT. ***Detection and Identification of Erythrocyte Antibodies in Sera.*** Anti-IgG and anti-C3d are recommended, although a polyspecific AGS may be sufficient for routine use. Anti-IgM and anti-IgA should be available in a reference laboratory.

Typing of Erythrocyte Antigens. Many antigens require specific antisera followed by the antiglobulin test; usually, only anti-IgG is required.

Incompatibility Testing. Polyspecific antiglobulin sera are generally used.

Special Studies. In addition to the antiglobulin consumption test and mixed agglutination reactions, AGS has been useful in the detection of antibodies against leukocytes and platelets.

The use of anti-lymphocyte globulins (ALG) in recipients of kidney transplants introduces new serological problems for blood banks. Both direct and indirect antiglobulin tests may be positive in these cases. To alleviate the typing and crossmatching difficulties, AGS absorbed with red blood cells coated with ALS is recommended (Swanson, 1982).

TYPING OF ERYTHROCYTE ANTIGENS

Manual ABO and Rh_0 Typing. Antisera, reagent red blood cells, and diluent controls are well standardized and readily available. ABO grouping includes cell (forward) and plasma or serum (reverse) grouping. Anti-A and anti-B are normally used for cell grouping. In addition, anti-A,B (from a group O person) is used to differentiate A_1 cells from A_2 cells. For serum typing, A_1 and B cells are normally used; A_2 cells may be used if anti-A_1 is suspected. While the results of red cell grouping are often clear-cut, the reactions of serum grouping may vary greatly in strength. An additional period of incubation or incubation at 4°C. may be required to demonstrate the presence of weak agglutinins. Group O cells are usually included for the antibody detection (screening) procedure. The room temperature results of these cells may be helpful when discrepancies with serum grouping arise.

For Rh_0 typing, only anti-Rh_0(D) is required. Many laboratories also use anti-CD or anti-DE to supplement the typing. All Rh_0-negative tests should be followed by the antiglobulin test to detect D^u variants. When the DAT is positive, saline-reacting anti-D should be used. Cells positive with anti-C or anti-E should not be considered Rh_0-positive. Since all anti-Rh_0 sera contain a potentiating medium, a diluent control should be used rather than an albumin control.

Automated ABO and Rh_0 Typing. Currently, a number of large blood centers use one of two types of machines: the continuous-flow system or the batch processing system.

The continuous-flow system (e.g., Technicon AutoAnalyzer) consists of a sampler, a proportioning pump, a manifold, a moving filter strip, and a vacuum pump. Plasma and cell aliquots are aspirated into the system through the sampler. Additional reagents, cells, and plasma are pumped into the manifold. After mixing and incubation, any aggregates formed decant out through the T-shaped decanter and deposit on the filter paper. Excess liquid is removed by the vacuum apparatus. The presence and absence of aggregates can be visualized on the filter paper. In addition to antisera and reagent red blood cells needed for cell and serum typing, Bromelin and PVP are usually used to enhance the reactivity. The presence of air bubbles in the system is essential to segregate the blood samples and to keep the system clean (Sturgeon, 1963). This system can also be used for automated reagin test (ART) (Schoeter, 1970) and, with modification, for antibody screening (Lalezari, 1968; Lee, 1970) and antibody identification and quantitation (Lee, 1977). Modification of the AutoAnalyzer system to provide sample identification and printing capabilities by a computer is evolving (Lee, 1980b; Rechsteiner, 1981).

The batch system (Groupamatic) consists of a sample identification device, aspirators, dilutors, a disk with 144 specially designed sample cups, a hydraulic transportation system, an agitator-centrifuge, photometers, and a computer. Twelve different tests can be carried out for each of 12 blood samples on one disk at one time. Each disk is transported from one station to the other for processing. Serologic reactivity is enhanced by agitation and centrifugation. Results are read by the colorimeters through cups with optically clear bottoms. The computer gathers the identification number and test results, makes an interpretation, and then prints out the final results (Muller, 1981).

Special Typings. Special typings are required in the following situations: (1) screening for compatible blood for recipients with irregular antibodies; (2) assisting in antibody identification; (3) determining zygosity of husbands of Rh_0-negative women; and (4) paternity testing or studies of twins. Special typing often requires several special antisera that are not standardized and may be very weak. These antisera should be tested with various techniques in order to determine which technique yields the best reaction. Then that particular technique should be adhered to strictly when using the antiserum. When many blood samples need to be screened, an AutoAnalyzer system is most helpful. Since some antigens have different frequencies among various ethnic groups, valuable time may be saved if selected blood samples are used. In larger blood centers, it is advisable to screen blood samples of all group O units for antigens such as D, Fy^a, Jk^a, K or others to suit the local demand. It is of equal importance to freeze all units of erythrocytes with specific antibodies, as these units would be suitable for patients with the same antibody(ies).

ANTIBODY DETECTION (SCREENING)

Reagent Red Blood Cells. Many antibodies react more strongly with cells having a double dose (homozygous) of the same antigens than with those having only a single dose (heterozygous) of antigen. Since it is impossible to obtain cells having all desirable antigens in the homozygous state, two different sample cells are normally recommended for critical antibody screening. These two samples should be complementary (supplementary) to each other in terms of antigenic composition to provide most of the desirable antigens. When these two types of cells are pooled, 50 per cent of them should contain all the antigens reacting with all the so-called "clinically significant antibodies," such as Rh, Kell, Fy^a, Jk^a, S, s, and others. Selected types of cells

Table 42–37. REACTIONS OF COMMON ERYTHROCYTE ANTIBODIES*

	Antibody For	Saline Medium	Albumin Medium	Antiglobulin Test	Enzyme Tests	In Vitro Hemolysis	Optimal C.°		
							4	*24*	*37*
Usually IgM	H, I	M	S	F	S	F	M	S	F
	i	M	S	F	S	S	M	S	F
	A, B, A,B	M	F	F	M	S	M	S	F
	Lu^a	M	S	F	F	N	M	S	M
	Lu^b	S	S	M	F	N	R	S	M
	M, N	M	S	S	F	N	M	M	F
	P_1	M	S	S	S	F	M	S	F
	PP_1P^k	M	M	M	M	M	S	M	M
	Le^a, Le^b	M	S	S	M	S	M	S	F
Usually IgG	S, s	S	S	M	S	N	F	S	M
	K, k, Js^a, Js^b	F	S	M	F	N	F	S	M
	C, D, E, c, e	S	S	M	M	N	F	S	M
	Fy^a, Fy^b	F	F	M	F	N	N	F	M
	Jk^a, Jk^b	F	S	M	M	F	N	S	M

*M = Most (>20%), S = Some (5–20%), F = Few (1–5%), R = Rare (<1%), N = Not reported.

may be included, such as I− and Le(a−b−), to meet local demands. Reactions of commonly seen erythrocyte antibodies are summarized in Table 42–37.

Procedures. Currently, none of the available techniques are capable of detecting all erythrocyte antibodies; it is unlikely that there will be such a technique in the future. It is also unfortunate that there is no general agreement about the so-called clinically significant antibodies. The best approach is to use at least two techniques for recipients and select the most practical one for blood donors.

Some laboratories use saline medium and room temperature incubation for 15 minutes, followed by centrifugation and reading. Other laboratories omit room temperature incubation completely. If results are negative, the tubes are incubated at 37° C. for an additional 30 minutes, centrifuged, and read again. If these results are negative, the cells are washed four times with saline and antiglobulin serum is added. An additional set of tubes using a one-stage enzyme test or high-protein medium followed by the antiglobulin test is also used to complement the first technique. However, there are antibodies that may react only with the two-stage enzyme test plus antiglobulin test; others react only with an AutoAnalyzer system; and still others react only with capillary methods. Only additional careful investigation may resolve some of these unusual findings.

As reviewed previously, LISS appears to shorten the length of time required for antibody association with erythrocytes and enhances the sensitivity for low affinity antibodies.

The patterns of antibody reactions commonly encountered in hospital blood banks are listed in Table 42–37. Several comments can be made from the results of the antibody detection (screening) test.

1. IgM antibodies normally react in saline medium at room temperature or lower, while IgG antibodies react best at 37°C. by the antiglobulin test.
2. Antibodies of the P and Lewis systems may react with all techniques and under all conditions.
3. Albumin medium and enzyme tests are particularly useful for detecting Rh and Kidd antibodies.
4. With rare exception the presence of hemolysis may normally exclude antibodies of Lutheran, MNSs, Kell, Duffy, and Rh systems.

Boral (1977), Henry (1977), and Mintz (1976) have reported on the safety of the type and screen as well as its use in terms of blood ordering strategy as a safe alternative to a two-unit crossmatch request for selected surgical procedures where the use of blood is unlikely or virtually nil.

ANTIBODY IDENTIFICATION

Using a Panel of Red Blood Cells. If we assume anti-D in the serum of Mrs. X, serum X would react with all D+ cells but would not react with D− cells. In other words, if another serum, Y, reacts similarly to that of serum X, we can assume that serum Y also contains anti-D. In order to accomplish this purpose, a panel of D+ and D− cells is required. Since each sample of erythrocytes possesses many other antigens in addition to D antigens, antibodies against other antigens can also be tentatively identified with the same panel of red blood cells. The following is a greatly simplified example:

CELLS IN A PANEL	KNOWN ANTIGENIC COMPOSITION					TEST SERUM	
	D	C	c	E	e	Y	Z
No. 1	+	+	+	−	−	+	−
No. 2	+	+	−	+	+	+	+
No. 3	+	−	+	−	+	+	−
No. 4	−	−	+	−	+	−	−
No. 5	−	+	−	−	+	−	−
No. 6	−	−	+	+	+	−	+

Serum Y, which reacts with 3 D+ cells but not with 3 D− cells, can be assumed to have anti-D; similarly, serum Z reacts with 2 E+ cells but not with 4 E− cells. Can we then assume serum Z to contain anti-E? The fundamental question is: what is the chance that antigens other than E are also present in the 2 E+ cells but absent in 4 E− cells? One can also question what the chance is of antigens other than D being present in all 3 D+ cells but not in 3 D− cells. Thus, the number of different cells with known antigenic composition in a panel becomes a critical issue.

Fortunately, the chance of such a coincidence can be estimated by Fisher's "exact method for 2 × 2 table" (Race, 1975b).

TOTAL NUMBER OF TYPE OF CELLS IN A PANEL	PROBABILITY OF COINCIDENCE WITH NUMBER OF CELL SAMPLES THAT REACT POSITIVELY				
•	1	2	3	4	5
6	1:6	1:15	1:20		
7	1:7	1:21	1:35		
8	1:8	1:28	1:56	1:70	
9	1:9	1:36	1:84	1:126	
10	1:10	1:45	1:120	1:210	1:252

Statistically, a chance of 1 in 20, or 5 per cent, is considered acceptable; a chance of less than 5 per cent is usually recommended (Mollison, 1983). From the listing, at least a total of seven cells with a minimum of two for each antigenic determinant is required to achieve such a statistic. In order to reduce the chance to less than 1 per cent for critical studies, a total of nine cells with a minimum of four for each antigenic determinant is needed.

For this reason, most of the commercially available panels consist of 8 to 10 reagent red blood cells. Since it is practically impossible to have four samples with the same determinant for each antigen, supplementary cells or panels should be available for a definitive study. In order to prepare a panel of cells capable of identifying many types of antibodies, each sample in the panel should be extensively typed for various known antigens.

The following simplified example is used to illustrate the identification of a single antibody.

CELLS IN A PANEL	KNOWN ANTIGENIC COMNPOSITION									TEST SERUM	
	D	C	c	E	e	K	k	Fy^a	Fy^b	37°C.	AGT
No. 1	+	+	+	−	+	−	+	+	+	−	+
No. 2	+	+	−	−	+	−	+	+	−	−	+
No. 3	+	−	+	+	+	+	+	−	+	−	−
No. 4	−	+	+	−	+	+	+	−	+	−	−
No. 5	−	−	+	−	+	−	+	+	−	−	+
No. 6	−	−	+	+	−	−	+	−	+	−	−
No. 7	−	+	+	−	+	−	+	+	+	−	+
No. 8	−	−	+	−	+	−	+	−	+	−	−

Since the test serum reacts negatively with cell No. 3, one can rule out all antigens present on the No. 3 cell except C and Fy^a; with No. 4 cell, the antigen C is excluded; with No. 6 and No. 8, Fy^a remains unexcluded. One can, then, tentatively identify the presence of anti-Fy^a in the test serum with a chance of coincidence of 1:70 or 1.5 per cent.

Table 42–38 shows an actual antibody identification sample. Several conclusions can be drawn from the results.

1. Since the auto control is negative, the serum contains no autoantibodies.

2. Since panel cells No. 2, No. 3, and No. 10 reacted negatively with the test serum, antibodies against antigens on those cells can be excluded (crossed-out), with only antibodies for c, f, V, M, Lu^a, and Js^a remaining unexcluded.

3. From the pattern of reactions, at least two antibodies may be involved; one reacts best at 4°C. while the other reacts by antiglobulin test.

4. Anti-M would react similarly to the pattern presented. Positive reactions are seen with 7 M+ cells but not with 3 M− cells, with the strongest being the two homozygous M cells (No. 5 and No. 10).

5. Anti-c would react more strongly with AGT, and reactions with 5 c+ cells but not with 5 c− cells are seen.

6. However, co-existence of antibodies against f, V, Lu^a, and Js^a cannot be excluded. Anti-Lu^a was excluded when the test serum did not agglutinate M−, c−, Lu(a+) cells. Anti-Js^a was excluded when the test serum did not agglutinate M−, c−, Js(a+) cells. Serum absorbed with M−, cDE cells was no longer reactive with f+ or V+ cells; the presence of anti-f and anti-V was ruled out.

7. The presence of anti-M and anti-c was confirmed by absorption and elution.

8. Cells of the patient were M− and c−, compatible with the presence of allo-anti-c and anti-M.

9. While anti-M is likely naturally occurring, previous pregnancies may be responsible for development of anti-c.

10. Although this serum contains only two antibodies, a considerable amount of work has to be done in order to establish unequivocally the antibodies identified. Not infrequently, coexisting antibodies cannot be ruled out because of the presence of several antibodies and the lack of cells of proper antigenic composition for such a discriminatory study.

Absorption. Absorption is a process used to remove or neutralize antibodies in sera. It can be accomplished by using (1) washed erythrocytes, (2) enzyme-treated erythrocytes, (3) formalinized erythrocytes, (4) stromata, or (5) soluble antigens (also known as neutralization). Each type of antigenic material has its advantages and disadvantages with its specific applications. The antigenic composition of the material used for absorption must be known and selected for a particular purpose.

The absorption temperature and time depend a great deal on the nature of the antibodies being absorbed. In general, the lower the ratio of antibody to antigen, the higher the efficiency of absorption. Agitation during the absorption period is always helpful.

Absorption has the following applications:

1. To confirm the specificity of an antibody, such as saliva with H or Le^a substance for anti-H and anti-Le^a, milk with I substance for anti-I, hydatid cyst fluid with P_1 substance for anti-P_1, urine with Sd^a substance for anti-Sd^a, and plasma with Ch^a substance for anti-Ch^a.

2. To remove cold or warm autoagglutinins for the evaluation of the possible presence of an alloantibody or antibodies. Cells from the patient are most useful, provided the patient has received no transfusions recently. Enzyme treatment of these cells is usually very effective.

3. To remove unwanted antibodies such as anti-A, anti-B, or others to prepare reagent antisera, Stromata and formalinized cells may be useful for this purpose in that hemolysis is avoided during the absorption procedure.

4. To remove a single antibody from a serum with multiple antibodies by the use of cells with appropriate antigens to assure the identity of the antibodies.

5. To sensitize cells for subsequent elution studies.

Elution. Elution is a process used to remove antibodies bound to erythrocytes. First, one must be certain that there are antibodies on the erythrocytes; this is usually ascertained with a positive antiglobulin test. Second, one must be certain that there are no unbound antibodies in the suspending medium. This is accomplished by checking the last saline fluid washing with appropriate cells reacting with the expected antibody. Eluates are usually made in saline and should be prepared and tested on the same day. When storage is anticipated, the eluate should be prepared in AB serum or 6 per cent albumin and kept at −20°C. or lower.

Elution can be accomplished in one of three ways: (1) By heating at 56° to 60°C. for 10 minutes with frequent agitation. Separation is accomplished by centrifugation in cups with prewarmed water to hold the test tubes. This procedure is most effective for IgM antibodies. (2) By the addition of 2 volumes of ether and 1 volume of saline to 1 volume of washed packed erythrocytes followed by inserting a stopper and shaking vigorously for 1 minute. The tube is centrifuged and the ether is removed by aspiration. Evaporation of residual ether is accomplished by placing the tube in a warm water bath. This procedure is useful for eluting IgG antibodies (Wiener, 1957), but is not particularly suitable for anti-S or anti-U antibodies. (3) While heat and ether elution procedures are being used in many laboratories, other chemicals, such as ethanol, chloroform, digitonin, xylene, and methylene chloride, have also been tried. Thus far, ethanol, chloroform, and digitonin are suitable for specific applications. Xylene gives excellent yields for many antibodies but not for anti-Jk^a or anti-Jk^b and is technically difficult to perform. Methylene chloride does not give as good a yield when compared to ether or xylene, but hardly misses any antibodies. Only additional studies will reveal which is the method of choice for a specific purpose.

Table 42–38. AN EXAMPLE OF ANTIBODY IDENTIFICATION
MOUNT SINAI HOSPITAL MEDICAL CENTER

Name: Case #7 (Problem #82-73) Age: 45 Sex: F Date: 8/18/1973
Diagnosis: Pregnancy Previous Transfusion: None Date: ______
Patient's Cell Type: O/DCCee Pregnancies: 3
Antibody: ______

	Rh-hr								MNS				LUTHERAN (Lu)		P	LEWIS (Le)		KELL						DUFFY (Fy)		KIDD (Jk)		SEX LINK	
Rh-hr Code	D	C	C^w	E	c	e	f	V	M	N	S	s	Lu^a	Lu^b	P_1	Le^a	Le^b	K	k	Kp^a	Kp^b	Js^a	Js^b	Fy^a	Fy^b	Jk^a	Jk^b	Xg^a	Vial No.
r′r′	0	+	0	0	0	+	0	0	+	+	0	0	0	+	+	0	0	0	+	0	+	0	+	0	0	+	+	+	1
R_1R_1	+	+	+	0	0	+	0	0	0	+	0	+	0	+	+	+	0	0	+	0	+	0	+	+	0	+	+	0	2
R_1R_1	+	+	0	0	0	+	0	0	0	+	+	+	0	+	+	0	+	+	+	+	+	0	+	+	+	0	+	+	3
$R_2'R_2$	+	0	0	+	+	0	0	0	+	+	+	+	+	+	+	0	+	0	+	0	+	0	+	+	+	+	+	+	4
r″r″	0	0	0	+	+	0	0	0	+	0	0	+	0	+	+	0	+	0	+	0	+	0	+	0	+	0	+	+	5
rr	0	0	0	0	+	+	+	+	+	+	0	+	0	+	+	0	+	0	+	0	+	0	+	0	0	+	0	0	6
rr	0	0	0	0	+	+	+	0	+	+	+	+	0	+	0	+	0	0	+	+	+	0	+	+	+	0	+	+	7
rr	0	0	0	0	+	+	+	0	+	+	+	0	0	+	+	0	+	+	+	0	+	0	+	0	+	0	+	+	8
R_ZR_1	+	+	0	+	0	+	0	0	+	0	0	+	0	+	+	0	+	0	+	0	+	0	+	+	0	0	+	+	9
r_yr_y	0	+	0	+	0	0	0	0	0	+	0	+	0	+	0	0	+	0	+	0	+	0	+	+	0	+	+	+	10
PATIENT	+	+	0	0	0	+	0		0	+	+	+	0	+	+	+	0	0	+	0	+	0	+	0	+	0	+	+	
R_1R_1	+	+	0	0	0	+	0	0	+	+	+	+	0	+	+	0	+	+	+	0	+	0	+	+	0	0	+	+	I
R_2R_2	+	0	0	+	+	0	0	0	0	+	+	+	0	+	+	+	0	0	+	0	+	0	+	0	+	+	+	+	II

VIAL NUMBER	1	2	3	4	5	6	7	8	9	10	I	II	AUTO
I. Saline: 4°C.	2+	0	0	2+	4+	2+	2+	2+	4+	0	2+	0	0
a. Immediate Spin	+w	0	0	+w	2+	+w	+w	+w	2+	0	+w	0	0
b. Room temp.—30 min	1+	0	0	1+	2+	1+	1+	1+	2+	0	1+	0	0
c. 37°C.—30 min	0	0	0	1+	1+	1+	1+	1+	0	0	0	1+	0
d. Saline 37°C. plus antiglobulin	0	0	0	1+	1+	1+	1+	1+	0	0	0	1+	0
II. Albumin:													
a. Immediate Spin	0	0	0	0	+w	0	0	0	+w	0	0	0	0
b. 37°C.—30 min	0	0	0	+w	+w	+w	+w	+w	0	0	0	+w	0
c. 37°C. plus antiglobulin	0	0	0	2+	2+	2+	2+	2+	0	0	0	2+	0
III. Enzyme (Cysteine Papain)													
a. 37°C.—30 min	0	0	0	+w	+w	+w	+w	+w	0	0	0	+w	0
b. 37°C. plus antiglobulin	0	0	0	2+	2+	2+	2+	2+	0	0	0	2+	0

5

Table 42–39. ANTIBODIES NOT IDENTIFIABLE WITH USUAL PANEL OF CELLS*

Antibody for	Erythrocytes Used for Detection			
	Own	*Type O*	*Donor*	*Specially Selected*
Auto: warm	+	+	+	Rh_{null}, LW−, D−−, U−
cold	+	+	+	A_1, O_h, p, i
Very frequent	−	+	+	U−, Lan−, Vel−, . .
Very infrequent	−	−	+	Husband, child, Wr^a, Di^a, Co^b. . .
Compound (Rh system)	−	+	+	ce, CE, Ce, cE, ce^s, (r^G for anti-G)
Complex (2 systems)	−	+	+	HI, Le^{bH}
Multiple	−	+	+	Positive for one antigen at one time
A or B	−	−	+	A or B but not O cells
Subtypes	−	+, −	+, −	A_1, M_1, Rh^b
Minus-minus phenotype	−	+, −	+, −	Fy(a−b−) for anti-Fy4, K_0 for anti-KL
Medicine, dye	+	−	+, −	Medicine or dye in the test system
Lactose	−	+	−	Preserved with or without lactose
Caprylate	−	+	+, −	Albumin with or without caprylate
Bromelin	−	+	−	Bromelin treated or untreated cells

*A positive reaction could also be due to presence of various types of polyagglutinable cells without specific antibody. Rouleaux must be excluded.

Elution has the following applications:

1. To confirm the presence of a single antibody in the presence of several antibodies suggested by the use of a panel of red blood cells.

2. To determine the specificity of antibodies bound to erythrocytes, such as in cases of autoimmune hemolytic anemia, hemolytic disease of the newborn, possible transfusion, reaction, and antibodies induced by medication.

3. To prepare a small amount of monospecific antibody by separation from other unwanted antibodies, such as anti-A, anti-B, and other irregular antibodies, which interfere with the monospecific antibody in special typings.

4. To demonstrate the presence of subgroups of A such as A_x, A_m, and A_{el}. Cells of these subgroups may not be agglutinated by anti-A or anti-A,B, but they will absorb large quantities of anti-A, and anti-A can then be eluted. This procedure confirms the presence of A antigen on these cells.

5. To prepare cells free of attached antibodies for additional studies, such as proper typing, which can then be carried out even by an antiglobulin test if required (partial elution).

Elution of antibodies can also be accomplished in an AutoAnalyzer system to characterize antibodies in a different manner (Lalezari, 1968). By increasing the temperature of the water bathing the coils containing sensitized erythrocytes, antibodies gradually elute from these cells. The temperature at which elution begins and at which complete elution takes place may be used to characterize a given antibody. For example, one might elute an anti-M between 21° and 35°C., while an anti-S may be eluted between 30° and 49°C.

Other Helpful Means for Antibody Identification. By use of a panel of cells, absorption and elution may identify most antibodies but may not do so in some other instances. Table 42–39 lists some of the antibodies that require the use of cells of a special type for their identification. It should be emphasized that the typing and direct AGT of patients' cells is of particular importance to evaluate the presence of one or more alloantibodies. Least incompatible blood can be successfully used in patients with autoantibodies, but this procedure must not be used for patients with alloantibodies. Some antibodies listed in Table 42–37 are uncommon but are seen in many laboratories. The list may serve as a check when unusual antibodies are encountered.

Absorption removes specific antibodies but may also remove non-specific antibodies (no homologous antigens of the erythrocytes used for absorption). This is known as the Matuhasi-Ogata phenomenon.

Eluates may require concentration before use. Excessive amounts of fluid can be removed by either vacuum evaporation or by dialysis against macromolecular concentration media, such as Carbowax* or Lyphogel†.

It becomes obvious that a large collection of different antisera with different specificities and of erythrocytes with various types of antigenic composition is essential in order to complete a more complicated antibody identification. Antisera aliquots can be kept in a frozen state. Special reagent red blood cells can also be kept in a frozen state either at −20°C. or in liquid nitrogen. To store erythrocytes at −20°C., increasing concentration of glycerin, from 4 to 8 per cent, and then to 16 per cent is required to be equilibrated with the cells. Before use, decreasing concentration of glycerol, 16 per cent, 8 per cent, and then 4 per cent, is required to process the cells prior to suspension in saline. Many methods are available to preserve rare cells in liquid nitrogen. The method reported by Behzad (1977) has been found to be uncomplicated and satisfactory.

Paternity Testing

TRENDS

Paternity testing in the United States has changed rapidly in recent years because of two major factors: demands from the government and advances in immunogenetics. The former is due to the enactment of Public Law 93–647 by Congress in 1975, requiring each state to develop an appropriate plan, in accordance with HEW standards, for the ascertainment of paternity and for child support enforcement (Abbott, 1976). This new ruling is aimed both at protecting the right of a child to have a father and at relieving the public of the burden of supporting illegitimate children. Although the "blood test" cannot determine absolutely who the father is, it does provide the best

*Union Carbide, New York, New York.
†Gelman, Ann Arbor, Michigan.

scientific evidence available to the court. This ruling has not only steadily increased the number of tests being done, but has also stimulated improvement of the efficiency of the test to better achieve the goal of ascertainment of paternity.

During this same time, good antisera for red blood cell antigens became widely available; HLA typing became reasonably standardized; and phenotyping of enzymes and serum proteins became practical. All these factors contributed to the high efficiency of paternity testing. The addition of isoelectrofocusing techniques, typing of restriction enzymes, and monoclonal antibodies will no doubt further improve the efficiency in the years to come. This subject has been reviewed by Lee (1975a), Polesky (1975), Sussman (1976), Silver (1978) and Lee (1979).

BLOOD GROUP GENETIC MARKERS

Genetic markers are inherited characteristics that differentiate individuals from each other. They could be physical signs such as the color of skin and eyes or the type of hair, or they could be differences demonstrable in the various blood constituents. The value of the former is rather limited in resolving the disputed parentages, while the latter consists of many identifiable markers and has thus become the most useful tool in assisting the judge in making his final decision.

All genetic markers are controlled by genes located on a pair of chromosomes. At any one time, only two genes are involved in the formation of a specific characteristic. However, there may be additional alternative genes at the same locus on a pair of chromosomes. From the inheritance point of view, each parent can contribute only one of the two genes to the child. In other words, a child cannot inherit both genes from a single parent and none from the other.

Based on this principle, the following rules of inheritance can be stated:

1. A child cannot have a genetic marker which is absent in both parents.
2. A child must inherit one of a pair of genetic markers from each parent.
3. A child cannot have a pair of identical genetic markers (aa) unless both parents have the marker (a).
4. A child must have the genetic marker (a or b) which is present as an identical pair in one parent (aa or bb).

Based on these rules, four types of exclusion of paternity are possible:

1. The child has a genetic marker (such as blood group B) which is absent in the mother and cannot be demonstrated in the alleged father.
2. In a system with more than two genetic markers (as ABO), the child lacks both genetic markers (type O, absence of both A and B) which are demonstrated in the alleged father (type AB).
3. A child is homozygous for a genetic marker (such as *E/E*) which is not present in both parents.
4. A child lacks a genetic marker (M negative), while the alleged father is homozygous for it. *(M/M)*.

The first two types of exclusion are based on the presence or absence of certain genetic markers demonstrable by direct examination and are known as *direct exclusions*. With extremely rare exceptions, these two types of exclusions can be accepted with great confidence.

The third and fourth types of exclusions, based on the inference of homozygous genotypes determined by a negative reaction in a particular test, are known as *indirect exclusions* and should be accepted with caution. The particular test should be repeated with the same and with different or alternative reagents, by a different technologist, or in a different laboratory. For some markers, zygosity may be determined by the use of the titration method or the study of family members. The use of other genetic markers may reveal additional exclusions. (For more details, see Lee, 1982.)

SELECTION OF GENETIC MARKERS FOR PATERNITY TESTING

Testing for all genetic markers demonstrable in the various constituents (cells and proteins) of blood is totally unrealistic.

There are far too many to make this approach practical and many are unsuitable for use in paternity testing. The guidelines discussed below should be taken into consideration before selecting particular genetic markers.

Inheritance. All markers used must follow the Mendelian laws of inheritance as established through family studies and studies of population genetics.

Polymorphism. Genetic markers which exhibit wide variation in a given population are most useful for paternity testing. On the other hand, genetic markers of very high or very low frequency are of limited value in differentiating one individual from another. However, the latter markers are valuable in estimating the chance of paternity. If, for instance, the alleged father shares a very low incidence marker with the child, he is most likely the father of the child.

Practicality. The availability and reliability of the reagents as well as procedures are of great importance. The cost in relation to information provided should also be taken into consideration. However, compared with the cost to a falsely accused man for supporting a child, the fee for paternity testing is minimal.

Bearing in mind the criteria mentioned, five groups of genetic markers have been commonly used. These include erythrocyte antigens, erythrocyte enzymes, HLA antigens, serum proteins other than immunoglobulins, and immunoglobulins.

PROPER IDENTIFICATION

Since proper identification of the individuals involved in a paternity case is of utmost importance, whenever feasible, all persons should be present at the same time to allow them to identify each other. Care should also be taken that the blood is drawn from the man identified as the alleged father and not from a male companion who might also be present.

Information kept in the records should include:

1. Name and location of the institution performing the testing.
2. Full name of each individual; identify the mother, the child, and the alleged father.

3. Age, sex, and race of each party, since they are pertinent in interpreting the results.

4. Address and telephone number (optional) of each party.

5. Signature of each adult and witness.

6. Thumb prints of the woman, the alleged father, and the child (foot prints if the child is less than one year old).

7. Initials of the person drawing the blood specimen.

In some laboratories, instant photographs are also being taken of all of the individuals. When this is done, each photograph should also bear the date and the signature of the person.

Whenever feasible, blood or saliva specimens should be obtained in duplicate so that any rechecking or duplicate testing can be done on a separate specimen. Whenever erythrocyte enzymes are being tested, a set of specimens must also be drawn in ACD or EDTA tubes. Another aliquot of specimen must also be collected if HLA testing is to be included. All tubes should be labeled with (1) the full name of the individual, (2) whether it is the mother or the alleged father or child, and (3) the date drawn. The label should be typed or marked in permanent ink and covered with transparent tape.

If the testing is not performed immediately, all specimens should be stored in a refrigerator or at room temperature for HLA typing, in a section with no other blood specimens. Any tubes or containers to be used for subsequent transfer of serum or cells must also be premarked with typed labels or permanent ink (Lee, 1979).

GENERAL COMMENTS ON LABORATORY TESTING FOR GENETIC MARKERS

1. *Technologist(s):* Testing of the blood group genetic markers should be performed only by qualified technologists well trained in handling the various procedures involved, as well as any problems which might arise.

2. *Reagents:* As much as is possible, licensed or certified reagents should be used. The use of any other reagents is acceptable only if proper controls are tested simultaneously.

3. *Controls:* Both negative and positive controls must be run for each reagent being used on the day of testing.

4. *Specimens:* Blood samples of all individuals in each case should be tested at the same time, with the same reagent, and by the same technologist(s) whenever possible.

5. *Procedures:* Since many procedures and techniques are available for testing blood group genetic markers, only those mastered by the technologist(s) performing the testing should be used. All testing should be reproducible and yield clear-cut definitive results.

6. *Recording results:* Results should be recorded as they are read, with any changes initialed by the one making the correction. The strength of the reactions should also be recorded whenever applicable. The source and lot number of the reagents must be included with the test results. In dealing with electrophoresis or microtiter plates, some laboratories take photographs of the patterns and keep these as records.

7. *Repeating tests:* Any time a doubtful result or an exclusion is obtained, the test should be repeated using different/additional reagents and by a different technologist.

8. In addition to selection of examinations as well as methods, a physician with special competence should not only supervise testing and observe reactions but also interpret results in a written format that is scientifically accurate and understood by other than medical personnel.

9. *Consultation:* In cases in which one laboratory encounters difficulty in testing or in interpretation, specimens may be mailed to a second laboratory which has more experience in dealing with the particular problem. Should the results disagree, a third laboratory should be consulted.

CRITERIA FOR EXCLUSION OF PATERNITY

One Genetic Marker (P). If the child is positive for a given genetic marker and both the mother and the alleged father are negative for the marker, then the alleged father is excluded from paternity. Exceptions to this type of an exclusion are extremely rare. This type of exclusion usually occurs (1) in a system in which the allelic marker is either unknown or not demonstrable, such as P_1, Xg^a, Se, $Rh_o(D)$, Glm(a), and Glm(x); (2) in a system with two allelic markers when only one is being tested for, such as K, Fy^a, Jk^a, Lu^a, and Km(1); and (3) in a system with a relatively high frequency of recombinants, such as the HLA-A and HLA-B markers.

Two Allelic Markers (P,Q). Exclusion of paternity can be concluded in each of the four combinations shown below. An example of each is included in parentheses.

MOTHER	CHILD	ALLEGED FATHER
1. P−Q+(M−)	P+Q+(M+)	P−Q+(M−)
2. P+Q−(N−)	P+Q+(N+)	P+Q−(N−)
3. any	P+Q−(*M*/*M*)	P−Q+(*N*/*N*)
4. any	P−Q+(*N*/*N*)	P+Q−(*M*/*M*)

In combinations 1 and 2, only one marker is involved as is described in the above section, whereas in combinations 3 and 4, the interpretation is based upon zygosity. Whenever this type of exclusion is being considered, possible variants must be kept in mind. Exclusions of this type are normally seen with the following allelic markers: M-N, S-s, C-c, E-e, K-k, Fy^a-Fy^b, Jk^a-Jk^b, Lu^a-Lu^b, PGM_1^1-PGM_1^2, AK^1-AK^2, ADA^1-ADA^2, $6PGD^A$-$6PGD^B$, GLO^1-GLO^2, EsD^1-EsD^2, GPT^1-GPT^2, Hp^1-Hp^2, Gc^1-Gc^2, $C3^1$-$C3^2$, Ag^x-Ag^y, G1m(f)-G1m(z), and Km(1)-Km(3).

More Than Two Allelic Markers (P,Q,R). Exclusion of paternity can also be obtained from combination of markers as shown below.

	MOTHER	CHILD	ALLEGED FATHER
	any	P−Q−R+	P+Q+R−
e.g.		Fy(a−b−4+)	Fy(a+b+4−)
		A−B−H+(0)	A+B+H−(AB)

In the AcP (acid phosphatase) system, all three of the common markers are demonstrable by electrophoresis. The presence of any two of these markers in the child, both of

Table 42–40. EVALUATION OF PATERNITY TESTING RESULTS

	Mother	Child No. 1	Child No. 2	Alleged Father	Comments
1. Phenotype	MNs	MSs	Ms	MNs	
Possible genotypes	*Ms/Ns*	*MS/Ms*	*Ms/Ms*	*MS/Ns*	Cannot have child No. 2
				Ms/NS	Cannot have child No. 1
2. Phenotype	K+k+ Js(a+b+) Kp(a−b+)	K+k+ Js(a+b+) Kp(a−b+)		K−k+ Js(a−b+) Kp(a−b+)	
Possible genotypes	KJs^{b}Kp^b/kJs^{a}Kp^b	KJs^{b}Kp^b/kJs^{a}Kp^b		kJs^{b}Kp^b/kJs^{b}Kp^b	Exclusion based on the genotype combinations
	KJs^{a}Kp^b/kJs^{b}Kp^b	KJs^{a}Kp^b/kJs^{b}Kp^b			No apparent exclusion, but Kjs^{a}Kp^b haplotype has never been reported
3. Phenotype	DCe	DCce		DCcEe	
Possible genotypes	DCe/DCe dCe/DCe	DCe/dce (Dce) DCe/dce(Dce) dCe/Dce		DCE/dce (Dce) DCe/DcE (dcE) dCe/DcE	If AF f pos, 0.2%; no exclusion If AF f neg, 99.8%; exclusion

4. In case No. 3 above, if the alleged father's mother and father were typed and the father was found to be DCe and the mother was found to be DcE, then the alleged father's genotype should be DCe/DcE and the alleged father would be excluded from paternity.

which are absent in the alleged father, constitutes an exclusion of paternity.

Genetic Markers on the X Chromosome. G6PD (for the black population only) and Xg^a can provide exclusion of paternity only if the child is a female, as in combinations 1 and 2 shown in the example below. In combination 3 of this example, the mother is excluded.

MOTHER	CHILD	ALLEGED FATHER
(1) Xg(a−)	fem. Xg(a+)	Xg(a−)
(2) any	fem. Xg(a−)	Xg(a+)
(3) Xg(a−)	male Xg(a+)	any

Haplotypes. This type of exclusion can be concluded when (1) more than one child is being tested, (2) certain haplotypes are unreported, (3) special antiserums for complex antigens are used, and (4) family members are studied. Examples of each of these cases are shown in Table 42–40.

Exclusion in the HLA system based on haplotypes should be reported with caution, since the frequency of recombination is rather high and there is also a problem with cross-reactivity in this system. The same precautions should also be kept in mind with the Gm system, since it too has a relatively high recombination frequency. When the mother is not available for testing, exclusion of paternity based on the phenotypes of the child and the alleged father can also be made in selected cases; of course, the chance of exclusion is reduced (Lee, 1980a).

VARIANTS IN HUMAN BLOOD GROUP GENETIC MARKERS

The Null or Minus-Minus Phenotypes. Table 42–41 is a review of the minus-minus phenotypes that have been reported for the blood group antigens, the red cell enzymes, and the serum proteins. The excellent review of this subject by Allen (1976) should be consulted for additional information.

All of the phenotypes listed in Table 42–41 can be

Table 42–41. NULL OR MINUS-MINUS PHENOTYPES

System	Phenotypes	System	Phenotypes
ABO	A−B−H+ (O) A−B−H− (Bombay, O_h^A, O_h^B)	Acid phosphatase	AcP_o
MNSs	M−N− (En(a−)) S−s− (S^u) M−N−S−s− (M^k)	Adenylate kinase Alanine aminotransferase	AK_o ALT $(GPT)_o$
Rh	E−e− (D−−,DC^w−,Dc−) D−C−c−E−e− (Rh null, −−−/−−−)	Esterase D	EsD_o
Duffy	Fy(a−b−)	Phosphoglucomutase	PGM_{1o}
Kidd	Jk(a−b−)	Globulin marker	Gm_o
Lutheran	Lu(a−b−)	Haptoglobin	Hp_o
Wright	Wr(a−b-, En(a−))	Complement	$C3_o$, Bf_o
Colton	Co(a−b−)	Group specific component	Gc_o
Scianna	Sc(−1−2)	Transferrin	Tf_o
Lewis	Le(a−b−)		
P	p		
Kell	K_o		

considered rare under normal circumstances except as follows: First, group O is fairly common in many populations. Second, Fy(a−b−) and Le(a−b−) are fairly common in the black populations, although they are considered rare in Caucasians. Similarly, the p phenotype is not uncommon in northern Sweden.

Two mechanisms have been postulated to explain the existence of these null phenotypes. The hypotheses are based on the assumption that at least two genes are required for the production of detectable genetic markers, the regulator and the structural gene. The purpose of the regulator gene is to produce or transform a precursor substance into a product on which the structural gene can act, thus producing a detectable genetic marker. Either of these two genes can be partially or totally non-functional, resulting in the null or minus-minus phenotype.

If the regulator gene is absent, not functioning properly, or being suppressed, there is no precursor substance being formed for the structural gene to act upon, with the end result of an incomplete or non-detectable genetic marker. In this case, the normal structural gene can be passed to the child. If the child then inherits a normal regulator gene from the other parent, a normal genetic marker will be produced. The Bombay phenotype, some of the Rh nulls, and the McLeod phenotype can all be explained by this hypothesis. In the ABO system, the H substance has been shown to be the precursor of A and B substances. Thus, in the Bombay type, the regulator H gene is absent, while the A or B structural gene capable of transforming precursor H substance to A or B substance is normal; in a group O person, both the A and B genes are absent. At the present time, no such biochemical evidence is available for other null phenotypes. There is, however, evidence to indicate that the regulator gene for the McLeod phenotype is located on the X chromosome. This type of abnormality is the rare exception to the direct exclusion, since it is possible for two seemingly group O individuals to have a group A or B child, just as it is possible for two Rh null individuals to have a child with normal Rh antigens.

A second mechanism by which minus-minus or null phenotypes can be produced is an absence or a malfunction of the structural gene. This is the case in phenotypes such as D--, DC^{w}-, and Dc-, where neither of the normal alleles E or e is expressed. If this defect were affecting only one of the two genes, the result would be a phenotype which appeared homozygous for the allele able to be expressed. An example of this would be *E*/- or *e*/-, which would be interpreted as *EE* or *ee*, respectively. These possibilities are what render an indirect exclusion less reliable than a direct exclusion.

A third possibility which should be kept in mind as an explanation for other null phenotypes is the presence of an alternate allele that results in an end product for which no antiserum is currently available. The recent demonstration of anti-Fy4 has shown that the majority of the blacks who are Fy(a−b−) are Fy^4/Fy^4, and that those who type as Fy(a−b+) or Fy(a+b−) are in actuality Fy^b/Fy^4 or Fy^a/Fy^4 and not necessarily Fy^b/Fy^b or Fy^a/Fy^a, as was generally assumed. Therefore, exclusion of paternity in blacks based on zygosity in the Duffy system is not valid. However, the Fy(a−b−) phenotype is extremely rare in Caucasians.

Similarly, one must remember that uncommon but demonstrable alleles also exist in other systems, such as C^w and e^s in the Rh system and M^g in the MNSs system. A person could be C/C^w and not *C/C*, E/e^s and not *E/E*, or N/M^g and not *N/N*, etc. In these cases, exclusion of paternity cannot be concluded unless these uncommon alternate markers have been tested for and ruled out as possibilities.

Crossing Over. Although several cases of crossing over in the MNSs system and one case in the Rh system have been reported, the incidence of such an occurrence is extremely rare and need not affect the interpretation of paternity testing in most instances. In the HLA and the Gm systems, the rate of crossing over is estimated between 1 and 2 per cent, allowing much less confidence to be placed in an indirect exclusion.

Trans- or Cis- Effects. When *C* is present in transposition (located on the other chromosome of the pair), the Rh_o(D) antigen is often typed as D^u, as in the genotype D^uCe/dCe. Thus, when the haplotype D^uCe is passed to a child who may inherit dce or other haplotypes without the *C* from the other parent, the child will be typed as DCce, not D^uce. Both *A* and *B* genes can be inherited as one unit on the same chromosome, known as cis-AB. About a dozen or so cases of this have been reported in the literature. In this rare exception, an AB parent may have an O child, normally considered as an exclusion of maternity or paternity. This variant can be recognized by both the weakness of the B antigen and a weak anti-B present in the serum.

Mutation. Theoretically, the presence of a genetic marker in the child not found in both parents can be explained on the basis of mutation. However, the mutation rate in man has been estimated as close to one in a million, and no convincing example of a mutation involved in paternity testing has ever been found (Race, 1975a).

Racial Difference. Differences in frequencies of various genetic markers in different races is well known and those of blood groups have been summarized by Mourant and his associates (1976). Quite often, the differences are small and balance out when many systems are being used. Some markers are much more prevalent in one race than in others; the following are examples: Little p is found in northern Sweden; Ul^a is found in the Finnish, Ge in Melanesians, and Sc 2 in the Mennonite population; Fy(a-b-), S-s-, Js^a, Hu, He, Gm^{agb}, Aw23, Aw34, Bw42, Bw53, and Bw58 are all rather common in blacks; and Di^a, St^a, and Bw54 are found in Orientals. While these are not absolute identification of certain races, they do help in the interpretation of test results. Consequently, the racial background of each party must be recorded.

Physiologic Variations. Many genetic markers are known to be poorly developed during infancy, such as A_1, I, P_1, Le^b, Xg^a, Lu^a, Gm, and Hp. Some of these markers are not fully developed until as late as 6 to 18 months of age. Other antigens such as D^u, C^u, E^u, c^v, e^i, M_2, and N_2 are expressed only very weakly in adults. It is not unusual, therefore, that these weak antigens may react with some antiserum and not with others of the same specificity; antisera specific for these weak antigens are unknown. Another consideration is the presence of mother's IgG in the infant's circulation. Thus, the results of a Gm typing of a young infant should be interpreted with caution.

Pathologic Variations. In addition to the physiologic variations discussed in the previous paragraph, it is necessary to remember that certain pathologic variations do occur that also influence test results. For instance, any conditions which result in hemolysis *in vivo* will lower the haptoglobin level significantly. Both the Gm and Km typings would be affected if the patient had abnormal immunoglobulin levels, such as agammaglobulinemia. Persons with abnormal markers in the Kell system, such as the McLeod phenotype, may have chronic granulomatous disease and/or acanthocytosis. Rh_{null} persons may have a compensated hemolytic anemia and have demonstrable stomatocytosis when a peripheral smear is reviewed. Adenocarcinoma of the upper gastrointestinal tract is often associated with an excess production of group-specific substance which may interfere with ABO grouping results. Bacterial infections of the large intestine may lead to persons having an acquired B antigen. Other conditions, such as intrauterine transfusions, bone marrow transplantation, or recent blood transfusions could lead to blood group chimerism.

THE EFFICIENCY OF A TEST SYSTEM IN THE EXCLUSION OF PATERNITY

If a man is not excluded from paternity by the "blood test," the court may rule that he must pay child support. Thus, he should have the right to ask how good the "blood test" is with regard to excluding a falsely accused man. In other words, the efficiency of a test system in the exclusion of paternity used by a particular laboratory becomes a very relevant issue.

There have been two types of expressions used for this purpose: the chance of exclusion (or power of exclusion) to represent the general efficiency, and random men not excluded (RMNE) to represent the individual efficiency for a given mother-child pair. The former is used to express the overall effectiveness among all cases and is an average value; the latter takes into consideration the phenotypes of the mother-child and is a specific value for each case.

Estimation of the general efficiency is based on the frequencies of paternal or obligatory genes. In a two allele co-dominant system with P and Q being the antithetical antigens and p and q being their gene frequencies, the chance of exclusion =pq4 when anti-P is used or p4q, when anti-Q is used, or pg(1-pq) when both antisera are used. The same principle is applied for multiple allele systems.

Cumulative Chance of Exclusion. Since genetic markers in one system are independent of those in other systems, a man could be excluded concurrently by markers in more than one system. However, since a man needs to be excluded from paternity only once, the cumulative chance is not equal to the sum of those individual systems, but can be calculated with the formula 1-(1-CE1) (1-CE2) (1-CE3). . .where CE1, CE2, and CE3. . .are the chance of exclusion of the individual systems.

RMNE is a relatively simple concept and is readily understandable by the medical and the legal professions. Its value is the sum of frequencies of compatible phenotypes as illustrated in the following example:

PHENOTYPE			
MOTHER'S	CHILD'S	COMPATIBLE MEN	RMNE VALUE
A	A	A, B, AB, O	1
A	O	A, B O	0.96
A	B, AB	B, AB	0.13

Similarly, the RMNE values can be derived for other blood group systems with the exception of the HLA system, in which there are too many compatible phenotypes. Fortunately, either formulas and/or computer programs have become available (Mayr, 1977; Allen, 1983). The cumulative value of all systems tested would be the products of the individual RMNE values.

RMNE values have been included in the report of paternity testing by several European investigators (Hummel, 1971; Mayr, 1977; Salmon, 1980). A low value would be indicative for paternity. It could be used as the only calculation or as an aid when the paternity index (see below) is inconclusive.

LIKELIHOOD OF PATERNITY

When the alleged father is not excluded from paternity, it does not mean that he is the father of the child, especially when the RMNE value is high. In these cases, estimation of likelihood of paternity can be very helpful. Again, there are two types of expressions for this purpose: the paternity index (PI) and relative chance of paternity (RCP).

Paternity index is usually expressed as X/Y where X is the chance of paternity of the alleged father while Y is the chance of paternity of the random man. Chance of paternity can be derived on the basis of genotype (see 2a and 3a in Table 42–42): the chance is 1 for homozygotes and 0.5 for heterozygotes; when zygosity is unknown, the chance is 100 per cent of the expected frequency of homozygotes and 50 per cent of the frequency of expected heterozygotes; gene frequencies are used for the random man (Lee, 1975b). PI of each trio in each genetic marker system can be predetermined to reduce repeated calculations (Lee, 1980a). The cumulative PI is the product of PIs in each individual system.

Estimation of paternity index can be readily accomplished by computer programs or by manual methods as illustrated in Table 42–42, using five simple steps:

Step 1: (a) List the phenotype of the child, mother, and alleged father. (b) List the possible genes or haplotypes for each phenotype. (c) Find the appropriate frequency of each gene or haplotype for the given race.

Step 2: (a) Identify the possible maternal genes of the child. (b) Estimate the frequency of each possible maternal gene (M) as in 2a of Table 42–42. (c) Identify the possible paternal gene(s) for each possible maternal gene.

5

Table 42–42. ESTIMATION OF PATERNITY INDEX FROM HLA TYPING RESULTS IN 5 STEPS*

Mount Sinai Hospital Blood Center, Chicago, Ill. 60608 Date ________ Tech ________ Case # ________

Attach labels or write in full name, age, sex, race, party, date of spe. & case code

	Child				Mother				Alleged Father			
Phenotype	2,x;44,18				2,x;44,y				2,x;8,18			
Possible haplotypes	2,44	2,28	x,44	x,18	2,44	2,y	x,44	x,y	2,8	2,18	x,8	x,18
Haplotype fre. (H, Use 0.0001 for 0 in the table)					.0662	.0147	.0036	.0006	.0102	.0087	.0008	.0012

Child's Haplotype From

Mother: Possible	Mother: Chance (M)	Father Possible
2,44	.8058	x,18;2,18
x,44	.0417	2,18

Paternity Index (X/Y) = 50.5408

Chance of Paternity

Alleged Father (M × F)	Random Man (M × H)
.8058X(.4443 + .0558) = .40298	.8058X(.0012 + .0087) = .00798
.0417X.4443 = .01853	.0417X.0087 = .00036
Sum (X) = .42151	Sum (Y) = = .00834

Mother's Genotype: Possible	Fre. (f)†	%	Chance to pass: 2,44	x,y	2,y	x,44
2,44/x,y	.000079	.0113	.0056	.0056		
2,y/x,44	.000106	.0152			.0076	.0076
2,44/2,y	.001946	.2784	.1392		.1392	
2,44/x,44	.000477	.0682	.0341			.0341
2,44/2,44	.004382	.6269	.6269			
Sum	.006990	100%	.8058	.0056	.1468	.0417

Alleged father's genotype: Possible	Fre. (f)†	%	Chance to pass: 2,8	x,18	2,18	x,8
2,8/x,18	.000024	.1116	.558	.0558		
2,18/x,8	.000014	.0651			.0326	.0326
2,18/2,8	.000177	.8233	.4117		.4117	
Sum	.000215	100%	.4657	.0558	.4443	.0326

*Form can be used for other blood group systems equally well.

†Homozygous: f = H × H, M or F = % × 1. Heterozygous: f = 2 × H1 × H2, M or F = % × ½.

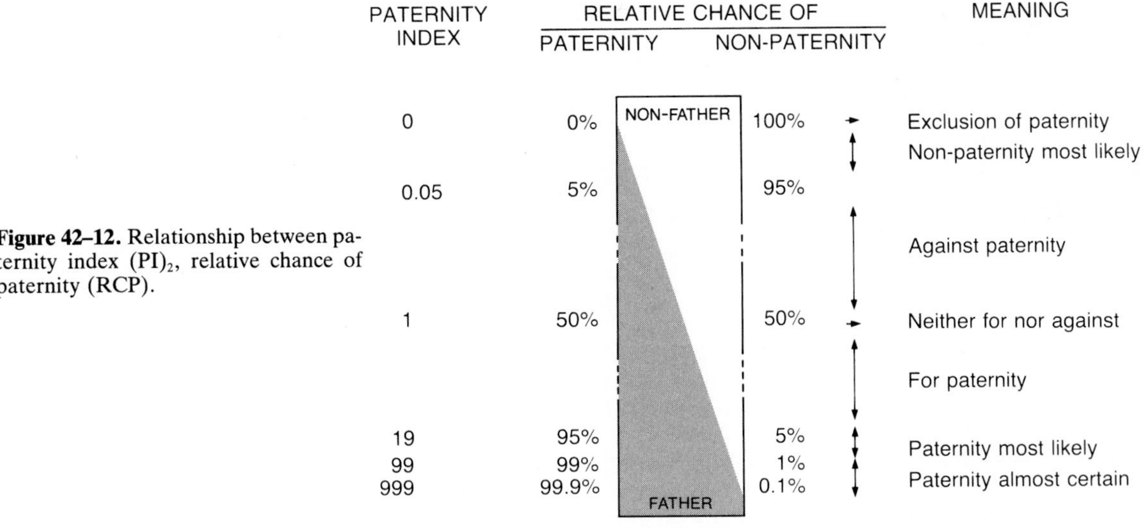

Figure 42–12. Relationship between paternity index $(PI)_2$, relative chance of paternity (RCP).

Table 42–43. SAMPLE REPORT OF PATERNITY TESTING, MOUNT SINAI HOSPITAL MEDICAL CENTER, CHICAGO

Genetic Marker System	Phenotype: *Child*	*Mother*	*Alleged Father*	Paternity Index
Name	Doe, Jennifer A.	Doe, Jane D.	Doe, John Allen	
ABO	A1	A1	0	0.9144
MNSs	Ns	MNs	MNs	1.3252
Rh	DCce	DCce	DCce	1.2091
Kell	K−k+	K−k+	K+k+	0.5235
Duffy	a+b+	a+b+	a+b+	0.9999
Kidd	a+b+	a+b+	a−b+	0.9998
AcP	A	AB	AB	1.2697
PGM1	1	1	1	1.3296
GLO	2	2	1−2	0.8724
GPT (ALT)	1−2	1−2	1−2	1.0000
EsD	1−2	1	1−2	5.1020
ADA	1	1	1	1.0499
AK	1	1	1	1.0284
PGD	A	A	A	1.0245
Hp	2	2	1−2	0.8573
Gc	1	1−2	1	1.3974
Tf	C	C	C	1.0061
Gm	fb	fb	fb	1.2887
Km	1−3+	1−3+	1−3+	1.1184
HLA−A, −B	2, −;7,13	2,24(9);7,13	2, −;13, −	13.0240
COMBINED PATERNITY INDEX				144.1964
RELATIVE CHANCE OF PATERNITY				99.3113%
RELATIVE CHANCE OF NON-PATERNITY				0.6887%

DATE: 11–29–82
BY L.K.L

REVIEWED BY: ____________

CASE NO. W749.EXP

5

Step 3: (a) Estimate the chance of passing each paternal gene (F) for the alleged father as in 3a of Table 42–42. (b) Obtain M × F values for each appropriate combination. (c) Sum all the M × F values, the X value.

Step 4: (a) Obtain the Y value as in step 3 by replacing the F values with the gene or haplotype frequencies.

Step 5: (a) PI = X/Y.

Although this example uses the HLA system, in which it is impractical to have all the PIs predetermined (Lee, 1980d), the same form can be used for any other genetic marker system.

Prior probability represents non-serological evidence in favor of paternity. When it is assigned to be 0.5, as in most laboratories, the PI value = X × 0.5/(Y × (1−0.5)) = X/Y remains unchanged. If the prior probability is p, then adjusted PI would be Xp/(Xp + Y(l-p)). Since the non-serological evidences are unknown to the medical profession, prior probability is the primary concern of the legal profession.

Relative chance of paternity is essentially the expression of PI in percentages. RCP = PI/(PI + 1) = X/(X+Y) or Xp/(Xp + Y(1-p)). RCP is also known in Europe as W or the plausibility of paternity. In expressing RCP, the negative aspect of the estimation is clearly indicated by the relative chance of nonpaternity to remind the court of the uncertain portion. Relationships between PI, RCP, and RCNP are illustrated in Figure 42–12.

To reduce human errors in printing and calculation, many laboratories which handle a large number of cases have computer programs to print out the report. One such example is shown in Table 42–43.

Abbott, J. P., Sell, K. W., Krause, H. D., et al.: Joint AMA-ABA guidelines: Present status of serologic testing in problems of disputed parentage. Fam. Law. Q., 9:3, 1976.

Allen, F. H.: Null types of the human erythrocyte blood groups. Am. J. Clin. Path., *66*:467, 1976.

Allen, F. H., Mayr, W. R., and Lee, C. L.: RMNE (random men not excluded). Calculation for 2-locus systems such as HLA. In International symposium on likelihood of paternity. Washington, D.C., AABB, 1983.

Anstee, D. J.: The blood group MNSs-active sialoglycoproteins. Semin. Hematol., *18*:13, 1981.

Behzad, O., and Lee, C. L.: A simple method for freezing reagent erythrocytes in liquid nitrogen. Transfusion, *17*:650, 1977.

Behzad, O., Lee, C. L., Gavin, J., and Marsh, W. L.: A new anti-erythrocytic antibody in the Duffy system: Anti-Fy4. Vox Sang., *24*:337, 1973.

Belzer, F. O., Kountz, S. L., and Perkin, H. A.: Red cell cold autoagglutinins as a cause of failure of renal allotransplantation. Transplantation, *11*:422, 1971.

Bird, G. W. G.: Lectins in blood banking: A brief review. Biotest Bull., *2*:2, 1977.

Boral, L. I., and Henry, J. B.: The type and screen: A safe alternative and supplement in selected surgical procedures. Transfusion, *17*:163, 1977.

Branch, D. R., and Petz, L. D.: Disulfide bonds are a requirement for Kell and Cartwright (Yt[a]) blood group antigen integrity. Transfusion, *22*:420, 1982.

Coombs, R. R. A., and Bedford, D.: The A and B antigens on human platelets demonstrated by means of mixed erythrocyte-platelet agglutination. Vox Sang., 5(O.S.):11, 1955.

Coombs, R. R. A., Mourant, A. F., and Race, R. R.: A new test for the detection of weak and "incomplete" Rh agglutinins. Br. J. Exp. Path., *26*:225, 1945.

Davidsohn, I.: Immunohematology, a new branch of clinical pathology. Am. J. Clin. Path., *124*:1333, 1954.

Donahue, R. P., Bias, W. B., Renwick, J. H., et al.: Probable assignment of the Duffy blood group locus to chromosome 1 in man. Proc. Natl. Acad. Sci. USA, *61*:949, 1968.

Fruitstone, M. J., Pygiel, S. A., and Clinton, B. A.: Manual polybrene vs. standard technics for antibody detection and identification. Transfusion, *22*:410, 1982.

Garratty, G.: The effects of storage and heparin on the activity of serum complement with particular reference to the detection of erythrocytic antibodies. Am. J. Clin. Path., *54*:531, 1970.

Gurner, B. W., and Coombs, R. R. A.: Examination of human leukocytes for the ABO, MN, Rh, Tj[a], Lutheran and Lewis systems of antigens by means of mixed erythrocyte-leukocyte agglutination. Vox Sang., *3*:13, 1958.

Hakomori, S. I.: Blood group ABH and Ii antigens of human erythrocytes: Chemistry, polymorphism, and their developmental change. Semin. Hematol., *18*:39, 1981.

Henry, J. B., Mintz, P. D., and Webb, W.: Optimal blood ordering for elective surgery. J.A.M.A., *237*:451, 1977.

Howell, E. D., and Perkin, H. A.: Anti-N like antibodies in the sera of patients undergoing chronic hemodialysis. Vox Sang., *23*:291, 1972.

Hughes-Jones, N. C., Gardner, B., and Telford, R.: The effect of pH and ionic strength on the reaction between anti-D and erythrocytes. Immunology, *7*:72, 1964.

Hummel, K., Ihm, P., Schmidt, V., and Wallisser, G.: Biostatistical Opinion of Parentage. Based upon the Results of Blood Group Tests. New York, International Publication Service, Vol. 1, Table-part 1, 1971.

Issitt, P. D.: Serology and Genetics of the Rhesus Blood Group System. Cincinnati, Montgomery Scientific Publications, 1979.

Issitt, P. D.: The MN Blood Group System. Cincinnati, Montgomery Scientific Publications, 1981.

Issitt, P. D., and Issitt, C. H.: Applied Blood Group Serology. 2nd ed. BCA, 1975.

Kitagawa, S., Lee, C. L., and Behzad, O.: Antibody detection using plasma in place of serum. Transfusion, *19*:60, 1978.

Klein, P. J., Bulla, M., Newman, R. A., et al.: Thomsen-Friedenreich antigen in hemolytic uremic syndrome. Lancet, *2*:1024, 1977.

Kornstad, L., and Heisto, H.: The frequency of formation of Kell antibodies in Kell-negative blood. Proc. 6th Cong. Europ. Soc. Haemat. Copenhagen, 1957, p. 754.

Lalezari, P.: A new method for detection of red cell antibodies. Transfusion, *8*:372, 1968.

Lalezari, P., and Jiang, A. F.: The Manual polybrene test: A simple and rapid procedure for detection of red cell antibodies. Transfusion, *20*:206, 1980.

Landsteiner, K. and Van der Scheer, J.: Serological differentiation of steric isomers (antigens containing tartaric acids). J. Exp. Med., *50*:407, 1929.

Lapinski, F., Crowley, K. M., Merrritt, C., and Henry, J. B.: Use of microplate methods in paternity testing. Am. J. Clin. Path., *70*:766, 1978.

Lee, C. L.: Current status of paternity testing. Family Law Quarterly, 9:615, 1975a.

Lee, C. L.: Estimation of likelihood of paternity. *In* Polesky, H. F. (ed.): Paternity Testing. Chicago, ASCP, 1975b, p. 28.

Lee, C. L.: Quantitation of antibodies to erythrocytes. *In* Schwartz, L., et al.: Blood Bank Technology, Baltimore, Williams and Wilkins, 1977, p. 3.

Lee, C. L.: Numerical expression of paternity test results using predetermined indexes. Am. J. Clin. Path., *73*:522, 1980a.

Lee, C. L., Behzad, O., Froker, A., and Mandin, B.: Identification of erythrocyte antibodies with an autoanalyzer. Adv. Automated Anal., *1*:317, 1970.

Lee, C. L., and Henry, J. B.: Laboratory evaluation of disputed parentage. *In* Henry, J. B. (ed.): Clinical Diagnosis and Management by Laboratory Methods. 16th ed. Philadelphia, W. B. Saunders Co., 1979, pp. 1409–1579.

Lee, C. L., and Ho, E.: A three-step test for rapid detection of erythrocyte antigens and antibodies. Lab. Med., *5*:47, 1974.

Lee, C. L., and Lebeck, L. K.: Derivation of random men not excluded values: A practical solution. *In* Walker, R. (ed.): Inclusion Probabilities in Parentage Testing. Virginia, AABB, 1983, pp. 525–534.

Lee, C. L., and Lebeck, L. K.: A fully automated blood processing system. Abstracts of 1980 Hematology-Transfusion joint meeting at Montreal, 1980b, p. 207.

Lee, C. L., Lebeck, L. K., and Pothiawala, M.: Exclusion of paternity without testing the mother. Am. J. Clin. Path., *74*:809, 1980c.

Lee, C. L., Lebeck, L. K., and Wong, C.: Estimating paternity index from HLA-typing results. Am. J. Clin. Path., *74*:218, 1980d.

Lee, C. L., and Williams, G.: How to deal with an indirect exclusion of paternity. Am. J. Clin. Path., *77*:204, 1982.

Lenny, L. L., Goldstein, J., and Rowe, A. W.: Cryopreservation of enzymatically converted B to O erythrocytes with and without metabolic rejuvenation. Transfusion, *22*:420, 1982.

Levin, S., Russell, E. D., et al.: Receptors of peanut agglutinin *(Arachus hypogea)* in childhood acute lymphocytic leukemia: Possible clinical significance. Blood, *55*:37, 1980.

Löw, E., and Messeter, L.: Antiglobulin test in low-ionic strength salt solution for rapid antibody screening and crossmatching. Vox Sang., *26*:53, 1974.

Marcus, D. M., Kundu, S. K., and Suzuki, A.: The P blood group system: Recent progress in immunochemistry and genetics. Semin. Hematol., *18*:63, 1981.

Marsh, W. L., Oyen, R., and Nichals, M. E.: Kx antigen; the McCloud phenotype and chronic granulomatous diseases: Further studies. Vox Sang., *31*:356, 1976.

Masouredis, S. P.: Quantitative and ultrastructural aspects of red cell membrane Rh antigens. *In* Henn, R. L. (ed.): A Seminar on Recent Advances in Immunohematology. Washington, D.C., AABB, 1973.

Mayr, W. R., and Pausch, V.: Calculation of the chance of paternity exclusion for the HLA system. Z. Immun. Forsch. Bd., *150*:447, 1977.

McGinniss, M. A.: The albumin agglutination phenomenon. *In* Seminar on Problems Encountered in Pretransfusion Tests. Washington, D.C., AABB, 1972.

McGinniss, M. A., and Dean, A.: K562 erythroid precursor cells and human red cell antigen expression: New findings. Transfusion, *22*:404, 1982.

Miller, L. H., Mason, S. J., et al.: Erythrocyte receptors for *(Plasmodium knowlesi)* malaria: Duffy blood determinants. Science, *189*:561, 1975.

Milstein, C.: Monoclonal antibodies. Sci. Am., *243*:66, 1980.

Mintz, P. D., Nordine, R. B., Henry, J. B., and Webb, W. R.: Expected hemotherapy in elective surgery. N.Y. J. Med., *76*:532, 1976.

Mollison, P. L.: Blood Transfusion in Clinical Medicine. 6th ed. Oxford, Blackwell Scientific Publications, 1983.

Mourant, A. E., Kopec, A. C., and Domaniewskia-Sobczak, K.: The Distribution of Human Blood Groups and Polymorphisms. 2nd ed. London, Oxford University Press, 1976.

Muller, A., Garretta, M., and Hebert, M.: Groupamatic system: Overview, history of development and evaluation of use. Vox Sang., *40*:201, 1981.

Myhre, B. A.: Antibody screening with the Autoanalyzer using donors' plasma in place of sera. Am. J. Clin. Path., *58*:698, 1972.

O'Neill, G. J.: The genetic control of Chido and Rodgers blood group substances. Semin. Hematol., *18*:32, 1981.

Polesky, H. F.: Paternity Testing. Chicago, American Society of Clinical Pathologists, 1975.

Polesky, H. F., and Hanson, M.: AABB-CAP survey data on hepatitis—incidence, surveillance, and prevention. Am. J. Clin. Path., *74*:565, 1980.

Pollack, W., and Reckel, R. P.: The zeta potential and hemagglutination with Rh antibodies. Int. Arch. Allergy, *38*:482, 1970.

Race, R. R., and Sanger, R.: Blood group polymorphism. *In* Ikkala, E., and Nykanen, A. (eds.): Transfusion and Immunology. Vammala, Vammalan Kirjapaino Oy, 1975a.

Race, R. R., and Sanger, R.: Blood Groups in Man. 6th ed. Oxford, Blackwell Scientific Publications, 1975b.

Rechsteiner, J., Lockyer, W. J., and Friedman, L. I.: Overview, history, evaluation and future development of the AutoGrouper 16-C. Vox Sang., *40*:192, 1981.

Roitt, I.: Essential Immunology. 4th ed. London, Oxford, Blackwell Scientific Publications, 1980.

Rosenfield, R. E., Shaikh, S. H., et al.: Augmentation of hemagglutination by low ionic conditions. Transfusion, *19*:499, 1979.

Salmon, D., and Salmon, C.: Blood groups and genetic markers: Polymorphism and probability of paternity. Transfusion, *20*:684, 1980.

Schoeter, A. L., Taswell, H. F., and Sweatt, M.: Adaptation of the single channel automated reagin test for syphilis to a multichannel automated blood grouping machine. Adv. Automated Analysis, *1*:265, 1970.

Schwartz, B. D.: The human major histocompatibility HLA complex. *In* Fudenberg, H. H., et al. (eds.): Basic and Clinical Immunology. Los Altos, Cal., Lange, 1982, p. 52.

Silver, H. (ed.): Paternity Testing. Washington, D.C., AABB, 1978.

Sturgeon, P., Cedergre, B., and McQuiston, O.: Automation of blood typing procedure. Vox Sang., *8*:438, 1963.

Sussman, L. N.: Paternity Testing by Blood Grouping. 2nd ed. Springfield, Ill. Charles C Thomas, 1976.

Swanson, E. W., Mann, R. M., et al.: Resolution of crossmatching problems associated with patients receiving anti-lymphocyte globulin. Transfusion, *22*:415, 1982.

Terasaki, P. I., Domenico, B., et al.: Microdroplet testing for HLA-A, -B, -C and -D antigens. Am. J. Clin. Path., *69*:103, 1978.

Westerveld, A., Jongsma, D., et al.: The assignment of AK_1, ABO linkage group to human chromosome 9. Proc. Acad. Natl. Sci. USA, *73*:895, 1976.

Widmann, F. K.: Technical Manual. 8th ed. Washington, D.C., AABB, 1981.

Wiener, W.: Eluting red-cell antibodies: A method and its application. Br. J. Haematol., *3*:276, 1957.

Wiener, W., and Vos, G. H.: Serology of acquired hemolytic anemias. Blood, *22*:606, 1963.

43

BLOOD BANKING AND HEMOTHERAPY

CHANG LING LEE, M.D., and JOHN BERNARD HENRY, M.D.

With a Section on Therapeutic Hemapheresis by Ronald A. Sacher, M.D., and Thomas A. Ruma, M.D.

Hemotherapy concerns infusion or removal of blood or blood elements to or from a patient for therapeutic purposes. Blood elements are known as either components or derivatives. Blood components, such as RBCs, WBCs, platelets, fresh frozen plasma, or cryoprecipitate, are prepared by many blood banks, while blood derivatives, such as albumin, immunoglobulins, concentrated antihemophiliac factor (AHF), or interferon, are commercially available or may be prepared by institutions that are specially equipped.

When mostly whole blood was used, many hospitals drew their own donors for their own patients. As use of more blood components became feasible and regulations became more rigid, preparation of blood components became a highly specialized profession. Currently, over 80 per cent of blood supplies in the United States come from fewer than 100 centers, which have the capability to recruit blood donors, collect blood, separate single units into components, process and store each component accordingly, and distribute them to hospitals as needed. People in these blood centers are truly the blood bankers.

On the other hand, since many hospitals now rely upon the supply of blood from community blood centers, their own hospital blood bank has become known as a "transfusion service." After the introduction of therapeutic apheresis, the term "transfusion service" will gradually be replaced by the term "hemotherapy." Hemotherapists ensure an adequate supply of blood components in the hospital, store them properly, and select and match the proper component for each patient. They act as consultants to physicians and provide maximal benefit with minimal risk to the patient.

Immunization associated with pregnancy may affect the unborn as well as the newborn. The mechanism is an immunological one. The diagnosis and prognosis of these conditions are based upon blood grouping and antibody workups; the treatment and prevention rely on blood components or derivatives. Logically, this subject should also be discussed under "hemotherapy."

BLOOD BANKING

Procurement of Blood and Blood Components

RECRUITMENT OF BLOOD DONORS

In recent years, two fundamental changes in donor recruitment have taken place. A shift from individual responsibility to community responsibility for blood replacement has occurred in some areas of our nation and from paid donors to voluntary donors throughout the United States.

For many years, motivation for blood donation has focused on individual responsibility to ensure that present and future blood needs of the donor and/or his family are met. This approach may create a hardship for those who are not qualified for blood donation or for those who have no one else to donate for them. In addition, record keeping is required, which can increase the costs. Hence blood replacement as a community responsibility has become more acceptable. Motivation based on group or community responsibility has been successful in some countries and to a variable extent in this country. A pluralistic approach to donor recruitment embracing individual and community responsibility is favored by many, since it utilizes both forms of motivation that have been demonstrated to be effective. Indeed, there appears to be a need for both individual and/or community responsibility to provide an adequate blood supply in response to demands throughout the United States (geographically or regionally) and at all times throughout the year.

Based on present usage, if about 4 per cent of the population (approximately 10 million) donated one unit of blood each year, the nation's required blood needs would be met. However, a variable but significant percentage of blood donors donate two or more times per year. Organized institutions or groups are rich sources of qualified blood donors.

Voluntary donors are defined as blood donors who receive no direct monetary compensation, while paid donors receive such remuneration.

The seriousness of post-transfusion hepatitis has attracted a great deal of attention for the past 10 years. Sufficient evidence indicates that for the most part the chance of contracting hepatitis from blood obtained from paid donors is greater than from that obtained from voluntary donors. Results of testing for hepatitis B surface antigen support this view for hepatitis B. Similar findings are true for non-A, non-B hepatitis which is responsible for the majority of post-transfusion hepatitis. Since currently available tests can detect and prevent only about 20 per cent of transfusion-associated hepatitis (Prince, 1975), blood from voluntary donors is preferred.

It should be stressed, however, that not all blood from voluntary donors is free of hepatitis and not all blood from paid donors is infectious. However, elimination of paid donors with increasing use of voluntary blood appears to be a definite trend, and labeling the source of blood units accordingly as a paid donor has been required by the FDA (Food and Drug Administration) since May, 1978.

SELECTION OF BLOOD DONORS

In order to protect the donor as well as the recipient, each blood donor must be screened prior to each blood donation by medical history and limited physical examination on the day of donation. This is to ensure that no harm will come to the donor by giving blood and that the unit when transfused will not in any way harm the recipient (Technical Manual of AABB, Widmann, 1981). Whenever a decision is made regarding acceptance or rejection of a blood donor, these two goals should be kept in mind, i.e., safety of donor and safety of patient.

Basic Qualifications

1. Age: Between the 21st and 66th birthday and between the 17th and 21st birthday depending on local law (age of majority) and consent of a guardian.
2. Body weight: 110 lb or more for 450 ($\pm$ 45) ml of blood collected in 63 ml of CPD anticoagulant plus up to 30 ml for additional tubes.
3. Temperature: Less than 37.5°C., or 99.5°F.
4. Pulse: Between 50–100 beats per minute, regular.
5. Blood pressure: systolic between 90–180 mm Hg; diastolic between 50–100 mm Hg.
6. Minimum hemoglobin: 13.5 g/dl (male), 12.5 g/dl (female); or minimum hematocrit: 41% (male), 38% (female).
7. Specific gravity (copper sulfate often used as a rapid hemoglobin screen). > 1.055 (male) > 1.053 (female)

Deferral

1. Permanent: history of viral hepatitis, history of jaundice of unknown cause, the only donor implicated in post-transfusion hepatitis, malignant tumors, leukemia, convulsion after infancy, fainting spells, abnormal bleeding tendency, known positive HBsAg test, serious cardiopulmonary disease.
2. Temporary: conditions requiring rest or medication: cold, flu, diabetes, tuberculosis, syphilis, and other infections, and diseases of the heart, lungs, kidney, stomach, or liver.
3. For 3 years: After prior residence in areas endemic for malaria or after cessation of antimalaria prophylaxis or

therapy provided the donors have been asymptomatic in the interim.

4. For 1 year: Severe illness, therapeutic rabies vaccine.

5. For 6 months: close contact with viral hepatitis, tattoo, injection of blood or components, donors implicated in post-transfusion hepatitis, major surgery, and travel to areas endemic for malaria without symptoms or suppressive medication.

6. For 2 months: German measles (rubella) vaccine.

7. For 8 weeks: previous blood donation.

8. For 6 weeks: after termination of pregnancy.

9. For 2 weeks: smallpox, measles (rubeola), mumps, and yellow fever vaccines, oral polio vaccine, animal serum products.

10. For 72 hours: dental or minor surgery, hyposensitization injections for allergy, symptomatic bronchial asthma.

11. For 48 hours: plasmapheresis, aspirin consumption by donor who is to be the only source of platelets for a patient.

12. For 24 hours: other types of vaccines.

Other Important Considerations

1. Identification: Full name, address, telephone number, age, sex, race (helpful for special typing), and social security number or driver's license number are very helpful.

2. Consent: A written consent of the prospective donor is required.

3. Preparation before donation: Eat a regular meal, avoid fatty food, and no alcohol within 12 hours prior to donation.

4. Exceptions: Exceptions can be made by a physician, especially for therapeutic bleeding, autotransfusions, immunization and hyperimmunization, and especially rare blood donors.

PHLEBOTOMY

1. Phlebotomists should be well-trained in aseptic techniques.

2. Materials used should be sterile (30 minutes at 121.5°C. by steam under pressure, or 2 hours at 170°C.). Disposable materials are preferred whenever feasible.

3. The donor blood bag, sample tube, and donor record should be properly identified and labeled before drawing blood.

4. The venipuncture site should be free of skin lesions of an infectious nature. Arms should also be inspected for needle marks, a sign of drug addiction.

5. Iodophor compounds (e.g., PVP-iodine or poloxamer-iodine complex) are preferred because they leave less odor and stain than does tincture of iodine. In addition, they do not cause skin reactions, and removal of iodine by additional washing is not required.

6. Plastic blood bags with additional satellite bags should be selected according to need. For instance, a single bag may be used for whole blood, double bags for red blood cell concentrates, triple bags for platelets or cryoprecipitate, and quadruple bags for both platelets and cryoprecipitate from the same donation.

7. Each bag should be examined for defects and the anticoagulant inside inspected.

8. For a donor over 110 pounds, the amount of blood drawn should be 450 ± 45 ml for 63 ml of CPD or CPDA-1, which is equivalent to 425 to 520 gm (weight of bag and anticoagulant not included).

9. A maximum of 30 ml in pilot sample is allowed for additional testing. Thorough mixing of the blood and anticoagulant in the bag and tubing is essential. Stripping the tubing several times before sealing is important.

10. After phlebotomy, establish that there is no leaking from the puncture site and that the donor is in satisfactory condition before leaving the room. A compress or adhesive bandage should be applied to the phlebotomy site.

HEMAPHERESIS

Hemapheresis is a procedure in which blood is removed from a donor, separated, and a portion retained, with the remainder being returned. The component removed may be plasma, platelets, leukocytes, or erythrocytes, and the processes are known respectively as plasmapheresis, plateletpheresis, leukapheresis, or erythrocytapheresis. An excellent discussion on this subject can be found in Chapter 10 of *Practical Blood Transfusion* (Huestis, 1981).

Apheresis donors should have the same general qualifications as whole blood donors. In addition, the body weight, total serum protein, platelet counts, and white blood cell counts should be monitored before and after the procedure whenever applicable or as indicated by the nature of the procedure. Usually not more than 15 per cent of the donor's blood volume should be extracorporeal at any time. Both the Code of Federal Regulations (640.2 and 640.6) and AABB Standards for Blood Banks and Transfusion Services (1976) should be consulted for further details pertaining to apheresis procedures.

Plasmapheresis. Plasmapheresis may be performed for two reasons: (1) for collection of plasma for fractionation into therapeutic components such as single donor plasma, fresh frozen plasma (FFP), and cryoprecipitate or derivatives such as albumin, gamma globulin, antihemophilic factor, and other factors (e.g., prothrombin complex, blood group typing sera); and (2) for therapeutic reasons.

Technically, plasmapheresis is performed using manual bag systems or centrifugal separation devices (p. 0000). With the use of manual bag systems, usually 500 ml of blood is drawn from the donor, and after the plasma is removed following centrifugation, the erythrocytes are returned to the donor. The process is usually repeated once more. Such a procedure may be repeated after 72 hours, but not more than four units (500 ml) of blood may be processed within seven days from the same blood donor. An eight-week interval is required for plasmapheresis following a whole blood donation. A plasmapheresis donor can donate a unit of whole blood 48 hours after the apheresis procedure.

Since the unit of blood is removed from the donor for centrifugation, proper identification of the unit is extremely important so that one avoids the reinfusion of the wrong unit of blood. Unit identification is usually done by a combination of a numerical system and either the donor's signature or a photo of the donor or both to ensure that the donor receives back his own blood.

Plasmapheresis can also be accomplished by mechanical devices. Currently, there are many types of these devices available. (1) Those designed primarily for harvesting platelets and/or granulocytes are based on the principle of centrifugal separation. (2) Those designed primarily for plasmapheresis are based on the principle of membrane filtration (TPE by Cobe Laboratory Inc. of Lakewood, Col., Cryomax by Parker Biomedical, Irvine, Cal., and PS-400 by Fenwall Laboratory, Deerfield, Ill.). The first group of machines includes semiautomatic, discontinuous systems, while the second group consists of continuous closed-loop systems. Both groups have the advantage of onsite return of cellular components (no misidentification problems) and therefore require less time for each procedure.

Plateletpheresis. Plateletpheresis is aimed at harvesting several times (approximately 10) the number of platelets that can be derived from one unit of blood from a single donor. In this way, not only is the chance of transmitting hepatitis reduced, but also the selection of HLA-compatible platelets becomes possible for particular recipients who are refractory to transfusion of random platelets (see Chap. 33). Donors for plateletpheresis should have a minimal platelet count of 150,000/μl and should not take any aspirin for the previous 48 hours.

Six to eight units of platelets can be collected from a single donor by a manual technique, as in plasmapheresis. This technique requires several hours, but requires no special instruments.

A machine (Haemonetics Model 30) has been developed to collect blood and anticoagulant into a centrifuge which separates whole blood into plasma, platelet, leukocyte, and erythrocyte fractions. From 400 to 700 ml of blood can be processed in each pass or batch depending on the size of the centrifuge bowl and the hematocrit of the donor. Normally six to eight passes can be processed in two to three hours. Approximately 6×10^{11} total platelets can usually be collected this way. In addition to a decrease in platelet count (between 40,000 and 90,000/μl) the donor also loses about 350 ml of plasma and 25 to 30 ml of erythrocytes per donation (in addition to pilot sample). Machines designed for leukapheresis can be used to harvest platelets.

Leukapheresis. Aggressive use of a large number of granulocytes has been successful in combating some infections unresponsive to antibiotics (Schiffer, 1974). Two types of procedures are currently available to harvest a large number of granulocytes: filtration technique and centrifugation technique.

In filtration leukapheresis, the calcium-dependent adhesion of granulocytes to nylon fibers is exploited. Granulocytes retained by the nylon filters can be eluted by flushing with a calcium-chelating citrated plasma. A continuous process is achieved by the use of a proportioning pump, and 6 to 8 L of blood can be pumped through the filters in a three- to four-hour donation period with a harvest of about 3×10^{10} granulocytes. A relatively large dose of heparin is used as the anticoagulant, and protamine sulfate is sometimes used to neutralize the effect of heparin at the end of a run. Side effects of both chemicals cause concern for some investigators. The effectiveness of granulocytes eluted from nylon fibers is a controversial subject at present.

In centrifugation leukapheresis, two automated techniques are available. However, the manual pheresis method described previously for platelets is less than ideal to collect adequate numbers of granulocytes efficiently.

Discontinuous Centrifugation. Essentially this is the same technique as that used for plateletpheresis. A red blood cell sedimenting agent, hydroxyethyl starch, is used routinely to enhance erythrocyte-granulocyte separation.

Continuous Centrifugation. These rather expensive machines (IBM 2997,* Celltrifuge II,† and Fenwal CS-3000‡) are designed for this purpose. Blood is drawn continuously from a donor into a centrifuge-cell separator which isolates the leukocytes from other blood components. The leukocytes are retained, while the remainder is continuously returned to the donor through a second venipuncture. Again, hydroxyethyl starch is often used as a sedimenting agent.

The yield from centrifugation leukapheresis is less than from filtration leukapheresis, about 10^{10} leukocytes per run. Improved methods have been used to augment the yield by increasing the circulating leukocytes and by enhancing red cell sedimentation. Etiocholanolone (a steroid metabolite) causes a granulocytosis by stimulating release of mature granulocytes from the bone marrow, while dexamethasone (a corticosteroid) increases the circulating granulocytes by decreasing the accumulation of granulocytes in the marginal pool. Both drugs, when given to a donor, can double the yield of granulocytes.

Prednisone and dexamethasone are the corticosteroids most commonly used. They should be given from 2 to 18 hours before the leukapheresis procedure to obtain maximum effect. A scheme used by Huestis (1981) is that of three 20 mg doses of prednisone given at 15, 12, and 2 hours, respectively, before leukapheresis. Corticosteroids are contraindicated in donors with peptic ulcers, diabetes, hypertension, or tuberculosis.

Hydroxyethyl starch (HES), a glycopyranone, promotes erythrocyte rouleau formation and allows clearer delineation of the white and red blood cell layers. The use of HES in all types of centrifugation leukaphereses can also double the yield of granulocytes. HES may improve the yield by sedimentation and thus make the procedure feasible in many small hospitals (Djerassi, 1977). The use of etiocholanolone or dexamethasone and HES increases the yield of leukocytes about six-fold and granulocytes six- to eight-fold. These agents exhibit little if any adverse effect on the donor. The number of erythrocytes and the amount of plasma lost by the donor are comparable to those from plateletpheresis. The donor must be monitored before each donation. The postdonation leukocyte count is usually slightly increased. Transfusion of manually collected granulocytes from patients with untreated chronic myelogenous leukemia has achieved favorable clinical responses in many recipients (Freireich, 1964). This latter method, however, is no longer used.

DONOR REACTIONS

Common Blood Donor Reactions

1. Donor feels faint. Stop the blood donation and ask the donor to inhale aromatic spirits of ammonia.

2. Fainting, weakness, perspiration, pallor, unconsciousness, slow pulse rate, nausea, vomiting, low blood pressure. Stop the donation and place the donor's head in a low

*International Business Machine Corp., Princeton, N.J.
†Haemonetics Corporation, Natick, Mass.
‡Fenwal Laboratory, Deerfield, Ill.

position. Be sure the donor has an adequate airway and apply cold compresses to forehead. If the needle is still in the donor's arm vein, the blood may be reinfused; otherwise, the needle should be removed.

3. Tetany or paresthesia and hyperventilation. Have the donor breathe several times into a paper bag.

4. Hematoma. Every effort should be made to prevent infiltration by inadvertent needle motion. Elevate the arm and apply compression locally, preferably cold.

5. Convulsions. Restrain the donor, remove the phlebotomy needle and use a tongue blade depressor or simple mouth airway to prevent biting. Maintain an adequate airway.

Reactions Observed During Apheresis

1. Chills. Cover the donor with a blanket and connect a blood warmer to the return channel.

2. Paresthesia and muscle cramping related to calcium binding by citrate (in centrifugal procedures). Slow the reinfusion and delay the next cycle until symptoms disappear.

3. Air embolus. Chest pain, shortness of breath, shock, pallor, sweating, mental confusion, and syncope. Although every effort should be made to prevent this from happening, if it does occur, place the donor on his left side with head down. Administer oxygen and transport promptly to an appropriate medical facility.

4. Sensitivity to heparin or protamine. Epistaxis or bleeding, chills, urticaria, or signs of anaphylactic shock. Discontinue infusion of heparin or protamine and treat anaphylaxis with epinephrine and steroids; transport promptly to an appropriate medical facility.

5. Bleeding from venipuncture site (heparinized donors). Remove needle if light pressure will not control it, then apply pressure and cold. If unusually troublesome, administer protamine.

6. Fever, chest pain, cough, shortness of breath, or other severe untoward reactions prompt stopping the procedure immediately for a physician's review and institution of appropriate measures.

Reactions 3, 4, and 6 are uncommon. However, adequate facilities should be available to handle all common reactions at the donor sites. A physician should be readily available to deal with reactions of apheresis donors.

Preparation of Blood Components

The development of plastic bags with integral tubing and of refrigerated centrifuges capable of handling large volumes at high speed makes possible splitting or separating a unit of whole blood into many components (red blood cells, platelets, cryoprecipitate, plasma, and leukocytes) and/or derivatives (plasma fraction subjected to physiochemical methods to generate albumin, coagulation concentrates such as antihemophilia factor [AHF], and prothrombin complex, plasma protein fraction [PPF], fibrinogen and immune globulins) for most appropriate effective and efficient hemotherapy. Thus, we are able to supply the exact components and/or derivatives to meet the needs of each patient and, at the same time, to avoid certain elements in the blood that a patient should not receive.

Plastic Bags. Plastic bags are available in many forms, and each is designed for a specific purpose. When the unit is to be used as whole blood, a single bag is suitable. If packed red blood cells (red blood cells or erythrocyte concentrate) are to be prepared, double bags connected by integral tubing should be used. When the unit is to be used for preparation of platelet concentrate, a pack of triple bags is suitable. Special bags with multiple satellite bags are also available for pediatric patients and for frozen storage at ultra low temperatures. These bags are designed in such a way that transfer of the contents may be accomplished within a closed system to avoid contamination. Should a bag have to be entered for transfer purposes, sterile technique must be followed, and the contents of the bag used within 24 hours.

Segments of plastic tubing connected to the bag, which are used for testing, should have the same identification as the bag. Should the identification number be different from that on the bag, the segment closest to the bag with the same number as the other segments must not be removed.

CENTRIFUGATION

The outcome of centrifugation depends on two factors, the relative centrifugal force and the duration of centrifugation. The relative centrifugal force (RCF-g) is the product of $0.00001118 \times r \times N^2$, where r is the radius of the rotor in centimeters and N is the number of revolutions per minute. Since different rotors have different radii, different speeds are used to achieve the same RCF in different centrifuges (see Chap. 1). The following RCF/minutes combinations are useful in the preparation of blood components: 5000 g/5 min for preparation of erythrocyte or platelet concentrate; 4170 g/10 min for preparation of cryoprecipitate; 5000 g/7 min for preparation of leukocyte-poor erythrocytes or cell-free plasma. All three combinations are referred to as heavy spin, while 4170 g/2 minute for preparation of platelet-rich plasma is referred to as light spin. However centrifugation at 5000 g is known as a plasma heavy spin.

For preparation of a platelet concentrate, centrifugation is done at 22°C., while for all other blood components, centrifugation is carried out between 1 and 6°C. Balancing the material in opposite sides is important and can be easily done with rubber disks of different weights. A protective plastic bag is very useful. The ports and tubings attached to the bag should be protected from breakage. Manual braking which disturbs the final bag content of blood should be avoided. All safety precautions should also be observed.

RED BLOOD CELLS (HUMAN)

Red blood cells are also known as packed cells. However, *erythrocyte concentrate* may be a more appropriate term. Blood should be drawn in a double bag. It can be prepared by transferring the plasma from the top of the unit to a satellite bag with the aid of a plasma expressor. The amount of plasma transferred to the satellite bag can be measured with a scale. Usually 225 ml of plasma is removed and the resultant erythrocyte concentrate has a hematocrit of about 70 per cent. When leukocyte-poor erythrocytes are needed (see below), the unit should be centrifuged and the buffy coat layer removed. The resultant erythrocyte concentrate would have a hematocrit of about 90 per cent and is also known as super-packed red blood cells. Erythrocyte concentrates can be prepared from whole blood at any time before the expiration date. If the unit has to be entered to remove the plasma, the cells must be used within 24 hours.

WASHED RED BLOOD CELLS

Properly washed erythrocytes contain: (1) A small number of leukocytes and platelets, reducing the chance of HLA immunization (sensitization) and a febrile reaction. (2) Very few microaggregates. This may be important as a suitable preparation for patients with pulmonary dysfunction or those undergoing cardiopulmonary bypass or massive transfusion. (3) Trace amounts of plasma. Thus, they are virtually devoid of regular and irregular antibodies, including plasma proteins as well as anticoagulants or unwanted metabolites such as ammonia and lactate.

Erythrocytes can be washed by multiple batch processing through centrifugation and decanting of the supernatant fluid. It is more convenient but expensive to use machines designed for deglycerolization of frozen red blood cells. The efficiency of washing depends a great deal on the amount of fluid and the method used. Washed erythrocytes should be used within 24 hours, because they are prepared in an open system.

LEUKOCYTE-POOR RED BLOOD CELLS

The majority of febrile non-hemolytic transfusion reactions can be alleviated by transfusing leukocyte-poor erythrocytes (with less than 25 per cent of the original leukocytes).

Leukocyte-poor erythrocytes can be prepared by several techniques: (1) Double centrifugation: Light spin followed by a heavy spin with the bag in the inverted position. The supernatant from the light spin can be used to prepare platelet concentrate and fresh frozen plasma. After the heavy spin, only the lower 80 per cent of erythrocytes is used for transfusion. (2) Inverted centrifugation: One heavy spin is required, and again only the lower 80 per cent of erythrocytes is used for transfusion. (3) Filtration: Passing the blood through a nylon filter is an efficient method for removal of granulocytes. Only blood collected in heparin can be used for this procedure. It therefore is seldom used. The cotton filters used in Europe remove lymphocytes as well as granulocytes (Diepenhorst, 1975). Preparations made from the above three methods contain from 5 to 30 per cent of the leukocytes and platelets in the original blood. (4) Sedimentation with HES (Donner, 1975): This provides a 90 per cent yield of erythrocytes with only about 10 per cent of the original number of leukocytes or platelets. (5) Washing: Washing erythrocytes stored in the liquid or frozen state provides good recovery of erythrocytes with a low number of leukocytes and platelets. (6) Frozen deglycerolized red blood cells. The freeze-thaw and wash methodologies described below result in a product with the least content of plasma, platelets, and leukocytes. It is used when maximally leukocyte-poor red blood cells are needed.

NEOCYTES

Some patients, such as those with thalassemia major or dyserythropoietic anemia, require repeated transfusion. Since each milliliter of erythrocytes theoretically could deposit 1 mg of iron in the tissue, hemochromatosis is likely to develop in these cases. If young RBCs (neocytes) with a 90-day life instead of conventional RBCs with a 60-day life are transfused, the number of transfusions could be reduced by one third. This in turn decreases the amount of iron deposits in the tissue.

Neocytes can be prepared by apheresis (Corash, 1981) or from an ordinary unit of blood (Graziano, 1982). Neocytes have a half-life of about 48 days (29 days for normal), a reticulocyte count of about 5 per cent (1 per cent for normal), and higher pyruvate kinase activity (1.3 times the normal).

PLATELET CONCENTRATES

These have several characteristics and requirements. Single units are prepared from units of whole blood before refrigeration. Platelet-rich plasma is separated by a light spin from the erythrocytes. A platelet concentrate is then obtained by a heavy spin of the platelet-rich plasma. Centrifugation should be done at 22°C. The separation must be performed within four hours after the blood is drawn. Therefore, the plasma portion can be frozen and used as fresh frozen plasma. Between 30 and 50 ml of plasma should be left with the platelets when the concentrate is stored at 20 to 24°C. However, only 20 to 30 ml of plasma is required when the concentrate is stored at 1 to 6°C. A unit should contain more than 5.5×10^{10} platelets (75 per cent of units tested after storage for 48 hours at 1 to 6°C. and for 72 hours at 22°C.) Multiple units of platelets from a single donor can be prepared by repeated bleeding using a manual method or an automated pheresis technique as described previously.

FRESH FROZEN PLASMA (FFP)

FFP can be prepared from a single heavy spin or from a double centrifugation to prepare platelet concentrate at the same time. Each unit contains about 225 ml of plasma. FFP should be frozen in a protective container within six hours after collection by placing it in a dry ice–alcohol bath or in a freezer at −30°C. or below. Bags should be frozen in a horizontal position and stored in a vertical position so that any inadvertent thawing will be apparent. When stored at −18°C. or less, the shelf-life is 12 months. When requested, FFP can be thawed with agitation in a 37°C. water bath and should be used within two hours.

CRYOPRECIPITATE (CRYO) OR CRYOPRECIPITATED ANTI-HEMOPHILIC FACTOR (AHF)

Plasma should be separated from erythrocytes within four hours of collection by a heavy spin. The plasma should be frozen within two hours of separation (or six hours of collection) in a mechanical freezer at −30°C. or less or in a dry ice–alcohol (95 per cent) bath. Frozen plasma should then be thawed between 1 and 6°C. overnight in a refrigerator or more quickly in a water bath at 4°C. The AHF-poor plasma is separated from the cryoprecipitate after light centrifugation, leaving about 10 ml of plasma with the cryoprecipitate. The precipitate should be frozen within four hours and stored at −18°C. or below in such a manner that thawing will be apparent. A bag of cryoprecipitate should contain on the average about 80 to 100 units of AHF per unit. When stored at

5

− 18°C. or below, the shelf-life is 12 months. When requested, cryoprecipitate may be thawed in a 37°C. water bath and then should be maintained at room temperature and used as soon as possible or within six hours of thawing.

OTHER BLOOD COMPONENTS

Single donor plasma can be separated from whole blood within 40 days after collection. If stored at − 18°C., the shelf-life is five years. It is mainly used for fractionation purposes by specially equipped institutions. Plasma from which cryoprecipitate has been removed must be so designated.

Whole blood (human) with cryoprecipitate removed is occasionally used as is whole blood (human) with platelets removed.

Processing and Distribution

PROCESSING OF BLOOD

Tests for Each Unit of Blood or Blood Component

ABO and RH$_0$ Typing. ABO grouping includes typing of cells (forward) and typing of serum or plasma (reverse). Anti-A,B should be included in cell typing to detect weak A variants, while A_2 cells should be included to confirm the presence of Anti-A_1 in the serum or reverse grouping. Typing for Rh_0 should also include a diluent control or albumin control. Anti-DC or anti-DE may be included as a double check. Cells negative for anti-D must be examined by the antiglobulin test for the detection of the D^u variant. Manual methods are usually used for a small number of donors, while automated procedures are usually used in large centers. Confirmation of all ABO and Rh_0 negative types is required on receipt of whole blood or red blood cell–containing components from another institution.

Antibody Screening (Detection). Emphasis on screening for irregular antibodies of donor blood has diminished in recent years for two reasons: (1) antibodies other than anti-A or anti-B in donor's blood have not been reported to cause a hemolytic transfusion reaction (Mollison, 1983); (2) as erythrocyte concentrates are being widely used for transfusion, the antibodies in the remaining small amount of plasma become less significant.

In some countries, an acceptable practice is to pool plasma of several donors in a preliminary screening. Since only about 1 to 2 per cent of donor serum is expected to have irregular antibodies, the amount of antiglobulin serum used can then be greatly reduced. Since human body temperature is close to 37°C., testing of antibodies at room temperature or at 4°C. may not be a valid approach.

Test for Syphilis. The wisdom of testing blood donors for syphilis by serologic methods has been questioned recently. If the donor has spirochetemia, serologic tests are usually negative, whereas, in the presence of anti-spirochetal antibodies, the donor blood is usually not infectious. VDRL or RPR tests are usually used for a small number of donors, while ART (automated reagin test) is usually used in large blood centers (see Chap. 47).

Tests for Hepatitis. Although viral hepatitis has been reviewed in Chapters 13 and 39, a brief review of testing is in order. Post-transfusion hepatitis has been found associated with type B (about 10 per cent), one documented case of type A, and the remaining with non-A non-B. However, antigen or antibodies related to type A hepatitis can be demonstrated only in selected, specially equipped laboratories. Very little information is available for the non-A and non-B types of hepatitis. Type B hepatitis is caused by Dane particles which consist of DNA core and a protein coat. Anti-core antibodies and DNA polymerase can be demonstrated during the acute stage of infection and occasionally post infection in selected laboratories. The protein outer coat has the same specificity as HBsAg (hepatitis B surface antigen). HBsAg itself is probably not infectious. HBsAg has several determinants: ayw1, ayw2, ayw3, ayw4, ayr, adw2, adw4, adr, adyw, and adyr. Only ad and ay can be determined easily for epidemiologic purposes. Persons with HBsAg are often positive for HBeAg or anti-HBe, which do not normally occur simultaneously. The presence of HBeAg may indicate infectivity, while the presence of anti-HBe usually indicates non-infectivity. More tests are available for HBsAg than perhaps for any other disease. Only the third generation tests are allowed for testing blood donors. Those tests capable of detecting all the antigens in the Bureau of Biologics (BOB) panel 2-C are qualified as third generation tests, i.e., RIA (radioimmunoassay), EIA (enzyme immunoassay), RPHA (reverse passive hemagglutination), and latex agglutination. All third generation tests are highly sensitive, but none of them is completely specific. Confirmatory tests such as neutralization are normally required. Third generation tests can detect a majority of donors who are capable of transmitting type B hepatitis. The fact that only about 10 per cent of post-transfusion hepatitis individuals are positive for HBsAg and that the percentage of reduction in post-transfusion hepatitis owing to testing is about 20 per cent tends to support this conclusion (Prince, 1975; Barker, 1970). According to a CAP survey, RIA is used by a majority of laboratories and offers the highest sensitivity and specificity (Polesky, 1980).

TESTS FOR SELECTED COMPONENTS

Platelet Count. Platelet counts are used to establish the yield and efficiency of plateletpheresis. Occasional platelet counts from units of platelet concentrates are also required. The number of platelets in relation to the volume of plasma in the bag determines the pH and hence the viability of platelets. The pH of a platelet preparation must be 6.0 or greater at the time of expiration. The plasma-to-platelet count ratio, as well as storage temperatures, are important in this regard. Sterility should be checked periodically on expired units.

Leukocyte Count. A leukocyte count is useful in determining the yield and proficiency of a leukapheresis procedure. A differential count, including percentage of granulocytes, should also be done in order to derive an absolute granulocyte count.

HLA Typing. In recipients refractory to platelet transfusion, the use of HLA-compatible donors may be helpful (Chap. 33). The benefit of using ABO and HLA-compatible donors for granulocyte transfusion has not been well established (Schiffer, 1974).

AHF Assay. Determination of AHF activity on selected units of cryoprecipitate is required. An average of 80 units of AHF (Factor VIII) per unit is required.

Total Protein. Determination of the donor's total serum protein is required for plasmapheresis programs.

LABELING OF BLOOD COMPONENTS

Each unit of blood or blood component should be labeled *correctly and clearly* with the nature of the contents in the bag and the date of expiration. Results of routine testing—ABO, Rh_0, antibody screening, and tests for syphilis and hepatitis—should also be included. Sufficient information should be on the unit so one can trace the donor and the institution where the unit was drawn and processed. With advances in computer technology, labels readable by a scanner as well as by the human eye have been proposed to reduce human transcription errors (Technical Manual of AABB, Miller, 1977, Chap. 6). In the United States, labels should satisfy the requirements set forth by the FDA (Food and Drug Administration) and the American Association of Blood Banks (AABB) or the Red Cross. For details, one should consult the most recent information from the Code of Federal Regulations, AABB Standards for Blood Banks and Transfusion Services, Technical Manual of AABB (Widmann, 1981), Red Cross Blood Service Directives, and American Blood Commission (Hubbell, 1981).

SHIPPING OF BLOOD COMPONENTS

All blood components are potentially hazardous and carry the possibility of transmitting hepatitis. Hence, they should be handled with meticulous care and respect. All components stored at 1 to 6°C. should be shipped with ice to ensure a temperature of 1 to 10°C. Materials which melt at 10°C. may be used as monitoring devices. Platelet concentrates stored at 20 to 24°C. should be shipped at temperatures as close as possible to 22°C. Fresh frozen plasma and frozen erythrocytes stored at −80°C. should be shipped with dry ice. Frozen erythrocytes stored in liquid nitrogen (low glycerol technique) should be shipped in a liquid nitrogen container; however, this may be impractical for long-distance transportation.

INVENTORY CONTROL

Ideally, no blood or blood components should be allowed to outdate. Although this is impractical or even impossible in small hospitals, every effort should be made to reduce such waste. Effective inventory control and an efficient transportation system can be of great help to improve the shelf-life. Computerized inventory control was intensively investigated about 10 years ago without success, largely because of high cost hardware and inadequate technology at that time. With advances in telecommunication systems and reductions in the cost of data processing, there is no doubt that effective inventory control will soon be available in many hospitals. Several regional blood centers as well as regional associations of blood service units already provide such inventory control. The Red Cross Blood Program has such a computer facility in Washington, D.C., for its 57 blood programs. Like the National Clearinghouse programs of the AABB, such inventory control assists immeasurably in responding to local variations in blood supply and demand by facilitating shipments of blood to meet patient care requirements and reduce outdating of blood. Although accurate figures for the entire nation are not available, outdating of blood probably approaches 10 per cent. Most of the blood in the United States is transfused within the first two weeks of storage. Therefore, the recent extension of duration of preservation from 21 days with CPD to 35 days for CPD adenine may or may not have a significant impact on outdating of blood with associated waste of red blood cells.

Preservation of Blood Components

STORAGE OF ERYTHROCYTES IN THE LIQUID STATE

Criteria. Erythrocytes which are infused into a recipient must be viable and functioning properly. Viability can be measured by tagging the erythrocytes with ^{51}Cr and estimating the number of tagged cells remaining in circulation 24 hours after transfusion. The 70 per cent viability criterion was chosen as the minimal requirement for limiting the shelf-life to 21 days when erythrocytes are stored between 1 and 6°C. (Fig. 43–1). This type of assay requires the use of radioactive isotopes and has to be done *in vivo:* however, an alternative *in vitro* method has been found to approximate the survival rate by measuring the level of adenosine triphosphate (ATP) in erythrocytes. ATP plays an important role in the glycolytic process of the erythrocyte by providing 8000 calories/mole as energy when it is split into adenosine diphosphate or adenosine monophosphate. The percentage of ATP after different periods of storage shows excellent correlation with values obtained by the *in vivo* measurement (Table 43–1).

It is of equal importance that transfused erythrocytes function properly, i.e., release oxygen to the tissue cells. Recently, 2,3–DPG (diphosphoglycerate) has been shown to play an important role in erythrocyte capability of releasing oxygen (Fig. 28–2). 2,3-DPG is an intermediate metabolite in the glycolytic cycle of erythrocytes and has a strong affinity for hemoglobin; thus it promotes the release of oxygen from oxygenated hemoglobin (2,3-DPG + $HbO_2 \rightarrow$ 2,3-DPG Hb + O_2). Consequently, the level of 2,3-DPG has become a useful index for measuring the function of erythrocytes. The 2,3-DPG level in ACD (acid-citrate-dextrose) blood begins to decrease after two days at 4°C., whereas in CPD (citrate-phosphate-dextrose) blood the decrease begins after one week. However, after transfusion, erythrocytes regenerate 2,3-DPG after three to eight hours, and normal levels are restored within 24 hours. The importance of 2,3-DPG levels is thus limited to those recipients who require oxygen supply urgently. Other criteria for successful preservation include a minimal accumulation of undesirable metabolites such as ammonia, plasma potassium, or acid equivalents (decrease in pH value). Some important changes in CPDA-1 blood are listed in Table 43–1.

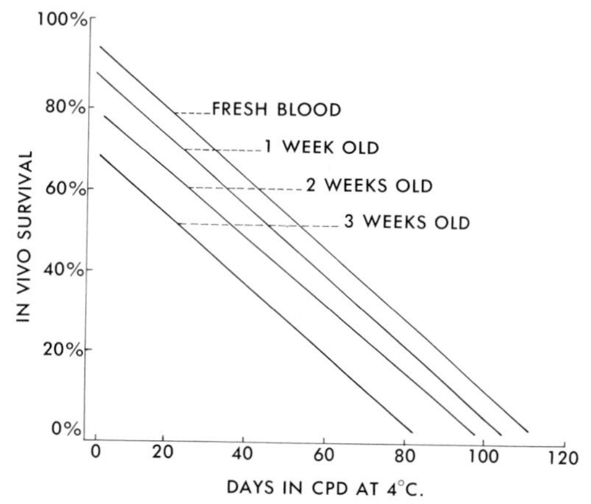

Figure 43–1. *In vivo* survival of erythrocytes stored at 4°C. (Modified from Huestis, 1981.)

Table 43–1. IMPORTANT CHANGES IN STORED CPDA-I BLOOD

		Days at 4°C.					
		0	*7*	*14*	*21*	*28*	*35*
Plasma	Glucose (mg/dl)	405	300	236	186	142	116
	Hgb (mg/dl)	37	53	103	204	353	477
	K^+ (mEq/L)	4	59	77	88	95	102
	Na^+ (mEq/L)	173	125	111	102	94	87
	Ammonia (μg/ml)	1.3	6.3	9.8	13	16	20
	pH at 37°C.	7.04	6.92	6.80	6.65	6.58	6.55
	ATP (μmol/g Hg)	4	3.73	3.88	3.50	2.87	2.28

Temperatures. The metabolic processes of erythrocytes are retarded at low temperatures. For liquid storage, 1° to 6°C. has been selected; for transportation 1° to 10°C. has been selected. For frozen storage, −65° to −95°C. for electric freezers and − 150° to − 196°C. for liquid nitrogen freezers have been designated.

Glycolytic metabolism is very slow between 1 and 6°C., practically at a standstill between −65° and −85°C., and virtually non-existent between − 150° and − 196°C.

Preservatives. The following are used for storage of erythrocytes in the liquid state (Table 43–2).

1. Heparin is an anticoagulant but not a preservative. Blood collected in heparin must be used within 48 hours and preferably within 24 hours. Heparin, which had been used for blood collected for cardiopulmonary bypass surgery and for exchange transfusion, is rarely used now except for removal of leukocytes by filtration leukapheresis. In addition to the short shelf-life of heparinized blood, heparin activates lipoprotein lipase, producing free fatty acids; these substances compete with bilirubin for binding sites on albumin. It also produces *in vivo* anticoagulation. These aspects should be taken into consideration when heparinized blood is used for exchange transfusion in newborns.

2. ACD (acid-citrate-dextrose) has been the standard solution for collecting blood for transfusion since 1943 (Mollison, 1983). Citrate chelates calcium and serves as an anticoagulant, while dextrose provides the source of energy and citric acid gives the solution a pH of about 5 (at room temperature). After the addition of blood, the plasma-ACD mixture has a pH value of about 7.1 at room temperature and about 7.4 at 4°C. The composition of ACD is listed in Table 43–2.

3. CPD (citrate-phosphate-dextrose) has essentially replaced ACD in the past few years, at least in the United States. The presence of phosphate contributes to the adenosine phosphate pool and thus improves the viability of erythrocytes. CPD has a slightly higher pH than ACD (5.5 alone, 7.5 at 4°C. with blood) and thus maintains the 2,3-DPG level for about one week with a lesser decrease in pH at 4°C.

4. CPD-Adenine (CPDA-1). The addition of 0.025 mmol/L adenine to the CPD solution as a preservative for blood collection can extend the shelf life to at least 35 days (Dawson, 1977). Adenine is required for the formation of ATP. CPD-adenine maintains the 2,3-DPG level about as well as CPD does; CPD-adenine (A1) as a preservative is available in the United States.

5. In Sweden, blood is collected into ACD-adenine solution. After centrifugation the plasma, WBCs, and platelets are transferred into a satellite bag and the RBCs are reconstituted with a saline-adenine-glucose solution from another satellite bag (Högman, 1978). The RBCs preserved with this solution have a shelf life of 35 days or longer. This product has the desired hematocrit with a very low incidence of febrile and urticarial reactions following transfusion. At the same time, additional blood components can be prepared for other patients. In the United States, a similar system (ADSOL), with the reconstituting solution containing 2 g of glucose, 750 mg of mannitol, 900 mg of NaCl, and 75 mg of adenine per 100 ml, will be available.

When RBC concentrates are preserved in CPDA-1, the hematocrit should be kept below 80 per cent and preferably below 75 per cent to maintain greater viability of the red blood cells. CPDA-2, with increased amounts of glucose and adenine, prolongs the shelf life of RBCs beyond 35 days. However, not too many physicians like to transfuse their patients with blood which has been preserved *in vitro* for such an extended period of time, since the *in vivo* life remains to be determined (Fig. 43–1).

6. Other preservatives. The addition of inosine, pyruvate, ascorbate, and methylene blue to CPD-adenine is a subject of intensive study.

STORAGE OF ERYTHROCYTES IN THE FROZEN STATE (Lukomskyj, 1974)

Cryoprotectives. In order to keep erythrocytes in the frozen state, a cryoprotective agent must be added to prevent injury from freezing and thawing. There are two types of cryoprotectives, intracellular (penetrating) and extracellular (non-penetrating). Glycerol and DMSO (dimethyl sulfoxide) belong to the first category, while HES (hydroxyethyl starch) belongs to the second. Currently only glycerol is used to keep erythrocytes in frozen state for hemotherapy. High concentrations of glycerol, about 40 to 47 per cent, are required for cells kept in an electric freezer, while low concentrations of glycerol, about 14 to 17 per cent, are required for cells kept in liquid nitrogen.

Glycerolization. Erythrocytes should be frozen within six days of collection. The unit should be equilibrated at room

Table 43–2. ANTICOAGULANTS FOR BLOOD COLLECTION

Constituent	Heparin	ACD Formula A	CPD	CPD Adenine
Heparin sodium	75000 U	—	—	—
Sodium chloride to make	1000 ml	—	—	—
Trisodium citrate	—	22.0 g	26.3 g	26.3 g
Citric acid	—	8.0g	3.27 g	3.27 g
Dextrose	—	24.5 g	25.5 g	31.9 g
NaH_2PO_4	—	—	2.22 g	2.22 g
Adenine	—	—	—	0.275 g
Water to make		1000 ml	1000 ml	1000 ml
Volume/100 ml blood	6 ml	15 ml	14 ml	14 ml

Table 43–3. TWO TYPES OF PROCEDURES FOR FREEZING RED BLOOD CELLS

Procedures	"High Glycerol–Slow Freeze"		"Low Glycerol–Rapid Freeze"	
	Tullis-Meryman-Valeri (1972, 1973)	*Huggins (1973)*	*Krijnen-Rowe (1964, 1968)*	*Åkerblom-Högman (1974)*
Glycerol (w/v)				
Initial	57%	79%	35%	35%
Final	40%	47%	17.5%	14%
Stages	2	2	1	1
Storage				
At	−65°C. to −85°C.		−150°C. to −196°C.	
Freezer	Electric		Liquid nitrogen	
Deglycerolization				
Number of solutions	3	4	2	2 3
Total volume in liters	2.5	6.6	1.5–2	1.2 3.6
Time in minutes	20 to 25	25 to 30	15 to 20	16 16
Methods of washing				
Centrifugation	Yes	No	Yes	Yes
Agglomeration	No	Yes	No	Yes

temperature with the plasma removed prior to the addition of glycerol. The glycerol should be added slowly, with constant agitation to ensure even and slow penetration of glycerol into the cells and to avoid a sudden change of osmotic pressure inside and outside the cells. After reaching equilibrium, the bag should be properly labeled and protected before being placed in a freezer. The excess glycerol may be removed to reduce space for storage and to improve the efficiency of deglycerolization. The exact procedure of glycerolization is determined by the method of storage and the techniques used for deglycerolization. Table 43–3 summarizes four protocols currently used for glycerolization of erythrocytes.

Deglycerolization. Erythrocytes to be deglycerolized should be thawed in a 37°C. water bath. Additional steps vary with the washing system in an institution. Table 43–4 summarizes the three systems used in the United States. While erythrocytes prepared by all protocols can be deglycerolized by centrifugation techniques, only erythrocytes glycerolized by the Huggins and Akerblom-Högman protocol can be deglycerolized by the agglomeration technique. It is important to remove glycerol slowly from the erythrocytes to avoid excessive hemolysis with a loss of cells. Incomplete removal of glycerol may be tested by measuring the intracellular glycerol concentration, by checking the freezing point (osmolality) of supernatant fluid, or simply by detecting presence of free hemoglobin when a few drops of washed erythrocytes are placed in a tube full of normal saline. Transfusion of erythrocytes with excessive glycerol may cause hemolysis *in vivo*.

REJUVENATION OF LIQUID-STORED ERYTHROCYTES

Red blood cells, in the liquid state, show many changes upon storage (Table 43–1). Their 2,3-diphosphoglycerate level decreases markedly after 10 days and their post-transfusion survival is reduced to below 70 per cent at the end of their shelf life. Both can be restored by incubation with media containing pyruvate, inosine, glucose, and phosphate with or without adenine (Valeri, 1972). The red cells can be frozen in the presence of glycerol and stored until needed. The same process can be applied to fresh red blood cells to increase the 2,3-DPG level to about 160 per cent; thus, two units of such modified blood can have the functional effect of three conventional units. Such a rejuvenation solution is commercially available in the United States.

STORAGE OF PLATELETS

Platelets can be stored at three different temperatures: 1 to 6°C., 22 to 24°C., and −80 or −150°C. (1) Between 20 and 24°C., continuous gentle agitation is required for warm storage platelets. Horizontal back and forth agitation may be the method of choice. Excessive agitation may cause aggregation of platelets. Between 30 and at least 50 ml of plasma is required to keep the pH above 6 for the 72 hours of shelf life.

Table 43–4. TYPES OF MACHINES FOR WASHING RED BLOOD CELLS

Machines	Blood Processes	Cytoglomerator	Cell Washer
Manufacturer	Haemonetics	Cryosan	IBM
Mode of washing	Continuous	Batch	Batch
Centrifugation	Yes	No	Yes
Agglomeration	No	Yes	No
Continuous-attention	No	Yes	No
Units washed at one time	1	5(WS 5) 1(WS 1)	1

(2) Between 1 and 6°C., only 20 to 30 ml of plasma is required and no agitation is necessary for the 48 hours of shelf life. Before use, platelets stored at 1 to 6°C. should be warmed to room temperature and resuspended. A new non-polyvinyl plastic container has been developed to extend platelet storage to five days. These new containers allow the CO_2 to escape, thus maintaining the pH level about 6.5 and consequently lengthening the shelf life of platelets. The increment in the recipient platelet counts is usually lower from platelets stored at 4°C., than those stored at 22°C. Some investigators believe that platelets stored at 4°C. may shorten the recipient's bleeding time more promptly. (3) Using 4 to 6 per cent DMSO or 5 to 14 per cent glycerol as a cryoprotective agent, platelets can be kept either at −80°C. or at −150°C. Owing to the many steps involved, the recovery rate is low; hence, this process is not yet practical for regular use.

STORAGE OF OTHER BLOOD COMPONENTS

Fresh frozen plasma (FFP) and cryoprecipitate are stored at −18°C. for a period of one year. Freezers with temperatures lower than −18°C. preserve better the activity of the coagulation factors. Both products should be thawed in a 37°C. water bath and used as soon as possible, e.g., FFP within two hours and cryoprecipitate within six hours. Gentle agitation of FFP while thawing reasonably rapidly in a 37°C. water bath allows less fibrinogen to precipitate, since fibrinogen precipitates from plasma at about 13°C. Reagent lymphocytes can be stored in the frozen state. No clinical method is available for freezing leukocytes for transfusion purposes.

Other blood products such as albumin, gamma globulin, or Rh immune globulin are prepared and supplied mainly by commercial firms. Instructions for each derivative should be followed before use.

Blood Substitutes

Blood components and derivatives are products from individual donors; they are subject to biological variations and possible contamination with unwanted agents and require extensive matching before transfusion. Blood substitutes can alleviate most of these problems. In addition, reasonably pure preparations can be made in amounts to suit our needs; thus, a standard or reference material can be made available. For these reasons, many investigators have been working on blood substitutes or so-called "artificial blood" for many years. From a functional point of view, these substitutes can be divided into two groups: (1) volume expanders and (2) oxygen carriers. Two promising oxygen carriers are hemoglobin and perfluorochemicals.

Plasma Volume Expanders. Plasma can be replaced at least temporarily by crystalloid or colloid solutions. These solutions are readily available, relatively inexpensive, stored at room temperature, and hepatitis free; furthermore, they require no compatibility testing. Consequently, these solutions are valuable in the initial treatment of hemorrhage and burn shock until definitive component therapy is available.

Among the crystalloid solutions, normal saline and Ringer's lactate are widely used. Normal saline is less expensive, while the lactate offers buffering effect and balanced electrolytes. Both will restore the blood volume only temporarily; additional supportive treatment is usually required.

Among the many colloid solutions which have been tried, only dextran and hydroxyethyl starch (HES) are available commercially in the United States. Dextrans are polysaccharides. The popular form, Dextran 70, has a molecular weight of 70,000 daltons with a half-life of six hours circulating time. Side effects such as urticaria, anaphylactic hypotension, and prolongation of bleeding time have been reported.

HES is derived from waxy starch composed almost entirely of amylopectin, with an average molecular weight of 450,000 daltons. HES metabolizes slowly and is excreted in the urine; hence, its plasma expansion effect lasts more than 24 hours. Thus far, in a few years of clinical trial, fewer bleeding tendencies have been reported than with dextran. Anaphylactic or long term side effects have not been reported. HES is available as a 6 per cent solution in normal saline. This product plays an important role in leukapheresis through its rouleau-inducing property. HES is the oncotic agent in Fluosol DA, an oxygen carrier.

Hemoglobin. Hemoglobin is the logical substitute for red blood cells because of its capacity to carry oxygen. It was soon found, however, that stromata with hemoglobin could cause hypercoagulopathy. As techniques for obtaining stromata-free hemoglobin became available, it was found that the free hemoglobin had only a two- to four-hour *in vivo* life span. While the last problem has been overcome by cross-linkage of hemoglobin molecules, the use of hemoglobin as an oxygen carrier is still in the experimental stages. Its major application would be for the military since it could be lyophilized and stored at room temperature in any amount required.

Perfluorochemicals. After systematic research, perfluorochemicals were found to have a high affinity and avidity for oxygen, to be biologically inert, and to have a very low level of toxicity. However, perfluorochemicals require 100 per cent oxygen (high Po_2) to function well, require storage in a frozen state, and are insoluble in water. One can theoretically accommodate the first two conditions and solve the third problem with the use of emulsifiers such as pluronic F-68 and yolk phospholipids. Other specific problems remain, such as one compound, perfluorotributylamine, remaining in the tissue for a long time, while another, perfluorodecalin, escapes from the lungs rapidly but does not form a stable emulsion if used alone. The currently available product, Fluosol-DA, consists of 14 per cent perfluorodecalin and 6 per cent perfluorotributylamine that must be stored in a frozen state until it is needed.

Fluosol-DA is prepared by Green Cross of Osaka, Japan. In addition to two perfluorochemicals, it also contains the two emulsifying agents mentioned above,

HES as the oncotic agent and Ringer's solution to supply electrolytes. About 40 per cent of these particles are less than 0.1 μ in size, 92 per cent are less than 0.2 μ, and all are smaller than 0.4 μ. Fluosol-DA has an oxygen carrying capacity of 7.2 volumes per volume at 37°C., about one third the capacity of red blood cells. Its half-life is from 7.5 hours for a 500 ml dose to 22 hours for a 1500 ml dose. A dose of 20 ml/kg is generally recommended.

Based on animal experimentation, Fluosol-DA showed negligible toxicity. Over 500 patients have been transfused with Fluosol-DA in Japan and no significant side reactions were observed. The five patients treated with Fluosol-DA in the United States were under close observation, and, except for a transient decrease in WBC count with the test dose, there were no significant side effects (Tremper, 1982). At present, Fluosol-DA is available at only a few selected centers by special request.

Although the clinical use of perfluorochemicals should proceed cautiously, their potential applications should be mentioned (Geyer, 1982):

1. Because of their inert nature, perfluorochemicals may be the treatment of choice for carbon monoxide poisoning.
2. Because of their small size, perfluorochemicals may circulate around thrombi in arteries to the ischemic heart or brain or to relieve a sickle cell crisis. Some animal experiments support this possibility.
3. Because of a lack of immunological incompatibility, many acute bleeders from trauma or surgery can be helped quickly, as well as patients requiring uncommon blood. Thus, the transfusion service may be changed drastically.
4. Transfusion-associated infections may be under better control.
5. Preservation of organs could be improved.
6. The inert nature of perfluorochemicals can also facilitate research of the circulatory system.

Additional research is required to make perfluorochemicals stable at room temperature and deliver oxygen under lower pressure. It should also be noted that perfluorochemicals may solve only the oxygen carrying problem; many other functions of blood probably can never be substituted.

BLOOD TRANSFUSION AND THERAPEUTIC HEMAPHERESIS

Selection of Blood Components

Hemotherapy employs blood components (red blood cells, platelets, granulocytes, plasma, cryoprecipitate) and derivatives (albumin, plasma protein fraction, Factor VIII concentrate, prothrombin complex* concentrate, and immune serum globulin) for treating patients. Blood transfusions may greatly benefit patients, but certain risks are also involved, such as transmission of infection, immunization (sensitization) to foreign antigens, and the possibility of a transfusion reaction. The physician must weigh the expected benefits against the potential danger before requesting blood for his patient. The following are useful recommendations:

1. Don't order a blood transfusion unless it is definitely indicated. Avoid "cosmetic" transfusions.
2. When a transfusion is indicated, use as little blood as possible. The incidence of hepatitis and other complications increases proportionately with the number of units transfused. Although demand for the "one unit transfusion" has been questioned, there are times when it is more appropriate to transfuse one unit than two.
3. Transfuse only the components needed by the patient, reducing complications due to unwanted components in whole blood and saving the other components for other recipients. Common blood components and derivatives with quantity expected from each unit, shelf-life (preservation or storage interval), and main indications are listed in Table 43–5. The values are approximate and may vary from unit to unit.

Some blood components are not listed in Table 43–5. For instance, leukocyte-poor blood has been largely replaced by thawed frozen or washed erythrocytes, which offer many additional theoretical advantages. Single-donor plasma has essentially been replaced by fresh frozen plasma or albumin preparations. Quite often, patients may need platelets and granulocytes; combined apheresis can harvest both at the same time.

The risk of transmitting hepatitis is a serious consideration. Albumin, immune serum globulin, and anti-Rh_0(D) immune globulin are practically hepatitis free. Factor II, VII, IX, and X preparations, which carry a high incidence of transmitting hepatitis, are not recommended. Cryoprecipitate can be used as a substitute for fibrinogen, and FFP can be substituted for Factors II, VII, IX, and X. All other blood components can transmit hepatitis; furthermore, washed erythrocytes (fresh or frozen) are believed to have less risk of hepatitis because of the dilution factor.

In summary, indications for transfusion of blood components and derivatives embrace the following: (a) Volume replacement for acute blood loss, i.e., hemorrhage, trauma, burns. (b) Red blood cell mass deficiency (chronic anemia with symptoms). (c) Coagulation factor deficiencies. (d) Leukocyte or platelet defect or decreased number. (e) Cardiopulmonary bypass (open heart surgery). (f) Exchange transfusion.

4. The selection of blood components or derivatives for various clinical conditions is dependent on the judgment of the clinician to provide for the needs of each patient. However, according to current knowledge, some general guidelines can be made, as summarized in Table 43–6. A number of clinical conditions which may not need any blood components or derivatives but which require the assistance of blood bank personnel are listed in Table 43–7.
5. It is important to request blood for transfusion well in advance so that appropriate components can be prepared and tests can be performed properly. Table 43–8 lists the approximate time required for pretransfusion examination and preparation.

*Factor IX.

Table 43–5. BLOOD COMPONENTS AND DERIVATIVES USED IN HEMOTHERAPY

Blood or Blood Components	Quantity	Shelf Life	Indications
Whole blood	450 ml blood 63 ml CPD 60 g hemoglobin 40% hematocrit	21 days at 4°C. (CPD, ACD) 35 days at 4°C. (CPD-adenine)	Brisk active bleeding.
Red blood cells (erythrocyte concentrate)	280 ml volume 60 g hemoglobin 70% hematocrit	Same as whole blood (1 day if opened)	Anemias, slow blood loss.
Washed red blood cells	250 ml volume 57 g hemoglobin 70% hematocrit	1 day (4°C.)	Prevention of febrile non-hemolytic transfusion reaction. Prevent HLA and protein sensitization. Reduce risk of hepatitis.
Frozen-thawed red blood cells (washed)	250 ml volume 54 g hemoglobin 60% hematocrit	3 years in freezer 1 day after washing	Supply of rare blood, autotransfusion, inventory control. Prevention of HLA and protein immunization as well as febrile nonhemolytic transfusion reaction.
Platelet concentrate	30–50 ml 20–30 ml 5.5×10^{10}	5 days (22° C.) 2 days (4° C.)	Hemorrhage, quantitative or qualitive platelet disorder.
Plateletpheresis	350 ml 5×10^{11}	1 day (22°C.) or (4° C.)	HLA-compatible recipient possible.*
Granulocyte concentrate pheresis	400 ml 2×10^{10}	Should be transfused immediately (4°C.)	Infections unresponsive to antibiotics in granulocytopenic patients.
Fresh frozen plasma	225 ml 13 g protein	1 year (−18°C.)	Supply coagulation factors, maintain blood volume, supply plasma for exchange transfusion.
Cryoprecipitate	10 ml 80 AHF units	1 year (−18°C.)	Supply factor VIII and fibrinogen (hemophilia A, von Willebrand's disease, and hypofibrinogenemia).
Factor VIII concentrate (lyophilized)	Up to 1000 units	2 years (2–8°C.)	Hemophiliacs.
Factor IX concentrate (lyophilized Factors II, VII, IX, X)	500 ml	Up to 2 years (2–8°C.)	Factor IX deficiency (hemophilia B).
†Albumin 5% 25%	250–500 ml 50–100 ml	3 years below 30°C.	Hypovolemia, burns, for binding bilirubin. Cerebral edema, hypoalbuminemia.
Plasma protein fraction 5%	250–500 ml	3 years below 30°C.	Hypovolemic shock, hypoproteinemia.
Immune serum globulin	2–10 ml	3 years (2–8°C.)	Prevent and modify type A hepatitis and certain other infections. Prophylactic use in patients with hypogammaglobulinemia.
Anti-Rh_0 (D) immune globulin	300 μg	1½ years (2–8°C.)	Prevent Rh_0 (D) immunization (e.g., postpartum or postabortion) and after inadvertent transfusion of Rh_0 (D)-positive red blood cell–containing components to an Rh_0 (D)-negative person.

*With less exposure to hepatitis and red cell antigen.
†Practically no risk of hepatitis.

Table 43–6. BLOOD COMPONENTS AND DERIVATIVES RECOMMENDED FOR VARIOUS CLINICAL CONDITIONS

Clinical Conditions	Preparation(s) Recommended and Comments
Active bleeding	Whole blood, less than three days old, if possible, for massive bleeding; red blood cells* or erythrocyte concentrate (EC)* and fresh frozen plasma (FFP) plus platelets can also be used.
Anemia: Transient Aplastic	Red blood cells (RBC) or EC within 7 days to reduce frequency of transfusion and exogenous iron.
Routine surgery	Whole blood, RBC,* or EC* of any age; fresh whole blood for unusual or massive bleeding; RBC, FFP, and platelets in lieu of fresh whole blood.
Cardiopulmonary bypass	Fresh RBC and non-colloid solution, washed RBC and colloid solution, fresh whole blood.
Repeated febrile/allergic transfusion reactions	Washed frozen or fresh erythrocytes; leukocyte-poor blood for febrile reaction.
Intrauterine transfusion	Washed erythrocytes (erythrocytes without lymphocytes).
Exchange transfusion for newborn	Fresh whole blood for Rh_0 sensitization, EC of mother's group + FFP (child's group) for ABO sensitization; albumin may replace FFP.
Hemodialysis, renal or hepatic failure	Frozen-thawed RBC or washed erythrocytes, red blood cell concentrate.
Anti-IgA requiring transfusion	Washed erythrocytes, frozen-thawed preferred; blood from IgA deficient donors.
Thrombocytopenia with hemorrhage or impending hemorrhage	Platelet concentrate (PC), HLA compatible in refractory patients.
Granulocytopenia with infection or impending infections	Granulocyte concentrate for antibiotic refractory cases.
Agammaglobulinemia or preventing hepatitis A	Immune serum globulin, recommended for laboratory accidental needle sticks.
Hemophilia or von Willebrand's disease	Cryoprecipitate or AHF concentrate (not in von Willebrand's disease).
Afibrinogenemia or hypofibrinogenemia	Cryoprecipitate, FFP, no commercial concentrate available.
Other coagulopathy	FFP or FFP deficient in Factor VIII.
Shock without hemorrhage	Albumin, colloid or non-colloid solutions.
Cerebral edema	25% albumin.
Prevention of Rh_0 sensitization	Anti-Rh_0 (D) immune globulin for Rh_0 (D)-negative women in pregnancy or after accidental transfusion with Rh_0 (D)-positive blood.

*The terms *erythrocyte concentrate* (EC) and *red blood cells* (RBC) are used interchangeably.

6. Consider autotransfusion for elective surgery, especially for female children and women in child-bearing age groups and for patients requiring blood from rare donors.

WHOLE BLOOD TRANSFUSION

Indications. Whole blood transfusion is rarely indicated except in cases of active bleeding that cannot be stopped immediately and in some exchange transfusions.

Limitations. When whole blood is stored at 4°C., the majority of granulocytes lose their phagocytic activity in three days, and practically all phagocytic activity is lost after four days. The number of granulocytes in one unit of blood (approximately 2.5×10^9) is too small to be of therapeutic value, even when all are alive and functioning. Whole blood cannot provide any meaningful number of granulocytes even when the blood is fresh.

Platelets in whole blood lose most of their viability after 12 hours, and almost all viability is lost in 24 hours. Whole blood is thus not a reliable or effective substitute for platelets.

There are changes in plasma proteins in stored blood. The half-life of factors V, VIII, and XI is about one week. Therefore, whole blood is not the best substitute for these three factors.

When whole blood is used for transfusion, only ABO type-specific blood should be used; otherwise, strong anti-A or anti-B in donor's blood plasma can cause a severe hemolytic transfusion reaction.

Since whole blood cannot be relied upon to provide meaningful numbers of platelets, granulocytes, or coagulation factors, the major consideration is eryth-

Table 43–7. THERAPEUTIC PROCEDURES RELATED TO BLOOD BANK

Clinical Conditions	Procedures Used and Comments
Elective surgery, rare blood type, many antibodies	Autotransfusion of liquid or frozen stored blood; avoids many other complications
Polycythemia, hemosiderosis	Therapeutic phlebotomy to reduce viscosity or exogenous iron
Macroglobinemia, undesirable elements in plasma	Plasmapheresis or plasma exchange to reduce viscosity or harmful agents in plasma
Selected types of leukemia	Leukapheresis (in experimental stages only)
Aplastic bone marrow	Bone marrow transplantation requires HLA compatible donors
End-stage renal disease	Kidney transplantation requires HLA- and ABO-compatible donors

Table 43–8. APPROXIMATE TIME REQUIRED FOR PREPARING FOR A BLOOD TRANSFUSION*

Procedures	Time in Minutes
1. Collecting the blood specimen	10
2. ABO and Rh_0 typing	10
3. ABO and Rh_0 typing plus antibody screening	45
4. Typing, antibody screening, and crossmatching	60
5. Antibody identification, additional	60 + (up to several days)
6. Fresh frozen plasma, thawing and testing	40
7. Cryoprecipitate, thawing and testing	20
8. Washing erythrocytes	45
9. Thawing and washing of frozen erythrocytes	60

*Excluding pick-up and delivery.

rocyte storage. The survival rate of erythrocytes stored in CPD at 4°C. for one week is about 98 per cent, and their 2,3-DPG level is about 99 per cent, both of which are essentially the same as in one- to two-day-old blood. The accumulation of metabolites or change in pH is also minimal. Thus, one can define fresh blood as blood less than seven days old. However, the *in vivo* survival rate decreases as the duration of storage of erythrocytes at 4°C. increases (Fig. 43–1). This fact should be taken into consideration for those patients with aplastic anemia, sickle cell anemia, thalassemia and other chronic anemias, who require repeated transfusions. The use of fresh red cells will reduce the number of transfusions and, hence, decrease the chance of hemosiderosis.

TRANSFUSION OF RED BLOOD CELLS

Indications. In chronic anemia, patients may have a hemoglobin as low as 4 g/dl without symptoms. On the other hand, virtually no surgeon is willing to accept a patient for major surgery with a hemoglobin below 8 g/dl except under special conditions. In a newborn child, a hemoglobin level of 14 g/dl is considered anemic. An average adult can afford to lose up to 1 L of blood and have it replaced with a crystalloid or colloid solution (Table 43–9), while a loss of 2 L of blood may be critical to life. These are only general guidelines to orient blood bankers. Each patient's particular condition must be judged by his own physician.

Conventional erythrocyte concentrates with 60 to 70 per cent hematocrits are satisfactory in most conditions; those with about 90 per cent hematocrit are difficult to infuse and are suitable only under selected conditions in which blood volume is a critical issue. For minimizing febrile transfusion reactions, leukocyte-poor erythrocytes have essentially been replaced by frozen-thawed or washed erythrocytes whenever feasible.

Freezing and Washing. The use of frozen washed erythrocytes increased five-fold from less than 1000 in 1970 to 5000 in 1975 in the American Red Cross system (Meryman, 1975). However, when medical conditions are analyzed for its usage, over 90 per cent of frozen-thawed erythrocytes were used for conditions not necessarily requiring frozen cells (Fig. 43–2). In other words, the same benefit at less cost could probably have been achieved by washing alone in the majority of these cases.

It should be stressed that the frozen state does not reduce the infectivity of type B viral hepatitis, but that dilution does (Barker, 1970). In that classic experiment, high concentrations (10^{-4} to 10^{6}) of

Table 43–9. PLASMA EXPANDERS DERIVED FROM BLOOD

	Fresh Frozen Plasma	5% Albumin	25% Salt-Poor Albumin	Plasma Protein Fraction
Unit volume	230 ml	250 ml	50 ml	250 ml
Sodium (mEq/L)	128+	100–160	100–160	130–160
Approximate cost/unit (1982)	$44.00	$75.00	$75.00	$75.00
Protein content	16 g (approx.)	12.5 g	12.5 g	12.5 g
Cost/g protein	$2.75	$6.00	$6.00	$6.00
Hepatitis risk	Same as whole blood	Near zero	Near zero	Near zero

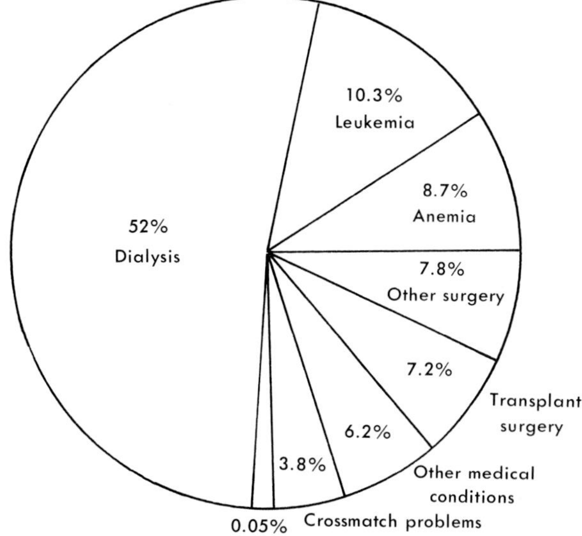

Figure 43–2. Use of frozen thawed erythrocytes in the American Red Cross System, 1974. (Data from Meryman, 1975.)

infectious agents (in the frozen state for years) produced clinical hepatitis in volunteers, lower concentrations (10^{-5} to 10^{-7}) produced antigenemia (HBsAg+), while very low blood concentrations (10^{-8}) produced neither hepatitis nor antigenemia. It should be mentioned further that the titer of HBsAg may not be parallel to the assumed infectious agent—Dane particles. Washing with large amounts of fluid dilutes infectious agents; although it may not completely prevent the infection, it appears to reduce the severity as reported in chimpanzees (Alter, 1978). For reducing the infectivity of viral hepatitis, washing is obviously the main factor. From an economic point of view, washing erythrocytes costs much less than washing frozen erythrocytes. In addition to reducing the incidence of hepatitis, febrile and urticarial reactions may be minimized with washed erythrocytes. For patients with anti-IgA, washed erythrocytes or compatible blood from an IgA-deficient donor should be used. In at least one case, frozen-thawed washed erythrocytes worked better than washed erythrocytes as transmembranous passage of glycerol may completely remove the IgA on the surface of erythrocytes (Miller, 1975).

Compatibility. ABO compatibility is an absolute requirement in erythrocyte transfusion. The majority of fatal transfusion reactions are due to ABO incompatibility. Group O erythrocytes can be used in the form of erythrocyte concentrate for other groups, and group A or B can be used for an AB recipient when group-specific blood is not available (Table 43–10). Since the Rh_0(D) antigen is very antigenic, one should use erythrocytes which are Rh_0(D)-specific. While Rh_0(D)-negative cells can be used for Rh_0-positive recipients, the reverse is true only in emergency situations (Table 43–10). If the recipient is a female of child-bearing age, Rh_0(D) immune globulin (RIG) can be used to prevent immunization (300 μg for each 15 ml of erythrocytes). Hence, large volumes of RIG are required to prevent immunization to only one unit of Rh_0(D)-positive blood. Matching Rh antigens other than D is impractical at present. However, should the patient have or have had IgG irregular antibodies against antigens such as K, Fy^a, Jk^a, c, or E, erythrocytes negative for such antigens should be used, even if these irregular antibodies are no longer in the patient's serum.

When a patient with group A_1 or A_1B blood has anti-HI active above room temperature, A_1 (or A_1B) erythrocytes should be used, as this antibody has been known to cause rapid destruction of incompatible erythrocytes. When an A_2 or A_2B patient has anti-A_1 active at 37°C., A_2 erythrocytes should be transfused (Mollison, 1983); frozen-thawed group O erythrocytes may also be used when A_2 erythrocytes are not available; this is especially true when additional irregular antibodies are present, e.g., anti-M.

Post-transfusion Increment of Hemoglobin. The post-transfusion increment of hemoglobin is inversely related to the blood volume of the patient and directly

Table 43–10. ABO AND RH_0 COMPATIBILITY IN BLOOD TRANSFUSION

Blood Type of Recipient	Blood Type of Donor					
	O	*A*	*B*	*AB*	*D−*	*D+*
O	Yes	No	No	No		
A	S	Yes	No	No		
B	S	No	Yes	No		
AB	S	S	S	Yes		
D−					Yes	E
D+					Yes	Yes

S = substitute as erythrocyte concentrates without high titer anti-A or anti-B or in form of washed erythrocytes.

E = only under extreme emergency conditions, especially if the recipient is a young female.

5

related to the volume of red blood cells transfused. The popular guideline that one unit of blood will increase the recipient's hemoglobin by about 1 g/dl should be qualified in two ways: it is applicable only for recipients who weigh about 100 lb and for erythrocyte concentrate (not whole blood). Table 43–11 may illustrate this point.

The patient's blood volume (approximately 8 per cent of body weight of an adult) after hemotherapy will eventually return to pretransfusion values, so that the hematocrit rise with EC (erythrocyte concentrate) and WB (whole blood) will ultimately be the same but may require 24 hours or longer.

Irradiated RBCs. The transfusion of alive lymphocytes into immunologically incompetent patients may induce a graft-versus-host reaction which often results in a fatal outcome. Living lymphocytes can be found not only in RBC and WBC preparations, but also in platelet concentrates and even frozen washed RBCs. It is therefore recommended to irradiate blood components before transfusion into recipients who have had intensive radiation treatment or large doses of immunosuppressive drugs. A range of 1500 to 2500 rads is usually used in these cases.

PLATELET TRANSFUSION

Effective platelet transfusion became practical when platelet concentrates could be stored for 72 hours and a large number of platelets could be harvested from a single donor. Platelet transfusion has successfully prevented death from hemorrhage in many leukemic patients. In general, platelet transfusion is useful in thrombocytopenia due to poor production (leukemia or aplastic anemia) and in patients with platelet dysfunction. Platelets are less effective in idiopathic thrombocytopenia and in hypersplenic thrombocytopenia. Platelets are ineffective and may be harmful in (1) disseminated intravascular coagulation (prior to heparinization) and (2) thrombotic thrombocytopenic purpura.

Whenever feasible, ABO-compatible platelets should be used, although ABO-incompatible platelets are effective. However, the presence of strong anti-A or anti-B in large volumes (300 to 350 ml) of plasma may cause positive direct antiglobulin test and shortened red cell survival (including a hemolytic transfusion reaction) and therefore cannot be ignored. Hence, plasma compatibility is more important than erythrocyte compatibility in platelet transfusion therapy if the platelets are relatively free of red blood cells. Rh_0 antigen is an important consideration only for the female recipient of child-bearing age or where the number of transfused Rh_0-positive erythrocytes is large. In such cases, anti-Rh_0 immune globulin may be used concurrently to prevent immunization. In patients refractory to platelet transfusion, HLA-compatible donors should be used.

Patients who are HLA-A2 positive have a less favorable response than those who are HLA-A2 negative. Platelets having HLA antigens cross-reacting with the antigens of the recipient may give the same satisfactory results as the matched platelets. However, some patients may not respond to platelets completely matched for HLA-A and -B antigens. This problem may not be resolved until reliable procedures for typing and crossmatching for platelet specific antigens have become available.

Autologous platelets are suitable for patients with solid tumors without bone marrow involvement and in patients with leukemia who are in remission. Their platelets can be kept frozen for future use.

Patients undergoing major surgery with a platelet count of 30,000/μl seldom bleed; furthermore, bedridden patients seldom bleed with platelet counts of 10,000/μl. Therefore, to prepare a patient for major surgery, the patient should have a platelet count above 30,000/μl or perhaps 50,000/μl according to some surgeons. For patients with platelet counts below 20,000/μl, preventive platelet transfusion has been found very useful.

Guidelines for matching and volume considerations for infusion warrant further consideration. Rh_0 compatibility is of primary importance for young females who have child-bearing potential. Rh_0 incompatibility will not influence the platelet response and Rh-positive platelets will not harm an Rh-negative recipient. There is a small risk of developing anti-Rh_0(D), which is harmless except during pregnancy with an Rh_0-

Table 43–11. VARIABLES AFFECTING POST-TRANSFUSION INCREMENT OF HEMOGLOBIN

	Blood Volume*		Hemoglobin		
	ml	*Increment (%)*	*g/dl*	*Total (g)*	*Increment (g/dl)*
Pretransfusion					
Recipient No. 1, 100 lb	3200		10	320	
No. 2, 150 lb	4800		10	480	
Whole blood (WB)	510		14	63	
Erythrocyte concentrate (EC)	280		22.5	63	
Post-transfusion					
Recipient No. 1 infused with WB	3710	16	10.3	383	0.3
EC	3480	9	11	383	1
No. 2 infused with WB	5310	11	10.2	543	0.2
EC	5080	6	10.7	543	0.7

*Recipient's blood volume is estimated by body weight in lb × 32.

positive fetus. Given the current inability to transfuse *all* Rh_o-negative recipients with Rh_o-negative platelets, Rh_o-negative platelets should be reserved when possible for this group whose immunization to the Rh_o(D) antigen would have the most impact.

Pooling of platelets of different ABO groups has certain theoretical disadvantages (soluble antigen-antibody complexes may induce platelet clumping) and therefore should be avoided.

We use the following guidelines for platelet matching:

1. A or AB platelets should be given to group A or AB patients if available.
2. Any group platelets can be given to O patients.
3. Although B platelets are preferable, supply situations often dictate that any platelets may be given to a B recipient. Alternatively, plateletpheresis of a B donor can be performed.
4. Rh_o-negative female patients under 45 will be given Rh_o-negative platelets *if* available. If not available, the options are to order an Rh_o-negative pheresis collection, to give Rh_o-positive platelets, or to give Rh_o-positive platelets followed by Rh_o immune globulin. If Rh_o-negative platelets are not available, further medical consultation about the available options is in order. Rh_o-negative patients other than females under 45 may be given platelets without regard to Rh type.
5. Pooling platelets should be done only within ABO groups. If, for example, 5 "O" and 5 "B" platelets are available for a B recipient, two separate pools should be forwarded. Therefore, a single platelet order may consist of more than one bag.

There will be occasions when these guidelines cannot be followed, mainly because of an inability to supply the needed product. Consultation with the transfusion service physician experienced in hemotherapy is necessary in these cases to determine the most appropriate course of action.

When volume involved is of clinical concern, the platelet order should be reduced or the daily dose divided into two or more transfusion episodes. In addition, pheresis platelet concentrates can be utilized. They provide the equivalent of 10 units of platelets in a 250 to 300 ml volume. Since they outdate in 24 hours, they must be used promptly.

One unit of platelet concentrate usually contains more than 5.5×10^{10} platelets. When a unit is transfused into a recipient with a blood volume of 5500 ($5.5 \times 10^6/\mu l$ of blood) the increment is about $5.5 \times 10^{10}/5.5 \times 10^6 = 10{,}000/\mu l$. In practice, only about half of the expected number is demonstrated one hour after transfusion. As a rough guide, one unit of platelet concentrate would produce an increment of 10,000/μl in a 100-pound patient. The remaining platelets may be retained by the spleen or used up at the bleeding sites. The consumption of platelets is usually increased if the patient has a fever, sepsis, or splenomegaly. For an average adult bleeding case, 4 to 8 units of random donor platelets is a reasonable quantity to transfuse initially. If the platelet increment is not adequate, this process may be repeated every six to eight hours until the bleeding stops. Chills and febrile reactions are common in patients receiving repeated platelet transfusions and are related to immunization through previous platelet or leukocyte transfusions. These symptoms can be relieved by an injection of meperidine hydrochloride or by pretreatment with corticosteroids.

GRANULOCYTE TRANSFUSION

Before platelet transfusions became a routine procedure, many leukemic patients died from hemorrhage. Although hemorrhage can now be largely controlled by platelet transfusion, the aggressive use of chemotherapy and radiation often leads to severe infections in leukemic patients. By repeated transfusions of large numbers of granulocytes, some of these infections unresponsive to antibiotics can be brought under control.

When the absolute granulocyte count is below 500/μl, the patient's chance of contracting infection is great, and with counts of 100/μl or below, infection is almost inevitable. In granulocytopenic patients with sepsis refractory to antibiotic therapy, granulocyte transfusion is indicated. Herzig (1977) has reported granulocyte transfusion for gram-negative septicemia to be effective in a controlled clinical study. For those patients with a count less than 100/μl, preventive granulocyte transfusion has been recommended, although the prophylactic use of granulocytes has not yet been demonstrated to be effective in most clinical situations.

Since the half-life of granulocytes in the circulation is only about six to eight hours, the therapeutic effect may not be obtained unless a minimum of 10^{10} granulocytes is transfused daily to an average adult for at least four to five days. A significant rise in circulating granulocyte level post-transfusion is usually not observed. ABO-compatible granulocytes appear to be essential for a successful therapeutic response, while the importance of HLA compatibility remains unclear. Because preformed leukoagglutinins in the recipient's plasma have been found in some studies (Herzig, 1975) to result in negligible intravascular recovery of transfused granulocytes, a crossmatch for leukoagglutinating antibodies has been used by some investigators to exclude donor-recipient pairs.

Granulocytes should be transfused as soon as possible after collection. Granulocytes should be infused via a standard administration set, ordinarily over three to four hours to minimize reactions. Careful observation of the patient by nursing personnel, with a physician readily available for reactions, is necessary. Since post-transfusion increments in WBC counts are rarely above 5 per cent, the presence of an increment more than 12 hours after transfusion suggests endogenous production due to bone marrow recovery rather than successful transfusion.

Granulocyte transfusion is often accompanied by chills and fever and sometimes by severe hypotension. These reactions can be minimized by giving no more than 10^{10} cells/hour and by administering to the patient meperidine hydrochloride (25 to 50 mg parenterally to an adult) or protecting him with corticosteroids (e.g., Solu-Cortef IV prior to infusion). Less commonly, pulmonary reactions (dyspnea, cough, cyanosis, pulmonary infiltrates) may be observed; these are attributed to leukocyte adherence or clumping in pulmonary capillaries. Other reactions can also occur, e.g., urticaria, bacterial contamination causing sepsis, hemolytic reactions due to incompatible red blood cells in the granulocyte concentrate, hepatitis, and delayed graft-versus-host disease. The fact that 80 to 85 per cent of all infections can be controlled by broad-spectrum antibiotics in addition to the possible induction of alloimmunization or CMV infection by granulocyte transfusions has markedly reduced their use.

TRANSFUSION OF PLASMA COMPONENTS AND/OR DERIVATIVES

Fresh Frozen Plasma (FFP). FFP is indicated in patients with hypovolemia and/or a deficiency in coagulation factors (see Chap. 32). FFP is often used to treat shock and to supplement massive transfusions and exchange transfusions. FFP has the risk of transmitting viral hepatitis and requires 20 minutes or more for thawing. If Factor VIII has been removed in the preparation of cryoprecipitate, the unit should be so labeled.

Cryoprecipitate (Cryo). Cryoprecipitate is indicated in patients with Factor VIII deficiency, such as hemophiliacs and those with von Willebrand's disease, as well as patients with hypofibrinogenemia from various causes. The potency of each unit of cryo varies greatly, but the average value must be 80 units of Factor VIII (the majority range from 60 to 120 units). Lyophilized AHF concentrate, which may contain up to 1000 units/vial, is available and is suitable when many units are required to prevent or to stop hemorrhage. The lyophilized form does not require a freezer for storage but has a greater risk of transmitting hepatitis and may contain strong anti-A and anti-B.

About a 30 per cent Factor VIII activity level is required for major surgery. Since the half-life *in vivo* is about 12 hours, a level of 50 to 60 per cent may be required several hours before the surgery. If a patient has only a 20 per cent activity and a 60 per cent activity is desirable, then the increase is 60 per cent minus 20 per cent = 40 per cent. If the patient is about 50 kg in weight, the plasma volume should be approximately 50 × 40 = 2000 ml, and the total number of units required would be 2000 × 40 per cent = 800 units. If the activity of each bag is roughly 100 units, then 8 bags of cryo are required. As a rough guide, one bag of cryo with about 100 units of AHF activity will increase the AHF activity about 5 per cent in a 100-lb recipient. In the case of a patient with inhibitors to AHF who is hemorrhaging, larger doses may have to be tried. If unsuccessful, plasma exchange or other experimental therapy may be attempted to remove the AHF inhibitor.

Since many factors are involved, namely, actual blood volume, activity in each bag, and response of the patient, this type of estimation is only approximate. Determination of AHF activity post transfusion or a bleeding time in von Willebrand's patients is the best guide for the amount of cryo required.

Albumin. Albumin is probably the most widely used plasma derivative. It is indicated in patients with hypovolemia, especially in shock, with severe burns, with cerebral edema, and with hyperbilirubinemia. Albumin preparations that have been heated at 60°C. for 10 hours have no risk of transmitting hepatitis. Since albumin is readily available, it is often used for treatment of shock. Albumin contains 96 per cent albumin and is available in 5 per cent and 25 per cent solutions. Plasma protein fraction (PPF), which contains 83 per cent albumin and 17 per cent globulin, is available in 5 per cent preparations.

Plasma albumin with a half-life of about 17 days represents 50 to 60 per cent of circulating plasma protein and 80 per cent of plasma colloid osmotic pressure. Twenty-five grams (100 ml of a 25 per cent w/v solution) is the osmotic equivalent of 500 ml (2 units) of citrated plasma. It is also used to correct hypoproteinemia states with hypoalbuminemia secondary to (1) decreased or impaired protein intake, (2) excessive protein loss into gastrointestinal tract lumen or via kidneys, (3) decreased hepatic synthesis, (4) repeated removal of large amounts of transudates from peritoneal or pleural spaces, or (5) draining exudative wounds and transudation from large weeping surfaces, e.g., pemphigus or burns. In general, however, there is only mild improvement of patients with nephrotic syndrome and virtually none with protein-losing enteropathies after transfusion of albumin. Furthermore, albumin offers virtually no demonstrable value in the general supportive management of the hypoproteinemia of cirrhosis.

Immune Serum Globulin (ISG). ISG is used to prevent or modify type A hepatitis and other infections. Since type A hepatitis can also be transmitted parenterally and since ISG may be effective in prevention of hepatitis B, ISG is recommended for accidental needle sticks in the laboratory. ISG is also used to supplement globulins in patients with hypogammaglobulinemia. ISG is available in a 16.5 per cent solution. It must be administered intramuscularly.

Specific Immunoglobulins. Anti-Rh_o(D) immunoglobulin (RIG) is widely used for the prevention of Rh_o(D) immunization in Rh_o-negative women with an Rh_o-positive baby or for those Rh_o-negative persons who have been accidentally transfused with Rh_o-positive erythrocytes or who have received Rh_o(D)-positive platelets. One vial contains 300 μg anti-Rh_o(D) and is recommended for 15 ml of packed erythrocytes or 30 ml of whole blood. Patients receiving multiple doses of anti-Rh_o(D) immunoglobulin may have a mild febrile reaction and a slight increase in bilirubin level. Additional discussion will be found in "Immunization Associated with Pregnancy" (p. 1058).

Specific anti-HBsAg hyperimmune serum is available, but its effectiveness in preventing or modifying type B hepatitis has not yet been fully established. It is believed to be useful in needle stick exposures to hepatitis B, but its use in other situations is less clearly indicated.

Transfusions in Special Conditions

AUTOLOGOUS TRANSFUSION

The only 100 per cent compatible blood is one's own blood or blood from an identical twin. Receiving one's own blood is known as autologous transfusion (versus homologous transfusion—receiving blood from others). In an autologous transfusion, the problem of introducing foreign antigens, antibodies, or infectious or toxic agents is eliminated. Multiple phlebotomies usually stimulate erythrocyte production; the resultant mild anemia is thought to improve capillary blood flow.

Autologous transfusions can be achieved by (1) predeposit, (2) intraoperative deposit, or (3) intraoperative salvage.

Predeposit. A patient can donate several units of blood, which can be stored at 4°C. or in the frozen state for future use such as elective surgery or for unexpected needs. This type of practice is particularly suitable for patients with multiple antibodies or for those who require rare blood types or have religious beliefs prohibiting acceptance of homologous blood. Individuals at risk for a nuclear accident with excessive radiation exposure should also consider the feasibility of such frozen storage of their own red blood cells.

The candidate should be in good health with a hemoglobin of at least 11 g/dl. While age and body weight can differ from the requirements for routine blood donation, the amount of anticoagulant in the bag must be adjusted according to the amount of blood drawn. Since only three days after donation are required to re-establish the original volume (often 24 hours is sufficient), one donation every four days is acceptable. Thus, at least four units could be available for 21-day storage. The unit should be processed routinely, and crossmatching is recommended as a check for unit identification. Unit identification should be done as in a manual apheresis procedure to ensure against the error of misidentification. In case there is an unexpected delay in surgery, the unit can be re-infused and another unit drawn to avoid outdating. However, this so-called "leapfrog" technique may be too involved to be of any practical benefit.

Intraoperative Deposit. This is known as hemodilution. Phlebotomy is performed immediately after induction of anesthesia. Lost blood volume is replaced with either saline, lactated Ringer's solution, or serum albumin. Hemodilution has been widely used in cardiopulmonary bypass. With this procedure, proportionately fewer erythrocytes are lost per volume of blood shed during surgery and less homologous blood replacement is required.

Intraoperative Salvage. In many types of surgery, such as for a ruptured ectopic pregnancy, chest and abdominal trauma, neurosurgery, and joint surgery, large volumes of blood may be recovered and given back to the patient. To avoid microaggregates, tissue fragments and clots, the blood must be filtered and preferably washed before reinfusion to the patient. This procedure should not be used in patients with malignancy, contaminated wounds, severe hepatitis, renal failure, or a coagulopathy. The theoretical risk of disseminated intravascular coagulation from red cell fragments is reduced by using appropriate microaggregate filters (Table 43–12).

MASSIVE TRANSFUSIONS

For patients with severe trauma or burns, and those requiring cardiac and vascular surgery or exchange transfusions, the amount of blood transfused may approach or exceed the recipient's blood volume. The following factors should be taken into consideration:

1. For active bleeding, whole blood is preferred. However, red blood cells (erythrocyte concentrate) and fresh frozen plasma (FFP) are excellent substitutes.
2. A large-bore needle or even a catheter may be required to increase the rate of infusion.
3. A blood warmer is usually required.
4. For extreme emergencies, ABO type-specific blood should be infused without crossmatching; however, O Rh_0-negative blood may be given (sometimes even O Rh_0-positive may be necessary) with crossmatching performed after the transfusion. Oberman (1978) has proposed the feasibility of a modified crossmatch.
5. The platelet count may drop sharply to 40,000 to 70,000/μl. However, replacement with platelets may not be required until the count is below 15,000/μl, although bleeding time may be prolonged below 100,000/μl.
6. Two units of FFP are recommended for every 10 units of stored blood infused.
7. There is no evidence that citrate and potassium in stored blood create a serious problem in massive transfusion. One ampule of sodium bicarbonate (44.5 mEq) for every 5 units of blood is recommended by some physicians (Greenwalt, 1977, p. 13).
8. Filters designed to retain microaggregates are recommended except in cases where the infusion rate must be fast, and when either fresh whole blood (as a source of viable platelets) or platelet concentrates are to be infused. Such filters should be changed after every 2 to 3 units infused to prevent reduction in flow rate and saturation of filter with particles. Table 43–12 shows several filters used with infusion sets for blood and blood components.

TRANSFUSION IN CARDIOPULMONARY BYPASS

Cardiopulmonary bypass is an essential system for open heart surgery. The patient's heparinized venous blood is drained into a 37°C. chamber where the partial pressure of O_2 is restored to the level of arterial blood and the excess O_2 and CO_2 are removed. Then the blood is pumped back to the patient. A cardiotomy aspiration system is also used to pump blood salvaged from the chest cavity back to the oxygenation chamber to be reused. With the bypass system, significant extracorporeal blood space, about 10 ml/lb body weight of patient, is created and can be compensated for by using either blood or crystalloid solutions. In patients with a body weight less than 10 kg or with a hemoglobin level less than 10 g/dl, blood is used; otherwise, 5 per cent glucose in lactated Ringer's solution is preferred by many physicians. The latter process is known as hemodilution and has the advantages of conserving blood and reducing the complications of blood transfusion. However, with this technique, the patient's hemoglobin may drop temporarily by 2 to 4 g/dl. Some degree of anemia exists even 24 hours later when equilibrium has been reached. To partially overcome this problem, red blood cells remaining in the pump system can be centrifuged, washed, and reinfused to the patient.

Table 43–12. FILTERS FOR INFUSION OF BLOOD AND BLOOD COMPONENTS

Blood Filters	Pore Size	Filter Material	Use	Contraindications
Standard				
Fenwal STD Blood Filter (large and reg. size surface area)	170 μ	Lexan plastic nylon mesh	All blood components	None
McGraw STD Blood Filter	170 μ	Nylon mesh	All blood components	None
Special				
Fenwal 4C2100	170 μ	Nylon mesh with smaller "dead" space	Fresh whole blood, platelets, AHF, cryoprecipitate	
Microaggregate (Micropore)				
Pall 40μ Ultipor Disposable Blood Filter (Pall) Corp., Glen Cove, Long Island, N.Y.)	40 μ	Pleated polyester mesh	Essentially all blood components (see contraindications) and where massive transfusions are indicated or after third unit infused within a 24-hour period	Do not use for platelet concentrates or fresh whole blood infusions.
Bentley Disposable Blood Filter (PF127, Bentley) Lab., Inc., Irvine, Cal.)	27 μ	Polyester urethane foam		
Swank In-Line Blood Filter (IL-200 Pioneer Filters, Inc., Beaverton, Ore.)	20 μ	Dacron wool		
Fenwall Microaggregate Blood Filter (Fenwal Lab., Morton Grove, Ill.) 4C2423 or 4C2131 (with tubing)	20 μ	Polyester nonwoven fiber		
Intersept Blood Filter (Johnson & Johnson Co., New Brunswick, N.J.)	20 μ	Woven Dacron mesh		
Imguard (Terumo Amer.)	25 μ	Cotton and nylon fibers	In-line removal of leukocytes.	

With a newly modified centrifuge, this process can be accomplished in three to four minutes (Yawn, 1982).

When blood is indicated, red blood cells are preferred to whole blood. Fresher blood should be used whenever feasible. When many units are required, especially Rh_0-negative blood, there is no reason that older blood cannot also be used. Although screening the patient for high titer cold agglutinins is done routinely for open heart surgery in some hospitals, its value remains to be documented. When many units of blood are transfused in a short time, warming the blood is definitely recommended.

Transient thrombocytopenia is often associated with cardiopulmonary bypass. Whether prophylactic or therapeutic platelet transfusions should be given is a controversial issue, and each individual patient should be evaluated separately. Quite often, mild and occasionally severe coagulopathies are associated with major cardiovascular surgery. Again, each case should be considered individually. Milam (1979) has presented an excellent review of transfusion in open heart surgery.

NEONATAL HEMOTHERAPY

Neonatology embraces the art and science of diagnosis and management of disorders of the newborn infant. Neonates are a special challenge to a blood transfusion service. Although exchange transfusions for hemolytic disease of newborn have diminished over the past decade, the volume of blood used by newborns in the United States remains essentially unchanged (Oski, 1977).

Normal blood volume for a neonate or newborn is approximately 10 per cent of body weight. A newborn weighing 1500 g would have a blood volume of 150 ml, while a newborn of 1000 g would have a blood volume of 100 ml. This relatively small blood volume makes the newborn liable to significant volume depletion after a minimal absolute amount of blood loss. For example, the loss of 10 ml in a 1000-g infant with 100 ml blood volume would be equivalent to a loss of a full unit of blood, or 500 ml, in an adult. In other words, more than 10 to 20 ml of blood loss in such a small infant may result in incipient or overt shock associated with volume depletion.

Neonates are subjected to multiple laboratory measurements and examinations requiring blood collection, e.g., blood gases, chemical pathologic determinations, and hematologic measurements. When such measurements, even with microsampling techniques, are frequent, with blood loss in excess of 7 to 10 ml per day, a neonate's blood volume can be depleted rapidly. These losses and resulting iatrogenic anemia require blood replacement. Newborn infants may need minimal blood volume replacement therapy in the form of 7 to 10 ml or 10 to 20 ml blood transfusions per day to maintain their total blood volume. Neonates are also susceptible to hypovolemia from a variety of causes. Hence, the need for more frequent blood transfusions in neonatology today can be appreciated.

In addition to exchange transfusions for disorders shown in Table 43–13, blood transfusions in the newborn may be considered for the following:

1. Iatrogenic anemia.
2. Newborn infants requiring surgery for such entities as cardiac defects and necrotizing enterocolitis.
3. Many circumstances associated with infants born hypovolemic, usually identified in terms of obstetrical procedures or other factors associated with labor and delivery.
4. Respiratory distress syndrome and prematurity where blood transfusions, including exchange transfusions, may be beneficial.

The term infant has blood with an increased affinity for oxygen. The P_{50} gradually increases and the increase is related both to the concentration of fetal hemoglobin and to the concentration of 2,3-DPG (Delivoria-Papadopoulos, 1976). Infants with respiratory distress syndrome have a lower P_{50} than term infants or other infants without respiratory distress. This is primarily due to decreased intracellular 2,3-DPG, as shown in Figure 28–2 (p. 632).

Exchange transfusion is performed in anticipation that blood with less oxygen affinity (higher P_{50} and increased 2,3-DPG) will promote more release of oxygen to the tissues.

In the immediate post-transfusion period, the P_{50} of infused blood depends on the storage time and anticoagulant of the unit transfused.

Exchange transfusion has been shown to increase the survival of low birth weight infants and those with RDS, although the mechanism may be unrelated to tissue oxygenation (Delivoria-Papadopoulos, 1976). Arterial oxygen concentration rises shortly after exchange transfusion, and there may be an improvement in pulmonary ventilation and perfusion that is not related to the properties of the transfused erythrocytes.

Practical and safe approaches to transfusion of neonates include the following (Kevy, 1977):

1. Collect a unit of blood into a CPD-quadruple donor pack. This can be aseptically separated into four units of 125 ml each. Each of these smaller units can then be further subdivided, provided that all the blood is utilized within 24 hours of the procedure. With this technique, the neonate need not be cross-matched more than once throughout a seven-day period, during which time he can receive as many as 16 transfusions. Also, several infants may be cross-matched to a single donor unit, i.e., "cow" method.
2. Use of donor blood drawn to a volume of 225 ml into a CPD triple pack with an appropriate reduction of the anticoagulant volume. In this manner, the donor can again donate up to 225 ml within a few days.
3. Satellite bags attached to a small volume of packed red blood cells or whole blood.
4. Use of small aliquots of group O,RH-compatible frozen red blood cells (Staples, 1976).

Additional donor requirements for neonatal blood transfusion may include freedom from sickle cell disease and glucose 6-phosphate deficiency in blacks, as well as direct antiglobulin, hemoglobin, hematocrit, and peripheral smear examination to exclude congenital erythrocytic abnormalities.

Some neonatal intensive care units have attempted to solve the problem of replacing blood in neonates with the so-called "walking donor" method. Traditionally, O negative hospital personnel volunteer a syringe-full of blood for injection into the neonatal patient. Oberman (1975) has summarized forcefully the disadvantages of the "walking donor" system:

1. Control of the blood transfusion is removed from the hospital transfusion service.
2. It is administratively difficult to maintain proper documentation of the source of blood in such programs.
3. In some instances, compatibility testing has been waived and hepatitis testing ignored.
4. The amount of heparin in the syringe may lead to inadvertent heparinization of the infant.
5. The hospital-based donor population has a higher incidence of hepatitis than the population at large.

Although we are opposed to a "walking donor" program, others believe that it is the most viable alternative in certain well-defined clinical situations. Hattersley (1976), for example, claims that the "walking donor" program may prove to be a useful "adjunct" to the intensive care nursery for premature infants with hyaline membrane disease requiring three or more transfusions.

BONE MARROW TRANSPLANTATION (BMT)

Bone marrow transplantation has changed the prognosis of certain cases of aplastic anemias and leukemias in recent years. At present, patients less than 40 years old with an HLA, MLC compatible sibling donor have a good chance to be cured of such diseases by BMT.

Just over a decade ago, the majority of severe aplastic anemia patients died within one year despite aggressive treatment and repeated transfusion support.

Table 43–13. CLINICAL DISORDERS OF NEONATES TREATED WITH EXCHANGE TRANSFUSION*

1. Hemolytic disease of the newborn secondary to blood group incompatibility
2. Neonatal hyperbilirubinemia resulting from
   a. Hereditary red cell and bilirubin metabolism defects
   b. Hemorrhage into enclosed spaces
   c. Prematurity
   d. Hyaline membrane disease (Gottuso, 1976)
   e. Intrauterine or neonatal infection
3. Respiratory distress syndrome (Delivoria-Papadopoulos, 1976)
4. Diffuse intravascular coagulation (DIC) secondary to abruptio placentae asphyxia, toxemia of pregnancy, sepsis, and generalized viral infections
5. Hypermagnesemia
6. Adenosine deaminase deficiency with severe combined immunodeficiency
7. Congenital isoimmune thrombocytopenic purpura

*Modified from Kevy (1977) and others.

5

Now, close to 80 per cent of unsensitized patients undergoing BMT will be alive and well without supportive therapy (Storb, 1980).

BMT also may offer a greater chance of survival for a child with lymphoblastic leukemia on a second or subsequent remission than does conventional chemotherapy. T-cell acute lymphocytic leukemia patients having a high risk of relapse are also candidates for BMT (Thomas, 1979).

Acute myelogenous leukemia patients with high white cell counts and totally abnormal chromosomal karyotypes or massive organomegaly will relapse within 15 months, and there appears to be no curable treatment. Results of BMT in such cases have been very successful (Kersey, 1982).

Bone marrow transplantation requires extensive support from the blood bank. Selection of compatible donors is of vital importance. In fact, the availability of HLA compatible sibling donors is one of the key factors in planning for BMT. ABO compatibility is less critical. Blood or blood components used pre-transplantation should not come from the potential BMT donor; in contrast to kidney transplantation, pre-transplantation sensitization reduces the chance of graft implantation.

For a period of 6 to 12 weeks post-transplantation, supportive treatment with blood components is essential to develop the hematopoietic system. Irradiated and washed RBCs are recommended to maintain the hematocrit level between 25 and 30 per cent. Irradiated platelets from random or single donors are needed to maintain the platelet count at about 20,000/μl. Granulocyte transfusions should be given when the granulocyte level falls below 200/μl or with uncontrollable infection. Peripheral lymphocytes and stem cells from the compatible donor have been helpful in reconstituting the patient's immune system.

BMT is a procedure with considerable risk; about 20 per cent mortality is common in most major institutions. However, with advances in the control of infection and graft-versus-host reactions, the outlook of BMT is continually improving. The collection of the patient's own stem cells, peripheral or bone marrow, during the remissions and transfusing them back to the patient after intensive suppressive therapy may alleviate many complications derived from homologous cell transplantations.

KIDNEY TRANSPLANTATION

For many years, nephrologists have tried to avoid giving blood transfusions to potential kidney recipients in order to avoid immunization of the patient. However, there is now overwhelming evidence from more than 40 independent studies that recipients who have had blood transfusions prior to transplantation have higher renal transplant survival rates than non-transfused recipients. In fact, of all the variables whose influence on cadaver transplant outcome has been studied, transfusion has the strongest effect. Sixty-nine per cent of patients having had more than 20 transfusions have a one-year graft survival rate compared to 42 per cent of patients without any transfusions. On the other hand the difference between zero and four HLA-A, -B antigens or DP mismatch, is only 9 per cent (Opelz, 1979). Blood from the kidney donor (DST or donor-specific transfusion) gave equally satisfactory results (First, 1982). The mechanism for this type of influence is not completely known. Preselection of responders may play some part. Potential recipients undergoing hemodialysis have a greater chance of contracting hepatitis. This hepatitis is usually of the "ay" subtype, whereas blood donor carriers are usually of the "ad" subtype. Therefore this hepatitis is unlikely to be related to blood transfusions. The increasing risk of CMV infection has also been repeatedly reported, especially at the time of graft rejection in some recipients (Betts, 1977). Anti-N is not an uncommon finding among the candidates undergoing dialysis. Some of them may have severe anemia and require transfusion of erythrocytes. For many years frozen-washed RBCs (50 per cent of the time) were used for these patients. This practice is still maintained in some hospitals. Until we know more about renal transplant survival, we must keep our minds open to various possible approaches.

PATIENTS RECEIVING CHEMOTHERAPY OR RADIATION

Patients with leukemia or advanced stages of malignancies often have associated thrombocytopenia and/or anemia. With the aggressive use of chemotherapy and radiation therapy, patients often become immunologically incompetent; hence, infection and graft-versus-host reactions may occur. Consequently, blood bankers are involved in the following areas: platelet transfusion for treatment or to prevent hemorrhage, a serious and sometimes fatal complication; transfusion of erythrocytes to correct severe anemia; and granulocyte transfusion to combat infection or prophylactic selection of blood components to prevent the development of infection. Finally, immunologically competent lymphocytes can be found in red blood cells or in platelet preparations and should be inactivated by irradiation. A 2000-rad dose is normally used at the Memorial Sloan-Kettering Cancer Center for such preparations given to immunodeficient patients (Mayer, 1982).

PATIENTS WITH HEART FAILURE

Patients with heart failure may also have severe anemia and require transfusion. In such cases, red blood cell concentrates, *not* whole blood, should be used. These units should be given at a slower rate and only one unit at a time. Treatment for heart failure should be continued. Diuretics before transfusion and warming the patient during transfusion are recommended. Skin capillaries which are dilated at warmer temperatures can retain about 300 ml of blood and therefore relieve some of the burden on the heart.

AUTOIMMUNE HEMOCYTOPENIA

Autoimmune diseases not infrequently cause hemolytic anemia, occasionally thrombocytopenia, and rarely leukocytopenia. Unless it is absolutely necessary, transfusions should be avoided. Antibodies responsible for autoimmune hemocytopenia can be of the cold or warm type. Cold autoantibodies to erythrocytes are usually associated with anti-I and rarely anti-P specificity. I-negative or P-negative donors are hard to find, and these hemolytic processes are often self-limiting. Simply keeping the patient warm may solve the problem. If transfusion is absolutely indicated and compatible blood is not available, the least incompatible blood may be used. Plasma exchange for anti-I may also be attempted to lower the titer. Warm autoantibodies causing hemolytic anemia may have anti-total Rh or "e" or other specificities. When transfusion is definitely required, the least incompatible blood or RBCs reacting more weakly than the autocontrol are often found to be satisfactory. Rh null donors are very rare, and these cells are abnormal *in vivo* anyway. The use of "e"-negative cells showed longer *in vivo* survival than "e"-positive cells in cases with anti-e specificity. When a larger amount of blood is required such as in surgery, trial transfusion of small amounts of chromium-labeled cells may be helpful. Checking the count at 3, 10, and 60 minutes postinjection may be worthwhile. If the survival rate at 60 minutes is 70 per cent or greater than that at 3 minutes, the donor would be acceptable; if it is less than 70 per cent, the level of acceptability should be judged by the needs of each individual case. It should be remembered that the transfusion of a small aliquot is different from a one unit transfusion, and that the result from the trial aliquot is much more amplified than the true condition. Platelet transfusion is of little value in cases of idiopathic thrombocytopenia.

Pretransfusion Testing

BLOOD SPECIMENS FROM THE RECIPIENT

1. The recipient must be positively identified by his or her first and last name plus hospital number or other available identifying number. This must correspond to the name on the wristband. In some hospitals, an additional wristband is used to identify the recipient from whom the blood has been drawn for compatibility testing.
2. Specimens must be labeled at the bedside with the full name of the patient, date, identification number, and the initials of the person drawing blood.
3. If the blood sample has to be drawn from intravenous (IV) tubing, it should be flushed with saline and the first 5 ml of blood discarded.
4. When additional transfusions are requested, a new specimen should be obtained at each 48-hour interval to identify an incompatibility from an antibody developed by an anamnestic response.
5. Hemolyzed blood samples should be avoided because they may mask hemolysis of donor erythrocytes in the crossmatch.
6. Normally a clotted specimen is used; however, if the patient has been heparinized, the blood specimen should be treated with protamine or glass beads to induce clotting.
7. The patient's erythrocytes may have to be washed if the patient has been receiving dextran or PVP or if there are protein abnormalities or strong cold agglutinins. It is good practice to wash red blood cells routinely before testing.
8. If the patient is going to be heparinized or receive PVP or dextran, a blood specimen should be drawn before such treatment.

ABO AND RH$_0$ TYPING, AND ANTIBODY SCREENING

ABO and Rh$_0$ typing should be done on every recipient before blood is issued. Under extreme emergency conditions we recommend ABO group-specific blood, but a physician may use O Rh$_0$-negative whole blood or preferably red blood cells (when there is inadequate time to determine ABO). The pretransfusion testing should then be completed subsequently as soon as possible (Oberman, 1978). ABO and Rh$_0$ typing can be performed the same way as for blood donors. However, in this case the D^u test is unnecessary because the patient would receive Rh$_0$-negative blood.

Antibody detection or screening in patients is much more important than it is for donors because the patient has 2 to 3 L of plasma, a much greater amount than that found in one unit of blood. Furthermore, weak reacting antibodies can become stronger after blood transfusion owing to a secondary (anamnestic) immune response. Antibody screening for patients must be done with two separate screening red blood cells in order to detect the commonly encountered and clinically significant antibodies (Boral, 1977b). The antiglobulin test should be included routinely for antibody screening. An additional enzyme or albumin technique is commonly used. A negative antibody screening procedure does not exclude the presence of irregular antibodies in a patient's serum. For instance, low incidence and narrow thermal range cold antibodies may be missed (Oberman, 1978; Boral, 1977b; Mintz, 1982).

Many investigators do not believe that antibodies reacting at room temperature or below are clinically significant, provided that the patient is not under hypothermia or being transfused rapidly with cold blood (Giblett, 1977).

ABO and Rh$_0$ typing and antibody detection (screening) should be done as early as possible, particularly for patients who are going to receive multiple transfusions. In this way, the blood bank can have sufficient time to identify the antibody, if present, and secure the special units of blood required. However, ABO and Rh$_0$ typing with antibody screening may be used without crossmatch for patients who are undergoing the type of surgery which normally requires no blood transfusion. A list of such elective operative procedures and a strategy for ordering blood, which we have advocated and found both acceptable and cost efficient, are shown in Table 43–14.

If the patient's erythrocytes exhibit a positive direct antiglobulin (DAGT) test or if spontaneous agglutination in albumin occurs, partial elution at 45°C. may be attempted to remove some of the attached antibodies for successful phenotyping of the patient. The eluted antibodies should also be identified.

COMPATIBILITY TESTING

1. Compatibility testing in a real sense reveals only detectable incompatibility between the recipient

Table 43–14. PROCEDURES FOR WHICH BLOOD IS USUALLY CROSSMATCHED BUT FOR WHICH TYPE AND SCREEN WOULD APPEAR ADEQUATE*

Type of Surgery	Procedure
General	Cholecystectomy; exploratory laparotomy; thyroidectomy; parathyroidectomy; parotidectomy; colostomy; vein stripping
Gynecologic	Hysterectomy; uterine suspension; tuboplasty; ovarian wedge resection
Neurosurgery	Laminectomy; ventriculoperitoneal shunt
Orthopedic	Total knee; medial meniscectomy; leg amputation; arthroscopy; removal of hip pin
Otolaryngology	Transantral ethmoidectomy; Caldwell-Luc
Plastic	Reduction mammoplasty; skin flap; skin graft
Urologic	Transurethral resection of the prostate; pyelolithotomy; ureterolithotomy; cystotomy; transurethral resection of bladder tumor; fulguration of bleeding bladder tumor; orchiectomy; orchiopexy; ureteral reimplantation

*From Mintz, 1976.

and the donor. Except in identical twins and autologous transfusions, no blood can be 100 per cent compatible. Consequently, the term incompatibility testing may be more appropriate.

2. Compatibility testing or crossmatching consists of a major and a minor test.

3. The minor crossmatch is no longer used in many hospitals for erythrocyte transfusions because of the popular use of erythrocyte concentrates and routine antibody screening of donor blood. However, when a large volume of plasma is used, as may be the case with platelet or granulocyte pheresis concentrates or with fresh frozen plasma, especially for children, a minor crossmatch is desirable. Advocates of the minor crossmatch also point out that it confirms ABO typing, reflects a positive DAT, and may permit recognition of a new blood group factor.

4. The minor crossmatch consists of testing the donor's plasma or serum against erythrocytes of the patient. As noted previously, it is useful to double check the ABO compatibility and occasionally to test for strong or hemolytic anti-A or anti-B (antibodies) in group O blood. The minor crossmatch may also reveal the presence of donor antibodies against low incidence antigens such as anti-C^W, anti-Wr^a, and anti-Lv^a.

5. The major crossmatch consists of testing the patient's serum or plasma against the donor's erythrocytes. Serum is normally preferable except under certain conditions where only plasma is available. In such cases, plasma can be converted into serum by the addition of calcium, thrombin, or glass beads. Patient's serum for crossmatch should not be inactivated.

6. It is recommended that donor erythrocytes be washed before testing. The possible presence of soluble antigens such as Le^a, Le^b, Rg^a, Ch^a, Cs^a, Yk^a, Bg^a, Bg^b, Bg^c, and Sd^a, which may interfere with the testing, will then be minimized.

7. Segments from the blood bag are recommended rather than tubes attached to the bag, as these segments are the true representative of the bag's contents.

8. The two-tube crossmatch is preferable to the one-tube crossmatch. In the former, one tube is incubated at room temperature in saline medium while the other is incubated at 37°C. in an albumin medium or with a one-stage enzyme technique. After 15 to 30 minutes' incubation, the tubes are centrifuged and read. If negative, the second tube is converted to the antiglobulin test and read microscopically.

9. In an incompatible crossmatch, the presence of rouleau should be ruled out before additional studies are conducted.

10. The autocontrol must be set up at the same time to differentiate alloantibodies from autoantibodies, a very important consideration in the selection of blood for transfusion.

11. When the autocontrol is negative, alloantibodies are suspected in an incompatible crossmatch. Anti-A_1 or anti-HI may be suspected if antibodies are reacting strongly at room temperature or below. Warm alloantibodies of many varieties may be suspected among those reacting strongly at 37°C. or with the antiglobulin test. They should be identified if possible before the patient receives any transfusions.

12. In emergency situations, random crossmatches may be performed at the same time as the antibody identification.

13. When the autocontrol is positive, autoantibodies or a positive antiglobulin test (often due to medication) should be suspected.

14. The possible presence of alloantibodies masked by autoantibodies should be ruled out before transfusion of a patient is attempted. This is best accomplished by autoabsorption when a sufficient number of erythrocytes are available. However, autoabsorption should be utilized only if the patient has not been transfused in the previous four months. Absorbed serum or specific eluates should be used for antibody identification or crossmatching.

15. Should the patient have previously identified antibodies, such as anti-K, -Fy^a, -Fy^b, -Jk^a, -Jl^b, -S, -s, -D, -E, -C, -c, or -e, the compatible units should be typed for the specific antigen(s) to avoid a delayed transfusion reaction. Only units negative for the appropriate antigen should be used. This caution is not as necessary for ordinary room temperature or cold-reacting antibodies such as anti-Le^a, -Le^b, -P_1, -M, -N, or others.

16. Should the patient have autoantibodies without alloantibodies, transfusion of least incompatible units selected by titration crossmatch and reacting less strongly than the autocontrol may be attempted.

Patients can usually tolerate such transfusions unless an underlying alloantibody is present but missed.

17. Patients with strong cold autoagglutinins should not be subjected to hypothermia, since this can induce a hemolytic transfusion reaction.

18. The compatibility test *in vivo* may be attempted under special conditions when the patient requires blood in the presence of an incompatible crossmatch and elucidation of the nature of the incompatibility has not been achieved or compatible blood cannot be found. Red cell survival studies using erythrocytes tagged with radioactive chromium (^{51}Cr) have been attempted in the more sophisticated hospitals.

There is no question that in many surgical patients there is no need for blood transfusion. For them, the *type* and *screen* without crossmatch are obviously sufficient. However, some blood bankers advocate the omission of compatibility testing completely (Mayer, 1982). To examine this important issue, data summarized by Walker (1982) may be very useful (Table 43–15). When random blood is used without any testing, almost two thirds of these transfusions would be compatible. When ABO groups are matched, over 99 per cent would be compatible. Matching of Rh improves the odds another 0.4 per cent, while antibody screening improves it only 0.14 per cent. The crossmatch increases the safety only 0.01 per cent. Therefore, do we need the crossmatch? First, we must be aware that crossmatching is designed not only for irregular antibodies but also for ABO incompatibility, which is by far the most important cause of fatality (Schmidt, 1980) and is not included in the above-mentioned estimation. Any financial saving from omitting crossmatching can hardly compensate for a single fatality! Second, 0.01 per cent is a small number in terms of statistics, but if you are the patient in that 0.01 per cent or the physician of that patient, the size of the number is no longer an issue. Based on these two simple facts, at least an immediate spin crossmatch is recommended before a unit of blood is released under urgent circumstances.

For platelet concentrates that have a large volume of plasma when stored at room temperature, not only must volume be considered in terms of recipient's condition and blood volume, but ABO matching becomes more important for the plasma than the few red blood cells present; then anti-A is more important than anti-B.

Table 43–15. PROBABILITY OF SAFE BLOOD TRANSFUSION*

Procedure	Compatibility	
	Individual	*Cumulative*
None	64.4%	64.4%
ABO grouping	35.0%	99.4%
Rh typing	0.4%	99.8%
Antibody screening	0.14%	99.94%
Crossmatching	0.01%	99.95%
Autotransfusion	100%	100%

*Modified from Walker, 1982.

Infusion of Blood Components

PROPER IDENTIFICATION

Although a great deal of attention has been given to ensure that a unit of blood is correctly identified, correct identification of a recipient has not been so emphasized. Before a unit of blood is transfused, many people are involved. Consequently, transcription error may occur in one of the many steps. The patient's full name, hospital number, and transfusion number (in some hospitals) must be clearly identified in each step of the transaction.

The majority of fatal transfusion reactions are due to *ABO incompatibility*. Therefore, ABO grouping of the patient from the correct specimen is of vital importance. In some hospitals, additional ABO grouping is done at the bedside and the patient is also checked by his or her ABO group. It should be re-emphasized that ABO compatibility is of utmost importance. The wrong patient may receive ABO-compatible blood, while the right patient cannot receive ABO-incompatible blood. This of course does not mean that the identification of the patient should be ignored. An identification of the patient by ABO group, especially as part of the armband, is highly recommended. Finger stick ABO typing as a double check for the ABO group has been found valuable in hospitals where new personnel are often involved.

Before a unit of blood component is infused into the patient, the full name of the patient, identification code(s) identical to that on the transfusion request, the ABO group of the component, and Rh must be checked with that of the patient. In rare cases, under emergency conditions, Rh_o-positive blood can be given to an Rh_o-negative person (p. 1031).

Emergency situations (often in ER, OR, or intensive care units) are most commonly associated with a failure in proper identification. Personnel involved in blood specimen collection for crossmatching and in blood infusion must be particularly cautious at these times.

CONDITIONS AFFECTING THE INFUSION OF BLOOD COMPONENTS

Intravenous Fluid. Only normal saline is suitable for use in blood transfusion. It is used to start the blood transfusion and can be used to dilute erythrocyte concentrates. Five per cent dextrose in water may cause red blood cell aggregation or hemolysis, while lactated Ringer's solution may cause clotting. Neither can or should replace normal saline. No medication should be added to or administered in the same line with blood or components. Blood components except platelets and thawed cryoprecipitate or fresh frozen plasma should be stored in a monitored blood bank refrigerator until immediately before transfusion. Therefore, one should not ask for a blood component from the blood bank until the infusion is underway or intravenous fluid has been started (Kienle, 1978).

Filters. Blood components should be transfused through a filter to eliminate infusion of fibrin clots and other particulate debris (see Table 43–12). Most standard blood and platelet transfusion sets have filters with a pore size of approximately 170 microns. Wide

5

variations exist in the surface area of the filter and the arrangement of the filter and drip chamber. Under normal conditions one filter can be used for two to four units of blood; however, one must judge the condition of the filter and the total time involved and change the filter accordingly.

Microaggregates which form progressively in whole blood or packed red blood cells after one week of storage at 4°C. consist of platelets, cell fragments, and nuclei of granulocytes ranging from 13 to 100 μ in diameter. Although the effect of these microaggregates remains unsettled, no one believes that a recipient should receive a large number of microaggregates. Special filters with pore sizes between 20 and 40 μ for screening out particulate material have been developed (see Table 43–12).

Microaggregate filters are available in two basic types, using the adhesiveness of Dacron or Nylon fibers or the filtration effect of polyurethane foam or polyester mesh (see Table 43–12). There are filters using both fibers and mesh. The most effective filter is the Dacron wool filter (Swank In-Line Blood Filter, IL-200 Pioneer Filters, Inc., Beaverton, Oregon) (Greenwalt, 1977; Solis, 1972) and the cotton wool filter (Diepenhorst, 1975). Microaggregate filters are recommended in cardiopulmonary bypass (to prevent cerebral embolism), in massive transfusions with blood more than one week old (large numbers of microaggregates), and in patients with pulmonary dysfunction. Microaggregate filters should not be used with platelet concentrates or fresh whole blood because viable platelets will be filtered out (excluded) from the infusion.

Filters with cotton and nylon, designed to remove leukocytes during transfusion, have become available and are useful in special conditions when other preparations of leukocyte-poor RBCs are not available.

Blood Warmers. Rapid infusion of large volumes of cold blood may precipitate ventricular arrhythmia and even death of the patient (Dybkjaer, 1964). A blood warmer is recommended for patients receiving many units of cold blood in a short period of time, in exchange transfusions and transfusion of premature infants, and for patients with strong cold autoagglutinins. The temperature of the blood warmer should be maintained at about 37°C. No hemolysis or increase in plasma potassium level will result at this temperature; however, when the blood temperature exceeds 40°C., hemolysis may occur. We have found the Fenwal dry heat blood warmer (No. 4R4305) incorporating blood warming bag (4C2416) acceptable for precise regulation of blood temperature and flow rate. This system warms blood from 4°C. and maintains a range of 32 to 37°C. at flow rates up to 150 ml per minute. Other equally satisfactory blood warmers are also available. When more than 20 units of blood are transfused into a patient, in addition to a blood warmer, $NaHCO_3$ infusion may be used and may reduce the mortality (Howland, 1957). Warming the patient is recommended for those with cold agglutinin disease and in transfusion of patients with circulatory overload (dilation of peripheral blood vessels can accommodate over 200 ml of blood) (Mollison, 1983).

Speed of Infusion. In most administration sets, 15 drops equals 1 ml. At a rate of 60 drops/min, $60/15 \times 60 = 240$ ml of blood can be transfused in one hour. The duration of transfusion can thus be estimated by the rate of infusion. Under normal conditions for an average adult without cardiopulmonary dysfunction, one unit of blood should be infused within one to two hours (Boral, 1977a). Blood transfusion should not be used to keep intravenous lines open, and extended time for infusions—unless critical for a patient with congestive heart failure—should be avoided. Blood is an ideal culture medium and when it warms up over several hours at room temperature while being infused may allow growth of bacteria that may enter the system during blood collection and/or infusion. In massive bleeding, the rate of infusion can be accelerated by the use of large needles at more than one site. In patients with severe anemia or heart failure, the rate of infusion should be reduced. The concurrent use of diuretics and/or digitalis may be useful. For the average size adult, furosemide, 20 to 40 mg intravenously for one to two units of red blood cells, has been most effective in our experience. However, it may be necessary to transfuse only half of one unit at one time. The remaining half should be stored in a blood bank refrigerator and used later within 24 hours. As a rule, during the first 15 minutes of transfusion, the rate of infusion should be slow in order to observe any patient reaction, especially when an incompatible or least incompatible unit is being transfused or when previous transfusion reactions have been reported.

MONITORING THE PATIENT

Transfusion is a serious and potentially hazardous treatment. Reactions can be fatal if proper precautions are not observed. In the United States, any fatal transfusion reaction must be reported immediately (within 24 hours) to the Food and Drug Administration. Most transfusion reactions develop within 30 minutes of transfusion. If the patient is being monitored carefully by medical or nursing personnel, the majority of fatal transfusion reactions can be avoided by prompt, early, and appropriate action. A patient's vital signs should be taken and recorded immediately before the transfusion to serve as a baseline, then every 15 minutes after the beginning of the transfusion for at least three times, and at the end of the transfusion. When the patient is under general anesthesia, hypotension, hemoglobinuria, and unexplained oozing may be the only signs of a hemolytic transfusion reaction.

We have reported favorable experience with an outpatient transfusion clinic in a hospital based blood bank and transfusion service which is responsive to increasing demands for ambulatory medical care, as well as cost-effective and satisfying to patients (Boral, 1977a).

THERAPEUTIC HEMAPHERESIS

Ronald A. Sacher, M.D.,
and Thomas A. Ruma, M.D.

Therapeutic hemapheresis implies an exchanging of "diseased" blood or components and replacement by "healthy" blood or components. Plasmapheresis (plasma removal) has been used and reported as successful therapy in such widely differing diseases as asthma and aluminum poisoning. Established indications do exist and are outlined in Table 43–16, which also shows some probable and possible indications. Cytapheresis is the term to describe removal of cellular components (viz., thrombocytopheresis—platelets; leukapheresis—white cells; and erythropheresis—red cells). The application of these procedures in component preparation has been discussed earlier in the chapter.

The pathogenesis of tissue injury in certain diseases involves the presence of harmful circulating plasma or cellular factors. Examples include hyperviscous plasma and quantitatively or qualitatively abnormal leukocytes or toxins. In some situations, therefore, patient benefit could be expected from discarding the undesirable plasma and reinfusing patients' red cells with an innocuous fluid as volume replacement. The efficiency or therapeutic benefit is likely to be greater when the harmful factor is distributed predominantly intravascularly and when the rate of accumulation of the harmful factors is "low."

In this situation, a single exchange may remove up to 90 per cent of the factor (e.g., hyperviscosity syndrome due to macroglobulinemia). However, in many clinical conditions in which plasmapheresis has been used, the pathogenesis of the disease is unclear and/or the serological markers of the disease are not well correlated with disease activity or therapeutic response. Controlled studies are needed to define appropriate indications.

METHODS

Plasma exchange may be accomplished either manually or mechanically by means of cell separators. Manual removal involves removal of a unit of whole blood, plasma removal by centrifugation, and then reinfusion of the red blood cells minus the plasma (or resuspended in saline or albumin). This is a laborious procedure and four to five hours may be required to remove a liter of plasma. Mechanical removal using a cell separator can achieve the same rate of removal in 45 minutes. The major limiting factors are the vascular access and the cardiovascular dynamics of the patient. The instruments may be either intermittent flow separators (Haemonetics, Natick, Mass.) or continuous flow separators (IBM 2997, Princeton, N.J., or Fenwal CS 3000, Travenol, Chicago, Ill.). Blood

Table 43–16. INDICATIONS FOR THERAPEUTIC HEMAPHERESIS

Benefit	Disease	Component Removed
Plasmapheresis		
Definite	Hyperviscosity syndromes	Abnormal protein
	Myasthenia gravis	Anti-cholinesterase antibody
	Goodpasture's syndrome	Anti-glomerular basement membrane antibody
Probable	Hyperlipidemia	Excess lipids and abnormal lipoproteins
	Renal transplant rejection	Antibody/cytotoxic lymphocytes
	Thrombotic thrombocytopenic purpura	? Platelet aggregating toxic factors
Possible	Rheumatoid arthritis	Immune complexes (IC)
	Systemic lupus erythematosus	Immune complexes
	Polyneuropathy	Antibody/IC
	Rh isoimmunization	Anti-Rh antibodies
	Immune thrombocytopenic purpura	Anti-platelet antibody
	Auto-immune hemolytic anemia	Anti-RBC antibody
	Essential cryoglobulinemia	Cryoglobulins
	Protein-bound toxins (e.g., mushroom poisoning)	Toxin bound to plasma proteins
	Rapidly progressive nephritis (without anti-GBM)	Immune complexes
Cytapheresis		
Definite	Hyperleukocytosis with leukostasis (AML and CML)	Excessive myeloid precursors
	Hemorrhagic thrombocythemia	Excess abnormal platelets
Probable	Renal transplant rejection	Cytotoxic lymphocytes
	Sickle cell complications	Sickled erythrocytes
Possible	Chronic lymphocytic leukemia	Abnormal lymphocytes

is separated by centrifugal force into its various components, which can then be directed into collection channels by instrument manipulation. Simultaneous withdrawal and reinfusion are usually performed and consequently require a withdrawal port on one arm and an infusion port on the other arm. (Usual plasma exchange involves 2 to 3 L of plasma!) Similar principles are applied to removal of cellular components.

INDICATIONS (see Table 43–16)

Plasmapheresis

Hyperviscosity Syndromes. The most established indication for plasma exchange is hyperviscosity syndromes associated with immunoglobulin abnormalities. This condition may occur with several immunoproliferative diseases (Waldenström's macroglobulinemia—85 per cent; IgA myeloma—10 per cent; IgG myeloma—5 per cent) that have in common an elevated plasma viscosity (normally less than 1.8). Viscosity is the property of fluids to resist flow, and for protein solutions this is dependent upon concentration of the protein and intrinsic viscosity of the individual protein molecule, which in turn is dependent on the molecular shape and size. In this respect, IgM molecules have a large molecular size and unusual molecular configuration. Furthermore, the molecular shape may enhance the tendency to aggregate and thereby increase viscosity. Viscosity is also dependent upon the interaction of protein molecules with blood cells and the formation of rouleau. Certain immunoglobulin molecules have the property of polymerizing (e.g., IgG_3) or of being insoluble in cold temperatures (cryoglobulins). These properties may enhance plasma viscosity under unfavorable circumstances, e.g., cold exposure (Bloch, 1973).

Clinical effects are mostly manifest from blood vessels with a sluggish circulation or in poorly supported or easily traumatized vessels. The usual clinical features of hyperviscosity are seen in such sites as retina (venous engorgement, sausage-linked vessels), ear (tinnitus, hearing loss, vertigo), nasal mucosa (epistaxis), and gingival and oral mucosa (dental bleeding). Furthermore, microcirculatory disturbances may be affected by abnormal platelet function.

Plasmapheresis as a therapeutic measure in multiple myeloma was introduced by Adams (1952) and in Waldenström's macroglobulinemia by Skoog (1959). The usual regimen is daily plasmapheresis (manual removal of two to three units of plasma) to achieve rapid lowering of plasma viscosity; and for maintenance, biweekly or alternate-weekly procedures in which two units are removed. Using the automated procedure currently available (either Haemonetics 30 or IBM 2997), 2 to 3 L of plasma can be removed in two hours, and the necessity for more frequent procedures is reduced to weekly or biweekly.

As mentioned, recurrence rate is dependent on distribution and route of production of the protein. In this regard, IgM paraprotein, which is mostly intravascular, can be effectively cleared with one passage. Repeat pheresis may not be needed for two to three weeks. Plasmapheresis does not influence the basic disease process, and therefore cessation of pheresis in the absence of other treatment may result in recurrence of hyperviscosity after two to three weeks. Effective chemotherapy may subsequently eliminate the need for plasmapheresis.

Myasthenia Gravis. In myasthenia gravis, antibodies directed against the motor end plate acetylcholine receptor protein (AchR) are considered important in the disease pathogenesis (Lindstrom, 1976). Lindstrom's data suggest that the titer of the antibodies increases with the degree of weakness, although no definite correlation is evident. Antibody titer is often markedly elevated in chronic disease refractory to conventional therapy. Conceivably, then, removal of this "circulating toxin" by means of plasmapheresis may produce improvement in the clinical manifestations by alleviating the "immunopharmacological blockage."

Plasma exchange has proved effective in controlling acute symptoms as a short-term control modality while other treatments (thymectomy, immunosuppressive drugs, etc.) become effective and also in the control of refractory patients in whom repeated plasmapheresis may be useful (Dau, 1977).

Goodpasture's Syndrome (Rapidly Progressive Glomerulonephritis with Anti-glomerular Basement Membrane). In this syndrome, characterized by hemoptysis, lung infiltrates, and glomerulonephritis, antibodies to basement membrane antigens are deposited in pulmonary and glomerular capillary walls (anti-GBM). Renal function may be improved and pulmonary hemorrhage ameliorated by plasmapheresis. Those patients with mild to moderate impairment, i.e., those with some normal glomeruli on renal biopsy, are most likely to respond to plasmapheresis.

ADDITIONAL APPLICATIONS OF THERAPEUTIC PLASMAPHERESIS

Several other conditions have been managed by therapeutic plasmapheresis to remove supposedly detrimental antibodies or antigen-antibody complexes in excess (Wenz, 1982).

Removal of antigen-antibody complexes in SLE has yielded variable clinical results (Moran, 1977; Jones, 1976). While plasmapheresis can remove immune complexes successfully in SLE, several studies have not demonstrated consistent clinical benefit in addition to medical treatment (Schlansky, 1980).

In hemophilia A patients refractory to factor VIII concentrates because of a high titer factor VIII inhibitor, plasmapheresis has been of significant benefit and, on occasion, lifesaving (Edson, 1973). Antileukocyte and antiplatelet antibodies that may arise in patients who must receive repeated platelet and leukocyte transfusions or in idiopathic thrombocytopenic purpura, may be removed by plasmapheresis. In autoimmune hemolytic anemia, circulating antibodies or antigen-antibody complexes capable of inflicting damage to red blood cells may be removed. Anti-Rho (D) antibodies in severe Rh hemolytic disease of the newborn (HDN) have been removed from the mother's plasma. Plasmapheresis reduced the amniotic fluid bilirubin and Rho (D) antibody titers significantly in seven of eight patients (Graham-Poole, 1977). While it has been possible to decrease maternal antibody levels in various other studies (Fraser, 1976; Robinson, 1980), the effectiveness of improving fetal viability is unclear.

Therapeutic plasmapheresis has occasionally been performed in many other disease states; however, a discussion of these is beyond the scope of this section. The miscellaneous conditions include essential cryoglobulinemia, post-transfusion purpura, hereditary errors of metabolism (Refsum's disease), homozygous familial hypercholesterolemia, ABO incompatible bone marrow transplants, Raynaud's disease, rheumatoid arthritis, multiple sclerosis, and the removal of circulating toxic substances in acute hepatic failure. Therapeutic plasmapheresis has been reported as beneficial in TTP (Bukowski, 1977; Myers, 1980); however, it is unclear whether this is due to the removal of a circulating toxic substance or the correction of some deficient factor by providing normal plasma to the patient during therapeutic plasmapheresis (Byrnes, 1977).

THERAPEUTIC CYTAPHERESIS

Therapeutic leukapheresis has been performed in acute myelocytic (AML) and chronic myelocytic leukemia (CML). Patients with AML are susceptible to leukostasis phenomena if white blood cell counts are greater than 100,000/μl. Leukostasis causes sluggish circulation and may precipitate vaso-occlusive problems leading to fatal pulmonary and cerebral insufficiency and intracerebral hemorrhage. Leukapheresis has been reported to result in rapid cytoreduction in these patients (Eisenstadt, 1978). In CML, leukostasis is a less frequently encountered problem; however, short-term cytoreduction has been achieved (Lowenthal, 1975). Chronic lymphocytic leukemia has also been treated by leukapheresis, but as with AML and CML, chemotherapy is the modality of choice, and leukapheresis should be reserved for the small fraction of patients with leukostasis.

Therapeutic plateletpheresis (thrombocytapheresis) and erythropheresis (red blood cell exchange) have been utilized much less frequently than therapeutic leukapheresis. Therapeutic plateletpheresis has been beneficial in achieving a short-term reduction of elevated platelet counts in chronic myeloproliferative disorders (Taft, 1977). Chemotherapy may take days to weeks to reduce platelet counts in these disorders. Erythropheresis has been used occasionally in the treatment of sickle cell disease complications, including hemolytic and pain crises, preparation for surgery, and priapism (Kernoff, 1977). Abnormal sickled red cells can be replaced by normal red cells in a short time period.

COMPLICATIONS

Repeated plasma exchange of normal donors at the rate of two units once or twice weekly (500–1000/ml plasma) produces a decrease in total serum protein during the initial six months (Friedman, 1975). This is mainly due to decreased immunoglobulins. However, the level of immunoglobulins usually remains in the normal range. With more intensive plasma exchange, using centrifugal blood separators, thrombocytopenia may be a problem.

Table 43–17. LABORATORY DETERMINATIONS COMMONLY MONITORED DURING PLASMAPHERESIS

CBC with differential white count
Platelet count
Serum calcium
Prothrombin time
Partial thromboplastin time
Serum viscosity
Serum electrolytes
Serum protein electrophoresis
Hepatitis B surface antigen (HbsAg)

Plasmapheresis is not an innocuous procedure. Very rare fatalities have been reported. Immediate complications include transient hypotension, bradycardia, urticarial reactions, and hypocalcemia. The transient hypotension occurs most frequently at the end of the procedure and can be ameliorated with fluid replacement. Hypocalcemia may occur from the citrate anticoagulation used for the procedure (ACD) and the replacement of CPD anticoagulated fresh frozen plasma. Allergic urticarial reactions are usually due to plasma protein allergens. Viral hepatitis from the use of FFP as replacement therapy is another potential complication. The use of albumin or plasma protein fraction (PPF) as replacement therapy rather than FFP reduces the likelihood of these complications but is more costly (See Table 43–9). Therapeutic leukapheresis and plateletpheresis are associated with fewer complications than therapeutic plasmapheresis since the quantity of blood removed is small, and specific replacement components are unnecessary. Erythropheresis, however, requires donor red cell replacement which carries the risk of hepatitis and red cell alloimmunization.

Prior to and following each hemapheresis, several parameters have been monitored in studies using centrifugal blood separators (Israel, 1977) (Table 43–17).

* * *

Transfusion Reactions

Since the transfusion of blood is accompanied by significant morbidity and mortality estimated to be about 0.5 per cent of transfusions (with more than 10 million transfusions dispensed annually in the United States), a review of the untoward reactions to transfusion is warranted (Myhre, 1978).

HEMOLYTIC TRANSFUSION REACTIONS

Causes

1. The blood and recipient are mismatched, usually owing to clerical errors.

2. An incompatible crossmatch is missed by the technologist (much less often).

3. The crossmatch may be compatible under normal conditions but the patient has been subjected to hypothermia, activating potent cold agglutinins which lyse his own or transfused erythrocytes.

4. The antibody level of the recipient may be undetectable at the time of crossmatch but increases

and becomes potent after the transfusion of erythrocytes with homologous antigens (anamnestic response) and hemolyzes the transfused cells. This is called a delayed hemolytic transfusion reaction because the shortened erythrocyte survival (hemolysis) follows the transfusion after a time interval of several days to two weeks. Such patients have most often received multiple transfusions, especially with trauma, but it may also occur in children with chronic anemia receiving intermittent hemotherapy.

5. Erythrocytes of the recipient may be defective, as in paroxysmal nocturnal hemoglobinuria; the erythrocytes hemolyze in the presence of complement in the transfused plasma.

6. The recipient may have a malfunctioning heart valve prosthesis causing hemolysis. Distilled water may enter the circulation as a result of irrigation of the bladder during prostate surgery. If the patient is also receiving a transfusion simultaneously, this may lead one to suspect erroneously a hemolytic transfusion reaction.

7. Erythrocytes of the patient may be hemolyzed by certain toxins such as those resulting from *Clostridium welchii* infection coincidental with transfusion.

8. Erythrocytes of the donor or patient may be defective in G6PD. If medication such as vitamin K, sulfonamide, or phenacetin is given, hemolysis may result.

9. Frozen-thawed erythrocytes, which may contain high levels of residual glycerol after inadequate washing, will hemolyze after being transfused.

10. The unit of blood may contain hemoglobin as a result of freezing (improper storage), contamination, or other mistreatment which may occur in collection, storage, and transportation.

Pathologic Physiology of Immune Hemolysis in Vivo. Hemolytic reactions due to antigen-antibody reactions are designated immune hemolysis. Immune hemolysis *in vivo* is divided into two basic types (Table 43–18 and Fig. 43–3), intravascular and extravascular. Antibodies, such as anti-A, anti-B, anti-I, anti-Le^a, and anti-P_1, which can activate complement can cause intravascular hemolysis if sufficiently active *in vivo* at body temperature, i.e., wide thermal range. Symptoms such as flushing, pain at injection site, shock, and hypotension may be related to activation of complement and the subsequent release of histamine, serotonin, or kinins. Hemoglobin released from the lysed erythrocytes combines with haptoglobin and usually deposits in the liver, where it is subsequently split into iron and bilirubin. Since the amount of haptoglobin is limited, hemoglobin can also be handled in alternative ways. The heme released can combine with albumin to form methemalbumin or combine with hemopexin. It is then processed in the liver into bilirubin and free iron. In the laboratory, one can demonstrate the presence of free plasma hemoglobin (or in the urine when plasma level is above the renal threshold), a decrease in haptoglobin, hemopexin, and albumin binding capacity with an increase in lactate dehydrogenase, hemoglobinuria, hemosiderinuria, and a positive DAT with a minor population of agglutinates. Serum bilirubin may be increased four to six hours later (Fig. 43–4).

Most IgG antibody–coated erythrocytes are destroyed extravascularly, mainly through phagocytosis in the reticuloendothelial system of the spleen. Complement-coated erythrocytes are similarly destroyed, but primarily in the liver. Some IgG antibodies may activate complement *in vivo,* such as some anti-K, anti-Fy^a, and anti-Jk^a and cause the complement and IgG-coated erythrocytes to be destroyed predominantly in the liver. As stated previously, other IgG antibody-coated erythrocytes are destroyed primarily in the spleen (Mollison, 1983). Recent evidence indicates IgG-coated erythrocytes can be destroyed through lymphocytes with Fc receptors. Hemolytic transfusion reactions may not be evident until 7 to 10 days post-transfusion. Anti-E and anti-c are not infrequent causes, and anti-M, anti-Lu^a, anti-K, anti-Ce, anti-Jk^b, anti-Jk^a, anti-k, and anti-U have also been implicated (Mollison, 1972). Such delayed he-

Table 43–18. MECHANISM OF IMMUNE HEMOLYTIC TRANSFUSION REACTIONS

Key Factors	Possible Mechanism	Laboratory Findings	Symptoms and Signs
IgM antibodies	Primarily intravascular hemolysis (activation of complement)	Plasma Hgb ↑ Haptoglobin ↓ Hemopexin ↓ Methemalbumin ↑ Hemoglobinuria +	Chill, fever Hemoglobinuria* Oliguria Anuria
IgG antibodies	Primarily extravascular hemolysis (phagocytosis)	Direct AGT + Bilirubin ↑ (Liver function ↓) (Hematocrit ↓)	 Jaundice
C3a C5a	Hemodynamic alternation	Histamine Serotonin Kinins	Flushing Pain Shock Hypotension*
Platelets Hageman factor	Disseminated intravascular coagulation	Coagulation factors ↓	Bleeding*

*Only signs under general anesthesia.

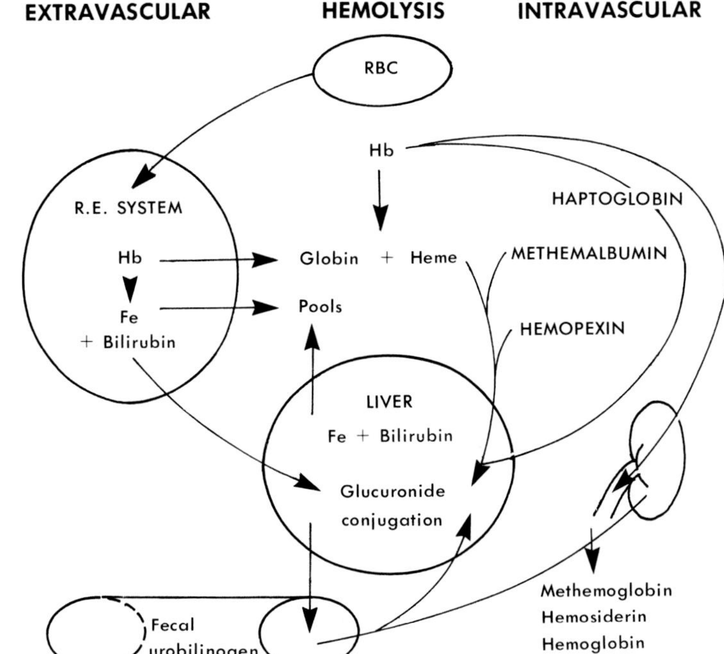

Figure 43–3. Two types of hemolysis *in vivo*.

molytic transfusion reactions are often manifested solely or primarily by an unexplained post-transfusion decrease in hematocrit (Solanki, 1978). Pineda (1978b) has reviewed the Mayo Clinic experience with 23 cases of delayed hemolytic transfusion reaction over a 10-year period. Death occurred in three patients and in one case hemolysis led to disseminated intravascular coagulation syndrome. Fever was the most frequent presenting symptom in this series, and all but one demonstrated a positive DAT.

TRANSFUSION REACTIONS RELATED TO LEUKOCYTES AND PLATELETS

Chills and fever are the most common symptoms of a transfusion reaction and are usually due to leukocytes contained in blood components. They are usually mild. However, since fever may be part of the symptomatology of a hemolytic transfusion reaction as well, chills and fever should be evaluated as a potential hemolytic transfusion reaction. Fever is more common in patients receiving granulocytes, particularly if prepared by filtration pheresis. Leukoagglutinins and cytotoxic antibodies can often be demonstrated in patients with febrile reactions; the use of leukocyte-poor blood or frozen-thawed red blood cells will usually alleviate these symptoms.

Immunization to HLA antigens and other white cell antigens seems to be the logical explanation for febrile reactions. Patients having repeated platelet transfusions also have a high incidence of febrile reactions. This fact tends to support the above assumption and indicates that platelet-poor erythrocytes may be just as important as leukocyte-poor preparations in preventing this type of reaction. Antipyretics, steroids, and meperidine may be used to relieve symptoms. Hypotension, dyspnea, and pulmonary

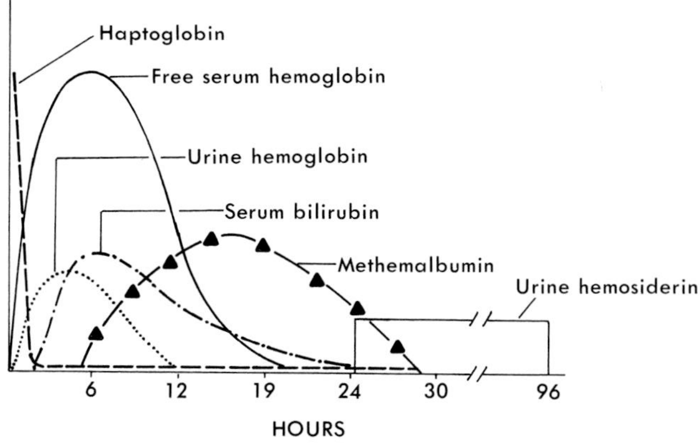

Figure 43–4. Laboratory findings in intravascular hemolysis. Positive direct antiglobulin test and presence of minor population of agglutinates are not listed. (Modified from Huestis, 1976.)

infiltration have also been related to the presence of leukocyte antibodies (Andrews, 1976) and may further complicate severe chill and fever reactions.

TRANSFUSION REACTIONS RELATED TO PLASMA PROTEINS

1. The second most common transfusion reaction referred to as allergic is manifested by urticaria, which can be controlled by antihistamines. When unusually extensive or involving oral, pharyngeal, or laryngeal edema, it is also known as an anaphylactoid reaction.

2. The more severe anaphylactic reaction, characterized by dyspnea, hypotension, and flushing of skin, is rare following transfusion. It is also believed to be due to plasma protein hypersensitivity in the recipient.

3. Anti-IgA antibodies have been demonstrated in 86 per cent of subjects who have had anaphylactic or anaphylactoid reactions (Mollison, 1983). There is little evidence that other classes of immunoglobulins cause this type of reaction.

4. Patients lacking plasma IgA are at increased risk of forming anti-IgA antibodies and often have anti-IgA even without known stimulation. These persons should be transfused only with IgA-deficient blood or with frozen-thawed red blood cells or washed erythrocytes from normal donors. When factor VIII or fibrinogen is required for such patients, cryoprecipitate prepared from an IgA-deficient donor is indicated.

5. The anaphylactoid reaction is not uncommon following intramuscular injection of serum immune globulins that contain 95 per cent IgG but also a detectable amount of IgA.

6. Treatment of urticarial reactions: When urticaria is not extensive, the patient may be given diphenhydramine hydrochloride (Benadryl) intramuscularly or intravenously (10 to 50 mg for an adult). Prophylactic use of diphenhydramine hydrochloride (50 mg p.o. 1 hour in advance of hemotherapy) will prevent or ameliorate such an allergic reaction to blood or plasma in adult patients with a known history of such reactions. When the urticaria is under control, the transfusion may be resumed.

For more extensive urticaria or an anaphylactoid reaction, blood transfusion should be discontinued and more aggressive therapy begun in the form of Benadryl plus epinephrine and even steroids. Appropriate evaluation of such a patient for IgA status and other forms of hypersensitivity phenomena should be completed before resuming hemotherapy.

OTHER COMPLICATIONS OF BLOOD TRANSFUSION

Circulatory Overload. A volume of 2 units of whole blood is more than 1 L, which is about 20 to 25 per cent of the blood volume of an average-sized person. Utilization of red blood cells as erythrocyte concentrate can deliver the same red cell mass in nearly half the volume. This should be considered carefully before a transfusion is attempted. Similar precautions should be followed with the use of albumin (each gram of albumin can retain about 20 ml of fluid in the circulatory system) as well as with infusions of a large volume of plasma, either fresh frozen or as suspension medium for large numbers of platelets. Sudden increases in the blood volume may precipitate congestive heart failure, particularly in infants and in persons with chronic anemia with underlying heart disease or with renal failure. In such cases, slow infusion of erythrocyte concentrate is definitely recommended; concurrent use of diuretics (pp. 1038 and 1042), and digitalis, and warming the patient may prevent circulatory overload.

Diseases Transmissible through Blood Transfusion

Viral Hepatitis. Viral hepatitis is by far the most important disease transmitted through blood transfusion. The incidence varies with the source of blood donors, the number of units transfused, and the type of component used.

Accumulated evidence indicates that the incidence of hepatitis in recipients of voluntary blood is lower than that of paid donor blood. As expected, the incidence increases as the number of transfusions increases, such as in patients undergoing open-heart surgery or surgical burn therapy.

Among the various blood components, albumin and globulin preparations are free of agents causing hepatitis if properly prepared (heated at 60°C. for 10 hours). Components or derivatives prepared from multiple donors have a higher incidence of causing hepatitis, especially factor II-VII-IX-X complex. There is some preliminary evidence that plasma derivatives from multiple donors may be associated with acquired immune deficiency syndrome (AIDS).

Among preparations from a single donor, the incidence varies with the amount of plasma in the preparation; the larger the amount of plasma, the greater the chance of hepatitis. Consequently, washed or frozen-thawed erythrocytes which contain only trace amounts of plasma have a minimal chance of transmitting hepatitis. Needless to say, the concentration of the infectious agents (not HBsAg) and the total amount of fluid used for washing play an important role in reducing infection. At least 5 types of viruses have been implicated in post-transfusion hepatitis (PTH). Hepatitis A virus was documented in only one case. Hepatitis B virus, which was thought to be responsible for all so-called "serum hepatitis," has been found recently in only about 7 per cent of the cases. Non-A and non-B are responsible for about 78 per cent of the cases. About 15 per cent are CMV, and a few are EBV.

Hepatitis B Virus. The use of blood from voluntary donors who have been screened with third generation tests for HBsAg, has decreased PTH due to HBV from between 20 and 30 per cent to less than 10 per cent. The use of a monoclonal antibody which can detect 0.1 ng/μl of antigen may further reduce the incidence of HBV infection. The availability of hyperimmune HBIg and a specific vaccine may help protect blood banking personnel, who are among the high risk populations.

Non-A and Non-B Virus. There is much evidence indicating the presence of non-A and non-B (NANB) hepatitis following blood transfusion. Serologically, it is neither A nor B. It has no cross-immunity to A or

B infection in man or in chimpanzees. An incubation period of 2 to 26 weeks is somewhat between those of A and B. Clinically, it is usually mild, with one third of the cases becoming chronic. Additional evidence, based on the incubation period, enzyme levels, different types of particles seen, and the lack of cross-immunity between cases, indicates the possible presence of at least two types of NANB hepatitis. Although there are many diagnostic tests reported, none are beyond the experimental stage at this time. The use of ALT levels to screen blood donors is a highly controversial issue (Aach, 1981; the reduction of 3.1 per cent of potential donors by screening would reduce NANB hepatitis by 31 per cent); it is similar to the AST issue reported over 20 years ago (Bang, 1959; the reduction of 9 per cent of the potential donors would reduce PTH by 75 per cent). Since the criterion of NANB hepatitis is mostly based on the elevation of ALT and only a very small number of cases have been confirmed by liver biopsy, the development of specific tests is essential in order to resolve this problem (Alter, 1981, 1982).

Cytomegalovirus (CMV). CMV has been known to produce post-transfusion syndrome—fever, splenomegaly, neutropenia, and atypical lymphocytes (Lang, 1969). This syndrome has been observed in patients receiving many units of blood, such as those undergoing open heart surgery. CMV has been estimated to be responsible for about 15 per cent of non-A and non-B post-transfusion hepatitis (Alter, 1981) and a cause of death in premature infants less than 28 weeks old and below 1200 g of weight (Yeager, 1980). CMV infection can also occur in immunologically incompetent patients such as recipients of bone marrow transplants at the time of graft rejection.

CMV infection can be established by a positive culture, presence of antibodies, or the demonstration of inclusion bodies. The best source of material for culture is leukocytes isolated by density gradient methods. Cultures of CMV may take about three weeks. Demonstration of inclusion bodies in leukocytes in urinary sediment is an insensitive technique. Serological methods, such as indirect immunofluorescent antibody, indirect hemagglutination, and enzyme immunoassay, are commonly used for this purpose. The demonstration of IgM anti-CMV or an increase of IgG anti-CMV of at least four-fold indicates a current infection; otherwise, a past infection is indicated.

Since CMV is located in leukocytes, they may remain there even after the development of anti-CMV. The use of CMV-negative blood has been recommended for transfusion of selected premature babies and in recipients of bone marrow grafts.

Epstein-Barr Virus (EBV). Transfusion-associated EBV infection is a relatively infrequent event. Only two of these patients following blood transfusion had evidence of infectious mononucleosis. One case followed a bone marrow transplantation and the other followed a renal transplantation (Tegtmeier, 1981).

Although there are many tests for EBV, only IgM anti-VCA indicates a current infection. While more than 90 per cent of recipients and donors have had previous exposure to EBV and screening for EBV serologically is a complicated procedure, screening for anti-EBV is also not suitable for routine use. On the other hand, transfusion of washed RBCs which contain few lymphocytes may reduce the chance of EBV infection in selected cases.

Malaria. A total of 55 cases have been reported in the United States related to blood transfusion between 1958 and 1978 (Huestis, 1981, p. 277). Only two of the implicated donors had been away from an endemic area for malaria for more than three years. A careful history may help to reduce this complication. Current donor standards exclude donors likely to transmit malaria.

Syphilis. Spirochetes do not appear to survive in citrated blood at 4°C. for more than 72 hours. Very few cases have been reported following blood transfusion in recent years. When a unit with high-titer antispirochete antibodies is transfused, the recipient may become seropositive for a short time (Mollison, 1983, p. 777). For this reason, donors with a false positive serologic test for syphilis should not be utilized.

Other Infections. Isolated cases have been reported for brucellosis, filariasis, infectious mononucleosis, and toxoplasmosis following blood transfusion. They are extremely rare. Transmission of babesiosis is also a theoretical possibility.

Undesirable Rare Complications Other than Infections

1. Anticoagulants, especially citrate in high concentration, may produce muscle tremor and electrocardiographic changes. This is a rare complication of massive transfusion.

2. Excessive potassium, which increases in plasma of stored whole blood (approximately 1 mmol/L/day after the first week, i.e., 23 mmol/L at 21 days) when administered to patients with poor renal function may also produce EKG changes and be harmful.

3. Ammonia and lactic acid accumulated during storage require detoxification in the liver and excretion by the kidneys. Precautions should be taken in patients with hepatorenal deficiency to minimize the use of whole blood and transfuse recently packed red blood cells when necessary.

4. Microaggregates have been discussed previously under the use of filters (p. 1042). Bredenberg (1977) has reviewed the relationship between massive blood transfusions and the adult respiratory distress syndrome, noting that clinical evidence is remarkably limited and experimental data controversial.

5. Air embolism is extremely rare since the introduction of plastic bags without an air vent.

6. Hemosiderosis. Each unit of blood contains about 250 mg of iron, while the physiologic loss of iron is only 1 mg/day. Repeated transfusions introduce excessive amounts of exogenous iron which deposit in the reticuloendothelial system, a condition known as hemosiderosis. In the case of hypoplastic anemia requiring repeated blood transfusions (e.g., sickle cell anemia, thalassemia) fresher blood (less than seven days of storage) should be used so that fewer transfusions are given to the same patient. In severe cases of

Table 43–19. INFORMATION ESSENTIAL TO AN INVESTIGATION OF TRANSFUSION REACTION

Patient's name________ Age______ Sex______ Race______

Admission No.______ Transfusion No.______ Rm No.______ Bed No. ______

Physician's name________ Diagnosis ________

Surgery________ Hypothermia______ Irrigation of bladder with ______

Medication: Penicillin______ Glucose/water______ Dextran______ Vit. K______ Alpha methyldopa ______

Others ________

Previous: Transfusions______ Pregnancies______ Allergy ______

Blood group: Patient______ Donor (No. ______) ______

Crossmatching: Major________ Minor ________

Transfusion: Started______ Stopped______ ml infused ______

Pain______ Dyspnea______ Cyanosis______ Vomiting______ Urticaria______ Chills______ Others____

	Before transfusion	During transfusion 15′	30′	60′	others
Temperature	______	______	______	______	______
Pulse rate	______	______	______	______	______
Blood pressure	______	______	______	______	______

Under anesthesia: Untoward oozing ______Tachycardia ______Hypotension______

Urine output ______ ml in ______ hours Hematuria ______ Others ______

hemosiderosis, therapeutic phlebotomy has been successful (Mollison, 1983, p. 780). More recently, iron chelating agents have been used in research protocols.

INVESTIGATION OF TRANSFUSION REACTIONS

Documentation. The physician in charge of the patient must be consulted to obtain as much information as possible to define the type of reaction and to guide the investigation. A useful check list is presented in Table 43–19.

Clerical Check. If the patient is suspected of having received the wrong unit of blood, the very first step is to check any possible clerical errors (Table 43–19).

Check the patient's full name, hospital number, transfusion number, and ABO group on the arm band against the information on the blood bag, crossmatching specimens, and blood bank records.

Laboratory Investigation (Table 43–20)

1. Routine tests for every transfusion reaction include (a) observation of any abnormal signs such as hemolysis, hemoglobinemia and/or hemoglobinuria,

Table 43–20. LABORATORY INVESTIGATION OF TRANSFUSION REACTIONS

	Patient's Blood			Donor's Blood	
	Pretransfusion	*Postransfusion*	**Urine**	*Tube or Segment*	*Container*
Routine for each case					
Abnormal signs: hemolysis, jaundice, not clotting, others	X	X	X		X
ABO and Rh_0 typing	X	X		X	X
Direct antiglobulin test	X	X			
Crossmatching	X	X		X	X
Whenever indicated					
Isoagglutinin titer/hemolysin	X			X	
Irregular antibodies	X	X		X	
Others		A, C	B		C

For A: 1. Free hemoglobin, haptoglobin, methemalbumin, hemopexin, bilirubin
2. Hemoglobin or hematocrit, differential count, white cell count
3. Platelet count, factor VIII, fibrinogen, fibrin-split products
4. Urea, creatinine, and other indicators for renal function
5. IgA and anti-IgA, antileukocyte antibodies
6. G6PD

For B: Hemoglobinuria, hemosiderinuria, urobilinogen

For C: Smear and culture for microorganisms

jaundice, poor clotting or bleeding, cloudy serum or plasma, or foul odor in blood specimens of the patient and the donor; (b) repeat of the ABO and Rh_o typing, direct antiglobulin test, and crossmatching.

2. Special tests are often required for selected cases, but each case should be dealt with individually to determine which additional tests are needed. The presence of strong or hemolytic donor plasma anti-A or anti-B should be ruled out first in a case of a hemolytic transfusion reaction. The presence of irregular antibodies in the patient, including those against leukocytes or platelets, should not be ignored.

In severe cases, it may be necessary to determine the extent of hemolysis as indicated by the presence of free hemoglobin in the plasma, ahaptoglobinemia, increase of methemalbumin, and bilirubin level (Fig. 43–4). Occasionally it may be necessary to check the extent of renal damage as indicated by serum urea and creatinine levels. If disseminated intravascular coagulation is suspected, a complete coagulation profile is warranted (see Chap. 32). If the reaction is of the anaphylactic type, determination of IgA and anti-IgA as well as anti-leukocyte antibodies may clarify the nature of the reaction. The possibility of G6PD deficiency and medication should be kept in mind. Microorganisms and bacterial toxins should not be forgotten. When deglycerolized erythrocytes are used, the presence of high residual glycerol may hemolyze the transfused erythrocytes.

PREVENTION OF TRANSFUSION REACTIONS

Prevention of transfusion reactions cannot be accomplished by the blood bank personnel alone; cooperation by other medical staff members is vital to its success. Figure 43–5 is an outline distributed to medical staff members at the Mount Sinai Hospital Medical Center. It is designed to review the 10 most important issues in the prevention of blood transfusion reactions; they are supplementary to what has already been discussed in different parts of the text.

Match the patient and blood (specimen and components)
(Absolute identification)
ABO compatibility is absolutely essential for RBCs
(Main cause of fatal reaction)
Transfuse patient only when it is definitely indicated
(Documentation for each case)
Component therapy to meet the specific needs
(No shotgun therapy!)
Hepatitis complication should be avoided by all means
(Second cause of fatal reaction)

Monitoring the patient during transfusion
(Severe reactions can be aborted)
Autotransfusion should be considered in selected patients
(The best blood is your own)
Transfuse washed RBCs whenever feasible
(Reduces many complications)
Condition of each patient should be considered
(Heart, kidney, liver, and lung)
History of previous immunization should be known
(Avoid delayed reactions)

Figure 43–5. Ten commandments of blood transfusion.

Hospital Transfusion Committee

REQUIREMENTS

A transfusion committee is required in every hospital where a transfusion service exists. This is not only to observe government regulations and to meet the criteria of accreditation agencies but also to promote communication and to serve as an educational pivot among the various parties involved in blood transfusion practice. Such education can contribute to improved patient care through optimal hemotherapy.

COMMITTEE

All parties deeply involved in transfusion practice should be represented; namely, blood bank director, other physicians including surgeons, anesthesiologists, hematologists, nephrologists, nursing staff, and administrators. The chairman should be someone who uses blood extensively and is interested in transfusion problems. The committee should meet not less than once every three months. An example of a review form is shown in Table 43–21.

ACTIVITIES

1. To assure adequate supplies of quality blood components and to maintain a cooperative relationship with the local supplier.
2. To establish transfusion policies and guidelines on the proper use of blood, blood components, and derivatives.
3. To prepare forms for adequate documentation of transfusion practice.
4. To review transfusion reactions and to improve the safety of blood transfusion.
5. To promote continuing education programs for various staff members and to inform them of any scientific advances or changes in regulatory policies.
6. To ensure the proper use of each blood component through a reviewing mechanism.

IMMUNIZATION ASSOCIATED WITH PREGNANCY

Maternal Immunization

With the exposure of the mother's immune apparatus to fetal blood, a maternal immune response with isoimmunization of fetus may ensue. The outcome of such isoimmunization may be hemolytic disease of the unborn or the newborn.

5

FACTORS AFFECTING MATERNAL IMMUNIZATION

Transplacental Hemorrhage (TPH). The presence of fetal erythrocytes in the mother's circulation can be demonstrated by the presence of erythrocytes containing fetal hemoglobin (Kleihauer, 1960), by a positive D^u test in Rh_o negative (D −) mothers (Polesky, 1971), or by a rosetting technique (Sebring, 1982). While none of these methods are very sensitive, they are the best available at present. Data from different laboratories indicate that TPH is negligible during the first and second trimesters; however, it may occur

Table 43–21. AN EXAMPLE OF A REVIEW FORM FOR TRANSFUSION COMMITTEE

BLOOD BANK AND TRANSFUSION SERVICE ANNUAL REPORT (19xx)

	Medicine	Neuro-Surgery	Gynecol-ogy	Ortho-pedics	Pediatrics	Surgery	Open Heart	Urology	Otorhino-laryngol-ogy	Renal Transplant	Burns	Total
No. of units crossmatched	4009	1475	1125	1865	732	4255	4475	610	371	624	759	20,300
No. of units transfused	2416	369	554	854	568	2020	2220	204	150	388	499	10,242
Crossmatch/transfusion ratio (C/T)	1.6	4.0	2.0	2.2	1.3	2.1	2.0	3.0	2.5	1.6	1.5	2.0
Transfusion reactions												94
Allergic	7	2	1	3	10	9	6	1			1	40
Febrile	26	2	2	5		6	2				1	44
Hemolytic	1											1
Delayed												
Other	2		2			3		1	1			9

during the third trimester and is fairly common at the time of delivery.

Up to 50 per cent of D− mothers with a D+ fetus may have demonstrable fetal erythrocytes at the time of delivery. About 20 per cent of these women may have 0.1 ml or more of fetal red cells, 1 per cent may have 3 ml or more, and up to 0.3 per cent may have 15 ml or more (Mollison, 1983, p. 340). The minimal dose of D+ erythrocytes capable of inducing a primary immunization is probably less than 0.1 ml (Mollison, 1983, p. 354). As expected, cesarean section and manual removal of the placenta are often associated with a considerable increase in TPH. Amniocentesis also increases the risk of TPH.

Maternal-fetal bleeding has been demonstrated in D− infants whose blood contains D+ erythrocytes from the mother. This has been implicated in the development of anti-D in a D− person without known antigenic stimulation; however, such a hypothesis has not been well established (Jennings, 1976).

Responder and Non-responder. A successful immunization of D− mothers is dependent not only on the dosage of D+ erythrocytes, but also on the mother's ability to respond to D+ antigens. An immunized mother can be recognized by the presence of anti-D in her serum or by the shortened survival of injected D+ erythrocytes. About one third of D− persons are non-responders and fail to form anti-D despite repeated injections of D+ erythrocytes (Mollison, 1983, p. 353).

Antigens Responsible for Immunization. The mother must be negative for an antigen(s) which the fetus inherits from the father in order to be immunized. Although Rh_o(D) antigen is by far the most important one involved in severe hemolytic disease of the newborn, other erythrocyte as well as leukocyte and platelet antigens can also induce maternal immunization by the formation of IgG antibodies. According to Giblett (1964), anti-D or anti-DC was found in 93 per cent of cases and anti-E, anti-c, or anti-Ce was found in 6 per cent of the cases. The remaining 1 per cent consisted of antibodies of other specificities. Anti-K, anti-k, anti-Fy^a, anti-Fy^b, anti-Kp^a, anti-Jk^a, anti-Jk^b, anti-M, anti-S, anti-s, anti-U, anti-Yt^a, anti-Di^a, anti-Di^b, anti-Co^a, anti-Wr^a, and many antibodies against low incidence antigens have been implicated in hemolytic disease of the newborn. In fact, many low incidence antigens were first recognized through the careful study of hemolytic disease of the newborn.

A or B antigens of the fetus can also immunize a group O mother, and the incidence is far greater than that induced by Rh antigens. However, clinically, the newborn presents a much milder disease and rarely requires the intensive treatment as in hemolytic disease of the newborn due to anti-D.

As early as 1943 Levine noted that ABO incompatibility between the mother and the fetus reduced the chance of Rh_o sensitization. His observation has been confirmed by many others. In general, Rh immunization occurs in only about half as many ABO-incompatible matings as ABO-compatible matings. Group O females offer stronger protection than those of other groups. For instance, in the mating of group B males with group O females, protection against Rh immunization was almost twice that found in the mating of group B males with group A females. The proportion of ABO compatible infants is approximately 0.8 (Mollison, 1983, p. 360).

The zygosity of the father of the infant also plays an important part in the immunization of the mother during subsequent pregnancies. If he is a homozygote, all their children are expected to be positive for that antigen; if he is a heterozygote, only 50 per cent of their children are expected to be positive when the mother is negative for that antigen. When zygosity is unknown, the gene frequency (approximately 0.6 for D) divided by phenotype frequency (approximately 0.84 for D), $0.6/0.84 = 0.71$, represents the chance that their children will be positive for that antigen (applied only to a two-allele system).

Thus, the chance for a Rh_o(D)-negative (−) woman (0.16) with a D+ husband (0.84) to be ABO compatible (0.8), to have a D+ fetus (0.71), to have sufficient transplacental hemorrhage to immunize the mother (0.2), and to be immunized again by a D+ fetus (0.71) is $0.16 \times 0.84 \times 0.8 \times 0.71 \times 0.2$

× 0.71 = 0.011. In other words, about 1 per cent of all women (or 6 per cent of D− women), in the absence of suppressive therapy and pregnant for the second time, may have an affected infant. This figure is close to what has been observed clinically.

Previous Immunization. Except in rare instances, the infant from the first pregnancy is seldom affected. If it is affected, the disease is usually very mild. However, if the mother has been immunized previously either through pregnancies or transfusions, the immunizing dose may be very small and the immune response may be much greater than that found in the primary immunization. Hence, a history of previous transfusions or other possible sources of immunization, such as abortion, as well as other normal pregnancies, should be established in a prenatal work-up.

History of Affected Infant(s). Murray (1957) showed that the risk of stillbirth in an existing pregnancy is greatly influenced by the condition of previous infants at time of delivery. When previous infants were delivered without anemia or only mild anemia, the risk was below 7 per cent. Those with moderate anemia showed 20 per cent; with severe anemia, 55 per cent; with one stillbirth, 70 per cent; and with more than one stillbirth, 80 per cent.

Previous Treatment. The incidence of hemolytic disease of the newborn due to anti-D has been greatly reduced since the advent of suppressive treatment employing anti-D globulin or Rh_o immune globulin (IgG Rh_o antibodies).

PRENATAL TESTING

Blood Specimen of the Mother

1. ABO and Rh_o typing of mother's blood should be done early in pregnancy.
2. Antibody screening (detection) should be performed not only against routine reagent red blood cells but also against the erythrocytes of the father whenever feasible. If anti-D is present, repeated comparative titers should be performed to see whether there is any increase in titer. If no antibodies are detected, it is advisable to repeat screening of a patient's serum one month prior to delivery to assure that no unexpected antibodies have developed in the latter part of the pregnancy.
3. Proper antibody identification employing a panel of reagent red blood cells must be performed if the screening is positive.
4. A serologic test for syphilis and possibly one for hepatitis B antigen should also be performed, as both diseases may affect the fetus.

Blood Specimen of the Father

1. ABO grouping is useful information to predict the ABO group of the fetus and, hence, the chance of ABO compatibility with the mother.
2. Complete Rh phenotyping regardless of whether he is D+ or D − is important. If he is D+, the chance for him to be a homozygote or heterozygote for D can be estimated as in Table 43–22.

If he is DccEe, or DccEE instead of DCcee, the chance of having a severely affected DccEe fetus is greater. If he is D−, other erythrocyte antigens may be inherited by the fetus and immunize the mother, especially E and c.

Table 43–22. LIKELIHOOD OF BEING HOMOZYGOUS FOR $Rh_0(D)$*

Phenotype	Whites	Blacks
Rh_0(Dce)	5%	48%
Rh_1rh(DCce)	10%	58%
Rh_2rh(DcEe)	10%	65%
Rh_1Rh_1(DCe)	95%	100%
Rh_2Rh_2(DcE)	92%	100%
Rh_1Rh_2(DCcEe)	96%	88%

*Based on New York Population (Wiener, 1969).

HEMOLYTIC DISEASE OF THE UNBORN

The passage of IgG Rh antibodies into the fetal circulation induces immune hemolysis and anemia in varying degrees of severity. In mild cases, the fetus can usually survive to term for natural delivery. In moderately severe cases, the fetus may live to near maturity and be delivered by early induction of labor, usually after 32 weeks of gestation. In very severe cases, the fetus may develop heart failure associated with other factors (anemia, asphyxia, and depressed serum protein concentration) with resulting massive edema and anasarca, known as "hydrops fetalis." Death *in utero* usually occurs in the latter instance. In a study of 1300 Rh-immunized women, the stillbirth rate was found to be approximately 12 per cent (Walker, 1956). In some cases with early diagnosis, the anemic fetus can be treated successfully by intrauterine transfusion. Repeated removal of antibodies from the mother's circulation by plasma exchange (Mollison, 1983, p. 687) has been attempted with successful results and may be used in selected cases. To establish the severity of disease in the affected fetus, the study of amniotic fluid described in Chapter 21 provides useful information.

AMNIOCENTESIS (see Chap. 21)

Transabdominal insertion of a needle into the amniotic cavity has long been used for injection of radiopaque material for amniography and for injection of hypertonic saline solution in order to terminate pregnancy. For the past decade, it has been widely used in prenatal diagnosis, assessment of fetal well-being or jeopardy, and prognosis of hemolytic disease of the newborn caused by Rh antibodies.

Indications

1. Serum titer of anti-D of 16 or higher by antiglobulin test in a pregnant woman with a history of previous stillbirth due to Rh immunization.
2. Serum titer of anti-D of 32 or higher in a pregnant woman with history of previous child who received exchange transfusions.
3. Progressive rise of anti-D serum titer to 64 or higher in a pregnant woman without history of affected fetus or child.

The initial amniocentesis is usually done between 24 and 28 weeks of gestation, or six to eight weeks before gestational age of previous fetal loss caused by Rh immunization. Meaningful information usually requires at least two amniocenteses, at one to two weeks' interval, in order to confirm and compare the results of each tap.

The amniotic fluid should be protected against light, which affects the level of pigments. The fluid portion should be separated as soon as possible from cellular and other sediment. Turbid fluid should be clarified by high-speed

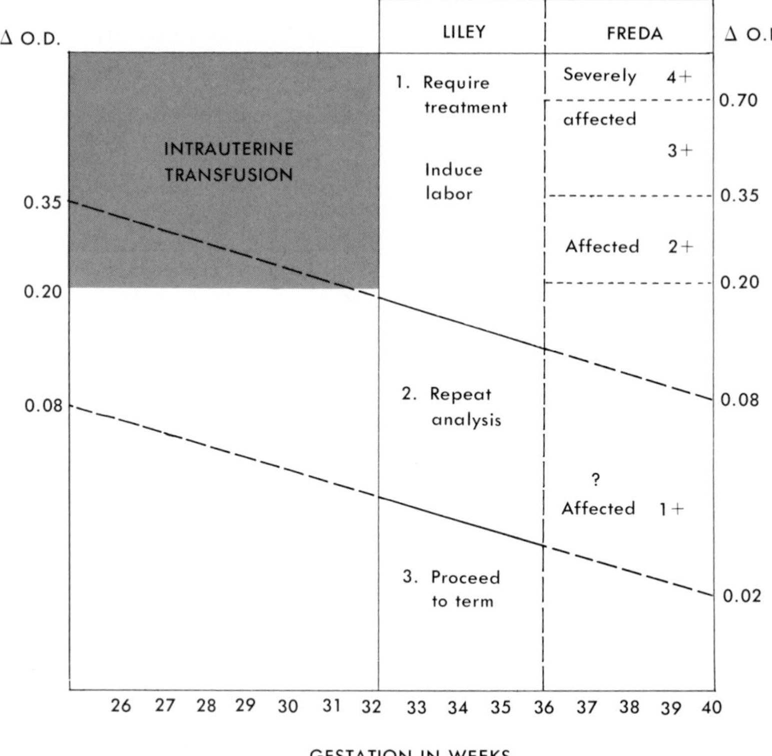

Figure 43–6. Methods of Liley and Freda on the assessment of fetal prognosis by the values of ΔO.D. at 450 nm of bilirubinoid in amniotic fluid. (Modified from Dito, 1975, p. 52.)

centrifugation or by filtration before being tested (see Chap. 21).

Testing

Bilirubin Pigment. The level of bilirubinoid is by far the most important determination. The exact nature of this pigment and its pathway into the amniotic cavity are not yet known. Results of bilirubinoid determination provide a high degree of accuracy in predicting the outcome of the pregnancy in Rh immunization. Presence of bilirubin pigment leads to an abnormal elevation of optical density at 450 nm in a spectrophotometric scan. The difference in optical density between baseline and peak of elevation is known as delta (Δ) O.D. The normal value of the Δ O.D. varies with gestational age; consequently, any value expressed must state the age of the fetus. As shown in Figures 43–6 and 21–1 (p. 504), Liley grouped all Δ O.D. values into three zones: Zone 1 requires immediate treatment with either exchange transfusion or the induction of labor. Zone 2 indicates a repeat analysis, while Zone 3 can proceed to term. In the same figure, Freda grouped all Δ O.D. into four zones. Basically, the three upper zones (4+, 3+, 2+) are equivalent to Zone 1 of Liley, while the lower zone is equivalent to Liley's Zones 2 and 3.

Increased optical density in a spectrophotometric scan of amniotic fluid may be due to material other than bilirubin. Blood, which is present in various amounts in about 50 per cent of the taps, produces a peak at 415 mμ; meconium gives high Δ O.D. below 425 mμ; urine shows a very high Δ O.D. below 400 mμ. A mixture of blood and bilirubin pigment can be differentiated by repetition of the scan after extraction of bilirubin with chloroform (Fig. 43–7 and p. 504).

Maturity of the Fetus (see Chap. 21). As the fetus approaches maturity, the lecithin/sphingomyelin (L/S) ratio increases in value. An L/S ratio of 2 or greater suggests that pulmonary maturity is sufficient for extrauterine survival and one can anticipate no respiratory disease syndrome neonatally. L/S ratios between 1.5 and 1.9 indicate a transitional state of pulmonary maturity, and a mild respiratory disease syndrome may be expected. When L/S ratios are less than 1.5, severe respiratory disease syndrome is the usual outcome.

Creatinine concentration in amniotic fluid reflects the increase of fetal muscle mass and fetal glomerular filtration. A value of 2 mg/dl or greater indicates sufficient fetal maturity. Other indices have also been used in selected laboratories (Dito, 1975—an excellent monograph on amniotic fluid which is recommended for additional information with our Chapter 21).

Anti-D Titer. Comparison with the anti-D titer of the maternal serum has been reported to be useful as a prognostic index for viability of the fetus.

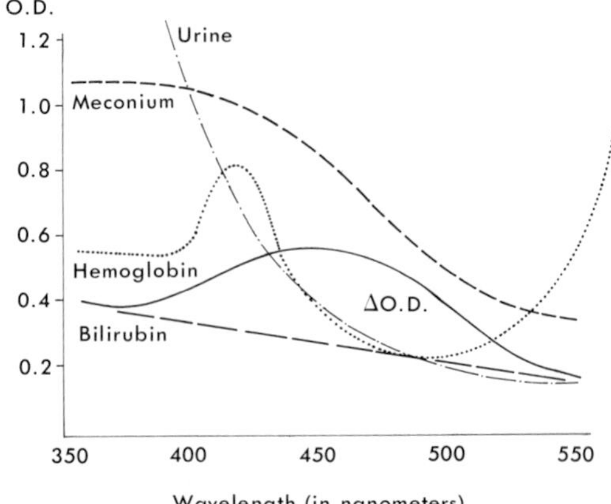

Figure 43–7. Differentiation of pigments commonly found in amniotic fluid by spectrophotometric scan.

ABO Typing. This can be done in three ways: (1) mixed agglutination of fetal epithelial cells using red blood cells of known group; (2) detection of soluble A, B, and H substances; or (3) direct erythrocyte typing, provided the red cells have been shown to be of fetal origin by means of the Kleihauer test. Rh typing and direct antiglobulin test can also be done with fetal red blood cells.

Sex Determination. Presence of sex chromatin (Barr body) in desquamated fetal cells indicates a female fetus.

Complications

1. Fetal or maternal bleeding and fetal death following amniocentesis have been reported.
2. Fetal-maternal hemorrhage, inducing additional immunization of the mother.
3. Infection, essentially preventable.

INTRAUTERINE TRANSFUSION

Intrauterine transfusion was made possible on the basis of (1) absorption of functional red blood cells from the peritoneal cavity into the general circulation; and (2) ability of the fetus to swallow radiopaque material, permitting visualization of the fetal peritoneal cavity by radiographic amniography. It offers a means of correcting severe fetal anemia *in utero,* thus preventing development of hydrops fetalis. However, it should be applied only in critically selected cases following timely and accurate diagnosis.

Indications. The following factors must be considered in making the decision for intrauterine transfusion: (1) previous history of stillbirth or exchange transfusion due to Rh immunization; (2) comparison of gestational age of previous fetal loss (stillbirth) with weeks of gestation of the current pregnancy; intrauterine transfusion, as a rule, is given between 20 and 33 weeks of gestation; (3) anti-D titer of maternal serum and bilirubin level in the amniotic fluid; and (4) when amniography discloses definite signs of hydrops, this is considered a contraindication. In these considerations it is not enough simply to decide which fetuses need transfusion, but more important, which do not.

Selection of Blood. Group O Rh-negative packed red blood cells are generally used for intrauterine transfusion. Frozen red blood cells have also been recommended owing to the fact that the washing process used for removal of the cryoprotective agent also reduces the chance of (1) transmitting hepatitis, (2) potassium intoxication, and (3) graft-versus-host reaction because of removal of most immunocompetent leukocytes. Very recently, automated machines for obtaining washed fresh red blood cells with few leukocytes have become available; such fresh washed cells may be the choice for intrauterine transfusion. Radiation of the blood before infusion may be helpful in preventing a graft vs. host reaction. The recommended volume to be injected depends on the individual's peritoneal size such as the following (Queenan, 1977):

Weeks of Gestation	20–22	23–24	25–26	27–29	30–31	32	33
Red blood cells (ml) (Hematocrit 70%)	20	30	35	40	50	60	70

During the initial transfusion, a self-retaining Teflon catheter is inserted to facilitate subsequent transfusions, which are usually repeated every two weeks until the infant can survive after delivery (more than 32 weeks of gestation).

Results. The general survival rate of infants receiving intrauterine transfusion is about 30 per cent; in fetuses with some signs of hydrops, survival is less than 14 per cent, while it is 45 per cent in those without signs of hydrops (Queenan, 1977). However, the value of intrauterine transfusion is doubtful in the presence of hydrops fetalis (Queenan, 1977).

Complications

Fetal. The mortality related to the procedure is about 14 per cent. Since premature labor is a common complication, many instances of fetal loss result from prematurity and associated respiratory distress syndrome. Injury to various parts of the fetus is not uncommon. Potassium intoxication, serum hepatitis, and graft-versus-host reaction have been reported. Exposure to x-ray should be reduced to minimal amounts.

Maternal. Infections may develop in about 10 per cent of women and bleeding in about 5 per cent (Queenan, 1977).

Hemolytic Disease of the Newborn

Rh INCOMPATIBILITY

The exact mechanism by which IgG antibodies pass through the placenta is not yet known. Since other immunoglobulins of size comparable to IgG do not pass through the placenta, size is obviously not the only determining factor. All four subclasses of IgG are able to pass the placenta, although some IgG2 may fail to do so (see Table 42–7, p. 977).

Anemia is probably the result of extravascular hemolysis. In a stillborn fetus, marked erythrophagocytosis is often found in the reticuloendothelial system, especially in the spleen. As a result of anemia, a large number of nucleated cells and reticulocytes can often be seen in the peripheral blood; hence, the term *erythroblastosis fetalis* has been used for this condition.

Before birth, the excessive amount of bilirubin (up to 22 mg/dl) derived from hemolysis is normally bound to albumin and then forms conjugated bilirubin in the mother's liver through the action of glucuronidase. In newborns, the glucuronidase levels in the liver are low and the amount of albumin is limited; therefore, a considerable amount of free (indirect) bilirubin accumulates. Free bilirubin has a high affinity for basal ganglia of the central nervous system and produces a yellow stain in brain tissue. Thus, the term *kernicterus* has been used to describe this condition. In severe cases, the infant becomes increasingly lethargic and exhibits opisthotonos and eventually respiratory failure, and death occurs. In milder cases, the infant may appear to be normal but may exhibit mental retardation later (Fig. 43–8).

According to the survey of Mollison (1983), when the bilirubin concentration in the plasma was 18

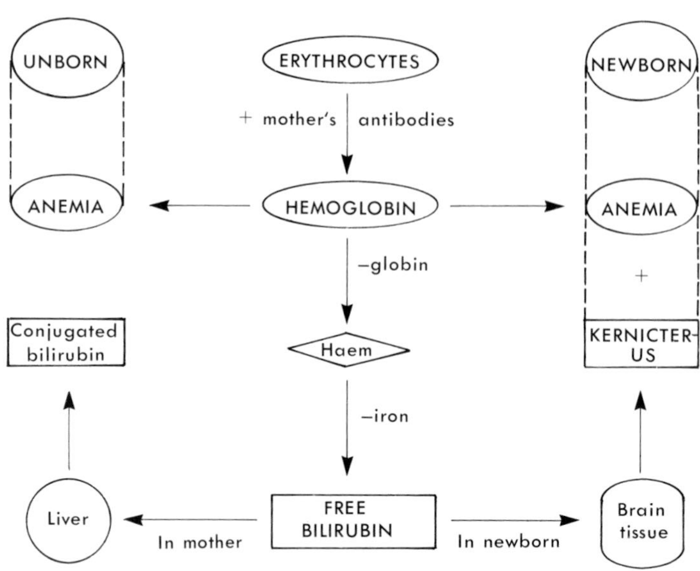

Figure 43–8. The effect of immune hemolysis in the unborn (anemia only) and in the newborn (anemia and kernicterus). This difference is due to the fact that the newborn's liver has insufficient glucuronidase to conjugate free bilirubin, which has a high affinity for brain tissue, thus producing kernicterus.

mg/dl or below, kernicterus was not observed. However, the incidence increased as bilirubin levels approached 19 mg/dl or higher. At a level of over 30 mg/dl, 8 out of 11 patients developed kernicterus. In many hospitals, a concentration of 16 mg/dl is used as the critical level to begin aggressive treatment regardless of the cause of the elevation. This lower level of bilirubin as a cut-off may be crucial and is attributed to variability in albumin binding capacity for bilirubin (measured by reserve albumin binding capacity), relative amount of free bilirubin in proportion to conjugated total serum bilirubin, and the possible existence of other facets of bilirubin transport and metabolism.

ABO INCOMPATIBILITY

ABO incompatibility is expected when the mother's blood is type O and the fetus has type A or B erythrocytes, or when the mother is A or B and the fetus is B or A, respectively. The theoretical chance of such combinations would be the mother's phenotype frequency multiplied by the gene frequency of the incompatible antigen, as follows:

MATERNAL PHENOTYPE	PHENOTYPE FREQUENCY	FETAL PHENOTYPE	GENE FREQUENCY	CHANCE OF SUCH COMBINATION
O	0.44	A	0.27	0.12
O	0.44	B	0.07	0.03
A	0.44	B	0.07	0.03
B	0.1	A	0.27	0.03
Total Chance				0.21

Clinically, hemolytic disease of the newborn is usually found only in infants of group A or B with group O mothers. Infants with mild jaundice as a sign of ABO incompatibility have been observed in only about 1 in 150 births (Mollison, 1983, p. 690). Many factors could be involved in the finding of such a low incidence; the presence of A or B antigens in soluble form as well as in the tissues may spare the erythrocytes from being the only target. Qualitative and/or quantitative ABH modifications of fetal erythrocytes making such cells potentially less antigenic and the lack of well-defined criteria for making such a diagnosis may also play an important role.

Jaundice developing within 24 hours after birth is frequently associated with ABO incompatibility, and the term *icterus praecox* has been used for this syndrome. The presence of high titer immune anti-A or anti-B in the mother's serum does not indicate that the fetus or the infant is affected. The direct antiglobulin test of infant's erythrocytes is not always positive in spite of the fact that anti-A or anti-B may be recovered in the eluate of the infant's erythrocytes. Spherocytosis, reticulocytosis, and mild anemia are often encountered. In general, only rare cases are severe enough to require treatment. While hemolytic disease of the newborn due to Rh incompatibility is rarely seen in the firstborn, it is not unusual to have the firstborn affected by ABO incompatibility.

DIAGNOSIS: NEONATAL TESTING

Direct Antiglobulin Test. The direct antiglobulin test of the cord blood sample is usually strongly positive. However, the strength of this reaction is not correlated with the severity of the disease. An infant with a strongly reacting test may have very mild or no disease at all. When the test is weak, it may indicate the presence of antibodies other than anti-D, although the mother may be D−. In cases of ABO incompatibility, the eluate study of the cord blood cells is more useful than the direct antiglobulin test which is often weakly reactive or negative.

Hemoglobin Concentration. The normal concentration of cord and venous blood samples of newborns ranges from 15 g/dl to over 20 g/dl. When the hemoglobin values are around 14 g/dl, the infant may suffer from severe disease and even kernicterus. When the hemoglobin concentration is below 14 g/dl, the infant is usually affected; the lower the concentration, the more severely affected the infant and the greater the incidence of kernicterus and hydrops fetalis.

Bilirubin Concentration. The bilirubin concentration of the cord specimen is probably the best index for prognosis. The level of bilirubin represents the combined result of hemolysis and liver function of the infant. Normal cord total serum bilirubin values are between 1 and 3 mg/dl, and a cord value of 5 mg/dl is generally considered an indication for exchange transfusion. The significance of bilirubin level is closely related to the age of the infant. The recommendation made by Allen (1957) serves as a useful guide for the management of hemolytic disease of the newborn (Fig. 43–9).

Other Helpful Measurements and/or Examinations. Erythroblastemia and reticulocytosis are often found in $Rh_0(D)$ incompatibility, whereas spherocytosis is seen in ABO incompatibility. Hyperbilirubinemia from other causes may be found in newborns. Some examples would include prematurity with insufficient hepatic glucuronidase, congenital syphilis, hepatitis, cytomegalic inclusion disease, toxoplasmosis, other bacterial infections, G6PD deficiency, galactosemia, hereditary hemolytic anemia, or that associated with a diabetic mother. Appropriate determinations should be made to exclude such possibilities.

MANAGEMENT

In addition to exchange transfusion for hemolytic disease of the newborn secondary to blood group incompatibility, other clinical disorders of newborns may be treated as shown in Table 43–13.

Rationale. The purpose of exchange transfusion is four-fold: (1) remove bilirubin to prevent injury to the brain tissue, (2) supply erythrocytes to correct the anemia, (3) remove erythrocytes coated with antibodies, and (4) remove free antibody which may cause additional hemolysis.

Indications. A bilirubin level above 5 mg/dl at birth, above 11.5 mg/dl 12 hours after birth, or above 16 mg/dl after 24 hours is definite indication for exchange transfusion. Hemoglobin concentrations below 14 g/dl or prematurity of the newborn are two important factors and should be taken into consideration.

Blood to be Used. If the infant is affected by anti-$Rh_0(D)$, ABO type- specific and Rh_0 (D−) blood should be used. If the infant is affected by anti-A or anti-B, group O erythrocytes with A or B or AB plasma are recommended. If compatible blood cannot be found, incompatible blood can be used under emergency conditions. Blood of the mother without the plasma is a practical alternative. When whole blood is used, it is desirable to remove part of the plasma to reduce the side effects and to provide a higher hemoglobin concentration. Blood should be warmed before it is transfused, especially in the case of a premature baby.

Frozen-thawed red blood cells have also been advocated for exchange transfusion (Grajwer, 1976; Staples, 1976). In addition to excellent red cell recovery, including adequate levels of 2,3-diphosphoglycerate, there is decreased antigenic stimulation from leukocytes and platelets. Theoretically, lymphocytes transfused into a neonate might induce a graft-versus-host (GVH) disease (see Chap. 33); radiation of fresh blood before use has thus been proposed to destroy lymphocytes and minimize the likelihood of GVH disease (Kevy, 1977). Such red cell transfusions may be combined with albumin or FFP to enhance bilirubin binding and removal.

Compatibility testing for exchange transfusion can be done in three ways: The first choice is to use mother's serum against the donor's erythrocytes. The mother's serum is readily available and contains antibodies of higher titer than that in the infant's serum. However, the mother's serum may contain IgM antibodies such as anti-Le^a, anti-I, and anti-HI, which

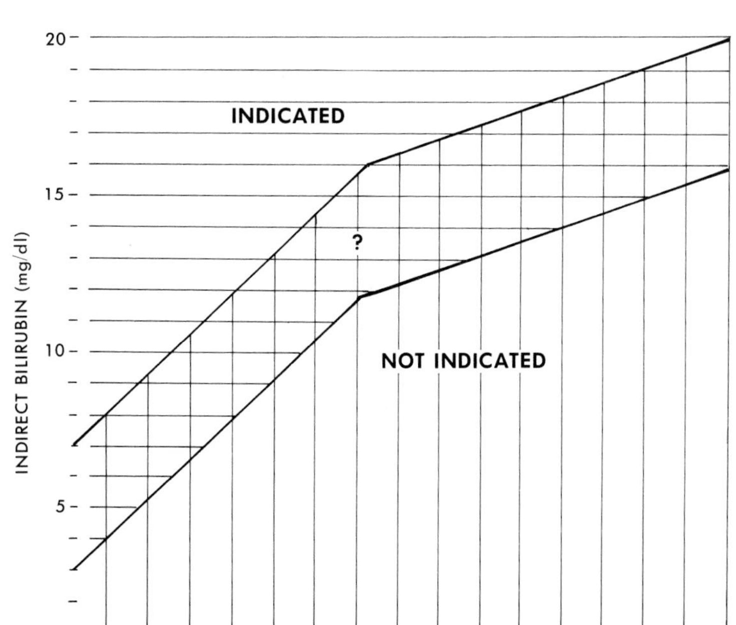

Figure 43–9. The use of the indirect bilirubin level of the newborn at different ages in hours as guide for exchange transfusion. (Adapted from Allen, 1957.)

5

may confuse the crossmatching. The treatment of mother's serum with 2-mercaptoethanol before crossmatch may be necessary. Using the eluate from the cord erythrocytes is the second best choice; it is particularly useful when the mother's serum has IgM type of antibodies and blood specimen from the mother is not available, or the ABO group of the donor is not compatible with mother's serum. When the eluate is not reactive, maternal and/or infant serum must also be used. Finally, it may sometimes be necessary to use serum of the newborn.

At the end of the first exchange transfusion, a blood specimen should be saved for crossmatches in possible additional exchange transfusions; the mother's serum serves as a useful double check for compatibility.

About 90 ml of blood per pound (infant weight) is a useful guideline for determining the amount required for exchange transfusion. In case of technical difficulties, at least 60 ml/lb should be given in order to achieve beneficial effects. In infants with heart failure, a larger amount of blood could be withdrawn than the amount infused, but the exchange should be done slowly. To counteract the effect of citrate, 1 ml of a 10 per cent solution of calcium gluconate is usually given for each 100 ml of blood exchanged. To avoid the use of citrate, heparinized blood was commonly used; since heparinized blood has only a two-day shelf life, it is impractical to have it readily available. In addition, heparin activates lipase to produce fatty acids which compete with bilirubin for albumin, an obvious disadvantage, as well as result in systemic anticoagulation.

In order to reduce the amount of potassium, lactate, or ammonia in stored blood, fresher blood should always be used for exchange transfusion.

Effect of Exchange Transfusion. Hemoglobin concentration is increased. The level of bilirubin and antibodies is usually decreased, but to a much lesser extent because both components are also distributed extravascularly. In severe cases, a second or even a third exchange is required to lower the bilirubin level.

Exchange transfusion can be hazardous; toxic effects of the anticoagulant, high levels of potassium or ammonia, technical problems, and infections have been reported. In general, it is a safe and useful procedure and lives of many newborns have thus been saved.

Other Treatment. Phototherapy may reduce the bilirubin levels in serum by acceleration of bilirubin catabolism through the skin. This has proved to be helpful in mild cases. Phenobarbital, which induces the formation of glucuronidase in the liver, has been used to reduce the serum bilirubin level of the infants by giving it either to the mother prenatally or to the infant neonatally. Both types of treatment can be used to supplement but not replace exchange transfusion.

PREVENTION OF Rh IMMUNIZATION

Rationale. It had been noted that when Rh_o(D)-negative volunteers were injected with D+ erythrocytes that had been coated *in vitro* with anti-D, they did not develop anti-D (Stern, 1961). When anti-D was administered to volunteers shortly after receiving D+ erythrocytes, the latter were removed rapidly from the circulation and no anti-D formed subsequently (Finn, 1961; Freda, 1964, 1978). On the basis of these observations, immune anti-Rh_o(D) has been used routinely to prevent Rh immunization of Rh_o(D)-negative mothers or other persons receiving D+ erythrocytes under various conditions. The exact mechanism of anti-Rh_o(D) remains to be established.

Indications. Rh_o(D) immune globulin is recommended for D− mothers without demonstrable anti-D in their plasma who deliver a D+ infant, or those who have had a miscarriage, abortion, ectopic pregnancy, or amniocentesis where the Rh of the fetus is unknown. It is also recommended for any women of childbearing age receiving D+ erythrocytes. Immune anti-D should not be given to a D+ person or to a D− person with anti-D. Mothers who receive antenatal RhIg have demonstrable anti-D in their sera but need another dose of RhIg at the time of parturition.

Dosage. Immune anti-D preparations in the United States contain about 300 μg of antibody/vial, which is sufficient to suppress antigenicity of about 15 ml of D+ erythrocytes (30 ml of blood). Since fetal maternal bleeding is seldom over 30 ml, one vial is adequate under normal conditions. When a larger amount of bleeding is suspected, the amount of fetal blood in the mother's circulation can be estimated by the fetal-maternal cell ratio using the acid elution technique. Taking all factors into consideration, a fetal-maternal cell ratio of 1:100 (1 per cent) in a 100 lb mother is equivalent to about 30 ml of fetal blood in the mother's circulation. Thus, regardless of any deviation from these two reference numbers, the number of vials of anti-D required can be readily calculated. For instance, if the fetal-maternal cell ratio is 2 per cent and the mother is 150 lb, $2 \times 1.5 = 3$ vials would be needed. To ensure complete protection, Walker recommends doubling the calculated dose (1977)

Since fetal-maternal hemorrhage happens also during pregnancy, investigators in Canada and Australia have been giving immune anti-D during the last trimester of pregnancy. The first injection is given during the 28th week of gestation and, in some cases, an additional injection is given sometime around the 33rd week of gestation. The results obtained seem better than those from their control groups (Davey, 1976; Bowman, 1976).

Administration. To test the mother's erythrocytes with immune anti-D prior to injection is not essential but is recommended for two purposes: to make sure that the mother is D− and to check for the possible presence of a large fetal maternal bleed, which would require an additional amount of immune anti-D. A large number of fetal cells in the mother's circulation can be revealed at the antiglobulin test phase (same as D^u test) in the form of a minor population of agglutinates. Should the D^u test be positive and the mother known to be D−, the fetal-maternal cell ratio could then be determined by the acid elution technique (Kleihauer, 1960) and the amount of immune anti-D adjusted according to the test results. A number of techniques are available for detecting a minor population of Rh_o(D+) fetal red cells (Polesky, 1981). Immune anti-D is normally given intramuscularly as soon as possible after delivery. However, beneficial effect has been observed even if it is administered after the recommended time limit of 72 hours under special situations. Mild local reactions at the injection site and a slight elevation in temperature are not infrequent. Fever, myalgia, lethargy, splenomegaly, and hyperbilirubinemia have been observed in persons receiving large doses of immune anti-D.

Specially prepared immune anti-D can be given intravenously, but this must be done slowly. These types of products have been used in Europe for years. The intravenous route is advisable for the recipient of a large dose. It not only relieves the painful effect of intramuscular injection but also provides a better clearance of D+ erythrocytes in the circulation (Mollison, 1983, p. 382).

After routine use of immune anti-D for D− mothers in the past decade, immunization to D antigen has been steadily decreasing. Morbidity and mortality of unborns (fetuses) or newborns due to Rh_o immunization have been greatly reduced. Exchange transfusion, a procedure which had been used very frequently for hemolytic disease of newborn, is now used only occasionally in many hospitals. Although the figures vary in different locations, the efficiency of immune anti-D in the prevention of Rh_o immunization is extremely high (Freda, 1978).

Since the discovery of Rh_o immunization in the early 1940's, diagnosis was advanced in the 1950's, effective management was achieved in the 1960's, and finally prevention became successful in the 1970's. The history of Rh_o immunization illustrates well the rapid achievements in the field of basic and applied immunohematology (Freda, 1978).

Aach, R. D., Szmuness, W., Mosely, J. W., et al.: Serum alanine aminotransferase of donors in relation to the risk of non-A, non-B hepatitis in recipients. N. Engl. J. Med., *304*:989, 1981.

Adams, N. S., Bland, W. H., and Bassett, S. H.: A method of human plasmapheresis. Proc. Soc. Exp. Biol. Med., *80*:377, 1952.

Akerblom, O., and Högman, C. F.: Frozen blood: A method for low-glycerol. Liquid nitrogen freezing allowing different post-thaw deglycerolization procedures. Transfusion, *14*:6, 1974.

Allen, F. H., and Diamond, L. K.: Erythroblastosis Fetalis. Boston, Little, Brown and Co., 1957.

Alter, H. J.: Posttransfusion hepatitis: Prologue, progress and prospects. *In* Keating, L. J., and Silvergleid, A. J. (eds.): Hepatitis. Washington, D.C., AABB, 1981.

Alter, H. J., Solomon, R. E., Hoofnagle, J. H., and Melpolder, J.: The clinical significance of elevated serum transaminase (ALT) in healthy donors. Transfusion, *22*:404, 1982.

Alter, H. J., Tabor, E., et al.: Transmission of hepatitis B virus infection by transfusion of frozen-deglycerolized red blood cells. N. Engl. J. Med., *298*:637, 1978.

Andrews, A. T., Zmijewski, C. M., et al.: Transfusion reaction with pulmonary infiltration associated with HLA specific leukocyte antibodies. Am. J. Clin. Path., *66*:483, 1976.

Bang, N. V., Ruegsegger, P., and Ley, A. B.: Detection of hepatitis carriers by serum glutamic oxalacetic transaminase activity. J.A.M.A., *171*:2303, 1959.

Barker, L. F., Shulman, N. R., and Murray, R.: Transmission of serum hepatitis. J.A.M.A., *211*:1509, 1970.

Betts, R. F., Freeman, R. B., Douglas, R. G., Jr., and Tally, T. E.: Clinical manifestations of renal allograft derived primary cytomegalovirus infection. Am. J. Dis. Child., *131*:759, 1977.

Bloch, K. J., and Maki, D. G.: Hyperviscosity syndromes associated with immunoglobulin abnormalities. Sem. Hematol., *10*:113, 1973.

Boral, L. I., Crowley, L. M., and Henry, J. B.: Adult transfusion outpatient clinic in a hospital-based blood bank. Transfusion, *17*:607, 1977a.

Boral, L. I., and Henry, J. B.: The type and screen: A safe alternative and supplement in selected surgical procedures. Transfusion, *17*:163, 1977b.

Bowman, J.: Winnipeg antenatal prophylaxis trial. *In* Scientific Symposium—Rh Antibody Mediated Immunosuppression. Raritan, N.J., Ortho Research Institute, 1976.

Branda, R. F., Moldow, C. E., McCullough, J. J., and Jacob, H. S.: Plasma exchange in the treatment of immune disease. Transfusion, *15*:570, 1975.

Bredenberg, C. E.: Does a relationship exist between massive blood transfusion and the adult respiratory distress syndrome? If so, what are the best preventive measures? Vox Sang., *32*:211, 1977.

Bukowski, R. M., King, J. W., and Hewlett, J. S.: Plasmapheresis in the treatment of thrombotic thrombocytopenic purpura. Blood, *50*:413, 1977.

Byrnes, J. J., and Khurana, M.: Treatment of thrombotic thrombocytopenic purpura with plasma. N. Engl. J. Med., *297*:1386, 1977.

Corash, L., Klein, H., et al.: Selective isolation of young erythrocytes for transfusion support of thalassemia major patients. Blood, *57*:599, 1981.

Dau, P. C., Lindstrom, J. M., Cassel, C. K., Denys, E. H., Shev, E. E., and Spitler, L. E.: Plasmapheresis and immunosuppressive drug therapy in myasthenia gravis. N. Engl. J. Med., *297*:1137, 1977.

Davey, M. G.: Antenatal administration of anti-Rh: Australia 1969–1975. *In* Scientific Symposium—Rh Antibody Mediated Immuno-suppression. Raritan, N.J., Ortho Research Institute, 1976.

Dawson, R. B.: Blood storage XIII: 2,3-DPG maintenance for six weeks in CPD-adenine-inosine preservative with and without methylene blue. Transfusion, *17*:238, 1977.

Delivoria-Papadopoulos, M., Miller, L. D., and Oski, F. A.: The role of exchange transfusion in the management of low-birth weight infants with and without severe respiratory distress syndrome. I. Initial observations. J. Pediatr., *89*:273, 1976.

Diepenhorst, P., and Engelfriet, C. P.: Removal of leukocytes from whole blood and erythrocyte suspensions by filtration through cotton wool. V. Results after transfusion of 1820 units of filtered erythrocytes. Vox Sang., *29*:15, 1975.

Dito, W. R., Patrick, C. W., and Shelly, J.: Clinical Pathological Correlations in Amniotic Fluid. Chicago, American Society of Clinical Pathologists, 1975.

Djerassi, I.: Gravity leukapheresis—a new method for collection of transfusable granulocytes. Exp. Hematol., *5*:139, 1977.

Donner, I., Moore, F. A., and Collins, F. A.: Efficacy of leukocyte-poor red blood cell suspensions prepared by sedimentation in hydroxyethyl starch. Transfusion, *15*:439, 1975.

Dybkjaer, E., and Elkjaer, P.: The use of heated blood in massive blood replacement. Acta Anaesth. Scand., *8*:271, 1964.

Edson, J. R., McArthur, J. R., Branda, R. F., McCullough, J. J., and Chou, S. N.: Successful management of a subdural hematoma in a hemophiliac with an anti–factor VIII antibody. Blood, *41*:113, 1973.

Eisenstadt, R. S., and Berkman, E. M.: Rapid cytoreduction in acute leukemia. Management of cerebral leukostasis by cell pheresis. Transfusion, *18*:113, 1978.

Finn, R., Clark, C. A., Donahue, W. T., et al.: Experimental studies on the prevention of Rh hemolytic disease. Br. Med. J., *1*:486, 1961.

First, M. R., Balakrishnan, K., Alexander, J. W., et al.: Pretransplant donor specific transfusions, sensitization and outcome in renal transplants. Transfusion, *22*:403, 1982.

Fraser, I. D., Bothamley, J. E., Bennett, M. O., and Airth, G. R.: Intensive antenatal plasmapheresis in severe rhesus immunization. Lancet, *1*:6, 1976.

Freda, V. J., Gorman, J. G., and Pollack, W.: Successful prevention of experimental Rh sensitization in man with an anti-Rh gamma globulin antibody preparation: A preliminary report. Transfusion, *4*:26, 1964.

Freda, V. J., Pollack, W., and Gorman, J. G.: Rh disease: How near the end? Hospital Practice, June, 1978.

Freireich, E. J., Levin, R. J., and Whang, J.: The function and fate of transfused leukocytes from donors with chronic myelocytic leukemia in leukopenic recipients. Ann. N.Y. Acad. Sci., *113*:1081, 1964.

5

Friedman, B. A., Schork, M. A., Mocniak, J. L., and Oberman, H. A.: Short-term and long-term effects of plasmapheresis on serum proteins and immunoglobulins. Transfusion, *15*:467, 1975.

Geyer, R. P.: Oxygen transport in vivo by means of perfluorochemical preparations (editorial). N. Engl. J. Med., *307*:304, 1982.

Giblett, E. R.: Blood group antibodies causing hemolytic diseases of the newborn. Clin. Obstet. Gynecol., 7:1044, 1964.

Giblett, E. R.: Blood group antibodies: An assessment of some laboratory practices. Transfusion, *17*:299, 1977.

Gottuso, M. A., Williams, M. L., and Oski, F. A.: The role of exchange transfusions in the management of low birth-weight infants with and without severe respiratory distress syndrome. II. Further observations and studies of mechanisms of action. J. Pediatr., *89*:279, 1976.

Graham-Poole, J., Barr, W., and Willoughby, M. L. N.: Continuous flow plasmapheresis in management of severe rhesus disease. Br. Med. J., *1*:1185, 1977.

Grajwer, L. A., Pildes, R. S., Zarif, M., et al.: Exchange transfusions in the neonate. A controlled study using frozen-stored erythrocytes resuspended in plasma. Am. J. Clin. Path., *66*:117, 1976.

Graziano, J. H., et al.: A simple technique for preparation of young red cells for transfusion from ordinary blood units. Blood, *59*:865, 1982.

Greenwalt, T. J. (ed.): General Principles of Blood Transfusion. Chicago, American Medical Association, 1977.

Hattersley, P. G., Goetzman, B. W., Gross, S., and Blankenship, W. J.: A walking blood donor program for seriously ill premature infants. Transfusion, *16*:366, 1976.

Henry, J. B., Mintz, P. D., and Webb, W.: Optimal blood ordering for elective surgery. J.A.M.A., *237*:451, 1977.

Herzig, G. P., and Graw, R. G.: Granulocyte transfusion for bacterial infections. Prog. Hematol., *10*:207, 1975.

Herzig, R. H., Herzig, G. P., Graw, R. G., et al.: Successful granulocyte transfusion for gram-negative septicemia. N. Engl. J. Med., *296*:701, 1977.

Högman, C. F., Hedlund, K., Akerblom, O., and Venge, P.: Red blood cell preservation in protein-poor media. I. Leukocyte enzymes as a cause of hemolysis. Transfusion, *18*:233, 1978.

Howland, W. S., Bellville, J. W., et al.: Massive blood replacement. V. Failure to observe citrate intoxication. Surg. Gynecol. Obstet., *105*:529, 1957.

Hubbell, R. C., and Henry, J. B.: New blood product label requirements. J. Clin. Lab. Automation, *1*:122, 1981.

Huestis, D. W., Bove, J. R., and Bush, S.: Practical Blood Transfusion. 3rd ed. Boston, Little, Brown & Co., 1981.

Huggins, C. E.: Practical preservation of blood by freezing. *In*: Red Cell Freezing. AABB, 1973, pp. 31–54.

Israel, L., Edelstein, R., Mannoni, P., Radot, E., and Greenspan, E. M.: Plasmapheresis in patients with disseminated cancer: Clinical results and correlation with changes in serum protein. Cancer, *40*:3146, 1977.

Jennings, E. R.: Maternal-fetal hemorrhage. *In* Scientific Symposium—Rh Antibody Mediated Immunosuppression. Raritan, N.J., Ortho Research Institute, 1976.

Jones, J. V., Bucknall, R. C., Cumming, R. H., Asplin, C. M., Fraser, I. D., Bothamley, J., Davis, P., and Hamblin, T. J.: Plasmapheresis in the management of acute systemic lupus erythematosus. Lancet, *1*:709, 1976.

Kaspersin, D., and Sanders, G.: Reported at the 4th Annual Apheresis Meeting in Chicago, Oct. 1982.

Kernoff, L. M., Botha, M. B., and Jacobs, P.: Exchange transfusions in sickle cell disease using a continuous-flow blood separator. Transfusion, *17*:269, 1977.

Kersey, J. H., Ramsay, N. K., et al.: Allogenic bone marrow transplantation in acute nonlymphocytic leukemia: A pilot study. Blood, *60*:400, 1982.

Kevy, S. V.: Pediatric transfusion therapy. Technical Improvement Service, Number 29, Immunohematology. Chicago, American Society of Clinical Pathologists, 1977.

Kienle, P. C.: Methods of administration of blood and its components. Infusion, *1*:26, 1978.

Kleihauer, E., and Betke, K.: Praktische Anwendung des Nachweises von Hb F-haltigen Zellen in fixierten Blutausstrichen. Internist, *1*:292, 1960.

Krijnen, H. W.: Glycerol treated human red blood cells frozen with liquid nitrogen. Vox Sang., *9*:559, 1964.

Lang, D. J., and Hanshaw, J. B.: Cytomegalovirus infection and the post transfusion syndrome: Recognition of primary infections in four patients. N. Engl. J. Med., *280*:1145, 1969.

Lasky, L. C., Ash, R. C., et al.: Collection of pluripotential hemopoietic stem cells by cytapheresis. Blood, *59*:822, 1982.

Lindstrom, J. M., Lennon, V. A., and Seybold, M. E.: Experimental autoimmune myasthenia gravis and myasthenia gravis: Biochemical and immunochemical aspects. Ann. N.Y. Acad. Sci., *274*:254, 1976.

Lockwood, C. M., and Peters, D. K.: The role of plasma exchange and immunosuppression in the treatment of Goodpasture's syndrome and glomerulonephritis. Plasma Ther., *1*(1):19, 1979.

Lowenthal, R. M., Buskard, N. A., Goldman, J. M., Spiers, A. S. D., Bergier, N., Graubner, M., and Galton, D. A. G.: Intensive leukapheresis as initial therapy for chronic granulocytic leukemia. Blood, *46*:835, 1975.

Lukomyskyj, L., and Lee, C. L.: Some aspects of frozen red blood cells. Lab. Med., *5*:42, 1974.

Mayer, K.: A different view of transfusion safety-type and screen, transfusion of Coombs incompatible cells, and fetal transfusion-induced graft versus host disease. *In* Polesky, H. F., and Walker, R. H. (eds.): Safety in Transfusion Practices. Skokie, Ill., CAP, 1982.

McGrath, M. A., and Penny, R.: Paraproteinemia: Blood hyperviscosity and clinical manifestations. J. Clin. Invest., *58*:1155, 1976.

Meryman, H. T.: Preservation of blood by freezing. *In* Ikkala, E., and Nykanen, A. (eds.): Transfusion and Immunology. Vammala, Vammala Kirjapaino Oy., 1975.

Milam, J. D., and Austin, S. F.: Red cell salvage in open-heart surgery. *In* Hemotherapy in Trauma and Surgery. Washington, D.C., AABB, 1979, pp. 67–75.

Miller, W. V. (eds.): AABB Technical Manual. 7th ed. Washington, D.C., AABB, 1977.

Miller, W. V., Holland, P. V., et al.: Anaphylactic reactions to IgA: A difficult transfusion problem. Am. J. Clin. Path., *54*:618, 1975.

Mintz, P. D., Haines, A. L., and Sullivan, M. F.: Incompatible crossmatch following nonreactive antibody detection test. Frequency and cause. Transfusion, *22*:107, 1982.

Mintz, P. D., Lauenstein, K., Hume, J., and Henry, J. B.: Expected hemotherapy in elective surgery: A followup. J.A.M.A., *239*:623, 1978.

Mintz, P. D., Nordine, R. B., Henry, J. B., and Webb, W. R.: Expected hemotherapy in elective surgery. N.Y. J. Med., *76*:532, 1976.

Mollison, P. L.: Blood Transfusion in Clinical Medicine. 5th ed. Oxford, Blackwell Scientific Publication, 1983.

Moran, C. J., Parry, H. F., Mowbray, J., Richards, J. D. M., and Goldstone, A. H.: Plasmapheresis in systemic lupus erythematosus. Br. Med. J., *1*:1573, 1977.

Murray, W., Murray, S., and Russel, J. K.: Stillbirth due to hemolytic disease of the newborn. J. Obstet. Gynecol., *44*:573, 1957.

Myers, T. J., Wakem, C. J., Ball, E. D., and Tremont, S. J.: Thrombotic thrombocytopenic purpura: Combined treatment with plasmapheresis and antiplatelet agents. Ann. Intern. Med., *92*:149, 1980.

Myhre, B., and Worthen, W.: Untoward response to blood transfusion. Lab. Med., *9*:29, 1978.

Oberman, H. A.: Replacement transfusion in the newborn infant: A commentary. J. Pediatr., *86*:586, 1975.

Oberman, H. A., Barnes, B. A., and Friedman, B. A.: The risk of abbreviating the major crossmatch in urgent or massive transfusion. Transfusion, *18*:137, 1978.

Opelz, G., and Terasaki, P. I.: Cadaver kidney transplants in North America. Analysis 1978. Dial. Transplant., *8*:167, 1979.

Oski, F. A.: Personal communication, 1977.

Pineda, A. A., Brazica, S. M., and Taswell, H. F.: Hemolytic transfusion reaction. Mayo Clin. Proc., *53*:378, 1978a.

Pineda, A. A., Taswell, H. F., and Brzica, S. M.: Delayed transfusion reactions: An immunologic hazard of blood transfusion. Transfusion, *18*:1, 1978b.

Polesky, H. F.: Reported at the 4th Annual Apheresis Meeting in Chicago, Oct. 1982.

Polesky, H. F., and Hanson, M.: AABB-CAP survey data on hepatitis—incidence, surveillance, and prevention. Am. J. Clin. Path., *74*:565, 1980.

Polesky, H. F., and Sebring, E. S.: Detection of fetal maternal hemorrhage: An evaluation of serological tests related to Rh_0(D) immune globulin (human). Transfusion, *11*:162, 1971.

Polesky, H. F., and Sebring, E. S.: Evaluation of methods for detection and quantitation of fetal cells and their effect on RhIgG usage. Am. J. Clin. Path., 76:525, 1981.

Prince, A. M.: Post transfusion hepatitis: Etiology and prevention. *In* Ikkala, E., and Nykanen, A. (eds.): Transfusion and Immunology. Vammala, Vammala Kirjapaino Oy., 1975.

Queenan, L. T.: Modern Management of the Rh Problem. 2nd ed. Hagerstown, Md., Hoeber Medical Division, Harper and Row, 1977.

Robinson, E. A. E., and Tovey, L. A. D.: Intensive plasma exchange in the management of severe Rh disease. Br. J. Haematol., *45*:621, 1980.

Rowe, A. W., Eyster, E., and Kellner, A.: Liquid nitrogen preservation of red blood cells for transfusion, a low glycerol-rapid freeze procedure. Cryobiology, *5*:119, 1968.

Schiffer, C. A., and McCredie, K. B.: Cell component therapy for patients with cancer. *In* Dawson, R. B. (ed.): A Technical Workshop of AABB, 1974.

Schlansky, R., DeHoratius, R. J., Pincus, T., Tung, K., and Ballas, S.: Plasmapheresis therapy in systemic lupus erythematosus (SLE). Clin. Res., *28*:150A, 1980.

Schmidt, P. J.: Transfusion mortality: With special reference to surgical and intensive care facilities. J. Fla. Med. Assoc., *67*:151, 1980.

Sebring, E. S., and Polesky, H. F.: Detection of fetal maternal hemorrhage in Rh immune globulin candidates: A rosetting technique using enzyme-treated Rh_2Rh_2 indicator erythrocytes. Transfusion, *22*:468, 1982.

Skoog, W. A., and Adams, W. S.: Plasmapheresis in a case of Waldenström's macroglobulinemia. Clin. Res., 7:96, 1959.

Solanki, D., and McCurdy, P. R.: Delayed hemolytic transfusion reaction reactions. An often missed entity. J.A.M.A., *239*:729, 1978.

Solis, R. T., and Gibbs, M. B.: Filtration of the microaggregates in stored blood transfusion. Transfusion, *12*:245, 1972.

Staples, J. W., and Fritz, G. E.: Development and use of pediatric frozen red cell packs. Transfusion, *16*:566, 1976.

Stern, K., Goodman, H. S., and Berger, M.: Experimental isoimmunization to hemoantigens in man. J. Immunol., *87*:189, 1961.

Storb, R., and Thomas, E. D.: Marrow transplantation in thirty "untransfused" patients with severe aplastic anemia. Ann. Intern. Med., *92*:306, 1980.

Taft, E. G., Babcock, R. B., Scharfman, W. B., and Tartaglia, A. P.: Platelet pheresis in the management of thrombocytosis. Blood, *50*:927, 1977.

Tegtmeier, G. E., and Bayer, W. L.: Those other agents in the differential diagnosis of post transfusion hepatitis. *In* Keating, L. J., and Silvergleid, A. J. (eds.): Hepatitis. AABB, 1981, pp. 67–98.

Thomas, F. D.: Current status of marrow transplantation of aplastic anemia and acute leukemia. Am. J. Clin. Path., *72*:887, 1979.

Tremper, K. K., et al.: The preoperative treatment of severely anemic patients with a perfluorochemical oxygen-transport fluid, Fluosol-DA. N. Engl. J. Med., *307*:277, 1982.

Valeri, C. R.: Principle of cryobiology: High glycerol and storage at 80°C and low glycerol and storage at 150°C. Red Cell Freezing. AABB, 1973, pp. 1–30.

Valeri, C. R., and Zaroulis, C. G.: Rejuvenation and freezing of outdated stored human red cells. N. Engl. J. Med., *187*:1307, 1972.

Walker, R. H.: On the safety of the abbreviated crossmatch. *In* Polesky, H. F., and Walker, R. H. (eds.): Safety in Transfusion Practices. Skokie, Ill., College of American Pathologists, 1982, pp. 71–106.

Walker, R. H.: Fetal-maternal hemorrhage. *In* Baer, D. M. (ed.): Blood Banking for Hospital Laboratory. Chicago, ASCP, 1977.

Walker, W., and Murray, S.: Haemolytic disease of the newborn as a family problem. Br. Med. J., *1*:187, 1956.

Wenz, B., and Barland, P.: Therapeutic intensive plasmapheresis. Sem. Hemat., *18*:147, 1982.

Widmann, F. K. (ed.): Technical Manual. 8th ed. Washington, D.C., AABB, 1981.

Wiener, A. S.: Problems and pitfalls in blood grouping tests for non parentage. I. Distribution of the blood groups. Am. J. Clin. Path., *51*:9, 1969.

Williams, W. J.: Serum viscosity. *In* Williams, W. J., Beutler, E., Erslev, A. J., and Rundles, R. W. (ed.): Textbook of Hematology. 2nd ed. New York, McGraw-Hill Book Co., 1977.

Yawn, D. H., et al.: An improved intraoperative red cell salvage system for rapid auto-transfusion. Transfusion, *22*:413, 1982.

Yeager, A. S., Grumet, F. C., and Hafleigh, E. B., et al.: Prevention of transfusion-acquired cytomegalovirus infections in newborn infants. J. Pediatr., *98*:281, 1981.

Part VI

MEDICAL MICROBIOLOGY

EDITED BY JOHN A. WASHINGTON II, M.D., and JOHN BERNARD HENRY, M.D.

44

MEDICAL MICROBIOLOGY

JOHN A. WASHINGTON II, M.D.

The laboratory diagnosis of an infectious disease is contingent upon prior determination of a differential diagnosis on the basis of the patient's history and physical examination, a consideration of those organisms most likely to have caused the disease, and the selection of those tests and procedures that are most likely to lead to the organism's detection and identification by means of microscopic examination, cultures, or immunologic techniques. Because infectious diseases may involve any body surface, system, and organ and because infectious diseases may be due to a wide variety of microorganisms, including bacteria, fungi, parasites, and viruses, selection of the proper specimen for the laboratory to examine is a critical but often neglected component of the diagnostic process.

The specimen for examination should be representative of the disease process and should be adequate in quantity for complete examination. It should be collected in such a way as to avoid contamination with the microflora that is indigenous to the skin and mucous membranes. Invasive techniques, such as transtracheal or suprapubic aspiration, may be required to obviate contamination of specimens by indigenous microflora. Specimens should, in general, be forwarded promptly to the laboratory for processing so that fastidious organisms do not perish or are not overgrown during storage. In some cases, special provisions may have to be made to ensure survival of organisms, such as the use of transport media or anaerobic containment. Recommendations regarding specimen selection, collection, and transport are made in the chapters that follow according to categories of etiologic agents causing infectious diseases.

In many instances, close cooperation between the microbiologist and histopathologist is essential for establishing the diagnosis of an infectious disease. Material removed surgically is obtained at considerable expense and some risk to the patient, and every effort should be made to ensure that it is examined microbiologically and histologically as carefully and completely as possible. Histologic examination shows whether the lesion is malignant or inflammatory and, if the latter, whether it is suppurative or granulomatous. Often, the material's histopathology will suggest a microbial etiology other than that originally suspected and additional special stains, cultures, and immunologic studies must be performed. Multiple specimens should be obtained from a large lesion and when several lesions are present. Tissue should be minced with sterile scissors and ground with a sterile abrasive, such as alundum, for microbiologic studies. Residual tissue should be stored at 5°C. for at least two weeks, pending the results of initial microbiologic and histopathologic examination, in case further studies are indicated.

The value of postmortem bacteriology is limited because of the poor correlation between ante- and postmortem culture results and because of the frequency of positive cultures and their lack of correlation with clinical or autopsy evidence of infectious disease. Because of the selectivity of the procedures used for their isolation and identification, mycobacteria, fungi, and viruses should be sought only when their presence was suspected clinically ante mortem or considered likely on the basis of postmortem findings.

Not all laboratories provide the same microbiologic services. The variety and extent of services provided by a laboratory depend on multiple factors, including the size of inpatient and outpatient facilities served, the interests and expertise of those directing and supervising the laboratory, the availability of tests and procedures in nearby or distant reference laboratories, and the cost-effectiveness of each procedure as determined by the clinical need and justification for its performance on-site, its test volume and cost, and the laboratory's ability to maintain its proficiency in performing the test. Basic bacteriologic procedures, such as preparing Gram's stained smears and inoculating media, are required of nearly all hospital laboratories. Whether or not specimens are examined for the presence of mycobacteria, fungi, viruses, and parasites and the extent of identification of microorganisms must be determined by each laboratory director on the basis of factors mentioned above.

Many specialized microbiologic services are provided by city, state, and regional laboratories and by other reference laboratories. Shipment of specimens to these laboratories must comply with Federal regulations (Section 72.25 of Part 72, Title 42). Services are also provided by the Centers for Disease Control (CDC), Atlanta, Georgia; however, the Centers' primary responsibility is to serve as a resource for state and regional laboratories, and physicians seeking CDC assistance should do so through their own state health departments. Specific notations are made in the text of subsequent chapters when direct consultation with CDC is recommended. *In vitro* diagnostic reference products are available from the Biologic Products Division of CDC to other federal agencies; international, state, regional, and local public health agencies; public health service grantees when the products are required by their grants; commercial producers of *in vitro* diagnostic products for use in evaluating production lots; collaborating researchers; and when there is a public health need for diagnostic products that can be neither purchased nor prepared in commercial laboratories.

In the chapters that follow, emphasis has been placed on specimen requirements, organism descriptions, and interpretation of findings. Detailed descriptions of techniques, stains, reagents, media, and methods of identification of organisms have not been included, since there are several excellent published books and manuals covering these aspects of medical microbiology. These resources are listed as general references at the end of each chapter. When a procedure considered to be particularly important and useful could not be located in the general references, citation of the specific reference describing the procedure was added.

In conclusion, there is no area of the clinical laboratory except microbiology in which the sources and varieties of specimens are so diverse; the process of selection, collection, and transport of the specimen so important; and the communication between physician and laboratory personnel so essential to the diagnosis of a disease. The laboratory needs to know what disease and etiologic agent are suspected. The laboratory requires a properly selected and collected specimen. An understanding by the clinician of the pathogenetic properties of microorganisms is essential for the correct interpretation of the laboratory's findings. The mere isolation of an organism or the demonstration of an immunologic response to a particular microbial antigen does not always constitute definitive evidence of its role in causing disease.

45

MEDICAL BACTERIOLOGY

JOHN A. WASHINGTON II, M.D.

An understanding of the locations, varieties, and roles of the bacterial flora indigenous to the skin and mucous membranes is essential to the proper selection and collection of material for cultures. The isolation and identification by the laboratory of a large number of bacteria from a specimen contaminated with indigenous flora is extraordinarily time-consuming and defies rational interpretation and therapy. The complexity of the problem posed by indigenous flora can best be illustrated in Table 45–1, in which are listed those bacteria commonly encountered on healthy human body surfaces. The magnitude of the problem

Table 45–1. BACTERIA COMMONLY FOUND ON HEALTHY HUMAN BODY SURFACES*

Bacteria	Skin	Conjunctiva	Upper Respiratory Tract	Mouth	Lower Intestine	Genitourinary Tract		
						External Genitalia	*Anterior Urethra*	*Vagina*
Aerobic and facultatively anaerobic								
Staphylococci	+	+	+	+	±	+	+ +	+
Streptococci								
viridans	±	±	+	+ +	+	+	±	+
group A			±	±				
group D			±	+	+	+	+	+
S. pneumoniae		±	+	+				
Neisseriae		±	±	+			+	±
Corynebacteria	+	+	+	+	+	+	+	+
Haemophili		±	+	+				
Enterobacteriaceae			±	±	+ +	+	+	±
Anaerobic								
Clostridia				±	+ +		±	±
Propionibacteria	+ +		+	±	±		±	
Actinomycetes			+	+	±			
Lactobacilli				+	+		±	+ +
Bifidobacteria				+	+ +			+ +
Bacteroides			+	+ +	+ +	+	+	+
Fusobacteria			+	+ +	+	+	+	±
Cocci								
gram-positive	+		+	+ +	+ +	+	±	+
gram-negative			+	+ +	+		±	+

*Adapted from Rosebury, 1962, and Sutter, 1980. ±, irregular; +, common; + +, prominent.

can best be illustrated by the fact that the number of bacteria on some areas of the skin, in the mouth, and in the descending colon may reach 10^6 organisms/sq cm, 10^9 organisms/ml, and 10^{11} organisms/g, respectively.

A specimen for bacterial culture that has been contaminated with indigenous flora has limited utility unless only specific organisms, e.g., group A streptococci in the throat, are being sought or certain precautions are taken. These precautions include disinfection of the area through which the specimen is aspirated or passes, as with a phlebotomy for blood culture or collection of a clean-voided midstream specimen for urine culture; bypassing the area, as with a transtracheal aspiration of lower respiratory secretions or with a suprapubic aspiration for bladder urine; or quantitation to establish the probability of disease, e.g., significant bacteriuria. Given these precautionary steps, the laboratory needs to define specimen requirements and instructions for microbiologic examination. A suggested list of instructions is shown in Table 45–2.

Table 45–2. INSTRUCTIONS FOR SPECIMEN COLLECTION AND TRANSPORT FOR BACTERIOLOGIC CULTURE*

Specimen	Container or Transport Device	Volume (ml)	Other Considerations
Blood			
Bacteria	Vacuum blood culture bottles containing liquid medium with SPS	Adults: 10 ml/100 ml bottle Infants: 1–3 ml/100 ml bottle	A minimum of 2 separate collections per 24 hr period is required; more than 3 per 24 hr period are rarely needed and should be collected only following consultation with laboratory consultant.
Catheters	Sterile, screw-capped or anaerobe tube	–	Disinfect surrounding entry site, remove catheter, and aseptically clip off tip into tube.
Exudates			
Transudate, drainages, ulcers	Swab or sterile, screwcapped tube	–	Such specimens are rarely suitable for anaerobic culture.
Eye	See "Other Considerations"	–	Cultures of patients with conjunctivitis are rarely useful. With corneal lesions swab material and scrapings should be applied directly to slides for smears and to media for culture.
Fecal material	Screw-capped jar	–	Freshly passed or collected material recommended. Transport medium should be used when delay anticipated.
Fluids			
Cerebrospinal	Sterile, screw-capped tube	1–5	Must be delivered to laboratory *immediately;* refrigeration of fluid may be deleterious to survival of certain bacteria.
Other (e.g., synovial, pleural, peritoneal)	Anaerobe vial	1–5	Collect with sterile needle and syringe; expel air bubbles before injection into vial.
Genitourinary			
For *Neisseria gonorrhoeae*	Swab or modified Thayer-Martin agar	–	*Women:* Cervix—moisten speculum with water before inserting into vagina; insert swab into cervical canal. Anal canal—insert swab approximately 2 cm and move from side to side to sample crypts. Urethra or vagina—cultures indicated when cervical not possible. *Men;* Urethra—swab may be used when a discharge is present; otherwise, a sterile bacteriologic loop is inserted to obtain scrapings for smear and culture. Anal canal—as for women.

*Adapted from Washington, 1981.

Table continued on following page

Table 45–2. INSTRUCTIONS FOR SPECIMEN COLLECTION AND TRANSPORT FOR BACTERIOLOGIC CULTURE (*Continued*)

Specimen	Container or Transport Device	Volume (ml)	Other Considerations
Cervix, vagina for other bacteria	Swab	–	These specimens are unsuitable for anaerobic culture.
Urine			
Midstream or catheterized	Sterile, screw-capped tube or jar	1–10	Specimen should be delivered to the laboratory immediately or, if delay (>2 h) is anticipated, refrigerated during transport.
Suprapubic aspirate	Anaerobe tube	1–10	Collect with sterile needle and syringe; expel air bubbles before injection into tube. This is the *only* type of urine specimen that is acceptable for anaerobic culture.
Abscess, wound	Anaerobe vial	–	Collect with sterile needle and syringe; expel air bubbles before injection into vial.
Respiratory tract			
Nasopharynx	Flexible wire calcium alginate–tipped swab	–	Useful for detecting carrier states of *Neisseria meningitidis, Corynebacterium diphtheriae,* and *Bordetella pertussis,* although nasopharyngeal aspirate with soft rubber catheter is better for detecting *B. pertussis.*
Throat	Swab	–	Tonsillar areas, pharynx, and areas of purulence, ulceration, inflammation, or capsule formation must be swabbed with minimal oral contamination. Ordinarily, cultures for group A streptococci suffice; however, the laboratory must be notified when diphtheria, pertussis, or gonococcal infection is suspected clinically so that appropriate selective media can be inoculated.
Sputum	Sterile, screw-capped jar	–	Subunit fresh specimen resulting from deep cough as soon after collection as possible. Specimens with >25 squamous epithelial cells/lpf are not acceptable for culture.
Transtracheal aspirate	Anaerobe vial	–	Collect with sterile needle and syringe or in trap; expel air bubbles before injection into vial.
Bronchial washings	Sterile, screw-capped vial	–	These specimens are unsuitable for anaerobic culture unless collected with a plugged telescoping catheter brush.
Tissue	Sterile, screw-capped jar or anaerobe tube	–	Samples representative of disease process must be submitted.

Having established these general guidelines, the next and probably more difficult step for the laboratory is to define criteria for rejection of certain requests for bacteriologic studies. Obvious criteria include discrepancies between patient identification data on the request form and on the specimen container or the absence of identification data on a container that arrives in the laboratory separated from a request form. Although erroneous reports are certainly intolerable, pinning the diagnosis of gonorrhea, tuberculosis, or hepatitis on the wrong patient has social and epidemiologic connotations of incredible magnitude. Dried-out specimens on swabs or swab specimens accompanied by requests for bacterial, mycobacterial, fungal, and viral cultures are clearly unacceptable unless it is simply impossible to obtain additional material. Under such circumstances the report should certainly bear the message that the specimen was unsatisfactory. Leaking containers bearing normally sterile body fluids should be reported as such.

SPECIMEN SELECTION AND COLLECTION

BLOOD

The indications for obtaining blood cultures are manifold but are basically the occurrence of a sudden relative change in pulse rate and temperature, with or without chills, prostration, and hypotension; a history of mild, intermittent, and persistent fever in association with a heart murmur; and generally any time sepsis is suspected. Bacteremia is generally intermittent, with the notable exception of that associated with endocarditis; therefore, it is imperative that more than one set of cultures be performed. Because bacteria indigenous to the skin can be associated with infectious processes of prosthetic material, careful antisepsis of the phlebotomy site with iodine or an iodophor is essential, as is the collection of more than one set of blood cultures. In nearly all cases of endocarditis two sets of blood cultures are sufficient to isolate the etiologic agent; in other types of bacteremias three sets, collected separately, usually suffice. The collection of a single set of blood cultures only is clearly unacceptable, and the laboratory should establish a policy that a minimum of two sets within a 24-hour interval be required. Conversely, the collection of more than three sets of cultures within this time interval is rarely indicated and should be performed only following consultation with the laboratory director.

Because the order of magnitude of bacteremia is very low in adults, the isolation rates of bacteria from blood are directly related to the volume of blood cultured. It is recommended, therefore, that between 20 and 30 ml (minimum, 10 ml) of blood be collected for each set of cultures. In infants the order of magnitude of bacteremia is considerably greater so that between 1 and 3 ml of blood should be adequate for each set of cultures. The volume of blood and the number of blood culture sets collected are independent variables reflecting the low order of magnitude of bacteremia on the one hand and its intermittency on the other.

Ordinarily, blood is inoculated at the bedside directly into bottles containing media; alternatively, it can be transported to the laboratory in a sterile tube containing sodium polyanethol sulfonate (SPS) and then inoculated into bottles containing media. It is suggested that the blood be diluted at least 10 per cent vol/vol in liquid medium. A suitable medium is soybean-casein digest (e.g., Tryptic soy, Difco Laboratories, Detroit, Mich.; Trypticase soy, BBL, Cockeysville, Md.), but brain-heart infusion, brucella, or supplemented peptone broth appears to represent a satisfactory alternative. In most cases media with lower oxidation-reduction potentials (E_h) do not provide better recovery of anaerobes than do commercially prepared, unvented vacuum blood culture bottles containing soybean-casein digest or brain-heart infusion broth; however, this equivalency in performance may vary according to the manufacturer of the bottled media. Certainly, media with low E_h values, such as Thiol and thioglycollate broths, should not be relied upon exclusively for blood cultures, since they are distinctly inferior to other media for recovering pseudomonads and yeasts. Among commercially produced blood culture bottles, those containing 100 ml of media are preferred.

Whether or not media made hypertonic by the addition of sucrose yield higher isolation rates than nonhypertonic media remains a controversial issue. Similarly, the potential advantages of prereduced anaerobically sterilized (PRAS) blood culture bottles may be medium- and system-dependent.

Blood should be anticoagulated with sodium polyanethol sulfonate (SPS), either in its transport tube or in the blood culture medium itself. Concentrations of SPS ranging from 0.025 to 0.05 per cent are satisfactory. SPS also possesses antiphagocytic and anticomplementary properties, and it inactivates aminoglycosidic antibiotics.

The value of adding penicillinase to blood culture media is uncertain; however, it is probably worthwhile when patients are receiving penicillins parenterally at the time the blood is collected.

Blood cultures should be incubated at 35° C. In a two or three vacuum bottle system, one should be incubated unvented while the other bottle(s) should be transiently vented prior to incubation. This procedure is necessary because of the mutually incompatible atmospheric requirements of anaerobes on the one hand and *Pseudomonas* and yeasts on the other. These requirements exist despite the recommended routine use of subcultures.

Cultures should be incubated for a minimum of seven days prior to their being discarded as negative.

In special circumstances, e.g., patients suspected of having endocarditis with negative cultures, incubation should be prolonged for two or three weeks.

Bottles should be examined macroscopically later in the day on which they were inoculated and daily thereafter for evidence of turbidity, hemolysis, gaseousness, and colony formation. In the presence of any of these signs or, in the case of radiometric devices, a growth index beyond recommended threshold, subcultures should be made to media appropriate to the isolation of the organism seen in a Gram's stained smear of the medium. Subcultures should routinely include a blood agar plate to be incubated anaerobically. Nearly 10 per cent of bacteremias are polymicrobial so that suitable differential media should be used for subcultures. In the absence of macroscopic or radiometric evidence of growth, each bottle should be routinely subcultured between 6 and 18 hours after it was inoculated by withdrawing an aliquot of the blood-broth mixture through the rubber stopper with a sterile needle and syringe and inoculating the mixture onto a quadrant of a chocolate blood agar plate that is incubated at 35° C. in 5 to 10 per cent CO_2 for 48 hours. A biphasic medium bottle is a suitable alternative. Neither additional subcultures nor routine anaerobic subcultures are necessary. Routine microscopic examination of an acridine orange stained smear may be performed instead of routine subculture.

Unless isolated from multiple cultures, the isolation of *Bacillus, Corynebacterium, Propionibacterium,* and *Staphylococcus epidermidis* represents contamination; however, because of the fact that these organisms commonly cause infections of prosthetic material, e.g., valves, joints, and shunts, their presence in blood cultures should not be casually dismissed or ignored prior to discussing the findings with the patient's physician. All other positive blood cultures should be reported promptly by phone to a physician as soon as the results of Gram's stained smears become available. Isolates should undergo antimicrobial susceptibility testing as expeditiously as possible so that appropriate adjustments in the antibiotic regimen can be made.

A lysis-centrifugation system (ISOLATOR, DuPont Co.) has recently become available and is undergoing evaluation. Early results suggest that this system detects significantly more bacteria and fungi than conventional broth methods.

A detailed guideline for blood culture procedures has recently been published by the American Society for Microbiology (Reller, 1982).

STERILE BODY FLUIDS

Cerebrospinal

Meningitis is a medical emergency requiring early therapy to prevent death or serious neurologic sequelae. Children between the ages of six months and one year are at greatest risk, with the majority of cases occurring during the first five years. Beyond the neonatal period of life when gram-negative bacilli and group B streptococci are the principal etiologic agents, *Haemophilus influenzae, Streptococcus pneumoniae,* and *Neisseria meningitidis* are the predominant causes of acute bacterial meningitis.

Partial therapy prior to hospital admission of patients with meningitis does modify the cerebrospinal fluid findings somewhat (Kaplan, 1980). In some situations in which the initial puncture yields normal results a second one may be required for proper diagnosis and therapy.

As for the collection of blood for culture, careful skin antisepsis is mandatory in preparation for a lumbar puncture. Since bacteremia is frequently associated with meningitis, cultures of blood should be made. Moreover, since the number of bacteria present in infected cerebrospinal fluid may be as few as 10/ml, it is important to provide the laboratory with an adequate ("as much as possible") volume for culture. This is even more important in cases of suspected mycobacterial or fungal meningitis in which the numbers of organisms are frequently few.

Specimens for microbiologic examination should be placed into sterile, screwcapped, and airtight tubes. It behooves the laboratory to examine specimen tubes included in lumbar puncture trays for sterility, the absence of stainable microorganisms, and the adequacy of the seal formed by the cap.

Cerebrospinal fluid should be transported to the laboratory promptly without refrigeration because of the sensitivity of *Haemophilus influenzae* and *Neisseria meningitidis* to prolonged transportation and temperature variations. Fluid should be examined microscopically by preparing a Gram's stained smear of spun sediment. Bearing in mind the fact that one organism will be seen per oil immersion field ($\times$ 1000) when there are 10^5 colony-forming units/ml and that concentrations of organisms below this level occur frequently, prolonged examinations of multiple fields in stained smears are required. When organisms resembling *Haemophilus, Neisseria,* or *Streptococcus* are seen, their identity can be confirmed rapidly with immunological tests. Reports of the accuracy of the Gram's stained smear vary but range from 60 to 80 per cent.

Two rapid diagnostic techniques have received increasing attention. These techniques include the detection by countercurrent immunoelectrophoresis (CIE) of specific polysaccharide antigens in cerebrospinal fluid, blood, and urine (Kaplan, 1980) and the detection of endotoxin in cerebrospinal fluid in gram-negative bacterial meningitis by the limulus lysate test (Nachum, 1973). These tests are usually unaffected by prior partial therapy and may, therefore, be helpful when bacterial meningitis is suspected on the basis of clinical and laboratory data other than cultures. Their speed of performance makes them a useful adjunct to the Gram's stained smear. Alternatives to CIE include latex agglutination, coagglutination, and immunofluorescent antibody techniques (Kaplan, 1980).

The principle of CIE is that a negatively charged bacterial antigen and a neutral or slightly charged antibody are placed in two opposed wells on an agarose-coated slide. Although the two will migrate slowly toward one another in alkaline (pH 8.2 to 8.6) media, electrophoresis causes the antigen to move rapidly toward the positive electrode. The antibody moves rapidly in the opposite direction because of the normal flow of buffer from the positive to the negative electrode. The two enter a zone of reaction and, if they combine into an antigen-antibody complex, form a precipitin line between the two wells.

With cerebrospinal fluid from a patient suspected of having meningitis serving as the antigen, electrophoresis is carried out with the following: *Haemophilus influenzae* type b antiserum, polyvalent pneumococcal antiserum, and *Neisseria meningitidis* antisera (poly A-D, poly X-Z). Because pneumococcal types VII and XIV are neutral and do not migrate toward the positive electrode, it is necessary to incorporate a sulfonated derivative of phenylboronic acid in the buffer system to ensure their detection (Anhalt, 1975). In suspected neonatal meningitis, streptococcal group B antiserum is included. Of note is the fact that *Neisseria meningitidis* group B antiserum will react with the Kl antigen of *Escherichia coli,* which is a frequent cause of neonatal meningitis.

The principle of the limulus lysate test is that a lysate prepared from amebocytes of the horseshoe crab, *Limulus polyphemus,* undergoes gelation when exposed to endotoxin. The assay of cerebrospinal fluid is rapid and provides a high level of sensitivity in the diagnosis of meningitis due to *Neisseria meningitidis, Haemophilus influenzae,* and other gram-negative bacteria.

Because of the small numbers of organisms that may be present in cerebrospinal fluid, some method of concentration prior to culture is usually performed. In many laboratories centrifugation at 2500 rpm for 15 minutes is used. This procedure is probably effective when there are numerous leukocytes present; however, in some cases the cell counts may be normal, especially early in the course of meningitis, and a force of 10,000 × g may be required to sediment bacteria. It is our practice, therefore, to concentrate the specimen by filtering it through a 0.45 μm membrane filter contained in a sterile, disposable unit (Swinnex, Millipore Corporation) and then to remove the filter and apply it directly to the surface of chocolate blood agar for culture (Washington, 1981).

Other fluids require no special instruction or precautions except for the use of careful aseptic technique in their collection and processing. Although anticoagulation of joint and pleural fluids may be desirable, it should be pointed out that heparin usually contains the preservative, benzyl alcohol, that may adversely affect the recovery of microorganisms.

TISSUE

Surgical

Whereas specimens such as blood and cerebrospinal fluid usually reflect medically urgent situations, those obtained surgically are done at great expense and at considerable risk to the patient. It therefore behooves the surgeon to obtain an amount of material that is adequate both for histopathologic and for microbiologic examination. Swabs are rarely adequate for this purpose. The histopathology of the lesion may not only serve to differentiate between infection and malignancy but also can help to distinguish between a suppurative and a granulomatous process. In some cases special stains are helpful in establishing the etiology of the process. In chronic lesions the differential diagnosis includes disease due to actinomycetes, brucellae, mycobacteria, and fungi, any one of which may be present only in small numbers, again emphasizing the need for obtaining adequate samples for examination.

Biopsies of ulcers and curettings of sinus tracts should be obtained to recover organisms that might be present only on the ulcer or sinus tract wall. Cultures of the drainage from such lesions are apt to be contaminated with flora indigenous to the skin or adjacent mucous membranes or with secondary invaders. Aspirations of closed abscesses are preferable to obtaining material on a swab after such lesions have been opened. Local anesthetics may be necessary for the collection of specimens; however, it must be remembered that these agents possess antimicrobial activity (Schmidt, 1970).

Tissue obtained surgically for culture should be placed into a sterile, wide-mouthed, screw-capped jar. Pus should be injected into an anaerobe vial for transport to the laboratory, or it can be sent in the syringe into which it was aspirated by plugging the needle with a sterile rubber stopper. When an abscess cavity is opened and drained, a portion of its wall should also be submitted for culture. As a general rule, tissue should be bisected aseptically by the surgeon in the operating room and material representative of the pathologic process submitted for both histopathologic and microbiologic examination. Good communication between histopathologist and microbiologist is important, especially in cases with fever of unknown origin for which an exploratory laparotomy is being done and multiple biopsies are taken.

Tissue received by the laboratory should be examined and its characteristics described on a work card before processing. It should then be finely minced with sterile scissors into a mortar where it is mixed with a sterile abrasive (alundum) in broth and ground with a pestle to render a 20 per cent suspension. This suspension is most conveniently transferred into a sterile dropper bottle that can be used to inoculate all of the necessary culture media and is then stored under refrigeration for at least two weeks before being discarded. We use the histopathology to determine what cultures should be made of each specimen we receive and perform special stains when necessary to try to elucidate the etiology of an infectious process. Our approach to tissue microbiology has been outlined elsewhere (Brewer, 1976).

Postmortem

The value of postmortem bacteriology is limited. Most studies have demonstrated that cultures performed on a single organ obtained post mortem rarely, if ever, provide sufficient information to determine the significance of a positive culture, even in the presence of histologic evidence of infection; that, in selected cases, postmortem cultures of multiple organs may be of value in identifying the etiologic agent of an infectious process, especially in cases of well-recognized clinical entities caused by a single organism or in cases of overwhelming sepsis; and that human tissues are not necessarily sterile at any given time (Wilson, 1972). A high percentage of postmortem bacterial cultures of lung, liver, and spleen from patients without apparent infection are positive. Routine postmortem cultures of any kind should be discouraged and should be reserved for selected cases in which a closed lesion or space can be sampled aseptically or in which material from multiple organs can be obtained.

EYE

Microbiologic studies of the eye in patients with conjunctivitis are of limited utility in establishing the etiologic diagnosis in many cases and are, therefore, probably seldom warranted. The most important step in the management of bacterial corneal ulcers, however, is prompt and meticulous laboratory investigation (Jones, 1981). Because of the small amount of material that can be obtained for culture, the laboratory should have certain materials available for the ophthalmologist to use. These are sterile calcium alginate, cotton, or Dacron-tipped swabs, a Kimura platinum spatula, glass microscopic slides, an alcohol lamp, and media including chocolate blood agar, fluid thioglycollate, Sabouraud dextrose agar, and Lowenstein-Jensen agar. The procedure for laboratory investigation of a corneal ulcer is to obtain material from the conjunctivae with a swab which is used to inoculate a chocolate blood agar plate and a Sabouraud dextrose agar, to anesthetize the cornea with proparacaine hydrochloride, and then to scrape the ulcer with the spatula to obtain material for smears and cultures (Jones, 1981). The slides are used for preparing Gram's stained smears and potassium hydroxide (KOH) preparations. Other slides may be used for acid-fast smears or for staining with Gomori methenamine silver for fungi. Corneal scrapings are spot inoculated onto chocolate blood agar and Sabouraud dextrose agar and into fluid thioglycollate medium. Lowenstein-Jensen agar can be inoculated in cases of suspected mycobacterial disease.

RESPIRATORY TRACT

Ear

Since the organisms associated with acute otitis media have been quite consistent and limited to only a few species, there is little reason in uncomplicated cases to perform tympanocentesis in order to obtain material for culture. In patients with severe pain and bulging tympanic membranes and in those who have impaired host defenses or fail to respond to therapy, tympanocentesis and culture are probably indicated. The correlation between cultures of the middle ear and of the nasopharynx is sufficiently poor that there is little reason to culture the latter site. In most cases the etiologic agent is *Streptococcus pneumoniae, S. pyogenes,* or *Haemophilus influenzae;* however, in neonates it is more frequently *Staphylococcus aureus, Escherichia coli,* or *Klebsiella pneumoniae,* and in chronic infections *Staphylococcus aureus* and *Pseudomonas aeruginosa* are predominant.

Nasopharynx

Nasal cultures are frequently performed to detect carrier states of *Staphylococcus aureus,* a procedure which is seldom indicated, however, because of the high incidence of carriers in the normal population and especially among hospital personnel and because of the generally poor correlation between phage types found in the nose and those isolated from wound infections. Phage typing of staphylococci is performed in a small number of medical centers and at the Centers for Disease Control, but generally only in epidemic situations.

Nasopharyngeal swabs may be used for the detection of carriers of *Streptococcus pyogenes, Corynebacterium diphtheriae, Bordetella pertussis,* and *Neisseria meningitidis.* A flexible wire Dacron, calcium alginate, or cotton-tipped swab should be passed gently through the nose into the nasopharynx and rotated to obtain material for culture. In clinically suspected cases of pertussis it is preferable to aspirate material from the nasopharynx by using a suction catheter (16 in. No. 8 French) attached to a syringe.

Those bacteria that produce pharyngitis are *Streptococcus pyogenes* (or a group A), *Neisseria gonorrhoeae, Corynebacterium diphtheriae,* and *Bordetella pertussis.* As has already been stated, nasopharyngeal aspirates represent the specimen of choice in cases with suspected pertussis. A swab of the membrane itself should be taken in cases of suspected diphtheria. Otherwise, an attempt should be made to swab with minimal oral contamination the posterior pharynx, the tonsils or tonsillar pillars, and any areas of purulence, exudation, or ulceration. The laboratory must be notified when gonorrhea, diphtheria, or pertussis is suspected so that cultures with suitable selective media are performed; otherwise, the laboratory is unlikely to recognize these pathogens or even be able to find them if a delayed request is made for their cultivation. In cases of suspected diphtheria, smears can be prepared for staining with Loeffler alkaline methylene blue to determine whether or not typical coryneform bacteria containing metachromatic granules are present. Pertussis may be rapidly diagnosed in many cases by staining smears directly with fluorescein-conjugated anti-*Bordetella pertussis* antiserum. Swabs from patients with suspected meningococcal carrier state or gonococcal pharyngitis are best inoculated directly onto modified Thayer-Martin agar that has been brought to room temperature prior to its use. If contained in a Transgrow bottle or in a biologic environmental chamber (JEMBEC), this medium should be incubated overnight prior to its shipment to the laboratory.

In cases of group A streptococcal pharyngitis, certain precautions should be observed to ensure that the diagnosis of this disease is accurately made. First, a diagnosis of streptococcal pharyngitis cannot be made reliably on clinical grounds alone and, therefore, requires that a throat culture be made. Second, the posterior pharynx, tonsils, or tonsillar pillars, and any areas of purulence, inflammation, or ulceration should be cultured, since sampling does affect the outcome of cultures. Third, the swab is used to inoculate a soybean-casein digest agar containing 5 per cent sheep blood. Such plates are available from a variety of commercial sources, but they must be stored in sealed plastic wrappers or bags under refrigeration to prevent deterioration. Their performance must be controlled by inoculation of each lot on a regular basis with a known group A streptococcus. Fourth, the area of primary inoculation must be streaked out for isolation with a sterile wire loop, and the surface of the agar must be stabbed in several areas to ensure detection of rare strains producing oxygen-sensitive hemolysin only. Fifth, the bacitracin disk test for presumptive identification of group A streptococci is unreliable when it is placed directly onto the primary plate and should be performed only with a purified subculture. Finally, the blood agar plates should be incubated at 35°C. for 18 to 24 hours in an atmosphere of room air to minimize growth of β-hemolytic streptococci belonging to Lancefield groups other than A. Cultures that are negative after 24 hours of incubation should probably be reincubated for an additional day before being discarded as negative.

Sputum

Bacterial cultures of sputum represent a major problem because they are commonly collected carelessly, frequently consist predominantly of saliva, usually contain large numbers of bacteria indigenous to the oral cavity, and in seriously ill hospitalized patients often contain gram-negative bacilli that have colonized the oropharynx shortly after hospitalization. Such cultures lack sensitivity and specificity and are, therefore, difficult to interpret. At the very least, the laboratory should impose a microscopic screening procedure for specimens submitted for culture in which the relative numbers of leukocytes, macrophages, and squamous epithelial cells can be assessed. Specimens should not get cultured unless there are fewer than 25 squamous epithelial cells per low power field (× 100). A report as to the unsatisfactory nature of a specimen and a request for another specimen is made both by phone and in writing. For those specimens deemed acceptable for culture, a report of the Gram's stained smear is issued stating the morphology of those organisms observed and their relative numbers (e.g., gram-positive cocci resembling pneumococci—many) and the relative numbers of white blood cells (>25/lpf = many, <25/lpf = few).

In years past, attempts were made to quantify bacterial isolates from sputum following its digestion on the principle that those organisms present in large numbers (> 10^5/ml) were more likely to be significant than were those present in small numbers; however, these results have been of little clinical value and have correlated poorly with the results of transtracheal aspiration.

In the patient with serious pulmonary infection and with multiple potentially pathogenic bacteria in cultures of sputum, it may then be necessary to consider performing bronchoscopy with aspiration or biopsy, transtracheal aspiration, thoracentesis, transthoracic needle biopsy, or open lung biopsy to establish the diagnosis. It must be pointed out that unless a plugged telescoping catheter brush is used, inner channel aspirates obtained by fiberoptic bronchoscopy have been found to be contaminated with oropharyngeal flora and do not, therefore, reliably reflect the bacteriology of the lower respiratory tract (Wimberley, 1982). While associated with certain definite risks, transtracheal aspiration can generally be done safely by a person experienced in its performance. Indications for its performance include cases of suspected anaerobic or gram-negative pneumonia or patients from whom an adequate expectorated sample cannot be obtained. Transthoracic needle aspiration may provide more valuable information than transtracheal aspiration but is probably associated with a higher frequency of complications.

GENITOURINARY TRACT

Genital

The bacteria most commonly found to be associated with sexually transmitted disease are *Neisseria gonorrhoeae* and *Chlamydia trachomatis,* the latter of which will be dealt with in another chapter in this section. It is not possible to distinguish on the basis of clinical signs and symptoms between urethritis due to these organisms. Cultures must be made; however, since the isolation of chlamydiae requires the use of cell culture techniques, most laboratories are unable to detect them.

In the male, Gram's stained smears of urethral exudates are both sensitive and specific in establishing the diagnosis of gonorrhea. In males with negative smears, cultures should be made. In the female, Gram's stained smears of vaginal or cervical smears lack sensitivity and specificity and are definitely *not* recommended as a means of establishing or ruling out the diagnosis of gonorrhea. Urethral exudate or scrapings obtained with a small, smooth platinum wire loop should be obtained routinely from males suspected of having gonorrhea. However, since gonococcal pharyngitis and proctitis are not uncommon manifestations of the disease in those practicing fellatio or homosexuality, cultures of the throat or of the anal crypts may also be be indicated. In the female, cultures of the cervical os and of the anal crypts should be performed routinely. Adequate visualization of the cervix must be obtained by means of a speculum lubricated with water. Swabs should be inoculated directly onto modified Thayer-Martin agar which has been prewarmed to room temperature. Thayer-Martin agar plates may be used, provided they can be placed shortly thereafter into an environment with increased CO_2. A candle extinction jar method is quite satisfactory for this purpose. Alternatively, the swab may be inoculated onto modified Thayer-Martin agar in a bottle containing CO_2 (Transgrow) or in a rectangular dish to which a CO_2-generating tablet is added and which is then placed into a ziplock bag (JEMBEC). Cultures that are mailed into the laboratory for processing must first be incubated overnight; otherwise, a significant number of cultures will fail to become positive.

A rare form of sexually transmitted disease in the United States is chancroid, which is caused by *Haemophilus ducreyi*. Cultivation of this organism requires inoculation of material from the lesion onto chocolate agar containing IsoVitaleX (BBL) and vancomycin (Hammond, 1978). Gram's stained smears of freshly expressed exudate from the edges of the lesion will often display pairs and short chains of gram-negative coccobacilli, while in cultures tangled chains and long parallel rows of bacilli are more frequently seen.

The presence of other bacteria in cultures of the urethra and vagina is of questionable clinical significance because of the enormous variety of flora indigenous to these sites. The role of *Gardnerella vaginalis* is not clear cut. Although its inoculation into the vagina of asymptomatic volunteers has produced disease, its presence in vaginal cultures of many asymptomatic females beclouds the issue.

Because of its prominence in causing neonatal meningitis, there has been much interest lately in identifying vaginal carriers of group B streptococci; however, there is as yet no consensus about the clinical management of this problem in pregnant females.

Anaerobic bacteria play a prominent role in severe infections of the female genital tract, including pelvic abscesses, septic abortions, puerperal sepsis, tubo-ovarian abscess, and endometritis. Because of the large number and variety of anaerobes in the vagina, cultures of material draining into the vagina are rarely of value in establishing the etiology of the infection. Attempts should be made to aspirate closed lesions with a sterile needle and syringe or to aspirate endometrial material with a needle or syringe or catheter following careful disinfection of the vagina and cervix. Since it is difficult to disinfect the cervical os, some have devised systems whereby sterile catheters or swabs can be inserted into the uterine cavity through the lumen of a large catheter placed in the cervical canal. Culdocentesis and laparoscopy have also been successfully used for obtaining material for culture. Pus obtained surgically from pelvic infections should always be placed into an anaerobic vial for transport and cultured for anaerobes.

Urinary

There are three categories of urinary specimens that may be collected for bacterial culture. The most frequently submitted one is the clean-voided midstream specimen. This approach should be used whenever possible, since it is relatively easy and can be taught to ambulatory patients and paramedical personnel, is safe, and, when properly performed, provides accurate results in the great majority of instances. Since the vagina and urethra harbor indigenous bacterial flora that can multiply rapidly in urine stored at room temperature and produce spurious results in cultures, every effort should be made to obtain a properly collected clean-voided midstream specimen by procedures described elsewhere in detail (Kunin, 1979). This effort will result in a very low incidence of contaminated cultures and produce results that are interpretable. It is desirable, particularly in larger hospitals, to train a team of paramedical personnel to collect all urine specimens for cultures. This responsibility may be one of several duties assigned to this team, the other responsibilities of which may include urinary catheter care and replacement. The value of a properly collected specimen more than offsets the costs of multiple poorly collected ones, not to mention the fact that the patient's management is more likely to be appropriate.

The second category of urinary specimen is the suprapubic aspiration, the indications for which include the collection of urine from infants and small children, adults in whom cultures of repeated clean-voided specimens have yielded equivocal results, and patients with suspected anaerobic bacteriuria. Bacteriuria due to anaerobes is rare and may be suspected when negative cultures of specimens with positive Gram's stained smears occur. In such cases the only acceptable specimen for anaerobic culture is that aspirated suprapubically.

The third category of specimen is that obtained by instrumentation, most commonly catheterization or cystoscopy. Although there are many indications for catheterization, the insertion of a catheter for the sole purpose of collecting urine for culture is discouraged because of the risk of development of bacteriuria associated with the procedure. This risk has been reported to be in the vicinity of 1 per cent in healthy ambulatory men and women and as high as 20 per cent when performed in women during labor. In patients with chronic indwelling catheters the urine should be collected by needle aspiration through a disinfected portion of the wall of the catheter and *not* from the drainage bag or by disconnecting the catheter from the collection tube.

Urine should be cultured within two hours of its collection or refrigerated during storage. Either of these precautions will help to ensure the accuracy of the results of quantitative cultures. Because of the difficulties encountered in getting specimens to the laboratory promptly, some have resorted to the direct inoculation of microcultures at the time the specimen is collected.

The simplest and most rapid method for detecting significant bacteriuria is to examine microscopically ($\times$ 1000) a Gram's stained smear of well-mixed, uncentrifuged urine. The presence of at least two bacteria per high power field correlates with the presence of significant bacteriuria in over 90 per cent of instances in experienced hands. An alternative procedure is to examine a wet mount, with or without methylene blue, of centrifuged urinary sediment with the high-dry objective (×400) under reduced light.

Quantitative cultures of urine should always be performed by inoculating a measured volume of urine into molten agar which is mixed and poured into a Petri dish or onto the surface of agar in a Petri dish. For practical purposes, the calibrated loop (0.001 or 0.01 ml) streak-plate technique is most rapid and convenient.

Quantitation is the essential parameter used for determining the presence of significant bacteriuria. Colony counts of 10^5/ml or greater are indicative of infection, while those exceeding 10^4/ml are indicative of probable infection. Colony counts between 10^3 and 10^4/ml indicate probable contamination, while fewer colonies are considered to represent contaminants. Obviously, if the specimen was improperly collected and transported to the laboratory, these interpretative criteria become less reliable. Low colony counts that are clinically significant may occur in urine from patients receiving antimicrobial therapy, or those with an obstructed ureter or with infections due to fastidious organisms (e.g., anaerobes). Colony counts may be reduced slightly by hydration. As a rule, the presence of an organism in any quantity in urine obtained by suprapubic aspiration is significant. Because of the importance of quantitation in urine bacteriology, cultures of urine in liquid media or of urinary sediment are unsuitable procedures yielding uninterpretable results.

There are a variety of commercially prepared microculture techniques for detecting bacteriuria (Kunin, 1979). These devices have their greatest utility in screening programs, in office practice, and in reducing numbers of contaminants resulting from delays in transporting urine specimens from the ward to the laboratory. A number of chemical screening methods have also been described; however, they tend to have less sensitivity and specificity than do the microbiologic methods.

FECES

Salmonellae, shigellae, *Vibrio cholerae, Staphylococcus aureus,* clostridia, and certain serotypes of *Escherichia coli* comprised the list of enteric pathogens for many years. The etiology of most cases of diarrheal disease remained obscure. The importance of *Campylobacter jejuni, Clostridium difficile,* and enterotoxigenic and invasive strains of *E. coli* has only been recognized for a few years, as has the lack of correlation between these two pathogenic properties and serotypes of *E. coli* previously called "enteropathogenic." Other bacteria are now recognized as causing diarrhea (Table 45–3). To complicate the picture further, reovirus-like (rotavirus) and parvovirus-like (Norwalk) agents have been clearly associated in recent years with diarrhea.

Despite all of these advances in our understanding of diarrheal disease, the clinical laboratory is pretty well limited to the diagnosis of salmonellosis, shigellosis, yersiniosis, and campylobacteriosis because the techniques used to determine enterotoxigenicity and invasiveness are complex and time consuming. The heat-labile enterotoxin of *Vibrio cholerae* and of some strains of *E. coli* induces morphologic changes in adrenal tumor or Chinese hamster ovary cells. The heat-stable enterotoxin produced by some strains of *E. coli* cannot be detected by an in vitro system. Its detection, as well as that of invasiveness by other strains of *E. coli,* requires animal inoculation.

Table 45–3. PATHOGENIC MECHANISMS OF BACTERIA CAUSING DIARRHEA

Mechanisms	Organisms
Preformed toxins	*Staphylococcus aureus* (enterotoxins A, B) *Clostridium botulinum* A, B, E
Enterotoxins following colonization	*Vibrio cholerae* *Vibrio parahaemolyticus* (?) *Escherichia coli* *Bacillus cereus* *Clostridium perfringens* A *Shigella dysenteriae* 1 *Aeromonas hydrophila* (?)
Invasiveness	*Salmonella* *Shigella* *Escherichia coli* *Staphylococcus aureus* *Yersinia enterocolitica* (?) *Campylobacter jejuni* (?) *Clostridium difficile*

Because most bacterial diarrheas are self-limited, stool cultures are generally limited to cases with severe diarrhea requiring hospitalization, persistent or recurrent diarrhea, and a dysentery-like clinical presentation.

Microscopic examination of diarrheal stool may be helpful in certain circumstances. In patients with suspected staphylococcal enterocolitis, an uncommon entity today, the finding of large numbers of gram-positive cocci resembling staphylococci is virtually diagnostic and may expedite the initiation of appropriate therapy. A methylene blue stain for leukocytes may be helpful in differentiating invasive and enterotoxigenic causes of diarrhea (Harris, 1972).

In the evaluation of a patient with diarrhea, a history of recent dietary intake and travel should be elicited. *Vibrio cholerae* has been encountered in patients who have recently traveled or resided in areas in which disease due to this organism is endemic. Disease due to *Vibrio parahaemolyticus* has been clearly associated with the ingestion of raw or incompletely cooked seafood or shellfish. Most laboratories do not inoculate media suitable for the isolation of vibrios unless specifically requested to do so.

A history of recent antibiotic therapy, particularly with ampicillin or amoxicillin, should suggest the diagnosis of antibiotic-associated colitis secondary to *C. difficile.* Proctoscopic examination of such cases often demonstrates pseudomembranous colitis.

In view of what has been stated about the lack of correlation between enterotoxigenicity or invasiveness and "enteropathogenic" serotypes of *Escherichia coli,* laboratories should no longer screen rectal swabs or stool material from infants for these organisms. Although most invasive strains of *E. coli* belong to a few serotypes, they are different from those that were formerly classified as "enteropathogenic." Although enterotoxigenicity is determined by a plasmid that is transferable by means of conjugation to other strains, it does nonetheless appear that this property may be limited to a relatively small number of serotypes which, however, do not correspond to the "enteropathogenic" serotypes identifiable with currently available methodology. One additional consideration is that it now appears that the capability of enterotoxigenic strains to produce disease may be related to another plasmid-determined property, a colonization factor. This subject is an area of intense interest and research so that further data will surely be forthcoming. It seems likely that other in vitro systems for detecting heat-labile toxin will become available in the near future.

Invasive forms of *Escherichia coli* diarrhea have thus far been rare. Enterotoxigenic forms of *E. coli* are frequent causes of travellers' diarrhea; however, their frequency of distribution in the United States remains unclear. Shigellosis and salmonellosis are global in distribution with the former being most common in young children and the latter affecting all age groups. Campylobacteriosis has been recognized in the United States and in many other parts of the world. Yersiniosis is common in Scandinavian countries and has only recently been recognized in this country. Diarrhea due to enterotoxigenic strains of *Bacillus cereus* or *B. subtilis* is common in Eastern Europe and is but rarely recognized in the United States. Enterotoxigenic strains of *Aeromonas hydrophila* have been reported from Asian and near Eastern countries but have not yet been confirmed here.

PROCESSING

Each laboratory must organize the processing of its specimens so that none of the efforts devoted to their proper selection, collection, and transport are wasted. Certain specimens, such as cerebrospinal fluid, must be processed immediately, since the results of stained smears or of immunological tests can have a major impact on therapy. Other specimens with lower orders of priority can be processed as time becomes available, provided that suitable steps are taken to ensure their integrity during periods of temporary storage. Small numbers of bacteria in urine do proliferate just as rapidly on a laboratory bench as at a nursing station unless refrigerated! Stained smears of medically urgent specimens should be prepared, examined, and reported as quickly as possible. Requests for additional material or for specimens to replace unsuitable ones must be made quickly, as should the notification of specimen rejection. In other words, the laboratory must establish a system of priorities based not only upon the urgency with which results are expected but also upon the feasibility of obtaining suitable material before therapy is instituted.

SMEARS

The laboratory should institute a system for routinely examining stained smears of certain types of specimens. Usually sterile body fluids, pus, urine, and material from wounds should be examined microscopically on a regular basis, primarily to provide preliminary results for clinical purposes and secondarily as a quality control measure. One should ordinarily expect to culture bacteria compatible morphologically with those observed in the stained smear.

Great care must be taken in preparing Gram's stained smears to prevent distortion of the organisms and to ensure accuracy of the staining reactions. A thin smear of an aliquot of the specimen that is representative of the infectious process should be prepared on a clean microscopic slide, allowed to dry, gently heat fixed, and then stained. Since 10^5 organisms/ml must be present for there to be at least one per oil immersion field ($\times$ 1000), most normally sterile body fluids must be examined microscopically for 15 to 30 minutes in order to detect small numbers of organisms. The relative numbers of white blood cells and squamous epithelial cells per low power field are useful in assessing the quality of certain specimens, e.g., sputa, wounds. Technologists should be encouraged to be as descriptive in their interpretation of Gram's stained smears as possible. Reporting that gram-positive cocci occur in pairs that resemble pneumococci can be very helpful. Pleomorphic gram-negative bacilli usually represent anaerobes and may be presumptively reported as such. Obviously, the reliability of such reports will be directly related to the experience and expertise of the technologist.

A Gram's stained smear of a drop of well-mixed uncentrifuged urine will provide a rapid and accurate determination of whether or not significant bacteriuria ($\geq 10^5$ colonies/ml) is present. The drop of urine should be placed on a clean microscopic slide, allowing it to dry without spreading, and then heat fixing and staining it. The finding of at least two bacteria per oil immersion field ($\times$ 1000) is indicative of significant bacteriuria, and the smear should, therefore, be reported as positive. Fewer than two bacteria per field constitute a borderline finding, while no bacteria per field should be reported as negative.

Another technique for examining bacteria is with fluorescent antibody microscopy. Although it is useful in examining specimens directly for the presence of *Bordetella pertussis, Listeria monocytogenes, Legionella,*

Brucella, and *Yersinia pestis,* its more common applications are for the detection of group A streptococci in throat swabs, either after a short period of incubation of the swab in broth or after the growth of β-hemolytic streptococci on blood agar; for the rapid presumptive identification of organisms resembling *Haemophilus influenzae, Streptococcus pneumoniae,* and *Neisseria meningitidis* seen in Gram's stained smears of cerebrospinal fluid; and for rapid identification of colonies resembling *Neisseria gonorrhoeae* growing on Thayer-Martin agar. Examples of fluorescent antibody staining of various microorganisms are seen in Figure 45–1. The sensitivity and specificity of this technique vary according to the conjugate and whether it is used for the direct or indirect fluorescent antibody stain.

MEDIA

Media should be selected carefully to provide the optimal conditions for growth of pathogens commonly encountered in a particular site or type of specimen. Consideration must be given to special growth requirements of bacteria associated with a particular type of infection or to the necessity of selecting out certain pathogenic bacteria from a mixed population of indigenous flora. In addition to the standard nutrient broth or agar media, therefore, one will often also inoculate differential or selective media. Guidelines for the selection of media to be used with different types of specimens are shown in Table 45–4. For each medium shown there are acceptable alternatives and, obviously, the list of potential types of specimens is far from complete.

INCUBATION

Bacterial cultures are generally incubated at 35°C. and examined initially after 18 to 24 hours of incubation. Added CO_2 in concentrations of 5 to 10 per cent enhances the growth of many bacteria and should be used whenever feasible. Exceptions to this recommendation are those cultures on differential and selective media in which pH alteration is used to differentiate colony types (e.g., xylose-lysine-deoxycholate [XLD] agar, Hektoen enteric [HE] agar). CO_2 is either essential or stimulatory to the growth of certain bacteria, e.g., *Neisseria gonorrhoeae, Haemophilus influenzae.*

Certain types of specimens should probably be stored following their inoculation onto culture media in case additional studies become necessary. Of greatest importance are tissues removed surgically, cerebrospinal and other normally sterile body fluids, foreign objects, intravascular cannulae, and prosthetic materials. Many laboratories store other types of specimens overnight under refrigeration in case of a mix-up or other problem requiring repetition of the culture. In many such instances, however, requesting another specimen is preferable to reculturing an old specimen.

Anaerobic Incubation Systems

Specimens submitted from appropriate sources and in proper containers for anaerobic culture should be processed expeditiously (Fig. 45–2), although it now appears that clinically significant anaerobes in large volumes of pus or in anaerobe transport vials do survive for 24 hours without difficulty. It is probably important, however, for media that have already been inoculated to be incubated anaerobically or to be placed into a CO_2 flush jar for storage until they can be transferred into an anaerobic incubation system.

There are three types of anaerobic culture systems in use in clinical laboratories today. The most convenient and widely used is the anaerobic jar (GasPak, BBL, Cockeysville, Md.) in which water is added to a CO_2 and H_2 generator package and O_2 is catalytically converted with H_2 to water with palladium-coated alumina pellets contained in a lid chamber. There are also evacuation-replacement jars on the market; however, these are somewhat less convenient for routine use in the clinical laboratory. A modification of this system is a transparent plastic bag containing its own gas generator and palladium catalyst and designed to hold a Petri dish (Bio-Bag Environmental Chamber, Type A, Marion Scientific, Kansas City, Mo.).

A second anaerobic system is the roll tube technique, in which prereduced anaerobically sterilized (PRAS) medium is distributed under anaerobic conditions as a thin layer around the internal surface of test tubes. Air is excluded from the tube during inoculation and subculture by displacement with an oxygen-free gas, such as CO_2, and by keeping it stoppered at all other times. This method has been adapted for clinical laboratory purposes by the Anaerobe Laboratory at the Virginia Polytechnic Institute (Holdeman, 1977). The advantages of this approach are that each tube becomes its own incubation system and each tube can be examined without disturbing the anaerobic conditions within. Its disadvantages are that the tubes are more cumbersome and time-consuming to work with and the colonial morphology may be less distinct on the agar layer within the tube than on agar plates.

The third approach to anaerobic culture is the anaerobic glove box or chamber which consists of a large, clear plastic, airtight bag or chamber filled with an oxygen-free gas mixture of nitrogen, hydrogen, and carbon dioxide. Specimens, plates, and tubes are introduced into or removed from the chamber through a gas interchange lock. Anaerobiosis in the chamber is maintained by palladium catalysts and the hydrogen gas in the chamber. All manipulations within the chamber are done with neoprene gloves sealed to the chamber wall. The chamber can function as its own incubation system by placing heating units in it. Alternatively, incubators can be placed into the chamber; however, they occupy a lot of space and are less desirable than the units which heat the whole chamber. Like the roll tube, the chamber permits examination of cultures at any time without interruption of anaerobiasis. In contrast to the roll tube,

Text continued on page 1082

6

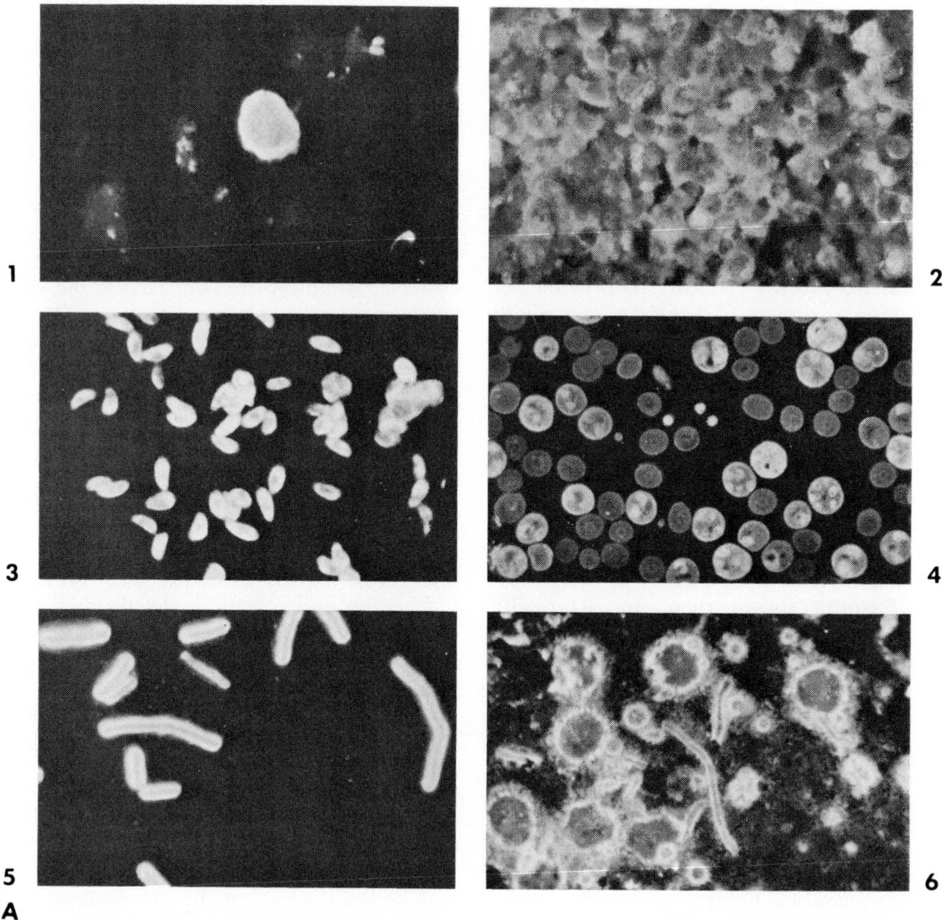

Figure 45–1. *A,* Fluorescent antibody staining* of microorganisms. *1, Entamoeba histolytica* in dried smear from culture (×1050). *2, Toxoplasma gondii* in spleen of infected mouse. Tissue fixed in alcohol–acetic acid and embedded in paraffin (×1050). *3, Toxoplasma gondii* in peritoneal exudate of infected mouse (× 1050). *4, Plasmodium berghei,* a parasite of rodents, as seen in rat blood during preliminary studies of human malaria. *5, Bacillus anthracis* is an impression smear from the liver of a mouse. Homologous antibody was prepared by injecting whole encapsulated antigen. Note both encapsulated and stripped forms (×600). *6, Pasteurella pestis* in smear of fluid aspirated from bubo of a fatal case of plague. Homologous antibody prepared by injecting whole-cell antigen. Note bizarre forms of plague bacilli and specifically stained soluble antigen surrounding tissue cells (×1050). (From Cherry, W. B., Goldman, M., and Carski, T. R.: Fluorescent Antibody Techniques. U.S. Department of Health, Education, and Welfare, 1960).

*By the direct method.

Illustration continued on opposite page

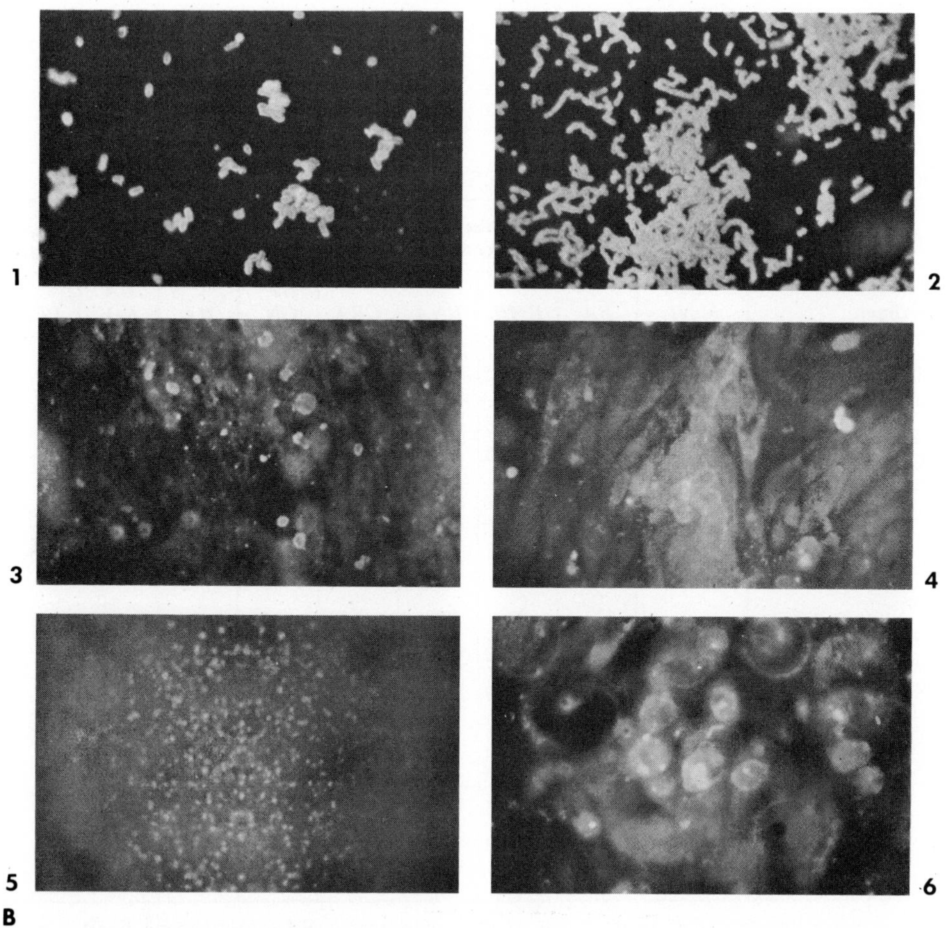

Figure 45–1. *Continued. B,* Fluorescent staining* of microorganisms. *1, Escherichia coli* in feces from a case of infantile diarrhea. Stained with pooled antibodies for enteropathogenic types of *E. coli* (×600). *2,* Group B streptococci in pure culture (×600). *3,* Rabies virus in impression smear of the brain of a mouse infected with street virus. Note the large aggregates of stained antigen (Negri bodies) and the numerous smaller particles that stain (×210). *4,* Simian foamy agent in a culture of monkey-kidney tissue on a coverslip. Two days after inoculation. Note stained antigen in nuclei of the multinucleated cells whose formation was induced by the infection (×210). *5, Rickettsia prowazekii* (epidemic typhus) in a smear of egg yolk sac. Stained with homologous antibody (×210). *6,* Poliovirus type I in monkey-kidney tissue cultures, 12 hours post-inoculation. Stained by complement method, using antipolio monkey serum and guinea pig complement followed by labeled anti-guinea pig complement (×210). (From Cherry, W. B., Goldman, M., and Carski, T. R.: Fluorescent Antibody Techniques. U.S. Department of Health, Education, and Welfare, 1960.)

*By the direct method except for polio virus in 6.

Table 45–4. GUIDELINES FOR MEDIA SELECTION FOR VARIOUS SPECIMENS*

	Media for Recovery of Aerobic and Facultatively Anaerobic Bacteria						Media for Recovery of Anaerobic Bacteria†			
Specimen	***Suppl thiogly***	***BA***	***EMB***	***CNA***	***CBA***	***HE, GN***	***BA***	***BA K-V***	***PEA***	***Suppl thiogly***
Fluids										
Cerebrospinal	X	X			X					
Abdominal	X	X	X	X			X	X	X	X
Pleural	X	X	X	X	X		X	X	X	X
Synovial	X	X	X	X	X		X	X	X	X
Wound										
Swab	X	X	X	X						
Aspirate	X	X	X	X			X	X	X	X
Tissue	X	X	X	X			X	X	X	X
Respiratory tract										
Throat		X								
Sputum		X	X		X					
Transtracheal aspirate	X	X	X	X	X		X	X	X	X
Bronchial washings	X	X	X	X	X					
Genitourinary										
Cervix, vagina		X		X	X‡					
Uterus, cul-de-sac	X	X	X	X	X		X	X	X	X
Prostate	X	X	X	X	X					
Urethra					X‡					
Urine										
Clean-voided		X	X							
Suprapubic aspirate	X	X	X				X	X	X	X
Fecal material		X	X			X				

*Abbreviations: Suppl thiogly = fluid thioglycollate + 10% rabbit serum; BA = blood agar; EMB = eosin methylene blue; CNA = colistin-nalidixic acid blood agar; CBA = chocolate blood agar; HE = Hektoen enteric agar; GN = enrichment broth; K-V = kanamycin-vancomycin; PEA = phenylethyl alcohol blood agar.

†Only for specimens from suitable source and received in anaerobe vial.

‡Modified Thayer-Martin agar.

Adapted from Washington, 1981.

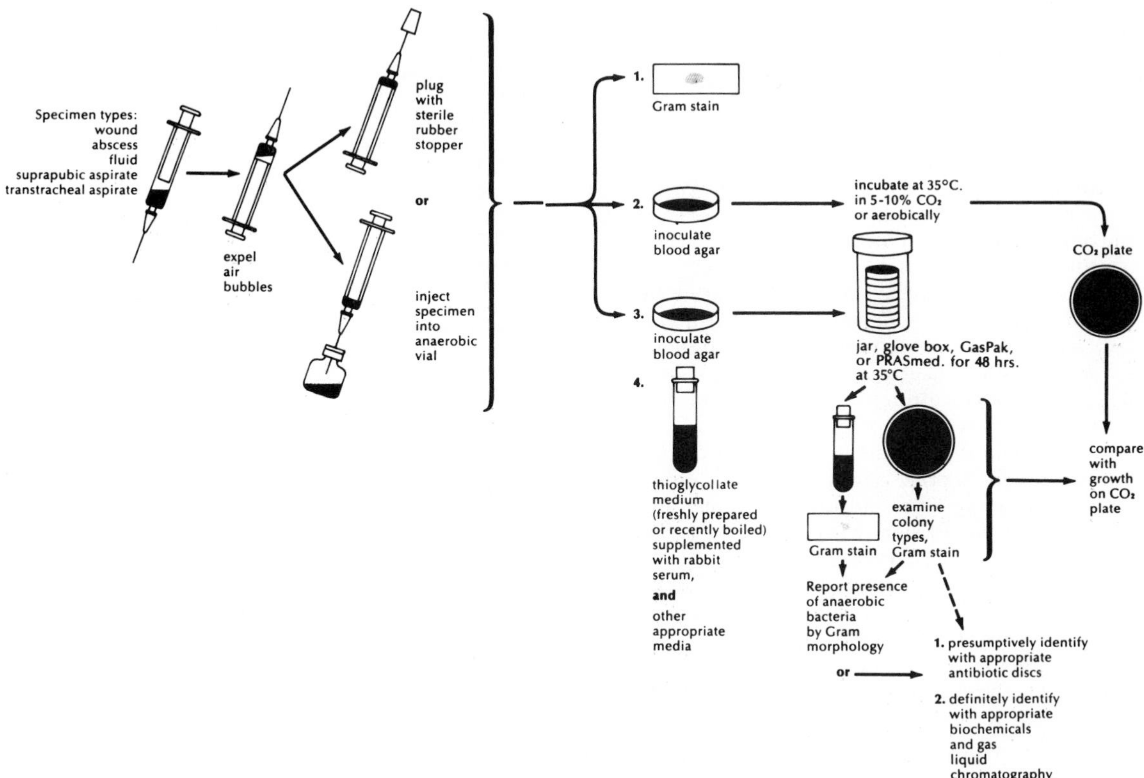

Figure 45–2. Flow chart for processing anaerobic specimens. (By permission of The Upjohn Company, Kalamazoo. Michigan, and J. A. Washington and L. LeBeau.)

conventional isolation and subculture techniques are used. The chamber itself requires a substantial amount of space.

Each of the three anaerobe systems has its advantages and disadvantages, but they are all equally effective for isolating clinically significant anaerobic bacteria from specimens. The selection of one of these systems for routine purposes depends upon many factors ranging from economic to technical. It is important to emphasize, however, the necessity of incubating cultures for at least 48 hours, since many anaerobic bacteria will not be evident after only 24 hours of incubation.

EXAMINATION OF CULTURES

All bacterial cultures should be examined routinely after 18 to 24 hours of incubation. The suggested duration of different types of cultures are listed in Table 45–5. In general, cultures of normally sterile body fluids, wounds, abscesses, tissues, and anaerobic cultures are retained for one week, although in most instances the plates are discarded in 48 hours and only the broth cultures are reincubated for the longer period of time. Stool cultures and subcultures are each examined for the presence of lactose-negative colonies and are discarded if none are present. Urine cultures that have no growth or only a few colonies after 18 to 24 hours of incubation are discarded as being negative. Throat cultures are examined for the presence of β-hemolytic streptococci after 18 to 24 hours of incubation; if none are present, the cultures are reincubated for another day. Identification procedures for colonies in sputum and urine cultures can begin after a day's incubation with no added incubation being necessary.

With positive cultures it is a good idea to develop a system of preliminary reports, since identification procedures may take as long as several days to complete. Although the timing of a preliminary report will vary according to the type of culture performed and the importance of the bacteria isolated, it is a good general rule to issue a preliminary report within the first 48 hours after receipt of the specimen. In some cases this report can be sooner and in some (e.g., blood, cerebrospinal fluid) it should be by phone as soon as any information becomes available.

Table 45–5. DURATION OF INCUBATION AND FREQUENCY OF EXAMINATION OF CULTURES

Type of Culture	Incubation Time Before Negative Culture Report (Days)	Frequency of Examination
Blood	14	Daily for 7 days and after 14 days
Fluids	7*	Daily
Abscesses, wounds	7*	Daily
Tissue	7*	Daily
Respiratory tract		
Throat	2	Daily
Sputum	1	Once
Transtracheal aspirate	7*	Daily
Bronchial washings	7*	Daily
Genitourinary		
Cervix, vagina	2	Daily
Uterus, cul-de-sac	7*	Daily
Prostate	2	Daily
Urethra	2	Daily
Urine	1	Once
Fecal material	1†	Once
Anaerobic	7*	Daily
Brucella	30	3 × weekly
Actinomyces	21	1 × weekly

*Plates are discarded after 48 hours, but tubes with supplemented fluid thioglycollate are kept for time specified in column.

†Initial cultures and subcultures of enrichment broth are examined after 18 to 24 hours for presence of lactose-negative colonies; if none are present, the cultures are reported as negative for salmonellae and shigellae.

MEDICALLY IMPORTANT BACTERIA

PYOGENIC COCCI

Gram-Positive

STAPHYLOCOCCUS

Definitions and Characteristics. Staphylococci are catalase-positive spherical cocci, often appearing in grape-like clusters in stained smears. They grow well on any peptone-containing nutrient medium under aerobic and anaerobic conditions and may produce hemolysis of various species of animal blood and yellow or orange pigment on agar. Growth of staphylococci is readily detected on blood agar plates or in various types of nutrient broths. A selective medium for the isolation of *Staphylococcus aureus* is one containing 7.5 to 10 per cent NaCl with mannitol.

Staphylococci have generally been distinguished from micrococci on the basis of their ability to produce acid anaerobically from glucose; however, this test has been difficult to interpret in some people's hands and criticized by others as providing an indistinct division between the two genera. Other test systems have, therefore, been described that are based on the ability of staphylococci to produce acid aerobically from glycerol in the presence of 0.4 μg/ml of erythromycin and on their sensitivity to lysostaphin (Schleifer, 1975). These tests provide more clearcut separation of the genera, are simpler to perform, and yield more rapid results than those dependent upon the production of acid from glucose under anaerobic conditions.

Staphylococcus aureus is differentiated from other species of staphylococci principally by its production of coagulases. Two antigenically distinct forms of coagulase have been recognized, one being bound to the cell wall and the other being released by or free from the cell wall. Although its mechanism has not been completely elucidated, it is thought that a plasma factor or coagulase-reacting factor reacts with cell-bound coagulase to form a coagulase-thrombin complex which, in turn, acts upon fibrinogen to form a fibrin clot. Cell-bound coagulase is called clumping factor by some and forms the basis of the slide coagulase test. Cell-free or unbound coagulase appears to form a complex with prothrombin to give a thrombin-like product. This form of coagulase serves as the basis for the tube coagulase test. Human and rabbit plasmas have been shown to be suitable for both of these tests; however, the appropriate dilution of plasmas must be determined for the optimal detection of coagulase, since their performance is affected by the presence of inhibitory and accessory factors. Under these circumstances it is more practical to use plasma prepared commercially for coagulase testing. Provided that a very dense, homogeneous bacterial suspension is mixed with a loopful of reconstituted rabbit plasma, clumping should be observed in nearly 99 per cent of instances with *Staphylococcus aureus*. Inoculation of a few colonies of *S. aureus* into a tube containing 0.5 ml of the same reconstituted rabbit plasma should produce a clot in over 99 per cent of instances and in nearly all cases within a four-hour period of incubation. The utilization of human plasma from normal, healthy donors requires careful quality control and titration to determine the dilution most suitable for routine use. The arbitrary selection of a specific dilution of donor plasma for routine purposes will result in a serious loss of sensitivity and of specificity in either coagulase test.

Pathogenesis and Virulence Factors. Most strains of *Staphylococcus aureus* produce α-, β-, and δ-toxins and a variety of other extracellular proteins, including leukocidin, urease, lipase, gelatinase, and phosphatase. Whereas the α-, β-, and δ-toxins are hemolytic, only the α- and β-toxins are considered to exert lethal and dermonecrotic activities. An epidermolytic toxin, which can be separated from the β-, α-, and δ-hemolysins, has been identified among phage group II staphylococci as the cause of the scalded skin syndrome. Otherwise, the roles of each of these toxins in the pathogenicity of staphylococci are unclear because of often contradictory data. Some staphylococci produce enterotoxins that produce vomiting and diarrhea. Five such enterotoxins have been identified thus far from strains of *S. aureus;* however, enterotoxin production by rare strains of coagulase-negative staphylococci has been reported. Toxic shock syndrome has been associated with strains of *S. aureus* which elaborate exotoxin C or enterotoxin F.

Factors of importance in the development of infections due to *S. aureus* include breaks in the continuity and integrity of mucosal and cutaneous surfaces, the presence of foreign bodies or implants, prior viral diseases, antecedent antimicrobial therapy, and underlying diseases with defects in cellular or humoral immunity. *S. aureus* may be present among the indigenous flora of the skin, eye, upper respiratory tract, gastrointestinal tract, urethra, and, infrequently, vagina. Infection may, therefore, arise from an endogenous or an exogenous source, involve local sites, spread contiguously, or invade the bloodstream with, possibly, the development of metastatic sites of infection (Fig. 45–3). Staphylococcal food poisoning, characterized by the occurrence of vomiting and diarrhea between one and six hours following ingestion of food containing enterotoxins, is not at all uncommon, although its true incidence is poorly defined, since it is not a reportable disease. The pathogenesis of toxic shock syndrome remains obscure, although the risk of incurring the disease appears to be related in women to tampon fluid capacity or absorbency. Vaginal cultures of most cases yield toxigenic strains of *S. aureus.*

Infections due to *Staphylococcus epidermidis* usually occur in patients with foreign bodies and especially in those with implanted prosthetic valves, joints, and shunts. *Staphylococcus saprophyticus* is an important cause of bacteriuria, particularly in sexually active young women. The pathogenicity of micrococci is uncertain owing to a great extent to problems associated with their identification.

Laboratory Diagnosis. The observation microscopically of typical rounded, gram-positive cocci in clusters in smears of material taken from previously unopened or undrained lesions is indicative of staphylococcal infection. Care should be taken in the interpretation of Gram's stained smears when only single or paired organisms are seen because of their possible confusion with pneumococci and streptococci.

In addition to collecting material from the infected lesion for smear and culture, consideration should be given in more seriously ill patients to performing blood cultures.

It is recommended that a slide coagulase test be performed initially, provided there is a sufficient number of colonies available to prepare a dense emulsion. The formation of clumping within 30 seconds is sufficient for the identification of *Staphylococcus aureus.* In the absence of clumping within 30 seconds or if only a few isolated staphylococcal colonies are present, several colonies should be transferred with a wire loop into a tube containing 0.5 ml of plasma that is incubated at 35°C. for four hours and then examined for clot formation. If no clot has formed, the tube should be reincubated and re-examined after a total of 20 hours of incubation. Examination of the test after only four hours of incubation is necessary because the vast majority of isolates of *S. aureus* will produce a clot within this time interval and because some strains produce a fibrinolysin that can lyse the clot and thereby produce a false-negative reaction if the test is only observed after 20 hours of incubation. Many species of coagulase-negative staphylococci have been proposed; however, with the exception of *S. saprophyticus,* which is resistant to novobiocin, speciation of such strains in the clinical laboratory is not practical. Until it is, it is probably sufficient for the clinical laboratory to call these coagulase-negative staphylococci.

Staphylococci may be classified on the basis of their

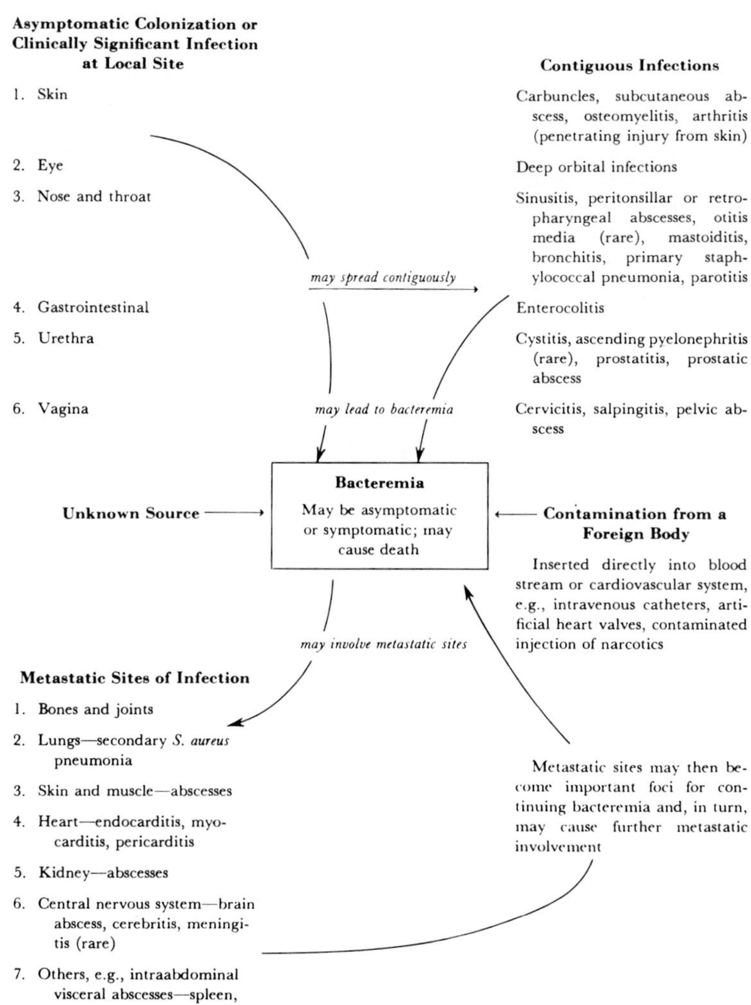

Figure 45–3. Pathogenic sequence of *Staphylococcus aureus* infection. (From Cohen, J. O.: The Staphylococci. New York, John Wiley & Sons, Inc., 1972.)

susceptibility to different bacteriophages. This classification is used for epidemiologic purposes in attempting to identify common source infections. Bacteriophage typing is generally available only through reference laboratories.

Antimicrobial Susceptibility. Whereas most staphylococci associated with community-acquired infections used to be susceptible to penicillin and most of those associated with nosocomially acquired infections were resistant to penicillin, this difference between susceptibility of strains according to their mode of acquisition has largely disappeared. It therefore behooves the laboratory to perform antimicrobial susceptibility tests. Penicillin, if the organism is susceptible to it, remains the antibiotic of choice in the therapy of staphylococcal infections. Methicillin resistance occurs in 5 to 20 per cent of isolates of *Staphylococcus epidermidis* and increasingly, among isolates of *S. aureus* in large, medical school–affiliated tertiary referral hospitals in the United States.

Penicillin resistance (minimal inhibitory concentration $\geq 0.2\ \mu g/ml$) is due to the production of a β-lactamase (penicillinase) associated with a plasmid in staphylococci. Methicillin resistance, on the other hand, is not related to a plasmid, and its mechanism appears to be related to differences in the penicillin-binding proteins of such strains. Plasmid-related resistance of staphylococci to aminoglycosides, especially gentamicin, is being reported. Staphylococci are generally quite susceptible *in vitro* to cephalosporins, erythromycin, chloramphenicol, and the lincomycins.

Prevention. A variety of measures have been attempted to prevent staphylococcal disease. Various types of vaccines have been tried with conflicting results in the literature. Clinical laboratories are often requested to prepare autogenous vaccines; however, this practice is discouraged because of the unstandardized nature of such vaccines, the existence of federal regulations surrounding the preparation of vaccines, and the absence of objective, carefully controlled trials substantiating their efficacy.

In some instances the application of bacterial interference has been successful in eliminating a virulent strain of *S. aureus* by replacing it with a less virulent strain (502A). Occasional reports of disease associated with *S. aureus* 502A have served to limit the use of this technique.

In the hospital the most successful means of prevention of staphylococcal disease has been careful surveillance and infection control measures. Containment and the proper disposal of infected materials, implementation of methods to prevent cross-contamination, institution of standardized antiseptic techniques, and improved operating room design represent some of the measures that have been used to prevent the spread of staphylococcal infections.

STREPTOCOCCUS

Definitions and Characteristics. Streptococci are catalase-negative, gram-positive, spherical, ovoid, or lancet-shaped cocci often seen in pairs or chains. Their minimal nutritional requirements are rather complex, with considerable interspecies variability. They are facultatively anaerobic. Some strains require added CO_2 for their initial isolation but may lose this requirement in subcultures. These CO_2-dependent strains have often been called "microaerophilic"; however, use of this term is discouraged because of its imprecision and the fact that most such strains can be classified into recognized species.

Streptococci can be broadly classified according to at least three schemes that unfortunately overlap and are, therefore, potentially confusing. One scheme places the streptococci into physiologic divisions: pyogenic, viridans, lactic, and enterococcal. In another they are categorized according to serologically active carbohydrates ('C" substance) into Lancefield groups. In the third scheme they are categorized according to their hemolytic reactions. Those strains that completely hemolyze the red cells about their colonies are called β-hemolytic, those that produce partial hemolysis are α-hemolytic, and those that do not hemolyze at all are γ-hemolytic. Four examples of the overlapping nature of these three schemes are given. A gamma-hemolytic *Streptococcus* may belong serologically to Lancefield's group D and physiologically be an enterococcus. α-Hemolytic strains are generally non-groupable serologically but physiologically represent viridans streptococci. β-Hemolytic streptococci belong to a Lancefield group and are pyogenic. Group D streptococci are usually γ-hemolytic but may be α- or β-hemolytic.

Each of these schemes for classifying streptococci serves a useful purpose so that it is generally not possible to eliminate any one of them completely. From the clinical standpoint, the separation of streptococci isolated from the blood of patients with subacute bacterial endocarditis into the physiologic divisions of viridans or enterococcus is of considerable importance in determining both the selection and the duration of antimicrobial therapy. The patient with viridans streptococcal endocarditis requires but two weeks of intramuscularly administered penicillin and aminoglycoside, while the patient with enterococcal streptococcal endocarditis requires three or four weeks of intravenously administered penicillin with intramuscularly administered aminoglycoside. It is essential for the laboratory to distinguish between group A streptococci and those belonging to other Lancefield groups in throat cultures, since the therapy in cases with group A streptococcal pharyngitis is directed toward the prevention of non-suppurative sequelae.

From the laboratory's point of view, the hemolytic reactions on blood agar produced by streptococci represent a useful point of departure for purposes of classification (Table 45–6). The methodology employed for classifying streptococci will be outlined in the section on laboratory diagnosis. It should be pointed out that most group D streptococci are not β-hemolytic and that this reaction is generally limited to a small percentage of isolates of *Streptococcus faecalis* and of *S. faecium.* These represent enterococcal group D streptococci, while *S. bovis* and *S. equinus* are non-enterococcal group D streptococci. Commonly included among the viridans streptococci are *S. pneumoniae, S. mutans, S. sanguis, S. mitis, S. salivarius,* and *S.* MG. Of as yet uncertain taxonomic status are nutritionally variant (pyridoxal-, B_6-, or thiol-dependent, satelliting) streptococci.

Group A streptococci may be typed according to their M and T protein antigens, the former of which represent essential virulence factors and convey type-specific immunity and the latter of which are unrelated to virulence and do not stimulate formation of protective antibodies. M antigens are often undetectable in unselected collections of group A streptococci; therefore, typing by the T agglutination system is also usually performed. Pneumococci are typable into more than 80 antigenic types on the basis of their capsular polysaccharide.

Pathogenesis and Virulence Factors. Group A streptococci elaborate more than 20 distinct exotoxins, including streptolysins O and S, which are hemolytic; erythrogenic toxin, which produces the rash in scarlet fever; streptokinase, which is fibrinolytic; hyaluronidase, which is a spreading factor; and diphosphopyridine nucleotidase, which is cardiotoxic. The M pro-

Table 45–6. CLASSIFICATION OF STREPTOCOCCI*

Hemolytic Reaction	Group	Species
β	A	*S. pyogenes*
	B	*S. agalactiae*
	C	*S. equisimilis*
		S. zooepidemicus
		S. equi
	D	*S. faecalis*
	F	*S. anginosus*
	G	unnamed
	E,L,M,P,U	–
α or γ	D	*S. faecalis*
		S. faecium
		S. bovis
		S. equinus
	F	*S. anginosus*
	none of above	*S. pneumoniae*
		S. mutans
		S. sanguis
		S. mitis
		S. salivarius
		S. MG
		S. uberis
		S. acidominimus
		S. morbillorum

*Based on Facklam, 1977.

6

tein inhibits phagocytosis. The pneumococcal capsule inhibits or prevents phagocytosis.

The common clinical manifestations of streptococcal diseases and their pathogenesis are listed in Table 45-7.

Laboratory Diagnosis. The diagnosis of streptococcal infection is usually made by culture of the organism from an infected site; however, documentation of an etiologic role of group A streptococci in its nonsuppurative sequelae, acute rheumatic fever and glomerulonephritis, must often be made serologically for two reasons. First, the organism may no longer be present in the pharynx or the skin at the time these sequelae appear, and, second, the recovery of group A streptococci from the upper respiratory tract does not always represent true infection (Kaplan, 1980). True group A streptococcal infection is documented by an antibody response to one or more antigens, including streptolysin O (ASO), deoxyribonuclease B (anti-DNase B), nicotinamide adenine dinucleotide (anti-NADase), hyaluronidase (AH), and a composite of "extracellular products" (antibodies to which are detected in the Streptozyme agglutinin test [Wampole Laboratories]). In a study of the serologic response in group A streptococcal pharyngitis, Kaplan and Huew (1980) found that the ASO, anti-DNase B, and Streptozyme tests displayed comparable sensitivity but that the Streptozyme test was slightly less specific than the other two tests. Of particular importance was their finding that each test detected significant antibody rises missed by at least one of the other two tests. Also important is the fact that the majority of children with streptococcal skin infections do not develop significant ASO titers. It is therefore recommended that two or three antibody tests be performed for maximal accuracy.

The signs and symptoms of group A streptococcal pharyngitis are highly variable and nonspecific; therefore, despite the lack of an immune response in approximately half of children with pharyngitis and group A streptococci isolated from their upper respiratory tracts (Kaplan, 1980), diagnosis usually depends on culture. The posterior pharynx, tonsillar pillars or tonsils, and areas of exudation, inflammation, or ulceration should be swabbed vigorously with minimal oral contamination. Group A streptococci on a swab in transport medium, e.g., Stuart's, will survive at room temperature for at least five days and usually longer. The swab should be inoculated onto a quarter to a third of a Petri dish containing 5 per cent sheep blood agar. A wire loop is then used to streak the inoculum for isolation over the remaining agar surface and for stabbing the surface of the agar in areas of the heaviest and lightest inocula. Cultures should be incubated for 18 to 24 hours at 35°C. in an atmosphere of room air. The presence of added

Table 45–7. COMMON CLINICAL MANIFESTATIONS AND PATHOGENESIS OF STREPTOCOCCAL DISEASE

Disease	Reservoir	Etiology
Group A		
Local and invasive forms		
Pharyngitis	Open lesions, normal skin, upper respiratory tract, perianal area; ?domestic animals, fomites, insect vectors	Intimate contact, minor trauma, insect bites, scratching; surgery, burns, wounds
Skin and soft tissue infections		
Superficial pyodermas		
Deeper skin and soft tissue		
Erysipelas		
Omphalitis		
Septicemia		
Poststreptococcal diseases		
Rheumatic fever	–	?Autoimmunity, cross-reactivity between streptococcal components and mammalian tissue
Acute glomerulonephritis	–	
Group B		
Neonatal sepsis and meningitis	Upper respiratory tract, vagina, nosocomial	?
Group D		
Endocarditis	Oral cavity, intestinal tract, vagina	Instrumentation of oral cavity and urinary tract resulting in transient bacteremia; abdominal or pelvic surgery; pre-existing valvular disease, prosthetic valve.
Urinary tract infection		
Intra-abdominal, pelvic abscess		
Viridans streptococci		
Endocarditis		
Intra-abdominal, pelvic, pulmonary, brain abscess		(As for group D)
Streptococcus pneumoniae		
Pneumonia	Upper respiratory tract	Prior viral infection of upper or lower respiratory tract, respiratory tract injury, pulmonary congestion, malnutrition, debility, sickle cell disease
Sinusitis		
Otitis		
Mastoiditis		
Meningitis		

Table 45–8. PRESUMPTIVE TESTS FOR GROUPING STREPTOCOCCI

Test	Group			
			D	
	A	***B***	***Enterococcal***	***Non-enterococcal***
Bacitracin inhibition*	+	−	−	−
Hippurate hydrolysis†	−	+	−	−
Esculin hydrolysis in presence of 40% bile	−	−	+	+
Growth in 6.5% NaCl	−	−	+	−

*Approximately 10% of non-group A β-hemolytic streptococci are inhibited by bacitracin.

†Some enterococci hydrolyze hippurate; therefore, hippurate-positive streptococci should have a negative bile-esculin reaction before being reported as belonging to group B.

CO_2 or anaerobiosis does not enhance the recovery of group A streptococci but does increase significantly the recovery of non-group A β-hemolytic streptococci. Incubation of agar plates in an atmosphere of room air does improve the specificity of throat cultures for group A streptococci.

Presumptive identification of group A streptococci by the bacitracin differentiation disk test is best accomplished with a pure subculture of β-hemolytic colonies, since the direct application of the disk to the primary culture plate may provide unreliable results. Nearly 10 per cent of non–group A β-hemolytic streptococci will be inhibited by bacitracin, while fewer than 1 per cent of group A strains will fail to be inhibited.

Other presumptive grouping tests for streptococci include those for determining the hydrolysis of sodium hippurate and the hydrolysis of esculin in the presence of 40 per cent bile (Table 45–8). In contrast to bacitracin differentiation, the bile-esculin test is highly sensitive and specific for group D streptococci. This is important because some strains of enterococcal group D streptococci hydrolyze hippurate, a reaction which is otherwise very sensitive and specific for group B. Bile-esculin positive strains can be further subdivided into enterococcal and non-enterococcal group D streptococci by determining their ability to grow in 6.5 per cent NaCl. A simple and reliable presumptive test for identifying group B streptococci is the CAMP reaction, which is a lytic phenomenon that occurs when group B streptococci are grown in the presence of β-toxin–producing staphylococci (Darling, 1975).

Definitive grouping of streptococci is usually performed by serologic means. The group-specific "C" substance can be extracted from cells by acid treatment, autoclaving, or enzymatic action. The extract and antiserum usually are combined in a capillary tube, and a white, flocculent precipitate forms at the antigen-antibody interface when the two are homologous. Counterimmunoelectrophoresis with and without (Hill, 1975) extraction procedures have also been successfully used for grouping streptococci and are both rapid and accurate. Protein A containing stabilized staphylococci coated with group-specific antibody have provided another rapid and accurate approach to grouping (Christensen, 1973; Edwards, 1974).

Immunofluorescence has been used for identifying group A and group B streptococci. With group A streptococci both direct and indirect techniques have been used. In the former a throat swab is incubated in Todd-Hewitt broth for between two and four hours, and a smear of spun sediment is stained with fluorescein-labeled anti-group A streptococcal reagent. This test is rapid, sensitive, and specific. Fluorescent microscopy (indirect) of smears of isolated β-hemolytic colonies stained with group-specific fluorescein-labeled conjugate is a rapid, sensitive, and specific method for identifying group A and group B streptococci.

Identification of groups other than A, B, and D is not necessary for routine clinical purposes. The majority will be streptococci belonging to Lancefield groups D, F, and G.

The identification of α- and γ-hemolytic streptococci has been discussed by Facklam (1977). For practical purposes, it is important to identify the group D streptococci, and it is helpful to distinguish between enterococcal and non-enterococcal strains, especially when they are isolated from the blood. It is also important to identify *Streptococcus pneumoniae.* This may be readily accomplished by use of a disk containing ethyl hydrocupreine hydrochloride (optochin) or of a bile solubility test with 10 per cent sodium deoxycholate. In the former test an inhibitory zone of at least 18 mm is indicative of susceptibility and that the organism is a pneumococcus. Direct application of 10 per cent deoxycholate solution will produce lysis of α-hemolytic colonies which are pneumococci. In clinical practice it is seldom necessary to provide further identification of the α- and γ- or viridans streptococci, and it is satisfactory to report them according to their hemolytic reactions or as viridans streptococci.

Antimicrobial Susceptibility. β-Hemolytic streptococci are inhibited by 0.005 to 0.01 μg/ml of penicillin with the exceptions of group B streptococci, which require up to eight times as much penicillin for inhibition, and enterococcal group D streptococci, which require 0.8 to 6.25 μg/ml for inhibition and nearly none of which are killed by as much as 100 μg/ml. At any rate, susceptibility testing with penicillin of group A streptococci isolated from patients with persistent or recurrent infection is not indicated. Among other orally administered antibiotics, resis-

6

tance of group A streptococci to erythromycin and cephalexin is rare, but to the tetracyclines it is relatively frequent (10 to 30 per cent), so that susceptibility testing of isolates from penicillin allergic patients is indicated.

Relative resistance of pneumococci to penicillin (0.1 to 0.5 μg/ml) has been reported in the United States, Australia, and New Guinea. Penicillin resistance in South Africa (≥ 2 μg/ml) was first reported in 1977; however, the incidence of such strains remains extremely low. Susceptibility testing of pneumococci from blood and cerebrospinal fluid with penicillin is warranted at this time. As with the group A streptococci, erythromycin resistance occurs rarely and tetracycline resistance not infrequently in pneumococci.

One of the best examples of the requirement for combined antimicrobial therapy is provided by the enterococcal group D streptococci which are not killed by high concentrations of penicillins or aminoglycosides and which cause endocarditis that cannot be cured by either of these classes of antibiotics alone. Combinations of a penicillin and an aminoglycoside are synergistic both *in vitro* and *in vivo* against these organisms. Although usually very susceptible to penicillin, the viridans streptococci are also synergistically affected by a combination of an aminoglycoside and penicillin. Susceptibility testing of some viridans streptococci can be difficult because of their fastidious nature and their requirement for CO_2.

Prevention and Control. Much thought has been devoted to the detection of streptococcal pharyngitis and to the prevention of its non-suppurative sequelae without, however, the achievement of a totally satisfactory solution. Many of the problems precluding satisfactory solution have been reviewed by Wannamaker (1972). Among these is the fact that group A streptococci account for but a small proportion of all respiratory illnesses and for approximately a third of acute pharyngitides. Many from whom group A streptococci are isolated are carriers and do not represent true infections (Kaplan, 1980). Acute nephritis is often not prevented by early treatment of pharyngitis and is clearly related to skin infection with a nephritogenic strain. Finally, approximately a third of children developing rheumatic fever give no antecedent history of upper respiratory tract infection. The value, therefore, of massive community or statewide programs of culturing all sore throats in school children and requiring treatment of all from whom group A streptococci were recovered remains unclear and requires further objective study.

There is general agreement on the need for a streptococcal vaccine to protect against acute nephritis and rheumatic fever in high risk groups; however, much work and many problems remain in this area. Type-specific and polyvalent pneumococcal vaccines have been evaluated successfully in clinical trials; however, geographic and temporal variations in the incidence of pneumococcal infections and types, as well as the identification and vaccination of high-risk populations, pose significant problems in vaccine use.

Gram-Negative

NEISSERIA AND BRANHAMELLA

Definitions and Characteristics. These genera are non-motile, catalase-, and oxidase-positive, aerobic gram-negative cocci which are often arranged in pairs with flattened adjacent surfaces. The genus *Branhamella* was separated from the neisseriae on the basis of differences in DNA base composition. It consists of the species *Branhamella catarrhalis,* although it has been proposed that *Neisseria caviae* and *Neisseria ovis* also be placed in the genus *Branhamella.* Recognized species of *Neisseria* are *N. meningitidis, N. gonorrhoeae, N. sicca, N. subflava, N. flavescens,* and *N. mucosa.*

Closely resembling *Neisseria* and *Branhamella* are the genera *Moraxella* and *Acinetobacter,* which can produce rods, however, in contrast to *Neisseria* and *Branhamella,* which produce only cocci. These rod forms, sometimes referred to as coccobacillary, will be considered in a later section dealing with non-fermenting gram-negative bacilli.

With the exception of *Acinetobacter,* all of these organisms are somewhat fastidious in their growth requirements, requiring in some instances the addition of blood, serum, cholesterol, or oleic acid to the medium to counteract growth inhibitors. Gonococci and meningococci generally require prompt incubation in CO_2 for growth; however, this requirement is strain-dependent, varies with the phase of the organism's growth curve, and is often lost in subcultures. Meningococci and most gonococci are not inhibited by the presence of vancomycin or lincomycin, colistin, and nystatin, a characteristic that is particularly useful in their selective isolation from specimens contaminated with other bacteria. Vancomycin-susceptible gonococci have been encountered in significant numbers of patients in some parts of the country and are inhibited on media containing this antibiotic.

Pathogenesis and Virulence Factors. Although opportunistic infections due to species of *Branhamella* and of *Neisseria* other than *N. gonorrhoeae* and *N. meningitidis* have occasionally been reported in compromised hosts, these species are generally non-pathogenic.

Meningococci may colonize the mucous membranes of the upper respiratory tract, an event that is usually followed in 7 to 10 days by the formation of bactericidal and hemagglutinating antibodies which, however, may not eliminate the carrier state but which convey group-specific immunity. In a few cases, however, disease results shortly after colonization, most frequently in the form of meningococcemia and meningitis (Fig. 45–4). The organism also has a tendency to invade serous membranes and joint tissues with the development of pleuritis, pericarditis, and arthritis. Carriage of meningococci in the nasopharynx is not uncommon; however, a direct correlation between carrier rates and incidence of meningococcal disease has not been established, with the possible exception of members of large households or households with an infant or childhood case during epidemics of

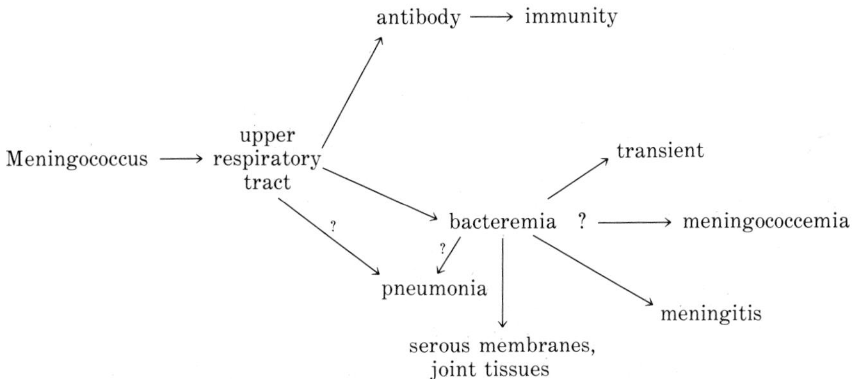

Figure 45–4. Pathogenesis and clinical aspects of meningococcal disease.

meningococcal disease. Meningococci have also been isolated from genital sources, where their clinical significance remains uncertain but where they may be readily misidentified as gonococci unless appropriate tests for distinguishing these two species are carried out.

The principal virulence factor of meningococci is a lipopolysaccharide-endotoxin complex, which in experimental animals activates the clotting cascade, depositing fibrin in small vessels, producing hemorrhage in the adrenals and other organs, and altering peripheral vascular resistance, leading to shock and death.

The pathogenesis and clinical manifestations of gonococcal infections differ somewhat from those of the meningococci (Fig. 45–5). Pathogenic types (1 and 2) of *Neisseria gonorrhoeae* adhere by means of pili, which nonpathogenic types (3 and 4) lack, to various human cells. These pili, which represent one of the principal virulence factors of the gonococcus, also may inhibit phagocytosis, are antigenically heterogeneous, and stimulate strain-specific antibody formation. Other possible virulence factors of *N. gonorrhoeae* are less clearly defined at this time.

Both gonococci and meningococci produce an IgA_1 protease which may also be important in their pathogenesis, since IgA is the antibody class which predominates in secretions on mucous membranes.

Laboratory Diagnosis. The single most important element in the laboratory diagnosis of meningo- and gonococcal diseases is the specimen, its proper selection, collection, and transport to the laboratory. The pathogenic species are sensitive to drying and extremes of temperature, and material should be cultured promptly for their recovery. They are mesophilic and grow poorly, if at all, at room temperature. Many require prompt incubation in CO_2 (2 to 18 per cent) for primary isolation. Media containing chocolatized blood are commonly used for cultures and should contain antibiotics, i.e., vancomycin or lincomycin,

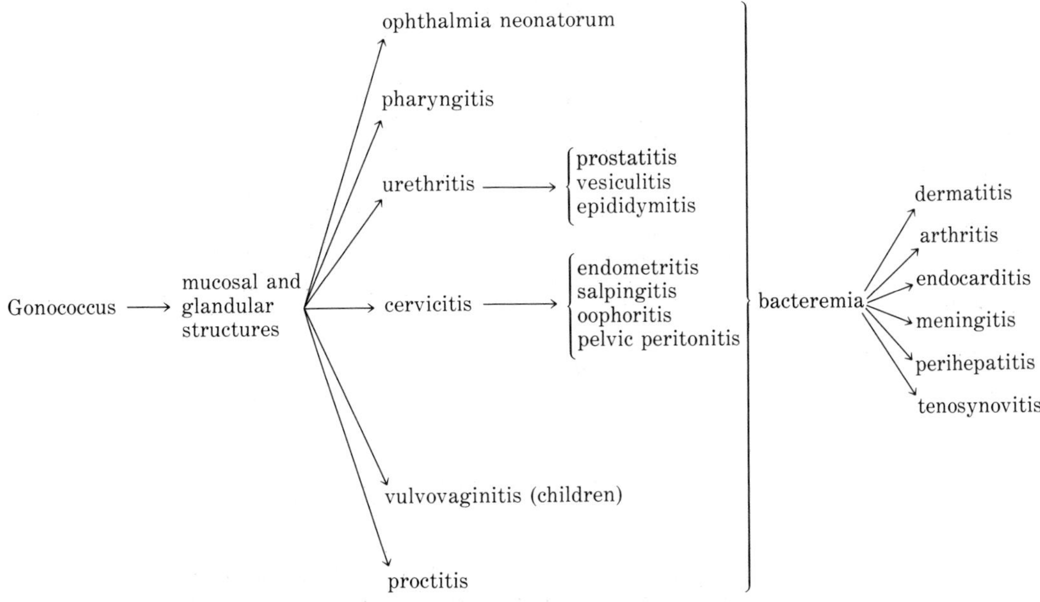

Figure 45–5. Pathogenesis and clinical manifestations of gonococcal disease.

as well as colistin, nystatin, and trimethoprim, if the specimen is contaminated with indigenous flora. Vancomycin-susceptible gonococci will grow on media containing lincomycin; however, because of the synergistic interaction of lincomycin and trimethoprim, the latter must be omitted from media containing lincomycin. It is suggested that specimens from genital sites be inoculated onto biplates containing Thayer-Martin medium with vancomycin and trimethoprim in one half of the plate and Thayer-Martin medium with lincomycin and without trimethoprim in the other half of the plate. Colistin should be incorporated in both media, but nystatin, which is unstable, should be replaced with anisomycin. Direct inoculation of specimens "at the bedside" is, therefore, often performed. This can be accomplished in several ways: the inoculation of Thayer-Martin medium with prompt incubation at 35°C. in CO_2, most frequently a candle jar; or the inoculation of modified Thayer-Martin medium in a bottle or chamber containing CO_2 (Transgrow) or in which CO_2 can be generated from a citric acid-bicarbonate tablet (JEMBEC). If any of these culture systems must be mailed to a reference laboratory for processing, they must first be incubated overnight to ensure growth of the organisms.

Cerebrospinal fluid from patients with bacterial meningitis should be rapidly transported to the laboratory for culture and must not be stored under refrigeration under any circumstances. Synovial and pericardial fluids should also be handled expeditiously. In these cases contamination of the specimen with indigenous flora is rarely a problem and selective media, such as Thayer-Martin, need not be used; however, chocolatized blood agar supplemented with yeast extract should be used not only for the recovery of meningococci but also for that of other pathogenic bacteria which can cause infection of these sites.

Characteristics that may be useful in differentiating the species of *Neisseria* and *Branhamella* are listed in Table 45–9. The isolation from a genital source of oxidase-positive gram-negative diplococci from Thayer-Martin medium constitutes presumptive identification of *Neisseria gonorrhoeae.* Confirmatory tests are, however, recommended because of the occasional isolation of *N. meningitidis* and *N. lactamica* from such sources. In cultures of the oropharynx carriage of these other two species is more frequent so that confirmatory tests must always be made with oxidase-positive gram-negative diplococci isolated from these sources on Thayer-Martin medium. As a rule, confirmatory tests may be limited to those for detecting the production of β-galactosidase and of acid from glucose, maltose, and sucrose. Immunofluorescence of colonies of *N. gonorrhoeae* is sufficiently specific to be used for the identification of this species.

Antimicrobial Susceptibility. Meningococci have remained susceptible to the penicillins and chloramphenicol to date, so that determining their susceptibility to these agents for therapeutic reasons is seldom necessary. Testing the inhibitory activity of sulfonamides, however, is indicated at the present time because of the proven efficacy of sulfonamides in eradicating the carriage of susceptible strains (minimal inhibitory concentration ≤ 10 μg/ml) from close contacts. All are susceptible to rifampin, the agent recommended in the United States for prophylaxis among household contacts unless susceptibility to sulfonamides is demonstrated.

Despite the fact that the concentrations of penicillin required to inhibit gonococci have increased somewhat in recent years, leading to recommendations that probenecid and increased dosages of penicillin be administered, outright penicillin resistance of gonococci due to β-lactamase was not reported until 1976. The prevalence of these strains is increasing throughout the world. They can be rapidly detected by testing for β-lactamase by any one of several acidimetric or iodometric methods. In the United States gonococci have remained susceptible to spectinomycin and tetracycline, which are the recommended alternatives to the penicillins in the treatment of gonorrhea.

Prevention. Polysaccharide vaccines against *Neisseria meningitidis* serogroups A and C have been licensed in this country and may be of value for travelers in countries known to have epidemic meningococcal disease, as an adjunct to antibiotic prophylaxis in household contacts of patients with meningococcal disease, and in populations at risk in epidemic situa-

Table 45–9. DIFFERENTIATION OF SPECIES OF *NEISSERIA* AND *BRANHAMELLA**

	N. gonorrhoeae	***N. meningitidis***	***N. lactamica***†	***N. sicca***	***N. subflava***	***N. flavescens***	***N. mucosa***	***B. catarrhalis***
Growth								
Thayer-Martin medium	+	+	+	–	–	–	–	–
Nutrient agar, 25° C.	–	–	d	d	d	+	+	+
Oxidase	+	+	+	+	+	+	+	+
β-Galactosidase	–	–	+	–	–	–	–	–
Reduction of nitrate	–	–	–	–	–	–	+	+
Production of acid from								
Glucose	+	+	+	+	+	–	+	–
Maltose	–	+	+	+	+	–	+	–
Lactose	–	–	+	–	–	–	–	–
Sucrose	–	–	–	+	v	–	+	–
Fructose	–	–	–	+	v	–	+	–

*+, ≥90% of strains positive; –, ≥90% of strains negative; d, some strains positive and others negative; v, inconstant reaction within strain.

†Species incertae sedis.

tions. A satisfactory serogroup B vaccine has not been developed. Antibiotic prophylaxis should be limited to household contacts and those who have had contact with patients' oral secretions. Rifampin, 600 mg every 12 hours for two days, is the drug of choice currently unless susceptibility to sulfonamides can be demonstrated. Some prefer to observe contacts carefully when sulfonamide resistance is demonstrated. One of the most common dilemmas occurring in laboratories is the isolation and identification of meningococci from throat swabs taken from patients with pharyngitis who coincidentally are carriers of this organism. Since reporting such findings is rarely of any clinical value and usually creates considerable consternation, it is recommended that the species designation of neisseriae from throat cultures not be reported unless (1) it is requested for purposes of identifying carriers or (2) it is *Neisseria gonorrhoeae,* the isolation of which is virtually always of clinical importance When specific requests are made for culture of meningococci and gonococci, the specimen should be inoculated onto modified Thayer-Martin medium.

The use of pre-exposure antibiotics to prevent gonococcal diseases is discouraged because of the potential risks of sensitization and the emergence of resistant strains. The sole exception to this rule is the application of silver nitrate solution or antibiotic ointment to the eyes of newborns to prevent gonococcal ophthalmia.

CORYNEFORM AND RELATED BACTERIA

The term coryneform has been used to describe gram-positive, non-spore–forming, non-filamentous rods which may exhibit pleomorphic morphology. In its broadest sense, the term might include *Actinomyces, Propionibacterium, Mycobacterium,* and *Nocardia,* as well as *Corynebacterium, Listeria,* and *Erysipelothrix;* however, taxonomists disagree as to the proper limits of the term. For purposes of simplicity of organization in this book, the term will be limited to *Corynebacterium, Listeria,* and *Erysipelothrix.* No endorsement, implied or otherwise, is intended by this approach.

CORYNEBACTERIUM

Definitions and Characteristics. The corynebacteria or "diphtheroids," as they are sometimes called, are widely distributed in nature and on the mucous membranes and skin of man and animals. Most species are rarely pathogenic in humans, with the notable exceptions of *Corynebacterium diphtheriae* and its closely related species or varieties, *C. diphtheriae* var. *ulcerans* and *C. pseudotuberculosis. C. pyogenes* and *C. haemolyticum* have been associated with diseases in humans; however, other than in their microscopic morphology, they share few characteristics in common with *C. diphtheriae,* and their taxonomic status remains uncertain at this time. Other species of *Corynebacterium,* particularly those belonging to group JK, have been clearly associated with infections of implanted prosthetic materials, e.g., heart valves, cerebrospinal fluid shunts, joints, have caused subacute bacterial endocarditis, and have been involved in a variety of opportunistic infections. Their etiologic role in causing such infections is established with considerable difficulty and often only after their repeated isolation from a particular source.

Pathogenesis and Virulence. Lysogenic strains of *Corynebacterium diphtheriae* harboring prophages carrying the TOX^+ gene excrete a toxin which enters the body of susceptible persons through lesions in epithelial surfaces or by attachment to and transport into epithelial cells, whence it is transported via the blood and lymphatics to a variety of organs, including the heart, kidneys, liver, pancreas, lungs, and peripheral nervous system. The exotoxin is a protein with a molecular weight of about 62,000, 25 ng of which injected subcutaneously will kill a 250 g guinea pig in four or five days. The organisms and their exotoxin produce a serum exudate and cellular infiltrate of the mucous membrane in the pharynx, leading to formation of a grayish pseudomembrane. Although toxin production and pathogenicity are often considered to be synonymous, pseudomembranes may form in persons infected with non-toxigenic strains. Extension of the pseudomembrane superiorly into the nasopharynx or inferiorly into the larynx may be so marked as to produce respiratory obstruction. Although *C. diphtheriae* infections of other parts of the body do occur, the most frequent ones observed in the United States today are those of the skin.

Transmission of *C. diphtheriae* is by droplet nuclei from the respiratory tract or by contact from cutaneous foci of infection.

Laboratory Diagnosis. Because of the relative rarity of diphtheria in the United States today, the diagnosis may be overlooked clinically and the laboratory may easily fail to recognize its causative agent in cultures. A tentative diagnosis must always be provided to the laboratory so that the specimen will be inoculated onto suitable media for isolation of the organism. Cystine-tellurite (CT) blood agar is the preferred medium for isolation of the organism, while the more nutritionally deficient Loeffler's (coagulated serum) or Pai's (coagulated egg) medium is more useful for microscopic morphology. The cells are often pleomorphic in appearance, are characteristically arranged side by side in palisade formation, and frequently display metachromatic granules. On CT medium colonies of *C. diphtheriae* are grayish black after 48 hours of incubation. Three colony types can be encountered: *gravis,* which are large, flat, dark gray, and have irregular edges with radial striations; *mitis,* which are black, convex, and moist; and *intermedius,* which are quite small and black.

Strains of corynebacteria can be speciated with biochemical tests (Table 45–10), but it is necessary to establish the virulence of isolates suspected of being *C. diphtheriae* by determining whether or not they produce exotoxin. This can be done by inoculating a broth culture subcutaneously into two guinea pigs, one of which has received diphtheria antitoxin intraperitoneally two hours previously. The unprotected

Table 45–10. DIFFERENTIAL CHARACTERISTICS OF SOME SPECIES WITHIN THE GENUS *CORYNEBACTERIUM**

Test	*C. diphtheriae*	*C. ulcerans*	*C. pseudotuberculosis*	*C. xerosis*	*C. pseudodiphtheriticum*	*Group JK*	*C. haemolyticum*	*C. pyogenes*
Catalase	+	+	+	+	+	+	−	−
Hemolysis	+	+	+	−	−	−	+	+
Gelatinase	−	+	−	−	−	−	−	+
Urease	−	+	+	−	+	−	−	−
NO_3 reduction	+	−	d	+	+	−	−	−
Sucrose fermentation	−	+	d	+	−	−	d	+

*d = variable.

guinea pig will die within one to four days if the inoculated strain was toxigenic. Alternatively, the elaboration of toxin may be detected *in vitro* by streaking the culture to be tested at right angles to a paper strip impregnated with antitoxin and embedded in agar and observing the formation of precipitin lines at 45 degree angles to the paper strip. Many modifications of this test have been described resulting from the failure of toxigenic strains to produce precipitin lines or from the formation of non-specific lines by nontoxigenic strains. The potency of the antitoxin, the inoculum size, the type of enrichment serum, and the duration of incubation all affect the outcome of this test.

The classification of the oral and skin corynebacteria or diphtheroids is difficult and confusing. Multiple approaches have been proposed and are based on characteristics such as oleate dependence, fluorescence, nitrate reduction, urease activity, and carbohydrate fermentations. Published fermentation reactions are highly variable, often conflicting, and reflect, among other things, the organisms'growth characteristics and whether or not the basal medium has been supplemented with serum or a source of oleate, e.g., Tween-80.

Antimicrobial Susceptibility. Although antitoxin remains the only specific method of treatment of diphtheria, antibiotics are administered to patients with disease and to asymptomatic carriers of toxigenic strains. *Corynebacterium diphtheriae* is usually inhibited by ≤0.5 μg/ml of penicillin, ≤0.05 μg/ml of erythromycin, and ≤0.3 μg/ml of clindamycin. Because of its activity and because it is well tolerated, erythromycin is often used for this purpose; however, benzathine penicillin may be useful in instances in which patient cooperation is suspect.

The antimicrobial susceptibilities of other species of corynebacteria or diphtheroids are far less predictable. Group JK, which has been isolated from immunocompromised patients with bacteremia and from patients with infective endocarditis, is often resistant to the penicillins and cephalosporins, variably susceptible to most other antibiotics, and almost uniformly susceptible to vancomycin. The therapy of infections due to these organisms is often complicated by the presence of compromised host defenses and of implanted prosthetic materials.

Prevention. The methods of prevention of diphtheria are almost exclusively active and passive immunization programs with supplemental antibiotics to eliminate the carrier state of toxigenic strains during epidemics. Immunity can be determined by the Schick test in which a small amount of toxin is injected intradermally on one forearm and toxoid into the other. The absence of erythema, induration, and necrosis 120 hours later in either forearm is indicative of immunity.

LISTERIA

Definitions and Characteristics. The pathogenic species for man and an intracellular parasite, *Listeria monocytogenes,* is most successfully isolated from tissue by culture of finely ground material. Fluids and swabs are directly plated on conventional bacteriologic media. The organism's growth is optimal at temperatures of 30 to 37°C.; however, growth does occur between 3 and 45°C. and does, in fact, appear to be enhanced in some instances after storage of the specimen under refrigeration.

L. monocytogenes is a facultatively anaerobic, catalase- and Voges-Proskauer–positive, gram-positive, non–spore-forming, non–acid-fast organism which may appear coccoid, coccobacillary, or bacillary microscopically. Rods may arrange themselves into palisades with V and Y forms typical of other coryneform bacteria. A narrow zone of β-hemolysis is produced on blood agar by fresh isolates. A characteristic tumbling motility occurs at room temperature but rarely at 35°C. This same temperature-dependent motility is also noted in semisolid media.

Pathogenesis and Virulence. *L. monocytogenes* is a rare or rarely recognized cause of meningitis and septicemia, predominantly in newborns, although it has a predilection for causing serious disease in patients with lymphoproliferative disorders. Cases of brain abscess, endocarditis, oculoglandular fever, pneumonia, urethritis, infectious mononucleosis–like disease, and habitual abortion have been associated with *Listeria.* A number of cases of *Listeria* sepsis and meningitis in renal transplant recipients have been described.

Intraperitoneal injection of the organism is fatal to rabbits and mice, with autopsy findings of foci of necrosis in the liver, spleen, lungs, adrenals, tonsils, and intestinal tract. The inflammatory infiltrate is predominantly mononuclear. The organism is an intracellular parasite; however, relatively little is known about its mechanisms of pathogenicity. Its hemolysin is lethal when injected into mice and may function by disrupting membranes. Its mode of transmission has not yet been clearly established.

Laboratory Diagnosis. Since listeriosis is a rare disease, it is rarely suspected clinically and the organism is often disregarded in the laboratory as being a diphtheroid or *Corynebacterium,* which it resembles microscopically. The isolation, especially from cerebrospinal fluid or blood, of small grayish-blue colonies surrounded by a narrow zone of β-hemolysis on blood agar should make one think of *L. monocytogenes* and lead one to perform a test for motility at 25°C. It does produce catalase and acid from glucose, trehalose, and salicin. A rapid presumptive diagnosis can also be made by immunofluorescence.

The organism resembles *Erysipelothrix rhusiopathiae;* however, there are several distinguishing characteristics between these two species (Table 45–11).

Antimicrobial Susceptibility. *L. monocytogenes* is usually inhibited by ≤0.5 μg/ml of penicillin or ampicillin, ≤6 μg/ml of chloramphenicol, ≤4 μg/ml of tetracycline, ≤16 μg/ml of kanamycin, and ≤4 μg/ml of gentamicin. Considerably higher concentrations of these antimicrobial agents are required for bactericidal activity, although substantially increased killing has been demonstrated in studies with combinations of penicillin or ampicillin with an aminoglycoside. Ampicillin, alone or in combination with

Table 45–11. DIFFERENTIAL CHARACTERISTICS OF *LISTERIA MONOCYTOGENES* AND *ERYSIPELOTHRIX RHUSIOPATHIAE*

Test	*L. monocytogenes*	*E. rhusiopathiae*
β-Hemolysis	+	−
Growth at 4° C.	+	−
Catalase	+	−
Motility	+	−
Esculin hydrolysis	+	−
Gluconate utilization	+	−
Voges-Proskauer	+	−
H_2S in TSI	−	+

an aminoglycoside, has been used successfully in the treatment of infections due to *Listeria monocytogenes*.

ERYSIPELOTHRIX RHUSIOPATHIAE

Definitions and Characteristics. *Erysipelothrix* is a catalase-negative, non–spore-forming, non-motile, facultatively anaerobic gram-positive bacillus which has a world-wide distribution. Cells from smooth phase colonies are small, straight, or slightly curved rods, while those from rough colonies are long and filamentous.

Pathogenesis and Virulence. *Erysipelothrix* infection is usually transmitted to man from animals by means of skin wounds produced with contaminated objects or in contact with blood, flesh, viscera, or feces of infected animals. The organism can be present in many species of mammals, birds, and fish; however, its most important animal reservoir is in domestic swine in which it can produce acute, subacute, subclinical, and chronic infection. Erysipeloid is principally an occupational disease of individuals in contact with animals and their products or by-products and wastes. The most common form of erysipeloid is a local cutaneous infection manifested by pain, swelling, and a cutaneous eruption characterized by a slowly progressive, slightly elevated, violaceous zone around the site of inoculation. The swelling and erythema migrate peripherally and the lesion involutes without desquamation. Systemic disease is rare, but there are numerous case reports of septicemia and endocarditis. Also rarely reported have been cases of arthritis and brain abscess.

Laboratory Diagnosis. Since positive cultures infrequently result from swab specimens of a local cutaneous lesion, biopsy or tissue aspirates represent the specimens of choice and should be placed into an infusion broth containing 1 per cent glucose followed by subculture onto blood agar. *Erysipelothrix* is rapidly fatal to mice when injected intraperitoneally and can be isolated in pure culture from the heart blood. Conventional blood culture media are suitable for its isolation from blood.

Erysipelothrix is oxidase- and catalase-negative. Characteristically, it produces H_2S in triple sugar iron agar (TSIA). It is non-motile, does not reduce nitrates to nitrite, and ferments glucose and lactose. It can be readily distinguished from *Listeria* (Table 45–11).

Antimicrobial Susceptibility. *Erysipelothrix* is susceptible to the penicillins, cephalosporins, erythromycin, clindamycin, chloramphenicol, and tetracyclines but resistant to sulfonamides and aminoglycosides.

Prevention. Preventive measures include an awareness on the part of those occupationally or recreationally (e.g., hunters) exposed to infected animals and their observance of simple hygienic practices; rodent control; and regular disinfection of fish tanks. Immunization is ineffective.

AEROBIC SPORE-FORMING BACILLI

BACILLUS

Definitions and Characteristics. The cells of members of this genus are strictly aerobic or facultatively anaerobic, rod-shaped, spore-forming, gram-positive, and catalase-positive. With the notable exception of the anthrax bacillus, they are usually motile by means of lateral or peritrichous flagella. Some strains will stain gram-negatively and because of their variable oxidase reactions are confused with gram-negative bacilli. The most reliable diagnostic characteristic of the genus is spore formation which occurs optimally and on a variety of media under aerobic conditions at 25 to 30°C. In Gram's stained smears endospores are detectable by the presence of unstained defects or holes within the cell. The spores themselves can be stained by any one of several methods.

Pathogenesis and Virulence Factors. Of the 48 distinct species of *Bacillus, Bacillus anthracis* is the only one that is uniformly and highly pathogenic. Great care must be exercised when handling material suspected of harboring this species. Work should be performed in biologic safety cabinets by gloved, gowned, masked, and immunized personnel; work surfaces must be disinfected with 5 per cent hypochlorite or 5 per cent phenol; and all supplies, materials, and equipment must be decontaminated. Animals should be inoculated only by properly attired and immunized personnel, should be housed separately, and should be autoclaved and incinerated after death.

There are three forms of anthrax which are recognized: cutaneous, inhalation, and intestinal. In its cutaneous form, anthrax produces a small, red, macular lesion that progresses on to a vesicle and finally necrosis with formation of a characteristic black eschar. Regional lymphadenopathy and septicemia may occur. The mortality in untreated cases with this form of disease is approximately 20 per cent. Inhalation of anthrax spores can lead to acute bronchopneumonia, mediastinitis, and septicemia. The mortality in recognized cases with this form of disease is nearly 100 per cent. Intestinal anthrax follows the ingestion of contaminated food and is manifested by nausea, vomiting, and diarrhea. In some cases there is gastrointestinal bleeding, followed by prostration, shock, and death. Septicemia can occur in all three forms of anthrax and may lead to a fatal purulent meningitis.

A major factor in the organism's pathogenic capabilities is its glutamyl polypeptide capsule that inhibits phagocytosis but antibodies to which are not protective against the disease. A complex toxin with three components is responsible for the signs and symptoms of anthrax.

Man becomes infected with anthrax by contact with and inhalation or ingestion of infected animals, their carcasses, or their by-products. Cattle, sheep, horses, and goats are the animals most frequently infected and provide a ready source of vegetative organisms which sporulate and perpetuate the environmental contamination.

Although usually saprophytic, other species of *Bacillus* have been recognized as causing disease. *B. cereus* has been associated with eye and ear infections, pneumonias, post-traumatic wound infections, septicemias, and endocarditis. Patients with pneumonias and septicemias are often immunosuppressed.

Acute diarrheal disease due to *B. cereus* has been reported in the European literature for many years but has been scarcely recognized in this country. The organism is widely distributed in foods, ordinarily in low numbers; however, it can reproduce rapidly to levels as high as 10^7 to 10^8/g of food. This almost invariably results from bulk preparation of foods followed by storage at room temperature with or without modest reheating prior to their being served. An illness characterized mostly by vomiting has been described in association with the consumption of cooked rice in Chinese restaurants. Illness in either case follows a brief incubation period of less than 18 hours. Diarrhea is due to an enterotoxin similar in activity to that of *Vibrio cholerae* and *Escherichia coli* which produces fluid accumulation in the rabbit ileal loop preparation.

Laboratory Diagnosis. Swabs of the vesicles and under the edge of the eschar in the cutaneous form of anthrax should be taken for smear and culture. Sputum in the inhalation form should be collected for smear and culture. Cultures of stool should be made in the intestinal form. Smears and cultures should be made of cerebrospinal fluid in suspected meningitis. In the septicemic stage, cultures of blood should be prepared.

The finding of large, boxcar-shaped, gram-positive cells in smears of any of these specimens should suggest the diagnosis. Fluorescent microscopy, available in some state health laboratories and at the Centers for Disease Control, can provide a rapid presumptive diagnosis. Cultures can be made on blood agar or, in the case of blood cultures, in conventional blood culture media.

Colonies of *B. anthracis* are usually flat, with an irregular margin ("Medusa head"), appear off-white with a ground glass surface, and are non-hemolytic. When touched with an inoculating loop, the colonies are tenacious and will stand up like beaten egg white. Anthrax bacilli are non-motile in either a hanging drop test or in semisolid media. Both *B. anthracis* and *B. cereus* ferment glucose, maltose, and sucrose and produce a positive Voges-Proskauer reaction. Other distinguishing features of *B. anthracis* are listed in Table 45–12.

Virulence tests may be performed by inoculating mice with either 0.2 ml subcutaneously or 0.5 ml

Table 45–12. DIFFERENTIAL CHARACTERISTICS OF *BACILLUS ANTHRACIS* AND *BACILLUS CEREUS*

Test	*B. anthracis*	*B. cereus*
Hemolysis	–	+
Motility	–	+
Capsulation	+	–
Fluorescent antibody	+	–
Animal pathogenicity	+	–
Gelatin liquefaction	–,(+)*	+
Lecithinase	–	+
Peptonization of milk	–	+
Salicin, acid	–,(+)*	+

*(+) = delayed reaction.

intraperitoneally of a barely turbid saline suspension prepared from colonies on agar. A broth culture should not be used for virulence testing because of the toxigenic products formed in broth by other *Bacillus* species. The mice will die in 24 to 72 hours, and the organisms can be demonstrated in smears and cultures of heart blood, liver, and spleen.

The detection of enterotoxin-producing strains of *B. cereus* depends upon the injection of sterile culture filtrates into the rabbit ileal loop preparation with resulting fluid accumulation. It is uncertain at this time how closely the *Bacillus* enterotoxin resembles that of *Vibrio cholerae* and *Escherichia coli;* however, the elaboration of other toxins that are cytotoxic to tissue culture interferes with the use of this enterotoxin detection method.

Antimicrobial Susceptibility. Although susceptible to a variety of agents, the antibiotic therapy of anthrax has centered on the use of penicillin with or without streptomycin. Both of these agents are highly active against *B. anthracis;* however, some strains do elaborate a β-lactamase.

The antimicrobial susceptibility of other species of *Bacillus* to the penicillins and cephalosporins is highly variable. Most strains are, however, inhibited by tetracycline, aminoglycosides, and chloramphenicol at low concentrations.

Prevention. Prevention of anthrax in humans ideally depends upon its control in animals. Prompt diagnosis of sick animals, their isolation and therapy, and cremation of carcasses are indicated when sporadic outbreaks occur. In enzootic areas vaccination with non-encapsulated spore preparations is used. Occupationally exposed persons should also be immunized.

Acute diarrheal disease due to *B. cereus* may be prevented by properly cooking and refrigerating foods prepared in bulk to prevent proliferation of vegetative forms of the bacteria and formation of the enterotoxin.

GRAM-NEGATIVE AEROBIC AND FACULTATIVELY ANAEROBIC RODS

For strictly functional reasons the laboratory classifies these organisms according to their manner of utilization of glucose (Fig. 45–6) and whether or not special growth factors or conditions are required.

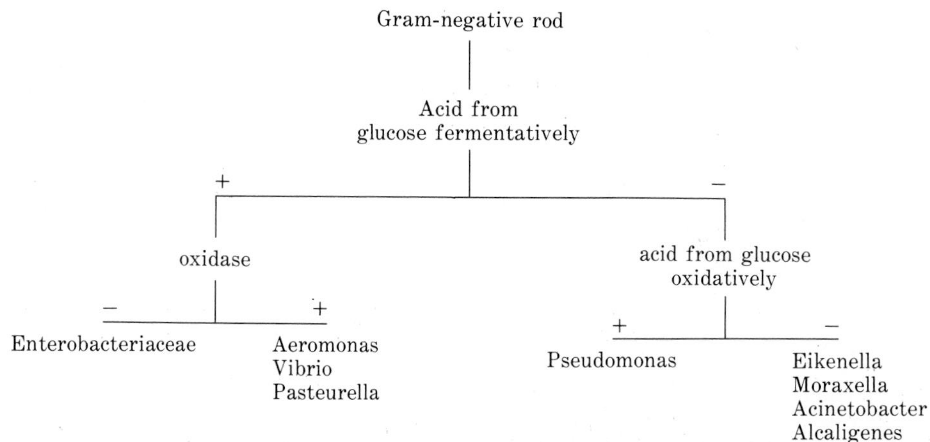

Figure 45–6. Brief functional classification of aerobic and facultatively anaerobic gram-negative bacilli growing on simple media.

Enterobacteriaceae

Definitions and Characteristics. The Enterobacteriaceae are aerobic and facultatively anaerobic, non-spore-forming, non-motile or peritrichously flagellated, oxidase-negative gram-negative bacilli which produce acid fermentatively from glucose and reduce nitrates to nitrites.

Pathogenesis and Virulence Factors. Endotoxins which are present within the cell walls of the Enterobacteriaceae, as well as other gram-negative bacilli, are responsible for the most part for the morbidity and mortality resulting from infections associated with these bacteria. Endotoxins consist of lipid and polysaccharide moieties with small amounts of amino acids. They may produce fever, granulocytosis, thrombocytopenia, disseminated intravascular coagulation, and activation of both the classic and alternate complement pathways (Elin, 1976). Endotoxin shock is the result of gram-negative septicemia with endotoxemia reacting with leukocytes, platelets, complement, and other serum proteins to increase the blood levels of proteolytic enzymes and vasoactive substances and resulting in pooling of blood, increased peripheral vasoconstriction, and diminution in cardiac output. Endotoxin also has effects on the endocrine, reticuloendothelial, and immunologic systems, as well as on metabolism of carbohydrates, lipids, proteins, and minerals.

There are three recognized pathogenetic mechanisms of bacterial diarrheas of acute onset (Table 45–3). Two types of enterotoxin have been found to be elaborated by *Escherichia coli:* a heat-stable toxin which is non-antigenic and is detectable primarily by quantitation of fluid accumulation in the gastrointestinal tract of infant mice, and a heat-labile toxin which is antigenic and is detectable primarily by quantitation of fluid accumulation in the rabbit ileal loop or by morphologic alterations in mouse adrenal tumor or Chinese hamster ovary cells in tissue cultures.

Other pathogenetic factors of the Enterobacteriaceae include the K1 antigen, which is associated with a high percentage of strains of *Escherichia coli* causing neonatal meningitis; the capsule of *Klebsiella pneumoniae,* which, like that of the pneumococcus, inhibits phagocytosis; and the Vi antigen of *Salmonella typhi,* which may interfere with intracellular killing of this organism.

The distribution of species of Enterobacteriaceae encountered in various diseases varies considerably. In the urinary tract those most frequently isolated are *Escherichia coli, Proteus mirabilis,* and *Klebsiella pneumoniae. Providencia* occurs almost exclusively in the urinary tract and most frequently in patients with chronic indwelling catheters. Gram-negative pneumonias associated with the Enterobacteriaceae are most frequently due to *K. pneumoniae.* Gram-negative bacteremias related to the Enterobacteriaceae are most frequently due to *Escherichia coli, Klebsiella pneumoniae,* and *Proteus mirabilis.* Infections acquired in the hospital are apt to be due to the more highly resistant groups, such as *Citrobacter, Enterobacter,* and *Serratia.* Shigellae are but rarely isolated from sources other than the gastrointestinal tract, while salmonellae are not infrequently isolated from other sources, such as urine or blood.

Laboratory Diagnosis

Isolation. The isolation of gram-negative bacilli, including the Enterobacteriaceae, is greatly facilitated by and in some instances requires the use of differential and selective media (Table 45–13). Eosin methylene blue (EMB) and MacConkey agar can be used interchangeably as differential media, as can xylose-lysine-deoxycholate (XLD) and Hektoen enteric (HE) agars as selective media for salmonellae and shigellae. Both XLD and HE are superior to Salmonella-Shigella (SS) agar for the isolation of enteric pathogens. Bismuth sulfite (BS) is especially useful for the detection of salmonellae in endemics or epidemics.

For specimens other than feces a differential medium should usually be inoculated in addition to a non-inhibitory, general-purpose nutrient agar medium, e.g., soybean-casein digest agar with 5 per cent sheep blood. For fecal specimens a differential medium and a selective medium should be inoculated, as well as an enrichment medium, such as selenite-F

Table 45–13. ENTERIC DIFFERENTIAL AND SELECTIVE MEDIA

Medium	Gram-Positive Bacteriostatic Agent	Fermentable Carbohydrate	Indicator	Colony Color		Category*
				Fermenter	*Non-fermenter*	
Eosin methelene blue (EMB)	Eosin Y Methylene blue	Lactose†	Eosin Y Methylene blue	Red or black with sheen	Colorless	D
MacConkey	Crystal violet Bile salts	Lactose	Neutral red	Red	Colorless	D
Xylose-lysine-deoxycholate (XLD)	Bile salts	Xylose Lactose Sucrose	Phenol red	Yellow	Red	S
Hektoen enteric (HE)	Bile salts	Salicin Lactose Sucrose	Bromothymol blue	Yellow-orange	Green, blue-green	S
Salmonella-shigella (SS)	Bile salts	Lactose	Neutral red	Red	Colorless	S
Bismuth sulfite (BS)	Brilliant green	Glucose	Bismuth sulfite	‡	‡	S
Thiosulfate citrate Bile salts sucrose (TCBS)§	Bile salts citrate pH 8.6	Sucrose	Thymol blue Bromothymol blue	Yellow	Colorless	S

*D = differential, S = selective.
†Levine's formulation.
‡H_2S-producing salmonellae have black colonies.
§Used for isolation of vibrios.

or gram-negative (GN) broth. With cultures of specimens other than feces, portions of colonies with distinct colonial morphologies should be inoculated into identification media. With cultures of feces, it is necessary only to identify colorless colonies on EMB or MacConkey agar (red on XLD and green to blue-green on HE). Salmonellae will often produce colonies with black centers owing to their production of H_2S.

Identification. Innumerable schemes based on the use of conventional biochemical media and of a variety of diagnostic kits have been described for the identification of the Enterobacteriaceae. It is beyond the scope of this chapter to describe them all, and the reader is referred to the laboratory procedure manuals listed in the general references (Lennette, 1980; Washington, 1981) or to the manuals prepared by the diagnostic kit manufacturers for more specific details. Most laboratories inoculate an initial series of tests usually including lysine and ornithine decarboxylases, deaminase, indole, citrate, urease, hydrogen sulfide, and motility. Additional tests are required for more specific identification of isolates. The selection and number of additional tests are predicated on factors including cost, interest, and skill. Precision increases with the number of tests performed but the advantages of performing an increasing number of tests can be offset by practicality and the skill of the technologists doing the work. A series of 20 tests, for example, to identify a gram-negative bacillus, colonies of which produce a green metallic sheen on EMB agar, is carrying precision to the point of absurdity, since a positive rapid indole test will provide the identification of *Escherichia coli* with equivalent precision in skilled hands. Even in unskilled hands the appropriate reactions in a series of five or six tests will provide the same level of precision in identifying this species under the conditions described above. Performing a sufficient number of tests to speciate an organism precisely often has little clinical value. Variabilities in individual biochemical test reactions, moreover, reduce the reliability of applying biotypes to epidemiologic investigation.

There are a variety of diagnostic kits on the market today for identifying the Enterobacteriaceae. Most of these or modifications thereof have published records of accuracy so that a laboratory's selection of any one of them for routine purposes can be based on personal preference and cost. All should be used according to manufacturers' recommendations.

Classification. The Classification of the Enterobacteriaceae has undergone considerable revision in recent years as the result of DNA hybridization and relatedness studies by investigators at the Centers for Disease Control and elsewhere. Based on genetic studies, a number of new genera and species have been proposed (Tables 45–14 to 45–17). Since phenotypic groupings on the basis of biochemical reactions are not always consistent with their DNA relatedness, the use of tribes (e.g., Klebsielleae, Proteeae) for grouping species within the Enterobacteriaceae has been discontinued in this chapter. Because of their uncertain taxonomic status or clinical importance, the genera *Erwinia* and *Pectobacterium* have been omitted from the tables of differential characteristics of the Enterobacteriaceae (Tables 45–14 to 45–17).

In the past it was customary to determine whether or not *E. coli* isolated from fecal material from infants belonged to an "enteropathogenic" serotype. Although epidemiologically associated with newborn nursery outbreaks of diarrhea, strains belonging to these serotypes have been found not to elaborate enterotoxin or to invade. Routine serotyping of strains isolated from fecal material of infants is, therefore, unnecessary and should not be done. Testing for agglutination in serogroups A, B, C, or D of a suspension of colonies suspected of representing *Shigella* should be performed.

The species designations of the salmonellae remain

Text continued on page 1102

Table 45–14. DIFFERENTIAL CHARACTERISTICS OF *ESCHERICHIA, CITROBACTER, KLUYVERA, ENTEROBACTER, HAFNIA,* AND *TATUMELLA**

		Escherichia			Citrobacter				Enterobacter						
Test	Shigella	*E. coli*	*E. hermanni*	*E. vulneris*	*C. freundii*	*C. diversus*	*C. amalonaticus*	Kluyvera	*E. cloacae*	*E. aerogenes*	*E. gergoviae*	*E. sakazakii*	*E. agglomerans*	*Tatumella ptyseos*	*Hafnia alvei*
Indole	–	+	+	–	–	+	+	+ or –	–	–	–	– or +	– or +	–	–
Methyl red	+	+	+	+	+	+	+	+	–	–	d	– or +	d	–	– or +
Voges-Proskauer	–	–	–	–	–	–	–	–	+	+	+	+	d	– (O'Meara) + (Coblenz)	+ or –
Citrate, Simmons'	–	–	–	–	+	+	+ or –	+	+	+	+	+	d	+ (25°C) – (36°C)	d
H_2S (TSI)	–	–	–	–	+	–	–	–	–	–	–	–	–	–	–
Urease	–	–	–	–	d	+ or –	+ or –	–	d	–	+	–	– or +	–	–
Phenylalanine deaminase	–	–	–	–	–	–	–	–	–	–	–	–	– or +	+	–
Lysine decarboxylase	–	+ or –	– or +	+	–	–	–	+ or –	–	+	+	–	–	–	+
Arginine dihydrolase	–	– or +	–	(+)	d	d	+ or –	–	+	-	–	+	–	–	–
Ornithine decarboxylase	d	d	+	–	– or +	+	+	+	+	+	+	+	–	–	+
Motility	–	+ or –	+	+	+	+	+	+	+	+	+	+	+ or –	+ (25°C) – (36°C)	+
KCN	–	–	+	d	+	–	+	+	+ or –	+	+	– or +	d	–	+
Malonate	–	–	–	+	–	+	–	+	+	+	+	+	+	–	+ or –
Lactose	–	+	d	(+)	(+)	d	d	+	d	+	d	+	d	–	d
Sucrose	–	d	d	d	d	– or +	– or +	+	+	+	+	+	+ or –	+	–
Mannitol	+ or –	+	+	+	+	+	+	+	+	+	+	+	+	–	+
Adonitol	–	–	–	–	–	+	–	–	– or +	+	–	–	–	–	–
Sorbitol	d	+	–	–	+	+	+	d	+	+	–	–	d	–	–
Raffinose	–	d	d	+	d	–	–	+	+	+	+	+	d	– or +	–
Cellobiose	–	–	+	+	d	+	+	+	+	+	+	+	+	–	d
Yellow pigment	–	–	+	d	–	–	–	–	–	–	–	+	+ or –	–	–

*Symbols: +, ≥90% positive reactions within 2 days; –, ≥90% negative reactions; (+), positive reactions in 3 to 7 days; + or –, reactions of most strains positive; – or +, reactions of most strains negative; $+^{w}$, weakly positive reaction; d, different reactions.

Table 45–15. DIFFERENTIAL CHARACTERISTICS OF *EDWARDSIELLA, SALMONELLA,* AND *ARIZONA**

Test	Edwardsiella		Salmonella			*Arizona hinshawii*
	E. tarda	*E. hoshinae*	*S. choleraesuis*	*S. typhi*	*S. enteritidis*	
Indole	+	+	–	–	–	–
Methyl red	+	+	+	+	+	+
Voges-Proskauer	–	–	–	–	–	–
Citrate, Simmons'	–	–	(+)	–	+ or (+)†	+
H_2S (TSI)	+	+	d	+	+†	+
Urease	–	–	–	–	–	–
Phenylalanine	–	–	–	–	–	–
Lysine decarboxylase	+	+	+	+	+	+
Arginine dihydrolase	–	–	(+)	+	+ or (+)	(+) or +
Ornithine decarboxylase	+	+	+	–	+	+
Motility	+	+	+	+	+	+
KCN	–	–	–	–	–	–
Malonate	–	+	–	–	–	+
Lactose	–	–	–	–	–	d
Sucrose	–	+	–	–	–	–
Mannitol	–	+	+	+	+	+
Dulcitol	–	–	d	d	+	–
Adonitol	–	–	–	–	–	–
Inositol	–	–	–	–	d	–
Sorbitol	–	–	+ or (+)	+	+	+
Arabinose	–	–	–	–	+	+
Raffinose	–	–	–	–	–	–
Rhamnose	–	–	+	–	+	+
Xylose	–	–	+	+	+†	+
Trehalose	–	+	–	+	+	+

*Symbols: As in Table 45–14.
†Reactions usually negative for *S. enteritidis* ser Paratyphi A.

6

Table 45–16. DIFFERENTIAL CHARACTERISTICS OF *KLEBSIELLA, CEDECEA,* AND *SERRATIA**

Test	Klebsiella				Cedecea			Serratia						
	K. pneumoniae	*K. oxytoca*	*K. ozaenae*	*K. rhinoscleromatis*	*C. davisae*	*C. lapagei*	*C. neteri*	*S. marcescens*	*S. liquefaciens*	*S. rubidaea*	*S. ficaria*	*S. plymuthica*	*S. odorifera*	*S. fonticola*
Indole	−	+	−	−	−	−	−	−	−	−	−	−	(+)[w]	−
Methyl red	− or +	d	+	+	+	d	+	− or +	+ or −	− or +	−	− or +	(+)	+
Voges-Proskauer	+	+	−	−	−	+ or −	+	+	− or +	+	+	+	d	−
Citrate, Simmons'	+	+	d	−	+ or −	+	+	+	+	+ or (+)	+	+	(+)	+
H_2S (TSI)	−	−	−	−	−	−	−	−	−	−	−	−	−	−
Urease	+	+	d	−	−	−	−	d	d	d	−	−	−	−
Phenylalanine deaminase	−	−	−	−	−	−	−	−	−	−	−	−	−	−
Lysine decarboxylase	+	+	d	−	−	−	−	+	+ or (+)	+ or (+)	−	−	+	+
Arginine dihydrolase	−	−	−	−	+ or −	+ or −	+	−	−	−	−	−	−	−
Ornithine decarboxylase	−	−	−	−	+	−	−	+	+	−	−	−	d	+
Motility	−	−	−	−	+	+ or −	+	+	+	+ or −	+	+	+	+
KCN	+	+	−	+	+ or −	+	+ or −	+	+	− or +	+	d	d	+
Malonate	+	+	−	+	+ or −	+	+	−	−	+ or −	−	−	−	+
Lactose	+	+	d	d	− or +	+ or −	(+)	−	d	+	−	(+)	(+)	+
Sucrose	+	+	− or +	+ or −	+	−	+	+	+	+	+	+	d	(+) or −
Mannitol	+	+	+	+	+	+	+	+	+	+	+	+	+	+
Dulcitol	− or +	− or +	−	−	−	−	−	−	−	−	−	−	−	+
Adonitol	+	+	+	+	−	−	−	d	d	+ or (+)	(+)	−	d	+
Inositol	+	+	d	+	−	−	−	d	+ or (+)	d	+	d	(+)	+
Sorbitol	+	+	+ or −	+	−	−	+	+	+	−	+	d	+	+
Arabinose	+	+	+	+	−	−	−	−	+	+	+	+	+	+
Raffinose	+	+	+	+ or −	−	−	−	−	+	+	+	+	d	+
Rhamnose	+	+	d	+	−	−	−	−	d	−	+	−	+	+ or −
Xylose	+	+	+	+	+	−	+	d	+	+	+	+	+	+ or −
Cellobiose	+	+	+	+	+	+	+	−	+	+	+	+	+	(+)
DNase	−	−	−	−	−	−	−	+	+ or −	+	+	+	+	−

*Symbols: As in Table 45–14.

Table 45–17. DIFFERENTIAL CHARACTERISTICS OF *PROTEUS, MORGANELLA, PROVIDENCIA,* AND *YERSINIA**

Test	Proteus				Providencia			Yersinia						
	P. vulgaris	*P. mirabilis*	*P. penneri*†	*Morganella morganii*	*P. rettgeri*	*P. alcalifaciens*	*P. stuartii*	*Y. pestis*	*Y. pseudo-tuberculosis*	*Y. entero-colitica*	*Y. inter-media*	*Y. kristen-seni*	*Y. frederick-seni*	*Y. ruckeri*
Indole	+	–	–	+	+	+	+	–	–	d	+	d	+	–
Methyl red	+	+	+	+	+	+	+	+	+	+ or (+)	+	+	+	+
Voges-Proskauer	–	– or +	–	–	–	–	–	– (28°C.) – (37°C.)	– (25°C.) – (37°C.)	+ (25°C.) – (37°C.)	+ (25°C.) – (37°C.)	– (25°C.) – (37°C.)	+ (25°C.) – (37°C.)	– or +^{w} (25°C.)
Citrate, Simmons'	d	(+)	–	–	+	+	+	–	– (25°C.)	– (25°C.)	d (25°C.)	– (25°C.)	d (25°C.)	(+)
H_2S (TSI)	+	+	–	–	–	–	–	–	–	–	–	–	–	–
Urease	+	+	+	+	+	–	d	–	+	+	+	+	+	–
Phenylalanine deaminase	+	+	+	+	+	+	+	–	–	–	–	–	–	–
Lysine decarboxylase	–	–	–	–	–	–	–	–	–	–	–	–	–	+ or (+)
Arginine dihydrolase	–	–	–	–	–	–	–	–	–	–	–	–	–	–
Ornithine decarboxylase	–	+	–	+	–	–	–	–	–	+‡	+	+	+	+
Motility	+	+	+	+	+	+	+	– (28°C.) – (37°C.)	+ (25°C.) – (37°C.)	+ (25°C.) – (37°C.)	+ (25°C.) – (37°C.)	+ (25°C.) – (37°C.)	+ (25°C.) – (37°C.)	+ or – (25°C.)
Gelatin liquefaction	+	+	(+)	–	–	–	–	–	–	–	–	–	–	+ or (+)
KCN	+	+	+	+	+	+	+	–	–	–	–	–	–	d
Malonate	–	–	–	–	–	–	–	–	–	–	–	–	–	–
Lactose	–	–	–	–	–	–	–	–	–	d	–	d	d	– or (+)
Sucrose	+	d	+	–	d	d	d	–	–	+‡	+	–	+	–
Mannitol	–	–	–	–	d	–	d	+	+	+	+	+	+	–
Adonitol	–	–	–	–	+	+	–	–	+	–	–	–	–	–
Rhamnose	–	–	–	–	d	–	–	–	+	–	+	–	+	–
Maltose	+	–	+	–	–	–	–	+	+	+	+	+	+	+
Xylose	–	+	+	–	d	–	–	+	+	d	+	+	+	–
Trehalose	d	+	(+)	d	–	–	+	+	+	+‡	+	+	+	+
Melibiose	–	–	–	–	–	–	–	–	+	–	+	–	–	–
Sorbitol	–	–	–	–	–	–	–	–	–	+‡	+	+	+	–
Raffinose	–	–	–	–	–	–	–	–	d	–	+	–	–	–
Cellobiose	–	–	–	–	–	–	–	–	–	+	+	+	+	–

*Symbols: As in Table 45–14.
†Formerly *P. vulgaris* biogroup 1 or indole-negative.
‡Most biotype 5 strains are negative.

in a state of some controversy. Classically, each new serotype has been given a new species designation, more recently derived from the town, region, or country of origin, e.g., *Salmonella minnesota.* With over 1500 serotypes already described, this system of nomenclature has been confusing and has been largely supplanted in this country by the recognition of only three species (Ewing, 1972): *S. choleraesuis, S. typhi,* and *S. enteritidis* (Table 45–15). All salmonellae, with the exceptions of those representing the first two species, are thereby considered to be serotypes or bioserotypes of *S. enteritidis* and are given infrasubspecific designations, e.g., *S. enteritidis* ser Typhimurium.

Grouping of the Enterobacteriaceae is based upon the slow and granular agglutinability of the "O" antigens, which are heat-stable, somatic antigens with intergeneric cross-reactivity, antibodies to which are frequently of the IgM class. They are predominantly lipopolysaccharide in content. The "H" antigen is the heat-labile, flagellar, protein antigen, antibodies to which are predominantly IgG and agglutination with which is rapid and fluffy. This antigen provides type-specificity to a strain. The "Vi" antigen is a heat-labile, surface or capsular, principally polysaccharide antigen which is generally associated with virulence and the presence of which is usually determined with isolates suspected of representing *S. typhi.*

Complete characterization of serotypes of salmonellae is impractical except in certain reference laboratories. It is, however, practical for clinical laboratories to test isolates for agglutination in the more commonly encountered group-specific antisera (A through E), as well as in a polyvalent grouping antiserum and Vi antiserum. Strains should then be submitted to a reference laboratory, usually a state health department laboratory, for serotyping for epidemiologic purposes.

Agglutinins (Widal) to *Salmonella* O (somatic) and H (flagellar) antigens may arise in the serum following typhoid immunization and current or past infections due to salmonellae or other Enterobacteriaceae sharing common antigens. Agglutinins, on the other hand, may not arise in patients receiving effective antibiotic therapy early in the course of salmonellosis. The prevalence and diagnostic value of agglutinins, therefore, varies widely in different populations. Hence, the diagnostic value of the Widal test, particularly of a single serum sample, is quite limited, and the test should never be used without concurrent bacteriological studies. Because of its poor sensitivity and specificity, the Widal test has been largely abandoned as a diagnostic tool in clinical laboratories in this country. The concept of a panel of "febrile agglutinin" tests for patients with fever of unknown etiology is both semantically and clinically inappropriate.

Antimicrobial Susceptibility. The susceptibility of the Enterobacteriaceae to various antimicrobial agents is highly variable. As a rule, therefore, clinically significant isolates require susceptibility testing to assist in their proper therapy. The frequency with which chromosome- and plasmid-mediated resistance is encountered, particularly in organisms responsible for hospital-acquired infections, further diminishes the predictability of susceptibility of a given species to a particular antibiotic.

Antibiotic resistance by the Enterobacteriaceae can be related to enzymatic inactivation, to altered permeability of components of the cell wall, to an altered structural target, to an altered metabolic pathway bypassing a reaction inhibited by the drug, or to alteration of an enzyme which remains functional but is less affected by the drug.

Although usually susceptible to a variety of antimicrobial agents, non-typhoidal, uncomplicated enteric infections due to salmonellae are generally not treated with antibiotics, since there are data demonstrating that such therapy may actually prolong the carrier state. Infections due to susceptible strains of *Salmonella typhi* are preferentially treated with chloramphenicol, despite this organism's susceptibility to other agents. Therapy with amoxicillin, ampicillin, or co-trimoxazole should be used in instances of chloramphenicol resistance.

It is desirable to treat patients with shigellosis in order to eliminate shedding of the organism in feces as rapidly as possible; however, the frequency of resistance of shigellae to ampicillin and other antimicrobial agents in several parts of the United States has forced some modifications in this practice. While ampicillin remains the drug of choice for the treatment of susceptible strains, co-trimoxazole appears to be a satisfactory alternative for ampicillin-resistant strains.

Prevention. The prevention of infections due to the Enterobacteriaceae is closely allied with infection control in hospitals, a topic covered in considerable detail in Chapter 54.

OXIDASE-POSITIVE GLUCOSE FERMENTERS OF MEDICAL SIGNIFICANCE

VIBRIO

Definitions and Characteristics. Vibrios are facultatively anaerobic, oxidase-positive, short, curved, or straight gram-negative bacilli which are usually motile by means of polar flagella, ferment carbohydrates, and reduce nitrates to nitrites. Several species are medically important (Table 45–18). Other vibrios (*V. cholerae* non O group 1) are also medically important. Organisms formerly known as *V. fetus* have been reclassified into the genus *Campylobacter.*

Pathogenesis and Virulence Factors. Cholera manifests itself by massive intestinal fluid loss secondary to stimulation of the adenyl cyclase system of cells in the small intestine with production of cyclic AMP. In this respect the enterotoxin acts in a manner similar to that of the heat-labile toxin of *Escherichia coli.* The mechanism of pathogenicity of *V. parahaemolyticus* appears to be related to invasiveness rather than to enterotoxin production. This halophilic organism is widely distributed in marine environments and has been found to contaminate fish and shellfish. Outbreaks of acute diarrheal disease following ingestion of contaminated food have been especially common in Japan but have also occurred in this and other countries. Wound infections and septicemias have been associated with non-cholera halophilic vibrios.

Table 45–18. DIFFERENTIAL CHARACTERISTICS OF *VIBRIO* SPECIES*

Test	Vibrio								
	V. cholerae	*V. mimicus*	*V. damsela*	*V. parahaemolyticus*	*V. alginolyticus*	*V. vulnificus*	*V. fluvialis*	*V. metschnikovii*	*V. hollisae*
Indole	+	+	−	+ or −	d	+	− or +	d	+
Voges-Proskauer	− or +	−	+	−	+	−	−	+	−
Lysine decarboxylase	+	+	+	+	+	+	−	d	−
Ornithine decarboxylase	+	+	−	+ or −	d	d	−	−	−
Arginine dihydrolase	−	−	+	−	−	−	+	d	−
Lactose	(+)	− or (+)	−	−	−	+	−	d	−
Sucrose	+	−	−	−	+	− or +	+	+	−
Mannitol	+	+	−	+	+	d	+	+	−
Maltose	+	+	+	+	+	+	+	+	−
Arabinose	−	−	−	+ or −	−	−	+	−	+
Salicin	−	−	−	−	−	+	−	− or +	−
Cellobiose	−	−	−	−	−	+	d	− or +	−
$NO_3 \rightarrow NO_2$	+	+	+	+	+	+	+	−	+
Oxidase	+	+	+	+	+	+	+	−	+
Growth in nutrient broth plus NaCl (%)									
0	+	+	−	−	−	−	$+^{w}$ or −	−	−
1	+	+	+	+	+	+	+	+	+
6	− or (+)	− or (+)	+	+	+	+	+	+	(+)
8	−	−	−	+	+	−	−	d	−
10	−	−	−	−	+	−	−	d	−
12	−	−	−	−	−	−	−	−	−

*Symbols as in Table 45–14.

Laboratory Diagnosis. Laboratories in the United States are unaccustomed to isolating vibrios from fecal material. Nonetheless, because cholera is pandemic in many other countries, its importation by travelers into western countries does occur. Moreover, the increasing recognition of non-cholera halophilic vibrios means that laboratories should be familiar with the techniques required for the isolation and identification of vibrios. Obviously, the laboratory must be informed that infection due to *V. cholerae* or vibrios is suspected on the basis of travel or dietary history so that the appropriate media can be inoculated. These include a selective agar, such as thiosulfate-citrate bile salts (TCBS). TCBS should not be autoclaved, and its final pH should be 8.4. An enrichment broth, such as alkaline peptone water, should also be inoculated and subcultured in 6 to 12 hours to a second set of TCBS plates. Yellow colonies on TCBS (due to sucrose fermentation) should be selected for further study with biochemical and serologic tests. The vibrios can be differentiated among themselves and from other enteric gram-negative bacilli according to reactions listed in Table 45–18. It may be necessary to carry out biochemical testing of the halophilic vibrios in media supplemented with 1 to 3 per cent NaCl. If triple sugar iron agar (TSIA) and lysine iron agar (LIA) are inoculated for screening purposes, their reactions will be acid slant/acid butt with no gas (A/A-) or H_2S and alkaline slant/alkaline butt (K/K), respectively. Agglutination of a saline suspension of the organism by polyvalent antiserum against *V. cholerae* should occur within a minute if the organism is present.

Antimicrobial Susceptibility. *V. cholerae* and the non-cholera halophilic vibrios are susceptible to a variety of agents, including tetracyclines, chloramphenicol, ampicillin, cephalosporins, and trimethoprim/sulfamethoxazole. *V. parahaemolyticus* is resistant to the penicillins but is otherwise susceptible to the other agents which are active against *V. cholerae.*

Prevention. The primary means of transmission of cholera is contaminated water. Otherwise, the disease itself is not particularly communicable, provided thorough handwashing and careful handling of patients' excreta are properly enforced. Simple enteric precautions in any general hospital should be adequate. Although the risk of contracting the disease is small, travelers to infected areas should be vaccinated, preferably within two months of their travel to such areas. Two vaccinations at one week's to one month's interval are recommended. Booster vaccinations should be given every three to six months if periods of exposure continue.

AEROMONAS

Definitions and Characteristics. Members of this genus are facultatively anaerobic, oxidase- and catalase-positive, rod-shaped gram-negative bacilli that are motile by means of polar flagella and form acids from carbohydrates by respiratory and fermentative metabolism. There are three species: *A. hydrophila, A. punctata,* and *A. salmonicida.* Another species, formerly *A. shigelloides,* is now classified as *Plesiomonas.*

Pathogenesis and Virulence Factors. *Aeromonas* has been isolated from tap water, rivers, soil, marine animals, and various foods. It has been isolated from feces of healthy persons and from patients with diarrheal disease of otherwise unexplained origin. Its role in producing diarrheal disease is possibly related to the production of an enterotoxin by some strains. A hemolysin and a cytopathic factor have also been described.

Aeromonas may cause infection of traumatically acquired wounds which are contaminated with soil or water. It may also cause septicemia in patients with acute leukemia.

Laboratory Diagnosis. The isolation of a fermenting, oxidase-positive, gram-negative bacillus should suggest strongly the possibility of *Aeromonas.* It grows readily on conventional laboratory media and produces colonies that resemble those of *Pseudomonas,* have a greenish ground glass appearance, and give off a fruity odor.

Antimicrobial Susceptibility. *Aeromonas* is susceptible to the aminoglycosides, chloramphenicol, and tetracyclines but produces a β-lactamase mediating resistance to the penicillins and cephalosporins. *Aeromonas* has been found to maintain R plasmids of both the Enterobacteriaceae and *Pseudomonas.*

PASTEURELLA

Definitions and Characteristics. The pasteurellae are facultatively anaerobic, oxidase- and catalase-positive, non-motile gram-negative bacteria that may range morphologically from coccobacilli to long filamentous rods. Four species are recognized: *P. multocida, P. pneumotropica, P. haemolytica,* and *P. ureae.*

Pathogenesis and Virulence Factors. Encapsulated strains are usually pathogenic for mice, and virulence has been found to be enhanced by free iron in various forms. The cell wall contains endotoxin but no exotoxin has been identified.

The pasteurellae are indigenous to many animals and are isolated frequently from wounds resulting from animal bites or scratches. Local infections can become systemic, and there have been a number of reports of septicemia, osteomyelitis, and meningitis. Pasteurellae have been associated with respiratory tract infections, including sinusitis, peritonsillar abscess, mastoiditis, pulmonary abscess, pneumonia, empyema, bronchitis, and bronchiectasis, usually in patients with chronic pulmonary disease.

Laboratory Diagnosis. Pasteurellae grow well on blood agar but are, with the exception of *P. haemolytica,* unable to grow on gram-negative differential agar media, such as eosin methylene blue (EMB) or MacConkey agar. The finding of a gram-negative bacillus that grows on blood agar only and is oxidase- and indole-positive and ONPG negative, strongly constitutes presumptive evidence for the isolation of *P. multocida,* the most frequently encountered species.

Antimicrobial Susceptibility. Characteristic of *P. multocida* is its susceptibility to penicillin G. Other agents with excellent activity *in vitro* against the organism include the cephalosporins and tetracyclines.

Prevention and Control. Primary attention should be devoted to proper wound care with close observation of those secondary to animal bites. The value of penicillin G as prophylaxis is uncertain.

GLUCOSE OXIDIZERS

PSEUDOMONAS

Definitions and Characteristics. Pseudomonads are strictly aerobic, catalase-positive, usually oxidase-positive gram-negative bacilli whose metabolism is respiratory and never fermentative and whose motility is by polar flagella. At least 29 species have been well characterized; however, only those deemed to be medically important will be considered here (Table 45–19). Other species have occasionally been isolated from clinical material and have been reported as causes of opportunistic infection. *P. testosteroni* and *P. acidovorans* have been included by some into the species *Comamonas terrigena,* which resembles *P. diminuta* and *P. alcalifaciens* except that it does not produce deoxyribonuclease and usually has two to four polar flagella.

Because of the fact that the pseudomonads are very adaptable and can use a large number of organic compounds for growth, they are essentially free-living and can be found in a tremendous variety of habitats (Table 45–20). Moreover, they are more resistant to antiseptic agents and disinfectants than most vegetative forms of bacteria.

Pathogenesis and Virulence Factors. The species causing the greatest morbidity and mortality today is *P. aeruginosa.* As has already been stated, it is nearly ubiquitous in the hospital environment, existing almost anywhere there is any moisture. The organism is more resistant than most vegetative bacteria to many disinfectants and antimicrobial agents. Although it produces a variety of enzymes and toxins, in addition to a slime polysaccharide and endotoxin, the mechanisms by which *P. aeruginosa* produces disease remain unclear. Its surface polysaccharide is released from cells multiplying *in vitro,* as are small amounts of endotoxin. It produces proteases that inactivate components of complement, thereby inhibiting to some degree opsonization and the inflammatory response and perhaps contributing to its invasiveness. Exotoxin A promotes cellular damage and tissue invasion and is toxic for macrophages. The organism produces infection in patients with burn, traumatic, and operative wounds; following urinary tract manipulation; in patients with diseases of the hematopoietic, reticuloendothelial, and lymphoid systems; and in those with impaired cellular or humoral defenses. Pulmonary infection occurs commonly in patients with cystic fibrosis. The mortality rate is highest in severely leukopenic (<1000 PMN/cu mm) patients.

P. pseudomallei is endemic in Southeast Asia, where asymptomatic or subclinical infection is frequent. A pulmonary form resembling tuberculosis or a mycotic infection occurs less frequently and has a relatively good prognosis. Its septicemic form is highly lethal.

P. mallei causes glanders, which may present as an acute fulminating and frequently fatal septicemic form, as an acute pneumonia with or without septicemia, as an acute or chronic suppurative infection, as a latent infection with eventual acute manifestations of the disease, or in an occult form with encapsulated nodules in various organs and especially the lungs.

Other species of *Pseudomonas,* although often isolated from clinical specimens, are only occasionally involved in disease (Table 45–20).

Laboratory Diagnosis. The presence of *P. aeruginosa* in cultures can often be suspected because of its musty odor, the rough or ground glass appearance of its colonies, and the presence of pigment or metallic sheen in its colonies. Its identification can be made easily with a positive oxidase reaction, an alkaline slant/neutral butt reaction in triple sugar iron agar (TSIA), and the formation of sheen and/or pigment on the slants of TSIA and Pseudomonas P agar. If all of these reactions do not occur, additional tests should be performed (Table 45–19). Tests of carbohydrate utilization should be carried out in O-F basal medium which contains a minimal quantity of peptone and a relatively large quantity of carbohydrate and which will provide detection of the very small quantities of acid formed by this group of bacteria. Reactions are usually complete within 48 hours but may require as long as seven days in some instances.

There are numerous as yet unnamed groups of organisms resembling *Pseudomonas* that are classified according to a numerical designation (Manual of Clinical Microbiology, 1980). Their clinical significance, as well as their taxonomy and nomenclature, remains obscure.

Antimicrobial Susceptibility. As a general rule, *P. aeruginosa* is susceptible to gentamicin, tobramycin, and amikacin. Most isolates are also susceptible to carboxy- and ureido-penicillins. Hospital epidemics of strains resistant to gentamicin and tobramycin have, however, occurred owing to aminoglycoside acetylating and, less often, adenylylating enzymes. Resistance to anti-pseudomonadal penicillins may also occur, owing to R plasmid mediated β-lactamase.

The susceptibility of other species of *Pseudomonas* varies considerably. Kanamycin, which is essentially inactive against *P. aeruginosa,* inhibits most strains of *P. stutzeri* and the *P. fluorescens* group. *P. cepacia* is usually resistant to aminoglycosides but is often susceptible to chloramphenicol and trimethoprim/sulfamethoxazole. Many isolates of *P. maltophilia* are resistant to aminoglycosides, but they are more frequently inhibited by gentamicin than by amikacin or tobramycin.

P. pseudomallei is usually susceptible to tetracycline, chloramphenicol, sulfonamides, and trimethoprim/sulfamethoxazole but not to penicillins, cephalosporins, polymyxins, or aminoglycosides. Antimicrobial susceptibility data on *P. mallei* are limited owing to the eradication of glanders in many parts of the world; however, sulfonamides have generally been considered to represent the agents of choice in the treatment of the disease.

Prevention and Control. With the exceptions of *P. pseudomallei* and *P. mallei,* prevention of disease due to pseudomonads is highly dependent upon hospital infection control and surveillance programs.

6

ACINETOBACTER

Definitions and Characteristics. Organisms in this genus are rod-shaped, sometimes nearly spherical,

Table 45–19. DIFFERENTIAL CHARACTERISTICS OF PSEUDOMONADS ISOLATED FROM CLINICAL MATERIAL*

Test	*P. aeruginosa*	*P. fluorescens grp.*	*P. maltophilia*	*P. stutzeri*	*P. cepacia*	*P. alcaligenes*	*P. diminuta*	*P. mallei*	*P. pseudomallei*	*P. putrefaciens*
Oxidase	+	+	−	+	+	+	+	+	+	+
Decarboxylase										
Lysine	−	−	+	−	+	−	−	−	−	−
Ornithine	−	−	−	−	− or +	−	−	−	−	+
Arginine dihydrolase	+	+	−	−	−	−	−	+	+	−
Acid (oxidatively) from										
Glucose	+	+	+ or (+)	+	+	−	−	+	+	d
Maltose	−	+ or −	+	+	+	−	−	(+)	+	d
Xylose	+	+	+ or −	+	+	−	−	−	+	−
Denitrification	+	−	−	+	−	−	−	−	+	−
Deoxyribonuclease	− or +	−	+	−	−	−	+	−	−	+
Citrate, Simmons	+	+	− or +	+	+	+ or −	−	−	+	− or +
Fluorescein	+	+	−	−	−	−	−	−	−	−
Pyocyanin	+	−	−	−	−	−	−	−	−	−
Growth at 42°C.	+	−	+	+	+ or −	+ or −	+	−	+	+
Flagella (No.)	1	>1	>1	1	>1	1	1	0	>1	1

*Symbols: See Table 45–14.

Table 45–20. RESERVOIRS AND CLINICAL MANIFESTATIONS OF CERTAIN PSEUDOMONADS

Species	Reservoir	Clinical Manifestations
P. aeruginosa	Soil, floors, sinks, baths, soaps, benzalkonium chloride, humidifiers, respirators, utensils, vases, salads, and other items used or present in hospitals; skin, feces	Wound infection, bacteriuria, pneumonia, bacteremia, and other opportunistic infections; chronic otitis media, ophthalmic infection
P. fluorescens	Soils, floors, baths, sinks, respirators, soaps, contaminated blood or blood products	Rarely, causes opportunistic infection
P. maltophilia } *P. stutzeri*	Ubiquitous (water, sewage, soil, raw milk, lower animals)	Rarely, causes opportunistic infection
P. cepacia	Water, soil, respirators, detergents, lubricants	Wound infection, foot rot, pneumonitis, bacteremia, endocarditis, bacteriuria
P. pseudomallei	Soil and water in endemic areas	Melioidosis
P. mallei	Warm-blooded animals	Glanders

non-motile, oxidase-negative, strictly aerobic, and gram-negative. Their metabolism is oxidative and those which form acid from carbohydrates do so by oxidation of aldehyde groups to produce aldobionic acids. Such organisms lack β-galactosidase and are, therefore, ONPG negative.

The taxonomy and nomenclature of these organisms have been in a state of turmoil for years. Acid-producing strains have been known as *Bacterium anitratum* and *Herellea vaginicola* and non–acid-producing strains as *Mima polymorpha*. The tribe Mimeae has, however, lost its standing in nomenclature, and both acid- and non–acid-producing strains are currently called *Acinetobacter calcoaceticus*. Two biotypes are recognized, *anitratum* and *lwoffi,* the former to include acid-producing and the latter to include non–acid-producing strains.

Pathogenesis and Virulence Factors. *Acinetobacter* is commonly found in soil and water and uncommonly found on the skin and mucous membranes of healthy people. Little is known about virulence factors in this group of organisms, but they do appear to form small amounts of endotoxin. Although usually non-pathogenic, they have been associated with a wide variety of diseases, including septicemia, bacteriuria, pneumonia, and abscesses. They are frequently encountered in mixed cultures of wounds or respiratory tract material without any clear-cut relationship with disease.

Laboratory Diagnosis. *Acinetobacter* can be distinguished readily from the pseudomonads on the basis of its lack of motility, inability to reduce nitrates, and its negative oxidase reaction. The ability by some strains to oxidize various carbohydrates and 10 per cent lactose agar slants provides ready identification of *A. calcoaceticus* var. *anitratus* (Table 45–21); however, non–acid-forming strains var. *lwoffi* require differentiation from the similarly inactive moraxellae (Table 45–21).

Antimicrobial Susceptibility. *Acinetobacter* is usually susceptible to aminoglycosides, including kanamycin, gentamicin, tobramycin, and amikacin. It is moderately susceptible to tetracycline but usually quite susceptible to minocycline. Most strains are inhibited by nalidixic acid. Other antimicrobial agents are usually inactive.

Table 45–21. DIFFERENTIAL CHARACTERISTICS OF *ACINETOBACTER* AND *MORAXELLA**

	A. calcoaceticus		
Test	***anitratrum***	***lwoffi***	**Moraxella**
Oxidase	–	–	+
Nitrate reduction	–	–	d
Carbohydrate metabolism	Oxidative	Inactive	Inactive
Acid from			
Dextrose	+	–	–
Maltose	(+) or –	–	–
Xylose	+	–	–
Acid on 10% lactose slant	+	–	–
Phenylalanine deaminase	–	–	d
Citrate utilization	+	+	d
Urease	(+) or –	(+) or –	d
Penicillin	Resistant	Resistant	Originally susceptible

*Symbols: See Table 45–14.

6

GRAM-NEGATIVE AEROBIC AND FACULTATIVELY ANAEROBIC RODS REQUIRING SPECIAL GROWTH FACTORS OR CONDITIONS (Table 45–13)

CAMPYLOBACTER

Definitions and Characteristics. Campylobacters are small, oxidase-positive, gram-negative, microaerophilic, curved to spiral rods with single, polar flagella. Growth is optimal in an atmosphere containing 5 per cent O_2, 10 per cent CO_2, and 85 per cent N_2.

Some confusion exists over the classification of *Campylobacter* species. Those classified as *Campylobacter fetus* subsp. *intestinalis* or as *C. fetus* subsp. *fetus* have been associated with septicemia, infective endocarditis, meningitis, septic arthritis, and other systemic infections, while those classified as *C. fetus* subsp. *jejuni* or simply as *C. jejuni* or *C. coli* have been associated with diarrhea. Not much is known about virulence factors of *Campylobacter,* although diarrhea due to *C. jejuni* appears to be due to an invasive rather than a toxigenic mechanism.

Laboratory Diagnosis. *C. fetus* subsp. *fetus* can be readily isolated from blood culture media, thioglycollate medium, or any peptone-yeast extract medium. Because it requires a lower concentration of oxygen than is present in air, growth of this organism is unlikely to occur on solid media under conventional incubation conditions.

The isolation of *C. jejuni* from fecal material is strictly dependent upon the use of a selective medium, a microaerophilic atmosphere of incubation, and incubation at 42°C. Selective media containing a variety of antibiotics, usually including vancomycin, polymyxin B, trimethoprim, and a cephalosporin, are commercially available for this purpose. Some workers advocate a brief (≤8 hours) period of incubation of the specimen at 5°C. in thioglycollate medium containing antibiotics before subculture onto a selective agar medium. Inoculation of specimens onto Thayer-Martin medium which is then incubated at 35 to 37°C. in a candle jar is not suitable for isolation of *C. jejuni* from feces.

In some cases, visualization of curved rods with characteristic corkscrew type of motility upon direct dark-field or phase-contrast microscopic examination of the feces offers a rapid means of detecting *C. jejuni.* The isolation of a catalase- and oxidase-positive small, slender, curved, motile gram-negative bacillus from a selective medium incubated at 42°C. constitutes strong presumptive evidence of *C. jejuni.* Confirmation can be made simply by demonstrating that the organism hydrolyzes hippurate and is susceptible to nalidixic acid. Strains of *C. fetus* subsp. *fetus* are resistant to nalidixic acid, fail to hydrolyze hippurate, and do not ordinarily grow at 42°C.

Antimicrobial Susceptibility. Both *C. fetus* subsp. *fetus* and *C. jejuni* are usually susceptible to aminoglycosides, chloramphenicol, clindamycin, and erythromycin. Pencillins are usually poorly active. Approximately 5 to 10 per cent of strains are resistant to tetracyclines. Although often self-limited, diarrhea due to *C. jejuni* may persist or recur; therefore, erythromycin treatment is usually advised in such cases.

BRUCELLA

Definitions and Characteristics. Brucellae are small, gram-negative coccobacilli, non-motile, strictly aerobic, catalase- and usually oxidase-positive rods. Growth is often enhanced by the presence of 5 to 10 per cent CO_2. Although growth may occur on ordinary media, it is usually optimal on a soybean-casein digest agar (trypticase soy, tryptic soy, tryptone soya, etc.) or in its liquid counterpart. Of the recognized species, *B. melitensis, B. abortus, B. suis,* and *B. canis* are those of medical importance in man.

Pathogenesis and Virulence Factors. The preferential hosts for brucellae are sheep and goats for *B. melitensis,* cattle for *B. abortus,* swine for *B. suis,* and dogs for *B. canis;* however, each species may occasionally infect other animals. Infection is acquired by man by direct contact with infected material, including animal carcasses, fetal membranes, vaginal discharges, fetuses, skin or mucous membranes, as well as by ingestion of unpasteurized milk or milk products from infected animals. Local lymphadenopathy often occurs with dissemination and secondary localization in the reticuloendothelial system and formation of granulomas in the spleen, bone, genitourinary tract, lungs, and soft tissues. Organisms may be seen within phagocytes.

Signs and symptoms are often variable and nonspecific with chills, fever, sweats, and anorexia occurring frequently. The fever is characteristically diurnal ("undulant"). Diagnosis of the disease beyond the acute bacteremic phase is difficult to establish.

The most common sources of infection in the United States in recent years are cattle and swine, and the majority of reported cases of brucellosis are in individuals working in packing plants. Infections due to *B. canis* have been acquired predominantly by contact with infected dogs or by accidental exposure to cultures of the organism in laboratories.

Laboratory Diagnosis. Blood cultures in a biphasis bottle (Castaneda technique) containing soybean-casein digest medium have been shown to be highly effective in detecting the presence of bacteremia in the early stages of brucellosis. Other normally sterile body fluids should be concentrated by filtration through a 0.45 μm membrane filter which is then placed onto a soybean-casein digest blood agar plate for culture. Tissue should be minced and then ground with a sterile abrasive in broth to produce a 20 per cent suspension which is then inoculated onto the appropriate medium. Specimens contaminated with other bacteria should be inoculated onto the more selective "W" or Wisconsin medium (Washington, 1981). Guinea pig inoculations subcutaneously or intraperitoneally may also be helpful. Cultures should be incubated in an atmosphere containing 5 to 10 per cent CO_2 and should be retained for three or four weeks before being discarded as negative. Blood cultures in Castaneda bottles should be tipped twice weekly so that the blood-broth mixture flows over the agar surface.

Smears of specimens may be examined by the

fluorescent antibody technique, as may colonies suspected of being *Brucella* which have grown in cultures. Colonies appear slowly and may initially be very small and difficult to see. The advantage of a biphasic medium for blood cultures is that it obviates the need for routine subcultures, a step that is otherwise quite important because of the lack of turbidity usually imparted to broth by *Brucella*.

Urease activity is manifested rapidly by *B. suis* and slowly or not at all by *B. melitensis* and *B. abortus*. *B. canis* shares some characteristics with *B. suis* so that its standing as a separate species is provisional. Dye inhibition tests with basic fuchsin and thionin are usually used in the identification process (Table 45–22). As has already been mentioned, the serologic confirmation at the genus level can be made with fluorescein-conjugated antiserum. Monospecific antisera can be used to distinguish between the *B. abortus*–*B. suis* complex and *B. melitensis;* however, such antisera are not widely available.

The diagnosis of brucellosis is often made serologically. A minimum titer of 1:160 in a standard tube agglutination test should lead one to suspect the diagnosis; however, evidence of recent brucellosis can be accepted only when a four-fold or greater rise in titer occurs during the first month or two of illness. Inhibitory prozones can occur in patients with titers as high as 1:640 so that all sera from patients with suspected disease should be diluted to at least 1:1280. Cross-reactivity with *Francisella tularensis* and with *Vibrio cholerae,* including cholera vaccination, occurs. The tube agglutination test is very sensitive and yields the most standardized results, in contrast to the more rapid slide agglutination tests which may give both falsely positive and falsely negative results.

Antimicrobial Susceptibility. The drugs of choice in the treatment of brucellosis are tetracycline, with or without streptomycin, or trimethoprim/sulfamethoxazole.

Prevention and Control. Since the major reservoirs of brucellae are livestock and milk and meat, eradication programs have been oriented to breaking the chain of infection and have included immunization, testing and disposal of infected animals, and pasteurization of milk and its by-products.

BORDETELLA

Definitions and Characteristics. Bordetellae are strictly aerobic, non-fermentative, minute coccobacilli requiring nicotinic acid, cysteine, and usually methionine but not hemin (X factor) or coenzyme I (V factor) for growth. Excess fatty acids are formed during growth and are inhibitory to further growth so that blood, charcoal, starch, or ion-exchange resins must be added to the medium to act as an adsorbent. Phase variation from smooth virulent strains to rough avirulent strains occurs after cultivation on artificial media.

Pathogenesis and Virulence Factors. The proposed pathogenetic sequence of infection due to *Bordetella pertussis* has been reviewed extensively by Olson (1975). The organism attaches to the ciliated epithelium of the respiratory tract, multiplies, and releases toxins with a variety of proposed effects which result, though not necessarily in sequence, in inflammation and epithelial necrosis, leukocytosis and lymphocytosis, accumulation of secretions, cough, and ultimately bronchopneumonia, hypoxic episodes, and encephalopathy. *B. pertussis* contains a protective antigen which when combined with antibody abolishes its infectivity. It appears, however, that both cellular and humoral immunity are needed to eradicate the organism.

B. parapertussis may infrequently cause a pertussis-like illness. *B. bronchiseptica,* on the other hand, is isolated from humans after contact with guinea pigs, rabbits, dogs, cats, and rodents in which it may represent a component of their indigenous flora or it may actually cause disease. Its role in causing human infection is much less clear cut.

Laboratory Diagnosis. The rate of isolation of *B. pertussis* from patients declines with the duration of illness. Normal healthy individuals are not carriers of the organism so that its isolation always represents disease.

The most commonly recommended specimen is the nasopharyngeal swab; however, nasopharyngeal aspirates with a soft rubber catheter have provided higher rates of isolation in some peoples' hands. In general, swabs or aspirates should be inoculated onto suitable media, e.g., charcoal or Bordet-Gengou agar, as quickly as possible; however, Stuart's transport medium has been found to be satisfactory for storage purposes for up to 24 hours. Other suitable transport media have been described but are less widely available. Swabs or aspirates may be inoculated into semisolid charcoal agar for mailing purposes.

Direct examination of smears stained with fluorescein-conjugated *B. pertussis* antiserum represents a rapid diagnostic test. Cultures are recommended, however, because a low rate of falsely positive and falsely negative smears does occur.

Table 45–22. DIFFERENTIAL CHARACTERISTICS OF SPECIES OF *BRUCELLA**

				Growth on		
				Basic Fuschsin	***Thionin***	
Species	**CO_2 Required**	**H_2S**	**Urease**	***1:50,000***	***1:25,000***	***1,50,000***
B. melitensis	–	–	– or (+)	+	–	+
B. abortus	d	+	(+) or –	+	–	+
B. suis	–	+ or –	+	– or +	+	+
B. canis	–	–	+	–	+	+

*Symbols: See Table 45–14.

6

Specimens should be inoculated onto Bordet-Gengou or charcoal agar with added (20 per cent) rabbit, sheep, or horse blood. One plate with and one without antibiotic should be used. Although penicillin (0.5 U/ml) is most frequently used, overgrowth by indigenous flora is better prevented by cephalexin (40 μg/ml), which has a broader spectrum of activity than penicillin. The cultures should be incubated at 36°C. and examined daily for up to six days.

Colonies suspected of representing *B. pertussis* can be presumptively identified by examining a smear stained with fluorescein-labeled specific antiserum. *B. pertussis* is rather inactive and will not grow on blood-free media, usually requires three to four days to grow on charcoal or Bordet-Gengou agar, and does not reduce nitrates, produce urease, or utilize citrate. *B. parapertussis* will grow on blood-free media, grows rapidly on charcoal or Bordet-Gengou agar, utilizes citrate, produces urease, but does not reduce nitrates. *B. bronchiseptica* is the most active of the three and grows readily on conventional nutrient media, reduces nitrates, utilizes citrate, and rapidly (≤4hours) hydrolyzes urea.

Antimicrobial Susceptibility. Antimicrobial agents probably play no role in the therapy of pertussis but do render negative nasopharyngeal cultures within one or two days which may prevent bacterial complications in patients with the disease and may be effective in preventing spread of the disease to non-immune contacts. Although several groups of agents are active *in vitro* against *B. pertussis,* erythromycin has been the only one consistently shown to be rapidly effective *in vivo.*

Prevention and Control. Vaccination represents the most effective means of control of pertussis in children, and current recommendations are to begin immunization at two months of age and to restrict it to the first six years because of the risks of neurologic complications. Workers in the health care fields probably should, however, also be immunized because of their greater risk of exposure and acquisition of the disease.

HAEMOPHILUS

Definitions and Characteristics. Members of the genus are small gram-negative rods or coccobacilli with a requirement for haemin or other porphyrins (X factor) and/or nicotinamide adenine di- or trinucleotides (V factor). The medically important species, as classified by Kilian (1976), are listed in Table 45–23. *Haemophilus parahaemolyticus* is not listed because it loses its hemolytic property rapidly in subcultures and becomes indistinguishable from *H. parainfluenzae. H. aegyptius* is omitted because of its close similarity to *H. influenzae* and doubts among taxonomists about the justification for differentiating these two species.

Pathogenesis and Virulence Factors. The virulence factors of species of *Haemophilus* are as yet poorly understood. Endotoxin is not produced by *H. influenzae,* and this species is rapidly killed once ingested by macrophages unless antibody, complement, or the phagocytes are deficient. The role of antibodies in immunity is also poorly understood. Antibodies develop with age, presumably following natural infection with *H. influenzae* or with cross-reacting antigenic organisms, so that most persons older than 15 years have antibodies. Which antibody and what level of that antibody are protective remain unknown.

Most *Haemophilus* species are indigenous to the upper respiratory tract and the oral cavity, and the encapsulated strains of *H. influenzae,* particularly those belonging to group B, are most often responsible for diseases due to *Haemophilus,* including meningitis, bacteremia, endocarditis, epiglottitis, otitis, conjunctivitis, and pneumonia. *H. parainfluenzae* has been associated with meningitis, while it, *H. paraphrophi-*

Table 45–23. DIFFERENTIAL CHARACTERISTICS OF MEDICALLY IMPORTANT *HAEMOPHILUS* SPECIES*

Species	Tests					
	δ-ALA† *Utilization*	*V-Factor Requirement*	*Indole*	*Urease*	*Ornithine Decarboxylase*	*CO_2 Enhancement*
H. influenzae						
biotype I	–	+	+	+	+	–
II	–	+	+	+	–	–
III	–	+	–	+	–	–
IV	–	+	–	+	+	–
V	–	+	+	–	+	–
H. haemolyticus	–	+	d	+	–	–
H. ducreyi	–	–	–	–	–	–
H. parainfluenzae		+				–
biotype I	+	+	–	–	+	–
II	+	+	–	+	+	–
III	+	+	–	+	–	d
H. paraphrophilus	+	+	–	–	–	d
H. aphrophilus	+	–	–	–	–	d

*Adapted from Kilian, 1976. Symbols: See Table 45–14.
†δ-Aminolevulinic acid.

lus, and *H. aphrophilus* have been associated with subacute bacterial endocarditis. *H. ducreyi* is responsible for chancroid.

Laboratory Diagnosis. The isolation of *Haemophilus* usually requires the presence of haemin (X factor) and/or nicotinamide adenine nucleotides (V factor) in the culture medium. The former is most frequently supplied by the incorporation of heat-lysed ("chocolatized") blood cells in agar, although it may also be provided by whole human, horse, or rabbit blood cells. The V factor is commonly supplied either by the incorporation of yeast extract or other appropriate supplements in the medium or by a *Staphylococcus* which is streaked across the agar surface and about which satellite colonies of V-dependent strains of *Haemophilus* grow. The differential characteristics of members of this genus are listed in Table 45–23.

The requirements for X and V factors are determined by placing paper disks or strips impregnated with each and with both factors onto a soybean-casein digest agar surface that has been streaked with the test strain. There are a number of difficulties posed by this approach. First of all, carry-over of haemin from the original isolation plate is almost unavoidable so that growth of an X- and V-dependent strain, such as *H. influenzae,* about the V strip or disk may occur, leading to an erroneous identification of *H. parainfluenzae* or *H. paraphrophilus.* One way of minimizing this transfer of haemin is to place a colony of the test strain into 1 to 2 ml of soybean-casein broth, mix the suspension thoroughly, and then use a swab to inoculate the surface of the agar on which the X and V factor requirements are to be tested. Despite this precaution, traces of haemin may still be transferred and lead to an erroneous test result. Therefore, although X factor is commonly listed among tests required to identify haemophili, it is suggested that a different test system be used for separating V-dependent species from the others. One such test which is simple and very reliable was described by Kilian (1974) and determines the ability of V-dependent species to use δ-aminolevulinic acid in the biosynthesis of porphobilinogen and porphyrins. The formation of porphobilinogen can be detected by adding Kovac's reagent to the reaction mixture and observing the development of a red color in the aqueous phase. Alternatively, the formation of porphyrins in the reaction mixture can be demonstrated by red fluorescence under a Wood's lamp. Hemolytic properties of human isolates of haemophili can be determined on rabbit or horse blood agar; however, neither taxonomic nor clinical considerations justify the performance of this test.

H. aphrophilus must often be distinguished from species such as *Actinobacillus actinomycetemcomitans, Cardiobacterium hominis,* and *Eikenella corrodens* (Table 45–24), all of which have been associated with subacute bacterial endocarditis.

The cultivation of *H. ducreyi* from chancroid lesions has been problematical. A Gram's stained smear of material from the lesion may be helpful if gram-negative bacilli in pairs or in rows ("schools of fish") are seen. Material may be inoculated onto GC medium base plus 1 per cent hemoglobin, 5 to 10 per cent fetal calf serum, 1 per cent IsoVitaleX (BBL Microbiology Systems), and 3 μg/ml of vancomycin.

The presence of typable strains of *H. influenzae* in smears can be rapidly confirmed microscopically by fluorescent antibody methods. They can also be detected rapidly in normally sterile body fluids, such as cerebrospinal or synovial fluid, by counterimmunoelectrophoresis (CIE). While fluorescent microscopy is usually reserved for situations in which organisms are seen in Gram's stained smears and rapid confirmation of their identity is sought, CIE is useful for screening the fluid directly for bacterial antigen in the absence of visible organisms in the smear. Another rapid detection method is to test the agglutinability of

Table 45–24. DIFFERENTIAL CHARACTERISTICS OF *HAEMOPHILUS APHROPHILUS, ACTINOBACILLUS ACTINOMYCETEMCOMITANS, CARDIOBACTERIUM HOMINIS,* AND *EIKENELLA CORRODENS**

Test	*H. aphrophilus*	*A. actinomycetemcomitans*	*C. hominis*	*E. corrodens*
Oxidase	−	−	+	+
Catalase	−	+	−	−
δ-ALA utilization†	+	+	+	+
V-requirement	−	−	−	−
Indole	−	−	+	−
Urease	−	−	−	−
Lysine decarboxylase	−	−	−	+
Ornithine decarboxylase	−	−	−	+
Acid from				
Glucose	+	+	+	−
Sucrose	+	−	+	−
Lactose	+	−	−	−
Mannitol	−	+	d	−
Xylose	−	d	−	−

*Symbols: See Table 45–14.
†δ-Aminolevulinic acid.

6

protein A–rich staphylococci coated with *H. influenzae* antiserum in the presence of soluble bacterial antigen in body fluids.

Antimicrobial Susceptibility. Since approximately 15 to 20 per cent of clinical isolates of *H. influenzae* are resistant to ampicillin because of β-lactamase production, it is necessary for the susceptibility of isolates from normally sterile body fluids or spaces to be tested. A variety of rapid acidimetric and iodometric tests for determining the elaboration of β-lactamase by bacteria have been described (see Chap. 52) and usually suffice for clinical purposes. Although a few cases of infections due to chloramphenicol-resistant *H. influenzae* have been reported, chloramphenicol, either alone or in combination with ampicillin, is recommended for the initial therapy of patients with diseases suspected to be due to haemophili. With β-lactamase-negative strains ampicillin remains the drug of choice.

GARDNERELLA

Definitions and Characteristics. Formerly classified as *Haemophilus vaginalis* or *Corynebacterium vaginale, Gardnerella vaginalis* is a pleomorphic gram-negative to gram-variable bacillus which is usually isolated from the human genital/urinary tract. The organism requires neither X nor V factors for growth.

Pathogenesis and Virulence Factors. Although originally considered a cause of non-specific vaginitis, *G. vaginalis* is found in the vaginas of 25 to 35 per cent of asymptomatic women. On the other hand, non-specific vaginitis is usually not present in the absence of the organism in vaginal cultures. Hence, the etiological role of *G. vaginalis* in non-specific vaginitis remains uncertain. Cases of puerperal fever associated with *Gardnerella* bacteremia have been reported, as have cases of bacteriuria.

Laboratory Diagnosis. *G. vaginalis* may sometimes be detected microscopically in either wet mounts or stained smears of vaginal secretions in "clue cells," which are finely granulated epithelial cells surrounded by masses of small, pleomorphic bacilli. Media containing proteose peptone no. 3 (e.g., Casman agar and proteose peptone-starch-dextrose [PSD] agar) have most often been used for isolation of *G. vaginalis.* Columbia colistin–nalidixic acid (CNA) agar has been found to be a useful selective medium. Since *G. vaginalis* produces β-hemolysis of human (but not sheep) blood, detection of the organism is enhanced by incorporating human (instead of sheep) blood into Columbia CNA agar. *G. vaginalis* is catalase- and oxidase-negative; it produces acid from glucose, maltose, and starch; and it neither reduces nitrates nor produces urease.

Antibiotic Susceptibility. Although *G. vaginalis* is susceptible to ampicillin, metronidazole has been found to be more effective in eradicating the organism from the vagina.

EIKENELLA

Definitions and Characteristics. Formerly classified as *Bacteroides corrodens,* the "corroding bacilli" that are facultatively anaerobic have been assigned to the species *Eikenella corrodens.* Strictly anaerobic corroding bacilli, which differ in several important respects from the facultatively anaerobic bacilli, remain classified as *Bacteroides corrodens.* Strains of *E. corrodens* are the same as King's subgroup Hb-1. They are oxidase-positive, catalase-negative, non-fermentative gram-negative bacilli, colonies of which may corrode or pit agar. Growth is enhanced by 5 to 10 per cent CO_2 and usually requires the presence of haemin (X factor) in the medium.

Pathogenesis and Virulence Factors. Little is known about factors contributing to the organism's virulence, and it has a low level of pathogenicity for animals. *Eikenella* resides predominantly in the nasopharynx and is isolated frequently from the upper respiratory tract. It has been recovered from abscesses and other types of infections in almost any site, may invade the bloodstream, and may cause endocarditis. Infections are usually mixed.

Laboratory Diagnosis. The most striking feature of *Eikenella* in cultures is its ability to pit the agar; however, pitting does not occur with all strains. The colonies appear slowly and are generally small (0.5 to 1.0 mm in diameter). It must usually be distinguished from other fastidious, slowly growing gram-negative bacilli (Table 45–24).

Antimicrobial Susceptibility. *Eikenella* is susceptible to the penicillins and chloramphenicol. Its susceptibility to aminoglycosides is variable, but it is resistant to clindamycin.

ACTINOBACILLUS ACTINOMYCETEMCOMITANS

Definitions and Characteristics. Other than the sesquipedalian character of its name, this organism currently occupies an uncertain taxonomic position. It is small, coccoid to bacillary in shape microscopically, grows aerobically and somewhat better in CO_2, and anaerobically, and may grow in broth in the form of small granules adhering to the walls of the tube. Colonies on blood agar appear slowly and are small.

Pathogenesis and Virulence Factors. *Actinobacillus actinomycetemcomitans* has a low level of pathogenicity. It derives its name from its frequent association with actinomycotic lesions. In recent years, however, it has most frequently been reported as a cause of subacute bacterial endocarditis.

Laboratory Diagnosis. The most frequently reported source of the organism in recent years is in blood cultures from patients with endocarditis. It appears to grow slowly in most currently used blood culture media. It must be differentiated from other slowly growing, somewhat fastidious gram-negative bacilli (Table 45–24).

Antimicrobial Susceptibility. Although not consistently susceptible to the penicillins, ampicillin alone has been successfully employed in the treatment of a number of reported cases. Ampicillin and streptomycin have been found to be bactericidal but not synergistic against the organism and have also been used in the therapy of endocarditis associated with it. Other active antimicrobial agents include the tetracyclines and chloramphenicol.

CALYMMATOBACTERIUM GRANULOMATIS

Description and Characteristics. Previously known as *Donovania granulomatis, Calymmatobacterium* is a gram-negative, non-motile, encapsulated, pleomorphic rod that may be cultured in yolk sacs or on fresh egg yolk medium. The organism possesses antigenic determinants similar to those of *Klebsiella,* leading some authors to classify it among the Enterobacteriaceae.

Pathogenesis and Virulence Factors. The organism does not produce disease in animals. In humans it causes granuloma inguinale characterized by ulcerogranulomatous lesions of the skin and mucosa of the genital and inguinal areas.

Laboratory Diagnosis. A fragment of tissue removed from the margin of an ulcer is pressed and rubbed against a glass slide and stained with Wright's or Giemsa's stain. The finding of small, straight or curved, pleomorphic rods with rounded ends and characteristic polar granules giving a safety pin appearance within mononuclear cells is the most effective way of establishing the diagnosis.

Antimicrobial Susceptibility. The tetracyclines, erythromycin, ampicillin, and chloramphenicol are active against *Calymmatobacterium.* Resistance may develop to streptomycin.

STREPTOBACILLUS MONILIFORMIS

Description and Characteristics. *Streptobacillus* is a facultatively anaerobic, fermentative, non-encapsulated, and non-motile gram-negative rod, frequently in chains and filaments, and often with a series of oval to elongated bulbous swellings giving a string-of-beads appearance. Blood, serum, or ascitic fluid is needed for growth in agar or broth. The microscopic morphology varies with time, being more homogeneously filamentous in young cultures and becoming fragmented into irregular coccobacilli with age. L-phase colonies may occur spontaneously on agar, have a "fried egg" appearance, become stabilized if penicillin is incorporated in the medium, and are indistinguishable from L-phase colonies of other bacteria and from mycoplasmas.

Pathogenesis and Virulence Factors. *Streptobacillus* occurs as indigenous flora in the upper respiratory tract of wild and laboratory rodents. Infection (Haverhill disease) in humans follows rodent bites, ingestion of contaminated food, or traumatic injury. Local lymphangitis and lymphadenitis may develop up to three weeks later, followed by the onset of fever, chills, malaise, and later by a general morbilliform maculopapular or petechial rash. Some patients develop a migratory polyarthritis. Endocarditis has been reported.

The histopathology is non-specific and demonstrates a chronic inflammatory reaction.

Laboratory Diagnosis. Sedimented red blood cells can be used to prepare pour plates by adding them to molten heart infusion (HI) agar supplemented with yeast extract. Red cells and sterile body fluids can also be plated on HI agar supplemented with yeast extract and with heat-inactivated sterile horse serum. Normally sterile body fluids should be examined microscopically after staining with Gram's and Giemsa's stains. Material should also be inoculated into HI broth containing the supplements described above.

The identification of *Streptobacillus* is rather complex. Colonies in broth form as fluff balls, while those on agar are small and slightly translucent to opaque with a slightly irregular edge. L-phase variants may form on agar. Subcultures are made from broth with pipets or by agar block transfers. Biochemical tests must be performed in HI agar or broth supplemented with yeast extract and horse serum.

Antimicrobial Susceptibility. Penicillin alone and in combination with streptomycin is active against *Streptobacillus.*

Prevention and Control. Since 10 to 65 per cent of rats are infected with the organism, their control and precautions against bites represent the only effective methods of control of the disease.

FRANCISELLA

Definitions and Characteristics. Formerly classified as *Pasteurella tularensis, Francisella tularensis* is a very small, strictly aerobic, coccoid to pleomorphic rod-shaped, gram-negative bacillus which requires cystine or cysteine for its growth. Faint bipolar staining occurs with aniline dyes.

Pathogenesis and Virulence Factors. Virulence appears to be related to a smooth colonial morphology. Repeated subcultures result in an alteration from smooth to rough colonies with a concomitant loss of virulence. Highly virulent strains for humans have citrulline ureidase activity and ferment glycerol and are most often associated with tickborne disease in rabbits. Toxins have not been recognized.

Tularemia may manifest itself after an incubation period of one to 10 days in various forms. Headache, fever, chills, vomiting, and myalgias characteristically occur at the onset. In the ulceroglandular type of disease, lymphadenitis and lymphadenopathy occur in the region draining the primary lesion. The lesion is initially papular and later ulcerative. A variation of this form of disease, the oculoglandular type, is characterized by inflammation of the conjunctiva and usually a papule of the lower lid with lymphadenitis of the preauricular, parotid, submaxillary, and anterior cervical nodes. An ingestion form of tularemia is characterized by ulcerative lesions of the mouth, throat, and upper gastrointestinal tract. Pneumonia may result from inhalation or secondary to bacteremia from another focus of infection.

Tularemia should be suspected in anyone who has been in an endemic area, has had contact with wild animals or livestock, has been engaged in farming operations, has drunk impure water, or has been exposed to cultures or infected animals in the laboratory. Trappers, hunters, fur and meat industry workers, agricultural workers, and laboratory personnel are at greatest risk. Because of its protean manifestations, tularemia is readily confused with many other diseases, such as brucellosis, anthrax, sporotrichosis, typhoid fever, tuberculosis, histoplasmosis, and syphilis.

Laboratory Diagnosis. Material suitable for examination includes fluid or curettings from the primary lesion, aspirates of enlarged regional nodes, sputum, pharyngeal washes, and gastric aspirates. Microscopic examination of clinical material or of colonies stained with specific fluorescein-labeled conjugate constitutes the most rapid and reliable means of identifying *Francisella*. Cultures may be made on glucose-cysteine agar supplemented with 5 per cent defibrinated rabbit blood. If the clinical material is contaminated with other bacteria, 1 ml each of penicillin, 100,000 U/ml; polymyxin B, 100,000 U/ml; and cycloheximide, 0.1 mg/ml, should be included in each liter of medium. Special care must be exercised in handling infected material to prevent aerosolization or direct contact with the skin. Cultures are incubated at 35°C. in an environment with or without added CO_2. Colonies usually appear within 24 hours and their identification or immunofluorescence with specific antiserum.

The diagnosis can also be established serologically. Agglutination titers as low as 1:40 in the absence of previous disease are diagnostic and may rise within the first three weeks to levels of 1:640 or greater. Brucella agglutinins may also rise non-specifically but usually to a significantly lower level.

Antimicrobial Susceptibility. Streptomycin is bactericidal while the tetracyclines and chloramphenicol are bacteriostatic to *Francisella*. Since relapses are not infrequent after treatment with these bacteriostatic agents, streptomycin is the agent of choice.

Prevention and Control. The most common methods of acquiring tularemia are insect bites by blood-sucking arthropods and contact with or ingestion and inhalation of infected material. A variety of vertebrates and invertebrates have been reported to be infected with *Francisella*, the most frequent mammalian species of which are rabbits, beavers, muskrats, voles, and sheep. Vectors include ticks, deerflies, and mosquitoes. Preventive measures, therefore, have been directed toward increasing public awareness, developing protective measures for persons at risk, decreasing the vector population, and controlling vertebrate sources.

LEGIONELLA

Definitions and Characteristics. *Legionella* organisms are fastidious, non–spore-forming, pleomorphic gram-negative bacilli. Seven species have been established (Table 45–25). The majority of clinical cases have been due to *L. pneumophila*, serogroup1.

Pathogenesis and Virulence Factors. A variety of extracellular enzymes, including protease, phosphatase, lipase, deoxyribonuclease, a cytotoxin, and endotoxin-like activity have been identified in *L. pneumophila*. Infection is usually manifested as an acute fibrinopurulent pneumonia, which is usually lobular in distribution. Histologically, there is an alveolar infiltrate of neutrophils and macrophages, accompanied by fibrin and red blood cell extravasation. *Legionella* organisms may be found in large numbers within alveolar macrophages. *L. pneumophila* has been isolated from blood, which presumably accounts for the disease's protean manifestations.

Laboratory Diagnosis. The diagnosis of legionellosis may be made by isolating the organism in

Table 45–25. CLASSIFICATION OF THE GENUS *LEGIONELLA**

Species	Original Designations (Year of Isolation)	Human Isolations	Environmental Isolations
Legionella pneumophila	OLDA (1948); Legionnaires' disease bacillus (1977)	Lung tissue, respiratory secretions, pleural fluid, hemodialysis shunt, pericardial fluid	Cooling towers, riparian soil, plumbing fixtures, tap water
L. micdadei	TATLOCK (1944); HEBA (1959); Pittsburgh pneumonia agent (1979); *L. pittsburgensis, Tatlockia micdadei*	Lung tissue, respiratory secretions, pleural fluid	Cooling tower, shower head, tap water
L. bozemanii	WIGA (1959); Mi-15 (1979); Legionella-like organism, LLO 1 and 2; *Fluoribacter bozemanae*	Lung tissue	None
L. dumoffii	NY-23 (1978); Tex-KL (1979), LLO 4	Lung tissue	Cooling tower
L. gormanii	LS-13 (1979)	None†	Riparian soil
L. longbeachae	LB-4 (1981)	Lung tissue, respiratory secretions	None
L. jordanis	BL-540 (1978)	None†	Riparian soil, treated sewage
L. oakridgensis	OR-10	None	Cooling towers

*Courtesy of A. William Pasculle, Ph.D.

†While no isolations of these organisms have been reported from humans, organisms staining with direct fluorescent antibody reagents prepared against these organisms have been detected in human lung tissue. In addition, antibody to these organisms has been detected in human serum specimens.

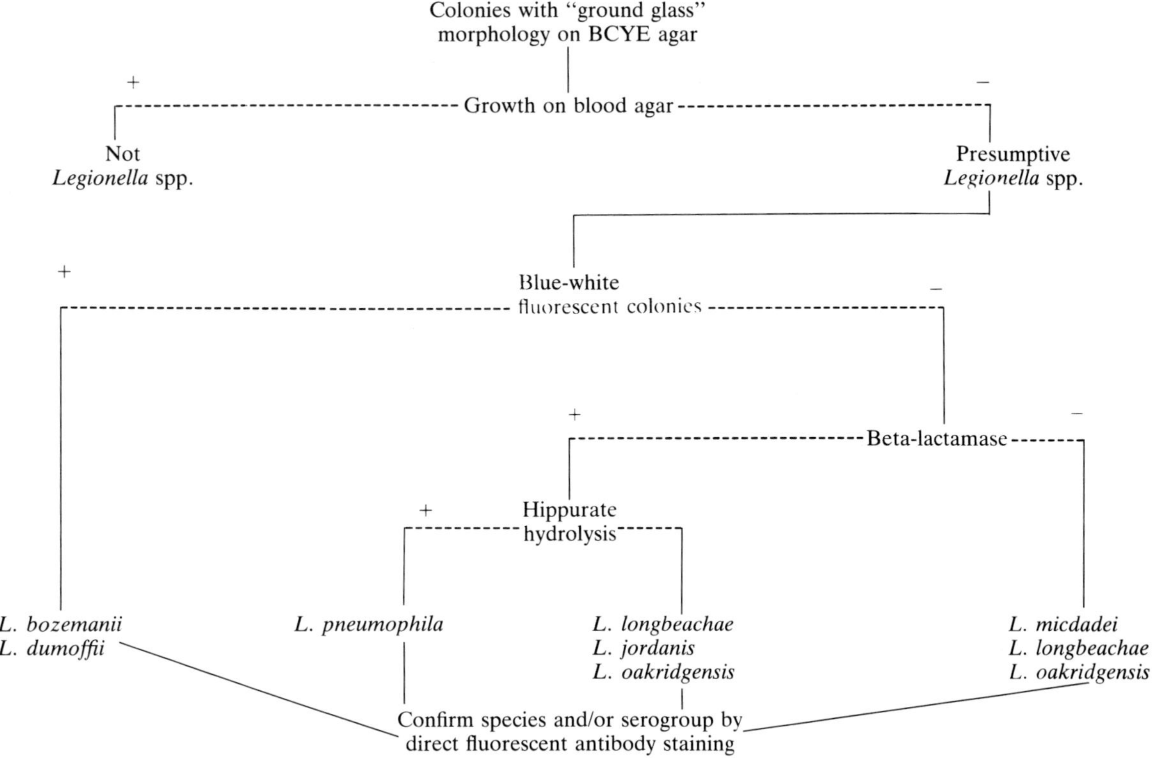

Figure 45–7. Identification of *Legionella* species. (Courtesy of A. William Pasculle, Ph.D.)

culture, detecting the organism in specimens by immunofluorescence, and demonstrating rising species or type-specific antibody titers.

Legionella may be isolated on a buffered charcoal yeast extract (BCYE) agar which contains essential growth factors, including L-cysteine and a ferric salt, and which must be incubated at 35°C. in an atmosphere containing 2 to 3 per cent CO_2. A flow chart for initial evaluation of isolates is shown in Figure 45–7. Confirmation and speciation is made according to phenotypic characteristics and by staining with fluorescein-labeled species- or type-specific conjugate (Table 45–26).

Legionella may be detected or identified by direct fluorescent-antibody (DFA) staining of specimens or colonies in cultures. The sensitivity of the DFA examination of respiratory specimens is approximately 45 per cent but is considerably higher in open lung biopsies. Although cross-reactions have been reported between *L. pneumophila* and other *Legionella* species, as well as with some strains of *Pseudomonas fluorescens* and *Bacteroides fragilis,* the DFA examination appears to be reasonably specific and certainly expedites diagnosis of the disease when positive.

The diagnosis of legionellosis can also be established serologically by a four-fold or greater rise in antibody titer to at least 1:128. A single antibody titer of 1:256 is presumptive evidence of past infection.

The sensitivity and specificity of culture, DFA examination, and serological diagnosis of legionellosis have been extensively reviewed by Winn and Pasculle (1982).

Antibiotic Susceptibility. Despite their susceptibility in vitro to a wide variety of antimicrobial agents, clinical response of infections due to the *Legionella* species is largely limited to erythromycin and rifampin.

ANAEROBIC BACTERIA

It is important to re-emphasize that anaerobes represent a major component of the indigenous flora of the skin and mucous membranes (Table 45–1) and, therefore, that their isolation and identification should be contingent upon the proper selection and collection of specimens, as well as upon their proper transport to the laboratory. Anaerobic infections are frequently mixed, consisting either of several species of anaerobes or of anaerobes with facultatively anaerobic bacteria. Mixed cultures commonly consist of an average of two facultatively anaerobic and three anaerobic species. The first task, therefore, in examining an anaerobic culture is to separate facultatively anaerobic from anaerobic bacteria. With experience, the more commonly isolated anaerobes can often be recognized on the basis of their colonial and microscopic morphologies and presumptively identified on the basis of a few additional tests, including their inhibition by certain antibiotics. Definitive identification is based

Table 45–26. PHENOTYPIC PROPERTIES OF *LEGIONELLA* SPECIES*

Characteristic	*L. pneumophila*	*L. longbeachae*	*L. micdadei*	*L. jordanis*	*L. oakridgensis*	*L. bozemanii*	*L. dumoffii*	*L. gormanii*
Require iron and cysteine for *primary* isolation (CYE,BCYE agar)	+	+	+	+	+†	+	+	+
Brown pigment from tyrosine	+	+	+	+	+	+	+	NG‡
Fluorescence (Woods' lamp)	Dull yellow	Dull yellow	Dull yellow	Dull yellow	Dull yellow	Blue-white	Blue-white	Blue-white
Catalase§	+	+	+	+	+	+	+	+
Oxidase	+	+	+	+	–	–	–	–
Gelatinase (Kohn method)¶	+	+	+	+	+	+	+	+
Hippurate hydrolysis	+	–	–	–	–	–	–	–
β-Lactamase (nitrocefin)	+	V**	–	+	V	V	V	+
Number of serogroups	8	2	1	1	1	1	1	1

*Courtesy of A. William Pasculle, Ph.D.
†*L. oakridgensis* may rapidly lose its requirements for cysteine.
‡*L. gormanii* does not grow on this medium.
§These reactions may be weak and difficult to demonstrate.
¶As employed in the API 20E test strip.
**Reactions of some strains may be either weak or variable.

Table 45–27. MEDICALLY IMPORTANT ANAEROBIC BACTERIA*

Description	Genus	Species
Gram-positive bacilli, spore-forming	*Clostridium*	*C. perfringens*
		C. ramosum
		C. septicum
		C. novyi
		C. histolyticum
		C. sporogenes
		C. sordellii
Gram-positive bacilli, non-spore-forming	*Actinomyces*	*A. israelii*
	Arachnia	*A. propionica*
	Eubacterium	*E. lentum*
		E. limosum
		E. alactolyticum
	Bifidobacterium	*B. eriksonii*
	Propionibacterium	*P. acnes*
	Lactobacillus	*L. catenaforme*
Gram-positive cocci	*Peptococcus*	*P. magnus*
		P. asaccharolyticus
		P. prevotii
	Peptostreptococcus	*P. anaerobius*
		P. intermedius
		P. micros
Gram-negative cocci	*Veillonella*	*V. parvula*
Gram-negative bacilli	*Bacteroides*	*B. fragilis group*
		B. melaninogenicus asaccharolyticus group
	Fusobacterium	*F. nucleatum*
		F. necrophorum
		F. varium
		F. mortiferum

*Adapted from Finegold, 1977.

upon biochemical reactions, physiologic and genetic characteristics, and pathogenicity and toxin neutralization tests.

The extent to which anaerobes are identified varies according to the facilities and expertise available, the interest of the laboratory personnel and clinical staff, and the clinical utility of the information available from the laboratory. In a small hospital laboratory, preliminary information based on colonial and microscopic morphology and aerotolerance studies is probably adequate. Presumptive identification based on morphology, antibiotic inhibition patterns, and a few other tests should be adequate for most clinical purposes. Definitive identification of isolates on a routine basis is probably unnecessary except in large reference laboratories or for investigational purposes.

Definitions and Characteristics. The term *anaerobe* can be defined as a bacterium that requires an atmosphere with reduced oxygen tension for its growth and that fails to grow on the surface of solid media in an atmosphere of room air with 10 per cent CO_2. A facultatively anaerobic bacterium will grow in either the presence or absence of room air. The term *microaerophile* has not been strictly defined and is commonly applied to bacteria, usually campylobacters and streptococci, that grow only or preferentially in an atmosphere with reduced oxygen and with increased carbon dioxide. Whether or not the so-called microaerophilic or air-tolerant streptococci should be classified as anaerobes or as viridans streptococci remains unsettled (Facklam, 1977).

The major groups of anaerobic bacteria which are encountered in clinical infections are listed in Table 45–27. Many additional species representing indigenous flora in humans and occasionally associated with disease are known.

Pathogenesis and Virulence Factors. Little is known about the factors responsible for the pathogenic and virulence properties of most anaerobes other than the histotoxic clostridia. Endotoxic, proteolytic, and heparinase activity have been identified among the Bacteroidaceae. The polysaccharide capsule of *Bacteroides fragilis* promotes abscess formation. The clostridia, on the other hand, elaborate potent exotoxins, including lethal and necrotizing toxins, hemolysins, lecithinases, gelatinases, hyaluronidases, and so on.

While clostridial infection may be either exogenous or endogenous in origin, disease due to the other anaerobes usually originates endogenously from the normal indigenous anaerobic flora of a contiguous mucous membrane, the integrity of which has been disrupted by surgery, instrumentation, trauma, or malignancy. Essential to the establishment of anaerobes in the infectious process is a decrease in the oxidation-reduction potential (E_h) of the area, which may result from a failure of its blood supply or from the presence or multiplication of other bacteria at the site.

Much of the older literature on anaerobic infections dealt almost exclusively with the histotoxic clostridial infections and with the clostridial intoxications, tetanus and botulism. Although these infections and intoxications are unquestionably of major medical importance, the role of other anaerobes in causing cellulitis and myonecrosis has been recognized only relatively recently.

Most isolates of *Clostridium perfringens* in hospital-practice today are the result of simple contamination of a wound. In such instances, the clostridia may multiply in cellular debris, a hematoma, or necrotic tissue without observable clinical symptomatology. Anaerobic cellulitis is a necrotizing process of the soft tissues. Its onset is gradual, but it can progress rapidly and extensively. Gas is produced; however, the process typically does not involve muscle. In addition to or instead of clostridia, the bacteriology of anaerobic cellulitis may involve anaerobic cocci and anaerobic gram-negative bacilli.

In contrast to anaerobic cellulitis, gas gangrene or clostridial myonecrosis is an acute and rapidly progressive invasive process producing marked changes in muscles. Distinguishing between anaerobic cellulitis and gas gangrene is critical in order to avoid performing unnecessarily aggressive and mutilating surgery in the former condition.

The histotoxic clostridia associated with gas gangrene include *C. perfringens, C. novyi, C. septicum, C. histolyticum, C. sporogenes,* and *C. bifermentans.* While *C. perfringens* has been the species most frequently involved in most reports of gas gangrene, the prevalence of the other species in this process has varied widely.

Tetanus and botulism are described as intoxications rather than infections because their manifestations are related to the elaboration of potent neurotoxins. Botulism is most frequently related to the ingestion of home-processed foods which have been improperly preserved or canned; however, sporadic outbreaks of the disease have been related to commercially processed food and to wounds infected with the organism. The incubation period for botulism is short, and signs and symptoms usually occur between 18 and 36 hours following ingestion of contaminated food. Of the seven antigenic types of botulinus toxin known, type A is the most common, followed by types B, E, and F in cases of food poisoning in North America. The toxin is absorbed from the intestinal tract and, rarely, from an infected wound and attaches ultimately to motor nerve terminals, thereby preventing acetylcholine release at the nerve endings.

Tetanus typically occurs in non-immunized persons within the first two weeks following a traumatically acquired puncture, laceration, or abrasion. Cases have been reported to occur postoperatively; following dental work, childbirth, and abortion; or in association with stasis and decubitus ulcers. The toxin, tetanospasmin, is transported to gangliosides in the central nervous system via the lymphatics and blood stream and by migration through the perineural spaces of peripheral nerves.

As has already been mentioned, other anaerobic bacteria, particularly the anaerobic cocci and gram-negative bacilli, have been associated with anaerobic cellulitis in addition to or instead of the histotoxic clostridial species. These organisms are part of the indigenous flora of the mucous membranes of the oral cavity and of the gastrointestinal and genitourinary tracts. As such, they are encountered in aspiration pneumonias, lung abscesses, empyemas, intra-abdominal infections and abscesses, pelvic abscesses, brain abscesses, and bacteremias. Anaerobic intra-abdominal infections commonly follow abdominal and especially colon surgery and are most frequently associated with the *Bacteroides fragilis* group. Clinically significant anaerobic bacteremias are also most frequently due to this species.

Laboratory Diagnosis. Although the extent of identification of anaerobes may vary considerably, certain basic and simple grouping procedures can be performed with a pure culture or subculture of an anaerobic organism: Gram's stained smear, motility, and antibiotic disk identification (Tables 45–28 and 45–29). It should be pointed out that the antibiotic content in each of the disks differs from that of disks used in the standard antimicrobial susceptibility test.

Propionibacterium acnes is catalase-positive and indole-positive and is the only non-spore-forming gram-positive bacillus that can be reliably identified without further tests. *Clostridium perfringens* usually produces a characteristic double zone of hemolysis and produces lecithinase on egg yolk agar.

Much can, therefore, be done to group the anaerobic bacteria with a few simple tests. Definitive identification requires the performance of many additional tests, including gas-liquid chromatography for end-product analysis. Approaches to the identification of anaerobic bacteria in clinical specimens have been published by Rosenblatt (1981), Sutter (1980), and Holdeman (1977).

Because of their rapid progression and considerable morbidity and mortality, the initial diagnosis and management of disease due to the clostridia must be based upon their clinical presentation and manifestations. In some patients with tetanus, no primary wound is evident. When a wound is present, organisms typical of *Clostridium tetani* are seldom seen in stained smears even though they may be recovered from cultures. Moreover, because of this organism's widespread distribution in nature, its isolation from a wound is not necessarily indicative of the diagnosis of tetanus. Laboratory confirmation of botulism requires detection of the toxin in serum, wounds, gastric contents, feces, or the food suspected of causing the disease. Procedures for extracting the toxin and for performing mouse neutralization tests are complex; therefore, it is suggested that the appropriate materials be referred to the Centers for Disease Control, Atlanta, Ga., for examination. Telephone consultation should be made in such instances to ensure that the requisite specimens are properly collected and transported to the Centers and that the appropriate authorities are alerted about the situation.

In cases with suspected anaerobic cellulitis or gas gangrene, the laboratory can be helpful by examining

Table 45–28. GROUP IDENTIFICATION OF GRAM-NEGATIVE ANAEROBES*

Organism	Cellular Morphology	Kanamycin† Disk (1000 μg)	Vancomycin† Disk (5 μg)	Colistin Disk (10 μg)	Pigment	Fluorescence	Pitting	Lipase	Lecithinase	Indole	Catalase	Nitrate Reduction	20% Bile (Growth)	Esculin Hydrolysis	Gelatin Liquefaction	Motility	Formate-Fumarate Stimulation
B. fragilis group	B	R	R	R	–	–	–	–	–	V	$+^{-}$	–	+	+	+	–	
Other saccharolytic *Bacteroides*	B CB	R	R^{S}	V	–	$-^{+}$	–	–	–	–	–	$-^{+}$	–	$+^{-}$	V	–	
B. melaninogenicus–B. asaccharolyticus group	B CB	R	R^{S}	S^{R}	+	+	–	V‡	–	V	–	–	–	$+^{-}$	+	–	
B. ureolyticus	B	S	R	S	–	–	$+^{-}$	–	–	–	$-^{+}$	$+^{-}$	–	–	–	–	+
F. nucleatum	B	S	R	S	–	$+^{-}$	–	–	–	+	–	–	–	–	–	–	
F. necrophorum	B	S	R	S	–	$+^{-}$	–	$+^{-}$	–	+	–	–	–	–	–	–	
F. mortiferum	B	S	R	S	–	–	–	–	–	–	–	–	+	+	–	–	
F. varium	B	S	R	S	–	–	–	–	–	$+^{-}$	–	–	+	–	–	–	
Other *Fusobacterium* sp.	B	S	R	S	–	$-^{+}$	–	–	–	$-^{+}$	–	–	V	V	–	–	
Veillonella	C	S	R	S	–	$-^{+}$	–	–	–	–	V	+	–	–	–	–	
Other gram-negative cocci	C	S	R	S	–	–	–	–	–	–	–	–	$-^{+}$	–	–	–	

*From Sutter, V. L., Citron, D. M., and Finegold, S. M.: Wadsworth Anaerobic Bacteriology Manual. 3rd ed. St. Louis, C. V. Mosby Co., 1980.

†Available from Baltimore Biological Laboratories.

‡+ Lipase indicates *B. melaninogenicus* ss. *intermedius*.

Table 45–29. GROUP IDENTIFICATION OF GRAM-POSITIVE ANAEROBES*

Organism	Cellular Morphology	Spores	Vancomycin Disk† (5 μg)	Colistin Disk (10 μg)	Kanamycin Disk† (1000 μg)	SPS	Pigment	Fluorescence	Lipase	Lecithinase	Nagler	Indole	Catalase	Nitrate Reduction	Gelatin Liquefaction	Motility
Peptococcus sp.	C		S	R	V	R	$-^{+}$	–	–	–		$-^{+}$	$-^{+}$	$-^{+}$	$-^{+}$	–
P. asaccharolyticus	C		S	R	V	R	–	–	–	–		+	$-^{+}$	–	–	–
Peptostreptococcus sp.	C		S	R	V	R	–	–	–	–		–	–	$-^{+}$	–	–
P. anaerobius	C CB		S	R	V	S	–	–	–	–		–	–	$-^{+}$	–	–
Propionibacterium sp.	B	–	S	R	S		$-^{+}$	–	$-^{+}$	–		V	V	V	V	–
P. acnes	B	–	S	R	S		$-^{+}$	–	–	–		$+^{-}$	$+^{-}$	$+^{-}$	+	–
Eubacterium sp.	B CB	–	S	R	V		–	–	$-^{+}$	$-^{+}$		$-^{+}$	$-^{+}$	$-^{+}$	$-^{+}$	$-^{+}$
Actinomyces sp.	B	–	S	R	S		$-^{+}$	–	$-^{+}$	–		–	$-^{+}$	$+^{-}$	$-^{+}$	–
Lactobacillus sp.	B	–	S^{R}	R	S^{R}		–	–	–	–		–	–	$-^{+}$	$-^{+}$	–
Bifidobacterium sp.	B	–	S	R	S^{R}		–	–	–	–		–	–	–	–	–
C. perfringens	B	–	S	R	S		–	–	–	+	+	–	–	$-^{+}$	+	–
Other Nagler-positive *Clostridum* sp.	B	+	S	R	V		–	–	–	+	+	+	–	$-^{+}$	$+^{-}$	V
Nagler-negative *Clostridum* sp.	B	+	S^{R}	R	V		–	V	V	V	–	V	–	V	V	V

*From Sutter, V. L., Citron, D. M., and Finegold, S. M.: Wadsworth Anaerobic Bacteriology Manual. 3rd ed. St. Louis, C. V. Mosby Co., 1980.

†Available from Baltimore Biological Laboratories.

6

exudate or tissue microscopically. The finding of numerous, large, "boxcar"-shaped, gram-positive bacilli provides presumptive confirmation of the diagnosis. Stained smears may also be diagnostic of anaerobic streptococcal myositis. Cultures of exudate, tissue, and blood should also be performed. Once again, the level or extent of identification varies considerably among laboratories; however, *Clostridium perfringens* may be easily identified by its Gram's stained morphology, the production of double zones of hemolysis on blood agar, and a positive Nagler reaction on egg yolk agar.

Antimicrobial Susceptibility. With the notable exception of the *Bacteroides fragilis* group, the anaerobic bacteria are usually susceptible to the penicillins and cephalosporins. The *B. fragilis* group is inhibited *in vitro* by high concentrations of the penicillins and cephalosporins. Nearly all anaerobes are susceptible to clindamycin, chloramphenicol, and metronidazole. For the past several years most anaerobes have been resistant to tetracycline. Although its analogs, minocycline and doxycycline, are more active, significant numbers of anaerobes remain resistant to them. Resistance to clindamycin by rare strains of *B. fragilis* and species of clostridia other than *C. perfringens* has been reported.

By and large, the lack of standardized disk diffusion susceptibility testing method for anaerobes and the largely predictable nature of their susceptibility to various agents obviate the necessity for performing susceptibility tests on a routine basis. Testing should be reserved, therefore, for problem cases. Larger laboratories should regularly monitor the susceptibility of clinically significant anaerobes in order to determine whether or not any significant alterations are occurring.

Prevention and Control. The prevention and control of anaerobic infections remains most effectively directed against the histotoxic clostridial infections and the clostridial intoxications in which debridement, wound care, immunization, and care in food handling play important roles.

Immunization with tetanus toxoid remains the most effective means of prevention of tetanus itself. The prevention of botulism hinges on the use of proper canning techniques, both commercially and in the home. In suspected cases consultation and laboratory assistance are available on a 24-hour basis at the Centers for Disease Control, Atlanta, Ga. A trivalent ABE antitoxin (Connaught) is also available through the Center.

The prevention of gas gangrene hinges on prompt surgical wound care, including thorough debridement. Antibiotics appear to play an important ancillary role to surgery in the management of traumatically acquired wounds. The therapy of gas gangrene is also largely surgical. As in prevention, antimicrobial therapy is also important. Of less certain value in the treatment of gas gangrene are antitoxin and hyperbaric oxygen.

Since other anaerobic infections are largely of endogenous origin, prevention is more difficult to accomplish. Perioperative antibiotic therapy in preparation for colon surgery and for pelvic surgery has been shown in controlled trials to reduce the incidence of postoperative infections which are due for the most part to anaerobes.

General References

Buchanan, R. E., and Gibbons, N. E. (eds.): Bergey's Manual of Determinative Bacteriology, 8th ed. Baltimore, Williams and Wilkins Co., 1974.

Finegold, S. M.: Anaerobic Bacteria in Human Disease. New York, Academic Press, 1977.

Hubbert, W. T., McCulloch, W. F., and Schnurrenberger, P. R. (ed.): Diseases Transmitted from Animals to Man. 6th ed. Springfield, Ill., Charles C Thomas, 1975.

Lennette, E. H., Balows, A., Hausler, W. J., Jr., and Truant, J. P. (eds.): Manual of Clinical Microbiology. 3rd ed. Washington, D.C., American Society for Microbiology, 1980.

Mandell, G. L., Douglas, R. G., and Bennett, J. E.: Principles and Practice of Infectious Diseases. New York, John Wiley and Sons, 1979.

Rose, N. R., and Friedman, H. (eds.): Manual of Clinical Immunology. 2nd ed. Washington, D.C., American Society for Microbiology, 1980.

Washington, J. A., II (ed.): Laboratory Procedures in Clinical Microbiology. New York, Springer-Verlag, 1981.

Specific References

Anhalt, J. P., and Yu, P. K. W.: Counterimmunoelectrophoresis of pneumococcal antigens: Improved sensitivity for the detection of types VII and XIV. J. Clin. Microbiol., *2*:510, 1975.

Brewer, N. S., and Weed, L. A.: Diagnostic tissue microbiology methods. Hum. Path., 7:141, 1976.

Christensen, P., Kahlmeter, G., Jonsson, S., and Kronvall, G.: New method for the serological grouping of streptococci with specific antibodies adsorbed to protein A-containing staphylococci. Infect. Immun., 7:881, 1973.

Darling, C. L.: Standardization and evaluation of the CAMP reaction for the prompt, presumptive identification of *Streptococcus agalactiae* (Lancefield group B) in clinical material. J. Clin. Microbiol., *1*:171, 1975.

Edwards, E. A., and Larson, G. L.: New method of grouping beta-hemolytic streptococci directly on sheep blood agar plates by coagglutination of specifically sensitized protein A-containing staphylococci. Appl. Microbiol., *28*:972, 1974.

Elin, R. J., and Wolff, S. M.: Biology of endotoxin. Ann. Rev. Med., *27*:127, 1976.

Facklam, R. R.: Physiological differentiation of viridans streptococci. J. Clin. Microbiol., *5*:184, 1977.

Hammond, G. W., Lian, C. J., Wilt, J. C., and Ronald, A. R.: Comparison of specimen collection and laboratory techniques for isolation of *Haemophilus ducreyi*. J. Clin. Microbiol. 7:39, 1978.

Harris, J. C., DuPont, H. L., and Hornick, R. B.: Fecal leukocytes in diarrheal illness. Ann. Intern. Med., 76:697, 1972.

Hill, H. R., Riter, M. E., Menge, S. K., Johnson, D. R., and Matsen, J. M.: Rapid identification of group B streptococci by counterimmunoelectrophoresis. J. Clin. Microbiol., *1*:188, 1975.

Holdeman, L. V., Cato, E. P., and Moore, W. E. C.: Anaerobe Laboratory Manual. 4th ed. Blacksburg, Va., Virginia Polytechnic Institute and State University, 1977.

Jones, D. B., Liesegang, T. J., and Robinson, N. M.: Laboratory diagnosis of ocular infections. *In* Washington, J. A., II (coordinating ed.): Cumitech 13. Washington, American Society for Microbiology, 1981, pp. 1–27.

Kaplan, E. L.: The group A streptococcal upper respiratory tract carrier state: An enigma. J. Pediatr., 97:337, 1980.

Kaplan, E. L., and Huew, B. B.: The sensitivity and specificity of an agglutination test for antibiodies to streptococcal extracellular antigens: A quantitative analysis and comparison of the Streptozyme test with the anti-streptolysin O and anti-deoxyribonuclease B tests. J. Pediatr., *96*:367, 1980.

Kaplan, S. L., and Feigin, R. D.: Rapid identification of the invading microorganism. Pediatr. Clin. N. Am., *27*:783, 1980.

Kilian, M.: A rapid method for the differentiation of *Haemophilus* strains. Acta Path. Microbiol. Scand., *82*(B):835, 1974.

Kilian, M.: A taxonomic study of the genus *Haemophilus,* with the proposal of a new species. J. Gen. Microbiol., *93*:9, 1976.

Kunin, C. M.: Detection, Prevention and Management of Urinary Tract Infections. 3rd ed. Philadelphia, Lea and Febiger, 1979.

Nachum, R., Lipsey, A., and Siegel, S. E.: Rapid detection of gram-negative bacterial meningitis by the limulus lysate test. N. Engl. J. Med., *289*:931, 1973.

Olson, L. C.: Pertussis. Medicine, *54*:427, 1975.

Reller, L. B., Murray, P. R., and MacLowry, J. D.: Blood Cultures II. *In* Washington, J. A. II (ed.): Cumitech 1A. Washington, D.C., American Society for Microbiology, 1982, pp. 1–11.

Rosebury, T.: Microorganisms Indigenous to Man. New York, McGraw-Hill Book Co., 1962.

Rosenblatt, J. E.: Anaerobic bacteria. *In* Washington, J. A., II (ed.): Laboratory Procedures in Clinical Microbiology. New York, Springer-Verlag, 1981, pp. 309–364.

Schleifer, K. H., and Kloos, W. E.: A simple test system for the separation of staphylococci from micrococci. J. Clin. Microbiol., *1*:337, 1975.

Schmidt, R. M., and Rosenkranz, H. S.: Antimicrobial activity of local anesthetics: Lidocaine and procaine. J. Infect. Dis., *121*:597, 1970.

Shulman, J. A., and Nahmias, A. J.: Staphylococcal infections: Clinical aspects. *In* Cohen, J. O. (ed.): The Staphylococci. New York, John Wiley and Sons, 1972, pp. 457–481.

Sutter, V. L., Citron, D. M., and Finegold, S. M.: Wadsworth Anaerobic Bacteriology Manual. 3rd ed. St. Louis, C. V. Mosby Co., 1980.

Wannamaker, L. W.: Perplexity and precision in the diagnosis of streptococcal pharyngitis. Am. J. Dis. Child., *124*:352, 1972.

Washington, J. A., II (ed.): Laboratory Procedures in Clinical Microbiology. New York, Springer-Verlag, 1981.

Wilson, W. R., Dolan, C. T., Washington, J. A., II, Brown, A. L., Jr., and Ritts, R. E., Jr.: Clinical significance of postmortem cultures. Arch. Pathol., *94*:244, 1972.

Wimberley, N. W., Bass, J. B., Boyd, B. W., Kirkpatrick, M. B., Serio, R. A., and Pollock, H. M.: Use of a bronchoscopic protected catheter brush for the diagnosis of pulmonary infections. Chest, *81*:556, 1982.

Winn, W. C., Jr., and Pasculle, A. W.: Laboratory diagnosis of infections caused by *Legionella* species. *In* Winn, W. C., Jr. (ed.): Symposium on Respiratory Infections. Clinics in Laboratory Medicine. Philadelphia, W. B. Saunders Co., 1982, pp. 343–369.

6

46

MYCOBACTERIAL DISEASES

HERBERT M. SOMMERS, M.D.

Before the introduction of streptomycin, the diagnosis of tuberculosis was often made on the basis of clinical symptoms, including cough, weight loss, and night sweats, an abnormal chest x-ray, and the finding of acid-fast bacilli in the sputum. Cultures were not always obtained, as there was little to be gained by recovering the organism. Therapy for all forms of mycobacterial disease was essentially the same and was based on putting the patient and the diseased organ at rest.

With introduction of streptomycin, it soon became apparent that resistance could develop rapidly, but to be able to detect resistance it was necessary to recover the organism. As more and more cultures were taken, improvements were made in both digestion and concentration procedures and culture media. Many of the cultures yielded "atypical" strains in that they were acid-fast but had colonial and/or other characteristics that differentiated them from *Mycobacterium tuberculosis.* As more and more of these atypical strains were isolated, many were found to have similar characteristics and have subsequently been classified in well-defined species. Not surprisingly, the control of tuberculosis has resulted in a relative increase in patients with disease from mycobacterial species other than *M. tuberculosis.*

SPECIMEN COLLECTION AND PREPARATION

Specimens from patients with tuberculosis usually contain mixed bacterial flora. The successful recovery of mycobacteria depends on properly collected specimens and on suppression of contaminating bacteria that might otherwise overgrow the mycobacteria. Therefore, methods for the collection of specimens should be directed toward minimizing the number of contaminating bacteria.

Sputum specimens containing *Mycobacterium tuberculosis* show faster growth with fewer contaminants when collected early in the morning with an ultrasonic or similar nebulizing device. Although it has been reported that pooled 24-hour sputum collections will yield more positive cultures than early morning specimens (Krasnow, 1969), growth is usually slower and the contamination rate is significantly higher in sputum pools (Kestle, 1967). Depending on whether there is minimal or advanced disease, there will be intermittent or continual shedding of tubercle bacilli. A minimum of three and not more than five early morning specimens will usually be sufficient to identify the patient with active disease (Krasnow, 1969).

Single clean-voided specimens collected early in the morning are preferred for the diagnosis of urinary tract tuberculosis. Three to five specimens are usually sufficient. Although 24-hour urine collections can be obtained, some laboratory workers believe tubercle bacilli can suffer irreversible injury with prolonged exposure to urine.

Cerebrospinal fluid should be inoculated to Middlebrook 7H9 broth or other types of non-inhibitory culture media after centrifugation.

If a pellicle is present in the cerebrospinal fluid, divide it into pieces for inoculation to several different types of culture media, saving a small fragment for an acid-fast stain. Portions of tissue from surgical biopsies or autopsies should be cut into small fragments and then either ground in a mortar and pestle with sterile sand or alundum powder or homogenized with a ground glass or Teflon homogenizer. The homogenized tissue should be inoculated to both selective and non-inhibitory culture media to provide optimal growth and control of contaminating bacteria.

Recovery of mycobacteria from a suspected tuberculous draining sinus is best from exudate or biopsies. Swabs taken from sinuses should be placed directly on culture media or in broth. Growth of mycobacteria from swab specimens is often inhibited by the hydrophobic nature of the lipid-containing mycobacterial cell wall, the mycobacteria preferring the interstices of the swab to the water-containing culture medium. Under these conditions growth of contaminating bacteria often masks the presence of mycobacteria.

Gastric washings are obtained at considerable discomfort to the patient and are frequently contaminated with commensal mycobacteria. Therefore, this method of specimen collection should be reserved for clinical situations in which more suitable specimens cannot be obtained. The frequent occurrence of commensal mycobacteria renders direct staining procedures of questionable value and necessitates complete identification of mycobacteria isolated. When required, specimens should be collected after an overnight fast and promptly neutralized with sodium carbonate before transport to the laboratory (Runyon, 1980).

DIGESTION AND CONCENTRATION

The isolation of mycobacteria from sputum and other clinical specimens poses a problem for the laboratory. The doubling time for *Mycobacterium tuberculosis* is approximately 20 to 22 hours, while other types of bacteria that can be present in the specimen may have doubling times of only 40 to 60 minutes. This disproportionate rate of growth between the two types of microorganisms can result in the accumulation of metabolic waste products from the rapidly growing bacteria and thereby make the culture medium unsatisfactory for the growth of mycobacteria. Therefore, the successful isolation of mycobacteria is dependent upon selective suppression of non-mycobacterial contaminating bacteria.

The high lipid content of mycobacterial cell walls makes them more resistant than contaminating bacteria to killing by strong acid and alkaline solutions. Specimens submitted for culture of mycobacteria which originate from sites normally colonized with other organisms are first treated with a chemical decontaminating agent to reduce bacterial overgrowth and liquefy mucus in order to facilitate concentration by centrifugation. After a carefully timed exposure during mechanical shaking, the acid or alkaline solution is neutralized and then centrifuged at 3000 to 4000 relative centrifugal force (RCF) for 30 minutes to concentrate the mycobacteria. The RCF should be as high as possible, as the lipid content of the mycobacterial cell wall provides a buoyant effect to tubercle bacilli, making their specific gravity close to unity. This makes selective sedimentation of mycobacteria in a thick, viscous sputum specimen difficult.

In the past, decontaminating solutions were often so strong that if exposure times were not carefully controlled, large numbers of mycobacteria were either killed or so seriously injured that they did not grow or grew only very slowly. Decreasing the strength of decontamination solutions has resulted in the improved survival and recovery of mycobacteria but frequently at the price of a higher incidence of culture contamination. Exposure of specimens to strong decontaminating agents, such as 4 per cent NaOH, 5 per cent oxalic acid, and 3 per cent NaOH, must be carefully timed (no more than 15 minutes) to prevent excessive chemical injury. Neutralization of a strong decontaminating solution requires an equally strong acid or alkaline solution, but often titration to a neutral endpoint is incomplete, with the specimen concentrate remaining either strongly alkaline or acid. Although the culture medium can act as a buffer for a moderate pH shift, an inadequately neutralized specimen can destroy the culture medium and prevent growth of any mycobacteria present. The use of decontaminating agents milder than 4 per cent NaOH or 5 per cent oxalic acid, such as trisodium phosphate (TSP) or TSP with benzalkonium chloride (Zephiran), has become an alternative in some laboratories. Specimens containing large numbers of *M. tuberculosis* can withstand the action of these agents for periods of time as long as 16 to 24 hours and still grow out as positive cultures. All specimens treated with TSP–benzalkonium chloride should be inoculated to egg-base culture media to neutralize the growth inhibition characteristics of benzalkonium chloride. The concentrate can also be neutralized by adding lecithin if it is to be inoculated to agar-base media (Runyon, 1980).

In response to the increased need to recover mycobacteria for susceptibility testing, Kubica (1963) developed a concentrating solution containing 2 per cent NaOH and N-acetyl-L-cysteine (NALC). NALC is a mucolytic agent that can liquefy mucus by splitting disulfide bonds. It does not have any antibacterial activity. Mild decontamination is effected by 2 per cent NaOH, and with the mucus liquefied, the mycobacteria are sedimented by centrifugation. Occasionally the concentration of NaOH has to be increased to 3 per cent during periods of warm weather or for specimens from patients with large pulmonary cavities associated with persistent non-mycobacterial contamination. One advantage of the NALC decontamination procedure is neutralization of the specimen by the addition of a large volume of a slightly acid, pH 6.8 phosphate buffer. The use of the buffer makes strong pH shifts less likely and, in addition, acts as a "wash" during centrifugation, diluting any toxic substances as well as decreasing the specific gravity of the specimen to make sedimentation of mycobacteria more effective. Following centrifugation, the sediment is resuspended in 0.2 per cent bovine albumin, which has a buffering and detoxifying effect on the sedimented concentrate. A second mucolytic agent, also very useful for concentrating mycobacteria, is dithiothreitol. Dithiothreitol (Sputolysin) is similar in action to NALC, splitting disulfide bonds to liquefy mucin (Shah, 1966). Cetyl-pyridium chloride with NaCl has recently been shown to be an effective decontaminating agent for specimens transported through the mail. Mycobacteria have withstood transit

Table 46–1. AGENTS FOR DIGESTION AND CONCENTRATION OF SPECIMENS CONTAINING MYCOBACTERIA

	Comments
N-acetyl-L-cysteine (NALC) + 2% NaOH	Mild decontamination solution with mucolytic agent—NALC—to free mycobacteria entrapped in mucus. NaOH may have to be increased to 3% to control contamination on occasion. NALC should be discarded after 24 to 48 hours. Do not expose specimen to NaOH for more than 15 minutes.
Dithiothreitol (Sputolysin, Calbiochem, La Jolla, Cal.) + 2% NaOH*	Very effective mucolytic agent used with 2% NaOH. Reagent more expensive than NALC, but has the same advantages as NALC.
13% Trisodium phosphate + benzalkonium chloride (Zephiran)	Preferred by laboratories that cannot always control time of exposure to decontamination solution. Benzalkonium chloride should be neutralized with lecithin if not inoculated to egg base culture medium.
1% Cetyl-pyridium chloride + 2% NaCL†	Effective as a decontamination solution for sputum specimens mailed from outpatient clinics. *M. tuberculosis* has survived 8-day transit without significant loss of viability.
4% NaOH	Traditional decontamination and concentration solution. Time of exposure must be carefully controlled. 4% NaOH will effect mucolytic action to promote concentration by centrifugation. Do not expose specimen to NaOH for more than 15 minutes.
4% Sulfuric acid	The use of 4% sulfuric acid when decontaminating urine specimens has improved recovery for many laboratories.
6% Oxalic acid	Most useful in the processing of specimens that contain *Pseudomonas aeruginosa* as a contaminant.

*See Shah, 1966.
†See Smithwick, 1975b.

times of eight days without significant loss of viability using this agent (Smithwick, 1975b).

Table 46–1 lists decontamination and concentration agents. The selection of one or more agents by a laboratory will depend on the number and types of specimens it receives and the time and technical staff available to process the specimens. The decontaminating procedures useful in laboratories receiving specimens from hospitalized patients may differ from those serving outpatient clinics. The specimens from some patients may require the use of different types of decontaminating agents if persistent contamination occurs; e.g., specimens containing *Pseudomonas aeruginosa* may survive 2 per cent NaOH-NALC and require concentration with 5 per cent oxalic acid.

CULTURE MEDIA

Culture media for mycobacteria can be classified as those solidified from coagulated eggs—"egg-base media"; those solidified with agar—"agar-base media"; liquid media; and media containing antimicrobial agents—"selective media."

Early attempts to recover mycobacteria by culture were only partially successful until a medium solidified with coagulated eggs was used. A large number of "egg-base" media have been developed, each differing slightly from the others. Most egg-base media are composed of varying combinations of whole eggs, potato flour, salts, and glycerol. Egg-base media are solidified by heating to 85 to 90°C. for 30 to 45 minutes (inspissation). Contaminating bacteria, particularly gram-positive bacteria, are controlled in part by the addition to the medium of aniline dyes such as crystal violet and malachite green. The concentration of aniline dye in a medium is important, as slight increases over the specified amount can result in significant inhibition of mycobacterial growth.

EGG-BASE CULTURE MEDIA

Numerous types of egg-base culture media have been described and are currently in use. The most commonly used egg-base medium for primary isolation of mycobacteria is Lowenstein-Jensen (see Table 46–2). Petragnani medium is more inhibitory and should be reserved for specimens known to contain large numbers of contaminants. A less inhibitory egg-base medium is the American Thoracic Society (ATS) medium. ATS is particularly helpful in the primary isolation of mycobacteria from specimens not likely to be contaminated, e.g., cerebrospinal fluid, pleural fluid, tissue biopsies, etc.

AGAR-BASE CULTURE MEDIA

During the 1950's Cohen and Middlebrook developed a series of mycobacterial culture media. These media were synthesized from salts, a series of organic compounds, glycerol, and albumin. Agar containing Middlebrook media is transparent and when scanned with a dissecting microscope can yield growth of *M. tuberculosis* after 12 to 14 instead of 18 to 24 days of

Table 46–2. NON-SELECTIVE MYCOBACTERIAL ISOLATION MEDIA

Medium	Components	Inhibitory Agent
Lowenstein-Jensen	Coagulated whole eggs, defined salts, glycerol, potato flour	0.025 g/100 ml malachite green
Petragnani	Coagulated whole eggs, egg yolks, whole milk, potato, potato flour, glycerol	0.052 g/100 ml malachite green
American Thoracic Society Medium	Coagulated fresh egg yolks, potato flour, glycerol	0.02 g/100 ml malachite green
Middlebrook 7H10	Defined salts, vitamins, co-factors oleic acid, albumin, catalase, glycerol, dextrose	0.0025 g/100 ml malachite green
Middlebrook 7H11	Defined salts, vitamins, co-factors oleic acid, albumin, catalase, glycerol, 0.1% casein hydrolysate	0.0025 g/100 ml malachite green

incubation. Middlebrook 7H9 broth is a popular liquid culture medium, and both 7H10 and 7H11 agar are widely used for primary isolation and susceptibility testing. The 7H11 medium differs from 7H10 only by the addition of 0. 1 per cent casein hydrolysate, which was found to improve the rate and amount of growth of mycobacteria resistant to isoniazid (Cohn, 1968). Both 7H10 and 7H11 contain malachite green but in much smaller quantities than in egg-base media. Although most culture media will yield more and larger colonies of mycobacteria when incubated in 5 to 10 per cent CO_2, the Middlebrook media must be incubated in CO_2 for recovery of equivalent numbers and size of colonies.

Agar media may be used in slanted culture tubes or poured in whole or divided Petri plates. The use of Petri plates permits the use of microscopy for early detection of growth and observation of colonial morphology, facilitates the isolation of individual colonies, and is helpful in detecting mixed cultures. Some commercially available 7H11 medium has been modified to increase the amount of malachite green. Laboratory workers should be careful to determine this, for while the increased content of aniline dye retards growth of contaminating bacteria, it can also inhibit the growth of mycobacteria.

Exposure of 7H10 to strong light or storage of the media at 4°C. for more than four weeks can be associated with deterioration and release of formaldehyde. The presence of formaldehyde results in a very inhibitory medium with little or no growth of mycobacteria (Miliner, 1969).

Both Middlebrook 7H10 and 7H11 can be used for mycobacterial drug susceptibility testing, although 7H11 is preferred. Incorporation of antimycobacterial agents into the medium after sterilization and just before it solidifies reduces the loss of drug activity that can occur with some agents during the long heating period used in preparing inspissated egg-based media. The components of non-selective culture media are listed in Table 46–2.

SELECTIVE CULTURE MEDIA

Mycobacterial culture media containing antimicrobial agents to suppress bacterial and fungal contamination have been used for many years. Although certain antimicrobial agents will reduce bacterial contamination, they can also exert a significant growth inhibition on mycobacteria. Despite the inhibition of growth of some mycobacterial species, the use of selective culture media can result in greatly improved recovery of mycobacteria. The names and components of several selective culture media are listed in Table 46–3.

One of the more commonly used selective culture media was developed by Gruft, who added penicillin,

Table 46–3. SELECTIVE MYCOBACTERIAL ISOLATION MEDIA

Medium	Components	Inhibitory Agents		
Gruft modification of Lowenstein-Jensen	Coagulated whole eggs, defined salts, glycerol, potato flour, RNA—17mg/100 ml	0.025	g/100 ml	malachite green
		50	units/ml	penicillin
		35	μg/ml	naldixic acid
Mycobactosel Lowenstein-Jensen	Coagulated whole eggs, defined salts, glycerol, potato flour	0.0025	g/100 ml	malachite green
		400	μg/ml	cycloheximide
		2	μg/ml	lincomycin
		35	μg/ml	nalidixic acid
Middlebrook 7H10	Defined salts, vitamins, co-factors, oleic acid, albumin, catalase, glycerol, and dextrose	0.0025	g/100 ml	malachite green
		360	μg/ml	cycloheximide
		2	μg/ml	lincomycin
		20	μg/ml	nalidixic acid
Selective 7H11 (Mitchison's medium)	Defined salts, vitamins, co-factors, oleic acid, albumin, catalase, glycerol, dextrose, and casein hydrolysate	0.0025	g/100 ml	malachite green
		50	μg/ml	carbenicillin
		10	μg/ml	amphotericin B
		200	units/ml	polymyxin B
		20	μg/ml	trimethoprim lactate

6

nalidixic acid, and RNA to Lowenstein-Jensen medium (Gruft, 1971). Subsequently, it was found that a medium containing cycloheximide, lincomycin, and nalidixic acid was also effective in the control of fungal and bacterial contaminants (Petran, 1971). By varying the amount of each of these three agents, the medium could be prepared in either a Lowenstein-Jensen or 7H10 base (Table 46–3).

The culture medium Selective 7H11 is a modification of an oleic acid agar medium first described by Mitchison. It contains four antimicrobial agents and was originally developed to be used for sputum specimens without exposure to a decontaminating agent. McClatchey (1976) suggested that the carbenicillin be reduced from 100 to 50 μg/ml and that 7H11 medium be used instead of oleic acid agar, calling this modification Selective 7H11. Several reports comparing Selective 7H11 medium with Lowenstein-Jensen and 7H11 have shown a distinct increase in recovery of mycobacteria when used with the NALC-2 per cent NaOH decontamination and concentration procedure. A recent report indicates Selective 7H10 medium can be used quite successfully on concentrated but non-decontaminated sputum specimens (Rothlauf, 1981).

STAINING FOR ACID-FAST BACILLI

The lipid-containing cell walls of mycobacteria have a unique characteristic in binding carbolfuchsin stain so tightly that it resists destaining with strong decolorizing agents such as alcohols and strong acids. This "acid-fast" staining reaction of mycobacteria, along with their unique beaded and slightly curved shape, is a valuable aid in the early detection of infection and monitoring of therapy. The finding of acid-fast bacilli in the sputum, combined with a history of cough, weight loss, and a chest x-ray showing a pulmonary infiltrate, is considered presumptive evidence of active tuberculosis and is sufficient to initiate therapy.

It has been estimated that there must be 10,000 acid-fast bacilli per milliliter of sputum to be detected by microscopy. Patients with extensive disease will shed large numbers of mycobacteria and show a good correlation between a positive smear and a positive culture. In patients with minimal or less advanced disease, the correlation of positive smears to positive cultures may range from 30 to 80 per cent (Rickman, 1980).

Acid-fast stains performed on a weekly basis are also useful in following the response of patients to drug therapy. After drugs are started, cultures will become negative before smears, indicating that the bacilli are injured sufficiently to prevent replication but not to the point of preventing binding of the stain. With continued drug treatment, more organisms are killed and fewer shed, so that following the number of stainable organisms in the sputum during treatment can provide an early objective measure of response. *It should be noted that in patients receiving antimycobacterial therapy not all stainable organisms are viable.* Should the number of organisms fail to decrease after therapy is started, the possibility of drug resistance must be considered. Additional cultures should be taken and drug susceptibility studies obtained.

Two types of acid-fast stains are frequently used:

1. The carbolfuchsin stains, so called because of the reagent formed by mixing the stain fuchsin with the disinfectant phenol (carbolic acid). Two procedures using carbolfuchsin stains are in common use: (a) the Ziehl-Neelsen, or "hot stain," and (b) the Kinyoun or "cold stain."

2. The fluorochrome dye, auramine 0, sometimes used in combination with a second fluorochrome stain, rhodamine.

Both stains bind to mycolic acid in the mycobacterial cell wall. Because of the small size of the organism and the low contrast in the color of the organism and the bright background, smears stained by carbolfuchsin must be scanned with the 100 × oil immersion objective, thereby restricting the area of a slide that can be viewed in a given period of time. In comparison, smears stained with auramine 0 can be scanned using a 25 × objective. Fluorochrome-stained mycobacteria appear bright yellow against a dark background obtained by counterstaining with potassium permanganate, thereby permitting the slide to be scanned under the lower magnification without losing sensitivity. The sharp visual contrast between the brightly colored mycobacteria and the dark background offers a distinct advantage in scanning a much larger area of the slide during the same time necessary for looking at the carbolfuchsin stain. For this reason, the fluorochrome stain will often result in the detection of mycobacteria in smaller numbers per slide than when using a carbolfuchsin stain. Fluorochrome-stained smears require a strong blue light source for illumination, either a 200 watt mercury vapor burner or a strong blue light source with a fluorescein isothiocyanate (FITC) filter. Modifications of the auramine fluorochrome staining procedure include the addition of rhodamine to give a more golden appearance to the mycobacteria or the use of potassium permanganate or acridine orange (Runyon, 1980; Vestal, 1975) as a counterstain to stain the background red to orange.

Enthusiasm for the carbolfuchsin and fluorochrome staining methods varies between laboratories, with different workers strongly partial to one method or the other. Specificity for mycobacteria seems to be the same for both, with the exception of a series of 15 strains of *Mycobacterium fortuitum,* in which 5 of the 15 did not stain with auramine but all 15 stained with carbolfuchsin (Joseph, 1967). Reports differ as to which of the two types of stain will bind to non-viable bacilli for the longest period of time. These differences probably reflect the care devoted to staining and microscopy by individual laboratories. As mentioned above, when using the auramine stain, a significantly larger area of the smear can be scanned in the same period of time used to scan a carbolfuchsin-stained smear. For this reason the fluorochrome stain offers the possibility of greater sensitivity. Because some workers are still hesitant to give up carbolfuchsin stains, some laboratories scan smears by the fluorochrome method and then confirm positive slides by destaining and restaining with a carbolfuchsin stain. Once laboratory workers have become familiar with the auramine stain, they usually prefer the fluorochrome method to carbolfuchsin stains.

Reports from examination of smears should provide some quantitation of the number of organisms present on a smear, inasmuch as there can be a relationship to the number of acid-fast bacilli present and the degree of activity of the disease. The American Thoracic Society recommends the method shown in Table 46–4.

The use of the sputum smear as a screening procedure for the diagnosis of pulmonary tuberculosis has recently been criticized following the finding by several large laboratories that up to 55 per cent of specimens that had positive smears failed to grow in culture. A review of the clinical symptoms and chest x-rays of many of these patients failed to show supporting clinical evidence for tuberculosis. The point has been made that as the incidence of tuberculosis decreases, the predictive value of a positive smear will also decline. When carried to the extreme, if there were no tuberculosis, 100 per cent of the positive smears would be false positives (Boyd, 1975; Pollock, 1977). As techniques for detecting mycobacteria become more sensitive, the finding of commensal mycobacteria that may be more susceptible than *M. tuberculosis* to the decontamination and concentrating procedures will result in a higher incidence of positive smears and negative cultures. Important factors in the predictive value of the smear include the presence or absence of abnormal findings on a chest x-ray, the clinical history, the patient's symptoms, and the number of bacilli present on a slide, with a correlation between increasing numbers of bacilli and the incidence of active infection.

Table 46–4. METHOD FOR REPORTING NUMBERS OF ACID-FAST BACILLI OBSERVED IN STAINED SMEARS*

Number AFB Observed/Field(F)	CDC Method Report	
0	Negative for AFB	(−)
1–2/300 F	Number seen†	(±)
1–9/100 F	Average No./100 F	(1 +)
1–9/10 F	Average No./10 F	(2 +)
1–9/F	Average No./F	(3 +)
> 9/F	> 9/F	(4 +)

*Examination at 800 to 1000 × is assumed. Magnifications less than 800 × should be clearly stated. If microscopist uses consistent procedure for smear examination, relative comparisons of multiple specimens should be easy for the clinician, regardless of magnification used. To equate numbers of bacilli observed at less than 800 × with those seen under oil immersion, adjust counts as follows: for magnifications about 650 ×, divide count by 2 near 450 × divide by 4, near 250 ×, divide by 10; e.g., if 8 AFB per 10 F were seen at 450 ×, the count at 1000 × would be about 2/10 F (8 ÷ 4).

†Counts less than 3/300 F at 800–1000 × are not considered positive; another specimen (or repeat smear of same specimen) should be processed if available.

American Thoracic Society: Diagnostic standards and classification of tuberculosis and other mycobacterial diseases. Am. Rev. Resp. Dis., *123*:343, 1981.

Table 46–5. EFFECT OF INCREASING CENTRIFUGAL FORCE ON POSITIVE SMEARS AND CULTURES FOR MYCOBACTERIA*

	Relative Centrifugal Force		
	1260	***3000***	***3800***
Positive smears	1.8%	4.5%	9.6%
Positive cultures	7.1%	11.2%	11.6%
Correlation of positive smears/cultures	25%	40%	82%

*Adapted from Rickman T. W., and Moyer N. P.: J. Clin. Microbiol., *11*:618, 1980.

Improved correlation between specimens showing a positive smear for acid-fast bacilli and a positive culture has been demonstrated by increasing the relative centrifugal force applied to a specimen following decontamination. All specimens producing a positive culture were usually detected by an RCF of 3000, although improved correlation between a positive smear and a positive culture continued up to an RCF of 3800 (Table 46–5), the highest RCF used in this study (Rickman, 1980). A method for filtration of sputum specimens treated with sodium hypochlorite has been described and perhaps is the most sensitive procedure for detecting acid-fast bacilli (Smithwick, 1981) but may be cumbersome for many laboratories.

The similarities and differences between the Ziehl-Neelsen, Kinyoun, and fluorochrome stains are listed in Table 46–6. For further details on preparing and interpreting these stains, please consult Runyon (1980), Vestal (1975), and Smithwick (1975a). It should be remembered that the auramine and auramine-rhodamine fluorochrome stains are not fluorescent antigen-antibody reactions. Fluorescent tagged antibodies, which are helpful for the identification of individual species of mycobacteria, have been described but are not in widespread use.

INCUBATION OF CULTURES

Most mycobacteria show growth stimulation when incubated in an atmosphere of increased concentration of carbon dioxide. Studies have suggested that the optimal concentration of CO_2 is between 8 and 12 per cent (Fig. 46–1). Increased CO_2 tension is a requirement for the proper use of 7H10, 7H11, and selective 7H11 culture media, and will also improve the number and size of colonies of mycobacteria on egg-base culture media. Candle extinction jars are not acceptable for this purpose, which is best served by a CO_2 incubator. The CO_2 concentration in the incubator should be monitored and recorded in the quality control chart on a daily basis.

M. tuberculosis will grow most rapidly when cultures are incubated at 37°C. In contrast, *M. marinum* and

Table 46–6. COMPARISON OF THE COMPONENTS OF ACID-FAST STAINS

Ziehl-Neelsen	Kinyoun's "Cold" Stain	Auramine Fluorochrome
Carbolfuchsin: 3.0 g of basic fuchsin in 10.0 ml of 90–95% ethanol dissolved in 90 ml of 5% aqueous solution of phenol.	*Carbolfuchsin:* 4.0 g of basic fuchsin in 20 ml of 90–95% ethanol added to 100 ml of a 9% aqueous solution of phenol.	*Phenolic auramine:* 0.1 g auramine 0 in 10 ml of 90–95% ethanol added to 3 g of phenol in 87.0 ml of distilled water.
Acid-alcohol: 3.0 ml of concentrated HCl in 97.0 ml of 90–95% ethanol.	*Acid-alcohol:* 3 ml of concentrated HCl in 97.0 ml of 90–95% ethanol.	*Acid-alcohol:* 0.5 ml of concentrated HCl in 100 ml of 70% alcohol.
Methylene blue counterstain: 0.3 mg of methylene blue chloride in 100 ml of distilled water.	*Methylene blue counterstain:* 0.3 mg of methylene blue chloride in 100 ml of distilled water.	*Potassium permanganate counterstain:* 0.5 g potassium permanganate in 100 ml of distilled water.

M. ulcerans, organisms causing disease of the skin, should be incubated at 30 to 32°C. for optimal recovery. Incubation of cultures at 37°C. for the recovery of *M. marinum, ulcerans,* or *haemophilum* will greatly delay or even prevent their growth. Similarly, cultures containing *M. xenopi* will show optimal growth and recovery when incubated at 42°C. If incubators for 30 to 32°C. are not available, cultures from skin infections or other sources thought to contain *M. marinum* can be placed in a temperature-monitored box or container at 24°C., away from heating or cooling air currents. A 42°C. incubator can be shared with other sections of the laboratory. Incubation of cultures at this temperature can offer a valuable identification characteristic for other types of bacteria *(Pseudomonas aeruginosa)* as well as for mycobacteria.

IDENTIFICATION

Laboratories receiving only occasional clinical specimens for mycobacteria may find the technical effort required to maintain competence for all services in the mycobacterial laboratory to be expensive and not cost effective. Other laboratories will find the number of specimens and patients seen in their institution requires complete identification as well as susceptibility testing of all mycobacterial isolates. In order to help each laboratory decide how far it should go in establishing mycobacterial services, the College of American Pathologists has suggested four "Extents" of service. A similar list of "Levels of Service" has subsequently been suggested by the American Thoracic Society. When these two lists are compared (Table 46–7), the similarities are readily apparent.

Inasmuch as *Mycobacterium tuberculosis* is the most common cause of mycobacterial disease in man, most laboratories will want to be able to identify this organism. The recommended procedures for the identification of *M. tuberculosis* are as follows:

1. The determination of rate of growth and the optimal temperature for isolation.
2. Photoreactivity.
3. Niacin accumulation.
4. Reduction of nitrates to nitrites.

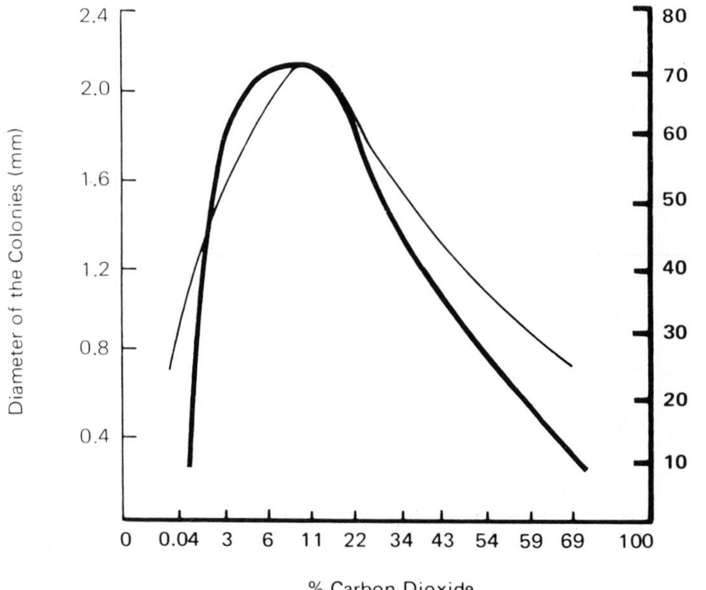

Figure 46–1. Effect of CO_2 on the growth (colony size and number of colonies) of *M. tuberculosis* on primary isolation from sputum. (Reprinted from David, H. L.: Bacteriology of the Mycobacterioses. U.S. Public Health Service, HEW Publication, 1976.)

Table 46–7. LABORATORY SELF-DETERMINED EXTENTS OR LEVELS OF SERVICE AS PROPOSED BY THE COLLEGE OF AMERICAN PATHOLOGISTS AND THE AMERICAN THORACIC SOCIETY

College of American Pathologists: Extents of Service for Participation in Mycobacterial Interlaboratory Comparison Surveys	American Thoracic Society: Levels of Service for Mycobacterial Laboratories
1. No mycobacterial procedures performed.	*Level I:* 1a. Collect adequate clinical specimens, including aerosol-induced sputa. 1b. Transport specimens to a higher level laboratory for isolation and identification. 1c. May prepare and examine smears for presumptive diagnosis and/or as a means of following the progress of diagnosed patients on chemotherapy.
2. Acid-fast stain of exudates, effusions, and body fluids, etc., with inoculation and referral of cultures to reference laboratories for further identification.	*Level II:* 2a. May perform all functions of Level I laboratories, and process specimens as necessary for culture on standard agar- and/or egg-base media. 2b. Identify *Mycobacterium tuberculosis.* 2c. May perform drug susceptibility studies against *M. tuberculosis* with 1° antituberculous drugs. 2d. Retain mycobacterial cultures for a reasonable time
3. Isolation of mycobacteria; identification of *Mycobacterium tuberculosis* and preliminary identification of the atypical forms as photochromogens, scotochromogens, non-photochromogens, and rapid growers. Drug susceptibility testing may or may not be performed.	*Level III:* 3a. May perform all functions of laboratories at lower levels, and identify all *Mycobacterium* species from clinical specimens. 3b. Perform drug susceptibility studies against mycobacteria. 3c. Retain mycobacterial cultures for a reasonable time. 3d. May conduct research and provide training.
4. Definitive identification of mycobacteria isolated to the extent required to establish a correct clinical diagnosis and to aid in the selection of safe and effective therapy. Drug susceptibility testing may or may not be performed.	

5. Catalase production—heat stable and semiquantitative.

6. Pyrazinamidase.

7. Growth inhibition by thiophene-2-carboxylic acid hydrazide (T_2H).

The details for determining these characteristics are available in standard laboratory manuals and will not be repeated here (Vestal, 1975; Runyon, 1980; Finegold, 1982). Although it is not always necessary to determine pyrazinamidase and T_2H growth inhibition on all isolates of *M. tuberculosis,* similarities between certain strains of the bacille Calmette Guérin (BCG) mutants of *M. bovis* and *M. tuberculosis* can best be resolved by these characteristics. Growth of *M. bovis* is inhibited by 1 to 5 μg/ml of T_2H, while that of *M. tuberculosis* is not. Another test, easy and reliable, distinguishing between *M. tuberculosis* and *M. bovis* identifies those organisms producing pyrazinamidase (Wayne, 1974). The use of BCG in the immunotherapy of malignant melanoma with subsequent isolation of the organism from regional lymph nodes and other clinical specimens from such patients has made the need to distinguish between these two species a more common problem today than in the past.

Identification of the other species of the clinically significant mycobacteria can be accomplished by use of the characteristics listed in Table 46–8. It can be seen that with the addition of the Tween 80 hydrolysis, urease, and three-day arylsulfatase tests, most species can be identified or placed in clinically relevant species complexes. Laboratories interested in developing special competence in the speciation of mycobacteria should consult more detailed manuals (Vestal, 1975; David, 1976; Sommers, 1979; Runyon, 1980; Finegold, 1982).

CLASSIFICATION OF MYCOBACTERIA

As more cultures were taken and increasing numbers of "atypical" mycobacteria isolated, there was a need for some form of classification of these organisms. In 1954, after studying a series of these "atypical" strains, Timpe proposed a classification of four groups of organisms based on (1) the rate of growth at 37°C., and (2) the presence or absence of pigmented colonies when grown in the dark and then exposed to light. Runyon (1959) further refined this classification, which is summarized briefly here:

I. Group I organisms are characterized by the ability to make a yellow carotene pigment when viable mycobacteria are exposed to a strong light. Because

Table 46–8. IDENTIFICATION CHARACTERISTICS OF MYCOBACTERIA*

Organism	Optimum Isolation Temperature and Rate of Growth	Pigmentation Growth in:		Niacin Test	Nitrate Reduction	Catalase		Tween 80 Hydrolysis 10 Days	Arylsulfatase 3 days	Urease	Resistance to T_2H 1 μg/ml	Growth on 5% NaCl 28°C.	Iron Uptake	Pyrazinamidase
		Light	*Dark*			*Semi-quantitative*†	*pH 7.0 68°C.*							
M. tuberculosis	37°C. 12–25 days	Buff	Buff	+	3–5+	<40‡	−	∓	−	+	+	−	−	+
M. africanum	37°C. 31–42	Buff	Buff	V	V	V	−	−	−		+	−	−	
M. bovis	37°C. 24–40	Buff	Buff	V	−	<20	−	−	−	+	−	−	−	−
M. ulcerans	32°C. 28–60	Buff	Buff	−	−	>50	+	−	−		+			−
M. kansasii	37°C. 10–20	Yellow	Buff	−	+	>50	+	+§	−	+	+	−	−	−
M. marinum	31–32°C. 5–14	Yellow	Buff	V	−	<40	−	+	∓	+	+	−	−	+
M. simiae	37°C. 7–14	Yellow¶	Buff	+	∓	>50	+	−	−	+	+	−	−	−
M. asiaticum	37°C. 10–21	Yellow	Buff	−	−	>45	+	+	−	−	+	−	−	−
M. szulgai	37°C. 12–25	Yellow to orange	Yellow – 37°C. Buff – 25°C.	+	+	>50	+	∓	−	+	+	−		−
M. scrofulaceum	37°C. 10+	Yellow	Yellow	−	−	>50	+	−	−	+	+	−	−	±
M. gordonae	37°C. 10+	Yellow to orange	Yellow	−	−	>50	+	+	−	−	+	−	−	V
M. flavescens	37°C. 7–10	Yellow	Yellow	−	+	>50	+	+	−	+	+	+	−	+
M. xenopi	42°C. 14–28	Yellow	Yellow	−	−	<40	+	−	±	−	+	−	−	+
M. intracellulare-avium complex	37°C. 10–21	Buff to pale yellow	Buff to pale yellow	−	−	<40	+	−	−	−	+	−	−	+
*M. haemophilum***	30°C. 14–28	Buff to gray	Buff to gray	−	−	<40	−	−	−	−	+	−	−	+
M. malmöense	37°C. 14–28	Buff	Buff	−	−	<45	±	+	−	±	+		−	±
M. gastri	37°C. 10–21	Buff	Buff	−	−	<40	−	+	−	+	+	−	−	−
M. terrae complex	37°C. 10–21	Buff	Buff	−	V	>50	+	+	±	−	+	−	−	±
M. triviale	37°C. 10–21	Buff	Buff	−	1–5+	>50	+	+	∓	−	+	+	−	
M. fortuitum	37°C. 3–5	Buff	Buff	−	2–5+	>50	+	±	+	+	+	+	+	+
M. chelonei ss *chelonei*	28°C. 3–5	Buff	Buff	V	−	>50	+	−	+	+	+	−	−	+
ss *abscessus*	37°C. 3–5	Buff	Buff	V	−	>50	+	V	+	+	+	+	−	+
M. smegmatis	37°C. 3–5	Buff to yellow	Buff to yellow	−	1–5+	>50	±	+	−		+	+	+	

Key to results: + = 84% of strains +; ± = 50–84%; ∓ = 16–49%; − = 16% of strains +; V = variable; blank spaces = little or no data.

*Modified from Sommers, H. M.: The identification of mycobacteria. *In* Baer, D. M. (ed.): Technical Improvement Service Number 28. Chicago, American Society of Clinical Pathologists, 1977. Used by permission.

†Numbers indicate millimeters of bubbles.

‡INH-resistant strains may be negative.

§Positive (most) in 24–48 hours.

¶Photochromogenicity unstable with repeated subcultures.

**Requires blood or ferric ammonium citrate for growth.

they make pigment only when exposed to light, these organisms are called photochromogens. Photochromogenic mycobacteria include *M. kansasii, M. simiae,* and *M. marinum.*

II. Group II mycobacteria produce bright yellow pigmented colonies when grown in either the light or the dark, although in some species of *M. scrofulaceum* the pigment may be intensified on exposure to light. This group of organisms is called "scotochromogens" for their characteristic to generate pigment in the dark. Species in the Group II scotochromogens include *M. scrofulaceum, M. gordonae,* and *M. flavescens.*

III. Runyon's third group of mycobacteria include a number of species, some producing small amounts of pale yellow pigment. Exposure of these organisms to bright light does not intensify the color, and hence they are designated "non-photochromogens." Species in this group include members of the *M. avium-intracellulare* complex, *M. haemophilum, M. malmoense, M. gastri,* and a group of organisms showing little or no pathogenicity for man termed the *M. terrae-nonchromogenicum-triviale* complex.

IV. The last of Runyon's four groups of atypical mycobacteria are characterized by the ability to grow more rapidly than the other three groups, often showing mature colonies in three to five days. These organisms are called "rapid growers." While some species of the "rapid growers" show an intense yellow pigmentation, the two species that are known to cause infection in man, *M. fortuitum* and *M. chelonei,* are non-pigmented.

Although Runyon's classification was helpful in organizing many of the "atypical" mycobacterial isolates into some form of order, it has become apparent that it is now necessary to speciate all isolates to determine their clinical significance and to avoid the confusion and misunderstanding that can occur with the terms photochromogen, scotochromogen, etc. The need for speciation of isolates rather than use of the Runyon group designation can be illustrated by *M. szulgai,* a mycobacterial species recently recognized to be associated with disease in humans. *M. szulgai* is scotochromogenic when incubated at 37°C. but photochromogenic when grown at 22 to 24°C. In contrast to most scotochromogenic mycobacteria, *M. szulgai* has been found to be associated with active, progressive disease in almost all instances (Davidson, 1976). Identification to species can help to either establish or exclude the probable role of the isolate in causing infection.

CLINICAL SIGNIFICANCE OF MYCOBACTERIAL SPECIES

MYCOBACTERIUM TUBERCULOSIS

The clinical significance of the different mycobacterial species in infection in humans depends in large part on the state of the host's immune system. *Mycobacterium tuberculosis* is the most common cause of pulmonary tuberculosis and remains the most virulent of all mycobacterial species. The disease is highly contagious and with the diagnosis of a new case of tuberculosis, careful investigation of close family contacts usually reveals additional cases of active disease. Although the disease may involve all susceptible individuals, there appears to be higher incidence of infection among disadvantaged minorities than in middle or upper class groups. This is considered likely because of the increased incidence of crowded housing and the possibility of nutritional deprivation. Outbreaks frequently involve multiple members of closed population groups, such as teachers and students in classrooms, sailors on ships, and family units living in limited housing. Such outbreaks are all too common and have established the value of intensive epidemiologic investigations in patients with newly recognized infections.

MYCOBACTERIUM BOVIS

Infection with *M. bovis* in the United States today is uncommon, owing in large part to the highly effective campaign to control tuberculosis in dairy herds and mandatory pasteurization of milk. Recently the use of a mutant strain of *M. bovis,* bacille Calmette Guérin (BCG), in the immunotherapy of malignant melanoma has resulted in occasional isolates from the regional lymph nodes or other sites of dissemination in patients who have been injected with the organism. Laboratories should be able to identify *M. bovis,* as a clinical history is not always available.

In contrast to the other mycobacterial species, *M. bovis* does not show growth stimulation with added glycerol, and, in fact, may be inhibited. Such specimens should be inoculated to media without added glycerol, such as 7H10 or 7H11, prepared by the processing laboratory. Petragnani medium contains a lower glycerol content than most other egg-base media and will show preferential recovery of some strains of *M. bovis* and BCG. The addition of 0.2 per cent $NaCO_2COCH_3$ (pyruvate) to culture media for specimens suspected to contain *M. bovis* results in stimulation to the number and size of colonies of *M. bovis* (Dixon, 1967).

Disease from mycobacteria other than *M. tuberculosis* (sometimes referred to by the acronym MOTT) is becoming more apparent clinically, probably not on an absolute basis, but rather as a reflection of decreasing incidence of infection from *M. tuberculosis* and improvement in the sensitivity of detection and identification of other mycobacterial species.

MYCOBACTERIUM ULCERANS

M. ulcerans, the cause of "Buruli ulcer," is a very slowly growing, non-pigmented organism responsible for chronic skin ulcers in patients living in the tropics. The incidence of the disease in the United States is very low, and infection seen here was usually acquired in the tropics (Tsang, 1973). The ulcers are indolent and may progress to significant destruction of skin and underlying tissue (Connor, 1966). Primary recovery of the organism on culture is difficult but works best when incubated at 30 to 33°C. A culture may take as long as six to nine months to become positive. Incubation at 37°C. may delay or prevent isolation.

MYCOBACTERIUM KANSASII

Clinical infection from *M. kansasii* may occur in all age groups and at any site in the body. In contrast to *M. tuberculosis,* pulmonary disease from *M. kansasii* is not highly contagious, with only rare reports of infection in more than one member of a family. In one epidemiologic study, pulmonary disease from *M. kansasii* was most frequently seen in middle-aged white males living in middle-class residential neighborhoods (Lichtenstein, 1965). This is in sharp contrast to infection from *M. tuberculosis,* in which many of the patients live in crowded slum housing. The lack of communicability and the predominance of middle-aged males, as well as abnormal pulmonary function studies in patients with *M. kansasii* infection (Ahn, 1976), have suggested that disease with this organism may be an opportunistic infection. Disseminated infection occurs infrequently and is usually associated with some defect in host defense. Clinically, isolates of *M. kansasii* exhibiting a strong catalase reaction are more frequently associated with pathogenicity than those showing only a weak reaction (Wayne, 1962). *M. kansasii* infections will usually respond to therapy with three or more antituberculous drugs, despite *in vitro* resistance to low levels of INH, ethambutol, and frequently other primary antituberculous drugs (Harris, 1975). The organism has been noted to cause infection in a number of patients with renal homografts, and can present as a cellulitis in patients on active immunosuppressive therapy (Fraser, 1975). A switch to alternate day corticosteroid therapy modified the host inflammatory response from cellulitis to a more characteristic granulomatous tissue reaction. Disseminated infection from *M. kansasii* is usually associated with either an underlying defect in the host defense mechanism or active immunosuppression (Fraser, 1975).

MYCOBACTERIUM MARINUM

M. marinum, formerly known as *M. balnei,* is a photoreactive mycobacterium growing best at 30 to 33°C. and is usually associated with chronic ulcerating granulomas of the skin. The organism can live in fresh or salt water, and infections are usually associated with minor trauma to the skin before or during immersion in water. Infections following skin abrasions in swimming pools ("swimming pool granulomas") have been reported (Schaefer, 1961), as well as infections in patients who are scratched on the hand or arm while caring for fish in aquariums (Heineman, 1972). Recovery of the organism by culture can be rapid (7 to 12 days) when incubated at skin temperature, 30 to 33°C. Growth is slow or may not occur when incubated at 37°C.

MYCOBACTERIUM SIMIAE

M. simiae was first described in 1965 during an investigation of spontaneous mycobacterial disease of monkeys (Karassova, 1965). Subsequently the organism was isolated from humans. In 1971, similar bacteria were isolated from the sputum of 35 patients in Havana (Valdivia, 1971). Studies by agglutination antibodies and immunodiffusion have shown the two organisms to have identical surface antigens. The name *Mycobacterium simiae* has been proposed, as it has precedence over *Mycobacterium habana* (Weiszfeiler, 1976).

Mycobacterium simiae has been recovered from a number of patients, but in only a few has it been shown to be associated with a granulomatous tissue reaction. The organism is resistant to many of the standard antimycobacterial drugs *in vitro.* Association of the organism in infection of monkeys and the appearance of disease in humans caring for monkeys raises certain epidemiologic questions. A hospital in Tucson was able to recover organisms similar to *M. simiae* from tap water in the building. This hospital had its own well as a source of water (Wolinsky, 1979).

MYCOBACTERIUM SZULGAI

Mycobacterium szulgai is a scotochromogenic mycobacterium when incubated at 37°C. and photochromogenic when grown at 24°C. It was first recognized because of its unique pattern of cell wall lipids demonstrated by thin-layer chromatography (Marks, 1972).

M. szulgai is known to cause granulomatous infection in the lung, lymph nodes, olecranal bursae, and palmar tendon sheaths (Davidson, 1976).

Most isolates have been recovered from patients who have had active infection. Patients who repeatedly yield scotochromogenic mycobacteria on culture and show evidence of active or progressive infection should be considered to have infection with *M. szulgai* until proven otherwise.

Mycobacterium szulgai is more susceptible to rifampin, ethionamide, ethambutol, and a higher concentration of isoniazid than other scotochromogens (Davidson, 1976). Seroagglutination and agglutination-absorption tests are specific and provide one means of identification (Schaefer, 1973).

MYCOBACTERIUM SCROFULACEUM

M. scrofulaceum (M. marianum) is a scotochromogenic mycobacterium widely distributed in the environment. Although it has been recovered from more than half of a series of soil specimens, the serotypes were different from those associated with human disease so that the source of the organism in human disease is not readily apparent (Wolinsky, 1968). The high incidence of skin sensitivity to PPD prepared from the Gause strain (PPD-G) of this organism suggests that it is widely available in our environment, although the incidence of clinical infection is low. *M. scrofulaceum* is one of the most common causes of cervical lymphadenitis in children ("scrofula") (Prissick, 1957). In contrast, scrofula in adults is usually due to *M. tuberculosis. M. scrofulaceum* is known to colonize old tuberculous cavities, but in such patients it is not thought to be clinically significant. Primary pulmonary disease with *M. scrofulaceum* occurs, but it is distinctly uncommon. The organism can sometimes be isolated from the sputum of patients with carcinoma of the lung or patients with other chronic pulmonary disease. When this occurs it is usually not associated with a granulomatous inflammatory response and may represent commensal colonization.

MYCOBACTERIUM XENOPI

First described in 1959 by Schwabacher, who cultured it from a skin lesion of the South African toad *Xenopus laevis, M. xenopi* has been found to cause pulmonary disease in England, France, and the United States. It has been shown to colonize the hot water systems of hospitals in the United States (Bullin, 1970; Gross, 1976) and Britain. The organism is usually pigmented bright yellow and was initially considered to be a scotochromogenic mycobacterium. For reasons which are not too clear, it can usually be isolated from cultures incubated at 42°C. more rapidly and with better growth than from cultures incubated at 35 to 37°C. Although Gross (1976) isolated *M. xenopi* at least three or more times from each of 105 patients, pulmonary disease could be attributed to the organism in only 11. It is important to differentiate the organism from the similar-appearing *Mycobacterium intracellulare* or scotochromogenic mycobacteria, as *M. xenopi* is much more responsive to drug therapy. Infection may also occur in immunosuppressed patients (Koizumi, 1980).

MYCOBACTERIUM INTRACELLULARE

M. intracellulare ("Battey bacillus") is very closely related to *M. avium*. Differentiation between the two and a series of closely related organisms can be difficult and may not be clinically significant. With this in mind, the term *M. avium-intracellulare* complex has been proposed to emphasize the similarities and the differences in this group of organisms.

For many years the organism causing disease of this type was called the "Battey bacillus" for the Battey State Hospital in Rome, Georgia. Like *M. kansasii, M. avium-intracellulare* causes disease more frequently in middle-aged men than in other groups. Quite often, patients with infection from *M. avium-intracellulare* have evidence of an underlying chronic pulmonary disease (Ahn, 1976). Infections with *M. avium-intracellulare* are not highly contagious, and infection in more than one member of a family is distinctly uncommon. This organism is responsible for more clinical infectious diseases than any other mycobacterium with the exception of *M. tuberculosis* (Good, 1980).

Infection with *M. avium-intracellulare* is usually seen in the lung, although other sites may be involved and disseminated infection has been reported. Disseminated infection from *M. avium-intracellulare* has been a rather striking finding in homosexual males demonstrating the acquired immunodeficiency syndrome (AIDS) (Zakowski, 1982). Infection with this organism among AIDS patients appears to be out of proportion to the normal distribution of infection with the agent for reasons not apparent at this time (Masur, 1982). In contrast to infection with many of the other species of mycobacteria, *M. avium-intracellulare* causes an indolent, chronic infection that is particularly difficult to treat. Therapy with three or four and five or six drugs may be only partially successful, with slowly progressive disease resulting (Dutt, 1977). Surgical resection combined with aggressive drug therapy has provided the best clinical results.

M. SCROFULACEUM AND MAIS GROUP

M. scrofulaceum shares certain traits with members of the *M. avium-intracellulare* group as determined in part by surface antigen agglutinin tests. Because of these similarities, it has been proposed that the two species be referred to as MAIS (Resnikov, 1973). Inasmuch as most typical strains of *M. avium-intracellulare* and *M. scrofulaceum* can be easily distinguished from each other on the basis of pigmentation, catalase activity, and urease production, not all workers endorse the proposal at this time (see Wolinsky [1979] for a more complete discussion). Hawkins (1977) has called attention to a group of organisms showing biochemical characteristics intermediate between those of *M. avium-intracellulare* and *M. scrofulaceum* for which she has proposed the term, "MAIS intermediate." Members of the MAIS intermediate group are usually yellow-pigmented, are not typable by surface antigen agglutinating antisera, and are rarely, if ever, associated with human disease (see Table 46–9 for distinguishing characteristics). Note that the terms "MAIS" and "MAIS intermediate" refer to two separate groups of organisms.

M. HAEMOPHILUM

A recently described species isolated from skin infections in patients who have lymphoma or renal transplants and who are consequently immunosuppressed, *M. haemophilum* is unique in that good growth requires ferric ions derived either from blood agar or ferric ammonium citrate added to egg base or agar media. Specimens should be incubated at 30 to 32°C. (Sompolinski, 1978). Although most cases have been found in Israel or Australia, the organism has also been isolated in Cleveland, Ohio (Davis, 1982).

M. MALMÖENSE

Another recently described species of mycobacterium, this organism is usually associated with pulmonary disease (Schröder, 1977). It has been found in patients in Sweden, Germany, Wales, Australia,

Table 46–9. CHARACTERISTICS OF "MAIS" INTERMEDIATE STRAINS*

Test or Property	Pigmented *M. avium-intracellulare* complex†	*M. scrofulaceum*	Pro Tempore "MAIS"‡ Intermediate	
Pigment	+	+	+	+
Catalase > 45 mm	−	+	+	−
Urease	−	+	−	+ (rare)

*Reproduced with permission from Hawkins, J. E.: Am. Rev. Resp. Dis., *116*:963, 1977.

†Other characteristics typical of the species.

‡MAIS = *M. avium-intracellulare-scrofulaceum.*

and now the United States (Good, 1980). *M. malmoense* is slowly growing, is non-pigmented and may initially appear similar to the non-photochromogenic mycobacteria.

MYCOBACTERIUM FORTUITUM AND MYCOBACTERIUM CHELONEI

Both *Mycobacterium fortuitum* and *M. chelonei* are closely related members of Runyon's group IV rapidly growing mycobacteria. Because of similarities between the two species, both in the cultural characteristics and in the type of disease caused in humans, it has been proposed in the past that the term *M. fortuitum-chelonei* complex be used instead of the individual species. *M. fortuitum* can be differentiated from *M. chelonei* without difficulty by nitroreductase activity. The two subspecies of *M. chelonei, M. chelonei* ss *chelonei* and *M. chelonei* ss *abscessus,* can be separated by the ability of the latter to grow on Lowenstein-Jensen medium containing 5 per cent NaCl. More recently, the demonstration *in vitro* of greater susceptibility of *M. fortuitum* to a wide range of antimicrobial agents has emphasized other differences between the two species and suggested that *M. fortuitum* be distinguished from *M. chelonei* and its two subspecies (Silcox, 1981). Of the two subspecies of *M. chelonei, M. chelonei* ss *abscessus* is more often associated with disease.

Infections from the *Mycobacterium fortuitum-chelonei* complex organisms usually involve the skin or epidermal derivatives. Skin abscesses resulting from vaccinations have been reported (Borghans, 1973), and eye infections, usually involving the cornea, have been described following trauma (Zimmerman, 1969).

Members of the *Mycobacterium fortuitum-chelonei* complex can be recovered from sputum, frequently without evidence of pulmonary disease, but lung infections do occur and when present are a difficult therapeutic problem. Most of the antimycobacterial drugs in current use are not effective against the *M. fortuitum-chelonei* complex. *M. fortuitum* has also been found as a postoperative infectious complication of cardiac valve replacement. Contamination from porcine valves has been documented, resulting in a myocardial abscess (Levy, 1977). More recently the laboratory characteristics of a large number of *M. fortuitum-chelonei* strains have been reported from organisms isolated from a series of outbreaks of infection involving cardiac prosthetic valves, mammary augmentation prostheses, and a renal dialysis center. Careful study has strongly implicated a third subspecies of *M. chelonei* (Silcox, 1981). The *M. fortuitum-chelonei* organisms are now the second most common group of non-tuberculous mycobacteria associated with infection in man (Good, 1980).

NON-PATHOGENIC MYCOBACTERIA

Mycobacterium gordonae ("tap-water bacillus," *M. aquae)* is a scotochromogenic mycobacterium that has not been clearly shown to be the cause of disease in humans. *M. gordonae* can colonize water taps and stills and, like *M. xenopi,* offers a challenge to the laboratory to determine its clinical significance. *M. gordonae* should be distinguished from *M. scrofulaceum* and *M. xenopi,* both of which are more likely to be the cause of active infection. Similarly, *M. flavescens* is not known to cause disease and should be identified to differentiate it from one of the more pathogenic scotochromogenic mycobaceria.

Non-pathogenic mycobacterial species in the non-photochromogenic Runyon group III, include *Mycobacterium gastri* and a poorly defined group termed the *M. terrae-nonchromogenicum-triviale* complex. It is generally believed that this group of organisms is without pathogenic potential unless there has been some serious defect in the patient's host defense mechanisms.

With the exception of *Mycobacterium fortuitum* and *M. chelonei,* very few, if any, mycobacteria of group IV cause clinical disease in humans. Most rapidly growing mycobacteria are pigmented yellow with the exception of *M. fortuitum* and *M. chelonei.* Both species are buff in color.

INCIDENCE OF TUBERCULOSIS AND MYCOBACTERIA OTHER THAN TUBERCULOSIS (MOTT)

Wide variation exists between hospitals in the same geographic region as to the relative incidence of MOTT and *M. tuberculosis* strains; this may, in part, depend on the population served by individual hospitals.

In reporting her experience in the recovery of mycobacteria in the Seattle region, Pollock (1977) found that *M. tuberculosis* made up 39 per cent of mycobacterial isolates from the University of Washington Hospital, a tertiary care referral institution, while the same organism accounted for 84 per cent of all acid-fast isolates at the local Veterans Hospital and 93 per cent at Harborview Medical Center, the city and county hospital for Seattle and King County.

SUSCEPTIBILITY TESTING OF MYCOBACTERIA

Random drug resistance in mycobacteria is independent of exposure to the agent. The frequency of drug-resistant mutants in a culture of tubercle bacilli has been estimated to be between 1 in 10^5 bacteria for isoniazid and 1 in 10^6 for streptomycin. If two drugs, isoniazid and streptomycin, are both given, the incidence of resistance will be the product of the two separately, or 1 of every 10^{11} organisms. The importance of the incidence of spontaneously resistant mutants becomes apparent when it is known that patients with an open pulmonary cavity may have a total bacillary population of 10^7 to 10^9 bacteria. If such patients are treated with a single antituberculous agent, their cultures will soon be populated only with resistant organisms and treatment will fail. For this reason, patients with tuberculosis must be treated with two or preferably three drugs. Failure to take all drugs may lead to the rapid emergence of drug-resistant tubercle bacilli.

Clinically, it has been found that if more than 1 per cent of a patient's tubercle bacilli are resistant to a drug *in vitro,* therapy with that drug will not be effective *in vivo*. Therefore, the susceptibility test must determine the *number* of bacilli susceptible and resistant. The inoculum should be adjusted so that the number of naturally resistant mutants will not mislead the laboratory worker to interpret the culture as resistant. At the same time, there must be a sufficiently dilute inoculum so that the incidence of drug resistance in the range of 1 per cent can be determined. For optimal results, such an inoculum will result in 100 to 300 colony-forming units on each quadrant of a four quadrant Petri plate. Because it is difficult to standardize an inoculum of mycobacteria, particularly *M. tuberculosis,* it is usually necessary to inoculate two sets of susceptibility test plates, the first with a 10^{-2} or 10^{-3} dilution of a barely turbid broth culture and the second set with a 100-fold dilution of the inoculum used for the first set. This procedure is known as the proportional susceptibility testing method.

Ten drugs are used in the treatment of tuberculosis. Four are considered "primary" and include streptomycin, isoniazid, rifampin, and ethambutol, while the remaining six, ethionamide, capreomycin, kanamycin, cycloserine, para-aminosalicylic acid, and pyrazinamide, are considered secondary and used only when resistance develops to the primary drugs. The suggested concentrations of the drugs used for mycobacterial susceptibility testing are listed in Table 46–10 for both egg base and agar base media.

The test is performed in plastic Petri plates divided into four quadrants. Five milliliters of agar is placed in each quadrant. The medium in the first quadrant does not contain any antimycobacterial agent and acts as a growth control. The other three quadrants contain dilutions of the drugs to be tested. Although drugs have been incorporated in inspissated egg-base media in the past, most laboratories now prefer using either 7H11 or 7H10 as a base medium, adding the drugs after cooling the agar to 45°C. Adding the drugs to the agar medium after autoclaving decreases the loss of activity that can occur in egg-base medium during inspissation. An additional loss of drug activity may

Table 46–10. DRUG CONCENTRATIONS FOR PROPORTION METHOD OF SUSCEPTIBILITY TESTING USING VARIOUS CULTURE MEDIA*

	Drug Concentrations (μg/ml)		
Drug	***7H10***	***7H11***	***Lowenstein-Jensen***
Isoniazid	0.2, 1.0	0.2, 1.0	0.2, 1.0
p-Aminosalicylic acid	2.0	8.0	0.5
Streptomycin	2.0	2.0	4.0
Rifampin	1.0	1.0	40.0
Ethambutol	2.0	7.5	2.0
Ethionamide	5.0	10.0	20.0
Kanamycin	5.0	6.0	20.0
Capreomycin	10.0	10.0	20.0
Cycloserine	20.0	30.0	30.0
Pyrazinamide	50	—	—

*Reproduced with permission from McClatchy, J. K.: *In* Lorian, V. (ed.): Antibiotics in Laboratory Medicine. Baltimore, Williams & Wilkins, 1974.

Table 46–11. DISTRIBUTION OF DRUG-CONTAINING DISKS FOR SUSCEPTIBILITY TESTS*

Plate No.	Quadrant No.	Amount of Drug per Disk (μg)	Final Drug Concentration (μg/ml)
1	I Control # 1	—	0
	II Isoniazid	1	0.2
	III Isoniazid	5	1.0
	IV Rifampin	5	1.0
2	I Streptomycin	10	2.0
	II Streptomycin	50	10.0
	III Ethambutol	25	5.0
	IV Ethambutol	50	10.0
3	I Para-aminosalicylic acid	10	2.0
	II Para-aminosalicylic acid	50	10.0
	III Control #2	—	0
	IV —	—	—

*Reproduced with permission of Kubica, G. P., et al.: Am. Rev. Resp. Dis., *112*:773, 1975.

occur in egg-base media with binding of some agents to egg albumin and other proteins.

A simplified method for preparing drug susceptibility plates has been developed which does not require weighing and dilution of each drug. This method uses filter paper disks containing the primary antituberculous drugs. Disks are available from microbiologic supply sources. With this method, preparation of drug-containing media is facilitated by placing a drug-containing disk in one quadrant of the plate and adding 5 ml of 7H10 or 7H11 agar. The drug diffuses into the medium and results in the recommended concentration of drug to be tested. Since each disk is marked with the name and concentration of drug it contains, labeling errors are eliminated, as well as errors that can occur in weighing, dilution, and measuring of drug solutions (Wayne, 1966). A suggested schedule for the use of drug-containing paper disks is given in Table 46–11.

To perform the test, susceptibility plates are inoculated with three drops in each quadrant of a 10^{-2} and 10^{-4} dilution of a barely turbid broth culture. Plates are incubated in CO_2 at 37°C. and interpreted between two and three weeks. Incubation of ethambutol-containing media for more than three weeks may result in the appearance of microcolonies following the inactivation of the drug. Interpretation of the inoculated plates should include either an estimate or a direct count of the total number of colonies on the control and drug-containing media. All colonies, even those showing inhibition of growth on drug-containing media, should be counted and related to the number of colonies on the control quadrant. Since the control quadrant should contain the same number of colonies inoculated to the test quadrants, the percentage of resistant colonies can be readily calculated from the two sets of plates inoculated with dilutions of organisms 100-fold apart.

The *direct mycobacterial susceptibility* test is inoculated from digested and concentrated sputum found to be positive for acid-fast bacilli. The *indirect susceptibility test* is inoculated from colonies isolated from a primary culture. The direct test will usually give good results only if large numbers of mycobacteria are present in the specimen. The advantage of the direct susceptibility test is an earlier report (three to four weeks) in contrast to the indirect test, which may take up to six to eight weeks. The disadvantage of the direct susceptibility test is that it usually requires a large number of mycobacteria for successful growth and is often overgrown by large numbers of contaminating bacteria.

PRIMARY DRUG RESISTANCE

Primary drug resistance in mycobacteria, defined as resistance to a drug by an organism isolated from a patient who has never received antituberculous therapy, was for years thought not to exceed 2 to 5 per cent of all isolates. In 1975 the United States Public Health Service initiated an ongoing surveillance program, designed to sample primary drug resistance in mycobacteria from different populations and geographic areas that have not been represented in previous surveys. Somewhat surprisingly, the first (Kopanoff, 1978) and second (Centers for Disease Control, 1980) summaries of this program have shown considerable variation in the incidence of primary drug resistance between different geographic areas of the country and various ethnic groups, ranging from as high as 15 per cent in Los Angeles and 19 per cent in Harlington, Texas, to 3.4 per cent in Detroit. Another striking finding was a marked difference in the incidence of resistance between ethnic groups, including 12.7 per cent in Asians, 15 per cent in Hispanics, and 5.8 per cent in Caucasians. The rate of primary drug resistance in all ethnic/racial groups in 1977 was 8.6 per cent (Kopanoff, 1978). A subsequent report in 1980 showed a decrease in the overall rate to 7.1 per cent, but still showed higher rates in Hispanics and Asians, as well as in their characteristic geographic locations in Texas and Los Angeles (Centers for Disease Control, 1980). The decision to offer drug susceptibility testing for mycobacteria may, therefore, vary from one laboratory to another, depending on location and population served, as well as on the volume of strains and availability of special facilities. If recent mycobacterial isolates are not tested for drug susceptibility, the organism should be retained in the refrigerator for a minimum of 6 to 12 months should evidence of drug resistance appear.

SHORT COURSE THERAPY FOR TUBERCULOSIS

Isoniazid and rifampin are both bactericidal to mycobacteria in the neutral or slightly alkaline environment of large pulmonary cavities, as well as in the acid environment of phagolysosomes in pulmonary macrophages. In many patients, administration of these two drugs has led to sterilization of the mycobacterial load in nine months, a much shorter time than was previously possible. Not only can therapy be reduced from 24 to 9 months, but administration of the drugs can be reduced from daily to twice weekly without interfering with therapeutic results. The ability to give the medication biweekly facilitates patient compliance as well as a reduction of drug costs to approximately one third of that needed for daily administration (Stead, 1981). Should resistance to one of these two drugs develop, the use of both streptomycin and pyrazinamide as an alternative for either isoniazid or rifampin is recommended. Streptomycin is active in the neutral to slightly alkaline environment of large cavities, while pyrazinamide is active in the acid environment of phagolysosomes and closed, small nodules (Grosset, 1980).

"RAPID" METHODS IN MYCOBACTERIOLOGY

The objective of adapting different types of technology and instruments to shorten the time for isolation, identification, and susceptibility testing of bacteria and other microorganisms has been particularly relevant for mycobacteria. *M. tuberculosis* has a generation time of approximately 18 to 22 hours, although other species of mycobacteria may grow more rapidly. If alternative methods to the standard procedures now used could be developed to provide culture and susceptibility information in a shorter time interval, significant cost savings might be effected by a reduction in hospitalization and return of the patient to a productive career.

INCREASED SENSITIVITY OF ACID-FAST SMEARS

As discussed earlier, improved correlation of positive acid-fast smears with positive cultures, as may be seen by using higher centrifugal forces during specimen concentration, provides one of the most "rapid" methods for the presumptive diagnosis of mycobacterial disease (Rickman, 1980).

THIN-LAYER CHROMATOGRAPHY

The detection of characteristic cell wall lipids specific or partially specific for different mycobacterial species by thin-layer chromatography (TLC) has been done since the mid-1960s. Extracts from control cultures and unknown isolates can be chromatographed concurrently using colonies obtained from primary cultures. TLC can provide a species identification for many but not all mycobacteria. This procedure is currently undergoing further evaluation as another aid for identification (Jenkins, 1981).

GAS-LIQUID CHROMATOGRAPHY

Gas-liquid chromatography (GLC) with and without mass spectrometry has been used for a number of years to detect and identify long-chain fatty acids extractable from the cell walls of mycobacteria. Tisdall (1982) developed a procedure for saponifying organisms in methanolic NaOH and reported correct grouping or speciation of 320 of 335 mycobacteria using chromatograms and colonial characteristics. More recently, studies have been most encouraging for the use of pyrolysis mass spectrometry in the identification and classification of mycobacteria (Wieten, 1981). At present, such approaches to identification are restricted to research centers. Further application of this type of instrumentation has been proposed to identify mycobacteria from primary specimens, such as sputum.

METABOLISM OF ^{14}C-LABELED SUBSTRATES (BACTEC)

One of the more promising methods to detect growth of mycobacteria rapidly is the use of ^{14}C-tagged metabolic intermediates (^{14}C palmitic-1 acid and formic ^{14}C acid). The finding of free $^{14}CO_2$ above the liquid culture phase indicates growth and active metabolism of the substrate; conversely, the lack of $^{14}CO_2$ can indicate the inhibition of growth by an agent such as antimycobacterial drugs (Middlebrook, 1977). Initial trials have shown this method to offer promise in the recovery and isolation of mycobacteria from clinical specimens, such as sputum previously shown to be positive by acid-fast smear. Vials of culture medium with sputum are incubated at 37°C. and tested for $^{14}CO_2$ every three to four days for the first two weeks and then every week for the remaining six to eight weeks. Detection of $^{14}CO_2$ correlates with utilization of the substrate and is specific for growth of mycobacteria. Application of ^{14}C-tagged substrates to the detection of growth of mycobacteria from smear-negative specimens is currently under study. Selective growth of mycobacteria in mixed cultures containing other respiratory tract bacteria found in sputum can be accomplished in part by incorporation of antibiotics in the culture vial.

The same principle of selective metabolism of ^{14}C substrate has also been applied to the rapid testing of *M. tuberculosis* for susceptibility to first-line antituberculous drugs. A growth control vial is used, and the inhibitory activity of the individual drugs is determined by the suppression of growth of a standard inoculum of the organism and the subsequent lack of evolution of $^{14}CO_2$. Initial results are encouraging, and further studies are in progress.

AGAR DISK DIFFUSION SUSCEPTIBILITY TESTING

As a result of recent outbreaks of infections from organisms in the *M. fortuitum-chelonei* complex (Centers for Disease Control, 1978; Hoffman, 1982), some workers have attempted to determine drug susceptibility by the Bauer-Kirby procedure, using Mueller-Hinton agar and drug-impregnated filter paper disks (Welch, 1979; Wallace, 1979). While susceptibility tests of this type can be completed within 48 to 72 hours, the method is not yet standardized and needs further study. In addition, correlation of the Bauer-Kirby susceptibility test results with clinical response is not well established. Preliminary studies using disk susceptibility tests have suggested that a number of antibiotics not previously used for treating infections caused by the drug-resistant members of the *M. fortuitum-chelonei* group may have clinical application (Dalovisio, 1981; Irwin, 1982).

Ahn, C. H., Nash, D. R., and Hurst, G. A.: Ventilatory defects in atypical mycobacteriosis. A comparison study with tuberculosis. Am. Rev. Resp. Dis., *113*:273, 1976.

Borghans, S. G. A., and Stanford, J. L.: *Mycobacterium chelonei* in abscesses after injection of diphtheria-pertussis-tetanus-poliovaccine. Am. Rev. Resp. Dis., *107*:1, 1973.

Boyd, J. C., and Marr, J. J.: Decreasing reliability of acid-fast smear techniques for detection of tuberculosis. Ann. Intern. Med., *82*:489, 1975.

Bullin, C. H., and Tanner, E. I.: Isolation of *Myobacterium xenopi* from water taps. J. Hyg. (Camb.), *68*:97, 1970.

Centers for Disease Control: Mycobacterial infections associated with augmentation mammoplasty—Florida, North Carolina, Texas. Morbid. Mortal. Weekly Rep., *27*:513, 1978.

Centers for Disease Control: Primary resistance to antituberculous drugs—United States. Morbid. Mortal. Weekly Rep., *29*:345, 1980.

Cohn, M. L., Waggoner, R. F., and McClatchy, J. K.: The 7H11 medium for the culture of mycobacteria. Am. Rev. Resp. Dis., *98*:295, 1968.

Connor, D. H., and Lunn, H. F.: Buruli ulceration. Arch. Pathol., *81*:183, 1966.

Dalovisio, J. R., Paukey, G. A., Wallace, R. J., and Jones, D. B.: Clinical usefulness of amikacin and doxycycline in the treatment of infection due to *Mycobacterium fortuitum* and *Mycobacterium chelonei*. Rev. Infect. Dis., *3*:1068, 1981.

David, H. C.: Bacteriology of the Mycobacterioses. U.S. Department of Health, Education and Welfare, Public Health Service Publication No. (CDC) 76–8316, 1976.

Davidson, P. T.: *Mycobacterium szulgai*. A new pathogen causing infection of the lung. Chest, *69*:799, 1976.

Davis, B. R., Brumbach, J., Sanders, W. J., and Wolinsky, E.: Skin lesions caused by *Mycobacterium haemophilum*. Ann. Intern. Med., *97*:723, 1982.

Dixon, J. M. S., and Cuthbert, E. H.: Isolation of tubercle bacilli from uncentrifuged sputum on pyruvic acid medium. Am. Rev. Resp. Dis., *96*:119, 1967.

Dutt, A. K., and Stead, W. W.: Results of treatment of patients infected with *M. intracellulare*. Am. Rev. Resp. Dis., *115*(Suppl.):396, 1977.

Finegold, S. M., and Martin, W. J.: Bailey and Scott's Diagnostic Microbiology. 6th ed. St. Louis. C. V. Mosby, 1982.

Fraser, D. W., Buxton, A. E., et al.: Disseminated *Mycobacterium kansasii* infection presenting as cellulitis in a recipient of a renal homograft. Am. Rev. Resp. Dis., *112*:125, 1975.

Good, R. C.: Isolation of nontuberculous mycobacteria in the United States. 1979. J. Infect. Dis., *142*:779, 1980.

Gross, W., Hawkins, J. E., and Murphy, D. B.: Water as a source of contamination. Am. Rev. Resp. Dis., *113*:(Part 2) 78, 1976.

Grosset, J.: Bacteriologic basis of short course chemotherapy for tuberculosis. Clin. Chest Med., *1*:231, 1980.

Gruft, H.: Isolation of acid-fast bacilli from contaminated specimens. Health Lab. Sci., *8*:79, 1971.

Harris, G. D., Johanson, W. G., and Nicholson, D. P.: Response to chemotherapy of pulmonary disease due to *Mycobacterium kansasii*. Am. Rev. Resp. Dis., *112*:31, 1975.

Hawkins, J. E.: Scotochromogenic mycobacteria which appear intermediate between *Mycobacterium avium-intracellulare* and *Mycobacterium scrofulaceum*. Am. Rev. Resp. Dis., *116*:963, 1977.

Heineman, H. S., Spitzer, S., and Pianphongsant, T.: Fish tank granuloma. A hobby hazard. Arch. Intern. Med., *130*:121, 1972.

Hoffman, P. C., Fraser, D. W., Robsicsek, F., et al.: Two outbreaks of sternal wound infections due to organisms of the *M. fortuitum* complex. J. Infect. Dis., *143*:533, 1982.

Irwin, R. S., Pratter, M. R., Corwin, R. W., Farrugia, R., and Teplitz, C.: Pulmonary infection with *Mycobacterium chelonei:* Successful treatment with one drug based on disk diffusion susceptibility data. J. Infect. Dis., *145*:722, 1982.

Jenkins, P. A.: Lipid analysis for the identification of mycobacteria: An appraisal. Rev. Infect. Dis., *3*:862, 1981.

Joseph, S. W.: Lack of auramine-rhodamine fluorescence of Runyon Group IV mycobacteria. Am. Rev. Resp. Dis., *95*:114, 1967.

Karassova, V., Weiszfeiler, J., and Krasznay, E.: Occurrence of atypical mycobacteria in *Macacus rhesus.* Acta Microbiol. Acad. Sci. Hung., *12*:275, 1965.

Kestle, D. G., and Kubica, G. P.: Sputum collection for cultivation of mycobacteria. An early morning specimen or the 24- to 72-our pool? Am. J. Clin. Path., *48*:347, 1967.

Koisumi, J. H., and Sommers, H. M.: *Mycobacterium xenopi* and pulmonary disease. Am. J. Clin. Path., *73*:826, 1980.

Kopanoff, D. E., Kilburn, J. O., Glassroth, J. L., et al.: A continuing survey of tuberculous primary resistance in the United States, March 1975 to November 1977. A United States Public Health Service Cooperative Study. Am. Rev. Resp. Dis., *118*:835, 1978.

Krasnow, I., and Wayne, L. G.: Comparison of methods for tuberculosis bacteriology. Appl. Microbiol., *18*:915, 1969.

Kubica, G. P., Dye, W. E., et al.: Sputum digestion and decontamination with N-acetyl-L-cysteine-sodium hydroxide for culture of mycobacteria. Am. Rev. Resp. Dis., *87*:775, 1963.

Kubica, G. P., Gross, W. M., et al.: Laboratory services for mycobacterial diseases. Am. Rev. Resp. Dis., *112*:883, 1975.

Levy, C., Curtin, J. A., et al.: *Mycobacterium chelonei* infection of porcine heart valves. N. Engl. J. Med., *297*:667, 1977.

Lichtenstein, M. R., Takimura, Y., and Thompson, J. R.: Photochromogenic mycobacterial pulmonary infection in a group of hospitalized patients in Chicago. II. Demographic studies. Am. Rev. Resp. Dis., *91*:592, 1965.

Marks, S., and Jenkins, P. A.: *Mycobacterium szulgai*—a new pathogen. Tubercle, *53*:210, 1972.

Masur, H.: *Mycobacterium avium-intracellulare:* Another scourge for individuals with the acute immunodeficiency syndrome. J.A.M.A., *248*:3013, 1982.

McClatchy, J. K.: Susceptibility testing of mycobacteria. *In* Baer, D. M. (ed.): Technical Improvement Service. Chicago, Commission on Continuing Education, American Society of Clinical Pathologists, No. 29, 1977.

McClatchy, J. K., Waggoner, R. F., Kanes, W., et al.: Isolation of mycobacteria from clinical specimens by use of selective 7H11 medium. Am. J. Clin. Path., *65*:412, 1976.

Middlebrook, G., Reggiardo, Z., and Tiggertt, W. D.: Automatable radiometric detection of growth of *Mycobacterium tuberculosis* in selective media. Am. Rev. Resp. Dis., *115*:1066, 1977.

Miliner, R. A., Stottmeir, K. D., and Kubica, G. P.: Formaldehyde: A photothermal activated toxic substance produced in Middlebrook 7H10 medium. Am. Rev. Resp. Dis., *99*:603, 1969.

Petran, E. I., and Vera, H. D.: Media for selective isolation of mycobacteria. Health Lab. Sci., *8*:225, 1971.

Pollock, H. M., and Wieman, E. J.: Smear results in the diagnosis of mycobacterioses using blue light fluorescence microscopy. J. Clin. Microbiol., *5*:329, 1977.

Prissick, F. H., and Masson, A. M.: Yellow-pigmented pathogenic mycobacteria from cervical lymphadenitis. Can. J. Microbiol., *3*:91, 1957.

Resnikov, M., Dawson, D. J.: Serological examination of some strains that are in the *Mycobacterium avium-intracellulare-scrofulaceum* complex but do not belong to Schaefer's serotypes. Appl. Microbiol., *26*:470, 1973.

Rickman, T. W., and Moyer, M. P.: Increased sensitivity of acid-fast smears. J. Clin. Microbiol., *11*:618, 1980.

Rothlauf, M. V., Brown, G. L., and Blair, E. B.: Isolation of mycobacteria from undecontaminated specimens with selective 7H10 medium. J. Clin. Microbiol., *13*:76, 1981.

Runyon, E. H.: Anonymous mycobacteria in pulmonary disease. Med. Clin. North Am., *43*:273, 1959.

Runyon, E. H., Karlson, A. G., et al.: Mycobacterium. *In* Lennette, E. H., Balows, A., Hausler, W. J., Jr., and Truant, J. P. (eds.): Manual of Clinical Microbiology. 3rd ed. Washington, D.C., American Society for Microbiology, 1980, p. 150.

Schaefer, W. B., and Davis, C. L.: A bacteriologic and histopathologic study of skin granuloma due to *Mycobacterium balnei.* Am. Rev. Resp. Dis., *84*:837, 1961.

Schaefer, W. B., Wolinsky, E., Jenkins, P. A., and Marks, J.: *Mycobacterium szulgai*—a new pathogen. Serologic identification and report of five new cases. Am. Rev. Resp. Dis., *108*:1320, 1973.

Schröder, K. H., and Juhlin, I.: *Mycobacterium malmöense* sp. nov. Int. J. Syst. Bacteriol., *27*:241, 1977.

Schwabacher, H.: A strain of mycobacterium isolated from skin lesions of a coldblooded animal, *Xenopus laevis,* and its relation to atypical acid-fast bacilli occurring in man. J. Hyg. (Camb.), *57*:57, 1959.

Shah, R. R., and Dye, W. E.: The use of dithiothreitol to replace N-acetyl-L-cysteine for routine sputum digestion-decontamination for the culture of mycobacteria. Am. Rev. Resp. Dis., *94*:454, 1966.

Silcox, U. A., Good, R. C., and Floyd, M. M.: Identification of clinically significant *Mycobacterium fortuitum* complex isolates. J. Clin. Microbiol., *14*:686, 1981.

Smithwick, R. W.: Laboratory Manual for Acid-fast Microscopy. U.S. Department of Health, Education and Welfare, Public Health Service Center for Disease Control, Mycobacterial Reference Section, Atlanta, Ga., 1975a.

Smithwick, R. W., and Stratigos, C. B.: Acid-fast microscopy on polycarbonate membrane filter sputum sediments. J. Clin. Microbiol., *13*:1109, 1981.

Smithwick, R. W., Stratigos, C. B., and David, H. L.: Use of cetylpyridium chloride and sodium chloride for the decontamination of sputum specimens that are transported to the laboratory for the isolation of *Mycobacterium tuberculosis.* J. Clin. Microbiol., *1*:411, 1975b.

Sommers, H. M.: Mycobacteria. *In* Koneman, E. W., Allen, S. D., Dowell, V. R., and Sommers, H. M. (ed.): Color Atlas and Textbook of Diagnostic Microbiology. Philadelphia, J. B. Lippincott Co., 1979.

Sompolinsky, D., Laziel, A., Maveh, D., and Yakilevitz, T.: *Mycobacterium haemophilum* sp. nov., a new pathogen of humans. Int. J. Syst. Bacteriol., *28*:67, 1978.

Stead, W. W., and Dutt, A. K.: What's new in tuberculosis? (editorial). Am. J. Med., *71*:1, 1981.

Timpe, A., and Runyon, E. H.: The relationship of "atypical" acid-fast bacteria to human disease. J. Lab. Clin. Med., *44*:202, 1954.

Tisdall, P. A., DeYoung, D. R., Roberts, G. D., and Anhalt, J. P.: Identification of clinical isolates of mycobacteria with gas liquid chromatography: A 10 month follow-up study. J. Clin. Microbiol., *16*:400, 1982.

Tsang, A. Y., and Farber, E. R.: The primary isolation of *Mycobacterium ulcerans.* Am. J. Clin. Path., *59*:688, 1973.

Valdivia, A., Mendez, J. S., and Font, M. S.: *Mycobacterium habana:* Probable nueva especie dentro de las micobacterias no classificadas. Bol. Hig. Epidemiol. Habana, *9*:65, 1971.

Vestal, A. L.: Procedures for the Isolation and Identification of Mycobacteria. U.S. Department of Health, Education and Welfare, Public Health Service Publication No. (CDC) 75–8230, 1975.

Wallace, R. D., Dalvisio, J. R., and Pankey, G. A.: Disk diffusion testing of susceptibility of *Mycobacterium fortuitum and chelonei.* Antimicrob. Agents Chemother., *16*:611, 1979.

Wayne, L. G.: Simple pyrazinamidase and urease tests for routine identification of mycobacteria. Am. Rev. Resp. Dis., *109*:147, 1974.

Wayne, L. G.: Two varieties of *Mycobacterium kansasii* with different clinical significance. Am. Rev. Resp. Dis., *86*:651, 1962.

Wayne, L. G., and Krasnow, I.: Preparation of tuberculosis drug susceptibility testing media using drug impregnated discs. Tech. Bull. Reg. Med. Tech., *36*:57, 1966.

Weiszfeiler, J. G., and Karczag, E.: Synonymy of *Mycobacterium simiae* Krasseva et al. 1965 and *Mycobacterium habana* Valdivia et al. 1971. Int. J. Syst. Bacteriol., *26*:474, 1976.

Welch, D. F., and Kelly, M. T.: Antimicrobial susceptibility testing of *Mycobacterium fortuitum* complex. Antimicrob. Agents Chemother., *15*:754, 1979.

Wieten, G., Haverkamp, J., Engel, H. W. B., and Berwald, L. G.: Application of pyrolysis mass spectrometry to the classification and identification of mycobacteria. Rev. Infect. Dis., *3*:871, 1981.

Wolinsky, E.: Nontuberculous mycobacteria and associated diseases. Am. Rev. Resp. Dis., *119*:107, 1979.

Wolinsky, E., and Rynearson, T. K.: Mycobacteria in soil and their relation to disease-associated strains. Am. Rev Resp. Dis., 97:1032, 1968.

Zakowski, P., Fligiel, S., Berlin, G. W., and Johnson, L.: Disseminated *Mycobacterium avium-intracellulare* infection in homosexual men dying of acquired immunodeficiency. J.A.M.A., *248*:2980, 1982.

Zimmerman, L. E., Turner, L., and McTigue, J. W.: *Mycobacterium fortuitum* infection of the cornea. Arch. Ophthalmol., *82*:596, 1969.

47

SPIROCHETES AND SPIRAL BACTERIA

RICHARD T. KELLY, M.D.

Spirochetes are motile, spiral-shaped organisms that divide by binary fission. Organisms pathogenic for man are found in three genera: Treponema, Borrelia, and Leptospira. Most of the spirochetes are so narrow that they cannot be visualized by conventional microscopy when stained with common bacteriologic stains. Special staining methods by which the width of the organisms is increased by the deposition of metallic salts allow visualization with the ordinary light microscope. Spirochetes are easily seen with darkfield microscopy, and this technique is usually employed when screening clinical specimens or evaluating cultures.

All pathogenic treponemes are morphologically indistinguishable from one another as well as from some non-pathogenic organisms. Because of this and the inability to cultivate any pathogenic treponemes *in vitro,* great care is required in interpreting clinical specimens. In addition to being morphologically identical, the three species of treponemes are immunologically identical. Thus, an individual with yaws or pinta has reactive serologic tests for syphilis. All treponemal infections respond to penicillin therapy. The amount and duration of antibiotic therapy varies with the stage of disease (Musher, 1981).

TREPONEMA

Treponemes are considered to be anaerobic microorganisms. Several non-pathogenic treponemes can be cultivated, but only under anaerobic conditions. Although pathogenic treponemes have not been cultured *in vitro,* survival studies (based on retention of motility) have shown that survival is greatly prolonged when the microorganisms are incubated in an oxygen-free environment and in the presence of reducing agents.

Syphilis

The etiologic agent of syphilis, *Treponema pallidum,* is a thin, spiral-shaped organism measuring 6 to 15 μ in length but only 0.2 μ in width (Fig. 47–1). The spirals vary in number from 4 to 14 and are rather uniform in appearance when compared with those of certain saprophytic organisms.

Following World War II, the reported incidence of early syphilis in the United States declined each year until 1958, when the rate once again began to progressively rise. In 1980, the number of reported cases of primary and secondary syphilis increased by 9.4 per cent over the total reported for 1979. At present, syphilis is the third most common of the specified reportable infectious diseases in the United States (Centers for Disease Control, 1981).

Syphilis is usually acquired by the venereal route. After a variable incubation period of 10 days to several months, the primary lesion or chancre appears. This begins as a small, usually solitary nodule that with enlargement and subsequent necrosis of the overlying epithelium results in the formation of a relatively painless ulcer. In contrast to other bacterial infections

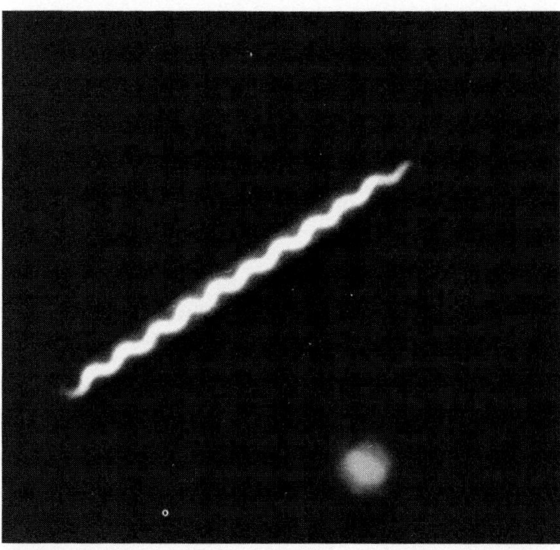

Figure 47–1. *Treponema pallidum,* darkfield preparation ×3500.

6

of the skin, pus is usually absent unless the lesion has become secondarily infected with other bacteria. Lesions are most frequently seen on the external genitalia; however, in women lesions may occur in the vagina and cervix. Chancres heal spontaneously without specific therapy. The systemic nature of the disease becomes apparent six to eight weeks after the appearance of the initial chancre when a generalized rash involving both skin and mucous membranes occurs. During this secondary phase of syphilis, there may also be involvement of the central nervous system, eyes, bones and liver. After a period of weeks to months, the lesions of secondary syphilis resolve spontaneously and the individual enters the latent phase of the disease. In latent syphilis, serologic tests for syphilis are reactive but clinical signs or symptoms are absent. Approximately one third of individuals with untreated latent syphilis will subsequently develop signs of tertiary syphilis—gummas, cardiovascular syphilis, or neurosyphilis.

Gummas are localized areas of granulomatous inflammation which may be found in any organ or tissue in the body. The gumma varies in size from microscopic up to 10 cm in diameter. On histologic examination, the lesions are found to be composed of caseous material surrounded by lymphocytes, plasma cells, and areas of perivascular inflammation. Spirochetes are rarely seen in the lesions, and it is therefore believed that gummas result from tissue hypersensitivity.

The basic lesion in cardiovascular syphilis is aortitis, which results from necrosis of the media secondary to endarteritis of the vasa vasorum of the vessel wall. This may lead to (1) narrowing of the coronary ostia, which is manifested clinically as angina pectoris, (2) dilatation of the aortic commissure and thickening of the valve leaflets, resulting in aortic regurgitation, or (3) aneurysm formation, most frequently of the ascending aorta, due to destruction of the elastic fibers in the wall and fibrosis.

The manifestations of neurosyphilis are highly variable and depend on whether involvement is predominantly meningovascular or parenchymatous. Tabes dorsalis results from degeneration of dorsal roots and columns at the lumbosacral and lower thoracic levels of the spinal cord. In paresis, the brain is shrunken and there is dilatation of the lateral ventricles. Silver impregnation staining techniques will demonstrate *Treponema pallidum* in the brain tissue. In neurosyphilis, the cerebrospinal fluid is reactive for reagin antibody. In addition, the cerebrospinal fluid has an increased cell count (over 4 lymphocytes per cu mm) and protein is elevated above 40 mg per 100 ml.

After the eighteenth week of pregnancy, an infected pregnant woman with early or early latent syphilis will transmit treponemes to the fetus with resultant infection. This may result in stillbirth or congenital syphilis. A diagnosis of congenital syphilis can be readily made in the newborn if treponemes can be demonstrated in mucus from the nasopharynx or lesions. Because of transplacental transfer of maternal antibodies, serologic tests for syphilis in the newborn must be carefully evaluated.

A diagnosis of syphilis and its stage is determined by evaluating three factors: (1) clinical findings, (2) demonstration of spirochetes in clinical specimens, and (3) presence of antibodies in blood or cerebrospinal fluid.

The demonstration of typical, motile treponemes by darkfield microscopy in properly prepared specimens is diagnostic in primary and secondary syphilis. Particular care is required in obtaining specimens from the mouth and oropharynx because of the presence of non-pathogenic treponemes that occur as part of the normal flora. Surgical gloves should be worn to protect the examiner from possible infection when obtaining specimens for darkfield microscopy. Lesions to be sampled are repeatedly cleansed with saline-soaked gauze sponges after removal of any surface crusts and then dried with a dry gauze sponge. The surface of the lesions is then abraded with a dry sponge or swab until bleeding occurs. Excess blood is removed with a sponge until a serous exudate is observed. Pressure applied to the base of the lesion is helpful in increasing the volume of exudate. A coverslip is touched to the surface of the lesion to pick up the exudate and is then inverted onto a microscope slide. The edges of the coverslip should be sealed with Vaspar or lanolin to prevent evaporation and contact with oxygen in the air. As rapidly as possible, preparations are examined with the darkfield microscope at a magnification of about 450×. Erythrocytes are invariably present and serve as a convenient guide to measuring the length of observed organisms. The length of *Treponema pallidum* averages one to two times the diameter of the red cell. The coils of *Treponema pallidum* are uniform and rather tightly wound when compared with those of saprophytic organisms. Marked directional motility is not seen with pathogenic treponema but may be seen in non-pathogenic organisms. If many bacteria other than spirochetes are present, it may indicate that the site was not sufficiently cleansed before sampling, or the lesions may be due to a different infectious process.

Serodiagnosis of Syphilis. Two types of tests are available for the serologic diagnosis of syphilis. One group uses a non-specific antigen which is lipoidal in character. Since 1906 when the first test of this type was developed, a large number of different tests using essentially the same type of antigen have been developed. Collectively, they are known as reagin tests. The term reagin as applied to syphilis serology is unfortunate in that it is easily confused with antibodies of the IgE class, which are also called reagin antibodies. Reagin tests for syphilis are tests which detect antibodies (IgG or IgM) produced by the infected host as a result of the interaction of lipids from either the host or spirochetes, or both, with the immune system of the host. The antigen originally described by Wassermann was an aqueous extract of liver. Current tests use as antigens defined mixtures of cardiolipin, cholesterol, and lecithin.

At present, two reagin tests are commonly performed in the clinical laboratory. These are the VDRL (developed by the Venereal Disease Research Laboratory) and the RPR (rapid plasma reagin). A variant of the RPR, the ART (automated reagin test), permits the test to be done on a large scale by automated equipment.

The VDRL test is performed by adding heat-inactivated serum to antigen, usually on a glass slide. After rotation for four minutes at room temperature, the test is read microscopically for agglutination, which is indicative of a reactive serum.

The RPR circle card test uses a modified VDRL antigen also containing choline and charcoal. The test is commonly done with unheated serum which is added with RPR antigen to a white plastic-coated card. Following rotation for eight minutes at room temperature, the tests are read macroscopically. A reactive test shows black clumps against the white background in contrast to a non-reactive serum, which results in an even light gray color.

All sera reactive with either reagin test should be subsequently tested with a specific treponemal antigen test to rule out biologic false positive reactions.

Specific Treponemal Antigen Tests. The first specific treponemal antigen test, the *Treponema pallidum* immobilization test (TPI), was developed in 1949 and has served as the standard against which all subsequent tests have been compared. The basis for this test was the immobilization of live, motile *Treponema pallidum* organisms by specific antibodies in serum from individuals with syphilis. The test is expensive to perform and is no longer available in the United States for diagnostic purposes.

At present, two specific treponemal antigen tests are available for confirmation of reactive reagin screen tests. The fluorescent treponemal antibody absorption test (FTA-ABS) uses as antigen a killed suspension of *Treponema pallidum* spirochetes obtained from infected rabbits. An aliquot of organisms is applied to a microscope slide and air-dried. The heat inactivated serum to be tested is diluted with sorbent, which is an extract of a non-pathogenic cultivatable treponeme to eliminate non-specific reactions, and applied to the slide. Following incubation and washing, fluorescein-conjugated anti-human globulin is added to the slide. After additional incubation and washing, the slide is examined with the fluorescent microscope. Sera containing antibody will result in fluorescent staining of the spirochetes. The FTA-ABS test is very specific but requires technically skilled and experienced personnel who meticulously adhere to the established protocol. For this reason, many laboratories in recent years have changed to the less technically demanding microhemagglutination assay for *Treponema pallidum* antibodies (MHA-TP). This test is based upon agglutination by specific antibodies in serum with lyophilized, formalinized, tanned sheep erythrocytes sensitized with *Treponema pallidum* antigen. As in the FTA-ABS test, sera (heat inactivation not required) to be tested are treated with an absorbing diluent to remove non-specific reactions. The test is done in microtitration trays; reactive sera produce a smooth mat of agglutinated cells in the wells of the tray.

Interpretation of Serologic Tests. Specific treponemal antigen tests are not recommended for screening purposes since 0.3 per cent of sera will give false positive reactions. By using one of the reagin tests for screening and reserving the treponemal antigen tests for confirmation, the incidence of true false positive reactions is markedly diminished.

The serologic response in the different stages of syphilis is summarized in Table 47–1. In primary syphilis, the RPR test is more sensitive than the VDRL; similarly, the FTA-ABS becomes reactive before the MHA-TP.

Quantitative RPR or VDRL titrations by two-fold dilutions of serum are of assistance in evaluating the extent of the disease process and response to treatment. High titers are indicative of active disease, whereas titers of less than 1:8 suggest latent infection, previous treatment, or late syphilis. Reagin tests should become non-reactive within one year following therapy in primary syphilis and two years when treated in the secondary stage. Reactivity after these intervals suggests inadequate treatment, re-infection, or a biologic false positive reaction. Therapy initiated during the later stage of the disease, however, usually does not result in a reversion of reactivity.

Reagin tests are reactive in a number of patients who do not have syphilis. These biologic false positive reactions may be acute or chronic. Transient false positive reactions are seen in a variety of bacterial and viral illnesses. Chronic false positive reactions frequently occur in patients with lupus erythematosus and other autoimmune diseases. False positive reactions occur also in drug addicts, during pregnancy, and in individuals over the age of 70. Usually, the problem of biological false positive reagin tests can be readily resolved by subsequent testing of sera by one of the specific treponemal antigen tests. A problem occasionally occurs when an individual has a reactive

Table 47–1. COMMONLY USED SEROLOGIC TESTS*

Test	Stage		
	1°	*2°*	*Late*
Nontreponemal (reaginic) tests			
Venereal Disease Research Laboratory test (VDRL)	70%†	99%†	1%‡
Rapid plasma-reagin card test (RPR); automated reagin test (ART)	80%	99%	0%
Specific treponemal tests			
Treponemal immobilization tests (TPI)	50%	97%	95%
Fluorescent antibody absorbed test (FTA-ABS)	85%	100%	98%
T. pallidum hemagglutination assay (TPHA-TP)	65%	100%	95%

*From Tramont, E. C.: *In* Mandell, G. L., Douglas, R. E., and Bennett, J. E. (eds.): Principles and Practice of Infectious Diseases. New York, John Wiley and Sons, 1979, p. 1831.

†Percentage of patients with positive serologic tests in treated or secondary syphilis.

‡Treated late syphilis.

6

reagin test and a borderline FTA-ABS or MHA-TP and there is no history or suggestion of infection. In this situation, the tests are repeated at monthly intervals. Most false positive borderline reactions will usually revert to negative over a several-month period.

Reagin tests in tertiary syphilis are highly variable, ranging from non-reactive to reactive at high dilutions. In neurosyphilis, serum reagin tests may be negative in as many as 50 per cent of cases. Because of exposure to antibiotics for treatment of unrelated infections, or inadequate treatment of primary or secondary syphilis, many cases of neurosyphilis do not present with classic signs or symptoms. The diagnosis must be clinically suspected and confirmed by serologic testing of serum and cerebrospinal fluid. The serum FTA-ABS test is reactive in 95 per cent of cases of neurosyphilis. In the cerebrospinal fluid, reagin tests are more likely to be reactive than the FTA-ABS.

A diagnosis of congenital syphilis is difficult to establish by serologic methods in the newborn because of transplacental transfer of IgG antibodies. The FTA-ABS (IgM) test was developed specifically for detecting immunoglobulins of the IgM class produced as a result of active infection in infected infants. Although initial reports of the use of this test in diagnosing congenital syphilis were favorable, subsequent studies have been disappointing and the test is not recommended. In suspected cases of congenital syphilis, serial monthly quantitative reagin tests (VDRL or RPR) should be performed on the infant's serum. If the reagin antibodies are a result of maternal transfer, titers will drop, whereas with true infection, titers will remain the same or increase.

Yaws and Pinta

The etiologic agents of yaws, *Treponema pertenue,* and pinta, *Treponema carateum,* are morphologically and immunologically identical to *Treponema pallidum.* Yaws is a disease of skin and bone affecting primarily children in tropical and subtropical countries. The initial lesion or mother yaw develops three to four weeks after exposure. This begins as an erythematous nodule and subsequently ulcerates. Disseminated secondary lesions of a similar nature develop six weeks to three months after the initial lesion and may continue for months to years. Tertiary lesions consisting of gummatous lesions of skin and bone do occur, but visceral lesions are rare. Pinta is found primarily in children in Central and South America. It affects only the skin and initially is manifested as red and blue lesions that later become depigmented. Both yaws and pinta are acquired by contact with infected persons; it is also possible that flies serve as vectors of transmission. Diagnosis is established by darkfield microscopy of material from suspect lesions.

Lyme Disease

Lyme disease was first described in 1975 in a group of patients from Lyme, Connecticut. Prominent features of the disease include expanding, annular erythematous skin lesions (erythema chronicum migrans) and recurrent episodes of arthritis. Some patients have also had symptoms of aseptic meningitis, encephalitis, cardiac abnormalities, and neuropathies. Patients respond to penicillin therapy, and the etiological agent was believed to be due to a penicillin sensitive agent transmitted by Ixodes species of ticks. Recently, Burgdorfer and associates isolated a treponeme-like spirochete from *Ixodes dammini* ticks, which reacted in high titers to sera from individuals convalescing from the disease but not from a control group (Burgdorfer, 1982). The organism, as yet unnamed, has also been isolated from the blood of two patients in the acute phase of illness by inoculating blood into media originally developed for the cultivation of borreliae (q.v.) (Benach, 1983). Lyme disease cases have been reported from 12 states, predominantly in Eastern and Midwestern parts of the United States; however, recent data suggest a larger geographical distribution.

BORRELIA

Borreliae are loosely coiled, spiral-shaped organisms that measure 10 to 20 μ in length and 0.2 to 0.4 μ in width. In contrast to other spirochetes, borreliae can be visualized by staining with aniline dyes (Fig. 47–2). A number of borrelia species have been successfully grown *in vitro* in complex enriched media.

Relapsing Fever

Two varieties of relapsing fever based on the arthropod vector transmitting the disease are recognized (Kelly, 1981). *Borrelia recurrentis* is the sole etiologic agent of louse-borne relapsing fever and is transmitted from man to man by the human body louse, *Pediculus humanus.* Tick-borne relapsing fever is caused by a variety of different species of borrelia, each of which is transmitted by and named for the species of Ornithodoros tick that acts as vector for the organisms. Rodents serve as natural reservoirs for tick-borne borreliae, and, in addition, borreliae are transmitted transovarianly in the tick, thus increasing the number of infected ticks. In the United States, the principal species of tick-borne borreliae are *B. hermsi, B. turicatae,* and *B. parkeri.*

Relapsing fever develops 2 to 15 days after infected lice are crushed during scratching or following the bite of an infected tick. It is a septicemic illness and is characterized by high fever and prostration that persist for three to seven days. An afebrile interval of days to weeks then occurs, followed by relapse. In untreated individuals, the number of sequential relapses may be as high as five. During the acute phases of the disease, borreliae can be seen in blood smears stained by the Wright or Giemsa method, or in darkfield preparations of wet mounts. During afebrile periods, the number of organisms present may be inadequate for microscopic detection, and animal inoculation or cultures may be necessary to recover borreliae. Young mice are inoculated intraperitoneally

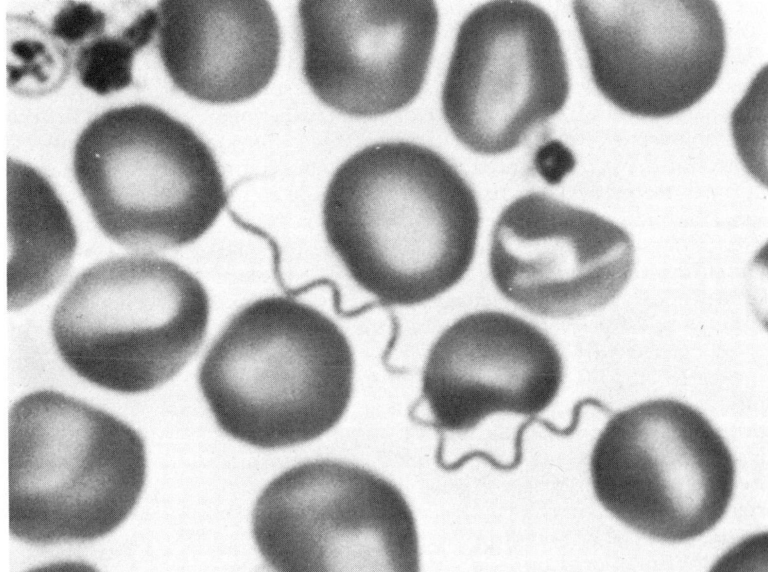

Figure 47–2. *Borrelia hermsi* in blood, Giemsa stain ×3500.

with 1 ml of citrated blood. At daily intervals, the tips of the tails are snipped with scissors to obtain a drop of blood that is either smeared and stained or examined by darkfield microscopy. Borreliae will not grow in conventional blood culture media and until recently could not be cultured *in vitro.* Complex media have been developed that permit isolation and growth of a number of species, including those found in the United States (Kelly, 1976).

Because of the lack of commercially obtainable reagents, serologic methods are not helpful in establishing a diagnosis of relapsing fever.

Relapsing fever responds well to treatment with a number of antibiotics. Tetracycline therapy is frequently employed.

Fusospirochetal Infection

In acute necrotizing ulcerative gingivitis (trench mouth, *Vincent's angina),* a number of species of anaerobic bacteria have been implicated as etiologic agents. Fusobacteria, bacteroides, and various spirochetes including *Borrelia (Treponema) vincenti* have been isolated or observed in smears. The various anaerobes apparently act synergistically in the pathogenesis of the disease process. The diagnosis is established by examining Gram's stains of smears from clinical infection that will demonstrate fusiform bacteria and numerous spirochetes. Penicillin or tetracycline therapy is effective.

LEPTOSPIRA

Leptospires are 6 to 20 μ long but only 0.1 μ wide. The organisms usually have hooked ends and are tightly coiled (Fig. 47–3). Two species of leptospires are recognized. *Leptospira biflexa* is a saprophyte found in fresh water. Over 100 different serotypes of the pathogenic species, *Leptospira interrogans,* are known. Human infections are most commonly due to organisms in the canicola, icterohaemorrhagiae, pomona, and autumnalis serogroups. Many different mammals serve as reservoir hosts for leptospira. Organisms are localized in the kidneys of chronically infected animals and are passed in the urine. Human infection results from contact with animal urine or water which has been contaminated with urine. Leptospirosis develops after an incubation period of 10 to 12 days. The signs and symptoms vary from a mild fever to severe illness, including jaundice, kidney failure, and meningitis.

Leptospirosis is an uncommon disease with only 85 cases being reported in the United States during the year 1980. Because of this and the relative non-

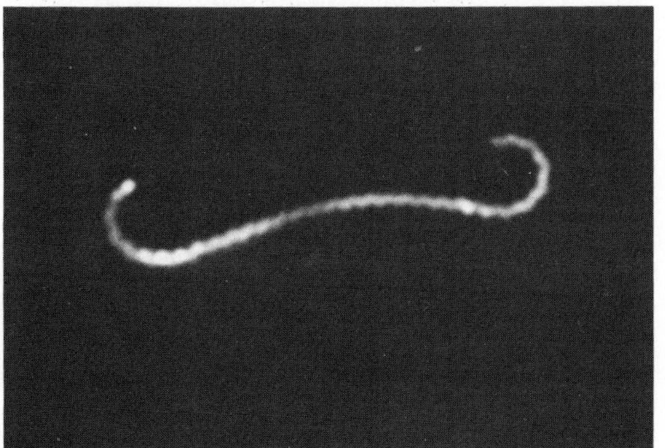

Figure 47–3. *Leptospira interrogans,* serovar *icterohaemorrhagiae,* darkfield preparation ×4000.

specificity of clinical symptoms, a diagnosis of leptospirosis may at times be difficult to establish. Although frequently requested by clinicians, darkfield examination of blood for the presence of leptospires is unreliable because of the presence of artifacts that may resemble leptospires. During the first week of illness, leptospira may be cultured from the blood. Urine cultures are more likely to be positive in the second week of illness, and organisms may be seen in darkfield preparations of urine. Special culture techniques and enriched media are required for recovery of leptospira from clinical specimens. Fletcher's or Stuart's medium containing 10 per cent heat-inactivated rabbit serum is inoculated with one or two drops of blood and incubated at 30°C. (Alexander, 1980). The incorporation of 5-fluorouracil, 200 μg/ml, in media for urine cultures inhibits the growth of contaminating bacteria but does not affect growth of leptospira. Because of the presence of possible inhibitory substances in urine, it is advisable to inoculate tubes of media with one or two drops of urine diluted 1 to 10 as well as undiluted urine. Cultures should be examined weekly by darkfield microscopy for six weeks before discarding as negative.

Serologic tests are very helpful in establishing a diagnosis of leptospirosis, particularly when cultures are negative. Agglutination tests using as antigen commercially available suspensions of pooled, killed leptospires will show rising titers by the second or third week of illness.

Although penicillin and other antibiotics inhibit the growth of leptospira *in vitro,* treatment of clinical cases with antibiotics does not appreciably alter the course of the disease (Stoenner, 1976).

SPIRILLUM

Spirillum minor is the only species pathogenic for man in the genus *Spirillum.* This spiral-shaped, gram-negative organism contains bipolar flagella and measures 0.5 μ in width and 1.7 to 5.0 μ in length. *Spirillum minor* and *Streptobacillus moniliformis* are both etiologic agents of rat-bite fever. The disease that occurs in man following exposure to *Spirillum minor* is termed sodoku and develops approximately two weeks after one has been bitten by a rat, mouse, or other rodent, or by rodent-eating animals such as cats. Sodoku is more common in Asia, and cases in the United States are quite rare. *Spirillum minor* has not been successfully grown *in vitro,* and diagnosis is dependent on demonstrating organisms in clinical specimens or by animal inoculation. Both forms of the disease respond to penicillin therapy (Ericsson, 1982).

Alexander, A. D.: Leptospira. *In* Lennette, E. H., Balows, A., Hausler, W. J., and Truant, J. P.: Manual of Clinical Microbiology. 3rd ed. Washington, American Society for Microbiology, 1980, p. 376.

Benach, J. L., Bosler, E. M., Hanrahan, J. P., Coleman, J. L., Habicht, G. S., Bast, T. F., Cameron, D. J., Ziegler, J. L., Barbour, A. G., Burgdorfer, W., Edelman, R., and Kaslow, R. A.: Spirochetes isolated from the blood of two patients with Lyme disease. N. Engl. J. Med., *308*:740, 1983.

Burgdorfer, W., Barbour, A. G., Hayes, S. F., Benach, J. L., Grunwald, T. E., and Davis, J. D.: Lyme disease—a tick borne spirochetosis. Science, *216*:1317, 1982.

Centers for Disease Control: Reported morbidity and mortality in the United States. Morbid. Mortal. Weekly Rep., *29*:78, 1981.

Ericsson, C. D.: Rat-bite fever. *In* Conn, H. F. (ed.): Current Therapy. Philadelphia, W. B. Saunders Company, 1982, p. 59.

Kelly, R. T.: Cultivation and physiology of relapsing fever borreliae. *In* Johnson, R. C. (ed.): The Biology of Parasitic Spirochetes. New York, Academic Press, 1976, p. 87.

Kelly, R. T.: The genus Borrelia. *In* Starr, M. P., Stolp, P. H., Trüper, H. G., Balows, A., and Schlegel, H. G. (eds.): The Prokaryotes. Berlin, Springer-Verlag, 1981, p. 578.

Musher, D. M.: Syphilis of the genital tract. *In* Braude, A. I. (ed.): Medical Microbiology and Infectious Diseases. Philadelphia, W. B. Saunders Company, 1981, p. 1216.

Stoenner, H. G.: Treatment and control of leptospirosis. *In* Johnson, R. C. (ed.): The Biology of Parasitic Spirochetes. New York, Academic Press, 1976, p. 375.

48

MYCOTIC DISEASE

ELMER W. KONEMAN, M.D., and GLENN D. ROBERTS, PH.D.

Interest in medical mycology has been on the upswing in the United States for the past decade. To some degree, attention to medical mycology has been a necessity because of the dramatic increase in the number of compromised patients who are receiving long-term courses of broad-spectrum antibiotics, corticosteroids, antimetabolites, or anticancer drugs or who are undergoing complex surgical procedures that require intensive postoperative life support. General improvement in medical care has led to a large population of individuals who are living to an older age with chronic diseases, such as diabetes mellitus, but who also are more susceptible to opportunistic fungal infections.

To a greater extent, however, this resurgent interest in mycology reflects a new discovery among general microbiologists and medical technologists that the study of mycology is innately fascinating. To a large degree, this has been brought about through the circulation of unknown fungal samples to clinical laboratories participating in various survey and proficiency test programs where technologists have the opportunity to study fungal species not frequently encountered in routine practice. The development of practical identification schemata that have recently been published in the literature and discussed in detail in mycology workshops throughout the country has served to remove some of the fear of approaching a subject that until recently was considered difficult and obscure.

Although this laboratory enthusiasm has to some extent had its effect in improving the diagnosis of mycotic disease, many primary care practitioners are still woefully lacking in their understanding of the basic principles of clinical mycology and how to properly approach a patient with potential fungal disease. There is a great need to increase physician awareness of the various clinical signs and symptoms of mycotic disease and of how to properly collect specimens and have them transported to the laboratory. Clinical pathologists, microbiologists, and medical technologists have a unique opportunity, even an obligation, to participate frequently in infectious disease conferences, grand rounds, and other teaching activities in which the clinical and laboratory diagnosis of mycotic disease can be openly discussed.

Therefore, the approach to the discussion of mycotic diseases in this chapter will take a somewhat different turn from the presentations in most current textbooks. The discussion will follow a natural sequence paralleling the manner in which the diagnosis of fungal disease is made in actual clinical practice.

There are three major areas of diagnostic activity, as outlined in Figure 48–1.

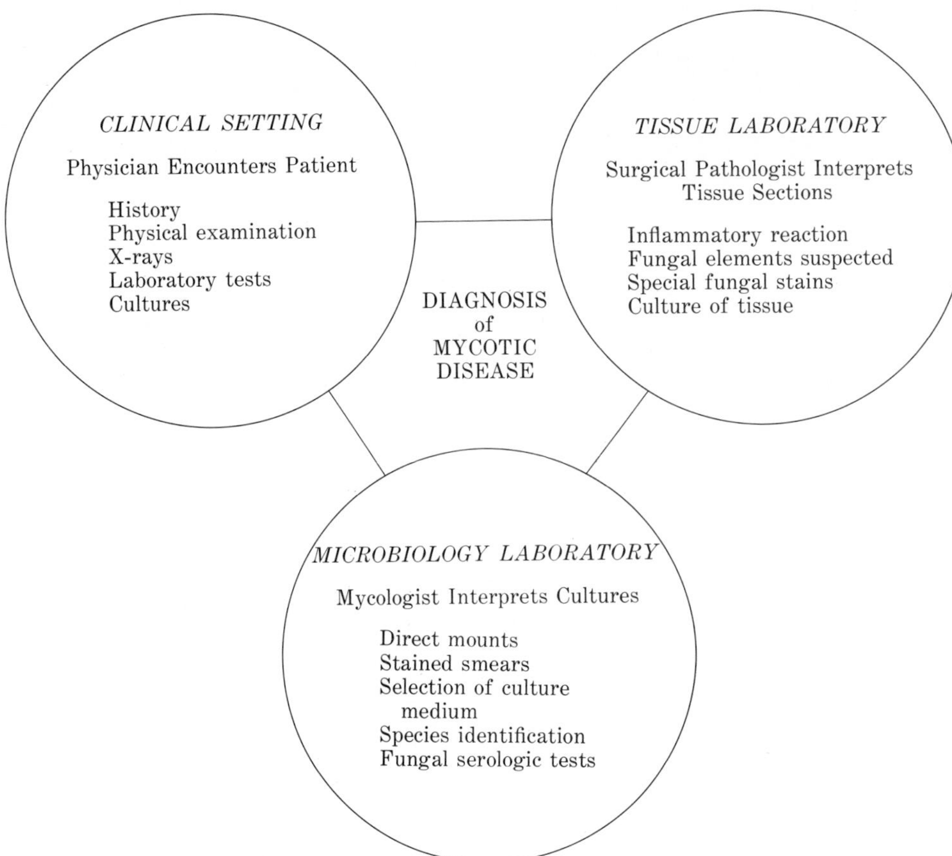

Figure 48–1. Diagnosis of fungal disease: spheres of activity.

1. *The Clinical Setting:* The physician encounters a patient with certain symptomatology, takes a history, performs a physical examination, requests x-rays and diagnostic laboratory tests, and obtains appropriate cultures.

2. *The Tissue Laboratory:* The surgical pathologist examines tissues submitted to the laboratory, prepares tissue sections, and examines them microscopically for characteristic tissue reactions and fungal elements. Special stains may be required. Portions of tissue are submitted for culture.

3. *The Microbiology Laboratory:* The microbiologist or mycologist processes and interprets cultures and makes a final species identification of any fungal organisms recovered.

The effectiveness with which any given patient with potential mycotic disease is evaluated and properly treated is dependent upon how well the communications are maintained among these three activities. If the physician is not alert to leading signs and symptoms of fungal infection or fails to obtain proper specimens, perhaps sending them to the laboratory in improper containers or fixed in formalin; if the surgical pathologist fails to recognize tissue reactions or the presence of structures suspicious for fungal infection or does not submit a portion of the tissue for culture; or if the mycologist fails to prepare direct mounts or stained smears or does not select appropriate culture media for the recovery of certain species of fungi, either by omission or because he was not informed of the physician's clinical impression, the ability to make a final diagnosis may be lost or severely compromised.

Figure 48–2 is an algorithm serving to illustrate the clinical and laboratory approach to the diagnosis of mycotic disease and also to outline the subsequent discussion in this chapter.

CLINICAL PRESENTATION OF MYCOTIC DISEASE

The time-honored taxonomy of the mycoses, based on clinical presentation of fungal diseases—namely (1) superficial mycoses, (2) subcutaneous mycoses, and (3) disseminated (deep-seated) mycoses—must now be viewed from a somewhat different perspective. The many situations in which host defenses are now compromised, as discussed above, has made the practical implementation of this classification difficult.

Fungi formerly considered non-pathogenic or limited to only one organ system, under proper circumstances and in a compromised host, can cause disease.

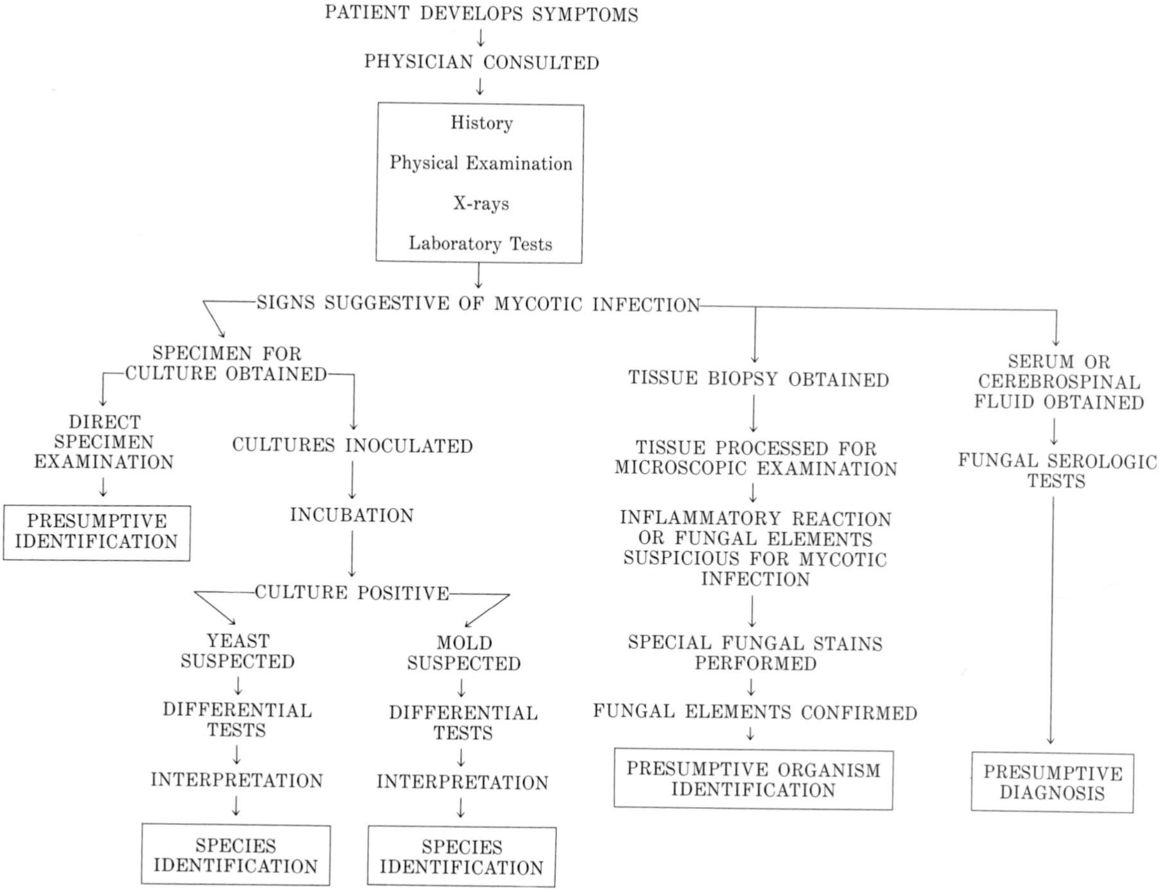

PATIENT DEVELOPS SYMPTOMS
↓
PHYSICIAN CONSULTED
↓
History
Physical Examination
X-rays
Laboratory Tests
↓
SIGNS SUGGESTIVE OF MYCOTIC INFECTION

SPECIMEN FOR CULTURE OBTAINED
→ DIRECT SPECIMEN EXAMINATION → PRESUMPTIVE IDENTIFICATION
→ CULTURES INOCULATED → INCUBATION → CULTURE POSITIVE
→ YEAST SUSPECTED → DIFFERENTIAL TESTS → INTERPRETATION → SPECIES IDENTIFICATION
→ MOLD SUSPECTED → DIFFERENTIAL TESTS → INTERPRETATION → SPECIES IDENTIFICATION

TISSUE BIOPSY OBTAINED → TISSUE PROCESSED FOR MICROSCOPIC EXAMINATION → INFLAMMATORY REACTION OR FUNGAL ELEMENTS SUSPICIOUS FOR MYCOTIC INFECTION → SPECIAL FUNGAL STAINS PERFORMED → FUNGAL ELEMENTS CONFIRMED → PRESUMPTIVE ORGANISM IDENTIFICATION

SERUM OR CEREBROSPINAL FLUID OBTAINED → FUNGAL SEROLOGIC TESTS → PRESUMPTIVE DIAGNOSIS

Figure 48–2. Algorithm for approach to diagnosis of fungal disease.

The clinician must be aware that the recovery of certain fungal species from the skin, mucous membranes, or other sites may not represent localized disease but a manifestation of disseminated involvement. Further studies, including culture of several secretions, especially sputum and urine, are required to determine the extent of involvement. The mucocutaneous presentation of *Histoplasma capsulatum, Blastomyces dermatitidis,* and *Cryptococcus neoformans* in particular most commonly indicates disseminated disease. Therefore, except in cases of classic superficial cutaneous dermatophyte infections which are known to remain localized, it is probably wise to assume that virtually any fungus species recovered in a symptomatic host potentially can represent disseminated disease, and a complete evaluation of the patient is indicated.

General Symptoms of Mycotic Disease

Deep-seated or disseminated fungal diseases may clinically mimic a number of other generalized diseases, such as tuberculosis, brucellosis, syphilis, sarcoidosis, and disseminated carcinomatosis, to name a few. It is necessary to recover the etiologic agent in culture or demonstrate it in biopsy specimens before a final diagnosis can be made.

Such non-specific complaints as fever, night sweats, weight loss, lassitude, easy fatigability, cough, chest pain, and so forth may be common to all of these conditions. Abnormal laboratory test results, such as leukocytosis (neutrophilia, lymphocytosis, and monocytosis), elevation in the erythrocyte sedimentation rate, or elevation in serum enzymes or protein fractions, indicate only that some type of inflammatory response is present, but are of little aid in making a differential diagnosis. Positive x-ray findings, such as pulmonary infiltrates or evidence of inflammatory processes in other organs, are rarely specific. In some patients with severely compromised host resistance, these general symptoms may be minimal, if present at all.

Therefore, the initial clue to the presence of possible fungal disease in a given patient often must come from the recognition of more specific signs and/or symptoms or from information derived from the clinical history. Since fungal diseases are rarely if ever transmitted from man to man, but rather are contracted from the environment, it is important that the physician elicit important historical information from the patient, such as past or recent travel into

6

geographic areas known to be endemic for certain fungi, or exposure to soil, dust, or other materials having a high probability of contamination.

Specific Signs and Symptoms of Fungal Disease

Tables 48–1 to 48–4 outline the clinical types of fungal diseases, specific symptomatology, modes of infection, and some of the differential diagnoses to be considered for the fungi most commonly causing human infections. The mycotic diseases included in Tables 48–1 to 48–4 are listed in Table 48–5. Table 48–1 includes those fungi that routinely cause deep-seated mycoses and can be generally considered pathogenic whenever isolated from a human host. Table 48–2 lists those fungi that are opportunistic pathogens, causing localized organ disease or, rarely, disseminated mycoses in hosts with compromised immune resistance. Table 48–3 includes those fungi that are most commonly incriminated in various types of subcutaneous diseases, although reported cases of deep visceral or disseminated diseases can be found in the literature. Table 48–4 lists those fungi that cause only superficial cutaneous disease limited to the keratinized integument and are not known to cause invasive or disseminated mycotic disease.

These tables have been constructed to provide the physician with a quick review of the fungal diseases most commonly encountered in clinical practice. These tables are in no way complete, and other references are recommended for more detailed coverage. It is hoped, however, that this manner of presentation will provide those symptoms and epidemiologic factors necessary to formulate inductively a working diagnosis when confronted by a patient with certain leading signs and symptoms, as outlined in these tables.

The morphologic characteristics by which the laboratory diagnosis for each of the fungi discussed can be made will be presented in later sections of this chapter.

APPROACH TO THE DEEP-SEATED MYCOSES

The various clinical parameters of the deep-seated mycoses are summarized in Table 48–1. One of these mycotic diseases must be considered in the differential diagnosis of any patient who presents with signs and symptoms of chronic inflammatory or debilitating disease. Symptoms such as low grade fever, weight loss, malaise, or persistence of single organ symptoms should draw one's attention to the potential for mycotic disease, although tuberculosis, systemic bacterial infections, and neoplasm must be ruled out.

If one of the deep-seated mycoses is suspected, it is important that the physician carefully examine the skin and mucous membranes. Histoplasmosis, for example, may first manifest itself with non-healing ulcerating lesions of the buccal mucosa, tongue, or posterior pharynx. Purulent material must be obtained from any suspicious lesion, direct mounts or stained smears for microscopic examination prepared, and a portion submitted for culture. Direct microscopic examination of purulent or serous material may provide an immediate diagnosis if "sulfur granules," budding yeasts, hyphal forms, or other fungal structures are identified.

If exudative material cannot be obtained from the lesion, a biopsy may be necessary. It is important that the physician alert the tissue laboratory if he suspects mycotic disease so that the biopsy specimen can be handled properly and small portions of tissue submitted for culture. Tissue biopsy specimens should be submitted to the laboratory in a sterile 4 by 4 inch gauze. Larger specimens should be submitted in sterile containers, and formalin fixative or "saline for injection," to which antibacterial substances have been added, should be avoided.

More than one specimen should be obtained from any patient in whom a deep-seated mycotic disease is suspected. For example, if spinal fluid is obtained from a patient with suspected fungal meningitis, sputum, urine, and possibly blood should also be submitted for culture. It is not uncommon for *Cryptococcus neoformans* to be recovered from the blood or urine when spinal fluid cultures fail to yield organisms.

Patients should be carefully questioned concerning travel to known endemic areas or about exposure to materials that may be potentially contaminated with fungal spores. History of a recent traumatic injury involving breaks in the skin or mucous membrane may be an extremely important point of information. The epidemiology of the fungal species causing deep-seated mycoses is outlined in Table 48–1.

APPROACH TO THE OPPORTUNISTIC MYCOSES

Table 48–2 outlines the clinical parameters of the more commonly encountered fungi that may be incriminated in the mycoses caused by certain species of opportunistic fungi. The various species of *Aspergillus, Candida, Geotrichum,* and Zygomycetes, as well as the bacteria *Actinomyces* and *Nocardia,* are widely distributed in nature and often are found as commensal inhabitants of the skin, respiratory passages, or gastrointestinal tract. Therefore, whenever one of these species is recovered from a patient with suspected infectious disease, it is necessary that the organism be isolated on repeated cultures directly from the site of infection before any given isolate can be considered pathogenic.

Physicians should be on the alert for opportunistic fungal infection in any patient whose immunologic response is compromised. The prolonged administration of broad-spectrum antibiotics or treatment with anticancer drugs inhibits both cellular and immune responses so that the usual symptoms and signs of infection may be obscure. Therefore, culture of secretions may be indicated even in the absence of clinical signs of infection. However, the recovery of an opportunistic fungal species from an immunosuppressed host should not preclude a thorough examination of the patient in search for a second microorganism of potentially greater significance that may be masked by the more rapidly growing opportunist.

Text continued on page 1163

Table 48–1. CLINICAL PARAMETERS OF THE DEEP-SEATED MYCOSES

Fungal Disease	Etiologic Agents	Clinical Disease Manifestations: Signs and Symptoms	Epidemiology and Modes of Infection	Differential Considerations
Blastomycosis	*Blastomyces dermatitidis*	*Primary Pulmonary Blastomycosis* *Self-Limited Disease:* Symptoms of non-specific respiratory disease—non-productive cough, intermittent chest pain, low grade fever, joint and muscle aches. *Progressive Disease:* Onset may be insidious, acting as a persistent "chest cold." Weight loss and progressive disability may be first signs. Cough productive of purulent or blood-tinged sputum, dyspnea, chest pain may increase in severity. Lung consolidation, pneumonia, and hilar adenopathy become evident on x-ray. *Primary Cutaneous Blastomycosis* *Gilchrist's Disease:* Rare. Lesions first appear on unclothed areas of skin, hands, face, and forearms. Firm, coalescing skin nodules first appear, with suppuration of their centers. Lesions become wartlike, spreading over the surface with verrucous borders. Cutaneous involvement usually means disseminated disease, which must always be ruled out. *Disseminated Blastomycosis* Patient experiences increase in fever, night chills, sweating, and progressive weakness. Skin is involved in large proportion of cases. Bone lesions occur in ⅔ of patients, usually in ribs or vertebrae. Spinal cord compression may result from vertebral collapse. Liver, spleen, kidneys, and prostate are the viscera most commonly involved; central nervous system lesions occur in ⅓ of patients.	No known animal to man or man to man transmission. Soil is thought to be the most probable source, although *B. dermatitidis* has only rarely been cultured from that source. Endemic disease in patients living in the Mississippi and Ohio river valleys, particularly those in close contact with the soil. Pulmonary disease is most common manifestation, presumably from inhalation of spores. Primary cutaneous disease results from inoculation of traumatic breaks in the skin with contaminated soil, dung, or other material.	*Pulmonary* -Tuberculosis -Aspiration pneumonia -Carcinoma of the lung -Other mycoses: Histoplasmosis Coccidioidomycosis Nocardiosis *Cutaneous* -Basal cell carcinoma -Leishmania: tropical sore -Other mycoses *Disseminated* -Tuberculosis -Metastatic carcinomatosis -Kala-azar -Other mycoses
Coccidioidomycosis	*Coccidioides immitis*	*Primary Pulmonary Coccidioidomycosis* 60% of infected individuals are asymptomatic. Remainder have "grippe" or influenza-like symptoms: fever, chills, headache, arthralgia, and dyspnea ("valley fever"). Chest pain aggravated by breathing, or sharp pleuritic pains simulating traumatic rib fracture or myocardial infarction. Cough usually non-productive and hemoptysis is rare. 2% of infected individuals ultimately present with residual cavitary or solid "coin lesions." Cavities are thin-walled, peripheral in location, and can closely simulate tuberculosis. *Primary Cutaneous Coccidioidomycosis* Primary skin lesions are rare, usually self-limited, and heal without sequelae. Erythema multiforme and erythema nodosum are common complications and are thought to portend a good prognosis. Erythematous rash is a frequent manifestation, secondary to a hypersensitivity reaction.	*C. immitis* is endemic in the dry desert regions of the southwestern United States and in Mexico. Man acquires the disease from exogenous sources, after contact with infected soil or inhalation of dust-laden spores. One reported incidence of man to man transmission occurred in six medical staff members attending a patient with osteolytic coccidioidomycosis where the infective mycelial form developed in the plaster cast. Spores disseminated in air currents were inhaled by the attendees (Emmons, 1977).	Clinical manifestations are protean, and primary disease can simulate many other bacterial, mycotic, or disseminated neoplastic diseases. Cavitary lesions may simulate tuberculosis, particularly when the lesions involve the upper lobes of the lungs. "Coin" lesions are often surgically removed, since they cannot be distinguished radiologically from solitary bronchiolar carcinoma or metastatic neoplasm.

(Table continued on following page)

Table 48–1. CLINICAL PARAMETERS OF THE DEEP-SEATED MYCOSES *(Continued)*

Fungal Disease	Etiologic Agents	Clinical Disease Manifestations: Signs and Symptoms	Epidemiology and Modes of Infection	Differential Considerations
		Disseminated Coccidioidomycosis Fever, rapidly progressing weight loss, and weakness are usual manifestations. Headache may be severe with CNS involvement, secondary to hydrocephalus. Cutaneous lesions are usually due to disseminated disease; destructive lymphadenopathy, osteomyelitis meningitis, and visceral involvement often seen in fatal cases.		
Cryptococcosis	*Cryptococcus neoformans*	*Central Nervous System Cryptococcosis* Insidious or abrupt onset of neurologic symptoms usually bring patient to physician: headache, increasing in frequency and severity; ataxia and vertigo; vomiting; memory lapses; and, less commonly, seizures of the jacksonian type. *Pulmonary Cryptococcosis* Symptoms often less than extent of disease: fever is usually mild or absent; cough is usually minimal, with production of scanty mucoid, blood-tinged sputum. Pleural pain occasionally present; pleural effusion rare. Rales and rhonchi are minimal because there is little exudation into the bronchial tree. *Disseminated Cryptococcosis* All viscera and organ systems may be involved. Cutaneous manifestations in 5% of cases: papules and vesicles of the face. Widely disseminated osseous lesions occur in 10% of cases. Weight loss, malaise, and persistence of fever often seen. Headache, vomiting, dizziness, restlessness, hallucinations, and personality changes simulating psychosis may be initial manifestations.	Cryptococci have a natural habitat in the soil. *C. neoformans* may be particularly found in the dust of pigeon droppings due to the alkaline medium rich in nitrogen which promotes growth. Man is particularly susceptible to infection when cleaning up dung-infested areas. Pigeons act as carriers of the organism but do not develop primary disease, presumably because of their high body temperature. The possibility of endogenous infection is still debated. Development of virulence in latent yeast cells inhaled at some previous time is a possibility.	*CNS* -Tubercular meningitis -Meningeal carcinomatosis *Pulmonary* -Tuberculosis -Other mycoses. The cavitary lesions of cryptococcosis can be distinguished from tuberculosis and histoplasmosis in that the thick wall or areas of calcification do not develop. *Disseminated* -Tuberculosis -Other mycoses -Mucin secreting carcinoma. It may be particularly difficult to differentiate gelatinous cysts of cryptococcus from mucin-secreting carcinoma.
Histoplasmosis	*Histoplasma capsulatum*	*Pulmonary Histoplasmosis* *Acute Form:* Disease usually mild or may be asymptomatic. Process usually self-limited. Nonproductive cough, shortness of breath, chest pain, hoarseness, hemoptysis, and cyanosis may be present. *Chronic Form:* Chronic cavitary lesions may develop in adults. Symptoms may include chronic cough, low-grade fever, and occasional hemoptysis. X-rays may be diagnostic if a radiodense, thick, laminated and calcified "histoplasmoma" is present.	Infections in the United States are most prevalent in the Mississippi River valley and its tributaries. Source of human infection is probably the soil. Soil laden with excreta of chickens, turkeys, birds, and bats ("cave fever") may have a high concentration of *H. capsulatum* organisms. Human infections most commonly result from inhalation of spore-laden dust. Serious acute infections have	*Pulmonary* -Tuberculosis -Viral pneumonia -Lipoidal pneumonia -Hamman-Rich syndrome -Interstitial fibrosis -Sarcoidosis *Disseminated* -Hodgkin's disease

		Disseminated Histoplasmosis Pulmonary symptoms may be minimal. Hepatosplenomegaly and diffuse lymphadenopathy are usually present in varying degrees of severity due to propensity of fungus to invade the cells of the reticuloendothelial system. Fever, anemia, leukopenia, weight loss, and lassitude often portend disseminated disease. Solitary or multiple ulcerations of the skin, mucous membranes, or intestinal lining may be initial indication of disseminated disease. Any of the viscera may be involved; adrenal gland disease leading to Addison's disease may lead to fatal outcome.	been reported following clean-up of chicken houses or turkey pens or removal of the dung from city squares under trees inhabited by starlings or other birds.	-Lymphosarcoma -Kala-azar
Paracoccidioidomycosis	*Paracoccidioides brasiliensis*	*Mucous Membrane Paracoccidioidomycosis* Ulcerating lesions present in the nasal or oral mucosa, gingivae; less commonly in the conjunctiva or anorectal mucosa. The ulcerations spread slowly and have a mulberry-like reddened appearance with yellow speckles. Extension to the tonsils is common. Lymphadenitis of the face and neck is severe. *Cutaneous Paracoccidioidomycosis* Lesions occur most commonly on the face, particularly in a perioral distribution, in association with oral mucous membrane disease. The lesions characteristically are ulcerative, have a crusted surface and a serpiginous border. Cervical lymph nodes are involved early in the disease. *Pulmonary Paracoccidioidomycosis* Pulmonary disease occurs in a high percentage of cases and the lungs may represent the portal of entry. Signs and symptoms often less than degree of involvement would indicate. Productive cough, hemoptysis, dyspnea, fever, malaise, weight loss, and easy fatigability are experienced in varying degrees. *Disseminated Paracoccidioidomycosis* The lymphatic system, spleen, intestines, and liver are most commonly involved. Extensive pulmonary disease, central nervous system disease, adrenal insufficiency, or perforation of intestinal ulcers is a more common cause of death.	Paracoccidioidomycosis is limited to the South American continent. Prevalence is highest in Brazil, Venezuela, and Colombia; the disease has not been reported in Chile, Guyana, and Surinam in South America, or in El Salvador, Nicaragua, or Panama in Central America. Most common portal of entry is still debated; however, current theory implicates the lungs. Infections through traumatic areas in the nasal mucosa, gums, oral mucosa, or pharynx have not been totally discounted. Primary inoculation may result from eating of raw vegetables. Inhalation of spores results in primary lung infections.	*Mucocutaneous* -Cutaneous tuberculosis -Syphilis -Yaws -Cutaneous leishmaniasis (tropical sore) -Sporotrichosis -Basal cell carcinoma *Pulmonary* -Tuberculosis -Other mycoses *Disseminated* -Tuberculosis -Tuberculous adenitis -Tertiary syphilis

Table 48–2. CLINICAL PARAMETERS OF THE OPPORTUNISTIC MYCOSES

Fungal Disease	Etiologic Agent	Clinical Disease Manifestations: Signs and Symptoms	Epidemiology and Modes of Infection	Differential Considerations
Aspergillosis	*Aspergillus fumigatus* *Aspergillus flavus* *Aspergillus niger* *Aspergillus terreus* Other *Aspergillus* species	*Pulmonary Aspergillosis* *Invasive:* Chief symptom is hemoptysis, resulting from necrotizing bronchopneumonia and pulmonary infarction (thromboses occur because of the propensity of the fungal hyphae to invade blood vessels). Dyspnea, fever, and tachypnea occur in progressive disease. *Allergic:* Most commonly develops in asthmatics who develop hypersensitivity to aspergilli antigens. Wheezing, cough, fever, and pleuritic pain are common symptoms. The presence of mucous plugs containing eosinophils and Charcot-Leyden crystals in expectorated sputum samples is highly suggestive of this form of the disease. *Fungus Ball:* Congenital bronchial cysts or cavitary lesions caused by tuberculosis, bronchiectasis, or carcinoma may become colonized with one of the aspergilli, notably *A. fumigatus*. The fungus colony tends to remain localized to the cyst cavity, only rarely invades into the adjacent pulmonary tissue, and is most commonly asymptomatic. *Otomycotic Aspergillosis* An aspergillus, notably *A. niger*, becomes colonized within a cerumen plug in the external auditory canal. Irritation of the canal mucosa occurs, resulting in itching, superficial erosion of the tympanic membrane, and impaired hearing. The exudate is usually foul smelling.	The spores of aspergilli are ubiquitous in nature, produced from mycelial forms that grow as saprobic fungi on decaying vegetation. Since aspergillus spores are commonly inhaled, aspergilli of various strains may be recovered from the upper respiratory passages of asymptomatic individuals. In the presence of suspicious symptoms, the same strain of *Aspergillus* must be recovered from multiple samples of respiratory secretions before the diagnosis can be accepted. *Aspergillus fumigatus* most commonly causes invasive pulmonary aspergillosis; *A. flavus* is usually incriminated in allergic bronchopulmonary disease; *A. fumigatus* and *A. niger* most commonly are recovered from cavitary fungus ball infections, and *A. niger* is most commonly implicated in otomycosis.	*Zygomycosis (Phycomycosis)* Hyphal fragments may be detected in direct mounts of sputum or other material. Those of aspergilli are slender, tend to have parallel walls, are septate, and branch dichotomously at 45 degree angles. Those of the Zygomycetes are irregularly broad, ribbon-like, aseptate, and branch at irregular angles. *Candidosis* Pneumonitis in compromised hosts caused by *Candida* species or other yeasts can closely simulate aspergillosis. Budding blastoconidia and focally constricted pseudohyphae are characteristic of *Candida*.
Candidosis	*Candida albicans* *Candida* species	*Cutaneous Candidosis* Generalized cutaneous, intertriginous, paronychia, onychia: redness, edema, scaling. *Mucous Membrane Candidosis* Vulvovaginal and oropharyngeal thrush: redness, edema, soft white patches on tonsils, gums, tongue, and vaginal mucosa. *Pulmonary Candidosis* Bronchial and bronchopulmonary varieties: cough, sputum production at times tinged with blood, pleuritis, and pleural effusion *Endocarditis and Septicemia* Fever, splenomegaly, heart murmur, congestive heart failure, and anemia may be seen in varying combinations.	Infections with *Candida* are endogenous. Various species of *Candida* colonize the skin and mucous membranes. Clinical disease may arise in conditions in which there is an alteration in host defenses or suppression of the normal bacterial flora. Conditions predisposing to candidosis are: -Pregnancy -Diabetes mellitus -Indwelling venous catheters -Chronic debilitating diseases -Prolonged therapy with broad-spectrum antibiotics	*Cutaneous and Mucous Membrane* -Bacterial infections -Avitaminosis -Contact dermatitis -Trichomonas (vaginal) -Vaginal gonorrhea *Pulmonary* -Aspergillosis -Geotrichosis -Other yeast infections *Septicemia* -Bacterial endocarditis
Geotrichosis	*Geotrichum candidum*	*Respiratory Geotrichosis* Acute bronchitis and tracheitis: Cough productive of mucoid or purulent sputum. Pulmonary: Cough, low grade fever, pleuritis.	Common environmental saprobe on tomatoes and other fruit, in soil, and in dairy products. Infections probably endogenous since	Geotrichosis cannot be clinically differentiated from other yeast infections, notably those caused by *Candida*

		Allergic variant causing wheezing and asthma-like attacks. Thin-walled cavities form rarely. Oral: Simulates candidal thrush. *Gastrointestinal Geotrichosis* Colitis	*Geotrichum* may colonize skin, mucous membranes, and gastrointestinal tract. Disease most commonly occurs in debilitated patients with primary diseases, such as diabetes mellitus, leukemia, lymphoma, and other neoplasms.	Allergic bronchopulmonary disease closely simulates a similar disease caused by aspergilli.
Zygomycosis (Phycomycosis) (Mucormycosis)	*Rhizopus* sp. *Absidia* sp. *Mucor* sp.	*Orbitocerebral Zygomycosis* *Nasal:* A thick, dark, blood-tinged nasal discharge may be found. The nasal turbinate appears black, malar anesthesia may be present, and a necrotic palatal ulcer may be observed. Signs of sinusitis. *Ocular:* Edema of the eyelids and retina, proptosis and signs of retinal artery thrombosis. Complete internal and external ophthalmoplegia may occur in severe cases. *Cerebral:* Cerebral zygomycosis usually occurs as a direct extension of nasal, sinus, or orbital disease. Headache, drowsiness, or semistupor portend possible cerebral involvement. Nuchal rigidity indicates meningeal involvement. This form can be rapidly fatal, with symptoms suggesting cerebrovascular accident due to propensity for hyphae to invade and cause thrombosis of cerebral vessels. *Pulmonary Zygomycosis* Onset may be insidious or sudden. Chest pain, hemoptysis, sputum production, and cough are seen in varying degrees of severity. Sudden development of chest pain and development of a pleural friction rub are found when the pleura is invaded. *Disseminated Zygomycosis* Rare occurrence, almost always in immunodepressed hosts. Virtually all organs may be involved, and the gastrointestinal tract in particular may be invaded, particularly the gastroesophageal region. Fever, weight loss, lassitude, and somnolence are common manifestations. Disease is rapidly fatal.	*Orbitocerebral* Diabetes mellitus is the most common predisposing condition. Uremic acidosis is less commonly a predisposing cause. *Pulmonary and Disseminated* Usually contracted as a nosocomial, hospital-acquired infection in patients being treated for leukemia or other disseminated neoplastic disease; or in those receiving corticosteroids for chronic renal disease or other immune related diseases. The Zygomycetes (Phycomycetes) comprise a group of fungi that are widely distributed in nature in soil and dung, and on vegetable matter. Spores are readily disseminated in the air. Portal of entry in man is by inhalation, either into the nasal passages or into the lungs. Gastrointestinal disease may occur from ingestion of contaminated foodstuffs. In disease, the fungus tends to invade blood vessels, causing extensive thrombosis and necrosis.	The triad of diabetic acidosis, ophthalmoplegia, and signs of diffuse cerebral vascular disease is virtually diagnostic of zygomycosis (phycomycosis). The nasal or external ocular exudation may become secondarily infected and simulate bacterial disease. It is important that the disease not be mistaken for bacterial infection. Since the fungus often does not exfoliate into the secretions, a tissue biopsy may be required to confirm the diagnosis. Pulmonary disease must be differentiated from other mycoses, particularly candidosis and aspergillosis.
Actinomycosis*	*Actinomyces israelii*	*Facial Actinomycosis* "Lumpy jaw" is the classic disease. There is painful induration and swelling of the subcutaneous tissue of the jaw and upper neck. As the disease progresses, deeply penetrating fistulae that break out on the skin surface develop, and exuding purulent material within which "sulfur granules" may be seen. *Thoracic Actinomycosis* Disease develops as a pneumonitis in the hilar or basal regions of the lung. The disease spreads by direct extension into the pleura, and adhesions are prominent. There may be direct extension through the thoracic wall with	Various speces of *Actinomyces* are harbored in the oral cavity, within carious teeth, or in tonsilar crypts. This accounts for the source of most infections. Facial disease often follows tooth extraction, oral surgery, or breaks in the oral mucosa either from stabbing the lining with bits of straw or other vegetative matter or from compound fractures of the mandible. Pulmonary disease also is thought to be endogenous, following aspiration	Actinomycosis may resemble many other suppurative inflammatory diseases. Cervical, pulmonary, and intestinal tuberculosis must be ruled out. Syphilitic gumma may closely resemble actinomycotic lesions. Appendicitis, carcinoma of the cecum, and amebiasis are all abdominal diseases which may simulate actinomycosis.

Table continued on following page

6

Table 48–2. CLINICAL PARAMETERS OF THE OPPORTUNISTIC MYCOSES *(Continued)*

Fungal Disease	Etiologic Agent	Clinical Disease Manifestations: Signs and Symptoms	Epidemiology and Modes of Infection	Differential Considerations
		formation of suppurative cutaneous fistulae. Cough, spiking fever, pleural pain, and production of a mucopurulent blood sputum may be observed *Abdominal Actinomycosis* Disease commonly occurs in the right lower abdomen, simulating appendicitis. The appendix and adjacent organs may be involved in a dense, suppurative fibrosing lesion. Right lower abdominal pain and presence of a cecal tumor mass are common symptoms. Penetration of the abdominal wall with development of suppurative cutaneous fistulae may occur. Rarely, disease may result from perforation of a gastric ulcer, with involvement of the liver and extrahepatic biliary system. Jaundice may occur. Salpingitis, cystitis, pyelonephritis, psoas muscle abscess, and direct extension into the spine are other complications of abdominal actinomycosis.	of infected materials from the tonsils or other areas in the oral cavity. Abdominal disease most commonly occurs secondary to a perforation of the gastrointestinal tract, either from ulceration or rupture of the appendix.	
Nocardiosis†	*Nocardia asteroides*	*Pulmonary Nocardiosis* Cough is the most common symptom, usually productive of a thick, at times bloody sputum. As the disease progresses chest pain, dyspnea, malaise, weight loss, low grade fever, and night sweats may be seen in varying degrees of severity. Cavitary disease, closely simulating tuberculosis, may lead to massive hemoptysis. Sinus tracts, simulating actinomycosis, may penetrate the chest wall. Suppurative pneumonia with consolidation of one or more lobes of the lungs is common in some patients, complicated by pleuritis. *Cerebral Nocardiosis* Nearly one third of patients with progressive pulmonary disease develop metastatic brain abscesses. Brain lesions often are multiple. Severe headache and localizing sensory or motor disturbances often have an acute onset. *Disseminated Nocardiosis* The kidney is the next most frequently involved organ in disseminated disease. Involvement of the spleen, liver, and adrenal glands occurs; bone disease is rare. Endocarditis, myocarditis, and pericarditis also may occur. The disseminated form is usually fatal within months to a few years. *Subcutaneous Nocardiosis* See Table 48–3: Mycetoma	*Nocardia asteroides* has a natural habitat in the soil. The portal of entry is through the respiratory tract through inhalation of dustborne spores. Susceptibility to infection increases in certain debilitating diseases such as Cushing's syndrome, in alveolar proteinosis, and in subjects with leukemia or lymphoma who are under chemotherapy. The recovery of *Nocardia asteroides* from pulmonary secretions usually indicates disease, although the organism has been recovered as a saprophyte from asymptomatic subjects. Nocardiosis occurs in all parts of the world, has no racial or occupational predilection, and has its highest age incidence at 30 to 50 years.	Pulmonary nocardiosis mimics tuberculosis and can be clinically difficult to differentiate. The organism does withstand the digestion and decontamination procedure and, if viable, can grow on Lowenstein-Jensen culture medium. Nocardia filaments may be missed in Ziehl-Neelsen stained smears because they are only partially acid fast. Pleural or chest wall involvement must be differentiated from actinomycosis. Disseminated disease is most commonly mistaken for carcinomatosis, particularly in the presence of brain lesions.

*Actinomycosis is currently classified as a bacterial and not a fungal disease.
†Nocardiosis is currently classified as a bacterial and not a fungal disease.

Table 48–3. CLINICAL PARAMETERS OF THE SUBCUTANEOUS MYCOSES

Fungal Disease	Etiologic Agent	Clinical Disease Manifestations: Signs and Symptoms	Epidemiology and Modes of Infection	Differential Considerations
Chromoblastomycosis	*Fonsecaea pedrosoi* *Fonsecaea compactum* *Phialophora verrucosa* *Cladosporium carrionii*	*Subcutaneous Chromoblastomycosis* With few exceptions, chromoblastomycosis is limited to the skin and subcutaneous tissue, most commonly involving the feet and legs. The initial lesion is a small papular or pustular ulcer, probably representing the site of inoculation, that exudes a serous exudate and forms a crust on the surface. As the disease becomes more chronic, the ulcer is replaced by a dry, crusted, warty, violaceous lesion that spreads locally but tends to remain restricted to the area of infection for months or years. In time the lesions become raised to form a cauliflower-like tumor having a dark brown or violaceous appearance, and in time the entire extremity may be covered. There is little pain. Secondary infections with bacteria may lead to lymphatic stasis and varying degrees of elephantiasis. *Cerebral Chromoblastomycosis* A few cases of cerebral chromoblastomycosis have been reported, probably representing hematogenous spread from primary subcutaneous sites of infection. Cerebral chromoblastomycosis is indistinguishable clinically from other types of brain abscess.	The organisms causing chromoblastomycosis have their natural habitat in the soil, and human infections occur secondary to skin penetration by infected thorns, splinters, or traumatic wounds contaminated with soil. Agricultural workers, field and jungle laborers, and mine workers make up a high percentage of reported cases, particularly individuals who work without protection of shoes. *F. pedrosoi* is the most common agent, and since this species prefers warm, moist conditions, most infections occur in the tropics. *F. pedrosoi* has been isolated from tree branches, bark, and trunks, rotten vegetative matter, and soil. *C. carrionii* and *P. verrucosa*, on the other hand, survive well in drier, colder conditions and can cause chromoblastomycosis in more temperate climates.	*Cutaneous blastomycosis:* The early lateral spread with a tendency to heal centrally with a flat, thin scar that is commonly seen in cutaneous blastomycosis is not seen in the lesions of chromoblastomycosis. *Cutaneous tuberculosis:* Recovery of the etiologic agent may be needed to make an early diagnosis. Tuberculosis usually does not form the advanced cauliflower tumors. *Leishmaniasis:* Lymphadenopathy is usually far more prominent. *Tertiary syphilis* *Yaws*

Table continued on following page

Table 48–3. CLINICAL PARAMETERS OF THE SUBCUTANEOUS MYCOSES *(Continued)*

Fungal Disease	Etiologic Agent	Clinical Disease Manifestations: Signs and Symptoms	Epidemiology and Modes of Infection	Differential Considerations
Mycetoma	Eumycotic *Pseudallescheria (Petriellidium) boydii* (Imperfect form: *Scedosporium apiospermum)* *Exophiala* *(Phialophora) jeanselmei* *Madurella grisea* Actinomycotic *Nocardia asteroides* *Nocardia brasiliensis* *Nocardia caviae* *Actinomyces israelii* *Actinomyces bovis* *Actinomadura* species *Streptomyces* species	Lesions most commonly occur on the foot. The neck or back (pack carriers), the hand, the scalp, or rarely other body sites may also be infected where traumatic breaks in the skin may occur. The initial lesion is a small area of swelling, usually on the sole or the dorsum of the foot, presumably at the primary site of inoculation. Swelling, suppuration, and healing occur in a cyclic pattern, but with slow progression until in severe cases the entire foot may be involved. Swelling can become so pronounced that the sole of the foot assumes a convex curvature. Multiple sinus tracts develop, exuding purulent material from cutaneous ostia onto the surface of the skin. Often a variety of "grains" or "granules" composed of aggregates of microorganisms mixed with purulent and necrotic debris may be observed within the exudate, at times helpful in making a genus identification. Hematogenous spread to other parts of the body does not occur; however, secondary bacterial infections may lead to bacterial septicemia. Although eumycotic mycetomas caused by a number of fungal species are separated from actinomycotic mycetomas caused by the Actinomycetes (Schizomycetes), they cannot be distinguished clinically.	The organisms causing mycetomas have their natural habitat in the soil and enter the body through traumatic breaks in the skin. The disease is not contagious. Mycetomas are more common in males, generally rural farmers. Most cases have been reported from Mexico, Africa, and South America, although cases have been reported from the southern United States. There are geographic differences in species distribution. Actinomycotic mycetomas tend to be more universal in distribution; eumycotic mycetomas predominate in tropical countries. *Pseudallescheria (Petriellidium) boydii* is the most common cause of mycetomas in the United States.	-*Bacterial cellulitis:* Subcutaneous staphylococcal abscesses (so called botryomycosis) may cause confusion; however, they rarely reach the severity of involvement as with the mycetomatous agents. -Elephantiasis secondary to filariasis. -Chromoblastomycosis where mycetomas taken on a more verrucous appearance.

		Experienced mycologists can separate the two by microscopically examining the grains and granules that form in the exudates. Actinomycosis is excluded from the actinomycotic mycetomas because the granules are more minute and the microaerophilic actinomycetes are endogenous in habitat and the mode of infection is different (Emmons, 1977).		
Sporotrichosis	*Sporothrix schenckii*	*Cutaneous Lymphatic Sporotrichosis* Following a penetrating wound of the skin with a splinter or thorn infected with spores, a small ulcerated lesion develops within one or two weeks, gradually enlarging into a sporotrichotic chancre which is slow to heal. Fever is uncommon. The lymphatics commonly become secondarily involved. As the fungus spreads up the lymphatic channels, a series of secondary subcutaneous nodules form. These become fixed to the skin, undergo necrosis, and ultimately surface to form secondary chancroid ulcers. Lesions often become infected with bacteria. *Cutaneous Non-lymphatic Sporotrichosis* Rarely, the primary lesion remains localized without lymphatic spread. The lesions may appear ulcerative, papu-	The classic method of infection is through traumatic puncture of the skin by a prick from a thorn, piece of shrub, or hay. The fungus may also be present on wood, barks, straw, soil, and even on insects. Insect bites may cause infections. The rose gardener is particularly vulnerable, or nursery workers who handle sphagnum moss. Alcoholic gardeners are also highly susceptible because of a diminution in peripheral pain sensation. The fungus also lives under old brick or masonry stone and can infect masonry workers by entering through cracks or fissures in the hands. In the United States most infections occur in the midwest, particularly in the states adjoining the Missouri and Mississippi River valleys.	The classic clinical presentation of a slow-to-heal ulcer on a finger or the hand, with a string of secondary lesions associated with a chain of enlarged lymph nodes extending up the arm is virtually diagnostic of sporotrichosis. Tularemia is a far more acute disease, with acute necrosis of the lymphatics and lymph nodes. Fever commonly accompanies tularemia infections. Infections with *Mycobacterium marinum* may mimic sporotrichosis.

Table continued on following page

Table 48–3. CLINICAL PARAMETERS OF THE SUBCUTANEOUS MYCOSES *(Continued)*

Fungal Disease	Etiologic Agent	Clinical Disease Manifestations: Signs and Symptoms	Epidemiology and Modes of Infection	Differential Considerations
		lar, or acneform. The neck, trunk, and arm are other sites besides the fingers and hand that may be involved.		
		Disseminated Sporotrichosis		
		Despite the propensity for primary lesions to spread via lymphatics, disseminated disease is rare. Constitutional symptoms are marked and the disease may be rapidly fatal. Widespread nodular and papular skin lesions, involvement of oral and nasal mucous membranes, and dissemination to the viscera have been seen. The central nervous system is not involved; pulmonary disease, lesions of bone (periostitis and osteomyelitis), joints, (synovitis) and muscle are the most common extracutaneous sites of infection.		Disseminated sporotrichosis must be differentiated from other systemic mycoses, from miliary tuberculosis, glanders, anthrax, or chronic disseminated bacterial diseases of other types.

Table 48–4. CLINICAL PARAMETERS OF THE SUPERFICIAL MYCOSES

Fungal Disease	Etiologic Agent	Clinical Disease Manifestations: Signs and Symptoms	Epidemiology and Modes of Infection	Differential Considerations
Dermatophytosis	*Microsporum audouinii* *Microsporum canis* *Microsporum gypseum* *Epidermophyton floccosum* *Trichophyton mentagrophytes* *Trichophyton rubrum* *Trichophyton tonsurans* *Trichophyton verrucosum* *Trichophyton schoenleinii* *Trichophyton violaceum*	The dermatophytes are a group of fungi that infect the superficial keratinized portion of the integument—skin, hair, and nails—without spread into the deeper skin, viscera, or dissemination. Various clinical types have only a rough correlation with specific dermatophyte species with considerable overlapping between types. *Tinea Pedis* (dermatophytosis of the foot) Ringworm of the foot or athlete's foot, the most common type of dermatophytosis, begins as a weeping, peeling lesion between the web of the 4th and 5th toes. Lesions extend to involve other toe webs and the subdigital and interdigital surfaces of the toes. In chronic cases, spread as a dry scaling condition over the sole, arch, heel, and even dorsum of the foot may occur. Acute lesions are pruritic; chronic disease may be asymptomatic. *T. rubrum*, *T. mentagrophytes*, and *E. floccosum* are most common species. *Tinea Corporis* (dermatophytosis of the body) Most common in children, involving the glabrous portions of the face, shoulders, arms, or other exposed surfaces. The lesions vary in size, are	Dermatophytic infections may be contracted in a variety of ways. Dermatophytes have been recovered from floors of shower stalls and locker rooms. It is probable that tinea pedis infections are incurred exogenously by walking barefoot over these contaminated areas. *M. audouinii*, the most frequent cause of inflammatory tinea capitis, can be transmitted from man to man by direct contact, or through contaminated fomites such as hair brushes, combs, or caps. *T. tonsurans* may be similarly transmitted. *E. floccosum*, *T. violaceum*, and *T. schoenleinii* may be directly transmitted from man to man through contaminated towels or clothes. Zoophilic sources are numerous. Tinea corporis is commonly secondary to *M. canis* transmitted from an infected cat or dog which is fondled by the patient. *T. verrucosum*, a cause of tinea barbae, is most commonly contracted from cattle. Farmers who hand-milk cows have the habit of resting the bearded surface of their face against the side of the cow. Dogs, chinchillas, guinea pigs, mice, horses, and other animals have been incrimated as sources for human ringworm infections.	Allergic dermatitis of the hands and feet can simulate dermatophytosis. These usually lack the reddened serpiginous margin of a classic ringworm lesion. Dermatophytid ("id") reactions are vesicular eruptions of the fingers caused by circulating antigens from a focus of mycotic infection elsewhere. These are allergic lesions and are not primary sites of fungal infection. Onychomycosis must be differentiated from *Candida* spp. infections, which can appear quite similar. It is essential that direct mounts be made to establish the correct etiology before dermatophyte therapy is instituted. Skin and nail lesions must also be differentiated from psoriasis, which can produce similar appearing alterations. Seborrhea of the scalp can also be mistaken for tinea capitis.

Table continued on following page

Table 48–4. CLINICAL PARAMETERS OF THE SUPERFICIAL MYCOSES *(Continued)*

Fungal Disease	Etiologic Agent	Clinical Disease Manifestations: Signs and Symptoms	Epidemiology and Modes of Infection	Differential Considerations
		circular, and exhibit a raised, red, serpiginous margin, accounting for the anachronistic term "ringworm." *M. canis, M. gypseum, T. mentagrophytes,* and *T. rubrum* most common.		
		Tinea Barbae (dermatophytosis of the beard) A severe pustular folliculitis involving the beard or other hairy areas of the face and neck. *T. verrucosum* and *T. mentagrophytes* are the most common species.		
		Tinea Cruris (dermatophytosis of the groin) Chronic, severely pruritic involvement of the groin and perineal and perianal areas. May be in epidemic form on shipboard or in locker rooms where community towels may transmit the disease. Lesions may remain localized *(E. floccosum)* or may spread widely over the buttocks or waist *(T. rubrum)*.		
		Lesions are sharply demarcated, marginated, centrally red, and usually dry.	*M. gypseum* is the most important geophilic fungus that causes ringworm in man. The soil is its natural habitat, where the fungus grows on keratinous debris. Children may become infected by direct contact during play (mudpies, etc.)	
		Tinea Capitis (dermatophytosis of the scalp) Classic type: *M. audouinii* Primary involvement of the hairs of the scalp in which the fungus invades the hair follicle, forming a sheath of spores around the hair shaft (ectothrix invasion).		

Hairs often break 1 to 2 mm above the surface and produce a bright green-yellow fluorescence under an ultraviolet Wood's lamp. Varying degrees of inflammation of the skin are noted, particularly severe with *M. canis*.

Black dot type: *T. tonsurans* and *T. violaceum*

Dry, diffuse scaly lesions of the scalp in which the hair shaft is invaded internally (endothrix invasion) with destruction of the keratin. The hair becomes fragile and breaks off beneath the surface of the skin, producing a "black dot." Boggy lesions known as kerions may develop in this type. *T. tonsurans* and *T. violaceum* are most common causes of black dot hair infection. *T. verrucosum* and *T. mentagrophytes* cause kerions.

Onychomycosis *(Tinea Unguium)*

Ringworm of the nails may involve either the feet or the hands, or both. The infected nails have a chalky, crumbling consistency or "moth-eaten" appearance or may become hypertrophic and project above a thickened nail bed and keratinized cells and debris. *T. rubrum* and *T. mentagrophytes* are the most common causes.

Table continued on following page

6

Table 48–4. CLINICAL PARAMETERS OF THE SUPERFICIAL MYCOSES *(Continued)*

Fungal Disease	Etiologic Agent	Clinical Disease Manifestations: Signs and Symptoms	Epidemiology and Modes of Infection	Differential Considerations
Tinea Nigra Palmaris	*Exophiala (Cladosporium) werneckii*	Superficial fungus infection of the skin, most commonly involving the palms of the hands but rarely other sites, with asymptomatic brown or black macules which may be discrete or become confluent. The dark pigmentation has been likened to skin stained with silver nitrate. Pigmentation is often most intense at the periphery of the macule, simulating a ringworm. Inflammation is not a feature, and pruritus is mild if present at all.	The disease is prevalent in South and Central America, but has been reported in the coastal southeastern United States. The fungus resides as a saprophyte in nature, and man presumably contracts the disease by direct contact with infected materials. Familial spread of the disease is a possibility.	Tinea nigra differs from tinea versicolor by its distinct dark pigmentation. The pigmented lesions of pinta can cause confusion, as can pigmented lesions of Addison's disease and syphilis. Laboratory examinations are required.
Pityrosporum (Tinea) Versicolor	*Malassezia (Pityrosporum) furfur*	The disease is recognized as an asymptomatic cream-tan discoloration of the superficial skin, most commonly of the chest or trunk, but may also involve groin, thighs, arms, face, and scalp. The lesions are non-inflammatory and covered by thin scales and generally are sharply marginated. The fungus interferes with sun tanning and may appear as light blotches in exposed areas.	The fungus exists as a free-living saprophyte and probably spreads from person to person by exposure to desquamated scales. Lack of personal hygiene facilitates development of skin lesions.	Tinea corporis can usually be distinguished by its distinct border and presence of inflammatory reaction. Seborrhea, secondary syphilis, and pinta must be considered and ruled out by laboratory examination.
Piedra Black Piedra White Piedra	*Piedraia hortae* *Trichosporon beigelii*	Infection of hairs, characterized by the presence of firmly adherent black, hard, gritty nodules (black piedra) or soft, mucilaginous nodules (white piedra). Scalp, beard, mustache, and genital hairs may be involved. The patient suffers no discomfort, since the lesion is limited to the hairs.	Prevalent in South America and tropical Africa. Reservoir may be in primates. White piedra is also found in Central Europe, England, and Japan.	The only major differential problem is in the recognition of nits of pediculosis capitis and bacterial trichomycoses that are not true "mycoses."

Table 48–5. MYCOTIC DISEASES INCLUDED IN TABLES 48–1 TO 48–4

Table 48–1, Deep-Seated Mycoses	Table 48–2, Opportunistic Mycoses	Table 48–3, Subcutaneous Mycoses	Table 48–4, Cutaneous Mycoses
Blastomycosis	Actinomycosis*	Actinomycosis*	Dermatomycoses
Coccidioidomycosis	Aspergillosis	Chromoblastomycosis	Piedra
Cryptococcosis	Candidosis	Mycetoma	Tinea versicolor
Histoplasmosis	Geotrichosis	Nocardiosis*	Tinea nigra palmaris
Paracoccidioidomycosis	Nocardiosis*	Sporotrichosis	
	Zygomycosis (Phycomycosis)		

*The actinomycetes, including *Actinomyces* sp. and *Nocardia* sp., are not fungi, but rather are bacteria belonging to the *Schizomycetes.*

APPROACH TO THE SUBCUTANEOUS MYCOSES

Table 48–3 outlines the clinical parameters of several fungi that are known to cause subcutaneous mycoses. In the United States, *Sporothrix schenckii, Pseudallescheria (Petriellidium) boydii,* and the members of the Actinomycetes *(Nocardia* and *Actinomyces)* will be the organisms most commonly recovered from cases of subcutaneous mycosis. A few cases of *Exophiala (Phialophora) jeanselmei* infections have been reported from the southeastern United States. The agents of chromoblastomycosis are endemic only in the tropical regions of the world.

In suspected mycetomatous disease, serous or purulent material from the draining sinuses should be directly examined for the presence of granules or grains, and a presumptive diagnosis can often be made. The morphology of these grains is discussed later in this chapter. Specimens should be cultured both aerobically and anaerobically, in that *Actinomyces* grows only anaerobically.

The clinical parameters of sporotrichosis, as outlined in Table 48–3, are virtually diagnostic. This disease should be suspected when any non-healing ulcers of the fingers, hand, foot, or leg are clinically encountered, particularly if there is concomitant involvement of the lymphatics draining the limb. Direct examination of any exudate that may be present or review of tissue sections of biopsy specimens will usually not reveal the characteristic yeast-like organisms. Therefore, the diagnosis can be confirmed only by recovering the causative organism in culture.

APPROACH TO THE SUPERFICIAL MYCOSES

Table 48–4 outlines the clinical parameters of the superficial mycoses. Ringworm infections caused by several species of dermatophytes are the most common mycoses encountered in clinical practice.

A variety of tinea infections may be encountered, as outlined in Table 48–4. The advent of griseofulvin has to some degree precluded the necessity to make a species identification, and fewer cutaneous cultures are referred to laboratories. However, physicians must confirm their clinical impression of dermatophyte infection by performing a direct potassium hydroxide mount of skin scales, hairs, or nail scrapings, because other microorganisms, notably species of *Candida,* can closely simulate tinea infections.

In collecting specimens for culture, the growing outer serpiginous border of typical ringworm lesions should be scraped with a blade, and the scales collected in a sterile Petri dish. Before cultures are taken, the skin should be cleansed with 70 per cent alcohol or other suitable disinfectant to remove contaminating surface bacteria. In collecting specimens from infected nails, some of the softened material from beneath the nail surface should be selected. The use of a Wood's lamp is useful in selecting infected hairs when *M. audouinii* or *M. canis* are the agents involved, since they produce a bright yellow-green fluorescence.

Dermatophyte infections remain confined to the keratinized portion of the integument, and subcutaneous or visceral invasion does not occur.

The other superficial mycoses listed in Table 48–4 have little clinical significance. Pityriasis versicolor is relatively frequent, and is most commonly diagnosed by direct examination of KOH mounts of superficial skin scales. The other conditions are only rarely encountered in the United States.

MISCELLANEOUS MYCOTIC DISEASES

A number of other fungal species, many commonly recovered as saprobic contaminants in the laboratory, can occasionally cause mycotic disease. Species of *Aspergillus, Fusarium, Candida,* and *Acremonium (Cephalosporium)* can cause mycotic keratitis, following corneal trauma or postoperatively. Keratitis begins as a small corneal ulcer which develops into a slightly raised, gray-white nodule with an opaque halo around the center. The cornea may become inflamed. Scarring may develop and the disease can progress to invade the anterior chamber if not treated. Corneal scrapings should be taken and microscopically examined for fungal mycelial elements.

Otomycosis was discussed above and is commonly caused by *A. fumigatus* and *A. niger.* Species of *Scopulariopsis, Rhizopus, Candida,* and some of the dermatophytes have also been recovered. The tympanic membrane is rarely perforated.

A condition known as cerebral chromomycosis can be caused by generally non-pathogenic species of *Cladosporium,* notably *C. bantianum.* This fungus species has been recovered from brain abscesses and focal parenchymal lesions.

Rhinosporidiosis is a chronic granulomatous infection of the nasal passages resulting in the production of polyps or a hyperplastic mucous membrane. The etiologic agent is *Rhinosporidium seeberi*. The eyes, ears, larynx, and occasionally the mucous membranes of the vagina or penis may be involved, where the disease must be differentiated from warts or condylomata.

Aflatoxins, toxic products of a number of fungal species that may cause gastrointestinal, neurologic, or allergic manifestations in man and animals, may be encountered more frequently than suspected. Many foodstuffs or commercial products made from vegetative by-products (sugar cane refuse, for example) may become infected with aflatoxin-producing species of fungi during storage. The toxic products accumulate in these foodstuffs and may be either ingested or inhaled. Gastrointestinal upset, transient neurologic symptoms such as headache, dizziness or neuromuscular manifestations, or allergic interstitial pulmonary disease simulating Hamman-Rich syndrome (bagassosis, byssinosis) may be encountered. A careful history of exposure to any of these materials must be elicited when encountering these clinical syndromes.

HISTOPATHOLOGY OF FUNGAL INFECTIONS

Surgical pathologists often play an important role in the diagnosis of mycotic disease. The referring physician should always inform the pathologist when he suspects one of the fungal diseases so that the biopsy or surgical specimen can be properly prepared for study and a portion can be submitted for culture.

Unfortunately, the specimen request slip does not routinely have this information, and the presence of fungal disease may be suspected only when suspicious fungal forms are detected in routine hematoxylin and eosin (H & E) sections of surgical or autopsy tissue. Often cultures have not been obtained, and it may be difficult to make a definitive identification based on tissue section morphology alone. The use of special stains that have a specific avidity for the carbohydrate-rich cell walls, capsules, or hyphal forms of fungi, such as the periodic acid–Schiff (PAS), Gomori methenamine silver (GMS), or mucicarmine stains, can be helpful. However, it should be pointed out that fungal forms can often be well visualized in routine H & E sections, and in many instances the use of special stains merely confirms an initial impression.

The discussion in this section will include a practical approach that surgical pathologists may find helpful in making a presumptive diagnosis when fungal elements are observed in tissue sections. Unfortunately, fungal forms are often distorted beyond recognition by the host's inflammatory response, making a diagnosis other than "fungal disease" difficult. Nevertheless, the approach outlined here will prove helpful in many instances in which fungal elements are present in tissue sections, and occasionally a definitive diagnosis may be possible.

Assessment of Inflammatory Tissue Reactions

The invasion of organs or tissues by fungi produces a variety of inflammatory reactions. Although these reactions are often non-specific, fungal diseases should be suspected when certain inflammatory patterns are recognized. The presence of granulomatous inflammation, caseous necrosis, or infiltration with multinucleated giant cells is highly suggestive of fungal disease.

In the following paragraphs are reviewed commonly encountered tissue inflammatory reactions and a brief discussion of some of the specific fungi that may be associated with each.

Suppurative Inflammation. The term *suppurative* refers to an inflammatory reaction in which polymorphonuclear leukocytes predominate (Fig. 48–3). Suppurative inflammation indicates the presence of pus, which may be loculated within walled-off abscesses, may cover the surface of mucous membranes, or may exude from the stomas of fistulae or sinus tracts.

Actinomycosis or nocardiosis should always be sus-

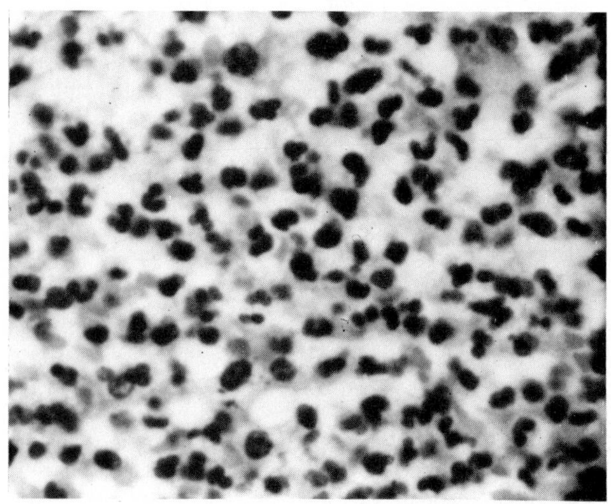

Figure 48–3. Suppurative inflammatory reaction showing dense infiltration with neutrophils. ×450. Hematoxylin-eosin stain.

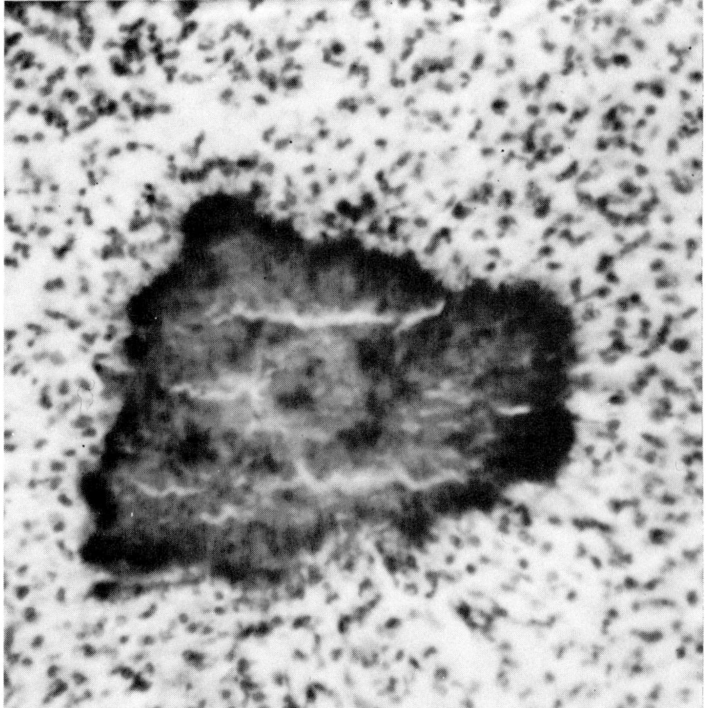

Figure 48–4. Suppurative inflammatory reaction including an actinomycotic "sulfur granule." ×250. Hematoxylin-eosin stain.

pected when a dense suppurative inflammatory response is seen in tissue sections from patients in whom fungal disease is suspected. Direct mounts of the purulent exudate or the stained tissue sections should be carefully examined for the presence of sulfur granules (Fig. 48–4). A Gram stain or silver stain may be necessary to make the final diagnosis by demonstrating the characteristic delicate, branching filamentous forms within the sulfur granule (Fig. 48–5).

Blastomyces dermatitidis also frequently produces suppurative inflammation, particularly within the characteristic intraepithelial microabscesses that are found

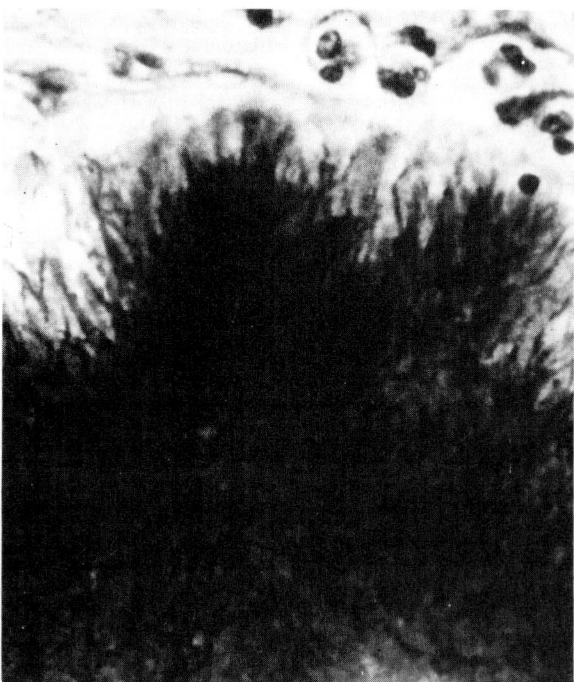

Figure 48–5. Margin of "sulfur granule" showing delicate branching filaments. ×950. Hematoxylin-eosin stain.

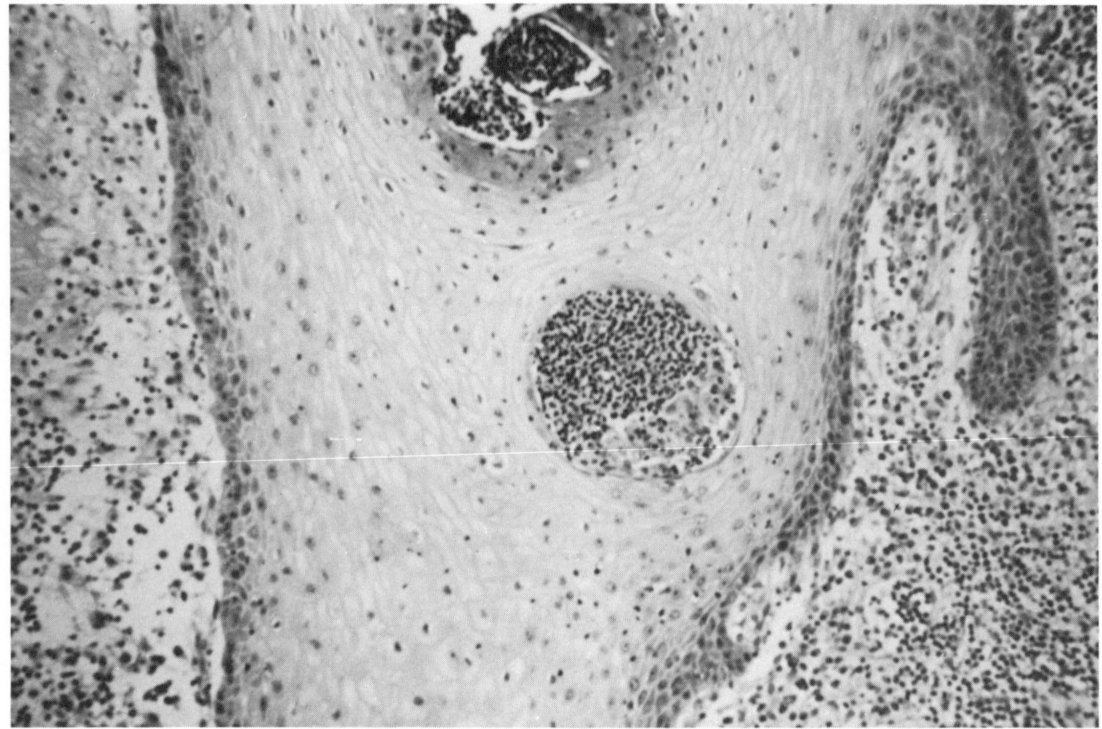

Figure 48–6. Section of skin showing hyperplastic squamous epithelium including epithelial microabscess. ×100. Hematoxylin-eosin stain. (From Dolan, C. T., Funkhouser, J. W., Koneman, E. W., Miller, N. G., and Roberts, G. D.: Atlas of Clinical Mycology II. Chicago, American Society of Clinical Pathologists, 1975.)

in primary or secondary cutaneous disease (Fig. 48–6). The additional detection of yeast forms 8 to 15 μ in diameter, with some having the single bud attached by a broad base, is virtually diagnostic (Fig. 48–7).

Chronic "Round Cell" Inflammation. If an acute suppurative inflammatory reaction does not resolve with healing in a relatively short time, the exudate begins to take on a different appearance, and a predominance of lymphocytes, monocytes, or other mononuclear inflammatory cells will be noted (Fig. 48–8). Polymorphonuclear leukocytes are either few in number or totally absent. This "round cell" response is referred to as chronic inflammation. This reaction is non-specific and may be seen in many different fungal infections and other chronic inflammatory responses as well.

An admixture of eosinophils in an inflammatory reaction often suggests an allergic or hypersensitivity response; a preponderance of plasma cells usually indicates an adequate immunologic response with production of type-specific proteins.

Granulomatous Inflammation. The term *granulomatous* is used to describe a specific type of chronic inflammation in which the cellular response is almost entirely composed of large macrophages or histiocytes, which often aggregate to form multinucleated giant cells.

The prototype of granulomatous inflammation is the tubercle, a focal collection of large mononuclear inflammatory cells surrounded by a cuff of lymphocytes, with varying degrees of caseous necrosis and infiltration with varying numbers of giant cells (see Fig. 48–11). Although most commonly produced by various species of mycobacteria, notably *M. tuberculosis,* tubercle-like reactions may also be seen with many fungal diseases.

The characteristic multinucleated giant cell in tuberculosis is the Langhans giant cell, characterized by the arrangement of the cell nuclei around the periphery of the cytoplasm, simulating a spoke wheel (Fig. 48–9). These are to be distinguished from foreign body or tumor giant cells, in which the nuclei are arranged irregularly throughout the cytoplasm (Fig. 48–10). Although tuberculosis is suspected when Langhans' giant cells are seen in inflammatory reactions, they may also be seen in a number of mycotic infections as well.

Caseation necrosis is another feature that often accompanies granulomatous inflammation. *Caseation* is a term that is used to designate a degenerative tissue response in which there develops a cheese-like consistency. When examined microscopically, areas of caseation necrosis are devoid of viable cells, but rather consist entirely of a homogeneously staining, finely granular material, within which Langhans' giant cells are often scattered (Fig. 48–11). Caseation necrosis is also one of the hallmarks of tuberculosis, thought to represent a hypersensitivity reaction to antigenic sub-

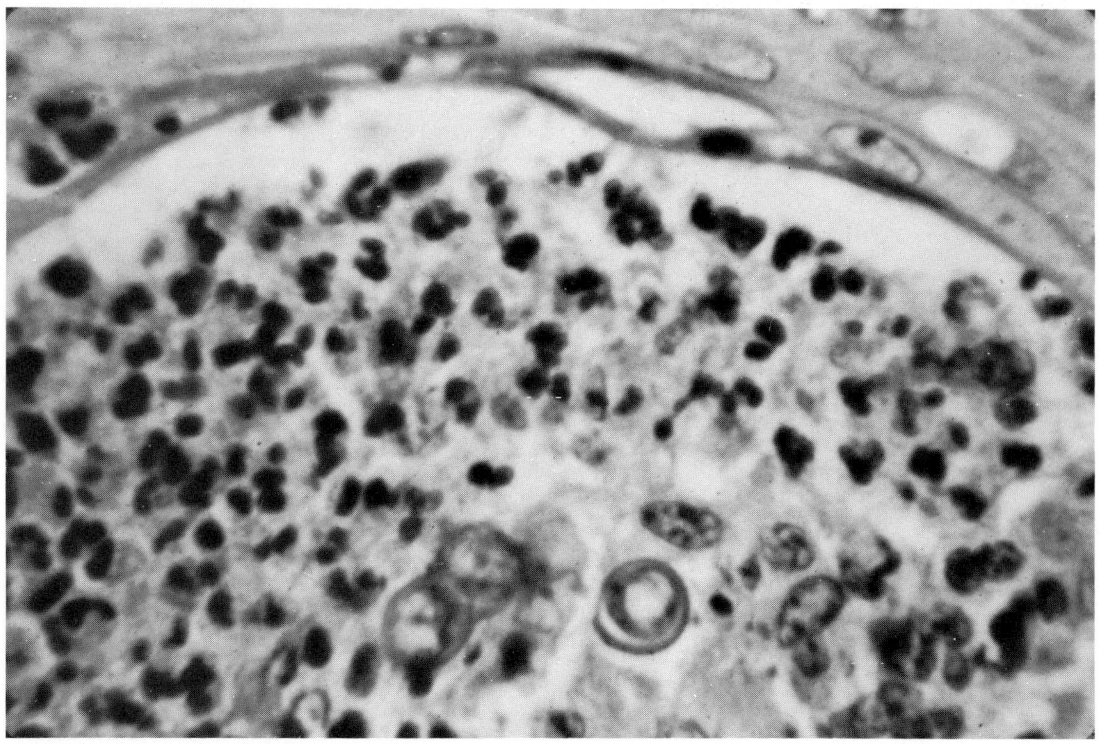

Figure 48–7. Cutaneous microabscess including broad-based budding yeast forms of *Blastomyces dermatitidis*. ×450. Hematoxylin-eosin stain. (From Dolan, C. T., Funkhouser, J. W., Koneman, E. W., Miller, N. G., and Roberts, G. D.: Atlas of Clinical Mycology II. Chicago, American Society of Clinical Pathologists, 1975.)

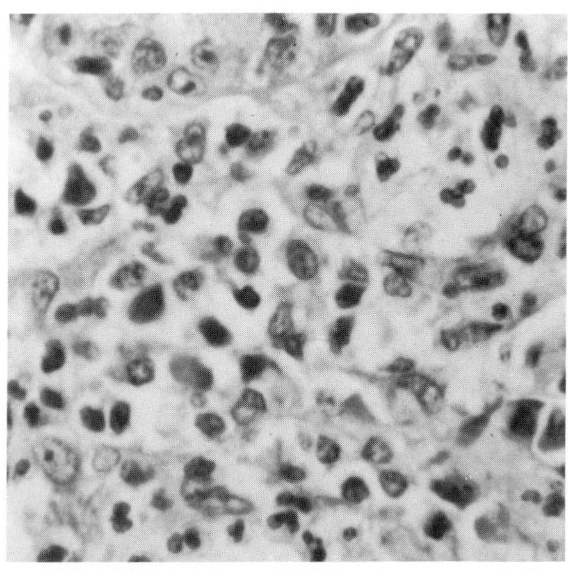

Figure 48–8. Chronic "round cell" inflammation showing reaction composed of mononuclear inflammatory cells. ×450. Hematoxylin-eosin stain.

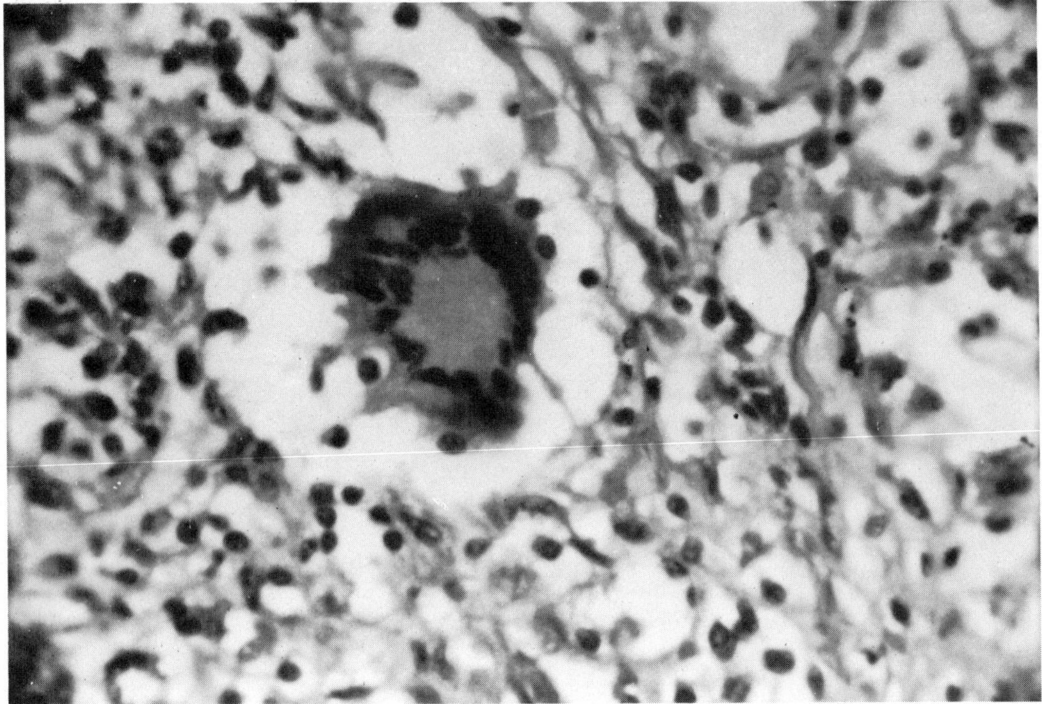

Figure 48–9. Inflammatory reaction including a Langhans giant cell with characteristic peripheral arrangement of nuclei. ×250. Hematoxylin-eosin stain.

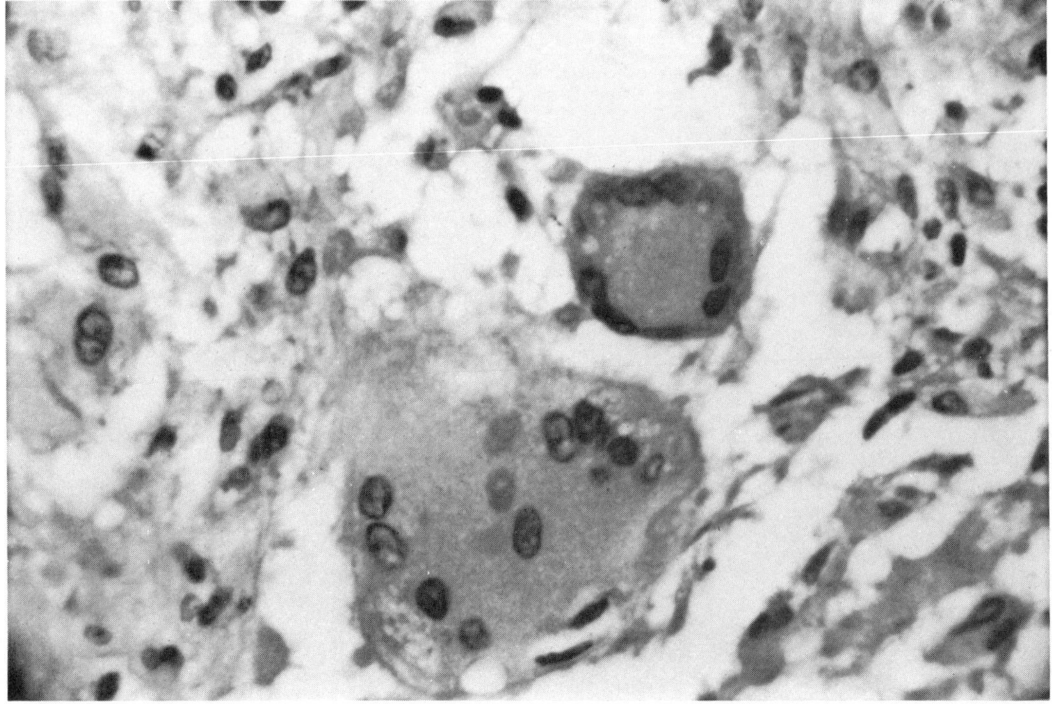

Figure 48–10. Comparison of Langhans' giant cell (top) with tumor giant cell (bottom). ×250. Hematoxylin-eosin stain.

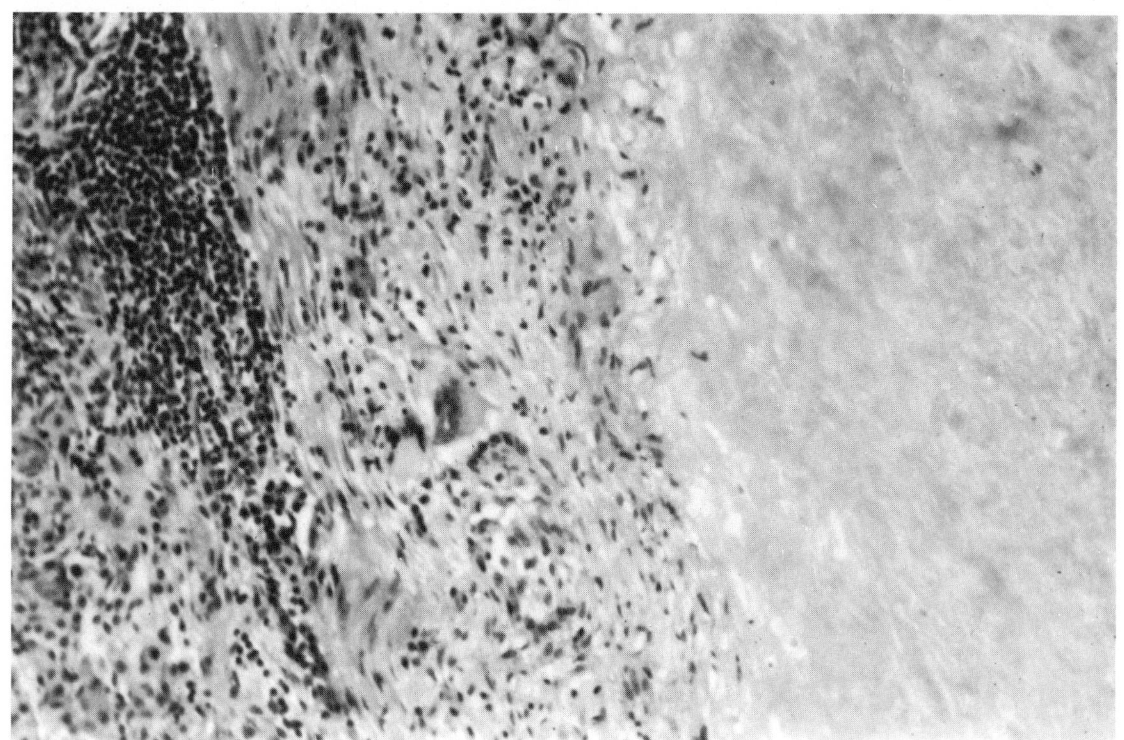

Figure 48–11. Portion of a "tuberculoma." Caseation necrosis is present on the right, adjacent to a band of fibrosis including giant cells and a collection of lymphocytes on the left. ×100. Hematoxylin-eosin stain.

stances produced by the tubercle bacilli. However, caseation necrosis is not infrequently seen in mycotic infections, notably *Histoplasma capsulatum* and *Coccidioides immitis,* and Langhans' giant cells may be seen as well.

Necrotizing Inflammation, With or Without Infarction. *Infarction* is a term used to describe that process by which a portion of an organ or segment of tissue undergoes cellular death due to sudden loss of blood supply. Infarctions are commonly observed in mycotic infections caused by *Aspergillus fumigatus* or one of the Zygomycetes (Phycomycetes) species of fungi because of their peculiar predilection for directly invading blood vessels (Fig. 48–12), causing vascular occlusion (thrombosis).

Necrosis is a term used to describe the "mopping up" cellular reaction in response to focal infarction. Virtually every type of inflammatory cell may be present in necrotizing inflammation, and a large amount of degenerate cellular debris is present. A large number of vacuolated, lipid-containing histiocytes are often present. Varying degrees of hemorrhage with the deposition of hemosiderin pigment in the areas of necrosis are seen. It is this type of reaction that produces the burned eschar appearance of tissue specimens that have been obtained from areas of necrosis secondary to Zygomycete infections.

Inert Response. Patients with immune deficiency disease or individuals under immunosuppressive therapy often do not produce a cellular inflammatory response to invading fungi or other microorganisms. So-called agranulocytic pneumonia is a prime example. For reasons not totally understood, *Cryptococcus neoformans* characteristically does not elicit a cellular inflammatory response, even in patients who are immunologically competent (Fig. 48–13). The lack of cellular response, together with the production of abundant polysaccharide capsular substance by *C. neoformans,* may lead to a misdiagnosis of mucin-secreting carcinoma.

In summary, fungal infections should be considered in the differential diagnosis of any of the tissue reactions described above, and special stains may be necessary to make an identification if either the yeast or hyphal forms cannot be recognized in routine H & E sections.

Presumptive Identification of Fungi in Tissue Sections

Fungi may assume one of two basic forms in tissues: (1) A mycelial form, characterized by the presence of filamentous structures called hyphae. (2) A yeast or "tissue" form in which only yeast cells are present. Tissue forms of commonly encountered fungi are listed in Table 48–6.

Some fungi produce only a yeast form in tissues,

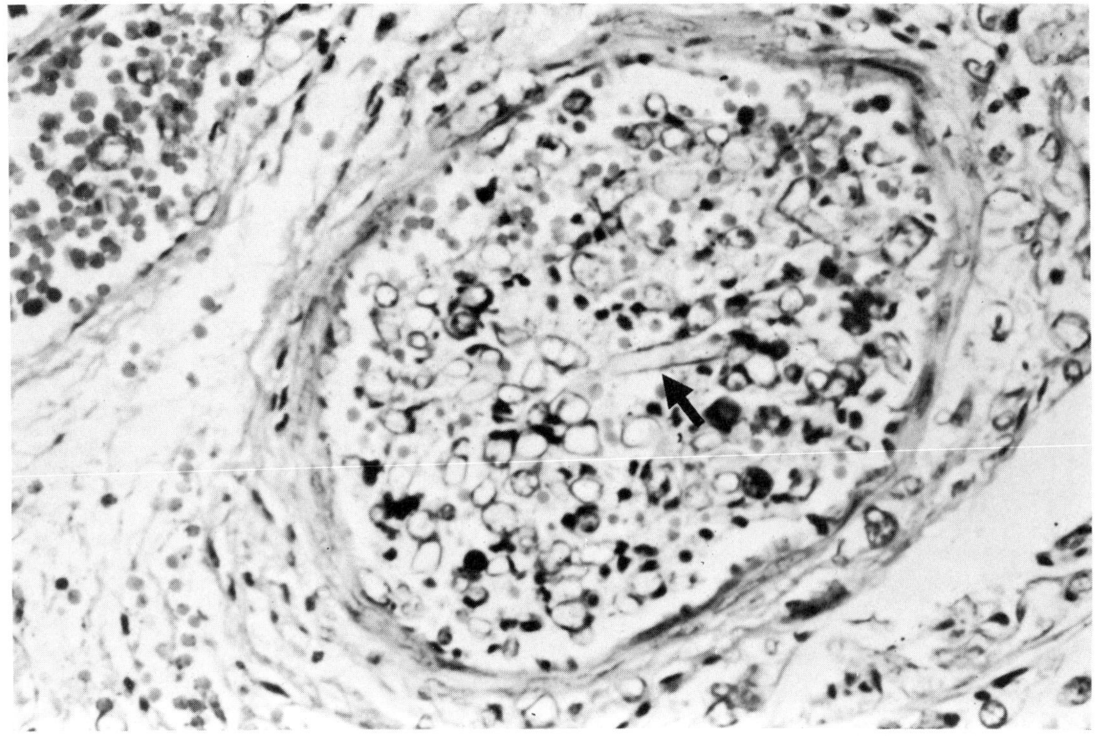

Figure 48–12. Arteriole showing a lumen occluded by aseptate hyphae (zygomycosis). ×250. Hematoxylin-eosin stain.

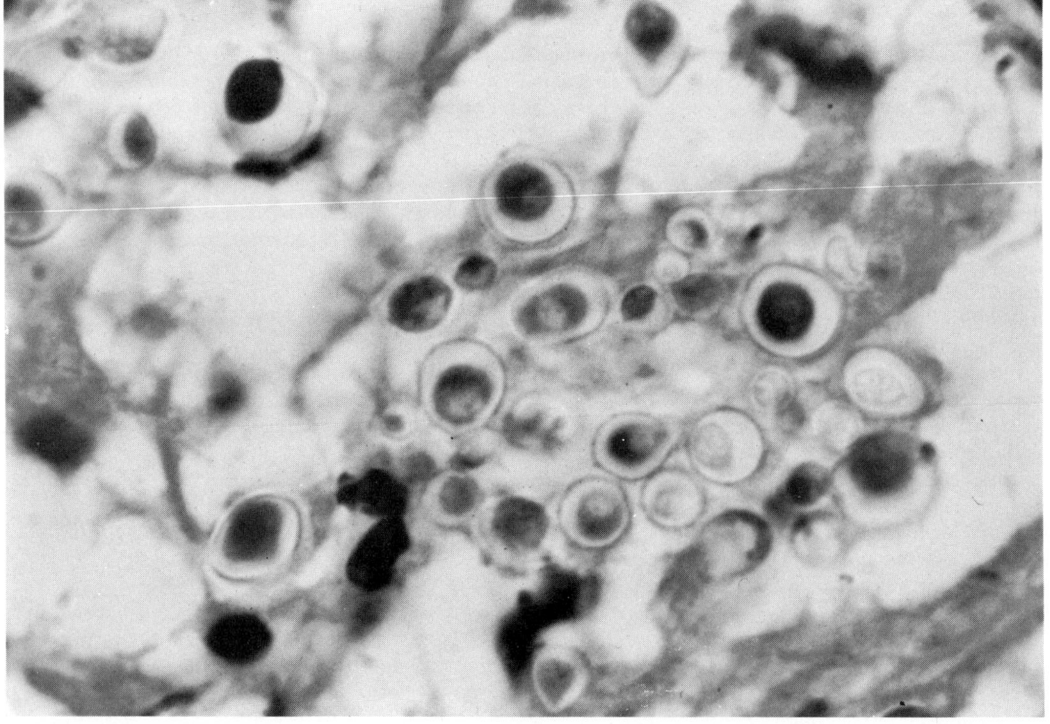

Figure 48–13. Tissue invasion with encapsulated yeast cells of *Cryptococcus neoformans*. Note lack of cellular inflammatory response and extreme variation in the size of the spherical yeast cells. ×250. Hematoxylin-eosin stain.

Table 48–6. TISSUE FORMS OF FUNGI OF MEDICAL IMPORTANCE TO MAN

Etiologic Agent	Diagnostic Tissue Form	Size	Comments
I. Deep-seated Mycoses			
Blastomyces dermatitidis	Thick-walled, double-contoured yeast cells, producing single bud attached by a broad base.	8–20 μ	
Coccidioides immitis	Thick-walled spherules enclosing numerous non-budding endospores.	10–60 μ	Rudimentary mycelium may rarely develop in open cavitary lesions.
Cryptococcus neoformans	Irregularly sized yeast cells, budding singly and attached by a hair-like neck, surrounded by a thick mucoid capsule.	4–15 μ	*Cryptococcus neoformans* may rarely form pseudohyphae.
Histoplasma capsulatum	Small yeast cells located within reticuloendothelial cells. Pseudocapsules account for the species name.	2–4 μ	True capsules do not form.
Paracoccidioides brasiliensis	Large yeast cells producing multiple buds arranged in the form of a mariner's wheel.	8–20 μ	
II. Opportunistic Mycoses			
Aspergillus species	Hyaline, septate hyphae, dichotomously branching and regular in diameter with parallel opposing walls.	5–10 μ	Rarely, conidial-bearing fruiting bodies may develop in fungus ball cavities.
Candida species	Pseudohyphae composed of elongated blastoconidia, showing regular points of constriction simulating link sausages. Budding oval or spherical blastospores also present.	5–10 μ (Pseudohyphae) 3–4 μ (Blastoconidia)	
Geotrichum candidum	Hyphae producing arthrocondia.	10–30 μ	
Zygomycetes *Mucor* sp. *Rhizopus* sp. *Absidia* sp.	Broad, aseptate, irregularly branching, ribbon-like hyphae with non-parallel opposing walls.		Rarely, sporangial fruiting bodies may form in fungus ball cavities.
Actinomyces israelii	Delicate, branching, minute filaments often within "sulfur granules."	Less than 1 μ	*A. israelii* is an anaerobic bacterium.
Nocardia asteroides	Delicate, branching, minute filaments often within "sulfur granules."		Branching filamentous, "partially" acid-fast bacterium.
III. Subcutaneous Mycoses Chromoblastomycosis group: *Fonsecaea pedrosoi* *Fonsecaea compactum* *Phialophora verrucosa* *Cladosporium carrionii*	Dark yellow or brown, septate, hyphal segments. Also, rounded or crescent-shaped, thick-walled deep yellow or brown sclerotic bodies.	5–8 μ (Hyphae) 8–15 μ (Sclerotic bodies)	
Pseudallescheria (Petriellidium) boydii	Production of yellow-gray granules containing wide mycelial forms often clubbed at the periphery of the granule.	6–8 μ	10–12 μ oval to round conidia may be produced in fungus ball cavities.
Actinomycetes	Delicate, branching filaments within "sulfur granules."	Less than 1 μ	*Nocardia* sp. filaments are partially acid-fast.
Sporothrix schenckii	Tiny, irregular, elongated cigar-shaped yeast forms.	3–5 μ	Yeast forms are extremely difficult to demonstrate in human tissues.
IV. Superficial Mycoses Dermatophyte group: *Microsporum* sp. *Epidermophyton* sp. *Trichophyton* sp.	Slender hyphal forms, often breaking into arthrospore-like segments in the stratum corneum of the skin. Endothrix and ectothrix minute spores in hair infections.	3–5 μ (Hyphae) 1–2 μ (Spores)	Fungal forms best demonstrated in direct KOH mounts of infected skin scales, nail scrapings, or plucked hairs.
Exophiala (Cladosporium) werneckii	Delicate, twisting, tortuous hyphal segments confined to the stratum lucidum.	1–2 μ	Fungal elements best demonstrated in direct KOH mounts.
Malassezia (Pityrosporum) furfur	Many short, stubby hyphal segments, admixed with budding spheroidal cells, limited to the stratum corneum.	3–5 μ (Hyphae) 4–6 μ (Cells)	Fungal elements best demonstrated in direct KOH mounts.

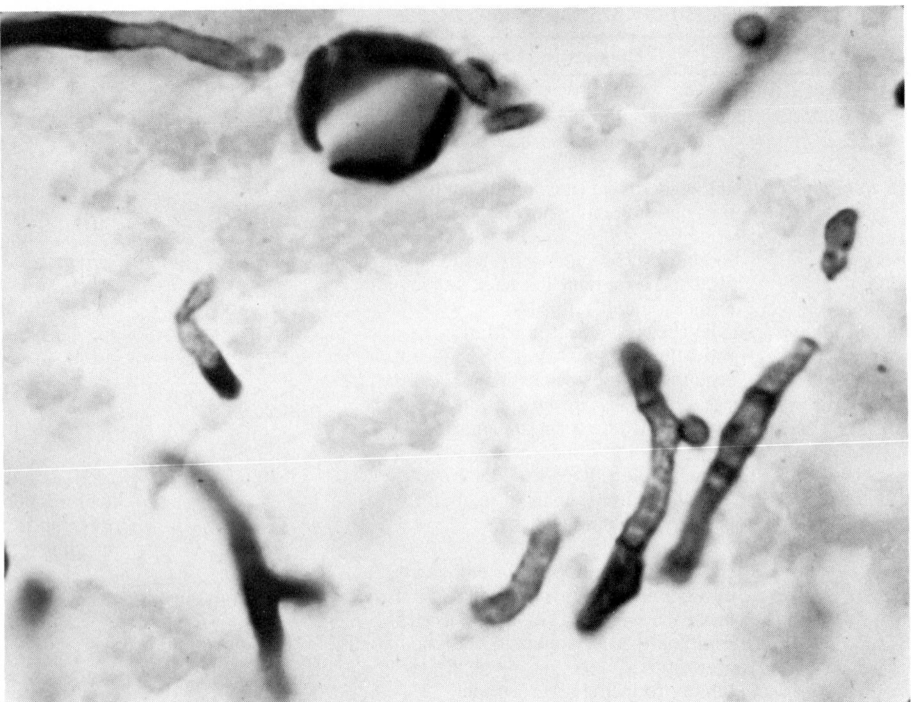

Figure 48–14. Tissue invasion with *Coccidioides immitis* showing rare occurrence of both spherule and hyphal forms. ×450. Gomori methenamine silver stain.

others only a mycelial form. Rarely do the two occur together in the same organ or tissue. The dimorphic fungi, which include most of the species causing deep-seated mycotic disease in man, are called "dimorphic" because they can assume either a mycelial or a yeast form depending upon environmental temperature.

The mycelial form is produced at temperatures less than 37°C. This is the natural form of filamentous fungi in the environment, is the form most commonly used for culture identification in the laboratory, and is the form that is most commonly infective for men.

The yeast form of the dimorphic fungi is assumed at 37°C. incubation, the normal body temperature of man. Only in rare instances will a dimorphic fungus assume the mycelial form in tissues. One example is shown in Figure 48–14, a case of cavitary *Coccidioides immitis* infection in a lung. Note that both the spherule and the mycelial forms are present. This situation occurs most commonly when a pulmonary cavity is in open communication with a bronchus and the fungus is exposed to atmospheric air.

Similarly, fungi that have only a mycelial form do not produce fruiting bodies when present in tissues, except in fugus ball infections when sporulation may occur. Figure 48–15 is an example of how fruiting bodies of *Aspergillus* species may appear in tissue sections. Shown are two vesicles with radiating phialides and a few brown conidia at the periphery. A definitive diagnosis of aspergillosis is possible when these structures are observed in tissue sections.

Therefore, the initial observation that should be made by the surgical pathologist when suspected fungal elements are seen in tissue sections is to determine whether the form being observed is mycelia or yeast, or, if possible, if one of the dimorphic pathogenic species might be present.

Identification of Yeast Forms in Tissues

Fungi that do not produce hyphae in tissue, rather remaining in the yeast form only, can be presumptively identified by evaluating the following: (1) the size of the individual yeast cells; (2) the arrangement and location of the yeast cells; and (3) the number and mode of attachment of buds (blastoconidia) that may be present.

Table 48–7 is a guide to the identification of the yeast forms most commonly observed in tissue sections. Note that these yeasts have been divided into two major groups based on the size of their individual cells: small yeasts ranging from 1 to 7 μ and large yeasts ranging from 8 to 20 μ.

Once it has been determined that the yeast cells being observed are small, generally between 1 and 4 μ, ascertain if any cells are intracellular. This assessment can be made on H & E stained tissue sections, as shown in Figure 48–16. Intracytoplasmic yeast cells, such as those seen in Figure 48–16, that appear to be encapsulated are highly suggestive of *Histoplasma*

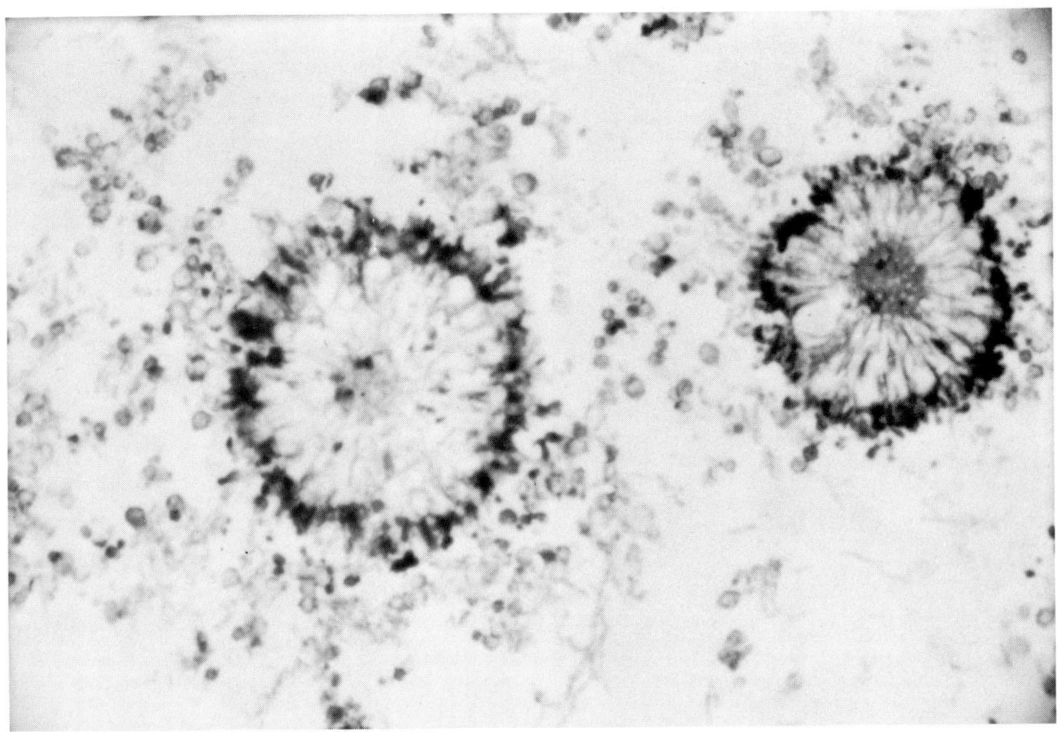

Figure 48–15. Transverse section of aspergillus "fruiting heads" seen in tissue section of lung with a fungus ball infection. ×450. Hematoxylin-eosin stain. Fruiting heads are easier to visualize when seen from the side, as illustrated in Figure 48–29.

Table 48–7. IDENTIFICATION OF TISSUE YEAST FORMS

Yeast Species	Size of Yeast Cells	Identifying Characteristics
I. Yeast cells of small size (1–4 μ)		
Coccidioides immitis (endospores)	Regular: 2–4 μ	Spherical, easy to identify when contained within characteristic spherule.
Cryptococcus neoformans (non-encapsulated)	Irregular size: range from 1–7 μ	Easy to identify when surrounded by thick mucinous capsule. Budding forms may be present, with daughter cell attached by narrow thread.
Histoplasma capsulatum	Regular: 2–4 μ	Have a characteristic pseudocapsule when observed within reticuloendothelial cells. May be extremely difficult to differentiate from coccidioides endospores or non-encapsulated cryptococcal cells when lying free in tissues.
Candida (Torulopsis) glabrata	Tiny: less than 1–2 μ	Cells usually lie in compact clusters within tissue spaces. Identification may be suspected on basis of extremely small size.
II. Yeast cells of large size: (8–20 μ)		
Blastomyces dermatitidis	Irregular 8–20 μ	Characteristic thick, doubly refractile wall, forming single bud attached with a broad base.
Coccidioides immitis (spherules)	Irregular: immature spherules 5–20 μ; mature 50 μ and greater	Immature spherules may simulate yeast cells of *B. dermatidis* due to thick refractile wall. Identification is made when endospores are identified within the spherule space.
Cryptococcus neoformans (encapsulated)	Irregular: 5–20 μ if capsule is measured	Thick mucinous capsule is virtually diagnostic. Look for small buds attached by hair-like threads.
Paracoccidioides brasiliensis	Irregular: 8–20 μ or more	Mature yeast cells have thick capsule, with multiple daughter buds around the periphery, simulating a mariner's wheel.

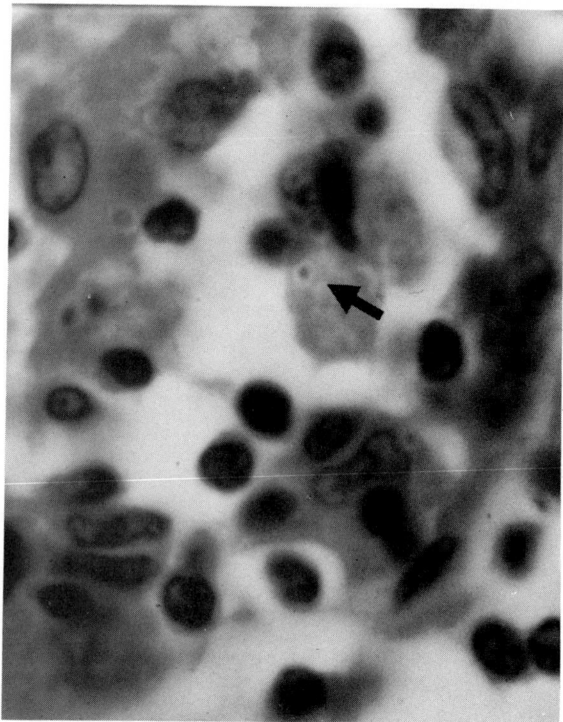

Figure 48–16. Section of an inflammatory reaction showing aggregates of large reticuloendothelial histolytic cells within the cytoplasm of which are contained small pseudoencapsulated yeast forms of *Histoplasma capsulatum.* ×950. Hematoxylin-eosin stain.

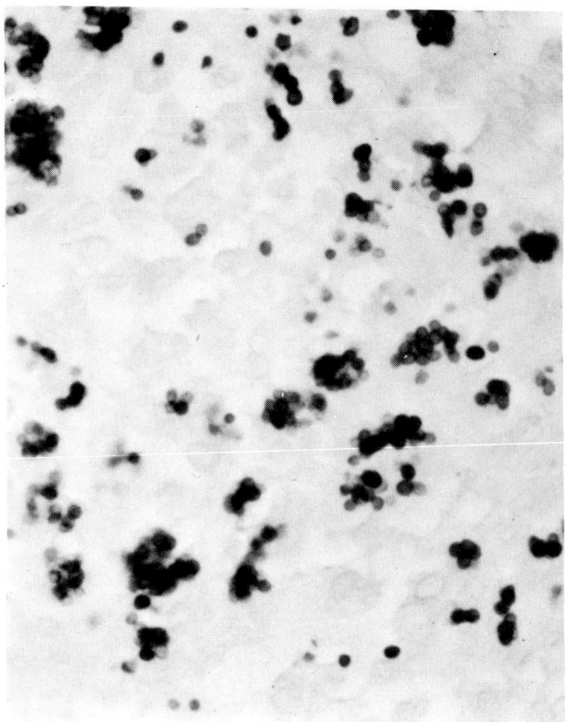

Figure 48–17. Section of lung showing intracellular clusters of tiny (2 to 4 μ) yeast forms of *Histoplasma capsulatum.* ×450. Gomori methenamine silver stain.

capsulatum. H. capsulatum, despite its species name, does not possess a true capsule; rather, the pseudoencapsulated effect is produced in stained preparations from the shrinkage of the yeast cell from the outer membrane during the fixation process. Figure 48–17 is a photomicrograph of a silver-stained section showing clusters of the tiny (2 to 4 μ) yeast forms of *H. capsulatum.*

The yeast forms of *Cryptococcus neoformans* can generally be readily identified by the presence of a thick, mucinous capsule (Fig. 48–13). The small central yeast cells vary from 2 to 7 μ in diameter; however, the presence of the capsule makes them appear as much as 20 μ in diameter. Variation in cell size is one helpful characteristic by which *C. neoformans* can be distinguished from other yeast cells of similar size. This feature is best demonstrated in silver-stained preparations. Figure 48–18 shows marked differences in size of the individual yeast cells.

The endospores of *Coccidioides immitis* are not difficult to identify when they are enclosed within the characteristic spherules to be described below. However, when 2 to 4 μ individual yeast cells are seen lying free in tissues (Fig. 48–22), it may be extremely difficult to differentiate extracellular forms of *H. capsulatum,* non-encapsulated forms of *C. neoformans* (irregularity in size may be one aid), and endospores of *C. immitis* that have been released from their spherules. In such instances, an extensive search

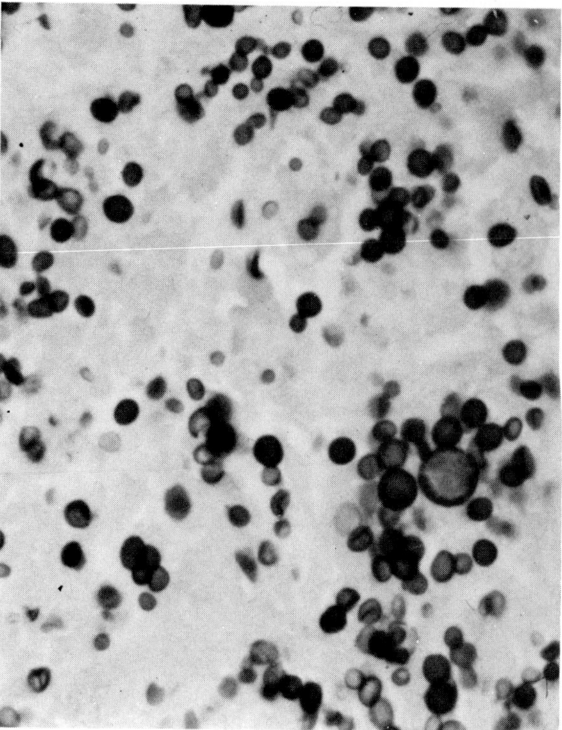

Figure 48–18. Section of lung illustrating the marked variation in size of cells of *Cryptococcus neoformans,* a helpful differential clue in the identification of this yeast. ×450. Gomori methenamine silver stain.

throughout the tissue sections may be necessary to locate a few yeast forms that may still be intracellular, a few forms that have retained a mucinous capsule, or remnants of a spherule before a presumptive identification can be made. In the absence of any of these, the final diagnosis may be possible only by recovering the causative agent in culture.

Candida glabrata is another yeast that is encountered in human infections with increasing frequency. *C. glabrata* may be suspected in tissue sections because of the small size of the yeast cells (2 to 5 μ) and their tendency to cluster together (Fig. 48–19). However, *C. glabrata* may on occasion be intracellular within non-nuclear inflammatory cells, and because of tissue shrinkage, may also appear pseudoencapsulated, closely simulating *H. capsulatum*. In these instances, recovery of the etiologic yeast in culture may be the only means for making a definitive identification.

The yeast forms of *Sporothrix schenckii* are also small but are rarely seen in human tissue. They can be demonstrated in animal tissue as illustrated in Figure 48–20. Characteristic cells are 2 to 5 μ, are oval to "cigar-shaped," and produce one or more buds at either or both poles.

The group of yeasts producing larger cells are generally identified in tissue sections with less difficulty than the smaller forms.

Blastomyces dermatitidis produces yeast cells that vary from 8 to 20 μ in diameter and have thick, doubly contoured walls that appear refractile. A definitive identification can be made if yeast cells having a single bud attached by a broad base are identified (Fig. 48–21). If budding forms cannot be found, there may be difficulty in distinguishing *B. dermatitidis* from immature spherules of *Coccidioides immitis* which are devoid of endospores. In these instances, additional tissue sections should be screened for mature spherules containing endospores or for broad-based budding forms. If not found, the final diagnosis may have to await positive culture results.

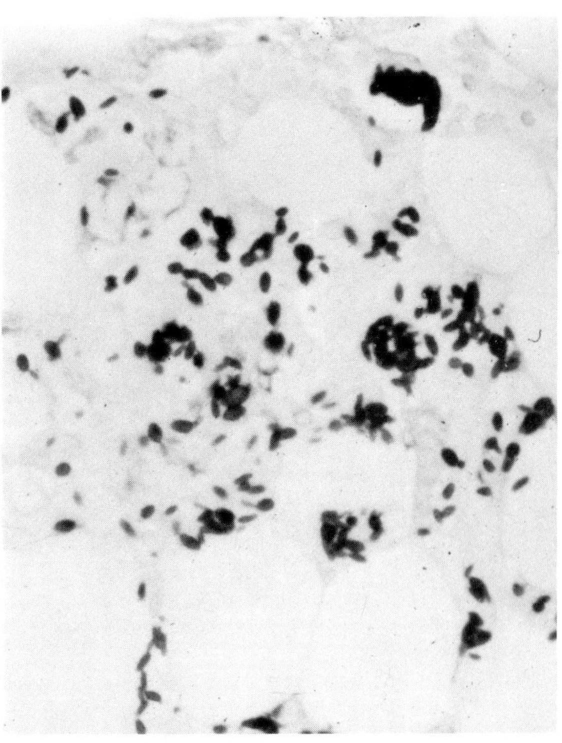

Figure 48–20. Section of animal tissue showing small (2 to 5 μ) oval to elongated (cigar bodies) yeast cells of *Sporothrix schenckii*. ×450. Gomori methenamine silver stain.

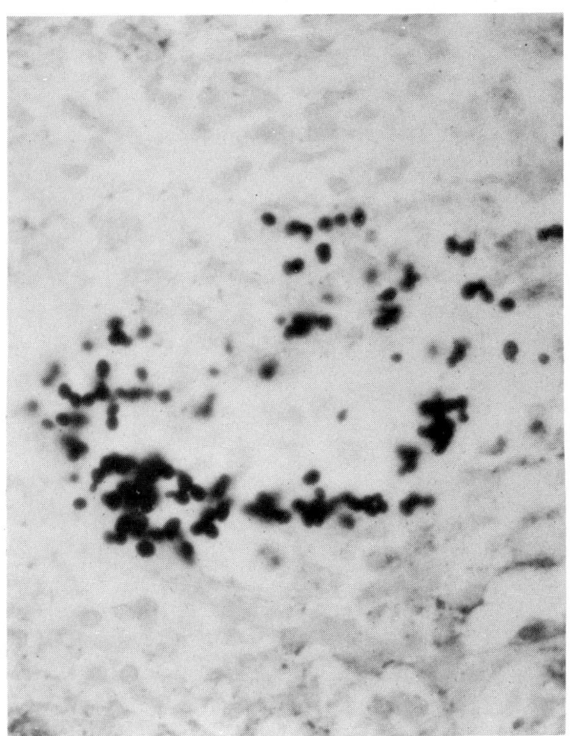

Figure 48–19. Inflammatory reaction showing clusters of small yeast forms of *Candida glabrata*. ×450. Gomori methenamine silver stain.

A typical spherule of *C. immitis* containing mature endospores is shown in Figure 48–22. Spherules are generally greater than 20 μ in diameter, reaching as much as 60 μ. Figure 48–22 is virtually diagnostic when observed in tissue sections.

Although the encapsulated yeast forms of *C. neoformans* may approach the size of *B. dermatitidis* in tissue sections, identification is usually not difficult. The mucicarmine stain is virtually specific for the capsular material of *C. neoformans* and can be useful if confusion should arise. The presence of the thick capsule, together with the narrow attachment of the budding cell, is usually sufficient to make a presumptive identification of *C. neoformans* in tissues. Because of the frequent lack of a cellular response and the dense infiltration of tissues with encapsulated *C. neoformans*, the differential diagnosis of mucin-secreting carcinoma may at times be difficult. However, the small central yeast cells and the lack of large pleomorphic nuclei are generally sufficient to suspect *C. neoformans*.

The large yeast forms of *Paracoccidioides brasiliensis* are not difficult to identify in tissue sections when the

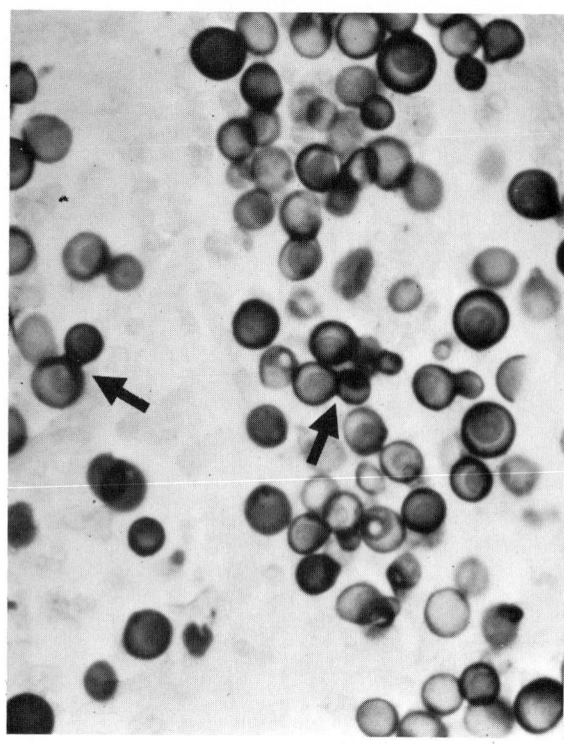

Figure 48–21. Section of lung showing large (8 to 15 μ) yeast cells of *Blastomyces dermatitidis*. Note broad-base budding forms. ×450. Gomori methenamine silver stain.

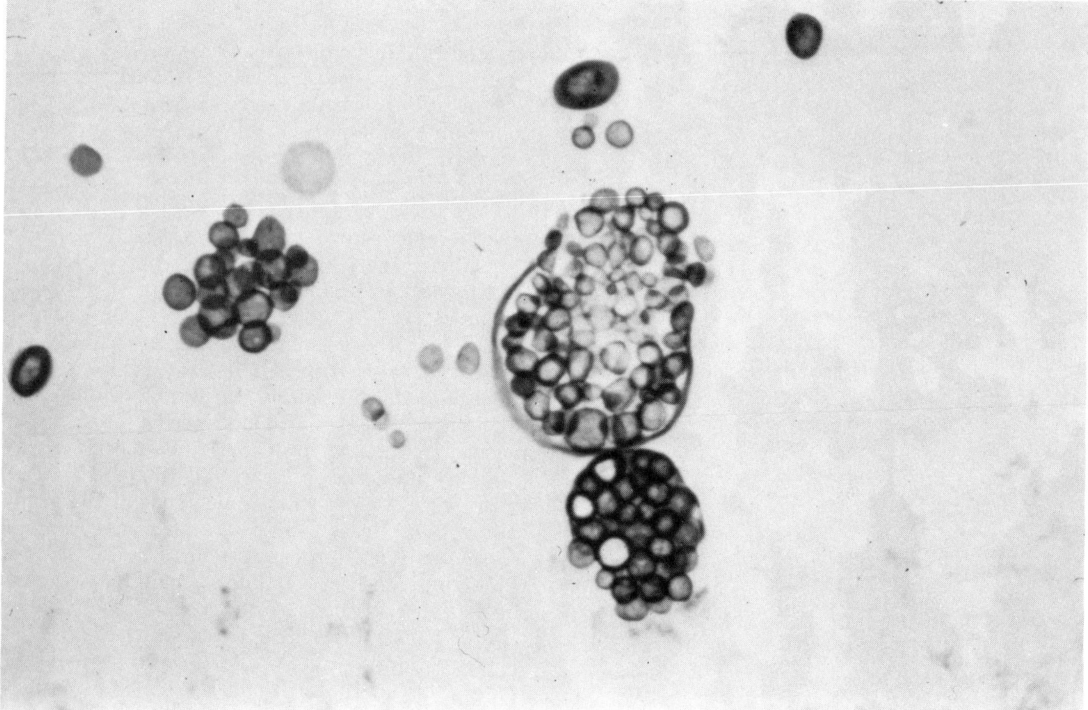

Figure 48–22. Section of lung showing a classic spherule of *Coccidioides immitis* containing numerous endospores. ×450. Gomori methenamine silver stain.

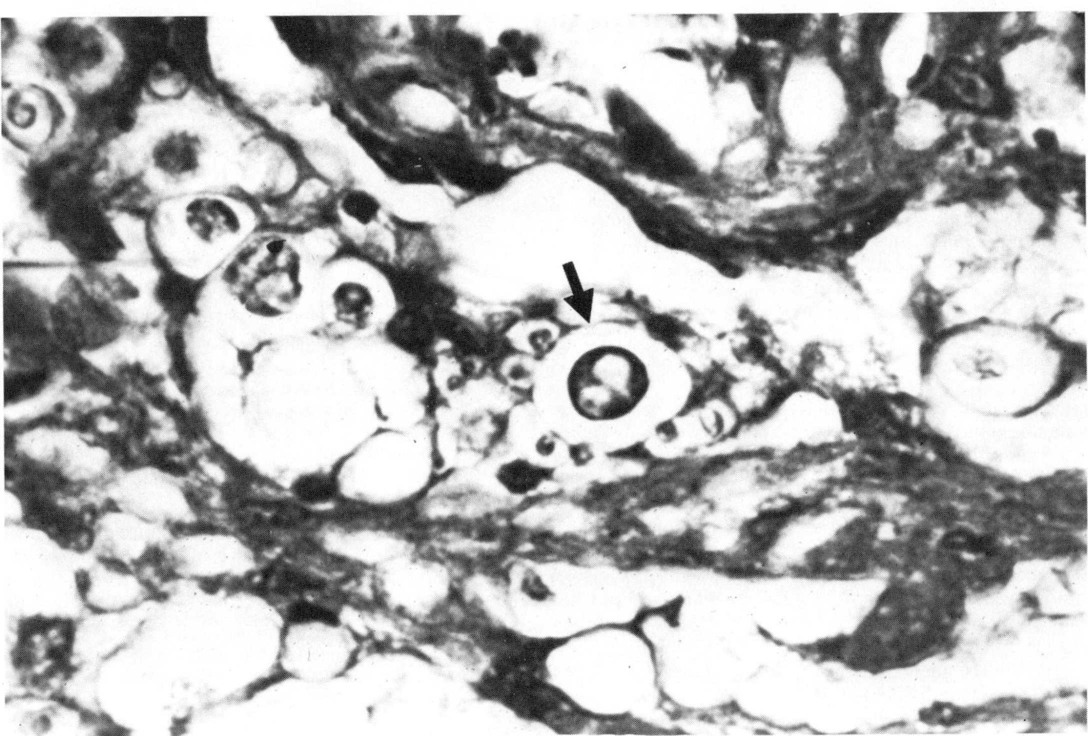

Figure 48–23. Tissue section showing *Paracoccidioides brasiliensis.* Note the characteristic large yeast cell (arrow) with multiple buds simulating a "mariner's wheel." ×450. Hematoxylin-eosin stain. (From Dolan, C. T., Funkhouser, J. W., Koneman, E. W., Miller, N. G., and Roberts, G. D.: Atlas of Clinical Mycology II. Chicago, American Society of Clinical Pathologists, 1975.)

multiple peripheral budding cells simulating a mariner's wheel are seen (Fig. 48–23). However, in the absence of multiple buds, the large mother yeast cells may be impossible to distinguish from *B. dermatitidis* in tissue sections, and cultures may be required to make the final identification. The clinical history and geographic location of the patient would also be helpful in making the differentiation.

Identification of Mycelial Forms in Tissues

The detection of delicate filaments or hyphal strands in tissue sections suggests one of the etiologic agents outlined in Table 48–8.

If the hyphal forms appear irregular in diameter, ranging between 10 and 60 μ, are ribbon-like, branch irregularly, and are devoid of septa, one of the fungal species belonging to the Zygomycetes (Phycomycetes) should be suspected (Fig. 48–24). In older lesions, the tissue reaction may distort the hyphae to the point that recognition becomes difficult (Fig. 48–25). Silver-stained preparations may not be useful, since the stain may not penetrate the hyphae (Fig. 48–26).

All other filamentous fungi produce septate hyphae in tissue sections. The mycelium of *Candida* species is actually composed of pseudohyphae, recognized by regular points of constriction along the strands, closely resembling link sausages (Fig. 48–27). Pseudohyphae are elongated blastoconidia, and the points of constriction represent the residual points of attachment of the primitive buds. The ability to recognize pseudohyphae is helpful in differentiating *Candida* from *Aspergillus. Candida* also commonly produce budding yeast cells along with the pseudohyphae, structures never formed by *Aspergillus* (Fig. 48–27).

When observing septate hyphae in tissue sections, an initial determination should be made whether or not arthroconidia are being formed. *Coccidioides immitis* is the most common pathogenic fungus that forms arthroconidia; however, as discussed above, these rarely form at 37°C. Therefore, the presence of arthroconidia in tissue sections is virtually diagnostic of geotrichosis. Geotrichosis, caused by *Geotrichum candidum,* is a relatively rare disease, and arthroconidia do not always form in tissues. The dermatophytic fungi also may produce arthroconidia; however, they are limited to the superficial corneum of the skin, and tissue biopsies are rarely procured to diagnose dermatophytoses.

Aspergillus is the most common fungal agent that will be observed in tissue sections. Unless there is considerable tissue distortion, the hyphae of *Aspergillus* species can be readily identified. They are distinctly septate (the septa appear more prominent in special fungal stained preparations), are uniform in diameter, range from 5 to 10 μ wide, have parallel walls, and

Table 48–8. IDENTIFICATION OF TISSUE HYPHAL FORMS

Hyphal Morphology Observed	Etiologic Agent Suspected	Comments
Hyphae aseptate, irregularly broad, and ribbon-like, 10–30 μ in diameter, irregularly branching, opposing hyphal walls not parallel.	Zygomycetes (Phycomycetes) Mucor species *Rhizopus* species *Absidia* species	In fungus ball cavities also look for diagnostic sporangial fruiting heads.
Hyphae appear septate, with points of constriction at septations, simulating link sausages. Oval 3–5 μ budding yeast cells may also be seen.	*Candida* species *Candida albicans*	Diagnostic chlamydospores do not form in tissues.
Hyphae clearly septate, regular in diameter, breaking into distinct arthrospores.	*Geotrichum candidum* Dermatophyte species: keratin skin only.	*Coccidioides immitis* only rarely forms rudimentary mycelial structures in tissues. Spherules usually can be found.
Hyphae, distinctly septate, hyaline, branch regularly and dichotomously at 45 degree angles, regular in diameter (5–10 μ) with opposite walls parallel.	*Aspergillus* species *Aspergillus fumigatus* *Aspergillus flavus* *Aspergillus niger*	In fungus ball cavities also look for diagnostic vesicular, conidia-bearing fruiting heads.
Hyphae distinctly septate, dark yellow or brown in color (dematiacious), in short segments without branching.	Chromoblastomycosis group: *Fonsecaea pedrosoi* *Fonsecaea compactum* *Phialophora verrucosa* *Cladosporium carrionii*	Also search the inflammatory areas for the presence of spherical, multi-celled, dark yellow or brown sclerotic bodies.
Hyphae in form of delicate, gram-positive, branching filaments, either free in the inflammatory infiltrate or confined within "sulfur granules" ("ray fungus").	Actinomycetes: *Actinomyces* species *Nocardia* species *Streptomyces* species	If *Actinomyces* species is suspected, tissue must be submitted for anaerobic culture. *Nocardia* sp. filaments are "partially" acid-fast.

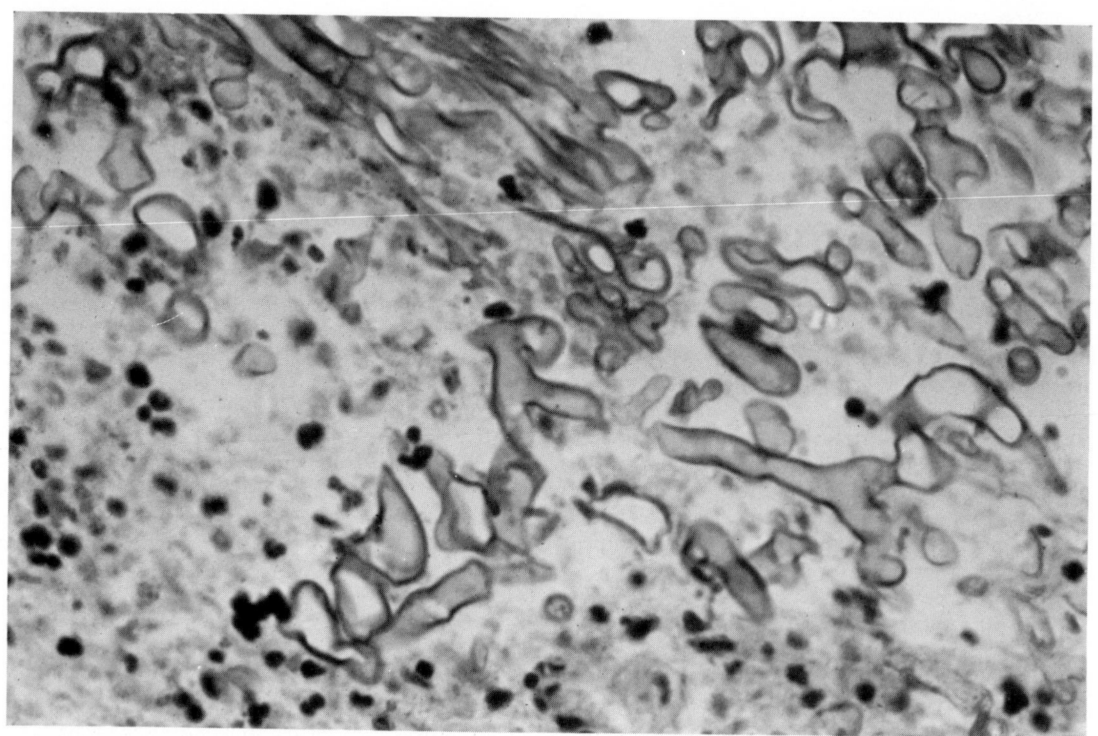

Figure 48–24. Tissue section showing broad, irregularly branching, ribbon-like aseptate hyphae of a Zygomycete. ×450. Hematoxylin-eosin stain.

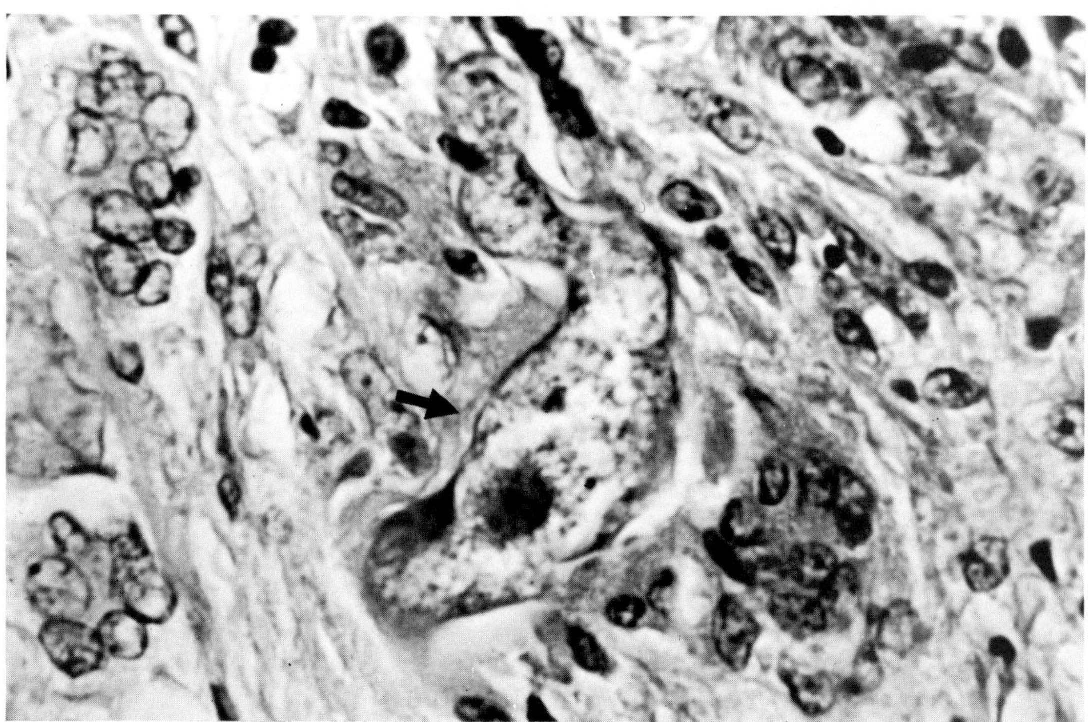

Figure 48–25. Tissue section exhibiting Zygomycete infection. Illustrated is a giant cell granulomatous reaction and a distorted ribbon-like hyphal fragment with severe cystic degeneration that makes identification difficult. ×450. Hematoxylin-eosin stain.

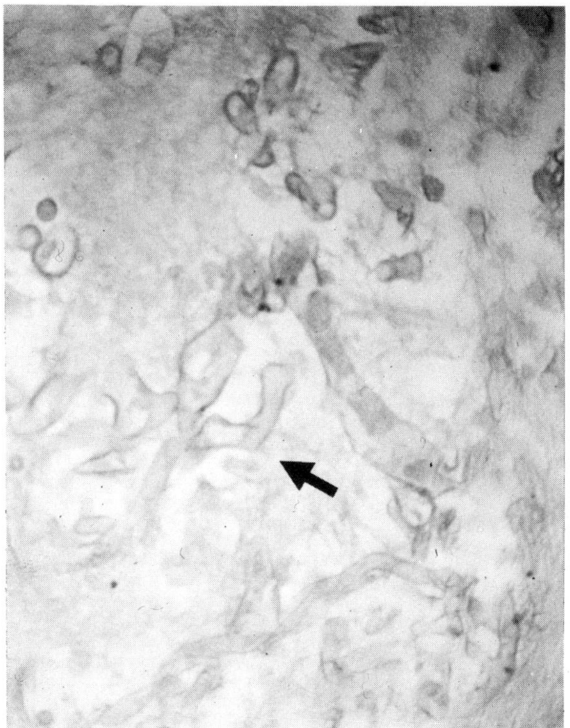

Figure 48–26. Section of lung tissue showing poor penetration of the hyphal forms of a Zygomycete by the silver stain. ×450. Gomori methenamine silver stain.

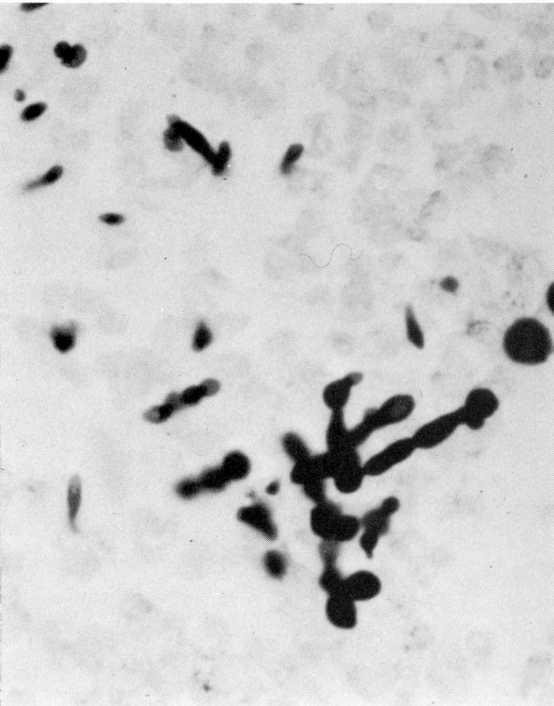

Figure 48–27. Tissue section showing infection with *Candida albicans.* Pseudohyphae with sausage-like points of constriction and a few budding cells are illustrated. ×450. Gomori methenamine silver stain.

6

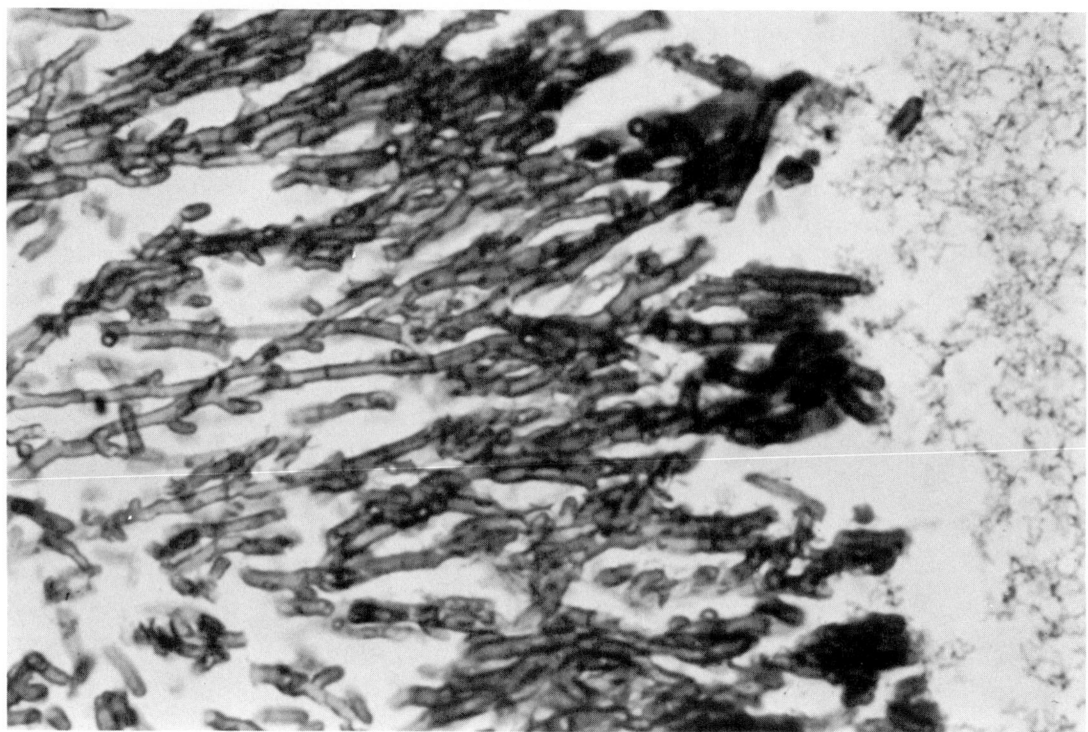

Figure 48–28. Tissue section showing invasion with septate, dichotomously branching hyphae of *Aspergillus* species. ×450. Gomori methenamine silver stain.

branch dichotomously at 45 degree angles (Fig. 48–28). Sporulation does not occur except in cavitary fungus ball infections, and the detection of the vesicular fruiting heads with radiating phialides and chains of spores can lead to a definitive diagnosis. A species identification may also be possible if the vesicle is club shaped and sporulation is seen to take place only from the top half of the vesicle (Fig. 48–29). These features are characteristic of *A. fumigatus,* the species most commonly causing aspergillosis in man. Globose vesicles covered with densely packed, black conidia are highly suggestive of *A. niger* infection.

Septate hyphae that have a distinctly dark yellow or brown appearance in H & E stained tissue sections suggest infection with one of the dematiacious fungal agents responsible for chromoblastomycosis (Fig. 48–30). Hyphae are generally short and fragmented and may appear distorted by the inflammatory reaction. The presumptive diagnosis of chromoblastomycosis in tissue sections of suspected lesions can be strengthened by detecting the characteristic spherical, multicelled brown-staining sclerotic bodies (Fig. 48–31).

The presence of thin, delicate filaments that average no more than 1 μ in diameter and are freely branching is highly suspicious for infection with *Actinomyces* species, *Nocardia* species or *Streptomyces* species (Fig. 48–32). These forms are actually bacterial in nature and may lie free within a purulent exudate or be confined within "sulfur granules."

Nocardia species can be presumptively identified by demonstrating that the branching filaments are partially acid-fast. By "partially acid-fast" is meant that a dilute mineral acid, such as 1 per cent H_2SO_4, was used as the decolorizer, rather than the more potent acid alcohol solutions used in the routine Ziehl-Neelsen acid-fast stain. These filamentous forms can be confused with the rapidly growing species of mycobacteria. However, mycobacteria rarely if ever branch, an important feature in distinguishing them from the Actinomycetes. In some instances, however, culture may be necessary before a definitive diagnosis can be rendered.

When examining tissue sections from suspected cases of subcutaneous mycetoma infection, careful examination of the grains and granules is important in rendering a presumptive diagnosis. The sulfur granules characteristic of the Actinomycetes have been described above. A gray-white granule in which club-shaped, true hyphae are present is highly suggestive of infection with *Pseudallescheria (Petriellidium) boydii,* the most common cause of eumycotic mycetomatous infections in the United States (Fig. 48–33).

Pathologists are urged to collect as many tissue sections containing fungal structures as possible. These serve not only as a means for self study and instruction of others, but as a valuable reference resource for comparing new cases of presumptive fungal infections. These reference slides are particularly useful for comparing new slides from those fungal infections that are only rarely encountered.

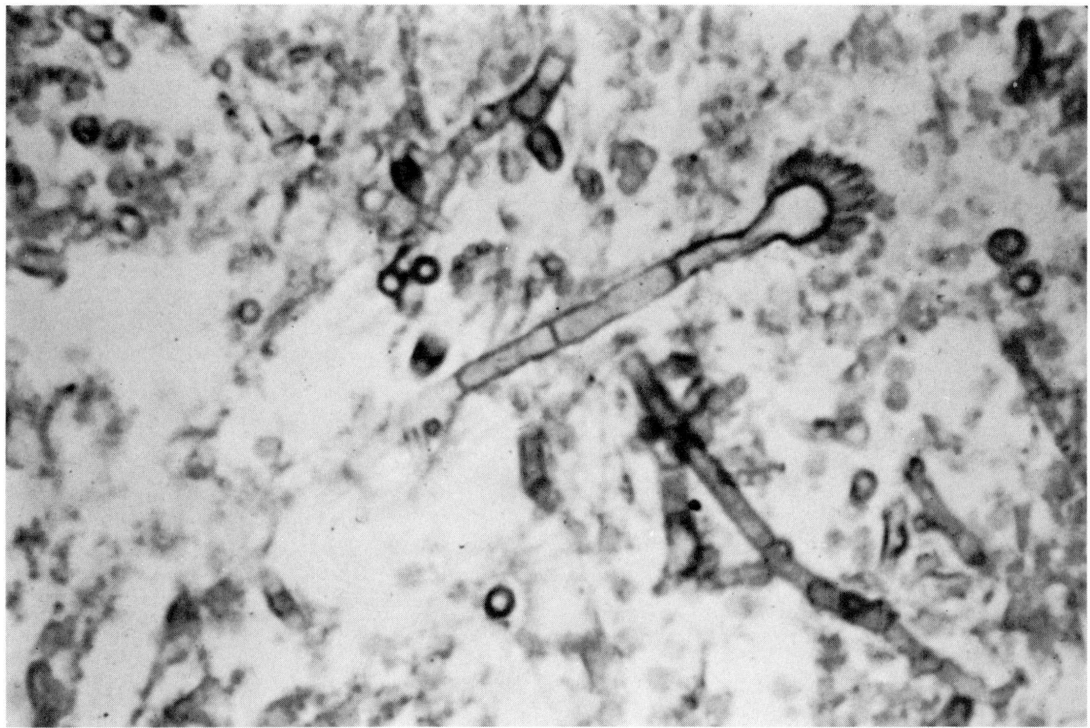

Figure 48–29. Tissue section showing portion of a fungus ball with a fruiting head having a club-shaped vesicle characteristic of *Aspergillus fumigatus*. ×100. Periodic acid–Schiff stain. (From Dolan, C. T., Funkhouser, J. W., Koneman, E. W., Miller, N. G., and Roberts, G. D.: Atlas of Clinical Mycology III. Chicago, American Society of Clinical Pathologists, 1975.)

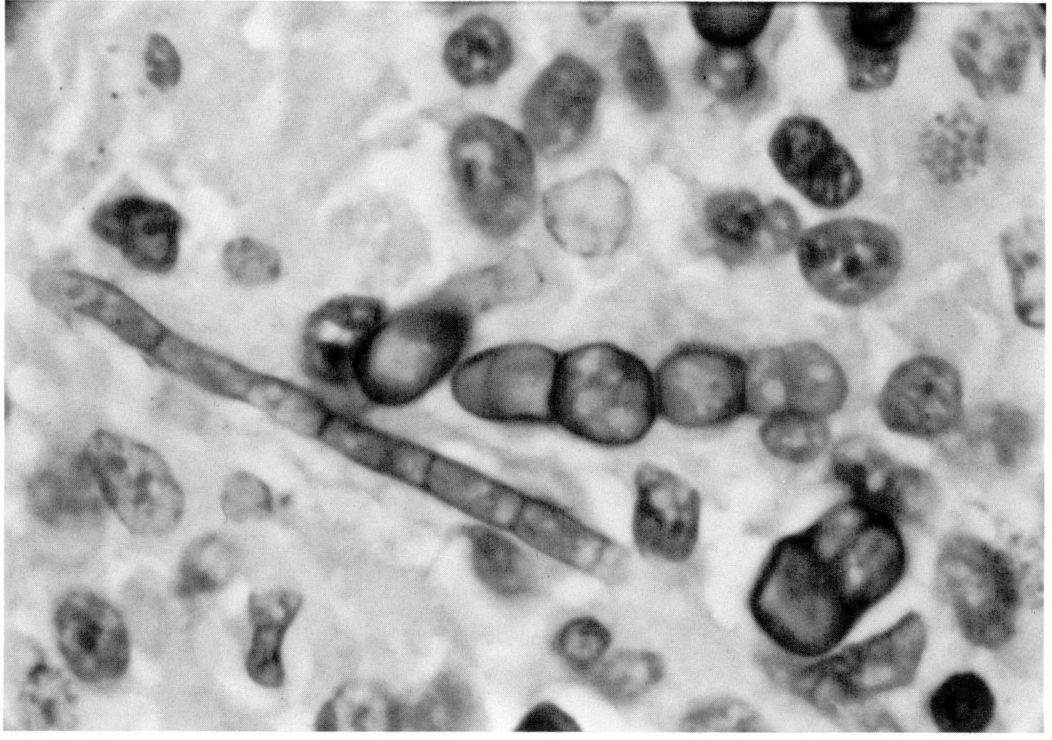

6

Figure 48–30. Inflammatory tissue reaction including short brown hyphal fragments suggestive of chromoblastomycosis infection. ×950. Hematoxylin-eosin stain.

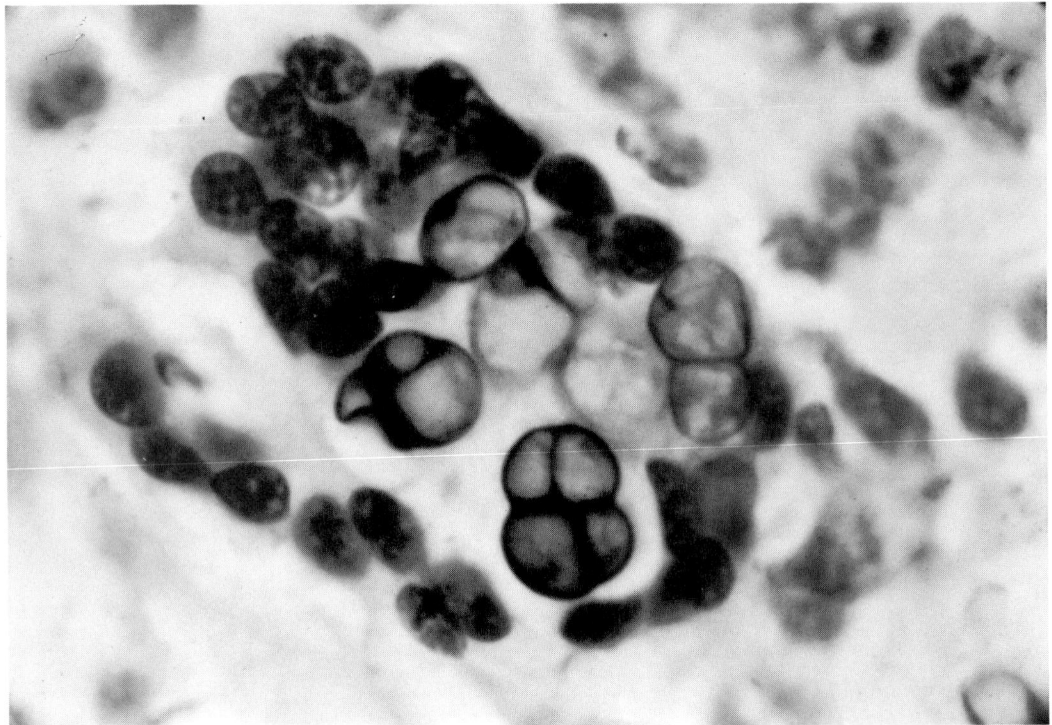

Figure 48–31. Multicelled brown sclerotic bodies characteristic of chromoblastomycosis infection. ×950. Hematoxylin-eosin stain.

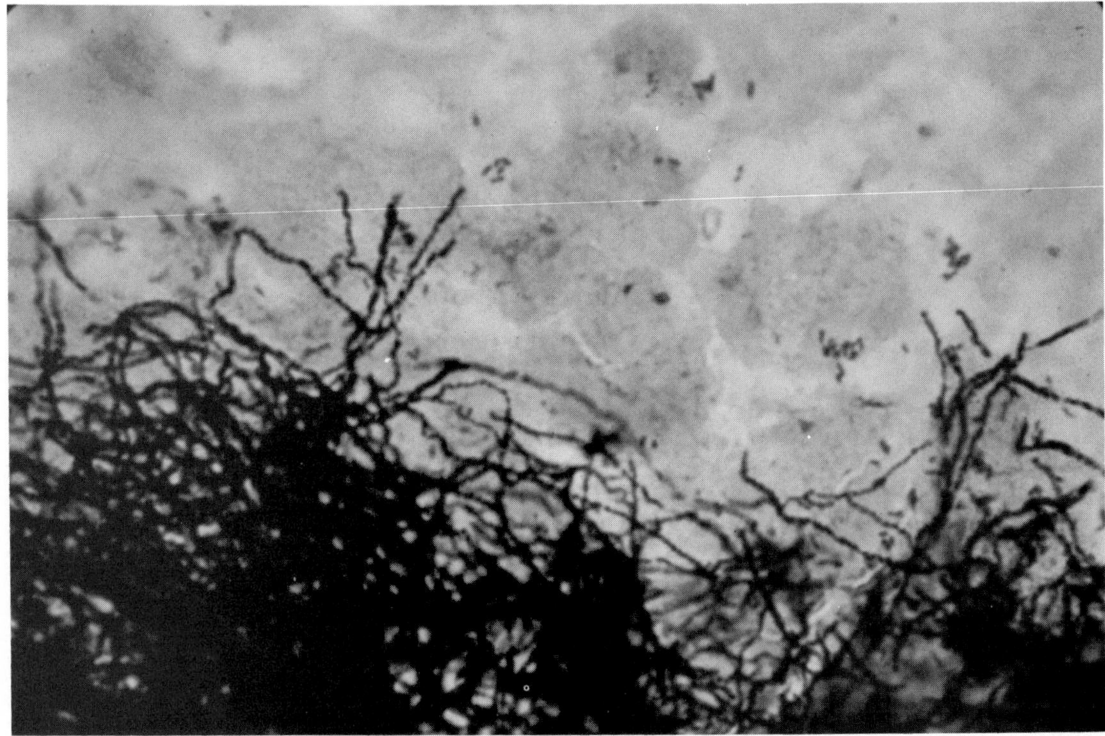

Figure 48–32. Tissue section showing infection with one of the aerobic actinomycetes. Note presence of delicate (1 μ) branching filaments. ×950. Gram stain.

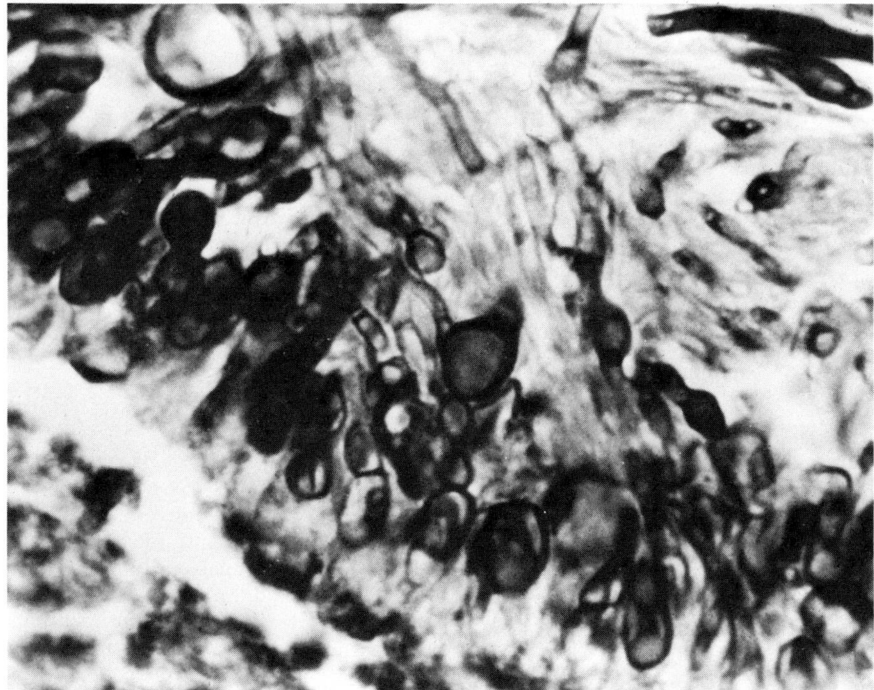

Figure 48–33. Section through a subcutaneous granule of *Pseudallescheria boydii* showing swollen cells at periphery. ×450. Gomori methenamine silver stain.

LABORATORY DIAGNOSIS OF FUNGAL INFECTIONS

The recovery of fungi from clinical specimens depends on the collection of an appropriate specimen and its rapid transport to the laboratory. If rapid transportation to the laboratory is impossible, the specimens should be refrigerated at 4°C. to prevent overgrowth by contaminating bacteria and yeasts which may be present. Once received by the laboratory, the specimen should be examined and inoculated onto appropriate culture media. The following section will be devoted to the processing and culturing of clinical specimens for mycologic examination.

Cerebrospinal Fluid

One to 3 ml of freshly collected cerebrospinal fluid should be filtered through a 0.45 μ Swinnex filter (Millipore Corporation) attached to a sterile syringe. The filter is removed and placed on an appropriate culture medium so that the side containing the concentrate touches the agar surface. Cultures should be examined daily and the filter pad moved to another location on the medium surface. If more than 3 ml of specimen is collected, equal amounts of 2 ml or more should be separately filtered and cultured onto the appropriate media. If less than 2 ml of sample is collected, the cerebrospinal fluid should be centrifuged for 10 minutes and one-drop aliquots of the sediment should be placed onto several areas on the agar surface. This method is preferable to streaking the sample onto the agar surface with a loop, since it allows the organism to acclimate more easily to environmental conditions. Cultures should be examined daily for visible evidence of growth.

Media which are suitable for culturing cerebrospinal fluid specimens include brain-heart infusion agar, chocolate agar, Sabouraud's dextrose agar, Sabhi agar, and inhibitory mold agar. Cerebrospinal fluid specimens should not be cultured onto media which contain cycloheximide, since some important pathogens are known to be inhibited by this antifungal agent.

Blood

Blood culture bottles containing soybean-casein digest (e.g., Trypticase or Tryptic soy) broth or Columbia broth are satisfactory for the recovery of fungi from blood. It is recommended that these be vented with a sterile cotton-plugged needle throughout the duration of incubation. However, it is recommended that a biphasic brain-heart infusion agar–brain-heart infusion broth bottle be used, since the recovery rate of fungi is somewhat quickened using this system. Blood culture bottles should be examined daily for visible evidence of growth. If the biphasic brain-heart infusion agar-broth bottle is used, the surface of the agar should be flooded with the blood and cultures should be examined daily. All blood culture bottles should be incubated at 30°C. for a minimum of 30 days. Growth may appear either on the agar slant or in the broth. If either Columbia broth or soybean-casein digest broth is used, subcultures after 24 and 48 hours should be made onto brain-heart infusion agar or Sabouraud's dextrose agar. Small laboratories may prefer to inoculate 5 to 10 ml of blood onto the surface of Sabouraud's dextrose agar or brain heart infusion agar. Although not as efficient as those previously described, this method is adequate.

Recent studies have shown that a lysis-centrifugation system (Isolator, DuPont Clinical Systems, Wilmington, Delaware) is superior to conventional blood culture media for the recovery of fungi (Bille, 1982).

Urine

Currently there is debate concerning the value of quantitating urine cultures, and it is not recommended. All urine samples should be centrifuged and the sediment inoculated onto an appropriate medium. Specimens should be streaked with a loop to ensure adequate isolation of colonies. Contamination by gram-negative bacteria is often observed, making it necessary to use media containing antibacterial antibiotics.

Respiratory Secretions

Properly collected, respiratory secretions (sputum, bronchial washings, and transtracheal aspirations) are among the most important of all clinical specimens received for fungal cultures. Many mycotic infections have pulmonary manifestations, and respiratory secretions often provide the only microbiologic evidence of infection.

Respiratory secretions are commonly contaminated with bacteria and rapidly growing molds which may suppress or overgrow the slower growing true mycotic pathogens. It is necessary that culture media containing antibacterial antibiotics be included in the battery of media to be used. Cycloheximide, an antifungal antibiotic which prevents the rapid overgrowth of cultures by rapidly growing molds, should also be incorporated into one of the culture media used. As much specimen as possible (up to 0.5 ml) should be inoculated onto the surface of appropriate media. Cultures should be incubated at 30°C. and examined every other day for visual evidence of growth.

Tissue, Bone Marrow, and Body Fluids

All biopsy tissues should be minced or ground before being cultured. As much specimen as possible should be inoculated onto the surface of appropriate culture media. If a zygomycete infection is suspected, the tissue should be minced and not ground, as the former reduces the destruction of hyphal elements. Currently the optimal system for processing tissue is the Stomacher (Tekmar, Cincinnati), which expresses cytoplasmic contents of cells by pressure exerted by the action of rapidly moving paddles. Five-tenths ml of tissue homogenate should be placed onto the surface of appropriate media, and cultures should be examined daily for visual evidence of growth.

Corneal Scrapings and Ear Cultures

Mycotic keratitis and external otomycosis are most often caused by the rapidly growing saprobic molds. For the recovery of these organisms, it is necessary that media be used which contain no antifungal antibiotics. As much specimen as possible should be inoculated onto the surface of appropriate media. Cultures should be examined daily for visual evidence of growth.

Oral Mucosa

Material from lesions in the mouth or pharynx should be cultured onto media which contain antibacterial and antifungal antibiotics. Cultures should be incubated for a minimum of 30 days before being reported out as negative, since slower growing pathogens (e.g., *H. capsulatum)* are commonly recovered from oropharyngeal lesions.

Skin Scrapings, Nails, and Hair

Most specimens submitted for dermatophyte culture are contaminated with bacteria and rapidly growing molds. It is necessary that a medium be used which contains antibacterial and antifungal antibiotics. The specimen should be inoculated onto the surface of the appropriate culture medium and incubated for a minimum of 30 days. Cultures should be examined periodically for visual evidence of growth.

MEDIA REQUIREMENTS AND INCUBATION CONDITIONS

Table 48–9 provides a description of specimen types and culture requirements for the recovery of fungal etiologic agents. The selection of appropriate culture media may be based upon the information presented in this table.

The culture media used for the recovery of fungi need not be elaborate or complex. Obviously one can enhance the recovery rate by using a number of media; however, the problem of economics arises. The combinations of penicillin (20 units/ml) and streptomycin (40 units/ml) or gentamicin (5 μg/ml) and chloramphenicol (16 μg/ml) have proved satisfactory to prevent most bacterial overgrowth. Cycloheximide (Actidione) in a concentration of 0.5 mg/ml is satisfactory for the prevention of overgrowth by rapidly growing molds; however, some pathogens, including *Cryptococcus neoformans* and *Aspergillus fumigatus,* may be totally or partially inhibited, and it is necessary to include a medium lacking cycloheximide in the battery of media used.

Table 48–9. SPECIMEN AND MEDIA REQUIREMENTS FOR THE RECOVERY OF FUNGI FROM SPECIFIC MYCOTIC INFECTIONS

Infection	Specimen Type	Common Culture Media
Histoplasmosis	Respiratory secretions; blood; bone marrow; urine; cerebrospinal fluid; mucocutaneous ulcers	Sabouraud's dextrose agar;* brain-heart infusion agar; inhibitory mold agar; Sabhi agar; brain-heart infusion blood agar with antibiotics;† brain-heart infusion blood agar with antibiotics and cycloheximide;‡ DuPont Isolator recommended for blood cultures.§
Blastomycosis	Respiratory secretions; skin; bone; urine; mucocutaneous ulcers	Sabouraud's dextrose agar;* brain-heart infusion agar; inhibitory mold agar; Sabhi agar; brain-heart infusion blood agar with antibiotics;† brain-heart infusion blood agar with antibiotics and cycloheximide.‡
Coccidioidomycosis	Respiratory secretions; skin; cerebrospinal fluid; urine; mucocutaneous ulcers	Sabouraud's dextrose agar;* brain-heart infusion agar; inhibitory mold agar; Sabhi agar; brain-heart infusion blood agar with antibiotics;† brain-heart infusion blood agar with antibiotics and cycloheximide.‡
Paracoccidioidomycosis	Respiratory secretions; mucocutaneous ulcers; skin; intestine	Sabouraud's dextrose agar;* brain-heart infusion agar; inhibitory mold agar; Sabhi agar; brain-heart infusion blood agar with antibiotics;† brain-heart infusion blood agar with antibiotics and cycloheximide.‡
Cryptococcosis	Respiratory secretions; cerebrospinal fluid; bone; urine; skin; pleural fluid; bone marrow; blood	Sabouraud's dextrose agar;* inhibitory mold agar; brain-heart infusion agar; Sabhi agar; brain-heart infusion blood agar with antibiotics.† Media containing cycloheximide inhibit the growth of *Cryptococcus neoformans*. DuPont Isolator recommended for blood cultures.§
Candidosis	Respiratory secretions; urine; mucocutaneous lesions; blood; stool; vagina; nails	Most common fungal and bacterial culture media are satisfactory; however, those containing cycloheximide inhibit some species. DuPont Isolator recommended for blood cultures.§
Aspergillosis	Respiratory secretions; mucous plugs; external ear	Sabouraud's dextrose agar;* brain-heart infusion agar; inhibitory mold agar; Sabhi agar; brain-heart infusion blood agar containing antibiotics.† Media containing cycloheximide are unsatisfactory and inhibit the growth of aspergilli.
Nocardiosis¶	Respiratory secretions; blood; cutaneous abscesses	Sabouraud's dextrose agar;* brain-heart infusion agar; Sabhi agar; DuPont Isolator recommended for blood cultures.§ Media containing antibiotics inhibit the growth of nocardiae.
Zygomycosis (Phycomycosis)	Respiratory secretions; rhino-orbital lesions; skin	Sabouraud's dextrose agar;* brain-heart infusion agar; inhibitory mold agar; Sabhi agar; brain-heart infusion blood agar with antibiotics.† Media containing cycloheximide inhibit the growth of zygomycetes.
Geotrichosis	Respiratory secretions; oropharynx; stool	Sabouraud's dextrose agar;* brain-heart infusion agar; inhibitory mold agar; Sabhi agar; brain-heart infusion blood agar with antibiotics;† brain-heart infusion blood agar with antibiotics and cycloheximide.‡

Table continued on following page

6

Table 48–9. SPECIMEN AND MEDIA REQUIREMENTS FOR THE RECOVERY OF FUNGI FROM SPECIFIC MYCOTIC INFECTIONS *(Continued)*

Infection	Specimen Type	Common Culture Media
Sporotrichosis	Respiratory secretions; lymphocutaneous abscesses; synovial fluid; nasal sinuses	Sabouraud's dextrose agar;* brain-heart infusion agar; inhibitory mold agar; Sabhi agar; brain-heart infusion blood agar with antibiotics;† brain-heart infusion blood agar with antibiotics and cycloheximide.‡
Mycetoma	Draining cutaneous sinuses; bone	*Eumycotic mycetoma:* Sabouraud's dextrose agar;* brain-heart infusion agar; inhibitory mold agar; Sabhi agar; all media should contain antibiotics and cycloheximide.‡ *Actinomycotic mycetoma:* Sabouraud's dextrose agar;* brain-heart infusion agar; Sabhi agar. Media containing antibiotics inhibit the growth of aerobic actinomycetes.
Chromoblastomycosis	Skin; brain	Sabouraud's dextrose agar;* brain-heart infusion agar; inhibitory mold agar; Sabhi agar. All media should contain antibiotics and cycloheximide.‡
Dermatomycosis	Hair; skin; nails	Mycosel agar or mycobiotic agar.**
Mycotic keratitis	Corneal scraping	Sabouraud's dextrose agar;* brain-heart infusion agar; Sabhi agar. Media containing antibiotics or cycloheximide are unsatisfactory.
Otomycosis	External ear	Sabouraud's dextrose agar;* brain-heart infusion agar; inhibitory mold agar; Sabhi agar; brain-heart in fusion blood agar containing antibiotics.† Media containing cycloheximide are unsatisfactory and inhibit the growth of several etiologic agents.

*Contains 2% dextrose, pH 7.0.

†Contains gentamicin, 5 μg/ml, and chloramphenicol, 16 μg/ml, or penicillin, 20 units/ml, and streptomycin, 40 units/ml.

‡Contains gentamicin, 5μg/ml, and chloramphenicol, 16 μg/ml, or penicillin, 20 units/ml, and streptomycin, 40 units/ml, and cycloheximide, 0.5 mg/ml.

§See Roberts (1975).

¶Not a mycotic infection; however, organisms are often recovered on fungal culture media.

**Contains chloramphenicol, 50 μg/ml, and cycloheximide, 0.5 mg/ml.

A number of commercially prepared culture media are available for the cultivation of fungi from clinical specimens. Included are Sabouraud's dextrose, Sabouraud's dextrose (Emmon's modification) containing 2 per cent dextrose, Sabhi, inhibitory mold, brain-heart infusion, and mycobiotic and mycosel agars. It is recommended that at least one culture medium be supplemented with 5 to 10 per cent sheep blood. This enhances the chances of recovery of some fastidious pathogens. It should be kept in mind that media containing blood, e.g., brain-heart infusion containing 5 to 10 per cent sheep blood, are excellent isolation media; however, they are not adequate as identification media. It is necessary to subculture the organisms that are recovered on media containing blood onto other media that will allow characteristic sporulation to occur. Media suitable for subculture include corn-meal agar, Sabouraud's dextrose agar, inhibitory mold agar, brain-heart infusion agar, or any of the previously mentioned media.

Cultures should be incubated only at 25 to 30°C.; incubation of duplicate cultures at 37°C. is unnecessary and costly. The recovery rate of the dimorphic pathogens is not significantly enhanced by incubating cultures at 37°C. All cultures should be incubated at 30°C. (optimal) for a minimum of 30 days before being discarded. Six weeks of incubation is optimal; however, limitation of space often prevents this.

Petri dishes or culture tubes are satisfactory for the recovery of fungi. For those laboratories not thoroughly acquainted with the handling of fungi, it is suggested that large screw-capped tubes be used. The slants should be thick and, after inoculation, the caps should be screwed on but left slightly loose. The disadvantages of this method include relatively poor aeration of cultures and a reduced surface area, which results in poorly isolated colonies. Culture tubes are more easily stored, require less space, are obviously safer for small laboratories, and have a lower dehydration rate. Although somewhat more hazardous, culture dishes may be used by those laboratories which are familiar with the handling of fungal cultures; however, they are not recommended for the inexperienced laboratory. The advantages include better aeration of cultures, a large surface area which provides better isolation of colonies, and greater ease of examination and subculture of fungal colonies. The disadvantages include an increased dehydration rate and an increased chance of laboratory contamination. Dehydration may be reduced by preparing the culture dishes to contain at least 40 ml of medium; lids should be taped down in two locations to prevent inadvertent opening, and dishes should be incubated in an atmosphere containing 30 to 40 per cent relative humidity.

DIRECT EXAMINATION OF CLINICAL SPECIMENS

In many instances the direct microscopic examination of a clinical specimen allows one to make a rapid tentative diagnosis. All laboratories will find the direct examination of a clinical specimen practical, since most already examine skin and nail scrapings microscopically for the presence of dermatophytes. The use of the direct examination may be extended to include all clinical specimens except blood.

The procedure is simple and consists of mixing a small amount of the specimen with a drop of 10 per cent potassium hydroxide on a microscope slide. A coverslip is positioned and the slide may be gently flamed and examined microscopically. Brightfield microscopy is satisfactory if the light is reduced; however, phase contrast microscopy is optimal because it provides more detail. Figures 48–34 to 48–41 present organisms commonly seen on direct microscopic examination with a detailed description of their characteristic features.

The India ink preparation is commonly used for the detection of *Cryptococcus neoformans* in cerebrospinal fluid. Although only positive in less than 50 per cent of the cases of cryptococcal meningitis, this examination is diagnostic when encapsulated organisms are present. A drop of India ink is mixed with a drop of sediment from centrifuged cerebrospinal fluid and is observed microscopically for the presence of encapsulated yeast cells. Cells of *C. neoformans* are usually encapsulated, may be budding, and are variable in size (Fig. 48–42). In most instances only a few cells are seen on direct examination.

IDENTIFICATION OF FILAMENTOUS FUNGI

Until recently, the filamentous fungi were considered to be either pathogens or saprobes. Saprobes previously thought to be non-pathogenic have been implicated as the etiologic agents of severe, often fatal, infections in compromised patients. Currently, it is necessary to consider all filamentous fungi as potential pathogens, and they should be handled with extreme caution in the laboratory.

The laboratory identification of the filamentous fungi should be performed in those laboratories equipped with biologic safety cabinets to prevent laboratory-acquired infection. Laboratories which do not have adequate facilities for handling filamentous fungal cultures should send suspected pathogens to a reference laboratory for proper identification.

Generally, the growth rate for the strict pathogens, including *Blastomyces dermatitidis, Histoplasma capsulatum,* and *Coccidioides immitis,* is slow, and one to six weeks are required before colonies become apparent; however, most appear within three to four weeks. *Coccidioides immitis* in some instances may produce visible growth within three to five days. When specimens contain an exceptionally high number of organisms, the growth rate may be somewhat shortened, e.g., *Blastomyces dermatitidis* may be seen within six days of incubation. It is recommended that all fungal cultures be kept for a minimum of 30 days before being discarded.

The colonial morphology is of little value in identifying the filamentous fungi due to natural variation among isolates and variation which is culture medium dependent. *Histoplasma capsulatum,* for example, on primary isolation often appears yeast-like on a blood-enriched medium, but on Sabouraud's dextrose agar or a similar medium it grows as a white tan fluffy colony. The growth rate usually provides more helpful information than colonial morphology. The definitive identification of the filamentous fungi is based on the characteristic microscopic morphology (type and arrangement of spores) and demonstration of both the saprobic and parasitic forms of the dimorphic fungi. The ability to identify visually the filamentous fungi is based on experience and exposure to a wide variety of fungi which occur in nature.

The fungi may be prepared for microscopic observation by several methods. The procedure most familiar to clinical microbiology laboratories is the wet mount, which is prepared by adding a small portion of the culture and supporting agar to a drop of lactophenol aniline blue on a microscope slide. A coverslip is positioned on the slide and gentle pressure is applied to disperse the sample so that microscopic features are easily observed. This method is helpful if characteristic spores are found; however, it is unsuitable for the detection of characteristic spore arrangements. The most helpful procedure to use is the adhesive transparent plastic tape (Scotch tape) method of preparing cultures for microscopic examination. The adhesive side of the tape is gently touched to the surface of a colony and then is adhered to a slide on which a drop of lactophenol aniline blue has been placed. (The mounting medium consists of 15 grams of polyvinyl alcohol, 100 ml of distilled water, 39 ml of lactic acid, 39 ml of phenol [melted], and 0.1 g of aniline blue. The polyvinyl alcohol is added to the

Text continued on page 1192

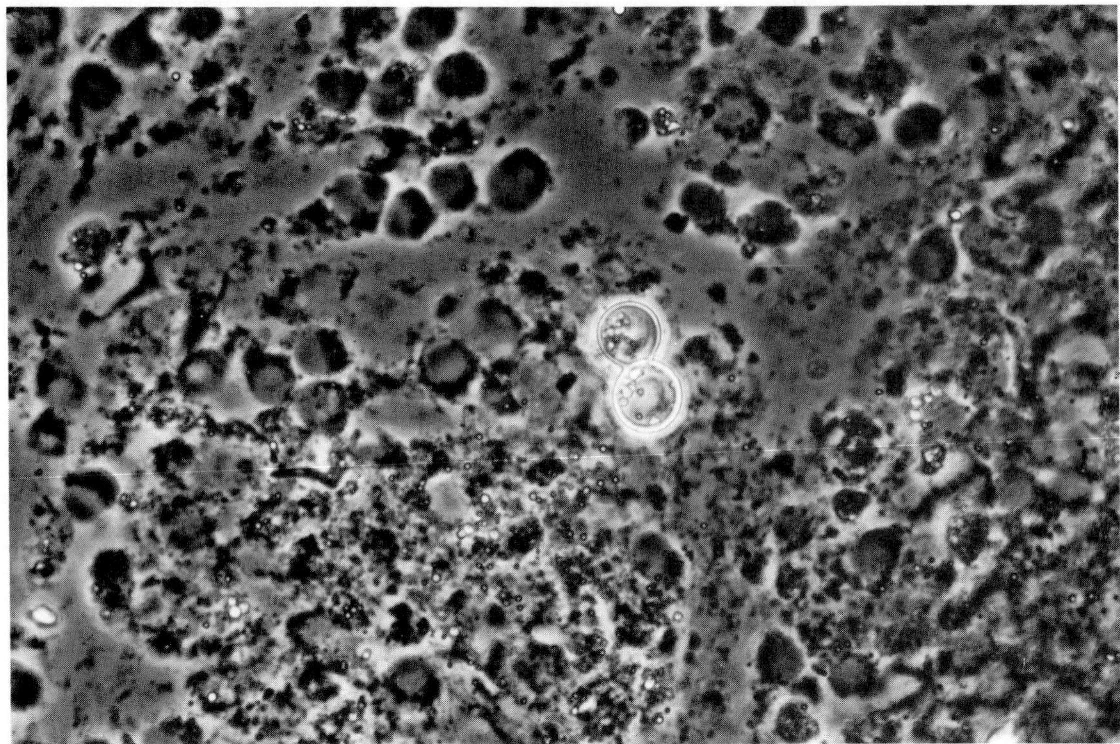

Figure 48–34. *Blastomyces dermatitidis* in sputum. Characteristic yeast form has budding cell attached by broad base. Also note "double contoured" appearance of cell wall and large size of cell. Phase contrast. ×450. (From Roberts, G. D.: J. Clin. Microbiol., *2*:261, 1975.)

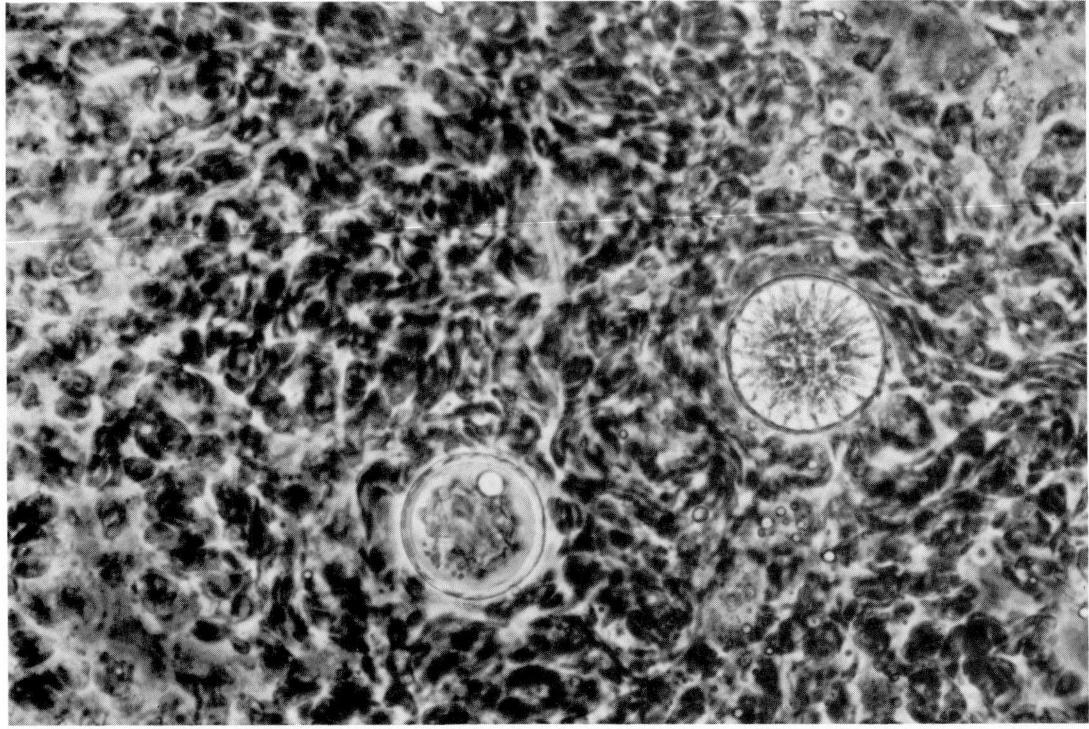

Figure 48–35. *Coccidioides immitis* in sputum. Large thick-walled spherules with a few endospores scattered within interior of spherule or cleavage furrows developing along periphery to form endospores. Phase contrast. ×450. (From Roberts, G. D.: J. Clin Microbiol., *2*:261, 1975.)

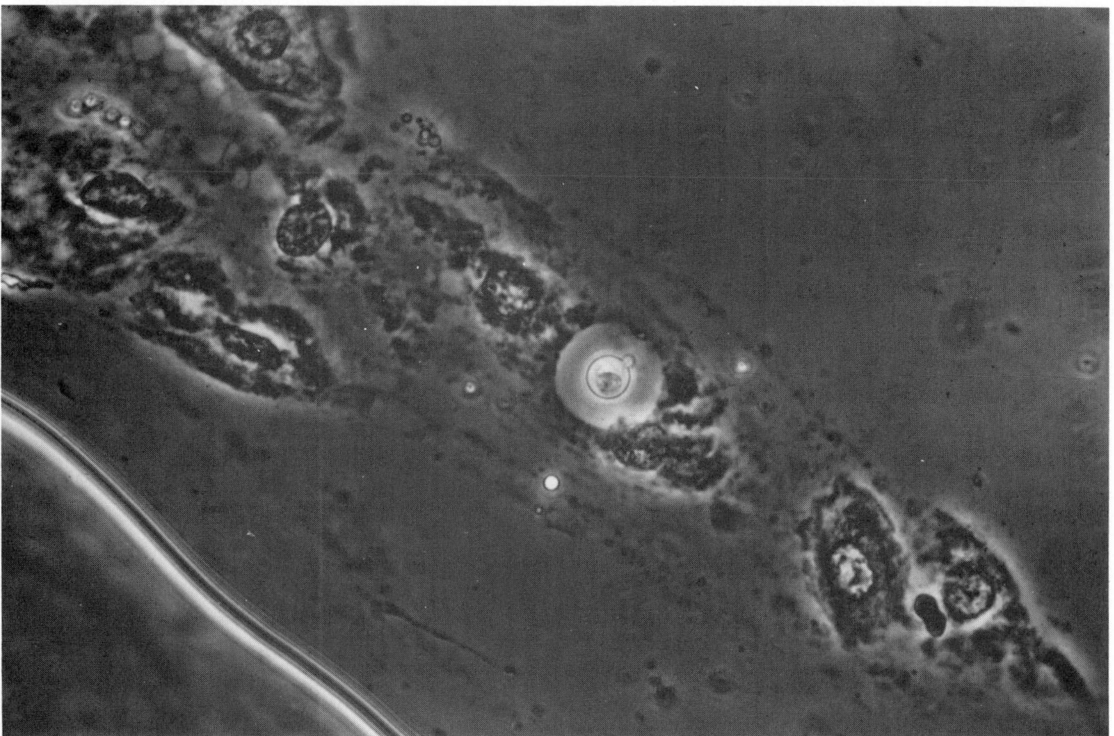

Figure 48–36. *Cryptococcus neoformans* in sputum. Spherical yeast cell is surrounded by large capsule with small bud arising from parent cell. Phase contrast. ×450. (From Roberts, G. D.: J. Clin. Microbiol., *2*:261, 1975.)

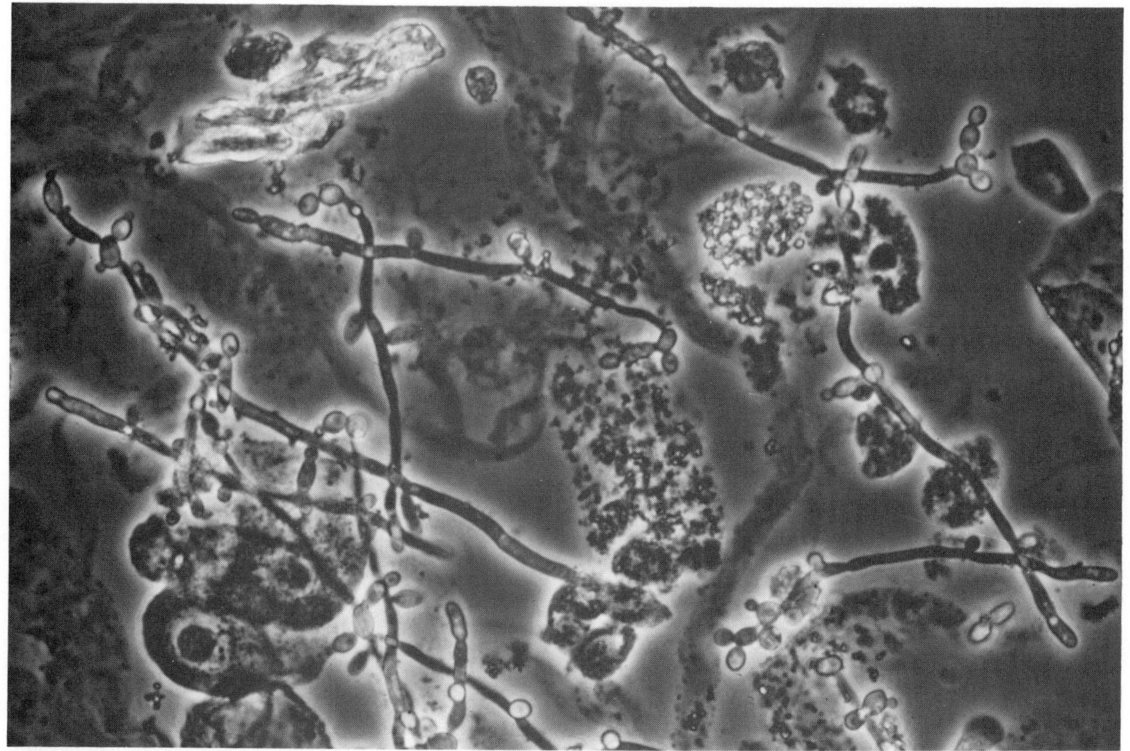

Figure 48–37. *Candida albicans* in urine. Hyphae and budding yeasts appear among epithelial cells. Phase contrast. ×450. (From Roberts, G. D.: J. Clin. Microbiol., *2*:261, 1975.)

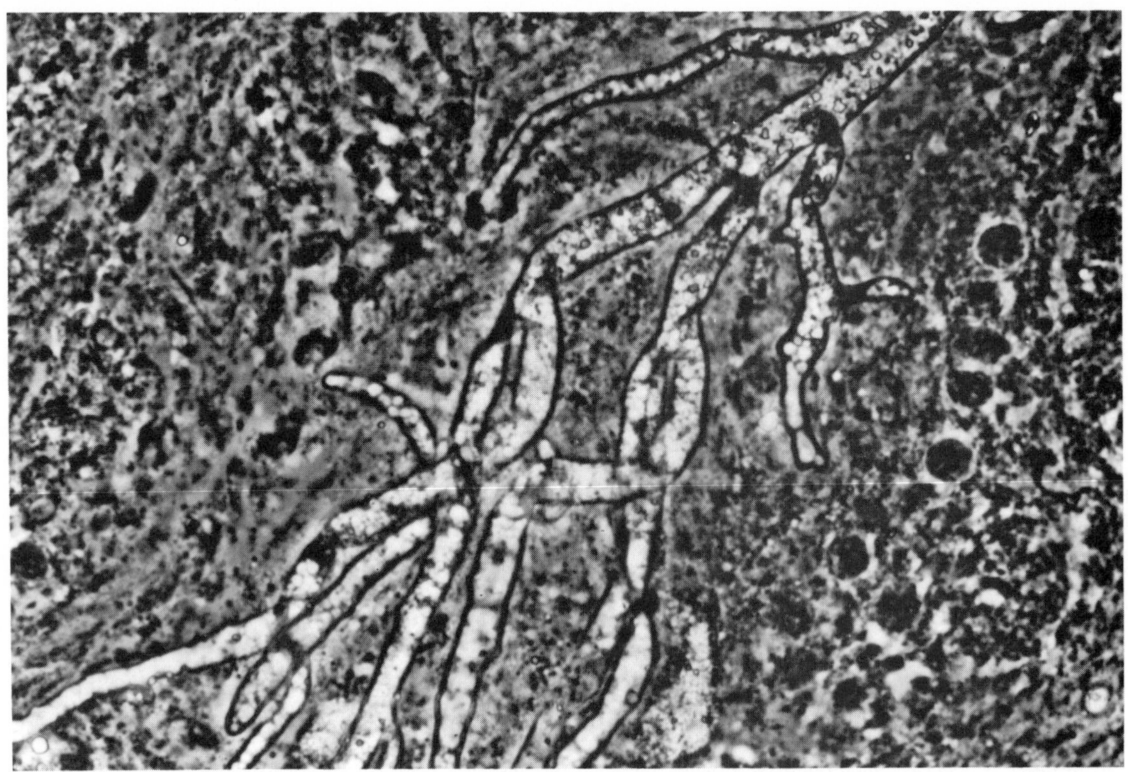

Figure 48–38. *Mucor* species in pus from skin lesion. The large, branching, ribbon-like aseptate hyphae are characteristic of a Zygomycete. Phase contrast. ×450. (From Roberts, G. D.: J. Clin. Microbiol., *2*:261, 1975.)

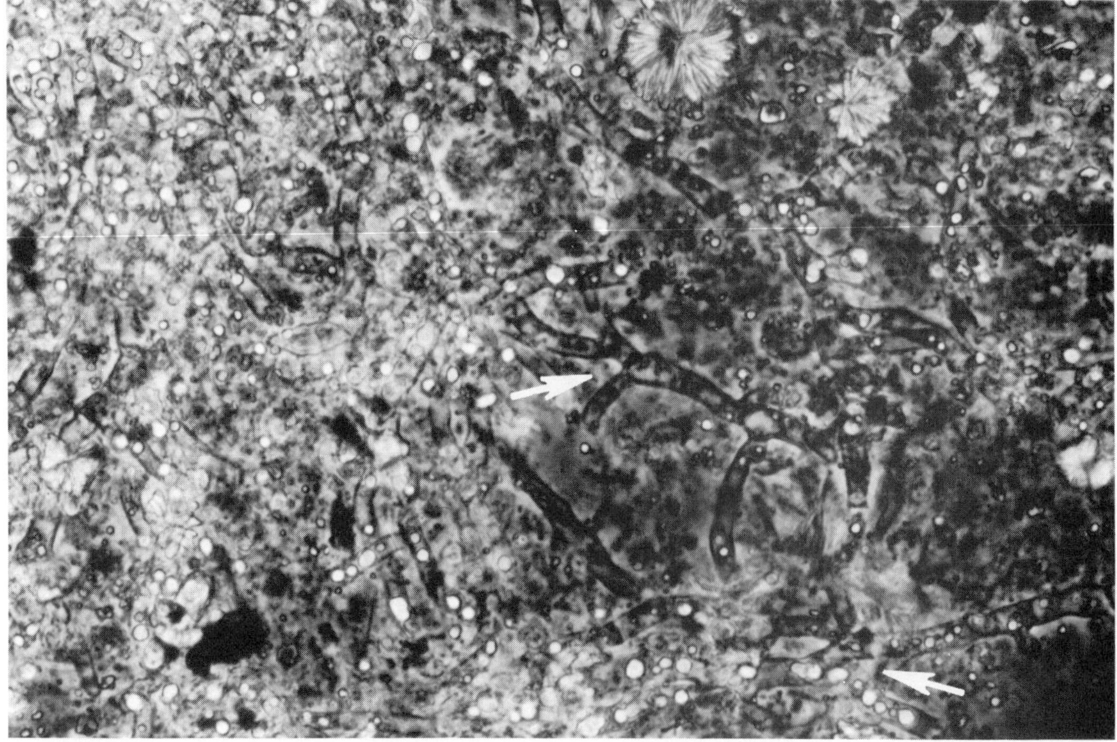

Figure 48–39. *Aspergillus fumigatus* in sputum. The septate hyphae show dichotomous branching (arrows). Phase contrast. ×450. (From Roberts, G. D.: J. Clin. Microbiol., *2*:261, 1975.)

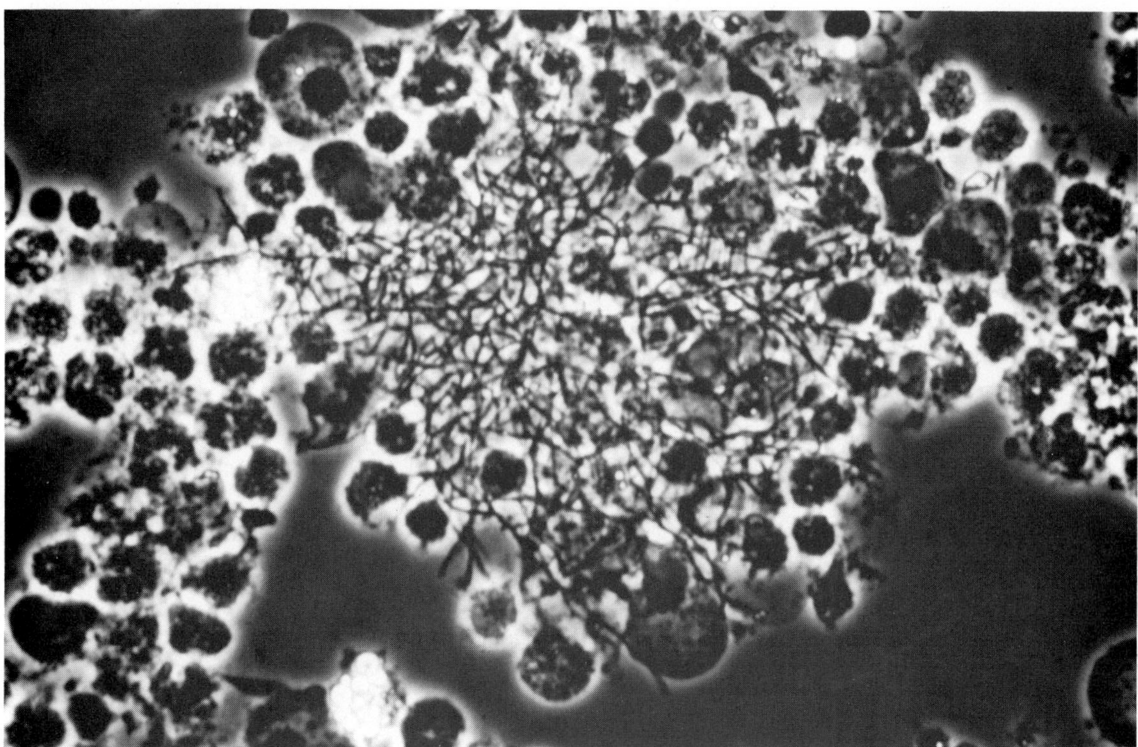

Figure 48–40. *Nocardia asteroides* in sputum. Small branching filaments are interpositioned among leukocytes. Phase contrast. ×450.

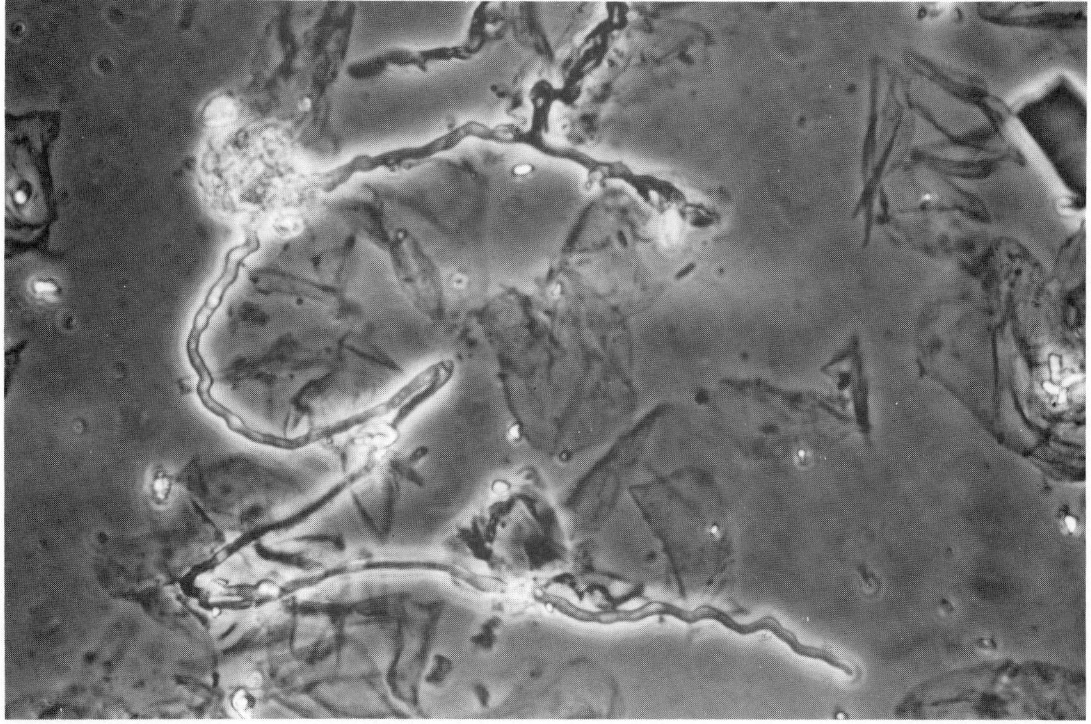

Figure 48–41. Dermatophyte in skin scraping. Septate hyphae intertwine among squamous cells. Phase contrast. ×450. (From Roberts, G. D.: J. Clin. Microbiol., *2*:261, 1975.)

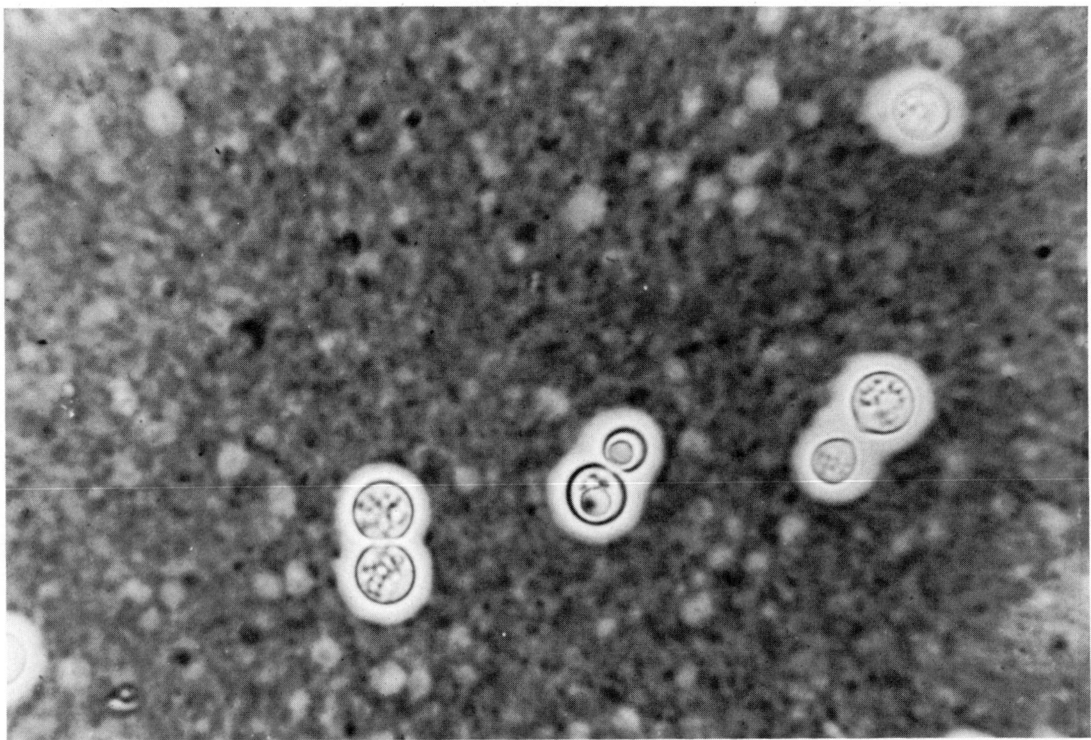

Figure 48–42. *Cryptococcus neoformans* in cerebrospinal fluid. India ink preparation shows encapsulated cell with "pinched off" buds. Also note that cells are spherical and vary in size. Phase contrast. ×450. (From Dolan, C. T., Funkhouser, J. W., Koneman, E. W., Miller, N. G., and Roberts, G. D.: Atlas of Clinical Mycology I. Chicago, American Society of Clinical Pathologists, 1975.)

water and is heated at 80°C. until clearing occurs. The lactic acid is added, followed by the phenol and aniline blue.) This technique allows one to observe the spores and supporting structures arranged somewhat as they were when part of the original colony. This method is inexpensive, rapid, and simple for observing the filamentous fungi and is preferred by most laboratories.

The most important feature required for the identification of filamentous fungi is the characteristic arrangement of spores. As has been previously mentioned, the wet mount is unsuitable for this purpose. The Scotch tape method, in most instances, allows one to visualize the characteristic arrangement of spores. However, in some instances no characteristic arrangements can be seen, and it is necessary to prepare a microslide culture as follows: a small agar block is placed on a sterile microscope slide; the four corners are lightly inoculated, and a coverslip is placed on top. The culture is incubated in a moist chamber and after adequate growth occurs, the coverslip is removed and placed on a slide to which a drop of lactophenol aniline blue has been added. This allows the undisturbed spores to be observed as they were arranged during growth under the coverslip. It is recommended that two microslide cultures be made concurrently, since it is often difficult to determine when the culture is mature enough for examination. If necessary, the agar block may be removed and a drop of lactophenol aniline blue and a coverslip are added to the microscope slide. Often, the characteristic arrangement of spores may be observed in this manner. This provides another opportunity to observe an organism using a single microculture.

All these techniques allow one to observe the microscopic features of the filamentous fungi. Initially, the hyphae should be examined to determine if they are septate. If no septa are present, the organism may be classified as a Zygomycete, e.g., *Rhizopus, Mucor,* or *Absidia.* The size of the hyphae is important also; Zygomycetes have large, ribbon-like, twisted hyphae which are quite distinct. The strict pathogens exhibit hyphae which are septate but quite small in diameter. Many of the other fungi, including *Aspergillus* and *Penicillium,* etc., have hyphae of intermediate size between those of the Zygomycetes and the strict pathogens. In many instances when a characteristic arrangement of spores is absent, a tentative identification of a potential pathogen may be made based strictly on the growth rate and the size of the hyphae present as seen by microscopic examination. Usually, it is necessary to subculture the organism to another medium to induce sporulation.

The definitive identification of the dimorphic fungi, including *Blastomyces dermatitidis, Sporothrix schenckii, Histoplasma capsulatum,* and *Coccidioides immitis,* may be made by using one of several methods after the characteristic mold form has been observed. *In vitro* conversion from the saprobic filamentous form to the parasitic form may be accomplished placing a large inoculum of the filamentous form onto the surface of a fresh, moist slant of an enriched medium containing blood. Brain-heart infusion agar containing 5 to 10 per cent sheep blood is preferred as the best conversion medium. Cultures are incubated at 37°C., and transfers are made to fresh media as soon as growth is apparent. Rarely, conversion may be completed overnight or within two to three days; however, usually several transfers are necessary for complete conversion, and this may require 7 to 21 days. The *in vitro* conversion procedure is most satisfactory for *Sporothrix schenckii* and *Blastomyces dermatitidis* when cottonseed agar is used for the latter. This procedure is not satisfactory for demonstrating the spherules and endospores of *Coccidioides immitis*.

The exoantigen method (Standard, 1979) is based on the principle that *B. dermatitidis, C. immitis,* and *H. capsulatum* produce cell-free exoantigens in culture that react with specific antibodies produced in animals immunized with the homologous antigens. Antigens are extracted by covering a culture with sterile distilled water containing merthiolate. After 24 hours, the water containing the exoantigen, if present, is filtered through a 0.45 μ filter and concentrated 25 to 50× in a Minicon B-15 concentrator (Amicon Corp., Lexington, Mass.). The concentrated fluid is reacted in microimmunodiffusion plates against antisera prepared against *H. capsulatum, B. dermatitidis,* and *C. immitis*. Plates are incubated for 24 hours at 25°C. and examined for precipitin bands of identity. This method is regarded as specific for the identification of the aforementioned dimorphic fungi (Kaufman, 1978).

Recognition of the characteristic microscopic features is determined by experience. It requires a careful comparison of the microscopic features of fungi with photographs and descriptions available in current texts and laboratory manuals. Figure 48–43 presents the microscopic features of filamentous organisms commonly encountered in the clinical microbiology laboratory; it is not within the scope of this chapter to present a detailed description of each organism (see general references).

The clinical significance of the presence of most filamentous fungi in clinical specimens is undetermined. The laboratory has an obligation to identify and to report all organisms that are present in clinical specimens, and the clinician then must determine the significance of the organisms to the patient. In many instances the presence of the filamentous fungi is unimportant; however, the same fungi recovered from a compromised patient may play an important role in causing infection. Table 48–10 presents filamentous fungi commonly recovered in clinical specimens, time required for their identification, probable recovery sites, and infections with which they have been associated.

IDENTIFICATION OF YEASTS AND YEAST-LIKE ORGANISMS

During recent years there has been a definite increase in the number of yeast infections caused by *Candida albicans* and *Cryptococcus neoformans;* moreover, other species previously thought to be non-pathogenic have also been implicated. This has resulted from the clinical alteration of host defense mechanisms by underlying disease processes and chemotherapeutic agents, including steroids, antibiotics, and immunosuppressive agents. Many infections are the result of long-term intravenous therapy combined with inadequate catheter care. It is well documented that infections produced by yeasts and yeast-like organisms occur primarily in the compromised patient.

The identification of yeasts and yeast-like organisms from clinical specimens is currently of interest to most laboratories; however, the significance of these organisms is questionable. Since yeasts are considered to be normal flora in the oropharynx and gastrointestinal tract, their recovery might be expected from most clinical specimens, including respiratory secretions, gastric washings, vaginal secretions, stool specimens, and throat cultures. Other sites where yeasts are commonly recovered include urine, skin, and nail scrapings. Yeasts and yeast-like organisms are not usually recovered from normally sterile body fluids, including blood, cerebrospinal fluid, and synovial fluid, where their presence should be considered an abnormal finding. Table 48–11 lists the most common yeast-like organisms that are encountered in the clinical microbiology laboratory and infections with which they have been associated.

Since many yeasts and yeast-like organisms are considered normal flora and others under appropriate circumstances are pathogens, the question of whether all laboratories should identify them is a valid one. Their repeated recovery from multiple specimens from the same patient indicates either colonization or infection with the organism. When this occurs, the clinical microbiology laboratory should speciate the organisms, since this information is often important in making a decision concerning which therapeutic agent is to be used for treatment. Other situations which warrant the complete identification of yeasts and yeast-like organisms include their recovery from patients who are compromised from an underlying disease process or by chemotherapy. The laboratory should always identify an organism from any site which the clinician feels is important.

Many different procedures are available for the identification of yeasts and yeast-like organisms, and the decision concerning which method should be used must be made by each individual laboratory. Obviously, some methods are better suited for large laboratories that have extensive experience and other methods are suitable for smaller laboratories. Representative methods which may be utilized by laboratories of all sizes will be presented in the following paragraphs.

Text continued on page 1202

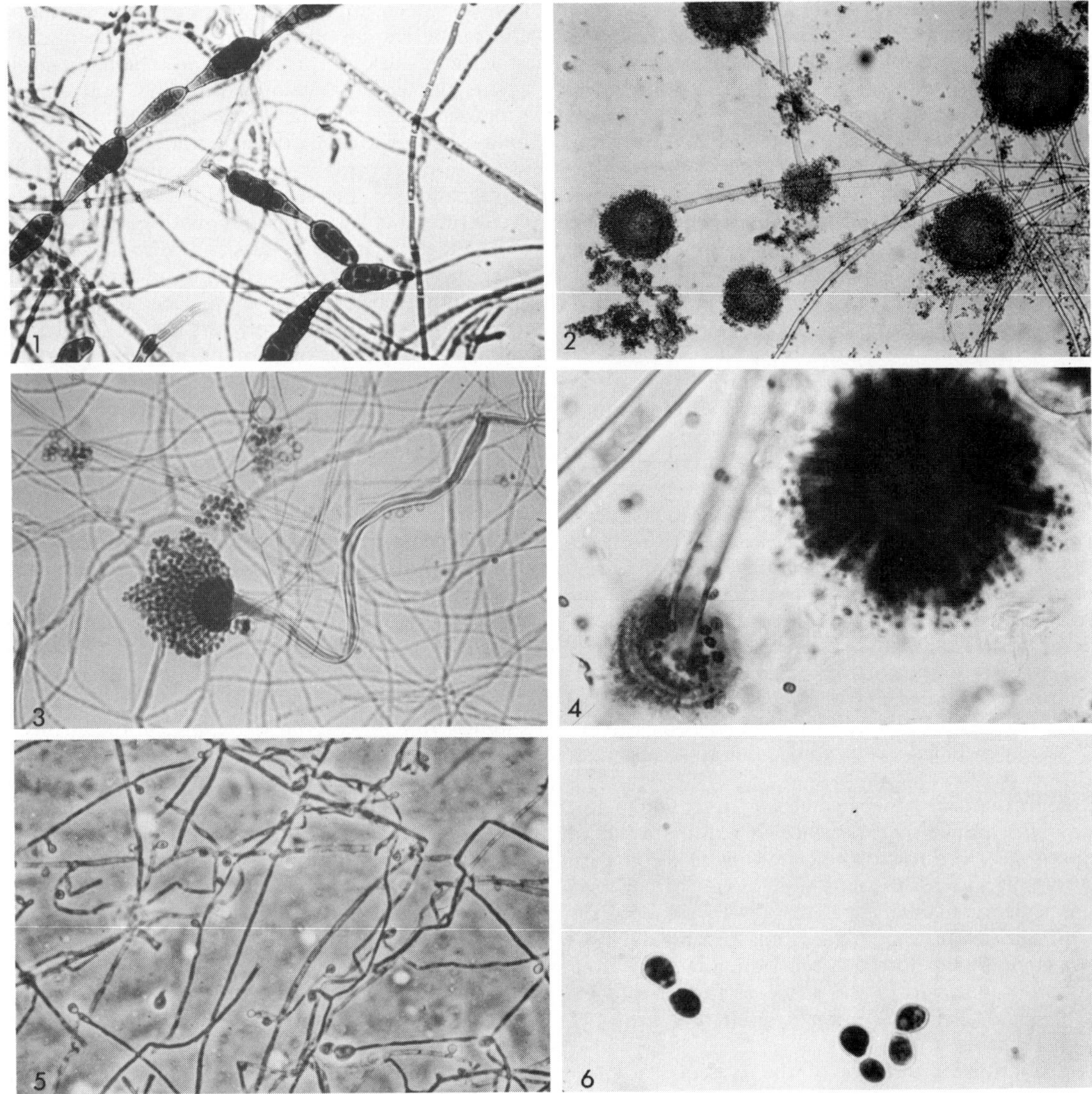

Figure 48–43. Common filamentous fungi which may be recovered from clinical specimens, microscopic features, lactophenol cotton blue preparation. ×450. (From Dolan, C. T., Funkhouser, J. W., Koneman, E. W., Miller, N. G., and Roberts, G. D.: Atlas of Clinical Mycology V and VI. Chicago, American Society of Clinical Pathologists, 1975.)

1. *Alternaria* species, conidia
2. *Aspergillus flavus,* conidial heads
3. *Aspergillus fumigatus,* conidial head
4. *Aspergillus niger,* conidial head
5. *Blastomyces dermatitidis,* filamentous form, conidia
6. *Blastomyces dermatitidis,* yeast form

Illustration continued on opposite page

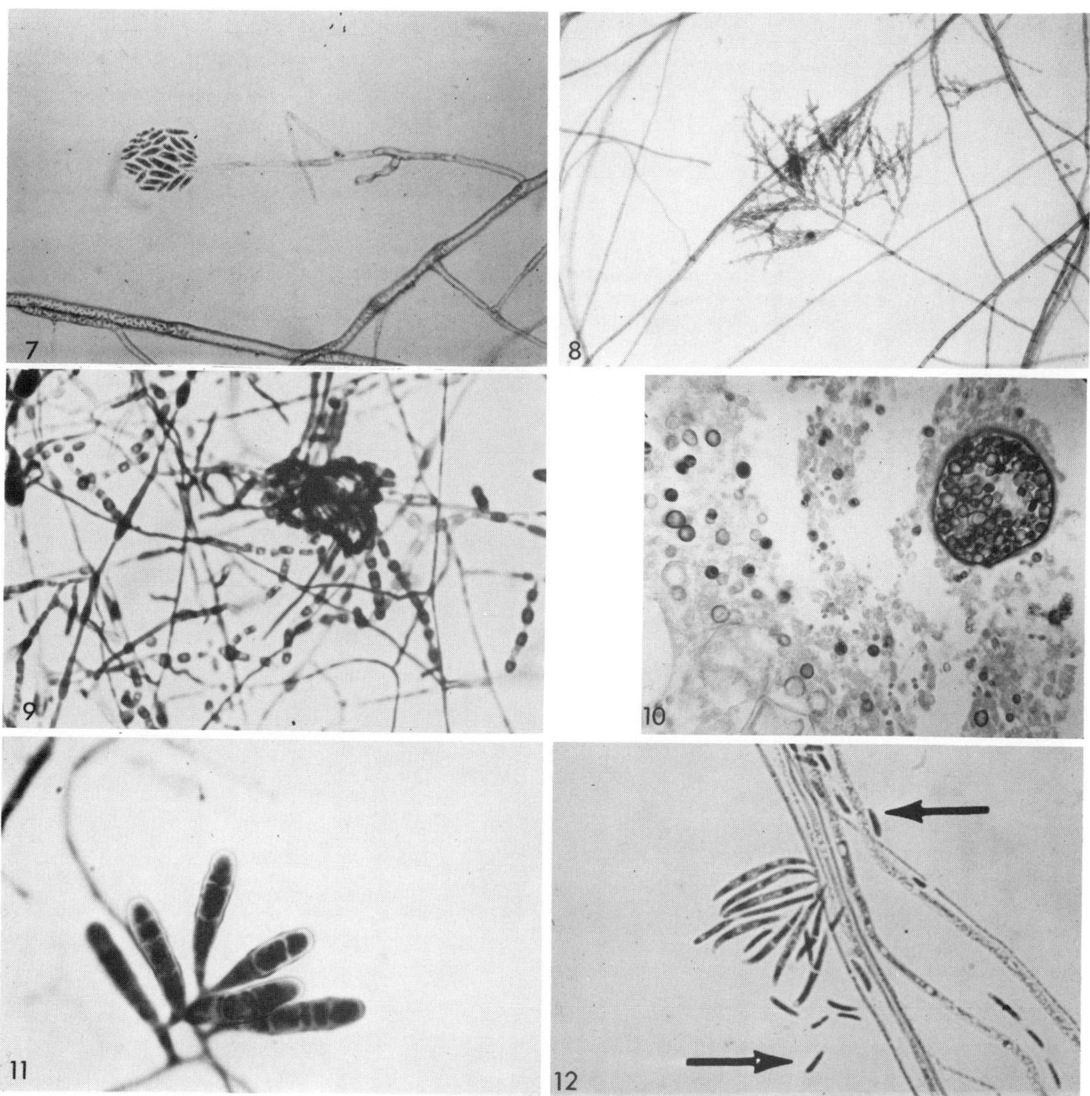

Figure 48–43 *Continued.*
7. *Acremonium* species, conidia
8. *Cladosporium* species, conidia
9. *Coccidioides immitis,* filamentous form, arthroconidia
10. *Coccidioides immitis,* spherule form
11. *Epidermophyton floccosum,* macroconidia
12. *Fusarium* species, macroconidia

Illustration continued on following page

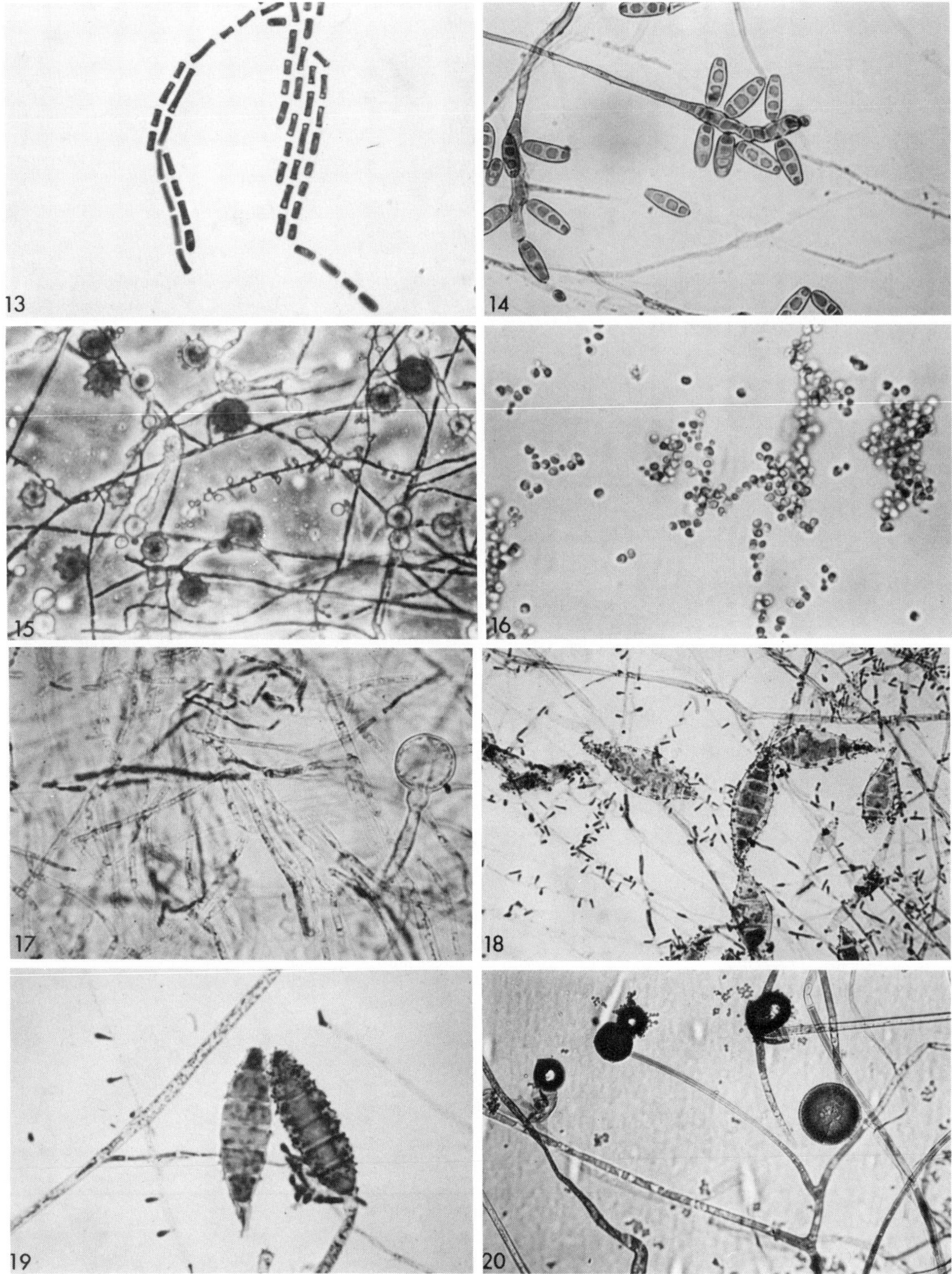

Figure 48–43 *Continued.*
13. *Geotrichum* species, arthroconidia
14. *Dreschlera* species, conidia
15. *Histoplasma capsulatum,* filamentous form, macroconidia and microconidia
16. *Histoplasma capsulatum,* yeast form
17. *Microsporum audouinii,* terminal chlamydospore
18. *Microsporum canis,* macroconidia and microconidia
19. *Microsporum gypseum,* microconidia and macroconidia
20. *Mucor* species, sporangia

Illustration continued on opposite page

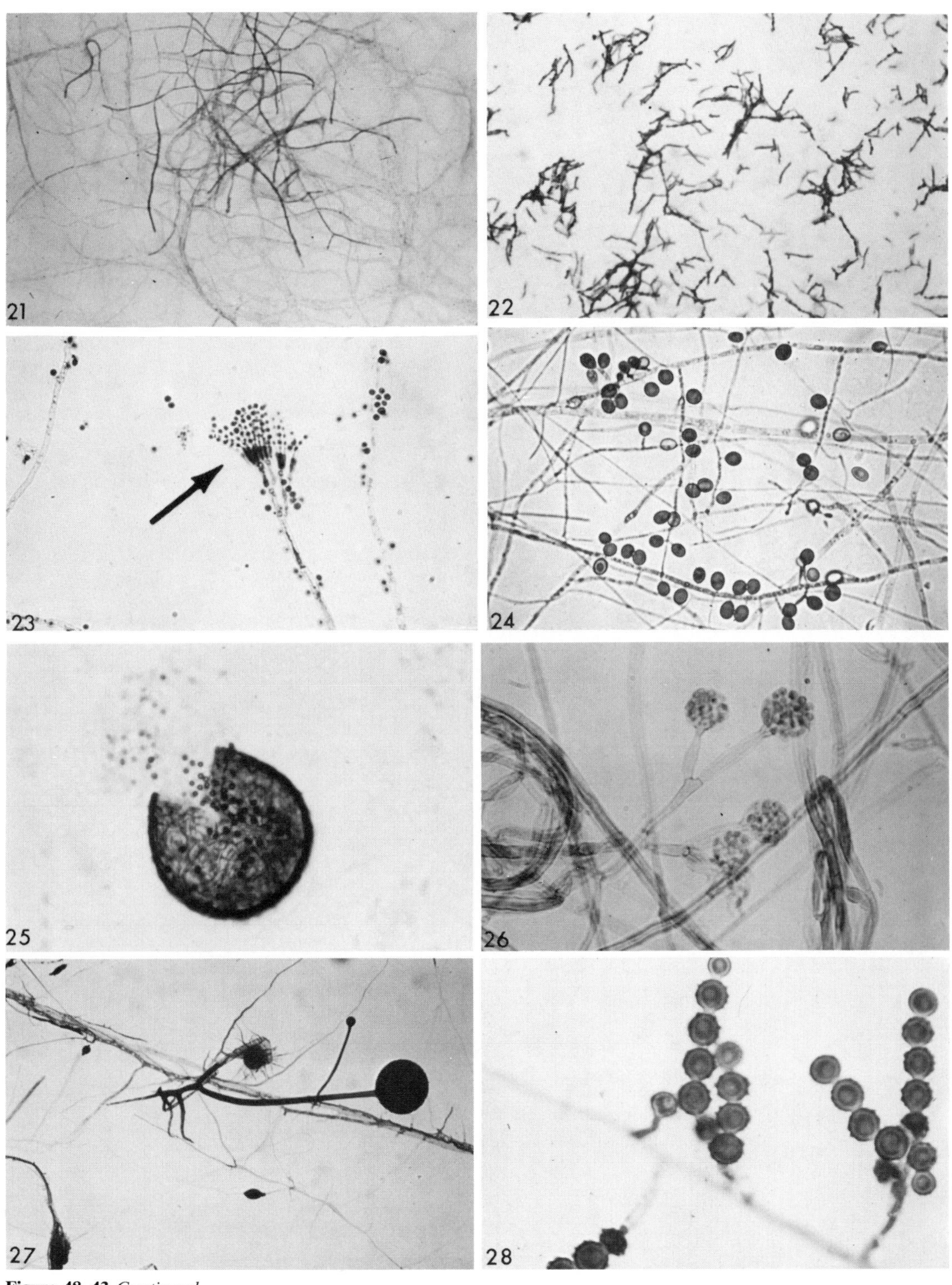

Figure 48–43 *Continued.*
21. *Nocardia asteroides,* branching filaments
22. *Nocardia asteroides,* coccobacillary form
23. *Penicillium* species, conidial head
24. *Pseudallescheria boydii,* conidial stage
25. *Pseudallescheria boydii,* cleistothecium
26. *Phialophora verrucosa,* flask-shaped phialide
27. *Rhizopus* species, sporangia and rhizoids
28. *Scopulariopsis* species, conidia

6

Illustration continued on following page

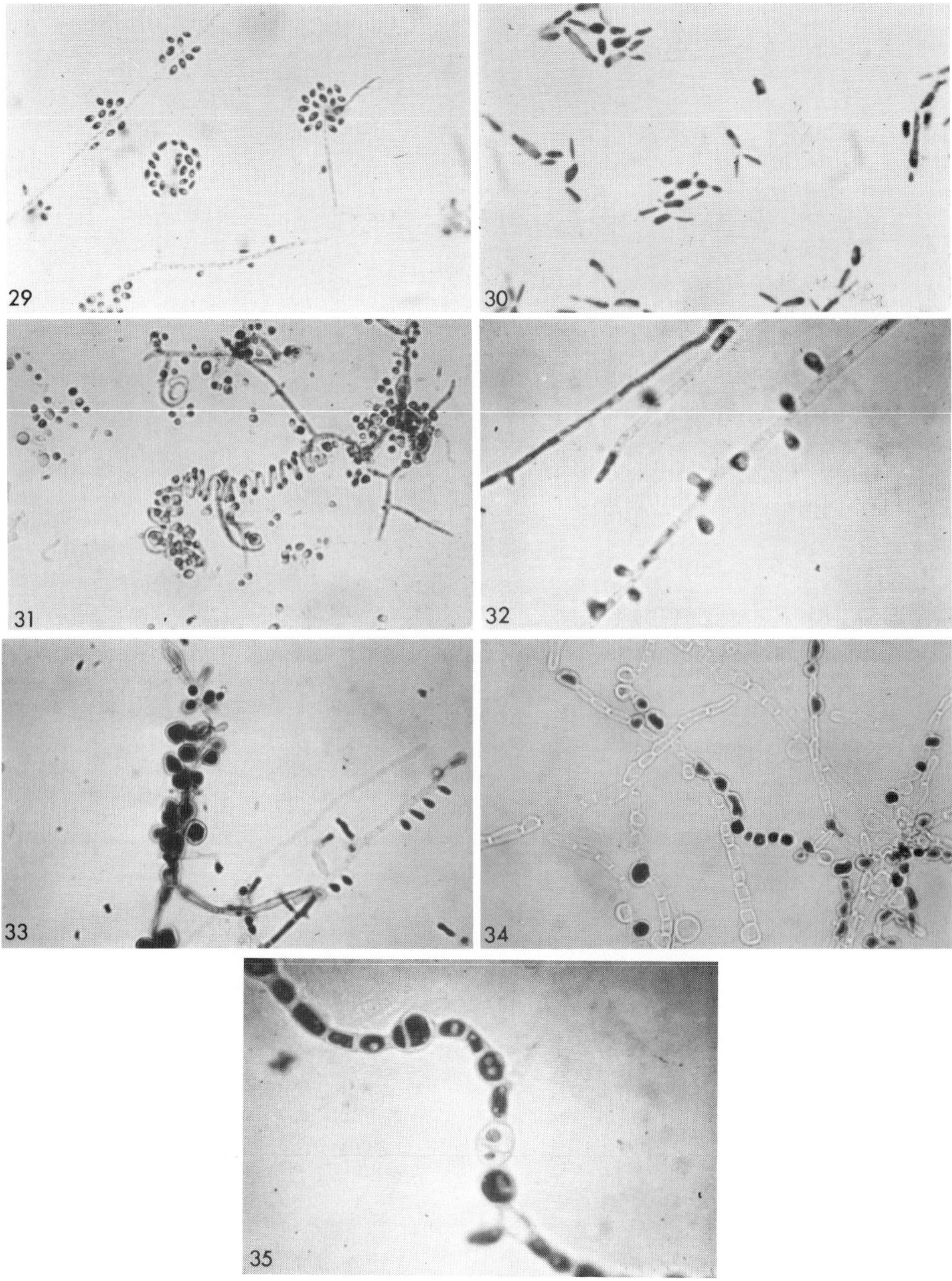

Figure 48–43 *Continued.*
29. *Sporothrix schenckii,* filamentous form, flowerette and sleve arrangements of conidia
30. *Sporothrix schenckii,* yeast form, cigar bodies
31. *Trichophyton mentagrophytes,* microconidia and spiral hyphae
32. *Trichophyton rubrum,* tear-shaped microconidia
33. *Trichophyton tonsurans,* swollen (balloon forms) microconidia
34. *Trichophyton verrucosum,* chains of chlamydospores at 37°C.
35. *Trichophyton violaceum,* swollen hyphae containing cytoplasmic granules

Table 48–10. COMMON FILAMENTOUS FUNGI IMPLICATED IN HUMAN MYCOTIC INFECTIONS

Etiologic Agent	Time Required for Identification	Probable Recovery Sites	Clinical Implication(s)
Acremonium (Cephalosporium) species	2–6 days	Skin, nails, respiratory secretions, cornea, vagina, gastric washings	Skin and nail infections, mycotic keratitis
Alternaria species	2–6 days	Skin, nails, conjunctiva, and respiratory secretions	Skin and nail infections, conjunctivitis, hypersentivity pneumonitis
Aspergillus flavus	1–4 days	Skin, respiratory secretions, gastric washings, nasal sinuses	Skin infections, allergic bronchopulmonary infection, sinusitis, myocarditis, disseminated infection, renal infection, subcutaneous mycetoma
Aspergillus fumigatus	2–6 days	Respiratory secretions, skin, ear, cornea, gastric washings, stool, nasal sinuses	Allergic bronchopulmonary infection, fungus ball, invasive pulmonary infection, skin and nail infections, external otomycosis, mycotic keratitis, sinusitis, myocarditis, renal infection
Aspergillus niger	1–4 days	Respiratory secretions, gastric washings, ear, skin	Fungus ball, pulmonary infection, external otomycosis, mycotic keratitis
Blastomyces dermatitidis	6–21 days (recovery time) [additional 3–14 days required for confirmatory identification]	Respiratory secretions, skin, oropharyngeal ulcers, bone, prostate	Pulmonary infection, skin infection, oropharyngeal ulceration, osteomyelitis, prostatitis, arthritis, CNS infection
Cladosporium species	6–10 days	Respiratory secretions, skin, nails, nose, cornea	Skin and nail infections, mycotic keratitis. Chromblastomycosis, brain abscess and tinea nigra palmaris caused by *Cladosporium carrionii, C. trichoides,* and *E. werneckii,* respectively
Coccidioides immitis	3–21 days	Respiratory secretions, skin, bone, cerebrospinal fluid, synovial fluid, urine, gastric washings	Pulmonary infection, skin infection, osteomyelitis, meningitis, arthritis, disseminated infection
Dreschlera species	2–6 days	Respiratory secretions, skin	Pulmonary infection (rare)
Epidermophyton floccosum	7–10 days	Skin, nails	Tinea cruris, tinea pedis, tinea corporis, onychomycosis
Fusarium species	2–6 days	Skin, respiratory secretions, cornea	Mycotic keratitis, skin infection (in burn patients)
Geotrichum species	2–6 days	Respiratory secretions, urine, skin, stool, vagina, conjunctiva, gastric washings, throat	Bronchitis, skin infection, colitis, conjunctivitis, thrush
Histoplasma capsulatum	10–45 days (recovery time) [additional 7–21 days required for confirmatory identification]	Respiratory secretions, bone marrow, blood, urine, adrenals, skin, cerebrospinal fluid, eye, pleural fluid, liver, spleen, oropharyngeal lesions, vagina, gastric washings, larynx	Pulmonary infection, oropharyngeal lesions, CNS infection, skin infection (rare), uveitis, peritonitis
Microsporum audouinii	10–14 days (recovery time) [additional 14–21 days required for confirmatory identification]	Hair	Tinea capitis

Table continued on following page

Table 48–10. COMMON FILAMENTOUS FUNGI IMPLICATED IN HUMAN MYCOTIC INFECTIONS *(Continued)*

Etiologic Agent	Time Required for Identification	Probable Recovery Sites	Clinical Implication(s)
Microsporum canis	5–7 days	Hair, skin	Tinea corporis, tinea capitis, tinea barbae, tinea manuum
Microsporum gypseum	3–6 days	Hair, skin	Tinea capitis, tinea corporis
Mucor species	1–5 days	Respiratory secretions, skin, nose, brain, stool, orbit, cornea, vitreous humor, gastric washings, wounds, ear	Rhinocerebral infection, pulmonary infection, gastrointestinal infection, mycotic keratitis, intraocular infection, external otomycosis, orbital cellulitis
*Nocardia asteroides**	4–25 days	Respiratory secretions, skin, urine, blood, brain, conjunctiva, bone, cornea, gastric washings	Pulmonary infection, mycetoma, brain abscess, conjunctivitis, osteomyelitis, mycotic keratitis
Penicillium species	2–6 days	Respiratory secretions, gastric washings, skin, urine, ear, cornea	Pulmonary infection, skin infection, external otomycosis, mycotic keratitis, endocarditis
Pseudallescheria (Petriellidium) boydii	2–6 days	Respiratory secretions, gastric washings, skin, cornea	Pulmonary fungus ball, mycetoma, mycotic keratitis
Phialophora species	6–21 days	Respiratory secretions, gastric washings, skin, cornea, conjunctiva	Some species produce chromoblastomycosis or mycetoma; mycotic keratitis, conjunctivitis, intraocular infection
Rhizopus species	1–5 days	Respiratory secretions, skin, nose, brain, stool, orbit, cornea, vitreous humor, gastric washings, wounds, ear	Rhinocerebral infection, pulmonary infection, mycotic keratitis, intraocular infection, orbital cellulitis, external otomycosis
Scopulariopsis species	2–6 days	Respiratory secretions, gastric washings, nails, skin, vitreous humor, ear	Pulmonary infection, nail infection, skin infection, intraocular infection, external otomycosis
Sporothrix schenckii	3–12 days (recovery time) [additional 2–10 days required for confirmatory identification]	Respiratory secretions, skin, subcutaneous tissue, maxillary sinuses, synovial fluid, bone marrow, bone, cerebrospinal fluid, ear, conjunctiva	Pulmonary infection, lymphocutaneous infection, sinusitis, arthritis, osteomyelitis, meningitis, external otomycosis, conjunctivitis, disseminated infection
Trichophyton mentagrophytes	7–10 days	Hair, skin, nails	Tinea barbae, tinea capitis, tinea corporis, tinea cruris, tinea pedis, onychomycosis
Tirichophyton rubrum	10–14 days	Hair, skin, nails	Tinea pedis, onychomycosis, tinea corporis, tinea cruris
Trichophyton tonsurans	10–14 days	Hair, skin, nails	Tinea capitis, tinea corporis, onychomycosis, tinea pedis
Trichophyton verrucosum	10–18 days	Hair, skin, nails	Tinea capitis, tinea corporis, tinea barbae
Trichophyton violaceum	14–18 days	Hair, skin, nails	Tinea capitis, tinea corporis, onychomycosis

*Although *N. asteroides* is a bacterium, it is commonly recovered on fungal culture media due to its slow growth rate.

Table 48–11. COMMON YEAST-LIKE ORGANISMS IMPLICATED IN HUMAN INFECTION*

Etiologic Agent	Probable Recovery Sites	Clinical Implication(s)
Candida albicans	Respiratory secretions, vagina, urine, skin, oropharynx, gastric washings, blood, stool, transtracheal aspiration, cornea, nails, cerebrospinal fluid, bone, peritoneal fluid	Pulmonary infection, vaginitis, urinary tract infection, dermatitis, fungemia, mycotic keratitis, onychomycosis, meningitis, osteomyelitis, peritonitis, myocarditis, endocarditis, endophthalmitis, disseminated infection, thrush, arthritis
Candida (Torulopsis) glabrata	Respiratory secretions, urine, vagina, gastric washings, blood, skin, oropharynx, transtracheal aspiration, stool, bone marrow, skin (rare)	Pulmonary infection, urinary tract infection, vaginitis, fungemia, disseminated infection, endocarditis
Candida tropicalis	Respiratory secretions, urine, gastric washings, vagina, blood, skin, oropharynx, transtracheal aspiration, stool, pleural fluid, peritoneal fluid, cornea	Pulmonary infection, vaginitis, thrush, endophthalmitis, endocarditis, arthritis, peritonitis, mycotic keratitis, fungemia
Candida parapsilosis	Respiratory secretions, urine, gastric washings, blood, vagina, oropharynx, skin, transtracheal aspiration, stool, pleural fluid, ear, nails	Endophthalmitis, endocarditis, vaginitis, mycotic keratitis, external otomycosis, paronychia, fungemia
Saccharomyces species	Respiratory secretions, urine, gastric washings, vagina, skin, oropharynx, transtracheal aspiration, stool	Pulmonary infection (rare), endocarditis
Candida krusei	Respiratory secretions, urine, gastric washings, vagina, skin, oropharynx, blood, transtracheal aspiration, stool, cornea	Endocarditis, vaginitis, urinary tract infection, mycotic keratitis
Candida guilliermondii	Respiratory secretions, gastric washings, vagina, skin, nails, oropharynx, blood, cornea, bone, urine	Endocarditis, fungemia, dermatitis, onychomycosis, mycotic keratitis, osteomyelitis, urinary tract infection
Rhodotorula species	Respiratory secretions, urine, gastric washings, blood, vagina, skin, oropharynx, stool, cerebrospinal fluid cornea	Fungemia, endocarditis, mycotic keratitis
Trichosporon species	Respiratory secretions, skin, oropharynx, stool	Pulmonary infection, brain abscess, disseminated infection, piedra
Cryptococcus neoformans	Respiratory secretions, cerebrospinal fluid, bone, blood, bone marrow, urine, skin, pleural fluid, gastric washings, transtracheal aspirations, cornea, orbit, vitreous humor	Pulmonary infection, meningitis, osteomyelitis, fungemia, disseminated infection, endocarditis, skin infection, mycotic keratitis, orbital cellulitis, endophthalmic infection
Candida pseudotropicalis	Respiratory secretions, vagina, urine, gastric washings, oropharynx	Vaginitis, urinary tract infection
Cryptococcus albidus/albidus	Respiratory secretions, skin, gastric washings, urine, cornea	Meningitis, pulmonary infection
Cryptococcus luteolus	Respiratory secretions, skin, nose	Not commonly implicated in human infection
Cryptococcus laurentii	Respiratory secretions, cerebrospinal fluid, skin, oropharynx, stool	Not commonly implicated in human infection
Cryptococcus albidus/diffluens	Respiratory secretions, urine, cerebrospinal fluid, gastric washings, skin	Not commonly implicated in human infection
Cryptococcus terreus	Respiratory secretions, skin, nose	Not commonly implicated in human infection

*Arranged in order of occurrence in the clinical laboratory.

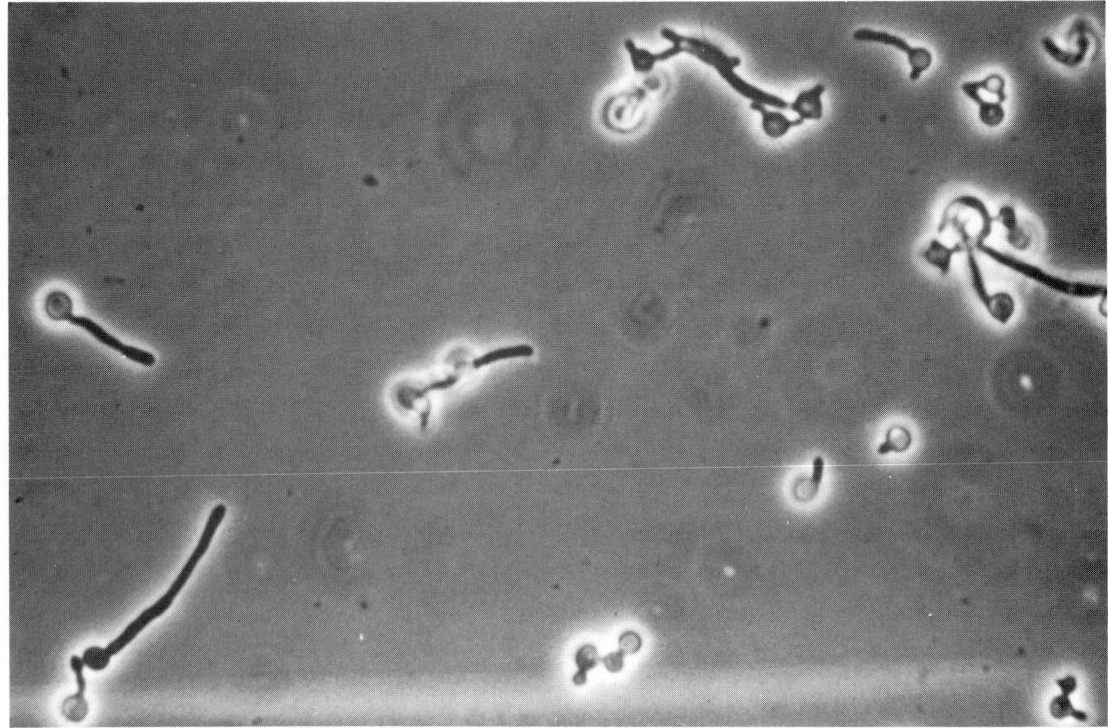

Figure 48–44. *Candida albicans,* green tube formation in normal human serum after incubation at 37°C. for three hours. Phase contrast. ×450. (From Dolan, C. T., Funkhouser, J. W., Koneman, E. W., Miller, N. G., and Roberts, G. D.: Atlas of Clinical Mycology I. Chicago, American Society of Clinical Pathologists, 1975.)

Germ Tube Test

The germ tube test is the most widely used test for the identification of *Candida albicans.* A very small inoculum from an isolated colony is suspended in a tube containing 0.5 ml of sterile normal human serum or another suitable substrate. The suspension is incubated for three hours at 37°C. and is observed microscopically for the presence of germ tubes. A germ tube is characterized by the production of an appendage one half the width of and three to four times the length of the cell from which it extends (Fig. 48–44). The presence of a germ tube provides a definitive identification of *Candida albicans* if the test is performed as described above. Some laboratories prefer to make the distinction between *Candida albicans* and *Candida stellatoidea,* although most laboratories consider *C. stellatoidea* to be a variant of *Candida albicans. Candida stellatoidea* may be differentiated from *Candida albicans* by its inability to assimilate sucrose. When performing the germ tube test, *Candida albicans* should be included as a positive control and *Candida tropicalis* as a negative control. If the germ tube test is incubated longer than three hours, *Candida tropicalis* may produce pseudogerm tubes which appear much wider and more hypha-like than true germ tubes.

Many other substrates, including sheep serum, fetal calf serum, Trypticase soy broth, Sabouraud's dextrose broth, and others, have been utilized for the germ tube test. Most of these substrates are satisfactory; however, extensive quality control testing should be performed to ensure reliable results. This method is recommended for all laboratories.

Urease Test

Urease production is most helpful for the detection of cryptococci. All common species of cryptococci produce urease; however, *Candida krusei,* members of the genus *Rhodotorula, Sporobolomyces,* and *Trichosporon* also exhibit this characteristic.

Urease production may be detected by placing a large inoculum from a single colony onto the surface of the upper portion of the slant in a tube of Christensen's urea agar. The tube is incubated at 37°C. for at least 72 hours. More rapid methods of detecting urease production include the urea broth (Roberts, 1978) and the selective urease tests (Zimmer, 1979). Most members of the genus *Cryptococcus* will produce urease within 15 minutes to 3 hours, and this is indicated by the production of a pink to red color. The urease test is best utilized as a screening tool for the detection of *Cryptococcus neoformans* when characteristic colonies are observed.

Carbohydrate Utilization (Assimilation)

Carbohydrate utilization tests are the most widely used methods for the definitive identification of clinically important yeasts and yeast-like organisms. Most laboratories are prepared to perform these tests; however, little standardization of methods exists. Generally, all methods utilize a basal medium (yeast nitrogen base) which supports the growth of yeasts when an appropriate carbohydrate substrate is added. The medium is observed for the presence of growth, which indicates utilization of a particular carbohydrate substrate by the organism.

Many methods have been developed for detecting carbohydrate utilization patterns: auxanographic plate methods utilizing carbohydrate-impregnated disks (Roberts, 1976) or carbohydrate nutrient–impregnated disks (Huppert, 1975); agar slant utilization methods involving individual carbohydrate sources contained within yeast nitrogen base agar slants (Adams, 1974); and broth tube methods containing individual carbohydrate sources within yeast nitrogen base broth (Wickerham, 1948). Numerous commercially prepared systems which contain carbohydrate utilization tests are available for yeast identification (Bowman, 1976; Buesching, 1979) and are recommended for most laboratories.

Carbohydrate utilization patterns for yeasts commonly encountered in the clinical laboratory are presented in Table 48–12.

Carbohydrate Fermentation

Carbohydrate fermentation tests are useful to supplement carbohydrate utilization test results when there is difficulty in making the definitive identification of an organism. Fermentation tests are less reliable when used alone and are most commonly used as supplementary tests.

Fermentation media contain peptone, beef or yeast extract, an indicator (bromcresol purple), and individual carbohydrate sources. Fermentation is detected by the production of gas only. Acid production (carbohydrate utilization), as indicated by a change in color of the indicator, is not an indication of fermentation. Most fermentation tests require an extended incubation period of 6 to 10 days before final results can be reported. Characteristic fermentation reactions are also presented in Table 48–12.

Nitrate Utilization

Nitrate utilization tests are most helpful for the identification of cryptococci. Basically most methods consist of placing an organism in an environment which contains potassium nitrate as the only inorganic nitrate source. This substrate can be reduced to nitrite and be detected using sulfanilic acid and α-naphthylamine reagents (Rhodes, 1975). The rapid nitrate reduction test (swab method) (Hopkins, 1977) is currently the method of choice for most clinical laboratories. The test is simple to perform, reagents are easy to prepare, and results are available within 10 minutes. This test is particularly helpful in making a rapid, tentative identification of *Cryptococcus neoformans* which does not reduce nitrate.

Pigment Production Media for the Identification of Cryptococcus Neoformans

Cryptococcus neoformans is known to possess an enzyme, phenoloxidase, which reacts with caffeic acid to produce a brown to black pigment. The thistle seed or niger seed agar modified by Paliwal and Randhawa (1978) is commonly used for the detection and identification of *Cryptococcus neoformans*. Most isolates of *Cryptococcus neoformans* produce the characteristic brown pigment within one to three days of incubation. A commercially available screening medium (CN Screen) for *Cryptococcus neoformans* (Flow Laboratories, Roslyn, N.Y.) was evaluated and found to be useful for the identification of this organism (Cooper, 1980). Also, a method utilizing L-β-3,4-dihydroxyphenylalanine has been recently described (Kaufman, 1982) and provides an identification of *C. neoformans* within three hours. Its use in the clinical laboratory is being evaluated.

Cornmeal Agar Morphology

Cornmeal agar has been successfully used for the detection of chlamydospores produced by *Candida albicans* and *Candida stellatoidea*. This method is currently satisfactory for the definitive identification of *Candida albicans* and *Candida stellatoidea* if sucrose assimilation testing is incorporated. However, it has been shown that distinct characteristic microscopic morphologic features of several common species of the genus *Candida* may be observed on cornmeal agar (Dolan, 1971). The morphology is distinct enough to provide a presumptive identification of the following members of the genus Candida: *Candida albicans, Candida glabrata, Candida krusei, Candida parapsilosis, Candida tropicalis,* and *Candida pseudotropicalis*. Microscopic features are also helpful in distinguishing between members of the genera *Cryptococcus* and *Saccharomyces,* although their definitive identification cannot be made on the basis of microscopic morphology on this medium. It is necessary to use biochemical tests to provide confirmation for the latter organisms. Cornmeal agar morphology is often difficult to determine, and perhaps its use should be limited to those laboratories with large volumes of yeasts submitted for identification.

It is not within the scope of this chapter to provide detailed descriptions of all methods useful for the identification of yeasts. Appropriate general references are provided which will allow a laboratory to select and perform those methods appropriate for each laboratory setting. Kits are commercially available for the identification of yeasts and most appear to be satisfactory. However, such factors as cost, stability of reagents, and adaptability to the laboratory setting should be considered before they are purchased. In most instances commercially available yeast identification kits are preferable to individually selected tests after germ tube and urease screening tests have been performed.

Text continued on page 1207

Table 48–12. CHARACTERISTIC BIOCHEMICAL FEATURES OF YEASTS COMMONLY RECOVERED FROM CLINICAL SPECIMENS

Organism	Utilization (Assimilation)							Fermentation*					Urease Production	Nitrate Utilization
	Dextrose	*Maltose*	*Sucrose*	*Lactose*	*Raffinose*	*Trehalose*	*Inositol*	*Dextrose*	*Maltose*	*Sucrose*	*Lactose*	*Galactose*		
Cryptococcus neoformans	+	+	+	−	±	+	+	−	−	−	−	−	+	−
C. albidus var. *albidus*	+	+	+	+†	+	+†	+	−	−	−	−	−	+	+
C. albidus var. *diffluens*	+	+	+	−	+	+	+	−	−	−	−	−	+	+
C. luteolus	+	+	+	−	−†	+	+	−	−	−	−	−	+	−
C. laurentii	+	+	+	+	+†	+	+	−	−	−	−	−	+	−
Candida albicans‡	+	+	+‡	−	−	+	−	G	G	−†	−	G	−	−
C. tropicalis	+	+	+†	−	−	+	−	G	G	G	−	G	−	−
C. parapsilosis	+	+	+	−	−	+	−	G	−	−	−	G†	−	−
C. krusei	+	−	−	−	−	−	−	G	−	−	−	−	+†	−
C. guilliermondii	+	+	+	−	+	+	−	G	−	G	−	G	−	−
C. pseudotropicalis	+	−	+	+	+	−	−	G	−	G	G	G	−	−
Rhodotorula rubra	+	+	+	−	+	+	−	−	−	−	−	−	+	−
Candida (Torulopsis) glabrata	+	−	−	−	−	+	−	G	−	−	−	−	−	−
Geotrichum candidum	+	−	−	−	−	−	−	−	−	−	−	−	−	−
Trichosporon beigelii	+	+†	+†	+	+†	+†	+†	−	−	−	−	−	+	−

*G = Fermentation detected by gas production.
†Strain variation.
‡*Candida stellatoidea* is included with *C. albicans* here; the only difference is in sucrose assimilation.

Table 48–13. COMMONLY AVAILABLE FUNGAL SEROLOGIC TESTS

Infection	Antigen(s)	Test(s)	Interpretation
Aspergillosis	*Aspergillus fumigatus* *Aspergillus niger* *Aspergillus flavus*	Immunodiffusion	One or more precipitin bands suggestive of active infection. Precipitin bands shown to correlate with complement-fixation titers—the greater the number of bands, the higher the titer. When cultural proof is presented in the presence of a positive test, it is diagnostic of active infection. Precipitins can be found in 95% of the fungus ball cases and 50% of the allergic bronchopulmonary cases. Sometimes positive in invasive infection, depending on the immunologic status of the patient.
Blastomycosis	*Blastomyces dermatitidis*		
	Yeast form	Complement-fixation	Titers of 1:8 to 1:16 are highly suggestive of active infection; titers of 1:32 or greater are indicative. Cross-reactions occur in patients having coccidioidomycosis or histoplasmosis; however, titers are usually lower. A decreasing titer is indicative of regression. Most patients (75%) having blastomycosis have negative tests.
	Yeast culture filtrate	Immunodiffusion	Preliminary results show that it is more sensitive than complement-fixation—80% detection rate.
Candidosis	*Candida albicans*	Immunodiffusion, Counterimmuno-electrophoresis	Test difficult to interpret because precipitins are found in 20–30% of the normal population, and reports in the literature are conflicting. Clinical correlation must exist for the test to be useful.
Coccidioidomycosis	Coccidioidin	Complement-fixation	Titers of 1:2 to 1:4 gave been seen in active infection. Low titers should be followed by repeat testing at 2–3 week intervals. Titers of greater than 1:16 are usually indicative of active infection. Cross-reactions occur in patients having histoplasmosis, and false-negative results occur in patients with solitary pulmonary lesions. Titer parallels severity of infection.
	Coccidioidin	Immunodiffusion	Results correlate with complement-fixation test and can be used as a screening test—should be confirmed by performing complement-fixation test.
	Coccidioidin	Latex agglutination	Precipitins occur during first three weeks of infection and are diagnostic, but not prognostic. Useful as a screening test for precipitins in early infection. False-positive tests frequent when diluted serum or cerebrospinal fluid specimens are used.

Table continued on following page

Table 48–13. COMMONLY AVAILABLE FUNGAL SEROLOGIC TESTS *(Continued)*

Infection	Antigen(s)	Test(s)	Interpretation
Cryptococcosis	No antigen—latex particles coated with hyperimmune anticryptococcal globulin	Latex agglutination for cryptococcal antigen	Presence of cryptococcal polysaccharide in body fluids is indicative of cryptococcosis. Rheumatoid factor presents false-positive reactions and RA test must be performed as a control. Decrease in antigen titer indicates regression. Positive tests (in CSF) have been seen in 95% of cryptococcal meningitis cases and 30% of non-meningitis cases. Serum is less frequently positive than CSF. Disseminated infections usually present positive results in serum. Test may be performed using serum, CSF, and urine. Test more sensitive than India ink preparation.
Histoplasmosis	Histoplasmin and yeast form of *Histoplasma capsulatum*	Complement-fixation	Titers of 1:8 to 1:16 are highly suspicious of infection; however, titers of 1:32 or greater are usually indicative of active infection. Cross-reactions occur in patients having aspergillosis, blastomycosis, and coccidioidomycosis, but titers are usually lower. Several follow-up serum samples should be tested—drawn at 2–3 week intervals. Rising titers indicate progressive infection and decreasing titers indicate regression. Some disseminated infections are non-reactive to the complement-fixation test. Recent skin tests in persons who have had prior exposure to *H. capsulatum* will cause an elevation in the complement-fixation titer. This occurs in 17–20% of persons tested. The yeast antigen gives positive reactions in 75–80% of cases, and the histoplasmin gives positive reactions in 10–15% of cases. In 10% of cases both are positive simultaneously.
	Histoplasmin	Immunodiffusion	H and M bands appearing simultaneously are indicative of active infection. M band may appear alone and can indicate early infection or chronic infection. Also the M band may appear after a recent skin test. The H band appears later than the M band and disappears earlier, and its disappearance may indicate regression of the infection.
	Histoplasmin	Latex agglutination	Test is unreliable. Many false-positive and negative tests may be observed. Any positive test should be confirmed by the complement-fixation test.
Sporotrichosis	Yeast of *Sporothrix schenckii*	Agglutination	Titers of 1:80 or greater usually indicative of active infection. Some cutaneous infections present negative tests; however, extracutaneous infections present positive tests.

Fungal Serologic Tests

The definitive diagnosis of mycotic infections is based on the successful recovery and identification of the etiologic agent from a clinical specimen. However, there are instances in which cultural proof cannot be obtained and other laboratory information must be utilized. Fungal serologic tests play an important role in the diagnosis of mycotic infections, although they often provide only tentative evidence of infection. These tests are helpful to supplement cultural or histopathologic evidence of etiology. Many of the tests used in fungal serology require difficult reagent preparation and precise technical expertise and are useful only in reference laboratories. Recently, commercial sources for reagents have become available, making fungal serologic testing feasible for laboratories other than reference laboratories. Demand, costs, expiration rates of reagents, and technical expertise requirements should be considered by individual laboratories before making a decision to institute such a testing program.

As with other serologic tests, false-negative results may occur when blood is drawn at an inappropriate time or if blood is drawn from a patient who is immunosuppressed by chemotherapy or underlying disease and whose antibody production is therefore diminished. Many of the antigens used for testing are crude extracts of the fungi and contain many common components that cross-react with other fungi to give false-positive results. For example, the antigens of *Histoplasma capsulatum* are similar to those of *Blastomyces dermatitidis* and *Coccidioides immitis*. Occasionally, a patient with histoplasmosis will have serologic tests that are positive to all the antigens. In most instances, however, the antibody titer is greater to the antigen from the organism which is the actual cause of infection, *H. capsulatum* in this instance. In addition, it is preferable to repeat serologic tests at two to three week intervals to detect a rise in titer to the antigen of the responsible etiologic agent.

Since most laboratories find it necessary to refer serum samples submitted for serologic testing to reference laboratories, it is necessary to discuss the collection and transport of those samples. Serum aseptically collected from at least 10 ml of blood is adequate for most serologic testing. Samples should be as fresh as possible; however, if short-term storage is required, 4°C. is satisfactory. If longer term storage within the laboratory is necessary, then temperatures of −20°C. to −60°C. are recommended.

When serum or cerebrospinal fluid samples are sent by mail, they should be packed in dry or wet ice to prevent bacterial contamination. Another suitable alternative is to add a preservative, e.g., merthiolate, so that the specimen contains a final concentration of 1:5000. Samples containing the preservative may be mailed without refrigeration.

All samples should be properly packaged and labeled according to governmental regulations before shipping. Air mail or air express routes of shipping are recommended to reduce the transit time.

Table 48–13 presents commonly utilized serologic tests and an interpretation of each. Used properly, these serologic tests can provide very helpful diagnostic information to the clinician in a much shorter time than is required for fungal cultures to become positive. In most instances fungal serologic tests provide enough information when combined with the clinical presentation and can provide a presumptive diagnosis of mycotic infection; their use is highly recommended.

Specific References

Adams, E. D., Jr., and Cooper, B. H.: Evaluation of a modified Wickerham medium for identifying medically important yeasts. Am. J. Med. Technol., *40*:377, 1974.

Bille, J., Roberts, G. D., Horstmeier, C. D., and Ilstrup, D. M.: Evaluation of a lysiscentrifugation system for the recovery of yeasts and filamentous fungi from blood. J. Clin. Microbiol., *18*:469, 1983.

Bowman, P. I., and Ahearn, D. G.: Evaluation of commercial systems for the identification of clinical yeast isolates. J. Clin. Microbiol., *4*:49, 1976.

Buesching, W. J., Kurek, K., and Roberts, G. D.: Evaluation of the modified API 20C system for identification of clinically important yeasts. J. Clin. Microbiol., *9*:565, 1979.

Cooper, B. H.: Clinical laboratory evaluation of a screening medium (CN screen) for *Cryptococcus neoformans*. J. Clin. Microbiol., *11*:672, 1980.

Dolan, C. T.: A practical approach to identification of yeast-like organisms. Am. J. Clin. Path., *55*:580, 1971.

Hopkins, J. M., and Land, G. A.: Rapid method for determining nitrate utilization by yeasts. J. Clin. Microbiol., *5*:497, 1977.

Huppert, M., Harper, G., Sun, S. H., and Delanerolle, V.: Rapid methods for identification of yeasts. J. Clin. Microbiol., *2*:21, 1975.

Kaufman, C. S., and Merz, W. G.: Two rapid pigmentation tests for identification of *Cryptococcus neoformans*. J. Clin. Microbiol., *15*:339, 1982.

Kaufman, L., and Standard, P.: Improved version of the exoantigen test for identification of *Coccidioides immitis* and *Histoplasma capsulatum* cultures. J. Clin. Microbiol., *8*:42, 1978.

Paliwal, D. K., and Randhawa, H. S.: Evaluation of a simplified *Guizzotia abyssinicia* seed medium for differentiation of *Cryptoccoccus neoformans*. J. Clin. Microbiol., *7*:346, 1978.

Rhodes, J. C., and Roberts, G. D.: Comparison of four methods for determining nitrate utilization by cryptococci. J. Clin. Microbiol., *1*:9, 1975.

Roberts, G. D.: Laboratory diagnosis of fungal infections. Human Path., *7*:161, 1976.

Roberts, G. D., Horstmeier, C. D., Land, G. A., and Foxworth, J. H.: Rapid urea broth test for yeasts. J. Clin. Microbiol., *7*:584, 1978.

Roberts, G. D., and Washington, J. A., II: Detection of fungi in blood cultures. J. Clin. Microbiol., *1*:309, 1975.

Staib, F., and Senska, M.: Der Braunfarbeffekt (BFE) bei *Cryptococcus neoformans* auf Guizzotia abyssinica-kreatinin-agar in Abhängigkeit vom Ausgangs-pH-wert. Zentralbl. Bakteriol. [Orig. A], *225*:113, 1973.

Standard, P. G., and Kaufman, L.: Manual for the immunological identification of pathogenic fungus cultures. U.S. Department of Health, Education and Welfare, Public Health Service, Center for Disease Control, 1979.

Wickerham, L. J., and Burton, K. A.: Carbon assimilation tests for the classification of yeasts. J. Bacteriol., *56*:363, 1948.

Zimmer, B. L., and Roberts, G. D.: Rapid selective urease test for presumptive identification of *Cryptococcus neoformans*. J. Clin. Microbiol., *10*:380, 1979.

General References

Ajello, L.: Epidemiology of human fungous infections. *In* Dalldorf, G. (ed.): Fungi and Fungous Diseases. Springfield, Ill., Charles C Thomas, Publisher, 1962, p. 69.

Baker, R. D.: Human Infection With Fungi, Actinomycetes and Algae. New York, Springer-Verlag, 1971.

6

Braude, A. I.: Diseases caused by fungi. *In* Thorn, G. W., Adams, R. D., Braunwald, E., Isselbacher, K. S., and Petersdorf, R. G. (eds.): Harrison's Principles of Internal Medicine. 8th ed. New York, McGraw-Hill Book Co., 1977, p. 937.

Chandler, F. W., Kaplan, W., and Ajello, L.: Color Atlas and Text of the Histopathology of Mycotic Disease. Chicago, Year Book Medical Publishers, 1980.

Conant, N. F., Smith, D. T., Baker, R. D., and Callaway, J. L.: Manual of Clinical Mycology. 3rd ed. Philadelphia, W. B. Saunders Company, 1971.

Emmons, C. W., Binford, C. H., Utz, J. P., and Kwon-Chung, K. J.: Medical Mycology. 3rd ed. Philadelphia, Lea and Febiger, 1977.

Kaufman, L.: Serodiagnosis of fungal diseases. *In* Rose, N. R., and Friedman, H. (eds.): Manual of Clinical Immunology. 2nd ed. Washington, D.C., American Society for Microbiology, 1980, p. 553.

Kersting, D. W.: The pathology of deep fungous infections. *In* Robinson, H. M. (ed.): The Diagnosis and Treatment of Fungal Infections. Springfield, Ill., Charles C Thomas, Publisher, 1974, p. 277.

Koneman, E. W., Roberts, G. D., and Wright, S. F.: Practical Laboratory Mycology. 2nd ed. Baltimore, Williams and Wilkins Company, 1978.

Rippon, J. W.: Medical Mycology: The Pathogenic Fungi and the Pathogenic Actinomycetes. 2nd ed. Philadelphia, W. B. Saunders Company, 1982.

Schwartz, J.: The pathogenesis of histoplasmosis, *In* Ajello, L., Chick, E. W., and Furcolow, M. F. (eds.): Histoplasmosis. Springfield, Ill., Charles C Thomas, Publisher, 1971, p. 244.

Silva-Hutner, M., and Cooper, B. H.: Medically important yeasts. *In* Lennette, E. H., Spaulding, E. H., and Truant, J. P. (eds.): Manual of Clinical Microbiology. 3rd ed. Washington, D.C., American Society for Microbiology, 1980, p. 562.

Wilson, J. W., and Plunkett, O. A.: The Fungous Diseases of Man. Berkeley, University of California Press, 1965.

49

MEDICAL PARASITOLOGY

JAMES W. SMITH, M.D.,
and YEZID GUTIERREZ, M.D., PH.D.

Parasitic diseases contribute significantly to medical, economic, and social problems of the world. In the United States, the incidence of most endemic parasitic infections has decreased, but for some, such as giardiasis and pneumocystosis, it has increased. In underdeveloped countries, incidence of some infections has increased in recent years. Relaxation of control efforts, development of insecticide resistance by mosquitos, and chemotherapy resistance by parasites have led to a resurgence of malaria. Modification of the environment by the building of dams, such as the Aswan dam, has increased the incidence of schistosomiasis. In the United States, parasitic diseases may be endemic or may have been acquired in foreign countries by immigrants, students, or visitors from these countries or by United States citizens who have been in endemic areas. A person may have entered the United States weeks or months before clinical disease develops.

This chapter emphasizes parasitic diseases as seen in the United States, whether acquired here or abroad. Incidence, seriousness of the infection to the patient, and importance of the laboratory for diagnosis determine the amount of discussion for each parasite.

Diagnosis of parasitic diseases is generally established by morphologic demonstration of parasites or by detecting immune response to parasites. Occasionally, culture or animal inoculation may be used. Proper diagnosis requires that (1) the physician consider that a parasite might be a cause of the disease, (2) appropriate specimens be obtained and properly transported to the laboratory, (3) the laboratory competently examine the specimens, (4) the laboratory results be effectively communicated to the physician, and (5) these results be correctly interpreted and applied to the care of the patient. A basic knowledge of the natural cycle of the disease is important in determining the diagnostic approach. Parasites may cause clinical disease at a time when diagnostic forms are not yet present in the usual site; for example, *Ascaris* larval migration may cause symptomatology weeks before eggs are present in feces. The overall expansion of medical knowledge has led to a decrease in the time devoted to parasitic diseases during physician training. In addition, most laboratories in the United States see few positive parasitology specimens from patients. Results of proficiency testing programs suggest that some laboratories have difficulty detecting and correctly identifying parasites, especially intestinal protozoa (Smith, 1979). To use the laboratory optimally, the clinician must have an understanding of the adequacy of the methods and personnel in the laboratory.

Figures on parasite prevalence in the United States are difficult to obtain. Laboratory methods used, populations studied, and criteria for diagnosis vary. A recent review of the incidence of various intestinal parasites in fecal specimens examined by state health department laboratories (CDC, Aug. 1979) (Table 49–1) gives some indication of the relative importance of various infections. In interpreting these data, the following should be considered. These specimens were submitted for parasite examinations, and thus are not prevalence figures. There are variations from state to state in methods used, proficiency of laboratories, and patient population examined. The figures do not

Table 49–1. INCIDENCE OF INTESTINAL PARASITES IN 322,735 FECAL SPECIMENS EXAMINED BY STATE HEALTH DEPARTMENT LABORATORIES, 1978*

Parasite	Number	Per Cent of Specimens
Protozoa		
Giardia lamblia	12,947	4.0
Entamoeba histolytica	2409	0.8
Dientamoeba fragilis	1880	0.6
Balantidium coli	7	
Isospora spp.	1	
Non-pathogenic	21,120	6.5
Nematodes		
Trichuris trichiura	5481	1.7
Ascaris lumbricoides	4630	1.4
Enterobius vermicularis	4344	1.4
Hookworm	2035	0.6
Strongyloides stercoralis	602	0.2
Trichostrongylus spp.	14	
Trematodes		
Clonorchis/opisthorchis	205	0.06
Schistosoma mansoni	48	
Fasciola hepatica	1	
Paragonimus westermani	1	
Cestodes		
Hymenolepis nana	1068	0.3
Taenia spp.	251	0.08
Diphyllobothrium latum	20	
Hymenolepis diminuta	12	
Dipylidium caninum	7	

*Adapted from Center for Disease Control: Intestinal Parasite Surveillance. Annual Summary, 1978. Issued August, 1979. Does not include laboratories in Guam, Puerto Rico, or Virgin Islands. One or more parasites were found in 14.7 per cent of specimens. Percentages are not calculated for parasites identified less than 100 times.

reflect accurately the incidence of enterobiasis, as fecal examination is a poor way to diagnose this infection. The incidence of specific parasites varies in different parts of the country. Nationwide, 14.7 per cent of specimens were positive for fecal parasites, with the frequency of positive specimens, in individual states, varying from 4 to 39 per cent.

Parasitic life cycles may be simple, as in amebae and pinworms, or complex, as in malaria and schistosomiasis. If there are multiple hosts, the definitive host harbors the sexual stage of the life cycle and the intermediate host(s) the asexual stage(s). A reservoir host is a host other than man that may also be parasitized by the same stage(s) of the parasite as man and thus serve as a source of infection. Man is an incidental host of some animal parasites.

The transmission of parasitic diseases is often influenced by sanitation, housing, diet, cooking, and social customs. In addition, geographic factors, such as lakes and rivers, climate, and altitude may play a significant role. Control efforts are aimed at breaking the life cycle in one or several places; for instance, eliminating a host, removing the reservoir of infection, assuring a safe water supply, or developing sanitary means of disposal of feces.

In this section, emphasis is on laboratory diagnosis. Sufficient information is given about parasitology, epidemiology, clinical disease, and pathology to provide a basic understanding of the disease. For more detailed information, the reader is referred to books listed under General References or to specific references.

In parasitology, as in other areas of biologic science, there are disagreements about taxonomy, pathogenesis, and methodology. We have not attempted to resolve these but have attempted to take a middle ground. Laboratory results that are not of direct diagnostic value will not be discussed.

LABORATORY METHODS

Numerous methods for diagnosis of parasitic diseases have been described; some are useful in detecting a wide variety of parasites, and others are useful for one or a few parasites. It is better for the laboratory to offer a limited number of procedures competently performed than a wide variety of infrequently and poorly performed tests. The methods described are widely used and should provide good results in the hands of proficient laboratory personnel. Some methods useful in special situations are briefly described or referenced. Descriptions of a variety of procedures of general and limited usefulness may be found in various parasitology and tropical medicine books and in books emphasizing methodology (Garcia, 1979; Lennette, 1980; Melvin, 1982).

The type of specimen collected will depend upon the species and form of parasite suspected. Knowledge of the life cycle of the parasite aids in determining the type, number, and frequency of specimens for diagnosis.

Calibration of an Ocular Micrometer

Measurement of size of parasites is important for accurately identifying both protozoa and helminths and should be done using an ocular micrometer that has been properly calibrated for each objective of each microscope with which it is to be used. (Fig. 49–1). For example, the similarly shaped eggs of *Diphyllobothrium latum, Paragonimus westermani,* and *Fasciola/Fasciolopsis* are readily differentiated by accurate measurement (Smith, 1979).

1. An ocular micrometer is inserted into the ocular element so that the scale is in focus when the microscope is in focus.

2. A ruled stage micrometer is placed on the microscope stage, the iris diaphragm is partially shut to reduce light, and the ruled scale is brought into focus.

3. The ocular micrometer scale and the stage micrometer scale are moved until the O's align. Then the ocular micrometer is examined until a division is found which also aligns with a division on the stage micrometer. Each large division of the stage micrometer equals 0.1 mm (100 microns) and each small division equals 0.01 mm (10 microns).

4. Distance between small ocular units is calculated by determining the distance in microns between two aligned divisions on the stage micrometer and dividing by the number of small ocular units between the same aligned divisions. The result is the distance between ocular units in

CALIBRATION OF OCULAR MICROMETER

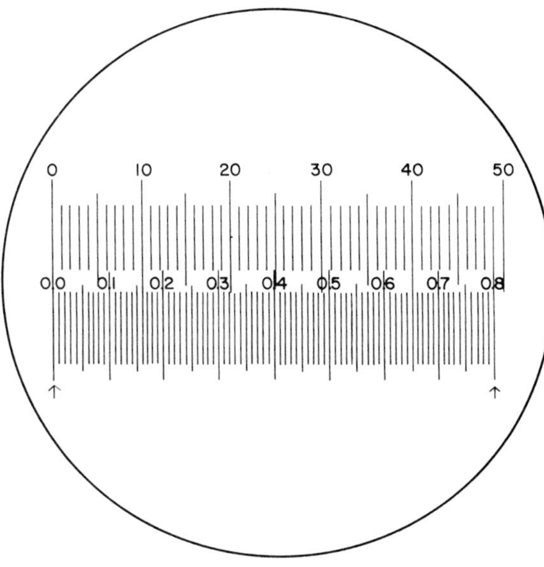

Ocular Micrometer–Top Scale
Stage Micrometer–Bottom Scale

Figure 49–1. Example of calibrated ocular micrometer. (From Melvin, 1982. 2nd ed.)

microns. In the example in Figure 49–1, 10 ocular units = 0.16 mm (160 μl); therefore, one ocular unit = 0.016 mm or 16 μ.

5. Record the unit value of an ocular micrometer division (in microns) using each objective of the microscope. Each microscope must be calibrated separately and must be recalibrated each time an objective or ocular is changed.

6. To determine the size of an object, count the number of ocular units that represent the dimension to be measured and multiply this number by the value calculated in Step 4 for the magnification used.

Blood Examination

Examination of blood films is the usual method for diagnosing blood parasites, although special, more sensitive procedures have been described for microfilaria (Knott, 1939; Desowitz, 1974), African trypanosomes (Lanham, 1968), and malaria (Keffer, 1966). Two types of blood films are prepared for diagnosis of blood parasite infections: thin films and thick films. In the thin film, the blood is spread over the slide in a thin layer and the red blood cells are intact after staining. In the thick film, the blood is concentrated in a small area and is many cell layers deep. During staining, the red cells are lysed, and only white blood cell nuclei, platelets, and parasites (if present) will be visible. The thick film is preferred for diagnosis, since it contains 16 to 30 times as much blood per microscopic field as does the thin film, thus increasing the chances of detecting minimal ("light") infections and decreasing the time needed for a reliable examination. Approximately the same amount of blood can be examined with the oil immersion lens in a thick film in five minutes as can be examined in a thin film in 30 minutes.

Parasite species can usually be determined from thick films by an experienced examiner. However, since morphologic characteristics, particularly those of the malarial parasites, are more definitive in thin films, these preparations may sometimes be needed for definite species identification. For routine examination both thick and thin films should be prepared.

PREPARATION OF SLIDES

Blood for examination may be obtained by finger stick, ear lobe puncture, or venipuncture. If obtained by venipuncture, the first drop of blood (anticoagulant-free) from the needle is used to prepare the films. Films, especially for diagnosis of malaria, should *not* be prepared from anticoagulated or clotted blood. Anticoagulants may cause distortion of the organisms and interfere with staining, particularly of the older malarial stages that may stain palely and appear degenerate. Anticoagulants do not interfere with the staining of microfilariae. If 70 per cent alcohol is used to disinfect the site of the stick, it must be wiped off or allowed to dry to assure that it does not fix blood cells and prevent dehemoglobinization of thick films.

A thin film is prepared in the manner described in the hematology section. Thick films may be prepared by touching the undersurface to a drop of blood on a stuck finger and rotating the slide to cover an area the size of a dime (1.5 cm). An alternative method is to puddle several small drops of blood with the corner of a slide. A proper thick film should be thin enough that newspaper print may be read through it. If too thick, the film may peel from the slide.

Thick and thin films may be prepared on separate slides or on a combination slide with a thin film on one end and thick film on the other. In such instances, only the thin film should be fixed with methyl alcohol (30 seconds) and contact of the thick film with alcohol fumes must be avoided. Thick films should be allowed to dry flat at room temperature, usually overnight. Excess heat may fix erythrocytes and prevent dehemoglobinization.

STAINING

Blood begins to lose its affinity for stain in about three days, and older thick films do not dehemoglobinize well. Staining is best performed with Giemsa stain. Wright's stain may be used for thin films but stains parasites less well than Giemsa. It is unsatisfactory for thick films because it fixes the erythrocytes. Fresh working Giemsa stain solution must be made each day by diluting stock Giemsa stain (commercially available) with M/15 phosphate buffered water, pH 7.0 to 7.2.* One part stock is added to 50 parts water in a Coplin jar and slides are stained for 50 minutes. (Thin films may alternatively be stained for

*Buffered water for Giemsa stain—pH 7.0–7.2
Acid buffer M/15 NaH_2PO_4—39 ml
Alkaline buffer M/15 Na_2PO_4—61 ml
Distilled water—900 ml
Check pH

20 minutes with a stain of one part Giemsa stock added to 20 parts buffered water.)

After staining, thin films are rinsed by briefly dipping the slide in buffered water. Thick film should be rinsed an additional three to five minutes in buffered water. Slides are allowed to air dry and are then examined with low power for microfilariae and with high power and oil immersion for blood and tissue protozoa.

Fecal Specimens

Infection with intestinal helminths can in most instances be diagnosed by demonstration of eggs or larvae in feces. Intestinal protozoan infections are diagnosed by finding trophozoites or cysts in feces. Some helminths produce many eggs per day and others produce few. It is advisable to select methods for routine examination that will allow identification of both helminth and protozoan parasites (Markell, 1977a), with use of other methods only when special situations require. As a minimum, laboratories performing fecal examinations for parasites should be capable of performing direct wet-mount examination, a concentration procedure, and a permanent stain method. Many protozoan infections will be missed unless permanent stains are examined (Garcia, 1979b).

SPECIMEN COLLECTION AND HANDLING

Detection and identification of parasites depend upon properly collected and handled specimens. Old, poorly preserved, or contaminated specimens are of little value. Specimens should not be collected for one week after the patient has been taking materials which leave crystalline residue, such as anti-diarrheal compounds, antacids, bismuth, and barium. In addition, oily laxatives, such as mineral oil, may interfere with examination. Antibiotics and contrast media may decrease the numbers of organisms, particularly protozoa, in the stool for two to three weeks. Specimens should be free of urine and should not be contaminated with toilet water or soil, as these may contain free living protozoa and helminths or may destroy trophozoites. Water stored in the laboratory may also become contaminated with free-living parasites. Specimens may be collected directly into clean, dry paper cartons, or may be collected in bed pans or, if not diarrheic, by squatting over wax paper. They should be submitted to the laboratory in containers with tight-fitting lids.

Because the numbers of diagnostic forms of some parasites (i.e., *Giardia, Strongyloides)* may vary with time, it is advisable to examine specimens obtained every second or third day with a total of three specimens being a minimum to reasonably assure freedom from infection.

When amebiasis is suspected and a series of normally passed stools has been negative, purged specimens may be desirable. The laboratory must be notified prior to submitting a purged series. Saline purgatives, such as sodium sulfate or buffered phosphosoda, are recommended. Each specimen should be collected separately and submitted to the laboratory within minutes of collection.

All fecal specimens must be labeled with proper identification information and must include the date and time of collection. Specimens should be submitted to the laboratory as soon as possible and should be handled expeditiously on arrival in the laboratory. Time is particularly important for loose and watery specimens because protozoan trophozoites degenerate rapidly. Liquid specimens should be examined or placed in fixatives within one hour after passage. Specimens that cannot be processed immediately should be left at room temperature or refrigerated and should not be placed in an incubator, as this only speeds disintegration of parasites. Placing specimens in appropriate fixatives immediately in the patient care area improves the yield of protozoa (Markell, 1977b).

If specimens must be collected at home or must be mailed to the laboratory, it is advisable to use a two-vial preservation technique with one portion of the specimen being fixed in three parts of 5 to 10 per cent buffered formalin and another portion of the specimen being fixed in three parts of polyvinyl alcohol (PVA) fixative. The specimen must be thoroughly mixed when placed in these fixatives. Specimens that arrive in the laboratory late in the day or during evening hours or that cannot be examined promptly may also be preserved by this two-vial technique. Other systems of preservation have been described (see Melvin, 1982), but most do not provide material with which to make permanently stained slides.

GROSS EXAMINATION

Fecal specimens should be examined grossly. The consistency of the specimen should be recorded as formed, soft, loose, or watery. Protozoan trophozoites are most likely to be found in watery, loose, or soft specimens and cysts in formed, soft, or loose specimens. Proglottids or adult worms may be detected by gross examination and, in addition, flecks of blood or mucus may be specifically selected for examination.

Many parasites are uniformly distributed in the stool as a result of the mixing action of the cecum (Martin, 1965); however, eggs that enter the fecal stream in the lower colon and rectum (such as schistosomes) may be unevenly distributed, as may taenia eggs and pinworm eggs that are released by rupture of parasites. Protozoan trophozoites may be more numerous in the last portion evacuated.

MICROSCOPIC EXAMINATION

Specimens may be examined microscopically by direct wet mounts of fresh or preserved material, wet mounts of concentrates, or permanent stains. Each procedure has specific advantages. Direct saline wet mounts of fresh feces allow detection and observation of motile protozoan trophozoites and helminth larvae. Direct mounts of preserved feces may allow detection of parasites that do not concentrate well. Concentration procedures increase the ability to detect protozoan cysts and helminth eggs and larvae, but generally are unsatisfactory for detecting protozoan trophozoites.

Permanent stains are useful for detection and morphologic examination of protozoan trophozoites and cysts.

At a minimum, formed stool specimens should be examined by concentration; soft and loose stools should be examined by direct wet mounts, concentration, and permanent stain procedures, and watery stools should be examined by permanent stains and direct wet mounts. If desired, watery specimens may be concentrated by simple centrifugation rather than by the special procedures described below.

It is best to preserve a portion of each specimen, including formed specimens, in a fixative for permanent staining. Permanent stains may aid in identification of protozoa detected by direct wet mounts or concentration.

Wet Mounts. Direct wet mounts or wet mounts of concentrated material are best made using 3 by 2 inch slides (rather than 3 by 1 inch) and 22 mm No. 1 coverslips. This prevents leaking of specimen onto the microscope and allows room to seal the coverslip with vaspar if desired (see below). Fecal preparations should be dense enough that newspaper print can just be read through them. Large particles should be avoided, as they prevent a proper fit of the coverslip. Air bubbles should also be avoided. Generally a double mount will be made, one unstained and one stained with a drop of iodine solution. The iodine should be that of Dobell and O'Connor* or a 1:5 dilution of Lugol's iodine. An overly strong iodine solution, such as straight Lugol's or Gram's iodine, will cause clumping of material, which will obscure organisms. Iodine makes nuclear structure of protozoan cysts more evident and stains glycogen masses; however, chromatoid bodies are less visible than in saline mounts and cysts are less refractile and thus may be more difficult to find. The unstained mount of fresh feces should be made in physiologic saline (0.85 per cent). For preserved feces, diluent is needed only if the preparation is too dense. Wet mounts may be used to examine a variety of body fluids in addition to feces.

Sealing of the wet mount with vaspar allows use of the oil immersion objective to examine the slide and prevents drying of the preparation. Vaspar is a 50/50 mixture of petroleum jelly and paraffin, which is heated on a hotplate till melted. A camel's-hair brush or cotton-tipped applicator is dipped in the melted vaspar and touched to opposite corners of the coverslip to attach it to the 3 by 2 inch slide, then with even strokes, vaspar is applied to the edges of the coverslip until it is completely sealed. This may require several dips.

Microscopically examine the entire mount in a systematic fashion. A good method is to begin in one corner and, using the stage, methodically scan each field of the coverslip with the 10× objective, going to high magnification to examine suspicious objects more carefully. It may be worthwhile also to scan across the coverslip several times with the high dry or oil immersion objective to ensure that small protozoa are not missed. Identification of protozoa should be with the 40× or 100× oil immersion objective. 20× dry and 50× oil immersion objectives, in addition to the usual 10× and 40× dry and 100× oil, may be useful in parasitology.

Concentration Procedures. Concentration procedures increase the ability to detect protozoan cysts and helminth eggs and larvae by decreasing the amount of background material in the preparations and by an actual concentration of organisms. Concentration procedures may be performed on fresh or preserved specimens. A wide variety of methods and modifications have been described, some of which are useful only for specific parasites (Melvin, 1982; Garcia, 1979b). For routine use, a method should be selected that will allow reliable detection of both protozoan cysts and helminth eggs. Concentration methods generally employ sedimentation or flotation. In sedimentation the heavier parasites settle to the bottom owing to gravity or centrifugation. In flotation, the parasites rise to the surface of a solution of high specific gravity.

The two most widely used procedures in the United States are the zinc sulfate centrifugal flotation technique of Faust and the formalin-ether sedimentation technique of Ritchie or modifications of them. Methods are described below for performing each technique on fresh specimens or formalin-preserved feces. The formalin-ether sedimentation technique has somewhat greater sensitivity in detecting most parasites but requires the use of ether, which may present storage, handling, and disposal problems. Ethyl acetate may be substituted for diethyl ether with comparable results (Young, 1979). The formalin–zinc sulfate method described is also effective (Bartlett, 1978), because formalin fixation decreases distortion of eggs, cysts, and larvae and prevents popping of opercula. There are problems using zinc sulfate concentration on fresh specimens. Schistosome eggs do not concentrate well with flotation methods. Centrifugation in both concentration procedures should be done in a free-swinging rather than an angle centrifuge.

Formalin-Ethyl Acetate Procedure. This concentration procedure is efficient in recovering most protozoan cysts and helminth eggs and larvae, including operculate eggs, and is moderately effective for schistosome eggs. Less distortion of cysts occurs with this technique than with the zinc sulfate method. *Hymenolepis nana* eggs may be missed, however, and concentration of *Giardia lamblia* and *Iodamoeba bütschlii* cysts may not be very good.

Technique for Fresh Specimens
(Adapted from Melvin, 1982)

1. Comminute a portion of stool about 2 cm diameter in sufficient saline so that 10 ml of suspension will yield about 1 ml of sediment upon centrifugation.

2. Strain about 10 ml of the suspension through a small funnel containing wet gauze or cheesecloth into a 15 ml conical centrifuge tube. (To conserve glassware, a cone-shaped paper cup [about a 4-ounce size] with the point cut off can be substituted for a funnel.)

---

*Dobell and O'Connor's Iodine Solution

Iodine (powdered crystals)	1g
Potassium iodide	2g
Distilled water	100 ml

Dissolve potassium iodide in water. Add iodine crystals and shake thoroughly. Filter or decant into dark bottle. Store away from light. Solution should be color of medium strong tea. Shelf life is at least two weeks.

6

3. Centrifuge at 650 g for one to two minutes. Decant supernatant. About 1 to 1.5 ml of sediment should be present. If the amount is much larger or smaller, adjust to the proper quantity in the following manner. (a) *Amount too large:* Resuspend the sediment in saline (or water) and pour out a portion. For example, if the amount is twice the desired quantity, pour out about half of the suspension and then add saline (or water) to bring the fluid level to about 10 ml and centrifuge again. (b) *Amount too small:* Pour off the supernatant and strain a second portion of the original fecal suspension into the tube. The amount to be strained can be determined from the amount of sediment; that is, if about half of the quantity necessary is obtained with the first centrifugation, strain another 10 ml into the tube. Centrifuge again. It is not necessary to have an exact quantity of sediment in the tube, but the quantity should approximate the amount indicated above.

4. Resuspend the sediment in fresh saline (or water), centrifuge, and decant as before.

5. Add about 9 ml of 10 per cent formalin to the sediment, mix thoroughly, and allow to stand for five minutes or longer. At this point, the formalin-feces mixture may be stoppered and saved until a later time. *Note:* Plastic squeeze bottles for saline and formalin will facilitate dispensing these solutions into the tubes.

6. Add 3 ml of ethyl acetate, stopper the tube, and shake vigorously in an inverted position for at least 30 seconds. Remove the stopper with care.

7. Centrifuge at 450 to 500 g for one minute. Four layers should result as follows: (1) layer of ethyl acetate, (2) plug of debris, (3) layer of formalin, and (4) sediment.

8. Free the plug of debris from the sides of the tube by ringing with an applicator stick and carefully decant and discard the top three layers. Use a cotton swab to clean debris from the walls of the tube.

9. With a pipette, mix the remaining sediment with the small amount of fluid that drains back from the sides of the tube and prepare iodine and unstained mounts for microscopic examination. If not enough fluid is left in the tube, a drop of saline or 10 per cent formalin can be added to the sediment.

10. If examination of the specimen is delayed, add 1 or 2 ml of 10 per cent formalin to the sediment and stopper the tube. Formalinized sediments may be kept for some time if they do not dry. Remove the excess formalin before making mounts.

Technique for Formalin-Preserved Specimens

1. Thoroughly stir the formalinized specimen.

2. Depending on the size and density of the specimen, strain a sufficient quantity through wet gauze into a conical 15 ml centrifuge tube to give 0.5 to 0.75 ml of sediment. Usually 4 to 5 ml is sufficient unless the fecal suspension is thin. In formalin-preserved specimens, the formalin has clarified the feces to some extent, and further clarification is caused primarily by the ethyl acetate. Therefore, the sediment volume during concentration is not as great as with fresh feces, and the initial quantity must be less.

3. Add tap water to make 10 ml of suspension, mix thoroughly, and centrifuge at 500 to 650 g for one to two minutes.

4. Decant supernatant and, if desired, wash again with tap water. The amount of sediment should be about 0.5 to 0.75 ml. If too much or too little is present, adjust the quantity by the method described for fresh material.

5. Add 9 ml of 10 per cent formalin (preferably buffered) to the sediment and mix thoroughly.

6. Add 4 ml of ethyl acetate, stopper the tube, and shake vigorously in an inverted position for at least 30 seconds. Remove the stopper with care.

7. Proceed as with fresh specimen.

Formalin-Zinc Sulfate Flotation Procedure (Bartlett, 1978). Formalin helps to clear the specimen and prevents popping of opercula and distortion of parasites. The method is unsatisfactory for detecting schistosome eggs.

Procedure

1. Strain a well-mixed fecal suspension through one layer of gauze into a round-bottomed 100 by 16 mm tube to within 2 cm of the rim (the specimen must have been fixed in formalin for at least 30 minutes).

2. Centrifuge at approximately 750 g for 3½ minutes. A free-swinging centrifuge must be used. Allow the centrifuge to come to a full stop without braking before lifting the lid.

3. Decant the supernatant from each tube, draining the last drop against a clean section of paper towel, and place upright in a test tube rack.

Steps 4 through 10 must be done without interruption.

4. Add zinc sulfate to within 2.5 cm of the rim of each tube. To prepare the zinc sulfate solution, dissolve about 400 g of $ZnSO_4$ in 1 L of water. Check the specific gravity with a good hydrometer and adjust as necessary to between 1.195 and 1.200, preferably closer to 1.200. Store in tightly stoppered container. Specific gravity should be checked at least once a week.

5. Mix the packed sediment thoroughly with two applicator sticks until no coarse particles remain.

6. Immediately centrifuge at 500 g for one and one half minutes in a free-swinging centrifuge.

7. As soon as the centrifuge comes to a full stop (without braking), very carefully transfer the tubes to a rack. Avoid disturbing the surface films, which now contain the floating parasites.

8. Allow the tubes to stand undisturbed for one full minute; then with a wire loop in which the loop is at a right angle to the stem, carefully transfer two loops of the surface film to the corresponding drops of saline or Dobell and O'Connor's iodine on a 3 by 2 inch glass slide. Touch the loop carefully to the surface film without dipping below the surface and deposit the drop in the loop beside a drop of saline or iodine. Then, using the heel of the loop, mix the fecal drops first in the saline then in the iodine.

9. Place a clean 22 by 30 mm, No. 1 coverslip on the fluid mount, avoiding trapped air bubbles.

10. Flame the wire loop, then proceed with steps 8 and 9 on the next tube.

11. Place each prepared slide mount in a Petri dish containing a moist paper towel to retard evaporation.

12. Examine the mounts immediately or at least within the hour. A longer holding period may make the identification of some stages more difficult.

Permanent Stain Technique. A variety of different permanent stains have been described and have advantages and disadvantages (Melvin, 1982). The most widely used technique in the United States is the Wheatley trichrome method, and it is the only stain which will be described. Iron hematoxylin and phosphotungstic acid hematoxylin stains are other widely used stains for fixed fecal smears. Chlorazol black E is also a satisfactory stain but can only be used on fresh fecal material.

Films for permanent staining may be prepared on clean 1 by 3 inch glass slides. Fresh films are made by smearing the unfixed fecal sample on a slide with applicator sticks in an even uniform smear, then fixing immediately in Schaudinn's fixative (slides must not be allowed to dry). After fixation of one hour or longer at room temperature, staining may be performed. PVA-fixed material should be well mixed and then smeared on the slide as described above, being sure the smear extends to the edges of the slide to prevent peeling. Leave smears at room temperature or in an incubator overnight to ensure they are dry before staining.

Wheatley Trichrome Stain (Melvin, 1974). Trichrome stain is relatively simple and rapid and uses reagents that are stable. It may be used with either fresh or PVA-fixed material, the only difference being in the timing of some staining steps. The method is simple in that overstaining and differentiation are not necessary to bring out the morphologic details of the parasites, nor is it necessary to treat with a mordant before staining. However, destaining the smears gives better differentiations of the organisms, and this step should be included. The stain solution is stable and may be used repeatedly, the lost volume being replaced by adding stock solution. Staining over 15 smears daily (in 50 ml of stain), however, tends to weaken the stain. If stain is allowed to evaporate, strength will return. This can be accomplished by leaving the cover off the staining dish for several hours or overnight. The staining of Schaudinn's fixed and PVA-fixed material differs chiefly in the increased times in various reagents required for the latter and in the omission of the fixative step, since the material in the PVA fixative is already fixed. Both procedures are given below. Each numbered step indicates a different Coplin jar. Control slides of known staining quality should be run with each batch of slides stained. Positive material is preferred, but negative material is satisfactory.

Staining Technique with Schaudinn's Fixed Smears

1. Schaudinn's fixative (Solution No. 1) ....5 min at 50°C. or 1 hr at room temperature. Do not allow smear to dry before placing it in Schaudinn's
2. 70% alcohol plus iodine (Solution No. 3) ....1 min (to remove mercuric chloride)
3. 70% alcohol ....1 min
4. 70% alcohol ....1 min
5. Stain (trichrome) (Solution No. 4) ....2-8 min
6. 90% alcohol, acidified (Solution No. 5) ....5-10 sec, total; usually a brief dip (in and out) is sufficient.

Since the acid alcohol continues to destain as long as it is in contact with the material, the time allowed *should include the few seconds between the time the slide is removed from the destain and rinsed in 95 per cent alcohol* (step 7). For more effective removal of the acid destain, two 95 per cent alcohol washes are suggested instead of one. These should be changed frequently to prevent them from becoming so acid that the destaining process will continue. Prolonged destaining in acid alcohol (over 20 seconds) may cause the organisms to be poorly differentiated, although larger trophozoites, particularly those of *Entamoeba coli,* may require slightly longer periods of decolorization.

Note: If several slides are being stained simultaneously, they should be destained separately. Remove only one slide at a time from the stain, destain it, rinse in the 95 per cent alcohols, and place it in the carbol-xylene (step 9).

7. 95% alcohol ....Rinse briefly
8. 95% alcohol ....Rinse twice
9. 100% alcohol or carbol-xylene ....1 min
10. Xylene ....1-3 min
11. Mount with coverslip using Permount or other mounting medium.

Staining Technique with PVA Fixed Smears

1. 70% alcohol plus iodine (Solution No. 3) ....10-20 min
2. 70% alcohol ....3-5 min
3. 70% alcohol ....3-5 min
4. Trichrome stain (Solution No. 4) ....8 min
5. 90% alcohol, acidified (Solution No. 5) ....10-20 sec, total (See previous paragraph on destaining.)
6. 95% alcohol ....Rinse to remove acid destain
7. 95% alcohol ....5 min
8. Carbol-xylene ....5-10 min
9. Xylene ....10 min
10. Mount with coverslip using Permount or other mounting medium.

Trichrome Stain Reactions. The ctyoplasm of thoroughly fixed and well-stained cysts and trophozoites is blue-green tinged with purple. Occasionally, *Entamoeba coli cysts* may stain slightly more purplish than cysts of other species. The nuclear chromatin, chromatoid bodies, and ingested red cells and bacteria stain red or purplish red. Other ingested particles, such as yeasts or molds, generally stain green, but variations frequently occur in the color reaction of ingested particles. Background material usually stains green, thus contrasting with the protozoa.

Non-staining cysts and those staining predominantly red are most frequently associated with incomplete fixation. Unsatisfactorily stained organisms obtained from specimens submitted in PVA-fixative usually indicate incomplete fixation associated with poor mixing of feces with fixative or delay in placing feces in fixative. Thorough mixing will yield critically stained cysts and trophozoites. Organisms, especially trophozoites, in soft or liquid specimens often stain better than those from formed specimens. Degenerate forms stain pale green, although understained or overstained organisms may also appear green.

Eggs and larvae stain red and contrast strongly with the green background. Thin-shelled eggs often collapse when placed in mounting medium, although some diagnostic features may be retained, especially if the smear is examined immediately.

Mononuclear and polymorphonuclear leukocytes must be differentiated from protozoa. The nuclei of pus cells and tissue cells stain red and the cytoplasm green. However, the cytoplasm of these cells does stain more greenish than that of the protozoa.

Occasionally, as with proficiency testing specimens, stains will be unsatisfactory when additional smears are not available. In such instances, destaining and restaining may produce a satisfactory stain. Slides are destained by removing the coverslip, then going from xylene to 90 per cent and then 70 per cent alcohols. Destain overnight or for several hours in strong acidified 70 per cent alcohol (1 ml glacial acetic acid in 40 ml 70 per cent alcohol). Wash well in 70 per cent alcohol to remove all acid. Restain, using the regular procedure, beginning with the 70 per cent alcohol. It may be helpful to shorten or eliminate the destain step.

Preparation of Solutions

Solution No. 1—Schaudinn's fixative

Ethyl alcohol, 95% .... 1 part
Saturated aqueous mercuric chloride .... 2 parts

Prepare saturated aqueous mercuric chloride by adding 90 g of mercuric chloride crystals to 1 L of distilled water. Dissolve by heating and then let cool (excess mercuric chloride will crystallize out). Filter the clear solution and store in a glass-stoppered bottle. Before use, add 5 ml of glacial acetic acid per 100 ml of solution.

Solution No. 2—PVA fixative

1. Stirring constantly, slowly add 5 g polyvinyl alcohol (PVA) powder to 100 ml modified Schaudinn's fixative at room temperature. (Modified Schaudinn's fixative contains 1.5 ml glycerol per 100 ml in addition to the other ingredients described above.)

2. Heat (to approximately 75° C.) while stirring until powder dissolves and solution clears (do not boil).

3. Cool to room temperature. Material should not be cloudy and should not gel. It is stable for months if visual examination is satisfactory. Prepared PVA fixative may be obtained from commercial sources.

Solution No. 3—Iodine alcohol

Prepare a stock solution by adding enough iodine crystals to 70 per cent alcohol to make a dark, concentrated solution. Either ethyl or isopropyl alcohol may be used. For use, dilute some of the stock with 70 per cent alcohol until a strong tea-colored solution is obtained. The exact concentration is not important, but the solution should not be too dark, since the iodine may stain the protozoa and interfere with subsequent hematoxylin or trichrome staining. If it is too light, the mercuric chloride in the fixative will not be removed and mercuric chloride crystals in the finished preparation will interfere with examination.

Solution No. 4—Trichrome stain

Chromotrope 2R	0.6 g
Light green SF	0.15 g
Fast green FCF	0.15 g
Phosphotungstic acid	0.7 g
Acetic acid (glacial)	1.0 ml
Distilled water	100.0 ml

Put the dry stains into a clean, dry flask. Add the glacial acetic acid, stir to mix, and dampen all of the stain powder. Allow the mixture to stand ("ripen") for 30 minutes. Add the distilled water. Shake to mix thoroughly. The stain is stable and is used without diluting. Good stain is deep purple, almost black.

Solution No. 5—Acidified alcohol

Acetic acid	0.45 ml
90% ethyl alcohol	99.55 ml

CELLULOSE TAPE TECHNIQUE FOR PINWORMS

Eggs of *Enterobius* are deposited in the perianal area and are detected by using this technique. Follow the directions in Figure 49–2 as described below:

1. Apply a strip of transparent cellulose tape 2½ to 3 inches in length to a glass slide so that the tape is wrapped around one end of the slide. (Frosted or opaque tape is not satisfactory.) A small portion of the end should be folded on itself to provide a non-sticky surface for handling the tape.
2. To obtain a sample, pull the folded tab so that the sticky side of the tape is freed, still leaving some of it stuck to the back of the slide.
3. Carry the freed tape over the end of a tongue blade so that the sticky side is out.
4. Hold the tape and slide against the tongue depressor.
5. Press the sticky surface onto the right and left perianal folds but do not insert the blade into the rectum.
6. Replace the tape onto the slide (these slides can be carried or sent by mail to the laboratory).
7. In the laboratory, pull tape back from the slide, leaving a small portion attached.
8. Add a drop of toluene and replace the tape on the slide. (The toluene clears everything except the eggs and adults, if present.)
9. Smooth out the tape with a piece of gauze, which should be disinfected and discarded. Examine for the eggs and female adults under the low power objective. In old or mailed-in specimens sometimes only empty egg shells are seen. (Other helminth eggs, especially *Taenia,* may occasionally be seen on the cellulose tapes.)
10. Remember that pinworm eggs are infectious, and specimens must be handled carefully to prevent infection.

CULTURE METHODS

Culture methods have been developed for a wide variety of protozoan parasites of man and for development of larvae of *Strongyloides stercoralis* and hookworm. Some, such as those for amebae (Melvin, 1982) may be of diagnostic aid, although they are not widely used. Procedures have been developed for culturing malaria, leishmania, and pneumocystis. Infection of experimental animals is not widely used for diagnosis.

IMMUNODIAGNOSTIC METHODS

Immunodiagnostic procedures for detecting antigen or antibody in parasitic diseases are numerous and are changing rapidly. It is beyond the scope of this chapter to discuss these in detail (see Kagan, 1980a and b).

Antigenic structure of parasites is complex and cross-reactions in serologic tests are common. Newer tests using different or more purified antigens are giving better results. Various types of tests have been described. Agglutination tests use whole organisms or antigen-coated particles such as in bentonite flocculation, indirect hemagglutination (IHA), and latex agglutination. Complement fixation tests have been widely used but are being superseded by newer tests. Precipitin tests include capillary precipitin, double gel diffusion, counterimmunoelectrophoresis (CIE), and circumlarval precipitin. Indirect immunofluorescence (IIF) has been widely applied to parasitic serology and is readily adapted to detect IgM antibody. Recent test development has emphasized enzyme-linked immunoassay (ELISA) and soluble antigen fluorescent antibody (SAFA), such as the FIAX system, although some improved tests are based on modifications of older methods such as IFA, CIE, or IIF. Thus, improvements in serologic methods and antigens are causing rapid changes in parasitic serology.

Most tests are infrequently needed in the United States and are generally sent to the Centers for Disease Control via the state health department laboratory. The laboratory may wish to perform some of the more commonly requested tests, such as those for toxoplasmosis, amebiasis, trichinosis, and perhaps echinococcosis. Reagents for these and a number of other parasites are available from commercial sources.

Interpretation of serologic tests must be based on interpretive criteria for the specific test used. In this chapter, tests and interpretive criteria will be those of the Centers for Disease Control (Table 49–2). The "diagnostic" titers given are highly suggestive of

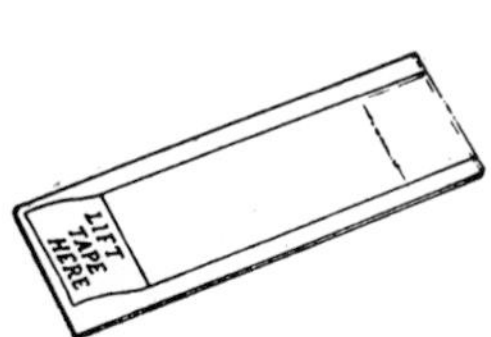

a. Cellulose-tape slide preparation

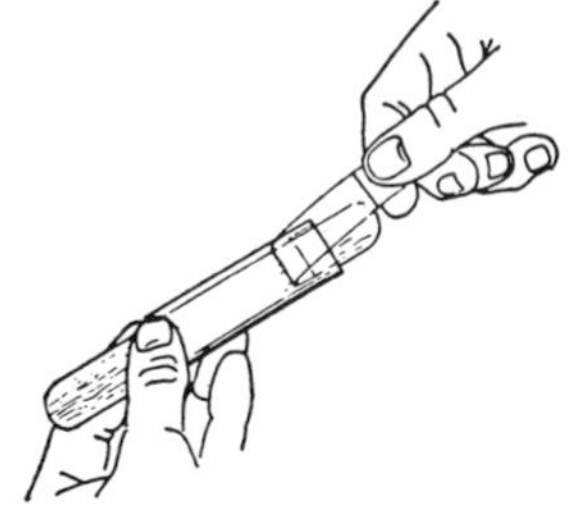

b. Hold slide against tongue depressor one inch from end and lift long portion of tape from slide

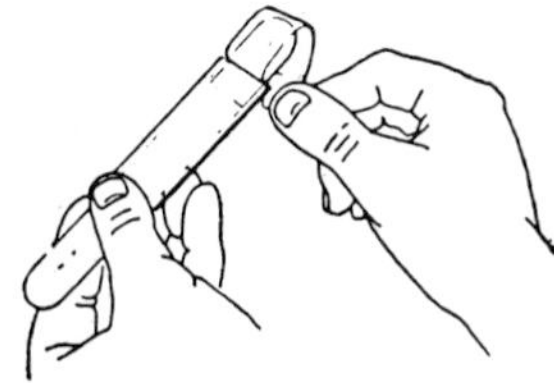

c. Loop tape over end of depressor to expose gummed surface

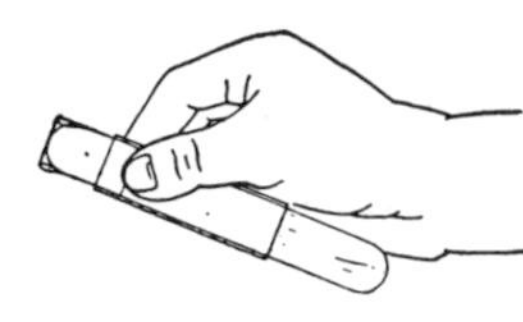

d. Hold tape and slide against tongue depressor

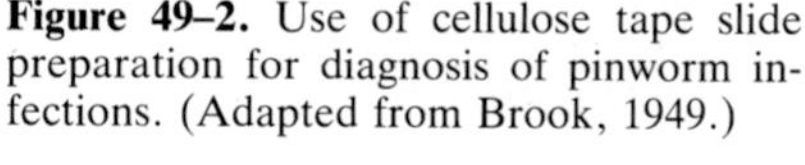

Figure 49–2. Use of cellulose tape slide preparation for diagnosis of pinworm infections. (Adapted from Brook, 1949.)

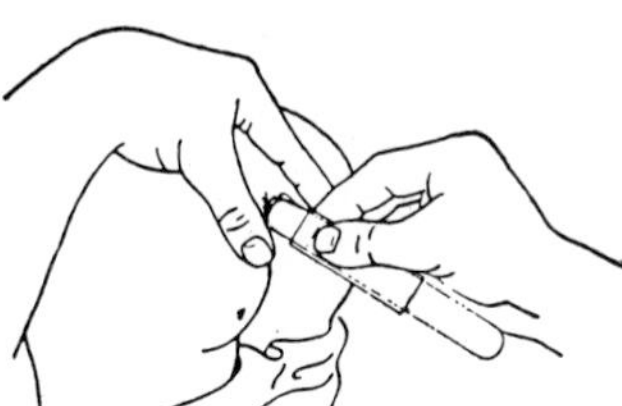

e. Press gummed surfaces against several areas of perianal region

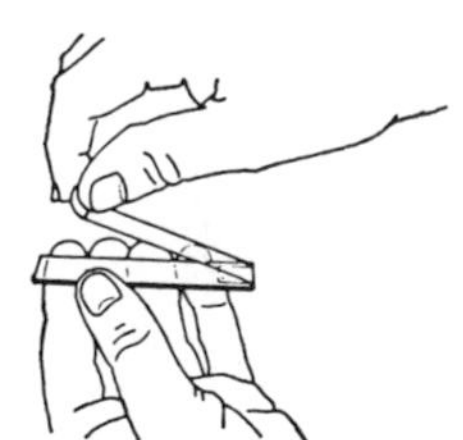

f. Replace tape on slide

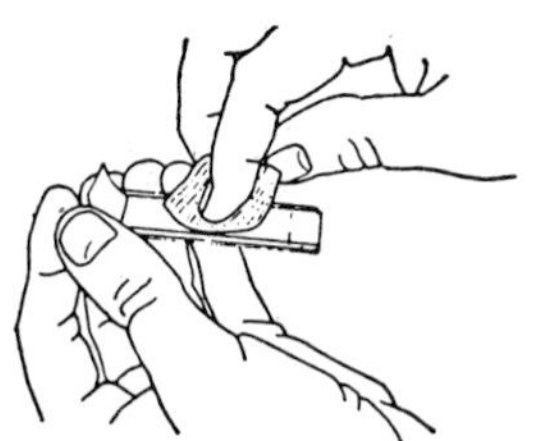

g. Smooth tape with cotton or gauze

Note: Specimens are best obtained a few hours after the person has retired, perhaps at 10 or 11 P.M., or the first thing in the morning before a bowel movement or bath.

6

Table 49–2. SEROLOGIC TESTS FOR PARASITIC DISEASES PERFORMED AT THE CENTERS FOR DISEASE CONTROL

Diseases	Tests*	Respective Diagnostic Titer(s)
Amebiasis	IHA	≥ 1:256
Ascariasis	ELISA	≥ 1:128
Babesiosis	IIF	≥ 1:16
Chagas' disease	CF	≥ 1:8
Cysticercosis	IHA	≥ 1:128
Echinococcosis	IHA	≥ 1:256
Filariasis	IHA	≥ 1:128
Leishmaniasis	DAT	≥ 1:64
Malaria	IIF	≥ 1:64
Paragonimiasis	CF	≥ 1:8
Pneumocystosis	IIF	≥ 1:16
Schistosomiasis	IIF	Positive
Strongyloidiasis	IHA	≥ 1:64
Toxocariasis	ELISA	≥ 1:32
Toxoplasmosis	IIF, IIF–IgM	≥ 1:256, 1:64†
Trichinellosis	BFT	≥ 1:5

*IHA—Indirect hemagglutination. CF—Complement fixation. DAT—Direct agglutination. IIF—Indirect immunofluorescence. BFT—Bentonite flocculation. ELISA—Enzyme-linked immunoassay.

†Any IFF–IgM titer to toxoplasmosis in an infant less than two years old is strongly suggestive of infection.

clinical infection, but a four-fold rise in titer is stronger evidence.

Cross-reactions are common and sensitivity and/or specificity of some tests may be poor. In addition, serology may not distinguish between previous and active infection; thus, for some infections serology may be helpful in screening persons who have visited an endemic area, whereas they are of little value in diagnosing infection in residents of the endemic area. The presence of antibody does not necessarily indicate immunity.

Serologic tests are most helpful when diagnostic forms cannot be readily demonstrated, as in tissue infections such as amebic liver abscess, trichinosis, visceral larva migrans, and toxoplasmosis.

Immunodiagnostic tests to detect parasite antigen have been described for a number of infections and could eventually replace morphologic diagnosis for many. Monoclonal antibodies may be particularly helpful in developing sensitive and specific antigen detection tests.

QUALITY CONTROL AND SAFETY

Quality control in parasitology is similar to quality control in other areas of the laboratory in that reagents and equipment must be monitored to assure that they perform properly. In addition, performance of personnel should be monitored periodically with internal and/or external unknown specimens. Ready availability and use of reference materials such as positive slides and fecal specimens, printed atlases (Spencer, 1982; Peters, 1977; Ash, 1980), or slide atlases (Smith, 1976a, b, and, c) containing diagnostic stages will aid in maintaining proficiency.

Unpreserved specimens submitted for parasitic examination should be considered potentially infectious, and in fact some preserved specimens may be infectious, (e.g., *Ascaris* eggs may survive and embryonate in 5 per cent formalin). Cysts of fecal protozoa, eggs of *Taenia solium, Enterobius Vermicularis,* and *Hymenolepis nana,* and larvae of *Strongyloides stercoralis* may be infective in fresh specimens. *Trichuris trichiura, Ascaris lumbricoides,* and hookworm may be infective in older specimens. Malaria and hemoflagellates in blood or tissues may be infective. Parasites are not the only potentially infective forms in specimens; feces submitted for parasitic examination may contain pathogens such as *Salmonella, Shigella,* or viruses. Strict observance of proper technique and proper disposal of contaminated material is essential. Personnel should not eat, drink, or smoke in the laboratory and should wash hands before doing any of these. Ether must not be used near a flame and should be purchased in small containers. Open containers should be stored on an open shelf in a well-ventilated room, but unopened containers should be stored in approved storage cabinets for flammable solvent. Ether, which has a very low flash point (−49°F.), should not be stored in a refrigerator, not even an "explosion proof" refrigerator. Fumes may accumulate in the refrigerator and be released when the door is opened. If an ignition source is present in the room, an explosion may result. Use of ethyl acetate rather than diethyl ether in concentration procedures is recommended.

PROTOZOA

Malaria

Malaria may be acute or chronic protozoal infection which is characterized by fever, anemia, and splenomegaly. It generally occurs between 45° North and 40° South latitude (Coatney, 1971). The sporozoan parasites of the genus *Plasmodium* are spread by female anopheline mosquitoes. Four species of plasmodia cause human malaria: *P. vivax, P. falciparum, P. malariae,* and *P. ovale. P. falciparum* infection occurs principally in tropical areas, whereas *P. vivax* infections occur in a wider area, including temperate zones. *P. ovale* is the lest frequent of the malarias, with most cases being acquired on the west coast of Africa.

Because of increasing world travel, malaria must be considered as a cause of fever even in malaria-free countries, and history of travel in endemic geographic areas should be sought. *P. falciparum* is becoming increasingly resistant to routine prophylaxis and therapy. Diagnosis is usually established by demonstrating parasites in blood films.

LIFE CYCLE

Malaria parasites have a sexual phase termed sporogony in *Anopheles* mosquitoes and an asexual stage termed schizogony in man (Fig. 49–3). The female anopheline mosquito, when feeding on an infected individual, obtains microgametocyte (male) and ma-

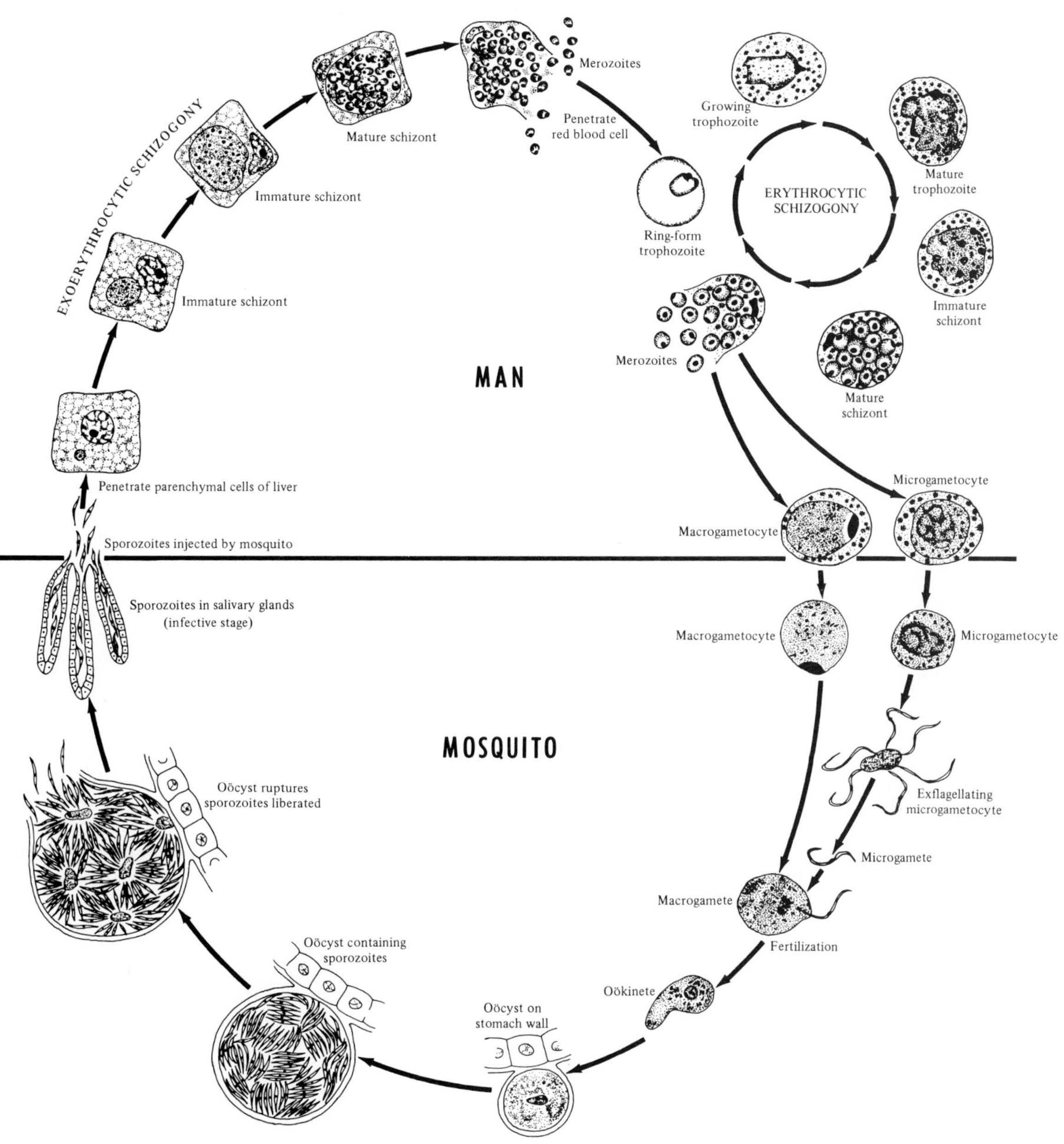

Figure 49–3. Life cycle of malaria. (Courtesy of the Centers for Disease Control, Parasitology Training Branch, Atlanta, Ga.)

6

crogametocyte (female) sex cells of the malaria parasites. In the mosquito, these gametocytes mature and fertilization occurs. An oocyst is then formed on the stomach of the mosquito, and within the oocyst numerous spindle-shaped sporozoites are formed. The mature oocyst ruptures into the body cavity, releasing the sporozoites, which then migrate through the tissues to the salivary glands from which they are injected into the vertebrate host as the mosquito feeds. The time required for development in the mosquito ranges from 8 to 21 days.

The sporozoites injected into the vertebrate host reach the hepatic parenchymal cells, in which they undergo extensive proliferation. This stage is known as the pre-erythrocytic phase of the disease. The parasites of *P. falciparum* and possibly *P. malariae* do not persist within the hepatic cells, whereas those of *P. vivax* and *P. ovale* may persist in liver cells in a recently described stage known as the hypnozoite (Krotoski, 1982). *P. vivax* and *P. ovale* may have relapses arising from activation of these hypnozoites in the liver, whereas *P. falciparum* and *P. malariae* do not. Any recurrences of the latter are termed recrudescences and are felt to arise from persisting blood forms. The liver cells are infected only by the sporozoites from the mosquito; this, transfusion-acquired *P. vivax* or *P. ovale* infection will not relapse. The infected liver cells rupture, releasing numerous merozoites which then infect erythrocytes. *P. vivax* primarily infects young erythrocytes, *P. malariae* primarily infects old erythrocytes, and *P. falciparum* infects erythrocytes of all ages (Figs. 49–4 to 49–7).

The stages seen in the erythrocytes are trophozoites (growing forms), schizonts (dividing forms), and gametocytes (sexual forms). The youngest trophozoites have a globose shape with a central vacuole, a red chromatin mass, and blue cytoplasm. In slides they appear to be rings and are generally referred to as rings or ring forms. Growing trophozoites beyond the ring stage have more abundant cytoplasm but still a single chromatin mass and may be irregular (ameboid) or compact. Mature trophozoites are usually compact but still have only one chromatin mass. Hemozoin (hematin) pigment from metabolized hemoglobin is not usually evident in ring forms but becomes evident in growing trophozoites. Immature schizonts have two or more chromatin masses and an undivided cytoplasm, and mature schizonts have both cytoplasm and chromatin completely divided so that individual merozoites are evident. The mature schizont ruptures the erythrocyte, and the merozoites infect additional red cells. This erythrocytic cycle takes 48 hours in *P. falciparum, P. ovale,* and *P. vivax* infections and 72 hours in *P. malariae* infections. Gametocytes (sex cells) develop directly from some merozoites. Those of *P. vivax, P. malariae,* and *P. ovale* are rounded, whereas those of *P. falciparum* are elongated (sausage-shaped). Macrogametocytes (female) are characterized by a compact chromatin mass, whereas microgametocytes (male) have chromatin that is more dispersed. Developing gametocytes are more compact than growing trophozoites.

EPIDEMIOLOGY

Endemic spread of malaria requires a reservoir of infection, an appropriate mosquito host, and a susceptible host. Control of malaria is directed at elimination of appropriate mosquitoes, removal of the reservoir of active cases, and prophylaxis of susceptible persons. However, emergence of mosquitoes resistant to insecticides, development of resistance to prophylaxis and therapy by *P. falciparum,* and lack of adequate funding have made control difficult in many areas. Blacks with sickle cell trait are less susceptible to *P. falciparum* malaria, and persons who lack certain Duffy blood group determinants show protection against *P. vivax* infections (Miller, 1976). Most patients who develop *P. falciparum* infection become symptomatic within one month, whereas there may be a delay of six months or more with other species of malaria. In 1980 only 21 per cent of *P. vivax* infections in the United States were manifest within one month, whereas 59 per cent of *P. falciparum* infections had onset within one month. Transfusion-induced malaria may occur when blood donors have subclinical malaria and, if not recognized, may be fatal. The number of civilian cases of malaria reported in the United States increased from 151 in 1970 to 1838 in 1980 but dropped to 1082 in 1981 (Centers for Disease Control, 1982b; Fig. 49–8). Approximately two thirds have been males, and the peak age group has been 20 to 29 years old. Of the 13 cases indigenous to the United States, two were transfusion induced, ten were congenital, and one was autochthonous. Species infecting United States civilians in 1980 were *P. vivax,* 44 per cent; *P. falciparum,* 31 per cent; *P. malariae,* 8 per cent; *P. ovale,* 2 per cent; mixed, 2 per cent; and undetermined, 13 per cent (Centers for Disease Control, 1982a).

CLINICAL DISEASE

The common presenting symptoms of malaria are chills and fever which are often associated with splenomegaly. In the early stages of the disease, the temperature spikes may occur in irregular fashion but become more periodic, with repeated spikes assuming a tertian (48 hour) pattern in *P. vivax, P. falciparum,* and *P. ovale,* and a quartan (72 hour) pattern in *P. malariae* infections. Patients with malaria may develop anemia, and may have variable manifestations, such as diarrhea, abdominal pain, headache, and muscle aches and pains. *P. falciparum* malaria can have high density parasitemias with as many as 50 per cent of the red cells being parasitized, which can lead to severe hemolysis with hemoglobinuria and severe anemia. Erythrocytes infected with growing trophozoites and schizonts of *P. falciparum* become sequestered in small vessels of the body and may lead to occlusion of these vessels, causing symptoms related to capillary obstruction. If there is obstruction of small vessels in the brain, there may be "cerebral malaria," in which the patient becomes disoriented and progresses to delirium and often death. Exchange transfusion may be lifesaving in severe *P. falciparum* infections (Nielson, 1979).

Text continued on page 1225

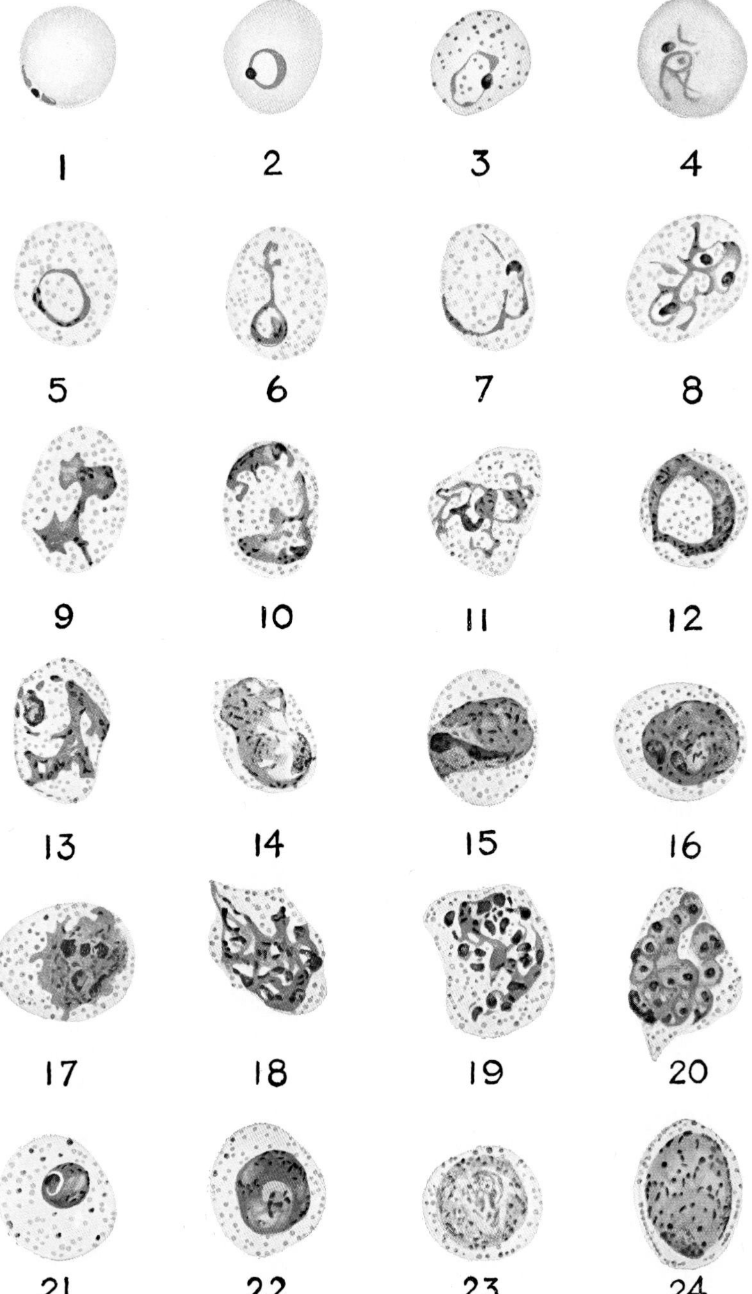

Figure 49–4. *Plasmodium vivax. 1,* Normal-size erythrocyte with marginal ring form trophozoite. *2,* Young signet ring form of trophozoite in macrocyte. *3,* Slightly older ring form trophozoite in erythrocyte showing basophilic stippling. *4,* Polychromatophilic erythrocyte containing young tertian parasite with pseudopodia. *5,* Ring form of trophozoite showing pigment in cytoplasm of an enlarged cell containing Schüffner's stippling. This stippling does not appear in all cells containing the growing and older forms of *Plasmodium vivax,* but it can be found with any stage from the fairly young ring form onward. *6* and *7,* Very tenuous medium trophozoite forms. *8,* Three ameboid trophozoites with fused cytoplasm. *9, 11, 12,* and *13,* Older ameboid trophozoites in process of development. *10,* Two ameboid trophozoites in one cell. *14,* Mature trophozoite. *15,* Mature trophozoite with chromatin apparently in process of division. *16, 17, 18,* and *19,* Schizonts showing progressive steps in division (presegmenting schizonts). *20,* Mature schizont. *21* and *22,* Developing gametocytes. *23,* Mature microgametocyte. *24,* Mature macrogametocyte. (From Wilcox, A.: Manual for the Microscopical Diagnosis of Malaria in Man. Bulletin No. 180, National Institute of Health, 1942.)

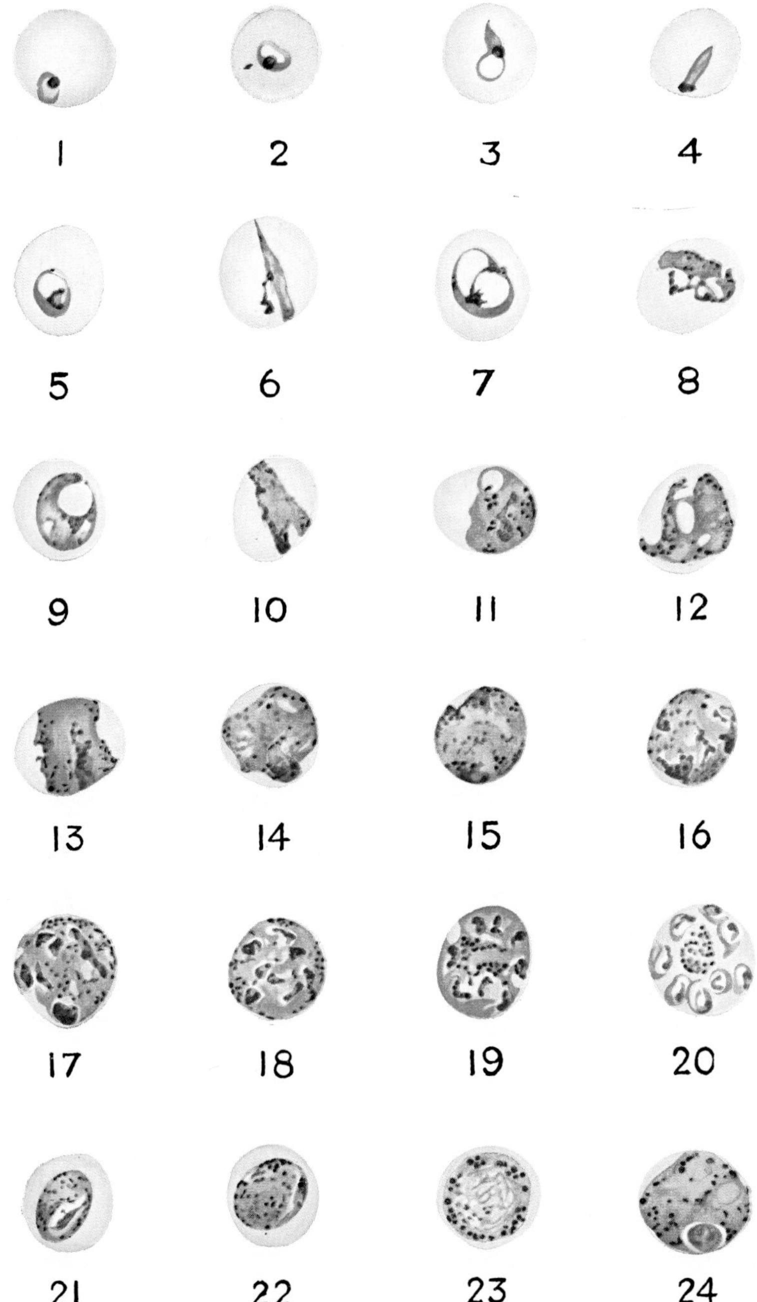

Figure 49–5. *Plasmodium malariae. 1,* Young ring form trophozoite of quartan malaria. *2, 3,* and *4,* Young trophozoite forms of the parasite showing gradual increase of chromatin and cytoplasm. *5,* Developing ring form of trophozoite showing pigment granule. *6,* Early band form of trophozoite—elongated chromatin, some pigment apparent. *7, 8, 9, 10, 11,* and *12,* Some forms which the developing trophozoite of quartan may take. *13* and *14,* Mature trophozoites—one a band form. *15, 16, 17, 18,* and *19,* Phases in the development of the schizont (presegmenting schizonts). *20,* Mature schizont. *21,* Immature microgametocyte. *22,* Immature macrogametocyte. *23,* Mature microgametocyte. *24,* Mature macrogametocyte. (From Wilcox, A.: Manual for the Microscopical Diagnosis of Malaria in Man. Bulletin No. 180, National Institute of Health, 1942.)

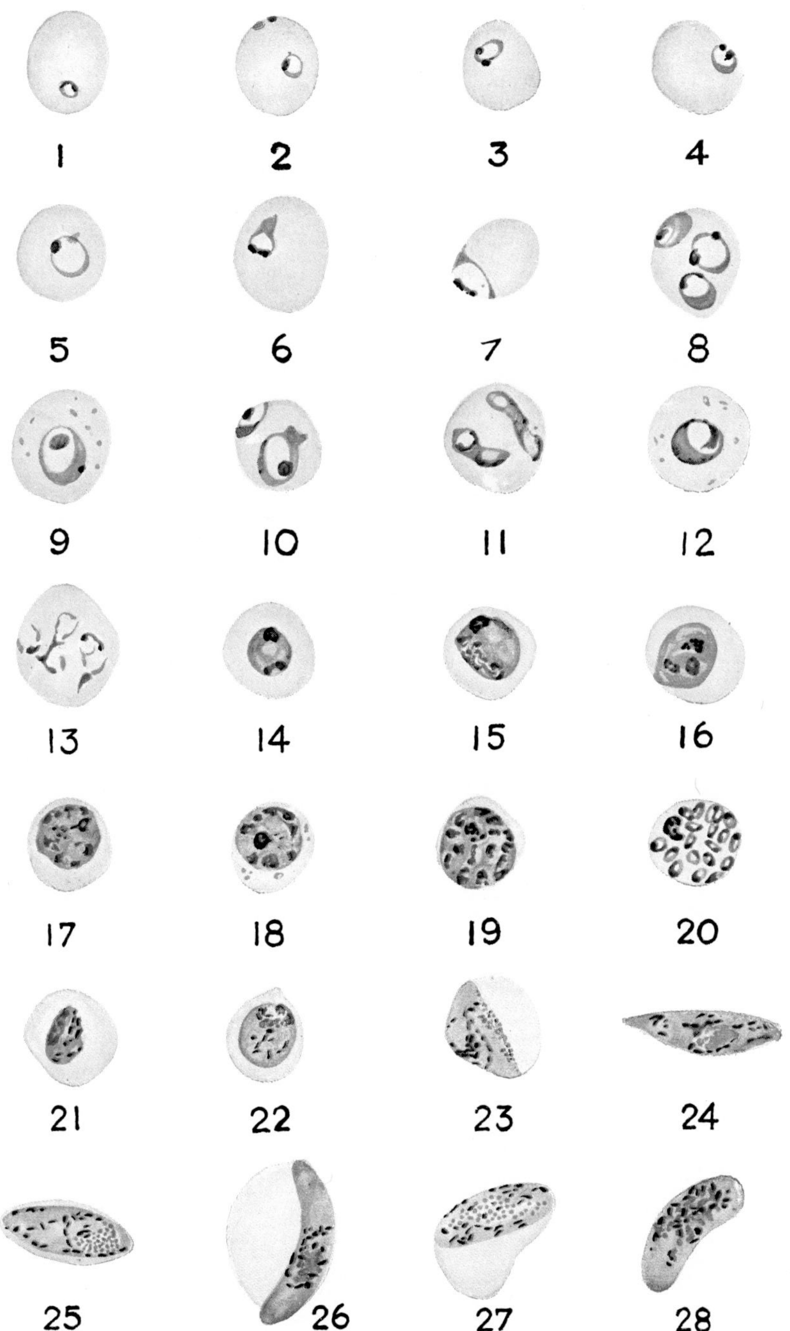

Figure 49–6. *Plasmodium falciparum. 1,* Very young ring form trophozoite. *2,* Double infection of single cell with young trophozoites, one a "marginal form," the other "signet ring" form. *3, 4,* Young trophozoites showing double chromatin dots. *5, 6, 7,* Developing trophozoite forms. *8,* Three medium trophozoites in one cell. *9,* Trophozoite showing pigment, in a cell containing Maurer's dots. *10, 11,* Two trophozoites in each of two cells, showing variation of forms which parasites may assume. *12,* Almost mature trophozoite showing haze of pigment throughout cytoplasm. Maurer's dots in the cell. *13,* Estivo-autumnal "slender forms." *14,* Mature trophozoite, showing clumped pigment. *15,* Parasite in the process of initial chromatin division. *16, 17, 18, 19,* Various phases of the development of the schizont (presegmenting schizonts). *20,* Mature schizont. *21, 22, 23, 24,* Successive forms in the development of the gametocyte—usually not found in the peripheral circulation. *25,* Immature macrogametocyte. *26,* Mature macrogametocyte. *27,* Immature microgametocyte. *28,* Mature microgametocyte. (Courtesy National Institutes of Health, U.S.P.H.S.)

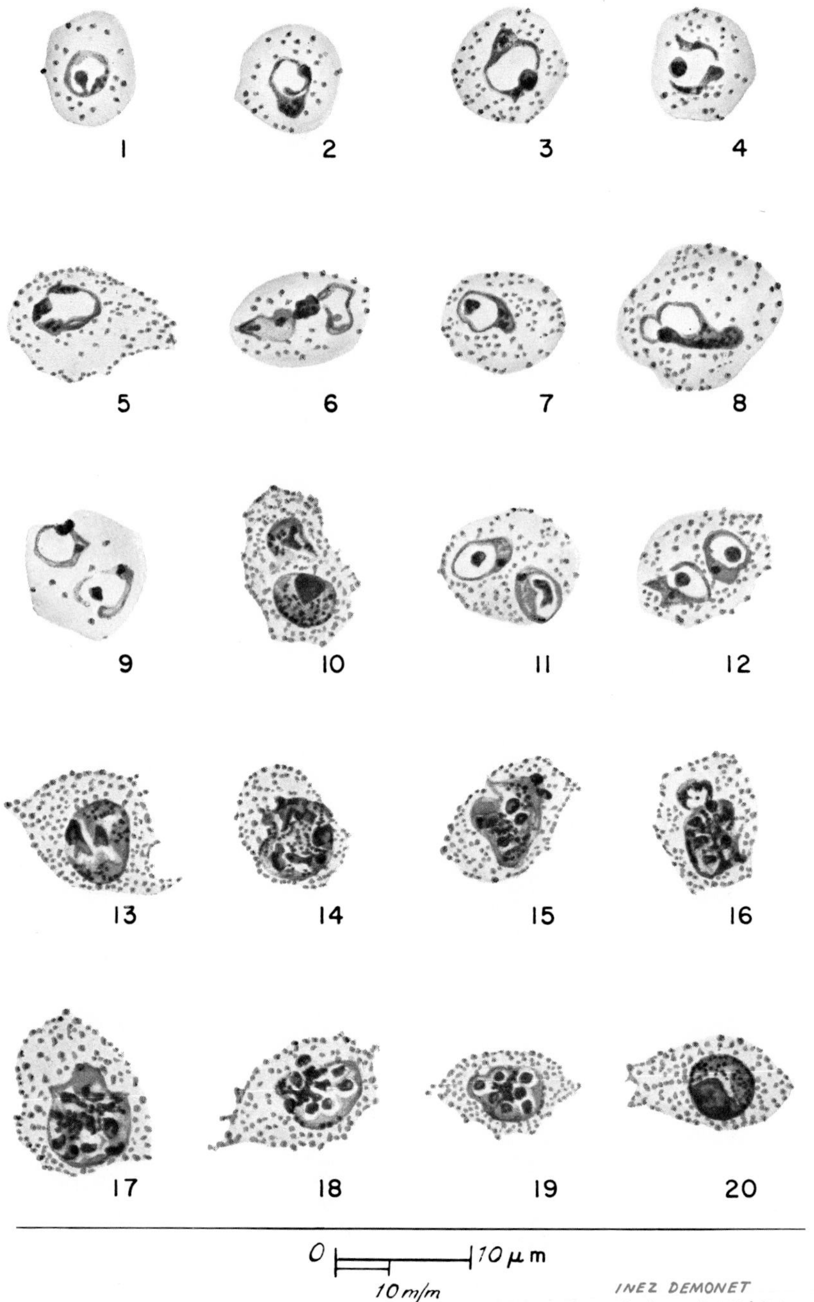

Figure 49–7. *Plasmodium ovale. 1,* Young ring-shaped trophozoite. *2, 3, 4, 5,* Older ring-shaped trophozoites. *6, 7, 8,* Older ameboid trophozoites. *9, 11, 12,* Doubly infected cells, trophozoites. *10,* Doubly infected cell, young gametocytes. *13,* First stage of the schizont. *14, 15, 16, 17, 18, 19,* Schizonts, progressive stages. *20,* Mature gametocyte.

Free translation of legend accompanying original plate in "Guide pratique d'examen microscopique du sang appliqué au diagnostic du paludisme" by Georges Villain. Reproduced with permission from "Biologie Medicale" supplement, 1935.

(Courtesy of Aimee Wilcox, National Institutes of Health Bulletin No. 180, U.S.P.H.S.)

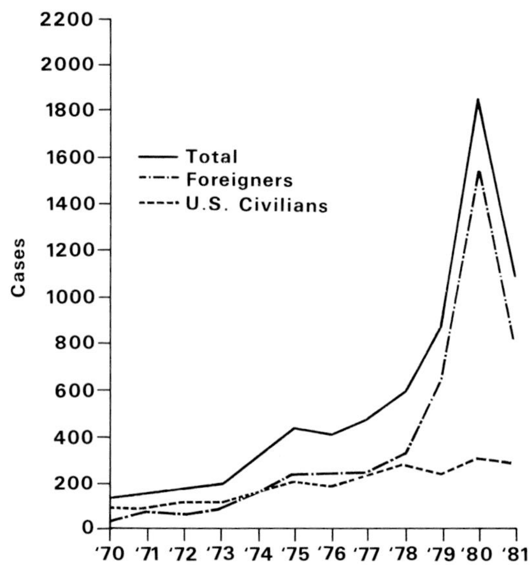

Figure 49–8. Malaria in the United States, 1970–1981. (Centers for Disease Control, 1982.)

The course of untreated malaria depends on the species. Most fatal cases of malaria are due to *P. falciparum.* With time, in non-fatal cases, the febrile paroxysms become less severe and the disease gradually subsides. Patients with *P. vivax* or *P. ovale* infection may have relapses arising from the latent exoerythrocytic stages after months or even years. Persons with *P. malariae* infection often have a low-grade parasitemia and may be asymptomatic with recrudescences occurring sporadically. Relapses and recrudescences may be associated with changes in the host's defense mechanisms or possibly with antigenic changes in the infecting organisms.

Patients with malaria may have biologically false positive serologic tests for syphilis and peripheral smears may show leukocytes that contain malaria pigment. Increased reticulocyte counts may be associated with the rapid erythrocyte turnover.

Therapy and prophylaxis of malaria have become more difficult because *P. falciparum* resistant to chloroquine has emerged in Southeast Asia, South and Central America, and Africa, and resistance to other drugs has been noted, particularly in Southeast Asia (Centers for Disease Control, 1982c). Persons with *P. vivax* or *P. ovale* infections who are no longer in endemic areas require therapy with primaquine to eradicate the hypnozoites and prevent relapses. Use of primaquine may be dangerous in patients who have glucose 6-phosphate dehydrogenase (G6PD) deficiency and in whom the drug may cause hemolysis of older erythrocytes.

DIAGNOSIS

Malaria should be included in the differential diagnosis of fever. History of travel, drug addiction, and blood transfusion should be sought. Diagnosis is generally established by demonstrating parasites in blood films. Both thin and thick blood films should be made. Blood films several hours apart may sometimes be required to demonstrate infection or to diagnose the species, as the number and morphologic stages of parasites vary during the cycle. Parasites can be seen in blood of almost all patients with clinical malaria by examining thick films.

Identification of malaria parasites in thin blood films requires a systematic approach. There are three major factors to be considered: appearance of infected erythrocytes, appearance of parasites, and stages found. Table 49–3 summarizes diagnostic characteristics of the species, and they are illustrated in Figures 49–4 to 49–7. Erythrocytes infected by *P. vivax* and *P. ovale* become enlarged. Those infected with early ring forms may be of normal size but, as growing trophozoites and schizonts develop they enlarge. Erythrocytes in *P. malariae* and *P. falciparum* infection are of normal size. Erythrocytes infected with *P. ovale* are often oval or fimbriated (have irregular projections of the cell margins). Erythrocytes infected with *P. vivax* may occasionally (less than 6 per cent) be oval, whereas in *P. ovale* infection over 20 per cent of the parasitized erythrocytes are oval or fimbriated. Schüffner's stippling, numerous small uniform pink granules in the erythrocyte, is usually present in erythrocytes infected with *P. vivax* and *P. ovale,* although it may not be evident in cells infected with ring forms or in improperly stained slides. When present, it is helpful as it is not seen in *P. malariae* or *P. falciparum* infection. As trophozoites grow in the infected cells, the amount of hemoglobin in the erythrocyte decreases and hemozoin pigment accumulates. The amount and appearance of the pigment varies among the species. Ring forms of all parasites may have a similar appearance and if only occasional ring forms are found, the species may not be identifiable. Young rings of *P. falciparum* are smaller than those of the other species (one sixth the diameter of the red blood cell, as opposed to one third the diameter of the red blood cell for the other species). Rings of *P. falciparum* that have grown will be similar in size to those of the other species. Marginal forms (spindle-shaped parasites with a central red chromatin mass that appear to be lying on the surface of the erythrocyte) are often seen in *P. falciparum* infection but are rarely seen in other types of infection. Infections of erythrocytes by multiple organisms and double chromatin dots in rings are most common in *P. falciparum* infections but can occur with the other species.

Growing trophozoites of *P. vivax* have irregular shapes and are termed ameboid. Those of *P. malariae* and *P. ovale* are compact. Growing trophozoites and schizonts of *P. falciparum* are not seen in the peripheral blood except in very severe infections. The number of merozoites in the mature schizont stage is helpful in identifying the various species.

The gametocytes of *P. falciparum* are distinctive because of their sausage shape. The gametocytes of *P. vivax, P. malariae,* and *P. ovale* are difficult to differentiate based on parasite morphology, although characteristics of infected red cells can aid identification.

The varieties of developmental stages in the peripheral blood aid in diagnosis. In *P. falciparum* there will

Table 49–3. COMPARISON OF PLASMODIUM SPECIES AFFECTING MAN*

	Appearance of Erythrocyte		Appearance of Parasite			
Species	***Size***	***Schüffner's Stippling***	***Cytoplasm***	***Pigment***	***Number of Merozoites***	**Stages Found in Circulating Blood**
Plasmodium vivax	Enlarged. Maximum size (attained with mature trophozoites and schizonts) may be 1½–2 times normal erythrocyte diameter.	+ With all stages except early ring forms.	Irregular, ameboid in trophozoites. Has "spread-out" appearance.	Golden-brown inconspicuous.	12–24 Average is 16.	All stages. Wide range of stages may be seen on given film.
Plasmodium malariae	Normal	– (Ziemann's dots rarely seen.)	Rounded, compact trophozoites with dense cytoplasm. Band-form trophozoites occasionally seen.	Dark-brown, coarse, conspicuous.	6–12 Average is 8. "Rosette" schizonts occasionally seen.	All stages. Wide variety of stages usually not seen. Relatively few rings or gametocytes generally present.
Plasmodium ovale	Enlarged. Maximum size may be 1¼–1½ times normal red blood cell diameter. Approximately 20% or more of infected red blood cells are oval and/or fimbriated (border has irregular projections).	+ With all stages except early ring forms.	Rounded, compact trophozoites. Occasionally slightly ameboid. Growing trophozoites have large chromatin mass.	Dark-brown conspicuous.	6–14 Average is 8.	All stages.
Plasmodium falciparum	Normal. Multiply-infected red blood cells are common.	– (Maurer's dots occasionally seen.)	Young rings are small, delicate, often with double chromatin dots. Gametocytes are crescent or elongate.	Black. Coarse and conspicuous in gametocytes.	6–32 Average is 20–24.	Rings and/or gametocytes. Other stages develop in blood vessels of internal organs but are not seen in peripheral blood except in severe infections.

*From Smith, J. W., Melvin, D. M., Orihel, T. C., et al.: Diagnostic Parasitology—Blood and Tissue Parasites. Chicago, American Society of Clinical Pathologists, 1976.

usually be only ring forms, and finding numerous ring forms without more mature stages is good evidence of *P. falciparum* infection. In *P. vivax, P. malariae,* and *P. ovale* infections, various stages of parasites will be found with some predominance of one stage depending on the part of the cycle.

Thick films are preferred for detecting malaria infections. Erythrocytes will be lysed so that the background will consist of white cell nuclei and platelet debris (Fig. 49–9). Ring forms will often have the appearance of punctuation marks rather than complete rings, and the presence of red chromatin and blue cytoplasm should be required to identify them as parasites. Schüffner's stippling may still be a helpful identifying characteristic, and it may be recognized around growing trophozoites as a pink halo rather than the distinct granules seen in thin films. The ameboid character of *P. vivax* trophozoites is not as evident in thick films, but the number of merozoites in mature schizonts is helpful. Macro- and microgametocytes usually cannot be differentiated. The distinctive sausage shape of *P. falciparum* gametocytes is still evident, although they may be more stubby than in thin films.

Mixed infections occur occasionally, but caution should be used in making such diagnoses unless there is definite evidence of two species. The most common mixed infections are *P. falciparum* and *P. vivax.* Finding gametocytes of *P. falciparum* in a person obviously infected with *P. vivax* is diagnostic.

There are multiple artifacts that may be confused with malaria parasites in thick and thin films. Malaria parasites should have deep red chromatin mass, blue cytoplasm, and (except for rings) some pigment. Probably the most commonly confused artifacts in thin films are blood platelets that are superimposed on red cells. These should be readily differentiated because they do not have a true ring form, do not show the differentiation of the chromatin and cytoplasm, and do not contain pigment. Clumps of bacteria or platelets may be confused with schizonts. At times, masses of fused platelets may resemble gametocytes of *P. falciparum* but once again do not show the differential staining or the pigment. Precipitated stain and contaminating bacteria, fungi, or spores may also be confused with parasites.

A variety of serologic tests have been developed for malaria but are not usually used to diagnose clinical infections. They are particularly useful for epidemiologic surveys and detection of infected blood donors. Those most commonly used are the indirect immunofluorescent (IIF) and the indirect hemagglutination (IHA) tests. IIF titers equal to or greater than 1:64 are suggestive of recent infection with malaria. These serologic tests show a false positive rate of 1 per cent or less and have a sensitivity of over 95 per cent.

Babesia

These sporozoan intraerythrocytic parasites of animals are spread by the bite of tick vectors and cause disease known as babesiosis or piroplasmosis. Man may occasionally be infected by various species, and fatal infections have occurred, especially in splenectomized individuals. Patients develop fever, malaise, and anemia. An outbreak that occurred on Nantucket Island off the coast of New England was caused by *Babesia microti,* which normally infects field and deer mice. Investigation showed that some patients har-

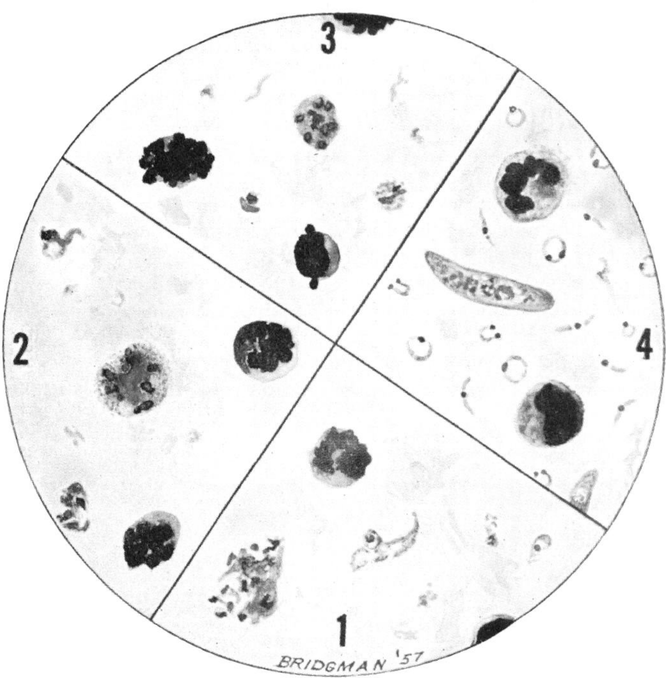

Figure 49–9. The human plasmodia as seen in thick film: *1, Plasmodium vivax:* young and older trophozoites and schizont; *2, P. ovale:* developing trophozoite and schizonts, one within a "ghost cell"; *3, P. malariae:* trophozoites and schizont; *4, P. falciparum:* young trophozoites and gametocyte. (From Markell, E. K., and Voge, M.: Medical Parasitology. Philadelphia, W. B. Saunders Company, 1976.)

6

bored the parasite for months and that some individuals showed serologic evidence of infection without a history of clinical disease. Thus, as with many other infections, the first cases recognized were severe, but with investigation, mild and subclinical cases were recognized. Babesiosis has also occurred in other areas of the United States (Rubush, 1980).

This parasite divides by schizogony. The trophozoites of many species are pear shaped, but those of *B. microti* usually look like rings and may be confused with malaria, especially *P. falciparum* (Fig. 49–10) (Healy, 1980). As a result of division of the organisms, erythrocytes may have multiple rings, often tetrads with the rings touching in the center. *Babesia* can be differentiated from malaria by the lack of blood pigment in the schizogony stage and absence of large growing trophozoites and gametocytes. History of travel to Nantucket or of a recent tick bite might suggest this infection. Malaria serology is negative. A serologic test for babesiosis is available from the Centers for Disease Control via the state health department laboratory.

Pneumocystis Carinii

Pneumocystis carinii is a parasite of uncertain taxonomy, probably a sporozoan. It was first recognized as a cause of interstitial pneumonia in malnourished and premature infants but is now most commonly seen in severely immunosuppressed patients, such as leukemic patients on chemotherapy and transplant recipients. It has become a major problem in homosexual males and others with the acquired immunodeficiency syndrome (Masur, 1981). Rapid diagnosis and early institution of therapy are important in improving survival.

The epidemiology is not completely understood. The organism can spread by the respiratory route (Walzer, 1977), and the infection is subclinical in most individuals. Clinical infection results from activation of latent infection or by acquiring the primary infection when the patient is immunosuppressed.

The organisms have two stages, trophozoites and cysts. Proliferation occurs in both stages, with up to eight organisms in mature cysts.

The infection may produce an interstitial pneumonia with alveoli filled with foamy exudate containing numerous extracellular and occasional intracellular *Pneumocystis* organisms. The amount of cellular reaction varies depending on the underlying disease and the duration and severity of infection. Malnourished infants have extensive interstitial plasma cell infiltration. Immunosuppressed patients often show little cellular infiltration. Patients present with fever and an interstitial pneumonia; Po_2 is low, often out of proportion to the degree of radiologic change. Although organisms have been described in other organs, the disease primarily affects the lung.

The principal means of diagnosis is demonstration of organisms in pulmonary material (Smith, 1982). The best specimen is an open lung biopsy, although in some cases the diagnosis can be established in transthoracic lung aspirates, transbronchial biopsies, or occasionally bronchial washings. Examination of sputum is generally unrewarding, and most experts refuse to examine sputum specimens. Open lung biopsies have the advantages that, when negative for *Pneumocystis* and other infectious agents, they more reliably exclude infectious etiologies and may allow diagnosis of neoplastic infiltration or reaction to chemotherapy. For tissue specimens, impression smears, in addition to sections, are helpful. They are often faster (two to three hours) and allow study of internal cyst morphology in Giemsa stains. In Giemsa stains, trophozoites and individual organisms within cysts have red nuclei and pale blue cytoplasm; cyst walls do not stain (Fig. 49–11). Cysts are generally 5 to 7μ in diameter and trophozoites are 1.5 to 4 μ. Methenamine silver stains the cyst wall and does not stain trophozoites. If organisms are numerous, methenamine silver stains show non-budding cysts that are often cup shaped and frequently have a darker staining central area. However, if only occasional organisms are seen, it may not be possible to differentiate cysts and yeast cells. The Gram-Weigert stain may also be used on imprints, frozen sections, or permanent sections to detect the presence of cysts (or fungi). It stains the cyst wall and takes only 20 minutes. A cresyl echt violet stain for cysts has been described (Bowling, 1973) which is relatively simple to perform. Another rapid stain for *P. carinii* in impression smears is toluidine blue O (Chalvardjian, 1963).

Immunodiagnostic tests for detecting antibody and antigen have been described but are of little assistance clinically because of lack of sensitivity and specificity. Tissue culture techniques are useful for studying the biology of *Pneumocystis* but are not useful clinically (Smith, 1984).

Toxoplasma Gondii

This sporozoan of the coccidian group has a worldwide distribution in man and in domestic and wild animals, especially those that are carnivorous. It

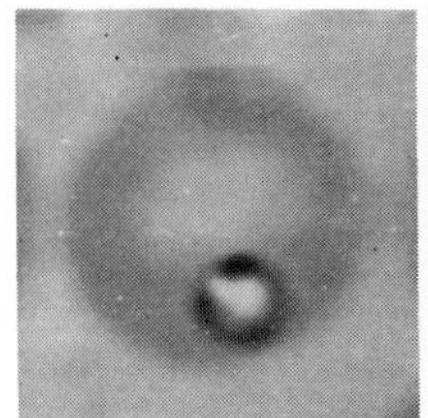
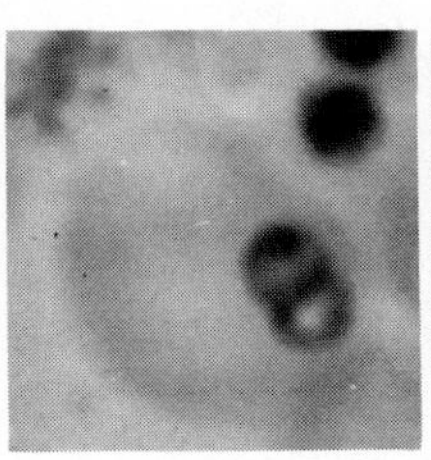
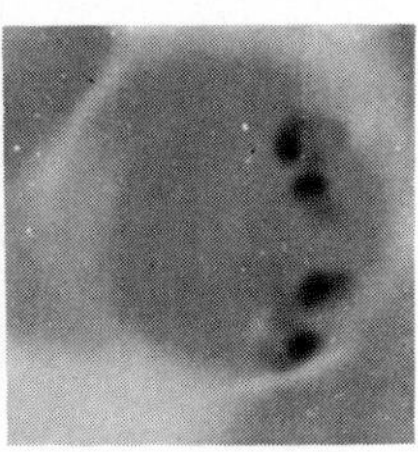

Figure 49–10. *Babesia microti.* The cell on the left contains one ring, that in the center has two rings, and the cell on the right has four small pyriform organisms.

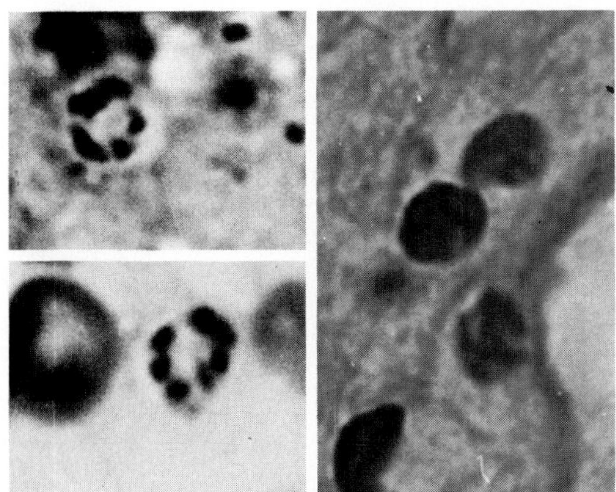

Figure 49–11. *Pneumocystis carinii.* Two Giemsa stained mature cysts are present on the left and are slightly smaller than an erythrocyte. Methenamine silver stain on the right stains only cyst walls.

generally produces an asymptomatic or mild infection but may cause serious congenital and ocular infections and acute, severe infections in immunosuppressed patients (Remington, 1976).

The life cycle has a sexual phase in the intestinal epithelium of cats and other feline definitive hosts. This phase is similar to *Isospora* intestinal infections. In the intestinal epithelium, asexual schizogony or sexual gametogony may occur. The latter leads to the development of immature oocysts that are passed in the feces and mature to the infective stage in one to five days. Ingestion of these sporocysts by a wide variety of susceptible intermediate hosts may cause infection in which the trophozoites (tachyzoites) may infect any nucleated cells. Proliferation of these trophozoites may lead to cell death or, if immunity has developed, to the formation of tissue cysts containing up to 3000 organisms. This cyst stage is seen in chronic infections. All stages of the life cycle occur in felines, but only the trophozoite and cyst stages occur in man and other intermediate hosts. Man may acquire infection by ingestion of inadequately cooked tissues of other infected intermediate hosts or ingestion of infective oocysts from material contaminated by cat feces. Recent outbreaks have occurred from inhaling contaminated dust in an indoor riding stable (Centers for Disease Control, 1977) and from drinking contaminated water (Benenson, 1982).

Most infections are asymptomatic, but there may be fever and lymphadenopathy with an illness resembling infectious mononucleosis. The most significant infections in man are congenital infections. Intrauterine death, microcephaly, or hydrocephaly with intracranial calcifications may develop if infection is acquired in the first half of pregnancy. Infections in the second half of pregnancy are usually asymptomatic at birth, although there may be fever, hepatosplenomegaly, and jaundice at the time of birth. Chorioretinitis or central nervous system manifestations may develop months or years later. Congenital toxoplasmosis is a significant cause of blindness, psychomotor retardation, and convulsive disorders.

Severe toxoplasmosis may develop in immunosuppressed hosts, either as a result of acquiring acute infection or by reactivation of latent infection. The disease usually presents with central nervous system manifestations, myocarditis, or pneumonitis.

Diagnosis of toxoplasmosis is usually established by serologic tests. Occasionally organisms may be demonstrated by inoculating appropriate material into tissue culture or uninfected mice (Fig. 49–12). Trophozoites are oval and measure approximately 3×7 μ. They are rarely demonstrated morphologically in human infections. The infection may be suspected on the basis of the histologic appearance of lymph nodes. Cysts also are rarely seen in sections of infected tissues.

Serology is the most common way to establish the diagnosis. The Sabin-Feldman dye test and indirect immunofluorescent (IIF) test are the standards to which other tests are compared, although the former is rarely used now. Recently described ELISA and FIAX tests give results similar to IIF. Reagents are commercially available. Antibodies appear in one to two weeks and titers peak at six to eight weeks. An IIF test for IgM may be helpful in diagnosing congenital and acute infection. An indirect hemagglutination (IHA) cannot replace the IIF. Because of the large number of persons who have had asymptomatic infections, low titers are of little significance. IIF titer interpretation is outlined in Table 49–4. Titers in patients with chronic ocular infections may be lower.

Hemoflagellates

The hemoflagellates of man and animals belong to the kinetoplastida because all have a kinetoplast, which is a mitochondrium containing DNA. Two genera are important in human disease, and both have

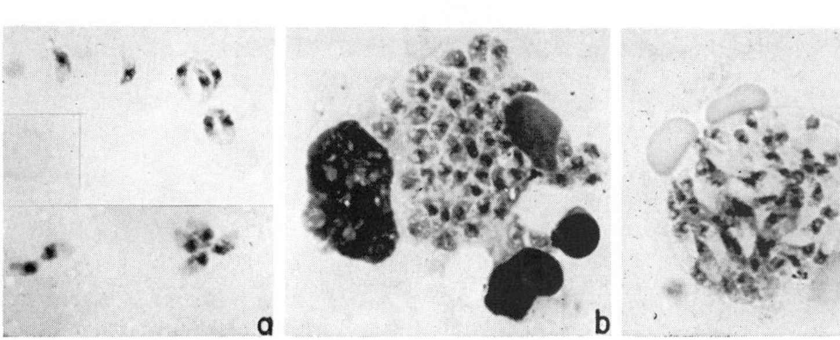

Figure 49–12. Toxoplasmata as seen *(a)* free in stained films of peritoneal exudate or tissue, *(b)* intracellularly, and *(c)* as pseudocyst in film of brain. Wright's stain (×800) reduced from a photomicrograph with a magnification of 1000 diameters. (Courtesy of Dr. A. B. Sabin and J.A.M.A.)

6

Table 49–4. INTERPRETATION OF INDIRECT IMMUNOFLUORESCENCE TITERS IN TOXOPLASMOSIS (AS PERFORMED AT CENTERS FOR DISEASE CONTROL)

IIF	IIF–IgM*	Interpretation
≤ 8	≤ 8	Negative
16–256	≤ 8	Past exposure (20% of population)
256	16–64	Questionable, obtain follow-up
≥ 1024	≤ 16	Recent infection over 3 months ago (< 1% of population)
≥ 1024	≥ 64	Recent infection 3 months ago (< 0.1% of population)

*Rheumatoid factor may interfere with IIF–IgM. Any non-rheumatoid IIF–IgM antibody in newborns is significant.

an arthropod in their life cycles. *Trypanosoma* may have human or animal reservoirs, and *Leishmania* have principally animal reservoirs.

The kinetoplastida have a variety of stages in man and their insect vectors (Fig. 49–13). These are named as described by Hoare (1966). The amastigote measures 2 to 5 μ with a nucleus, a kinetoplast, and an axoneme but no external flagellum. The promastigote is elongated and slender with a central nucleus, an anteriorly located kinetoplast axoneme, and a flagellum extending from the anterior end. The epimastigote is similar to the promastigote, but the kinetoplast is closer to the nucleus, and there is a small undulating membrane with axoneme, then flagellum. The trypomastigote has the kinetoplast at the posterior end and an undulating membrane and axoneme extending the entire length, emerging as a flagellum at the anterior end. *Leishmania* spp. have only amastigotes (vertebrate hosts) and promastigotes (insect vectors) in their life cycles. *Trypanosoma* spp. may have all four stages.

The amastigote is intracellular. In some *Trypanosoma* spp. the amastigotes may occur in any cell type of the vertebrate, whereas in *Leishmania* spp. amastigotes occur only in macrophages. Both promastigotes and epimastigotes are found in cultures and in vectors but are not significant stages in man. Promastigotes from the insect vectors are the infective stages of *Leishmania* spp. for the vertebrate host. For *Trypanosoma* spp., trypomastigotes occur in the vertebrate's blood and are the infective stages from the insect vector.

TRYPANOSOMES

There are two main infections with trypanosomes, geographically classified as African trypanosomiasis and American trypanosomiasis. Both are of great

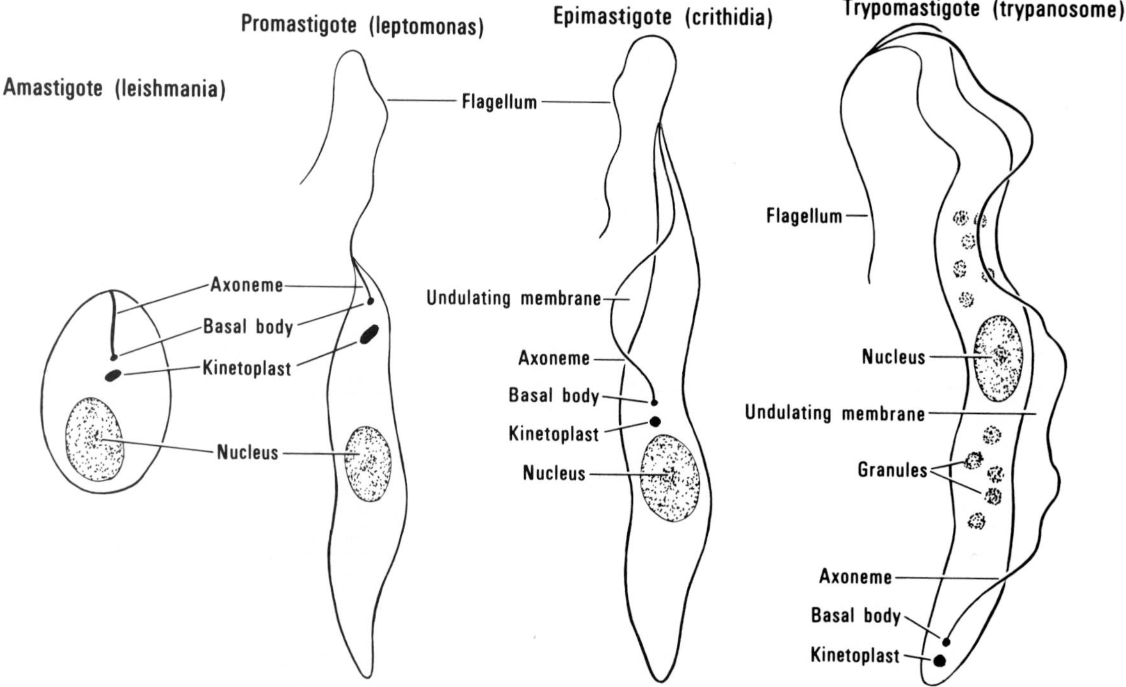

Figure 49–13. Morphology of hemoflagellates.

importance in endemic areas but are rarely seen in the United States. Infection of man with a third species, *T. rangeli,* has been described, but it does not cause clinical illness. Trypomastigotes of *T. brucei* (Fig. 49–14) are up to 30 μ long with graceful curves and a small kinetoplast, whereas those of *T. cruzi* are shorter (20 μ) with "S" and "C" shapes and a larger kinetoplast.

African trypanosomiasis is caused by the *Trypanosoma brucei* group which may infect both animals and man and is transmitted by tsetse flies of the genus *Glossina.* These flies are limited to equatorial Africa, and therefore the disease is found only in these areas. The infection in eastern Africa is caused by *T. brucei rhodesiense* and is characterized by an acute febrile illness with lymphadenopathy which is rapidly progressive. Patients die before central nervous system involvement is prominent. There are a number of animal reservoir hosts.

The infection in western Africa is caused by *T. brucei gambiense* and is called African sleeping sickness. The disease has a more chronic course with prominent central nervous system involvement. Somnolence, confusion, and fatigue progress, leading to stupor, coma, and eventual death. Man is the reservoir for this disease.

The diagnosis is suspected on the basis of geographic history and clinical findings. Patients show high IgM levels in blood and cerebrospinal fluid. There is pleocytosis with 50 to 500 mononuclear cells per cubic millimeter in cerebrospinal fluid. The diagnosis is established by demonstrating the parasites in films of peripheral blood (Fig. 49–14). A concentration method utilizing a resin column is more sensitive (Lanham, 1968).

American trypanosomiasis or Chagas' disease is caused by *T. cruzi.* In its sylvatic form the parasite occurs in the United States, Central America, and most of South America. Human infections are common in parts of Mexico and Central and South America. It is transmitted by a reduviid bug (kissing bug) with several genera and species in different countries and ecological niches. Some reduviids are responsible for maintaining the sylvatic cycle in animal reservoirs, whereas others are adapted to a domiciliary life in the poorly constructed houses of Latinoamerican peasants. At the time of feeding, the reduviid bug defecates. The bug feces contain the infective forms which, as a result of scratching or rubbing, enter the body at the bite site or through intact mucosa of the mouth or conjunctiva. The infective forms actively enter the cells, where they transform into amastigotes, the reproductive stage. When the infected cell is filled with amastigotes, transformation to trypomastigotes occurs; trypomastigotes are released into the peripheral blood and thus reach different tissues where they can start the reproductive cycle *de novo.*

Chagas' disease may cause acute or chronic infections. Acute disease is most common in infants and is characterized by malaise, chills, fever, hepatosplenomegaly, and myocarditis. In older individuals, the acute course is milder or often asymptomatic. After the acute stage, the patient remains infected for life. Chronic manifestations of the infection are related to the destruction of the effector cells of the parasympathetic system. Alterations in the conduction system of the heart, megaesophagus, and megacolon are usual clinical manifestations.

Diagnosis in the acute stage is established by demonstrating the parasite in blood films or cultures. In the chronic stage, serodiagnosis is used. Complement fixation and indirect hemagglutination are most widely used, but a number of newer tests are being studied. The infection can be transmitted by blood transfusion, and quiescent infections may be exacerbated by immunosuppression.

LEISHMANIA

There are three classic forms of leishmaniasis—cutaneous, visceral, and mucocutaneous—produced by different species or species complexes of *Leishmania.* Taxonomy is complex and controversial. These diseases are zoonoses transmitted by sandflies belonging to the genus *Phlebotomus* in the Old World and *Lutzomyia* in the American continent. All are infections of the reticuloendothelial system.

Cutaneous leishmaniasis, or Oriental sore, occurs in southern Europe, northern Africa, the Middle East, Iran, Afghanistan and southern Russia, and is caused by *L. tropica.* The infection consists of a benign ulcer, usually on an exposed area of the body, which usually heals spontaneously and confers longlasting immunity.

Visceral leishmaniasis, or kala-azar, is caused by *L. donovani* in the Old World (south Europe, north Africa, Afghanistan, Pakistan, India, and China) and *L. chagasi* in Brazil, Venezuela, and, sporadically, in

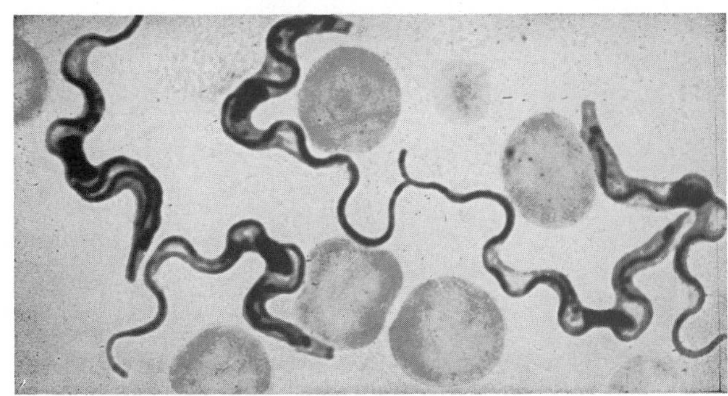

Figure 49–14. *Trypanosoma brucei* in stained blood film; ×about 2000. (Krall.)

6

other countries of the American continent. In some persons, the infection is benign and not manifest clinically. In overt cases, there is marked involvement of the reticuloendothelial system of liver, spleen, lymph nodes, and bone marrow. Without treatment, the disease is progressive, resulting in death in 75 per cent of the cases. Diagnosis is established by demonstrating the organisms in liver, spleen, or bone marrow biopsies. Serological tests (complement fixation and IIF) may assist in diagnosis.

Mucocutaneous leishmaniasis has several clinical forms produced by several different species and subspecies as defined by epidemiological, clinical, and biochemical studies (Lainson, 1978). *L. braziliensis* has three subspecies: *L. b. braziliensis* is responsible for cutaneous and mucocutaneous lesions in Brazil; *L. b. guyanensis* in northern South America and *L. b. panamensis* in Colombia, Panama, and Central America produce cutaneous lesions. *L. mexicana* has also three subspecies: *L. m. mexicana* is responsible for cutaneous lesions, especially in the ear (chiclero ulcer), in Central America; *L. m. amazonensis* produces cutaneous lesions in the Amazon region; and *L. m. pifanoi* causes simple cutaneous lesions in Venezuela. All three members of the *mexicana* group may cause disseminated cutaneous leishmaniasis in anergic patients. The last species, *L. peruviana,* produces a cutaneous lesion, "uta," in people living on the slopes of the western Peruvian Andes and Argentine highlands. These infections are generally self-limited and follow a rather benign course. Extension to the cartilage of the naso-oropharynx by *L. braziliensis* produces a more devastating disease with disfigurement. Rarely, it may be fatal if the pharyngeal area is involved.

The diagnosis is established by finding the parasites in histological sections or imprints of biopsies from the ulcer border (Fig. 49–15). Species cannot be distinguished morphologically. The presence of the kinetoplast allows differentiation from *Histoplasma capsulatum* and *Toxoplasma*. Absence of methenamine silver staining will also aid in distinguishing from *Histoplasma*. Serology (direct agglutination test) may aid in diagnosis or epidemiologic surveys.

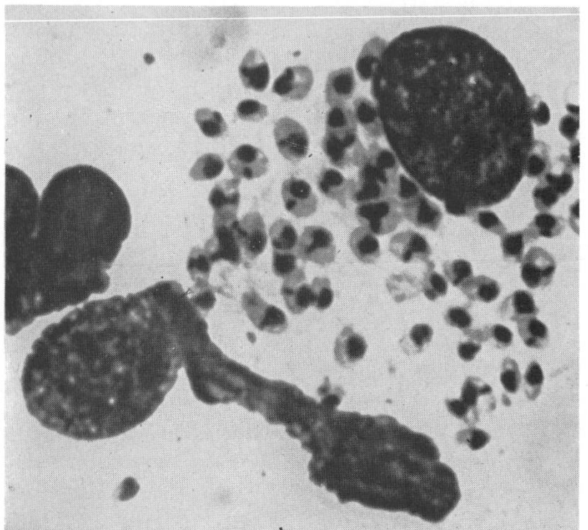

Figure 49–15. *Leishmania donovani* in stained smear from spleen puncture. (From Hunter, G. W., Swartzwelder, J. C., and Clyde, D. F.: A Manual of Tropical Medicine. Philadelphia, W. B. Saunders Company, 1976.)

Soil Amebae

Amebic encephalitis is now recognized as being two different disease entities produced by two different genera of free-living amebae. *Primary amebic meningoencephalitis* (Martinez, 1980) is produced by amebo-flagellates belonging to the genus *Naegleria,* of which *N. fowleri* is the principal agent in man. The disease runs an acute course, and there is usually a history of swimming in rivers or lakes (sometimes in heated swimming pools) 48 to 72 hours before the first symptoms appear. The patient first complains of headache, followed by signs of meningeal irritation which progress to coma and death within six to eight days. The parasite lives in the bottom of lakes or rivers and is accidentally aspirated into the nose while swimming. It invades the olfactory neuroepithelium and gains access to the brain through the cribiform plate. Histopathologically, there is macroscopic hemorrhage and inflammation in the base of the brain with marked mononuclear cellular infiltrate and numerous amebae. The parasites are 10 to 15 μ in diameter and have a nucleus with a clear space between the nuclear membrane and a large conspicuous central karyosome. There are no cysts in tissues. Diagnosis is established by finding the organism in the cerebrospinal fluid. Only trophozoites are found and have blunt pseudopodia. The cerebrospinal fluid findings are similar to those of bacterial meningitis with pleocytosis, high protein, low glucose, and hemorrhage.

Granulomatous amebic encephalitis (Martinez, 1980) is apparently produced by several species of the *Acanthamoeba* genus. It is a subacute to chronic infection generally seen in immunosuppressed patients who present with signs of meningism progressing to coma and death. The gross pathological findings are focal necrosis, hemorrhage, and inflammation grossly resembling hemorrhagic infarcts. Microscopically, there is chronic granulomatous encephalitis with necrosis and giant cells. Parasites are numerous, measuring 25 to 35 μ in diameter. The nuclei are similar to those of *Naegleria,* but double-walled cysts are also present in the tissues. The portal of entry is not well established, but the lungs, skin ulcers, and olfactory bulb have been incriminated. The diagnosis is established by finding trophozoites and cysts in the cerebrospinal fluid. Trophozoites are larger than those of *Naegleria* and have spine-like pseudopodia. *Acanthamoeba* may also cause eye and respiratory infections.

Culture or animal inoculation may be used to detect *Naegleria* or *Acanthamoeba* in infected spinal fluid (Visvesvara, 1980a).

Intestinal and Atrial Protozoa

Protozoa inhabiting the intestinal tract of man are generally amebae and flagellates, although occasional ciliate and coccidian infections are seen. In a review of fecal specimens submitted to state health department laboratories (see Table 49–1), non-pathogenic protozoa were found in 6.5 per cent of specimens with the potential pathogens *Giardia lamblia* in 4.0 per cent, *Entamoeba histolytica* in 0.8 per cent and *Dientamoeba fragilis* in 0.6 per cent. Most of the intestinal infections (except some coccidia) are acquired by fecal/oral contamination, either directly, as by food handlers, or indirectly via contaminated water.

For most laboratories, identification of intestinal protozoa is the most difficult aspect of parasitology. The parasites are small and the pathogenic organisms must be differentiated from the non-pathogenic organisms, as well as from inflammatory cells, epithelial cells, and other confusing objects. There are a number of characteristics that assist in identifying intestinal protozoa. Size is helpful (Fig. 49–16), and a properly calibrated ocular micrometer must be available. Amebae must be differentiated from flagellates. This is relatively easy in wet mounts of fresh material where the amebae move in the typical ameboid fashion, whereas flagellates move more rapidly and in a "falling leaf," darting, or tumbling fashion.

Number and size of nuclei and pattern of chromatin distribution in nuclei are helpful and are best seen in permanently stained preparations.

Helpful cytoplasmic characteristics include fibrils and special structures in flagellates, ingested materials in trophozoites, and glycogen masses and chromatoid bodies in amebic cysts. Flagellates will generally have a long axis with a nucleus or nuclei at one end and tapering at the opposite end.

Organisms may degenerate before or after feces are passed, and some organisms may be too degenerated to be identified. Multiple organisms should be examined, and both nuclear and cytoplasmic characteristics assessed. It may not be possible to identify definitively each individual parasite. In addition, before identifying two species, there should be two distinct populations of organisms, not just an occasional organism with an atypical appearance.

Direct wet mounts of fresh material are helpful for identification of trophozoites or cysts, whereas formalin-fixed material is helpful primarily for detection of cysts. Permanently stained preparations are useful for detection and accurate identification of trophozoites and cysts.

AMEBAE

There are three genera of amebae that may inhabit the intestinal tract of man: *Entamoeba, Endolimax,* and *Iodamoeba.* The life cycles of the amebae are similar (except for *Entamoeba gingivalis,* which does not have a cyst stage). Cysts are ingested and excyst in the small intestine. The resulting trophozoites proliferate in the lumen of the colon. Cysts and/or trophozoites may be passed in feces. Mature cysts are the infective stage.

The genus *Entamoeba,* characterized by having chromatin on the nuclear membrane, is the most important and includes *E. histolytica,* the etiologic agent of amebiasis, *E. hartmanni* and *E. coli,* which are commonly found, and *E. polecki,* which is occasionally found in people who have contact with pigs (Levin, 1970). *Entamoeba gingivalis* may inhabit the oral cavity of people with poor oral hygiene. *Endolimax nana* and *Iodamoeba bütschlii* are non-pathogenic. *Dientamoeba fragilis* is now recognized to be a flagellate without flagella. It is included under the flagellates in the text

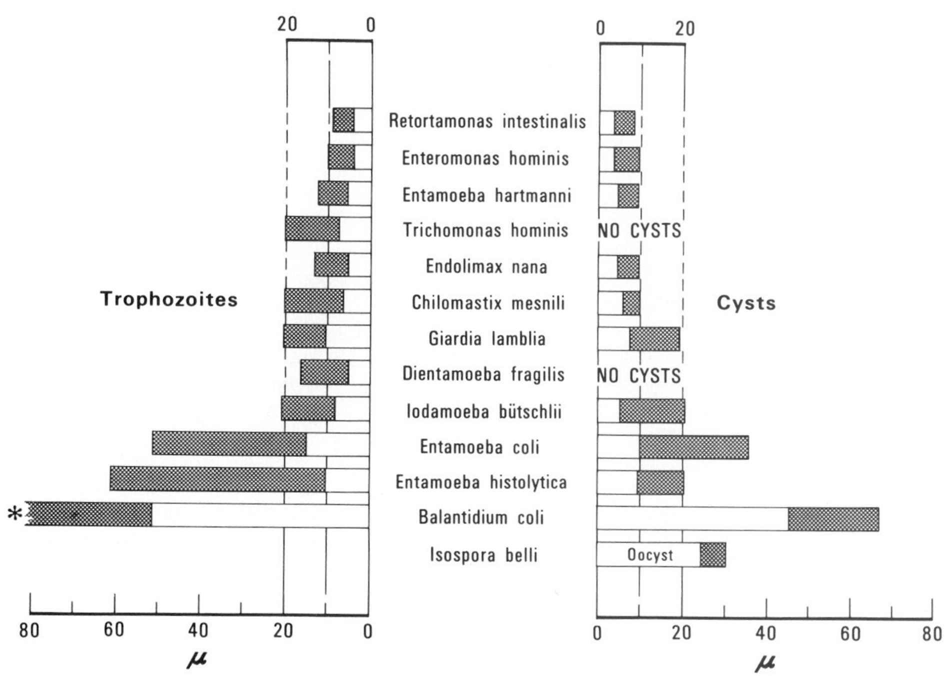

Figure 49–16. Size ranges of intestinal protozoa. *B. coli* trophozoites may measure up to 2000 μ.)

6

but remains with the amebae in tables and figures because the laboratory problem is to distinguish it from the amebae.

Entamoeba histolytica. *E. histolytica* may cause various clinical diseases, most commonly amebic dysentery, amebic colitis, and liver abscesses (Adams, 1977a and b). General host defense mechanisms, previous contact with parasite, diet, and the strain of *E. histolytica* may influence the manifestations of infection in the individual. Recent work (Sargeaunt, 1980) analyzing isoenzyme patterns (zymodemes) has shown that only certain strains are pathogenic. Most strains lead a commensal existence in the intestinal lumen.

Amebic dysentery is a severe acute disease characterized by bloody diarrhea with abdominal cramping. There is extensive invasion of the mucosa with ulceration that may lead to perforation and peritonitis, severe hemorrhage, or secondary bacterial infection. Amebic dysentery is infrequent in the United States. The more common form in this country is amebic colitis, which may have various symptoms such as diarrhea, constipation, abdominal cramping, and weight loss but without the severe dysentery with blood and mucus seen in amebic dysentery. There are small, pinpoint mucosal ulcerations that may expand in the submucosa to form flask-shaped ulcers. All of the colon may be involved or only a portion, most commonly the cecum, rectosigmoid, or ascending colon.

The most common form of extraintestinal amebiasis is amebic abscess of the liver, which occurs in approximately 5 per cent of symptomatic patients. Symptoms are fever and right upper quadrant pain. These liver abscesses are usually diagnosed by radiographic scans, ultrasound, and serologic tests. Amebae are present in the stool in less than half the patients at the time liver abscess is manifest. Another condition known as amebic hepatitis may occur in some cases and is characterized by an enlarged, tender liver in someone with intestinal amebiasis. It is debatable whether this state is a result of bacterial, toxic, or direct amebic involvement of the liver. Rarely, amebic abscesses may appear in other organs, such as the lung and brain, either by direct spread from the intestinal disease or by secondary spread from a liver abscess.

Rarely there may be granulation tissue masses, known as amebomas, formed in response to amebae. In the intestine, they may cause "napkin ring" lesions and be confused with carcinomas. Very rarely amebic ulcerations may occur in perianal or other areas of skin.

Epidemiology. Most infections with *E. histolytica* are acquired by ingestion of contaminated food or water (Elsdon-Dew, 1968), although a recent outbreak was caused by a contaminated colonic irrigation machine (Istre, 1982). In a recent review of outbreaks of amebiasis in the United States, Krogstad (1978) noted that pseudo-outbreaks have occurred as a result of laboratory misidentification of inflammatory cells, other amebae, and fecal debris as *E. histolytica*. Many infections in United States citizens have been acquired in foreign countries such as Mexico.

Diagnosis. Examination of a series of stool specimens will allow diagnosis of the intestinal infection in most cases. If the patient has been given antibiotics or gallbladder dyes, the amebic infection may be suppressed for a period of time. If there is a strong suspicion of amebiasis and stool examinations are negative, collection of a purged series is recommended. Some laboratories use culture procedures to grow the amebae. Culture is essential if zymodemes are to be determined to see if the strain is pathogenic. Serologic tests are positive in approximately 70 per cent of patients with invasive intestinal amebiasis but in only 5 per cent of patients with commensal infection.

Aspirated material from liver abscesses can be examined microscopically to detect trophozoites. The last material aspirated is most likely to contain trophozoites and may be examined by direct microscopic examination or permanently stained slides. If tissue is available, sections may show organisms. Culture procedures may be attempted, but since bacteria are not present in the liver abscesses they (e.g., *Clostridium perfringens*) will need to be added to the culture. Serologic tests are positive in over 95 per cent of patients with amebic liver abscess.

The trophozoites of *Entamoeba histolytica* vary from 10 to 60 μ, with the commensal forms usually 15 to 20 μ and the invasive forms over 20 μ in greatest dimension (Table 49–5; Figs. 49–17 to 49–19). In direct wet mounts, the trophozoites show progressive motility with hyaline pseudopodia that are rapidly formed by sharp demarcation between endoplasm and ectoplasm, but unstained nuclei are not visible. In severe disease, some trophozoites may contain ingested erythrocytes, a feature diagnostic of *E. histolytica* infection. The peripheral nuclear chromatin is typically distributed evenly as fine granules which generally appear to be a smooth layer of chromatin material. The karyosome is small and centrally located, with fine fibrils attaching it to the nuclear membrane; however, these fibrils are not generally visible. Nuclei vary, and eccentric karyosomes and irregularly distributed peripheral chromatin may be seen. The appearance of amebae may vary, and there is no single characteristic that is pathognomonic except the phagocytosis of erythrocytes, which very rarely occurs with other species. The cytoplasm is finely granular, and in invasive organisms there are either no inclusions or only erythrocyte inclusions. Non-invasive organisms may occasionally contain ingested bacteria. In degenerating organisms, the cytoplasm may become vacuolated and nuclei may show abnormal chromatin clumping. Cysts of *E. histolytica* are spherical and 10 to 20 μ in diameter, with the usual range being 12 to 15 μ (Table 49–6; Figs. 49–17, to 49–19). The precyst stage has a single nucleus and is rounded but does not have a refractile cyst wall. As it matures the cyst develops four nuclei, each of which is approximately one sixth the diameter of the cyst. The nuclei show characteristics similar to those of trophozoite nuclei, but it should be emphasized that nuclear characteristics are not as helpful in differentiation of *Entamoeba* cysts as they are in differentiation of tro-

Text continued on page 1238

Table 49–5. MORPHOLOGY OF TROPHOZOITES OF INTESTINAL AMEBAE*

Species	Size (in Diameter or Length)	Motility	Nucleus			Cytoplasm	
			Numbers	*Peripheral Chromatin*	*Karyosomal Chromatin*	*Appearance*	*Inclusions*
Entamoeba histolytica	10–60 μ. Usual range,† 15–20 μ—commensal form. ‡Over 20 μ—invasive form.	Progressive, with hyaline, finger-like pseudopods.	1 Not visible in unstained preparations.	Fine granules. Usually evenly distributed and uniform in size.	Small, discrete. Usually central but occasionally eccentric.	Finely granular.	Erythrocytes occasionally. Non-invasive contain bacteria.
Entamoeba hartmanni	5–12 μ. Usual range, 8–10 μ.	Usually non-progressive, but may be progressive occasionally	1 Not visible in unstained preparations.	Similar to *E. histolytica.*	Small, discrete, often eccentric.	Finely granular.	Bacteria
Entamoeba coli	15–50 μ. Usual range, 20–25 μ.	Sluggish, non-progressive, with blunt pseudopods.	1 Often visible in unstained preparations.	Coarse granules, irregular in size and distribution.	Large, discrete, usually eccentric.	Coarse, often vacuolated.	Bacteria, yeasts, other materials.
Endolimax nana	6–12 μ. Usual range, 8–10 μ.	Sluggish, usually non-progressive, with blunt pseudopods.	1 Visible occasionally in unstained preparations.	None.	Large, irregularly shaped.	Granular, vacuolated.	Bacteria.
Iodamoeba bütschlii	8–20 μ. Usual range, 12–15 μ.	Sluggish, usually non-progressive.	1 Not usually visible in unstained preparations.	None.	Large, usually central. Surrounded by refractile, achromatic granules. These granules are often not distinct even in stained slides.	Coarsely granular, vacuolated.	Bacteria, yeasts, or other material.
Dientamoeba fragilis¶	5–15 μ. Usual range, 9–12 μ.	Pseudopodia are angular, serrated, or broad lobed and hyaline, almost transparent.	2 (In approximately 20% of organisms only 1 nucleus is present.) Nuclei invisible in unstained preparations.	None.	Large cluster of 4–8 granules.	Finely granular, vacuolated.	Bacteria.

*Adapted with permission from Brooke, M. M., and Melvin, D. M.: Morphology of Diagnostic Stages of Intestinal Parasite of Man, USDHEW PHS Publication No. 1966, 1969.

†Usually found in asymptomatic or chronic cases; may contain bacteria.

‡Usually found in acute cases; often contain red blood cells.

§Visibility is for unfixed material. Nuclei may sometimes be visible in fixed material.

¶A flagellate (see text).

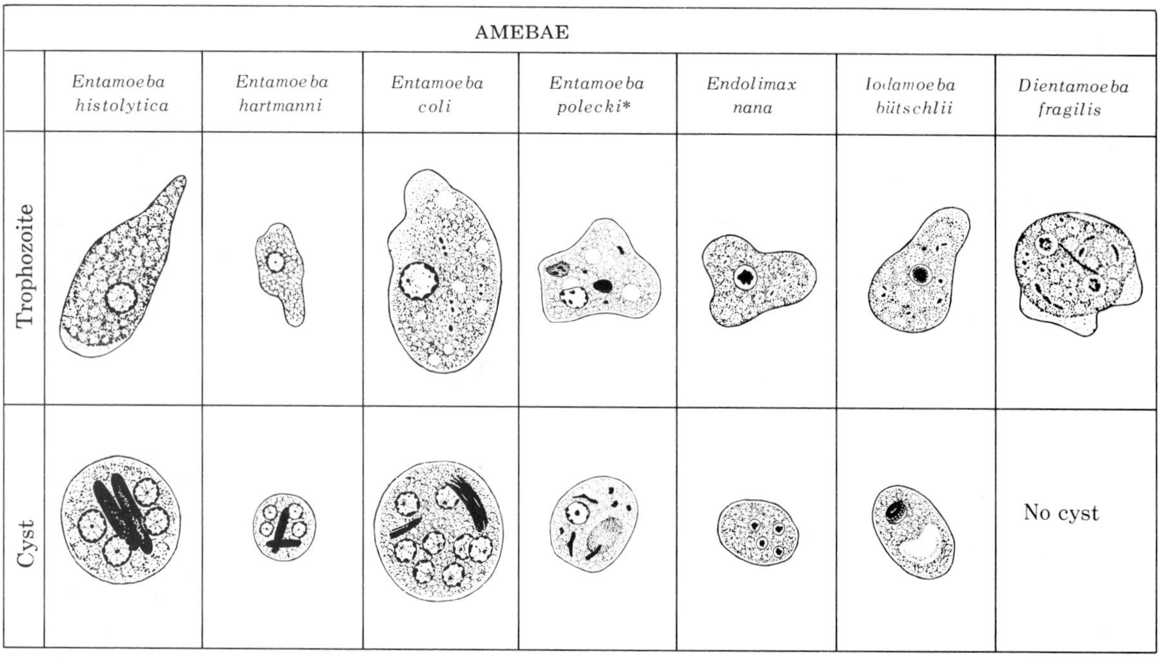

AMEBAE							
	Entamoeba histolytica	*Entamoeba hartmanni*	*Entamoeba coli*	*Entamoeba polecki**	*Endolimax nana*	*Iodamoeba bütschlii*	*Dientamoeba fragilis*
Trophozoite							
Cyst							No cyst

*Rare, probably of animal origin

Figure 49–17. Amebae found in stool specimens of man. (*Dientamoeba fragilis* is a flagellate; see text.)

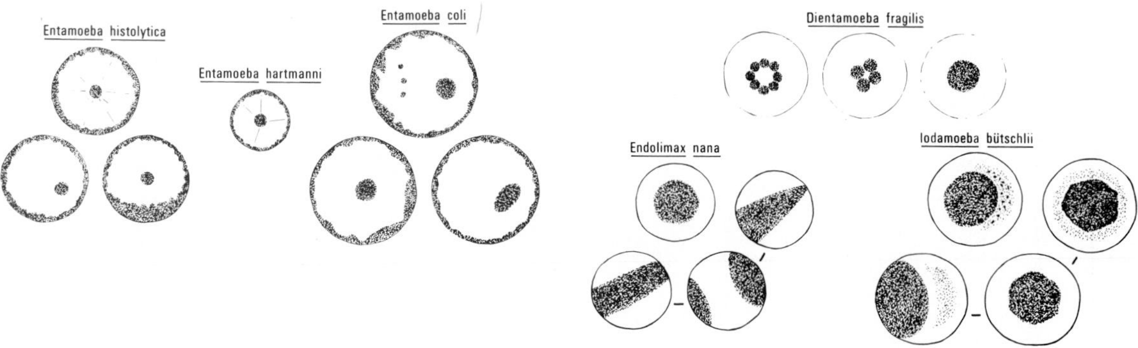

Figure 49–18. Nuclei of amebae. This drawing shows some of the various appearances of amebic nuclei in stained preparations. (*Dientamoeba fragilis* is a flagellate; see text.)

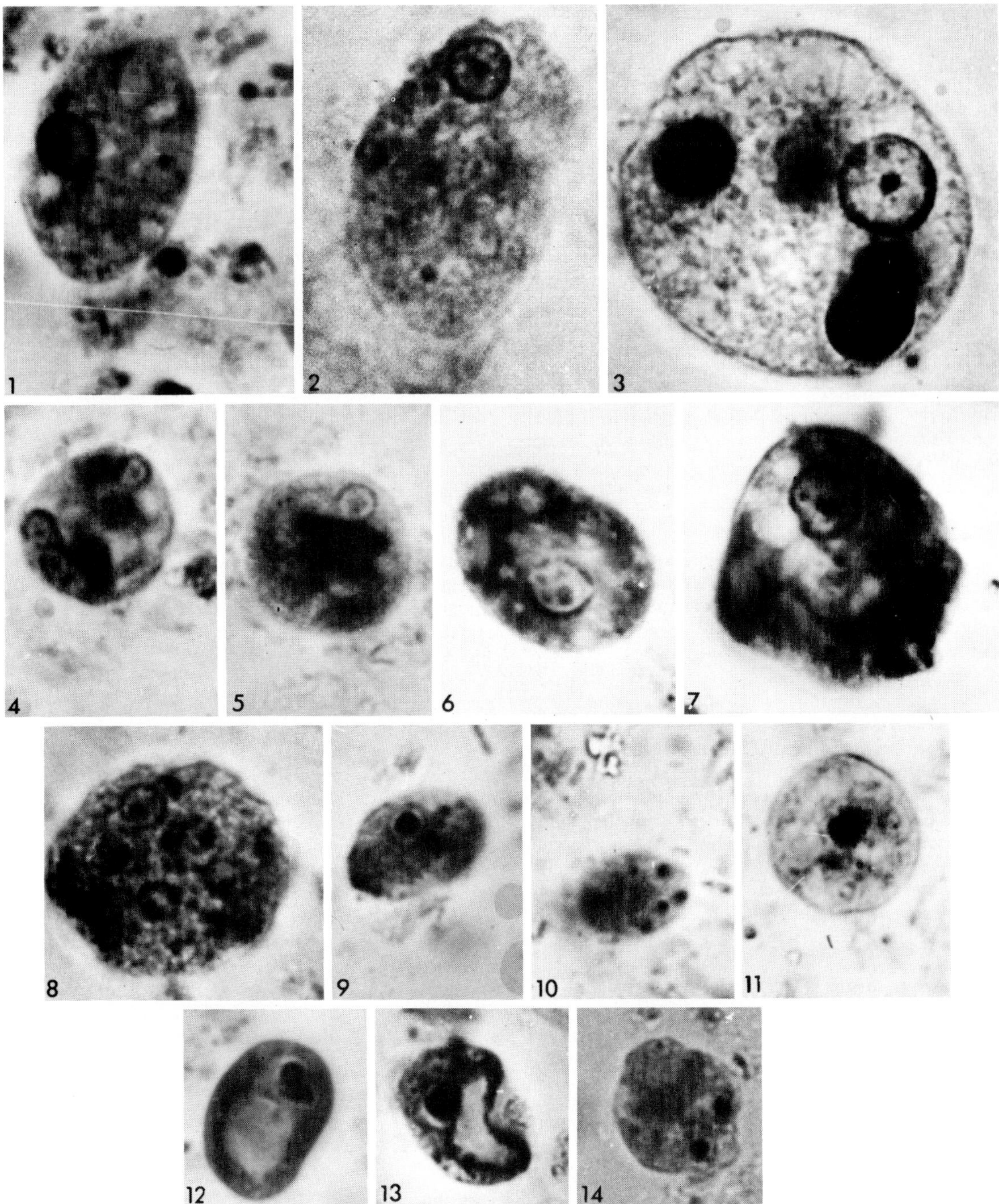

Figure 49–19. Amebae, trichrome stain, oil immersion. *1* and *2, Entamoeba histolytica* trophozoites. *3, E. histolytica* trophozoite with ingested erythrocytes. *4, E. histolytica* cyst with three nuclei visible, chromatoid bodies, and glycogen vacuoles. *5, E. histolytica* cyst with chromatoid bodies. *6* and *7, E. coli* trophozoites. *8, E. coli* cyst. *9, Endolimax nana* trophozoite. *10, E. nana* cyst with four nuclei. *11, Iodamoeba bütschlii* trophozoite and achromatic granules above karyosome. *12, I. bütschlii* cyst with achromatic granules below karyosome and glycogen vacuole. *13, I. bütschlii* cyst without evident achromatic granules and with glycogen vacuole and irregular shape. *14, Dientamoeba fragilis* trophozoite.

phozoites. The cytoplasm of the cyst may contain glycogen vacuoles and chromatoid bodies with blunted or rounded ends. The number and size of nuclei and the appearance of chromatoid bodies are good diagnostic criteria for cysts.

Non-pathogenic amebae. Laboratory personnel must be able to differentiate the non-pathogenic intestinal amebae from *E. histolytica* and *Dientamoeba fragilis* (a flagellate), which are potential pathogens. Identification characteristics are summarized in Tables 49–5 and 49–6 and Figures 49–16 to 49–19. Identification of trophozoites is based on size and nuclear and cytoplasmic characteristics. Identification of cysts is based on size, number and characteristics of nuclei, and presence and character of chromatoid bodies and glycogen masses. Characteristics are best visualized in permanent stained sections.

E. hartmanni has morphologic characteristics similar to those of *E. histolytica* except that the trophozoites have a maximum diameter of 12 μ and the cysts have a maximum diameter of 10 μ. Differentiation is based on measurement with a properly calibrated ocular micrometer.

E. coli is a common lumen-dwelling ameba and may be difficult to differentiate from *E. histolytica*. The cytoplasm stains somewhat more darkly than the cytoplasm of *E. histolytica* and is more vacuolated, containing numerous ingested bacteria, yeasts, and other materials. Occasional *E. coli* nuclei may have evenly distributed chromatin and/or central karyosomes.

Cysts of *E. coli*, when mature, contain eight nuclei, with occasional supernucleate cysts containing 16 or more nuclei. Immature cysts with four nuclei are not common and, when present, the individual nuclei are larger (one fourth the diameter of the cyst) than those of *E. histolytica* (one sixth the diameter of the cyst). Distribution of peripheral chromatin and karyosomes should not be given great emphasis in identification of *Entamoeba* cysts. Chromatoid bodies, when present, are irregular in shape, with fibrillar, splintered, or pointed ends rather than the rounded ends seen in *E. histolytica*. Glycogen may be present in immature cysts.

E. polecki is an infrequently seen parasite and is not further described (Fig. 49–17).

E. nana trophozoites often have atypical nuclei that contain a triangular chromatin mass, a band of chromatin across the nucleus, or two discrete masses of chromatin on opposite sides of the nuclear membrane (Fig. 49–18). These atypical forms may be helpful in differentiating *E. nana* from *Iodamoeba bütschlii*. The karyolymph space of *E. nana* is usually quite clear and halo-like, in contrast to the more "muddy" karyolymph space of *I. bütschlii*. Cysts with less than four nuclei are infrequently seen. Chromatoid bodies as such are rarely seen, but there may be small, irregular portions of chromatoid material. Glycogen, when present, is usually diffuse rather than a discrete mass. Cysts are usually not hard to differentiate from those of other amebae but may be confused with *Blastocystis hominis* organisms, which show granules but do not have the distinct karyolymph space around these granules as seen in *E. nana* nuclei and have variable sizes and numbers of granules. (*Blastocystis hominis* is thought by some to be a protozoan. It is frequently found in stools and may occasionally be associated with diarrhea [Phillips, 1976; Zierdt, 1967].)

The nuclei of *I. bütschlii* have a large, centrally located karyosome that is frequently surrounded by achromatic granules which may not be distinct but appear only as a muddy karyolymph space. In some nuclei, the karyolymph space will be clear without evident achromatic granules and thus be indistinguishable from *E. nana* (Fig. 49–19).

Cysts of *Iodamoeba bütschlii* (Figs. 49–17 to 49–19) usually contain only one nucleus in which the karyosome is often eccentric with a nearby crescent of achromatic granules. The cyst is characterized by a prominent vacuole of glycogen that stains reddish brown in iodine-stained wet mounts, thus the name of the organism. Glycogen is dissolved by aqueous fixatives and thus may not be demonstrable in material that has been stored.

FLAGELLATES (Table 49–7; Fig. 49–20)

Dientamoeba fragilis. *D. fragilis* is an ameboid pathogen without a cyst stage which infects the colon and has been associated with diarrhea (Yang, 1977; Spencer, 1979). It was formerly considered to be an ameba and has this appearance in man but is now correctly classified as a flagellate. It must be differentiated from the amebae and is included in tables and figures for amebae (Table 49–5; Figs. 49–17 to 49–19). Symptoms include diarrhea and abdominal pain. Pathogenesis is not well defined, but some feel that there is mucosal damage. Recent evidence suggests that dientamebiasis is a more frequent cause of diarrhea than previously thought, with 4.2 per cent of patients in a recent study harboring this organism. Approximately 25 per cent of persons infected with this parasite have symptomatic disease. In contrast to amebiasis, this infection is not usually associated with other fecal protozoa, but it shows a 10 to 20 times greater than expected association with enterobiasis (pinworms). This association and some experimental evidence suggest that *D. fragilis* infection may be spread by ingestion of pinworm eggs infected with *D. fragilis* (Burrows, 1956). The infection may easily be overlooked unless permanently stained slides are examined. The number of parasites in feces may vary from day to day and the number of parasites is greater in the last than in the first portion of a bowel movement.

Two thirds to four fifths of the organisms will contain two nuclei. These nuclei do not have peripheral chromatin but do have a cluster of four to eight karyosomal granules, which may appear to be one large irregular karyosome in some instances; thus, a uninucleate *D. fragilis* may be confused with an *E. nana* or *I. bütschlii* trophozoite. The cytoplasm of *D. fragilis* is delicate; therefore, trophozoites may be easily overlooked. The finely granular cytoplasm often contains ingested bacteria. Although it is taxonomically a flagellate, it has no flagella.

Giardia lamblia. *G. lamblia* is a pathogenic intes-

Table 49–6. MORPHOLOGY OF CYSTS OF INTESTINAL AMEBAE*

			Nucleus			Cytoplasm	
Species	**Size**	**Shape**	***Number***	***Peripheral Chromatin***	***Karyosomal Chromatin***	***Chromatoid Bodies***	***Glycogen***
Entamoeba histolytica	10–20 μ. Usual range, 12–15 μ.	Usually spherical.	4 in mature cyst. Immature cysts with 1 or 2 occasionally seen.	Peripheral chromatin present. Fine, uniform granules, evenly distributed.	Small, discrete, usually central.	Present. Elongated bars with bluntly rounded ends.	Usually diffuse. Concentrated mass often present in young cysts. Stains reddish brown with iodine.
Entamoeba hartmanni	5–10 μ. Usual range, 6–8 μ.	Usually spherical.	4 in mature cyst. Immature cysts with 1 or 2 often seen.	Similar to *E. histolytica.*	Similar to *E. histolytica.*	Present. Elongated bars with bluntly rounded ends.	Similar to *E. histolytica.*
Entamoeba coli	10–35 μ. Usual range, 15–25 μ.	Usually spherical. Occasionally oval, triangular, or of another shape.	8 in mature cyst. Occasionally, supernucleate cysts with 16 or more are seen. Immature cysts with 2 or more occasionally seen.	Peripheral chromatin present. Coarse granules irregular in size and distribution, but often appear more uniform than in trophozoites.	Large, discrete, usually eccentric, but occasionally central.	Present. Usually splinter-like with pointed ends.	Usually diffuse, but occasionally well-defined mass in immature cysts. Stains reddish brown with iodine.
Endolimax nana	5–10 μ. Usual range, 6–8 μ.	Spherical, ovoid, or ellipsoidal.	4 in mature cysts. Immature cysts with less than 4 rarely seen.	None.	Large, usually centrally located.	Occasionally, granules or small oval masses seen, but bodies as seen in *Entamoeba* species are not present.	Usually diffuse. Concentrated mass seen occasionally in young cysts. Stains reddish brown with iodine.
Iodamoeba bütschlii	5–20 μ. Usual range, 10–12 μ.	Ovoid, ellipsoidal, triangular, or of another shape.	1 in mature cyst.	None.	Large, usually eccentric. Refractile, achromatic granules on one side of karyosome.	Granules occasionally present, but bodies as seen in *Entamoeba* species are not present.	Compact, well-defined mass. Stains dark brown with iodine.

*Adapted with permission from Brooke, M. M., and Melvin, D. M.: Morphology of Diagnostic Stages of Intestinal Parasites of Man, USDHEW PHS Publication No. 1966, 1969.

6

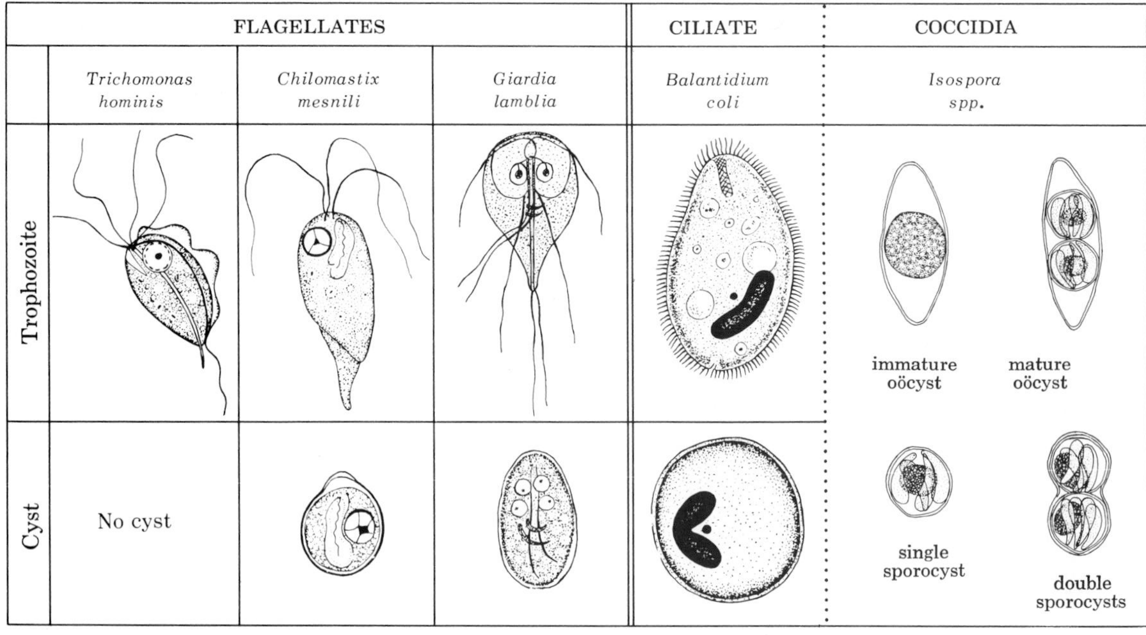

Figure 49–20. Flagellates, ciliate, and coccidia. (Adapted from Brooke and Melvin, 1964.)

tinal protozoan that causes both endemic and epidemic disease (Meyer, 1979), with recent water-borne outbreaks described in Aspen, Colorado, Leningrad, Russia, and Rome, New York, and in campers in the western United States (Smith, 1980). This organism may also cause infections in children, particularly those in day-care facilities (Black, 1977). It was the most frequent pathogenic parasite identified in fecal specimens by state health laboratories during 1978 (4.0 per cent). It appears that some of the large outbreaks have been related to problems in the water supply. Pathogenic protozoa are not killed by the usual concentrations of chlorine in municipal water supplies and thus, unless the water supply is filtered, it may serve as a source of infection as it did in the Rome, New York, outbreak.

G. lamblia causes an infection of the small intestine. There are often asymptomatic individuals, and the disease may vary from mild diarrhea with vague abdominal complaints to a full malabsorption syndrome with diarrhea and steatorrhea, similar to sprue. The exact mechanism by which *G. lamblia* causes disease is not known. It does not infect other organs of the body. The disease occurs worldwide and is increasingly recognized in the "developed" areas of the world. Giardiasis should be considered in any patient presenting with diarrhea of over ten days' duration.

Diagnosis is established by demonstration of *Giardia* trophozoites and/or cysts in fecal specimens. The passage of organisms may vary from day to day; therefore, multiple specimens, collected over a period of time, must be examined. Direct wet mounts are particularly helpful for demonstrating the motile trophozoites, although they may also be used to show cysts. Cysts can be demonstrated by concentration techniques, and both trophozoites and cysts may be demonstrated and carefully studied in permanently stained slides. In some cases, the organisms cannot be demonstrated in fecal specimens, and aspirates of small bowel material may be required to demonstrate them. In such instances, the laboratory should be advised ahead of time so that it will be able to perform a direct wet mount when the specimen is received. An IIF serologic test has recently been developed and appears promising (Visvesvara, 1980b).

G. lamblia is shaped like half a pear (Table 49–7; Figs. 49–20 and 49–21). When viewed in its broad dimension, it is pear shaped with a tapered posterior end and has two nuclei giving the appearance of a smiling face with prominent eyes. When viewed from the side, the anterior end of the organism is thicker and tapers, posteriorly, with the anterior half to three fourths consisting of a sucking disk. The flagella are not usually evident in wet mounts or in stained preparations.

Cysts of *G. lamblia* are oval, and the cytoplasm is often retracted from the wall. *G. lamblia* is readily differentiated from other protozoa of man by the binucleate trophozoite with its distinctive structures and the quadrinucleate cyst with fibrils. Generally when organisms are missed, it is because they are overlooked rather than because they are misidentified.

Chilomastix mesnili. *C. mesnili* (Table 49–7; Figs. 49–20 and 49–22) is a non-pathogenic lumen-dwelling flagellate of man which must be differentiated from trophozoites of amebae in stained smears. The consistent location of the *C. mesnili* nucleus at one end of the organism and the tapering of the end opposite the nucleus are helpful. If multiple organisms are examined, the cytostome will be visible in some. The flagella are usually not visible in stained or

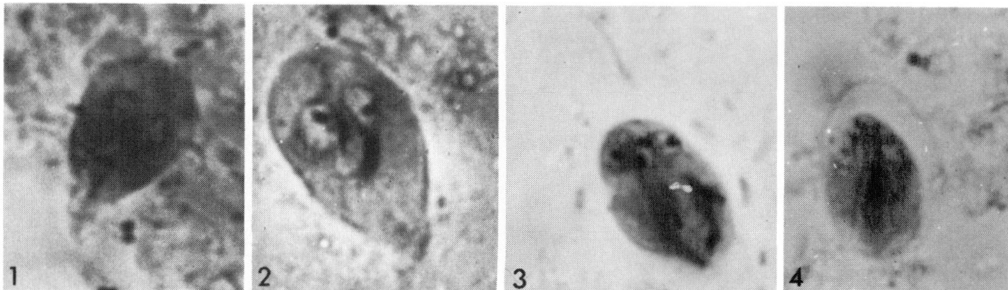

Figure 49–21. *Giardia lamblia,* trichrome stain, oil immersion. *1* and *2,* Trophozoites with prominent nuclei, median bodies, and tapered posterior ends. *3* and *4,* Cysts with nuclei and fibrils. The cyst on the right has retracted from the cyst wall.

formalin-fixed preparations. The lemon-shaped cysts contain various curved cytostomal fibers that have a "safety-pin" appearance.

Trichomonas. *T. hominis* (Table 50–7; Fig. 50–20) is a less frequent non-pathogenic flagellate, which does not have a cyst form. The organisms do not stain particularly well but have a nucleus with a small karyosome and unevenly distributed chromatin in stained material. They may be confused with *Entameoba hartmanni* or small *E. histolytica* trophozoites. The axostyle may be visible and aids in identification. Several organisms may have to be examined in order to demonstrate the undulating membrane, flagella, axostyle, or cost.

T. vaginalis causes a common vaginal infection characterized by inflammation with itching and vaginal discharge. Occasionally the urinary tract may be involved. The infection may be spread by sexual intercourse. Males may have asymptomatic infections or occasionally symptomatic prostatitis or urethritis. *T. vaginalis* infections are usually diagnosed by the physician in his office using the simple procedure of direct wet mount to look for the typical jerky motile organisms. Direct wet mounts are positive in about 70 per cent of infected women. Cultures may increase the diagnostic accuracy to over 90 per cent (Levett, 1980).

Morphologically, *T. vaginalis* resembles *T. hominis* but is larger (30 μ), and the undulating membrane extends only half the length of the body. Because of the differences in habitat, it is generally not necessary to differentiate these trichomonads morphologically.

Two small infrequently found intestinal flagellates, *Enteromonas hominis* and *Retortamonas intestinalis,* will not be described other than in Table 49–7. *Trichomonas tenax* is a trichomonad that occasionally infects the oral cavity but does not cause disease.

CILIATES

Balantidium coli. The ciliate *B. coli* (Fig. 49–20) may cause a severe intestinal infection similar to the intestinal phase of amebiasis with colonic ulcerations, but it does not cause liver abscesses and other systemic lesions. It appears that man acquires the infection from association with hogs, which are commonly infected. The trophozoites vary greatly in size, from 40 to over 200 μ in greatest dimension, with most measuring 40 to 70 μ. The body is uniformly covered with cilia that are slightly longer at the anterior end adjacent to the cytostome. There is a larger macronucleus, which is readily seen, and a smaller micronucleus, which is infrequently visible. There are numerous food vacuoles and contractile vacuoles in the cytoplasm. The encysted organism is rounded and when young, will still show cilia that disappear as the cyst ages. This organism does not present diagnostic problems other than sometimes being overlooked because of its large size. Specimens contaminated with stagnant water may contain other ciliates, which can usually be distinguished from *B. coli* by differences in their ciliary pattern.

COCCIDIA

Coccidia of the genera *Toxoplasma, Isospora, Sarcocystis,* and *Cryptosporidium* may infect man. All have

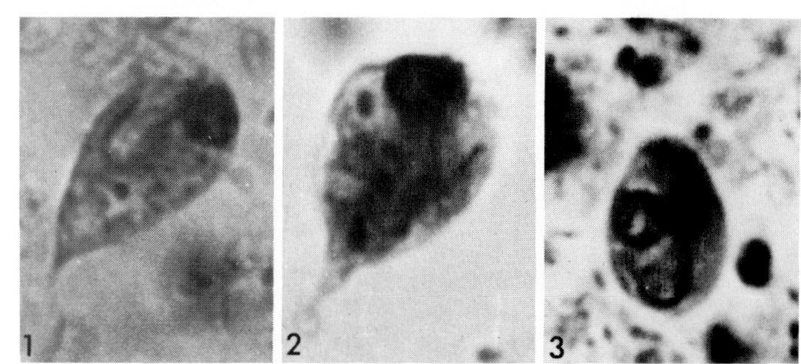

Figure 49–22. *Chilomastix mesnili,* trichrome stain, oil immersion. *1* and *2,* Trophozoites with anterior nuclei and tapered posterior ends. The cytostome is to the left of the nucleus in *1* and to the right of the nucleus in *2. 3* is a cyst with the typical lemon shape. Nucleus is on the left. Curved fibrils are prominent at the bottom of the cyst.

Table 49–7. MORPHOLOGY OF INTESTINAL FLAGELLATES*

TROPHOZOITES

Species	Size (Length)	Shape	Motility	Number of Nuclei	Number of Flagella†	Other Features
Trichomonas‡ hominis	8–20 μ. Usual range, 11–12 μ.	Pear-shaped.	Rapid, jerking.	1 Not visible in unstained mounts.	3–5 anterior. 1 posterior.	Undulating membrane extending length of body.
Chilomastix mesnili	6–24 μ. Usual range, 10–15 μ.	Pear-shaped.	Stiff, rotary.	1 Not visible in unstained mounts.	3 anterior. 1 in cytostome.	Prominent cytostome extending ⅓–½ length of body. Spiral groove across ventral surface.
Giardia lamblia	10–20 μ. Usual range, 12–15 μ.	Pear-shaped.	"Falling leaf."	2 Not visible in unstained mounts.	4 lateral. 2 ventral. 2 caudal.	Sucking disk occupying ½–¾ of ventral surface.
Enteromonas hominis	4–10 μ. Usual range, 8–9 μ.	Oval.	Jerking.	1 Not visible in unstained mounts.	3 anterior. 1 posterior.	One side of body flattened. Posterior flagellum extending free, posteriorly or laterally.
Retortamonas intestinalis	4–9 μ. Usual range, 6–7 μ.	Pear-shaped or oval.	Jerking.	1 Not visible in unstained mounts.	1 anterior. 1 posterior.	Prominent cytostome extending approximately ½ length of body.

CYSTS

Species	Size	Shape	Number of Nuclei	Other Features
Chilomastix mesnili	6–10 μ. Usual range, 8–9 μ.	Lemon-shaped, with anterior hyaline knob or "nipple."	1 Not visible in unstained preparations.	Cytostome with supporting fibrils. Usually visible in stained preparations.
Giardia lamblia	8–9 μ. Usual range, 11–12 μ.	Oval or ellipsoidal.	Usually 4. Not distinct in unstained preparations. Usually located at one end.	Fibrils or flagella longitudinally in cyst. Cytoplasm often retracts from a portion of cell wall.
Enteromonas hominis	4–10 μ. Usual range, 6–8 μ.	Elongated or oval.	1–4, usually 2 lying at opposite ends of cyst. Not visible in unstained mounts.	Resembles *E. nana* cyst. Fibrils or flagella are usually not seen.
Retortamonas intestinalis	4–9 μ. Usual range, 4–7 μ.	Pear-shaped or slightly lemon-shaped.	1 Not visible in unstained mounts.	Resembles *Chilomastix* cyst. Shadow outline of cytostome with supporting fibrils extends above nucleus.

*Adapted with permission from Brooke, M. M., and Melvin, D. M.: Morphology of Diagnostic Stages of Intestinal Parasites of Man, USDHEW PHS Publication No. 1966, 1969.

†Not a practical feature for identification of species in routine fecal examinations.

‡*Trichomonas hominis* does not have a cyst form.

become better understood during the last decade. *Toxoplasma* has already been discussed.

Isospora have a sexual cycle in the epithelial cells of the small intestine of man and animals. The oocysts passed with the stools are the infective stages which produce an infection in another host. A tissue phase with tachyzoites and bradyzoites (cysts) may occur, but direct transmission is usually via the oocysts.

There is only one species, *I. belli,* which is known in man and which has been associated with diarrhea and malabsorption (Brandborg, 1970). The diagnosis is established by finding the unsporulated oocyst measuring 12 × 30 μ in direct stool examinations or in concentrations. If feces are left at room temperature for 24 to 48 hours, sporulation will occur. The infectious oocyst contains two sporocysts each with four sporozoites (Fig. 49–20).

Sarcocystis species require two hosts. In the definitive host the sexual cycle occurs in the epithelial cells of the small intestinal mucosa (similar to the *Isospora*). In the intermediate host, cystic stages develop in the muscles after a complicated cycle. There are two forms of parasitism by *Sarcocystis* in man. In the first form, man is an intermediate host of several unnamed species of *Sarcocystis,* with cysts occurring in the muscles (Beaver, 1979). The second is intestinal infection (Fig. 49–23) produced by *Sarcocystis hominis* and *S. suishominis* (formerly *I. hominis).* Man and other primates are the definitive hosts, and cattle and pigs are the respective intermediate hosts. The infection is acquired by eating poorly cooked infected meat. There are usually no symptoms, but occasional patients have transient diarrhea, abdominal pain, or anorexia. The diagnosis is established by recovering the sporulated 25 × 33 μ oocysts in the stools.

Cryptosporidium has one host in its life cycle. Parasites develop intracellularly just beneath the surface of large and small intestinal epithelial cells, often in the brush border. The gallbladder and pancreas may also be infected. Patients may have malaise, fever, abdominal cramps, anorexia, and diarrhea. Most reported infections have occurred in immunocompromised patients in whom profuse watery diarrhea may last for months. In a recent report on 21 patients with acquired immunodeficiency syndrome who had the infection, 14 died (Centers for Disease Control, 1982d). No effective therapy is known. Infection in immunocompetent persons has a self-limited course of one to two weeks (Reese, 1982; Current, 1983).

Diagnosis may be established by small intestine or colon biopsy or by examination of the stool to detect the 4 to 6 μ refractile organisms (Garcia, 1983; Current, 1983) (Fig. 49–23). Because of their small size they are easily overlooked.

The best concentration procedure is said to be Sheather's sugar flotation, although other concentration methods appear useful. Various stains may be used (Garcia, 1983; Current, 1983) including Giemsa, modified acid-fast (similar to that for *Nocardia*), or carbol-fuchsin. A serologic test has recently been described (Campbell, 1983).

Non-parasitic Objects. There are various inflammatory and tissue cells, yeasts, and other substances that may be seen in feces. Table 49–8 lists characteristics that may aid in their differentiation from protozoa.

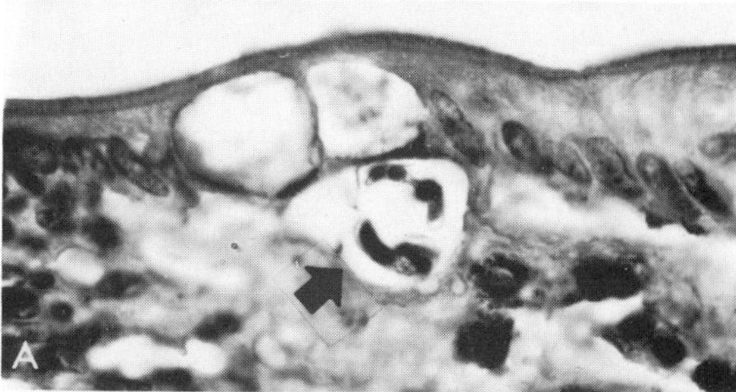

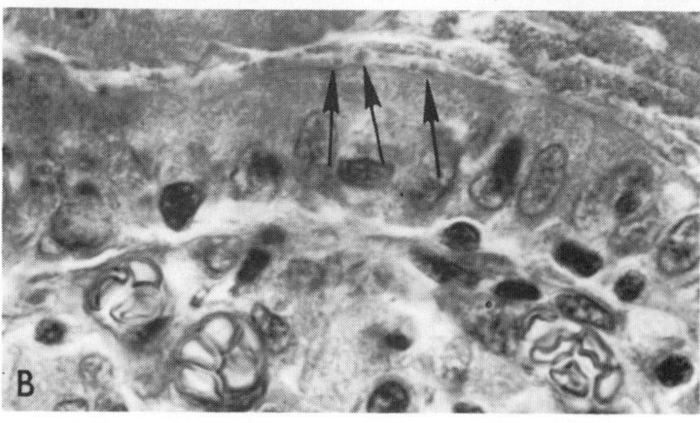

Figure 49–23. Coccidia in human intestine. *A, Sarcocystis* sp. mature oocyst (arrow) in epithelial cell (×800). *B, Cryptosporidium* sp. Note the very small oocysts (arrows) maturing within the brush border of the epithelial cells (×800).

INTESTINAL HELMINTHS

Helminths are classified into nematodes (roundworms) and platyhelminths (flat worms). Platyhelminths in turn are divided into trematodes (flukes) and cestodes (tapeworms). The adult worms vary in size from barely visible to the naked eye to 10 meters in length.

Helminth life cycles may be direct or indirect. Direct development requires only one host which harbors the adult worms, and eggs or larvae are passed in the stools. In some instances, the eggs are infective when passed and, in others, require a soil maturation period to reach the infective stage. Indirect cycles are more complex and include intermediate hosts, in which the larval stages develop, and definitive hosts, which harbor the adults. Adult and larval stages occur in intestinal lumen or tissues of the host. Most living organisms, including man, serve as definitive and/or intermediate hosts for many parasitic helminths.

Signs and symptoms of helminth infections are caused by adults, larvae or eggs, or host reactions to them or their products. Eosinophilia is common, especially in early stages of infection in which parasites are in tissue.

If parasitic infection is to be suspected and diag-

Table 49–8. NON-PARASITIC OBJECTS THAT MAY BE CONFUSED WITH INTESTINAL PROTOZOA*

Artifact	Resemblance	Saline Mount	Differential Characteristics of Artifact Permanent Stain	
			Cytoplasm	*Nucleus*
Polymorphonuclear leukocytes (Seen in dysentery and other inflammatory bowel diseases.)	*E. histolytica* cyst	Usually not a problem. Granules in cytoplasm. Cell border irregular.	Less dense, often frothy. Border less clearly demarcated than that of ameba.	More coarse. Larger, relative to size of organism. Irregular shape and size. Chromatin unevenly distributed. Chromatin strands may link nuclei.
Macrophages (Seen in dysentery and other inflammatory bowel diseases. May be present in purged specimens.)	Amebic trophozoite, especially *E. histolytica*	Nuclei larger and of irregular shape, with irregular chromatin distribution. Cytoplasm granular; may contain ingested debris. Cell border irregular and indistinct. Movement irregular and pseudopodia indistinct.	Coarse. May contain inclusions.	Large and often irregular in shape. Chromatin irregularly distributed.
Squamous epithelial cells (from anal mucosa)	Amebic trophozoite	Nucleus refractile and large. Cytoplasm smooth. Cell border distinct.	Stains poorly.	Large and single. Large chromatin mass may resemble karyosome.
Columnar epithelial cells (from intestinal mucosa)	Amebic trophozoite	Nucleus refractile and large. Cytoplasm smooth. Cell border distinct.	Stains poorly.	Large with heavy chromatin on nuclear membrane. Often large central chromatin mass resembling karyosome.
Yeasts (Normal constituent of feces.)	Protozoan cyst	Oval. Thick wall. No internal structure. Budding forms may be seen.	Oval. Little internal structure. Refractile cell wall. Budding forms may be seen.	None.
Starch granules	Protozoan cyst	Rounded or angular. Very refractile. No internal structure. Stain pink to purple in iodine mounts.	Not a problem in permanently stained slides.	

Note: Other artifacts, such as contaminating plant cells and pollen grains, are occasionally seen. These should not be difficult to differentiate.
*From Smith, 1976.

nosed, a clear understanding of the life cycle, the tissues likely to be compromised, and the geographic distribution is necessary. Final diagnosis usually depends upon the morphologic identification in feces, blood, or tissue of a stage of the parasite (egg, larva, embryo, or adult). However, in some infections only a clinical diagnosis is possible, or diagnosis is established indirectly by serologic methods.

Identification of helminth eggs in feces is particularly important and should be approached systematically. Size of eggs is particularly important and requires use of a properly calibrated ocular micrometer (Fig. 49–24). Shape and thickness of the shell should be noted. Special structures, such as a mamillated covering, operculum, shoulders adjacent to the operculum, abopercular knob, polar plugs, or spines should be noted. Eggs should be examined to determine if they are undeveloped, developing, or embryonated. Hooklets should be sought if certain cestode eggs are suspected. If these various characteristics are considered and the examiner is familiar with the background material in feces, there should be no difficulty detecting and identifying eggs.

Nematodes

Nematodes are the most common helminths in man. The intestinal nematodes are diagnosed by finding eggs, larvae, or adult worms in the feces.

Enterobius vermicularis. Enterobiasis or oxyuriasis (pinworms) is the most common helminthic infection in children of all social strata in the United States. The prevalence is unknown, but there are estimates of 30 and 16 per cent in children and adults, respectively. Rates are often higher in institutions (Warren, 1974).

The normal habitat is the lumen of the cecum and adjacent areas where both males and females live. The female worm measures up to 13 mm in length and has a pointed posterior end which gives the common name pinworm. A characteristic of both adult worms is a cephalic knob which is seen as alae (Fig. 49–25).

The gravid female migrates to the perianal area, usually during the evening, and deposits eggs in the folds of the perianal skin. The eggs (Fig. 49–26) are ovoid with one side flattened, measure 50 to 60 by 20 to 30 μ, are embryonated when laid, and are infective within hours. If eggs are ingested by the appropriate host, the life cycle is completed.

Clinically, in most cases enterobiasis is asymptomatic or causes very mild disease. There may be *pruritus ani,* usually at night, which is related to the migration of the parasites to the perianal area, and there may be irritability. Pinworms may be found in surgical specimens of the appendix, either in the lumen or buried in the mucosa. They are identified by their size and typical morphology with lateral alae (Fig. 49–27). It appears that in most cases the worm is just an incidental bystander.

Adult females may migrate to unusual sites, such as the uterus, fallopian tubes, or peritoneal cavity, and granulomatous reaction to eggs or dead adults may be found (Symmers, 1950). Eggs may be seen in Papanicolaou smears when adults migrate to the vagina.

Diagnosis is usually made by recovery of typical eggs from the perianal folds. This is best accomplished with the cellulose tape technique (see p. 1217) because only 5 to 10 per cent of the cases are detected with

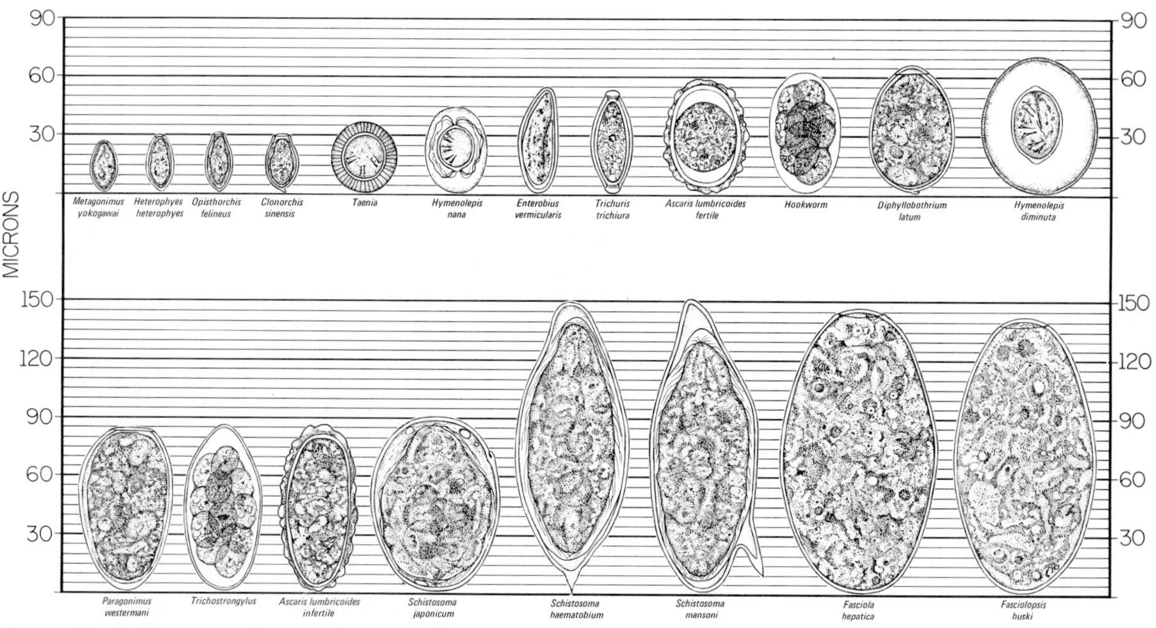

Figure 49–24. Relative sizes of helminth eggs. (From Parasitology Training Branch, Centers for Disease Control, Atlanta, Ga.)

6

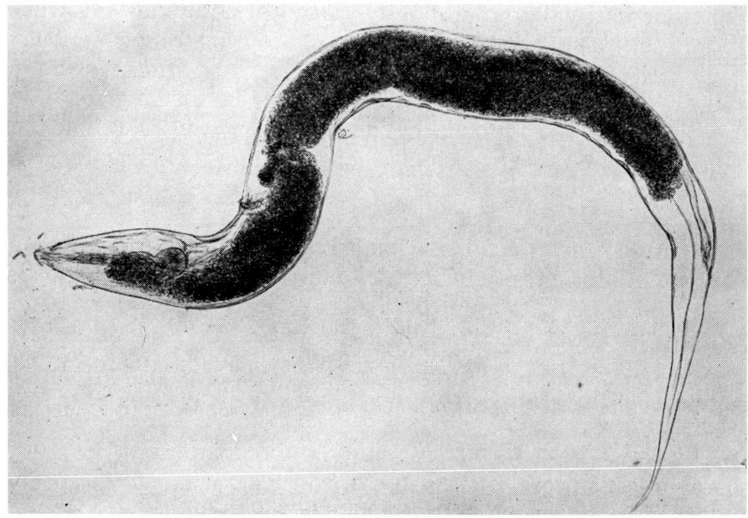

Figure 49–25. Adult female *E. vermicularis* showing bulb behind esophagus, vulva, egg mass, anus, and pointed posterior end. (From Hunter, C. W., Swartzwelder, J. C., and Clyde, D. F.: A Manual of Tropical Medicine. Philadelphia, W. B. Saunders Company, 1976.)

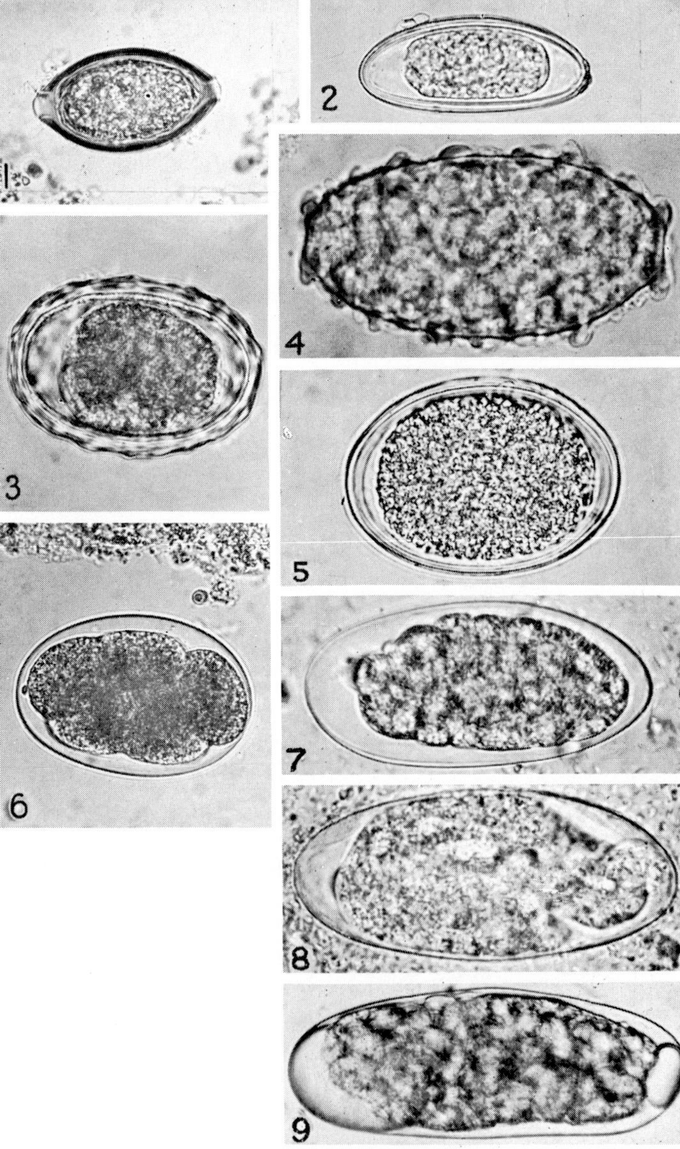

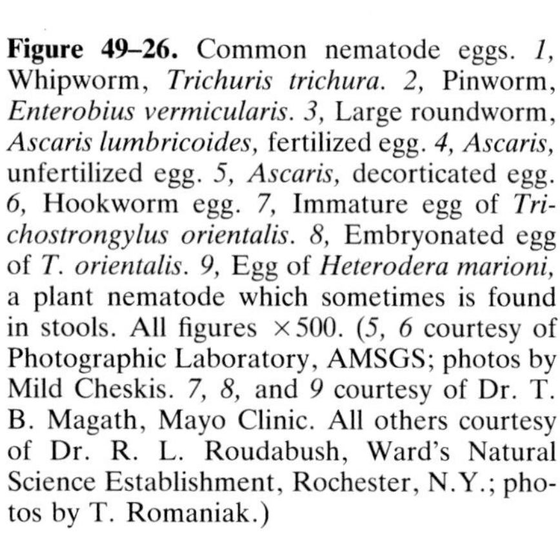

Figure 49–26. Common nematode eggs. *1,* Whipworm, *Trichuris trichura. 2,* Pinworm, *Enterobius vermicularis. 3,* Large roundworm, *Ascaris lumbricoides,* fertilized egg. *4, Ascaris,* unfertilized egg. *5, Ascaris,* decorticated egg. *6,* Hookworm egg. *7,* Immature egg of *Trichostrongylus orientalis. 8,* Embryonated egg of *T. orientalis. 9,* Egg of *Heterodera marioni,* a plant nematode which sometimes is found in stools. All figures ×500. (*5, 6* courtesy of Photographic Laboratory, AMSGS; photos by Mild Cheskis. *7, 8,* and *9* courtesy of Dr. T. B. Magath, Mayo Clinic. All others courtesy of Dr. R. L. Roudabush, Ward's Natural Science Establishment, Rochester, N.Y.; photos by T. Romaniak.)

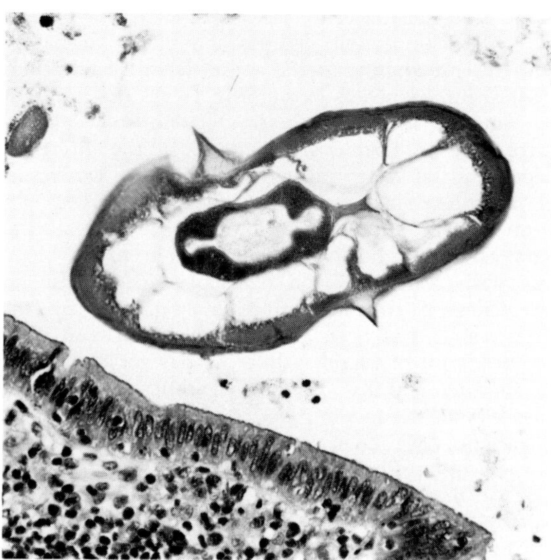

Figure 49–27. *Enterobius vermicularis.* Adult in appendix. Note the characteristic lateral alae (×250).

routine stool examination. The sample should always be taken at night after the child has gone to sleep or in the morning before a bath. Diagnosis may require examination of several samples taken on different days before the eggs can be found (Sadun, 1956). Visual examination of the anal area may allow detection of adult worms.

Trichuris trichiura. A common nematode, especially in tropical and subtropical areas, *Trichuris* is the causative agent of trichuriasis (whipworm infection) in man.

Trichuris adults are found in the large intestine, especially the cecum, but in more severe infections they can be found in the entire colon and rectum. The worms are easily identified because the anterior portion is long and slender, with a thicker posterior end, thus the name whipworm (Fig. 49–28). Adults measure up to 50 mm in length and live attached to the colonic mucosa by their slender anterior portions. Like most nematodes, the posterior end of the male is curved ventrally. *Trichuris* is one of the soil-transmitted helminths with a direct life cycle. The unembryonated eggs (Figs. 49–24 and 49–26) passed with the stools require several weeks in appropriate soil to mature to the infective stage. When embryonated eggs are swallowed, the larvae are released and mature into adults in the colon. Attachment to the mucosa occurs early, and the worms apparently remain attached during their lifetime (estimated to be four to five years).

The clinical manifestations of trichuriasis in man depend upon the number of worms present (Jung, 1951). In light to moderate infections (most cases) there are no symptoms. However, with larger numbers (300 worms) there may be diarrhea, and in the most severe cases there is dysentery, clinically indistinguishable from that caused by amebae, with mucus and blood in the stools. A common complication in children is rectal prolapse, a consequence of the patient's repeated efforts to void when there is diarrhea.

The diagnosis is made by finding the typical eggs measuring 52 to 57 by 22 to 23 μ (Figs. 49–24 and 49–26) in direct fecal smears or with the concentration techniques. The eggs are barrel-shaped with refractile polar plugs at both ends. If eggs are found in the direct mount, they may be quantified in various ways. A simple method is to determine the number of eggs in a standard smear (equivalent to 2 mg of stool). Light infections will have less than 5 eggs per slide and heavy infections over 25 eggs. Watery stools or those containing large amounts of mucus or undigested food are not suitable for egg counts. The egg size varies under normal conditions. Oversized eggs or eggs with atypical shape may result from previous treatment with anthelmintics.

Ascaris lumbricoides. This is the largest nematode of the human intestinal tract. The infection (ascariasis) is common in many parts of the world, with over half a billion people infected. This soil-transmitted helminth occurs mainly in areas where sanitation is poor (WHO, 1964). Like *Trichuris,* it is especially common in children, who are also more likely to have heavy infections.

The female measures up to 35 cm in length by 6 mm in diameter. The male is smaller and has the posterior end curved ventrally. The adult parasites live in the duodenum and proximal jejunum. Each female lays approximately 200,000 non-embryonated eggs per day. They measure 45 to 70 by 35 to 50 μ. When the eggs are deposited in a satisfactory environment, they become infective in four to six weeks. If the infective eggs are swallowed, they will hatch in the intestine and release larvae. These penetrate the intestinal mucosa and enter the bloodstream, which carries them to the lungs where they develop for several days in the alveolar capillary bed. When the larvae have developed to the proper stage, they break into the alveoli, migrate upward in the respiratory tree to the epiglottis, are swallowed, and grow to adulthood in the small intestine. The entire development from embryonated egg to adult takes approximately two months.

Ascariasis varies from asymptomatic infection to severe disease. In the intestine a few worms will not usually cause noticeable symptoms, but heavy infections may produce pain, abdominal discomfort, and diarrhea. A mass of worms may cause intestinal obstruction, especially in young children, and migra-

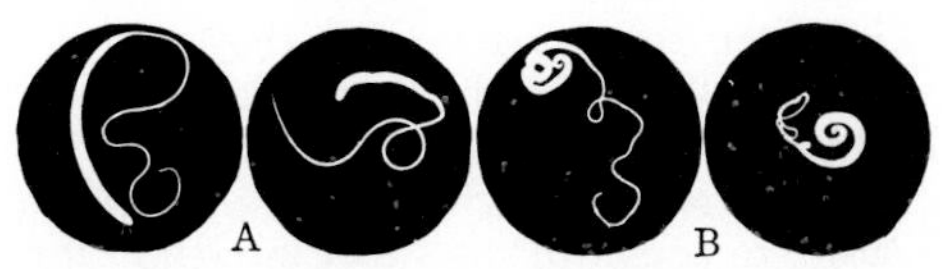

Figure 49–28. Whipworms *(Trichuris trichiura). A,* Females; *B,* males. The posterior portion of the male is usually coiled as is shown at the right. Photographs of mounted specimens. Natural size.

tion to the common bile duct may cause biliary colic and obstruction, leading to cholangitis and intrahepatic abscesses. Migration to the appendix may cause appendicitis and to the stomach, emesis. Fever or drug therapy (especially anesthetics) may stimulate migration.

Migration of large numbers of larvae through the lungs causes Loeffler's syndrome, characterized by diffuse mottled infiltrates of both lungs in radiographs, peripheral eosinophilia, and mild bronchitis. The syndrome is rarely diagnosed even in endemic areas, and only seldom have patients come to autopsy (Spillmann, 1975).

Diagnosis is established by demonstrating eggs in feces or occasionally by examining an adult which has been passed or vomited. The direct smear will almost always reveal infection even if there is only one female worm. The 200,000 eggs that one female produces every 24 hours will give at least five eggs per slide of 2 mg of feces. Counts of less than 20 eggs per slide indicate light infections and over 100, heavy infections.

Fertile *Ascaris* eggs are round to slightly oval with a yellow-brown, irregular external mamillated layer and a thick shell. In fresh specimens the egg is undeveloped, and there is a clear space beneath the shell at each end. Sometimes the egg is decorticate (the mamillated layer is missing) and the egg may be confused with hookworm eggs (Fig. 49–26), but the *Ascaris* egg has a much thicker shell. Unfertilized eggs are larger, up to 94 by 44 μ, more elongated with a thinner, more irregular external layer, and have irregular globules of yolk material filling the egg without clear areas at the ends (see Fig. 49–26).

Hookworms. These nematodes commonly infect the small intestine of man. The two principal species causing disease in man are *Ancylostoma duodenale* and *Necator americanus.* The infection is most frequent in the tropics but also occurs in subtropical areas. In Europe, hookworms were once very prevalent, and in the United States there are still some endemic areas in the Southeast.

The female measures up to 12 mm in length and the male slightly less. The males are easily distinguished by the fan-shaped copulatory bursa at the posterior end. Male and female parasites attach to the small intestinal mucosa but often change attachment site (in contrast to *Trichuris,* which do not change sites).

The females lay the characteristic eggs which are passed in feces (Fig. 49–26). In soil, they develop in one or more days (depending on conditions) and release rhabditiform larvae that develop to the infective filariform stage in about seven days. If these larvae contact the skin of an appropriate host, they will actively penetrate, gain access to the host's circulation, travel to the lungs where they penetrate into the alveoli, move up the tracheobronchial tree to be swallowed, and mature to adults in the small intestine. Ingested *A. duodenale* larvae can develop into adults in the intestine without tissue migration.

Hookworms may produce various clinical manifestations in man. In the skin, if the host has been previously sensitized to the parasite, there may be marked inflammation, redness and blister formation with intense itching at the site of larval penetration, a condition known as "ground itch." In the lungs, if the number of larvae migrating at one time is large, there may be Loeffler's syndrome. In the intestine, depending on worm burden, the infection can result in gastrointestinal symptoms, such as diarrhea, abdominal pain, and nausea. However, the main clinical manifestation of hookworm infections is chronic blood loss with secondary iron deficiency anemia due to laceration of the small intestinal mucosa by the parasites. It has been estimated that between 0.15 and 0.25 ml of blood is lost per day for each adult *A. duodenale* and 0.03 ml for each adult *N. americanus.* The blood loss and number of worms in hookworm infections have been shown to correlate with the number of eggs per gram of stool, so that egg counts may aid in determining need to treat (Layrisse, 1964a and b).

The diagnosis is made by finding the characteristic eggs in the stools. The eggs measure 58 to 76 μ long by 36 to 40 μ wide and have a thin shell. The egg

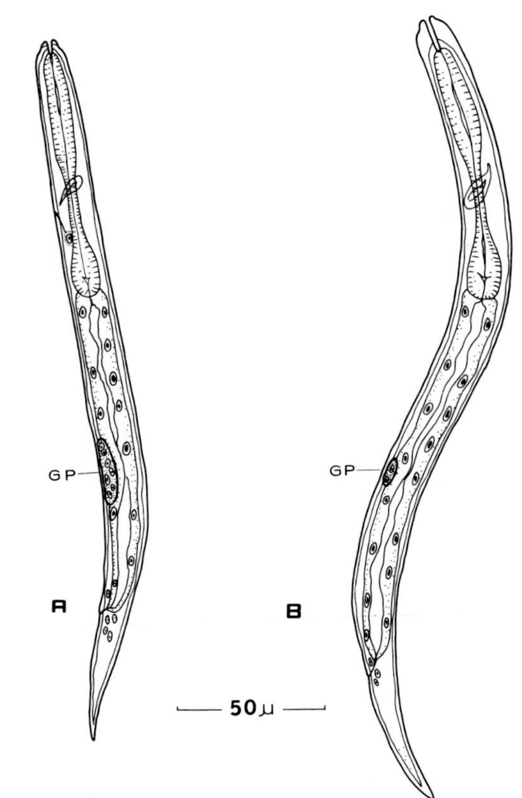

Figure 49–29. Hookworm and *Strongyloides stercoralis* larvae. *A, S. stercoralis* rhabditoid larva in human stools. Note the short size of the buccal cavity and the large genital primordium (GP). *B,* Hookworm rhabditoid larva as seen in a few instances in stools left for at least 24 hours at room temperature. The buccal cavity is longer and the genital primordium is smaller.

is usually in the four to eight cell segmented stage when passed but may vary from unsegmented to embryonated, the latter in specimens from constipated patients. Embryonated eggs or free larvae may be found in unpreserved specimens not examined promptly. Hookworm rhabditiform larvae can be differentiated from those of *Strongyloides stercoralis* because of their longer buccal chamber and inconspicuous genital primordium (Fig. 49–29). Filariform hookworm larvae have a pointed posterior end and an esophagus approximately one fourth the length of the larva. If specimens are contaminated with soil, the larvae must also be differentiated from larvae of free-living nematodes. Hookworm eggs must be differentiated from eggs of *Trichostrongylus* species (which are longer and more pointed) and of *Meloidogyne (Heterodera)* spp., which are longer and narrower, have blunt ends, and are often asymmetrical. *Meloidogyne* spp. are plant parasitic nematodes, the eggs of which are accidentally ingested when eating root vegetables such as potatoes, carrots, and onions (Fig. 49–26).

In direct wet mounts, egg counts of less than 5 eggs per slide denote light infections, which are unlikely to cause symptoms or anemia, whereas more than 25 denote heavy infections. Eggs from different human hookworm species cannot be differentiated; therefore, "hookworm eggs" should be reported.

Adults of human hookworms can be differentiated on the basis of the types of mouth parts. *Ancylostoma* have teeth, whereas *N. americanus* adults have a pair of cutting plates. Configuration of the male copulatory bursa and other characteristics are also used to identify species.

Trichostrongylus spp. These small nematodes live with their anterior ends embedded in the small intestinal epithelium of man and animals. Several species may infect man, including *T. colubriformis, T. axei, T. orientalis,* and *T. brevis. Trichostrongylus* infections in man have been described mainly in the Far East, India, and Russia, with sporadic cases in Latin America and the United States (Faust, 1975).

The females lay eggs that are passed with the stools. After a short period of maturation in the soil, larvae emerge, then develop to the infective stage, crawl on soil and vegetation, and infect a new host when ingested with contaminated food or water. They develop to adults in the intestine without migration through the lungs. The disease is usually asymptomatic, but heavy infections may produce abdominal pain and diarrhea, usually with a mild eosinophilia. The diagnosis is made by finding the typical eggs in the patient's stools. Eggs resemble those of hookworm but are narrower and longer (Fig. 49–26), measuring 78 to 98 μ by 40 to 50 μ, and have somewhat pointed ends. Eggs from different species of *Trichostrongylus* cannot be differentiated; therefore, only a generic identification is made.

Strongyloides stercoralis. *S. stercoralis* is a small nematode which lives buried in the mucosa of the duodenum and jejunum (Fig. 49–30). The infection is more common in warm climates, but also occurs in temperate zones.

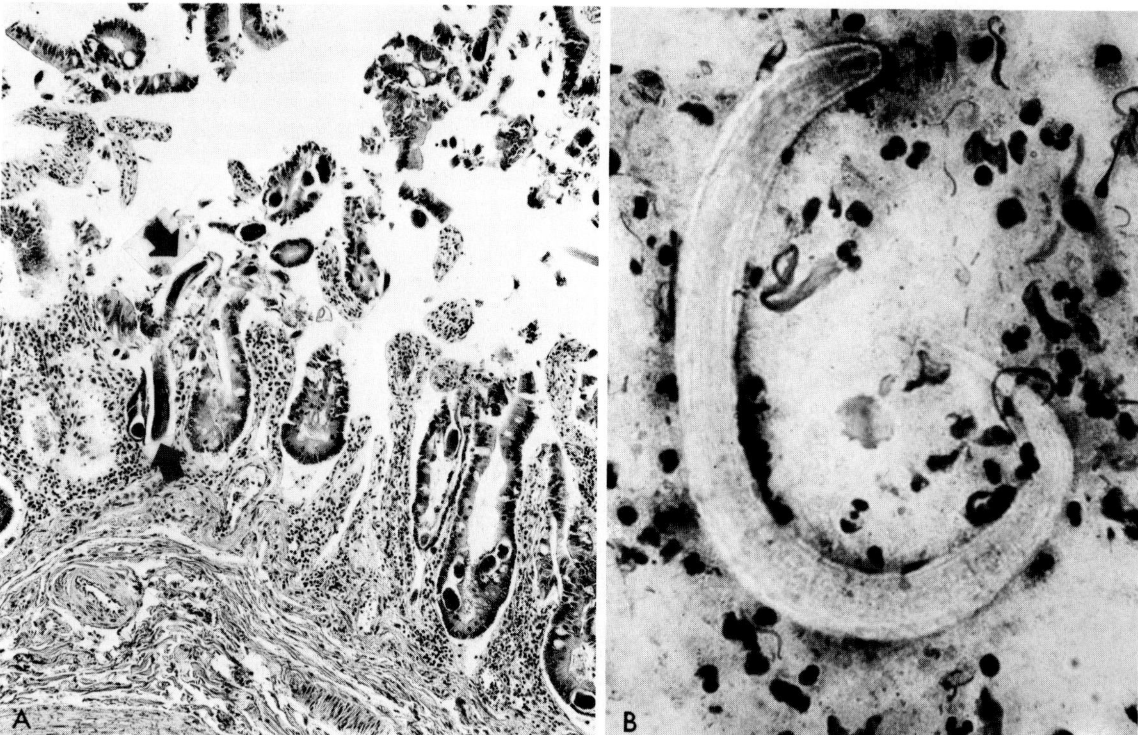

Figure 49–30. *Strongyloides stercoralis.* Patient with massive strongyloidiasis. *A,* Adult female (arrows) and eggs in the duodenal mucosa (×80). *B,* Larva in sputum smear (×470).

6

The small parasitic female is 2 mm long and reproduces parthenogenetically. There is no parasitic male in the vertebrate phase of the cycle. The female lays eggs deep in the mucosa. These develop rhabditiform larvae, which hatch and find their way into the intestinal lumen to be passed with the patient's stools. Therefore, eggs are almost never found in the stools. Larvae, if deposited in appropriate areas, will mature to infective filariform larvae in a short time. Infective larvae, penetrate the skin and migrate via the circulatory system to the lungs, then migrate to the small intestine and grow to adult females. Under certain circumstances, larvae in soil may develop a free-living generation in which there are male and female adults, eggs, and larvae.

The clinical manifestations of strongyloidiasis are variable (Milder, 1981). As with hookworm, parasites in the skin may produce irritation with pruritus and redness at the site of entry, and migration of large numbers of larvae through the lungs may produce a Loeffler syndrome with peripheral eosinophilia (Purtilo, 1974).

The intestinal phase of the infection produces no symptoms in the great majority of cases. However, some patients may have gastrointestinal symptoms varying from a mild to severe diarrhea, and some may develop a malabsorption syndrome.

Strongyloidiasis may persist for over 40 years and recently has been recognized as a continuing problem in allied troops who were prisoners of the Japanese during World War II (Gill, 1979; Grove, 1980). The females live for several months; thus, persistence of infection for years is a result of autoinfection. Rhabditiform larvae in intestinal contents sometimes develop into infective filariform larvae which penetrate the mucosa, reach the circulation, and complete the life cycle. A second mechanism is for filariform larvae to develop in fecal material in the perianal area and penetrate the skin. In the normal patient, the chronic infection is not heavy, and principal symptoms are urticaria or linear cutaneous rashes (larva currens).

In immunocompromised patients, internal autoinfection may become quite severe (hyperinfection) and is often fatal (Igra-Siegman, 1981). Severe pneumonitis is often the presenting manifestation and septicemia is a frequent complication. There may be marked diarrhea and enteritis. Patients who have lived in endemic areas should be screened for *Strongyloides* before receiving immunosuppressive therapy.

Strongyloidiasis is generally diagnosed by the recovery and identification of the typical rhabditiform larvae in the stools (Fig. 49–29). Morphology of larvae must be carefully studied to be certain that they are *Strongyloides* larvae. *Strongyloides* rhabditiform larvae have a short buccal cavity and a prominent genital primordium, whereas hookworm rhabditiform larvae have a long buccal cavity and an indistinct genital primordium. *Strongyloides* filariform larvae have a notched tail and an esophagus approximately half the length of the body. In fresh saline mounts the moving parasites may be easily detected under low power. If infective larvae are found in a recently passed stool sample, then the diagnosis of superinfection is warranted (Eveland, 1975).

Finally, there are cases in which the infection is suspected clinically and the laboratory cannot demonstrate the parasite in repeated fecal examinations. In these cases, examination of duodenal aspirates or duodenal material scraped from a swallowed string (Beal, 1970) may be helpful, or the Baerman concentration technique for stools may be used (Melvin, 1982). In hyperinfection, larvae may be found in smears of pulmonary secretions (Yassin, 1980).

Trematodes

Trematodes or flukes are platyhelminths (flattened dorsoventrally). They are hermaphroditic except for the schistosomes, which have separate sexes. Mature worms vary in length from 1 mm *(Metagonimus)* to 70 mm *(Fasciolopsis)*. There are two suckers: one oral, through which the digestive tract opens, and one ventral for attachment. There are male and female reproductive organs and the cuticle may be smooth or rough depending on species.

The adult hermaphroditic flukes infecting man live in intestine, lungs, or biliary tree. The eggs are operculate and may be unembryonated or contain larvae when laid depending on the species. Eggs reach the exterior environment in the stool, urine, or sputum. Trematodes complete their life cycles in fresh water and require two intermediate hosts. The first are usually specific molluscs and the second are plants, crabs, fish, ants, etc. Disposal of feces so that trematode larval stages reach water, as well as availability of appropriate intermediate hosts, are important factors in perpetuating the infections. Dietary customs must allow the infective stages to be ingested by man for the life cycle to be completed.

Human trematode infections occur in the tropical and subtropical areas of the world, with different areas having different types of trematodes. There is no single place where all of these infections co-exist in man. In spite of control campaigns, some are spreading because of man-made environmental changes, such as dams and irrigation systems. The symptomatology varies depending upon the number of worms parasitizing the host at a given time, the tissues and organs involved, and the host response. Many infections are asymptomatic.

Diagnosis is established by demonstrating eggs in fecal specimens. Direct mounts and formalin-ether concentration are useful for all trematodes. Zinc sulfate flotation methods are less satisfactory for fluke eggs.

Fasciolopsis buski. This trematode occurs naturally in pigs, other animals, and man in China and some other countries of Southeast Asia. The parasite is a fleshy worm measuring up to 70 mm long by 20 mm wide and 3 mm thick.

The worms live attached to the duodenal and jejunal mucosa. The characteristic eggs are found in the stools (Fig. 49–31) and require a long maturation period in fresh water, after which they release an embryo that seeks a particular species of snail. In the snail, the parasite gives rise to numerous larval forms that leave the molluscan and encyst on water plants. When these plants are ingested by appropriate hosts, the parasites

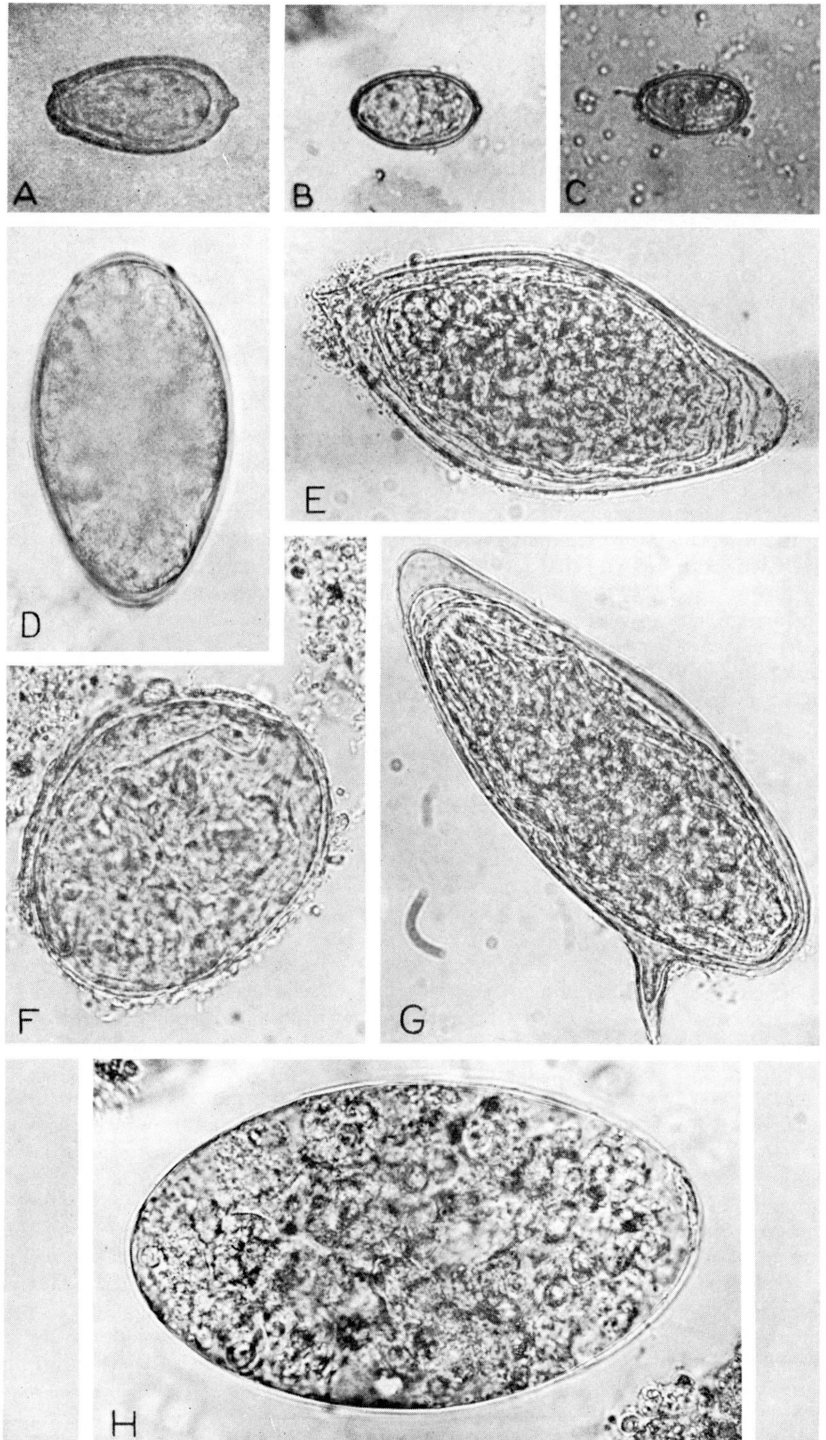

Figure 49–31. Trematode eggs. *A,* Liver fluke, *Clonorchis sinensis. B, Heterophyes heterophyes. C, Metagonimus yokogawai. D,* Lung fluke, *Paragonimus westermani. E,* Blood fluke, *Schistosoma haematobium. F,* Oriental blood fluke, *Schistosoma japonicum. G,* Manson blood fluke, *Schistosoma mansoni. H,* Large intestinal fluke, *Fasciolopsis buski.* All figures ×500 except *A,* which is ×830. (*A* courtesy of Dr. E. C. Faust, in Brenemann: Practice of Pediatrics, W. F. Prior Co.; *B* and *C* courtesy of Lt. L. W. Shatterly, MSC, School of Aviation Medicine, Gunter AFB, Alabama. All others courtesy of Dr. R. L. Roudabush, Ward's Natural Science Establishment, Rochester, New York; photos by T. Romaniak.)

grow to adulthood in the intestine in approximately three months.

The symptomatology is related to the number of worms. Ulceration of the superficial mucosa and obstruction can occur if there are enough worms, but apparently most of the symptomatology is due to "toxic" effects. Diarrhea and epigastric pain are the main presenting symptoms, but anorexia, nausea, and vomiting can occur accompanied by eosinophilia. The infection may be asymptomatic.

The diagnosis is made by finding eggs in the stools. The oval, operculate eggs measure 130 to 140 μ by 80 to 85 μ and are unembryonated. The shell is of moderate thickness and does not have other distinctive structures. Differentiation from *Fasciola* eggs (see below) is generally not possible, but they can be differentiated from *Echinostoma* spp. eggs because the latter are smaller.

Heterophyes spp. and Metagonimus spp. These two genera of trematodes include a number of species represented by minute worms measuring 1 to 3 mm long. Both groups have several species that may infect man, usually living attached to the mucosa of the small intestine by means of the ventral sucker. The operculate eggs are passed with the stools. The life cycle requires a molluscan as the first intermediate host and a fresh water fish as the second. Infection occurs after ingestion of uncooked fish.

The clinical manifestations vary with the number of worms present. There are minute areas of inflammation at the attachment sites, and diarrhea and abdominal pain may be present.

The diagnosis is established by finding the embryonated, operculate eggs which measure less than 30 by 17 μ. These eggs may be difficult or impossible to differentiate from those of *Clonorchis* and *Opisthorchis* spp. (Fig. 49–31).

Fasciola spp. There are at least two species of *Fasciola* that parasitize man: *F. hepatica* and *F. gigantica*. Both are parasites of domestic and wild animals, such as cattle, sheep, and goats, and accidentally of man. *F. hepatica* has a worldwide distribution, while *F. gigantica* is restricted to Africa, Asia, and Hawaii.

The adult parasites live in the biliary tree where they lay eggs that are passed in feces. After developing in water and following a life cycle similar to that of *Fasciolopsis* (see above), the infective larvae encyst on aquatic plants such as water chestnuts. When ingested, the infective larvae are released from their cysts and penetrate through the intestinal wall into the peritoneal cavity. They migrate to the liver, bore through the liver capsule and parenchyma, and finally reach the bile ducts, where they mature and live.

The young larvae produce little or no symptomatology during migration. In the liver they elicit an inflammatory response in the biliary ducts with hyperplasia of the epithelium and eventually fibrosis of the ducts. The bile drainage may be slowed and bile salt precipitation may result in stone formation. Eosinophilia may be present in the early stages, especially during larval migration.

The diagnosis is established by finding eggs in stools. The unembryonated, operculate eggs measure 130 to 150 μ by 63 to 90 μ and cannot be distinguished from those of *Fasciolopsis* (Fig. 49–31). Care must be taken to differentiate between a real parasitism and a spurious presence of eggs resulting from ingestion of infected liver. These can be differentiated by advising the patient to abstain from ingesting liver for three days or more and then repeating the stool examination. If eggs are still found, infection is present.

Clonorchis sinensis and Opisthorchis spp. These closely related trematodes inhabit the biliary system of man and other carnivorous mammals, such as cats and dogs. Many authors consider *Clonorchis* to be synonymous with *Opisthorchis* and call all *Opisthorchis*. *Clonorchis sinensis* occurs mainly in Japan, Korea, China, Taiwan, and Vietnam. *Opisthorchis* spp. are found mainly in central and eastern Europe, as well as in Turkey and Siberia, but there are also foci in Vietnam, and they have been recorded sporadically in India and Japan. The parasites are up to 25 mm long and produce small eggs that enter the duodenum with the bile and are passed in stools. After a cycle in the molluscan first intermediate host, the parasite enters muscles of one of several species of fresh water fish, where infective larvae develop. Infection is acquired by the ingestion of uncooked fish. After excystation in the duodenum, the infective larvae migrate via the ampulla of Vater and common bile ducts into bile ducts of the liver where they mature and live.

The infection in man is generally asymptomatic or very mild (Strauss, 1962); however, large numbers of parasites produce a variety of gastrointestinal disturbances.

The diagnosis is made by recovering the embryonated eggs from stools (Fig. 49–31). Eggs measure 23 to 35 μ by 12 to 20 μ, and the eggs of *Opisthorchis* cannot be differentiated from those of *Clonorchis*. These eggs are difficult to differentiate from those of the *Heterophyes/Metagonimus* group. Eggs of *Clonorchis/Opisthorchis* often have a hook on the abopercular end and are narrower at the end with the flattened operculum. *Heterophyes/Metagonimus* do not have the hook and are wider and more rounded at the opercular end. Specific differentiation of the eggs is not always possible, and a generic diagnosis of *Clonorchis/Opisthorchis/Heterophyes/Metagonimus* spp. may be reported.

Paragonimus spp. There are several species of *Paragonimus* that may parasitize the lungs of man and other carnivores. The first species to be described was *P. westermani,* which is found in Japan, Korea, Formosa, China, Manchuria, the Philippines, and Southeast Asia. Isolated cases of *Paragonimus* infection have been reported in other places such as Africa and South, Central, and North America. Some of these cases have been caused by *Paragonimus* spp. other than *P. westermani.*

The adult parasites measure up to 12 mm by 6 mm and live in the lungs, where they are encapsulated by the host's fibrous reaction. Usually each "capsule" measures less than 20 mm in diameter and contains two or three adult worms bathed by fluid. There is usually a communication between the capsule and the bronchi through which the eggs find their way into the respiratory tree. The eggs are generally passed in the stools, but may reach the environment in expectorated sputum. The parasite needs a molluscan as first intermediate host and crabs or crayfish as the second. Infective larvae encyst in the muscles of these second intermediate hosts and, if uncooked, infection follows their ingestion. Larvae are released in the stomach and migrate through the intestinal wall into the peritoneal cavity, reaching the lungs after boring through the diaphragm.

Symptoms may be caused by larvae migrating through the tissues or by adults established in the lungs. Light infections are generally asymptomatic. The onset of the disease is usually associated with slight chills, fever, and high eosinophilia. Once the worms are well established in the lungs, the main symptoms are those of chronic cough with abundant mucus production and episodes of hemoptysis. Radiographs vary considerably but may show nodular shadows, calcifications, or patchy infiltrations. If the eggs are not passed via the bronchial tree, they are deposited in the pulmonary parenchyma where they may cause an extensive granulomatous reaction. The parasites do not always successfully reach the lungs and have been found in many other locations, including peritoneum, subcutaneous tissues, and brain.

Diagnosis is made by finding the typical eggs in either stools or sputum (Fig. 49–31). The operculate, unembryonated eggs measure 80 to 120 μ by 48 to 60 μ and have a moderately thick shell. The operculum is flattened and is usually set off from the rest of the shell by prominent shoulders. The abopercular end is sometimes thickened but does not have a knob. Size allows ready distinction from the eggs of *D. latum* and *Fasciola* or *Fasciolopsis*.

Schistosomes. These trematodes inhabit blood vessels of many animals, including man. They have separate male and female worms. Man is infected by at least four species or species complexes *(S. mansoni, S. japonicum, S. mekongi,* and *S. haematobium).* Each species complex constitutes several related species, which are difficult to differentiate morphologically. Schistosomes are the most important trematodes in man in terms of incidence and severity of infection.

The adult female parasites are slender, measuring up to 26 mm by 0.5 mm. The males are slightly shorter and have a longitudinal canal resulting from the infolding of the lateral aspects of the body toward the center. The female takes up residence in this canal early in development, and the worms stay together in this fashion for the rest of their lives. The adult parasites live in the smaller venules of the mesenteric and vesicle plexuses (Fig. 49–32) where they elicit little or no inflammatory reaction. The female deposits eggs in the smallest venules of the intestine or the bladder wall near the superficial layers of the mucosa. The eggs elicit a marked inflammatory reaction with both mononuclear and polymorphonuclear cellular infiltrates and formation of microabscesses. These usually rupture into the lumen allowing the eggs to be excreted in feces or urine.

The eggs develop as they move through the tissues

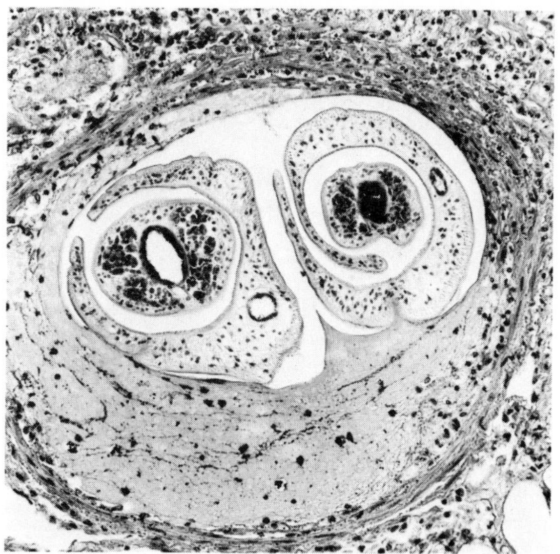

Figure 49–32. *Schistosoma mansoni.* Cross-section of adults in mesenteric vein. Note the female at the center, in the male's gynecophorous canal (×120).

and are fully embryonated when they are passed. After reaching fresh water, they hatch; then the swimming larvae must find an appropriate fresh water snail as intermediate host. In the snail, a complicated proliferative life cycle occurs, ending with the liberation of many thousands of small larvae known as cercariae. Cercariae swim freely in the water for only a few hours. If they contact susceptible hosts, they actively penetrate through the skin.

After penetration, the parasites enter the circulation and pass through the lungs to establish themselves in the liver for a short period of maturation, then migrate via the portal system to the mesenteric or vesicle venules where sexual maturity occurs and oviposition starts.

The infection is similar for all species of human schistosomes in that disease results from the eggs rather than from the adult worms. The parasite attempts to shed as many eggs as possible into the external environment; however, some eggs are trapped in the tissues, and the host's reaction to the egg antigens results in microabscesses that can progress to granulomas and eventual fibrosis. The granuloma formation has been related to hypersensitivity reaction in the host. Moreover, some eggs may be carried by the portal vein to the liver (Fig. 49–33), where they lead to the development of granulomas that can coalesce, resulting in so-called "pipe stem" fibrosis of the liver and eventually in portal hypertension with its associated manifestations.

Diagnosis is usually established by demonstrating eggs in fecal or urine specimens by direct mount or formalin-ether concentration. Zinc sulfate concentration is not satisfactory for the heavy schistosome eggs. Eggs may sometimes be demonstrated in biopsies of rectal or bladder tissue either by crush preparation or

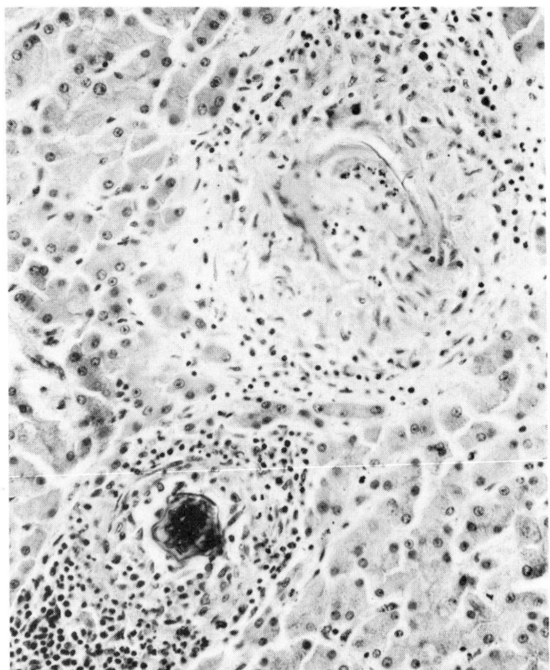

Figure 49–33. *Schistosoma mansoni.* Recent granuloma with egg in liver. Note the miracidium inside the egg and collapse of the shell due to fixation. The upper granuloma corresponds to an older one, and there are only rests of the egg (×200).

by section, and they may sometimes be found in liver biopsies. Eggs may be difficult to speciate in sections because of folds and shrinkage. If eggs are not found by routine fecal or urine examination, hatching may be attempted. This method may be especially helpful in light infections or in chronic infections in which many eggs are trapped in fibrous tissue and few reach the lumen. Feces mixed with distilled water are placed in a flask that is painted black or wrapped with foil to keep out light, with only the neck or a side arm exposed to a bright light. In the presence of water, the eggs hatch and the swimming larvae seek light in the neck or side arm. With a hand lens they can be detected swimming near the surface and removed with a capillary pipette for more detailed examination. Species cannot be identified with this technique.

Serologic tests may be helpful in screening persons who have returned to the United States from endemic areas or in patients with negative stool or urine examinations. Many serologic techniques have been studied, but currently the indirect immunofluorescence (IIF), using frozen sections of male adult worms, is used by the Centers for Disease Control (CDC). A titer of 1:16 is considered significant. The test is reported as positive or negative because there is no correlation between titer and stage of the disease. In occasional patients, the circumoval precipitation tests (COP) may be helpful.

Tests to detect schistosome antigens have recently been described, but it is too early to know how useful they will be.

Schistosoma mansoni. *S. mansoni* occurs in Africa, especially in the tropical areas and the Nile delta. In the Western Hemisphere it occurs in Brazil, Venezuela, Surinam, and the West Indies. Puerto Rico has several foci, and there are many infected Puerto Ricans who have moved to the United States.

S. mansoni adults live in the mesenteric venous plexuses of the large intestine, and the symptomatology they produce depends on the stage of the infection. During the prepatent period, there may be urticarial skin rash, fever, eosinophilia, or diarrhea, and the liver may be enlarged and tender. After the parasites lodge in the mesenteric veins, there may be abdominal pain and dysentery with abundant blood and mucus in the stools. During this period, the characteristic eggs are usually found in stools. These symptoms eventually subside and the chronic phase of the disease with granuloma formation and fibrosis ensues. The chronic phase can last for many years depending on the number of worms present, occasionally resulting in liver fibrosis and the portal hypertension syndrome. Eggs measure 116 to 180 μ by 45 to 58 μ and are oval, with a large distinctive lateral spine that protrudes from the side of the egg near one end (Fig. 49–31). If the spine is not visible, the egg may be rotated by tapping the coverslip. Movement of the larva within the egg may be evident in unfixed material if the larva is viable.

Schistosoma japonicum. *S. japonicum* occurs in Japan, China, Korea, and the Philippines and causes disease that is clinically similar to *S. mansoni* in most aspects. Eggs readily reach the liver, and fibrosis with portal hypertension is a common complication of chronic *S. japonicum* infection.

The eggs are broadly oval, measuring 75 to 90 μ by 60 to 68 μ and often have a characteristic rudimentary lateral spine, which may be difficult to demonstrate.

Schistosoma mekongi. This is a newly recognized species that occurs only in the lower Mekong River basin (Bruce, 1980). It is differentiated from *S. japonicum* by several biological characteristics and egg morphology. The eggs are generally smaller (60 to 70 μ by 52 to 62 μ) than those of *S. japonicum,* but they are otherwise indistinguishable.

Schistosoma haematobium. This trematode occurs on the African continent, where its distribution includes both the tropical and subtropical areas. The Nile river banks and delta have a particularly high incidence. There are also foci in the Middle East and Madagascar.

The parasites migrate via the hemorrhoidal veins to the venous plexuses of the urinary bladder, prostate, uterus, and vagina. One of the earliest and most common symptoms of the infection is hematuria, especially at the end of micturition. In the chronic stages there may be pelvic pain and bladder colic with increased desire to urinate. Accumulation of eggs in the bladder wall results in hypertrophy of the epithelium, squamous metaplasia, and marked fibrosis, which are responsible for the above symptoms and may lead to urinary obstruction. An association between urinary schistosomiasis and squamous cell carcinoma of the urinary bladder has been repeatedly noted, but there is not as yet conclusive proof of a cause-and-effect relationship.

The eggs are elongated, measuring 112 to 180 μ by 40 to 70 μ, and have a terminal spine (Fig. 49–31). Examining urine sediment may allow detection of eggs. Late morning specimens are usually best.

Swimmer's Itch. This entity, also known as schistosome cercarial dermatitis, is produced by the cutaneous penetration of cercariae of non-human schistosomes. Generally, they are cercariae of blood flukes of birds and mammals and may affect persons exposing skin to fresh or salt water. In all these cases, man is a non-compatible host and the life cycle cannot be completed. Probably some degree of prior sensitization to the cercariae is required. The cercariae apparently cannot penetrate beyond the superficial layers of the skin. The disease is a dermatitis with erythema and urticaria which can progress to the formation of papules. The reaction is most intense within 48 to 72 hours after exposure to contaminated waters and eventually subsides spontaneously. The disease has a worldwide distribution, and it is well known in the United States. The diagnosis is established on clinical grounds.

Cestodes

Cestodes (tapeworms) are platyhelminth parasites characterized by a body or strobila composed of segments called proglottids and an anterior portion known as a scolex. Tapeworm scolices have various structures for attachment to the intestinal mucosa depending on species. These include suckers, grooves or bothria, and a rostellum with hooks. Behind the scolex is the neck from which new proglottids develop. Each proglottid has one or two complete sets of male and female organs. Proglottids develop from immature to mature egg-producing, with those farthest from the neck being most developed. In some species there is active oviposition, but in most species eggs are stored in the uterus, which thus becomes gravid. A prominent structure usually visible with the naked eye is the genital pore where the male and female organs meet. The adults parasitize the small intestine of vertebrates. Size varies considerably from species barely visible with the naked eye to species 20 to 25 feet long. Adult and larval stages of cestodes contain basophilic laminated bodies known as calcareous corpuscles, which aid in recognition of cestode tissue (Wardle, 1952).

Eggs are passed with the stools and usually require one, two, or more intermediate hosts for the asexual larval stages to develop. Intermediate hosts include both invertebrates and vertebrates.

Cestode larval stages of various types develop to the infective stage in the tissues of the intermediate host. The life cycle is completed when infective larvae are ingested by the appropriate definitive host. The types of cestode larval stages that may infect man are cysticercus, hydatid, coenurus, and sparganum, and the infections in man are known as cysticercosis, hydatidosis, coenurosis, and sparganosis.

Taeniarhynchus saginatus (=Taenia saginata) and Taenia solium. Man is the sole definitive host for *T. saginatus,* the beef tapeworm, and *T. solium,* the pork tapeworm. *T. solium* is common in Eastern Europe, Latin America, China, Pakistan, and India, and cases found in the United States are imported. *T. saginatus* has a wider distribution with a greater incidence in the Middle East, Africa, Europe, and Latin America, and it occurs occasionally in the United States.

Both parasites live in the small intestine and produce large numbers of eggs that are stored in the uterus. Eggs reach the stools and the outside when gravid proglottids drop from the strobila. Proglottids either rupture in the intestine, freeing the eggs (usual in *T. solium),* or are passed with the stools intact and still active (usual in *T. saginatus).* When the appropriate intermediate hosts, such as cattle in *T. saginatus* and pigs in *T. solium,* swallow the eggs, the larvae (cysticerci) develop in the tissues. After ingestion of poorly cooked contaminated meat, the cysticercus develops into an adult in the small intestine of man, the definitive host (usually only one adult in each infection).

The symptomatology produced by both of these parasites in man is minimal, but gastrointestinal disturbances have been described. A striking biological difference of practical importance is that *T. solium* eggs, if ingested by man, can develop into cysticerci (see below).

Diagnosis is established by finding eggs in the stools using direct or concentration techniques, or in the perianal folds with the cellophane tape technique. The eggs are spherical and measure 31 to 43 μ in diameter (Fig. 49–34). The shell is thick, radially striated, and contains a six-hooked embryo. Unfortunately, the eggs of *T. saginatus* and *T. solium* cannot be differentiated morphologically and are reported as "*Taeniarhynchus* or *Taenia* eggs."

Grossly, both parasites have a similar strobila up to 7 meters in length. However, on close examination the uterus of *T. saginatus* has 15 to 20 lateral branches, whereas *T. sodium* has 7 to 13 lateral branches (Fig. 49–35). Microscopically, the scolex of *T. solium* has a rostellum with two rows of hooks, while that of *T. saginatus* has no rostellum and no hooks.

In many instances passed proglottids are brought to the laboratory for identification. Careful handling and clearing of these specimens overnight in glycerol should be done so that the branches of the uterus can be counted and a specific identification can be made.

Dipylidium caninum. This tapeworm is worldwide in distribution, and dogs are usually the definitive hosts.

The life cycle involves an arthropod intermediate host, usually a flea, which ingests the eggs and in which the infective larvae develop. The definitive host acquires the infection by ingesting a flea infected with the larval stage. Larvae attach to the small intestinal mucosa and mature to adult parasites, which measure approximately 70 cm in length. The proglottids are barrel-shaped with a genital pore and sex organs on each side. The uterus of the gravid proglottid consists of numerous small capsules each containing 8 to 20 eggs (Fig. 49–35).

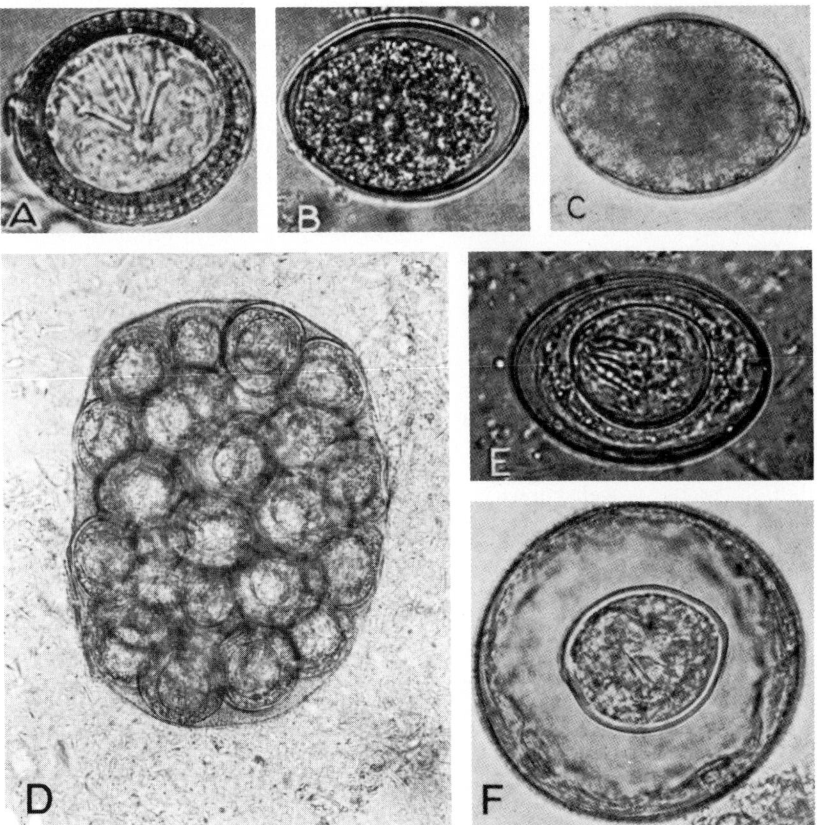

Figure 49–34. Cestode eggs in stools. *A, Taeniarhynchus saginatus* or *Taenia solium* (×750). *B* and *C,* Broad tapeworm or fish tapeworm of man, *Diphyllobothrium latum* (×500). *D, Dipylidium caninum* egg pack; Note the membrane surrounding the eggs (×300). *E,* Dwarf tapeworm, *Hymenolepis nana* (×750). *F,* Rat tapeworm, *Hymenolepis diminuta* (×650). (*B* courtesy of Lt. L. W. Shetterby, School of Aviation Medicine, Gunter AFB, Alabama; *A, C, E,* and *F,* courtesy of Dr. R. L. Roudabush, Ward's Natural Science Establishment, Rochester, New York; photos by T. Romaniak.)

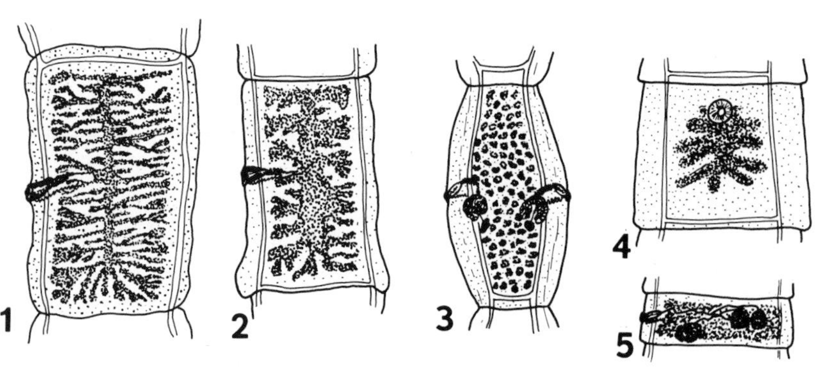

Figure 49–35. Gravid proglottids of different human tapeworms. *1, Taeniarhynchus saginatus. 2, Taenia solium. 3, Dipylidium caninum. 4, Diphyllobothrium latum. 5, Hymenolepis spp.*

The parasitism results in little or no symptomatology. The diagnosis is made by finding the spherical eggs, measuring 24 to 40 μ, singly or in packets, and containing a six-hooked embryo (Fig. 49–34). Sometimes a segment of the strobila is passed, and it can be identified by the double genital pores and the egg packets.

Hymenolepis nana. *H. nana,* known as the dwarf tapeworm of man, has worldwide distribution and is the most frequently found tapeworm in the United States. The parasite has a delicate strobila measuring up to 40 mm in length, genital pores are located on one side, and the scolex has a rostellum with hooks. The life cycle has a dual pathway, which is of practical importance. The first is a direct type of development occurring when the host ingests freshly passed eggs. After the embryos are released from the eggs in the intestine, they penetrate the mucosal villi, where development to infective larvae occurs. The larvae drop into the lumen and develop to adults in a number that correlates with the number of eggs ingested. The tissue phase, though only of a few days' duration, is apparently sufficient to confer a strong immunity in the host (Heyneman, 1963).

The second type of development is infrequent and is similar to that of *H. diminuta* in that infection is acquired by ingesting an infected arthropod (see below). Therefore, the host does not develop immunity to the larval parasite and when adults start oviposition, the eggs may hatch in the intestine, invade the mucosa, and undergo a development similar to that described above, with infection by many thousands of worms. This mechanism has been demonstrated in experimental animals and has been proposed as an explanation for the massive infections sometimes seen in man.

Symptomatic infection develops in patients with large numbers of worms attached to the small intestinal mucosa, with non-specific general and gastrointestinal symptoms. The diagnosis is made by the recovery from stools of the oval colorless eggs, which measure 30 to 43 μ in diameter (Fig. 49–34) and have a medium-thick shell. They contain a six-hooked embryo when passed and have polar thickenings at each end from which polar filaments arise. Portions of the strobila or complete worms may occasionally be passed.

Hymenolepis diminuta. This cestode infects rats, mice, and other rodents, and is found throughout the world. Sporadic cases have been reported in man in almost every country.

Embryonated eggs passed in stools are ingested by several species of insect larvae in which the infective *H. diminuta* larvae develop. Accidental ingestion of infected insects results in infection. Adults develop in the small intestine and measure up to 60 cm in length. The strobila is delicate, and all genital pores are located on one side (Fig. 49–35). The scolex has no hooks. Eggs are released when the gravid proglottids detach from the body of the adult worm. Infections are usually asymptomatic, although occasional cases with intestinal symptoms have been reported. The diagnosis is made by finding the characteristic eggs in the feces, 60 to 82 μ by 72 to 86 μ (Fig. 49–34). They are almost spherical with an inner membrane with two rudimentary polar thickenings, but there are no polar filaments. They contain a six-hooked embryo.

Diphyllobothrium spp. This group is composed of large cestodes that infect many wild and domestic carnivores in addition to man (Vik, 1964). They are widely distributed in the temperate zones, especially in central and northern Europe, northern USSR, and central Siberia. In Asia they occur in Manchuria and Japan. In North America the main endemic areas are in the vicinity of the lakes in the northern United States and Canada. An outbreak was recently described in San Francisco (Centers for Disease Control, 1981a). There are isolated foci in Chile, Uganda, and the Middle East.

The parasite inhabits the small intestine and can reach a length of up to 10 meters. The scolex is elongated with a pair of deep longitudinal grooves (bothria) that are distinctive for this group of tapeworms. There is a genital pore located medially and ventrally, and next to it is an opening for oviposition from which unembryonated eggs are passed (Fig. 49–35). They are elongate, measuring 58 to 76 μ by 40 to 51 μ and have an operculum (in contrast to other cestodes). They often have a small, round, knob-like protrusion of the shell on the abopercular (posterior) pole (Fig. 49–34). There are no shoulders adjacent to the operculum.

Eggs are passed in stools and must reach a fresh water stream or lake to continue the life cycle. A first intermediate host may be one of many species of small aquatic arthropods. The second intermediate host is a small fish that ingests the arthropods, and the third intermediate host is a larger fish that ingests the smaller fish. In the muscles of the large fish the larva (sparganum) develops to the infective stage, and the life cycle is completed when it is ingested by any of the definitive hosts in raw or inadequately cooked fish.

There are several species of *Diphyllobothrium* that may parasitize man, but the most common is *D. latum.* These parasites are closely related and differentiation cannot be made on egg morphology.

The symptomatology produced by *Diphyllobothrium* infections is variable. Usually the worms are harbored for many years without appreciable symptomatology. Passage of a portion of the strobila may be what brings the patient to the physician. In northern Europe where the parasite is endemic a small percentage of patients develop findings of vitamin B_{12} deficiency, including megaloblastic anemia. The parasite selectively competes with the host for vitamin B_{12}, which thus accumulates in the worm tissues in large amounts. This syndrome is rarely seen in North America or in endemic foci other than northern Europe.

The diagnosis is made by finding portions of strobila in fecal specimens or by finding eggs in the stools by either direct or concentration methods.

TISSUE HELMINTHS

Nematodes

Filariae. These nematodes are widely distributed in nature, with representatives occurring in almost every vertebrate species. The adults are long and slender, measuring many centimeters in length, and may inhabit almost any tissue (i.e., subcutaneous tissues, lymphatics, blood vessels, peritoneal and pleural cavities, heart, brain, etc.). Some species wander about in tissues, whereas others remain stationary and become encased in a nodular fibrous tissue reaction. Usually, both male and female worms are found together in these tissues. The progeny are microfilariae which are slender, motile embryos found either in the circulating blood or wandering in the subcutaneous tissues, depending upon the species. Microfilariae are not infective to vertebrates but must be ingested by a biting arthropod, usually a mosquito or fly, in which they mature to the infective stage. These infective larvae enter the definitive hosts when the arthropod takes another meal. The larvae migrate to the appropriate location and develop into adults. Maturation requires from two months to a year.

Diagnosis of Filariasis. Geographic location, type of disease, and time of obtaining a specimen may aid in diagnosis, but the actual diagnosis is usually based on identification of microfilariae in blood or material obtained from the skin. Species identification of blood microfilariae is particularly important, as some may cause serious disease while others rarely do. Diagnostic laboratory identification usually uses Giemsa- or hematoxylin-stained thick films, although special, more sensitive procedures, such as membrane filter, Knott's concentration, or saponin lysis, may be useful in some cases. Microfilariae may sometimes be seen moving in direct mounts of blood or tissue fluid.

There are numerous anatomic landmarks in microfilariae, some of which may be demonstrated with special stains, but all of these are not needed for routine identification of common human species.

The principal characteristics that are used in diagnostic laboratories are the presence of a sheath and its staining characteristics, the shape and nuclear distribution in the tail, the size of the cephalic space, and the appearance of the nuclear column. The length is helpful, but it is difficult to measure and is rarely needed in the routine clinical laboratory. *Wuchereria* and *Brugia* microfilariae usually have a nocturnal periodicity, so the blood sample should be drawn between 10 P.M. and 2 A.M. *Loa loa* has a diurnal periodicity, and microfilariae are best found in blood at around noon. *Dipetalonema* and *Mansonella* are characteristically non-periodic. Serologic tests using extracts of *Dirofilaria immitis* as antigen include indirect hemagglutination and flocculation tests, but they allow only a diagnosis of the filarial group rather than the species. Moreover, there is frequent cross-reactivity with other parasites (false positives), as well as many false negatives (Kagan, 1980a, 1980b).

Wuchereria bancrofti. This filarial worm lives in the lymphatic channels (Fig. 49–36), usually those draining the lower extremities (Sasa, 1976). It occurs mainly in central and north Africa, Southeast Asia, India, northern South America, the West Indies, and some South Pacific Islands.

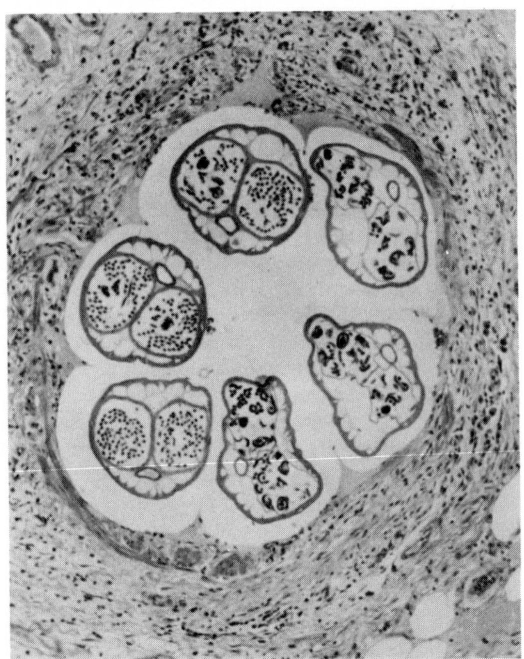

Figure 49–36. *Wuchereria bancrofti.* Cross-section of adult in human lymph node. Note fibrosis surrounding the worm (×120).

The female worms produce microfilariae that enter the blood stream and circulate mainly during the hours of 10 P.M. to 2 A.M. This nocturnal periodicity corresponds to the peak activity of the mosquitoes that serve as vectors, usually species of *Culex, Aedes, Anopheles,* or *Mansonia.* In some Pacific Islands *W. bancrofti* microfilaremia is continuous, although it is higher in the afternoon and is called subperiodic. The clinical manifestations of *Wuchereria* infection vary. People who are in endemic areas for only a short time and get infected usually suffer a few acute bouts of transient lymphangitis and lymphadenopathy, which resolve in a short time without microfilaremia (Beaver, 1970). People who live in endemic areas are continuously re-exposed to the parasite over many years and develop heavy infection. The infection can become a chronic condition with protracted lymphadenopathy and lymphangitis, which may progress to lymphedema and fibrosis with resultant elephantiasis, usually most severe in the lower extremities and male or female genital organs.

Specimens for diagnosis must be obtained at the time when microfilaremia would be expected to occur. The microfilaria of *W. bancrofti* has a sheath that does not stain well with Giemsa stain. The tail is pointed, and there are no nuclei in the tip. The cephalic space is not as long as it is wide and the nuclei in the nuclear column are distinct (Fig. 49–37).

Brugia malayi. This is similar in most respects to *W. bancrofti* but has a more restricted geographical

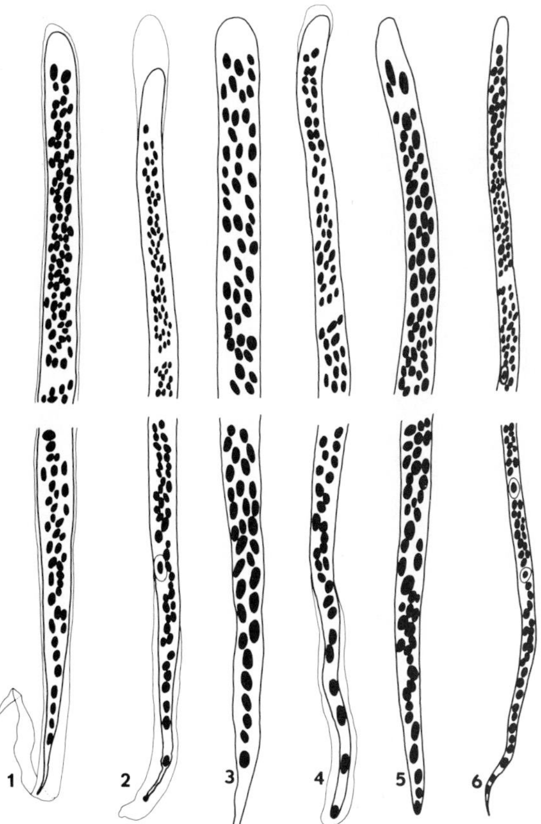

Figure 49–37. Anterior and posterior ends of microfilariae most commonly found in man. *1, Wuchereria bancrofti. 2, Brugia malayi. 3, Onchocerca volvulus. 4, Loa loa. 5, Dipetalonema perstans. 6, Mansonella ozzardi.* All camera lucida drawings.

distribution, occurring mainly in India, Southeast Asia, Korea, the Philippines, and Japan. The disease in man is usually milder and more frequently involves the lymphatics of the upper extremities (Sasa, 1976).

The microfilaria of *B. malayi* has a sheath that stains well with Giemsa stain. The tail has a swelling at the tip and has two solitary nuclei in the tail, beyond the end of the nuclear column, which may be called terminal and subterminal nuclei. They may be smaller than other nuclei and are not always seen. The cephalic space may be much longer than it is wide, and the nuclear column may be blurred in Giemsa stains (Fig. 49–37).

Loa loa. The agent of "loaisis" or "fugitive swellings" is found primarily in the rain forests of Africa, where horse flies of the genus *Chrysops* are the vectors (Sasa, 1976).

The adult worms live in the subcutaneous tissues, where they seem to move freely and produce repeated swellings less than 30 mm in diameter that last two to three days. The parasite elicits high eosinophilia, and the infection has been seen in the United States in people with a history of travel to Africa. The microfilaria of *Loa loa* has a sheath that does not stain with Giemsa stain. The tail has nuclei to the rounded tip. The nuclear column is distinct, and the cephalic space is short (Fig. 49–37).

Dipetalonema perstans and Mansonella ozzardi. Infections by both of these filarial worms are usually asymptomatic in man. *Dipetalonema* infections are found in Africa and the northern part of South America, whereas *Mansonella* is restricted to Central and South America, as well as the West Indies. The vectors of both of these nematodes are "gnats" belonging to the genus *Culicoides.* The adult parasites live in the peritoneal, pleural, or pericardial cavities, and the microfilariae (Fig. 49–37) appear in the peripheral blood at all hours of the day and night. Microfilariae of both species are unsheathed. *M. ozzardi* microfilariae have a thin, pointed tail without nuclei, whereas the tail of *D. perstans* is broad and blunt with nuclei extending to the tip.

Onchocerca volvulus. The filaria causing onchocerciasis lives in the subcutaneous tissues of man, and the microfilariae inhabit the skin. The vectors are small flies belonging to the genus *Simulium. Onchocerca* occurs mainly in Africa, but there are some endemic foci in Central America (Mexico and Guatemala), Colombia, Venezuela, Ecuador, and Brazil (Sasa, 1976).

There are various clinical manifestations of the disease. The adult parasites in the subcutaneous tissues are tightly coiled upon themselves and elicit a host response of fibrosis and inflammation that results in the formation of a hard subcutaneous nodule measuring up to 40 mm in diameter (Fig. 49–38). In general, these nodules are on the upper half of the body in patients in Central America and in the lower half of those in Africa. The main complications arise from the microfilariae that migrate throughout the skin, with greatest numbers near the nodules. There is itching, which can be accompanied by changes in the skin represented by several forms of dermatitis. The microfilariae may damage the eyes, causing keratitis, corneal opacity, and damage to the anterior chamber and iris, thus leading to blindness in a significant percentage of the infected population.

In *Onchocerca* (Fig. 49–37) infections the microfilariae are detected in teased skin snips coverslipped in saline or stained sections. Cases with skin microfilariae in the Western Hemisphere (Central and South America) are usually *Onchocerca.* Those from Africa present more problems, as there are other filaria with skin microfilariae that may infect man but usually do not cause disease.

Dirofilaria spp. Zoonotic filariases have become important in this country because they can result in potentially expensive hospitalization and surgery in some patients. Although several species have caused disease, only the two most likely to be found are discussed here (Beaver, 1965; Orihel, 1965; Gutierrez, 1984).

Dirofilaria immitis, commonly known as the dog heart worm, has a life cycle similar to that of the other filarial worms and is widely distributed in the tropics and subtropics. In the United States it is endemic, especially in the Southeast and Mississippi River basin, although it is also present in other parts

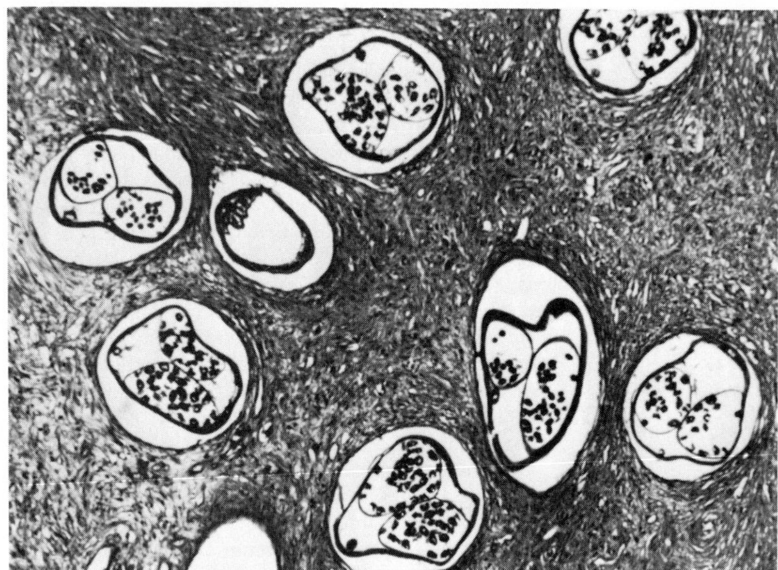

Figure 49–38. *Onchocerca volvulus* nodule. Section showing fibrous tissue with several cross-sections of adult parasite (× 48).

of the country (Ciferri, 1982). In the dog, the adult worm usually lives in the right ventricle and the major branches of the pulmonary artery and may cause chronic heart failure.

In man, accidental infections are probably acquired by the bite of the intermediate host and result in one worm, seldom more, usually lodged in the right heart or pulmonary artery. In man, the worm does not mature and microfilariae are not produced. When the worm dies, it is embolized to a smaller branch of the pulmonary artery, resulting in an infarct that heals and may appear as a coin lesion in a chest radiograph. The patient may undergo resection of the lesion because of suspicion of a malignancy. Microscopic examination reveals the typical cross-sections of the parasite, and if enough morphologic characteristics are evident in the dead parasite, the specific diagnosis can be made (Fig. 49–39). The cuticle is thick and is smooth in the sense that the outer surface has no longitudinal ridges (see below for comparison). The diameter of the worm varies considerably, but it is generally less than 0.4 mm (Beaver, 1965).

Dirofilaria tenuis is usually found in the subcutaneous tissues of the raccoon in the southeastern part of the United States. Accidental infections occur in man and are manifest as small subcutaneous inflammatory nodules. These may be removed surgically. On section the parasite is encased in a marked inflammatory reaction with granulation tissue. The worm usually is dead before its removal. The cuticle measures 5 to 8 μ thick, is delicate, and has characteristic longitudinal ridges that are spaced at about 10 μ intervals. The transverse diameter is usually less than 0.3 mm (Fig. 49–39) (Orihel, 1965).

Trichinella spiralis. Trichinosis in man occurs mainly in temperate zones of the Northern and Southern Hemispheres. In the United States the incidence of trichinosis has been in steady decline, and currently less than 150 cases are reported per year (Centers for Disease Control, 1981b).

The adult *Trichinella* lives in the mucosa of the small intestine of man and other carnivorous animals. The female measures 3 to 4 mm long and deposits larvae measuring 80 to 120 μ, which enter the lymphatics and venules, reach the general circulation, and are distributed throughout the body. In striated muscles, the larvae invade muscle fibers and mature to the infective stage. The larvae will be curled and measure up to 1.0 mm long. They produce muscle damage, and the host's inflammatory response leads to the formation of a fibrous capsule around each larva. Such larvae are often referred to as encysted, though the "cyst" is of host origin. Larvae may remain viable for extended periods of time (years), and "cysts" may eventually become calcified. Ingestion of muscle containing infective larvae by an appropriate host will complete the life cycle. Larvae mature to adults rapidly, and larviposition begins in about one week. Pork and pork products, especially various cured sausages, are the main source of human infection, although bear meat or beef that has been adulterated with pork may be sources. Adequate cooking or extended freezing will destroy larvae.

Symptoms principally relate to intestinal tract, skeletal muscle, or allergic manifestations. The intestinal phase of the infection begins following ingestion of infected meat and may cause nausea, vomiting, diarrhea, and pain depending upon the patient's susceptibility and the number of worms present and may last for several days. Migration of larvae into muscles begins in 10 to 14 days and results in high eosinophilia, fever, muscle pain, and, in some cases, difficulty in breathing, swallowing, and speech. Periorbital edema is frequent and may be associated with photophobia. After the parasites are encysted, there is little symptomatology. Adult worms are usually eliminated from the intestine after two to three weeks by the host's immune response, although corticosteroid therapy may delay this elimination and thus prolong larviposition.

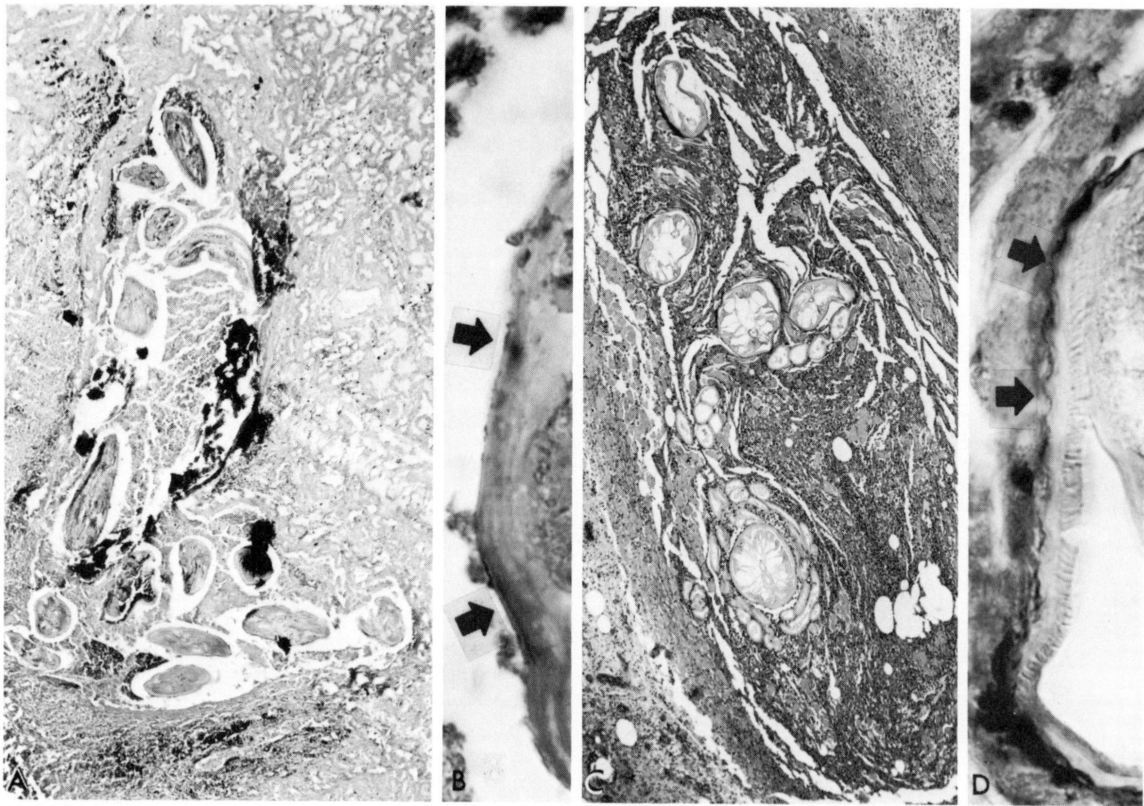

Figure 49–39. Zoonotic filariae in man. *A* and *B*, *Dirofilaria immitis*. *A*, Cross-section of embolized adult worm in human pulmonary artery (×50). *B*, Parasite cuticle showing the smooth outer surface (arrows) (×800). *C* and *D*, *D. tenuis*. *C*, Cross-section of adult in subcutaneous tissue abscess (×50). *D*, Cuticle with characteristic longitudinal ridges (arrows) (×800). (*D. tenuis*, case of Dr. J. Suarez-Hoyos, Tampa, Florida.)

The diagnosis is usually made clinically in the acute stage. Larvae or adults are rarely recovered from stools during the diarrheic phase. During the migration stage, larvae have been occasionally recovered from blood by using a technique such as Knott's concentration.

Clinically, the best clues are a history of exposure, clinical findings of intestinal symptoms, muscle pain, periorbital edema, and eosinophilia. Creatine phosphokinase and other serum enzymes may be elevated. There are often "clusters" of cases with a common infection source. After larval migration to the muscles, the diagnosis may be established by a muscle biopsy, but in light infections larvae may not be detected in multiple sections (Fig. 49–40).

Diagnosis is often established indirectly by serologic tests; some are commercially available. The most commonly used are bentonite flocculation (BF), fluorescent antibody (IIF), and complement fixation (CF). The bentonite flocculation test is very sensitive and usually becomes negative two to three years after an infection; thus, a positive test usually indicates active infection. The test becomes positive after the third week of infection and is most helpful when a fourfold rise in paired sera can be demonstrated. The CF test detects antibodies slightly earlier than the BF test, and the FA is considered to be as good as the BF (Kagan, 1980a, 1980b).

Larva migrans. Larva migrans is produced by the prolonged wandering through the tissues of nematode larvae. If this migration occurs within the layers of the skin where tracks may be seen, then the entity is called cutaneous larva migrans. The syndrome is produced by several human and non-human species of hookworm and *Strongyloides* and is manifested by tortuous, markedly pruritic red tracks on the skin.

Visceral larva migrans is produced by larvae from non-human nematodes, especially the dog ascarid, *Toxocara canis,* but also occasionally *T. cati.* When man accidentally ingests infective eggs, the larvae hatch and penetrate into the circulation. In man, an abnormal host, the larvae are unable to complete their cycle, and there is prolonged migration of the larvae through various tissues and organs (Beaver, 1952, 1969). The patient is usually a child between 1½ and 4 years of age who presents with a clinical picture of failure to thrive, low-grade fever, hepatomegaly, and sometimes pulmonary infiltrates. Laboratory studies reveal hypergammaglobulinemia and high eosinophilia (up to 80 per cent in half of the cases) with absolute eosinophil counts greater than 20,000/cu mm.

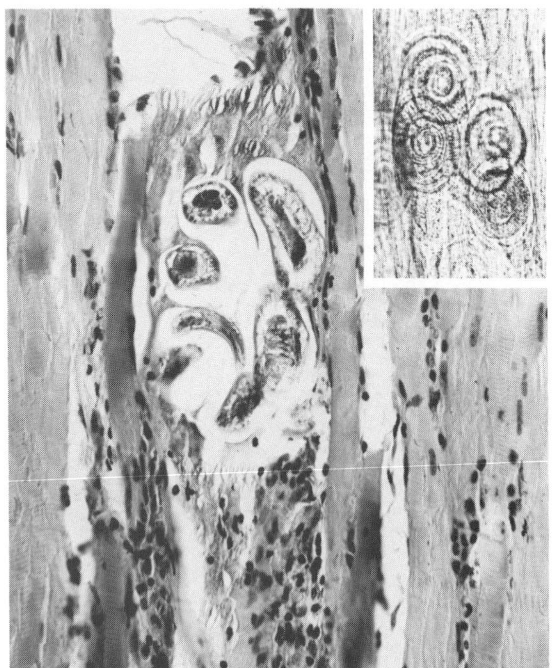

Figure 49–40. *Trichinella spiralis,* cross-section of larva in deltoid muscle (×200). Inset shows whole larvae in wet muscle preparation (×63).

The diagnosis is difficult to confirm because the parasite usually cannot be recovered. Open liver biopsy may show larvae of 18 μ diameter surrounded by an inflammatory granuloma (Fig. 49–41), but this procedure is seldom done because of the risk.

Serologic tests may aid in establishing the diagnosis. Different methods vary in sensitivity and specificity. The enzyme-linked immunoassay (ELISA) using embryonated egg extracts as antigen (Cypess, 1977) offers much better sensitivity and specificity, and cross-reacting *Ascaris* antibodies can be removed by preadsorption. In visceral larva migrans, a significant titer is 1:32, whereas if ocular toxocariasis is suspected, a titer of 1:8 is significant (Kagan, 1980a, 1980b).

Angiostrongylus cantonensis. The agent of angiostrongyloidiasis or eosinophilic meningoencephalitis in man is a nematode up to 25 mm in length that usually lives in the pulmonary artery of rodents. Man is an incidental host. The parasite occurs mainly in Southeast Asia and the Pacific Islands, including Hawaii.

Female worms lay eggs in the pulmonary parenchyma, where they hatch. Larvae migrate up the trachea to the gastrointestinal tract and the stools. The larvae develop to the infective stage in slugs or land snails. Ingestion of the molluscan by the rodent results in the infection. Larvae enter the circulation, then migrate to the brain, where they mature. They then migrate to the lungs.

In man, who acquires the infection by eating the uncooked molluscan on contaminated vegetables, the entire life cycle is usually not completed, but central nervous system invasion occurs. Infection produced by the larvae may present as meningitis with a high spinal fluid eosinophilia. It is seldom fatal. The few cases that have been autopsied have shown typical immature *Angiostrongylus* worms in the brain and spinal cord. The diagnosis is made clinically and the spinal fluid eosinophilia is highly suggestive. The infection may occur in epidemic form if there has been a common exposure.

A new species, *Angiostrongylus costaricensis,* has been recognized in Central and South America (Loria-Cortez, 1980). It lives in the mesenteric arteries of the ileum and cecum and produces an acute disease, usually in children. Adults, eggs, and larvae are found in surgical specimens and larvae in stools.

Cestodes

Several diseases, sometimes serious, may result from the development of cestode larval stages in tissues of man.

Cysticercus. This is a cyst with a single inverted scolex representing the larval stage of a large number of tapeworms, including *Taenia* spp. The cysticerci of *T. saginatus* develop in cattle and those of *T. solium* in pigs and are known as *Cysticercus bovis* and *C. cellulosae,* respectively. They may be differentiated because the cysticercus of *T. solium* has a characteristic rostellum with hooks, similar to the adult, and *T.*

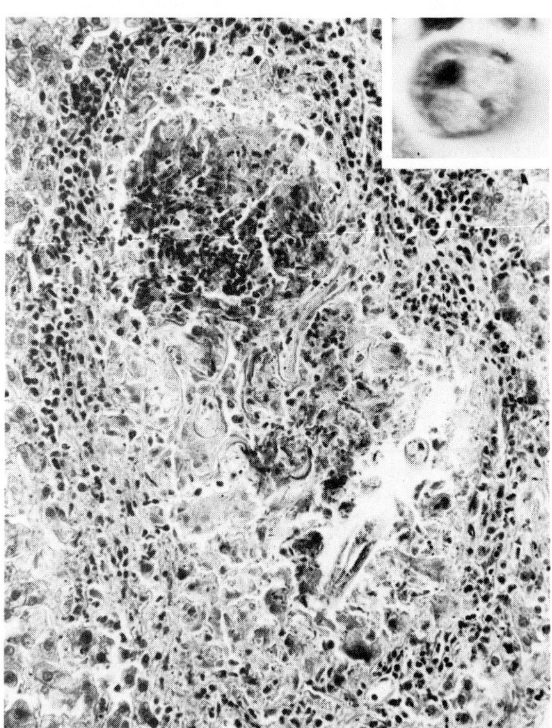

Figure 49–41. *Toxocara canis* granuloma in human liver with cross and oblique section of larva (×200). Inset is high magnification of larva on cross-section (×800).

saginatus does not. Most cysticerci in man are morphologically indistinguishable from those of *T. solium* (i.e., they have a rostellum) so that all have been ascribed to this species. However, it is possible that related species of animal tapeworms with similar cysticerci could exist in man. This would explain some of the epidemiologic inconsistencies between the distribution of *T. solium* (adult) and *C. cellulosae* (larva) in man. *T. saginatus (C. bovis)* does not develop cysticerci in man.

Infection in man results from the accidental ingestion of eggs with food or water. The embryos hatch from the eggs, penetrate the intestinal mucosa, and reach other organs of the body via blood. Infections range from a single cysticercus to thousands of them. The usual location is in the skeletal muscles, but they can be found in almost any organ, including heart, brain, eye, etc. (Fig. 49–42). Symptomatology is related to the number of cysticerci, their location, and the amount of host reaction. In the brain, the infection can cause seizures or symptoms of a space-occupying lesion.

In endemic areas, diagnosis is usually made clinically. In non-endemic areas, diagnosis may be difficult. Serologic tests, such as indirect hemagglutination (IHA), may be helpful depending on the clinical disease, but there are cross-reactions with other diseases. The newer radiologic techniques such as CAT scans have made diagnosis much easier but are not readily available in most endemic areas. Radiographs have been used to demonstrate calcified cysticerci but are not effective in diagnosing recent infections. Definitive diagnosis may be established by identification of larvae removed by surgery.

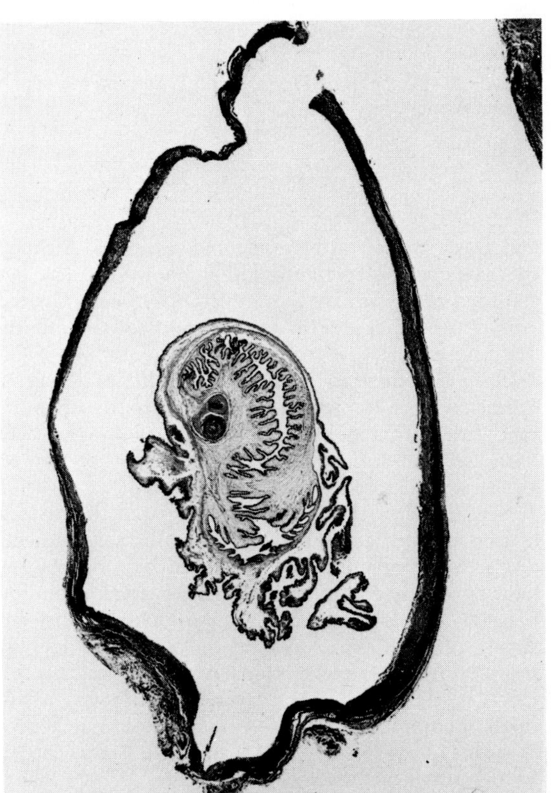

Figure 49–42. *Cysticercus* sp. from subcutaneous tissues. The larva has a tightly invaginated scolex in the bladder (×11). (Case of Dr. H. Estrada, Manizales, Colombia).

Hydatid. Hydatidosis or hydatid cysts in man are caused by the larval stages of various species of cestodes belonging to the genus *Echinococcus.*

Various wild and domestic carnivores, including dogs, are definitive hosts. The adults live attached to the mucosa of the small intestine, measure up to 6 mm in length, and are usually composed of a scolex with a rostellum plus three segments. Eggs are passed in the stools and are ingested by the intermediate hosts, which include sheep, cattle, pigs, rodents, etc. (considered to be the main reservoirs in nature). Man is occasionally an accidental intermediate host.

In the intermediate host the eggs hatch in the intestine; embryos penetrate the intestinal wall and then migrate to different organs where growth of the hydatid cyst begins. Development is slow, taking many years for the formation of a cyst 10 to 15 cm in diameter. The cyst is lined by a germinal membrane consisting of a single cell layer from which numerous infective larvae grow. The cyst lumen is filled with clear fluid. The larvae number in the thousands and may be attached to the germinal membrane but can also be found free in the cyst fluid. External to the germinal membrane is an acellular friable membrane called the laminated layer. On the outside of this layer is the host's fibrous reaction surrounded by normal tissue.

Symptoms in man are those of a slowly growing space-occupying lesion, usually in the liver, lungs, or brain, but other organs can be involved.

Several species of *Echinococcus* may cause hydatid cysts in man. The most common is *E. granulosus,* which is found mainly in countries with large sheep and cattle industries, such as Australia, the southern part of South America, northern and eastern Europe, northern China, the Middle East, and southern and northern Africa. In the United States occasional cases, usually imported but occasionally autochthonous, are reported.

The next most frequent species is *E. multilocularis,* which produces the multiloculated or alveolar hydatid disease. It is found principally in southern Germany, Switzerland, USSR, France, Italy, Argentina, Uruguay, New Zealand, Australia, and Alaska. The usual intermediate hosts are small rodents such as mice.

A third species, *E. vogeli,* may infect man in parts of Central and South America (D'Alessandro, 1979). Wildcats are the definitive hosts.

The diagnosis of the infection is usually made serologically. The serologic tests used include the indirect hemagglutination (IHA) bentonite flocculation (BF), and latex agglutination. An IHA titer of 1:256 is considered significant and is positive in 88% of people with non-calcified hepatic cysts. Low titers with any of these tests do not necessarily mean infection, since sera from patients with other conditions, such as liver cirrhosis and collagen diseases, cross-react. Cross-reactions with other cestode larvae such as cysticercus are also common. In addition, patients with calcified hepatic cysts or cysts of lung frequently have negative serology.

In surgical and autopsy material there are morphologic differences among the *Echinococcus* cysts mentioned above. *E. granulosus* is unilocular (Fig. 49–43), while *E. multilocularis* and *E. vogeli* are composed of many different compartments.

Coenurus. This is the agent of coenurosis, a sporadic, accidental infection of man following ingestion of eggs of a tapeworm belonging to the genus *Multiceps*. The adult parasites live in the intestine of dogs. Goats, cattle, and occasionally man are the intermediate hosts (Templeton, 1971).

The larval coenurus stage usually develops in the brain or spinal cord of the intermediate hosts, but other organs can be involved. It is a transparent large cyst up to 10 cm in diameter filled with clear fluid and containing up to several hundred larvae growing on the inner side of the cyst membrane. The diagnosis is made clinically and by study of cyst morphology after its removal. Species identification is not possible based on examination of the cyst alone.

Sparganum. Sparganosis in man is caused by larval stages of various *Spirometra* species, which are tapeworms closely related to *Diphyllobothrium* (Swartzwelder, 1964). *Spirometra* are widely distributed in many domestic and wild animals, including both cats and dogs, which are the definitive hosts. Although the life cycle is not completely known, it has been assumed to be similar to that of *Diphyllobothrium* with vertebrates other than fish serving as second intermediate hosts.

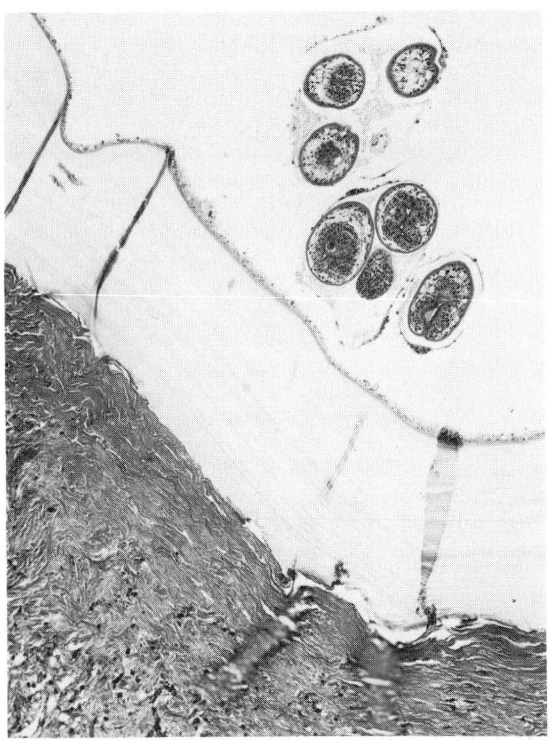

Figure 49–43. *Echinococcus granulosus.* Hydatid cyst in human liver. There are several protoscolices, a thin germinal membrane, a thick laminated membrane, and fibrous host reaction (×100).

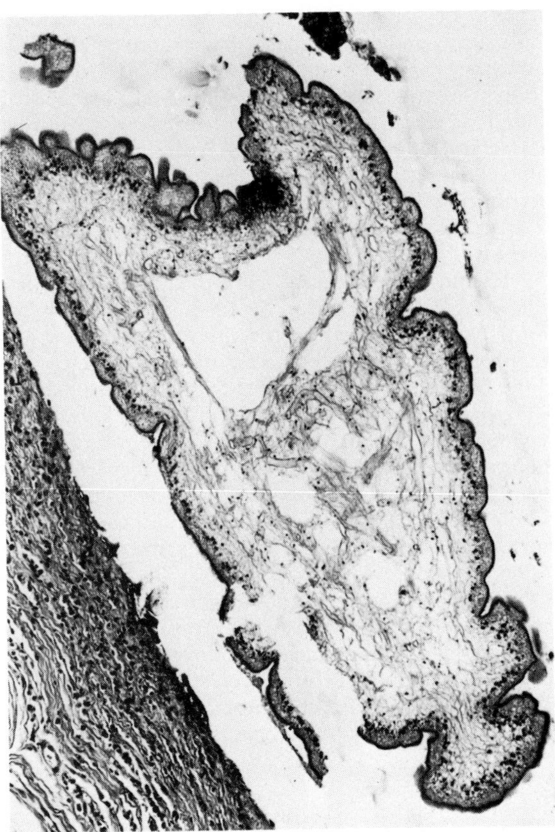

Figure 49–44. *Sparganum.* Larva of *Spirometra* spp. in human tissues.

The infection in man is thought to occur by ingestion of water contaminated with the arthropod first intermediate host harboring the larvae. The *Sparganum* larva develops in man, who therefore acts as the second intermediate host.

Symptoms of the infection are related to the localization of the larva, which is usually subcutaneous. An area of inflammation with redness, edema, and pain is usually the main presentation. Removal of the parasite reveals a delicate, slender, white worm measuring 60 to 80 mm long by 1 to 2 mm wide. The morphology in cross-sections is typical of that of a larval cestode with thick layered cuticle and a basement membrane (Fig. 49–44). There is not a cavity as seen in the nematodes, and the larva contains numerous calcareous corpuscles.

Other Helminth Infections. In addition to the diseases described in this chapter, occasional humans have been infected with a number of other helminths (see General References).

MEDICAL ENTOMOLOGY

Arthropods are of great medical importance because they transmit a wide variety of infectious agents, including parasites, viruses, rickettsia, and bacteria. Arthropods are widespread in the environment, and excrement and fragments (frass) of various arthropods are present in soil and dust of various types. Persons may become hypersensitive to these arthropod materials and develop allergic manifestations, such as asthma and "hay fever." Chemical substances in the bodies of some arthropods may be irritating to persons who come in contact with them, as by crushing the arthropod.

Many of the biting arthropods are attempting to obtain a blood meal, which is essential for their development. In contrast, stinging arthropods use their caudal stingers as a defense mechanism. Reaction to the arthropods may result from mechanical damage, toxic substances produced by the arthropod, or hypersensitivity to various arthropod antigens. In addition, there may be secondary mechanical damage from scratching or secondary infection from microorganisms borne by the arthropod or arising from the host's environment.

The arthropods may have egg, larval, nymph, and adult stages, and their effect on man may be caused by one or more of these. Identification of these parasites is dependent on morphologic recognition of the arthropod in one of its stages. Identification is based on various structural characteristics described in many books and manuals (CDC, 1969; Smith, 1973; Harwood, 1979). If the laboratory is not proficient, the specimens may be referred to a competent entomologist.

Small arthropods, such as mosquitoes, flies, lice, and fleas, may be submitted live or dead without preservative, but the morphology of larval stages and larger arthropods will be better preserved in 10 per cent formalin or 70 per cent alcohol. Examination with a hand lens, dissecting microscope, or light microscope will allow study of the characteristics of the parasite.

The arthropods that will be emphasized in this section are those that live on man in the United States and which the laboratory is most likely to be asked to identify. For more complete coverage of medical entomology, see specialized books (Smith, 1973; Harwood, 1979) or general parasitology books.

Class Arachnida

This class includes mites, scorpions, spiders, and ticks and represents those arthropods with adults having a cephalothorax, abdomen, and eight legs.

Mites. Mites are of microscopic size, most measuring less than 1 mm in length. They are widely distributed in the environment. Allergens from mites in the environment may be responsible for allergy to "dust" in some individuals. Various species of mites parasitize the skin of animals, including man, and cause a disease called mange. Man is commonly

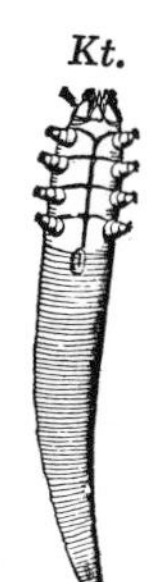

Figure 49–45. The "face insect," *Demodex folliculorum* (×100); *Kt.*, biting jaws. (After R. Blanchard in Brumpt.)

infested by three mites: *Demodex* spp. the follicle mite; *Sarcoptes scabiei,* the itch mite, which causes a disease known as scabies; and larval trombiculid mites, called red bugs, chiggers, or harvest mites. Man may occasionally be an accidental host for various animal mites in the environment.

Demodex species (Fig. 49–45) parasitize hair follicles or sebaceous glands, particularly of the face, and are widespread in man, probably infesting over half of middle-aged adults. The infestation is usually asymptomatic but may be associated with skin problems such as blackheads and acne in some cases. These parasites may often be seen as an incidental finding in histologic sections of facial skin. They are recognized by their elongated shape and stubby legs.

S. scabiei females (Fig. 49–46) tunnel in the superficial layers of skin, particularly in the interdigital areas and the flexor surfaces of the wrists and forearms, but they may also infest other areas. The female lays eggs in the tunnels which embryonate and larvae

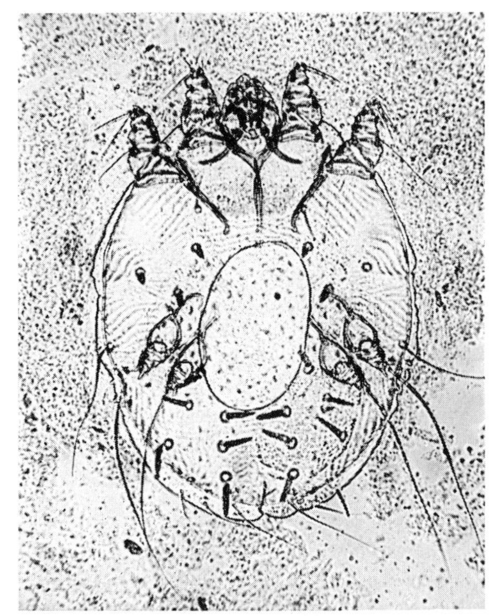

Figure 49–46. *Sarcoptes scabiei,* adult female. (From Markell, E. K., and Voge, M.: Medical Parasitology. Philadelphia, W. B. Saunders Company, 1976.)

6

hatch (Fig. 49–47). The disease is spread by person-to-person contact, as in sleeping in the same bed or holding hands or contact with contaminated clothing or other articles. The itching results from a sensitization reaction to the parasites and their products and varies in severity from patient to patient. There may be itching in areas in which there are no mites. Lesions often become secondarily infected (Orkin, 1975). The diagnosis is established by dissecting organisms or eggs from the tunnels, placing them in 20 per cent potassium hydroxide or mineral oil for clearing, and examining them under the microscope. Eggs, six-legged larvae, eight-legged nymphs, or adults may be detected and are diagnostic. Unfortunately, these cannot be readily demonstrated in all patients.

When scabies has been detected in a place, such as a school, there are often numerous individuals who develop itching without evidence of disease, probably of psychological origin. Care must be taken to properly diagnose the disease to prevent such pseudoepidemics. A particularly severe form of the disease may occur, especially in institutionalized patients, and is called "Norwegian scabies."

Trombiculid mites infest grasses and bushes, and their six-legged larvae, chiggers (red bugs, harvest mites), may attack man. The larvae attach to the skin, usually in areas of tight clothing such as elastic bands or belts. In sensitive individuals there is reaction to the secretions of the larvae with swollen itching areas at the sites of attachment which persist for days. Excoriations may become secondarily infected. Diagnosis is established on clinical grounds. Other trombiculid mites may be vectors of scrub typhus caused by *Rickettsia tsutsugamushi*.

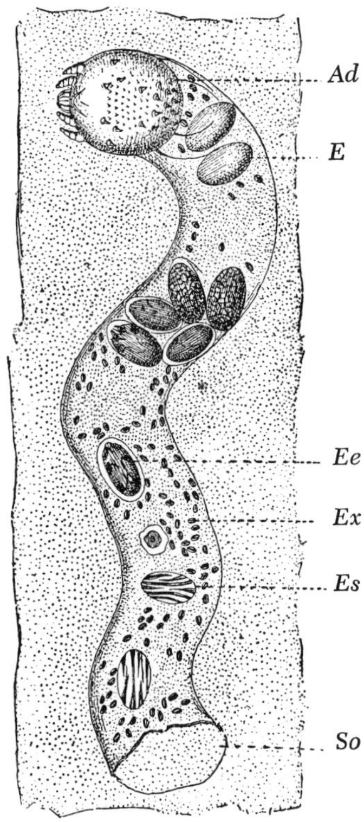

Figure 49–47. *Sarcoptes scabiei.* Diagram of a subcutaneous burrow; *A,* adult female; *E,* eggs; *Ee,* embryo egg; *Ex,* excrement; *Es,* egg shell; *So,* skin orifice. (After Railliet in Brumpt.)

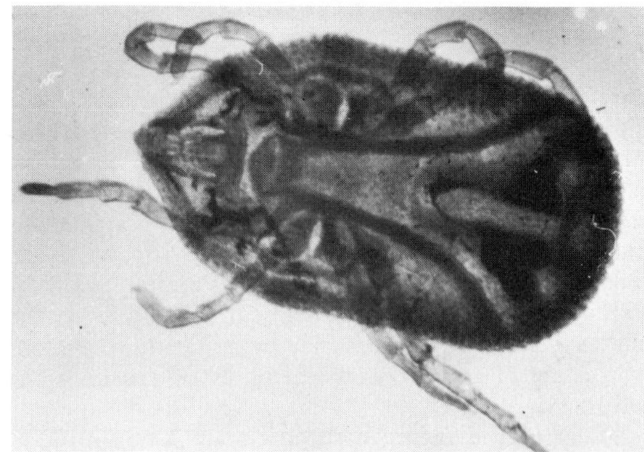

Figure 49–48. *Ornithodoros kellyi,* a soft tick, photographed with transmitted light.

Ticks. Ticks belong to the superfamily *Ixodoidea* and are important as vectors in infectious diseases, but in addition may cause local damage from bites and may cause tick paralysis. There are two groups of ticks. Soft ticks belonging to the family *Argasidae* (Fig. 49–48) have a soft leathery body, and mouthparts are not visible from above. Hard ticks belonging to the family *Ixodidae* have a hard dorsal plate, and mouth parts are visible from above (Fig. 49–49). The dorsal plate covers the entire dorsum of the male, but only the anterior portion of the female, allowing the body to swell when engorged. Unengorged ticks are generally 3 to 4 mm long, but engorged ticks may be up to 1.5 cm long. The stages in development are egg, larva, nymph, and adult. Blood meals are essential for the development of ticks. Infestation is acquired in grassy or bushy areas where the ticks reside between blood meals on various mammals.

Tick paralysis is an ascending paralysis that develops in occasional patients, especially children, bitten by various ticks and is due to a toxic substance introduced

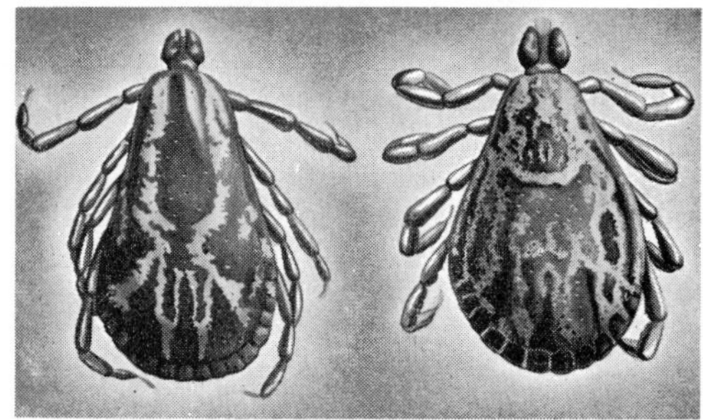

Figure 49–49. *Dermacentor andersoni* and *Dermacentor variabilis;* vectors of Rocky Mountain spotted fever rickettsiae. (Courtesy of Merck, Sharp & Dohme, Inc.)

by the tick. This disease may be confused with Guillain-Barré syndrome, poliomyelitis, botulism, and other paralytic diseases. Removal of ticks results in recovery.

Class Insecta

Members of the class Insecta are characterized by a body divided into head, thorax, and abdomen and having three pairs of legs. There are usually two pairs of wings. Insects of medical importance include lice, fleas, bugs, mosquitoes, and flies. Bees and wasps may cause severe reactions, particularly in sensitive individuals, but will not be further described.

Lice. Lice are flattened dorsoventrally and are wingless. There are three lice that infest man and obtain nourishment by biting and sucking on the human host. They are named according to the region of the body that they usually (but not exclusively) inhabit. *Pediculus humanus capitis* is the head louse and is 1 to 2 mm long. *P. humanus corporis* is the body louse and is 2 to 4 mm long, and *Phthirus pubis* is the pubic or crab louse and is approximately 1 mm long (Fig. 49–50). The body louse is particularly important as the vector of epidemic typhus. Infections with lice usually occur when people live in crowded conditions with little opportunity for bathing and laundering. Infestation may be spread by intimate contact, as in bed partners, or by contaminated hats, clothing, blankets, or furniture. Eggs of *P. humanus capitis* and *P. pubis* are attached to hairs and are known as "nits" (Fig. 49–51). Eggs of *P. humanus corporis* are laid in clothing. Diagnosis is suspected from finding bites but established by finding adults, usually in hairy areas, such as the head, eyebrows, armpits, and genital areas, or by detecting "nits" attached to hairs *(P. humanus capitis* and *P. pubis)* or eggs in clothing *(P. humanus corporis).* "Nits" should be examined microscopically to be certain they are truly eggs and not globs of hair spray or some other material.

Fleas. Fleas are bloodsucking wingless insects that are laterally compressed and have large hind legs for jumping. They average 2 to 4 mm long and have bloodsucking mouthparts. The oriental rat flea *(Xenopsylla cheopis)* is the vector of plague, and fleas may be associated with other infections. Flea bites cause little trouble to some persons but are quite irritating to others, probably as a result of sensitization of the host. Man may be infected by the human flea *(Pulex irritans)* (Fig. 49–52) or may be an incidental host for fleas of other animals, particularly the dog flea *(Ctenocephalides canis)* and the cat flea *(C. felis).* Eggs develop in dog and cat bedding and in carpets and furniture. They usually cause little difficulty for man unless the pet is no longer present, for then they will bite man. This usually occurs after moving, boarding, or death of pets.

Bugs. Reduviid bugs are bloodsucking bugs that are vectors of South American trypanosomiasis and will not be discussed further.

The bed bug, *Cimex lectularius* (Fig. 49–53) is reddish brown and about 5 mm long and has short wing pads but cannot fly. Bites of these bloodsucking insects vary in severity depending on the degree of sensitivity the host has developed. In some individuals they may cause wheals up to 3 mm in diameter with intense itching; in others they cause almost no reaction. During the day the bugs live in mattresses, bedsteads, cracks in walls, furniture, etc., and at night come out to bite the sleeping victim. Diagnosis is established by identifying the adult bugs or on clinical grounds.

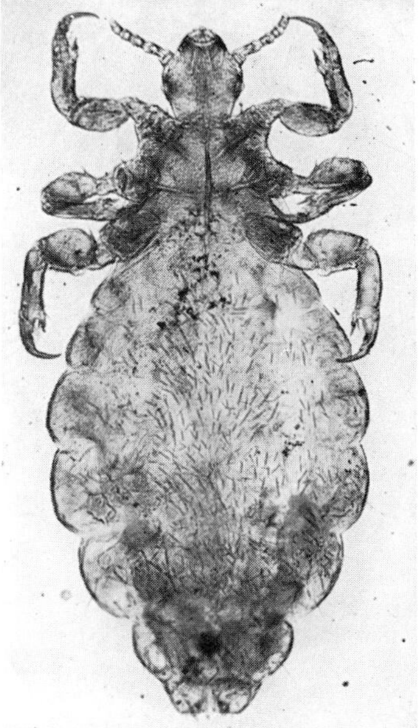

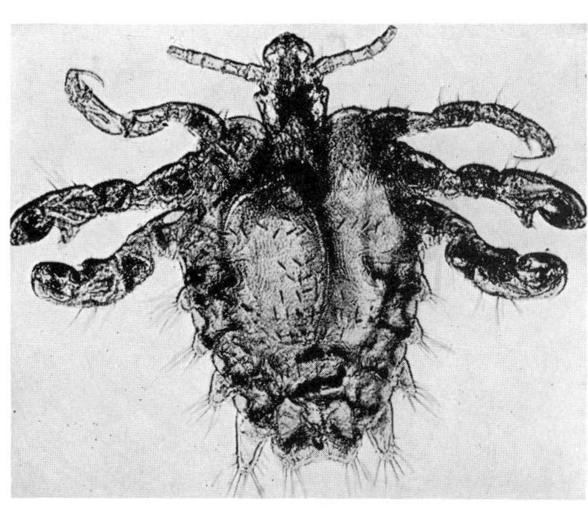

Figure 49–50. *Pediculus humanus* (left) and *Phthirus pubis* (right).

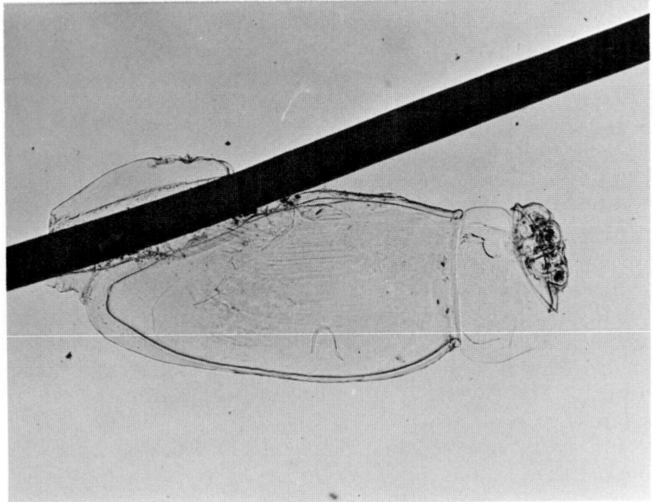

Figure 49–51. *Pediculus capitis.* Empty egg case ("nit") attached to hair (×60). (From Raphael, S. S.: Lynch's Medical Laboratory Technology. Philadelphia, W. B. Saunders Company, 1976.)

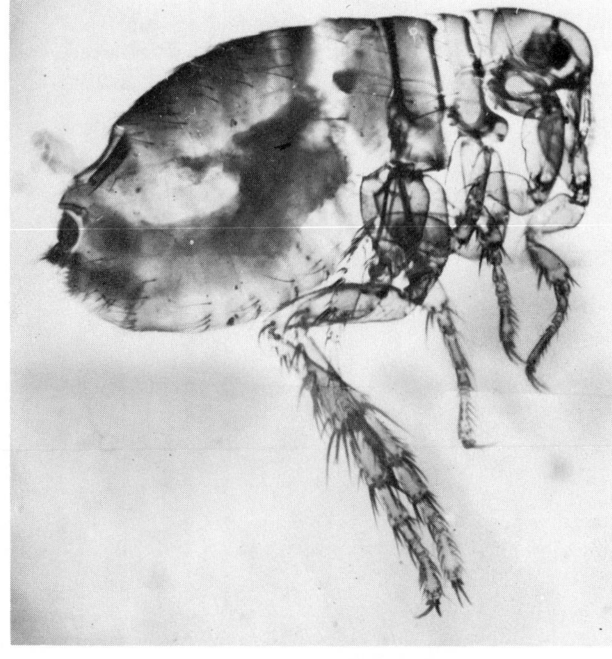

Figure 49–52. *Pulex irritans* female flea. Note the powerful hind legs.

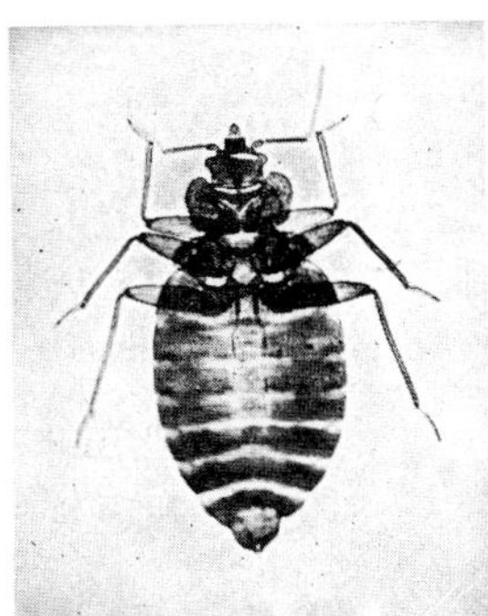

Figure 49–53. The common bedbug, *Cimex lectularius,* male (×5). In the female the posterior end of the abdomen is more rounded. (Cleared with sodium hydroxide to bring out the structure more clearly.)

Flies. Mosquitoes are flies with two pairs of wings with scales and a proboscis for sucking. They are important in transmission of a number of serious infectious diseases. In addition, they are a nuisance, since their bites make living in some environments quite uncomfortable. The severity of reaction to their bite is related to the degree of sensitivity in the host.

Bloodsucking flies of various types may be important as vectors of infectious diseases or may be important only as pests that inflict painful wounds. Other flies (filth flies) may spread a variety of infectious diseases, such as salmonellosis, typhoid fever, shigellosis, and poliomyelitis, by mechanical means.

Larvae of various flies (maggots) may be seen in a variety of conditions and are often brought to the laboratory as "worms." There are characteristics that allow their identification by experienced entomologists, although sometimes they must be allowed to develop to adult flies for specific identification.

Specific myiases are caused by flies that deposit eggs on the tissues of specific hosts. The larvae invade the host and are thus truly parasitic. These are usually infestations of other animal species. For example, the primary screw-worm, *Cochliomyia hominivorax,* is a serious economic problem to the cattle industry in the southern United States. When man is infected, the disease may be particularly severe if the larvae invade the eye, nose, or mouth.

Semispecific myiases are caused by flies which usually lay their eggs on dead animals or rotting vegetation but which may lay eggs on open wounds or around the nose or other mucous membranes. The larvae usually live a saprophytic existence on necrotic material or secretions and on occasion have been proposed as agents for debridement of wounds. The larvae may be irritating, especially in the nasal areas, where they cause increased mucus flow.

Accidental myiasis involving the gastrointestinal tract occurs when eggs or larvae are accidentally ingested and survive the digestive juices. They may be asymptomatic or may be associated with nausea, abdominal pain, and diarrhea. The maggots are usually found in vomitus or feces and submitted to the laboratory as "worms." Care should be taken to assure that the larvae were present in the specimen when passed and did not develop later. The latter is particularly common in larvae detected when the mother is washing diapers.

General References

Adams, A. R. D., and Maegraith, B. G.: Clinical Tropical Diseases, 6th ed. Oxford, Blackwell Scientific Publications, 1976.

Ash, L. R., and Orihel, T. C.: Atlas of Human Parasitology. Chicago, American Society of Clinical Pathologists, 1980.

Brooke, M. M., and Melvin, D. M.: Morphology of Diagnostic Stages of Intestinal Parasites of Man (Publication No. [CDC] 74–8116). Washington, D.C., United States Department of Health, Education, and Welfare, 1969.

Brown, H. W.: Basic Clinical Parasitology. 4th ed. New York, Appleton-Century-Crofts, 1975.

Bruce-Chwatt, L. J.: Essential Malariology. London, Heinemann, 1980.

Centers for Disease Control: Pictorial Keys to Arthropods, Reptiles, Birds and Mammals of Public Health Significance. 2nd ed. (Publication No. 1955). Washington, D.C., U.S. Government Printing Office, 1969.

Coatney, G. R., Collins, W. E., Warren, M., and Contacos, P. G.: The Primate Malarias. Washington, D.C., U.S. Government Printing Office, 1971.

Edington, G. M., and Gilles, H. M.: Pathology in the Tropics. London, Edward Arnold (Publishers), 1969.

Faust, E. C., Beaver, P. C., and Jung, R. C.: Animal Agents and Vectors of Human Disease. 4th ed. Philadelphia, Lea & Febiger, 1975.

Faust, E. C., Russel, P. F., and Jung, R. C.: Craig and Faust's Clinical Parasitology. 8th ed. Philadelphia, Lea & Febiger, 1970.

Garcia, L. S., and Ash, L. R.: Diagnostic Parasitology: Clinical Laboratory Manual. 2nd ed. St. Louis, The C. V. Mosby Company, 1979a.

Harwood, R. F., and James, M. T.: Entomology in Human and Animal Health. 7th ed. New York, Macmillan, 1979.

Hunter, G. W., III, Swartzwelder, J. C., and Clyde, D. F.: Tropical Medicine. 5th ed. Philadelphia, W. B. Saunders Company, 1976.

Keusch, G. T. (eds.): The biology of parasitic infection; workshop on interactions of nutrition and parasitic diseases. Rev. Infect. Dis., *4*:735, 1982.

Kreier, J. P. (ed.): Malaria 1. Epidemiology, chemotherapy, morphology and metabolism. Malaria 2. Pathology, vector studies, and culture. Malaria 3. Immunology and immunization. New York, Academic Press, 1981.

Lennette, E. H., Balows, A., Hausler, W. J., Jr., and Truant, J. P.: Manual of Clinical Microbiology. 3rd ed. Washington, D.C., American Society for Microbiology, 1980.

Manson-Bahr, P. E. C., and Apted, F. I. C.: Manson's Tropical Diseases. 18th ed. London, Baillière Tindall, 1982.

Marcial-Rojas, R. A.: Pathology of Protozoal and Helminthic Diseases with Clinical Correlation. Baltimore, Williams and Wilkins Company, 1971.

Markell, E. K., and Voge, M.: Medical Parasitology. 5th ed. Philadelphia, W. B. Saunders Company, 1981.

Melvin, D. M., and Brooke, M. M.: Laboratory Procedures for the Diagnosis of Intestinal Parasites. 3rd ed. (DHEW Publication [CDC] 82–8282). Atlanta, Laboratory Training and Consultation Division, Centers for Disease Control, 1982.

Peters, W., and Gilles, H. M.: A Colour Atlas of Tropical Medicine and Parasitology. London, Wolfe Medical Publications, 1977.

Sasa, M.: Human Filariasis: A Global Survey of Epidemiology and Control. Baltimore, University Park Press, 1976.

Smith, J. W., Ash, L. R., Thompson, J. H., McQuay, R. M., Melvin, D. M., and Orihel, T. C.: Diagnostic Parasitology—Intestinal Helminths. Chicago, American Society of Clinical Pathologists, 1976a.

Smith, J. W., McQuay, R. M., Ash, L. R., Melvin, D. M., Orihel, T. C., and Thompson, J. H.: Diagnostic Parasitology—Intestinal Protozoa. Chicago, American Society of Clinical Pathologists, 1976b.

Smith, J. W., Melvin, D. M., Orihel, T. C., Ash, L. R., McQuay, R. M., and Thompson, J. H.: Diagnostic Parasitology—Blood and Tissue Parasites. Chicago, American Society of Clinical Pathologists, 1976c.

Smith, K. G. V.: Insects and Other Arthropods of Medical Importance. London, British Museum of Natural History, 1973.

Spencer, F. M., and Monroe, L. S.: The Color Atlas of Intestinal Parasites. 2nd ed. Springfield, Ill., Charles C Thomas, 1982.

Spencer, H., Dayan, A. D., Gibson, J. B., Huntsman, R. G., Hutt, M. S. R., Jenkins, G. C., Koberle, F., Maegraith, B. G., and Salfelder, K.: Tropical Pathology. Berlin, Springer-Verlag, 1973.

Wardle, R. A., and McLeod, J. A.: The Zoology of Tapeworms. Minneapolis, University of Minnesota Press, 1952.

Warren, K. S., and Mahmoud, A. A. F.: Geographic Medicine for the Practitioner: Algorithms in the Diagnosis and Management of Exotic Diseases. Chicago, University of Chicago Press, 1978.

Specific References

Adams, E. B., and MacLeod, I. N.: Invasive amebiasis. I. Amebic dysentery and its complications. Medicine, *56*:315, 1977a.

Adams, E. B., and MacLeod, I. N.: Invasive amebiasis. II. Amebic liver abscess and its complications. Medicine, *56*:325, 1977b.

Barlett, M. S., Harper, K., Smith, N., Verbanac, T., and Smith, J. W.: Comparative evaluation of a modified zinc sulfate flotation technique. J. Clin. Microbiol., *7*:524, 1978.

Beal, C. B., Viens, P., Grant, R. G. L., and Hughes, J. M.: A new technique for sampling duodenal contents. Am. J. Trop. Med. Hyg., *19*:349, 1970.

Beaver, P. C.: The nature of visceral larva migrans. J. Parasitol., *55*:3, 1969.

Beaver, P. C.: Filariasis without microfilaremia. Am. J. Trop. Med. Hyg., *19*:181, 1970.

Beaver, P. C., Gadgil, R. K., and Morera, P.: *Sarcocystis* in man: A review and report of five cases. Am. J. Trop. Med. Hyg., *28*:819, 1979.

Beaver, P. C., and Orihel, T. C.: Human infection with filariae of animals in the United States. Am. J. Trop. Med. Hyg., *14*:1010, 1965.

Beaver, P. C., Snyder, C. H., Carrera, G. M., Dent, J. H., and Lafferty, J. W.: Chronic eosinophilia due to visceral larva migrans: Report of three cases. Pediatrics, *9*:7, 1952.

Benenson, M. W., Takafuji, E. T., Lemon, S. M., Greenup, R. L., and Sulzer, A. J.: Oocyst-transmitted toxoplasmosis associated with ingestion of contaminated water. N. Engl. J. Med., *307*:666, 1982.

Black, R. E., Dykes, A. C., Sinclair, S. P., and Wells, J. G.: Giardiasis in day-care centers: Evidence of person-to-person transmission. Pediatrics, *60*:486, 1977.

Bowling, M. C., Smith, I. M., and Wescott, S. L.: A rapid staining procedure for *Pneumocystic carinii*. Am. J. Med. Technol., *39*:267, 1973.

Brandborg, L. L., Goldberg, S. B., and Breidenbach, W. C.: Human coccidiosis—a possible cause of malabsorption. N. Engl. J. Med., *283*:1306, 1970.

Bruce, J. I., and Sornmani, S.: The Mekong Schistosome. Malacological Review, Suppl. #2. Whitmore Lake, Michigan, 1980.

Burrows, R. B., and Swerdlow, M. A.: *Enterobius vermicularis* as a probable vector of *Dientamoeba fragilis*. Am. J. Trop. Med. Hyg., *5*:258, 1956.

Campbell, P. N., and Current, W. L.: Demonstration of serum antibodies to *Cryptosporidium* sp. in normal and immunodeficient humans with confirmed infections. J. Clin. Microbiol., *18*:165, 1983.

Centers for Disease Control: Toxoplasmosis. Morbid. Mortal. Weekly Rep., *26*:408, 1977.

Centers for Disease Control: Intestinal Parasite Surveillance. Annual Summary, 1978. Issued August 1979.

Centers for Disease Control: Diphyllobothriasis associated with salmon—United States. Morbid. Mortal. Weekly Rep., *30*:331, 1981a.

Centers for Disease Control: Trichinosis Surveillance. Annual Summary, 1980, Issued November 1981b.

Centers for Disease Control: Malaria Surveillance. Annual Summary, 1980. Issued January 1982a.

Centers for Disease Control: Malaria Surveillance. Annual Summary, 1981. Issued November 1982b.

Centers for Disease Control: Prevention of malaria in travelers, 1982. Morbid. Mortal. Weekly Rep., *21*:15, 1982c.

Centers for Disease Control: Cryptosporidiosis: Assessment of chemotherapy of males with acquired immunodeficiency syndrome (AIDS) Morbid. Mortal. Weekly Rep., *31*:589, 1982d.

Chalvardjian, A. M., and Grawe, L. A.: A new procedure for the identification of *Pneumocystis carinii* cyst in tissue sections and smears. J. Clin. Path., *16*:383, 1963.

Ciferri, F.: Human pulmonary dirofilariasis in the United States: A critical review. Am. J. Trop. Med. Hyg., *31*:302, 1982.

Current, W. L., Reese, N. C., Ernst, J. V., Bailey, W. S., Heyman, M. B., and Weinstein, W. M.: Human cryptosporidiosis in immunocompetent and immunodeficient persons. N. Engl. J. Med., *308*:1252, 1983.

Cypress, R. H., Karol, M. H., Zidian, J. C., Glickman, L. T., and Gitlin, D.: Larvae-specific antibodies in patients with visceral larva migrans. J. Infect. Dis., *135*:633, 1977.

D'Alessandro, A., Rausch, R. L., Cuello, C., and Aristizabal, N.: *Echinococcus vogeli* in man, with a review of polycystic hydatid disease in Colombia and neighboring countries. Am. J. Trop. Med. Hyg., *28*:303, 1979.

Desowitz, R. S., and Hitchcock, J. C.: Hyperendemic bancroftian filariasis in the Kingdom of Tonga: The application of the membrane filter technique to an age-stratified blood survey. Am. J. Trop. Med. Hyg., *23*:877, 1974.

Elsdon-Dew, R.: The epidemiology of amebiasis. Adv. Parasit., *6*:1, 1968.

Eveland, L. K., Kenney, M., and Yermakov, V.: Laboratory diagnosis of autoinfection in strongyloidiasis. Am. J. Clin. Path., *63*:421, 1975.

Garcia, L. S., Brewer, T. C., and Bruckner, D. A.: A comparison of the formalin-ether concentration and trichrome-stained smear methods for the recovery and identification of intestinal protozoa. Am. J. Med. Tech., *45*:932, 1979b.

Garcia, L. S., Bruckner, D. A., Brewer, T. C., and Shimizu, R. Y.: Techniques for the recovery and identification of *Cryptosporidium* oocysts from stool specimens. J. Clin. Microbiol., *18*:185, 1983.

Gill, G. V., and Bell, D. R.: *Strongyloides stercoralis* infection in former Far East Prisoners of war. Br. Med. J., *2*:572, 1979.

Grove, D. I.: Strongyloidiasis in allied ex-prisoners of war in Southeast Asia. Br. Med. J., *1*:598, 1980.

Gutierrez, Y.: Diagnosis of zoonotic filarial infections in tissue sections. Human Path., in press, 1984.

Healy, G. R., and Rubush, T. K.: Morphology of *Babesia microti* in human blood smears. Am. J. Clin. Path., *73*:107, 1980.

Heyneman, D.: Host-parasite resistance patterns—some implications from experimental studies with helminths. Ann. N.Y. Acad. Sci., *113*:114, 1963.

Hoare, C. A., and Wallace, F. G.: Developmental stages of trypanosomatid flagellates: A new terminology. Nature, *212*:1385, 1966.

Igra-Siegman, Y., Kapila, R., Sen, P., Kaminski, Z. C., and Louria, D. B.: Syndrome of hyperinfection with *Strongyloides stercoralis*. Rev. Infect. Dis., *3*:397, 1981.

Istre, G. R., Kreiss, K., Hopkins, R. S., Healy, G. R., Benziger, M., Canfield, T. M., Dickinson, P., Englert, T. R., Compton, R. C., Mathews, H. M., and Simmons, R. A.: An outbreak of amebiasis spread by colonic irrigation at a chiropractic clinic. N. Engl. J. Med., *307*:339, 1982.

Jung, R. C., and Beaver, P. C.: Clinical observations on *Trichocephalus trichiurus* (whipworm) infestation in children. Pediatrics, *8*:548, 1951.

Kagan, I. G.: Serodiagnosis of parasitic diseases. *In* Lennette, E. H., Balows, A., Hausler, W. J., Jr., and Truant, J. P.: Manual of Clinical Microbiology. 3rd ed. Washington, D.C., American Society for Microbiology, 1980a, p. 724.

Kagan, I. G.: Serodiagnosis of parasitic diseases. *In* Rose, N. R., and Friedman, H.: Manual of Clinical Immunology. 2nd ed. Washington, D.C., American Society for Microbiology, 1980b, p. 573.

Keffer, J. H.: Malarial parasites, concentration by saponin hemolysis. Am. J. Clin. Path., *46*:155, 1966.

Knott, J. A.: A method for making microfilarial surveys on day blood. Trans. R. Soc. Trop. Med. Hyg., *33*:191, 1939.

Krogstad, D. J., Spencer, H. C., Healy, G. R., Gleason, N. N., Sexton, J. J., and Herron, C. A.: Amebiasis: Epidemiologic studies in the United States. Ann. Intern. Med., *88*:89, 1978.

Krotoski, W. A., Garnham, P. C. C., Krotoski, D. M., Killick-Kendrick, R., Draper, C. C., Targett, G. A. T., and Guy, M. W.: Observations on early and late post-sporozoite tissue stages in primate malaria. 1. Discovery of a new latent form of *Plasmodium cynomolgi* (the hypnozoite), and failure to detect hepatic forms within the first 24 hrs. after infection. Am. J. Trop. Med. Hyg., *31*:24, 1982.

Lainson, R., and Shaw, J. J.: Epidemiology and ecology of leishmaniasis in Latin-America. Nature, *273*:595, 1978.

Lanham, S. M.: The separation of trypanosomes from blood cells and their behavior on TEAE- and DEAE-cellulose and DEAE-Saphadex. Trans. R. Soc. Trop. Med. Hyg., *62*:129, 1968.

Layrisse, M., Blumenfeld, N., Carbonell, L., Desenne, J., and Roche, M.: Intestinal absorption tests and biopsy of the jejunum in subjects with heavy hookworm infection. Am. J. Trop. Med. Hyg., *13*:297, 1964a.

Layrisse, M., and Roche, M.: The relationship between anemia and hookworm infection: Results of surveys of rural Venezuelan population. Am. J. Hyg., *79*:279, 1964b.

Levett, P. N.: A comparison of five methods for the detection of *Trichomonas vaginalis* in clinical specimens. Med. Lab. Sci., *37*:85, 1980.

Levin, R. L., and Armstrong, D. E.: Human infection with *Entamoeba polecki*. Am. J. Clin. Path., *54*:611, 1970.

Loria-Cortez, R., and Lobo-Sanahuja, J. F.: Clinical abdominal angiostrongylosis. A study of 116 children with intestinal eosinophilic granuloma caused by *Angiostrongylus costaricensis*. Am. J. Trop. Med. Hyg., *29*:538, 1980.

Markell, E. K., Ash, L. R., Melvin, D. M., Moore, D. V., Sogandares-Bernal, F., and Voge, M.: Procedures suggested for use in examination of clinical specimens for parasitic infection: A statement by the Subcommittee on Laboratory Standards, Committee on Education, American Society of Parasitologists. J. Parasitol., *63*:959, 1977a.

Markell, E. K., and Quinn, P. M.: Comparison of immediate polyvinyl alcohol (PVA) fixation with delayed Schaudinn's fixation for the demonstration of protozoa in stool specimens. Am. J. Trop. Med. Hyg., *26*:1139, 1977b.

Martin, L. K.: Randomness of particle distribution in human feces and the resulting influence on helminth egg counting. Am. J. Trop. Med. Hyg., *14*:747, 1965.

Martinez, A. J.: Is *Acanthamoeba encephalitis* an opportunistic infection? Neurology, *30*:567, 1980.

Masur, H., Michelis, M. A., Greene, J. B., Onorati, I., Vande-Stouwe, R. A., Holzman, R. S., Wormser, G., Brettman, L., Lange, M., Murray, H. W., and Cunningham-Rundles, S.: An outbreak of community-acquired *Pneumocystis carinii* pneumonia. N. Engl. J. Med., *305*:1431, 1981.

Meyer, E. A., and Radulescu, S.: Giardia and giardiasis. Adv. Parasitol., *17*:1, 1979.

Milder, J. E., Walzer, P. O., Kilgore, G., Rutherford, I., and Klein, M.: Clinical features of *Strongyloides stercoralis* infection in an endemic area of the United States. Gastroenterology, *80*:1481, 1981.

Miller, L. H., Mason, S. J., Clyde, D. F., and McGinniss, M. H.: The resistance factor to *Plasmodium vivax* in blacks, the Duffy-blood-group genotype, FyFy. N. Engl. J. Med., *295*:302, 1976.

Nielson, R. L., Kohler, R. B., Chin, W., McCarthy, L., and Luft, F. C.: The use of exchange transfusions: A potentially useful adjunct in the treatment of fulminant falciparum malaria. Am. J. Med. Sci., *277*:325, 1979.

Orihel, T. C., and Beaver, P. C.: Morphology and relationship of *Dirofilaria tenuis* and *Dirofilaria conjunctivae*. Am. J. Trop. Med. Hyg., *14*:1030, 1965.

Orkin, M.: Today's scabies (editorial). Arch. Dermatol., *111*:1431, 1975.

Phillips, B. P., and Zierdt, C. H.: *Blastocystis hominis:* Pathogenic potential in human patients and in gnotobiotes. Exp. Parasit., *39*:358, 1976.

Purtilo, D. T., Meyers, W. M., and Connor, D. H.: Fatal strongyloidiasis in immunosuppressed patients. Am. J. Med., *56*:488, 1974.

Reese, N. C., Current, W. L., Ernst, J. V., and Bailey, W. S.: Cryptosporidiosis of man and calf: A case report and results of experimental infections in mice and rats. Am. J. Trop. Med. Hyg., *31*:226, 1982.

Remington, J. S., and Desmonts, G.: Toxoplasmosis. *In* Remington, J. S., and Klein, J. P.: Infectious Diseases of the Fetus and Newborn Infant. Philadelphia, W. B. Saunders Company, 1976, p. 191.

Rubush, T. K.: Human babesiosis in North America. Trans. R. Soc. Trop. Med. Hyg., *74*:149, 1980.

Sadun, E. H., and Melvin, D. M.: The probability of detecting infections with *Enterobius vermicularis* by successive examination. J. Pediatr., *48*:438, 1956.

Sargeaunt, P. G., and Williams, J. E.: A comparative study of *Entamoeba histolytica* (NIH: 200, HK9, etc.) "*E. histolytica*-like" and other morphologically identical amoebae using isoenzyme electrophoresis. Trans. Roy. Soc. Trop. Med. Hyg., *74*:469, 1980.

Smith, J. W.: Identification of fecal parasites in the special parasitology survey of the College of American Pathologists. Am. J. Clin. Path., *72*:371, 1979.

Smith, J. W., and Bartlett, M. S.: Laboratory diagnosis of *Pneumocystis carinii* infection. Clin. Lab. Med., *2*:393, 1982.

Smith, J. W., and Bartlett, M. S.: In vitro cultivation of *Pneumocystis*. *In* Young, L. S. (ed.): *Pneumocystis carinii* Pneumonia; Pathogenesis, Diagnosis, and Therapy. New York, Marcel Dekker, 1984.

Smith, J. W., and Wolfe, M. S.: Giardiasis. Ann. Rev. Med., *31*:373, 1980.

Spencer, M. J., Garcia, L. S., and Chapin, M. R.: *Dientamoeba fragilis,* an intestinal pathogen in children. Am. J. Dis. Child., *133*:390, 1979.

Spillman, R. K.: Pulmonary ascariasis in tropical communities. Am. J. Trop. Med. Hyg., *24*:791, 1975.

Strauss, W. G.: Clinical manifestations of clonorchiasis: A controlled study of 105 cases. Am. J. Trop. Med. Hyg., *11*:625, 1962.

Swartzwelder, J. C., Beaver, P. C., and Hood, M. W.: Sparganosis in southern United States. Am. J. Trop. Med. Hyg., *13*:43, 1964.

Symmers, W. St. C.: Pathology of oxyuriasis, with special reference to granulomas due to the presence of *Oxyuris vermicularis (Enterobius vermicularis)* and its ova in tissues. Arch. Path., *50*:475, 1950.

Templeton, A. C.: Anatomical and geographical location of human coenurus infection. Trop. Geogr. Med., *23*:105, 1971.

Teutch, S. M., Juranek, D. D., Sulzer, A., Dubey, J. P., and Sikes, R. K.: Epidemic toxoplasmosis associated with infected cats. N. Engl. J. Med., *300*:695, 1979.

Vik, R.: The genus *Diphyllobothrium:* An example of the interdependence of systematics and experimental biology. Exp. Parasitol., *15*:361, 1964.

Visvesvara, G. S.: Free-living pathogenic amoebae. *In* Lennette, E. H., Balows, A., Hausler, W. J., Jr., and Truant, J.: Manual of Clinical Microbiology. 3rd ed. Washington, D.C., American Society for Microbiology, 1980a, p. 704.

Visvesvara, G. S., Smith, P. D., Healy, G. R., and Brown, W. R.: An immunofluorescent test to detect serum antibodies to *Giardia lamblia*. Ann. Intern. Med., *93*:802, 1980b.

Walzer, P. D., Schnelle, V., Armstrong, D., and Rosen, P. P.: Nude mouse: A new experimental model for *Pneumocystis carinii* infection. Science, *197*:177, 1977.

Warren, K. S.: Helminthic diseases endemic in the United States. Am. J. Trop. Med. Hyg., *23*:723, 1974.

WHO Expert Committee on Helminthiasis: Soil-transmitted helminths. WHO Tech. Rep. Ser. No. 277, 1964, pp. 1–70.

Yang, J., and Scholten, T.: *Dientamoeba fragilis:* A review with notes on its epidemiology, pathogenicity, mode of transmission, and diagnosis. Am. J. Trop. Med. Hyg., *26*:16, 1977.

Yassin, S. M. A., and Garret, M.: Parasites in cytodiagnosis: A case report of *Strongyloides stercoralis* in Papanicolaou smears of gastric aspirate with a review of the literature. Acta Cytol., *24*:539, 1980.

Zierdt, C. H., Rude, W. S., and Bull, B. S.: Protozoan characteristics of *Blastocystis hominis*. Am. J. Clin. Path., *48*:495, 1967.

6

50

VIRUSES, RICKETTSIA, AND CHLAMYDIA

C. GEORGE RAY, M.D., MARY JANE HICKS, M.D., and LINDA L. MINNICH, M.S.

VIRAL INFECTIONS

Virology is a relatively new discipline when compared with bacteriology. The beginning of the modern era of virology can best be credited to Walter Reed, who demonstrated in 1901 that yellow fever was caused by a viral agent. Since 1949, when John Enders and his collaborators reported the growth of viruses in tissue culture with resultant cytopathic effects, both our knowledge of viral infections in humans and the ability to identify them have increased in logarithmic fashion.

It is now reasonable, and indeed, important to consider wider application of diagnostic virology for direct patient management in the community-based hospital. In addition to public health and epidemiologic benefits, diagnosis can aid the clinician greatly in considering further diagnostic and therapeutic maneuvers—the result of a rapid viral diagnosis can be consideration for fewer other tests and therapies, and even shortening of hospitalization times in many cases. Furthermore, the results can aid the physician in prognostication and in understanding the clinical behavior of such infections. Specific antiviral therapy is available for a few infections, but an armamentarium comparable to that presently available for bacterial diseases will probably not be realized for several years. Nevertheless, the prospects are clear: in each future year there will be a greater demand on the diagnostic laboratory to make rapid etiologic diagnoses of viral infections with the possibility of specific therapy in mind. This has already been shown to be true for herpes simplex, varicella-zoster, and perhaps influenza A infections.

Our present experience has been in a community-based diagnostic laboratory, where we have found that it is not unreasonable to expect a 30 to 40 per cent diagnostic yield for viral infections among all patients studied. Such a laboratory, of course, includes specimens accompanied by a specific request to rule out certain viral possibilities and others from patients with illnesses of obscure nature for which viral cultures are included as part of the screening process; therefore, in a competent laboratory, negative results can also be of value.

We have also found, as have others, that rapid diagnosis is often a possibility. With standard cell culture methods alone, 59 per cent of infections can be detected within 48 hours, and over 90 per cent are found within five days or less. In addition, special rapid diagnostic procedures, including cytology, immunofluorescence, immunoperoxidase, and electron microscopy, can sometimes yield definitive positive answers within a few hours, and many of these are not beyond the scope of a well-equipped hospital laboratory.

We would point out, however, that diagnostic virology does require a reasonable degree of technical expertise and an adequate volume of specimens to sustain a quality operation and yet be economical. Therefore, we recommend that such diagnostic services not be considered a necessity in every laboratory in a given community. It is preferable to consider the potential volume involved, and designate one laboratory in a given population sector to serve as the regional virology diagnostic laboratory (Ray, 1982).

The specific approaches to viral diagnosis include (1) serologic studies, in most cases requiring acute and convalescent sera; (2) cytologic studies, with particular attention to intracellular inclusions, and possible giant-cell formation; (3) direct examination by electron microscopy; (4) isolation of viruses from tissue or body fluids in appropriate tissue culture, animal, or avian host systems; and (5) demonstration of viral components in clinical samples or host cell systems by immunologic or molecular methods. Any or all of these approaches may be considered in the workup of a patient, and require knowledge of the possible agents that might be associated with the illness in question, as well as their behavior in the laboratory. At the present time, greatest emphasis is placed upon direct isolation and demonstration of the agent in host cell systems, but this should not discount the other approaches, which may complement or even speed diagnosis. Chlamydia and rickettsia, which are more like bacteria in their biology, do share a property common with viruses in that they require living cells in order to replicate. This property, and the fact that the principles of diagnosis are similar for these agents and for viruses, make it logical to include them in this chapter.

SELECTION AND COLLECTION OF SPECIMENS

C. R. Madeley, in his excellent discussion of collection and transport of specimens (1977), has appropriately emphasized the need for careful communication between the physician caring for the patient and the laboratory prior to collection of specimens. The decision regarding which types of specimens are to be obtained and how they should be transported and processed requires clinical and epidemiologic considerations, as well as an understanding of the biology of the agents which are to be sought. For these reasons, we would urge that such studies not be undertaken until after there has been a discussion with the virologist in charge.

The agents most commonly sought in the major syndrome categories encountered in a diagnostic laboratory, and the yield of the agents from various specimens (on a relative scale of − to + + + +) are listed in Table 50–1. In addition, it is usually advisable to request 3 to 10 ml of clotted blood in the acute phase of illness, separate the serum, and store it frozen (at least −20°C) for possible reference in serologic testing, if it later becomes apparent this will be useful. Table 50–2 lists the serologic tests which are most commonly used.

The relationship of stage of illness to the expected laboratory diagnostic yield is shown in Table 50–3. It is apparent that the best chances for viral detection will exist when specimens are taken and processed as early in the acute phase of illness as is possible.

There are some simple guidelines concerning specimen collection. For swabs and other samples which may dry out during transport to the laboratory, a virus transport medium (VTM) is necessary. Buffered saline with protein as a stabilizer and added antibiotics, such as penicillin or vancomycin (Forrer, 1982), gentamicin, and amphotericin B, to suppress bacterial and fungal overgrowth, is commonly used. Veal infusion broth, 1 per cent bovine serum albumin, and even skimmed cow's milk are all usable alternatives; most bacteriologic media, particularly reducing media and semisolid vehicles, should be avoided. It should be remembered that antibiotic-containing media should not be used to moisten swabs applied to denuded skin or mucosal surfaces if the patient has a history of allergy to any of the components. The VTM can be dispensed in 2 ml aliquots into screw-capped tubes or vials with non-toxic cap liners, and kept frozen at −20°C. until used. Following collection, specimens should be kept at 2 to 8°C. prior to and during transport.

The following comments are useful to remember when collecting samples for different viral agents.

Respiratory Syndromes. The primary sampling site is the respiratory tract. Cotton-tipped throat swabs, well saturated with pharyngeal secretions, and nasopharyngeal swabs are preferred, both immersed into a single vial of VTM. The ends may be broken off from transport to the laboratory. Alternative methods which have produced high yields of respiratory viruses are nasopharyngeal washings, using buffered saline, or, in patients able to cooperate, pharyngeal washings after gargling with antibiotic-free VTM. Some investigators have reported excellent results when nasopharyngeal washings are immediately inoculated into cell cultures without further processing.

Central Nervous System Syndromes. Feces, throat swabs, and cerebrospinal fluid should be obtained from patients with aseptic meningitis or encephalitis. If mumps is suspected, urine may also be of value. Feces, 5 to 10 g collected in screw-capped bottles, are preferred for enterovirus isolation, but this may delay workup while one waits for the patient to defecate. A useful alternative is a rectal swab, immersed in VTM; however, it must be emphasized that rectal swabs are greatly inferior to feces unless the swab is well soiled with fecal material. In patients with suspected herpes simplex encephalitis, a brain biopsy is usually required to establish a timely and accurate diagnosis (Nahmias, 1982).

Cerebrospinal fluid, 1 to 3 ml, is collected in a sterile tube and held at 2 to 8°C. without further processing until inoculation.

Exanthems and Enanthems. Throat and rectal swabs or feces should be obtained; in addition, any

Table 50–1. APPROPRIATE SPECIMENS FOR VIRUS ISOLATION*

Disease Category and Agents Generally Sought	Specimens					
	Throat	*Stool*	*CSF*	*Urine*	*Vesicle Fluid*	*Other*
Meningitis-encephalitis						
Mumps	+ + + +	– –	+ + +	+ +	– –	
Enteroviruses	+ + +	+ + + +	+ + +	– –	– –	
Herpes simplex	±	– –	±	– –	+‡	Brain biopsy + + + +
Arboviruses†	– –	– –	+	– –	– –	Brain + + +
						Blood +
Respiratory disease						
Myxoviruses, paramyxoviruses, and rhinoviruses	+ + + +	– –	– –	– –	– –	
Adenoviruses	+ + + +	+ + + +	– –	– –	– –	
Exanthems and enanthems						
Rubella†	+ + + +	– –	– –	+	– –	
Measles	+ + +	– –	– –	+ +	– –	
Vaccinia	– –	– –	– –	– –	+ + + +	
Varicella-zoster	– –	– –	– –	– –	+ + + +	
Herpes simplex	+ + +	– –	– –	– –	+ + + +	
Enteroviruses	+ + +	+ + + +	– –	– –	+	
Myocarditis-pericarditis						
Enteroviruses†	+ +	+ + +	– –	– –	– –	Pericardial fluid ±
Myxoviruses†	+ + +	– –	– –	– –	– –	
Paramyxoviruses†	+ + +	– –	– –	– –	– –	
Other						
Cytomegalovirus	+ +	– –	– –	+ + +	– –	Leukocytes + Lung, liver biopsy + + +

*In general, it is important to remember that virus shedding often diminishes rapidly after the onset of illness; therefore, it is important to attempt to collect specimens as early as possible, including an acute serum sample for future testing.

†Because it is frequently very difficult to isolate and/or associate these agents with the disease in question, it is emphasized that serologic tests are particularly important in order to ensure a diagnosis.

‡Meningitis associated with primary genital (type 2) herpes simplex virus infection may be accompanied by virus-positive genital lesions and CSF.

– – = no yield; ± to + + + + = relative yield on culture.

Table 50–2. APPROPRIATE SEROLOGIC TESTS*

Meningoencephalitis		Respiratory Syndromes		Miscellaneous	
Agent	***Serologic Test***	***Agent***	***Serologic Test***	***Agent***	***Serologic Test***
Echovirus	Neutralization	Influenza	CF, HI, or neutralization	Varicella	CF or IFA
Coxsackievirus	Neutralization	Respiratory syncytial	CF, IFA, or neutralization	Rubella	HI, CF, EIA, or IFA
Polio	Neutralization, CF	Parainfluenza	CF, HI, or neutralization	Measles	CF or HI
Herpes	Neutralization, CF	Adenovirus	CF or neutralization	Cytomegalovirus	CF, IFA, or EIA
Mumps	CF, HI, or neutralization	Psittacosis	CF		
Arboviruses	HI, CF, or neutralization	Mycoplasma	CF		

*CF = Complement fixation. HI = Hemagglutination-inhibition. IFA = Indirect immunofluorescence. EIA = Enzyme-linked immunoassay.

ulcerated lesions should be directly swabbed and the swabs placed in VTM. If vesicular or bullous lesions are present, these can be aspirated into a tuberculin syringe or capillary tube, the contents discharged into VTM, followed by rinsing of the tube or syringe with VTM. The base of the lesion should also be swabbed and the swab placed in the same vial of VTM. Smaller lesions can be gently unroofed, and the fluid obtained by thorough soaking of a swab. It is often useful to sample several lesions and pool the sample into one vial of VTM in order to increase the virus yield. In addition, the fluid may be collected for direct electron microscopic examination, and it may be desirable to scrape the base of the lesion for cytologic study or immunofluorescent staining.

Table 50–3. RELATION OF STAGE OF ILLNESS TO PRESENCE OF VIRUS IN TEST MATERIAL AND TO APPEARANCE OF ANTIBODY*

Stage of Illness	Virus Demonstrable in Appropriate Test Material	Specific Antibody Present in Serum
Incubation period	Rarely	—
Prodromal period	Rarely	—
Onset	Frequently	—
Acute phase	Frequently	Frequently or generally†
Recovery phase	Rarely	Generally
Convalescence	Very rarely	Usually

*From Lennette, E. H., and Schmidt, N. J., (eds.): Diagnostic Procedures for Viral and Rickettsial Infections. 4th ed. New York, American Public Health Association, 1969, p. 31.

†In certain widespread endemic diseases, antibody representing prior experience with the agent is generally encountered in acute-phase blood (e.g., influenza, herpes simplex). In other instances (Western equine encephalomyelitis, poliomyelitis), antibody is frequently present in acute-phase serum; antibody formation apparently is well under way by the time the acute-phase specimen is taken.

Whether antibody is encountered will also depend upon the type of antibody (neutralizing, CF, IFA, PHA, EIA, or HI), because of temporal differences in persistence after infection.

Ophthalmologic Syndromes. Conjunctivitis is best approached by obtaining a swab of conjunctival exudate and epithelial cells and immersing it in VTM. Conjunctival scrapings for cytologic examination can also be of value, particularly when evidence of chlamydial infection is sought. Occasionally, corneal scrapings or aqueous humor may be submitted for study by the ophthalmologist.

Congenital Infections. Viral agents most commonly involved in congenital or perinatal infections include cytomegalovirus, rubella, herpes simplex, and enteroviruses. Cultures to be considered include throat, stool or rectal swab, cerebrospinal fluid, urine, and vesicle fluid.

Other Specimens. Urine is often a useful culture source for acquired or congenital cytomegalovirus infection, acute hemorrhagic cystitis associated with adenoviruses, and possibly other agents. Occasionally mumps or measles virus may also be detected in the urine for up to two weeks after onset of illness. Clean-voided specimens, 5 to 10 ml, are preferred, with transport to the laboratory as quickly as possible. Some laboratories prefer, if there is to be a delay of several hours before processing, to alkalinize the urine to a pH of 7.0; however, the evidence that this is crucial is not convincing. Other body fluids, such as pleural fluid, tracheobronchial washings, joint fluid, etc., are collected in sterile containers without further processing before transport.

Blood is usually not cultured for viruses; however, it is worthwhile to consider doing so in some situations, such as suspected viral hemorrhagic fevers, certain arboviral infections, and in situations of special interest to both the clinician and the virologist. While not wishing to completely discourage blood culture for viremia, we would point out that the yield of such cultures is usually quite low in contrast to the expense and effort of performing the studies. This is most

Table 50–4. POSTMORTEM SPECIMENS OF CHOICE

Syndrome	Specimens
Respiratory	Lung, tracheal swab
Central nervous system	Brain, spinal cord, cerebrospinal fluid, feces
Undiagnosed febrile illnesses	Brain, liver, lung, spleen, kidney, blood, feces, skin lesions, pharyngeal swab
Cardiovascular	Myocardium, pericardium and pericardial fluid, feces
Hepatitis	Liver, blood, feces

likely due to the fact that the detectable viremic phase in many acute viral infections is often gone by the time the illness is manifest and cultures are considered. Isolation attempts can be made on serum or on buffy coat material from heparinized or citrated blood samples.

Biopsy materials can also be handled with relative ease by simply placing the tissue in a sterile screw-capped bottle or vial for transport. In general, 1 to 3 g of tissue are preferred. If only very small pieces of tissue are available, these should be placed in a vial of VTM to keep them from drying out.

Postmortem specimens, 2 to 3 g of each tissue, are obtained with separate, sterile instruments in order to prevent cross-contamination, and handled in the same way as biopsy tissues. The selection of sites for sampling depends on the individual case and the viral agents suspected. Table 50–4 serves as a general guide in this selection.

Transport of Specimens. In general, prompt transport to the laboratory gives the best assurance of viral detection. If there is a delay of more than a few minutes, it is best to keep the specimens cooled to approximately 4°C., *but not frozen.* Freezing can destroy the infectivity of some viruses quickly, and should be done only if there is to be a prolonged delay of more than a day between collection and processing of specimens. Table 50–5 summarizes the relative stability of various viral agents in clinical samples.

Table 50–5. STABILITY OF VIRUSES IN CLINICAL SPECIMENS

Relatively stable*	Adenoviruses, enteroviruses
Variably stable†	Influenza, parainfluenza, arboviruses, herpes simplex, measles, mumps, rubella, rhinoviruses.
Unstable‡	Respiratory syncytial, varicella-zoster, cytomegaloviruses

*Stable at room temperature for several hours or more. All can be frozen at −70°C. without significant loss of infectivity.

†Stable at room temperature for at least one to three hours; freezing at −70°C. can result in variable loss of infectivity.

‡Unstable at room temperature; specimens should be kept cool and inoculated as soon as possible; infectivity can be totally lost on freezing.

Transport to the laboratory in the cool, unfrozen state can be accomplished in several ways, including the use of sealed, frozen ice packs in insulated or styrofoam containers, wet ice in bags, or, if short distances are involved over a brief time, placement of the sealed vials into a carton of crushed ice. When freezing is unavoidable, such as for shipment that may take many hours, the best alternative is to "snap-freeze" the samples in dry ice, dry ice and alcohol, or liquid nitrogen and transport the specimens in either dry ice or liquid nitrogen. It must be remembered that specimens that are being shipped by air or by mail must be appropriately labeled as infectious material and properly packaged according to federal guidelines.

TISSUE CULTURE TECHNIQUES

The cornerstone of diagnostic virology is the establishment and maintenance of tissue cultures. There are several cell culture techniques, including organ cultures and co-cultivation methods, that are applicable to special situations in medical virology. However, monolayer cell cultures are most commonly used in the clinical laboratory, and this discussion will focus on these. Excellent, detailed instructions and discussion of the monolayer methods can be found in the text by Lennette (1979). Kruse (1973) also has edited a thorough text dealing with both simple and complex cell and organ culture methods, which serves as a useful laboratory reference.

Monolayer cultures are prepared by dispersing tissue cells, usually with a proteolytic enzyme such as trypsin, suspending in a nutrient growth medium, and aliquoting into stationary tubes or bottles. The cells settle to the most dependent surface, adhere, and proliferate until a monolayer one cell in thickness develops. When this has occurred, the growth medium is replaced with maintenance medium (a liquid with only enough nutrients to keep the cells viable and containing no viral inhibitors). These cells are then ready for virus isolation and, depending upon the cell type, can remain viable for up to several weeks.

Types of Cell Cultures

There are three basic types of monolayer cell cultures. *Primary cultures* are derived directly from the parent tissue, such as human embryonic kidney, rhesus monkey kidney, human amnion, etc. These epithelial cells may be subcultured once, by trypsinizing and dispersing a primary monolayer, giving *secondary cultures,* which usually have similar appearance and virus sensitivity. Often, when one has an organ which has been minced and treated with trypsin to disperse the cells, many more cells are obtained than may be needed immediately. The excess cells in suspension can be placed in a freezing medium and kept frozen in liquid nitrogen until needed, then thawed and dispensed into bottles or tubes for use.

Diploid cell lines are usually derived from human embryonic lung or tonsil tissues. They are prepared in a manner similar to primary cultures, or by explantation of small (1 sq mm) fragments of tissue in bottles with growth medium to allow outgrowth of fibroblast cells. The resultant fibroblast monolayers retain a diploid chromosome number, and can be subcultured 20 to 50 times before they lose viability.

Heteroploid cell lines are, for practical purposes, "immortalized" cells which can be subcultured indefinitely. Most are derived from human epithelial carcinomas or otherwise transformed cells. The most popular are HeLa from a cervical carcinoma, KB from a carcinoma of the nasopharynx, Hep-2, and HL cells. These cells grow rapidly, and have a heteroploid chromosome count.

Selection of Culture Systems

Each of these cell types has distinctive uses in the virus laboratory, much as special and selective media do in bacteriology. They differ significantly in their susceptibility to various viruses, and these differences will be mentioned in the sections to follow. In general, it is preferable to have representatives of all three types available for use, and when a variety of possible agents are being sought in an individual patient all three are often inoculated simultaneously.

Primary (or secondary) rhesus or cynomolgus monkey kidney (MK) cells are good cell culture courses because of their broad sensitivity to human viruses, especially influenza, parainfluenza, mumps, many of the enteroviruses, and some adenoviruses.

Human diploid fibroblasts complement primary MK, extending the viral spectrum to particularly include herpes simplex, varicella-zoster, cytomegaloviruses, rhinoviruses, and some enteroviruses and adenoviruses.

Heteroploid cell lines have been particularly useful in the detection of respiratory syncytial virus, many adenoviruses, and some herpes simplex and enterovirus isolates.

There are many other cell cultures to choose from that have excellent broad-spectrum viral sensitivity (e.g., primary human embryonic kidney), or special sensitivity (e.g., primary African green monkey kidney for rubella virus isolation). However, the problems of cost and availability must be weighed against the relative usefulness of the culture systems in a clinical laboratory; for example, acute rubella infection can often be diagnosed serologically with paired sera obtained 10 to 14 days apart, while rubella virus isolation and identification, which is somewhat less sensitive, may take 8 to 20 days.

Other culture systems that should be available to the clinical laboratory include mice and embryonated hen's eggs. Suckling mice less than 24 hours of age are sensitive indicators of coxsackievirus A or B infection; in fact, many group A coxsackieviruses will be missed if newborn mice should be used frequently in the diagnostic laboratory, but when clinical and epidemiologic findings suggest such infections, and other culture systems do not yield an answer, mice can be valuable. Newborn mice are also susceptible to rabies, herpes simplex, and most arboviruses.

Embryonated hen's eggs are very sensitive to most strains of influenza A and B viruses, sometimes allowing isolation of these agents when cell culture attempts have failed. They are also useful in the isolation and identification of variola and vaccinia viruses, and are susceptible to herpes simplex viruses, but not to other agents of the herpesvirus group.

Table 50–6 summarizes the relative virus sensitivity of the different major culture systems in current use; however, this serves only as a rough guideline. Different strains of viruses, even within a given serotype, sometimes behave variably in different systems, or even in different laboratories. Some infections, including several not listed in Table 50–6, are better diagnosed by serologic or other methods that will be discussed in their specific sections.

Media

While a variety of culture media can be used, only a few are required in the clinical laboratory. These can be purchased ready for use as a concentrated (10×) solution or as a powder that is mixed with deionized distilled water and then sterilized by pressure filtration through a Millipore or nucleopore filter. Autoclavable minimal essential medium (MEM) is also available. The powder can be stored in the refrigerator in a desiccator for many months, and the liquid

Table 50–6. VIRUS CULTURE SYSTEMS AND THEIR SENSITIVITY TO DIFFERENT VIRUSES*

Virus	PMK	HDF	HET	Mice	Eggs
Adenoviruses	+ (var)	+ (var)	+ + (var)	–	–
Herpes simplex	0	+ +	+ (var)	+	+
Cytomegalovirus	–	+ +	–	–	–
Varicella-zoster	–	+ +	–	–	–
Vaccinia	+	+	+	–	+ +
Echoviruses	+ +	+ + (var)	0	–	–
Polioviruses	+ +	+ +	+ +	–	–
Coxsackievirus A	0(var)	0(var)	–	+ +†	–
Coxsackievirus B	+	–	+ +	+ +†	–
Arboviruses	–	–	–	+ +†	–
Influenza	+ +	–	–	–	+ +
Parainfluenza	+ +	–	–	–	0
Respiratory syncytial	+	0	+ +	–	–
Rhinoviruses	0	+ +	0	–	–
Mumps	+ +	0	0	0	+
Measles	+ +	0	0	–	–
Rubella‡	–	–	–	–	–
Rabies	–	–	–	+ +†	–

*PMK = Primary monkey kidney; HDF = human diploid fibroblast cell strains; HET = heteroploid cell lines; var = variable. A + + means maximum sensitivity for a virus; + means that the system is usually satisfactory for routine use; 0 means that the system is not reliable by itself for routine use; – means that the system is completely insensitive to the virus.

†Newborn mice required.

‡Special culture systems usually required (see text).

media are usually stable for one year at 2 to 8°C. if glutamine or antibiotics have not been added. All media should be checked for sterility before use.

Hanks' and Earle's balanced salt solutions serve as the base for most media and are excellent general diluents in the virology laboratory. They differ in buffering capacity, with Earle's solution being a stronger buffer for use in maintenance media where established cells produce large amounts of acid. Hanks' solution is useful in growth media where minimal acid is produced by the growing cultures. Tris or tricine buffers are useful alternatives when additional buffering capacity is needed (e.g., microtiter neutralizations), and reduce the need for frequent changing of media after inoculation.

Phenol red, a non-toxic pH indicator, is also a useful component of media. It is purple at a pH of 8.4 or greater, which is above that tolerated by most cell cultures, yellow at a pH of 6.8 or below, and orange to red in the physiologic range of 7.0 to 7.4.

Serum is required for growth and often is also necessary in maintenance media. It should have the properties of preservation of cell viability, and relative absence of antibodies or non-specific inhibitors of viruses. Fetal, neonatal, or agamma calf serum is generally useful in this regard, and is used at a 5 to 10 per cent concentration in growth media, depending upon the needs of the cell type. For maintenance or viral isolation, the serum concentration should be reduced as much as possible to a point which allows cell viability and minimizes the risk of serum inhibition of viruses. For respiratory agents, particularly influenza or parainfluenza virus, the less serum the better. In general, a 1 to 2 per cent serum concentration in maintenance media works well for routine use.

Bicarbonate ion is necessary for cell growth, and almost all media use a carbonic acid–sodium bicarbonate buffer system. Since the carbonic acid is volatile, cell cultures must be tightly sealed to avoid an excessive rise in pH. For tissue work in microtiter plates or other semi-open systems, a CO_2 incubator can be used to compensate the buffer system, or non-volatile buffers such as tricine can be added. We have found, even in closed culture systems, that adding approximately 10 ml of 1 M tricine buffer and 10 ml of 8.8 per cent $NaHCO_3$ to 500 ml of media serves to maintain an optimum pH and is not deleterious to the cells or viruses. Leibovitz Medium No. 15 contains galactose instead of glucose and is useful when a low bicarbonate concentration is required, such as for isolation of some rhinoviruses.

Of the various chemically defined media available, Eagle's minimum essential medium (MEM) and Medium 199 are the most popular in the virology laboratory. We prefer MEM because of its lesser cost and its proven performance. In summary, we currently suggest that MEM with added tricine and sodium bicarbonate and 5 to 10 per cent fetal calf serum be used for growth purposes, and MEM with tricine, sodium bicarbonate, and 1 to 2 per cent fetal calf serum be used for maintenance and virus isolation.

Reagents

The selection of water for use in tissue culture work is important. We prefer sterile distilled water which has been deionized to a resistance of greater than 1 million ohms. In some areas, double distilling or the use of simple deionizing units can achieve this level of purity.

There are a number of satisfactory antibiotic combinations for use in treating bacterial, fungal, and mycoplasmal contaminants in inoculated tissue cultures and clinical samples. Our preference is Hanks' BSS containing aqueous penicillin G at a concentration of 1000 units per ml, gentamicin at 0.5 mg per ml, and amphotericin B at a concentration of 10 μg per ml. This solution is stable for months when frozen.

Sodium bicarbonate, 8.8 per cent, is prepared in water, filter sterilized or autoclaved, and stored at room temperature.

Other essential reagents include trypsin, 0.25 per cent solution with EDTA, and GKN (glucose, KCl, NaCl) solution for rinsing cell monolayers prior to trypsinization; phosphate buffered saline (PBS) at a pH of 7.0 is a useful general diluent, and 2 per cent phosphotungstic acid at pH 7.0 for electronic microscopy preparations.

Our virus transport medium consists of veal or heart infusion broth with 0.1 per cent gelatin and antibiotics added to a final concentration of 2000 units/ml penicillin G, 0.2 mg/ml gentamicin, and 5 μg/ml amphotericin B. The pH is adjusted to 7.2 to 7.4 and the solution dispensed in 2-ml aliquots and frozen until used.

Preparation of Specimens

Swabs. Swabs of throat, rectum, and other sites are vigorously agitated in 2 ml of transport media, wrung out on the side of the tube, and discarded. If it is expected that bacterial or fungal contamination of the specimen will be a problem, the solution can be left at room temperature for 30 minutes to allow the added antibiotics to be effective, or else filtered through a 0.45- or 0.22-micron syringe filter. In some situations, such as use of rectal swabs, 0.5 to 1.0 ml of Hanks' BSS with antibiotics can be added, followed by centrifugation at 3500 rpm for 10 minutes to clarify the medium. Aliquots of 0.2 ml are inoculated into tissue culture tubes which have been drained of media. Inoculated tubes are placed in a roller drum for one hour to allow adsorption of virus, then replenished with maintenance media.

Feces. Approximately 2g of feces are thoroughly mixed with 12 ml of Hanks' BSS with antibiotics in a centrifuge tube and held at room temperature for 30 minutes. The suspension is then centrifuged at 3500 rpm in a refrigerated centrifuge for 15 minutes, and 0.2 ml of the supernatant inoculated into each tissue culture tube as above.

Urine. While some authorities recommend adjustment of urine pH to 7.0 to 7.2 with sodium bicarbonate, we have not found this to be particularly advantageous unless there is going to be an unavoidable delay of several hours before inoculation. It is preferable to obtain a fresh, clean-voided morning urine, add 0.5 ml of Hanks' BSS with antibiotics to 2 ml of the sample, and inoculate 0.2 ml into the tissue culture tubes as described for swab specimens. The pH of the tubes may then be adjusted if the specimen is too acid. It is advisable to change the media 16 to 24 hours after inoculation.

Cerebrospinal Fluid. Aliquots of 0.2 ml of CSF are placed directly into tissue culture tubes without prior treatment and handled as described above.

Tissues. When biopsy tissue or autopsy materials are received, 1 to 2 g are ground in a mortar and pestle with sterile sand, and a 10 per cent suspension (w/v) prepared in Hanks' BSS with antibiotics. Alternatively, a Pyrex glass tissue grinder may be used.

In either case, special care must be taken to avoid aerosol contamination of the work area; such preparation must be done in a biologic safety cabinet. The suspension is centrifuged at 3500 rpm for 15 minutes, and 0.2 ml of supernatant is inoculated into each tissue culture tube as described for swabs. The media should be changed after 16 to 24 hours of incubation, since many such inocula are toxic to tissue cultures.

In special situations, such as herpes simplex encephalitis, the virus yield is often enhanced by careful trypsinization of the biopsy tissue and co-cultivation of the resultant cell suspension by inoculation directly on the tissue culture monolayer. This requires care in allowing the viable cells to attach to the monolayer, then later changing the media to remove unattached, non-viable material and toxic products. Methods such as this, as well as explant cultures, are also particularly useful when seeking fastidious, highly cell-associated viruses or attempting to detect latent virus infection; however, their use in the routine clinical laboratory is limited.

Blood. While attempts to culture blood or bone marrow are not often made, there are occasions when this may be desirable. Serum, buffy coat, or anticoagulated whole blood (0.05 to 0.2 ml) can be inoculated directly into tissue culture tubes or mice. The tubes should be kept stationary for two to four hours to allow adsorption of free virus or leukocytes; then the medium is changed, followed by a second change the following day.

INOCULATION INTO OTHER HOST SYSTEMS

It may be desirable to inoculate the prepared specimens directly into mice or embryonated eggs, in addition to tissue culture tubes. Newborn mice, less than 24 hours of age, are preferable for most virus work, because of their greater susceptibility to infection. When seeking arboviruses, rabies, or herpes simplex virus, 0.015 ml of suspension is inoculated intracerebrally with a tuberculin syringe and the mice are observed for 21 to 28 days for mortality or encephalitic signs. If group A or B coxsackieviruses are suspected, we prefer several routes of inoculation: 0.015 ml intracerebrally, 0.05 ml intraperitoneally, and 0.03 ml subcutaneously. They are observed for 14 days for mortality, encephalitic signs with spastic paralysis (coxsackievirus B), or flaccid paralysis and cyanosis (coxsackievirus A). Deaths in the first postinoculation day are considered as nonspecific or post-traumatic and can be disregarded.

Inoculation into embryonated hen's eggs can be into the amnionic, allantoic, or yolk sacs, or onto the chorioallantoic membrane. Of these sites, the amnionic sac is most commonly used for influenza virus isolation. The chorioallantoic membrane is particularly useful in isolation and identification of variola and vaccinia viruses.

Recognition of Viruses in Cell Cultures

There are several ways in which viruses affect cell cultures. The most common is induction of morphologic changes in the cell cultures, called cytopathic effect (CPE), as the viruses replicate. The type of CPE induced varies with the viral agent involved and the cells affected. These changes can usually be easily seen on low-power (40 ×) microscopic inspection, and the different appearances are often distinctive enough to permit a tentative virus group identification. These will be illustrated in the appropriate sections in this chapter.

Some agents, such as influenza and parainfluenza viruses, may or may not induce CPE; however, they induce hemagglutination antigens on the tissue culture cell surface which will adsorb red blood cells from various animal and avian species. As infection progresses, these hemagglutinins are released into the media, as part of the envelope of intact virions. Virus infection of the cell culture can be detected after 24 hours to a few days of incubation by adding guinea pig red blood cells to the cell cultures, incubating at 4°C. for 45 to 60 minutes, then reading the tubes microscopically to determine if the red cells have become adherent to the cell culture surface (*hemadsorption*) or have agglutinated in the medium (*hemagglutination*). Incubation in the cold enhances this phenomenon, except for parainfluenza type 4 virus, where incubation at room temperature is preferred for detection of hemadsorption.

Another method, called the *interference* test, is more tedious, but has been found useful for rubella virus detection. Rubella virus infects and replicates well in primary African green monkey kidney; however, no CPE or hemadsorption occurs. The presence of rubella virus is demonstrated by incubating the infected cell cultures for seven days or more, then adding another "challenge" virus (usually an enterovirus) which is known to infect the cell culture and produce CPE. If the challenge fails to cause CPE, it is likely that rubella virus is present and has interfered with the replication of the second virus, probably by stimulating interferon production.

Sometimes, despite careful precautions and media changes, specimens will be toxic to tissue culture cells, producing what appears to be CPE. This is particularly a problem with feces, urine, blood, and tissue homogenates. The changes usually occur within 24 hours, and toxicity can be recognized by transferring a small amount of material to new cell cultures. Toxic products are usually diluted by this method so that no change occurs; if a virus is responsible for the effect, it will again produce CPE on transfer.

Occasions frequently arise when cell infection is either equivocal, definite but so minimal that it appears it will be difficult to further identify the virus, or undetectable after prolonged incubation of a specimen which was felt to have a high probability of being positive. In any of these situations, the culture can be "passed" by subculturing 0.2 ml of the contents into fresh tissue culture tubes. This can be done by transfer of media, media and scraped or trypsinized cells, or media and cells disrupted by sonication or freeze-thawing, depending upon the viral agent suspected. Passing cultures enhances the propagation of viruses with the development of greater and often more rapid and recognizable CPE or hemadsorption. It also serves to "adapt" the viruses to the cell culture, making it easier to identify them by serologic methods.

Identification of an Isolate

Preliminary virus group identification of an isolate can often be made quickly, on the basis of differential growth in certain cell cultures, mice or eggs, type of CPE produced, or ability to induce hemagglutination or hemadsorption. In many situations, the site from which the isolate was obtained and the clinical syndrome further aid in definitive early identification. For example, an isolate from the respiratory tract of an infant with bronchiolitis, which produces syncytia in heteroploid cell cultures and does not hemadsorb, is most likely to be respiratory syncytial virus. An isolate from the urine of a newborn infant with suspected congenital infection, growing only in human diploid fibroblasts and producing multiple foci of groups of rounded cells, is most likely to be a cytomegalovirus.

Utilizing these principles mentioned above, the laboratory can then proceed to specific confirmation and serotyping, as needed. The most common method employed is *neutralization* of the effect of the virus in the culture system in which it was detected. Briefly stated, this involves mixing a standard amount of the unknown virus with type-specific antisera, incubating the serum-virus and positive control (virus-PBS) mixtures at 35°C. for 45 to 60 minutes, and inoculating into the appropriate cultures. Identity of the isolate is confirmed when the specific antiserum inhibits the effect of the virus as compared with the positive control.

6

This principle can be applied to inhibition of CPE, hemadsorption, hemagglutination, or illness in animals.

Other, less commonly employed methods include identification by complement fixation, immunodiffusion, or immune electron microscopy. In some instances, immunofluorescence or immunoperoxidase methods may be directly applied to the infected cells for rapid identification (Gardner, 1980; Kawamura, 1977).

In the sections that follow, identification of specific viruses is discussed in more detail.

Other Systems of Virus Detection

Besides cell cultures, suckling mice, and embryonated eggs, there are several other methods which are useful for viral diagnosis. Of these, one of the oldest, and still occasionally useful, is histologic or cytologic examination. While not nearly so sensitive as virus isolation, such findings can guide the laboratory and sometimes be of immediate help to the clinician. For example, cytologic examination of the base of a vesicle may reveal intranuclear inclusions and multinucleated giant cells, indicating a herpes simplex or varicella-zoster infection. There are numerous examples, which will be considered in sections dealing with specific viruses.

Direct and indirect immunofluorescence methods have also become increasingly popular in the virology laboratory and have the advantages of speed and flexibility. These methods can be employed for rapid detection of viral antigens in cells obtained directly from the patient, such as exfoliated nasopharyngeal cells, urine sediment, vesicle scrapings, or biopsy tissues, and have been particularly successful in the rapid diagnosis of infections due to mumps, measles, herpes simplex, varicella-zoster, respiratory syncytial, influenza, parainfluenza, and adenoviruses (Minnich, 1980). As mentioned before the same methodology can also be applied to identification of an isolate in cell cultures.

Enzyme-linked immunosorbent assays (EIA) and immunoperoxidase methods have also been used by some virologists for detection of antigens in clinical samples and cell cultures. The EIA systems have been especially useful for detection of respiratory syncytial virus (McIntosh, 1982) and rotavirus (Yolken, 1982). Although EIA, immunoperoxidase, and immunofluorescence provide the potential for rapid diagnosis and detection of viral antigen when the virus is not cultivable, these systems require careful quality control and technical expertise to provide accurate diagnosis.

Radioimmunoassay for the detection of viral antigen in body fluids and secretions is rapid and sensitive. It is often used for the detection of hepatitis B viral infections, and may eventually be useful in several other infections.

Direct electron microscopy has further extended the capability of viral diagnosis. For years, it has been an excellent method for discerning between poxvirus and herpesvirus infections in vesicular eruptions. More recently, it has become particularly helpful in diagnosing infections due to viral agents which grow poorly, or not at all, in present culture systems. For example, rotaviruses and several other agents responsible for acute diarrhea in infants and young children have been detected by direct examination of the diarrheal stool. A positive result can often be found in two hours by this method, and it can also be used to group viral isolates from tissue cultures where CPE is unusual. A further refinement, immune electron microscopy, has been used to identify viral serotypes and to detect antibodies in human sera. This method allows visualization of virus-antibody aggregates when specific reactions have occurred.

SERODIAGNOSIS

While the emphasis on viral diagnosis has shifted somewhat away from serology and emphasized direct demonstration of viruses or their antigens, serodiagnosis continues to have significant value. In general, it is wise to obtain a sample of serum from most patients being cultured, and make plans to collect a convalescent serum, usually after two to three weeks. There are two important reasons to do this:

1. The viral agent may be missed on culture for a variety of reasons, and serodiagnosis may be the only method of detecting it. In some diseases, such as coxsackievirus B myopericarditis, virus shedding may have ceased by the time clinical disease is apparent, and serology is particularly valuable. Other infections, such as rubella, infectious mononucleosis, and arbovirus encephalitis, represent situations where routine culture is difficult to particularly slow, and serology is the preferred method of diagnosis.

2. In some instances, a viral isolate may be obtained, but it is unclear whether that agent is temporally or causally related to the illness in question. For example, an enterovirus isolated only from the feces of a patient with encephalitis may be involved in the illness or may represent a transient "carrier" state of several weeks' duration, related to asymptomatic infection, but not to the current illness. If a significant rise in antibodies to that agent is demonstrated, it becomes likely that the virus was causative. However, one must be careful of over-interpretation of such data; dual viral infections can occur, and if the epidemiologic and clinical data are suggestive, one may even wish to do serologies for other viral agents on the same sera to rule out other possible infections.

The interpretation of serologic data is easiest when paired, acute and convalescent sera are tested simultaneously. A *four-fold or greater rise* in antibody titer or conversion from seronegative to seropositive strongly supports a current infection. A four-fold or greater fall in titer, when the first serum is collected late in the source of an acute illness, assumes some significance, but must be interpreted with caution; similarly, single, late acute or convalescent sera with high titers may occasionally be useful, but one must be careful about over-interpretation. In some diseases, e.g., arbovirus infections, a "presumptive" diagnosis based on a single high titer may be made. This is based on a knowledge of the duration and level of specific antibodies in these infections, and the fact that persons with infections months to years in the past do not have antibody titers approaching those found in the patient. Another special instance is mumps virus infection, wherein antibodies to the "S" (soluble) antigen and a modest titer to the "V" antigen would be considered as presumptive evidence of recent mumps infection. Finally, antibody responses to primary viral infections usually follow classic patterns in that much of the early antibody is of the IgM class, which will later be replaced almost totally by IgG antibodies. In critical situations where only a single serum is available, it may be possible to determine whether the specific antiviral antibody is primarily IgM or IgG. If it is determined to be mostly IgM, this suggests a close temporal association to the disease in question. However, we do not recommend this as a routine test for the clinical virology laboratory. While the methodology for removal or quantitation of specific IgM or IgG antibodies appears to be simple, there are potential pitfalls and strict quality control is mandatory.

The most common serologic test employed in a routine laboratory is the complement fixation (CF) test. Others include hemagglutination-inhibition (HI), neutralization, and indirect immunofluorescent antibody tests. These and other tests are discussed further in the sections dealing with specific viruses.

A particularly vexing problem encountered in both public health and clinical laboratories is the receipt of paired sera (or, worse yet, a single serum) with an order marked "viral serology." It is very important to emphasize to the ordering physician the need to provide vital data, including the age of the patient, type of illness and date of onset, and the dates the sera were drawn. If no viral isolates were obtained from the patient, a decision can still be made regarding the choice of tests, based on these data. Most laboratories design serologic "batteries" to test these sera accordingly. For example, if a respiratory illness is involved, the "battery" might include influenza A and B, adenoviruses, respiratory syncytial, parainfluenza, and *Mycoplasma pneumoniae;* if the diagnosis is encephalitis, mumps and herpes simplex would be tested for; and, if the illness occurred in the summer or autumn, arbovirus serologies might be added, including those agents known to exist in the area.

SPECIFIC VIRAL AGENTS

Virus Classification

Virus classification is constantly undergoing extensive revision. Classification has previously been attempted on the basis of means of transmission (arboviruses), sites of isolation (adenoviruses), disease produced (poxviruses), and more recently on the basis of morphologic, chemical, and immunologic properties. There have been numerous important advances in viral taxonomy, including comprehensive decisions made at the meetings of the International Committee on Taxonomy of Viruses (ICTV). The ICTV study groups continue to define and describe virus groups and report their decisions periodically in *Intervirology* (Matthews, 1982). These reports form the basis for the viral classification and taxonomy presented here (Tables 50–7 and 50–8). The present classification is based primarily on physical, morphologic, and chemical data to the family level, and immunologic criteria and natural host range are utilized primarily for division at the genus and species levels. The remainder of this discussion will primarily involve viruses known to infect and cause disease in man. Not included in this classification are the unconventional viruses, such as scrapie, Creutzfeldt-Jakob, and Kuru agents, since little is currently known of their physical and chemical nature.

Table 50–7. DNA VIRUSES

Family and Genus	Representative Species
Parvoviridae	
Parvovirus	Gastroenteritis virus of humans*
Adeno-associated group (vernacular name)	Human adeno-associated virus
Densovirus	
Papovaviridae	
Papillomavirus	Papillomavirus of man
Polyomavirus	BK virus and JC virus SV40 (monkey)
Adenoviridae	
Mastadenovirus	Human adenovirus
Aviadenovirus	
Iridoviridae (not known to infect man)	
Iriovirus	
Herpetoviridae (Herpesviridae)	
Herpes simplex virus	Herpes simplex types 1 and 2, cytomegalovirus, Epstein-Barr virus, and varicella
Poxiviridae	
Orthopoxvirus (vaccinia subgroup)	Vaccinia, variola, cow pox virus
Avipoxvirus	
Capripoxvirus (sheep pox subgroup)	
Lepori pox virus (Myxoma subgroup)	
Parapoxvirus (Orf subgroup)	Orf virus, milker's nodule virus
Entomopox virus	
Hepadnavirus	Hepatitis B virus

*Possible species.

Adenoviruses

Initially isolated from adenoid tissue by Rowe in 1953, adenoviruses have since become recognized as important causes of disease. There are at least 39 different antigenic types which affect humans, of which types 1, 2, 3, 5, and 7 constitute the bulk of isolates.

It has been estimated that adenoviruses are responsible for up to 10 per cent of all febrile illnesses occurring in the first two years of life, and 5 per cent of febrile episodes in the 2- to 4-year age group. In older schoolchildren and young adults, sharp outbreaks are not unusual. Table 50–9 lists the recognized adenovirus-associated syndromes and the serotypes that have been usually associated with these. The most common illnesses include undifferentiated febrile illnesses in younger children, and upper or lower respiratory syndromes, often associated with tonsillitis and occasionally also with conjunctivitis (pharyngoconjunctival fever). The upper respiratory illnesses sometimes mimic acute streptococcal pharyngitis and tonsillitis with exudates and cervical lymphadenopathy. Pneumonia can be severe and occasionally fatal. It sometimes resembles an acute bacterial process that is unresponsive to antibiotics and may persist for several weeks. In some instances, chronic pulmonary disease has resulted. Pertussis-like illnesses have also been well described, with episodes of severe paroxysmal cough associated with lymphocytosis.

Aside from the febrile respiratory syndromes, eye infections are also commonly associated with adenoviruses, particularly acute follicular conjunctivitis and the more severe keratoconjunctivitis, which may produce symptoms lasting for three weeks or more. Some of these infections occur in sharp outbreaks related to inadequately chlorinated swimming pools ("swimming-pool conjunctivitis"), and other outbreaks have been attributed to such items as contaminated eye droppers or tonometers in ophthalmology clinics and sharing of cloth towels.

In addition, adenoviruses have occasionally been associated with urethritis, cervicitis, maculopapular or petechial exanthems, and disseminated illnesses which may include encephalitis, myocarditis, hepatitis, and diarrhea. The association between most of the recognized serotypes and primary viral diarrhea per se is largely unproven. However, adenovirus type 38, which is exceedingly difficult to cultivate in the laboratory, is now considered to cause 5 to 15 per cent of cases of infantile enteritis in some areas of the world (Hierholzer, 1982). There is evidence, mostly circumstantial, that adenoviruses may also be important in the

Table 50–8. RNA VIRUSES

Family and Genus	Representative Species
Reoviridae	
Orbivirus	Colorado tick fever
Reovirus	Human reovirus
Rotavirus	Acute diarrhea virus of young children
Picornaviridae	
Enterovirus	Polio, coxsackievirus A, coxsackievirus B, echovirus, enterovirus 68–71, hepatitis A (enterovirus 72)
Rhinovirus	Human rhinovirus
Calicivirus*	
Togaviridae	
Alphavirus (arbovirus group A)	WEE, EEE, Venezuelan encephalitis
Flavivirus (arbovirus group B)	Yellow fever virus, dengue, St. Louis encephalitis, Japanese B encephalitis
Rubivirus	Rubella virus
Pestivirus	
Retroviridae	
Oncovirinea† (leukovirus)	
Type C oncovirus group‡	
Mammalian type C oncovirus group§	Murine sarcoma and leukemia virus, feline sarcoma and leukemia viruses
Avian type C oncovirus group§	
Reptilian type C oncovirus group§	
Retroviridae (*Continued*)	
Type B oncovirus group‡	Mouse mammary tumor viruses
Spumavirinae† (genera not defined)	Human foamy virus group
Lentivirinae† (genera not defined)	
Orthomyxoviridae	
Influenza virus	Influenza A, B; Influenza C
Paramyxoviridae	
Paramyxovirus	Parainfluenza virus, mumps virus, Newcastle disease virus
Pneumovirus	Respiratory syncytial virus
Morbillivirus	Measles virus
Rhabdoviridae	
Lyssavirus	Rabies virus
Vesiculovirus	Chandipura virus
Arenaviridae	
Arenavirus	Lymphocytic choriomeningitis virus, Lassa virus, Argentinian and Bolivian hemorrhagic fever viruses
Coronaviridae	
Coronavirus	Human coronaviruses, avian infectious bronchitis virus
Bunyaviridae (previously designated Togaviridae)	
Bunyavirus	Bunyamwera virus, California encephalitis virus

*Possible family (Caliciviridae).
†Subfamilies.
‡Genera.
§Subgenera.

Table 50–9. CLINICAL SYNDROMES SHOWN TO BE ASSOCIATED WITH ADENOVIRUS INFECTIONS

Syndromes	Serotypes Associated*
Childhood febrile illness; pharyngoconjunctival fever	1, 2, 3, 5, 6, 7, 7a, (14, 21)
Pneumonia in infants; acute respiratory illness and pneumonia in adults	1, 2, 3, 5, 7, 7a, (21)
Pertussis-like illness	1, 2, 3, 5, 19, 21.
Conjunctivitis	2, 5, 7, 8, 19, (1,4,6,9,10,11,15, 16,17,20,22)
Keratoconjunctivitis	3, 8, 9, 19, (2,7a)
Acute hemorrhagic cystitis	11, (21)
Gastroenteritis	38 (36)

*Underlined serotypes are those which have more commonly been associated with outbreaks; serotypes in parentheses are only occasionally associated with the syndrome.

pathogenesis of childhood intussusception, acute appendicitis, and mesenteric adenitis. One syndrome of interest is acute hemorrhagic cystitis. This has been associated with adenovirus type 11 in particular, usually lasts two weeks or less, and most commonly affects children aged 5 to 15 years.

Aside from direct or indirect contact with infected secretions, most adenovirus infections are spread via respiratory droplets. Fecal-oral spread is also possible.

LABORATORY DIAGNOSIS

The majority of these viruses can be isolated from throat swabs and rectal swabs, as well as other clinically affected sites (conjunctiva, lung, urine). While primary embryonic human kidney cell cultures are considered very sensitive for isolation, most types will also grow more or less readily in human heteroploid or diploid fibroblast cell cultures, and some also produce CPE in RMK cultures. The CPE is characteristic (Fig. 50–1) with rounded, often uniformly swollen cells that tend to form grapelike clusters. As CPE progresses, the cell sheet often appears lacy and later detaches from the tube wall. The spread with which CPE develops varies from strain to strain and may take from two days to three weeks.

The viruses contain both group-specific and type-specific

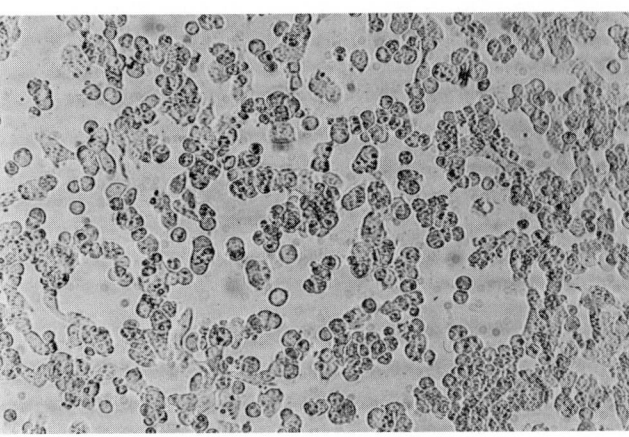

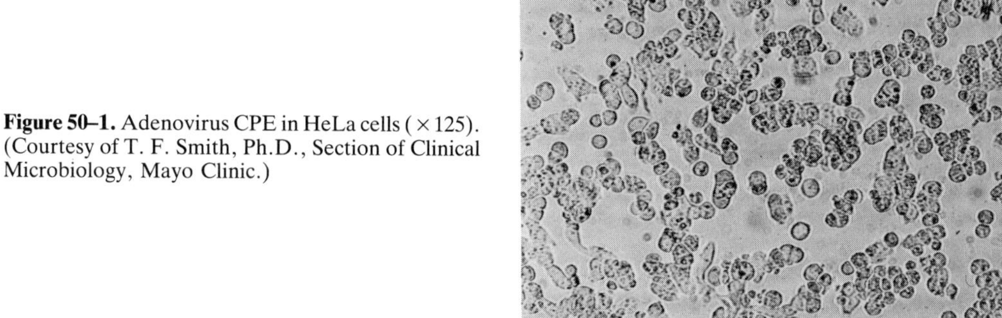

Figure 50–1. Adenovirus CPE in HeLa cells (×125). (Courtesy of T. F. Smith, Ph.D., Section of Clinical Microbiology, Mayo Clinic.)

antigens. The former is sometimes used in either a complement-fixation or gel-diffusion procedure for serologic confirmation of the isolate as an adenovirus; however, specific serotyping requires neutralization by type-specific antiserum. Our usual approach is to select specific antisera for typing of the unknown isolate, based upon the clinical syndrome and known epidemiology. Table 50–9 serves as a useful guideline in this regard. For isolates which are not readily identified by a limited battery of antisera to common types, it is possible to classify them into one of three groups, depending on their ability to agglutinate rat or monkey erythrocytes, then proceed to neutralization tests, or hemagglutination-inhibition tests, depending upon their behavior. However, before expending a great deal of time and effort on specific serotyping of all adenovirus isolates, it should be determined whether such identification could have significant relevance to the patient, the illness, or the epidemiologic situation.

Serologic diagnosis, using paired sera, is useful in situations where the virus was not detected, or as further confirmation that the virus isolated was temporally associated with the illness in question. The usual test utilizes the group antigen in a CF test, which is convenient and sometimes helpful. However, the CF serology is not as sensitive as a neutralization test. Portnoy (1967) showed that in patients with adenovirus isolates the neutralizing antibody titer to the homologous virus rose significantly at least twice as often as did the CF antibody titer to the group antigen.

INTERPRETATION OF LABORATORY FINDINGS

There is little difficulty in associating an adenovirus with a disease if it has been directly isolated from a biopsy of clinically affected tissue, e.g., lung. The association is even more firm if "smudgy" intranuclear inclusions typical of adenoviruses are also seen on histologic examination.

In other situations, epidemiologic evidence has been sufficiently convincing to allow rather firm conclusions about the association of some adenovirus isolates with specific clinical syndromes. For example, the isolation of adenovirus type 11 from the urine of a child with acute hemorrhagic cystitis would be considered significant; similarly, any adenovirus isolate from a conjunctival swab from a patient with acute conjunctivitis, in the absence of evidence for bacterial, chlamydial, or other concomitant viral infection, would strongly suggest an etiologic association.

The difficulties in interpretation which commonly arise are related to several facts. Adenoviruses are extremely ubiquitous, particularly in patients between the ages of four months and four years, and subclinical infections with seroconversions are common. Furthermore, these agents can lead to persistent, asymptomatic infections of the adenoid and tonsillar tissues as well as the lymphoid tissues of the small bowel. As a result, intermittent virus shedding into the respiratory secretions or the feces may last for as long as 6 to 18 months after primary infection, and such shedding may be enhanced by stress, such as other viral or bacterial infections. For these reasons, adenovirus isolates from throat or fecal samples must be interpreted with caution, even when supported by antibody seroconversions. This dilemma is particularly difficult in the younger age groups (under four years).

Extensive epidemiologic studies (Brandt, 1969; Fox, 1977) have helped our understanding of these problems, but the interpretive difficulties remain. Based upon the epidemiologic findings relevant to the recognized adenoviral febrile and respiratory syndromes, we have developed the following rough guidelines for interpretation: simultaneous isolation from both throat and feces has approximately a 70 to 85 per cent probability of etiologic association with the illness, based upon the ability also to demonstrate a significant seroconversion. Isolation from the throat, and not the feces, has approximately a 50 to 60 per cent probability of such an association, and isolation only from the feces drops this figure to between 20 and 35 per cent. The interpretation of the significance of the isolates or serologies can be further aided if the laboratory has made an attempt to exclude other common viral agents, such as enteroviruses and parainfluenza and influenza viruses, and if bacterial pathogens have also been reasonably excluded. Also, the finding of such isolates in older children and adults with compatible illnesses assumes somewhat greater significance, since chronic carriage appears to diminish with advancing age.

Herpesviruses

HERPES SIMPLEX VIRUS (HSV, OR HERPESVIRUS HOMINIS)

The common cold sore, or fever blister (herpes labialis), the most usual manifestation of HSV infection, has been described since antiquity. The virus was first isolated in 1919 by inoculation of herpes labialis vesicle fluid into a rabbit cornea, and transmissibility was demonstrated by reinoculation from the infected rabbit cornea to the cornea of a blind man. Following the successful growth of HSV in tissue culture the virus was shown to be etiologically related to a wide variety of clinical syndromes, as well as subclinical infection, occurring with either primary or recurrent disease. Immunologic investigation in the early 1960's established two broadly cross-reacting antigenic types of HSV: herpes simplex virus type 1 (HSV-1) and herpes simplex virus type 2 (HSV-2). In general HSV-1 is found primarily in and around the oral cavity and in skin lesions above the waist, while HSV-2 is isolated primarily from the genital tract and skin lesions below the waist. Neonatal disease usually results from HSV-2 infection, and HSV encephalitis in adults is usually caused by HSV-1 infection. The vast majority (approximately 99 per cent) of all primary HSV infections are asymptomatic, and the host-parasite relationship can be seen in Figure 50–2. Recurrent HSV disease usually occurs at the site of primary infection, but other distant sites may be involved. Recurrence with cell-to-cell spread of virus occurs in the presence of serum-neutralizing antibodies. Fever, sunlight, environmental temperature extremes, infection, physical trauma, emotional stress, neoplasia, and pregnancy are some of the factors noted to trigger recurrent HSV disease. Recurrent infection is usually the result of reactivation of latent virus residing in paraspinal or cranial nerve ganglia innervating the site of primary infection. The activated virus presumably travels down the axon to the skin (or other site) and induces disease. However, in some instances exogenous reinfection cannot be ruled out.

Epidemiology. The HSV are widespread, and man is the only natural host or known reservoir of infection for the human herpesviruses (herpesviruses of other vertebrates occur). The incubation period usually lasts 2 to 12 days, and there is no apparent sexual or seasonal predilection for infection. Based on serologic evidence, by age 25 years approximately 70 to 80 per cent have experienced contact with virus, and by 45 years this rises to nearly 100 per cent in some populations. However, the range of antibody prevalence in adults varies greatly with socioeconomic class. Approximately 30 to 50 per cent of upper socioeconomic class adults compared to 80 to 100 per cent of adults in lower socioeconomic groups have detectable antibody to HSV. HSV can be cultured from the oropharynx in about 1 per cent of healthy adults and from the genital tract of slightly less than 1 per cent of non-pregnant, asymptomatic adult women.

Malnutrition, concurrent debilitating disease, a variety of acute childhood illnesses, and prematurity all predispose to disseminated primary infections in infants and young children.

The transmission of HSV-1 is usually non-venereal but probably requires close contact, i.e., hand-to-mouth and kissing. HSV-2 is venereally transmitted and is most often acquired by newborns passing through an infected birth canal (perinatal transmission). Mechanisms of antenatal transmission are less well understood. Beyond the neonatal period, young children and preadolescents are infected almost exclusively with HSV-1, while HSV-2 is isolated most commonly from the 15- to 30-year age group, usually from genital lesions.

Clinical Aspects. Acute gingivostomatitis is the most common manifestation of primary HSV-1 infection and is most frequent in the one- to four-year age group. The differential diagnosis includes aphthous stomatitis and herpangina. Other manifestations of primary HSV infections include rhinitis, keratoconjunctivitis, meningoencephalitis, eczema herpeticum (Kaposi's varicelliform eruption), traumatic herpes, e.g., herpetic whitlow, and generalized infection. Primarily acquired HSV-1 infection in young adults may frequently produce an acute upper respiratory illness with pharyngitis and tonsillitis (Glezen, 1975). Primary HSV-1 infection may also cause follicular conjunctivitis with chemosis, edema, and corneal ulcers. The ulcers may progress from small dendritic ulcers to large "geographic" ulcers. Secondary bacterial infection may then lead to opacification of the lens. Herpes labialis and dendritic corneal ulcers are the most common manifestations of symptomatic, recurrent HSV-1 infection.

Immunosuppressed patients with primary or recurrent disease show a predilection for esophageal ulceration and interstitial pneumonitis as well as disseminated disease.

Occasionally, HSV-1 will also cause a severe necrotizing encephalitis usually affecting the temporal or frontal lobes. It is often fatal (average mortality of about 50 per cent), and more than half of the survivors are left with significant neurologic sequelae. However, a specific antiviral agent, adenine arabinoside, has provided a good therapeutic index, and a newer antiviral, acyclovir, may also be useful. There appears to be no age, sex, or socioeconomic predilection for HSV encephalitis. About 15 per cent have a history of recurrent herpes labialis, which is similar to the frequency observed in the general population, and about one third of patients with encephalitis will manifest herpes labialis during the course of encephalitis.

The most common form of HSV-2 primary and recurrent disease has been recognized for approximately 200 years, but reawakened interest is related to the discovery of

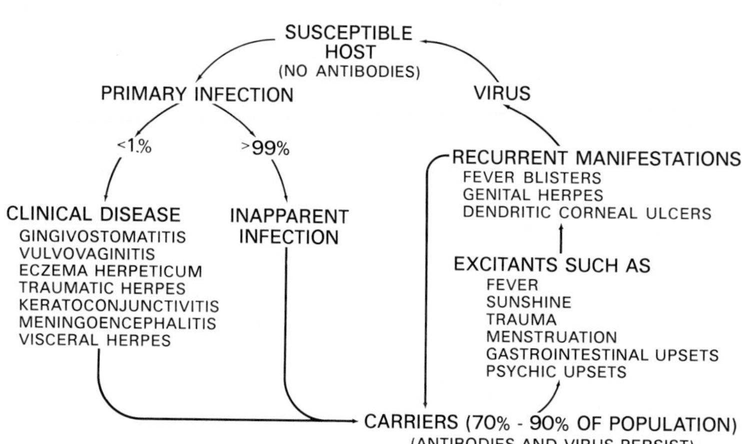

Figure 50–2. The host-parasite relationship of herpes simplex virus in man. (From Krugman, S., and Ward, R.: Infectious Diseases of Children. St. Louis, C. V. Mosby Co., 1968.)

widespread venereal transmission, neonatal infection, and a possible, but unproved, association with carcinoma of the cervix. HSV-2 is the most common cause of genital vesicular lesions in men and women.

Occasionally during primary HSV-2 genital infection in adults, a concurrent, usually benign aseptic meningitis develops, either from neuronal ascent or via hematogenous spread. Transient myelitis or myeloradiculitis can also occur.

Neonatal HSV infections may be acquired in the antenatal (intrauterine) or perinatal period. The majority, however, are acquired perinatally as the result of exposure to an infected birth canal during delivery. The greatest risk (approximately 40 per cent) to the fetus occurs as a result of primary acquired HSV infection in the mother's genital tract late in pregnancy, with active lesions present at the time of birth. If primary genital infection occurs at 32 weeks gestation or later, without active lesions at birth, the neonatal risk of infection is about 10 per cent. The risk of neonatal infection in a pregnant woman with recurrent genital herpes, active or not, at the time of delivery is unknown. When virus is present in the vagina or cervix and if membranes have been ruptured for four hours or greater prior to delivery, there is an increased chance that ascending virus may have infected the infant. Approximately half of clinically infected infants are born to asymptomatic mothers.

The mode of transmission of intrauterine infection is less well defined and probably involves hematogenous, transplacental spread, as well as ascending infection with associated chorioamnionitis. The spectrum of disease in an infected neonate varies from subclinical to severe, with symptoms and signs reflecting the organs of involvement, i.e., lungs, liver, adrenals, brain, retina, and skin. In overwhelming generalized infection encephalitis and respiratory and/or heptic failure with increasing jaundice and adrenal insufficiency may occur. Infants that survive infection are often, but not always, left with some degree of neurologic damage and may manifest recurrent vesicular skin lesions for years.

Although HSV-1 and HSV-2 generally have different modes of transmission and associated clinical disease, there is overlap. HSV-2 infection may occur in the oral cavity and HSV-1 may infect the genital tract. When HSV-1 genital disease occurs in pregnant women, it may cause neonatal disease as well. Both types of virus may cause cutaneous vesicular eruptions indistinguishable from varicella-zoster; also, erythema multiforme, probably the result of an immune reaction to HSV, has been associated with both HSV-1 and HSV-2.

Laboratory Diagnosis. Viral isolation is the best means of documenting HSV infection. The virus has been isolated from vesicular fluid, ulcer scrapings, throat swabs, saliva, cervical secretions, CSF, paraspinal and cranial nerve ganglia, and clinically infected tissues. Other sites from which virus is isolated less frequently include buffy coat, urine, and rectal cultures. The virus grows rapidly *in vitro*, with cytopathogenic effects (CPE) often apparent by 24 hours. The human diploid fibroblast and primary rabbit kidney are the tissue culture systems of choice, and HSV produces a rather specific pattern of CPE with large, round, "balloon" cells (Fig. 50–3). Less commonly there is formation of multinucleated syncytial giant cells.

A HSV isolate from a typical lesion is diagnostic with regard to the etiology of the lesion. Isolates from normally sterile, clinically infected tissues from patients with compatible syndromes, such as brain, lung, or liver, are also highly significant, especially in the absence of other etiologic possibilities. However, isolation of HSV from throat cultures or vesicular lesions of patients with undifferentiated febrile illness could result from reactivation of HSV without being causally related to the acute disease process. In fact, the potential reactivation of a HSV at any site during another febrile illness must be considered in interpreting a HSV isolate.

Differentiating a HSV isolate into type 1 or 2 is rarely clinically indicated, and the available HSV typing sera show extensive cross-reactivity, as would be expected. Immunofluorescent, immunoperoxidase, and indirect hemagglutination inhibition methods have been used to type HSV isolates (Stewart, 1976). More precise typing of HSV strains can be accomplished by newer methods, such as the use of restriction endonucleases or highly specific monoclonal antibodies.

Serology is a useful epidemiologic tool for determining prevalence of exposure to HSV and for diagnosing primary infection when a four-fold or greater rise in antibody titer is demonstrated. However, in the adult population the prevalence of previous virus exposure is so great that detection of antibody gives no information as to when disease was first acquired, and since most primary infections are asymptomatic, there is little opportunity to demonstrate

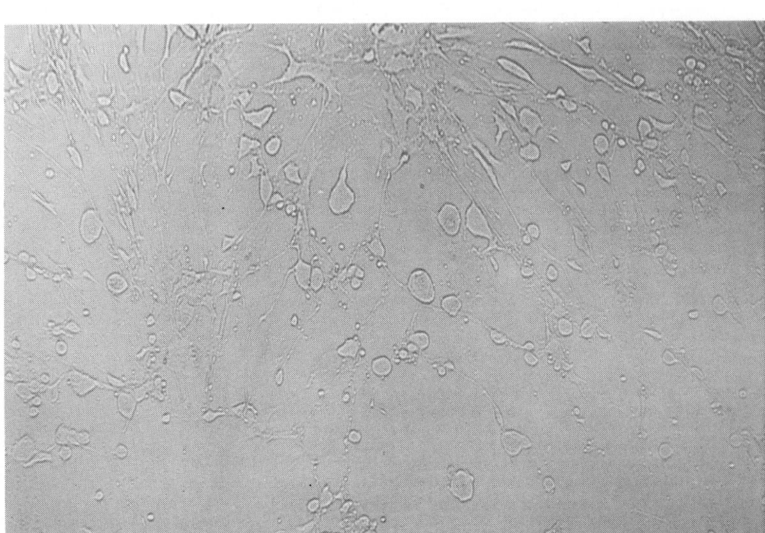

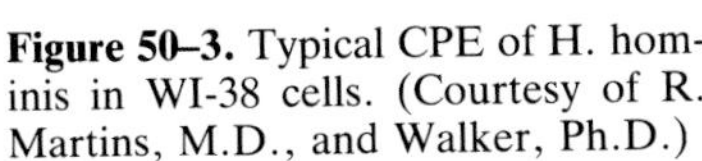

Figure 50–3. Typical CPE of H. hominis in WI-38 cells. (Courtesy of R. Martins, M.D., and Walker, Ph.D.)

the initial titer rise. Early recurrent infections may significantly boost antibody titers, but following multiple recurrences, titers usually become stabilized at moderately high levels, as measured by complement fixation (CF), neutralization (NA), or other techniques.

CF antibodies are sensitive, stable, and long lasting, but they are reactive against broadly held antigens in both HSV-1 and HSV-2, making it impossible to distinguish type 1 from type 2 primary or recurrent infection. This difficulty in serodifferentiation of type 1 versus type 2 infections extends to other serologic techniques, including NA and indirect hemagglutination (IHA). All three methods are more sensitive for HSV-1 than for HSV-2 infections, but CF and NA tests are more sensitive than IHA for HSV-1 infections. However, IHA appears slightly more sensitive than the other methods in early HSV-2 infections, but titers are often already high by the time acute serum is drawn, making demonstration of a significant titer rise difficult (Back, 1974).

To further complicate matters, primary or recurrent infection by either HSV-1 or 2 usually causes elevation of antibody titer to both strains of HSV, and the greatest titer rise may be heterotypic. Therefore, serologic determination of which virus induced a recent infection is extremely difficult. Neutralization (NA) kinetics and plaque reduction techniques have been employed (Plummer, 1973). The indirect immunofluorescence and enzyme immunoassay (EIA) methods are useful in determining the immunoglobulin class of antibody responding to infection. These can be used in detecting a primary IgM response, but sera containing rheumatoid factor may give a false positive reaction.

Cytology and histology can be diagnostically supportive in the proper clinical setting, but neither is as sensitive as viral culture. Papanicolaou staining of cervical or vesicle lesion scrapings may reveal cells characteristic of HSV infection. In primary disease the uninucleated or multinucleated viral infected cells show occasional intranuclear inclusions with a ground glass nuclear appearance (Fig. 50–4). In recurrent genital herpes, tight aggregates of multinucleated cells demonstrating intranuclear inclusions are frequently seen (Fig. 50–5). However, it is extremely difficult, if not impossible, to distinguish primary from recurrent herpes genitalis by this method. Infected tissues stained with hematoxylin and eosin may also reveal Cowdry type A intranuclear inclusions identical to those seen in Figure 50–5 and support a diagnosis of HSV infection in the proper clinical setting.

CYTOMEGALOVIRUS

Human cytomegalovirus (CMV) is indistinguishable by negative staining electron microscopy from its close relatives, herpes simplex and varicella. CMV infection results in distinctive histologic changes characterized by striking epithelial cell cytomegaly with a single, large, red intranuclear inclusion surrounded by a halo, giving the cell the appearance of an owl's eye (Fig. 50–6).

CMV infections have a long incubation period (weeks to months) which parallels the slow replicative cycle in tissue culture. Infections may be local or systemic and can be either active or latent.

Epidemiology. CMV infection is endemic worldwide with

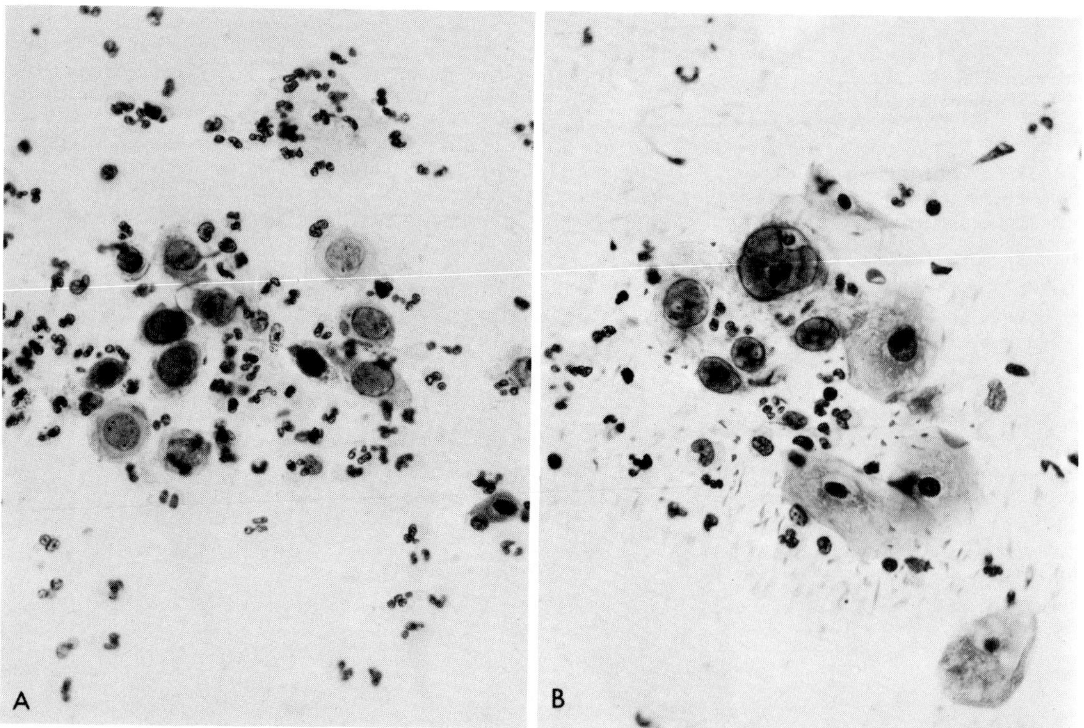

Figure 50–4. *A,* Early primary herpes genitalis. Infected squamous cells with intranuclear vacuolization and "ground glass" nuclear appearance (×500). *B,* Multinucleated viral infected cells with a predominantly "ground glass" nuclear appearance. Intranuclear inclusions are identified in some of the cells (×500). (From Ng, A. B. P., Regan, J. W., and Lindner, E.: Acta Cytol., *14*:125, 1970.)

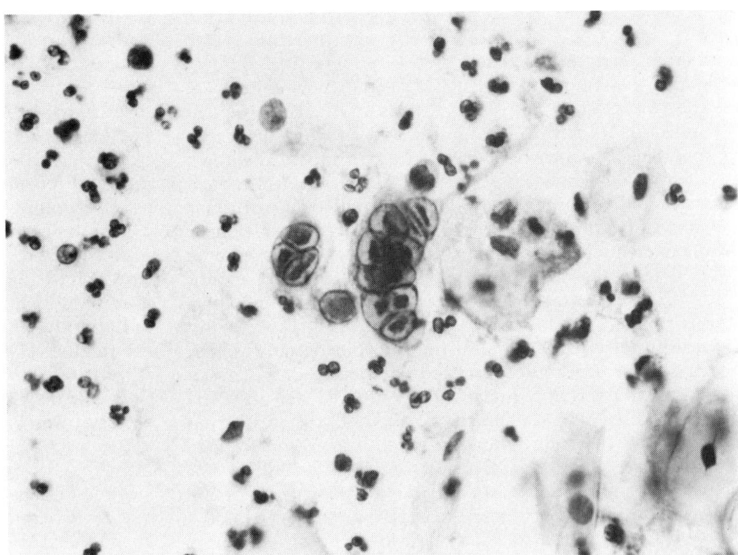

Figure 50–5. Recurrent herpes genitalis. Tight aggregates of infected cells with intranuclear acidophilic inclusions ($\times$500). (From Ng, A. B. P., Regan, J. W., and Lindner, E.: Acta Cytol., *14*:126, 1970.)

the highest prevalence rates among very young children, particularly those living under crowded, intimate conditions. The infection may be congenital, but it is most often acquired in the perinatal or postnatal periods. The prevalence of viral excretion in the urine, reflecting active infection, varies from 0.5 to 2.0 per cent at birth to 10 to 56 per cent at six months of age, depending upon the population studied. By one year of age the prevalence of viral excretion usually stabilizes or declines, and less than 1 per cent of normal, healthy adults excrete virus in the urine. The rate of viruria, however, increases during pregnancy to 4 to 13 per cent in the third trimester, and the incidence of positive cervical cultures has been reported to be as high as 28 per cent in late pregnancy. On the other hand, the rate of serologic positivity, also reflecting experience with CMV, increases slowly through childhood. During adolescence the infection rate rises significantly, until 35 to 100 per cent of adults have detectable complement fixation (CF) antibodies by age 35. The incidence of seropositivity varies greatly depending on the socioeconomic status and living conditions of the population surveyed. Serologic evidence also indicates that adult women have higher rates of CF positivity than men of the same age.

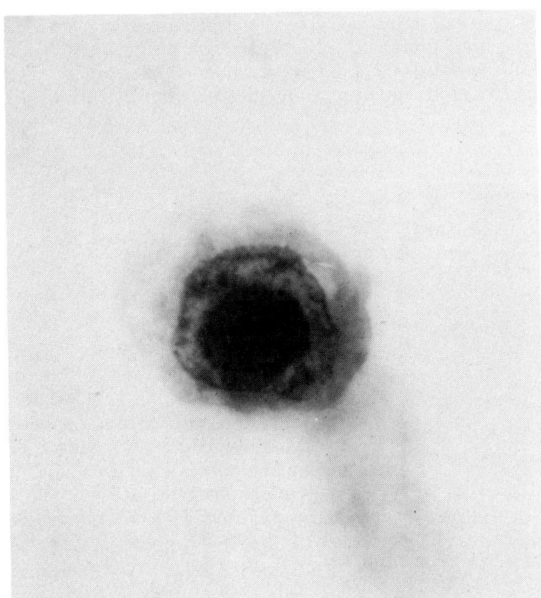

Figure 50–6. Intranuclear inclusion in a renal epithelial cell. Urinary sediment from a child with congenital cytomegalovirus disease. (From Blanc, W. A., and Goetz, R.: Pediatrics, *29*:61, 1962.)

Congenital Infection. CMV is probably the most common cause of congenital infection in humans. The mode of natural transmission of virus from mother to fetus is ill defined because of the usual lack of either maternal or fetal signs or symptoms. Maternal CMV infections, like herpes simplex virus infections, are subject to recurrence, especially in the genital tract, and the role of recurrent infection in intrauterine transmission is poorly understood. More often, a congenitally infected infant is a first child of a younger mother, suggesting a relationship to a primarily acquired maternal infection, but sequentially infected children born to the same mother have been occasionally reported. The frequency of congenital CMV infection varies with socioeconomic class (greater frequency in less affluent classes) and is more prevalent in low birth weight infants.

The vast majority of congenital CMV infections are asymptomatic or characterized by mild hepatomegaly with moderately abnormal liver functions and jaundice. However, symptoms vary from these minor manifestations to severe, disseminated disease with growth retardation, chorioretinitis, pneumonitis, thrombocytopenic purpura, maculopapular or hemorrhagic skin rash, and hemolytic anemia. Congenitally infected infants sometimes excrete extremely high titers of infectious CMV in the urine for periods as long as a year or more after birth, and, therefore, could function as a source of acquired infection for others. It is estimated that 10 per cent of newborn virus excretors are neurologically damaged, but this is probably a conservative figure.

Acquired Infections and Reactivated Latent Infections.

By adulthood most persons have experienced asymptomatic contact with CMV as evidenced by the presence of CF antibodies. Persons experiencing acquired infection, reinfection with the same or different CMV strains, or reactivation of a latent infection can excrete virus in titers as high as 10^6 infective units/ml in the urine and/or saliva for weeks or months. Dissemination of infection to others is known to occur and can be via oral, respiratory, or venereal routes, or parenterally by organ transplantation or blood transfusion.

Clinical manifestations reflect the organ(s) of involvement with preferential targets being liver, spleen, hematopoietic system, kidney, and lungs. A heterophile negative mononucleosis-like syndrome with fever, splenomegaly, and atypical lymphocytosis following open-heart surgery utilizing extracorporeal circulation and multiple blood transfusions, and a similar syndrome unrelated to transfusion and seen mostly in adults (rarely under 20 and usually over 30 years) are both caused by CMV infection. Studies of the acquisition rate of CMV infection following blood transfusion suggest a 5 to 12 per cent blood donor CMV carrier rate. The risk of transfusion-acquired CMV infection also appears to be high among ill newborn infants of CMV-seronegative mothers who receive blood transfusions from seropositive donors (estimated at 12.5 per cent). Such infected infants can become severely ill, with symptoms including pneumonia and hepatitis (Yeager, 1981).

Cases of anicteric and icteric hepatitis have also been related to acquired CMV infection. Despite the frequent histologic evidence of renal involvement, symptomatic renal disease is not seen. Reactivation or primary CMV infections are known to complicate a wide variety of chronic debilitating diseases, in particular hematopoietic and lymphoreticular malignancies, post-allograft transplantation patients, and others undergoing immunosuppressive therapy. In immunosuppressed patients, the lungs appear to be the primary target organ, accompanied by frequent liver involvement. Asymptomatic involvement is common and is often diagnosed only by the distinctive histologic changes. The nonspecific symptoms and chest x-ray findings, when they occur, are those of an interstitial pneumonitis of variable severity.

Prospective studies of renal transplant patients receiving immunosuppressive therapy have shown that the majority developed active CMV infection, and reactivation of latent infection appeared to be the most probable pathogenetic mechanism. However, recent data indicate that the highest mortality risk for such patients occurs when tissue from a seropositive donor is transplanted into a seronegative recipient. This suggests that primary CMV infection is more severe than reactivation in this group. Symptoms may include fever, arthralgia, pneumonitis, leukopenia, and hepatitis. Other diseases in the post-transplant patients included retinitis and glial-nodule encephalitis. The majority of immunosuppressed patients with CMV infection have a normal serum antibody response to the virus. Therefore, it seems more likely that the CMV infection (primary or reactivated) may be related to defective cell-mediated immunity.

Laboratory Diagnosis and Interpretation. Viral culture is the method of choice for confirming CMV infection. Virus is most often recovered from the urine during active infection, but may also be isolated from blood leukocytes, saliva, semen, cervix, and other infected tissues (lung, liver, kidney). CMV exhibits strict species-specific growth requirements, and viral replication occurs best in human diploid fibroblasts. The virus exhibits somewhat unpredictable thermal and chemical instability. Some workers report that the virus is stable at 4°C. for as long as seven days and that freezing causes complete loss of virus infectivity. However, if stored at −80°C. or lower, the virus is relatively stable. For best results, a fresh specimen from any source should be inoculated into tissue culture as soon as possible. The virus is highly cell-associated and sometimes slow growing, occasionally requiring four to six weeks for primary isolation. Human CMV are identified by distinctive cytopathogenic effects in tissue culture (Fig. 50–7). Small nests of enlarged, rounded, refractile cells surrounded by normal fibroblasts are scattered throughout the cell sheet. In patients who are shedding large quantities of CMV (e.g., some congenitally infected neonates), the viral particles can often be detected rapidly by direct electron microscopy of ultracentrifuged urine sediment.

Isolation of CMV from clinically infected tissues is etiologically significant. However, one must remember that other opportunistic organisms, especially *Pneumocystis carinii,* may simultaneously infect a compromised host and may be contributing significantly to the symptomatology. In view of the high prevalence of CMV viruria during infancy and in institutionalized children, caution is necessary in these populations in equating viral isolation from the urine with

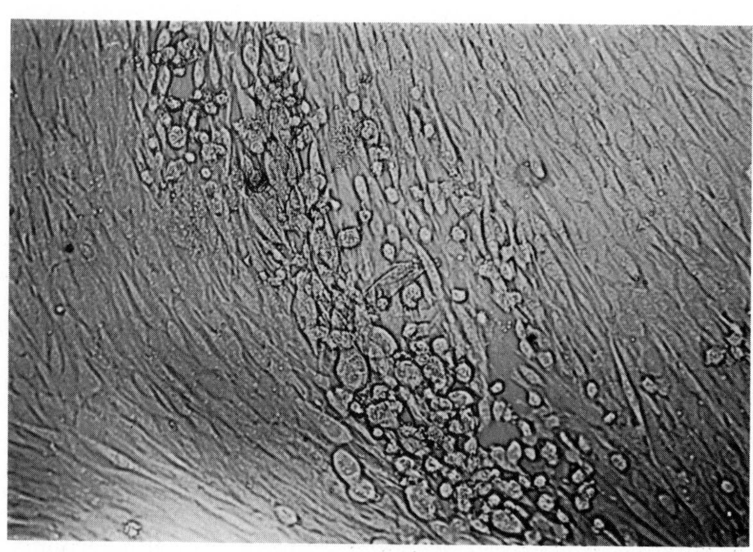

Figure 50–7. Cytopathic effect of CMV in human embryonic lung fibroblasts; focal lesion, strain C87. Unstained preparation (×140). (From Lennette, E. H., and Schmidt, N. J. [eds.]: Diagnostic Procedures for Viral and Rickettsial Infections. 4th ed. New York, American Public Health Association, 1969.)

acute disease. In older, immunologically normal children and adults viruria assumes greater diagnostic importance. Isolation of CMV from the blood leukocytes also requires some interpretive caution, since asymptomatic carriage of virus has been demonstrated. However, when associated with a compatible clinical syndrome for which no other cause can be demonstrated, the significance of the isolation increases.

Serology plays a supportive role in diagnosing CMV infection. There is a qualitative and quantitative antigenic heterogeneity within human CMV with several different strains being recognized. This becomes important when interpreting serologic data based on the use of a single antigenic strain of CMV.

A microtiter CF test is a commonly used method for determining the presence of CMV antibodies. Although a broadly reactive CMV antigen (strain AD169) is used, some degree of strain specificity is still demonstrated. The CF test measures IgG antibody, and a titer of 1:8 or greater is considered evidence of prior exposure to CMV. In association with compatible clinical and virologic isolation data, a fourfold or greater rise in CF titer is good evidence for acquired or reactivated CMV infection. Following acquired infection and seroconversion, CF titers have declined to undetectable levels and, to further complicate interpretation, wide, spontaneous fluctuations in CF titers have been observed prospectively in apparently normal, healthy adults (Waner, 1973). Therefore, both the absence of a CF titer and a fourfold change in the titer must be interpreted with caution. The indirect fluorescent antibody and EIA tests are also relatively easy to perform and allow measurement of antibodies of specific immunoglobulin classes; unfortunately these methods have not yet become either adequately sensitive or specific for the detection of IgM antibodies. At present, the best serologic method in use for the detection of CMV-specific IgM antibodies is the radioimmunoassay (RIA). Detection of these antibodies by this method appears to correlate well with recent primary infection, and also may support the diagnosis of symptomatic congenital infection (Griffiths, 1982). The CMV IgM antibody test has shown cross-reactivity with Epstein-Barr (heterophile-positive infectious mononucleosis), varicella, and herpes simplex viruses. Therefore, the IgM antibody appears to detect broadly held antigens of the human herpesvirus group. Also, sera containing rheumatoid factor may give a false positive IgM reaction. Neutralizing antibodies show greater strain specificity and are detected by cumbersome plaque reduction techniques.

Examination of a stained (hematoxylin-eosin, Giemsa, or Papanicolaou) urinary sediment of a fresh, filtered (membrane filter with 0.5 μ pore size) urine specimen for typical inclusion bearing cells (Fig. 50–6) is rarely helpful, being 60 to 80 per cent less sensitive than urine culture and not entirely specific. Infected cells are shed only intermittently. Tissue biopsy for histologic examination is also less sensitive than culture of the infected tissue. Typical histologic changes are rarely seen in absence of a positive culture. However, positive cultures (for example, postmortem lung) can occur in the absence of any typical histologic changes, i.e., epithelial cytomegaly and intranuclear inclusions. In the latter instance it may be difficult to interpret the significance of the CMV isolate, especially when it occurs unassociated with recognizable symptomatology.

VARICELLA-ZOSTER VIRUS

Man is the only known natural host of varicella-zoster (V-Z) virus. The name reflects the two diseases associated with the virus, i.e., varicella (chickenpox) and zoster (shingles). Primary infection with V-Z virus results in the clinical manifestations of chickenpox. Following this the virus enters a latent phase, presumably within nuclei of neurons in dorsal root ganglia. Reactivation of virus results in the clinical manifestations characteristic of zoster.

Epidemiology. Varicella is endemic with superimposed winter or spring epidemics every two to five years. The two- to eight-year age group is primarily affected, but susceptible individuals of any age may become infected. The disease is highly contagious, with an 80 to 90 per cent clinical attack rate. Immunity to varicella is lifelong. The presumed mode of transmission is via the respiratory tract, but virus is only occasionally isolated from this site.

Zoster is a sporadic disease most commonly occurring in persons over 45 years of age, and there is no sex, racial, geographic, or seasonal predilection for infection.

Zoster is less communicable than varicella, probably because it is usually a more localized disease, but infected persons can transmit typical varicella infection to exposed susceptible persons. Humoral immunity to varicella does not protect against reactivation and clinical zoster. Depressed host immune response is associated with reactivation of V-Z virus, and the following specific factors have been associated with triggering the onset of zoster: manipulation of the spinal cord, local radiation therapy, and underlying diseases or therapy which suppress cellular immunity.

Clinical Aspects. The incubation period of varicella is usually 14 to 17 days. There may be a one- to three-day prodromal period of fever, headache, and malaise prior to eruption of the red macular rash that progresses to papules, vesicles, and pustules that crust over and are shed without scarring. The vesicle is described as a "dew drop on a rose petal." The eruption is centripetal, involving the trunk more heavily than the extremities, palms and soles, in contrast to the eruption in smallpox. Successive crops of lesions continue to appear in the same area for 2 to 6 days, leading to lesions in different stages of development at one time.

Complications of varicella include an interstitial, nodular pneumonitis, especially in adults. This occurs concomitantly with the typical skin rash and follows a course of variable severity depending on the host's immune competence. There are several rare hemorrhagic varicella syndromes which may complicate primary infection. Febrile purpura occurs in both children and adults, usually within a few days of the onset of eruption, and is characterized by thrombocytopenia with hemorrhage into the vesicles. Postinfectious purpura is another complication also characterized by thrombocytopenia with gastrointestinal, genitourinary, cutaneous, and mucous membrane hemorrhage, beginning one to two weeks after appearance of the rash. More severe hemorrhagic manifestations include malignant varicella with purpura, and purpura fulminans.

Encephalitic complications of varicella most commonly include acute cerebellar ataxia, which has an excellent prognosis, and cerebral involvement. Other complications include Reye's syndrome, nephritis, nephrosis, hepatitis, arthritis, and myocarditis. Immune-suppressed susceptible individuals have an increased risk of complications following exposure to V-Z virus.

Zoster infection is heralded by neuralgia for a few days to weeks, followed by the characteristic eruption typically confined to one or two adjacent dermatomes. Occasionally the distribution involves multiple dermatomes or may cross the midline. Severity of the infection increases with advancing age. Older patients have a greater tendency to develop persistent neuralgia, which is often severe and may last several months to a year. Zoster usually involves the thoracic dermatomes, followed in frequency by lumbar, cervical, and trigeminal nerve distributions. When cranial nerve roots are involved, encephalomyelitis may develop; pleural inflammation may accompany a thoracic eruption.

Cell-mediated immunity (CMI) correlates best with immunity to zoster. Patients with Hodgkin's disease have a greatly increased risk (25 per cent) of zoster, especially those with advanced, recurrent disease or those recently finishing radiation therapy, and up to 70 per cent with zoster may develop disseminated disease. Between 5 and 10 per cent of non-Hodgkin's lymphoma and leukemia patients may also develop zoster.

Neonatal varicella occurs and may be acquired *in utero* or in the perinatal period. A few reports have associated primary V-Z virus infection in pregnant women with congenital anomalies in their infants. The greatest risk to the infant appears to be when the onset of maternal illness occurs within four days or less prior to delivery (Meyers, 1974).

Approximately 9 per cent of parturient women in one study (Gershon, 1976a) lacked antibodies to varicella, thus making their newborn infants likewise susceptible to varicella infection.

Laboratory Diagnosis. Clinical diagnosis of typical varicella infection in children and zoster infection in adults can be made with great accuracy. However, herpes simplex virus infection can cause a vesicular eruption identical to V-Z virus infection, and should be strongly suspected in patients with "recurrent" zoster. The best way to confirm infection is to recover the virus in human diploid fibroblast cell cultures. Vesicle fluid is the most reliable source of virus for isolation attempts. Rapid diagnosis can also be made by direct immunofluorescence to detect viral antigens in vesicular lesions (Drew, 1980).

Serologic methods have been employed for epidemiologic surveys for determining prevalence of past exposure to infection as well as documenting recent infection. The CF test is often used for determining V-Z virus antibody. The major disadvantage is its relative insensitivity, especially after a year or more following infection. Therefore, CF is most useful for confirming recent infection. Heterologous antibody response following infection with another herpesvirus can also interfere with the CF test. An indirect immunofluorescent technique for detecting antibodies directed against specific membrane antigens (FAMA) acquired by infected tissue culture cells is a more sensitive and specific serologic technique which is useful in determining susceptibility to infection in epidemiologic studies (Williams, 1974). This method is also rapid and hence particularly useful in determining susceptibility to infection in immunosuppressed patients exposed to varicella. The FAMA method can usually detect antibody within two days after onset of rash, unless the patient is immunosuppressed. Other frequently employed serologic methods include indirect immunofluorescence for detection of antibodies to intercellular antigens, anti-complement immunofluoresence (Prissner, 1982), and immune adherence hemagglutination (Gershon, 1976b).

Other methods for presumptively diagnosing V-Z virus infection include scraping the base of a vesicular lesion and histologically observing multinucleated giant cells containing intranuclear inclusions or observing herpesvirus particles by electron microscopy; however, these techniques will not differentiate between V-Z and herpes simplex virus infections.

EPSTEIN-BARR VIRUS

Epstein-Barr virus (EBV) was first discovered in 1964 when Dr. M. A. Epstein and associates demonstrated a herpes-like virus by EM in cell cultures from a Burkitt's lymphoma. Subsequently, EBV antibody was later demonstrated in the sera of nearly all patients with African Burkitt's lymphoma and nasopharyngeal carcinoma. However, unexpectedly, EBV antibody was shown to be highly prevalent within the general population as well.

EBV was serendipitously linked to infectious mononucleosis (IM) in 1967, when a laboratory technician working with EBV developed classic heterophile-antibody positive IM. During the course of the disease, antibodies to EBV appeared and rose to high titer. The virus can be demonstrated *in vitro* by its ability to transform lymphocytes into indefinitely propagating lymphoblastoid cell lines, and the transformed cells contain EBV antigen demonstrable by immunofluorescent staining.

Epidemiology. EBV is present worldwide and, based upon seroepidemiologic survey data, it is apparent that EBV infection during childhood is quite frequent, especially in less affluent socioeconomic groups. In socioeconomically deprived areas 80 per cent of five-year-old children are seropositive, while 40 to 50 per cent of five-year-old children from higher socioeconomic groups are seropositive (Andiman, 1980). By 40 years of age most persons have acquired EBV infection. In young children EBV infection is usually asymptomatic or associated only with an undifferentiated febrile illness or mild upper respiratory symptoms. If EBV infection is acquired by an adolescent or adult, which happens in 40 to 50 per cent of persons who missed childhood exposure, the IM syndrome develops. Infectious mononucleosis shows no seasonal trends in the general population, but early fall and spring are periods of high frequency among college students.

The evidence linking IM to EBV etiology is as follows: (1) IM occurs only in persons lacking prior EBV antibody; (2) all patients with classical heterophile-positive IM have high antibody titers to EBV; (3) IM does not occur in persons with pre-existing EBV antibody; (4) EBV antigen can be detected in lymphocytes; (5) throat washings from IM patients contain a lymphocyte-transforming agent which induces lymphocyte proliferation and the appearance of EBV-like antigens in susceptible cells; and (6) no other infectious agent has been consistently linked to heterophile-positive IM.

The evidence linking EBV to both African Burkitt's lymphoma and nasopharyngeal carcinoma includes demonstration of EBV-associated antigens in cultured lymphoblasts from both tumors. Proof of etiologic involvement in these tumors is difficult, but some species of animals inoculated with EBV or EBV-containing lymphoid cells develop malignant lymphomas. Supportive evidence includes the fact that EBV can transform lymphoid cells into permanent cell lines.

Clinical Aspects. Infectious mononucleosis is characterized by a three- to five-day prodromal period of non-specific symptoms including fever, asthenia, fatigue, and anorexia. This is followed most commonly by severe pharyngitis, lymphadenitis, and splenomegaly. Other less common manifestations include mild hepatitis, conjunctivitis, and a fleeting maculopapular rash. This stage of illness usually lasts 10 to 20 days. Fatigue and asthenia persist throughout the illness into the convalescent stage which may extend for months.

Infectious mononucleosis is usually a self-limited benign disease, but occasionally severe complications and rarely death have occurred. Complications include severe hepatic involvement, neurologic manifestations with encephalitis, pneumonitis, thrombocytopenia, splenic rupture, hemolytic anemia, airway obstruction, and transient cutaneous hypersensitivity to ampicillin. On rare occasions, some patients with immunodeficiency disorders have developed a severe, often lethal lymphoproliferative syndrome.

IM appears to be transmitted primarily by close contact with infective oropharyngeal secretions. Other reported routes of transmission include blood transfusion and transplacental spread.

As occurs with the other herpesviruses, there is a persistent viral carrier state after primary infection, which may be followed by asymptomatic reactivation of endogenous

EBV. Immunosuppressed patients have a higher prevalence (35 to 47 per cent) of oropharyngeal excretion of EBV as compared to healthy controls (17 per cent) (Strauch, 1974).

Laboratory Diagnosis. Since *in vitro* systems for isolation and identification of the EBV are difficult, expensive, and time-consuming, the usual diagnosis of IM is based primarily on clinical, hematologic, and serologic data. In the adolescent and young adult the clinical signs and symptoms can strongly suggest the diagnosis of IM. The peripheral blood picture usually shows an absolute lymphocytosis with 10 to 20 per cent or more atypical lymphocytes. Early, the lymphocytosis results from increased B- and T-lymphocytes, but later there is a predominance of T-lymphocytes. The EBV appears to infect only B-lymphocytes, while the atypical lymphocytes are uninfected T-lymphocytes.

Heterophile antibody usually, but not always, appears in patients with IM. There are multiple types of heterophile antibodies, all of which agglutinate sheep red blood cells (RBC) and are IgM immunoglobulins. The heterophile antibody produced during IM can be differentiated from the Forssman type by differential absorption techniques. Forssman antigen (found in guinea pig or horse kidney cells) will not absorb IM-induced heterophile antibody from serum, but the non-specific antisheep RBC agglutinins found in normal persons and in serum sickness patients are absorbed by Forssman antigen. Beef RBC will absorb IM-induced heterophile antibody and serum sickness antibody. Therefore, a patient's serum with IM heterophile antibodies differentially absorbed with both antigens will show little or no reduction in sheep RBC agglutination activity following absorption with Forssman antigen, but will show loss of agglutinating activity following absorption with beef RBC's. A patient with serum sickness will show loss of activity following absorption with both cell types. During the first two weeks of EBV infection, approximately 60 per cent of patients develop a positive classic heterophile test with titers of 1:56 or greater. This increases to 80 to 90 per cent by one month, then declines to undetectable levels in most cases by three to six months.

Formaldehyde-treated horse RBC, ox RBC, and enzyme treated and untreated sheep cells are also acceptably sensitive and specific for detection of IM heterophile antibodies and can be used in rapid, qualitative "spot" screening tests. The horse RBC agglutination test stays positive at a titer of 1:40 or greater for 12 months or more in 75 per cent of cases. Sheep and beef cell hemolysin tests are each 81 to 85 per cent sensitive for the diagnosis of IM.

The classic heterophile antibody test will be negative in about 10 per cent of IM cases subsequently shown to have acute EBV infection by specific EBV serology. The false negative rate is even higher in young children. In comparison with the classic heterophile test, the Monospot test has a 2 per cent false negative rate and a 6 to 13 per cent false positive rate. A positive Monospot correlates with a heterophile titer of 1:29 or greater. False positives have been associated with hepatitis A, hepatitis B, leukemia, lymphomas, and pancreatic carcinoma. It is estimated that of all IM-like illnesses, as many as one fourth will be heterophile negative. Of these, 20 to 45 per cent will demonstrate EBV antibodies suggestive of infection. Cytomegalovirus and *Toxoplasma gondii* infections probably account for most of the remainder.

During primary infection with EBV, antibodies develop to a wide variety of antigens including the viral capsid antigen (VCA), early antigens (EA), membrane antigens (MA), and nuclear antigens (NA). Antibodies to early antigens have been subdivided into diffuse (D) and restricted (R) types based upon the location in infected cells. More broadly reactive antibodies to crude extracts of lymphoblastoid cell lines can also be detected by complement fixation, immunoprecipitation, and neutralization techniques. Indirect immunofluorescence, using EBV-infected lymphoblastoid cells and fluorescein-conjugated immunoglobulin, is employed for detecting antibodies to the VCA and EA, and anti-complement immunofluorescence is used to detect antibodies to the NA (Andiman, 1980).

During primary EBV infection, early acute phase sera often already contain IgG-VCA antibodies in high titers, and paired sera will demonstrate a significant titer rise in only about 20 per cent. IgG anti-VCA titers then slowly decline to low levels, but persist for life. Anti-EBNA antibody appears two to eight weeks after onset of infection and also usually persists for life. Anti-EA antibody, usually of the D type, generally appears and persists only during the active phase of infection (weeks to months). In the early phase of acute infection, IgM-specific anti-VCA titers are elevated; however, reactivation of infection may also cause this antibody to reappear (Henle, 1974). The R form of anti-EA appears much less commonly, and its continuing presence has been correlated with a persistent IM-like syndrome (Horwitz, 1975).

Guidelines for the interpretation of EBV serologic tests are shown in Table 50–10. The diagnosis of active EBV infection is usually based on any one or a combination of the following: Positive IgG-VCA and IgM-VCA; seroconversion of anti-EBNA from negative to positive; and elevated anti-EA titers ($\geq$1:10) (Henle, 1974). Four-fold or greater increases in anti-VCA or anti-EBNA titers in serial sera also help support the diagnosis.

It should also be mentioned that high anti-VCA titers as well as antibodies to EA are often found in patients with African Burkitt's lymphoma and nasopharyngeal carcinoma. However, diagnosis of these tumors is based upon biopsy and demonstration of typical histologic patterns.

Poxviruses

Historically, the most important poxvirus affecting humans was variola, the cause of smallpox. There are two

Table 50–10. GUIDELINES FOR THE INTERPRETATION OF EPSTEIN-BARR VIRAL SEROLOGIES

	Antibodies			
Clinical Situation	***IgG-VCA***	***EBNA***	***EA***	***IGM-VCA***
No past infection	–	–	–	–
Acute infection	+	–	+ (usually D)	+
Convalescent phase	+	+	+ or –	+ or –
Past infection	+	+	–	–
Chronic or reactivated infection	+	+	+ (D or R)	– (see text)

+ = Antibody present. – = Antibody absent.

variants of this agent—variola major, which is a severe disease with mortality rates ranging as high as 35 per cent, and variola minor (also called alastrim), a milder disease with mortality rates of only 1 to 2 per cent. The two strains are not distinguishable from one another in the laboratory. At the present time, smallpox has been totally eradicated throughout the world, and interest in this virus is now primarily historical and scientific.

Vaccinia virus is closely related antigenically to variola and cowpox viruses. Its exact origin is obscure; some believe it is an attenuated variola strain, others believe it is a variant of cowpox, and still others have proposed that it is a hybrid of both. Regardless of its origin, it was used for many years for effective immunization against smallpox. Unfortunately, vaccinia virus can sometimes produce severe, disseminated disease or progressive local necrosis, particularly in patients with atopic dermatitis or immunodeficiency. Use of vaccinia virus for immunization is no longer recommended.

Both variola and vaccinia viruses could be isolated in routine cell cultures, such as the heteroploid cell lines, and they also grow well and can be distinguished from one another on the basis of pock development on chorioallantoic membranes in embryonated eggs.

Other methods used to distinguish these viruses from other cases of vesicular, vesiculopustular, or papular eruptions (e.g., herpes simplex, varicella-zoster viruses) include direct examination of the vesicular fluid or crusts by electron microscopy and cytologic examination of scrapings taken from the base of the lesions. In the latter method, air-dried and fixed smears are stained with methyl violet (Gutstein's method), or Giemsa stain. The presence of intranuclear inclusions and/or multinucleated giant cells suggests the diagnosis of a herpes group infection and tends to rule out poxvirus. Poxvirus infections are characterized by swollen epithelial cells containing intracytoplasmic inclusions surrounded by a halo (Guarnieri bodies). Poxvirus antigens may also be detected in skin lesions by agar gel precipitation or complement fixation methods.

Cowpox and paravaccinia (milker's nodules) are bovine poxviruses which are occasionally transmitted to humans in direct contact with infected cows or calves. Cowpox is characterized in humans by low grade fever and multiple papular lesions on the fingers and hands which later become vesicular and pustular, resolving after several weeks. Paravaccinia is somewhat similar, except that the lesion is usually solitary, progressing to a firm nodule 1 to 2 cm in diameter in 10 days, then crusting and healing in another two to three weeks. A clinical picture nearly identical to paravaccinia is also seen with orf, a poxvirus of sheep (ecthyma contagiosum), and is an occupational hazard among sheep farmers (Fig. 50–8).

The diagnosis of these diseases is usually made on clinical and epidemiologic grounds; confirmation of orf infection can be made by determining specific CF antibody responses, a special procedure not generally available except in some public health laboratories.

Molluscum contagiosum, a poxvirus disease affecting humans only, produces smooth, "pearly" skin papules, averaging about 4 mm in diameter. This agent cannot be cultured in the laboratory. Diagnosis is by clinical and histologic examination.

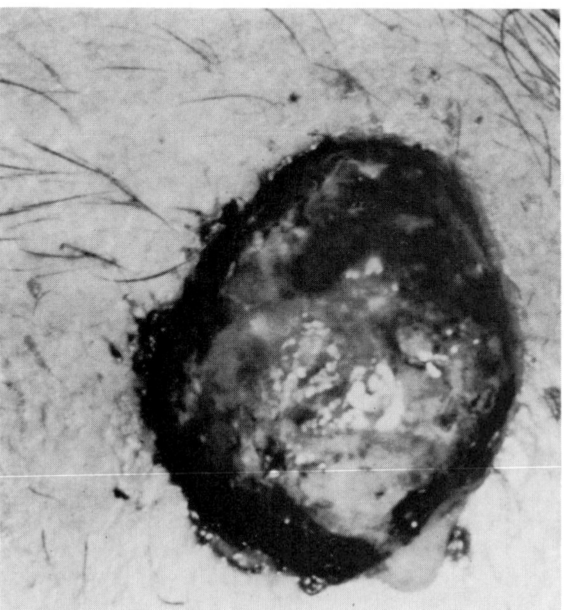

Figure 50–8. The acute stage of orf showing a nodule with a weeping, ulcerated surface. (From Leavell, U. E., et al.: J.A.M.A., *204*:660, 1968.)

Enteroviruses

Enteroviruses include poliovirus, coxsackievirus, and echovirus species, for which man is the only known natural host. At present, there are at least 70 different recognized serotypes. Poliovirus was the first virus to be described and propagated in tissue culture in 1949 by Enders, Weller, and Robbins. During the peak incidence of poliomyelitis in the United States in the mid-twentieth century, about 150 deaths and 7000 cases of residual paralysis occurred annually. This, plus the successful growth of virus in tissue culture, provided a great stimulus for vaccine research which resulted in the Salk and Sabin vaccines. The use of these vaccines has nearly eradicated poliomyelitis from developed countries. There are three distinct poliovirus serotypes recognized, and all grow well in tissue culture.

Another two enterovirus groups were discovered during intense epidemiologic studies of poliomyelitis. Coxsackieviruses were first recovered in 1948 in suckling mice inoculated with the fecal extracts from two children with a paralytic poliomyelitis-like syndrome. They derive their name from the fact that both isolates were discovered in Coxsackie, New York. Two groups of coxsackieviruses were later defined on the basis of unique clinical and pathologic effects on suckling mice: group A coxsackieviruses cause flaccid paralysis, myositis, and death within a week, whereas group B viruses produce encephalitis with a spastic paralysis, myocarditis, and other visceral inflammatory changes. All the group B coxsackieviruses, but only a few group A coxsackieviruses, grow in tissue culture; therefore, inoculation into suckling mice is necessary for isolation of most of the latter. No single antigen is common to all coxsackieviruses, although there may be some heterotypic cross-reactivity between group A viruses. There is a common coxsackievirus B antigen, however, which is also shared with one group A coxsackievirus. Currently, 24 group A and 6 group B coxsackievirus serotypes are recognized.

Beginning in 1950, many new non-polio, non-coxsackievirus human enteric viral isolates were discovered. These viruses were initially called "ophans" because they were often not associated with recognized disease. All the isolates grew well in tissue culture, producing cytopathogenic changes. Subsequently in 1955 the name was changed to ECHO, an abbreviation for "enteric cytopathogenic human orphans." There is no common echovirus group antigen, and 34 different echovirus serotypes were originally recognized. Echovirus 10, however, has been reclassified as a reovirus and echovirus 28 is now classified as a rhinovirus. Echovirus 9 is now reclassified as coxsackievirus A23 because of its behavior in suckling mice.

In recent years, higher-numbered enteroviruses have been described, which have overlapping biologic characteristics with echo- and coxsackieviruses. These are classified separately as enterovirus types 68–72.

Enteroviruses are ubiquitous agents that are spread primarily by fecal-oral contamination, but respiratory transmission also occurs. The viruses initially colonize the alimentary tract, growing in the lymphoid tissues of the nasopharynx and intestinal tract. Viremia subsequently occurs, allowing secondary localization in other viscera and lymphoid tissues. Infection is often asymptomatic (30 to 90 per cent), but a wide variety of notable syndromes may also occur, including paralytic disease, aseptic meningitis, encephalitis, pleurodynia, pericarditis, herpangina, and lymphonodular pharyngitis. However, the most common clinical picture is that of an undifferentiated febrile illness with malaise, headache, myalgia, and sore throat. Enteroviruses may also cause a generalized disease of variable severity in newborn infants. Table 50–11 shows which non-polio enteroviruses are most commonly associated with the various syndromes.

POLIOVIRUS

Polioviruses are found in a worldwide distribution. In many underdeveloped countries poliomyelitis is still endemic and nearly all infections are subclinical. When symptomatic disease occurs it primarily involves infants and children. With improved sanitation the age distribution changes to include older children and adults. In temperate climates, the wild viruses are most commonly isolated during the summer and autumn months.

Clinical disease usually occurs in one of three forms: (1) non-specific febrile illness, (2) aseptic meningitis, or (3) poliomyelitis, which is classically an asymmetrical, flaccid paralysis of variable extent. Maximum involvement is evident within a few days after onset of paralysis, and is followed by gradual recovery of temporarily damaged motor neurons which may continue for up to six months.

Laboratory diagnosis is based on viral isolation in tissue culture followed by identification by neutralization techniques using type-specific antisera. The virus is readily isolated from throat swabs early in the infection and from feces after onset of symptoms. It is rarely isolated from the CSF. Following oral polio vaccination with the live attenuated virus, fecal excretion may be observed for up to 18 weeks. In countries where there is widespread vaccination with live attenuated vaccine, a polio isolate from a patient with a compatible clinical syndrome and recent vaccine exposure should be forwarded to a reference laboratory to determine if it is a wild virus strain or a vaccine strain. A four-fold or greater rise in complement fixation antibody titer is indicative of recent infection or polio vaccination. However, CF titers may decline to undetectable levels, and neutralization techniques may be required to determine immune status.

COXSACKIE- AND ECHOVIRUSES

These viruses have the same pathogenesis, mode of spread, and seasonal occurrence that poliovirus infections demonstrate. In contrast, however, these viruses produce a wider variety of clinical syndromes (Table 50–11) and have a greater tendency to infect the meninges and cerebrum with only rare involvement of motor neurons of the spinal cord. Also, these infections can pursue a relapsing course for several weeks, manifesting a variety of different clinical syndromes. Recurrent infection by some coxsackievirus B serotypes and rarely by echovirus serotypes may occur.

Table 50–11. CLINICAL SYNDROMES ASSOCIATED WITH ENTEROVIRUS INFECTIONS: RELATIVE FREQUENCIES AND COMMON SEROTYPES INVOLVED

	Enterovirus Serotypes		
	Coxsackievirus		
Syndrome	***Group A***	***Group B***	***Echovirus and Enterovirus (E)***
Aseptic meningitis	+ 2,4,7,9,10	+ + 1,2,3,4,5,6	+ + + + most serotypes
Muscle paralysis and weakness	+ 7*,9	+ 2,3,4,5	+ + 2,4,6,9,11,30, E71
Encephalitis and radiculitis	+ 2,5,6	+ + + + 1,2,3,4,5	+ 2,6,9,10,E70,E71
Pleurodynia (epidemic myalgia)	−	+ + + + 1,2,3,4,5	+ 1,6,9
Pericarditis, myocarditis	+ 4,16	+ + + + 1,2,3,4,5	+ 1,6,8,9,19
Rashes	+ + + 4,5,6,9,16	+ + 2,3,5	+ + + 2,4,6,9,11,16,18
Respiratory illness	+ + 9,16,21,24	+ + 1,3,4,5	+ + + 4,9,11,20,25
Hand-foot-and-mouth disease	+ + + + 16,5,10	+ 2,5	−
Herpangina	+ + + + 1,2,3,4,5,6,8,10,22	+ 1,2,3,4,5	+ 9,16,17
Conjunctivitis	24	1,5	7,E70
Generalized disease (infants)	+ 9	+ + + 1,2,3,4,5,	+ 5,11,16,19

Code: − = not reported + = uncommon.
+ + to + + + + = relative frequencies of isolation.
*Coxsackievirus A 7 is second to poliovirus as a cause of neuromuscular disease.

6

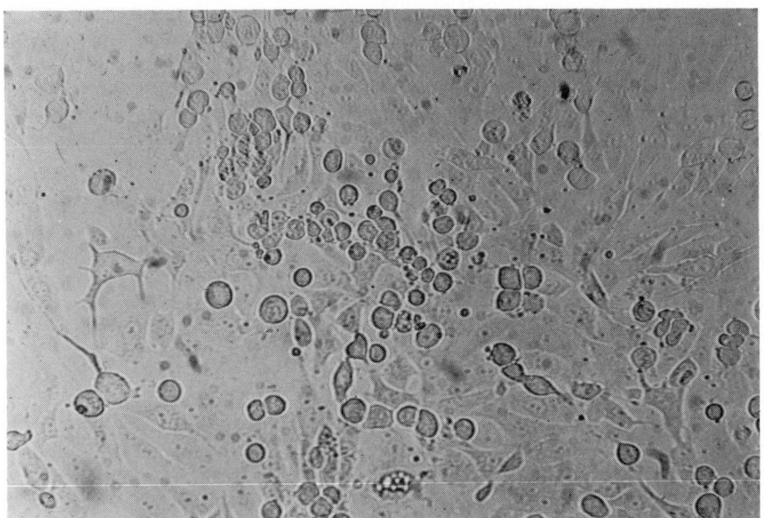

Figure 50–9. Typical CPE of enteroviruses in primary monkey kidney culture (coxsackievirus B) (×125). (From Herrmann, E. C., Jr., et al.: Mayo Clin. Proc. *47*:577, 1972.)

Additional diseases that have been etiologically linked to enteroviruses include hepatitis, transverse myelitis, cranial nerve palsies, and acute hemorrhagic conjunctivitis (AHC). AHC was epidemic in Africa, Asia, India, and parts of Europe from 1969 to 1974. It is now endemic in these areas, and the viral isolate from affected persons has been called enterovirus 70. Coxsackieviruses have been implicated in a wide variety of other syndromes, including acute cerebellar ataxia, hemolytic-uremic syndrome, hepatitis, nephritis, and chronic myopathies.

Both coxsackie- and echoviruses have been implicated in occasionally fatal, generalized infections of newborns manifested by fever, meningitis, rash, diarrhea, or shock. This occurs primarily in the summer and fall and is often associated with recent maternal infection with the same virus. Sometimes the infected infant exhibits only signs of sepsis and shock with a negative bacteriologic workup, thus emphasizing the need to include these agents in the differential diagnosis of neonatal sepsis.

Laboratory Diagnosis. These viruses can be grown best in primary monkey kidney cell cultures in which they produce distinctive cytopathic effects (Fig. 50–9) or in suckling mice (coxsackievirus A). Most enteroviruses will become apparent in tissue culture within a few days, allowing a rapid presumptive identification, which is followed by confirmation techniques using type-specific antisera.

The pattern of growth in multiple tissue culture systems often suggests the species of enterovirus being isolated (Table 50–12). Since there are so many serotypic possibilities within species, pools of several different antisera are used, often in an intersecting pattern (Fig. 50–10) for viral neutralization studies. For confirmation of these results, a neutralization test using a single specific antiserum is then performed to identify the isolate.

Table 50–12. PATTERN OF ENTEROVIRUS GROWTH IN SELECTED CULTURE SYSTEMS

	RMK*	HDF†	HET‡	Mice
Poliovirus	+§	+	+	−
Echovirus	+	+	−	−
Coxsackievirus A	±	±	−	+
Coxsackievirus B	+	−	+	+

*Primary rhesus monkey kidney.
†Human diploid fibroblasts.
‡Human heteroploid cells.
§+ = growth.
± = growth in some strains.
− = no growth.

During the course of an enteroviral infection, the virus is present in the oropharynx and often in the feces at the onset of disease. After one or two weeks the virus disappears from the throat but will continue to be excreted in the feces for as long as 16 to 18 weeks. Virus may also be isolated from specimens taken from clinically infected sites, i.e., CSF, blood, or tissues. Recovery of virus from these ordinarily sterile sites is diagnostic. Isolation of virus from the throat only or from both the throat and feces early in the course of a compatible illness also supports an etiologic relationship. Viral recovery from the feces alone, with or without seroconversion (discussed below), however, must be interpreted with caution, since viral excretion and gradual decline of antibody titers may continue for several weeks beyond initial infection. This is particularly a diagnostic problem with young children in whom the prevalence of asymptomatic fecal excretion may range from 3 to 4 per cent in the northern United States to 30 per cent in the Gulf states during the summer and early fall. Therefore, a fecal isolate may not necessarily be etiologically related to the acute disease being investigated. This becomes less of a diagnostic problem with adults because of the somewhat lower incidence of asymptomatic fecal excretion.

Serum-neutralizing antibodies develop rapidly, often reaching high titers shortly after the onset of symptoms, and may persist at high titers for years, sometimes making demonstration of a four-fold or greater change in titer difficult. Neutralizing antibodies are the most serotypically specific, but because of the large numbers of viral serotypes, performing neutralizing antibody titers on paired sera becomes a laborious and time-consuming technique. Use of information contained in Table 50–11, as well as local epidemiologic data, aids in determining which viruses one should select for use in neutralization serology.

Complement fixation antibodies develop more slowly and decline to low levels, rarely being detectable after three years. Also, CF serologies are insensitive and rather nonspecific owing to heterotypic cross-reactivity. They are of little practical value except in poliovirus serodiagnosis. Only a few enteroviral serotypes produce hemagglutination inhibition antibodies, thus limiting the usefulness of this serologic technique. To further complicate the situation,

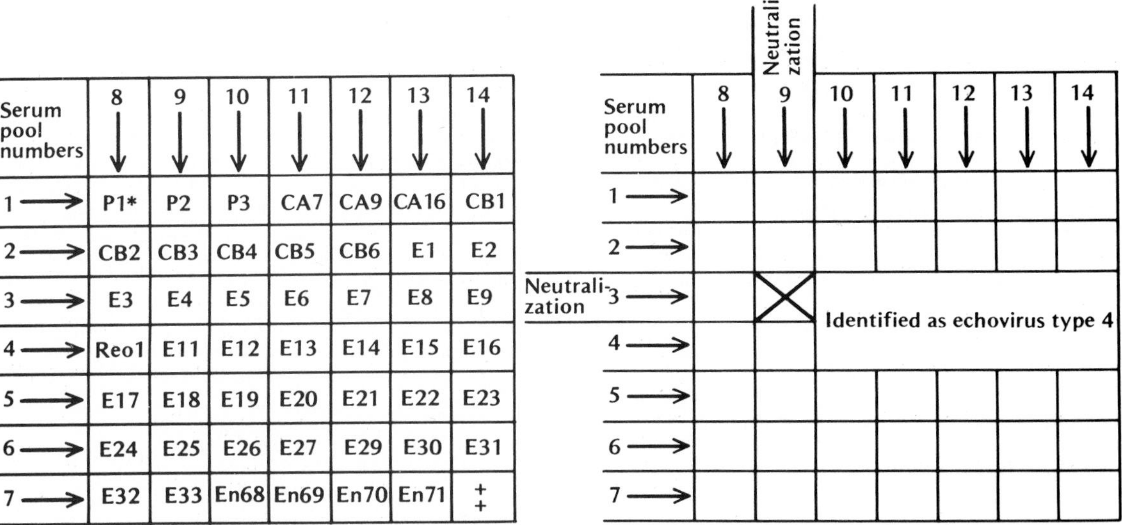

COMPOSITION OF SERUM POOLS

Serum pool numbers	8 ↓	9 ↓	10 ↓	11 ↓	12 ↓	13 ↓	14 ↓
1 ⟶	P1*	P2	P3	CA7	CA9	CA16	CB1
2 ⟶	CB2	CB3	CB4	CB5	CB6	E1	E2
3 ⟶	E3	E4	E5	E6	E7	E8	E9
4 ⟶	Reo1	E11	E12	E13	E14	E15	E16
5 ⟶	E17	E18	E19	E20	E21	E22	E23
6 ⟶	E24	E25	E26	E27	E29	E30	E31
7 ⟶	E32	E33	En68	En69	En70	En71	‡

*P = poliovirus immune serum; CA = group A coxsackievirus; CB = group B coxsackievirus; E = echovirus; En = enterovirus immune serum type

‡ Immune serum to enterovirus candidate strain

Figure 50–10. Fourteen-pool intersecting serum scheme for identification of enteroviruses. (From Lennette, E. H., and Schmidt, N. J. [eds.]: Diagnostic procedures for Viral, Rickettsial and Chlamydial Infections. 5th ed. New York, American Public Health Association, 1979.)

there may be considerable variability in antibody response; therefore, a lack of seroconversion does not exclude the possibility of a coxsackie- or echovirus infection. Despite these disadvantages, a four-fold or greater rise or fall in antibody titer is considered significant when interpreted in the context of the clinical syndrome and epidemiologic data.

In some enterovirus infections, such as myocarditis or pericarditis due to group B coxsackieviruses, virus isolation rates are usually less than 10 per cent, even when affected tissue or pericardial fluid is cultured. The clinical and experimental data would suggest that the syndrome is immunologically mediated, particularly by T-lymphocytes (Woodruff, 1974), and virus excretion may have ceased or considerably diminished by the time symptoms are manifest. In these situations, diagnosis by neutralization antibody testing of paired sera is usually much more sensitive than culture.

Arboviruses

The term *arbovirus* indicates those agents which share in common a similar mode of transmission by hemophagous insects, especially ticks and mosquitoes. There are over 250 viruses in this category, including representatives from the Togaviridae, Bunyaviridae, Reoviridae (Orbivirus), and Rhabdoviridae families, as well as some unclassified agents. The arboviruses which have been found associated with disease in the United States are summarized in Table 50–13.

The major syndromes are loosely categorized as (1) fever, malaise (any of these viruses); (2) fever, encephalitis, or aseptic meningitis (the encephalitis agents, California, Powassan, and occasionally Colorado tick fever); (3) fever, myalgia, and headache (Colorado tick fever); (4) fever, myalgia, headache, rash, lymphadenopathy (dengue); and (5) fever, hemorrhagic diathesis (yellow fever, sometimes dengue).

The most important of these agents in the United States are St. Louis encephalitis, western equine encephalitis, Colorado tick fever, and California (La Crosse) virus. Eastern equine encephalitis infections are identified only occasionally; Powassan infections of humans appear to be rare.

Virus isolation attempts are only occasionally successful in these infections. The most common method used is

Table 50–13. IMPORTANT ARBOVIRUSES IN THE UNITED STATES

TOGAVIRIDAE FAMILY
Alphavirus group
Eastern equine encephalitis
Western equine encephalitis
Venezuelan equine encephalitis*
Flavivirus group
St. Louis encephalitis
Yellow fever*
Powassan
Dengue types 1, 2, 3, 4*
BUNYAVIRIDAE FAMILY
California group
California (La Crosse)
REOVIRIDAE FAMILY (ORBIVIRUS)
Colorado tick fever

*Venezuelan equine encephalitis, yellow fever, and dengue are not now indigenous to the continental United States; however, imported cases from adjacent tropical and subtropical areas are occasionally diagnosed, and the potential vectors for these agents do exist in North America.

6

inoculation of serum (whole blood is preferable for Colorado tick fever), CSF, or brain homogenates into suckling mice. Confirmation and identification of isolates usually require the aid of a public health laboratory. However, serologic diagnosis has been shown to be a much more practical approach and is preferable. A knowledge of the epidemiologic behavior of these viruses, coupled with the clinical history, helps one to select the appropriate serologies to be done.

The seasonal distribution parallels the activity of the insect vector—the encephalitides are common from midsummer through early autumn (usually July through September), then disappear; Colorado tick fever is more common during late spring and early summer, the period of greatest tick activity.

Eastern equine encephalitis is confined primarily to wooded, swampy areas along the eastern seaboard, from New England to Florida. Young children are most commonly affected. Serologic diagnosis is by CF or HI antibody titer rises between acute and convalescent sera.

St. Louis and western equine encephalitis viruses have been responsible for outbreaks of central nervous disease in many areas of the United States and are not at all as geographically restricted as the names suggest. Interestingly, the highest attack and sequelae rates are among individuals over 40 years of age with St. Louis encephalitis, while infants and young children are more severely affected during western equine encephalitis outbreaks.

In both of these infections, HI and CF antibodies are usually significantly elevated within two to three weeks after onset, and serologic confirmation is based upon a fourfold or greater antibody titer rise between acute and convalescent sera. If the first serum sample has been obtained later than seven days after onset, a diagnosis is considered likely if the HI titer is $\geq$1:80 or the CF titer is $\geq$1:16 for either antigen ("presumptive" case). Single HI titers of 1:40 are suggestive of recent infection but are usually regarded as "equivocal" or inconclusive cases.

California virus is a major cause of encephalitis during the summer season in Minnesota, Ohio, Indiana, and Wisconsin, but is actually very rare in the western states. It most commonly affects children between the ages of five and nine years and is associated with suburban or rural environments (Balfour, 1973). Serologic diagnosis can be made on paired sera utilizing either a CF or HI test. However, the CF titer tends to rise more slowly in this infection, reaching a peak usually by three to five weeks after onset. Precipitating antibody to the La Crosse strain of California virus has also been shown to appear during the infection and to disappear within one year. Balfour (1974) has shown that counterimmunoelectrophoresis of the patient's serum, using the La Crosse strain as the antigen, will detect precipitating antibody in 41 per cent of acute phase sera and 100 per cent of convalescent sera in proved cases. This method appears sensitive and can be completed in 1.5 hours.

Colorado tick fever (mountain fever, tick fever) is found in brushy, wooded mountain areas in the western United States, corresponding to the habitat of the vector *Dermacentor andersoni*. It is usually an acute febrile illness with headache and myalgia beginning three to five days after the tick bite. Occasionally, encephalitis and hemorrhagic complications may also develop. The diagnosis is usually made serologically by CF or indirect immunofluorescence testing, but antibody develops slowly and a significant rise may not be detected until four to six weeks after the onset of illness. The viral antigen can also be detected by direct immunofluorescence of erythrocytes from infected patients. This cell-associated viremia can persist for as long as 20 weeks.

Influenza Viruses

Influenza viruses exist as three distinct types, A, B, and C, based on immunologically different soluble nucleoprotein antigens. These viruses are characterized by hemagglutinin (HA) and neuraminidase (NA) protein spikes projecting from the surface of the lipid-containing envelope. The HA attaches to specific glycoprotein receptors on a variety of cell surfaces including erythrocytes. The neuraminidase destroys these receptor sites, releasing the absorbed virus from the surface of cells. This activity may facilitate the spread of virus within the infected host. There are antigenically variable HA ($H_{1,2,3}$) and neuraminidase ($N_{1,2}$) antigens which are used for subtyping and determining specific immunity to human influenza A subtypes. Within each subtype there are strains which show minor serologic differences and are designated in the following example: A/Hong Kong/68 (H_3N_2), i.e., virus type/site of original isolation/year of initial isolation, followed by H, N notation. The HA and NA of influenza B viruses are less well characterized and are therefore not used in the nomenclature (Table 50–14).

The outstanding characteristic of influenza viruses (primarily type A) is the tendency to cause periodic local epidemics and major pandemics owing to their ability to undergo minor and major antigenic changes. Probable influenza epidemics have been described for several centuries; at least four major pandemics have occurred within the past century.

Epidemiology. Influenza A infections occur most frequently during the winter in temperate climates and cause

Table 50–14. CLASSIFICATION AND EPIDEMIOLOGY OF INFLUENZA VIRUSES

Nucleoprotein Type	Hemagglutinin Subtype	Neuraminidase subtype	Representative Strain	Epidemic Year
A	H_1	N_1	Swine-like agent	1918*
A	H_1	N_1	A/PR/34 (formerly A_0)	1933
A	H_1	N_1	A/FM/47	1947
A	H_2	N_2	A/Singapore/57 (formerly A_2; Asian)	1957*
A	H_3	N_2	A/Hong Kong/68	1968*
			A/England/72	1972
B			B/Mass/66	
			B/Vic/70	
			B/Hong Kong/72	
C			C/Taylor/47	

*Pandemics occurred at these times.

major epidemics every two to four years. Influenza B occurs more sporadically or in localized outbreaks. Influenza C usually causes mild or undetected disease, but serologic evidence reveals a high prevalence of infection.

The periodicity of influenza A infection results from the antigenic drifts and shifts which occur, leaving the population susceptible to reinfection by different strains or different subtypes when they occur. Antigenic drifts involve no major change in HA or NA antigens, but antisera prepared in animals against specific strains vary in ability to inhibit hemagglutination of similar strains isolated from differing geographic locations or time periods. Major antigenic shifts occur when there is a major change in HA and/or NA types. This occurs approximately every 10 to 15 years and is responsible for severe pandemics (Table 50–14).

Influenza A epidemics develop rapidly over three to six weeks, with the peak prevalence of infection occurring within two to three months, and then subside rapidly. From 10 to 50 per cent of an urban population may be affected, and serologic testing suggests that up to 25 per cent may experience subclinical infection. The highest attack rates often occur in children, and serologic evidence indicates that by school age most persons have been infected at least once. Influenza B spreads more slowly but otherwise behaves similarly to type A. Influenza C probably never causes significant epidemics.

Clinical Aspects. During outbreaks of influenza A or B, the disease manifests the typical pattern of rapid onset, following an incubation period of one to three days, with headache, myalgia, fever, chills, and marked prostration accompanied by rhinitis, sore throat and often a cough with chest pain. The acute disease usually lasts three days to a week, but convalescence with fatigue, malaise, and cough may last an additional two to three weeks. The disease in infants can be very severe, associated with febrile convulsions and/or severe croup, occasionally requiring tracheostomy.

A more serious form of influenza infection is primary viral pneumonia which occurs within the first one to three days after onset of initial symptoms. During the pandemic of 1918 there was a high mortality in young adults due to influenza pneumonia. Other respiratory complications include a mixed bacterial and viral pneumonia also occurring within one to three days of onset, or a superimposed bacterial pneumonia developing later in the illness or during the convalescent period.

Another problem complicating influenza infection is congestive heart failure and pulmonary edema in persons with marginal cardiovascular or respiratory status. Some additional described complications include disseminated intravascular coagulation with hemolytic-uremic syndrome, severe myositis with elevated muscle enzymes, Reye's syndrome, acute renal failure, encephalopathy, and pericarditis.

Laboratory Diagnosis. Influenza A and B viruses are readily isolated from nasopharyngeal-throat swabs taken during the first three days of acute illness and inoculated into primary monkey kidney cell cultures or amnionic sacs of embryonated hen's eggs. The presence of virus is indicated by hemadsorption of guinea pig erythrocytes to infected tissue culture cells (see section on parainfluenza viruses) or detection of hemagglutinating activity in the amnionic or allantoic fluid. Both systems are often used simultaneously to increase the sensitivity of detection. Further identification is based on neutralization of this activity by specific antisera *in vitro*. Influenza C is isolated best by inoculation of the amnionic sac of embryonated eggs.

Serologic diagnosis is useful when a four-fold or greater rise in antibody titer to a specific, currently infecting strain of influenza is demonstrated. However, a single elevated titer to a totally new antigenic strain in convalescent sera during an outbreak caused by the same virus offers supportive evidence of infection.

There may be variable antibody responses to any of the four major influenza antigens: matrix (M) protein, nucleoprotein (NP), neuraminidase (NA), and hemagglutinin (HA). The M and NP antigens are stable in contrast to NA and HA antigens. Antibodies to M antigen usually occur only following severe illness and hence are rarely sought, but antibody rises to NP antigens are more predictable, and tests for NP antibody are quite sensitive.

Complement fixation (CF) techniques may be utilized for serodiagnosis in laboratories already equipped for CF procedures. Either the NP antigen or whole virion (HA and NA) may be used as the antigen in the system, thereby affording the degree of specificity desired. Results using the whole virion compare with those obtained by hemagglutination inhibition (HI). However, the HI test system is simpler and less technically demanding than CF and hence is the most common serologic technique employed for both serodiagnosis and epidemiologic studies. The choice of antigen in the HI test should be a strain most closely related antigenically to the suspected current epidemic strain. Another serologic method less commonly employed is single radial immunodiffusion (Mostow, 1975).

Parainfluenza (PI) Viruses

First discovered in 1953, the PI viruses are now recognized as four distinct serologic types, designated as types 1, 2, 3, and 4. They share some common antigens among themselves, as well as with some other human and animal viruses. Most notable is the antigenic sharing between PI type 2 and mumps, as well as simian virus-5 (SV-5). The latter agent is a common contaminant of monkey kidney cell cultures; it causes hemadsorption and occasionally is misidentified as a parainfluenza virus in clinical samples. This mistake can be prevented by including appropriate cell culture controls when identifying suspected human hemadsorbing agents, and, when SV-5 is specifically suspected as a contaminant, neutralization by specific antiserum to SV-5 should also be checked when typing an isolate.

All four serotypes are primarily respiratory tract pathogens. Of these, type 4 is the least frequent, and generally associated with only mild upper respiratory symptoms. Types 1, 2, and 3 are extremely important and common agents, particularly among infants and young children, producing croup, tracheobronchitis, bronchiolitis, pneumonia, or a combination of these syndromes. In older children and adults, the symptoms are more often those of a "common cold," pharyngitis, or laryngitis. Infections may occur in any season, but are generally more common in the autumn and winter.

Virus shedding from the respiratory tract can be detected for up to a week after onset, then disappears rapidly. Pooled nasopharyngeal and throat swabs or nasopharyngeal washings are the best sources for isolation attempts.

Primary or secondary rhesus monkey kidney cell cultures are preferred for isolation. The PI viruses are recognized by the fact that infected cultures will produce hemagglutinin on the cell surfaces, and eventually release this into the media. After one day of incubation, and at one- to two-day intervals thereafter, the cell cultures are tested for the presence of hemadsorption by the addition of 0.1 ml of a 0.5 per cent suspension of guinea pig red blood cells in PBS. A fresh suspension of guinea pig cells is usually stable for up to seven days at 4°C. The tubes are incubated horizontally at 4°C. with the cell culture down for 45 to

6

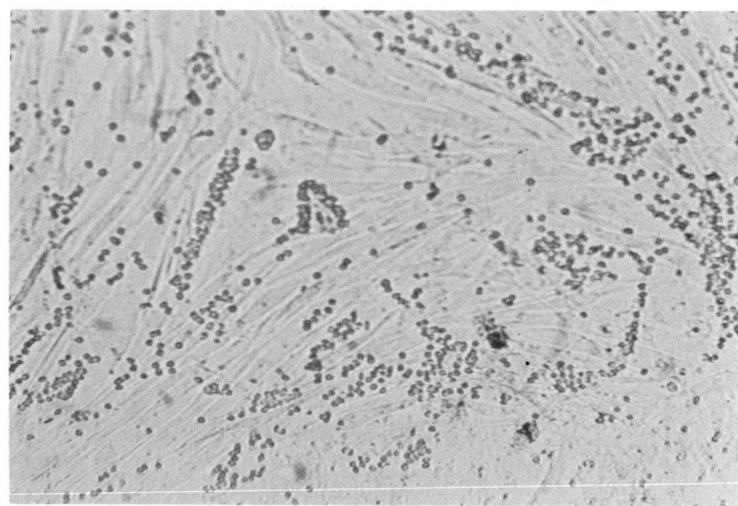

Figure 50–11. Hemadsorption with guinea pig erythrocytes in monkey kidney cells infected with parainfluenza 3. (From Herrmann, E. C., Jr., and Hable, K. A.: Mayo Clin. Proc., *45*:185, 1970.)

60 minutes, then examined microscopically for hemadsorption (Fig. 50–11). The tubes should also be inspected to determine if hemagglutination has occurred in the media as a result of excess free hemagglutinin release. This may block the hemadsorption phenomenon, but nevertheless indicates virus presence. Types 1, 2, and 3 hemadsorb at 4°C., with reversal above 25°C. for types 1 and 3; type 4 hemadsorbs only at 25 to 37°C. If cultures are negative at 4°C., reincubation at 25°C. for 30 minutes will detect type 4. If the cultures are hemadsorption- or hemagglutinin-positive, they can be passed into fresh culture tubes for further identification, or the infected cells may be directly examined by immunofluorescent or immunoperoxidase methods for rapid typing (Benjamin, 1974). If the cultures are read as negative, the medium is removed and fresh maintenance medium added, followed by reincubation. Virus detection in cell cultures is usually made in one to five days. Cytopathic effect is often nondescript or absent, with the exception of PI type 2, which will often produce syncytia (Fig. 50–12).

The classic methods of PI virus identification are hemadsorption-inhibition (HadI) or neutralization. Antisera for either test must first be treated with receptor-destroying enzyme and heat inactivated to remove non-specific inhibitors. In the HadI test, infected cell cultures are washed three times with PBS or Hank's BSS, then 0.5 ml of diluted antiserum is added. After 30 minutes incubation at 35°C., 0.2 ml of 0.4 per cent guinea pig red blood cells is added, and the cultures are reincubated at 4°C. for 30 minutes. The serum which inhibits hemadsorption as compared with controls identifies the isolate. The neutralization test differs only in that the fluid harvest from infected cell cultures is first incubated at 35°C. with treated antisera, then inoculated into fresh cell cultures and tested periodically for hemadsorption.

Interpretation of the significance of clinical isolates is usually not difficult, since asymptomatic carriers of PI viruses are rare. However, if the diagnosis of PI infection is suspected but cannot be confirmed by isolation, serologic testing may be desired. Either the HI or neutralization tests are preferred.

Respiratory Syncytial Virus (RSV)

RSV is considered the single most important respiratory virus affecting infants and young children. Infection with severe illness can occur as early as the first week of life and

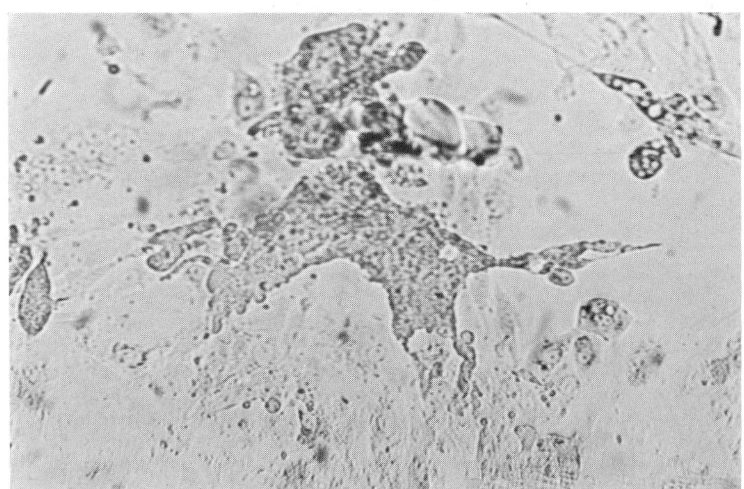

Figure 50–12. Typical syncytial pattern of cytopathic effect produced in monkey kidney cells by parainfluenza virus. (From Herrmann, E. C., Jr., and Hable, K. A.: Mayo Clin. Proc., *45*:184, 1970.)

is manifested primarily in infants as bronchiolitis, pneumonia, or both. Older children and adults are also susceptible, and reinfection is common. This latter group usually develops mild coryza and cough in response to infection, but croup and tracheobronchitis can also occur. RSV has also been associated with acute flare-ups of asthmatic bronchitis or chronic bronchitis in older individuals.

Infections are most commonly seen during the winter and early spring. Outbreaks among infants in a community usually last 8 to 12 weeks, and are often associated with a high degree of morbidity. Mortality in hospitalized infants is estimated to be as high as 2 per cent, and epidemic spread in a hospital setting is recognized as a serious problem. The virus is extremely labile and does not tolerate freezing well at all. The usual method of diagnosis is to obtain pooled nasopharyngeal and throat swab specimens (some workers prefer nasopharyngeal washings), and inoculate these as quickly as possible into cell cultures. As with parainfluenza viruses, shedding of virus is most prominent in the first week of illness.

RSV will grow in the three basic types of cell cultures, but is most reliably isolated in human heteroploid cell cultures. The cytopathic effect (CPE) is characteristically fusion of cells to form multinucleated syncytial or "giant" cells (Fig. 50–13) and may appear anytime from 2 to 14 days after inoculation. RSV does not possess or produce a hemagglutinin. The characteristic CPE, the lack of hemadsorption with guinea pig red blood cells, and the usual syndromes associated with RSV often allow the laboratory to make a presumptive etiologic diagnosis and distinguish this virus from other agents which produce syncytia, such as parainfluenza type 2, mumps, and measles viruses. Definitive identification, if necessary, can be done by immunofluorescent or immunoperoxidase, neutralization, or complement fixation tests.

Rapid identification of RSV infections has also been made by immunofluorescent examination of infected epithelial cells shed from the respiratory tract (Minnich, 1980).

As with parainfluenza viruses, interpretation of the significance of a clinical isolate of RSV is usually not difficult, since asymptomatic carriage is exceedingly rare. Serologic diagnosis, if deemed necessary, is usually by CF or neutralization; however, there are difficulties. Young infants do not always respond serologically to such infections; therefore, absence of a significant antibody response does not rule out infection. There is also a disparity between CF and neutralizing antibody responses, in that as many as 50 per cent of sera containing CF antibody may have no detectable neutralizing antibody (Fulginiti, 1974).

Rhinoviruses

Over 89 serotypes of rhinoviruses are currently recognized. They are acknowledged as important causes of the common cold, but are very rarely and questionably associated with more severe disease, such as lower respiratory illnesses. Rhinovirus infections have also been blamed for some acute exacerbations of illness in asthmatics and patients with chronic bronchitis.

While they are important causes of morbidity in the general population, the nature of the illness produced is usually such that a diagnostic virology laboratory is only occasionally requested to specifically seek them by culture. The highest yield of virus isolation from nasopharyngeal and throat specimens is in the first three to five days of illness.

The rhinoviruses have been isolated in monkey kidney, human embryonic kidney, human diploid fibroblasts, and occasionally in heteroploid cell lines. Of these, the human diploid fibroblasts, particularly WI-38 cells, have been the most sensitive. Most rhinoviruses grow best at 33°C. incubation, a factor which is also likely to explain their growth and pathology as limited primarily to the cooler environment of the upper respiratory tract in humans. In addition, continuous rotation of cultures in roller drums is usually required for primary isolation. These special incubation requirements are usually not all met in a diagnostic laboratory unless there is a special interest in rhinovirus infections. The CPE produced consists of irregular-sized, rounded cells which often glisten like dewdrops when fine focusing adjustment is made microscopically. As CPE progresses, cell disintegration and granularity become more apparent (Fig. 50–14). The CPE bears a close resemblance to that seen with some enterovirus isolates.

Because of the multiplicity of serotypes, neither specific serotyping nor serologic diagnosis is feasible in other than a research laboratory. If an isolate is suspected of being a rhinovirus, it can be confirmed by demonstrating resistance to chloroform or ether inactivation (ruling out herpesviruses) and by acid lability. In the latter test, rhinovirus infectivity

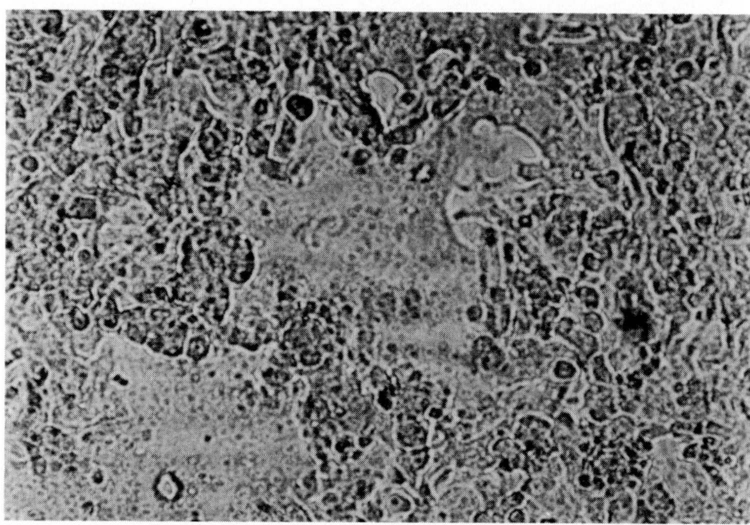

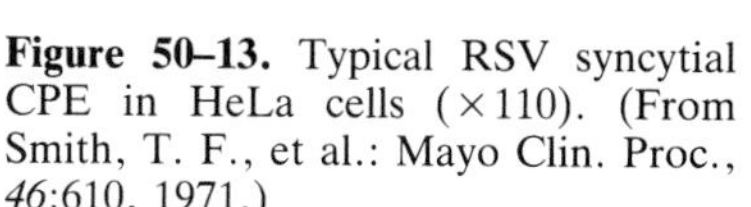

Figure 50–13. Typical RSV syncytial CPE in HeLa cells (×110). (From Smith, T. F., et al.: Mayo Clin. Proc., *46*:610, 1971.)

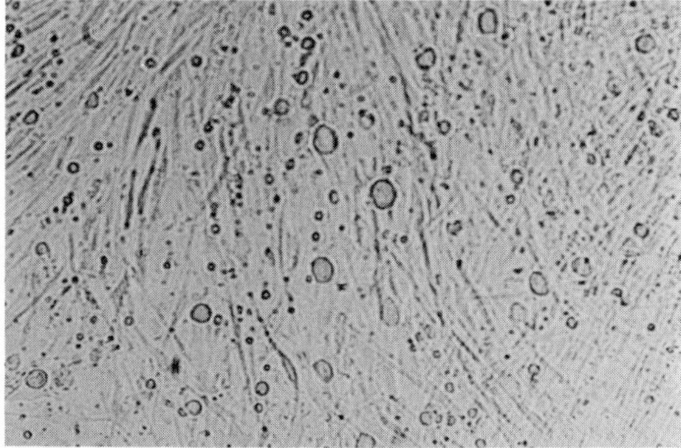

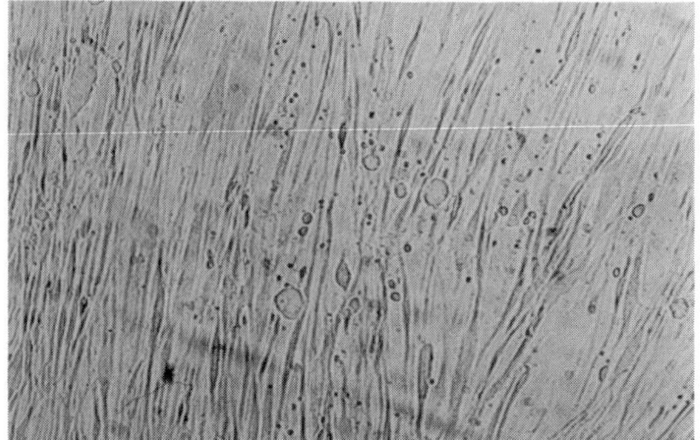

Figure 50–14. Rhinovirus CPE in WI-38 cell culture (×125). (From Person, D. A., and Herrmann, E. C., Jr.: Mayo Clin. Proc., *45*:521, 1970.)

is lost when the harvest is diluted at 1:10 in a solution at a pH of 2.0 to 2.2 and held at room temperature for two hours. Enteroviruses, which can be confused with rhinoviruses, are not inactivated by this procedure.

Coronaviruses

Like the rhinoviruses, coronaviruses are considered to be important causes of mild upper respiratory illnesses, particularly among adults. Also, based on serologic surveys, they may be associated with some cases of lower respiratory disease in young children (McIntosh, 1974).

The number of serotypes is unknown; two strains (229E and OC43) have been studied to some extent epidemiologically, and their overall contribution to human disease is presently not known. Coronaviruses are rarely, if ever, specifically sought in a hospital or public health laboratory. They have been isolated with some difficulty on human diploid lung fibroblasts, human embryonic trachea organ cultures, and in human embryonic intestinal fibroblasts. Some strains have been adapted to grow in human cell lines with plaque production. Most coronavirus isolates have been identified by electron microscopy or immune electron microscopy of culture supernatant fluids (Kapikian, 1973).

Most infections have been identified serologically, using either CF or HI tests, but these have not yet been routinely employed for clinical diagnosis.

Mumps Virus

There is only one serotype of mumps virus, although minor antigens are shared with other paramyxoviruses. Man is the only known host and reservoir of infection. The typical parotitis syndrome was accurately described by Hippocrates in the fifth century. The name *mumps* was derived from the mumbling speech of patients whose jaws were too painful to move.

The virus contains a hemagglutinin (HA), neuraminidase (NA), and hemolysin associated with the viral envelope. Two antigens elicit immunologic responses in an infected host. These are the soluble S antigen derived from the nucleocapsid and the V antigen derived from the surface hemagglutinin.

Epidemiology. The infection is endemic worldwide and primarily affects the 6- to 10-year age group. Infections occur predominantly in the spring, with mumps virus infection being the most common case of aseptic meningitis during this time period. Approximately 85 per cent of exposed susceptible contacts become infected, but 25 to 40 per cent of infections are asymptomatic. Seroepidemiologic surveys indicate that 80 to 90 per cent of adults have evidence of prior mumps virus infection. Virus is transmitted by infective salivary secretions and possibly by urine. Oral secretions contain virus for about six days before onset of parotitis until as long as two weeks afterwards. Viruria may persist for two to three weeks. The incubation period ranges from two to four weeks. Symptomatology coincides with onset of viremia, and multiple organ systems may be subclinically seeded with virus. Direct spread from the respiratory tract to the parotid gland is also a possibility.

Clinical Aspects. Onset of parotitis is typically sudden and may or may not be preceded by non-specific prodromal symptoms. Often there are few systemic manifestations of disease. The parotid swelling usually resolves within a week. Twenty to 35 per cent of postpubertal men who acquire mumps develop epididymoorchitis within one to two weeks following parotitis. Only 1 to 12 per cent of cases are bilateral; hence sterility is an uncommon late sequela. Pancreatitis complicating mumps may be difficult to diagnose, since both conditions may cause hyperamylasemia.

Approximately half of patients with mumps show CSF pleocytosis, but meningeal symptoms are less common. Conversely, 30 to 40 per cent of proven cases of mumps meningitis are unassociated with parotitis. Encephalitis is an unusual complication, but may lead to a variety of neurologic sequelae. Other rare CNS complications include a mild poliomyelitis-like syndrome, transverse myelitis, cerebellar ataxia, and Guillain-Barré syndrome. Additional complications include oophoritis, myocarditis, hepatitis, thrombocytopenic purpura, lower respiratory tract disease, polyarthritis, and thyroiditis.

Laboratory Diagnosis. The typical parotitis syndrome can be diagnosed clinically with great accuracy by physicians and laymen alike. Diagnosis by viral isolation or serologic techniques is most useful when the patient presents with a non-parotitis syndrome in which mumps virus infection is part of the differential diagnosis. Viral isolation from blood, CSF, oropharyngeal secretions, and urine confirms the diagnosis of current mumps virus infection. Best isolation results are obtained by using primary monkey kidney cell cultures. Characteristic CPE with large syncytial giant cells (Fig. 50–15) may or may not be produced; therefore, hemadsorption, employing guinea pig erythrocytes, should be performed periodically as described for the parainfluenza viruses. Specific identification is based on hemadsorption inhibition or neutralization using mumps virus antiserum.

Complement fixation (CF), neutralization, hemagglutination inhibition (HI), and radioimmunoassay (Daugharty, 1973) methods have all been employed for serologic diagnosis. The CF method is most widely used. The S and V antigens elicit characteristic specific CF antibody responses. The S antibody develops early, rises rapidly, and often peaks within the first week of symptoms. Afterward the S antibody

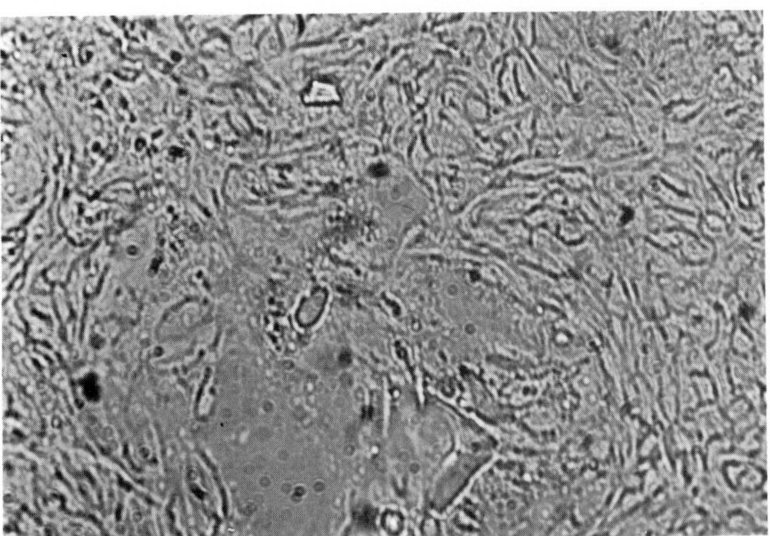

Figure 50–15. Typical syncytial CPE produced by mumps virus in RMK cells. (From Person, D. A., Smith, T. F., and Herrmann, E. C., Jr.: Mayo Clin. Proc., *46*:544, 1971.)

declines to undetectable levels within 6 to 12 months. The V antibody rises more slowly, peaking in two to three weeks, and then usually persists for a lifetime. Therefore, an acute serum demonstrating an elevated S antibody titer suggests acute or very recent disease. For definitive diagnosis of acute disease, a four-fold or greater change in antibody (usually V antibody) is required. Serum demonstrating only a V antibody titer indicates past infection and immunity. The V antigen elicits a delayed hypersensitivity reaction when used as an intradermal skin test in persons previously infected with mumps virus. However, the skin test has not been shown to be sufficiently specific to be used as a sole criterion for immunity or susceptibility.

Measles Virus

Measles virus or morbillivirus (previously called rubeola) has man as the only known natural host, but serologically related viruses infect animals, e.g., canine distemper and rinderpest viruses. Infection is characterized by the formation of large syncytial giant cells in tissues both *in vivo* and *in vitro*.

Epidemiology. Prior to widespread vaccination practices, measles epidemics occurred approximately every two years, usually in the late winter and spring, and primarily affected children. The disease is highly contagious, with secondary infections occurring in approximately 90 per cent of susceptible contacts, and the clinical attack rate of infected persons is greater than 95 per cent. By age 20 years about 95 per cent of persons in populous areas have been infected. The disease is communicable from five days before to five days after onset of the rash, and the infection is transmitted by oropharyngeal secretions introduced into the respiratory tract. The incubation period ranges from 7 to 18 days.

Clinical Manifestations. There is an initial three- to four-day prodromal period characterized by malaise, high fever, rhinitis, cough, and conjunctivitis. The pathognomonic Koplik spots appear on the buccal mucosa one to two days before onset of the red maculopapular rash which begins on the forehead and extends downward over the face, trunk, and lower extremities. The rash resolves in the same sequence, lasting approximately six days.

Infections may extend into the lower respiratory tract, causing croup, bronchitis, bronchiolitis, and rarely a giant cell interstitial pneumonia, particularly in immunocompromised children. Other complications include myocarditis, thrombocytopenia, mesenteric lymphadenitis with abdominal pain, and superimposed bacterial pneumonia and otitis media. Encephalomyelitis occurs in about 0.1 per cent of cases. Subacute sclerosing panencephalitis (SSPE), also called Dawson's encephalitis or inclusion encephalitis, is a rare later CNS complication.

Transplacental infection results in an increased frequency of abortion and stillbirth, but a suggested increased incidence of congenital malformation lacks confirmation.

Laboratory Diagnosis. Clinical diagnosis of a typical case of measles can be made with a high degree of accuracy, but demonstration of the virus or seroconversion is necessary to confirm the diagnosis. Best isolation results are achieved from specimens taken within the first few days of illness. Virus is present in the peripheral blood buffy coat during the first day of illness, in nasopharyngeal secretions during the first four to five days, and may be present in urinary sediment for as long as one week. Measles virus grows slowly in primary monkey or human kidney and human amnion cell cultures, producing characteristic multinucleate, syncytial giant cells after seven to ten days of incubation. The absence of hemadsorption with non-simian erythrocytes is useful to distinguish this virus from other paramyxoviruses, especially mumps. Identification is based on neutralization of cytopathic effects (CPE) with measles virus antiserum or by specific immunofluorescence of infected cell cultures.

Hemagglutination inhibition (HI), neutralization (NA), and complement fixation (CF) methods have all been employed for the serodiagnosis of measles. The HI test is usually the most rapid and useful method, having sensitivity and specificity comparable to NA and greater than CF. Antibody detected by all three methods appears within one to two days after the onset of rash and titers peak ten days to two weeks later. Antibody titers decline very gradually, making serodiagnosis after the first week of illness often difficult. The presence of specific IgM antibody also documents recent infection. Serodiagnosis is based on a four-fold rise in antibody titer.

The diagnosis of suspected SSPE is supported by extremely high serum and CSF measles antibody titers. Titers in this disease are characteristically ten-fold greater than titers in normal patients one year following typical measles. A serum HI titer of 1:1000 or greater in the proper clinical

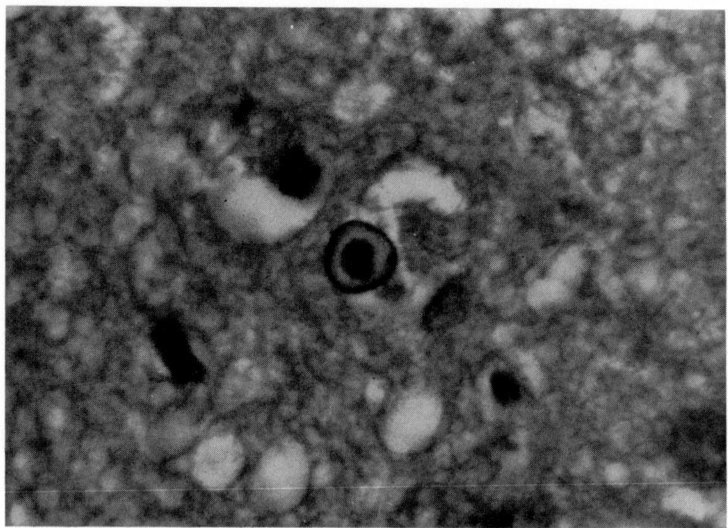

Figure 50–16. Cowdry type A intranuclear inclusion from a case of subacute sclerosing panencephalitis. (Courtesy of John Budinger, M.D.)

setting and without a history of recent measles is suggestive of SSPE; detectable CSF antibody further supports the diagnosis. Histologically, there are Cowdry type A intranuclear inclusions within neurons and glial cells of the brain (Fig. 50–16).

During measles, giant cells are characteristically formed at many sites of infection, including the skin, buccal mucosa, respiratory and occasionally urinary epithelium and within reticuloendothelial cells of lymph nodes or spleen. (Warthin-Finkeldey cells). During active disease, histologic examination of immunofluorescent staining of affected tissues, tissue scrapings, or urinary sediment may reveal the characteristic giant cells or antigen.

Rubella Virus

Clinical rubella (three-day measles or German measles) was first described in Germany about 200 years ago and was called *rötheln.* In the late 1930's the viral agent was transmitted to man and monkeys, but the virus was not isolated *in vitro* until 1962. In tissue culture systems used at that time the rubella virus produced no cytopathic effect, and hence was undetected until the interference or exclusion technique for identification was devised.

Rubella virus infection causes a benign, usually mild exanthematous illness when acquired postnatally; however, severe congenital anomalies can be produced in infants following maternal infection in the first trimester.

Epidemiology. Major epidemics of rubella have occurred in six- to ten-year cycles, in the winter and spring, primarily involving school age children; however, this pattern has been altered by the widespread use of the live attenuated vaccine. The disease has now become more common in older children and adolescents.

Rubella is probably transmitted by inhalation of infective droplets into the oropharynx. It is highly communicable, but less so than measles infections. Approximately 15 to 20 per cent of adults have escaped infection. The incubation period varies from two to three weeks with an average of about 18 days, and the contagious period extends from a week before to a week after onset of the rash.

The incidence of congenital birth defects varies with time of maternal infection. Estimates of risk of fetal malformations following infection in the first month of gestation vary from 50 to 80 per cent, decreasing to approximately 25 per cent in the second month and 17 per cent in the third month. The overall risk following exposure in the first trimester is about 25 per cent. The incidence of viral excretion by congenitally infected infants declines with age, but some still excrete virus for up to three years, serving as reservoirs of infection.

Clinical Aspects. Infection acquired by children is a mild disease characterized by generalized lymphadenopathy which is particularly prominent in the posterior cervical, suboccipital, and posterior auricular locations. This is followed by a macular rash which varies in intensity, starting on the forehead and face and spreading downward over the trunk and extremities. It usually lasts for three days. An infected older individual may have prodromal symptoms of malaise, headache, and fever. Complications are few but include postinfectious encephalitis, thrombocytopenia, arthritis, and arthralgias. Since many other infectious agents can produce rubella-like illness, the proof of rubella infection can only be established with certainty by laboratory studies.

Congenital rubella traditionally was thought to be manifested by congenital heart disease (patent ductus arteriosus, ventricular septal defect, and pulmonary stenosis), corneal clouding, cataracts, chorioretinitis, microcephaly, mental retardation, and deafness. Following the 1964 epidemic, additional manifestations were described, leading to the term "expanded rubella syndrome." These include hepatosplenomegaly, thrombocytopenic purpura, intrauterine growth retardation, interstitial pneumonia, myocarditis, and metaphyseal bone lesions. Table 50–15 outlines the relative

Table 50–15. FREQUENCY OF MAJOR FINDINGS IN SYMPTOMATIC CONGENITAL RUBELLA INFECTIONS

Frequency	Manifestations
75% +	Congenital heart disease (patent ductus arteriosus, pulmonary stenosis, etc.)
50–75%	Eyes—cataracts, chorioretinitis, cloudy cornea, microphthalmia, glaucoma
75% +	Deafness
30–40%	Hepatosplenomegaly
40–60%	Thrombocytopenic purpura
40–60%	Intrauterine growth retardation

frequencies of the major findings in congenital infections. A delayed onset progressive panencephalitis has also been described as a result of congenital rubella (Townsend, 1975).

Laboratory Diagnosis. The diagnosis of current or remote rubella infection is important in two circumstances: (1) diagnosis of congenital rubella, and (2) determination of immune status of women of reproductive age. Serodiagnosis of acute infection is indicated in a susceptible pregnant woman possibly exposed to rubella. Attempts to isolate the virus are most often indicated for the diagnosis of congenital infection, in which case viral excretion from the oropharynx and feces may continue for up to three years. Following postnatally acquired infection, virus can be isolated from the oropharynx for about seven days before to approximately two weeks after appearance of the rash and from the blood for a few days prior to onset of the rash. It may also be isolated occasionally from the feces, urine, and placental and fetal tissues of abortuses.

The virus can be grown in several continuous cell lines, including rabbit kidney (RK-13), rabbit cornea (SIRC), and green monkey kidney (VERO) in which microfoci of CPE have been described, but the usual way to demonstrate a rubella isolate is by the interference or exclusion method. By this technique primary African green monkey kidney cells are inoculated with a specimen, and after seven to ten days the cell culture and uninoculated control tubes are challenged by inoculation with another virus, usually an echovirus, and observed for the CPE characteristic of the superinfecting virus. Presence of CPE in control tubes and absence of CPE in the inoculated tubes indicate the possible presence of rubella virus. Absolute identification requires specific neutralization of interference with rubella antiserum. The presence of virus is diagnostic for congenital infection; however, the vaccination history must be considered in interpreting isolates from older infants or children. A reliable way to differentiate wild from vaccine strains has not been developed.

Serologic techniques, usually quicker and simpler than viral isolation, are used primarily for the diagnosis of postnatally acquired infection and for determining immune status. Hemagglutination, EIA, or complement fixation methods may be employed. Single radial hemolysis is used by some as a screening test for immunity. The virologic and serologic sequence of events following infection can be seen in Figure 50–17. HI or EIA antibodies usually become detectable about 14 to 17 days after primary exposure or about two to three days after onset of the rash. Peak titers are reached in about two weeks, slowly decline for a few years, and then persist for life. CF antibodies demonstrate a slower onset and peak, and then become undetectable after a few years. Neutralization and immunofluorescence tests are demanding and therefore not commonly performed.

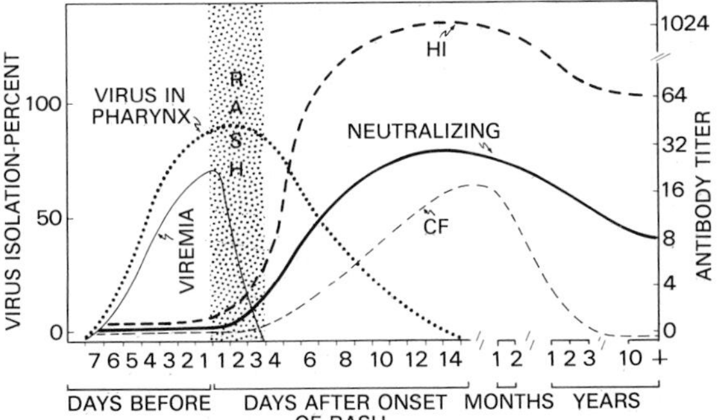

Figure 50–17. Virologic and serologic events with acute postnatal rubella infection. (From Krugman, S., and Ward, R. A.: Infectious Diseases of Children. 4th ed. St. Louis, C. V. Mosby Co., 1968.)

The presence of any detectable titer in the absence of disease indicates previous infection and hence immunity to reinfection. However, re-exposure to rubella virus has resulted in an asymptomatic anamnestic rise in antibody titers, but viremia has not been demonstrated to accompany this phenomenon. Therefore, a fetus would appear to be at little or no risk under these circumstances. A rubella titer is often routinely performed as part of a prenatal workup of pregnant women. If antibody is undetected, the woman is considered potentially susceptible and is followed accordingly. However, if a pregnant woman first comes to medical attention after a history of exposure to possible rubella, a titer done within the first two weeks after exposure will accurately reflect the woman's immune status prior to exposure. If antibodies are detected at any titer within this time frame, risk of damage to the fetus is assumed to be negligible. If no antibody is detected, a subsequent sample two weeks later should be obtained to determine whether a four-fold rise in HI or EIA antibody titer has occurred. If the woman has recently had a clinical syndrome compatible with rubella, it may be too late to demonstrate an antibody rise by HI or EIA methods, but CF antibodies, which develop more slowly, may still demonstrate a significant titer rise. The presence of specific IgM antibodies by indirect immunofluorescence or other methods may also be useful in diagnosing primary disease. It must be emphasized that paired sera should always be examined simultaneously in the same test run if reliable interpretations of quantitative antibody responses are to be made.

Rabies

Rabies is a worldwide zoonotic disease, affecting a wide variety of warm-blooded mammals and bats. Man is usually infected by contact with saliva or infected tissues through skin wounds (usually bites), and occasionally via the respiratory route by inhaling highly infectious aerosols. The incubation period in man and animals is usually one to three months, but can range from 10 days to 16 months or perhaps longer. There have been only three documented human survivors of clinical rabies to date—two infected with wild ("street") virus, and one laboratory worker presumably infected by an attenuated, live vaccine strain.

Because of the potential danger of lethal infection, and the obvious public health importance attached to this disease, it is recommended that *all rabies diagnostic work involving animals and humans be performed at a public health laboratory with special isolation facilities and trained, rabies-immunized personnel.*

In humans, the diagnosis is suggested by a history of possible or proved exposure (not always elicited), and a prodromal phase of non-specific complaints, hyperesthesia, and emotional changes progressing in two to four days to an "excitation" phase. This phase is characterized by increasing emotional lability, multiple cranial nerve weaknesses, spasmodic contractures of the muscles of swallowing and respiration, particularly when the patient attempts to swallow liquids (hydrophobia), and increased muscle tone. This is followed by progression to flaccid muscle paralysis, coma, and usually death.

The diagnosis of rabies in humans can be confirmed by culture, immunofluorescent, histologic, and serologic methods.

Culture of 20 per cent suspensions of brain biopsy or postmortem brain tissue is done by intracerebral inoculation of one- to two-day-old mice, and observing for neurologic signs or death for 28 days. Virus has also been isolated from salivary secretions, myocardium, skeletal muscles, lung, liver, and kidney in fatal human cases.

The diagnosis of rabies in humans can be confirmed by culture, immunofluorescent, histologic, and serologic methods.

Culture of 20 per cent suspensions of brain biopsy or postmortem brain tissue is done by intracerebral inoculation of one- to two-day-old mice, and observing for neurologic signs or death for 28 days. Virus has also been isolated from salivary secretions, myocardium, skeletal muscles, lung, liver, and kidney in fatal human cases.

Direct immunofluorescence to demonstrate the antigen is also a reliable diagnostic method and may be used on brain smears; it has also been reported that antigen may be detected by examination of skin biopsy material taken from the nape of the neck.

Intracytoplasmic inclusions in neurons, measuring 2 to 10 μm in diameter (Negri bodies), can be demonstrated in fixed brain sections or impression smears by staining with eosin and methylene blue, Giemsa, or Seller's stains; however, these methods are not as sensitive as culture or immunofluorescence.

Serologic diagnosis can be made by mouse-neutralization, indirect fluorescent antibody, fluorescent focus inhibition, or CF methods. Rabies antibody testing and advice concerning immunization can be obtained from the Centers for Disease Control through individual state health department laboratories.

Hepatitis

The clinical diagnosis of viral hepatitis is usually not difficult, supported by elevations of SGOT or SGPT enzymes and bilirubin, a moderate increase in the serum alkaline phosphatase, and variable prolongation of the prothrombin time. While toxic, metabolic, obstructive, and bacterial causes need to be ruled out, the clinician is usually able to narrow the possibilities down to a viral etiology. The problem then is, which virus?

A number of different viral agents can cause acute hepatitis, either as an isolated infection or as part of a systemic illness. These include Epstein-Barr virus, cytomegalovirus, adenoviruses, enteroviruses, and yellow fever, as well as some others. However, the majority of cases of hepatitis are due to three different agents, which will be discussed in further detail. These are hepatitis A, hepatitis B, and a third candidate virus, called "non-A, non-B hepatitis," which may actually represent two or more different agents. Recently, another agent, "delta antigen," has been described. This is thought to be a small, defective RNA virus which replicates only in the presence of infection by hepatitis B virus, and has most often been detected in drug addicts and hemophiliacs with chronic hepatitis B infections (Raimondo, 1982).

While the clinical behavior of these three viruses is usually indistinguishable, they have some differentiating characteristics, summarized in Table 50–16. There is no cross-immunity between these agents, and none have been grown in culture systems other than humans and other primates. It has been increasingly recognized that specific etiologic diagnosis in individual cases has important implications in terms of both patient management and epidemiologic control.

HEPATITIS A

Hepatitis A is ubiquitous, and is often associated with subclinical infection. Based on serosurveys, approximately 40 to 45 per cent of adults have evidence of prior infection. Outbreaks are not uncommon, often involving family members or groups exposed to a common source of food or water contamination. The illness tends to be milder and of shorter duration than hepatitis B, but fatalities have been recorded.

Hepatitis A probably rarely if ever spreads by parenteral mechanisms, even though transient viremia has been noted during infection. There is also no evidence that either a chronic viremic or intestinal carrier state exists. Cases are generally considered infectious from one to two weeks before the onset of abnormal enzyme levels to two weeks after the peak levels have been attained.

In the past, hepatitis A has been diagnosed after hepatitis B infection was excluded by appropriate laboratory tests; however, with the recognition that non-A, non-B hepatitis may be more common than originally thought, this assumption becomes less tenable. Hepatitis A virus antigen has been identified in feces, and occasionally in serum, by somewhat laborious electron microscopic and radioimmunoassay methods, but these are not readily adapted to the clinical laboratory.

Serologic tests utilizing antigen extracts from infected marmoset livers or infectious human feces have been devised. A CF test or a modification of the CF test, the immune adherence hemagglutination assay (IAHA), have both been used to demonstrate antibody titer responses to hepatitis A in paired sera obtained two or more weeks apart. More recently, RIA or EIA methods have been developed for the serodiagnosis of hepatitis A virus infection. IgM-specific antibodies appear early in illness, and can persist for four to six months (average is 80 days). The detection of these antibodies in a single serum sample supports the diagnosis of a recent primary infection (Snydman, 1981). The presence of IgG-specific antibodies alone indicates more remote past infection and immunity to reinfection.

Table 50–16. CHARACTERISTICS OF HEPATITIS VIRUSES

Characteristic	Hepatitis Agent		
	A	***B***	***Non-A, Non-B***
Agent type	Enterovirus 72	Hepadnavirus type 1	Unknown
Culture systems	Man, subhuman primates	Man, subhuman primates	Man, subhuman primates
Primary modes of transmission	Fecal-oral, urine, ?respiratory	Parenteral, sexual	Parenteral, ?fecal-oral
Epidemiology	Sharp outbreaks common	Often sporadic	Sporadic
Incubation period	2–6 weeks	6 weeks–6 months	2–15 weeks
Chronic carriage	Not shown	Yes—chronic viremia	Yes—chronic viremia
Chronic hepatic disease	No	Yes	Yes
Gamma-globulin prophylaxis	Effective	Probably effective	Not known

HEPATITIS B

Initially thought to be the major cause of post-transfusion hepatitis (serum hepatitis), hepatitis B has now assumed major public health importance in a number of other situations. In the United States, 0.5 to 0.9 per cent of adults are potentially infectious carriers of the virus, and 8 to 12 per cent of adults are antibody-positive, indicating a relative ubiquity of the agent. These rates increase to significantly higher levels in some groups, such as individuals repeatedly exposed to blood or blood products (surgeons, dentists, immunosuppressed patients, and patients and staff in hemodialysis units), institutionalized groups, illicit drug users, and homosexual males. While parenteral infection is considered to be the most important mode of spread, infections can be acquired by rather casual contact with infective blood or serum, whereby inoculation may occur through often trivial or even unnoticed breaks in skin or mucous membranes. Sexual transmission is also strongly suggested, particularly by the studies of male homosexuals, and arthropod spread (mosquitos, bedbugs) is suspected in some tropical areas. All ages are susceptible; maternal transmission to the fetus or newborn is recognized, and frequently leads to chronic infection of the infant. While nearly all body secretions have been shown to contain the viral surface antigen (e.g., saliva, urine, semen, sweat, and colostrum), it still appears that the most dangerous source of infection is blood and its byproducts. The infectivity titer of human serum which contains the surface antigen (HB_sAg) has been shown to be as high as $10^{7.5}$ ID_{50}/ml in primates, and very likely is similar in humans. The implications for the laboratory are clear: all bloods and sera must be handled with great care to avoid spillage or aerosolization, and disposal should be done so as not to endanger others who might come into contact with these samples.

Hepatitis B infection can be severe and prolonged, in contrast to the usual hepatitis A–associated illnesses. The usual course of infection is shown in Figure 50–18. After exposure, and approximately 1 to 7 weeks before illness or enzyme elevations appear, the viral surface antigen (HB_sAg) is detectable in the blood. The antigenemia persists for 1 to 12 weeks, then usually disappears after symptoms and laboratory evidence of hepatic dysfunction have resolved. CF antibody to the viral "core" antigen (anti-HB_c) usually appears at the time enzyme elevations are first seen, and disappears within a few years after antigenemia is no longer detectable. Antibody to the surface antigen (anti-HB_s) usually appears later, sometimes being delayed by 6 to 12 months after the acute episode. It appears to be relatively protective against reinfection. In some patients with acute infection, HB_sAg has declined to an undetectable level and the presence of anti-HB_c may be the only marker of acute hepatitis B. When this occurs and the anti-HB_s has not yet developed, the patient is said to be in the "core window." Other findings include the frequent detection of complete infectious virions (HB virus, formerely called Dane particles) and HB virus–associated DNA polymerase during the active phase of disease (Robinson, 1976). Another antigen, HB_eAg, has also been described, which is sometimes detected in acute serum as well as in chronic carriers and seems associated with a higher degree of infectivity (Sherlock, 1976; reviewed also by Robinson, 1976).

In some individuals, HB_sAg is not eliminated, and antigenemia can persist indefinitely (chronic infection). In these patients, anti-HB_c, DNA polymerase activity, and sometimes HB_eAg or antibody to HB_e (anti-HB_e) will also persist, and anti-HB_s is not detectable. These persons are not only potentially infectious to others, but can go on to develop either chronic persistent hepatitis (generally considered a benign, asymptomatic condition) or the more aggressive chronic active hepatitis, which may progress to cirrhosis. The various possible results of hepatitis B infection are illustrated in Figure 50–19. This demonstrates the importance of establishing whether or not a patient has hepatitis B, as well as to obtain appropriate follow-up to determine what the individual prognosis might be in proven cases. (See also Chaps. 15 and 39.)

Hepatitis B infection can also lead to extrahepatic manifestations. These can take the form of a serum sickness syndrome during the prodrome of an acute infection, or immune complex vasculitis, affecting a variety of organs and tissues, in chronic infections (Duffy, 1976).

The primary laboratory tests for diagnosis are those designed to detect HB_sAg in the serum. These are used to detect active infections as well as to screen potential blood donors. Of these, immunodiffusion, counterimmunoelectrophoresis, complement fixation, and radioimmunoassay (RIA) have all been used. The relative sensitivities of these tests for detection of HB_sAg are approximately 1, 10, 100, and 1000, respectively. Reversed passive hemagglutination, using antibody-sensitized sheep, turkey, or human red blood cells, has also been used as a rapid screening test, with a sensitivity claimed to be near that of RIA (Vandervelde, 1974), but false-positive results have been a problem in many laboratories.

Our current preference is to use either the RIA or EIA tests, which appear to be of equal sensitivity. These tests will detect nearly all cases of acute hepatitis B and most chronic carriers. It has been suggested that adding an RIA or EIA test to detect anti-HB_c will enhance the sensitivity of detection, particularly for chronic carriers.

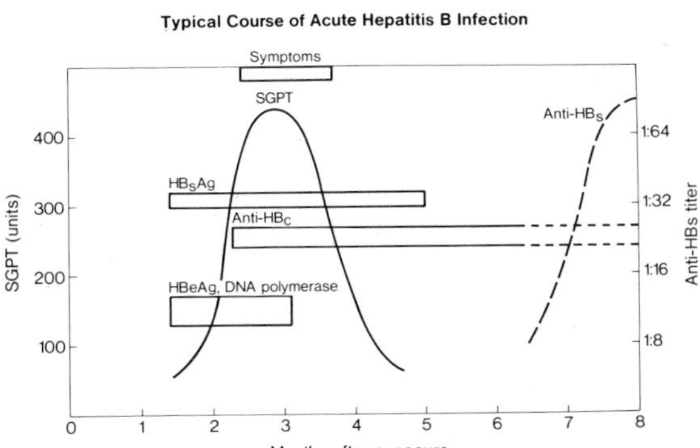

Figure 50–18. Typical course of acute hepatitis B infection.

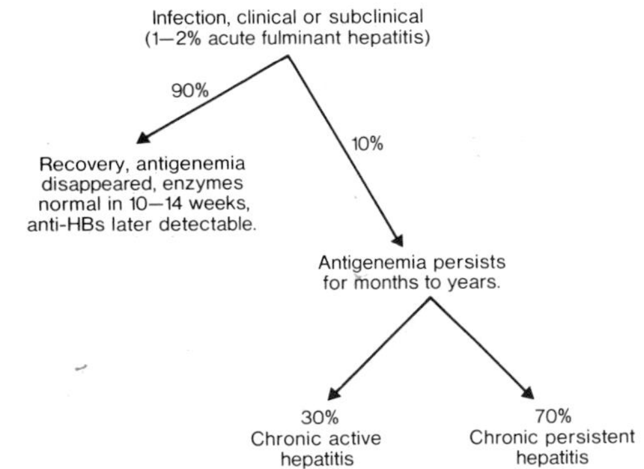

Figure 50–19. Outcome of hepatitis B infection.

6

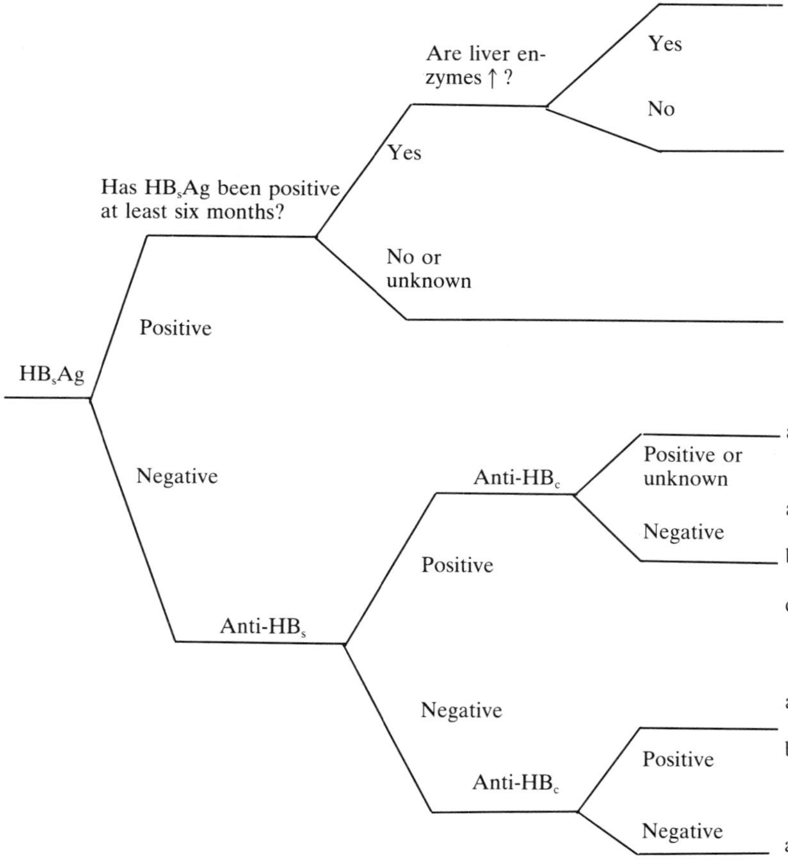

HB_sAg	Has HB_sAg been positive at least six months? / Anti-HB_s	Are liver enzymes ↑ ? / Anti-HB_c	Interpretation	Immune to further HBV infection	Potentially infectious to others for HBV
Positive	Yes	Yes	a) Chronic persistent hepatitis, or	Yes	Yes
			b) Chronic active hepatitis[1]	Yes	Yes
Positive	Yes	No	a) Chronic carrier of HBV (As symptomatic)	Yes	Yes
Positive	No or unknown		a) Acute HBV infection, or	Yes	Yes
			b) Chronic carrier of HBV	Yes	Yes
Negative	Positive	Positive or unknown	a) Normal immune response to prior HBV infection	Yes	No
Negative	Positive	Negative	a) Response to immunization with HBV vaccine, or	Yes	No
			b) Passive immunity after HBIG vaccination, or	Yes/no[2]	No
			c) Normal immune response to prior HBV infection, many years later	Yes	No
Negative	Negative	Positive	a) "Window phase" convalescence of HBV infection, or	Yes	No
			b) "Low level carrier" in non-acute setting[3]	Yes	No/yes[4]
Negative	Negative	Negative	a) No evidence of HBV infection	No	No

[1]Liver biopsy is needed to make definitive diagnosis between "A" and "B."
[2]Passive protection is of limited duration.
[3]May be infectious in a transfusion setting.
[4]HB_sAg level below level of detection.

Figure 50–20. Interpretation of hepatitis B serology results. (From Centers for Disease Control: Hepatitis Surveillance Report No. 47, Issued December 1981.)

Serologic testing for anti-HB_s is usually not helpful for diagnosis, since the antibody often appears weeks to months after antigenemia has subsided. It can be detected rather simply by passive hemagglutination of antigen-sensitized red blood cells, RIA, or EIA. Such testing is primarily useful in determining past infection and possible immunity in individuals who may have been exposed to infection, or who are likey to work in situations where exposure risks are high, e.g., hemodialysis unit personnel.

An algorithmic approach to the use and interpretation of HB_sAg, anti-HB_c, and anti-HB_s is shown in Figure 50–20. Mushawar (1981) has also published an excellent summary of interpretive approaches to such serologic data.

HB_eAg and anti-HB_e can be detected by immunoprecipitation, or more sensitive hemagglutination or RIA methods. While there may be prognostic implications of such detection, it cannot yet be strongly recommended that these be sought in a routine setting.

There are also antigenic determinants of HB_sAg that can be discerned with specific antisera. These include the "a" determinant, which is group-specific and found in all HB_sAg samples, and subdeterminants, such as "d," "y," "w," and "r," which are type-specific. In all, there may be as many as 18 such subdeterminants. These are not clinically useful, but subtyping does occasionally play a very helpful role in epidemiologic investigations. Such testing is available in special situations by consultation with the Centers for Disease Control through state health laboratories.

NON-A, NON-B HEPATITIS

Until recently, most viral hepatitis that could not be proved to be associated with hepatitis B, cytomegalovirus, or Epstein-Barr virus infection has been presumed to be due to hepatitis A. With the advent of specific diagnostic methods for all these other agents, this has been shown to be an erroneous assumption. Non-A, non-B hepatitis has been shown to be quite common. It is estimated that as many as 90 per cent of the cases of post-transfusion hepatitis now seen in the United States may be related to this agent. Furthermore, chronic antigenemic carrier states exist and may be associated with chronic active hepatitis. Sporadic cases have also been documented without known exposure to blood or blood products. It is estimated that non-A, non-B hepatitis may account for 25 per cent of non-transfusion-associated hepatitis in the United States (Robinson, 1982).

The diagnosis of non-A, non-B hepatitis is currently made only by excluding other known causes of hepatitis by appropriate laboratory tests. Little is currently known of the nature of the infectious agent, or even whether a heterogeneous group of viruses may be involved. Similarly, the epidemiology is as yet obscure, except for the known risk of transmission via transfusion. The disease produced is somewhat comparable to hepatitis A, usually being relatively mild, but the risks of chronic carriage and possible progressive liver disease are of great concern.

Viral Gastroenteritis Agents

Gastroenteritis accounts for approximately 12 per cent of all pediatric hospital admissions and is second only to the common cold as a cause of disease in infants and children. Overall, only approximately 30 per cent of cases in the United States and western Europe can be associated with bacterial pathogens. A viral etiology was first postulated in 1931, but studies in the 1940's attempting to demonstrate the communicability of the disease by using bacteria-free stool filtrates for oral ingestion by animals and human volunteers gave variable results.

Enteroviruses and adenoviruses which can be readily isolated in the laboratory have been suggested as possible etiologic agents of diarrhea, but subsequent studies have failed to show significantly different rates of isolation of most of these viruses from healthy controls versus patients with diarrhea.

With the use of immune-electron microscopy (IEM), Kapikian (1972) demonstrated 27 nm virus particles (later called the Norwalk agent) resembling parvoviruses in diarrheal stools and etiologically associated these with an acute non-bacterial gastroenteritis syndrome. Subsequently, several other parvovirus-like agents which were antigenically unrelated to the Norwalk agent have also been detected in diarrhea outbreaks. Later, 70 nm virus particles resembling reoviruses but antigenically different were demonstrated in duodenal mucosa by negative stain electron microscopy. This same virus was subsequently repeatedly demonstrated with high frequency in feces from patients with acute non-bacterial gastroenteritis, while it was consistently absent from healthy controls. This reovirus-like agent was subsequently called duovirus, orbivirus, and rotavirus. The most recent recommendation is to use the term rotavirus. It is possible that at least four antigenic types involve humans. Adenovirus type 38 (and perhaps other high-numbered serotypes) are also recognized causes of gastroenteritis. Like the parvovirus-like agents and rotaviruses, they are not reliably cultivated in routine tissue culture systems. In addition to the above viruses, extensive electron microscopic studies of feces from children with non-bacterial gastroenteritis have revealed several additional candidate viruses: "minireovirus," morphologically similar to reoviruses but only about 30 nm in diameter; caliciviruses; and "astroviruses," measuring about 28 to 30 nm in diameter and having a star-shaped periphery (Appleton, 1975; Middleton, 1977). The etiologic significance of these agents is still unclear. Coronavirus-like agents have also been suggested as possible etiologic agents (Caul, 1975; Vaucher, 1982). Of these agents, the rotavirus appears to be the most frequent cause of gastroenteritis. It is estimated that between 60 and 80 per cent of cases in infants and young children are due to this agent, and parvovirus-like agents are the next most common.

Epidemiology and Clinical Aspects. The rotavirus is associated with sporadic, moderate to severe diarrhea occurring most often in the 3- to 23-month age group, primarily during the winter. The incubation period is estimated to be 72 hours or greater. The diarrhea lasts 2 to 11 days and may be associated with mild to moderate vomiting for 1 to 5 days and fever for 2 to 4 days. Dehydration requiring hospitalization frequently occurs. When an infant with this disease is hospitalized, strict isolation techniques are mandatory because of the high incidence of nosocomial infection in children on the same ward. One seroepidemiologic survey (Gomez-Barreto, 1976) revealed that about 60 per cent of the 6-month to 4-year age group, 30 per cent of those 4 to 10 years, 50 to 60 per cent of those 10 to 30 years, and 45 per cent of those over 30 years of age had complement fixing antibodies to the rotavirus. The significance of serum antibody is unknown because reinfection apparently can occur in the presence of antibodies.

The parvovirus-like agents cause an explosive, rapidly spreading epidemic disease manifested primarily by nausea, vomiting, abdominal cramps, malaise, and a mild to moderate diarrhea, with complete recovery usually within 24 to 48 hours. This disease can affect all ages during all seasons. The incubation period is estimated to be 4 to 77 hours, and reinfection in the presence of humoral immunity may occur.

Enteric adenovirus-associated illnesses in infants and young children are similar to those described for rotaviruses, but the mean duration of symptoms is somewhat more prolonged (8.0 days).

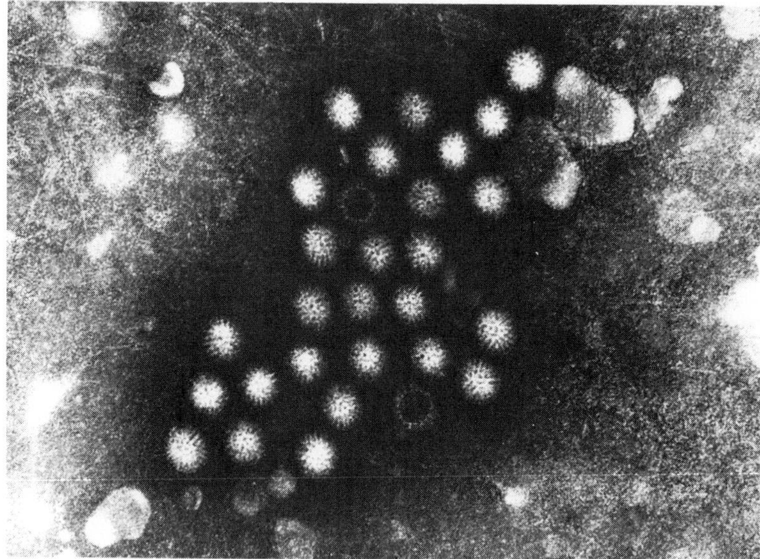

Figure 50–21. Rotavirus particles demonstrated by direct electron microscopy of diarrheal stool negatively stained with 2 per cent phosphotungstic acid. (Courtesy of Dr. Claire Payne.)

Laboratory Diagnosis and Interpretation. The clinical syndromes and epidemiology of these virus infections are quite helpful in suggesting the correct etiology, but definitive diagnosis requires demonstration of the virus. These viruses do not grow in routine tissue culture; therefore, direct electron microscopic examination of fluid extracts of diarrheal stools which have been negatively stained (Fig. 50–21) is the usual way to demonstrate their presence. However, an enzyme-linked immunosorbent assay (Yolken, 1977) and radioimmunoassay techniques have been developed for their detection. During convalescent stages virus is usually not detectable, further strengthening the diagnostic association of the agents with acute disease.

Complement fixation (CF) and EIA have been used to study antibody to the rotavirus. The antigen is prepared from stool filtrates of infected persons or calves infected with an antigenically similar virus. Antibody titers have been shown to rise by four-fold or greater following acute rotavirus infections, but this is a variable observation. Furthermore, the significance of humoral immunity to this agent is unknown.

The usual method for demonstrating antibody to the parvovirus-like agents is by immune electron microscopy (Kapikian, 1972) which was used initially to demonstrate the virus in stools and to relate the agent serologically to acute disease. Reinfection frequently occurs in individuals with humoral antibodies, which questions their importance in disease prevention. There appear to be two kinds of immunity to the parvovirus-like agents: a short-term immunity which appears protective for one to two months and longer-term immunity lasting at least two to four years (Parrino, 1977). However, both forms of immunity appear to be imperfect and the mechanisms of each are unknown.

Other, Less Commonly Encountered Viral Agents

REOVIRUSES

Originally identified as ECHO virus type 10, reoviruses are now known to be double-stranded RNA viruses, totally unrelated to enteroviruses. They have been perhaps appropriately named, since they can be found in the respiratory and enteric tracts of humans and other mammals, and their association with disease in humans is still largely obscure. These features led to the term "respiratory-enteric orphans."

Reoviruses have been frequently isolated from healthy subjects, as well as from infants and children with fevers and exanthems or diarrhea. (These viruses should not be confused with the reovirus-like rotaviruses described in the section on gastroenteritis). There have also been isolated reports of encephalitis, hepatitis, and pneumonia associated with reovirus infections, and virus has been isolated from affected tissues in some of these cases. Nevertheless, their overall role and importance in human disease remains uncertain.

Three serotypes are known to infect humans (types 1, 2, and 3). They grow well in a variety of cell types, with rhesus monkey kidney cells being most commonly used. Cytopathic effects are often slow to develop, usually taking 10 to 21 days, and often appear only as a granular, nonspecific degeneration. Serial passages of cultures are often necessary, and staining of the infected tissue culture cells is often helpful to distinguish the typical small cytoplasmic inclusions in a perinuclear array. Reoviruses will agglutinate human "O" erythrocytes, and identification of isolates as well as serologic determination of antibody responses can be made by HI testing or by neutralization.

LYMPHOCYTIC CHORIOMENINGITIS VIRUS

Lymphocytic choriomeningitis virus is an arenavirus that is usually transmitted to humans from chronically infected rodents by aerosol, fomites, or contact with infected tissues. In the United States, most cases have been traced to contact with rodent breeding colonies in research or pet supply centers, and to pet hamsters in the home. The illness is usually febrile and flu-like with myalgia. Occasionally, meningitis or meningoencephalitis will also occur and has been associated with transient hydrocephalus, elevated CSF protein values to 290 mg/dl, and CSF lymphocyte counts to 8300/cu mm.

The diagnosis is suggested by a history of rodent contact. The virus can be isolated in the early stages of disease by intracerebral injection of CSF and whole blood into suckling or weanling mice or young guinea pigs. Serodiagnosis is most commonly employed, using either CF or indirect immunofluorescence testing.

ARENAVIRUSES ASSOCIATED WITH HEMORRHAGIC FEVERS

These viruses, like lymphocytic choriomeningitis, are thought to be transmitted primarily from infected rodents to humans, although person-to-person transmission has also been documented for most of them. They include the agents of the South American hemorrhagic fevers (Junin and Machupo viruses) and Lassa virus, the cause of Lassa fever in Africa. All are associated with severe, febrile illnesses usually accompanied by hemorrhagic manifestations, neurologic disturbances, bradycardia, and shock. Lassa fever also causes an exudative pharyngitis and frequently myocarditis and hepatitis. Mortality rates are estimated as 10 to 50 per cent for Lassa fever, and 5 to 30 per cent for the others. All are considered highly infectious and extremely dangerous. Imported cases to non-endemic areas have occurred with a significant risk of spread to medical and laboratory personnel. The virus can be isolated during illness from blood, respiratory secretions, urine, feces, and vomitus (Woodruff, 1973).

The diagnosis is suggested primarily by the clinical syndrome and the recent travel history of the patient. If one of these agents is suspected, *strict isolation precautions are mandatory, and public health officials should be immediately notified.* While virus isolation from blood and other sites can be made in suckling mice, hamsters, and some tissue cultures, and CF antibodies can be determined, *these attempts should not be made in a hospital diagnostic laboratory.* All specimens should be forwarded to a well-equipped isolation facility after consultation with public health authorities.

MARBURG AND EBOLA VIRUSES

In 1967, 26 cases of severe hemorrhagic fever occurred in Germany and Yugoslavia among persons caring for a group of African green monkeys imported from central Uganda. A smaller cluster of three cases was documented in South Africa in 1975. The agent in both instances was subsequently identified as Marburg virus.

In 1976, severe outbreaks of hemorrhagic fever appeared in northern Zaire and southern Sudan and were later found to be due to an agent now known as Ebola virus, named after a small river in Zaire.

While both agents produce a similar, highly fatal (30 to 80 per cent mortality) contagious disease and both have a similar physical appearance in cultures (filamentous particles averaging 100 nm in diameter and 300 to 1500 nm in length, with budding from cell membranes), each appears to be antigenically distinctive. The ecology and epidemiology of these agents is currently not well understod (Johnson, 1977; Heymann, 1980).

Like the arenavirus-associated hemorrhagic fevers, the travel history of the patient and the hemorrhagic fever syndrome suggest the diagnostic possibilities, and precautions with regard to the patient and handling and processing of specimens are the same. The viruses have been grown in Vero cells (a continuous African green monkey kidney cell line), mice, and guinea pigs, but *this should never be attempted in a hospital diagnostic laboratory.*

RICKETTSIAL INFECTIONS

Tribe *Rickettsieae* are fastidious, obligate intracellular parasites with the exception of *Rochalimaea quintana.* They are pleomorphic coccobacillary organisms possessing both RNA and DNA and both synthetic and energy-producing enzyme systems. These organisms are characterized by their natural proclivity to infect arthropods and other mammals (except for *R. quintana*), which serve as vectors and reservoirs of disease for incidental human infection.

Rickettsial disease, especially epidemic typhus, has historically been a major cause of worldwide morbidity and mortality and has been estimated as second only to malaria as a cause of human death from infectious disease. In the early twentieth century, Ricketts, for whom the microorganisms are named, successfully transmitted Rocky Mountain spotted fever, incriminated the wood tick as a vector, and observed the organisms in smears of tick tissue. Shortly thereafter, other rickettsial vectors were incriminated and further transmission studies performed. In 1926, rodents were recognized as natural reservoirs of infections. Brill recognized a mild form of epidemic typhus unassociated with the louse vector in 1910, and Zinsser in 1934 postulated that the disease was a recrudescent form of typhus occurring following stress or declining immunity. This was subsequently confirmed. In 1915 Weil and Felix recognized that agglutinins from typhus fever patients reacted with certain strains of *Proteus* sp., and this discovery led to the widely used but non-specific Weil-Felix reaction.

The human pathogens can be divided into five antigenic groups: the typhus group, spotted fever group, scrub typhus, Q fever, and trench fever. The species within these groups as well as the epidemiology and natural cycles are outlined in Table 50–17. Rocky Mountain spotted fever (RMSF) and Q fever are the most common rickettsial diseases in the continental United States, but Brill-Zinsser disease, murine typhus, and rickettsialpox are also found occasionally.

Organisms enter through the skin or respiratory tract and probably replicate locally during the incubation period. This is followed by a rickettsemia, which coincides with initial symptoms and needs organisms throughout the vascular system to infect endothelial cells, leading to the characteristic rash. Later, immunologic mechanisms may be important in enhancing vasculitis, and the toxic febrile state may be related to type-specific toxins. Rickettsial diseases in general are characterized by sudden onset of fever, chills, moderate to severe headache, malaise, and a variable degree of prostration and toxicity. In contrast to the other rickettsial infections, there is no rash in Q fever, and pneumonia is found in approximately half of the cases. An eschar or local skin lesion may be seen at the site of initial entry of the organism in rickettsialpox or scrub typhus infections. There is usually prominent lymphadenopathy in the region draining the area of the eschar of scrub typhus.

Epidemic typhus is caused by *R. prowazekii* and the vector is the body louse (*Pediculus humanus*). The disease is usually maintained in a man-to-louse-to-man cycle. Man is infected by rubbing infected feces deposited by the louse into broken skin. Epidemic typhus may be accompanied by circulatory distur-

Table 50–17. RICKETTSIAL DISEASES OF MAN

Group and Type	Species	Disease Synonyms	Geographical Distribution	Natural Cycle		Transmission to Man
				Arthropod	*Mammal*	
Typhus						
Epidemic	*R. prowazekii*	Louse-born typhus, exanthematous typhus	Worldwide except Australia	Body louse	Man, flying squirrel (USA)	Infected louse feces into broken skin
Brill's disease	*R. prowazekii*	Recrudescent typhus, sporadic typhus	North America, Europe		Recurrence years after original attack of epidemic typhus	
Endemic	*R. typhi*	Murine typhus, endemic typhus, flea-borne typhus	Worldwide	Rat flea	Rats	Infected flea feces into broken skin
Spotted Fever						
Rocky Mountain spotted fever	*R. rickettsii*	Fiebre manchada, São Paulo typhus	Western Hemisphere	Ticks	Wild rodents, dogs, birds	Tick bite
Boutonneuse fever	*R. conorii*	Marseilles fever, South African tick bite fever, Kenya tick typhus, Indian tick typhus	Africa, Europe, Middle East, India	Ticks	Wild rodents, dogs	Tick bite
Queensland tick typhus	*R. australis*		Australia	Ticks	Marsupials, wild rodents	Tick bite
North Asian tick-borne rickettsiosis	*R. siberica*	Siberian tick typhus	Siberia, Mongolia	Ticks	Wild rodents	Tick bite
Rickettsialpox	*R. akari*	Vesicular rickettsiosis	North America, Europe	Bloodsucking mite	House mouse and other rodents	Mite bite
Scrub typhus	*R. tsutsugamushi*	Mite-borne typhus, tropical typhus, rural typhus	Asia, Australia, Pacific Islands	Trombiculid mites	Wild rodents, birds	Chigger bite
Q fever	*C. burnetii*	Balkan grippe	Worldwide	Ticks	Small mammals, cattle, sheep and goats	Inhalation of dried, infected material
Trench Fever	*Rochalimaea quintana*	Wolhynian fever, five-day fever	Europe, Africa, North America, Middle East	Body louse	Man	Infected louse feces into broken skin

bances, peripheral vascular collapse, and hepatic, renal, and CNS disturbances. The southern flying squirrel, *Glaucomys volans,* is the only known extrahuman vertebrate reservoir for *R. prowazekii* (Bozeman, 1975), and sporadic cases of "epidemic" typhus have been recently reported in areas where this squirrel is indigenous (Duma, 1981). Brill-Zinsser disease, the recurrent form, is usually milder, but the disease is characterized by rickettsemia and is communicable to others if the proper vector is present.

Endemic (murine) typhus is caused by *R. typhi,* and the vector is primarily the rat flea (*Xenopsylla cheopis*). Again, disease is transmitted to man by rubbing infected feces from the vector into broken skin. Disease is maintained in nature by small rodents, and man is only an incidental host. This is one of the most benign of the rickettsioses and occurs in the southeastern and Gulf Coast areas of the United States primarily in the summer and fall.

Scrub typhus is caused by *R. tsutsugamushi,* and a larval mite (usually *Leptotrombidium akamushi* or *L. deliense*) is the vector. Infection is transmitted when the chigger burrows beneath the skin to obtain a tissue fluid meal. Small rodents are the natural hosts, with only incidental human infection. Complications of disease are similar to those of epidemic typhus, but myocarditis more often occurs with scrub typhus. The disease occurs primarily in Asia, India, Australia, and the South Pacific islands.

Rocky Mountain spotted fever is caused by *R. rickettsii,* and the wood tick (*Dermacentor andersoni*) and the dog tick. (*D. variabilis*) are the vectors. Small mammals serve as natural hosts and reservoirs of infection, and man is incidentally infected by the bite of the tick. The disease may be quite severe, with delirium, shock, and renal failure complicating the usual clinical manifestations. However, recent serologic studies on children living in endemic areas suggest that subclinical infections may also occur (Marx, 1982). The disease occurs throughout the United States and the Western Hemisphere.

Rickettsialpox, caused by *R. akari* and transmitted by the bite of a mite vector (*Allodermanyssus sanguineus*), is maintained in nature in small rodents and mice and occasionally infects house mice. It produces a mild, non-fatal, febrile illness lasting about one week, and occurs sporadically in the United States.

Q fever, caused by *Coxiella burnetii,* has an extensive wild and domestic animal host range, and is transmitted in nature to small wild mammals by ticks. However, man is infected by inhalation of droplets contaminated by salivary secretions or placental tissues of infected animals. Transmission among cattle, sheep, or goats may occur without an arthropod vector. Farm workers and slaughterhouse employees are at greatest hazard for infection, which is characterized by an interstitial pneumonitis. This organism also can cause a subacute bacterial endocarditis. There is no rash, and Weil-Felix agglutinins are not produced. The disease occurs worldwide, including the United States.

Trench fever is caused by *R. quintana,* which has been cultivated *in vitro* on blood agar. This characteristic makes one question the proper classification of this organism. The body louse (*P. humanus*) functions as the vector, and man is the only vertebrate host and reservoir of infection. Trench fever, primarily a disease of the military, is characterized by severe muscle, joint, and bone pains, primarily in the shins, and may pursue a relapsing course with persistent rickettsemia for several years. The disease has occurred in troops in Europe, Africa, and North America.

Laboratory Diagnosis. Isolation of these organisms is extremely hazardous and should be attempted only by experienced, well-equipped reference laboratories. Aseptically collected tissues or whole blood that is flash frozen and maintained at −70°C. or lower during shipment maintain organism viability. Animal or embryonated egg inoculation methods are employed for isolation of *Rickettsia* spp., as well as tissue culture techniques for isolating *R. rickettsii* from blood or ticks (Wike, 1972). Smears of tissues infected *in vivo* or *in vitro* can be specially stained with Giménez, Macchiavello, or Giemsa stains. None of the above stains reliably differentiate these organisms from bacteria. *Rickettsia* sp. are usually seen in the cytoplasm of cells except for *R. rickettsii,* which may also be present within nuclei. Organisms in infected tissues, ticks, and tissue culture cells may also be demonstrated by direct immunofluorescence using specific antisera (Burgdorfer, 1970; Hanon, 1966).

The complement fixation (CF) test is useful for serodiagnosis of nearly all the rickettsioses except scrub typhus, in which a mutually exclusive antigenic multiplicity of strains makes CF serodiagnosis too antigenically specific and hence impractical. For the other rickettsioses, CF tests detect group-reactive antibodies (see Table 50–18), and hence may not be entirely specific. Therefore, one must use caution in interpretation. Past immunizations and previous exposure in endemic areas may cause persistent low CF antibody titers that are uninterpretable. Nevertheless, the CF test on paired sera may be a useful serodiagnostic tool. CF antibodies first appear one to two weeks after onset of symptoms, and a four-fold or greater titer rise can usually be detected during convalescence. Demonstration of significant seroconversions in the proper clinical context is diagnostic for rickettsial group infection.

The Weil-Felix reaction depends on agglutination of OX-19, OX-2, of OX-K strains of *Proteus vulgaris* by antibody produced during typhus or spotted fever rickettsial infections. The usual pattern of reactions can be seen in Table 50–18. They vary in sensitivity and are frequently non-specific. False positive results are common, and may be the result of other infections, including urinary tract bacterial infections, leptospirosis, borreliosis, or severe hepatic or biliary tract disease.

Indirect immunofluorescence shows promise for the diagnosis of scrub typhus infections because the antibody detected by this method is more group-reactive toward the multiple *R. tsutsugamushi* strains. Direct immunofluorescent methods for specifically identifying *R. rickettsii* in frozen and paraffin-embedded infected tissues have been described (Walker, 1978,

Table 50–18. CLASSIFICATION AND ANTIGENIC COMPOSITION OF RICKETTSIEAE

Group and Type	Species	Soluble CF*	MICRO-IF†	Agglutination	Weil-Felix Agglutinin
Typhus group	*R. prowazekii*	GS‡	SS§	SS	OX-19
	R. typhi	GS	SS	SS	OX-19
Spotted fever group	*R. rickettsii*	GS	SS	SS	OX-19 or OX-2
	R. conorii	GS	SS	SS	OX-19 or OX-2
	R. australis	GS	SS	ND	OX-19 or OX-2
	R. siberica	GS	SS	ND	OX-19 or OX-2
	R. akari	GS	SS	SS	None
Scrub typhus group	*R. tsutsugamushi*	SS¶	SS	ND	OX-K
Q fever	*Coxiella burnetti*	None	SS	SS	None
Trenchfever	*Rochalimaea quintana*	SS	ND	ND	None

*Complement fixation.
†Immunofluorescence.
‡Group specific.
§Species specific.
¶There are at least eight immunotypes.

1980). Tissue immunofluorescence is more sensitive and specific than serologic methods and is currently the best procedure for early diagnosis.

Agglutinin titers may be useful in diagnosis of Q fever. In general, these antibodies appear and rise earlier to higher titer than CF titers, but both may persist for many years afterward. Since antibodies to *C. burnetii* do not cross-react with other rickettsiae, a significant rise in titer is considered diagnostic (except in recent vaccinees). This would make the test particularly useful for diagnosing subacute endocarditis caused by *C. burnetii.* In general, rickettsial agglutination tests (Fiset, 1969) appear to be more species-specific than the CF tests. This would be particularly useful in identifying murine typhus infection in individuals who have received epidemic typhus vaccine. A specific, rapid latex agglutination test for *R. rickettsii* has been described (Hechemy, 1980).

CHLAMYDIAL INFECTIONS

Formerly referred to as bedsonia, and originally thought to be viruses because of their obligate intracellular parasitism, the chlamydiae are now recognized as a unique, bacteria-like group of organisms. They possess a gram-negative cell wall, divide by binary fission, contain both RNA and DNA, are unable to grow outside an animal cell, and are susceptible to a variety of antibiotics. While chlamydiae affect a wide range of animal and avian hosts, this discussion will center on the agents known to affect humans. Table 50–19 represents a current classification of these and the syndromes with which they have been associated.

C. trachomatis has been distinguished from *C. psittaci* by the observation that the intracellular inclusions in the former are compact, contain glycogen, and are stained by iodine (Fig. 50–22), whereas *C. psittaci* inclusions are diffuse and are not stained by iodine.

All the chlamydiae have a common CF antigen. In

Table 50–19. CHLAMYDIAE AFFECTING HUMANS, AND DISEASES THEY PRODUCE

Genus	Species	Disease	Immunotypes Involved
Chlamydia			
	psittaci	Psittacosis (ornithosis)	
	trachomatis	Trachoma	A, B, Ba, C
		Inclusion conjunctivitis	
		Non-gonococcal urethritis	
		Cervicitis	D, E, F, G
		Salpingitis	H, I, J, K
		Pneumonia in infancy	
		Lymphogranuloma venereum	L_1, L_2, L_3

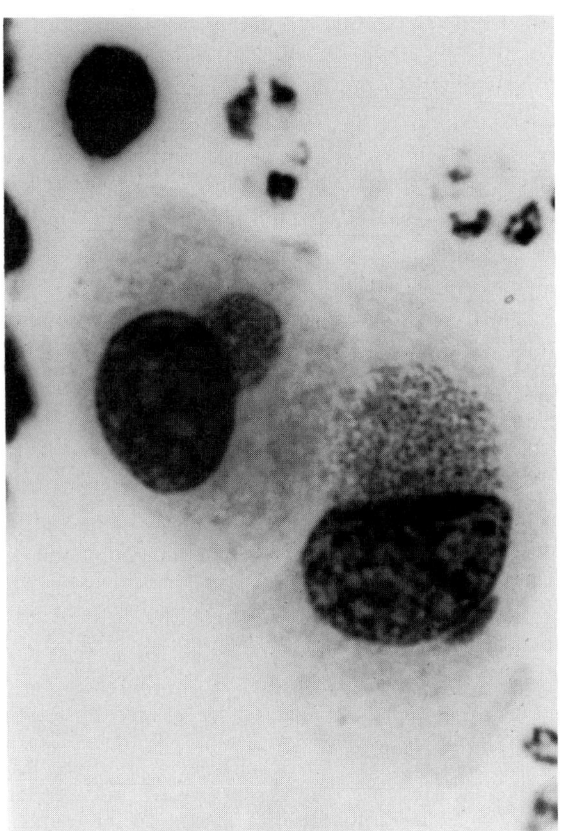

Figure 50–22. Chlamydial agent in conjunctival scraping (×1100). (Courtesy of Z. Naib, M.D.).

addition, there are several immunotypes of *C. trachomatis* which have some correlation with the diseases produced and their epidemiology (Table 50–19).

CLINICAL ASPECTS

Psittacosis (Ornithosis)

Psittacosis, a disease of psittacine birds such as parrots, parakeets, and cockatoos, is not as restricted in its host range as the name implies. The organisms can also infect pigeons, turkeys, chickens, and other avians, and the name ornithosis is currently preferred. Birds can infect humans via inhalation of contaminated aerosols or fomites, and person-to-person transmission has also been documented. There is an incubation period of 7 to 14 days, and the syndrome is usually characterized by chills, fever, malaise, and pneumonia. Hepatosplenomegaly, jaundice, and myopericarditis may also occur.

The diagnosis is suggested by a history of bird contact and is a particular hazard for pet-shop workers, avian pet owners, and poultry workers. The diagnosis is usually confirmed by demonstrating a significant rise in CF antibody titers in paired acute and convalescent sera.

Lymphogranuloma Venereum (LGV)

Lymphogranuloma venereum is venereally transmitted. The initial lesion is a small, painless 2 to 3 mm genital vesicle or ulcer which often goes unnoticed and heals in a few days. This is followed by inguinal adenopathy, which can be extensive, and may be associated with systemic signs of meningitis or meningoencephalitis, pneumonia, keratoconjunctivitis with eyelid edema and preauricular adenopathy, or polyarthritis. Erythema nodosum or erythema multiforme is also frequently associated with infection. Occasionally, severe proctitis or proctocolitis can develop, and rectal or urethral strictures may result from infection. The Frei test, a delayed hypersensitivity skin test using purified "Lygranum" chlamydial antigen, becomes positive as early as 10 days after infection and remains positive indefinitely. However, it does not necessarily distinguish recent LGV infection from past infection with this or other members of the Chlamydia genus, and a negative test does not rule out such infection. CF or immunofluorescent testing is most commonly used for serodiagnosis. The antibody response has usually reached a peak titer before the diagnosis is considered, which often negates the opportunity to detect a rising titer during illness. A CF antibody titer of 1:16 or greater usually supports the clinical diagnosis. Specimens of choice for isolation purposes are usually lymph node aspirate or rectal biopsy.

Trachoma and Other Chlamydia Trachomatis Infections

Endemic trachoma is present in many areas of the world, including some parts of the United States. It is usually spread by direct contact and begins as a conjunctivitis, which may persist for months to years and which can spread to the cornea, causing vascularization, scarring, and blindness. Immunotypes A, B, Ba, and C are most commonly involved.

The diagnosis can be made by examination by immunofluorescence, iodine, or Giemsa staining of methanol or acetone-fixed conjunctival scrapings, looking for intracytoplasmic inclusions in epithelial cells, as shown in Figure 50–22. Culture is a much more sensitive method, and is currently done more commonly in cell cultures than by other means.

Other immunotypes of *C. trachomatis,* such as types D, E, F, G, H, I, J, and K, are being increasingly recognized as important disease-producing agents in humans. While these are thought to be spread primarily from a venereal reservoir, contact transmission by non-venereal reservoir routes is also possible. Inclusion conjunctivitis can occur at all ages. This is similar to trachoma, but is generally milder and usually self-limiting. In the United States, this is most often seen in infants, with onset at any time after three days of age. It can closely mimic acute neonatal gonococcal conjunctivitis. These strains have also been implicated as causes of non-gonococcal urethritis in adults and are thought to account for as many as 40 per cent of male cases.

In addition, some episodes of cervicitis, as well as salpingitis, have been associated with genital *C. trachomatis* infection in females. Similar immunotypes have been isolated from respiratory tract secretions, associated with high type specific antibody titers in serum, nasal, and lacrimal secretions, in infants from three weeks to six months of age with a protracted "pertussoid" pneumonia syndrome (Beem, 1977). Only about half of these infants had a history of preceding or concurrent conjunctivitis.

LABORATORY DIAGNOSIS

Diagnosis of infection with *Chlamydia psittaci* is commonly made by demonstration of a four-fold or greater rise in CF antibody titer. The agent can be cultivated in the yolk sac of embryonated eggs, by intraperitoneal inoculation of mice, or by inoculation into HeLa 229 or other cell cultures. Inclusions in cell culture are demonstrated with Giemsa or methyl green–neutral red stains, but not iodine.

Chlamydia trachomatis has been isolated in cell cultures, in yolk sacs, and in mice after intracerebral or intraperitoneal inoculation.

For isolation purposes, specimens may be collected as biopsy samples (e.g., lung), as whole secretions, or as calcium alginate swabs from affected sites (e.g., eye, respiratory tract, cervix, urethra), and placed in a sucrose-phosphate buffer (2SP) described by Gordon (1972), containing 50 μg of streptomycin per ml and 25 units of nystatin per ml, for transport to the laboratory. Specimens should contain epithelial cells, not just exudate. The organisms can withstand freezing at −70°C or lower, but should not be kept frozen at higher temperatures. Tissue homogenates are prepared by grinding tissue in 2SP and inoculated as 20, 2, and 0.2 per cent suspensions. While several methods for isolation in cell culture have been described, a common method is the use of cycloheximide-treated McCoy cells (a strain of mouse heteroploid cells). In this procedure, McCoy cells are trypsinized and seeded into sterile flat-bottomed 1 or 2 dram vials containing 12 mm circular or 9 mm^2 rectangular coverslips. The cells are grown to confluence on the coverslips (one to two days) using MEM with 10 per cent fetal calf serum and *without* penicillin. The medium is aspirated, and 0.2 to 0.3 ml of specimen in 2SP is inoculated onto the cells. Vials are centrifuged at 3500 rpm for one to two hours at 30°C. Vials are refilled with MEM with 10 per cent fetal calf serum, 1 μg/ml cycloheximide, and 0.5 per cent glucose. After two to four days of incubation at 35°C., the medium is aspirated, coverslip-fixed in methanol, stained with filtered Jones' iodine solution, and examined for the presence and quantity of chlamydial inclusions. Against the background of yellow staining cells, the inclusions are cytoplasmic and perinuclear, and stain light to dark brown. Care must be taken to avoid confusion of inclusions with artifacts such as cell debris, starch granules from examination gloves, and red blood cells. Positive specimens may be detected as early as 48 hours post-inoculation.

Alternative staining methods include Giemsa, acridine-orange, methyl-green–neutral red (Woodland, 1982) and immunofluorescence (Stephens, 1982). The McCoy cell–cycloheximide culture system may be adapted to a micro-test system (Yoder, 1981) or to use of rapidly produced monolayers by treating coverslips with gluteraldehyde-activated γ-aminopropyltriethoxy silane (Evans, 1980).

Sensitivity of this culture system may be affected by the fetal calf serum (Evans, 1980) and cycloheximide concentration (La Scolea, 1981). All lots of fetal calf serum must be screened for inhibitors, and concentrations of cycloheximide activity will vary from lot to lot. Antibiotics such as penicillin and ampicillin must be strictly avoided in the culture system. Because of inhibitors, newborn calf serum should not be substituted for fetal calf serum (La Scolea, 1982). When culturing *C. psittaci,* the Giemsa, immunofluorescence, or methyl-green–neutral red stain must be used, as the inclusions will not stain with Jones' iodine. HeLa 229 cells are preferred for isolation of *C. psittaci.*

Antibody titers to *C. trachomatis* in serum, and even tears, can be measured by neutralization or microimmunofluorescent methods (Wang, 1975). Commercial reagents are available for indirect immunofluorescence testing. This is useful in detection of IgM-specific antibody. IgM-specific antibody to *C. trachomatis* is present in infants with pneumonia caused by this organism, but is not usually found in the asymptomatic carrier state. The CF test is useful in the diagnosis of LGV and psittacosis. Serologies have not been found to be particularly helpful in diagnosis of pelvic inflammatory disease and non-gonococcal urethritis because there is a high prevalence of antibody to *C. trachomatis* in the general population.

General References

Chernesky, M. A., Ray, C. G., and Smith, T. F.: Laboratory diagnosis of viral infections. *In* Drew, W. L. (ed.): Cumitech 15. Washington, D.C., American Society for Microbiology, 1982.

Gardner, P. S., and McQuillin, J.: Rapid Virus Diagnosis. Application of Immunofluorescence. 2nd ed. London, Butterworth and Company, Ltd., 1980.

Kawamura, A. (ed.): Fluorescent Antibody Techniques and Their Applications. 2nd ed. Baltimore, University Park Press, 1977.

Kruse, P. F., and Patterson, M. K.: Tissue Culture. Methods and Applications. New York, Academic Press, 1973.

Lennette, E. H., Balows, A., Hausler, W. J., Jr., and Truant, J. P. (eds.): Manual of Clinical Microbiology. 3rd ed. Washington, D.C., American Society for Microbiology, 1980.

Lennette, E. H., and Schmidt, N. J.: Diagnostic Procedures for Viral, Rickettsial, and Chlamydial Infections. 5th ed. New York, American Public Health Association, Inc., 1979.

Madeley, C. R.: Guide to the Collection and Transport of Virological Specimens. Geneva, World Health Organization, 1977.

Rose, N. R., and Friedman, H. (eds.): Manual of Clinical Immunology. 2nd ed. Washington, D. C., American Society for Microbiology, 1980.

Schachter, J., and Dawson, C. R.: Human Chlamydial Infections. Littleton, PSG Publishing Company, Inc., 1978.

Specific References

Andiman, W. A., et al.: Epstein-Barr virus. *In* Rose, N. R., and Friedman, H. (eds.): Manual of Clinical Immunology. Washington D.C., American Society of Microbiology, 1980.

Appleton, H., and Higgins, P. G.: Viruses and gastroenteritis in infants. Lancet, *1*:1297, 1975.

Back, A. F., et al.: Indirect hemagglutinating antibody response to *Herpesvirus* types 1 and 2 in immunized laboratory animals and natural infections in man. Appl. Microbiol., *28*:392, 1974.

Balfour, H. H., Jr., et al.: California arbovirus infections. Pediatrics, *52*:680, 1973.

Balfour, H. H., Jr., and Edelman, C. K.: Diagnosis of California (La Crosse) encephalitis by precipitin techniques: A prospective study. Appl. Microbiol., *28*:807, 1974.

Beem, M. O., and Saxon, E. M.: Respiratory-tract colonization and a distinctive pneumonic syndrome in infants infected with *Chlamydia trachomatis*. N. Engl. J. Med., *296*:306, 1977.

Benjamin, D. R., and Ray, C. G.: Use of immunoperoxidase for the rapid identification of human myxoviruses and paramyxoviruses in tissue culture. Appl. Microbiol., *28*:47, 1974.

Bozeman, F. M., et al.: Epidemic typhus rickettsiae isolated from flying squirrels. Nature, *225*:545, 1975.

Brandt, C. D., et al.: Infections in 18,000 infants and children in a controlled study of respiratory tract disease. 1. Adenovirus pathogenicity in relation to serologic type and illness syndrome. Am. J. Epidemiol., *90*:484, 1969.

Burgdorfer, W.: Hemolymph test. A technique for detection of rickettsia in ticks. Am. J. Trop. Med. Hyg., *19*:1010, 1970.

Caul, E. O., and Clarke, S. K. R.: Coronavirus propagated from a patient with nonbacterial gastroenteritis. Lancet, *2*:953, 1975.

Daugharty, H., Warfield, D. T., Hemingway, W. D., and Casey, H. C.: Mumps class-specific immunoglobulins in radioimmunoassay and conventional serology. Infect. Immunol., *7*:380, 973.

Drew, W. L., and Mintz, L.: Rapid diagnosis of varicella-zoster infection by direct immunofluorescence. Am. J. Clin. Path., *73*:699, 1980.

Duffy, J., et al.: Polyarthritis, polyarteritis, and hepatitis B. Medicine, *55*:19, 1976.

Duma, R. J., et al.: Epidemic typhus in the United States associated with flying squirrels. J.A.M.A., *245*:2318, 1981.

Evans, R. T.: Suppression of *Chlamydia trachomatis* inclusion formation by fetal calf serum in cyclohexamide-treated McCoy cells. J. Clin. Microbiol., *11*:424, 1980.

Evans, R. T., and Taylor-Robinson, D.: Detection of *Chlamydia trachomatis* in rapidly produced McCoy cell monolayers. J. Clin. Path., *33*:591, 1980.

Fiset, P., et al.: A microagglutination technique for the detection and measurement of rickettsial antibodies. Acta Virol., *13*:60, 1969.

Forrer, C. B., et al.: Comparison of vancomycin and penicillin for viral isolation. J. Clin. Microbiol., *16*:295, 1982.

Fox, J. P., et al.: The Seattle virus watch VII. Observations of adenovirus infections. Am. J. Epidemiol., *105*:362, 1977.

Frommell, G. T., et al.: Isolation of *Chlamydia trachomatis* from infant lung tissue. N. Engl. J. Med., *296*:1150, 1977.

Fulginiti, V. A., and Stahl, M.: Parainfluenza and respiratory syncytial viruses. *In* Lennette, E. H., Spaulding, E. H., and Truant, J. P. (eds.): Manual of Clinical Microbiology. 2nd ed. Washington, D.C., American Society for Microbiology, 1974.

Gershon, A. A., et al.: Antibody to varicella-zoster virus in parturient women and their offspring in the first year of life. Pediatrics, *58*:692, 1976a.

Gershon, A. A., et al.: Detection of antibody to varicella zoster virus by immune adherence hemagglutination. Proc. Soc. Exp. Biol. Med., *151*:637, 1976b.

Glezen, W. P., et al.: Acute respiratory disease of university students with special reference to the etiologic role of *Herpesvirus hominis*. Am. J. Epidemiol., *101*:111, 1975.

Gomez-Barreto, J., et al.: Acute enteritis associated with reovirus-like agents. J.A.M.A., *235*:1857, 1976.

Gordon, F. B., et al.: Effect of ionizing radiation on susceptibility of McCoy cell cultures to *Chlamydia trachomatis*. Appl. Microbiol., *23*:123, 1972.

Griffiths, P. D., et al.: Infection with cytomegalovirus during pregnancy: Specific IgM antibodies as a marker of recent primary infection. J. Infect. Dis. *145*:647, 1982.

Hanon, N., et al.: Assay of *Coxiella burnetii* by enumeration of immunofluorescent infected cells. J. Immunol., *97*:492, 1966.

Hechemy, K. E., et al.: Detection of Rocky Mountain spotted fever antibodies by a latex agglutination test. J. Clin. Microbiol., *12*:144, 1980.

Henle, W., et al.: Epstein-Barr virus specific tests in infectious mononucleosis. Hum. Path., *5*:551, 1974.

Heymann, D. L., et al.: Ebola hemorrhagic fever: Tandala, Zaire, 1977–1978. J. Infect. Dis., *142*:372, 1980.

Hierholzer, J. C., et al.: New Human adenovirus associated with respiratory illness: Candidate adenovirus type 39. J. Clin. Microbiol., *16*:15, 1982.

Horwitz, C. A., et al.: Clinical evaluation of patients with infectious mononucleosis and antibody to the R form of EB virus early antigen. Am. J. Med., *58*:330, 1975.

Johnson, K. M., et al.: Isolation and partial characterization of a new virus causing acute hemorrhagic fever in Zaire. Lancet, *1*:569, 1977.

Kapikian, A. Z., et al.: Detection of coronavirus strain 692 by immune electron microscopy. Infect. Immunol., *7*:111, 1973.

Kapikian, A. Z., et al.: Visualization by immune electron microscopy of a 27-nm particle associated with acute infectious nonbacterial gastroenteritis. J. Virol., *10*:1075, 1972.

Kuo, C. C., et al.: Primary isolation of TRIC organisms in HeLa 229 cells treated with DEAE-dextran. J. Infect. Dis., *125*:665, 1972.

La Scolea, L. J., Jr., and Baldigo, S. M.: Infectivity of *Chlamydia trachomatis* in tissue culture with newborn calf serum. J. Clin. Microbiol., *15*:951, 1982.

La Scolea, L. J., Jr., and Keddell, J. E.: Efficacy of various cell culture procedures for detection of *Chlamydia trachomatis* and applicability to diagnosis of pediatric infections. J. Clin. Microbiol., *13*:705, 1981.

Marx, R. S., et al.: Rocky Mountain spotted fever. Am. J. Dis. Child., *136*:16, 1982.

Matthews, R. E. R.: Classification and nomenclature of viruses. Intervirology, *17*:1, 1982.

McIntosh, K., et al.: Coronavirus infection in acute lower respiratory tract disease of infants. J. Infect. Dis., *130*:502, 1974.

McIntosh, K., et al.: Enzyme-linked immunosorbent assay for detection of respiratory syncytial virus infection: Application to clinical samples. J. Clin. Microbiol., *16*:329, 1982.

Meyers, J. D.: Congenital varicella in term infants: Risk reconsidered. J. Infect. Dis., *129*:215, 1974.

Middleton, P. J., et al.: Viruses associated with acute gastroenteritis in young children. Am. J. Dis. Child., *131*:733, 1977.

Minnich, L. L., and Ray, C. G.: Comparison of direct immunofluorescent staining of clinical specimens for respiratory virus antigens with conventional isolation techniques. J. Clin. Microbiol., *12*:391, 1980.

Mostow, S. R., et al.: Application of the single radial immunodiffusion test for assay of antibody to influenza type A virus. J. Clin. Microbiol., *2*:351, 1975.

Mushawar, I. K., et al.: Interpretation of various serological profiles of hepatitis B virus infection. Am. J. Clin. Path., *76*:773, 1981.

Nahmias, A. J., et al.: Herpes simplex virus encephalitis: Laboratory evaluations and their diagnostic significance. J. Infect. Dis., *145*:829, 1982.

Osborn, M. D., and Johnson, A. P.: Effect of various analgesics and lubricants on isolation of *Chlamydia trachomatis* and *Neisseria gonorrhoeae*. J. Clin. Microbiol., *15*:522, 1982.

Parrino, T. A., et al.: Clinical immunity in acute gastroenteritis caused by the Norwalk agent. N. Engl. J. Med., *297*:86, 1977.

Plummer, G.: A review of the identification and titration of antibodies to herpes simplex viruses type 1 and 2 in human sera. Cancer Res., *33*:1469, 1973.

Portnoy, B., et al.: The sensitivity of the CF test for the detection of adenovirus infections in infants and children with lower respiratory disease. Am. J. Epidemiol., *86*:362, 1967.

Preissner, C. M., et al.: Evaluation of the anticomplement immunofluorescence test for detection of antibody to varicella-zoster virus. J. Clin. Microbiol., *16*:373, 1982.

Raimondo, G., et al.: Multicentre study of prevalence of HBV-associated delta infection and liver disease in drug-addicts. Lancet, *1*:249, 1982.

Ray, C. G., and Minnich, L. L.: Regional diagnostic virology services. Are satellite laboratories necessary? J.A.M.A., *247*:1309, 1982.

Robinson, W. S.: The enigma of non-A, non-B hepatitis. J. Infect. Dis., *145*:387, 1982.

Robinson, W. S., and Lutwick, L. I.: The virus of hepatitis, type B. N. Engl. J. Med., *295*:1168, 1232, 1976.

Schachter, J.: Chlamydial infections. N. Engl. J. Med., *298*:428, 1978.

Schoenbaum, S. C., et al.: Epidemiology of influenza in the elderly: Evidence of virus recycling. Am. J. Epidemiol., *103*:166, 1976.

Sherlock, S.: Predicting progression of acute type-B hepatitis to chronicity. Lancet, *2*:354, 1976.

Snydman, D. R., et al.: Use of IgM-hepatitis A antibody testing. J.A.M.A., *245*:827, 1981.

Stephens, R. S., et al.: Sensitivity of immunofluorescence with monoclonal antibodies for detection of *Chlamydia trachomatis* inclusions in cell culture. J. Clin. Microbiol., *16*:4, 1982.

Stewart, J. A., et al.: Herpes simplex virus. *In* Rose, N. R., and Friedman, H. (eds.): Manual of Clinical Immunology. Washington, D. C., American Society for Microbiology, 1976.

Strauch, B., et al.: Oropharyngeal excretion of Epstein-Barr virus by renal transplant in immunosuppressed patients. Lancet, *1*:1234, 1974.

Townsend, J. J., et al.: Progressive rubella panencephalitis-onset late after congenital rubella. N. Engl. J. Med., *292*:990, 1975.

Vandervelde, E. M., et al.: User's guide to some new tests for hepatitis B antigen. Lancet, *2*:1066, 1974.

Vaucher, Y. E., et al.: Pleomorphic enveloped virus-like particles associated with neonatal gastrointestinal disease.. J. Infect. Dis., *145*:27, 1982.

Walker, D. H., and Cain, B. G.: A method for specific diagnosis of Rocky Mountain spotted fever on fixed paraffin-embedded tissue for immunofluorescence. J. Infect. Dis., *137*:206, 1978.

Walker, D. H., et al.: Laboratory diagnosis of Rocky Mountain spotted fever. South. Med. J., *73*:1443, 1980.

Waner, J. L., et al.: Patterns of cytomegalovirus complement-fixing antibody activity: A longitudinal study of blood donors. J. Infect. Dis., *127*:538, 1973.

Wang, S. P., et al.: Simplified microimmunofluorescence test with Trachoma-Lymphogranuloma venereum (*Chlamydia trachomatis*) antigens for use as a screening test for antibody. J. Clin. Microbiol., *1*:250, 1975.

Wentworth, B. B., and Alexander, E. R.: Isolation of *Chlamydia trachomatis* by use of 5-iodo-2-deoxyuridine-treated cells. Appl. Microbiol., *27*:912, 1974.

Wike, D. A., et al.: Plaque formation in tissue cultures by *Rickettsia rickettsi* isolated directly from whole blood and tick hemolymph. Infect. Immunol., *6*:736, 1972.

Williams, V., et al.: Serologic response to varicella-zoster membrane antigens measured by indirect immunofluorescence. J. Infect. Dis., *130*:669, 1974.

Woodland, R. M., et al.: A rapid method for staining inclusions of *Chlamydia psittaci* and *Chlamydia trachomatis*. J. Clin. Path., *35*:642, 1982.

Woodruff, A. W., et al.: Lassa fever in Britain: An imported case. Br. Med. J., *3*:616, 1973.

Woodruff, J. F., et al.: Involvement of T lymphocytes in the pathogenesis of coxsackie virus B3 in heart disease. J. Immunol., *113*:1726, 1974.

Yeager, A. S., et al.: Prevention of transfusion-acquired cytomegalovirus infections in newborn infants. J. Pediatr., *98*:281, 1981.

Yoder, B. L., et al.: Microtest procedure for isolation of *Chlamydia trachomatis*. J. Clin. Microbiol., *13*:1036, 1981.

Yolken, R. H.: Enzyme immunoassays for the detection of infectious antigens in body fluids: Current limitations and future prospects. Rev. Infect. Dis., *4*:35, 1982.

Yolken, R. H., et al.: Enzyme-linked immunosorbent assay (ELISA) for detection of human reovirus-like agent of infantile gastroenteritis. Lancet, *2*:263, 1977.

51

MYCOPLASMAL INFECTION

GEORGE E. KENNY, PH.D.,
and HJORDIS M. FOY, M.D., PH.D.

BIOLOGY OF THE ORGANISMS

Mycoplasmata are the smallest (0.3 to 0.5 μm) free-living organisms known and differ from bacteria especially in their lack of a cell wall. They are unlike cell wall–defective bacteria (L-forms) in that the latter revert to their normal morphology when cultured on the appropriate media. Although the size and pliability of mycoplasmata allow them to pass filters that retain bacteria, they resemble bacteria more than viruses. Thus, they contain both RNA and DNA, grow on artificial media, and carry out their own replication processes. The biologic characteristics of human Mycoplasma are outlined in Table 51–1.

Mycoplasmata were originally designated as "PPLO," "*p*leuro*p*neumonia-*l*ike *o*rganisms," because the agent first discovered in 1898 caused pleuropneumonia in cattle. The human species belong to two families, Mycoplasmataceae and Acholeplasmataceae, which are classified in the order Mycoplasmatales, class Mollicutes. *Mycoplasma* require sterols (cholesterol) for growth; *Acholeplasma* do not. The only *Acholeplasma* species found in humans, *Acholeplasma laidlawii,* is probably a saprophyte and is commonly found in sewage. The family Mycoplasmataceae is divided into two genera, *Mycoplasma* and *Ureaplasma;* the latter requires urea for growth. The ten species of mycoplasmata isolated from humans are described in Table 51–1. *Mycoplasma* species can be distinguished by their ability to ferment glucose and utilize arginine or by their requirements for urea. Serologically, they are heterogeneous and can be divided into five quite dissimilar groups (Kenny, 1979). A large number of *Mycoplasma* species have also been isolated from animals, but these do not infect humans. However, they do pose problems as contaminants in tissue culture systems used for isolation of viruses (Barile, 1979).

NORMAL FLORA AND ROLE IN DISEASE

Four species, *Mycoplasma orale* (formerly *Mycoplasma pharyngis* or *Mycoplasma orale type 1*), *Mycoplasma buccale* (formerly *Mycoplasma orale type 2*), *Mycoplasma faucium* (formerly *Mycoplasma orale type 3*), and *Mycoplasma salivarium,* inhabit the oral cavity and are considered normal flora (Table 51–1). *M. salivarium* is found in large quantities in periodontal crevices and is absent in edentulous persons; it may possibly play a role in periodontal disease.

Mycoplasma pneumoniae, formerly called Eaton agent after its discoverer, is a definite human pathogen, best known as a cause of pneumonitis (Grayston, 1969). The disease previously was called "atypical pneumonia" because it does not respond to penicillin. However, it is but one of the atypical pneumonias. It is popularly known as "walking pneumonia" because the patient may appear only moderately ill, despite widespread pulmonary infiltrates. Indeed, mycoplasmal pneumonia may be associated with lobar infiltrates resembling those of pneumococcal pneumonia. Attack rates are highest among older children and young adults. The spectrum of manifestations comprises pharyngitis, bronchitis, tracheobronchitis, and bronchiolitis. Complications include hemolytic anemia, pleuritis, a variety of skin rashes, Stevens-Johnson syndrome, meningitis, encephalitis, and temporary arthritis. Death is a rare sequel but occasionally occurs in persons developing hemolytic anemia with thromboembolism or in those developing respiratory failure (Foy, 1981).

Mycoplasma hominis and *Ureaplasma urealyticum* normally inhabit the urogenital tract in sexually mature men and women; higher isolation rates are obtained from women than from men, possibly reflecting more favorable growth conditions in the vaginal tract. The degree of colonization with these species is related to sexual activity and to the number of sexual partners (Taylor-Robinson, 1979). The isolation rate of *U. urealyticum* approaches 100 per cent for female prostitutes. A much stronger association of ureaplasmata with certain diseases is now evident because the organisms have been isolated in pure culture from blood (postpartum fever), bladder and ureter urine (pyelonephritis), prostatic secretions (prostatitis), and lungs from children dying in infancy. Isolation of ureaplasmata in pure culture is associated with about

Table 51–1. SPECIES OF MYCOPLASMATA FOUND IN HUMANS, THEIR LABORATORY CHARACTERISTICS, NORMAL SOURCES, AND ROLE IN DISEASE

Species	Serologic Group*	Glucose Fermentation	Arginine Utilization	Urea Utilization	Optimum pH	Growth† in Air	Growth† in 95% N_2 5% CO_2	Normal Source	Role in Disease
A. laidlawii	2	+	–	–	7.0–8.0	+ + + +	+ + + +	Skin, mouth, sewage	Unknown
M. orale (M. pharyngis)	7	–	+	–	6.0–7.0	+	+ + +	Mouth	None known
M. buccale (M. orale type 2)	7	–	+	–	6.0–7.0	+	+ + +	Mouth	None known
M. faucium (M. orale type 3)	7	–	+	–	6.0–7.0	+	+ + +	Mouth	None known
M. salivarium	7	–	+	–	6.0–7.0	+	+ + +	Periodontal crevices, mouth	Periodontal disease?
M. hominis	7	–	+	–	6.0–7.5	+ + +	+ + +	Genital tract, mouth	Opportunistic in pelvic inflammatory disease
M. pneumoniae	5	+	–	–	6.5–7.5	+ + + +	+	Repiratory tract	Pneumonitis, bronchitis, pharyngitis
M. fermentans	6	+	+	–	7.0–8.0	+ +	+ + +	Genital tract	Rare, none known
U. urealyticum (T-strains)	?	–	–	+	5.5–6.5	+ + +	+ + +	Genital tract (rarely throat)	Urethritis?
M. genitalium	?	+	?	–	6.5–7.5	?	?	Genital tract	Unknown

*According to Kenny, 1970.
†+ = Marginal growth; + + + + = maximal growth.

10 per cent of these diseases. *M. hominis* has been isolated in pure culture from salpingitis. Thus, it appears that both organisms are opportunistic invaders and the organisms can be isolated in pure culture from blood and may not necessarily be associated with disease. Although *Chlamydia trachomatis* is the most important cause of non-gonococcal urethritis, *U. urealyticum* may cause a proportion of this disease, particularly among previously sexually inexperienced males (Bowie, 1977), and experimental infection of humans results in demonstrable disease (Taylor-Robinson, 1979). Little is known of the prevalence of the new organism *Mycoplasma genitalium* (Tully, 1981).

COLLECTION OF SPECIMENS

Since mycoplasmata are surface parasites, various secretions and body fluids, such as urine, vaginal discharge, saliva, and sputum are adequate for isolation attempts (Kenny, 1980a). Sputum samples are frequently diluted 1:10 and 1:100 to avoid toxic effects. Similarly, washings of tissues are more useful for isolation than minced tissues. Pharyngeal swabs in respiratory infections and vaginal and urethral swabs in urogenital infections are also adequate. The tip of the swab is broken into the collection medium. Patients with *M. pneumoniae* pneumonia seldom have a productive cough at onset of illness; however, throat swabs are a good substitute for sputum, since the organisms colonize the pharynx, particularly in children. The organism is recovered even after treatment with tetracycline or erythromycin has been initiated, despite the fact that these drugs are known to shorten the duration of illness. The collection media commonly used contain 0.5 per cent bovine albumin with soybean-casein digest (e.g., Trypticase soy) broth (Grayston, 1969). Penicillin (100 U/ml) is usually added to control bacterial contamination. Specimens can be stored refrigerated at −4°C. for several days, and most mycoplasmata withstand transportation and freezing at −70°C. well.

ISOLATION OF ORGANISMS

Mycoplasmata require special agar plates and broth cultures. The latter are especially advantageous for large inocula with small numbers of organisms (Kenny, 1980a). Growth may cause faint turbidity or small spherules or colonies in fluid medium, but is better demonstrated by pH changes of indicators when appropriate substrates are used (Table 51–1). Subculture to agar plates is necessary for identification. *Mycoplasma* media contain fresh yeast extract, peptone, and animal serum. Penicillin is added to suppress bacterial growth; thallium acetate is also used for this purpose but is toxic for *U. urealyticum.* The organisms form small colonies that grow both on the agar surface and into the agar, with the resulting appearance of "fried eggs," or they may have a granular appearance (Fig. 51–1). For subculture, small blocks of agar have to be cut out and smeared face down on the surface of fresh plates. Most human *Mycoplasma* species can be seen with magnification within a couple of days, but it may take two to four weeks for *M. pneumoniae* colonies to become visible. Diphasic media, consisting of an agar base overlaid with a fluid medium with a pH indicator for glucose fermentation, are particularly useful for isolation of *M. pneumoniae* (Kenny, 1980a). Although mycoplasmata can be separated by their ability to ferment glucose and utilize arginine, species identification is carried out by inhibition with specific antisera, according to the method of Clyde (1964). *U. urealyticum,* discovered in the 1960's, forms minute colonies on agar media (Shepard, 1974). Thus they were first called T-strains for tiny. They are detected readily in well-buffered urea broth where their presence is recognized by alkaline changes (Kenny, 1980a). Subculture must be done as soon as the pH

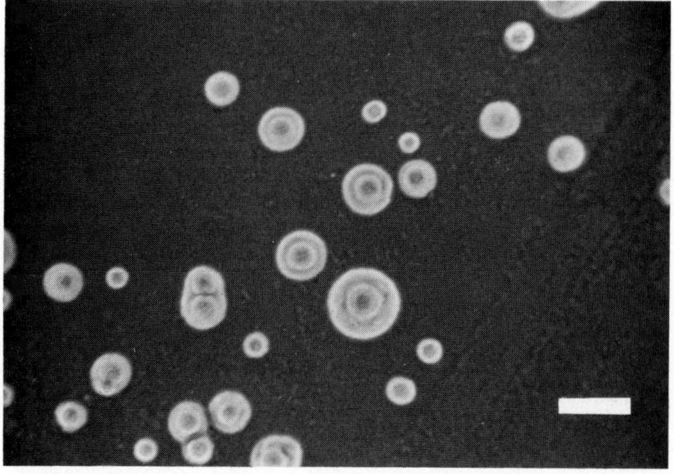

Figure 51–1. Colonies of *Mycoplasma pneumoniae* strain AP-164 on agar at 10 days of incubation. Bar = 100 μm.

increases, since the organisms die off rapidly. Lincomycin, 30 μg/ml, can be incorporated into the culture medium to suppress the growth of *M. hominis,* whose large colonies may obscure detection of ureaplasmata.

SEROLOGY

Serology of Mycoplasma pneumoniae Infections

Detection of antibody in persons infected with *M. pneumoniae* is accomplished by three methods: (1) complement fixation with lipid or whole organism antigen, (2) fluorescent antibody, and (3) metabolic inhibition testing (Kenny, 1980b). *M. pneumoniae* is unusual among microorganisms in that glycolipids are the major complement-fixing antigen and the major antigen toward which humans respond in infections. Serodiagnosis by complement fixation using lipid extracts of the organisms gives both greater titer rises and lower background antibody than the use of whole organism antigen. Antibody also has been measured by the indirect fluorescent antibody technique, which requires less antigen but is more tedious. The metabolic inhibition test measures the ability of antibody to stop growth of the organism as indicated by the prevention of appearance of a metabolic product (i.e., acid from glucose [Taylor-Robinson, 1966]). Metabolic inhibition tests are simple to perform and require little antigen but have the disadvantage that the endpoint changes from day to day. Metabolic inhibition tests correlate well with complement fixation testing. The complement-fixation test is most likely to be used in reference laboratories because of the commercial availability of antigen. The enzyme-linked immunosorbent assays (ELISA) developed so far correlate very well with complement-fixing antibody testing and thus may measure lipid antigens but give the capability of distinguishing IgM and IgG antibodies. Development of tests to measure protein antigens is urgently needed. Serodiagnosis is best accomplished by testing acute and convalescent sera for four-fold antibody rises. Determining a "diagnostic" titer is of doubtful utility because of the long persistence of antibody. A rise of cold agglutinin antibody titers is suggestive of recent infection, but significant cold agglutinin rises are found in diseases of other etiology.

Serology of Mycoplasma hominis and Ureaplasma urealyticum Infections

No routine methods for detection of antibodies to *M. hominis* or *U. urealyticum* have yet been generally accepted. ELISA methodology is being developed in several laboratories and no doubt will be the method of choice. Use of more conventional methods, such as metabolic inhibition tests (Purcell, 1966a and b) and the complement-mediated mycoplasmacidal tests, has been largely unsuccessful because of the antigenic heterogeneity detected by these tests (*U. urealyticum* has 11 serotypes [Robertson, 1982] and *M. hominis* shows a number of cross-reacting specificities). The ELISA tests, particularly for *U. urealyticum,* appear to show group reactivity for the various types, a result which, if confirmed, would simplify serological testing.

INTERPRETATION AND CLINICAL SIGNIFICANCE OF LABORATORY RESULTS

Isolation of mycoplasmata requires experience among the laboratory personnel and cannot be carried out by most routine hospital laboratories. Because any constituents of the growth media, especially the serum, can have mycoplasmacidal components, new batches of media should be tested not only with known *Mycoplasma* stock strains but also with clinical materials (Kenny, 1980a). Sometimes artifacts in the agar are mistaken for *Mycoplasma* colonies.

A throat culture is positive for *M. pneumoniae* in about two thirds of patients who by multiple diagnostic tests are shown to be infected with this organism. Since shedding ceases one to two months following onset of illness, a positive throat culture is practically diagnostic.

Genital mycoplasmata isolated from the vagina or cervix should be considered normal flora in sexually active persons. Isolation from the male urethra may have more significance. Isolation of the organisms from blood, pelvic abscesses, or laparotomy specimens has considerable significance, provided that it is proved that bacteria (particularly anaerobes) and *C. trachomatis* are not present. Quantitation of the number of organisms is important and has been important in deriving some of the potential association of the organisms with non-gonococcal urethritis and prostatitis. The role of *U. urealyticum* in fetal loss, low birth weight, and dysfertility is doubtful.

Although serological results become available only after the patient has recovered, the data are important in epidemic situations. In family spread, the case-to-case interval averages three weeks. Correlation between four-fold antibody rises and isolation of the organism is excellent (60 to 70 per cent) in pneumonia patients. However, it has been clearly demonstrated that false-positive antibody increases can be observed in pancreatitis (Leinikki, 1978) and in infections of the central nervous system with bacteria (Kleemola, 1982). These false-positive reactions may result from cross-reactions between glycolipids and polysaccharides and/or polyclonal activation. Thus, caution must be used in associating unusual diseases with *M. pneumoniae* infection in the absence of respiratory symptoms. The cross-reactivity of the present serodiagnostic methods underscores the need for development of ELISA to protein antigens which ought to be more specific. In pneumonia cases, cold agglutinin titers (greater than 1:32) are found in about two thirds of *M. pneumoniae* patients, particularly those with more severe disease. However, cold agglutinins may also appear in several other infectious diseases, so the test is not specific. Cold agglutinins and anti-MG (antibodies) are reviewed in Chapter 42.

The presence of tetracyclines and macrolides in serum may interfere with the interpretation and reading of metabolic inhibition antibody titers by giving false-positive reactions.

Serologic diagnosis for other human mycoplasmal infection has not advanced sufficiently to be of assistance in the routine management of patients.

Barile, M. F.: Mycoplasma–tissue cell interactions. *In* Tully, J. G., and Whitcomb, R. F. (eds.): The Mycoplasmas, Vol. II. New York, Academic Press, 1979, p. 425.

Bowie, W. R., Wang, S. P., Alexander, E. R., Floyd, J., Forsyth, P. S., Pollock, H. M., Lin, J. S., and Holmes, K. K.: Etiology of nongonococcal urethritis. Evidence for *Chlamydia trachomatis* and *Ureaplasma urealyticum*. J. Clin. Invest., *59*:735, 1977.

Clyde, W. A., Jr.: Mycoplasma species identification based upon growth inhibition by specific antisera. J. Immunol., *92*:958, 1964.

Foy, H. M.: Pneumonia, *Mycoplasma pneumoniae*. *In* Top, F. H., and Wehrle, P. F. (eds.): Communicable and Infectious Diseases. 9th ed. St. Louis, The C. V. Mosby Company, 1981, p. 504.

Grayston, J. T., Foy, H. M., and Kenny, G. E.: The epidemiology of Mycoplasma infections of the human respiratory tract. *In* Hayflick, L. (ed.): The Mycoplasmatales and L-phase of Bacteria. New York, Appleton-Century-Crofts, 1969, p. 651.

Kenny, G. E.: Antigenic determinants. *In* Barile, M. F., and Razin, S. (eds.): The Mycoplasmas, Vol. I. New York, Academic Press, 1979, p. 351.

Kenny, G. E.: Mycoplasmata. *In* Lennette, E. H., Balows, A., Hausler, W. J., Jr., and Truant, J. P. (eds.): Manual of Clinical Microbiology. 3rd ed. Washington, D. C., American Society for Microbiology, 1980a, p. 365.

Kenny, G. E.: Serology of mycoplasmic infections. *In* Rose, N. R., and Friedman, H. (eds.): Manual of Clinical Immunology. 2nd ed. Washington, D.C., American Society for Microbiology, 1980b, p. 547.

Kleemola, M., and Kahty, H.: Increase in antibodies to *Mycoplasma pneumoniae* in patients with purulent meningitis. J. Infect. Dis., *146*:284, 1982.

Leinikki, P. O., Panzar, P., and Tykka, H.: Immunoglobulin M antibody response against *Mycoplasma pneumoniae* lipid antigen in patients with acute pancreatitis. J. Clin. Microbiol., *8*:113, 1978.

Purcell, R. H., Taylor-Robinson, D., Wong, D., and Chanock, R. M.: Color test for the measurement of antibody to T-strain mycoplasmas. J. Bacteriol., *92*:6, 1966a.

Purcell, R. H., Taylor-Robinson, D., Wong, D. C., and Chanock, R. M.: A color test for the measurement of antibody to the nonacid-forming human *Mycoplasma* species. Am. J. Epidemiol., *84*:51, 1966b.

Robertson, J. A., and Stemke, G. W.: Expanded serotyping scheme for *Ureaplasma urealyticum* strains isolated from humans. J. Clin. Microbiol., *15*:873, 1982.

Shepard, M. C., Lunceford, C. D., Ford, D. K., Purcell, R. H., Taylor-Robinson, D., Razin, S., and Black, F. T.: *Ureaplasma urealyticum* gen. nov. sp. nov.: proposed nomenclature for the human T (T-strain) mycoplasmas. Int. J. Syst. Bacteriol., *24*:160, 1974.

Taylor-Robinson, D., and McCormack, W. M.: Mycoplasmas in human genitourinary infections. *In* Tully, J. G., and Whitcomb, R. F. (eds.): The Mycoplasmas, Vol. II. New York, Academic Press, 1979, p. 307.

Taylor-Robinson, D., Purcell, R. H., Wong, D. C., and Chanock, R. M.: A color test for the measurement of antibody to certain Mycoplasma species based upon the inhibition of acid production. J. Hyg., *64*:91, 1966.

Tully, J. G., Taylor-Robinson, D., Cole, R. M., and Rose, D. L.: A newly discovered mycoplasma in the human urogenital tract. Lancet *1*:1288, 1981.

52

BACTERIAL SUSCEPTIBILITY TESTING AND ASSAYS

JOHN M. MATSEN, M.D.

GENERAL PRINCIPLES AND CONSIDERATIONS

HISTORICAL PERSPECTIVES

In the period antedating the development of the first agents of the modern era of antimicrobial therapy, namely the sulfonamides, medical scientists utilized the first forms of *in vitro* testing to determine the potency of antiseptic agents. Fleming (1924), the discoverer of penicillin, reported on a "slide cell," which he used to test the effects of various antiseptics on bacterial agents. Fleming (1938) also later described a similar technique for studying the effect of various sulfonamide derivatives on *Streptococcus pneumoniae.*

Reddish (1929) described a diffusion susceptibility test for testing antiseptics, ointments, etc. At the same time, Fleming (1929) used a gutter cut into an agar plate, which he filled with the compound to be tested. Organisms were streaked at right angles to the gutter and susceptibility was determined by the distance of inhibition. The first susceptibility testing for systemically used antimicrobials was carried out with the sulfonamides in the 1930's. In 1939 Rose and Miller attempted to standardize the multiple testing variables present in the plate diffusion method by addressing the inoculum size, the composition of media, organisms tested, etc. Subsequently, various methods were described, first for the sulfonamides and penicillins and, later, for other agents as they were discovered, utilizing various broth dilution techniques or techniques incorporating antimicrobials in varying concentrations directly into agar media. The principle of the diffusion test was first described, as noted above, by Fleming (1929). By placing the agent to be tested in a "gutter" or well in an agar plate, he was then able to measure the margin of inhibition against the organism to be tested. Others subsequently modified this principle by filling cylinders placed on the surface of the agar, placing a drop of an antimicrobial on the surface of the agar, and applying absorbent paper disks as reservoirs of known amounts of antimicrobial agents on the surface of the agar plate, which was seeded with the test organism.

Subsequently, all of the above tests have been refined in order to obviate problems which initially affected the precision of the methodologies. It is the purpose of this chapter to define currently used techniques for antimicrobial susceptibility testing and assay, and to outline the advantages, difficulties, and comparison factors. Each of the methods thus described has historical precedents dating back 30 to 50 years. Even the automated methods are based upon principles related to conventional techniques that were modified from the ideas first explored many years ago.

DEFINITION OF TERMS

The vocabulary of antimicrobial susceptibility testing includes several terms with which the reader should become conversant.

Susceptibility. The level of antimicrobial at which the growth of a given strain or microorganism is inhibited or killed by an antimicrobial compound.

A Susceptible Organism. An organism which is inhibited or killed by the concentration of the antimicrobial usually achieved in the serum, other body fluids, and tissues of the patient who has been given the usual dose of the antimicrobial by the usual route of administration.

Resistance. An organism is resistant to an antimicrobial when its level of susceptibility is beyond that normally achieved in the human body by the usual dose given by the usual route of administration.

Intermediate Susceptibility. Sometimes referred to as indeterminate or equivocal susceptibility, this category includes strains that are not clearly resistant or susceptible to a given antimicrobial agent but for which an *in vivo* response is probable if the agent were given in high dosages (see Group II, p. 1326).

Minimal Inhibitory Concentration (MIC). In simplest terms, the lowest concentration of antimicrobial at which no bacterial growth occurs for a given bacterial strain.

Minimum Lethal Concentration (MLC) or Minimum Bactericidal Concentration (MBC). The lowest concentration of antimicrobial at which no viable bacterial cells remain for a given strain.

Antimicrobial Assay. The determination of the concentration of an antimicrobial present in serum or other body fluid.

Serum Bactericidal Assay. The determination of the titer of serum which will, in combination with the antibiotic present in the serum, kill 99.9 per cent of the inoculum in the serum sample.

WHICH ORGANISMS SHOULD BE TESTED FOR ANTIMICROBIAL SUSCEPTIBILITY?

Bacteria for which susceptibility testing should be performed are potential pathogens or those which are likely pathogens in unusual situations, such as in the compromised patient. Susceptibility testing should be avoided for organisms with predictable susceptibility patterns, as the chance of a laboratory error is greater than the potential presence of a resistant organism among some species. This point is demonstrated in susceptibility testing of Group A streptococci with penicillin. Any potential pathogen with a significant proportion of resistant strains will require appropriate susceptibility testing. Organisms that develop resistance rapidly on exposure to antimicrobial agents should be tested again if isolated during therapy, as should certain antimicrobial agents for which a propensity exists for the development of resistance during their clinical use. Organisms not usually considered to be pathogenic may be pathogenic in patients with immune deficiencies where the antibiotic must act alone, and, in that context, isolates in those clinical circumstances may well require susceptibility testing that would not otherwise be necessary. Caution should be exercised to avoid susceptibility testing of organisms representing normal flora that are not acting as pathogens in the clinical setting and of mixed organism cultures. In the latter instance, susceptibility testing should be delayed until the organisms have been separated on isolation plates.

Generally speaking, the following organism groups are currently tested:

Staphylococcus aureus.

Staphylococcus epidermidis (when associated with clinical disease).

The Enterobacteriaceae.

Pseudomonas species and other gram-negative nonfermentative bacilli.

Haemophilus influenzae (ampicillin).

Neisseria gonorrhoeae (in treatment failure situations or where resistant organisms are endemic).

Other infrequently isolated organisms with unpredictable susceptibility.

ANTIMICROBIALS TO BE TESTED

Recommendations of the National Committee for Clinical Laboratory Standards (1975) and recommendations promulgated by the Centers for Disease Control (Thornsberry, 1977b) generally include the grouping of antimicrobials for susceptibility testing into those being used for gram-positive organisms and those being used for gram-negative organisms. A further subgrouping of the gram-negative organism panel into one for gram-negative infections and urinary tract isolates and one for the *Pseudomonas* and nonfermenter group of organisms may be desirable. It is this latter approach that will be outlined here for the reader's consideration (Table 52–1).

USE OF SUSCEPTIBILITY TESTING

Susceptibility tests, in the clinical setting, are justified in terms of the guidance that they provide for the physician. Where specific susceptibility testing results are not available, the physician, under ideal conditions, bases his or her approach to therapy upon accumulated knowledge regarding the organisms likely to be present in the specific disease entity, as well as the most likely susceptibility profile based upon past experience. Some organisms, such as Group A *Streptococcus,* are almost absolutely predictable with respect to their susceptibility to penicillin. Other organisms may have very little predictability of susceptibility. Such is the case with some of the gram-negative organisms, such as *Proteus rettgeri*. The majority of organisms with which the physician must deal in clinical settings have greater or lesser predictability depending upon the antibiotic being considered.

Susceptibility testing results, when available, should help the physician to select the most effective

Table 52–1. PROPOSED ANTIMICROBIALS FOR ROUTINE TESTING

Gram-Positive Organisms	Enterobacteriaceae	Other Gram-Negative Organisms
Amikacin	Amikacin	Amikacin
Ampicillin	Ampicillin	Carbenicillin
Cephalothin	Carbenicillin	Colistin (or polymyxin B)
Chloramphenicol	Cephalothin	Gentamicin
Clindamycin	Chloramphenicol	Tobramycin
Erythromycin	Colistin (or polymyxin B)	Chloramphenicol‡
Gentamicin	Gentamicin	Kanamycin‡
Methicillin, nafcillin, or oxacillin	Tetracycline	Sulfonamide‡
Penicillin	Tobramycin	Tetracycline‡
Tetracycline	Nitrofurantoin*	
Vancomycin	Sulfonamide*	
	Trimethoprim-sulfamethoxazole*†	
	Kanamycin§	
	Nalidixic acid§	

*Reported for urinary tract isolates only.
†Trimethoprim-sulfamethoxazole may be effective against organisms isolated from other sites.
‡Reported for non-fermentative bacilli other than *Pseudomonas aeruginosa*.
§May be substituted for other agents, depending upon physician use and preference.

and preferred agent for the organism in question. In most instances, the physician will also have a number of other considerations to take into account when choosing the antimicrobial to be administered. Factors relating both to the antimicrobial and to the patient's underlying circumstances must be taken into consideration. The physician must also consider economic factors in administering antimicrobial agents, either in the hospital or in the office or clinic setting.

In many respects, the narrower the spectrum of the antimicrobial, the more preferred is its use when one knows specifically the organism being treated. However, the converse is true when one thinks in terms of approaching an unknown infection, where one may or may not know the susceptibility pattern. In that context, the broader spectrum antibiotics have great value. In gram-negative sepsis, the more common approach is to use an aminoglycoside antibiotic in conjunction with one of the cephalosporin or semisynthetic penicillin agents. This allows for the broad coverage necessitated by the unknown status of the organism's susceptibility.

In an ideal setting, susceptibility data should also provide some indication to the physician as to what level of antimicrobial is necessary. With the existing high content disk diffusion methodology, the values that have been established for the "susceptible" category take into consideration the usual dosage of antimicrobial, administered by the usual route, in systemic infections. For those agents for which toxicity is not a factor, an intermediate or indeterminate reading allows the physician to increase the dosage with some degree of confidence. However, for most antimicrobials the values reported for the disk diffusion method do not completely reflect the high concentration of antimicrobial in the urine owing to its excretion through the kidney. The level of susceptibility should ideally provide some correlation and provide some understanding as to the level of antimicrobial necessary to treat the specific infection effectively.

The degree of susceptibility of an organism at times can assist in determining the length of therapy. It has been suggested that viridans streptococci, in cases of endocarditis, inhibited by less than 0.2 μg/ml of penicillin, can be treated in one half to two thirds the time normally required for treatment of those organisms demonstrating a lesser degree of susceptibility. However, in most circumstances the degree of susceptibility of an organism is not the determining factor in the length of therapy. Rather, it is the specific clinical condition and the identity of the organism that provide the more appropriate guidelines for that decision.

In those settings where it is desirable to use a combination of antimicrobials, the classic approach to dilution or diffusion susceptibility testing will only infrequently provide assistance regarding the preferred antimicrobial combination. However, special testing can be performed, in which antimicrobials are tested in combination and in varying concentrations against the organism to be treated. These tests, however, can be rather expensive for the patient because of their complexity.

An age-old dilemma of the physician, that of receiving susceptibility results for a patient who is already receiving antimicrobial therapy, requires a decision as to whether or not susceptibility test results warrant a change in therapy. This dilemma is lessened when the patient is not doing well or when susceptibility results indicate resistance to the compound being used. However, in those instances in which susceptibility tests demonstrate susceptibility to the agent being used and to another agent or agents that are less expensive or less toxic, the physician will be required to exercise clinical judgment in determining the therapeutic approach. Our experience indicates that the physician will alter therapy in 20 to 30 per cent of such instances.

THE NEED FOR ASSAY INFORMATION

The physician, for the support of antimicrobial therapy, often requires information relating to the pharmacokinetics of an antimicrobial agent in serum, urine, or other body fluids. Assays of antimicrobial levels may be helpful in predicting the likelihood of success of antimicrobial usage and as a means of attempting to prevent the potential toxicity which accompanies the use of a number of antimicrobial agents.

Both the estimation of therapeutic success and the prevention of toxicity may be important in the patient with normal excretory function but are of more frequent concern in the patient who has compromised renal function. One is much more likely to perform assays in patients in whom kidney or liver failure or dysfunction is present. Examples would include the use of an aminoglycoside antibiotic in a patient in whom the serum creatinine values were elevated, or the use of chloramphenicol in a newborn infant in whom the liver-conjugating enzymes are immature.

Another consideration in the use and the need for antimicrobial assays is whether or not the sample should be tested at the anticipated trough or peak level. To measure maximum effect, peak levels become an obvious choice; however, there is evidence to indicate that the trough level of aminoglycoside antibiotics may assist in preventing both oto- and nephrotoxicity.

Antimicrobial assays may also be used to resolve quandaries relating to the failure of therapy where *in vitro* susceptibilities would have predicted response.

All in all, the assay of antimicrobial agents becomes an important part of most clinical microbiology laboratories. The methodology and specific approaches will be discussed later in this chapter.

Serum 'cidal assays, or serum bactericidal titers, have become increasingly important in many clinical microbiology laboratories. Another name for this test is the Schlichter (1947) test, which is used primarily in the management of endocarditis, osteomyelitis, or other serious bacterial infections. The methodology of this test will also be explained subsequently in this chapter. For introductory purposes, it is sufficient to explain that this test provides a quantitation of the combined effect of serum (or other body fluid) and the antibiotic which the patient is receiving. The assumption may be made, in the absence of an implanted prosthesis or other foreign material, that therapy can be anticipated to be successful if bactericidal activity has been demonstrated in a dilution of serum of 1:8 or 1:16 or greater. In staphylococcal endocarditis it is preferable to have activity of 1:32 or greater. Again, this test is used as a predictor of success in antimicrobial usage and also to monitor the appropriateness of therapy.

TIMELINESS OF RESULTS

The potential exists for rapid answers in both susceptibility testing and antimicrobial assays. Currently, for example, instrumentation and other methodology exists which will allow for rapid susceptibility information within three to six hours following the isolation of an organism. In other circumstances, studies have demonstrated that with urine and other body fluids, where assessment by Gram stain has indicated the probable presence of a single organism, susceptibility results can be generated within a shorter time frame.

In part, the challenge to the pathologist is to coordinate susceptibility and culture information. A laboratory locked into set protocols at times is unresponsive to the individual cases in which this particular information becomes very important to the physician. Certain kinds of cultures such as those of blood or cerebrospinal fluid, carry with them the greater likelihood that information received from the laboratory with regard to organism susceptibility may have an impact on patient care, on success of therapy, and on the length of hospital stay. In that context, one hopes that the clinical laboratory will be responsive to processing these cultures as rapidly as possible. Studies we have performed would indicate that there is a substantial impact on patient care when the susceptibility information is received simultaneously with preliminary culture information or within a short time after the beginning of therapy. The longer the result is in arriving, the less chance the physician will use the data in altering or modifying therapy.

The pressure for rapid susceptibility and assay testing results has its practical considerations, and if physicians know that rapid answers can be forthcoming, they will learn to expect this service and will plan their therapeutic decisions accordingly. In our own hospital, for example, where radioimmunoassay is currently used for gentamicin and bioassay for tobramycin, physicians indicate that they are much more likely to use gentamicin than tobramycin, largely on the basis of having access to the more rapid assay information provided by radioimmunoassay. They can determine trough levels and anticipate that within one hour they will know the dose they should provide the patient. In the case of peak levels, additional doses of antimicrobials can be given should these levels not be sufficient in terms of the current dosage, or the dosage can be reduced if these levels approach toxic ranges.

The clinical laboratory, along with providing rapid answers, should also pay attention to the details of result transmission and reporting. Just as the laboratory usually calls results of positive cultures of body fluids and tissues, it should also call results of priority susceptibility or assay tests, alterations in susceptibility or abnormal assay results, or in instances of resistance to an antimicrobial agent that is listed as therapy on the laboratory request slip.

In general, susceptibility results that do not become available until physicians have made their late afternoon rounds may have less impact on physicians' antimicrobial usage than if they are transmitted as quickly as possible for the physician to review on the same day that test results become available.

REGULATING AGENCIES, STANDARDIZATION, AND "APPROVED" METHODS

Valid and accurate results are more likely to be received from any clinical laboratory today than at any time previously. The regulation of antimicrobial susceptibility testing in the past has been very loose and has resulted in considerable variation in test methodology and test results. In 1966 Bauer et al. published their classic paper on the high content disk diffusion technique. This served as the basis for a number of recommendations for standardization and led to its recognition and promulgation by the Food and Drug Administration (Federal Register, 1972, 1973), to whom responsibility for antimicrobial susceptibility testing materials and methodology has been given. Other groups, such as the National Committee for Clinical Laboratory Standards (1975), have essentially agreed to this methodology and described it in greater detail. Textbooks and other manuals, such as the Manual of Clinical Microbiology for the American Society for Microbiology (Matsen, 1974), have also promulgated this methodology, adding emphasis to the desirability and necessity of uniform testing approaches.

It is anticipated that further standardization will occur for the alternative susceptibility methods, as has occurred with the diffusion method noted above and with the agar dilution methodology as advocated by the International Collaborative Study Group (Ericsson, 1971). It is of note that the latter group has achieved almost universal acceptance of this agar dilution methodology.

QUANTITATIVE VS. QUALITATIVE TESTING

Historically, clinical laboratories have been restrained in their ability to do quantitative susceptibility testing because of practicality and economics. Until a standardized agar dilution method was available, only a very few institutions, such as the Mayo Clinic, performed agar dilution susceptibilities on a routine basis (Washington, 1969). The advent of the Steers (1959) replicator and the practical approach, as developed by the Mayo Clinic (Washington, 1974a), has made this a very useful quantitative method for those institutions with high volumes of susceptibility tests. Broth dilution capability, while always available to the routine laboratory, was very prohibitive because of the cumbersome nature of the individual dilution sets for each antibiotic. With the advent of microbroth dilution techniques, this approach has become convenient and economical (Gavan, 1970, 1974; Gerlach, 1974, 1977; Goss, 1968; MacLowry, 1968, 1970; McMaster, 1978). In essence, microdilution costs are close enough to those of the disk diffusion test to make this method economically feasible. In addition, the advent of instrument-generated laboratory or commercially produced microbroth dilution plates, conveniently provided in bulk quantities, has made this a practical method as well (Tilton, 1973).

If a laboratory chooses to provide quantitative results to the physician, it is obliged to provide a ready reference for understanding the meaning and interpretation of the results being reported. In this context, it is important to determine whether the physician population one serves even desires to have quantitative data. Most commercial firms now producing the microdilution plates provide tables and reference data sufficient for appropriate physician education.

Disk diffusion testing, if carefully standardized, can provide quantitative information by extrapolating the MIC from zone diameters on the basis of previously derived regression plots. For an explanation of regression analysis and the uses to which it can be put, refer to page 1334.

In conjunction with the usage of the susceptible, intermediate, and resistant categories, it is pertinent to explain the four categories of susceptibility proposed by the International Collaborative Group (Ericsson, 1971). Group I includes high degrees of bacterial susceptibility, which would provide a strong likelihood of *in vivo* response if mild to moderately severe systemic infections were treated with the usual (orally administered where applicable) dosage of antibiotic. This group could be defined as "susceptible" without further qualifications.

Group II would include a level of susceptibility which would make the *in vivo* response probable in systemic infections if the antimicrobial were given in high dosage or up to the limits ot toxicity. Group III would comprise that level of susceptibility which would make *in vivo* response probable in the treatment of localized infections at sites where the agent could be concentrated by the physiologic processes or by direct local application. Group IV, then, would include organisms of a degree of resistance which would make the *in vivo* response improbable. This group would be designated as resistant. The International Collaborative Group further advocated that the application of these categories would be antimicrobial-specific, with various modifications to fit each agent's unique pharmacokinetic features.

Susceptibility testing results usually reflect inhibition, rather than destruction or killing, of growth. This result can be of concern in certain types of infections, such as those due to staphylococci, where there may be a rather marked difference between the inhibitory and the killing or bactericidal concentration for several antibiotics, even with those which are ordinarily considered to be bactericidal in nature. For most infections, the inhibitory result is sufficient to direct the therapeutic choice of an antimicrobial agent. However, as indicated above, certain categories of infections may require determination of bactericidal concentrations.

One of the major problems in the use of susceptibility data is its relationship to anticipated urinary antimicrobial concentrations. It is generally acknowledged that urinary tract infections respond to the concentrations of antimicrobial in the urine which significantly exceed those generally present in the serum. The standardized disk diffusion method does not provide the physician with appropriate information regarding achievable urine levels. Unless the physician determines that the intermediate or indeterminate interpretive criteria are applicable to the urinary tract, the therapeutic approach may be far too conservative in terms of achievable antimicrobial levels in the urine, where they tend to be highly concentrated. In most instances, concentrations of antimicrobials tested by dilution methods range from those attainable in urine to those attainable in serum. Quantitative data, as provided by dilution testing, also has potential value, clinically, in the management of bacterial endocarditis, as well as in serious infections of compromised patients. Furthermore, it is becoming apparent that both quantitative inhibitory and bactericidal information can be of considerable help with staphylococcal infections, in which up to 40 per cent of the strains isolated from clinically significant infections may be termed "tolerant," with a considerable spread between the inhibitory and bactericidal concentrations (Sabath, 1977). Broth dilution testing allows determination of bactericidal endpoints.

MEDIA: TYPE AND CONTENT

One of the major problems in performing susceptibility tests is not only the variation among different formulations but also lot-to-lot and manufacturer-to-manufacturer variations of specific formulations. Whereas Mueller-Hinton medium has been chosen for standardized diffusion and dilution testing purposes because of its growth-potentiating properties for *Neisseria* and other fastidious organisms, it continues to be vulnerable to lot-to-lot and manufacturer-to-manufacturer variations. Our own experience would indicate that over the past three years there have been substantial problems in susceptibility testing media performance, and at almost all times one or more antibiotics will be outside the limits of quality control as established by regulating agencies and advisory committees. We have explored the susceptibility of one of the new cell wall active antimicrobials in six different media, and the MIC's varied by as much as ten-fold with the same strain depending upon which medium was used. Some of this variation relates to cation differences and some relates to the digestion process necessary for the production of the protein components of the media. Much remains to be done in terms of providing a stoichiometrically precise medium which can be manufactured uniformly to provide a consistent end-product.

It is important, therefore, that the performance of media to be used by a laboratory be regularly assessed by appropriate quality control means. It is also hoped that media manufacturers will be placed under the constraints to adhere to performance standards of media in order to assure more uniform results in the clinical laboratories of this country.

DILUTION TESTING

General Considerations

Stock Solutions. The preparation of stock solutions necessitates obtaining standard preparation either from the manufacturer or from laboratory supply firms* which can provide the testing material. In most instances, antimicrobial preparations intended for clinical use are not acceptable as laboratory testing reagents, as they may be chemically impure and inaccurate as to stated activity. Laboratory testing materials should:

1. Have a date of expiration clearly visible on the container.
2. Have a readily apparent statement of activity in μg or IU per mg or ml of preparation.
3. Be dated on arrival in the laboratory.
4. Be dated when opened.
5. Be stored in a desiccator after opening.
6. Be carefully weighed in an analytical balance or measured with pipettes of appropriate volumetric capacity.
7. Be sterilized by membrane filtration if necessary.
8. Be stored at −20°C. or colder.
9. Be dissolved or diluted in the appropriate solvent and diluent (see Table 52–2).

Inoculum Standardization. The use of a barium sulfate standard for standardization of inoculum has become routine for most susceptibility procedures. It should be stressed that this step is vulnerable to inefficient use of time, to errors in formulation and, therefore, determinations of turbidity, and to visual aberrations due to improper mixing. To ensure the maximum efficiency and accuracy, the following measures should be considered:

1. The turbidity standard is prepared by adding 0.5 ml of 0.048 M $BaCl_2$ (1.175 per cent, w/v, $BaCl_2 \cdot 2H_2O$) to 99.5 ml of 0.36 N H_2SO_4 (1 per cent, v/v). This is then equivalent to one half the density of a MacFarland No. 1 barium sulfate standard.
2. The standard should be placed in a sealed tube to avoid fluid loss by evaporation (Washington, 1973).
3. The standard should be agitated with a vortex mixer prior to each use.
4. The actual process of inoculum standardization can be enhanced and time conserved by utilizing the modified Rh view box apparatus described by Stemper and Matsen (1970). This reference provides both a narrative description of use and a blueprint of design.
5. The use of a black on white background, either as a feature of the apparatus referred to above or separately, will also facilitate turbidity comparison.

AGAR DILUTION SUSCEPTIBILITY TESTING

The agar dilution method, as described initially by the International Collaborative Study Group (Ericsson, 1971) and later in greater detail by Washington (1974b), has been used on a routine clinical basis primarily for research purposes and in larger clinical laboratories. To make this particular method economical on a day-to-day basis, at least 20 organisms should probably be tested daily. If the laboratory is performing more than 20 tests per day, then this method is the most economical of all of the susceptibility test methodologies.

Instrumentation. In order to achieve the economical advantage described above, this method requires an inoculum-replicating device, such as that of Steers (1959). Modifications of the instrumentation are possible by using a spring-loaded device which allows for more rapid and potentially more uniform application of the inoculum to the individual plates. In addition, the Steers device (Melrose Machine Shop, Woodlyn, Pa.) has been modified for use with a larger, square plate which provides for 36 inoculum

*These compounds are also available from United States Pharmacopeia Convention, Inc., 12601 Twinbrook Parkway, Rockville, Md., 20852.

Table 52–2. PREPARATION AND STORAGE OF ANTIMICROBIAL AGENTS*

The following table indicates the solvents and diluents to be used in the preparation of stock antibiotic solutions from antibiotic powder.

Antimicrobial	Solvent	Dilution
Amikacin	[3]Water	Water
Amphotericin B	Dimethylsulfoxide	Water, adjust to pH 9.0 with NaOH
Ampicillin	[1]Phosphate buffer, pH 8.0, 0.1 M	Phosphate buffer, pH 6.0, 0.1 M
Carbenicillin	Water	Water
Cephalothin	Phosphate buffer, pH 6.0, 0.1 M	Water
Chloram-	Ethanol	Water
phenicol	Water	Water
Clindamycin	Water	Water
Cycloserine	Ethanol	Water
Erythromycin	Water	Water
Ethambutol	Saline, 0.85%	Saline, 0.85%
5-Fluorocytosine	[3]Water	Water
Gentamicin	Water	Water
Isoniazid	[3]Water	Water
Kanamycin	1N NaOH	Water
Nalidixid acid	Dimethylformamide	Water
Nitrofurantoin	Water	Water
Oxacillin	Water	Water
Penicillin	Water	Water
Polymyxin B	Dimethylsulfoxide	Phosphate buffer, pH 7.0
Rifampin	Water	Water
Streptomycin	10% NaOH + hot water	Water
Sulfonamides	Water	Water
Tetracyclines	Water	Water
Tobramycin	Water	Water
Vancomycin		

COMMENTS:
1. Phosphate buffers should be kept in the refrigerator for use as diluents.
2. Stock solutions are stored in the freezer at —35°C. At this temperature, stock solutions of most antibiotics (except pencillins, which should be replaced monthly) are stable for approximately six months.
3. The aminoglycoside antibiotics may also be dissolved in the phosphate buffer pH 8.0, 0.1 M.

*Modified from Washington (1974b).

implants. Though the seed plate and inoculating prongs can be made out of either aluminum or stainless steel, the aluminum construction is more vulnerable to erosion and pitting. The care of the instrumentation is important. Washington (1974a) advocates soaking the seed plate and inoculating prongs overnight in 70 per cent ethyl alcohol, after scrubbing them clean with a brush. They are then wrapped in a cloth towel and this pack is placed in a large glass Petri dish and autoclaved prior to use. Glass rings, called by some "Raschig" rings, can be placed around the inoculum of spreading *Proteus* strains in order to inhibit their dispersion across the agar test plate. These rings can be cleaned by boiling in water for 20 minutes and then soaking in 70 per cent ethyl alcohol prior to use.

Medium. Mueller-Hinton agar (MHA) or other agar media may be used for this method. One may also add whole, chocolatized, lysed, or peptic digest of blood, usually in a 5 per cent v/v amount for those organisms that require this enrichment. Brain-heart infusion or Wilkins-Chalgren (1976) agar with 5 per cent sheep blood can be used for testing anaerobic organisms.

One should establish performance standards for each of the several antimicrobials to be used. It is important to note that cation differences can be substantial among the three media mentioned above, and in this context, performance, especially with the aminoglycoside antibiotics, can vary from lot to lot and from manufacturer to manufacturer, as well as from medium to medium (Reller, 1974; Washington, 1978).

Antimicrobial Preparations. Individual antimicrobials are prepared in sterile distilled water for later addition to the melted agar medium. The simplest approach to this task is to follow a systematized guide such as that presented in Table 52–3, as modified from Ericsson (1971). By preparing concentrations in this manner, 1.5 ml of antimicrobial solution can be added to 13.5 ml agar suspension or, alternatively, 2 ml of antimicrobial solution to 18 ml suspension for pouring into 100 mm plates.

Use of the scheme in Table 52–3 is made additionally practical in that only one pipette need be used for each series of three dilutions. Furthermore, this method is not as vulnerable to the cumulative error which can pose a serious problem in fixed and repetitive serial dilution methods.

The general approach, in the past, to tube dilution testing has been strictly in terms of two-fold dilutions. Whereas this does provide considerable information with respect to the level of antimicrobial susceptibility, in actuality it provides more information than is needed in most clinical circumstances. Therefore, institutions such as the Mayo Clinic (Washington, 1974a) have developed an abbreviated set of concentrations to be used for agar dilution susceptibility testing. In most instances, this set includes only three or four concentrations. The determination of the concentrations of antimicrobial to be tested is based upon an assessment of the levels in serum likely to be attained in the treatment of systemic infection with the usual dose by the usual route of administration, and levels relating to

Table 52–3. MODIFIED GUIDE FOR DILUTION OF ANTIMICROBIALS IN AGAR

Antimicrobial Solution		Volume of Sterile Water to Be Added	Concentration as Added to Melted Agar 1:9 or for Further Dilution on Lines Below	Final Concentration in Agar	
μg or IU/ml	*Stock vol. (in ml.)*	(in ml)	*μg or IU/ml*		Log$_2$
2000	6.4	3.6	1280	128	7
1280	2	2	640	64	6
1280	1	3	320	32	5
1280	1	7	160	16	4
160	2	2	80	8	3
160	1	3	40	4	2
160	1	7	20	2	1
20	2	2	10	1	0
20	1	3	5	0.5	−1
20	1	7	2.5	0.25	−2

expected urinary tract concentrations. This abbreviated scheme has obvious economic advantages over a ten- or twelve-level two-fold dilution approach.

Preparation of Plates. The medium, once it has been prepared according to the manufacturer's directions, is allowed to cool to approximately 45 to 50°C. in an appropriately adjusted waterbath. The medium is usually prepared in screw-cap bottles, as these allow for ease of mixing.

Considerations in the preparation of plates include the ability to produce a plate which is level and uniform in consistency. In addition, the antimicrobials should be evenly distributed throughout the agar medium. Therefore, one should take care to add the antibiotic quickly in order that the agar medium not cool below 45°C. This prevents partial coalescence of the agar, which can result not only in uneven plates but also in non-uniform distribution of the antimicrobial. Similarly, adding an antimicrobial prior to cooling to 50°C. can be detrimental in that the increased temperature can have an adverse effect on the activity of some antimicrobials. In mixing the antimicrobial and agar, one should take care not to introduce bubbles by being too vigorous in the mixing process. Bubbles can result in an uneven surface, and the usual method of handling these bubbles, that of flaming the surface of the plate, can also have an adverse effect with respect to certain antimicrobials.

A separate plate of Mueller-Hinton agar without added antibiotics should also be poured for each dilution series in order to provide an appropriate growth control.

Once plates have been allowed to harden, they should be carefully marked as to the type and concentration of antimicrobial agent present. These plates can then be used within a short period of time or can be packaged in plastic bags and stored at 4°C. Studies by Ryan (1970) have shown that most antimicrobial agents in agar can be stored in this fashion for four weeks. The exceptions are the penicillins and nitrofurantoin. These should not be stored longer than one week. For reference work and other investigational studies, plates should be used within 24 hours of preparation.

Because of the need for uniformity and to obviate the possibility of inoculum spot coalescence on the agar, plates should be dried sufficiently to remove surface moisture before use.

A special note should be made at this point that blood products are usually added to the agar after the antimicrobial has been added and thoroughly mixed. Once the blood has been added, the plates should be poured immediately in order to avoid the possibility of coalescence of agar.

Inoculum is prepared as for other susceptibility tests. Between four and six morphologically identical colonies are touched with an inoculating loop or needle and suspended in 2 ml of an appropriate sterile medium. Either soybean-casein digest broth (e.g., Trypticase Soy Broth [TSB]) or Mueller-Hinton Broth (MHB) is usually used. One should be aware that streptococci do not generally grow well in MHB and that TSB should routinely be used for these organisms. There are several approaches to the standardization of the density of the inoculum (Ericsson, 1971; Washington, 1974a). A suitable approach is as follows: after inoculating 2 ml of sterile broth, the organisms are allowed to grow for 2 to 4 hours at 35°C. or are allowed to incubate overnight at the same temperature, and the turbidity of the broth culture is then adjusted to match that of the 0.5 MacFarland standard, by diluting the suspension with similar broth. A 1:200 dilution of the standardized organism suspension is made so that the final inoculum is in the range of 5 × 10^6 CFU/ml. An alternative approach to achieving this inoculum size is either to perform a 1:200 dilution of an overnight broth culture or to use a 0.5 ml broth culture that has been heavily inoculated and allowed to incubate for four hours.

Once the inoculum has been standardized, it should be transferred to the test medium without delay before organism replication occurs.

The whole process of inoculum preparation is facilitated if one uses a rack for the inoculated tubes with the same configuration as that of the replicator device's seed plate (Washington, 1974a). This will also facilitate the recording of specimen numbers onto a grid sheet marked in such a way that the location of each organism being tested can be easily noted.

Transfer of Inoculum. The first step in preparing for the transfer of inoculum from the standardized broth cultures into the seed plate wells should be to fill one well, usually in a corner, with India ink to define clearly the orientation of the organisms being tested. From the standardized broth tubes, an amount of inoculum approximately equivalent to one half to two thirds the potential volume of each well in the seed plate well is transferred to that well. Individual pipettes must be used for each organism; however, the amount to be transferred need only be approximate, so that less expensive Pasteur pipettes can be used. The head of the replicating device, containing the individual inoculation prongs corresponding with the wells in the seed plate, is then lowered into the seed plate, raised, and lowered onto the agar surface. The prongs are constructed so as to deliver approximately 0.001 to 0.003 ml or approximately 1 × 10^4 colony-forming units (CFU). The size of the inoculum spot on the agar surface is approximately 5 to 8 mm.

As one transfers the inoculum from a seed plate to the agar surface with any replicator device, one should be careful to use smooth hand movements to prevent splatter. One should avoid pressure on the agar surface with the inoculating head and should allow it to remain on the agar for 3 to 5 seconds prior to returning it to the seed plate. One should move from the least concentrated antimicrobial plate toward the most concentrated in the series in order to avoid the possibility of transfer of antimicrobial either to the seed plate or to subsequent dilutions in the series.

As has already been mentioned, 12 × 12 mm Raschig rings (Scientific Glass Apparatus, Bloomfield, N.J.) can be used to prevent spreading by *Proteus*. Once inoculation has taken place, these rings should be set on the agar. After the transfer of inocula has been completed, the plate is covered and allowed to stand until the inoculum droplets are absorbed into the agar; however, the surface of the agar should be carefully examined immediately after inoculum transfer in order to ensure that there is an inoculum droplet at each location where this transfer should have occurred. One can use a 0.001 ml calibrated loop for the transfer, on a single specimen basis, of inoculum from the appropriate seed plate well to the location on the agar surface where any droplets were not transferred.

Incubation. The plates are incubated at 35°C. in an inverted position for 16 to 20 hours. The atmosphere of incubation is usually ambient air, although, for those organisms requiring increased CO_2, incubation in CO_2 is possible as long as one tests appropriate controls in the same environment. In testing anaerobic organisms, these plates can be incubated in an anaerobic environment.

Results. According to the report of the International Collaborative Study (Ericsson, 1971), a barely visible haze of growth or a single colony is disregarded; if several colonies are found extending more than one dilution beyond an obvious endpoint, the purity of this strain is checked and the test repeated. The results are recorded on the grid which has been used to define the geographic location, both in the seed plate and on the agar surface, of the several specimens being tested.

Haemophilus influenzae. Because of the advent of ampicillin-resistant *H. influenzae,* the need has arisen for testing of this organism either by dilution or disk diffusion techniques or by determining beta-lactamase production. When several strains of *Haemophilus* are to be tested simultaneously, the agar dilution method facilitates this evaluation.

A stock antibiotic solution of ampicillin and the medium is prepared according to procedures already described. The test medium is Mueller-Hinton agar with added sterile horse blood or 1 per cent hemaglobin and IsoVitaleX (BioQuest, Cockeysville, Md.). The inoculum is prepared by scraping the growth from a pure culture (on chocolate or other suitable medium) of the *Haemophilus* with a sterile platinum loop into 4 ml of TSB to a density matching the 0.5 MacFarland turbidity standard (approximately 10^8 CFU/ml). This standardized suspension is then diluted 1:100. A suitable control *(Escherichia coli,* ATCC 25922) should be prepared and tested concurrently. If several strains are tested, the inoculating apparatus of Steers (1959) may be used; however, for few strains it is easier to spot inoculate the agar with a sterile 0.001 ml calibrated loop. It is suggested that an atmosphere with increased CO_2 should not be used unless it is required for the growth of a specific strain.

Results are determined in the same way as that described above for the agar dilution method. This procedure can be very helpful in those situations in which there is equivocation about the results of disk diffusion testing. It can also be of value in those situations in which ampicillin resistance is suspected despite the absence of beta-lactamase production. It should be stressed that some strains of *Haemophilus influenzae* that are resistant to ampicillin are not beta-lactamase producers.

MACROBROTH DILUTION METHODS

The details of this procedure are described elsewhere (Ericsson, 1971; Washington, 1974b). Because of the necessity of preparing dilution series singly, macrobroth dilution methods are quite cumbersome and time-consuming.

Medium. The medium is usually Mueller-Hinton broth, although many other media have been used, including those resulting from soy digests, tryptose phosphate, nutrient, Eugon, brain-heart infusion, etc. Comparative studies have clearly indicated that the MIC and MBC values for test organisms can vary widely depending upon the type of media used, pH, osmolality, and electrical conductivity. Results can vary with certain antimicrobials by more than ten-fold by employing different test media for determining the MIC in broth. This variation should be of major consideration in attempting to provide data that can be of value to the physician and that can be compared among laboratories. It is the position of the author that, for the present time, media other than Mueller-Hinton should be used only when organisms fail to grow well in Mueller-Hinton medium.

Antimicrobial Preparation. The method of arriving at stock solutions for broth dilution testing has been previously described in this section. As for agar dilution, a table modified from the International Collaborative Study Report by Ericsson (1971) is included (Table 52–4) for use in the preparation of these dilutions.

Dilutions either can be two-fold, with a wide or narrow range, or can be set at various predetermined levels in order to derive an appropriate analysis of high and low susceptibility. It has been our experience that when macrobroth dilution testing is done in the laboratory, it is often done for single organism determinations; however, it is still necessary to test control organisms concurrently.

Inoculum. The inoculum in the macrobroth method is in the range of 10^5 to 10^6 CFU/ml. One can use a 1:1000 or 1:2000 dilution of either an overnight broth culture, a 4 to 6 hour, 0.5 ml broth culture, or a 1:200 dilution of a broth culture adjusted to match the turbidity of a MacFarland 0.5 standard. It is customary to add 1 ml of standardized organism suspension to 1 ml of antibiotic solution in each tube. Tubes are incubated, with caps or plugs, in order to obviate evaporation and contamination, at 35°C.

Results. Since Mueller-Hinton broth has a slight turbidity, one must be careful to compare it with an uninoculated control. The MIC is determined as the least amount of antibiotic that results in complete inhibition of growth as judged by visual examination.

One advantage of this type of dilution test is that one can proceed to transfer aliquots from those tubes which demonstrate no visible growth to agar plate surfaces in order to determine the minimal bactericidal concentration, a concept discussed on page 1344.

MICROBROTH DILUTION TESTING

Microbroth dilution or microdilution technology has gained great acceptance over the past few years. Whereas microdilution trays, made of molded plastic, have been

Table 52–4. MODIFIED GUIDE FOR DILUTION OF ANTIMICROBIALS IN BROTH

Antimicrobial Solution: *μg or IU/ml*	Antimicrobial Solution: *Stock vol. (in ml.)*	Volume of Sterile Water to Be Added	Concentration as Added to Melted Agar 1:9 or for Further Dilution on Lines Below (*μg or IU/ml*)	Final Concentration in Agar (*μg or IU/ml*)	Log_2
2000	2	13.62 ml	256	128	7
256	2	2 vols	128	64	6
256	1	3	64	32	5
256	1	7	32	16	4
32	2	2	16	8	3
32	1	3	8	4	2
32	1	7	4	2	1
4	2	2	2	1	0
4	1	3	1	0.5	−1
4	1	7	0.5	0.25	−2
0.5	2	2	0.25	0.125	−3
0.5	1	3	0.125	0.063	−4
0.5	1	7	0.063	0.031	−5

available for serologic determinations for a number of years, it is only in recent years that this methodology has taken hold for use with antimicrobial susceptibility testing. The method has some very real advantages in terms of the availability of commercially prepared trays containing prefrozen and diluted antimicrobials, and, for the larger clinical laboratories, instrumentation can be purchased for producing plates (Tilton, 1973).

The basic methodology, therefore, will vary, depending upon the amount of equipment available in that laboratory and whether or not the laboratory purchases the preprepared dilution trays. Although the description provided in this section includes the entire methodology, it should be recognized that one can step into this process at any step along the way.

Available Equipment. The basic unit of the microdilution system is the molded plastic tray or plate which contains 8 rows of 12 small, either flat bottomed or V-shaped cups to which can be delivered a small volume (usually 0.1 ml) of inoculum. These trays can be purchased from several commercial manufacturers, and the author knows of no reason why one particular tray should be favored over another. Of consideration in the use of the trays is whether or not they can be reused. It should be pointed out that whereas it might be economically advantageous to wash and reuse trays, scratching of plastic surfaces, as will occur on the outer surface of the bottom of the individual wells, can interfere with the reading of broth dilution tests.

It is helpful, when performing microdilution tests, to have some way of dispensing the transparent tape for sealing the individual trays once the inoculum and the antimicrobial have been delivered; therefore, a small device for dispensing transparent tape may facilitate this procedure. In addition, one should also consider obtaining a reading rack with mirror to facilitate determination of the results.

Other factors to be considered are the specially calibrated loops that can be used for the dilution of antimicrobial solutions, and the specially constructed pipettes that can be used for the delivery of inoculum. Several levels of mechanization are available, including inoculating heads, much like those used for agar dilution testing, which can be used either manually or in a mechanized fashion for the delivery of inoculum into the antimicrobial-containing plates. It is not within the scope of this chapter to review all of the equipment available for the microdilution method; however, potential users should carefully consider the various alternatives in instrumentation that are available.

Media. The microdilution test can be performed with Mueller-Hinton broth; however, because of the deficiency of cations in formulations of this medium, it is suggested that it be supplemented with cation to assure appropriate susceptibility results (Thornsberry, 1977a). Reller (1974) recommends a final concentration of 50 mg of calcium and 25 mg of magnesium per liter of Mueller-Hinton broth to obviate this problem. This can be accomplished by preparing Mueller-Hinton broth, according to the manufacturer's directions, and adding the appropriate concentrations of calcium and magnesium with $CaCl_2$ and $MgCl_2$. As has been noted previously, the concentration of these divalent cations in Mueller-Hinton broth is so small that one can add these cations as though none were present originally.

Antimicrobials. Commercial firms have now developed the capacity for local distribution of prefrozen or lyophilized antimicrobial-containing trays for use in the clinical laboratory. The Food and Drug Administration has developed criteria for the quality control of these commercially prepared dilution sets, and the clinical laboratory can be assured that these trays will perform appropriately. The trays come individually or multiply packaged.

In preparing one's own trays, dilutions can be prepared by using the dilution schedule shown in Table 52–4, or one can use specially calibrated microdilution loops for serially diluting these trays. If one uses the fully instrumented approach to the preparation of trays, then the manufacturer's directions should be closely followed.

To be considered in the preparation of microdilution trays is the matter of using frozen stock solutions. Barry (1976) has suggested that allowing a stock solution to freeze, thawing it for preparing the dilutions, transferring these dilutions to the trays, and then refreezing them for storage, despite two freeze-thaw cycles, may be acceptable.

These trays, once prepared, can be frozen and stored in plastic bags for at least two weeks. If plates are purchased commercially, one should follow the manufacturer's outdate suggestions carefully.

Inoculation. The desired density of organisms is 5000

CFU per 0.1 ml of final volume in the tray wells. The inoculators deliver approximately 5 to 10 μl per prong or loop or 1 to 3 μl per pin. Therefore, the final inoculum delivered will depend upon the type of delivery system used. A final concentration in the well should be 10^5 CFU/ml. Another variable to be considered is that instruments deliver various volumes of antimicrobial solutions. Therefore, one must have a carefully defined protocol for delivery of the antimicrobial solutions into the trays and for diluting the inoculum. Once the inoculum has been delivered to the tray, it is sealed with transparent tape and incubated for 16 to 20 hours at 35°C.

Results. The MIC is defined as the lowest concentration without visible turbidity or a button of cells at the bottom of the well. Gerlach (1974) has demonstrated 95 per cent reproducibility in MIC determinations, a value which is consistent with the reproducibility of other susceptibility tests.

Rapid Results. Preliminary information (Bartlett, 1976) indicates that the addition of tetrazolium can expedite determination of the MIC in microdilution tests; however, the reproducibility of this procedure remains to be established, and it appears that an adjustment in inoculum must be made to assure reproducibility. It would seem best to assume that the microdilution method requires a 16- to 20-hour incubation period until more studies become available regarding rapid techniques.

Special Considerations. It is tempting to stack microdilution trays in order to conserve incubator space; however, uniformity in temperatures of individual trays within an incubator depends on the circulation of air. Stacking trays, therefore, may well prevent trays from arriving at the appropriate temperature within the 16- to 20-hour incubation period. The longer the incubation time, the less impact this variable would have on the final result.

Thornsberry (1977a) has reported that some beta-lactamase–producing strains of *Staphylococcus aureus* may give spuriously low penicillin or ampicillin MIC's in microdilution tests despite their production of beta-lactamase and probable resistance to penicillins in severe infections. It is suggested that all *Staphylococcus aureus* determined to be susceptible in the microdilution method be evaluated for the production of beta-lactamase.

Newer Automated Broth Dilution Adaptations

Special Considerations in Automation. The advent of automation brings with it some very intriguing possibilities for clinical microbiology, but also presents potential problems. Because of automation, it is very likely that we will need to redefine certain performance guidelines. Yet, at the same time, the only meaningful way to evaluate these newer methods is to compare them with the reference or standard methods. Currently, therefore, newer methods may be compared with the agar dilution method, as described by the International Collaborative Study (Ericsson, 1971); however, it may be more meaningful, if the automated method procedurally resembles the broth dilution test, to equate performance to standard or reference broth dilution methods.

Any automated approach ought to have the same degree of precision or reproducibility that we expect from the other methods, and one would anticipate that these new techniques should approach 95 per cent reproducibility.

Cost should be taken into account in the overall evaluation of the practicality and use of instrumentation. Increased costs may be acceptable if precision, objectivity in determining results, convenience, uniformity, economy of time, and speed in obtaining results are enhanced and if there is a potential interface with a computer for both quality control and data processing. Automation does add another variable to quality control related to the maintenance and performance of instrumentation.

Instrumentation alone is difficult to justify, and it is to be hoped that automated, semiautomated, and mechanized procedures will be critically evaluated and the results reported to the profession to provide a reasonable basis for all of us to make a judgment regarding the incorporation of these innovations into our own clinical laboratories.

Devices

Autobac I (Pfizer, Inc.). Autobac I is a semiautomated system for measuring antimicrobial susceptibilities of bacteria within a three- to five-hour time period. Although the basic system is adaptable to several aspects of clinical microbiology, the discussion here will be limited to its performance of susceptibility tests.

Instrumentation. The system comprises four separate components (McKie, 1974; Praglin, 1974). The central component of the system is a light-scattering photometer which also possesses the electronic capability to alter the evaluation mode and to be umbilicized to a free-standing computer unit that will become more important in future uses of this instrument (Matsen, 1977).

The second component is a cuvette comprising 12 individual test chambers and a thirteenth control chamber. This cuvette is molded so a broth inoculum tube can be firmly attached to it. It has a removable thick plastic manifold allowing access to the individual control chambers for the delivery of individual paper disks containing the antimicrobial substances.

The third component is a dispenser which delivers the antimicrobial disks to the individual chambers of the cuvette. The order of alignment of the antimicrobial substances is predetermined and cannot be randomly varied by the operator. The disks serve as the vehicles for delivering the antimicrobial agents by the principle of disk elution.

The fourth component is a dedicated, combined incubator and shaker. The internal housing within this incubator-shaker is designed to firmly hold the individual cuvettes.

An additional component of this system is a calibration wedge, by which the photometer is adjusted and can be checked. Finally, there is a multi-copy report form which is fed into the photometer housing for printing of results.

Susceptibility Testing Procedure. As the manufacturer provides complete testing procedures, the instructions will not be repeated here. Basically, the method involves selecting an organism from an initial isolation plate or directly from what appears to be a unimicrobially infected fluid specimen, and standardizing its inoculum density in saline with the light-scattering photometer. Newer models of the

Autobac have the capacity for varying the meter reading in order that different inocula may be used. An aliquot of the standardized inoculum is then transferred into a tube of eugonic broth which is then screwed into the cuvette and firmly seated. The cuvette is then inverted on a level surface so that all the broth is distributed to a holding chamber situated at one end of the cuvette. Further manipulations of the cuvette are made so as to distribute the broth evenly along the length of the cuvette. Thus, 1.5 ml aliquots are delivered into each of the individual chambers of the cuvette, which have been previously loaded with the antimicrobial disks by the disk dispenser.

The cuvette is then placed in the incubator-shaker for approximately three hours. The cuvette is then placed on a holding bar or carriage in the light-scattering photometer housing and the photometer lid is closed. A report form is inserted to record the result and the machine begins its computation. Sufficient growth must be obtained in the control chamber for the photometer to accept the report slip. If growth is insufficient, the cuvette is returned to the incubator-shaker for an additional period of time. If there is sufficient growth in the control chamber, a light-scatter index is calculated by means of a minicomputer within the photometer housing. This index is a numerical value between 0 and 1 with 0.01 subdivisions. An interpretation of susceptible, intermediate, or resistant is calculated for each antimicrobial agent in the control chamber and in each chamber containing antimicrobial (light-scatter index, or LSI). Modifications of the antimicrobial content of the disks and of the instrument's program can be made. For example, disks containing two or three amounts of each antimicrobial may be tested, and a result (MIC) formulated either from the absolute LSI derived from each chamber or by using a mathematical calculation based on a regression analysis of the LSI from the high and low antimicrobial disks used in the series.

Problem Areas. A seven-laboratory collaborative study evaluated the Autobac instrument and compared it to disk diffusion and the ICS agar dilution methods (Thornsberry, 1975). There was an overall agreement of about 90 per cent between the automated results and those of the other two methods. The principal difficulties were encountered with testing *Enterobacter* against ampicillin and cephalothin, and with *Pseudomonas aeruginosa* tested against chloramphenicol, tetracycline, and gentamicin. It has also been shown that the Autobac instrument is unlikely to detect methicillin- or nafcillin-resistant strains of *Staphylococcus;* therefore, it is suggested that when multiply resistant strains of staphylococci are encountered, they should be considered potentially resistant to the penicillinase-resistant semisynthetic penicillins and tested by another acceptable procedure (Cleary, 1978). Experience also demonstrates that ampicillin-resistant enterococci should be rechecked for susceptibility by a dilution or diffusion method. As with the disk diffusion method, one should also run a purity check on any specimen being tested in the Autobac.

Other Devices. Other forms of automation currently being marketed are limited to those used for the microdilution test. However, under evaluation are instruments manufactured by the McDonnell Douglas Astronautics Company (AutoMicrobic System or AMS), Abbott Laboratories (MS-2), and Cathra (Repliscan). In addition, testing has been done of radiometric, laser-light scattering, and electrical impedance devices; however, none of these three systems is currently projected for marketing within the near future.

It is very likely that the Automicrobic, the MS-2, and the Repliscan devices will become available for susceptibility testing purposes in the near future. Since published results of clinical trials of these devices are not yet available, it seems premature to review their operation or instrumentation further.

DIFFUSION TESTING

Principles

The observation that an antibiotic that diffused from antibiotic-impregnated material or from a reservoir cut in the surface of an agar plate inhibited the growth of a susceptible organism led ultimately to the development of a standardized antibiotic-impregnated paper disk diffusion method of susceptibility testing (Bauer, 1966). Historically many methods were employed, and a number are still in use or are being proposed for use in clinical laboratories. However, it is of major significance that the U.S. Food and Drug Administration, given the responsibility in this area by the United States Supreme Court, has recently recommended similar methodology for use in all laboratories (Federal Register, 1972, 1973). A subcommittee of the National Committee for Clinical Laboratory Standards (1975) has also recommended essentially the same method.

In brief, this method involves placing a known amount of antibiotic in a small, absorbent paper disk measuring 6 mm in diameter. The placement of this disk on an agar surface previously inoculated with the organism to be tested will result in a concentric zone of inhibited growth for susceptible organisms. The zone of inhibition for the great majority of antimicrobial agents has been shown to relate linearly to the minimal inhibitory concentration (MIC) of the antibiotic as measured by dilution susceptibility testing (Matsen, 1970; Ericsson, 1971).

This relationship is of great importance in understanding the principle of the disk diffusion susceptibility test and the genesis of the interpretive criteria. The relation between MIC and zone diameter of inhibition can be expressed by regression analysis (Fig. 52–1). A sample of at least 100 to 150 organisms, representing the species of bacteria for which the antimicrobial agent might be used, is tested by both disk diffusion and agar or broth dilution. Organisms are selected to provide MIC values that are fairly evenly spread over the clinically relevant ranges of concentrations. Any values representing no zone of inhibition are excluded from the graphs and from the calculations of the regression lines. The ordinate or Y-axis denotes the MIC on a logarithmic scale, whereas the abscissa or X-axis represents zone diameters of inhibition on an arithmetic scale (Fig. 52–1). Since the distribution of plots with most antimicrobials is linear, application of the formula of least squares results in the mathematical computation of the "regression line" (line of best fit) shown in the figure. In those situations in which the relationship is not linear, this line has diminished significance. The calculated line is not, however, the "true" regression line. This is because, in the two-fold dilution

6

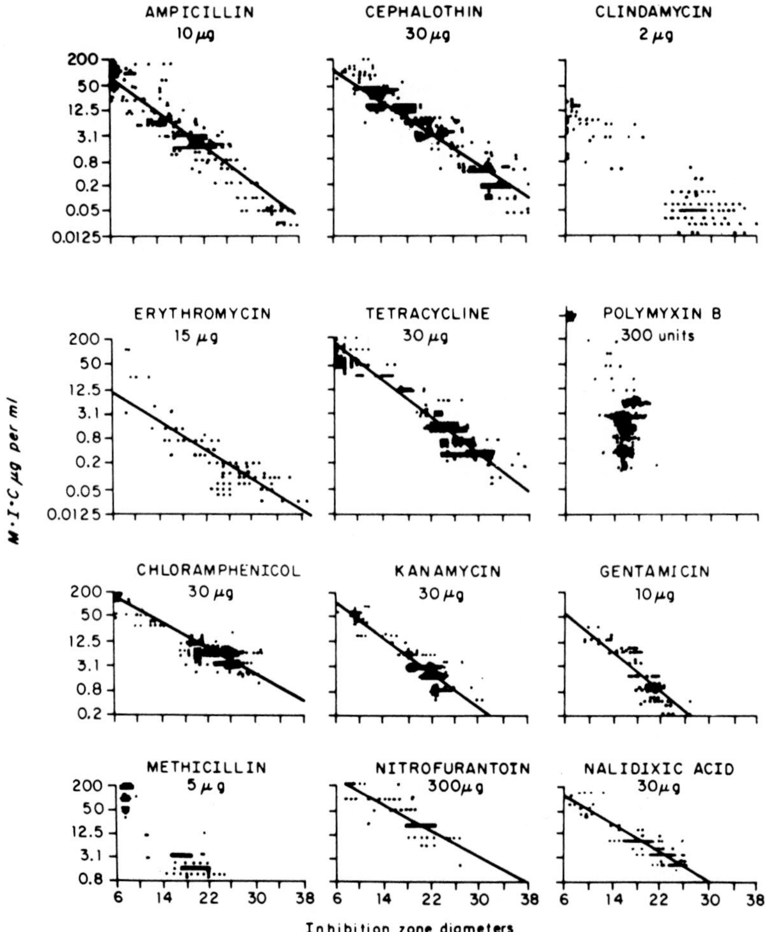

Figure 52–1. Relationship of zone diameter to agar dilution MIC with some commonly used antimicrobials. All except polymyxin and gentamicin show combined data from clinical laboratories of the Universities of Minnesota and Washington. The disk content is shown below each antimicrobial. Polymyxin MIC's are in units per milliliter. (From Matsen, 1974.)

test, as used in this graph, the *average* true value of the MIC is one half of a two-fold dilution lower than the observed value. Organism values, as derived from the dual test evaluation, are distributed on either side of these regression lines, and the pattern of organism scatter must be considered in arriving at susceptibility category breakpoints.

By defining the serum levels of the antibiotic achievable with the recommended dosages given by the usual routes of administration, one derives the MIC values in micrograms per ml (µg/ml) which would be expected to be inhibitory *in vivo*. The zone diameter interpretive criteria for susceptibility are then based on the zone of inhibition corresponding to this MIC value, while the criteria for defining intermediate susceptibility and resistance are based on considerations of toxicity and pharmacokinetics of the individual compounds, as well as the scatter or organisms on the histogram, as shown in Figure 52–1. The intermediate zone, in addition to providing an indication for maximum dosage if that particular antimicrobial is to be used, also serves as a buffer zone to minimize false susceptible or resistant interpretations related to the scatter of organisms.

Disk Content Selection

The proper disk content for each antimicrobial should be based upon a number of experimentally derived factors, among which are the following:

1. Zone sizes of very susceptible organisms should preferably be in the range of 20 to 30 mm and no more than 35 mm. When larger zone sizes occur, reproducibility becomes increasingly difficult. Examples of large zone sizes are those occurring with susceptible staphylococci and the 10 unit penicillin disk.

2. Zone sizes should be large enough that the test maintains discriminating capability for organisms with intermediate levels of susceptibility, i.e., an intermediate-resistant zone diameter partition greater than 12 mm. There is an interesting corollary which holds true for certain antibiotics: the regression line usually crosses the Y-axis at

a point where the MIC value is three to five times the stated content of the disk.

3. The stability of the antibiotic under routine storage conditions has a bearing on disk content. The smaller the disk content of unstable antimicrobial agents, the more crucial is the proportional deterioration of the antibiotic. The concept of the high content disk was an important feature of the standardized method originally proposed by Bauer (1966). The higher the disk content, the less likely is antimicrobial deterioration to be significant in the test.

4. Other considerations include the linearity and slope of the regression line and the standard deviation of organism plots about the line of regression. An error rate–bounded method for examining the relationship between zone diameter and MIC was described by Metzler (1974), who recommended limiting the rates of false susceptibles and false resistants obtained by the disk diffusion technique to 1 and 5 per cent, respectively.

The content of the disks is under the regulation of the Food and Drug Administration. Currently, the content of the disks must be not more than 150 per cent or less than 67 per cent of their stated content. Therefore, there is a possibility of considerable variation in content, and many large disk manufacturers aim for a modest overfill.

Indications and Limitations

Indications for disk diffusion susceptibility testing are similar to the indications for susceptibility testing in general. In addition, it is important to understand that the standardized disk diffusion method should be used only for rapidly growing organisms for which an end-point can be determined within an 18- to 24-hour period. Continued incubation beyond that time interval may sufficiently alter the interaction between organism and antimicrobial to give erroneous results. Furthermore, certain organisms or antibiotics require special test conditions. *Haemophilus influenzae,* as has already been discussed, requires the addition of special nutrients to the medium. Streptococci grow poorly on Mueller-Hinton medium and require the addition of 5 per cent sheep blood. In testing sulfonamides or the combination of sulfamethoxazole and trimethoprim, blood additives cannot be used owing to the antagonistic effect of para-aminobenzoic acid present in blood. When sulfonamides are tested against *Neisseria meningitidis,* special factors must be considered. Disk diffusion susceptibility testing of penicillin is not standardized for *Neisseria meningitidis;* therefore, susceptibility testing of this antibiotic-organism pair should be carried out with agar dilution methods. Susceptibility testing should not be done with either methenamine mandelate or methenamine hippurate, as there is not sufficient analogy between the *in vivo* and *in vitro* conditions.

The disk diffusion method can be used for susceptibility testing of some anaerobic bacteria; however, the test procedures differ substantially from those used with rapidly growing aerobic and facultatively anaerobic bacteria (see p. 1340).

Recommended Antimicrobials

Currently, it is recommended that only one agent from each class of closely related antimicrobials be tested. Generally, this is the only agent available owing to Food and Drug Administration regulations. Although the class representative is usually sufficient for most testing situations, a few circumstances do exist wherein one cannot extrapolate susceptibility results to other agents within the class. Dilution testing is indicated in the unusual cases where this differentiation is clinically important. Two examples within the cephalosporin group illustrate this point. *Haemophilus influenzae* is usually susceptible to cephalothin, the class disk representative of the cephalosporin group, but is resistant to cephalexin. Therefore, one cannot extrapolate susceptibility to cephalexin from the cephalothin results in this instance. Cefazolin is usually more active *in vitro* than cephalothin against *Escherichia coli* and a zone diameter of 13 mm with the cephalothin disk can be used to indicate *E. coli* susceptibility to cefazolin. With few exceptions, however, the general guidelines in Table 52–1 should be used for selecting antimicrobials to be tested routinely against rapidly growing aerobic and facultatively anaerobic bacteria.

Recommended Methods for Disk Diffusion Testing

AGAR DIFFUSION SURFACE-STREAK METHOD

This method of susceptibility, as proposed in 1966 by Bauer, Kirby, Sherris, and Turck, is the basis for the methods recommended by the United States Food and Drug Administration (Federal Register, 1972, 1973) and the National Committee for Clinical Laboratory Standards (1975). The method described here is essentially that of the latter group and is given here because it encompasses the details of the method recommended by the Food and Drug Administration and emphasizes a few additional details which the author feels are important in the performance of the disk diffusion test. The method should be followed closely if accurate, reproducible results are to be anticipated.

Medium and Preparation of Plates. Mueller-Hinton medium is the recommended medium, and emphasis should be made that the interpretive chart (Table 52–5) is valid only when this medium is used in the prescribed manner. For justification of the use of Mueller-Hinton medium, the reader is referred to the report of the International Collaborative Study (Ericsson, 1971). Although Mueller-Hinton supports the growth of most organisms for which susceptibility testing will be done, 5 per cent defibrinated sheep, horse, or other animal blood should be added to ensure adequate growth of streptococci and other fastidious organisms, and 5 per cent laked horse blood. Fildes digest, or other similar nutrient additive should be added for testing *Haemophilus.*

In general, it is advisable to use 150 mm Petri plates, although current recommendations do allow use of 100 mm plates instead. Agar depth should be in the range of 4 to 6 mm (Barry, 1973a) (20 to 25 ml of agar for the 100 mm plates and 79 to 80 ml for the 150 mm plates). After plates are prepared, they are best stored at 4°C. in cellophane wrapping, and should be used within a two-week period. Immediately prior to use plates should be "dried" in an incubator for 30 minutes to facilitate removal of excess surface moisture.

Preparation of Inoculum. An inoculating needle or loop is used to transfer portions of four or five colonies of the organism into 4 or 5 ml of a suitable broth medium

Table 52–5. ZONE DIAMETER INTERPRETIVE STANDARDS[1, 2]

Antimicrobial Agent		Disk Potency	Zone Diameter (mm)			Approximate MIC Correlates	
			Resistant	*Intermediate*	*Susceptible*	*Resistant*	*Susceptible*
Amikacin[3,4]		30 µg	≤14	15–16	≥17	>16 µg/ml	≤8 µg/ml
Ampicillin[5]	Enterobacteriaceae &				≥14		
	Enterococci	10 µg	≤11	12–13	≥29	≥32µg/ml	≤8 µg/ml
	Staph/Pen susc. orgs.	10 µg	≤20	21–28		≥2.0 µg/ml penicillinase[6]	≤0.2 µg/ml
	Haemophilus	10 µg	≤19	—	≥20	—	≤2.0 µg/ml
Carbenicillin	*Proteus & E. coli*	100 µg	≤17	18–22	≥23	≥32 µg/ml	≤16 µg/ml
	P. aeruginosa[7]	100 µg	≤11	12–14	≥13	≥250 µg/ml	≤125 µg/ml
Cephalothin[8]		30 µg	≤14	15–17	≥18	≥32 µg/ml	≤ 10 µg/ml
Chloramphenicol		30 µg	≤12	13–17	≥18	≥25 µg/ml	≤12.5 µg/ml
Clindamycin[9]		2 µg	≤14	15–16	≥17	≥ 2 µg/ml	≤1 µg/ml
Colistin[10]		10 µg	≤8	9–10	≥11	—	—
Erythromycin		15 µg	≤13	14–17	≥18	≥8 µg/ml	≤2 µg/ml
Gentamicin		10 µg	≤12	13–14	≥15	≥6 µg/ml	≤6 µg/ml
Kanamycin		30 µg	≤13	14–17	≥18	≥25 µg/ml	≤ 6 µg/ml
Methicillin[11]		5 µg	≤9	10–13	≥14	—	≤3 µg/ml
Nafcillin[12]		1 µg	≤10	11–12	≥13	—	≤ 3 µg/ml
Naldixic acid[13]		30 µg	≤13	14–18	≥19	≥32 µg/ml	≤12 µg/ml
Neomycin		30 µg	≤12	13–16	≥17	—	≤10 µg/ml
Nitrofurantoin[13]		300 µg	≤14	15–16	≥17	≥100 µg/ml	≤25 µg/ml
Penicillin G[14]	Staphylococci	10 units	≤20	21–28	≥29	penicillinase[6]	≤0.1 µg/ml
	Other organisms	10 units	≤11	12–21	≥22	≥32 µg/ml	≤1.5 µg/ml
Polymyxin B[10]		300 units	≤8	9–11	≥12	≥50 units/ml	
Streptomycin		10 µg	≤11	12–14	≥15	≥15 µg/ml	≤6 µg/ml
Sulfonamides	*N. mening.* only	250/300 µg			≥40		
	Other organisms[13]	250/300 µg	≤12	13–16	≥17	≥350 µg/ml	≤100 µg/ml
Tetracycline[15]		30 µg	≤14	15–18	≥19	≥12 µg/ml	≤4 µg/ml
Tobramycin		10 µg	≤12	13–14	≥15	≥6 µg/ml	≤6 µg/ml
Trimethoprim-sulfamethoxazole[13]		1.25 µg/23.75 µg	≤10	11–15	≥16	≥200 µg/ml	≤35 µg/ml
Vancomycin		30 µg	≤9	10–11	≥12	—	≤5 µg/ml

[1]Bauer (1966).
[2]NCCLS Subcommittee on Antimicrobial Susceptibility Testing (1975); Federal Register (1972, 1973).
[3]Tentative standards from Bristol Laboratories.
[4]Kelly, M.T., and Matsen, J. M.: In vitro activity, synergism, and testing parameters of amikacin, with comparisons to other aminoglycoside antibiotics. Antimicrob. Agents Chemother., 9:440, 1975.
[5]Class disk for ampicillin, hetacillin, and amoxicillin.
[6]Resistant strains of *S. aureus* produce penicillinase. There are significant reports of ampicillin-resistant strains which produce penicillinase.
[7]Tentative standards from UUMC Clinical Microbiology Laboratory.
[8]Class disk for cephalothin, cephaloridine, cephalexin, cefazolin, cephacetrile, cephradrine, and cephapirin.
[9]The clindamycin disk is used to test susceptibility to both clindamycin and lincomycin. Owing to the greater activity of clindamycin, separate interpretive categories of zone diameters are recommended when reporting susceptibility to lincomycin as follows: ≤16 = R, 17–20 = I, ≥21 = S.
[10]Colistin and polymyxin B diffuse poorly in agar, and thus the accuracy of diffusion tests is less than that found with other antimicrobics, and MIC correlates cannot be calculated reliably from regression analysis.
[11]Class disk for penicillinase-resistant penicillins (i.e., methicillin, cloxacillin, dicloxacillin, oxacillin, and nafcillin).
[13]Urinary tract infections only.
[14]Class disk for penicillin G, phenocymethyl penicillin, and phenthicillin.
[15]Class disk for tetracyclines.

(soybean-casein digest or tryptose phosphate broths are suggested) which is allowed to incubate at 35°C. until the turbidity of the culture compares to that of the recommended turbidity standard (see p. 1327). The standard is agitated on a vortex mixer immediately prior to use. Unless the standard is contained in heat-sealed glass tubes, it should probably be replaced every six months. If appropriately sealed, the standard may last indefinitely (Washington, 1973). The turbidity of the culture, if excessive, may be adjusted by the addition of sterile saline or broth or, if inadequate, by the addition of colonies, provided they are well isolated and are morphologically identical to those originally selected. The modified laboratory view box previously described (Stemper, 1970) enhances the process of handling the culture tubes and the standard during turbidity adjustment. The standardized inoculum suspension should be inoculated within 15 to 20 minutes.

Inoculation of Medium. A sterile cotton swab on a wooden applicator stick is dipped into the standardized inoculum suspension. Excess broth is expressed by pressing and rotating the swab against the inside of the suspension tube. The swab is then streaked evenly in three directions on the surface of the agar plate. A final sweep is made of the agar rim with the cotton swab. This inoculum is allowed to dry for three to five minutes and disks are then applied, either by a mechanical dispenser or by hand using sterile forceps. After placement, disks are pressed firmly but gently onto the agar surface. The spatial arrangement of the disks should preclude the development of overlapping zones of inhibition and, therefore, limits the number of disks that can be placed to 12 or 13 (9 in the outer ring) on a 150 mm plate.

Quality Assurance. Quality assurance should extend to all phases of the testing procedure. The Mueller-Hinton medium should be of proper depth (4 to 6 mm), should not be allowed to dry out excessively (store refrigerated, in cellophane wrapping, and use within two weeks), and should be checked for appropriate pH. Disks should be stored frozen (−12 to −20°C.) and should be removed from the freezer as individual cartridges; the cartridge in use should be kept in a desiccated container at 4°C. and allowed to equilibrate to room temperature prior to use each day. Disks should be purchased through a local distributor whose storage conditions (4°C.) are known or directly from the manufacturer. The practice of receiving disks from pharmaceutical representatives is to be avoided because of the unknown storage conditions prior to receipt. A representative disk from each cartridge should be tested with control bacterial strains (*Staphylococcus aureus* ATCC 25923 for antimicrobials to be tested against gram-positive organisms, *Escherichia coli* ATCC 25922, and *Pseudomonas aeruginosa* ATCC 27853 for agents to be tested against gram-negative bacilli) prior to the routine use of other disks from that cartridge. The control strains should be tested frequently and, ideally, each time a set of susceptibility tests is performed. An easily accessible, easily readable chart is recommended to facilitate recording and interpretation of quality assurance testing. Limits of excursion for the control *S. aureus, E. coli,* and *P. aeruginosa* are given in Table 52–6; however, it should be stressed that these limits are rather broad, and ideally each laboratory would establish its own, narrower limits of control.

A separate sheep blood agar plate should be streaked in quadrants, with the swab used for streaking the surface of each Mueller-Hinton plate to check for purity of inoculum.

Results. Zone diameters are measured under reflected light with a ruler or calipers on the undersurface of the Petri dish. If blood has been added to the Mueller-Hinton agar, the zones are measured from the surface of the agar after removing the cover. The end-point is complete inhibition of growth as determined visually, except in the case of sulfonamides, where organisms may grow through several generations before inhibition occurs. In this instance, slight growth (80 per cent or greater inhibition) is disregarded, and the margin of heavy growth is measured. The swarming of *Proteus* is also disregarded, and the margin of heavy growth which is usually clearly apparent is measured.

While preliminary readings may be obtained as soon as growth patterns become apparent (usually 6 to 8 hours), readings made at this time should be verified at 18 to 20 hours. Measurement of zones should include the entire diameter of the zone, including the disk. Should colonies be seen within the zone of inhibition, the purity check plate should be analyzed. If it is obvious that more than one organism is present, the test should be repeated. If the culture is pure, the colonies are regarded as significant and included in zone diameter measurement. Fortunately, this is not a frequent occurrence.

The zone diameter interpretive criteria, along with the MIC correlates, are shown in Table 52–5. This table contains a compilation of data from the Centers for Disease Control (Thornsberry, 1977b) and from the National Committee for Clinical Laboratory Standards recommendations (1975).

Should a physician desire quantitative information, these MIC correlates can be referred to, as can the regression line plots such as that shown in Figure 52–1. One may give a

Table 52–6. SUSCEPTIBILITY OF CONTROL STRAINS*

		Zone Diameter of Inhibition (mm)		
Antibiotic	**Disk Potency**	***S. aureus* *(ATCC 25923)***	***E. coli* *(ATCC 25922)***	***P. aeruginosa* *(ATCC 27853)***
Amikacin	10 μg	18–24	18–24	15–22
Ampicillin	10 μg	24–35	15–20	—
Bacitracin	10 U	17–22	—	—
Carbenicillin	100 μg	—	24–29	20–24
Cephalothin	30 μg	25–37	18–23	—
Chloramphenicol	30 μg	19–26	21–27	6
Clindamycin	2 μg	23–29	—	—
Colistin	10 μg	—	11–15	12–16
Erythromycin	15 μg	23–30	8–14	—
Gantrisin	250 or 300 μg	23–27	22–26	6
Gentamicin	10 μg	19–27	19–26	16–21
Kanamycin	30 μg	19–26	17–25	6
Methicillin	5 μg	17–22	—	—
Nalidixic acid	30 μg	—	21–25	—
Neomycin	30 μg	18–26	17–23	—
Nitrofurantoin	300 μg	—	20–24	—
Penicillin G	10 U	26–37	—	—
Polymyxin B	300 U	7–13	12–16	—
Streptomycin	10 μg	14–22	12–20	—
Tetracycline	30 μg	19–28	18–25	9–14
Trimethoprim-sulfamethoxazole	1.25 μg 23.75 μg	24–32	24–32	—
Tobramycin	10 μg	19–29	18–26	19–25
Vancomycin	30 μg	15–19	—	—

*From Thornsberry (1977b).

range of MIC values for any given zone size based upon these regression line plots if one strictly adheres to the standard method.

AGAR OVERLAY DIFFUSION METHOD

An acceptable alternative method of inoculating disk diffusion test plates is the agar overlay method (Barry, 1970). This method is also applicable only to tests with commonly isolated, rapidly growing aerobic and facultatively anaerobic bacteria, such as *S. aureus,* Enterobacteriaceae, *P. aeruginosa,* and other non-fermentative gram-negative bacilli.

Preparation of Plates. Mueller-Hinton agar is poured to a depth of 4 mm in 150 × 15 mm plastic Petri dishes.

Preparation and Incorporation of Inoculum. Four to five isolated colonies of the same morphologic type are selected from a primary isolation plate. A turbid suspension is prepared in 0.5 ml of brain-heart infusion broth in a 13 × 100 mm tube, which is then incubated in a 35 to 37°C. waterbath or heating block for four to eight hours. This suspension is well mixed after incubation, and a 0.001 loopful is transferred to a 9 ml aqueous solution of agar that has been held no longer than 8 hours in a 45 to 50°C. heating block (16 × 125 mm screw-capped tubes are routinely used). Tubes not used within this time interval are discarded. The melted agar, now inoculated with the test organism, is mixed by inverting several times before being poured over the surface of Mueller-Hinton agar in the 150 × 15 mm plastic Petri plate. The thin layer of melted agar will solidify too quickly on the Mueller-Hinton agar unless it is first brought to room temperature. Plates should be left for 3 to 5 minutes on a flat surface so that the agar overlay can harden properly before the disks are placed on the surface as described above.

Incubation. After the disks have been placed on the agar surface, the plates are inverted and incubated at 35°C. within 15 minutes for 16 to 18 hours.

Results. The plates are read in a manner similar to that employed with the surface streak disk diffusion method. The interpretive criteria are those listed in Table 52–5.

Interpretation of Results

If the standard method is followed closely, results are reliable and reproducible. Interpretation is based upon the establishment, for each antimicrobial, of zone diameters which correlate with MIC values and which, in turn, relate to achievable levels of antimicrobial in body fluids and tissues. The categories of susceptible, intermediate, and resistant apply to systemic infections (except for nitrofurantoin, sulfonamides, and nalidixic acid). In situations in which an antibiotic dose may be safely increased, concentrations far in excess of the levels considered in the establishment of these interpretive criteria may be reached. Similarly, the concentration of certain antimicrobials in the urine is many-fold higher than that considered as the upper limit of susceptibility in systemic infection. The interpretive criteria and MIC correlates presented in Table 52–5 are rough guidelines which provide, in most situations, a certain margin of safety to cover biologic differences among organisms and differences in the human host's response to the organism and to the antibiotic. Furthermore, the disk producing the greatest zone of inhibition does not necessarily indicate that that particular agent is the agent of choice for a given pathogen.

Regression Information for Commonly Used Therapeutics

Each antibiotic varies somewhat or greatly from other agents in its regression analysis. For this reason, and because of the added information these analyses provide, regression lines for all of the currently commonly used antibiotics are helpful for reference purposes. While these regression plots can be used as already described elsewhere in this chapter, each laboratory desiring to use these plots in this manner should verify by control organism plots that these results are reproducible in their own laboratory. For further information on regression plots, the reader is referred to more detailed sources of information (Chabbert, 1949; Matsen, 1970, 1974).

Common Errors

Though the disk diffusion method is a fairly forgiving method, there are errors that occur which compromise accuracy and reliability, and one error can obviously compound another. Included below is a list of what might be considered "common errors" occurring in clinical microbiology laboratories.

1. Failure to use Mueller-Hinton medium.
2. Use of outdated medium or plates.
3. Failure to test the pH of Mueller-Hinton medium or committing other media preparation mistakes.
4. Failure to standardize the inoculum or to use proper density standardization procedures.
5. Use of an inaccurate turbidity reference standard (usually due to incorrect preparation, leakage, or evaporation).
6. Failure to express excess fluid from swab used for plate inoculation.
7. Excessive time lapse between inoculum standardization and plate inoculation.
8. Use of outdated or improperly stored disks.
9. Prolonged time lapse in applying disks after plates have been inoculated.
10. Delay in incubation following inoculation and disk placement, thus allowing antibiotic "prediffusion" prior to optimal organism growth conditions.
11. Failure to use quality control strains or the use of improper quality control strains.
12. The testing of mixed cultures.
13. Transcription errors.
14. The testing of organisms which require anaerobic incubation, or which are so slow in their growth as to preclude a zone reading within a 18- to 24-hour time frame.

It is apparent that problems in each of these situations can be obviated by closely adhering to the prescribed methods.

INDICATIONS FOR DIRECT SUSCEPTIBILITY TESTING ON CLINICAL MATERIALS

While permissible in emergency situations in which cerebrospinal fluid or other body fluid specimens with gram-stained smears indicating that a pure culture may be expected, direct susceptibility testing of clinical material on a routine basis is to be avoided and discouraged. Mixtures or organisms, common in many specimens, may produce inaccurate interpretations (Shahidi, 1969). It may also be difficult to standardize the inoculum from direct clinical material (Ellner, 1976; Hollick, 1976; Wegner, 1976). The use of a purity check will be of great assistance in these emergency situations, as will an assessment of the nature of the "lawn" of inoculum on the susceptibility test plate. Results reported from such emergency tests should, unless a pure culture results and the appropriate inoculum has been achieved, be reported as preliminary or tentative and should be repeated and confirmed using one of the recommended methods (Barry, 1973b).

QUALITY CONTROL

As indicated in the preceding section, adherence to the prescribed methodology is important in the performance of the disk diffusion test. Attention to these detailed instructions is the best approach to quality control. The actual approach to quality assurance in the laboratory is geared to the various test materials (Mueller-Hinton medium, barium-sulfate turbidity standard, and antimicrobial disks), to the use of control organisms, and to the appropriate reading, interpretation, and transcription of zone sizes (Blazevic, 1972).

SPECIAL CONSIDERATIONS

Anaerobes. Because of the unusual features associated with the growth of anaerobic organisms, which include the requirements for an anaerobic environment, wide variations in replication times, as well as other organism-specific features, the susceptibility testing of anaerobic organisms poses special problems for the clinical microbiology laboratory. In this context, the methodologies that have been previously described do not have the same broad applicability for this group that they do for the aerobic or facultatively anaerobic and rapidly growing organisms. However, modifications of each of the susceptibility systems previously described have been worked out either for anaerobes in general or for specific groups of anaerobic organisms.

Problems with anaerobic susceptibility testing have been related to the polymicrobial nature of anaerobic infections, which also pose problems in the approach to therapy. In addition, delays in reporting anaerobic susceptibilities have led to less than optimal application of results to the therapy of the patient. Furthermore, the vast majority of anaerobic organisms are predictably susceptible to penicillin G, carbenicillin, and ticarcillin (*Bacteroides fragilis* and some *Bacteroides melaninogenicus* excepted) and chloramphenicol and clindamycin (*B. fragilis* and *B. melaninogenicus* included), and are variably susceptible to the tetracyclines and erythromycin. Newer cephalosporin-like antimicrobials, such as the cephamycins, are potentially useful in treating anaerobic infections, as may be newer agents now being investigated, e.g., piperacillin.

Anaerobic susceptibility testing, in our experience, has been of limited utility. We specifically inquire of the physician submitting any non–body fluid anaerobic isolate as to whether or not susceptibility testing is desired. In almost all instances, the physician elects to forego the susceptibility testing. This area, therefore, represents one of the most selective ones in all of clinical microbiology with respect to the need and clinical usefulness of susceptibility testing.

Physicians at times will order anaerobic susceptibility tests, and there is no question about their utility in certain specific clinical instances, especially those in which the clinical disease is still present after two or three days of therapy. It should, however, be realized that just as anaerobic infections can develop insidiously, they may be slow in demonstrating clinical and laboratory evidence of response to therapy.

Of considerable potential utility because of its simplicity in a wide spectrum of clinical laboratories is the broth-disk method of Wilkins (1973), which was carefully evaluated by Blazevic (1975) and found to be very reproducible and comparable to standard methodology. The test is based on the principle of disk elution; however, the disks are not specially prepared but rather are multiples of the disks used in the standard disk diffusion test. Therefore, the availability of disks presents, for most laboratories, no problem, and the quality control of the performance of the disks can be tied in with the quality control of the standard methodology.

Materials. The medium is pre-reduced brain-heart infusion broth supplemented with 0.005 per cent hemin, 0.002 per cent menadione, and 0.05 per cent yeast extract (BHI-S). The amount of broth per tube is important, as one is dealing with a quantitative dilution of antimicrobial agents.

Inoculum. The inoculum is one drop of a turbid 18- to 24-hour culture grown in pre-reduced chopped meat broth, chopped meat glucose broth, or peptone-yeast-extract-glucose broth.

Procedure. The test is conducted in an anaerobic environment, either in a glovebox or in roll tubes inoculated with the Virginia Polytechnic Institute Cannula Apparatus. The appropriate number of antimicrobial disks is added to each tube of BHI-S (Table 52–7). When large numbers of disks are to be added they should be incubated anaerobically prior to addition to the broth (to avoid false sensitivities of strict anaerobes). In addition to the tubes containing antimicrobials, a tube without antimicrobials is inoculated as a growth control. One drop of inoculum is added to each tube, which is then sealed with a rubber stopper and incubated for 18 to 24 hours at 35°C. After incubation, a gram-stained smear should be made of the growth control to check for purity of the test suspension.

Table 52–7. BROTH-DISK METHOD FOR ANAEROBIC SUSCEPTIBILITY TESTING

Antimicrobial	Disk Content	No. of Disks per Tube	Final Concentration (μg/ml)
Ampicillin	10 μg	2	4
Carbenicillin	100 μg	5	100
Cephalothin	30 μg	1	6
Chloramphenicol	30 μg	2	12
Clindamycin	2 μg	4	1.6
Clindamycin	4 μg	8	3.2
Doxycycline	5 μg	3	3
Erythromycin	15 μg	1	3
Gentamicin	10 μg	3	6
Penicillin G	10 units	1	2 units
Tetracycline	30 μg	1	6

Test Interpretation. The interpretation of this particular susceptibility test differs from that used in the standard broth dilution test. In this particular test the end-point is determined by comparing the growth in each tube with that of the control. Susceptibility is defined by concentrations of antimicrobial yielding turbidity less than 50 per cent of that found in the growth control. Resistance is the presence of turbidity greater than 50 per cent of that in the growth control. Kurzynski (1976) has described a modification of this method in which the test is performed in thioglycollate broth incubated in air rather than anaerobically. This modification requires that the tubes be left at room temperature for two to three hours to ensure elution of the antimicrobial agent from the disks, since diffusion occurs more slowly because of the 0.05 per cent agar usually present in thioglycollate. The incubation time and determination of end-points are similar to those above, although with the more fastidious organisms 48 hours of incubation may be necessary.

Anaerobic Agar Dilution Testing. The basic principles of this test are the same as those previously described for routine agar dilution testing. However, there are several modifications due to the unique nature of the anaerobic organisms.

Medium. Brucella or brain-heart infusion agar with vitamin K_1, 10 μg/ml and 5 per cent whole or laked sheep blood, has been used by many investigators in the past; however, a subcommittee of the National Committee for Clinical Laboratory Standards, which has been developing a standard method for testing anaerobic bacteria, is recommending the Wilkins-Chalgren (1976) medium for this purpose.

The inoculum can be brought to desired density in thioglycollate-135 C without an indicator (Bio-Quest, Cockeysville, Md.) and enriched with hemin (0.005 per cent), menadione (0.002 per cent), and $NaHCO_3$ (1 mg/ml).

Inoculum. A 24- to 48-hour incubation is required to bring organism turbidity to the equivalent of a MacFarland 0.5 standard. There is no further dilution of the broth suspension, and inoculation is made onto the agar as described previously. Incubation is at 35°C. for 48 hours in an anaerobic jar or chamber. The remaining test procedure is carried out as described for the ICS agar dilution methodology.

Antimicrobials. The antimicrobials usually tested are those listed in Table 52–7 for the broth-disk method. The plates should be prepared within 18 to 24 hours of use and should be stored at room temperature to delay absorption of oxygen, which occurs more rapidly at lower temperatures.

Whenever this test is performed, a plate containing no antibiotics should be inoculated and incubated simultaneously with the test plates, in the same environment.

The agar dilution method lends itself very readily to the testing of large numbers of organisms; hence, its principal uses in testing anaerobes are in the evaluation of new antimicrobial agents and in epidemiologic surveys of collections of strains to determine whether or not alterations in susceptibility have occurred.

Anaerobic Micro Broth Dilution. The basic methodology, again, for testing anaerobes with the micro broth method is similar to that employed for regular aerobic organisms. The limitations of this method relate to the fact that the work should be performed, ideally, in an anaerobic chamber, which limits the ability of many laboratories to perform these tests.

Medium. Brucella or brain-heart infusion broth supplemented with menadione (0.005 per cent) and hemin (0.001 per cent) or Schaedler broth should be used for both inoculum preparation and for dilution of antimicrobials.

Disk Diffusion Susceptibility Testing for Anaerobic Organisms. Sutter (1975) has provided guidelines for disk diffusion testing of anaerobes. Freshly prepared *Brucella* agar containing 5 per cent defibrinated sheep blood and 0.5 μg/ml menadione is used in 90 × 15 mm Petri dishes. The agar is poured to a depth of 5 to 6 mm, and not more than 4 antibiotic disks are applied to each plate. A few colonies or a 3 mm loopful from a broth culture of each strain to be tested is inoculated into a tube containing thioglycollate 135-C medium to which is added 5 mg/ml hemin prior to autoclaving and 1 μg/ml $NaHCO_3$ plus 0.5 μg/ml of filter-sterilized menadione after autoclaving. These tubes are incubated for 4 to 6 hours and then diluted to the density of a 0.5 MacFarland standard.

Streaking of the agar surface is done according to the method of Bauer (1966) with cotton swabs (Acme Cotton Company, Valley Stream, Long Island, N.Y.), and the plates are incubated at 37°C. in anaerobic incubators. Results are read after approximately 24 hours by measuring the diameter of the zone of inhibition around the antibiotic disks. Interpretation of results is made according to criteria published by Sutter (1975). An anaerobic control strain, selected for its susceptibility to penicillin, should be tested simultaneously with the test bacteria in order to demonstrate appropriate function of the test.

The Category Method for Anaerobic Bacteria. The category test (Thornsberry, 1977a) has been shown to be simple and reproducible and is another method which will be mentioned in order to give appropriate alternatives for anaerobic susceptibility testing. This method tests anaerobes with two or three concentrations of appropriate antimicrobials that have been selected to conform generally to the categories of susceptibility suggested by the International Collaborative Study (p. 1326).

Medium. The concentrations of antimicrobial agents specified in Table 52–8 are prepared in pre-reduced Schaedler broth.

As with the broth-disk method of Wilkins (1973), the antimicrobial agents may also be added by means of paper disks; however, the authors (Thornsberry, 1977a) are careful to point out that it is impractical to use commercial disks, and advocate that disks of the proper concentrations can be easily prepared in the laboratory by adding the proper amount of antimicrobial to blank disks, drying them, and storing them with a desiccant at −70°C.

Table 52–8. CONCENTRATIONS OF ANTIMICROBIAL AGENTS TO BE USED IN CATEGORY TEST

Antimicrobial Agent	Concentration (μg/ml)
Penicillin G	0.25, 16, 128
Tetracycline	2, 8, 32
Clindamycin	2, 8, 64
Erythromycin	2, 4, 64
Chloramphenicol	1, 8

Inoculum. The inoculum is prepared by removing an amount of overnight growth from a Schaedler agar plate and suspending it in Schaedler broth in order to adjust the turbidity to that of a 0.5 MacFarland standard. Alternatively, an overnight broth culture can be adjusted to the same turbidity.

Test Performance. Antimicrobial solutions or disks are added to Schaedler broth so that the final concentrations are those listed in Table 52–8. A calibrated dropper is used to add 0.25 ml of the adjusted inoculum to each tube containing the antimicrobial and to a tube containing broth but no antimicrobial. The tubes are incubated anaerobically for 18 to 24 hours at 35°C. The end-point is the lowest concentration without macroscopic growth, and one should be careful to ensure that there is adequate growth in the control broth. The results can be reported as MIC's or as categories of susceptibility. For all but chloramphenicol three concentrations are tested, which allows interpretation as shown in Table 52–9.

Susceptibility Testing of *Haemophilus influenzae*. Susceptibility testing with *Haemophilus influenzae* has assumed increased significance in that this organism has also demonstrated the capacity to produce beta-lactamase and manifest absolute resistance to the penicillin and semi-synthetic penicillin compounds. For most serious infections, such as meningitis, determination of the MIC is desirable. One can also test for the production of beta-lactamase and in most circumstances this information is sufficient. There are rare strains of *H. influenzae* that demonstrate resistance to penicillin by mechanisms other than beta-lactamase; therefore, susceptibility testing assumes increased significance with this particular organism. Agar dilution testing of *H. influenzae* has already been described in this chapter (see p. 1328).

Broth Dilution Testing for Haemophilus influenzae. Schaedler's broth supplemented with 5 per cent Fildes reagent is used in either the microbroth or the macrobroth procedure (Thornsberry, 1977a), as has already been described. The inoculum can be prepared by suspending organisms taken from a chocolate agar plate, in Schaedler broth, to equal the density of a 0.5 MacFarland standard.

Interpretation. Susceptible strains of *H. influenzae* are inhibited by 1 μg/ml or less of ampicillin. Ampicillin-resistant strains generally have MIC's of 8 μg/ml or higher, although occasional ones may have an MIC value of 4 μg/ml. Strains from patients with meningitis with MIC values of 2 μg/ml or greater should be considered ampicillin-resistant (Thornsberry, 1977a).

Table 52–9. INTERPRETIVE GUIDELINES FOR CATEGORY METHOD OF SUSCEPTIBILITY TESTING

	Growth in Four Tubes			
Category	***Control***	***Low***	***Medium***	***High***
I	+	–	–	–
II	+	+	–	–
III	+	+	+	–
IV	+	+	+	+

Disk Diffusion Testing with Haemophilus influenzae. Mueller-Hinton agar (pH 7.2) should be supplemented with 1 per cent IsoVitaleX (BBL) and 1 per cent hemoglobin (Thornsberry, 1974). This preparation is superior to one with chocolatized sheep blood because the zones on chocolatized blood agar are very difficult to read. The disk diffusion test is carried out exactly as that described for the standard method, except that for ampicillin a zone diameter of 20 mm or greater defines susceptibility. Some ampicillin-resistant strains produce zone diameters close to 19 mm; however, there will almost always be varying numbers of colonies within this zone. Thornsberry (1977a) indicates that a 10-unit penicillin disk can also be used, as it discriminates between ampicillin-resistant and susceptible strains very well with the same zone diameter interpretive criteria as those described for ampicillin.

The susceptibility of *H. influenzae* to other antimicrobial agents can be determined by using the interpretive criteria listed in Table 52–5 (Thornsberry, 1977a).

Susceptibility Testing of *Staphylococcus aureus*. Problems associated with susceptibility testing of staphylococci fall into three main categories:

1. Detection of resistance to the semi-synthetic, penicillinase-resistant penicillins requires an incubation temperature of 35°C. Alternatively, detection of this resistance can be enhanced by using a heavy inoculum, extending the incubation time to 48 hours, or adding 5 per cent NaCl to the testing medium. For all practical purposes, unless there is a specific epidemiologic problem requiring added surveillance, an incubation temperature of 35°C. suffices.

2. Resistance to the semi-synthetic, penicillinase-resistant penicillins will not be reliably detected with cloxacillin or dicloxacillin (Drew, 1972). Susceptibility testing by the disk diffusion method should be done with methicillin, nafcillin, or oxacillin. Methicillin is probably the most widely used, but is also the least stable of the three compounds. Because resistance to methicillin is still uncommon in the United States, finding a resistant strain should prompt confirmation of its identity to be sure that it is *S. aureus* and repeat testing because of the possibility of reduced potency of the disk.

3. Staphylococci exist in which there is a large discrepancy between the MIC and MBC values when they are tested against the semi-synthetic penicillinase-resistant penicillins (Sabath, 1977). This phenomenon has been called "tolerance" and has led to a significant increase in the number of laboratory requests for both MBC and MIC determinations. It is estimated that as many as 40 per cent of the isolates of *Staphylococcus aureus* from clinically significant infections in hospital settings may demonstrate "tolerance." Both *Staphylococcus aureus* and enterococci may appear to be fully susceptible to a penicillin by MIC criteria, but they may be very resistant when one assesses the MBC of the penicillin or related compound.

Tolerance may be important in some patients and should be taken into account by the physician in the approach to the therapy of staphylococcal disease. It also has ramifications in the laboratory, not only in terms of additional requests for MBC testing, but also in the potential usage of combinations of antibiotics, i.e., an aminoglycoside and a semi-synthetic penicillinase-resistant penicillin, and the monitoring of therapy with aminoglycosides.

It should be noted at this point that *Staphylococcus epidermidis* is often resistant to the penicillinase-resistant, semi-synthetic penicillins (methicillin, nafcillin, and oxacillin).

Susceptibility Tests for *Neisseria gonorrhoeae*. Two types of resistance exist with *Neisseria gonorrhoeae.* One is a relative resistance which has been present for many years and seems to have reached a peak and remained stable over the recent years. This type of resistance has led to the current use of 4.8 million units of penicillin, in contrast to much lower dosages which at one time were uniformly effective in treating gonorrhea. A second type of resistance has manifested itself in recent years and is mediated through the production of penicillinase. Therefore, one can approach the assessment of susceptibility of *Neisseria gonorrhoeae* in two ways. One can test for its absolute susceptibility by means of the agar dilution test. Moreover, one can test for the production of beta-lactamase or penicillinase, as will be described in this section. A disk diffusion test was described by Ronald (1968) in which a zone diameter of 20 mm was equivalent to susceptibility of less than 1 unit of penicillin. This method did not gain wide acceptance; however, a modified disk diffusion test with the same zone diameter interpretive criterion has been shown to correlate with beta-lactamase production (Thornsberry, 1977a). In this test, an inoculum equivalent in density to a 0.5 MacFarland standard is applied, as for the standard disk diffusion method, to GC base agar supplemented with 1 per cent IsoVitaleX. A single 10 U penicillin disk is placed on the agar surface. Strains that produce beta-lactamase produce zone diameters of less than 19 mm. This method allows most laboratories to test for gonococcal susceptibility patterns and the likelihood of beta-lactamase production. Other than testing for beta-lactamase, there is seldom a need for susceptibility testing of *Neisseria gonorrhoeae,* except in instances of treatment failure, in epidemiologic investigations, or in studies of *in vitro* antibiotic susceptibility. In such instances, agar dilution studies can be performed. The growth from four to five colonies of the organism, grown on chocolate agar or modified Thayer-Martin medium, is suspended in TSB and adjusted to the appropriate density by comparison to a MacFarland 0.5 standard. A 1:20 dilution is made in broth and is streaked directly onto GC medium containing hemoglobin (1 g/100 ml), 1 per cent IsoVitaleX (BioQuest), or Supplement C (Difco) and the appropriate concentrations of antimicrobial. These plates should be used within 48 hours of preparation. They are incubated at 35°C. in an environment of increased CO_2 and are read at 24 hours if sufficient growth has occurred.

One should also test a control strain of *Neisseria gonorrhoeae* with known susceptibility, and it is recommended that *Sarcina lutea* be included to provide additional technical control. Barry (1976) stresses that the density of the inoculum is an important variable and suggests checking the adjusted cell suspension by diluting it by a factor of 50 and streaking it onto a chocolate agar plate with a 0.001 ml calibrated loop. If the inoculum is correct, from 10 to 100 colonies should grow on the agar.

Susceptibility Testing of *Neisseria meningitidis*. Susceptibility testing of *Neisseria meningitidis* is rarely required because beta-lactamase production by this species has not yet been demonstrated. Testing is usually carried out for research or epidemiologic purposes. However, since sulfonamides can prevent meningitis in close contacts of patients with meningococcal meningitis and because sulfonamide resistance is not uncommonly present in meningococci, susceptibility testing of sulfonamides may be necessary. A slight modification of the disk diffusion methodology, as described by Bennett (1968), is used with a zone diameter of 40 mm defining susceptibility. Susceptibility testing by the agar dilution method can also be carried out as described for *Neisseria gonorrhoeae.*

THE DETERMINATION OF BETA-LACTAMASE PRODUCTION

Beta-lactamase production is primarily determined with *H. influenzae, N. gonorrhoeae,* and *S. aureus.* Several methods exist that are applicable for testing these three organisms. Whereas the production of beta-lactamase is usually very rapidly demonstrated with *Haemophilus* and *Neisseria,* it can take longer to manifest itself with staphylococci, so that the tests should be allowed to incubate for at least one hour. Staphylococcal beta-lactamases are inducible, while the beta-lactamases of *H. influenzae* and *N. gonorrhoeae* are not.

Four tests will be described for the production of beta-lactamase. Each has its advantages and disadvantages (Thornsberry, 1977c). The reagents for each of the tests, with the exception of the chromogenic cephalosporin, are widely available and easy to prepare. For the purposes described above, the sensitivity and specificity of these tests are equivalent; however, the chromogenic cephalosporin test is more sensitive than the others for investigating the presence of beta-lactamases in other gram-negative bacilli, e.g., Enterobacteriaceae. Each of the tests can be performed rapidly and will provide results within minutes. The selection of one of these tests for routine purposes depends on various factors, including availability of reagents, stability of reagents, personal experience and expertise, ease of performance of the test, and clarity of end points.

CHROMOGENIC CEPHALOSPORIN TEST (O'Callaghan, 1972)

Reagents

Cephalosporin 87/312*
Dimethylsulfoxide (DMSO)
Phosphate buffer, pH 7

Monopotassium phosphate, M/15	39.2 ml
Disodium phosphate, M/15	60.8 ml

Dissolve cephalosporin in DMSO and mix in phosphate buffer to final concentration of 500 μg/ml.

Test

Microdilution Plate or Small Tube. Add 0.05 ml cephalosporin substrate to a well of a microdilution plate (or to a small tube). With a loop, remove the growth from several colonies of the test organism. Make a heavy turbid suspension in the cephalosporin solution. Mix for 1 minute. Observe for color change immediately, after 10 minutes, and after 1 hour. If the culture produces beta-lactamase, the color of the substrate will change from yellow to red. Beta-lactamase–producing *H. influenzae* or *N. gonorrhoeae* usually turn the solution red in less than 10 minutes, but staphylococci may require an hour. Run the test with a known beta-lactamase– and a non-beta-lactamase–producing strain of *N. gonorrhoeae, H. influenzae,* or *S. aureus.*

Agar Plate Modification. The agar plate should contain the organism in pure culture. Place a drop (approximately 0.05 ml) of the cephalosporin reagent on an area of bacterial growth: Tilt the plate slightly to permit the drop to spread across the plate. If the organism produces beta-lactamase, the reagent will turn red along the streak; if it is beta-lactamase–negative, the reagent will be yellow along the streak. Because the red color is not as easily seen as in the test done in the microdilution well, the test should be repeated in a microdilution well or small tube if there is any doubt about the result. Usually a positive test can be read immediately, but the plate should be re-examined after 10 minutes. Experience with staphylococci in this test is very limited.

---

*Glaxo, Ltd., Greenford, Middlesex UB6 OHE England.

Precautions

1. Primary isolation media (e.g., modified Thayer-Martin medium) may contain beta-lactamase–producing bacteria in addition to those of interest (e.g., *N. gonorrhoeae*) and may cause a false-positive test.

2. Clinical specimens (e.g., urethral discharge, vaginal secretion) cannot be tested directly with the chromogenic cephalosporin test.

RAPID MICROTUBE IODOMETRIC TEST (Catlin, 1975)

Reagents

Penicillin G powder
Phosphate buffer, pH 6
  Monopotassium phosphate, M/15 87.7 ml
  Disodium phosphate, M/15 17.7 ml
Starch
Iodine
Potassium iodide

Solution. Add sodium or potassium penicillin G powder (most readily available as sodium or potassium penicillin G for intravenous human use) to freshly prepared pH 6.0 phosphate buffer to obtain a solution with a concentration of 6000 μg/ml. Small aliquots of the penicillin solution can be dispensed into vials that can be tightly sealed and frozen in non–frost-free freezers. Frost-free freezers are unsuitable because repeated thawing cycles cause deterioration of the penicillin. Aliquots can be thawed and used for up to one week or as long as correct results are obtained with control cultures of known reactivity.

Starch Solution. Add 1.0 g of soluble starch to 100 ml of distilled water. Place in boiling water bath until the starch goes into solution. Prepare fresh or store in refrigerator for no more than one week. Smaller volumes of this 1 per cent solution can be made because 10 ml is enough for over 100 tests. Starch designated for use in iodometric tests is commercially available.

Iodine. Dissolve 2.03 g of iodine and 53.2 g of potassium iodide in 100 ml of distilled water. Store at room temperature in brown glass bottle. Prepare fresh when the solution develops excessive precipitate (usually several months). Run the test with known beta-lactamase–positive and beta-lactamase–negative strains of *N. gonorrhoeae, H. influenzae,* or *S. aureus.*

Test Procedure. Dispense 0.1 ml of the penicillin solution into a well of a microdilution plate or a small test tube. Remove several colonies of an 18- to 24-hour pure culture with a loop and make a *heavy* turbid suspension in the penicillin solution in the well. Stir for 30 seconds and *let the mixture stand for one hour at room temperature to allow time for the beta-lactamase to break down the penicillin to penicilloic acid. H. influenzae* and *N. gonorrhoeae* usually do not require an hour of incubation, but staphylococci may. Add 2 drops of starch solution to the suspension of bacteria and penicillin. Mix. Add 1 drop of iodine reagent. The solution will immediately turn blue because of the reaction of the iodine and the starch. If the iodine is added prematurely, the enzymatic reaction may stop and a false-negative test may result. Stir the mixture for one minute. Rapid decolorization indicates the production of beta-lactamase. If the solution remains blue for longer than 10 minutes, the organism did not produce the enzyme.

Precautions

1. Primary isolation medium (e.g., modified Thayer-Martin medium) may contain beta-lactamase–producing bacteria in addition to the bacteria of interest (e.g., *N. gonorrhoeae*) and cause a false-positive test.

2. Clinical specimens (e.g., urethral discharge, vaginal secretions) cannot be tested directly with the iodometric test.

RAPID SLIDE IODOMETRIC TEST (Rosenblatt, 1978)

Penicillin Solution. Dissolve penicillin (penicillin G, potassium, for injection U.S.P. [buffered], one million units per vial) in 1 ml sterile water and remove 0.15 ml aliquots for freezing at −20°C. (frozen vials may be used for as long as 30 days, but should be discarded after use, once thawed).

Iodine. Dissolve 1.5 g potassium iodine and 0.3 g iodine in 100 ml of 0.1 M phosphate buffer at pH 6.4. This buffer is prepared by the addition of 60 ml pH 6.0 buffer to 40 ml pH 7.0 buffer. The iodine solution is stored in a brown bottle at 4°C.

Starch Solution. Dissolve 0.4 g soluble starch (Difco) in 100 ml distilled water. Autoclave and store at 4°C.

A penicillin-iodine mixture is prepared by adding 1.1 ml of the iodine solution to a vial containing 0.5 ml of thawed penicillin G. Once this mixture has been prepared it should be used within one hour. A loopful of test organisms is removed from growth on the surface of an agar plate and emulsified in 1 drop of the penicillin-iodine mixture on an ordinary glass microscope slide. Immediately, one drop of starch solution is added. A negative test for penicillinase is indicated by the development of a purple or lavender color which remains for 5 minutes.

A white color indicates a positive test. Most reactions will be complete by 30 seconds, with a final reading taken at 5 minutes for the detection of small amounts of penicillinase.

RAPID ACIDIMETRIC TEST FOR BETA-LACTAMASE PRODUCTION IN BACTERIA (Thornsberry, 1977c)

Reagents

Phenol red solution, 0.5%
Penicillin G
Sodium hydroxide, 1 M

Two ml of 0.5 per cent phenol red solution is added to 16.6 ml of sterile distilled water. This solution is then added to a vial containing 20 million units of potassium penicillin G (Pfizer). Sodium hydroxide (1 M) is added drop by drop until the test solution turns violet (pH 8.5). The test solution is either used immediately or divided into portions in screwcapped tubes and frozen at −60°C. for as long as one week.

Test Procedure. Dip a capillary tube (0.7 to 1.0 mm OD) into the test solution and allow liquid to flow by capillary action for a distance of 1 to 2 cm into the tube. The tip of the capillary tube is scraped lightly across several *H. influenzae* colonies from an agar plate (chocolate agar plus 1 per cent IsoVitaleX [BioQuest]) that has been incubated 24 hours, so that a plug of bacteria fills the bottom of the tube. Allow no air to be trapped between the test solution and the bacteria, since the two must be in contact. The filled capillary tubes are incubated at room temperature in a vertical position. This is achieved by sticking the empty end of the capillary tube into clay and letting it hang straight down. If the organism produces beta-lactamase, the test solution turns a bright yellow in 5 to 15 minutes. In the tests with organisms that do not produce beta-lactamase, the test solution either does not change color at all or changes to no more than a pale pink color. Include a penicillin-resistant *S. aureus* as a positive control and a penicillin-susceptible *S. aureus* as a negative control with each *Haemophilus* tested.

SPECIAL TESTS

Bactericidal Activity Testing. The majority of bacterial susceptibility testing is to determine inhibitory end-points. While antimicrobials may exert a killing effect in their action on bacteria and the concentration of antibiotic required for this lethal or bactericidal activity may, in fact, be very close to that of the inhibitory concentration, there may be situations, as with some staphylococci and enterococci, in which the inhibitory and bactericidal concentrations vary considerably. In addition, the assessment of an antimicrobial's bactericidal activity becomes all the more important in the patient whose immune defense mechanisms are compromised. In this circumstance an adjustment of antimicrobial therapy may well be warranted on the basis of the bactericidal test result.

Recently, the "minimal lethal concentration" (MLC) has been proposed for the effect previously known as the minimal bactericidal concentration (MBC). The reader should be aware that the terms are analogous.

In order to establish the MBC or MLC of an antimicrobial, one begins by performing a standard broth dilution test, as for determining the MIC. For this test, however, it is necessary to quantitate the inoculum; this may be done by streaking 0.1 ml of 1:100 and 1:1000 dilutions of the inoculum over an agar surface. After the inhibitory phase of the test has been completed, a 0.01 ml calibrated loop is used to subculture from each tube to a quadrant of a blood agar plate. The plates are then incubated overnight, and the MBC or MLC is the lowest concentration (in μg/ml) of antimicrobial, subculture of which is lethal to 99.9 per cent of the original inoculum.

This method provides the greatest efficiency for the clinical laboratory. Were one to perform bactericidal testing for reference or investigational purposes, a more carefully defined and volumetrically determined procedure should be used.

Combination Testing. Therapy in serious infections is very often approached with combinations of antimicrobials. In the compromised patient and in unusual clinical circumstances, testing of the combined action of antimicrobials may be warranted. There are several ways in which this testing can be accomplished, although what is described here is meant to be a practical method that can be used efficiently and economically in the clinical laboratory. An approach to testing combinations of three or more antimicrobials has been described by Berenbaum (1978).

Materials. The test procedure outlined here requires two microdilution plates, a set of 15 μl pipette droppers, and 50 μl diluters. Mueller-Hinton broth is used, and the antimicrobials to be tested are made up in solutions so that they can be utilized alone and in various combinations. The inoculum density should be standardized with a 0.5 MacFarland standard and then diluted 1:100 in Mueller-Hinton broth.

Procedure. Two microdilution plates are placed side by side, and the first four rows of the second plate are relabeled I through L. Only four rows are used in this second plate (Fig. 52–2). Fifty μl of MHB is dispensed to all wells except A-1 with a 50 μl pipette dropper. The antibiotic solutions are labeled No. 1 and No. 2 and are diluted to contain concentrations equivalent to four times those finally desired. One hundred μl of antibiotic solution No. 1 is added to well A-1, and 50 μl to the rest of the wells in column No. 1 (B through L) with the pipette dropper. The antibiotic in the first well (column 1) of each row is then serially diluted across the plates through column 11 (do not dilute into wells in column 12). With the 50 μl pipette dropper, dispense 50 μl of antibiotic solution No. 2 into each well in row A (1 through 12). Again, with the 50 μl diluters, dilute serially down each column from each well in row A through wells in row K (do not dilute into wells in row L). Add 50 μl of the standardized inoculum to each of the 144 wells using a 50 μl pipette dropper. Cover the plate with a plastic tape and incubate. The MIC for antimicrobial No. 1 can be obtained from the wells in row L and the MIC for antimicrobial No. 2 from the wells in column 12. Well L-12 contains no antimicrobial and serves

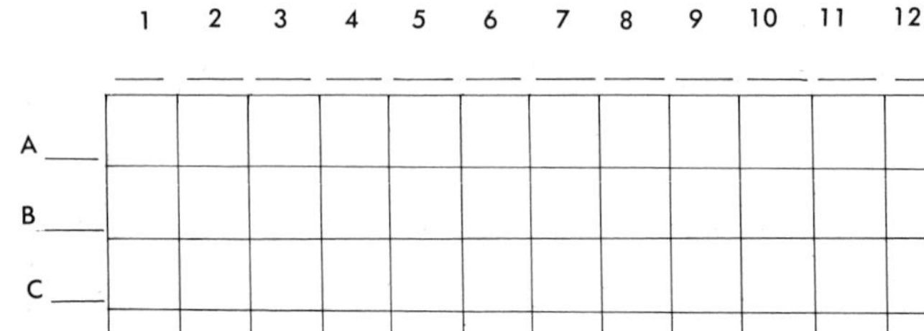

Figure 52–2. Arrangement of tubes and chart for results of combination study of two antimicrobial agents.

as the growth control. Results are recorded on a chart as shown in Figure 52–2. This chart serves as a laboratory work sheet and for plotting an isobologram. A straight line is drawn between the MIC values of each antimicrobial. A curve is constructed from the MIC of the combinations of the two antimicrobials. If the curve falls below the line that has been drawn between two MIC values of each antimicrobial, a synergistic effect has been demonstrated (Fig. 52–3). If the curve is outside this line, then antagonism has been demonstrated. A detailed discussion of the mathematical considerations involved in the determination of synergy can be found elsewhere (Berenbaum, 1978).

QUALITY CONTROL OF SUSCEPTIBILITY TESTING

Quality control is extremely important in antimicrobial susceptibility testing and for the other tests performed in the support of antimicrobial therapy. All of the various parameters of each test should be regularly evaluated in order to ensure confidence in the performance of the test.

This section will outline an overall quality control program for the various tests that have been described.

STOCK CULTURES

One should maintain a collection of all organisms needed for quality control of the media, the actual tests themselves, and any reagents that may be needed. Stock cultures of most organisms may be maintained on sealed agar deeps at 25°C. in the dark, at −70°C., or in a lyophilized state. Stock cultures of organisms with ATCC designation may be obtained from the American Type Culture Collectin (12301 Parklawn Drive, Rockville, Md. 20852): *Staphylococcus aureus* ATCC 25923, *Escherichia coli* ATCC 25922, and *Pseudomonas aeruginosa* ATCC 27853 for disk diffusion susceptibility testing; *S. aureus* ATCC 29213 and *Streptococcus faecalis* ATCC 29212 for dilution susceptibility testing; *S. aureus* ATCC 25923, *P. aeruginosa* ATCC 27853, and *E. coli* ATCC 29194 for Autobac I; and *Bacillus subtilis* ATCC 6633, *Klebsiella pneumoniae* ATCC 27799, and *Clostridium perfringens* UUMC 9758 for antimicrobial assays.

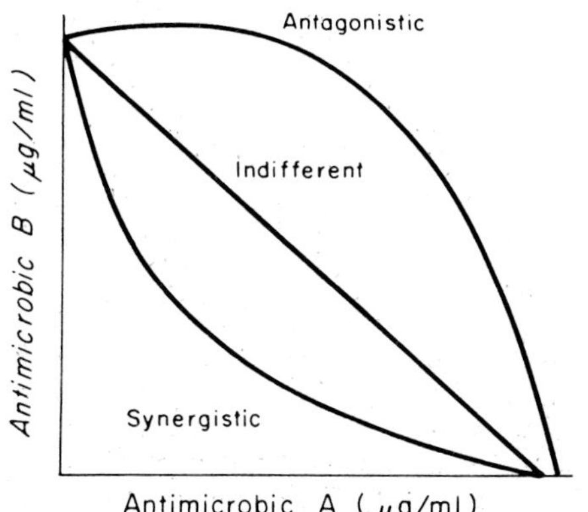

Figure 52–3. Isobologram portraying three possible results when two antimicrobials (A and B) are tested singly and in various combinations; either MIC or MLC endpoints may be plotted. A straight line joining the values obtained with each drug separately represents an isobol which indicates indifference. Antagonism is indicated by an isobol which bows upward away from the coordinates, and a bowing toward the coordinates indicates synergism. (With permission from Barry, A. L., and Sabath, L. D.: *In* Lennett, E. H., Spaulding, E. H., and Truant, J. P. [eds.]: Manual of Clinical Microbiology. 2nd ed. Washington, D.C., American Society for Microbiology, 1974. p. 431.)

Stock Culture Storage

Gram-Negative Bacilli. These can be stored on small soybean-casein digest agar slants at room temperature in the dark and should be transferred weekly or twice monthly to new slants. Reference strains of these organisms should be kept in a lyophilized or frozen state in the event that the performance of the organisms on slants should change. Both the *E. coli* (ATCC 25922) and the *K. pneumoniae* (ATCC 27799) have proved to be extremely stable over many years. The *P. aeruginosa* (ATCC 27853) control strain, if subcultured daily, has a tendency to develop colonies resistant to carbenicillin. It is suggested that subculturing of this strain on a daily basis be limited to one week and that a fresh subculture be obtained from a lyophilized or frozen stock culture (Thornsberry, 1977a).

Gram-Positive Cocci. The *S. aureus* (ATCC 25923) and *S. faecalis* (ATCC 29212) are maintained on sheep blood agar at room temperature or transferred weekly or when new sheep blood plates are tested. Again, reference cultures are maintained in a lyophilized or frozen state in case questions arise about organism performance.

Clostridium perfringens. *Clostridium perfringens* can be maintained at room temperature in chopped meat medium and needs to be transferred to new chopped meat medium only every three months.

Media

Sterility. A sample of each lot of plated medium prepared in the clinical laboratory should be incubated to check for sterility. Plates containing media from commercial sources should also be checked for sterility.

Performance. Mueller-Hinton agar plates are tested with both *E. coli* (ATCC 25922) and *S. aureus* (ATCC 25923). These are incubated in an aerobic environment for 24 hours at 35°C. The pH of the medium should be 7.2 to 7.4 at 25°C., and the agar depth should be 4 to 5 mm. The surface of the agar should be even and the depth of the agar uniform. Mueller-Hinton broth is also tested with the same control organisms as the Mueller-Hinton agar plates.

Antimicrobial Disks and Stock Solutions. Stock antimicrobial solutions are frozen in readily usable aliquots. Once thawed they are not to be reused. Control organisms should be tested each time a new lot of antimicrobial is prepared or each time a new vial of antimicrobial disks is to be used. The vial of disks should be tested the day prior to its being used on a routine basis. All antimicrobial materials should be labeled as to the date of expiration, the date received in the laboratory, and the date opened. Unused lots of stock solutions should be discarded after the expiration date. Stock solutions can be stored at −20°C. or below for six months, with the exception of the penicillins and nitrofurantoin. All antimicrobial disks should be frozen at −20°C. in containers with desiccant. After removal from the freezer, disks should be allowed to equilibrate to room temperature before the containers are opened.

Procedural Checks. Each procedure has its own quality control checks. These are listed in the order that they have been presented in this chapter.

Dilution Testing. Dilution test series should be inoculated with the control strains listed above for dilution testing. At the Mayo Clinic, *E. coli* (ATCC 25922), *S. aureus* (ATCC 25923), and a strain of *P. aeruginosa* are used on a daily basis for quality control of agar dilution tests. The means and ranges of minimal inhibitory concentrations with these organisms are published elsewhere (Washington, 1974a). In agar dilution testing, it is important to inoculate an agar plate without antimicrobials in order to verify the viability of the test organism. In addition, each well of the seed plate should be subcultured to a quadrant of a blood agar plate in order to verify the purity of the inoculum. Dilution testing, in general, presents some special quality control problems. With all but the category or abbreviated methods of dilution testing, each dilution set will contain 8 to 12 twofold dilution steps. Control organisms should ideally provide a means of evaluating the performance of each antimicrobial agent by providing MIC values that are at least one two-fold (log_2) dilution from either end of the dilution scale for each antimicrobial being evaluated. Since the selection of the control strains for disk diffusion testing was made on the basis of their susceptibility (vs. resistance) to various antimicrobials, it has been suggested that *S. aureus* ATCC 29213 and *S. faecalis* ATCC 29212 be used for quality control of dilution tests. These strains are more likely to yield MIC values above the lowest level of susceptibility tested (Thornsberry, 1977a). It should be noted that the only difference between *S. aureus* ATCC 25923 and *S. aureus* ATCC 29213 is that the former does not produce beta-lactamase, whereas the latter does and is, therefore, resistant to penicillin. Extensive data regarding the MIC values of various antimicrobials with these strains are not yet available.

The two control strains described above should be tested with each set of dilutions performed. Since most laboratories will perform susceptibility tests of a number of organisms each day, it is to be expected that, in order to control the performance of dilution tests, control organisms should be run with each group of organisms tested. This is especially important with broth dilution tests because of their vulnerability to inoculum size variations.

Since the 0.5 MacFarland turbidity standard is used for adjusting the inoculum of all antimicrobial susceptibility tests, it should be carefully maintained, as has already been described in this chapter.

Autobac I. Because disks are used as the source of antimicrobial and because of the number of test variables, including instrument function, control strains should be tested regularly in the Autobac. The manufacturer provides detailed quality control guidelines for those who purchase this instrument.

Disk Diffusion Testing. Considerable work has been done with the quality control of the disk diffusion methodology, and the performance of the three ATCC strains used for quality control has been carefully defined. The control limits for the zone diameters of inhibition of the control strains are listed in Tables 52–10 to 52–12. These are important tables for those using the disk diffusion method and should be maintained for reference purposes. Some antimicrobials are tested against two or three of the control strains. This overlap provides a double check on the performance of most antimicrobials and on the test itself.

The control strains should be tested daily or at least each time the test is conducted, and the zone diameters should be recorded on a quality control chart for easy visualization. Should the zone diameters fall outside the expected ranges, an investigation must be made to determine what has gone wrong.

Pretest monitoring of the performance of new vials of antimicrobial disks must be performed to detect any potential problems with the disks in this vial. This step is highly recommended, as it will obviate the necessity of having to repeat all of the susceptibility tests any time a disk from a new vial might perform poorly. At least in some instances, it will assist in making a decision as to whether or not to report susceptibility testing results if the zone diameters of the control strain(s) are not within the control limits on a particular day's run. If problems do occur, a log should be kept as to what they are and their disposition.

Table 52–10. CONTROL LIMITS FOR MONITORING PRECISION AND ACCURACY OF INHIBITORY ZONE DIAMETERS OBTAINED IN GROUPS OF FIVE SEPARATE OBSERVATIONS WITH ESCHERICHIA COLI ATCC 25922*

Antimicrobial Agent	Disk Content (μg)	Individual Test Control (Zone Diam. mm)	Accuracy Control (Zone Diam. mm)[a]	Precision Control (Range of Five Values[b])	
				Maximum	*Average*[c]
Ampicillin	10	15–20	15.8–19.2	6	2.9
Carbenicillin	100	24–29	25.0–28.0	7	3.5
Cephalothin	30	18–23	18.8–22.2	6	2.9
Chloramphenicol	30	21–27	22.0–26.0	7	3.5
Colistin	10	11–15	11.7–14.3	4	2.3
Erythromycin	15	8–14	9.0–13.0	7	3.5
Gentamicin	10	19–26	20.2–24.8	8	4.1
Kanamycin	30	17–25	18.3–23.7	9	4.7
Neomycin	30	17–23	18.0–22.0	6	3.5
Polymyxin B	300 U	12–16	12.7–15.3	4	2.3
Streptomycin	10	12–20	13.3–18.7	9	4.7
Tetracycline	30	18–25	19.2–23.8	8	4.1
Tobramycin	10	18–26			
Trimethoprim-sulfamethoxazole	1.25 / 23.75	24–32	25.3–30.7	9	4.7

*From Thornsberry (1977c).

[a]Mean of five values.

[b]Maximum value minus minimum value obtained in a series of five consecutive tests should not exceed the listed maximum limits, and the mean should fall within the range listed under "accuracy control."

[c]In a continuing series of ranges from consecutive groups of five tests each, the average range should approximate the listed value.

Table 52–11. CONTROL LIMITS FOR MONITORING PRECISION AND ACCURACY OF INHIBITORY ZONE DIAMETERS OBTAINED IN GROUPS OF FIVE SEPARATE OBSERVATIONS WITH STAPHYLOCOCCUS AUREUS ATCC 25923*

Antimicrobial Agent	Disk Content (μg)	Individual Test Control (Zone Diam. mm)	Accuracy Control (Zone Diam. mm)[a]	Precision Control (Range[b] of Five Values)	
				Maximum	*Average*[c]
Ampicillin	10	24–35	25.8–33.2	13	6.4
Cephalothin	30	25–37	27.0–35.0	14	7.0
Chloramphenicol	30	19–26	20.2–24.8	8	4.1
Clindamycin	2	23–29	24.0–28.0	7	3.5
Erythromycin	15	23–30	23.3–28.7	9	4.7
Gentamicin	10	19–27	20.3–25.7	9	4.7
Kanamycin	30	19–26	20.2–24.8	8	4.1
Methicillin	5	17–22	17.8–21.2	6	2.9
Neomycin	30	18–26	19.3–24.7	9	4.7
Penicillin G	10 U	26–37	27.8–35.2	13	6.4
Polymyxin B	300 U	7–13			
Streptomycin	10	14–22	15.3–20.7	9	4.7
Tetracycline	30	19–28	20.5–26.5	11	5.2
Tobramycin	10	19–29			
Vancomycin	30	15–19	15.7–18.3	4	2.3
Trimethoprim-sulfamethoxazole	1.25 23.75	24–32	25.0–31.0	7	3.5

*From Thornsberry (1977c).
[a]See footnote a in Table 52–10.
[b]See footnote b in Table 52–10.
[c]See footnote c in Table 52–10.

Other Susceptibility Testing. Currently, there are no established reference strains for control of susceptibility tests of anaerobic bacteria, haemophili, and neisseriae. Therefore, the laboratory should attempt to maintain stock cultures of each of these organisms for control purposes. *Neisseria* and *Haemophilus* species are very difficult to maintain in a clinical laboratory setting short of freezing at −70°C., and, even there, there is considerable risk of loss of viability, especially during the freezing and thawing processes themselves.

Proficiency Testing. Proficiency testing for clinical laboratories is an important part of monitoring of actual performance. It may be carried out with well-characterized internal unknowns or with external unknowns provided by the proficiency testing program conducted by the College of American Pathologists or by the Centers for Disease Control.

Table 52–12. SUGGESTED QUALITY CONTROL LIMITS FOR INHIBITORY ZONE DIAMETERS WHEN TESTING WITH PSEUDOMONAS AERUGINOSA ATCC 27853*

Antimicrobial Agent	Disk Content (μg)	Individual Test Control Zone Diameter (mm)
Carbenicillin	100	19–25
Gentamicin	10	16–22
Tobramycin	10	19–25
Polymyxin B	300 U	13–18
Colistin	10	11–15
Tetracycline	30	6–14
Chloramphenicol	30	6–12

*From Thornsberry (1977c).

ASSAYS OF ANTIMICROBIAL AGENTS

Indications for Assays. Basically, the assessment of the concentration of an antimicrobial in the serum or a body fluid of a patient is made in order to determine potential effect of that agent or the likelihood of toxicity. The circumstances in which antimicrobial assays are ordered, therefore, are those in which a low therapeutic-toxic ratio may exist, as in the case of the aminoglycosides or of chloramphenicol in newborn infants. A second circumstance would be in a patient in whom the anticipated clinical effect has not occurred, possibly owing to individual variations in the pharmacokinetics of the antimicrobial in the patient or to particular characteristics of the patient, organism, or antimicrobial that interfere with the activity of the antimicrobial. It is not within the scope of this chapter to go into all of the factors that can lead to the failure of antimicrobial therapy; however, it should be pointed out that these factors must be assessed because something can often be done to obviate their effects in the patient. A third circumstance in which antimicrobial assays become important is in the treatment of severe local infections, where fluid specimens may be available for assay, or in situations where the underlying disease of the patient is such that the antibiotic must do more of the job of eradicating the organism than would be the case in a normal patient with appropriately functioning host defense capabilities.

There are many methods for performing antimicrobial assays, including chemical, turbidimetric, agar diffusion, pH alteration and inhibition, enzymatic, radioimmunoassay, hemoglobin reduction, chromatographic, and many other techniques. Radioimmunoassay (RIA) and high pressure liquid chromatography (HPLC) have opened a new era in the assay of antimicrobials; however, not only is there a substantial investment in the equipment to perform these tests, but a certain level of expertise is required. These tests, nonetheless, will become more and more available in the future. In the interim and for those clinical laboratories where the availability of this instrumentation will continue to be a problem, there are several bioassay means that can be used very effectively to assay most antimicrobials. In addition, there are several innovations being used which will allow for greater ease in testing for antimicrobials in the presence of other agents being used in combination therapy. The three test organisms listed in Table 52–13 cover well over 90 per cent of the assay requests at the University of Utah Medical Center. Currently, for the high volume assay requests (for gentamicin) we use the radioimmunoassay (RIA) during the daytime hours and utilize the bioassay for single test requests in the evening and on weekends. For the less frequently used aminoglycosides, we continue to do the bioassay, as it is more economical. If more than three aminoglycoside assays can be done on a daily basis, RIA is cost-justifiable. The organisms used in the bioassay of antibiotic levels in serum and body fluids are listed in Table 52–13. It is not within the scope of this chapter to discuss the radioimmunoassay procedures in detail, as they are discussed elsewhere in this volume.

***Bacillus subtilis* Assay.** The *Bacillus subtilis* assay can be used for antimicrobials listed in Table 52–13 when no other antibiotics are present. It can also be used as a general method for assaying the aminoglycoside antibiotics in the presence of beta-lactam antibiotics if beta-lactamase is added to inactivate the cephalosporins and penicillins. Therefore, it has broad applicability and is presented here not only to provide an alternative for the testing of the aminoglycosides but also as a method for assaying antibiotics not covered by the other assay methods. The method outlined here is based on the description by Sabath (1974a).

Preparation of Assay Strain. The assay organism is the spore form of *Bacillus subtilis* ATCC 6633, which can be used as a lyophilized preparation (Difco Laboratories, Detroit, Mich.) or prepared spores as described elsewhere (Sabath, 1974a).

Preparation and Storage of Assay Plates. Plates for assay are prepared by adding 0.1 ml of the *B. subtilis* spore suspension to 100 ml of molten medium (Difco antibiotic assay medium No. 5 or Grove and Randall medium No. 5) at 48 to 65°C. and pouring 5 ml of the seeded agar into 100 mm plastic Petri dishes, which are allowed to remain on a level surface (check with spirit level) at room temperature until the agar has hardened. The plates can be used immediately, or they can be stored at 4°C. in sealed plastic bags: plates stored for less than 2 weeks provide results after 2 hours of incubation, while those stored for 2 to 6 weeks require 4 to 5 hours of incubation before readings can be made.

Procedure. The assay of a single serum sample requires two assay plates and 16 0.25 inch (0.6 cm) paper disks No. 740-E (Schleicher and Schuell Company, Keene, N.H.). The disks are arranged in four rows of four disks inside the lid of one of the assay plates, and 0.02 ml of the sample is placed on each of the four disks in the top row. Normal human sera (previously checked to be sure it does not contain antibacterial activity) are prepared with 12, 6, and 1.5 μg/ml for the gentamicin serum assay (suggested standards for other assays are streptomycin, 25, 12.5, and 3.1 μg/ml; vancomycin, 40, 20, and 10 μg/ml; kanamycin, 27, 9, and 3 μg/ml; and tobramycin and neomycin, 12, 6, 1.5 μg/ml), and 0.02 ml of each standard is placed on each of the four paper disks in the bottom row. A reference mark should be made on the bottom of each assay plate to designate the location of the 12-μg standard on the surface of the seeded agar. Disks with samples for assay are placed on the surface of the agar in a clockwise sequence. The duplicate disks containing samples are placed on the agar surface of the same plate so that pairs containing the same fluid are opposite each other. The other eight disks are placed in identical fashion to form a ring on the surface of the seeded agar in the second plate, and the two assay plates are placed on a level shelf at 37°C.

Incubation and Reading. Zone diameters of inhibition can be measured with a ruler or, for greater accuracy, with a vernier caliper after approximately four hours of incubation. The rapidity of formation of zones depends upon how long the plates have been stored.

Calculation. The results are calculated by plotting a dose response ("standard") curve (Fig. 52–4) on semilogarithmic paper, relating the concentration (μg/ml) of antibiotic in

Table 52–13. ORGANISMS TO BE USED IN BIOASSAY OF ANTIBIOTICS IN SERUM AND BODY FLUIDS

Antimicrobial	Test Organism	Antimicrobials that Do Not Interfere with Test Results
Ampicillin	*Clostridium perfringens*	Aminoglycosides
Amikacin	*Klebsiella pneumoniae* ATCC 27799	Ampicillin, carbenicillin, cephalothin, chloramphenicol, clindamycin, other penicillins
Carbenicillin	*C. perfringens*	Aminoglycosides
Cephalothin	*Bacillus subtilis* ATCC 6633	
Cephazolin	*B. subtilis* ATCC 6633	
Clindamycin	*C. perfringens*	Aminoglycosides
Chloramphenicol	*C. perfringens*	Aminoglycosides
Gentamicin	*K. pneumoniae* ATCC 27799	See amikacin above
Nafcillin	*B. subtilis* ATCC 6633	
Penicillin	*B. subtilis* ATCC 6633	
Tobramycin	*K. pneumoniae* ATCC 27799	See amikacin above
Vancomycin	*C. perfringens*	Aminoglycosides

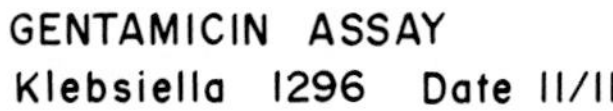

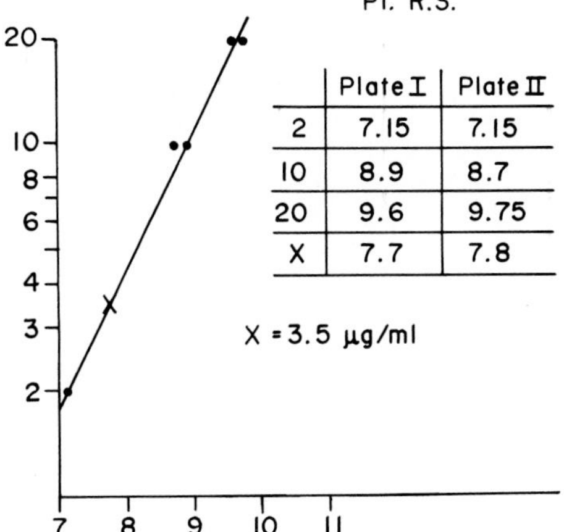

Figure 52–4. Standard curve of *Klebsiella pneumoniae* ATCC 27799 with gentamicin in bioassay.

the standard sera (log scale) to the zone diameter (mm) of inhibition. A separate curve is plotted for each of the two plates. Each point plotted represents the mean of the duplicate standards, as do diameters of the zones of inhibition around the two sample disks on each plate. The concentration in the unknown serum being assayed is extrapolated from the standard curve.

Assay of Samples Containing More Than One Antibiotic. The agar diffusion assay described above can be used to measure gentamicin or other aminoglycosides in the presence of any other penicillin or cephalosporin currently in use in the United States by simply adding 0.02 ml of beta-lactamase II (Whatman Biochemicals, Maidenhead, Surrey, England) to 0.1 ml of the serum for assay a few minutes before loading the disks (in calculating results, allow for dilution of sample by enzyme fluid by increasing "apparent" gentamicin value by 20 per cent). Alternatively, a beta-lactamase II may be prepared by simply growing *Bacillus cereus* 569 (ATCC 27348) at 37°C. for 18 hours in Difco brain-heart infusion broth containing 20 µg of cephalothin per ml and using the supernatant fluid as a crude beta-lactamase II. Should a non–beta-lactam antibiotic, such as tetracycline or clindamycin, be present, the assay should be performed with a test organism highly resistant to the interfering antibiotic.

Another bioassay, developed by Lund (1973), for the rapid measurement of aminoglycosides in blood and other body fluids, especially for those in which there are other antimicrobial agents, utilizes a multiply resistant *Klebsiella pneumoniae* (ATCC 27799) (Table 52–14). The basic principles of this test are the same as those described for the *B. subtilis* assay; however, the advantages of using the *Klebsiella* are that non–beta-lactam antibiotics do not interfere with the bioassay of aminoglycosides. The reader should consult the description by Lund (1973) for details of performing this bioassay.

Assay for Antibiotics Other Than Aminoglycosides. There are numerous bioassay procedures described for antibiotics other than aminoglycosides; however, the presence of aminoglycosides in the fluid to be assayed usually interferes with reliable measurement of the non-aminoglycosidic antibiotic. In these instances, one may use *Clostridium perfringens* as the test organism for bioassays of penicillins (except nafcillin), clindamycin, chloramphenicol, and vancomycin (Sabath, 1974b), since *C. perfringens* is resistant to the aminoglycosides.

Table 52–14. SUSCEPTIBILITY OF KLEBSIELLA ATCC 27799 TO 19 ANTIBIOTICS

Antibiotic	MIC*	Zone Size†
Ampicillin	>1000	6
Amikacin	0.8	
Carbenicillin	>2000	6
Cephalothin	300	6
Chloramphenicol	>2000	6
Clindamycin	500	6
Colistin	3.1	14
Erythromycin	800	8
Gentamicin	1.5	20
Kanamycin	>1000	6
Methicillin	>1000	6
Nalidixic acid	12.5	16
Nitrofurantoin	500	7
Penicillin G	>2000	6
Polymyxin B	1.5	15
Streptomycin	>1000	6
Tetracycline	>2000	6
Tobramycin	0.2	6
Vancomycin		6

*Minimum inhibitory concentration in µg/ml (U/ml for penicillin G and polymyxin B).

†Inhibition zone diameter in mm from disk diffusion method.

Interpretation of Assay Results. Interpretation of results of antimicrobial assays requires a knowledge of the pharmacokinetics of the agent in question, the timing of collection of the sample for assay, the status of the patient's renal and hepatic function, and the potential interactions of antimicrobial combinations. Anticipated peak serum and urine concentrations with moderate doses of antimicrobials are listed in Table 52–15.

Serum Bactericidal Testing. The serum bactericidal or Schlichter test is often used to monitor the therapy of patients with endocarditis and osteomyelitis and for evaluating therapy in other serious infections (Jawetz, 1962; Klastersky, 1974; Pien, 1974; Schlichter, 1947). Much confusion about this test exists in the literature because of the lack of a standardized method for performing it (Pien, 1974). In fact, the original test described by Schlichter (1947) was a serum inhibitory titer at the anticipated nadir or trough antimicrobial level. In principle, it involves serial dilution of the patient's serum during antimicrobial therapy to determine the maximum dilution or titer of antimicrobial activity of the serum/antibiotic combination against the organism isolated from an infectious process in the patient being studied. The inoculum should be quantitated in order to give an indication of the sensitivity of the test and also to provide a means by which one may assess the reproducibility or precision of the test should repeat determinations be necessary. The interpretation of this test should not be generalized to all infections. One may anticipate that the effect achieved in the patient is adequate if a peak level of bactericidal activity has been demonstrated in a serum dilution of 1:8 or greater. In staphylococcal endocarditis, a titer of 1:32 or greater is desirable. Whereas this test may be extremely helpful in predicting the outcome of osteomyelitis and endocarditis, it has been our experience that

Table 52–15. ANTICIPATED PEAK ANTIBIOTIC SERUM LEVELS (MODERATE DOSE)

Antimicrobial	Serum Concentration (μg/ml)	Urine Concentration (μg/ml)
Amikacin (I.M.)	10–25	150–250
Amoxicillin (P.O.)	5–7	1000–1500
Ampicillin (P.O.)	2–4	100–600
(I.V.)	3–7	100–600
Carbenicillin (P.O.)	5–15	600–1200
(I.V.)	100–200	600–1500
Cefazolin (I.M.)	25–50	1500–3000
Cephalexin (P.O.)	6–20	800–2000
Cephalothin (I.V.)	10–60	1000–1500
Chloramphenicol (P.O.)	4–14	50–120
Clindamycin (P.O.)	2–5	8–25
(I.V.)	10–20	20–45
Colistimethate	4–8	50–250
Erythromycin (P.O.)	1–4	15–50
(I.V.)	5–15	50–200
Gentamicin (I.M.)	4–7	100–300
Kantamycin (I.M.)	12–30	150–300
Methicillin (I.V.)	10–20	50–120
Penicillin G (P.O.)	0.5	70–100
Polymyxin B (I.M.)	2–6	15
Tetracyclines (P.O.)	1–4	1200
(I.M.)	4–6	100–300
Tobramycin (I.M.)	4–7	100–300

the test is not as predictive of outcome when prosthetic devices are present. In certain kinds of infections, therefore, the serum bactericidal test is an indicator of therapeutic effect and a predictor of therapeutic success.

To perform the test, it is necessary to use the organism isolated from the patient's site of infection. If the patient has endocarditis, then the organism is taken from the blood. If the patient has osteomyelitis, then the organism is either a blood stream isolate or an isolate aspirated directly from the lesion. The organism is inoculated into 4 ml of Trypticase soy broth, which is incubated at 35°C. for four hours or until its turbidity matches that of an 0.5 MacFarland standard. It should be noted that endocarditis may be caused by slow-growing organisms, such as viridans streptococci, which may require the addition of 5 per cent horse serum to TSB and overnight incubation. Where serum has been added, as a facilitator of growth, it should be used throughout the entire test in order to enhance the growth of the organism.

A sample of blood is obtained from the patient, usually at the anticipated peak antimicrobial level. The serum is separated aseptically and stored at −20°C. until used. If the patient has a positive blood culture, the serum should be filtered prior to use.

Sterile TSB, 0.5 ml, is pipetted into each of 7 tubes. The patient's serum is thawed and mixed, and 0.5 ml is added to a tube without broth. This serves as an undiluted test tube. A half milliliter of serum is added to the first tube containing TSB; it is mixed and 0.5 ml is then serially diluted through all of the remaining tubes; 0.5 ml is discarded from tube 6, and tube 7 serves as the organism growth control and contains only broth.

The adjusted inoculum of the test organism is diluted 1:1000, and 0.5 ml of this dilution is added to each tube in the series, mixed, and incubated at 35°C. for 24 hours. With a 0.001 ml calibrated loop, duplicate blood agar plates are streaked with the inoculum and also incubated at 35°C. After 24 hours of incubation, the number of organisms present is determined and should approximate 10^5CFU/ml (the actual number will vary from 5×10^4 to 5×10^5CFU/ml). After 24 hours' incubation, the test series of tubes are shaken and the results recorded as "growth" or "no-growth" for each tube. All tubes without visible growth are subcultured with a 0.01 ml calibrated loop on a quadrant of a sheep blood agar plate which is incubated overnight at 35°C. The next day the number of colonies subcultured from each tube is recorded, and the results reported as the highest dilution or titer of serum resulting in complete or 99.9 per cent killing of the original inoculum.

Barry, A. L.: The Antimicrobic Susceptibility Test: Principles and Practices. Philadelphia, Lea and Febiger, 1976.

Barry, A. L., and Fay, G. D.: The amount of agar in antimicrobic disk susceptibility test plates. Am. J. Clin. Pathl., *59*:196, 1973a.

Barry, A. L., Garcia, F., and Thrupp, L. D.: An improved single-disk method for testing the antibiotic susceptibility of rapidly growing pathogens. Am. J. Clin. Path., *53*:149, 1970.

Barry, A. L., Joyce, L. J., Adams, A. P., and Benner, E. J.: Rapid determinations of antimicrobial susceptibility for urgent clinical situations. Am. J. Clin. Path., *59*:693, 1973b.

Bartlett, R. C., Mazens, M., and Greenfield, B.: Acceleration of tetrazolium reduction by bacteria. J. Clin. Microbiol., *3*:327, 1976.

Bauer, A. W., Kirby, W. M. M., Sherris, J. C., and Turck, M.: Antibiotic susceptibility testing by a standardized single disk method. Am. J. Clin. Path., *45*:493, 1966.

Bennett, J. V., Camp, H. M., and Eickhoff, T. C.: Rapid sulfonamide disc sensitivity test for meningococci. Appl. Microbiol., *16*:1056, 1968.

Berenbaum, M. C.: A method for testing for synergy with any number of agents. J. Infect. Dis., *137*:122, 1978.

Blazevic, D. J.: Evaluation of the modified broth-disk method for determining antibiotic susceptibilities of anaerobic bacteria. Antimicrob. Agents Chemother., *7*:721, 1975.

Blazevic, D. J., Koepcke, M. H., and Matsen, J. M.: Quality control testing with the disc antibiotic susceptibility test of Bauer-Kirby-Sherris-Turck. Am. J. Clin. Path., *57*:592, 1972.

Catlin, B. W.: Iodometric detection of *Haemophilus influenzae* beta-lactamase: Rapid, presumptive test for ampicillin resistance. Antimicrob. Agents Chemother., *7*:265, 1975.

Chabbert, Y.: Titrage de la sensibilite des germes aerobies aux antibiotiques par la methode de la cupule en gelose. Ann. Inst. Pasteur (Paris), *76*:68, 1949.

Cleary, T. J., and Maurer, D.: Methicillin-resistant *Staphylococcus aureus* susceptibility testing by an automated system. Autobac I. Antimicrob. Agents Chemother., *13*:837, 1978.

Drew, W. L., Barry, A. L., O'Toole, R., and Sherris, J. C.: Reliability of the Kirby-Bauer disc diffusion method for detecting methicillin-resistant strains of *Staphylococcus aureus*. Appl. Microbiol., *24*:240, 1972.

Ellner, P. D., and Johnson, E.: Unreliability of direct antibiotic susceptibility testing on wound exudates. Antimicrob. Agents Chemother., *9*:355, 1976.

Ericsson, H. M., and Sherris, J. C.: Antibiotic sensitivity testing. Report of an international collaborative study. Acta. Path. Microbiol. Scand., Sect. B., Suppl. 217, p. 1, 1971.

Federal Register, Rules and Regulations: Antibiotic susceptibility discs. *37*:20525, 1972.

Federal Register, Rules and Regulations: Antibiotic susceptibility discs: Correction. *38*:20076, 1973.

Fleming, A.: The antibacterial action *in vitro* of 2-(*p*-aminobenzenesulphonamido) pyridine on pneumococci and streptococci. Lancet, *2*:74, 1938.

Fleming, A.: A comparison of the activities of antiseptics on bacteria and on leukocytes. Proc. R. Soc. Lond. (Biol.), *96*:171, 1924.

Fleming, A.: On the antibacterial action of cultures of penicillium, with special reference to their use in the isolation of *B. influenzae*. Br. J. Exp. Path., *102*:226, 1929.

Gavan, T. L., and Butler, D. A.: An automated microdilution method for antimicrobial susceptibility testing. *In* Balows, A. (ed.): Current Techniques for Antibiotic Susceptibility Testing. Springfield, Ill., Charles C Thomas, Publisher, 1974, p. 88.

Gavan, T. L., and Town, M. A.: A microdilution method for antibiotic susceptibility testing: An evaluation. Am. J. Clin. Path., *53*:880, 1970.

Gerlach, E. H.: Dilution test procedures for susceptibility testing. *In* Bondi, H., Bartola, J. T., and Prier, J. E. (eds.): The Clinical Laboratory as an Aid in Chemotherapy of Infectious Diseases. Baltimore, University Park Press, 1977, p. 45.

Gerlach, E. H.: Microdilution I: A comparative study. *In* Balows, A. (ed.): Current Techniques for Antibiotic Susceptibility Testing. Springfield, Ill., Charles C Thomas, Publisher, 1974, p. 63.

Goss, W. A., and Cimijotti, E. B.: Evaluation of an automatic diluting device for microbiological applications. Appl. Microbiol., *16*:1414, 1968.

Hollick, G. E., and Washington, J. A., II: Comparison of direct and standardized disk diffusion susceptibility of testing urine cultures. Antimicrob. Agents Chemother., *9*:804, 1976.

Jawetz, E.: Assay of antibacterial activity in serum. Am. J. Dis. Child., *103*:113, 1962.

Klastersky, J., et al.: Antibacterial activity in serum and urine as a therapeutic guide in bacterial infections. J. Infec. Dis., *129*:187, 1974.

Kurzynski, T. A., Yrios, J. W., Helstad, A. G., and Field, C. R.: Aerobically incubated thioglycolate broth disk method for antibiotic susceptibility testing of anaerobes. Antimicrob. Agents Chemother., *10*:727, 1976.

Lund, M. E., Blazevic, D. J., and Matsen, J. M.: Rapid gentamicin bioassay using a multiple antibiotic-resistant strain of *Klebsiella pneumoniae*. Antimicrob. Agents Chemother., *4*:569, 1973.

MacLowry, J. D., Jaqua, M. J., and Selepak, S. T., Detailed methodology and implementation of a semiautomated serial dilution microtechnique for antimicrobial susceptibility testing. Appl. Microbiol., *20*:46, 1970.

MacLowry, J. D., and Marsh, H. H.: Semiautomatic microtechnique for serial dilution-antibiotic sensitivity testing in the clinical laboratory. J. Lab. Clin. Med., *72*:685, 1968.

Matsen, J. M., and Barry, A. L.: Susceptibility testing: Diffusion test procedures. *In* Lennette, E. H., Spaulding, E. H., and Truant, J. P. (eds.): Manual of Clinical Microbiology. 2nd ed. Washington, D.C., Am Soc. Microbiol., 1974, p. 418.

Matsen, J. M., Koepcke, M. J. H., and Quie, P. G.: Evaluation of the Bauer-Kirby-Sherris-Turck single-disc diffusion method of antibiotic susceptibility testing. Antimicrob. Agents Chemother., 1969. Am. Soc. Microbiol., Washington, D.C., p. 445, 1970.

Matsen, J. M., Sielaff, B. H., and Buck, G. E.: Rapid automated bacterial identification with computerized programming of augmented Autobac I results. *In* Sharpe, A. N., and Clark, D. S. (eds.): Mechanizing Microbiology. Springfield, Ill., Charles C Thomas, Publisher, 1977, p. 240.

McKie, J. E., Jr., Borovoy, R. J., Dooley, J. F., Evanega, G. R., Mendoza, G., Meyer, F., Moody, M., Packer, D. E., Praglin, J., and Smith, H.: Autobac 1-A 3-hour automated, antimicrobial susceptibility system: II. Microbiological studies, *In* Heden, C., and Illeni, T. (eds.): Automation in Microbiology and Immunology. New York, John Wiley & Sons, Inc., 1974.

McMaster, P. R. B., Robertson, E. A., Witebsky, F. C., and MacLowry, J. D.: Evaluation of a dispensing instrument (Dynatec MIC-2000) for preparing microtiter antibiotic plates and testing their potency during storage. Antimicrob. Agents Chemother., *13*:842, 1978.

Metzler, C. M., and Dettaan, R. M.: Susceptibility tests of anaerobic bacteria: Statistical and clinical considerations. J. Infect. Dis., *130*:588, 1974.

National Committee for Clinical Laboratory Standards. Performance standards for antimicrobial disc susceptibility tests. Approved Standard ASM-2, Villanova, Pa., 1975.

O'Callaghan, C. H., Morris, A., Kirby, S. M., and Shingler, A. H.: Novel method for the detection of β-lactamases by using a chromogenic cephalosporin substrate. Antimicrob. Agents Chemother., *1*:283, 1972.

Pien, F. D., and Vosti, K. L.: Variation in performance of the serum bactericidal test. Antimicrob. Agents Chemother., *6*:330, 1974.

Praglin, J., Curtis, A. C., Longhenry, D. K., and McKie, J. E., Jr.: Autobac 1—A 3-hour automated antimicrobial susceptibility system: I. System description: *In* Heden, C., and Illeni, T. (eds.): Automation in Microbiology and Immunology. New York, John Wiley & Sons, Inc., 1974.

Reddish, G. F.: Methods of testing antiseptics. J. Lab Clin. Med., *14*:649, 1929.

Reller, L. B., Schoenknecht, F. D., Kenny, M. A., and Sherris, J. C.: Antibiotic susceptibility testing of *Pseudomonas aeruginosa:* Selection of a control strain and criteria for magnesium and calcium content in media. J. Infect. Dis., *130*:454, 1974.

Ronald, A. R., Eby, J., and Sherris, J. C.: Susceptibility of *Neisseria gonorrhoeae* to penicillin and tetracycline. Antimicrob. Agents Chemother., p. 431, 1968.

Rose, S. B., and Miller, R. E.: Studies with the agar cup-plate method I. A standardized agar cup-plate technique. J. Bacteriol., *38*:525, 1939.

Rosenblatt, J. E., and Neuman, A. M.: Laboratory suggestions—A rapid slide test for penicillinase. Am. J. Clin. Path., *69*:351, 1978.

Ryan, K. J., Needham, G. M., Dunsmoor, C. L., and Sherris, J. C.: Stability of antibiotics and chemotherapeutics in agar plates. Appl. Microbiol., *20*:447, 1970.

Sabath, L. D., and Matsen, J. M.: Assay of antimicrobial agents (Antibiotic Section). *In* Lennette, E. H., Spaulding, E. H., and Truant, J. P. (eds.): Manual of Clinical Microbiology. 2nd ed. Washington, D.C., Am. Soc. Microbiol., 1974a.

Sabath, L. D., and Toftegaard, I.: Rapid microassays for clindamycin and gentamicin when present together and the effect of pH and of each on antibacterial activity of the other. Antimicrob. Agents Chemother., *6*:54, 1974b.

Sabath, L. D., Wheeler, N., Laverdiere, M., Blazevic, D., and Wilkinson, B. J.: A new type of penicillin resistance of *Staphylococcus aureus*. Lancet, *1*:443, 1977.

Schlichter, J. G., and Maclean, H. A.: A method of determining effective therapeutic level in the treatment of subacute bacterial endocarditis with penicillin. Am. Heart J., *34*:209, 1947.

Shahidi, A., and Ellner, P. D.: Effect of mixed cultures on antibiotic susceptibility testing. Appl. Microbiol., *18*:766, 1969.

Steers, E., Foltz, E. L., and Graves, B. S.: An inocula replicating apparatus for routine testing of bacterial susceptibility to antibiotics. Antibiot. Chemother. (Basel), *9*:307, 1959.

Stemper, J. E., and Matsen, J. M.: Device for turbidity standardizing of cultures for antibiotic sensitivity testing. Appl. Microbiol., *19*:1015, 1970.

Sutter, V. L., Vargo, V. L., and Finegold, S. M.: Wadsworth Anaerobic Bacteriology Manual. 2nd ed. The Regents of the University of California, Los Angeles, 1975.

Thornsberry, C.: Rapid laboratory tests for β-lactamase production by bacteria. U.S. Dept. of Health, Education and Welfare, Public Health Service, Center for Disease Control, Atlanta, Ga., 1977c.

Thornsberry, C., Gavan, T., and Gerlach, E. H.: New developments in antimicrobial agent susceptibility testing. *In* Sherris, J. C. (ed.): Cumitech 6. Am. Soc. Microbiol., Washington, D.C., 1977a.

Thornsberry, C., Gavan, T. L., Sherris, J. C., Balows, A., Matsen, J. M., Sabath, L. D., Schoenknecht, F., Thrupp, L. D., and Washington, J. A., II.: Laboratory evaluation of a rapid, automated susceptibility testing system: Report of a collaborative study. Antimicrob. Agents Chemother., *7*:466, 1975.

Thornsberry, C., and Hawkins, T. M.: Agar disc diffusion susceptibility testing procedure. U.S. Dept. of Health, Education and Welfare, Publ. Health Serv., Center for Disease Control, Atlanta, Ga., 1977b.

Thornsberry, C., and Kirven, L. A.: Antimicrobial susceptibility of *Haemophilus influenzae*. Antimicrob. Agents Chemother., *6*:620, 1974.

Tilton, R. C., Lieberman, L., and Gerlach, E. H.: Microdilution antibiotic susceptibility testing: Examination of certain variables. Appl. Microbiol., *26*:658, 1973.

Washington, J. A., II.:Antimicrobial susceptibility of *Enterobacteriaceae* and nonfermenting gram-negative bacilli. Mayo Clin. Proc., *44*:811, 1969.

Washington, J. A., II, Snyder, R. J., Kohner, P. C., Wiltse, C. G., Ilstrup, D. M., and McCall, J. T.: Effect of cation content of agar on the activity of gentamicin, tobramycin and amikacin against *Pseudomonas aeruginosa*. J. Infect. Dis., *137*:103, 1978.

Washington, J. A., II., Warren, E., Dolan, C. T., and Karlson, A. G.: Antimicrobial susceptibility tests of bacteria. *In* Washington, J. A., II (ed.): Laboratory Procedures in Clinical Microbiology. Boston, Little, Brown and Company, 1974a, p. 286.

Washington, J. A., II, and Barry, A. L.: Dilution test procedures. *In* Lennette, E. H., Spaulding, E. H., and Truant, J. P. (eds.): Manual of Clinical Microbiology. 2nd ed. Washington, D.C., American Society for Microbiology, 1974b, p. 410.

Washington, J. A., II., Warren, E., and Karlson, A. G.: Stability of barium sulfate turbidity standards. Appl. Microbiol., *24*:1013, 1972.

Wegner, D. L., Mathis, C. R., and Neblett, T. R.: Direct method to determine the antibiotic susceptibility of rapidly growing blood pathogens. Antimicrob. Agents Chemother., *9*:861, 1976.

Wilkins, T. D., and Thiel, T.: Modified broth-disk method for testing the antibiotic susceptibility of anaerobic bacteria. Antimicrob. Agents Chemother., *3*:350, 1973.

Wilkins, T. D., and Chalgren, S.: Medium for use in antibiotic susceptibility testing of anaerobic bacteria. Antimicrob. Agents Chemother., *10*:926, 1976.

53

QUALITY CONTROL IN MICROBIOLOGY

THOMAS L. GAVAN, M.D.

During the past 20 years quality control and quality assurance procedures have been increasingly emphasized. Procedures that provide information useful in the diagnosis of human disease are subject to variables that may lead to errors in test results and subsequently to diagnostic errors. Clinical chemistry and hematology lend themselves easily to well-established statistical quality control procedures because of the quantitative nature of many of the tests performed. In contrast, clinical microbiology is primarily a qualitative discipline, which, in addition, requires subjective interpretation. The variables of specimen collection and transport, selection and use of appropriate isolation media, incubating conditions, identification criteria, antimicrobial susceptibility testing, and reporting methods contribute to the list of possible sources of error that can lead to the production of irrelevant or (worse) misleading information (Dolan, 1977). Therefore, a quality assurance program in clinical microbiology must encompass all these aspects so that the limits of accuracy and reproducibility of microbiologic procedures can be determined and maintained at levels that can consistently and reliably provide, at reasonable expense, clinically relevant diagnostic information.

The degree of effort expended on a quality assurance program will vary widely, depending upon the size of the laboratory and the variety of procedures employed. However, the program instituted must encompass all procedures in use. In larger laboratories a specific technologist may be assigned responsibility for quality control on a full-time basis; in small laboratories this may be a part-time assignment.

The laboratory director should plan the quality assurance program, and, if he or she does not take personal charge, should delegate responsibility and authority for its implementation. Quality control records must be reviewed at least monthly to assure that deficiencies noted are corrected.

The essential areas to be considered in implementing a comprehensive quality assurance program are as follows:

1. Personnel
2. Documentation of procedures
3. Specific areas of quality control
   a. Media
   b. Antimicrobial susceptibility tests
   c. Equipment
   d. Stock organisms, source and storage
4. Proficiency testing

PERSONNEL

Because of the high level of subjective interpretation required at nearly every step in processing specimens submitted for microbiologic evaluation, the qualifications, experience, and motivation of the personnel must be of the highest level. Individuals who aspire to perform a useful service in a microbiology laboratory must have not only a broad education in the basic fundamentals of the discipline but also adequate training in practical laboratory work under the supervision of an experienced microbiologist. It has been shown that errors resulting in erroneous laboratory reports are closely related to the type of training, experience, and supervisory ability of the technologist immediately responsible for the microbiology section (Barry, 1968). New employees must be taught simple basic principles and continually supervised to discourage the all-too-common tendency of adopting more expedient but less effective methods.

Continuing education of the microbiology laboratory worker is essential if high levels of quality are to be maintained. This can take the form of seminars, journal clubs, and laboratory rounds where current developments can be presented and discussed. Because the handling of many microbiologic specimens may be dependent upon a particular clinical situation, microbiological-clinical correlations should be stressed. Personnel should be encouraged to attend meetings and seminars and to read current literature in clinical microbiology. Up-to-date reference books as well as appropriate journals should be available in the laboratory library.

DOCUMENTATION OF PROCEDURES

A detailed procedure manual is a necessary first step in developing a comprehensive quality control program. In such a manual are included all the policies which will guide the operation of the laboratory.

The organization of the laboratory should be outlined, with the responsibility and authority of all personnel at various levels clearly defined. Availability of services during regular working hours as well as evenings, nights, weekends, and holidays should be stated. Instructions for appropriate specimen collection, labeling, and transport to the laboratory, as well as criteria for specimen acceptability, are especially important. The above information should also be included in a manual for physicians and nurses and should be readily available to them to minimize the frequency of inappropriate specimens and to define clearly the laboratory's policy when such specimens are submitted.

For intralaboratory specimen handling, there should be instructions for appropriate accessioning procedures and internal laboratory communication for each specimen type (e.g., urine, blood, etc.). Worksheets, log books, and result reporting are included. For each category of specimen there should be an outline providing the technologist with instructions for processing. This includes specimen requirements, media to be inoculated, incubation conditions (temperature and atmosphere), criteria for initial culture review, criteria for the selection of colonies to be further isolated and identified, the extent to which identification should be carried out, and criteria for the reporting of test results (e.g., under what circumstances immediate telephone reports are required).

Laboratory safety should be a part of every procedure manual. This section should stress biologic, chemical, mechanical, and electrical hazards that may be encountered in the laboratory and how each employee is expected to handle situations involving these hazards. Special attention should be given to proper procedures for the safe disposal of contaminated materials.

The procedure manual should include a concise systematic description of all serologic procedures, biochemical tests, reagents, and media prepared in or used by the laboratory. This description should include the principles involved, source of materials, instructions for preparation and for use, significance of test results, and references where appropriate.

The quality control section should include a description of the program for monitoring equipment function, media, reagents, and stains, as well as the criteria for judging these items acceptable. The details of such a program are the subject of subsequent sections of this chapter. Finally, the procedure manual, once developed, must be reviewed at least annually to ensure that it is consistent with current operating procedures. As new procedures or changes in existing procedures are approved and introduced into the laboratory, appropriate entries must be made in the procedure manual. These should be initialed by the laboratory supervisor and/or the laboratory director. At the time of the annual review, a cover letter signed by the laboratory director should be included in the manual, indicating that the contents were reviewed and that they reflect the approved operating procedures of the laboratory.

SPECIFIC AREAS OF QUALITY CONTROL

Media

Sterility and intended performance of all culture media must be established before use in the clinical laboratory. This applies both to media prepared in house from individual ingredients or dehydrated materials and to media received from commercial manufacturers already prepared and ready for use. The latter category also includes those commercially available "kit" products consisting of fixed batteries of media to be used in the identification of various groups of microorganisms. One can argue that commercially prepared media do not require the same degree of quality control as those that are prepared in the laboratory (Nagel, 1973). In recent years the Food and Drug Administration has established regulations for manufacturers of prepared media, which requires them to adhere to manufacturing, labeling, and quality control practices that yield a high quality finished product. These control measures ensure that these products are satisfactory for the stated shelf life of the product when stored under stated conditions. The greatest variables in this situation can occur during transport of the product from manufacturer to consumer, at times due to storage for varying lengths of time by intermediaries. Although most manufacturers strive to provide appropriately insulated shipping containers, exposure to excessive heat or cold can damage a medium to the point that reliable results may not be obtained. It is prudent, therefore, to monitor sterility and performance of these media, at least in the case of those most sensitive to deterioration and at least concurrently with clinical use.

Laboratory Prepared Media. Media preparation should be scheduled so that all required quality control testing can be performed and evaluated prior to use. Raw materials should be dated upon receipt, and when the container is opened, the suppliers' recommendations for storage and expiration dates should be rigidly followed. When a batch of medium is prepared, a production record should be kept. This will include the name of the medium, volume produced, formulation, manufacturer and lot numbers of ingredients, expiration date, and sterilization, dispensing, packaging, and labeling requirements. This information can be very useful for resolving problems that may occur. Sources of error in preparation of media from commercial dehydrated products include:

1. Improper storage
2. Outdated materials
3. Incorrect weighing
4. Incorrect measurement of water
5. Use of tap water, or use of water from a malfunctioning still
6. Use of glassware or stainless steel containers contaminated with detergents or chemicals
7. Incomplete mixing of ingredients or incomplete solution of ingredients
8. Overheating at any time during preparation or sterilization
9. Remelting solid media more than once
10. Improper determination of pH

Sterility Testing. Sterility testing must be applied to all batches of tubed or plated media, whether manufactured in-house or purchased ready for use. This is especially true with those media to which one or more sterile components are added after sterilization of the basal medium. It is obvious that the entire lot cannot be checked for sterility because of the possibility of deterioration. Therefore, a reasonable sample must be selected. When batches consist of 100 units or less, a 5 to 10 per cent sample should suffice. With batches of more than 100 units, 10 plates or tubes taken at random will usually detect batch contamination. Even though the batch has passed this sterility check, the technologist should be aware that random surface contamination can occur and should examine each plate at the time of inoculation for visible colonies. Growth of a specific colonial type beginning partway through the streaked area of a plate should alert the technologist to the possibility of contamination.

Special sterility problems can be seen with a selective medium. In this case the inhibiting properties of the medium may suppress growth of a contaminating organism to the extent that visible colonies are not produced, but at the same time viable organisms may make their appearance when isolated colonies are picked and transferred to a non-inhibiting medium. If aliquots of the finished medium are inoculated into 10 to 20 volumes of a noninhibiting broth medium, contamination can be detected and subsequent problems eliminated.

In addition to sterility testing, all media prepared or received should be examined visually, and the color, clarity, and state of hydration determined. These characteristics also should be observed by technologists as part of their preinoculation inspection of all tubes and plates. Unless the medium contains some insoluble component (e.g., starch in Mueller-Hinton medium), the presence of turbidity or a precipitate indicates a defect on the medium. This may occur after storage. If the precipitate fails to disappear upon heating the medium to the temperature of incubation, the lot should be rejected. Media containing pH indicators provide a degree of built-in control. The color of each new lot should be compared with that of a previous satisfactory lot, and if the color differs, the pH should be rechecked. The pH of most media should fall ± 0.2 of the pH specified by the manufacturer. The pH of all media should be determined electrometrically at room temperature. Media should not be tested when hot, because the pH tends to rise on cooling and the amount of change varies with the formulation.

To prevent dehydration of prepared or purchased media, proper storage conditions should be maintained. Problems should not occur with liquid or solid media stored in sealed, screw-capped containers. Dehydration of plated media cannot be completely prevented even when sealed in plastic bags. Media which show surface cracks or separation from the edge of the plate are not satisfactory for use and should be discarded.

Performance Tests of Media. The ability of isolation, selective, and differential media to perform as expected must be determined. Full scale performance testing of media prepared in house is essential. With commercially prepared media, which has been subjected to extensive quality control during manufacture, a modified system for performance testing may be satisfactory. It is recommended that before omitting pre-use performance testing, all media obtained ready for use be subjected to an extensive control program for at least several consecutive batches to ascertain reliability.

For purposes of this discussion, a quantity of medium prepared in the laboratory at one time is considered to be a batch. A "batch" of commercial medium is defined as a shipment of a common lot number received at one time. If a "batch" is not used in one month, the medium should be rechecked.

A collection of stable stock cultures with known characteristics is essential. Table 53–1 provides a list of quality control organisms for a wide variety of media and their expected reactions. These recommendations have been found useful in a large diagnostic laboratory, but may not be applicable to all laboratories, and some additional tests or media may be added to reflect local evaluation and identification practices. The source and storage of stock strains are discussed later.

Media intended for isolation should be tested using the most fastidious organism expected to be isolated. If more than one bacterial characteristic is to be demonstrated, multiple organisms may have to be used. For example, sheep blood agar plates are almost universally employed as a routine isolation medium. Both the ability to detect small numbers of fastidious organisms and the ability to demonstrate characteristic hemolysis must be manifest. This requires the use of several test organisms (Table 53–1). Furthermore, the inoculum chosen for testing isolation media must be light. Plates are inoculated with a 1:10 dilution in broth of suspension of the test organism(s) adjusted to the density of a McFarland 0.5 standard. This provides a relatively standardized inoculum for obtaining isolated colonies. The colony counts, particularly on highly enriched isolation media, with or without inhibitors, can serve as a guide for evaluation

Table 53–1. RECOMMENDED CHALLENGING ORGANISMS FOR USE IN PERFORMANCE TESTING OF PLATED AND TUBED CULTURE MEDIA

Medium	Positive Control	Expected Result	Negative Control	Expected Result	Frequency Tested
Bile-Esculin	Enterococcus	Growth; medium turns black	Group A streptococcus	No change in color of medium	Each lot
Bird seed agar	*Cryptococcus neoformans*	Colonies turn brown	*Candida albicans*	Colonies do not turn brown	Each lot
Chocolate agar	*Neisseria gonorrhoeae*	Enhanced growth	None		Each lot
	Neisseria meningitidis	Enhanced growth	None		Each lot
	Haemophilus influenzae	Enhanced growth	None		Each lot
Columbia blood agar	*Escherichia coli*	Growth and typical colonial morphology	None		Each lot
	Pseudomonas aeruginosa	Growth and typical colonial morphology	None		Each lot
	Acinetobacter calcoaceticus var. *anitratus*	Growth and typical colonial morphology	None		Each lot
	Group A streptococcus	Typical colonial morphology and growth, beta-hemolysis	None		Each lot
	Streptococcus pneumoniae	Typical colonial morphology and growth, alpha-hemolysis	None		Each lot
	Enterococcus	Growth and typical colonial morphology	None		Each lot
Corn meal agar	*Candida albicans*	Production of chlamydospores and pseudohyphae	*Cryptococcus neoformans*	No production of chlamydospores or pseudohyphae	Each lot
Citrate agar slant	*Enterobacter cloacae*	Growth—slant turns Prussian blue	*Escherichia coli*	No growth	Each lot
Cystine trypticase agar	*Escherichia coli* and dextrose disk	Growth, fermentation, acid (yellow) production	*Escherichia coli* (no dextrose disk)	Growth, no fermentation or acid production	Each lot
Decarboxylase broth	None		*Escherichia coli*	Growth is indicated by the yellow color of the broth	Each lot
Fletcher's medium	*Leptospira interrogans* ser. *ictero-haemorrhagiae*	Growth	None		
Hippurate broth	Group B streptococcus (hemolytic and nonhemolytic strains)	Medium turns purple on addition of Ninhydrin	Group D streptococcus	Medium does *not* turn purple on addition of Ninhydrin	Each lot
Indole-nitrate-motility media	*Bacteroides thetaiotaomicron*	Indole produced	*Bacteroides fragilis*	No indole produced	Each lot
	Clostridium novyi Type A	Positive motility	*Bacteroides fragilis*	Negative motility	

Lysine-iron agar	*Edwardsiella tarda*	Alkaline/alkaline/(+) H_2S*	*Proteus rettgeri*	Red/alkaline/(−)H_2S*	
Lowenstein-Jensen agar	*Mycobacterium tuberculosis*	Characteristic growth	None		Each lot
Lowenstein-Jensen-Gruft	*Mycobacterium tuberculosis*	Characteristic growth	*Klebsiella pneumoniae* *Staphylococcus* species	No growth No growth	Each lot
Malonate broth	*Enterobacter aerogenes*	Prussian blue color change	*Escherichia coli*	No color change (stays green)	Each lot
Motility (BHI)	*Escherichia coli*	Growth out from stab	*Klebsiella pneumoniae*	No growth out from stab	Each lot
Methyl red broth	*Escherichia coli*	Color change from yellow to red with addition of reagent	*Enterobacter aerogenes*	No color change	Each lot and weekly
Mycobiotic agar	*Candida albicans*	Growth	*Cryptococcus neoformans* *Escherichia coli*	Growth inhibition	Each lot
Phenyl-ethyl-alcohol agar	*Staphylococcus aureus*	Enhanced growth	*Proteus mirabilis* stab *Pseudomonas aeruginosa*	Growth inhibition Growth inhibition	Each lot
Sabouraud dextrose agar	*Candida albicans* *Cryptococcus neoformans*	Growth Growth	None		Each lot
Sabouraud dextrose agar w/gentamicin	*Candida albicans* *Cryptococcus neoformans*	Growth Growth	*Escherichia coli* *Staphylococcus aureus* *Klebsiella pneumoniae*	Growth inhibition Growth inhibition Growth inhibition	Each lot
Thayer-Martin or Martin-Lewis agar	*Neisseria gonorrhoeae* *Neisseria meningitidis*	Growth Growth	*Staphylococcus aureus* *Candida albicans* *Escherichia coli* *Proteus mirabilis* stab	Growth inhibition Growth inhibition Growth inhibition Growth inhibition	Each lot
Tryptic soy agar	*Staphylococcus aureus* Enterococcus	Growth Growth	None		Each lot
Rabbit blood agar	*Haemophilus haemolyticus*	Beta-hemolysis and growth	*Haemophilus influenzae*	Growth and no hemolysis	Each lot
Xylose-lysine-desoxycholate agar	*Shigella sonnei* *Salmonella typhi* *Escherichia coli*	Colorless colonies Growth—H_2S production Yellow colonies	*Staphylocuccus aureus*	Growth inhibition	Each lot
Brain-heart-infusion broth	*Staphylococcus aureus* *Escherichia coli*	Growth Growth	None		Each lot
Chocolate agar slants	*Haemophilus influenzae* *Neisseria gonorrhoeae*	Growth Growth	None		Each lot
Tryptic soy broth with 6.5% NaCl	Enterococcus	Turbid growth	Group B streptococcus	No growth	Each lot
Triple sugar iron agar	*Proteus vulgaris*	Acid/acid/+H_2S*	*Pseudomonas aeruginosa*	Alkaline/alkaline/ −H_2S*	Each lot
Tryptic soy broth blood bottles	*Clostridium novyi* Group A	Growth	None		Each lot

Table continued on following page

6

Table 53–1. RECOMMENDED CHALLENGING ORGANISMS FOR USE IN PERFORMANCE TESTING OF PLATED AND TUBED CULTURE MEDIA (*Continued*)

Medium	Positive Control	Expected Result	Negative Control	Expected Result	Frequency Tested
	Bacteroides fragilis *Haemophilus influenzae*	Growth			
Urea agar slants	*Cryptococcus neoformans*	Medium changes to pink color	*Candida albicans*	No change to pink color in medium.	Each lot
Voges-Proskauer broth	*Enterobacter aerogenes*	Broth changes from yellow to red with addition of reagents	*Escherichia coli*	Broth remains yellow, i.e., no color change	
Nitrate agar slants	*Escherichia coli*	Red color when reagents are added	*Acinetobacter calcoaceticus* var. *anitratus*	No color change when reagents are added	Each lot
O-F dextrose	*Pseudomonas aeruginosa* (open)	Acid production (yellow)	*Pseudomonas aeruginosa* plus oil overlay	No acid production in fermentative tube	Each lot
	Klebsiella pneumoniae (open)	Acid production (yellow)	*Alcaligenes faecalis* plus oil overlay	No acid production in fermentative tube	
	Klebsiella pneumoniae plus oil overlay	Acid production (yellow)	*Alcaligenes faecalis* (open)	No acid production in oxidative tube	
O-F plain	*Pseudomonas aeruginosa* + dextrose disk	Acid production (yellow) oxidative positive	*Pseudomonas aeruginosa* + dextrose disk + oil	No acid production in fermentative tube	Each lot
			Pseudomonas aeruginosa	No acid production in oxidative tube	
			Pseudomonas aeruginosa + oil	No acid production in fermentative tube	
Phenylalanine deaminase agar slant	*Proteus mirabilis*	Reagent ferric chloride changes from yellow to green	*Escherichia coli*	Reagent ferric chloride stays yellow	New lot
Sorbitol phenol-red broth	*Enterobacter aerogenes*	Acid production (yellow)	*Proteus mirabilis*	No acid production, broth remains red in color	Each lot
Selenite F broth	*Shigella sonnei* *Salmonella typhi*	Enhanced growth Enhanced growth	None		Each lot
Thioglycollate broth	*Clostridium novyi* Type A	Growth	None		Each lot

Todd-Hewitt broth	Enterococcus	Growth	None		Each lot
	Group A streptococcus	Growth			
	Group B streptococcus	Growth			
	Group C streptococcus	Growth			
	Group D streptococcus	Growth			
	Group G streptococcus	Growth			
Colistin-nalidixic acid agar	Enterococcus	Enhanced growth	*Escherichia coli*	Growth inhibition	Each lot
	Staphylococcus aureus	Growth	*Pseudomonas aeruginosa*	Growth inhibition	
	Group A streptococcus	Enhanced growth			
Deoxyribonuclease agar	*Serratia marcescens*	Red colored zone around growth	*Escherichia coli*	No red colored zone around growth	Each lot
	Staphylococcus aureus	Red colored zone around growth	*Staphylococcus epidermidis*	No red colored zone around growth	
Egg yolk agar	*Clostridium novyi* Type A	Lecithinase positive, i.e., zone of precipitation in agar around colony	*Bacteroides fragilis*	Lecithinase negative, i.e., no zone of precipitation	Each lot
		Lipase positive, i.e., formation of an iridescent "pearly" luster over and around the colony		Lipase negative, i.e., no iridescent "pearly" luster over or around the colony	
MacConkey agar	*Escherichia coli*	Lactose positive—pink colonies	*Proteus mirabilis* stab	Inhibition of swarming growth	Each lot
	Shigella sonnei	Lactose negative—colorless colonies	Enterococcus	Growth inhibition	
			Staphylococcus aureus	Growth inhibition	
Mueller-Hinton agar	*Escherichia coli* ATCC 25922				Each lot, then daily
	Staphylococcus aureus ATCC 25923				
	Pseudomonas aeruginosa ATCC 27853				

*The reactions are listed in the following order: slant/butt/H_2S production.

of batch-to-batch reproducibility. In these cases a 1:1000 dilution (or one which yields 10^5 cfu/ml) of the McFarland adjusted suspension would be more appropriate. The inoculum and method of inoculation for biochemical or other differential tests should be that actually used in the laboratory. Rapid identification "kit" systems should be controlled according to the recommendation of the manufacturer.

In some laboratories highly specialized media, such as Bordet-Gengou, are made up and stored until the occasion for use when the basal medium is remelted, appropriate enrichments added, and plates poured. In these instances quality control prior to use may not be practical, but should be carried out concurrently with inoculation of clinical material. Similarly, media for the isolation of fungi and mycobacteria may require concurrent testing. Tables 53–2 and 53–3 list recommendations for expiration dating of plated and tubed media prepared and stored in the laboratory.

Reagents

Reagents used in the microbiology laboratory include stains, chemicals, antimicrobials, impregnated paper disks or strips, and antisera. All must be monitored for effective performance. Stains and chemicals obtained from reputable sources should be labeled with lot number, dates of preparation or receipt, opening, and expiration. Freshness and stability can be assured if relatively small quantities are purchased or prepared at one time. Performance tests of each batch should be carried out prior to use and at appropriate intervals during the lifetime of the batch. These intervals are dependent upon the inherent stability of the reagent or stain and the frequency with which they are used. For example, Gram's stain may be checked on preparation and at weekly intervals, whereas less frequently used stains, such as flagella stain, should be tested concurrently with use with control organisms having known flagellar characteristics. Also, stable chemical reagents such as Kovacs' reagent for the indole test should be tested on preparation and at weekly intervals. Unstable reagents, such as hydrogen peroxide for the catalase test or tetramethyl-*p*-phenylenediamine dihydrochloride for the oxidase test, should be tested on each day of use. Table 53–4 lists recommended challenge organisms for use in the control of a variety of reagent materials and the maximum intervals for testing. These organisms provide both positive and negative reactions for each reagent.

Reagent-impregnated paper disks or strips obtained from reputable manufacturers should be stored with a

Table 53–2. EXPIRATION DATING FOR PLATED MEDIA, CALCULATED FROM DATE OF PRODUCTION*

Medium	Expiration Date
Bile-esculin agar	6 weeks
Bird seed agar	6 weeks
Brain-heart infusion agar	6 weeks
Brain-heart infusion w/blood	1 month
Brain-heart infusion w/gentamicin	6 weeks
Chocolate agar	1 month
Columbia blood agar	1 month
Columbia CNA agar	1 month
Corn meal agar w/Tween 80	6 weeks
DNase agar w/methyl green	6 weeks
DNase test agar w/toluidine blue	6 weeks
EMB agar	1 month
Hektoen agar	1 month
Mycobiotic agar	6 weeks
MacConkey agar	1 month
Phenylethyl alcohol agar w/blood	1 month
Potato dextrose agar	6 weeks
Rabbit blood agar	1 month
Sabouraud dextrose agar	6 weeks
Sabouraud dextrose agar w/gentamicin	6 weeks
Schaedler blood agar w/vitamin K	1 month
TB sensitivity plates	3 weeks
Thayer-Martin medium	1 month
Tryptic soy agar	6 weeks
XLD agar	1 month

*Stored in airtight wrappers at 2 to 8°C.

Table 53–3. EXPIRATION DATING OF TUBED MEDIA CALCULATED FROM DATE OF PRODUCTION*

Medium	Expiration Date
Bordet-Gengou agar base	6 months
Biphasic fungal blood culture bottles	6 months
Brain-heart infusion broth	6 months
Brain-heart infusion agar	6 months
CTA medium plain	6 months
CTA medium w/carbohydrate	6 weeks
Fletcher's medium	3 months
Hippurate substrate (Frozen at −20°C.)	3 months
Indole-nitrate broth	1 month
Indole-nitrate motility medium	1 month
KCN broth base	6 months
KCN broth w/KCN	2 weeks
Lysine iron agar	6 months
Malonate broth	6 months
Middlebrook 7H9 broth	3 months
Middlebrook 7H11S agar (Mitchison)	1 month
Motility GI medium	6 months
Mueller-Hinton broth bottles	6 weeks
MR-VP medium	6 months
Nitrate agar	6 months
Nutrient agar	6 months
Nutrient broth	6 months
OF medium plain	3 months
OF medium w/carbohydrate	6 weeks
Selenite broth	6 months
Sabouraud dextrose agar	6 months
SF broth	6 months
Simmons citrate agar	3 months
Thioglycollate broth	1 month
Todd-Hewitt broth	6 months
Tryptic soy broth w/6.5% NaCl	6 months
Trichophyton agars 1–7	6 months
Triple surgar iron agar	6 months
Urea agar	6 months

*Stored at 2 to 8 °C. (except hippurate substrate) with tubes tightly capped.

desiccant (usually supplied with the original packaging) under the conditions described by the manufacturer. Suitable organisms for testing these items are listed in Table 53–4. Antimicrobial impregnated disks are covered under susceptibility testing control.

Antisera

Antisera for organism grouping and typing should be dated when received and when reconstituted. Storage at refrigerator temperatures is mandatory, with minimal exposure to room temperature at the time of use. Antisera must not be used beyond the manufacturer's expiration date and, when used, should be carefully inspected for turbidity or precipitate which may indicate contamination. Such sera must be discarded as unsatisfactory.

Each antiserum should be tested with organisms that produce a positive reaction and no reaction (negative). Table 53–5 lists suggested organisms that may be used with commonly used antisera. Each new vial of antiserum should be checked prior to initial use and at monthly intervals thereafter until the expiration date is reached. Saline should not be substituted for a negative control.

Antimicrobial Susceptibility Tests and Assays

Disks for antimicrobial susceptibility testing must be stored and used carefully after they are received in the laboratory and must not be used beyond the manufacturer's expiration date. They must be stored with a desiccant at temperatures less than 8°C. If possible, all disks, but especially those of the penicillin family, should be stored at −14°C. or less with desiccation. When a working supply of disks is removed from storage, the container should be allowed to warm to room temperature before opening to prevent condensation of moisture on the disk surfaces. Disk cartridges not used can be stored in the refrigerator at 2 to 8°C. Disks should be arranged on the plates to avoid overlapping of inhibitory zones or distortion of zones by synergistic or antagonistic drugs.

Disks used with automated susceptibility testing systems may have a different antimicrobial content, as well as tighter tolerance limits than those manufactured for the diffusion test. In no instance should disks for diffusion testing be used with these systems unless so recommended by the manufacturer.

Antimicrobials to be used in dilution tests should be assayed materials rather than preparations manufactured for clinical administration. Appropriate standards assayed for specific drug activity can be obtained from the drug manufacturer or purchased from the United States Pharmacopeia (USP-NF Reference Standards, 12601 Twinbrook Parkway, Rockville, Md. 20852).

Unopened powder standards may be stored for several years at room temperature. Once opened they should be stored with a desiccant in an anhydrous jar. Synthetic penicillins and cephalosporins should be stored at 2 to 8°C. Solutions of aminoglycosides, tetracycline, erythromycin, and clindamycin are stable at room temperature. Synthetic penicillins and cephalosporins may be stored at −20°C. for up to one month.

Because of the large number of variables affecting all types of susceptibility tests, it is not practical to monitor each one. A program to monitor endpoint reproducibility and accuracy is sufficient to detect when significant changes have been introduced. When results depart significantly from the expected, then factors known to be sources of error, such as inoculum density, medium pH, disk storage, etc., can be considered individually to resolve the problem.

Endpoint surveillance programs, regardless of the test method to be controlled, involve the repetitive testing of "standard" strains of bacteria. With the disk diffusion test, the following reference strains have been designated: *Staphylococcus aureus* ATCC 24923; *Escherichia coli* ATCC 25922; and *Pseudomonas aeruginosa* ATCC 27853. Expected inhibitory zone diameters have been determined for these organisms. The *P. aeruginosa* has been recommended as a reference strain to monitor tests with aminoglycoside antibiotics because the other reference cultures do not readily detect the effects of divalent cations in the medium on these agents (Thornsberry, 1977).

Currently the best estimate of the true inhibitory zone diameters to be expected with the standard reference cultures of *S. aureus, E. coli,* and *P. aeruginosa* are contained in the National Committee for Chemical Laboratory Standards (NCCLS) publication, "Performance Standards for Antimicrobic Disc Susceptibility Tests M2-T3" and its periodic supplements and revisions (available from NCCLS, 771 E. Lancaster Ave., Villanova, Pa 19085).

Standards for evaluating precision and accuracy of broth or agar dilution susceptibility testing procedures have not been developed to the extent that has been established for the disk diffusion test. Reproducibility of broth and agar dilution procedures is said to be on the order of $\pm \log_2$ dilution interval. In addition to the standard reference cultures of *S. aureus, E. coli,* and *P. aeruginosa,* other organisms must be used when monitoring dilution tests. Suitable reference cultures are listed in Table 53–6.

Reference standard cultures appropriate for monitoring each drug tested should be employed with each run of tests. The minimum inhibitory concentration (MIC) of the reference standard is then recorded and plotted. After 10 such tests have been made, a trend toward a median MIC value will be noted. These can be considered out of control if the MIC departs from the median by more than one $\log_2$ dilution.

Disk diffusion assay methods have widespread application in clinical laboratories for determining the levels in serum and other body fluids of potentially toxic antimicrobial agents and should be subjected to quality control. Serum assay procedures can be controlled by testing frozen aliquots of a pool of serum to which has been added the antimicrobial being tested in a concentration equivalent to the peak serum

Table 53–4. RECOMMENDED CHALLENGING ORGANISMS FOR USE IN PERFORMANCE TESTING OF REAGENTS, STRIPS, AND DISKS

Medium	Positive Control	Expected Result	Negative Control	Expected Result	Frequency Tested
Arginine decarboxylase	*Enterobacter cloacae*	Broth with arginine and test organism is purple; growth control is yellow	*Enterobacter aerogenes*	Broth with arginine and test organism is yellow; growth control is yellow	New lot, then weekly
Bacitracin disk	Group A streptococcus	Zone of inhibition measuring 10–18 mm around the disk	Group B streptococcus	No zone of inhibition around the disk	New lot, then weekly
Carbohydrate disks	Use appropriate positive controls	Acid production (yellow color)	Use appropriate negative controls	Acid production (yellow color)	New lot, then each test
Coagulase plasma	*Staphylococcus aureus*	Plasma clotted	*Staphylococcus epidermidis*	Plasma not clotted	New lot, then daily
Cytochrome oxidase strips	*Pseudomonas aeruginosa* ATCC 27853	Bacteria on strip turns blue-black	*Escherichia coli* ATCC 25922	No change in color of bacteria on strip	New lot, then daily
Ehrlich's reagent	*Escherichia coli*	A red ring will develop just below the xylene layer	*Enterobacter aerogenes*	Red ring does not develop	New lot, then weekly
Factor strips on tryptic soy agar plates "X"	*Haemophilus aphrophilus*	Growth around strip	*Haemophilus influenzae*	No growth around strip	New lot, then weekly
			Haemophilus parainfluenzae	No growth around strip	
"V"	*Haemophilus parainfluenzae*	Growth around strip	*Haemophilus influenzae*	No growth around strip	New lot, then weekly
"XV"	*Haemophilus influenzae*	Growth around strip	None		New lot, then weekly
	Haemophilus parainfluenzae	Growth around strip			New lot, then weekly
	Haemophilus aphrophilus	Growth around stip			
Ferric chloride	*Proteus mirabilis*	Slant of phenylalanine deaminase agar turns green	*Escherichia coli*	Slant of phenylalanine deaminase agar does not change color	New lot, then weekly
Gelatin strips	*Pseudomonas aeruginosa*	Organism liquefies the gelatin, leaving the clear blue supporting base, within 48 hours	*Pasteurella multocida*	Organism does *not* liquefy the gelatin revealing the clear blue supporting base	New lot, each test
Germ tube serum	*Candida albicans*	Germ tube production in 2 hours	*Candida tropicalis*	No germ tube production in 2 hours	New lot
			Candida parapsilosis		

Gram stain reagents	*Staphylococcus aureus* ATCC 25923	Purple organisms	*Escherichia coli* ATCC 25922	Red organisms	Daily
Hydrogen peroxide	*Staphylococcus aureus* ATCC 25923	Bacteria "bubbles" on glass slide	Group A streptococcus	No bubbles produced by bacteria on glass slide	Daily
KCN broth base with potassium cyanide	*Proteus vulgaris*	Growth	*Shigella sonnei*	No growth	Each test
Kovacs	*Escherichia coli*	Tryptophane broth will turn a deep red color after the addition of 5 drops of reagent	*Enterobacter aerogenes*	Tryptophane broth will *not* change color after the addition of 5 drops of reagent	New lot, then weekly
Methyl red	*Escherichia coli*	Broth turns red	*Enterobacter aerogenes*	Broth remains yellow	New lot, then weekly
Ninhydrin	Group B streptococcus	1% aqueous sodium hippurate substrate turns purple with addition of reagent	Group A streptococcus	1% aqueous sodium hippurate substrate does *not* turn purple with addition of reagents, i.e., remains cloudy	New lot, then each test
Nitrate Nitrate I (0.8 % sulfanilic acid) Nitrate II (0.5% N,N,dimethyl-1-naphthy-lamine)	*Escherichia coli*	Nitrate agar slant turns red on addition of reagents	*Acinetobacter calcoaceticus* var. *anitratus*	Nitrate agar slant produces *no* color change when reagents are added	New lot, then weekly
ONPG (beta-galactosidase) tablets	*Shigella sonnei*	Water around dissolved tablet turns yellow in 6 hours or less	*Salmonella typhi*	No color change in water around dissolved tablet	New lot, each test
Optochin disk	*Streptococcus pneumoniae*	Zone of inhibition measuring greater than 15 mm around the disk	Alpha hemolytic (viridans) streptococcus	No zone of inhibitor around the disk	New lot, then weekly
Ornithine decarboxylase	*Enterobacter hafniae*	Broth with ornithine and test organism is purple; growth control is yellow	*Proteus vulgaris*	Broth with ornithine and test organism is yellow; growth control is yellow	New lot, then weekly
Sodium desoxycholate	*Streptococcus pneumoniae*	Colonies on blood agar plate lyse	Alpha hemolytic (viridans) streptococcus	Colonies remain unchanged	New lot, then weekly
Voges-Proskauer Voges-Proskauer I (alpha napthol) Voges-Proskauer II (potassium hydroxide)	*Enterobacter aerogenes*	VI broth changes from yellow to red with addition of reagents	*Escherichia coli*	VP broth produces *no* color change with addition of reagents	New lot, then weekly

6

Table 53–5. CHALLENGE ORGANISMS FOR USE IN QUALITY CONTROL OF DIAGNOSTIC ANTISERA

Antiserum	Challenge Organism	Expected Reaction
Arizona	*Arizona hinshawii*	Agglutination
Alkalescens—dispar	Alkalescens—dispar	Agglutination
Arizona—mono	*Arizona hinshawii*	Agglutination
Bethesda—Ballerup	*Citrobacter freundii*	Agglutination
Escherichia coli	*Escherichia coli*	
Poly A	$026{:}B_6$	Agglutination
Poly B	$086{:}B_7$	Agglutination
Poly C	$018{:}B_{21}$	Agglutination
Haemophilus influenzae	*Haemophilus influenzae*	Capsular swelling (Quellung)
*Herellea vaginicola**	*Herellea vaginicola*	Agglutination
Mima polymorpha†	*Mima polymorpha*	Agglutination
Neisseria meningitidis	*Neisseria meningitidis*	Agglutination
Salmonella		
Polyvalent	*Salmonella* sp.	Agglutination
Polyvalent H	*Salmonella paratyphi*	
Salmonella		
Group A	*Salmonella paratyphi A*	Agglutination
Group B	*S. typhimurium*	Agglutination
Group C_1	*S. thompson*	Agglutination
Group C_2	*S. virginia*	Agglutination
Group D	*S. enteriditis*	Agglutination
Group E	*S. newington*	Agglutination
Group Vi	*S. typhi*	Agglutination
Shigella		
A	*Shigella dysenteriae*	Agglutination
B	*S. flexneri*	Agglutination
C	*S. boydii*	Agglutination
D	*S. sonnei*	Agglutination
Streptococcus pneumoniae	*Streptococcus pneumoniae*	Capsular swelling (Quellung)

**Acinetobacter calcoaceticus* var. *anitratus*.
†*Acinetobacter calcoaceticus* var. *lwoffi*.

Table 53–6. EXPECTED MINIMUM INHIBITORY CONCENTRATION (MIC) ENDPOINTS* FOR QUALITY CONTROL OF DILUTION ANTIMICROBIAL SUSCEPTIBILITY TESTS

	Minimum Inhibitory Concentration (μg/ml)			
Antimicrobial Agent	***E. coli* ATCC 25922**	***Enterococcus* ATCC 29212**	***S. aureus* ATCC 29213**	***P. aeruginosa* ATCC 27853**
Clindamycin	>16	8	≤0.25	>16
Erythromycin	>16	2	≤0.25	>16
Methicillin	>16	>16	1	>16
Nafcillin	>16	4	≤0.25	>16
Penicillin G	>4	2	0.5	>4
Ampicillin	2	1	0.5	>16
Cephalothin	8	32	≤1	>64
Tetracycline	1	16	0.5	8
Carbenicillin	≤8	32	≤8	32
Chloramphenicol	4	4	4	>32
Vancomycin	>64	2	1	>64
Kanamycin	2	32	≤1	>64
Gentamicin	0.5	8	≤0.25	0.5
Tobramycin	0.5	16	≤0.25	<0.25
Amikacin	1	>64	≤1	≤1
Nitrofurantoin	≤8	≤8	16	>512
Nalidixic acid	≤2	>128	32	128
Trimethoprim-sulfamethoxazole	≤0.5/9.5	≤0.5/9.5	≤0.5/9.5	16/304

*Endpoints are based on broth microdilution test. Differences of one or two dilutions may be anticipated with broth macrotube dilution or agar dilution tests. Tests are considered in control if observed MIC is ± one dilution interval from the above listed mean.

level obtained with normal doses. The serum pool should be tested for non-specific or antibiotic inhibition before antimicrobials are added. A blank control consisting of serum pool without antimicrobial should be run with each serum assay. Frozen aliquots of previously tested patient serum may also be retested.

Aliquots of the control serum must be kept frozen at −20°C. until used. Sera containing cephalosporins and penicillins should be stored at −70°C. Such pools should remain stable for six months if they are not thawed and refrozen.

One is often asked to assay one antimicrobial when a second antimicrobial is present. In some instances agents such as beta-lactamase, which inhibit the undesired drug but have no effect on the drug to be assayed, are added to the test system. In other situations, a test organism susceptible to the desired drug but resistant to the undesired drug may be used. In either case, the fact that the test conditions have actually suppressed the activity of the undesired drug should be demonstrated. This can be accomplished simply by placing an ordinary susceptibility testing disk containing the undesired drug on the test medium along with the standards, unknowns, and controls. Since each 6-mm assay disk will absorb 20 μl, the equivalent serum concentration in μg or units/ml represented by a susceptibility disk is 50 times the disk content. For example, if the test assay system successfully suppresses the inhibitory effect of a 10-unit penicillin disk, then one can assume the test system can suppress the equivalent of 500 units/ml of penicillin in the serum specimen. This can be reassuring when reporting levels of toxic agents.

Equipment

Properly functioning equipment is essential. A quality control program should include routine surveillance of all temperature-controlled mechanical and electrical apparatus. Preventive maintenance schedules should be established according to the recommendations of the equipment manufacturers. A maintenance manual listing the frequency and nature of the maintenance required should be attached to or located near each piece of equipment. These should be reviewed periodically to ascertain that the required maintenance has actually been performed and actions to correct defects noted. The maintenance manual should clearly define who is responsible for each maintenance item. In larger institutions these functions should be carried out by maintenance or engineering personnel.

Temperatures of incubators, refrigerators, freezers, water baths, heating blocks, and ovens should be recorded daily. Preferably, this should be done at the beginning and end of each day or on the day of use in the case of equipment used intermittently. It is good practice to make it a habit among personnel to check the temperature each time the equipment is used throughout the day. Recording these intermediate observations is not necessary. Thermometers vary widely in their calibration accuracy. All thermometers used should be calibrated against a National Bureau of Standards thermometer, and the correction factor, if any, should be noted on a tag attached to the thermometer. Since thermometers in air can respond to transient temperature fluctuations when incubator or refrigerator doors are opened, the thermometer should be immersed in propylene glycol or water (if temperature range permits). A temperature log or graph should be attached in a prominent position to each piece of equipment for convenience in recording and as an obvious reminder to observe and record the temperature. The acceptable temperature range should be indicated and space should be provided to record the source of trouble and corrective action taken when temperatures fall outside the established limits. Temperature chart recorders and thermostatic devices that sound an alarm locally or at a remote location should be considered to prevent loss of cultures or materials due to excessively large temperature changes as a result of thermostat malfunction or electrical failure, particularly at night. Continuous monitoring is not practical or even desired for all pieces of temperature-controlled equipment. Commonly available high-low thermometers are relatively inexpensive and establish the range of temperature fluctuation that has occurred since the last reading and resetting.

The interiors of incubators, refrigerators, freezers, and water baths must be periodically cleaned. Freezers should be defrosted at appropriate intervals. The use of frost-free freezers in clinical laboratories is subject to question, since the temperature may rise above the melting point of some of the stored materials during the defrost cycle. Appropriate back-up storage facilities are required so that the above maintenance can be carried out.

Autoclaves should be equipped with temperature chart recorders so that the operation has evidence and documentation that appropriate temperatures were maintained during the entire sterilizing cycle. In addition, a suspension of or strips impregnated with spores of *Bacillus stearothermophilus* should be used regularly to monitor sterilization. Ampules or strips may be placed in a test pack. An indicator should be placed in the coolest part of the chamber, usually the front of the lowest shelf. In large autoclaves or ones with large loads, several locations should be checked to assure an even distribution of sterilizing conditions. These biologic checks should be made *at least monthly.* The use of tape with heat-sensitive dye markers is useful for monitoring each load, but does not supersede the biologic tests. It is essential that autoclave operators understand the principles of steam sterilization and follow standardized procedures.

The atmosphere in carbon dioxide incubators and anaerobic jars and chambers requires continued surveillance. Carbon dioxide can be accurately measured by trapping a sample in a syringe or balloon and measuring the CO_2 with the instruments used to measure expired CO_2 in a pulmonary function laboratory. This degree of accuracy is seldom required and a more practical method is to use a CO_2 analyzer (American Scientific Products Cat. No. G1725). This apparatus, originally intended for measurement of furnace flue gases, is easy to use and provides measurements of CO_2 satisfactory for clinical laboratory purposes. These checks should be made daily. The concentration of CO_2 should not exceed 10 per cent after flushing the chamber and should not fall below 5 per cent overnight. When a new CO_2 incubator is put into service, frequent checks during the CO_2 cycling process should be made to determine the characteristics of the system. In addition to direct measurement of CO_2, biologic indicators such as a CO_2-dependent strain of *Neisseria gonorrhoeae* are recommended. This procedure should be controlled by a parallel culture incubated without CO_2 to verify CO_2 dependency.

Each time anaerobic jars are used, a freshly activated cold catalyst should be installed. Used catalyst can be reactivated by heating in an oven at 160°C. for one and a half to two hours. Reactivated catalyst should be stored in an air-tight container with a desiccant. Chemical indicators, such as methylene blue or resazurin, and/or biologic indicators (e.g., a culture of *Clostridium novyi*) should be included in each jar to confirm that anaerobic conditions were achieved. Similar controls and precautions with catalyst are required with anaerobic chambers.

Biologic safety cabinets are required, especially for handling specimens or cultures containing mycobacteria and pathogenic fungi. The air flow across the face of the hood should be checked periodically to determine that it meets the manufacturer's specifications. The air flow velocity should not be less than 100 feet per minute. Filters should be replaced after appropriate decontamination according to the manufacturer's instructions. A qualified technician should certify that it is free of leaks and that original specifications are met. Ultraviolet lamps used in hoods or elsewhere in the laboratory for decontamination purposes must be checked for efficiency at three-month intervals or replaced according to the schedule provided by the lamp manufacturer. Ultraviolet lamps must be kept free of dust which markedly reduces their efficiency.

All balances, particularly analytical balances, must be protected against temperature variation, vibration, and humidity. Knife edges must be smooth and the pans scrupulously clean. National Bureau of Standards Class S weights should be available and used to check the accuracy of analytical balances monthly.

A regular schedule of cleaning and maintaining microscopes should be followed. All personnel must be instructed in the proper procedures for microscope alignment, usage, and cleaning. Without careful attention to these details, the finest microscope will give mediocre performance.

Glassware used in the laboratory must be inspected, and chipped or cracked pieces should be discarded. Glassware must be free of all detergents. Volumetric glassware, especially pipettes and pipettors, should be subjected to a routine checking procedure to verify their calibration accuracy.

Stock Organisms, Source and Storage

As indicated previously, a collection of stable organisms with reliable morphologic, biochemical, physiologic, and serologic characteristics is essential to a quality control program. The desired characteristic(s) for each organism in the collection must be reproducible when maintained under proper conditions. Stock organisms can be obtained from a variety of sources, e.g., (1) The American Type Culture Collection, Rockville, Maryland; (2) Bactrol Discs, Difco Laboratories; (3) Bact-Chek Discs, Roche Diagnostics, Hoffman La Roche; (4) proficiency testing programs; (5) reference laboratories or public health laboratories; and (6) your own laboratory. Tables 53–1 and 53–4 list the kinds of organisms that should be included.

Three methods can be used to store stock cultures: (1) lyophilization (freeze drying); (2) ultra freezing; and (3) use of appropriate storage media at room temperature, in the refrigerator or incubator. Lyophilization is the most reliable method but also the most elaborate. Most laboratories will lack the facilities for this process, although cultures may be obtained from outside sources in the lyophilized state.

Ultrafreezing may be used for aerobic and anaerobic organisms. A loop full of a log phase culture can be suspended in 0.5 to 1.0 ml of sterile defibrinated sheep blood in a screw cap vial. These vials can be quick frozen in a dry ice ethanol bath, in liquid nitrogen, or in an ultrafreezer and then stored at −40°C. or lower. Organisms can be recovered after thawing at 37°C. in a water bath for several minutes. A modification of this method is to include sterile glass beads in the vial so that each bead is uniformly coated with the organism blood suspension (Nagel, 1972). Individual beads can be quickly removed from the vial and placed in a tube of an appropriate broth medium for growth. The remaining unused beads are returned promptly to the freezer before they have a chance to thaw.

The simplest methods involve the use of solid, semisolid, or broth media for storage. These media should preserve the viability and stability of the organism without excessive growth or metabolic activity. Table 53–7 lists several suitable media and the organisms which can be stored.

PROFICIENCY TESTING

Proficiency testing, required by certain government and private accrediting or auditing agencies, provides a valuable adjunct to a laboratory's quality control program as a means of judging overall quality. Satisfactory performance indicates that all procedures, equipment, media, reagents, and personnel involved in the processing of these samples are working as expected. For optimal use as a quality control measure, these external unknowns should be introduced to the laboratory as clinical specimens and not identified as test samples. Similarly, internally fabricated specimens using organisms from the laboratory's own culture collection can be submitted as a "blind" to evaluate performance problems. These "blind" unknowns present several problems which must be overcome. The quality control technologist must introduce the samples in a form indistinguishable from routine clinical specimens. Care must be taken that reports are not included inadvertently in any real

Table 53–7. RECOMMENDED MEDIA FOR STORAGE OF STOCK CULTURES

Medium	Organisms	Storage Time*
Cystine-trypticase agar (CTA)	Enterobacteriaceae Non-fermenters Staphylococci Streptococci Pneumococci *Listeria*	2–3 months
Soybean casein digest agar (deeps or semisolid)	Enterobacteriaceae Staphylococci	1 year
Blood or chocolate agar slants	Fastidious organisms Pneumococci Streptococci *Haemophilus influenzae* *Neisseria gonorrhoeae* *Neisseria meningitidis*	variable
Cooked meat medium	Anaerobes Facultative anaerobes	2–3 months
Lowenstein-Jensen	Mycobacteria	3 months

*At 4 to 8°C.

patient's record, and where organisms are used that will prompt a telephone call to the "requesting physician," he be notified in advance or the culture labeled as an autopsy. A mechanism should be worked out with the hospital business office so that there will be no confusion over laboratory charges.

Proficiency testing programs provided by external agencies (e.g., College of American Pathologists, Centers for Disease Control, or state or local health departments) in general provide information which allows comparisons of the performance of the laboratory with that of all other participants in the program. In addition, these programs as a rule provide a considerable amount of timely educational material which addresses problems in evaluation and identification procedures that may be encountered by participants when dealing with clinical specimens similar to the test sample. Some programs provide data regarding the results obtained by participants from the important differential tests used in identifying the test organism(s). This information can be valuable in several ways. It can verify that the test procedures used in the laboratory are adequate and that the individual test results are in agreement. When misidentification occurs, specific defective differential tests can be pinpointed. In addition, these data document the differential characteristics of the test organism(s), making it extremely valuable for future use as internal blind unknown organisms or as organisms to be implemented into the laboratory's media and reagent control program.

Results of internal and external testing programs should be reviewed on a regular basis and discussed with all personnel. These discussions should be an educational exercise with emphasis on laboratory and personnel improvement.

DOCUMENTATION OF QUALITY CONTROL

The quality control program should be completely described in the laboratory procedure manual. This should include a definition of the person or persons responsible for carrying out the program, as well as the mechanism whereby information obtained as a result of the program is communicated to the laboratory director. Each procedure, medium, reagent, item of equipment, etc., to be controlled should have the control methods defined, as well as the frequency of testing, limits for acceptability, and action to be taken when not acceptable. Appropriate work forms should be developed to assist persons making the control observations to record these results. For example, simple logs or graphs for daily temperature recordings of refrigerators and incubators can be attached to the unit. It is important to include in these records the limits of acceptability and to provide a place to record the reasons for the unacceptable result (if known), and the action taken to correct the defect.

These working records must be reviewed at least monthly by the person responsible for the quality control program, the laboratory director, or a supervisor. If the laboratory director does not personally inspect all control records, a summary report should be prepared which lists the item controlled, the number of control observations made, the number of times out of control, a summary of the reasons (if known), and the corrective actions taken. All records should be signed or initialed by the person making the observation as well as by the supervisor reviewer. Bartlett (1974, 1975) describes and illustrates numerous forms and recording methods which provide excellent assistance in developing the documentation aspects of a control program.

Barry, D. L., and Bernsohn, K. L.: The role of quality control in the clinical bacteriology laboratory. Am. J. Med. Tech., *34*:195, 1968.

Bartlett, R. C.: Functional quality control. *In* Prier, J. E., Bartola, J., and Friedman J. (eds.): Quality Control in Microbiology. Baltimore, University Park Press, 1975, p. 145.

Bartlett, R. C.: Medical Microbiology: Quality, Cost and Clinical Relevance. New York, Wiley-Interscience, 1974.

Blazevic, D. J., Hall, C. T., and Wilson, M. E.: Cumitech 3. Practical Quality Control Procedures for the Clinical Microbiol-

6

ogy Laboratory, Washington, D.C., American Society for Microbiology, 1976.

Dolan, C. T., Gavan, T. L., King, J. W., Marymont, J. H., Smith, J. W., and Sommers, H. M.: Clinical Relevance in Microbiology. Chicago, College of American Pathologists, 1977.

Lennette, E. H., Spaulding, E. H., and Truant, J. P. (eds.): Manual of Clinical Microbiology. 2nd ed., Washington, D.C., American Society for Microbiology, 1974.

Nagel, J. G., and Kunz, L. J.: Needless retesting of quality-assured, commercially prepared culture media. Appl. Microbiol., *26*:31, 1973.

Nagel, J. G., and Kunz, L. J.: Simplified storage and retrieval of stock cultures. Appl. Microbiol., *23*:837, 1972.

National Committee for Clinical Laboratory Standards. Approved Standard M2-T3. Performance Standards for Antimicrobial Disc Susceptibility Tests. Villanova, Pa., 1980.

Prier, J. E., Bartola, J. T., and Friedman, H. (eds.): Quality Control in Microbiology. Baltimore, University Park Press, 1975.

Russell, R. L.: Quality control in the microbiology laboratory. *In* Lennette, R. H., Spaulding, E. H., and Truant, J. P. (eds.): Manual of Clinical Microbiology. 2nd ed. Washington, D.C., American Society for Microbiology, 1974, p. 862.

Russell, R. L., Yoshimori, R. S., Rhodes, T. F., Reynolds, J. W., and Jennings, E. R.: A quality control program for clinical microbiology. Tech. Bull. Reg. Med. Tech., *39*:195, 1969.

Thornsberry, C., Gavan, T. L., and Gerlach, E. A.: Cumitech 6. New Developments in Antimicrobial Agent Susceptibility Testing. Washington, D.C., American Society for Microbiology, 1977.

Vera, H. D., and Dumoff, M.: Culture media. *In* Lennette, E. H., Spaulding, E. H., and Truant, J. P. (eds.): Manual of Clinical Microbiology. 2nd ed. Washington, D.C., American Society for Microbiology, 1974, p. 881.

54

HOSPITAL INFECTION CONTROL

THOMAS F. KEYS, M.D.

Historical Perspective

The communicability of infectious diseases was clearly recognized four centuries ago by Fracastorius, an Italian, who wrote in his book *Contagion* that "there are, it seems, three fundamentally different types of contagion: the first infects by direct contact only; the second does the same, but in addition leaves fomes . . . ; thirdly, there is a kind of contagion which . . . also infects at a distance" (Fracastorious, 1930). Florence Nightingale uttered a prophetic statement over 100 years ago in her classic text on the design, construction, and facilities of hospitals: "It may seem a strange principle to enunciate as the very first requirement in a hospital that it should do the sick no harm" (Nightingale, 1863).

In the nineteenth century, Ignaz Semmelweiss, a Hungarian physician, emerged as a tragic figure in the control of a serious hospital infection, puerperal sepsis (childbed fever). Semmelweiss conducted classic studies on the cause and prevention of childbed fever shortly after graduating from medical school in Vienna and then upon his return to Hungary several years later. Unfortunately, he did not publish his studies until 1861, several years before his death. Throughout his professional career, Semmelweiss was opposed in his theories about this infectious disease. He died at the age of 47, ironically of streptococcal sepsis after performing an autopsy on a victim of the disease. Semmelweiss's bitterness was expressed in an open letter to one of his colleagues, Professor Scanzoni of Wurzburg, in 1862: "You have proved, Sir, that one can murder exceedingly well in your new and well-equipped maternity hospital, if one is properly qualified" (Antall, 1973).

With the advancement of techniques for surgical procedures and anesthesia, it was Joseph Lister, an Englishman who lived from 1827 to 1912, who stressed his concern about wound infections: "You must be able to see with your mental eye the septic ferments as one sees flies and other insects with the corporal eye. If you can, you will be properly on your guard against them" (Guthrie, 1949).

Lister was the first physician to use a phenol (carbolic acid) locally following repair of open compound fractures to prevent serious wound infections. He later extended this application to silk, catgut, and even to a carbolic steam spray for the operating room!

The genius of Louis Pasteur, his discovery of fermentation, and the germ theory prompted him to discuss avoidance of wound sepsis in a talk to Paris physicians in the late 1870's:

> If I had the honor of being a surgeon, convinced as I am of the dangers caused by the germs of microbes scattered on the surface of every object, particularly in the hospitals, not only would I use absolutely clean instruments, but after cleansing my hands with the greatest care and putting them quickly through a flame, I would only make use of charpie, bandages and sponges which had previously been raised to a heat of 130 to 150 degrees centigrade. . . . All that is easy to practice, and, in that way, I should still have to fear the germs suspended in the atmosphere surrounding the patient; but observation shows us every day that the number of those germs is almost insignificant compared to that of those which lie scattered on the surface of objects or in the cleanest, ordinary water (Vallery-Radot, 1916).

Pasteur's statements remain lucid and exceedingly to the point as one examines our approach to prevention of wound sepsis in today's hospitals.

Significance

Hospital-associated infections have been estimated to occur in 3 to 13 per cent of all inpatients (Barrett-Connor, 1972). Lower rates are reported in patients residing in community hospitals, whereas higher rates are noted in major medical centers. In 1976 Altemeier estimated that over two million cases of wound infections had occurred in the United States alone. There is no reason to believe the problem has become less frequent in the intervening years. The financial burden of hospital infections is enormous. There is a direct expense borne by both patient and hospital estimated at six to nine thousand dollars per infection. In addition, there is loss of gainful employment as well as associated pain and discomfort from the infection. Mortality is high in patients with hospital-associated infections. Lorian (1972) has stated that excess mortality is either coincidental or an expression of the debility of this patient population. One must realize that patients with terminal disease may succumb to infection during hospitalization, often from bacteria in their own gastrointestinal tract. It is always difficult to "blame" the hospital for such an infection associated with a disease that has a hopeless prognosis.

Perhaps one of every three doctors in the United States is subjected to legal investigation related to possible malpractice. Unless negligence is proved on the part of the physician, other staff, and the hospital, most cases are not justified (Dornette, 1973). Successful legal action might occur if a newly operated patient is moved into a room shared by a patient with an obvious wound infection. Other examples might be not culturing a wound when pus is clearly present; not examining a wound when there is pain and fever; and not obtaining a chest x-ray if a patient is suspected of having pneumonia. Unfortunately, standards of hospital care are so high in the public mind that complications are simply not expected. Therefore, it is important that all individuals working in the hospital conform to procedures and practices that are currently acceptable and in keeping with professional standards of the community. In short, it is necessary that any conditions that might cause hospital infection be remedied by an active infection control program.

There are few objective data currently available to support a highly structured infection-control program. Nevertheless, some program must be adapted to the needs of the individual hospital. This must include a system for the recognition and control of infection hazards. Established guidelines by the Joint Commission on Accreditation of Hospitals (1981) clearly state that there must be an effective infection control program within the hospital. Unfortunately, the program by itself does not generate an income, and it is often difficult for administrators to justify this expense. In 1970 Edwards (1971) estimated the cost of a surveillance program for a 600-bed hospital in Chicago. The cost to the hospital was approximately $100,000 per year, which amounted to less than $3.00 per patient admission. Comparing this cost with an anticipated expense of six to nine thousand dollars for a serious hospital infection, a surveillance program appears justified. Or phrased another way, if such a program were available and might spare the possibility of a serious hospital infection, would you as a patient be willing to spend several dollars to maintain it? I doubt if many of us would decline to participate.

ORGANIZATION

The purpose of the infection control program is to develop and maintain effective measures for the recognition and prevention of hospital-associated (nosocomial) infections. If the following goals or objectives are met, the program will be successful:

A practical surveillance system to detect nosocomial infections.

Written procedures for controlling all infection hazards to patients, employees, and visitors.

A strong employee health program, including orientation of new employees to the hazards of hospital infections.

An effective continuing education program for all staff.

The Hospital Infection Committee

According to guidelines established by the Joint Commission on Accreditation of Hospitals (1981) the following criteria should be applied in staffing the hospital infection committee:

> Responsibility for monitoring the infection control program shall be vested in a multidisciplinary committee. . . Its membership shall include representation from the medical staff, administration, nursing services, and where available, the microbiology section of the laboratory. Any individual employed in a surveillance or epidemiologic capacity shall be a member of the committee.

The hospital infection committee must receive enthusiastic support from administration and all staff personnel. It is not a policeman, but it must have the authority to conduct epidemiologic investigations when appropriate, and it must be objective in making decisions and firm in implementing them. It is vital that the infection committee be well represented by members of the medical and surgical staff. If the committee is heavy with administrators, nurses, and members of support facilities, it will have serious problems in initiating policies that affect professional activities of the medical and surgical staff. In addition to the chairperson and surveillance officer (who should also be the committee's secretary), other members should include:

Nursing service—two members: one responsible for inservice training; the other supervisory for general ward nursing.

Medical staff—one member, preferably involved in the care of immunologically compromised patients.

Surgical staff—two members: a general surgeon and either an orthopedic surgeon, a cardiac surgeon, or a neurosurgeon.

Pediatric staff—one member, preferably involved in the newborn nursery and neonatal intensive care unit.

Clinical laboratory—one member with knowledge of clinical microbiology (if not already the chairperson, surveillance officer, or environmental officer).

Employee health—one member, preferably nursing supervisor of the area.

Administration—one member, preferably knowledgeable about the nursing and support facilities for patient care.

The chairperson is the key to the success of the committee and to the entire infection control program. An individual whose "credentials document knowledge of and special interest or experience in infection control" is suited for the role (Joint Commission, 1981). Preferably, this might be a physician specializing in infectious diseases or a pathologist-microbiologist, or a surgeon. However, of greater importance is the personality of the individual and an ability to handle tactfully individuals engaged in medical, surgical, nursing, and support activities in the hospital. It is desirable that the chairperson remain in the position for at leave five years and be remunerated financially for time and effort. Financial reimbursement proportional to the time spent in infection-control activities should be provided by the hospital administration.

The committee should meet at least every one to two months and more frequently if necessary, depending on the complexities of the institution and the nature of the day-to-day problems. There is no point in meeting regularly without a well-conceived and prepared agenda, despite the attractiveness of having a fancy lunch in a quiet dining room for a change! It is important for the committee to seek advice and counsel from additional individuals representative of dietary, pharmacy, central supply, engineering, and housekeeping when the need arises. If a problem develops in a special area, the chairperson may designate a subcommittee or an *ad hoc* committee composed of individuals expert therein to review the situation in detail and present the problem and possible solutions to the entire committee at a later date.

The responsibilities of the hospital infection committee include:

1. To review nosocomial infections in regard to their management and epidemic potential.
2. To review and make recommendations regarding infection control procedures throughout all areas in the hospital, such as pharmacy, central supply, housekeeping, laundry, surgery, anesthesia, nursing, dietetics, engineering, surgical pathology, clinical pathology, radiology, respiratory therapy, physical medicine, and employee health.
3. To implement policies to control community epidemic problems as they might affect the hospital.
4. To review antibiotic usage both for prophylaxis and therapy as related to appropriateness, cost, toxicity, and emergence of antibiotic-resistant bacteria.
5. To review and endorse ongoing educational programs in infection control for staff and hospital employees.
6. To review and endorse studies involving infection control.

The Infection Control Team

The team is composed of individuals who are regularly active on the hospital infection committee and includes the chairperson, individual(s) performing surveillance, and a member of the clinical laboratory. The team may expand with individuals expert in certain areas, as during an investigation of a possible outbreak or epidemic problem.

The Infection Control Officer. Qualifications are the same as those for chairperson of the hospital infection committee. Responsibilities include:

1. Chairmanship of the hospital infection committee.
2. Effective communication among all professional and non-professional staff working in the hospital environment.
3. Regular review of recognized nosocomial infection cases and, as well, autopsy cases for possible unrecognized infection.
4. Information relay of potential epidemiologic significance from the laboratory to appropriate staff (for example, informing a ward nurse that a patient's sputum smear has just been reported as positive for acid-fast bacilli or that a patient's serum sample is positive for hepatitis B surface antigen).
5. Consultation with administration to discuss problems and policies of infection control, especially with new construction, remodeling, and purchase of any items that present infection hazards.
6. Evaluation of the effectiveness of other infection control team members.
7. Consultation with Employee Health Service as needed, especially with regard to potential communicable disease in employees.
8. Epidemiologic investigation and, if necessary, request for assistance from state and federal health authorities.
9. Educational programs on infection control for medical staff and other employee groups.
10. Clinical laboratory research to better understand the problems and improve the quality of infection control procedures.

The Surveillance Officer. This individual is usually a nurse or other qualified person who has a special interest, dedication, and training in practical matters of hospital infection control. Like the infection control officer, the surveillance officer must know the hospital and relate well to administration, staff, and patients at all levels. Responsibilities include:

1. Surveillance according to procedures approved by the hospital infection committee.
2. Instruction on practices and procedures of infection control to nursing service (including the operating room), dietetics, employee health, and other hospital departments (physical medicine, radiology, etc.)
3. Orientation of new employees on infection control, including personal hygiene and their attentiveness to the existing policies and procedures.
4. Written guidelines regarding isolation and care of patients with communicable diseases as recommended by the hospital infection committee.
5. Regular follow-up of patients with communicable diseases and recommendations for isolation procedures and other precautions as indicated.

It is obvious that more than one surveillance officer

or infection control nurse will be required to discharge these responsibilities if the hospital is of significant size and complexity. Current recommendations are that one individual be employed full time for every 300 acute medical and surgical beds.

The Environmental Officer. This individual must be knowledgeable about the practical applications of microbiology to the infection control program. In general, a clinical microbiologist or laboratory technologist would be considered for this position. The responsibilities include:

1. Assistant to director in performance of duties and investigations.
2. Guidelines and instruction on infection control in hemodialysis, pharmacy, clinical pathology, central supply, housekeeping, and engineering. In conjunction with engineering, the environmental officer should provide guidelines and recommendations for the maintenance of adequate ventilation and waste disposal.
3. Collection and interpretation of environmental cultures as approved by the hospital infection committee.

Excellent training programs on hospital infection control are available at Centers for Disease Control in Atlanta and through the Association for Practitioners in Infection Control (APIC). I would strongly recommend these courses for any fledgling members on the Infection Control Team.

Responsibilities of the Infection Control Team

The responsibilities of the Infection Control Team include maintenance of approved isolation standards, surveillance of hospital-associated infections, collection and interpretation of environmental cultures, and investigation of a suspected outbreak or epidemic of hospital infection. Each one of these responsibilities is described in detail below.

Isolation Procedures. Sir William Osler was once quoted as saying that "Soap and water and common sense are the best disinfectants" (Bean, 1930). This simple statement illustrates well the basic approach to handling patients admitted to the hospital or those who develop infections of a communicable nature while within the hospital. The purpose of isolation is to prevent access of infectious particles from air and contact to patients, sources recognized by Fracastorius in 1565 and Florence Nightingale in 1863. Unfortunately, well-designed controlled studies have not been possible to determine the beneficial aspects of certain isolation procedures. However, the theory is with us, and until our knowledge expands, the somewhat conservative isolation measures recommended by the American Hospital Association and Centers for Disease Control should be adhered to. Despite the deficiencies in any plan for isolating patients with potentially communicable disease, it is critical that a program be simple and applicable to the day-to-day problems of a hospital. The standards must apply equally to physicians, nurses, visitors, housekeepers, technicians, and so forth. On occasion, physicians will not adhere to established isolation procedures and a gentle reprimand by the chairperson of the infection committee is necessary. In a sense, physicians, like patients, are guests of the hospital and must abide by established guidelines for infection control. An invitation to attend an infection committee meeting sometimes is advisable so that the situation or problem may be aired more fully. Modification of an existing isolation policy can even be considered. It is important to realize that isolation procedures must not isolate the patient from the devotion, attention, evaluation, and therapy of health care providers. In addition, the need for isolation must be reviewed with the patient and with his family and other visitors not only by the nurse who is fulfilling the request by a physician, but by that physician as well. If the need arises, any member of the infection control team should be available for counsel.

We have used as a guide, "Isolation techniques for use in hospitals," developed by the Centers for Disease Control (CDC), Atlanta, Georgia (CDC, 1975). A copy of this very valuable booklet is available directly from the Centers. Modification of their isolation standards may be necessary, depending on the complexity and uniqueness of an individual hospital. Guidelines should be available at every nursing station for review on the wards. At our institution, physicians are provided with an abbreviated outline of isolation protocol that is conveniently carried in a pocket calendar notebook (Table 54–1). Guidelines for these categories are elaborated below:

Strict Isolation. This form of isolation is used principally for patients with severe burns, disseminated herpes infections, and well-documented staphylococcal pneumonia. A private room is required, with gown, mask, and gloves for direct patient contact. When the degree of contagiousness lessens, strict isolation is no longer necessary. For example, when a patient with staphylococcal pneumonia is responding clinically to appropriate antibiotic therapy and secretions can be adequately contained, strict isolation is no longer required. Similarly, after disseminated herpes lesions have resolved to the crusting and healing stages, the same principle holds.

Respiratory Isolation. Candidates for respiratory isolation include patients with suspected or culturally documented active pulmonary tuberculosis, influenza, and several other acute respiratory infections. Although the justification for placing patients with meningitis in respiratory isolation is poorly documented, this is done until a preliminary diagnosis is established and the patient is on appropriate antimicrobial therapy, generally within 24 to 48 hours. On the other hand, it is important for patients admitted with measles to be in respiratory isolation because of viable viral particles in their respiratory secretions. Respiratory isolation should include a private room, preferably with ventilation exhausted to the outside. Although masks only trap large particulate matter and do not prevent entry of respiratory droplet nuclei, they heighten the awareness of staff for a patient's respiratory infection. For pulmonary tuberculosis, duration of isolation after therapy has commenced is not

Table 54–1. HOSPITAL ISOLATION PROCEDURES

Categories	Criteria	Precautions
STRICT ISOLATION (Yellow card)	Burns, extensive Staphylococcal pneumonia Diphtheria Chickenpox Disseminated herpes Congenital rubella Rabies	Private room Gown Mask Gloves for patient contact Scrupulous handwashing Disinfection of patient-associated articles
RESPIRATORY ISOLATION (Red card)	Tuberculosis, pulmonary suspected or sputum-positive Influenza pneumonia Meningitis (meningococcal) Measles Pertussis Mumps Rubella	Private room Mask Scrupulous handwashing Disinfection of articles contaminated with secretions
ENTERIC PRECAUTIONS (Dark brown card)	Diarrhea, acute or until etiology established Salmonella Shigella *Camplyobacter jejuni* *Clostridium difficile*	Private room Gown and gloves for contact with patient or articles likely contaminated with fecal material Scrupulous handwashing Disinfection of articles contaminated with feces.
HEPATITIS PRECAUTIONS (Light brown card)	Hepatitis; viral (B or non-B) Hepatitis B antigen positive patients	Same as above plus special blood precautions
WOUND AND SKIN PRECAUTIONS (Green card)	Burns, moderate Pyogenic wound and skin infections where drainage cannot be contained in dressing Puerperal sepsis Eruptive herpes	Private room Gown Mask and gloves for direct wound contact Scrupulous handwashing Disinfection of contaminated articles
CJ PRECAUTIONS (Gray card)	Suspected Creutzfeld-Jakob disease	Private room Special precautions for blood and CSF
PROTECTIVE ISOLATION (Blue card)	Bone marrow or heart transplant patients	Private room with $\geq$ 15 air exchanges/hr Mask, gown, and gloves at discretion of service Scrupulous handwashing

clear cut. Communicability appears to be higher in patients with active open cavitary disease, as well as in those with tracheobronchial and vocal cord involvement. As a rule, therapy should be continued for at least seven to ten days before taking patients with pulmonary tuberculosis out of respiratory isolation, provided the patient is cooperative and capable of containing respiratory secretions.

Enteric Precautions. This isolation category applies principally for patients with acute diarrhea (often caused by *Campylobacter, Clostridium difficile, Salmonella, Shigella,* and parvoviruses). A private room and gloving and gowning by staff who may come in contact with contaminated excretions are recommended. Duration of isolation depends to a great extent on the clinical illness and infecting agent. Some patients may be in the hospital for days before an infectious etiology of diarrhea is considered. Ideally, they should be placed on Enteric Precautions at the time of admission and continued until an infectious cause has been ruled out. On the other hand, patients with gastrointestinal salmonellosis may remain infected long after they have become asymptomatic. The need for prolonged isolation in this case has not been established.

Viral Hepatitis Precautions. This category, formerly a portion of Enteric Precautions, was separated to avoid confusion and to emphasize clearly the need for needle and blood precautions with hepatitis B virus. A private room is recommended and special attention directed toward collecting and processing blood and urine specimens as well as disposing of intravascular infusion devices. These precautions apply also to patients with acute non-A–non-B hepatitis and asymptomatic carriers of hepatitis B surface antigen.

Wound and Skin Precautions. This isolation category generally applies to purulent postoperative wound infections with drainage that cannot be contained within a simple, dry dressing. The category is also useful for patients with local herpes infections until the lesions are in a final stage of healing. A private room is recommended, and patients are generally confined to their room until drainage is under control. When caring for a patient's wound, disposable gloves must be worn with scrupulous handwashing afterward. For patients with mild to moderate burn wounds, we have used a modified form of wound isolation. This allows a more liberal approach to ambulation and greater interaction with staff, other patients, family, and visitors. Such an approach reduces the incidence of deprivation problems, especially in pediatric burn wound cases after youngsters are on prolonged rigorous isolation.

Creutzfeldt-Jakob Precautions. Creutzfeldt-Jakob disease (CJD) is a progressive infection of the central nervous system thought to be due to a slow virus like that causing kuru. Although there is very little evidence that CJD is transmissible except after contact with brain tissue, some precautions appear reasonable (Jarvis, 1982). A private room is desirable but not necessary. Special attention is given to collecting blood and cerebrospinal fluid. Specimens are double bagged and labeled "CJD Precautions." All used needles and syringes are autoclaved before being incinerated. The same applies for disposable lumbar puncture equipment and EEG electrodes. Reusable manometers are autoclaved before reuse.

Protective Isolation. At our institution, only bone marrow and cardiac transplant recipients qualify for this category. A private room with at least 15 air exchanges per hour is used; gowns, masks, and gloves are worn at the discretion of the attending physician. Scrupulous hand washing is enforced. Simple protective isolation for neutropenic patients has recently been shown to be of no value in protecting them from infection (Nauseef, 1981). A private room close to a

NAME ______________________ I.D. No. ______________________

AGE ______________ TODAY'S DATE ______________ ROOM NO. ______________

ADM ______________ DISM ______________ SERVICE ______________

DIAGNOSIS ____

SURGERY THIS ADMISSION:

Date	Procedure	Doctor	O.R.

PATHOGEN(S)

Site	Lab No.	Date	Organism	Antibiotic Susceptibility
________	________	________	________	________
________	________	________	________	________

INFECTION SITE

☐ Surg Wound ☐ Super ☐ Deep ☐ Clean ☐ Clean-Contam

☐ Foreign body ☐ Prophy Antibiotics

☐ Urinary ☐ Asx ☐ Other ☐ Cath Date ______________ to ______________

☐ Pneumonia ☐ Trach ☐ Intub ☐ IPPB Date ______________________

☐ Skin ☐ IV ☐ Biopsy ☐ Angio ☐ Cardiac Cath ☐ Other

☐ Bacteremia ☐ Secondary ☐ Primary ☐ Indeterm

☐ Other ______________________

☐ Hospital Infection Ward ______________ Room ______________ ☐ Endogenous

☐ Exogenous

Figure 54–1. Hospital infection surveillance card.

nursing station but remote from clinically infected cases, with careful hand washing between patient contacts, is our only recommendation.

Surveillance of Hospital Infections. Although arguments exist about the usefulness of surveillance, at least some prospective information on the types of infections occurring within the hospital is essential for an infection control program. Surveillance allows the infection control team to appreciate the cause and origin of hospital infections. It provides a data base that can be readily reviewed if a potential epidemic or outbreak situation develops. Furthermore, surveillance stimulates a greater awareness of infection control problems and provides a format of continuing education for medical and nursing staff. In addition, if the surveillance system is comparable with that of other hospitals, causes and solutions to problems may be found simply by reviewing others' experience, either in the literature or by direct communication.

On the other hand, surveillance must not totally consume the energies of the infection control team. Many hospitals cannot afford surveillance of all their infections, but give priority to high risk areas such as intensive care units (Landry, 1982). It is important for each hospital to determine the need for and degree of surveillance essential for its own infection control program. In my opinion, no more than 40 per cent of the team's effort should be spent on surveillance, with the remainder used for educational, administrative, and research activities.

In order for surveillance of hospital infections to be useful, definitions of infection must be clear, and basic epidemiologic data must be collected, reviewed weekly, and disseminated regularly to the hospital infection committee. Detection of hospital infections involves assessment of both laboratory culture results and the patient's clinical condition.

A data collection card (epi-card) is ideal for recording basic surveillance information (Fig. 54–1). The card must be easy to use and carry. It is hardly necessary, in fact superfluous, to record a wealth of detail on the epi-card. Only information necessary to document a hospital-associated infection is needed. By and large, most hospital-associated infections occur after a patient has been hospitalized for at least 48 to 72 hours. Bacteriologic data as reported by the clinical laboratory are entered on the central portion of the epi-card. On the top portion of the card, the patient's name, identification number, room number, admission date, service, and working diagnosis are recorded. The surveillance officer, working with laboratory and clinical clues, makes the diagnosis of hospital infection. Afterward, the remainder of the card is filled out with facts related to the infection site. Our definition of infection is in keeping with that established by the Centers for Disease Control (Garner, 1970).

Wound Infection. A surgical wound with purulent drainage is infected. If it develops or extends below the fascial plane, it is considered a deep infection. If it is confined to the subcutaneous space, the infection is superficial. It is important in reporting wound infections that they all be accurately classified at the time of surgery. Altemeier's categories of clean, clean-contaminated, contaminated, and dirty serve this purpose (Table 54–2). Most meaningful "attack rates" are derived by considering only the clean and clean-contaminated wound categories. Wound infections may not necessarily present during the same hospitalization as for surgery. Those following insertion of prosthetic devices, including cardiac valves and hip appliances, may not emerge until weeks, months, or sometimes years after operation.

Urinary Infection. Hospital urinary tract infections are usually associated with urologic instrumentation such as urethral catheterization. While often asymptomatic, catheter-associated bacteriuria may become symptomatic later during hospitalization or after dismissal. A count of at least 10,000 to 100,000 colony forming units per ml of urine is generally diagnostic of infection.

Pneumonia. Hospital-associated pneumonia is often exceedingly difficult to diagnose. Symptoms, signs, x-rays, and laboratory findings of pneumonia may be confused with those of pulmonary infarction, edema, atelectasis, and the shock lung syndrome. Ideally, diagnostic criteria should include a cough productive of purulent sputum, fever, and evidence

Table 54–2. CLASSIFICATION OF OPERATIVE WOUNDS IN RELATION TO CONTAMINATION AND INCREASING RISK OF INFECTION

Clean
- Non-traumatic
- No inflammation encountered
- No break in technique
- Respiratory, alimentary, genitourinary tracts not entered

Clean-contaminated
- Gastrointestinal or respiratory tracts entered without significant spillage
- Appendectomy
- Oropharynx entered
- Vagina entered
- Genitourinary tract entered in absence of infected urine
- Biliary tract entered in absence of infected bile
- Minor break in technique

Contaminated
- Major break in technique
- Gross spillage from gastrointestinal tract
- Traumatic wound, fresh
- Entrance of genitourinary or biliary tracts in presence of infected urine or bile

Dirty and infected
- Acute bacterial inflammation encountered, without pus
- Transection of "clean" tissue for the purpose of surgical access to a collection of pus
- Perforated viscus encountered
- Traumatic wound with retained devitalized tissue, foreign bodies, fecal contamination and/or delayed treatment, or from dirty source

of pneumonia on chest x-ray that was not present on admission.

Other Infection Sites. These include the skin, which may be the point of entry of an intravascular line or biopsy tool, burn wounds, gastroenteritis, meningitis, and endometritis.

Bloodstream. All bacteremias should be noted on the epi-cards. They may occur secondarily from wound, urinary, lung, and skin infections. Bacteremias cannot be taken lightly, since they carry significant morbidity and mortality for the hospitalized patient. When the source of bacteremia is uncertain, it may be designated as either indeterminate or primary if it may have resulted from direct inoculation of contaminated material into the bloodstream.

Synthesis of Surveillance Data. Surveillance cards should be reviewed at least weekly by the infection control officer. In addition, the cards may be used for line-listing certain infections, such as wound infections, urinary infections, and bacteremias. While line-listings do not indicate attack rates of hospital infections, because they lack denominator data (number of cases at risk), they are still helpful if a trend toward a certain type of infection is developing in the hospital environment.

As noted previously, surveillance data must fulfill a greater role than occupying the surveillance officer's filing cabinet. Data must be organized in such a fashion that they can be reviewed and understood by all members of the hospital infection committee. In this way, surveillance will help in recognizing a need to change a policy, practice, or procedure. Such data must also be available for instant retrieval if review is necessary during investigation of a possible outbreak or epidemic of hospital infection.

Surveillance data gathered at our institution are routinely organized in several forms. First, a line-listing for all clean and clean-contaminated wound infections is prepared on a monthly basis for review by members of the hospital infection committee. To illustrate, the following heading is used to prepare the line-listing sheet of surgical wound infections:

> Date (week, month) Hospital
> *Organism/Surgeon/Procedure Date/ O.R./Date and Ward Cultured/Patient ID*

Secondly, the surveillance data are organized for a monthly nosocomial infection report, which provides a summary of cases with infections over cases at risk during the same period, usually by procedures or dismissals, for computation of hospital infection attack rates or "percentages" (Fig. 54–2). This basic report contains enough information for regular review by the hospital infection committee. If an increased number of certain infections is noted, it may be necessary to collect more denominator information before one can accurately assess the problem. For example, if during a reporting period an increased number of urinary tract infections was noted, one also must know how many patients during that same period underwent urologic instrumentation, especially urethral catheterization. Antibiotic susceptibility data are recorded on a monthly basis for all bacteremias, allowing for inspection of changing patterns of antibiotic susceptibility. This information may also be correlated with intrahospital antibiotic usage.

Although monthly surveillance reports are intended for review mainly by the hospital infection committee, they may also be useful for educating physicians, nurses, and other staff about principles and practices of infection control. It is possible to condense surveillance data to those applicable only on certain wards or in certain sections of the hospital. The ward or "unit" report can be forwarded to the nursing supervisor on a regular basis. This reporting system is best adapted for high-risk patient areas such as medical and surgical intensive care units. A regular review of the unit report by the infection control team to the medical and nursing staff not only makes them aware of potential epidemic problems but also provides them with essential inservice training.

Environmental Cultures. For several decades hospitals dutifully collected a large variety and number of bacterial cultures from their environment. This labor contributed greatly to the cost and also, it was believed, to the effectiveness of an infection control program. Specimens came from floors, sinks, walls, ceilings, staircases, air, water, and linen on a routine basis. These microbiologic data accumulated in hospital files and served no useful purpose, except perhaps to satisfy the requirements of certain regulatory agencies. With strong support from the American Public Health and American Hospital Associations (1974, 1975), the trend of excess environmental culturing has now been reversed. As a general guideline, environmental cultures should be taken only during an investigation of an outbreak or for research purposes. Routine monitoring is indicated only for hospital steam and gas sterilizers (weekly or with every load of implantable objects), dry heat ovens (monthly), and water used for dialysis (monthly).

Investigation of an Outbreak. Emotions run high when word leaks out that a certain hospital has an epidemic. The term, defined by Webster as "common to, or affecting at the same time, many in a community," is usually misused and not truly representative of the problem at hand. Nevertheless, an investigation may be required, and this can only be done through the hospital infection committee with firm support by administration and staff. Occasionally, a complex problem, which may be scientific or political, may require outside resources for assistance. Public health authorities, beginning at the local level, should first be consulted. If necessary, state agencies may ask for assistance from the federal government through the Epidemiological Investigation Service, a branch of the CDC.

It is crucial to establish first whether or not a "problem" (avoid the word epidemic) really exists. As a rule, two or more cases of a clinical infection of identical cause or circumstance appearing within a limited time qualify for an investigation (Castle, 1977). The etiology must be determined as rapidly as possible by a competent clinical microbiology laboratory.

1. *TOTALS* Infections ______ Dismissals ______ Attack Rate ______ %

   Wounds ______ Skin ______

   Urinary ______ Primary bacteremias ______

   Pneumonia ______ Other ______

2. *OPERATIVE WOUNDS* (Clean and Clean-Contaminated cases only)

Service	*Infections*	*Total Cases*	*Attack Rate* (%)
General Surgery	______	______	______
Orthopedics	______	______	______
Cardiac	______	______	______
Etc.	______	______	______

3. *NON-WOUNDS*

Service	*Urinary*	*Pneumonia*	*Skin*	*Other*	*Total*	*Dism*	*Attack Rate* (%)
Medicine	______	______	______	______	______	______	______
Surgery	______	______	______	______	______	______	______
Pediatrics	______	______	______	______	______	______	______
Obstetrics	______	______	______	______	______	______	______
Nursery	______	______	______	______	______	______	______
Etc.	______	______	______	______	______	______	______

4. *BACTEREMIAS*

Service	*Ward*	*Date Cultured*	*Organism*	*Focus*	*Antibiotic Susceptibility*
Hematology	______	______	______	______	______
Nephrology	______	______	______	______	______
Surgery	______	______	______	______	______
Etc.	______	______	______	______	______

Figure 54–2. Hospital-associated monthly infection report.

The next task is to identify all other clinical cases that have been recognized by routine surveillance within the past several months. Review of line-listing sheets, monthly surveillance reports, and details as recorded on the epi-cards is extremely helpful. In addition, it is desirable to locate additional cases that may not have been recognized by routine surveillance, since this usually reflects only 60 to 70 per cent of actual hospital infections. An intensified surveillance in areas where the index of suspicion is high may provide more cases. Even though they may not be definite, they should at least be examined to assess their epidemiologic significance. All suspected and confirmed cases are entered on a special line-listing sheet that is constructed to assess the clinical and epidemiologic features of the problem. For example, if there was concern about an increased incidence of operative wound infections, the following line listing might be used:

Culture results/Date/Ward
Operation/Date/Room/Team
Pre-op diagnosis/Patient identification

The next step in the investigation is to develop an attack rate for the recognized infections:

$$\text{Attack rate } (\%) = \frac{\text{number of infected cases}}{\text{number of cases at risk}} \times 100$$

Although it may not be completely accurate, the denominator figure in this formula usually represents the number of patients operated on, instrumented, or dismissed during the study period. Attack rates can be computed by the week, month, quarter, or year, depending on the nature of the investigation. A comparison of these data with those generated during a comparable period when there did not appear to be a problem is done using simple statistical analysis (Chi square) (Hill, 1971). If a significant difference in attack rates is documented, the investigation is continued. If there is not, the investigation is usually terminated. Often, however, review of the case material and epidemiologic features of the suspected outbreak generate significant concern among staff and administrators. Certain flaws and problems in existing infection control programs and policies can be recognized and hopefully remedied. On the other hand, if there is firm statistical support for an epidemic problem, the investigation must continue. A critical analysis of all procedures, including dates and locations of operations and use of catheters (urinary and vascular) and inhalation equipment, must take place. This information can also be line-listed and compared with those of a control population without infection but subjected to the same variables as the case population. After the data have been further refined, an hypothesis or tentative explanation of the problem is offered. It is extremely important to consult outside resources, including the literature, before formulating an hypothesis. Hypothesis testing may be done by instituting appropriate control measures for variables that the investigation has determined might have influenced the outcome of the population at risk. Once the hypothesis is verified, a corrective policy or procedure must be quickly drafted by the infection committee, approved by administration, and implemented. A strong educational program is essential to guarantee its effectiveness. Staff simply have to know about the problem before cooperation and adherence to a new policy will take place.

Environmental Services (Housekeeping)

Hospital staff, particularly physicians, often fail to recognize the responsibility that housekeeping has in maintaining an effective infection control program. While it is obviously impossible to maintain a totally "germ-free" hospital environment, effective cleaning measures do greatly reduce the germ load to a susceptible patient population. Details of cleaning procedures are well outlined in recent publications (Altemeier, 1976).

It is important for housekeeping personnel to understand the reasons behind the cleaning procedures and their key role in prevention of hospital infections. They will work harder with this knowledge if it is tactfully presented. Furthermore, employees must be cautioned regarding their exposure to potentially contaminated materials and wastes in the course of their duties. Of greatest concern at present is the possibility of hepatitis B infection after accidental inoculation from contaminated needles, syringes, and glassware in loose refuse. Such materials must be secured in a firm, clearly designated container to reduce this possibility. Needle sticks and other wounds should be promptly reported to the Employee Health Service for evaluation and follow-up.

The housekeeping department is frequently assaulted by detailmen who are in the business of selling items allegedly helpful in infection control. While it is important to be tactful and courteous, all such inquiries should be channeled through the hospital's purchasing service and administration prior to consideration by the infection control committee. For example, a variety of disinfectants are currently available for cleaning floors, but their overall usefulness has not been well established. It may be argued that germicidal cleaners are even not necessary in operating rooms and intensive care units because bacterial counts on floors rapidly increase within 20 to 30 minutes after application of germicides. Furthermore, certain germicides may prove so toxic to the housekeeping staff that their cleaning procedures become less effective. The plain fact is that the liberal application of a good detergent with generous amounts of water is the surest and most economical method for general cleaning. It is also important to realize that incompatibilities may exist between detergents and germicides, particularly with the quaternary ammonium compounds (QUATS). QUATS have themselves been associated with outbreaks of infections due to gram-negative bacteria, and they probably serve no useful purpose in a modern-day hospital (Dixon, 1976).

Last, the Housekeeping Department has the responsibility for maintaining adequate handwashing facilities for staff, patients, and visitors. The recent promotion of handwashing as a sound practice (Steere, 1975), which it certainly is, has resulted in the availability of many handwashing preparations. Soap products ranging from dispensable, impregnated dry soap leaves to foam compounds containing hexachlorophene, alcohol, and emollients are now produced. Liquid soaps are often said to be superior to bar soaps, but there is no good scientific evidence to support this. In fact, contaminated liquid soap dispensers have been implicated in outbreaks of hospital infections. If bar soap is adequately maintained, it should be satisfactory in most areas of the hospital, provided that people know how to wash their hands. Plain soap without germicides does not promote the growth or transmission of bacteria (Bamran, 1965). For handwashing in the operating room theater, prior to performing other invasive procedures, and when caring for isolation patients, germicidal soaps are recommended. They are also indicated for staff working in high-risk areas, such as intensive care units and the nursery.

Employee Health Service

The hospital employee health service is integral to infection control. It protects employees from acquiring infections at work by offering immunization and surveillance for infections likely to occur in the susceptible population. It ensures that other employees and patients are not exposed to potential communicable diseases by clearing employees with infections before they return to work. The infection control officer should be available for consultation and education to all employees. Common infections communicable to employees include tuberculosis and hepatitis B virus infection. In addition, employees may also be susceptible to rubella and cytomegalovirus infections.

Tuberculosis is not nearly as prevalent now as it was 25 years ago. Even though the classic features of the disease may be present on admission, the diagnosis may not be suspected by a physician unfamiliar with the disease (Furey, 1976; MacGregor, 1975). Such patients often reside on a general medical ward for several weeks before the diagnosis is considered. During this time, liberal exposure with infected respiratory droplet nuclei may occur to other patients and staff. Therefore, the health service must provide an active surveillance program for the early detection of tuberculosis for all their employees (Craven, 1975). Those who are tuberculin negative with the two step procedure (Thompson, 1979) should have skin tests repeated at least every several years and more frequently with continuous exposure to suspected or proven tuberculosis (workers in respiratory intensive care units and bronchoscopy and respiratory wards). Additional surveillance may be necessary after inadvertent exposure from a highly contagious patient. Knowledge of an employee's prior tuberculin test always makes the job easier.

With the commercial availability of serologic tests, hepatitis B virus (HBV) can be recognized and distinguished from other types of liver disease (Walsh, 1970). Employees working in clinical laboratory areas, emergency rooms, operating and recovery areas, dialysis units, hematology-oncology wards, pathology laboratories, gastrointestinal/hepatitis units, and blood bank are at risk of acquiring HBV (Maynard, 1981). If concern exists about control measures in these areas, surveillance of employees using antibody tests to HBV is recommended (Mosley, 1982.) When inadvertent exposure to HBV by needle stick, other sharp object, or mucous membrane contact occurs, an employee is a candidate for immune globulin prophylaxis. If antibody to HBV is already present, immunoprophylaxis is not needed. Otherwise, hepatitis B immunoglobulin (HBIG) or, if not available, standard immune globulin (SIG) is indicated (Centers for Disease Control, 1982a). If the source of a needle stick is unknown, it is our practice to give SIG shortly after exposure. Needle stick recipients of HBV should receive a booster injection in 30 days. A newly developed hepatitis B vaccine has recently been marketed (Centers for Disease Control, 1982b). Among candidates for vaccination are health care workers who have frequent blood contact. Hospitals are currently developing priority systems for vaccine allocation. High priority candidates would include hospital employees in hemodialysis, blood bank, and laboratory areas as well as IV nurses, ICU nurses, and phlebotomists.

Both male and female hospital employees are now candidates for rubella vaccination (Centers for Disease Control, 1981). This change was prompted by an outbreak of rubella among hospital employees in a large medical center (Polk, 1980). At our institution, all new employees and those already working in Obstetrics, Gynecology, and Pediatrics are screened for rubella antibody. Those who are non-immune are offered vaccination.

A pregnant employee may express concern or fear about acquiring cytomegalovirus (CMV) infection from patients. It is our practice to have such employees avoid direct contact with cases of acute or persistent CMV infection. However, many patients such as infants and renal transplant recipients may be excreting CMV without symptoms. The only way to prevent contact would be to transfer the employee away from a newborn nursery, pediatric, or transplantation care area (Klein, 1981).

Employees must be knowledgeable about infections that they may bring into the hospital. These include skin and acute respiratory infections and diarrhea. The health service must be consulted promptly to assess the significance of these problems. Active skin lesions due to *Staphylococcus aureus, Streptococcus pyogenes,* and *Herpes simplex* will restrict employees from working in patient care areas until healing has occurred. Similarly, employees with streptococcal pharyngitis must not work around patients until they have received effective treatment for this disease. Influenza is a highly contagious respiratory infection; employees should always be reminded about this at the beginning of every "flu" season; they also should be encouraged to participate in annual influenza vaccination. While most cases of gastroenteritis are non-specific, they may be due to communicable pathogens such as *Salmonella, Shigella,* and parvovirus-like agents (for example, Norwalk agent) (Flewett, 1975). It would be neither wise nor prudent for an employee to return to work until after gastrointestinal symptoms have subsuded.

Antibiotic prophylaxis has been advised to employees, usually physicians or nurses, who have had significant exposure to patients with acute meningococcal meningitis (McCormick, 1975). Indication should include only intimate contact with potentially infected respiratory secretions, as might occur during mouth-to-mouth resuscitation. Rifampin, 300 mg by mouth twice daily for two days, is the antibiotic currently recommended unless the organism is known to be susceptible to sulfa drugs (Pickering, 1976).

CONCLUSION

In conclusion, the fundamental principles of infection control are not difficult to understand. As our knowledge of hospital-associated infections advances, new methods of prevention must be devised. Concern is currently directed at controlling spread of infection from the animate and inanimate environment of the hospital. Reasonably sound practices have been established for the care of operative wounds (Subcommittee on Aseptic Methods, 1968; Cruse 1973), urinary catheters (Stamm, 1975), inhalation equipment (Pierce, 1973), and intravascular devices (Maki,

1973). However, many infections in hospitalized patients arise from their own endogenous flora. More knowledge about patient host defenses is required before a solution to this problem can be found. Polyvalent vaccines against aerobic gram-negative bacteria have been proposed to protect the susceptible hospitalized patient (Hewitt, 1974). Replacement of host flora with less virulent and yet protective organisms has also been suggested (Feingold, 1970).

For the present time there is much we can do to educate ourselves and colleagues about the merits of already established practices and procedures of infection control. Special presentations to employees working in housekeeping and dietetics are necessary because they are not as knowledgeable about medical topics as are physicians and nurses. Of the latter, it is unfortunate but true that some physicians are less inclined to follow established infection control practices, simply because they fail to realize their importance and significance. An occasional stimulating, clinically oriented presentation to the medical and surgical staff about the hazards of hospital infections can be quite helpful in this regard. Although physicians are rarely incriminated outside of the operating room as a source of hospital infection, they are objects of scrutiny by all other hospital employees, as well as by patients and visitors. Physicians' words and actions can do much to improve rather than detract from a hospital infection control program.

Altemeier, W. A., Burke, J. F., Pruitt, B. A., et al.: Manual on Control of Infection in Surgical Patients. Philadelphia, J. B. Lippincott, 1976.

American Hospital Association, Committee on Infections Within Hospitals: Statement on microbiologic sampling in the hospital. Hospitals, *48*:125, 1974.

American Public Health Association, Committee on Microbial Contamination of Surfaces: Environmental microbiologic sampling in the hospital. Health Lab. Sci., *12*:234, 1975.

Antall, J., and Szebelledy, G.: Pictures from the History of Medicine: The Semmelweis Medical Historical Museum. Budapest, Corvina Press, 1973, p. 15.

Bamran, E. A., et al.: Bacteriologic studies relating to handwashing. I. The inability of soap bars to transmit bacteria. Am. J. Publ. Health, *55*:915, 1965.

Barrett-Connor, E.: Control and prevention of hospital-acquired infection. Prevent. Med., *1*:195, 1972.

Bean, W. B.: Sir William Osler: Aphorisms from his bedside teachings and writings collected by Robert Bennett Bean. New York, Henry Schuman, 1930, p. 130.

Castle, M., and Mallison, G. F.: Effective investigations of nosocomial outbreaks. Assoc. Prac. Infec. Control, *5*:13, 1977.

Centers for Disease Control: Isolation Techniques for Use in Hospitals. Washington, U.S. Government Printing Office, 1975.

Centers for Disease Control: Recommendations of the Immunization Practices Advisory Committee. Rubella prevention. Morbid. Mortal. Rep., *30*:37, 1981.

Centers for Disease Control: Recommendations of the Immunization Practices Advisory Committee. Immune globulins for protection against viral hepatitis. Ann. Intern. Med., *96*:193, 1982.

Centers for Disease Control: Recommendations of the Immunization Practices Advisory Committee. Inactivated hepatitis B virus vaccine. Morbid. Mortal. Rep., *31*:317, 1982b.

Craven, R. B., Wenzel, R. P., and Atuk, N. O.: Minimizing tuberculosis risk to hospital personnel and students exposed to unsuspected disease. Ann. Intern. Med., *82*:628, 1975.

Cruse, P. J. E., and Foord, R.: A 5 year prospective study of 23,649 surgical wounds. Arch. Surg., *107*:206, 1973.

Dixon, R. E., Kaslow, R. A., Mackel, D. C., et al.: Aqueous quaternary ammonium antiseptics and disinfectants. J.A.M.A., *236*:2415, 1976.

Dornette, W. H. L.: Legal aspects of hospital-acquired infection. J. Legal Med., 1973, p. 37.

Edwards, L. D., Levin, S., and Lepper, M. H.: Descriptive epidemiology. Environ. San., *45*:75, 1971.

Feingold, D. S.: Hospital-acquired infections. N. Engl. J. Med., *283*:1384, 1970.

Flewett, T. H., Bryden, A. S., Davies, H., et al.: Epidemic viral enteritis in a long-stay children's ward. Lancet, *1*:4, 1975.

Fracastorius, H.: Contagion—History of Medicine Series II. New York, G. P. Putnam's Sons, 1930, p. 7.

Furey, W. W., and Stefancic, M. F.: Tuberculosis in a community hospital. J.A.M.A., *235*:168, 1976.

Garner, J. S., Bennett, J. V., Scheckler, W. E., et al.: Surveillance of nosocomial infection. Proceedings of the International Conference on Nosocomial Infections, Atlanta, 1970, p. 277.

Grady, G. F., and Lee, V. A.: Hepatitis B immune globulin—prevention of hepatitis from accidental exposure among medical personnel. N. Engl. J. Med., *293*:1067, 1975.

Guthrie, D.: Lord Lister, His Life and Doctrine. Edinburgh, E. S. Livingstone, 1949, p. 55.

Hewitt, W. L., and Sanford, J. P.: Workshop on hospital-associated infections. J. Infect. Dis., *130*:680, 1974.

Hill, A. B.: Principles of Medical Statistics. New York, Oxford University, 1971.

Jarvis, W. R.: Precautions for Creutzfeldt-Jakob disease. Infect. Control, *3*:238, 1982.

Joint Commission on Accreditation of Hospitals: Infection Control—Standards Adopted by Board of Commissioners, 1981.

Klein, J. O.: Management of infections in hospital employees. Am. J. Med., *70*:919, 1981.

Landry, S. L., Donowitz, L. G., and Wenzel, R. P.: Hospital-wide surveillance: Perspective for the practitioner. Assoc. Prac. Infect. Control. *10*:66, 1982.

Lorian, V., and Topf, B.: Microbiology of nosocomial infections. Arch. Intern. Med., *130*:104, 1972.

MacGregor, R. R.: A year's experience with tuberculosis in a private urban teaching hospital in the postsanatorium era. Am. J. Med., *58*:221, 1975.

Maki, D. G., Goldmann, D. A., and Rhame F. S.: Infection control in intravenous therapy. Ann. Intern. Med., *79*:867, 1973.

Maynard, J. E.: Nosocomial viral hepatitis. Am. J. Med., *70*:439, 1981.

McCormick, J. B., and Bennett, J. V.: Public health considerations in the management of meningococcal disease. Ann. Intern. Med., *83*:883, 1975.

Mosley, J. W.: Prevention of intrahospital transmission of HBV. Viral Hepatitis. 1981 International Symposium. Philadelphia, Franklin Institute Press, 1982, p. 555.

Nauseef, W. M., and Maki, D. G.: A study of the value of simple protective isolation in patients with granulocytopaenia. N. Engl. J. Med., *304*:448, 1981.

Nightingale, F.: Notes on Hospitals. London, Longman, Roberts and Green, 1863, preface p. iii.

Pickering, L. K.: Chemoprophylaxis against *Neisseria meningitidis*. J.A.M.A., *236*:1882, 1976.

Pierce, A. K., and Sanford, J. P.: Bacterial contamination of aerosols. Arch. Intern. Med., *131*:156, 1973.

Polk, B. F., White, J. A., DeGirolami, P. C., et al.: An outbreak of rubella among hospital personnel. N. Engl. J. Med., *303*:541, 1981.

Stamm, W. E.: Guidelines for prevention of catheter-associated urinary tract infections. Ann. Intern. Med., *82*:386, 1975.

Steere, A. C., and Mallison, G. F.: Handwashing practices for the prevention of nosocomial infections. Ann. Intern. Med., *83*:683, 1975.

Subcommittee on Aseptic Methods in Operating Theatres: Preparation of the patient and performance of the operation. Lancet, *1*:834, 1968.

Thompson, N. J., Glassroth, J. L., Snider, D. E., et al.: The booster phenomenon in serial tuberculin testing. Am. Rev. Resp. Dis., *119*:587, 1979.

Vallery-Radot, R.: The Life of Pasteur. New York, Garden City, 1916, p. 274.

Walsh, J. H., Yalow, R., and Berson, S. A.: Detection of Australia antigen and antibody by means of radioimmunoassay techniques. J. Infect. Dis., *121*:550, 1970.

Part VII

ADMINISTRATION OF THE CLINICAL LABORATORY

EDITED BY WILLIAM W. McLENDON, M.D., and JOHN BERNARD HENRY, M.D.

55

ORGANIZATION AND MANAGEMENT OF THE CLINICAL LABORATORY

WILLIAM W. MCLENDON, M.D., and CHARLIE C. BARNES, JR., B.A.

The efficient operation of a clinical laboratory and the effective delivery of medical laboratory services to clinicians and their patients require a complex interdigitation of expertise in medical, scientific, and technical areas; resources in the form of personnel, laboratory and data processing equipment, supplies, and facilities; and skills in organization, management, and communication. Laboratory directors and supervisors must also be aware of the many accreditation standards and governmental regulations which apply to laboratory practice and must assure quality laboratory performance. The increasing costs of medical care mandate that those in clinical laboratories and their clinical colleagues be concerned as well with the effective utilization of laboratory services in medical care.

Although the medical, scientific, and technical expertise covered in preceding sections of this text are an essential prerequisite for the provision of medical laboratory services, success in applying these techniques to benefit patient care is vitally dependent on the management and communication skills of laboratory directors, supervisors, and technologists.

The relationship of these aspects of laboratory practice to science and medicine can be best understood in reference to Figure 55–1. The discipline of laboratory medicine can be viewed as a bridging endeavor linking the basic medical, biologic, and physical science with medical practice. Those working in clinical laboratories have the exciting opportunity and challenge to apply advances in the sciences to assist their clinical colleagues in making diagnostic, therapeutic, and prognostic decisions. In this role the laboratorian serves as a clinical consultant to the clinician and the patient.

As shown in the same illustration, however, this purely scientific and clinical approach to laboratory medicine is no longer sufficient. The bridge between the basic sciences and clinical medicine is now buttressed by essential support derived from computer science, management techniques, and industry. In recent years the relationship between laboratory medicine and industry has become bi-directional as individuals move from one to the other and as new methods and instruments are developed and evaluated jointly. Increasingly all of these service activities in laboratory medicine are guided and, to an ever greater extent, restricted by the proliferation of accreditation standards, governmental regulations, and financial constraints.

In addition to the patient care service role, most individuals in laboratory medicine also have roles as educators and many have roles as research and developmental scientists.

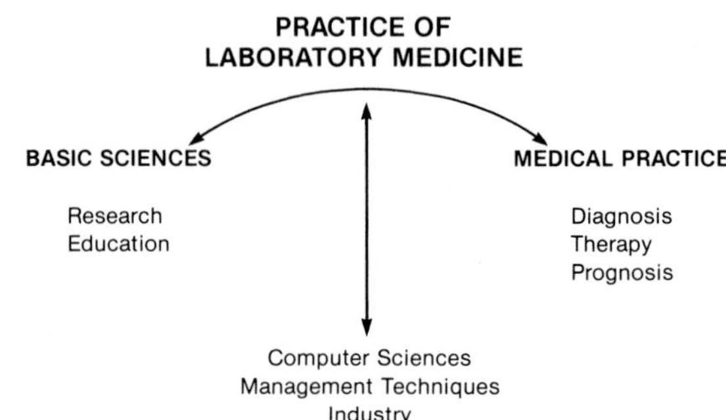

Figure 55–1. A concept of the practice of laboratory medicine.

To be successful, persons in laboratory medicine today must be skilled in all these functions and be aware of all those external influences affecting the practice of laboratory medicine. They must assume other complimentary roles as well—those of managers and executives. Managers are those who manage the work of others, while executives are all those in a modern organization who, by virtue of position and knowledge, are responsible for contributions that significantly affect the capacity of the organization to perform and obtain results (Drucker, 1967). By this definition, all the key persons in a modern clinical laboratory are executives—that is, laboratory directors, managers, supervisors, and technologists.

Dorsey (1969) has summarized the most prominent indicators of a lack of management and communication skills on the part of clinical laboratory executives:

1. Inability to maintain an adequate staff. The deficiency may be due to an insufficient number of trained workers or inefficient use of the personnel available.
2. Recurring or persistent misunderstandings with the hospital administration.
3. Frequent or recurrent confusion concerning requisitions or reports of laboratory work. It makes little difference how accurately a technologist performs a test if the report doesn't reach the doctor until 48 hours later, or if the result is reported on the wrong patient's chart.
4. Frequent "rush" orders for supplies.
5. Low morale in the laboratory.
6. Requests for deserved pay raise by competent workers (when funds are available).
7. Excessive cost of operation.
8. Ignorance of the cost of operation.
9. Expenditure of much of the director's time in making minor decisions.
10. Inability to do one or more tests when a key individual has a day off.

Success as an executive in a clinical laboratory is dependent upon the acquisition of management knowledge and skills as well as the development of certain personal characteristics. Scheer provides five such characteristics essential to success for an executive, whether one is in business or in laboratory medicine (Dorsey, 1969):

1. *Motivation.* The executive's value is in direct proportion to his ability to motivate himself and his workers.
2. *Vision.* Every executive is a supervisor. The word supervisor carries the connotation of someone possessed with "super" vision; hence, one capable of seeing over and beyond the obvious.
3. *Decision-making ability.* The individual who cannot make decisions must yield authority to one who can.
4. *Good health.* In this case good health embodies more than physical fitness. It means living a balanced life physically, emotionally, and spiritually as the best antidote to the tensions, frustrations, strain, and effort which are the lot of the executive.
5. *Humility.* This implies the recognition that we each have shortcomings, that we are not self-sufficient, and that we need the help of our subordinates just as much as they need our help.

General guidelines for operation of laboratories with consideration of their organization and management are considered in this chapter, while fiscal management and information management are discussed in Chapters 56 and 57, respectively.

Space limitations preclude a thorough coverage of these and related topics, and the reader is referred to the works cited in the references of each chapter. The recent volumes on clinical laboratory management, as well as the more general works on management, particularly those of Peter Drucker, are highly recommended. *The Effective Executive* by Drucker is a readable introduction to the problems and challenges of being an executive with practical suggestions for becoming a more effective executive. Every laboratory director and supervisor should also be familiar with the latest regulations of the Joint Commission on Accreditation of Hospitals (JCAH) in regard to pathology services and the applicable local, state, and federal governmental regulations. *The Laboratory Regulation Manual,* a publication of the Health Law Center with quarterly supplements and newsletter, provides detailed current information on laboratory regulations at the local, state, and federal level. The Standards for Accreditation of Medical Laboratories, the Inspection Checklists, and the Inspection and Accreditation Newsletter, all available from the College of American Pathologists, are particularly valuable, since they provide a distillation of laboratory regulations from a variety of sources.

SETTING GOALS AND OBJECTIVES

The first step in a systematic approach to the organization and management of the clinical laboratory begins with the establishment of general goals (also known as the mission statement) and specific objectives by the laboratory staff. The use of such objectives for purposes of management is known as *management by objectives* or MBO (Bennington, 1977). In order to achieve these objectives, the clinical laboratory must have adequate facilities, equipment and supplies, and an adequate number of qualified personnel; each of these three areas is briefly considered in the following sections of this chapter. As used here, *goals* are those general and qualitative statements of overall philosophy of the organization. An example of a goal is: "a commitment by the hospital laboratories to be a vital component of a hospital whose goal is to provide a patient care environment of excellence, to serve the community, and to serve as a setting for clinical teaching."

The goals should be consistent with the organizational structure, the management style of the laboratory director, and the available resources. In turn, such goals should influence the future programs of the laboratory and the activities of the director and the laboratory staff.

The types of goals set for a laboratory will vary greatly. For instance, the goals for the operation of an office laboratory with two physicians are vastly different from those of a reference laboratory serving thousands of physicians and patients over a large geographic area. Similarly, a great difference in goals may exist for laboratories in hospitals of the same size, depending upon the types of patients served, the nature of the hospital (acute care versus chronic care; secondary care versus tertiary care), and the nature of the educational and research commitments.

A useful exercise for a new laboratory, or periodically for an existing laboratory, is to put into writing the overall *goals* of the laboratory after discussions with the appropriate persons in the organization. As a part of this process, laboratory directors should encourage written input from each organizational level toward the development of the goals and objectives. Such written goals may be organized as follows:

1. A statement of the primary external goals of the laboratory. Most laboratories exist within the framework of some other institution such as a hospital, clinic, practice, or corporation. The goals of the laboratory should thus be a subset of the overall goals of that organization or institution. As pointed out by Drucker (1967), "what happens inside any organization is only effort and cost while the results of those efforts and costs are on the outside." Specifically, a hospital or laboratory has results only with respect to the patient, who is not a member of the hospital or laboratory organization. Without a stated primary commitment to the patient, Lundberg (1975) has commented that "in a complicated health-care organization the patients' true needs are often lost in the clamor of special interests."

2. A statement of the primary internal goal of the laboratory in reference to service, research, or education.

3. A statement as to the secondary and tertiary goals of the laboratory in reference to service, research, and education.

4. A statement in reference to the management philosophy and need for cost effectiveness.

5. A statement as to what kind of environment is desired in the laboratory with respect to interpersonal relationships, working conditions, and attitudes toward teaching and scholarly activities.

Such overall goals, once established, should be reviewed every year and appropriate modifications made. However, if the goals have been thoughtfully composed, such modifications should be minimal unless a major change has been made in the parent organization or in the leadership of the laboratory. Such a review can be done most effectively at the time of the year when the current year's accomplishments are being reviewed and the objectives for the next budget year are being established (see Chap. 56).

In contrast to the more general goals mentioned above, *objectives* should be quantifiable statements which are achievable over a designated period of time. An example of an objective might be "to evaluate available approaches to automation of antibiotic susceptibility testing and to implement the optimal approach by the end of the fiscal year." Allowing affected personnel to have input into formulating such objectives generally enhances the success of this approach of management by objectives. Priority ranking of objectives based on organizational goals is essential, since resources often limit the ability to implement all objectives within a designated planning period. Therefore, periodic review of these priorities is encouraged as a means of compensating for changing needs and circumstances. Finally, a careful assessment of results is necessary, preferably in a graphic, quantifiable manner.

Management by objectives is a process of formulation, performance and assessment, and as such it provides means of focus on pertinent factors and issues that affect the practice of laboratory medicine. As a tool of management, management by objectives encourages discussion, interaction, and consensus decision-making among all organizational levels of the laboratory.

LABORATORY FACILITIES AND ORGANIZATION

This discussion of laboratory design is intended as an outline of the considerations necessary in preparing a functional design for a clinical laboratory. A *Manual for Laboratory Planning and Design* should be consulted for details, specific suggestions, examples of laboratories, and an excellent bibliography (Thomas, 1977).

The successful design of a functional clinical laboratory, either new or renovated, requires the close cooperation of several groups of professionals. First, the laboratory director and the entire laboratory staff need to be intimately and continually involved with the process. The laboratory director should have a clear understanding with the appropriate administrative personnel concerning the right to final review of all plans and any changes. In order to prevent misunderstandings, all recommendations and changes must be documented in writing. Second, outside consultants or designers of laboratories may be utilized, although this is not an essential feature. Third, an architect or architectural firm is essential in preparing the various drawings and specifications, the final approved copies of which will be used in the bidding process and by the contractor for construction. Fourth, a contractor is needed to construct the facility.

Functional Considerations in Laboratory Design

The laboratory director having the opportunity to design a new laboratory or make major renovations in an older laboratory should think in functional terms about the laboratory operation and its facility needs.

Traditionally laboratories have been organized in relationship to techniques or historical accident rather than in relationship to clinical problems, disease orientation, or functional efficiency. It has been pointed out that traditional laboratories have a mixture of approaches: for example, clinical chemistry is technique oriented; clinical microbiology is technique and disease oriented; urinalysis is specimen oriented; hematology is specimen and organ system oriented; and blood bank is product oriented. Such an organizational approach may continue to be of value in the future, but alternative functional approaches might also be considered. These include laboratories organized on the basis of the turn-around time (TAT) of procedures (Lundberg, 1975); laboratories based on disease- or problem-oriented panels (Henry, 1977); automated laboratories organized for production-line techniques and the generation of clinician-oriented reports (Reece, 1974); laboratories organized to provide a screening function with automatic definitive testing of the same samples as a follow-up of the initial findings (the Pali concept of Altshuler, 1972); and laboratories designed to provide decentralized services to meet special patient needs for the clinic or office practice (Benjamin, 1982; Fisher, 1983).

Spatial Considerations in Laboratory Design

Spatial Relationships Within the Institution. If the laboratory director has the opportunity to design a laboratory for an entirely new building or hospital, or to relocate a laboratory in an existing hospital or building, it is critical that the location of the laboratory be studied in relationship to the other hospital services, to traffic, to supporting services, and to users. For example, the blood bank and the critical care laboratory procedures should be readily accessible to the emergency room, operating rooms, and intensive care unit. The location of the blood bank should allow rapid access and egress of donors and adequate parking for donors if the blood bank is responsible for donor procurement, phlebotomy, and/or apheresis. A phlebotomy and specimen collection area should be planned in the proximity of the ambulatory care facility and the admitting office. The relationship to the central supply and other supporting areas should be considered. If the laboratory is serving an inpatient population, accessibility to corridors and elevators providing access to the main patient care units is essential.

Intralaboratory Relationships. The relationship of various laboratories to each other and to supporting areas such as phlebotomy, specimen receipt, data processing, glass washing, and storage should be taken into account. A workable arrangement is to have a specimen receiving, data processing, and reporting center serve as the hub of the laboratory. Radiating from this could be the various laboratories. The critical care laboratories and large volume laboratories (such as hematology and chemistry) might be most closely related to these central areas. Those laboratories with greater turn-around time and/or less volume, as well as those requiring special safety features (such as clinical microbiology and radioassay laboratories), might be more removed from the central area.

A systematic approach to determining the optimal internal layout of laboratories is available (Gonzales-Menocal, 1973). The same system may be used when designing a hospital to determine the best location for a laboratory in relationship to other hospital services.

Traffic Flow. It is very important to plan the traffic flow so that intralaboratory traffic is separated from outside traffic. Provisions should be made for ambulatory patients and blood bank donors coming into the laboratory.

Specimen and Data Flow. A diagram of specimen and data flow through the proposed laboratory will be helpful in arranging a schematic layout. Questions which should be considered include: (1) Do all specimens come to a central processing area or to the individual laboratory section? (2) Are pre-analytical processing and storage of specimens to be done centrally or by each laboratory? (3) Are telephone inquiries and reporting to be done centrally or by each laboratory? (4) Are routine and stat (emergency) specimens to be treated in the same manner?

Specific Design Considerations

Square Footage. The gross square footage of laboratory space can be calculated by using the outside dimensions of laboratory sections or of an entire laboratory to determine the square footage. However, a more important consideration is the net square footage. This represents the gross square footage less the square footage occupied by halls, stairways, walls, chases, elevators, restrooms, and other common spaces. The net square footage thus gives one an indication of the actual square footage available for laboratory use. Depending on the design of the laboratory, the net square footage in modern clinical laboratories varies from approximately 65 per cent to 90 per cent of the gross square footage, according to a recent survey (Thomas, 1977).

Mechanical Services. Proper planning of mechanical services is essential for any laboratory. Special attention should be paid to temperature control and air handling, especially in reference to staff comfort and safety. Noise control is also of vital importance for the morale and productivity of the laboratory staff.

Casework and Interior Design. One of the most important decisions the laboratory director has to make in regard to a new or renovated laboratory is the nature of the casework (laboratory benches and cabinets) which will be used in the laboratory. In a small laboratory it may be appropriate simply to design the casework as part of the internal planning for the laboratory and to have the casework constructed and installed by a contractor. In the larger laboratory with multiple laboratory sections, however, it is generally preferable to obtain standard casework from some reputable manufacturer. Because it is impossible to anticipate completely the future needs of the laboratory, many manufacturers offer modular designs for laboratory casework. This approach may provide utilities along the outer walls of the laboratory with some flexibility in the cabinet components which can be attached to supporting framework. Such a system allows the laboratory to make future changes in one or more laboratory sections by exchanging component parts or obtaining additional component parts from the manufacturer. It also tends to minimize the amount of plumbing and carpentry work which is necessary as changes are made. Such cabinet work generally adds a higher cost initially; hence, this must be weighed against the likelihood that this flexibility will be required in the future.

On a larger scale, the laboratory director should also investigate the desirability of a modular approach to interior walls within the laboratory. Such a system has to be carefully designed by the architect to coordinate with a modular or grid system in the ceiling and floor utilities. This can be very expensive, but may be worthwhile if the laboratory anticipates major changes. Another approach is to have the laboratory built with rigid outside walls and the interior divided by partial or complete modular walls as part of the casework.

Communications. By the nature of its activity, a clinical laboratory has as one of its primary functions the process of communication of information, both within the laboratory and between the laboratory and the physician (see also Chap. 58). In the one- or two-room laboratory, a telephone with one or two extensions and one or two incoming lines may suffice. The problem is much more complex in the multi-section laboratory. Here a decision must be made as to whether there will be a central answering service with the ability to transfer calls to the individual sections or whether each section will have its own lines. The use of communication consultants such as those available from the local telephone company in the planning stage can be very helpful to the laboratory director in making these plans. Larger institutions may employ a communication staff and engineer to provide this consultation.

Intercom systems are essential within larger laboratories and may be of two types. One type, private communication, can be a part of the telephone system. This has the advantages that additional equipment is not needed, telephone conversations can be private, switching from the intercom to telephone lines is convenient, and private conversations may minimize lab noise and confusion.

For laboratory areas where persons are performing tests and may not be able to answer a telephone, a public address intercom system may be desirable. This has the disadvantage of contributing significantly to the noise level of the laboratory environment, but it provides easy location of an individual within the laboratory. In any event, the trade-off in terms of efficiency of operation may be necessary.

Since most larger laboratories today, or in the not-too-distant future, will have automated data processing, planning should include consideration of the installation and location of conduits and terminal boxes for data processing equipment. Even if a system does not exist in the laboratory, advice can be obtained concerning the nature of conduits and the location of terminal boxes for future systems. If one is planning to build an entire institution, of which the laboratories are a part, consideration should also be given to the necessity for conduits connecting the laboratory and hospital computer systems with nursing stations and other hospital areas. A dedicated laboratory information system located within the laboratory area will require special attention to air conditioning and humidity (see also Chap. 57).

Safety. During the planning stage the laboratory director should become thoroughly familiar with both federal Occupational Safety and Health Act regulations and state and local regulations. The current checklists of the College of American Pathologists Inspection and Accreditation Program offer a convenient guide to safety requirements, since they are designed to highlight the major safety requirements of the laboratory. The Joint Commission on Accreditation of Hospitals also offers a useful self-evaluation form on Safety and Sanitation.

The fire safety measures will be determined to a large extent by local regulations; however, planners should devote attention to locations of fire extinguishers, safety showers, eyewashes, and evacuation routes and exits. Biologic, toxic, and radioactive hazards also have to be considered. Design of hoods and ventilation systems should be based on the anticipated use of toxic or biologic hazards in the various laboratory areas. The storage of large quantities of flammable or toxic reagents requires special precautions and thorough planning.

Offices. It is desirable to have the administrative offices of the department located near the laboratories. These offices provide space for the laboratory directors, department administrators, and support staff. Spatial organization will vary with the available space. As the organizational center of the department, however, this area should be designed to accommodate its various functions (providing information and management assistance, consultation, and a site for departmental resources).

General Laboratory Support Functions. The following are some of the general laboratory support functions which are frequently neglected in laboratory planning.

Storerooms. It should be determined whether the major storage will be handled outside of the laboratory or whether a central laboratory storeroom will be needed. Regardless of this decision, sufficient storage should be available within each laboratory to handle several days' to several weeks' supply of critical material. Modular storage cabinets which can be filled in a central storeroom and then transported to the laboratory areas should be investigated. Special consideration should be given to the storage of flammables and compressed gases.

Glassware Washing. Glassware washing and appropriate sterilization facilities should be included in any laboratory design. They may be centralized or made available in individual laboratories. Media and reagent preparation facilities may also be needed, requiring special exhaust and temperature control for autoclaves.

Staff Facilities. Lounges, lockers, and toilets are essential for the comfort and morale of the employees and must be included in any plans. Appearance and aesthetic design is important and interior designers may be consulted. Local building codes generally will specify the minimum toilet facilities which must be made available.

Blood Collecting Area and Examining Rooms. If the laboratory provides blood collection for ambulatory patients, adequate facilities including waiting rooms and restrooms for patients should be included in the design. Many laboratories are finding that this can be most effectively planned as part of a central receiving and processing area. Data processing terminals should be available in this area for verification of patient identity, entry of patient test requisitions, and preparation of blood collection labels.

Library and Conference Rooms. These facilities are essential for all levels of the laboratory staff. Teaching programs, continuing education presentations, seminars, and large conferences require adequate space and audio-visual capabilities. Smaller groups may require less space and less sophisticated equipment. The departmental library can serve as a source of selected reference books and professional journals to supplement the resources available in the institutional or regional reference library.

Space for Research and Development. Depending upon the goals and needs of the laboratory, space may be allotted for research and development work.

Stages in Laboratory Design and Building

Preparation of a Functional Program. The functional program is defined as a written document giving the purposes of the laboratory, the functions which are necessary to achieve these purposes, and the various interrelationships of functions within the laboratory. The program should not include square footage estimates as such, but should include detailed information concerning the current and proposed figures for the number of patients to be served and specimens to be processed; the number of technical, clerical, and supervisory personnel; and the number of clinical scientists and pathologists. A detailed listing of bench space required per technologist is desirable as well as a detailed listing of the present and anticipated bench top and freestanding equipment. If teaching programs exist, the number of students to be housed in the laboratory for both lecture and bench-type instruction should be taken into consideration.

During the development of the functional program, the temptation to sketch out the laboratory design should be resisted. However, it is essential to generate functional flow diagrams of the processes proposed for the laboratory; this is invaluable to the architect.

One should also avoid the temptation to adopt some standardized square footage figure or to copy some other laboratory. It is, however, useful to visit other laboratories, especially recently constructed or renovated laboratories, to profit by their successes and mistakes. Prior to the visit, broadly based discussions among as many of the laboratory personnel as possible are very helpful in developing an outline or checklist of questions to use at the site visit.

In the preparation of the functional program, general statements about flexibility and the potential need for expansion in the future are essential. The architects should be aware of budget limitations and time constraints.

Schematic Design Drawing. In this stage the laboratory personnel responsible for planning the new or renovated laboratory should meet with the architects to help them develop an understanding of the relationships of one laboratory to another and that of the laboratories to other services in the institution. The architect will use the functional program narrative at this point to translate the specific functional requirements into an architectural program which assigns space to the functions. From this point simple line drawings are developed to show the possible arrangements of laboratories and their divisions with suggested corridors, stairways, elevators, lounges, and other common areas.

Design Development Drawing. These drawings represent the next stage of architectural design and provide the detailed location of doors, windows, partitions, fixed and movable equipment, bench space, seats, furniture, and associated support facilities. They also include details of the proposed mechanical, electrical, and plumbing needs. At this point it is extremely important for the laboratory to furnish the architect with a complete list of present and proposed equipment, including specific electrical requirements, size, and estimated BTU output. The last of these is of extreme importance, since too often air conditioning systems are designed for the number of personnel in an area, neglecting the much greater output of heat by modern automated laboratory equipment. Special requirements for venting and exhaust, air flow, and utilities are indicated in this stage.

Working Drawings and Specifications. These drawings represent the final or contract documents and give the detailed information necessary for construction of the proposed laboratory. Architectural drawings of the structure are supplemented by detailed drawings of the plumbing, electrical, and mechanical services. A set of specifications is also prepared to document the quality of materials, in contrast to the working drawings which delineate the location of materials.

Period of Construction. After bids are let and the contractor is chosen, the laboratory director will have to deal through the owner's representative or the architect. It is important that the progress of the building be monitored and that the problems be called to the attention of the appropriate person. Change orders must be in writing and must go through the architect or owner's representative to the contractor. The director should be aware that change orders may be very expensive and should be avoided except where absolutely necessary. The more comprehensive the planning prior to construction, the less the need for change orders during construction.

At the conclusion of the construction, the owner or person responsible makes a final inspection, with documentation of those items which must be corrected before the building is accepted. The laboratory director or designee should be involved in this process.

PURCHASING

In a manner similar to a business, clinical laboratories require raw materials for successful operation. Whereas equipment idled by breakdowns or lack of supplies is an economic loss for business, the same situation in the clinical laboratory can seriously interfere with the delivery of patient care.

Responsible people must decide what supplies they need, when they need them, and in what quantities. Much time can be wasted in the purchasing procedure unless a workable procurement system is developed. In the larger medical centers, the process may involve many people with elaborate systems for obtaining and evaluating bids, selecting vendors, awarding contracts, shipping, and receiving. In contrast, in the physician's office laboratory, the entire process may be handled by the technologist dealing directly with the vendors.

Whatever the environment, two essential components are common to most purchasing systems. Product research and well-developed specifications help assure adequate quality of materials, while inventory control helps assure adequate quantity of materials for the laboratory operation.

Product Specifications

Since the basis for any purchasing process is the need to procure goods to meet specific needs, time must be spent on product research leading to the development of product specifications. The medical laboratory supply market is very competitive, with many similar items available for each need; only through product investigation can the best product for the available funds be determined.

This process can be accomplished by comparative evaluations within the laboratory, by consultation with other users, or by reference to publications, such as the *Journal of Clinical Laboratory Automation,* offering comparative studies of equipment and supplies. Product specifications prepared after such a study help assure adequate quality of purchased reagents and supplies.

A similar process of evaluation and product specification is necessary prior to purchase of major equipment. In addition, the following considerations are important:

1. Written specifications must include a detailed description of the required equipment; specifications should never be communicated verbally.

2. On-site visits to see equipment operating in other laboratories are encouraged. More valuable is the trial installation of the equipment within the laboratory. This allows operation of the equipment under the particular conditions of the laboratory; equally important, it gives personnel an opportunity to test the equipment and have input into the purchase decision.

3. An environment necessary to accommodate the equipment must be prepared in advance. Such special requirements as high amperage, special gases, controlled humidity, unusual weight loads, or high BTU output are but a few of the considerations. Not infrequently laboratories receive much-needed equipment which then lies idle for weeks or months while an adequate area is belatedly prepared.

4. A more complicated decision, but one that must be made, is whether to lease, rent, or buy major equipment. See Chapter 56 for discussion of this issue.

5. If a certificate of need is required, this process can usually be accomplished in parallel with the product evaluation and development of specifications.

6. Complete instruction manuals should be obtained with the instrument and preventive maintenance schedules established (Hamlin, 1982).

7. If the equipment is to be interfaced to a laboratory computer system for on-line data acquisition, consideration should be given to requiring the interface (hardware and software) as a part of the purchase agreement.

Purchasing of Supplies

Orders should be placed only by authorized staff members who are familiar with the quality of service and reliability of the suppliers. Delivery schedules are a major factor in determining whether a purchasing system is out of control. High-use items should be delivered frequently. Release orders and standing orders are excellent methods of doing this and can save laboratory time and money. Release orders are annual contracts in which the vendor agrees to deliver goods at a predetermined price as notified by the laboratory. The standing order is an annual contract in which the vendor agrees to deliver goods at a predetermined price and on an established schedule.

Receiving and Accounts Payable

Three documents are usually involved in the purchasing process. The purchase requisition or order states the desired goods or services with an estimate of the cost. The packing slip accompanies the shipped goods, and the invoice may be included or follow. Payment is made from the invoice which should be checked for correlation with the original order and the packing slip.

Goods should be unpacked and inspected as soon as possible to ensure that everything is delivered or that some acknowledgment of back-ordered items is made. Damaged or defective goods should be identified early in order to assure replacement or credit. Reagents and supplies can be dated, catalogued, and labeled at this time.

Records and Inventory Control

Much has been written about inventory control, and there are elaborate formulas for deciding inventory size and reordering time, but for most laboratories simpler methods will serve as well. One of these methods is through the use of an inventory system using stock record cards. Computerized inventory systems are also available.

In an inventory system, levels are set at low and high points. The low level is that point at which on-hand supplies are sufficient to carry the laboratory through until goods on order are received. The upper limit is that level which will meet the laboratory's requirements for a longer period of time, such as several months to a year. The primary factors determining these limits are the anticipated delivery time for each item, the available storage space, the shelf life of the item, and the anticipated rate of usage.

An effective inventory control system requires excellent communications between all sections of the laboratory and the person(s) responsible for purchasing. The latter must be made aware of anticipated increases or decreases in requirements for all items and must closely monitor delivery times and vendor performance and response.

PERSONNEL

A clinical laboratory should have goals and objectives and must have facilities, supplies, and equipment. However, the most essential component in any health care activity is people. Consider that employees' salaries and related benefits constitute 60 to 70 per cent of most laboratory expense budgets. Thus, the responsible laboratory director should be concerned with developing this human resource to its optimal level, as management has been defined as "getting things done through the efforts of other people." This requires an understanding of those factors affecting personnel motivation and performance as well as those techniques available for personnel management.

Motivation

The day-to-day operation of a laboratory and the motivation of the persons in that laboratory will be determined to a large extent by the management style of those responsible for directing the institution, the laboratory, and the various laboratory sections. Such management styles are determined by a person's personality and previous experience and training, but can be modified if a conscious effort is made.

Current understanding of the influence of leadership and management styles on the operation of organizations and the motivation of personnel has been derived from the work of a number of persons, particularly Maslow (1954), McGregor (1960), and Herzberg (1968).

Maslow developed a theory of human motivation based on the belief that man is a wanting animal, that his behavior is determined by unsatisfied needs, and that these needs form an internal hierarchy. He identified five needs and arranged them in a hierarchy of importance from the most fundamental to the ones providing the most satisfaction. These are as follows: bodily needs such as food, clothing, and shelter; the need to feel secure; the need to feel loved or wanted; the ego need to feel important; and the self-actualization need, or the need to feel that one is doing well and is developing one's ability. For those who have a job with a reasonable salary and working conditions, the first three levels of internal needs are usually reasonably well satisfied. It is the satisfaction of their needs at the fourth and fifth levels which determine how well persons perform on a job and how well they are motivated.

Based on the work of Maslow, McGregor (1960) has described two extreme management styles: Theory X style, which unfortunately still exists in many medical care settings, is based on the assumption that people dislike work; that they have to be driven, threatened, and punished to achieve organizational goals (such as "good patient care"); and that they lack ambition and want only security. Such an approach worked reasonably well in a time when the average employee was uneducated and dependent on orders from an authority who had almost unlimited power. In today's medical care institutions, where well-educated, highly motivated, and professional staff are essential for medical care, such a management style can be disastrous.

At an opposite pole is McGregor's Theory Y management style. This is based on the assumptions that work is as natural as rest or play; people don't have to be threatened or forced to work; they will commit themselves to the external organization only to the extent that they can see ways of satisfying their own internal ego and developmental needs; and people want responsibility in the proper environment when given the opportunity.

The degree of delegation of authority and sharing of responsibility will be a reflection both of the size of the laboratory and of the management style of the persons in charge. A Theory X organization will have little delegation of authority and sharing of responsibility. A Theory Y organization, however, is characterized by a decentralized type of organization with greater delegation of authority and sharing of responsibility and therefore more staff participation. As the laboratory organization becomes larger, the need for more delegation should be apparent; failure to acknowledge this will generally lead to major organizational problems. One of the most common management failures in clinical laboratories is the reluctance to share responsibility, thus resulting in the underutilization of talented persons. In situations in which responsibility is delegated and shared, prospective supervisors and managers are identified and trained.

The need for delegated authority and shared responsibility is related to the concept of *span of control:* that is, how many persons or operations can one person effectively direct? The traditional view is that one person can direct the activities of some four to eight other persons or groups, although exceptions obviously exist.

Although Theory X and Theory Y may be considered as "extremes" in styles of management, other theories are based on the general premises of motivating individuals. A new approach is found in the book *Theory Z,* in which William Ouchi suggests that the involvement of workers is a key for increased productivity. According to Ouchi, motivation of employees may be enhanced by a combination of trust, subtlety, and intimacy provided by management style and the organization. In a Theory Z approach, employees are encouraged to seek common societal goals through participation, incentives, and collective values that reward all of the employees in a like manner. Managers are responsible for providing an atmosphere of discussion, stability, involvement, and corporate satisfaction.

It is important to remember that no one style is appropriate in all situations in any one laboratory or organization; the director or supervisor must be able to use the appropriate style for the situation or person with which one is dealing at the moment. Proper understanding and use of these observations on human motivation, however, can lead to better motivated and more productive personnel in the laboratory. In our experience the most effective way to accomplish this is to begin with a mutual commitment by all those in the clinical laboratories to create a working environment in which there is concern for each patient served, mutual respect for each co-worker, and enthusiasm for teaching and advancement of the field of laboratory medicine.

Personnel Management

The more tangible aspects of dealing with personnel in the clinical laboratory setting are addressed in the discussion of personnel management. Personnel policies, procedures, and records are vital to the smooth operation of any laboratory and are necessary to meet accreditation and legal requirements.

Policy Manual. All laboratories should have readily available administrative policy manuals which state the laboratory and institutional policy for the guidance of those working in the laboratory. Recurrent crises concerning the same problems are symptomatic of a laboratory that has no clearly understood and documented policies.

The policy should reflect the philosophy and overall goals of the larger organization as well as those of the laboratory. They should be written in consultation with the persons involved and reviewed by the appropriate persons in the institution (e.g., the personnel department) to be certain they are consistent with institutional policy. Like the laboratory procedure manuals, policies should be dated and approved by the laboratory director. Because of the rapidly changing nature of most laboratory operations, they should be reviewed and updated at least annually, with a signature or initials and a date to document this review.

Job Description. A job description is a summary of all the important or significant facts about a particular job. It is a useful tool in classifying positions, determining pay grades, recruitment, orientation of new employees, and setting employee performance standards.

Generally, institutions formulate guidelines to assist in job description preparation. It is important to prepare job descriptions that are clear and concise, as well as thorough, so that duties and responsibilities are easily understood by both the employee and management. It is also helpful to define the purpose of the job and to show its relationship to other jobs in the organization.

Position Classification. In most organizations, a method for position classification has been developed. This involves determining the different kinds or "classes" of positions existing in the institution. The duties and responsibilities of the positions (job descriptions) are the basis upon which the individual positions are assigned at the appropriate class (levels).

Each class consists of all positions (e.g., medical technologist), regardless of departmental location, that are sufficiently alike in duties and responsibilities to have the same descriptive title, to have the same pay scale, and to require substantially the same qualifications. Within each class, such as Medical Technologist I, a number of pay steps are established. This provides a means to compensate the experienced employee at job entry. The steps also facilitate annual and merit raises, when available.

Recruitment and Selection of Employees. The recruitment and selection of new employees is one of the most crucial management tasks performed in the laboratory, since each person added to the staff influences positively or negatively the future of the laboratory. In addition, the legal requirements for personnel recruitment and management require a considerable knowledge of Affirmative Action, equal employment regulations, and appropriate job qualifications. An excellent review of these factors can be found in *Law for Personnel Managers: How to Hire the People You Need Without Discrimination,* by Robert L. Brady.

After assessing staffing requirements and making the decision to fill a vacant position, the first step in the selection process is the initial screening. Minimum criteria should be defined for each position, and all applicants should be compared to these criteria. The criteria should include such things as minimum education and experience and any required licensure, certification, or specialized training. This initial screening can be accomplished by the personnel department; only those candidates meeting the minimum qualifications should be referred to the laboratory for interviewing. Although the laboratory director may elect to delegate the selection of the personnel to supervisors or others, the final responsibility for the choice rests with the director. Therefore, laboratory directors and supervisors should agree on the personnel requirements and the acceptable qualifications for a position.

It is much easier to ensure that important considerations are not overlooked if the interviewer prepares in advance an informal list of established criteria and interview questions based upon the job description. In the case of a supervisory position these criteria may be qualitative. Such things as problem solving aptitude, ability to communicate, creativity, and innovation may be more important and harder to define than the applicant's technical expertise. This approach also ensures that all candidates are compared equitably. Informal notes about the interview should be made to assist in the selection process.

As the selection process narrows to serious contenders, it is appropriate to check the candidates' past employment records. It is helpful to structure questions to past employers around those criteria used in the interview. This gives excellent comparison between the candidates' responses and proven work habits. Through such a standardized screening and interviewing process, the laboratory should be able to recruit quality personnel.

Orientation. The important step of introducing the employee to his or her new environment comes after the selection and hiring process. An orientation program is probably one of the most overlooked tools available to the manager.

Apart from an institutional orientation program, each laboratory should have a program of orientation for new employees to make them aware of the policies, procedures, and standards of performance used in the particular laboratory. Even though a new employee may be a registered technologist, his or her experience with the particular procedures in use in the new environment may be limited. During this orientation it should be emphasized that suggestions for changing procedures or methods are welcome and will be given due consideration, but that each employee must follow the laboratory method and procedure exactly as prescribed. Individual initiative in modifying laboratory determinations without consultation and proper documentation cannot be tolerated.

Done correctly, orientation can establish early in the employee's career an understanding of the philosophy of the laboratory and the institution. It can correct those misunderstandings that are so often present with new employees and can establish in the beginning an open channel of communication between the supervisor and the new employee.

In-Service Continuing Education. Because of the rapidly changing nature of laboratory medicine, it is also desirable to have regular continuing education sessions for laboratory staff. These can be developed and presented by the laboratory staff and directors, with outside participants as needed. Content of continuing education programs should be developed to meet varying needs of each staff level. In all cases, staff input and involvement should be encouraged. In addition, the staff should be given the time and encouraged to attend appropriate medical staff meetings in the institution as well as continuing education programs in laboratory medicine elsewhere. Documentation of attendance at such meetings, as well as topics covered, should be maintained to meet accreditation requirements.

Intralaboratory Staff Meetings. Intralaboratory communications are enhanced and crises minimized when regularly scheduled meetings of laboratory directors, associates, supervisors, and staff are held. Meetings of the supervisors and laboratory director should be held on a regular basis to discuss administrative, professional, and technical problems. Periodic full laboratory staff meetings are also useful as a forum for discussing problems, new policies and procedures, and planning. Such meetings, if properly organized and directed, tend to promote teamwork in the laboratory and to bring problems to light before they become crises. Documentation of staff meetings is desirable, and minutes of the meetings provide a record for communication of factual data, discussion, and conclusions.

Personnel Records. All institutions maintain some employee personnel records, but the laboratory may wish to keep a duplicate set of records for their use. If so, consideration should be given to what information should be and legally can be kept in these records.

The question of employee privacy has become a much-discussed issue recently, and court cases have been brought relative to this question. Since laws pertaining to this are changing rapidly, the reader is encouraged to determine what current organizational, state, and federal guidelines exist relative to this matter. Access to confidential and personal information should be limited to appropriate individuals. Before duplicating existing personnel records, thought should be given to the implications and responsibilities related to such an act, and counsel with appropriate personnel authorities is advised.

Evaluations. An important part of employee development is feedback, whether negative or positive. This can be accomplished through random meetings, memoranda added to the file, or a structured evaluation system. The last of these offers the opportunity for the employee and supervisor to take time to review past performance as well as to project future expectation. It provides both parties the framework within which constructive criticism can be given and provides the vehicle by which relationships can be redefined.

As with other management tools, the format of the evaluation forms can vary according to preference. For fairness and uniformity, the same form should be used for all employees. The form need not be complex, and frequently measured aspects of performance are attendance, adaptability, job knowledge and skill, quality and quantity of work, and working relationships.

Discipline and Dismissal. Some employees will fall short of expected standards. When this situation arises decisive action is imperative. "No action" is not an acceptable approach; how much action to take will depend upon the type of infraction and the circumstances surrounding it. Institution policies on discipline and dismissal should be used to establish acceptable procedures for written and oral warning and the dismissal process.

Because of the seriousness of some acts, the laboratory director or supervisor may elect to recommend dismissal of the employee immediately rather than following the sequences noted above. In most hospitals, however, the procedure for such dismissals would include consultation with the personnel department.

Success in handling disciplinary problems comes with consistency of approach, promptness, and equity in dealing with all personnel. The importance of thorough documentation of personnel problems and resulting actions cannot be overemphasized. With proper employee recruitment, selection, orientation, and motivation, disciplinary problems should be minimized.

Altshuler, C. H., et al.: The PALI and SLIC Systems. CRC Critical Reviews in Clinical Laboratory Sciences, Vol. 3, no. 3, pp. 379–402, 1972.

Becan-McBride, K.: Textbook of Clinical Laboratory Supervision. New York, Appleton-Century-Crofts, 1982.

Benjamin, D. R.: The "third wave" laboratory. Am. J. Clin. Path., 78:324, 1982.

Bennington, J. L.: Management by objectives. *In* Bennington, J. L., et al. (eds.): Management and Cost Control Techniques for the Clinical Laboratory. Baltimore, University Park Press, 1977.

Brady, R. L.: Law for Personnel Managers: How to Hire the People You Need Without Discrimination. Stamford, Conn., Bureau of Law and Business, Inc., 1980.

Dorsey, D. B., et al. (eds.): Administration in the Pathology Laboratory, rev. ed. Skokie, Ill. College of American Pathologists, 1969.

Drucker, P. F.: The Effective Executive. New York, Harper and Row, 1967.

Drucker, P. F.: Management: Tasks, Responsibilities, Practices. New York, Harper and Row, Publishers, 1974.

Feegel, J. R.: Legal Aspects of Laboratory Medicine. Boston, Little, Brown and Co., 1973.

Fisher, P. M., et al.: The Office Laboratory. East Norwalk, Conn., Appleton-Century-Crofts, 1983.

Gonzales-Menocal, P., et al.: A quantitative approach to the solution of laboratory layout problems. Laboratory Medicine, Vol. 4, no. 11, p. 17, 1973.

Hamlin, W. B., et al. (ed.): Laboratory Instrument Maintenance and Function Verification. 3rd ed. Skokie, Ill., College of American Pathologists, 1982.

Henry, J. B.: Introduction to Organ Panels. *In* Henry, J. B., and Giegel, J. L. (eds.): Quality Control in Laboratory Medicine. New York, Masson Publishing USA, 1977.

Herzberg, F.: One more time: How do you motivate employees? Harvard Business Review, January-February, 1968.

JCAH Hospital Staff-Evaluation Survey, Safety and Sanitation, 1982. May be obtained from the Joint Commission on Accreditation of Hospitals.

Joint Commission on Accreditation of Hospitals: Pathology Services. In Accreditation Manual for Hospitals, Chicago, 1982.

Laboratory Regulation Manual. Health Law Center, Aspen Systems Corporation, 20010 Century Boulevard, Germantown, Md. 20767. Loose-leaf manual of laboratory regulations with quarterly newsletter and supplements.

Levey, S., and Loomba, N. P. (eds.): Health Care Administration: A Managerial Perspective. Philadelphia, J. B. Lippincott Co., 1973.

Lundberg, G. D.: Managing the Patient-Focused Laboratory. Oradell, N.J., Medical Economics Company, 1975.

Maslow, A. H.: Motivation and Personality. New York, Harper and Row, Publishers, 1954.

McGregor, D.: The Human Side of Enterprise. New York, McGraw-Hill Book Co., 1960.

Ouchi, W.: Theory Z. Reading, Mass., Addison-Wesley, 1981.

Reece, R. L.: The screening laboratory of 1980. Perspect. Biol. Med., *17*:227, 1974.

Selected Readings in Laboratory Management. A loose-leaf binder available from the College of American Pathologists. Skokie, Ill., 1982.

Snyder, J. R., Larsen, A. L., et al. (eds.): Administration and Supervision in Laboratory Medicine. Philadelphia, Harper and Row, 1983.

Shuffstall, R. M., and Hemmaplardh, B.: The Hospital Laboratory. St. Louis, C. V. Mosby Company, 1979.

Thomas, R. G. (eds.): Manual for Laboratory Planning and Design. Rev. ed. Skokie, Ill., College of American Pathologists, 1977.

Veterans Administration, Department of Medicine and Surgery: Chapter 240, Laboratory Services, *In* Planning Criteria for Medical Facilities. Manual M-7. Washington, D.C., US Government Printing Office, 1974.

56

FISCAL MANAGEMENT

WILLIAM W. MCLENDON, M.D., and HELEN DOERPINGHAUS, B.A.

7

The ability of the laboratory to meet the goals and objectives as discussed in Chapter 55 (p. 1383) depends on the availability and management of fiscal resources for the optimal provision of facilities, equipment, supplies, and personnel. In this chapter we will address external factors which influence fiscal decisions, tools which are available for fiscal decision-making, and techniques available for developing and monitoring laboratory budgets utilizing the concept of responsibility budgeting.

FACTORS INFLUENCING FISCAL DECISIONS

Government. With the passage of various federal health legislation, the degree of external control over hospital and laboratory fiscal decisions has increased tremendously since the 1960's in parallel with increasing governmental funding of medical care in the United States. We will not attempt to review these influences in detail since the legislation and regulations are changing rapidly. Laboratory directors, supervisors, and administrators, however, should be familiar with such programs and the controls which they bring to the financing of hospital and laboratory services. In addition, laboratory directors in institutions financed by cities, counties, states, or other governmental entities should also be aware of the financial constraints imposed by such entities.

Non-governmental Third-Party Payers. Since the 1930's an extensive system of private health care financing has also developed in the United States. This is generally of two types. One is the many non-profit health and hospital insurance plans such as Blue Cross and Blue Shield which are available in every state. The second type is the commercial, for-profit health insurance companies.

Private insurance companies and other agencies concerned with rising costs of health care have established means of reviewing costs and charges for laboratory and hospital services, to ensure the optimal expenditure of health and medical care funds. Representatives of business, labor, and consumer groups have also become increasingly concerned about these issues. These reviewing authorities and interest groups will influence the laboratory director's program and fiscal planning and should be considered in making such plans.

Centralized vs. Decentralized Laboratory Services. Because of concern with cost containment, increasing pressure has been placed upon laboratories to prevent inappropriate duplication and to stimulate regionalization of services, particularly in the area of the specialized and non-emergency laboratory services.

Multi-institutional efforts to reduce unnecessary duplication of laboratory services can take many forms, ranging from simple sharing of services to the merging of institutions or the formation of consortia. The decision as to which laboratory procedures should be done locally and which might be done in a regional laboratory or on a shared basis is a very complex one and should be made only after due consideration of the many factors involved. One method is to use the criteria proposed by Hain (1972). Although he was concerned with those procedures which should be done in a physician's office and those which could be done in a centralized laboratory facility, the criteria could be useful in a more general context:

> The procedures which can be done more reliably or at less cost centrally and for which the turn-around time from collection of the specimen to reporting of results to the attending physician will not impede the immediate effective care of the patient should be done in the [regional or shared laboratory]. All others would be done in the peripheral facility [hospital or office laboratory].

In theory this approach is attractive, but in actual practice it may break down, since different measurements can become critical, depending on the patient rather than some other criteria. As a result, laboratories must still maintain back-up capability for a wide range of measurements.

Brown (1975) provides practical guidelines for those considering regional or shared laboratory services, with a checklist of questions to be considered in the planning stages of such a venture. These include turnaround time, cost, transportation, communication, need for 24-hour-a-day service, stat requirements, method dependence of results, and continuity of interpretation.

More recently, with the development of microelectronics, an opposite trend toward decentralization of laboratory services has evolved. This parallels the development of the concept of distributed processing in the computer field whereby small computers provide for the immediate, local data processing needs while the large centralized computer serves a coordinating role for communications, data base management, and complex computations. In the laboratory field, this trend is manifested by the use of bedside testing, home testing (e.g., pregnancy tests and blood glucose monitoring), and the resurgence of the physician's office laboratory. Benjamin (1982) points out the similarities of the current centralized clinical laboratories to the industrial age factory model. He quotes Alvin Toffler's book *The Third Wave,* in which the current dying industrial society is seen as being replaced by a more diversified and decentralized society. He projects that clinical laboratories will follow the same pattern as we approach the 21st century. While retaining the advances in standardization of technique and quality assurance, such a decentralized approach would allow more customized service to assist physicians in the diagnosis and management of individual patients, rather than focusing entirely on generating numbers.

TOOLS FOR FISCAL DECISION-MAKING

One of the basic premises of management is that one cannot manage that which one cannot measure. Although this is not entirely true of a service-oriented professional function such as a medical laboratory, the laboratory director needs certain quantitative management tools to deal rationally with the development and monitoring of budgets and the utilization of fiscal resources.

Laboratory Workload Recording Method

Until relatively recently, laboratories had no standard method of workload measurement related to the time expended by laboratory technologists in performing laboratory measurements and examinations. Utilizing the experience of the workload system developed by the Canadian Association of Pathologists, and working in conjunction with the U.S. Veterans Administration and other groups, the College of American Pathologists (CAP) has developed a standardized workload recording method for clinical laboratories (CAP, 1983). This method is now recognized as a means of recording laboratory workload by the American Hospital Association and other organizations.

A laboratory utilizing this method makes a *raw count,* which is a simple tally of all procedures performed. This may be done by procedure name and/or by a numerical system such as CPT-4. The CAP workload recording method provides each determination or procedure with a *unit value,* weighted according to the methodology used and to the degree of automation involved. As a result, the system is applicable to both the large, highly automated laboratory and the small laboratory using manual procedures. The official unit value for each procedure was derived after the performance of time-motion studies in a sufficient number of laboratories to provide a statistically meaningful data base. Temporary unit values may be assigned to new or infrequent procedures after a standardized time study is performed by the laboratory and submitted to CAP.

Each *unit* in the workload recording method represents one minute of technical, clerical, and aide time. The *unit value* of a particular procedure includes the time for specimen processing and testing, clerical work including logging and recording of results, and supportive activities such as solution preparation and glassware washing. It does not include the interpretation of results by pathologists, or their assistance to clinical colleagues in terms of what to order and in what order to request it; nor does it include the time for specimen collection, quality control samples, or reports. Specimens used for quality assurance, standards, and repeat measurements may be given the same unit value as a patient specimen and considered as additional procedures. When specimen collection is performed by the laboratory, additional units of work are credited to the laboratory. Monthly totals of the raw counts of procedures are collected by the laboratory and then multiplied by the appropriate unit value of each procedure to produce the total unit value.

Although the system may be used locally by an individual laboratory, the greatest value and ease of operation are provided when the monthly figures are submitted to the CAP Computer Assisted Workload Program on standardized workload reporting forms. In addition to workload figures, the laboratory submits the number of worked, paid, and specified man hours of technical, clerical, and aide time during the month. The *worked man hours* are defined as the actual number of hours employees worked in the laboratory during the month, whereas *paid man hours* reflect the total number of paid hours and include holiday, sick leave, and vacation hours. *Specified man hours* are total hours worked minus hours spent on untimed activities. Utilizing these monthly inputs, the computer program then provides reports giving the laboratory workload in raw count and total units by sections, along with the listing of paid and worked hours plus calculated productivity figures. See Figure 56-1 for definitions.

Since the workload unit is defined as one minute of technical, clerical, and aide time, in an ideal situation there should be a productivity of 60 workload units (that is, 60 minutes of productive work) for each hour of worked time. In actual practice, the average workload productivity in most laboratories is in the range of 30 to 55 workload units per hour. Because of the many variables that enter into the calculation of this figure, one should not interpret it as an absolute indication of productivity. On the other hand, it can be of great value in comparing current with previous productivity, in comparing sections within a laboratory, and in comparing one laboratory

CAP workload unit = 1 minute of technical, clerical, and aide time

Productivity (units/hr) $= \frac{\text{total workload units}}{\text{hours}}$

Paid productivity $= \frac{\text{total workload units}}{\text{paid hours}}$

Worked productivity $= \frac{\text{total workload units}}{\text{worked hours}}$

Specified productivity $= \frac{\text{total workload units}}{\text{specified hours}}$

Figure 56–1. Definitions of terms used in the CAP Workload Reporting System (CAP, 1983).

with other comparable laboratories (such data are provided by the CAP computerized service). If a laboratory section consistently has a workload productivity in the range of 20 to 30, for example, then one must assume a low productivity for this laboratory, probably indicating an overstaffing of the laboratory. On the other hand, if a laboratory's productivity consistently runs over 60, then the laboratory may well be understaffed and need additional personnel support. Both of these judgments assume that the workload units are reasonable for the laboratory's methods and that input errors are excluded.

The utilization of this tool provides a well-standardized and relatively flexible approach to documenting workload and determining productivity. Laboratories are encouraged to utilize this tool, since it provides useful information for budget forecasting and determining future staffing levels. It should be emphasized, however, that the workload figures are *not a direct measure of the cost* of performing a laboratory procedure since they are an estimate only of time expended and take no account of the reagent use, equipment cost, or overhead. Additional information on the workload system and its use in financial management in the clinical laboratory is presented by Sattler (1980).

In projecting workload figures for purposes of future planning, one should take into account two types of growth. One is the *intrinsic growth* in the utilization of laboratory services resulting from improvements in the available laboratory services and from physicians' greater utilization of these services. Such intrinsic growth in the 1970's was 20 per cent or greater per year for areas such as clinical chemistry, with an overall growth of clinical laboratory procedures 10 per cent or greater per year during this same time. Because of increasingly limited resources for health care expenditures and resulting restrictions on use of health care services, it is very unlikely that this rate of growth will continue in the 1980's. Such growth is in addition to the *growth due to increased volume*—that is, growth related to new beds or different types of beds (e.g., intensive care) or to expanded outpatient or other services (e.g., transplantation, oncology, burn unit). Both the intrinsic growth and the growth due to new services are obviously influenced by many factors. Thus a laboratory should not base planning on growth figures such as those cited above, but must utilize data from its own experience. Realistic projections of future volume must also take into account the negative effect of changing patterns of reimbursement for laboratory services. Tools available for workload forecasting are presented in much greater detail by Westlake (1977).

7

Cost Finding

Cost finding is the means by which a laboratory documents its costs for performing a particular procedure and then establishes its charges based on the involved direct and indirect costs.

Ideally, cost finding should be done by laboratory personnel in consultation with the fiscal staff of the hospital. This combination is necessary, since the laboratory staff can analyze steps involved in performing procedures, while fiscal personnel are needed to provide the indirect (or overhead) expenses and to assist in preparing the data for submission to the hospital administration, board of trustees, and third party payers for approval.

Direct vs. Indirect Costs. Two general types of costs are involved in the operation of a laboratory or in costing any single procedure. The first of these is *direct costs,* which are the costs of materials, supplies, and personnel time directly attributable to the specific measurement or examination. Equipment depreciation may be included as part of direct or indirect costs, depending upon the accounting method in use. Equipment leasing is generally considered a direct cost. *Indirect costs* are those costs necessary to operate a laboratory that are not directly attributable to specific measurements or examinations. Such costs include allocated portion of utilities, laboratory and institutional administrative expenses, building depreciation, and janitorial service. The allocation of the costs to the laboratory may be done by various approaches. One (known as step down allocation method) is to take the cost of operating the non-revenue-producing services in a hospital and then allocate this cost to the revenue-producing department on the basis of some formula, such as the number of personnel employed by the area (in the case of the personnel department expense) or the number of square feet in an area (in the case of the janitorial services). Another approach is to determine total expenses for the non-revenue-producing departments as a percentage of the total expenses for operating the hospital or institution. This percentage, representing the indirect expenses, would then be added to the direct expenses for any test procedure to determine the total charge.

Fixed vs. Variable Costs. The concept of fixed and variable costs is useful in analyzing the effects of changing volumes of determinations on expenses and revenue. The *fixed costs* in a laboratory are constant over time regardless of volume of determinations. Depreciation, supervisor salaries, and rental charges are examples. The laboratory will incur these charges at a fixed rate that should not vary with reasonable changes in work volume. On the other hand, *variable costs* are those costs (for items such as supplies and reagents) which will vary in a relationship to the volume of determinations. Fixed costs are much larger, since personnel costs usually account for about 60 to 70 per cent of the total budget of most hospitals. In general, therefore, the greater the workload performed by the laboratory, the less the per unit cost. Decreases in per unit cost, however, are eventually limited regardless of further increases in volume because of the necessity for incremental additions of personnel and/or equipment.

Revenue is traditionally also dependent on volume, so that the *break-even point* for a laboratory is attained at the time revenue exceeds total expenses (that is, the sum of the fixed expenses and the variable expenses). This is graphically shown in Figure 56–2. By use of such a diagram with the current and historical data from a laboratory, one may predict the effect of changing total volume, increasing or decreasing charges, or changing the fixed expenses by adding personnel or equipment (Louvau, 1977). This approach is not applicable to those laboratories where revenue is based upon a predetermined reimbursement rather than upon the volume of work performed. Thus, if the hospital or laboratory is reimbursed a fixed sum of money for its operations, an increased volume of work only adds to the variable expenses and will not affect the revenue.

Development of Charges. The development of charges is a necessary part of most laboratory operations if the patient or a third-party is to be billed a fee for laboratory determinations. The actual method of development of charges will vary from institution to institution depending on the fiscal structure of the institution and the external controls. We will not review these procedures in detail because of the currently rapidly changing procedures for reimbursement for laboratory determinations. When comparing charges from a non-hospital laboratory with those from a hospital laboratory, however, one should be aware of increased overall costs necessary to operate a "full service" laboratory in a large community hospital or a medical center with its requirements for emergency services, specialized services, and training programs.

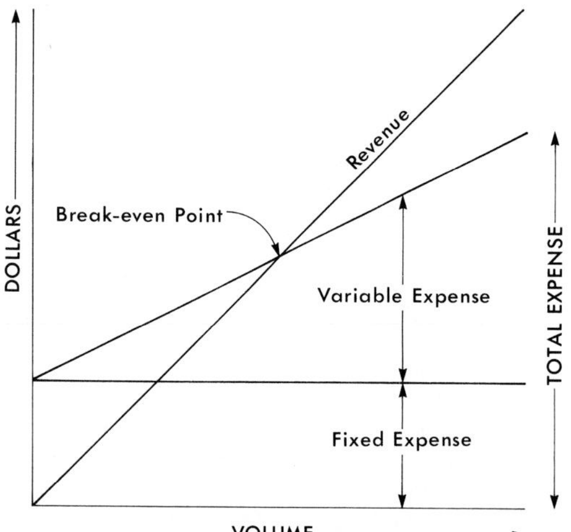

Figure 56–2. Relationships of expenses and revenues to the break-even point. (Modified from Bennington, J. L., et al. [eds.]: Management and Cost Control Techniques for the Clinical Laboratory. Baltimore, University Park Press, 1977.)

RESPONSIBILITY BUDGETING

A budget is an itemized statement of estimated income and/or expenses which is prepared as a financial plan for the coming year. Once prepared, it is then used as a guideline for fiscal management and cost control on an ongoing basis. In order to do this one must have a means of comparing on a regular basis the projected budget with the actual expenses and making adjustments where necessary during the year.

In the past most budgets have been formulated on the basis of negotiating for additional funds for growth and expansion with little attention directed to the base (or continuing) budget from the previous year. *Zero-base budgeting,* in contrast, is founded on the assumption that no base budget is carried forward to the next year and that existing as well as proposed expenditures must be justified. It should be observed, however, that a zero-base budget approach is time-consuming and expensive to institute properly and that alternative ways exist to achieve the same goal. The discussion which follows will be applicable to either the usual budget procedure or the zero-base budget procedure.

Responsibility budgeting follows the philosophy of placing the accountability for the budget at the lowest level of management possible. It is generally recognized that in order for this approach to be successful, five concepts basic to this form of budgeting must be followed (Bennington, 1977):

1. Planned and actual expenses are to be charged to the lowest level of the organization from which they are incurred.
2. No expense item is to be charged to a department unless the department can exercise control of that expense item.
3. All departments included in the budget must be headed by someone who can be held responsible for the costs of that department.
4. Every item of expense can be controlled by someone in the total organization.
5. The department head must participate in the budget formulation process and agree that the planned expenditure of his or her organizational unit is realistic.

Budget Development

Table of Organization and Chart of Accounts. Before a laboratory can introduce the concept of

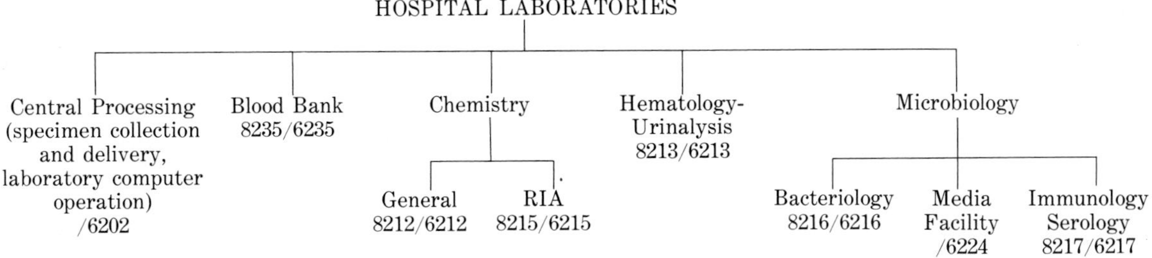

Figure 56–3. Hypothetical budgetary organizational chart for responsibility budgeting. Each budget center is given a cost center number (62– – series) and a revenue code (82– – series) if the center is revenue generating.

responsibility budgeting, an organizational chart which accurately reflects the actual budget centers in the laboratory must be developed. The financial or *budgetary organizational chart* (Fig. 56–3) does not necessarily have to agree with the administrative organizational chart, but it must recognize all areas within the laboratory which incur expenses, which generate income, and for which a separate budget is developed. In most accounting systems each area will be given a unique cost center code and a unique revenue code. It is also important to identify clearly the person responsible for the budget in each of these areas.

The *chart of accounts* is developed for each budget center by listing the expense items for that center broken down into the usual categories such as salaries, fringe benefits, overtime, supplies, reagents, and equipment repairs. Within each major category, there are further subdivisions, each assigned a unique code number for ease of computerization. See Figure 56–4 for an example of a portion of a typical chart of accounts.

The design of such an organizational chart and the development of a chart of accounts thus gives the laboratory the information necessary to monitor trends in expenses and revenues by budget centers within the laboratory and to project such expenses and revenues for budget preparation.

The actual budget process should allow adequate time to review past performance compared with planned performance, to establish plans for the next year, and to convert these plans into quantitative financial data for review and approval of the next year's budget. The steps to accomplish this process are outlined in the following section.

Objectives. As noted in Chapter 55, objectives should be made annually for each section having responsibility for development of the budget, as well as for the entire laboratory. Such objectives should be achievable, quantifiable, and consistent with the in-

CHART OF ACCOUNTS

120—SALARIES & WAGES—SIA

1210 Salaries—SIA. Compensation for services of employees regularly employed on a permanent basis (permanent full time and permanent part time).

1211 Shift Differential. Additional compensation to employees who work on the evening or night shift.

1213 On-Call Pay. Additional compensation paid to those employees who stand by and remain ready to perform their normal duties on a specific pre-determined date when called upon.

1220 Salaries—Overtime. Additional compensation paid to those employees who are subject to the Fair Labor Standards Act whenever those employees work in excess of 40 hours during the hospital's work week.

1250 Holiday Premium Pay. Additional compensation paid to SIA employees who are required to work on days designated as "Holiday Premium" days.

1255 Longevity Pay. Additional compensation recognizes the long term service of Permanent Full Time Staff employees who have at least fifteen years of aggregate hospital service.

1290 Workmen's Compensation. Wage continuation payments to those employees who sustain job-related illness or accidents.

Figure 56–4. Portion of a typical chart of accounts.

stitutional philosophy and developed with as broad an input as is reasonable. They should include projections of growth and new programs and reflect needs for personnel and capital equipment. We have found that objectives can be best developed as a response to observed needs and can be best evaluated when coupled with a strategy for implementation.

Expense Projections. When a decision is first made to implement responsibility budgeting in the laboratory, it may be difficult to find detailed fiscal information on expenses for preceding years in the records of either the laboratory or the accounting department. After the chart of accounts has been established for a year or so, such records will become available and will be useful tools for future budget preparation.

The projection of expenses for the coming year is ordinarily based on at least six to nine months of actual expense data, which are then annualized to serve as a baseline for the preparation of the next year's budget. The projected expenses for the next 12 months are then derived from the annualized current data, taking into account anticipated changes in the following areas: inflation, workload, inpatient census, outpatient visits, and new or deleted hospital programs which would affect the laboratories. For example, the data for seven months' actual expenses and revenue can be multiplied by 12/7 to estimate the annual figures. Such figures, however, can be misleading if revenue and/or expenses are not relatively evenly distributed during the year in question (e.g., if service contracts or large purchases are paid once a year rather than being paid during the year). In addition, input should be obtained from the various sections of the laboratory concerning addition of new services, deletion of obsolete measurements, introduction of automated equipment, and anticipated changes in vendors' prices.

Revenue Projections. Revenue projections are best made by projecting the number of procedures to be performed during the budget year and calculating the revenue based on the current charges. The same projected variables considered in estimating expenses should also be considered in estimating revenue. Part of the budget process usually consists of determining whether the proposed expense budget will be covered by the revenues to be generated at the current level of charges. If this appears unlikely, and if the expenses cannot be trimmed further without compromising patient care, then part of the budget recommendation may be that certain or all charges are increased. On the other hand, if new services and equipment significantly reduce the cost of certain measurements, the budget planning may lead to recommendations that selected charges be reduced. In either case, the projection of new charges as anticipated revenue must be made and incorporated into the budget. This approach is not universally applicable since increasingly hospitals are receiving predetermined amounts of revenue or have severe controls on upward pricing of services.

Capital Equipment Budget. In most institutions a capital equipment budget is a separate budget, prepared in parallel with the operating budget. Capital budget requests are obviously closely related to the short- and long-range goals of the institution and the laboratories.

The decision as to whether major capital equipment should be purchased outright or financed through leasing or rental must be made. The principal advantages of leasing are the low capital outlay and the ability to surrender the equipment when it becomes obsolete. The decision, however, is a complex one, involving not only institutional fiscal policy but also outside influences. Boer (1977) provides a more detailed discussion.

If equipment is to be purchased, then the operating budget usually shows the anticipated annual depreciation of this equipment, as either a direct cost or an indirect cost, depending upon the accounting procedure used by the particular institution. If the equipment is to be leased or rented, then the annual lease or rental amount for the equipment usually is shown in the appropriate line as a direct operating expense for the year.

A justification for new equipment generally is based on one or more reasons. Replacement equipment is best justified by thorough documentation of the extent of the down time and cost of repairs of current equipment as well as enhancements of the new instrument itself. This can be done by maintaining a log listing the type and duration of such problems; most current accreditation standards require such documentation.

A second type of justification for capital equipment is based on the projection that the new equipment will provide labor savings and greater efficiency for the laboratory and possibly greater revenue. If the laboratory is not willing to give up positions as a trade for such equipment, then the laboratory director must be prepared to justify with workload statistics the fact that the personnel are currently overworked and/or document that the persons freed from one task will be assigned to other needed tasks.

Capital expenses also may be justified on the basis of new or improved services. Such justification usually is based on the medical necessity to improve the quality or efficiency of services or the variety and complexity of measurements and examinations offered.

Budget Monitoring

No budgeting system is complete without consistent financial feedback during the budget year. This is usually accomplished through the use of some type of accounting report. Such reports come in many different formats but have as their basic goal the presentation of current monthly and year-to-date data on revenue, expenses, and statistics as compared with the previously projected budget figures. Stadler (1982) discusses the development of such a report.

An example of a simple format to accomplish a monthly monitoring for a single laboratory section is shown in Figure 56–5. A microcomputer with an electronic spread sheet program (of the type originally known as Visi Calc) is used to tabulate the data and

	This Yr	Last Yr	Variance	% Var :	Budget	Variance	% Var
PERSONNEL				:			
FTE Positions	12	12	0	.00 :	12	0	.00
FTE Filled	11	10	1	10.00 :	12	−1	−8.33
Filled/Total	.92	.83	.08	10.00 :	1	−.08	−8.33
Hours Work	1500	1389	111	7.99 :	1400	100	7.14
Hours Paid	2019	1910	109	5.71 :	1800	219	12.17
HrWk/HrPd	.74	.73	.02	2.16 :			
Hours Specif	1291	1185	106	8.95 :			
VOLUME & PRODUCTIVITY				:			
Billed Tests	2757	2555	202	7.91 :	2800	−43	−1.54
CAP Count	7178	7029	149	2.12 :			
Units	70399	69022	1377	2.00 :			
Worked Prod	46.93	49.69	−2.76	−5.55 :	48	−1.07	−2.22
Paid Prod	34.87	36.14	−1.27	−3.51 :	36	−1.13	−3.14
Specif Prod	90.88	97.08	−6.19	−6.38 :			
REVENUE				:			
Billed Revenue	82302	79036	3266	4.13 :	85000	−2698	−3.17
Less Uncol	8230	7900	330	4.18 :	8500	−270	−3.18
Net Rev	74072	71136	2936	4.13 :	76500	−2428	−3.17
NetRev/Test	26.87	27.84	−.97	−3.50 :	27.32	−.45	−1.66
EXPENSES				:			
Sal&Benif	19785	18225	1560	8.56 :	19000	785	4.13
OtherDir	18870	17890	980	5.48 :	18500	370	2.00
Indirect	14766	13469	1297	9.63 :	12500	2266	18.13
TotExp	53421	49584	3837	7.74 :	50000	3421	6.84
Exp/Test	19.38	19.41	−.03	−.16 :	17.86	1.52	8.51
EXP/NET REV	.72	.70	.02	3.47 :	.65	.07	10.34

Prepared by HLD Date 10/24

NOTES: Negative variance = less than last year or budgeted.
Positive variance = greater than last year or budgeted.

Figure 56–5. Hypothetical management monthly report for RIA endocrine laboratory, prepared using an electronic spreadsheet program and a personal computer.

make the necessary calculations. This particular report summarizes data available to the laboratory director or administrator from several sources, including the monthly hospital patient activities report, the monthly hospital financial reports, the laboratory's workload report, and the laboratory's current personnel status report. The average cost for a procedure, the average charge for the procedure, and the ratio of expenses to net revenue have been found to be very useful indicators of activity in a section. Other useful reports give year-to-date figures and provide a summary of data from all lab sections.

The ready availability of such computers and software has given the laboratory director, supervisor, and administrator a relatively inexpensive and powerful tool for budget monitoring. Such programs are also ideally suited for making projections of changes in revenue, expenses, and/or volume of determinations. With Visi Calc or other electronic spread sheet programs, it is a simple task to determine the effect on the total budget of, for example, a 10 per cent salary increase or 5 per cent decrease in revenue. As a change is made in one area, all related volumes are automatically recalculated so that one can easily go through a series of "what if?" exercises with minimal expenditures of time and effort (after the initial format or "template" is established).

These reports are most useful when they are monitored on a regular basis by meetings of persons from each responsibility center with the laboratory director. At such meetings the data can be checked for accuracy, and unexpected variances from the budgeted projections can be investigated to determine the cause and to implement corrective action.

In summary, responsibility budgeting provides laboratory directors and supervisors with a way to have meaningful input into fiscal decisions being made on their behalf and a mechanism to monitor and control the fiscal operation of the laboratory. The process requires a plan, as outlined previously, as well as regular monitoring of the results during the budget year. With each succeeding month and year of the use of this system, the preparation of budgets and accurate projection of income and revenue should become less difficult and more accurate. Furthermore, sound fiscal management of the laboratory contributes to improved and expanded patient care services within the confines of inevitable financial constraints.

Benjamin, D. R.: The "third wave" laboratory. Am. J. Clin. Path., *78*:324, 1982.

Bennington, J. L.: Responsibility budgeting. *In* Bennington, J. L., Boer, G. B., Louvau, G. E., and Westlake, G. E. (eds.): Management and Cost Control Techniques for Clinical Laboratory. Baltimore, University Park Press, 1977.

Boer, G. B.: Cost analysis. *In* Bennington, J. L., et al. (eds.): Management and Cost Control Techniques for Clinical Laboratory. Baltimore, University Park Press, 1977.

Brown, M., McCool, B., Matti, L., and Shipley, L.: Shared laboratory services? What to consider. Hospitals, *49*(9):48, 1975.

CAP: Manual for Laboratory Workload Recording Method. Skokie, Ill., College of American Pathologists, 1983.

Hain, R. F.: The community core laboratory: The laboratory of the future. South. Med. J., *65*:379, 1972.

Louvau, G. E.: Break-even and bivariate linear regression analysis. *In* Bennington, J. L., et al.: (eds.): Management and Cost Control Techniques for Clinical Laboratory. Baltimore, University Park Press, 1977.

Sattler, J.: A Practical Guide to Financial Management of the Clinical Laboratory. Oradell, N.J., Medical Economics Company Book Division, 1980.

Stadler, S. L.: Developing computerized lab management reports. Medical Laboratory Observer, December 1982, pp. 75–79.

Westlake, G. E.: Forecasting and test volume projection. *In* Bennington, J. L., et al. (eds.): Management and Cost Control Techniques for Clinical Laboratory. Baltimore, University Park Press, 1977.

57

INFORMATION MANAGEMENT

DAVID CHOU, M.D., and WILLIAM W. MCLENDON, M.D.

7

The interchange of information between the laboratory and the clinician is a daily occurrence and is an essential component of the practice of laboratory medicine. The transmission of information has frequently been called communications. The data generated by the laboratory has been called potential information and is not actual information until it has been utilized in patient care (Levey, 1973). One of the roles of the laboratory in information management lies in ensuring the exchange of valid data in a timely fashion between the laboratory and those utilizing its data. Other important roles of those in laboratory medicine are education and consultation to help ensure proper utilization of these data in patient care.

The typical cycle of communications necessary to completely process a request for laboratory procedures is shown in Figure 57–1. In a physician's office laboratory, only the patient, the physician, and the

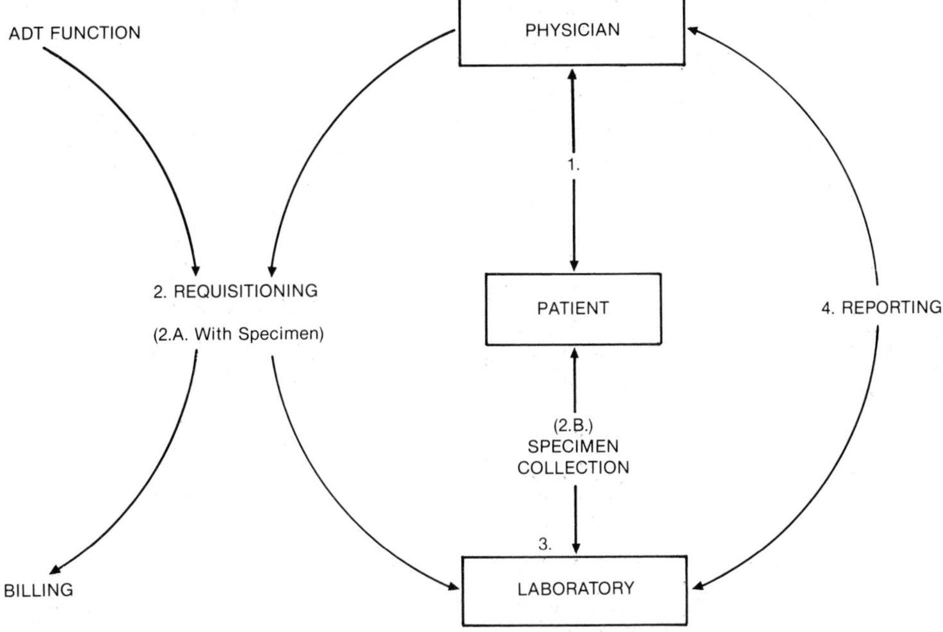

Figure 57–1. Cycle of communications in processing a typical clinical laboratory determination. The intralaboratory component of this cycle comprises only step 3 (the data acquisition from performance of the requested determination) plus step 2.B., when the laboratory performs the specimen collection. All the other essential components (patient-physician encounter, requisitioning, and reporting) are extralaboratory activities.

laboratory technologist may be involved in the cycle. In a large medical center, however, more than 30 persons and many more steps may be involved in completing this cycle. With each additional step or person, an additional potential source of error, confusion, or delay is introduced. In order to contribute effectively to medical care, those in the modern clinical laboratory must concern themselves with the ramifications of this entire cycle rather than confining their interest only to the generation and dissemination of laboratory results.

The first step in the cycle of physician-laboratory interaction is the encounter between the patient and the physician, resulting in a decision for a laboratory test. The physician's decision is translated into a written requisition for laboratory measurements or examinations. The requisition includes the requested determinations as well as basic demographic information about the patient. Following collection of the specimen by the physician or laboratory personnel, the requisition and appropriately labeled specimen are sent to the laboratory.

The requested measurements and/or examinations are performed, the resulting data are processed and checked for validity, and a report is returned to the physician. Although this simplified cycle highlights the essential information interchange involving a clinical laboratory, many other interactions are necessary, especially in larger laboratories. Some of these functions are reviewed subsequently.

This chapter will discuss the essential factors in the dissemination and management of information within and outside the laboratory. In particular, it will try to examine some of the tools available to the clinical laboratory for the management of information. Some of these, such as laboratory manuals, are traditional, whereas others, such as the computer and associated automated telecommunications, have been extensively utilized only recently.

COMMUNICATIONS

Standard II for Laboratory Accreditation (CAP, 1982) states in part: ". . .the laboratories shall have methods for communication to insure prompt, reliable reporting and appropriate record storage and retrieval." The interpretation of the standard includes the comment that "facilities for communication. . . shall be appropriate for the size and complexity of the organization."

In settings such as the physician's office laboratory, the intralaboratory and extralaboratory information exchange is essentially the same. In a large institution the requirements for both intralaboratory and extralaboratory information interchange increase greatly, frequently resulting in significant increases in response time to the physician's request for laboratory support in caring for the patient. In a biologic analogy, Drucker (1967) has pointed out that an organization, like an animal, has to devote an ever greater portion of its resources to internal tasks of circulation and information transfer as the mass of the organization grows. This same problem occurs as laboratories and medical institutions grow. Additional insights concerning laboratory communications are provided in a study by Krieg (1978).

Intralaboratory Communications

Policy Manual. All laboratories should have administrative policy manuals which state the laboratory and institutional policy for the guidance of those working in the laboratory. The policy should reflect the mission statement, organizational structure, and philosophy of the institution as well as those of the laboratory. Appropriate persons in the institution (e.g., the personnel department) should review such documentation to ensure that it reflects institutional policy. Like the laboratory procedure manuals, policies should be dated and approved by the laboratory director, with an annual documented review and update by the appropriate persons. Policy manuals should be readily available to all laboratory employees, including new employees.

Procedure Manual. Standard IV of the College of American Pathologists Commission on Laboratory Inspection and Accreditation (CAP, 1982) states that "each laboratory. . . shall have a quality control system to assure the reliability and medical usefulness of laboratory data." The explanatory notes state, "Procedure manuals should follow a standard format and indicate test sources, dates of adoption and evidence of ongoing review." Federal and many state regulating bodies concerned with clinical laboratory practice have similar requirements.

Orientation, continuing in-service education, and *intralaboratory staff meetings* provide additional methods for dissemination of information. These topics have been covered in Chapter 55.

Extralaboratory Communications

Manual of Procedures and Collection Instructions. The interpretation of CAP Standard IV states that (CAP, 1982):

> Written instructions shall be available which provide, in detail, the methods for procuring, transporting, and processing appropriate specimens. There shall be a written description of the system for the timely reporting of patient data to the physician and of the safeguards taken to ensure the correctness of that data.

At a minimum, such manuals should be available at every patient unit. A loose-leaf format with each page dated allows sections to be updated without having to reprint the entire volume. A list of locations of all notebooks should be maintained by the laboratory and one person designated to update the manuals as changes are made. Dedicated word processors or microcomputers with word-processing software greatly facilitate the updating and printing of revisions.

Laboratory Users' Manual. In addition to a detailed manual of laboratory procedures and collection instructions, many laboratories provide physicians with a pocket-sized manual. A users' manual of two sections has been found to be most useful. The first section contains a directory of the laboratory sections (e.g., hematology, chemistry) with listings of the key resource personnel, the laboratory location, telephone numbers, operating hours, and special instructions. The second half of the manual consists of an alphabetical listing of laboratory measurements and examinations.

Laboratory Bulletins. Periodic laboratory bulletins or newsletters, circulated to the medical staff, are a useful means of communicating information about new laboratory services or policies. These are generally most effective when issued in a standard format on a regular basis. Optimally, these should be concisely written and carefully edited discussions of topics of current interest. An effective approach is to use a one-page or multiple-page issue on one major topic with brief general announcements at the end. Misunderstandings can be avoided if a draft of the proposed bulletin is reviewed in advance by those staff physicians most knowledgeable or most affected by the subject.

Other Extralaboratory Communications. One of the most important functions of laboratory directors is availability for verbal consultations from users. It is by such communications that the laboratory staff becomes aware of its failure or success in meeting the needs of the users. As emphasized by Drucker (1967), "There are no results within the organization. All the results are on the outside. . . ." A negative or defensive attitude about constructive criticisms frequently results in their cessation. This will result in the unrealistic impression that no problems exist; it will become apparent that communications have failed only when a major crisis arises.

The importance of open communications and mutual respect between the laboratory staff and the nursing and clerical staffs throughout the hospital is frequently overlooked. The work of these persons in collecting specimens, transmitting orders, completing requisitions, and charting laboratory reports has a direct impact on the laboratory's ability to perform its function. As a result, orientation programs and in-service education by laboratory staff covering these subjects can promote good will and minimize misunderstandings between these various groups in the hospital.

Requisitioning and Reporting

REQUISITIONING

Proper requisitioning procedures assure adequate identification of the patient and the specimen, indicate the measurements or examinations desired, and facilitate reporting of the results. An additional important function is the provision of administrative and billing data.

The CAP Standards for Accreditation of Medical Laboratories (CAP, 1982) and The Joint Commission on Accreditation of Hospitals (JCAH, 1982) both recognize the key role of requisitioning and require that specimens be accompanied by the following information:

Laboratory procedure number or other identification.

Identification of the patient (name and hospital number).

Room number or address of patient.

Age of patient.

Sex of patient.

Status (stat, pre-op, etc.).

Name of the practitioner.

Date and time the specimen was collected.

Date and time the specimen was received.

In addition, the following information must be maintained by the laboratory and/or reported:

Date, time, and by whom the specimen was examined.

Condition of any unsatisfactory specimen.

Type of test or procedure performed.

Results and date of reporting.

The format of laboratory requisitions varies considerably from hospital to hospital. Although various sizes of requisitions have been used, many requisitions today are either the size of a computer card (3¼ by 7⅜ inches, or 8.3 by 18.7 cm) or medical record size (8½ by 11 inches, or 21.5 by 28 cm). The former are generally multipart forms, one of which is usually a computer card for the business office. The top sheet is used as the report copy, with other sheets used as laboratory and physician copies.

The larger, medical-record size requisitions can be used for both the physician's order and the requisition, thus preventing transcription errors in ordering. The original is sent to the laboratory as a requisition, and the second copy is left in the chart as a record of the order. In general, these types of requisitions are used with computerized systems where reports will be given on other forms. Such a requisition, however, can also serve as a manual back-up report for an automated reporting system.

In order to facilitate the use of requisitions by nursing, clerical, and laboratory personnel, the design should be such that each requisition has specific areas reserved for the required information, such as patient identification, the date and time of specimen collection, identification of the person who collected the specimen, and the measurement or examination requested. When the same requisition form is to be used for reporting, appropriate space should be provided for the results, date and time of reporting, the initials of the technologist performing the determination, and the identification of the laboratory performing the test. In order to facilitate feedback, it is also desirable to have imprinted on the form the name of the director of the laboratories and/or the director of the laboratory section in which the requisition is used.

If the laboratory has different requisitions for different sections, the general layout of the forms should be the same in order to simplify their use by clerical and nursing personnel. The requisition itself should use black ink on white paper for best results if medical records containing these reports are to be microfilmed; the requisitions for different sections can be color coded and tabbed for quick identification.

PATIENT AND SPECIMEN IDENTIFICATION

At this time no completely reliable, generally acceptable, and cost-effective system of positive patient and specimen identification is available. This area remains one of the major unsolved problems in the clinical laboratories, since reliable patient and specimen identification is an essential feature of any accurate laboratory testing and reporting system. The bar-coded label used in grocery stores and other businesses has been applied to managing blood bank products and may be useful for patient identification in the future.

Laboratory professionals must take utmost care with the manual system and insist on proper identification of patients and specimens. Most hospitals apply an armband on inpatients at admission, and laboratory personnel should check this armband with the requisition. A useful additional check is to ask the patient for his or her name and birthdate and to check this against the data available on the armband and the requisition. If the patient is not lucid or if the proper identification is not on the patient (identification on the bed or in the room is not acceptable, since patients are moved without changing such identification), laboratory personnel should be instructed to seek positive identification by other persons who know the patient. Such identification should be documented on the requisition. Each specimen should be labeled immediately by the person collecting the specimen with the patient's full name (correctly spelled), hospital numbers, and date. Blood specimens for crossmatching should also show the name of the phlebotomist on the label. When specimens are collected by other than laboratory personnel, these data should be verified; improperly labeled or unlabeled specimens should not be accepted by the laboratory.

It is anticipated that, in the next decade, reliable and cost-effective methods of patient and specimen identification will be available. A laboratory considering such an approach should coordinate plans in a hospital-wide effort. Any identification system being used for laboratory purposes should be the same as that used for admitting, nursing, pharmacy, radiology, and other services. Otherwise the expense will be prohibitive and great confusion may result.

REPORTS

Written Reports. The College of American Pathologists states that the laboratory director is responsible for all laboratory reports and that "the laboratories shall have methods for communication to insure prompt, reliable reporting and appropriate record storage and retrieval" (CAP, 1982).

General Qualities of a Laboratory Report. A subcommittee of the College of American Pathologists reported in 1974 on general qualities of a good laboratory report (Burns, 1974). These considerations are of value in designing either a manual or a computer-generated reporting system. They are as follows:

1. Compactness.
2. Consistency of terminology, format, and usage of abbreviations and symbols.
3. Clearly understandable.
4. Logical and accessible location in medical chart.
5. Statement of date and time of collection.
6. Gross description and source of specimen when pertinent.
7. Sharp differentiation of reference or normal and abnormal values.
8. Sequential order of multiple results on single specimen.
9. Identification of patient, patient location, and physician.
10. Assurance of accuracy of transcription of request.
11. Ease of preparation.
12. Administrative and record-keeping value.

Verbal Reports. Verbal reports constitute a major problem for many laboratories. It is essential that verbal or telephone reports be given in order to facilitate medical care, particularly in an emergency situation. On the other hand, this is a major potential source of errors and resulting medical liability. At a minimum, the laboratory should require proper identification of the person receiving the report and of the patient. The person giving the report should repeat the patient's name, identification number, and location along with the results in order to further confirm the identification.

As an alternative to verbal reports, many laboratories are using various transmission devices from the laboratory to key areas, such as the emergency room and intensive care unit, that require immediate reports. One type allows a handwritten result on either blank paper or a preprinted form to be transmitted electronically and generated in a similar form at the receiving end. This has the advantage of being reliable and relatively inexpensive, but it is subject to transcription errors at the time of input. Another approach is facsimile transmission. This has the advantage of giving an exact facsimile of the original test report, but has the disadvantage of being more expensive, generally slower, and in some cases less reliable. In most cases, the computer has supplanted the need for such devices through the availability of remote terminals and printers.

MANUAL SYSTEMS FOR TEST REQUISITIONING AND REPORTING

Most manual systems are based on combined test requisitioning and reporting forms. Although a requisitioning and reporting system may meet the needs of the laboratory, it is important that the laboratory director be aware of the need of the clinician for a concise, readable, and chronologic presentation of laboratory data. Traditionally this has been performed by shingling the laboratory reports in the patient record. If these reports are color coded by originating laboratory and the reports from a single laboratory are put together on a carrier page, this can provide a chronologic reporting system. This can be facilitated by using reports designed in a vertical format so that the date and time of collection are seen across the top and the results are written vertically.

An alternative method exists for providing a chronologically oriented type of report that simulates a computerized cumulative report (Henry, 1964). The laboratory has an 8½ by 11 inch or larger master card (cumulative report card or CRC) on which the patient's demographic data are written or imprinted at the time of admission or of first laboratory activity. A simple disposable requisition is used to request testing and for billing purposes. After the determinations are performed in the laboratory, the results are written in the proper position on the master card (CRC) in the laboratory along with the date and time of collection at the head of the column. If the laboratory is large and organized in sections, each section may have a separate CRC for its data. After the laboratory data are placed on the CRC, a dated photocopy is made; this copy is sent to the physician or chart as the report. As subsequent data are added to the card and copies made, the earlier copies in the chart are removed and replaced by the updated photocopy of the CRC. This system has the advantage of providing a cumulative report to both the physician and the laboratory and of allowing the laboratory to check the current data against the previous data to determine if the results are reasonable. It can be used either as a totally manual system or as a temporary manual back-up approach for a computerized reporting system. The disadvantages of the system relate to the investment of clerical time and photocopying, as well as the possibility of transcription errors. Also, if the patient volume is high, the cost of filing and retrieving the master cards can be considerable.

DATA PROCESSING AND TELECOMMUNICATIONS

Data processing refers to the process whereby raw data are entered into a computer, stored, manipulated, and outputted. Telecommunications refers to the transmission of information by any of a number of electromagnetic methods. In the most general sense, the telephone is one such telecommunications device. Increasingly, telecommunications involves the transmission of data between computer-related devices.

Within the last decade the computer has emerged as a major tool within the clinical laboratory. Its impact on information management in the laboratory is potentially as great as the impact of automated analyzers on the analytical process of the laboratory. A large number of factors contributed to the migration of computers into the mainstream of laboratory information management. First, the computer has emerged because of the need for most laboratories to manage their growth during the last decade. Many facilities tripled their workload within ten years, making management and staffing a difficult task. In many cases, the computer has stabilized personnel requirements in this period of growth through improved productivity of existing personnel. Second, the complexity of providing certain types of information, such as management reports on laboratory utilization and productivity, has made the computer a virtual necessity in most larger laboratories. Third, the computer is able to transmit large amounts of laboratory data rapidly to remote locations. Last, all of these applications have become increasingly cost effective with decreasing computer prices.

These factors, however, do not imply that computerization should be a goal for every laboratory. A manual system can frequently yield as many benefits as a fully computerized system without the capital investment and high support costs. The test volume at which a laboratory will benefit significantly from a computer system differs depending on the environment. If the laboratory director intends to computerize, he should closely evaluate the benefits versus the liabilities and anticipate this development through implementing manual systems which allow for the smooth transition to an automated system.

Definition of Terms and Concepts

Knowledge of basic data processing and computer terms will be useful for communication with computer specialists and vendors. Unfortunately, there is no easy way to determine what constitutes adequate knowledge, but the following basic terms and concepts provide useful background information.

HARDWARE

Electronic computer systems comprise *software* and *hardware*. Hardware includes all the tangible physical or "hard" parts of a computer. Software is the instructions which the machine follows to perform a task.

Recent advances in electronic device technology have dramatically influenced the evolution of computers. The electronic tubes of first generation computers produced in the 1950's were rapidly replaced by more reliable transistors in the second generation computers of the early 1960's. Transistors were in turn replaced by the simple integrated circuits (ICs) which appeared in third generation computers manufactured during the mid to late 1960's. Current fourth generation computers are manufactured from ICs having as many as several hundred thousand transistors. No more than 10,000 transistors are needed to make a small computer.

The central processing unit, or *CPU*, is considered to be the brain of the computer system. It consists of a control unit, the arithmetic logic unit, or *ALU*, and central memory. The control unit makes changes in program flow as a result of program conditions. The ALU performs all arithmetic operations and tests the logical conditions set up in programs. *Central memory* provides storage and rapid access for data and programs.

Most parts of a CPU are manufactured today from ICs. A *microprocessor* is a special case whereby almost the entire CPU and sometimes small amounts of central memory are manufactured from a single piece of silicon. This profound simplification has been the main contributor to decreasing the cost and increasing the reliability of the modern computer.

In most cases, central memories are manufactured from separate ICs, called semiconductor memories. Semiconductor memories fall into at least two categories. One class, commonly called *RAM* (for random access memory), serves as storage for data and programs that are frequently altered. Information stored in RAMs is lost if there is an electrical power interruption. A second type of semiconductor memory is a *ROM* (for read only memory), which is characterized by its ability to store information in a manner unaffected by the loss of power. Both ROMs and RAMs are random access devices, characterized by a uniform time requirement for data to be written or retrieved from any storage location in a memory. Programs stored in ROMs are called *firmware,* since such programs may be altered only with special equipment.

Two types of RAMs are currently in general use. The first type, *dynamic* RAMs, has generally been used in larger computers because of its low cost. This memory, however, requires complex support circuitry to rewrite information into the RAMs every 1 to 2 milliseconds to avoid loss of data, since the data will "fade" with time. *Static* RAMs, on the other hand, are more costly but do not require *refreshing* of memory contents and generally tend to be more reliable at the integrated circuit level. Many machines with dynamic memories incorporate error correction schemes to circumvent problems of unreproducible or *soft errors* which sometimes occur. It is possible to design reliable systems around either static or dynamic RAMs.

At least four types of ROMs are in widespread use. A mask programmed ROM is loaded with its contents, or "programmed," at the time of manufacturing. *PROMs* (programmable ROMs) can be programmed after manufacturing. Fusible PROMs are programmed by selectively burning away parts of the chip. Both types can be programmed only once. *EPROMs* (electrically programmed PROMs) may be erased by UV light. *EAPROMs* (electrically alterable PROMs) are erased by a high voltage signal and also programmed electrically. Both EPROMs and EAPROMs can be programmed many times.

Additional types of memory, such as tapes and disks, are used by most computers for storage of less frequently accessed data. Most such devices require more time for retrieving data but also cost considerably less than central memory. These fall into a class of *on-line storage* devices.

Magnetic tapes similar to those used in audio recorders are the most inexpensive form of data storage. With magnetic tape, access to a given piece of information is often slow, since access time is dependent on the position of the read-write head relative to the desired information on the tape. Data stored on a tape are said to be *sequential,* since we must serially pass over all information whether we utilize it or not. Access time for a given piece of data may take minutes under the worst conditions. Tapes, however, are the standard method for transporting information between computers and for archival storage of data no longer needed on-line to the computer.

Disk memory consists of a rotating record-like device covered with a magnetic surface that can be easily accessed with either a movable or fixed read/write head positioned close to its flat surface. Data are recorded in concentric circles, called *tracks,* and access to a given piece of information is more rapid than tapes. Positioning the head over the desired track and waiting for the information to rotate under the head is a fairly rapid process, taking milliseconds. The cost of a disk and its associated hardware is usually considerably higher than that of tape. A single reel of tape costs less than 20 dollars and a disk pack costs up to 1000 dollars. Transferring information stored on disk to another computer is usually not possible, since the format of data on disks is not standardized. *Floppy disks* (also called diskettes) are similar to the hard disks described above and have been used in many microcomputer-based instruments and word processors because of their low cost (less than five dollars).

Winchester disk technology, introduced by IBM in 1973, has gained popularity in the microcomputer/minicomputer market. This type of disk utilizes a special read/write head in a sealed case ventilated through microscopic filters to remove dust and other particles floating in the air. This filtering of air allows the head to travel closer to the magnetic media and, consequently, permits greater density of information (White, 1980). Such storage devices have already decreased the cost of information storage by an order of magnitude.

Optical devices for data storage have been designed. These devices currently allow data to be written only once but do have the advantage of permitting vastly increased amounts of data storage. When such optical disks come into wide use, they will significantly alter the current limitations on the cost of mass data storage.

The most common unit of measure for computer memories and storage is the *byte.* The byte is defined as eight *bits* (one bit is a single *bi*nary dig*it*.). This is a convenient size since one character (such as the letter "A") is usually represented in one byte. One kilobyte or K-byte of memory represents 1024 bytes (or 2^{10}), and one megabyte equals 1,048,576 (or 2^{20}) bytes. Currently, computer memories range from tens of kilobytes to tens of megabytes. Most tapes and disks store between 1 and 500 megabytes.

Input and output devices include those which are designed to support communications between man and machine as well as devices such as tapes and disks which are used for communications between computers. Traditionally, keyboards, terminals, and printers are the most highly visible I/O devices.

The most common I/O device in laboratory systems is the CRT terminal, or cathode-ray tube terminal. This is a television-like device designed to output characters and, occasionally, graphics to a user and usually has a keyboard attached. Keyboards are the most frequent form of direct input into a computer. Most keyboards are a variation of the common typewriter keyboard. Special keyboards, similar to touch-tone telephone keyboards, may be used for special input stations, such as those for a differential leukocyte count in the hematology laboratory.

Card readers, where data were entered through punched "IBM" or Hollerith cards, were popular in the past. Most newer laboratory systems avoid card readers owing to their high cost when compared to keyboards and CRT terminals.

Mark sense document and card readers are frequently used in laboratory systems and are preferred by some over keyboard terminals. The user blackens appropriate boxes on a card with a pencil in order to enter a given result. Other formats include punching holes in cards to indicate results. Possible advantages of this approach are as follows: (1) no typing experience is needed by the user; (2) one input device might service an entire laboratory, resulting in lower initial hardware costs; and (3) the method offers an intrinsic information backup in case of machine failure. Disadvantages include (1) less flexibility in changing tests or test formats, since new documents or cards must be printed up each time; and (2) lack of feedback from the input device, possibly promoting user errors that are difficult to detect.

Hand-held bar code and character readers similar to those seen in some department stores have been used to read labels on blood products. Other light pens which read specially formed letters have also been utilized to read test request forms. Such devices have also been used for specimen identification by some laboratory instrument manufacturers.

The most common output device for laboratory systems is the printer. Slow-speed *character printers* generally fall into three categories: impact character, dot matrix character, and matrix thermal character printers. Impact character printers are typewriter-like devices which usually give high-quality printout but are expensive, noisy, and slow. Matrix printers use dots to form characters and offer higher speed, lower costs, and less noise at the expense of legibility. Neither type of printer is quiet enough to use in an office or patient setting without special acoustical isolation. Thermal printers are similar to impact matrix printers, except that they use heat to burn an image onto specially treated paper. Although thermal printers are almost noiseless, the special paper does have the disadvantage of image degeneration over time and high expense when compared to conventional paper. Newer non-impact matrix printers use ink jet technology to squirt dots onto, or lasers to burn images into, paper. These methods are quieter than impact methods, but currently are either expensive or unreliable when compared with impact technology. Many matrix type printers also support graphics output.

Line printers are high-speed output devices which typically print an entire line at once and output information at more than 10 to 100 times the rate of the previously described character printers. Because of their higher speed, large outputs such as ward summary reports are frequently sent to these printers rather than the slower character units. These units may be quite expensive and noisy and cannot be readily placed on a patient ward.

CRT terminals are appearing which offer high speed graphics when a hard copy capability is not necessary. The more expensive devices can offer exceptional quality, detail, and even color for displaying graphs. These terminals are uncommon at this time in laboratory computer systems owing to their high costs but should appear in the near future.

Voice input and output devices have recently gained some interest but have not achieved wide acceptance. The practicality of voice computer output for general use appears promising as a consequence of low cost devices recently introduced by several manufacturers. Voice recognition computers have been under development. Devices with a limited vocabulary are already being produced for use in special environments. One editorial in an industry journal predicts that voice response typewriters capable of accepting a common business vocabulary will be commonplace by the end of the decade. Such devices have the potential for solving many man-machine interface problems.

The direct input and output of data to and from laboratory instruments is not as straightforward as from previously described I/O devices. Laboratory instrumentation does not function in a strictly digital fashion. Until recently, most instruments provided continuous, or *analog,* signals which are not compatible with most computers. The fundamental difference between analog and digital signals lies in the way numbers are electrically represented. Analog signals, in their expression of numbers, can theoretically represent any value within a given continuum, whereas numbers in digital computers can only take on certain discrete values. Through the use of low cost IC analog-to-digital (A/D) and digital-to-analog (D/A) converters, signals can be converted from one form to another. Newer laboratory instruments usually have built-in A/D and D/A converters and frequently incorporate a microcomputer to find peaks and provide appropriate digital signals for the laboratory computer.

Such progress, however, has not altered the fact that interfacing instruments to a computer is not automatic. The lack of standardization among instrument and computer manufacturers has often made it difficult to interface instruments to computers. Even if an instrument is electronically and mechanically compatible, it may take much effort before data can be transferred automatically from an instrument to a patient file owing to the lack of software standards.

A *microcomputer* is defined as a computer whose CPU had been constructed from a microprocessor. Single chip ICs are the most common form of microprocessors and are widely available. Some laboratories have manipulated and stored quality control information, for example, with such machines. Most small desk top microcomputers, also called personal computers, fill a niche between calculators and larger computers. However, they have limitations for use in applications requiring the management and storage of large amounts of data.

Most larger laboratory systems are designed from larger computers, typically called *minicomputers.* Most computers in the future may be technically microcomputers, even though their capabilities will be equivalent to today's larger minicomputers. Most hospital information systems are designed to operate on *mainframe* computers, which have even larger computational capabilities than minicomputers.

Microprocessors are available today for under five dollars. One goal envisioned by futurists is to develop a hierarchy of computers, from microcomputers at the bottom controlling instruments to a mainframe computer at the top handling the hospital information system. Minicomputers in the laboratory, pharmacy, and other areas will service local requirements and feed data to the central unit as necessary. Such an approach is called *distributed processing* and will greatly improve reliability of computer systems through modularity. Unfortunately, intercomputer communications grows rapidly in complexity as the number of systems increases. The current promise of distributed processing lies in the ability of the system designer to partition a problem in such a fashion that the communications requirement is minimized. Perhaps some breakthroughs in computer science will solve this difficulty in the future. This communications problem partially explains why computer systems with more than three or four CPUs are rarely found in practice. Many users and vendors use the term distributed processing inappropriately. The simple interconnection of two or more computers does not imply distributed processing but only that some form of computer *networking* has been implemented.

COMPUTER TELECOMMUNICATIONS

Computer telecommunications has grown rapidly over the last several years, especially intercomputer communications. Although this form of communication may be important if several computers are used within the hospital, most communications problems associated with laboratory computers lie within the realm of input/output terminals communicating with one computer. Similar problems can be encountered in both types of communication, but intercomputer data transfer usually demands higher speeds and greater reliability owing to the lack of a human interpreter at one end. Virtually any electromagnetic media can be used to transfer digital information, including wires, cables, light, radio, microwave, and satellite systems.

Acoustic couplers can be used for data transmission over dialed telephone lines. These devices consist of a microphone and a loudspeaker connected to a device which converts digital pulses to and from audible tones. By dialing up a computer and placing a telephone handset into the acoustic coupler, a user can communicate with a computer. The advantage of this dial-up approach is that a number of widely separated laboratories can share a single computer line and minimize initial computer costs. Telephone lines can be expensive to maintain, however, and computer security may pose serious problems with such open accessibility. In addition, such communication, by computer standards, is relatively slow. *Modems* are similar to acoustic couplers except that they are wired into the telephone line instead of using the handset.

Most low-speed computer devices operate with a binary character set standard, called *ASCII* (for *A*merican *S*tandard *C*ode for *I*nformation *I*nterchange), consisting of seven bits used to represent one character. IBM has also developed a separate eight-bit character set, called *EBCDIC* (for *E*xtended *B*inary *C*oded *D*ecimal *I*nformation *C*ode). Both forms are in common use. Most terminals adhere to a mechanical and electrical interface standard, called *RS-232C*, originally established by EIA (the Electronics Industry Association). This standard is also being used by most instrument manufacturers for their computer interfaces.

The speed at which a computer communicates with a remote printer or terminal is usually measured in *baud* (for *b*its *aud*io). In most cases, a baud corresponds to a transmission rate of one bit per second. For most terminals, one character requires the transmission of ten bits. The two additional bits, called the start and stop bits, are additional overhead imposed by the communications system in addition to the eight bits (one byte) needed to transmit the character. Most dial-up telephone modems operate at 1200 baud, or 120 characters per second.

For short distances (usually less than 500 feet), most instruments and terminals adhering to the RS-232C standard can be directly wired to a computer possessing a similar interface. For longer distances or for situations requiring the convenience of dialed telephone lines, modems or acoustic couplers will frequently be needed.

The communications between a remote terminal and the computer may occur in a number of different forms. Most terminals support a *half-duplex* mode where either the computer or the terminal can use the communications line (but not both simultaneously). If the user needs to interrupt a computer transmission, he must interrupt the circuit by sending a *break* character. In the *full-duplex* mode, both the computer and the terminal can transmit data simultaneously without interference with each other.

Intercomputer communications must be far more complex in order to ensure data integrity. Error detection is largely ignored on low-speed devices, since the assumption is that users will detect them. Extensive error detection is present in almost all computer communications protocols. Error checking and, occasionally, error correction schemes are used.

SOFTWARE

Both data and program are pieces of information stored in the memory of a computer. Specifically, data are information which is being moved, manipulated, or tested. A program is a set of instructions which directs a machine how to behave in handling the data. Software collectively refers to all programs used in computers.

Currently, programming requires large amounts of time, effort, and skilled personnel. One of the frequently quoted axioms in the computer industry has been that software constituted only 30 per cent of the total system costs in the 1950's and over 80 per cent of the costs in the 1970's (Branscomb, 1982). Although the sharing of computer software among users may modify these percentages, increasing software complexity and inflation will probably continue to drive up software costs, even as hardware costs drop. The most important point is that most software should not be considered disposable, and both users and manufacturers should ensure that programs are transferable to newer hardware.

Early electronic computers were programmed in *machine language*. Instructions were entered by inputting numbers, usually in a binary format, into the machine through switches. Because of the obvious inconvenience of associating binary numbers with instructions and inputting them through switches, a symbolic *assembly language* was developed which performed some of the more tedious tasks associated with programming. Many laboratory systems designed in the mid to late 1960's were programmed using assembly language because it resulted in systems which efficiently utilized expensive hardware resources. Unfortunately, this approach frequently results in systems with limited flexibility because of the time needed for any programming changes. In addition, resulting programs cannot be transported to another machine. A more detailed discussion of software development problems and the use of assembly language can be found in Brooks (1979).

Because of the limitations of assembly language, FORTRAN (*For*mula *Tran*slation) rapidly gained acceptance. FORTRAN represented an early attempt to develop *higher level computer languages*, languages which were more English-like in nature. Early approaches to high level languages usually involved a translater, called a *compiler*, which converted the instructions written in the higher-level language, the source code, into machine language. Once the machine language output, the *object code*, is produced, it can be stored and used without the compiler itself. Some manufacturers attempt to maintain the proprietary nature of their programs by not making source codes available to the user. If the source code is lost for any reason, such as a manufacturer going bankrupt, the user will not be able to make any programming changes. Later developments in high level languages include COBOL (*Com*mon *B*usiness *O*riented *L*anguage), Algol (*Algo*rithmic *L*anguage), and Pascal.

As utilization of computers increased, programs called *operating systems* (also frequently called *monitors* or *executives*) were developed which supervised the orderly execution of programs and provided for certain basic functions utilized by all programs. For a laboratory system, these functions might include data acquisition from instruments, management of CRTs and printers, and the management and control of disks.

Early operating systems were *batch* oriented. Programs or jobs were stored in the sequence in which they were to be run and were executed one at a time. Most recent operating systems are *timeshared*. In this type of system, a number of user programs are executed simultaneously, and all users appear as if they have the entire machine available to themselves as a result of the speed of the machine. For laboratory systems, a *real-time* capability is necessary for operating systems. This term refers to the need to capture data from instruments and process it without delay. Instruments will not wait for the computer, but most computers today are so much faster than laboratory instruments that this is not usually a problem.

Faster machines have also resulted in changes in higher level languages. The inconvenience of going through a compilation from source to object code, and the necessary restriction imposed on the language by this process, prompted the development of *interpreted languages*. In interpreted languages, no object code is produced. Instead a program, the interpreter, examines each character in the source code and executes the instruction as soon as it is decoded. In general, interpreters are less efficient than compilers, since they may repeatedly examine a program statement rather than convert it directly to machine code. One popular interpreted language in the laboratory field is *MUMPS* (*M*assachusetts General Hospital *U*tility *M*ulti-*P*rogramming *S*ystem). Its popularity stems from its ability to simplify the building of patient data bases. Another popular language, *BASIC* (*B*eginners *A*ll-Purpose *S*ymbolic *I*nstruction *C*ode) is usually interpreted, although it may be compiled. The tradeoffs between compilers and interpreters will depend on applications and personal preferences.

One way to view the interaction of software and hardware is that software essentially layers over a hardware core, providing the final interfaces to the user and computer applications (Fig. 57–2). The software itself may also be designed in a layered manner where the more basic functions are supported by primary software, such as an operating system, as well as the hardware, and more sophisticated software utilizes functions provided by less sophisticated software. The outermost software layer, which interfaces with the user, runs applications programs, such as those supporting test requisition, result entry, and result reporting. Advances in hardware technology have permitted an increase in the complexity of this software layering. Although this layering results in machines which run less efficiently than those ma-

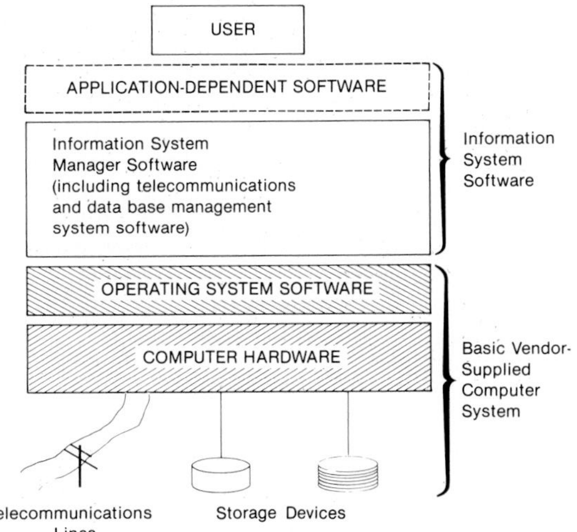

Figure 57–2. Contemporary information system structure. (Modified from Madnick: Science, *195*:1191–1199, 1977.)

chines with less layering, it allows programmers greater productivity. Many studies have shown that the average person can produce only between 10 and 40 lines of computer code per day. This productivity rate appears to be relatively independent of the computer language used (Brooks, 1979). Since higher level languages condense the information content per line of code and more complex higher level languages can be developed through layering, this software approach increases programmer productivity but decreases hardware performance, an attractive tradeoff. Large operating systems, compilers, and interpreters may all be utilized by user application programs during operations. One direct consequence of this layering can be that application programs are more user oriented.

DATA

Programs generally operate on information that may be included within the program itself or on information acquired from sources external to the program. In either case, such information is called *data*, and the organization of such information is called the *data structure*. Data stored on disks, tapes, and other devices external to the main memory or the CPU are called a *file*. Although files and data structures may contain some explicit information about the purpose and type of information which is stored, additional information needed to meaningfully interpret the data is usually implicit to minimize disk or tape space requirements. For example, an accounting system will almost always omit the dollar sign ($) and the decimal point. In other words, 15.25 will appear as 1525 in a disk file. Such implicit information makes the use of data in files nearly impossible without some prior knowledge of the data structure. A program without the appropriate information could potentially substitute one patient's laboratory results for another patient's results because of errors in recognizing the format for a patient identification number.

Data structures are critical to the design of programs. First, the input data and the output data will frequently occupy the majority of the disk and central memory storage. In a laboratory system, for example, the size of the laboratory easily exceeds the size of programs by an order of magnitude. The design of the data structure may impose limitations on the stored information. A system might be limited to storing information on 256 patients in a certain category, while a second system might be limited to 64,000 patients. The smaller system, if programmed properly, will run faster and more efficiently within its limitations than the larger system, assuming comparable resources. Since it requires fewer software and hardware resources, it will be less expensive to purchase and use than the larger system. But all these points on efficiency will be irrelevant if the user's needs exceed 256 patients or, at some future date, grow beyond 256 patients.

Unanticipated growth always seems to be a difficulty with computer systems, especially since the installation process for computers frequently requires years. Unfortunately, if the program or software does not allow for growth, the results can be disastrous. Data structures may also be sufficiently rigid that growth is basically impossible. At this point, the user has little alternative except to discard all old software and data and start over, an alternative which may be more expensive than the initial difference between the purchase price of the larger and smaller system.

During the last ten years or so, progress in improving hardware performance has permitted the evolution of specialized software systems known as *database management systems* (DBMS). Such systems can allow the user to tailor the data organization to specific applications with greater ease. A DBMS may be viewed as a very high-level programming language. Although such systems have not been widely used in the laboratory computer field, their appearance in other areas has greatly speeded up programming of new systems and has made database expansion and alteration much easier. Such systems may be designed so that end users without programming experience can perform inquiries or *queries* of the database. Such systems are complex and inefficient and usually require the use of very high performance computers.

In spite of the rapid progress that has occurred with computer hardware, basic concepts in software have progressed slowly (Brooks, 1979). Those closely following the computer field have observed that few major breakthroughs have actually occurred in programming concepts. Improved laboratory computers have largely resulted from a better understanding of how the computer fits into daily laboratory operations.

Scope of Hospital and Laboratory Data Processing

Planning for the data processing needs of clinical laboratories, especially those in a hospital setting, involves consideration of many issues both inside and outside the laboratories. As shown in Figure 57–1, many of the essential components for the interaction between the physician and the laboratory exist outside the laboratory. In addition, obtaining financial and administrative information needed for the laboratory computer frequently requires interaction with hospital management and administrative data processing facilities. For example, the laboratory is dependent on others for the assignment of a unique medical record number, an important consideration in any laboratory computerization.

Hospital information systems (HIS) is the term used to describe collectively the operation of one or more computers that provide information handling and processing for patient data on a hospital-wide basis. The term hospital information systems can describe an entire spectrum of computer systems ranging from those limited to handling simple interdepartmental communications to those designed to computerize the entire patient chart. Most hospital information systems support financial transactions; more recently such systems include support for patient care–related information.

Because of the broad range of the HIS, the exact nature of the information interchange varies considerably. Figure 57–3 outlines a substantial portion of

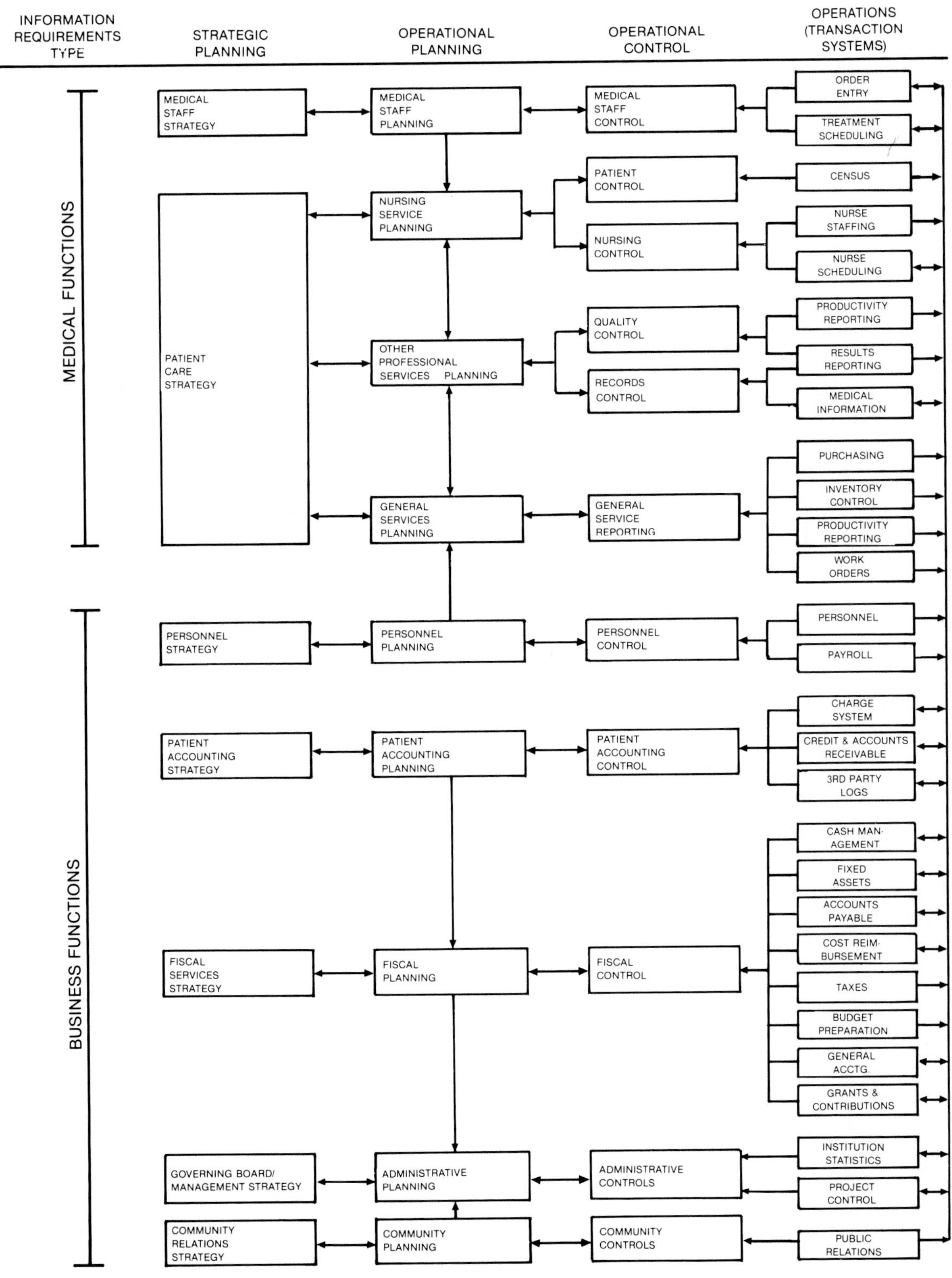

Figure 57–3. Hospital information systems. (Modified from Shaffert, 1978.)

the information flow within the hospital setting. This information is divided into four major categories which fall into a rather traditional view of management as summarized by Anthony (1980). Upper management performs strategic planning, using data for defining institutional goals. Middle management uses information for operational planning, integrating the institutional goals and the daily operations. The lowest management level uses information for operational control, that is, to manage the day-to-day operations of an organization. The daily operations occur at the lowest information level and simply consist of the transactions occurring between individuals. Almost all transactions at the lowest level have been computerized in some fashion; almost none of the information categories at the strategic planning level have been computerized.

Hospital information systems almost always differ only in the number of functions which they implement. The simplest computer-based communications systems, for example, implement a patient census system and a charge system which bills for services and supplies. More complex systems process and store patient medical information in some form.

Laboratory information system (LIS) is the term used to describe a computer system designed for supporting the information management in the clinical laboratory. Such a system may be a submodule of an HIS or may be free standing. In a free standing LIS, ultimate integration of the LIS into the HIS is an important consideration. The interaction of the HIS with the LIS lies in four general areas: (1) the exchange of requests for tests (order/entry), (2) the location of the patient (patient census), (3) the return of laboratory results (results reporting and medical information), and (4) a charge for the test ordered (charge system). The exchange of patient census information has frequently been called admission/discharge/transfer or *ADT*.

In a totally integrated system, ADT information can be acquired from the admissions office through terminals placed in the admissions office. Physician orders can also be made through terminals placed in patient care areas. The laboratory receives the request and integrates it with the specimen. The LIS contributes to the organization of the laboratory workload. If an assay is performed on an automated instrument, the results are entered directly into the computer with results verification as the only human interaction with the data. As soon as the data are verified, terminals and printers in patient care areas can be used by nurses and physicians to retrieve results.

An institutional commitment is necessary to develop a totally integrated HIS and LIS. This process usually requires careful, long-range planning. Because of differences between computers and poor standardization within the computer field, this goal of integrating the database may be difficult and expensive. The non-integrated approach can also result in some organizationally undesirable results, such as the placement of multiple printers and terminals on each patient unit. Continued parallel development of independent computer systems may result in situations in which later integration becomes impossible.

A recent study of the HIS at the National Institutes of Health Clinical Center suggests that the totally integrated approach provides significant clinical benefits (Analytical Services, 1982). The most important factor in the NIH study was that clinicians do use remote terminals for results retrieval. In surveys, physicians considered laboratory results retrieval to be the most important use of the HIS, accounting for an average of 16 minutes per day of physician-computer interaction. Some institutions have substituted terminals in patient care areas for paper printouts from the computer with considerable success. These experiences basically underscore the importance of being able to provide an integrated HIS, in spite of the costs of integration.

Both HIS and LIS systems can be very cost effective. In the past, justifications for such systems frequently argued that, when compared with manual methods, computer systems recover lost charges, frequently estimated to be at 5 per cent or more of gross revenues. Recent studies on the HIS at the Clinical Center (Analytical Services, 1982) and LIS elsewhere (Lincoln, 1980; Henricks, 1982) also show significant improvements in productivity. These quantitative factors do not include the intangible benefits resulting from improved accessibility and accuracy of the data.

Features of a Laboratory Information System

The features of a laboratory information system can be divided into two categories. Features essential for the operation of a basic laboratory system are as follows: (1) Method for requisition of tests requested, either preceded by or with the concurrent entry of patient administrative data such as name, identification number, age, sex, physician, and location. (2) The preparation of lists, generally in the form of gummed labels, for blood drawing team use. (3) Preparation of worklists. (4) Manual and on-line methods for entry of laboratory data with procedures for verification of the data entry and hard copy printouts of check lists. (5) The generation of reports for the physician's use. At a minimum, these should include location reports, with the data sorted by all patients for a particular location (i.e., clinic or floor), and patient interim and cumulative reports. (6) Billing data available for either manual or on-line transmission to the hospital billing computer. (7) Feedback to laboratory management as to performance of the system, usually in the form of a discrepancy report.

Other features which are desirable may not be essential in the first stage of development. Many of these are by-products of the database provided by the essential features noted above. The additional features are as follows: (1) Detailed quality control reports. (2) Workload reports, preferably in the format of the College of American Pathologists standardized workload reporting system. (3) Other statistical and management reports, tailored for the needs of the specific laboratory. (4) More sophisticated billing, either by the laboratory computer or by on-line transmission of data to the hospital computer. (5) Epidemiologic reports as a by-product of the clinical microbiology laboratory system. (6) Ability to retrieve laboratory data for educational or research purposes (for example, "all patients with an MCV greater than 100 and a hematocrit of 20 per cent or less" or "all patients over 50 years of age having a positive blood culture with *Staphylococcus aureus* for the previous six months"). (7) Data communications capabilities to remote locations served by the laboratories. (8) Instructions to nursing personnel in regard to collection of specimens and preparation of patients. (9) Graphic display or reporting of data. (10) Interpretative reporting of data with suggested follow-up laboratory studies. (11) Reports on physician utilization of laboratory services.

Approaches to Laboratory Computerization

The practical use of computer techniques in the routine clinical laboratory began in earnest in the mid-1960's and has shown a maturation during the 1970's. In the first decade of this development, the laboratory director planning a laboratory information system generally had two possible approaches to consider. The first was a "do-it-yourself" approach, generally utilizing local personnel and equipment. The second was the purchase of a "turnkey" computer system developed by a commercial vendor. More recently, microcomputers have also been used to solve specific data acquisition and reporting needs in the laboratory, although many are not suitable for a total laboratory information system. No one approach is ideal for all laboratories. The laboratory director considering computerization of the clinical laboratory should examine all approaches and combinations of approaches. Special local needs and resources should be considered before making a decision.

IN-HOUSE DEVELOPMENT OF A LABORATORY INFORMATION SYSTEM

The development of a laboratory information system utilizing personnel and hardware of an existing hospital business computer system formerly was the first suggestion of the hospital administrator or member of the hospital board when approached about laboratory computerization. This is a result of a belief that a computer system which can serve the business needs of a bank, hospital, or industrial concern should be able to handle the data processing needs of a clinical laboratory. In addition, such an approach *seems* to be most cost effective, since it makes use of computer equipment, programs, and expertise already present in the hospital. Unfortunately, far more failures than successes have resulted to date from such an approach (Johnson, 1975). The failures can be attributed in part to the great difference in needs between the simultaneous on-line processing of multiple automated instruments and the production of various laboratory reports on demand versus the batch processing of payrolls and patient billing. Such an approach also overlooks the fact that software development now may account for up to 90 per cent of the costs of a computer system. A reason frequently cited for a laboratory undertaking to develop its own laboratory information system is that "its needs are unique and cannot be met by a more standard approach." Johnson (1975) has documented the failure of many of these unique in-house developments and answers this rationale for their development as follows:

> The laboratory with so called unique requirements—which, consequently *must* develop its own automated information system, is a laboratory with a director who is incapable of defining correct objectives and/or who is on an ego trip. "Unique requirements" and "maximum flexibility because the laboratory needs are changing" is the last refuge of the incompetent. Those unique requirements are the very tip of the iceberg. With regards to the changing needs of the laboratory which no one can anticipate, it is said in the *Rubaiyat,* "If you don't know where you're going, any road will take you there."

Successful examples of in-house developed systems do exist where the resources and talent were available to see the task to completion. In most cases, these have been stand-alone systems developed in the laboratory environment.

TURNKEY LABORATORY INFORMATION SYSTEMS

The most popular approach to computerization is to acquire a vendor-developed system LIS. Such systems have been called "turnkey systems," since in theory one can purchase the system and "turn the key" to make it operational. In practice, the laboratory director and staff must make substantial decisions about laboratory operations and the computer system before it can be installed. The installation period itself will also involve substantial work, since both the old system and the computerized system will be used in parallel until the testing of the new system is complete.

For most institutions, however, the advantages of this approach far outweigh its disadvantages, and generally there is a greater assurance of success and predictability of cost. The extremely high cost of system development can be distributed among several or many installations rather than borne by a single site. Furthermore, if the company remains in business and has a continuing commitment to the laboratory system, the user will have access to improved programs, usually at a fairly modest cost. A large users group may also contribute ideas for improvements and supply user-generated programs. The availability of convenient hardware and software support should be an important consideration in the selection of any computer system. Finally, inspection of the vendor-developed system at other sites can be made by the user for evaluation of suitability for his own site and proof that the vendor does have an operational system.

The disadvantages of a turnkey system must also be considered. One is the apparent inflexibility of some commercial systems. Early systems required reprogramming for even minor changes. Most modern systems have modular designs where common changes are made through tables. These table-driven systems allow the user to add, delete, and change features without vendor support or reprogramming. Some features, even in modular systems, will require additional programming. In most cases, commercial systems will satisfy only 80 to 90 per cent of the needs of any given institution. It is important that the laboratory decide on the importance of those missing features and whether the vendor should be asked to customize the system to support these needs.

A laboratory computer system should be expected to last about five years before needing replacement or a major upgrade. If the laboratory intends to use the vendor for support and ongoing development, the prospective purchaser should investigate the ability of the company to survive in a competitive marketplace as well as its attitude toward user support. Such an evaluation will be, at best, quite subjective, since much information is usually hidden or unavailable. In cases in which the company supplying the system does not manufacture the hardware, the support for the hardware and software may come from separate sources. In such cases, the user should investigate support by both vendors. The computer industry is highly volatile; thus, having a large company as a base is no assurance that a laboratory system will survive.

The acquisition of any computer usually involves the issue of a formal document, a request for proposal or *RFP*, soliciting proposals from vendors. Included in such a document should be a detailed description of the laboratory and institutional environment as well as the goals that the laboratory seeks for the computer system. Many institutions include detailed requirements for the hardware. Preferably RFPs should address the information processing and handling requirements of a laboratory, allowing the vendor to specify the hardware. In some cases, several RFPs may be issued as the user becomes more aware of his actual requirements (Shaffert, 1978). Additional information on the acquisition of laboratory information system may be found in a brochure written by the American Society of Testing Materials in conjunction with the College of American Pathologists (ASTM, 1981).

Planning for a Laboratory Computer: Systems Analysis

One of the most common errors of laboratory directors in regard to data processing for their laboratories has been the assumption that the introduction of a computerized system to the laboratory will automatically solve all of their organizational, workload, and workflow problems. Experience has shown that the introduction of a computer system into a poorly organized and chaotic laboratory situation only increases chaos.

The technique of systems analysis can be utilized in order to avoid this problem (Grams, 1972). By this technique, a systematic study of the present system, a review of available methods to solve the laboratory's problems, and a proposal for a new system for the laboratory can be made. As part of this process, a manual back-up system for the proposed computer system can be designed and implemented prior to the actual implementation of the computerized system. In many instances, this process provides benefits to the laboratory's operations almost equal to those provided by the ultimate installation of the computer system.

The laboratory director may receive professional assistance from systems analysts, although analysis itself should be done by the laboratory staff with guidance from available materials. The steps to be undertaken can be briefly summarized as follows (Grams, 1972):

1. *Descriptive phase:* In the first step of this phase, the exact *definition of the problem* to be solved is stated in a single statement with qualifiers to define, in order of importance, the various components of the major problem statement. Problems must be concise. Frequently, statements are so global in nature that determining whether a solution has been reached is impossible. As pointed out by Grams, such a problem statement is a preliminary statement and should be re-evaluated and reconfirmed after each successive stage in the systems analysis.

A second and very important step in the descriptive phase of systems analysis is a *description of the operational system,* that is, a description of the current approach to the flow of specimens and data within the laboratory and institution. In this description, the use of charts will greatly facilitate the process. At the end of the operational systems description, the problem statement should be reconfirmed and modified as necessary.

2. *Investigative phase (research):* In this phase, the laboratory director and the project team research the current literature, consult vendors, make personal contacts, and make on-site visits to determine the *relevant existing systems* which might be available to solve the laboratory's problems. The material gathered in this phase will generally consist of a description of more than one system, but an attempt should be made to describe only those systems which have been successful or have great promise for success in the near future. The description should be limited to those systems which are readily available, which are not unique, and which may be able to be utilized in solving the current problem. At the end of this phase, the initial problem statement should again be reconfirmed and modified if necessary.

3. *Creative phase:* After study and documentation of the present system and of relevant existing systems elsewhere, the laboratory director and his team are now ready to describe the proposed system for the laboratory. The *proposed system description* is done in similar fashion to the description of the existing system and the relevant outside systems. In addition, one must list ways in which the proposed system can be evaluated after implementation and provide justifications for the proposed system.

4. *Implementation phase:* A description of the planned implementation schedule for the proposed system is developed (see below).

5. *Evaluation phase:* An evaluation of the proposed system is developed in order to determine if the system is meeting the desired goals.

Implementation and Evaluation

Although the most visible parts of the implementation of a computer system take only weeks to months, the steps involved in the planning leading to the implementation will often take months to years. The following are examples of multiple plans leading to the final implementation. These assume that necessary analyses have been performed and specific operation decisions have been completed. Some considerations for discussion include the following:

1. Remodeling, if necessary, of space for the computer with special consideration given to air conditioning (including humidity control), electrical requirements, fire suppression, etc.

2. Many laboratories have centralized the computer operations into a central receiving and dispatch center. With such a concept, a single physical location serves to support the computer and a central receiving area. Telephone calls may also be directed to this location with appropriate equipment.

3. The necessary personnel needed to support the computer operations should be funded, recruited, and trained.

4. Report forms should be designed and purchased. Computer supplies should be purchased which are sufficient for startup operations. Storage cabinets for tapes and disks should be available. Some laboratories have used this period as an opportunity to redesign requisition forms.

5. Computer systems have reached a high index of reliability, but they do fail. A manual back-up system should be designed which will allow for operations in event of machine failure.

6. A graduated program of in-service education should be started. Many commercial vendors provide substantial support for this training. This should initially involve laboratory personnel, followed by physicians and clerks, since they will usually be involved as users. The laboratory and hospital staff should be kept informed about progress of the system. Physicians should be consulted about report format options and be given the opportunity to assist in decisions in such areas.

7. Because of the wide availability of the information in a computerized database, thought must be given to ways to restrict access to patient information. In particular, extralaboratory access of information must be such that unauthorized personnel cannot readily access laboratory results. Regulations issued by the CAP and other regulatory agencies view the criteria used for maintaining medical chart security in nursing areas as insufficient when applied to computer systems. A terminal in a nursing station with no access restrictions is considered inappropriate. One of the most frequently overlooked security problems lies in the dial-in telephone port used by service and programming personnel. Such lines can easily be disconnected during periods of inactivity by a mechanical switch.

During the installation phase, the laboratory will go through a phase of parallel operations during which both the old and new systems are being used. This can be a difficult period, since personnel will be doing twice the work without any benefits from the computer. If this phase is handled well, however, the excitement of the new system will reduce the psychological impact of this additional work. This testing phase is critical in shaking out problems which may not have been obvious earlier.

Evaluation of the system must continue long after implementation. The ultimate goal of any computer operation must center on the continued refinement of the computer programs to match laboratory needs. Although implementation of a system has the highest visibility, the continued review and refinement ultimately have much greater impact on its success. A successful computer system which remains static during its lifetime is rare.

American Society for Testing Materials: Standard Guide for Computer Automation in the Clinical Laboratory, Designation E792–81, in Annual Book of ASTM Standards. Philadelphia, 1981.

Analytical Services: Evaluation of the Medical Information System at the NIH Clinical Center, Vol. I & II, 1982, sections 1.0 and 2.1 (NIH-79-302-1 through 6). National Technical Information Services PB82-190075.

Anthony, R., and Herzlinger, R.: Management Control in Nonprofit Organizations. Homewood, Ill., Irwin, 1980, pp. 2–3.

Branscomb, L. M.: Electronics and computers: An overview. Science, *215*:755, 1982.

Brooks, F.: The Mythical Man-Month. Essays on Software Engineering. Reading, Mass., Addison-Wesley, 1979.

Burns, E. L., Hanson, D. J., Schoen, I., Barnett, R. N., Minckler, T., and Winter, S.: Communication of laboratory data to the clinician. Am. J. Clin. Path., *61*:900, 1974.

College of American Pathologists: Standards for Laboratory Accreditation. Pathologist '82, *36*:641, 1982.

Computer Management Series. Reprints from Harvard Business Review, order number 21054, 1969.

Computers and electronics. Science, *215*:4534, 1982.

Drucker, P. F.: The Effective Executive. New York, Harper & Row, Publishers, 1967.

The electronics revolution. Science, *195*:4283, 1977.

Grams, R. R.: Problem Solving, Systems Analysis and Medicine. Springfield, Ill., Charles C Thomas, 1972.

Henricks, E. J., and Langhofer, L. A.: Community hospital laboratory information system. An eight-year longitudinal study of economic impact. Am. J. Clin. Path., *77*:297, 1982.

Henry, J. B., and Pruitt, C. T.: This report system reduces lab errors. Mod. Hosp., *104*:118, 1964.

JCAH Accreditation Manual for Hospitals. Chicago, 1982.

Johnson, J. L.: Achieving the Optimum Information System for the Laboratory. Northbrook, Ill., J. Lloyd Johnson Associates, 1975.

Krieg, A. F.: Laboratory Communication, Getting Your Message Through. Medical Economics Co., 1978.

Levey, S., and Loomba, N. P.: Health Information Systems in Health Care Administration: A Managerial Perspective. Philadelphia, J. B. Lippincott Co., 1973.

Lincoln, T., and Korpman, R. A.: Computers, health care, and medical information science. Science, *210*:257, 1980.

Management Information Series. Reprints from Harvard Business Review, order number 21114, 1976.

Shaffert, T. K. (ed.): Hospital information systems. *In* Topics in Health Care Financing. Germantown, Md., Aspen Systems Corporation, 1978.

Vacrous, A.: Microcomputers. Sci. Am., *232*:32, 1980.

White, R. M.: Disk storage technology. Sci. Am., *243*:138, 1980.

APPENDIX 1

PHYSIOLOGIC SOLUTIONS, BUFFERS, ACID-BASE INDICATORS, STANDARD REFERENCE MATERIALS, AND TEMPERATURE CONVERSIONS

PHYSIOLOGIC SOLUTIONS

A physiologic solution is one that contains various salts in concentrations that closely approximate the composition of fluids in the human body. The simplest of these is physiologic saline, which has the same osmotic pressure as the blood. There are more elaborate solutions, for example, to maintain tissues in a metabolically active state for longer periods of time. The table below gives formulas of solutions that are isotonic with respect to blood.

BUFFERS*

Buffers have the ability to resist changes in pH. Buffers usually consist of a weak acid and its salt or a weak base and its salt. The Henderson-Hasselbalch equation is useful in calculating the acid (or base) to salt ratio required to establish a desired pH from a buffer system. For example, if 1 L of 0.1 M acetic acid buffer (total molarity of acetate ion plus acetic acid) at pH 4.90 is desired, use the expression

$$(1)\ \text{pH} = \text{pK} + \log \frac{[\text{A}^-]}{[\text{HA}]}$$

(Henderson-Hasselbalch equation)

Substituting for pH = 4.90 and pK = 4.76 (for acetic acid),

$$(2)\ 4.90 = 4.76 + \log \frac{[\text{acetate}]}{[\text{acetic acid}]},$$

$$(3)\ \log \frac{[\text{acetate}]}{[\text{acetic acid}]} = 0.14,$$

$$(4)\ \frac{[\text{acetate}]}{[\text{acetic acid}]} = 1.38.$$

$$(5)\ [\text{acetate}] + [\text{acetic acid}] = 0.1\ \text{M}$$

$$(6)\ \text{and}\ \frac{[\text{acetate}]}{[\text{acetic acid}]} = 1.38$$

$$(7)\ \text{or}\ [\text{acetate}] = 1.38\ [\text{acetic acid}]$$

$$(8)\ 1.38\ [\text{acetic acid}] + [\text{acetic acid}] = 0.1\ \text{M}$$

*For a comprehensive discussion, including preparation of buffer solutions of a definite ionic strength, consult Bates, R. G.: Determination of pH—Theory and Practice. 2nd ed. New York, John Wiley & Sons, Inc., 1973.

PHYSIOLOGIC SOLUTIONS

	Saline	Locke's Solution	Ringer's* Solution	Tyrode's Solution
Sodium chloride	0.85 g	0.9 g	0.7 g	0.8 g
Calcium chloride		0.024 g	0.0026 g	0.02 g
Potassium chloride		0.042 g	0.035 g	0.02 g
Sodium bicarbonate		0.01–0.03 g		0.1 g
D-Glucose		0.1–0.25 g		0.1 g
Magnesium chloride				0.01 g
Monosodium phosphate				0.005 g
Distilled water	100 ml	100 ml	100 ml	100 ml

*Porter modification.

(9) [acetic acid] = 0.042 M = 2.52 g acetic acid/liter

(10) [acetate] = 0.058 M = 4.76 g sodium acetate/liter

Similarly, if 648 ml of 0.025 molar diethylbarbituric acid and 10 ml of 0.5 molar sodium diethylbarbiturate are mixed and diluted to 1 L, the approximate pH of the solution is calculated, knowing that the pK for diethylbarbituric acid = 7.98.

(1) Molar concentration $= \frac{\text{moles}}{\text{liter}}$

(2) liters $\left(\frac{\text{moles}}{\text{liter}}\right) = \text{moles}$

For diethylbarbituric acid

(3) (0.648)(0.025) = 0.0162 mole

(4) which diluted to 1 L = 0.0162 mole/liter

For sodium diethylbarbiturate

(5) (0.010)(0.5) = 0.005 mole

(6) which, diluted to 1 L = 0.005 mole/liter

(7) $\text{pH} = \text{pK} + \log \frac{[\text{salt}]}{[\text{acid}]} = \text{pK} - \log \frac{[\text{acid}]}{[\text{salt}]}$

(8) $= 7.98 - \log \frac{0.0162}{0.005}$

(9) $= 7.98 - \log 3.24$

(10) $= 7.98 - 0.51$

(11) $\therefore \text{pH} = 7.47$

The maximum buffering capacity is at the pK value of the weak acid or base. For instance, for acetic acid with a pH value of 4.76, more acid will be required to change the pH of an acetate buffer from 4.76 to 4.66 than from 4.20 to 4.10. Efficient buffering capacity covers a pH range of about 1 unit on either side of the pK value of the weak acid or base. For acetic acid, this would be from about pH 3.8 to 5.8.

Sorensen's Phosphate Buffers

These buffer solutions are generally useful, since the range of the mixtures is from pH 5 to 8.

Fifteenth Molar Monobasic Potassium Phosphate Solution (KH_2PO_4). Weight 9.0727 g of monobasic potassium phosphate. Dissolve it in distilled water and dilute to exactly 1 L with distilled water. The solution must be absolutely clear and should yield no test for chloride or sulfates. Phosphate salt solutions should be kept in the refrigerator.

Fifteenth Molar Dibasic Sodium Phosphate Solution (Na_2HPO_4). Expose dibasic sodium phosphate containing 12 moles of water of crystallization to ordinary atmosphere for two weeks. It should then contain 2 moles of water of crystallization. Dissolve 11.867 g of disodium phosphate duohydrate in distilled water and dilute to exactly 1 L with distilled water. The solution must be absolutely clear and should yield no test for chloride or sulfates.

SORENSEN'S TABLE OF BUFFER MIXTURES

Na_2HPO_4 Solution (ml)	KH_2PO_4 Solution (ml)	pH
0.25	9.75	5.288
0.5	9.5	5.589
1.0	9.0	5.906
2.0	8.0	6.239
3.0	7.0	6.468
4.0	6.0	6.643
5.0	5.0	6.813
6.0	4.0	6.979
7.0	3.0	7.168
8.0	2.0	7.381
9.0	1.0	7.731
9.5	0.5	8.043

*Tris(Hydroxymethyl)Aminomethane Buffer**

Tris(hydroxymethyl)aminomethane buffer can be used for a pH range between 7.0 and 9.0, but its best buffer capacity is between 7.5 and 8.5. It is practically ineffective below pH 7.0 and above pH 9.0. One advantage of the buffer is its excellent stability. The buffer can be prepared by weighing the desired amount of tris(hydroxymethyl)aminomethane, dissolving it in water and adjusting the pH to the desired value with HCl. For example, if 100 ml of 0.05 M buffer is desired, place 0.6057 g of tris(hydroxymethyl)aminomethane into a 100 ml volumetric flask. This is dissolved in approximately 50 ml of distilled water. Add 0.1 N HCl, as indicated in the table at the top of p. 1419, and fill up to the mark with distilled water. The table shows the pH values obtained when 0.6057 g of tris(hydroxymethyl)aminomethane dissolved in water is mixed with the indicated amounts of 0.1 N HCl and diluted to 100 ml.

ACID-BASE INDICATORS†

An acid-base indicator is a weak acid or a weak base, the undissociated form of which has a color and constitution other than the iogenic form. Color change takes place over a certain narrow range of hydrogen ion concentrations. This range is called the color change interval and is expressed in terms of pH (the negative logarithm of the hydrogen ion concentration). A great number of substances show indicator properties, although relatively few of them are practically applied for neutralization reactions and pH determinations. In general, weak acids should be titrated in the presence of indicators that change in slightly

*If buffers of a higher molarity are desired, the 0.1 N HCl may have to be replaced by a 1.0 N HCl.

†Based on Lange, N. A.: Handbook of Chemistry. Revised 11th ed. New York, McGraw-Hill Book Company, Inc., 1973.

ml 0.1 N HCl Added	Resulting pH at 23°C.	Resulting pH at 37°C.
5.0	9.10	8.95
7.5	8.92	8.78
10.0	8.74	8.60
12.5	8.62	8.48
15.0	8.50	8.37
17.5	8.40	8.27
20.0	8.32	8.18
22.5	8.23	8.10
25.0	8.14	8.00
27.5	8.05	7.90
30.0	7.96	7.82
32.5	7.87	7.73
35.0	7.77	7.63
37.5	7.66	7.52
40.0	7.54	7.40
42.5	7.36	7.22
45.0	7.20	7.05

ACID-BASE INDICATORS

Indicator	pH Range	Quantity of Indicator per 10 ml	Color	
			Acid	*Alkaline*
Thymol blue (A)*†	1.2–2.8	1–2 drops 0.1% soln. in aq.	Red	Yellow
Methyl orange (B)	3.1–4.4	1 drop 0.1% soln. in aq.	Red	Orange
Bromphenol blue (A)†	3.0–4.6	1 drop 0.1% soln. in aq.	Yellow	Blue-violet
Bromcresol green (A)†	4.0–5.6	1 drop 0.1% soln. in aq.	Yellow	Blue
Methyl red (A)†	4.4–6.2	1 drop 0.1% soln. in aq.	Red	Yellow
Bromcresol purple (A)†	5.2–6.8	1 drop 0.1% soln. in aq.	Yellow	Purple
Bromthymol blue (A)†	6.2–7.6	1 drop 0.1% soln. in aq.	Yellow	Blue
Phenol red (A)†	6.4–8.0	1 drop 0.1% soln. in aq.	Yellow	Red
Neutral red (B)	6.8–8.0	1 drop 0.1% soln. in 70% alc.	Red	Yellow
Thymol blue (A)†‡	8.0–9.6	1–5 drops 0.1% soln. in aq.	Yellow	Blue
Phenolphthalein (A)	8.0–10.0	1–5 drops 0.1% soln. in 70% alc.	Colorless	Red
Thymolphthalein (A)	9.4–10.6	1 drop 0.1% soln. in 90% alc.	Colorless	Blue

The letters A or B following the name of the indicator signify, respectively, that the compound is an indicator *acid* or *base*.

*For the acid range.

†Sodium salt.

‡For the alkaline range.

COMMONLY USED ACIDS AND ALKALIES*

Solution	Mol. Weight	Spec. Gravity†	gm. per Liter†	Molarity†	Normality†	Approx. Number of ml Required to Make 1000 ml of 1 N Solution
Conc. HCl	36.46	1.19	440	12	12	83
Conc. H_2SO_4	98.08	1.84	1730	18	36	28
Conc. HNO_3	63.02	1.42	990	16	16	64
Conc. lactic acid	90.08	1.21	1030	11	11	87
Glacial acetic acid	60.08	1.06	1060	17.5	17.5	57
Conc. NH_4OH	35.05	0.90	250	15	15	67

*Commercially available.
†Figures may vary slightly according to the lot or manufacturer.

STANDARD REFERENCE MATERIALS FOR CLINICAL MEASUREMENTS*†

SRM No.	Name	Purity (%)	Property Certified	Amount (g)	Date Issued
40h	Sodium oxalate	99.95	Reductometric standard	60	April 24, 1969
83c	Arsenic trioxide	99.99	Reductometric standard	75	April 16, 1970
84h	Acid potassium phthalate	99.993	Acidimetric standard	60	July 9, 1969
136c	Potassium dichromate	99.98	Oxidation standard	60	March 24, 1970
186Ic	Potassium dihydrogen phosphate	99.9	pH	30	Sept. 1, 1970
186IIc	Disodium hydrogen phosphate	99.9	pH	30	Sept. 1, 1970
350	Benzoic acid	99.98	Acidimetric standard	30	April 15, 1958
911a	Cholesterol	99.4	Identity and purity	2.0	June 6, 1974
912	Urea	99.7	Identity and purity	25	Sept. 24, 1968
913	Uric acid	99.7	Identity and purity	10	Sept. 24, 1968
914	Creatinine	99.8	Identity and purity	10	Sept. 24, 1968
915	Calcium carbonate	99.9	Identity and purity	20	March 4, 1969
916	Bilirubin	99	Identity and purity	0.1	March 10, 1971
917	D-Glucose	99.9	Identity and purity	25	Nov. 18, 1970
918	Potassium chloride	99.9	Identity and purity	20	Jan. 22, 1971
922	tris(Hydroxymethyl)amino-methane	99.9	pH	25	Dec. 13, 1973
923	tris(Hydroxymethyl)amino-methane hydrochloride	99.7	pH	35	Dec. 13, 1973
930b	Glass filters for spectrophotometry		Absorbance	3 filters	Feb. 24, 1975
933	Clinical laboratory thermometers		Temperature	Set of 3	August 23, 1974
937	Iron metal	99.9		50	Summer, 1978
1571	Orchard leaves		Major and trace constituents	75	Oct. 1, 1971
2201	NaCl	99.9	pNa pCl	120	Feb. 22, 1971
2202	KCl	99.9	pK pCl	160	Feb. 22, 1971

*Orders and requests for information about these SRM's should be directed to the Office of Standard Reference Materials, Institute for Materials Research, National Bureau of Standards, Washington, D.C. 20234.
†NBS Spec. Publ. 260, Catalog of NBS Standard Reference Materials, 1975–1976 edition.

TEMPERATURE CONVERSIONS

Centigrade	Fahrenheit	Centigrade	Fahrenheit
110°	230°	38	100.4°
100	212	37.5	99.5
95	203	37	98.6
90	194	36.5	97.7
85	185	36	96.8
80	176	35.5	95.9
75	167	35	95
70	158	34	93.2
65	149	33	91.4
60	140	32	89.6
55	131	31	87.8
50	122	30	86
45	113	25	77
44	111.2	20	68
43	109.4	15	59
42	107.6	10	50
41	105.8	+5	41
40.5	104.9	0	32
40	104	−5	23
39.5	103.1	−10	14
39	102.2	−15	+5
38.5	101.3	−20	−4

0.54°C = 1°F
1°C = 1.8°F

To convert Fahrenheit into centigrade, subtract 32 and multiply by 0.555.
To convert centigrade into Fahrenheit, multiply by 1.8 and add 32.

alkaline solutions. Weak bases should be titrated in the presence of indicators that change in slightly acid solutions.

The availability of precision pH meters allows titration to a selected endpoint (pH) and may replace use of indicators for several applications.

Lange, N. A., and Dean, I. A. (eds.): Handbook of Chemistry. 11th ed. New York, McGraw-Hill Book Company, 1973.
Long, C. (ed.): Biochemists' Handbook. Princeton, N.J., D. Van Nostrand Co., Inc., 1961.
Meinke, W. W.: Standard Reference Materials for Clinical Measurements. Anal. Chem., *43*:31A, 1971.
The Merck Index; an Encyclopedia of Chemicals and Drugs. 10th ed. Rahway, N.J., Merck & Co., Inc., 1983.

APPENDIX 2

DESIRABLE WEIGHTS AND BODY SURFACE AREA

1983 METROPOLITAN HEIGHT AND WEIGHT TABLES*

Height	Small Frame	Medium Frame	Large Frame
		MEN	
Height	**Small Frame**	**Medium Frame**	**Large Frame**
5′2″	128–134	131–141	138–150
5′3″	130–136	133–143	140–153
5′4″	132–138	135–145	142–156
5′5″	134–140	137–148	144–160
5′6″	136–142	139–151	146–164
5′7″	138–145	142–154	149–168
5′8″	140–148	145–157	152–172
5′9″	142–151	148–160	155–176
5′10″	144–154	151–163	158–180
5′11″	146–157	154–166	161–184
6′0″	149–160	157–170	164–188
6′1″	152–164	160–174	168–192
6′2″	155–168	164–178	172–197
6′3″	158–172	167–182	176–202
6′4″	162–176	171–187	181–207
		WOMEN	
Height	**Small Frame**	**Medium Frame**	**Large Frame**
4′10″	102–111	109–121	118–131
4′11″	103–113	111–123	120–134
5′0″	104–115	113–126	122–137
5′1″	106–118	115–129	125–140
5′2″	108–121	118–132	128–143
5′3″	111–124	121–135	131–147
5′4″	114–127	124–138	134–151
5′5″	117–130	127–141	137–155
5′6″	120–133	130–144	140–159
5′7″	123–136	133–147	143–163
5′8″	126–139	136–150	146–167
5′9″	129–142	139–153	149–170
5′10″	132–145	142–156	152–173
5′11″	135–148	145–159	155–176
6′0″	138–151	148–162	158–179

*Weight in pounds at ages 29–59 years according to build. In shoes and 3 pounds of indoor clothing for women and 5 pounds for men. (Sources: Society of Actuaries, Build Study, 1979, Society of Actuaries and Association of Life Insurance Medical Directors of America, Chicago, 1980, p. 127. Metropolitan Life Insurance Company, New York, 1983.)

OPTIMAL WEIGHTS FOR MEN AND WOMEN*

Height	Fogerty Center Acceptable Weight† in Pounds		Range of Acceptable Weights‡ in Pounds	
			25% Under- to 5% Overweight	*15% Under- to 5% Overweight*
	Men	***Women***	***Men***	***Women***
5 ft 0 in	—	95–125	—	106–131
5 2	—	102–131	—	111–138
5 4	120–149	108–137	112–156	118–145
5 6	126–157	114–145	119–166	122–152
5 8	133–166	121–153	125–175	129–160
5 10	141–175	129–161	132–185	135–167
6 0	149–184	137–171	140–195	142–175
6 2	157–194	—	148–207	—
6 4	165–204	—	156–218	—

*Height and weight in street clothing.

†Recommended by the Fogerty International Center Conference on Obesity, Washington, D.C., October 1973; adapted from the Metropolitan Life Insurance desirable weight tables, adjusted for height and weight to street clothing. (Sims, E. A. H.: *In* Bray, G. A. [ed.]: Obesity in America. U.S. Dept. Health, Education, and Welfare, NIH Publication No. 79–359. Washington, D.C., 1979, p. 7.)

‡From tables of the Build Study, 1979. Mortality rates equal to or less than the average, adjusted for age, were obtained in the range of 25% underweight to 5% overweight for men and 15% underweight to 5% overweight for women. (Build Study, 1979. Chicago, Society of Actuaries and Association of Life Insurance Medical Directors of America, 1980, p. 127.)

NOMOGRAM FOR THE DETERMINATION OF BODY SURFACE AREA OF CHILDREN AND ADULTS*

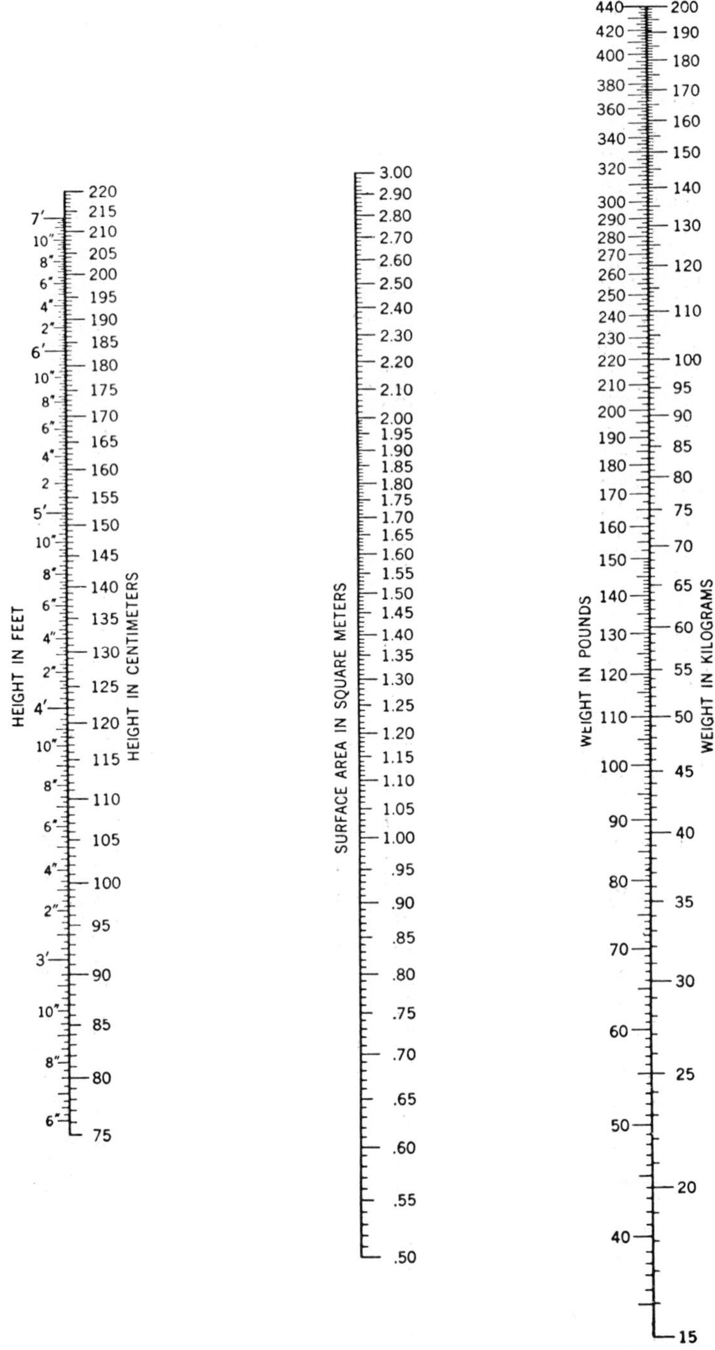

*From Boothby, W. M., and Sandiford, R. B.: Boston Med. Surg. J., *185*:337, 1921.

NOMOGRAM FOR THE DETERMINATION OF BODY SURFACE AREA OF CHILDREN*

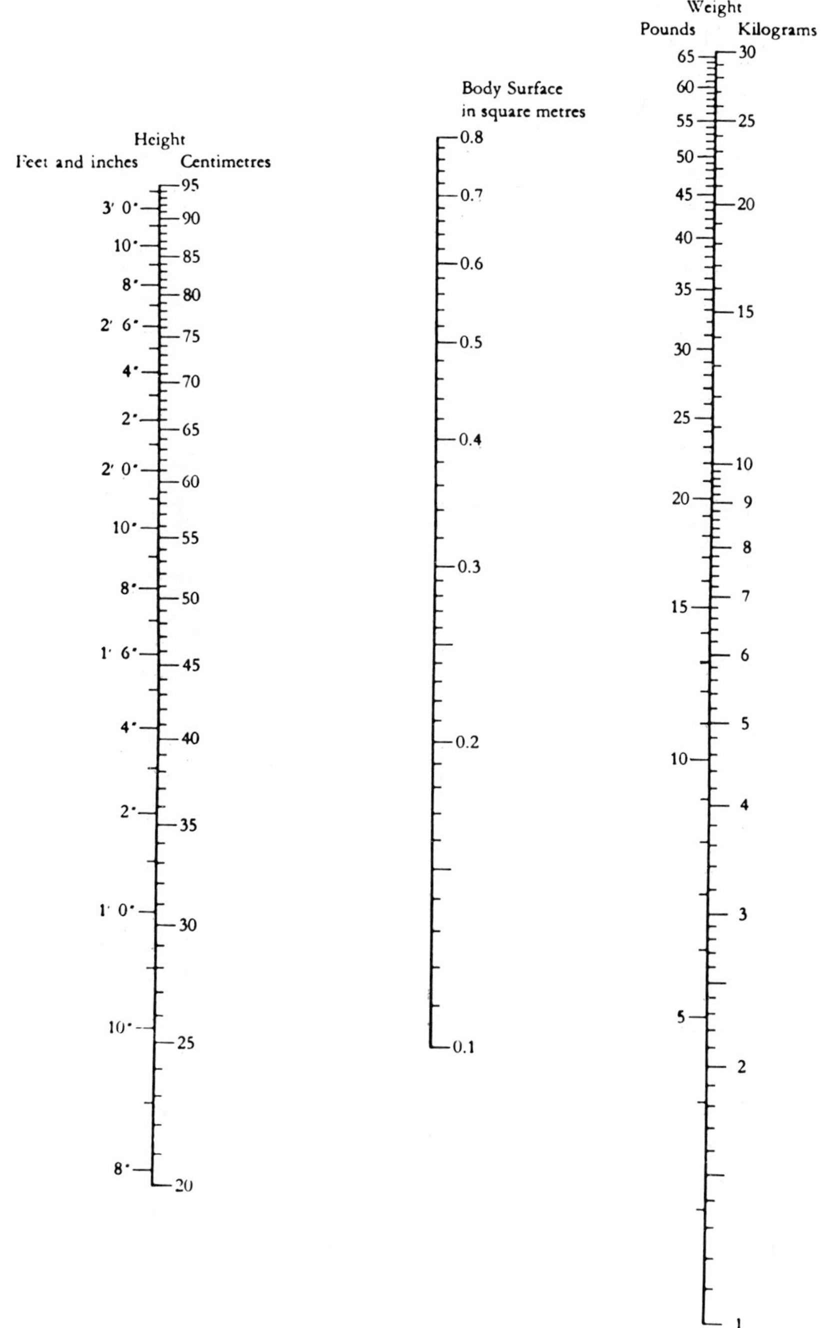

*From DuBois, E. F.: Basal Metabolism in Health and Disease. Philadelphia, Lea & Febiger, 1936.

APPENDIX 3

PERIODIC CHART OF THE ELEMENTS*

*From The Merck Index, An Encyclopedia of Chemicals, Drugs, and Biologicals. 10th ed. Rahway, N.J., Merck & Co., Inc. , 1983.

PERIODIC CHART OF THE ELEMENTS

KEY

Oxidation States →	+1 +3	**79**	← Atomic Number
	Au		← Atomic Symbol
Atomic Weight →	196.9665		
Electron Configuration →	-32-18-1		

Orbital	IA	IIA	IIIB	IVB	VB	VIB	VIIB	VIIIB			IB	IIB	IIIA	IVA	VA	VIA	VIIA	VIIIA
	±1 **1** **H** 1.0079 1																	0 **2** **He** 4.00260 2
	+1 **3** **Li** 6.941 2-1	+2 **4** **Be** 9.01218 2-2											+3 **5** **B** 10.81 2-3	+2 ±4 **6** **C** 12.011 2-4	±1 ±2 ±3 +4 +5 **7** **N** 14.0067 2-5	-2 **8** **O** 15.9994 2-6	-1 **9** **F** 18.998403 2-7	0 **10** **Ne** 20.179 2-8
	+1 **11** **Na** 22.98977 2-8-1	+2 **12** **Mg** 24.305 2-8-2											+3 **13** **Al** 26.98154 2-8-3	+2 ±4 **14** **Si** 28.0855 2-8-4	±3 +5 **15** **P** 30.97376 2-8-5	+4 +6 -2 **16** **S** 32.06 2-8-6	±1 +5 +7 **17** **Cl** 35.453 2-8-7	0 **18** **Ar** 39.948 2-8-8
2	+1 **19** **K** 39.0983 -8-8-1	+2 **20** **Ca** 40.08 -8-8-2	+3 **21** **Sc** 44.9559 -8-9-2	+2 +3 +4 **22** **Ti** 47.88 -8-10-2	+2 +3 +4 +5 **23** **V** 50.9415 -8-11-2	+2 +3 +6 **24** **Cr** 51.996 -8-13-1	+2 +3 +4 +7 **25** **Mn** 54.9380 -8-13-2	+2 +3 **26** **Fe** 55.847 -8-14-2	+2 +3 **27** **Co** 58.9332 -8-15-2	+2 +3 **28** **Ni** 58.69 -8-16-2	+1 +2 **29** **Cu** 63.546 -8-18-1	+2 **30** **Zn** 65.38 -8-18-2	+3 **31** **Ga** 69.72 -8-18-3	+2 +4 **32** **Ge** 72.59 -8-18-4	±3 +5 **33** **As** 74.9216 -8-18-5	+4 +6 -2 **34** **Se** 78.96 -8-18-6	±1 +5 **35** **Br** 79.904 -8-18-7	0 **36** **Kr** 83.80 -8-18-8
2-8	+1 **37** **Rb** 85.4678 -18-8-1	+2 **38** **Sr** 87.62 -18-8-2	+3 **39** **Y** 88.9059 -18-9-2	+4 **40** **Zr** 91.22 -18-10-2	+3 +5 **41** **Nb** 92.9064 -18-12-1	+6 **42** **Mo** 95.94 -18-13-1	+4 +6 +7 **43** **Tc** (98) -18-13-2	+3 **44** **Ru** 101.07 -18-15-1	+3 **45** **Rh** 102.9055 -18-16-1	+2 +4 **46** **Pd** 106.42 -18-18-0	+1 **47** **Ag** 107.868 -18-18-1	+2 **48** **Cd** 112.41 -18-18-2	+3 **49** **In** 114.82 -18-18-3	+2 +4 **50** **Sn** 118.69 -18-18-4	±3 +5 **51** **Sb** 121.75 -18-18-5	+4 +6 -2 **52** **Te** 127.60 -18-18-6	±1 +5 +7 **53** **I** 126.9045 -18-18-7	0 **54** **Xe** 131.29 -18-18-8
2-8-18	+1 **55** **Cs** 132.9054 -18-8-1	+2 **56** **Ba** 137.33 -18-8-2	**57-71** See Lantha-nides	+4 **72** **Hf** 178.49 -32-10-2	+5 **73** **Ta** 180.9479 -32-11-2	+6 **74** **W** 183.85 -32-12-2	+4 +6 +7 **75** **Re** 186.207 -32-13-2	+3 +4 **76** **Os** 190.2 -32-14-2	+3 +4 **77** **Ir** 192.22 -32-15-2	+2 +4 **78** **Pt** 195.08 -32-16-2	+1 +3 **79** **Au** 196.9665 -32-18-1	+1 +2 **80** **Hg** 200.59 -32-18-2	+1 +3 **81** **Tl** 204.383 -32-18-3	+2 +4 **82** **Pb** 207.2 -32-18-4	+3 +5 **83** **Bi** 208.9804 -32-18-5	+2 +4 **84** **Po** (209) -32-18-6	±1 +5 +7 **85** **At** (210) -32-18-7	0 **86** **Rn** (222) -32-18-8
2-8-18-32	+1 **87** **Fr** (223) -18-8-1	+2 **88** **Ra** 226.0254 -18-8-2	**89-103** See Acti-nides	+4 **104** (261) -32-10-2	**105** (262) -32-11-2	**106** (263) -32-12-2												

Transition Elements (groups IIIB–IIB)

Noble Gases (group VIIIA)

Lanthanides	+3 **57** **La** 138.9055 -18-9-2	+3 +4 **58** **Ce** 140.12 -20-8-2	+3 **59** **Pr** 140.9077 -21-8-2	+3 **60** **Nd** 144.24 -22-8-2	+3 **61** **Pm** (145) -23-8-2	+2 +3 **62** **Sm** 150.36 -24-8-2	+2 +3 **63** **Eu** 151.96 -25-8-2	+3 **64** **Gd** 157.25 -25-9-2	+3 **65** **Tb** 158.9254 -27-8-2	+3 **66** **Dy** 162.50 -28-8-2	+3 **67** **Ho** 164.9304 -29-8-2	+3 **68** **Er** 167.26 -30-8-2	+3 **69** **Tm** 168.9342 -31-8-2	+2 +3 **70** **Yb** 173.04 -32-8-2	+3 **71** **Lu** 174.967 -32-9-2
Actinides	+3 **89** **Ac** 227.0278 -18-9-2	+4 **90** **Th** 232.0381 -18-10-2	+4 +5 **91** **Pa** 231.0359 -20-9-2	+3 +4 +5 +6 **92** **U** 238.0289 -21-9-2	+3 +4 +5 +6 **93** **Np** 237.0482 -22-9-2	+3 +4 +5 +6 **94** **Pu** (244) -24-8-2	+3 +4 +5 +6 **95** **Am** (243) -25-8-2	+3 **96** **Cm** (247) -25-9-2	+3 +4 **97** **Bk** (247) -27-8-2	+3 **98** **Cf** (251) -28-8-2	+3 **99** **Es** (252) -29-8-2	+3 **100** **Fm** (257) -30-8-2	+2 +3 **101** **Md** (258) -31-8-2	+2 +3 **102** **No** (259) -32-8-2	+3 **103** **Lr** (260) -32-9-2

Note: Atomic weights are those of the most commonly available long-lived isotopes based on the 1979 IUPAC Atomic Weights of the Elements. A value given in parentheses denotes the mass number of the longest-lived isotope.

APPENDIX 4

SI UNITS

H. PETER LEHMANN, PH.D. AND JOHN BERNARD HENRY, M.D.

Recommendations for the standardized presentation of clinical laboratory data based on the International System of Units (SI Units) were first proposed in 1967 by the Commission on Clinical Chemistry of the International Union of Pure and Applied Chemistry (IUPAC) and Expert Panel on Quantities and Units of the International Federation of Clinical Chemistry (IFCC) (Dybkaer, 1967). Revisions of the original recommendations were published in 1974 as provisional proposals (Recommendation 1973, IUPAC/IFCC, 1974) and as final recommendations in 1979 (Recommendation 1978, IUPAC/IFCC, 1979). Support for these proposals came from the International Committee for Standardization in Hematology and the World Association of (Anatomic and Clinical) Pathology Societies, who, along with the International Federation of Clinical Chemistry, agreed to recommend to all concerned with health services throughout the world that, with regard to units of measurements for medical laboratory results, the International System of Units be accepted in its broad application (International Committee for Standardization in Hematology et al., 1973). The World Health Organization, at the 30th World Health Assembly in 1977, recommended the adoption of the SI by the entire scientific community, and particularly the medical community, throughout the world (World Health Organization, 1977a). Thus, the recommendations for the use of SI units in medicine has resulted in adoption and use of the suggested units by the medical community in a number of countries (often prompted by national legislation in this regard), and the expectation is that the system will be adopted worldwide over the next few years for reporting clinical laboratory data. The feasibility of rigid adoption of the SI to all clinical laboratory measurements has been discussed in a number of editorials and articles in the medical literature, that have been reviewed and summarized (Lehmann, 1979).

The SI consists of seven dimensionally independent base units that are listed in Table 1, along with the symbols to be used to denote these units. Table 2 lists a number of derived units of the SI that are used in the clinical laboratory. There are two kinds of derived units: coherent units, which are derived directly from the base units without the use of conversion factors, and non-coherent units, which are constructed from the base units and contain a numerical factor in order to make the numbers more convenient to use. The approved prefixes to denote fractions or multiples of base and derived SI units are given in Table 3. A complete description of the SI and its application in medicine may be found in the World Health Organization publication, The SI for the Health Professions (World Health Organization, 1977b).

Table 1. SI BASE UNITS

Quantity	Name	Symbol
Length	meter	m
Mass	kilogram	kg
Time	second	s
Electric current	ampere	A
Thermodynamic temperature	kelvin	K
Luminous intensity	candela	cd
Amount of substance	mole	mol

In making the conversion to recommended SI units (Tables 4 to 12), the following guidelines were followed:

1. All reference intervals have been converted to SI units except in cases where the measurements are not quantitative.
2. Chemical names have not been changed; e.g., urea is retained instead of changing to carbamide.
3. Factors were calculated on the basis of relative masses for atoms corrected to conform to the 1967 (amended 1973) values of the Commission on Atomic Weights of the International Union of Pure and Applied Chemistry.
4. Factors were calculated to the base unit for volume of one liter in accordance with Recommendation 1978.
5. The order of magnitude of the factors were calculated to make the values in SI units convenient numbers, i.e., with prefixes, a number not greater than 1000 or smaller than 0.001.
6. The number in "Recommended SI Units" is equal to the number in "Conventional Units" times the "Factor."
7. For compounds where relative molecular masses are not definitely known, e.g., proteins, reference intervals are converted to mass amounts per liter.
8. For mixtures of indeterminate composition, e.g., 17-ketosteroids, reference intervals are converted to mass amounts per liter.
9. Quantities of a relative nature which are usually expressed as percentages, e.g., fractions of LDH isoenzymes, are given as fractions.
10. Enzyme units are given as the International Unit per liter (U/L). Although the coherent SI unit for catalytic activity (including enzymes), the katal,

Table 2. SI DERIVED UNITS

Quantity	Unit Name	Unit Symbol
Area	square meter*	m^2
Volume	cubic meter*	m^3
	liter†	L = dm^3‡
Concentration		
Mass	kilogram/liter†	kg/L
Substance	mole/liter†	mol/L
Molality	mole/kilogram	mol/kg
Density	kilogram/liter†	kg/L
Mass fraction	kilogram/kilogram	kg/kg
Mole fraction	mole/mole	mol/mol
Number concentration	number/liter	L^{-1}
Temperature	degree Celsius*	°C = °K-273.15
Pressure	Pascal*	Pa = kg/m s^2
Frequency	Hertz*	Hz = 1 cycle/s
Clearance	liter/second†	L/s
Electrical potential	volt*	V = kg m^2/s^3A
Energy	Joule*	J = kg m^2/s^2

*Derived coherent unit.
†Derived non-coherent unit.
‡"L" has been accepted by IUPAC and the General Conference on Weights and Measures as the symbol for the liter, and may be used instead of the traditional and recommended symbol "l."

has been defined as the number of moles of substrate converted per second under defined conditions, its adoption is limited.

11. The pH scale is retained for measurement of hydrogen ion concentrations.

Table 3. PREFIXES

Prefix	Prefix Symbol	Factor
exa	E	10^{18}
peta	P	10^{15}
tera	T	10^{12}
giga	G	10^{9}
mega	M	10^{6}
kilo	k	10^{3}
hecto	h	10^{2}
deca	da	10^{1}
deci	d	10^{-1}
centi	c	10^{-2}
milli	m	10^{-3}
micro	μ	10^{-6}
nano	n	10^{-9}
pico	p	10^{-12}
femto	f	10^{-15}
atto	a	10^{-18}

Dybkaer, R., and Jørgensen, K.: Quantities and Units in Clinical Chemistry, Including Recommendation 1966 of the Commission on Clinical Chemistry of the International Union of Pure and Applied Chemistry and of the International Federation of Clinical Chemistry. Copenhagen, Munksgaard, 1967.

International Committee for Standardization in Hematology, International Federation of Clinical Chemistry, and World Association of (Anatomic and Clinical) Pathology Societies: Recommendations for use of SI units in clinical laboratory measurements. Br. J. Haematol., *23*:787, 1972; Clin. Chem., *19*:135, 1973.

International Union of Pure and Applied Chemistry and International Federation of Clinical Chemistry: Recommendation 1973. Quantities and units in clinical chemistry. Pure Appl. Chem., *37*:519, 1974. List of quantities in clinical chemistry. Pure Appl. Chem., *37*:549, 1974.

International Union of Pure and Applied Chemistry and International Federation of Clinical Chemistry: Approved Recommendation (1978). Quantities and units in clinical chemistry. Clin. Chim. Acta, *96*:157F, 1979. List of quantities in clinical chemistry. Clin. Chim. Acta, *96*:185F, 1979.

Lehmann, H. P.: SI units. CRC Rev. Clin. Lab. Sci., *10*:147, 1979.

Tietz, N. W. (ed.): Clinical Guide to Laboratory Tests. Philadelphia, W. B. Saunders Company, 1983.

Triplett, D. A., and Harms, C. S.: Procedures for the Coagulation Laboratory. Chicago, American Society of Clinical Pathologists, 1981.

World Health Organization: Use of SI units in medicine. WHO Official Records No. 240, p. 21, 1977a.

World Health Organization: The SI for the Health Professions. Geneva, WHO, 1977b.

NOTES TO TABLES 4 THROUGH 12

a. It is recommended (World Health Organization, 1977) that the units mm Hg be retained for pressures (P_{CO_2}, P_{O_2}) at the present time.

b. Percentages are expressed as fractions in the SI, where a fraction is a dimensionless quantity given by: the number of defined particles constituting a specified component divided by the total number of defined particles in the system.

c. Unit base on hydrogen ion concentration.

d. One (1) International Unit of insulin corresponds to 0.04167 mg of the 4th International Standard (a mixture of 52% beef insulin and 48% pig insulin).

e. Factor based on relative molecular mass of triolein (885.4).

f. One (1) International Unit of luteinizing hormone corresponds to 0.2296 mg of 2nd reference preparation (1964).

g. One (1) is equivalent to the turbidity of a solution containing 0.65 mmol/L of $BaSO_4$.

h. Factor based on the relative molecular mass of cysteine, 121.16.

Table 4. WHOLE BLOOD, SERUM, AND PLASMA CHEMISTRY

Component	System	Typical Reference Intervals: *Conventional Units*	*Factor**	*Recommended SI Units*†
Acetoacetic acid:				
qualitative	Serum	Negative	—	Negative
quantitative	Serum	0.2–1.0 mg/dl	98	19.6–98.0 μmol/L
Acetone:				
qualitative	Serum	Negative	—	Negative
quantitative	Serum	0.3–2.0 mg/dl	172	51.6–344.0 μmol/L
Albumin:				
quantitative	Serum	3.2–4.5 g/dl (salt fractionation)	10	32–45 g/L
		3.2–5.6 g/dl (electrophoresis)		32–56 g/L
		3.8–5.0 g/dl (dye binding)		38–50 g/L
Alcohol, ethyl	Serum or whole blood	Negative—but presented as mg/dl	0.22	Negative—but presented as mmol/L
Aldolase	Serum:			
	adults	3–8 Sibley-Lehninger U/dl at 37°C.	7.4	22–59 mU/L at 37°C.
	children	Approximately 2 times adult levels		Approximately 2 times adult levels
	newborn	Approximately 4 times adult levels		Approximately 4 times adult levels
Alpha-amino acid nitrogen	Serum	3.6–7.0 mg/dl	0.714	2.6–5.0 mmol/L
δ-Aminolevulinic acid	Serum	0.01–0.03 mg/dl	76.3	0.76–2.29 μmol/L
Ammonia	Plasma	20–120 μg/dl (diffusion)	0.554	11.1–67.0 μmol/L
		40–80 μg/dl (enzymatic method)		22.2–44.3 μmol/L
		12–48 μg/dl (resin method)		6.7–26.6 μmol/L
Amylase	Serum	60–160 Somogyi units/dl	1.85	111–296 U/L
Argininosuccinic lyase	Serum	0–4 U/dl	10	0–40 U/L
Arsenic‡	Whole blood	<7 μg/dl	0.13	<0.91 μmol/L
Ascorbic acid (vitamin C)	Plasma	0.6–1.6 mg/dl	56.8	34–91 μmol/L
	Whole blood	0.7–2.0 mg/dl		40–114 μmol/L
Barbiturates	Serum, plasma, or whole blood	Negative	—	Negative
Base excess	Whole blood:			
	male	−3.3 to +1.2 mEq/l	1	−3.3 to +1.2 mmol/L
	female	−2.4 to +2.3 mEq/l		−2.4 to +2.3 mmol/L
Base, total	Serum	145–160 mEq/l	1	145–160 mmol/L
Bicarbonate	Plasma	21–28 mM	1	21–28 mmol/L
Bile acids	Serum	0.3–3.0 mg/dl	10	3.0–30.0 mg/L
Bilirubin:	Serum			
direct (conjugated)		Up to 0.3 mg/dl	17.1	Up to 5.1 μmol/L
indirect (unconjugated)		0.1–1.0 mg/dl		1.7–17.1 μmol/L
total		0.1–1.2 mg/dl		1.7–20.5 μmol/L
newborns total		1–12 mg/dl		17.1–205.0 μmol/L

Blood gases: (Chapter 7)	Whole blood			
pH		7.38–7.44 (arterial)	1	7.38–7.44
		7.36–7.41 (venous)		7.36–7.41
P_{CO_2}	Whole blood	35–40 mm Hg (arterial)	0.133	4.66–5.32 kPa[a]
		40–45 mm Hg (venous)		5.32–5.99 kPa[a]
P_{O_2}	Whole blood	95–100 mm Hg (arterial)	0.133	12.64–13.30 kPa[a]
Bromide	Serum	0–5 mg/dl	0.125	0–0.63 mmol/L
BSP (Bromsulphalein) (5 mg/kg)	Serum	less than 6% retention 45 min. after injection	0.01[b]	fraction retention <0.06 at 45 min after dye injection
Calcium:				
ionized	Serum	4–4.8 mg/dl	0.25	1.0–1.2 mmol/L
		2.0–2.4 mEq/l	0.5	
		30–58% of total	0.01[b]	0.30–0.58 of total
total	Serum	9.2–11.0 mg/dl	0.25	2.3–2.8 mmol/L
		4.6–5.5 mEq/l	0.5	23–28 mmol/L
Carbon dioxide (CO_2 content)	Whole blood (arterial)	19–24 mM	1	19–24 mmol/L
	Plasma or serum (arterial)	21–28 mM		21–28 mmol/L
Carbon dioxide	Whole blood (venous)	22–26 mM	1	22–26 mmol/L
	Plasma or serum (venous)	24–30 mM		24–30 mmol/L
CO_2 combining power	Plasma or serum (venous)	24–30 mM	1	24–30 mmol/L
CO_2 partial pressure (P_{CO_2})	Whole blood (arterial)	35–40 mm Hg	0.133	4.66–5.32 kPa[a]
	Whole blood (venous)	40–45 mm Hg		5.32–5.99 kPa[a]
Carbonic acid (H_2CO_3)	Whole blood (arterial)	1.05–1.45 mM	1	1.05–1.45 mmol/L
	Whole blood (venous)	1.15–1.50 mM		1.15–1.50 mmol/L
	Plasma (venous)	1.02–1.38 mM		1.02–1.38 mmol/L
Carboxyhemoglobin (carbon monoxide hemoglobin)	Whole blood:			
	suburban nonsmokers	<1.5% saturation of hemoglobin	0.01[b]	fraction hemoglobin saturated: <0.015
	smokers	1.5–5.0% saturation		0.015–0.050
	heavy smokers	5.0–9.0% saturation		0.050–0.090
Carotene, beta	Serum	40–200 μg/dl	0.0186	0.74–3.72 μmol/L
Ceruloplasmin	Serum	23–50 mg/dl	10	230–500 mg/L
Chloride	Serum	95–103 mEq/l	1	95–103 mmol/L
Cholesterol				
total (Chapter 11)	Serum	150–250 mg/dl (varies with diet, sex, and age)	0.026	3.90–6.50 mmol/L
esters	Serum	65–75% of total cholesterol	0.01[b]	fraction of total cholesterol: 0.65–0.75
Cholinesterase (Pseudocholinesterase)	Erythrocytes	0.65–1.3 pH units	1	0.65–1.3 units[c]
	Plasma	0.5–1.3 pH units		0.5–1.3 units
		8–18 IU/l at 37°C.	1	8–18 U/L at 37°C.
Citrate	Serum or plasma	1.7–3.0 mg/dl	52	88–156 μmol/L
Copper	Serum, plasma:			
	male	70–140 μg/dl	0.157	11.0–22.0 μmol/L
	female	80–155 μg/dl		12.6–24.3 μmol/L

Table 4. WHOLE BLOOD, SERUM, AND PLASMA CHEMISTRY *(Continued)*

Component	System	Typical Reference Intervals		
		Conventional Units	***Factor****	***Recommended SI Units*†**
Cortisol	Plasma:			
	8 A.M.–10 A.M.	5–23 µg/dl	27.6	138–635 nmol/L
	4 P.M.–6 P.M.	3–13 µg/dl		83–359 nmol/L
Creatine as creatinine	Serum or plasma:			
	male	0.1–0.4 mg/dl	76.3	7.6–30.5 µmol/L
	female	0.2–0.7 mg/dl	76.3	15.3–53.4 µmol/L
Creatine kinase (CK)	Serum:			
	male	55–170 U/l at 37°C.	1	55–170 U/L at 37°C.
	female	30–135 U/l at 37°C.	1	30–135 U/L at 37°C.
Creatinine (Chapter 9)	Serum or plasma	0.6–1.2 mg/dl (adult)	88.4	53–106 µmol/L
		0.3–0.6 mg/dl (children <2 yr.)		27–54 µmol/L
Creatinine clearance (endogenous) (Chapter 8)	Serum or plasma and urine:			
	male	107–139 ml/min.	0.0167	1.78–2.32 ml/s
	female	87–107 ml/min.		1.45–1.79 ml/s
Cryoglobulins	Serum	Negative	—	Negative
Electrophoresis, protein (Chapter 12)	Serum	per cent:		
Albumin		52–65% of total protein	0.01[b]	fraction of total protein: 0.52–0.65
Alpha-1		2.5–5.0% of total protein	0.01	0.025–0.05
Alpha-2		7.0–13.0% of total protein	0.01	0.07–0.13
Beta		8.0–14.0% of total protein	0.01	0.08–0.14
Gamma		12.0–22.0% of total protein	0.01	0.12–0.22
	Serum	Concentration		
Albumin		3.2–5.6 gm/dl	10	32–56 g/L
Alpha-1		0.1–0.4 gm/dl		1–4 g/L
Alpha-2		0.4–1.2 gm/dl		4–12 g/L
Beta		0.5–1.1 gm/dl		5–11 g/L
Gamma		0.5–1.6 gm/dl		5–16 g/L
Fats, neutral (see Triglycerides)				
Fatty acids:				
total (free and esterified)	Serum	9–15 mM	1	9–15 mmol/L
free (non-esterified)	Plasma	300–480 µEq/l	1	300–480 µmol/L
Ferritin	Serum			
male		15–200 ng/ml		15–200 µg/L
female		12–150 ng/ml		15–150 µg/L
Fibrinogen	Plasma	200–400 mg/dl	0.01	2.00–4.00 g/L
Fluoride	Whole blood	<0.05 mg/dl	0.53	<0.027 mmol/L
Folate	Serum	5–25 ng/ml (bioassay)	2.27	11–56 nmol/L
		>2.3 ng/ml (radioassay)		>5.2 nmol/L
	Erythrocytes	166–640 ng/ml (bioassay)		376–1452 nmol/L
		>140 ng/ml (radioassay)		>318 nmol/L

Galactose	Whole blood:			
	adults	none	—	none
	children	<20 mg/dl	0.055	<1.1 mmol/L
Gamma globulin	Serum	0.5–1.6 gm/dl	10	5–16 g/L
Globulins, total	Serum	2.3–3.5 gm/dl	10	23–35 g/L
Glucose, fasting	Serum or plasma	70–110 mg/dl	0.055	3.85–6.05 mmol/L
	Whole blood	60–100 mg/dl		3.30–5.50 mmol/L
Glucose tolerance	Serum or plasma:			
oral	fasting	70–110 mg/dl	0.055	3.85–6.05 mmol/L
(See Table 10–5,	30 min.	30–60 mg/dl above fasting		1.65–3.30 mmol/L above fasting
p. 173, for	60 min.	20–50 mg/dl above fasting		1.10–2.75 mmol/L above fasting
criteria employed)	120 min.	5–15 mg/dl above fasting		0.28–0.83 mmol/L above fasting
	180 min.	Fasting level or below		Fasting level or below
	Serum or plasma:			
intravenous	fasting	70–110 mg/dl		3.85–6.05 mmol/L
	5 min.	Maximum of 250 mg/dl		Maximum of 13.75 mmol/L
	60 min.	Significant decrease		Significant decrease
	120 min.	Below 120 mg/dl		Below 6.60 mmol/L
	180 min.	Fasting level		Fasting level
Glucose 6-phosphate dehydrogenase (G6PD)	Erythrocytes	250–500 units/10^6 cells	1	250–500 μunits/cell
		1200–2000 mIU/ml packed erythrocytes	1	1200–2000 U/L packed erythrocytes
γ-Glutamyl transferase	Serum	5–40 IU/l	1	5–40 U/L at 37°C.
Glutathione	Whole blood	24–37 mg/dl	0.032	0.77–1.18 mmol/L
Growth hormone	Serum	<10 ng/ml	1	<10 μg/L
Guanase	Serum	<3 nM/ml/min	1	<3 U/L at 37 °C.
Haptoglobin	Serum	60–270 mg/dl	0.01	0.6–2.7 g/L
Hemoglobin	Serum or plasma:			
	qualitative	Negative	—	Negative
	quantitative	0.5–5.0 mg/dl	10	5–50 mg/L
	Whole blood:			
	female	12.0–16.0 g/dl	10	1.86–2.48 mmol/L
	male	13.5–18.0 g/dl		2.09–2.79 mmol/L
α-Hydroxybutyrate dehydrogenase	Serum	140–350 U/ml	1	140–350 kU/L
17-Hydroxycorticosteroids	Plasma:			
	male	7–19 μg/dl	10	70–190 μg/L
	female	9–21 μg/dl		9–21 μg/L
	after 24 USP units of ACTH I.M.	35–55 μg/dl		350–550 μg/L
Immunoglobulins:	Serum			
IgG		800–1801 mg/dl	0.01	8.0–18.0 g/L
IgA		113–563 mg/dl		1.1–5.6 g/L
IgM		54–222 mg/dl		0.54–2.2 g/L
IgD		0.5–3.0 mg/dl	10	5.0–30 mg/L
IgE		0.01–0.04 mg/dl		0.1–0.4 mg/L

Table 4. WHOLE BLOOD, SERUM, AND PLASMA CHEMISTRY *(Continued)*

Component	System	Typical Reference Intervals: *Conventional Units*	*Factor**	*Recommended SI Units*†
Insulin	Plasma:			
	bioassay	11–240 μIU/ml[d]	0.0417	0.46–10.00 μg/L
	radioimmunoassay	4–24 μIU/ml		0.17–1.00 μg/L
Insulin tolerance (0.1 unit/kg) (See Table 10–4, p. 170)	Serum:			
	fasting	Glucose of 70–110 mg/dl	0.055	Glucose of 3.85–6.05 mmol/L
	30 min.	Fall to 50% of fasting level	0.01[d]	Fall to 0.5 of fasting level
	90 min.	Fasting level		Fasting level
Iodine:				
butanol-extraction (BEI)	Serum	3.5–6.5 μg/dl	0.079	0.28–0.51 μmol/L
protein bound (PBI)	Serum	4.0–8.0 μg/dl		0.32–0.63 μmol/L
Iron, total	Serum	60–150 μg/dl	0.179	11–27 μmol/L
Iron binding capacity	Serum	250–400 μg/dl	0.179	54–64 μmol/L
Iron saturation	Serum	20–55%	0.01[b]	fraction of total iron binding capacity: 0.20–0.55
Isocitric dehydrogenase	Serum	50–240 units/ml at 25°C. (Wolfson-Williams Ashman units)	0.0167	0.83–4.18 U/L at 25°C.
Ketone bodies	Serum	Negative	—	Negative
17-Ketosteroids	Plasma	25–125 μg/dl	0.01	0.25–1.25 mg/L
Lactic acid (as lactate)	Whole blood:			
	venous	5–20 mg/dl	0.111	0.6–2.2 mmol/L
	arterial	3–7 mg/dl		0.3–0.8 mmol/L
Lactate dehydrogenase (LDH)	Serum	(lactate → pyruvate) 80–120 units at 30°C.	0.48	38–62 U/L at 30°C.
		(pyruvate → lactate) 185–640 units at 30°C.	0.48	90–310 U/L at 30°C.
		(lactate → pyruvate) 100–190 U/l at 37°C.	1	100–190 U/L at 37°C.
Lactate dehydrogenase isoenzymes:	Serum			fraction of total LDH:
LDH_1 (anode)		17–27%	0.01[b]	0.17–0.27
LDH_2		27–37%		0.27–0.37
LDH_3		18–25%		0.18–0.25
LDH_4		3–8%		0.03–0.08
LDH_5 (cathode)		0–5%		0.00–0.05
Lactate dehydrogenase (heat stable)	Serum	30–60% of total	0.01[b]	fraction of total LDH: 0.30–0.60
Lactose tolerance	Serum	Serum glucose changes similar to glucose tolerance test	—	Serum glucose changes similar to glucose tolerance test
Lead	Whole blood	0–50 μg/dl	0.048	0–2.4 μmol/L
Leucine aminopeptidase (LAP)	Serum:			
	male	80–200 U/ml (Goldbarg-Rutenberg)	0.24	19.2–48.0 U/L
	female	75–185 U/ml (Goldbarg-Rutenberg)		18.0–44.4 U/L
Lipase	Serum	0–1.5 U/ml (Cherry-Crandall)	278	0–417 U/L
		14–280 mIU/ml	1	14–280 U/L

Lipids, total	Serum	400–800 mg/dl	0.01	4.00–8.00 g/L
cholesterol (see Chap. 11)		150–250 mg/dl	0.026	3.9–6.5 mmol/L
triglycerides (see Chap. 11)		10–190 mg/dl	0.109	1.09–20.71 mmol/L
phospholipids		150–380 mg/dl	0.01	1.50–380 g/L
fatty acids (free)		9.0–15.0 mM/l	1	9.0–15.0 mmol/L
		300–480 μEq/l	0.01	300–480 μmol/L
phospholipid phosphorus		8.0–11.0 mg/dl	0.323	2.58–3.55 mmol/L
Lithium	Serum	Negative	—	Negative
Therapeutic interval		0.5–1.4 mEq/l	1	0.5–1.4 mmol/L
Long-acting thyroid-stimulating hormone (LATS)	Serum	None	—	None
Luteinizing hormone (LH)	Serum:			
	male	6–30 mIU/ml	0.23	1.4–6.9 mg/L
	female	Mid cycle peak: 3 times baseline value		Mid cycle peak: 3 times baseline value
		Premenopausal <30 mIU/ml		Premenopausal <5 times baseline value
		Postmenopausal >35 mIU/ml		Postmenopausal >5 times baseline value
Macroglobulins, total	Serum	70–430 mg/dl	0.01	0.7–4.3 g/L
Magnesium	Serum	1.3–2.1 mEq/l	0.5	0.7–1.1 mmol/L
		1.8–3.0 mg/dl	0.41	0.7–1.1 mmol/L
Methemoglobin	Whole blood	0–0.24 g/dl	10	0.0–2.4 g/L
		<1% of total hemoglobin	0.01[b]	fraction of total hemoglobin <0.01
Mucoprotein	Serum	80–200 mg/dl	0.01	0.8–2.0 g/L
Muramidase	Serum	4–13 mg/l		4–13 mg/L
Non-protein nitrogen (NPN)	Serum or plasma	20–35 mg/dl	0.714	14.3–25.0 mmol/L
	Whole blood	25–50 mg/dl		17.9–35.7 mmol/L
5′Nucleotidase	Serum	0–1.6 units at 37°C.	1	0–1.6 units at 37°C.
Ornithine carbamyl transferase	Serum	8–20 mIU/ml at 37°C.	1	8–20 U/L at 37°C.
Osmolality	Serum	280–295 mOsm/kg	1	280–295 mmol/L
Oxygen: (Chapter 7)				
pressure (Po_2)	Whole blood (arterial)	95–100 mm Hg	0.133	12.64–13.30 kPa[a]
content	Whole blood (arterial)	15–23 volume %	0.01[b]	volume fraction: 0.15–0.23
saturation	Whole blood (arterial)	94–100%		0.94–1.00
pH	Whole blood (arterial)	7.38–7.44	1	7.38–7.44
	Whole blood (venous)	7.36–7.41		7.36–7.41
	Serum or plasma (venous)	7.35–7.45		7.35–7.45
Phenylalanine	Serum:			
	adults	<3.0 mg/dl	0.061	<0.18 mmol/L
	newborns (term)	1.2–3.5 mg/dl		0.07–0.21 mmol/L

Table 4. WHOLE BLOOD, SERUM, AND PLASMA CHEMISTRY *(Continued)*

Component	System	Typical Reference Intervals		
		Conventional Units	*Factor**	*Recommended SI Units†*
Phosphatase				
acid phosphatase	Serum	0.13–0.63 U/l at 37°C. (paranitrophenyl-phosphate)	16.67	2.2–10.5 U/L at 37°C.
alkaline phosphatase	Serum	20–90 IU/l at 30°C. (paranitrophenyl-phosphate in AMP buffer)	1	20–90 U/L at 30°C.
Phospholipid phosphorus	Serum	8–11 mg/dl	0.323	2.6–3.6 mmol/L
Phospholipids	Serum	150–380 mg/dl	0.01	1.50–3.80 g/L
Phosphorus, inorganic	Serum:			
	adults	2.3–4.7 mg/dl	0.323	0.78–1.52 mmol/L
	children	4.0–7.0 mg/dl		1.29–2.26 mmol/L
Potassium	Plasma	3.8–5.0 mEq/l	1	3.8–5.0 mmol/L
Prolactin	Serum: female	1–25 ng/ml	1	1–25 μg/L
	male	1–20 ng/ml		1–20 μg/L
Proteins: (Chapter 12)	Serum			
total		6.0–7.8 g/dl	10	60–78 g/L
albumin		3.2–4.5 g/dl		32–45 g/L
globulin		2.3–3.5 g/dl		23–35 g/L
Protein fractionation		See electrophoresis		See electrophoresis
Protoporphyrin	Erythrocytes	15–50 μg/dl	0.018	0.27–0.90 μmol/L
Pyruvate	Whole blood	0.3–0.9 mg/dl	114	34–103 μmol/L
Salicylates	Serum	Negative	—	Negative
therapeutic interval		15–30 mg/dl	0.072	1.44–1.80 mmol/L
		150–300 μg/ml	0.0072	1.08–2.16 mmol/L
Sodium	Plasma	136–142 mEq/l	1	136–142 mmol/L
Sulfate, inorganic	Serum	0.2–1.3 mEq/l	0.5	0.10–0.65 mmol/L
		0.9–6.0 mg/dl as SO_4^{--}	0.104	0.09–0.62 mmol/L as SO_4^{--}
Sulfhemoglobin	Whole blood	Negative	—	Negative
Sulfonamides	Serum or whole blood	Negative	—	Negative
Testosterone	Serum or plasma:			
	male	300–1200 ng/dl	0.035	10.0–42.0 nmol/L
	female	30–95 ng/dl		1.1–3.3 nmol/L
Thiocyanate	Serum	Negative	—	Negative
Thyroid hormone tests: (Chapter 16)	Serum			
a) Expressed as thyroxine:				
T_4 by column		5.0–11.0 μg/dl	13.0	65–143 nmol/L
T_4 by competitive binding—Murphy-Pattee		6.0–11.8 μg/dl		78–153 nmol/L
T_4 RIA		5.5–12.5 μg/dl	13.0	72–163 nmol/L
free T_4		0.9–2.3 ng/dl		12–30 pmol/L

b) Expressed as iodine:				
T_4 by column		3.2–7.2 μg/dl	79.0	253–569 nmol/L
T_4 by competitive binding—Murphy-Pattee		3.9–7.7 μg/dl		308–608 nmol/L
free T_4		0.6–1.5 ng/dl	79.0	47–119 pmol/L
T_3 resin uptake		25–38 relative % uptake	0.01[b]	relative uptake fraction: 0.25–0.38
Thyroxine-binding globulin (TBG)	Serum	10–26 μg/dl	10	100–260 μg/L
TSH	Serum	<10μU/ml	1	$<10^{-3}$ IU/L
Transferases				
aspartate amino transferase (AST or SGOT)	Serum	10–40 U/ml (Karmen) at 25°C. 16–60 U/ml (Karmen) at 30°C.	0.48	8–29 U/L at 30°C. 8–33 U/L at 37°C.
alanine amino transferase (ALT or SGPT)	Serum	10–30 U/ml (Karmen) at 25°C. 8–50 U/ml (Karmen) at 30°C.	0.48	4–24 U/L at 30°C. 4–36 U/L at 37°C.
gamma glutamyl transferase (GGT)		5–40 IU/l at 37°C.	1	5.40 U/L at 37°C.
Triglycerides (Chapter 11)	Serum	10–190 mg/dl	0.011[c]	0.11–2.09 mmol/L
Urea nitrogen	Serum	8–23 mg/dl	0.357	2.9–8.2 mmol/L
Urea clearance:	Serum and urine			
maximum clearance		64–99 ml/min	0.0167	1.07–1.65 ml/s
standard clearance		41–65 ml/min, or more than 75% of normal clearance		0.68–1.09 ml/s or more than 0.75 of normal clearance
Uric acid	Serum:			
	male	4.0–8.5 mg/dl	0.059	0.24–0.5 mmol/L
	female	2.7–7.3 mg/dl		0.16–0.43 mmol/L
Vitamin A	Serum	15–60 μg/dl	0.035	0.53–2.10 μmol/L
Vitamin A tolerance	Serum:			
	fasting 3 hr. or 6 hr. after 5000 units	15–60 μg/dl	0.035	0.53–2.10 μmol/L
	vitamin A/kg	200–600 μg/dl		7.00–21.00 μmol/L
	24 hrs.	Fasting values or slightly above	—	Fasting values or slightly above
Vitamin B_{12}	Serum	160–950 pg/ml	0.74	118–703 pmol/L
Unsaturated vitamin B_{12} binding capacity	Serum	1000–2000 pg/ml	0.74	740–1480 pmol/L
Vitamin C	Plasma	0.6–1.6 mg/dl	56.8	34–91 μmol/L
Xylose absorption	Serum:			
	normal	25–40 mg/dl between 1 and 2 hr.	0.067	1.68–2.68 mmol/L between 1 and 2 h
	in malabsorption	Maximum approximately 10 mg/dl		Maximum approximately 0.67 mmol/L
Dose: adult		25 g D-xylose	0.067	0.167 mol D-xylose
children		0.5 g/kg D-xylose		3.33 mmol/kg D-xylose
Zinc	Serum	50–150 μg/dl	0.153	7.65–22.95 μmol/L

*Factor = Number factor (note that units are not presented).
†Value in SI units = Value in conventional units × factor.
‡Usually not measured in blood (preferred specimen in urine, hair, or nails except in acute cases where gastric contents are used).

Table 5. URINE

Component	Type of Urine Specimen	Typical Reference Intervals		
		Conventional Units	*Factor*	*Recommended SI Units*
Acetoacetic acid	Random	Negative	—	Negative
Acetone	Random	Negative	—	Negative
Addis count	12 hr. collection	WBC and epithelial cells:		
		1,800,000/12 hr.	1	1.8×10^6/12 h
		RBC 500,000/12 hr.	1	0.5×10^6/12 h
		Hyaline casts: 0–5000/12 hr.	1	5.0×10^3/12 h
Albumin:				
qualitative	Random	Negative	—	Negative
quantitative	24 hr.	15–150 mg/24 hr.	1	0.015–0.150 g/24 h
Aldosterone	24 hr.	2–26 μg/24 hr.	2.77	5.5–72.0 nmol/24 h
Alkapton bodies	Random	Negative	—	Negative
Alpha-amino acid nitrogen	24 hr.	100–290 mg/24 hr.	0.0714	7.14–20.71 mmol/24 h
δ-Aminolevulinic acid	Random:			
	adult	0.1–0.6 mg/dl	76.3	7.6–45.8 μmol/L
	children	<0.5 mg/dl		<38.1 μmol/L
	24 hr.	1.5–7.5 mg/24 hr.	7.63	11.15–57.2 μmol/24 h
Ammonia nitrogen	24 hr.	20–70 mEq/24 hr.		
		500–1200 mg/24 hr.	0.071	35.5–85.2 mmol/24 h
Amylase	2 hr.	35–260 Somogyi units/hr.	0.185	6.5–48.1 U/h
Arsenic	24 hr.	<50 μg/l	0.013	<0.65 μmol/L
Ascorbic acid	Random	1–7 mg/dl	0.057	0.06–0.40 mmol/L
	24 hr.	>50 mg/24 hr.	0.0057	>0.29 mmol/24 h
Bence Jones protein	Random	Negative	—	Negative
Beryllium	24 hr.	<0.05 μg/24 hr.	111	<5.55 nmol/24 h
Bilirubin, qualitative	Random	Negative	—	Negative
Blood, occult	Random	Negative	—	Negative
Borate	24 hr.	<2 mg/l	16	<32 μmol/L
Calcium:				
qualitative (Sulkowitch)	Random	1+ turbidity	1	1+ turbidity
quantitative	24 hr.:			
	average diet	100–240 mg/24 hr.	0.025	2.50–6.25 mmol/24 h
	low calcium diet	<150 mg/24 hr.		<3.75 mmol/24 h
	high calcium diet	240–300 mg/24 hr.		6.25–7.50 mmol/24 h
Catecholamines	Random	0–14 μg/dl	10	0–140 μg/L
	24 hr.	<100 μg/24 hr. (varies with activity)	1	<100 μg/24 h
Epinephrine		<10 ng/24 hr.	5.46	<55 nmol/24 h
Norepinephrine		<100 ng/24 hr.	5.91	<590 nmol/24 h
Total free catecholamines		4–126 μg/24 hr.	1	4–126 μg/24 h
Total metanephrines		0.1–1.6 mg/24 hr.	1	0.1–1.6 mg/24 h
Chloride	24 hr.	140–250 mEq/24 hr.	1	140–250 mmol/24 h

Concentration test (Fishberg):	Random—after fluid restriction			
Specific gravity		>1.025	1	>1.025
Osmolality		>850 mOsm/l	1	>850 mmol/L
Copper	24 hr.	0–50 μg/24 hr.	0.016	0–0.48 μmol/24 h
Coproporphyrin	Random:			
	adult	3–20 μg/dl	0.015	0.045–0.30 μmol/L
	24 hr.:			
	adult	50–160 μg/24 hr.	0.0015	0.075–0.24 μmol/24 h
	children	0–80 μg/24 hr.	0.0015	0.00–0.12 μmol/24 hr
Creatine	24 hr.:			
	male	0–40 mg/24 hr.	0.0076	0–0.30 mmol/24 h
	female	0–100 mg/24 hr.		0–0.76 mmol/24 h
		Higher in children and during pregnancy	—	Higher in children and during pregnancy
Creatinine	24 hr.:			
	male	20–26 mg/kg/24 hr.	0.0088	0.18–0.23 mmol/kg/24 h
		1.0–2.0 g/24 hr.	8.8	8.8–17.6 mmol/24 h
	female	14–22 mg/kg/24 hr.	0.0088	0.12–0.19 mmol/kg/24 h
		0.8–1.8 g/24 hr.	8.8	7.0–15.8 mmol/24 h
Cystine, qualitative	Random	Negative	—	Negative
Cystine and cysteine	24 hr.	10–100 mg/24 hr.	.0083[h]	0.08–0.83 mmol/24 h
Diacetic acid	Random	Negative	—	Negative
Epinephrine	24 hr.	0–20 μg/24 hr.	0.0055	0.00–0.11 μmol/24 h
Estrogens				
total	24 hr.:			
	male	5–18 μg/24 hr.	1	5–18 μg/24 h
	female:			
	ovulation	28–100 μg/24 hr.		28–80 μg/24 h
	luteal peak	22–80 μg/24 hr.		22–105 μg/24 h
	at menses	4–25 μg/24 hr.		4–25 μg/24 h
	pregnancy	Up to 45,000 μg/24 hr.		Up to 45,000 μg/24 h
	postmenopausal	Up to 10 μg/24 hr.		Up to 10 μg/24 h
fractionated	24 hr., non-pregnant, midcycle			
Estrone (E^1)	—	2–25 μg/24 hr.	3.7	7–93 nmol/24 h
Estradiol (E^2)	—	0–10 μg/24 hr.	3.7	0–37 nmol/24 h
Estriol (E^3)	—	2–30 μg/24 hr.	3.5	7–105 nmol/24 h
Fat, qualitative	Random	Negative	—	Negative
FIGLU (N-formiminoglutamic acid)	24 hr.	<3 mg/24 hr.	5.7	<17.0 μmol/24 h
	after 15 g of L-histidine	4 mg/8 hr.	5.7	23.0 μmol/8 h
Fluoride	24 hr.	<1 mg/24 hr.	0.053	0.053 mmol/24 h
Follicle-stimulating hormone (FSH)	24 hr.:			
	adult	6–50 Mouse uterine units (MUU)/24 hr.	1	4–25 mIU/ml
	prepubertal	<10 MUU/24 hr.	1	4–30 mIU/ml
	postmenopausal	>50 MUU/24 hr.	1	40–50 mIU/ml
	midcycle	2× baseline		

Table 5. URINE *(Continued)*

Component	Type of Urine Specimen	Typical Reference Intervals: *Conventional Units*	*Factor*	*Recommended SI Units*
Fructose	24 hr.	30–65 mg/24 hr.	0.0056	0.17–0.36 mmol/24 h
Glucose:				
qualitative	Random	Negative	—	Negative
quantitative:	24 hr.			
copper-reducing substances		0.5–1.5 g/24 hr.	1	0.5–1.5 g/24 h
total sugars		average 250 mg/24 hr.	1	average 250 mg/24 h
glucose		average 130 mg/24 hr.	0.0056	average 0.73 mmol/24 h
Gonadotropins, pituitary (FSH and LH)	24 hr.	10–50 MUU/24 hr.	1	10–50 IU/24 h
Etiocholanolone	24 hr.:			
	male	1.4–5.0 mg/24 hr.	3.44	4.8–17.2 μmol/24 h
	female	0.8–4.0 mg/24 hr.		2.8–13.8 μmol/24 h
Dehydroepiandrosterone	24 hr.:			
	male	0.2–2.0 mg/24 hr.	3.46	0.7–6.9 μmol/24 h
	female	0.2–1.8 mg/24 hr.		0.7–6.2 μmol/24 h
11-Ketoandrosterone	24 hr.:			
	male	0.2–1.0 mg/24 hr.	3.28	0.7–3.3 μmol/24 h
	female	0.2–0.8 mg/24 hr.		0.7–2.6 μmol/24 h
11-Ketoetiocholanolone	24 hr.:			
	male	0.2–1.0 mg/24 hr.	3.28	0.7–3.3 μmol/24 h
	female	0.2–0.8 mg/24 hr.		0.7–2.6 μmol/24 h
11-Hydroxyandrosterone	24 hr.:			
	male	0.1–0.8 mg/24 hr.	3.26	0.3–2.6 μmol/24 h
	female	0.0–0.5 mg/24 hr.		0.0–1.6 μmol/24 h
11-Hydroxyetiocholanolone	24 hr.:			
	male	0.2–0.6 mg/24 hr.	3.26	0.7–2.0 μmol/24 h
	female	0.1–1.1 mg/24 hr.		0.3–3.6 μmol/24 h
Lactose	24 hr.	14–40 mg/24 hr.	2.9	41–116 μmol/24 h
Lead	24 hr.	<100 μg/24 hr.	0.0048	<0.48 μmol/24 h
Magnesium	24 hr.	6.0–8.5 mEq/24 hr.	0.5	3.0–4.3 mmol/24 h
Melanin, qualitative	Random	Negative	—	Negative
3-Methoxy-4-hydroxymandelic acid (VMA)	24 hr.:			
	adults	1.5–7.5 mg/24 hr.	5.05	7.6–37.9 μmol/24 h
	infants	83 μg/kg/24 hr.	0.0051	0.4 μmol/kg/24 h

Mucin	24 hr.	100–150 mg/24 hr.	1	100–150 mg/24 h
Muramidase (lysozyme)	24 hr.	1.3–36 mg/24 hr.		1.3–36 mg/24 h
Myoglobin				
qualitative	Random	Negative	—	Negative
quantitative	24 hr.	<4 mg/l	1	<4 mg/L
Osmolality	Random	500–800 mOsm/kg water	1	500–800 mmol/kg
Pentoses	24 hr.	2–5 mg/kg/24 hr.	1	2–5 mg/kg/24 h
pH	Random	4.6–8.0	1	4.6–8.0
Phenosulfonphthalein (PSP)	Urine timed after 6 mg PSP IV			
	15 min.	20–50% dye excreted	0.01[b]	fraction dye excreted: 0.2–0.5
	30 min.	16–24% dye excreted		0.16–0.24
	60 min.	9–17% dye excreted		0.09–0.17
	120 min.	3–10% dye excreted		0.03–0.10
Phenylpyruvic acid, qualitative	Random	Negative	—	Negative
Phosphorus	Random	0.9–1.3 g/24 hr.	32	29–42 mmol/24 h
Porphobilinogen:				
qualitative	Random	Negative	—	Negative
quantitative	24 hr.	0–1.0 mg/24 hr.	4.42	0–4.4 μmol/24 h
Potassium	24 hr.	40–80 mEq/24 hr.	1	40–80 mmol/24 h
Pregnancy tests	Concentrated morning specimen	Positive in normal pregnancies or with tumors producing chorionic gonadotropin	—	Positive in normal pregnancies or with tumors producing chorionic gonadotropin
Pregnanediol	24 hr.:			
	male	0–1.5 mg/24 hr.	3.12	0–4.7 μmol/24 h
	female	1–8 mg/24 hr.		3–25 μmol/24 h
	peak	1 week after ovulation	—	1 week after ovulation
	pregnancy	<50 mg/24 hr.		156 μmol/24 h
	children	Negative	—	Negative
Pregnanetriol	24 hr.:			
	male	0.4–2.4 mg/24 hr.	2.97	1.2–7.1 μmol/24 h
	female	0.5–2.0 mg/24 hr.		1.5–5.9 μmol/24 h
	children	Up to 1 mg/24 hr.		Up to 3 μmol/24 h
Protein, qualitative	Random	Negative	—	Negative
	24 hr.	40–150 mg/24 hr.	1	40–150 mg/24 h
Reducing substances, total	24 hr.	0.5–1.5 mg/24 hr.	1	0.5–1.5 mg/24 h
Sodium	24 hr.	75–200 mEq/24 hr.	1	75–200 mmol/24 h
Solids, total	24 hr.	55–70 g/24 hr.	1	55–70 g/24 h
		Decreases with age to 30 g/24 hr.	—	Decreases with age to 30 g/24 h
Specific gravity	Random	1.016–1.022 (normal fluid intake)	1	Relative Density (U 20°C./water 20°C.) 1.016–1.022 (normal fluid intake)
		1.001–1.035 (range)		1.001–1.034 (range)

Table 5. URINE *(Continued)*

Component	Type of Urine Specimen	Typical Reference Intervals		
		Conventional Units	***Factor***	***Recommended SI Units***
Sugars (excluding glucose)	Random	Negative	—	Negative
Titratable acidity	24 hr.	20–50 mEq/24 hr.	1	20–50 mmol/24 h
Urea nitrogen	24 hr.	6–17 g/24 hr.	0.0357	0.21–0.60 mol/24 h
Uric acid	24 hr.	250–750 mg/24 hr.	0.0059	1.48–4.43 mmol/24 h
Urobilinogen	2 hr.	0.3–1.0 Ehrlich Units	—	
	24 hr.	0.05–2.5 mg/24 hr. or	1.69	0.09–4.23 μmol/24 h
		0.5–4.0 Ehrlich units/24 hr.	—	
Uropepsin	Random	15–45 units/hr. (Anson)	7.37	111–332 U/h
	24 hr.	1500–5000 units/24 hr. (Anson)		11–37 kU/h
Uroporphyrins:				
qualitative	Random	Negative	—	Negative
quantitative	24 hr.	10–30 μg/24 hr.	0.0012	0.012–0.037 μmol/24 h
Vanillylmandelic acid (VMA)	24 hr.	1.5–7.5 mg/24 hr.	5.05	7.6–37.9 μmol/24 h
Volume, total	24 hr.	600–1600 ml/24 hr.	0.001	0.6–1.6 L/24 h
Zinc	24 hr.	0.15–1.2 mg/24 hr.	15.3	2.3–18.4 μmol/24 h

Table 6. SYNOVIAL FLUID

Component	Typical Reference Intervals		
	Conventional Units	***Factor***	***Recommended SI Units***
Blood-serum-synovial fluid glucose difference	<10 mg/dl	0.055	<0.55 mmol/L
Differential cell count	Granulocytes <25% of nucleated cells	0.01[b]	Granulocyte number fraction: <25% of nucleated cells
Fibrin clot	Absent	—	Absent
Mucin clot	Abundant	—	Abundant
Nucleated cell count	<200 cells/μl	10^6	<2 × 10^8 cells/L
Viscosity	High	—	High
Volume	<3.5 ml	0.001	<0.0035L

Table 7. SEMINAL FLUID

Component	Typical Reference Intervals		
	Conventional Units	***Factor***	***Recommended SI Units***
Liquefaction	within 20 min.	1	within 20 min
Sperm morphology	>70% normal, mature spermatozoa	0.01[b]	number fraction: >0.7 normal, mature spermatozoa
Sperm motility	>60%	0.01[b]	number fraction: >0.6
pH	>7.0 (average 7.7)	1	>7.0 (average 7.7)
Sperm count	60–150 million/ml	10^3	60–150 × 10^9/L
Volume	1.5–5.0 ml	0.001	0.0015–0.005L

Table 8. GASTRIC FLUID

Component	Typical Reference Intervals		
	Conventional Units	***Factor***	***Recommended SI Units***
Fasting residual volume	20–100 ml	0.001	0.02–0.10L
pH	<2.0	1	<2.0
Basal acid output (BAO)	0–6 mEq/hr.	1	0–6 mmol/h
Maximum acid output (MAO) (after histamine stimulation)	5–40 mEq/hr.	1	5–40 mmol/h
BAO/MAO ratio	<0.4	1	<0.4

Table 9. HEMATOLOGY

Component	Typical Reference Intervals		
	Conventional Units	*Factor*	*Recommended SI Units*
Red cell volume:			
male	20–36 ml/kg body weight	0.001	0.020–0.036 L/kg body weight
female	19–31 ml/kg body weight	—	0.019–0.031 L/kg body weight
Plasma volume:			
male	25–43 ml/kg body weight	0.001	0.040–0.050 L/kg body weight
female	28–45 ml/kg body weight	—	0.040–0.050 L/kg body weight
Coagulation and hemostatic tests:			
Bleeding time			
Mielke template	2–8 minutes		2–8 min
Simplate	3–8 minutes		3–8 min
Antithrombin III			
Immunologic	21–30 mg/dL		210–310 mg/L
Functional	80–120%		0.8–1.2
Clot retraction	40–94% of serum extruded in one hour at 37°C		
Euglobulin clot lysis time	Clot lyses between 2 and 4 hours at 37°C		
Factor assays (procoagulant)	0.5–1.5 U/mL		0.5–1.5
Factor VIII antigen (Factor VIIIR:Ag; Laurell)	0.5–1.5 U/mL		0.5–1.5
Ristocetin cofactor (Factor VIIIR:RCoF)	0.5–1.5 U/mL		0.5–1.5
Factor XIII (screening test)	Clot insoluble in 5M urea at 24 hours		
Fibrinogen	200–400 mg/dL		2–4 g/dL
Fibrinogen split products	10 ug/mL		10 mg/L
Partial thromboplastin time (PTT)	Depends upon phospholipid reagent used, typically 60–85 seconds		
Activated PTT	Depends upon activator and phospholipid reagents used, typically 20–35 seconds		
Plasminogen			
Immunologic	10–20 mg/dL		100–200 mg/L
Functional	2.2–4.2 CTA U/mL*		
Prothrombin time	Depends upon thromboplastin reagent used, typically 9.5–12 seconds		
Thrombin time	Depends upon concentration of thrombin reagent used, typically 20–29 seconds		
Whole blood clot lysis time	None in 24 hours		
Complete blood count (CBC)			
Hematocrit:			
male	40–54%	0.01[b]	volume fraction: 0.40–0.54
female	38–47%		0.38–0.47
Hemoglobin:			
male	13.5–18.0 g/dl	0.155	2.09–2.79 mmol/L
female	12.0–16.0 g/dl		1.86–2.48 mmol/L
Red cell count:			
male	4.6–6.2 × 10^6/µl	10^6	4.6–6.2 × 10^{12}/L
female	4.2–5.4 × 10^6/µl		4.2–5.4 × 10^{12}/L
White cell count	4.5–11.0 × 10^3/µl	10^6	4.5–11.0 × 10^9/L

Table 9. HEMATOLOGY *(Continued)*

Component	Typical Reference Intervals: *Conventional Units*			*Factor*	*Recommended SI Units*		
Erythrocyte indices:							
Mean corpuscular volume (MCV)	80–96 cu. microns			1	80–96 fl		
Mean corpuscular hemoglobin (MCH)	27–31 pg			1	27–31 pg		
Mean corpuscular hemoglobin concentration (MCHC)	32–36%			0.01[b]	concentration fraction: 0.32–0.36		
White blood cell differential (adult):	Mean per cent	Range of absolute counts			Mean number fraction†	Range of absolute count	
Segmented neutrophils	56%	1800–7000/μl		10^6	0.56	1.8–7.8 × 10^9/L	
Bands	3%	0–700/μl		10^6	0.03	0–0.70 × 10^9/L	
Eosinophils	2.7%	0–450/μl		10^6	0.027	0–0.45 × 10^9/L	
Basophils	0.3%	0–200/μl		10^6	0.003	0–0.20 × 10^9/L	
Lymphocytes	34%	1000–4800/μl		10^6	0.34	1.0–4.8 × 10^9/L	
Monocytes	4%	0–800/μl		10^6	0.04	0–0.80 × 10^9/L	
Hemoglobin A_2	1.5–3.5% of total hemoglobin			0.01[b]	mass fraction: 0.015–0.035 of total hemoglobin		
Hemoglobin F	<2%			0.01[b]	mass fraction: <0.02		
Osmotic fragility	% NaCl	% Lysis: Fresh	% Lysis: 24 hr. at 37°C.	% NaCl—171 % Lysis—0.01[b]	NaCl mmol/L	Lysed Fraction: Fresh	Lysed Fraction: 24 h at 37°C.
	0.2	—	95–100		34.2	—	0.95–1.00
	0.3	97–100	85–100		51.3	0.97–1.00	0.85–1.00
	0.35	90–99	75–100		59.8	0.90–0.99	0.75–1.00
	0.4	50–95	65–100		68.4	0.50–0.95	0.65–1.00
	0.45	5–45	55–95		77.0	0.05–0.45	0.55–0.95
	0.5	0–6	40–85		85.5	0–0.06	0.40–0.85
	0.55	0	15–70		94.1	0	0.15–0.70
	0.6	—	0–40		102.6	—	0–0.40
	0.65	—	0–10		111.2	—	0–0.10
	0.7	—	0–5		119.7	—	0–0.05
	0.75	—	0		128.3	—	0
Platelet count	150,000–400,000/μl			10^6	0.15–0.4 × 10^{12}/L		
Reticulocyte count	0.5–1.5%			0.01[b]	number fraction: 0.005–0.015		
	25,000–75,000 cells/μl			10^6	25–75 × 10^9/L		
Sedimentation rate (ESR) (Westergren)							
Men under 50 yrs.	<50 mm/hr			1	<15 mm/h		
Men over 50 yrs.	<20 mm/hr				<20 mm/h		
Women under 50 yrs.	<20 mm/hr				<20 mm/h		
Women over 50 yrs.	<30 mm/hr				<30 mm/h		
Viscosity	1.4–1.8 times water			1	1.4–1.8 times water		
Zeta sedimentation ratio	41–54%			0.01	fraction: 0.41–0.54		

*CTA = Committee on Thrombotic Agents.
†All percentages are multiplied by 0.01[b] to give fraction.

Table 10. AMNIOTIC FLUID

Component	Typical Reference Intervals		
	Conventional Units	*Factor*	*Recommended SI Units*
Appearance:			
early gestation	Clear	—	Clear
term	Clear or slightly opalescent	—	Clear or slightly opalescent
Albumin:			
early gestation	0.39 g/dl	10	3.9 g/L
term	0.19 g/dl		1.9 g/L
Bilirubin:			
early gestation	<0.075 mg/dl	17.1	<1.28 μmol/L
term	<0.025 mg/dl		<0.43 μmol/L
Chloride:			
early gestation	Approximately equal to serum chloride	—	Approximately equal to serum chloride
term	Generally 1–3 mEq/l lower than serum chloride	1	Generally 1–3 mmol/L lower than serum chloride
Creatinine:			
early gestation	0.8–1.1 mg/dl	88.4	70.7–97.2 μmol/L
term	1.8–4.0 mg/dl (generally > 2 mg/dl)		159.1–353.6 μmol/L (generally > 176.8 μmol/L)
Estriol:			
early gestation	<10 μg/dl	0.035	<0.35 μmol/L
term	>60 μg/dl		>2.1 μmol/L
Lecithin/sphingomyelin		1	
Early (immature)	<1:1	1	<1:1
Term (mature)	>2:1	1	>2:1
Osmolality:			
early gestation	Approximately equal to serum osmolality	1	Approximately equal to serum osmolality
term	230–270 mOsm/l	1	<230–270 mmol/L
P_{CO_2}:			
early gestation	33–55 mm Hg	0.133	4.39–7.32 kPa[a]
term	42–55 mm Hg (increases toward term)		5.59–7.32 kPa[a] (increases toward term)
pH;			
early gestation	7.12–7.38	1	7.12–7.38
term	6.91–7.43 (decreases toward term)		6.91–7.43
Protein, total:			
early gestation	0.60 ± 0.24 g/dl	10	6.0 ± 2.4 g/L
term	0.26 ± 0.19 g/dl		2.6 ± 1.9 g/L
Sodium:			
early gestation	Approximately equal to serum sodium	—	Approximately equal to serum sodium
term	7–10 mEq/l lower than serum sodium	1	7–10 mmol/L lower than serum sodium
Staining, cytologic:			
Oil red O:			
early gestation	<10%	0.01[b]	stained fraction: <0.1
term	>50%		>0.5
Nile blue sulfate:			
early gestation	0	0.01[b]	stained fraction: 0
term	>20%		>0.2
Urea:			
early gestation	18.0 ± 5.9 mg/dl	0.166	2.99 ± 0.98 mmol/L
term	30.3 ± 11.4 mg/dl		5.03 ± 1.89 mmol/L
Uric acid:			
early gestation	3.72 ± 0.96 mg/dl	0.059	0.22 ± 0.06 mmol/L
term	9.90 ± 2.23 mg/dl		0.58 ± 0.13 mmol/L
Volume:			
early gestation	450–1200 ml	0.001	0.45–1.2 L
term	500–1400 ml (increases toward term)		0.5–1.4 L (increases toward term)

Table 11. CEREBROSPINAL FLUID

Component	Typical Reference Intervals		
	Conventional Units	***Factor***	***Recommended SI Units***
Albumin	10–30 mg/dl	10	100–300 mg/L
Calcium	2.1–2.7 mEq/l	0.5	1.05–1.35 mmol/L
Cell count	0–5 cells/μl	10^6	0–5 × 10^6/L
Chloride:			
adult	118–132 mEq/l	1	118–132 mmol/L
Glucose	50–80 mg/dl	0.055	2.75–4.40 mmol/L
Lactate dehydrogenase (LDH)	Approximately 10% of serum level	—	activity fraction: approximately 0.1 of serum level
Protein:			
total CSF	15–45 mg/dl	10	150–450 mg/L
ventricular fluid	5–15 mg/dl		50–150 mg/L
Protein electrophoresis:			
Prealbumin	2–7%	0.01[b]	fraction: 0.02–0.07
Albumin	56–76%		0.56–0.76
Alpha-1 globulin	2–7%		0.02–0.07
Alpha-2 globulin	4–12%		0.04–0.12
Beta globulin	8–18%		0.08–0.18
Gamma globulin	3–12%		0.03–0.12
Xanthochromia	Negative	—	Negative

Table 12. MISCELLANEOUS

Component	Specimen	Typical Reference Intervals		
		Conventional Units	***Factor***	***Recommended SI Units***
Bile, qualitative	Random stool	Negative in adults Positive in children	— —	Negative in adults Positive in children
Chloride	Sweat	4–60 mEq/l	1	4–60 mmol/L
Clearances:	Serum and urine (timed)			
creatinine, endogenous		115 ± 20 ml/min.	0.0167	1.92 ± 0.33 ml/s
Diodrast		600–720 ml/min.		10.02–12.02 ml/s
inulin		100–150 ml/min.		1.67–2.51 ml/s
PAH		600–750 ml/min.		10.02–12.53 ml/s
Diagnex blue (tubeless gastric analysis)	Urine	Free acid present	—	Free acid present
Fat:	Stool, 72 hr.			
total fat		<5 g/24 hr. 10–25% of dry matter	0.01[b] 0.01	<5 g/24 h mass fraction: 0.1–0.24 of dry matter
neutral fat		1–5% of dry matter	0.01	0.01–0.05 of dry matter
free fatty acids		5–13% of dry matter	0.01	0.05–0.13 of dry matter
combined fatty acids		5–15% of dry matter	0.01	0.05–0.15 of dry matter
Nitrogen, total	Stool, 24 hr.	10% of intake 1–2 g/24 hr.	0.01[b] 0.071	mass fraction: 0.1 of intake 0.071–0.142 mol/24 h
Sodium	Sweat	10–80 mEq/l	1	10–80 mmol/L
Trypsin activity	Random, fresh stool	Positive (2+ to 4+)	—	Positive (2+ to 4+)
Thyroid ^{131}I uptake		7.5–25% in 6 hr.	0.01[b]	fraction uptake: 0.075–0.25 in 6 h
Urobilinogen:				
qualitative	Random stool	Positive	—	Positive
quantitative	Stool, 24 hr	40–200 mg/24 hr. 80–280 Ehrlich units/24 hr.	0.00169	0.068–0.34 mmol/24 h

SELECTED PEDIATRIC REFERENCE VALUES*

S†-Acid phosphatase

Newborn: 7.4–19.4 U/L
2–13 yrs: 6.4–15.2 U/L

S-Aldolase

Newborn: to 4 × adult value
Child: to 2 × adult value

S-Alkaline phosphatase

Newborn: 40–300 U/L
Child: 60–270 U/L

S-Alpha fetoprotein:

Newborn: up to 100 mg/L
2 weeks: undetectable

S-Amylase

Newborn: little, if any, amylase activity
1 year: adult values

S-Aspartate aminotransferase

Newborn: 16–74 U/L
1–3 yrs: 6–30 U/L

S-Bilirubin

Newborn:

	PRE-TERM	FULL-TERM
24 h	17.1–102.8 μmol/L (10–60 mg/L)	34.2–102.8 μmol/L (20–60 mg/L)
48 h	102.8–137.0 μmol/L (60–80 mg/L)	102.8–119.9 μmol/L (60–70 mg/L)
3–5 d	171.0–266.5 μmol/L (100–150 mg/L)	68.6–205.2 μmol/L (40–120 mg/L)

S-Calcium

Pre-term, first week: 1.5–2.5 mmol/L (60–100 mg/L)
Full-term, first week: 1.75–3.00 mmol/L (70–120 mg/L)
1–2 yrs: 2.5–3.0 mmol/L (100–120 mg/L)
2–16 yrs: 2.25–2.88 mmol/L (90–115 mg/L)

U†-Catecholamines

	NOREPINEPHRINE	EPINEPHRINE
1 yr:	29.5–86.8 nmol/d (5.4–15.9 μg/d)	0.6–25.4 nmol/d (0.1–4.3 μg/d)
1–5 yrs:	44.2–168.1 nmol/d (8.1–30.8 μg/d)	4.7–53.8 nmol/d (0.8–9.1 μg/d)
6–15 yrs:	103.7–388.1 nmol/d (19.0–71.1 μg/d)	7.7–62.1 nmol/d (1.3–10.5 μg/d)
>15 yrs:	188.8–474.8 nmol/d (34.4–87.0 μg/d)	20.7–78.0 nmol/d (3.5–13.2 μg/d)

U-Chloride

Infant: 1.7–8.5 mmol/d
Child: 17–34 mmol/d

S-Cholesterol

Cord blood: 1.2–2.5 mmol/L (460–980 mg/L)
1–2 yrs: 1.8–4.9 mmol/L (700–1900 mg/L)
2–16 yrs: 3.5–6.5 mmol/L (1350–2500 mg/L)

U-Cortisol (free)

4 mos–10 yrs: 2–27 μg/d 5.5–74.5 nmol/d
11–20 yrs: 0.7–55 μg/d 1.9–151.8 nmol/d

*Information based on: Meites, S. (ed.): Pediatric Clinical Chemistry. Washington, D.C., American Association for Clinical Chemistry, 1977.
†*S* = serum; *U* = urine.

S-Creatine kinase

Newborn:	3 × adult values
3 wks–3 mos:	1.5 × adult values
>1 yr:	at adult values

S-Creatinine

Upper reference value:

Up to 5 yrs:	44 μmol/L (5.0 mg/L)
Up to 6 yrs:	53 μmol/L (6.0 mg/L)
Up to 7 yrs:	62 μmol/L (7.0 mg/L)
Up to 8 yrs:	70 μmol/L (8.0 mg/L)
Up to 9 yrs:	79 μmol/L (9.0 mg/L)
Up to 10 yrs:	88 μmol/L (10.0 mg/L)
>10 yrs:	106 μmol/L (12.0 mg/L)

S-Estradiol

0–2 yrs:	0–7 pg/ml	0–24 pmol/L
2–4 yrs:	0–7 pg/ml	0–24 pmol/L
4–6 yrs:	0–14 pg/ml	0–49 pmol/L
6–8 yrs:	0–10 pg/ml	0–35 pmol/L
8–10 yrs:	0–100 pg/ml	0–347 pmol/L
10–12 yrs:	0–100 pg/ml	0–347 pmol/L
12–14 yrs:	0–100 pg/ml	0–347 pmol/L
14–16 yrs:	7–105 pg/ml	24–364 pmol/L
16–25 yrs:	7–320 pg/ml	24–1110 pmol/L

Fecal Fat:

Pre-term newborn:	up to 40% excreted
Full-term newborn:	up to 20% excreted
3 mos–1 yr:	up to 15% excreted
1 yr:	up to 8.5% excreted

P-Nonesterified fatty acids

Newborn:	0–1845 mmol/L
4 mos–10 yrs:	300–1100 mmol/L

S-Glucose

Pre-term newborn:	1.2–3.6 mmol/L (200–656 mg/L)
Full-term newborn:	1.1–6.0 mmol/L (200–1100 mg/L)
Child:	3.3–5.8 mmol/L (600–1050 mg/L)

S-γ-Glutamyltransferase

Premature newborn:	56–233 U/L
Newborn–3 wks:	10–103 U/L
3 wks–3 mos:	4–111 U/L
1–5 yrs:	2–23 U/L
6–15 yrs:	2–23 U/L
16 yrs–adult:	2–35 U/L

S-Haptoglobin

Newborn:	detectable haptoglobin in only 10–20%
1 yr and older:	at adult values

S-Immunoglobulin IgG

0–5 wks:	7500–15,000 mg/L
6 mos:	1500–7000 mg/L
1 yr:	1400–10,300 mg/L
5 yrs:	3700–15,000 mg/L
10 yrs:	4400–15,500 mg/L

S-Immunoglobulin IgA

0–5 wks:	none
6 mos:	200–1300 mg/L
1 yr:	200–1300 mg/L
5 yrs:	300–2000 mg/L
10 yrs:	500–2300 mg/L

S-Immunoglobulin IgM

0–5 wks:	less than 200 mg/L
6 mos:	300–600 mg/L
1 yr:	300–1600 mg/L
5 yrs:	200–2200 mg/L
10 yrs:	300–1700 mg/L

Inulin clearance

<1 mo:	29–88 ml/min per 1.73 m^2 of body surface
1–6 mos:	40–112 ml/min per 1.73 m^2 of body surface
6–12 mos:	62–121 ml/min per 1.73 m^2 of body surface
>1 yr:	78–164 ml/min per 1.73 m^2 of body surface

U-17-Ketosteroids

0–3 days:	0–0.5 mg/d	
1–3 yrs:	<2.0 mg/d	
3–6 yrs:	0.5–3.0 mg/d	
6–9 yrs:	0.8–4.0 mg/d	
10–12 yrs:	male:	0.7–6.0 mg/d
	female:	0.7–5.0 mg/d
Adolescent:	male:	3–15 mg/d
	female:	3–12 mg/d

S-Lactate dehydrogenase

1–3 days:	up to 2 × adult values

S-Phosphorus (inorganic)

	PRE-TERM	FULL-TERM
Newborn:	1.8–2.6 mmol/L (56.0–80.0 mg/L)	1.6–2.5 mmol/L (50.0–78.0 mg/L)
6–10 days:	2.0–3.8 mmol/L (61–117 mg/L)	1.6–2.9 mmol/L (49–89 mg/L)

4 mos:	1.6–2.6 mmol/L (48–81 mg/L)
1 yr:	1.25–2.1 mmol/L (39–60 mg/L)
2–16 yrs:	0.9–1.5 mmol/L (26–50 mg/L)

S-Potassium

Pre-term newborn:	4.5–7.2 mmol/L
Full-term newborn:	5.0–7.7 mmol/L
2 d–2 wks:	4.0–6.4 mmol/L
2 wks–3 mos:	4.0–6.2 mmol/L
3 mos–1 yr:	3.7–5.6 mmol/L
1–16 yrs:	3.6–5.2 mmol/L

S-Testosterone

AGE	MALE	FEMALE
0–2 yrs:	0.14–1.28 nmol/L	0.24–0.62 nmol/L
2–4 yrs:	0.17–5.55 nmol/L	0.24–0.69 nmol/L
4–6 yrs:	0.28–1.39 nmol/L	0.35–0.69 nmol/L
6–8 yrs:	0.21–9.72 nmol/L	0.52–1.04 nmol/L
8–10 yrs:	0.31–1.74 nmol/L	0.69–1.39 nmol/L
10–12 yrs:	0.29–10.06 nmol/L	0.69–1.74 nmol/L
12–14 yrs:	0.17–26.37 nmol/L	1.04–2.43 nmol/L
14–16 yrs:	3.12–19.43 nmol/L	1.21–3.30 nmol/L
16–18 yrs:	9.02–25.33 nmol/L	1.39–3.30 nmol/L
18–20 yrs:	13.88–24.98 nmol/L	1.39–3.30 nmol/L
20–25 yrs:	11.80–38.86 nmol/L	1.39–3.30 nmol/L

S-Thyroxine

1–3 days:	142–296 nmol/L (11–23 μg/dl)
1 wk–1 mo:	116–232 nmol/L (9–18 μg/dl)
1–4 mos:	97–212 nmol/L (7.5–16.5 μg/dl)
4–12 mos:	71–187 nmol/L (5.5–14.5 μg/dl)
1–6 yrs:	71–174 nmol/L (5.5–13.5 μg/dl)
6–10 yrs:	64–161 nmol/L (5.0–12.5 μg/dl)

INDEX

Note: Page numbers in *italic* type refer to illustrations and tables. Page numbers in **boldface** type indicate color illustrations.

GUIDELINES FOR ORDERING BLOOD FOR ELECTIVE SURGERY

General Surgery

Procedure	Units
Amputation A/K, B/K	T&S
Cholecystectomy and CD exploration	T&S
Gastrectomy with/without vagotomy:	
Subtotal	1
Total	1
Gastric bypass	T&S
Splenectomy	1
Sympathectomy	T&S
*Exploratory laparotomy	T&S
Esophageal resection	2–4
Breast biopsy	T&S
Mastectomy:	
Simple	T&S
Radical	1
Radical with immediate reconstruction	1
Pancreatectomy:	
Partial	2
Radical (Whipple)	4
Thyroidectomy:	
Partial	T&S
Total	T&S
Parathyroidectomy	T&S
Parotidectomy	T&S
Colon resection:	
Total large colon	2
Hemicolectomy	2
Sigmoidectomy	2
Anterior resection	2
Small bowel segment	1
Abdominal-perineal resection	2
Colostomy, gastrostomy	T&S
Hemorrhoidectomy	T&S
Pilonidal cyst	T&S
Hernia:	
Inguinal	T&S
Incisional	T&S
Umbilical	T&S
Ventral	T&S
Hiatal	T&S
Vein stripping	T&S
Aneurysm resection	6
Femoropopliteal bypass	3
Portacaval shunt	4
Hepatectomy	6

Cardiopulmonary

Procedure	Units
Resection of ascending aortic aneurysm	10
Resection of descending aortic aneurysm	10
Partial or complete A-V canal repair	6
Closure of patient ductus arteriosus	4
Pulmonary valvulotomy	3
Pericardectomy	8
Open mitral commissurotomy	4
Closed mitral commissurotomy	4
Valve replacement:	
Aortic	6
Mitral	6
Double valve	6
Vein graft with other procedure	6
Valve replacement plus single vein grafts	6
Coarctation of the aorta, correction	4
Aortic valvulotomy or annuloplasty	4
Thoracotomy:	
Pneumonectomy	2
Wedge resection	2
Esophagectomy	2
Bronchopleural fistula	2
Pectus excavatum	1
Tracheostomy	T&S
Embolectomy	2
Vascular tumors	4
Thoracic aneurysm	10
Coronary vein graft:	
Single	4
Double	4
Triple	4
All reoperations	8
Repair of tetralogy of Fallot	6
Repair of atrial septal defect	3
Repair of ventricular septal defect	4
Resection of ventricular aneurysm	6
Bronchoscopy	0
Coronary artery bypass graft	4
Pacemaker	0
Quadruple vein graft	4

Otolaryngology

Procedure	Units
Branchial cleft cyst	T&S
Glossectomy	2
Laryngectomy	2
Laryngectomy w/radical neck	4
Mandibulectomy	2
Ethmoidectomy	T&S
Caldwell-Luc	T&S
Orbital exploration	T&S
Mastoidectomy	T&S
Septoplasty/rhinoplasty	T&S
Tumor of plate	T&S
Maxillectomy	2
Jaw, neck, tongue dissection	4
Temporal bone resection	6
Angiofibroma resection	6
Radical neck dissection	2
Carotid body tumor resection	4
Larynogoscopy	0
Myringotomy w/PE tube	0
Tympanoplasty	0

Neurosurgery

Procedure	Units
Carpal tunnel procedures	0
Cranioplasty	T&S
Craniotomy:	
Aneurysm	4–6
Subdural, epidural hematoma	2
Tumor	4–6
Cordotomy	T&S
Laminectomy	T&S
Lumbar laminectomy (single level)	T&S
Nerve repair	T&S
Hypophysectomy	T&S
Scalp and skull lesions (no intracranial communications)	T&S
Transsphenoidal hypophysectomy	T&S
Ulnar nerve transportation	0
Ventricular peritoneal shunt	T&S